MATERNAL-CHILD NURSING

• • • • • • • • • • • •

Emily Slone McKinney, MSN, RN, C

Lecturer, Louise Herrington School of Nursing

Baylor University

Dallas, Texas

Formerly, Education Coordinator, Women's Services

Baylor Medical Center at Irving

Irving, Texas

Jean Weiler Ashwill, MSN, RN

Director, Center for Continuing Nursing Education

School of Nursing

University of Texas at Arlington

Arlington, Texas

Sharon Smith Murray, MSN, RN, C

Professor, Health Professions

Golden West College

Huntington Beach, California

Susan Rowen James, MSN, RN

Associate Professor, Division of Nursing and Health Studies

Curry College

Milton, Massachusetts

Trula Myers Gorrie, MN, RN, C

Professor Emeritus

Golden West College

Huntington Beach, California

Susan Colvert Droske, MSN, RN, CPN

Associate Professor of Nursing

Texarkana College

Texarkana, Texas

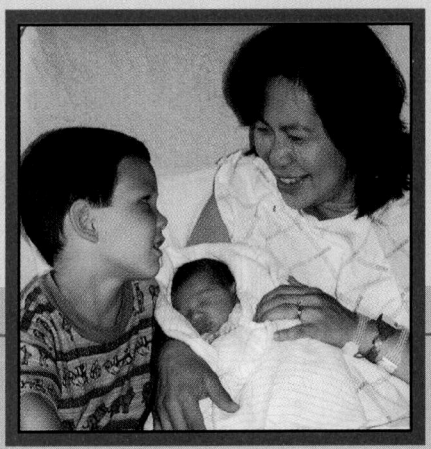

Maternal-Child
Nursing

♦ ♦ ♦ ♦ ♦ ♦ ♦

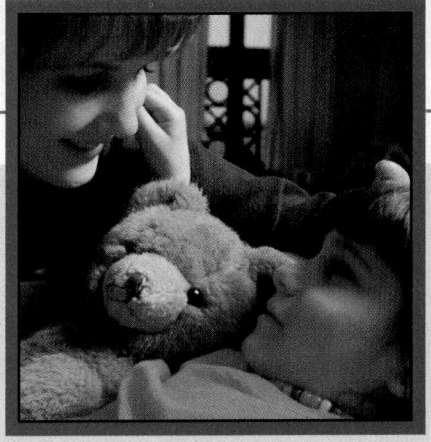

W.B. SAUNDERS COMPANY
A Harcourt Health Sciences Company
Philadelphia London New York St. Louis Sydney Toronto

W.B. SAUNDERS COMPANY

A *Harcourt Health Sciences Company*

The Curtis Center
Independence Square West
Philadelphia, Pennsylvania 19106

Library of Congress Cataloging-in-Publication Data

Maternal-child nursing / Emily Slone McKinney . . . [et al.]. — 1st ed.
  p.   cm.
  Includes bibliographical references.
  ISBN 0–7216–8138–7
  1. Maternity nursing.   2. Pediatric nursing.   I. McKinney, Emily
Slone.
  [DNLM: 1. Maternal-Child Nursing—methods. 2. Pediatric Nursing—
methods.   WY 157.3 M4253 2000]
RG951.M38   2000
610.73′678—dc21
DNLM/DLC
for Library of Congress   99–31878
                                                                CIP

Nursing Editorial Director: Sally Schrefer
Editorial Manager: Thomas Eoyang

MATERNAL-CHILD NURSING   ISBN 0–7216–8138–7

Bottom cover photo courtesy of Cook Children's Health Care System, Forth Worth, Texas.

Printed in the United States of America

Last digit is the print number: 9   8   7   6   5   4   3   2   1

◆ ◆ ◆ ◆ ◆ ◆ ◆ ◆ ◆ ◆

To my husband, Michael, for his faithful love and support.

To our daughters, Cathy and Amy.

To the many nursing students who have taught me so much.

E.S.M.

For my husband, Skip, who is always there to help and support.

For my children, Vicki, Holly, and Shannon, for their love and understanding.

For Marina and Nicholas, who keep us entertained as only children can.

S.S.M.

To my husband, Vince, whom I love and cherish, and to my children and their families, who bring me tremendous joy.

J.W.A.

To my husband, Bob, for his continuing encouragement and support and for his patience.

To Elena and Carolyn, for all their help with the day-to-day things while my concentration was elsewhere, and to Richard, whose curiosity and interest in this project helped me see it in a different light.

S.R.J.

Madoka Armstrong, MSN, RN, GPMHNP
Psychiatric Mental Health Nurse Practitioner
The Holiner Psychiatric Group
Dallas, Texas
    Chapter 53: The Child with a Psychosocial Disorder
    Chapter 54: The Child with a Cognitive Deficit

Carol Bolinger, RN, MSN, CPNP, CPON
Oncology Pediatric Nurse Practitioner
Primary Children's Medical Center
Salt Lake City, Utah
    Chapter 48: The Child with Cancer

Cam Brandt, RN, MS
Education Coordinator
Cook Children's Health Care System
Fort Worth, Texas
    Chapter 42: The Child with a Fluid and Electrolyte Alteration

Debbie Calligaro-Wharton, RN, MS
Clinical Nurse Specialist—Neurology
Children's Medical Center of Dallas
Dallas, Texas
    Chapter 52: The Child with a Neurologic Alteration

Marilyn Cox, MSN
Endocrine Clinical Nurse Specialist
Children's Medical Center
Dallas, Texas
    Chapter 51: The Child with an Endocrine Alteration

Stephanie Eckstein, RN, MSN, CNS
Education Coordinator for Continuing
    Professional Education
Cook Children's Health Care System
Fort Worth, Texas
    Chapter 35: The Ill Child in the Hospital and Other
    Care Settings

Dayna Joy Greene, RN, MSN, CPNP
Oncology Pediatric Nurse Practitioner
Primary Children's Medical Center
Salt Lake City, Utah
    Chapter 48: The Child with Cancer

Linda Lewis Lai, RN, MSN, CCRN
Texas Christian University, Harris College of Nursing
Staff Nurse, Pediatric Intensive Care Unit
Cook Children's Health Care System
Fort Worth, Texas
    Chapter 46: The Child with a Cardiovascular Alteration

Contributors

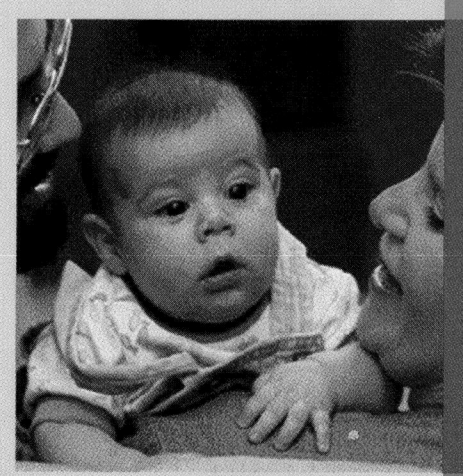

Nancy Noonan, MS, APRN
Clinical Nurse Specialist
Primary Children's Medical Center
Salt Lake City, Utah
    Chapter 47: The Child with a Hematologic Alteration

Cheryl Ann Sams, RN, MSN
Clinical Nurse Specialist
Hospital for Sick Children
Clinical Tutor
University of Toronto
Toronto, Ontario
    Chapter 43: The Child with a Gastrointestinal Alteration

The authors gratefully acknowledge, once again, the work of the chapter contributors to
Ashwill and Droske, *Nursing Care of Children*:

Jane A. Ahlrichs, BSN, MEd, RN
Director, Nursing Services
Pediatric Rehabilitation/Transitional Care
Children's Hospital Medical Center
Cincinnati, Ohio

Susan Allen, RN, MSN
Clinical Director/Clinical Nurse Specialist
Emergency Department
Blank Children's Hospital
Des Moines, Iowa

Jean Weiler Ashwill, MSN, RN
Director of Continuing Nursing Education
University of Texas at Arlington School of Nursing
Arlington, Texas

Ann Aurigemma, RN, BS, MA
Head Nurse, Pediatrics
New York University Medical Center
New York, New York

Karen Bernardy, RN, MSN
Child Health Consultant
Conyers, Georgia

Marilyn Cox Borgersen, MSN, RN
Endocrine Clinical Nurse Specialist
Children's Medical Center
Dallas, Texas

Susan Burkett, RN, MSN, CPNP, CPN
Administrator
T. C. Thompson Children's Hospital
Chattanooga, Tennessee

Nancy H. Busen, PhD, RN, C-FNP
Associate Professor of Nursing
Coordinator, Graduate Pediatric Nurse Practitioner Program
University of Texas Houston Health Science Center
School of Nursing
Houston, Texas

Dolores W. Clark, RN, BSN, MSN, FNP
Specialist
University of Texas at Arlington School of Nursing
Arlington, Texas
Advanced Pediatric Nurse
Community Oriented Primary Care Clinic
Parkland Memorial Hospital
Dallas, Texas

Joan Marie Cutrone, BSN, MA, RN
Head Nurse, Neonatal ICU
New York University Medical Center
New York, New York

Bernadette Daborn, RN, MA
Head Nurse, Pediatrics
New York University Medical Center
New York, New York

Kimberly L. Davies, BS, RN, CEN
Pediatric Trauma Coordinator
Children's Medical Center of Dallas
Dallas, Texas

Susan Colvert Droske, MSN, RN, CPN
Associate Professor of Nursing
Texarkana College
Texarkana, Texas

Dallas Estey, RNC, MSN
Neonatal Nurse Practitioner
Woman's Hospital
Baton Rouge, Louisiana

Joan Holter Gildea, MA, RNC
Clinical Assistant Director of Nursing
New York University Medical Center
New York, New York

Judith W. Gross, PhD, RN
Assistant Professor
College of Nursing
Medical University of South Carolina
Charleston, South Carolina

Julie F. Gwin, BSN, RN, MN
Assistant Professor
Department of Nursing
Tarrant County Junior College
Staff Nurse
Cook Children's Medical Center
Fort Worth, Texas

Deborah Parkman Henderson, PhD, RN
Lecturer
UCLA School of Medicine
University of California Los Angeles
Harbor-UCLA Medical Center
Torrance, California

Jill Howie-Stites, RN, MN
Nurse Practitioner
Children's Hospital of Orange County
Orange, California

Sylvia H. Imhoff, RN, MSN, JD
Attorney
Slack & Davis
Austin, Texas

Stephen Jones, MS, RNC, PNP, ET
Assistant Professor
Clinical Nursing Education
Albany Medical College
Albany, New York
Adjunct Clinical Instructor
Russell Sage College
Troy, New York

Kathleen A. Koszarek, RNC, MSN
Neonatal Nurse Practitioner
Ochsner Foundation Hospital
New Orleans, Louisiana

Melva Kravitz, PhD, RN
Director, Research & Education
Division of Nursing
Yale-New Haven Hospital
New Haven, Connecticut

Gwendolyn T. Martin, RN, BSN, MSN, CNS, CPN
Pediatric Coordinator
Community Hospice of Texas
Fort Worth, Texas

Sharon M. McLeod, MS, CCLS, CTRS
Director, Child Life Department
Children's Hospital Medical Center
Cincinnati, Ohio

Michele Michael, PhD, CRNP
Assistant Professor
School of Nursing
University of Maryland
Baltimore, Maryland

Maribeth Moran, MSN, RN, CPN
Assistant Professor
College of Nursing
University of Oklahoma
Oklahoma City, Oklahoma

Donna Nash Parnell, RN, BSN, MNSc
Trauma Coordinator
Arkansas Children's Hospital
Little Rock, Arkansas

Therese L. Polacek, RN, MSN. CPNP
Assistant Professor
College of St. Scholastica
Duluth, Minnesota

Mary C. Rathlev, RN, MSN
Program Manager
Program CHAMP (Children's HIV/AIDS Model Program)
Children's National Medical Center
Washington, D.C.

Leslie M. Reed, RN, MSN
Renal Transplant Nurse Specialist
Children's Mercy Hospital
Kansas City, Missouri

Janice G. Sample, BSN, MNSc, CNRN
Certified Neuroscience Registered Nurse
American Association of Neuroscience Nurses
Assistant Professor
Texarkana College
Texarkana, Texas

Anne Scott, PhD, RN
Per Diem Staff Nurse—Pediatrics
Bulloch Memorial Hospital
Director of Nursing Research
Associate Professor
Georgia Southern University
Statesboro, Georgia

Mary Ellen Sheldon, RNC, MA, CCRN
Pediatric Staff Development Instructor
New York University Medical Center
New York, New York

Nedra Skale, MS, MJ, RN, CAN
Nurse Associate
Midwest Orthopaedics
Chicago, Illinois

Dotty Volz, RN, MSN
Clinical Nurse Specialist
T. C. Thompson Children's Hospital
Chattanooga, Tennessee
CEO, Dotty Volz & Associates
Hixson, Tennessee

Brenda J. Wagner, RN, BSN, MSN, PhD
Clinical Psychologist
Scottish Rite Children's Medical Center
Atlanta, Georgia

Anne Weir, RNP, C, MSN
Clinical Instructor
Arkansas Children's Hospital
Little Rock, Arkansas

Sharon Whalen, RN, MS
Clinical Nurse Specialist
Huntington Beach, California

Vicki L. Zeigler, RN, MSN
Pediatric Arrhythmia Case Manager
Cardiology Department
Cook Children's Medical Center
Forth Worth, Texas

Reviewers

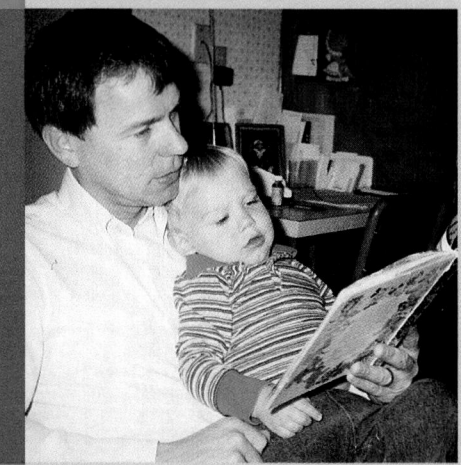

Megan Archer, BSN, RN, CEN, MICN, NREMT-P
Emergency Department
Carolinas Medical Center
Charlotte, North Carolina

Roselyn Holloway, MSN, RN
Methodist Hospital School of Nursing
Lubbock, Texas

Sherry Neil-Urban, RN, PhD, RNC
University of Nevada–Reno
Reno, Nevada

Ruth H. Robillard, EdD, RN
Assistant Professor
Department of Nursing
University of North Florida
Jacksonville, Florida

Antonia Scacco-Neumann, MSN, RN
Instructor
Kent State University School of Nursing
Kent, Ohio

Barbara Weintraub, MSN, RN, MPH, CEN
Clinical Educator
Children's Memorial Hospital
Chicago, Illinois

Jeanne Whalen, BSN, RN, CEN
Union Regional Medical Center
Monroe, North Carolina

Children are a precious gift. Some of the most satisfying nursing roles involve helping families bring their children into the world, being a resource as they rear them, and supporting families during times of illness. In addition to providing care to young families as they bear and raise children, nurses play a crucial role in women's health care from the teen years through postmenopausal life. *Maternal-Child Nursing* is written to provide a foundation for care of these individuals and their families to the nursing student or the nurse entering maternity or pediatric nursing from another area of nursing.

Maternal-Child Nursing builds on two other successful texts to combine maternity, women's health, and pediatric nursing. *Nursing Care of Children: Principles and Practice* by Jean Weiler Ashwill and Susan Colvert Droske, and *Foundations of Maternal-Newborn Nursing* by Trula Myers Gorrie, Emily Slone McKinney, and Sharon Smith Murray form the foundation of this text.

Maternal-Child Nursing emphasizes evidence-based nursing care throughout. The scientific base of maternity and pediatric nursing care is demonstrated in the narrative and features in which the nursing process is applied. Physiologic and pathophysiological processes are presented so the reader can understand why problems occur and the reasons behind nursing care. Current references, many of them from Internet sources for maximum timeliness, provide the reader with the latest information that applies to the clinical area. National standards and guidelines, such as those from the Association of Women's Health, Obstetric, and Neonatal Nurses (AWHONN), Society of Pediatric Nurses, and American Nurses Association, are used when they apply.

Maternity, women's health, and pediatric nursing may be practiced in a wide variety of settings. Where appropriate, our text discusses care of clients in settings as diverse as acute and chronic care facilities, the community, schools, and the home. Methods to ease transition among facilities and improve continuity of care are highlighted when appropriate.

Legal and ethical issues add to the complexity of practice for today's nurse. Our book discusses the legal obligations of maternal-child nurses and how to meet those obligations to provide optimum client care. Ethical principles and decision-making are discussed in the first chapter of the text. Ethical issues, such as issues involving very early gestation babies or the end of life, are discussed in other chapters when appropriate.

Nursing students have time demands from work, family, and community activities in addition to their nursing education. A significant number of nurses use English as a second language. With those realities in mind, we have written a text to effectively convey necessary information that focuses on critical elements and that is concise without the use of unnecessarily complex language. Important terms are defined on the first page of the chapter for ready access as the student studies the chapter.

Concepts

Several conceptual threads are woven into our book. The *family* is a concept that is incorporated in both the maternity and pediatric sections as a vital part of maternal-child nursing care. Family considerations appear in every step of

Preface

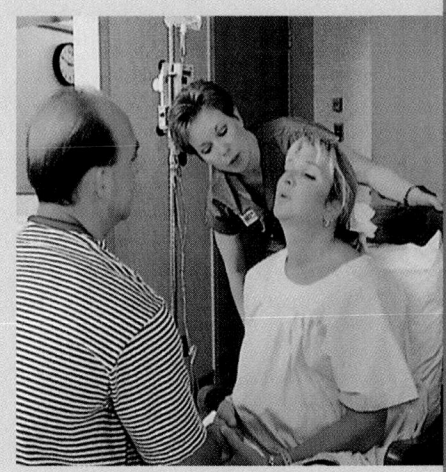

the nursing process. The family may be the conventional mother-father-child arrangement or might be a single-parent or multigenerational family. We consider several types of family styles as we present nursing care. We sometimes ask the reader to use critical thinking to examine his or her own assumptions and biases about families while studying.

Without *communication*, nursing care would be inadequate and sometimes unsafe. Teaching effective communication skills is incorporated into several features of the text as well as into the main narrative. Separate boxes within the narrative are communication cues to give tips about verbal and nonverbal communication with clients and their families. Children are not little adults and nowhere is this more true than in communicating with children. Therefore, communicating with children is presented in a separate chapter to supplement information given in other pediatric chapters.

Health promotion is obvious in chapters covering normal childbearing and child rearing, but we also incorporate it into the chapters covering various disorders. Health promotion during illness may be as simple as reminding the reader that a technology-laden woman in labor is still having a baby and thus needs human contact or that sick children need activities to promote their normal growth and development as much as they need the high-tech procedures that return them to physical wellness.

Teaching is closely related to health promotion. Teaching is an expected part of nursing care to empower clients and their families to maintain health or return to health after illness or injury. Several features discussed later help the reader provide better teaching to clients in an understandable form.

Cultural variety characterizes nursing practice today as the lines between individual nations become more blurred. The nurse must assess for unique cultural needs and incorporate them into care as much as possible to promote acceptance of nursing care by the client. Cultural influences are examined in many ways in our text, including critical thinking exercises to help the student "think outside the box" of his or her own culture.

Growth and development are concepts that appear throughout the book. We cover physical growth and development as the child is conceived and matures before birth and throughout childhood, and as the woman matures through the childbearing years and into the climacteric. Specific chapters in the pediatric section focus on growth and development issues, including anticipatory guidance, specific to each age group from infancy through adolescence.

Advocacy is emphasized in our text. Whether it is advocacy for a woman or family to be informed about their rights or advocacy for child and adult victims of violence, the concept is incorporated in relevant places.

Features

Maternity and women's health nursing care differs from nursing care of children and their families in several important respects. Because of this fact, some features in the text appear in one part but not in the other. Other features appear in both parts of the text.

Visual appeal characterizes many features in the text. Beautiful illustrations and photographs convey clinical information and also capture the essence of care for maternity and pediatric clients.

LEARNING OBJECTIVES
Learning objectives provide direction for the reader to understand what is important to glean from the chapter. Many objectives ask that the learner use critical thinking and apply the nursing process—two crucial components of professional nursing—to care of clients with the conditions discussed in that chapter. Other features within the chapters reinforce these two components of care.

NURSING PROCESS
Several methods help the learner use the nursing process in care of maternity, women's health, and pediatric clients. Steps of the nursing process include assessment, formulating nursing diagnoses after analysis of the assessment data, planning care, providing nursing interventions, and evaluating the nursing interventions, expected outcomes or goals, and appropriateness of nursing diagnoses as care proceeds. We address these steps in three different ways in our book, depending on whether the process is discussed in the maternity/women's health or the pediatric section. The three approaches show the student that there is more than one way to communicate the nursing process. These different approaches to the nursing process also provide teaching tools to meet the needs of students' varied learning styles.

In the maternity and women's health section, the nursing process is presented in two ways. Nursing care is first presented as a *text discussion* that would apply to a typical client with the condition. In addition, a *nursing care plan* that applies to a client created in a specific scenario is constructed for many common conditions. This technique helps the student see individualization of nursing care. Many nursing care plans list *additional nursing diagnoses to consider* to encourage the reader to think of other client needs. The approach of scenario-based care plans is especially useful for showing learners how to apply the nursing process in dynamic conditions such as labor and birth.

In the pediatric section, the nursing process is applied to care of the most common childhood conditions by a blend of a text discussion similar to the maternity/women's health section and a generic rather than scenario-based nursing care plan. The student thus has the benefit of seeing typical nursing diagnoses, expected outcomes, and interventions with their rationales discussed in a manner similar to standard care plans the learner may encounter in clinical facilities. The evaluation step of the nursing process provides sample questions the nurse would need to answer to determine whether the expected outcomes were achieved and whether further actions or revisions of nursing care are needed. The pediatric application of the nursing process provides a framework for the nursing instructor to help students individualize nursing care for their specific clients based on a generic plan of care.

CRITICAL THINKING EXERCISES
Critical thinking is encouraged in multiple ways in *Maternal-Child Nursing,* but specific Critical Thinking Exercises present typical client scenarios or other real-life situations and ask the reader to solve nursing care problems that are not always obvious. We use the exercises to help the student learn to figure out the answer, choose the best interventions, or determine possible meanings or importance of signs and symptoms. Answers are provided at the end of the chapter so the student can check his or her solutions to these problems.

CRITICAL TO REMEMBER
Students always want to know, "Will this be on the test?" The authors cannot answer that question, but Critical to Remember boxes provide a condensed summary of very important information needed to provide safe care.

WANT TO KNOW BOXES
Because teaching is an essential part of nursing care, we give students teaching guidelines for common client needs in terms that most lay people can understand. The Want to Know boxes provide sample answers for questions that clients are most likely to ask, such as when to go to the birth center or methods of managing type I diabetes mellitus at home.

CLINICAL REFERENCE PAGES
Clinical Reference pages provide a resource for the reader when studying pediatric conditions. This feature provides the reader with basic information related to a group of disorders such as a compact review of related anatomy and physiology, differences between children and adults in the system

being studied, commonly used drugs, lab values, and diagnostic tests and procedures that apply to the conditions discussed in that chapter.

PATHOPHYSIOLOGY BOXES

Also present in many pediatric chapters are pathophysiology boxes. These boxes give the reader a brief overview of how the illness occurs. The boxes provide a scientific basis for understanding the therapeutic management of the illness and its nursing care.

PHOTO STORIES

"A picture is worth a thousand words" applies to the photo stories that appear in the pediatric section. Photo stories help the reader see well-child checks and assessments of growth and development. Some photo stories take the reader through the experience of care for a specific condition.

PROCEDURES

Clinical skills are presented in procedures throughout the text. Procedures related to maternity and women's health are presented in the chapters to which they apply. Because many procedures are common to care of several pediatric conditions, they are covered in a chapter devoted to procedures, Chapter 37.

DRUG GUIDES

Drug information may be presented in two ways: tables for related drugs used in the care of various conditions and drug guides for specific common drugs. Drug guides provide the nurse with greater detail for commonly encountered drugs in maternity and women's health care.

KEY CONCEPTS

Key concepts summarize important points of each chapter. They provide a general review for the material just presented to help the reader identify areas in which more study is needed.

Appendixes

Thirteen appendices provide a reference source for both the reader and the teacher. Some appendixes apply to maternity, women's health, and pediatric nursing. Others apply to a single specialty. Appendix L, Resources for Health Care Providers and Families, gives information about professional organizations, support groups, and sources of assistance that may be helpful. Internet web pages are listed for many of these resources. Additional important information that re-lates to drug ingestion during pregnancy and lactation appears in Appendix C.

Ancillaries

Materials that complement *Maternal-Child Nursing* include an *Instructor's Electronic Resource*, which is a single CD-ROM containing three separate teacher support programs: (a) a full instructor's manual in the most common word processing formats; (b) a computerized testbank using the Saunders *EXAMaster™* 99 program; and (c) *LectureView*, an innovative combination of word slides and selected images from the text, all suitable for classroom projection through PowerPoint.

The *Study Guide for Maternal-Child Nursing* will be available on-line for students using the text, and can be found on the book's dedicated website:

www.wbsaunders.com/SIMON/McKinney/mat-ch/

Interactive learning activities with helpful feedback will give students both guidance and reinforcement to aid learning.

Acknowledgments

Many people in addition to the authors made *Maternal-Child Nursing* a reality. Thomas Eoyang, Editorial Manager for Nursing Books at W. B. Saunders, first proposed that the authors build on the success of their separate maternity and pediatric books to write a combined text. Thomas has remained a regular consultant as we wrote *Maternal-Child Nursing*. Editorial assistants Gina Hopf and Adrienne Simon helped us many times with various details required to bring the project to fruition.

Developmental editors who refined and organized our manuscript and made it ready for production included Debi Osnowitz, Hope Steele, and Sue Bredensteiner. Peggy Gordon, production editor, managed the book as it made its transition from manuscript to bound volume. Peggy often encouraged us when the parade of paper seemed as if it would never end.

Our acknowledgments would not be complete without thanking two people who were coauthors for the parent texts, Trula Gorrie and Susan Droske. Although they did not directly participate in writing *Maternal-Child Nursing*, their work is evident in many of its chapters. Susan was both an editor and a contributor to Ashwill and Droske, *Nursing Care of Children: Principles and Practice*. Trula, lead author of Gorrie, McKinney, and Murray, *Foundations of Maternal-Newborn Nursing*, remains a valued colleague after her retirement and continues to encourage us as we write for maternity and pediatric nurses of the future.

Brief Contents

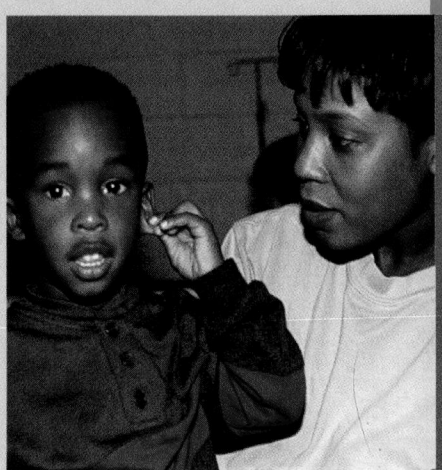

Contents

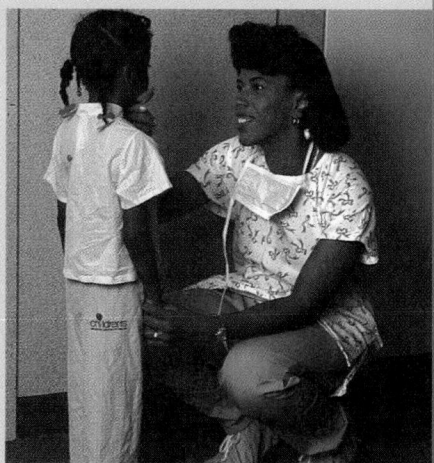

I

Introduction to Maternal-Child Nursing

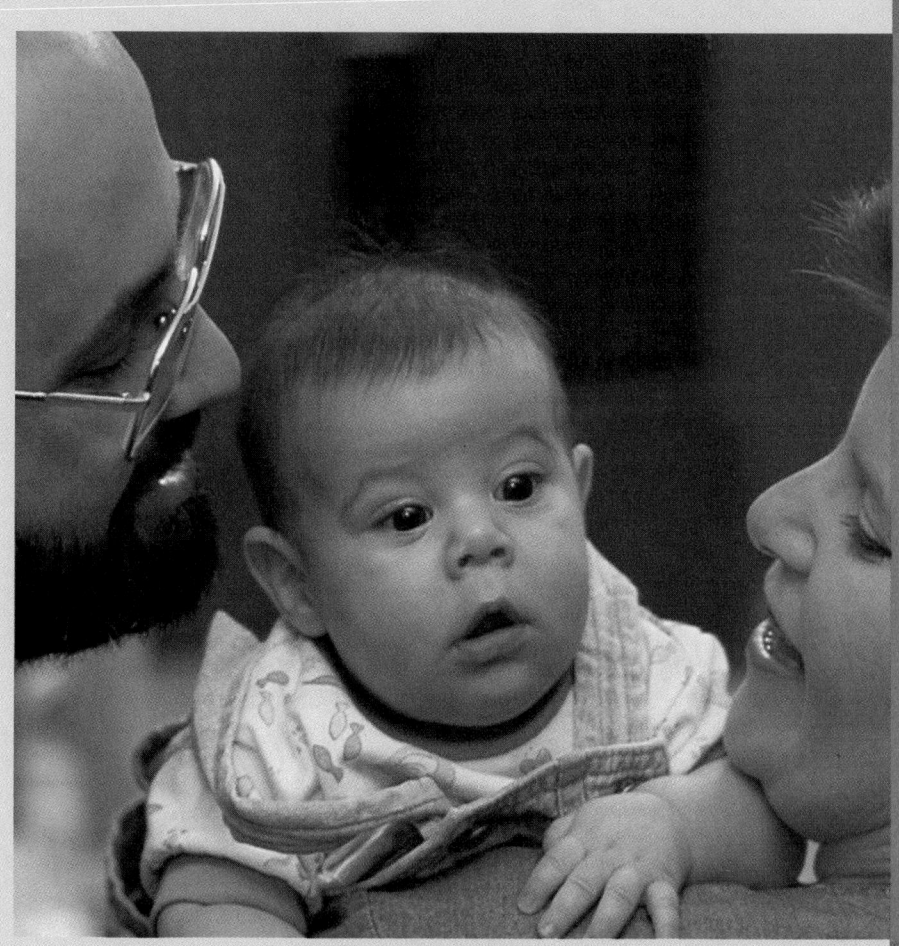

1

⋄ ⋄ ⋄ ⋄ ⋄ ⋄ ⋄ ⋄ ⋄ ⋄ ⋄

Foundations of Maternity and Pediatric Nursing

LEARNING OBJECTIVES

After studying this chapter, you should be able to:

- Describe the historical background of maternity and pediatric care.
- Compare current settings for childbirth both within and outside the hospital setting.
- Identify trends that led to the development of family-centered maternity and pediatric care.
- Describe current trends that affect perinatal and pediatric nursing, including cost containment, outcomes management, home care, and advances in technology.
- Discuss trends in maternal, infant, and childhood mortality rates.
- Compare current infant mortality rates for specific ethnic groups and nations.
- Identify some of the effects of poverty and violence on the well-being of children and families.
- Apply theories and principles of ethics to ethical dilemmas.
- Discuss ethical conflicts that the nurse may encounter in maternal and pediatric nursing practice.
- Relate how major social issues, such as poverty and access to health care, affect maternal-child nursing.
- Describe the legal basis for nursing practice.

- Identify measures used to defend malpractice claims.
- Identify current trends in health care and their implications for nursing.

DEFINITIONS

advocacy Speaking or arguing in support of a policy or a person's rights.

antepartum Term referring to the period before the onset of labor.

bioethics Rules or principles that govern right conduct, specifically those that relate to health care.

case management A practice model that uses a systematic approach to identify specific client needs and to manage client care to ensure optimal outcomes.

deontologic theory Ethical theory holding that the right course of action is the one dictated by ethical principles and moral rules.

ethical dilemma A situation in which no solution seems completely satisfactory.

ethics Rules or principles that govern right conduct and distinctions between right and wrong.

infant mortality rate Number of deaths per 1,000 live births that occur within the first 12 months of life.

intrapartum Term describing the time of labor and childbirth.

lactation Secretion of milk from the breasts; also describes the time when a child is breast-fed.

malpractice Negligence by a professional person.

maternal mortality rate Number of maternal deaths from childbirth and the complications of pregnancy, childbirth, and the puerperium (the first 42 days after the end of the pregnancy) per 100,000 live births.

morbidity Ratio of sick to well persons in a defined population.

negligence Failure to act in the way a reasonable, prudent person of similar background would act in similar circumstances.

neonatal mortality rate Number of deaths per 1,000 live births that occur at birth or within the first 28 days of life.

nurse practice acts Laws that determine the scope of nursing practice in each state.

postpartum Term denoting the first 6 weeks following childbirth.

standard of care Level of care that can be expected of a professional. This level is determined by laws, professional organizations, and health care agencies.

standardized procedures Procedures determined by nurses, physicians, and administrators that allow nurses to perform duties usually part of the medical practice.

utilitarian theory Ethical theory holding that the right course of action is the one that produces the greatest good.

WIC A Special Supplemental Food Program for Women, Infants, and Children that provides nutritious food and nutrition education to low-income pregnant and postpartum women and their children.

To better understand contemporary maternity and pediatric nursing, the nurse needs to understand the history of these fields, trends and issues affecting contemporary practice, and the ethical and legal frameworks within which maternity and pediatric nursing care is provided.

Historical Perspectives

Maternity Nursing

Major changes in maternity care occurred in the first half of the twentieth century as childbirth moved out of the home and into a hospital setting. Rapid change continues as health care reform attempts to control the rising cost of care while advances in expensive technology accelerate. Despite changes, health care professionals attempt to maintain the quality of care.

"GRANNY" MIDWIVES
Before the twentieth century, childbirth usually occurred in the home with the assistance of a "granny" midwife whose training came through an apprenticeship with a more experienced granny midwife. Physicians were involved in childbirth only if there were serious problems.

Although many women and infants fared well when a lay midwife assisted with birth in the home, maternal and infant death rates resulting from childbearing were high. The primary causes of maternal death were postpartum hemorrhage, postpartum infection, also known as puerperal sepsis (or "childbed fever"), and toxemia, now known as pregnancy-induced hypertension. The primary causes of infant death were prematurity, dehydration from diarrhea, and contagious diseases.

EMERGENCE OF MEDICAL MANAGEMENT
In the late nineteenth century, technological developments that were available to physicians but not to midwives led to a decline in home births and an increase in physician-assisted hospital births. Important discoveries that set the stage for a change in maternity care included the following:

- The discovery by Semmelweis that puerperal infection could be prevented by hygienic practices
- The development of forceps to facilitate birth
- The discovery of chloroform, which was used to control pain during childbirth
- The use of drugs to initiate labor or to increase uterine contractions
- Advances in operative procedures, such as cesarean birth

By 1960, 90% of all births in the United States occurred in hospitals. Maternity care became highly regimented. All antepartum, intrapartum, and postpartum care was managed by physicians. Lay midwifery became illegal in many areas, and nurse-midwifery was not well established. The woman had a passive role in childbirth, as the physician "delivered" her baby. Nurses' primary functions were to assist the physician and to follow prescribed medical orders after childbirth. Teaching and counseling were not valued nursing functions at that time.

Unlike home births, early hospital births hindered bonding between parents and infant. During labor, the woman often received medication, such as "twilight sleep," a combination of a narcotic and scopolamine, that provided pain relief but left her disoriented, confused, and heavily sedated. Because of this practice and because little was known of the importance of early contact between parents and child, many mothers did not see the infant for several hours after the delivery. The father was relegated to a waiting area and was not allowed to see the mother until some time after the birth of their infant.

Despite the technological advances and the move from home birth to hospital birth, maternal and infant mortality declined only slowly. The slow decline was primarily due to problems that could have been prevented, such as poor nutrition, infectious diseases, and inadequate prenatal care. These stubborn problems remained because of inequalities in health care delivery. Whereas affluent families could afford comprehensive medical care that began early in the pregnancy, poor families had very limited access to care or to information about childbearing. Two concurrent trends, federal involvement and consumer demands, led to additional changes in maternity care.

GOVERNMENT INVOLVEMENT IN MATERNAL-INFANT CARE
The high rates of maternal and infant mortality among indigent women provided the impetus for federal involvement in maternity care. The Sheppard-Towner Act of 1921 provided funds for state-managed programs for mothers and children. Although this act was later repealed, it set the scene for future allocation of federal funds. Today, the federal government supports several programs to improve the health of mothers, infants, and young children (Table 1–1). Although projects supported by government funds partially solved the problem of maternal and infant mortality, the *distribution* of health care remained unequal. Most physicians practiced in urban or suburban areas where the affluent could afford to pay for medical services, but women in rural or inner city areas had difficulty obtaining care. The distribution of health care services is a problem that persists today.

The ongoing problem of providing health care for poor women and children left the door open for nurses to expand their roles, and programs emerged to prepare nurses for advanced practice (see Chapter 2).

IMPACT OF CONSUMER DEMANDS ON HEALTH CARE
In the early 1950s, consumers began to insist on their right to be involved in the health care they received. Pregnant women were no longer willing to accept only what was of-

TABLE 1-1

Federal Projects for Maternal-Child Care

Program	Purpose
Title V of Social Security Act	Provides funds for maternal-child health programs
National Institute of Health and Human Development	Supports research and education of personnel needed for maternal and child health programs
Title V Amendment of Public Health Service Act	Established the Maternal and Infant Care (MIC) projects to provide comprehensive prenatal and infant care in public clinics
Title XIX of Medicaid program	Provides funds to facilitate access to care by pregnant women and young children
Head Start	Provides educational opportunities for low-income children of preschool age
National Center for Family Planning	A clearinghouse for contraceptive information
Women, Infants, and Children (WIC) program	Provides supplemental food and nutrition information

fered. They wanted information about planning and spacing their children, and they wanted to know what to expect during pregnancy. The father, siblings, and grandparents wanted to be part of the extraordinary events of pregnancy and childbirth. Parents also wanted more say in how the birth of their child was accomplished.

A growing consensus among child psychologists and nurse researchers, moreover, indicated that the benefits of early, extended parent-newborn contact far outweighed the risk of infection. Parents began to insist that their infant remain with them, and the practice of separating the infant from the family was abandoned.

DEVELOPMENT OF FAMILY-CENTERED MATERNITY CARE

Family-centered maternity care is the term used to describe safe, quality care that recognizes and adapts to both the physical and psychosocial needs of the family, including those of the newborn. The emphasis is on fostering family unity while maintaining physical safety.

The basic principles of family-centered care are as follows:

- Childbirth is usually a normal, healthy event in the life of a family.
- Childbirth affects the entire family, and restructuring of family relationships is required.
- Families are capable of making decisions about care, provided that they are given adequate information and professional support.

Family-centered care greatly increased the responsibilities of nurses. It is no longer enough for nurses to provide only physical care and to assist physicians. Nurses now assume a major role in teaching, counseling, and supporting families in their decisions.

Current Settings for Childbirth

As family-centered maternity care has emerged, settings for childbirth have changed to meet the needs of new families.

TRADITIONAL HOSPITAL SETTING

In traditional hospitals of the past, labor often took place in a functional hospital room. When birth was imminent, the mother was moved to a delivery area similar to an operating room. After giving birth, the mother was transferred to a recovery area for 1 to 2 hours of observation and then taken to the postpartum unit, which resembled a standard hospital room. The infant was usually moved to the newborn nursery when the mother was transferred to the recovery area. Mother and infant were reunited when the mother was settled in the postpartum unit. Beginning in the 1970s, the father or another significant support person could usually remain with the mother throughout labor, birth, and recovery.

Although birth in a traditional hospital setting was safe, the setting was impersonal and uncomfortable. Having to move from room to room, especially during late labor, was a major disadvantage. Each move was uncomfortable for the mother, disrupted the family's time together, and often separated the parents from the infant. Because of these disadvantages, hospitals began to devise settings that were more comfortable and that facilitated family participation.

Labor, Delivery, and Recovery Rooms.   Today, most hospitals offer alternative settings for childbirth. The most common is the labor, delivery, and recovery (LDR) room. In an LDR room, normal labor, childbirth, and recovery from childbirth take place in one setting. The homelike furniture can quickly be transformed into a well-equipped delivery room. A typical LDR room is illustrated in Figure 1-1.

During labor, the woman's significant others are al-

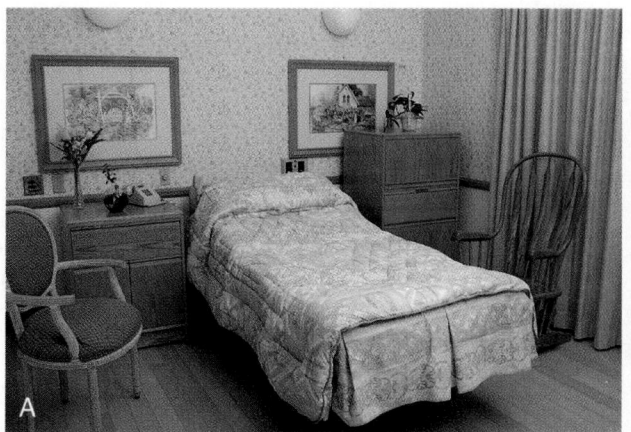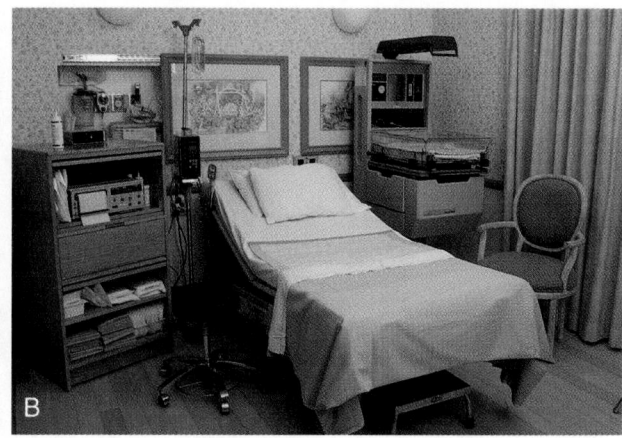

FIGURE 1–1
. . . .
A typical labor, delivery, and recovery room. Home-like furnishings (A) can be adapted quickly to
reveal needed technical equipment (B).

lowed to remain with her. Once she has given birth, the
mother typically remains in the LDR room for 1 to 2 hours,
after which she is transferred to the postpartum unit. The
infant may remain with the mother throughout her stay in
the LDR room. When she is transferred to the postpartum
unit, the infant may be transferred to the nursery or may
remain with the mother.

The major advantages of LDR rooms are that the setting is more comfortable and home-like and the family can
remain with the mother throughout. Disadvantages for the
family include the routine (rather than selective) use of
technology, such as electronic fetal monitoring and the administration of intravenous fluids.

Labor, Delivery, Recovery, and Postpartum Rooms.
Some hospitals offer rooms that are similar to LDR rooms
in layout and in function, but the mother is not transferred
to a postpartum unit. She and the infant remain in the labor, delivery, recovery, and postpartum (LDRP) room until
discharge. Fathers are encouraged to stay with the mother
and infant, and many facilities provide beds so they can stay
through the night.

BIRTH CENTERS
Free-standing birth centers provide maternity care to low-
risk women outside the hospital setting. In addition to care
during childbirth, birth centers also provide antepartum and
postpartum care. Both the mother and infant continue to
receive follow-up care during the first 6 weeks. This may
include help with breast-feeding problems, a postpartum examination at 4 to 6 weeks, family planning information,
and examination of the newborn. Birth is often assisted by
certified nurse-midwives who have provided care for the
woman throughout her pregnancy and will continue to provide primary care for both the mother and the infant after
birth.

Birth centers generally charge less than traditional hospitals, which provide advanced technology that may be unnecessary for low-risk clients. Moreover, women who want
a safe, home-like birth in a familiar setting with staff they

have known throughout their pregnancies express a very
high rate of satisfaction.

The major disadvantage is that most free-standing birth
centers are not equipped for obstetric emergencies. Should
unforeseen difficulties develop during labor, the woman
must be transferred by ambulance to a nearby hospital to
the care of a backup physician who has agreed to perform
this role.

HOME BIRTHS
In the United States, only a small number of women have
their babies at home. Because malpractice insurance for
midwives attending home births is expensive and difficult
to obtain, the number of midwives who offer this service
has decreased greatly. Many have moved their practices to
hospitals or birth centers.

Home birth provides the advantages of keeping the
family together in their own environment throughout the
childbirth experience. Bonding with the infant is unim-
peded by hospital routines, and breast-feeding is highly encouraged and supported. Women maintain a feeling of control because they actively plan and prepare for each detail
of the birth.

Giving birth at home also has disadvantages. Women
who plan a home birth must be screened carefully to make
sure that they have a very low risk for complications. If
transfer to a nearby hospital becomes necessary, the time
required may be too long. Other problems of home birth
include the need for the parents to provide a setting and
adequate supplies for the birth. Moreover, the mother must
take care of herself and the infant without the professional
help she would have in a hospital setting.

Pediatric Nursing

Pediatric nursing has been influenced by factors similar to
those affecting maternity care.

SOCIETAL CHANGES
On the North American continent, as European settle-
ments expanded during the seventeenth and eighteenth

centuries, children were valued as assets to the community because of the desire to increase the population and to share the work to be done. Public schools were established, and the courts began to view children as minors and to protect them accordingly. Devastating epidemics of smallpox, diphtheria, scarlet fever, and measles took their toll on children in the eighteenth century. Children often died of these virulent diseases within 1 day.

The high mortality rate in children led some physicians to examine common child care practices. In 1748, William Cadogan's "Essay on Nursing" discouraged unhealthy child care practices, such as swaddling infants in three or four layers of clothing and feeding them thin gruel within hours after birth. Instead, Cadogan urged mothers to breast-feed their infants and identified certain practices that were thought to contribute to childhood illness. Unfortunately, despite the efforts of Cadogan and others, child care practices were slow to change. Later in the eighteenth century, the health of children improved with the development of certain advances, such as inoculation against smallpox.

In the nineteenth century, with the flood of immigrants to eastern American cities, infectious diseases flourished as a result of crowded living conditions, inadequate and unsanitary food, and harsh working conditions for men, women, and children. Twelve- and 14-hour work days were common for children working in factories, whose earnings were essential to the survival of the family. The most serious child health problems during the nineteenth century were caused by poverty and overcrowding. Infants were fed contaminated milk, sometimes from tuberculosis-infected cows; milk was carried to the cities and purchased by mothers with no means to refrigerate it. Infectious diarrhea was a common cause of infant death.

During the late nineteenth century, conditions began to improve for children and families. Lillian Wald initiated public health nursing at Henry Street Settlement House in New York City, where nurses taught mothers in their homes. In 1889, a milk distribution center opened in New York City to provide uncontaminated milk to sick infants.

HYGIENE AND HOSPITALIZATION

Knowledge of the discoveries of scientists, such as Pasteur, Lister, and Koch, who proved that many diseases were caused by bacteria, became widespread. The use of hygienic practices in hospitals and foundling homes gradually increased. Hospitals began to require personnel to wear uniforms and to limit contact between children in the wards. In an effort to prevent infection, hospital wards were closed to visitors. Because parental visits were noted to cause distress, particularly when parents had to leave, parental visitation was considered to be emotionally stressful to hospitalized children. In an effort to prevent such emotional distress and the spread of infection, parents were prohibited from visiting hospitalized children. As hospital care focused on preventing disease transmission and curing physical diseases, the emotional health of hospitalized children received little attention.

During the twentieth century, as knowledge about nutrition, sanitation, bacteriology, pharmacology, medication, and psychology increased, dramatic changes in child health occurred. In the 1940s and 1950s, the introduction of penicillin, corticosteroids, and vaccines against many communicable diseases saved the lives of tens of thousands of children. Technological advances in the 1970s and 1980s led to more children surviving conditions that had previously been fatal (e.g., cystic fibrosis), resulting in more children with chronic disabilities. An increase in societal concern for children brought about the development of federally supported programs, such as school lunch programs, the Supplemental Food Program for Women, Infants, and Children (WIC), Medicare, and Medicaid (see p. 10), under which the Early Periodic Screening, Diagnosis, and Treatment program, WIC, and Project Head Start were implemented.

DEVELOPMENT OF FAMILY-CENTERED PEDIATRIC CARE

Family-centered care in pediatrics was born out of the recognition that the emotional needs of hospitalized children were in most cases unmet. Parents were not involved in the direct care of their children. Children were often unprepared for procedures and tests, and visiting was severely controlled and even discouraged.

Family-centered care is based on a philosophy that recognizes and respects the pivotal role of the family in the lives of children with special health needs. It strives to support families in their natural caregiving roles and promotes patterns of living at home and in the community. Finally, parents and professionals are viewed as equals in a partnership committed to excellence at all levels of health care (Shelton & Stepanek, 1994).

In health care settings that have a family-centered philosophy, families are given choices, provide input, and are provided information that is understandable by them. The family is respected and its strengths are recognized.

The Association for the Care of Children's Health (ACCH), an interdisciplinary organization, was founded in 1965 to provide a forum for sharing experiences and common problems and to foster growth in children who must undergo hospitalization. Today the organization has broadened its focus on pediatric health care to include the community and the home.

Through the efforts of ACCH and other organizations, increasing attention has been paid to the psychological and emotional effects of hospitalization during childhood. In response to greater knowledge about the emotional effects of illness and hospitalization, hospital policies and health care services for children have changed. Twenty-four-hour parental visitation, sibling visitation policies, and home care services have become commonplace. The psychological preparation of children for hospitalization and surgery has become standard nursing practice. In many hospitals, child life programs have been established to help children and their families cope with the stress of illness. Shorter hospital stays, home care, and day surgery have also helped to minimize the emotional impact of hospitalization and illness on children.

Current Trends in Maternity and Pediatric Care

In the past few years there has been a concerted effort by the government, insurance companies, hospitals, and health care providers to reform health care delivery in the United States. One goal of this reform movement is to control the ever-increasing costs of health care. This trend has involved a change in where and how money is spent. In the past, most of the health care budget was spent in acute care settings, where the facility charged for services after the services were provided. Because hospitals were paid for whatever services they provided, they had no incentive to be efficient or cost-conscious.

Cost Containment

One way in which those paying for health care have attempted to control costs is by shifting to a *prospective* form of payment. In this arrangement, clients no longer pay whatever charges the hospital decides on for service provided. Instead, a fixed amount of money is agreed to in advance for necessary services for specifically diagnosed conditions. One example of this approach is *diagnosis-related groups* (DRGs).

DIAGNOSIS-RELATED GROUPS
Diagnosis-related grouping is a method of classifying related medical diagnoses based on the amount of resources that are generally required by the client. This method became a standard in 1987, when the federal government set the amount of money that would be paid by Medicare for each DRG. If the facility delivers more services or has greater costs than what it will be reimbursed for by Medicare, the facility must absorb the excess costs. Conversely, if the facility delivers the care at less cost than the payment for that DRG, the facility keeps the remaining money. Obviously, health care facilities working under this arrangement benefit financially if they can reduce the client's length of stay and thereby reduce the costs for service. Although the DRG system originally applied only to Medicare clients, most states have adopted the system for Medicaid payments, and many insurance companies use a similar system.

MANAGED CARE
Health insurance companies also examined the cost of health care and instituted a health care delivery system that has been called *managed care*. Examples of managed care organizations are health maintenance organizations (HMOs), point of service plans (POSs), and preferred provider organizations (PPOs). In return for a set fee or premium, HMOs provide relatively comprehensive health services for persons enrolled in the organization. Similarly, PPOs are groups of health care providers who agree to provide health services to a specific group of clients at a discounted cost. When the client needs medical treatment, managed care includes strategies such as payment arrangements and preadmission authorization to control costs.

CAPITATED CARE
Capitation may be incorporated into any type of managed care plan. In a pure capitated care plan, the employer (or government) pays a set amount of money each year to a network of primary care providers. This amount might be adjusted for age and sex of the client group. In exchange for access to a guaranteed client base, the primary care providers agree to provide general health care and to pay for all aspects of the client's care, including laboratory work, specialist visits, and hospital care.

Capitated plans are of interest to both employers and the government because they allow a predictable amount of money to be budgeted for health care. Clients do not have unexpected financial burdens from illness. However, clients lose most of their freedom of choice regarding who will provide their care. Primary care providers can lose money if they refer too many clients to specialists, who may have no restrictions on their fees, or if they order too many diagnostic tests. Some health care providers and consumers fear that cost constraints might affect treatment decisions.

Effects of Cost Containment

Prospective payment plans have had major effects on maternity care, primarily in relation to the length of stay. Mothers who have a normal vaginal birth may leave the birth facility within 24 to 48 hours, and mothers who give birth by cesarean section may go home within 72 hours. This policy of early discharge has been intensely criticized because problems have developed with mothers or infants who have needed to be readmitted to the birth facility. As a result, legislation has been passed that mandates a minimum 48-hour length of stay for vaginal births and 4 days for cesarean births, unless the woman and her health care provider choose an earlier discharge time.

Reduced length of stays have also affected caregivers, particularly nurses. Since the mid-1990s nurses have become increasingly concerned with meeting the needs of families who leave the hospital a short time after the birth of an infant. Nurses find it especially difficult to provide adequate information about self-care and infant care within the first 24 hours, when the mother is still recovering from childbirth.

The American Academy of Pediatrics has raised several concerns related to managed care and the care of children. Some of the concerns include appropriate pediatric referrals and delays in treatment authorization; limited coordination with community health, education, and social services; and a general lack of research related to children in managed care (AAP Committee on Child Health Financing, 1995).

Managed care, provided appropriately, can increase access to a full range of health care providers and services, but it must be closely monitored. Pediatric nurses serve as child advocates in the areas of preventive, acute, and chronic pediatric care. The teaching timelines for preventive and home care have been shortened drastically, and the call to "begin teaching the moment the child enters the health care system" has taken on a new meaning. Parents and other caregivers are being asked to do procedures at home that were once done by professionals in a hospital setting. Systems must be in place to monitor compliance, understanding, and the total care of the child. Assessment and communication skills must be keen, and the nurse must be able to work with specialists in other disciplines.

CASE MANAGEMENT
Case management is a practice model that uses a systematic approach to identify specific clients and to manage care to ensure optimal outcomes (Ignatavicius & Hausman, 1995). In this model, the services needed by the client and family

are coordinated by a case manager or case coordinator, who focuses on both quality and cost outcomes. Inherent to case management is the coordination of care by all members of the health care team. The guidelines established in 1995 by the Joint Commission on the Accreditation of Healthcare Organizations require an interdisciplinary, collaborative approach to client care. This concept is at the core of case management.

Clinical practice guidelines are an important tool in developing guidelines for safe, effective care. The Agency for Health Care Policy and Research has developed several guidelines related to adult and child care. Currently, guidelines for the following areas of pediatric health have been released: acute pain management, sickle cell disease, management of cancer pain, and otitis media with effusion. Continued research and sharing of information in this area are needed to ensure quality case management.

OUTCOMES MANAGEMENT

The determination to lower health care costs while maintaining the quality of care has led to a clinical practice model called *outcomes management*. This is a systematic method to identify client outcomes and to focus care on interventions that will accomplish the stated outcomes for specific case types, such as the woman who has just given birth or the child with asthma. The planning tools used by the health care team to identify and meet stated outcomes are *clinical pathways*. Other names for clinical pathways include *critical or clinical paths*, *care paths*, *care maps*, *collaborative plans of care*, *anticipated recovery paths*, and *multidisciplinary action plans*.

CLINICAL PATHWAYS

Clinical pathways are a tool for measuring outcomes. Clinical pathways are interdisciplinary plans of care that outline the optimal sequencing and timing of interventions for clients with a particular diagnosis, procedure, or symptom (Ignatavicius & Hausman, 1995). Although the concept of clinical pathways is not new, it has only recently been widely accepted as the use of case management has become widespread in various health care settings. The purpose, as in managed care and case management, is to provide quality care while controlling costs.

Clinical pathways identify client outcomes, specify time lines, promote collaboration, and involve a comprehensive approach to care. They are characterized by the following:

- Expected client outcomes by the time of discharge are listed.
- Specific time lines for sequencing interventions are outlined.
- Clinical pathways are jointly developed by multiple health care professionals, including physicians, to reflect interdisciplinary interventions.
- The approach to care is comprehensive and includes nutrition, diagnostic tests, treatments, medications, mobility and activity, teaching, and discharge planning (Ignatavicius & Hausman, 1995).

Clinical pathways can be used in settings other than the hospital. Home health agencies use clinical pathways, which may be developed in collaboration with hospital staff.

Facilities differ in how they use clinical pathways. For instance, they may be used for change-of-shift reports to indicate information about length of stay, individual needs, and priorities of the shift for each client. They may also be used as an adjunct to, or instead of, nursing care plans and to document the client's progress in meeting the desired outcomes. Many pathways are particularly helpful in identifying families that need follow-up care.

Variances. Deviations, often called *variances*, may occur, either in the time line or in the expected outcomes. A variance is the difference between what was expected and what actually happened. A variance may be positive or negative. A positive variance occurs when a client progresses faster than expected and is discharged sooner than planned. A negative variance occurs when progress is slower than expected, outcomes are not met within the designated time frame, and the length of stay is prolonged.

Students Using Clinical Pathways. Clinical pathways are guidelines for care. Although a pathway provides insight into the scheduling of assessments and care, it is not meant to teach nursing skills and procedures. One purpose of this book is to provide ample information so that students can *use* clinical pathways in a clinical setting. This involves teaching *why and how to perform assessments* and interpreting the significance of the data obtained. Moreover, the book emphasizes ways of providing information, care, and comfort for clients and their families as they progress along a clinical pathway. Sample clinical pathways are provided throughout the text.

▌ *Home Care*

Home nursing care has experienced dramatic growth since 1990. Advances in portable technology, such as state-of-the-art electronic fetal monitors or infusion pumps for the administration of intravenous nutrition or subcutaneous medications, allow nurses to perform complicated procedures in the home. In addition, consumers often prefer home care because of decreased stress on the family when the client is able to remain at home rather than be separated from the family support system because of the need for hospitalization.

Home care services may be provided in the form of telephone calls, home visits, information lines, and lactation consultations, among others. Infants with congenital anomalies, such as cleft palate, may need care that is adapted to their condition. Moreover, increasing numbers of technology-dependent infants and children are now cared for at home. The numbers include those needing ventilator assistance, total parenteral nutrition, intravenous medications, apnea monitoring, and other device-associated nursing care.

Because care is given in an environment that is physically separated from an acute care institution, nurses must be able to function independently and must be confident of their clinical skills. They should be proficient at interviewing, counseling, and teaching. They often assume a leadership role in coordinating all the services a family may require, and they frequently supervise the work of other care providers.

▌ *Health Insurance*

The number of uninsured children in the United States continues to grow. About 85% of children have some form of health insurance, whether it be private or publicly funded. Public health insurance for children is provided primarily through Medicaid, but it also is provided through Medicare and the Civilian Health and Medical Program of the Uniformed Services (CHAMPUS). The number of children covered by private health insurance decreased from 74% in 1987 to 66% in 1996. During the same period, the proportion of children covered by public health insurance increased from 19% to 25% (Centers for Disease Control and Prevention [CDC], 1998a). This means that more than 10.6 million children (15%) are less likely to receive preventive care or to use health care services, and are at increased risk for health problems (Holl et al., 1995).

Latino children are less likely to have health insurance than either white or black children (Fig. 1–2). Young children ages birth to 5 years are more likely to have coverage than older children (CDC, 1998a).

Uninsured children may live in families with incomes below the poverty level or they may be dependents of working parents who do not have insurance for a variety of reasons.

- Increasing numbers of children now live with single mothers who work in low-paying service jobs without medical insurance.
- Employer health care benefits have declined over the past decade.
- If family coverage is offered, the employee may decline it because of the high cost of the premiums (Carnegie Corporation of New York, 1994).

Besides the obvious implication of not having health insurance—the inability to pay for health care during illness—there is another very important effect on children and adults who are not insured: they are less likely to receive preventive care. This places them at increased risk for preventable illnesses and, because preventive health care is a learned behavior, these children are more likely to become adults who are less healthy.

The uninsured pregnant woman is less likely to have prenatal care than the insured woman or will seek care later in her pregnancy. Complications are more likely to be severe if they occur, and the health of her fetus is threatened.

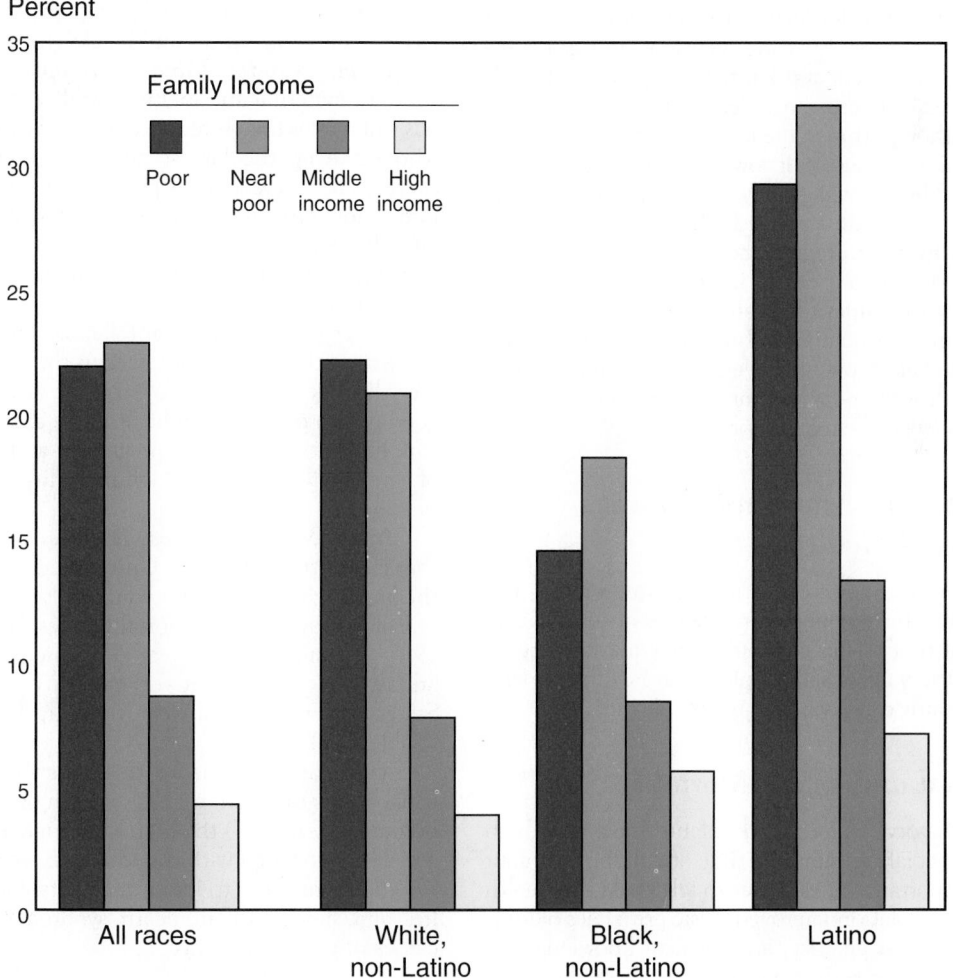

FIGURE 1–2

Percentage of children under 18 years of age with no health insurance, by family income and race. (From Centers for Disease Control and Prevention, National Center for Health Statistics, National Health Interview Survey.)

Therefore, the lack of health insurance for a pregnant woman is likely to cost society more.

Health Care Assistance Programs

Many programs, some funded privately, others by the government, assist in the care of mothers, infants, and children. The supplemental food program known as the WIC program, which was established in 1972, provides supplemental food supplies to low-income women who are pregnant or breast-feeding and to their children up to the age of 5 years. The WIC program has long been heralded as a cost-effective program that not only provides nutritional support but also links families with other services, such as prenatal care and immunizations.

Medicaid's Early and Periodic Screening, Diagnosis, and Treatment Program was developed to provide comprehensive health care to Medicaid recipients from birth to 21 years of age. The goal of the program is to prevent health problems before they become severe. This program pays for well-child examinations and for the treatment of any medical problems diagnosed during such checkups.

Public Law 99–457 is part of the Individuals with Disabilities Act that provides financial incentives to states to establish comprehensive early intervention services for infants and toddlers with, or at risk for, developmental disabilities. Services include screening, identification, referral, and treatment. Although this is a federal law and entitlement, each state bases coverage on its own definition of developmental delay. Thus, coverage may vary from state to state. Some states provide care for at-risk children.

The Healthy Start Program, begun in 1991, is a major initiative to reduce infant deaths in communities with disproportionately high infant mortality rates. Strategies used include reducing the number of high-risk pregnancies, reducing the number of low-birth-weight and preterm births, improving birth-weight-specific survival, and ameliorating specific causes of postneonatal mortality.

Statistics on Maternal, Infant, and Child Health

Statistics is the science of collecting and interpreting numeric data. Statistics are important sources of information about the health of groups of people. They may also be an indication of the value a society places on health care and the kind of health care available to the people.

Maternal and Infant Mortality

Throughout history, women and infants have had high death rates, especially around the time of childbirth. Infant and maternal mortality rates began to fall when the health of the general population improved, basic principles of sanitation were put into practice, and medical knowledge increased. A further large decrease was a result of the widespread availability of antibiotics, improvements in public health, and better prenatal care. Today, mothers seldom die in childbirth and infant mortality rates continue downward. The downward trend in maternal and infant mortality rates, however, is greater for whites than for nonwhite groups.

MATERNAL MORTALITY

In 1995, the maternal mortality rate was 7.1 per 100,000 live births for all women in the United States. African-American women are more likely to die from birth-related causes than white women. The maternal mortality rate for African-American women is 22.1, whereas for white women it is 4.2 (U.S. Department of Health and Human Services [USDHHS], 1998).

INFANT MORTALITY

Infant mortality rates have improved somewhat slower than maternal mortality rates. Between 1950 and 1990, infant mortality dropped from 29.2 to 9.8 deaths per 1,000 live births. In 1997 the infant mortality rate (death before the age of 1 year) was 7.1 per 1,000 live births, the lowest ever recorded in the United States (CDC, 1998c). Moreover, the neonatal mortality rate (death before 28 days of life) dropped to 4.7 deaths per 1,000 live births (National Center for Health Statistics [NCHS], 1998).

Although infant mortality rates in the United States have declined overall, rates have declined faster for whites than for African-Americans. In 1997 the mortality rate for white infants was 6.0. For black infants the rate was 13.7 (NCHS, 1998). Figure 1–3 compares the rates of infant mortality among whites and blacks since 1940.

Disparity Across Minority Groups.   The racial differences in maternal and infant mortality rates are most obvious when rates for whites are compared with rates for blacks, who make up the largest minority group in the United States. The discrepancy is primarily due to increases in the rate of low-birth-weight infants (below 2,500 g). Black infants have twice the risk for low birth weight than other newborns, and they are twice as likely to die before their first birthday.

Poverty is an important factor. Proportionally more nonwhites than whites are poor in the United States. People who live below the poverty line are unlikely to be in good health or to get the health care they need. Obtaining care becomes vital during pregnancy and infancy, and lack of care is reflected in the high mortality rates in all categories.

Infant Mortality Across Nations.   One would expect that a country such as the United States, which has one of the largest gross national products in the world, would have one of the lowest infant mortality rates. However, data from 1997, the most recent year for which comparative data are available, show that the mortality rate in the United States was worse that year than in 18 other countries (Table 1–2).

The major reasons for this poor showing are (1) unequal access to health care for women of different socioeconomic levels and (2) the high rate of adolescent pregnancy, which is associated with the low birth weight and prematurity that contribute to infant mortality. Congenital anomalies and sudden infant death syndrome are also leading causes of infant mortality.

Adolescent Pregnancy

In the United States, adolescent pregnancy rates are high, with approximately 1,465 teens giving birth each day (March of Dimes, 1995). Although the rate has decreased

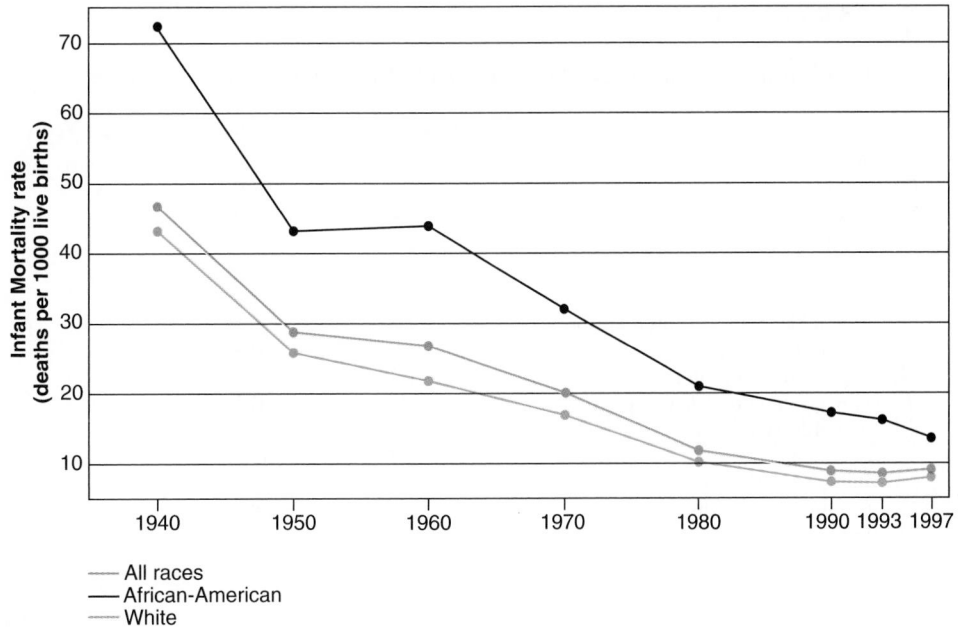

— All races
— African-American
— White

FIGURE 1–3

Infant mortality rates from 1940 to 1997 based on deaths per 1,000 live births. Data based on advance report on final mortality statistics. (National Center for Health Statistics, U.S. Department of Health and Human Services, Public Health Service, Centers for Disease Control and Prevention, 1994. *Monthly Vital Statistics Report 43*[2], Supplement; and Centers for Disease Control. [1998c]. Births and deaths: Preliminary data for 1997. *National Vital Statistics Reports.)*

TABLE 1–2

Infant Mortality Rates for Selected Countries

Country	Infant Mortality (per 1,000 Live Births)
Japan	4.25
Singapore	4.34
Hong Kong	4.43
Sweden	4.45
Finland	4.72
Switzerland	5.12
Norway	5.23
Denmark	5.45
Germany	5.60
Netherlands	5.64
Ireland	5.93
Australia, Northern Ireland	6.05
England, Wales, Scotland	6.20
Austria	6.25
Canada*	6.30
France*	6.47
Italy	6.63
Spain*	6.69
United States	7.1

* 1993 data.

From U.S. Department of Health and Human Services. (1998). *Health, United States, 1998, with socioeconomic status and health chartbook.* Washington, DC: Author; and Centers for Disease Control and Prevention. (1998c). Births and deaths: Preliminary data for 1997. *National Vital Statistics Reports, 47*(4), 1–42.

from 62.1 per 1,000 teenagers 15 to 19 years old in 1991 to 54.4 in 1996, the number of teenagers is increasing (Guyer et al., 1996; USDHHS, 1998). This change in the population will further increase adolescent pregnancies.

Childhood Mortality

The leading cause of infant mortality is congenital anomalies, with anomalies of the heart having the highest incidence of death. Disorders related to short gestation and unspecified low birth weight make up the second leading cause of death in infants. Sudden infant death syndrome, which accounted for 10% of all infant deaths, is showing a steady decline (CDC, 1998e).

Death rates for children have significantly declined over the past 20 years. Table 1–3 shows the leading causes of death in children. Although death rates attributed to unintentional injury have also dropped, accidents are still the leading cause of death in children ages 1 to 19 years. Homicide is the fourth leading cause of death for children ages 1 to 4 years, the third leading cause for children ages 5 to 14 years, and the second leading cause for children more than 14 years old (CDC, 1998e). Other common causes of death in children include cancer, chronic obstructive pulmonary diseases, and human immunodeficiency virus (HIV) infection.

Morbidity

Morbidity is the ratio of sick to well persons in a community. This ratio is presented as rates per 1,000 population. This term is used in reference to acute and chronic illness

TABLE 1–3

Death Rates for the 10 Leading Causes of Death in Specific Age Groups

Cause	1–4 Years	5–14 Years	15–24 Years
All causes	35.6	21.7	84.6
Accidents	12.8	8.6	35.4
Motor vehicle	4.9	5.0	27.1
All other	7.8	3.6	8.3
Congenital anomalies	3.9	1.1	1.0
Malignant neoplasms	3.0	2.6	4.3
Homicide and legal intervention	2.2	1.1	15.8
Diseases of the heart	1.3	0.8	2.8
Pneumonia and influenza	1.1	0.4	0.6
Human immunodeficiency virus infection	—	0.3	0.8
Septicemia	0.4	—	—
Benign neoplasms	0.4	0.2	—
Cerebrovascular diseases	0.3	—	0.5
Suicide	—	0.8	11.3
Chronic obstructive pulmonary disease	—	0.3	0.5
All other causes	9.7	4.6	11.5

Excerpted from a table of deaths and death rates for the 10 leading causes of death in specified age groups: United States, preliminary data for 1997. Centers for Disease Control and Prevention. (1998). Births and deaths: Preliminary data for 1997. *National Vital Statistics Reports, 47*(4), 32.

as well as disability. Because morbidity statistics are collected and updated less frequently than mortality statistics, it is difficult to present current data in all areas of pediatrics.

Respiratory tract–related illnesses are the leading cause of morbidity in children. Children experience an average of six respiratory tract infections per year. Infectious diseases are the most common cause of school absenteeism (Feigin & Cherry, 1998). Statistics regarding morbidity related to particular disorders are presented throughout this book as the disorders are discussed.

The Youth Risk Behavior Surveillance System has identified six categories of health risk behaviors among youth that contribute to increased morbidity: tobacco use; unhealthy dietary behaviors; inadequate physical activity; alcohol and other drug use; sexual behaviors that may result in HIV infection, other sexually transmitted diseases, and unintended pregnancies; and behaviors that result in intentional injuries (violence and suicide) and unintentional injuries (motor vehicle crashes) (CDC, 1998d).

There is a link between children living in poverty and poorer health outcomes. Children who live in families of higher income and higher education have a better chance of being born healthy and remaining so. Access to health care, the health behaviors of parents and siblings, and exposure to environmental risks are among the factors contributing to the disparity in children's health (National Institute of Child Health and Human Development [NICHHD], 1998).

Ethical Perspectives on Maternal and Child Nursing

Maternal-child nurses often struggle with ethical and social dilemmas that affect families. Nurses must know how to approach these issues in a knowledgeable and systematic way.

Ethics and Bioethics

Ethics involves determining the best course of action in a certain situation. Ethical reasoning is the analysis of what is morally right and reasonable. Bioethics is the application of ethics to health care. Ethical behavior for nurses is discussed in various codes, such as the American Nurses' Association Code for Nurses. Ethical issues have become more complex as developing technology has allowed more options in health care. These issues are controversial because there is lack of agreement over what is right or best and because moral support is possible for more than one course of action.

Ethical Dilemmas

An ethical dilemma is a situation in which no solution seems completely satisfactory. Opposing courses of action may seem equally desirable, or all possible solutions may seem undesirable. Ethical dilemmas are among the most difficult situations in nursing practice. Finding solutions involves applying ethical theories and principles and determining the burdens and benefits of any course of action.

ETHICAL THEORIES

Two major theories guide ethical decision making. Few people use one theory exclusively. Instead, they make decisions by examining both theories and trying to determine which one is more appropriate for the circumstances.

Deontologic Theory. The deontologic approach determines what is right by applying ethical principles and moral rules. It does not vary the solution according to individual situations. One example is the rule "life must be maintained at all costs and in all circumstances." Strictly used, the deontologic approach would not consider the quality of life or weigh the use of scarce resources against the likelihood that the life maintained would be near normal.

Utilitarian Theory.   The utilitarian theory approaches ethical dilemmas by analyzing the benefits and burdens of any course of action to find one that will result in the greatest amount of good. With this theory, the appropriate actions may vary according to the situation. It is a pragmatic approach concerned with the consequences of actions more than the actual actions themselves. In its simplest form, this is an end-justifies-the-means approach. If the outcome is positive, the method of arriving at that outcome is less important.

ETHICAL PRINCIPLES

Ethical principles are also important in solving ethical dilemmas. Four of the most important principles are beneficence, nonmaleficence, autonomy, and justice. Although principles guide decision making, in some situations it may be impossible to apply one principle without encountering conflict with another. In such cases, one principle may outweigh another in importance.

For example, treatments designed to do good may also cause some harm. A cesarean birth may prevent permanent harm to a fetus in distress. However, the surgery that saves the fetus also harms the mother, causing pain, temporary disability, and possible financial hardship. Both mother and health care providers may decide that the principle of beneficence outweighs the principle of nonmaleficence. A third possibility is that if the mother does not want surgery, the principles of autonomy and justice must also be considered. Is the mother's right to determine what happens to her body more or less important than the right of the fetus to fair and equal treatment?

SOLVING ETHICAL DILEMMAS

Although using a specific approach does not guarantee a right decision, it provides a logical, systematic method for going through the steps of decision making.

Decision making in ethical dilemmas may seem straightforward, but it may not result in answers agreeable to everyone. Many agencies, therefore, have bioethics committees to formulate policies for ethical situations, provide education, and help make decisions in specific cases. The committees include a variety of professionals such as nurses, physicians, social workers, ethicists, and clergy members. The client and family also participate, if possible. A satisfac-

. . . .
Ethical Principles

Beneficence.   One is required to do or promote good for others.

Nonmaleficence.   One must avoid risking or causing harm to others.

Autonomy.   People have the right to self-determination. This includes the right to respect, privacy, and the information necessary to make decisions.

Justice.   All people should be treated equally and fairly regardless of disease or social or economic status.

. . . .
CRITICAL THINKING EXERCISE 1–1

The parents of an infant with anencephaly state that they would like to donate the organs from their dying infant to another infant who might live as a result. They feel that in this way their own infant will live on as a part of another baby. Although these transplants have been performed in the past, they are not currently performed because of the ethical concerns involved.

1. What is the deontologic view of this decision?
2. How does the utilitarian view differ?
3. What ethical principles are involved? If such transplants became routine, what potential problems might arise?

tory solution to ethical dilemmas is more likely to occur when a variety of people work together.

Ethical dilemmas may also have legal ramifications. For example, although the American Medical Association has stated that anencephalic organ donation is ethically permissible, it may be illegal. In many states, the legal criteria for death include both cardiopulmonary and brain death. Anencephalic infants do not meet those criteria, so that donation of their organs would be illegal, even if it were ethical (Rhodes, 1996a).

Ethical Issues in Reproduction

Reproductive issues often involve conflicts in which a woman behaves in a way that may cause harm to her fetus or that is disapproved of by some or most members of society. Conflicts between a mother and fetus occur when the mother's needs, behavior, or wishes may injure the fetus. The most obvious instances are those involving abortion, substance abuse, or a mother's refusal to follow the advice of caregivers. Health care workers and society in general may respond to such a woman with anger rather than support. The rights of both mother and fetus must be examined, however.

ELECTIVE ABORTION

Abortion was a volatile legal, social, and political issue even before the *Roe v. Wade* decision by the U.S. Supreme Court in 1973. Before that time, states could prohibit abortion, making the procedure illegal. In *Roe v. Wade* the court stated that abortion was legal anywhere in the United States and that existing state laws prohibiting abortion were unconstitutional because they interfered with the mother's constitutional right to privacy. The Supreme Court decision stipulated that (1) a woman could obtain an abortion at any time during the first trimester, (2) the state could regulate abortions during the second trimester only to protect the woman's health, and (3) the state could regulate or prohibit abortion during the third trimester, except when the mother's life might be jeopardized by continuing the pregnancy.

For many, a woman's constitutional right to privacy conflicts with a fetus's right to life. The Supreme Court did not rule, however, on when life begins. This omission provokes debate between those who believe life begins at conception and those who believe life begins when the fetus is viable, or capable of living outside the uterus. Those who believe life begins at conception may be opposed to abortion at any time during pregnancy. Those who believe life begins when the fetus is viable (20 to 26 weeks of gestation) may oppose abortion after that time. Nurses need to be knowledgeable about past Supreme Court decisions related to abortion and about the conflicting beliefs that divide society on this issue.

Conflicting Beliefs About Abortion.   Perhaps no issue creates greater division or incites more powerful emotions among Americans than that of elective abortion. Some people believe abortion should be illegal at any time because it deprives the fetus of life. In contrast, others believe that women have the right to control their reproductive function and that political discussion of reproductive rights is an invasion of the most private decisions of women.

Belief That Abortion Is a Private Choice.   At the heart of political action to keep abortion legal is the conviction that women have the right to make decisions about their reproductive function on the basis of their own ethical and moral beliefs and that the government has no place in these decisions.

In 1995, the rate of legal abortions was 31.1 abortions for every 100 live births. Many abortions are obtained by minors (USDHHS, 1998). Advocates of the legal right to abortion point out that abortion, either legal or illegal, has always been a reality of life and will continue to be so, regardless of legislation or judicial rulings. Advocates express concern about the unsafe conditions that accompany illegal abortion, citing the deaths that occurred as a result of illegal abortions performed before the *Roe v. Wade* decision.

Belief That Abortion Is Taking a Life.   Many people believe that legalized abortion condones taking a life, and feel morally bound to protect the lives of fetuses. Persons opposed to abortion have demonstrated their commitment by organizing to become a potent political force. They have willingly been arrested for civil disobedience when they attempted to prevent admissions to clinics that perform abortions.

Legal Aspects of Roe v. Wade.   Abortion has been a complex legal issue since 1973, and the U.S. Supreme Court has made major decisions that affect abortion law since that time. Some decisions have strengthened the original *Roe v. Wade* ruling, and others have weakened it. Because nurses should know about the legal history of abortion, some of these decisions are enumerated in the accompanying box. Legislation introduced in 1995 banning late-term abortions received a presidential veto because it did not provide an exception for when the mother's health is at risk. Other versions of this bill will probably be introduced in the future and, if passed, may come before the Supreme Court.

Implications for Nurses.   As health care professionals, nurses are involved in the conflict between differing beliefs about abortion. Nurses have several responsibilities that cannot be ignored. First, they must be informed about the complexity of the abortion issue from a legal and ethical standpoint and know the exact regulations and laws in their state. Second, they must realize that, for many, abortion is an ethical dilemma that results in confusion, ambivalence, and personal distress. Next, they must also recognize that

• • • • • • • • • • •
Supreme Court Decisions on Abortion Since Roe v. Wade

1976: States cannot give a husband veto power over his spouse's decision to have an abortion.

1977: States do not have an obligation to pay for abortions as part of government-funded health care programs (considered by abortion rights advocates to be unfair discrimination against poor women who are unable to pay for an abortion).

1979: Physicians have broad discretion in determining fetal viability, and states have leeway to restrict abortions of viable fetuses.

1979: States may require parental consent for minors seeking abortions as long as an alternative, such as the minor getting a judge's approval, is also available.

1989: Upheld a Missouri law barring abortions performed in public hospitals and clinics or performed by public employees. Also required physicians to conduct tests for fetal viability at 20 weeks of gestation.

1990: States may require notification of both parents before a person under the age of 18 years has an abortion. A judge can authorize the abortion without parental consent.

1992: Validated Pennsylvania law imposing restrictions on abortions. The restrictions upheld include the following:

A woman must be told about fetal development and alternatives to abortion.
She must wait at least 24 hours after this explanation before having an abortion.
Unmarried women under the age of 18 must obtain consent from their parents or a judge.
Physicians must keep detailed records of each abortion, subject to public disclosure.

Struck down only one requirement of the Pennsylvania law: that a married woman must inform her husband before having an abortion.

1993: Rescinded the so-called gag rule, which restricted the counseling that health care professionals (with the exception of physicians) could provide at federally funded family planning clinics.

1995: Upheld a ruling that states cannot withhold state funds for abortions in case of pregnancies resulting from rape or incest or when the mother's life is in danger.

the issue is not a dilemma for many but is a fundamental violation of the personal or religious views that give meaning to their lives. Finally, it is absolutely essential that nurses acknowledge the sincere convictions and the strong emotions of people on all sides of the issue.

Personal Values.   Nurses respond to abortion in ways that illustrate the complexity of the issue and the ambivalence that it often produces. For instance, some nurses have no objection to participating in abortions. Others do not assist with abortions but may care for women after the procedure. Some nurses assist with a first-trimester abortion but may object to later abortions. Many nurses are comfortable assisting in abortion if the fetus has severe anomalies but are uncomfortable in other circumstances. Some nurses feel that they could not provide care before, during, or after an abortion but that they are bound by conscience to try to dissuade a woman from the decision to abort.

Professional Obligations. Nurses have no obligation to support a position with which they disagree. Many states have laws that allow nurses to refuse to assist with the procedure if abortions violate ethical, moral, or religious beliefs. Nurses are obligated, however, to disclose this information before they are employed in an institution that performs abortions. It would be unethical for a nurse to withhold this information until assigned to care for a woman having an abortion and then refuse to provide care. As always, nurses must respect the decisions of women who look to nurses for care. If nurses feel that they are not able to provide compassionate care because of personal convictions, they must inform a supervisor so that appropriate care can be arranged.

MANDATED CONTRACEPTION

The availability of long-term contraceptive devices that are injected or implanted under the skin has led to speculation about whether certain women should be forced to use them. In fact, the procedure has already been used as a condition of probation, allowing women accused of child abuse to avoid jail terms. Legislative efforts have been made to require women who receive public assistance to use the implants.

Some feel that forced contraception is a way to prevent additional births to women considered unsuitable parents and a way to decrease government expenses for dependent children. This punitive approach to social and ethical problems, however, does not provide long-term solutions. In addition, coercing the poor to use birth control to limit the money spent supporting them is questionable both legally and ethically.

Such a practice would interfere with a woman's constitutional rights to privacy, to reproduction, to refusal of medical treatment, and to freedom from cruel and unusual punishment. In addition, the implants may pose health risks to the woman. Other methods of limiting unwanted pregnancies, such as access to free or low-cost information on family planning, would be more appropriate.

FETAL INJURY

If a mother's actions cause injury to her fetus, the question of whether she should be restrained or prosecuted has both legal and ethical implications. In some instances, courts have issued jail sentences to women who have caused or who may cause injury to the fetus. This response punishes the woman and places her in a situation in which she cannot further harm the fetus. In other cases, women have been forced to undergo cesarean births against their will when physicians have testified that such a procedure was necessary to prevent injury to the fetus.

The state has an interest in protecting children, and the Supreme Court has ruled that a child has the right to begin life with a sound mind and body. Many states have laws requiring the reporting of evidence of prenatal drug exposure, which is considered child abuse. Women have been charged with negligence, involuntary manslaughter, delivering drugs to a minor, and child endangerment.

Yet forcing a woman to behave in a certain way because she is pregnant violates the principles of autonomy, self-determination of competent adults, bodily integrity, and personal freedom. Because of fear of prosecution, this practice could impede health care during pregnancy instead of advancing it. Women are unlikely to seek prenatal care or treatment for substance abuse unless they feel safe.

The punitive approach to fetal injury also raises the question of how much control the government seeking to protect the fetus should have over a pregnant woman. Laws could be passed mandating fetal testing, the use of tocolytics for preterm labor, intrauterine surgery, or even the foods a pregnant woman eats. It could be hard to decide just how much control should be allowed in the interests of fetal safety.

FETAL THERAPY

Fetal therapy is in its early phases but may become more widespread as techniques improve. Although intrauterine blood transfusions are relatively standard practice in some areas, most fetal surgery is far from routine.

The risks and benefits of surgery for major fetal anomalies must be considered in every case. Even when surgery is successful, the fetus may not survive, may have other serious problems, or may be born preterm. The mother may need weeks of bed rest and a cesarean delivery. Yet in spite of the risks, successful surgery may result in the birth of an infant who could not otherwise have survived.

Parents need help in balancing the potential risks to the mother with the best interests of the fetus. There is a danger that they might feel pressured to have surgery or other fetal treatment they do not understand. As with any situation involving informed consent, women need adequate information before making a decision. They should understand whether procedures are still experimental, what the chances of success are, and what alternatives are available.

ISSUES IN INFERTILITY

Infertility Treatment. Perinatal technology has found ways for some infertile couples to bear children (see Chapter 10). There are many happy results from such practices when infertile couples are finally able to give birth, but there have been some ethical concerns as well.

Concerns include the high cost and overall low success of various treatments. Because the costs are usually not covered by insurance, their use is limited to the affluent. The high price of research on techniques that will benefit only a few has also been questioned. Some think that the money should be spent on research that will help a greater number of people. Even with high-technology treatments, many infertile couples will never give birth. Success rates for these procedures are still low. Also, when treatment is successful, there is a high risk of multiple births and premature infants, leading to extensive complications and expensive care associated with preterm birth.

Other ethical concerns focus on the fate of unused embryos. Should they be frozen for later use by the woman or someone else, or could they be used in genetic research? Who should make these decisions? In multiple pregnancies with more fetuses than can be expected to survive intact, reduction surgery may be used to destroy one or more fetuses for the benefit of those remaining. The ethical and long-term psychological implications of this procedure are also controversial.

Assisted reproductive techniques now allow postmenopausal women to become mothers. What are the ethical implications of giving birth to children who may very well be orphaned at an early age? Should the age and health of the parents be a factor in determining whether this treatment is offered? Should the risk these women face for developing complications that might result in low-birth-weight infants be considered?

Surrogate Parenting. In surrogate parenting, a woman agrees to bear an infant for another woman. Cases in which the surrogate mother has wanted to keep the child have been controversial. There are no standard regulations governing these cases, which are decided on an individual basis. Ethical concerns involve who should be a surrogate mother, what her role should be after birth, and who should make these decisions. Screening of parents as well as surrogates may be necessary to determine whether they are suitable for their roles. But who should do the screening? Should it be left to the private interests of those involved, or should the government become involved? There are no definite answers to these questions at this time.

Cessation of Treatment. The decision to cease treatment is always a difficult one and seems to be compounded when the client is an infant or child. Children who would have died in the past can now have their lives extended through the use of life support. Parents must be involved in the decision-making process immediately and informed about available options. Laws in some states permit parents to provide advance directives for their minor children. When an older child is involved, their views are considered.

In this age of resource allocation, debate centers on how to manage critical care resources. Many believe that these decisions should not be made at the bedside. The American Academy of Pediatrics, in its statement Ethics and the Care of Critically Ill Infants and Children (1996), encouraged society to engage in a thorough debate about the economic, cultural, religious, social, and moral consequences of imposing limits on which patients should receive intensive care.

Social Issues

Nurses are exposed to many social issues that influence health care and often have legal or ethical implications. Some of the issues that affect maternity and pediatric care include poverty, homelessness, access to care, and allocation of funds.

Poverty

Poverty is an underlying factor in problems such as inadequate access to health care and homelessness. The number of children living in households with cash incomes below the poverty level has stayed around 20% since 1981. Children under age 6 are more often found in families with incomes below the poverty line than are older children. Children in female-headed households are more likely to be living in poverty (CDC, 1998a).

Poverty becomes a health issue because it affects access to health care and decreases opportunities linked with health promotion. Poverty rates in the United States are geographic. The southern and western portions of the country have disproportionately more of the nation's poor population.

Nurses can play a role in meeting the health care needs of mothers and their infants and children by recognizing the adverse effect of poverty on health and identifying poverty as a practice concern. Several goals in the U.S. Public Health Service's *Healthy People 2000* have implications for maternal-child nurses:

- To reduce the infant mortality rate to no more than 7 per 1,000 live births, and the mortality among black infants to no more than 11 per 1,000 live births.
- To reduce the incidence of low birth weight to no more than 5% of live births and no more than 9% of black infants.
- To ensure that 90% of all pregnant women receive prenatal care in the first trimester of pregnancy.
- To ensure that at least 90% of children younger than 2 years of age complete the basic immunization series.
- To reduce vaccine-preventable diseases as follows: (1) measles and rubella to zero cases, (2) mumps to no more than 500 cases per year, and (3) pertussis to no more than 1,000 cases per year.

Revised objectives to be released in early 2000 set health goals for 2010.

Poverty tends to breed poverty. In poor families, children may leave the educational system early, making them less likely to learn skills necessary to obtain good jobs. Childbearing at an early age is common and interferes with education and the ability to work. The cycle of poverty (Fig. 1–4) may continue from one generation to another as a result of hopelessness and apathy.

Homelessness

Families, many of which are composed of single women and their children, are the fastest-growing group of homeless people. Some homeless women are substance abusers. Both homeless women and their children are poorly nourished and are exposed to tuberculosis, HIV infection, and sexually transmissible diseases. Rape and assault are problems, with a high rate of pregnancy among homeless girls. Infants born to homeless women are subject to a lower birth weight and a greater likelihood of neonatal mortality (Beal & Redlener, 1995).

Pregnancy and birth, especially among teenagers, are important causes contributing to homelessness. Pregnancy interferes with a woman's ability to work and may decrease her income to the point at which she loses her housing. Without child care or a home address, she may have less chance of obtaining and keeping employment. In addition, her children are more likely to be sick because of inadequate food and shelter. Without money to pay for insurance or early health care, there is an increased chance that children will need hospitalization.

Federal funding has provided assistance with shelter and health care for homeless people. The homeless, however, have the same difficulties in obtaining health care as

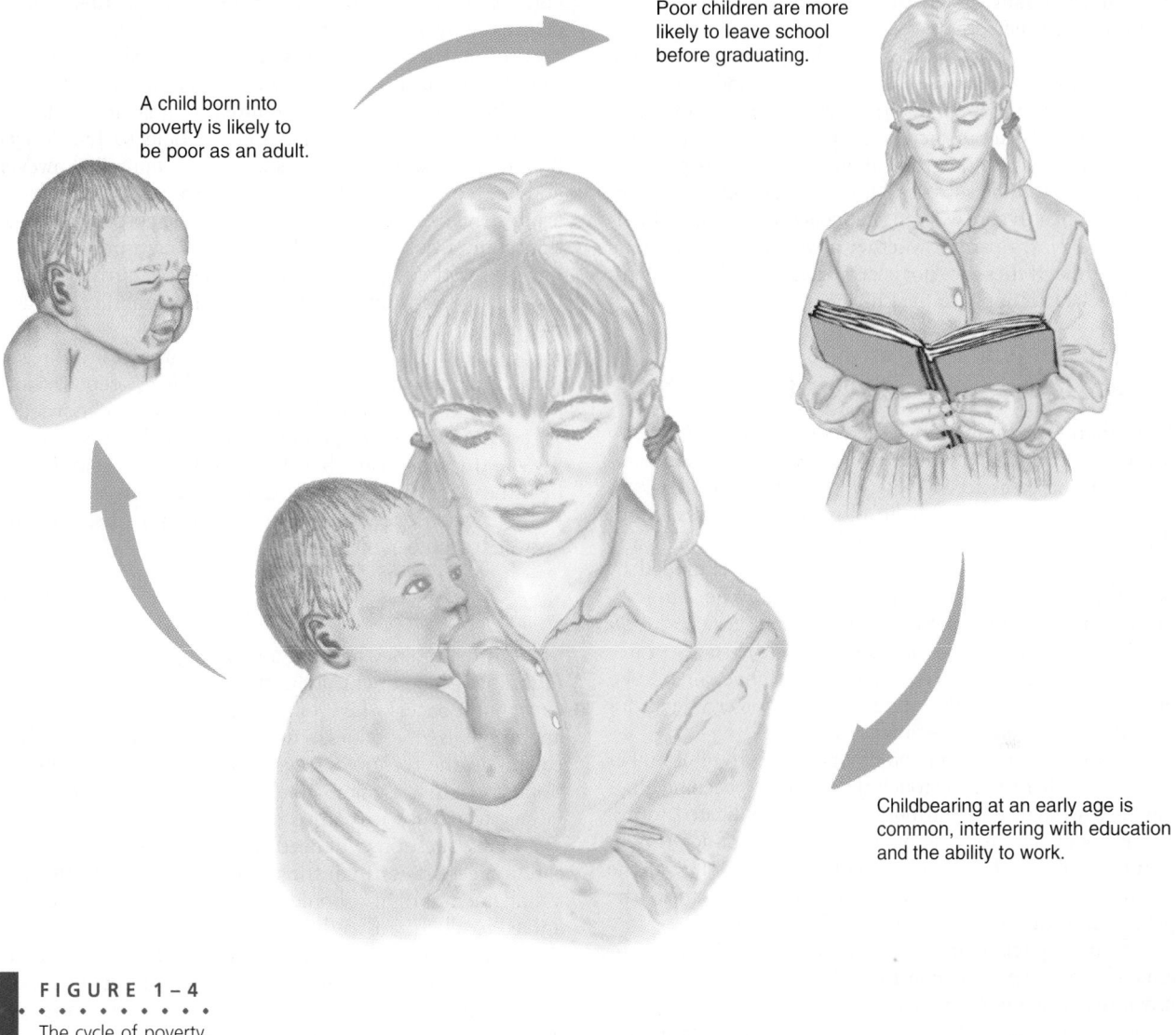

A child born into poverty is likely to be poor as an adult.

Poor children are more likely to leave school before graduating.

Childbearing at an early age is common, interfering with education and the ability to work.

FIGURE 1–4

The cycle of poverty.

other poor people because of lack of transportation, inconvenient hours, and lack of continuity of care.

Access to Health Care

Even people with incomes above the poverty level may not be able to pay for health care. The working poor have jobs but receive wages that barely meet their day-to-day needs. They have little opportunity to save for emergencies such as serious illness. In 1995, 16.5% of the population younger than 65 years in the United States had no health insurance (NCHS, 1997). Millions of others have only limited insurance and would not be able to survive financially should serious illness occur. People without insurance seek care only when absolutely necessary. Health maintenance and illness prevention may seem costly and unnecessary to them. Some receive no health care during pregnancy until they arrive at the hospital for birth.

The number of uninsured American children has also increased, owing to a decline in private, employer-paid coverage. This has had a tremendous impact on the low-income worker who does not have employer-paid coverage and is unable to afford individually purchased insurance. Although Medicaid (see p. 18) has expanded its coverage, there are millions of children who live in households with incomes just above the Medicaid eligibility level and whose families cannot afford to purchase private insurance.

Prenatal Care in the United States

Prenatal care is widely accepted as an important element in improving the health of mothers and infants. In 1996 in the United States, 4% of live births were to mothers who did not have prenatal care until the third trimester or who did not have prenatal care at all (DHHS, 1998). Poor prenatal care often occurs because care is not easily available.

Lack of access to care is a major reason for the high infant mortality rate and the large number of low-birth-weight infants born each year in the United States. Because preterm infants form the largest category of those needing intensive care, millions of dollars could be saved each year by ensuring adequate prenatal care. Even a small improvement in an infant's birth weight decreases complications and hospital time.

In some situations, women can obtain prenatal care but choose not to do so. These women may not understand the importance of the care or may deny they are pregnant. Some have had such unsatisfactory past experiences with the health care system that they avoid it as long as possible. Others want to hide substance use or other habits from disapproving health care workers. Language and cultural differences also play a part in whether a woman seeks prenatal care. Although these are not access issues as such, they must be addressed to improve health care.

Government Programs for Health Care: Medicaid

More than 44% of all money spent on health care in 1995 was publicly funded (NCHS, 1997). One government program that increases access to health care is Medicaid, which has existed since 1965. Medicaid provides health care for the poor, aged, and disabled, with pregnant women and young children especially targeted. Medicaid is funded by both the federal and the state governments. The states administer the program and determine which services are offered. Although there is variation among the states in just how poor one must be to qualify for assistance, all women at less than 133% of the current federal poverty level for income are eligible for perinatal care.

Medicaid has a number of problems. It often takes weeks for a client to go through the process to become eligible. The woman must fill out lengthy, complicated forms, provide documentation of income, then wait for determination of eligibility. If a woman is not already enrolled at the beginning of her pregnancy, she is unlikely to finish the process in time to receive early prenatal care.

Some physicians are unwilling to care for Medicaid clients who are likely to be at high risk. Many are especially unwilling if reimbursement is slow and less than that paid by other insurers. With their continual concern about malpractice suits, physicians may be less inclined to accept high-risk, lower-paying clients.

However, the distinction between public and private health coverage are becoming less distinct. Medicaid may now reimburse as well as or better than some private insurers. Providers will then eagerly care for clients covered by Medicaid.

Allocation of Health Care Resources

In 1995, the United States spent $988.5 billion on health care. This amount is $3,621 per person (NCHS, 1997). Expenditures continue to climb every year. Methods of reforming health care financing have drawn increasing attention in recent times, and many changes are occurring. How to provide care for the poor, the uninsured or underinsured, and those with long-term care needs are areas that must be addressed. The distribution of the limited funds available for health care among all these areas is a major concern.

Care versus Cure

One problem to be addressed is whether the focus of health care should be on preventive and caring measures or on cure of disease. Medicine has traditionally centered more on treatment and cure than on prevention and care. Yet prevention not only avoids suffering but is also less expensive than treating diseases once they are diagnosed.

The focus on cure has resulted in great technological advances that have enabled some people to live longer, healthier lives. Financial resources are limited, however, and the costs of expensive technology must be balanced against the benefits obtained. Indeed, the cost of one organ transplant would pay for the prenatal care of many low-income mothers, possibly preventing the births of many low-birth-weight infants who may suffer disability throughout life.

In addition, quality of life issues are important in regard to technology. Neonatal nurseries are able to keep very-low-birth-weight babies alive because of advances in knowledge. Some of these infants go on to lead normal or near-normal lives. Others gain time but not quality of life. Families and health care professionals face difficult decisions about when to treat, when to terminate treatment, and when suffering outweighs the benefits.

Health Care Rationing

Modern technology has had a great impact on health care rationing. Some might argue that such rationing does not exist, but it occurs when some people have no access to care and there is not enough money for all people to share equally in the technology available. Health care is also rationed when it is more freely given to those who have money to pay for it than to those who do not.

Many questions will need answers as the costs of health care increase faster than the funds available. Is health care a fundamental right? Should a certain level of care be guaranteed to all citizens? What should that care entail? Should the cost of treatment and its effectiveness be considered when one is deciding how much government or third-party payers will cover? Nurses will be instrumental in finding solutions to these vital questions.

Violence

In today's society, women and children are the victims and sometimes the perpetrators of violence. Violence is not only a social problem, it is also a health problem. Acts of violence can include child abuse, domestic abuse, and murder. Children who live in an environment of violence feel helpless and ineffective. These children have difficulty sleeping and show increased anxiety and fearfulness. They may perpetuate the violence they see in their homes when they are adults because they have known nothing else in family relationships.

Violence in schools continues to rise, and for many children it is a daily stressor. Experts in the field of education have cited socioeconomic disparity, language barriers, diverse cultural upbringing, lack of supervision and behavioral feedback, domestic violence, and changes within the family as possible causes for the increased violence. Traditional approaches to aggressive behavior in the school, such as suspension, detention, and being sent to the principal's office, have been ineffective in changing behavior, and serve only to exclude the student from education, leading to an increased dropout rate. Nurses must educate themselves on the issue of violence and, in turn, work with schools and parents to combat the problem. In addition, they should not ignore the child who is afraid to go to school or is having other school-related problems.

Children and adolescents are also exposed to violence via television, movies, video games, and youth-oriented music. Nurses should make this issue a part of anticipatory guidance. Parents should be encouraged to monitor their children's media exposure and limit their children's television viewing to 2 hours or less per day.

The American Academy of Pediatrics encourages clinicians to be concerned about adolescents who display aggressive or acting-out behaviors, such as lying, stealing, temper outbursts, vandalism, excessive fighting, and destructiveness. It further recommends that health care providers promote the responsibility of every family to create a gun-safe home environment, including asking about the presence of guns in the home and counseling patients, parents, and relatives on the importance of firearm safety and the dangers of having a gun, especially a handgun.

Nurses working with children should ask them about violence in their school, home, or neighborhood, and whether they have had any personal experience with violent behavior. In some cases it may be necessary to contact parents, human resource departments, police, or other authorities in order to protect children and adolescents who are either in violent situations or at risk for violence.

Legal Issues

The legal foundation for the practice of nursing provides safeguards for health care and sets standards by which nurses can be evaluated. Nurses need to understand how the law applies specifically to them. When nurses do not meet the standards expected, they may be held legally accountable.

Safeguards for Health Care

Three categories of safeguards determine how the law views nursing practice: (1) nurse practice acts, (2) standards of care set by professional organizations, and (3) rules and policies set by the institution employing the nurse. Additional information about nursing responsibilities is presented in Chapter 2.

NURSE PRACTICE ACTS

Every state has a nurse practice act that determines the scope of practice of registered nurses in that state. Nurse practice acts define what the nurse is and is not allowed to do in caring for clients. Some parts of the law may be very specific. Others are stated broadly enough to allow interpretation of the law that permits flexibility in the role of nurses. Nurse practice acts vary from state to state, and nurses must be knowledgeable about these laws wherever they practice.

Laws relating to nursing practice also delineate methods, called *standardized procedures*, by which nurses may assume certain duties commonly considered part of medical practice. The procedures are written by committees of nurses, physicians, and administrators. They specify the nursing qualifications required for practicing the procedures, define the appropriate situations, and list the education required. Standardized procedures allow for changing the role of the nurse to meet the needs of the community and to reflect expanding knowledge.

STANDARDS OF CARE

Courts have generally held that nurses must practice according to established standards and health agency policies, although these standards and policies do not have the force of law. Standards of care are set by professional associations and describe the level of care that can be expected from practitioners. For example, perinatal nurses are held to the standards published by the Association of Women's Health, Obstetric, and Neonatal Nurses (AWHONN, formerly NAACOG), a widely respected organization for nurses in this field. The Society of Pediatric Nurses is the primary organization that sets standards for pediatric nurses. See Chapter 2 for additional information about professional organizations for maternity and pediatric nurses.

Other regulatory bodies, such as the Occupational Safety and Health Administration (OSHA), the Food and Drug Administration (FDA), and the Centers for Disease Control and Prevention (CDC), also provide guidelines for practice. Accrediting agencies, such as the Joint Commission on Accreditation of Healthcare Organizations and the Community Health Accreditation Program, give their approval after visiting facilities and observing whether standards are being met in practice.

AGENCY POLICIES

Each health care agency sets specific policies, procedures, and protocols that govern nursing care. All nurses should be familiar with those that apply in the agencies in which they work. Nurses are frequently involved in writing nursing policies and procedures and in revising them when necessary.

Accountability

Nursing accountability involves a knowledge of current laws. Accountability in pediatric nursing requires special consideration because the nurse must be accountable to the family as well as the child.

In 1984, the subject of handicapped infants was addressed by the Child Abuse Amendments and delegated to state child protective agencies to investigate allegations of necessary medical care being denied. These regulations come into play when caring for children with symptoms of acquired immunodeficiency syndrome (AIDS).

Both federal and state legislative bodies have addressed the issue of child abuse. Considerable variation exists among state laws in the investigative authority and procedures granted to child protective workers. When child abuse is suspected, issues often arise as to whether a health care provider may investigate the home situation and obtain relevant records.

A recent issue pertaining to nursing accountability is inadequate hospital staffing due to budget cuts. A nurse has a duty to communicate concerns about staffing levels immediately through established channels. A nurse will not be excused from responsibility (e.g., late medication administration or injury resulting from inadequate supervision of a client), just as a hospital will not be excused for insufficient staffing because of budget cuts.

Accountability also involves competency. If a nurse is not competent to perform a particular nursing task (e.g., to administer a new chemotherapeutic drug), or if a client's status worsens to the point at which the care needs are beyond the nurse's competency level (e.g., a client requiring hemodynamic monitoring), the nurse must immediately communicate this fact to the nursing supervisor or physician. The fact that a client's transfer to the intensive care unit (ICU) was requested but denied because the ICU was at full capacity is an insufficient defense in a charge of nursing negligence. Additionally, the fact that a call was placed to a physician but there was no return call is no excuse for harm caused to a client because of delayed treatment. The nurse has an obligation to pursue needed care through the chain of command at the facility.

Malpractice

Negligence is failure to perform the way a reasonable, prudent person of similar background would act in a similar situation. Negligence may consist of doing something that should not be done or failing to do something that should be done.

Malpractice is negligence by professionals, such as nurses or physicians, in the performance of their duties. Nurses may be accused of malpractice if they do not perform according to established standards of care and in the manner of a reasonable, prudent nurse with similar education and experience. Four elements must be present to prove negligence. They are duty, breach of duty, damage, and proximate cause.

PREVENTION OF MALPRACTICE CLAIMS
Malpractice claims have escalated in recent years. As a result of awards from such claims, the cost of malpractice insurance has risen for all health care workers. In addition, more health care workers practice defensively, accumulating evidence that they are acting in the client's best interest. For example, nurses must be careful to include detailed data when they chart. This responsibility is especially important in perinatal nursing, because this is the area in which most suits occur.

There are many reasons why perinatal nurses may be-

come defendants in lawsuits. Complications are usually unexpected because parents view pregnancy and birth as normal. The birth of a child with a problem is a tragic surprise, and they may look for someone to blame. Although very small preterm infants now survive, some have long-term disabilities that require expensive care. Statutes of limitations vary in different states, but plaintiffs often have more than 20 years for lawsuits that involve a newborn. Therefore, there is a longer period during which a malpractice suit may be filed.

Prevention of claims is sometimes referred to as *risk management* or *quality assurance*. Although it may not be possible to prevent all malpractice claims, nurses can help prevent malpractice judgments against themselves by following guidelines for informed consent, refusal of care, and documentation; acting as a client advocate; and maintaining their level of expertise.

Informed Consent. When clients receive adequate information, they are less likely to file malpractice suits. Informed consent is an ethical concept that has been enacted into law. Clients have the right to decide whether to accept or reject treatment options as part of their right to function autonomously. To make wise decisions, they need full information about treatments offered. Without proper informed consent, assault and battery charges can result.

The law mandates what procedures require informed consent. The same laws govern both adults and children. The law mandates what to inform about as "risks" specific to each procedure. Nurses must be familiar with those procedures requiring consent.

Competence. Certain requirements must be met before consent can be considered informed. The first requirement is that the client be competent, or able to think through a situation and make rational decisions. A client who is comatose or severely mentally retarded is incapable of making such decisions. Minors are not allowed to give consent; however, children should have procedures explained to them in terms appropriate for their age. A client who has received drugs that impair ability to think is temporarily incompetent. In these cases, another person is appointed to make decisions for the client.

Most states allow some exceptions for parental consent in cases involving emancipated minors. An *emancipated minor* is a minor child who has the legal competency of an adult because of circumstances involving marriage, divorce, parenting of a child, living independently without parents, or enlistment in the armed services. Legal counsel may be consulted to verify the status of the emancipated minor for consent purposes.

Most states allow minors to obtain treatment for drug or

alcohol abuse or sexually transmitted diseases, and to have access to birth control without parental consent. At present, laws governing adolescent abortion vary widely from state to state.

Full Disclosure.   The second requirement is that of full disclosure of information, including what the treatment entails and the expected results. The risks, side effects, and benefits as well as other treatment options must be explained to clients. The client must also be informed as to what would happen if no treatment were chosen.

For example, the National Childhood Vaccine Injury Act mandates that explanations about the risks of communicable diseases and the risks and benefits associated with immunizations should be given to all parents to enable them to make informed decisions about their child's health care. Parents need to know the common side effects and what to do in an emergency if any occur. The law stipulates that children injured by the vaccine must go through the administrative compensation system (funds from an excise tax levied on the vaccines) and reject an award before attempting to sue in a civil suit either the manufacturer or the person who gave the vaccine. Furthermore, the law mandates certain record-keeping and reporting requirements for nurses.

Understanding of Information.   The client must comprehend information about proposed treatment. Health professionals must explain the facts in terms the person can understand. If a client does not speak English, an interpreter may be necessary. Nurses must be client advocates when they find that a client does not fully understand a treatment or has questions about it. If it is a minor point, the nurse may be able to explain it. Otherwise, the nurse must inform the physician so that the client's misconceptions can be clarified.

Voluntary Consent.   Clients must be allowed to make choices voluntarily without undue influence or coercion from others. Although others can give information, the client alone makes the decision. Clients should not feel pressured to choose in a certain way or feel that their future care depends on their decision.

REFUSAL OF CARE

Sometimes clients decline treatment offered by health care workers. Clients may refuse treatment when they believe that the benefits of treatment do not outweigh the burdens of the treatment or the quality of life they can expect after that treatment. Clients have the right to refuse care, and they can withdraw agreement to treatment at any time. When a person makes this decision, a number of steps should be taken.

First, it should be established by the physician or nurse that the client understands the treatment and the results of refusal. The physician, if unaware of the client's decision, should be notified by the nurse. The nurse documents the refusal, explanations given to the client, and notification of the physician on the chart. If the treatment is considered vital to the client's well-being, the physician discusses the need with the client and documents the discussion. Opinions by other physicians may be offered to the client as well.

Clients may be asked to sign a form indicating that they understand the possible results of rejecting treatment. This measure is to prevent a later lawsuit in which a client claims lack of knowledge of the possible results of a decision. If there is no ethical dilemma, the client's decision stands.

When parents refuse to give consent for what is deemed necessary treatment of a child, the state may be petitioned to intervene. The court may place the child in the temporary custody of the government or a private agency. The nurse may be asked to witness such a transaction when physicians act in cases of emergencies, such as a life-saving blood transfusion for a child despite parental objections based on religious beliefs.

In cases of an ethical dilemma, a referral may be made to the hospital ethics committee. In rare situations, the physician may seek a court ruling to force treatment. One example is a woman's refusal of a cesarean birth, even though her refusal is likely to cause grave harm to the fetus. This situation is the only legal instance in which a person is forced to undergo surgery for the health of another. Court action is avoided if possible, however, because it places the client, family, and caregiver in adversarial positions. In addition, it invades the client's privacy and interferes with her autonomy and right to informed consent.

TERMINATING LIFE SUPPORT

Decisions to terminate life support systems continue to present gut-wrenching situations to nurses, especially when an infant or child is involved. Contrary to the common belief that such decisions should be determined by what is termed "quality of life," the legal system plays a major role in this area of health care.

Frequently, parents become attached to a primary care nurse and request that the nurse participate in the decision as to whether or not to terminate life support for their child. A nurse might be faced with such a situation in the neonatal ICU with a teenage parent of a premature infant with a congenital defect, or in a chronic care oncology unit with a terminally ill child.

In such instances, a team conference should be arranged with the parents, primary nurse, physician, and a hospital staff attorney who is knowledgeable about applicable laws in that particular state. Problems may arise when there is a discrepancy between what families, physicians, and nurses think is best.

The issue of when first to discuss with adolescents the idea of cardiopulmonary resuscitation, mechanical ventilation, and do-not-resuscitate (DNR) orders is always sensitive. Adolescent patients who have reached majority age must give consent if they are of sound mind. In most states, minority status ends at the age of 18 years.

ADOPTION

Nurses may care for infants involved in adoptions. The nurse may need to consult with the birth parents, adoptive parents, social workers, obstetrician, or pediatrician to determine the various rights of the child, birth parents, and adoptive parents (e.g., in matters concerning visitation rights, informed consent, or discharge planning).

In open adoptions, the birth mother may opt to room in with the baby during hospitalization. The birth mother and adoptive parents typically have had contact prior to the delivery and have an informal agreement regarding shared responsibility for the baby. The birth parent may even participate in discharge planning because she may have extended rights to visit the child after adoption.

Issues may develop as to the state of mind of the birth

mother at the time of relinquishing parental rights (which cannot occur until after birth, unlike the relinquishment of the birth father's rights). State laws vary as to the legal time period necessary (1 day to several weeks after the birth of the child) before a birth mother can lawfully relinquish her rights to the child.

Some state laws allow the birth mother to relinquish her rights immediately after birth. In such cases, the nurse has the responsibility of protecting the birth mother and child to ensure that the birth mother is not coerced into making a decision while under the effects of anesthesia. Factual documentation of such circumstances may be requested if the birth mother later asserts her rights to the child, claiming "undue influence" or "coercion."

Although birth fathers rarely participate in the care of the baby during hospitalization, they have the same rights as the birth mother. Unless the birth father relinquishes his legal rights to the child, the adoptive parents are taking a risk when taking custody of the child at the time of discharge from the hospital. The birth father may later assert his rights to the child after attachment has occurred with the adoptive parents.

DOCUMENTATION

Documentation is especially important when there is a question of liability because it is the best evidence that a standard of care has been maintained. All information recorded about a client should reflect that standard of care. This information includes nurses' notes, fetal monitoring strips, flow sheets, and any other data recorded in the chart. In many instances, notations on hospital records are the only proof that care has been given. Unfortunately, deficiencies in accurate and thorough documentation are common (Simpson & Chez, 1996). When documentation is not present, juries tend to assume that care was not given. Although documentation is not listed as a step in the nursing process, it is an integral part of the process.

It is especially important that documentation be specific and complete in perinatal and pediatric nursing. Nurses are unlikely to be able to remember situations that happened years in the past and, if sued, must rely on their documentation to explain their care. Documentation must show that the client was assessed appropriately, that continuing monitoring of problems was provided, that problems were identified and correct interventions were instituted, and that changes in the client's condition were reported to the primary care provider.

Documenting Discharge Teaching. With the length of hospital stay becoming shorter, discharge teaching becomes increasingly important to ensure that new mothers know how to take care of themselves and their infants and that parents know how to care for their child. To prevent lawsuits, nurses must document the teaching they perform as well as the client's understanding of that teaching. It is important to include information about the parents' degree of understanding of the teaching. The nurse should also note the need for reinforcement and how that reinforcement was provided. If follow-up home care is planned, teaching can be continued at home and documented on forms by the home care nurse.

Documenting Incidents. Another form of documentation used in risk management is the incident report, sometimes called a quality assurance report or a variance report. The nurse completes a report when something occurs that might result in legal action, such as in injury to a client. The report warns the agency's legal department that there may be a problem. It also identifies situations that might endanger clients in the future. Incident reports are not a part of the client's chart and should not be referred to on the chart. When an incident occurs, documentation on the chart should include the same type of factual information about the client's condition that would be recorded in any other situation.

THE NURSE AS CLIENT ADVOCATE

Malpractice suits may be brought if nurses fail in their role of client advocate. Nurses are ethically and legally bound to act as the client's advocate. This means that the nurse must act in the client's best interests at all times. When nurses feel that the client's best interests are not being served, they are obligated to seek help for the client from appropriate sources. This usually involves taking the problem through the normal chain of command. The nurse consults a supervisor and the client's physician. If the results are not satisfactory, the nurse continues through administrative channels to the director of nurses, hospital administrator, and chief of the medical staff, if necessary. All nurses should know the chain of command for their workplaces.

In seeking help for clients, nurses must document their efforts. For example, if a postpartum patient experiences excessive bleeding, the nurse documents what was done to control the bleeding. The nurse also documents each time the physician was called about the problem, what information was given the physician, and the response received. When nurses cannot contact the physician or do not receive adequate instructions, they should document their efforts to seek instruction from others, such as the supervisor. They should also complete an incident report. It is essential that they continue in their efforts until the client receives the care needed.

MAINTAINING EXPERTISE

Maintaining expertise is another way for nurses to prevent malpractice liability. To ensure that nurses maintain their expertise to provide safe care, many states require proof of continuing education for renewal of nursing licenses. Nursing knowledge grows and changes rapidly, and it is essential that all nurses keep current. Incorporating new information learned by attending classes or conferences and reading nursing journals can help nurses perform the way a reasonably prudent peer would perform. Journals provide information from nursing research that may be important in updating nursing practice. It is important for all nurses to analyze research articles to determine whether changes in client care are indicated.

Employers often provide continuing education classes for their nurses. Many workshops and seminars are available on a wide variety of nursing subjects. Membership in professional organizations, such as state branches of the American Nurses' Association or specialty organizations such as AWHONN and the Society of Pediatric Nurses, gives nurses access to new information through publications as well as nursing conferences and other educational offerings.

Maintaining expertise may be a concern when nurses "float" or are required to work with clients who have needs different from those of their usual clients. In these situations, the employer must provide orientation and education so that the nurse can perform care safely in new areas. Nurses who work outside their usual expertise must assess their own skills and avoid performing tasks or taking on responsibilities in areas in which they are not competent. Many nurses learn to provide care in two or three different areas and are floated only to those areas. This system meets the need for flexible staffing while providing safe client care.

Current Trends and Their Legal and Ethical Implications

Recent health care changes have affected the way nurses give care and may have legal and ethical implications as well. These changes result from efforts to lower health care costs. Two of special concern are the use of unlicensed assistive personnel and early discharge.

Use of Unlicensed Assistive Personnel

In an effort to reduce health care costs, many agencies have increased the use of unlicensed assistive personnel to perform direct client care, and have decreased the number of nurses who supervise them. An unlicensed person may be trained to do everything from housekeeping tasks to drawing blood and performing other diagnostic testing to giving medications, all in the same day. This practice raises grave concerns about the quality of care clients receive when the nurse becomes responsible for the care of more clients but must rely on unlicensed persons to perform much of the care formerly provided by professionals.

Nurses must be aware of their legal responsibilities in these situations. They must know that the nurse is always responsible for client assessments and must make the critical judgments that are necessary to ensure client safety. Nurses must know what each unlicensed person caring for clients is able to do and must supervise them closely enough to ensure that they perform delegated tasks competently. The American Nurses Association and state boards of nursing have issued statements to help nurses understand their role in working with unlicensed assistive personnel (American Nurses Association, 1994).

Concerns About Early Discharge

Health care professionals are concerned about the ability of women to care for themselves or their infant or child when discharge occurs very early. Women may be exhausted from a long labor or illness and unable to take in all the information that nurses attempt to teach before discharge. Once home, many women must care for other children as well, often without family members or friends to help them.

During the time that clients remain in the birth or acute care facility, nurses are able to detect indications of complications that may not be apparent to lay people. Mothers at home may not recognize the developing signs of serious maternal or neonatal infection or of jaundice, and care may be delayed until the illness is severe. There may be legal implications if a client develops a complication after early discharge.

Dealing with the Problem of Early Discharge

Nurses must establish ways of helping clients who go home soon after birth or parents who must take their child home when only slightly less ill or very soon after surgery. New teaching tactics may be necessary, with more teaching taking place during pregnancy when the mother's physical needs do not interfere with her ability to assimilate new knowledge. Parent teaching can be done before actual admission of a child for surgery. If a child is admitted when acutely ill, parent teaching begins almost immediately after admission.

Careful documentation and notification of the primary care provider are essential when abnormal findings develop so that clients are not discharged inappropriately. Methods of follow-up such as home visits, phone calls, or return visits by the families to the birth facility for nursing assessments in the first 24 to 48 hours after discharge have become increasingly important.

KEY CONCEPTS
. . . .

- Changes in maternity and pediatric care in the United States came about as a result of technological advances, increased knowledge, government involvement, and consumer demands.
- Family-centered maternity and pediatric care, based on the principle that families can make decisions about health care if they have adequate information, has greatly increased the responsibility of nurses.
- Prospective payment plans such as

preferred provider organizations (PPOs) or health maintenance organizations (HMOs) control health care costs by negotiating reduced charges with providers such as facilities and physicians and by restricting client access to any provider of choice.

- Capitated plans are those in which a group of providers agrees to provide all services for a client for a set annual fee. If the client requires more costly care, the provider network pays those added

charges. If the client requires less care than the annual fee, the network keeps the additional money.

- Case management and outcomes management, which came about as a result of cost-containment strategies, have resulted in new tools to reduce the length of stay for mothers and infants in the birth facility. Teaching of mothers, children, and families begins as soon as they enter the health care system.

- Clinical pathways are interdisciplinary guidelines for assessments and interventions that will accomplish the identified outcomes in the shortest time.
- Home care of maternity and pediatric clients has increased because of the need to control costs and because of the availability of portable technology.
- The number of uninsured children continues to rise, reducing their chances of receiving preventive health care.
- Infant and maternal mortality rates have declined dramatically in the last 50 years; however, the United States continues to rank well below other industrialized nations, and there is still wide variation in mortality rates across ethnic groups.
- Accidents are the leading cause of death in children ages 1 to 19 years.
- Nurses must examine their beliefs and come to a personal decision about abortion before they are faced with the situation in their own practice. Nurses are obligated to share objections related to abortion care with their employer before the need to provide that care arises.
- Punitive approaches to ethical and social problems may prevent clients from seeking care, particularly preventive care.
- Poverty is a major social issue that leads to questions about allocation of health care resources, access to care, government programs to increase health care to indigent women and children, and health care rationing.
- To give informed consent, the client must be competent, receive full information, understand that information, and consent voluntarily. The parents usually give consent for a minor child, although adolescents may be able to consent to their own treatment related to sexually transmitted diseases, contraception, alcohol and drug abuse, and sometimes abortion.
- Nurses are accountable for their practice and must be acquainted with laws, standards and guidelines, and agency policies that affect their practice.
- Nurses can help to prevent malpractice claims by following guidelines for informed consent, refusal of care, and documentation, and by maintaining their level of expertise.
- Documentation is the best evidence that the standard of care was met in client care. Therefore, nurses must ensure that their documentation accurately reflects the care given.
- The nurse is the professional who decides what tasks may safely be delegated to unlicensed assistive personnel. In making such decisions, the nurse is guided by recommendations of the state licensing board, standards of care, and agency policy.

ANSWERS TO CRITICAL THINKING EXERCISE 1–1

1. The deontologic view is that it is wrong to take organs necessary for life from one human being to give to another, even when the donor cannot survive. This view disapproves of aggressive treatment necessary to maintain perfusion of the organs until a recipient is located because treatment does not help the dying infant and may increase suffering. This concern invokes the principle of nonmaleficence.
2. The utilitarian view is that anencephalic infants cannot survive but that their organs could provide great benefit to other infants (beneficence). Because this family feels strongly that helping other infants allows good to come from their own tragedy, the greatest good would be for an organ transplant.
3. Potential problems include the possibility that transplants might someday be required, even against the parents' will (and might deny them autonomy). A woman might be forced to carry a pregnancy to term so that the organs can be harvested, even if the parents would rather terminate the pregnancy. If anencephalic infants are used for organ donation, perhaps people with profound mental retardation or in persistent vegetative states might be placed in the same situation. Choosing infants to benefit would also be a concern, involving principles of justice. An overriding concern would be determining who would make the decisions necessary.

REFERENCES AND READINGS

Alfaro-LeFevere, R. (1995). *Critical thinking in nursing*. Philadelphia: Saunders.

American Academy of Pediatrics & American College of Obstetricians and Gynecologists. (1997). *Guidelines for perinatal care* (4th ed.). Elk Grove Village, IL, and Washington, DC: Author.

American Academy of Pediatrics Committee on Bioethics. (1996). *Ethics and the care of critically ill infants and children*. Elk Grove Village, IL: American Academy of Pediatrics.

American Academy of Pediatrics Committee on Child Health Financing. (1994). Medicaid policy statement. *Pediatrics, 93*(1), 135–36.

American Academy of Pediatrics Committee on Child Health Financing. (1995). *Guiding principles for managed care arrangements for the health care of infants, children, adolescents, and young adults*. Elk Grove Village, IL: American Academy of Pediatrics.

American Academy of Pediatrics Committee on Communications. (1995). *Media violence*. Elk Grove Village, IL: American Academy of Pediatrics.

American Nurses Association. (1994). *Registered professional nurses and unlicensed assistive personnel*. Washington, DC: Author.

Association of Women's Health, Obstetric, and Neonatal Nurses. (1994a). *Shortened maternity and newborn hospital stays* [Position statement]. Washington, DC: Author.

Association of Women's Health, Obstetric, and Neonatal Nurses. (1994b). *Didactic content and clinical skills verification for profes-*

sional nurse providers of perinatal home care. Washington, DC: Author.

Association of Women's Health, Obstetric, and Neonatal Nurses. (1995). *The role of the nurse in clinical ethical decision making.* Washington, DC: Author.

Attenborough, R. (1997). The Canadian health care system: Development, reform, and opportunities for nurses. *Journal of Obstetric, Gynecologic, and Neonatal Nursing, 26*(2), 229–234.

Beal, A. C., & Redlener, I. (1995). Enhancing perinatal outcome in homeless women: The challenge of providing comprehensive health care. *Seminars in Perinatology, 19*(4), 307–313.

Bendell, Abbe. (1997). Health care in the 1990s: Changes in health care delivery models for survival. *Journal of Obstetric, Gynecologic, and Neonatal Nursing, 26*(2), 212–216.

Blendon, R., Altman, D., Benson, J., Brodie, M., James, M., & Chervinsky, G. (1995). The public and the welfare reform debate. *Archives of Pediatric and Adolescent Medicine, 149,* 1065–1069.

Bower, K. A. (1997). Case management and clinical paths: Strategies to support the perinatal experience. *Journal of Obstetric, Gynecologic, and Neonatal Nursing, 26*(3), 329–333.

Brent, N. J. (1997). *Nurses and the law: A guide to principles and applications.* Philadelphia: Saunders.

Broome, M. E., & Stieglitz, K. A. (1992). The consent process and children. *Research in Nursing and Health, 15,* 147–152.

Bruce, B., & Ritchie, J. (1997). Nurses' practices and perceptions of family-centered care. *Journal of Pediatric Nursing, 12*(4), 214–222.

Callister, L. C. (1995). Cultural meanings of childbirth. *Journal of Obstetric, Gynecologic, and Neonatal Nursing, 24*(4), 327–334.

Carnegie Corporation of New York. (1994). *Starting points: Meeting the needs of our youngest children.* New York: Author.

Carpenito, L. (1997). *Nursing diagnosis: Application to clinical practice* (7th ed.). Philadelphia: Lippincott.

Cascio, H. (1998). Medicaid experiments in capitation: What they can teach us about capitation in private managed care. What physicians and patients should know. Available from Internet address home1.gte.net/hcascio/flmchmo/capitate.htm.

Centers for Disease Control and Prevention. (1996). Monthly immunization table. *Morbidity and Mortality Weekly Report, 45*(1), 10.

Centers for Disease Control and Prevention. (1998a). *America's Children 1998.* Hysattsville, MD: National Center for Health Statistics.

Centers for Disease Control and Prevention. (1998b). Report of final natality statistics, 1996. *Monthly Vital Statistics Report, 46*(11), 1–19.

Centers for Disease Control and Prevention. (1998c). Births and deaths: Preliminary data for 1997. *National Vital Statistics Reports, 47*(4), 1–42.

Centers for Disease Control and Prevention. (1998d). Youth risk behavior surveillance—United States. *Morbidity and Mortality Weekly Report, 47*(SS-3), 1–3.

Centers for Disease Control and Prevention. (1998e). *Monthly Vital Statistics Report, 46*(12), 1–42.

Cox, R. P. (1997). Family healthcare delivery for the 21st century. *Journal of Obstetric, Gynecologic, and Neonatal Nursing, 26*(1), 109–118.

Doenges, M., Moorhouse, M., & Burley, J. (1995). *Application of nursing process and nursing diagnosis: An interactive text for diagnostic reasoning.* Philadelphia: Davis.

Dolan J., Fitzpatrick M., & Hermann, E. (1983). *Nursing in society: A historical perspective* (15th ed.). Philadelphia: Saunders.

Doolittle, D. (1998). Welfare reform: Loss of supplemental security income (SSI) for children with disabilities. *Journal of Society of Pediatric Nurses, 3*(1), 33–44.

Driscoll, K. M. (1998). Legal aspects of perinatal care. In C. Kenner, J. W. Lott, & A. A. Flandermeyer (Eds.), *Comprehensive neonatal nursing: A physiologic perspective* (pp. 32–45). Philadelphia: Saunders.

Elder, K. N. (1998). Managed care: The value you bring. *American Journal of Nursing, 98*(6), 34–39.

Evans, C. J. (1995). Postpartum home care in the United States. *Journal of Obstetric, Gynecologic, and Neonatal Nursing, 24*(2), 180–186.

Feigin, R., & Cherry, J. (1998). *Textbook of pediatric infectious diseases.* Philadelphia: Saunders.

Fleschler, R. G., & King, B. P. (1995). Perinatal outcomes management: Balancing quality with cost. *Journal of Perinatal-Neonatal Nursing, 9*(2), 21–28.

Gardner, S. L., & Hagedorn, M. E. (1997). Holding nurses accountable. *AWHONN's Lifelines, 1*(1), 55–56.

Gupton, A. (1995). The Canadian perspective on postpartum home care. *Journal of Obstetric, Gynecologic, and Neonatal Nursing, 24*(2), 173–179.

Guyer, B., Martin, J., MacDorman, M., Anderson, R., & Strobino, D. (1997). Annual summary of vital statistics—1996. *Pediatrics, 95*(6), 905–918.

Guyer, B., Strobino, D. M., Ventura, S. J., MacDorman, M., & Martin, J. A. (1996). Annual summary of vital statistics—1995. *Pediatrics, 98*(6), 1007–1020.

Hayes, J. (1997). Coordinated systems of community-based health care delivery: A vehicle for health care reform. *Journal of Pediatric Nursing, 12*(5), 288–291.

Henry, J. K. (1997). Community nursing centers: Models of nurse-managed care. *Journal of Obstetric, Gynecologic, and Neonatal Nursing, 26*(2), 224–228.

Holl, J., Szilagyi, P., Rodewald, L., Byrd, R., & Weitzman, M. (1995). Profile of uninsured children in the United States. *Archives of Pediatric Adolescent Medicine, 149,* 398–406.

Horton, J. A. (Ed.). (1995). Demographic classification. *The women's health data book* (2nd ed.). Washington, DC: Jacobs Institute of Women's Health.

Ignatavicius, D., & Hausman, K. (1995). *Clinical pathways for collaborative practice.* Philadelphia: Saunders.

Johnson, M. (1996). Television violence and its effect on children. *Journal of Pediatric Nursing, 11*(2), 94–98.

Kachoyeanos, M. K. (1995). Maintaining an ethical stand without jeopardizing your job. *MCN: American Journal of Maternal/Child Nursing, 20*(5), 243–248.

Keppler, A. B. (1995). Postpartum care center: Follow-up care in a hospital-based clinic. *Journal of Obstetric, Gynecologic, and Neonatal Nursing, 24*(1), 17–21.

Kjervik, D. K. (1996). Legal and ethical issues. In J. Cookfair (Ed.), *Nursing care in the community.* St. Louis: Mosby.

Ladebauche, P. (1995). Limiting liability to avoid malpractice litigation. *The American Journal of Maternal/Child Nursing, 20*(6), 339.

Lannon, C., Brack, V., Stuart, J., Caplow, M., McNeill, A., Bordley, W. C., & Margolis, P. (1995). What mothers say about why poor children fall behind on immunizations. *Archives of Pediatric and Adolescent Medicine, 149,* 1070–1075.

Lescale, K. B., Inglis, S. R., Eddleman, K. A., Peeper, E. Q., Chervenak, F. A., & McCullough, L. B. (1996). Conflicts between physicians and patients in nonelective cesarean delivery: Incidence and the adequacy of informed consent. *American Journal of Perinatology, 13*(3), 171–176.

Lobar, S., Phillips, S., & Simunek, L. (1997). Legal issues in nonrelated infant adoption: Nursing implications. *Journal of Society of Pediatric Nurses, 2*(3), 116–124.

Lindgren, K. (1996). Maternal-fetal conflict: Court-ordered cesarean section. *Journal of Obstetric, Gynecologic, and Neonatal Nursing, 25*(8), 653–656.

Locher, A.W. (1996). Ethics, women with HIV, and procreation: Implications for nursing practice. *Journal of Obstetric, Gynecologic, and Neonatal Nursing, 25*(6), 465–469.

Lund, P. Z. (1997). Changing times, shifting paradigms. *Lifelines, 1*(6), 38–42.

Maloni, J. A., Cheng, C. Y., Liebl, C. P., & Maier, J. S. (1996). Transforming prenatal care: Reflections on the past and present with implications for the future. *Journal of Obstetric, Gynecologic, and Neonatal Nursing, 25*(1), 17–23.

March of Dimes Birth Defects Foundation. (1993). *Toward improving the outcome of pregnancy: The 90's and beyond.* White Plains, NY: Author.

March of Dimes Birth Defects Foundation. (1995). *March of Dimes Birth Defects Foundation Mission.* White Plains, NY: Author.

McGregor, L. A. (1998). Unlicensed assistive personnel: Getting it right from the beginning. *MCN: American Journal of Maternal/Child Nursing, 23*(2), 65–69.

Meissner-Cutler, S., & Gardner, S. L. (1997). Maternal-child nursing and the law. In S. L. Gardner & M. I. E. Hagedorn (Eds.), *Legal aspects of maternal-child nursing practice* (pp. 25–50). Menlo Park, CA: Addison-Wesley.

National Center for Health Statistics. (1997). *Healthy people 2000 review, 1997.* Hyattsville, MD: Public Health Service.

National Center for Health Statistics. (1998). *Health, United States, 1998, with socioeconomic status and health chartbook.* Hyattsville, MD: Author.

National Health Law Program and National Center for Youth Law. (1997). EPSDT update for child health insurance and Medicaid advocates. Los Angeles, CA: Author.

National Institute of Child Health and Human Development. (1998). *America's children: Key national indicators of well-being.* Hyattsville, MD: Author.

Newacheck, P., Jameson, W., & Halfon, N. (1994). Health status and income: The impact of poverty on child health. *Journal of School Health, 64*(6), 229–233.

Pence, M. (1997). Patient-focused models of care. *Journal of Obstetric, Gynecologic, and Neonatal Nursing, 26*(3), 320–326.

Penticuff, J. (1996). Ethical dimensions in genetic screening: A look into the future. *Journal of Obstetric, Gynecologic, and Neonatal Nursing, 25*(9), 785–789.

Piotrowski, K. (1996). Caring for the maternal-infant client. In J. Cookfair (Ed.), *Nursing care in the community.* St. Louis: Mosby.

Plotnick, J., & Presler, B. (1996). Rugged individualism and compassion: The foundation of public policy. *Maternal and Child Nursing, 21,* 20–33.

Pridham, K., Broome, M., & Woodring, B. (1996). Education for the nursing of children and their families: Standards and guidelines for prelicensure and early professional education. *Journal of Pediatric Nursing, 11*(5), 273–279.

Proctor, S. (1998). What determines quality in maternity care? Comparing the perceptions of childbearing women and midwives. *Birth, 25*(2), 85–93.

Rachuba, L., Stanton, B., & Howard, D. (1995). Violent crime in the United States. *Archives of Pediatric and Adolescent Medicine, 149,* 953–960.

Rhodes, A. M. (1996a). Anencephalic organ donation. *MCN: American Journal of Maternal/Child Nursing, 21*(1), 15.

Rhodes, A. M. (1996b). Drug use during pregnancy. *MCN: American Journal of Maternal/Child Nursing, 21*(3), 127.

Rhodes, A. M. (1996c). Testing the standards of death. *MCN: American Journal of Maternal/Child Nursing, 21*(2), 109.

Rhodes, A. M. (1997). Viable fetus vs. drug-abusing mother. *MCN: American Journal of Maternal/Child Nursing, 22*(3), 127.

Robinson, C. (1997). Early intervention services. *Journal of Society of Pediatric Nurses, 2*(4), 191–192.

Ryan, C., Schober, S., & Turczyn, K. (1997).

Operational definitions for year 2000 objectives: Priority area 20, immunization and infectious diseases. Hyattsville, MD: Centers for Disease Control and Prevention/National Center for Health Statistics.

Shelton, T., & Stepanek, J. (1994). *Family-centered care for children needing specialized health and developmental services.* Washington, DC: Association for the Care of Children's Health.

Silber, K., & Dorner, P. M. (1990). *Children of open adoption.* San Antonio, TX: Corona.

Simkin, P. (1989). Childbearing in social context. *Women and Health, 15*(3), 5–21.

Simpson, K. R. (1997). What nurses need to know. *Lifelines, 1*(3), 26–31.

Simpson, K. R., & Chez, B. F. (1996). Professional and legal issues. In K. R. Simpson & P. A. Creehan (Eds.), *AWHONN's perinatal nursing.* Philadelphia: Lippincott.

Singh, G. K., Mathews, T. J., Clarke, S. C., Yannicos, K., & Smith, B. L. (1995). A summary of births, marriages, divorces, and deaths, 1994. *Monthly Statistics Report, 43*(13).

Singh, G. K., & Yu, S. M. (1995). Infant mortality in the United States: Trends, differentials, and projections, 1950 through 2010. *American Journal of Public Health, 85*(7), 957–964.

Sklan, M. L. (1994, Winter). Medicine and law: Recent developments. *Tort & Insurance Law Journal, 22*(2), 347–348.

Solar, J. M. (1994). Analysis of legal issues, pharmaceutical cases. Part II. Over-the-counter medications and drug samples. In *Medical device and pharmaceutical litigation.* Houston, TX: University of Houston Law Foundation.

Southwell, S. M., & Archer-Dusté, H. (1998). Ethical aspects of perinatal care. In C. Kenner, J. W. Lott, & A. A. Flandemeyer (Eds.), *Comprehensive neonatal nursing: A physiologic perspective* (pp. 13–31). Philadelphia: Saunders.

Spence, A. (1995). Family instability leaves children vulnerable. *AAP News, 11*(8), 10–12.

Steinbock, B. (1984). Baby Jane Doe in court. *Hastings Report, 40*(1), 13–19.

Taylor, D. L., & Woods, N. F. (1996).

Changing women's health, changing nursing practice. *Journal of Obstetric, Gynecologic, and Neonatal Nursing, 25*(9), 791–802.

Torres, J. L., & Blair, T. M. (1992). Administering emergency medical care to minors. *Topics in Emergency Medicine, 14*(4), 20–23.

U.S. Bureau of the Census. (1995). *Statistical abstract of the United States* (115th ed., pp. 87–90). Washington, DC: Author.

U.S. Department of Health and Human Services. (1990). *Healthy People 2000.* Washington, DC: Author.

U.S. Department of Health and Human Services. (1998). *Health, United States, 1998, with socioeconomic status and health chartbook.* Washington, DC: Author.

Ward, S. L. (1998). Caring and healing in the 21st century. *MCN: American Journal of Maternal/Child Nursing, 23*(4), 210–215.

Weese, C. B., Drauss, M. R. (1995). A "barrier-free" health care system does not ensure adequate vaccination of 2-year-old children. *Archives of Pediatric and Adolescent Medicine, 149,* 1130–1135.

Wegman, M. E. (1996). Infant mortality: Some international comparisons. *Pediatrics, 98*(6), 1020–1027.

Wertz, R., & Wertz, D. (1992). *Lying-in: A history of childbirth in America* (2nd ed.). New Haven, CT: Yale University Press.

White, C. C. (1995). Migrant farmworker children suffer inferior health care. *AAP News, 11*(10), 8–25.

Woodring, B. (1998). *Standards and guidelines for pre-licensure and early professional education for the nursing care of children and their families* (Rev. ed.). Denver, CO: Society of Pediatric Nurses.

Yoos, H. L., Kitzman, H., Olds, D. L., & Overacker, I. (1995). Community: Implications for culturally competent pediatric care. *Journal of Pediatric Nursing, 10*(6), 343–353.

York, R., Grant, C., Gibeau, A., Beecham, J., & Kessler, J. (1996). A review of problems of universal access to prenatal care. *Nursing Clinics of North America, 31*(2), 279–292.

Yudkowsky, B., & Tang, S. (1997). Children at risk: Their health insurance status by state. *Pediatrics, 99*(5), e2.

2

The Nurse's Role in Maternity and Pediatric Nursing

LEARNING OBJECTIVES

After studying this chapter, you should be able to:

- Explain roles the nurse may assume in maternity and pediatric nursing practice.
- Explain the roles of nurses with advanced preparation for maternity and pediatric nursing practice.
- Explain the incorporation of critical thinking into nursing practice.
- Describe the steps of the nursing process and relate them to maternity and pediatric nursing.
- Discuss the importance of nursing research in clinical practice.

DEFINITIONS

advocacy Speaking or arguing in support of a policy or a person's rights.

ambiguity (ambiguous) Lack of clarity or certainty; having more than one meaning.

assumptions Beliefs taken for granted without examination.

baseline data Information that describes the status of the client before treatment begins.

bias A prejudice that sways the mind.

cesarean birth Surgical birth of the fetus through an incision in the abdominal wall and uterus.

delegated nursing interventions Physician-prescribed nursing actions that require nursing judgment because nurses are accountable for correct implementation. See also *independent nursing interventions*.

fetus The developing baby from 9 weeks after conception until birth. In everyday practice, the term is often used to describe a developing baby during pregnancy, regardless of age.

independent nursing interventions Nurse-prescribed actions used in both nursing diagnoses and collaboratively addressed problems. See also *delegated nursing interventions*.

inference The act of drawing a conclusion or making a deduction.

judgment An opinion.

nursing diagnosis A clinical judgment about individual, family, or community responses to actual or potential health problems or life processes.

reflection Meditation, attentive consideration.

skepticism Doubt in the absence of conclusive evidence.

suspend To delay or to bring to a stop temporarily.

validate To make certain that the information collected during assessment is accurate.

As nursing care changed from the category-specific care of the mother, newborn, or child to family-centered care, maternity and pediatric nursing entered a new era of autonomy and independence. Nurses today must be able to communicate with and teach effectively clients of many ages and levels of development and education. They must be able to think critically and use the nursing process to develop a plan of care that meets the unique needs of each client and family. They are expected to use current research to solve problems and to collaborate with other health care providers.

The Role of the Professional Nurse

The professional nurse has a responsibility to provide the highest quality care to every client. The American Nurses Association (ANA) Code for Nurses provides guidelines for ethical and professional behavior. The code emphasizes the nurse's accountability to the client, the community, and the profession. The nurse should understand the implications of this code and strive to practice accordingly. Professional nurses have a legal obligation to know and understand the standard of care imposed on them. It is critical that nurses maintain competence and a current knowledge base in their areas of practice.

Standards of practice describe the level of performance expected of a professional nurse as determined by an authority in the practice. For example, perinatal nurses are held to the standards published by the Association of Women's Health, Obstetric, and Neonatal Nurses (AWHONN). AWHONN recently published the fifth edition of its *Standards and Guidelines* to guide practice and shape institutional guidelines.

The ANA and the Society of Pediatric Nurses formed a task force to develop *Standards of Care and Standards of Professional Performance for Pediatric Nurses*. These standards can be used as a guide for practice by nurses who care for children in all clinical settings. Other standards of practice for specific clinical areas, such as pediatric oncology nursing or emergency nursing, are available from nursing specialty groups.

As health care moves to family-centered and community-based health services, all nurses should expect to care for children, adolescents, and their families. *Standards and Guidelines for Prelicensure and Early Professional Education for the Nursing Care of Children and Their Families* have been developed by academic and clinical educators to meet this need. These published standards are stated in the form of 11 goals, based on issues central to the health of children and their families. The issues are child, family, and societal areas; clinical problems; and care delivery (Woodring, 1998).

Maternity and pediatric nurses function in a variety of

roles, including those of care provider, teacher, collaborator, researcher, advocate, and manager.

Care Provider

The nurse provides direct nursing care to women, infants, children, and their families in times of childbearing, illness, injury, recovery, and wellness. Nursing care is based on the nursing process. The nurse obtains health histories, assesses client needs, monitors growth and development, performs health screening procedures, develops comprehensive plans of care, provides treatment and care, makes referrals, and evaluates the effects of care. Pediatric care is especially based on an understanding of the child's developmental stage and is aimed at meeting the child's physical and emotional needs at that level. Developing a therapeutic relationship with and providing support to clients and their families are essential components of nursing care. Maternity and pediatric nurses practice family-centered care, embracing diversity in family structures and cultural backgrounds. These nurses strive to empower families, encouraging them to participate in their care and the care of their child.

Teacher

Education is an essential role of today's nurse. Client teaching begins early, during a woman's prenatal care, and continues through her recovery from childbirth (Fig. 2–1). Pediatric nurses prepare children for procedures, hospitalization, or surgery, using knowledge of growth and development to teach children at various levels of understanding. Families need information as well as emotional support so that they can cope with the anxiety and uncertainty of a child's illness. Nurses teach family members how to provide care, watch for important signs, and increase the client's comfort. They also work with new parents and parents of ill children so that the parents are prepared to assume responsibility for care at home after the child has been discharged from the hospital.

Education is essential for promotion of health. The nurse applies principles of teaching and learning to change the behavior of family members. Nurses motivate women,

children, and families to take charge of and make responsible decisions about their own health. For teaching to be effective, it must incorporate the family's values and health beliefs.

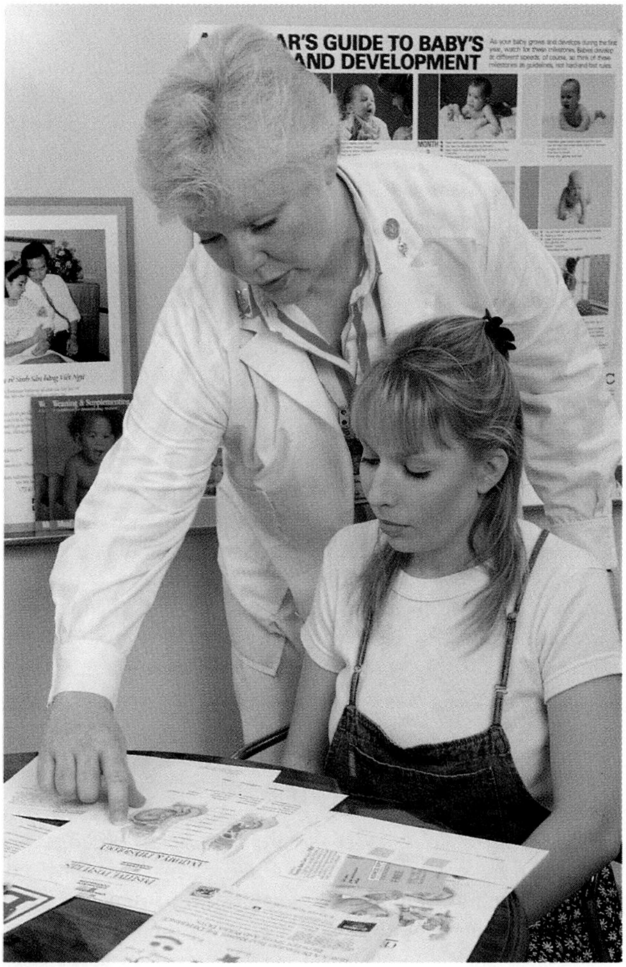

Pediatric nurses play an important role in the prevention of illness and injury through education and anticipatory guidance. Teaching about immunizations, safety, dental care, socialization, and discipline is a necessary component of care. Nurses offer guidance to parents with regard to child-rearing practices and preventing potential problems. They also answer questions about growth and development and assist families in understanding their children. Teaching often involves providing emotional support and counseling to children and families.

FACTORS INFLUENCING LEARNING

A number of factors influence learning at any age. These factors include the following:

- *Developmental level.* Teenage parents often have very different concerns than older parents. Developmental level also influences whether a person learns best by reading printed material, watching videos, participating in group discussions, play, or other means.
- *Language.* The ability to understand the language in which teaching is done determines how much the family learns. Families for whom English is not their primary language may not understand idioms, nuances, medical words, or slang terms. An interpreter for the deaf may be necessary for the client who is hearing impaired.
- *Culture.* People tend to forget content with which they disagree. The nurse's teaching can be most effective if cultural considerations are weighed and incorporated into the education.
- *Previous experiences.* Parents who have other children may need less education about pregnancy care or infant and child care. They may, however, have additional concerns about meeting the needs of several children and about sibling rivalry.
- *Physical environment.* The nurse must consider privacy when discussing sensitive issues such as adolescent sexuality or domestic violence. A group discussion, on the other hand, may prompt participants to ask questions of concern to all members of the group, such as the experiences they can expect in labor.
- *Organization and skill of the teacher.* The teacher must determine the objectives of the teaching, develop a plan to meet the objectives, and gather all materials before teaching. The nurse must determine the best way to present the material for the intended audience. A summary of the information is helpful when concluding a teaching session.

PRINCIPLES OF TEACHING AND LEARNING

Applying the following principles will help nurses become effective teachers in the childbearing setting.

- Real learning depends on the readiness of the family to learn and the relevance of the content.
- Active participation increases learning. Whenever possible, the learner should be involved in the educational process and not act as a passive listener or viewer. A

FIGURE 2–1

In the prenatal clinic, the nurse teaches a woman one-on-one.

discussion format in which all can participate stimulates more learning than a straight lecture.

- Repetition of a skill increases retention and promotes a feeling of competence.
- Praise and positive feedback are powerful motivators for learning. They are particularly important when the family is trying to master a frustrating task, such as breastfeeding an unresponsive infant.
- Role modeling is an effective method for demonstrating behavior. Nurses must be aware that their behavior is scrutinized carefully at all times and that it may be copied later.
- Conflicts and frustration impede learning, and they should be recognized and resolved for learning to progress.
- Learning is enhanced when teaching is structured to present simple tasks before more complex material. For instance, the nurse teaches how to care for the umbilical cord, which is simple, before teaching how to bathe and shampoo the newborn, which is more difficult.
- A variety of teaching methods is necessary to maintain interest and to illustrate concepts. Posters, videos, and printed materials supplement lectures and discussion. Models may be especially useful for teaching family planning or the processes of labor.
- Information is retained better when it is presented in small segments over a period of time. Abbreviated hospital stays do not support this practice, making follow-up care particularly important.

Collaborator

Nurses collaborate with other members of the health care team, often coordinating and managing the client's care. Care is improved by an interdisciplinary approach as nurses work together with dieticians, social workers, physicians, and others.

Managing the transition from a hospital or any other acute care setting to the client's home or another facility involves discharge planning and collaboration with other health care professionals. The trend toward home care makes collaboration increasingly important. The nurse must be knowledgeable about community resources, appropriate home care agencies for the type of client or problem, and financial resources. Cooperation and communication are essential as clients, including parents of children, are encouraged to participate in their care.

Researcher

Nurses contribute to their profession's knowledge base by systematically investigating theoretical or practice issues in nursing. Nursing does not merely "borrow" scientific knowledge from medicine and basic sciences. Nursing generates and answers its own questions based on research of its unique subject matter. The responsibility for research within nursing is not limited to nurses with graduate degrees. It is important that all nurses apply research findings to their practice, rather than basing care decisions merely on intuition or tradition. Nurses can contribute to the body of professional knowledge by demonstrating an awareness of the value of nursing research and assisting in problem identification and data collection. Nurses should keep their knowledge current by networking and sharing research findings at conferences, by publishing, and by reading research journal articles.

Advocate

An advocate is one who speaks on behalf of another. As the health care environment becomes increasingly complex, care can become impersonal. The wishes and needs of children and families are sometimes discounted or ignored in the effort to treat and to cure. As the health professional who is closest to the client, the nurse is in an ideal position to humanize care and to intercede on the client's behalf. As an advocate, the nurse considers the family's wishes in planning and implementing care. The nurse informs families of treatments and procedures, ensuring that the families are involved directly in decisions and activities related to their care. The nurse must be sensitive to the values, beliefs, and customs of families.

Nurses must be advocates for health promotion for vulnerable groups such as children or victims of domestic violence. Nurses can promote the rights of children and families by participating in groups dedicated to the welfare of children and families, such as professional nursing societies, parent support groups, religious organizations, and voluntary organizations. Through involvement with health care planning on a political or legislative level, and by working as consumer advocates, nurses can initiate changes for better quality health care. Nurses possess unique knowledge and skills and can make valuable contributions in developing health care strategies to ensure that all clients receive optimal care.

Manager of Care

As a result of the decreased length of stay in acute care facilities, nurses often are not able to provide total direct client care. Instead, they delegate concrete tasks, such as giving a bath or taking vital signs, to others. As a result, nurses spend more time teaching and supervising nonlicensed personnel, planning and coordinating care, and collaborating with other professionals and agencies. Moreover, nurses are expected to understand the financial squeeze resulting from cost-containment strategies and to contribute to their institutions' economic viability. At the same time, they must continue to act as client advocates and to maintain a standard of care.

▌ Advanced Preparation for Maternity and Pediatric Nurses

The increasing complexity of care and a focus on cost containment have led to a greater need for nurses with advanced preparation. Advanced practice nurses may practice as certified nurse-midwives, nurse practitioners, or clinical nurse specialists, among other possibilities. Advanced practice nurses may also work as nurse administrators, nurse educators, and nurse researchers. Preparation for advanced practice involves obtaining a master's or doctoral degree.

Certified Nurse-Midwives

Certified nurse-midwives (CNMs) are registered nurses who have completed an extensive program of study and clinical experience. They must pass a certification test administered by the American College of Nurse-Midwives. CNMs are qualified to provide complete care during pregnancy, childbirth, and the postpartum period in uncomplicated pregnancies. They provide information about preventive measures and preparation for normal pregnancy and childbirth. They spend a great deal of time counseling and supporting the childbearing family. The CNM also provides gynecological services as well as family planning information and counseling.

Despite the proven effectiveness of nurse-midwives, for many years they were restricted in the scope and location of their practice. In 1970, however, many of these restrictions were alleviated when the American College of Obstetricians and Gynecologists, together with the Nurses Association of the American College of Obstetricians and Gynecologists—now known as the Association of Women's Health, Obstetric, and Neonatal Nurses—issued a joint statement that admitted nurse-midwives as part of the health care team. In 1981, Congress authorized Medicaid payments for the services of CNMs. This measure has greatly increased use of nurse-midwives, particularly by health maintenance organizations (HMOs), in birthing centers, and in some hospitals.

Nurse Practitioners

Nurse practitioners are advanced practice nurses who work according to protocols. Most nurse practitioners collaborate with a physician, but, depending on their scope of practice and their individual state's board of nursing mandates, they may work independently. Nurse practitioners provide care for specific groups of clients in a variety of settings (primary care facilities, schools, acute care facilities, rehabilitation centers). They may address occupational health, women's health, family health, and the health of the elderly or the very young.

Maternity nurse practitioners, or women's health nurse practitioners, assess a pregnant woman at prenatal appointments and evaluate the progress of the pregnancy. Although they do not usually assist with childbirth, nurse practitioners provide information and care during the postpartum period.

Family planning nurse practitioners often work in family planning clinics or with physicians in private practice. Major responsibilities include performing pelvic examinations and screening procedures for sexually transmitted diseases and providing family planning services.

Pediatric nurse practitioners use advanced skills to assess and treat ill children according to established protocols. The health care services they provide range from physical examinations to the treatment of common illnesses and injuries. It is becoming more common for newborn nurseries to be staffed by pediatric or neonatal nurse practitioners.

Family nurse practitioners are prepared to provide care for all family members. They care for women during uncomplicated pregnancies and provide follow-up care for the mother and infant after childbirth. Unlike certified nurse-midwives, they do not assist with childbirth. They diagnose and treat clients holistically, with a strong emphasis on prevention.

Clinical Nurse Specialists

Clinical specialists are registered nurses who, through study and supervised practice at the graduate level (master's or doctorate), have become expert in the care of childbearing families or pediatric clients. Four major subroles have been identified for clinical nurse specialists: expert practitioner, educator, researcher, and consultant. These professionals often function as clinical leaders, role models, client advocates, and change agents. Unlike nurse practitioners, clinical nurse specialists are not prepared to provide primary care.

■ Implications of Changing Roles for Nurses

As nursing care has changed, so also have the roles of maternity and pediatric nurses with both basic and advanced preparation. Nurses now work in a variety of areas. Although they previously worked almost exclusively in the hospital setting, many now provide home care and community-based care. Some of the settings for care of maternity and pediatric clients include:

- Acute care settings: general hospital units, intensive care units, surgical units, postanesthesia care units, emergency care facilities, and on board emergency transport craft
- Clinics and physician offices
- Home health agencies
- Schools
- Rehabilitation centers or long-term care facilities
- Summer camps and day care centers
- Hospice programs or respite care programs
- Psychiatric centers

Therapeutic Communication

Therapeutic communication is a skill nurses must have to carry out the many roles expected within the profession. Therapeutic communication, unlike social communication, is purposeful, goal directed, and focused. Although it may seem simple, therapeutic communication requires conscious effort and considerable practice.

GUIDELINES FOR THERAPEUTIC COMMUNICATION

Therapeutic communication requires flexibility and cannot depend on a particular set of learned techniques. Certain guidelines, however, may prove helpful.

- A calm setting that provides privacy, reduces distractions, and minimizes interruptions is essential.
- Interactions should begin with introductions and clarification of the nurse's role. The nurse might say, "My name is Claudia Lyall. I am here to complete the discharge teaching that was started yesterday." This introduction acknowledges the nurse's purpose and sets the

stage for a discussion of the client's concerns about what happens when the family is discharged from the hospital.

- Therapeutic communication should be focused because it is directed toward meeting the needs expressed by the family. Beginning the interaction with an open-ended question, such as "How do you feel about going home today?" is one method of focusing the interaction. It may also be necessary to redirect the conversation. For instance, the nurse might say, "Thanks for showing me the beautiful pictures of the baby. I understand you are having a bit of trouble getting him to nurse."

- Nonverbal behaviors may communicate more powerful messages to the client than the spoken word. For example, facial expressions and eye movements can confirm or contradict what is said. Repetitive hand gestures, such as finger tapping or twirling a lock of hair, may indicate frustration, irritation, or boredom. Body posture, stance, and gait can convey energy, depression, or discomfort. Voice tone, pitch, rate, and volume may indicate joy, anger, or fear. Communicating with a young child may require that the nurse sit or squat to get to the child's level. Grooming also conveys messages about the nurse's self-image.

- Active listening requires that the nurse attend to what is being said as well as to the nonverbal clues. Attending behaviors that convey the nurse's interest and a sincere desire to understand include the following:
  - Eye contact, which signals a readiness to interact.
  - Relaxed posture, with the upper portion of the body inclined toward the client.
  - Encouraging cues, such as nodding, leaning closer, and smiling. Verbal cues include "Uh huh, go on," "Tell me about that," or "Can you give me an example?"
  - Touch, which can be a powerful response when words would break a mood or fail to convey the depth of feeling experienced between the woman and the nurse.
  - Cultural differences influence communication. In some cultures, such as Chinese and Southeast Asian, prolonged eye contact is considered confrontational. People from Middle Eastern or Native American cultures are sometimes uncomfortable with touch and would be disturbed by unsolicited touching.
  - Clarifying communication involves a unique process of the listener receiving the message as the sender intended. It may be necessary for the nurse to ask questions if the meaning of a statement is unclear. For instance, the nurse might say, "I'm not sure I understand."
  - Emotions are part of communication, and nurses must often reflect feelings that are expressed verbally or nonverbally. The nurse might suggest, "You looked forward to delivery in a birth center and are disappointed that you needed a cesarean birth?"

THERAPEUTIC COMMUNICATION TECHNIQUES

Therapeutic communication involves responding as well as listening, and nurses must learn to use responses that facilitate rather than block communication. These facilitative responses, often called communication techniques, focus on both the content of the message and the feeling that accompanies the message. Communication techniques include clarifying, reflecting, being silent, questioning, and directing. A brief review of these and other communication techniques can be found in Table 2–1. In addition to being aware of effective communication techniques, nurses must be aware of blocks to communication. These are listed with examples and alternatives in Table 2–2. Chapter 32 describes in more detail methods of communicating with pediatric clients and their families.

Critical Thinking

In recent years critical thinking has received widespread attention in nursing. Clearly, nurses must be concerned with the development of critical thinking skills, which are needed not only to pass the National Council Licensure Examination but also to function clinically.

DEFINITIONS

Unlike undirected thinking, during which the mind wanders freely, critical thinking is controlled and directed toward finding solutions or forming opinions. To do this effectively, people must gain insight into their own thought processes. This process means analyzing one's own thinking by taking it apart to examine and criticize it. It includes recognizing and acknowledging specific habits and responses that can interfere with productive thinking.

Critical thinking is based on reason rather than on preference or prejudice. Moreover, critical thinking seeks to examine feelings so that one can understand how emotions affect thinking. Last but not least, critical thinking requires that one suspend judgment until there is adequate evidence to support inferences or conclusions.

THE PURPOSE OF CRITICAL THINKING

The purpose of critical thinking is to identify and then to overcome habits or impulses that can result in poor decisions or inappropriate actions. The primary purpose of critical thinking in nursing is to help nurses make the best clinical judgments. The process begins when nurses realize that it is not enough to accumulate a fund of knowledge from texts and lectures. They must also be able to *apply* the knowledge to specific clinical situations and thus to reach conclusions that provide the most effective care in each situation.

In addition to acquiring knowledge and learning to apply that knowledge, nurses must also examine their own thought processes for flaws that can lead to inaccurate conclusions or poor judgments. Although this examination requires a great deal of self-analysis, a series of steps makes the process easier. Critical thinking exercises are presented throughout this book to help students develop skill in critical thinking and applying knowledge.

STEPS IN CRITICAL THINKING

A series of steps may help clarify how critical thinking is learned. These steps may be called the ABCDEs of critical thinking. They include a recognition of *assumptions*, an examination of personal *biases*, an analysis of how much pres-

TABLE 2–1
• • • • • • • • • • •

Communication Techniques

Definition	Examples
Clarifying	
Clearing up or following up to understand both content and feelings expressed, to check the accuracy of how the nurse perceives the message.	"I'm confused about your plans. Could you explain?" "Tell me what you mean when you say you don't feel like yourself." "Are you saying that _____?" "Can you tell me more about _____?"
Paraphrasing	
Restating in words other than those used by the client what the client seems to express; this is a form of clarification.	**Example No. 1** CLIENT: "My boyfriend won't even come into the room for the birth. I am furious with him." NURSE: "You want him with you and you are angry because he won't be here?" **Example No. 2** CLIENT: "My baby cries all of the time. We aren't getting any sleep." NURSE: "You are feeling exhausted and it seems like your baby cries a great deal? Can you tell me what a typical day is like?"
Reflecting	
Verbalizing comprehension of what the client said and what the client seems to be feeling. It is important to link content and feeling and to reflect the client as a mirror reflects a person. The opinion, values, and personality of the nurse should not be in the reflected image.	**Example No. 1** CLIENT: "I don't know what to do. My husband doesn't think a cesarean is needed, but the doctor says the baby is showing some stress." NURSE: "You're confused and frightened because they don't agree?" **Example No. 2** CLIENT (woman in early labor): "It was my husband's idea for me to become pregnant. I wasn't too excited about it at first." NURSE: "I'll bet the dad will be a pushover as a father." The nurse's statement reflects the nurse's opinion and fails to acknowledge the mother's statement. A better response might be: "Your husband was more excited early in the pregnancy than you?"
Silence	
Waiting and allowing time for the client to continue. Verbal communication need not be constant.	The nurse waits quietly for the client to continue.
Structuring	
Creating guidelines or setting priorities.	"You said you don't know how to take care of the baby and also that you are afraid of getting pregnant again. What should we talk about first?"
Pinpointing	
Calling attention to differences or inconsistencies in statements.	Nurse talking to an 8-year-old child: "You said you didn't want your mother to spend the night with you, but you cry every night after she leaves. It can be scary being alone. I will sit with you and we can talk about asking your mother to stay tomorrow night."
Questioning	
Eliciting information directly; using open-ended questions to avoid yes or no answers and to prevent controlling the answers.	"How do you feel about being pregnant?" instead of "Are you happy to be pregnant?"
Directing	
Using nonverbal responses or succinct comments to encourage the client to continue.	Nodding. "Um mm." "You were saying _____." "Please go on."
Summarizing	
Reviewing the main themes or issues that were discussed.	"You had two major concerns today _____." "We have talked about breast-feeding and how to bathe the baby today."

TABLE 2-2
• • • • • • • • • • •

Behaviors That Block Communication

Behavior	Example	Alternative
Conveying lack of interest	Looking away, fidgeting	Attending behaviors such as eye contact, nodding
Conveying sense of haste	Checking the time, standing near the door	Sitting at bedside
Closed posture	Arms crossed over chest, holding clip board in front of body	Leaning forward with arms relaxed
Interrupting, finishing sentences	WOMAN: "I'm not sure how _____." NURSE: "We will have a bath demonstration later."	"Go on _____." "You were saying _____."
Providing false reassurance	"You're going to be okay."	"I sense you are concerned about how to care for the baby. I will help you give the bath today."
Inappropriate self-disclosure	To woman in labor: "I was in labor 12 hours, then had a cesarean."	"What concerns you most about labor?"
Giving advice	"You should _____." "If I were you, I would _____."	"How do you feel about that?" "What do you think is most important?"
Failure to acknowledge comments or feelings	MOTHER: "Being a parent is hard work. I never have time for myself." NURSE: "It is going to get worse before it gets better. Parenting is hard work."	"Parenting is hard work. Let's talk about some ways that you might get a break."

sure one has for *closure*, an examination of how one collects and analyzes *data*, and an evaluation of how *emotions* and *environmental factors* may interfere with one's ability to think critically.

A. Recognizing Assumptions. *Assumptions* are ideas, beliefs, or values that are taken for granted. Assumptions may lead to unexamined thoughts or unsound actions. For instance, consider the consequences of the following assumptions: "Anyone who wants a job can get one." "Teenagers don't listen." "Every woman wants a baby." "Children should be seen but not heard."

When attempting to identify assumptions, it may be helpful to make a list of everything known about a specific situation. Then each item on the list should be analyzed to determine which is true, which could be true, and which is either untrue or lacks enough evidence to determine whether it is true or not.

B. Examining Biases. *Biases* are prejudices that sway an individual toward a particular conclusion or course of action on the basis of personal theories or stereotypes. Biases are based on unexamined beliefs, and many are widespread. Some examples are "fat people are lazy," "women are bad drivers," and "men are insensitive."

People are often biased toward those of different races, religions, or lifestyles. When faced with a predisposition to judge a person or a group of persons, it may be wise to ask oneself (or a co-worker) a series of questions: "Why do you think that?" "What if this person were a different client?" "What if there were different circumstances?" "What might someone who disagrees say?" "What is influencing my thinking?"

C. Analyzing the Need for Closure. Many people look for immediate answers and experience a great deal of anxiety until a solution is found for any problem. In other words, they have very little tolerance for doubt or uncertainty, sometimes called ambiguity. As a result, they feel pressure to come to a decision, or to reach *closure*, as early as possible. This is one of the most important aspects of critical thinking because those who feel pressure to come to an early decision, or to find a quick solution, often do so with insufficient data.

To overcome the pressure to reach an early conclusion, a conscious effort must be made to suspend judgment. This is sometimes called *reflective skepticism*. The first step is to acknowledge the anxiety that postponing decisions creates. The next step involves deliberately waiting to make a decision.

People who jump to conclusions often stop with one answer. To overcome this tendency, they should always look for a second right answer. They could also imagine the problem from the perspective of someone else. They might also ask a series of questions, such as "What alternatives do we have?" "What else might work?" "What information supports this?" "What effect would that have?" "Is there good evidence to support that decision?" "Is there reason to doubt that evidence?"

Unlike those who feel pressure for closure, some people can tolerate a great deal of doubt and uncertainty. They are comfortable with data collection and analysis but feel uncomfortable making decisions. They may procrastinate or put off coming to a decision for as long as possible. Failure to make a decision in the clinical area may have serious consequences for clients and their families. Several questions may help overcome the tendency to put off coming to a decision. Some of these questions are "What signs indicate something is wrong?" "Do I need to do something about it?" "How much time do I have?" "What happens if I don't do something about this?" "What could happen if I do?" "What should I do first?" "What resources can help me?" This step might also be called *priority setting;* it is one of the most important aspects of critical thinking.

D. Managing Data.   Expertise in collecting, organizing, and analyzing data involves developing an attitude of *inquiry* and learning to live with questions. Questions to ask for data management include "Why?" "What if?" "What else?" "Is this relevant?" "How does it relate to that?" "How can I organize the data?" "Does it form patterns?" "What can I infer from those patterns?"

Collecting Data.   To obtain complete data, one must develop skill in verbal communication. Asking open-ended questions elicits more information than asking questions that require only a one-word answer. Follow-up questions are often needed to clarify information or to pursue a particular train of thought.

Validating Data.   Information that is unclear or incomplete should be validated. This process may involve rechecking physical signs, collecting additional information, or determining whether a perception is accurate. For instance, the comment "You seem uncomfortable" may result in the client's denying or acknowledging discomfort.

Organizing and Analyzing Data.   Data are more useful when organized into patterns or clusters. The first step is to separate data that are relevant from data that may be interesting but that are not related to the current situation.

The next step is to compare one's data with expected norms to determine what is within the expected range (normal) and what is not within the expected range (abnormal). Abnormal results provide cues that can be grouped or clustered so that conclusions can be made. For example, grouping all data that may indicate excessive bleeding, such as pulse rate, blood pressure, amount of visible bleeding, and skin color, may make the information more meaningful. Organizing data into clusters often reveals that additional data are needed before a decision can be reached.

E. Evaluating Other Factors.   A variety of *emotions* and *environmental factors* can influence critical thinking. For instance, the clinical area is often a noisy, fast-paced, hectic environment with time limitations and distractions that make calm reflection and reasoning difficult. Moreover, fatigue may reduce one's ability to concentrate at the end of a 10- or 12-hour shift. The nurse may desperately want to reassure anxious parents about their sick child. Inexperienced nurses and students may lack confidence in their knowledge and experience. As a result, they often feel anxious, which can reduce their ability to think critically.

Many nurses, both experienced and inexperienced, have a strong need to protect their self-image. As a result, they become very defensive when they have said or done something wrong. This response is a serious barrier to critical thinking and requires that all health care professionals learn to acknowledge mistakes and to feel comfortable with constructive criticism.

Extreme emotions, such as anger or frustration, impede

critical thinking by narrowing the focus to only data that support the intense feeling. For example, people who are extremely frustrated may repeat the perceived cause of their frustration over and over and may be unable to move on to other information so the problem can be addressed.

The first step in dealing with factors or emotions that impede thinking is to recognize and acknowledge them. To develop critical thinking skills, one must learn to admit mistakes and become comfortable saying, "I was wrong." Asking for assistance, verification, or validation is wise when fatigue is a problem or when lack of confidence creates anxiety.

It is essential for the person who experiences intense frustration or anger to recognize the emotions and their impact on rational thought. It may be helpful to ask a trusted colleague to point out when signs of these emotions, such as repetitive vehement comments, occur. Some people use other methods of control, such as visualizations, a series of breathing exercises, or, when possible, a brief, self-imposed "time-out" from the precipitating situation.

The Nursing Process in Maternity and Pediatric Care

The nursing process forms the basis for all of nursing. The nursing process consists of five distinct steps: (1) assessment, (2) nursing diagnosis, (3) planning, (4) implementation of the plan (interventions), and (5) evaluation. Despite the apparent complexity of the process, the nurse soon learns to use the steps of the nursing process in order when caring for clients.

In maternal-newborn nursing, the nursing process must be adapted to a population that is generally healthy and that is experiencing a life event that holds the potential for growth as well as for problems. Much maternal-newborn nursing activity is devoted to assessing and diagnosing client strengths and healthy functioning and to supporting adaptive responses. This focus differs somewhat from providing care for clients who are ill, and it presents some difficulty for maternal-newborn nurses when they use the list of largely problem-oriented nursing diagnoses provided by the North American Nursing Diagnosis Association (NANDA).

Pediatric nursing, including care of a newborn, presents another problem for many nursing students. Whereas use of the nursing process when caring for adults may involve only the client, in caring for infants and children it must involve their family as well. Therefore, it is not uncommon for planning and interventions to state what the parent is expected to do or to specify interventions such as teaching a parent. The involvement of a third party (the family) may be different to the nursing student who has applied the nursing process only to care of adults in the past.

Assessment

Nursing assessment is the systematic collection of relevant data to determine the client's and family's current health status, coping patterns, needs, and problems. The data collected include not only physiologic data but also psychological, social, and cultural data relevant to life processes.

Developing Individualized Nursing Care Through the Nursing Process

Although the nursing process is the foundation for maternal-child nursing, initially it is a challenging process to apply in the clinical area. It requires proficiency in focus assessments of the new mother and infant as well as the ability to analyze data on, and plan nursing care for, individual clients and families. It may be helpful to pose questions at each step of the nursing process.

ASSESSMENT

1. Were there data that were not within normal limits or expected parameters? For example, the client states that she feels "dizzy" when she tries to ambulate.
2. If so, what else should be assessed? (What else should I look for? What might be related to this symptom?) For instance, what are the blood pressure, pulse, skin color, temperature, and amount of lochia if the client feels "dizzy"?
3. Did the assessment identify the cause of the abnormal data? What are the hemoglobin value, hematocrit, and estimated blood loss during childbirth?
4. Are there other factors? What medication is the client taking? How long has it been since she has eaten? Is the environment a related factor (crowded, warm, unfamiliar)? Is she reluctant to ask for assistance?

ANALYSIS

1. Are adequate data available to reach a conclusion? What else is needed? (What do you wish you had assessed? What would you look for next time?)
2. What is the major concern? (On the basis of the data, what are you worried about?) The client who is "dizzy" may fall as she ambulates to the bathroom.
3. What might happen if no action is taken? (What might happen to the client if you do nothing?) She may suffer an injury or a complication.
4. Is there a NANDA-approved diagnostic category that reflects your major concern? How is it defined? Suppose that during analysis you decide the major concern is that the client will faint and suffer an injury. What diagnostic category most closely reflects this concern? High Risk for Injury? Definition: "The state in which an individual is at risk for harm because of a perceptual or physiologic deficit, a lack of awareness of hazards, or maturational age."
5. Do this category and definition fit this client? Is she at greater risk for a problem than others in a similar situation? Why? What are the additional risk factors?

6. Is this a problem that nurses can manage independently? Are medical interventions also necessary?
7. If the problem can be managed by nurses, is it an actual problem (defining characteristics are present), at-risk problem (risk factors are present), or possible problem (you have a hunch and some data, but not enough)?

PLANNING

1. What outcomes are desired? That the client will remain free of injury during hospital stay? That she will demonstrate position changes that reduce the episodes of vertigo?
2. Would the outcomes be clear, specific, and measurable to anyone reading them?
3. What nursing interventions should be initiated and carried out to accomplish these goals or outcomes?
4. Are your written interventions specific and clear? Are action verbs used (*assess, teach, assist*)? After you have written the interventions, look them over. Do they define exactly what is to be done (when, what, how far, how often)? Will they prevent the client from suffering an injury?
5. Are the interventions based on sound rationale? For instance, dehydration that may occur during labor causes weakness that may result in falls; loss of blood during delivery often exceeds 500 ml, which results in hypotension that is aggravated when the client stands suddenly.

IMPLEMENTING NURSING INTERVENTIONS

1. What are the expected effects of the prescribed intervention? Are there potential adverse effects? What are they?
2. Are the interventions acceptable to the client and family?
3. Are the interventions clearly written so that they can be carefully followed?

EVALUATION

1. What is the status of the client right now?
2. What were the goals and outcomes? Are they specific? Can they be measured?
3. Compare the current status of the client with the stated goals and outcomes.
4. What should be done now?

Abbreviation: NANDA, North American Nursing Diagnosis Association.

Nurses must assess the belief systems, available support, perceptions, and plans of other family members in an effort to provide the best nursing care.

During the assessment phase, three activities take place: collecting data, grouping findings, and writing the nursing diagnoses. Data can be collected through interview, physical examination, observation, review of records, and diagnostic reports, as well as through collaboration with other health care workers and the family. Two levels of nursing assessment are used to collect comprehensive data: (1) database assessment and (2) focus assessments.

DATABASE ASSESSMENT

The database assessment is usually performed during the initial contact with the client. Its purpose is to gather information about all aspects of the client's health. This information, called *baseline data*, describes the client's health status before interventions begin. It forms the basis for identifying both strengths and problems.

A variety of methods may be used to organize the assessment. For example, information may be grouped according to body systems. Assessment can also be organized around nursing models that are based on nursing theory, such as

Roy's adaptation model, Gordon's Functional Health Patterns, NANDA's Human Response Patterns, or Orem's self-care deficit theory.

FOCUS ASSESSMENT

A focus assessment is used to gather information that is specifically related to an actual health problem or a problem that the client or family is at risk for acquiring. A focus assessment is often performed at the beginning of a shift and centers on areas relevant to the client's diagnosis and current status. For example, the nurse would perform a focus assessment of the respiratory system for the child with acute asthma several times during the child's hospitalization.

Nursing Diagnosis

The data gathered during assessment must be analyzed to identify problems or potential problems. Data are validated and grouped in a process of critical thinking so that cues and inferences can be determined. A *nursing diagnosis* is a clinical judgment about the response of an individual, family, or community to actual and potential health problems or life processes. Nursing diagnoses provide the basis for selecting nursing interventions to achieve outcomes for which the nurse is accountable (North American Nursing Diagnosis Association, 1996). At this time more than 100 nursing diagnoses have been identified by NANDA (see Appendix A).

There are three types of nursing diagnoses. An *actual nursing diagnosis* describes a human response to a health condition or life process affecting an individual, family, or community. It is supported by defining characteristics (manifestations, signs and symptoms) that can be clustered in patterns of related cues or inferences. *Risk nursing diagnoses* describe human responses to health conditions or life processes that may develop in a vulnerable individual, family, or community. They are supported by risk factors that contribute to increased vulnerability. *Wellness nursing diagnoses* describe human responses to levels of wellness in an individual, family, or community that have a potential for enhancement to a higher state.

Each nursing diagnosis is a concise term or phrase that represents a pattern of related cues or signs and symptoms. One problem that nurses often encounter is writing nursing diagnoses that nursing actions cannot address. For example, a medical diagnosis, such as pyloric stenosis, cannot be treated by a nurse. It is appropriate, however, to say that there are nursing actions that can decrease the fluid volume deficit associated with pyloric stenosis.

A nursing diagnosis consists of two sections joined by the phrase "related to." The statement begins with the client's response to the current problem and then describes the causative factor or factors. An example is *Altered Family Processes* related to *the diagnosis of a child with cancer*. The causative factors can be physiologic, psychological, sociocultural, environmental, or spiritual. They assist the nurse in identifying nursing interventions as planning takes place.

Planning

The nurse next plans care for problems that were identified during assessment and are reflected in the nursing diagnoses. During this step, nurses set priorities, develop goals or outcomes that state what is to be accomplished by a certain time, and plan interventions to accomplish those goals.

SETTING PRIORITIES

Setting priorities includes (1) determining what problems need immediate attention (i.e., life-threatening problems) and taking immediate action; (2) determining whether there are potential problems that call for a physician's orders for diagnosis, monitoring, or treatment; and (3) identifying actual nursing diagnoses, which take precedence over at-risk diagnoses.

ESTABLISHING GOALS AND EXPECTED OUTCOMES

Although the terms *goals* and *outcomes* are sometimes used interchangeably, they are different. Generally, broad goals do not state the specific outcome criteria and are less measurable than outcome statements. If broad goals are developed, they should be linked to more specific and measurable outcome criteria. For example, if the goal is that the parents will demonstrate effective parenting by discharge, *outcome criteria* that serve as evidence might be prompt, consistent responses to infant signals and competence in bathing, feeding, and comforting the infant.

Certain rules should be followed when writing outcomes:

- Outcomes should be stated in client terms. This wording identifies who is expected to achieve the goal (the woman, infant or child, or family).
- Measurable verbs must be used. For example, "identify," "demonstrate," "express," "walk," "relate," and "list" are verbs that are observable and measurable. Examples of verbs that are difficult to measure are "understand," "appreciate," "feel," "accept," "know," and "experience."
- A time frame is necessary. When is the person expected to perform the action? After teaching? By 1 day after hospitalization? Before discharge?
- Goals and outcomes must be realistic and attainable by nursing interventions only.
- Goals and outcomes are worked out in collaboration with the client and family to ensure their participation in the plan of care.

Implementation

Implementation is the action phase of the nursing process. Once the goals and desired outcomes are developed, it is necessary to devise nursing interventions that will help the client meet the established outcomes. During this phase, the nurse is constantly evaluating and reassessing to determine that the interventions remain appropriate. As the client's condition changes, so does the plan of care.

The type of nursing interventions implemented depends on whether the nursing diagnosis was an actual, risk, or wellness diagnosis. Nursing interventions for actual nursing diagnoses are aimed at reducing or eliminating the causes or related factors. Interventions for risk nursing diagnoses are aimed at (1) monitoring for onset of the problem, (2) reducing or eliminating risk factors, and (3) preventing the problem. For a wellness nursing diagnosis, interventions focus on supporting the individual's or family's coping mechanisms and promoting a higher level of wellness.

A major problem with implementing nursing interventions is that written interventions often are not specific and do not spell out exactly what should be done. A well-written nursing intervention should be specific: "Provide 200 ml of fluid (water or juice of choice) q2h while the woman is awake." Poorly written interventions, such as "assist with breast-feeding," provide generalizations rather than specific steps to follow.

Evaluation

The evaluation determines how well the plan worked or how well the goals or outcomes were met. To evaluate, the nurse must assess the status of the client and compare the current status with the goals or outcome criteria that were developed during the planning step. The nurse then judges how well the client is progressing toward goal achievement and makes a decision. Should the plan be continued? Modified? Abandoned? Are the problems resolved or the causes diminished? Is another nursing diagnosis more relevant?

The nursing process is dynamic, and evaluation frequently results in expanded assessment and additional or modified nursing diagnoses and interventions. Nurses are cautioned not to view lack of goal achievement as a failure. Instead, it is simply time to reassess and to begin the process anew.

Collaborative Problems

In addition to nursing diagnoses, which describe problems that respond to independent nursing functions, nurses must also deal with problems that are beyond the scope of independent nursing practice. These are sometimes termed *collaborative problems*—physiologic complications that usually occur in association with a specific pathologic condition or treatment.

Nurses monitor to detect the onset of the complication and collaborate with physicians to manage changes in client status. Both physician-prescribed and nursing-prescribed interventions are necessary to minimize complications (Carpenito, 1997).

PLANNING
It is inappropriate to identify client-centered goals for a collaborative problem because the goals cannot be achieved by independent nursing action. Collaborative problems should reflect the nurse's responsibility in situations requiring physician-prescribed interventions. The nurse's responsibility includes the following:

- Monitoring for signs of complications
- Managing the complications with nursing- and physician-prescribed interventions (Carpenito, 1997)

INTERVENTIONS
Nursing interventions for collaborative problems include (1) performing frequent assessments to monitor the status of the client and detect signs and symptoms of complications, (2) communicating with the physician when signs and symptoms of complications are noted, (3) performing physician-prescribed interventions, including standing orders and protocols, to prevent or correct the complication, and (4) performing nursing interventions described in the standards of care or policy and procedure manuals.

EVALUATION
Although client-centered goals or outcomes are not developed for collaborative problems, the nurse collects data, compares the data with established norms, and judges whether the data are within normal limits. If the data are not within normal limits, the nurse asks the physician for additional direction and implements physician-prescribed interventions as well as nursing interventions.

▮ Nursing Research

As nursing and the health care system change, nurses will be challenged to demonstrate that what they do improves client outcomes and is cost-effective. To meet this challenge, nurses must participate in research and encourage the utilization of research. With the establishment of the National Institute of Nursing Research as a full-fledged member of the National Institutes of Health, nurses now have an infrastructure in place to ensure that nursing research is supported and that a group of well-prepared nurse researchers will be educated.

The amount of clinically based nursing research conducted is increasing rapidly as nurse researchers strive to develop an independent body of knowledge that demonstrates the value of nursing interventions. Although knowledge is being generated, there is a gap between knowledge acquired by researchers and application of that knowledge to care of the client in the clinical area.

Although students and inexperienced nurses may not participate in research projects, they must take advantage of the knowledge obtained by the research team. Professional journals are the best sources of new information that can help nurses provide improved care and demonstrate that what they do makes a difference in client outcomes.

▮ KEY CONCEPTS

- Maternal-newborn and pediatric nurses function in a variety of roles, including care provider, teacher, collaborator, researcher, advocate, and manager.
- The care settings in which maternity and pediatric nurses may practice include acute care settings, clinics, physicians' offices, home health agencies, schools, rehabilitation centers, summer camps, day care centers, and hospices.
- Registered nurses with advanced education are prepared to provide primary care for women and children as certified nurse-midwives and nurse practitioners.
- Clinical nurse specialists function as educators, researchers, and consultants to provide in-depth interventions for many problems en-

countered in maternity and pediatric care.

■ Nurses must be adept at communicating and at removing blocks to communication to meet their responsibilities as educators and counselors.

■ A primary responsibility of nurses is to provide information to childbearing families and to children and their families; nurses must know the principles of teaching and learning to fulfill the role of educator.

■ Nurses must learn to think critically by examining their own thought processes for flaws that can lead to inaccurate conclusions or poor clinical judgments.

■ The nursing process begins with assessment and includes analysis of data that may result in nursing diagnoses. Nursing diagnoses are problems that nurses are legally accountable for identifying and managing independently.

■ Collaborative problems are usually physiologic complications that require both physician-prescribed and nurse-prescribed interventions.

■ Professional journals are the best sources of information about research projects that demonstrate the effectiveness of nursing interventions.

REFERENCES AND READINGS

Alfaro-LeFevre, R. (1995). *Critical thinking in nursing: A practical approach*. Philadelphia: Saunders.

American Nurses' Association and the Society of Pediatric Nurses (1996). *Statement on the scope and standards of pediatric clinical practice* (pp. 25–35). Washington, DC: American Nurses Publishing.

Arnold, E., & Boggs, K. (1995). *Interpersonal relationships: Professional communication skills for nurses* (2nd ed.). Philadelphia: Saunders.

Association of Women's Health, Obstetric, and Neonatal Nurses. (1997). *Standards and guidelines for professional nursing practice in the care of women and newborns* (5th ed.). Washington, DC: Author.

Carpenito, L. J. (1997). *Handbook of nursing diagnosis* (7th ed.). Philadelphia: Lippincott.

Case, B. (1994). Walking around the elephant: A critical-thinking strategy for decision making. *Journal of Continuing Education in Nursing, 25*(3), 101–109.

Doenges, M., Moorhous, M., & Burley, J. (1995). *Application of nursing process and nursing diagnosis: An interactive text for diagnostic reasoning*. Philadelphia: Davis.

Fitzgerald, S. M., & Wood, S. H. (1997). Advanced practice nursing: Back to the future. *Journal of Obstetric, Gynecologic, and Neonatal Nurses, 26*(1), 101–107.

Katz, J. R. (1997). Back to basics: Providing effective client teaching. *American Journal of Nursing, 97*(5), 33–36.

Kramer, M. K. (1993). Concept clarification and critical thinking: Integrated processes. *Journal of Nursing Education, 32*(9), 406–414.

National League for Nursing. (1992a). *Criteria for the evaluation of associate degree programs in nursing*. New York: Author.

National League for Nursing. (1992b). *Criteria for the evaluation of baccalaureate and higher degree programs in nursing*. New York: Author.

North American Nursing Diagnosis Association. (1996). *Nursing diagnoses: Definitions & classification (1997–1998)*. Philadelphia: Author.

Pless, B., & Clayton, G. (1993). Clarifying the concept of critical thinking in nursing. *Journal of Nursing Education, 32*(9), 425–428.

Roux, G. M., Haas, P., & Sandefur, J. A. (1998). Advanced practice nursing: Two NPs reflect on their roles & responsibilities. *AWHONN Lifelines, 2*(2), 39–42.

Rubenfeld, M. G., & Scheffer, B. K. (1995). *Critical thinking in nursing: An interactive approach*. Philadelphia: Lippincott.

Sams, L., & DeGeorges, K. M. (1998). Seize the evidence and the opportunity. *AWHONN Lifelines, 2*(3), 15–17.

Sinclair, B. P. (1997). Advanced practice nurses in integrated health care systems. *Journal of Obstetric, Gynecologic, and Neonatal Nurses, 26*(2), 217–223.

Sperhac, A., & Strodtbeck, F. (1997). Advanced practice nursing: New opportunities for blended roles. *MCN: American Journal of Maternal/Child Nursing, 22*(6), 287–293.

Tucker, D. A., & Flannery, J. (1996). The student process for success: The nursing care plan. *Nurse Educator, 21*(1), 47–50.

Woodring, B. (1998). *Standards and guidelines for pre-licensure and early professional education for the nursing care of children and their families* (Rev. ed.). Denver, CO: Society of Pediatric Nurses.

3

The Childbearing and Child-Rearing Family

LEARNING OBJECTIVES

After studying this chapter, you should be able to:

- Explain the importance of family when caring for maternity and pediatric clients.
- Describe different family structures and their impact on family functioning.
- Differentiate between healthy and dysfunctional families.
- List internal and external coping behaviors used by families when they face a crisis.
- Compare Western cultural values with those of other cultural groups.
- Describe the effect of cultural diversity on nursing practice.
- Describe different styles of parenting that you may encounter.
- Explain how variables in parent and child may affect their relationship.
- Discuss the use of discipline in a child's socialization.
- Evaluate the effects of an ill child on the family.

DEFINITIONS

coping Efforts directed toward managing and solving various problems, events, and stressors.

culture The sum of values, beliefs, and practices of a group of people that are transmitted from one generation to the next.

discipline The structure an adult sets for a child's life, designed to allow the child to fit happily and effectively into the real world; the training expected to produce a specific type or pattern of behavior.

egocentric Preoccupied with one's own interests and needs.

ethnic Pertaining to religious, racial, national, or cultural group characteristics, especially speech patterns, social customs, and physical characteristics.

ethnicity Condition of belonging to a particular ethnic group; also refers to ethnic pride.

ethnocentrism The opinion that the beliefs and customs of one's own ethnic group are superior to those of others.

family Two or more emotionally involved people living in close proximity and having reciprocal obligations with a sense of commonness, caring, and commitment (Friedman, 1986).

fatalism The belief that events are predestined.

nuclear family A family consisting of a two-generation relationship of parents and children, living together, and more or less isolated from other close relatives.

stress Any situation or condition, positive or negative, requiring adjustment on the part of the individual, family, or group.

No factor influences a person as profoundly as the family. Families protect and promote children's growth, development, health, and well-being until the children reach maturity. A healthy family provides children with love, affection, and a sense of belonging, and nurtures feelings of self-esteem and self-worth. Children need stable families to grow into happy, functioning adults. Family relationships continue to be important during adulthood. Family relationships influence, positively or negatively, people's relationships with others. Family influence carries over into the next generation as a person selects a mate, forms a new family, and often rears children.

For nurses in maternity and pediatric practice, the whole family is the client. The nurse cares for the client in the context of a dynamic family system, rather than caring for just a childbearing woman, an infant, or a child. The nurse is responsible for supporting families and encouraging healthy coping patterns as families experience the crisis of birth or illness.

The Family and Nursing Care

Family structures in the United States have changed considerably in the past 30 years. In 1998, married couples with children composed only 24.6% of families (U.S. Census Bureau, 1998). In addition, roles have changed within the family. Whereas the role of provider was once almost exclusively assigned to the father, both parents now may be providers, and many fathers are active in nurturing and disciplining their children.

Family Theories and Models

Scholars use different theories or models to explain the dynamics of family relations. For the past 20 years, the most commonly discussed theory in family literature has been von Bertalanffy's systems theory. According to von Bertalanffy (1968), any system is characterized by wholeness, feedback, equifinality (reaching a goal from several starting points), and boundaries.

A family can be viewed as a system, and a direct offshoot of von Bertalanffy's general systems theory is family systems theory. The family systems theory developed by Bowen (1976) is widely accepted today. Bowen described four processes that occur within families:

- Differentiation of self (distinguishing between feelings and thoughts)
- Multigeneration transmission process (how the family members socialize the child)

- Triangulation (two family members experiencing anxiety coerce a third member into joining them in order to decrease their anxiety)
- Family projection process (anxiety of one of the parents is decreased by becoming overly involved with one of the children)

The family systems theory gives nurses a way to organize their thinking about families. It helps nurses understand how families function and what happens when something goes wrong.

Theories help to organize facts in some sort of pattern. One analogy is a coat rack. A pile of clothes on the floor has no organization. Hung on a coat rack, however, the clothes can be organized. For instance, the shirts can be placed on one hook, the sweaters on another, the scarves on another, and the jackets on another. The theory is like a coat rack: it provides one way to organize facts.

TYPES OF FAMILIES

Family types are sometimes categorized into three groups: traditional, nontraditional, and high-risk. Nontraditional and high-risk families often need care different from the care needed by traditional families. Different family structures can produce varying stressors. For example, the single-parent family has as many demands placed on it for resources such as time and money as the two-parent family. There is only one parent, however, to meet these demands.

Traditional Families. Traditional families (also called nuclear families) are headed by two parents who view parenting as the major priority in their lives and whose energies are not depleted by many stressful conditions, such as poverty, illness, or substance abuse. Generally, traditional families are motivated to learn all they can about pregnancy, childbirth, and parenting (Fig. 3–1). Traditional families can be single-income or dual-income families.

Single-Income Families. In the 1950s and 1960s, the idealized single-income American family was depicted in several long-running television series, such as *Leave It to*

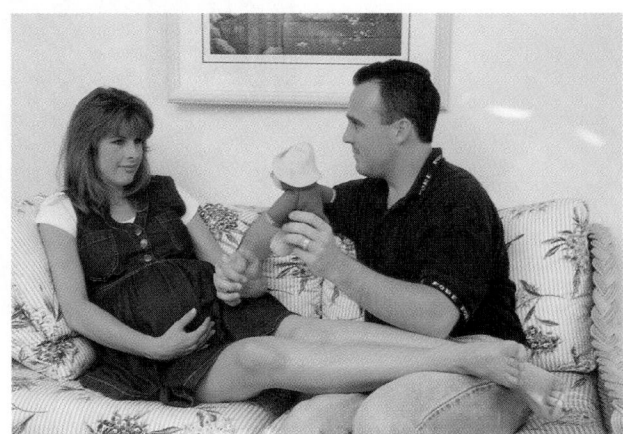

Figure 3 – 1
Traditional, two-parent families typically have the resources to prepare for childbirth and the needs of infants.

Beaver. This family was composed of a father who was the sole provider, a mother who was homemaker and caregiver, and two children. Today, this family structure represents a small minority of the nation's families.

Dual-Income Families. Most two-parent families now depend on two incomes. This economic reality has created a great deal of stress on parents, subjecting them to many of the same problems that single-parent families face. For instance, reliable, competent child care has become a major issue and has increased the stress traditional families experience.

Nontraditional Families. The growing number of nontraditional families includes single-parent families, blended families, adoptive families, unmarried couples with children, multigenerational families, and homosexual parent families (Fig. 3–2).

Single-Parent Families. Millions of families are now headed by a single parent, most often the mother, who not only must function as homemaker and caregiver but also is often the major provider for the family's financial needs. Divorce is the most common cause of single-parent families, although childbirth among unmarried women is also a major contributor.

Single-parent families are more likely to live below the poverty level than two-parent families and are vulnerable to a variety of problems. Single parents may feel overwhelmed by the prospect of assuming all child-rearing responsibilities and may be less prepared for illness or loss of a job than two-parent families.

Blended Families. Blended families are formed when single, divorced, or widowed parents marry and bring children from a previous union into the new relationship. Many times the couple desires children with each other, creating

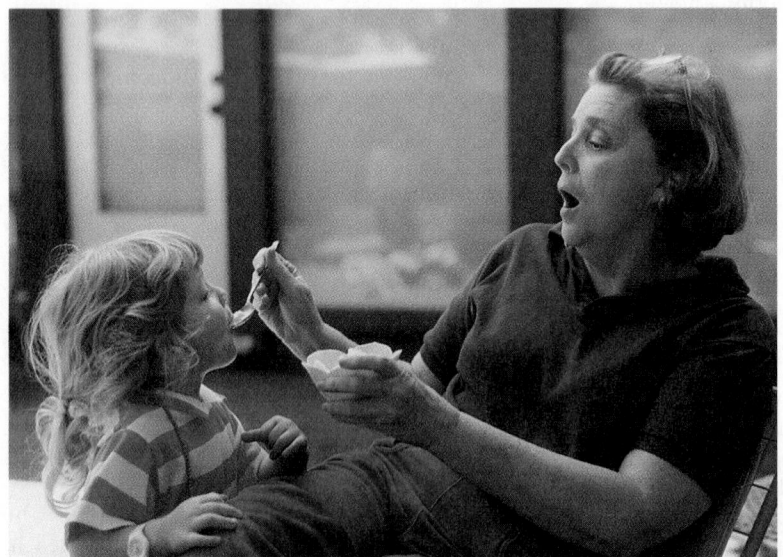

◄ Busy parents may rely on grandparents for child care or for an additional measure of love and attention for their children. Some grandparents raise grandchildren because of their own children's inability to do so.

Fathers are the primary child care providers in a growing number of families. Fathers who are not the primary caregivers often participate more actively in caring for their children than the fathers of previous generations.

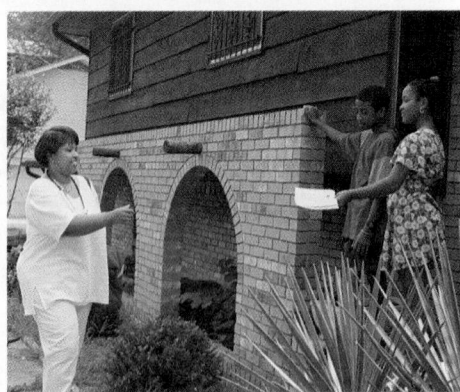

A single parent often experiences financial and time constraints. Children in single-parent families are often given more responsibility to care for themselves and younger siblings. ►

Figure 3–2
• • • • • • • • • •
The nurse caring for a child needs to know the child's family structure and the identity of the child's primary caregiver. This background becomes the context in which the nurse provides care. If family support is a concern, the nurse can provide information about local community resources. For example, in some communities, after-school programs and "warm lines" can help self-care children with schoolwork and alleviate loneliness and fear for some children.

a contemporary family structure commonly described as "yours, mine, and ours." These families may have difficulty forming a cohesive family unit unless they can overcome differences in parenting styles and values. Differing expectations of children's behavior and development as well as differing beliefs about discipline often cause family conflict.

Adoptive Families.   People who adopt a child may have problems that biologic parents do not face. Biologic parents have the long period of gestation and the gradual changes of pregnancy to help them adjust emotionally and socially to the birth of a child. Adoptive parents may add pressure to themselves by having an unrealistically high standard for themselves as parents. Adoptive parents as well as biologic parents need information, support, and guidance to prepare them to care for the infant or child and to maintain their own relationship.

Unmarried Couples with Children.   Unmarried couples with children may be similar to traditional and blended families although the couple is not married. The parents may have children from previous relationships, and they may have one or more children from their present relationship. Parents in a stable long-term relationship may head this type of family or the parental liaison may be recent.

Multigenerational Families.   The multigenerational or extended family includes members from three generations living under one roof. This family structure is becoming increasingly common in the United States. Elderly parents may be invited to live with their adult children, or in some cases adult children return to their parents' home, either because they are unable to support themselves or because they want the additional support that the grandparents provide for the grandchildren. This arrangement has given rise to the term *boomerang* families. Extended families are vulnerable to generational conflicts and may need education and referral to counselors to prevent disintegration of the family unit.

Grandparents, because of the inability of the parents to care for the children, are heading a growing number of households. The mother or father may be present physically but absent emotionally, or the parent may be absent physically for short or long periods. If the grandparents are elderly, and sometimes even if they are not, the strain of raising children a second time may cause tremendous physical, financial, and emotional stress.

Homosexual Parent Families.   Although families headed by same-sex parents are proportionately uncommon, they are recognized increasingly in the United States. The children in such families may be the offspring of previous heterosexual unions, or they may be adopted children or children conceived by therapeutic (sometimes called artificial) insemination of one or both members of a lesbian couple. This couple may face many challenges from a community that is unaccustomed to alternative lifestyles.

CHARACTERISTICS OF HEALTHY FAMILIES

In general, healthy families are able to adapt to changes that occur in the family unit. Pregnancy and parenthood create some of the most powerful changes that a family experiences.

Healthy families exhibit some common characteristics that provide a framework for assessing how all families function:

- Members of healthy families communicate openly with one another to express their concerns and needs.
- Healthy families remain flexible in role assignment so that if one person is unable to complete the usual tasks, another member offers assistance.
- Adults in healthy families agree on the basic principles of parenting so that there is minimal discord about such things as discipline and sleep schedules.
- Healthy families are adaptable and are not overwhelmed by changes that occur in the home and in relationships as a result of childbirth and parenthood.
- Members of healthy families volunteer assistance without waiting to be asked.

Factors That Interfere with Family Functioning

Factors that interfere with the family's ability to provide for the needs of its members include lack of financial resources, absence of adequate family support, birth of an infant who needs specialized care, an ill child, unhealthy habits such as smoking or abuse of other substances, and inability to make mature decisions that are necessary to provide care for the children.

HIGH-RISK FAMILIES

All families encounter stressors, but some factors add to the usual stress experienced by a family. The nurse must consider the additional needs of the family with a higher risk for being dysfunctional. Examples of these high-risk families are those experiencing marital conflict and divorce, those with adolescent parents, families affected by violence against one or more of the family members, those involved with substance abuse, and families with an ill child.

Marital Conflict and Divorce.   Although divorce is traumatic to children, research has shown that living in a home filled with conflict is even more traumatic. Divorce can be the outcome of many years of unresolved family conflict. It can result in disputes over child custody, visitation, and child support; changes in housing, lifestyle, cultural expectations, friends, and extended family relationships; diminished self-esteem; and changes in the physical, emotional, or spiritual health of the child and other family members.

Divorce is loss that needs to be grieved. The conflict and divorce may affect children, and young children may be unable to verbalize their distress. Nurses can help children through the grieving process with age-appropriate activities such as therapeutic play (see Chapter 35). Principles of active listening (see Chapter 2) are valuable for both adults and children to help them express their feelings. Nurses can also help newly divorced or separated parents through listening, encouragement, and referrals to support groups or counselors.

Adolescent Parenting. The pregnancy rate for teenagers in the United States is higher than in any other developed country. In 1996, 4.2% of all live births were to white teens under 18, while 10.3% of the live births were to black teens. Birth rates for Latino teens (of Mexican origin) are reported for selected states and are affected by immigration, but 7.3% of all live births in those states were to Latino girls under 18. Teen births to other groups, such as American Indians, Alaska Natives, various Asian or Pacific Islander groups, and other Latino groups (such as Puerto Rican or Cuban), make up the remaining numbers of teens giving birth in 1996 (Department of Health and Human Services, 1998). Most adolescent pregnancies are unplanned and unwanted.

Teenage parenting often has a negative impact on the health and social outcomes of the entire family. Adolescent girls are at increased risk for a number of pregnancy complications such as pregnancy-induced hypertension or fetal growth restriction. Those who become parents during adolescence are unlikely to attain a high level of education, and as a result are more likely to be poor and often homeless. The father of the child often does not contribute to the economic or psychological support of his children. Children of adolescent parents have a higher mortality rate and are more likely to suffer violence and neglect (DHHS, 1998). Moreover, the cycle of teen parenting and economic hardship is more likely to be continued because children of adolescent parents are themselves more likely to become teenage parents. Chapter 25 provides additional information about adolescent childbearing.

Violence. Violence is a constant stressor in some families. Violence can occur in any family of any socioeconomic or educational status. Women who suffer physical or emotional abuse frequently have poorer pregnancy outcomes than women who are not abused (see Chapter 25). Their children endure the psychological pain of seeing their mother victimized by the man who is supposed to love and care for her. Additionally, because of the role models they see in the adults, these children may repeat the cycle of violence when they are adults and become abusers or victims of violence themselves.

Abuse of the child may also be physical or emotional, or the abuse may be in the form of neglect (see Chapter 53). Often one child in the family is the target of abuse or neglect, while others are given proper care. As in adult abuse, children who witness abuse are more likely to repeat that behavior when they are parents themselves because they have not learned constructive ways to deal with their stress or to discipline children.

Substance Abuse. Substance abuse can adversely affect the health of the child before birth. The infant may suffer direct effects of the abused substances or may experience adverse effects from the mother's inadequate diet or lack of prenatal care during pregnancy (see Chapter 30).

Parents who abuse drugs may also neglect their children. Maintaining the drug habit has a stronger pull on the parents than does care of their children. Additionally, their children are more likely to live in poverty and to be homeless because so much money is spent maintaining the parent's substance habit.

The child may be the substance abuser in the home. The drug habit can lead a child into unhealthy friendships and may result in criminal activity to maintain the habit. School achievement is likely to plummet, and the older adolescent may drop out of school. Both children and adults can die as a result of their drug activity, either as a direct effect of the drugs or from associated criminal activity or risk-taking behaviors.

Child with Special Needs. When a child is born with a birth defect or has an illness that requires special care, the family is under additional stress. In most cases, their initial reactions of shock and disbelief gradually resolve into acceptance of the child's limitations. However, the parents' grieving may be chronic as they repeatedly see other children doing things that their child cannot—and perhaps will not ever—do.

These families often suffer financial hardship. Health insurance benefits may quickly reach their maximum. Even if the child has public assistance for health care costs, the family often experiences a fall in income because one parent must remain home with the sick child rather than working.

Strains on the marriage and the parents' relationships with their other children are inevitable under these circumstances. Parents have little time or energy left to nurture their relationship with each other, and divorce may add yet another strain to the family. Siblings may resent the parental time and attention required for care of the ill child, yet feel guilty if they express their resentment.

The outlook is not always pessimistic in these families, however. If the family learns skills to cope with the added demands imposed on it by this situation, there is potential for growth in maturity, compassion, and strength of character. See Chapter 36 for more information about families that have children with special needs.

Healthy versus Dysfunctional Families

Family conflict is unavoidable. It is a natural result of a perceived unequal exchange or an imbalance in the use of resources by individual members. Conflict should not be viewed as bad or disruptive because it is the management of the conflict, not the conflict itself, that may be problematic. Conflict can produce growth and improved family functioning if the outcome is resolution as opposed to dissolution or continued conflict. Three ingredients are required to resolve conflict:

- Open communication
- Accurate perceptions about the nature and degree of conflict
- Constructive efforts to resolve the conflict, such as willingness to consider the view of the other, consider alternate solutions, and compromise

Dysfunctional families have problems in any one or a combination of these areas. They tend to become trapped in patterns in which they maintain conflicts rather than resolving them. The conflicts create stress, and the family must cope with the resultant stress.

COPING WITH STRESS

Curran (1985) views the family as a delicately balanced system. Stressors are forces, either inside or outside the family,

• • • • • • • • • • •
Coping Strategies of Families

INTERNAL COPING STRATEGIES

- Reliance on the family group
- Use of humor
- Greater sharing of feelings, thoughts, time, and activities
- Controlling the meaning of the problem (reframing)
- Attributing a spiritual purpose to the event
- Optimism
- Selective ignoring of negatives
- Making the event less important
- Joint problem solving
- Role flexibility

EXTERNAL COPING STRATEGIES

- Seeking information
- Increasing links to the community
- Using social support systems (e.g., family, friends, experts, co-workers, professional services)
- Joining self-help groups
- Seeking spiritual support

Data from Cohen, F. (1984). Coping. In J. D. Matarazzo, S. Weiss, J. Herd, & S. Weiss (Eds.), *Behavioral health: A handbook of health enhancement and disease prevention* (pp. 261–274). New York: Wiley.

that contribute to fluctuations in the balance of the family system. Families respond in some manner to these stressors. Some families are able to mobilize their strengths and resources, thus effectively adapting to the stressors. Other families fall apart. Curran identified patterns of families who were coping effectively:

- Recognizing that stress is temporary and may be positive
- Working together to find solutions
- Developing new rules, including prioritizing time and sharing responsibility
- Expecting that some stress is normal
- Feeling accomplishment in dealing with stress

Families who dealt ineffectively with stress exhibited the following patterns:

- Feeling guilt for permitting stress to exist
- Looking for a place to lay blame rather than a solution to the problem
- Giving in to stress and giving up trying to master it
- Focusing on family problems rather than on strengths
- Feeling weaker rather than stronger after a normal stress experience
- Growing to dislike family life as a result of the accumulation of stress

COPING STRATEGIES
Some families adjust quickly to extreme crises, whereas other families become chaotic with relatively minor crises. Family functional patterns that existed before the crisis are probably the best indicators of how the family will respond to a crisis. Family coping strategies can be divided into internal (intrafamilial) and external (extrafamilial).

Cultural Influences on Maternity and Pediatric Nursing

Culture is the sum of the beliefs and values that are learned, shared, and transmitted from generation to generation by a particular group. Cultural values guide the thinking, decisions, and actions of the group, particularly in pivotal events such as birth, reaching sexual maturity, and death. *Ethnicity* is the condition of belonging to a particular group that shares race, language and dialect, religious faiths, traditions, values, and symbols, as well as food preferences, literature, and folklore. Cultural beliefs and values vary among different groups, and nurses must be aware that individuals often believe their cultural values and patterns of behavior are superior to those of other groups. This belief, termed *ethnocentrism*, forms the basis for many conflicts that occur when people from different cultural groups have frequent contact.

Nurses must be aware that culture is composed of visible and invisible layers that could be said to resemble an iceberg (Fig. 3–3). The observable behaviors can be compared with the visible tip of the iceberg. The history, beliefs, values, and religion are not observed, but they are the hidden foundation on which behaviors are based and can be likened to the large, submerged part of the iceberg. To comprehend cultural behavior fully, one must seek knowledge of the hidden beliefs that behaviors express.

Religious beliefs often have a strong influence on families as they face the crisis of illness. Specific beliefs about the causes, treatment, and cure of illness are important for the nurse to know to empower the family to deal with the immediate crisis. Table 3–1 describes how some religious beliefs affect health care.

Implications of Cultural Diversity for Nurses

Many immigrants and refugees are relatively young, which means that nurses in most localities will provide care for culturally diverse childbearing and child-rearing families. To provide effective care, nurses must be aware that culture is among the most significant factors that influence birth and parenthood, health and illness.

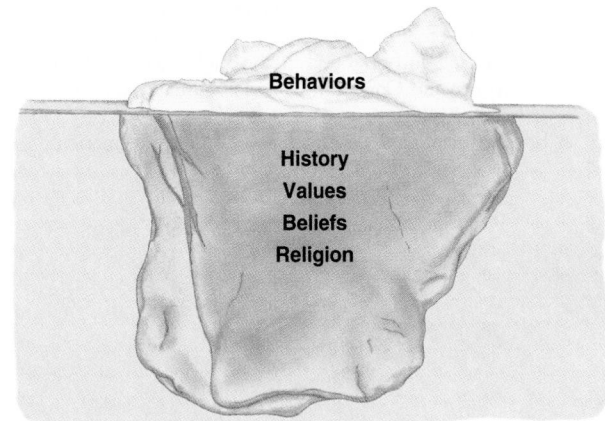

FIGURE 3–3
• • • • • • • • • •
Visible and hidden layers of culture are like the visible and submerged parts of an iceberg. Many cultural differences are hidden below the surface.

TABLE 3-1
• • • • • • • • • • • •

Religious Beliefs Affecting Health Care

Religion and Basic Beliefs	Practices
Christian Science	
Based on scientific system of healing. Beliefs based on Bible, science, and health with key to scriptures. Seek to overcome evil through prayer, belief, and Christian acts. Healing is divinely natural, not miraculous.	*Birth:* Use physician or midwife during childbirth. No baptism ceremony. *Dietary practices:* Alcohol and tobacco are considered drugs and are not used. Coffee and tea may also be declined. *Death:* Autopsy and donation of organs are usually declined. *Health care:* May refuse medical treatment. View health in a spiritual framework. Seek exemption from immunizations, but obey legal requirements. When Christian Science believer is hospitalized, parent or client may request that a Christian Science practitioner be notified to come.
Jehovah's Witness	
Believe in God and Son Jesus Christ. Expected to follow the example of Jesus Christ in daily living. Expected to preach house to house about the good news of God. Bible is doctrinal authority. No distinction made between clergy and laity.	*Baptism:* No infant baptism. Baptism by immersion of adults. *Dietary practices:* Use of tobacco and alcohol discouraged. *Death:* Autopsy decided by persons involved. Burial and cremation acceptable. *Birth control and abortion:* Use of birth control is a personal decision. Abortion opposed based on Exodus 21:22–23. *Health care:* Blood transfusions not allowed. May accept alernatives to transfusions, such as use of nonblood plasma expanders, careful surgical technique to minimize blood loss, and use of autologous transfusions. Nurses should check unconscious clients for identification that states that the person does not want a transfusion. Jehovah's Witnesses are prepared to die rather than break God's law. Respect the health care given by physicians, but look to God and His laws as the final authority for their decisions.
The Church of Jesus Christ of Latter-Day Saints (Mormon)	
Restorationism: True church of Christ ended with the first generation of apostles, but was restored with the founding of Mormon Church. Articles of faith: Mormon doctrine states that individuals are saved if they are obedient to God's divine ordinances (faith, repentance, baptism by immersion and laying on of hands, observance of Lord's Supper on Sunday). Word of God can be found in the Bible, Book of Mormon, Doctrine, and Covenants, Pearl of Great Price, and current revelations. Christ will return to rule in Zion, located in America.	*Baptism:* By immersion. Considered essential for the living and the dead. If a child older than 8 is very ill, whether baptized or unbaptized, a member of the church's priesthood should be called. *Holy Communion:* Hospitalized client may desire to have a member of the church's priesthood administer the sacrament. *Anointing of the sick:* Mormons frequently are anointed and given a blessing before going to the hospital and after admission by laying on of hands. *Dietary practices:* Tobacco and caffeine are not used. Mormons eat meat (limited), but encourage the intake of fruits, grains, and herbs. *Death:* Prefer burial of the body. A church elder should be notified to assist the family. *Birth control and abortion:* Abortion is opposed unless the life of the mother is in danger. Only natural methods of birth control are recommended. Other means are used only when the physical or emotional health of the mother is at stake. *Other practices:* Believe in the healing power of "laying on of hands." Cleanliness is very important. Believe in healthy living and adhere to health care requirements. Families are of great importance, so visiting should be encouraged. The church maintains a welfare system to assist those in need.

TABLE 3–1

Religious Beliefs Affecting Health Care Continued

Religion and Basic Beliefs	Practices
Roman Catholic	
Beliefs based on Bible, Apostolic tradition, and contemporary revelation.	*Baptism:* Infant baptism by affusion (sprinkling of water on head). Original sin is believed to be "washed away." If death is imminent or a fetus is aborted, anyone can perform the baptism by sprinkling water on the forehead, saying "I baptize thee in the name of the Father, Son, and Holy Spirit." Anointing of the sick encouraged for anyone who is ill or injured. Always done if prognosis is poor. *Dietary practices:* Fasting and abstinence from meat optional during Lent. No meat on Ash Wednesday and on Fridays during Lent strongly encouraged. Children and ill adults exempt from all fasting. *Death:* Organ donation permitted.
Hinduism	
Belief in reincarnation and Karma, Yoga. Nonviolent approach to living. Various deities worshiped: Vishnu, Shiva, Ganesh, Surya, Durgam Shati. Congregation worship is not customary.	*Dietary practices:* Dietary restrictions vary according to sect. *Death:* Death rituals specify practices and who can touch corpse. *Other practices:* Oppose artificial insemination. Circumcision is observed by ritual.
Islam	
Sunni (90%), Shiite (10%). Belief in one God. Based on the teaching of Muhammad. Five Pillars of Islam. Compulsory prayers are said at dawn, noon, afternoon, after sunset, and after nightfall.	*Dietary practices:* Prohibit eating pork and the use of alcohol. Fast during Ramadan (ninth month of Muslim year). *Death:* Oppose autopsy and organ donation. Death ritual prescribes the handling of corpse by only family and friends.
Judaism	
Beliefs are based on the Old Testament, the Torah, and the Talmud, the oral and written laws of faith. Belief in one God who is approached directly. Believe Messiah is still to come. Believe Jews are God's chosen people.	*Circumcision:* A symbol of God's covenant wih Israel. Done on eighth day after birth. *Bar Mitzvah:* Ceremonial rite of passage for boys (approximately 13 years of age) into manhood. *Death:* Remains are washed according to rite by members of the Ritual Burial Society. Burial occurs as soon as possible.

Data from Carson, V. B. (1989). *Spiritual dimensions of nursing practice* (pp. 100–102). Philadelphia: Saunders. Betz, C. L., Hunsberger, M., & Wright, S. (1994). *Family centered nursing care of children* (2nd ed., pp. 2230–2236). Philadelphia: Saunders.

Western Cultural Beliefs

Nursing practice in the United States is based largely on Western beliefs. Nurses must recognize that these beliefs may differ significantly from those of other societies and that the differences may cause a great deal of conflict.

Leininger (1978) identified seven dominant Western cultural values. These values greatly influence the thinking and action of nurses in the United States but may not be shared by their clients.

1. *Democracy* is a cultural value not shared by families who believe that elders or other higher authorities in the group make decisions. Fatalism, or a belief that events and results are predestined, may also affect health care decisions.
2. *Individualism* conflicts with the values of many cultural groups in which individual goals are subordinated to the greater good of the group.
3. *Cleanliness* is an American "obsession" viewed with amazement by many.
4. *Preoccupation with time,* which is measured by health care professionals in minutes and hours, is a major source of conflict with those who mark time by different standards, such as seasons or body needs.
5. *Reliance on machines and equipment* may intimidate families who are not comfortable with technology.
6. *The belief that optimal health is a right* is in direct conflict with beliefs in many cultures in the world in which health is not a major emphasis or even an expectation.
7. *Admiration of self-sufficiency and financial success* may conflict with the beliefs of other societies that place less value on wealth and more value on less tangible things such as spirituality.

Cultural Influences on the Care of Specific Groups

To provide the best care for all clients, the nurse should know common cultural beliefs and practices that influence nursing care. Because communication is an essential component of nursing assessment and teaching, the nurse must understand cultural influences that may form barriers to communicating with people from another culture.

ASIAN-AMERICANS

In Asian-American culture, the family is highly valued and often consists of many generations that remain close to each other. The elders of the family are highly respected. Self-sufficiency and self-control are highly valued. Asian-Americans place a high value on "face," or honor, and may be unwilling to do anything that causes another to "lose face." When medication or therapy is recommended, they seldom say no. They may accept the prescription or medication sample but not take the medicine, or they may agree to undergo a procedure but not keep the appointment. Stoicism may make pain assessment difficult.

Language is the greatest barrier to health care for those from Southeast Asia (Mattson, 1995). Besides the national languages of Vietnam, Cambodia, and Laos, numerous tribal languages are spoken in each country. Moreover, people from Southeast Asia speak softly and avoid prolonged eye contact, which they consider rude.

LATINOS

Latinos include those whose origin is Mexico, Central and South America, and Puerto Rico. Men are usually the head of household and considered strong (macho). Women are the homemakers. Latinos usually have a close extended family and place a high value on children.

Latinos tend to be polite and gracious in conversation. Preliminary social interaction is particularly important, and Latinos may be insulted if a problem is addressed directly without taking time for "small talk." This is counter to the Western value of "getting to the point" and may cause frustration for the client as well as for the health care worker.

There is a strong association between religion and health. The *curandero*, a folk healer, may be consulted for health care before an American health care worker is consulted.

AFRICAN-AMERICANS

African-Americans are often part of a close extended family, although many heads of household are single women. They have a sense of loyalty to their people and community, but they sometimes distrust the majority group.

African-Americans sometimes use a communication style that may cause conflict when they seek health care. They may use idioms, colloquial expressions, or speech patterns that are unfamiliar to health care workers. Nurses must often clarify what is being said so that misunderstandings can be avoided and teaching can be effective.

The black minister is highly influential, and religious rituals, such as prayer, are frequently used. Illness may be seen as the will of God.

NATIVE AMERICANS

Native Americans may consider a willful child to be strong and a docile child to be weak. They have close family relationships, and respect for their elders is the norm. Native Americans may consider health to be a state of harmony with nature, and may believe that supernatural influences have a great impact on health and illness. Native Americans may highly respect a medicine man, whom they believe to be given power by supernatural forces. The use of herbs and rituals is part of the medicine man's curative practice.

MIDDLE EASTERNERS

Middle Eastern immigrants come from several countries, including Lebanon, Syria, Saudi Arabia, Egypt, Turkey, Iran, and Palestine. Islam is the dominant religion in these countries. The man is typically the head of the household in Muslim families. Muslim women often prefer a female health care provider because of laws of modesty. Many Muslim women keep their head, arms to the wrists, and legs to the ankles covered. Islam requires believers to kneel and pray five times a day: at dawn, noon, afternoon, after sunset, and after nightfall. Muslims do not eat pork and do not use alcohol. Some are vegetarians.

Communication in these countries is elaborate, and obtaining health information may be difficult because Islam dictates that family affairs should be kept within the family. Personal information is shared only with personal friends, and the health assessment must be done gradually. When interpreters are used, they should be of the same country and religion, if possible, because of regional differences and hostilities. Because Muslim society tends to be paternalistic, it is wise to ask the husband's permission or opinion when family members need health care.

Cross-Cultural Health Beliefs

More than 100 different ethnocultural groups reside in the United States, and numerous traditional health beliefs are observed among these groups. For example, definitions of health are often culturally based. People of Asian origin may view health as the balance of yin and yang. Those of African or Haitian origin may define health as harmony with nature. Those from Mexico, Central and South America, and Puerto Rico often see health as a balance of hot and cold.

TRADITIONAL METHODS OF PREVENTING ILLNESS

The traditional methods of preventing illness rest in the person's ability to understand the cause of a given illness in the culture. These causes may include the following:

- Agents such as hexes, spells, or the evil eye, which may strike a person (often a child) and cause injury, illness, or misfortune
- Phenomena such as soul loss or accidentally provoking envy, jealousy, or hate of a friend or acquaintance
- Environmental factors such as bad air, and natural events such as solar eclipses

Practices to prevent illness developed from beliefs about the cause of illness. One must avoid those known to transmit hexes and spells. Elaborate methods are used to prevent inciting envy or jealousy of others and to avoid the evil eye. Protective or religious objects, such as amulets with magic powers or consecrated religious objects (talismans), are frequently worn or carried to prevent illness. There are also numerous food taboos and traditional combinations that are prescribed in traditional belief systems to prevent illness. For instance, people from many ethnic backgrounds eat raw garlic to prevent illness. Those of African origin may consume nonfood substances such as starch to make labor easier.

TRADITIONAL PRACTICES TO MAINTAIN HEALTH

A variety of traditional practices are used to maintain health. For instance, wearing proper clothing, such as a scarf, may prevent drafts and thus maintain the health of a woman who is pregnant and believes she must avoid cool air. Mental and spiritual health is maintained by activities such as silence, meditation, and prayer. Many people view illness as punishment for breaking a religious code and adhere strictly to religious morals and practices to maintain health.

TRADITIONAL PRACTICES TO RESTORE HEALTH

Traditional practices to restore health often conflict with Western medical practice. Some of the most common practices include the use of natural substances, such as herbs and plants, to treat illness. Religious charms, holy words, or traditional healers may be tried before an individual seeks a medical opinion. Wearing religious medals, carrying prayer cards, or performing sacrifices are other practices used to treat illness.

A variety of substances may be ingested for the treatment of illnesses. The nurse should try to identify what the woman or child is taking and to determine whether the active ingredient may alter the effects of prescribed medication. In the case of a pregnant woman, the effects of the traditional substance on the developing fetus must be considered as well.

Dermabrasion, the rubbing or irritation of the skin to relieve discomfort, is a common health care practice. The most popular form is *coining*, in which an area is covered with an ointment and the edge of a coin is rubbed over the area. All dermabrasion methods leave marks resembling bruises or burns on the skin and may be mistaken for signs of physical abuse (Mattson, 1995).

Cultural Assessment

All health care professionals must develop skill in performing a cultural assessment so they can understand the meaning of health and illness in the cultural groups they encounter. The following questions might be considered in making such an assessment:

- What is the family's ethnic affiliation?
- Is childbearing viewed as a normal process, a time of vulnerability, or a state of illness?
- What are the prescribed practices, customs, or rituals related to diet, activity, or behavior during pregnancy and childbirth or illness?
- What maternal restrictions or precautions are necessary

during pregnancy, childbirth, and after birth? Are women exempted from any religious practices at this time?
- Who provides support during pregnancy, childbirth, and parenthood?
- What are the prescribed practices and restrictions related to care of the newborn?
- Who in the family hierarchy makes health care decisions?
- How is time marked—in minutes and hours, or by seasons and body needs?
- How does the family view life and death? Are predestination and fatalism among the family's beliefs?
- How can health care professionals be most helpful?

After such an assessment, plans for care should show respect for cultural differences and traditional healing practices. Additional cultural information is presented throughout this book relating to specific areas in maternity and pediatric nursing care.

Parenting

Parenting implies the commitment of an individual or individuals to provide for the physical and psychosocial needs of a child. Many believe that parenting is the most difficult and yet rewarding experience an individual can have. Many parents assume this important job with little education in parenting or child rearing. If the parents themselves have had good parents as role models and seek resources, the transition to parenting is made easier.

Parenting Styles

Three major styles of parenting are authoritarian, authoritative, and permissive. These three styles represent a continuum of control exerted by the parents over the child, with the authoritarian parent exerting the most control and the permissive parent exerting the least.

Authoritarian parents have rules. They expect obedience from the child without any questioning about the reasons behind the rule. They also expect the child to accept the family beliefs and principles without question. Give and take is discouraged.

Children raised with this style of parenting are typically shy and withdrawn because of a lack of self-confidence. If the parents are somewhat affectionate, the child may be sensitive, submissive, honest, and dependable. If affection has been withheld, however, the child may exhibit rebellious, antisocial behavior.

Authoritative parents tend to show respect for the opinions of each of their children by allowing them to be different. Although there are rules in the household, the parents permit discussion if the children do not understand or agree with the rules. The parents make it clear to the children that although they (the parents) are the ultimate authority, some negotiation and compromise may take place. This style of parenting tends to result in children who have high self-esteem and are independent, inquisitive, happy, assertive, and highly interactive.

Permissive parents have little or no control over the behavior of their children. If any rules exist in the home, they are inconsistent and unclear. Underlying reasons for rules may be given, but the children are generally allowed to decide whether they will follow the rule, and to what extent. Limits are not set, and discipline is inconsistent. The children learn that they can get away with any behavior. Role reversal occurs: the children are more like the parents, and the parents are like the children.

Children who come from this type of home are typically disrespectful, disobedient, aggressive, irresponsible, and defiant. They tend to be insecure because of a lack of guidelines to direct their behavior. These children tend to be creative and spontaneous.

Research has supported the view that authoritative parents tend to be more effective than either rigid authoritarian or permissive parents. Parenting is more effective if individuals are able to adjust their behavior to meet the needs of their children at different developmental stages (Mrazek et al., 1995). In other words, the skills needed to support the autonomy of a toddler are very different from those needed to negotiate the individualism of an adolescent.

Parent-Child Relationship Factors

The parents' age, experience, and self-confidence affect the quality of the parent-child relationship, the stability of the marital relationship, and the interplay between the child's individualism and the parents' expectations of the child.

PARENTAL CHARACTERISTICS
Parenting is multidimensional. Studies have supported the development of key characteristics that can be used to assess the qualities of parenting. Mrazek et al. (1995) identified five key dimensions of parenting:

- Emotional availability (degree of emotional warmth)
- Control (degree of flexibility and permission)
- Psychiatric disturbance (presence, type, and severity of overt disorder)
- Knowledge base (understanding of emotional and physical development as well as of basic child care principles)
- Commitment (adequate prioritization of child care responsibilities)

In addition, parents who have had previous experience with children, whether through younger siblings, a career, or raising previous children, bring an element of experience to the art of parenting. Self-confidence and age can also be factors in a person's ability to parent. How an individual was parented has a major impact on how he or she will assume the role. The strength of the parents' relationship also affects their parenting skills, as does the presence or absence of support systems. Support can come from the family or community. Peer groups can provide an arena for parents to share experiences and solve problems. Parents with more experience are often an important resource for new parents.

CHARACTERISTICS OF THE CHILD
Characteristics that may affect the parent-child relationship include the child's physical appearance, sex, and temperament. At birth, the infant's physical appearance may not meet the parents' expectations, or the infant may resemble a disliked relative. As a result, the parent may subconsciously reject the child. If the parents desired a baby of a particular sex, they may be disappointed. If parents are not given the opportunity to talk about this disappointment, they may reject the infant. See Chapter 21 for additional information about bonding and attachment.

TEMPERAMENT AND PARENTAL EXPECTATIONS
Temperament can be described as the way individuals behave, or their behavioral style. Several researchers have studied temperament. Chess and Thomas (1996) developed three temperament categories based on nine characteristics of temperament they identified in children.

- *Easy:* These children are even-tempered, predictable, and regular in their habits. They react positively to new stimuli.
- *Difficult:* These children are highly active, irritable, moody, and irregular in their habits. They adapt slowly to new stimuli and often express intense negative emotions.
- *Slow to warm up:* These children are inactive, moody, and moderately irregular in their habits. They adapt slowly to new stimuli and express mildly intense negative emotions.

There has been some objection to the term *difficult* because it tends to have a negative connotation. That is the term established in temperament research, however, and it is important that parents recognize that a "difficult" child is very normal. As is true for other characteristics such as appearance, the parent-child relationship is likely to have less conflict if the child's temperament meets the parents' expectations.

DISCIPLINE
Children's behavior challenges most parents. The manner in which parents respond to a child's behavior has a profound effect on the child's self-esteem and future interactions with others. Children learn to view themselves in the same way that the parent views them. Thus, if parents view their children as wild, the children begin to view themselves as wild, and soon their actions consistently reinforce their self-image. In this way, the children will not disappoint the parents. This pattern is called a *self-fulfilling prophecy* and is a cyclic process.

Discipline refers to the system of teaching and nurturing that prepares children to achieve competence, self-control, self-direction, and caring for others (Howard, 1996). Discipline is designed to teach a child how to function effectively within society. It is the foundation for self-discipline. The primary goal of a parent should be to help the child feel lovable and capable. This goal is best accomplished by the parent setting limits to enhance a sense of security until the child can incorporate the family's values and is capable of self-discipline.

When a child is in the health care system, the nurse has the opportunity to aid in the socialization of the child to some degree. Through both formal instruction and informal role modeling, the nurse can help the parent learn how to discipline a child effectively. The accompanying box lists ways in which a parent or nurse can facilitate children's socialization and increase their self-esteem.

. . . .
Ways to Promote a Child's Socialization and Self-Esteem

PROMOTING A CHILD'S SENSE OF BEING LOVABLE

- Spend guaranteed time with the child.
- Be nonjudgmental and nondirective.
- Play with the child.
- Attend to the child through eye contact, touch, and active listening.
- Ignore minor transgressions.
- Convey positive regard; label the act, not the child.
- Offer positive feedback for positive behavior.
- Make verbal and nonverbal messages match. Avoid giving the child mixed messages.
- Warn the child 5 minutes before changing the activity.
- Offer thank-you messages.
- Give apologies, but not for punishment.

PROMOTING A CHILD'S SENSE OF BEING CAPABLE

- Establish and maintain routines.
- Role model for the child.
- Make instructions short, simple, and clear.
- Progressively increase expectations as the child ages.
- Allow role-taking opportunities.
- Offer praise and reward.
- Ensure appropriate consequences that are natural and logical.
- Promise but do not threaten.
- Carry out consequences immediately.
- Allow the child to make choices.

Adapted from Howard, B. (1991). Discipline in early childhood. *Pediatric Clinics of North America, 38*(6), 1351–1369.

DEALING WITH MISBEHAVIOR

A child's misbehavior may be defined as behavior outside the norms of acceptance within the family. Misbehavior stretches the limits of tolerance in all parents, even the most patient parent. A parent's response to the child's misbehavior can have minor consequences, such as short-term frustration, or major consequences, such as child abuse. To prevent these negative consequences, the nurse can help to teach parents various strategies for effective discipline. There are three essential components of effective discipline:

- A positive, supportive, loving relationship between the parent(s) and child
- Use of positive reinforcement strategies to increase desired behaviors
- Removing reinforcement or applying punishment to reduce or eliminate undesired behaviors (American Academy of Pediatrics, 1998).

Punishment is the application of a negative stimulus to reduce or eliminate a behavior. Punishment can be in the form of a verbal statement or it can be of a corporal nature that involves some form of physical pain.

Time-Out. Time-out is a method to remove the attention given to a child who is misbehaving. The child is placed in a nonstimulating environment where the parent can observe unobtrusively. For example, a chair could be placed facing a wall in a hall or bathroom. The child is told to sit on the chair for a predetermined time, usually 1 minute per year of age. If the child cries or fights, the timing is not begun until the child is quiet. The use of a kitchen timer with a bell is effective because the child knows when the time begins and when it has elapsed. At that time, the child is permitted to get up. After the child has calmed and the time is completed, it may be appropriate to discuss the behavior that prompted the time-out at a level appropriate to the child's age.

Corporal Punishment. Corporal punishment usually takes the form of spanking. It is highly controversial. The problems cited when corporal punishment is used include the following:

- The decrease in misbehavior is short term.
- Children learn that violence is acceptable.
- Children become accustomed to the pain, so some parents may feel that more severe pain is needed.
- Parents may experience rage and lose control, causing harm to the child.

Because of the negative consequences of spanking and because it is no more effective than other methods of discipline, the American Academy of Pediatrics (1998) recommends that parents be encouraged and assisted in developing methods of discipline other than spanking.

Behavior Modification. The behavior modification technique of discipline rewards positive behavior and ignores negative behavior. This technique requires parents to choose selected behaviors, preferably only one at a time, that they desire to stop. They choose others that they want to encourage. The basic technique is useful for any age from toddlerhood through adolescence. For a young child, the selected positive behaviors are marked on a chart and explained to the child. For an older child, a contract can be written. The negative behaviors are kept in mind by the parents, but are not recorded where the child can see them. A system of rewards is established. Stickers or stars on a chart for young children and tokens for older children are effective ways to record the behaviors. Children should receive a predetermined reward, for example, a movie, book, or outing, after they successfully perform the behavior a set number of times. This system should continue for several months until the behavior becomes a habit for the child.

CRITICAL TO REMEMBER
. . . .
Corporal Punishment as Discipline

Corporal punishment can lead to child abuse if the disciplinarian loses control. It can also lead to false accusations of child abuse by either the child or other adults. Because of the high cost and low benefit of this form of punishment, parents should think seriously before using it.

Children gain a sense of mastery and actually enjoy the process, often viewing it as a game.

Negative behaviors are simply ignored. If the parent refuses to give the child attention for the behavior, the child soon gives up that strategy. Consistency is the key to success for this technique, and many parents find this method difficult to enforce. Parents need to be warned that children frequently test the seriousness of this attempt by increasing their negative behavior soon after the parents begin ignoring it. If this technique is to be successful, the parents need to ignore the negative behavior every time.

Reasoning. Reasoning involves explaining why a behavior is not permitted. Younger children lack the cognitive skills and developmental abilities to comprehend reasoning fully. For example, a 4-year-old may better understand that he will have to spend time in his room if he breaks his brother's toy rather than understanding the concept of respecting the property of others.

When this technique is used with older children, it is important to focus on the behavior and not the child. The child should not be made to feel guilt and shame because these feelings are counterproductive and can damage the child's self-esteem. The parent can focus on the behavior most effectively by using "I" rather than "you" messages.

A "you" message is one that criticizes children and uses guilt in an attempt to get them to change their behavior. An example of a "you" message would be, "Don't take your little sister's toys away and make her cry. You're being a bad boy!"

By contrast, an "I" message focuses on the misbehavior by explaining its effect on others. An example of an "I" message would be, "Your little sister cries when you take her toys away because she doesn't know that you will give them back to her."

Consequences. This technique helps children learn the direct result of their misbehavior and can be used with toddlers through adolescents. If children must deal with the consequences of their behavior and the consequences are meaningful to them, they are less likely to repeat the behavior. There are three categories of consequences:

- *Natural:* Consequences that occur spontaneously. For example, a child loses a favorite toy after leaving it outside and the parent does not replace it.
- *Logical:* Consequences that are directly related to the misbehavior. For example, when two children are fighting over a toy, the parent removes the toy from both of them for a day.
- *Unrelated:* Consequences that are imposed purposely. For example, a child comes in late for dinner and, as a consequence, is not allowed to watch TV that evening.

Some parents have difficulty allowing their children to face the consequences of their actions. When parents choose to deny their children this experience, they lose an important opportunity to teach responsibility for one's actions.

KEY CONCEPTS

- Traditional families may be single-income or dual-income families. Two-income families are much more common at present.
- Nontraditional family structures may require different nursing care than traditional families. These families may include single-parent, blended, adoptive, unmarried with children, multigenerational (extended), and homosexual parent families.
- High-risk families have additional stressors that affect their functioning. Some high-risk families include families headed by adolescents; families affected by marital discord or divorce, violence, or substance abuse; or families with a severely or chronically ill member.
- All families experience stress. It is how the family deals with stress that is important.
- Identifying healthy versus dysfunctional family patterns can help the nurse implement effective strategies to care for the child and the family.
- Clients during health and illness are cared for within the framework of their family and their culture.
- Differing cultural beliefs and expectations can create conflict between health care providers and clients and their families.
- Traditional cultural beliefs may be used to prevent illness, maintain health, and restore health.
- The nurse can help parents learn effective discipline methods by teaching and role modeling.
- The effects of an ill child on a family may include fear, helplessness, anxiety, role confusion, and general stress on the parents. The siblings of the ill child may experience confusion, anger, resentment, and guilt.
- A knowledge of generally effective, healthy internal and external coping strategies can help the nurse offer the family specific suggestions for coping.

REFERENCES AND READINGS

American Academy of Pediatrics Committee on Community Health Services. (1997). Health care for children of immigrant families. *Pediatrics, 100*(1), 153–156.

American Academy of Pediatrics Committee on Psychosocial Aspects of Child and Family Health. (1998). Guidance for effective discipline. *Pediatrics, 101*(4), 723–728.

Bear, G., Minke, K., & Thomas, A. (1997). *Children's needs II: Development, problems and alternatives.* Bethesda, MD: National Association of School Psychologists.

Bowen, M. (1976). Theory in the practice of psychotherapy. In P. J. Guerin (Ed.), *Family therapy theory and practice* (pp. 42–89). New York: Gardner Press.

Boyle, J. S., Ferrell, J. A., Hodnicki, D. R., & Muller, R. B. (1997). Going home: African-American caregiving for adult children with human immunodeficiency virus disease. *Holistic Nursing Practice, 11*(2), 27–35.

Callister, L. C. (1995). Cultural meanings of childbirth. *Journal of Obstetric, Gynecologic, and Neonatal Nursing, 24*(4), 327–334.

Chess, S., & Thomas, A. (1996). *Temperament theory and practice.* New York: Brunner/Mazel.

Cohen, F. (1984). Coping. In J. D. Matarazzo, S. Weiss, J. Herd, & S. Weiss (Eds.), *Behavioral health: A handbook of health enhancement and disease prevention* (pp. 261–274). New York: Wiley.

Curran, D. (1985). *Stress and the healthy family.* Minneapolis: Winston.

Department of Health and Human Services. (1998). *Health, United States, 1998, with socioeconomic status and health chartbook.* Hyattsville, MD: Author.

Friedman, M. (1986). *Family nursing: Theory and assessment.* Norwalk, CT: Appleton-Century-Crofts.

Grusec, J., & Goodnow, J. (1994). Impact of parental discipline methods on the child's internalization of values: A reconceptualization of current points of view. *Developmental Psychology, 30,* 4–19.

Howard, B. (1996). Advising parents on discipline: What works. *Pediatrics, 98*(4), 809–815.

Hutchinson, M. K., & BaqiAziz, M. (1994). Nursing care of the childbearing Muslim family. *Journal of Obstetric, Gynecologic, and Neonatal Nursing, 23*(9), 767–772.

Lamberg, L. (1996). Nationwide study of health and coping among immigrant children and families. *Journal of the American Medical Association, 276*(18), 1455–1456.

Leininger, M. (1978). *Transcultural nursing: Concepts, theories, practices.* New York: Wiley.

Levine, M., Carey, W., & Crocker, A. (1999). *Developmental-behavioral pediatrics.* Philadelphia: Saunders.

Mattson, S. (1995). Culturally sensitive perinatal care for Southeast Asians. *Journal of Obstetric, Gynecologic, and Neonatal Nursing, 24*(4), 335–342.

Miller, M. A. (1995). Culture, spirituality, and women's health. *Journal of Obstetric, Gynecologic, and Neonatal Nursing, 24*(3), 257–263.

Mrazek, D., Mrazek, P., & Klinnert, M. (1995). Clinical assessment of parenting. *Journal of the American Academy of Child and Adolescent Psychiatry, 34*(3), 272–282.

Nance, T. A. (1995). Intercultural communication: Finding common ground. *Journal of Obstetric, Gynecologic, and Neonatal Nursing, 24*(3), 249–255.

Nicholson, B. C., Janz, P. C., & Fox, R. A. (1998). Evaluating a brief parental-education program for parents of young children. *Psychological Report, 82*(3 Pt. 2), 1107–1113.

Smikstein, G. (1978). The family Apgar: A proposal for a family function test and its use by physicians. *Journal of Family Practice, 6*(6), 1231–1239.

Spector, R. (1991). *Cultural diversity in health and illness* (3rd ed.). Norwalk, CT: Appleton & Lange.

Spector, R. E. (1995). Cultural concepts of women's health and health-promoting behaviors. *Journal of Obstetric, Gynecologic, and Neonatal Nursing, 24*(3), 241–245.

Thomas, A., & Chess, S. (1977). *Temperament and development.* New York: Brunner/Mazel.

U.S. Census Bureau. (1998). *March 1998 current population survey.* Hyattsville, MD: Author.

von Bertalanffy, L. (1968). *General systems theory.* New York: Braziller.

4

Health Promotion for the Developing Child

After studying this chapter, you should be able to:

- Define terms related to growth and development.
- Discuss principles of growth and development.
- Describe various factors, including genetics, that affect growth and development.
- Discuss the following theorists' ideas about growth and development: Piaget, Freud, Erikson, Kohlberg.
- Discuss theories of language development.
- Identify methods used to assess growth and development.
- Describe the classifications and social aspects of play.
- Explain how play enhances growth and development.
- Identify health-promoting activities that are essential for the normal growth and development of infants and children.
- Discuss recommendations for scheduled vaccines.
- Discuss the components of a nutritional assessment.
- Discuss the etiology and prevention of childhood injuries.

DEFINITIONS

cephalocaudal Progression from head to toe.

chronological age Age in years.

developmental age Age based on functional behavior and ability to adapt to the environment; does not necessarily correspond to chronological age.

dramatic play Play in which children act out roles and experiences that may have happened to them, that they fear will happen to them, or that they have observed happening to someone else.

familiarization play Use of materials that are commonly associated with health care situations in creative and playful activities.

growth spurts Brief periods of a rapid increase in growth rate.

heredity Transmission of genetic characteristics from parent to offspring.

learning Behavior changes that occur as a result of both maturation and experience with the environment.

nutrients Foods that supply the body with elements necessary for metabolism.

proximodistal Progression from the center outward or from the midline to the periphery.

recommended dietary allowance (RDA) Recommendations for the average amounts of nutrients that should be consumed daily by healthy people in the United States.

regression Appearance of behavior more appropriate to an earlier stage of development; often used to cope with stress or anxiety.

symbolic play Use of games and interactions that represent an issue or concern to be addressed.

Humans grow and change dramatically during childhood and adolescence. Normal growth and development proceed in an orderly, predictable pattern that provides the basis for assessing an individual's abilities and potential. Nurses provide health care teaching and anticipatory guidance about the growth and development of children in many settings, such as newborn nurseries, emergency departments, clinics, and pediatric inpatient units.

Overview of Growth and Development

Nurses are often the members of the health care team whom parents approach. Parents are often concerned that their children are not progressing normally. Nurses can reassure parents about normal variations in development and can also identify problems early so that developmental delays can be addressed as soon as possible. Nurses who work with ill children must have a clear understanding of how children differ from adults and from each other at various stages. This awareness is essential to allow nurses to create developmentally appropriate plans of care to meet the needs of their young patients.

Definition of Terms

Although the terms *growth* and *development* are often used together and interchangeably, they have distinct definitions and meanings. Growth generally refers to an increase in the physical size of a whole or any of its parts, or an increase in the number and size of cells.

Growth can be measured easily and accurately. For example, any observer can see that an infant grows rapidly during the first year of life. This growth can be measured readily by determining changes in weight and length. The difference in size between a newborn and a 12-month-old is an obvious sign of the remarkable growth that occurs during the first year of life.

Development is a more complex and subtle concept. Development is generally considered a continuous, orderly series of conditions that leads to activities, new motives for activities, and patterns of behavior.

Another definition of development is an increase in function and complexity that occurs through growth, maturation, and learning—in other words, an increase in capabilities. Development is illustrated by the process of language acquisition. The use of language becomes increasingly complex as the child matures. At 10 to 12 months of age, a child uses single words to communicate simple desires and needs. By age 4 to 5 years, complete and complex sentences are used to relate elaborate tales. Language development can be measured by determining vocabulary, articulation skill, and word use.

Maturity and learning also affect development. *Maturation* is the physical change in the complexity of body structures that enables a child to function at increasingly higher levels. Maturity is programmed genetically and may occur as a result of several changes. For example, maturation of the central nervous system depends on changes that occur throughout the body, such as an increase in the number of neurons, myelinization of nerve fibers, lengthening of muscles, and overall weight gain.

Learning involves changes in behavior that occur as a result of both maturation and experience with the environment. Predictable patterns are observed in learning, and these patterns are sequential, orderly, and progressive. For example, when learning to walk, babies first learn to control their heads, then to roll over, next to sit, then to crawl, and finally to walk. The child's muscle mass and nervous system must grow and mature as well.

These examples show how complex and interrelated the processes of growth, development, maturation, and learning are. Children must be monitored carefully to ensure that these complicated events and activities unfold normally. Wide variations occur as children grow and develop. Each child has a unique rate and pattern of development, although parameters are used to identify abnormalities. Nurses must be familiar with normal parameters so that delays can be detected early. The earlier that delays are discovered and treated, the less dramatic their effect will be.

Stages of Growth and Development

To simplify analysis and discussion of the complex processes and theories related to growth and development, researchers and theorists have identified stages or age groupings. These stages serve as reference points in describing various features of growth and development. Chapters 5 through 8 discuss the physical growth and cognitive, emotional, language, and motor development specific to each stage.

Parameters of Growth

Statistical data derived from research studies of large groups of children provide health care professionals with information about how children normally grow. Throughout infancy, childhood, and adolescence, growth occurs in bursts separated by periods when no growth occurs (Lampl, 1995).

Stages of Growth and Development

The following stages and age groupings refer to stages of childhood growth and development.

Newborn	Birth–1 month
Infancy	1 month–1 year
Toddlerhood	1–3 years
Preschool age	3–6 years
School age	6–11 or 12 years
Adolescence	11 or 12–21 years

Weight, height, and head circumference are parameters that are used to monitor growth. They should be measured at regular intervals during childhood. The weight of the average term newborn is approximately 7 to 8 lb (3.2 to 3.6 kg). Male infants are usually slightly heavier than female infants. Usually, the birth weight doubles by 6 months of age and triples by 1 year of age. Between 2 and 3 years of age, the weight quadruples. Slow, steady weight gain during childhood is followed by a growth spurt during adolescence.

The average newborn is approximately 20 inches (50 cm) long, with an average increase of approximately 1 inch (2.54 cm) per month for the first 6 months, followed by an increase of approximately ½ inch (1.27 cm) per month for the remainder of the first year. The child gains 3 inches (7.6 cm) per year from age 1 through 7 years, then 2 inches (5 cm) per year from age 8 through 15 years. Boys generally add more height during adolescence than do girls. Body proportion changes are shown in Figure 4–1.

Head circumference indicates brain growth. The normal occipital-frontal circumference of the term newborn head is 13 to 14 inches (33 to 35 cm). Average head growth occurs according to the following pattern: 4 inches (10 cm) during the first year; 1 inch (2.5 cm) during the second year; ½ inch (1.2 cm) per year from 3 to 5 years; and ½ inch (1.2 cm) per 5 years until puberty. The average adult head circumference is approximately 21 inches (53 cm).

Dentition, the eruption of teeth, also follows a sequential pattern. Primary dentition usually begins to emerge at approximately 6 to 8 months. Most children have 20 teeth by age 2½ years. Permanent teeth, 32 in all, erupt beginning at approximately age 6 years, accompanied by the loss of primary teeth (see Chapter 33). Although some parents place importance on eruption of the teeth as a sign of maturation, dentition is not related to the level or rate of development.

Principles of Growth and Development

Patterns of Growth and Development

Growth and development are directional and follow predictable patterns. The first direction of growth is *cephalocaudal*, or proceeding from head to tail (or toe). This means that structures and functions originating in the head develop before those in the lower parts of the body. At birth, the head is large, a full one fourth of the entire body length, the trunk is long, and the arms are longer than the legs. As the child matures, the body proportions gradually change, and by adulthood, the legs have increased in size from approximately 38% to 50% of the total body length (see Fig. 4–1).

Directional growth and development are illustrated further by myelinization of the nerves, which begins in the

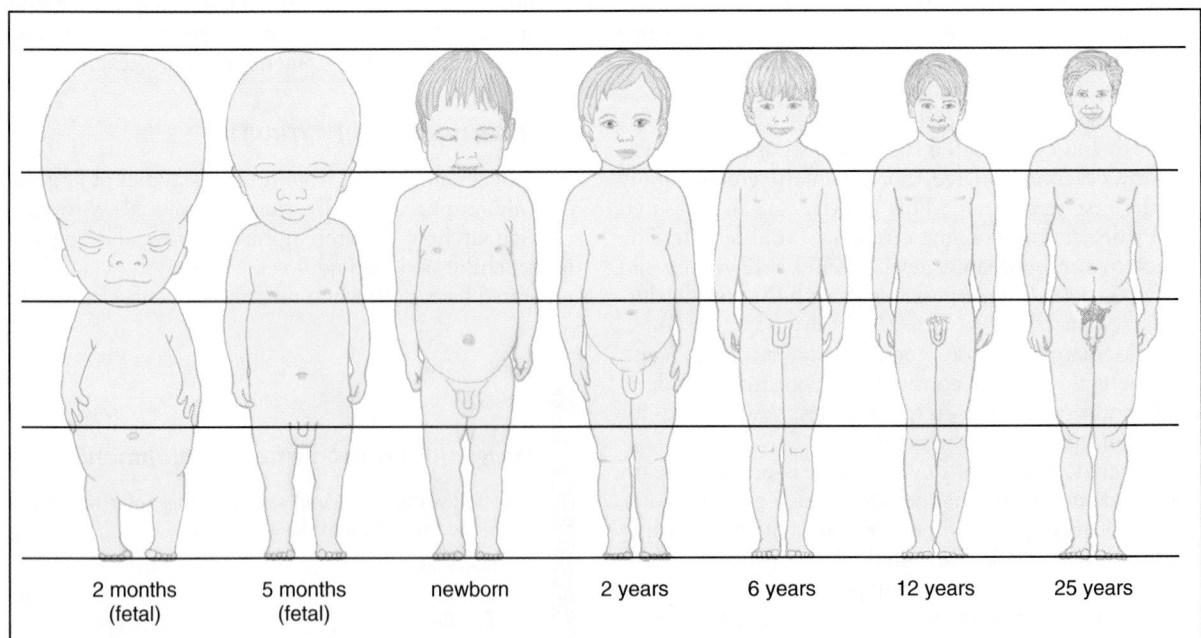

| 2 months (fetal) | 5 months (fetal) | newborn | 2 years | 6 years | 12 years | 25 years |

FIGURE 4–1
. . . .
Changes in body proportions with growth.

Directional Patterns of Growth and Development

CEPHALOCAUDAL PATTERN (HEAD TO TOE)

Examples

- Head initially grows fastest (fetus), then trunk (infant), then legs (child).
- Infant can raise the head before sitting and can sit before standing.

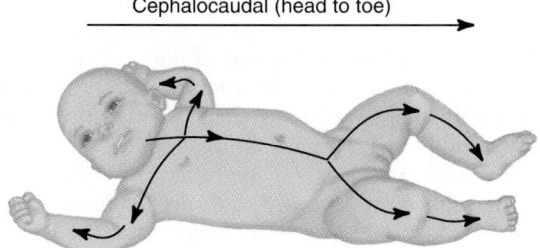

Cephalocaudal (head to toe)

Proximal distal (from the center outward)

PROXIMODISTAL PATTERN (FROM THE CENTER OUTWARD)

Examples

- In the respiratory system, the trachea develops first in the embryo, followed by branching and growth outward of the bronchi, bronchioles, and alveoli in the fetus and infant.
- Motor control of the arms comes before control of the hands, and hand control comes before finger control.

brain and spreads downward as the child matures. Growth of the myelin sheath and other nerve structures contributes to cephalocaudal development, which is illustrated by an infant's ability to raise the head before being able to sit and to sit before being able to stand.

A second directional aspect of growth and development is *proximodistal,* which means progression from the center outward, or from the midline to the periphery. The growth and branching pattern of the respiratory tract illustrates this concept. The trachea, which is the central structure of the respiratory tree, forms in the embryo by 24 days of gestation. Branching and growth outward occur in the bronchi, bronchioles, and alveoli throughout fetal life and infancy. Alveoli, which are the most distal structures of the system, continue to grow and develop in number and function until middle childhood.

Growth and development follow patterns, one of which is general to specific. As a child matures, activities become less generalized and more focused. For example, a newborn's response to pain is usually a whole-body response, with flailing of the arms and legs even if the pain is in the abdomen. As the child matures, the pain response becomes more localized to the stimulus. An older child with abdominal pain guards the abdomen. Another example is palmar grasp (use of the whole hand to grasp an object) at 4 to 5 months of age. At approximately 9 months of age, the palmar grasp

is gradually replaced by the pincer grasp (use of the thumb and forefinger). The pincer grasp requires more specific fine motor muscle control than does the palmar grasp.

Another pattern is the progression of functions from simple to complex. This pattern is easily observed in language development. A toddler's first sentences are formed simply, using only a noun and a verb. By age 5 years, the child constructs detailed stories using many complex modifiers.

The rate of growth is not constant as the child matures. *Growth spurts,* alternating with periods of slow or stagnant growth, are observed throughout childhood. Spurts are frequently seen as the child prepares to master a significant developmental task, such as walking. An increase in growth around a child's first birthday may promote the neuromuscular maturation needed for taking the first steps.

All facets of development (cognitive, motor, emotional, language) normally proceed according to these patterns. Knowledge of these concepts is useful when determining how a child's development is progressing and when comparing a child's development with normal patterns.

Mastery of developmental tasks is not static or permanent, and developmental stages do not always correlate with chronological age. Children progress through developmental stages at varying rates within normal limits and may master developmental tasks only to regress to earlier levels when ill or stressed. Also, people can struggle repeatedly with particular developmental tasks throughout life, even though they have achieved more advanced levels of development.

Critical Periods

After birth, critical or sensitive periods exist for optimal growth and development. Similar to times during embryologic and fetal life in which certain organs are formed and are particularly vulnerable to injury, critical periods are blocks of time during which children are ready to master specific developmental tasks. Children can master tasks outside of these critical periods, but some tasks are learned more easily during particular periods.

Many factors affect a child's sensitive learning periods, such as injury, illness, and malnutrition. For example, the sensitive period for learning to walk seems to be during the latter part of the first year and the beginning of the second year. Children seem to be driven by an irresistible urge to practice walking and display great pride as they succeed. If a child is immobilized, for instance for the treatment of an orthopedic condition from age 10 months to 18 months, the child may have difficulty learning to walk. The child can learn to walk, but the task may be more difficult than for others.

Factors Influencing Growth and Development

GENETICS

One of the factors with the greatest influence on a child's growth and development is genetics. Genetic potential is affected by many factors. Environment influences how and to what extent particular genetic traits are manifested. A more complete discussion of genetics is included in Chapter 9.

ENVIRONMENT

The environment is a significant determinant of growth and developmental outcome, both before and after birth. Prenatal environmental factors include maternal smoking, alcohol intake, and disease, such as diabetes. Socioeconomic status, interpersonal relationships, and environmental hazards are only a few of the factors that affect children both before and after birth. Environmental factors that affect children are discussed in each individual growth and development chapter and in Chapter 3.

CULTURE

Culture is the way of life of a people, including their habits, beliefs, language, and values. It is a significant factor influencing children as they grow toward adulthood.

When gathering data, nurses must recognize how the common family structures and traditional values of various groups affect children's performance on assessment tests. The child's cultural and ethnic background must be considered when assessing growth and development. Standard growth curves and developmental tests do not necessarily reflect the normal growth and development of children of various cultural groups. Growth curves for children of various racial and cultural backgrounds are increasingly available. Nurse researchers and others conduct studies to determine the effectiveness of measurement tools for culturally diverse populations. In addition, culturally sensitive instruments are being developed to gather data to determine appropriate nursing interventions. To provide quality care to all patients, nurses must consider the effect of culture on children and families. Chapter 3 provides a more in-depth look at families and the influence of culture.

NUTRITION

Because children are growing constantly and need a continuous supply of nutrients, nutrition plays an important role throughout childhood. Nutrition to support growth requires a minimum intake of energy, protein, and nutrients appropriate for age and body size (Trahms & Pipes, 1997). Good nutritional status is also needed for normal function of hormones, especially growth factor and sex hormones. The effect of nutrition on growth and development is discussed more in depth later in this chapter and in the growth and development chapters.

HEALTH STATUS

Overall health status plays an important part in the growth and development of children. At the cellular level, inherited or acquired disease can affect the delivery of nutrients, hormones, or oxygen to organs and also organ growth and function. Disease states that affect growth and development include digestive or malabsorption disorders, heart defects, and metabolic diseases.

FAMILY

A child is an inseparable part of a family. Family relationships and influences are major determinants of how children grow and progress. Because of the special bond and influence of the family on the child, there can be no separation of child from family in the health care setting. For example, to diminish anxiety in a child, nurses sometimes attempt to reduce parental anxiety, which may then reduce the stress on the child. Nursing care of children involves nursing care of the whole family and requires skill in dealing with both adults and children.

> Nurses might reduce parental anxiety about an ill child by saying, "Your child is in the best place possible here at the hospital. You brought him in at just the right time so that we can help him."

Family structures are in a constant state of change, and these dynamic states influence how children develop. Within the family, relationships change because of marriage, birth, divorce, death, and new roles and responsibilities. Societal forces outside the family, such as economics, population shifts, and migration, change how children are raised. These forces cause changes in family structures and the outcomes of child rearing that must be considered when planning nursing care for children. The family is discussed in Chapter 3.

Parental Attitudes.   Parental attitudes affect growth and development. Growth and development continue throughout life, and parents have stage-related needs and tasks that affect their children. Superimposed on these developmental issues are other factors influencing parental attitudes: educational level, childhood experiences, financial pressures, marital status, and available support systems. Parental attitudes are also affected by the child's temperament, the child's unique way of relating to the world. Temperament is discussed in Chapter 3, which describes the easy child, the slow-to-warm child, and the difficult child. These different temperaments affect parenting practices and whether a child's unique personality traits develop into assets or problems.

Child-rearing Philosophies.   Child-rearing philosophies, shaped by a myriad of life events, have an effect on how children grow and develop. For example, well-educated, well-read parents often provide their children with extra stimulation and opportunities for learning, beginning at a young age. This enrichment includes extra parental attention and interaction, not necessarily expensive toys. Generally, development progresses best when enriched opportunities for learning are provided.

Other parents may not recognize the need to provide a rich learning environment at home, may not have time, or may not value this type of parenting. Children of these parents may not progress at the same rate as those raised in a more enriched atmosphere.

A significant point for parents to remember is that children must be ready to learn. If motor and neurologic structures are not mature, no amount of added stimulation will produce new behavior. The result of an overzealous approach toward accomplishing a specific task is frustration for both child and parent. For example, a child who is 6 months old will not be able to walk alone, no matter how much time and effort the parent expends. However, at 12 to 14 months, a child usually is ready to begin walking and will do so with ease if given opportunities to practice.

Theories of Growth and Development

Many theorists have attempted to organize and classify the complex phenomena of growth and development. No single theory can adequately explain the wondrous journey from infancy to adulthood. However, each theorist contributes a piece of the puzzle. Theories are not facts, but merely attempts to explain human behavior. Table 4–1 compares and contrasts theories discussed in the text. The chapters on each age group provide further discussion of these theories.

Piaget's Theory of Cognitive Development

Jean Piaget (1896–1980), a Swiss theorist, made major contributions to the study of how children learn. His complex

TABLE 4–1

Theories of Growth and Development

	Piaget's Periods of Cognitive Development	Freud's Stages of Psychosexual Development	Erikson's Stages of Psychosocial Development	Kohlberg's Stages of Moral Development
Infancy	*Period 1 (Birth–2 Years): Sensorimotor Period*	*Oral Stage*	*Trust versus Mistrust*	*Stage 0 (0–2 Years): Naivete and Egocentrism*
	Reflexive behavior is used to adapt to the environment; egocentric view of the world; development of object permanence.	Mouth is a sensory organ; infant takes in and explores during oral passive substage (first half of infancy);infant strikes out with teeth during oral aggressive substage (latter half of infancy).	Development of a sense that the self is good and the world is good when consistent, predictable, reliable care is received; characterized by hope.	No moral sensitivity; decisions are made on the basis of what pleases the child; infants like or love what helps them and dislike what hurts them; no awareness of the effect of their actions on others. "Good is what I like and want."
Toddlerhood	*Period 2 (2–7 Years): Preoperational Thought*	*Anal Stage*	*Autonomy versus Shame and Doubt*	*Stage 1 (2–3 Years): Punishment-Obedience Orientation*
	Thinking remains egocentric, becomes magical, and is dominated by perception.	Major focus of sexual interest is anus; control of bodily functions is major feature.	Development of sense of control over the self and bodily functions; exerts self; characterized by will.	Right or wrong is determined by physical consequences: "If I get caught and punished for doing it, it is wrong. If I am not caught or punished, then it must be right."
Preschool Age		*Phallic or Oedipal/ Electra Stage*	*Initiative versus Guilt*	*Premorality or Preconventional Morality Stage 2 (4–7 Years): Instrumental Hedonism and Concrete Reciprocity*
		Genitals become focus of sexual curiosity; superego (conscience) develops; feelings of guilt emerge.	Development of a can-do attitude about the self; behavior becomes goal-directed, competitive, and imaginative; initiation into sex role; characterized by purpose.	Child conforms to rules out of self-interest: "I'll do this for you if you do this for me"; behavior is guided by an "eye for an eye" orientation. "If you do something bad to me, then it's OK if I do something bad to you."
School Age	*Period 3 (7–11 Years): Concrete Operations*	*Latency Stage*	*Industry versus Inferiority*	*Morality of Conventional Role Conformity Stage 3 (7–10 Years): Good-Boy/ Girl Orientation*
	Thinking becomes more systematic and logical, but concrete objects and activities are needed.	Sexual feelings are firmly repressed by the superego; period of relative calm.	Mastering of useful skills and tools of the culture; learning how to play and work with peers; characterized by competence.	Morality is based on avoiding disapproval or disturbing the conscience; child is becoming socially sensitive.
				Stage 4 (Begins at About 10–12 Years): Law and Order Orientation
				Right takes on a religious or metaphysical quality. Child wants to do duty, show respect for authority, and maintain social order; obeys rules for their own sake.

Table continued on following page

TABLE 4–1
• • • • • • • • • • •

Theories of Growth and Development Continued

	Piaget's Periods of Cognitive Development	Freud's Stages of Psychosexual Development	Erikson's Stages of Psychosocial Development	Kohlberg's Stages of Moral Development
Adolescence	**Period 4 (11 Years–Adulthood): Formal Operations**	**Puberty or Genital Stage**	**Identity versus Role Confusion**	**Morality of Self-Accepted Moral Principles Stage 5: Social Contract Orientation**
	New ideas can be created; situations can be analyzed; use of abstract thinking.	Stimulated by increasing hormone levels; sexual energy wells up in full force, resulting in personal and family turmoil.	Begins to develop a sense of "I"; this process is life-long; peers become of paramount importance; child gains independence from parents; characterized by faith in self.	Right is determined by what is best for the majority; exceptions to rules can be made if a person's welfare is violated; the end no longer justifies the means; laws are for mutual good and mutual cooperation.
Adulthood			**Intimacy versus Isolation**	
			Development of the ability to lose the self in genuine mutuality with another; characterized by love.	
			Generativity versus Stagnation	**Stage 6: Personal Principle Orientation**
			Production of ideas and materials through work; creation of children; characterized by care.	Achieved only by the morally mature individual; few people reach this level; these people do what they think is right, regardless of others' opinions, legal sanctions, or personal sacrifice; actions are guided by internal standards; integrity is of utmost importance; may be willing to die for their beliefs.
			Ego Integrity versus Despair	**Stage 7: Universal Principle Orientation**
			Realization that there is order and purpose to life; characterized by wisdom.	This stage is achieved by only a rare few; Mother Teresa, Gandhi, and Socrates are examples; these individuals transcend the teachings of organized religion and perceive themselves as part of the cosmic order; understand the reason for their existence and live for their beliefs.

theory provides a framework for understanding how thinking during childhood progresses and differs from adult thinking. Like other developmental theorists, Piaget postulated that as children develop intellectually, they pass through progressive stages. The ages assigned to these periods are only averages.

During the sensorimotor period of development, infant thinking seems to involve the entire body. Reflexive behavior is gradually replaced by more complex activities. The world becomes increasingly solid through the development of the concept of object permanence, which is the aware-

ness that objects continue to exist even when they disappear from sight. By the end of this stage, the infant shows some evidence of reasoning.

During the period of preoperational thought, language becomes increasingly useful. Judgments are dominated by perception and are illogical, and thinking is characterized, especially during the early part of this stage, by egocentrism. In other words, children are unable to think about another person's viewpoint and believe that everyone perceives situations as they do. Magical thinking, or the belief that events occur because of wishing, and animism, or the perception that all objects have life and feeling, characterize this period.

At the end of the preoperational stage, the child shifts from egocentric thinking and begins to be able to look at the world from another person's view. This shifting enables the child to move into the period of concrete operations, where the child is no longer bound by perceptions and can distinguish fact from fantasy. The concept of time becomes increasingly clear during this stage, although far past and far future events remain obscure. Although reasoning powers increase rapidly during this stage, the child cannot deal with abstractions or socialized thinking.

Normally, adolescents progress to the period of formal operations. In this period, the adolescent proceeds from concrete to abstract and symbolic, and from self-centered to other-centered. How the adolescent understands and perceives the world is affected by this period (Ford & Coleman, 1999). All of these stages of cognitive development are discussed in the chapters on each age group.

Nursing Implications of Piaget's Theory

Piaget's theory is especially significant to nurses as they develop teaching plans of care for children. Piaget believed that learning should be geared to the child's level of understanding and that the child should be an active participant in the learning process. For health teaching to be effective, nurses must understand the different cognitive abilities of children at various ages. Nurses also must know how to engage children in the learning process with developmentally appropriate activities.

Because illness and hospitalization are often frightening to children, especially toddlers and preschoolers, nurses must understand the cognitive basis of fears related to treatment and be able to intervene appropriately (see Chapter 35).

Freud's Theory of Psychosexual Development

Sigmund Freud (1856–1939) developed theories to explain psychosexual development. His theories were in vogue for many years and provided a basis for other theories. Freud postulated that early childhood experiences provide unconscious motivation for actions later in life. According to Freudian theory, certain parts of the body assume psychological significance as foci of sexual energy. These areas shift from one part of the body to another as the child moves through different stages of development. Freud's work may help to explain normal behavior that parents may confuse with abnormal behavior, and it also may provide a good foundation for sex education.

Freud believed that during infancy, sexual behavior seems to focus around the mouth, the most erogenous area of the infant body (oral stage). Infants derive pleasure from sucking and exploring objects by placing them in their mouths. During toddlerhood, when toilet training becomes a major developmental task, sensations seem to shift away from the mouth and toward the anus (anal stage). Psycho-

analysts see this period as a time of holding on and letting go. A sense of control or autonomy develops as the child masters bodily functions.

During the preschool years, interest in the genitalia arises (phallic stage). Children are curious about anatomic differences, childbirth, and sexuality. Children at this age often ask many questions, freely exhibit their own sexual organs, and want to peek at those of others. Children often masturbate, sometimes causing great concern in parents. Although it is not universal, a phenomenon described by Freud as the Oedipus complex in boys and the Electra complex in girls is seen in preschool children. This possessiveness of the child for the opposite-sex parent, marked by aggressiveness toward the same-sex parent, is considered normal behavior, as is a heightened interest in sex. To resolve these disturbing sexual feelings, the preschooler identifies with or becomes more like the same-sex parent. The superego (an inner voice that reprimands and evokes guilt) also develops. The superego is similar to a conscience (S. Freud, 1923/1960).

Freud describes the school-age period as the latency stage, when sexuality plays a less prominent role in the everyday life of the child. Best friends and same-sex peer groups are influential in the school-age child's life. Younger school-age children often refuse to play with children of the opposite sex, whereas prepubertal children begin to desire the companionship of opposite-sex friends.

During adolescence, interest in sex again flourishes as children search for identity (genital stage). Under the influence of fluctuating hormone levels, dramatic physical changes, and shifting social relationships, the adolescent develops a more adult view of sexuality. Their cognitive skills are not fully developed, however, and adolescents often make questionable judgments about sexual matters and may have questions and concerns about their behavior and feelings (A. Freud, 1974; Litt & Martin, 1999).

Nursing Implications of Freud's Theory

Both children and parents may have questions and concerns about normal sexual development and sex education. Nurses must understand normal sexual growth and development to help parents and children form healthy attitudes about sex.

Erikson's Psychosocial Theory

Born in 1902, Erik H. Erikson, inspired by the work of Sigmund Freud, proposed a popular theory about child development. He viewed development as a lifelong series of conflicts affected by social and cultural factors. Each conflict must be resolved for the child and adult to progress emotionally. There is wide variation in how individuals address the conflicts. According to Erikson, however, unsuccessful resolution leaves the individual emotionally handicapped.

Each of eight stages of development has a specific central conflict or developmental task. These eight tasks are described in terms of a positive or negative resolution. The actual resolution of a specific conflict lies somewhere along a continuum between a perfect positive and a perfect negative.

The first developmental task is the establishment of trust. The basic quality of trust provides a foundation for the personality. If an infant's physical and emotional needs are met in a timely manner through warm and nurturing interactions with a consistent caregiver, the infant begins to sense that the world is trustworthy. The infant begins to develop trust in others and a sense of being worthy of love. Through successful achievement of a sense of trust, the infant can move on to subsequent developmental stages.

According to Erikson, unsuccessful resolution of this first developmental task results in a sense of mistrust. If needs are consistently unmet, acute tension begins to appear in children. During infancy, signs of unmet needs include restlessness, fretfulness, whining, crying, clinging, physical tenseness, and physical dysfunctions such as vomiting, diarrhea, and sleep disturbances. All children exhibit these signs at times. If these behaviors become personality characteristics, however, unsuccessful resolution of this stage is suspected.

The toddler's developmental task is to acquire a sense of autonomy rather than a sense of shame and doubt. A positive resolution of this task is accomplished by the ability to control the body and bodily functions, especially elimination. Success at this stage does not mean that the toddler, even as an adult, will exhibit autonomous behavior in all life situations. In certain circumstances, feelings of shame and self-doubt are normal and may be adaptive.

Erikson's theory describes each developmental stage, with crises related to individual stages emerging at specific times and in a particular order. Likewise, each stage is built on the resolution of previous developmental tasks. During each conflict, however, the child spends some energy and time resolving earlier conflicts (Erikson, 1963).

Nursing Implications of Erikson's Theory

In stressful situations, such as hospitalization, children, even those with healthy personalities, evoke defense mechanisms that protect them against undue anxiety. *Regression*, a behavior used frequently by children, is a reactivation of behavior more appropriate to an earlier stage of development. This defense mechanism is illustrated by a 6-year-old boy who reverts to sucking his thumb and wetting his pants under increased stress, such as illness or the birth of a sibling. Nurses can educate parents about regression and encourage them to offer their children support, not ridicule. They can provide constructive suggestions for stress management and reassure parents that regression normally subsides as anxiety decreases. This phenomenon is discussed in Chapter 35.

Erikson's main contribution to the study of human development lies in his outline of a universal sequence of phases of psychosocial development. His work is especially relevant to nursing because it provides a theoretical basis for much of the emotional care that is given to children. The stages are further discussed in the chapters on each age group.

Kohlberg's Theory of Moral Development

Lawrence Kohlberg (1927–1987), a psychologist and philosopher, described a stage theory of moral development that closely parallels Piaget's stages of cognitive development. He discussed moral development as a complicated process involving the acceptance of the values and rules of society in a way that shapes behavior. This cognitive-developmental theory postulates that although knowing what behaviors are right and wrong is important, it is much less important than understanding and appreciating why the behaviors should or should not be exhibited (Bear, Richards, & Gibbs, 1997).

Guilt, an internal expression of self-criticism and feeling of remorse, is an emotion closely tied to moral reasoning. Most children 12 years old or older react to misbehavior with guilt. Guilt helps them realize when their moral judgment fails.

Building on Piaget's work, Kohlberg studied boys and girls from middle- and lower-class families in the United States and other countries. He interviewed them by presenting scenarios with moral dilemmas and asking them to make a judgment. His focus was not on the answer but on the reasoning behind the judgment (Kohlberg, 1964). He then classified the responses into a series of levels and stages, as described below.

LEVEL 1: PREMORALITY (PRECONVENTIONAL MORALITY)

The child demonstrates acceptable behavior because of fear of punishment from a superior force, such as a parent. At this stage of cognitive and moral development, children cannot reason as mature members of society. They view the world in a selfish, egocentric way, with no real understanding of right or wrong. They view morality as external to themselves, and their behavior reflects what others tell them to do, rather than an internal drive to do what is right. In other words, they have an external locus of control. A child who thinks, "I will not steal money from my sister because my mother will spank me" illustrates premorality.

Within this level are three stages:

- Stage 0 (0 to 2 years): The infant has no awareness of right or wrong and does not consider the effect of his or her actions on others.
- Stage 1 (2 to 3 years): The child obeys rules to avoid punishment, and acts to avoid displeasing those who are in power.
- Stage 2 (4 to 7 years): The child conforms to rules to obtain rewards or have favors returned. This type of behavior coincides with Piaget's preconceptual stage of cognition, in which thinking is dominated by perception and egocentrism.

LEVEL 2: MORALITY OF CONVENTIONAL ROLE CONFORMITY (CONVENTIONAL MORALITY)

The child conforms to rules to please others. The child still has an external locus of control, but a concern for social order begins to emerge and replace the more egocentric thinking of the earlier stage. The child has an increased awareness of others' feelings. In the child's view, good behavior is that which those in authority will approve. If behavior is not acceptable, the child feels guilty.

Within this level are Stage 3 (7 to 10 years), in which conformity occurs to avoid disapproval or dislike by others, and Stage 4 (10 to 12 years), in which the child has more concern with society as a whole. In these stages, emphasis is on obeying laws to maintain social order. This level of moral reasoning develops as the child shifts the focus of living from the family to peer groups and society as a whole. As the child's cognitive capacities increase, an internal sense of right and wrong emerges and the individual is said to have developed an internal locus of control. Along with this internal locus of control comes the ability to consider circumstances when judging behavior.

LEVEL 3: MORALITY OF SELF-ACCEPTED MORAL PRINCIPLES (POSTCONVENTIONAL MORALITY)

The person focuses on individual rights and principles of conscience during this stage. There is an internal locus of control. Concern about what is best for all is uppermost, and the person steps back from his or her own viewpoint to consider what rights and values must be upheld for the good of all. Because abstract thinking abilities are necessary for this type of reasoning, this level is not attained until adolescence. Some individuals never reach this point. Within this level is Stage 5, in which conformity occurs because individuals have basic rights and society needs to be improved. The adolescent in this stage gives as well as takes, and does not expect to get something without paying for it. In Stage 6, conformity is based on universal principles of justice and occurs to avoid self-condemnation (Colby, Kohlberg, & Kauffman, 1987; Feldman, 1998; Kohlberg, 1964).

Only a few morally mature individuals achieve Stage 6. These people, committed to a moral idea, live and die for their principles.

Kohlberg believes that children proceed from one stage to the next in a sequence that does not vary, although some people may never reach the highest levels. Even though children are raised in different cultures and with different experiences, he believes that all children progress according to his description.

Nursing Implications of Kohlberg's Theory

Nurses must be aware of how moral development progresses to provide anticipatory guidance to parents about expectations and discipline of their children. Parents are often distraught because their young children apparently do not understand right and wrong. For example, a 6-year-old girl who takes money from her mother's purse does not show remorse or seem to recognize that stealing is wrong. In fact, she is more concerned about her punishment than about her misdeed. With an understanding of normal moral development, the nurse can reassure the concerned parents that the child is showing age-appropriate behavior.

Theories of Language Development

Human language has a number of characteristics that are not shared with other species of animals that communicate with each other. Human language has meaning, provides a mechanism for thought, and permits tremendous creativity.

Because language is such a complex process and involves such a vast number of neuromuscular structures, brain growth and differentiation must reach a certain level of maturity before a child can speak. Language development closely parallels cognitive development and is discussed by most cognitive theorists as they explain the maturation of thinking abilities. The process of how language develops remains a mystery, however.

Passive or receptive language is the ability to understand the spoken word. Expressive language is the ability to produce meaningful vocalizations. In most people, the areas in the brain responsible for expressive language are close to motor centers in the left cerebral area that control muscle movement of the mouth, tongue, and hands. Humans use a variety of facial and hand movements as well as words to convey ideas.

Crying is the infant's first method of communication. These vocalizations quickly become distinct and individual and accurately convey such states as hunger, diaper discomfort, pain, loneliness, and boredom. Vowel sounds appear first, as early as 2 weeks of age, followed by consonants at approximately 5 months of age.

By age 2 years, children have a vocabulary of roughly 300 words and can construct simple sentences. By age 4 years, children have gained a sense of correct grammar and articulation, but several consonants, including *l* and *r*, remain difficult to pronounce. For example, the sentence "The red and blue bird flew up to the tree" might be pronounced by the preschooler as "The wed and boo bud fwew up to the twee!"

The language of school-age children is less concrete and much more articulate than that of the preschooler. Between the ages of 5 and 10 years, children begin to understand the structure of language. By 12 years the child has many of the cognitive and linguistic skills of adults (Kelly & Sally, 1999).

Infants learn much of their language from their parents. Children who are raised in homes where verbalization is encouraged and modeled tend to display advanced language skills. Also, in infancy, receptive ability (the understanding of language) is more developed than expressive skill (the actual articulation of words). This tendency persists throughout life and is important to realize when caring for children. In clinical situations, nurses must communicate what is happening to their young patients, using simple, age-appropriate words, even though the child may not verbalize understanding. Language development is discussed in more depth in chapters on each age group.

Influence of Heredity on Growth and Development

Heredity is the transmission of genetic characteristics from parent to offspring and is one of the most significant determinants of growth and development. Because all humans are products of the biologic composition of their parents, heredity must be considered when assessing a child's growth and developmental patterns and when caring for children with inherited diseases. Genetic disorders are common and have a significant effect on the growth and development of children. Because genetic diseases are complex, permanent, and chronic, children, families, and entire communities are affected.

Nurses need a working knowledge of how common genetic traits are transmitted, how common chromosomal abnormalities occur, and what effects these diseases have on children and families. Alert and skilled nurses in hospital, clinic, and home settings can provide early assessment and identification. Nurses should be knowledgeable about appropriate referral sources so that prompt genetic evaluation and counseling can be provided. After genetic counseling sessions, nurses can interpret, clarify, and reinforce information that is provided to families.

A significant role of nurses is offering families support in coping with genetic abnormalities. Nurses can act as child and family advocates, helping them maneuver through the complexities of the health care system. Finally, nurses are in an excellent position to educate families and communities about the causes of birth defects and the prevention of environmentally induced disorders. Refer to Chapter 9 for a discussion of heredity and environmental influences on development.

◼ *Assessment of Growth*

Because growth is an excellent indicator of physical well-being, accurate assessments must be made at regular intervals so that patterns of growth can be determined. Trained individuals using calibrated equipment and proper techniques should perform growth measurement. Methods of obtaining accurate measurements in children are described in Chapter 33. To minimize the chance of error, data should be collected on children under consistent conditions on a routine basis, and values should be recorded and plotted on growth charts immediately.

Standardized growth charts allow an individual child's growth to be compared with statistical norms. The most commonly used growth charts are those developed by the National Center for Health Statistics. Separate charts are available for boys and girls. One set of charts is used for children from birth to 3 years, and another set is used for children ages 2 years to 18 years (see Appendix H).

Because height and weight are the best indicators of growth, these parameters are measured, plotted on growth charts, and monitored over time. Brain growth can also be monitored by measuring infant frontal-occipital circumference at intervals and plotting the values on growth charts. It is important to relate head size to weight because larger babies have bigger heads. These measurements are routinely performed during the first 2 years of life.

Growth rate is measured in percentiles. The area between any two percentiles is referred to as a growth channel (see Growth Charts in Appendix H). Childhood growth normally progresses according to a pattern along a particular growth channel. Deviations from normal growth patterns may suggest problems. Any change of more than two growth channels indicates a need for more in-depth assessment.

Recognition of abnormal growth patterns is an important function of the nurse. The earlier that growth disorders are detected, diagnosed, and treated, the better the long-term prognosis.

◼ *Assessment of Development*

Assessment of development is a more complex process than assessment of growth. To assess developmental progress accurately, nurses must gather data from many sources, including observations and interviews, physical examinations, interactions with the child and parents, and various standardized assessment tools.

Observation is a valuable method most often used to obtain information about a child's *developmental age* (level of functioning). By watching a child during daily activities, such as eating, playing, toileting, and dressing, nurses gather a great deal of assessment data. Observation of the child's problem-solving abilities, communication patterns, interaction skills, and emotional responses can yield valuable information about the child's level of development. Similarly, interviews and physical examinations can provide much information about how the child functions.

In addition to these sources of data, many standardized assessment tools are available for nurses and other health care professionals to use for developmental assessment. Developmental assessment should be part of a newborn's assessment and of every well-child examination, for several reasons. One reason is that parents want to know how their child compares with others and whether development is normal, especially if they experienced a difficult pregnancy or have developmentally delayed children. Developmental assessment tends to allay fears. Another reason is that abnormal development must be discovered early to facilitate optimal outcomes through early intervention.

Newborn Assessment

Two newborn screening tools that are used are the Brazelton Neonatal Behavior Assessment Scale and the New Ballard Score, which is an adaptation of the Dubowitz tool for estimation of gestational age. These tools are described in Chapter 22.

Denver Developmental Screening Test II

The most widely used screening tool for infants and young children is the Denver Developmental Screening Test II (DDST-II; see Appendix I). The DDST-II provides a clinical impression of a child's overall development and alerts the user to potential developmental difficulties.

The DDST-II, designed to be used with children between birth and 6 years of age, assesses development based on the performance of a series of age-appropriate tasks. There are 125 tasks or items arranged in four functional areas:

1. Personal-social (getting along with others, caring for personal needs)
2. Fine motor (eye-hand coordination, problem-solving skills)

3. Language (hearing, using, and understanding language)
4. Gross motor (sitting, jumping)

Items for rating the child's behavior are also included at the end of the test.

The test form is arranged with age scales across the top and bottom (see Appendix I for a sample test form). After calculating the child's *chronological age* (age in years), the test administrator draws an age line on the form. Each of the 125 tasks or items is arranged on a shaded bar depicting at which ages 25%, 50%, 75%, and 90% of the children in the research sample completed that particular item. The child is presented with the assessment items clustered around the age line. The directions must be followed exactly during administration of the test. A score for performance on each item is recorded according to the following scale: pass (P), fail (F), no opportunity (NO), and refusal (R). At the completion of the test the screener scores test behavior ratings (located at the bottom left of the form).

Interpretation of the test is based first on individual items, then on the test as a whole. Individual items are considered as "advanced, normal, caution, delayed, or no opportunity."

The results of the test can be used to identify a child's developmental age and how a child compares with others of the same chronological age. This information can be used to alert health care providers to potential problems. To ensure that the results are accurate, only individuals who are trained to administer the test in a standardized manner should perform testing. Training is obtained through study of the testing manual, review of the accompanying videotape, and supervised practice with children of various ages.

Although the DDST-II is widely used, it is a screening test only, not an intelligence quotient (IQ) test. It is not a definitive predictor of future abilities, and it should not be used to determine diagnostic labels. It is, however, a useful tool for noting problems, validating hunches, monitoring development, and providing referrals.

PRINCIPLES GUIDING SCREENING WITH THE DDST-II

Preterm Delivery.   Up to age 24 months, allowance must be made for prematurity in calculating the age line. For example, a 9-month-old child who was born 2 months prematurely should be compared with a normal 7-month-old infant.

Optimum Performance.   A child's performance must be judged as the best of which the child is capable. Results obtained when a child is tired, hungry, bored, frightened, ill, or under the influence of medications cannot be considered reliable or valid.

Parental Input.   Parents provide important, useful information about their child's normal behavior and should be present during the screening. Their input also helps to determine whether the child's development is steady, accelerating, or slowing.

Gross Motor Development versus Fine Motor Development.   Assessment of large muscle development is less significant for overall evaluation than assessment of fine motor development. For example, developmentally delayed infants often sit and walk at appropriate ages; however, their use of their hands, especially the pincer grasp, is a much more reliable indicator of overall development.

IMPLICATIONS FOR NURSES

To ensure the child's best performance, nurses must first establish rapport and create a comfortable screening environment. The test should be administered in a comfortably warm room with the child dressed, but with restrictive clothing and shoes removed. Test materials should be located where the child can easily reach them. Only materials that are being used immediately for testing should be available to the child. All other materials should be out of sight. Young children may be held, but they should be able to rest their elbows on the testing table to manipulate objects.

Nurses should avoid making prejudgments about how a child will perform on the tests based on the child's or the parents' physical appearance. It is important to avoid being misled by a child's charm, facial features, small or large size, handicap, or oddly shaped head. Children should be given every opportunity to perform to the best of their ability.

As the testing progresses, it is important to avoid causing unnecessary worry in parents. Doubts should not be expressed until the screener is certain that the child should be seen for further evaluation. The slightest suggestion of concern, which may be communicated by even a casual facial expression, can create unnecessary concern and diminished trust. The role of the nurse is to gather valid assessment data, determine deviations from normal, make appropriate referrals, and provide support. Diagnosing developmental delay is a function of other health care professionals.

At the completion of the DDST-II, the nurse should ask the parents if the child acted in a normal and expected manner. If the parent responds negatively, the evaluation should be rescheduled. When explaining the results, emphasis should be placed on the items the child passed, those items the child failed but was not expected to pass, and finally those items the child failed and was expected to pass. Answer the parent's questions and if indicated refer for additional developmental testing.

The Nurse's Role in Promoting Optimal Growth and Development

Nurses are particularly concerned with preventing disease and promoting health. One aspect of preventive care is providing anticipatory guidance or basic information for parents about normal growth and development as their child reaches different age levels.

Brazelton (1992) describes "touchpoints" as predictable times during which health care professionals can reach into a family system and, through supportive help, diminish or prevent problems. These points generally occur just before a growth or developmental spurt in which the child's behavior changes and the parents' normal modes of handling behavior do not work. During these periods, the child becomes difficult to understand. The nurse can anticipate these predictable periods, which also provide a window of opportunity to offer information about normal growth and development as well as practical interventions to prevent problems characteristic of that age. Age-appropriate topics for anticipatory guidance are discussed further in the chapters on specific age groups.

ADMINISTERING THE DENVER DEVELOPMENTAL SCREENING TEST II

• • • • • • •

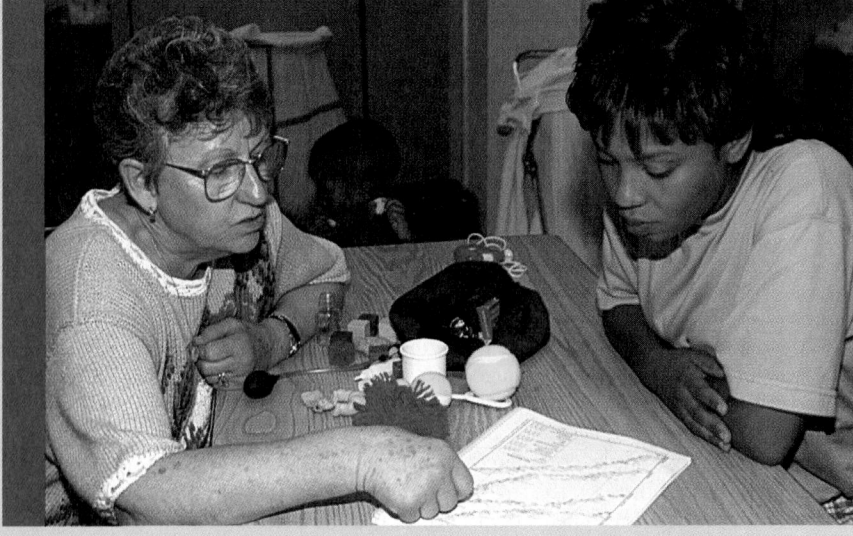

TeVonte ("T") is visiting the clinic for preventive health care shortly after his third birthday. The nurse will administer a Denver Developmental Screening Test II (DDST-II) to evaluate his development in each of four areas: personal-social, fine-motor-adaptive, language, and gross motor.

Before beginning T's DDST-II screening test, the nurse explains its purpose to his mother, Monifa Lee. The test assesses the child's performance of various age-appropriate tasks. The nurse emphasizes to the mother that the DDST-II is not an IQ test but rather compares her child's development with that of other children of the same age.

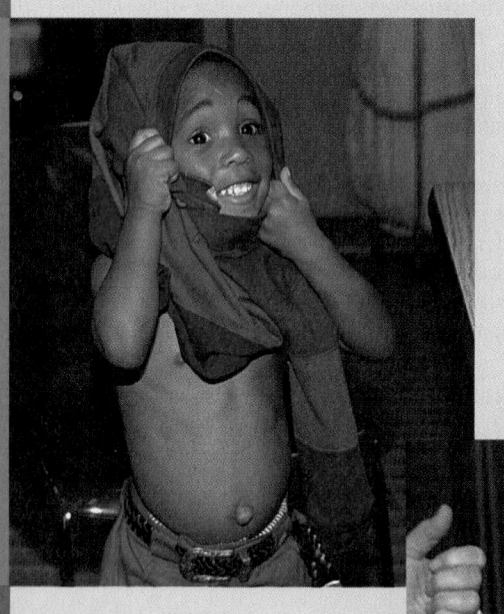

After verifying T's age, the nurse begins the test with personal-social items. After helping him remove his shirt, the nurse asks T to put it back on. T pulls the shirt over his head, then slips each arm into a sleeve.

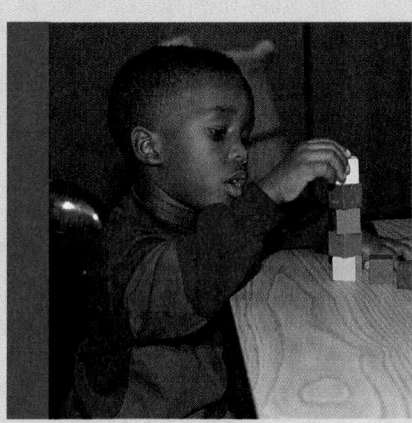

Colored cubes are used to evaluate T's ability to name colors and to build a tower. T is building a tower of eight blocks, which allows the tester to evaluate his fine-motor-adaptive development.

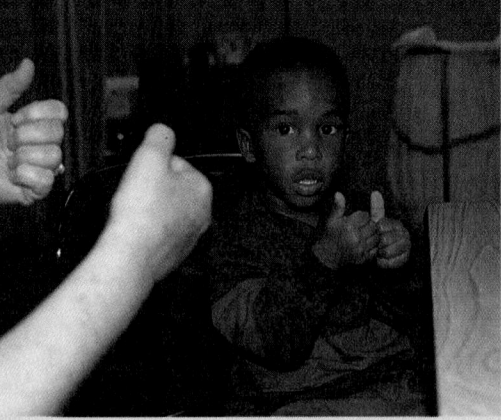

The nurse shows T how to wiggle his thumbs. T passes this part of the test because he keeps his fists closed and wiggles only his thumbs.

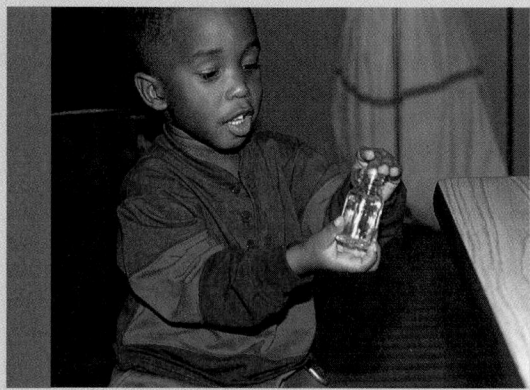

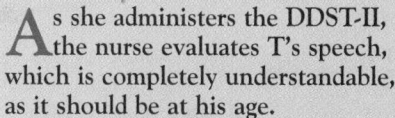
s she administers the DDST-II, the nurse evaluates T's speech, which is completely understandable, as it should be at his age.

An additional part of the language section of the test is to identify at least four of the pictures printed in the test manual. T correctly names the dog as well as the other objects.

T plays with a raisin in a jar as part of the fine-motor screening. The nurse observes to see whether T will pick up the raisin using his thumb and forefinger. T is really more interested in eating the raisin!

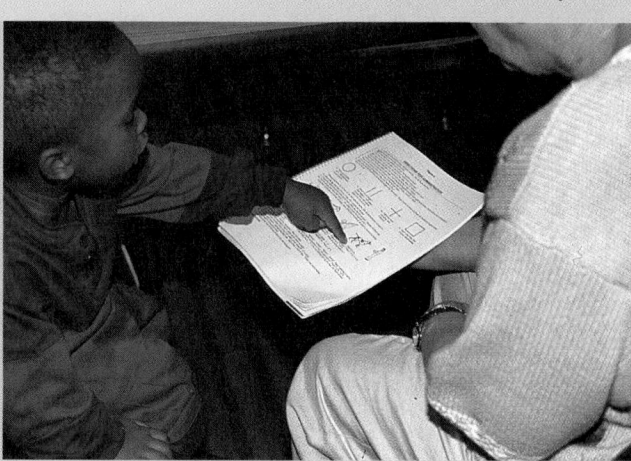

A s the nurse shows T how to hop, he hops quickly in response. T's expression shows that he enjoys the gross motor part of the DDST-II.

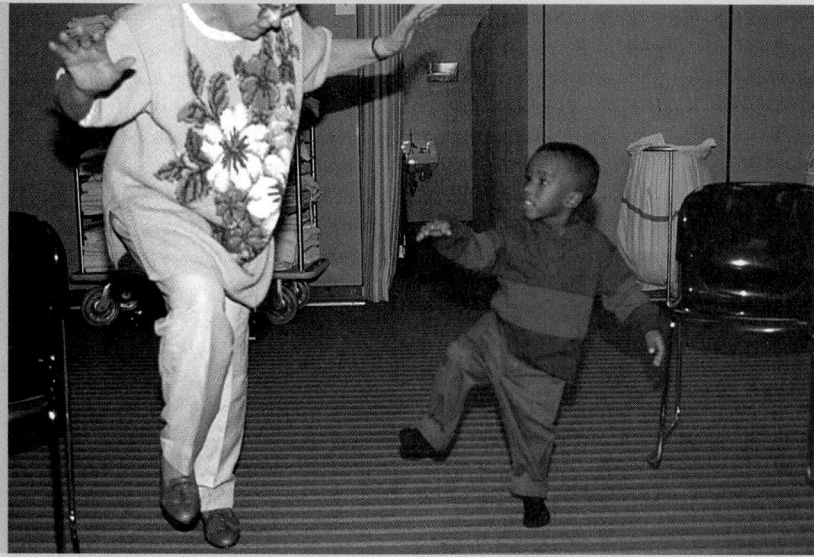

T eVonte shows the nurse that he can balance on each foot for 3 seconds. Note that he is effectively using his arms to help maintain his balance.

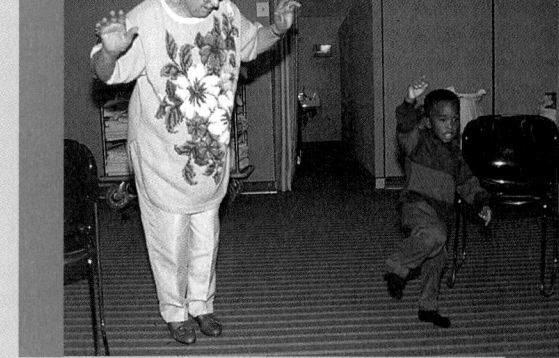

After completing the DDST-II, the nurse shares the results with T's mother. The screening indicates that T's development is appropriate for his age. The nurse recommends that TeVonte continue to have well-child screenings each year, including a DDST-II up to the age of 6 years.

The Developmental Assessment

Nursing care for children is not complete without addressing the developmental issues that are unique to each child. Because children grow and change rapidly, the nurse must use knowledge of theories of growth and development to create plans of care for both healthy and ill children. Assessment data are collected from a variety of sources, categorized, and analyzed with a theoretical knowledge base and clinical experience. A list of strengths and problems related to growth and development is generated. Nursing diagnoses are formulated with individualized goals, interventions, and evaluation to address specific problems that are related to, but differ from, physiologic and psychosocial needs.

Assessment

During the initial interview, the nurse asks questions about the child's cognitive, language, motor, and emotional development. The parents' emotional state, level of education, and culture must be considered when information is gathered. The nurse might use the following questions and statements when interviewing the parents of a 4-year-old child.

- What does the child like to do at home?
- Does the child know the days of the week?
- Describe the child's typical day.
- Does the child attend preschool?
- Can the child throw a ball, ride a tricycle, climb?
- Can the child draw pictures, color them?
- How effective is the child's use of language?
- How did development progress during infancy and toddlerhood?

The nurse also assesses the child's ability to think through situations and to communicate verbally. How the child interacts with other children and adults can also be a measure of cognitive abilities. The number, type, length, appropriateness, and correct use of words and sentences are also noted. Careful observation of the child in a variety of situations, including play, provides valuable information about cognitive development.

A child's stage of emotional development can be assessed in a number of ways. From Erikson's theory, it is expected that the major conflict of a 4-year-old would be developing a sense of initiative rather than a sense of guilt. If the child is hospitalized, however, regressive behaviors might be exhibited if the anxiety of hospitalization becomes overwhelming. Questions directed to the parents, such as those that follow, could help validate inferences about the child's psychosocial development.

- What types of play activities does the child like best?
- How does the child get along with other children? With adults?
- How does the child usually handle stressful situations?
- What do you do to help your child cope with problems?
- How does the child's ability to cope compare with your other children?
- Is the behavior exhibited the child's usual behavior?

The nurse can also obtain valuable information from careful observation of a child who is hospitalized. The nurse should note how the child deals with pain, intrusive procedures, and separation from parents.

Play

Although play is not work in the traditional sense, it is the work of children. Play is those tasks, done to amuse oneself, that have behavioral, social, or psychomotor rewards. To adult observers, children's play may appear unorganized, meaningless, and even chaotic. Anyone who watches carefully, however, quickly discovers that play is a rich activity, intricately woven with meaning and purpose. In adulthood, work is any activity during which one uses time and energy to create a product or achieve a goal. Play in childhood is similar to adult work in that it is undertaken by the child to accomplish developmental tasks and master the environment.

Play is also an important part of the developmental process. Play is how children learn about shape, color, cause and effect, and themselves. In addition to cognitive thinking, play helps the child learn social interaction and psychomotor skills. It is a way of communicating joy, fear, sorrow, and anxiety.

CLASSIFICATIONS OF PLAY

Piaget (1962) described three types of play that relate to periods of sensorimotor, preoperational, and concrete operational functioning:

Practice play, which is also known as functional or sensorimotor play, involves repetitive muscle movements and the introduction of a deliberate complication into the way of doing something. Children who are running, gathering, dumping, and manipulating objects are displaying practice play (Ross, 1997).

Symbolic play, as its name suggests, uses games and interactions that represent an issue or concern to be addressed. Garvey (1979) identified three elements of symbolic play: one or more objects, a theme or plan, and roles. As children play, they incorporate some object (a syringe), use a theme (getting an injection), and then play the roles each player will have (child, nurse). Because there are no rules in symbolic play, the child can use this play not only to reinforce or learn the good things in life, but also to alter those things that are painful.

Games include rules and usually are played by more than one person, although some games can be played by oneself. For example, the card game solitaire is played by one person, as are many video games. Games with rules rarely occur before age 4 years and are most common with the school-age child (Piaget, 1962). Games continue throughout life as adults play board games, cards, and sports.

Through games children learn to play by the rules and to take turns. One common way children accomplish this is through board games. Young children often make up games with unique sets of rules, which may change each time the game is played. Older children have games with specific rules; younger children tend to change the rules.

SOCIAL ASPECTS OF PLAY

As the child develops, there is more interaction with people. Certain types of play are associated with, but not limited to, specific age groups.

Solitary Play. Solitary play is characterized by independent play (Fig. 4–2). The child plays alone with toys that are very different from those chosen by other children in the area. This type of play begins in infancy and is common in toddlers because of their limited social, cognitive, and physical skills. It is important for children in all age groups, however, to have some time to play by themselves.

Parallel Play. Parallel play is usually associated with toddlers, although it can be found in any age group. Children play side by side with similar toys, but there is a lack of group activity.

Associative Play. Associative play is characterized by group play without group goals. Children in this type of play do not set group rules, and although they may all be playing with the same types of toys and may even trade toys, there is a lack of formal organization. This type of play can begin during toddlerhood and continue into the preschool age.

Cooperative Play. Cooperative play begins in the late preschool years. This type of play is organized and has group goals. There is usually at least one leader, and children are definitely in or out of the group.

Onlooker Play. Onlooker play is present when the child observes others playing. Although the child may ask questions of the players, there is no attempt to join the play (see Fig. 4–2). This type of play usually starts during the toddler years but can be observed at any age.

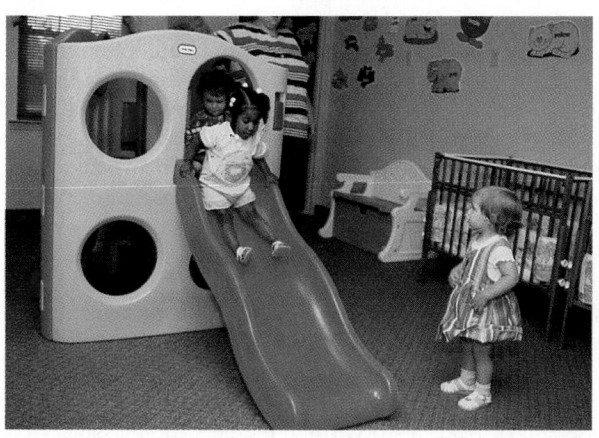

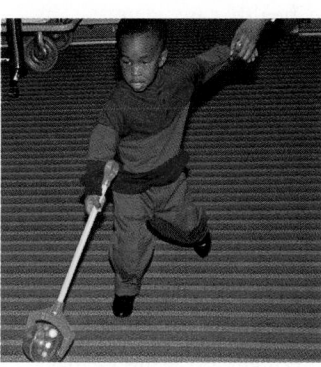

◀ When engaging in solitary play, the child is playing apart from other children and with different types of toys. (Courtesy of The University of Texas at Arlington School of Nursing, Arlington, Texas.)

The little girl at right demonstrates onlooker play. She is interested in what is going on and observes another girl playing on the slide, but she makes no attempt to join the youngster on the slide.

Playing safely with medical equipment (familiarization play) lessens its unfamiliarity to the child and can allay fears. A less fearful child is likely to be more cooperative and less traumatized by necessary care. (Courtesy of The University of Texas at Arlington School of Nursing, Arlington, Texas.) ▶

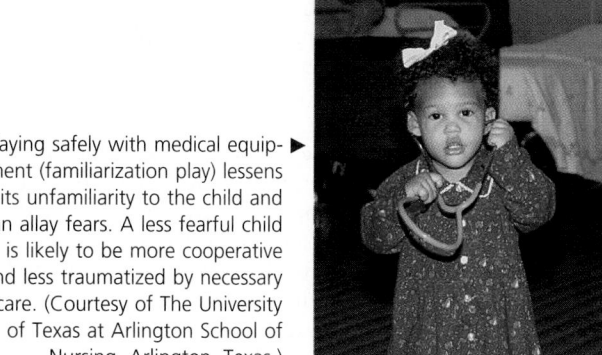

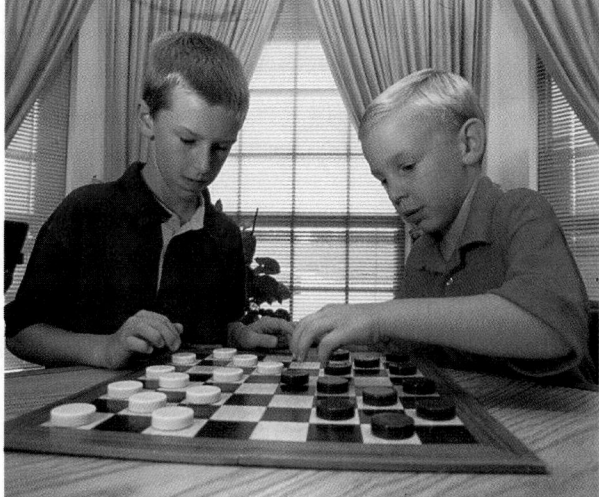

Games with rules, such as board games, help children learn boundaries, teamwork, taking turns, and competition. (Courtesy of Cook Children's Medical Center, Fort Worth, Texas.)

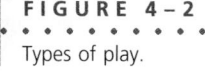

FIGURE 4–2
• • • • • • • • •
Types of play.

TYPES OF PLAY

Dramatic Play. Dramatic play allows children to act out roles and experiences that may have happened to them, that they fear will happen, or that they have observed in others. This type of play can be spontaneous or guided, and it often includes medical or nursing equipment. It is especially valuable for children who have or will experience multiple procedures or hospitalizations.

Hospitals and clinics with child life specialists on staff usually have a medical play area as part of the activity room. Nurses may provide opportunities for spontaneous as well as guided dramatic play. The nurse may choose to observe spontaneous play or be an active participant with the child. There will be occasions when nurses will want to structure the dramatic play to review a specific treatment or procedure. In guided play situations, the nurse directs the focus of the play. Specialized play kits may be developed for specific procedures, such as central line care, casting, bone marrow aspirations, lumbar punctures, and surgery, using supplies related to the hospital or clinic setting.

Familiarization Play. Familiarization play allows children to handle and explore health care materials in nonthreatening and fun ways (see Fig. 4–2). This type of play is especially helpful for, but not limited to, preparing children for procedures and the whole experience of hospitalization.

Examples of familiarization activities include using sponge mouth swabs as painting and gluing tools; making jewelry from Band-Aids, tape, gauze, and lid tops; creating mobiles and collages with health care supplies; making finger puppets using plaster casting material; filling a basin with water and using tubing, syringes, medicine cups, and bulb syringes for water play; decorating beds, wheelchairs, and IV poles with health care supplies; and using syringes for painting activities.

FUNCTIONS OF PLAY

Play enhances the child's growth and development. Some of the more common functions of play are physical development, cognitive development, emotional development, social development, and moral development.

Physical Development. Play aids in the development of both fine and gross motor activity. Children repeat certain body movements purely for pleasure, and these movements in turn aid in the development of body control. For example, an infant will first hit at a rattle, then will attempt to grasp it, and eventually will be able to pick up that same rattle. Next the infant will shake the rattle or perhaps bring it to the mouth.

The parent and child may make a game of repeating sounds such as "ma ma" or "da da," which increases the child's language ability. Repeating rhymes and songs can be a fun way for children to increase their vocabulary. Children love to color on a paper with a crayon and will scribble before being able to draw pictures and to color. This aids the child in eventually learning how to write letters and numerals.

Cognitive Development. Play is a key element in the cognitive development of children. Once a child has learned a general concept, further experiences with that concept expand from that beginning knowledge. Piaget gave the example of an infant learning to swing an object and then subsequently swinging other objects (Piaget, 1962). This could apply, for example, to things to be eaten, read, or ridden. Progression takes place as the child begins to have certain experiences and to test beliefs and to understand the surrounding world.

Children can increase their problem-solving abilities through games and puzzles. Pretend play can stimulate several types of learning. Language abilities are strengthened as the child models significant others in role-playing. The child must organize thoughts and be able to communicate with others involved in the play scenario. Children who play "house" create elaborate details of what the characters do and say.

Children also increase their understanding of size, shape, and texture through play. They begin to understand relationships as they attempt to put a square peg into a round hole, for example. Books and videos increase a child's vocabulary while increasing understanding of the world.

Emotional Development. Children who are experiencing an anxiety-producing situation are often helped through role-playing. Play can be a way of coping with emotional conflict. Play can be a way to determine what is real and what is not. Children may escape through play into a world of fantasy and make-believe in order to make sense out of a sometimes senseless world. Play can also increase a child's self-awareness as an event or situation is explored through role-playing or symbolic play.

As significant others in a child's life respond to the child's initiation of play, the child begins to learn that he or she is important and cared for. Whether the play is initiated by the child or the adult, when a significant person plays a board game with a child, shares a bike ride, plays baseball, or reads a story, the child gets the message, "You are more important than any other thing at this time." The child's self-esteem is increased.

Social Development. The newborn cannot distinguish self from others and therefore is narcissistic. As the infant begins to play with others and things, a realization of self and others begins to develop. The infant begins to experience the joy of interacting with others and soon initiates behavior that involves others. Infants discover that when they coo, their mothers coo back. Children will soon expect this response and make a game of playing with their mothers.

Playing make-believe aids the child in trying on different roles. When the child plays "restaurant" or "hospital," the rules that govern these settings are experimented with.

Of course, most games, from board games to sports, involve interaction with others. The child learns boundaries, taking turns, teamwork, and competition. Children also learn how to negotiate with different personalities and the feelings associated with winning and losing. They learn to share and to take turns (see Fig. 4–2).

Moral Development. When children engage in play with their peers and their families, they begin to learn which behaviors are acceptable and which are not. Quickly they learn that taking turns is rewarded and cheating is not. Group play assists the child in recognizing the importance of teamwork, sharing, and being aware of the feelings of others.

Health Promotion

Immunizations

Immunizations are effective in decreasing and, in some cases, eliminating childhood infectious diseases. Smallpox has been virtually eliminated, and the incidence of diphtheria, pertussis, tetanus, measles, mumps, rubella, and poliomyelitis has greatly declined in the United States. The incidence of diseases caused by *Hemophilus influenzae* type b (Hib) has been reduced by 95%. This pathogen was responsible for serious bacterial infections in infants and children (Dashefsky, 1999).

OBSTACLES TO IMMUNIZATIONS

Major reasons identified for low immunization rates during health care visits include providers who lack knowledge regarding contraindications to immunizations and providers who are unwilling to administer multiple vaccines. Other reasons are inadequate access to medical care and the lack of public knowledge regarding immunizations (Bell et al., 1997; Dashefsky, 1999; Udovic et al., 1998). Finally, in the 1980s the safety of the pertussis portion of the diphtheria-tetanus-pertussis (DPT) vaccine was questioned. Some parents elected not to immunize their children, which resulted in an increase in pertussis cases. Medical concern has led to the development of the accellular pertussis vaccine, which has fewer side effects (American Academy of Pediatrics Committee on Infectious Diseases [AAPCID], 1996, 1997a).

INFORMED CONSENT

The National Childhood Vaccine Injury Act of 1986 requires that the benefits and risks associated with immunizations be discussed with parents prior to immunizations. The act also requires that families receive vaccine information statements (VISs) prior to immunization.

All health care providers who administer immunizations are required by federal law to provide general information about immunizations to the child and parents, preferably in the family's native language. Before providers administer a vaccine, parents should read the federally required information about that vaccine and have the opportunity to ask questions. The providers must use either the VISs or a handout that provides all required information (AAPCID, 1997c). It is necessary that the parents feel comfortable with the information, as well as with the answers to any questions. It has been shown that the VISs do increase the knowledge level of the parents and are beneficial. Providing the information before scheduled vaccinations allows parents the time to read all the information. Providers are encouraged to obtain written informed consent for each vaccine administered. If signatures are not obtained, the patient's medical record should document that the vaccine information was reviewed.

IMMUNIZATION SCHEDULE

Recommendations regarding vaccinations in the United States are made by the Advisory Committee on Immunization Practices (ACIP) of the Centers for Disease Control, the American Academy of Pediatrics (AAP) Committee on Infectious Diseases, and the American Academy of Family Physicians (AAFP) each January.

All states require immunizations for children enrolled in licensed child care programs and school. Some states further require immunizations in the upper grades and at the time of college entrance. One group of children who may be overlooked are those who receive home schooling. It is of utmost importance, therefore, that immunization records be traced and that vaccinations be given over the course of the fewest visits possible. State requirements can be obtained from each state health department. Appendix F outlines the current recommendations for immunization of healthy children in the United States.

CHILDREN WITH AN UNCERTAIN HISTORY OF IMMUNIZATION

When a lapse in immunization occurs, the entire series does not have to be restarted. Charts of children should be flagged to remind health care providers of the immunization status of these children. For children of unknown or uncertain immunization status, appropriate immunization should be administered. Readministration of measles, mumps, and rubella (MMR) vaccine, Hib vaccine, oral poliovirus (OPV) vaccine, or hepatitis B vaccine to someone who is immune has no harmful effects. For children older than 7 years, the tetanus-diphtheria (Td) vaccine rather than the diphtheria-tetanus-pertussis (DTP) vaccine should be administered (AAPCID, 1997c).

International adoptees, refugees, and exchange students should be immunized according to recommended schedules for healthy infants and children. If written records of prior immunization are not available, the child begins the schedule for children not immunized during infancy. Table 4–2 presents recommendations for immunizing children who were not immunized during infancy.

Barriers to Immunization

Complexity of the health care system, which may lead to a delay in vaccinating children when parents become confused or frustrated with the health care system. Special barriers include

- Appointment-only clinics
- Excessively long waiting periods
- Inconvenient scheduling
- Inaccessible clinic sites
- The need for formal referral from a primary health care provider
- Language and cultural barriers

Expense of immunization services.

Parental misconceptions about disease severity, vaccine efficiency and safety, complications, and contraindications.

Inaccurate record-keeping by parents and health care workers.

Reluctance of the health care worker to give more than two vaccines during the same visit.

Lack of public awareness of the need for immunizations.

TABLE 4-2
• • • • • • • • • • •

Recommended Immunization Schedules for Children Not Immunized in the First Year of Life*

Recommended Time/Age	Immunization(s)†‡	Comments
Younger Than 7 Years		
First visit	DTaP (or DTP), Hib,‡ HBV, MMR, OPV‖	If indicated, tuberculin testing may be done at same visit. If child is 5 years of age or older, Hib is not indicated in most circumstances.
Interval after first visit		
1 mo (4 wk)	DTaP (or DTP), HBV, Var*	The second dose of OPV may be given if accelerated poliomyelitis vaccination is necessary, such as for travelers to areas where polio is endemic.
2 mo	DTaP (or DTP), Hib,‡ OPV§	Second dose of Hib is indicated only if the first dose was received when younger than 15 months.
≥8 mo	DTaP (or DTP), HBV, OPV§	OPV and HBV are not given if the third doses were given earlier.
Age 4–6 yr (at or before school entry)	DTaP (or DTP), OPV,§ MMR	DTaP (or DTP) is not necessary if the fourth dose was given after the fourth birthday; OPV is not necessary if the third dose was given after the fourth birthday.
7–12 Years		
First visit	HBV, MMR, Td, OPV	
Interval after first visit		
2 mo (8 wk)	HBV, MMR, Var,‖ Td, OPV§	OPV also may be given 1 month after the first visit if accelerated poliomyelitis vaccination is necessary.
8–14 mo	HBV, Td, OPV§	OPV is not given if the third dose was given earlier.

* Table is not completely consistent with all package inserts. For products used, also consult manufacturer's package insert for instructions on storage, handling, dosage, and administration. Biologics prepared by different manufacturers may vary, and package inserts of the same manufacturer may change from time to time. Therefore, the physician should be aware of the contents of the current package insert.

    Vaccine abbreviations: HBV indicates hepatitis B virus vaccine; Var, varicella vaccine; DTP, diphtheria and tetanus toxoids and pertussis vaccine; DTaP, diphtheria and tetanus toxoids and acellular pertussis vaccine; Hib, *Hemophilus influenzae* type b conjugate vaccine; OPV, oral poliovirus vaccine; IPV, inactivated poliovirus vaccine; MMR, live measles-mumps-rubella vaccine; Td, adult tetanus toxoid (full dose) and diphtheria toxoid (reduced dose), for children ≥7 years and adults.

† If all needed vaccines cannot be administered simultaneously, priority should be given to protecting the child against those diseases that pose the greatest immediate risk. In the United States, these diseases for children younger than 2 years usually are measles and *Hemophilus influenzae* type b infection; for children older than 7 years, they are measles, mumps, and rubella. Before 13 years of age, immunity against hepatitis B and varicella should be ensured.

‡ DTaP, HBV, Hib, MMR, and Var can be given simultaneously at separate sites if failure of the child to return for future immunizations is a concern.

§ IPV is also acceptable; however, for infants and children starting vaccination late (i.e., after 6 months of age), OPV is preferred in order to complete an accelerated schedule with a minimum number of injections.

‖ Varicella vaccine can be administered to susceptible children any time after 12 months of age.

From American Academy of Pediatrics Committee on Infectious Diseases. (1997). *Report of the Committee on Infectious Diseases*. Elk Grove, IL: American Academy of Pediatrics.

When taking an immunization history, the nurse should avoid asking the question, "Are your child's immunizations up to date?" This question will frequently be answered with a yes, but that does not give the nurse sufficient information. The nurse may gain more information by asking, "Can you tell me when and what was the last immunization your child had?"

ADMINISTRATION OF VACCINES

The manufacturer's packaging insert for each vaccine includes recommendations for handling, storage, administra-

tion site, dosage, and route. Personnel responsible for handling vaccines should be familiar with storage requirements to minimize the risk of vaccine failures. When multidose vials are used, sterile technique should be used to prevent contamination. To ensure safe administration, the vaccines should be given by the recommended route. In children whose gluteal muscle has not yet developed (those younger than 2 years), the preferred site for intramuscular (IM) injections is the anterolateral aspect of the thigh. The deltoid muscle can be used in children 18 months and older. The ventrogluteal site may be used in older children (see Chapter 38). Vaccines given by IM administration need to be

• • • • • • • • • •
Nursing Responsibility in Administering Vaccines

- Know the recommended immunization schedule and the recommended alternative schedule for those with lapsed immunizations or unknown immunization history.
- Acquire up-to-date information because recommendations are revised frequently.
- Assess the family's beliefs and values to assist in the education of the family as to the rationale for immunizations, the risks and side effects, and the risks of nonimmunization.
- Take a careful history to determine possible contraindications or precautions, and report any pertinent information to the practitioner. Educate the family as to the rationale for any contraindications.
- "Gloves are not required when administering vaccinations unless the persons who administer the vaccine will come in contact with potentially infectious body fluids or have open lesions" (AAPCID, 1997).
- Some vaccines come mixed in one syringe (e.g., DTP-Hib). Other vaccines should not be mixed. Check manufacturer's recommendations.
- Administer vaccines according to the manufacturer's recommended sites.

- Aspirate to make sure that the needle has not been placed in a blood vessel.
- Wash hands before vaccine administration and between children.
- Review with the parents common side effects and the signs of potential severe reactions that warrant contacting the practitioner.
- Administer prophylactic acetaminophen before or shortly after administration of DTP or DTaP. Instruct the parents to continue age-appropriate dosing every 4 to 6 hours for at least 24 hours.
- For painful or red injection sites, apply cold compresses for the first 24 hours, then use warm or cold compresses as long as needed.
- Give multiple administrations in different sites and record those sites in the medical record.
- Document parental consent in the medical record. Documentation should also include the type of vaccine, date of administration, manufacturer and lot number, expiration date, administration site, any data pertinent to risks and side effects, and the signature and title of the person administering the immunization.

injected deep into the muscle mass to avoid irritation and possible necrosis.

More than one immunization may be administered at the same age or time. Some vaccines, such as DTP and MMR, are given as a multiple vaccine. When more than one injection is to be given, vaccines should be administered using separate syringes, not mixed into one. They should be given at different sites (preferably in different thighs), and the site used for each vaccine should be recorded in order to identify possible reactions.

PRECAUTIONS AND CONTRAINDICATIONS
The main purpose of vaccination is to achieve immunity with the fewest possible side effects. Most vaccines have no side effects; when side effects do occur, they are usually mild. Fever and local irritation are common after administration of DTP vaccine, and fever and rash can occur 1 to 2 weeks after administration of live-virus measles vaccine.

Some severe side effects have been reported, however. These events are usually not predictable. There are reported cases of healthy children developing paralytic polio after administration of OPV. Reactions to the MMR vaccine

• • • • • • • • • •
Common Misconceptions About Administration and Safety of Vaccines

The following conditions or circumstances are *not* contraindications to the administration of vaccines:

- Mild acute illness with low-grade fever or mild diarrhea in an otherwise healthy child
- A reaction to a previous dose of DTP vaccine with only soreness, redness, or swelling in the immediate vicinity of the injection site

have included anaphylactic reactions, both in children with and in those without a history of egg allergy. This has prompted consideration of other possible causative agents. For instance, the MMR vaccine contains neomycin, which may be the cause of the sensitivity.

Before a second dose of any vaccine is given, it should be ascertained whether any side effects or possible reactions occurred after the previous dose. The National Childhood Vaccine Injury Act of 1986 requires health care providers who administer vaccines to maintain permanent vaccination records and to report occurrences of certain adverse events stipulated in the act. Anaphylaxis or anaphylactic shock and encephalopathy are examples of two reportable events associated with the tetanus and pertussis vaccines. Providers administering immunizations must be aware of reportable events and comply with the provisions of the act.

IMMUNOCOMPROMISED CHILDREN
Children who are immunologically compromised should not receive live bacterial or viral vaccines (e.g., OPV, MMR, or varicella vaccine). There are some exceptions related to children with human immunodeficiency virus (HIV) and in some specific instances of children in remission from cancer. Siblings and other household contacts of children who are immunocompromised should not receive OPV vaccine because the vaccine strains are transmissible. MMR vaccine can be given because the MMR vaccine does not shed the viruses.

EDUCATION
Immunization is a critical component of a child's health care. Knowledge of immunization schedules and an awareness of potential delays will aid the health care provider in identifying children who have not been fully immunized. Health care providers must provide parents with accurate information regarding immunizations, as immunizations are

the primary and safest means of managing preventable infectious diseases.

Nutrition

To provide care for infants and children, the nurse must have an understanding of the nutritional needs of the body. The body is nourished by food. Foods are comprised of six basic *nutrients*: carbohydrates, fats, proteins, water, vitamins, and minerals. Carbohydrates, fats, and proteins provide energy, which is required by the cells of the body to transport all substances across the cell membrane, to synthesize substances within the cell, and to dispose of waste products.

CARBOHYDRATES

Carbohydrates should be the major dietary source of energy. Foods that are good sources of carbohydrates are relatively inexpensive and easily obtained. Insufficient calorie intake causes the body to break down protein and fat for energy and glucose production. There is no recommended dietary allowance for carbohydrates. The National Research Council recommends that after infancy, at least 50% to 60% of the energy requirement should be provided by carbohydrates, especially complex carbohydrates (Food and Nutrition Board, 1989). Most *complex carbohydrates* are found in starch from cereal grains, roots, vegetables, and legumes. The more mature the vegetable, the higher the starch content.

FATS

Fats should serve as the secondary source of energy by providing 30% or less of daily calorie intake. Of this amount, 10% should be saturated, 10% polyunsaturated, and 10% monounsaturated fatty acids. Dietary fat allows the absorption of the fat-soluble vitamins (A, D, E, and K) and adds flavor to foods. The layer of fat beneath the skin plays a role in regulating body temperature. Fat is a component of cell membranes and acts as a protective padding of the internal organs. When excess calories are consumed, dietary fats are stored as excess body fat.

PROTEINS

Dietary *protein* is necessary for building and maintaining body tissues. Proteins are involved in homeostasis by working with other elements in the blood to maintain fluid balance. Many vitamins and minerals are bound to protein carriers for transport. Proteins, as antibodies, aid in the regulation of the body's immune system.

WATER

Water is essential for life. It transports nutrients to cells and waste products away from the cells. It assists in the regulation of body temperature and in chemical reactions. Water lubricates joints and provides form and structure to the cells and the medium for body fluids. Water is found in most foods, including solids. Water requirements can be estimated by a variety of methods. The child's activity level and ambient temperature influence the amount of water needed.

VITAMINS AND MINERALS

Vitamins and *minerals* are necessary in the regulation of metabolic processes. They are present in a wide variety of foods. Vitamins and minerals are added to processed formulas and to other foods such as cereals. It is generally not necessary for children to receive supplementation after infancy unless they are at nutritional risk (e.g., have anorexia or a chronic disease).

DIETARY GUIDELINES

Food Guide Pyramid. The guidelines for a healthful diet for Americans age 2 years or older were published by the United States Department of Agriculture (USDA) in 1992. The guidelines recommend that a variety of foods be eaten to get the energy, proteins, vitamins, minerals, and fiber needed for good health. The diet should be low in fat, saturated fat, and cholesterol. There should be ample vegetables, fruits, and grain products to provide needed vitamins, minerals, fiber, and complex carbohydrates. Sugars, salt, and sodium should be used in moderation.

Dietary Guidelines for Americans

- Eat a variety of foods.
- Maintain desirable weight.
- Avoid too much fat, saturated fat, and cholesterol.
- Eat foods with adequate starch and fiber.
- Avoid too much sugar.
- Avoid too much sodium.

Note: These guidelines apply to children age 2 years and older. Adapted from guidelines issued by the United States Department of Agriculture and the Department of Health and Human Services.

The Food Guide Pyramid was developed by the USDA to show what should be eaten each day (see Fig. 15–2). The pyramid focuses on eating a variety of foods to get the required nutrients and adequate energy. The importance of grains, fruits, and vegetables is evident in the pyramid.

Energy, Calories, and Servings. *Energy* is measured in calories. Energy or calorie needs depend on the person's age, sex, height, weight, and level of physical activity. Table 4–3 shows the recommended dietary allowances (RDAs) for energy and protein for children. Recommended dietary allowances are used as an assessment guide, and their use should be limited to healthy infants and children. Very active children and those going through rapid growth spurts have higher energy needs than more sedate children or those who are in periods when growth is slower.

CULTURAL AND RELIGIOUS INFLUENCES ON DIET

Dietary intake is profoundly affected by both cultural and religious beliefs. An understanding of these patterns will assist the nurse in both the assessment and implementation of nutrition-related behaviors. Hospitalized children who become stressed by being in a new and strange environment do not need the added stress of unfamiliar foods. Information regarding a child's food preferences can be obtained during a dietary history.

A child's religious beliefs may also have an impact on the types of foods eaten and the way in which they are served. Within religious groups there may be a variety of

TABLE 4–3

Recommended Dietary Allowances for Energy and Protein

Age	Calories Daily	Calories Per kg	Protein Daily	Protein Per kg
1–3 yr	1,300	102	16 g	1.2
4–6 yr	1,800	90	24 g	1.1
7–10 yr	2,000	70	28 g	1.0
11–14 yr (female)	2,200	47	46 g	
11–14 yr (male)	2,500	55	45 g	

From *Recommended dietary allowances* (ed. 10). Copyright © 1989 by the National Academy of Sciences. Courtesy of the National Academy Press, Washington, DC.

dietary observances. The nurse should assist and encourage the child and the child's family in communicating specific dietary needs.

ASSESSMENT OF NUTRITION

A nutritional assessment is an essential component of the health examination of infants and children. This assessment should include anthropometric data, biochemical data, clinical examination, and dietary history. From these data a plan of care can be developed. In addition, children at risk can be identified and areas of prevention pursued through teaching and further evaluation and follow-up.

Anthropometric Data. *Height* and *head circumference* reflect past nutrition or chronic nutritional problems. Weight, skin fold thickness, and midarm circumference better reflect present nutritional status. The nurse should always be aware of the roles of birth weight and ethnic, familial, and environmental factors when evaluating anthropometric measurements. Infants and children should be measured during each preventive health care visit.

Clinical Evaluation. The clinical evaluation includes a physical examination and complete history. Special attention is paid to the areas where signs of nutritional deficiencies appear: the skin, hair, teeth, gums, lips, tongue, and eyes. Clinical symptoms usually are not by themselves diagnostic but may suggest conditions, which are then confirmed by biochemical tests and diet histories. There may be more than one deficiency. (See also the section on Failure to Thrive in Chapter 53.)

Dietary History. Obtaining an accurate history of dietary intake is difficult. The knowledge that what the child is eating is being recorded can influence what the parent feeds the child or what the child eats. Children often cannot remember what they have eaten. If the child or parent is not committed to the process, incomplete information may be obtained. It is still a useful assessment process, however, and should be used. Patient teaching should include an understanding of the importance of recording the child's dietary intake and the need for accuracy. Common methods of assessing dietary intake include the following:

- 24-hour recall
- Food frequency questionnaire
- Food diary

Twenty-Four-Hour Recall. With the *24-hour recall* method, the child or parent is asked to recall everything the child has eaten in the past 24 hours. A questionnaire may be used, or the nurse may conduct an interview asking the pertinent questions.

The child or parent may have difficulty remembering the kinds and amounts of food eaten. Or, they may have had an atypical day on the previous day or may not feel comfortable relating what was eaten the day being evaluated. How the child or parent sees the nurse may influence the response; they may say what they think the interviewer wants to hear. Asking for information in relation to meals eaten as opposed to food groups may increase the accuracy of the assessment.

Food Frequency Questionnaire. The *food frequency questionnaire* elicits information on the intake of particular foods or food groups on a daily, weekly, or monthly basis. This tool can be used to validate the 24-hour recall data.

As for all methods of assessment, this requires the interviewer to be nonjudgmental and objective. Putting the information into a questionnaire may be less threatening to the child and family and will save time.

Food Diary. When keeping a *food diary*, the child or parent records everything consumed during a specified time period. Various sources recommend different lengths of time for keeping the diary; 3-day to 7-day records may be used. As in all nursing care, the nurse must evaluate what is a reasonable time to expect the family or child to keep the records. The time, place, and people present when the food was eaten may also be recorded. This provides the nurse with additional information, which may identify trends and other information related to the child's eating behaviors.

Safety

Unintentional injury is the most significant but underrecognized public health threat facing children today. Unintentional injury is the leading cause of death in children. Across the ages, motor vehicle traffic injuries and firearm injuries are the two major causes of injury (Guyer et al., 1998).

The number of childhood deaths is staggering, but it is only a fraction of the number of children who are hospitalized and require emergency treatment, and who suffer permanent disability as a result of injury.

The economic burden to society is equally staggering, reaching billions of dollars yearly. What cannot be quantified is the emotional loss, suffering, and pain the child and family must endure once an injury has occurred.

CHILDHOOD INJURIES: ETIOLOGY AND PREVENTION

All children are at risk for injury because of their normal curiosity, impulsiveness, and impatience. Everywhere they venture, they are exposed to potentially hazardous situations.

Injury Prevention. Injury prevention is a relatively new focus of health promotion. The term "accident," with its implied meaning of random chance or lack of responsi-

---

CRITICAL TO REMEMBER

Relationship Between Safety and Childhood Development

Developmentally, children are vulnerable to injury, for the following reasons:

• Children are naturally curious and enjoy exploring their surroundings.
• Children are driven to test and master new skills.
• Children frequently attempt activities before they have developed the cognitive and physical skills required to accomplish the task safely.
• Children often assert themselves and challenge rules.
• Children develop a strong desire for peer approval as they grow older.

What Nurses Can Do to Prevent Childhood Injuries

• Model safety practices in the home, work, and community.
• Educate parents and children through anticipatory safety guidance to help reduce needless injuries.
• Support legislative efforts that advocate prevention measures.
• Collaborate with other health care providers to promote safety and injury prevention.

---

bility, is being replaced with "injury," with its implication that injuries have causes that can be modified to prevent or lessen their frequency and severity. Safety education is a critical component of injury prevention. It increases awareness, attempts to modify human behavior, and reinforces changes implemented through legal mandates (i.e., seat belt laws) or product modification (i.e., crib design, air bags).

Nurses need to become proactive in childhood injury prevention by increasing children's and adults' awareness of safety issues. Nurses who care for children are acutely aware of the devastating effects and complex problems injuries cause. From their experiences, they become well-informed advocates for childhood safety.

Anticipatory Guidance. To be most effective in providing anticipatory safety guidance, nurses must gear educational strategies to the child's level of growth and development. Knowledge of growth and development also helps the nurse understand the risks associated with each age group and choose the educational strategy appropriate to a child's developmental level.

Early in their parenting experience, parents need to know how to provide a safe environment for their children as well as what behaviors they can expect at various developmental levels. Anticipatory guidance builds on the safety principles of the previous stage. Awareness of a child's changing capabilities allows the parent to be more alert and reactive to safety hazards that the child is likely to encounter. This awareness is especially important for first-time parents.

Simply telling parents to "watch your children" or to "childproof" the home, or telling a child to "be careful," has little educational impact. Educational efforts are much more likely to be effective if they focus on specific problems with specific solutions, rather than providing broad or vague advice.

Teaching Strategies. Teaching can be formal or informal, simple or elaborate, as long as it provides relevant safety information and coincides with the child's or parent's cognitive abilities. For children younger than 5 or 6 years, it is advisable to incorporate the parent into the teaching process so that the parents can assist with reinforcement or questions the child later has about the safety issue. With younger children, who are easily distracted, the information should be presented in short sessions.

Many local and national organizations have safety information available for distribution. This information can be used to supplement the teaching process. Prepared materials range from pamphlets, booklets, posters, and audiovisual materials to entire teaching programs that can assist in providing injury prevention education to all age groups. Some programs offer the materials free of cost. See Appendix L for a partial listing of organizations that provide safety information.

KEY CONCEPTS

- Growth, development, maturation, and learning are complex, interrelated processes that produce complicated series of changes in individuals from conception to death.
- Growth and development proceed from simple to complex, proximal to distal, and head to lower extremities.
- As children grow and develop, wide variations within normal limits occur.
- Weight, height, and head circumference, common parameters used to monitor growth, should be measured and evaluated at regular intervals.
- The earlier that delays and deviations from normal are treated, the less severe the effect will be on growth and developmental outcomes.
- Numerous factors, including genetics, environment, culture, nutrition, health status, and family structure, affect how children grow and develop.
- Piaget's theory of cognitive development describes how children learn to deal with their environment through thinking and reasoning. Progress in learning during various periods is based on the child's ability to create patterns of understanding and behavior.
- Freud's psychosexual theory attempts to explain how humans struggle in both conscious and unconscious ways to become individual beings. During each stage of sexual development in children, a different area of the body is the focus of attention and pleasure.
- Erikson's theory of psychosocial development describes a series of crises emerging at specific times and in a particular order. These stages occur throughout life, and each must be resolved for an individual to progress emotionally.
- Kohlberg discusses moral development as a complex process involving progressive acceptance of the values and rules of society in a way that determines behavior. A maturing individual becomes less concerned with avoiding punishment and more interested in human rights and universal justice.
- Language development, a complex process involving extensive neuromuscular maturation, begins as undifferentiated crying at birth and proceeds throughout life to provide a vehicle for communication, thought, and creativity.
- A variety of screening tools, such as the DDST-II, are used by nurses to gain an overall picture of a child's developmental progress and to alert the nurse to potential developmental delays.
- To provide high-quality, developmentally appropriate care to children and parents, nurses must be aware of normal patterns of growth and development.
- Piaget described three types of play, related to periods of sensorimotor, preoperational, and concrete operational functioning: practice play, symbolic play, and games.
- Play enhances the child's growth and development through physical, cognitive, emotional, social, and moral development.
- Personnel who administer and handle vaccines must be aware of recommendations for handling, storing, and administering the vaccines. Special attention should be given to the site of administration, dosage, and route.
- When a lapse in immunization occurs, the entire series does not have to be restarted.
- Children who are immunologically compromised should not receive live bacterial or viral vaccines.
- The six basic nutrients are carbohydrates, protein, fat, vitamins, minerals, and water.
- Components of a nutritional assessment are anthropometric data, biochemical data, clinical examination, and dietary history.
- Many childhood injuries and deaths are predictable and preventable.
- Understanding the developmental milestones of each age group is important for promoting safety awareness for parents, caregivers, and children.

REFERENCES AND READINGS

American Academy of Pediatrics Committee on Infectious Diseases. (1996). The relationship between pertussis vaccine and central nervous system sequelae: Continuing assessment. *Pediatrics, 97*(2), 279–281.
American Academy of Pediatrics Committee on Infectious Diseases. (1997a). Acellular pertussis vaccine: Recommendations for use as the initial series in infants and children. *Pediatrics, 99*(2), 282–288.
American Academy of Pediatrics Committee on Infectious Diseases. (1997b). Immuniza-

tion of adolescents: Recommendations of the Advisory Committee on Immunization Practices, the American Academy of Pediatrics, the American Academy of Family Physicians, and the American Medical Association. *Pediatrics, 99*(3), 479–488.
American Academy of Pediatrics Committee on Infectious Diseases. (1997c). *1997 red book:* Report *of the Committee on Infectious Diseases* (24th ed.). Elk Grove Village, IL: American Academy of Pediatrics.

American Academy of Pediatrics Committee on Infectious Diseases. (1999a). Poliomyelitis prevention: Revised recommendations for use of inactivated and live oral poliovirus vaccines. *Pediatrics, 103*(1), 171–172.
American Academy of Pediatrics Committee on Infectious Diseases. (1999b). Recommended childhood immunization schedule—United States, January–December 1999. *Pediatrics, 103*(1), 182–185.

American Academy of Pediatrics Committee on Nutrition. (1998). *Pediatric nutrition handbook*. Elk Grove Village, IL: American Academy of Pediatrics.

Bear, G. G., Richards, H. C., & J. C. Gibbs. (1997). Sociomoral reasoning and behavior. In G. C. Bear, K. M. Minke, & A. Thomas (Eds.), *Children's needs II: Development, problems and alternatives*. Bethesda, MD: National Association of School Psychologists.

Bell, L. M., Pritchard, M., Anderko, R., & Levenson, R. (1997). A program to immunize hospitalized preschool-aged children: Evaluation and impact. *Pediatrics, 100*(2), 192–196.

Brady, M. (1994). Educating youths and their parents about the prevention of firearm injury. *Journal of Pediatric Health Care, 8*(3), 120–129.

Brazelton, T. B. (1992). *Touchpoints*. Menlo Park, CA: Addison-Wesley.

Cagle, C. S., & Keen-Payne, R. (1996). Health promotion teaching in preschools. *MCN: American Journal of Maternal/Child Health, 21*, 96–99.

Chance, P. (Ed.). (1979). *Learning through play*. New York: Gardner Press.

Colby, A., Kohlberg, L., & Kauffman, K. (1987). Theoretical introduction to the measurement of moral judgement. In A. Colby & L. Kohlberg (Eds.), *The measurement of moral judgement: Vol. 1*. Cambridge, England: Cambridge University Press.

Crain, W. C. (1992). *Theories of development: Concepts and applications*. Englewood Cliffs, NJ: Prentice-Hall.

Dashefsky, B. (1999). Immunization practices. In F. D. Burg, E. R. Wald, J. R. Ingelfinger, & R. A. Polin (Eds.), *Gellis & Kagan's current pediatric therapy*. Philadelphia: Saunders.

Elkind, D. (1970). *Children and adolescents: Interpretive essays on Jean Piaget*. New York: Oxford University Press.

Emde, R. N. (1998). Early emotional development: New modes of thinking for research and intervention. *Pediatrics, 102*(5), 1236–1243.

Erikson, E. H. (1963). *Childhood and society* (2nd ed.). New York: Norton.

Feldman, R. S. (1998). *Child development*. Upper Saddle River, New Jersey: Prentice-Hall.

Flavell, J. (1963). *The developmental psychology of Jean Piaget*. Princeton, NJ: Van Nostrand.

Food and Nutrition Board, National Research Council. (1989). *Recommended dietary allowances* (10th ed.). Washington, DC: National Academy of Sciences.

Ford, C. A., & Coleman, W. L. (1999). Adolescent development and behavior: Implications for the primary care physician. In M. D. Levine, W. B. Carey, & A. C. Crocker (Eds.), *Developmental behavioral pediatrics*. Philadelphia: Saunders.

Frankenburg, W. K., & Dodds, J. B. (1992). *Denver II screening manual*. Denver, CO: Developmental Materials.

Freud, A. (1974). *Introduction to psychoanalysis*. New York: International Universities Press.

Freud, S. (1960). *The ego and the id*. (J. Riviere, Trans.). New York: Norton. (Original work published 1923)

Garvey, C. (1977). *Play*. Cambridge, MA: Harvard University Press.

Garvey, C. (1979). What is play? In P. Chance (Ed.), *Learning through play*. New York: Gardner Press.

Glascoe, F. P., Foster, E. M., & Wolraich, M. L. (1997). An economic analysis of developmental detection methods. *Pediatrics, 99*(6), 830–837.

Guyer, B., MacDorman, M. F., Martin, J. A., Peters, K. D., & Strobino, D. M. (1998). Annual summary of vital statistics—1997. *Pediatrics, 102*(6), 1333–1349.

Immunization Action Coalition/Hepatitis B Coalition (1998). Needle tips and the hepatitis B. *Coalition News, 6*(2), 1–3.

Jost, K. E. (1996). Nursing standards for child development. *MCN: American Journal of Maternal/Child Nursing, 21*, 67–71.

Kelly, D. P., & Sally, J. I. (1999). Disorders of speech and language. In M. D. Levine, W. B. Carey, & A. C. Crocker (Eds.), *Developmental behavioral pediatrics*. Philadelphia: Saunders.

Kohlberg, L. (1964). Development of moral character. In M. Hoffman & L. Hoffman (Eds.), *Review of child development research: Vol. 1*. New York: Russell Sage Foundation.

Kohlberg, L. (1984). *The psychology of moral development*. San Francisco: Harper & Row.

Lampl, M. (1995). Leaps and bounds: How children grow. *Pediatric Basics, 72*, 10–16.

Litt, I. F., & Martin, J. A. (1999). Development of sexuality and its problems. In M. D. Levine, W. B. Carey, & A. C. Crocker (Eds.), *Developmental behavioral pediatrics*. Philadelphia: Saunders.

Melmed, M. E. (1998). Talking with parents about emotional development. *Pediatrics, 102*(5), 1317–1326.

Piaget, J. (1962). *Play, dreams and imitation childhood*. New York: Norton.

Piaget, J. (1967). *Six psychological studies*. New York: Random House.

Richmond, P. G. (1971). *An introduction to Piaget*. New York: Basic Books.

Ross, R. P. (1997). Play. In G. G. Bear, K. M. Minke, & A. Thomas (Eds.), *Children's needs II: Development, problems and alternatives*. Bethesda, MD: National Association of School Psychologists.

Selekman, J. (1998). Infectious diseases and the immunizations of today and tomorrow. *Pediatric Nursing, 24*(4), 309–315.

Sparks, L., & Russell, C. (1998). The new varicella vaccine: Efficacy, safety and administration. *Journal of Pediatric Nursing, 13*(2), 85–94.

Trahms, C. M., & Pipes, P. L. (1997). *Nutrition in infancy and childhood*. New York: WCB/McGraw-Hill.

Udovic, S. L., Lieu, T. A., Black, S. B., Ray, P. M., Ray, G. T., & Shinefield, H. R. (1998). Parent reports on willingness to accept childhood immunizations during urgent care visits. *Pediatrics, 102*(4), e47.

United States Department of Agriculture & United States Department of Health and Human Services. (1992). *Dietary guidelines for Americans*. Hyattsville, MD: US Government Printing Office.

5

The Infant

LEARNING OBJECTIVES

After studying this chapter, you should be able to:

- Describe the physiologic changes that occur during infancy.
- Describe the motor, psychosocial, language, and cognitive development of the infant.
- Discuss common problems of infancy, such as separation anxiety, sleep, irritability, and colic.
- Discuss the importance of immunizations and recommended immunization schedules for infants.
- Provide parents with anticipatory guidance for common concerns during infancy, such as sleep problems, nutrition, play, safety, and immunizations.

DEFINITIONS

asphyxiation   A state of suffocation that severely compromises oxygen delivery to the body.

egocentrism   Complete absorption with self; an inability to understand that others have a different point of view.

mistrust   The negative resolution of the first developmental task, according to Erikson's theory. Mistrust results in acute emotional tension and behavioral signs of unmet needs.

object permanence   The realization that objects continue to exist even though they are out of sight.

parent-infant attachment   A sense of belonging to or connection between a parent and infant.

pincer grasp   The use of index finger and thumb to grip objects.

sensorimotor stage   Piaget's first stage of cognitive development, in which infants and young toddlers use mainly senses and movement to begin to understand and control their environment.

stranger anxiety   The ability of an infant to distinguish between caregivers and others, to prefer parents to other caregivers, and to become distressed when separation occurs.

trust   The basic emotion established during infancy as a result of satisfying interactions between child and caregiver. Trust provides the foundation upon which a healthy personality is built.

During no time after birth does a human being grow and change as dramatically as during infancy. Between the ages of 1 month and 1 year, the infancy period, a child grows and develops from a tiny bundle of physiologic needs to a dynamo capable of locomotion and language, ready to embark on the adventures of the toddler years.

Growth and Development of the Infant

Even though historically adults considered infants unable to do much more than eat and sleep, it is now well documented that even young infants can organize their experiences in meaningful ways and adapt to changes in the envi-ronment. Evidence shows that infants form strong bonds with their caregivers, communicate their needs and wants, and interact socially. By the end of the first year of life, infants can move about on their own, elicit responses from adults, communicate through the use of rudimentary language, and solve simple problems.

Infancy is characterized by the need to establish harmony between the self and the world. To achieve this harmony, the infant needs food, warmth, comfort, oral satisfaction, environmental stimulation, and opportunities for self-exploration and expression. Competent caregivers satisfy the needs of helpless infants, providing a warm, nurturing relationship so that the children experience a sense of trust in the world and in themselves. These challenges make infancy an exciting yet demanding period for both child and parents.

Nurses play an important role in the promotion and maintenance of health in infants. Providing parents with information about immunization, feeding, sleep, safety, and other common concerns is an important nursing responsibility. Nurses are in a good position to offer anticipatory guidance based on the infant's growth and development. Table 5–1 summarizes the growth and development of the infant.

TABLE 5-1

Summary of Growth and Development: The Infant

Physical	Motor	Psychosocial	Sensory/Cognitive	Language/Communication
1–2 Months				
Fast growth; weight gain of 1.5 lb (0.68 kg) per month and height gain of 1 inch (2.54 cm) per month during first 6 months. Upper limbs and head grow faster. Primitive reflexes present; strong suck and gag reflex. Obligate nose breather. Posterior fontanel closes by 8 weeks.	**Gross:** May lift head when held against shoulder. Head lag. **Fine:** Palmar grasp. 1 month: Immediately drops object placed in hand. Fist usually clenched (grasp reflex). 2 months: Holds objects momentarily. Hands often open (grasp reflex fading).	Erikson's stage of trust versus mistrust. Infant learns that world is good and "I am good." This stage is the foundation for other stages. Child is entirely dependent on parents and other caregivers. Needs should be met in a timely fashion. Touch is important.	Piaget's sensorimotor phase. 1 month: Notices bright objects if in line of vision. Vision 20/100. Reflexes dominate behavior. 2 months: Begins to follow objects.	Strong cry. Throaty sounds. Responds to human faces. 6–8 weeks: Begins to smile in response to stimuli.
3 Months				
Primitive reflexes fading.	**Gross:** Can get hand to mouth. Can lift head off bed when in prone position. Head lag still present but decreasing. **Fine:** Holds objects placed in hands. Grasp reflex absent.	Smiles in response to others. Uses sucking to soothe self.	Follows an object with eyes. Plays with fingers.	Babbles, coos. Enjoys making sounds. Responds to voices, watches speaker.

TABLE 5-1
. . . .

Summary of Growth and Development: The Infant Continued

Physical	Motor	Psychosocial	Sensory/Cognitive	Language/ Communication
4–5 Months				
Can breathe when nose is obstructed. Growth rate declines. Drooling begins. Moro, tonic neck, and rooting reflexes have disappeared.	**Gross:** Plays with feet; puts foot in mouth. Bears weight when held in a standing position. Turns from abdomen to back. **Fine:** Begins reaching and grasping with palm. Hits at object, misses.	Mouth is a sensory organ used to explore the environment. Attachment is an ongoing process throughout infancy. Has increased interest in parent, shows trust, knows parent. Shows emotions of fear and anger.	4 months: Brings hands together at midline. Vision 20/80. Begins to play with objects. Recognizes familiar faces. Turns head to locate sounds. Shows anticipation and excitement. Memory span is 5–7 min. Plays with favorite toys.	Crying becomes differentiated. Babbling is common. Begins consonant sounds: *H, N, G, K, P, B* (4 months). Makes vowel sounds: *ee, ah, ooh* (5 months).
6–7 Months				
Weight gain slows to 1 lb (0.45 kg) per month. Length gain of 0.5 inch (1.27 cm) per month. Birth weight doubles; tooth eruption begins; chewing and biting occur. Maternal iron stores are depleted.	**Gross:** Sits, leaning forward on both hands; when supine, lifts head off table. Turns from back to abdomen. **Fine:** Transfers objects from one hand to another. Picks up object well.	Smiles at self in mirror. Plays peek-a-boo. Begins to show stranger anxiety.	Can fixate on small objects. Adjusts posture to see. Responds to name. Exhibits beginning sense of object permanence. Recognizes parent in other clothes, places. Is alert for 1½–2 hours.	Produces vowel sounds and chained syllables. Begins to imitate sounds. Belly laughs. Babbles (one syllable) with pleasure. Calls for help. "Talks" to toys and image in mirror.
8–9 Months				
Continues to gain weight, length. Patterns of bladder and bowel elimination begin to become regular.	**Gross:** Sits steadily unsupported. Can crawl and pull up. **Fine:** Pincer grasp develops. Reaches for toys. Rakes for objects and releases objects.	Stranger anxiety is at its height. Separation anxiety is increasing. Follows parent around the house.	Beginning development of depth perception. Object permanence continues to develop. Uses hands to learn concepts of in and out.	Stringing together of vowels and consonants begins. First few words begin to have meaning (Mama, Daddy, bye-bye, baby). Begins to understand and obey simple commands, such as, "Wave bye-bye." Responds to "No!" Shouts for attention.
10–12 Months				
Birth weight triples; birth length increases by 50% (12 months). Head and chest circumference equal. Babinski reflex disappears.	**Gross:** Can walk with one hand held, but crawls to get places quickly. **Fine:** Releases hold on cup. Finger-feeds self (10 months). Feeds self with spoon (12 months). Holds crayon to mark on paper. Pincer grasp is complete (12 months).	Has mood changes. Quiets self. Is quieted by music. Tenderly cuddles toy.	Vision 20/40. Searches for hidden toy. Explores boxes, inserts objects in container. Symbol recognition is developing (enjoys books).	Can say 2 or more words. Says "Mama" or "Dada" specifically. Waves bye-bye. Begins to differentiate between words. Enjoys jabbering. Vocalization decreases when walking. Knows own name.

Physical Growth and Development

Growth is an excellent indicator of overall health during infancy. Although growth rates are variable, infants usually double their birth weights by 6 months and triple them by 1 year of age. During the first 5 to 6 months, the average weight gain is 1.5 lb (0.68 kg) per month. Throughout the next 6 months, weight increase is approximately 1 lb (0.45 kg) per month. Weight gain in formula-fed infants is slightly greater than in breast-fed infants.

During the first 6 months, infants increase their birth length by approximately 1 inch (2.54 cm) per month, slowing to 0.5 inch (1.27 cm) per month over the next 6 months. By 1 year of age, most infants have increased their birth length by 50%.

The head circumference growth rate during the first year is slightly less than 0.5 inch (1.27 cm) per month. Usually the posterior fontanel closes by 6 to 8 weeks of age, whereas the larger anterior fontanel may remain open until 18 months. Head circumference and fontanel measurements indicate brain growth and are obtained, along with height and weight, at each well-baby visit. Chapter 33 discusses growth rate monitoring throughout infancy.

MATURATION OF BODY SYSTEMS

In addition to height and weight, organ systems grow and mature rapidly in the infant. Even though body systems are developing rapidly, the infant's organs differ from those of older children and adults in both structure and function. These differences place the infant at risk for problems that might not be expected in older individuals. Knowledge of these differences provides the nurse with important rationales on which to base anticipatory guidance and specific nursing interventions.

Neurologic System.   Brain growth and differentiation occur rapidly during the first year of life and depend on nutrition and the function of the other organ systems. At birth, the brain accounts for approximately 10% to 12% of body weight. By 1 year of age, the brain has doubled its weight, with a major growth spurt occurring between 15 and 20 weeks of age and another between 30 weeks and 1 year of age. Increases in the number of synapses and expanded myelination of nerves contribute to maturation of the neurologic system during infancy. Primitive reflexes disappear as the cerebral cortex thickens and motor areas of the brain continue to develop, proceeding in a cephalocaudal pattern: arms first, then legs.

CRITICAL TO REMEMBER

· · · · · · · · · · · ·

Risks Caused by the Infant's Immature Body Systems

- An immature respiratory system places the infant at risk for respiratory infection.
- An immature immune system places the infant at risk for infection.
- An immature renal system places the infant at risk for fluid and electrolyte imbalances.

Respiratory System.   In the first year of life, the lungs increase to three times their weight and six times their volume at birth. In the newborn, alveoli number approximately 20 million, increasing to the adult number of 300 million by age 8 years. During infancy, the trachea remains small, supported only by soft cartilage.

The diameter and length of the trachea, bronchi, and bronchioles increase with age. These tiny, collapsible air passages, however, leave infants vulnerable to respiratory difficulties caused by infection or foreign bodies. The eustachian tube is short and relatively horizontal, placing the infant at risk for middle-ear infections.

Cardiovascular System.   The cardiovascular system undergoes dramatic changes in the transition from fetal to extrauterine circulation. Fetal shunts close, and pulmonary circulation increases drastically. During infancy, the heart doubles in size and weight, the heart rate gradually slows, and blood pressure increases.

Immune System.   Transplacental transfer of maternal antibodies supplements the infant's weak response to infection until approximately 3 to 4 months of age. Although the infant begins to produce immunoglobulins (Ig) soon after birth, by 1 year of age, the infant has only approximately 60% of the adult IgG level, 75% of the adult IgM level, and 20% of the adult IgA level. Breast milk transmits additional IgA protection. The activity of T lymphocytes also increases after birth.

Even though the immune system matures during infancy, maximum protection against infection is not achieved until early childhood. This immaturity places the infant at risk for infection.

Gastrointestinal System.   The stomach capacity of a newborn is only approximately 30 ml, but with feedings, the capacity increases rapidly to approximately 200 ml at 1 year of age. In the gastrointestinal system, enzymes needed for the digestion and absorption of proteins, fats, and carbohydrates mature and increase in concentration. Although the newborn's gastrointestinal system is capable of digesting protein and lactase, the ability to digest and absorb fat does not reach adult levels until approximately 6 to 9 months of age.

Renal System.   Kidney mass increases threefold during the first year of life. Although the glomeruli enlarge considerably during the first few months, the glomerular filtration rate remains low. Thus, the kidney is not effective as a filtration organ or efficient in concentrating urine until after the first year of life.

Because of the functional immaturity of the renal system, the infant is at great risk for fluid and electrolyte imbalance.

Motor Development

During the first few months after birth, muscle growth and weight gain allow for increased control of reflexes and more purposeful movement (see the photostory on pages 84–87). At 1 month, movement occurs in a random fashion, with the fists tightly clenched. Because the neck musculature is weak and the head is large, infants can lift their heads only briefly. By 2 to 3 months, infants can lift their heads 90° from a prone position and can hold them steadily erect in a sitting position. During this time, active grasping gradually replaces reflexive grasping and increases in frequency as eye-hand coordination improves (see Table 5–1).

The Moro, tonic neck, and rooting reflexes disappear at approximately 3 to 4 months. These primitive reflexes, which are controlled by the midbrain, probably disappear because they are suppressed by growing cortical layers. Head control steadily increases during the third month. By the fourth month, the head remains in a straight line with the body when the infant is pulled to a sitting position. Most infants play with their feet by 4 to 5 months, drawing them up to suck on their toes.

During the fifth and sixth months, motor development accelerates rapidly. Infants of this age readily reach for and grasp objects. They can bear weight when held in a standing position and can turn from abdomen to back. By 5 months, some infants rock back and forth as a precursor to crawling.

Six-month-old infants can sit alone, leaning forward on their hands. This ability provides them with a wider view of the world and creates new ways to play. Infants of this age can roll from back to abdomen and can raise their heads from the table when supine. At 6 to 7 months they transfer objects from one hand to another. In addition, they can grab objects, even small ones, and insert them into their mouths with lightning speed.

At 6 to 9 months, infants begin to explore the world by crawling. By 9 months, most infants have enough muscle strength and coordination to pull themselves up and cruise around furniture. These new methods of mobility enable the infant to follow a parent or caregiver around the house.

By 6 to 7 months, infants become increasingly adept at pointing to make their demands known. Six-month-olds grasp objects with all their fingers in a raking motion, but 9-month-olds use their thumbs and forefingers in a fine motor skill called the *pincer grasp*. This grasp provides infants with a useful yet potentially dangerous ability to grab, hold, and insert tiny objects into their mouths.

Nine-month-old infants can wave bye-bye or clap their hands together. They can pick up objects, but have difficulty releasing them on request. By 1 year of age, they can extend an object and release it into an offered hand. Most 1-year-old children can balance well enough to walk when holding another person's hand. They often resort to crawling, however, as a more rapid and efficient way to move about.

An increased ability to move about, reach objects, and explore their world places infants at great risk for accidents and injury. Nurses provide information to parents about how quickly infant motor skills develop.

Parents need anticipatory guidance about ways to prevent accidents by "baby-proofing" their homes before each motor development milestone is reached. The nurse might, for instance, explain, "Infants grow and mature very rapidly and you will be very busy with a new baby. Now is the time to 'baby proof' your home before Mary turns over and begins crawling and reaching for objects. By doing this now, you can prevent later injuries and worries."

Cognitive Development

Many factors contribute to the way in which infants learn about their world. Besides innate intellectual aptitude and motivation, the infants' sensory capabilities, neuromuscular control, and perceptual skills all affect how their cognitive processes unfold during infancy and throughout life. In addition, variables such as the quality and quantity of parental interaction and environmental stimulation contribute to cognitive development.

Cognitive development during the first 2 years of life begins with a profound state of egocentrism. *Egocentrism* is the child's complete self-absorption and the inability to view the world from anyone else's vantage point. As infants' cognitive capacities expand, they become increasingly aware of the outside world and their separateness from it. Gradually, with maturation and experience, they become capable of differentiating themselves from others and their surroundings.

According to Piaget's theory, cognitive development occurs in stages or periods (see Chapter 4). Infancy is included in the *sensorimotor stage* (birth to 2 years), during which infants experience the world through their senses and their attempts to control the environment. Learning activities progress from simple reflex behavior to trial-and-error experiments.

During the first month of life, infants are in the first substage, reflex activity, of the sensorimotor period. In this substage, behavior such as grasping, sucking, or looking is dominated by reflexes. Piaget believed that infants organize their activity, survive, and adapt to their world with the use of reflexes.

Primary circular reactions dominate the second substage, occurring from age 1 to 4 months. During this substage, reflexes become more organized and new schemata are acquired, usually centering on the infant's body. Sensual activities such as sucking and kicking become less reflexive and more controlled, and are repeated because of the stimulation they provide. The baby also begins to recognize objects, especially those that bring pleasure, such as the breast or bottle.

During the third substage, or the stage of secondary circular reactions, infants perform actions that are more oriented toward the world outside their own bodies. The 4- to 8-month-old infant in this substage begins to play with objects in the external environment, such as a rattle or stuffed toy. The infant's actions are labeled secondary because they are intentional (repeated because of the response that is elicited). For example, a baby in this substage intentionally shakes a rattle to hear the sound.

By age 8 to 12 months, infants in the fourth substage, coordination of secondary schemata, begin to relate to objects as if they realize that the objects exist even when they are out of sight. This awareness is referred to as *object permanence* and is illustrated by a 9-month-old infant seeking a toy after it is hidden under a pillow. In contrast, 6-month-olds can follow the path of a toy that is dropped in front of them; however, they will not look for the dropped toy or protest its disappearance until they are older and have developed the concept of object permanence.

Infants in the fourth substage solve problems differently than they do in earlier substages. Rather than randomly selecting approaches to problems, they choose actions that were successful in the past. This tendency suggests that they remember and can perform some mental processing. They seem to be able to identify simple causal relationships, and

Text continued on page 88

THE FIRST YEAR: GROWTH AND DEVELOPMENT MILESTONES

◆ ◆ ◆ ◆ ◆ ◆ ◆

During the first year after birth, the infant's development is dramatic as the child grows toward independence. Knowledge of developmental milestones helps caregivers determine whether the baby is growing and maturing as expected. One should remember that these markers are averages, and that healthy infants often vary. Some infants reach each milestone earlier than average, while other normal infants reach each milestone later than most. Knowledge of normal growth and development helps the nurse promote the safety of children. Parents should be taught to prepare for the child's safety before the child reaches each milestone.

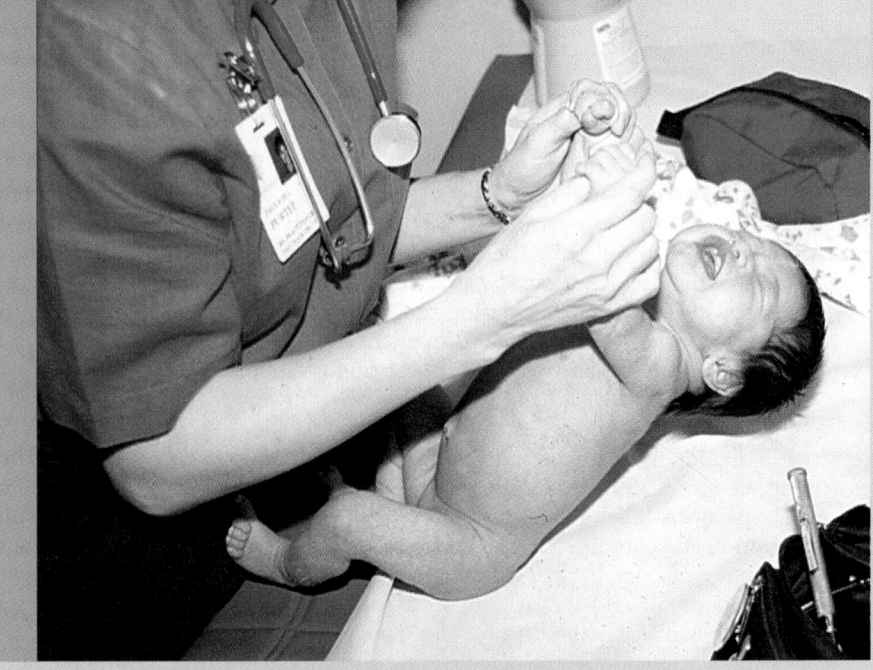

This 18-day-old infant demonstrates substantial head lag as the nurse lifts her trunk from the examining table. Weak neck muscles, combined with a large head, limit her ability to keep her head aligned with her spine as she is pulled toward a sitting position.

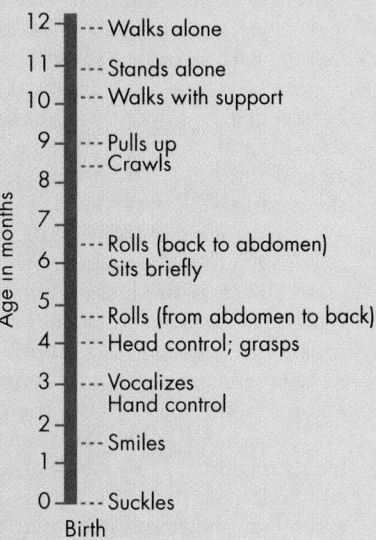

Age in months	
12	Walks alone
11	Stands alone
10	Walks with support
9	Pulls up
8	Crawls
7	
6	Rolls (back to abdomen) / Sits briefly
5	Rolls (from abdomen to back)
4	Head control; grasps
3	Vocalizes / Hand control
2	
1	Smiles
0 Birth	Suckles

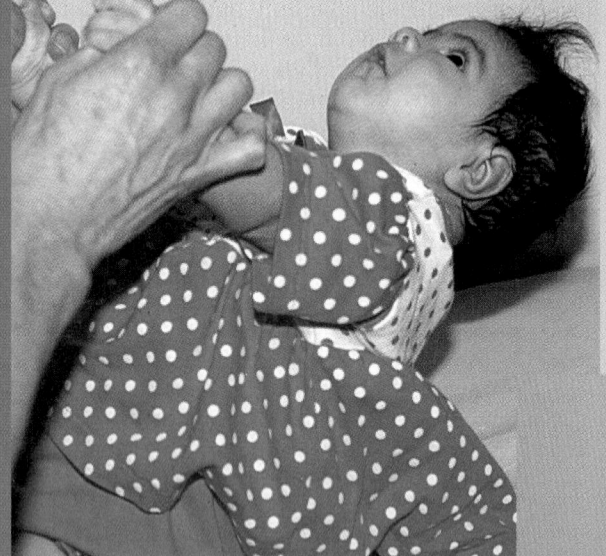

By 2 months, this infant has much less head lag as her neck muscles become stronger and better able to support her head.

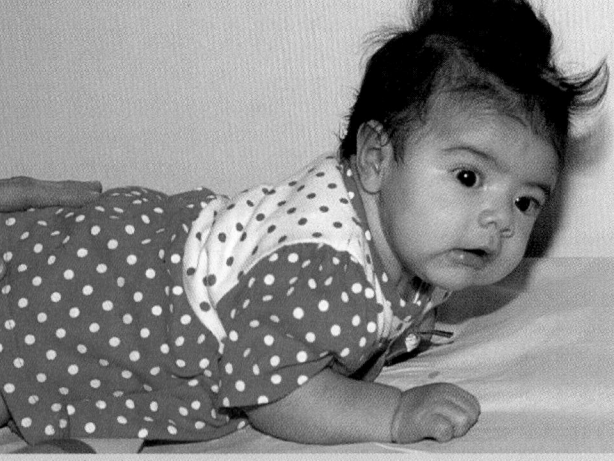

This 2-month-old infant can lift her head from the prone position and briefly hold it erect.

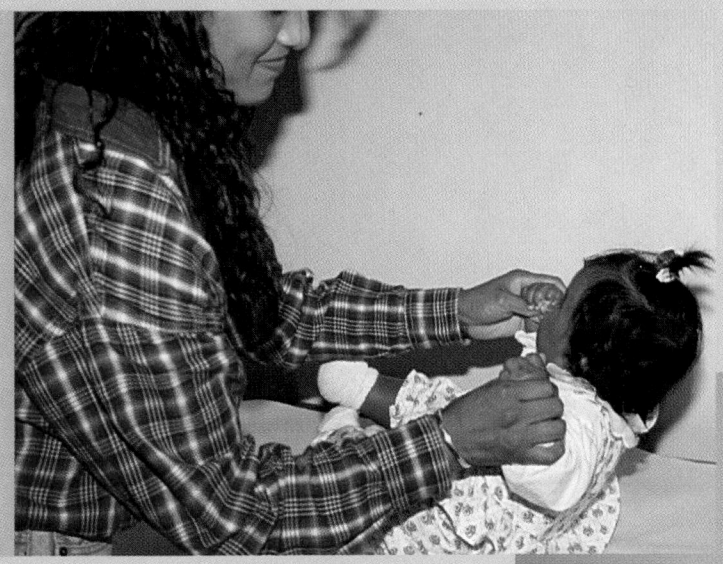

Head control steadily increases so that by 4 months, this infant keeps her head in a straight line as her mother pulls her to a sitting position.

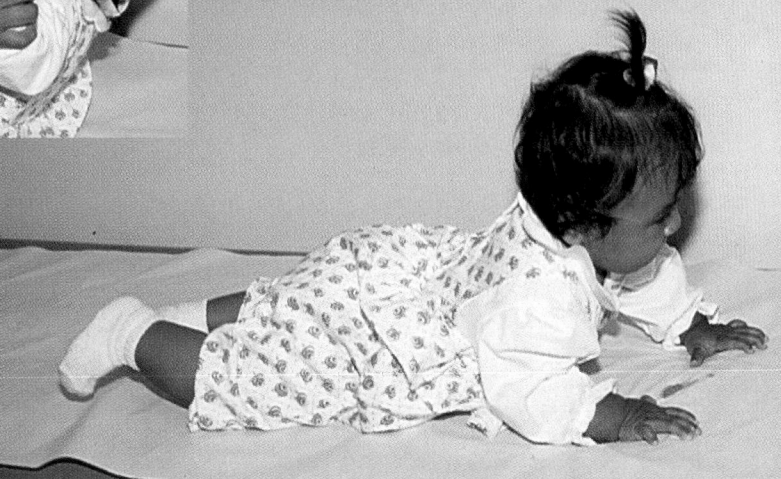

This 4-month-old infant can easily lift her head from a prone position and hold it steadily erect.

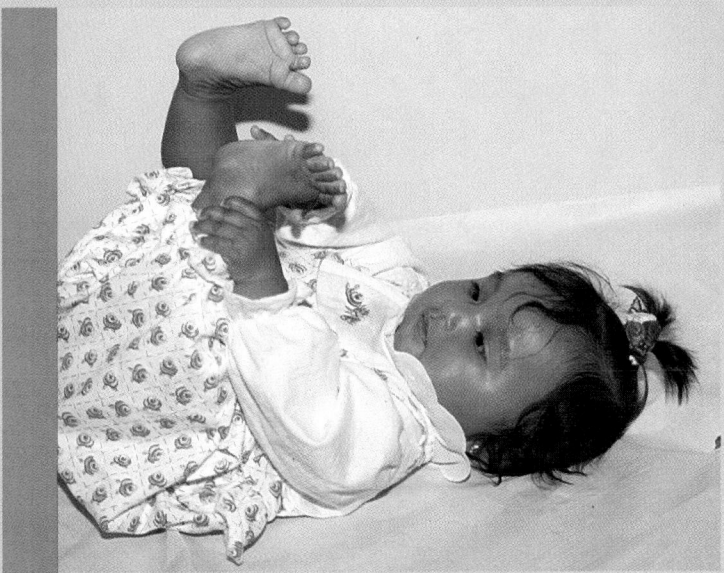

This 4-month-old infant takes pleasure in exploring her own body. She begins playing with her feet, and often puts her toes in her mouth.

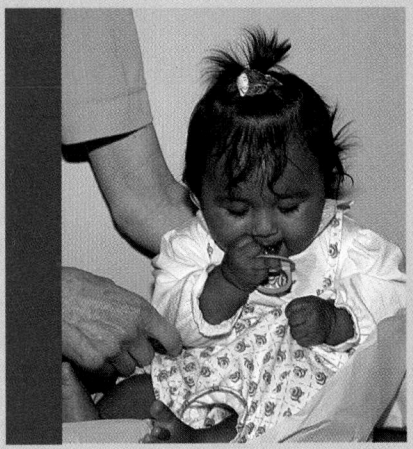

By 4 months, the infant can purposefully grasp objects with the palms of her hands.

CONTINUED

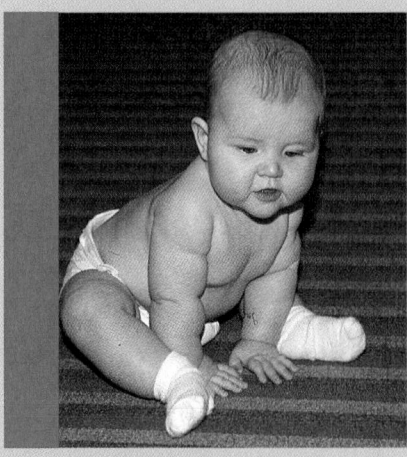

At 6 months, this infant can sit briefly if she leans forward on both hands for support.

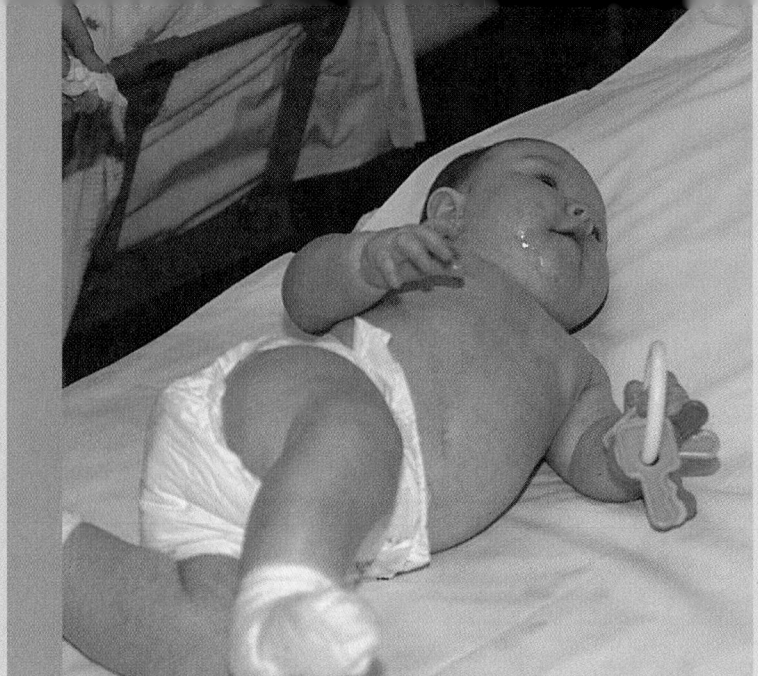

This 6-month-old infant can easily turn from her abdomen onto her back. An adult must be near if an infant of this age is on an elevated surface, such as an examining table or diaper-changing table. To reduce the risk of accidents, the nurse should teach parents about safety measures before the child reaches each developmental milestone.

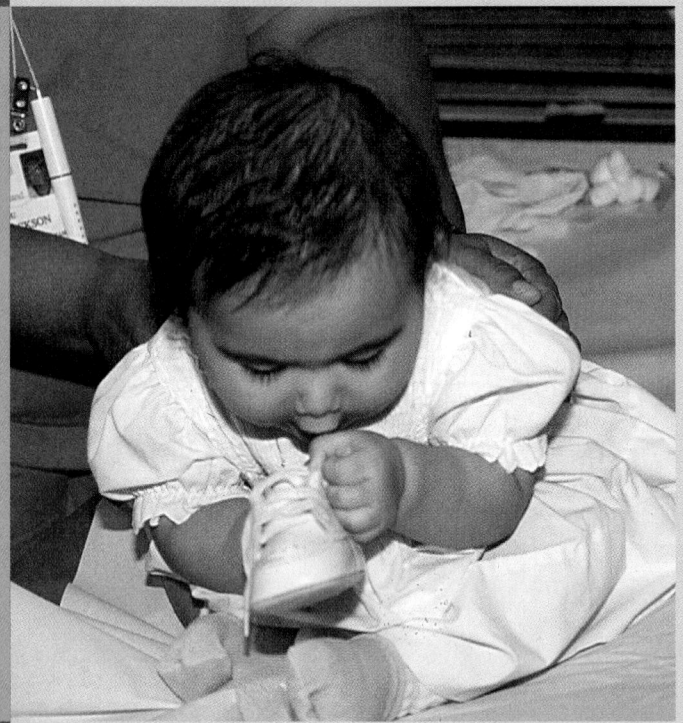

This 7-month-old infant can sit unsupported and hold her shoe. Note also that she explores it with her mouth. The nurse should teach parents that everything infants of this age can hold in their hands will go into their mouths. Parents must put dangerous materials, such as medications, cleaning solutions, and items small enough to swallow, well out of reach.

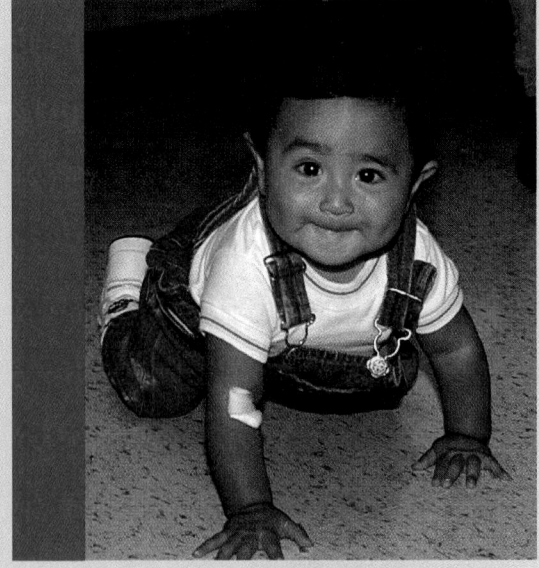

This 9-month-old infant crawls quickly, keeping his belly off the floor.

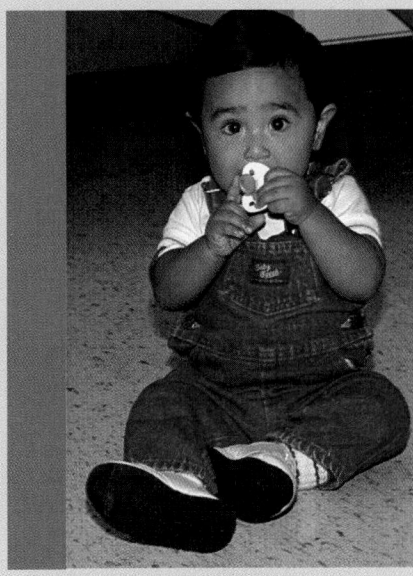

At 9 months, this infant can move easily from a crawling to a sitting position and can sit steadily with no support. He also begins grasping objects with the finer pincer grasp rather than the palmar grasp. If a parent tries to hide something, such as a pacifier, he will not forget the object and will search for it.

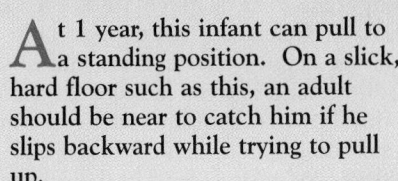

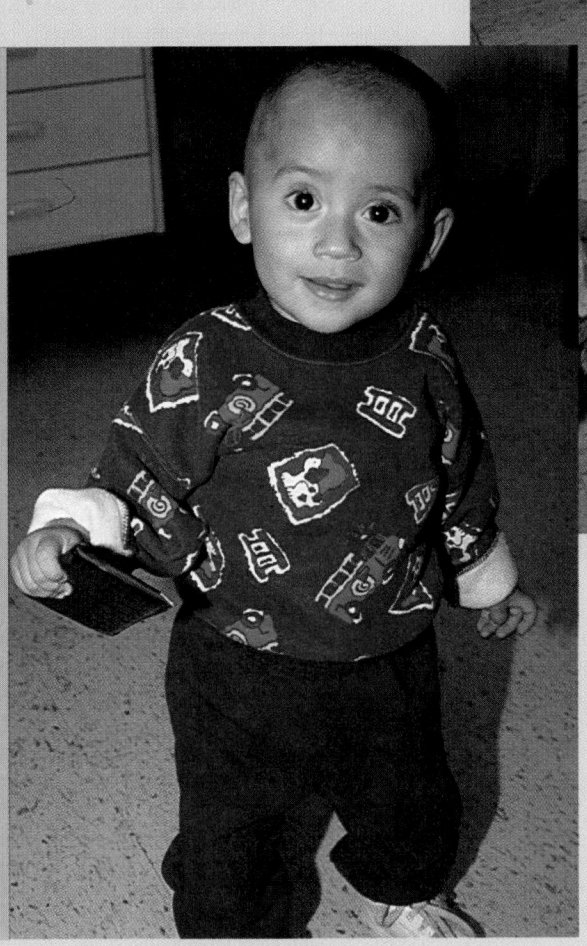

At 1 year, this infant can pull to a standing position. On a slick, hard floor such as this, an adult should be near to catch him if he slips backward while trying to pull up.

After pulling himself to a standing position, this 1-year-old can stand alone.

After the first year, motor development is less dramatic. Nevertheless, to promote the child's safety and normal development, nurses must prepare parents for new milestones.

Photos courtesy of Parkland Health and Hospital System Community Oriented Primary Care Clinic and The University of Texas at Arlington School of Nursing.

they show definite intentionality. For example, when an 11-month-old child sees a toy that is beyond reach, the child uses the blanket that it is resting on to pull it closer (Piaget, 1952; Flavell, 1964).

Cognitive development in the infant parallels motor development. It appears that motor activity is necessary for cognitive development and that cognitive development is based on interaction with the environment, not simply maturation. Infancy is the period when the child lays the foundation for later cognitive functioning. Nurses can promote the cognitive development of infants by encouraging parents to interact with their infants and provide them with novel, interesting stimuli. At the same time, parents should maintain familiar, routine experiences through which their infants can develop a sense of security about the world. Within this type of environment, infants will thrive and learn.

Sensory Development

VISION

The size of the eye at birth is approximately one-half to three-quarters the size of the adult eye. Growth of the eye, including its internal structures, is rapid during the first year. As infants grow and become more interested in the environment, their eyes remain open for longer periods. They show a preference for familiar faces and are increasingly able to fixate on objects. Visual acuity is estimated at approximately 20/100 to 20/150 at birth, but improves rapidly during infancy and toddlerhood. Infants show a preference for high-contrast colors, such as black and white and primary colors. Pastel colors are not easily distinguished until about 6 months of age.

Young infants may lack coordination of eye movements and extraocular muscle alignment, but should achieve proper coordination by age 4 to 6 months. Persistent lack of eye muscle control beyond the age of 4 to 6 months needs further evaluation. Depth perception appears to begin at approximately 7 to 9 months and contributes to the infant's new ability to move about independently.

HEARING

Hearing seems to be relatively acute, even at birth, as shown by reflexive generalized reactions to noise. With myelination of the auditory nerve tracts during the first year, responses to sound become increasingly more specialized. By 4 months, infants should turn their eyes and heads toward a sound coming from behind, and by 10 months, infants should respond to the sound of their names. The National Institutes of Health has recommended that all newborns be screened for hearing impairment. Several states have mandated newborn hearing screening (Schuman, 1998).

Language Development

The acquisition of language has its roots in infancy as the child becomes increasingly intrigued with sound, begins to realize that words have meaning, and eventually uses simple sounds to communicate. Although young infants probably understand tones and inflections of voice rather than words themselves, it is not long before repetition and practice of

---

> ### CRITICAL TO REMEMBER
> ### *Possible Signs of Developmental Delays*
>
> - Lack of eye muscle control after 4 to 6 months suggests vision impairments and the need for further evaluation.
> - Lack of a social smile by 8 to 12 weeks requires further evaluation and close follow-up.

---

sounds enables them to understand and communicate with words. Infants can understand more than they can express.

The social smile develops early in the infant, usually by 3 to 5 weeks of age (Fig. 5–1). This powerful communication tool helps to foster attachment and demonstrates that the infant can differentiate between people and objects within the environment. The infant who does not display a social smile by the age of 8 to 12 weeks needs further evaluation and close follow-up because of the possibility of developmental delay.

During infancy, connections form within the central nervous system, providing fine motor control of the numerous muscles required for speech. Maturation of the mouth, jaw, and larynx; bone growth; and development of the face help to prepare the infant to speak.

Vocalization does not appear to be reflexive but rather is a relatively high-level activity similar to conversation. Parents usually elicit vocalization in infants better than other adults can. Infants' brains process speech and language in the environment, using cues, structure, and distributional patterns to construct their native tongue (Karmiloff-Smith, 1995).

Although there is great variability, most children begin to make nonmeaningful sounds, such as "ma," "da," or "ah," by 4 to 6 months. The sounds become more meaningful and specific by 9 to 15 months, and by age 1 year, the child usually has a vocabulary of several words, such as "mama," "dada," and "bye-bye." Infants who have older siblings or who are

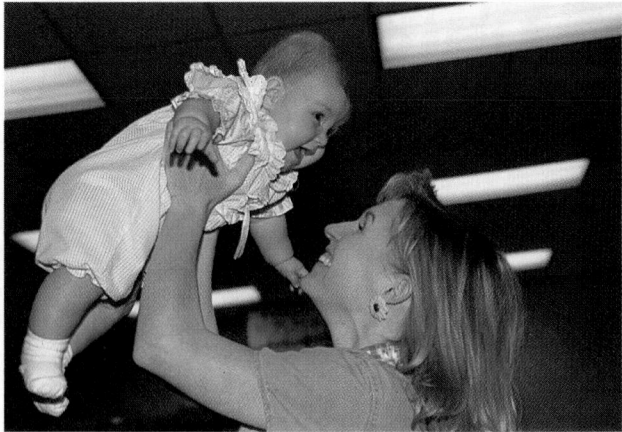

FIGURE 5–1

This 6-month-old infant responds delightedly to her mother with a true social smile. Such interactive responses between parent and child promote communication and emotional development.

••••••••••

Language and Communication: Developmental Milestones in Infancy

1–3 MONTHS

Reflexive smile at first, then smile becomes more voluntary; sets up a reciprocal smiling cycle with parent. Cooing.

3–4 MONTHS

Crying becomes more differentiated. Babbling is common.

4–6 MONTHS

Plays with sound, repeating sounds to self. Can identify mother's voice. May squeal in excitement.

6–8 MONTHS

Single consonant babbling occurs. Increasing interest in sound.

8–9 MONTHS

Stringing of vowels and consonants together begins. First few words begin to have meaning (Mama, Daddy, bye-bye, baby). Begins to understand and obey simple commands such as "Wave bye-bye."

9–12 MONTHS

Vocabulary of two or three words. Gestures are used to communicate. Speech development may slow temporarily when walking begins.

raised in verbally rich environments sometimes meet these developmental milestones earlier than other infants.

Psychosocial Development

Most experts agree that infancy is a crucial period during which children develop the foundation of their personalities and their sense of self. According to Erik Erikson's theory of psychosocial development (1963), infants struggle to establish a sense of basic *trust* rather than a sense of basic *mistrust* in their world, their caregivers, and themselves. If provided with consistent, satisfying experiences delivered in a timely manner, infants come to rely on the fact that their needs will be met and that, in turn, they will be able to tolerate some degree of frustration and discomfort until those needs are met. This sense of confidence is an early form of trust and provides the foundation for a healthy personality.

On the other hand, if infants' needs are ignored or met in a consistently haphazard, inadequate manner, they have no reason to believe that their needs will be met or that their environment is a safe, secure place. According to Erikson, without consistent satisfaction of needs, the individual develops a basic sense of suspicion or mistrust.

Parallel to this viewpoint is Freudian theory, which regards infancy as the oral stage. The mouth is the major focus of this stage. Observation of infants for a few minutes shows

that most of their behavior centers on their mouths. Sensory stimulation and pleasure as well as nourishment are experienced through their mouths. Sucking is an adaptive behavior that provides comfort and satisfaction while enabling infants to experience and explore their world. Later in infancy, as teething progresses, the mouth becomes an effective tool for aggressive behavior (see Chapter 4).

PARENT-INFANT ATTACHMENT

One of the most important aspects of infant psychosocial development is parent-infant attachment. Attachment is a sense of belonging to or connection with each other. This significant bond between infant and parent is critical to normal development and even survival. Initiated immediately after birth, attachment is strengthened by many mutually satisfying interactions between the parents and the infant throughout the first months of life.

For example, noisy distress in infants signals a need, such as hunger. The parents respond by providing food. In turn, the infants respond by quieting and accepting nourishment. The infants derive pleasure from having their hunger satiated, and the parents from successfully caring for the child. A basic reciprocal cycle is set in motion in which parents learn to regulate infant feeding, sleep, and activity through a series of interactions. These interactions include rocking, touching, talking, smiling, and singing. The infants respond by quieting, eating, watching, smiling, or sleeping.

Conversely, chronic inability or unwillingness of parents to meet the dependency needs of their infants fosters insecurity and dissatisfaction in the infants. A cycle of dissatisfaction is established in which parents become frustrated as caregivers and have further difficulty providing for the infants' needs.

If parents can adapt to the infants, meet their needs, and provide nurturance, attachment is secure. Psychosocial development can proceed based on a strong foundation of attachment. On the other hand, if parents' personalities and abilities to cope with infant care do not match their infants' needs, the relationship is considered at risk.

Although the establishment of trust depends heavily on the quality of the parental interaction, the infant also needs consistent, satisfying social interactions within a family structure. Family routines can help to provide this consistency. Touch is an important tool that can be used by all family members to convey a sense of caring.

STRANGER ANXIETY

Another important aspect of psychosocial development is stranger anxiety or separation anxiety. By 6 to 7 months, expanding cognitive capacities and strong feelings of attachment enable infants to differentiate between caregivers and strangers and to be wary of the latter. Infants display an obvious preference for parents over other caregivers and other unfamiliar people. Anxiety, demonstrated by crying, clinging, and turning away from the stranger, is manifested when separation occurs. This behavior peaks at approximately 7 to 9 months and again during toddlerhood, when separation may be difficult (see Chapter 6).

Although stressful for parents, stranger anxiety is a normal sign of healthy attachment and occurs because of cognitive development (object permanence). Nurses can reassure parents that although their infants seem distressed, leaving them for short periods does no harm. Separations should be accomplished swiftly, yet with care, love, and emphasis on the parents' return.

Health Promotion for the Infant and Family

Parents, particularly new parents, often need guidance in caring for their infant. Nurses can provide valuable information about health promotion of the infant. Specific guidance about everyday concerns, such as sleep, crying, and feeding, can be offered, as well as anticipatory guidance about injury prevention. An important nursing responsibil-

ity is to provide parents with information about immunizations and dental care. Nurses can offer support to new parents by identifying strategies for coping with the first few months with an infant. Table 5–2 presents an overview of health screening, health maintenance, and anticipatory guidance activities for infants.

Sleep, Rest, and Crying

Newborns may sleep as much as 17 to 20 hours per day. Sleep patterns vary widely, with some infants sleeping only 2 to 3 hours at a time. At approximately 3 to 4 months of age, most infants begin to sleep for longer periods during

---

TABLE 5–2

· · · · · · · · · · · ·

Health Screening, Health Maintenance, and Anticipatory Guidance for Infants

0–2 Months	*4 Months*	*6 Months*	*9 Months*	*12 Months*
Immunizations				
Hep B (birth to 2 months)		Hep B-3		
Hep B (1 month after first dose)				
DTaP (2 months)	DTaP	DTaP or DTP #3		
IPV (2 months)	IPV			May give IPV at 2, 4 months and OPV at 12–18 months and 4–6 years; *or* IPV at 2, 4, and 12–18 months and 4–6 years.
Rotavirus* (2 months)	Rotavirus	Rotavirus		
Hib (2 months)	Hib	Hib		
				Varicella (12–18 months)
				MMR (12–15 months)
Safety				
Secure in car seat in the back seat.	Guard infant on bed or changing table.	Remove chemicals, poisons, and plants from infant's reach.	Anticipate increased mobility.	Prevent burns and scalding.
Infants under 20 lb or 1 year of age must always ride in a rear-facing car seat in the back seat.	Be sure safety straps are used for infant seat.	Cover electric outlets.	Protect from falls.	Guard against falls.
Never put an infant in the front seat of a car with a passenger-side air bag.		Do not leave unattended in bath.	Use gates to protect infant from stairs.	Supervise child in or near water.
Be sure bathwater is no hotter than 120°F.			Remove hazardous objects from low places.	Keep older siblings' toys from infant.
Never shake or vigorously jiggle baby's head.			Keep syrup of ipecac and poison control telephone number on hand.	Lock poisons away.
Do not hold infant while drinking hot liquids.			Be sure toys have no small pieces.	
Baby-proof home.				
Nutrition				
Breast milk or formula is main food throughout infancy; no homogenized cow's milk.	May offer rice cereal mixed with breast milk or formula.	Introduce strained vegetables, fruits, and meats one at a time.	Table foods can be given when infant is sitting at the family table.	Self-feeding of table food is appropriate. Liquids can be given with a cup.

TABLE 5–2
. . . .

Health Screening, Health Maintenance, and Anticipatory Guidance for Infants Continued

0–2 Months	4 Months	6 Months	9 Months	12 Months
Nutrition continued				
Vitamin D and iron are not routinely given unless infant is in a high-risk group. Fluoride is not given during first 6 months; after 6 months it is given only if the water supply is severely deficient in fluoride.		Begin use of cup for juice and water. Give only water if bottle is taken to bed.	Self-feeding can begin. Avoid foods that might cause choking (e.g., popcorn, peanuts, hard candy, hot dogs, raw vegetables, raisins).	Weaning may be started. Breast or bottle should be gradually eliminated.
Vision and Hearing				
Check for response to sound of bell. Assess ability to follow light past midline.	Assess for strabismus. (see Chapter 55).		Assess for ability to look for objects.	Assess for ability to respond to name and other sounds. Assess ability to see and grasp.
Dental Care				
		Discuss teething and associated problems. When teeth erupt they may be cleaned with cotton swabs or a soft cloth.	Continue to discuss teething and associated problems. Compare with normal growth.	Continue to discuss teething and associated problems. Do not allow bottle in bed.
Screening				
Height, weight, and head circumference should be compared with normal limits at each well-child visit.	Height, weight, and head circumference should be monitored and compared with normal limits. Encourage parents to talk to infant.	Height, weight, and head circumference should be monitored and compared with normal limits. Hemoglobin and hematocrit screening for anemia is done (6–9 months). Urinalysis (1–12 months).	Height, weight, and head circumference should be monitored and compared with normal limits. Monitor deviations. Hemoglobin and hematocrit screening is done (6–9 months).	Monitor weight, height, and head circumference and compare with norms.
Teaching and Counseling				
Discuss irregular sleep patterns. Reinforce parents' desire to cuddle and play with infant. Discuss importance of development of trust. Discuss needs and behavior of siblings.	Encourage parents to play with infant and provide safe, age-appropriate toys. Reassure parents that holding infant will not result in a "spoiled" child.	Discuss sleep problems and interventions. Encourage playing and talking to infant. Discuss stranger anxiety. Reassure that thumb sucking is normal.	Discuss play and social games. Educate about normal behavior and expectations of growing infant. Discuss stranger anxiety. Encourage vocalization by talking to infant.	Discuss increasing mobility and growing need for autonomy. Encourage regular bedtime. Encourage vocalization and social play.

Abbreviations: DTaP, diphtheria-tetanus-acellular pertussis; Hib, *Hemophilus influenzae* type B conjugate vaccine; Hep-B, hepatitis B virus vaccine; OPV, oral poliovirus vaccine; IPV, inactivated poliovirus vaccine.

*At time of publication suspended until further research can determine whether the risks of the disease outweigh the risks of the vaccine.

the night, although some children do not sleep through the night consistently until the second year.

Often one of the most difficult tasks for new parents is the regulation of their infants' sleep-wake cycles. Parents need anticipatory guidance about what to expect regarding sleep, rest, and crying.

PATTERNS OF CRYING

Nurses can suggest that parents console their infants when they cry by holding them, talking softly, or humming. Gently stroking an infant's head, back, and arms may also be soothing. Infant massage techniques and simply "centering" are easily accomplished by positioning the infant's arms and legs toward the midline of the body. Swaddling a new infant is a consoling technique that assists the infant in centering. Some infants respond readily to attempts to comfort them, sleep a great deal, and fit easily into their family's lifestyle.

On the other hand, some infants cry more readily and for longer periods and spend more time in a fretful, restless state than others. These infants often experience more colic symptoms and sleep problems. This irritability may be caused by health problems, such as feeding difficulties, infection, or allergies, but often no clear cause emerges. In some cases, infant temperament or the combination of a sensitive, irritable infant and parents who have not yet learned to respond to the infant's needs correctly may be the cause (Carey, 1998).

STRATEGIES FOR SOOTHING INFANTS

Specific strategies to diminish infant irritability include activities such as taking the baby for a car ride, carrying the infant in a front pack close to the parent's chest, or swinging the baby in an infant swing. Vertical positioning and constant motion, such as that obtained when walking with the baby carried over the shoulder, are sometimes helpful. The football carry position, with gentle patting on the back, can also be tried. Sometimes irritable infants need to be left alone to cry. If parents choose this strategy, they must be cautioned to limit the crying time to 15 to 20 minutes and to check the baby frequently.

Few interventions are consistently successful because infant responses may be variable. Providing parents with strategies, however, helps to decrease their anxiety and increase their feelings of control and competence. As infants grow and develop, they are better able to regulate their sleep-wake cycles. Generally, during the third or fourth month of life, sleep problems and irritability improve.

The Infant with Colic

Colic usually refers to unexplained crying or fussing in infants, which may be characterized by infants pulling up their arms and legs. Periods of crying tend to occur at the same time of day, often in the late afternoon or evening. Colic occurs in 10% to 20% of infants younger than 3 months of age.

ETIOLOGY

The cause of colic is unknown, but several theories have been researched. The possibilities include but are not limited to allergy, cow's milk intolerance, maternal anxiety, familial stress, and too rapid feeding or overfeeding. It is highly likely that more than one factor may be involved. Colic is more common in infants with sensitive temperaments, who seem to need increased attention. Some have suggested that it may even be an extreme variant of normal crying (Berkowitz, 1996).

MANAGEMENT

It must be determined whether, in fact, the infant is crying because of colic and not because of an acute condition such as intussusception, otitis media, or a fracture. Symptoms of milk allergy other than crying should be present before formula changes are made. Anticholinergics, motility-enhancing agents, barbiturates, and antiflatulents may be prescribed. Many practitioners avoid using these drugs because of their limited success, lack of scientific data, and possible side effects. Chamomile tea has a calming and sedating effect and is effective in some infants. It has been used for thousands of years and is readily available in most grocery stores, and allergic reactions are rare. If parents are using such herbs, be sure they know the appropriate dose and are aware of possible allergic reactions (Kemper, 1996).

NURSING CONSIDERATIONS

Assessment. Because the etiology of colic and the care of an infant with colic are so individualized, it is very important that a thorough history be obtained. Provide a concerned and caring atmosphere during the assessment and reassure the parents that colic is not related to "bad parenting." Determine whether any other symptoms are associated with the crying. Discuss the infant's eating habits, including whether the infant is breast- or bottle-fed. Ask the parents if there are commonalities associated with the crying (time of day, associated activities, family members present). Ask what has been tried and what works and what does not work. If the parents are unsure, suggest they keep a diary for 48 to 72 hours to determine patterns. Assess the parents' stress level and support system.

Nursing Interventions. Educate the parents regarding the normal growth and development needs of infants related to sleep and awake times, feeding, soothing, and holding. Listen to the parents with an empathic ear. Encourage parents to soothe their infant by rocking and cuddling. Some infants will quiet when given a massage, pacifier, or warm bath. If the parent is busy, a swing may provide a soothing, rhythmic effect. Some of the same strategies for soothing infants may also be effective in quieting infants with colic.

Some infants seem most distressed during high-activity times when the family may be busy preparing meals, doing chores, gathering at the end of the day, and so forth. By assisting parents to see such trends, the nurse can help them establish alternative routines to decrease the infant's stimuli. The parent may choose to feed the infant away from all of the activity or to have a later dinner. Each family will be unique, and the nurse's role is to facilitate problem solving.

If, after 30 minutes, none of the interventions are effective, the infant should be placed in the crib. If crying continues for more than 15 to 20 minutes longer, pick the infant up again and try to soothe.

The Family's Need for Support. All families need extra support after the birth of an infant. If the infant has colic, the need increases. During the first few months after the addition of a new baby, demanding work schedules, lack of recovery time from childbirth, the needs of other family members, physical exhaustion, and sleep deprivation can combine with the presence of a fretful infant to create stressful situations for the entire family. Sometimes infant temperament and parental coping styles are not compatible.

The nurse might, for example, explain to new parents, "Parenting is very much a challenge even when parents care about their baby as much as you do. It is difficult at first even to discern what Avery is telling you when she cries. But you will feel more and more comfortable, even see that she has a different cry when she is hungry and when she is tired."

In validating the parents' feelings, the nurse recognizes that the infant's irritability or colic is real, not imagined, and that the infant is a challenge to handle. The nurse can reassure the parents that the infant is healthy, normal, and gaining weight and that the parents are competent in their nurturing role.

The emotional reserves of the parents can be restored through rest and pleasurable activities. Parents may need brief periods of relief from infant care responsibilities. Grandparents or other family members may be able to provide the parents with an evening out or a night of uninterrupted sleep. This direct support can help to restore the parents' energy to cope with daily activities and feel more relaxed and confident in their parenting.

CRITICAL THINKING EXERCISE 5-1

Mary Brown and her 4-week-old daughter, Heidi, are being seen for a well-baby checkup. Heidi is Mrs. Brown's first child. Mrs. Brown looks very tired and begins to cry when you ask her how she is doing.

1. What are some of the possible causes the nurse should explore?
2. How can you explore these possible causes?
3. What are some of the appropriate nursing measures?

Play

One sign of infants' cognitive development is the beginning evidence of play. Early signs of play are related to infants' motor and cognitive development. They mouth, shake, inspect, and reach for objects. Infants observe and engage other members of the family. In fact, human involvement is the most important component of play. A familiar game that we all have played is peek-a-boo. Not only is this game fun, but it is also associated with the development of object permanence. Table 5–3 outlines appropriate play activities and toys for the infant. See Chapter 4 for more information related to play.

FEEDING AND NUTRITION

Because infancy is a period of rapid growth, nutritional needs are of special significance. During infancy, eating progresses from a principally reflex activity to relatively sophisticated yet messy attempts at self-feeding. Because the infant's gastrointestinal system continues to mature throughout the first year, changes in diet, the introduction of new foods, and even upsets in routines can result in feeding problems.

TABLE 5-3

Age-Related Activities and Toys for Infants

General Activities	Toys and Specific Types of Play
The infant enjoys watching other members of the family, being rocked, being taken for a walk in a stroller, time spent in a swing, supervised time on a blanket on the floor, crawling, walking, and being sung and read to.	Oral movements (playing with the nipple of the bottle, lip movements unrelated to sucking); peek-a-boo; playing with the caretaker's fingers, hair, face, and the infant's own body parts; and playing in water.
Play is narcissistic; it is difficult, if not impossible, to direct play.	Soft stuffed animals, crib mobiles, squeeze toys, rattles, busy boxes, mirrors, musical toys, water toys during the bath, blocks, safe kitchen utensils, push toys (after infant begins to walk).
Human interaction is the most important component of play.	Contrasting colors for young infants (black-and-white mobiles).
	Large picture books.

CRITICAL TO REMEMBER

Essential Information for Infant Nutrition

- Breast milk or commercially prepared formula provides optimal nutrition throughout infancy.
- Formula must be prepared according to instructions, and leftover formula should be stored according to the manufacturer's directions.
- Some health care providers discourage the use of powdered formula until the infant is older than 6 weeks.

Parents often have many questions and concerns about nutrition. They are influenced by a variety of sources, including relatives and friends who may not be aware of current scientific practices regarding infant feeding. The nurse must have a clear understanding of gastrointestinal maturation and knowledge about breast-feeding and various infant formulas and foods to provide anticipatory guidance. Families and cultures vary widely in food preferences and infant feeding practices. The nurse must remain cognizant of these differences when providing anticipatory guidance related to infant nutrition.

BREAST-FEEDING
The American Academy of Pediatrics strongly recommends breast-feeding for all infants, including premature and sick newborns, with rare exceptions (American Academy of Pediatrics, 1997). Mothers who breast-feed need instruction and support as they begin. They are more likely to succeed if they are given practical information. Many facilities provide home visits or may call to assess the mother's needs. It is becoming increasingly common for hospitals to have nurses on staff who are certified lactation consultants. Lactation specialists are prepared to deal with more difficult problems. Mothers may also be referred to a lactation consultant or support group such as the La Leche League. La Leche Leagues are available in most communities and are listed in the telephone directory. Significant others are included in teaching to provide a support system for the mother. An in-depth discussion of breastfeeding can be found in Chapter 24.

BOTTLE FEEDING
Formula. Infant formula does not have the immunologic properties and digestibility of human milk, but it does meet the energy and nutrient requirements of infants. The Infant Formula Act of 1980, which was revised in 1986, establishes the standards for infant formulas. It also requires that the label show the quantity of each nutrient.

There are many reasons why some mothers choose to use formula. Some mothers simply do not want to breast-feed. Others may use formula to supplement an omitted breast-feeding, rather than pump their breasts. Infants with galactosemia or whose mother uses illegal drugs, is taking certain prescribed drugs, has untreated active tuberculosis, or is infected with the human immunodeficiency virus

(HIV) should not be breast-fed. In countries where there is an increased risk for other infectious diseases and nutritional deficiencies resulting in infant death, the risk associated with not breast-feeding may outweigh the possible risk of the infant acquiring HIV infection (AAP, 1997).

Mothers who choose not to breast-feed should never be forced to breast-feed or made to feel guilty because of their choice. Rather, support should be given for whatever feeding choice is selected.

Formulas are available as three types:

- Concentrated liquid, which is diluted with water according to instructions
- Powder, which is mixed with water according to instructions
- Ready-to-use formula, which can be poured directly into a bottle

It is very important that the parent understand preparation instructions and care of any leftover formula. Many manufacturers print instructions in several languages. Some health care providers discourage the use of powdered formula until the infant is past age 6 weeks. Chapter 24 provides more specific information regarding bottle-feeding and special formulas. Chapter 24 discusses feeding the normal infant, and Chapters 29 and 30 discuss feeding the high-risk newborn.

Cow's Milk. Cow's milk (whole, skim, 1%, and 2%) is not recommended in the first 12 months. Cow's milk contains too little iron and its high renal solute load and unmodified derivatives can put small infants at risk for dehydration. The tough, hard curd is difficult for infants to digest. In addition, skim milk and reduced fat milk deprive the infant of needed calories and essential fatty acids. The incidences of allergy and iron deficiency anemia are higher in infants who are given cow's milk than in those who receive breast milk or formula.

WEANING
Weaning is the replacement of breast- or bottle-feedings with drinking from a cup. Infants usually have a decreasing interest in the breast or bottle starting between ages 6 and 12 months. This varies from infant to infant, but, if solids and a cup have been introduced, the infant will probably begin to indicate a readiness for the cup. When weaning is begun after age 18 months, the infant may resist because of increased attachment to the breast or bottle.

Behaviors that might indicate a readiness to begin weaning include:

- Throwing the bottle down
- Chewing on the nipple
- Taking only a few ounces of formula
- Refusing the breast or dawdling

Weaning should not take place during times of change or stress (e.g., illness, starting child care, the arrival of a new baby). Weaning is a gradual process and should start with the replacement of one bottle- or breast-feeding at a time. If breast-feeding must be terminated before age 6 months, it should be replaced with bottle-feedings to meet the infant's sucking needs. The older infant who has learned to use a cup may not need to use a bottle.

The first bottle- or breast-feeding eliminated should be

the one the infant is least interested in. Initially the infant may accept the cup only after drinking some formula from the bottle or milk from the breast. The infant is next offered the cup before the feeding. In approximately 1 week another feeding can be eliminated if the infant is not resisting the change. The bedtime feeding is usually the last feeding to be eliminated.

The child is giving up time that had been spent being held in the parent's arms. The parent needs to respond to the infant's continued need to be held and cuddled. Infants should not be allowed to carry bottles around as toys, to take them to bed, or to use them as pacifiers. Infants who indicate sucking needs should be given pacifiers.

Juices. Citrus fruits and juices are introduced after age 6 months. This later introduction reduces the chance of allergies. In infants with a history of allergies, orange and tomato juice should be delayed until age 1 year. Some prepared foods and dinners contain orange juice and tomato juice. Parents should be taught to read labels. Juice is not warmed because heating destroys vitamin C. Juices should be kept in a covered container in the refrigerator to prevent the loss of the vitamin. Juices should not be given in the bottle to avoid the development of nursing-bottle caries.

Water. Sufficient water is provided in breast milk and in prepared formula during the nursing period. When solid foods are introduced, it may be necessary to add water because some foods (such as strained meats and high meat dinners) have a high renal solute load. Infants should be offered water as part of a feeding or during the day. Additional water is necessary when intake is low or the infant is experiencing fluid loss because of illness (fever, respiratory disease).

SOLID FOODS

The early introduction of solid food is associated with a higher incidence of food allergy. In addition, the solids the infant eats cannot be adequately digested and the nutrients in breast or formula milk will not be taken in because the infant's appetite has been satisfied. In contrast, failure to offer solids by age 6 months may result in difficulty accepting solid feedings at a later time (AAP, 1998).

The feeding of semisolid foods should be delayed until the infant's consumption of foods is no longer a reflexive process and the infant has the fine and gross motor skills needed to consume them (Trahms & Pipes, 1997). The infant goes through a so-called transitional period during which prepared foods are introduced and given together with human milk or formula. This usually occurs between ages 4 and 6 months. The growth and development of each infant vary, and there are milestones that indicate the infant's readiness for solid foods.

Solids should be introduced one at a time in small amounts (1 teaspoon to 2 tablespoons) for several days before introducing a new food. This is done to avoid confusion should a food intolerance be present. The order of introduction is not critical, but rice cereal is most often recommended as a first food because it is high in iron, is easily digested, and has a low allergenic probability. Other commercially available cereals include oatmeal, barley, mixed grain, and cereals with added fruit. When foods are first being introduced, mixed grains and cereals with added fruit should be avoided. Foods should never be mixed with for-

> ⋯⋯⋯⋯⋯
> ### *Readiness for Introduction of Solids*
>
> - Infant can sit.
> - Birth weight has doubled and infant weighs at least 13 lb.
> - Can reach for an object and maintain balance.
> - Reaches for objects and brings to mouth.
> - Indicates a desire for food by opening mouth and leaning forward.
> - Extrusion reflex has disappeared (4–5 months).
> - Moves food to back of mouth and swallows during spoon feedings.

mula and fed through a nipple with a large hole. This deprives the child of the chewing experience as well as changing the texture and taste of the food. There may be medical conditions (such as gastroesophageal reflux) in which an exception to this rule is made.

Several commercially prepared fruits and vegetables are available. In addition, fruits and vegetables can easily be steamed or boiled and then pureed in a blender or food processor at home. It is usually necessary to add a small amount of water during the blending process. As with cereals, mixed fruits should be avoided until the infant is older and has tolerated individual foods.

Although most sources indicate that the order of introduction of foods is arbitrary, the introduction of meat usually follows cereal, fruit, and vegetables after age 6 months. The infant may be given ground liver, lean beef, or a variety of commercially prepared meats.

Salt and sugar should not be added to commercially or home-prepared foods. Parents should avoid using canned foods or home-prepared foods that contain large amounts of sugar and salt. Feeding honey to infants under age 12 months has been associated with botulism and should therefore be avoided.

Finger Foods. Between age 8 and 10 months the infant can be introduced to finger foods. At this time the pincer grasp is developing and the infant can pick up foods. The infant will have a palmar grasp before this time and soft foods can be given, but the infant will mainly "play" with the food. This can be a positive experience that enables the infant to feel different textures and increase fine motor skills.

Finger foods should be bite-sized pieces of soft food. Arrowroot biscuits, cheese sticks, slices of canned peaches or pears, slices of bananas, and breads can be offered. As children's fine motor skills increase, they may enjoy eating some of the dry cereals, such as Cheerios.

Snacks. When the infant is on a three-meals-a-day schedule, small snacks are an appropriate addition to the nutritional intake. Because infants have small stomachs, they may not be content to wait until the next meal before eating. Snacks should be nutritious, and parents should resist the urge to give infants a bottle to satisfy their hunger. Some of the finger foods listed above are good nutritious snacks. If the infant is not hungry at mealtime, the snack should be given in a smaller portion or eliminated.

FOOD ALLERGIES

Food allergies can occur at any age, but the incidence for development of certain food allergies is increased before age

1 year. Some of the more common food allergies are allergies to milk, egg, soy products, peanuts, chocolate, corn, and wheat. Cow's milk protein intolerance is the most common food allergy during infancy, but this usually does not last past age 3 or 4 years.

Some of the common clinical manifestations of food allergies are abdominal pain, diarrhea, nasal congestion, cough, wheezing, vomiting, and rashes. Many children will "outgrow" their allergic response to certain foods; for example, 70% to 80% of infants with a milk allergy will tolerate milk by age 4 years. Children who develop food allergies after age 3 years tend not to outgrow them.

Safety

The rapidly growing infant becomes mobile seemingly overnight. With newfound mobility comes the potential for unintentional injury. As the infant's musculature strengthens and coordination improves, the infant has an insatiable desire to explore. Without the cognitive skills needed to differentiate danger from safety, the rolling, crawling, toddling infant is at great risk for accidents.

Infants are totally dependent on others for safety and protection. They are especially vulnerable to serious injury because of their relatively large head size. Motor development progresses to the point where they quickly master new skills to learn more about their environment. They begin impulsively to reach out and move toward interesting objects around them.

Because of an infant's dependence, parents and caregivers are the primary recipients of anticipatory safety guidance. From the first day of life, safety must be considered and incorporated into the infant's world. Providing a safe environment for a rapidly growing infant is challenging. Potential safety hazards multiply as the baby learns to creep, crawl, climb, and explore. Some parents may not have a complete awareness of the safety issues that must be addressed to protect the infant from injury.

MOTOR VEHICLE SAFETY

Injuries associated with automobile accidents constitute the single greatest threat to an infant's life and health. Restraining seats are the only practical means of reducing this risk. The crushing forces of a crash or sudden stop, even at low speed, can cause serious injury to the infant. Without a car safety seat, an infant involved in a collision or sudden stop becomes an unguided missile, colliding with the interior of the car or, worse, being ejected from the vehicle. In a collision, infants are usually thrust headfirst, placing them at greater risk for head, facial, or spinal injuries because of the weight of the head, high center of gravity, and open fontanel (Halpern, 1987).

Infant safety in motor vehicles depends entirely on adults. Parents must be informed that they cannot protect their child from injury in a crash by cradling or holding the infant in their laps. Adults are neither strong enough nor quick enough to prevent the sudden forward motions or to overcome the inertial forces (external forces of motion caused by impact) exerted in a crash. An unrestrained adult is propelled forward, trapping and crushing the infant between the adult's body and the hard surfaces inside the car on impact. The only way to prevent injuries and death to

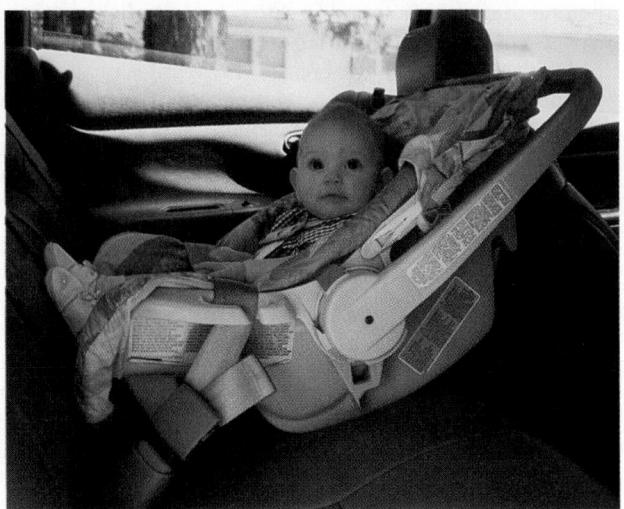

FIGURE 5–2
. . . .
The infant rides facing the rear of the vehicle, ideally in the middle of the back seat. The infant seat is secured to the vehicle with the seat belts; straps on the car seat adjust to accommodate the growing baby. The smaller infant will need a rolled blanket to prevent excess head movement.

an infant in a car is to use a car safety seat for each trip, no matter how short.

A lifelong practice begins with the newborn's first ride home. Getting a child accustomed to using a safety seat at a young age establishes a safety habit and may reduce resistance later (Fig. 5–2).

Some injuries and deaths have been associated with the deployment of air bags. Infants and children should not be restrained in the front seat of cars equipped with passenger-side air bags. When deployed, the air bag can severely jolt the car safety seat and harm the infant. The National Highway Traffic Safety Administration recommends placing all children age 12 and under in the rear seat with the appropriate restraint. Infants weighing less than 20 lb or younger than 1 year should always be in the back seat in rear-facing car seats (Huff, Bagwell, & Bachman, 1998). Children should be properly secured in the vehicle's back seat in a child safety seat, a booster seat, or shoulder/lap belt correct for the child's size (Fig. 5–3).

PROVIDING A SAFE ENVIRONMENT

During infancy and early childhood, when children are typically limited to the home environment, safety in and around the home is a top priority. With the exception of injuries and deaths related to motor vehicle crashes, the majority of childhood injuries occur in the home. Parents must also consider safety as a factor when selecting day care facilities for their child.

Burn Safety.   Infants are especially vulnerable to inflicted burns, particularly scald burns. Their limited mobility makes it impossible for them to escape from immersion in hot water. Parents should be instructed to decrease the setting on hot water heaters to 120°F. Infant skin is thin, causing burns to occur faster at lower temperatures than burns

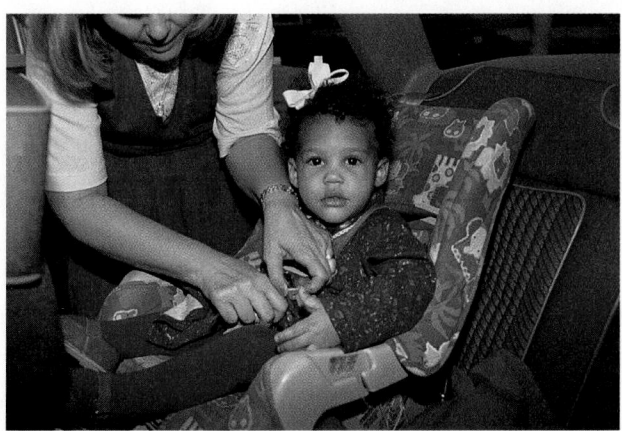

FIGURE 5-3

When an older infant easily sits alone, the car safety seat can be adjusted to a forward-facing, upright position. This seat is appropriate for the toddler until the child reaches about 40 pounds. The safety straps should be adjusted to provide a snug fit, and the seat should be placed in the back seat of the car, ideally in the middle.

- The distance between slats must be no more than 2⅜ inches wide to prevent entrapment of the infant's head or body.
- The interior of the crib must snugly accommodate a standard size mattress so that the gap is minimal, less than the width of two adult fingers. Excessive space could allow the infant to become wedged, potentially suffocating.
- Decorative enhancements on the crib are not recommended because they can break apart and be aspirated by the infant. Design cutouts can trap an infant's arm or neck, causing death or serious injury.
- Cornerposts or finials that rise above the end panels can snag garments and inadvertently strangle infants.
- The drop side must be impossible for an infant to release. Activating the drop side must take either a strong force (at least 10 lb) or a distinct action at each locking device.
- Wood surfaces should be free of splinters, cracks, and lead-based paint.

occur in adults. With water temperature settings of 140°F, it takes only 3 seconds for the child to suffer serious burns. When the temperature is lowered by 20°, it takes 8 to 10 minutes of submersion to cause the same degree of burn injury. An adult should test the water temperature before the infant is submerged to decrease the risk of accidental scald injuries.

Burn injuries in infants can also be caused by a variety of other sources. Exposure to sunlight can result in serious sunburn to their delicate skin. Parents should be encouraged to apply sunblock and sunscreens liberally and to protect the face and head with a hat when exposing the infant or toddler to sunlight, even for brief periods.

Parents should be advised to avoid smoking, drinking hot liquids, or cooking while holding an infant. As infants begin to crawl around on the floor, open electric sockets should be covered with appropriate socket protectors. Open stoves or fireplaces are especially intriguing to an exploring infant and should be outfitted with a guard or grid. Cool mist vaporizers should be used rather than steam vaporizers to prevent scald injuries to a curious infant.

Safe Baby Furnishings. Baby furniture, although seemingly benign, can present lethal hazards to a growing infant. Parents should be aware of safety considerations when planning or decorating the infant's room. Parents need to be aware that older furniture that has been handed down may not meet current safety regulations. In older cribs the gaps between slats may be large enough that infants could entrap their heads, or the paint may contain lead.

Hanging toys or mobiles placed over the crib should be positioned well out of the infant's reach to prevent entanglement and strangulation. Large toys in the crib should be avoided because an older infant may use them as steps to climb over the side, resulting in a serious fall injury. Cribs should be positioned away from curtains or blinds to prevent accidental entanglement in dangling cords.

Preventing Falls. Infants are often placed on surfaces at heights that are convenient for the adult, such as on changing tables, counters, or furniture. These surfaces often have no restraining barriers. Infants begin to roll over as early as 2 months, and as they begin to scoot or crawl, fall injuries from these elevations are common. There must be constant adult supervision when infants are placed at such heights (Fig. 5–4). If the parent or nurse must move away from the infant, the adult should either take the infant or, if supplies are close, place a hand on the infant while reaching. At home, parents may choose to place their child on the floor for changing diapers or providing other care.

Falls from infant seats or out of high chairs are common and can be prevented with supervision and the use of safety restraining straps to limit the mobility of the infant (see Fig. 5–4).

As infants begin to crawl, using gates at the top and bottom of stairs can prevent falls. Infant walkers are dangerous, and the American Academy of Pediatrics discourages their use (AAP, 1995). They allow infants mobility and the freedom to explore surroundings before they have developed the ability to interpret heights or protect themselves from falls.

Preventing Asphyxiation. *Asphyxiation* (suffocation) occurs when air cannot get into or out of the lungs and oxygen supplies are consequently depleted. Carbon dioxide levels then increase, causing life-threatening disruption of cardiac and cerebral functioning. Choking occurs when substances or objects are *aspirated* into the airway or into the branches of the lower airways, causing partial or complete obstruction of the lungs. Strangulation is typically thought of as a constriction of the neck, but it also includes blockage

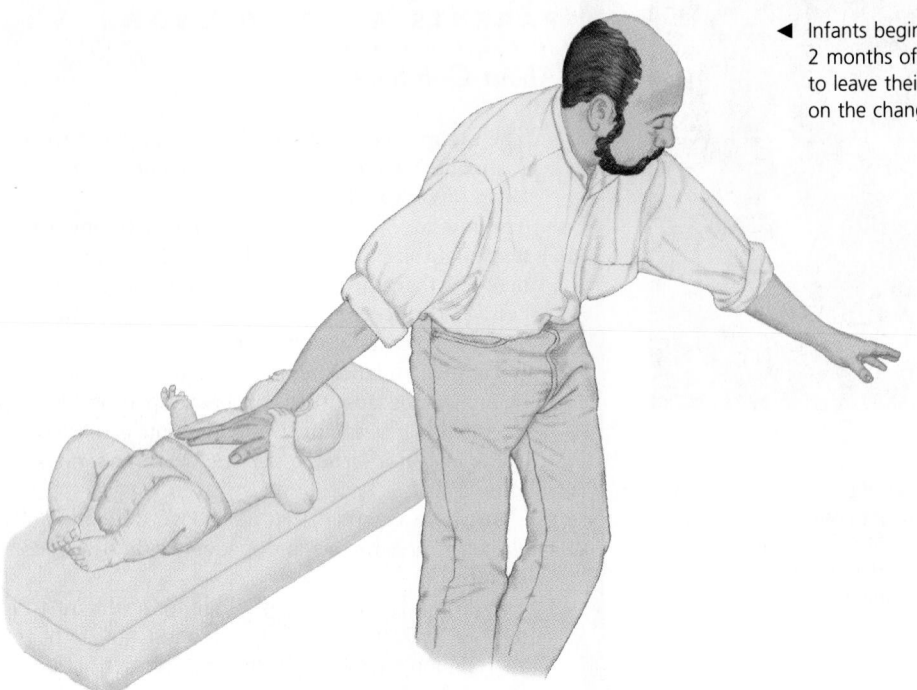

◀ Infants begin to roll over by themselves as early as 2 months of age. The nurse must warn parents not to leave their infant unattended, even for a second, on the changing table or other high surfaces.

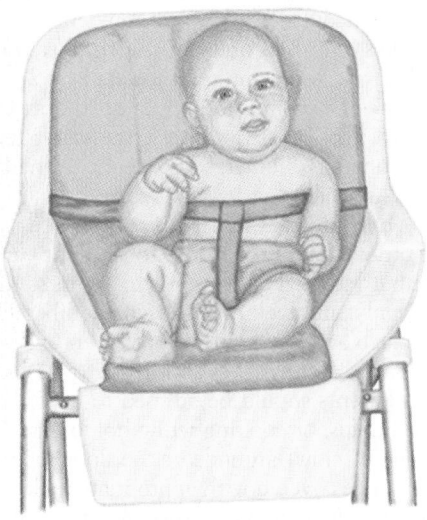

Close supervision and the use of restraining straps can ▶ prevent falls from high chairs, a common cause of injuries in children.

FIGURE 5-4
. . . .
Safety education for parents of infants should emphasize the need for constant supervision and the use of restraining devices to prevent falls.

of the nose and mouth by airtight materials, such as plastic. This blockage prevents air exchange. All plastic bags or covers should be stored out of the infant's reach. Choking is a major concern in the first few months of an infant's life, when aspiration of feedings or vomit can occur easily because of the immature swallowing mechanism. Parents should be taught to position infants on their sides after feedings and to avoid placing small infants in bed with a bottle propped in their mouths.

As infants grow, they begin to explore the world around them by placing anything and everything in their mouths. Size, shape, and consistency are major determinants of whether a food or object is likely to be aspirated by an infant. Food that is round or similar to the size of the airway is especially dangerous. Dangerous foods include sliced hot dogs, hard candy, peanuts, grapes, and chewing gum. These foods should be avoided until the child is able to chew thoroughly before swallowing. Food should be cut into small pieces and the child should be supervised while eating. Playing, singing, or other activities should be strongly discouraged while eating, to avoid choking. Infants are equally endangered by rattles, pieces of toys, ribbons from stuffed animals, and common household objects such as coins, buttons, pins, or beads found on the floor or within their reach.

Anticipatory guidance for parents includes performing a thorough inspection of the infant's surroundings to remove all potential items that infants could grasp, place in their mouths, and choke on. Parents can be encouraged to crawl through the home to gain a better perspective of the infant's environment. Parents can then substitute safe objects for exploration.

Ornaments or toys with detachable parts are not recommended for infants because of the aspiration risk. In 1979, the Consumer Product Safety Commission established a toy standard to prevent choking hazards in nonfood products targeted for children younger than 3 years of age. Parents should take extra care to note the presence of small detachable parts on toys before allowing the infant to play with the item. Although the government regulates the size of parts on infant's toys, older children's toys are not regulated by the same standard. As the infant explores an older sibling's or a playmate's territory, adult supervision is important.

To prevent strangulation injuries, parents should be cautioned against placing a pacifier on a string or cord around the infant's neck, putting an infant to sleep with a bib in place, or positioning a crib near blinds or curtain cords. Crib slats should comply with the 2⅜-inch width requirement to prevent head entrapment.

In addition to inspecting and providing a safe environment for the infant, parents should be instructed in the appropriate action to take if the infant chokes. (See Chapter 34 for a discussion of emergency procedures.)

Immunization

The importance of childhood immunization against disease cannot be overemphasized. Infants are especially vulnerable to infectious disease because their immune systems are immature. Term newborns are protected from certain infections by transplacental passive immunity from their mothers. Breast-fed infants receive additional immunoglobulins against many types of viruses and bacteria. Transplacental immunity is effective only for approximately 3 months, however, and for a variety of reasons, many mothers choose not to breast-feed. In any case, this passive immunity does not cover all diseases, and infection in the infant can be devastating. Immunization offers protection that all infants need.

Nurses play an important role in health promotion and disease prevention related to immunization. Nursing responsibilities include assessing current immunization status, removing barriers to receiving immunizations, tracking immunization records, providing parent education, and recognizing contraindications to the receipt of vaccines. Chapter 4 provides detailed information regarding immunizations and their schedule. See Table 5–2 for immunizations given during infancy.

Dental Care

Eruption of the infant's first teeth is a developmental milestone that has great significance for many parents. Deciduous or "baby" teeth usually erupt between 5 and 9 months of age. The first to appear are the lower central incisors, followed by the upper central incisors, then the upper lateral incisors. The next teeth to erupt are usually the lower lateral incisors, first primary molars, canines, and the second primary molars. The average child has six to eight teeth by the first birthday.

TEETHING

Although sometimes asymptomatic, teething is often signaled by behavior such as night wakening, daytime restlessness, an increase in nonnutritive sucking, excess drooling, and temporary loss of appetite. Some degree of discomfort is normal, but a health care professional should investigate elevated temperature, irritability, ear tugging, or diarrhea further.

To help parents cope with teething, nurses can suggest that they provide cool liquids and hard foods (such as dry toast, Popsicles, or frozen bagels) for chewing. Hard, cold teethers and ice wrapped in cloth may also provide comfort for inflamed gums. Nurses should explain to parents that over-the-counter topical medications for gum pain relief should be used only as directed. Home remedies, such as rubbing the gums with whiskey or aspirin, should be discouraged, but acetaminophen administered as directed for the child's age can be used to relieve discomfort. Although these interventions can be helpful, parents should understand that absolute relief comes only with tooth eruption.

CLEANING TEETH

Because the primary teeth are used for chewing until the permanent teeth erupt and because decay of the primary teeth often results in decay of the permanent teeth, dental care must begin in infancy. Cotton swabs or a soft washcloth can be used to clean the teeth with the child positioned in the parent's lap or on a changing table. Toothpaste is not recommended because infants tend to swallow it, possibly ingesting excessive amounts of fluoride. Too much fluoride can cause fluorosis, which results in staining of the teeth (Roberts et al., 1998).

Appropriate amounts of fluoride, however, are necessary for the development of healthy teeth. Infants receive fluoride when formula and cereal are mixed with water from fluoridated water supplies.

BOTTLE MOUTH CARIES

Bottle mouth caries or nursing-bottle caries is a well-described form of tooth decay that can develop in infants and children. The decay pattern usually involves the incisors initially, then spreads to other teeth. Decay may be so serious that tooth loss occurs prematurely. When the infant is allowed to fall asleep with a bottle containing milk or juice, the carbohydrate-rich solution bathes the teeth for a long period and may cause dental caries (Barnes, 1992).

Nurses should discourage parents from giving bedtime bottles of milk or juice to infants. If a nighttime bottle is necessary, plain water is an acceptable substitute for carbohydrate-rich liquids (Von Burg, Sanders, & Weddell, 1995). A pacifier is an acceptable alternative to a nighttime bottle, although the practice of dipping the pacifier in Karo corn syrup or honey to encourage acceptance poses the same problem. An additional danger of the use of honey in infancy is botulism.

KEY CONCEPTS

- During the first year of life, the infant's organs grow and mature at a rapid rate, yet organ systems of infants remain very different from those of older children and adults.
- Weight gain and muscle growth during infancy allow the infant to have increased control of reflexes and increasingly coordinated movement.
- Sensory capabilities, neuromuscular control, perceptual skills, the quality and quantity of parental interaction, and environmental stimulation all affect cognitive development during infancy.
- Infants develop language first by listening to sounds of caregivers, then by realizing that certain sounds have special meaning, and eventually by using simple words to communicate.
- Infancy is the period during which children develop the foundation of their personalities, struggling to establish a sense of basic trust rather than mistrust.
- One of the most important features of psychosocial development

during infancy is parent-infant attachment, or the sense of belonging with one another.
- Common problems during infancy such as separation anxiety, sleep disorders, and fretfulness cause parents concern and distress. Nurses should be available with information and support to provide anticipatory guidance.
- Colic can be very stressful for parents. The cause of colic is unknown, and care of the infant must be individualized. Support of the parents is very important.
- Play enhances the infant's growth and development.
- Because infancy is a period of very rapid growth and development, nutritional needs are of special significance. Parents frequently have many questions and concerns about nutrition.
- Breast milk or commercially prepared formulas provide the foundation of nutrition throughout infancy.
- Solid foods are usually introduced between 4 and 6 months of age in

small amounts, one food at a time, based on the infant's growth and development.
- Weaning usually begins between ages 6 and 12 months. It should never take place during stress, and the infant should receive breast milk or formula in the cup until age 12 months.
- Improved motor development coupled with a keen desire to explore the environment places the infant at great risk for unintentional injury.
- Nurses play an important role in health promotion and disease prevention related to immunizations.
- Teething usually begins between 5 and 9 months of age. Some degree of discomfort is normal, and parents often need suggestions for coping with teething.
- Bottle mouth caries or nursing bottle syndrome is a form of tooth decay that can develop in infants and children as a result of prolonged breast-feeding or bottle-feeding, especially at night.

ANSWERS TO CRITICAL THINKING EXERCISE 5–1

1. Since this is Mrs. Brown's first child, she might be insecure about caring for Heidi. She might not be aware of normal growth and developmental milestones for this age. Heidi may be awake for long periods at night or she may have colic, depriving Mrs. Brown of sleep. Mr. Brown may travel or need to be away from home with his job and may not be available to help with Heidi. Mrs. Brown may not have an extended family to help her with the care of the in-

fant. Mrs. Brown may be experiencing postpartum depression.
2. Trust must be established, and this can be accomplished by supporting Mrs. Brown and encouraging her to verbalize her concerns. Mothers of newborns often need reassurance that they are doing a good job, and they need to be given permission to ask any question, no matter how insignificant they or the nurse might think the question is. The nurse can validate Mrs. Brown's feelings of being overwhelmed.

3. The nurse must determine if Mrs. Brown has a support system and, if not, problem-solve with her to provide the support she needs. If Heidi is colicky, Mrs. Brown will need added support and the various interventions will need to be discussed. The nurse ends the visit by giving Mrs. Brown permission to contact her as questions and problems arise. The nurse also makes a note to contact Mrs. Brown by phone in a couple of days to see how she is doing.

REFERENCES AND READINGS

American Academy of Pediatrics. (1997). Breastfeeding and the use of human milk. *Pediatrics, 100*(6), 1035–1039.

American Academy of Pediatrics Committee on Injury and Poison Prevention. (1995). Injuries associated with infant walkers. *Pediatrics, 95*(5), 778–780.

American Academy of Pediatrics Committee on Nutrition. (1995). Fluoride supplementation for children: Interim policy recommendations. *Pediatrics, 95*(5), 777–778.

American Academy of Pediatrics Committee on Nutrition. (1998). *Pediatric nutrition*

handbook. Elk Grove Village, IL: American Academy of Pediatrics.

American Academy of Pediatrics Committee on Nutrition. (1998). Soy protein-based formulas: Recommendations for use in infant feeding. *Pediatrics, 101*(1), 148–153.

American Academy of Pediatrics Work Group on Breastfeeding. (1998). Breastfeeding and the use of human milk. *Pediatrics, 100*(6), 1035–1039.

American Public Health Association. (1990). *Healthy people 2000.* Washington, DC: U.S. Government Printing Office.

Balon, A. (1997). Management of infantile colic. *American Family Physician, 55*(1), 235–242.

Barnes, G. P. (1992). Ethnicity, location, age and fluoridation factors in baby bottle tooth decay and caries prevalence of Head Start children. *Public Health Reports, 107*(2), 167–173.

Behrman, R. E., & Kliegman, R. (1998). *Nelson essentials of pediatrics.* Philadelphia: Saunders.

Behrman, R. E., Kliegman, R., Arvin, A., & Nelson, W. E. (1996). *Nelson textbook of pediatrics.* Philadelphia: Saunders.

Berkowitz, C. (1996). *Pediatrics: A primary care approach.* Philadelphia: Saunders.

Carey, W. (1998). Let's give temperament its due. *Contemporary Pediatrics, 15*(5), 91–113.

Castiglia, P. T. (1987). Speech and language development. *Journal of Pediatric Health Care, 1*(3), 165–167.

Castiglia, P. T. (1992). Teething. *Journal of Pediatric Health Care, 6*(3), 153–154.

Chess, S., & Thomas, A. (1985). Temperamental differences: A critical concept in child health care. *Pediatric Nursing, 11*(3), 167–171.

Chess, S., & Thomas, A. (1996). *Temperament: Theory and practice.* New York: Brunner/Mazel.

Davis, J., & Sherer, K. (1994). *Applied nutrition and diet therapy for nurses.* Philadelphia: Saunders.

Erikson, E. H. (1963). *Childhood and society* (2nd ed.). New York: Norton.

Esquivel, M. (1997). Airbag safety issues examined. *AAP News, 13*(1), 1.

Flavell, J. H. (1964). *The developmental psychology of Jean Piaget.* New York: Van Nostrand.

Froese-Fretz, A. (1996). Ask the expert. *Journal of the Society of Pediatric Nursing, 1*(1), 41–42.

Graham, J., Goldie, S., Segui-Gomez, M., Thompson, K., Nelson, T., Glass, R., Simpson, A., & Woerner, L. (1998). *Pediatrics, 102*(1), e3.

Halpern, J. S. (1987). The misuse of child safety restraints. *Journal of Emergency Nursing, 13*(6), 365–368.

Henry, J. T. (1992). Routine growth monitoring and assessment of growth disorders. *Journal of Pediatric Health Care, 6,* 291–301.

Hill, D., Hudson, I., Sheffield, L., Shelton, M., Menahem, S., & Hosking, C. (1995). A low allergen diet is a significant intervention in infantile colic: Results of a community-based study. *Journal of Allergy and Clinical Immunology, 96*(6), 886–892.

Huff, G., Bagwell, S., & Bachman, D. (1998). Airbag injuries in infants and children: A case report and review of the literature. *Pediatrics, 102*(1), e2.

Karmiloff-Smith, A. (1995). The extraordinary cognitive journey from foetus through infancy. *Journal of Child Psychology and Psychiatry, 36*(8), 1293–1313.

Keefe, M. R., & Froese-Fretz, A. (1991). Living with an irritable infant: Maternal perspectives. *MCN: American Journal of Maternal/Child Nursing, 16*(5), 255–259.

Keefe, M. R., Kotzer, A. M., Froese-Fretz, A., & Curtin, M. (1996). A longitudinal comparison of irritable and nonirritable infants. *Nursing Research, 45*(1), 4–9.

Kemper, K. (1996). Seven herbs every pediatrician should know. *Contemporary Pediatrics, 13*(12), 79–90.

Levine, M., Carey, W., & Crocker, A. (1992). *Developmental-behavioral pediatrics.* Philadelphia: Saunders.

Mack, R. (1998). "Something wicked this way comes": Herbs even witches should avoid. *Contemporary Pediatrics, 15*(6), 49–64.

Mehl, A., & Thomson, V. (1998). Newborn hearing screening: The great omission. *Pediatrics, 101*(1), e4.

Moore, M. L., & Krowchuk, H. (1997). Parent line: Nurse telephone intervention for parents and caregivers of children from birth through age 5. *Journal of the Society of Pediatric Nursing, 2*(4), 179–184.

Muniz, A., & Joffe, M. (1997). Foreign bodies ingested and inhaled. *Contemporary Pediatrics, 14*(12), 78–100.

Olsen, R., Barbaresi, W., & Olsen, G. (1998). Development in the first year of life. *Contemporary Pediatrics, 15*(7), 81–115.

Piaget, J. (1952). *The origins of intelligence in children.* New York: International Universities Press.

Roberts, M., Keels, M., Sharp, M., & Lewis, J. (1998). Fluoride supplement prescribing and dental referral patterns among academic pediatricians. *Pediatrics, 101*(1), e6.

Schmitt, B. (1999). *Instructions for pediatric patients.* Philadelphia: Saunders.

Schuman, A. (1998). Universal newborn hearing screening: The time is right. *Contemporary Pediatrics, 15*(7), 49–59.

Sinclair, D. (1989). *Human growth after birth.* New York: Oxford University Press.

Stern, D. (1985). *The interpersonal world of the infant.* New York: Basic Books.

Sullivan, J. (1997). Learning the baby: A maternal thinking and problem-solving process. *Journal of the Society of Pediatric Nursing, 2*(1), 21–28.

Trahms, C. M., & Pipes, P. L. (1997). *Nutrition in infancy and childhood.* St. Louis: Mosby.

Von Burg, M. M., Sanders, B. J., & Weddell, J. A. (1995). Baby bottle tooth decay: A concern for all mothers. *Pediatric Nursing, 21*(6), 515–519.

Wilson, C. B. (1986). Immunologic basis for increased susceptibility of the neonate to infection. *Journal of Pediatrics, 108*(1), 1–12.

White, B. L. (1975). *The first three years of life.* Englewood Cliffs, NJ: Prentice-Hall.

Wright, A., Bauer, M., Naylor, A., Sutcliffe, E., & Clark, L. (1998). Increasing breastfeeding rates to reduce infant illness at the community level. *Pediatrics, 101*(5), 837–844.

6

The Toddler
and the
Preschooler

from a secure base of trust established during the first year. The preschool period, ages 3 through 5 years, is a time of relative tranquility after the tumultuous toddler period.

▋ Growth and Development of the Toddler and Preschooler

The toddler years are characterized by a struggle for autonomy as the child develops a sense of self separate from the parent. Boundless energy and insatiable curiosity drive the toddler to explore the environment and master new skills (Fig. 6–1). The combination of increased motor skills, im-

The developmental changes that mark the transition from infancy to early childhood are dramatic. During the toddler years (the period from 12 through 36 months of age), the child begins to strike out independently

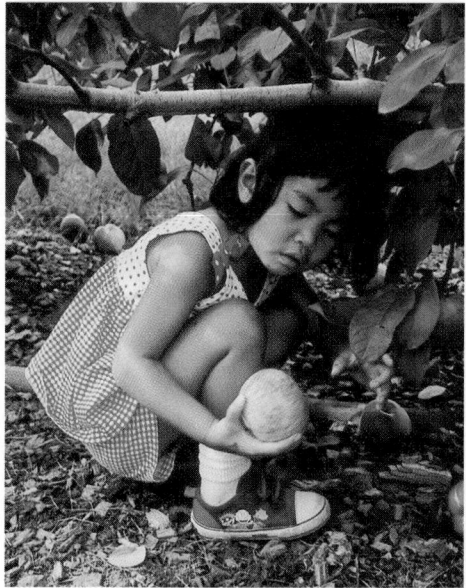

◄ The toddler is enchanted by a world filled with discovery. Curiosity provides resources for the tremendous cognitive growth that occurs during this period.

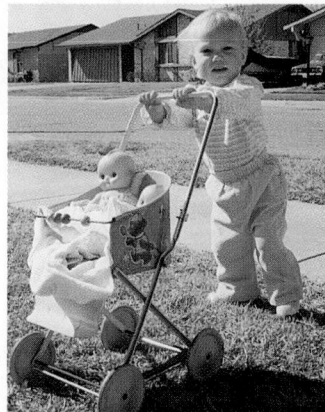

◄ Toddlers enjoy push-pull toys. Toys should be strong and sturdy; wheeled toys should not tip over easily.

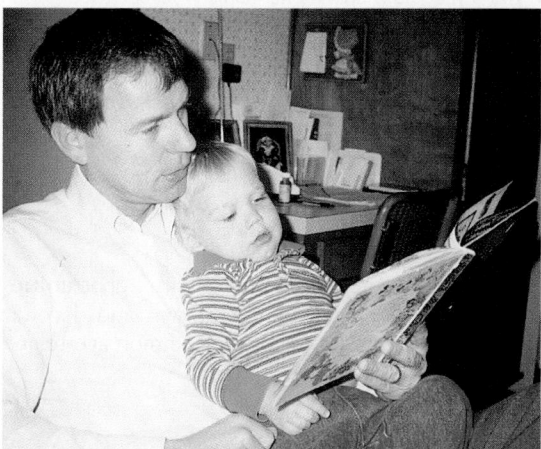

Reading simple stories provides quiet, enjoyable times for toddlers and parents and enhances speech and language development.

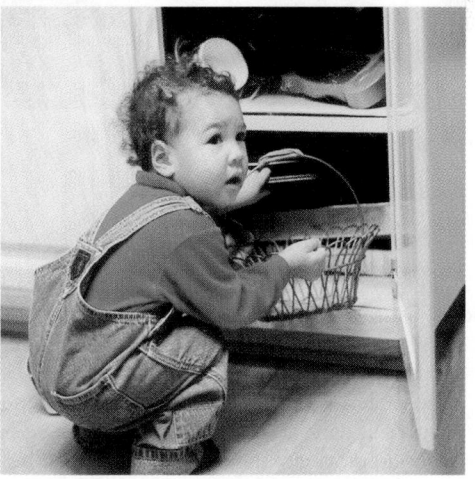

Pots and pans are popular toys for inquisitive toddlers. However, exploring cupboards can be a dangerous activity for toddlers. Toxic cleaning substances and other dangerous objects must be kept behind locked doors or otherwise out of reach.

▋
FIGURE 6–1
· · · · · · · · · ·
Growth and development of the toddler.

103

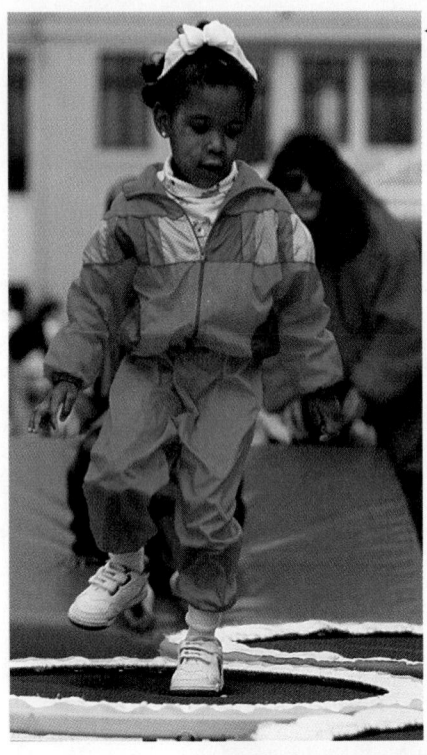

◀ As the brain matures, the preschool child's motor development matures. Opportunities for practice contribute to the development of motor skills. (Courtesy of Cook Children's Medical Center, Fort Worth, Texas.)

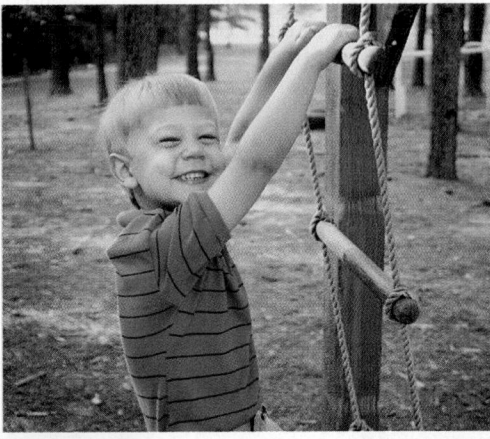

◀ This 4-year-old's motor development has increased to the point that he can jump and climb well. The 4-year-old can also throw a ball overhand and cut on a curved line with scissors.

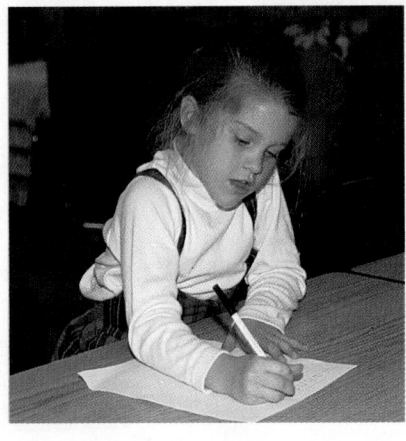

◀ This 5-year-old is printing her name in readable letters. Children of this age can usually skip and can both throw and catch a ball. (Courtesy of The University of Texas at Arlington School of Nursing, Arlington, Texas.)

FIGURE 6–2
• • • • • • • • • •
Growth and development of the preschooler.

maturity, and lack of experience place the toddler at risk for unintentional injury. Toddlers' egocentric and demanding behavior, often marked by temper tantrums and negativism, have given this age the label "the terrible twos."

The preschooler becomes increasingly independent, mastering many self-care and motor skills and developing greater social and emotional maturity (Fig. 6–2). The preschooler is imaginative, creative, and curious. Many parents describe this period as their favorite age as they watch the dramatic transformation of a chubby toddler into an agile, articulate child who is ready to enter the world of peers and school.

The growth and development of the toddler and preschooler are summarized in Table 6–1. The nurse's roles as health care provider, family counselor, and child advocate continue during the toddler and preschool years. Well-child checkups provide the nurse with opportunities for anticipatory guidance related to growth and development, safety, nutrition, and some of the common age-related concerns of parents.

Physical Growth and Development

THE TODDLER

Physical growth slows during the toddler years. The average weight gain is 2.25 kg (5 lb) per year. A child's birth weight has quadrupled by age 2 to 3 years. The rate of increase in height also slows, with the average toddler growing approximately 7.5 cm (3 inches) per year.

The brain grows at a slower rate during this period than during infancy. Head circumference reflects this growth, in-

Text continued on page 109

TABLE 6–1
• • • • • • • • • • •

Summary of Growth and Development: The Toddler and the Preschool Child

Physical	Motor	Psychosocial	Sensory/Cognitive	Language/ Communication
15 Months				
Toddler				
Gains 5 lb (2.25 kg) per year. Grows 3 inches (7.5 cm) per year. Twelve teeth erupt.	**Gross** Walks alone. Climbs stairs; slides down backward on abdomen. Enjoys throwing objects to the floor. May climb out of high chair, crib, or stroller. Constantly on the go. **Fine:** Builds a tower of two blocks. Drinks from a cup, holding the cup with both hands. Takes off socks and shoes. Puts a pellet in a bottle and pours it out. Wants to carry something in each hand.	Onset of negativism. Demands attention. Frequent mood swings. Begins to insist on doing things without help. Shows affection to parents. Recognizes self in photographs, mirror. Imitates housework. Easily distracted and entertained. May indicate wet diaper. Likes to take off shoes and socks.	Places a round block in a round hole. Unable to transfer knowledge to a new situation. Pats picture in a book. Imitates simple actions. Binocular vision well developed. Looks at picture books with parent. Enjoys feeling different textures; dislikes substances that stick to fingers.	Vocabulary of four to six words. Uses gestures and expressive jargon (few real words can be recognized). May say "bye-bye." Asks for objects by pointing. Understands simple directions ("no," "show me," "look"). Points to and names one body part.
18 Months				
Anterior fontanel closed.	**Gross:** Walks fast; seldom falls. Runs stiffly; falls. Pulls toys and large objects. Carries large toy while walking. Climbs. Walks up or down stairs with adult holding his hand. Squats fully and stands again without falling. Seats himself in a small chair. Jumps in place with both feet. **Fine:** Puts blocks in large holes, rings on peg. Scribbles; may attempt to draw horizontal lines. Can drink from a cup without much spilling. Feeds self partially. Builds tower of four to five blocks. Turns knob of radio or TV. Shows hand preference.	Demands attention. Opposes parents with "No!" Less afraid of strangers. Little toleration for frustration. Temper tantrums may be triggered by fatigue, frustration, or anger. Unable to share. Imitates housework. Treats other toddlers as if they were objects. May indicate readiness for toilet training. Tries to brush teeth. Likes to undress. Is an entertaining show-off. Balances desire for independence with desire for closeness (e.g., explores across the room and then comes back to cuddle).	Imitates people and things in the environment. Explores environment extensively. Searches for desired object (toy) in more than one place. Follows simple, one-part directions. Infers causes from observing effects; beginning to figure out how things work. Short attention span. Remembers where objects belong. Has 20/40 vision.	Vocabulary of 30 or more words. "No" is chief word. Holographic speech (uses a single word with accompanying gestures to express whole ideas). Asks for some wants by naming (e.g., juice, cookie, outside). Gets coat and says "bye-bye." May not talk yet.

Table continued on following page

TABLE 6-1

• • • • • • • • • • •

Summary of Growth and Development: The Toddler and the Preschool Child Continued

Physical	Motor	Psychosocial	Sensory/Cognitive	Language/ Communication
24 Months				
Adult height approximately double height at 2 years.	**Gross:** Runs fairly well. Walks up and down stairs holding on to handrail (two feet on each step). Throws ball with both hands without falling. Kicks ball. **Fine:** Opens doorknob. Drinks from a small cup using only one hand. Uses a spoon, spilling little. Turns pages of a book one at a time. Unzips large zipper; unbuttons large buttons. Puts on coat without help. Builds tower of six to seven blocks. Lines blocks up, making a train.	Negativistic, stubborn. Wants to do things for self. Likes to tell others what to do. Engages in pretend play. Still cannot share. May bite, slap, or hit. Wants own way in everything. Affectionate. Has a positive self-concept. Likes to dress and take off clothes. Brushes teeth with help. May demonstrate readiness for toilet training by anticipating a need to defecate or urinate. May be afraid of the dark or of animals.	Places a square block into the appropriate hole. Magical thinking. Matches simple shapes and colors. Names three body parts on request. Beginning to understand time ("after lunch"), but does not understand clock or calendar time. Is learning to wait; understands "soon." Attention span of approximately 2 minutes.	Vocabulary of 300 or more words. Uses two- to three-word sentences ("Go bye-bye." "More milk."). Telegraphic speech ("Me do." "Daddy push"). Egocentric speech, monologues. Uses pronouns (I, me). Talks constantly. Refers to self by first name. Listens to and enjoys simple stories.
30 Months				
	Gross: Stands on one foot alone for 1 second. Jumps with both feet. Can throw a large ball about 5 feet. Catches a large ball with both arms and body. Can walk on tiptoe. **Fine:** Likes to fill containers with objects. Puts on simple clothes independently, snaps large snaps, and buttons large buttons. Twists lid off a jar. Places simple shapes in correct hole. Uses fork. May use toilet, but still needs help. Builds tower of eight blocks.	Plays in an organized, focused manner for 20 minutes or longer. Beginning to think about the consequences of behavior. May sort blocks or dolls and pretend that they are members of a family (e.g., a big block is the head of the family).	Can think about the consequences of behavior. Names six body parts on request. Beginning to understand "tomorrow" and "yesterday."	Vocabulary increases; can name almost everything at home or on walks. More conversation with others; less monologue. Sentences of three or more words. Knows first and last name. Uses plurals.
3 Years				
Appears taller and thinner as body contours change. Growth occurs more in limbs than in trunk.	**Gross:** Pedals tricycle. Goes up stairs (alternating feet) without holding on. Jumps from bottom step.	Curious and energetic. Increasingly independent. Imitates role models. Wants to please.	Preconceptual phase. Egocentric in thought and actions (cannot appreciate another's viewpoint).	Talks incessantly whether anyone is listening or not. Uses telegraphic speech.

TABLE 6–1

• • • • • • • • • • •

Summary of Growth and Development: The Toddler and the Preschool Child Continued

Physical	Motor	Psychosocial	Sensory/Cognitive	Language/ Communication
Average growth 2–3 inches (6–8 cm) per year. Average weight gain 4–5 lb (1.8–2.3 kg) per year. Average weight 32 lb (14.6 kg). Average height 37.25 inches (95 cm). 20 teeth present.	Stands briefly on one foot. Walks well on uneven surfaces. Can walk a straight line. Walks backward. Throws ball with one hand. Catches large ball with both hands. **Fine:** Copies circle; copies cross. Draws a person with three parts (usually a circle with eyes). Can cut on a straight line with scissors. Strings large beads. Builds a tower of 10 cubes. Builds a bridge with three cubes.	Thrives on routine. Bedtime rituals are important. Jealous of siblings. Play is parallel and associative. Understands turn-taking and is capable of sharing, but does not always want to share. Occasional feelings of guilt and shame. Fears of the dark, animals, shadows, and strangers. Feeds self well. Can go to the toilet without help; usually stays dry at night. Can wash and dry hands; brush teeth; dress self completely, except for back buttons. Puts shoes on. Can help with simple household tasks (dusting, picking up toys, setting the table). Sexual curiosity is common. May masturbate, knows sex differences and own sex.	Magical thinking; shifts between reality and imagination. Animism (believes anything that moves is alive). Lacks reversibility. Has an attention span of 10 minutes. Has a slight understanding of past and future, but tomorrow and yesterday are still confusing. Thinks illogically. Understands simple reasoning. Sense of humor. Follows simple directions.	Constantly asks how and why questions. Speaks in sentences of three to four words. Vocabulary of 300 to 900 words. Uses pronouns (I, me, you). Talks to himself. Understands spatial relationships (in, on, under). Knows functions of common objects. Can count three objects. Can tell full name, age, and sex.

4 Years

Growth rate similar to previous year. Average weight 36.75 lb (16.7 kg). Average height 40.5 inches (103 cm). Birth length doubles.	**Gross:** Very active; constantly on the go. Runs well. Can catch and throw ball overhand. Jumps and climbs well. Swings. Goes up and down stairs without holding on. Hops on one foot. Heel-toe walks. **Fine:** Copies a square. Tries to print letters. Draws a person with two to four parts. Can cut on a curved line with scissors. Handedness is usually established.	Increasingly independent. Separates more easily from parent. Play is associative; cooperates with other children, but less likely to share than 3-year-old. May have an imaginary friend. Still jealous of siblings, but beginning to work through jealousy. Dresses and undresses self. Can button front and side of clothes, but needs help with zippers. Can lace shoes, but not tie them.	Intuitive thought stage. Beginning to be less egocentric, but still unable to take another's point of view. Highly imaginative. Still believes that thoughts cause events. Lacks reversibility. Has an attention span of 20 minutes. Improved understanding of time (tomorrow, this afternoon, next week). Can name one or more colors. Can complete an 8- to 10-piece puzzle.	Constantly asks questions. Vocabulary of 1,500 words. Speaks in sentences of four to five words. Tells stories mixing reality and fantasy. Uses "I" frequently. Counts to 5. Understands same and different. Knows days of the week. Stuttering fairly common (normal language variation).

Table continued on following page

TABLE 6-1 . . . .

Summary of Growth and Development: The Toddler and the Preschool Child Continued

Physical	Motor	Psychosocial	Sensory/Cognitive	Language/Communication
		Can brush teeth and bathe self. Bossy, name-calling. Boasts, brags, and exaggerates. May use profanity to get attention. May "run away from home." Increased ability to think without acting out; anticipates events. Sexual curiosity and exploration is common. Identifies with opposite-sex parent.	Has difficulty distinguishing reality from fantasy.	

5 Years

Physical	Motor	Psychosocial	Sensory/Cognitive	Language/Communication
Average weight 41.25 lb (18.7 kg). Average height 43.25 inches (110 cm). May begin to lose deciduous teeth. First permanent teeth (molars) may erupt.	**Gross:** Runs with more control and power. Throws and catches a ball well. Stands on one foot (10 seconds). Able to skip, roller skate, swing on a swing, and hit a ball with a bat. Can jump rope. Hops on either foot. **Fine:** Copies a triangle or diamond. Draws a person with a body and six parts. Prints first name and some letters. Cuts out simple shapes with scissors. Hits a nail on the head with a hammer.	Increasingly independent. Gets along well with parents. Industrious and proud of accomplishments. Play is associative; like rules, but may cheat to win. More generous with toys. Less imaginative, more realistic. Daydreams. Less argumentative and rebellious. Responsible; values rules. Fewer fears. Protective of younger siblings. May show tension by biting nails, picking nose, or whining. Aware of cultural differences. Dresses without help. Can tie shoelaces. Can put toys away neatly. Pours from a small pitcher. Spreads butter with a knife; can cut own meat. Identifies with same-sex parent and enjoys doing things together.	Beginning to understand others' viewpoints. Has an attention span of 30 minutes. Lacks reversibility. Better understanding of time. Can name four or more colors. Can count ten or more objects. May do simple addition, but cannot subtract. Can name a penny, nickel, and dime.	Asks questions and the meaning of words. Vocabulary of 2,100 words. Speaks in sentences of more than five words. Uses all parts of speech. Can define simple words by describing their use or shape. May use fantasy in stories, but is aware of distortions made. Counts to 10. Understands basic number concepts. Recalls parts of a story. Follows three-part commands. Knows the days of the week, seasons. Knows name and address.

creasing approximately 3.5 cm (1.8 inches) during the toddler years, compared with the growth of 12 cm (4.7 inches) in the first 12 months. By the age of 2 years, the brain has attained 90% of adult size.

Immature abdominal musculature gives the toddler a potbellied appearance, with an exaggerated lumbar curve. The child's short legs may appear slightly bowed, and the feet seem flat because of a plantar fat pad that disappears around the age of 2 years. During the toddler years, muscle tissue gradually replaces much of the adipose tissue (baby fat) present during infancy. As the musculoskeletal system matures and the child walks and runs more, the cherubic toddler disappears and the child grows into a taller, leaner preschooler.

THE PRESCHOOLER

The growth of the preschool child is slow and steady. Height and weight gain is minimal during this period. The average weight gain is about 2.25 kg (5 lb) per year, and the height gain averages 5.0 to 7.5 cm (2 to 3 inches) per year. Children attain half their adult height between the ages of 2 and 3 years. During this time, growth occurs more rapidly in the legs than in the trunk, accumulation of adipose tissue declines, and the child's appetite decreases. As a result, the preschooler loses the potbellied appearance of the toddler, becoming slimmer and more agile. Muscles grow faster than bones during the preschool period. Muscle strength is influenced by nutrition, genetic makeup, and the opportunity to exercise and use the muscles. Knock-knees are common in 3-year-olds and are often associated with occasional stumbling and falling. Maturation of the knee and hip joints usually corrects this problem by age 4 or 5 years.

As the lungs grow, the vital capacity increases and the respiratory rate slows. Respirations remain primarily diaphragmatic until age 5 or 6. The heart rate decreases and the blood pressure increases as the heart increases in size (see Chapter 33 for vital sign ranges). Cardiovascular maturation enables the preschooler to engage in more sustained and strenuous activity.

All 20 deciduous teeth are present by age 3. Deciduous teeth may begin to fall out at the end of the preschool period. The first permanent teeth to erupt, the back molars, usually appear in the early school-age years.

Motor Development

THE TODDLER

Learning to walk is the crowning achievement of the toddler period. The child is in perpetual motion, seemingly compelled to pull up, take a few steps, fall, and repeat the process over and over, oblivious to bumps and bruises. The toddler will repeat this performance hundreds of times, until the skill of walking has been perfected.

The age at which children learn to walk varies widely. Most children can walk alone by 15 months. By 18 months of age, toddlers walk well and try to run, but fall often. At approximately 15 months of age, many toddlers become avid climbers. Chairs, tables, and bookcases all present irresistible challenges and risks for injury. Parents may have difficulty keeping the toddler in a crib and may decide it is time to move the child to a regular bed.

Toddlers are also engaged in perfecting fine motor skills. Hand-eye coordination improves with maturity and practice. Mealtimes are still messy. Although most 18-month-olds can hold a cup with both hands and drink from it without much spilling, eating with a spoon is difficult. Most of the food conveyed in a spoon is spilled. Children need a great deal of practice with a spoon before they can feed themselves without spilling. Most toddlers can feed themselves with a spoon by their second birthday if they have been allowed to practice.

At 18 months of age, the toddler enjoys removing clothing. By 24 months the toddler can put on simple items of clothing, but cannot differentiate front from back. Children at this age also can zip large zippers, put on shoes, and wash and dry their hands. Two-year-olds brush their teeth, but need help in adequately removing plaque.

The toddler's increasing motor skills allow more independence in all areas of daily life. Feeding, dressing, and play provide opportunities for the child to develop autonomy. Motor development in this age group is far ahead of development of judgment and perception. This different timing of the development of different skills increases the risk for injury.

THE PRESCHOOLER

Coordination and muscle strength increase rapidly between the ages of 3 and 5. Increases in brain size and nerve myelinization enable the child to perfect fine and gross motor skills.

Motor abilities vary widely among children. Although motor skill is less influenced by environment than other areas of development, such as language, opportunities to practice may contribute to better motor skills. For example, a 4-year-old who often plays catch with a sibling or parent generally finds playing Little League baseball as a 7-year-old easier than a child without a similar experience.

Handedness begins to emerge at about 3 years and is usually clearly established by age 4. The nurse should encourage parents to provide left-handed children with appropriate tools, particularly left-handed scissors. Left-handed children should not be forced to use their right hands, because coordination is usually better when they use the dominant side. Eye-hand coordination is usually good enough by age 5 for a child to hit a nail on the head with a hammer. Increased coordination allows the child to perform many self-care skills and to become more independent.

By age 4 or 5, the child is independent and can dress, eat, and go to the bathroom without help (see Table 6–1). Unlike the toddler, who must be restrained to avoid injury, the older preschooler can usually be trusted to heed verbal warnings of danger.

Cognitive and Sensory Development

THE TODDLER

Toddlers are consumed with curiosity. Their boundless energy and insatiable inquisitiveness provide them with resources for the tremendous cognitive growth that occurs during this period.

Toddlers between the ages of 12 and 18 months are in Piaget's sensorimotor period (see Chapter 4). Learning in this stage occurs mainly by trial and error. Toddlers spend most of a busy day experimenting to see what will happen as they dump, fill, empty, and explore every accessible area of their environment. Between 19 and 24 months, the child enters the final stage of the sensorimotor period. Object permanence is firmly established by this age. The child has a beginning ability to use symbols and words when referring to absent people or objects and begins to solve problems mentally rather than by repeating an action over and over. A toddler at this stage is often seen imitating the parent of the same sex performing household tasks (termed domestic mimicry). Late in this stage, the child displays deferred imitation (e.g., imitating the parent putting on makeup or shaving hours after that parent has left for work). The 18-month-old has a beginning ability to wait, as evidenced by the toddler responding appropriately to a parent or caregiver who says, "just a minute." The child's concept of time is still immature, however, and "a minute" may seem like an hour to the toddler.

> Toddlers think in terms of the predictable routines of their daily schedule. When talking with the toddler, the nurse should use time orientation in relation to familiar activities. For example, a toddler understands "Your mother will be here after your nap" better than "Your mother will be here at 2 o'clock."

Many hours each day are spent putting objects into holes and smaller objects into each other as the child experiments with sizes, shapes, and spatial relations. Toddlers enjoy opening drawers and doors, exploring the contents of cabinets and closets, and generally wreaking havoc throughout the house as well as exposing themselves to potential danger.

At around 24 months, children enter the preconceptual phase of Piaget's preoperational period. This phase ends at age 4. The preoperational stage is characterized by an increased ability to think symbolically. Children begin to think and reason at a primitive level. Two-year-olds have a beginning ability to retain mental images. This ability allows them to internalize what they see and experience. Symbols in the form of words can be used to represent ideas. Increasing amounts of play time are spent pretending. A box may become a spaceship or a hat; pebbles may be money or popcorn. The child's rapidly increasing vocabulary enhances symbolic play. The toddler begins to think about alternative solutions to a problem and can even consider the consequences of an action without carrying it out (touching a hot stove, running too fast on a slippery sidewalk).

The toddler's thinking is immature, limited in its logic and bound to the present. Egocentrism, animism, irreversibility, magical thinking, and centration characterize the preoperational thought of the toddler (Table 6–2).

THE PRESCHOOLER

By age 3 years, the brain has reached two thirds of its adult size. Maturation of the central nervous system contributes to the child's increasing cognitive abilities.

According to Piaget, the preschool child is in the preoperational stage of cognitive development. This stage is divided into two phases, the preconceptual phase (2 to 4 years) and the intuitive phase (4 to 7 years). During the preconceptual phase, the child is beginning to use *symbolic thought*, the ability to allow a mental image (words or ideas) to represent objects or ideas. Mental symbols allow the child to remember the past and to describe events that happened in the past. The 3-year-old can retain a mental image of a loved one and can periodically "refuel" by thinking about that person. A photograph can help some children cope with separation by bridging the gap between physical presence and mental image. Preschoolers' ability to remember their parents and to recognize that their needs can be met

TABLE 6–2

Characteristics of Preoperational Thinking

Characteristic	Example
Egocentrism: Views everything in relation to self; is unable to consider another's point of view.	Toddler takes a toy away from another child and cannot understand that the other child wants (or has a right to) the toy, too.
Animism: Believes that inert objects are alive and have wills of their own.	Toddler trips over a toy and scolds the toy for hurting her. She believes that the toy hurt her on purpose.
Irreversibility: Cannot see a process in reverse order. Cannot follow a line of reasoning back to its beginning. Cannot hold on to two or more sequential thoughts simultaneously.	If the child takes a toy apart, the child cannot remember the sequence for putting it back together. If child is taken on a walk, child cannot retrace steps and find way home.
Magical thought: Believes that magical thought is the cause of events, that wishing something will make it so.	Toddlers often feel extremely powerful and believe that their thoughts cause events to happen. May believe that parents are all-powerful and can read minds or have magical powers.
Centration: Tends to focus on only one aspect of an experience, ignoring other possible alternatives. Focuses on the dominant characteristic of an object, excluding other characteristics.	May have difficulty putting together a puzzle, concentrating on only one detail of a piece (such as shape) and ignoring other qualities (such as color or detail). Cannot follow more than one direction at at time.

even though their parents are not present increases their ability to tolerate separation.

Because preschoolers still engage in *animism*, they often endow inanimate objects with lifelike qualities during play. A doll may become a crying baby, or a teddy bear may become a friend who listens sympathetically. *Symbolic play* is important for emotional development because it allows the child to work through distressing feelings. For this reason, it is therapeutic to allow a child to play with medical equipment after a painful procedure. Four-year-olds who have received injections may be found working out their feelings by giving their dolls "lots of shots."

During the preconceptual phase, reality may be distorted by *transductive reasoning*. The preschool child reasons from particular to particular, rather than from particular to general and vice versa, as adults do. The child cannot understand that relationships exist and cannot view the whole in relation to its parts. The preschool child has difficulty focusing on the important aspects of a situation. To a child, everything is important and interdependent. This type of thinking is called *field dependency*. For example, the preschooler may have difficulty falling asleep at night because the parent did not follow the usual bedtime routine. Objects, routine, and sameness are important to the preschool child. Rituals provide the preschool child with a feeling of control.

The intuitive phase is characterized by centration and lack of reversibility. *Centration* is the tendency to center or focus on one part of a situation and ignore the other parts. The child cannot understand logical relationships and is unable to focus on more than one aspect of a situation at a time. For example, the child may not be able to follow a sequence of directions, but will perform well if the directions are given one at a time.

The 4- or 5-year-old shows *irreversibility* in thought. Children this age cannot reverse a process or the order of events. They may be able to take a complex puzzle apart but have difficulty putting it back together. Likewise, the 4- or 5-year-old might understand that two identical glasses contain the same amount of water. However, if the water in one of the glasses is poured into a third container of a different shape, the child will believe that the third container holds a different amount of water. The child will not realize that if the water is poured back into the original glass, the glass will contain the original amount. The 4- or 5-year old also lacks reversibility for mathematical processes. The child may be able to add 3 and 1 and get 4, but reversing the problem ($4 - 1 = 3$) would be too difficult.

The preschool years are a period of rapid learning. The preschool child is curious and wants to know how things work. Preschoolers' thinking is still magical and egocentric (self-centered). Children at this age tend to understand events only as they are affected by them, believing that everyone else has had the same experience. Children seeing their mother in distress may bring her a doll, assuming that it would comfort the mother as it does the child.

Preschool children often think that their thoughts are powerful enough to cause things to happen. They may frighten themselves with some of their ideas, believing that they may become what they imagine they will be. Preschoolers may feel overwhelmed by guilt when a sibling is hospitalized because they believe that their hostile feelings caused the sibling's illness. Likewise, a child of this age may say, "I got sick because I was bad."

Language Development

THE TODDLER

The acquisition of language is one of the most dramatic developments of early childhood. Although the age at which children begin to talk varies widely, most can communicate verbally by their second birthday. The rate of language development depends on physical maturity and the amount of reinforcement that the child has received. The language characteristics of toddlers at various ages are summarized in Table 6–1. Between 15 and 24 months of age, language ability develops rapidly. Toddlers understand many more words than they can say because receptive language (what the child understands) develops sooner and more quickly than speech. Sometime after 18 months, many children experience a sudden spurt in speech production and comprehension, resulting in a vocabulary of 300 or more words at 24 months. By 2 years of age, roughly 60% to 70% of toddlers' speech should be understandable. Because children of 24 to 30 months are less egocentric and better able to consider another's point of view, they engage in more conversation with others and less monologue.

If language development is not progressing normally, parents should be advised to pursue follow-up care. Children of bilingual families, twins, and children other than firstborns may have slower language development.

Parents can promote language development by talking to their child and incorporating teaching into daily routines. Feeding, bathing, dressing, and going on outings to both new and familiar places offer opportunities for verbal interaction and the practice of growing language skills. The child should be encouraged to express needs rather than the parent anticipating and providing what the child wants before the child asks for it. Reading simple, entertaining stories with colorful pictures provides quiet, enjoyable times for toddlers and parents and enhances speech and language development.

THE PRESCHOOLER

A dramatic increase in language skill in the preschool period promotes self-control and increases the child's ability to direct and be directed by others. Children at this age may be heard talking to themselves about things they have heard or been taught.

The preschooler's vocabulary increases rapidly, from 200 words at age 2 to more than 2,100 words at age 5. In less than 3 years, the child grows from a toddler who knows only a few words into a child who skillfully uses an extensive vocabulary to describe events, share feelings, and ask questions. Three-year-olds speak in short, telegraphic sentences. They may talk to themselves or to imaginary friends. A delightful characteristic of young preschoolers is the tendency to engage in lengthy monologues, regardless of whether anyone is listening or even present. Such self-talk provides the child with opportunities to practice speech and is often accompanied by *symbolic play*.

By age 4, children talk incessantly and tend to boast and exaggerate. They enjoy rhymes and silly ways to use similar words. Four-year-olds expect more detailed answers to their questions. They may use speech aggressively and may use profanity to gain attention. "Bad" language should be ignored, thus depriving the child of reinforcement of the behavior. When children feel that they gain power over their parents by using bad language, these verbalizations will continue.

Five-year-olds speak in sentences of adult length and use all parts of speech. They usually are proficient storytellers who produce elaborate tales for anyone who will listen. Their tendency to mix fantasy with reality may be perceived as lying by adults. The child of 5 usually can recite the days of the week and can name the seasons.

Nurses can teach parents strategies to promote their child's language development. It is important for parents to talk with the child and respond to the child's attempts at communication. Reading to the child and making reading materials available can help build vocabulary and promote a lifelong love of reading. Watching educational television programs, such as *Sesame Street*, with their child may augment parents' communication skills with their child. Preschoolers spend a lot of time asking "how" and "why" questions, often taxing parents' patience. Short, simple, honest answers encourage vocabulary building and boost self-esteem.

Psychosocial Development

THE TODDLER

The toddler is developing a sense of *autonomy*, giving up the comfort of dependence enjoyed during infancy. If a basic sense of trust was established during the first year, the toddler can venture forward and separate from parents for short periods to explore and experience the world.

According to Erikson (1963), the toddler is struggling with the developmental task of acquiring a sense of autonomy while overcoming a sense of shame and doubt. Toddlers discover that they have wills of their own and that they can control others. Asserting their wills and insisting on their own way, however, often leads to conflict with those they love, whereas submissive behavior is rewarded with affection and approval. Toddlers experience conflict because they want to assert their own wills but do not want to risk losing the approval of loved ones. If the child continues to practice dependent behavior, doubt related to abilities develops. Toddlers may feel shame for independent impulses, particularly if there is frequent punishment associated with their actions.

CRITICAL TO REMEMBER

Important Tasks of the Toddler Period

- Recognition of self as a separate person, with own will
- Control of impulses and acquisition of socially acceptable ways to communicate wants and needs
- Control of elimination
- Toleration of separation from the parent

The toddler learns which behaviors gain approval and which result in censure and punishment. The 2-year-old does not have a conscience but avoids punishment by controlling his or her behavior. Right and wrong are determined by the consequences of actions.

At around 15 months, toddlers begin to demonstrate their developing autonomy with two almost universal behaviors: *negativism* and *ritualism*.

Negativism. Negativism, one of the most dramatic expressions of independence, is shown in a variety of ways. The toddler's favorite word seems to be "no." Unable to distinguish between requests and directives, the toddler seems to feel that saying "yes" would mean giving up free will. The child often seems to delight in this test of wills between parent and child. Negativism may result in screaming, kicking, hitting, biting, or breath holding. Parents often interpret the child's negative behavior as being bad or stubborn. Nurses can help parents understand their toddler's behavior as an important sign of the child's progress from dependency to autonomy and independence. Parents should be given support and encouraged to deal with the toddler's trying behavior with patience and a sense of humor. Although general permissiveness is not recommended, too much pressure and forceful methods of control often lead to defiance, tantrums, and prolonged negative behavior.

Ritualism and the Importance of Routine. Ritualism helps the child venture out and away from the safety of the parents by ensuring uniformity and security. Ritualism allows the toddler to have a sense of control. The child feels more confident with a secure home base. The toddler insists on sameness. Milk may have to be poured into the same cup, parents may have to sit in the same chairs at dinnertime, and a specified routine may have to be followed countless times throughout the day. The child may be unable to go to sleep unless a bedtime ritual is followed exactly (e.g., a drink of water, two stories, prayers, and a teddy bear). The child may experience distress if this routine is not followed exactly the next night. Failure to recognize the importance of such rituals may increase stress and insecurity.

Events such as hospitalization, where continuity of routine cannot be ensured, are difficult for the toddler. The nurse can decrease the stress of hospitalization by incorporating the child's usual rituals and routines from home into nursing care activities. Keeping hospital routines as similar to those of home as possible and recognizing ritualistic needs gives the toddler some sense of control and security and decreases feelings of helplessness and fear. See Chapter 35 for further discussion of the hospitalized child.

Separation Anxiety. Separation anxiety peaks again in the toddler period. Although the concept of object permanence is fully developed in the toddler, children at this stage have difficulty differentiating their own feelings from those of their parents. While the children experience a strong desire to be independent and leave their mothers, they fear that their mothers also want to leave them. A toddler may strike out independently across the room, only to rush back in tears to the mother, as if the child were frightened and angry with the mother for leaving. For a brief period, the parent may find it almost impossible to talk on the telephone without interruption or even to go into the bathroom without being followed. Leave-taking and brief separations are acceptable to a toddler if they are the toddler's idea, but the parent's departure may cause desperate clinging and crying. Games such as hide-and-seek help the child master fears of separation. By repeating separation under conditions the child can control, the toddler is helped to overcome the anxiety associated with separation. The child learns from experience that loved ones will return after separation.

Being left with a stranger can be stressful. Toddlers should be told honestly and clearly about a separation shortly before it occurs. The child should also be reassured that the parent is coming back. When a parent returns, the toddler often shows anger at being left by ignoring the parent or by pretending to be more interested in play than in going home. Parents of hospitalized toddlers are frequently distressed by such behavior when they visit their child (see Chapter 35).

Tolerating brief separations from parents is an important developmental task of the toddler. Transition objects, such as a favorite blanket or toy, provide comfort to the toddler in stressful situations such as separation, illness, or even bedtime. Such objects help children make the transition from dependency to autonomy. Toddlers may become so attached to an object that they can hardly bear to part with it, even for a quick run through the washing machine.

The nurse can offer support by explaining that the behavior is a normal growth and development milestone and telling the parents that plenty of affection and attention is needed to help the toddler cope with the stress of separation. The nurse should counsel parents to leave a toddler only briefly at first and, if possible, to delay extended separations until the toddler can handle them better. The nurse who helps parents understand normal toddler behavior in response to separation helps parents cope with the frustrations of this transition.

Play. Toddlers spend most of their time at play. Play is serious business to the toddler—it is the work of the child. Many hours are spent each day in play perfecting fine and gross motor skills, learning to control inner urges, and gaining self-esteem. Play during this period reflects the develop-

mental level of the egocentric toddler. The toddler engages in *parallel play,* in which children play alongside, but not with, other children (Fig. 6–3). Little regard is given to the feelings of others. Children engaged in this type of play frequently grab toys away from other children or may hit or fight to obtain a wanted toy. Because toddlers are egocentric, they do not realize that they are hurting the other child and feel no shame for aggressive actions.

Imitation or acting out of scenes of everyday life is common as the toddler begins to try out roles and identify with adults. Active, large-muscle play helps the toddler vent frustrations and dissipate excess energy. The nurse can help parents understand how play enhances the toddler's development. The nurse should encourage parents to play with their toddler and to provide opportunities for the toddler to play with other children. The nurse should teach parents that the house should be childproofed daily. Toys must be strong, safe, and too large to swallow or place in the ear or nose. Toddlers need supervision at all times. A variety of play materials, which need not be expensive, and a safe play environment enhance the toddler's development (Table 6–3).

Psychosexual Development. At around 18 months, toddlers enter Freud's anal stage. Freud theorized that as children focus on mastery of bowel and bladder functions, their attention is also directed to the genital area. Even before the age of 2, children are aware of their own sex and begin to develop a sense of gender identity. By 2½ or 3 years, toddlers can correctly identify anatomic pictures of boys and girls. It is not until age 5 that gender identity is fully established and the child understands gender as permanent (e.g., that gender does not change with the addition of a wig or a dress) (Kohlberg, 1966).

Children begin to be aware of expected sex role behaviors at an early age. By age 3, most toddlers show an awareness of sex role stereotypes and tend to imitate the same-sex parent during play. Sex role identification continues throughout the toddler and preschool years as the child incorporates the attitudes, roles, and values of the same-sex parent. Although sex role stereotypes have relaxed

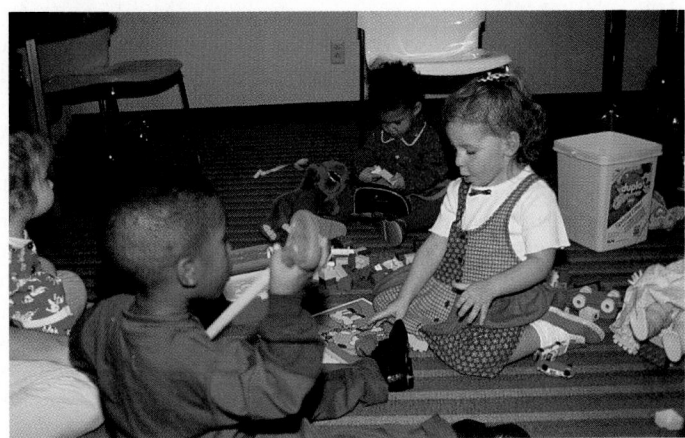

Parallel play occurs when children play side by side with similar toys, but there is no organized group activity. The children play *beside* each other but not *with* each other. (Courtesy of The University of Texas at Arlington School of Nursing, Arlington, Texas.)

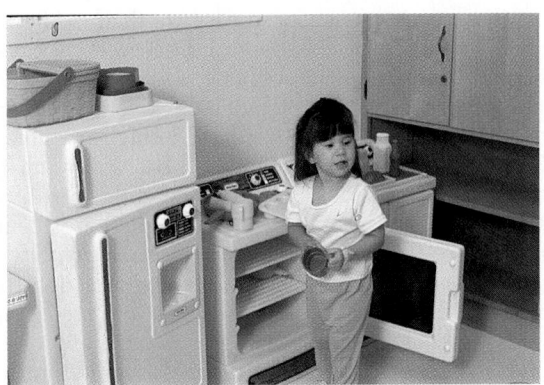

Symbolic play consists of activities that the child uses to express his or her perception of reality. This little girl is acting out a familiar adult scenario as she manipulates child-size toys that represent kitchen equipment.

FIGURE 6–3
• • • • • • • •
Types of play.

TABLE 6-3

Age-Related Activities and Toys for Toddlers and Preschoolers

General Activities	Toys and Specific Types of Play
Toddler	
The toddler fills and empties containers, begins dramatic play, has increased use of motor skills, enjoys feeling different textures, explores the home environment, imitates others, likes to be read to and to look at books and television that are age appropriate. Toys should meet the child's need for activity and inquisitiveness. Children in this age group also enjoy manipulating small objects such as toy people, cars, and animals.	Continued exploring of the body parts of self and others; mechanical toys; objects of different textures such as clay, sand, finger paints, and bubbles; push-pull toys; large ball; sand and water play; blocks; painting; coloring with large crayons; nesting toys; large puzzles; trucks; dolls. Therapeutic play can begin at this age.
Preschooler	
Dramatic play is prominent. Children of this age like to run, jump, hop, and in general increase motor skills. The child likes to build and create things, whether it be sand castles or mud pies. Play is simple and imaginative. Simple collections begin.	Riding toys, building materials such as sand and blocks, dolls, drawing materials, crayons, cars, puzzles, books, appropriate television and videos, nonsense rhymes, singing games, pretending to be something or somebody, dressing up, finger paints, clay, cutting, pasting, simple board and card games.

somewhat in recent years, children behave according to adult expectations. Children learn behavior by reinforcement and punishment as well as by imitation. If a boy repeatedly hears that boys don't play with dolls, he will spurn such "girl's toys" and will play with toys that his parents consider masculine, to gain their praise and approval. Nurses should be aware of their own biases about sex-typed behaviors and should support the parents in their choice of toys and activities for their child. The nurse can be most helpful by encouraging parents to make traditionally sex-typed toys available to both boys and girls if this approach is consistent with the parents' beliefs. Parents' expectations of appropriate sex role behavior differ according to their cultural backgrounds. In most cultures, boys and girls are treated differently and thus are taught "male" and "female" behaviors.

Parents are often concerned about their toddler's interest in and curiosity about sexual differences. Sex play and masturbation are common among toddlers. Nurses can reassure parents that self-exploration or exploration of another toddler's body is normal behavior during early childhood. Parents should respect the child's curiosity as normal without judging the child as "bad." The child should be told that touching private parts is something that is done only in private. When parents discover children involved in sex play, casually telling them to dress and directing them to another activity can limit sex play without producing feelings of shame or anxiety. The nurse should explain to parents that positive attitudes toward sexuality are learned from parents who are comfortable with their own sexuality. As young children learn about their bodies and explore anatomic differences, they frequently ask questions about where babies come from or why "Brian looks different from Emily." Honest, straightforward answers using the correct terminology satisfy the toddler's curiosity and lay the foundation for healthy sexual attitudes.

THE PRESCHOOLER

The preschool years are a critical period for the development of socialization. Children need opportunities to play with others to learn communication and social skills. They also need appropriate guidance to learn acceptable behavior.

According to Erikson, the developmental task of the preschooler is to achieve a sense of initiative. The preschooler is busy learning how to do things and takes great pride in new accomplishments. If the child acts inappropriately or is repeatedly criticized or punished for attempts to explore and learn, feelings of guilt, anxiety, shame, and fear may result. For example, an adult's comment, "That's nice, but it would look better if you did it this way," may cause the child to feel inferior. Such subtle criticism can make the child reluctant to try new activities. A feeling of inferiority may also develop if adults are always doing things for the child rather than encouraging independence. The child who does not achieve a sense of initiative will feel defeated, angry, and afraid of people and new situations. Nurses can promote the healthy psychosocial development of preschoolers and help them gain a sense of initiative by teaching parents the importance of providing the child with opportunities to explore in a safe, stimulating environment. Adults should encourage the preschooler's imagination and creativity and should praise appropriate behavior.

Play. Learning to relate to age-mates is another developmental task that is significant during the preschool period. Preschoolers need experience playing with other children to learn how to relate to other people. Three-year-olds are capable of sharing and are more likely to do so than the toddler. Four-year-olds tend to be more argumentative and less generous with playmates. Although this behavior may appear to be a step backward to parents, it is actually a sign of growth because the 4-year-olds feel more secure in a group and are testing their roles and communication skills. The 5-year-old enjoys playing with other children and generally can play with another child for longer periods before arguments develop.

Children between the ages of 3 and 5 years enjoy parallel and associative play. Children learn to share and cooperate as they play in small groups. During play, preschoolers learn simple games and rules, language concepts, and social roles. Play is often imitative, dramatic, and creative. Various roles are explored through play as children imitate significant adults. Preschoolers enjoy dress-up clothes, housekeeping toys, dollhouses, and other toys that encourage pretending (see Fig. 6–3). Tricycles and climbing toys help to develop muscles and coordination. Preschoolers also enjoy materials for cutting, pasting, and painting. Such manipulative and creative materials stimulate imagination and fine motor development (see Table 6–3).

Imaginary friends are common around the age of 3. Boundaries between reality and fantasy are blurred at this age, and "pretend" can seem real, especially during play. Imaginary friends serve many purposes. They may take the blame when the child misbehaves, allowing the child to save face when he feels guilty about his behavior. Imaginary friends may be companions during lonely times. They may accomplish a task that the child is struggling with or allow the child to practice roles. For example, the child may scold an imaginary friend and administer punishment, just as a parent would. Imaginary friends seem to be more common in highly imaginative and intelligent children.

Psychosexual Development. Sexual identity and body image are developing. Sexual curiosity and explorations are normal. Preschoolers are curious about anatomic differences and seek to investigate them. Preschoolers show interest in the differences between the sexes and often compare their bodies with those of others. "Playing doctor" and hiding with a friend to investigate anatomic differences are common activities during the preschool period. The nurse should reassure parents that the child is simply learning about his or her body and that the parents can direct the child to another activity. Preschoolers are interested in where they came from and how babies are made. Parents should be encouraged to assess what the child already knows about the subject and to determine why the child is asking the question. Questions should be answered simply, honestly, and matter-of-factly. The child usually neither wants nor understands detailed explanations.

A warm, accepting, matter-of-fact attitude toward sexual matters promotes a positive, healthy perspective in children. An atmosphere of acceptance can be created by parents in the early preschool years when the first questions arise. A parental attitude of "You can ask me anything" can set the stage for healthy interaction from early childhood on into adolescence, when parental guidance is so important.

Masturbation is common and may increase in frequency when the child is under stress. Parents are often concerned about such behavior. The nurse can help parents handle these situations by explaining that such self-comforting behaviors are normal for this age. If the parent discovers the child masturbating, it is best to simply redirect the child's attention without punishing, shaming, or reprimanding. Children should be taught that touching their genitals is not appropriate in public.

Children form ideas about sexuality based on the physical interactions between their parents. Positive signs of physical and emotional intimacy between parents send a positive signal to the child. Conversely, parents who constantly fight and are not mutually responsive can have the opposite effect (Tharinger & Lasser, 1997).

At this age, a sense of rivalry with the same-sex parent develops. It is common for a preschool boy to compete with his father for the attention of his mother. A girl likewise may become "Daddy's girl," often cuddling and flirting with her father while excluding her mother from the relationship. This rivalry is usually resolved early in the school-age period as the child identifies strongly with the same-sex parent and same-sex peers. According to Freudian theory, the oedipal stage is resolved when the child strongly identifies with the parent of the same sex. By the end of the preschool period, the child identifies with and imitates the same-sex parent. In single-parent homes, if the parent and child are not of the same sex it is important for the child to have a friendly, stable relationship with an adult relative or friend of the same sex who can serve as a role model. By age 3, children know sex differences. They imitate masculine and feminine behaviors in play, and gender identity is well established by age 6.

Spiritual and Moral Development

Learning the difference between right and wrong (the development of a conscience) is another important task of the preschool period. According to Kohlberg (1964), children between the ages of 4 and 7 years are in the second stage of the preconventional level of moral development. In this stage, children obey rules out of self-interest. They tend to believe that if the consequences of an action are personally advantageous, the action is right. An "eye-for-an-eye" orientation guides their behavior.

The preschooler begins to use self-control to resist temptation and tries to "be good" to avoid feelings of guilt. Preschoolers determine right from wrong by the consequences of disobeying their parents' rules. At this age, children have little understanding of the reason for a rule. For example, when asked why it is wrong to hit another child, the preschooler might reply, "Because my mother says so." Preschoolers adhere to parents' rules dogmatically, deciding whether to break a rule based on the resulting punishment.

Preschoolers often have difficulty applying rules in different situations. The child may know that it is wrong to hit a sibling but may not understand that it is also wrong to hit another child at day care. Because the preschooler is egocentric, understanding another's viewpoint is difficult. The child begins to develop a conscience as a result of consistent rewards for good behavior and punishment for bad behavior.

The preschool child's concept of God is concrete. The family's religious beliefs and customs, such as bedtime prayers, mealtime grace, and Bible stories, are important to preschoolers. Such rituals, practiced in an atmosphere of love, can be deeply meaningful and comforting to children of this age.

◼ Health Promotion for the Toddler or Preschooler and Family

Table 6–4 presents an overview of health screening, health maintenance, and anticipatory guidance activities for the toddler and the preschooler.

TABLE 6–4

Health Screening, Health Maintenance, and Anticipatory Guidance for Toddlers and Preschoolers

15 Months	18 Months	30 Months	3 Years	4 Years	5 Years
Immunization					
Two possible polio schedules: OPV or IPV at 12–18 months. DTaP or DTP at 15–18 months. MMR at 12–15 months. Varicella vaccine at 12–18 months. Hib at 12–15 months. Hep B-3 at 6–18 months.	See 15-month schedule.		Review immunization record; administer appropriate immunizations if not up to date.	DtaP or DTP at 4–6 years. OPV or IPV at 4–6 years. MMR at 4–6 years. Review reactions to previous immunizations.	Administer immunizations if not given at 4 years.
Safety					
Use toddler car seat. Supervise child near water. Keep poisons and sharp objects locked up and out of child's reach. Do not leave child unattended in bathtub. Cover electrical outlets. Supervise child near stove, fireplace.	Supervise child at playgrounds. Protect child from falling. Supervise child around pets: teach not to approach strange dogs. Keep poison control center number and syrup of ipecac available in home.	Supervise child near outdoor hazard (street, swimming pools, garages, power tools, pesticides). Never leave child unattended in the car. Use sunscreen. Provide safe toys.	Supervise child on street. Use car seat; or use booster seat and shoulder harness seat belt if child weighs more than 40 lb. Teach child not to play with matches, and how to escape from burning home. Supervise child when near a fireplace or grill. Teach safety around pets, and not to approach strange dogs. Avoid foods that may be aspirated.	Instruct child in street safety (wait at the curb until told to cross, avoid riding cycles near street or driveways). Use booster seat and safety belts in cars. Teach child to swim; supervise child near water. Teach child not to talk to strangers.	Instruct child in playground safety; teach child not to talk to strangers. Use booster seat and safety belts in cars. Child should know own name, address, and phone number, and how to seek help if lost.
Nutrition					
Do not give bottle as a substitute for solid foods. Feeding: offer finger foods, cup.	Physiologic anorexia. Do not force child to eat. Recognize ritualistic needs. Toddlers often go on food jags.	Serve small portions. Child needs approximately 1,300 calories per day. Avoid cariogenic foods.	Review vitamin and fluoride dosage. Discuss diet, feeding issues, and snacks.	Child needs approximately 1,700 calories per day.	Assess adequacy of diet and snacks. Avoid concentrated sweets.
Vision and Hearing					
Ask parents if child seems to hear and see well. Child should localize sounds. Child should accurately visualize small objects (i.e., raisins).	Assess speech and language. Ear infections may affect hearing.	Assess speech and language. Two thirds of child's speech should be intelligible.	Assess parental perceptions of child's vision and hearing. Assess readiness for objective screening.	Parental perception. Assess readiness for objective screening.	Perform vision and hearing screening. Address parental concerns.

TABLE 6-4
. . . .

Health Screening, Health Maintenance, and Anticipatory Guidance for Toddlers and Preschoolers Continued

15 Months	18 Months	30 Months	3 Years	4 Years	5 Years
Perform Hirschberg's light reflex test to detect overt strabismus.		Perform audiometric hearing screening (with parental practice beforehand). Perform HOTV vision test (with parental practice beforehand). Perform Hirschberg's light reflex test to detect overt strabismus and cover test to detect latent strabismus.	Speech should be 50%–75% intelligible. Address parental concerns. Stuttering is fairly common. Assess parents' reactions.	Assess speech intelligibility (most speech should be intelligible). Address parental concerns.	

Dental Care

15 Months	18 Months	30 Months	3 Years	4 Years	5 Years
Brush and floss twice daily with help from parents. Use fluoridated water or supplements. Do not allow child to have a bottle in bed.	Limit concentrated sweets.	First visit to dentist should occur when all primary teeth have erupted.	First dental visit, if not done previously. Does child brush teeth with supervision?	Well-balanced diet. Limit sweets. Brush and floss twice daily. Dental visit every 6–12 months.	Child should have dental visit every 6–12 months.

Screening

15 Months	18 Months	30 Months	3 Years	4 Years	5 Years
Monitor growth trajectory for deviations as indicated on growth chart. Evaluate hematocrit if not done at 9 months.	Screen for hypertension, iron deficiency anemia.	Screen for elevated cholesterol and triglyceride levels if there is a family history of obesity, cardiovascular disease, or elevated cholesterol levels.	Monitor height and weight for deviations as indicated on growth chart.	Review results of lead and tuberculosis screening if performed.	

Teaching and Counseling

15 Months	18 Months	30 Months	3 Years	4 Years	5 Years
Discuss limit setting, discipline. Assess child's readiness for toilet training: suggest waiting if possible. Reassure parents that negativism will pass.	Assess readiness for toilet training. Discuss negativism and ways to handle it.	*Toilet training:* nighttime wetting and daytime accidents are common. Discuss possible night fears; advise parents that these may soon appear. Discuss discipline (consistency, positive techniques).	Discuss child's fears (the dark, monsters) and the results of active imagination. Discuss thumb sucking and masturbation. Assess parents' reactions. Discuss TV viewing, violence. Discuss elimination (bowel and bladder control). Encourage enrollment in nursery school.	Discuss imaginary friends, fantasies. Discuss sleep patterns and concerns (nightmares, fear of the dark, difficulty falling or staying asleep). Assess child's ability to separate from parents. Recommend TV restrictions. Prepare parents for child's increasing sexual curiosity.	Assess school readiness: child's reactions, parent's expectations, and child's ability to tolerate separation from parents and to do schoolwork.

Abbreviations: Hep B-3, hepatitis B virus vaccine; DTaP, diphtheria and tetanus toxoids and acellular pertussis vaccine; DTP, diphtheria, tetanus toxoids, and pertussis vaccine; Hib, *Hemophilus influenzae* type B conjugate vaccine; OPV, oral poliovirus vaccine; IPV, inactivated poliovirus vaccine; MMR, measles, mumps, and rubella.

The Toddler and the Preschooler

Nutrition

The rate of growth slows during the toddler and preschool period, and so does the child's appetite. This is sometimes referred to as "physiologic anorexia." The child's food experiences during this period can have a lasting effect on how food and meals are viewed. The family is the primary influence at this time, although television plays an important role. Children should be discouraged from eating while watching television, and family mealtimes should be encouraged.

NUTRITIONAL REQUIREMENTS

Recommended dietary allowances per day for energy and protein vary according to the child's age (see Table 4–3). Fat and cholesterol intake should not be restricted in children less than 2 years old (American Academy of Pediatrics [AAP] Committee on Nutrition, 1998a). There are many similarities in the nutritional needs of the toddler and the preschooler. Children this age who eat well-balanced diets should not suffer from iron deficiency. If milk remains the primary food, however, it will replace foods rich in iron, vitamins, and minerals, such as dark green leafy vegetables, meats, and legumes. Three to four servings from the milk group each day are more than adequate for this age child. (See Chapter 47 for a discussion of iron deficiency anemia.) The child who is healthy does not need vitamin supplementation. However, giving a daily children's multivitamin containing 100% of the RDA is not harmful.

After 2 years of age, low-fat (2%) milk may be given. Milk intake should be limited to 2 to 3 cups per day. Yogurt and cheese are other milk-group sources. Poultry, fish, and lean meat are good sources of iron. Low-sugar breakfast cereals are sources of iron and vitamins. Snacks of fruits and vegetables assist in meeting the child's nutritional requirements.

SOLID FOODS

Children at this age are increasing their proficiency in using a spoon and cup. By age 2 years children can hold a cup in one hand and use a spoon well (Fig. 6–4). By age 12 months, most children are eating the same foods as the rest of the family. The child should be offered three meals and two snacks each day.

By age 3 to 4 years, the child begins to use a fork. The child continues to develop fine motor skills and by the end of the preschool period should be beginning to use a knife for cutting.

Nutritious Snacks

Fresh fruit
Celery sticks with peanut butter or cheese spread
Yogurt
Bagels
Carrot sticks
Graham crackers
Pretzels
Puddings

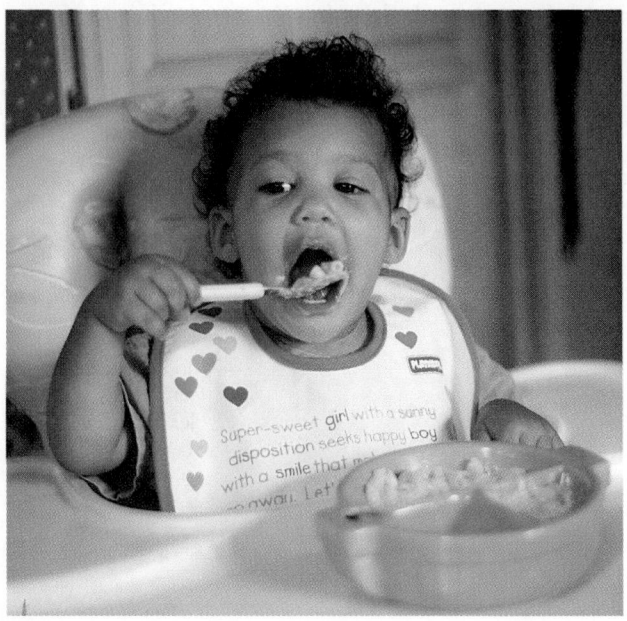

FIGURE 6–4

By age 1 year, most children are eating the same foods as the rest of the family. Toddlers should be offered three meals and two healthy snacks a day. Most 2-year-olds can drink from a cup and use a spoon well if given the opportunity to practice.

One method to determine serving size for children is 1 tablespoon of solid food per year of age. Children may be more likely to try new foods and eat nutritious meals if smaller portions are served. Foods of different textures, colors, consistencies, tastes, and temperatures should be offered. The child should sit in a chair that allows easy access to the food; the dishes should be small, nonbreakable, and, when possible, steady enough to prevent spilling. Thick, short-handled spoons and forks and shallow bowls increase the toddler's ability to eat successfully.

Foods that could be aspirated should continue to be avoided during the toddler period. Soft drinks and candy should be discouraged. Sugar is a source of calories and is naturally present in breast milk as lactose, in fruits as fructose, and in grain products as maltose. A diet with too much sugar, however, can replace other more nutritious foods and increase tooth decay. Artificial sweeteners and foods that contain artificial sweeteners are not recommended for children less than 2 years old.

AGE-RELATED NUTRITIONAL CHALLENGES

Food Jags. The volume of food the child eats may vary from day to day. The child may want the same food at every meal for several days and then suddenly reject the food completely. Children this age may refuse foods because of odor and temperature. They may not like mixing foods and therefore may not eat casseroles. This dislike does not seem to apply to foods such as pizza, spaghetti, and macaroni and cheese. Many children prefer juices over milk and water. Too much milk is not good, but neither is too much juice, because it can replace other foods and their nutrients. Parents and older siblings can affect how a child sees a food

Increasing Nutritious Intake

- Limit to two nutritious snacks per day and give only at toddler's request.
- Limit to 6 ounces of juice per day.
- Introduce to finger foods at age 8 to 10 months and continue to make these types of food available.
- Limit to 16 to 24 ounces of milk per day.
- Keep mealtimes pleasant.
- Do not force feed.
- Do not feed children who can feed themselves.

and should be careful about making negative comments about a certain food. Children should be assisted in developing tastes for new foods through role modeling and making the foods available.

Physiologic Anorexia. Parents should be taught appropriate ways to approach the child who is experiencing physiologic anorexia. Children should not be allowed to "fill up" with snacks, milk, and juices. Small portions should be offered so that the child does not feel overwhelmed by the amount of food. Mealtimes should be pleasant and not a time to discuss discipline problems or even the child's poor appetite. Children should never be made to sit at the table after the rest of the family has left. This will only create a negative association with mealtime. Parents need to maintain a balance between ignoring their child's nutritional intake and making it the focus of their parenting.

The nurse can encourage parents to focus more on the weekly nutritional intake of their child than on one day's intake. Frequently children are the best judge of what they need, and they may eat primarily fruit one day and peanut butter the next. Nutritional consumption tends to balance out over a week.

Dental Care

Most toddlers have a complete set of 20 deciduous teeth by the time they are 30 months old. Although the exact time of eruption of teeth varies, an approximate rule of thumb to assess the number of teeth is the age of the toddler in months minus 6. Usually, one tooth erupts for each month of age past 6 months up to 30 months of age.

Permanent teeth are calcifying during the toddler period, long before they are visible. Proper care of the deciduous teeth is crucial for the toddler's general health and for the health and alignment of the permanent teeth. Deciduous teeth play an important role in the growth and development of the jaws and face and in speech development. Premature loss of the deciduous teeth complicates eruption of the permanent teeth, often leading to malocclusion. Nurses need to be aware that some parents do not understand the value of preserving primary teeth.

Because toddlers do not have the manual dexterity to remove plaque adequately, parents must be responsible for cleaning their teeth (Fig. 6–5). Children can be encouraged to brush their teeth after the teeth have been thoroughly cleaned by a parent. Because toddlers like to imitate, watching parents brush their teeth can be motivating. A small, soft nylon bristle brush works best. Optimum access and

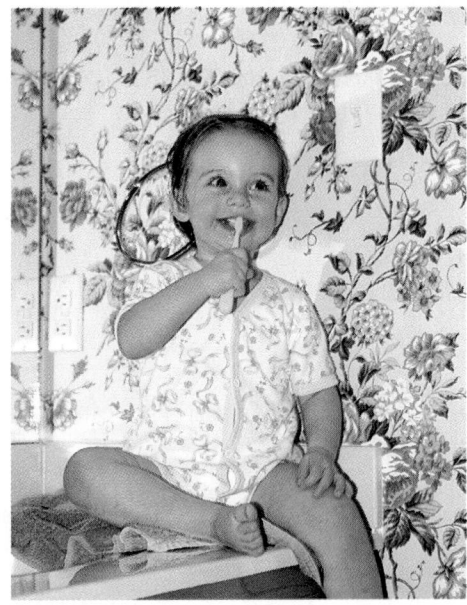

FIGURE 6–5

Care of the deciduous teeth promotes healthy development of the permanent teeth. Because 2-year-olds lack the manual dexterity to remove plaque adequately, parents must assume responsibility for cleaning the toddler's teeth.

visibility are provided if the parent sits on the floor or bed with the child's head in the parent's lap and the child's body perpendicular to the parent's. This position also gives the parent some control of the child's head movement. Toothpaste is not recommended for young children because they often do not like the taste or, if they do, tend to swallow it. If the child receives fluoride from other sources, such as water or supplements, excess amounts of fluoride may be ingested if fluoride toothpaste is swallowed. Ingestion of excessive amounts of fluoride may lead to fluorosis, which produces white speckles or brown discoloration of the enamel. Ideally, teeth should be brushed after every meal and especially at bedtime. Flossing between teeth helps remove plaque and should be done daily by the parent after the toddler's teeth are brushed.

Fluoride makes tooth enamel resistant to acid attack, preventing decay. Fluoride supplementation is no longer recommended from birth, and doses during the first 6 years of life have been decreased (Roberts et al., 1998). Supplements are recommended for children in some age groups living in areas with less than optimum fluoride in the drinking water supply (Table 6–5).

A diet that is low in sweets and high in nutritious food promotes dental health. Sweets are most likely to cause caries if they are sticky or if they are eaten between meals rather than with meals. Nutritious snacks, such as fresh fruit, yogurt, or cheese, should be offered instead of candy, soda, or cookies.

The first dental visit should be made 6 months after the first primary tooth erupts and no later than age 30 months. The first appointment should be made before any dental work needs to be done so that the visit is enjoyable and free from discomfort. This visit provides an opportunity

TABLE 6–5

Fluoride Supplementation Schedule for Infants and Children (Revised 1994)

Age of Child	Fluoride in Home Water (ppm)		
	<0.3	0.3–0.6	>0.6
Birth to 6 months	0	0	0
6 months to 3 years	0.25	0	0
3–6 years	0.5	0.25	0
6–16 years	1.0	0.5	0

Note: Numbers are milligrams of fluoride per day. Jointly endorsed by the American Academy of Pediatrics, the American Academy of Pediatric Dentistry, and the American Dental Association.

From American Academy of Pediatrics Committee on Nutrition. (1995). Fluoride supplementation for children. *Pediatrics,* 95(5), 777. Reproduced by permission.

Abbreviation: ppm, parts per million.

for early assessment of the child's dental health as well as for teaching parents good preventive dental health practices.

Because the enamel on primary teeth is thinner than on permanent teeth, preschoolers' teeth are prone to destruction from decay. The distance from the tooth surface to the pulp is shorter also, so that tooth abscesses from caries can occur rapidly. Untreated caries can lead to pain, abscess formation, and poor digestion because of ineffective chewing. Many parents do not realize that the deciduous teeth are important to protect the dental arch. If deciduous teeth are lost early (e.g., because of decay) the remaining teeth may drift out of position, block proper eruption of the permanent teeth, and lead to malocclusion.

Nurses play an important role in the promotion of dental health by teaching proper tooth cleaning, including the removal of plaque and the importance of adequate fluoride ingestion; encouraging a balanced diet, limited in sweets; and recommending twice yearly visits to the dentist. Preschoolers can usually brush their own teeth. Short back-and-forth or up-and-down strokes are easiest for the child to manage. Parents should monitor the child's toothbrushing and inspect the child's teeth to be sure that all plaque has been removed. Parents must help with flossing because it requires more manual dexterity than preschoolers have.

Sleep and Rest

During the second year, children require approximately 12 to 14 hours of sleep each day. Most 2-year-olds take one nap a day until the end of the second or third year, when many children give up the habit. Toddlers often resist going to bed, using dawdling or even temper tantrums to postpone separation from loved ones and the exciting events of the day. Firm, consistent limits are needed when toddlers try stalling tactics such as asking for one more drink of water.

Bedtime protests may be reduced by warning the child a few minutes before it is time for bed. Winding down with a quiet activity for 30 minutes before bedtime also helps

toddlers prepare for sleep. Bedtime offers an opportunity for some snuggle time, when the parent and toddler can read a story and share the events of the day. Children of this age often have trouble relaxing and falling asleep. A warm bath before bedtime promotes relaxation. Bedtime rituals are important and should be followed consistently. Transition objects, such as a favorite blanket or stuffed animal, are often an important part of the child's bedtime routine.

Because preschoolers expend so much energy growing and learning, they need adequate rest. The preschooler needs an average of 10 to 12 hours of sleep in a 24-hour period. Some preschoolers do well without a nap during the day, but others still need a nap. Resistance to naps is common at this age. The child usually does not want to leave his family or playmates, toys, and exciting activities to go into a darkened room to lie down and rest. A quiet time spent listening to music or looking at a favorite book may help the child relax and get some rest. Insufficient rest during the day may lead to irritability, decreased resistance to infection, and difficulty sleeping at night.

Sleep problems are more common during the preschool years than in any other period of childhood. Because of their active imaginations and immaturity, preschoolers often have nightmares and have trouble falling asleep at night. Because the boundaries between reality and fantasy are not well defined for children of this age, monsters and scary creatures that lurk in the preschooler's imagination become real to the child after the light is turned off. Patient reassurance from a caring parent may be needed again and again. Nightmares—frightening dreams that awaken the child from sleep—are common among preschoolers. A familiar environment and comforting with a hug and verbal reassurance from a parent usually enable the child to return to sleep. Night terrors differ from nightmares. Night terrors occur during deep sleep and the child remains asleep even though the eyes may be open. The child does not awaken but moans, screams, or cries and does not recognize parents. Efforts to comfort the child may lead to agitation. The child does not remember the episode in the morning, even if awakened during the night terror. Parents should be instructed not to attempt to comfort or awaken the child during a night terror, but allow the child to sleep.

The nurse should assess sleep patterns during well-child visits. Parental concerns should be addressed. The nurse can reassure parents that resistance to going to bed, fears, and nightmares are normal for children of this age. The nurse should assess the frequency of sleep problems and parents' reactions to them. If sleep problems occur often and are disruptive to the family, further investigation and intervention may be indicated.

Ritualistic techniques and transition objects that helped decrease bedtime resistance in the toddler are continued during the preschool period. Avoiding high-carbohydrate snacks and excitement before bedtime promotes relaxation. Children should not be forced to face their fear alone by sleeping in a completely dark room or with the door shut. Parents can search the room to reassure the preschooler that the room is safe. Progressive head-to-toe relaxation is an effective technique for helping preschoolers to fall asleep. A set bedtime promotes security and healthy sleep habits.

A child who has slept for a long time at the babysitter's

CRITICAL THINKING EXERCISE 6–1

Mr. and Mrs. Thomas have brought 2-year-old Todd to the clinic for his annual physical examination. The parents report that bedtime is a major production almost every night. They state that he cries, comes out of his room, and displays various other behaviors that delay sleep. They wonder if he has a sleep disorder. They relate that, other than an occasional temper tantrum, they do not have any other concerns.

1. What information do you need from the parents in order to assess the problem?
2. After you have the above information, what advice should you give the Thomases?

PARENTS WANT TO KNOW

Guidelines for Disciplining a Toddler

- Discipline must be consistent. Inconsistency is confusing and counterproductive. It is important to follow through every time.
- Discipline must be immediate. Consequences of behavior should occur as soon as possible after the behavior occurs. Threats such as "Just wait until your father gets home!" are confusing and ineffective for a child of this age.
- Discipline must be realistic and age-appropriate. Toddlers should not be expected to act like "little ladies" or "little gentlemen."
- Discipline must be related to the incident. Consequences that are logical results of a behavior are most effective.
- Limits must be clearly explained to the child.
- Toddlers must be given time to respond to instructions.
- Withdrawal of love should never be used as punishment. Comforting the child after discipline promotes positive feelings. Love is the key to effective discipline.
- Arguments and extensive explanations should be avoided.
- Praise for good behavior should be used to build self-confidence and self-esteem.
- The toddler must be separated from the behavior ("I love you very much. Hitting your sister needs to stop").

or at day care may not be ready to sleep again. Communication with the child's daytime caretaker is important to determine whether the child is maintaining a balance of activity, rest, and sleep.

Discipline

Effective discipline strategies should include a comprehensive approach that includes consideration of the parent-child relationship, reinforcement of desired behaviors, and consequences for negative behaviors (AAP Committee on Psychosocial Aspects of Child and Family Health, 1998). One goal of discipline and limit setting is to teach self-control. Eventually the child internalizes controls established by parental limits and begins to develop a conscience.

Toddlers need and want discipline to feel secure. They have little control over their behavior and need limits to learn how to behave and how to follow the rules and expectations of society. Toddlers' negativism, intense emotions, and curiosity place them at risk for injury. Because they are usually unaware of the consequences of their actions, vigilance and limits are needed for safety. Toddlers are frightened by a lack of limits and will deliberately test their parents until they are shown how far they can go. Firm discipline promotes the development of autonomy by giving the child a feeling of freedom within bounds.

Toddlers often repeat parental prohibitions to themselves while engaging in a forbidden activity. For example, a toddler may walk over to an electrical outlet, knowing that it is out of bounds, and mumble, "No, no, hurt!" while playing with the outlet. Although remembering the prohibition, the toddler lacks sufficient self-control to prevent the behavior.

Effective discipline techniques for children of this age include a time-out (1 minute per year of age), diversion, and positive reinforcement. Teaching parents how to discipline their child helps avoid problems related to the incorrect use of discipline. It is very important that the parent be consistent. Physical punishment, such as spanking, is one of the least effective discipline techniques (see Chapter 3).

Preschoolers are struggling to gain control over their strong inner impulses. To achieve this control, they need limits set on their behavior. When limits are set, the child feels more secure and can explore the environment and try out new roles in an atmosphere of freedom and safety. Appropriate limit setting helps the child learn self-confidence, self-control, and moral values. The child must be consistently disciplined for acts that are destructive, socially unacceptable, or morally wrong. Limits must be clearly defined and consistently enforced to be effective. To prevent confusion and anxiety, the consequences of misbehavior should be spelled out in advance and carried out immediately after misbehavior occurs. When the child is disciplined for misbehavior, a simple, truthful explanation of why the behavior was unacceptable should be given.

The focus of the explanation should be on the behavior rather than on the child. For example, "I don't like to see you throwing toys" is a better response than "I don't want to be around you when you act like that" or "You're a bad girl for doing that."

Discipline techniques that are effective with preschoolers include:

1. Time-out (removing the child from a situation for a short period and offering an explanation for the punishment).
2. Time-in (frequent, brief, nonverbal, physical contact when the child is acting appropriately. For example, the mother periodically strokes the child's hair or rubs

his back when he is quietly playing on the floor near his mother while she talks on the telephone. The child who receives this type of reinforcement is more likely to continue what he is doing and much less likely to interrupt the mother).

3. Offering restricted choices (e.g., "You may drink your juice in the kitchen or you may go into the living room without your juice").
4. Diversion (e.g., "You must stop marking on the wall with crayons. Here, mark on this paper instead").

Consistent positive reinforcement for desired behavior is a powerful tool. If the parent does not care or is too busy to enforce rules consistently, the child will not internalize rules and will not feel guilty about breaking them. The child will be unruly and will be unable to follow the rules set by society.

Spending enjoyable time with their children is another way parents can model positive behaviors. Having good times with children increases the children's self-esteem and reinforces good behavior. See Chapter 3 for more discussion of discipline.

Toddler Safety

Understanding the developmental changes a toddler undergoes helps the nurse and parent appreciate why children are more injury-prone in this stage of development than at any other time. Constant supervision is challenging for parents but is the most important factor in preventing injuries in this energetic age group.

CAR SAFETY

Motor vehicle injuries are a significant threat to the toddler. Although toddlers begin to develop more independent behaviors, they are still wholly reliant on an adult for protection while traveling in a car. Once a toddler is able to sit up alone, car safety seats can be adjusted to face forward in an upright position. Safety straps should be adjusted to provide a snug fit.

CRITICAL TO REMEMBER

Car Safety

- Toddlers should be restrained in an upright, forward-facing position in a car safety seat until they weigh 40 lb (18.14 kg) (usually 3 to 5 years of age).
- Car doors should be locked while the car is in motion to prevent a curious toddler from opening the door.
- Until passenger vehicles are equipped with air bags that are safe and effective for children, children under 13 years of age should not ride in a front passsenger seat that is equipped with an air bag (Centers for Disease Control, 1997).
- A booster seat is recommended for a preschooler who weighs more than 40 lb. It raises the child to accommodate the seat belt system of the car.

Because children begin to imitate their parents at an early age, parents should be encouraged to model safe behavior by consistently wearing their seat belts. As the toddler's cognitive and fine motor skills develop, some children wiggle free of the restraining system, despite releases that are designed to be difficult for a child to operate. Parents must insist on compliance in spite of temper tantrums.

Because of the short physical stature of the toddler, adults should visually inspect the area surrounding the automobile before placing it in gear. A toddler near the car may not be visible and can sustain serious crushing injuries if run over by the car or trapped between the car and a stationary object. There is always the potential for a toddler to dart out on foot into oncoming traffic. Parents should closely supervise play activities and remain physically close to the toddler to prevent these types of injuries.

Toddlers or infants should never be left unattended in a car, even for a moment. Exposure to extreme heat or cold is dangerous in this age group. Injuries have occurred when parents have left cars running for various reasons and curious toddlers have disengaged the gears, causing the car to roll and collide with other objects.

AIRPLANE SAFETY

There is ongoing concern regarding the lack of regulations to ensure that children under 2 years of age are restrained properly during airplane flights. Parents should be encouraged to use a forward-facing restraint for children weighing more than 20 lb (9.07 kg) and older than 1 year of age, until they are able to sit properly in a standard aircraft seat with the seat belt fastened securely and low across their laps (AAP, 1998).

FIRE AND BURN SAFETY

Toddlers, with their increased mobility and developing fine motor skills, can reach hot water, open fires, or hot objects placed on counters and stoves above their eye level. They may pull objects off stoves, pull down cords attached to small appliances, open oven doors, and place electric cords or frayed wires into their mouths. They may drink liquids that are dangerously hot. Parents should be encouraged to remain in the kitchen when preparing a meal and reminded to use the back burners on the stove and to turn pot handles inward and toward the middle of the stove to reduce the toddler's risk of burn injuries. Dangling cords from irons or other small appliances should not be accessible to toddlers. Open fires and heaters are also inviting. Sturdy guards fixed to the wall prevent young children from getting too close to these burn hazards. Additionally, the curious toddler is fascinated with matches and lighters; therefore, they must be kept out of reach.

Toddlers depend on adults for their protection in the event of a house fire. Anticipatory guidance should stress the importance of smoke detectors and escape plans. Parents should not use them to distract or amuse the toddler.

PREVENTING FALLS

Toddlers move quickly and climb everywhere. Toddlers can fall from playground equipment, off tricycles, and out of windows. Falls from above the first floor of a building can result in serious injury. A chair next to a kitchen counter or table allows the toddler easy access to dangerously high places. Because climbing and exploration are a normal aspect of the developmental process, safety education for the parent emphasizes constant supervision and some anticipatory planning, such as moving furniture, installing screen guards, or restricting access to potential climbing hazards.

WATER SAFETY

Toddlers love to play in water. Most drownings occur when a child is left alone in a bathtub or falls into a residential pool. Even when a child survives a submersion injury, the risk of permanent brain and lung damage is great. Parents should be educated never to leave a child alone in or near a bathtub, pail of water, wading or swimming pool, or any other body of water, even for a moment. A toddler can drown in as little as 1 inch of water. Toilet lids should remain closed. Toddlers can inadvertently fall headfirst into a toilet or bucket, and they lack the upper-body strength and coordination to remove themselves from submersion. Preventing drowning requires constant parental supervision of the toddler.

PREVENTING POISONING

Children younger than 5 years are the most common victims of poisoning, and children ages 1 to 3 years are at the highest risk. The home is the site of exposure in over 90% of cases (National Center for Health Statistics, 1997). With exploration, everything eventually finds its way to the child's mouth, even if it does not smell or taste good. Small children who are thirsty or hungry will ingest poisons that look or smell inviting.

Parents need to be educated on how to poison-proof the home. Child-resistant locks or catches should be placed on all cupboards that contain poisons. Parents should be taught the appropriate actions to take if an ingestion occurs: immediately contacting a poison control center or a physician. Parents should keep syrup of ipecac in the home and be familiar with its administration. However, they should not give syrup of ipecac to a child unless instructed to do so by the poison control center or a physician.

Parents and caregivers should not refer to medicine as candy, and, because young children often mimic their parents, adults should be discouraged from taking medicine in the child's presence. The same precautions should be taken when small children go to a grandparent's home to visit. Childproof caps slow the child but are not an absolute barrier. Labeling poisons with characteristic symbols, such as the skull and crossbones or "Mr. Yuk," helps provide visual cues to young children; however, labels are not absolute deterrents for a determined child. The best way to prevent toxic ingestions is by carefully storing all potential poisons in a place that is inaccessible to children.

Preschooler Safety

Preschoolers are active and inquisitive. They have greater self-control, but their understanding of danger is not fully developed. Safety becomes even more challenging for the parent because preschoolers are no longer content with their own backyards. Preschoolers are mesmerized by cartoons depicting make-believe situations. They see cartoon characters engaging in daring endeavors and walking away unharmed. Because of their magical thinking, preschoolers

Guidelines for the Administration of Syrup of Ipecac

INDICATIONS

To counteract the ingestion of a potentially toxic substance in the awake, alert child. It is most effective given in the first hour after the ingestion of the toxic substance. Administration should be followed by 10 to 20 ml/kg of clear fluids.

DOSAGES BY AGE

Younger than 6 months: none
6 to 12 months: 10 ml, do not repeat
1 to 12 years: 15 ml, may repeat once if vomiting has not occurred in 20 minutes
Older than 12 years: 30 ml, may repeat once if vomiting has not occurred in 20 minutes

CONTRAINDICATIONS

Nontoxic substances, acids, alkalis, petroleum distillates, hydrocarbons, loss of gag reflex, coma, or seizures.

Data from Barone, M. A. (1996). *The Harriet Lane handbook*. St. Louis: Mosby, and Behrman, R. E., & Kliegman, R. M. (1998). *Nelson essentials of pediatrics* (3rd ed.). Philadelphia: Saunders.

may believe that these feats are possible and may attempt them.

Safety education can now be directed toward the child as well as the parent. Children of this age have a strong sense of rhythm, and songs and rhymes about safety can enhance the learning process. Instruction should be simple, with one concept introduced at a time. Short stories, puppet shows, songs, coloring activities, and role-playing games are all suitable learning activities that help preschoolers learn safety-conscious behaviors.

CAR SAFETY

Preschoolers should remain in a car safety seat until they weigh 40 lb (18.14 kg). Once a child has outgrown the child car safety seat, a booster seat is strongly recommended (Fig. 6-6). Although preferable to no restraints at all, standard seat belts alone can contribute to injury because they fit poorly over the small frame of the preschooler. The standard shoulder harness often crosses the child's face or neck, and the lap belt is positioned across the midabdomen rather than across the bony structure of the pelvis. Booster seats are designed to raise the child high enough so that the restraining straps are correctly positioned over the child's smaller body frame.

Parents continue to have primary responsibility for ensuring that a child is safely restrained before the vehicle is started and in motion. Parents must insist that children remain restrained at all times and that seat belts be used correctly. Although it may seem fun and relatively harmless, riding in the open bed of a pickup truck or in the cargo area of a van or station wagon can be deadly in the event of a crash. It is outlawed in some states.

Childhood Poison Prevention

- Keep all poisons, medicines, cleaners, and toxic substances out of the reach of children. Never discard poisons in a wastebasket.
- Parents should be familiar with poisons commonly found in or near the home, including detergents, drain cleaner, dishwashing soap, furniture polish, cleaning agents, window cleaners, all medicines, vitamins, children's medications, sprays, powders, cosmetics, fingernail preparations, hair care products, sachets, mothballs, rodent poisons, fertilizers, gasoline, paints, glues, insecticides, cigarette butts, plants, and shrubs.
- Poisons should be stored in areas that are secured with locks or protected by child-resistant safety latches.
- Medicines and all harmful substances should be purchased in child-resistant packages.
- Alcoholic beverages should be kept out of the reach of children or locked in a separate cabinet. Parents should be discouraged from giving sips of alcohol to children because small amounts can be toxic to young children.
- Children should not be allowed to chew on plants or shrubs.
- Ashtrays should be kept empty and out of the reach of small children.
- Handbags and overnight luggage of guests in the home often contain medicines or other toxic substances and should be kept out of a child's reach.
- Poisons or harmful substances should always be stored in the original container. Parents should be discouraged from placing toxic substances in food or beverage containers for storage.
- Children should be taught to ask an adult before they touch a nonfood substance.
- Parents should poison-proof all areas of the home, especially the following areas: kitchen, bathroom, pantry, bedroom, garage, basement, and work areas. Grandparents and other caregivers should be encouraged to do the same.
- The telephone number of the local poison control center should be posted for immediate access in the event of a poisoning. Parents should be instructed, when contacting the poison control center, to have on hand the substance with the label for prompt identification of toxic ingredients.

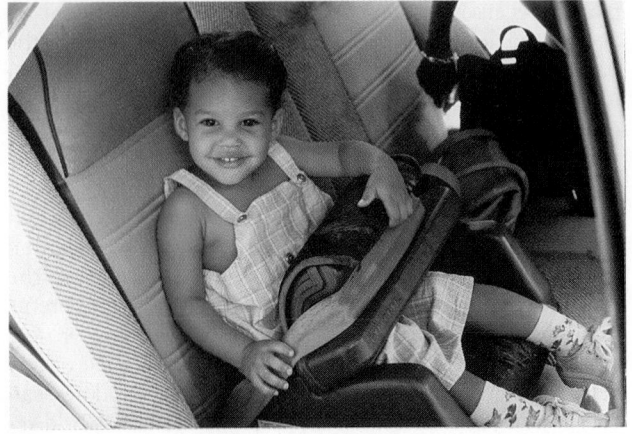

FIGURE 6–6

A booster seat with an abdominal shield is strongly recommended for children who have outgrown a child safety seat. Booster seats raise the young child high enough to allow the car seat belts to be correctly positioned over the child's chest and pelvis.

Children younger than 5 years are at the greatest risk for burn deaths in a house fire. They often panic and hide in closets or under beds rather than escaping safely. Parents should practice fire drills with their children to teach them what to do in the event of a house fire. Preschoolers should become familiar with the sounds emitted by the smoke alarms and taught to crawl under smoke and to check doors for heat.

Preschoolers are at an ideal age to learn what to do if their clothing ignites in flames. Preschoolers should be instructed to stop immediately if their clothes catch on fire and to cover their face and mouth with their hands. They should then drop to the ground and roll to smother the flames. This simple command (stop, drop, and roll) can help prevent severe burn injuries. Teaching specific behaviors educates children to remain calm and not panic.

FIREARM SAFETY

Many guns are kept in the home loaded and readily accessible to young children. Parents should be encouraged to evaluate critically their need for a firearm in the home. Do the potentially devastating risks outweigh any benefits of keeping a weapon in the home? Parents who choose to keep a gun in the home should receive anticipatory guidance about injury prevention. Guns kept in the home should always be unloaded, stored with trigger guards in place, securely locked in metal vaults, and inaccessible to all children (Brady, 1994).

PERSONAL SAFETY

Preschoolers have an interest in establishing relationships with others as they expand the boundaries of their world. With the child's increasing assertion of independence, parents are less able to provide the constant protection they once did.

Teaching children about personal safety encourages them to develop skills to detect danger and teaches appropriate ways to handle threatening situations. Strangers are often portrayed as evil characters, when in reality their

FIRE AND BURN SAFETY

Preschoolers imitate adults in all types of daily routines and activities. They may attempt these activities before they are able to manage the appliance safely (e.g., stove, iron, oven), increasing the risk of burn injuries. Matches and lighters continue to fascinate preschoolers. With their increased fine motor skills, preschoolers may be able to ignite a flame. Teaching a preschooler that lighters and matches are adult tools and instructing them to tell an adult immediately if they find these items can prevent burn injuries.

appearance and approach may be nonthreatening and friendly. Distinguishing a stranger from a well-intentioned person is challenging and often difficult for the preschooler. Basic guidelines that a child needs to know about personal safety include saying no, getting away, and telling an adult.

Children need to know how to access emergency help if they need it. Parents should help their children learn to identify safety officials and how to dial 911 or other locally appropriate emergency numbers. Children need to respond to emergency operators with their full name, address, parent's name, and other appropriate information, and should remain on the phone until help arrives. Parents can practice this safety skill with their children to ensure proper reactions in an emergency and to help the child understand what constitutes an emergency situation.

SEXUAL ABUSE

Sexual abuse is another threat to personal safety. Preventing sexual abuse begins with teaching children the normal, healthy boundaries of their bodies and what constitutes inappropriate behavior. Often the victimizers are known and trusted by the child. Abusers frequently intimidate the child into silence with threats of personal harm or suggestions that the child initiated the behavior. Children need to know that no matter how great the threat, if someone is touching their body in an inappropriate way, they should always tell an adult. If that adult cannot help them, they should tell as many adults as necessary until the inappropriate behavior is stopped (Chapter 53).

Selected Issues Related to the Toddler

Toilet Training

Control of elimination is one of the major tasks of toddlerhood. Successful toilet training depends on the readiness of both the child and the parent. The parent must be willing to spend the necessary time and emotional energy to encourage the child on a daily basis.

Toilet training is one of the most frustrating and time-consuming tasks that parents face. It can be so frustrating for some that researchers have linked toilet training accidents with many cases of child abuse. Parents who do not understand normal growth and development patterns often have unrealistic expectations and can become frustrated to the point of rage.

The nurse can assist parents by explaining developmental milestones and encouraging parents not to begin training until the child shows signs of readiness. Helping the parent recognize factors that interfere with toilet training, such as stress, can make the training easier. The parent may not have the necessary reserves of patience and energy for toilet training during stressful times, such as near the birth of another child or while moving to a new house. Training may be easier if it is postponed until routines return to normal.

The nurse can assist parents in toilet training the toddler by explaining the importance of maturation to successful toilet training. Parents need to know that both physical and psychological readiness are necessary for toilet training

Signs of Readiness for Toilet Training

PHYSICAL READINESS

Child can remove own clothing.
Child willing to let go of a toy when asked.
Child able to sit, squat, and walk well.
Child has been walking for 1 year.

PSYCHOLOGICAL READINESS

Child notices if diaper is wet.
Child may indicate that diaper needs to be changed by pulling on diaper, squatting, or repeating a word or phrase.
Child communicates need to go to the bathroom or can get there by self.
Child wants to please parent by staying dry.

to be successful. Myelinization of the spinal cord, which usually occurs between 12 and 18 months, must be complete before the child can voluntarily control bowel and bladder sphincters. The nurse can offer anticipatory guidance to parents by teaching them the signs that the toddler is ready for toilet training. The average toddler is not ready for toilet training to begin until 18 to 24 months of age. Waiting until the child is 24 to 30 months old makes the task considerably easier because toddlers of this age are less negative and usually are more willing to control their sphincters to please their parents.

There are no set rules or timetables for toilet training (Fig. 6–7). The age at which toilet training is usually begun varies from culture to culture. If the child resists, it is helpful

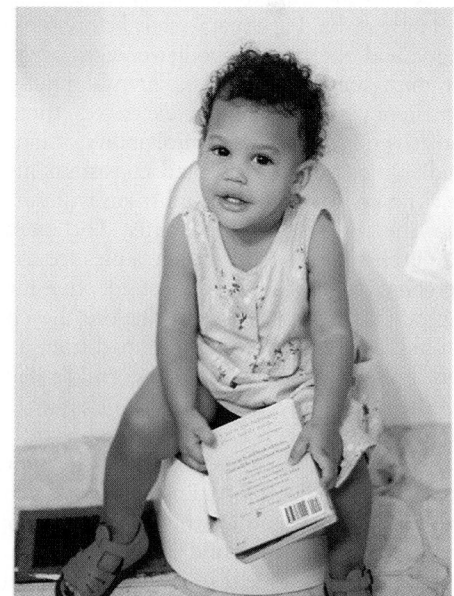

FIGURE 6–7

There are no set rules for toilet training. The nurse can help parents understand that both physical and psychological readiness are necessary for success.

to stop training and wait 30 to 60 days and begin again. Bowel control is usually achieved before bladder control. Daytime bladder control occurs before nighttime bladder control. Some children do achieve daytime bladder control before bowel control. This phenomenon is referred to as "toileting refusal," and it can be distressful to parents. Recent and past studies have shown that these children do have higher rates of constipation and painful defecation, but it is unknown if this is a cause or effect of stool toileting refusal (Blum, Taubman, & Osborne, 1997).

A relaxed, child-centered approach is most successful, with plenty of praise for each success. Punishment and coercive techniques cause feelings of shame and lead to power struggles. The child should never be forced to sit on the potty for long periods. Successful toilet training is a gradual process, and relapses must be expected. Accidents often occur when children are too busy playing to notice a full bladder until it is too late. Many children cannot remain completely dry until the age of 3 years. Parents should respond to accidents with tolerance instead of scolding or shaming the child.

Temper Tantrums

Temper tantrums are a common toddler response to anger and frustration and often result from thwarted attempts at mastery and autonomy. Tantrums may also occur as an emotional release of tension after a long, tiring day. Unable to express anger in more productive ways because of limited language and reasoning abilities, toddlers may react by screaming, kicking, throwing things, or even biting themselves or banging their heads. Tantrums occur more often when toddlers are tired, hungry, bored, or excessively stimulated.

The nurse can help parents by identifying strategies to decrease the frequency of tantrums. Limiting situations that are too much for the child to handle is helpful. Anticipating periods of fatigue, having a snack ready before the child gets too hungry, and offering the toddler choices when possible can minimize temper tantrums. Parental practices such as inconsistency, permissiveness, excessive strictness, and overprotectiveness increase the probability of tantrums.

Toddlers need appropriate and consistent limits. Letting the child know that temper tantrums will not be tolerated gives the child a sense of security. The intensity of a toddler's outburst almost seems to be a plea for someone to stop the behavior. Probably the most effective method for handling tantrums is to isolate and ignore the child. The child should learn that nothing is gained from a tantrum, not even attention. Giving in to the child's demands or scolding the child only increases the behavior. Toddlers stop using tantrums when they do not achieve their goals and as their verbal skills increase. Once the tantrum has subsided and the toddler has regained some self-control, the parent should comfort and let the child know that limits are necessary and that the child is loved. Acknowledging the child's angry feelings and rewarding more mature ways of expressing them assists the child to gain self-control.

Sibling Rivalry

Sharing parents' love and attention is difficult for most toddlers. Often toddlers have intense feelings of jealousy and

> ### CRITICAL TO REMEMBER
> #### Strategies to Decrease Sibling Rivalry
>
> - Including the toddler in preparations for the new baby
> - Explaining to the toddler what new babies are like
> - Letting the child feel the fetus move
> - Reading picture books about new siblings
> - Talking about changes that the newborn might create
> - Acknowledging the older child's feelings about these changes
> - Referring to the baby as "ours"

envy toward a new infant sibling. Toddlers' egocentrism makes it difficult for them to understand that a parent can love more than one child at a time.

Because the infant needs a great deal of time and attention, the toddler's routine is disrupted. The toddler has limited resources to cope with such stress and may react by treating the baby roughly, damaging property, or harming pets. The toddler may seem to regress by asking for a bottle or pacifier, or by using baby talk.

Any changes, such as moving the toddler to a new bedroom or beginning day care, should be made as far in advance as possible so that the toddler will not feel displaced by abrupt changes when the baby arrives. Many hospitals offer sibling preparation classes. When the mother and infant come home from the hospital, the mother's first concern should be greeting the older sibling. The father or another caregiver should carry the newborn, allowing the mother's arms to be free to hug the waiting toddler and to express how the child was missed. A toddler's jealous feelings can become intense when visitors lavish gifts and praise on the baby. These feelings can be minimized by giving an inexpensive gift to the toddler each time the baby receives one. Visitors should be encouraged to pay attention to the older child as well as the baby. Parents should anticipate behavior changes, even if the toddler has been prepared for the arrival of a new baby. The parents should be present when the toddler is with the infant to prevent the toddler from inadvertently harming the newborn sibling.

> It is important to help toddlers recognize and identify negative feelings toward a new sibling. Firm limits must be set, however, if the toddler tries to harm the baby. The child may be told "It's okay to feel jealous, but it's not okay to hurt the baby." Praise should be given for affectionate, cooperative behavior.

Planned, uninterrupted, private time is important to maintain feelings of closeness between parent and toddler. Even 10 or 15 minutes a day while the baby is sleeping is valuable. Allowing the toddler to choose an activity for this time with the parent makes it even more special. This special time should be given to the child each day, regardless of the child's behavior.

Selected Issues Related to the Preschooler

Stuttering

Stuttering or stammering is a disturbance in the flow and time patterning of speech. During the preschool years, children often have experiences they want to share but have difficulty putting the words together. It is common for children at this age to repeat whole words or phrases and to interject "uh" and "um" in their speech. As the child's communication skills develop, most children grow out of their normal *dysfluency*. Dysfluency tends to be more common during times of excitement, when formulating long and complex sentences, when trying to think of a particular word, and during times of stress.

Reactions to stuttering can increase the dysfluency. There are no definite clinical signs that clearly indicate the prognosis or need for referral of an individual child. Health care providers should intervene on the cautious side and refer the child to a fluency specialist for evaluation when

- The child shows any reaction to the dysfluency
- There is a physical struggle to get words out
- The frequency of dysfluency is excessive
- The parents are strongly concerned about possible stuttering (Wexler, 1996a).

Parents can help their child by focusing on the ideas the child is expressing, not on the way he or she is speaking.

PARENTS WANT TO KNOW

How to Help the Child Who Stutters

- Listen closely when your child speaks.
- Speak slowly and pause frequently. This provides a model for the child and gives the child more time to understand what is being said as well as to formulate thoughts.
- Provide opportunities for the child to talk without distractions or competition from other family members.
- Reduce pressure to communicate by limiting the number of questions asked that require an immediate answer.
- Limit time pressure. Don't ask a second question before the first question is answered.
- Observe situations that increase or decrease fluent behavior. Increase those times when the child is more fluent.
- Recognize that certain environmental factors may have a negative effect on fluency: competition to speak, excitement, time pressure, arguing, fatigue, new situations, unfamiliar listeners.
- Repeat or rephrase what your child says to verify that you have understood it.

Adapted from American Speech-Language-Hearing Association. (1998). Stuttering: Do's & Don'ts for Parents. *Healthtouch Online for Better Health.*

Parents should not complete their child's sentences or draw attention to their child's speech. They should not criticize or correct the child's speech.

Preschool and Day Care Programs

A quality day care program provides an environment in which the child can expand social and play skills as well as manipulate play materials unavailable at home.

Working mothers often express guilt and concern about the effect of day care on their child's emotional well-being and cognitive development. Some concerns about the effect of day care on the child's development can be minimized by careful selection of the day care facility.

The nurse is in an excellent position to advise parents about child care. Parents need specific advice about options that are affordable but will not compromise the child's health and development. It is imperative that parents visit the day care center to evaluate the quality of the program. They should evaluate the attitude and qualifications of the caregivers as well as operating procedures, costs, child care and disciplinary practices, meals, safety precautions, sanitary conditions, and the child-staff ratio.

The child needs preparation before beginning day care. The parent should tell the child what to expect in simple, concrete terms. Emphasizing the exciting parts of the experience will help the child view the experience positively. The parent should also explain the reason for separation. It is not uncommon for an imaginative preschooler to believe that he or she is being "sent away" because of some misdeed.

When parents must take their child to a babysitter or day care center, they should give the child an explanation for the separation. A statement such as "I have to work so I can buy food and clothes for the family and toys for you" is not adequate. In response to this explanation, one 3-year-old boy wailed, "But I have enough toys!" More effective would be to explain the separation by saying, "We both have work to do. My work is at my office, and your work is at school."

It is important for the parent to reassure the child ("I'm really going to miss you today and I wish you could be with me") and to let the child know that separation is painful for the parent as well, but necessary. At the end of the day, when picking up the child, it is equally important to let the child know how happy the parent is to see the child. By responding to the child's feelings, parents can lessen the stress of separation.

Transition objects may help the child adjust to the new environment. Providing the staff with information about the child's interests, home routine, special terms, and names of pets and siblings helps the new caregiver make the child feel more comfortable. Parents should always assure the child that they will return to take the child home at the end of the day.

Preparing the Child for School

Preparation for school begins long before the preschool period. The earliest interactions between parent and infant lay the foundation for school readiness. Research shows that the most important factor in the development of academic competency is the relationship between parent and child. Parents who are attuned to their child and who structure the environment to provide challenges as well as security facilitate the child's cognitive growth. An interesting environment, combined with parental encouragement and support, maximizes the child's potential.

Parents are the child's first and most important teachers. They structure the child's environment and offer opportunities for learning. Visiting a zoo, fire station, or museum and talking about the experience increases the child's general knowledge and vocabulary. Intellectual development is also fostered by cooking together, playing simple games, or putting together puzzles. Playing with clay, paint, and scissors promotes fine motor skills and provides opportunity for self-expression. Reading to the child is one of the most valuable activities for promoting school readiness. Listening to stories and discussing them can promote reading readiness. Dramatic play encourages reading readiness by providing opportunities for symbolic thinking and problem solving.

Preschool and day care programs can supplement the developmental opportunities provided by parents at home. Opportunities to play with other children and to learn how to share the attention of an adult are some benefits of a good preschool program. Head Start programs offer low-income children and their families opportunities for remedial and supportive activities. Kindergarten provides a transition between home and first grade through a structured learning environment. In kindergarten, children prepare for school by learning to cooperate with other children, developing listening skills, and forming a positive attitude toward school.

Nurses can provide parents with strategies designed to promote safety as part of preparation for school. Teaching children about street safety and dealing with strangers and ensuring that children know their telephone number and address are important aspects of preparation for school.

Not every 5-year-old is ready for kindergarten. Both chronological age and developmental maturity should be considered when assessing a child's readiness for school. At this age, boys tend to lag behind girls developmentally by about 6 months.

Checklist for School Readiness

- Child is physically healthy and strong enough to enjoy the challenge of going to school and to handle the increased stresses involved.
- Child attends to own toileting needs and washes hands independently.
- Child can separate from parent and spend several hours each day in an unfamiliar place with adults and children who are largely unknown at first.
- Child's attention span is long enough that child can sit for a fairly long period and concentrate on one thing at a time, gradually learning to enjoy the practicing and problem-solving activity involved.
- Child can listen to and follow two- or three-part instructions.
- Child can restrict talking to appropriate times.
- Child is able to tolerate the frustration of not receiving immediate attention from the teacher or others; can wait for and take turns.
- Child has some basic hand-eye skills necessary for learning to read and write.
- Child can hold a pencil properly and turn pages one at a time.
- Child knows the alphabet and can recognize some letters visually.
- Child counts to 10.
- Child recognizes the colors of the rainbow.

KEY CONCEPTS

- The slower physical growth rate of the toddler (in comparison with an infant) leads to a reduced demand for calories and decreased appetite (physiologic anorexia).
- The combination of increased motor skills, immaturity, and lack of experience places the toddler at risk for unintentional injury. Anticipatory guidance for the parents about childproofing the home is an essential nursing role.
- Children's coordination and muscle strength increase rapidly between the ages of 3 and 5. Increases in brain size and nerve myelinization enable the child to perfect fine and gross motor skills. The preschool child has the skills needed to engage in such activities as running, riding a tricycle, cutting with scissors, and drawing.
- Toddlers' behavior is characterized by negativism, ritualism, and egocentrism.
- The preschool years are a critical period for the development of socialization. Children need opportunities to play with others to learn communication skills and ways to get along with others. Preschool children learn to share and cooperate as they play in small groups. Their play is often imitative, dramatic, and creative.
- Preschoolers' thinking is still magical and egocentric. They tend to understand events only as those events affect them, believing that everyone else has the same experience. Preschool children may be overwhelmed by guilt feelings if a loved one is injured or becomes ill because they believe their thoughts are powerful enough to cause events to happen.
- Toddlerhood is characterized by the struggle for autonomy as the child develops a sense of self as separate from the parent. The Eriksonian task for the toddler is centered on autonomy versus shame and doubt.
- According to Erikson, the developmental task of the preschooler is to gain a sense of initiative. The preschooler is busy learning how to do things and takes great pride in new accomplishments.

- Sexual identity and body image are developing in the preschool period. Sexual curiosity, anatomic explorations, and masturbation are common. The nurse should encourage parents to answer the preschooler's questions simply and honestly. Children should not be shamed or punished for self-comforting behaviors or for investigating sexual differences.
- Food jags and physiologic anorexia are common occurrences in the young child.
- Toddlers need approximately 12 to 14 hours of sleep per day.
- The preschooler needs an average of 10 to 12 hours of sleep in a 24-hour period. Because of the preschooler's active imagination and immaturity, sleep problems are common.
- Firm, consistent discipline helps toddlers learn self-control. Effective discipline techniques include time-outs, diversion, and positive reinforcements.
- Preschool children need consistent discipline to learn acceptable behavior. Appropriate limit setting helps the child learn self-confidence, self-control, and moral values. Discipline techniques that are effective at this age include time-out, time-in, the use of restricted choices, and diversion.
- All 20 deciduous teeth are present by age 3 years. Proper care of deciduous teeth is crucial for the child's general health and for the health and alignment of permanent teeth. Nurses should teach parents the importance of good oral hygiene, adequate fluoride intake, good nutrition, and regular dental checkups.
- Nurses can help parents with toilet training by explaining the signs of physical and psychological readiness. Readiness depends on myelinization of the nerve pathways that enable the child to control the bowel and bladder sphincters.
- Sibling rivalry can be minimized with techniques such as including the toddler in preparations for the new baby, acknowledging the toddler's negative feelings while setting appropriate limits, and affirming the toddler as special and loved.
- The nurse plays an important role in helping parents prepare their children for school and in assessing children's readiness for school. Parents can help their child succeed in school by providing a stimulating environment and encouragement and support.
- Health promotion for the preschool child includes ensuring adequate sleep, optimal nutrition, dental care, immunizations, and prevention of injuries.

ANSWERS TO CRITICAL THINKING EXERCISE 6–1

1. The nurse needs to know if there is a bedtime ritual. If a ritual exists, the nurse determines what it is and whether it is implemented consistently. Even though the parents volunteered that they did not have any other concerns, the nurse should ask about Todd's daily routine. Questions related to his play activities, eating habits, and daily routine might be helpful. The parents should be asked what discipline methods they use and if they are effective (i.e., what the parents do when Todd resists their instructions). This information will give the nurse a general idea of what the child's environment is like.

The nurse is trying to determine whether the parents are supporting this child's need for structure while allowing him to venture out. The nurse is looking for balance and gathering information to determine whether consistent limits are set within the family.

2. Two-year-old children need limits set to feel secure. They do not have the maturity to control their behavior. They must be taught the rules. It is not unusual for toddlers to delay going to bed. The parents should be told that this behavior is part of normal growth and development. By providing a bedtime ritual, which may include quiet time,

a snack, a story, and perhaps a prayer, parents help children find security in a routine that is repeated night after night. Children begin to know that their parents expect them to stay in bed and that they cannot manipulate their parents. Children who "wear their parents down" are confused and are not given the sense of control that they need to explore and become autonomous. Parents should be assured that by creating a consistent environment, they will not only help their child, they will save themselves a good deal of frustration.

REFERENCES AND READINGS

American Academy of Pediatrics. (1998). Airline seats for infants. *AAP News, 14*(8), 5.

American Academy of Pediatrics Committee on Nutrition. (1995). Fluoride supplementation for children. *Pediatrics, 95*(5), 777.

American Academy of Pediatrics Committee on Nutrition. (1998a). Cholesterol in childhood. *Pediatrics, 101*(1), 141–147.

American Academy of Pediatrics Committee on Nutrition. (1998b). *Pediatric nutrition handbook* (4th ed.). Elk Grove Village, IL: American Academy of Pediatrics.

American Academy of Pediatrics Committee on Psychosocial Aspects of Child and Family Health. (1998). Guidance for effective discipline. *Pediatrics, 101*(4), 723–728.

Bernardo, L. M. (1996). Parent-reported injury-associated behaviors and life events among injured, ill, and well preschool children. *Journal of Pediatric Nursing, 11*(2), 100–119.

Bloom, L. (1998). Language development and emotional expression. *Pediatrics, 102*(5), 1272–1277.

Blum, N. J., Taubman, B., & Osborne, M. L. (1997). Behavioral characteristics of children with stool toileting refusal. *Pediatrics, 99*(1), 50–53.

Blum, N. J., Williams, G. E., Friman, P. C., & Christophersen, E. R. (1995). Disciplining young children: The role of verbal instructions and reasoning. *Pediatrics, 96,* 336–341.

Brady, M. (1994). Educating youths and their parents about the prevention of firearm injury. *Journal of Pediatric Health Care, 8*(3), 120–129.

Centers for Disease Control. (1997). Approval of installation of air bag on-off switches for certain motor-vehicle owners. *MMWR, 46,* 1098–1099.

Christophersen, E. (1997a). *Beyond discipline: Parenting that lasts a lifetime* (2nd ed.). Shawnee Mission, KS: Overland Press.

Christophersen, E. (1997b). *Guidelines for common sense child rearing.* Shawnee Mission, KS: Overland Press.

Crawley, T. (1996). Childhood injury: Significance and prevention strategies. *Journal of Pediatric Nursing, 11*(4), 225–231.

Emude, R. N. (1998). Early emotional development: New modes of thinking for research and intervention. *Pediatrics, 102*(5), 1236–1243.

Erikson, E. H. (1963). *Childhood and society* (2nd ed.). New York: Norton.

Fox, N. A. (1998). Temperament and regulation of emotion in the first years of life. *Pediatrics, 102*(5), 1230–1235.

Greenspan, S. (1995). *The challenging child.* Reading, MA: Perseus Books.

Gross, D., & Garvey, C. (1997). Scolding, spanking, and time-out revisited. *MCN: American Journal of Maternal/Child Nursing, 22,* 209–213.

Institute of Medicine, National Academy of Sciences, Food and Nutrition Board. (1989). *National Research Council recommended dietary allowances.* Washington, DC: National Academy Press.

Kennedy, C. M., & Lipsitt, L. P. (1998). Risk-taking in preschool children. *Journal of Pediatric Nursing, 13*(2), 77–84.

Kohlberg, L. (1966). A cognitive developmental analysis of children's sex-role concepts and attitudes. In E. E. Maccoby (Ed.). *The development of sex differences.* Stanford, CA: Stanford University Press.

Kohlberg, L. (1964). Development of moral character. In M. Hoffman & L. Hoffman (Eds.). *Review of child development research. Vol. 1.* New York: Russel Sage Foundation.

Meltzoff, A. (1995). Understanding the intentions of others: Re-enactment of intended acts by 18-month-old children. *Developmental Psychology, 31*(5), 838–850.

National Center for Health Statistics. (1997). *Health, United States, 1996–97 and injury chartbook.* Hyattsville, MD: Author.

Roberts, M. W., Keels, M. A., Sharp, M. C., & Lewis, J. L. (1998). Fluoride supplement prescribing and dental referral patterns among academic pediatricians. *Pediatrics, 101*(1), e6.

Rodgers, G. B. (1998). Let's welcome a new generation of child-resistant packaging. *Contemporary Pediatrics, 15*(3), 57–72.

Scholer, S. J., Mitchel, E. F., & Ray, W. A. (1997). Predictors of injury mortality in early childhood. *Pediatrics, 100*(3), 342–347.

Socolar, R. R., & Stein, R. E. (1995). Spanking infants and toddlers: Maternal belief and practice. *Pediatrics, 95*(1), 105–111.

Stein, M. T. (1998). Preparing families for the toddler and preschool years. *Contemporary Pediatrics, 15*(1), 88–110.

Taubman, B. (1997). Toilet training and toileting refusal for stool only: A prospective study. *Pediatrics, 99*(1), 54–58.

Tharinger, D., & Lasser, J. (1997). Sexual interest and expression. In Bear, G. G., Minke, K. M., & Thomas, A. (Eds.). *Children's needs: II. Development, problems and alternatives.* Bethesda, MD: National Association of School Psychologists.

Trahms, C. M., & Pipes, P. L. (1997). *Nutrition in infancy and childhood.* New York: WCB/McGraw-Hill.

Wexler, K. B. (1996a). Stuttering in children and adolescents: Part I. *Emergency and Office Pediatrics, 9*(3), 73–76.

Wexler, K. B. (1996b). Stuttering in children and adolescents: Part II. Evaluation. *Emergency and Office Pediatrics, 9*(5), 147–150.

Yoshinaga-Itano, C., Sedey, A. L., Coulter, D. K., & Mehl, A. L. (1998). Language of early- and later-identified children with hearing loss. *Pediatrics, 102*(5), 1161–1171.

Zurbrugg, E. B. (1998). When time-out fails, try plan B. *Contemporary Pediatrics, 15*(1), 79–84.

7

◆ ◆ ◆ ◆ ◆ ◆ ◆ ◆ ◆ ◆

The School-Age Child

LEARNING OBJECTIVES

After studying this chapter, you should be able to:

- Describe normal growth and development of the school-age child and assess the child for normal developmental milestones.
- Describe the maturational changes that take place during the school-age period and discuss implications for health care.
- Identify the stages of moral development of the school-age child and discuss implications for effective parenting strategies.
- Discuss the effect of schools on the development of the child and implications for teachers and parents.
- Discuss anticipatory guidance related to discipline techniques, nutrition, and safety for school-age children.
- Describe anticipatory guidance that the nurse can offer to decrease children's stress.

DEFINITIONS

caries Decay of the teeth.

conservation Ability to understand that certain properties of objects do not change simply because their order, form, or appearance has changed.

malocclusion Misalignment of the teeth or dental arches. Teeth may be crowded, crooked, or out of alignment.

menarche Onset of menstruation.

self-care children Children who care for themselves at home after school, formerly called latchkey children.

The school-age years, from 6 to 12, are one of the healthiest periods of life. Slow, steady physical growth and rapid cognitive and social development characterize this time. During these 6 years, the child's world expands from the tight circle of the family to include children and adults at school, at church or synagogue, and in the community. The child becomes increasingly independent. Peers become important as the child starts school and gradually moves away from the security of home. This period is a time of best friends, sharing, and exploring.

◼ Growth and Development of the School-Age Child

The school-age child develops a sense of industry and learns the basic skills needed to function in society. The child develops an appreciation of rules and a conscience. Cognitively, the child grows from the egocentrism of early childhood to more mature thinking. This maturity is characterized by the ability to solve problems and make independent judgments based on reason. The child is invested in the task of middle childhood: learning to do things and do them well. Competence and self-esteem increase with each academic, social, and athletic achievement. The relative stability and security of the school-age period prepare the child to enter the storm of adolescence.

TABLE 7-1

Summary of Growth and Development: The School-Age Child

Physical	Motor	Psychosocial	Sensory/Cognitive
6 Years			
Average weight gain: 2.5 kg (5.5 lb) per year. Average increase in height: 5.5 cm (2 inches) per year. Growth occurs in spurts; caloric needs increase during growth spurts. Growth of trunk, arms, and legs exceeds that of head. Posture becomes more erect. *Dentition:* Child loses the first primary teeth (usually lower central incisors). First molars erupt.	**Gross:** Full of energy; in constant motion. Need activities that require use of large muscles. Can skip, jump rope; some can ride two-wheel bicycle. Balance and rhythm are good. Gross motor skills better developed than fine motor coordination. **Fine:** Can tie shoelaces. Draws people with good detail. Prints; may reverse letters. Can cut with scissors; pastes. Can button and zip clothes; dresses without help. Draws a person with 12 parts.	Outgoing, boisterous, "know-it-all." Craves attention; insists on being first and will cheat to win. Loves new places, ideas, accomplishments. Has a good sense of humor. Loves parents; worries that something may happen to them. Argumentative. Uses tension outlets—wriggling, biting fingernails, twisting hair. Temper tantrums return.	Intuitive thought stage. Attends first grade. Learning to read. Knows right hand from left. Understands morning, afternoon, night. Understands numbers. Knows values of coins.
7 Years			
Boys are approximately 2.54 cm (1 inch) taller and 0.9 kg (2 lb) heavier on average than girls. Lymphatic tissue increases in size until age 9 years. Frontal sinuses develop. *Dentition:* Upper central incisors and lower lateral incisors erupt. *Skull:* Jaw begins to grow to accommodate permanent teeth; facial contours change. Brain attains 90% of adult size.	**Gross:** Quieter, more cautious than the 6-year-old. Jumps rope well. Plays "girl games" or "boy games" according to sex. **Fine:** Draws a person with 16 parts.	Perfectionist, self-critical. Becomes more sensitive, reflective, and quiet. Wants to be liked by peers. Likes to make things; often starts projects without finishing them. Aware of family roles and responsibility. Believes promises are important and should be kept. Strong sense of justice; may tattle.	Intuitive thought stage. Attends second grade. Understands clock time; can read time to the nearest quarter hour. Can copy a diamond. Visual acuity fully developed. Can read regular-size print.

TABLE 7–1

Summary of Growth and Development: The School-Age Child Continued

Physical	Motor	Psychosocial	Sensory/Cognitive
8 Years			
Flexible and limber; bones grow faster than ligaments. *Dentition:* Upper lateral incisors and lower cuspids erupt. *Eyes:* Myopia may appear.	**Gross:** More coordinated and graceful, but rapid growth of arms and legs may cause frequent stumbling and spills at the table. Rides bicycle well. Enjoys sports. Plays and works hard. **Fine:** Writes cursive.	Happy, cooperative with peers. Has a best friend. Prefers to play with same-sex peers. Dislikes being alone. Enjoys talking on the telephone. Enjoys dramatic play. Loves collections. Likes school. Enjoys running errands, helping. May insist on changing the rules of games to win. Strong sense of humor. Modest.	Concrete operations stage. Attends third grade. Knows the date. Can name months in order. Understands conservation of mass, reversibility. Likes riddles and jokes. Can count backward from 20.
9–10 Years			
Brain growth complete by age 10 years. IgA and IgG reach adult levels.	**Gross:** High energy; always on the go. Coordination improves. Enjoys team sports. **Fine:** Eye-hand coordination well developed; enjoys crafts.	Clubs at a peak; likes secret codes and rituals. Peers' opinions are more important than parents'; child questions parental values. Fairly responsible, dependable. Increasingly polite with adults. Hero worship continues. Anger may flare, but child usually can control it. Ready for camp away from home.	Understands conservation of weight. Attends fourth and fifth grades. Reads more; enjoys books and comics. Understands fractions. Enjoys collections. Makes detailed drawings. Interested in how things work. Less easily distracted.
11–12 Years			
Rapid growth spurt and menarche occur in girls. Girls are 2.54 cm (1 inch) taller and 0.9 kg (2 lb) heavier on average than boys. Boys have greater physical strength, may become overweight. Eruption of permanent teeth complete except for third molars. About 90% of facial growth is attained by age 12.	**Gross:** More awkward because of growth spurt. May drop out of team sports to avoid embarrassment. **Fine:** Fine motor control begins to approximate that of adults.	Loyal to friends, team. Has a best friend. Boys tease opposite sex; girls flirt with boys. Girls may become "boy crazy." Modest, secretive. Needs privacy and time alone. Critical of own work. Wants more independence; may begin to rebel against parents. Begins to think about social problems, prejudices.	Formal operations stage. Attends sixth and seventh grades. Likes to talk on the telephone. Understands conservation of volume. Enjoys reading mysteries, romances, adventure stories; also reads for practical purposes.

Abbreviations: IgA, immunoglobulin A; IgG, immunoglobulin G.

Growth and development of the school-age child are summarized in Table 7–1.

Physical Growth and Development

The school-age years are characterized by slow and steady growth. The physical changes that occur during this period are gradual and subtle. Although growth rates vary among children, average weight gain is 2.5 kg (5.5 lb) per year, and the average increase in height is approximately 5.5 cm (2 inches) per year. During the early school-age period, boys are approximately 1 inch taller and 2 lb heavier than girls are. At around age 10 or 12 years, girls begin to catch up in size as they experience the preadolescent growth spurt.

By age 12, girls are 1 inch taller than boys and 2 lb heavier. This growth spurt, which signals the onset of puberty, occurs 2 years later in boys than in girls, usually between 12 and 14 years.

BODY SYSTEMS

School-age children appear thinner and more graceful than preschoolers do. Musculoskeletal growth leads to greater co-ordination and strength. The muscles are still immature, however, and can be injured from overuse. Growth of the facial bones changes facial proportions. As the facial bones grow, the eustachian tube assumes a more downward and inward position, resulting in fewer ear infections than in the preschool years. Lymphatic tissues continue to grow until about age 9. Enlarged tonsils and adenoids are common during these years and are not always an indication of ill-

ness. Frontal sinuses develop at age 7. The respiratory system also continues to mature. During the school-age years, the lungs and alveoli develop fully, and fewer respiratory infections occur.

DENTITION

During the school-age years, all 20 primary (deciduous) teeth are lost and are replaced by 28 of the 32 permanent teeth. All permanent teeth, except the second and third molars, erupt during the school-age period. The order of eruption of permanent teeth and loss of primary teeth is shown in Figure 33–7. The first teeth to be lost are usually the lower central incisors, at around age 6. Most first graders are characterized by a snaggle-tooth appearance (Fig. 7–1), and visits from the "Tooth Fairy" are important signs of growing up.

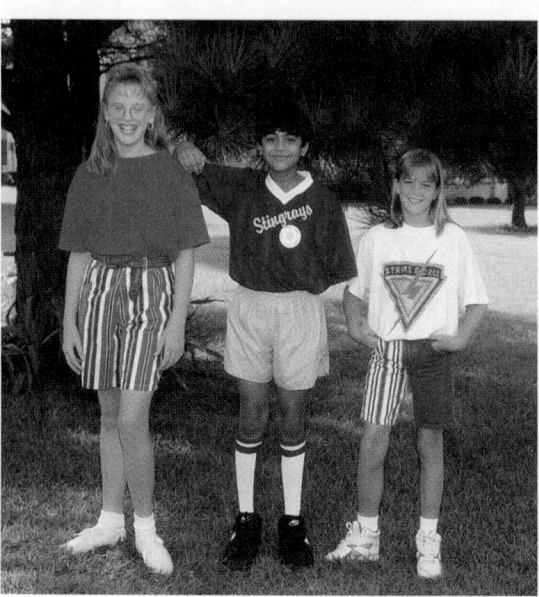

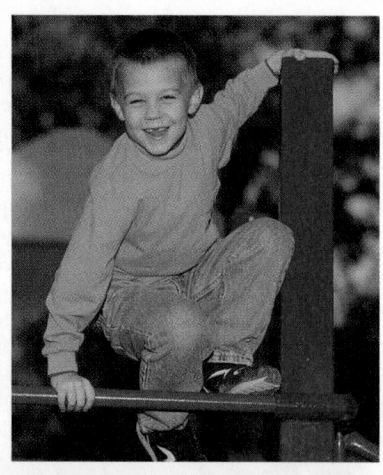

◀ Children of the same age can vary significantly in height and physical development.

◀ School-age children often have a snaggle-tooth appearance while they are losing their primary teeth.

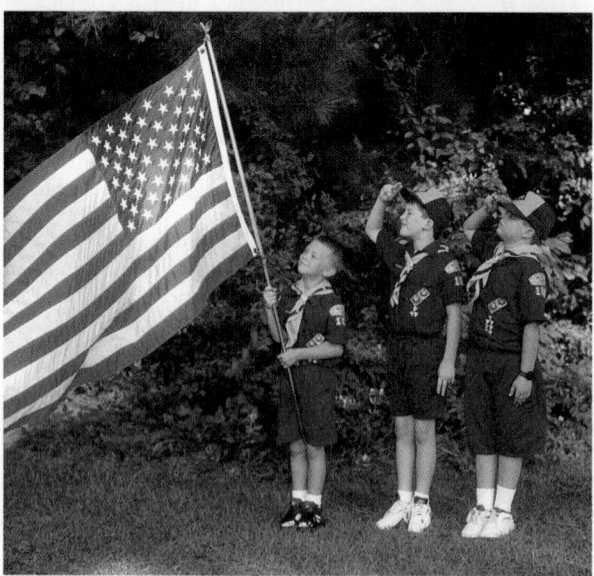

◀ Organizations such as Boy Scouts help to foster self-esteem and competence.

FIGURE 7–1
. . . .
Growth and development of the school-age child.

are less likely to feel embarrassed and anxious. Regardless of whether sex education is a part of a formal school curriculum, children need accurate information. Basic anatomy and physiology, information about bodily functions, and the expected changes of puberty should be introduced to children before the onset of puberty. Older school-age children need information about menstruation, nocturnal emissions, and reproduction. Sex education programs must also include information about responsible sexuality and other related issues, such as teenage pregnancy, human immunodeficiency virus (HIV), and sexually transmissible diseases.

SEXUAL DEVELOPMENT

Puberty is a time of dramatic physical change. It includes the growth spurt, development of primary and secondary sexual characteristics, and maturation of the sexual organs. The age at onset of puberty varies widely, and puberty is occurring at an earlier age than previously thought. On the average, African-American girls begin puberty between 8 and 9 years of age and white girls by 10 years of age (Herman-Giddens et al., 1997). The reason for the earlier development among African-American girls is not known. Puberty begins about 1½ to 2 years later in boys. *Menarche*, the onset of menstruation, occurs, on the average, during the 12th year. Females who are significantly overweight tend to have earlier onset of puberty and menarche (Slyper, 1998). Because puberty is occurring increasingly earlier, many 10- and 11-year-old girls have already experienced menarche. Wide variations in maturity at this age are a common cause of embarrassment because the school-age child does not want to appear different from peers. Children who mature either early or late may struggle with feelings of self-consciousness and inferiority. Table 8–1 describes the usual sequence of appearance of secondary sex characteristics during the school-age and adolescent periods.

Because of earlier onset of puberty, sex education programs should be introduced in elementary school. Nurses are in an excellent position to serve as resource persons for parents and teachers who are responsible for sex education. Children's questions about sexuality and related issues should be answered honestly and matter-of-factly. If sex education is presented within the context of learning about the human body, with its wonders and mysteries, children

Motor Development

THE IMPORTANCE OF ACTIVE PLAY

School-age children spend much of their time in active play, practicing and refining motor skills. They seem to be constantly in motion. Children of this age enjoy active sports and games as well as crafts and fine motor activities (Table 7–2). Activities requiring balance and strength, such as bicycle riding, tree climbing, and skating, are exciting and fun for the school-age child. Coordination and motor skills improve as the child is given an opportunity to practice.

Children should be encouraged to engage in physical activities. During the school-age years, children learn physical fitness skills that contribute to their health for the rest of their lives. Cardiovascular fitness, strength, and flexibility are improved by physical activity. Popular games such as tag, jump rope, and hide-and-seek provide a release of emotional tension and enhance the development of leader and follower skills.

Team sports, such as soccer and baseball, provide opportunities not only for exercise and refinement of motor skills, but also for the development of sportsmanship and teamwork. Nurses should advise parents on ways to prevent sports injuries. Sports activities should be well supervised, and protective gear (such as helmets for T-ball and shin guards for soccer) should be mandatory.

Obesity is the most common cause of abnormal growth acceleration in childhood in the United States (Slyper, 1998). Time spent watching television or playing computer games often diminishes a child's interest in active play outside. Nurses can help reverse this trend by advising parents to limit their children's television-watching time to 2 hours

TABLE 7–2

Age-Related Activities and Toys for the School-Age Child

General Activities	Toys and Specific Types of Play
Play becomes organized with more direction. The early school-age child continues dramatic play with increased creativity but loses some spontaneity. Awareness of rules when playing games. Begins to compete in sports.	Collections, drawing, construction, dolls, pets, guessing games, board games, riddles, physical games, competitive play, reading, bike riding, hobbies, sewing, listening to the radio, watching television and videos, cooking.

per day or less and to encourage them to engage in more active play. Parents should provide adequate space for children to run, jump, and scuffle. The child should have enough free time to exercise and play. Parents should role model both good nutrition and exercise.

PREVENTING FATIGUE AND DEHYDRATION

Because children enjoy active play and are so full of energy, they often do not recognize fatigue. Six-year-olds in particular will not stop an activity to rest. Parents must learn to recognize signs of fatigue or irritability and enforce rest periods before the child becomes exhausted. Because the child's metabolic rate is higher than an adult's and sweating ability is limited, extremes in temperature while exercising can be dangerous. Dehydration and overheating can pose threats to the child's health. Frequent rest periods and adequate hydration are essential for the child during physical exercise.

DEVELOPMENT OF FINE MOTOR SKILLS

Increased myelinization of the central nervous system is shown by refinement of fine motor skills. Balance and eye-hand coordination improve with maturity and practice. School-age children take pride in activities that require dexterity and fine motor skill, such as model building, playing a musical instrument, or drawing.

Cognitive Development

Thought processes undergo dramatic changes as the child moves from the intuitive thinking of the preschool years to the logical operations of the school-age years. The school-age child gains new knowledge and develops more efficient problem-solving ability and greater flexibility of thinking. The 6- and 7-year-old remain in the intuitive thought stage (Piaget, 1962) characteristic of the older preschool child. By age 8, the child moves into the stage of concrete operations, followed by the stage of formal operations at around age 12. See Chapter 8 for a discussion of formal operations; see Chapter 54 for a discussion of the child with cognitive defects, including mental retardation and developmental disabilities.

INTUITIVE THOUGHT STAGE

In the intuitive thought stage (6 to 7 years), thinking is based on immediate perceptions of the environment and the child's own viewpoint. Thinking is still characterized by egocentrism, animism, and centration (see Chapter 6). At 6 and 7 years old, children cannot understand another's viewpoint, form hypotheses, or deal with abstract concepts. The child in the intuitive thought stage has difficulty forming categories and often solves problems by random guessing.

CONCRETE OPERATIONS STAGE

By age 7 or 8, the child enters the stage of concrete operations. Children learn that their point of view is not the only one as they encounter different interpretations of reality and begin to differentiate their own viewpoints from those of peers and adults (Piaget, 1962). This newly developed freedom from egocentrism enables children to think more flexibly and to learn about the environment more accurately. Problem solving becomes more efficient and reliable as the child learns how to form hypotheses. The use of symbolism becomes more sophisticated, and children now can manipulate symbols for things in the way that they once manipulated the things themselves. The child learns the alphabet and how to read. Attention span increases as the child grows older, facilitating classroom learning.

Reversibility.   Children in the concrete operations stage grasp the concept of *reversibility*. They can mentally retrace a process, a skill necessary for understanding mathematical problems ($5 + 3 = 8$ and $8 - 3 = 5$). The child can take a toy apart and put it back together or walk to school and find the way back home without getting lost. Reversibility also enables a child to anticipate the results of actions, a valuable tool for problem solving.

The understanding of time gradually develops during the early school-age years. Children can understand and use clock time at around age 8 years. Although calendar time is understood and dates are memorized by age 8 or 9, mastery of historical time does not occur until later.

Conservation.   Gradually, the school-age child masters the concept of *conservation*. The child learns that certain properties of objects do not change simply because their order, form, or appearance has changed. For example, the child has mastered conservation of mass when the child recognizes that a lump of clay that has been pounded flat is still the same amount of clay as when it was rolled into a ball. The child understands conservation of weight when able to correctly answer the classic nonsense question, "Which weighs more, a pound of feathers or a pound of rocks?" The concept of conservation does not develop all at once. The simpler conservations, such as number and mass, are understood first, and more complex conservations are mastered later. An understanding of conservation of weight develops at age 9 or 10, and volume at age 11 or 12.

Classification and Logic.   Older school-age children are able to classify objects according to characteristics they share, to place things in a logical order, and to recall similarities and differences. This ability is reflected in the school-age child's interest in collections. Children love to collect and classify stamps, stickers, sports cards, shells, dolls, rocks, or anything imaginable. School-age children understand relationships such as larger and smaller, lighter and darker. They can comprehend class inclusion, the concept that objects can belong to more than one classification. For example, a man can be a brother, father, and son at the same time.

School-age children move away from magical thinking as they discover that there are logical, physical explanations for most phenomena. The school-age child is a skeptic, no longer believing in Santa Claus or the Easter Bunny.

Humor.   Children in the concrete operations stage have a delightful sense of humor. Around the age of 8, increased mastery of language and the beginning of logic enable children to appreciate a play on words. They laugh at incongruities and love silly jokes, riddles, and puns ("How do you keep a mad elephant from charging? You take away its credit cards!"). Riddle and joke books make ideal gifts for young school-age children.

Sensory Development

VISION

The eyes are fully developed by age 6. Visual acuity, ocular muscle control, peripheral vision, and color discrimination are fully developed by age 7. Just before puberty, some children's eyes experience a growth spurt, resulting in myopia. Children with poor visual acuity usually do not complain of vision problems because the changes occur so gradually that they are difficult to notice. The young child may never have had 20/20 vision and has nothing with which to compare the imperfect vision. For these reasons, yearly vision screening is important for school-age children.

HEARING

With maturation and growth of the eustachian tube, middle-ear infections occur less frequently than in younger children. However, chronic middle-ear infections are a problem for a few children, resulting in hearing loss. Annual audiometric screening tests are important to detect hearing loss before unrecognized deficits lead to learning problems.

Language Development

Language development continues at a rapid pace during the school-age years. Vocabulary expands, and sentence structure becomes more complex. By age 6, the child's vocabulary is approximately 8,000 to 14,000 words. There is an increase in the use of culturally specific words at this age. Bilingual children may speak English at school and a different language at home.

Reading effectively improves language skills. Regular trips to the library, where the child can check out books of special interest, can promote a love of reading and enhance school performance. School-age children enjoy being read to as well as reading on their own.

School-age children often go through a period in which they experiment with profanity and dirty jokes. Children may imitate parents who use such words as part of their vocabulary.

Psychosocial Development

DEVELOPMENT OF A SENSE OF INDUSTRY

According to Erikson (1963), the central task of the school-age years is the development of a sense of industry. Ideally, the child is prepared for this task with a secure sense of self as separate from loved ones in the family. The child should have learned to trust others and should have developed a sense of autonomy and initiative during the preceding years. The school-age child replaces fantasy play with "work" at school, crafts, chores, hobbies, and athletics. The child is rewarded with a sense of satisfaction from achieving a skill as well as with external rewards, such as good grades, trophies, or an allowance. School-age children enjoy undertaking new tasks and carrying them through to completion. Whether it is baking a cake, hitting a home run, or scoring 100 on a math test, purposeful activity leads to a sense of worth and competence. Successful resolution of the task of industry depends on learning to do things and do them well. School-age children learn skills that they will need later to compete in the adult world. A person's fundamental attitude toward work is established during the school-age years.

FOSTERING SELF-ESTEEM

The negative component of this developmental stage is a sense of inferiority. If a child cannot separate psychologically from the parent or if expectations are set too high for the child to achieve, the child develops feelings of inferiority. If a child believes that success is unattainable, confidence is lost and the child will not take pleasure in attempting new experiences. Children who have this experience will then have a pervasive feeling of inferiority and incompetence that will affect all aspects of their lives. The child who lacks a sense of industry has a poor foundation for mastering the tasks of adolescence. The reality is that no one can master everything. Every child will feel deficient or inferior at something. The task of the caring parent or teacher is to identify areas in which a child is competent and to build on successful experiences to foster feelings of mastery and success. Nurses can suggest ways in which parents and teachers can promote a sense of self-esteem and competence in school-age children.

At this age, the approval and esteem of those outside the family, especially peers, become important. Children learn that their parents are not infallible. As they begin to test parents' authority and knowledge, the influence of teachers and other adults is felt more and more. The peer group becomes the major socializing influence of the school-age child. Although parents' love, praise, and support are needed, even craved during stressful times, the child begins to prefer activities with friends to activities with the family. As the child becomes more independent, increasing time is spent with friends and away from the family.

The concept of friendship changes as the child matures. At 6 and 7 years old, children form friendships merely on the basis of who lives nearby or who has toys that they enjoy. By the time children are 9 or 10, friendships are based more on emotional bonds, warm feelings, and trust-building experiences. Children learn that friendship is more than just being together. Children at 11 and 12 years are loyal to their friends, often sharing problems and giving emotional support. School-age children tend to form friendships with peers of the same sex. Developing friendships and succeeding in social interactions lead to a sense of industry.

• • • • • • • • • • •

Tips for Promoting Self-Esteem in Children

- Provide children with opportunities for assuming responsibility.
- Provide opportunities for making responsible choices and solving problems.
- Offer encouragement and positive feedback.
- Encourage self-discipline by providing guidelines and consequences.
- Help children feel okay about mistakes and failures.

Data from Brooks, R. B. (1992). Self-esteem during the school years: Its normal development and hazardous decline. *Pediatric Clinics of North America, 39*(3), 537–550.

Friendships are important for the emotional well-being of school-age children. Friends teach children skills they will use in future relationships.

Children learn a body of rules, sayings, and superstitions as they enter the culture of childhood. Rules are important to children because they provide predictability and offer security. Learning the sayings, jokes, and riddles is an important part of social interaction among peers. Sayings such as "Step on a crack and you'll break your mother's back" or "Finders, keepers; losers, weepers" have been part of the lore of childhood for generations.

Children become sensitive to the norms and values of the peer group because pressure to conform is great. Children often find that it is painful to be different. Peer approval is a strong motivating force and allows the child to risk disapproval from parents.

The school-age years are a time of formal and informal clubs. Informal clubs among 6-, 7-, and 8-year-olds are loosely organized, with fluid membership. Membership changes frequently and is based on mutual interests, such as playing ball, riding bikes, or playing with dolls. Children learn interpersonal skills, such as sharing, cooperation, and tolerance, in these groups.

Clubs among older school-age children tend to be more structured, often characterized by secret codes, rituals, and rigid rules. A club may be formed for the purpose of exclusion, in which children snub another child for some reason.

Formal organizations, such as Boy Scouts, Girl Scouts, Campfire Boys and Girls, and 4-H, organized by adults, also foster self-esteem and competence as children earn ranks and merit badges. Transmission of societal values, such as service to others, duty to God, and good citizenship, are important goals of these organizations.

Spiritual and Moral Development

The school-age years are pivotal in the development of a conscience and the internalization of values. Tremendous strides are made in moral development during these 6 years. Several theorists have described the dramatic growth that occurs during this stage.

PIAGET
Piaget asserted that young school-age children obey rules because powerful, all-knowing adults hand them down. During this stage, children know the rules, but not the reasons behind them. Rules are interpreted in a literal way, and the child is unable to adjust rules to fit differing circumstances. The perception of guilt changes as the child matures. Piaget stated that up to about age 8, children judge degrees of guilt by the amount of damage done. No distinction is made between accidental and intentional wrongdoing. For example, the child believes that a child who broke five china cups by accident is guiltier than a child who broke one cup on purpose. By age 10, children are able to consider the intent of the action. Older school-age children are more flexible in their decisions and can take into account extenuating circumstances.

KOHLBERG
Kohlberg described moral development in terms of three levels containing six stages (see Chapter 4). According to Kohlberg's theory, children 4 to 7 years old are in stage 2 of the preconventional level, in which right and wrong are determined by physical consequences. The child obeys because of fear of punishment. If the child is not caught or punished for an act, the child does not consider the act wrong. At this stage, children conform to rules out of self-interest or in terms of what others can do in return ("I'll do this for you if you'll do that for me"). Behavior is guided by an "eye-for-an-eye" philosophy. Kohlberg describes children between the ages of 7 and 12 as being in stage 3 of the conventional level. A "good-boy" orientation characterizes this stage, in which the child conforms to rules to please others and avoid disapproval. This stage parallels the concrete operations stage of cognitive development. Around the age of 12, children enter stage 4 of the conventional level. There is an orientation toward respecting authority, obeying rules, and maintaining social order. Most religions place the age of accountability at approximately 12 years.

INFLUENCE OF THE FAMILY
Parents and teachers profoundly influence moral development. Parents can teach children the difference between right and wrong most effectively by living according to their values. A father who lectures his child about the importance of honesty gives a mixed message when he brags about fooling his boss or cheating on his income tax return. The moral atmosphere in the home is a critical factor in the personality development of the child. Children learn self-discipline and internalization of values through obedience to external rules. School-age children are legalistic, and they feel loved and secure when they know that firm limits are set on their behavior. They want and expect discipline for wrongdoings. For moral teaching to be effective, parents must be consistent in their expectations of their children as well as in administering rewards and punishment.

SPIRITUALITY AND RELIGION
Spiritually, school-age children become acquainted with the basic content of their faith. Children reared within a religious tradition feel a part of their religion. Although their thinking is still concrete, children begin to use abstract concepts to describe God and are able to comprehend God as a power greater than themselves or their parents. Because school-age children think literally, spiritual concepts take on materialistic and physical expression. Heaven and hell fascinate them. Concern for rules and a maturing conscience may cause a nagging sense of guilt and fear of going to hell. Younger school-age children still tend to associate accidents and illness with punishment for real or imagined wrongdoing. One 6-year-old child hospitalized for an appendectomy said, "God saw all the bad things I did, and He punished me." Reassurance that God does not punish children by making them sick reduces anxiety.

Health Promotion for the School-Age Child and Family

Table 7–3 presents an overview of health screening, health maintenance, and anticipatory guidance activities for school-age children.

Nutritional Requirements

Growth continues at a slow but regular pace, but the school-age child begins to have an increase in appetite. During the later school-age years energy needs increase. Children in this age group tend to have few eating idiosyncrasies and generally enjoy eating to satisfy appetite and as a social function. Children who developed dislikes for certain foods during earlier periods may continue to refuse those foods. A child of this age is influenced by family patterns and the limitations their activities put on them. They may rush through a meal in order to go out to play or watch a favorite program on television.

The caloric and protein requirements begin to increase at about age 11 years because of the preadolescent growth spurt. The requirements for males and females also begin to vary at this age. A gradual increase of food intake will also take place.

Age-Related Nutritional Challenges

At this age the child's schedule changes and more time is spent away from home. Most children eat lunch at school, and they usually have a choice of foods. Even if the parent packs a lunch for the child to take to school, there are no guarantees that the child will eat the lunch. Children sometimes trade foods with other children or may not eat a particular item. It is also during this period that the child becomes more active in clubs, sports, and other activities that interrupt the normal meal schedule.

The federal government funds the School Lunch Program, which provides approximately one third of the recommended dietary allowances for a child. This program provides lunches for low-income children either free or at reduced rates. Some schools also offer breakfast and milk programs.

School-age children usually request a snack after school and in the evening. Parents should be encouraged to provide their child with healthy choices for snacks. By not buying foods high in calories and low in nutrients the parent can remove the temptation for the child to choose the less healthy foods.

Unpredictable schedules, advertising, easy access to fast food, and peer pressure all have an effect on the foods a child chooses. The child may begin to prefer "junk foods," which do not have much nutritional value. Most of these foods are high in fat and sugar. The family plays an important role in modeling good eating habits for the child. Schools also have a responsibility to provide nutritious meals for children.

Obesity

When intake of food exceeds expenditure, the excess is stored as fat. Obesity is an excessive accumulation of fat in the body. There is an increase of weight beyond that considered desirable with regard to age, height, and bone structure.

Obesity can be a precursor of hyperlipidemia, sleep apnea, cholelithiasis (gallstones), orthopedic problems, hypertension, and diabetes. In addition, children who are obese can have psychosocial difficulties, eating disorders, and inappropriate expectations because their greater growth makes them appear older than they are (Dietz, 1998). Because the obese child develops increased numbers of fat cells, which are carried into adulthood, preventing obesity in childhood can reduce the risk of obesity in adulthood and plays a role in preventing disease.

ETIOLOGY

Cultural, genetic, environmental, and socioeconomic factors have been linked to childhood obesity. Children with low metabolic rates and an increased number of fat cells tend to gain more weight. Children with one or both parents overweight are at increased risk for obesity (Strauss & Dietz, 1999). It is often very difficult to separate out the factors in a family in which the parents are obese. When a parent lacks nutritional knowledge, it is reflected in the meals and snacks provided in the home. The child is at risk for developing the same habits. Obesity is more prevalent among children raised in urban communities and in smaller families. In addition, obesity varies among different ethnic groups, geographic regions, and socioeconomic classes (American Academy of Pediatrics Committee on Nutrition, 1998).

Unstructured meals, "meals on the run," and meals at fast food restaurants can also lack proper nutrition and be high in calories. Lack of exercise also contributes to obesity. Recent studies have shown that as children get older, they are less likely to be involved in regular physical education classes (Centers for Disease Control, 1998). The child who is given food for reward or punishment attaches more to eating than gaining nutrition. Some people still think that a fat baby is a healthy baby. This type of thinking leads to overfeeding.

Although the child may experience an initial weight loss, the long-term success rate for the elimination of obesity is poor. Positive outcomes are increased when the child has a support system and understands the importance of diet and exercise.

PREVENTION

Early identification of risk factors can target the child who needs special attention and support. All children should be taught healthy eating habits and the importance of exercise. Three critical periods appear to exist for the development of childhood obesity: early infancy (1 year or younger), middle childhood (4 to 7 years), and puberty (Strauss & Dietz, 1999). Special attention should be given during these periods so that early intervention can take place.

▌ NURSING CARE
· · · · · · · · ·
The Child with Obesity

Assessment

There is no generally accepted definition of obesity. The child who is obese looks overweight. In addition, graph the child's weight and height to determine in which percentile the child falls. A caliper measurement of skin fold thickness should be taken and compared with established guidelines. The best site for measurement is the triceps. The body mass index (BMI) provides another measurement of body fat that takes into account the child who is highly muscled.

TABLE 7–3
• • • • • • • • • • •

Health Screening, Health Maintenance, and Anticipatory Guidance for School-Age Children

6–7 Years	8–10 Years	10–12 Years
Immunization		
DTaP at 4–6 years OPV or IPV at 4–6 years MMR at 4–6 years Review immunization record; administer appropriate immunizations if not up to date. Review previous reactions and contraindications.	Review immunization record; administer appropriate immunizations if not up to date.	Those who have not previously received the second dose of MMR should complete the schedule no later than the 11–12-year visit. Hepatitis B vaccine given to 11–12-year-olds who have not previously received three doses of hepatitis B vaccine. Should initiate or complete the series. Td at 11–12 years if at least 5 years since last dose of DTP, DTaP, or DT. Varicella vaccine at 11–12 if child lacks a reliable history of chicken pox.
Safety		
Advise parents on use of child seat belts and fire and bicycle safety. Does child know how to swim? Is water play supervised at all times? Does child play sports? Is the sports program well supervised, and is protective gear mandatory (e.g., helmets for T-ball, shin guards for soccer)? Teach child safety around swings, skateboards, and playground equipment. Advise parents to protect child from sunburn with sunscreen.	Advise parents and child on use of child seat belts. Teach child not to ride in back of pickup trucks. Teach child safety around lawn tractors, farm equipment. Does child know how to swim? Does child take risks that concern or frighten parents? Does child know what to do if approached by a stranger? *Sex education:* Make child aware of "good touching" and "bad touching." Discuss dangers of fireworks, matches, and campfires. Advise child to wear a helmet when riding a bicycle or horse.	Advise child on use of car safety belts. Has there been any involvement in or discussion of drugs, smoking, and alcohol? Does child know how to swim? Teach gun safety.
Nutrition		
Assess usual diet: what do meals and snacks consist of? Discuss importance of breakfast to school performance. Discuss food pyramid and importance of a healthy diet. Does child or parent have any concerns about weight?	Appetite increases. Child needs approximately 2,400 calories per day. *Nutrition education:* Nutritious snacks, basic cooking skills, meal planning. Assess regularity of meals and snacks.	Assess adequacy of diet and snacks. Is child too busy to eat properly? Assess amount and frequency of junk food, fast food. Teach child to avoid concentrated sweets.
Vision, Hearing, and Speech		
Assess vision with Snellen charts and hearing with audiometry every 2 years. If child has been screened elsewhere, what were the results? Assess parents' and teacher's perceptions of child's vision and hearing. Is child's speech clear? Any dysfluency?	Assess vision with Snellen charts and hearing with audiometry every 2 years. Have corrective lenses been prescribed? Does child wear them? Teach child and parents not to remove earwax with cotton-tipped applicators or hairpins.	Assess vision with Snellen charts and hearing with audiometry every 2 years. Address parental concerns. Discuss effect on hearing of listening to loud music with headphones.
Dental Care		
Does child brush teeth and have regular dental checkups? Does parent assist child with flossing? Discuss importance of dental visits every 6 months to 1 year.	Does child brush teeth and have regular dental checkups? Many cavities? Malocclusion? Discuss importance of a well-balanced diet, limited sweets. Does child brush and floss twice daily? Discuss importance of good oral hygiene if child has braces.	Does child brush and floss twice daily? Discuss importance of a dental visit every 6 months to 1 year.

TABLE 7-3

Health Screening, Health Maintenance, and Anticipatory Guidance for School-Age Children Continued

6–7 Years	8–10 Years	10–12 Years
Screening		
Plot height and weight on growth charts.	Plot height and weight on growth charts. Assess if weight gain follows the curve (high-risk period for obesity).	Plot height and weight on growth charts.
Screen blood pressure yearly.		Assess for scoliosis.
Perform bacteriuria screen for girls.	Screen blood pressure yearly.	Screen blood pressure yearly.
Perform annual TB testing for high-risk children.	Perform bacteriuria screen for girls.	Perform bacteriuria screen for girls.
Screen blood cholesterol level if there is family history of hyperlipidemia or early myocardial infarction.	Perform annual TB testing for high-risk children.	Perform annual TB testing in high-risk children.
	Assess hemoglobin or hematocrit and perform urinalysis once during school-age years, more often if indicated.	
Teaching and Counseling		
Discuss TV viewing. Advise parents that child's TV viewing should be limited to 2 hours per day.	Assess parents' and child's reactions to school. How is child doing in school? If there are difficulties, have they been addressed by the school and parents? How many days has child been absent from school? Reasons?	Assess child's stress level. Help parents and child identify factors that produce stress and suggest ways to cope with its effects.
How does child get along with other children? How much time does child spend playing with other children? Does child have a best friend?		Discuss dangers of drug and alcohol use and sexual activiy.
Is gender identity fixed?	Child care arrangements for before and after school?	
If child has not started school, assess parents' and child's reactions to approaching school entry, parents' perceptions of child's readiness for school.	Have sexuality and sexual development been discussed with child? Any signs of puberty yet? Does child understand what is happening and what will happen in the future?	

Abbreviations: DTaP, diphtheria and tetanus toxoids and acellular pertussis vaccine; DTP, diphtheria, tetanus toxoids, and pertussis vaccine; Td, tetanus and diphtheria toxoids; OPV, oral poliovirus vaccine; IPV, inactivated poliovirus vaccine; MMR, measles, mumps, and rubella vaccine.

Take a dietary history and evaluate the child's eating habits and patterns. The child or parents (or both) should keep a food diary for 1 week. The diary should include the time, place, and type and amount of food eaten and the reason for eating. The general dietary habits of the family should also be assessed.

Take a psychosocial history of the child and family. The possibility of disease as a contributing factor must be evaluated. Increased weight gain has been associated with central nervous system tumors, hypothyroidism, Cushing syndrome, and Turner syndrome.

Also assess the child's exercise or lack of it. The amount of time spent watching television, at a computer, and playing video games is pertinent. Determine whether the child is participating in any regularly scheduled exercise.

Nursing Diagnosis and Planning

An appropriate nursing diagnosis is

- Altered Nutrition: More Than Body Requirements related to excessive intake.
  Expected Outcomes: The child or adolescent will show a commitment to changing behaviors that increase risk for weight gain, as evidenced by developing and implementing an exercise plan and altering diet to allow for weight loss while maintaining normal growth patterns.

Interventions

One of the key elements of successful weight reduction in the child or adolescent is ownership by the child of whatever plan is proposed. Care should be taken to avoid a power struggle between the parent and child. Obviously the young child will need more parental involvement than the older child or adolescent. The family should be willing to support the child but should not take on the role of watchdog.

Diet and Exercise

A child's caloric requirements vary depending on the age and sex of the child. By changing the obese child's lifestyle to include exercise and nutritional foods in smaller servings, the possibility of success is increased. Teach the family and child how to select and prepare foods that are tasteful and how to restrict serving size. The child's favorite foods should be identified and incorporated whenever possible. Since snacks are an important aspect in childhood nutrition, nutritious snacks should be identified. Involvement of the whole family will create family behaviors that support the child's new eating and activity behaviors.

Television time should be limited. Children should be involved in regular physical exercise at school and at home. Children can be encouraged to ride their bicycles or to walk rather than ride to a friend's house to play. Planned physical activities should be part of the child's after-school routine and on weekends.

Support Groups

Some older children and adolescents may find success in a support group such as Weight Watchers and Overeaters Anonymous. Some centers have a special group for children. There may be other support groups associated with schools, summer camps, and children's hospitals in the community.

A team approach is often necessary for successful weight reduction. Psychological support may be essential for the child and family to be successful. A registered dietician can provide expertise in the identification and planning of foods that not only are nutritional, but that the child also likes.

Parental Support

Parents can support the child by

- Praising the child.
- Never using food as a reward.
- Establishing daily family mealtimes and snack times.
- Offering only healthy options (ask the child to choose between an apple or popcorn, not an apple or a cookie).
- Removing temptations. Parents can control the food that is purchased.
- Being a role model by improving own eating habits and levels of activity.
- Being consistent (Barlow & Dietz, 1998).

For a discussion of other eating alterations such as anorexia nervosa and bulimia nervosa, see Chapter 53.

Evaluation

The child's weight loss is assessed at regular predetermined intervals. The log or diary is reviewed and areas of concern are discussed. This is also an excellent time for positive feedback related to changes in eating behaviors and adherence to an exercise program.

Feelings and goals should also be discussed. If the child is having difficulty losing weight, the plan should be assessed to determine if it is appropriate for the needs of that child.

Dental Care

Although the incidence of dental *caries* (tooth decay) has declined in recent years, tooth decay remains a significant health problem among school-age children. Unfortunately, many parents and school-age children consider dental hygiene to be of minor importance. Many parents erroneously believe that dental care, even brushing, is not important for primary teeth because they will all fall out anyway. However, premature loss of these deciduous teeth can complicate eruption of permanent teeth and lead to malocclusion.

School-age children are able to assume responsibility for their own dental hygiene. Good oral health habits tend to be carried into the adult years, reducing cavity formation for a lifetime. Thorough brushing with fluoride toothpaste followed by flossing between the teeth should be done after meals and especially before bedtime. Proper brushing and flossing and a well-balanced diet promote healthy gums as well as prevent cavities. Sugary or sticky between-meal snacks should be limited. Candy that dissolves quickly, such as chocolate, is less cariogenic than sticky candy, which stays in contact with teeth longer. Information related to fluoride supplementation is discussed in Chapter 6.

MALOCCLUSION

Good occlusion of the teeth is important for tooth formation, speech development, and physical appearance. Many school-age children need braces to correct *malocclusion*, a condition in which the teeth are crowded, crooked, or out of alignment. Factors such as heredity, cleft palate, premature loss of primary teeth, and mouth breathing lead to malocclusion. Thumb sucking is not believed to cause malocclusion unless it persists past the age of 5 or 6. Malocclusion becomes particularly noticeable between the ages of 6 and 12, when the permanent teeth are erupting.

Children with braces are at increased risk for dental caries and must be scrupulous about their dental hygiene. School nurses can encourage children who wear braces to brush after every meal and snack, eat a nutritious diet, and visit the dentist at least once every 6 months. Use of a Water Pik keeps gums healthy and helps remove food particles from around wires and bands.

Braces cause many children to feel self-conscious and may be difficult for a school-age child to accept. However, for some children, orthodontic appliances may be a status symbol. Parental support and encouragement are important to help the child adjust to orthodontic treatment.

PREVENTING DENTAL INJURIES

During the school-age years, injuries to the teeth can occur easily. Many injuries can be avoided by using mouth protectors. These resilient shields protect against injuries by cushioning blows that might otherwise damage teeth or lead to jaw fractures (American Dental Association, 1998). Children should wear a mouth protector when participating in contact sports, riding a bike, or doing in-line skating. Custom-made mouth protectors constructed by the dentist are more expensive than stock mouth protectors purchased in stores, but their better fit makes them more comfortable and less likely to interfere with speech and breathing.

DENTAL HEALTH EDUCATION

Health education curricula need to be designed to foster attitudes and behaviors among children that promote good personal oral hygiene practices and awareness of the risks of dental disease. The school nurse is in an excellent position to educate children about dental health as well as to detect problems such as untreated caries, inflamed gums, or malocclusion. The nurse should look for signs of smokeless tobacco use (irritation of the gums at the tobacco placement site, gum recession, and stained teeth) and should take this opportunity to explain to the child the risks of using tobacco. The use of snuff and chewing tobacco carries multiple dangers, including a greatly increased risk of oral cancer and heart disease.

Sleep and Rest

The number of hours spent sleeping decreases as the child grows older. Children ages 6 and 7 years need about 12 hours of sleep per night. Some children also continue to need an afternoon quiet time or nap to restore energy levels. The 12-year-old needs about 9 to 10 hours of sleep at night. More sleep is needed when the child enters the preadolescent growth spurt. Adequate sleep is important for school performance and physical growth. Inadequate sleep can cause irritability, inability to concentrate, and poor school performance.

To promote rest and sleep, a period of quiet activity just before bedtime is helpful. A leisurely bedtime routine, with adequate time for the child to read, listen to the radio or CDs, or just daydream, promotes relaxation. Children who do not obtain adequate rest often have difficulty getting up in the morning, creating family disturbance as they rush to get ready for school, perhaps skipping breakfast or leaving the house in the heat of frustration. A set bedtime and waking time, consistently enforced, promote security and healthful sleep habits. Bedtime offers an ideal opportunity for parent and child to share important events of the day or give a kiss and a hug, unthinkable in front of peers earlier in the day.

Discipline

Because school-age children possess a strong sense of justice and believe in the importance of rules, they want and expect limits to be set on their behavior. Firm, consistent limits increase children's sense of security and reinforce the message that an adult cares about them. Realistic expectations, clearly defined rules, and logical consequences help children to develop self-discipline and increased self-esteem. Some families have meetings where they discuss how responsibilities in the family will be shared. The child is made to feel more a part of the solution, rather than the problem.

Responsibility can be developed in children through the use of natural and logical consequences related to actions. Children become accountable for their actions. If a child leaves a toy outside and it is damaged, the parent is empathetic but does not replace the toy. The parent does not get in a power struggle, nor does the parent verbally attack the child. The child begins to understand that there are consequences to actions. Correctly used, the deed will be separated from the doer, moral judgment will not be passed, focus will be on the present, not the past, and respect and firm kindness will be shown. In addition, the child will be given choices and the consequence will relate to the logic of the situation (Dinkmeyer & McKay, 1996).

Teachers' disciplinary efforts are often thwarted when parents do not support them or show no concern about their children's misbehavior. Teamwork between parents and teachers is essential for effective discipline. Regular parent-teacher conferences help make discipline effective.

Safety

Approaches to safety education vary as the child grows older. Physically, this age is a period of great activity, with the child moving from the home environment and into the community. The school-age child experiences less fear in play activities and frequently imitates adult life by using tools and household items. Children in this age group enjoy helping with adult routines and chores around the home. Anticipatory guidance related to safety is very important, and in fact is a national health objective (Quinlan, Sacks, & Dresnow, 1998).

Safety education is best accomplished by simply stating safety rules and providing reinforcement through short projects and immediate rewards. Role-playing activities and error-detection picture games are excellent ways to reinforce safety lessons. Children in this age group are inquisitive and will frequently ask questions. The answers to their questions should contain concrete rationales. Group projects with safety topics help to foster independent thinking while promoting interactions with the child's peer group.

CAR SAFETY

The school-age child is large enough to use the vehicle's three-point restraining system. Compliance often is determined by family values, with use or nonuse reflecting parental practices. For the younger, smaller child, correct positioning of the seat belt is important. Parents should help adjust the belts so that the lap belt fits snugly over the bony pelvis and the shoulder harness is positioned across the chest.

FIRE AND BURN SAFETY

Parents should continue to reinforce safety procedures associated with fire safety. Routine fire drills should be practiced in the home. Repetition of family drills helps to ensure that the child will respond correctly and automatically to smoke alarms. Children of this age can better comprehend cause-and-effect relationships, so they can understand why they should not play with potentially flammable substances.

CRITICAL THINKING EXERCISE 7–1

Mrs. George states that Megan, age 11, has recently started to leave her belongings throughout the house and that her room is always a mess. Mrs. George states that she is frustrated and feels as if she is constantly asking Megan to pick her things up and to clean her room.

1. What assumptions might a nurse make based on Mrs. George's report about her daughter's behavior?
2. What other data does the nurse need to clarify to best help Mrs. George and Megan in this situation?
3. What are some possible approaches the nurse might suggest to Mrs. George?

CRITICAL TO REMEMBER

Fire Safety Rules

- Know two specific escape routes from each area in the home.
- Know how to access 911.
- Know how to crawl under the smoke to leave a burning house.
- Have a predetermined meeting area outside the house.
- Never return to a burning house.
- Practice fire drills.

School-age children are eager to help parents with daily chores such as cooking or ironing. Parents need to invest the time to teach their children how to use tools and appliances properly and must establish guidelines to avoid burn injuries as a result of the inexperience of the child.

Fireworks create another burn hazard for children. Each summer, many children are seriously burned or permanently scarred by fireworks. To prevent serious burn injuries, the federal government, under the Federal Hazardous Substance Act, prohibits the sale of the more dangerous fireworks to the general public. However, there is always a degree of risk associated with any fireworks. There are no absolutely safe fireworks for children or adults. Fireworks are best left to the experts and viewed from a safe distance. Encourage families to enjoy the many community-sponsored fireworks displays.

BICYCLE, IN-LINE SKATING, AND SKATEBOARD SAFETY

Mastering the ability to ride a bicycle is a milestone in a child's life, leading to independence. The bicycle is typically considered a toy but is actually a vehicle that is capable of speedy transportation. It is also a major cause of death and serious head trauma in children (Sosin, Sacks, & Webb, 1996). For this reason, the public health community sup-

ports the mandatory use of bicycle helmets. Research has demonstrated that the use of a helmet can reduce the incidence of head injury by as much as 85% when fitted properly (Logan et al., 1998).

Bicycle safety practices actually begin when the child learns to ride a tricycle and progressively build as the child becomes more skilled and begins to ride a bicycle. A helmet and other safety accessories are essential for protection, but they are only an adjunct to the child's skill level and knowledge of the rules of the road. A young cyclist is unpredictable and may be preoccupied with managing the bicycle itself. For this reason, parents should set limits on where, when, and how far the child may ride, until the child can competently maneuver the bicycle.

In-line skating and skateboarding are recreational activities that are popular with school-age children. Balancing, stopping, and turning are challenging and require motor skills similar to those required for bicycling. As the child begins to learn these skills, falls are frequent and protective gear is essential. Helmets and protective pads covering the knees and elbows help to protect the most vulnerable areas of the child's body from serious injury. Key educational points and an overview of safety principles are described in the accompanying box.

PARENTS WANT TO KNOW
· · · · · · · · · ·
About Bicycle, In-Line Skating, and Skateboard Safety

- Children should always wear a helmet when riding a bike, in-line skating, or skateboarding. This safety practice should begin when the child begins to learn these activities.
- Helmets should fit properly and snugly on the head. Helmets need to be lightweight and ventilated and have reflective trim.
- Children should be taught not to ride at dusk or in the dark. They should always call home for a ride if it is after dark.
- Children should never ride two on a bicycle.
- Children should not ride barefoot, in thongs, or in slippers. Audio headsets should be avoided while riding a bicycle because they can diminish hearing capabilities.
- Children should be encouraged to stay on sidewalks, paths, or driveways until they have mastered advanced biking skills and know the rules of the road.
- While riding or in-line skating, children should avoid uneven road surfaces, gravel, potholes, or bumps.
- Bicycles should be equipped with reflectors and lights. Children should routinely inspect their own bicycles with their parents' help to ensure that they are functioning properly (brakes, tires, lights, and so forth).
- Parents should be taught the importance of proper sizing when purchasing a bicycle for their child. Oversized bicycles are responsible for many injuries.
- The child should be able to place the balls of both feet on the ground when sitting on the seat with the hands on the handlebars.
- The child should be able to straddle the center bar

with both feet flat on the ground. There should be about 1 inch of clearance between the crotch and the bar.
- The handlebars should be within easy reach for the child.

Rules of the Road

- Children younger than 8 years should ride only with adult supervision, and never in the street. In-line skating or skateboarding should be limited to areas where there is no car traffic.
- Children should not ride bicycles on roads with heavy traffic.
- A bicycle should be ridden on the right side of the road, with the traffic. Bike riders must obey all traffic laws, traffic signs, and lights.
- Children should learn the appropriate hand signals and use them every time before turning.
- Bicycles should be walked across busy intersections, not ridden.
- Children need to learn to stop, look left, look right, and look left again before entering a street or leaving a driveway, alley, or parking lot.
- Children should stop at all intersections, marked and unmarked.
- Children riding bicycles should obey all stop signs and red lights.
- Children should look back and yield to traffic coming from behind before turning left at intersections.
- Basic bicycle safety rules apply to in-line skating and skateboarding.

PEDESTRIAN SAFETY

Children between the ages of 5 and 9 years are at the greatest risk for auto-pedestrian injuries. The tremendous forces of impact and the lack of protection for the pedestrian can lead to severe injury. Children are commonly struck when they dart into traffic, especially where parked cars obscure the driver's view of the child (e.g., crossing the street in front of a school bus, playing near cars in driveways or yards). Several factors predispose this age group to such injuries. Their smaller physical stature limits their visibility to drivers until too late. Additionally, children in this age group have the misconception that if they can see the car, the driver must be able to see them and will be able to stop instantly. Focused on play activities, they often impulsively dart into the street, oblivious to boundaries and potential traffic dangers.

Children learn traffic safety by watching and doing. Exposure to traffic increases as the child begins to walk to and from school and friends' houses. Parents have the responsibility of practicing pedestrian safety hundreds of times before the child is allowed to venture across streets alone.

WATER SAFETY

School-age children learn to swim well enough to keep their heads above water for a short time at about the age of 8. The length of time they can keep their heads above water and their swimming ability increase with age and experience. The incidence of drowning decreases in this age group; however, adult supervision is still needed to prevent a water-related injury. Children in this age group often overestimate their swimming capabilities and endurance. As their swimming abilities improve, anticipatory guidance can be directed toward general swimming safety. Children should be taught to stay away from canals and the fast-moving waters of creeks or rivers. Children need to be taught to wade into shallow water or to jump feet first into water of unknown depth to prevent neck injuries. Safety near the water includes never running, pushing, or jumping on others who are in the water.

Adjustment to School

Most children are eager to start school, particularly if they have older siblings. They even look forward to bringing home their books and doing "real" homework. This enthusiasm usually fades quickly, however. Most children adjust well to first grade, enjoying the opportunities it provides for peer interaction and stimulating experiences. First grade may be the child's first experience of being away from home. For these children, starting school may be a frightening experience. Even children who have attended preschool have some anxiety about beginning first grade. Adjustment to school depends on a variety of factors, including the child's physical and emotional maturity, the child's experiences, and the parents' ability to support the child and accept the separation (see Chapter 6).

INFLUENCE OF PEERS

School is often the first experience a child has with a large number of children of the same age. From peers children learn how to cooperate, compete, bargain, and follow rules. Peer approval is of major importance as children look to their friends for recognition and support. The influence of peers becomes stronger as the child grows older.

INFLUENCE OF TEACHERS

Teachers have a significant influence on the social and intellectual development of children. An effective teacher makes learning fun and capitalizes on the child's interests and talents. Teachers guide the child's learning by rewarding success and helping the child learn from and deal with failures. The teacher plays an important role in preventing feelings of inferiority in the child. By structuring the learning environment so that the child experiences success, the teacher bolsters feelings of industry.

The student-teacher relationship is a key factor in school success. Effective teachers motivate students by being warm and understanding, showing interest, and communicating at the child's level. Children value the opinion of such teachers and will work to gain their approval. Favorite teachers serve as role models and are often objects of hero worship by their students.

Even excellent teachers cannot do an effective job alone. They need the support of parents and school administration to maximize the learning potentials of children.

THE PARENTS' ROLE

Parents play a key role in their children's academic success. By taking an active interest in children's progress and encouraging them to do their best, parents can foster learning. Positive reinforcement should be given for honest efforts, not just good grades. Parents should enforce rules that encourage self-discipline and good study habits (e.g., no television until homework is finished). The child must create and adhere to a schedule for completing large assignments to prevent last-minute panic. If the child does not have a desk or another private place for homework, the kitchen table or another quiet, well-lighted area should be made available during study time. The television should be turned off during study time, and distractions should be kept to a minimum. Adequate sleep is important for school performance. Parents may need to enforce bedtime rules to meet the child's needs. Rewarding children for meeting deadlines and for being organized encourages them to take responsibility for their learning and fosters skills that are important for success in jobs as adults.

Parents need to communicate with teachers and stay informed about their children's progress. Visiting the classroom and attending parent-teacher conferences and school activities are important. Showing respect and support for the teacher facilitates learning.

SCHOOL REFUSAL

School refusal is a descriptive term for behavior that may indicate the presence of a specific phobia, separation anxiety, truancy, or social phobia (Kutcher, 1997). In the past, the term was used interchangeably with school phobia and school avoidance (Paige, 1997). There is much discussion over the diagnosis and treatment of children who refuse to attend school and the appropriate label for these children. School phobia needs to be defined both symptomatically and operationally to determine if its cause is related to anxiety (e.g., panic, phobic, and separation) or another cause (e.g., truancy) (Klykylo, Kay, & Rube, 1998).

School refusal has been defined as frequent absences from school or attendance at school under duress or following tantrums or noncompliance (Kearney & Beasley, 1994). Some school-refusing children show specific fears of school or school-related situations (tests, bullies, teacher reprimands, undressing for gym) (King, Ollendick, & Tonge, 1995). Because some children with school refusal behaviors have intense emotional distress related to school attendance, they are labeled phobic. The confusion over the use of these terms can make assessment and treatment of these children difficult. For a discussion of separation anxiety see Chapter 53.

Children may go to school unwillingly or may refuse and have temper tantrums if the parents insist on taking the child to school. Younger children may complain of stomachaches, headaches, nausea and vomiting. Older children may complain of palpitations and feeling faint. These symptoms typically resolve when the child is returned home.

HELPING A CHILD OVERCOME SCHOOL REFUSAL

In uncomplicated cases, the child should be returned to school as soon as possible. If symptoms are severe, a limited period of part-time or modified school attendance may be necessary. For example, part of the day may be spent in the counselor's or school nurse's office, with assignments obtained from the teacher. The child should be gently questioned about factors at school that cause worry or fear. Specific causes, such as a bully or an overly critical teacher, should be dealt with immediately. Parents must support each other because the child may play one parent against the other to avoid school. Parents should be empathetic, yet firm and consistent in their insistence that the child attend school. Parents should not pick the child up at school once the child is there. Positive reinforcement for school attendance is essential. Encouraging and maintaining peer contacts and emphasizing the positive aspects of school are helpful. The principal and teacher should be told about the situation so that they can cooperate with the treatment plan.

Self-Care Children

The number of children who let themselves into their homes after school and are left alone continues to grow as the number of dual-income and single-parent families increases. These children are called *self-care children*, previously referred to as latchkey children.

Parents often feel guilty about leaving children alone and may feel concern for their children's safety. Potential positive outcomes of this experience are learning to be independent and responsible. The quality of the parent-child relationship and parents who are emotionally supportive and establish firm rules play a role in moderating the effects on the child in self-care.

Self-care children living in high-crime urban areas seem more fearful and isolated than their peers who are in supervised child care. They are also at greater risk for drug and tobacco use. Interestingly, children in suburban and rural areas do not seem to have these negative effects of self-care. Some think it is related to fewer restrictions on outdoor play and fewer threats of physical harm (Lowe Vandell, Pierce, & Stright, 1997).

Support for Self-Care Children

Nurses can help families by offering support and education to parents and children to reduce the risks for self-care children. Parents need to know how to prepare their children for self-care, teaching them specific strategies for staying safe at home alone. Nurses can serve as child advocates by working to develop expanded after-school child-care programs in the community. A number of communities have established after-school telephone help lines to provide information, support, and assistance to self-care children.

Stress

Today's children are subjected to stress as no generation has been before. Alarming increases in drug abuse, childhood suicide, child abduction and murder, and school failure attest to the overwhelming stress that children experience. Rapid, bewildering social change and ever-increasing demands for achievement often pressure children to grow up too quickly.

Stressed children may not show serious symptoms during childhood but may develop patterns of emotional response that can lead to serious illness as adults.

SOURCES OF STRESS FOR CHILDREN

Growing up is stressful, even for well-adjusted children with loving, supportive families. Children experience stress from societal change, school, competitive athletics, rushed schedules, and the media.

• • • • • • • • • • •

Manifestations of Stress in Children

How children perceive stress influences its effects. It is not just the stress but how the child perceives and responds to the stress that determines whether the child experiences symptoms of stress.

Intervention is needed when a child shows the following signs of stress:

- Unhappiness, moodiness
- Irritability, increased aggressive behavior
- Fatigue, inability to concentrate
- Hyperactivity
- Changes in eating or sleeping habits
- Physical complaints (nausea, headaches, stomachaches)
- Bedwetting
- Substance abuse
- Diminished school performance
- Suicidal behavior

Middle-class children in particular are pressured to grow up quickly. Achievement-oriented parents, focused on success and financial gain, often view children as extensions of themselves and unwittingly expect too much of their children. Pressure on children to succeed, to win, and to be the best and brightest is great, especially when parents value academic achievement. Children are often pressured into a frenzied schedule of music, dance, sport, and art lessons and may have little time for family meals or playing with friends. Self-esteem and peer relationships often suffer.

Economically deprived children must cope with an even greater burden of stress. Faced with the dangers of violence, drug and alcohol addiction, and gangs, these children must fight daily for survival. Children from lower-income families travel dangerous streets to and from school and suffer from the insecurity and uncertainty of poverty. If the child happens to be homeless—as is increasingly common—they have the added stress of living on the street or in shelters. Both homeless and low-income children experience significant adversity in their lives, with homeless children having increased stress (Bassuk et al., 1997).

School Pressures. School can be a source of stress for children. Some children are unable to cope with the competitive, test-regulated curricula of school. They find it difficult to keep up with the unrelenting academic pressure. School imposes chronic stress on these children, and they tend to dislike school and stay home whenever they can. They are often tardy and may abuse alcohol and drugs. Eventually, they may drop out of school. These children rarely return to complete their education.

Other children, particularly those who are academically gifted, find school stressful because it is tedious. Boredom can be stressful. Meaningless, repetitive schoolwork can cause bright, talented children to become chronically fatigued, inattentive, and careless.

Physical Threats. Children also face other types of stress at school. Violence and theft in schools are national problems. Fears of being beaten up or held up are commonly voiced by school-age children. The child who leaves a bike unlocked or a watch or jacket unattended quickly learns the hazards of such carelessness. Students who abuse drugs or participate in gang activity create a pervasive attitude of wariness and fear and are a real source of stress for children.

Competitive Sports. Participation in competitive sports is stressful for some children. Fear of failure, especially in front of a cheering crowd, can be overwhelming. Some parents contribute to competitive stress by overemphasizing the importance of winning. Because of their own needs or interests, some parents push their children to participate in organized sports at an early age (Figure 7–2).

Tight Schedules and "Adaptation Overload." As the number of single parents and working mothers increases, so does the stress on children who must adapt to parents' work schedules. Many children are rushed from home to school to carpool to day care or a babysitter. Children must draw on their energy reserves to exercise self-control in these varying situations and may not be able to cope. Fatigue and exhaustion from such demands often result in behavioral problems and regression.

Family Pressures. In today's mobile society it is not unusual for families to move and for children to have to leave other family members and friends. Attending a new school, making new friends, and losing former support systems can be very stressful for children. This happens at a time when one or both parents are also making major adjustments in their lives and they may not have the time and energy to meet all of the needs of the child.

Overhearing parents quarrel produces anxiety and fear in children and erodes a child's sense of security. Some parents, although physically present, may be emotionally unavailable to children because of their own stresses. Divorce and separation are especially painful. Changes frequently caused by divorce, such as moving to a new house, attending a new school, and, usually the most stressful of all, separation from one of the parents, can cause great stress for children.

Influence of the Media. The media are a common source of stress for today's children. Sexual and violent material portraying loss of control may frighten children because it suggests that they may not be able to master their own sexual and aggressive impulses. Television exposes children to vivid portrayals of the problems of today's society for many hours of their day. It also tends to isolate children from their parents and peers. Hours spent watching television can limit children's participation in more creative play as well as contact and interaction with others.

INTERVENTIONS AND ANTICIPATORY GUIDANCE

The nurse is in an ideal position to help parents and children identify factors that produce stress and to suggest ways to cope with its effects. Parents can meet basic psychological needs, influence self-esteem, shape values, control exposure to stressful events and provide support (Hess & Copeland, 1997). Parents may need guidance about realistic expectations of their children. Parents should watch for behavior changes in their children that may indicate signs of stress and offer appropriate reassurance. If there is a significant tension in the home, parents can try to resolve conflicts by negotiating rather than continuing to build an emotionally charged atmosphere. Parents should examine the child's

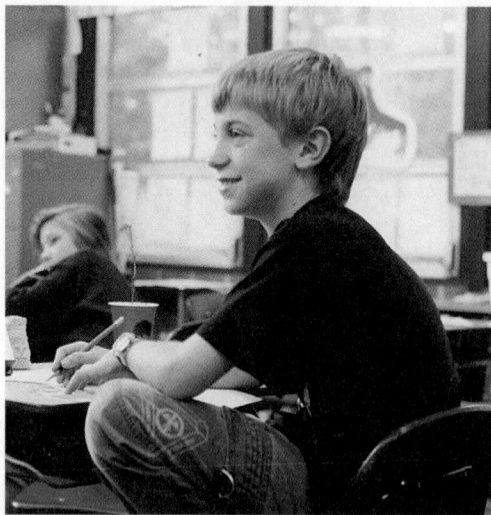

◄ Attention span increases during the school-age years, facilitating classroom learning.

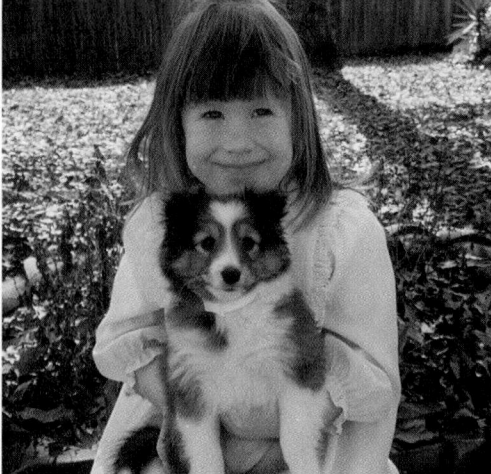

The nurse is in an excellent position to help parents and children identify factors that produce stress and to suggest ways to cope with its effects. Participation in competitive sports is stressful for some children, especially if parents push their child to play organized sports at an early age or overemphasize the importance of winning. Focusing on having fun and on the excitement of the game decreases competitive stress.

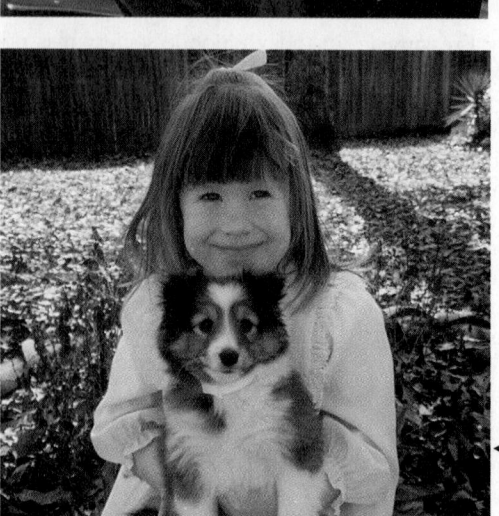

◄ Spending time playing with and caring for pets can be fun and relaxing. Children who are given time and encouragement to play are better able to deal with the stresses of life.

FIGURE 7–2
· · · · · · · · · ·
Health promotion for the school-age child and family.

schedule to make sure the child is not overburdened with school and extracurricular activities.

Close communication with teachers is important to prevent and deal with school-related stress. Becoming interested in and involved with the child's schoolwork conveys support and caring. Parents need to become active in parent-teacher associations and other community organizations to find solutions to the problems of violence and crime in the schools.

Children should be allowed to decide whether to participate in competitive athletics. It is important for parents to talk to coaches to determine what is expected of their children. Corrective instruction rather than punishment should be given for errors. Parents should serve as role models for good sportsmanship.

Limiting the number of hours that children watch television and helping them to select appropriate programs can decrease its negative effects. Watching television with

children and discussing the content of programs is also helpful.

Children need to have time just to play. Parents should recognize that play is the child's work. Whether it is shooting baskets in the driveway, working on a collection, or building a model, play reduces stress for children. Toys and games that provide the greatest opportunity to use imagination are the best stress relievers. Most children love animals. Spending time playing with and caring for pets can be relaxing and fun. Children who are given the time and encouragement to play are better able to deal with the stresses of life (see Chapter 4).

One of the most effective antidotes for childhood stress is a loving, attentive parent who takes the time to listen. A sympathetic adult who understands the stresses of childhood can offer valuable support. Discussion and modeling of ways to deal with the inevitable stresses of life can teach the child valuable lessons for living in today's society.

KEY CONCEPTS

■ Slow, steady physical growth and rapid social and cognitive development characterize the school-age years, from 6 to 12. Average weight gain in the school-age child is 2.5 kg (5.5 lb) per year, and the increase in height is approximately 5.5 cm (2 inches) per year. During the early school-age period, boys are approximately 2.54 cm (1 inch) taller and 0.9 kg (2 lb) heavier than girls.

■ During the school-age years, children gradually move away from home and parents as a primary source of support, and they enter the wider world of peers and school.

■ Physical changes include increased height and weight, increased muscle mass, maturation of body systems, and increased antibody production. During the school-age period, all 20 primary teeth are lost and are replaced by 28 of the 32 permanent teeth.

■ The age at onset of puberty varies widely, but puberty is occurring at an earlier age then in the past. On average, African-American girls enter puberty between 8 and 9 years of age and white girls by 10 years of age.

■ School-age children enjoy a variety of activities. Cooperative play and team sports are typical of this age group.

■ According to Erikson, the developmental task of this period is the development of a sense of industry.

■ The child develops a conscience and internalizes cultural and social values. The child is able to understand and obey rules.

■ Thinking becomes less egocentric as children learn to consider viewpoints different from their own. School-age children can solve problems, form hypotheses, and make judgments based on reason.

■ School-age children experience an increase in appetite, and older school-age children have increased energy needs as they approach puberty.

■ Sources of stress for school-age children include societal change, school, competitive athletics, rushed schedules, fear of violence from gangs or bullies, chaotic living conditions if homeless, and the media. Teaching children coping strategies can reduce the effects of stress.

■ Dental care is increasingly important as the primary teeth are replaced by permanent teeth.

■ Safety issues are related to the child moving more from the home environment to the community, less fear when playing, and the increased use of tools and household items.

ANSWERS TO CRITICAL THINKING EXERCISE 7–1

1. The nurse might assume that Mrs. George is inconsistent in her expectations. There may not be consequences associated with Megan's behavior. Mrs. George is engaging in a power struggle with Megan. Mrs. George's expectations of a clean room may be different from Megan's.

2. The nurse can begin to gather data by asking Mrs. George to describe a typical day when she feels upset with Megan's behavior. The nurse can further ask, "What is your re-sponse to her behavior?" Based on Mrs. George's response, the nurse can determine how the mother is reacting to Megan's behavior and begin to develop strategies. The nurse can determine if Mrs. George has an emotional response to the situation and reacts, or if she remains focused and has a plan of action.

3. Some children respond to family meetings where they are involved in the decision making related to the goals of the household. After the family agrees on a solution, there must be consequences to not following the plan. The family might discuss putting items left in a public area into a holding box for a period of time. Or, if Megan does not pick up her room and dirty clothes do not make it to the hamper, then her clothes will not be washed. Consistency and consequences are the foundation for making such a plan work. This is one way to develop a responsible child.

REFERENCES AND READINGS

American Academy of Pediatrics Committee on Injury and Poison Prevention and Committee on Sports Medicine and Fitness. (1998). In-line skating injuries in children and adolescents. *Pediatrics, 101*(4), 720–722.

American Academy of Pediatrics Committee on Nutrition. (1998). *Pediatric nutrition handbook.* Elk Grove Village, IL: Author.

American Academy of Pediatrics Committee on Psychosocial Aspects of Child and Family Health. (1998). American Academy of Pediatrics: Guidance for effective discipline. *Pediatrics, 101*(4), 723–728.

American Academy of Pediatrics Division of Child Health Research. (1997). Emphasis on bike helmet use yields desired results. *AAP News, 13*(4), 17.

American Dental Association. (1998, February). Teeth and gums change rapidly as kids go through the wonder years [News release]. Chicago: Author.

American Psychiatric Association. (1997). *Diagnostic and statistical manual of mental disorders* (4th ed.). Washington, DC: Author.

Barlow, S. E., & Dietz, W. H. (1998). Obesity evaluation and treatment: Expert com-mittee recommendations. *Pediatrics, 102*(3), 29.

Bassuk, E. L., Weinreb, L. F., Dawson, R., Perloff, J. N., & Buckner, J. C. (1997). Determinants of behavior in homeless and low-income housed preschool children. *Pediatrics, 100*(1), 92–100.

Berkowitz, C. (1996). *Pediatrics: A primary care approach.* Philadelphia: Saunders.

Birch, L. L., & Fisher, J. O. (1998). Development of eating behaviors among children and adolescents. *Pediatrics, 101*(3), 539–549.

Centers for Disease Control. (1998). Youth risk behavior surveillance—United States, 1997. *Morbidity and Mortality Weekly Report, 47*(No. SS-3).

Christophersen, E. R. (1998). *Beyond discipline: Parenting that lasts a lifetime.* Shawnee Mission, KS: Overland Press.

Dietz, W. H. (1998). Health consequences of obesity in youth: Childhood predictors of adult disease. *Pediatrics, 101*(3), 518–525.

Dinkmeyer, D., & McKay, G. (1996). *Raising a responsible child.* New York: Simon & Schuster.

Erikson, E. (1963). *Childhood and society* (2nd ed.). New York: Norton.

Feldman, R. S. (1998). *Child development.* Upper Saddle River, NJ: Prentice Hall.

Fontanesi, J. (1997). School health and behavioral and developmental pediatrics. *Pediatric Annals, 26*(12), 724–727.

Harrell, J. S., Gansky, S. A., Bradley, C. B., & McMurry, R. G. Leisure time activities of elementary school children. *Nursing Research. 46*(5), 246–253.

Herman-Giddens, M. E., Slora, E. J., Wasserman, R. C., Bourdony, C. J., Bhapkar, M. V., Koch, G. G., & Hasemeier, M. (1997). Secondary sexual characteristics and menses in young girls seen in office practice: A study from the pediatric research in office settings network. *Pediatrics, 99*(4), 505–512.

Hernandez, B., Uphold, C. R., Graham, M. V., & Singer, L. (1998). Prevalence and correlates of obesity in preschool children. *Journal of Pediatric Nursing, 13*(2), 68–76.

Hess, R. S., & Copeland, E. P. (1997). Stress. In G. G. Bear, K. M. Minke, & A. Thomas (Eds.), *Children's needs: II. Development, problems and alternatives* (pp. 293–314). Bethesda, MD: National Association of School Psychologists.

Jarvis, C. (1996). *Physical examination and health assessment.* Philadelphia: Saunders.

Kaplan, D. W., Brindis, C., Naylor, K. E., Phibbs, S. L., Ahlstrand, K. R., & Melinkovich, P. (1998). Elementary school-based health center use. *Pediatrics, 101*(6), 12.

Kearney, C. A., & Beasley, J. F. (1994). The clinical treatment of school refusal behavior: A survey of referral and practice characteristics. *Psychology in the Schools, 22,* 85–96.

King, N. J., Ollendick, T. H., & Tonge, B. J. (1995). *School refusal: Assessment and treatment.* Boston: Allyn & Bacon.

Klykylo, W. M., Kay, J., & Rube, D. (1998). *Clinical child psychiatry.* Philadelphia: Saunders.

Kutcher, S. P. (1997). *Child and adolescent psychopharmacology.* Philadelphia: Saunders.

Logan, P., Leadbetter, S., Gibson, R. E., Schieber, R., Branche, C., Bender, P., Zane, D., Humphreys, J., & Anderson, S. (1998). *Pediatrics, 101*(4), 578–582.

Lowe Vandell, D., Pierce, K., & Stright, A. (1997). Child care. In G. G. Bear, K. M. Minke, & A. Thomas (Eds.), *Children's needs: II. Development, problems and alternatives* (pp. 293–314). Bethesda, MD: National Association of School Psychologists.

Maguire, M. C. (1997). Tuberculosis skin testing at the end of a century. *Pediatric Nursing, 23*(2), 209–211.

Muscari, M. E., Catalino, C., & Faherty, J. (1998). Little women: Early menarche in rural girls. *Pediatric Nursing, 24*(1), 11–15.

Neff, J. A., & Dale, J. (1996). Worries of school-age children. *Journal of Society of Pediatric Nursing, 1*(1), 27–32.

Nelson, J. (1996). *Positive discipline.* New York: Ballantine Books.

Paige, L. Z. (1997). School phobia, school refusal, and school avoidance. In G. G. Bear, K. M. Minke, & A. Thomas (Eds.), *Chil-*

dren's needs: II. Development, problems and alternatives (pp. 339–347). Bethesda, MD: National Association of School Psychologists.

Piaget, J. (1962). *Play, dreams, and imitation in childhood* (C. Gattegno & F. M. Hodgson, trans.). New York: Norton.

Quinlan, K. P., Sacks, J. J., & Dresnow, M. (1998). Exposure to and compliance with pediatric injury prevention counseling—United States, 1994. *Pediatrics, 102*(5), 55.

Schor, E. L. (1998). Guiding the family of the school-age child. *Contemporary Pediatrics, 15*(3), 75–94.

Slyper, A. (1998). Childhood obesity, adipose tissue distribution, and the pediatric practitioner. *Pediatrics, 102*(1), 4.

Sosin, D. M., Sacks, J. J., & Webb, K. W. (1996). Pediatric head injuries and deaths from bicycling in the United States. *Pediatrics, 98*(5), 868–870.

Strauss, R. S., & Dietz, W. H. (1999). Obesity. In F. D. Burg, E. R. Wald, J. R. Ingelfinger, & R. A. Polin (Eds.), *Gellis and Kagan's current pediatric therapy* (pp. 8–10). Philadelphia: Saunders.

Trahms, C. M., & Pipes, P. L. (1997). *Nutrition in infancy and childhood* (6th ed.). New York: McGraw-Hill.

Troiano, R. P., & Flegal, K. M. (1998). Overweight children and adolescents: Description, epidemiology, and demographics. *Pediatrics, 101*(3), 497–504.

Varma, V. (1997). *Violence in children and adolescents.* Bristol, PA: Jessica Kingsley.

Weinreb, L., Goldberg, R., Bassuk, E., & Perloff, J. (1998). Determinants of health and service use patterns of homeless and low-income housed children. *Pediatrics, 102*(3), 554–562.

8

♦ ♦ ♦ ♦ ♦ ♦ ♦ ♦ ♦ ♦ ♦ ♦ ♦

The Adolescent

LEARNING OBJECTIVES

After studying this chapter, you should be able to:

- Describe the normal growth and development of the adolescent.
- Identify the sexual maturity rating and Tanner stages and recognize deviations from normal.
- Describe the developmental tasks of adolescence.
- Describe the concept of identity formation in relation to adolescent psychosocial development.
- Describe appropriate health-promoting behaviors for adolescents and young adults.
- Provide anticipatory guidance for adolescents and their families with respect to risk-taking behaviors, nutrition, and safety.
- Discuss the incidence of adolescent violence and strategies to deal with aggressive behavior.
- Discuss adolescent sexuality and related health risks.

DEFINITIONS

adolescence Period between the onset of puberty and the cessation of physical growth; the passage from childhood to adulthood.

autonomy Independent will and the capacity to be self-governing.

egocentrism Concerned with oneself; the lack of differentiation between one's own views and those of others.

identity formation The acquisition of psychosocial, sexual, and vocational identity.

primary sexual characteristics Internal and external reproductive organs in males and females (i.e., uterus, fallopian tubes, ovaries, vagina, vulva, penis, testes, spermatic cord).

puberty Period of time during which adolescents experience a growth spurt, develop secondary sexual characteristics, and achieve reproductive maturity.

pubescence Period of time prior to sexual maturity, characterized by the development of breast tissue and pubic hair in girls and genital growth and pubic hair in boys.

reproductive maturity The establishment of menstruation/ovulation in females and the development of spermatogenesis in males.

risk-taking behaviors Behaviors that predispose the adolescent to physical or psychosocial harm.

secondary sexual characteristics Physical characteristics of males and females influenced by reproductive hormones but having no direct role in reproduction (i.e., voice, body shape, pubic hair distribution, breasts).

sexual maturity rating (SMR) Stages of sexual maturation based on pubic hair and breast development in girls and pubic hair and genital development in boys.

Adolescence spans ages 11 to 21 years; the developmental tasks of early adolescence, as well as the beginning stages of sexual maturation, may overlap with the school-age years. Adolescence is a time of change for teenagers and their families, a transition from childhood to adulthood. During this transition period dramatic physical, cognitive, psychosocial, and psychosexual changes take place that are exciting and at the same time frightening.

Growth and Development of the Adolescent

The adolescent tries out many new roles during this time as part of the important developmental task of identity formation. The peer group is of the utmost importance as adolescents experiment with new roles outside the confines of the family unit. When identity formation is complete, the young adult is emancipated from the family and establishes independence.

The rapid rate of physical growth during adolescence is second only to that of infancy. Adolescents come in many shapes and sizes, and the changes that take place during the teen years are obvious and dramatic. With physical change come the development of secondary sexual characteristics and an intense interest in the opposite sex. Adolescents move from the same-sex friendships of childhood to the capacity for intimate, long-lasting relationships as young adults. Sexual orientation and gender identity are often recognized during adolescence as the teenager engages in exploration and self-discovery.

Parents as well as adolescents need the nurse's support and guidance in understanding and facilitating health-promoting behaviors. Nurses can assist adolescents and their families in the areas of health promotion, disease prevention, and management of common problems by using effective communication strategies, knowledge of normal growth and development, anticipatory guidance, and early identification of potential problems.

Growth and development of the adolescent are summarized in Table 8–1.

Physical Growth and Development

Physical development during the adolescent years is characterized by dramatic changes in size and appearance. Girls experience budding of the breasts followed by the appearance of pubic hair. About 1 year after breast development, there is a rapid increase in height. Growth in height in girls typically ceases 2 to 2.5 years after menarche.

Boys also experience physical changes, but those changes are not as obvious as in girls. Boys first experience testicular enlargement, followed in about a year by penile enlargement. Pubic hair usually precedes the growth of the penis. The growth spurt in boys occurs later than it does in girls, beginning between ages $10\frac{1}{2}$ and 16 years and ending between $13\frac{1}{2}$ and $17\frac{1}{2}$ years of age. Growth does continue at a much slower pace for several years after the spurt but usually ceases between 18 and 20 years of age.

Muscle mass increases in boys, and fat deposits increase in girls. Because of greater muscle mass, fully developed adolescent boys tend to be larger and stronger than adolescent girls.

TABLE 8–1

Summary of Growth and Development: The Adolescent

Physical	Motor	Psychosocial
Early Adolescence (11–14 Years)		
Girls:	Increase in gross muscle mass and fine motor coordination.	Often shy, awkward. More confident with same sex.
Breast tissue develops.	Prone to ligament tears.	Self-conscious.
Girls at this age are generally taller and slightly heavier than boys, and they begin to put on fat.	Awkward, gangly during and immediately after PHV.	Low self-esteem common.
PHV: 8.3 cm per year.	Physical contact sports not recommended before PHV is over.	Begin rebellious behavior.
Menarche, pubic hair, axillary hair.	Watch for exercise-induced asthma.	Struggle over dependence/independence issues.
Boys:		
PHV: 9.4 cm per year.		
Testes enlarge.		
Gynecomastia.		
Spermatogenesis.		
Boys may appear chunky before PHV.		
Both:		
Cardiovascular pump less mature.		
Appetite increases in response to rapid growth.		

TABLE 8-1

• • • • • • • • • • •

Summary of Growth and Development: The Adolescent Continued

Physical	Motor	Psychosocial
Middle Adolescence (15–17 Years)		
Girls: Increase in percentage of total body fat. Average height gain: 6–10.4 cm per year. Increase in breast size. Increase in pubic hair. Sexual maturation occurs. "Hourglass" body contour develops. Growth decelerates. Appetite declines. **Boys:** Genitalia enlarge. Gynecomastia begins to decline. Voice begins to change as larynx enlarges. Muscle mass increases. Facial hair appears. Rapid growth in height. 2–3 years after PHV. Appetite intense. **Both:** Dentition complete. Incidence of gingivitis increases; malocclusions present in 50% of adolescents. Sweat gland function increases. Acne peaks. Sensory and language development complete. Increasing capacity of cardiovascular pump.	Increased coordination in fine and gross muscle. More adept at sports. Greater physical endurance. Greater skill at drawing, sewing, etc.	Impulsive, impatient. Conflict with parents increases. Limit testing. Sexual experimentation begins. Narcissistic, moody. Intensely private. Peer group of utmost importance.
Late Adolescence (18–21 Years)		
Girls: Physically mature. Sexual maturation complete. **Boys:** Physically mature, although boys may continue to increase in height and weight. Rapid growth decelerates. Sexual maturation complete. Gynecomastia resolves. **Both:** Cardiovascular pump mature. Appetite relatively stable. Verbal and written expression becomes more sophisticated with additional education and experience.	Endurance for motor activity increases, especially with fitness training. Boys may continue to increase in muscle bulk for competitive sports.	Less emotionally labile. Idealistic but more realistic with respect to partner selection and goals. May continue sexual experimentation. Independent, yet maintains family ties. Engaged in education/employment.

Abbreviation: PHV, peak height velocity ("growth spurt").

Psychosexual Development, Hormonal Changes, and Sexual Maturation

The physical development, hormonal changes, and sexual maturation that occur during adolescence correspond to Freud's final stage of psychosexual development, the genital stage (see Chapter 4 for a discussion of Freud's stages of psychosexual development). The genital stage begins with the production of sex hormones and maturation of the reproductive system. Sexual tension and energy are manifested in the development of sexual relationships with others, and sexual gratification is sought. Freud's theory suggests that personality development is closely related to psychosexual development, with an emphasis on aggressive and sexual impulses as determining factors of personality. Freud's theories about male dominance, sexual repression, and the Oedipus complex and Electra complex make the psychosexual theory of development highly controversial even today.

Girls generally reach physical maturation before boys with the onset and establishment of *menstruation* (*menarche*). Menarche usually occurs between the ages of 9 and 15 years (average, 12.8 years). African-American girls experience menarche slightly earlier than whites (Herman-Giddens et al., 1997). Most young women achieve *reproductive maturity* 2 to 5 years after the start of menstruation. During the 2 to 5 years before reproductive maturity, the female sex hormones gradually increase, ovulation occurs more frequently, and menstrual periods become more regular.

Ultimately, the height, weight, and body build of adolescents are influenced by diet, exercise, and hereditary factors. Over the past three decades, adolescents have become taller and heavier than their ancestors, and the age of puberty has fallen. The earlier onset of puberty has implications for the timing of sex education programs and anticipatory guidance.

The physical growth of boys and girls is directly related to sexual maturation and occurs in a relatively predictable sequence. The secretion of sex hormones—estrogen in girls and testosterone in boys—influences the development of breast tissue, pubic hair, and genitalia. Hormonal secretion at the time of puberty is the result of a complex regulatory process between the environment, the central nervous system, the hypothalamus, the pituitary gland, the gonads, and the adrenal glands. *Puberty* is a biologic process that brings about the period of peak height velocity (PHV), or the "growth spurt," the changes in body composition, and the development of *primary* and *secondary sexual characteristics* in both sexes. Although variable in both sexes, the PHV occurs at approximately age 12 years in girls and age 13.5 years in boys. Table 8–2 describes five distinct stages in a *sexual maturity rating* (SMR) based on breast and pubic hair development in girls and genital and pubic hair development in boys, and includes approximate age ranges for early, middle, and late puberty (Tanner, 1962). The beginning Tanner stages frequently occur in the school-age child, and Tanner stages 3 to 5 occur in adolescence.

TABLE 8–2

Sexual Maturity Rating (SMR): Tanner Stages of Adolescent Sexual Development

Boys

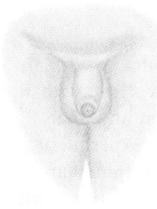 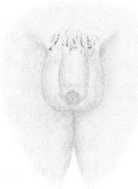 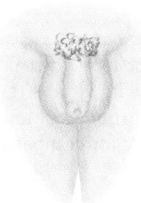 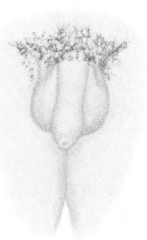 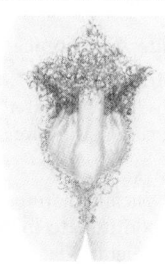

Stage 1	*Stage 2*	*Stage 3*	*Stage 4*	*Stage 5*
Pubic hair: None	*Pubic hair*: Slight, long, straight, slightly pigmented at the base of the penis	*Pubic hair*: Darker in color, starts to curl, small amount	*Pubic hair*: Coarse, curly, similar to adult but less quantity	*Pubic hair*: Adult distribution spread to inner thighs
Penis: Preadolescent	*Penis*: Slight enlargement	*Penis*: Longer	*Penis*: Larger, glans and breadth increase in size	*Penis*: Adult in size and shape
Testes: Preadolescent	*Testes*: Enlarged scrotum, pink, slight alteration in texture	*Testes*: Larger	*Testes*: Larger, scrotum darker	*Testes*: Adult

Early puberty: Testes, 9.5 to 13.5 years; penis, 10.5 to 14.5 years; pubic hair, 12 to 12.5 years

Middle puberty: Testes, 13.5 to 14.5 years; penis, 13.5 to 15 years; pubic hair, 12.5 to 14.5 years

Late puberty: Testes, 13.5 to 17 years; penis, 13.5 to 16 years; pubic hair, 13.5 to 16.5 years

TABLE 8–2

Sexual Maturity Rating (SMR): Tanner Stages of Adolescent Sexual Development Continued

*Breast Development in Girls**

   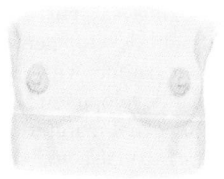 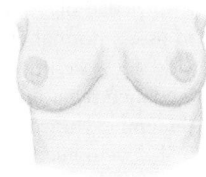

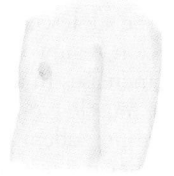   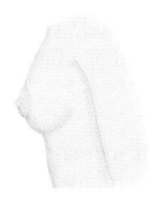 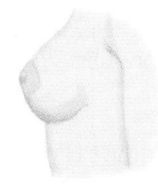

Stage 1	*Stage 2*	*Stage 3*	*Stage 4*	*Stage 5*
Preadolescent	Breast bud stage (thelarche): Breast and papilla elevated as small mound, areolar diameter increased	Breast and areola enlarged, no contour separation	Areola and papilla form secondary mound	Mature, nipple projects, areola part of general breast contour

Early puberty: 9 to 13 years

Middle puberty: 12 to 13 years

Late puberty: 14 to 17 years*

Pubic Hair Development in Girls

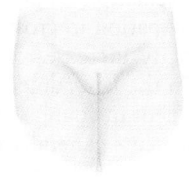 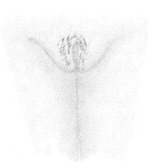 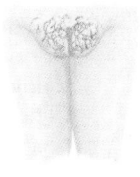 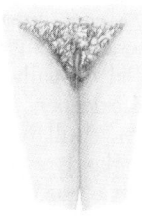 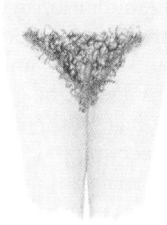

Stage 1	*Stage 2*	*Stage 3*	*Stage 4*	*Stage 5*
Preadolescent (none)	Sparse, lightly pigmented, straight medial border of labia	Darker, coarser, beginning to curl, increased over pubis	Coarse, curly, less in amount than adult, typical female triangle	Adult female triangle, adult quantity spread to medial surface of thighs

Early puberty: 10 to 11.5 years

Middle puberty: 11.5 to 13 years

Late puberty: 14.5 to 16.5 years

* Breast and pubic hair development may continue into late adolescence and increase with pregnancy.

Adapted from Tanner, J. M. (1962). *Growth at adolescence* (2nd ed.). Oxford: Blackwell Scientific Publications; and Marshall, W. A., & Tanner, J. (1969). Variations in pattern of pubertal changes in girls. *Archives of Disease of Children, 44,* 291–303. Adapted with permission from Blackwell Scientific Publications and The BMJ Publishing Group.

In boys, puberty is considered delayed if there is a lack of testicular enlargement or pubic hair development by the age of 14 years. Absence of breast budding or pubic hair development in girls by 13 years or lack of menses by 16 years requires referral (Allan, 1999). Some of the more common causes of delayed puberty are chronic illnesses, malnutrition, extreme exercise, and hypothyroidism.

FEMALE SEXUAL MATURATION

Sexual maturation in girls begins with the appearance of breast buds (*thelarche*), which is the first sign of ovarian function. Thelarche occurs at approximately age 9 to 11 years and is followed by the growth of pubic hair. The PHV is reached during thelarche, usually in Tanner stage 2 or 3. Linear growth slows and menarche begins approximately 1

Understanding the Use of Tanner Staging

Knowledge of Tanner staging is essential for nurses to assess normal growth and development and to provide adolescents and their parents with anticipatory guidance regarding sexual development. Nurses must remember, however, that sexual maturation and physical development are *highly variable* and that Tanner stages may overlap with one another. A description of the adolescent's sexual maturity rating provides greater information about the child's physical development than does chronological age (age in years).

Nursing Goals for Preparticipation Sports Physical Examination

- Assess the adolescent athlete's general health.
- Identify conditions that could limit participation or predispose to injury.
- Assess the adolescent athlete's physical and psychosocial maturity.
- Determine the athlete's fitness relative to performance requirements.
- Assess legal insurance requirements for participation.
- Provide wellness counseling and anticipatory guidance.

year after the PHV. As pubic hair increases in amount and becomes dark, coarse, and curly, axillary hair develops and the apocrine sweat glands reach secretory capacity in Tanner stage 3 or 4. Frequent showers and deodorants become important to the adolescent. With increasing hormonal activity, girls develop a more adult body contour by age 14 to 15 years. As breasts mature the nipples project more and the pubic hair extends to the medial thighs; the young female is estimated to be at Tanner stage 5. Ovulation may be established and conception can occur.

MALE SEXUAL MATURATION

The first sign of pubertal changes in boys is testicular enlargement in response to testosterone secretion, which usually occurs in Tanner stage 2. There is also some slight pubic hair and some alteration in the smooth skin texture of the scrotum. As testosterone secretion increases, the penis as well as the testes and scrotum enlarge. The PHV usually occurs during Tanner stages 3 and 4, and the voice deepens and "cracks" as the cartilage in the larynx enlarges. Axillary hair develops, and the eccrine and apocrine sweat glands respond to stressful or emotional stimuli. Skin surface bacteria metabolize secretions from the apocrine glands, and body odor develops. Gynecomastia (male breast enlargement) occurs in about 50% to 60% of young males during early adolescence and may be unilateral or bilateral (Kreipe & McAnarney, 1998). This phenomenon is often disturbing to boys, and they need considerable reassurance that the breast tissue will decrease. During Tanner stages 4 and 5 increasing levels of testosterone cause sebaceous glands to enlarge, and excessive sebum may result in acne. The voice continues to deepen, facial hair appears at the corners of the upper lip and chin, and ejaculation may occur. Nurses need to provide anticipatory guidance to adolescent boys regarding involuntary nocturnal emissions of seminal fluid ("wet dreams") and assure them that this occurrence is normal. By Tanner stage 5 genital maturation is complete, spermatogenesis is well established, facial hair is present on the sides of the face, and the male physique is adult-like in appearance. Gynecomastia significantly decreases or disappears, much to the adolescent male's relief.

Motor Development

Adolescents often engage in various forms of motor activity, from aerobic exercise to football. Motor activities such as sports and dancing provide an outlet for the adolescent's energy as well as an opportunity for competition, teamwork, and social relationships. Large muscle mass increases in adolescents, and coordination of gross and fine muscle groups improves. With practice, adolescents become more adept at athletics and also at art, music, sewing, and other activities using fine motor skills. The bones are not completely calcified until after puberty and are still fairly resistant to breaks in the young adolescent. Participants in sports activities should be grouped according to their size and their sexual maturity rating rather than their chronological age. A small, thin, late-maturing boy is less capable of competing with an early-maturing, muscular classmate, and injuries are more likely to occur.

Nurses, particularly schools nurses, may be helpful in assessing the growth and development of adolescents and counseling them about sports activities in which they can succeed, rather than those in which they will meet with physical and psychological failure.

The development of the cardiovascular pump plays an essential role in the adolescent's participation in gross motor activities. Cardiopulmonary capacity increases during adolescence and is relatively mature in the late adolescent. The cardiovascular pump is not as efficient in young adolescents, whose lungs are smaller. Adolescents generally cannot run as fast or as long as the young adult. The athlete's aerobic power, body composition, joint flexibility, and strength of skeletal muscles determine physical fitness.

Cognitive Development

Cognitive development influences every aspect of adolescent psychosocial development. Cognition moves from concrete to abstract thinking during the three phases of adolescent development (Table 8–3).

The Adolescent Who Is Involved in Athletics

Adolescents participating in athletics need

- Adequate equipment
- Appropriate training schedules
- Frequent rest periods
- Adequate fluids to prevent injury, dehydration, and exhaustion

TABLE 8–3

Adolescent Psychosocial Development

	Early Adolescence (11–14 Years)	Middle Adolescence (15–17 Years)	Late Adolescence (18–21 Years)
Cognitive Development	Concrete thinking, limited abstract thought. Appreciates here and now. Little sense of later consequences.	Early abstract thought; use of inductive/deductive reasoning. Able to understand later consequences of actions. Able to connect separate events and to project into the future. Self-absorbed/introspective; daydreams, fantasizes.	Abstract reasoning; able to abstract and conceptualize. Idealism about life, love, and society. Concern for society, politics, and religion.
Developmental Tasks			
Identity/Self-Perception	Reacts to imaginary audience; personal fable present. Self-conscious about bodily changes. Reacts to peers; conforms. Often experiences low self-esteem.	State of flux over body image. Narcissistic, introspective. Often moody, impulsive, impatient. Values group identity over family. Can be manipulative for self-gain. Begins to think of future.	Realistic body image. Generally positive outlook on future. Able to consider others' needs, less narcissistic. Able to reject group pressure in favor of own interests.
Emancipation from Family/ Independence	Transition from obedient to rebellious. Ambivalence about independence. Fluctuates between child and adult behavior. Rejection of parental rules but desire to please adults. Self-esteem declines when punished for poor behavior. Hero worship, crushes common with both sexes.	Independent, private. Limit testing maximal. Overt rebellion, withdrawal. Role-playing common, roles easily abandoned (moratorium). Separation from parents. Child-parent conflict often intense.	Emancipation from parents, but maintains ties with parents. Future-directed. Adult-like commitments to relationships/roles. Consideration of family. Educational/vocational goals related to physical and financial emancipation from parent.
Education/Vocation	Goals unrealistic, changing. Structured school setting. Role models important.	Begins to identify skills and interests. Self-esteem often tied to school achievements and popularity. Begins to consider long-term consequences of school performance. Role-playing with after-school activities and part-time jobs.	Realistic career plans. Less flux about future goals. Commitment to work and school, but career choices may change frequently.
Sexuality Social/Peers	Same-sex best friend. Group activity with same sex. Concern about "normal" body changes.	Peer acceptance of utmost importance. Intense preoccupation with physical appeal and body image.	More commitment to intimate relationships; long-term relationships. More realistic concept of partner's role.

Table continued on following page

TABLE 8-3

Adolescent Psychosocial Development Continued

	Early Adolescence (11–14 Years)	Middle Adolescence (15–17 Years)	Late Adolescence (18–21 Years)
Sexuality Social/Peers (cont.)	Boy-girl fantasy, often with peers and media stars. Sexual experimentation may occur, but not as common as in middle adolescence.	Intense interest in opposite sex. Sexual experimentation common. Relationships generally short-term. Serial partners. Role of partner often unrealistic. Decision about heterosexual/ homosexual orientation.	Peer group less important. Mate selection possible. Some continuation of sexual experimentation. Serial monogamous relationships for those uncommitted.
Professional Nursing Approach			
• Enjoy teens • Be patient • Be flexible • Know adolescent development • Be open • Listen	Be open, direct, supportive. Set limits, give concrete choices. Encourage self-responsibility and measures to enhance self-esteem. Orient to reality.	Be open, objective; negotiate choices. Consider how teen will look to peers. Encourage problem solving. Praise good decisions. Keep criticism to a minimum. Be an advocate, but don't take sides against parent. Set firm limits. Maintain confidentiality.	Encourage mutual decision making. Act as a resource and role model. Consider hidden agendas. Explore feelings about health care choices. Allow for questions and analysis of health care options.

According to Piaget, formal operations, or abstract thinking, characterizes the last stage of cognitive development. Early abstract thinking encompasses inductive and deductive reasoning, the ability to connect separate events, and the ability to understand later consequences. Abstract thinking in late adolescence is increasingly logical, and young adults are capable of scientific reasoning, understanding complex concepts, and using analytical methods. Because of logical reasoning, adolescents are able to differentiate between others' perceptions and their own, and to view social situations from a societal perspective.

For example, sex education for ninth graders is very different than it is for college freshmen or adolescents with their first full-time jobs. The college freshman should be able to appreciate the later consequences of sexual behavior, whereas the young adolescent is focused on the here and now. Ask the ninth grader and the college freshman how an unwanted baby will affect their lives and compare their answers.

For a variety of reasons (including poor comprehension ability, lack of education, and chronic substance abuse), some older adolescents remain concrete thinkers. Nurses and educators must know their audience and address them appropriately. Counseling a group of adolescent substance abusers may be ineffective if the consequence of their behavior is tied to the future when their thinking is in the present.

Sensory Development

The eyes and ears of adolescents are fully developed and, with the exception of refractive errors and occasional minor infections of the eyes, ears, and sinuses, the sensory system remains quite healthy. Myopia occurs in early adolescence between ages 11 and 13 years.

Because of increased participation in competitive sports and outdoor activities, eye injuries are common in adolescence. Boys are more prone to eye injuries than girls. Adolescents should always be required to wear safety or protective equipment when competing in sports or participating in any activity that may compromise eye safety.

Language Development and Communication

With the acquisition of formal operational thought and adequate intellectual capacity, adolescents are able to understand abstract concepts, process complex thoughts, and express themselves verbally. Adolescents who read extensively are generally more articulate and have a larger vocabulary than those who do not. Social development and self-confidence play a significant role in how well adolescents express themselves verbally to others. Shy, introverted adolescents may have difficulty speaking to a group or to members of the opposite sex, but may write expressively. Conversely, extroverted, social adolescents who have no trouble with verbal expression may lack the reading and writing skills for effective written communication.

Computer technology has added to the adolescent's avenues for creative expression. Adolescents are capable of expressing ideas in symbols and abstract concepts, and many enjoy interpreting or even developing complex computer programs. Computers have a symbolic language of their own that some adolescents find fascinating. Teens may become more proficient with computer technology than their parents. As well as teaching teens basic computer literacy, many high schools have computer clubs where students who excel in computer languages share ideas and knowledge of computer information systems.

Communicating with adolescents sometimes presents a challenge to parents and other adults. Although adolescents are capable of verbal expression, they are also intensely private and may not wish to divulge their thoughts and feelings to others. Developmentally, the verbally expressive 12-year-old may turn into a relatively uncommunicative 14-year-old. Conflict with parents increases tension in communication.

> Nurses who work with adolescents must develop communication skills that include assuring confidentiality, making no assumptions, remaining nonjudgmental, and posing open-ended questions. Questions such as "Tell me about your plans for the future" will glean more information than "Do you plan to go to college?" "Do you live with your parents?" makes an assumption about the living situation that could make the adolescent feel uncomfortable. "Describe where you live and who lives with you" gives the adolescent an opportunity to discuss the living situation.

Confidentiality is often an issue when adolescents are seen in the health care setting. Nurses should encourage adolescents to involve their parents, but it is not unusual for adolescents to ask that communication be kept confidential. The adolescent must understand that the nurse will respect this confidentiality unless the information shared suggests a potential life-threatening danger either to the adolescent or to others.

Screening tools are used in some settings to target areas of concern. Two of the more popular tools are HEADSS, which includes assessment of home, education, activities, drugs, sex, and suicide; and Guidelines for Adolescent Preventive Services (GAPS), which includes parenting, development, drugs, sex, learning problems, depression, abuse, safety, and diet and fitness. The GAPS is a comprehensive packet of services that includes not only screening but preventive services. The West Virginia University Adolescent

PARENTS WANT TO KNOW
About Communicating with Adolescents

Parents need encouragement to maintain open communication with their teenager while not appearing too intrusive. Plying adolescents with questions or going through their belongings causes feelings of invasion and a lack of trust. Adolescents get more out of discussions in which they participate than lectures, and are more likely to respond positively to adults who listen and appear interested in what they have to say.

CRITICAL THINKING EXERCISE 8–1

The nurse is caring for a 15-year-old girl, Heidi, who has been admitted to the hospital with dehydration. She is very quiet and answers questions with a simple yes or no. On the day Heidi is to be discharged she says, "I'll tell you something, but you can't tell anyone else."

1. What factors does the nurse have to consider in this situation?
2. What would be the nurse's best response?

Risk Score (WVUARS) includes the areas in the tools listed above but adds some other features, such as nutrition, exercise, friends/recreation, and self-perception. This particular tool assesses and also focuses on intervention and prevention (Perkins et al., 1997). Facility staff must identify which tool best suits their philosophy of care.

Some clinics send a questionnaire prior to the visit so that the adolescent can complete it at home and return it during the visit. Some settings display their policy on confidentiality, always underlining the need to share information only if someone is in danger. Four critical areas that need to be assessed are

- The adolescent's strengths and difficulties, as the family sees them
- The teenager's functioning at home
- The teenager's functioning at school
- Peer relationships (Prazer & Friedman, 1997)

Depending on the issues identified, it may be decided to set a time to meet with the adolescent alone. Issues related to the time it takes to do an adequate interview may arise in the present managed care environment. Nurses should be knowledgeable about communicating with adolescents and aware of when referral is warranted.

Psychosocial Development

Identity formation is the major developmental task of adolescence; other tasks include the formation of a sexual and vocational identity and the ability to emancipate oneself from the family or to become independent (Fig. 8–1). Energy is focused within the self, and the adolescent is described as egocentric or self-absorbed. Frustrated parents often describe teenagers during this phase as self-centered, lazy, or irresponsible. In fact, they just need time to think, concentrate on themselves, and determine who they are going to be. Erik Erikson (1968) described the conflict of this phase of psychosocial development as identity formation versus role confusion; this phase corresponds to Freud's genital stage of psychosexual development (see Chapter 4 for information on developmental theories).

In the transition period from childhood to adulthood, adolescents try on new roles and experiment with the environment until finding a role that fits. The phase of experimentation has been termed the *moratorium*, meaning a period of delay granted to someone not yet ready to make more than a tentative commitment (Erikson, 1968). The lack of commitment is illustrated by the adolescent's changing in-

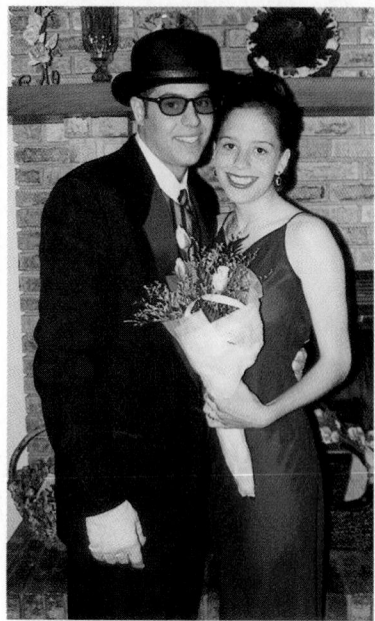

◄ Relationships with the opposite sex are more mature by late adolescence. Late adolescents have more realistic expectations of both themselves and those who are important to them. They devote many hours and much anxious thought toward making events such as prom night memorable for a lifetime. Some adolescents may be left out because they are "unpopular" or shy, or do not have the financial resources to participate in these special events.

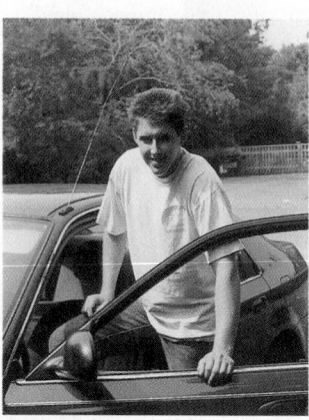

◄ With the freedom driving brings to the adolescent comes responsibility. The adolescent's inexperience and risk-taking behaviors can be a lethal combination.

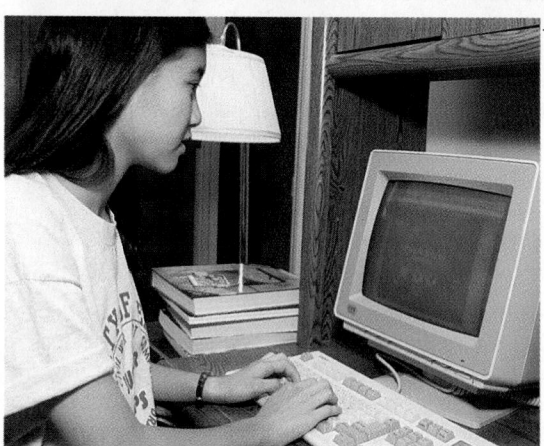

◄ Computers in school and in many homes provide the adolescent with opportunities for learning, creative expression, communication, and entertainment. Adolescents often enjoy "surfing" the Internet, which can provide them with information not readily available locally. Parents must monitor their computer connections, however, for these networks sometimes allow access to people and activities that conflict with family values.

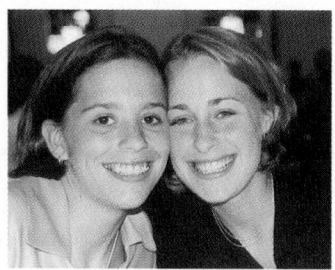

◄ Although teens often have friends of both sexes, they are more comfortable sharing many hopes, dreams, secrets, and even embarrassing incidents with friends of the same sex.

FIGURE 8–1
Growth and development of the adolescent.

terests from year to year. Parents may invest in expensive sports equipment or a musical instrument only to find it abandoned after a short time.

The peer group plays an essential role in adolescent identity formation. Teenagers take their cues on appearance, social behavior, and language from the peer group. The peer group serves as a safe haven as adolescents emo-tionally move away from the family and struggle to determine who they are. The peer group validates acceptable behavior, and teenagers feel secure in trying on new roles with peer group approval. It is not unusual for teens to spend all day with friends in school and all evening rehashing the day's events over the phone (Table 8–4). Changes in the adolescent's body image, psychosocial development, and peer group acceptance are closely related. Early and middle adolescents are particularly audience conscious and feel that they are the focus of everyone's attention. A bad hair day or a blemish may throw the adolescent into despair. Clothing, hairstyles, and material possessions that are accepted by the group attain the highest importance. Nurses should counsel parents to negotiate choices with teens but always to consider how peers will judge the child.

Early and middle adolescence are the periods when teens are prone to gang formation and activities. Peer modeling and peer acceptance, being of the utmost importance, lead some adolescents to form gangs that provide a collec-

---

CRITICAL TO REMEMBER

The Adolescent and Erikson

• Identity formation and establishment of autonomy
• Acquisition of abstract reasoning leading to
  • Analytical thinking
  • Problem solving
  • Planning for the future

TABLE 8-4

Age-Related Activities and Games for Adolescents

General Activities	Games and Special Types of Play
Games and athletics are the most common forms of play. Strict rules are in place. Competition is important.	Sports, videos, movies, reading, parties, hobbies, listening to favorite music on video or compact disc, experimenting with makeup and hairstyles

tive identity and give them a sense of belonging. Peer pressure, companionship, and protection are the most frequently reported reasons for joining gangs, particularly those associated with violent or criminal acts.

There are marked developmental differences between early and late adolescence. Each age group has unique reactions to the developmental tasks, which are influenced by the adolescent's cognitive thinking (see Table 8–3). According to Swiss psychologist Jean Piaget (1969), adolescent cognition is characterized by the transition from concrete operational thought to formal operational thought, the ability to think logically and use deductive and abstract reasoning (see Chapters 4 and 7 for further information on Piaget's theory of cognition). The acquisition of formal operational thinking allows the adolescent to draw on past experience and apply knowledge to the future by drawing on logical consequences from a set of observations. Adolescents are capable of using abstract symbols such as those derived from higher-order mathematics, making and testing hypotheses, and considering and arguing philosophical issues. Problem-solving and decision-making skills become more highly developed, although adolescents may still be conflicted about idealism versus reality.

EARLY ADOLESCENCE

The early adolescent (11 to 14 years) has intense feelings about body image and the many physical changes taking place. Less confident with members of the opposite sex, early adolescents tend to group together and have best friends of the same sex. One has only to visit the local mall or movie theater to see groups of young teens of the same sex, observing but rarely speaking to groups of the opposite sex.

The early adolescent is very egocentric and may go from obedience to rebellion with respect to parental authority. Parents are often shocked by the sudden turn of events and are hurt by the teen's rejection. Providing parents with anticipatory guidance regarding age-specific developmental changes is a primary nursing function. For example, the happy-go-lucky 11-year-old may turn into the shy, self-absorbed 12-year-old who seems comfortable only in the presence of friends. Young teens, who are developmentally egocentric, fail to differentiate between how others see them and their own mental preoccupations, thinking everyone is as obsessed with them as they are with themselves. Elkind (1993) describes this phenomenon as a reaction to the imaginary audience. The belief in the imaginary audience is probably why young teens are so self-conscious: they believe everyone is critical of them, and indeed teens are very critical of each other, especially of one who is different. Self-conscious behavior may also be the result of the physical and emotional transition to middle adolescence. The early adolescent is losing the familiar role of the child but does not yet feel comfortable with the role of the adult. Ambivalence toward independence is common, and the teen who feels too grown up for a good-night kiss still falls asleep with a favorite teddy bear.

Elkind (1993) believes that because young teens are so audience conscious, they see themselves as unique and tell themselves a "personal fable" that supports feelings of invulnerability. They believe bad things will happen to others, but not to them. Adolescent suicide attempts serve as a dramatic message to others, but young teens often do not realize the very final consequences of their actions.

MIDDLE ADOLESCENCE

Middle adolescence (15 to 17 years) is often described by parents as the most frustrating period of adolescent development. The real audience gradually replaces the imaginary audience, and teens become even more introspective and narcissistic. Conformity to peer group norms becomes even

Signs of Gang Involvement

- Associating with new friends while ignoring old friends. The child usually will not talk about the new friends or what they do together.
- A change in hairstyle or clothing, and associating with other youths with the same style. Usually some of the clothing, such as a hat or jacket, has the gang's initials or "street" name on it. Parents may note tattoos on the body.
- Unexplained source of money or possessions (stereos, jewelry, cars).
- Indications of drug, alcohol, or inhalant abuse (e.g., paint or correction fluid on the clothes, the smell of chemicals on the breath or clothes).
- Change in attitude toward activities such as sports, Scouts, or church. Discipline problems at school, in public, or at home. Youth no longer accepts parents' authority and challenges it frequently.
- Problems at school, such as failing classes, skipping school, or causing problems in class.
- Fear of the police.
- Unexplained signs of fighting, such as bruises, cuts, or complaints of pain.
- Graffiti on or around residence or possessions.
- Threats from rival gang members. Sometimes a family member is a victim of a drive-by shooting before the family realizes the youth is involved in a gang.

more important, and conflicts between teenagers and parents often escalate. Testing of limits, sulky withdrawal, and overt rebellion may occur over conflicts with regard to curfews, friends, activities, appearance, cars, and money. It is important for nurses to counsel parents to negotiate choices where possible and to set limits that are perceived as reasonable by the adolescent. Consistent discipline and structure actually make adolescents feel more secure and assist them with decision making. With parental guidance, adolescents are able to make decisions that will result in desirable outcomes. Adults must keep in mind that middle adolescents are impulsive and impatient, however. Parental concern may be seen as interference rather than guidance and may be met with resistance and resentment.

Feelings about self-image and social relationships are intense. Middle adolescence is a time of transition from same-sex friendships to an extreme interest in the opposite sex. The proportion of teens who are sexually experienced and sexually active has declined slightly, as has the teen pregnancy rate (Kaufmann et al., 1998). Explanations for this slight decrease generally fall into two schools: one school points to abstinence education, the other cites sex education that promotes more widespread and effective contraceptive use (Flinn & Hauser, 1998). Nurses and other health care providers cannot become complacent in response to this change in trends. The United States still has one of the highest adolescent pregnancy rates, and in a recent survey by the Centers for Disease Control (1998), 7.2% of adolescents had initiated sexual intercourse before age 13, and 48.4% of the 8th through 12th graders surveyed had had sexual intercourse during their lifetimes.

Sexual activity is often related to peer pressure and self-esteem issues. Adolescents with low self-esteem are more vulnerable and are apt to engage in negative risk-taking activities associated with sexuality. Decisions about sexual activity are often impulsive and made with little regard to later consequences or prior preparation. Nurses may help by providing accurate information to assist adolescents in making appropriate sexual choices. Parents need encouragement to maintain open communication and guide teenagers in sexual decision making. Providing parental guidance about sexual behavior is not easy during middle adolescence, when privacy is of extreme importance and communication with parents tends to decrease. Additionally, some parents may find sexual behavior a difficult topic to discuss and often avoid talking with teens regarding sexual issues altogether.

In the initial stages of establishing a vocational identity, adolescents are more likely to experience role diffusion and have unrealistic expectations of themselves. Some adolescents will identify a role that holds their interest, while others will experiment with many roles, moving quickly from one role to another. Overidentification with glamorous roles takes precedence over reality and is enriched by daydreams and fantasy. It is not unusual for a 15-year-old girl to spend time with her friends describing her future as a popular media star, while failing to fold the laundry or do the dishes.

During middle adolescence, some teens acquire part-time jobs and identify various skills and interests. Part-time jobs are often a source of income for material possessions and activities not provided by parents. Such experiences

---

CRITICAL TO REMEMBER

Elements of Adolescent Care

Nurses working with middle adolescents must

- Be approachable
- Maintain objectivity
- Encourage confidence
- Maintain parental authority
- Be a child advocate while not coming between adolescents and their parents
- Encourage the family to work as a mutually respectful unit

---

help adolescents set realistic expectations about work, become more independent, and develop their self-esteem. Those who are successful in the working world demonstrate a sense of responsibility and tend to have more positive social interactions. However, some adolescents may allow work to interfere with educational activity and have difficulty setting priorities. School nurses, in collaboration with parents and teachers, are in an excellent position to identify working students and to assist them in setting realistic guidelines for work and education.

LATE ADOLESCENCE (18 TO 21 YEARS)

Late adolescence is characterized by the ability to think abstractly, conceptualize verbally, and express one's thoughts and feelings about various aspects of life. Late adolescents tend to be idealistic about love, social issues, ethics, and lifestyles until their experiences modify their beliefs. Conformity becomes less important as teens progress through late adolescence. With the development of a unique identity, self-esteem increases and adolescents are able to resist group pressure if it is not in their best interest. Interactions with parents are less turbulent unless values clash, and relationships with both friends and family are maintained.

Emancipation (leaving home) is a major issue; late adolescents prepare themselves to meet this task through education or vocational training. Identifying realistic career goals is important, but many adolescents are not quite ready to make lifelong commitments. Changing career goals is not uncommon, but the nurse should watch for those adolescents who have set no career goals, who demonstrate apathy about the future, and who appear committed only to the present. Boredom and apathy are often symptoms of a greater problem, namely, depression.

Social relationships are more mature, although partner selection often continues to fluctuate. Friendships developed in late adolescence may last a lifetime, and expectations of friends and lovers become more realistic and less self-serving. The ability to consider others' needs increases, and recognition of societal needs is more apparent as the adolescent moves from adolescence to adulthood.

Failure to achieve identity formation may leave adolescents in role confusion and impede the successful mastery of the tasks of young adulthood. A positive ego identity depends on the adolescent's ability to accept the past, learn from experience, and become engaged in the future. Most adolescents move through the identity versus role confusion stage of development with minimal difficulty.

Moral and Spiritual Development

Children develop moral reasoning in a sequential manner, as described by American psychologist Lawrence Kohlberg (1984). As adolescents move from concrete to analytical thinking they advance to Kohlberg's stage 4 conventional level or Kohlberg's stage 5 postconventional level of moral development. Adolescents who remain concrete thinkers may never advance beyond Kohlberg's stage 3 of moral reasoning: conformity to please others and avoid punishment. The teenager's sense of justice is developed through interpersonal relationships with peers, family, and other adult role models. Behaviors that are modeled and rewarded, such as helping the less fortunate and showing loyalty to friends, contribute to the development of a conscience, which operates as a moral guide for subsequent behavior. The middle to late teenager can appreciate that stealing from others is wrong regardless of whether one is caught and punished.

Adolescents and young adults develop a respect for law and order and a society-maintaining orientation (Kohlberg's stage 4). Young adults may even advance to the societal-perspective stage (Kohlberg's stage 5), which honors the moral rules of right and wrong, contractual agreements, majority opinion, and overall utility or the greatest good for the greatest number. (See Chapter 4 for all stages of Kohlberg's theory of moral development.)

Older adolescents and young adults question the values of family and society and challenge existing moral codes before integrating their experiences and beliefs into a personal moral framework. Once the moral framework is developed, interpersonal relationships tend to be with those whose values and beliefs are similar.

Young adolescents in the stage of concrete operational thought are able to think logically. In this stage, children deal well with the observable, but also begin to see other points of view and to examine what they have learned. The young adolescent will accept religious teaching and examine how religious concepts relate to everyday life. Young adolescents are especially inclined to look to God for guidance when troubled.

Middle to late adolescents are capable of analytical thought and may begin to question the religious affiliation of the family, much as they question other family values. Older adolescents may explore different kinds of religion and share religious activities with the peer group.

▎ Health Promotion for the Adolescent and Family

Adolescence is generally a period of wellness. Young people may seek health care for school or sports physicals, skin conditions (acne, contact dermatitis), acute minor illnesses (colds and flu), conditions related to sexuality (birth control, pregnancy, and sexually transmissible diseases [STDs]), and the management of chronic illness (diabetes, epilepsy). Health promotion and disease prevention are achieved through adequate nutrition, rest, balanced exercise, and proper immunization against disease.

Table 8–5 presents an overview of health screening, health maintenance, and anticipatory guidance activities for adolescents.

Nutrition

The accelerated growth (in linear height, weight, and muscle mass) and sexual maturation during adolescence increase teenagers' nutritional needs, including needs for protein, calories, zinc, calcium, and iron. Periods of intense growth require increased caloric intake, and the adolescent appears constantly hungry. Snacks and regular meals must contain adequate nutrients to meet the body's anabolic needs. Adolescents are generally interested in nutrition and the effect food has on their bodies. Teenagers tend to be concerned about their weight, complexion, sexual development, and acceptance by their peers. These issues, together with the adolescent's increasing independence, can have nutritional implications.

Age-Related Nutritional Challenges

The adolescent's food habits are influenced by many factors. Unfortunately, this happens at a time when the body has increased nutritional needs. Boys tend to have fewer nutritional deficiencies than girls because they take in more food and are less likely to be dieting. Milk is frequently replaced by soft drinks. Fast foods and "junk foods" sometimes become the mainstay of the adolescent's diet. The social aspect of food consumption gains importance, and adolescents may prefer to eat meals with peers at social gatherings and restaurants of their choice. Parental supervision of meals declines as the adolescent spends more time away from home and engages in extracurricular activities with peers.

Nutritional Guidance for the Adolescent

The nurse must have an understanding of growth and development to be successful in counseling adolescents and their parents about nutrition. The adolescent's increasing need to be independent and to make his or her own choices should guide the nurse in teaching nutrition. The adolescent should always be involved in the planning.

The nurse should assess the adolescent's present diet and determine habits and eating patterns. The assessment should elicit how often the adolescent eats food from the different food groups and what foods the adolescent does not eat. Based on this information, nutritious foods for meals can be identified and a plan developed.

The nurse can also assist the adolescent by pointing out nutritious fast foods and snacks. An awareness of nutritious fast foods can also aid the adolescent in meal selection. Many fast food chains have salads with nonfat or low-fat dressings, grilled chicken sandwiches, pasta, and nonfat yogurt. Fat and salt content has been reduced and vegetable fats have replaced animal fats at some restaurants. Adolescents should be guided in mixing an occasional hamburger and fries with a regular selection of more nutritious foods.

TABLE 8-5

• • • • • • • • • • • • •

Health Screening, Health Maintenance, and Anticipatory Guidance for Adolescents

11–14 Years	*15–17 Years*	*18–21 Years*
Immunization		
Those who have not received second dose of MMR should complete the schedule by 11–12 years of age. Td is given at 11–12 years of age if at least 5 years have elapsed since the last dose of DTP, DTaP, or DT. Td boosters should be given every 10 years. Varicella: those who have not had chickenpox and who have not been immunized at 13 years of age should receive two doses of varicella vaccine given at least 4 weeks apart. Hep B may be given to all adolescents who have not been immunized against hepatitis B at any visit.	Hep B if not already vaccinated. Varicella vaccine if adolescent has not had prior infection with chicken pox or has not been immunized.	High-risk adolescents should receive influenza, pneumococcal, and hepatitis A vaccines. No OPV, IPV, or live-virus measles vaccines should be given to pregnant teens. Give hep B vaccine if not already vaccinated through 18 years of age.
Safety		
Counsel about seat belts, emergency numbers, and bicycle safety. Counsel about need for proper equipment during exercise and sports activities. Discuss use of sunscreens, diet, and fluids during exercise. Discuss water and pool safety. Discuss firearm and neighborhood safety. Discuss safety issues related to body piercing and tattooing. Discuss proper use of 911 emergency number.	Counsel about safety issues associated with sexual activity, drugs, and alcohol. Counsel about water safety and diving accidents. Discuss neighborhood safety. Discuss use of seat belts while driving any motor vehicle. Discuss driving under the influence of drugs and alcohol. Discuss firearm safety. Discuss proper use of safety equipment with sports. Counsel about use of 911, CPR, and Heimlich maneuver in emergencies. Discuss safety issues when babysitting. Discuss resisting peer pressure.	Counsel about safety issues associated with travel, school, and work. Counsel about use of 911, CPR, and Heimlich maneuver in emergencies. Discuss sexual activity and safe sex practices. Discuss alcohol and drug use, needle sharing. Discuss firearms and neighborhood safety.
Nutrition		
Counsel about appetite increases in response to body's needs for protein, calcium, iron, and zinc. Discuss concerns about weight and body build. Assess usual diet for basic nutrients. Assess height-to-weight ratio before and after "growth spurt." Counsel to continue to avoid concentrated sweets and high-fat foods for snacks. Assess food and fluid intake in relation to sports activities.	Assess usual diet and perception of body image in relation to peers. Discuss basics of nutrition relative to dieting. Assess potential for eating disorders: overeating, undereating, bingeing and purging. Assess eating as a coping mechanism. Assess consumption of fast and junk food. Assess food and fluids in relation to sports.	Need for calories declines, with the following exceptions: need for calories and protein increases with sports activities; need for calories, calcium, iron, and protein increases during pregnancy. Continue to avoid fad diets, junk food, and fast food. Assess basic cooking and meal-planning skills. Assist in choosing nutritious, low-fat foods in restaurants and other facilities.
Screening		
Advise vision screening yearly, refractive errors common. Counsel regarding proper use and care of glasses and contacts. Measure blood pressure. Do sports physicals. Check height and weight, do obesity screens.	Perform vision screening and assess need for prescription lens change as necessary. Measure blood pressure, height, and weight. Do sports physicals. Assess hemoglobin, hematocrit; do urinalysis at age 15 years.	Perform vision screening every 2 years or as needed. Perform TB testing if child is at high risk. Assess hemoglobin, hematocrit; do urinalysis at age 19 years. Measure height, weight, and blood pressure.

TABLE 8–5

Health Screening, Health Maintenance, and Anticipatory Guidance for Adolescents Continued

11–14 Years	15–17 Years	18–21 Years
Perform TB testing if child is at high risk.	Perform TB testing if child is at high risk. Perform pelvic exam and Pap smear for sexually active females. Obtain material for VDRL and STD culture as appropriate for sexually active males and females. Instruct in breast self-examination. Perform Pap smear for adolescent girls seeking contraception, regardless of sexual activity. Perform testicular screening for cancer beginning at age 15 years in males.	Do cardiac risk appraisal. Do pre-employment or school physical. Screen for HIV and hepatitis B as appropriate. Instruct in breast self-examination, do testicular screening. In both sexes, obtain material for gonorrhea and chlamydia culture and for VDRL test if sexually active. Do pelvic exam and Pap smear in girls.
Dental Care		
Counsel about brushing, flossing, and having regular check-ups every 6 months. Assess need for braces; counsel about low-cost dental facilities. Counsel about oral hygiene. Assess whether fluoridated water or fluoride supplements might be needed. Ask about diet, sweets, cavities, use of dental sealant.	Gingivitis is common. Advise on need to floss and correction of malocclusions. Assess whether fluoridated water or fluoride supplements may be needed (through age 16). Provide emergency care for avulsed or fractured teeth. Ask about diet, cavities. Good oral hygiene is necessary with braces.	Individuals of this age are less prone to dental accidents. Counsel to brush and floss twice daily. Braces are usually off. Advise dental visits every 6 months.
Sleep		
Adolescents of this age need 8 hours or more. Growth may be fatiguing. More difficulty waking in morning. May nap after school if tired and no activities are planned.	Adolescents of this age need 8 hours of sleep but often get less as activities increase. May be difficult to wake up in morning. Like to stay up late with friends or to watch TV shows.	Individuals of this age need 8 hours (some need less). Sleep time varies. May stay up later at night or weekends. May go to bed early for work. May stay up late with studies.
Exercise		
May fatigue quickly with exercise. Assess exercise program for safety, cardiovascular fitness, rest, fluids, and psychological well-being. Counsel adolescent and parents about appropriate sports before, during, and after "growth spurt."	May fatigue quickly without endurance training. Assess diet, exercise, and overall physical fitness. Counsel regarding competitive sports and stress. Encourage a balance in sport activities and studies. Counsel to consider physical stature and psychosocial readiness when selecting sport activities.	Capacity for endurance increases. Counsel on an appropriate long-term diet, exercise program. Assess cardiovascular risk factors. Encourage a balance in sport activities with work and studies.

Abbreviations: Hep B, hepatitis B virus vaccine; DTaP, diphtheria and tetanus toxoids and acellular pertussis vaccine; DTP, diphtheria, tetanus toxoids, and pertussis vaccine; Td, tetanus and diphtheria toxoids; OPV, oral poliovirus vaccine; IPV, inactivated poliovirus vaccine; MMR, measles, mumps, and rubella; Advisory Committee on Immunization Practices (ACIP); American Academy of Pediatrics (AAP); American Academy of Family Physicians (AAFP). TB, tuberculosis; STD, sexually transmissible disease; HIV, human immunodeficiency virus; Pap, Papanicolaou.

• • • • • • • • • •

Factors Influencing the Adolescent's Diet

- Busy schedule (sports, activities, jobs)
- Body image concerns, which can lead to undereating
- Skipping breakfast
- Eating away from home
- Eating fast food frequently
- Beginning to buy and prepare own food
- Peer pressure
- Psychological and emotional problems

Permission should be given to eat foods that may be somewhat untraditional at a particular meal, such as pizza for breakfast.

Body image is of particular importance to adolescents. The media reinforce the belief that "thin is in." Adolescents hold themselves to standards set by the entertainment and advertising worlds, which emphasize fitness, glamour, and sexuality. Products that promise a quick weight loss or enhanced muscle mass with a lean physique are appealing to adolescents. Weight management techniques may include fasting, diet pills and laxatives, self-induced vomiting, and fad diets instead of low-fat, low-calorie, nutritionally sound diets and more aerobic exercise. Adolescents may not realize that unsound nutritional habits often follow for a lifetime, or that growth and development may be delayed or permanently impaired. School nurses are in an excellent position to identify adolescents who have nutritional problems and to provide counseling or referral for adolescents and their families. (See Chapter 53 for information on eating disorders.)

Sleep and Rest

Along with increasingly independent activities, adolescents show a propensity for staying up late (particularly if working on a school project or attending a weekend party) and having difficulty waking up in the morning. Setting one's own bedtime and sleeping late on weekends are behaviors associated with gaining independence. Hours of sleep may vary from 6 to 8 hours during the week to 12 hours on the weekends, but an overall average of 8 hours per night is recommended for adolescents and young adults.

Rapid physical growth and increased activities contribute to the adolescent's fatigue, and frustrated parents may complain that their teenager has energy for everything but household and family chores. Nurses can educate teens and their parents to set realistic schedules that allow time for adequate rest and relaxation. Some teens may find themselves so overscheduled that they develop sleep disturbances from excess fatigue and anxiety. Adult sleep cycles are formed during adolescence, and sleep disturbances continue into the adult years. Persistent difficulty in falling asleep, wakefulness during the night, or early waking may be signs of emotional problems associated with tension, anxiety, or depression, and may warrant referral.

Exercise and Activity

Although adolescents are often involved in many activities, these activities don't always promote physical fitness. A re-

cent study found that only 48.8% of the students were enrolled in a physical education (PE) class and that the older the child, the less likely he or she was to be enrolled in a PE class (Centers for Disease Control [CDC], 1998). Regular exercise enhances physical and emotional development and promotes healthy sleep patterns. Healthy diet and exercise habits formed during adolescence can follow into adulthood and significantly reduce the risk of cardiovascular disease.

Adolescence is an ideal time to initiate an exercise program, either as a team sport or as an individual activity. Exercise need not always involve an athletic activity but should provide for a program that gradually increases exercise over a 1- to 3-week period with a goal of 30- to 60-minute sessions three to four times per week to enhance cardiovascular fitness (Rocchini, 1992). Nurses can assist adolescents in designing an exercise program that allows for gradual fitness and provides for warm-up and cool-down sessions. Exercise programs are highly personal and should be structured for enjoyment, with consideration of physical capabilities and limitations.

Safety

Injuries claim more lives during adolescence than all other causes of death combined. The predominance of injuries during adolescence results from a combination of factors: physical growth, psychomotor function, insufficient physical coordination for the task, energy, impulsivity, peer pressure, and inexperience. Impulsivity, inexperience, and peer pressure may place adolescents in unsafe situations. Feelings of invulnerability ("it can't happen to me") persist, and little thought may be given to the negative consequences of certain behaviors. Alcohol and other drugs that impair judgment are known to contribute to fatal injuries among adolescents, especially those involving firearms and motor vehicles. The sad fact is, most serious or fatal injuries involving adolescents are preventable.

Nurses must educate adolescents and their families about safety issues and injury prevention. Nurses in school and community action programs are becoming more focused on preventing firearm and traumatic head injuries. Factual information with supportive explanations should be provided. Expressing a genuine interest in adolescents as individuals and listening in a nonjudgmental way are also important steps to gain confidence and trust. Helping the adolescent recognize that there are choices when faced with difficult or potentially dangerous situations is an important component of safety promotion with this age group.

The adolescent period is also a frightening time for parents because they are aware of the risks predisposing the adolescent to injury or death. Parents may request guidance from health care professionals in setting appropriate limits and establishing methods of effective enforcement. Parents should be encouraged to model the safe behaviors that they expect from the adolescent.

CAR SAFETY

Obtaining a driver's license signifies a passage into adulthood and provides the adolescent with the means to explore and experience the world more freely. Driving is a complex activity, and proficiency requires skill, judgment, and experience. The adolescent's lack of judgment, opposition to authority, and need to express independence often result in a disregard for sound defensive driving practices. Risk-taking behaviors appear to play a major role in the high incidence of car-related injuries and deaths among teenagers. The young, inexperienced driver tends to drive faster and take more chances while operating a car than older drivers do. The Youth Risk Behavior Surveillance Survey of high school students found that 19.3% had rarely or never worn a seat belt, and during the 30 days preceding the survey, 36.6% had ridden with a driver who had been drinking alcohol (CDC, 1998).

There is an alarming association between the use of alcohol and motor vehicle crashes in adolescents. Despite legal drinking age laws, alcohol is easily accessible to adolescents. The greater social activity of the teenager, combined with the availability of alcohol, increases the incidence of impaired driving.

Nurses can promote car safety by supporting driver education programs for teenagers and the use of seat belts. Additionally, many schools and community organizations have developed prevention programs that are helpful in presenting the facts about drinking and driving to adolescents. Nurses should encourage teens and their parents to set up a ride-home agreement to discourage any driving after drinking alcohol. Adolescents need to know that they have an option available to them if they find themselves in a situation where the driver has been drinking. Dealing with the inconveniences of finding another ride home is much better than dealing with the injuries and damages of motor vehicle crashes.

WATER SAFETY

Drowning is a needless cause of death in teenagers. Most drowning deaths occur in lakes, rivers, and ponds, with the rest occurring in public or private swimming pools. Risk-taking behaviors contribute greatly to deaths from drowning and to spinal cord injuries. Adolescents are able to travel to areas that are free of adult supervision. Frequently, alcohol and drugs are contributing factors. Given the combination of freedom and alcohol, adolescents may inadvertently place themselves at risk for injury by exceeding the limits for safe swimming and diving.

Safety promotion includes the encouraging of swimming lessons, water safety classes, and the completion of a course in cardiopulmonary resuscitation. Adolescents need to know how alcohol and drugs impair their ability to perform activities at which they are usually competent.

SUICIDE

Suicide is the third leading cause of death for teenagers 15 to 19 years. Between 1979 and 1996, suicide rates increased by 13%, although they did decline by 2% between 1996 and 1997 (Guyer et al., 1998). The identification of adolescents at risk for suicide is a priority. Depression is a common finding among suicidal youths; other risk factors include declining mental health, poor impulse control, poor school performance, family disorganization, conduct disorders, substance abuse, homosexuality, and recent stress. A recent study has suggested that suicide attempts are associated with other problem behaviors and that potential antecedents to problem behaviors, such as a previous history of sexual abuse, life stressors, impulsive behavior, lack of optimism,

hopelessness, and depression, should be studied (Woods et al., 1997). Nurses must be involved in identifying high-risk adolescents through the scientific study of these phenomena. Adolescents identified as at risk for suicide and their families should be targeted for supportive guidance and counseling before a crisis situation. Nurses should counsel parents that *all* adolescent suicidal gestures should be taken very seriously. Many adolescents do not know what type of drug ingestion or action will actually harm them. The suicidal gestures may appear minor to adults, but the actions may have serious intent. (See Chapter 53 for more in-depth information on suicide and nursing interventions.)

VIOLENCE

Violence continues to threaten the health and well-being of adolescents and society as a whole (see Chapter 1). Homicide is the fourth leading cause of death in children ages 10 to 14, and for teens 15 to 19 years old it is the second leading cause of death after unintentional injury. The homicide rate increased by 24% between 1979 and 1997, but decreased by 18% between 1996 and 1997 (Guyer et al., 1998).

Violence against oneself is also a major issue with adolescents. As noted, suicide is one of the leading causes of death in teenagers.

Factors contributing to violence are multiple and complex. Contributing factors related to behavior provide the greatest opportunity for interventions initiated by health care professionals.

Nurses working with children, adolescents, and their families have the opportunity to include violence prevention as a component of anticipatory guidance. Ideally, prevention should begin when the child is young. Violence is a learned behavior. It is often reinforced by the actions of those closest to the child and by ever-increasing exposure to violence in the media. Assessing how a family deals with anger and resolves conflict provides insight into the way the child will be likely to react to similar situations. A family with violent tendencies should be referred to a counselor. Learning to react to anger or stress with nonviolent actions through conflict resolution is the goal for the youth. Unfortunately, intervention cannot be a one-time educational session. Efforts must be reinforced in multiple facets of the adolescent's life, such as in school, youth organizations, religious organizations, and home.

• • • • • • • • • • •

Factors Contributing to Adolescent Violence

- Low socioeconomic status
- Crowded urban housing
- Single-parent family or limited parental supervision
- History of family violence or child abuse
- Access to guns
- Peer pressure or gang involvement
- Limited education
- Racism
- Drug or alcohol use or abuse
- Low self-esteem and hopelessness about the future
- Aggression

Parents need to be aware of the amount and type of violence that their children are exposed to in the media. There is growing evidence suggesting that exposure to media violence does lead to aggressive behavior by the children who watch the programs (Strasburger and Donnerstein, 1999). It is unrealistic to expect parents to isolate their children from all media violence, but they can be encouraged to monitor and limit their children's TV viewing and to co-view and discuss the implications of violence with their children.

The availability of firearms is related to violent acts. In a survey of students in grades 9 through 12 conducted by the U.S. Centers for Disease Control and Prevention, it was found that 8.5% had carried a weapon within the 30 days preceding the survey (CDC, 1998). Carrying a weapon can establish a feeling of control or power, or it may be a response to fear of those with power. Regardless of the reasons, firearms in the hands of adolescents are impulsively used, before the ramifications of such actions can be logically considered.

As society urgently seeks a solution to the growing problem of violence, health care professionals must become advocates of violence prevention. Opportunities for adolescents to discover and use less violent means to express themselves or resolve day-to-day issues should be taught and promoted. Given the tragic effects of violence on the safety and health of American children, nurses should participate in efforts to resolve the complex issues of violence in our society. A product-oriented focus on firearms that incorporates several strategies, including legislation, education, regulation, litigation, and firearm modification, may be an effective approach to this problem (Freed, Vernick, & Hargbarten, 1998).

Dental Care

The incidence of dental caries decreases in adolescence, but dental hygiene remains very important. Most permanent teeth have erupted with the possible exception of the third molars (wisdom teeth), which erupt by late adolescence or remain impacted and may be removed surgically. Several dental conditions are prevalent during the adolescent years: gingivitis, malocclusion, and dental trauma. Gingivitis is the inflammation and breakdown of the gingival epithelium; the gums appear pale and swollen and bleed easily. Increased hormonal activity at the time of puberty, diets high in sugar and simple carbohydrates, and the use of dental braces and appliances that make cleaning less effective are thought to contribute to the development of gingivitis.

Malocclusion (improper contact) occurs in approximately 50% of adolescents due to facial and mandibular bone growth and dental crowding. Treatment varies but generally entails dental devices such as braces to correct tooth position and redirect facial growth. Adolescents may be self-conscious if their peers are no longer in braces, and may need reassurance that the condition is temporary. For economic reasons, some adolescents are unable to correct malocclusions and suffer the consequences indefinitely. Nurses help by referring adolescents with no dental care to free clinics or agencies providing dental care at low cost. People with uncorrected malocclusions are at greater risk for dental trauma.

PARENTS WANT TO KNOW

About Caring for a Child with an Avulsed Tooth

A tooth that has been completely knocked out of the mouth (avulsed) can sometimes be replanted. The sooner the replantation occurs, the greater is the likelihood of success. If the tooth can be recovered, it should be rinsed in lukewarm tap water and placed in the tooth socket. The tooth should not be scrubbed, and cleaning agents and disinfectants should be avoided. If the tooth cannot be repositioned, it should be placed in a container of milk and the child should proceed to the dentist *immediately*. If milk is not available, the tooth may be held in the child's or parent's mouth in saliva. Make sure to avoid sudden stops while driving to the dentist's office if the tooth is being held in the mouth. The prognosis is best if the injury is treated within 30 minutes.

A tooth that has been completely knocked out of the mouth (avulsed) can sometimes be replanted. The sooner the replantation occurs, the greater is the likelihood of success. The prognosis is best if the injury is treated within 30 minutes. School and clinic nurses may be the first health professionals to see a child with a complete tooth avulsion and should be aware of the proper procedure. Parents should also know how to care for their child if such an incident should occur.

Other Issues

BODY PIERCING

Ear piercing has been popular with teens for many years. Today the tongue, lip, eyebrow, nose, navel, and nipple are also common sites. Generally, body piercing is harmless, but nurses should caution teens about performing these procedures under less than sterile conditions and should educate teens about complications such as bleeding, infection, keloid formation, and allergies to metal. Qualified personnel using sterile needles should perform piercing procedures. The area needs to be cleaned twice a day (more often for a tongue piercing).

TATTOOS

Tattoos are increasingly popular among mainstream adolescents and are not necessarily a mark of gang membership (Armstrong, 1995). Like clothing and hairstyles, tattoos serve to define one's identity. Unfortunately, tattoos are often the result of an impulsive decision and are performed by amateurs who are not qualified to do the procedure. Because of the invasiveness of the tattoo procedure, it should be considered a health-risk situation. Little regulation exists in the tattoo industry, and nurses should educate adolescents about the risks of blood-borne infections, skin infections, and allergic reactions to dyes used in the tattoo process. Additionally, nurses need to be informed about tattoo removal to provide correct information to adolescents and their families. Impulsive decisions to tattoo are often regret-ted, and teens or their parents may want the tattoo re-moved. Laser therapy is available for tattoo removal but is costly and not usually covered by insurance. Amateur tat-toos are removed quite easily, but studio tattoos made with red and green dyes are quite difficult to remove. Tattoo re-moval requires several visits, and adolescents have to toler-ate the tattoo's presence during the removal process.

SUNTANNING

There is no such thing as a "good" tan. It is difficult, how-ever, to convince adolescents that tanning not only is harm-ful to their skin, but also is a risk factor for developing skin cancer later in life. The media (advertising, movies, and television) promote the image of beach glamour: young, well built, and tanned. Although most companies that man-ufacture tanning products promote the sun protection factor (SPF) in their products, the advertised image remains a bronzed, attractive young person. Most exposure to ultravio-let radiation occurs during childhood and adolescence, and skin cancers could be prevented with the appropriate and consistent use of sunscreens and sunblocks.

Nurses should educate teens about the benefits and side effects of different sun protection products and encourage use not only for water sports but also for all activities that involve sun exposure. Teens involved in athletic activities are often exposed to the sun for long periods without protec-tion. Teenagers may be cognizant of body exposure at a beach but may forget about the exposure of body parts dur-ing a long tennis match or a baseball game, especially on a cloudy day, when up to 80% of the sun's radiation reaches the ground. Nurses should caution teens receiving any type of medication about the side effects related to sun exposure. Some medications may potentiate the sun's ultraviolet rays, resulting in quicker burning. The side effects of sunscreen products include itching, burning, and redness immediately or up to 24 hours after the product is applied. Some people are allergic or sensitive to the sunscreen agent (such as PABA, PABA esters, cinnamates, anthranilates, or benzo-phenones) or to other ingredients used, such as fragrances or preservatives. Sunscreen use should be discontinued if an allergic dermatitis is noted and another type of sunscreen may be tried. There are numerous products on the market

with various ingredients that have sunscreening capabili-ties. Sun damage can be prevented and simple measures can minimize the effects of ultraviolet radiation on the skin.

Sexual Activity

ADOLESCENT SEXUALITY

Adolescent sexuality refers to the thoughts, feelings, and be-haviors related to the adolescent's sexual identity. Middle adolescence typically marks the initial period of dating and experimentation with heterosexual and homosexual behav-iors, although in some cultures sexual experimentation oc-curs much earlier. Initially, group dating may be popular, but this is quickly replaced by dating in couples, who may be sexual partners. Intimate relationships in middle adoles-cence are usually short-lived as adolescents experiment with their sexual identity. Of greatest concern to parents during the adolescent's stage of sexual experimentation are un-wanted pregnancy, STDs, and the teen's feelings of despair over failed relationships. Adolescents themselves are often impervious to the possibility of negative consequences of their sexual experimentation and believe that "it can't hap-pen to me."

Homosexual behavior in adolescence does not neces-sarily indicate that the adolescent will maintain a homosex-ual orientation. Gay and lesbian adolescents face many challenges growing up in a society that is often unaccepting. Those adolescents who self-identify their sexual preference as homosexual during high school are at increased risk for a variety of health risks and problem behaviors, including suicide, victimization, risky sexual behaviors, and multiple substance abuse (Garofalo et al., 1998).

Most very young teens have not had intercourse. The likelihood of teenagers having intercourse increases with age, however. The Youth Risk Behavior Surveillance Sys-tem showed that 7.2% of the group had sexual intercourse before age 13 years and that 48.4% of all adolescents had been involved in sexual activity (CDC, 1998). Adolescence is a period of risk taking, and many adolescents choose not only to be sexually active, but also to do so unprotected.

The initiation of sex and the application of healthy behaviors is driven by two themes: (1) seeing sex as danger-ous and as involving the risks of STDs, especially HIV, and (2) the risk of early pregnancy, with the recognition that intercourse should be postponed until later and, for many, until marriage (Monsen, Jackson, & Livingston, 1996).

The adolescent's limited cognitive abilities or lack of abstract thinking may influence contraceptive practices. Adolescents who feel invulnerable to pregnancy often can-not assimilate and apply to themselves information about sexual behavior, conception, and birth control. Lack of self-esteem and peer pressure also play a role in determining adolescents' sexual behavior. Teens may use sex to feel loved or desired, and they may fear abandonment by a part-ner if sex is refused. Some teens lack correct reproductive information and don't plan ahead for sexual encounters. Sexual activity is often impulsive, erratic, and unplanned, as the relationships are relatively short-term. Chapter 25 provides information related to adolescent pregnancy, in-cluding sex education.

Nurses in schools and community clinics are in a position to identify teens at risk for pregnancy and to provide guidance with appropriate information and referral in a confidential atmosphere. Nurses should strongly encourage adolescents to discuss sexuality, sexual behavior, and contraception with their parents whenever possible, but must guarantee confidentiality of communication.

The nurse's professional role is to ensure that adolescents have the knowledge, skills, and opportunities that enable them to make responsible decisions regarding sexual behavior. Education regarding sexuality and contraception should be oriented to the developmental level of the individual or group. Additionally, primary prevention must be emphasized by assisting adolescents to develop coping strategies to meet their needs in ways other than through sexual behavior.

ADOLESCENT CONTRACEPTION

Complete protection from pregnancy and STDs is achievable only through sexual abstinence. Because approximately half of adolescents between ages 15 and 19 years are sexually active, however, nurses need to feel comfortable with managing health concerns related to sexuality. Comprehensive health care includes providing services for sexually active adolescents. Health care providers should provide screening for and management of STDs, contraceptive services, and psychosocial counseling. When educating adolescents about birth control methods, it is ideal to see partners together. Open communication between partners is essential, and decisions about contraception should be mutual. Both male and female adolescents need to assume responsibility for sexual behavior. Regardless of the method of birth control selected, all adolescents need frequent follow-up to maintain consistent contraception behaviors. Counseling teens about sexuality and contraception requires nurses who are open, forthright, and respectful of the decisions teens make about sexual activity. See Chapter 31 for information on STDs and Chapter 10 for information related to contraception.

CRITICAL TO REMEMBER

Factors to Consider in Selecting Adolescent Contraception

- Cognitive development (concrete versus abstract thinking)
- Understanding and acceptance of attitudes and values
- Sexual maturity rating
- Communication between partners
- Opportunity to counsel both partners
- Use of more than one method
- Frequency of intercourse
- Appropriate information (three messages per visit)
- Problem-solving abilities (appeal to logic and feelings of power over body)
- Communication with parents or other adults
- Physical and mental health
- Motivation of both partners
- Concrete, graphic instruction in all methods
- Number and sex of partners
- Encouragement that abstinence is alright

KEY CONCEPTS

- Adolescence is a period of transition from childhood to adulthood that is marked by important biologic and psychological changes.
- Biologic development during adolescence is variable. Primary and secondary sexual characteristics are acquired through the influence of reproductive hormones in males and females.
- Sexual maturity ratings (SMR/Tanner stages) are somewhat variable but predictable stages of sexual maturation that are based on pubic hair and breast development in girls and pubic hair and genital development in boys.
- According to Erikson, the major developmental task in adolescence is the development of an identity/self-perception. Other developmental tasks include the development of a sexual identity, a

- vocational/educational identity, and independence/autonomy.
- Early and middle adolescents are egocentric and concerned with themselves.
- Cognitive thinking during adolescence moves from concrete to abstract reasoning.
- According to Kohlberg, adolescents and young adults develop a respect for law and order and a society-maintaining orientation.
- Adolescents question the values of family and society before integrating their experiences and beliefs into a personal moral framework.
- Adolescents may be emotionally labile, with extreme highs and extreme lows.
- The pace of physical growth during adolescence is second only to the pace of growth during infancy.

- Poor eating habits and lack of aerobic exercise contribute to obesity and decreased overall physical fitness.
- Suntanning, body piercing, and tattooing are behaviors associated with identity formation.
- Risk-taking behavior is considered part of normal growth and development.
- Safety issues related to sports activity, sexual activity, firearms, and the use of motor vehicles should be emphasized.
- Sexual maturation precipitates sexual activity; teen pregnancy and sexually transmissible diseases are related issues.

ANSWERS TO CRITICAL THINKING EXERCISE 8–1

1. The main issues will be confidentiality and trust. To establish trust, the nurse must be honest with Heidi. The nurse must be clear about the boundaries before the conversation continues. Depending on what Heidi tells the nurse, she may want to encourage Heidi to share the information with her parents. Finally, there should be no question that if the information has the potential to cause harm to either Heidi or others, it cannot be kept confidential.

2. A therapeutic response would be, "Heidi, I want you to feel comfortable talking with me. I will keep what you tell me confidential unless it is something that might be harmful to you or others."

REFERENCES AND READINGS

Allan, D. B. (1999). Precocious and delayed puberty. In F. D. Burg, E. R. Wald, J. R. Ingelfinger, & R. A. Polin (Eds.), *Gellis & Kagan's current pediatric therapy* (16th ed., pp. 759–761). Philadelphia: Saunders.

American Academy of Pediatrics Committee on Infectious Diseases. (1997). Immunization of adolescents: Recommendations of the Advisory Committee on Immunization Practices, the American Academy of Pediatrics, the American Academy of Family Physicians, and the American Medical Association. *Pediatrics, 99*(3), 479–488.

American Academy of Pediatrics Committee on Injury and Poison Prevention and Committee on Adolescence. (1996). The teenage driver. *Pediatrics, 98*(5), 987–990.

American Academy of Pediatrics Committee on Nutrition. (1998). *Pediatric nutrition handbook.* Elk Grove Village, IL: American Academy of Pediatrics.

American Medical Association, Department of Adolescent Health. (1996). Guidelines for adolescent preventive services (GAPS). Chicago: American Medical Association.

Armstrong, M. L. (1995). Adolescent tattoos: Educating vs. pontificating. *Pediatric Nursing, 21*(6), 561–564.

Armstrong, M. L. (1996). You pierced what? *Pediatric Nursing, 22*(3), 236–238.

Bear, G. G., Minke, K. M., & Thomas, A. (1997). *Children's needs II: Development, problems and alternatives.* Bethesda, MD: National Association of School Psychologists.

Centers for Disease Control. (1998). Youth risk behavior surveillance—United States, 1997. *Morbidity and Mortality Weekly Report, 47*(SS-3).

Elkind, D. (1993). *Parenting your teenager.* New York: Ballantine Books.

Erikson, E. (1968). *Identity: Youth and crisis.* New York: Norton.

Federal Interagency Forum on Child and Family Statistics. (1998). America's children: Key national indicators of well being. In *Federal Interagency Forum on Child and Family Statistics.* Washington, DC: US Government Printing Office.

Flinn, S., & Hauser D. (1998). *Teenage pregnancy: The Case for Prevention.* Washington, DC: Advocates for Youth.

Ford, C. A., & Coleman, W. L. (1999). Adolescent development and behavior: Implications for the primary care physician. In M. D. Levine, W. B. Carey, & A. C. Crocker (Eds.), *Developmental-behavioral pediatrics* (3rd ed., pp. 69–79). Philadelphia: Saunders.

Freed, L. H., Vernick, J. S., & Hargaarten, S. W. (1998). Prevention of firearm-related injuries and deaths among youth. *Pediatric Clinics of North America, 45*(2), 427–438.

Garofalo, R., Wolf, R. C., Kessel, S., Palfrey, J., & DuRant, R. H. (1998). The association between health risk behaviors and sexual orientation among a school-based sample of adolescents. *Pediatrics, 101*(5), 895–902.

Goldenring, J., & Cohen, E. (1988). Getting into adolescent heads. *Contemporary Pediatrics, 7*, 75–90.

Guyer, B., MacDorman, M. F., Martin, J. A., Peters, K. D., & Strobino, D. M. (1998). Annual summary of vital statistics—1997. *Pediatrics, 102*(6), 1333–1349.

Hennes, H., & Calhoun, A. D. (1998). Violence among children and adolescents. *Pediatric Clinics of North America, 45*(2).

Hergenroeder, A. C. (1998). Prevention of sports injuries. *Pediatrics, 101*(6), 1057–1063.

Herman-Giddens, M. E., Slora, E. J., Wasserman, R. C., Bourdony, C. J., Bhapkar, M. V., Koch, G. G., & Hasemeier, M. (1997). Secondary sexual characteristics and menses in young girls seen in office practice: A study from the pediatric research office settings network. *Pediatrics, 99*(4), 505–512.

Hern, M. J., Gates, D., Amlung, S., & McCabe, P. (1998). Linking learning with health behaviors of high school adolescents. *Pediatric Nursing, 24*(2), 127–131.

Hollen P. J., & Brickle, B. B. (1998). Quality parental decision making and distress. *Journal of Pediatric Nursing, 13*(3), 140–150.

Kaufmann, R. B., Spitz, A. M., Strauss, L. T., Morris, L., Santelli, J. S., Koonin, L. M., & Marks, J. S. (1998). The decline in US teen pregnancy rates, 1990–1995. *Pediatrics, 102*(5), 1141–1147.

Kohl, H. W., & Hobbs, K. E. (1998). Development of physical activity behaviors among children and adolescents. *Pediatrics, 101*(3), 549–554.

Kohlberg, L. (1984). *Essays on moral development.* San Francisco: Harper & Row.

Kreipe, R. E., & McAnarney, E. R. (1998). Adolescent medicine. In R. E. Behrman & R. M. Kliegman (Eds.), *Nelson essentials of pediatrics* (3rd ed.). Philadelphia: Saunders.

Lamb, J. M., Puskar, K. R., Sereika, S. M., & Corcoran, M. (1998). School-based intervention to promote coping in rural teens. *MCN: American Journal of Maternal/Child Nursing, 23*(4), 187–194.

Litt, I. F., & Martin, J. A. (1999). Development of sexuality and its problems. In M. D. Levine, W. B. Carey, & A. C. Crocker (Eds.), *Developmental-behavioral pediatrics* (3rd ed., pp. 457–470). Philadelphia: Saunders.

Marshall, W. A., & Tanner, J. (1969). Variations in pattern of pubertal changes in girls. *Archives of disease of children, 44*, 291–303.

Monsen, R. B., Jackson, C. P., & Livingston, M. (1996). Having a future: Sexual decision making in early adolescence. *Journal of Pediatric Nursing, 11*(3), 183–188.

Orr, D. P. (1998). Helping adolescents toward adulthood. *Contemporary Pediatrics, 15*(5), 55–76.

Perkins, K., Ferrari, N., Rosas, A., Bessette, R., Williams, A., & Hatim, O. (1997). You won't know unless you ask: The biopsychosocial interview for adolescents. *Clinical Pediatrics, 36*(2), 79–86.

Piaget, J. (1969). *The theory of stages in cognitive development.* New York: McGraw-Hill.

Prazer, G. E., & Friedman, S. B. (1997). An office-based approach to adolescent psychosocial issues. *Contemporary Pediatrics, 14*(5), 59–76.

Purcell, J. S., Hergenroeder, A. C., Kozinetz, C., Smith, E. O., & Hill, R. B. (1997). Interviewing techniques with adolescents in primary care. *Journal of Adolescent Health, 20*(4), 300–305.

Rew, L. (1997). Health-related, help-seeking behaviors in female Mexican-American adolescents. *Journal of the Society of Pediatric Nursing, 2*(4), 156–162.

Rocchini, A. (1992). Cardiovascular risk factors and prevention. In W. McAnarney, R. Kreipe, D. Orr, & G. Comerci (Eds.), *Textbook of adolescent medicine* (pp. 365–373). Philadelphia: Saunders.

Skiba, A., Loghmani, E., & Orr, D. (1997). Nutritional screening and guidance for adolescents. In *Adolescent health update.* Elk Grove Village, IL: American Academy of Pediatrics.

Stashwick, C. A. (1997). The pre-college visit. *Contemporary Pediatrics, 14*(7), 89–103.

Steom, K. F., Roeser, R., & Markus, H. R. (1998). Self-schemas and possible selves as predictors and outcomes of risky behaviors in adolescents. *Nursing Research, 47*(2), 96–106.

Strasburger, V. C., & Brown, R. T. (1997). Adolescent medicine. *Pediatric Clinics of North America, 44*(6).

Strasburger, V. C., & Donnerstein, E. (1999). Children, adolescents, and the media: Issues and solutions. *Pediatrics, 103*(1), 129–139.

Stuppy, D. J., Armstrong, M. L., & Casals-Ariet, C. (1998). Attitudes of health care providers and students towards tattooed people. *Journal of Advanced Nursing, 27*(6), 1165–1170.

Tanner, J. (1962). *Growth at adolescence* (2nd ed.). Oxford: Blackwell Scientific Publications.

Trahms, C. M., & Pipes, P. L. (1997). *Nutrition in infancy and childhood.* New York: McGraw-Hill.

Trickett, P. K., & Schellenbach, C. J. (1998). *Violence against children in the family and community.* Washington, DC: American Psychological Association.

United States Department of Health and Human Services. (1998). *America's adolescents: Are they healthy?* San Francisco: National Adolescent Health Information Center.

United States Department of Justice. (1998). *Bureau of Justice Statistics.* Washington, DC: US Department of Justice, Office of Justice Programs.

Villarruel, A. M. (1998). Cultural influences on the sexual attitudes, beliefs, and norms of young Latino adolescents. *Journal of the Society of Pediatric Nurses, 3*(2), 69–79.

Woods, E. R., Lin, Y. G., Middleman, A., Beckford, P., Chase, L., & DuRant, R. H. (1997). The associations of suicide attempts in adolescents. *Pediatrics, 99*(6), 791–796.

9

◆ ◆ ◆ ◆ ◆ ◆ ◆ ◆ ◆ ◆ ◆

Hereditary and Environmental Influences on Development

LEARNING OBJECTIVES

After studying this chapter, you should be able to:

■ Describe the structure and function of normal human genes and chromosomes.
■ Give examples of ways genes and chromosomes are studied.
■ Describe the transmission of single gene traits from parent to child.
■ Relate chromosomal abnormalities to spontaneous abortion and to birth defects in the infant.
■ Explain characteristics of multifactorial birth defects.
■ Identify environmental factors that can interfere with prenatal development, and explain how their effects can be avoided or reduced.
■ Describe the process of genetic counseling.
■ Explain the role of the nurse in caring for individuals or families with concerns about birth defects.

DEFINITIONS

allele   An alternate form of a gene.

autosome   Any of the 22 pairs of chromosomes other than the sex chromosomes.

birth defect   An abnormality of structure, function, or body metabolism that often results in a physical or mental handicap, shortens life, or is fatal (according to the March of Dimes Birth Defects Foundation).

congenital   Present at birth.

diploid   Having a pair of chromosomes (46, or 23 pairs, in humans) that represents one copy of every chromosome from each parent; the number of chromosomes normally present in body cells other than gametes.

familial   Presence of a trait or condition in a family more often than would be expected by chance alone.

gamete   Reproductive cell; in the female an ovum and in the male a spermatozoon.

genetic   Pertaining to the genes or the chromosomes.

genotype   Genetic makeup of an individual.

haploid   Having one copy of a chromosome from each pair (23 in humans, or half the diploid number). Gametes normally have a haploid number of chromosomes.

heterozygous   Having two different alleles for a genetic trait.

homozygous   Having two identical alleles for a genetic trait.

karyotype   A photomicrograph of a cell's chromosomes, arranged from largest to smallest pairs.

monosomy   Presence of only one of a chromosome pair in every body cell.

mutation   Variation in a gene that affects its function.

pedigree   A graphic representation of a family's medical and hereditary history and the relationships among the family members; may be called a genogram.

phenotype   The outward expression of one's genetic makeup.

polymorphism   Common variation in a gene that does not negatively affect its function or the individual's health.

polyploidy   Having additional full sets of chromosomes.

sex chromosome   The X or Y chromosome. Females have two X chromosomes; males have one X and one Y chromosome.

somatic cells   Body cells other than the gametes, or germ cells.

teratogen   An agent that can cause defects in a developing baby during pregnancy.

translocation   Attachment of all or part of a chromosome to another chromosome.

trisomy   Presence of three copies of a chromosome in each body cell.

Hereditary and environmental forces influence one's development from before conception until death. The nurse needs a basic knowledge of these forces to understand disorders evident at birth and those that develop later in life.

Hereditary Influences

Hereditary influences on development result from the directions for cellular functions provided by genes that make up the 46 chromosomes in every somatic cell. Disease or disorders can result if too much or too little genetic material is present in the cells, or if one or more genes are abnormal and provide incorrect directions.

Structure of Genes and Chromosomes

A review of the structure of genes and chromosomes aids in understanding how disorders occur. Chromosomes are composed of genes that in turn are composed of DNA (Fig. 9–1).

DNA

DNA (deoxyribonucleic acid) is the basic building block of genes and chromosomes. It has three units: (1) a sugar (deoxyribose), (2) a phosphate group, and (3) one of four nitrogen bases (adenine, thymine, guanine, and cytosine).

DNA resembles a spiral ladder, with a sugar and a phosphate group forming each side of the ladder and a pair of nitrogen bases forming each rung. The four bases of the DNA molecule pair with one another in a fixed way, allowing the DNA to be duplicated accurately during each cell division.

- Adenine pairs with thymine.
- Guanine pairs with cytosine.

The sequence of base pairs within the DNA determines which amino acids will be assembled to form a protein and the order in which they will be assembled. Some of these proteins form the structure of body cells; others are enzymes that control metabolic processes within the cell. If the sequence of nitrogen bases in the DNA is incorrect, or if some bases are missing or added, a defect in body structure or function may result.

GENES

A gene is a segment of DNA that directs the production of a specific product needed for body structure or function. Humans may have as many as 100,000 genes.

Genes that code for the same trait often have two or more alternate forms (alleles). Many alleles are normal, such as those that code for a person's blood type. Normal alleles, or polymorphisms, provide genetic variation and sometimes a biologic advantage. However, abnormal alleles (mutations) may harm function, such as those that cause the production of abnormal hemoglobin in sickle cell disease.

Genes are too small to be seen under a microscope, but many can be studied by some type of tissue analysis:

- By measuring the products that the genes direct cells to produce, such as an enzyme or other substance
- By studying the gene's DNA directly if its exact location is known
- By analyzing the gene's close association (linkage) with another gene that can be studied in one of the previous two ways.

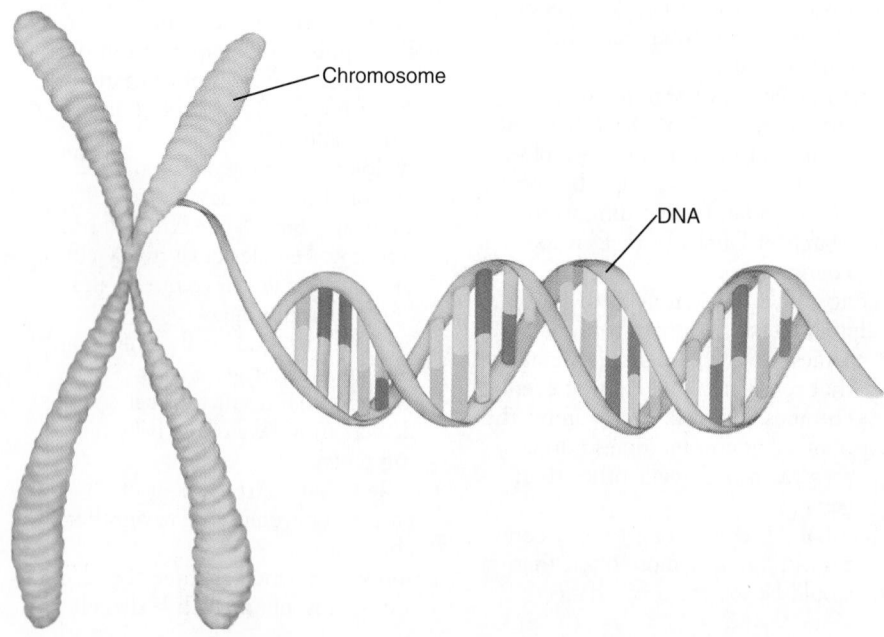

Chromosome

DNA

FIGURE 9–1

Diagrammatic representation of the DNA helix, which is the building block of genes and chromosomes.

The Human Genome Project is an international effort to identify all genes contained in the 46 human chromosomes. Information gained from this project may allow advances such as

- Genetic testing to determine the risk for, or presence of, a disorder
- Basing reproductive decisions on accurate and specific information
- Identifying genetic susceptibility to a disorder so that interventions to reduce risk can be instituted
- Using gene therapy to modify a defective gene.

The explosion of knowledge about the genetic basis for many diseases raises many legal and ethical issues for which we do not yet have answers. As our knowledge base grows, new issues are likely to emerge:

- Genetic information has implications for others in the person's family, raising privacy issues.
- Identification of genetic problems could lead to poor self-esteem, guilt, and excessive caution, or, conversely, a reckless lifestyle.
- Presymptomatic identification of genetically influenced illness would be a source of long-term anxiety.
- Genetic knowledge could affect one's choice of a partner.
- Discrimination may occur, such as the imposition of high insurance rates or the denial of insurance coverage, or the decision not to hire a qualified (but genetically compromised) person.

CHROMOSOMES

Genes are organized into 46 paired chromosomes in the nucleus of most somatic cells. Twenty-two chromosome pairs are autosomes, and the 23rd pair makes up the sex chromosomes. Added or missing chromosomes or structurally abnormal chromosomes are usually harmful.

Mature gametes have half the chromosomes (23) of other body cells. One chromosome from each pair is distributed randomly in the gametes, allowing variation of genetic traits among people. When the ovum and sperm unite at conception, the total is restored to 46 paired chromosomes.

Cells for chromosomal analysis must have a nucleus and must be living. Chromosomes can be studied using any of several types of cells: white blood cells, skin fibroblasts, bone marrow cells, and fetal cells from the chorionic villi (future placenta) or those suspended in amniotic fluid.

Unlike genes, chromosomes can be seen under the microscope, but only during division of live cells. Specimens must be obtained and preserved carefully to provide enough living cells for chromosomal analysis. Temperature extremes, clotting of blood, or adding improper preservatives can kill the cells and render them useless for analysis.

Chromosomes look jumbled when viewed under a microscope (Fig. 9–2). Photographing the chromosomes and then arranging them in that picture from largest to smallest pairs into a karyotype (Fig. 9–3) allows systematic study.

Transmission of Traits by Single Genes

Inherited characteristics are passed from parent to child by the genes in each chromosome. These traits are classified

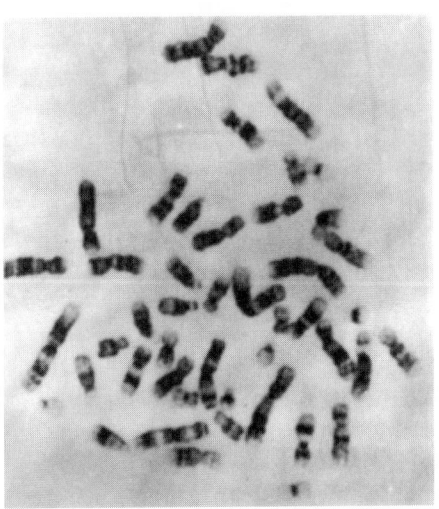

FIGURE 9–2

When viewed under a microscope, chromosomes appear jumbled. (From Thompson, M. W., McInnes, R. R., & Willard, H. F. [1991]. *Thompson and Thompson genetics in medicine* [5th ed., p. 16]. Philadelphia: Saunders. Courtesy of R. G. Worton, The Hospital for Sick Children, Toronto.)

according to whether they are dominant (strong) or recessive (weak) and whether the gene is located on one of the autosome pairs or on the sex chromosomes. Both normal and abnormal hereditary characteristics are transmitted by these mechanisms.

ALLELES

Because humans have a pair of matched chromosomes (except the sex chromosomes in the male), they have one allele for a gene at the same location on each member of the chromosome pair. The paired alleles may be identical (homozygous) or different (heterozygous).

Some alleles, both normal and abnormal, occur more frequently in certain groups than they do in the population as a whole. For example, the gene that causes Tay-Sachs disease is carried by about 1 of every 27 Ashkenazi Jews, whose families have their roots in Eastern Europe. However, only 1 of every 150 people outside this group carries the gene. Other disorders that are prevalent in certain ethnic groups are cystic fibrosis (primarily whites of northern European descent) and sickle cell disease (primarily people of African descent).

A new trait (harmful, neutral, or sometimes beneficial) may emerge because of a change in the gene within the gamete. The DNA in the gamete is then different from that in the person's somatic cells. The offspring who receives the new version of the gene will have it in all somatic cells and can transmit it to future generations.

DOMINANCE

Dominance describes how one's genetic composition is translated into the phenotype, or observable characteristics. In the case of a dominant gene, one copy is enough to cause the trait to be expressed. For example, in the ABO blood system, genes for type A and type B are dominant. There-

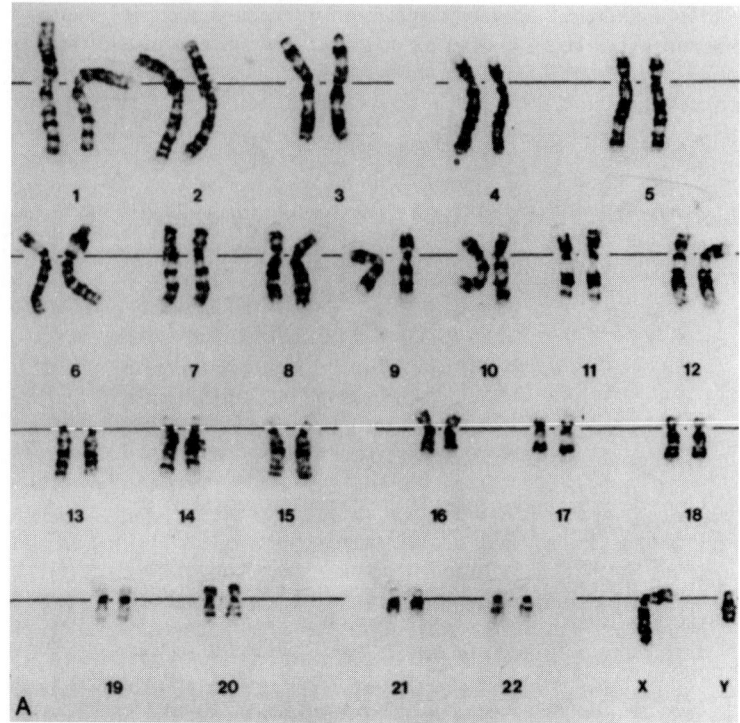

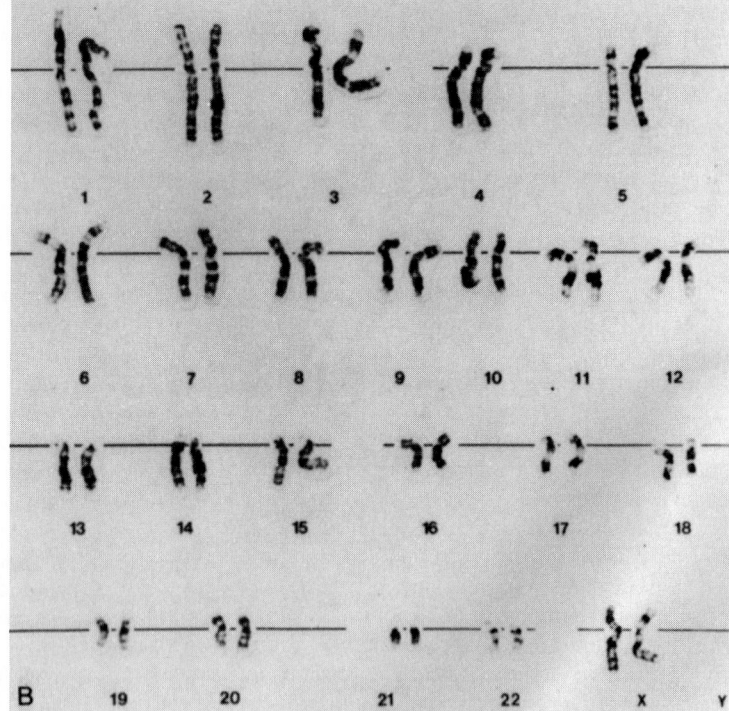

FIGURE 9–3

Chromosomes arranged in karyotypes. *A,* Normal male karyotype: 46,XY. *B,* Normal female karyotype: 46,XX. (From Knuppel, R. A., & Drukker, J. E. [1993]. *High-risk pregnancy: A team approach* [p. 666]. Philadelphia: Saunders. Courtesy of The Children's Hospital, Denver.)

fore, a single copy of either of these genes is enough to be expressed in the person's blood type.

Two identical copies of a recessive gene are required for the trait to be expressed. The gene for blood group O is recessive. Only if a person receives a gene for blood group O from both parents will laboratory testing identify his or her blood group as O. If the person receives a gene for group O from one parent and group A from the other parent, group A will be expressed in laboratory blood typing.

Other alleles are equally dominant. The person who receives a gene for blood group A from one parent and group B from the other will have type AB blood because both alleles are equally dominant and both are expressed in blood typing.

Dominance and recessiveness are not absolute for all genes. Some people with a single copy of an abnormal recessive gene (carriers) may have a lower-than-normal level of the gene product (such as an enzyme) that can be detected by laboratory methods. These people usually do not have the disease because the normal copy of the gene directs production of enough of the required product to allow normal or near-normal function.

CHROMOSOME LOCATION

Genes located on autosomes are either autosomal dominant or autosomal recessive, depending on the number of identical copies of the gene needed to produce the trait. However, genes located on the X chromosome are paired only in females because males have one X and one Y chromosome.

A female with an abnormal recessive gene on one of her X chromosomes usually has a normal gene on the other X chromosome that compensates and maintains relatively normal function. However, the male is at a disadvantage if his only X chromosome has an abnormal gene. The male has no compensating normal gene because his other sex chromosome is a Y. The abnormal gene will be expressed in the male because it is unopposed by a normal gene.

Patterns of Single-Gene Inheritance

Three important patterns of single-gene inheritance are (1) autosomal dominant, (2) autosomal recessive, and (3) X-linked. Table 9–1 summarizes characteristics and transmission of each pattern. The inheritance patterns are graphically illustrated with a pedigree to represent a family's history and the relationships among family members.

> Some people may be offended because they associate the word "pedigree" with animals. The nurse may need to interpret it for the client. For example, when taking a genetic family history, the nurse might say, "I'm going to use several symbols to depict your family tree and its members' health histories. This diagram is often called a pedigree."

Single-gene traits have mathematically predictable and fixed rates of occurrence. For example, if a couple has a child with an autosomal recessive disorder, the risk that future children will have the same disorder is one in four (25%) at every conception. It is not important how many of their children are affected; the *risk* is the same at every conception.

AUTOSOMAL DOMINANT TRAITS

An autosomal dominant trait is produced by a dominant gene on a non-sex chromosome. The expression of abnormal autosomal dominant genes may result in multiple and seemingly unrelated effects in the person. The gene's effects may vary substantially in severity, leading a family to think that a trait skips a generation. A careful physical examination may reveal subtle evidence of the trait in each generation. Some people may carry the dominant gene but may have no apparent expression of it in their physical makeup.

In some autosomal dominant disorders, such as Huntington's disease, the person having the gene will always have the disease if he or she lives long enough. In other disorders, only a portion of those carrying the gene will ever exhibit the disease.

New mutations account for the introduction of abnormal autosomal dominant traits into a family that has no prior history. Men who father children in their fifth decade or later are more likely to have offspring with a new autosomal dominant mutation.

The person who is affected with an autosomal dominant disorder is usually heterozygous for the gene—that is, the person has a normal gene on one chromosome and an abnormal gene on the other chromosome of the pair that overrides the influence of the normal gene. Occasionally, a person receives two copies of the same abnormal autosomal dominant gene. Such an individual is usually much more severely affected than someone with only one copy.

AUTOSOMAL RECESSIVE TRAITS

An autosomal recessive trait occurs when a person receives two copies of a recessive gene carried on an autosome. Everyone carries two to six abnormal autosomal recessive genes without manifesting the disorder because they have a compensating normal gene. Because the probability that two unrelated people will share even one of the same abnormal genes is low, the incidence of autosomal recessive diseases is relatively low in the general population.

Situations that increase the likelihood that two parents will share the same abnormal autosomal recessive gene are

- Consanguinity (blood relationship of the parents)
- Membership in groups that are isolated by culture, geography, religion, or other factors.

Many autosomal recessive disorders are severe, and affected persons may not live long enough to reproduce. Two exceptions are phenylketonuria and cystic fibrosis. Improved care of people with these disorders has allowed them to live into their reproductive years. If one member of the couple has the autosomal recessive disorder, all of their children will be carriers. Their risk for having similarly affected children is higher as well, depending on the prevalence of the abnormal gene in the general population.

X-LINKED TRAITS

X-linked recessive traits are more common than X-linked dominant ones, and are the only pattern discussed here. Sex differences in the occurrence of X-linked recessive traits and the relationship of affected males to one another distinguish these disorders from autosomal dominant or recessive disorders. In general, males are the only ones who show full effects of an X-linked recessive disorder because their only X chromosome has the abnormal gene on it. Females can show the full disorder in two uncommon circumstances:

- When a female has a single X chromosome (Turner's syndrome, p. 180)
- When a female child is born to an affected father and a carrier mother

X-linked recessive disorders can be relatively mild, such as colorblindness, or they may be severe, such as hemophilia. Those having the disorder may be affected with varying degrees of severity.

TABLE 9-1

• • • • • • • • • • •

Single-Gene Traits

Pedigree Symbols

A pedigree is a way to symbolically represent a family's medical history and the relationships of its members to one another. It can help identify patterns of inheritance that may help distinguish one type of disorder from another.

◻ Male

◯ Female

◇2 Sex not specified
(number indicates the number of persons represented by the symbol)

■ ● Affected

◧ ◑ Carriers (heterozygous) for an autosomal recessive trait

⊙ Female carrier of an X-linked recessive trait

⊘ Deceased

◻—◯ Mating/marriage

◻=◯ Consanguineous mating/marriage

I Roman numerals indicate generations

Autosomal Recessive

Characteristics

Two autosomal recessive genes are required to produce the trait.
Males and females are equally likely to have the trait.
There is often no prior family history of the disorder before the first affected child.
If more than one family member is affected, they are usually full siblings.
Consanguinity (blood relationship) of the parents increases the risk for the disorder.
Disorders are more likely to occur in groups isolated by geography, culture, religion, or other factors.
Some autosomal recessive disorders are more common in specific ethnic groups.

Transmission of Trait from Parent to Child

Unaffected parents are carriers of the abnormal autosomal recessive trait.
Children of carriers have a 25% (1 in 4) chance for receiving both copies of the defective gene and thus having the disorder.
Children of carriers have a 50% (1 in 2) chance of receiving one copy of the gene and being carriers like the parents.
Children of carriers have a 25% (1 in 4) chance of receiving both copies of the normal gene. They are neither carriers nor affected.

Examples

Normal traits: Blood group O; Rh-negative blood factor.
Abnormal traits: Tay-Sachs disease; sickle cell disease; cystic fibrosis.

Pedigree

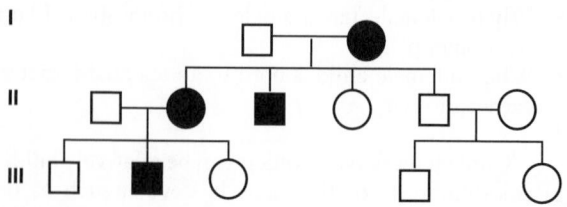

Autosomal Dominant

Characteristics

A single copy of the gene is enough to produce the trait.
Males and females are equally likely to have the trait.
Often appears in every generation of a family, although family members having the trait may have widely varying manifestations of it.
May have multiple and seemingly unrelated effects on body structure and function.

Transmission of Trait from Parent to Child

A parent with the trait has a 50% (1 in 2) chance of passing the trait to the child.
The trait may arise as a new mutation from an unaffected parent. The child who receives the mutated gene can then transmit it to future generations.

Examples

Normal traits: Blood groups A and B; Rh-positive blood factor.
Abnormal traits: Huntington's disease; neurofibromatosis.

Pedigree

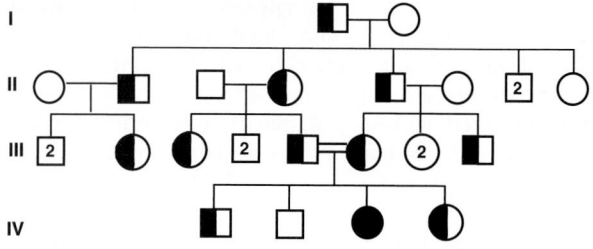

X-Linked Recessive

Characteristics

Although recessive, only one copy of the gene is needed to cause the disorder in the male, who does not have a compensating X without the trait.
Males are affected, with rare exceptions.
Females are carriers of the trait, but not usually adversely affected.
Affected males are related to one another through carrier females.
Affected males do not transmit the trait to their sons.

Transmission of Trait from Parent to Child

Males who have the disorder transmit the gene to 100% of their daughters and none of their sons.
Sons of carrier females have a 50% (1 in 2) chance of being affected. They also have a 50% chance of being unaffected.
Daughters of carrier females have a 50% (1 in 2) chance of being carriers like their mothers. They also have a 50% chance of being neither affected nor carriers.
An abnormal X-linked recessive gene also may arise by mutation.

Examples

Colorblindness; Duchenne's muscular dystrophy; hemophilia A

Pedigree

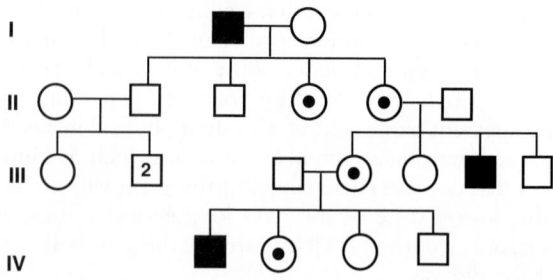

Single-Gene Abnormalities

- A person affected with an autosomal dominant disorder has a 50% chance of transmitting the disorder to each of his or her children.
- Two healthy parents who carry the same abnormal autosomal recessive gene have a 25% chance of having a child affected with the disorder caused by this gene.
- Parental consanguinity increases the risk for having a child with an autosomal recessive disorder.
- One copy of an abnormal X-linked recessive gene is enough to produce the disorder in a male.
- Abnormal genes can arise as new mutations that are then transmitted to future generations.

Chromosomal Abnormalities

Chromosomal abnormalities can be numerical or structural. They are quite common (50% or more) in the embryo or fetus that is spontaneously aborted. Chromosomal abnormalities often cause major defects because they involve many added or missing genes.

NUMERICAL ABNORMALITIES

Numerical chromosomal abnormalities are those involving added or missing single chromosomes and those with multiple sets of chromosomes. Trisomy and monosomy are numerical abnormalities of single chromosomes. Polyploidy describes abnormalities involving whole sets of chromosomes.

Trisomy. A trisomy exists when each body cell contains an extra copy of one chromosome, bringing the total number to 47 (Fig. 9–4). Each chromosome is normal, but there are too many in every cell. The most common trisomy is *Down syndrome*, or trisomy 21. In Down syndrome, each cell has three copies of chromosome 21. Trisomies of chromosomes 13 and 18 are less common and have more severe

effects. The incidence of trisomies increases with maternal age, so that most women who are 35 years old or older are offered prenatal diagnosis to determine whether the fetus has Down syndrome or another trisomy.

Infants with Down syndrome have characteristic features that are usually noticed shortly after birth (p. 535). Chromosomal analysis is done during the neonatal period to confirm the diagnosis and to determine whether Down syndrome is caused by trisomy 21 or a rarer chromosomal anomaly that involves a structural rather than a numerical abnormality.

Monosomy. A monosomy exists when each body cell has a missing chromosome, with a total number of 45. The only monosomy that is compatible with postnatal life is *Turner's syndrome*, or monosomy X (Fig. 9–5). People with Turner's syndrome have a single X chromosome and are always female.

Liveborn infants with Turner's syndrome have excess skin around the neck and edema that is most noticeable in the hands and feet. If Turner's syndrome is not identified and treated during infancy or childhood, an affected girl

Chromosome Abnormalities

Chromosome abnormalities are either numerical or structural.

Numerical	Structural
Entire single chromosome added (trisomy)	Part of a chromosome missing or added
Entire single chromosome missing (monosomy)	Rearrangements of material within chromosome(s)
One or more added sets of chromosomes (polyploidy)	Two chromosomes that adhere to each other
	Fragility of a specific site on the X chromosome

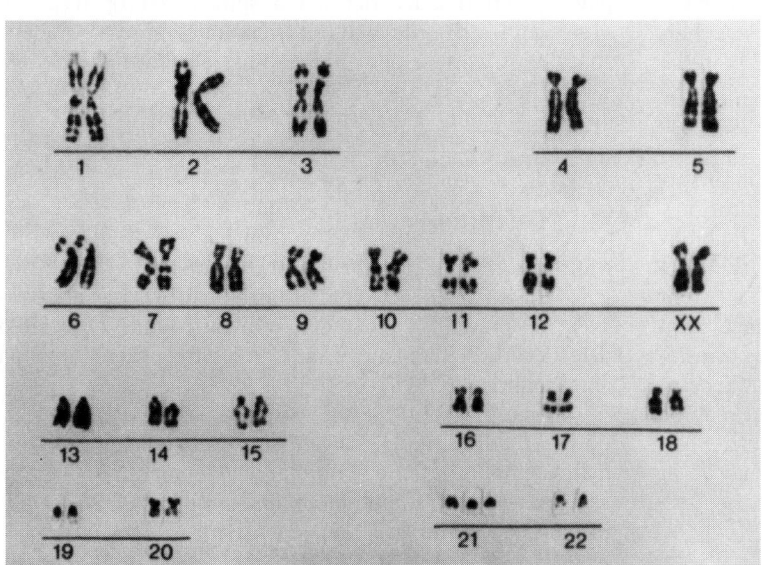

FIGURE 9–4

Karyotype of a female with trisomy 21 (Down syndrome: 47,XX, +21). (From Hacker, N., & Moore, J. G. [1992]. *Essentials of obstetrics and gynecology* [2nd ed., p. 95]. Philadelphia: Saunders.)

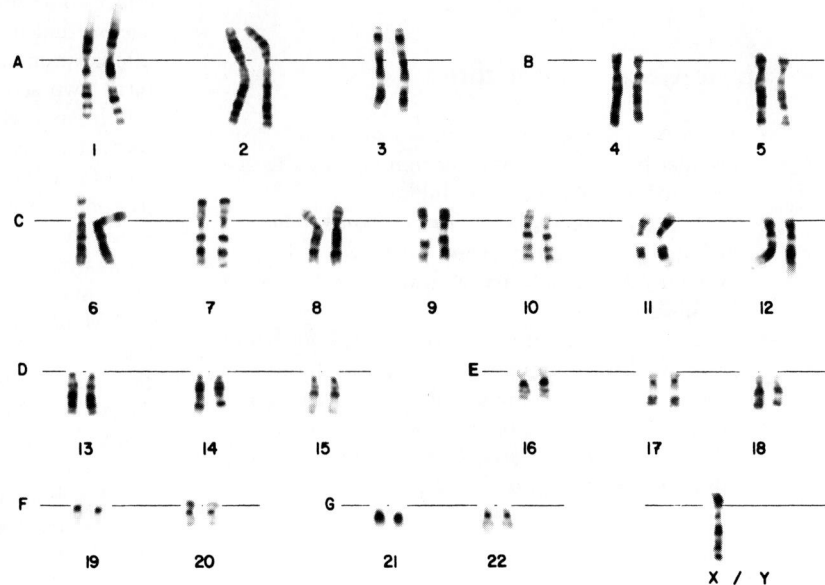

FIGURE 9-5

Karyotype of a female with monosomy X (Turner's syndrome: 45,X). (Courtesy of Dr. Mary Jo Harrod, University of Texas Southwestern Medical Center.)

will remain very short and will not have menstrual periods or develop secondary sex characteristics. Children with Turner's syndrome usually have normal intelligence, although they may have difficulty with spatial relationships or solving visual problems, such as reading a map.

Polyploidy. Polyploidy may occur when gametes do not halve their chromosome number during meiosis and retain both members of the pair, or when two sperm fertilize an ovum simultaneously. The result is an embryo with one or more extra sets of chromosomes. The total number of chromosomes is a multiple of the haploid number of 23 (69 or 92 total chromosomes). Polyploidy usually results in an early spontaneous abortion but is occasionally seen in a liveborn infant.

STRUCTURAL ABNORMALITIES

The structure of one or more chromosomes may be abnormal. Part of a chromosome may be missing or added, or DNA within the chromosome may be rearranged. Some of these rearrangements are harmless polymorphisms. Others are harmful, however, because important genetic material is lost or duplicated in the structural abnormality, or the position of the genes in relation to other genes is altered so that normal function is not possible.

Another structural abnormality occurs when all or part of a chromosome is attached to another (translocation). Many people with a translocation chromosomal abnormality are clinically normal because the total of their genetic material is normal, or balanced (Fig. 9–6). If a parent has a balanced translocation, the offspring may have completely normal chromosomes or may have a balanced translocation like the parent. However, the offspring may receive too much or too little chromosomal material and may be spontaneously aborted or may have birth defects. Either balanced or unbalanced chromosomal translocations may occur spontaneously in the offspring of parents who have no translocation.

X-linked mental retardation (fragile X syndrome) is a special type of structural abnormality that exists on the X chromosome. With this abnormality, a site on part of the X chromosome is more fragile than normal. As in X-linked recessive traits, males are more significantly affected than are females, who have a compensating X chromosome that is usually normal. Fragile X syndrome is the most common form of male mental retardation (Hall, 1996a).

Multifactorial Disorders

Multifactorial disorders are those resulting from an interaction of genetic and environmental factors. The genetic tendency toward the disorder is modified by the environment. These interactions may influence prenatal and postnatal development either positively or negatively. For example, two embryos may have an equal genetic susceptibility for the development of a disorder such as spina bifida (open spine). However, the disorder will not occur unless an environment that favors its development, such as deficient maternal intake of folic acid, also exists.

Characteristics of Multifactorial Disorders

Multifactorial disorders have two characteristics that distinguish them from other types of birth defects. They are typically (1) present and detectable at birth and (2) isolated defects rather than ones that occur with other unrelated abnormalities.

A multifactorial defect may *cause* a secondary defect, however. For example, infants with spina bifida often have hydrocephalus because abnormal development of the spine and spinal cord disrupts spinal fluid circulation, allowing it to build up within the brain's ventricular system.

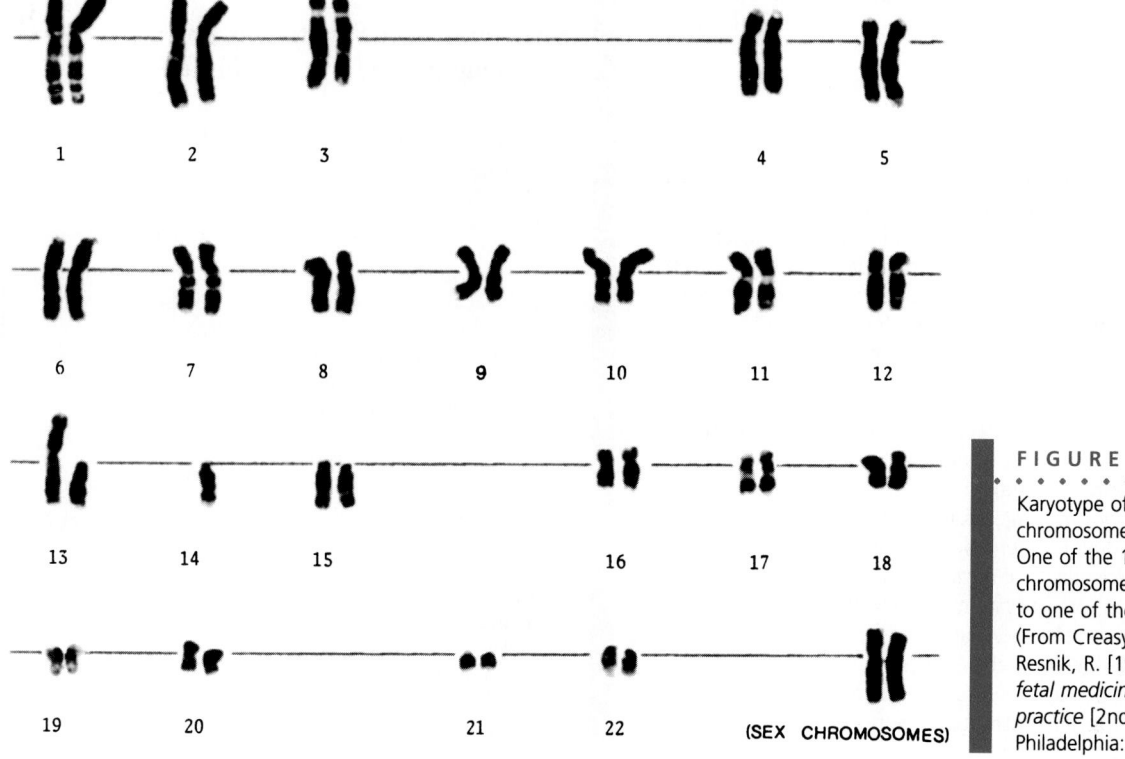

1   2   3   4   5

6   7   8   9   10   11   12

13   14   15   16   17   18

19   20   21   22   (SEX CHROMOSOMES)

FIGURE 9–6

Karyotype of a balanced chromosome translocation. One of the 14th chromosome pair is attached to one of the 13th pair. (From Creasy, R. K., & Resnik, R. [1989]. *Maternal-fetal medicine: Principles and practice* [2nd ed., p. 37]. Philadelphia: Saunders.)

The infant who has spina bifida plus defects other than those associated with disrupted central nervous system development probably does *not* have a multifactorial disorder. In this case, the spina bifida is more likely to be part of a syndrome that may pose a much different risk for recurrence in a future child.

Multifactorial disorders represent some of the most common birth defects that a maternal-child nurse encounters. Examples include

- Many heart defects
- Neural tube defects such as anencephaly (absence of most of the brain and skull) and spina bifida
- Cleft lip and cleft palate
- Pyloric stenosis

Risk for Occurrence

Unlike single-gene traits, multifactorial disorders are not associated with a fixed risk of occurrence or recurrence in a family. The risks are an average rather than a constant percentage. Factors that may affect the degree of risk are

- Number of affected close relatives
- Severity of the disorder in affected family members
- Sex of affected person(s)
- Geographic location
- Seasonal variations

Environmental Influences

Environment may influence prenatal development positively, as when good nutrition supplies all necessary raw ma-

---

CRITICAL TO REMEMBER

Multifactorial Birth Defects

- Multifactorial defects are some of the most common birth defects encountered in maternity and pediatric nursing practice.
- They are a result of interaction between one's genetic susceptibility and environmental factors during prenatal development.
- These are usually single, isolated defects, although the primary defect may cause secondary defects.
- Some occur more often in certain geographic areas.
- A greater risk of occurrence exists if
  - Several close relatives have the defect, whether mild or severe.
  - One close relative has a severe form of the defect.
  - The defect occurs in a child of the less frequently affected sex.
- Infants who have several major or minor defects, or both, that are not directly related probably *do not* have a multifactorial defect but have another syndrome, such as a chromosomal abnormality.

terials for fetal growth. Some environmental influences are harmful, however, such as teratogens or mechanical forces that disrupt development.

Teratogens

Teratogens are agents in the fetal environment that either cause or increase the likelihood that a birth defect will occur. People often ask whether a certain drug or other substance will harm the baby. Some drugs have been definitely established as either safe or harmful. For most agents, however, their potential for harming the fetus is not clear. Several factors make it difficult to establish the teratogenic potential of an agent:

- *Retrospective study.* Investigators must rely on the mother's memory about substances she ingested or was exposed to during pregnancy.
- *Timing of exposure.* Agents may be harmful at one stage of prenatal development but not at another.
- *Different susceptibility of organ systems.* Some agents affect only one fetal organ system, or they affect one system at one stage of development and another system at a different stage of development.
- *Noncontrolled fetal exposure.* Exposures cannot be controlled to eliminate extraneous agents or to ensure a consistent dose.
- *Placental transfer.* Agents vary in their ability to cross the placenta.
- *Individual variations.* Fetuses show varying susceptibility to harmful agents.
- *Nontransferability of animal studies.* Results of animal studies cannot always be applied to humans.

Teratogens typically cause more than one defect, which distinguishes teratogenic defects from multifactorial disorders. Children affected by single-gene and chromosome defects, however, are also likely to have multiple defects.

Hundreds of individual agents are either known or suspected teratogens. Types of teratogens include

- Maternal infectious agents (viruses or bacteria) that cross the placenta and damage the embryo or fetus
- Drugs and other substances used by the woman (therapeutic agents, illicit drugs, tobacco, alcohol)
- Pollutants, chemicals, or other substances to which the mother is exposed in her daily life
- Ionizing radiation
- Maternal hyperthermia
- Effects of maternal disorders, such as diabetes mellitus or phenylketonuria

It is theoretically possible to eliminate all or some of the risk to the developing fetus by avoiding exposure to the agent or changing the fetal environment in some way.

AVOIDING FETAL EXPOSURE

Ideally, avoiding exposure to harmful influences begins before conception because major organ systems develop early in pregnancy, often before a woman realizes she is pregnant. To avoid some agents, such as alcohol or illicit drugs, pregnant women must be committed to make substantial lifestyle changes.

• • • • • • • • • • •

Environmental Substances Known or Thought to Harm the Fetus

Alcohol
Aminoglycosides
Antineoplastic agents
Antithyroid drugs
Cocaine
Diethylstilbestrol
Diphenylhydantoin (phenytoin)
Folic acid antagonists
Infections
    Cytomegalovirus
    Herpes simplex virus
    Human immunodeficiency virus
    Rubella
    Syphilis
    Toxoplasmosis
    Varicella
Lithium
Mercury
Retinoic acid
Tetracycline
Tobacco
Trimethadione
Valproic acid
Warfarin

Infections. Rubella immunization at least 3 months before pregnancy virtually eliminates the risk that the mother will contract this infection, which can damage the fetus severely. For infections that cannot be prevented by immunization, the nurse can counsel the woman to avoid situations in which acquiring the disease is more likely.

Drugs and Other Substances. The U.S. Food and Drug Administration has established pregnancy categories for therapeutic drugs based on their potential to harm the fetus. The categories range from A through D, and X. Class A drugs have no demonstrated fetal risk in well-controlled studies. At the opposite end, pregnancy category X drugs are well established as being harmful. For about 80% of therapeutic drugs, it is unknown whether they are definitely safe or definitely unsafe. (See Appendix C for a list of common drugs and other substances that may affect the fetus adversely.) In deciding whether to prescribe a drug, the physician must often balance the woman's need for the drug's therapeutic effects against the fetal need to avoid exposure to it.

It is especially difficult to establish whether an illicit drug can cause prenatal damage, because women who use illegal drugs often have other problems that complicate analysis of fetal effects. For example, these women may use multiple drugs and often have poor nutrition, untreated diseases, inadequate prenatal care, and a stressful life. In addition, illicit drugs are unlikely to be pure, and the substances used to dilute them may themselves be harmful.

The best action is for the woman to eliminate use of nontherapeutic drugs and substances such as alcohol. If she takes therapeutic drugs, the physician may be able to prescribe an alternative drug with a lower risk to the fetus or may eliminate therapeutic drugs that are not essential.

Ionizing Radiation.   Nonurgent radiologic procedures may be done during the first 2 weeks after the menstrual period begins. This is usually before ovulation and thus before conception is possible. For urgent procedures, the lower abdomen should be shielded with a lead apron, if possible. The radiation dose is kept as low as possible to reduce fetal exposure.

Maternal Hyperthermia.   The mother's temperature may rise unavoidably during illness. However, pregnant women should be cautioned to avoid or limit exposure to heat such as saunas or hot tubs.

MANIPULATING THE FETAL ENVIRONMENT

Appropriate medical therapy can help a woman avoid fetal damage that could result from her illness. For example, a woman who has diabetes should try to keep her blood glucose levels normal and stable before and during pregnancy for the best possible fetal outcomes. A woman with phenylketonuria should return to her special low-phenylalanine diet before conception to avoid buildup of toxic metabolic products in her body that may damage the fetus.

Occasionally, a pregnant woman is given a drug to medicate her fetus—for example, digitalis for fetal cardiac arrhythmias. In these cases, it is the fetus who has the disorder, not the mother. The mother is the conduit for medicating the fetus to allow normal development and function.

Mechanical Disruptions to Fetal Development

Mechanical forces that interfere with normal prenatal development include oligohydramnios and fibrous amniotic bands.

Oligohydramnios, an abnormally small volume of amniotic fluid, reduces the cushion surrounding the fetus and may result in deformations such as clubfoot. Prolonged oligohydramnios can interfere with fetal lung development because it does not allow normal development of the alveoli. Oligohydramnios may not be the primary fetal problem but rather may be related to other fetal anomalies.

Fibrous amniotic bands may result from tears in the inner sac (amnion) of the fetal membranes and can result in fetal deformations or intrauterine limb amputation. Fibrous bands are usually sporadic and unlikely to recur. Because these bands can cause multiple defects, they may be confused with birth defects from other causes such as chromosome or single-gene abnormalities.

▮ Genetic Counseling

Genetic counseling provides services to help people understand the disorder about which they are concerned and the risk that it will occur in their family.

Availability

Genetic counseling is often available through university medical centers. State departments of mental health and mental retardation or rehabilitation services also may provide counseling services. Local chapters of the March of Dimes are an important source of information about birth defects and counseling sites. Also, organizations that focus on specific birth defects provide valuable support and assistance in obtaining needed services for individuals and families affected by that disorder.

Focus on the Family

Genetic counseling focuses on the family rather than on an individual. One family member may have a birth defect, but study of the entire family is often needed for accurate counseling. This may involve obtaining medical records or performing physical examinations or laboratory studies on numerous family members. Counseling is impaired if family members are unwilling to provide their medical records or agree to examinations or laboratory studies. Moreover, those who seek counseling may be unwilling to request cooperation from other family members or to share genetic information they acquire.

Process of Genetic Counseling

Genetic counseling is often a slow process that is not always straightforward. Several visits spread over months may be needed. In addition, some tests may be performed at only one or a few laboratories in the world, and several weeks may be needed to complete them. Despite a comprehensive evaluation, a diagnosis may never be established. An accurate diagnosis is crucial to provide families with the best information about the risks for a specific birth defect, the prognosis for one affected, and options available to avoid or manage the disorder. Advances in knowledge about birth defects may allow a definite diagnosis later, and families are encouraged to contact the center for updates. Table 9–2 lists examples of procedures that may be used before conception, prenatally, and after birth to establish an accurate diagnosis related to birth defects.

A genetic evaluation may include many factors, such as

- A complete medical history, including prenatal and perinatal history
- The medical history of other family members
- Laboratory, imaging, or other studies
- Physical assessment of a child with the birth defect and other family members as needed
- Examination of photographs, particularly for family members who are deceased or unavailable
- Construction of a pedigree to identify relationships among family members and their relevant medical history

If a diagnosis is established, genetic counseling educates the family about

- What is known about the cause of the disorder
- The natural course of the disorder
- Options for care of an affected person
- The likelihood that the disorder will occur or recur
- The availability of prenatal diagnosis for the disorder
- How a couple may be able to avoid having an affected child
- The availability of treatment and services for the person with the disorder

TABLE 9-2

. . . .

Diagnostic Methods That May Be Used in Genetic Counseling

Preconception Screening

Family history to identify hereditary patterns of disease or birth defects
Examination of family photographs
Physical examination for obvious or subtle signs of birth defects
Carrier testing
　Persons from ethnic groups with a higher incidence of some disorders
　Persons with a family history suggesting that they may carry a gene for a specific disorder
Chromosomal analysis
DNA analysis

Prenatal Diagnosis for Fetal Abnormalities

Chorionic villus sampling
Amniocentesis
Ultrasonography
Percutaneous umbilical blood sampling

Postnatal Diagnosis for an Infant with a Birth Defect

Physical examination and measurements
Imaging procedures (ultrasonography, radiography, echocardiography)
Chromosomal analysis
DNA analysis
Tests for metabolic disorders (phenylketonuria, cystic fibrosis)
Hemoglobin analysis for disorders such as sickle cell disease
Immunologic testing for infections
Autopsy

Genetic counseling is nondirective; that is, the counselor does not tell the individual or parents what decision to make but educates them about options for dealing with the disorder. Families often interpret the counseling subjectively, however. Some parents may regard a 50% risk of occurrence or recurrence as low, whereas others may think that a 1% risk is unacceptably high. The family's values and beliefs also influence whether they seek counseling and what they do with the information that is provided.

Supplemental Services

Comprehensive genetic counseling includes services of professionals from many disciplines, such as biology, medicine, nursing, social work, and education. These professionals provide added support for families; they may offer referral to parent support groups, grief counseling, and intervention for problems that accompany the birth of a child with a birth defect, such as socioeconomic or family dysfunction.

Nursing Care of Families Concerned About Birth Defects

Nurses have an important role in helping families that are concerned about birth defects. Some nurses work directly with family members who are undergoing genetic counseling. Many more nurses are generalists who bring their knowledge about birth defects and their prevention to those they encounter in everyday practice.

Nurses as Part of a Genetic Counseling Team

Genetic nursing may include

- Providing counseling (after having additional education)
- Guiding a woman or couple through prenatal diagnosis
- Supporting parents as they make decisions after receiving abnormal prenatal diagnostic results
- Helping the family deal with the emotional impact of a birth defect
- Assisting parents who have had a child with a birth defect to locate needed services and support
- Coordinating services of other professionals, such as social workers, physical and occupational therapists, psychologists, and dietitians
- Helping families find appropriate support groups to help them cope with the daily stresses associated with a child who has a birth defect

Nurses in General Practice

Nurses who work in women's health care and those who work in antepartum, intrapartum, newborn, or pediatric settings often encounter families who are concerned about birth defects. These families may include a member who has a birth defect. Other families may believe that they have an increased risk for having a child with a birth defect. Generalist nurses provide care and support that complements those of nurses who work on a genetic counseling team.

WOMEN'S HEALTH NURSES

The ideal time to provide counseling is before conception so the childbearing couple has more options if problems are identified. As in antepartum care, the primary nursing role is to identify families who might benefit from counseling before conception. Personal and family histories are commonly taken at primary health care visits, and the nurse may identify a history that could affect a future child that the couple might conceive.

ANTEPARTUM NURSES

During the initial antepartum interview, the nurse may identify the pregnant woman or family who may benefit from genetic counseling. The antepartum nurse also assists families with decision making, teaching, and emotional support.

Identifying Families for Referral. Nurses in antepartum settings often identify a woman or family who is appropriately referred for genetic counseling. The personal and family history of the woman and her partner may reveal factors that increase their risks for having a child with a birth defect. In addition to the usual medical history about disorders such as hypertension or diabetes, the woman should be questioned about a family history of birth defects, diseases that seem to "run in the family," mental retardation, or developmental delay.

About Birth Defects

How can this birth defect be genetic? No one else in our family has ever had anything like it.
Autosomal recessive disorders are carried by parents who themselves are unaffected. The abnormal gene may have been passed down through many generations, but there is no risk for an affected child until *two* carrier parents mate.

Isn't there only a one-in-a-million chance that this birth defect will happen to another of our children?
Autosomal recessive disorders have a 25% (1 in 4) chance of recurring in children of the same parents. Autosomal dominant disorders may pose a 50% risk for recurrence unless they resulted from a new mutation in the parental germ cells.

Isn't this birth defect very likely to recur? We'd better not have any more children.
Some birth defects are associated with a relatively high risk of recurrence; others have a relatively low risk. Prenatal diagnosis may offer parents a way to avoid having an affected child, or some disorders may be treated before birth.

Since we've already had a child with this birth defect [an autosomal recessive one], will the next three be normal?
If both parents are carriers for an autosomal recessive disorder, there is a 25% (1 in 4) risk that is constant with

each conception. The chance is the same (1 in 4) that their children will be neither affected nor carriers.

If I have an amniocentesis or other prenatal diagnostic test, can the test detect all birth defects?
Although many disorders can be prenatally diagnosed, not all can be diagnosed in the same fetus. Testing is offered for one or more specific disorders after a careful family history is taken to determine appropriate tests.

If the prenatal test is normal, will my baby be normal?
Normal results from prenatal testing exclude those disorders that were specifically tested for. Every healthy couple has about a 5% risk of having a child with a birth defect, some of which are not obvious at birth. This baseline risk remains even if all prenatal test results are normal.

Will I have to have an abortion if my prenatal tests show that my baby is abnormal?
Abortion may be an option for parents whose fetus is affected with a birth defect, but most parents are reassured by normal test results. If results are abnormal, some parents appreciate the time to prepare for a child with special needs. Better medical management can be planned for a newborn who is expected to have problems. Prenatal diagnosis gives many parents the confidence to have children despite their increased risk for having a child with a birth defect.

Some people are reluctant to disclose that they have a family member with mental retardation or a birth defect. The nurse can gently probe for sensitive information by asking questions about whether there are family members who have learning problems or who are "slow." Using words that are lay-oriented often elicits more information than using clinical terms that may seem harsh.

Helping the Family Decide About Genetic Counseling. If genetic counseling is appropriate, the physician usually discusses it with the woman and offers to refer her and her partner to an appropriate center. The final decision, however, rests with the couple. The nurse can help the family decide whether they want genetic counseling at all and weigh issues that are important to them.

Genetic counseling can raise issues that are uncomfortable, such as whether to undergo prenatal diagnosis, what to do if a condition cannot be prenatally diagnosed, and what options are acceptable if prenatal diagnosis shows abnormal results. Counseling may open family conflicts if information from other family members is needed or if family values differ on issues such as abortion of an abnormal fetus. In addition, the tests can show unexpected results (Table 9–3). The nurse must be careful not to allow personal values to influence the family's decision. It is the family members who must live with the decision they make.

Reasons for Referral to a Genetic Counselor

Pregnant women who will be 35 years of age or older when the infant is born
Men who father children after age 40
Members of a group with an increased incidence of a specific disorder
Carriers of autosomal recessive disorders
Women who are carriers of X-linked disorders
Couples related by blood (consanguineous relationship)
Family history of birth defect or mental retardation
Family history of unexplained stillbirth
Women who experience multiple spontaneous abortions
Pregnant women exposed to known or suspected teratogens or other harmful agents, either before or during pregnancy
Pregnant women with abnormal prenatal screening results, such as alpha-fetoprotein, triple screen, or suspicious ultrasound findings

Teaching About Lifestyle. Nurses can teach a pregnant woman about harmful factors in her lifestyle that can be modified to reduce the risk of defects to her offspring. The nurse can support the woman in making lifestyle changes that may be difficult, such as stopping alcohol con-

TABLE 9–3

• • • • • • • • •

Problems Encountered in Genetic Counseling and Prenatal Diagnosis

Inadequate Medical Records

Family members' refusal to share information
Records that are incomplete, vague, or uninformative

Inconclusive Testing

Too few family members available when family studies are needed
Inadequate number of live fetal cells obtained during amniocentesis
Failure of fetal cells to grow in culture
Ambiguous prenatal test results that are neither clearly normal nor clearly abnormal

Unexpected Results from Prenatal Diagnosis

Finding an abnormality other than the one tested for
Nonpaternity revealed

Inability to Determine the Severity of a Prenatally Diagnosed Disorder

Inability to Rule Out All Birth Defects

---

sumption, reducing or eliminating smoking, or improving her diet. Liberal praise can motivate a woman to continue her efforts to promote an optimal outcome. A negative attitude from nurses or other professionals may make her feel like a failure, and she may abandon her efforts to create a healthier lifestyle.

Providing Emotional Support. The time between prenatal testing and results sometimes spans several difficult weeks. In the meantime, the pregnancy is becoming more obvious and the woman may begin to feel fetal movement. Many women delay telling friends or family about their pregnancy until they know that prenatal test results are normal. They often delay investing emotionally in their pregnancy because it seems so tentative until test results are known. When results are abnormal, women face more difficult decisions about whether to terminate or continue the pregnancy.

Helping the Family Deal with Abnormal Results. Because prenatal diagnostic tests are performed to detect disorders involving serious physical and often mental effects, the woman or couple whose test results are abnormal must confront painful decisions. For many of these disorders, no effective prenatal or postnatal treatment exists. In many cases, there are only two choices: continue the pregnancy or terminate it. In addition, the decision to terminate a pregnancy must be made in a short time. Arriving at "no decision" is effectively a decision to continue the pregnancy. Although the physician or genetic counselor is the one who discusses abnormal results and available options, the nurse reinforces the information given to these anxious families.

When test results are abnormal, nurses can expect the couple to grieve. Even if a pregnancy was unplanned, the woman who reaches the time of prenatal diagnosis has already made the initial decision to continue the pregnancy.

If results are abnormal, she must decide all over again about terminating the pregnancy. Women who continue their pregnancies grieve over the expected normal infant.

INTRAPARTUM AND NEONATAL NURSES

Nurses working in intrapartum and neonatal settings encounter families who have given birth to an infant with a birth defect that was often unexpected. Stillborn infants sometimes have birth defects that contributed to their intrauterine death. Besides the loss of their baby, these parents face added pain because of the associated abnormality. An autopsy documents all anomalies and helps establish the most accurate diagnosis of the birth defect for counseling. Nursing care for families experiencing a perinatal loss, whether a result of the infant's death or the loss of the expected normal infant, is addressed in Chapter 25.

Nurses who care for these families in the intrapartum and neonatal settings will find the parents anxious, depressed, and sometimes hostile because of the unexpected event. The family's usual coping mechanisms may be inadequate for the situation, yet they have not developed new ones. Various diagnostic studies are often recommended soon after the birth of an abnormal infant to establish a diagnosis and to give parents accurate information about the disorder and their options. However, a high anxiety level reduces their ability to understand the often massive amount of information received. The nurse is in the best position to evaluate the family's perception of the problem, help them understand the diagnostic tests, reinforce correct information, and correct misunderstandings. Moreover, the nurse is often most therapeutic by just being an available, active listener, helping to ease the family's pain over the event.

Nurses should encourage families to contact lay support groups. These groups are a significant source of support because they understand fully the daily problems encountered when caring for a child with a birth defect. They can help the parents deal with the stress and chronic grief associated with prolonged care of these children. Support groups can also help the parents see the positive aspects and victories when caring for their special-needs child.

PEDIATRIC NURSES

Children with birth defects typically have numerous recurrent medical problems. They usually are hospitalized more often and for longer periods than children without birth defects. They may have to travel to specialized hospitals for care, adding to the family's stress. Their families often have large expenses for medical care and equipment that are not covered by insurance or public assistance programs. There may be lost income because one parent, usually the mother, stops working to care for the child.

Family dysfunction is common, and the strain of having a child with a serious birth defect may lead to divorce. Siblings of the child often feel left out of their parents' attention because the needs of the sick child demand so much of the parents' time.

The pediatric nurse can reduce the family's stress by helping them locate appropriate support services. The nurse can contact social services departments to help the family find financial and other resources needed to care for the child. If parents have not connected with a lay support group, the pediatric nurse can encourage them to do so.

KEY CONCEPTS

- The 46 human chromosomes are long strands of DNA, each containing up to several thousand individual genes.
- With the exception of those genes located on the X and Y chromosomes in males, genes are inherited in pairs that may be identical or different. Some genes are dominant, and some are recessive.
- Many genes can be analyzed by the products they produce, their DNA, or their close association with another gene that is more easily analyzed.
- Cells for chromosome analysis must be living. Specimens must be handled carefully to preserve their viability.

- Chromosome abnormalities are either numerical, with the addition or deletion of an entire chromosome or chromosomes, or structural, with deletion, addition, rearrangement, or fragility of the chromosome material.
- Single-gene disorders are associated with a fixed risk of occurrence or recurrence. The type of single-gene abnormality (autosomal dominant, autosomal recessive, or X-linked) determines the level of risk.
- Multifactorial disorders occur because of a genetic predisposition combined with environmental factors.
- Relatively few agents that can enter the fetal environment are

known to be either definitely teratogenic or definitely safe.
- The purpose of genetic counseling is to educate individuals or families, providing them with accurate information so they can make informed decisions about reproduction and appropriate care for affected members.
- The nurse cares for people with concerns about birth defects by identifying those needing referral, by teaching, by coordinating services, and by offering emotional support.

REFERENCES AND READINGS

American Academy of Pediatrics and American College of Obstetricians and Gynecologists. (1997). *Guidelines for perinatal care* (4th ed.). Elk Grove Village, IL, and Washington, DC: Author.

American College of Obstetricians and Gynecologists. (1995). Genetic technologies. *Technical bulletin 208.* Washington, DC: Author.

Grabowski, G. A., & Whitsett, J. A. (1996). Gene therapy. In W. E. Nelson, R. E. Behrman, R. M. Kliegman, & A. M. Arvin (Eds.), *Nelson textbook of pediatrics* (15th ed., pp. 321–326). Philadelphia: Saunders.

Guyton, A. C., & Hall, J. E. (1996). *Textbook of medical physiology* (9th ed.). Philadelphia: Saunders.

Hall, J. G. (1996a). Chromosomal clinical abnormalities. In W. E. Nelson, R. E. Behrman, R. M. Kliegman, & A. M. Arvin (Eds.), *Nelson textbook of pediatrics* (15th ed., pp. 312–321). Philadelphia: Saunders.

Hall, J. G. (1996b). Genetic counseling. In W. E. Nelson, R. E. Behrman, R. M. Kliegman, & A. M. Arvin (Eds.), *Nelson textbook of pediatrics* (15th ed., p. 327). Philadelphia: Saunders.

Kenner, C., Hilse, M. A., & Hetteberg, C. (1998). Human genetics. In C. Kenner, J. W. Lott, and A. A. Flandermeyer (Eds.), *Comprehensive neonatal nursing: A physiologic perspective* (2nd ed., pp. 87–111). Philadelphia: Saunders.

Milunsky, J., & Milunsky, A. (1997). Genetic counseling in perinatal medicine. In E. A. Reece (Ed.), *Obstetrics and gynecology clinics of North America* (pp. 1–17). Philadelphia: Saunders.

Moore, K. L. (1998). *Before we are born: Essentials of embryology and birth defects* (5th ed.). Philadelphia: Saunders.

Moore, K. L., & Persaud, T. V. M. (1998). *The developing human: Clinically oriented embryology.* Philadelphia: Saunders.

Penticuff, J. H. (1996). Ethical dimensions in genetic screening: A look into the future. *Journal of Obstetric, Gynecologic, and Neonatal Nursing, 25*(9), 785–789.

Parker, L. A. (1998). Ambiguous genitalia: Etiology, treatment, and nursing implications. *Journal of Obstetric, Gynecologic, and Neonatal Nursing, 27*(1), 15–22.

Rhodes, A. M. (1995). Liability for failure to offer prenatal AFP testing. *MCN: American Journal of Maternal/Child Nursing, 20*(3), 169.

Rogers, J., & Davis, B. A. (1995). How risky are hot tubs and saunas for pregnant women? *MCN: American Journal of Maternal/Child Nursing, 20*(3), 137.

Scanlon, C., & Fibison, W. (1995). *Managing genetic information: Implications for nursing practice.* Washington, DC: American Nurses Association.

Schmid, P. B. (1997). The truth about genetic testing: Understanding the capabili-

ties and limitations of molecular technologies. Presentation at the AWHONN Northeast Texas Section Meeting, May 3, 1997, Arlington, TX.

Sciosa, A. L. (1999). Prenatal genetic diagnosis. In R. K. Creasy & R. Resnik (Eds.), *Maternal-fetal medicine* (4th ed., pp. 40–62). Philadelphia: Saunders.

Shapiro, L. J. (1996a). Inheritance patterns. In W. E. Nelson, R. E. Behrman, R. M. Kliegman, & A. M. Arvin (Eds.), *Nelson textbook of pediatrics* (15th ed., pp. 308–312). Philadelphia: Saunders.

Shapiro, L. J. (1996b). The molecular basis of genetic disorders. In W. E. Nelson, R. E. Behrman, R. M. Kliegman, & A. M. Arvin (Eds.), *Nelson textbook of pediatrics* (15th ed., pp. 299–305). Philadelphia: Saunders.

Shapiro, L. J. (1996c). Molecular diagnosis. In W. E. Nelson, R. E. Behrman, R. M. Kliegman, & A. M. Arvin (Eds.), *Nelson textbook of pediatrics* (15th ed., pp. 305–308). Philadelphia: Saunders.

Slaughter, L. (1997). Ensuring protection from genetic discrimination in health insurance. *Lifelines, 1*(3), 23.

Williams, J. K., & Lea, D. H. (1995). Applying new genetic technologies: Assessment and ethical considerations. *Nurse Practitioner, 20*(7), 16–26.

II

Maternity
Nursing Care

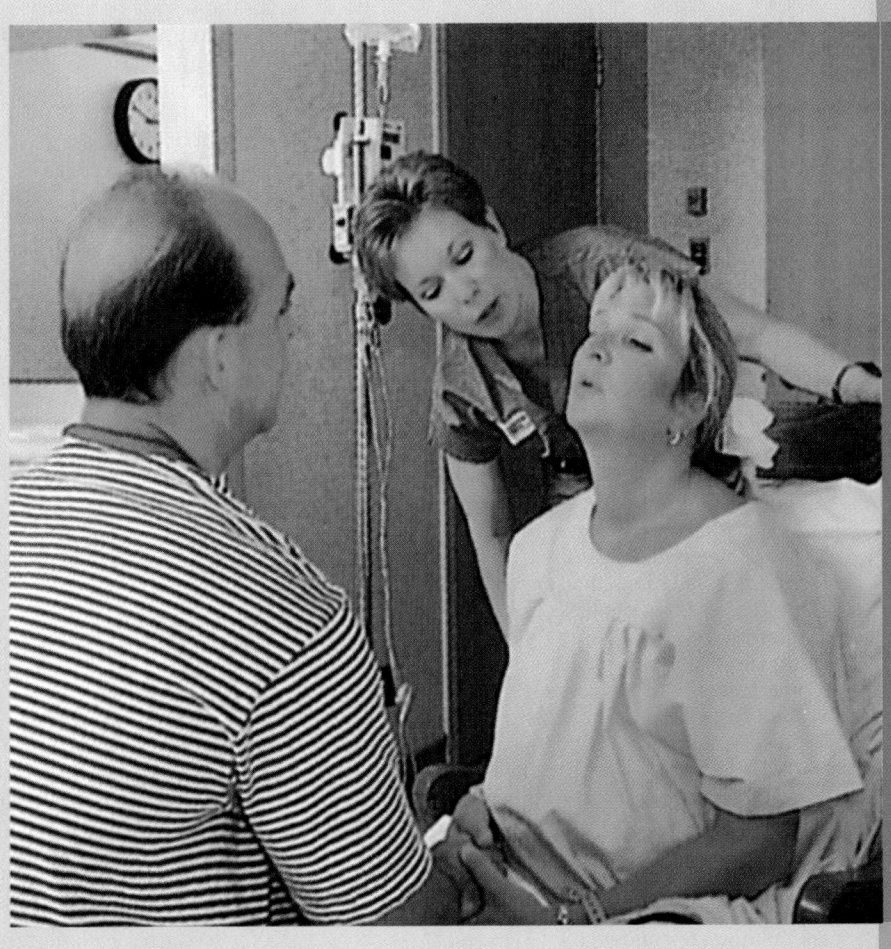

10

Management of Fertility and Infertility

LEARNING OBJECTIVES

After studying this chapter, you should be able to:

■ Describe the role of the nurse in helping couples choose contraceptive methods.

■ Compare and contrast contraceptive methods in terms of safety, effectiveness, convenience, education needed to use, interference with spontaneity, availability, expense, and preference.

■ Explain why informed consent is important for contraception.

■ Compare and contrast contraceptive needs of adolescent and perimenopausal women.

■ Explain the mechanism of action for each method of family planning available: sterilization, hormonal contraceptives, intrauterine devices, barrier, and natural family planning.

■ Explain factors that can impair a couple's ability to conceive.

■ Describe factors that may cause repeated pregnancy losses.

■ Specify evaluations that may be performed when a couple seeks help for infertility.

■ Explain the use of procedures and treatments that may aid a couple's ability to conceive and carry the fetus to viability.

■ Discuss the nurse's role for families needing care related to fertility or infertility.

DEFINITIONS

anovulatory (or anovular) Menstrual cycles occurring without ovulation.

azoospermia Absence of sperm in semen.

basal body temperature Body temperature at rest.

cervical cap A small cuplike device placed over the cervix to prevent sperm from entering, thus preventing pregnancy.

climacteric Endocrine, body, and psychic changes occurring at the end of a woman's reproductive period. Also informally called menopause.

coitus Sexual union between a male and a female.

coitus interruptus Withdrawal of the penis from the vagina before ejaculation.

condom Latex, polyurethane, or natural membrane shield covering the penis or lining the vagina to prevent sperm from entering the cervix or to prevent infection or both.

contraception Prevention of pregnancy.

diaphragm A contraceptive device consisting of a latex dome that covers the cervix and prevents entrance of sperm; must be used with a spermicide to be effective.

endometriosis Presence of endometrial tissue (uterine lining) outside the uterine cavity.

ferning (or fern test) Microscopic fernlike appearance of dried cervical mucus that is most apparent at the time of ovulation.

gametogenesis Development and maturation of the sperm and ova.

gestational surrogate A woman who carries the embryo of an infertile couple and relinquishes the child after birth.

hormone implant Small capsules of progestin inserted subcutaneously to provide contraception.

impotence Inability of a man to achieve or maintain an erection of the penis that is sufficiently rigid to permit successful sexual intercourse.

incompetent cervix Inability of the cervix to remain closed long enough during pregnancy for the fetus to survive.

infertility Inability of a couple to conceive after 1 year of regular intercourse (two or three times weekly) without using contraception; also the involuntary inability to con-

ceive and produce viable offspring when the couple chooses. Primary infertility occurs in a couple that has never conceived; secondary infertility occurs in a couple that has conceived at least once before.

intrauterine device (IUD) A mechanical device inserted into the uterus to prevent pregnancy.

libido Sexual desire.

mittelschmerz Low abdominal pain that occurs at ovulation.

natural family planning Method of predicting ovulation based on normal changes in a woman's body.

oligospermia A decreased number of sperm in semen, usually considered to be fewer than 20 million per milliliter.

oral contraceptive Drug that inhibits ovulation; contains progestins alone or in combination with estrogen.

progestin Any natural or synthetic form of progesterone.

retrograde ejaculation Discharge of semen into the bladder rather than from the end of the penis.

semen Spermatozoa with their nourishing and protective fluid, discharged at ejaculation.

sexually transmissible (or transmitted) disease (STD) A disease passed to others primarily through sexual contact. Also called sexually transmissible (or transmitted) infections (STI).

spermicide A chemical, such as nonoxynol-9, that kills sperm.

spinnbarkeit Clear, slippery, stretchy quality of cervical mucus during ovulation.

sterility Total inability to conceive.

surrogate mother A fertile woman inseminated with the purpose of conceiving and relinquishing a child to an infertile couple.

tubal ligation Occluding the fallopian tubes to prevent passage of ova or sperm, thus preventing pregnancy.

varicocele Abnormal dilation or varicosity of veins in the spermatic cord.

vasectomy Occluding the vas deferens to prevent passage of sperm, thus preventing pregnancy.

Family planning involves choosing the time to have children. It includes contraception—the prevention of pregnancy—as well as methods to achieve pregnancy. If both partners are fertile, approximately 90% of women will conceive within 1 year if they do not use contraception (Cunningham et al., 1997). Therefore, those who wish to control the timing of pregnancies cannot leave contraception to chance.

Role of the Nurse in Contraception

The nurse's role in family planning is that of counselor and educator. To fulfill this role, nurses need current, correct information about contraceptive methods. More than half of all pregnancies are unintended. About half of the unintended pregnancies occur in women who are using a contraceptive method but use it incorrectly or have a contraceptive failure.

Nurses must feel comfortable discussing contraception and be sensitive to the woman's concerns and feelings. In discussions of family planning, the woman's preferences take precedence. Nurses must be careful not to introduce their own biases toward or against specific methods. The nurse's personal experiences and choices regarding contraception are not pertinent. The needs and feelings of the woman and her partner must be the focus of counseling (Fig. 10–1).

Considerations When Choosing a Contraceptive Method

No contraceptive method is perfect. Each has advantages and disadvantages (Table 10–1). Women change contraceptive methods as circumstances in their lives change and may try several before finding one that is satisfactory. The rate at which women discontinue the use of their contraceptive method is shown in Table 10–2. Careful consideration of all factors can help women choose methods that best meet their needs.

Safety

The safety of the method is a primary consideration. Medical conditions may make some methods unsafe for certain women. For example, oral contraceptives (OCs) should not be used by women who have had thrombophlebitis or strokes because the hormones used may cause these conditions to recur. The diaphragm is unsafe for a woman with a history of toxic shock syndrome.

Protection from Sexually Transmissible Diseases

No contraceptive (other than abstinence) is 100% effective in preventing sexually transmissible diseases (STDs). The risk of exposure to STDs should be considered in counseling women about contraceptive choices. The male condom offers the best protection available. It should be used whenever there is a risk that one partner may have an STD, even when another form of contraception is practiced.

Effectiveness

The importance of avoiding pregnancy must be considered when choosing a contraceptive method. Effectiveness is determined by how often the method fails to prevent pregnancy (see Table 10–2). Failure rates reflect two different types of failure:

1. The ideal, perfect, or theoretic failure rate refers to perfect use of the method with every act of intercourse.
2. The typical, actual, or user failure rate refers to the occurrence of pregnancy in real people using the method.

The difference between the two rates of failure shows how forgiving a method is or how likely pregnancy is to occur

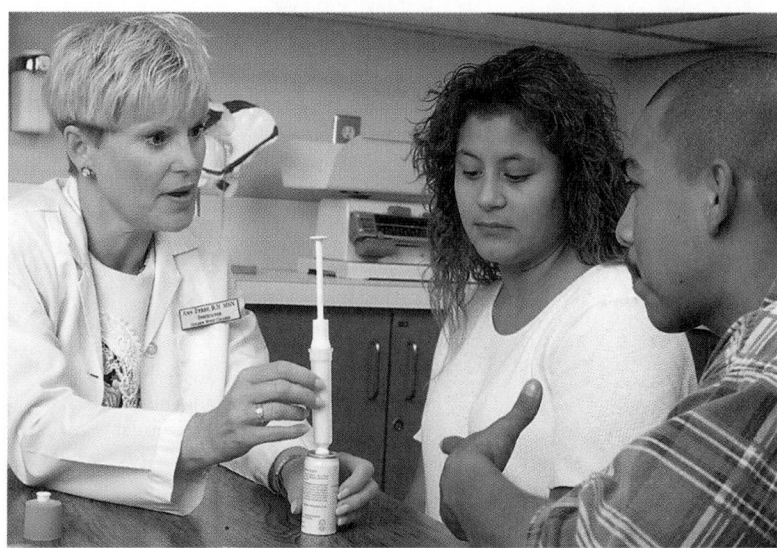

FIGURE 10–1

Success of contraception is more likely when both the woman and her partner are involved in discussions. The nurse demonstrates filling a foam applicator.

TABLE 10–1
· · · · · · · · · · · ·

Advantages and Disadvantages of Most Common Contraceptive Methods

Method	Advantages	Disadvantages
Sterilization (tubal ligation and vasectomy)	Ends concern about contraception. Tubal ligation can be performed during hospitalization for childbirth or at another time. Vasectomy may be performed in physician's office under local anesthesia. Although expensive initially, long-term cost is low.	Does not protect against STDs. Reversal is difficult, expensive, and potentially impossible. Requires surgery, with potential complications of all surgeries. Vasectomy requires another contraceptive method until semen is free of sperm.
Implant	In place at all times. Unrelated to coitus.	Does not protect against STDs. Expensive initially (although lower overall cost), requires minor surgery to implant and remove. Slightly visible. Side effects may lead to discontinuation.
Progestin injections (Depo-Provera)	Unrelated to coitus.	Must be repeated every 3 months. Side effects similar to other progestin contraceptives. Does not protect against STDs.
Oral contraceptives	Taken at time unrelated to coitus. See Table 10–3.	Must be taken at same time each day. May cause side effects and complications. Does not protect against STDs. See Table 10–3.
Intrauterine devices	In place at all times. Low long-term cost.	Does not protect against STDs. High initial cost. Can be expelled without woman's knowledge—must check for strings. Potential problems: menorrhagia, infection, ectopic pregnancy, abortion, perforation.
Barrier		
All methods	Avoids use of systemic hormones. Offers some protection against STDs.	Most coitus-related (must be used just before coitus). May interfere with sensation. Some people are sensitive to components of spermicide or latex.
Chemical (spermicides)	Quick and easy. No prescription needed. Inexpensive per single use.	Films and suppositories must melt to be effective. Usually effective for only 1 hr. May be messy. New application needed for subsequent intercourse.
Condoms	Quick and easy. No prescription needed. Best protection available for STDs. Inexpensive per single use. Can be carried discreetly. Vaginal condoms increase women's control over contraceptive use and protection from STDs.	Must be checked for expiration date and holes. Can break or slip off. Can be used only once. Vaginal condom may seem unattractive.
Diaphragm	Can be inserted several hours before coitus.	Initially expensive. Requires nurse practitioner, certified nurse-midwife, or physician to fit. Requires education on proper use. Some women have difficulty with correct insertion or removal. Added spermicide necessary for repeat coitus. Possibility of toxic shock or bladder infection. Must be refitted after each birth or weight change of 10 or more pounds.

TABLE 10–1
• • • • • • • • • • • •

Advantages and Disadvantages of Most Common Contraceptive Methods Continued

Method	Advantages	Disadvantages
Cervical cap	Smaller than diaphragm and may fit women who cannot wear a diaphragm. Requires less spermicide and no additional spermicide for repeated intercourse. No pressure against bladder. Less noticeable than diaphragm. Can remain in place 48 hr.	Sizes are limited. Initially expensive. Requires nurse practitioner or physician to fit. Requires education on proper use. Somewhat more difficult to insert than diaphragm. Can be dislodged during intercourse. Possibility of toxic shock. Must be refitted each year and after birth, abortion, or surgery.
Natural family planning		
All methods	Inexpensive. No drugs or hormones. Helps woman learn about her body. Acceptable to most religions. May be used to achieve pregnancy. Can combine with barrier methods to increase effectiveness.	Requires high level of motivation. Extensive education needed. Requires abstinence for large part of each cycle. High risk of pregnancy from error. Many factors may change ovulation time.

TABLE 10–2
• • • • • • • • • • • •

Contraceptive Effectiveness, Failure, and Discontinuation Rates

Method	Effectiveness Rate: Actual or Typical Use (%)	Failure Rate: Actual or Typical Use (%)	Failure Rate: Ideal or Perfect Use (%)	Discontinuation Rate at 1 Year (%)
Sterilization				
Tubal ligation	99.5	0.5	0.5	
Vasectomy	99.85	0.15	0.1	
Hormone implants	99.95	0.05	0.05	12
Injectable hormones	99.7	0.3	0.3	30
Oral contraceptives	95	5		29
Combined estrogen/progestin			0.1	
Progestin only			0.5	
Intrauterine devices				
Progesterone	98	2	1.5	19
Copper	99.2	0.8	0.6	22
Condoms				
Male	86	14	3	39
Female	79	21	5	44
Diaphragm	80	20	6	44
Cervical cap				
Parous women	60	40	26	58
Nulliparous women	80	20	9	44
Spermicides: gel, foam, films, suppositories	74	26	6	60
Natural family planning	75	25		37
Calendar			9	
Ovulation			3	
Symptothermal			2	
Coitus interruptus (withdrawal)	81	19	4	
No contraceptive use	15	85	85	

Percentage of women who may be expected to avoid pregnancy or become pregnant with use of each method from typical and perfect use during the first year. Discontinuation rate is the rate of women who do not wish to become pregnant and stop using a method by the end of 1 year of use. The discontinuation rate often rises with each year of use.

Modified from Hatcher, R. A., Trussell, J., Stewart, F., Cates, W., Stewart, G. K., Guest, F., & Kowal, D. (1998). *Contraceptive technology* (17th ed.). New York: Ardent Media, with permission.

if use is occasionally imperfect. Failure rates are listed as number of pregnancies in 100 women per year.

Effectiveness drops greatly when the user does not understand how to use the method. The failure rate commonly decreases after the first year of use because experience with the method leads to more accurate use. Combining two less reliable methods, such as a condom with a spermicide, increases effectiveness.

Convenience

Convenience is another important factor in choosing a contraceptive method. A contraceptive such as spermicide that seems "messy" may be considered inconvenient and unattractive. If the woman perceives her contraceptive as difficult to use, time-consuming, or too much "bother," she is unlikely to use it consistently. Women knowledgeable about the contraceptive technique are less likely to feel that the contraceptive is difficult to use.

Education Needed

Some methods of contraception, such as condoms, involve very little education, whereas others are more complicated. Women using natural family-planning methods need extensive education to practice these methods successfully.

Side Effects

Many methods of contraception have bothersome side effects that should be discussed. When women know what to expect, they are often more willing to tolerate side effects, especially if they know they do not indicate a health risk.

Interference with Spontaneity

Coitus-related contraceptive methods, such as spermicides and barrier methods, must be used just before sexual intercourse. They interrupt love making, increasing the chance that the method will not be used. Some couples remedy this problem by making placement of the contraceptive device a part of foreplay.

Availability

Condoms and spermicides are readily available without prescriptions. They can be purchased anonymously at any time. Their availability may be important to an adolescent who wants to hide her sexual activity or to women who are embarrassed to discuss contraception with a health care provider.

Expense

The cost of family-planning methods per use can be compared with long-term expense. The price of condoms and spermicides is relatively low, but frequent use makes them expensive over a period of years. The yearly cost of any contraceptive method is less than the cost of a pregnancy.

Methods that depend on periodic visits to a nurse practitioner or physician are more costly than over-the-counter methods. Although they require a health practitioner visit,

the copper-T IUD, implants, and injectable contraceptives are the most cost-effective reversible contraceptives available over a 5-year period because they prevent pregnancy so well (Trussell et al., 1995).

Preference

Consistent use of any method depends on whether it meets the needs of the woman and her partner. If the woman feels pressured into choosing a method or if the chosen method fails to live up to her expectations, use is likely to be inconsistent. Some women are uncomfortable with their bodies and embarrassed by methods that involve touching the vagina. Inserting a diaphragm or cervical cap or performing a daily assessment of cervical mucus may be unacceptable to them.

Religious and Personal Beliefs

Religious or other personal beliefs also affect the choice of contraceptives. Roman Catholics may not believe in the use of any contraceptives other than natural family planning.

Culture

Culture may also influence the method chosen. In African-American culture, OCs and female sterilization are most often chosen, and male sterilization is rare (Lethbridge, 1995). Hmong women may report that their husbands do not believe in contraception (Jambunathan & Stewart, 1995).

▌ Informed Consent

Because some methods have potentially dangerous side effects, the woman must sign an informed consent form to show that she received and understands information about risks and benefits. Written consent must be obtained from women choosing surgical sterilization, OCs, hormone implants or injections, and IUDs. Of course, whether or not a formal consent form is used, every woman should receive information about the chosen contraceptive method and its proper use, the risks and benefits, and the alternative methods available.

▌ Adolescents

Although the rate of adolescent pregnancies has diminished in recent years, adolescent pregnancy is still a major problem. Approximately a million teenaged girls become pregnant each year. Because of the severe impact of pregnancy on the teenager, finding methods to enhance contraception use among adolescents is extremely important. (See Chapter 25 for information about adolescent pregnancy.)

Adolescent Knowledge

Many adolescents have little knowledge about their own anatomy and physiology, including how and when conception occurs. They are likely to learn about contraception from other teenagers, who often pass on incorrect information. Even adolescents who have been pregnant misunder-

CRITICAL THINKING EXERCISE 10-1

A 15-year-old girl approaches the nurse with questions about contraception. She says she does not want to become pregnant, but her boyfriend does not want to use condoms, and she is too embarrassed to go to see a physician for other contraceptive methods.

How should the nurse handle the situation?

stand contraceptive techniques, and they may become pregnant again because of lack of information about family planning.

MISINFORMATION

Misinformation and erroneous beliefs cause adolescents to use ineffective methods of contraception or no method at all. Some teenagers think they cannot become pregnant the first time they have intercourse. Others think they must have an orgasm or must have been menstruating a certain length of time. Pregnancy, however, can result from any intercourse near ovulation. Although many adolescents have anovulatory menstrual cycles during the early months after menarche, they cannot depend on anovulation to prevent pregnancy.

Teenagers may douche (insert a solution into the vagina) after intercourse to prevent pregnancy. Douching, however, is ineffective because sperm may enter the cervix soon after ejaculation. Coitus interruptus (withdrawal) is another unreliable method used by teenagers. It requires more control over timing of ejaculation than most adolescent boys have. In addition, semen spilled near the vagina can enter and cause pregnancy even without penetration by the penis.

RISK-TAKING BEHAVIOR

Adolescents are more likely than adults to take risks in sexual activity because they believe that their chances of becoming pregnant are small. Often they do not plan intercourse and therefore are not prepared with contraceptives.

Their risk-taking behavior may lead to STDs as well as to pregnancy.

Counseling Adolescents

Nurses who counsel adolescents about sexuality must be sensitive to the feelings, concerns, and needs of the teenager. They must be prepared to be accepting of the teenager regardless of personal feelings about adolescent sexuality. The teenager may not ask about contraception because she does not want anyone to know that she is sexually active. Her need for secrecy may cause her to miss appointments for family planning.

Because of her youth and possible lack of knowledge about anatomy and physiology, the adolescent often needs more extensive teaching than the older woman. Liberal use of audiovisual materials, such as pictures, anatomic models, and samples of various methods, helps the teenager understand the information more easily. Using a banana and condom or showing her the packet of pills she will be using may be an important aid.

Using understandable terminology is especially important when teaching adolescents. The nurse must know street terms for body parts and sexual intercourse; they may be the only words with which the teenager is familiar.

Adolescents are most successful when they choose contraceptive methods that are easy to use and that seem unrelated to coitus. Many teenagers choose oral or injectable contraceptives. These methods are safe, seem unrelated to sex, and are not difficult or messy. Long-term OC use has not been found to cause problems in healthy women.

Adolescents may, however, be inconsistent in taking pills every day. They are more likely to discontinue any method for minor side effects, such as nausea or spotting. Their concerns should be taken seriously, and attempts should be made to alleviate side effects or they will stop using the method, with pregnancy as a possible result.

Condom use should be encouraged to help prevent STDs, even when using another contraceptive method (Fig. 10–2). In one study, consistent condom use with another

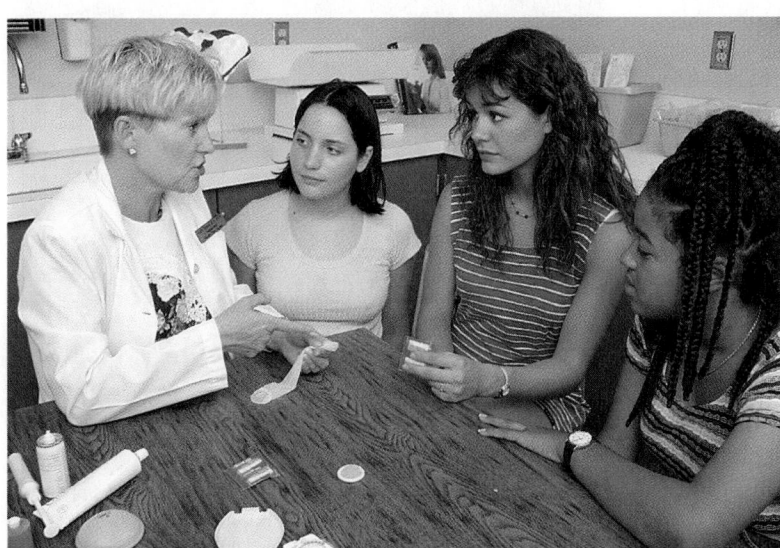

FIGURE 10-2

Although many adolescents choose oral contraceptives, the nurse emphasizes the need to use condoms for protection against sexually transmissible diseases. Demonstrating with actual contraceptives increases understanding.

method was reported to occur in only 37% of young women (Dinerman et al., 1995). Many young women are uneasy about asking a partner to use a condom. They benefit from learning to negotiate condom use with a partner.

Perimenopausal Women

Perimenopausal women may continue to ovulate as long as they have regular menstrual periods, and some ovulate even when indications of menopause are present. Pregnancy is rare after age 50, and contraception can be discontinued sooner if menstruation has ceased for at least 2 years (Cunningham et al., 1997). The mature woman who does not smoke and has no other contraindications can use any method of contraception.

Methods of Contraception

Sterilization

Sterilization is an extremely popular method of contraception for couples who have completed their families. In the United States, approximately 1 million sterilizations are performed annually (Stewart & Carignan, 1998). Although it is expensive at the time of surgery, sterilization ends all further contraceptive costs. It should always be considered a permanent end to fertility because reversal surgery is difficult, expensive, not always successful, and usually not covered by insurance.

Couples considering sterilization need counseling to ensure that they understand all aspects of the procedure. When surgery is planned for immediately after childbirth, the decision should be made well before labor begins. Future marriage, divorce, or death of a child may cause couples to regret their decision. Although pregnancy is rare after sterilization, the risk of failure should be discussed.

TUBAL LIGATION

Female sterilization is the method of contraception used by more than 10 million women in the United States (Stewart & Carignan, 1998). The effectiveness rate is 99.5%. The surgery is easiest during the first 48 hours after birth, when the fundus is located near the umbilicus and the fallopian tubes are just below the abdominal wall. For the woman who is not postpartum, the procedure is often performed in an outpatient surgery department. General anesthesia is most common, but regional or local anesthesia may be used.

The procedure can be performed in three ways. A mini-laparotomy incision is made near the umbilicus in the postpartum period or just above the symphysis pubis at other times. The surgeon brings the tubes through the incision, where a piece is removed and the ends are tied or cauterized or both. In the second method, surgery is performed through a laparoscope inserted through a small incision. The surgeon identifies the fallopian tubes and blocks them with clips or rings or destroys a portion of the tubes with electrocoagulation. The third method is performed during other surgery, generally along with cesarean birth, when a woman is sure that she wants the procedure regardless of the outcome of the birth.

VASECTOMY

Vasectomy, the male sterilization procedure, is 99.85% effective. It involves making a small puncture or incision in the scrotum and cutting the vas deferens, which carries sperm from the testes to the penis. Cautery may also be used. After vasectomy, semen no longer contains sperm.

Vasectomy involves lower morbidity rates than tubal ligation, and because it can be performed in a physician's office under local anesthesia, it is less expensive. After surgery, the man applies ice to the area and watches for excessive swelling or bleeding.

The couple should understand that complete sterilization does not occur until all sperm have left the system, a process that may take a month or more. The man should submit semen specimens for analysis until two specimens show no sperm present.

Hormonal Contraceptives

Hormonal contraceptives alter the normal hormone fluctuations of the menstrual cycle. They may be given by implant, by injection, or orally.

HORMONE IMPLANT

The progestin implant (Norplant and Norplant-2) is the most effective form of contraception available today (99.95% effective). Six flexible capsules about 1.5 inches long (the size of a match) are inserted subcutaneously into the upper inner arm under a local anesthetic (Fig. 10–3). This area is used because it is easily accessible and low in fat. The capsules are inserted in a fan-shaped configuration and are only slightly visible. They release progestin continuously at gradually decreasing levels over the 5 years they are effective.

The progestin implant is expensive at the time of insertion, although the long-term cost is relatively low. Medicaid covers the cost; other insurance plans often pay all or part. It has been used by approximately 1 million women in the United States and by more than 2.5 million women worldwide (AWHONN, 1995).

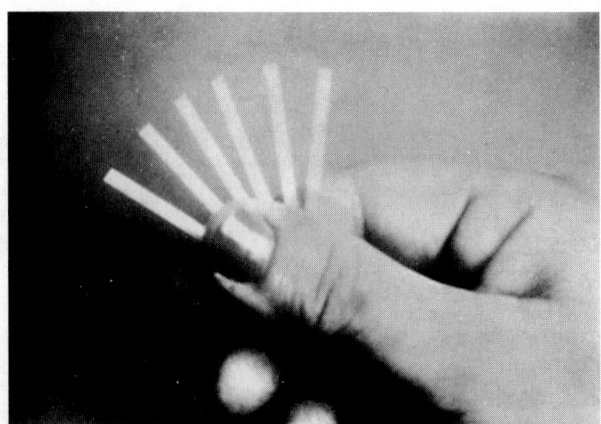

FIGURE 10–3

Norplant capsules are inserted under the skin of the upper arm and remain effective for 5 years. (Courtesy of Wyeth-Ayerst Laboratories, Philadelphia, Pennsylvania.)

Action. The action of the hormone implant is similar to that of progestin-only OCs. It inhibits ovulation and development of the endometrium and causes changes in cervical mucus that impede penetration by the sperm. Norplant can be inserted after delivery, but breastfeeding women should wait 6 weeks. Effectiveness is slightly reduced in women weighing more than 131 pounds. Fertility returns promptly after the capsules are removed.

Side Effects. Menstrual changes occur in more than 80% of women and are the most common cause for discontinuation of the method (Hatcher, 1998). Women may have irregular, midcycle, or prolonged bleeding, which usually decreases by 1 year of use. If necessary, bleeding may be treated with oral estrogen or ibuprofen. Some women have decreased bleeding or amenorrhea. Other side effects include headaches, breast tenderness, ovarian cysts, weight gain, acne, dizziness, and mood changes. Infection and expulsion of the implants are rare complications. Removal may be difficult if the capsules are deeply implanted. Practitioners must be trained in both insertion and removal.

HORMONE INJECTIONS

Depo-Provera (medroxyprogesterone acetate or DMPA) is an injectable progestin. It prevents ovulation for 14 weeks, although women are advised to repeat doses every 3 months to avoid decreases in hormone levels. It is 99.7% effective, it is convenient, and it does not contain estrogen. Action and side effects are similar to those of other progestin contraceptives. Menstrual irregularities are the major reason for discontinuation. Although spotting and breakthrough bleeding are common, amenorrhea occurs in 50% of women at 1 year. Weight gain averages about 4 pounds per year. Other side effects include headaches, depression, hair loss, and decreased bone density with long-term use.

Depo-Provera is given by deep intramuscular injection. The site should not be massaged after injection, because this action accelerates absorption. The first injection is best given within 5 days of the menstrual period. If given later in the cycle, an additional form of contraception should be used for 1 week. Women can use Depo-Provera at any age, if they are in good health. For breastfeeding women, it is often started 6 weeks after delivery, when lactation is well established. Fertility returns in approximately 6 to 12 months (Hatcher, 1998).

ORAL CONTRACEPTIVES

Oral contraceptives are the most widely used reversible contraceptive method in the United States (Trussell & Kowal, 1998). Combination OCs contain both estrogen and progestin, whereas "minipills" contain only progestin. Both types contain much lower hormone levels than the original OCs, thus decreasing the risk of long-term side effects. Oral contraceptives have a 95% typical effectiveness rate.

Combination. Estrogen and progestin combinations are the most common OCs and have an action similar to pregnancy in preventing ovulation. The high level of estrogen and progestin prevents the discharge of follicle-stimulating and luteinizing hormones from the pituitary. This process inhibits maturation of the follicle and ovulation. In addition, the endometrium becomes less hospitable to implantation.

Combination OCs are available in packets of 21 or 28 tablets. With 21-tablet packets, the woman takes one pill daily for 3 weeks, then stops for a week, during which menses occurs. Packets of 28 tablets include 7 tablets made of an inert substance that the woman takes during the fourth week. These extra pills avoid disrupting the everyday routine of taking pills.

Monophasic or multiphasic dosages are available. Monophasic pills have an estrogen and progestin content that remains constant throughout the cycle. With multiphasic pills, the estrogen dose may be constant or increased in the later part of the cycle. The progestin is low at the beginning of the cycle and is increased later. This change helps reduce side effects. Because there may be two or three phases of dosage changes, women must take the pills in the proper order.

Progestin Only. Oral contraceptives that contain progestin but no estrogen are called minipills. They are useful for women who cannot take estrogen. They are less effective at inhibiting ovulation but cause thickening of the cervical mucus, which helps prevent penetration by sperm and makes the endometrial lining unfavorable for implantation. These pills avoid the side effects and risk factors associated with estrogen. If the woman misses any pills or does not take them at the same time each day, however, chances of pregnancy increase. Breakthrough bleeding and higher risk of pregnancy have made these OCs less popular than the combination OCs.

Benefits, Risks, and Cautions. When choosing OCs, the balance between the benefits and the risks must be weighed for each individual (Table 10–3). Women often exaggerate the health risks and underestimate the health benefits of OCs (Tessler & Peipert, 1997). The method provides many benefits in addition to safe, reliable contraception. Although OCs were once thought unsafe for older women, studies show that women in good health who do not smoke can continue to take OCs until age 50. Smoking increases the incidence of complications for women of all ages. Other risk factors include hypertension, high cholesterol levels, obesity, and diabetes. With careful follow-up, however, diabetic women may use any contraceptive method, if they have no other contraindications (Kjos, 1996).

Although there are risks in using OCs, it is important for women to know that the chances of complications and death during pregnancy and childbirth are greater (Hatcher & Guillebaud, 1998). Oral contraceptives provide no protection against STDs and may increase susceptibility to chlamydia. A woman should be advised to use a condom and spermicide if her partner may be infected.

Side Effects. Approximately 29% of women who do not wish to become pregnant discontinue OCs within a year. A major reason is side effects. Most side effects are minor and often decrease after the first few months of use. They are less frequent in low-dose OCs. Decreasing the amount of estrogen helps relieve nausea, headaches, or breast tenderness, whereas increasing the estrogen content prevents breakthrough bleeding. Other side effects include weight gain or loss, fluid retention, amenorrhea, and chloasma.

Teaching. Education about proper use of OCs greatly increases their effectiveness. Because the instructions can be complicated, they should be written clearly and simply

TABLE 10-3

Potential Benefits and Risks of Oral Contraceptives

Benefits	Risks*
Highly effective contraception.	No protection against STDs.
Reduces ovarian and endometrial cancer by as much as 50%. Protection continues for years after use.	May affect carbohydrate metabolism and may affect diabetes.
Regulates menstrual cycles and reduces cramping, menstrual blood loss, and associated anemia.	May increase risk for breast and cervical cancer.
Decreased incidence of	Increased incidence of
benign breast disease	deep and superficial vein thrombosis
ovarian cysts	pulmonary embolism
pelvic inflammatory disease	myocardial infarction
ectopic pregnancy	stroke
Improves	hypertension
endometriosis	migraines
premenstrual syndrome (for some)	chlamydial infection
dysmenorrhea	benign liver tumors
fibroids (leiomyomata)	gallbladder disease
	depression
	growth of fibroids

* Incidence of many risks is significantly reduced with the low-dose oral contraceptives currently used. Avoiding oral contraceptive use in women who smoke or have other risk factors lowers the risk for cardiovascular disease significantly.

in her own language, if she can read. Almost one-third of the 3.5 million yearly unintended pregnancies that occur in the United States are due to failure to follow instructions correctly or failure or discontinuation of OCs (Rosenberg et al., 1995).

The nurse should listen carefully to women's concerns about side effects and help them find methods to relieve them. Accidental pregnancy occurs in almost 25% of women who discontinue OCs owing to side effects because these women did not use another method of contraception or used a less effective method (Rosenberg et al., 1995). Women should be instructed that they need a back-up contraceptive method readily available should they decide to stop taking their OCs.

Blood Hormone Levels. Because maintaining a constant blood hormone level is important for effectiveness, the woman must take the pills at the same time each day. Many women make them a part of their bedtime routine, whereas others take them with a meal to avoid nausea. Unless they begin the pills during the first 7 days of the menstrual cycle, women should use another contraceptive method during the first week of the first cycle until the blood hormone levels are established (Cunningham et al., 1997).

Missed Doses. The woman should follow instructions from her provider if she misses one or more doses of her OC. Usually another contraceptive method is recommended as additional protection if she misses doses.

If a woman misses a period and thinks she may be pregnant because she missed one or more doses, she should stop taking the pills and get a sensitive pregnancy test immediately. It is essential that she use another contraceptive method during this time. Although there is no established association with significant fetal anomalies, continued use of OCs during pregnancy is not advisable.

Nutrition. Low-estrogen OCs now used do not interfere with nutritional status. Women do not need to take vitamin supplements just because they are taking OCs (Mahan & Escott-Stump, 1996).

Postpartum and Lactation. Because of their increased risk of thrombosis, postpartum women who are not breastfeeding should wait 3 weeks to begin OCs (Kennedy & Trussell, 1998). Combination OCs reduce milk production in lactating women, and small amounts may be transferred to the milk. Progestin-only contraceptives may be a better

CRITICAL TO REMEMBER

Cautions in Using Oral Contraceptives

Oral contraceptives should not be used by women with a history of any of the following:

- Thrombophlebitis and thromboembolic disorders
- Cerebrovascular or cardiovascular diseases
- Any estrogen-dependent cancer or breast cancer
- Benign or malignant liver tumors

Oral contraceptives should not be used by women who currently have any of the following:

- Any of the above conditions
- Impaired liver function
- Suspected or known pregnancy
- Undiagnosed vaginal bleeding
- Heavy cigarette smoking (more than 20 per day in women older than 35). Any use of cigarettes is discouraged and should be evaluated individually.

TABLE 10-4

"ACHES" Warning Signs of Oral Contraceptive Complications

	Warning Sign	*Possible Complication*
A	Abdominal pain (severe)	Benign liver tumor, gallbladder disease
C	Chest pain, dyspnea, hemoptysis	Pulmonary emboli or myocardial infarction
H	Severe headache, weakness or numbness of extremities	Stroke
E	Eye problems (visual changes such as blurred or double vision or visual loss, speech disturbance)	Stroke
S	Severe leg pain or swelling (calf or thigh)	Deep vein thrombosis

Note: The acronym ACHES can be used to help women remember warning signs that may indicate complications when using oral contraceptives. Other signs include jaundice, a breast lump, and depression. The woman should contact her health care provider if any of these signs develop.

Data from Hatcher & Guillebaud, 1998.

choice because they do not affect milk production. They can be started at 6 weeks postpartum.

Other Medications. Oral contraceptives may interact with other medications, and the effectiveness of each may be changed. For example, antibiotics, such as ampicillin and tetracycline, and some anticonvulsants decrease the effectiveness of OCs. Therefore, the woman should always tell any health care provider prescribing medications for her what other drugs she is taking.

Follow-Up. The woman who takes OCs should have a yearly pelvic examination and a Papanicolaou (Pap) smear, breast examination, and blood pressure measurement. She should report any signs of adverse reaction immediately. Use of the acronym ACHES may help the woman to remember signs that may indicate complications (Table 10–4). Return of fertility usually occurs within 2 to 3 months after the pills are discontinued.

Postcoital Emergency Contraception. Postcoital contraception (often called emergency contraception or the "morning-after pill") is a method to prevent pregnancy after unprotected intercourse. This method may be used after contraceptive failure, such as a condom breaking during intercourse. It may also be used after rape or in situations when contraceptives were used incorrectly or not at all.

The most common method involves taking a larger-than-usual dose of an OC as soon as possible within 72 hours after unprotected intercourse. A second dose is taken 12 hours after the first. A kit (Preven) containing four contraceptive tablets and a pregnancy test is available by prescription. Treatment reduces the risk of pregnancy by 75%.

The high hormone levels prevent or delay ovulation to prevent fertilization and may have some effect on endometrial development. The treatment is ineffective if pregnancy has already occurred, and it does not harm a developing fetus. Antiemetics may be prescribed to treat the side effects of nausea and vomiting.

Progestin-only contraceptives may be preferable for women who cannot take estrogen or wish to decrease the nausea. Insertion of the copper-T 380A IUD within 5 days of intercourse may also be used; this is 99% effective.

Intrauterine Devices

Intrauterine devices are inserted into the uterus to provide continuous pregnancy prevention. The two types available in the United States, the copper-T 380A (ParaGard) and the progestin IUD (Progestasert), are both shaped like the letter T (Fig. 10–4). They are 98% to 99.2% effective. Although there was a concern about safety with early models, IUDs are considered very safe at this time. They are often inserted at the 6-week postpartum checkup and are safe during lactation.

ACTION

The exact mechanism of action is unknown, but IUDs appear to affect sperm and ova to prevent fertilization. Sperm are immobilized, and ova move through the fallopian tubes more quickly. A sterile inflammatory response of the endometrium may prevent implantation. The ParaGard IUD has copper wire wound around it and remains effective for 10 years. Progestin is continuously released from the Progestasert IUD, which must be replaced yearly.

SIDE EFFECTS

Side effects include cramping and bleeding with insertion. Menorrhagia (increased bleeding during menstruation) and

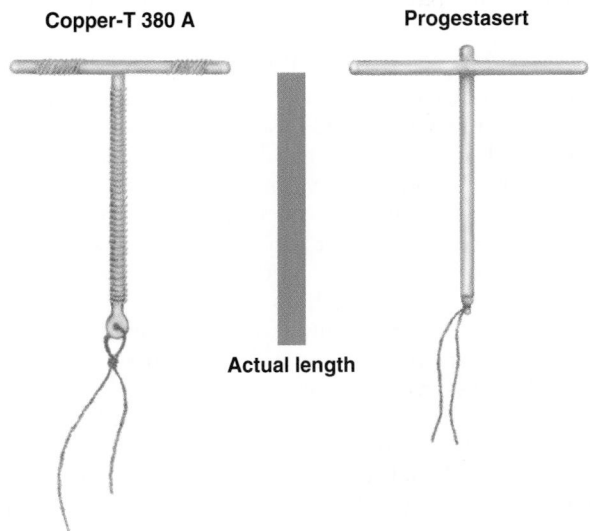

FIGURE 10-4

The Copper-T 380A (ParaGard) and progestin (Progestasert) intrauterine devices (IUDs). Currently, IUDs are considered a very safe method for preventing pregnancy.

dysmenorrhea (painful menstruation) are common reasons for removal. Pelvic infections are less common than with the original models. They occur most often in the first few weeks after insertion or from STDs. Therefore, only women in mutually monogamous relationships and at low risk for STDs should use IUDs.

Complications include expulsion and perforation of the uterus. Women who become pregnant using the IUD are more likely to have ectopic pregnancies or spontaneous abortions. Nulliparous women and those with recent or recurrent pelvic infections, a history of ectopic pregnancy, bleeding disorders, or abnormalities of the uterus should choose another contraceptive method.

TEACHING

Teaching the woman about side effects and about checking for the presence of the plastic strings, or "tail," extending from the IUD into the vagina is important. The woman should feel for the strings once a week during the first 4 weeks, then monthly after menses, and if she has signs of expulsion (cramping or unexpected bleeding). If the strings are longer or shorter than they were previously, she should see her health care provider. Signs of infection, such as unusual vaginal discharge, pain or itching, low pelvic pain, and fever, should prompt a call to the physician. Any signs of pregnancy should be reported to rule out ectopic pregnancy and to remove the device if pregnancy occurs. The woman should return yearly for a Pap smear and to check for anemia if menses are heavy.

Barrier Methods

The barrier methods of contraception involve chemicals or devices that prevent sperm from entering the cervix. All of the barrier methods are coitus related and may interfere with spontaneity. They avoid use of systemic hormones, however, and provide some protection from STDs.

CHEMICAL BARRIERS

Chemicals that kill sperm are called *spermicides* and come in many forms. Creams and gels are generally used with mechanical barriers such as the diaphragm or cervical cap. Foams, suppositories, and vaginal film may be used alone. They are inserted into the vagina just before sexual intercourse and are effective for about 1 hour. Vaginal films and suppositories must melt before they become effective. This process takes approximately 15 minutes.

Spermicides are readily available without a prescription, are inexpensive per use, and are easy to use. They may provide some protection against some STDs. Spermicides should be used with condoms. They increase lubrication, decreasing the risk of condom breakage.

Women should avoid douching for at least 6 hours after intercourse and should add more spermicide if coitus is repeated. Frequent use or sensitivity to the products may cause genital irritation, which could increase susceptibility to infection. Some women and their partners think that spermicides are messy and interfere with sensation during intercourse. When used alone, spermicides are 74% effective. Effectiveness is increased when spermicides are used with a mechanical barrier method.

MECHANICAL BARRIERS

Mechanical barriers include the condom, diaphragm, and cervical cap.

Male Condom. Condoms, one of the most popular contraceptive methods in the United States, cover the penis to prevent sperm from entering the vagina. They are most often made of latex and may be coated with spermicide. Some condoms are made from polyurethane or natural membrane. Polyurethane condoms are thinner than latex and can be used by people who are allergic to latex. They may require lubrication to avoid breakage. Natural membrane condoms do not prevent passage of viruses and do not provide protection from STDs caused by viruses. Latex condoms provide the best protection available (other than abstinence) against STDs. They should be used during any possible exposure to an STD, even if another contraceptive technique is practiced or if the woman is pregnant.

Although women are aware of the protection offered by condoms, those reporting use at last intercourse is low (Murphy et al., 1995; Hiltabiddle, 1996). In one large study, 52% of the women studied had not used condoms in the last 6 months, and only 12% reported that they always used condoms (Lauver et al., 1995).

Condoms are readily available, are inexpensive, and can be carried inconspicuously by the man or the woman. The typical failure rate of 14% can be decreased greatly by combining condom use with another method, such as a vaginal spermicide. Reservoir tips and water-based lubricants help prevent breakage. Some couples reject condoms because they interfere with spontaneity or sensation. People allergic to latex should avoid the use of latex condoms because severe reactions are possible. Condoms may be affected by vaginal medications and should not be used concurrently.

Female Condom. The female condom is a polyurethane sheath inserted into the vagina. A flexible ring fits over the cervix like a diaphragm, and another ring extends outside the vagina to cover the perineum partially (Fig. 10–5).

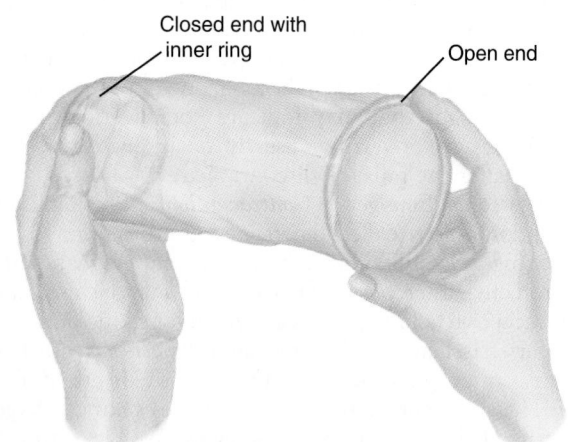

Closed end with inner ring   Open end

FIGURE 10–5
. . . .

The female condom. A woman can protect herself from sexually transmissible diseases without relying on use of the male condom.

What Is the Proper Way to Use Condoms?

Although condoms are easy to use, proper use increases their effectiveness.

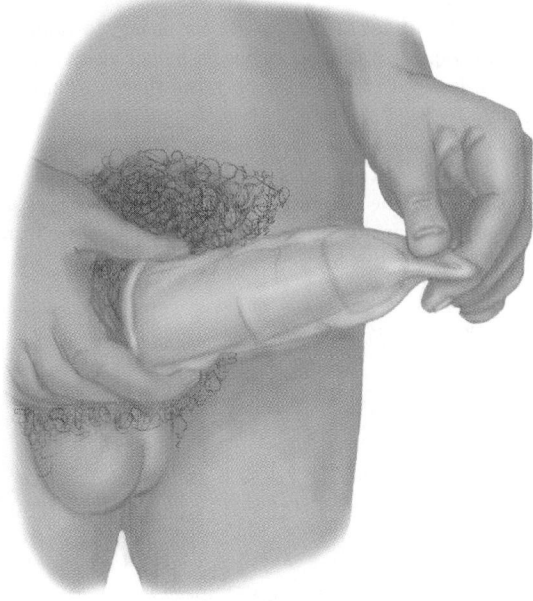

- Condoms are available in a variety of colors, textures, and materials, but those made of latex are most effective. Others may help protect against pregnancy but may not protect against STDs.
- Check the expiration dates on packages because condoms may deteriorate after 5 years.
- Lubrication may increase comfort for the woman and reduce the risk of breakage. Use a water-soluble lubricant or a spermicide because oil-based products (such as petroleum jelly or baby oil) cause deterioration.
- Because sperm may be present in pre-ejaculatory fluid, always apply the condom before there is any contact of the penis with the vagina.
- Squeeze the air out of the tip of the condom, and leave one-half inch of space at the tip as the condom is rolled onto the erect penis. This space allows a place for sperm to collect and helps prevent breakage.
- Withdraw the penis from the vagina before it becomes soft, and hold the condom in place so it does not slip off and no semen spills into the vagina.
- Use a new condom each time intercourse is repeated.

The female condom is the first contraceptive device that allows a woman some protection from STDs without relying on the male condom. It is less effective, however, and many women object to it on esthetic grounds. It has a typical failure rate of approximately 21%.

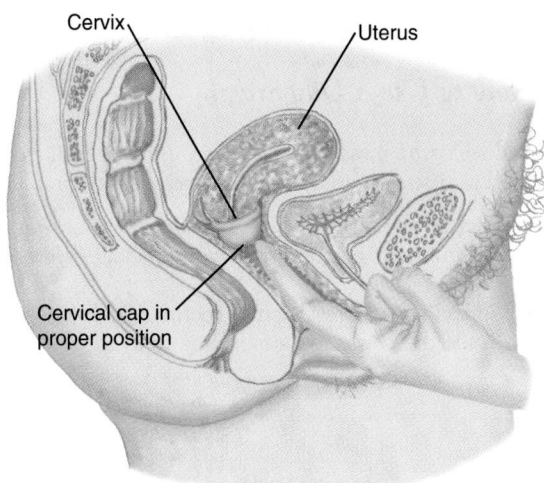

The cervical cap is inserted much like the diaphragm. The woman should check to be certain that it is placed over the cervix.

Diaphragm. The diaphragm is a latex dome surrounded by a spring or coil. The woman places spermicidal cream or gel into the dome and around the rim, then inserts it over the cervix by hand or with a plastic introducer. The diaphragm prevents passage of sperm into the cervix while holding spermicide in place for additional protection. It must be fitted by a nurse practitioner, nurse-midwife, or physician. The woman should be checked for size changes yearly, after a weight gain or loss of more than 10 pounds, and after each pregnancy or abortion.

Pressure on the urethra may cause irritation and urinary tract infections. An allergy to latex or a history of toxic shock syndrome precludes use. The diaphragm may be damaged by some medications used for vaginal infections and should not be used during treatment.

Cervical Cap. The cervical cap is similar to the diaphragm but smaller. The flexible latex cup fits over the cervix and remains in place by suction (Fig. 10–6). Women with cervical abnormalities may not be able to use it. It is 80% effective for nulliparous women but only 60% effective for women who have already given birth.

Because it is smaller than the diaphragm, the cervical cap is less noticeable and causes no pressure on the bladder. It can remain in place for 48 hours, and more spermicide is not needed if intercourse is repeated. It should not be removed for 6 hours after the last intercourse. The nurse should teach the woman to feel her cervix to check placement before and after intercourse, because the cap can be dislodged. It should not be used during menses or in women with a history of toxic shock syndrome (see Chapter 31). The fit should be checked yearly; after abortion, childbirth, or surgery; or if it dislodges frequently.

Natural Family-Planning Methods

Natural family-planning methods, also called fertility awareness or periodic abstinence methods, use physiologic cues to predict ovulation and avoid coitus when conditions are

How to Use a Diaphragm

Follow instructions carefully when using your diaphragm. Skill at insertion and removal increases with practice.

- Plan to insert the diaphragm during lovemaking or several hours before. Empty your bladder before insertion.
- Spread about a teaspoon of spermicidal cream or gel inside the dome and around the rim.

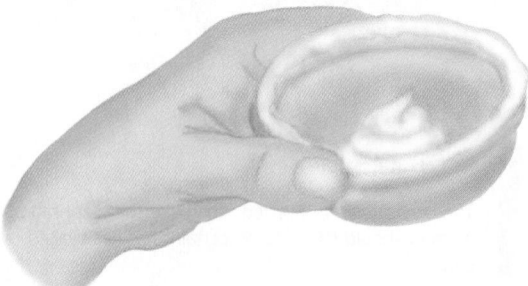

- Insert it into the vagina with the spermicide toward the cervix. A squatting position or placing one foot on a chair makes insertion and removal easier.

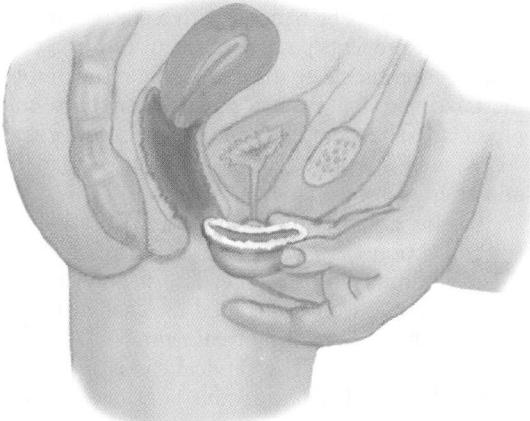

- Be sure that the front rim fits behind your pubic bone and that you can feel the cervix through the center of the diaphragm.

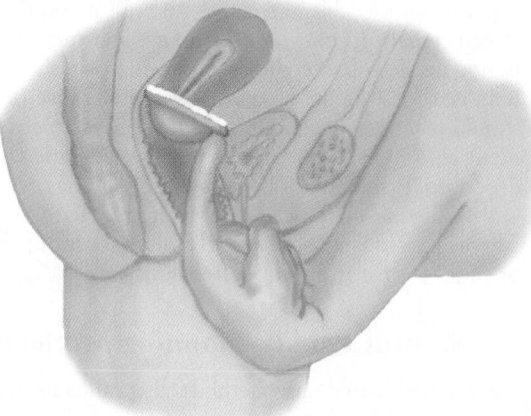

- If more than 6 hours elapse between insertion and intercourse or if you have intercourse again, insert more spermicide into the vagina without removing the diaphragm.
- Leave the diaphragm in place for at least 6 hours after the last intercourse, but to reduce risk of infection, leave it in place for no more than a total of 24 hours.
- Douching with the diaphragm in place is unnecessary and will lessen the effectiveness.
- To remove the diaphragm, assume a squatting position and bear down. Hook a finger around the front rim to break the suction and pull down.

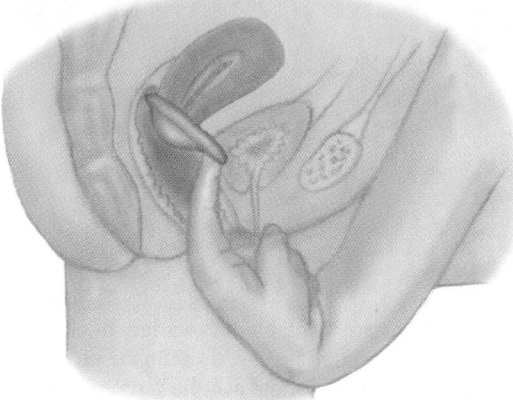

- Wash the diaphragm with mild soap and dry well after each use. Inspect it for holes by holding it up to a light. If you find one, use another contraceptive method and go to your health care provider for a new diaphragm.

favorable for fertilization. They can also help women who wish to become pregnant. The ovum may be fertilized for approximately 24 hours, and some sperm may live up to 72 hours in the female genital tract, although most live only 24 hours (Guyton & Hall, 1996). Some research indicates that fertilization is most likely to occur from coitus during the 6 days up to and including ovulation (Wilcox et al., 1995).

Natural family-planning helps women learn about how their bodies change throughout the menstrual cycle. It is acceptable to most religious groups and avoids the use of drugs, chemicals, and devices. Couples must be highly motivated, however, because they must abstain from intercourse during as much as half the menstrual cycle. Natural family-planning methods may be very effective if used perfectly. The method is very unforgiving, however, and errors in predicting ovulation or intercourse during the forbidden times carry a high risk of pregnancy. Some women use the method to determine when they are fertile and use a barrier contraceptive at that time.

CALENDAR

The calendar method is based on the timing of ovulation, approximately 14 days before the onset of menses. To determine the range in cycle length, the woman keeps track of the length of her cycles for 6 months. She subtracts 18 to 20 days from the shortest cycle and 10 days from the longest cycle to predict the time when fertilization is possible. The calendar method is unreliable because many factors, such as illness or stress, can affect the time of ovulation.

BASAL BODY TEMPERATURE

In the basal body temperature method, the woman charts her oral temperature each morning before getting out of bed or increasing her activity, which would cause her temperature to rise (see Procedure 10–1). Her temperature may drop slightly before ovulation and then rise approximately 0.2° to 0.45°C (0.4° to 0.8°F) with ovulation. The temperature remains higher throughout the second half of the cycle. The woman is no longer fertile on the third day after the rise in temperature.

Used alone, this method is not reliable because temperature changes are very small and the rise in temperature indicates that ovulation has already occurred. Intercourse the day before the temperature rise may well result in pregnancy.

CERVICAL MUCUS (OVULATION)

Also called the "ovulation" or Billings method, the cervical mucus technique is based on changes in cervical mucus. The woman assesses the cervical mucus by wiping it from the vaginal orifice with tissue each day. There is no mucus for the first 3 to 4 days after menses, and then thick, sticky mucus begins to appear. As estrogen increases, the mucus changes to clear, slippery, and stretchy, like egg white. This condition is called *spinnbarkeit* (see Procedure 10–1). After ovulation, mucus decreases in amount and becomes thick and sticky again.

To prevent pregnancy, couples must avoid intercourse from the time mucus is first present until the evening of the fourth day after the height of slippery mucus. Intercourse is allowed only every other day when there is no mucus, because semen interferes with mucus assessment.

SYMPTOTHERMAL METHOD

The symptothermal method combines the calendar, basal body temperature, and cervical mucus methods. In addition, symptoms that occur near ovulation, such as weight gain, abdominal bloating, mittelschmerz (pain on ovulation), or increased libido, are noted.

Least Reliable Methods of Contraception

The following methods of contraception are not considered reliable but are used by women who lack information about

---

PROCEDURE 10–1

. . . .

Teaching Women Fertility Awareness

PURPOSE: To identify whether ovulation occurs and the probable time of ovulation.

Basal Body Temperature

The basal body temperature (BBT) is designed to detect the slight elevation in temperature that accompanies increased progesterone secretion in response to the luteinizing hormone (LH) surge and ovulation.

1. Teach the woman the relationship between her BBT and ovulation:
   a. The BBT is the lowest, or resting, temperature of the body.
   b. During the first half of the woman's menstrual cycle, her temperature is lower than during the second half of the cycle.

c. The basal temperature often drops slightly just before ovulation. Not all women experience this fall in basal temperature.
d. Progesterone is secreted during the second half of the cycle, rising just after ovulation. The BBT rises after the slight drop near ovulation and remains higher during the second half of the cycle.
e. The BBT remains higher if conception occurs and falls about 2 to 4 days before menstruation if conception does not occur.

This method of fertility awareness requires careful assessment and recordkeeping by the woman. She is more likely to have an accurate record if she understands the relationship between her basal temperature and ovulation.

Procedure continued on following page

PROCEDURE 10–1 *Continued*

Teaching Women Fertility Awareness

2. Explain the occurrences that can interfere with the accuracy of her BBT. Examples include illness, restless or inadequate sleep (fewer than 6 hours), waking later than usual, traveling across time zones (jet lag), alcohol intake the evening before, sleeping under an electric blanket or on a heated waterbed, or performing any activity before taking the temperature. *Temperature changes are very slight at ovulation; these factors can cause the temperature to rise even if ovulation has not occurred.*

3. Show the woman a glass fever thermometer and a glass basal thermometer. Explain that the range of temperatures on the basal thermometer is smaller (96° to 100°F) and is marked in tenths of a degree. Explain how to read the marks on the thermometer. Electronic basal thermometers are available that digitally display tenths of a degree. These require less time for accurate assessment than glass ones. The woman should read the instructions that come with her specific thermometer. *The woman should see the differences between a fever thermometer, which may be familiar to her, and a basal thermometer. The temperature rise is very slight (about 0.4°F higher than during the first half of the cycle). A special thermometer is needed to detect the change more accurately. Some women may not know how to read a glass thermometer and should be taught. Reading and following instructions specific for the thermometer increases the accuracy of the assessment.*

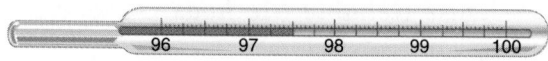

4. Basal temperatures with glass thermometers can be taken orally, rectally, or vaginally. The woman should use the same site for all readings. *Body temperatures vary when different sites are used. The basal temperature identifies very small fluctuations, and varying sites may show changes unrelated to ovulation.*

5. Show the woman the chart for recording her BBT and the symbols for marking relevant events, such as menstrual periods, intercourse, illness, or other occurrences that may alter her BBT. *The chart allows a consistent, more accurate interpretation of temperature fluctuations.*

6. Teach the woman how to take her basal temperature:
   a. If a glass thermometer is used, shake it down the night before.
   b. As soon as she awakens, but before any activity, the basal thermometer should be placed under her tongue and remain until the electronic thermometer beeps. A glass thermometer requires up to 10 minutes for an accurate reading if the oral site is used. The thermometer should remain still while it is registering the temperature.
   c. Record the reading on the chart provided. *Performing any activity before taking the basal temperature, including shaking the thermometer down, can alter the reading enough to cause inaccurate interpretation.*

7. Encourage the woman to demonstrate taking her temperature and recording the result. Ask her to list events other than ovulation that can alter the

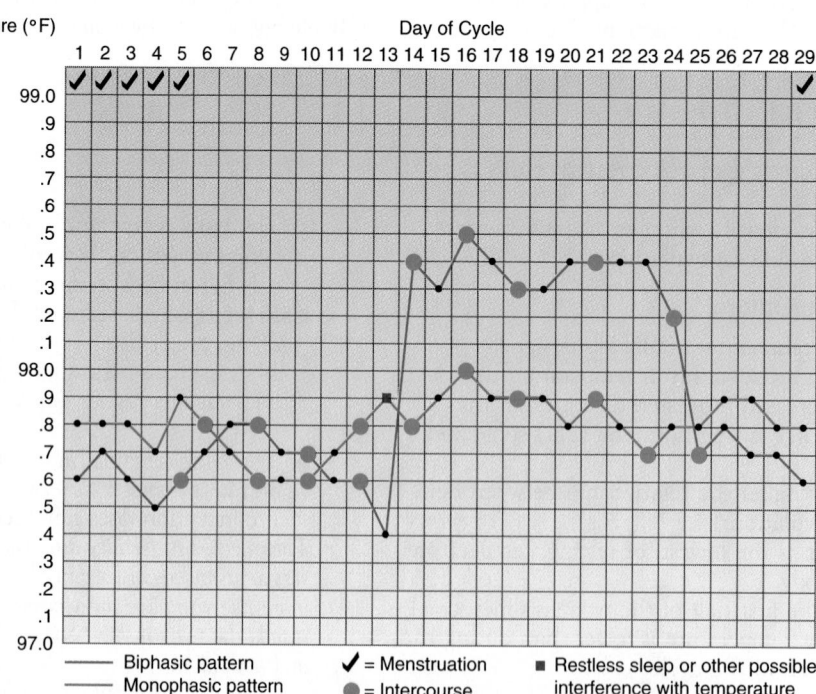

PROCEDURE 10–1 *Continued*

Teaching Women Fertility Awareness

BBT. *Discussion verifies that she has correctly understood the teaching and allows correction of misunderstandings.*

8. As a method to avoid pregnancy: Explain that for the greatest effectiveness, a woman should avoid intercourse from the onset of the menstrual period through the second day of elevated temperature. *The most conservative approach requires a long period of abstinence while a viable ovum could be present, because it primarily identifies that ovulation has already occurred. Not all women have a temperature drop at the time of ovulation, and the rise in BBT occurs after ovulation. Also, sperm can remain viable in the woman's reproductive tract for 72 or more hours, although most die within 24 hours. To reduce the time of abstinence, couples using fertility awareness as a method of contraception usually combine methods, such as BBT and the cervical mucus assessment.*

9. To enhance the chances of conception, the couple should have intercourse when the temperature falls: emphasize that the BBT primarily identifies that ovulation has already occurred and that progesterone secretion is adequate to prepare her endometrium during the second half of her menstrual cycle. The BBT is less effective for timing intercourse to coincide with ovulation because of the short life span of the ovum after ovulation. *Careful timing increases the likelihood that sperm will be available to fertilize the ovum while it is viable. The woman receiving infertility therapy should understand the limitations of the BBT in enhancing conception.*

Cervical Mucus Assessment

To facilitate survival of the sperm and promote their passage into the woman's uterus, the cervical mucus normally changes just before ovulation.

1. Teach the woman how her cervical mucus changes throughout the menstrual cycle. Spinnbarkeit describes how much the mucus can be stretched between her fingers or between a microscope slide and coverslip. Before and after ovulation, the cervical mucus is scant, thick, sticky, and opaque. It stretches less than 6 cm (2.3 inches). Just before and for 2 to 3 days after ovulation, the cervical mucus is thin, slippery, and clear

and is similar to raw egg white. It stretches 6 cm or more. When this ovulatory mucus is present, the woman has probably ovulated and could become pregnant. *As with the BBT, this method requires careful assessment and recordkeeping by the woman. She is more likely to perform the assessment and record changes in her cervical mucus accurately if she understands how the changes relate to fertility.*

2. Explain the factors that can interfere with the accuracy of her assessment. The mucus may be thicker if she takes antihistamines. Vaginal infections, contraceptive foams or jellies, sexual arousal, and semen can make the mucus thinner even if ovulation has not occurred. Tell her to record these factors.

3. Using raw egg white, demonstrate how to stretch mucus between the thumb and forefinger. Have the woman perform a return demonstration of the process. *Visual and tactile experiences enhance learning. A return demonstration allows the nurse to determine whether the woman has misunderstood the teaching.*

4. Teach the woman to wash her hands before and after assessing her mucus. *Hand washing reduces the chance of introducing infection into the reproductive tract and of transferring infectious organisms from the vagina to other areas.*

5. Teach the woman to obtain a small sample of mucus several times a day from just inside her vagina and to note the following:
   a. The general sensation of wetness (around ovulation) or dryness (not near ovulation) on her labia
   b. The appearance and consistency of the mucus: thick, sticky, and whitish or thin, slippery, and clear or watery
   c. The distance the mucus will stretch between her fingers, usually at least 6 cm (2.3 inches) at the time of ovulation.
   This measurement allows the woman to identify cyclic changes in her mucus over the entire duration of her menstrual cycle.

6. Have the woman record the day's typical mucus characteristics (often combined with the BBT recording). *Recording provides a means of evaluating signs and symptoms associated with ovulation during the entire cycle.*

7. As a method of contraception, the woman should avoid intercourse from the time the thin, stretchy ovulatory mucus appears until the fourth day after the height of the slippery mucus. *Avoiding intercourse reduces the chance that sperm are available for fertilization while the ovum is viable.*

8. As a method to enhance conception, the couple should have intercourse every 2 days during the period of ovulatory mucus (approximately days 12 to 16 if the woman has a 28-day cycle). *Timing intercourse makes sperm available to fertilize the ovum while it is viable.*

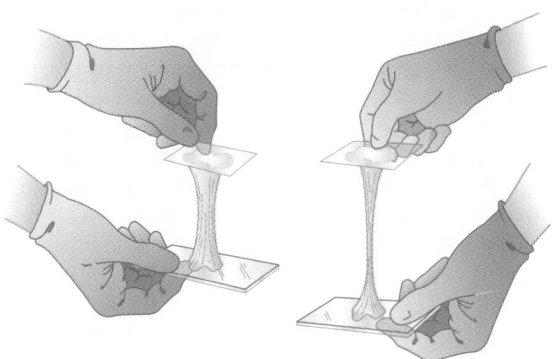

their risks and other options or who will not use other methods for medical or personal reasons. To help women understand the risks involved, the nurse needs to be familiar with these methods.

BREAST-FEEDING

Breast-feeding inhibits ovulation because suckling and prolactin interfere with secretion of gonadotropin-releasing hormone and luteinizing hormone. The frequency, intensity, and duration of suckling are very important in inhibiting ovulation.

Women who breast-feed completely (at least 10 times in 24 hours with no supplementary feedings) may avoid ovulation and resumption of menstrual cycles. The menstrual cycle generally resumes by 6 months. Another method of contraception should be used by this time.

COITUS INTERRUPTUS

Also called withdrawal, coitus interruptus is the removal of the penis from the vagina before ejaculation. Although it has an effectiveness rate of 81%, coitus interruptus requires great control by the man and may be unsatisfying for both partners. Fluid that escapes from the penis before ejaculation is not felt by the man or woman and may contain sperm. Sperm spilled on the vulva may enter the vagina and cause pregnancy.

■ NURSING CARE
Choosing a Contraceptive Method

Assessment

Perform the assessment in a quiet area where interruptions are unlikely. Assure the woman that her confidentiality will be maintained.

Introducing the Subject

In the postpartum setting, introduce the subject by asking the woman if she plans to have more children. Most women indicate a desire to wait a period of time before the next pregnancy. Identify problems that the woman has had in the past with contraception.

Determining the Woman's Understanding

Determine the woman's understanding of her contraceptive technique. For example, ask how she inserts her diaphragm or what time of day she takes her OC. The woman should know how to use her technique effectively and what to do in special circumstances, such as missing an OC pill. Explore any misinformation, concerns, or problems that she may have in regard to effectiveness, technique, or common side effects of the method.

Assessing the Woman's Satisfaction

Assess the woman's satisfaction with her contraceptive. Women may be unsure about their method in the early months until they gain comfort from repetitive use. Side effects also affect satisfaction. They may be severe enough to cause the woman to consider another method, or they may be relieved by simple techniques.

Discussing Available Choices

If the woman is considering a change in contraceptive method, assess for factors that would help determine the best method for her. Include history of medical conditions, childbearing history, cultural and religious beliefs, and intensity of desire to prevent pregnancy. The woman's ability to understand and follow complicated directions is important as well.

The relationship of the couple is important. If the relationship is mutually monogamous, there is no risk of STDs if neither partner is infected. If either of the couple has more than one partner, protection against STDs with a barrier method is essential, even if the woman uses another contraceptive method.

Nursing Diagnosis and Planning

Lack of knowledge about family planning is common. A nursing diagnosis that addresses this problem is

■ Risk for Altered Health Maintenance related to lack of understanding about contraceptive methods chosen and available.
  Expected Outcomes: The woman will correctly describe how to use her contraceptive method, including solving common problems, and will describe common side effects, indications of complications, and correct follow-up. The woman will report that she and her partner are satisfied with their contraceptive method.

Interventions

Increasing Understanding of the Chosen Method

Fill in gaps in the woman's knowledge about how her contraceptive method works, its effectiveness, advantages and disadvantages, common side effects and complications, and when to seek help. Teach with demonstrations and return demonstrations for using the method. Give suggestions for managing side effects and common problems.

Teaching about Other Methods

Provide information about other forms of contraceptives, if the woman wishes. Discuss aspects most important to the woman and her lifestyle. If a prescription or fitting is needed, discuss what may happen during the visit.

Protecting Against Sexually Transmissible Diseases

Address defense against STDs, particularly if the woman is using a method that does not provide protection. This is a delicate subject. A way to approach it might be to say, "The method you are using is very effective against pregnancy but does not protect you against diseases, like HIV, you might catch from a partner. If there is any chance that you or your partner might have sex with more than one person or that your partner might have an infection, you should protect yourself by using one of the barrier types of contraception. Let me explain about those further."

Including the Woman's Partner

Invite the woman to include her partner in discussions, if possible. If the partner understands the proper method of use, he may be more cooperative and willing to help ensure contraceptive success.

Evaluation
- Can the woman explain the proper use of her contraceptive technique?
- Can she describe side effects, complications, and how to solve common problems?
- Do she and her partner report satisfaction with their chosen method?

■ Role of the Nurse in Infertility Care

Although infertility care is a specialty, many general-practice nurses meet persons who are seeking help for infertility or who have had infertility treatment in varied settings, such as perioperative and maternity settings. In addition, parenthood after infertility is not always easy, and nurses who work in pediatric or psychosocial settings may counsel families needing help with parenting and changes in their personal relationships. Friends and family members often see the nurse as one who can answer questions and refer them to appropriate resources when they have problems conceiving.

Extent of Infertility

The extent of infertility depends on how the problem is defined. Infertility is not an absolute condition; it is a reduced ability to conceive. Infertility is strictly defined as the inability to conceive after 1 year of unprotected regular sexual intercourse. A more workable definition does not specify a time limit but recognizes that infertility is any involuntary inability to conceive at the time desired. The definition is commonly expanded to include couples who conceive but repeatedly lose a pregnancy (*pregnancy wastage*) before the fetus is old enough to survive. Couples with primary infertility have never conceived. Couples with secondary infertility may have conceived before but are unable to conceive again.

About 15% to 20% of U.S. couples cannot have a baby when they desire (Carcio, 1998; Edwards & Brody, 1995). Couples who delay childbearing until their middle to late 30s feel pressured by the approaching end of the woman's reproductive years.

Although the rate of infertility has not increased, more couples are seeking help for impaired conception. Some couples delay childbearing until their middle to late 30s, when a natural decline in fertility begins. Because of advances in diagnosis and treatment, couples who might have accepted childlessness may enter infertility therapy or resume therapy they had abandoned. In addition, women who want to have a child without a male partner may be served by infertility services.

Factors Contributing to Infertility

The ability to conceive depends not only on normal reproductive function in each partner but also on a sensitive interaction between the partners. For some couples, identification and treatment of infertility are simple; for other couples, complex evaluation and treatment are required.

Because some factors contributing to infertility remain unknown, treatment of an identified problem does not always lead to a successful pregnancy.

FACTORS IN THE MAN
The test of a man's fertility is his ability to initiate pregnancy in a fertile woman. Few absolute criteria distinguish normal from abnormal male fertility, although an adequate number of sperm having normal structure and function must be deposited near the woman's cervix. Problems may occur with the sperm, with erection or ejaculation, or with the seminal fluid that carries the sperm into the woman's reproductive tract.

Abnormalities of the Sperm. Many factors can impair the number, structure, or function of sperm. Some conditions, such as an acute illness, are temporary; other conditions, such as a genetic disorder, are permanent. A single finding or several findings may be abnormal. Further complicating evaluation of a man's fertility are the normal daily variations in semen.

Evaluation of the semen may reveal that the man has azoospermia or oligospermia. The average number of sperm released at ejaculation is 400 million. Twenty million sperm per milliliter of semen is considered the minimum number adequate for unassisted fertilization.

A sufficient number of normal sperm must move in a purposeful direction to reach the ovum in the fallopian tube. Abnormal sperm structure or movement may reduce fertility, regardless of the actual number of sperm. Inflammatory processes in the man's reproductive organs may cause the sperm to clump, inhibiting their motility and fertilizing ability. Other sperm may look normal but may be unable to penetrate the ovum.

Many factors can impair the number and function of the sperm, such as the following:

- Abnormal hormonal stimulation of sperm production
- Acute or chronic illness such as mumps, cirrhosis, or renal failure
- Infections of the genital tract
- Anatomic abnormalities, such as a varicocele or obstruction of the ducts that carry sperm to the penis
- Exposure to toxins, such as lead, pesticides, or other chemicals
- Therapeutic treatments, such as antineoplastic drugs or radiation for cancer
- Excessive alcohol intake
- Use of illicit drugs, such as marijuana or cocaine
- An elevated scrotal temperature resulting from febrile illness, repeated use of saunas or hot tubs, or sitting for prolonged periods
- Immunologic factors produced by the man against his own sperm (autoantibodies) or by the woman, causing the sperm to clump or be unable to penetrate the ovum

Abnormal Erections. Abnormal erections reduce the man's ability to deposit sperm-bearing seminal fluid in the woman's upper vagina near her cervix. Erections are influenced by both physical and psychological factors. Central nervous system dysfunction, which may be caused by drugs, psychiatric disturbance, or chronic illness, can interfere with erections. Spinal cord disorders and disorders or surgery affecting the autonomic nervous system may also disrupt normal erections. Peripheral vascular disease reduces the amount of blood entering the penis and thus reduces the ability to maintain an erection. Drugs, such as antihypertensives, may reduce the erection or shorten its duration.

Abnormal Ejaculation. Abnormal ejaculation prevents deposition of the sperm in the ideal place to achieve pregnancy. Retrograde ejaculation may occur in the man who has diabetes or neurologic disorders, has had surgery that impairs function of the sympathetic nerves, or takes drugs such as antihypertensives and psychotropics. Men who have suffered spinal cord injury may retain the ability to ejaculate, depending on the level of cord damage.

Anatomic abnormalities, such as hypospadias (urethral opening on the underside of the penis), may cause deposition of semen near the vaginal outlet rather than near the cervix.

Excessive alcohol intake or use of illicit drugs can adversely affect ejaculation as well as sperm number and function. Ejaculation may be slow, absent, or retrograde when a man takes drugs that affect the neurologic coordination of this event. Premature ejaculation is usually related to psychological disorders, such as performance anxiety or unresolved conflicts.

Abnormalities of Seminal Fluid. The seminal fluid nourishes, protects, and carries sperm into the vagina until they enter the cervix. Only sperm enter the cervix; the seminal fluid remains in the vagina. Semen coagulates immediately after ejaculation but liquefies within 30 minutes, permitting forward movement of sperm. Seminal fluid that remains thick traps the sperm, impeding their movement into the cervix. The pH of seminal fluid is slightly alkaline to protect the sperm from the acidic secretions of the vagina. Adequate fructose must be present to provide energy for the sperm. Seminal fluid that is abnormal in amount, consistency, or chemical composition suggests obstruction, inflammation, or infection. The presence of large numbers of leukocytes suggests infection.

FACTORS IN THE WOMAN

A woman's fertility depends on the following:

- Regular production of normal ova
- An open path from her cervix to the fallopian tube to permit fertilization and movement of the embryo into the uterus for implantation
- A uterine endometrium that supports the pregnancy after implantation

Disorders of Ovulation. Normal ovulation depends on delicately timed and balanced secretions from the hypothalamus and pituitary and an ovarian response to mature and release an ovum. The hypothalamus secretes gonadotropin-releasing hormone (GnRH) beginning at puberty. This hormone, in turn, stimulates the pituitary to release follicle-stimulating hormone (FSH) and luteinizing hormone (LH). Follicle-stimulating hormone stimulates maturation of several follicles in the ovary. As the follicles mature, the ovary secretes estrogen to thicken the endometrium. About 24 to 36 hours before ovulation, there is a marked surge of LH, which stimulates final maturation and release of one ovum from its follicle. The other follicles regress permanently. The collapsed follicle from which the ovum was released, now called a *corpus luteum*, produces progesterone and estrogen, which further prepare the endometrium for implantation and nourishment of the fertilized ovum.

Ovulation can be disrupted by the following:

- A dysfunction in the hypothalamus or pituitary gland that alters the secretion of GnRH, FSH, and LH
- Failure of the ovaries to respond to FSH and LH stimulation, preventing maturation and release of the ovum

Disruption of hormone secretion or of the ovarian response to hormone secretion can be caused by many factors, such as cranial tumors, stress, obesity, anorexia, systemic disease, and abnormalities in the ovaries or other endocrine glands. A few women have premature ovarian failure, also known as early menopause.

A woman does not produce new oocytes after her birth. Her existing oocytes are therefore vulnerable until the end of her reproductive life to cumulative toxic effects from therapeutic drugs, social or abused drugs, and environmental agents. Factors that may impair normal ovulation include cancer chemotherapeutic agents, excessive alcohol intake, and cigarette smoking.

Women with ovulation disorders often have abnormal menses because hormone levels do not permit normal development and shedding of the endometrium. Some women have absent, scant, or heavy menstrual periods, but others have no menstrual disorders; inability to conceive may be their only complaint.

As a woman approaches the end of her reproductive life, she ovulates and menstruates more erratically. Thus, her fertility naturally declines with age, falling dramatically after 40 years.

Abnormalities of the Fallopian Tubes. At least one open fallopian tube is needed for conception and implantation. Tubal obstruction may occur because of scarring and adhesions following reproductive tract infections. STDs, such as chlamydia and gonorrhea, are responsible for many cases of infertility from tubal obstruction.

Endometriosis may cause tubal adhesions, painful menstrual periods, and painful intercourse. Small lesions are unlikely to affect tubal function, but large lesions can distort tubal anatomy and lead to infertility.

Tubal obstruction also may occur if adhesions develop after pelvic surgery, ruptured appendix, peritonitis, or ovarian cysts. In addition, the fallopian tubes and other reproductive organs may have congenital anomalies that disrupt normal function.

The conditions that cause obstruction also may interfere with normal motility within the fallopian tube. Poor movement of the fimbriated (distal) end of the tube may prevent the pickup of the ovum from the ovarian surface after ovulation. Abnormal action of the cilia within the tube prevents normal transport of the ovum toward the uterine cavity.

Depending on the extent and location of the blockage, fallopian tube obstructions can prevent fertilization of the ovum or lead to an ectopic pregnancy. Complete tubal occlusion prevents fertilizing sperm from reaching the ovum, and the woman will be sterile without the use of advanced techniques, such as *in vitro* fertilization. Because sperm can reach the ovum to fertilize it but the embryo cannot reach the uterine cavity to implant, partial obstruction may result in a tubal pregnancy.

Abnormalities of the Cervix. Estrogen levels from the ovary peak twice during the menstrual cycle, once before ovulation and again about 1 week after ovulation. The first peak occurs about 2 days before ovulation and causes the woman's cervix to dilate slightly and produce the clear, thin, slippery mucus described on page 205. This mucus facilitates passage of sperm into the uterus and capacitation to ready one sperm for fertilization. Low estrogen levels prevent development of this mucus and are usually associated with anovulation.

Polyps or scarring from past surgical procedures, such as cauterization or conization, may obstruct the woman's cervix. Abnormal cervical mucus caused by estrogen deficiency, surgical destruction of the mucus-secreting glands, and cervical damage secondary to infection or other factors prevent normal capacitation and movement of the sperm into the uterus and fallopian tubes for fertilization.

Repeated Pregnancy Loss

Couples that repeatedly lose pregnancies have the same result as those unable to conceive: no living child. Repeated losses may result from abnormalities in the fetus or placenta or from maternal factors.

ABNORMALITIES OF THE FETAL CHROMOSOMES

Errors in the fetal chromosomes may result in spontaneous abortion, usually in the first trimester. Chromosomal abnormalities often disrupt development severely, and the embryo or fetus cannot survive to live birth.

ABNORMALITIES OF THE CERVIX OR UTERUS

Stenosis or congenital malformations of the cervix or uterine cavity may cause repeated loss of a normal embryo or fetus (Fig. 10–7). These malformations may prevent normal implantation of the fertilized ovum or may prevent normal prenatal growth of the placenta or fetus.

Women who were exposed prenatally to diethylstilbestrol are more likely to have uterine malformations or an incompetent cervix. Cervical or uterine abnormalities also may occur after surgery or trauma from a previous birth. Painless and premature cervical dilation, often early in the second trimester, is characteristic in women with an incompetent cervix.

Uterine myomas, or fibroids (benign tumors of the uterine muscle), and adhesions inside the uterine cavity may cause repeated fetal losses. These problems can alter the blood supply to the developing fetus or cause uterine irritability that results in preterm labor and birth.

ENDOCRINE ABNORMALITIES

Inadequate progesterone secretion by the corpus luteum (luteal phase defect) prevents normal implantation and establishment of the placenta. The embryo may not implant, or it may implant poorly. In other cases, the corpus luteum may develop and function properly, but the woman's endometrium may not respond to its progesterone secretion.

Hypothyroidism and hyperthyroidism may be associ-

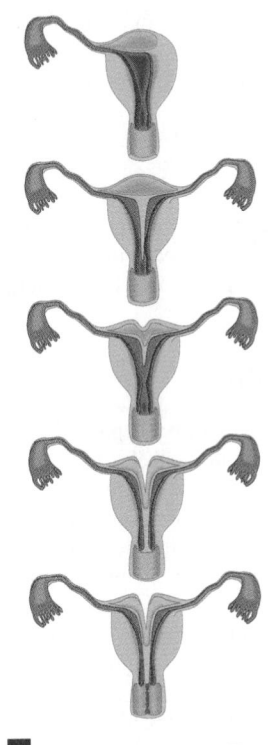

Uterus having a single horn (unicornuate) and only one fallopian tube

Single uterus with a midline septum

Uterus having two horns (bicornuate) with an indentation at the top

Double uterus with one vagina

Double uterus and vagina

FIGURE 10–7

Types of uterine malformations that may cause infertility or repeated pregnancy loss.

ated with the inability to conceive and with recurrent pregnancy loss. Because of its effects on maternal blood glucose levels and the vascular system, poorly controlled diabetes can result in repeated pregnancy loss as well as many other complications of pregnancy.

IMMUNOLOGIC FACTORS

Immunologic factors are implicated in some cases of recurrent pregnancy loss, although not all are established conclusively. The embryo has antigens different from those of the mother and ordinarily would be rejected as any other foreign tissue would be rejected. The mother's body, however, normally blocks this rejection response and tolerates the developing baby. Some women's bodies respond inappropriately to the embryo, rejecting it as foreign tissue. These women often have recurrent spontaneous abortions.

Women with autoimmune disease, such as systemic lupus erythematosus (SLE), are more likely to experience spontaneous abortion. Pregnancy loss in these women appears related to thrombosis or other damage in placental blood vessels. Women with SLE often have other complications during pregnancy, such as exacerbation of their symptoms, fetal heart block, fetal distress, and stillbirth.

ENVIRONMENTAL AGENTS

Some environmental agents have a well-established relationship to impairment of fertility and pregnancy loss. Examples of established toxins are ionizing radiation, alcohol, and isotretinoin (Accutane). Suspected toxins are numerous; among them are cigarette smoke, anesthetic gas, chemicals such as organic solvents or pesticides, and lead and mercury in occupational settings. These agents may be directly toxic to the embryo or fetus, causing its death, or they may interfere with normal placental function necessary to sustain the pregnancy.

INFECTIONS

Infections of the reproductive tract are associated with poor pregnancy outcomes in general, and they may be related to early pregnancy losses as well. These infections are often asymptomatic, making their link to pregnancy loss difficult to establish.

■ Evaluation of Infertility

When a couple seeks help to conceive, both partners are evaluated in a systematic, timely, and cost-effective manner. Couples are often in a hurry for definitive therapy, but a thorough assessment of their problem is essential for suitable treatment. Some tests, such as semen evaluation, must be repeated sequentially for an accurate picture. The prolonged evaluation process is frustrating to many couples, especially older ones who are anxious for a child before the end of the woman's reproductive years. Another frustration is that some diagnostic tests are investigational and their usefulness and normal values are not well established. Other tests are commonly used, but well-accepted normal values have not been established.

Numerous professionals may be involved in evaluation and care of infertile couples: nurses, physicians specializing in reproductive medicine, gynecologists, urologists, microsurgeons, embryologists, and ultrasonographers. In addition, general and specialized laboratory facilities may provide diagnostic services to enhance treatment. Nurses working in infertility clinics often coordinate communication among the many providers and help the couple negotiate the maze of evaluation and treatment.

Preconception Counseling

Couples may be offered preconception counseling to help them evaluate their risk for birth defects and perhaps reduce their risk for bearing a child with a serious birth defect. Many women seeking infertility care are older than 35, an age at which having an infant with a chromosome defect increases (see Chapter 9). A thorough history and physical examination of both members of the couple, including their family histories, may identify increased risk for having a child with a single-gene defect. Counseling can help the woman understand *before conception* the importance of an adequate diet and avoidance of teratogens that can harm the developing fetus even before she knows she is pregnant.

History and Physical Examination

A thorough history and physical examination of each partner can help identify the appropriate diagnostic tests and therapy and identify risks for birth defects in the couple's offspring.

HISTORY

The partners' general health history is reviewed to determine problems that affect their general health as well as their fertility. An extensive reproductive history is also taken. It includes the following:

- The woman's menstrual pattern
- Contraceptive history
- Any pregnancies and their outcomes
- Previous fertility of the man and woman with other partners
- Pattern of intercourse in relation to the woman's menstrual cycles
- Length of time the couple has had unprotected intercourse
- Any home tests the couple has used, such as basal body temperature or over-the-counter ovulation predictor kits

The medical history, including childhood illnesses and surgery and any exposure to toxins, provide clues to the possible cause of infertility. The couple's past and present occupations may identify toxin exposure, stressors, or other adverse influences on reproduction. Investigation of the couple's usual frequency and timing of intercourse may identify the need for a change in practice to promote conception.

PHYSICAL EXAMINATION

Couples that seek help for infertility are usually healthy. A thorough physical examination of each partner, however, may identify endocrine disturbances, cranial tumors, or undiagnosed chronic disease. Examination of the reproductive organs may reveal structural defects, infection, cysts, or other abnormalities. Chromosomal analysis may be performed for couples experiencing repeated pregnancy loss that is not explained by other factors.

Diagnostic Tests

Each couple's evaluation is individualized, but testing generally proceeds from the simple and less expensive to the more complex and expensive diagnostics. Simple evaluations are done simultaneously, but more complex tests are delayed until the need for them is established. Two methods of identifying ovulation, basal body temperature and assessment of cervical mucus, can be used as contraceptive measures in addition to their use in infertility care (see Procedure 10–1).

Five basic tests are common in early infertility evaluation:

- Semen analysis
- Basal body temperature and ovulation predictor kits
- Postcoital test
- Hysterosalpingogram
- Endometrial biopsy

Table 10–5 describes diagnostic tests that may be offered to the infertile couple and the nursing care associated with each.

■ Therapies to Facilitate Pregnancy

Evaluation of the couple identifies whether therapy might improve their chances to conceive and complete a pregnancy. A variety of procedures may be used, depending on the couple's initial and ongoing evaluations and on their

INFERTILE COUPLES WANT TO KNOW

What Is Infertility Treatment Like?

General

- Both members of the couple are evaluated.
- Simpler evaluations and therapies are done before more complex efforts are undertaken.
- A complete medical history and physical examination are done for each partner.
- The ages of the partners, particularly the woman's, are considered. Evaluations and therapy proceed more quickly if the woman is in her mid-30s or older.
- Costs may be partially covered by insurance; check to see what your insurance covers.
- Difficult decisions may be required at different times during evaluation and treatment. Decisions might include whether to proceed to more complex and expensive tests and therapies, whether to take a break from treatment, or whether to abandon treatment altogether.
- Infertility treatment can be stressful, can occupy many hours per week, and requires a substantial commitment to self-care.
- Infertility remains unexplained in about 20% of couples.

Men

- Semen analysis is usually the first test. Several semen specimens are obtained over a period of several weeks to obtain the best evaluation.
- Depending on your medical history, physical examination, and semen analysis, other diagnostic tests may be done (hormone assay, an ultrasonogram of your reproductive organs, a biopsy of your testicles, and specialized tests of sperm function).
- Corrective measures may include medications, surgery, and methods to reduce the scrotal temperature.

Women

- The first evaluation is usually to determine whether you are ovulating each month. You may be taught to take your basal body temperature each morning and to assess your cervical mucus as the first step. These assessments are often done at the same time as other tests.
- Other evaluations may include a postcoital test to determine how your partner's sperm react in your body, an ultrasound examination, a laparoscopy, and a hysterosalpingogram (x-ray of your uterus and tubes).
- For some tests and therapies, an operative procedure is required (hysteroscopy, laparoscopy, laser surgery, or microsurgery) on either an outpatient or an inpatient basis.
- Typically, infertility evaluations and treatments require more of the woman's time, energy, physical discomfort, and risk than the man's.
- Corrective measures depend on the problem identified. Examples include medications, surgery, and advanced reproductive techniques, such as *in vitro* fertilization.

TABLE 10–5

Selected Diagnostic Tests in Infertility

Test/Purpose	Nursing Implications
Male	
Semen Analysis	
Evaluates structure and function of sperm and composition of seminal fluid. Semen volume: 2.0–6.0 ml pH: 7.2–7.8 Sperm concentration: 20 million/ml or more Motility: 50% or more with normal forms Morphology: 60% or more with normal forms Viability: 50% or more live Liquefaction: within 30 min Leukocytes (white blood cells): fewer than 1 million/ml Fructose: 150–600 mg/dl	Explain purpose of semen analysis: three or more specimens are usually collected over several weeks' time for more accurate analysis. Explain to the man that he should collect the specimen by masturbation after a 2- to 3-day abstinence; semen may be collected in a condom if masturbation is unacceptable. Teach the man to note the time the specimen was obtained so the laboratory can evaluate liquefaction of the semen. To maintain warmth, the specimen should be transported near the body and should arrive in the laboratory within 1 hr.
Endocrine Tests	
Evaluate function of hypothalamus, pituitary gland, and the response of the testicles. Assays are made to determine testosterone, estradiol, luteinizing hormone (LH), and follicle-stimulating hormone (FSH) levels. Additional tests may be made on the basis of history and physical findings.	Teach the man about the relationship between hypothalamic and pituitary function and sperm formation; LH stimulates testosterone production by Leydig cells of the testes, and FSH stimulates Sertoli cells of the testes to produce sperm.

Table continued on following page

TABLE 10–5
• • • • • • • • • • • •

Selected Diagnostic Tests in Infertility Continued

Test/Purpose	Nursing Implications
Ultrasonography	
Evaluates structure of prostate gland, seminal vesicles, and ejaculatory ducts by use of a transrectal probe.	Teach the man that ultrasonography uses sound waves to evaluate these structures; no radiation is involved.
Testicular Biopsy	
An invasive test for obtaining a sample of testicular tissue; identifies pathology and obstructions.	Explain the purpose of the test; a local anesthetic is used, and there should be little discomfort.
Sperm Penetration Assay	
Evaluates fertilizing ability of sperm; assesses ability of sperm to undergo changes that allow penetration of a hamster ovum from which the zona pellucida has been removed.	Explain the purpose of the test; abnormal penetration does not necessarily mean that the sperm cannot fertilize a human ovum.
Female	
Ovulation Prediction	
Uses any of several methods to identify the surge of LH, which precedes ovulation by 24–36 hr; improves ability to time intercourse to coincide with ovulation, and identifies the absence of ovulation.	Explain the purpose of the tests (commercial ovulation predictor kits, basal body temperature, and cervical mucus assessment). Teach the woman to follow the instructions on the commercial product. Teach her how to do the basal body temperature and cervical mucus assessment (see Procedure 10–1).
Ultrasonography	
Evaluates structure of pelvic organs. Identifies ovarian follicles and release of ova at ovulation. Evaluates for presence of ectopic or multifetal pregnancy.	Teach the woman that ultrasonography uses sound waves to evaluate these structures; no radiation is involved. Explain preparations needed for specific evaluations.
Postcoital Test	
Evaluates characteristics of cervical mucus and sperm function within that mucus at time of ovulation. Ultrasonography ensures proper timing for test.	Explain that the test is performed 6 to 12 hours after intercourse; the woman may have to rearrange her personal or work commitments each time this test is done.
Endocrine Tests	
Evaluates functions of hypothalamus, pituitary gland, and ovary. Assays are made to determine LH, FSH, estrogen, and progesterone levels. Additional hormone evaluations may be done on the basis of the history and physical findings.	Explain the purpose of each test: FSH and LH stimulate ovulation; estrogen and progesterone prepare uterine endometrium for implantation of a fertilized ovum. Explain the importance of timing within the cycle to provide best information.
Hysterosalpingogram	
X-ray that uses contrast medium to evaluate the structure and patency of the uterus and fallopian tubes.	The test is performed after the menstrual period during the first half of the cycle to avoid flushing menstrual debris through the tubes into the pelvic cavity and to avoid disrupting a pregnancy that might be in place. Explain the purpose of the test. Contrast medium is injected through the cervix, and x-rays are made at the same time.
Endometrial Biopsy (Endometrial Sampling)	
An invasive test for obtaining a small sample of endometrial tissue; determines whether endometrium is responding properly to estrogen and progesterone stimulation from ovary.	Explain the purpose of the test. The test is done 2–3 days before the woman expects her menstrual period; some cramping may occur, but it should be relieved with mild analgesics, such as ibuprofen.
Hysteroscopy and Laparoscopy	
Examines uterine interior and pelvic organs with an endoscope; general anesthesia is used. Identifies abnormalities (polyps, endometrial adhesions). Some surgical procedures may be done via the endoscope.	Explain the purpose of the test and any procedures that will be done at the same time. The woman takes nothing by mouth and should urinate before the procedure. Carbon dioxide gas, used to separate pelvic organs for better visibility, may cause temporary shoulder pain.

personal choices. Some therapy, like timing intercourse to coincide with ovulation, is simple; other procedures may involve considerable expense, discomfort, or unpleasant side effects. Many couples need a combination of treatments to improve their chances of conception.

Identification of appropriate infertility therapy is not always straightforward. Many factors must be considered, including the couple's history, their medical evaluations, financial resources, age and other time constraints, and religious and cultural values. Generally, simpler treatments are indicated before more complex ones, but the needs of each couple are considered individually.

Medications

Medications may be used to improve semen quality, reduce endometriosis, induce ovulation, prepare the uterine endometrium, or support the pregnancy once it is established. Table 10–6 summarizes medications used in infertility therapy.

Ovulation Induction

Medications to induce ovulation may be prescribed for the woman who does not ovulate or who ovulates erratically. Medications may also be given to provide multiple ova if a woman plans to have *in vitro* fertilization, gamete intrafallopian transfer, or tubal embryo transfer. Clomiphene citrate is a drug often used to stimulate ovulation. Clomiphene has also been used to stimulate sperm production, although this use is unlabeled.

Ovulation induction increases the risk of multiple births because several ova may be released and fertilized. Another serious complication is *ovarian hyperstimulation syndrome*, which involves marked ovarian enlargement with exudation of fluid into the woman's peritoneal and pleural cavities. Careful adjustment of medication dosage and serial ultrasound examinations prevent most cases of high multifetal pregnancy (triplets or more) and ovarian hyperstimulation syndrome.

Surgical Procedures

In some men, correction of a varicocele improves sperm quality and quantity. Endoscopic procedures may be used to correct obstructions, with minimal invasiveness in either the man or the woman. The woman may need a laparotomy to relieve pelvic adhesions and obstructions caused by endometriosis, infection, or previous surgical procedures if these cannot be corrected via laparoscopy. Laser surgical techniques may be used to reduce adhesions because they are minimally invasive, precise, and less likely to cause formation of new adhesions. For surgical correction of obstructions in the fallopian tubes or tubal structures in the male genital tract, microsurgical techniques are needed because these structures are very narrow.

TABLE 10–6

Medications Used for Infertility Therapy

Drug	Use
Bromocriptine (Parlodel)	Corrects excessive prolactin secretion by anterior pituitary to induce ovulation and promote development of corpus luteum
Clomiphene (Clomid, Serophene)	Induction of ovulation by stimulating the pituitary production of FSH and LH Treatment of male infertility by increasing sperm production (unlabeled use)
Chorionic gonadotropin, human (hCG; Pregnyl)	Used with menotropins to stimulate ovulation in the female or sperm formation in the male; stimulates progesterone production by corpus luteum
Gonadotropin-releasing hormone (GnRH; Lutrepulse)	Stimulates release of FSH and LH from the pituitary gland in men and women who have deficient GnRH secretion by their hypothalamus; FSH and LH, in turn, stimulate ovulation in the female and stimulate testosterone production and spermatogenesis
Leuprolide (Lupron)	Reduces endometriosis; adjunct to drug given to stimulate ovulation
Menotropins (FSH and LH; Pergonal)	Promotes follicular growth and maturation; stimulates spermatogenesis (given with hCG)
Nafarelin (Synarel)	Reduces endometriosis
Progesterone	Promotes implantation of embryo
Urofollitropin (Metrodin)	Stimulates ovulation (given in conjunction with hCG)

Transcervical balloon tuboplasty may be used to unblock the fallopian tubes without more invasive procedures, such as laparoscopy or laparotomy. A thin catheter is threaded through the uterus into the fallopian tube, and the balloon is inflated to clear the blockage.

Therapeutic Insemination

The technique of therapeutic insemination (formerly called artificial insemination) may use either the partner's semen or that of a donor to overcome a low sperm count. Donor insemination also may be used if the man carries a genetic defect or if a woman wants a biologic child without having a relationship with a male partner. Intrauterine insemination (IUI) is a variation that allows the sperm to bypass cervical mucus and reduces some immunologic incompatibilities by injecting sperm directly into the uterus.

Sperm for therapeutic insemination or IUI are obtained from semen collected by masturbation. The sperm are washed in a series of solutions in the laboratory and then concentrated before they are used for inseminations. This process also removes many of the antibodies that interfere with sperm motility and ability to penetrate the ovum.

Men who donate semen for therapeutic insemination are screened to reduce the risk of transmitting diseases or genetic defects. They are questioned about their personal and family health history, including genetic disorders or birth defects. Questions about their social habits and personality can disclose high-risk behaviors and also give recipient parents information about traits their child might have. Physical and laboratory examinations are performed to evaluate the man's general health, determine his blood type and Rh factor, and screen for infections such as STDs or human immunodeficiency virus (HIV). Carrier testing for some genetic defects, such as sickle cell and Tay-Sachs diseases, reduces the risk of passing on these disorders. To reduce the risk of transmitting diseases that may not be apparent at the initial screening, donor semen is frozen and held for 6 months before use. The man is retested for diseases such as HIV several times during the 6 months.

Surrogate Parenting

A surrogate mother may enter the picture if the woman is infertile or if she cannot carry a fetus to live birth. Surrogacy is different from therapeutic insemination because it is not anonymous. In addition, the woman who carries the child inevitably forms bonds with the fetus during the months of pregnancy.

Money paid to the surrogate mother can raise issues of baby selling. Could a poor but fertile woman feel compelled to provide her body for a more well-to-do couple? Yet not compensating a woman for the real physical and emotional risks of this undertaking can be construed as exploitative as well.

Custody issues are clearer when the birth mother is a gestational surrogate than when she also donates her ovum to the child. Courts have more often recognized the genetic parents as the legal parents and upheld the contracts between them and the gestational surrogate. In surrogacy and other advanced techniques, the laws are behind the available technology.

Advanced Reproductive Techniques

One class of advanced reproductive technologies bypasses many natural obstacles to conception by placing intact gametes together to allow fertilization. This class includes *in vitro* fertilization (IVF), gamete intrafallopian transfer (GIFT), and tubal embryo transfer (TET). Each of these procedures begins with ovulation induction to permit retrieval of several ova, thus improving the likelihood of a successful pregnancy. Sperm are prepared and concentrated as they are for therapeutic insemination.

Another class of advanced reproductive technologies involves assisting fertilization with microsurgical techniques. These techniques bypass obstacles to fertilization by penetrating the ovum with tiny needles to allow placement of the sperm within the ovum or its surrounding zona pellucida.

Couples who have concerns about a specific genetic defect in the family may be offered preimplantation genetic testing of their embryo. This testing allows them to make informed decisions about whether they wish to implant the resulting embryo into the uterus.

IN VITRO FERTILIZATION

The technique of IVF involves bypassing blocked or absent fallopian tubes. The physician removes the ova by laparoscope or by ultrasound-guided transvaginal retrieval and mixes them with prepared sperm from the woman's partner or a donor. Two days later, up to four embryos are returned to the uterus to increase the likelihood of a successful pregnancy. Additional embryos may be transferred if the woman is older. The woman receives supplemental progesterone to enhance the receptivity of her endometrium to implantation.

GAMETE INTRAFALLOPIAN TRANSFER

For GIFT to take place, the woman must have at least one patent fallopian tube. The procedure begins in a manner similar to that of IVF, with retrieval of multiple ova and washed sperm. The retrieved ova are drawn into a catheter that also carries prepared sperm. Sperm and up to two ova per tube are injected into each fallopian tube through a laparoscope (Fig. 10–8). Additional prepared sperm may be injected into the uterus through the cervix to improve the chance of successful fertilization. Progesterone is given to enhance implantation of any fertilized ova.

TUBAL EMBRYO TRANSFER

Tubal embryo transfer, also called *zygote intrafallopian transfer (ZIFT)*, is a hybrid of IVF and GIFT. The woman's ova are fertilized outside her body as in IVF, but the resulting fertilized ova are placed in the fallopian tubes and enter the uterus naturally for implantation. The woman must have at least one patent fallopian tube.

COMPARISON OF *IN VITRO* FERTILIZATION, GAMETE INTRAFALLOPIAN TRANSFER, AND TUBAL EMBRYO TRANSFER

The primary advantage of GIFT and TET over IVF is a higher pregnancy rate. With IVF or TET, there is evidence of fertilization before placement in the uterus or tubes. The

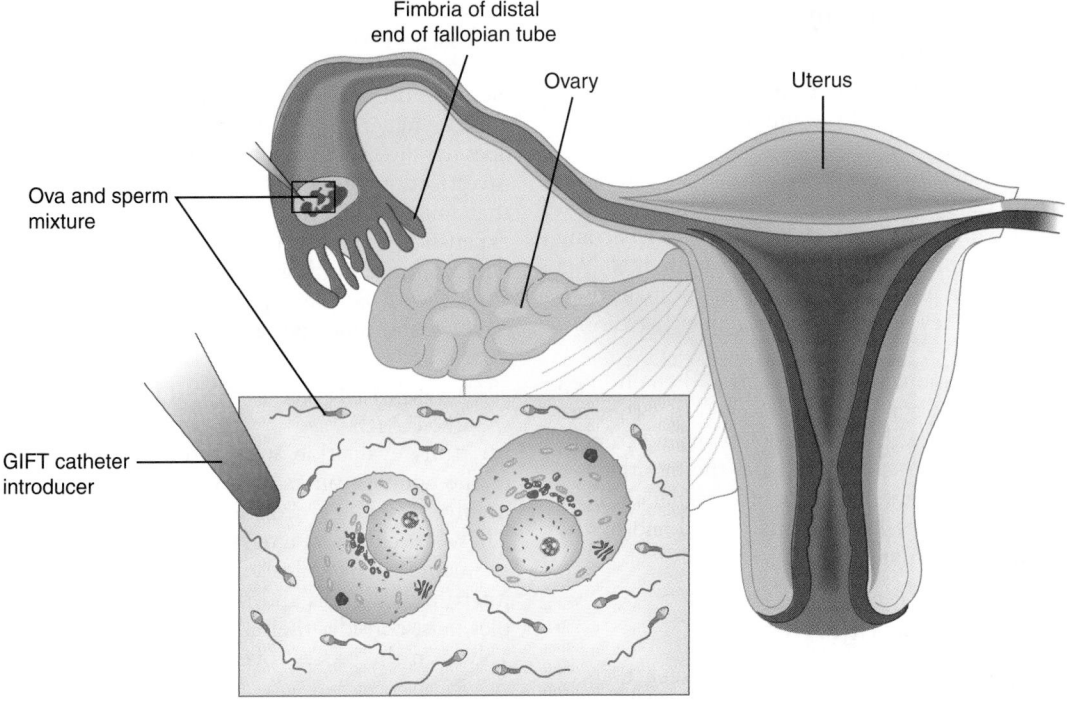

Fimbria of distal
end of fallopian tube

Ovary

Uterus

Ova and sperm
mixture

GIFT catheter
introducer

FIGURE 10–8

Gamete intrafallopian transfer (GIFT). Multiple ova and washed sperm are injected into the fallopian tube, where fertilization may occur.

disadvantage of these procedures is that the woman will need to have a laparoscopy to retrieve gametes (IVF) or to place the gametes (GIFT) or fertilized ova (TET) into the fallopian tube. Either GIFT or TET may result in a tubal pregnancy if the embryo cannot reach the uterine cavity to implant.

These reproductive techniques can result in multifetal pregnancy, sometimes high multiples. Pregnancies with more than twins carry a substantially higher risk to both mother and infants because of preterm labor and birth, placental insufficiency, and a high demand on maternal body systems. Selective reduction in the number of fetuses may give those remaining a better chance to progress to a live birth. Such a procedure is, of course, heavily laden with emotional and ethical concerns.

MICROSURGICALLY ASSISTED FERTILIZATION

Microsurgical techniques, related to IVF but considerably more complex, may help couples to conceive despite severe male infertility. Only one or a few sperm are required to use these procedures. The sperm may be obtained from ejaculated semen, by aspiration from the epididymis using microsurgical techniques, or by testicular biopsy.

One technique involves making small slits in the zona pellucida cells that surround the ovum to allow sperm to gain access to the ovum itself to achieve fertilization. A similar technique injects sperm into the space just under the zona pellucida. Direct injection of a spermatozoon into the cytoplasm of the ovum is called intracytoplasmic sperm injection. For these techniques, the retrieval of oocytes and

the placement of the resulting conceptus into the uterus are similar to those of IVF.

Responses to Infertility

The desire for children is strong in many couples. If a couple does not achieve pregnancy or produce a living child as expected, the man and woman often experience psychological distress and a threat to their self-images. Either or both partners may feel like failures. Their marital and family relationships may be stressed, and they may withdraw from relationships with others that they previously found satisfying.

Assumption of Fertility

Many couples practice contraception for a number of years before they decide to have a baby. When they do want a child, they discontinue contraception and assume that pregnancy will occur within a few months at most.

Either or both partners may experiment with the role of parent as they anticipate pregnancy. They develop a heightened awareness of children and parenting. Being with others who are expecting or who already have children is exciting because they plan to join their ranks shortly. They may discuss issues such as full-time parenting by one partner, child care, and future lifestyle changes. They may begin acquiring toys and furnishings a child will need. Both partners may develop a fantasy child or a concept of what their baby will be like.

Growing Awareness of a Problem

As the months pass, the couple gradually becomes concerned about the inability to conceive. If the woman is older, they feel the urgency of the limited time before her reproductive years end.

The couple begins to feel uneasy with child-related activities. Now they are not so sure when they will be parents. Events such as baby showers or christenings may become melancholy rather than joyful occasions. Family members and friends who are having children may feel guilty at their good fortune when they are around the couple that cannot conceive.

The potential grandparents may feel that their children are waiting too long to start a family or even that they are selfish. If they are aware that the couple is trying to conceive, they become even more worried as the months pass without the longed-for announcement of a pregnancy. They are twice saddened by the lack of a grandchild and by the hurt their adult children are enduring.

Seeking Help for Infertility

Eventually, couples must decide whether to seek help to conceive. They may reach this point after only a few menstrual cycles or, at the opposite extreme, may never seek help. Many factors enter into their decision. These include their ages (especially the woman's), how long they have been unable to conceive, how much they want a biologic child, how they regard adoption, and how they feel about a child-free life.

IDENTIFYING THE IMPORTANCE OF HAVING A BABY

Each partner may place a different priority on having a baby. Conflicts may arise when one partner wants help to conceive sooner than the other. In addition, cultural or religious beliefs influence how each feels about procreation and whether options such as assisted reproductive procedures or adoption are acceptable. How the couple resolves these differences is crucial to the stability of the relationship.

Men and women often differ in their reactions to infertility. Women may want to talk about their feelings and frustrations, but men often internalize their feelings or feel that they must be strong for their partner. The woman may interpret her partner's reluctance to express his feelings and his stoicism as disinterest or lack of concern and care for her.

SHARING INTIMATE INFORMATION

Although the infertility specialist will limit questions to those necessary, evaluation and treatment for infertility require that both partners reveal intimate information about their sexual relationship, such as the frequency and timing of intercourse. In addition, infertile couples may feel that the evaluation calls their sexual adequacy into question.

CONSIDERING FINANCIAL RESOURCES

Financial concerns enter into the couple's decision about whether to seek treatment and how far to carry it. Techniques such as basal body temperature assessment or ovulation predictor kits are fairly inexpensive but have limited usefulness in achieving a pregnancy when there are complex problems. Advanced techniques, such as IVF, are expensive and may have a very low likelihood of success for some couples. Health insurance may not cover infertility treatment at all or may not cover all procedures because the problem does not directly threaten the health of either partner. Also, investigational treatments are often not covered. The drugs that must be taken to achieve pregnancy are often quite expensive. Expense and restricted coverage limit treatment choices for many low-income or middle-income couples. Those who seek and pursue infertility treatment usually have greater financial resources than those who do not.

COMMITTING TO INVOLVEMENT IN CARE

Infertility evaluation and treatment require a commitment of the couple's time, energy, and money. Couples can be involved in this process for most or even all of a decade. They participate on a day-to-day basis as they do home assessments, take medications, and keep detailed records. For infertility diagnosis and therapy to be most effective, couples must consider their ability and desire to be directly involved in the process over a long period.

Reactions During Evaluation and Treatment

Couples undergoing infertility evaluation and treatment have different reactions to the process. In addition, their reactions may change as infertility care progresses.

INFLUENCES ON DECISION MAKING

If their evaluation shows that a treatment or procedure may enable them to conceive, the couple must then decide whether to proceed. The decision-making process begins early and must be repeated during therapy if pregnancy does not occur. A complex array of factors enters into their decisions about beginning and continuing treatment or whether to end their pursuit of pregnancy. These factors interact dynamically as the couple makes each decision. The nurse helps both partners examine each factor and arrive at a decision that is best for them.

Social, Cultural, and Religious Values. Some medically appropriate options may not be acceptable to every couple. Surrogate parenting, IVF, and therapeutic insemination (especially with donor sperm) are inconsistent with the personal or religious beliefs of many people. If a procedure offers the partners hope for a child but is incompatible with their beliefs, their choices are two: use the technology despite their beliefs or accept childlessness. Adoption may be a third alternative for some couples if the desire for a biologic child is not absolute. As in other decisions, couples must work out conflicting personal values about what therapy is acceptable.

Difficulty of Treatment. The couple must consider how difficult, risky, and uncomfortable therapy will be. The level of difficulty involves physical, psychological, geographic, and time factors. Employment constraints often affect treatment decisions as well.

Several infertility treatments involve invasive procedures or surgery. The person who undergoes the procedure must be the one who ultimately decides whether to do it. That person alone can decide whether the hope of a child is worth the risks and discomfort of the procedure.

Infertility treatment is stressful. Often partners feel or are willing to tolerate different levels of stress. To reduce the stress, they may abandon treatment completely or may take a vacation for a few months from the constant preoccupation with conceiving. Women nearing or in their 40s often do not feel that they have the luxury of skipping a treatment cycle.

Some couples encounter geographic difficulties if they must travel a long distance for therapy. Time stresses are substantial. The partners, particularly the woman, feel that achieving pregnancy is their new career. One or both partners may spend many hours every week in pursuit of pregnancy.

Employment constraints may be a barrier to infertility therapy because of the time required for treatment. The impact of time is usually greatest on the woman. Time away from work may burden the employer or coworkers. Stopping work may not be an option because the family needs the money and often needs the insurance coverage that comes with employment.

Probability of Success.   Couples often have a biased interpretation of their statistical probability of success, especially when they begin treatment with a new procedure. For example, if a procedure has a 15% likelihood of success with each cycle, they tend to expect that they will be in the successful group rather than in the 85% who do not meet with success. As time goes by, however, they must weigh the likelihood of success of any therapy against financial concerns and their own willingness to accept the discomfort and difficulty associated with it.

Financial Concerns.   Some couples, particularly those with ample resources and a strong desire for a biologic child, pursue expensive treatments and pursue them longer than others of more limited means. They may do so despite a low probability of success. Couples with financial limitations find that they must abandon treatment sooner than they want. Other couples go heavily into debt, adding financial strain to the other stresses of treatment in their quest for a child of their own.

PSYCHOLOGICAL REACTIONS

A couple's initial reaction to infertility is often one of shock because the partners are usually healthy and often have had no idea that they might have problems conceiving. Their reactions vary according to how easily their infertility is alleviated, their personalities and self-images, and the strength of their relationship.

Guilt.   A partner having the only identified problem might feel that he or she is depriving the other of children. This feeling may be compounded if the "normal" partner has children from another relationship. It may be difficult for this person to understand that not all factors affecting fertility can be detected and that what seems like the one partner's problem is often the couple's problem.

Either partner may feel guilty about past choices that now affect fertility. A woman with adhesions resulting from a sexually acquired infection may regret her past choices. The man who wanted to delay pregnancy longer than the woman may feel guilty if her age is now limiting the time she has for conceiving.

Isolation.   Infertile couples often feel different from friends and relatives who do not have difficulty conceiving. To insulate themselves from painful reminders of their infertility, they may withdraw from these relationships. Some couples develop supportive relationships with others who are also infertile, which somewhat diminishes their sense of isolation.

Depression.   One or both partners may experience depression as their sense of competence and control over their bodies is challenged, especially if therapy is not successful quickly. They often feel as if they are on a roller coaster of hope alternating with despair when the woman has her menstrual period each month. In an attempt to insulate themselves from disappointment, couples with long-term infertility try not to expect too much with each cycle.

The couple may feel envious of those who conceive easily. They may become judgmental and angry when they see those who seem to "have no business having a baby," such as an adolescent or a poor woman who has several children.

Stress on the Relationship.   Because infertility can challenge one's identity and self-esteem, the partners may find less satisfaction in their relationship. They may feel unlovable or unappealing to their mates.

The man may find it difficult to perform on demand for semen specimens and postcoital tests, feeling that others will judge his sexual function. The fact that semen samples are best obtained by masturbation is unacceptable to some men. Both partners are stressed when intercourse must be scheduled to coincide with specific evaluations or with ovulation. Intercourse can become a chore or a medical procedure more than an expression of love. It may come to be associated with failure rather than fulfillment.

If sperm from an anonymous donor is used for therapeutic insemination or other techniques, the man may feel that his masculinity is further threatened. He may have difficulty distinguishing fatherhood as a biologic achievement from fatherhood as a relationship.

The partners find their relationship strained if they disagree on which treatments are appropriate and how long they should be pursued. One partner may want to keep trying "one more month," and the other may want to abandon treatment. If they are considering adoption, their relationship may be strained if they differ on whether to adopt and what kind of child they are willing to accept.

Outcomes After Infertility Therapy

After infertility therapy, three outcomes are possible. Pregnancy may be achieved and then lost, causing mixed emotions of grief and optimism. The couple may become parents, either biologically or through adoption. Infertility therapy may be unsuccessful, and the couple must decide whether to pursue adoption.

PREGNANCY LOSS AFTER INFERTILITY THERAPY

Couples who suffer pregnancy loss after infertility therapy may interpret the experience with mixed feelings of loss and gain. Couples undergoing infertility evaluation and treatment are often aware of a pregnancy much earlier than fertile couples. They want to hope yet expect to be disappointed again. If a spontaneous abortion occurs, they may grieve profoundly for what they achieved and then lost.

Yet despite their grief about the pregnancy loss, the partners may be encouraged because they have proved that they can achieve a pregnancy. They may feel that if they succeeded once, they can do it again.

PARENTHOOD AFTER INFERTILITY THERAPY

Couples that achieve conception experience varied emotions. If they have been disappointed many times before, they may hardly believe the good news. Pregnancy after infertility therapy is emotionally tentative for many infertile couples, especially those who have been trying to conceive for a long time or those who have lost a pregnancy. They may distance themselves from the reality of the pregnancy until much later in gestation than would fertile couples. The woman has grown accustomed to sensing and reporting every symptom and may interpret normal physiologic changes of pregnancy as a threat.

The previously infertile couple may find little sympathy from those who do not understand their fear of investing in the pregnancy. Others may be annoyed because they expect the couple to be overjoyed at a successful and apparently normal pregnancy. Outsiders may feel that the partners are self-centered and cannot decide what they want. Other infertile couples, who were previously a source of mutual support, may withdraw from the couple that achieves a pregnancy.

The parents' anxiety may be heightened during labor. They are afraid that something will go wrong at the last moment. Even after the birth of a healthy infant, some parents have difficulty relaxing and enjoying their baby.

These new parents often need much nursing support as they gain experience with their child. Infertile couples who eventually have biologic or adopted children may have unrealistic expectations about parenting. After investing so much financial, physical, and emotional resources in having a child, they may be reluctant to express any unhappiness or frustration over the realities of childrearing.

CHOOSING TO ADOPT

Couples who consider adoption must confront their personal preferences, limitations, and biases. As much as they want a child, many couples are not willing to adopt *any* child. Most couples prefer to adopt a newborn or an infant of their race. Some prefer an infant but are also willing to adopt an older child, one with special needs, one of a mixed or different race, or a group of siblings. Other couples, for a variety of reasons, will not consider adopting these children. Couples, particularly older ones, may turn to foreign adoption because they are considered too old to be adoptive parents by most U.S. agencies.

Some couples fear adopting a child because the woman might become pregnant. Although pregnancy has been the goal for a long time, they may worry that they would love their adopted child differently from their biologic child.

Couples that decide to adopt face further scrutiny of their personal lives. Agencies investigate their home, financial means (which may have been seriously drained),

and fitness as parents. Once again, they may feel that their personal competence is questioned.

The couple that decides on adoption may have emotions similar to those who achieve a pregnancy. They may be slow to invest in the process emotionally because they expect disappointment again. In addition, the adopted child often comes to them suddenly and unexpectedly. Although they may have been waiting months for this happy event, they have little time to adjust to the reality that they are becoming parents.

▌ NURSING CARE
· · · · · · · · · · ·
The Infertile Couple

Nursing care of the infertile couple is challenging but can be most satisfying. Regardless of the setting where they are encountered, the nurse often addresses the couple's emotional needs associated with infertility evaluation, treatment, and outcomes of therapy.

Assessment

Most infertile couples have previously had a positive self-image and feelings of competence about themselves. The diagnosis of infertility shakes their positive view. The nurse should be aware that these feelings may underlie their physical concerns.

Determine at what point the couple is in their infertility treatment. Couples who have just discovered that they may have difficulty conceiving may be shocked yet optimistic that therapy will result in a baby for them. Couples with longstanding infertility may have a deeper sense of failure and a pessimistic outlook. Listen for remarks that are negative, expressing guilt or helplessness.

Evaluate how infertility has affected the partners' relationships with each other. Are there conflicts or differences in their values? Observing their body language, such as eye contact, may provide clues about how similarly or differently they are committed to diagnosis and treatment. Ask them how their relationship has changed. Are they more or less satisfied with their marital relationship than they were before they had problems conceiving?

Ask about support systems. Couples suffering from infertility often withdraw from old relationships but do not form new supportive ones. Do others who are significant in the partners' lives know that they are trying to conceive? Are family members and friends nearby, and are they supportive? Have they encountered others' assumptions that infertility is the "fault" of one partner or the other? Are they subjected to questions that invade their privacy, such as, "When are you two going to have a baby of your own?"

Elicit information about how the couple's culture or religion views infertility and the impact of these values on therapy. Are there therapies that are unacceptable to one or both partners?

Determine how the couple is coping with the stresses of treatment. How much has infertility cost them in time, money, and discomfort? Identify the successes and failures they have experienced. Their ages, especially the woman's, add another stressor that they cannot avoid.

If the woman is pregnant or has given birth recently or if the couple has adopted a child recently, observe for high levels of anxiety in either or both parents. Assess them for negative behaviors and comments, such as reluctance to feel joy or a sense that they will "fail" again.

Nursing Diagnosis and Planning

A nursing diagnosis commonly encountered is

■ Situational Low Self-Esteem related to perception of reproductive inadequacy.
   Expected Outcomes: The person(s) will express feelings about infertility and its evaluation and treatment, will explore ways to increase control within the situation of infertility, and will identify aspects of self that are positive.

Expected outcomes may apply to the man, the woman, or both partners.

Interventions

Assisting Communication

Use a variety of communication techniques, such as active listening and exploration, to encourage the partners to express their feelings honestly. Provide privacy and acceptance of their feelings.

Encourage the partners to accept their feelings, both positive and negative. For example, the couple that has finally achieved pregnancy may be living a lie to some extent. The partners may act elated because they believe they should feel happy yet inside feel cautious and hesitant to become attached to their baby. Explain that feelings are not right or wrong but simply exist. It may be helpful to open the subject of negative feelings (fear of attachment) within a successful situation (pregnancy or birth) to reinforce the normality of their mixed emotions. This technique gives them the opportunity to talk about emotional reactions that they or others feel are inappropriate and might otherwise be reluctant to discuss.

Discuss possible differences in ways the man and the woman communicate. For example, explain that the woman may feel more comfortable than the man in talking about their problem and concerns about treatment. Explain that these differences in communication style can cause misunderstandings because one partner believes that the other does not care as much about their problem. Encourage them to be open with each other for the best mutual support.

Increasing the Couple's Sense of Control

Explore how the couple has dealt with stressors in the past and how these techniques might be used to cope with the present crisis. Reinforce positive coping skills, such as learning more about infertility and the proposed therapy for it.

Couples that experience undue stress may benefit from relaxation techniques, such as visualization and moderate exercise. Frequent strenuous exercise may reduce the woman's ability to ovulate. Although a hot tub is relaxing for many people, it should be avoided because the high temperatures may inhibit spermatogenesis. In addition, the woman could become pregnant with any cycle, and high body temperatures have been associated with fetal anomalies.

Discuss behaviors that enhance the ability to handle stress and that provide a good environment for a pregnancy that might occur. Reinforce healthy choices, such as good nutrition and a balance between exercise and rest. Teach the couple ways to enhance general health if deficiencies are identified.

Explain any procedures and their purpose in language that the couple can understand. Reinforce any medical explanations they have been given. Encourage questions so that the couple is fully informed. Have the partners restate what was explained to reduce misunderstandings.

Help the couple explore options at each decision point. No one else can decide the best course of action, but the nurse can help identify pros and cons of each choice so that the partners can arrive at a decision appropriate for them. Be nondirective so that the choices are theirs and do not reflect the biases of the nurse or other caregivers.

Reducing Isolation

Because couples often distance themselves from friends and family relationships that they find painful, they may have few social supports. Refer them to available support groups to provide emotional outlets, a sense of belonging, and a source of information. Help them to identify ways they can improve communication with family and friends. Remind them that they have undergone significant shifts in self-image that have also affected those around them.

Promoting a Positive Self-Image

Explore with them areas of competence and activities that make them feel good about themselves. Reinforce positive attitudes and self-evaluations. Encourage them to maintain activities such as hobbies, sports, or volunteer work. The career of either partner may be a source of stress that needs relief, or it may be an avenue that fosters a positive self-perception.

Evaluation

• Did the partners express their feelings about their situation, usually over a period of time?
• Did the partners explore ways to increase personal control over their lives and express feelings of reduced helplessness and dependence?
• Did the partners identify one or more aspects of self perceived as positive and identify areas of competence?

KEY CONCEPTS
. . . .

■ The nurse plays an important role in educating women about contraceptive techniques available and their correct use.
■ In choosing the best contraceptive method for an individual woman, important issues include safety, protection from STDs, effectiveness, convenience, education needed, side effects, interference with spontaneity, availability, expense, preference, religious beliefs, and culture.
■ Because some methods have potential for serious complications,

- an informed consent form may be necessary.
- Adolescents often have erroneous beliefs and incorrect information about contraception that increase their risk of pregnancy and STDs.
- Adolescents feel more comfortable talking about contraception with a nurse who has an accepting attitude, provides extra time for education, and uses understandable terms and audiovisual materials.
- Contraception is necessary to prevent pregnancy until menstruation has ceased for 2 years. The healthy perimenopausal woman who does not smoke or have contraindications can use any method of contraception safely.
- Sterilization offers permanent contraception. A tubal ligation can be performed soon after birth or at any time. Vasectomy is less expensive and can be performed in an office under local anesthesia. Although surgery to reverse sterilization is possible, it is expensive and not always successful.
- Hormonal contraceptives include OCs, hormone injections, and the progestin implant. Hormonal contraceptives inhibit ovulation and make the cervical mucus unreceptive to sperm. Side effects and complications make these unsuitable for some women.
- Intrauterine devices are very effective and safe in women with no risk of STDs. Women must learn how to check for the device's strings and when to seek medical treatment.
- Barrier methods may be chemical or mechanical. They kill or prevent sperm from entering the cervix and provide some protection against STDs.
- Natural family-planning methods involve avoidance of coitus when physiologic cues suggest that ovulation is likely. They are acceptable to most religions but involve extensive education and high motivation and have a high risk of pregnancy should error occur.
- About 20% of infertile couples have no identified problem explained by current evaluation techniques.
- Because of the many unknown factors in reproduction, identification and correction of problems in one or both partners do not necessarily resolve their infertility.
- A variety of structural and functional abnormalities may contribute to a couple's infertility. The man may have abnormalities of the sperm or of the seminal fluid, or with ejaculation. The woman may have ovulation disorders, anatomic problems such as fallopian tube occlusion, or physiologic disorders such as hormone imbalances.
- A systematic evaluation of both partners, proceeding from simple to more complex, identifies therapy most likely to be successful and cost effective.
- Infertility is a crisis for the couple and often for the extended family. Either or both partners may feel that the inability to conceive represents a personal failure.
- Infertile couples must make choices at many points before and during evaluation and therapy. Some major factors that enter into their decisions involve social, cultural, and religious values; difficulty of treatment; probability of success; financial resources; and age, particularly the woman's.
- The possible outcomes after infertility therapy may present new challenges to the partners and their families: unsuccessful therapy and the choice of whether to pursue adoption, pregnancy loss after infertility, and parenthood after infertility.

ANSWER TO CRITICAL THINKING EXERCISE 10–1

Find a private place to talk without interruption. Use therapeutic communication to explore this girl's feelings further. Help her think through the ways a pregnancy might change her life and how she would feel about those changes. Discuss what happens when a woman is examined during a visit for contraceptive counseling. Explore what she feels would be most embarrassing about seeing a physician. Would a female nurse practitioner, midwife, or physician be more acceptable? Discuss common contraceptive methods and determine her understanding and feelings about them. Also discuss negotiation skills for condom use, because condoms are important for prevention of STDs as well as pregnancy. Try role playing with the adolescent acting the role of her partner and the nurse taking the role of the adolescent.

REFERENCES AND READINGS

American College of Obstetricians and Gynecologists. (1996). Emergency oral contraception. ACOG Practice Patterns, Number 2. Washington, DC: Author.

AWHONN. (1995). Wyeth-Ayerst offers legal aid to Norplant system prescribers. AWHONN Voice, 3(3), 2.

Beckman, L. J., & Harvey, S. M. (1996). Factors affecting the consistent use of barrier methods of contraception. Obstetrics and Gynecology, 88(3, suppl.), 65S–71S.

Balen, A. H., & Jacobs, H. S. (1997). Infertility in practice. New York: Churchill Livingstone.

Borgatta, L. (1998). Managing clinical complexities of long-term contraception. Medscape Women's Health, 3(1).

Boxer, A. S. (1996). Images of infertility. Nurse Practitioner Forum, 7(2), 60–63.

Carcio, H. A. (1998). Causes of infertility. In H. A. Carcio (Ed.), Management of the infertile woman (pp. 25–48). Philadelphia: Lippincott.

Cunningham, F. G., MacDonald, P. C., Gant, N. F., Leveno, K. J., Gilstrap, L. C., Hankins, G. D. V., et al. (1997). Williams obstetrics (20th ed.). Norwalk, CT: Appleton & Lange.

Dinerman, L. M., Wilson, M. D., Duggan, A. K., & Joffe, A. (1995). Outcomes of adolescents using levonorgestrel implants vs. oral contraceptives or other contraceptive methods. Archives of Pediatrics and Adolescent Medicine, 149, 967–972.

Edwards, R. G., & Brody, S. A. (1995). Principles and practices of assisted human reproduction. Philadelphia: Saunders.

Freda, M. C., Abruzzo-Fogarassy, M., Adams, N. V., Davini, D., DeVore, N., & Merkatz, I. R. (1996). Women's responses to Depo-Provera. MCN: American Journal of Maternal/Child Nursing, 21(4), 183–186.

Friedman, C. I. (1994). Male infertility: Intrauterine insemination. In F. A. Zuspan & E. J. Quilligan (Eds.). *Current therapy in obstetrics and gynecology 4* (pp. 83–86). Philadelphia: Saunders.

Geerling, J. H. (1995). Natural family planning. *American Family Physician, 52*(6), 1749–1756.

Gerchufsky, M. (1995). Updating family planning options. *Advance for Nurse Practitioners, 3*(5), 18–23.

Glasier, A., & Baird, D. (1998). The effects of self-administering emergency contraception. *New England Journal of Medicine, 339*(1), 1–4.

Guyton, A. C., & Hall, J. E. (1996). *Textbook of medical physiology* (9th ed.). Philadelphia: Saunders.

Hatasaka, H. (1995). Implantable levonorgestrel contraception: 4 years of experience with Norplant. *Clinical Obstetrics and Gynecology, 38*(4), 859–871.

Hatcher, R. A. (1998). Depo-Provera, Norplant and progestin-only pills (minipills). In R. A. Hatcher, J. Trussell, F. Stewart, W. Cates, G. K. Stewart, F. Guest, & D. Kowal. *Contraceptive technology* (17th ed., pp. 467–509). New York: Ardent Media.

Hatcher, R. A., & Guillebaud, J. (1998). The pill: Combined oral contraceptives. In R. A. Hatcher, J. Trussell, F. Stewart, W. Cates, G. K. Stewart, F. Guest, & D. Kowal. *Contraceptive technology* (17th ed., pp. 405–466). New York: Ardent Media.

Hesla, J. S., & Murphy, A. A. (1995). The effects of contraceptive agents on the endometrium. *Infertility and Reproductive Medicine Clinics of North America, 6*(2), 379–400.

Hiltabiddle, S. J. (1996). Adolescent condom use, the health belief model, and the prevention of sexually transmitted disease. *Journal of Obstetric, Gynecologic, and Neonatal Nursing, 25*(1), 61–66.

Hirsch, A. M., & Hirsch, S. M. (1995). The long-term psychosocial effects of infertility. *Journal of Obstetric, Gynecologic, and Neonatal Nursing, 24*(6), 517–522.

Hogsdon, B. B., & Kizior, R. J. (1998). *Saunders nursing drug handbook 1998.* Philadelphia: Saunders.

Jambunathan, J., & Stewart, S. (1995). Hmong women in Wisconsin: What are their concerns in pregnancy and childbirth? *Birth, 22*(4), 204–210.

Jirka, J., Schuett, S., & Foxall, M. J. (1996). Loneliness and social support in infertile couples. *Journal of Obstetric, Gynecologic, and Neonatal Nursing, 25*(1), 55–60.

Johnson, C. L. (1996). Regaining self-esteem: Strategies and interventions for the infertile woman. *Journal of Obstetric, Gynecologic, and Neonatal Nursing, 25*(4), 291–295.

Kennedy, K. I. (1999). Fertility, sexuality, and contraception during lactation. In J. Riordan & K. G. Auerbach. *Breastfeeding and human lactation* (2nd ed., pp. 675–705.)

Kennedy, K. I., & Trussell, J. (1998). Postpartum contraception and lactation. In R. A. Hatcher, J. Trussell, F. Stewart, W. Cates, G. K. Stewart, F. Guest, & D. Kowal. *Contraceptive technology* (17th ed., pp. 589–614). New York: Ardent Media.

Keye, W. R., Chang, R. J., Rebar, R. W., & Soules, M. R. (1995). *Infertility: Evaluation and treatment.* Philadelphia: Saunders.

Kipersztok, S. (1995). The new progestins. *Infertility and Reproductive Medicine Clinics of North America, 6*(1), 61–75.

Kjos, S. (1996). Contraception in diabetic women. *Obstetrics and Gynecology Clinics of North America, 23*(1), 243–258.

Lande, R. E. (1995). New era for injectables. *Population reports,* Series K, 23(5). Baltimore: Johns Hopkins University, Population Information Program.

Lauver, D., Armstrong, K., Marks, S., & Schwarz, S. (1995). HIV risk status and preventive behaviors among 17,619 women. *Journal of Obstetric, Gynecologic, and Neonatal Nursing, 24*(1), 33–39.

Lethbridge, D. J. (1995). Fertility management in Taiwanese and African-American women. *Journal of Obstetric, Gynecologic, and Neonatal Nursing, 24*(5), 459–463.

Lindberg, C. E. (1997). Emergency contraception: The nurse's role in providing postcoital options. *Journal of Obstetric, Gynecologic, and Neonatal Nursing, 26*(2), 144–152.

Mahan, L. K., & Escott-Stump, S. (1996). *Krause's food, nutrition, and diet therapy* (9th ed.). Philadelphia: Saunders.

Marquette, C. M., Koonin, L. M., Antarsh, L., Gargiullo, P. M., & Smith, J. C. (1995). Vasectomy in the United States, 1991. *American Journal of Public Health, 85*(5), 644–649.

Mastroianni, L. (1996). Forty years of infertility management: Exponential progress and a demanding future. *Nurse Practitioner Forum, 7*(2), 87–91.

Mishell, D. R. (1997). Family planning. In D. R. Mishell, M. A. Stenchever, W. Droegemueller, & A. L. Herbst. *Comprehensive gynecology* (pp. 283–352). St. Louis: Mosby–Year Book.

Murphy, P., Kirkman, A., & Hale, R. W. (1995). A national survey of women's attitudes toward oral contraception and other forms of birth control. *Women's Health Issues, 5*(2), 94–99.

Nelson, A. (1995). Patient selection key to IUD success. *Contemporary OB/GYN, 40*(10), 49–62.

O'Connell, M. L. (1996). The effect of birth control methods on sexually transmitted disease/HIV risk. *Journal of Obstetric, Gynecologic, and Neonatal Nursing, 25*(6), 476–480.

Potter, L. S. (1996). How effective are contraceptives? The determination and measurement of pregnancy rates. *Obstetrics and Gynecology, 88*(3, suppl.), 113S–123S.

Rosenberg, M. J., Waugh, M. S., & Long, S. (1995). Unintended pregnancies and use, misuse and discontinuation of oral contraceptives. *Journal of Reproductive Medicine, 40*(5), 355–360.

Schnare, S., & Mtsuda, K. J. (1997). Today's contraceptive choices. *RN, 60*(12), 30–37.

Schoener, C. J., & Krysa, L. W. (1996). The comfort and discomfort of infertility. *Journal of Obstetric, Gynecologic, and Neonatal Nursing, 25*(2), 167–172.

Sherrod, R. A. (1995). A male perspective on infertility. *MCN: American Journal of Maternal/Child Nursing, 20*(5), 269–275.

Stansberry, J. (1996). The infertile couple: An overview of pathophysiology and diagnostic evaluation for the primary care clinician. *Nurse Practitioner Forum, 7*(2), 70–86.

Stewart, G. K., & Carignan, C. S. (1998). Female and male sterilization. In R. A. Hatcher, J. Trussell, F. Stewart, W. Cates, G. K. Stewart, F. Guest, & D. Kowal. *Contraceptive technology* (17th ed., pp. 545–588). New York: Ardent Media.

Tessler, S. L., & Peipert, J. F. (1997). Perceptions of contraceptive effectiveness and health effects of oral contraception. *Women's Health Issues, 7*(6), 400–406.

Tietz, N. W. (1995). *Clinical guide to laboratory tests* (3rd ed.). Philadelphia: Saunders.

Timbers, K. A., & Feinberg, R. F. (1996). Recurrent pregnancy loss: A review. *Nurse Practitioner Forum, 7*(2), 64–75.

Treiman, K., Liskin, L., Kols, A., & Rinehart, W. (1995). IUDs: An update. *Population Reports* (Series B, No. 6). Baltimore: Johns Hopkins University, Population Information Program.

Trent, A. J. & Clark, K. (1997). What nurses should know about natural family planning. *Journal of Obstetric, Gynecologic, and Neonatal Nursing, 26*(61), 643–648.

Trussell, J., Ellertson, C., & Stewart, F. (1996). The effectiveness of Yuzpe regimen of emergency contraception. *Family Planning Perspectives, 28*(2), 58–64, 87–88.

Trussell, J., & Kowal, D. (1998). The essentials of contraception. In R. A. Hatcher, J. Trussell, F. Stewart, W. Cates, G. K. Stewart, F. Guest, & D. Kowal. *Contraceptive technology* (17th ed., pp. 211–247). New York: Ardent Media.

Trussell, J., Leveque, J. A., Koenig, J. D., London, R., Borden, S., Henneberry, J., LaGuardia, K. D., Stewart, F., Wilson, T. G., Wysocki, S., & Strauss, M. (1995). The economic value of contraception: A comparison of 15 methods. *American Journal of Public Health, 85*(4), 494–503.

Wilcox, A. J., Weinberg, C. R., & Baird, D. D. (1995). Timing of sexual intercourse in relation to ovulation. *New England Journal of Medicine, 333*(23), 1517–1521.

11

Reproductive Anatomy and Physiology

LEARNING OBJECTIVES

After studying this chapter, you should be able to:

- Explain female and male sexual development from prenatal life through sexual maturity.
- Describe normal anatomy of the female and male reproductive systems.
- Explain normal function of the female and male reproductive systems.
- Explain normal structure and function of the female breast.

DEFINITIONS

amenorrhea Absence of menstruation. Primary amenorrhea is a delay of the first menstruation. Secondary amenorrhea is cessation of menstruation after its initiation.

cilia Hairlike processes on the surface of a cell. Cilia beat rhythmically to move the cell or to move fluid or other substances over the cell surface.

climacteric Endocrine, body, and psychic changes occurring at the end of a woman's reproductive period. Also informally called menopause.

coitus Sexual union between a male and a female.

fornix (pl. fornices) An arch or pouchlike structure at the upper end of the vagina. Also called a cul-de-sac.

gamete Reproductive cell: in the female an ovum, and in the male a spermatozoon.

genetic sex Sex determined at conception by union of two X chromosomes (female) or an X and a Y chromosome (male). Also called chromosomal sex.

gonad Reproductive (sex) gland that produces gametes and sex hormones. The female gonads are ovaries; the male gonads are testes.

gonadotropic hormones Secretions of the anterior pituitary gland that stimulate the gonads, specifically follicle-stimulating hormone and luteinizing hormone. Chorionic gonadotropin is secreted by the placenta during pregnancy.

graafian follicle A small sac within the ovary that contains the maturing ovum.

menarche Onset of menstruation; average age is 13 years.

menopause Permanent cessation of menstruation during the climacteric.

puberty Period of sexual maturation accompanied by the development of secondary sex characteristics and the capacity to reproduce.

ruga (pl. rugae) Ridge or fold of tissue, as on the male's scrotum and in the female's vagina.

secondary sex characteristics Physical differences between mature males and females that are not directly related to reproduction.

somatic sex Gender assignment as male or female on the basis of form and structure of the external genitalia.

spermatogenesis Formation of male gametes (sperm) in the testes.

spinnbarkeit Clear, slippery, stretchy quality of cervical mucus during ovulation.

This chapter reviews basic prenatal development, sexual maturation, and structure and function of both female and male reproductive systems.

Sexual Development

Sexual development begins at conception, when the genetic sex is determined by union of an ovum and a sperm. During childhood, the sex organs are quiet.

Prenatal Development

The mother's ovum carries a single X chromosome. Each of the father's spermatozoa carries either an X chromosome or a Y chromosome. If an X-bearing spermatozoon fertilizes the ovum, the offspring's genetic sex is female. If a Y-bearing spermatozoon fertilizes the ovum, a male offspring results.

Although genetic sex is determined at conception, the reproductive system of both males and females is similar, or sexually undifferentiated, for the first 6 weeks of prenatal life. During the seventh week, differences between males and females appear in the internal structures. The external genitalia look similar until the ninth week, when these outer structures begin to change. Differentiation of the external sexual organs is complete at about 12 weeks.

During fetal life, both ovaries and testes secrete their primary hormones, estrogen and testosterone, respectively. Testosterone causes development of male sex organs and external genitalia, and its absence results in development of female sex characteristics. Although estrogen is secreted by the fetal ovary, this hormone is not required to initiate development of female sex structures. The trend for prenatal sexual development is to have female structures unless a Y chromosome is present.

Childhood

The sex glands of both girls and boys are inactive during infancy and childhood. At sexual maturity, the hypothalamus stimulates the anterior pituitary gland to produce hormones that, in turn, stimulate sex hormone production by the gonads.

Sexual Maturation

Puberty refers to the time during which the reproductive organs become fully functional. Puberty is not a single event but a series of changes occurring over several years during late childhood and early adolescence.

INITIATION OF SEXUAL MATURATION

Not all of the factors that initiate sexual maturation are known. Secretions of the hypothalamus, the anterior pituitary, and the gonads all play a part. The hypothalamus is capable of secreting gonadotropin-releasing hormone (GnRH) to initiate puberty during infancy and early childhood, but it does not do so in significant amounts until late childhood. Production of even tiny quantities of sex hormones by the young child's ovaries or testes inhibits secretions of the hypothalamus, avoiding premature onset of puberty. Maturation of another brain area, as yet unknown, probably triggers the hypothalamus to initiate puberty (Guyton, 1996).

The maturing child's hypothalamus gradually increases production of GnRH beginning at about 8 years of age. The level of GnRH increases slowly until it is adequate to stimulate the anterior pituitary to increase its production of follicle-stimulating hormone (FSH) and luteinizing hormone (LH). The ovaries and testes increase production of sex hormones and begin maturing gametes in response to higher levels of FSH and LH. The sex hormones also induce development of secondary sex characteristics. Table 11–1 presents the major hormones that play a role in reproduction.

There is individual variation in the age at which the changes of puberty begin and in the time required to complete these changes. Nutritional state can influence the start of puberty, with the well-nourished child having an earlier onset. Girls are about 6 months to 1 year younger than boys when hormonal changes of puberty begin, although the girl's growth spurt earlier in puberty makes it seem that she begins puberty about 2 years before boys of the same age. Changes of puberty occur in an orderly sequence in both sexes. Increases in height and weight are dramatic during puberty but slow after puberty until the mature height and weight are attained. Table 11–2 lists secondary sex characteristics of males and females.

FEMALE PUBERTY CHANGES

As the girl matures, the anterior pituitary gland secretes increasing amounts of FSH and LH in response to the hypothalamic secretion of GnRH. These two pituitary secretions stimulate secretion of estrogens and progesterone by the ovary, resulting in maturation of the reproductive organs and breasts and in development of secondary sex characteristics such as axillary and pubic hair. The first noticeable changes of puberty begin at about 10 to 11 years in girls, with the development of breast buds. The first menstrual period occurs 2 to 2.5 years later, when the girl is about 12 to 13 years old.

Breast Changes. The earliest outward changes of puberty occur in the breasts. First, the nipple enlarges and protrudes. The areola surrounding the nipple enlarges and becomes somewhat protuberant, although less so than the nipple. These changes are followed by growth of the glandular and ductal tissue. Fat is deposited in the breasts. During puberty, a girl's breasts often develop at different rates, resulting in a temporarily lopsided appearance.

Body Contours. The pelvis widens and assumes a rounded, basinlike shape that is favorable for passage of the fetus during childbirth. Fat is deposited selectively in the

TABLE 11–1
• • • • • • • • • • • •

Major Hormones in Reproduction

Produced by	Target Organs	Action in Female	Action in Male
Gonadotropin-Releasing Hormone (GnRH)			
Hypothalamus	Anterior pituitary	Stimulates release of FSH and LH, initiating puberty and sustaining female reproductive cycles; release is pulsatile	Stimulates release of FSH and LH, initiating puberty; release is pulsatile
Follicle-Stimulating Hormone (FSH)			
Anterior pituitary	Ovaries (female) Testes (male)	1. Stimulates production of estrogens, progesterone 2. Stimulates growth and maturation of graafian follicles before ovulation	Stimulates sperm formation in Sertoli cells of testes
Luteinizing Hormone (LH)			
Anterior pituitary	Ovaries (female) Testes (male)	1. Stimulates final maturation of follicle 2. Surge of LH about 14 days before next expected menstrual period causes ovulation 3. Stimulates transformation of graafian follicle into corpus luteum, which continues secretion of estrogens and progesterone for about 12 days if ovum is not fertilized. If fertilization occurs, placenta gradually assumes this function.	Stimulates Leydig cells of testes to secrete testosterone
Estrogens			
1. Ovaries and corpus luteum (female) 2. Placenta (pregnancy) 3. Formed in small quantities from testosterone in Sertoli cells of testes (male); other tissues, especially the liver, produce estrogen in the male	Internal and external reproductive organs; breasts (female) Testes (male)	1. Reproductive organs a. Maturation at puberty b. Stimulation of endometrium before ovulation 2. Breasts: induce growth of glandular and ductal tissue; initiate deposition of fat at puberty 3. Stimulate growth of long bones but cause closure of epiphyses, limiting mature height 4. Pregnancy: stimulate growth of uterus, breast tissue; inhibit active milk production; relax pelvic ligaments	Necessary for normal sperm formation
Progesterone			
Ovary, corpus luteum, placenta	Uterus, female breasts	1. Stimulates secretion of endometrial glands; causes endometrial vessels to become highly dilated and tortuous in preparation for possible embryo implantation	Not applicable

Major Hormones in Reproduction Continued

Produced by	Target Organs	Action in Female	Action in Male
Ovary, corpus luteum, placenta (*cont.*)		2. Pregnancy: induces growth of cells of fallopian tubes and uterine lining to nourish embryo; decreases contractions of uterus; prepares breasts for lactation but inhibits prolactin secretion	
Prolactin			
Anterior pituitary	Female breasts	Stimulates secretion of milk (lactogenesis); estrogen and progesterone from placenta have an inhibiting effect on milk production until after placenta is expelled at birth; sucking of newborn stimulates prolactin secretion to maintain milk production	Not applicable
Oxytocin			
Posterior pituitary	Uterus, female breasts	1. Uterus; stimulates contractions during birth and stimulates postpartum contractions to compress uterine vessels and control bleeding 2. Stimulates let-down, or milk-ejection reflex during breast-feeding	Not applicable
Testosterone			
Testes (male) Adrenal glands (female) Ovaries (female)	Sexual organs (male) Male body conformation after puberty	Small quantities of androgenic (masculinizing) hormones from adrenal glands cause growth of pubic and axillary hair at puberty. Most androgens, such as testosterone, are converted to estrogen.	1. Induces development of male sex organs in fetus 2. Induces growth and division of the cells that mature sperm 3. Induces development of male secondary sex characteristics

hips, giving them a rounder appearance than those of the male.

Body Hair. Pubic hair appears, downy at first but becoming thicker as puberty progresses. Axillary hair appears near the time of menarche. The texture and quantity of pubic and axillary hair vary among women and in different ethnic groups. Women of African descent usually have body hair that is coarser and curlier than that of white women. Asian women often have sparser body hair than women of other racial groups.

Skeletal Growth. In response to estrogen stimulation, the girl grows taller for several years during early puberty. The growth spurt begins about 1 year after initial breast development. Estrogen's other powerful effect on the skeleton is to cause the epiphyses (growth areas of the bone) to unite with the shaft of the bones; this development eventually stops growth in height.

Reproductive Organs. The girl's external genitalia enlarge as fat is deposited in the mons pubis, labia majora, and labia minora. The vagina, uterus, fallopian tubes,

TABLE 11-2

Comparison of Secondary Sex Characteristics in Females and Males

Females	Males
Development of glandular and ductal systems in the breast; deposition of fat selectively in the breast, buttocks, and thighs	Muscle mass 50% greater
Wide, round pelvis	Narrow, upright, and heavier pelvis
Pubic and axillary hair	Pubic and axillary hair; facial and chest hair; increased amount of hair on upper back in some males; male-pattern baldness, beginning on top of head
Soft, smooth skin texture	Coarser skin
Higher-pitched voice	Deeper voice

and ovaries grow larger. In addition, the vaginal mucosa changes, becoming more resistant to trauma and infection in preparation for sexual activity. Cyclic changes in the reproductive organs occur during each female reproductive cycle.

Menarche. Two to 2.5 years after a girl's breasts begin developing, she experiences her first menstrual period. Early menstrual periods are often irregular and scant. These early menstrual cycles are not usually fertile because ovulation occurs inconsistently. Fertile reproductive cycles require preparation of the uterine lining precisely timed with ovulation. Ovulation may occur during any female reproductive cycle, however, including the first. The sexually active girl can conceive even before her first menstrual period.

Delayed onset of menstruation is called *primary amenorrhea* if the girl's periods have not begun by the age of 16 years. It may also be considered if the girl is more than 1 year older than her mother or sisters were when their menarche occurred. *Secondary amenorrhea* describes absence of menstruation for at least three cycles after regular cycles have been established. Both primary and secondary amenorrhea are more common in females who are thin because they may have too little fat to produce enough sex hormones to stimulate ovulation and menstruation. Pregnancy is a common cause of secondary amenorrhea as well.

MALE PUBERTY CHANGES

Secretion of GnRH by the hypothalamus begins increasing at about the age of 10 to 13 years, stimulating secretion of LH and FSH from the anterior pituitary. LH and FSH then stimulate secretion of testosterone and eventually spermatogenesis. Testosterone stimulates development of a boy's reproductive organs and secondary sex characteristics. The outward changes of puberty begin at about 13 to 16 years of age.

Growth of the Testes and Penis. The first outward evidence of male sexual maturation is growth of the testes. Growth in circumference and lengthening of the penis follow about a year after testicular growth begins. The skin of the scrotum thins and darkens.

Nocturnal Emissions. Often called "wet dreams," nocturnal emissions commonly occur during the teenage years. The boy experiences a spontaneous ejaculation of seminal fluid during sleep, often accompanied by dreams with sexual content. It is important to prepare boys for this normal occurrence so that they do not feel abnormal or ashamed.

Body Hair. Pubic hair growth begins at the base of the penis. Gradually the hair coarsens and spreads upward and in the midline of the abdomen. About 2 years later, axillary hair appears. Facial hair begins as a fine, downy mustache and progresses to the characteristic beard of the adult male. In most boys, chest hair develops, and some have hair on their upper backs. The amount and character of body hair vary among men of different racial groups, with Asian and Native American men often having less than white or African men.

Body Composition. Testosterone causes the male to develop a greater muscle mass than the female. At maturity, the man's muscle mass exceeds the woman's by 50%.

Skeletal Growth. Testosterone causes boys to undergo a rapid growth spurt, especially in height. A boy's linear growth begins about a year later than a girl's and lasts for a longer time, resulting in the male's greater average height at maturity. Testosterone causes union of the epiphysis with the shaft of long bones, as estrogen does in girls. The height-limiting effect of testosterone, however, is not as strong as that of estrogen in females, so boys grow in stature for several years more than girls.

A boy's shoulders broaden as his height increases. His pelvis assumes a more upright shape, with a narrower diameter and heavier composition than the female's.

Voice Changes. Hypertrophy of the laryngeal mucosa and enlargement of the larynx cause the male's voice to deepen. Before reaching its bass tones at maturity, many boys experience an embarrassing "cracking" or "squeaking" of their voices when they speak.

Decline in Fertility

A woman's ability to reproduce decreases over a period of years called the climacteric. In most women, the climacteric occurs between the ages of 45 and 50. At this time, maturation of ova and production of ovarian hormones decline. The external and internal reproductive organs atrophy somewhat as well. Menopause is the term used to describe the final menstrual period. *Menopause* and *climacteric*, however, are often used interchangeably to describe the entire gradual process of change. *Perimenopause* is the time from onset of symptoms associated with the climacteric until at least 1 year after the last menstrual period.

Males do not experience a distinct marker event like menopause. Their production of testosterone and sperm gradually declines, but men in their 50s, 60s, and beyond may still be able to father children.

Female Reproductive Anatomy

External Female Reproductive Organs

Collectively, the external female reproductive organs are called the *vulva* (Fig. 11–1).

MONS PUBIS
The mons pubis is the rounded, fleshy prominence over the symphysis pubis that forms the anterior border of the external reproductive organs. It is covered with varying amounts of pubic hair.

LABIA MAJORA AND LABIA MINORA
The labia majora are two rounded, fleshy folds of tissue that extend from the mons pubis to the perineum. They have a slightly deeper pigmentation than surrounding skin and are covered with pubic hair. The labia majora protect the more fragile tissues of the external genitalia.

The labia minora run parallel to and within the labia majora. The labia minora extend from the clitoris anteriorly and merge posteriorly to form the fourchette, or posterior rim of the vaginal introitus. The labia minora do not have pubic hair. They are highly vascular and respond to stimulation by becoming engorged with blood.

CLITORIS
The clitoris is a small projection at the anterior junction of the labia minora. The clitoris is composed of highly sensitive erectile tissue that is similar to that of the penis. The labia majora merge to form a prepuce over the clitoris.

VESTIBULE
The vestibule refers to structures enclosed by the labia minora. The urinary meatus, vaginal introitus, and ducts of Skene's and Bartholin's glands lie within the vestibule. Skene's, or periurethral, glands provide lubrication for the urethra. Bartholin's glands provide lubrication for the vaginal introitus, particularly during sexual arousal.

The vaginal introitus is surrounded by erectile tissue. During sexual stimulation, blood flows into the erectile tissue, allowing the introitus to tighten around the penis. This process adds a massaging feeling that heightens the male's sexual sensations, encouraging release of semen.

The hymen is a thin fold of mucosa partially separating the vagina from the vestibule. The hymen may be broken with injury, with the use of tampons, during intercourse, or during childbirth. The intactness, or lack thereof, of the hymen is not a criterion of virginity.

PERINEUM
The perineum is the most posterior part of the external female reproductive organs. It extends from the fourchette anteriorly to the anus posteriorly and is composed of fibrous and muscular tissues that support pelvic structures.

Internal Female Reproductive Organs

The internal reproductive structures are the vagina, uterus, fallopian tubes, and ovaries (Figs. 11–2 and 11–3).

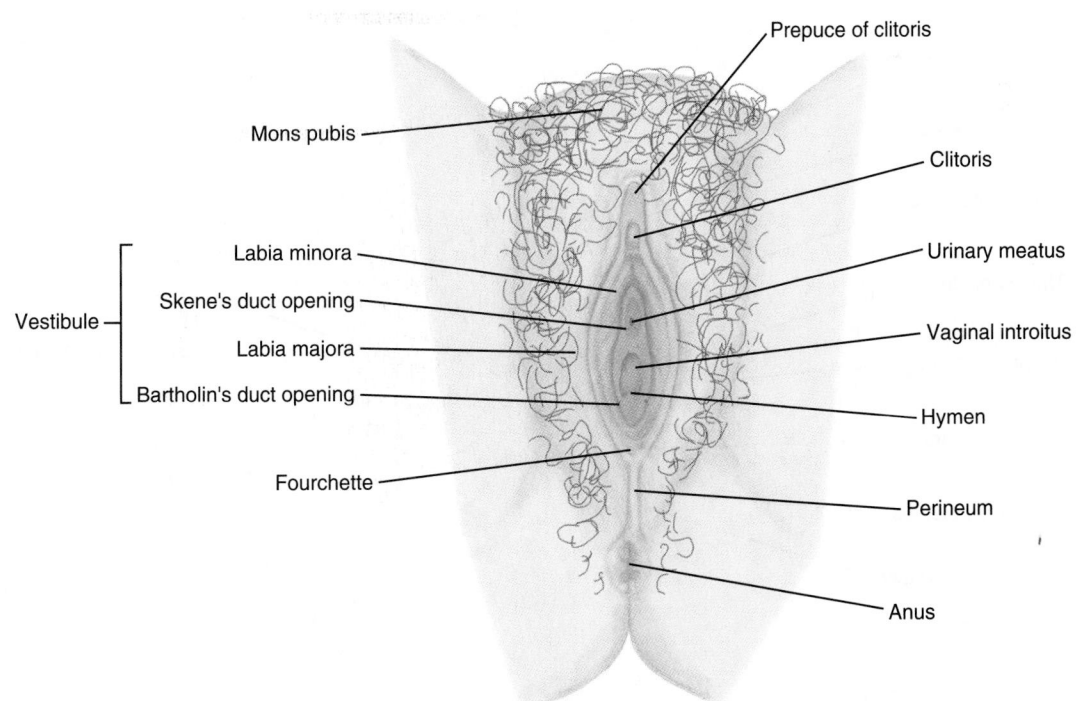

FIGURE 11-1
• • • • • • • • •
External female reproductive structures.

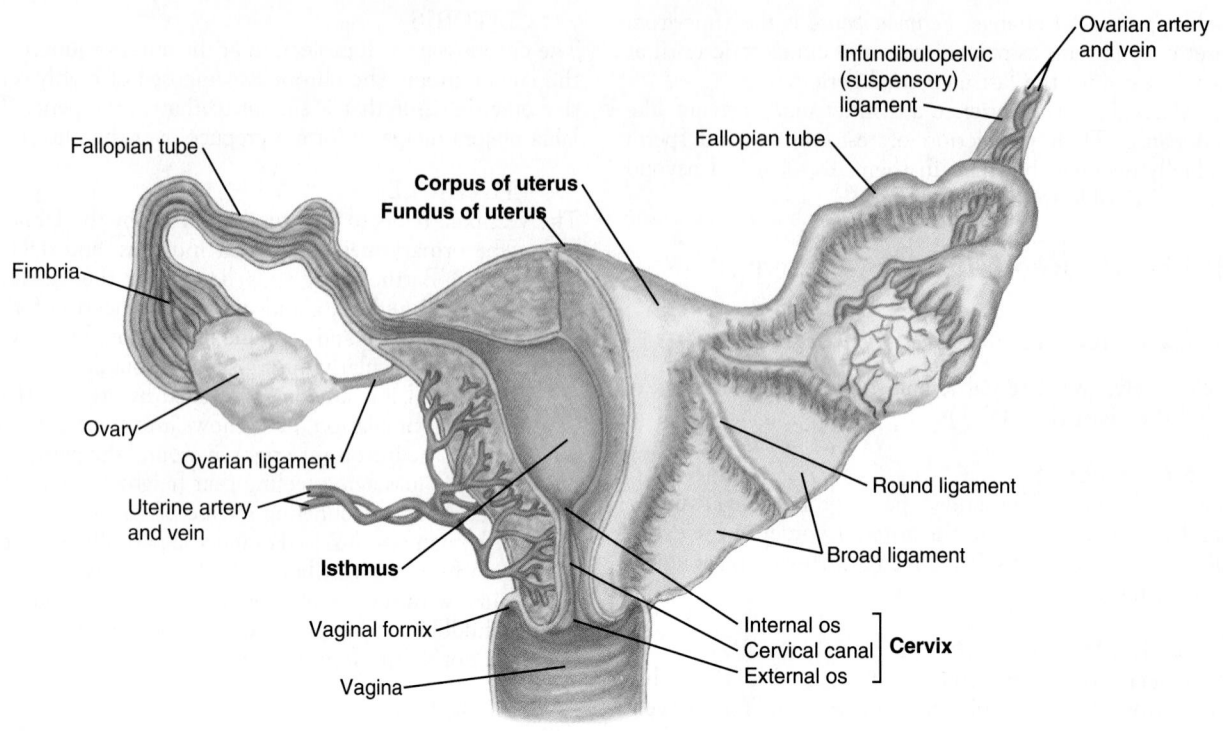

Internal female reproductive structures, anterior view.

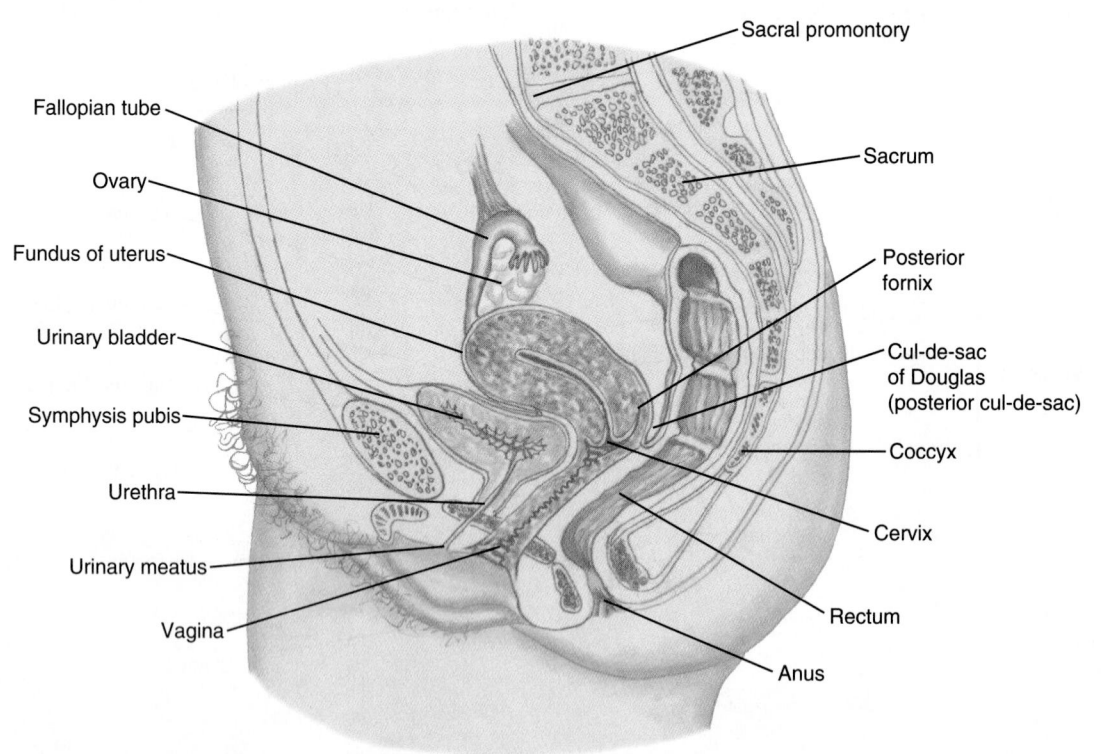

Internal female reproductive structures, midsagittal view.

VAGINA

The vagina is a tube of muscular and membranous tissue about 8 to 10 cm long, lying between the bladder anteriorly and the rectum posteriorly. The vagina connects the uterus above with the vestibule below. The vaginal lining has multiple folds, or rugae, and a muscular layer that are capable of marked distention during childbirth. The vagina is lubricated by secretions of the cervix, the lowermost part of the uterus, and by the Bartholin's glands.

The vagina does not end abruptly at the uterine opening but arches to form the vaginal fornix. Each fornix is described by its location: anterior, posterior, or lateral.

The three major functions of the vagina are

- To allow discharge of the menstrual flow
- As the female organ of coitus, to receive the male penis
- To allow passage of the fetus from the uterus

UTERUS

The uterus is a hollow, thick-walled, muscular organ that is shaped like a flattened upside-down pear. The uterus houses and nourishes the fetus until birth, then contracts rhythmically during labor to expel the fetus. Each month, the uterus is prepared for a pregnancy, whether or not conception occurs.

The uterus measures about 7.5 × 5 × 2.5 cm (3 × 2 × 1 inch) and is larger in a woman who has borne children than in one who has not. It is suspended above the bladder and is anterior to the rectum. Its normal position is anteverted (rotated forward) and slightly anteflexed (flexed forward).

Divisions of the Uterus.   The uterus is divided into three parts.

Corpus.   The upper part is the corpus, or body, of the uterus. The *fundus* of the uterus is the part of the corpus above the area where the fallopian tubes enter the uterus.

Isthmus.   A narrower transition zone, the isthmus, is between the corpus of the uterus and the cervix. During late pregnancy, the isthmus elongates and is known as the lower uterine segment.

Cervix.   The cervix is the tubular "neck" of the lower uterus and is about 2 to 3 cm long. The os is the opening in the cervix that runs between the uterus and the vagina. The upper part of the cervix is marked by the internal os, and the lower cervix is marked by the external os. The external os of a childless woman is round and smooth. After vaginal birth, the external os has an irregular, slitlike shape and may have tags of scar tissue.

Layers of the Uterus.   The uterus has three layers.

Perimetrium.   The perimetrium is the outer peritoneal layer of serous membrane that covers most of the uterus. Laterally, the perimetrium is continuous with the broad ligaments on either side of the uterus.

Myometrium.   The myometrium is the middle layer of thick muscle. Most of the muscle fibers are concentrated in the upper uterus, and their number diminishes progressively toward the cervix. The myometrium contains three types of smooth muscle fiber (Fig. 11–4). These types are

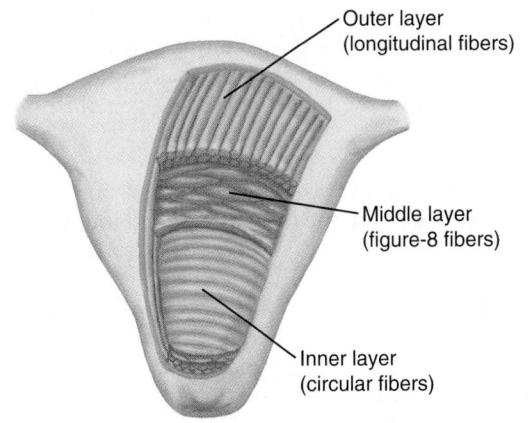

Outer layer (longitudinal fibers)

Middle layer (figure-8 fibers)

Inner layer (circular fibers)

FIGURE 11–4

Layers of the myometrium, showing the three types of smooth muscle fiber.

- *Longitudinal fibers*, which are found mostly in the fundus and are designed to expel the fetus efficiently toward the pelvic outlet during birth
- *Interlacing figure-8 fibers*, which make up the middle layer. These fibers contract after birth to compress the blood vessels that pass between them to limit blood loss.
- *Circular fibers*, which form constrictions where the fallopian tubes enter the uterus and surround the internal cervical os. Circular fibers prevent reflux of menstrual blood and tissue into the fallopian tubes, promote normal implantation of the fertilized ovum by controlling its entry into the uterus, and retain the fetus until the appropriate time of birth.

Endometrium.   The endometrium is the inner layer of the uterus. It is responsive to the cyclic variations of estrogen and progesterone during the female reproductive cycle (see p. 233). The two layers of the endometrium are

- The *basal layer*, which is nearest the myometrium, regenerates the functional layer of the endometrium after each menstrual period and after childbirth.
- The *functional layer*, which lies above the basal layer and contains the endometrial arteries, veins, and glands. This layer is shed during each menstrual period and after childbirth in the *lochia*.

FALLOPIAN TUBES

The fallopian tubes, also called *oviducts*, are 8 to 14 cm (3 to 5.6 inches) long and quite narrow (2 to 3 mm at their narrowest and 5 to 8 mm at their widest). They are a pathway for the ovum between the ovary and the uterus. The fallopian tubes are lined with folded epithelium containing cilia that beat rhythmically toward the uterine cavity to propel the ovum through the tube. Each fallopian tube enters the upper uterus at the *cornu*, or horn, of the uterus.

The four divisions of the tubes are

- The *interstitial* portion, which runs into the uterine cavity and lies within the uterine wall
- The *isthmus*, which is the narrow part of the tube adjacent to the uterus

- The *ampulla*, which is the wider area of the tube lateral to the isthmus, where fertilization occurs
- The *infundibulum*, which is the wide, funnel-shaped terminal end of the tube. *Fimbria* are fingerlike processes surrounding the infundibulum.

The fallopian tubes are not directly connected to the ovary. At ovulation, the ovum is expelled into the abdominal cavity. Wavelike motions of the fimbria draw the ovum into the tube. The tubal isthmus, however, remains contracted until 3 days after conception to allow the fertilized ovum to develop within the tube. Initial growth of the fertilized ovum within the fallopian tube promotes its normal implantation in the fundal portion of the uterine corpus.

OVARIES

The ovaries have two functions: to produce sex hormones and to develop an ovum to maturity during each reproductive cycle.

The ovaries secrete estrogen and progesterone in varying amounts during a woman's reproductive cycle to prepare the uterine lining for pregnancy. Ovarian hormone secretion gradually declines to very low levels during the climacteric.

At birth, the ovary contains all the ova that it will ever have. About 1 million immature ova are present at birth. Many of these degenerate until, at puberty, 200,000 to 400,000 remain. Many ova begin the maturation process during each reproductive cycle, but most never reach maturity. During the course of a woman's reproductive life, only about 400 of the ova ever mature enough to be released and fertilized. By the time a woman reaches the climacteric, almost all of her ova have been released during ovulation or have regressed. The few remaining ova are unresponsive to stimulating hormones and do not mature.

Support Structures

The bony pelvis supports and protects the lower abdominal and internal reproductive organs. Muscles and ligaments provide added support for the internal organs of the pelvis against the downward force of gravity and the increases in intra-abdominal pressure.

PELVIS

The bony pelvis is a basin-shaped structure at the lower end of the spine. Its posterior wall is formed by the sacrum. The side and anterior pelvic walls are composed of three fused bones: the *ilium*, the *ischium*, and the *pubis*. Figure 11–5 illustrates important anatomic landmarks on the pelvis.

The *linea terminalis*, also called the pelvic brim or ileopectineal line, is an imaginary line that divides the upper, or false, pelvis from the lower, or true, pelvis. The false pelvis provides support for the internal organs and the upper part of the body. The true pelvis is most important during childbirth, and its divisions and measurements are discussed in Chapter 17.

MUSCLES

Paired muscles enclose the lower pelvis and provide support for internal reproductive, urinary, and bowel structures (Fig. 11–6). In addition, a fibromuscular sheet, the *pelvic fascia*, provides support for the pelvic organs. Vaginal and urethral openings are in the pelvic fascia.

The *levator ani* is a collection of three pairs of muscles: the *pubococcygeus*, which is also called the *pubovaginal muscle* in the female; the *puborectal*; and the *iliococcygeus*. These muscles support internal pelvic structures and resist increases in the intra-abdominal pressure.

The *ischiocavernosus muscle* extends from the clitoris to the ischial tuberosities on each side of the lower bony pelvis. The two *transverse perineal muscles* extend from fibrous tissue

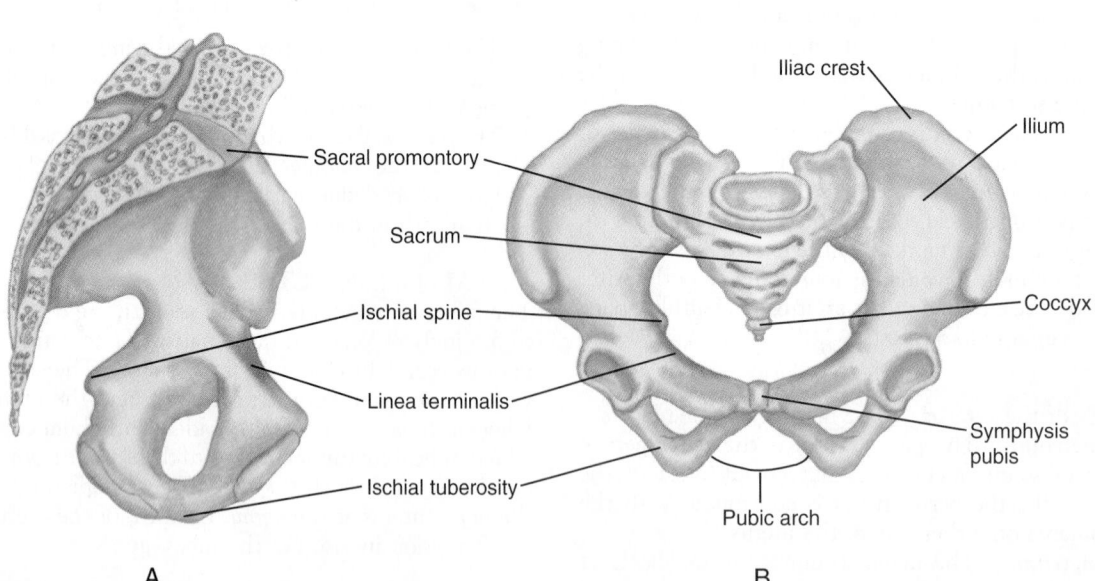

A   B

FIGURE 11–5

Structures of the bony pelvis, shown in lateral *(A)* and anterior *(B)* views.

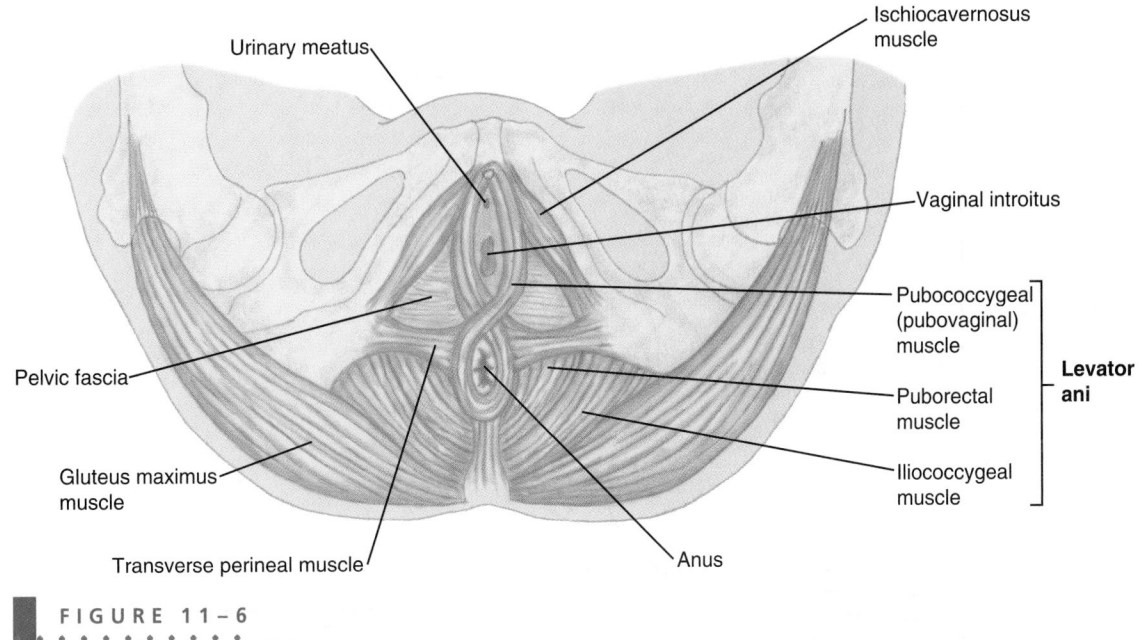

FIGURE 11-6

Muscles of the female pelvic floor.

of the perineum to the two ischial tuberosities, stabilizing the center of the perineum.

LIGAMENTS

Seven pairs of ligaments maintain the internal reproductive organs, with their nerve and blood supplies, in their proper positions within the pelvis (see Fig. 11–2).

Lateral Support.   Paired ligaments stabilize the uterus and ovaries laterally and keep them in the midline of the pelvis. The *broad ligament* is a sheet of tissue extending from each side of the uterus to the lateral pelvic wall. The *round ligament* and fallopian tube mark the upper border of the broad ligament; the lower edge is bounded by the uterine blood vessels. Within the two broad ligaments are the ovarian ligaments, blood vessels, and lymphatics.

The right and left *cardinal ligaments* provide support to the lower uterus and vagina. They extend from the lateral walls of the cervix and vagina to the side walls of the pelvis.

The two *ovarian ligaments* connect the ovaries to the lateral uterine walls. The *infundibulopelvic,* or *suspensory, ligaments* connect the lateral ovary and distal fallopian tubes to the pelvic side walls. The infundibulopelvic ligament also carries the blood vessel and nerve supply for the ovary.

Anterior Support.   Two pairs of ligaments provide anterior support for the internal reproductive organs. The *round ligaments* connect the upper uterus to the connective tissue of the labia majora. These ligaments maintain the uterus in its normal anteflexed position and help direct the fetal presenting part against the cervix during labor.

The *pubocervical ligaments* support the cervix anteriorly. They connect the cervix to the interior surface of the symphysis pubis.

Posterior Support.   The *uterosacral ligaments* provide posterior support, extending from the lower posterior uterus to the sacrum. These ligaments also contain sympathetic and parasympathetic nerves of the autonomic nervous system.

BLOOD SUPPLY

The uterine blood supply is carried by the *uterine arteries,* which are branches of the internal iliac artery. These vessels enter the uterus at the lower border of the broad ligament, near the isthmus of the uterus. The vessels branch downward to supply the cervix and vagina and upward to supply the uterus. The upper branch also supplies the ovaries and fallopian tubes. The vessels are coiled to allow for elongation as the uterus enlarges and rises out of the pelvis during pregnancy. Blood drains into the *uterine veins* and from there into the internal iliac veins.

Additional ovarian and tubal blood supply is carried by the *ovarian artery,* which arises from the abdominal aorta. The ovarian blood supply drains into the two *ovarian veins.*

NERVE SUPPLY

Most functions of the reproductive system are under involuntary, or unconscious, control. Nerves of the autonomic nervous system from the uterovaginal plexus and inferior hypogastric plexus control automatic functions of the reproductive system.

Sensory and motor nerves that innervate the reproductive organs enter the spinal cord at the T12 through L2 levels. These nerves are important during childbearing for pain management.

Female Reproductive Cycle

The female reproductive cycle describes the regular and recurrent changes in the anterior pituitary secretions, ovaries, and uterine endometrium that are designed to prepare the body for pregnancy (Figure 11–7). The female reproductive cycle is often called the *menstrual cycle* because menstruation provides a marker for each cycle's beginning and end if pregnancy does not occur.

The duration of the cycle is about 28 days, although it may range from 20 to 45 days (Guyton, 1996). Significant

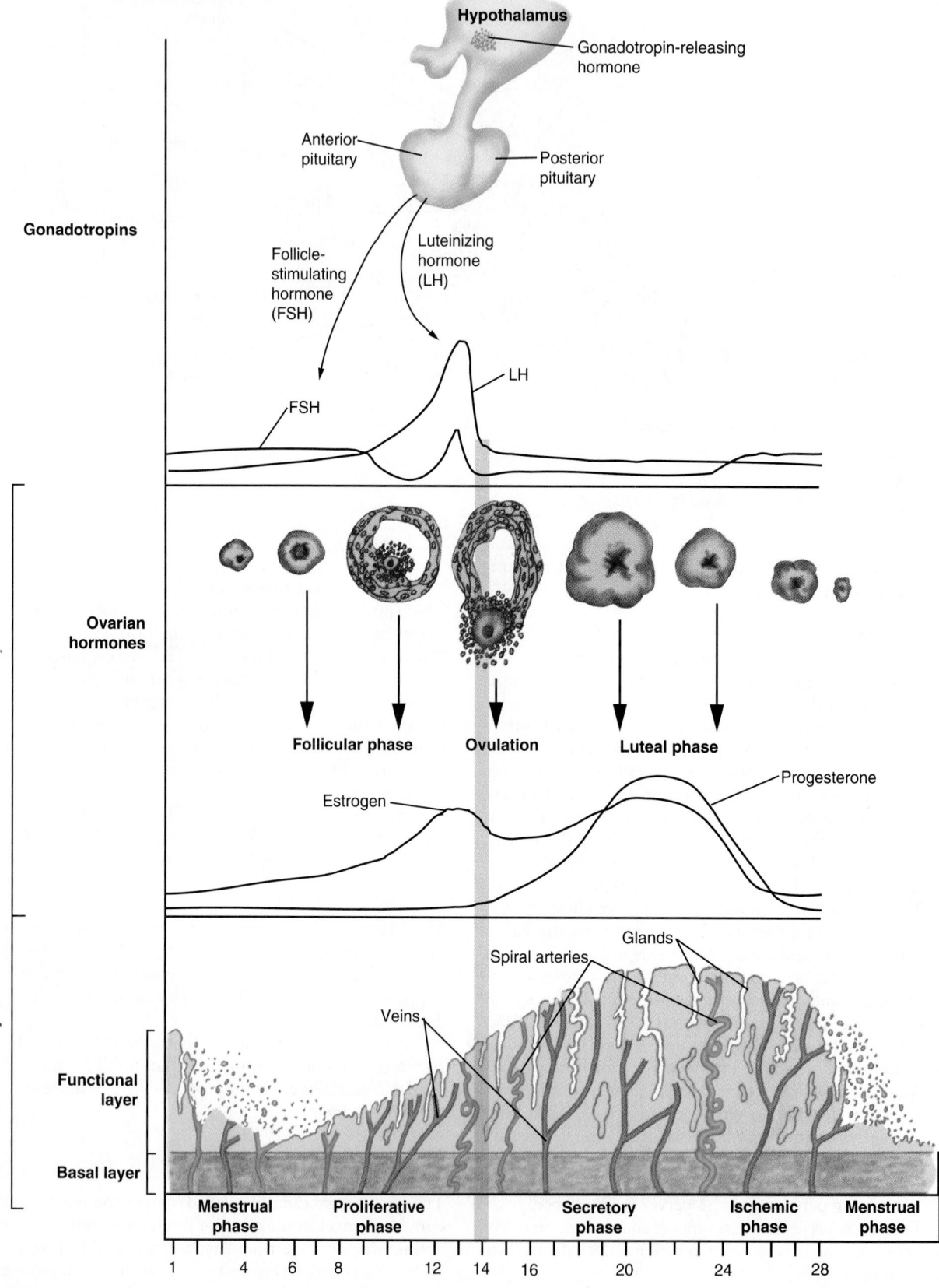

FIGURE 11–7

The female reproductive cycle, showing the changes in hormone secretion from the anterior pituitary and interrelated changes in the ovary and uterine endometrium.

deviations from the 28-day cycle are associated with reduced fertility. The first day of the menstrual period is counted as day 1 of the woman's cycle. The female reproductive cycle is further divided into two cycles that reflect changes in the ovaries and uterine endometrium.

Ovarian Cycle

In response to GnRH from the woman's hypothalamus, the anterior pituitary secretes FSH and LH. The FSH and LH stimulate the ovaries to mature an ovum, release it, and secrete other hormones that will prepare the endometrium for implantation of a fertilized ovum. The ovarian cycle consists of three phases: the follicular phase, the ovulatory phase, and the luteal phase.

FOLLICULAR PHASE
The follicular phase is the period during which an ovum matures. It begins with the first day of menstruation and ends about 14 days later in a 28-day cycle. The length of this phase varies more among different women than do the lengths of the other two phases. The decrease in estrogen and progesterone secretion by the ovary just before menstruation stimulates secretion of FSH and LH by the anterior pituitary. As the FSH and LH levels rise slightly, 6 to 12 graafian follicles, each containing an immature ovum, begin growing. Each follicle secretes fluid containing high levels of estrogen, which accelerates maturation by making the follicle more sensitive to the effects of FSH. Eventually, one follicle matures before the others. The mature follicle secretes large amounts of estrogen, which depresses FSH secretion. The brief dip in FSH secretion just before ovulation blocks further maturation of the less-developed follicles. Occasionally, more than one follicle matures and releases its ovum; this condition can lead to a multifetal pregnancy.

OVULATORY PHASE
Near the middle of a 28-day reproductive cycle, about 2 days before ovulation, LH secretion rises markedly. Secretion of FSH also rises, but less than LH does. These surges in LH and FSH cause a slight fall in follicular estrogen production and a rise in progesterone secretion, stimulating final maturation of a single follicle and release of its ovum. Ovulation marks the beginning of the luteal phase of the female reproductive cycle and occurs about 14 days before the next menstrual period.

The mature follicle is a mass of cells with a fluid-filled chamber. A smaller mass of cells houses the ovum within this chamber. At ovulation, a blisterlike projection, called a *stigma*, forms on the wall of the follicle, the follicle ruptures, and the ovum with its surrounding cells is released from the surface of the ovary. There it is picked up by the fimbriated end of the fallopian tube for transport to the uterus.

LUTEAL PHASE
After ovulation and under the influence of LH, the remaining cells of the old follicle persist for about 12 days as a *corpus luteum*. The corpus luteum secretes estrogen and large amounts of progesterone to prepare the endometrium for a fertilized ovum. Levels of FSH and LH decrease during this phase in response to higher levels of estrogen and pro-

gesterone. If the ovum is fertilized, it secretes a hormone (chorionic gonadotropin) that causes the corpus luteum to persist in order to maintain an early pregnancy. If the ovum is not fertilized, FSH and LH fall to low levels, and the corpus luteum regresses. Decline of estrogen and progesterone with the regression of the corpus luteum results in menstruation as the uterine lining breaks down.

The loss of estrogen and progesterone from the corpus luteum at the end of one cycle stimulates the anterior pituitary again to secrete more FSH and LH, initiating a new cycle. The old corpus luteum is replaced by fibrous tissue called the *corpus albicans*.

Endometrial Cycle

The uterine endometrium responds to ovarian hormone stimulation with cyclic changes. Three phases mark the changes in the endometrium: the proliferative phase, the secretory phase, and the menstrual phase.

PROLIFERATIVE PHASE
The proliferative phase takes place as the ovum matures and is released during the first half of the ovarian cycle. After completion of a menstrual period, the endometrium is very thin, with only the basal layer of cells remaining. These cells multiply to form new endometrial epithelium and endometrial glands under the stimulation of estrogen secreted by the maturing ovarian follicles. Endometrial spiral arteries and endometrial veins elongate to accompany thickening of the functional endometrial layer and to nourish the proliferating cells. As ovulation approaches, the endometrial glands secrete a thin, stringy mucus that aids entry of sperm into the uterus.

SECRETORY PHASE
The secretory phase occurs during the second half of the ovarian cycle as the uterus is prepared to receive a fertilized ovum. The endometrium continues to thicken under the influence of estrogen and progesterone from the corpus luteum, reaching its maximum thickness of 5 to 6 mm. The blood vessels and endometrial glands become twisted and dilated.

Progesterone from the corpus luteum causes the thick endometrium to secrete substances that nourish a fertilized ovum. Large quantities of glycogen, proteins, lipids, and minerals are stored within the endometrium, awaiting arrival of the ovum.

MENSTRUAL PHASE
If fertilization does not occur, the corpus luteum regresses, and its production of estrogen and progesterone falls. About 2 days before the onset of the menses, vasospasm of the endometrial blood vessels causes the endometrium to become ischemic and necrotic. The necrotic areas of endometrium separate from the basal layers, resulting in the menstrual flow. The duration of the menstrual phase is about 5 days.

During a menstrual period, women lose about 40 ml of blood. Because of the recurrent loss of blood, many women are mildly anemic during their reproductive years, especially if their diets are low in iron.

Changes in Cervical Mucus

During most of the female reproductive cycle, the mucus of the cervix is scant, thick, and sticky. Just before ovulation, cervical mucus becomes thin, clear, and elastic to promote passage of sperm into the uterus and fallopian tube, where they can fertilize the ovum. *Spinnbarkeit* refers to the elasticity of cervical mucus. A woman may assess the elasticity of her cervical mucus either to avoid or to promote conception.

The Female Breast

Structure

The breasts, or mammary glands, are not directly functional in reproduction, but they secrete milk after childbirth to nourish the infant. The small, raised nipple is at the center of each breast (Fig. 11–8). The nipple is composed of sensitive erectile tissue and can respond to sexual stimulation. Surrounding the nipple is a larger circular areola. Both the nipple and areola are darker than surrounding skin. Montgomery's tubercles are sebaceous glands in the areola. They are inactive and not obvious except during pregnancy and lactation, when they enlarge and secrete a substance that keeps the nipple soft.

Within each breast are lobes of glandular tissue that secrete milk. These lobes are arranged like spokes of a wheel around the hub. Fifteen to 20 of these lobes are arranged around and behind the nipple and areola. Fibrous tissue and

fat in the breast support the glandular tissue, blood vessels, lymphatics, and nerves.

Alveoli are small sacs that contain acinar cells to secrete milk. The acinar cells extract substances needed from the mammary blood supply to manufacture milk when the breasts are properly stimulated by the anterior pituitary gland. Myoepithelial cells surround the alveoli to contract and eject the milk into the ductal system when signaled by secretion of the hormone oxytocin from the posterior pituitary gland.

The alveoli drain into lactiferous ducts, which connect to drain milk from all areas of the breast. The lactiferous ducts become wider under the areola and are called *lactiferous sinuses* in this area. The lactiferous sinuses narrow again as they open to the outside in the nipple.

Function

The breasts are inactive until puberty, when rising estrogen levels stimulate growth of the glandular tissue. Fat is deposited in the breasts, resulting in the mature female contour. The amount of fat is the major determinant of breast size; the amount of glandular tissue is similar for all mature women. Breast size is therefore unrelated to the amount of milk a woman can produce during lactation.

During pregnancy, high levels of estrogen and progesterone, produced by the placenta, stimulate growth of the alveoli and ductal system to prepare them for lactation. Prolactin secreted by the anterior pituitary gland stimulates milk production during pregnancy, but this effect is inhib-

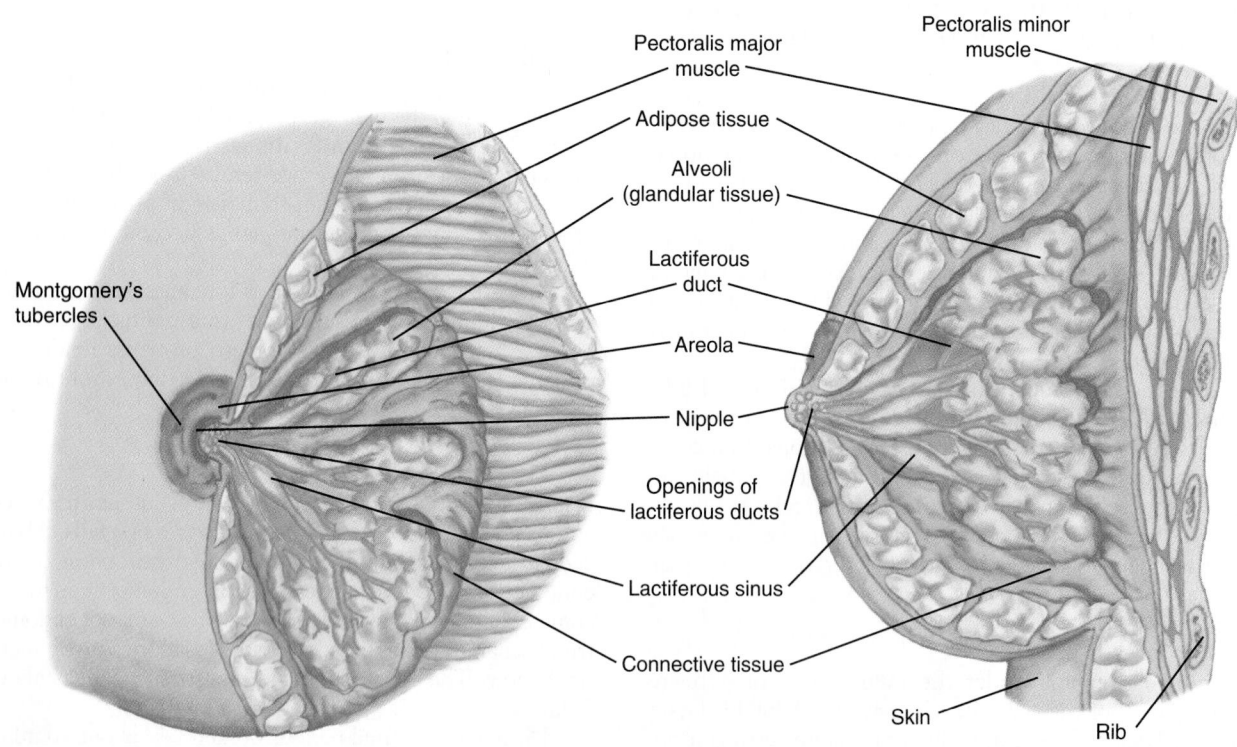

FIGURE 11–8

Structures of the female breast.

ited by estrogen and progesterone produced by the placenta. Inhibiting effects of estrogen and progesterone stop when the placenta is expelled after birth, and active milk production occurs in response to the infant's nursing.

Male Reproductive Anatomy and Physiology

External Male Reproductive Organs

The male has two external organs of reproduction: the penis and the scrotum (Fig. 11–9).

PENIS

The penis has two functions. As part of the urinary tract, it carries urine from the bladder to the exterior during urination. As a reproductive organ, the penis deposits semen into the female vagina during coitus.

The penis is composed mostly of erectile tissue, which is spongy tissue with many small spaces inside. There are three areas of erectile tissue: the corpus spongiosum, which surrounds the urethra, and two columns of the corpus cavernosum, one on each side of the penis.

The penis is flaccid most of the time because the small spaces within the erectile tissue are collapsed. During sexual stimulation, arteries within the penis dilate and veins are partly occluded, trapping blood in the spongy tissue. Entrapment of blood within the penis causes erection and enables the man to penetrate the vagina during sexual intercourse.

The glans is the distal end of the penis. The urinary meatus is centered in the end of the glans. Covering the glans is the loose skin of the prepuce, or foreskin. The prepuce may be removed during *circumcision.*

SCROTUM

The scrotum is a pouch of thin skin and muscle suspended behind the penis. The skin of the scrotum is darker than the surrounding skin and is covered with rugae. The scrotum is divided internally by a septum. One testicle is contained within each pocket of the scrotum.

The scrotum's main function is to keep the testes cooler than the core body temperature. Formation of normal sperm requires that the testes not be too warm. A cremaster muscle is attached to each testicle. This muscle can tighten, drawing the testes closer to the body and warming them, or it can relax, allowing the testes to fall away from the body and become cooler.

Internal Male Reproductive Organs

TESTES

The male gonads, or testes, have two functions: they serve as endocrine glands, and they produce male gametes, or sperm, also called spermatozoa. Androgens, which are the male sex hormones, are the primary endocrine secretions of the testes. Androgens are produced by Leydig cells of the testes. The primary androgen produced by the testes is testosterone.

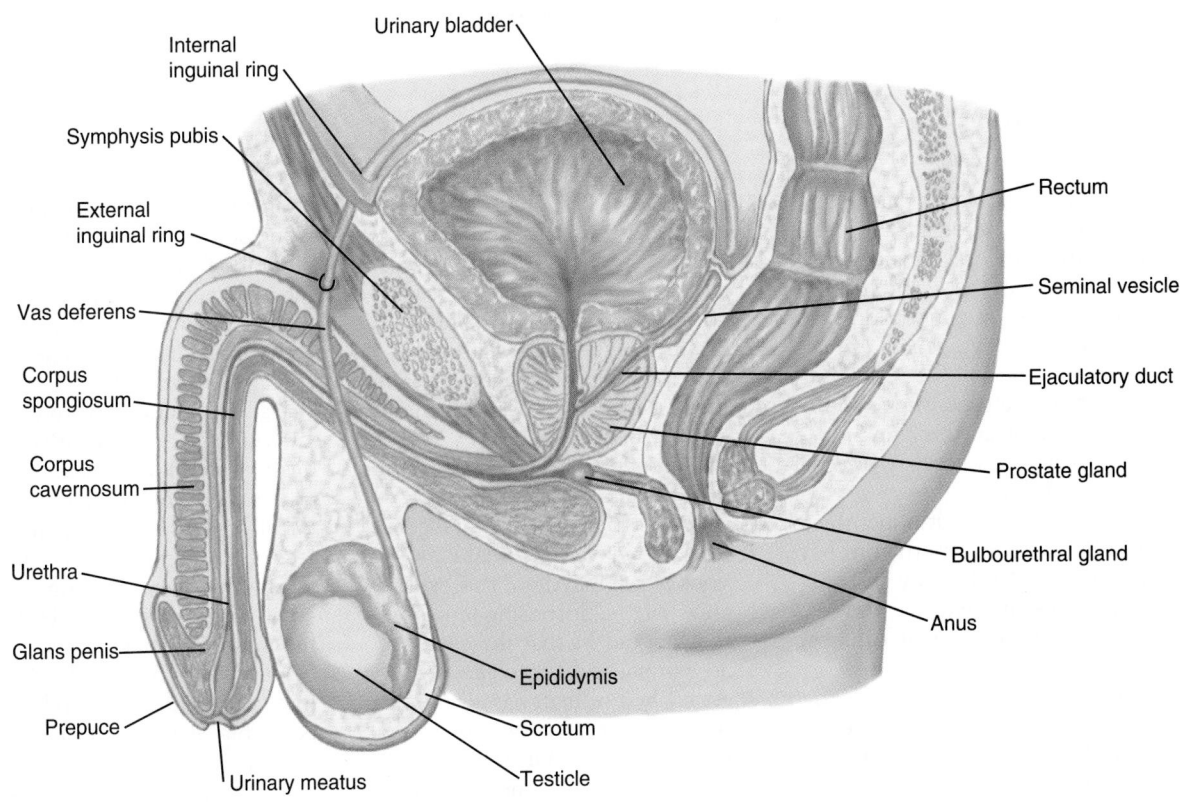

FIGURE 11–9

. . . .

Structures of the male reproductive system, midsagittal view.

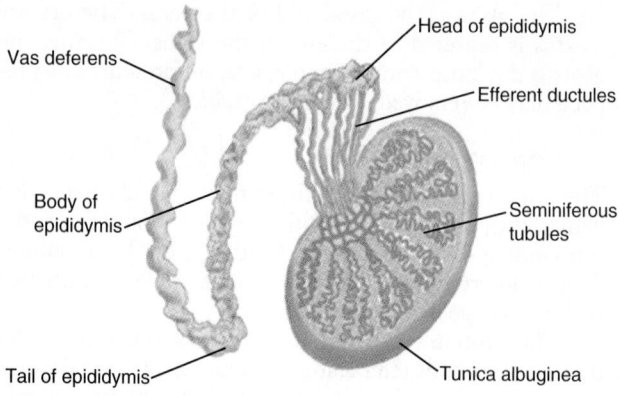

Vas deferens

Head of epididymis

Efferent ductules

Body of epididymis

Seminiferous tubules

Tail of epididymis

Tunica albuginea

FIGURE 11–10
• • • • • • • • • •
Internal structures of the testis. Production of sperm begins within the tiny, coiled seminiferous tubules. Immature sperm pass from the seminiferous tubules to the epididymis and then to the vas deferens. During their passage through these structures, the sperm mature and acquire the ability to propel themselves.

Unlike the female, who experiences a cyclic pattern of hormone secretion, the male secretes testosterone in a relatively even pattern. A small amount of testosterone is converted to estrogen in the male and is necessary for sperm formation.

Spermatogenesis occurs within tiny coiled tubes, called the seminiferous tubules, of the testes (Fig. 11–10). Leydig cells are interstitial cells that support the seminiferous tubules and secrete testosterone, a hormone necessary for forming new cells that will mature into sperm. Sertoli cells within the seminiferous tubules respond to FSH secretion by nourishing and supporting sperm as they mature. Unlike the female, who has a lifetime supply of ova in her gonads at birth, the male does not begin producing sperm until puberty. The normal male produces new sperm throughout life, although production declines with age.

At ejaculation, about 400 million sperm are deposited in the vagina. This large number is needed for normal fertility, although a single sperm fertilizes the ovum. Only a few sperm ever reach the fallopian tube, where an ovum may be available for fertilization.

ACCESSORY DUCTS AND GLANDS

From the seminiferous tubules, sperm pass into the epididymis within the scrotum for storage and final maturation. In the epididymis, sperm develop the ability to be motile. Secretions within the epididymis, however, inhibit actual motility until ejaculation occurs.

The epididymis empties into the vas deferens, where larger numbers of sperm are stored. The vas deferens then leads upward into the pelvis, then back down toward the penis through the internal and external inguinal rings. Within the pelvis, the vas deferens joins the ejaculatory duct before connecting to the urethra.

Three glands—the *seminal vesicles*, the *prostate*, and the *bulbourethral glands*—secrete seminal fluids that carry sperm into the vagina during intercourse. The seminal fluid (1) nourishes the sperm, (2) protects the sperm from the acidic environment of the vagina, (3) enhances the motility of the sperm, and (4) washes the sperm out of the urethra so that the maximum number are deposited in the vagina.

KEY CONCEPTS
• • • • • • • • • • •

- Initial prenatal development of the reproductive organs is similar for both males and females. If a critical part of the Y chromosome is not present at conception, female reproductive structures will develop.
- Puberty is the time when the reproductive organs become fully functional and secondary sex characteristics develop.
- Puberty begins about 6 months to 1 year earlier in girls than in boys, although the girl's early growth spurt makes it seem that she begins puberty much earlier than the boy.
- Females are generally shorter than males because they begin their growth spurt at an earlier age and complete it more quickly than boys.
- The onset of menstruation (menar-

che) is an obvious marker of puberty in girls.
- Girls often do not ovulate in early menstrual cycles, although it is possible for them to ovulate even before the first one. A girl can, therefore, become pregnant before her first menstrual period if she is sexually active.
- The onset of puberty is more subtle in boys than in girls, and begins with growth of the testes and penis.
- Boys may have nocturnal emissions of seminal fluid; this experience may be distressing unless they are taught that these events are normal and expected.
- At birth, a woman has all the ova she will ever have. New ova are not formed after birth; almost all are depleted when she reaches the climacteric.
- The female reproductive cycle is

often called the menstrual cycle. It includes changes in the anterior pituitary gland, ovaries, and uterine endometrium to prepare for a fertilized ovum. The character of cervical mucus also changes to encourage fertilization.
- Breast size is unrelated to glandular tissue or to the quantity or quality of milk a woman can produce for her infant after childbirth. Breast size is primarily related to the amount of fat present.
- For normal sperm to form, a man's testes must be cooler than his core body temperature.
- Seminal fluids secreted by the seminal vesicles, prostate, and bulbourethral glands nourish and protect the sperm, enhance their motility, and ensure that most sperm are deposited in the vagina during sexual intercourse.

REFERENCES AND READINGS

Cunningham, F. G., MacDonald, P. C., Gant, N. F., Leveno, K. J., Gilstrap, L. C., Hankins, G. D. V., et al. (1997). *Williams obstetrics* (20th ed.). Norwalk, CT: Appleton & Lange.

DiGeorge, A. M., & Garibaldi, L. (1996). Physiology of puberty. In W. E. Nelson, R. E. Behrman, R. M. Kliegman, & A. M. Arvin (Eds.), *Nelson textbook of pediatrics* (15th ed., pp. 1579–1580). Philadelphia: Saunders.

Georges, J. M. (1995). Structure and function of the female reproductive system. In L. C. Copstead (Ed.), *Perspectives on pathophysiology* (pp. 648–666). Philadelphia: Saunders.

Guyton, A. C. (1996). *Textbook of medical physiology* (9th ed.). Philadelphia: Saunders.

Mikkelsen, D. (1995). Structure and function of the male genitourinary system. In L. C. Copstead (Ed.), *Perspectives on pathophysiology* (pp. 612–633). Philadelphia: Saunders.

Moore, K. L., & Persaud, T. V. N. (1998). *Before we are born* (5th ed.). Philadelphia: Saunders.

Moore, K. L., & Persaud, T. V. N. (1998). *The developing human: Clinically oriented embryology* (6th ed.). Philadelphia: Saunders.

Preparation of Sperm for Fertilization

Sperm are not immediately ready to fertilize the ovum when they are ejaculated. While making the trip to the ovum, the sperm undergo changes that enable one of them to penetrate the protective layers surrounding the ovum. This process is *capacitation*. During capacitation a glycoprotein coat and seminal proteins are removed from the acrosome (tip of the sperm head). After capacitation, the sperm look the same but are more active and can better penetrate the corona radiata and zona pellucida that surround the ovum.

The sperm that reach the ovum release an enzyme (hyaluronidase) to digest a pathway through the corona radiata and zona pellucida. Their tails beat harder to propel them toward the center of the ovum. Eventually, one spermatozoon penetrates the ovum.

Fertilization

Fertilization occurs when one spermatozoon enters the ovum and the two nuclei containing the parents' chromosomes merge (Fig. 12–3).

Entry of One Spermatozoon into the Ovum

Entry of a spermatozoon into the ovum has two results:

- Changes in the zona pellucida surrounding the ovum prevent other sperm from entering.
- The ovum, which has been suspended in the middle of its second meiotic division since just before ovulation, completes meiosis.

The results are a nucleus with 23 chromosomes and expulsion of a second nonfunctional polar body. The mature ovum now contains 23 unpaired chromosomes, 22 autosomes and one X chromosome, in its nucleus.

Fusion of the Nuclei of Sperm and Ovum

Fusion of the nuclei of the sperm and ovum begins when the sperm enters the ovum. The sperm head enlarges, and the tail degenerates. The nuclei of the gametes move toward the center of the ovum, where the membranes surrounding their nuclei touch and dissolve. The 23 chromosomes from the sperm mingle with the 23 from the ovum, restoring the diploid number to 46. Fertilization is complete, and cell division can begin when the nuclei of the sperm and ovum unite.

Pre-Embryonic Period

The pre-embryonic period is the first 2 weeks after conception. Figure 12–4 illustrates the period from fertilization through implantation.

Initiation of Cell Division

The zygote divides into two cells, then four, then eight cells while in the fallopian tube. Up to the 16-cell stage, the cells become smaller with each division, so they occupy about the same amount of space as the original ovum. When the conceptus is a solid ball of 12 to 16 cells, it is called a *morula* because it resembles a mulberry.

The outer cells of the morula secrete fluid, forming a sac of cells with an inner cell mass placed off-center within the sac. This is the *blastocyst*. The inner cell mass develops into the fetus. Part of the outer layer of cells develops into the placenta and fetal membranes.

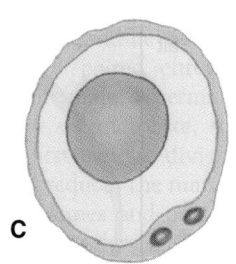

B

Mixing of cell nuclei and chromosomes of ovum and sperm

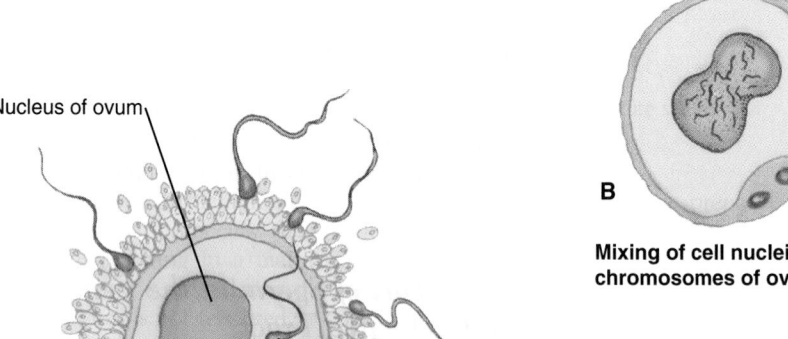

Fertilization complete

C

FIGURE 12–3

Process of fertilization. *A,* A sperm enters the ovum. *B,* The 23 chromosomes from the sperm mingle with the 23 chromosomes from the ovum, restoring the diploid number to 46. *C,* The fertilized ovum, now called a zygote, is ready for the first mitotic cell division.

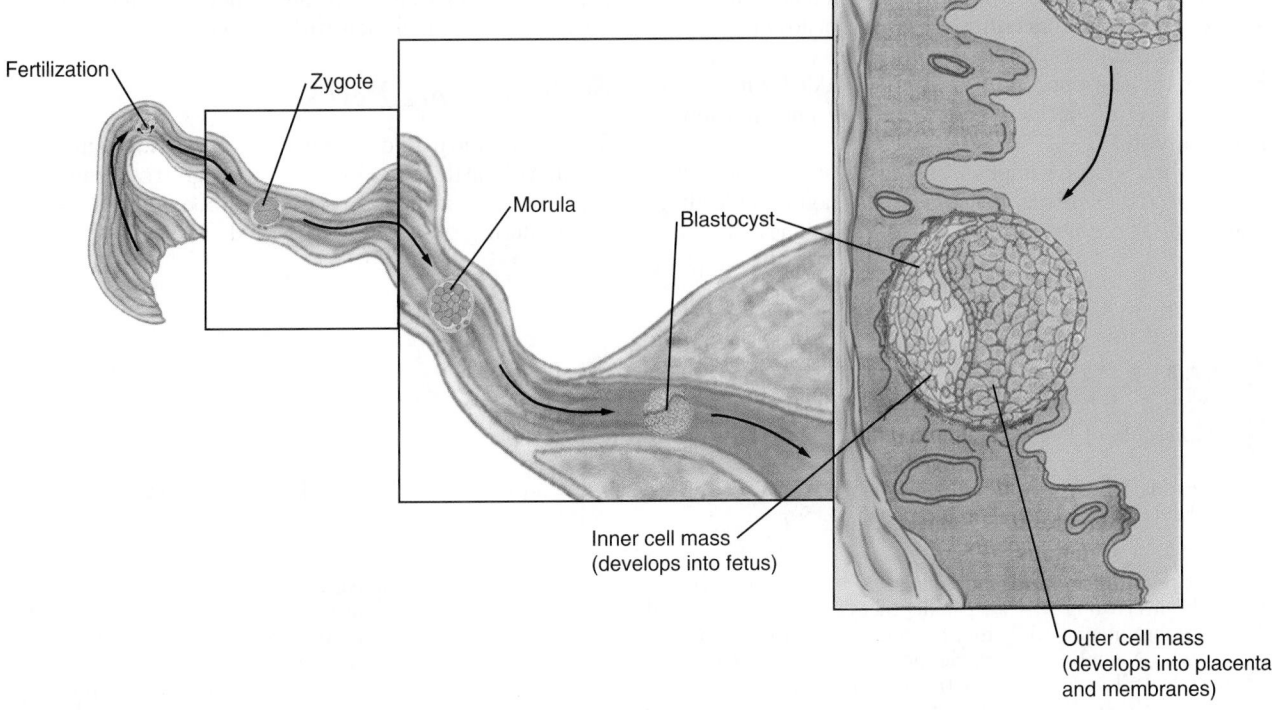

FIGURE 12-4

Prenatal development from fertilization through implantation of the blastocyst. Implantation gradually occurs from the 6th through the 10th day. Implantation is complete on the 10th day.

Entry of the Zygote into the Uterus

The conceptus enters the uterus about 3 days after conception, when it contains about 100 cells. It lingers in the uterus another 2 to 4 days before beginning implantation. The endometrium, now called the *decidua*, is in the secretory phase of the reproductive cycle, 1.5 weeks before the woman would begin her menstrual period. The endometrial glands are secreting at their maximum, providing rich fluids to nourish the conceptus before placental circulation is established. The endometrial spiral arteries are well developed in the secretory phase, providing easy access for developing the placental blood supply.

Implantation in the Decidua

The conceptus carries a small supply of nutrients for early cell division, but implantation (*nidation*) at the proper time and location in the uterus is crucial for continued development. Implantation is a gradual process that occurs between the 6th and 10th days. Embryonic structures also are developing during implantation.

Maintaining the Decidua

Implantation and survival of the conceptus are critically dependent on a continuing supply of estrogen and progesterone to maintain the decidua in the secretory phase. The zygote secretes human chorionic gonadotropin (hCG) to signal the woman's body that a pregnancy has begun. With continued hCG production by the conceptus, the corpus luteum persists and continues secreting estrogen and progesterone.

Location of Implantation

The conceptus must be in the right place at the right time for normal implantation to occur. The site of implantation is important because that is the place that the placenta develops. Normal implantation occurs in the upper uterus (fundus). The upper uterus is the best area for implantation and placental development for three reasons:

- The upper uterus is richly supplied with blood for optimal fetal gas exchange and nutrition.
- The uterine lining is thick in the upper uterus, preventing the placenta from attaching so deeply that it cannot be easily expelled after birth.
- Implantation in the upper uterus limits blood loss after birth because strong interlacing muscle fibers in this area compress open vessels after the placenta detaches.

Mechanism of Implantation

Enzymes produced by the conceptus erode the decidua, tapping maternal sources of nutrition. Primary chorionic villi are tiny projections on the surface of the conceptus. They extend into the decidua basalis that lies between the conceptus and the wall of the uterus. The chorionic villi eventually form the fetal side of the placenta; the decidua basalis forms the maternal side of the placenta (see p. 251).

At this early stage, nutritive fluid passes to the embryo

by *diffusion* (passive movement across a cell membrane from an area of higher concentration to one of lower concentration) because no circulatory system is yet established. By 10 days, the conceptus is fully embedded within the mother's uterine decidua, and the site of implantation is almost invisible.

As the conceptus implants, usually near the time of the next expected menstrual period, a small amount of bleeding may occur at the site. Implantation bleeding may cause in-

accurate calculation of a pregnancy's duration if it is counted as a normal menstrual period.

Embryonic Period

The embryonic period of development extends from the beginning of the third week through the eighth week after conception. Basic structures of all major body organs are completed during the embryonic period. Table 12–2 presents

TABLE 12–2

Timetable of Prenatal Development Based on Fertilization Age*

Nervous/Sensory System	Cardiorespiratory System	Digestive System	Genitourinary System	Musculoskeletal System	Integumentary System
3 Weeks: 1.5 mm CRL					
Flat neural plate begins closing to form neural tube. Neural tube still open at each end.	Heart consists of 2 parallel tubes that fuse into a single tube. Contractions of heart tube begin. Chorionic villi of early placenta connect with heart.	Endoderm (inner germ layer) will become digestive tract.		Paired, cube-shaped swellings (somites) appear and will form most of the head and trunk skeleton. Muscle, bone, and cartilage develop from mesoderm.	Epidermis (outer skin layer) will develop from ectoderm (outer germ layer). Dermis (deep skin layer) and connective tissue will develop from mesoderm (middle germ layer).
4 Weeks: 4.0 mm CRL					
Neural tube closed at each end. Cranial end of neural tube will form brain; caudal end will form spinal cord. Eye development begins as an outgrowth of forebrain. Nose development begins as two pits. Inner ear begins developing from hind brain.	Heart begins partitioning into 4 chambers and begins beating. Blood circulating through embryonic vessels and chorionic villi. Tracheal development begins as a bud on the upper gut and branches into two bronchial buds.	Development of primitive gut as embryo folds laterally. Stomach begins as a widening of the tube-shaped primitive gut. Liver, gallbladder, and biliary ducts begin as a bud from primitive gut.	Primordial germ (reproductive) cells are present on embryonic yolk sac.	Upper limb buds are present and look like flippers. Lower limb buds appear.	Mammary ridges that will develop into mammary glands appear.
6 Weeks: 13 mm CRL					
Development of pituitary gland and cranial nerves. Head sharply flexed because of rapid brain growth. Eyelid development beginning. External ear development begins in neck region as six swellings.	Blood formation primarily in liver. Three right and two left lung lobes develop as outgrowths of the right and left bronchi.	Most intestines are contained within the umbilical cord because the liver and kidneys occupy most of the abdominal cavity. Stomach nearing final form. Development of upper and lower jaws.	Kidneys are near bladder in the pelvis. Kidneys occupy much of the abdominal cavity. Primordial germ cells incorporated into developing gonads. Male and female gonads are identical in appearance.	Arms paddle-shaped, fingers webbed. Feet and toes develop similarly, but a few days later than arms and hands. Bones cartilaginous, but ossification of skull begins.	Mammary glands begin development. Tooth buds for primary (deciduous) teeth begin developing.

TABLE 12–2

Timetable of Prenatal Development Based on Fertilization Age* Continued

Nervous/Sensory System	Cardiorespiratory System	Digestive System	Genitourinary System	Musculoskeletal System	Integumentary System
8 Weeks: 30 mm CRL					
Spinal cord stops at end of vertebral column. Taste buds begin developing. Eyelids fuse. Ears have final form but are low-set.	Heart partitioned into 4 chambers. Heart beat detectable with ultrasound. Additional branching of bronchi.	Stomach has reached final form. Lips are fused. Intestines remain in umbilical cord.	Testes begin developing under influence of Y chromosome. Ovaries will develop if a Y chromosome is not present. External genitalia begin to differentiate but still appear quite similar.	Fingers and toes still webbed, but distinct by end of eighth week. Bones begin to ossify. Joints resemble those of adults.	
10 Weeks: 61 mm CRL; Weight, 14 g					
Head flexion still present, but straighter. Eyelids closed and fused. Top of external ear slightly below eye level.	May be possible to detect heartbeat with Doppler transducer. Blood produced in spleen and lymphatic tissue.	Intestines contained within abdominal cavity as growth of this cavity catches up with digestive system development. Digestive tract patent from mouth to anus.	Kidneys in their adult position. Male and female external genitalia have different appearance but are still easily confused.	Toes distinct; soles face each other.	Fingernails begin developing. Tooth buds for permanent teeth begin developing below those for primary teeth.
12 Weeks: 87 mm CRL; Weight, 45 g					
Surface of brain is smooth, without sulci (grooves) or gyri (convolutions). Nasal septum and palate complete development.	Heart beat should be detected with Doppler transducer.	Sucking reflex present. Bile formed by liver.	Kidneys begin producing urine. Male and female external genitalia can be distinguished by appearance.	Limbs are long and thin. Involuntary muscles of viscera develop.	Downy lanugo begins developing at end of this week.
16 Weeks: 140 mm CRL; Weight, 200 g					
	Pulmonary vascular system developing rapidly.	Fetus swallows amniotic fluid and produces meconium (bowel contents).	Urine excreted into amniotic fluid.	Lower limbs reach final relative length, longer than upper limbs. A woman who has been pregnant before may begin to feel fetal movements.	External ears have enough cartilage to stand away from head somewhat. Blood vessels easily visible through the delicate skin. Fingerprints developing.
20 Weeks: 160 mm CRL; Weight, 460 g					
Myelination of nerves begins, and continues through first year of postnatal life.	Heartbeat should be detectable with regular fetoscope.	Peristalsis well developed.	Over 40% of nephrons are mature and functioning. Testes contained in abdomen, but begin descent toward scrotum. Primordial follicles of ovary develop.	Fetal movements felt by mother and may be palpable by an experienced examiner.	Skin is thin and covered with vernix caseosa. Brown fat production complete. Nipples begin development.

Table continued on following page

TABLE 12–2
• • • • • • • • • • • •

*Timetable of Prenatal Development Based on Fertilization Age** Continued

Nervous/Sensory System	Cardiorespiratory System	Digestive System	Genitourinary System	Musculoskeletal System	Integumentary System
24 Weeks: 230 mm CRL; Weight, 820 g					
Spinal cord ends at level of first sacral vertebra because of more rapid growth of vertebral canal.	Primitive thin-walled alveoli (air sacs) have developed and are surrounded by capillary network. Surfactant production begins in lungs to reduce surface tension within alveoli. Respiration possible, but most fetuses die if born at this time.			Fetus is active. Fetal movements become progressively more noticeable to both mother and examiner.	Body appearance lean. Skin wrinkled and red. Fingerprints and footprints developed. Fingernails present. Eyebrows and lashes present.
28 Weeks: 270 mm CRL; Weight, 1300 g					
Major sulci and gyri are present. Eyelids no longer fused after 26 weeks. Responds to bitter substances on tongue.	Erythrocyte formation shifts completely to bone marrow. Sufficient alveoli, surfactant, and capillary network to allow respiratory function, although respiratory distress syndrome is common. Many infants born at this time survive with intensive care.		Testes begin descent into scrotum.		Skin slightly wrinkled, but smoothing out as subcutaneous fat is deposited under it.
32 Weeks: 300 mm CRL; Weight, 2100 g					
			Testes enter scrotum.		Skin smooth and pigmented. Large vessels visible beneath skin. Fingernails reach fingertips. Lanugo disappearing.
38 Weeks: 360 mm CRL; Weight, 3400 g					
Sulci and gyri developed. Visual acuity about 20/600 at birth.	Newborn infant has about one-eighth to one-sixth the number of alveoli of an adult. Well-developed ability to exchange gas.		Both testes usually palpable in scrotum at birth. The newborn girl's ovaries contain about 1 million follicles. No new ones are formed after birth.		Fetus plump and skin smooth. Vernix caseosa present in major body creases. Lanugo present on shoulders and upper back only. Fingernails extend beyond the fingertips. Ear cartilage firm.

* Fertilization age is about 2 weeks less than gestational age.
Abbreviation: CRL, crown-to-rump length.

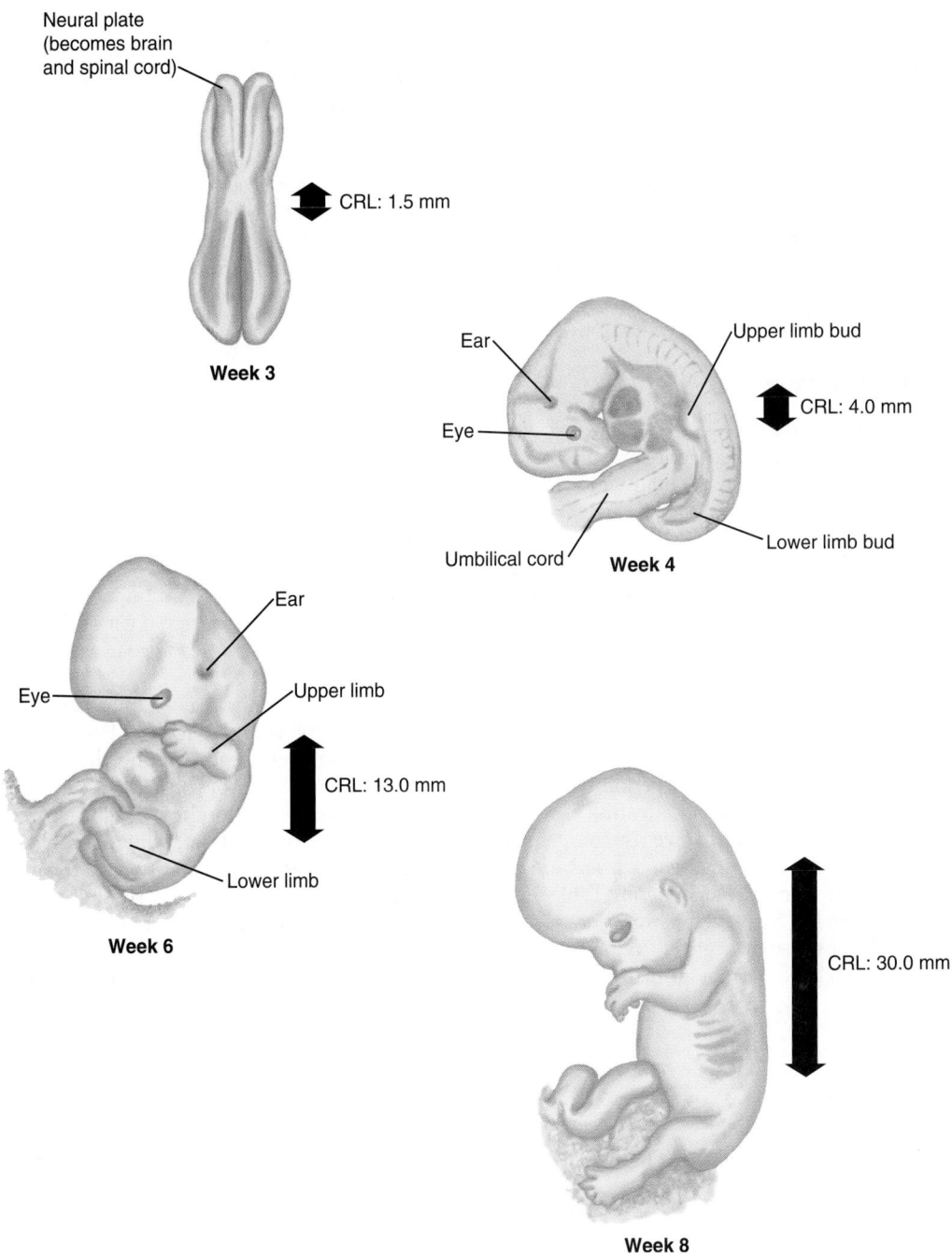

Neural plate (becomes brain and spinal cord)

CRL: 1.5 mm

Week 3

Ear

Upper limb bud

Eye

CRL: 4.0 mm

Umbilical cord   **Week 4**   Lower limb bud

Ear

Eye

Upper limb

CRL: 13.0 mm

Lower limb

Week 6

CRL: 30.0 mm

Week 8

FIGURE 12–5

Embryonic development from 3 weeks through the eighth week after fertilization. CRL is crown-to-rump length.

major developments in body systems during prenatal life. Figure 12–5 illustrates the external appearance of the embryo from the third through the eighth week after conception.

Differentiation of Cells

The embryo progresses from having cells with essentially identical functions (undifferentiated) to differentiated, or specialized, body cells. By the end of the eighth week, all major organ systems are in place, and many are functioning in a simple way.

Development of the specialized structures is controlled by three factors: (1) the genetic information in the chromosomes received from the parents, (2) interaction between adjacent tissues, and (3) timing. Although basic instructions are carried within the chromosomes, one tissue may induce change toward greater specialization in another, but only if a signal between the two tissues occurs at a specific time during development. In this way, structures develop with appropriate size and relationships to each other.

During the embryonic period, structures are vulnerable to damage from teratogens because they are developing rapidly. Normal development of one structure often requires normal and properly timed development of another. Unfortunately, a woman may not realize she is pregnant at this sensitive time. For this reason, the possibility of pregnancy should be explored with her before drugs or diagnostic procedures, such as radiography, are prescribed. Some agents may be damaging at one time during pregnancy but not at another. Others may be damaging at any time during pregnancy. Appendix C contains information about substances that may cause prenatal damage.

Weekly Developments

Development of the embryo and fetus proceeds in a cephalocaudal (head-to-toe) and a central-to-peripheral direction, a pattern that continues after birth in the infant and child.

SECOND WEEK

Implantation is complete by the end of the second week. The most growth occurs in the outer cells (*trophoblast*), which eventually become the fetal part of the placenta. The inner cell mass that will develop into the baby becomes flattened into the *embryonic disk*. Cells that eventually form part of the fetal membranes develop.

THIRD WEEK

Many women miss their first menstrual period during the third week of pregnancy. The embryonic disk develops three layers (*germ layers*) that, in turn, give rise to the major organ systems of the body. The three germ layers are the ectoderm, the mesoderm, and the endoderm. Table 12–3 lists structures that develop from each germ layer.

The central nervous system begins developing during the third week. A thickened flat neural plate appears, extending toward the end of the embryonic disk that will become the head. The neural plate develops a longitudinal groove that folds to form the neural tube. At the end of the third week, the neural tube is fused in the middle but is still open at each end.

Early heart development consists of a pair of parallel tubes that run longitudinally and join. The primitive heart begins beating at 21 to 22 days. Vessels developing in the chorionic villi and membranes join the heart tubes. Primitive blood cells arise from the endoderm lining the distal blood vessels.

FOURTH WEEK

The shape of the embryo changes. It folds at the head and tail end and laterally. The embryo resembles a C-shaped cylinder by the end of the fourth week. A "tail" is apparent during the embryonic period because the brain and spinal cord develop more rapidly than other systems.

The neural tube completes closure during the fourth week. If the neural tube does not close, defects such as anencephaly and spina bifida result.

Formation of the face and upper respiratory tract begins. Beginnings of the internal ear and the eye are apparent. The upper extremities appear as buds on the lateral body walls.

Because the embryo is sharply flexed anteriorly, the heart is near the embryo's mouth. Partitioning of the heart into four chambers begins during the fourth week and is completed by the end of the sixth week.

The lower respiratory tract begins growth as a branch of the upper digestive tract, which is tubular at this time. Gradually, the esophagus and trachea separate completely. The trachea branches to form the right and left bronchi. These bronchi in turn branch to form the three lobes of the right lung and two lobes of the left lung. Continued branching of the bronchi eventually forms the terminal air

---

TABLE 12–3

Derivatives of the Three Germ Layers

Ectoderm	Mesoderm	Endoderm
Developing Structures		
Brain and spinal cord	Cartilage	Lining of gastrointestinal
Peripheral nervous system	Bone	and respiratory tracts
Pituitary gland	Connective tissue	Tonsils
Sensory epithelium of the	Muscle tissue	Thyroid
eye, ear, and nose	Heart	Parathyroid
Epidermis	Blood vessels	Thymus
Hair	Blood cells	Liver
Nails	Lymphatic system	Pancreas
Subcutaneous glands	Spleen	Lining of urinary bladder
Mammary glands	Kidneys	and urethra
Tooth enamel	Adrenal cortex	Lining of ear canal
	Ovaries	
	Testes	
	Reproductive system	
	Lining membranes (pericardial,	
	pleural, peritoneal)	

Weeks 25

Because of matu
and central nerv
vive if born after
smoother-skinne
the skin. The ski
9 weeks, reopen.
shifts from the sp

During early
the amniotic sac
position during t

- The uterus is :
  the fetus in fle
  pole of the egg
  feet as the larg
- The fetal head
  the head to dri

Weeks 29

The skin is pigm
Larger vessels are
laries cannot be s
extend to the fin
fat, rounding the
this period, chanc

Weeks 33

Growth of all boc
rate of growth slc
mainly gaining w
enable efficient an

The well-nou
subcutaneous fat. I
upper back, and u
creases, such as th

The testes are
female infants are
neath the areola a

Full term ran
age, or 38 to 42 w
tion occurs about 2
strual period, the
about 2 weeks shor
age, however, is m
the last menstrual
most women do nc

■ Auxiliary

Three auxiliary stru
the pregnancy and
the placenta, the u

Placenta

The placenta is a t
major functions are
between mother an
is smooth, with bra
covered surface. Th
ches to the uterus (

sacs (*alveoli*). The alveoli proliferate and become surrounded by a rich capillary network that allows oxygen and carbon dioxide exchange at birth.

FIFTH WEEK

The head is very large because the brain grows rapidly during the fifth week. The heart is beating and developing four chambers. Upper limb buds are paddle-shaped, with obvious notches between the fingers. Lower limbs are also paddle-shaped, but the area between the toes is not as well defined as the division between the fingers.

SIXTH WEEK

The head is prominent because of rapid development and is bent over the chest. The heart reaches its final four-chambered form. Upper and lower extremities continue to become more defined.

The eye continues to develop, and the beginning of the external ear is apparent as six small bumps near each side of the neck. Facial development begins with eyes, ears, and nasal pits widely separated, aligned with the body walls. Gradually, the embryo grows so that the face comes together at the midline.

SEVENTH WEEK

Growth and refinement of all systems occur. The face becomes more human-looking. The eyelids begin to grow, and the extremities become longer and better defined. The trunk elongates and straightens, although a C-shaped spinal curve is still present at birth.

During the embryonic period, the intestines grow faster than the abdominal cavity. The relatively large liver and kidneys also occupy much of the abdominal cavity. Therefore, most of the intestines are contained within the umbilical cord while the abdominal cavity grows to accommodate them. By 10 weeks, the abdomen is large enough to contain all its normal contents.

EIGHTH WEEK

The embryo has a definite human form, and refinements to all systems continue. The ears are low-set but are approaching their final location. The eyes are pigmented but not fully covered by eyelids. Fingers and toes are stubby but well defined. The external genitalia begin to differentiate, but male and female characteristics are not distinct until after the 10th week.

■ Fetal Period

The fetal period begins 9 weeks after conception and ends with birth. Dramatic growth and refinement in the structure and function of all organ systems occur during the fetal period. Teratogens may damage already formed structures but are less likely to cause major structural alterations. The central nervous system is vulnerable to damaging agents through the entire pregnancy. Figure 12–6 illustrates growth and development during the fetal period.

Weeks 9 Through 12

At the beginning of this period, the head is large, about half the total length of the fetus. The body begins growing faster than the head. The extremities approach their final relative lengths, although the legs remain proportionally shorter than the arms. The first fetal movements begin but are too slight for the mother to detect.

The face is broad, with a wide nose and widely spaced eyes. The eyes close at 9 weeks and reopen at about 26 weeks. The ears appear low-set because the mandible is still small.

The intestinal contents that were partly contained within the umbilical cord enter the abdomen as the capacity of the abdominal cavity catches up with their size. Blood formation occurs primarily in the liver during the 9th week but shifts to the spleen by the end of the 12th week. The fetus begins producing urine during this period, excreting it into the amniotic fluid.

Internal differences in males and females become apparent in the seventh week. External genitalia look similar until the end of the ninth week. By the end of the 12th week, the fetal sex can be determined by the appearance of the external genitalia.

Weeks 13 Through 16

The fetus grows rapidly in length, so the head becomes smaller in proportion to the total length. Movements strengthen, and some women, particularly those who have been pregnant before, are able to detect them. Fetal movements produce the experience of *quickening*.

The face looks human because the eyes face forward. The ears approach their final position, in line with the eyes.

Weeks 17 Through 20

Fetal movements feel like fluttering, or "butterflies." Some women may not recognize these subtle sensations for what they are.

Changes in the skin and hair are evident. *Vernix caseosa*, a fatty cheeselike secretion of the fetal sebaceous glands, covers the skin to protect it from constant exposure to amniotic fluid. *Lanugo* is fine, downy hair that covers the fetal body to help the vernix adhere to the skin. Both vernix and lanugo diminish as the fetus reaches term. Eyebrows and head hair appear.

Brown fat is heat-producing fat deposited on the back of the neck, behind the sternum, and around the kidneys. Brown fat helps the neonate maintain temperature stability after birth.

Weeks 21 Through 24

The fetus continues growing and gaining weight but is thin and has little subcutaneous fat. The skin is translucent and looks red because the capillaries are close to its fragile surface.

The lungs begin to produce *surfactant*, a surface-active lipid that makes it easier for the baby to breathe after birth. Surfactant reduces surface tension in the lung alveoli and keeps them from collapsing with each breath.

The capillary network surrounding the alveoli is increasing but is still very immature, although some gas exchange is possible. A 22- to 25-week fetus may survive with intensive care, although the child is more likely to die during later infancy or have prematurity-related disabilities.

50.0 cm —

36.0 cm —

Size (crown-to-rump length)

30.0 cm —

27.0 cm —

23.0 cm —

16.0 cm —

14.0 cm —

8.7 cm —

5.0 cm —

9

11

FIGURE 1

Fetal developme
gestational age,
than the fertiliz

TABLE 12–4

Mechanisms of Placental Transfer

Mechanism	Description	Examples of Substances Transferred
Simple diffusion	Passive movement of substances across a cell membrane from an area of higher concentration to one of lower concentration	Oxygen and carbon dioxide Carbon monoxide Water Urea and uric acid Most drugs and their metabolites
Facilitated diffusion	Passage of substances across a cell membrane by binding with carrier proteins that assist transfer	Glucose
Active transport	Transfer of substances across a cell membrane against a pressure or electrical gradient, or from an area of lower concentration to one of higher concentration	Amino acids Water-soluble vitamins Minerals: Calcium, iron, iodine
Pinocytosis	Movement of large molecules by ingestion within cells	Maternal IgG class antibodies Some passage of maternal IgA antibodies

a higher average hemoglobin (14.5 to 22.5 g/dl) and hematocrit value (about 48% to 69%).

• Hemoglobin can carry more oxygen at low carbon dioxide partial pressure (Pco_2) levels than it can at high ones (Bohr effect). Blood entering the placenta from the fetus has a high Pco_2, but carbon dioxide diffuses quickly to the mother's blood, where the Pco_2 is lower, reversing the levels of carbon dioxide in maternal and fetal blood supplies. Therefore, the fetal blood becomes more alkaline, and the maternal blood becomes more acidic. This difference allows the mother's blood to give up oxygen and the fetal blood to combine with oxygen readily.

Nutrient Transfer. The growing fetus requires a constant supply of nutrients from the pregnant woman. Glucose, fatty acids, electrolytes, and vitamins pass readily across the placenta.

Waste Removal. In addition to carbon dioxide, urea, uric acid, and bilirubin are readily transferred from the fetus to the mother for disposal.

Antibody Transfer. Many of the immunoglobulin G (IgG) class of antibodies are passed from mother to fetus through the placenta. This process confers passive (temporary) immunity to the fetus against diseases such as measles if the mother is immune to them. The preterm infant has little protection offered by maternal antibodies because they are transferred during late pregnancy.

Passage of antibodies from expectant mother to fetus is not always beneficial. If maternal and fetal blood types are not compatible, the mother either may already have or may produce antibodies against fetal erythrocytes. The mother's antibodies may then destroy the fetal erythrocytes, causing fetal anemia or even fetal death.

Transfer of Maternal Hormones. Most maternal protein hormones do not reach the fetus in amounts sufficient to cause abnormalities.

ENDOCRINE FUNCTIONS

The placenta produces several hormones necessary for normal pregnancy. Human chorionic gonadotropin (hCG) causes the corpus luteum to persist and secrete estrogens and progesterone. As the placenta develops, it produces estrogens and progesterone, and the corpus luteum gradually regresses after 20 weeks. When a Y chromosome is present in the male fetus, hCG also causes the fetal testes to secrete testosterone necessary for normal development of male reproductive structures.

Human placental lactogen, also called human chorionic somatomammotropin, is a placental hormone that promotes normal nutrition and growth of the fetus and maternal breast development for lactation. The hormone decreases maternal insulin sensitivity and utilization of glucose, making more glucose available for fetal nutrition.

Steroid hormones secreted by the placenta include estrogens and progesterone. Estrogens cause enlargement of the woman's uterus, enlargement of the breasts, growth of the ductal system of the breasts, and enlargement of the external genitalia. Progesterone is essential for normal continuation of the pregnancy. Progesterone causes the endometrium to change into the decidua, providing nourishment for the early conceptus. Progesterone also reduces uterine contractions, thereby preventing spontaneous abortion. Progesterone acts with estrogens and other hormones to cause growth of the breasts, budding of the alveoli that will secrete milk, and development of secretory characteristics in the alveolar cells.

Other hormones produced by the placenta include human chorionic thyrotropin and human chorionic adrenocorticotropin.

Fetal Membranes and Amniotic Fluid

The two fetal membranes are the *amnion* (inner membrane) and the *chorion* (outer membrane). The two membranes are so close as to be one. (Together, they are often called the bag of waters.) The membranes can, however, be separated. If they rupture in labor, amnion and chorion usually rupture together, releasing the amniotic fluid within the sac.

The amnion is continuous with the surface of the umbilical cord, joining the epithelium of the fetus's abdominal skin. Chorionic villi proliferate over the entire surface of the gestational sac for the first 8 weeks after conception. A conceptus observed at this time looks like a shaggy sphere with the embryo suspended inside. As the embryo grows, it bulges into the uterine cavity. The villi on the outer surface gradually atrophy and form the smooth-surfaced chorion. The remaining villi continue to branch and enlarge to form the fetal side of the placenta.

Amniotic fluid protects the growing fetus and promotes normal prenatal development. Amniotic fluid protects the fetus by

- Cushioning against an impact to the maternal abdomen
- Providing a stable temperature

Amniotic fluid promotes normal prenatal development by

- Allowing symmetric development as the major body surfaces fold toward the midline
- Keeping the membranes from adhering to developing fetal parts
- Allowing room and buoyancy for fetal movement

Amniotic fluid is derived from two sources: fetal urine and fluid transported from the maternal blood across the amnion. Cast-off fetal epithelial cells and vernix are suspended in the amniotic fluid. The water of the amniotic fluid changes by absorption across the amnion, returning to the mother. The fetus also swallows amniotic fluid and absorbs it in the digestive tract; waste products are returned to the placenta through the umbilical arteries.

The volume of amniotic fluid increases during pregnancy, until it is about 500 to 1,500 ml at term (Guyton, 1996). An abnormally small quantity of fluid (less than 50% of the amount expected for gestation, or less than 500 ml at term) is called *oligohydramnios* and may be associated with poor fetal lung development and malformations that result from compression of fetal parts. Oligohydramnios may occur because the kidneys fail to develop, urine excretion is blocked, or placental blood flow is inadequate. *Hydramnios* (also called *polyhydramnios*) is the opposite situation, in which the quantity may exceed 2,000 ml. Hydramnios may occur when the fetus has a severe malformation of the central nervous system or gastrointestinal tract that prevents normal ingestion of amniotic fluid.

Fetal Circulation

The course of fetal blood circulation is from the fetal heart, to the placenta for exchange of oxygen and waste products, and back to the fetus for delivery to fetal tissues (Fig. 12–9A).

UMBILICAL CORD
The umbilical cord is the lifeline between the fetus and placenta. It has two arteries that carry deoxygenated blood and waste products away from the fetus to the placenta, where these substances are transferred to the mother's circulation for elimination. The umbilical vein carries freshly oxygenated and nutrient-rich blood from the placenta back to the fetus. The umbilical arteries and vein are coiled within the cord to allow them to stretch and prevent obstruction of blood flow through them. The entire cord is cushioned by a soft substance called *Wharton's jelly* to prevent obstruction due to pressure.

FETAL CIRCULATORY CIRCUIT
Because the fetus does not breathe air or metabolize substances in the liver, several alterations of the postbirth cir-

culatory route are needed. Three shunts in the fetal circulatory system divert most circulating blood away from the lungs and liver. These shunts are the ductus venosus, the foramen ovale, and the ductus arteriosus.

Oxygenated blood from the placenta enters the fetal body through the umbilical vein. About half the blood goes through the liver, and the rest bypasses the liver and enters the inferior vena cava through the first shunt, the *ductus venosus*. The blood then enters the right atrium. Most of the blood passes directly into the left atrium through the second shunt, the *foramen ovale*, where it mixes with the small amount of blood returning from the lungs. Blood is pumped from the left ventricle into the aorta to nourish the body. A small amount of blood from the right ventricle is circulated to the lungs to nourish the lung tissue. The rest of the blood from the right ventricle joins oxygenated blood in the aorta through the third shunt, the *ductus arteriosus*. The head and upper body receive the greatest amount of oxygenated blood.

The muscle wall of the right side of the fetal heart is thicker than that of the left because resistance to blood flow through the uninflated lungs is high. When the infant begins breathing after birth, resistance to pulmonary blood flow falls dramatically, and the right side of the heart does not need to be so thick. During infancy, the thickness of the right heart gradually decreases as its workload decreases.

CHANGES IN BLOOD CIRCULATION AFTER BIRTH
Fetal circulatory shunts are not needed after birth because the infant oxygenates blood in the lungs, metabolizes substances in the liver, and is not circulating blood to the placenta (see Fig. 12–9B). As the infant breathes, blood flow to the lungs increases, pressure in the right heart falls, and the foramen ovale closes. The ductus arteriosus constricts as the arterial oxygen level rises. The ductus venosus constricts when flow of blood from the umbilical cord stops.

Transition to the postnatal circulatory pattern is gradual. Functional closure occurs when the infant breathes. The foramen ovale and ductus venosus are permanently closed as tissue proliferates in these structures. The ductus venosus becomes a ligament, as do the umbilical vein and arteries.

Multifetal Pregnancy

Multifetal pregnancy is a deviation from the usual course of gestation. Twins occur *spontaneously* about once in 85 pregnancies, triplets about once in 8,100 pregnancies, quadruplets once in 729,000 pregnancies, and quintuplets only once in more than 65 million pregnancies (Moore & Persaud, 1998). Greater use of assisted reproductive techniques (see Chapter 10) has increased the number of multiples, especially higher-order multiples (triplets or more), dramatically in recent years.

Twinning is the most common form of multifetal pregnancy. The same processes that occur in twin pregnancies also may occur in other multiple gestations. Twins are often called "identical" or "fraternal" by laypeople. They are more accurately described by their genetic origin or by the number of ova and sperm involved. The two types of twins are monozygotic and dizygotic. Figure 12–10 illustrates these two mechanisms of twinning.

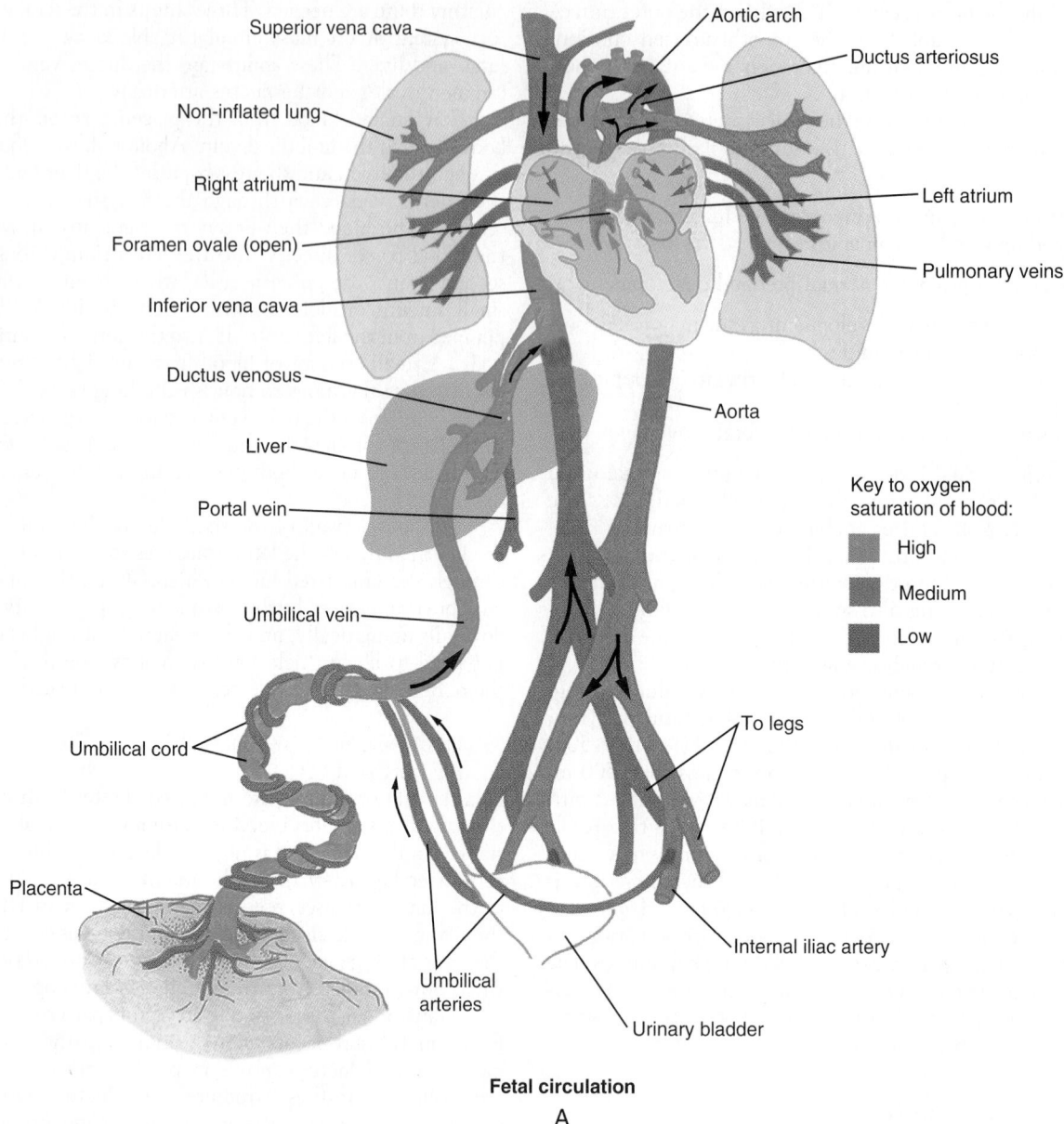

Superior vena cava

Non-inflated lung

Right atrium

Foramen ovale (open)

Inferior vena cava

Ductus venosus

Liver

Portal vein

Umbilical vein

Umbilical cord

Placenta

Umbilical arteries

Aortic arch

Ductus arteriosus

Left atrium

Pulmonary veins

Aorta

Key to oxygen saturation of blood:

High

Medium

Low

To legs

Internal iliac artery

Urinary bladder

Fetal circulation

A

FIGURE 12–9

A, Fetal circulation. Three shunts—the ductus venosus, the ductus arteriosus, and the foramen ovale—allow most blood from the placenta to bypass the fetal lungs and liver.

Monozygotic Twinning

Monozygotic twins are conceived by the union of a single ovum and spermatozoon, with later division of the conceptus into two. Monozygotic twins have identical genetic complements and are of the same sex. They may not always look identical at birth, however, because one twin may have grown much larger than the other, or one may have a birth defect, such as a cleft lip. Monozygotic twinning occurs essentially at random and is unrelated to the use of assisted reproductive techniques.

In monozygotic twinning, a single conceptus divides early in gestation. In most cases of monozygotic twins (65%), the formed *blastocyst* has two inner cell masses instead of one. With two inner cell masses, the fetuses have two amnions (inner membranes) but a single chorion (outer membrane).

If the conceptus divides earlier, two separate but identical morulas (and then blastocysts) develop and implant separately. These monozygotic twins have two amnions and two chorions. Although their placentas develop separately, they may fuse and appear as one at birth. Their chorions also may fuse during prenatal development. Therefore, examining the placenta and membranes after birth cannot always establish whether twins are monozygotic or dizygotic.

Late separation of the inner cell mass may result in twins with a single amnion and a single chorion. These twins often die because their umbilical cords become entangled. Incomplete separation of the inner cell mass may result in conjoined twins.

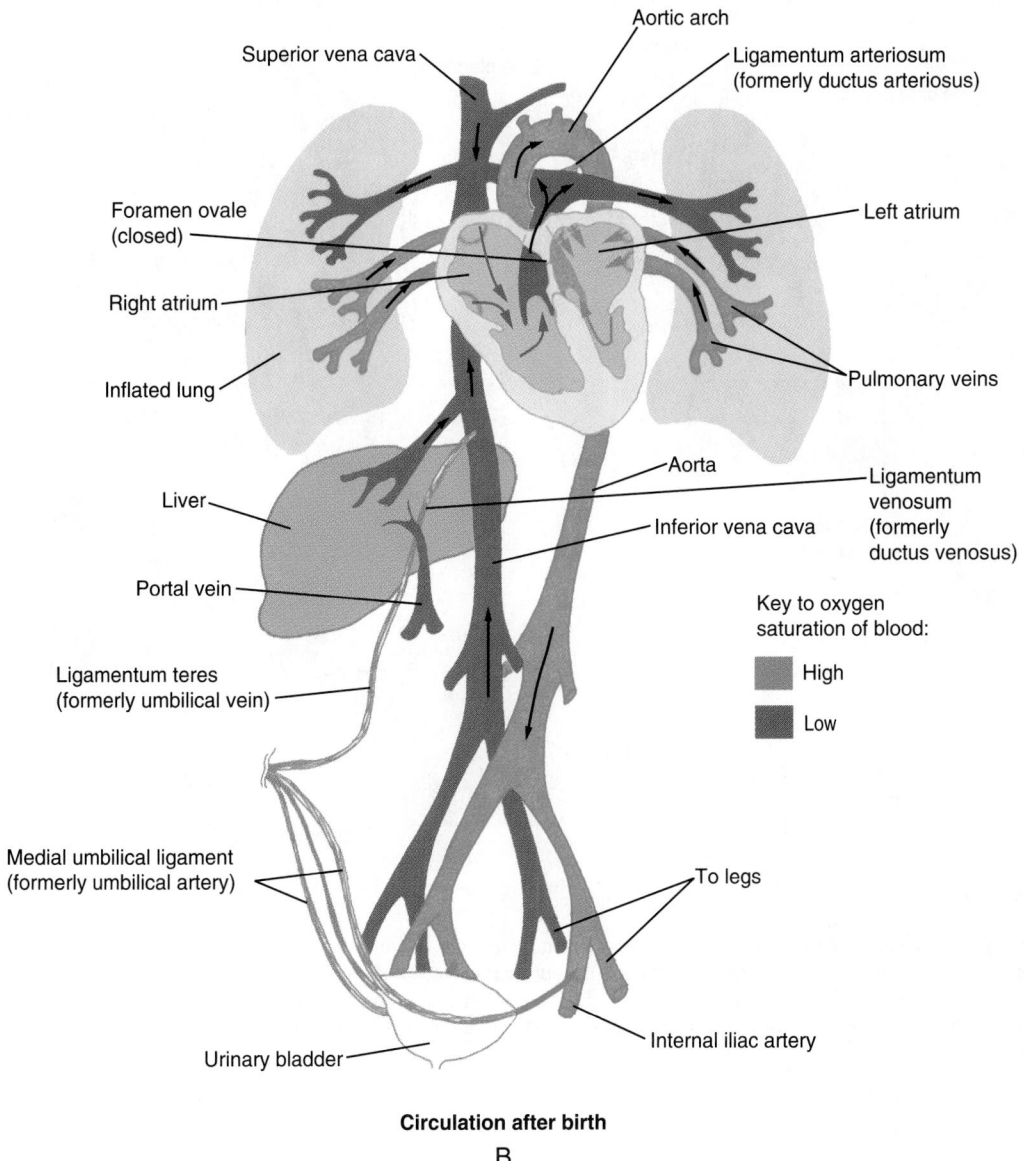

Circulation after birth

B

FIGURE 12–9

Continued. B, Circulation after birth. Note that the fetal shunts have closed. The umbilical vessels, the ductus venosus, and the ductus arteriosus have been converted to ligaments.

Dizygotic Twinning

Dizygotic twins arise from two ova that are fertilized by different sperm. Dizygotic twins may be the same or different sex, and they may or may not have similar physical traits. Dizygotic twins and higher-order multiples are associated with the use of assisted reproductive techiques because these therapies involve induction of multiple ovulation and implantation of multiple fertilized ova.

Dizygotic twinning may be hereditary in some families, presumably because of an inherited tendency of the women to release more than one ovum per cycle. Women of some races are more likely to have dizygotic twins as well:

- African: 1 in 20 births
- White: 1 in 125 births
- Asian: 1 in 500 births

Advancing maternal age is also associated with an increased incidence of dizygotic twin births.

Because dizygotic twins arise from two separate zygotes, their membranes and placentas are separate. The membranes, placentas, or both may fuse during development if they implant closely. Dizygotic twins are not conjoined because they do not involve division of a single cell mass into two, but arise from two separate conceptions.

Other Multifetal Gestations

Pregnancies resulting in more offspring than twins may arise from a single zygote or a combination of a single and multiple zygotes, or each may arise from a separate zygote. These higher-number pregnancies pose much greater hazards to both the expectant mother and fetuses. The incidence of long-term handicaps is higher as the number of fetuses increases.

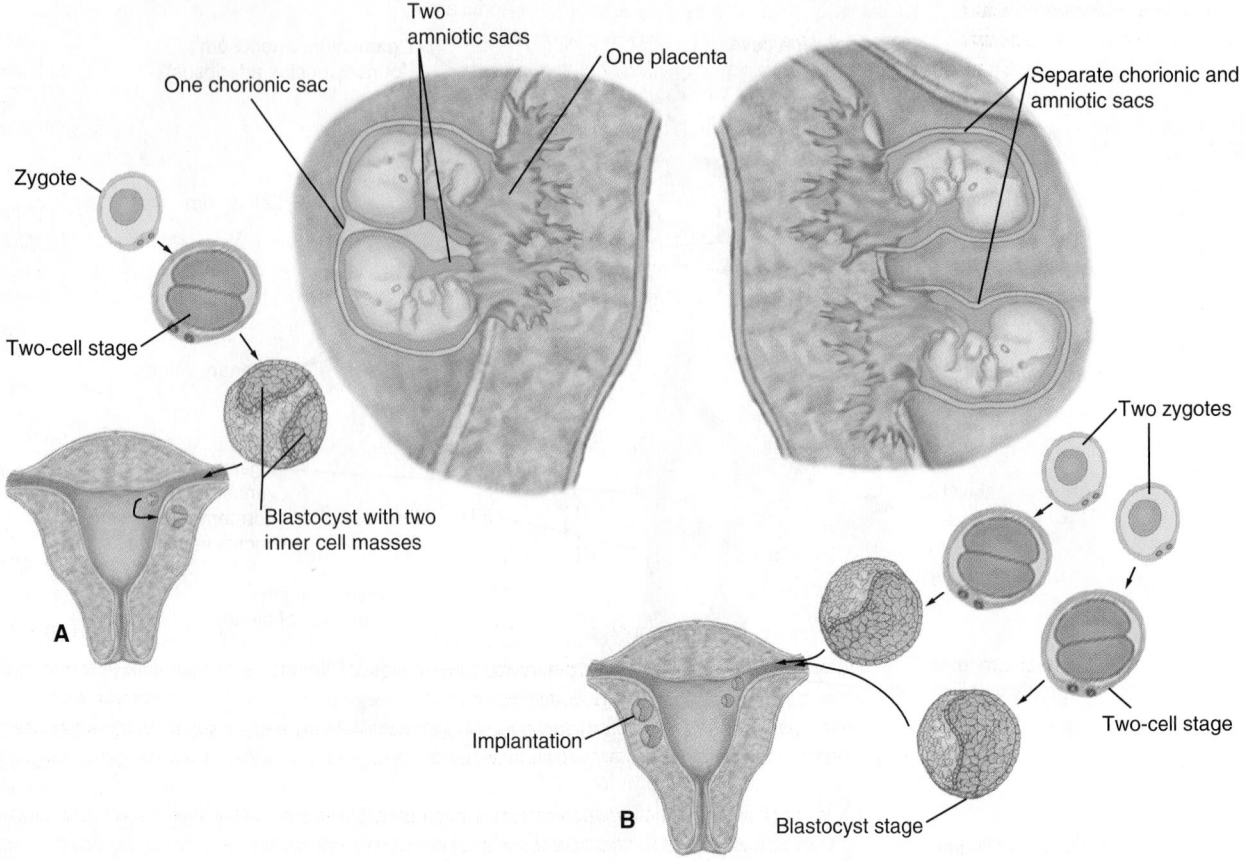

FIGURE 12–10

A, Monozygotic twinning. The single inner cell mass divides into two inner cell masses during the blastocyst stage. These twins have a single placenta and chorion, but each twin develops in its own amnion. *B,* Dizygotic twinning. Two ova are released during ovulation, and each is fertilized by a separate spermatozoon. The ova may implant near each other in the uterus, or they may be far apart.

KEY CONCEPTS

- The purpose of gametogenesis is to produce ova and sperm that have half the full number of chromosomes, or 23 unpaired chromosomes. When an ovum and a sperm unite at conception, the number is restored to 46 paired chromosomes.
- The female has all the ova she will ever have at 30 weeks of prenatal gestation. No other ova are formed after this time.
- One primary oocyte can mature into one mature ovum that contains 23 unpaired chromosomes (22 autosomes and an X chromosome).
- A male can continuously produce new sperm from puberty through the rest of his life, although fertility declines somewhat after age 40.
- One primary spermatocyte can result in production of four mature sperm. Two of the mature sperm have 22 autosomes and an X sex chromosome. Two have 22 autosomes and a Y sex chromosome.
- The male determines the baby's sex because only sperm carry either an X or a Y sex chromosome. The female can contribute only an X chromosome to the baby.
- The basic structure of all organ systems is established during the first 8 weeks of pregnancy. Teratogens during this period may cause major structural and functional damage to the developing organs.
- The fetal period is one of growth and refinement of already established organ systems. Teratogens can still damage the fetus but are less likely to cause major structural damage. They may, however, still cause major functional damage.
- The placenta is an embryonic or fetal organ with metabolic, respiratory, and endocrine functions.
- Transfer of substances between mother and embryo or fetus occurs by four mechanisms: simple diffusion, facilitated diffusion, active transport, and pinocytosis.

- Most substances in the maternal blood can be transferred to the fetus.
- The fetal membranes contain the amniotic fluid, which cushions the fetus, allows normal prenatal development, and maintains a stable temperature.
- The umbilical cord is the lifeline between the fetus and the placenta. Two umbilical arteries carry deoxygenated blood and waste products to the placenta for transfer to the mother's blood. One umbilical vein carries oxygenated and nutrient-rich blood to the fetus. Coiling of the vessels and enclosure in Wharton's jelly reduce the risk of obstruction of the umbilical vessels.
- The fetal circulatory system has three shunts that partially bypass the fetal liver and lungs. These are the ductus venosus, the foramen ovale, and the ductus arteriosus. These structures close functionally after birth but are not closed permanently until several weeks or months later.
- Multifetal pregnancy may be monozygotic or dizygotic. Twins are the most common form of multifetal pregnancy.
- Dizygotic twins are more likely to occur in certain families and racial groups, in older mothers, and in women who undergo fertility therapy.

REFERENCES AND READINGS

Benirschke, K. (1998). Multiple gestation: Incidence, etiology and inheritance. In R. K. Creasy & R. Resnik (Eds.), *Maternal-fetal medicine: Principles and practice* (pp. 598–615). Philadelphia: Saunders.

Benirschke, K. (1998). Normal development. In R. K. Creasy & R. Resnik (Eds.), *Maternal-fetal medicine: Principles and practice* (pp. 63–71). Philadelphia: Saunders.

Guyton, A. C. (1996). *Textbook of medical physiology* (9th ed.). Philadelphia: Saunders.

Moore, K. L., & Persaud, T. V. N. (1998). *Before we are born: Essentials of embryology and birth defects* (5th ed.). Philadelphia: Saunders.

Moore, K. L., & Persaud, T. V. N. (1998). *The developing human: Clinically oriented embryology* (6th ed.). Philadelphia: Saunders.

From the moment of conception, important chang[es oc]cur in the pregnant woman's body. These chang[es are] necessary to support and nourish the fetus and [to pre]pare the woman for childbirth and lactation. Nurse[s must] understand not only the physiologic changes but al[so the] ways these changes affect the daily lives of exp[ectant] mothers.

Changes in Body Systems

Pregnancy challenges each body system to adapt to [in]creasing demands of the fetus.

Reproductive System

UTERUS

Growth. Before conception the uterus is a [small] pear-shaped organ entirely contained in the pelvic [cavity.] It weighs approximately 60 g (2 ounces) and has a c[apacity] of about 10 ml (one third of an ounce). At the end [of preg]nancy, the uterus extends to the level of the xipho[id pro]cess, weighs approximately 1,000 g (2.2 lb), and has a [capac]ity of about 5,000 ml.

Uterine growth occurs as the result of both hyp[erplasia] and hypertrophy. During the first trimester, growth [is due] mainly to hyperplasia and the formation of new c[ells as a] result of stimulation of the myometrium by estroge[n (Res]nik, 1999). During the second and third trimesters, [uterine] growth is due to hypertrophy as the muscle fibers st[retch in] all directions. Fibrous tissue accumulates in the oute[r muscle] layer of the uterus, and the amount of elastic ti[ssue in]creases. These changes greatly increase the strengt[h of the] muscle wall.

Muscle fibers in the myometrium increase [in both] length and width. As a result, by the third trime[ster, the] uterine muscles are thin, and the fetus can be easily [palpated] through the abdominal wall. As the uterus expa[nds into] the abdominal cavity, it gradually displaces the i[ntestines] upward and laterally as it rotates to the right. The [rotation] is probably due to pressure of the rectosigmoid colo[n on the] left side of the pelvis.

Pattern of Uterine Growth.   The uterus grows [in a pre]dictable pattern that provides information abo[ut fetal] growth and helps to confirm the expected date of [delivery] (EDD), sometimes called the expected date of birt[h or EDB] (Fig. 13–1). By 12 weeks of gestation, the uteru[s can be] palpated above the symphysis pubis. At 16 weeks, [the fun]dus reaches midway between the symphysis pubis [and the] umbilicus. It is located at the umbilicus by 20 we[eks.]

The fundus reaches its highest level at the xiph[oid pro]cess at 36 weeks. Because it pushes against the di[aphragm,]

13

♦ ♦ ♦ ♦ ♦ ♦ ♦ ♦

Physiologic Adaptations to Pregnancy

LEARNING OBJECTIVES

After studying this chapter, you should be able to:

- Describe the physiologic changes that occur during pregnancy.
- Differentiate presumptive, probable, and positive signs of pregnancy.
- Compute gravida, para, and estimated date of delivery (birth).
- Describe initial antepartum assessments in terms of history, physical examination, and risk assessment.
- Identify subsequent antepartum assessments.
- Discuss maternal adaptations to multifetal pregnancy.
- Describe the common discomforts of pregnancy in terms of causes and measures that prevent or relieve them.
- Discuss nursing process and critical thinking skills needed to develop nursing care plans for the most common problems and discomforts of pregnancy.

DEFINITIONS

abortion In the United States, a spontaneous or elective termination of pregnancy before the 20th week of gestation, based on the date of the last menstrual period. Spontaneous abortion is frequently termed "miscarriage" by the lay public.

amenorrhea Absence of menstruation. Primary amenorrhea is a delay of the first menstruation. Sec-

ondary a
menstru
Braxton H
lar, mild
occur th
become
mester.
Chadwick
ation of
bia duri
increase
chloasma
the face
called "
colostrum
ing preg
days fol
diastasis r
gitudina
(rectus
nancy.
Goodell's
vix, ute
nancy.
gravida
been p
ration
hyperemi
of the
multigrav
been p
multipara
birth t
than 2
nullipara
compl
weeks
para N
have
delive
cate w
alive
not re
infant
(twins
parou
physiol
crease
by dil
pande
by an
cytes

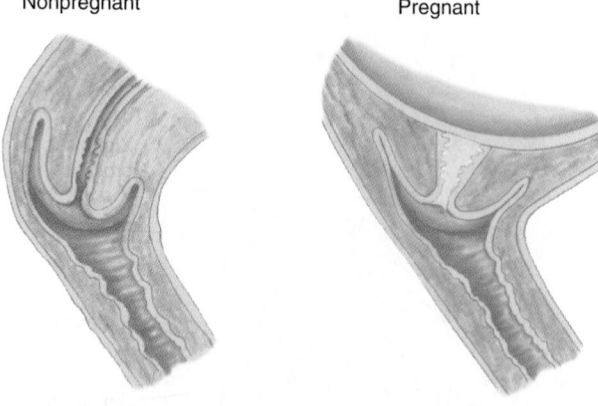

Nonpregnant   Pregnant

FIGURE 13–2

Cervical changes that occur during pregnancy. Note enlargement of spaces in cervical mucosa, which are filled with a thick mucous plug.

the cervix to soften. Before pregnancy, the cervix has a consistency similar to that of the tip of the nose. After conception, the cervix feels more like the lobe of the ear. The cervical softening is referred to as *Goodell's sign*.

The cervical glands proliferate during pregnancy, and the endocervical tissue resembles a honeycomb that fills with mucus. The mucus forms a plug in the cervical canal and blocks the ascent of bacteria from the vagina into the uterus during pregnancy (Fig. 13–2). One of the earliest signs of labor may be "bloody show," which consists of the mucous plug plus a small amount of blood produced by disruption of the cervical capillaries as the mucous plug is dislodged when the cervix begins to thin and dilate.

VAGINA AND VULVA

Increased vascularity of the vagina causes the vaginal walls, as well as the cervix, to appear bluish. Softening of the abundant connective tissue allows the vagina to distend during childbirth. The vaginal mucosa thickens, and vaginal rugae (folds) become very prominent.

Vaginal cells contain increasing amounts of glycogen, which causes rapid sloughing and increased vaginal discharge. The pH of the vaginal discharge is acidic because of the increased production of lactic acid that results from the action of *Lactobacillus acidophilus* on glycogen in the vaginal epithelium (Cunningham et al., 1997). The acidic condition works to prevent growth of harmful bacteria found in the vagina. The glycogen-rich environment, however, favors the growth of *Candida albicans*, so that persistent yeast infections (candidiasis) are common during pregnancy.

Increased vascularity, edema, and connective tissue changes make the tissues of the vulva and perineum more pliable. Pelvic congestion during pregnancy can lead to heightened sexual interest and increased orgasmic experiences.

OVARIES

After conception, the major function of the ovaries is to secrete progesterone for the first 6 to 7 weeks of the pregnancy. Progesterone is called the hormone of pregnancy, and if the pregnancy is to be maintained, adequate progesterone must be available from the earliest stages. The corpus luteum secretes progesterone until the placenta is developed. Once developed, the placenta secretes progesterone throughout pregnancy.

Ovulation ceases during pregnancy because the circulating levels of estrogen and progesterone are high, inhibiting the release of follicle-stimulating hormone (FSH) and luteinizing hormone (LH), which are necessary for ovulation.

BREASTS

During pregnancy, the breasts change in size and appearance because of the effects of estrogen and progesterone (Fig. 13–3). Estrogen stimulates the growth of mammary ductal tissue, and progesterone promotes the growth of lobes, lobules, and alveoli. The breasts become highly vascular, and a delicate network of veins is often visible. If the increase in breast size is extensive, striations ("stretch marks") may develop.

Characteristic changes in the nipples and areolae occur during pregnancy. The nipples increase in size and become more erect, and the areolae become larger and more pigmented. Women with very light complexions exhibit less

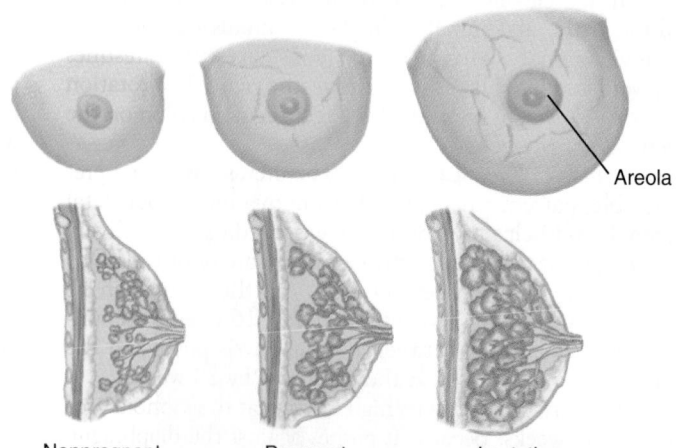

Areola

FIGURE 13–3

Breast changes that occur during pregnancy. The breasts increase in size and become more vascular, the areolae become darker, and the nipples become more erect.

Nonpregnant   Pregnant   Lactating

change in pigmentation than those who have darker skin. Sebaceous glands, called *tubercles of Montgomery*, become more prominent during pregnancy and secrete a substance that lubricates the nipples. In addition, a thin, yellowish breast fluid (*colostrum*) is present in greater or lesser amounts throughout pregnancy and can readily be expressed by the third trimester.

Cardiovascular System

HEART
Heart Size and Position. Cardiac changes are slight, and they reverse soon after childbirth. The muscles of the heart (myocardium) enlarge slightly because of an increased workload during pregnancy. The heart is pushed upward and toward the left as the uterus elevates the diaphragm during the third trimester. As a result of the change in position, the locations for auscultating heart sounds may be shifted upward and laterally in late pregnancy.

Heart Sounds. During pregnancy some heart sounds may be altered to the extent that they would be considered abnormal in a nonpregnant state. The changes are first heard between 12 and 20 weeks and continue for 2 to 4 weeks after childbirth. The most common variations in heart sounds include splitting of the first heart sound and a systolic murmur that is found in 90% of pregnant women (Cunningham et al., 1997). Diastolic murmurs occur in 20% of pregnant women and are thought to be due to increased blood flow through the tricuspid or mitral valve or to physiologic dilation of the pulmonary artery (Blackburn & Loper, 1992).

BLOOD VOLUME
Plasma Volume. Total blood volume is a combination of plasma and solutes, such as red blood cells (erythrocytes), white blood cells (leukocytes), and platelets (thrombocytes). Plasma volume increases progressively from 6 to 8 weeks' gestation to approximately 5,000 ml at 32 weeks. This is an increase of 45% (1,200 to 1,600 ml) above nonpregnant values (Monga, 1999). The increase may be related to estrogen stimulation of the renin-angiotensin-aldosterone system, which stimulates sodium and water retention.

The increased volume is needed for two reasons: (1) to transport nutrients and oxygen to the placenta, where they become available for the growing fetus, and (2) to meet the demands of the expanded maternal tissue in the uterus and breasts. The greater volume also provides a reserve to protect the pregnant woman from the adverse effects of the blood loss that occurs during childbirth.

Red Blood Cell Volume. Red blood cell mass increases by 250 to 450 ml, about 20% to 30% above pre-pregnancy values (Monga, 1999). The increase in plasma volume is more pronounced and occurs earlier than the increase in red blood cell volume. The resulting dilution of red blood cell mass causes a decline in maternal hematocrit. This condition is frequently called *physiologic anemia* or *pseudoanemia of pregnancy* because it reflects the dilution of red blood cells in a greatly expanded plasma volume and does not indicate true anemia.

Frequent laboratory examinations may be needed to distinguish physiologic anemia from true anemia. Generally, iron deficiency anemia does not exist unless the hemoglobin is 10.5 g/dl or lower (Duffy, 1999) or the hematocrit is less than 33%. Iron supplementation is necessary if the hemoglobin or hematocrit falls below these levels.

Dilution of red blood cells by plasma may also have a protective function. By decreasing blood viscosity, dilution may counter the tendency to form clots (thrombi) that can obstruct blood vessels and cause serious complications (see Chapter 28).

CARDIAC OUTPUT
The expanded vascular volume of pregnancy causes an increase in cardiac output, the amount of blood discharged from the heart each minute. It is based on stroke volume (the amount of blood pumped from the heart with each contraction) and heart rate (the number of times the heart beats each minute). Cardiac output rises rapidly during the first trimester and remains elevated throughout pregnancy. During pregnancy, the increase in cardiac output is due primarily to a gain in stroke volume, but the heart rate also rises about 15 to 20 beats per minute (BPM) (Blackburn & Loper, 1992).

PERIPHERAL VASCULAR RESISTANCE
Peripheral vascular resistance falls during pregnancy. This change is likely due to (1) smooth muscle relaxation in vessel walls due to the effects of progesterone; (2) the addition of the uteroplacental unit, which provides a greater area for circulation; (3) fetal heat production, which may cause vasodilation; and (4) an increased synthesis of prostaglandins that cause resistance to circulating vasoconstrictors, such as angiotensin II and norepinephrine.

BLOOD PRESSURE
As a result of decreased peripheral vascular resistance, blood pressure remains stable during pregnancy despite the increase in blood volume. Systolic pressure remains largely unchanged, although diastolic pressure may decrease (by about 10 mm Hg) during the first and second trimesters (Monga, 1999). During the third trimester, blood pressure rises slightly. Blood pressure should, however, remain at or near the normal levels of early pregnancy.

Effect of Position on Blood Pressure. Arterial blood pressure is affected by position during pregnancy. Pressure is lowest when the pregnant woman is in a lateral recumbent position. Pressures are significantly higher when she is standing than when she is sitting. Moreover, an increase in both systolic and diastolic pressure occurs when the arm is held in a dependent position.

Each agency needs to standardize the way blood pressure is taken and to document the position as well as the pressure so that the site of assessment remains consistent. Moreover, controversy continues over whether Korotkoff's fifth phase (disappearance of sound) correlates better with the true diastolic pressure than does the fourth phase (muffling). Facilities should select which phase is to be used and remain consistent throughout the prenatal, intrapartum, and postpartum periods. Blood pressures of 140/90 require additional assessment.

Mean Arterial Pressure. The mean arterial pressure (MAP) is the average pressure within an artery over a complete cycle of one heartbeat. The MAP is estimated by computing one third of the pulse pressure (systolic pressure minus diastolic pressure) and adding that figure to the diastolic pressure. According to some researchers, an elevated MAP (above 85 mm Hg) is predictive of hypertension.

Supine Hypotension. When the pregnant woman is in the supine position, particularly during the second and third trimesters, the weight of the *gravid* (pregnant) uterus partially occludes the vena cava and the descending aorta (Fig. 13–4). The occlusion impedes return of blood from the lower extremities and, as a consequence, reduces cardiac return, cardiac output, and blood pressure. This condition is called supine hypotensive syndrome or vena caval syndrome. Symptoms include faintness, lightheadedness, dizziness, and agitation. Some may experience syncope, a brief lapse in consciousness. Blood flow through the placenta also decreases if the woman remains in the supine position for a prolonged period, and decreased blood flow could result in fetal hypoxia.

Turning to a lateral recumbent position alleviates the pressure on the blood vessels and quickly corrects supine hypotension. Women should be advised to rest in a side-lying position to prevent supine hypotension. If they must assume a supine position for fetal surveillance testing, a wedge or pillow under the right hip is effective in decreasing supine hypotension.

BLOOD FLOW

Four major changes in blood flow occur during pregnancy:

- Blood flow is altered to include the uteroplacental unit. Approximately 500 ml/min is required to perfuse the placenta adequately.
- Approximately 30% more blood must circulate through the maternal kidneys to remove the increased metabolic wastes generated by mother and fetus.
- The woman's skin requires increased circulation to dissipate the heat generated by increased metabolism during pregnancy.
- The weight of the expanding uterus on the inferior vena cava and iliac veins partially obstructs blood return from veins in the legs, causing stasis of blood and venous distension. Prolonged engorgement of the veins of the lower legs may result in varicose veins of the legs, vulva, or rectum (hemorrhoids).

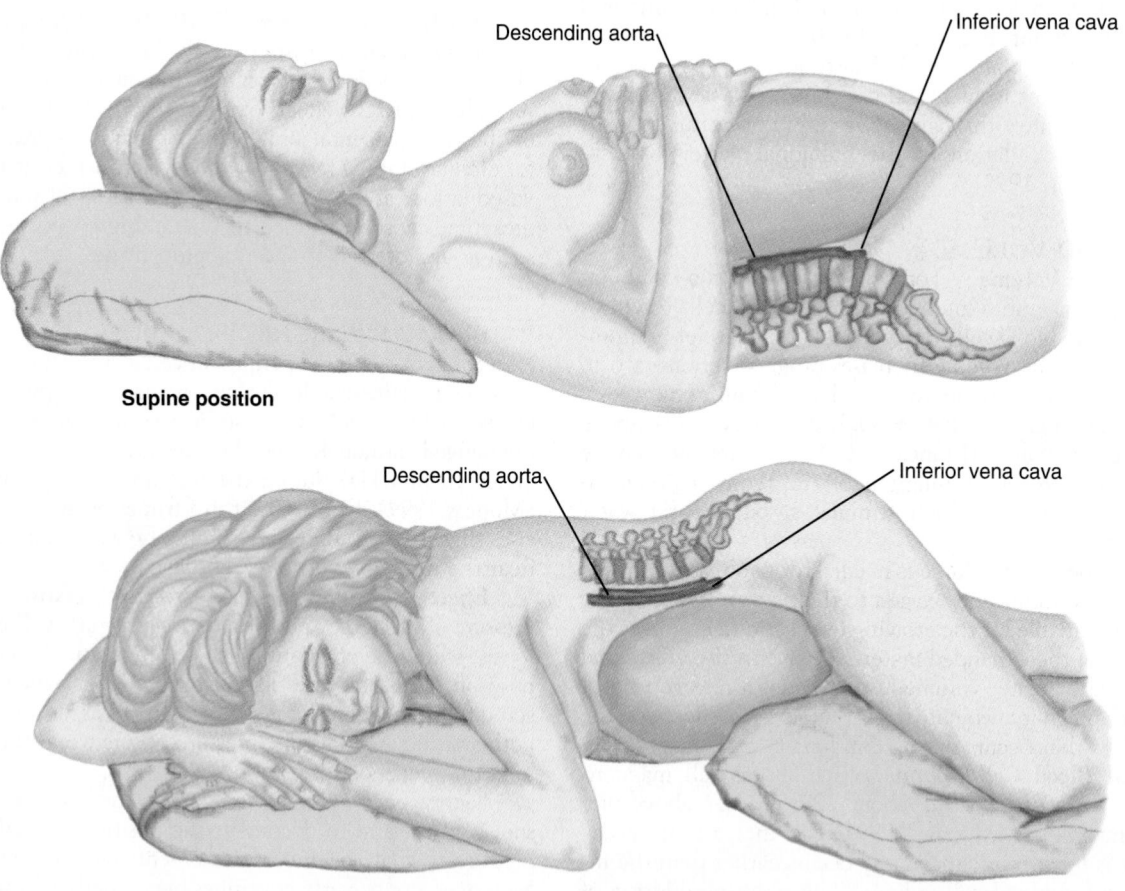

Supine position

Right lateral position

FIGURE 13-4

Vena caval syndrome, or supine hypotensive syndrome. When the woman is supine, the weight of the gravid uterus partially occludes the vena cava and the descending aorta. Turning to a lateral recumbent position corrects supine hypotension.

BLOOD COMPONENTS

During pregnancy, erythrocytes increase by 20% to 30%. The rise reflects accelerated production of erythrocytes rather than prolonged red cell life. The gain in erythrocytes greatly increases the maternal demand for iron, which is necessary for hemoglobin formation.

Although iron absorption and iron-binding power are increased during pregnancy, sufficient iron is not always supplied by diet. Iron supplementation may be needed to promote hemoglobin synthesis and ensure that erythrocyte production is sufficient to prevent iron deficiency anemia (see Chapter 26).

Leukocytes increase from an average prepregnancy level of 5,000 cells/mm³ to an average of 10,000 cells/mm³ (Baker, 1995). Leukocytes increase further during labor as a result of exertion and may reach 25,000 cells/mm³ by the early postpartum period.

During pregnancy, plasma fibrinogen (factor I) rises by about 50%. Elevated fibrinogen levels increase the ability to form clots. This offers some protection from hemorrhage during childbirth, but it also increases the risk of thrombus formation in the legs and the development of thrombophlebitis. The risk is a particular concern if the woman must stand or sit for prolonged periods, with stasis of blood in the veins of the legs. (See Appendix D for additional changes in blood components.)

Respiratory System

OXYGEN CONSUMPTION

Oxygen consumption increases by about 15% to 20% in pregnancy. Half the oxygen is used by the fetus and the rest is consumed by the uterus, the breast tissue, and the increased respiratory and cardiac demands. To compensate for the increased need for oxygen, the woman breathes more deeply, although her respiratory rate remains unchanged. As a result, the tidal volume (the volume of gas moved into or out of the respiratory tract with each breath) as well as the respiratory minute volume (the volume of air inspired or expired in 1 minute) increase by about 40%. As a consequence of the elevated minute volume, the partial pressure of carbon dioxide (Pco_2) is lowered. Renal excretion of bicarbonate partially compensates for the resulting respiratory alkalosis. Decreased partial pressure of Pco_2 also promotes the transfer of carbon dioxide from fetal to maternal circulation.

HORMONAL FACTORS

Progesterone. Progesterone plays a role in decreasing airway resistance by relaxing the smooth muscle in the respiratory tract. It is also believed to raise the sensitivity of the respiratory center (medulla oblongata) to carbon dioxide, thus stimulating the increase in minute ventilation and lowering the Pco_2. These two factors are responsible for the heightened awareness of the need to breathe experienced by many women during pregnancy.

Estrogen. Estrogen causes increased vascularity of the mucous membranes of the upper respiratory tract. As the capillaries become engorged, edema and hyperemia develop within the nose, pharynx, larynx, and trachea. This congestion may result in nasal and sinus stuffiness, epistaxis

(nosebleeds), and changes in the voice. Increased vascularity also causes edema of the eardrum and eustachian tubes, which may result in a sense of fullness in the ears or earaches.

PHYSICAL CHANGES

By the third trimester, the enlarging uterus lifts the diaphragm by about 4 cm (1.6 inches), which prevents the lungs from expanding fully. To compensate for the reduced space, the ribs flare, the substernal angle widens, and the circumference of the chest expands by about 6 cm (2.5 inches). Breathing becomes thoracic rather than abdominal, adding to the dyspnea many women experience.

Gastrointestinal System

MOUTH

Elevated levels of estrogen cause hyperemia of the tissues of the mouth and gums, which may lead to gingivitis and bleeding gums. Some women develop severe vascular hypertrophy of the gums, which appear reddened and swollen and bleed easily. The condition regresses spontaneously after childbirth.

Some women experience *ptyalism*, or excessive salivation, that is unpleasant and embarrassing. The cause appears to be stimulation of the salivary glands by the ingestion of starch (Cunningham et al., 1997). Small, frequent meals, gum chewing, and oral lozenges offer limited relief for some women. Contrary to common belief, the teeth are unaffected by pregnancy and do not lose minerals to the fetus.

ESOPHAGUS

The lower esophageal sphincter tone decreases during pregnancy, primarily because of the effect of progesterone on the smooth muscles. The reduced tone allows reflux of acidic stomach contents into the esophagus and produces heartburn (*pyrosis*).

STOMACH AND SMALL INTESTINE

Elevated levels of progesterone relax all smooth muscle, decreasing gastrointestinal tone and motility. The stomach and small intestine take longer to empty, allowing additional time for nutrients to be absorbed. This slowed process benefits the growing fetus, but it may contribute to the nausea many expectant mothers experience.

LARGE INTESTINE

Decreased motility in the large intestine allows time for more water to be absorbed, which may lead to constipation. Hemorrhoids may be caused or exacerbated by constipation if the expectant mother must strain to have bowel movements.

LIVER AND GALLBLADDER

Progesterone causes functional changes of the liver and gallbladder. The gallbladder becomes hypotonic and emptying time is prolonged, resulting in thicker bile, which can predispose to the development of gallstones. Reduced gallbladder tone also leads to a tendency to retain bile salts, which can lead to itching (pruritus).

During the last trimester, the liver is pushed upward

and backward by the enlarging uterus, and liver function is also altered. Serum alkaline phosphatase and serum cholesterol levels are almost doubled by the end of pregnancy, whereas levels of serum albumin fall gradually. These changes are due primarily to the effect of estrogen and to hemodilution.

Urinary System

BLADDER

During the first and third trimesters, pressure on the bladder from the uterus causes the woman to experience frequency and urgency of urination. The cause is uterine expansion within the pelvis in early pregnancy. Late in the third trimester, the fetus settles into the pelvis (lightening), again causing frequency, urgency, and nocturia.

The uterus extends into the abdominal cavity during the second trimester, so that pressure on the bladder is relieved and the urge to void decreases. In addition, bladder capacity almost doubles as the bladder, like all smooth muscle, relaxes in response to increasing levels of progesterone.

Bladder mucosa becomes congested with blood, and the bladder walls become hypertrophied as a result of stimulation from estrogen. Decreased drainage of blood from the base of the bladder makes the tissues edematous and susceptible to trauma and infection during childbirth.

KIDNEYS AND URETERS

Changes in Size and Shape of the Kidneys. During pregnancy, the kidneys change in both size and shape because dilation of the renal pelves, calyces, and ureters occurs above the pelvic brim. The dilation is caused by (1) the effect of progesterone, which makes the ureters more distensible, and (2) compression of the ureters between the enlarging uterus and the bony pelvic brim. As the flow of urine through the ureters is obstructed, particularly on the right side (the left ureter is cushioned by the sigmoid colon), the ureters and renal pelvis dilate. The resulting stasis of urine allows time for bacteria to multiply and increases the risk of urinary tract infection during pregnancy.

Functional Changes of the Kidneys. Renal plasma flow, the total amount of plasma to flow through the kidneys, increases by 35% to 60%. The rise is due to increases in plasma volume and cardiac output. The glomerular filtration rate, the rate at which water and dissolved substances are filtered in the glomerulus, increases by as much as 50%. This increase is due to the increase in renal plasma flow and to decreased colloid osmotic pressure caused by a reduction in the concentration of plasma proteins.

The increases in renal plasma flow and glomerular filtration rate are necessary to excrete additional metabolic waste from the mother and fetus, but they also affect the excretion of glucose. As the glomerular filtration rate increases, the filtered load of glucose exceeds the ability of the renal tubules to reabsorb it, and glucose spills into the urine. Therefore, glycosuria is common during pregnancy, particularly after the consumption of foods, such as candy or cookies, that are high in simple sugars. Furthermore, small quantities of amino acids and water-soluble vitamins are excreted. Bacteria thrive in urine that is rich in nutrients, so that glycosuria is one more reason why the incidence of urinary tract infections increases during pregnancy.

Tests of renal function may be misleading during pregnancy. As a result of increased glomerular filtration rate, plasma concentrations of both creatinine and urea normally decline.

Integumentary System

SKIN

Circulation to the skin increases during pregnancy and encourages activity of the sweat and sebaceous glands. Pregnant women feel warmer and perspire more, particularly during the last trimester. Accelerated activity of the sebaceous glands fosters the development of facial blemishes. Additional changes include hyperpigmentation and vascular changes in the skin.

Hyperpigmentation. Increased pigmentation may begin as early as the second month, when levels of melanocyte-stimulating hormone (MSH) become elevated because of the effects of estrogen and progesterone. Brunettes and dark-skinned women exhibit more hyperpigmentation than women with very light skin. Areas of pigmentation include brownish patches, called *chloasma* or the *mask of pregnancy*, over the forehead, cheeks, and bridge of the nose. A dark line of pigmentation (*linea nigra*) may also extend from the umbilicus to the symphysis pubis. Preexisting moles become darker, and the areolae become darker as pregnancy progresses. Hyperpigmentation usually disappears following childbirth, when the levels of estrogen and progesterone decline.

Cutaneous Vascular Changes. Blood vessels dilate and proliferate during pregnancy. This change is thought to be due largely to the effect of estrogen. Changes in surface blood vessels are obvious during pregnancy, especially in white women. These include angiomas that appear as tiny red elevations that branch in all directions. Commonly called *vascular spiders* or *telangiectasis*, they appear most often on the face, neck, upper chest, and arms. Redness of the palms or soles of the feet, known as *palmar erythema*, also occurs in many white women and in some African-American women. Although vascular changes may be emotionally distressing for the expectant mother, they are clinically insignificant and usually disappear shortly after childbirth.

CONNECTIVE TISSUE

Linear tears may occur in the connective tissue, most often on the abdomen, breasts, and buttocks, appearing as slightly depressed, pink to purple streaks called *striae gravidarum* or "stretch marks" (Fig. 13–5). Women are concerned about striae because they fade to silvery lines but do not disappear after childbirth. Laser therapy is sometimes used after childbirth to reduce or eliminate severe striae. Many women insist that striae can be prevented by massage with oil or vitamin E, but the effectiveness of this treatment has not been documented. Antipruritic ointments may be effective in controlling the itching that accompanies severe striae.

HAIR AND NAILS

Because fewer follicles are in the resting phase, hair grows more rapidly and less hair falls out during pregnancy. After childbirth, hair follicles return to normal activity, and many

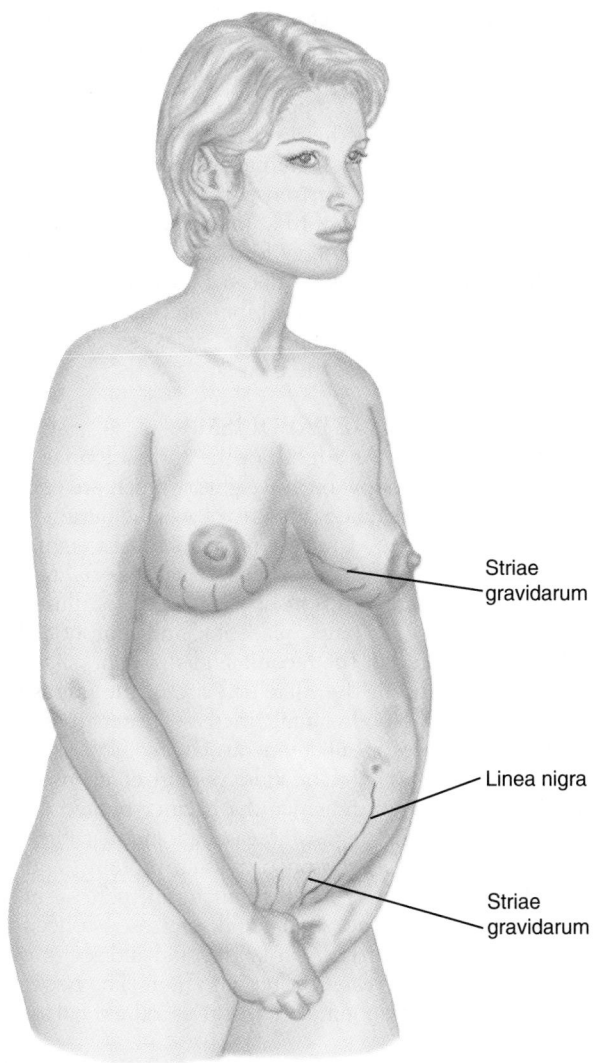

FIGURE 13–5
Striae gravidarum are linear tears that may occur in the connective tissue. Linea nigra, a dark line of pigmentation from the umbilicus to the symphysis pubis, may also appear.

women become concerned about the rate of hair loss. They need reassurance that more follicles have returned to the normal resting phase and that excessive hair loss will not continue.

Nail growth increases during pregnancy. Many women notice thinning and softening of the nails as pregnancy progresses, although the reasons for this change are unclear.

Musculoskeletal System

POSTURAL CHANGES

Musculoskeletal changes are progressive. They begin in the second trimester, when the hormones relaxin and progesterone initiate gradual softening of the pelvic ligaments and joints. This facilitates passage of the fetus through the pelvis at the time of birth. Relaxation of the pelvic joints creates pelvic instability, and the woman assumes a wide stance and

the waddling gait of pregnancy to compensate for a changing center of gravity.

During the third trimester, as the uterus increases in size, it becomes necessary for the expectant mother to lean backward to maintain her balance. This posture creates a progressive *lordosis*, or curvature of the lower spine, and may lead to backache.

ABDOMINAL WALL

During the third trimester the abdominal muscles may become so stretched that the rectus abdominis muscles separate (*diastasis recti*). The extent of the separation varies from slight, which is not clinically significant, to severe, when a large portion of the uterine wall is covered only by skin and fascia (see Figure 21–5).

Endocrine System

PITUITARY GLAND

During pregnancy, prolactin from the anterior pituitary increases to prepare the breasts to produce milk. The posterior pituitary secretes oxytocin, which stimulates the milk-ejection reflex after childbirth. Oxytocin also stimulates contractions of the uterus, but during pregnancy this action is inhibited by progesterone, which relaxes smooth muscle fibers of the uterus. After childbirth, progesterone levels decline, and oxytocin keeps the uterus contracted, preventing excessive bleeding.

THYROID GLAND

Early in the first trimester, a rise in total thyroxine (T_4) and thyroxine-binding protein occurs. The increased amounts of T_4 bind readily with the thyroxine-binding proteins, and the serum level of unbound T_4 remains stable. These changes produce slight enlargement in the size of the thyroid gland and an increase in basal metabolic rate (BMR). The BMR increases by 20% to 25% during pregnancy, causing greater cardiac output, pulse rate, and heat intolerance. The BMR returns to normal within a few weeks after childbirth.

PARATHYROID GLANDS

During pregnancy, fetal demands for calcium and phosphorus increase, and the maternal parathyroid glands produce additional parathyroid hormone. Parathyroid hormone improves absorption of calcium from the intestine, to decrease renal losses and to mobilize bone. During pregnancy, however, no loss of bone density occurs despite the increase in parathyroid activity. The skeleton appears to be protected by increased levels of calcitonin and by estrogen, which interfere with the action of parathyroid hormone on bone.

PANCREAS

Significant changes in the pancreas during pregnancy are due to alterations in maternal blood glucose concentrations and consequent fluctuations in insulin production. During the first trimester, the increasing glucose demand by the fetus causes a fall in maternal blood glucose. As a result, the islets of Langerhans produce less insulin.

During the second trimester, maternal tissue sensitivity to insulin begins to decline, mainly because of the effects of human placental lactogen, prolactin, progesterone, and cortisol. By the end of pregnancy, tissue sensitivity to insulin falls by as much as 80% (Baker, 1995). The resulting higher blood glucose level makes more glucose available for fetal energy needs and stimulates the pancreas of a healthy woman to produce additional insulin. Inadequate insulin production results in gestational diabetes, described in Chapter 26.

ADRENAL GLANDS

The adrenal glands produce a significant increase in cortisol and aldosterone. Cortisol regulates carbohydrate and protein metabolism. It stimulates gluconeogenesis (formation of glycogen from noncarbohydrate sources such as amino or fatty acids) whenever the supply of glucose is inadequate to meet the body's needs for energy.

Aldosterone regulates the absorption of sodium from the distal tubules of the kidneys. It increases during pregnancy to overcome the salt-wasting effects of progesterone to maintain the necessary level of sodium in the greatly expanded blood volume. Aldosterone is closely related to water metabolism.

CHANGES CAUSED BY PLACENTAL HORMONES

Human Chorionic Gonadotropin. In early pregnancy, human chorionic gonadotropin (hCG) is produced by the trophoblastic cells that surround the developing embryo. This hormone stimulates the corpus luteum to produce progesterone and estrogen until the placenta is sufficiently developed to assume that function. It also causes a positive pregnancy test.

Estrogen. After the sixth or seventh week of pregnancy estrogen is produced primarily by the placenta. Estrogen has numerous functions during pregnancy: (1) it stimulates uterine growth and increases blood supply to uterine vessels; (2) it aids in developing the ductal system in the breasts in preparation for lactation; and (3) it is associated with hyperpigmentation, vascular changes in the skin, increased activity of the salivary glands, and hyperemia of the gums and nasal mucous membranes.

Progesterone. Progesterone is produced first by the corpus luteum and then by the fully developed placenta. Progesterone is the most important hormone of pregnancy. The major functions include

- Maintaining the endometrial layer for implantation of the fertilized ovum
- Preventing spontaneous abortion by relaxing smooth muscles of the uterus
- Stimulating the development of the lobes and lobules in the breast in preparation for lactation
- Facilitating the deposit of maternal fat stores, which provide a reserve of energy for pregnancy and lactation

Progesterone relaxes not only the smooth muscle of the uterus but also all other smooth muscle. As a consequence, progesterone is associated with decreased motility of the bowel, dilation of the ureters, and increased bladder capacity. Progesterone raises the respiratory sensitivity to carbon dioxide and thus stimulates increased ventilation.

Human Placental Lactogen. Also called human chorionic somatomammotropin (hCS), human placental lactogen (hPL) increases the availability of glucose for the fetus, who needs a constant supply. Human placental lactogen does this by decreasing the sensitivity of maternal cells to insulin, which decreases maternal metabolism of glucose, thereby freeing glucose for transport to the fetus. In addition, under the influence of hPL, free fatty acids are quickly metabolized to provide energy for the pregnant woman.

Relaxin. Relaxin is produced by the corpus luteum and by the placenta. Relaxin inhibits uterine activity, softens connective tissue in the cervix, relaxes pelvic joints, and stimulates growth of the breasts.

CHANGES IN METABOLISM

Weight Gain. As a result of the correlation between infant mortality and low birth weights, women are encouraged to gain an adequate amount of weight during pregnancy. (See Table 15–1 for the recommended weight gain for women of normal weight and those with special needs.)

The normal composition of weight gain is illustrated in Figure 15–1. The fetus, placenta, and amniotic fluid make up less than half the recommended weight gain. The remainder is found in the increased size of the uterus and breasts, increased blood volume, increased interstitial fluid, and maternal stores of subcutaneous fat.

Water Metabolism. The kidneys must compensate for the many factors that influence the balance of fluid during pregnancy. For example, an increased glomerular filtration rate, decreased concentration of plasma proteins, and increased progesterone levels all result in an increase in sodium excretion. On the other hand, increased concentrations of estrogen, cortisol, prolactin, and aldosterone all tend to promote the reabsorption of sodium. The net effect of the combined hormonal action is that sodium balance is maintained.

Dependent Edema. Because of hemodilution, a slight decrease occurs in colloid osmotic pressure, which favors the development of edema during pregnancy. Edema is further increased toward term, when the weight of the uterus compresses the veins of the pelvis. This process delays venous return, causing the veins of the legs to become distended, and increases venous pressure, resulting in additional fluid shifts from the vascular compartment to interstitial spaces.

Edema of the feet and ankles is obvious at the end of the day, particularly if a pregnant woman stands for prolonged periods. Dependent edema is clinically insignificant. If edema of the face or hands is noted, however, further assessment for hypertension or proteinuria is essential to determine whether pregnancy-induced hypertension is developing.

Carpal Tunnel Syndrome. Fluid retention is also associated with carpal tunnel syndrome, believed to result when edema compresses the median nerve at the point where it goes through the carpal tunnel of the wrist. Symptoms include soreness, weakness, and tenderness of the muscles of the thumb. The condition usually resolves when the pregnancy ends.

Carbohydrate Metabolism. Carbohydrate metabolism changes markedly during pregnancy because more insulin is required as pregnancy progresses. As hormones such as progesterone and hPL cause maternal tissue to be resistant to insulin, insulinase, an enzyme produced by the placenta, speeds the breakdown of insulin.

Decreasing the mother's ability to use insulin is a protective mechanism to supply glucose for the fetus. The mother's pancreas produces more insulin so that she can metabolize enough glucose to meet her energy needs and to prevent hyperglycemia. In some women, however, insulin production cannot be increased, and these women experience periodic hyperglycemia. This condition is called *pregnancy-induced glucose intolerance*, or gestational diabetes (see Chapter 26).

▌ *Confirmation of Pregnancy*

Traditionally, the diagnosis of pregnancy has been based on symptoms experienced by the woman as well as on signs observed by a physician, nurse-midwife, or nurse practitioner. Figure 13–6 summarizes fetal and maternal changes that occur throughout pregnancy. These signs and symptoms are grouped into three classifications: presumptive, probable, and positive indications of pregnancy. A diagnosis of pregnancy cannot be made solely on the presumptive or probable signs. Table 13–1 lists other possible causes for these signs.

Presumptive Indications of Pregnancy

Presumptive indications can also be termed subjective changes because they are what the woman experiences and reports. Presumptive changes are the least reliable indicators of pregnancy because any one of them can be caused by conditions other than pregnancy.

AMENORRHEA

Absence of menstruation in a sexually active woman who regularly menstruates strongly suggests that conception has occurred. Menses cease after conception because progesterone and estrogen, secreted from the corpus luteum, maintain the endometrial lining in preparation for implantation of the fertilized ovum.

NAUSEA AND VOMITING

Many women experience nausea and vomiting, which generally begin about 6 weeks after the last menstrual period. Symptoms generally disappear by about 16 weeks (Cunningham et al., 1997). Nausea and vomiting are believed to be caused by the increased levels of hormones (hCG, estrogen), decreased gastric motility (an effect of progesterone), and the relative hypoglycemia that results from nightlong fasting.

FATIGUE

Fatigue and drowsiness during the first trimester are very common. The direct cause is unknown, but it may be related to the hypoglycemia that occurs periodically as glucose is transferred from the mother to the fetus.

URINARY FREQUENCY

Urinary frequency begins in the first few weeks of pregnancy, as pressure is exerted on the bladder by the expanding uterus. This symptom abates during the second trimester, when the uterus expands into the abdominal cavity. Late in the third trimester, the fetus settles into the pelvic cavity, and the woman once again experiences frequency and urgency of urination because the uterus presses against the bladder.

Gestational age 1–4 weeks

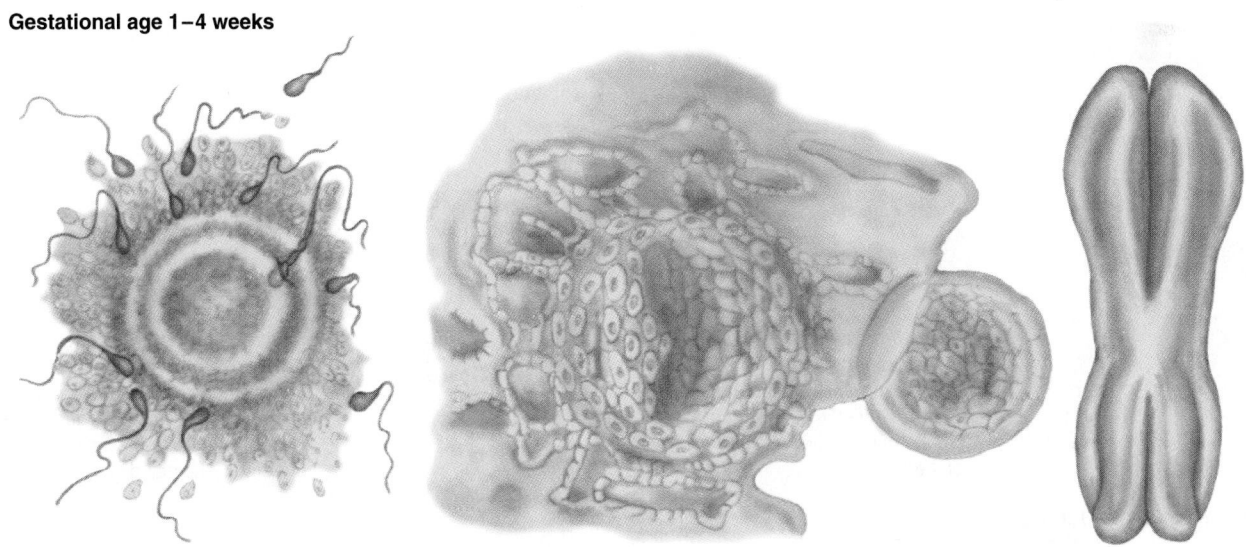

Woman's basal body temperature elevated; hCG elevated; pregnancy tests positive.

Crown-to-rump length 4 mm. Fertilization, implantation. Pre-embryonic stage.

▌ FIGURE 13–6
• • • • • • • • •
Fetal growth and development and maternal responses based on the date of the last menstrual period.

Illustration continued on following page

Gestational age 5–8 weeks

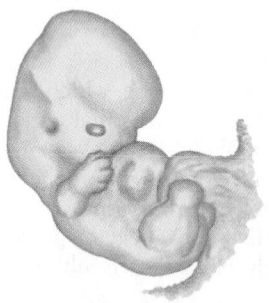

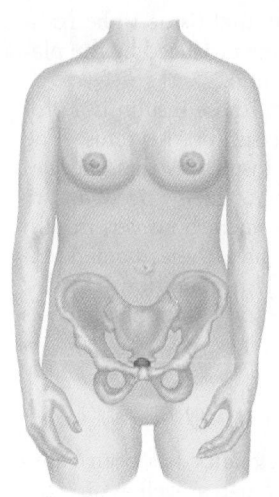

Crown-to-rump length 13 mm. Embryonic stage. Heart developed, beginning to pump. Arm and leg buds present. Head large, with facial features beginning to form.

Woman misses menstrual period. Nausea; fatigue. Tingling of breasts. Uterus is size of a lemon; positive Chadwick's, Goodell's and Hegar's sign. Urinary frequency as enlarging uterus presses on the bladder; increased vaginal discharge.

Gestational age 9–12 weeks

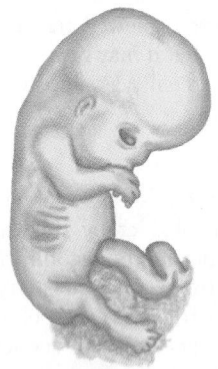

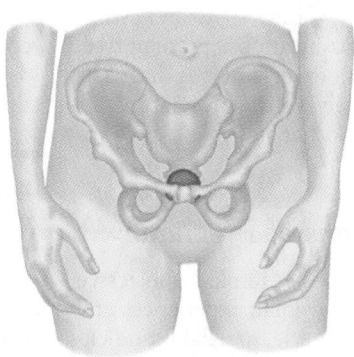

Crown-to-rump length 6–7 cm (2.4–3.8 in). Fetal stage begins at 10 weeks after last menstrual period. Extremities developed; fingers and toes differentiated; external genitalia show signs of male or female sex. Weight 14 g (0.5 oz).

Nausea decreases after 12 weeks. Uterus is size of an orange; palpable above symphysis pubis. Vulvar varicosities may appear.

Gestational age 13–16 weeks

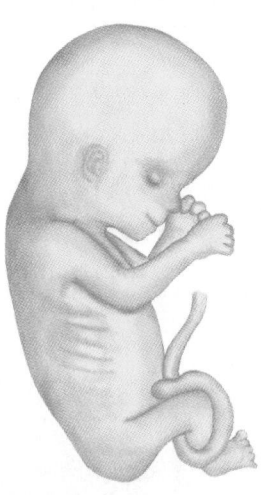

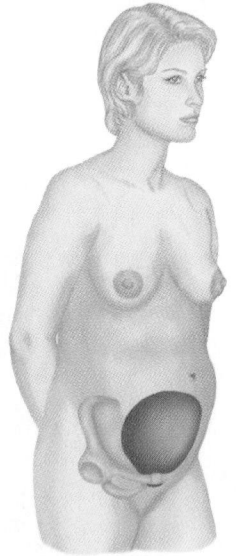

Crown-to-rump length 12 cm (4.7 in). Weight 110 g (4 oz). Fetus begins to move. Head and thorax can be identified by ultrasound; sexual organs formed. Urine formation begins.

Fetal movement may be felt. Uterus has risen into the abdomen; fundus midway between symphysis pubis and umbilicus. Urinary frequency decreases; blood volume increases; uterine souffle heard.

FIGURE 13–6
• • • • • • • • •
Continued

Gestational age 17–20 weeks

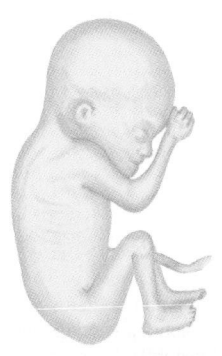

Crown-to-rump length 16 cm (6.3 in). Weight 320 g (11 oz). Heart beat can be heard with fetoscope or electronic device. Meconium begins collecting in bowel. Period of very rapid growth.

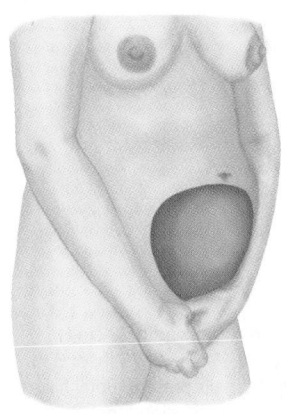

Fetal movements felt. Skin pigmentation increases: areolae darken; chloasma and linea nigra may be obvious. Colostrum may be expressed. Braxton-Hicks contractions palpable. Fundus at level of umbilicus.

Gestational age 21–24 weeks

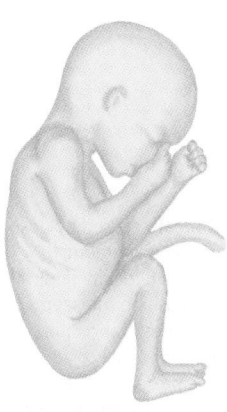

Crown-to-rump length 21 cm (8 in). Weight 630 g (1 lb, 6 oz). Skin wrinkled and red; vernix present; head and body covered with lanugo.

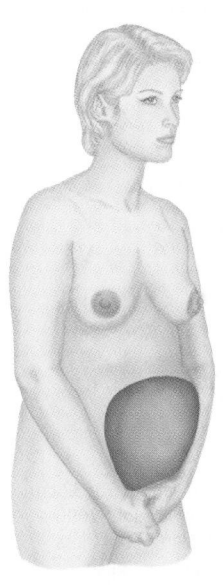

Relaxation of smooth muscles of veins and bladder increases the chance of varicose veins and urinary tract infections. Woman is more aware of fetal movements.

Gestational age 25–28 weeks

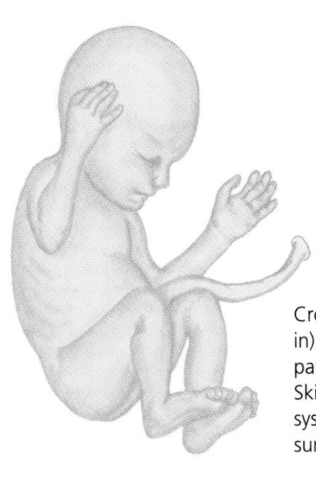

Crown-to-rump length 25 cm (9.8 in). Weight 1000 g (2 lb, 3 oz). Eyes partially open; eyelashes present. Skin covered with vernix. Respiratory system immature, but fetus may survive if born.

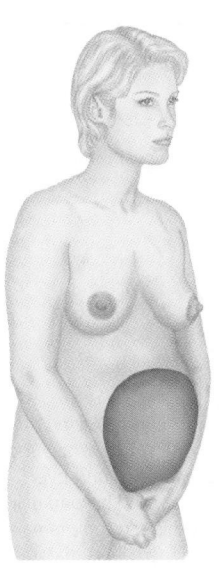

Period of greatest weight gain and lowest hemoglobin level begins. Fundal height is 3 to 4 fingerbreadths above umbilicus. Lordosis may cause backache.

FIGURE 13–6
• • • • • • • • •
Continued

Illustration continued on following page

Gestational age 29–32 weeks

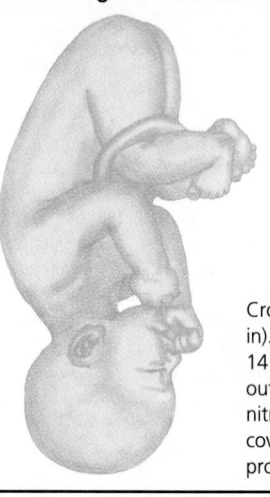

Crown-to-rump length 28 cm (11 in). Weight 1700 g (3.75 lb, or 3 lb, 14 oz). Toenails present. Body filling out, testes descending. Iron, nitrogen, calcium stored. Vernix covers body. Chances of survival improving.

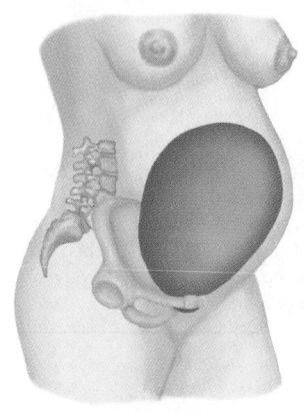

Heartburn common as uterus presses on diaphragm and displaces stomach. Braxton-Hicks contractions more noticeable. Lordosis increases; waddling gait develops as relaxin softens pelvic joints.

Gestational age 33–36 weeks

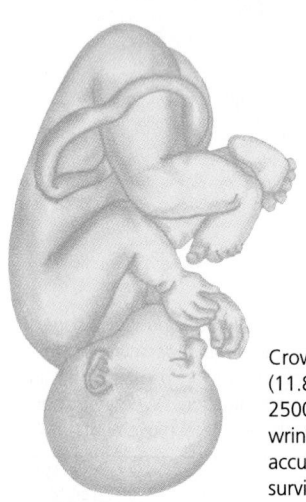

Crown-to-rump length 30–32 cm (11.8 to 12.6 in). Weight 2000–2500 g (4 lb). Skin thicker, less wrinkled as subcutaneous fat accumulates. Excellent chance for survival.

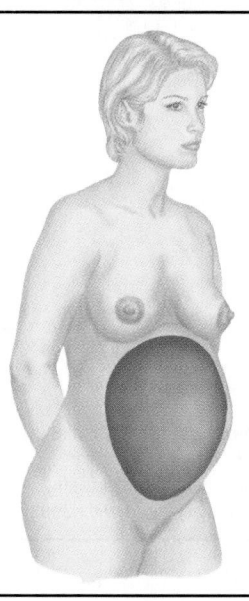

Shortness of breath caused by upward pressure on diaphragm; woman may have difficulty finding a comfortable position for sleep. Umbilicus protrudes. Varicosities more pronounced; pedal or ankle edema may be present. Urinary frequency noted following lightening when presenting part settles into pelvic cavity.

Gestational age 37–40 weeks

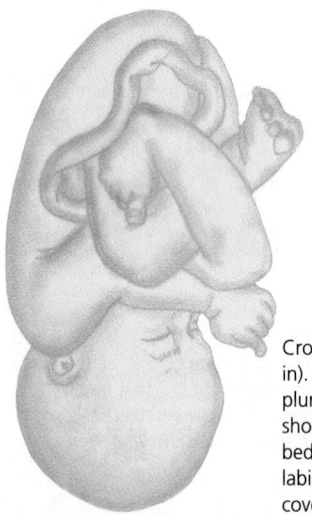

Crown-to-rump length 36 cm (14 in). Weight 3400 g (7 lb, 8 oz). Body plump; lanugo remains only over shoulders; nails extend beyond nail beds; testes within scrotum; female labia well developed; labia majora cover labia minora.

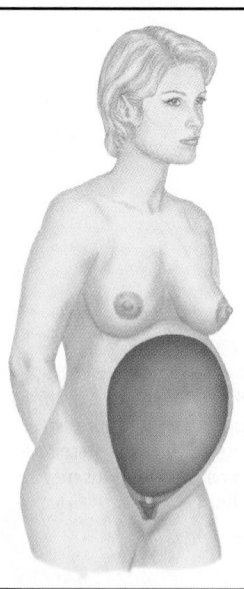

Woman is uncomfortable; looking forward to birth of baby. Cervix softens, begins to efface; mucus plug is often lost.

FIGURE 13–6
• • • • • • • •
Continued

TABLE 13-1

Indications of Pregnancy and Other Possible Causes

Sign	Other Possible Causes
Presumptive Indications	
Amenorrhea	Emotional stress, strenuous physical exercise, endocrine problems, chronic disease, early menopause
Nausea and vomiting	Gastrointestinal virus, food poisoning, emotional stress
Fatigue	Illness, stress, sudden changes in lifestyle
Urinary frequency	Urinary tract infections
Breast and skin changes	Premenstrual changes, use of oral contraceptives
Quickening	Abdominal gas, peristalsis, or pseudocyesis (false pregnancy)
Probable Indications	
Abdominal enlargement	Abdominal or uterine tumors
Cervical changes	Infection or hormonal imbalance
Ballottement	Uterine or cervical polyps
Braxton Hicks contractions	Soft uterine fibroids (myomas)
Palpation of fetal outline	Large myomas may feel like the fetal head; small, soft myomas may simulate small parts of the fetus
Pregnancy tests	Certain medications (antianxiety or anticonvulsant drugs), premature menopause, blood in urine, or malignant tumors that produce human chorionic gonadotropin may result in false-positive findings
Positive Indications	
Auscultation of fetal heart sounds	
Fetal movements felt by examiner	
Visualization of embryo or fetus	

BREAST AND SKIN CHANGES

Breast changes occur at about the sixth week of pregnancy. Breast tenderness, feelings of fullness, and increased size and pigmentation of the areolae are present. These changes are due to the influence of estrogen and progesterone.

Many women observe increased pigmentation of the skin (chloasma, linea nigra, darkening of the areolae of the breasts) during pregnancy. These skin changes are due to increased levels of melanocyte-stimulating hormone, one of the effects of estrogen.

FETAL MOVEMENT

Unlike other presumptive indications of pregnancy, fetal movement is not perceived until the second trimester. Although some women feel movement sooner, most expectant mothers first notice subtle fetal movements (quickening) between 16 and 20 weeks. These movements gradually increase in intensity.

Probable Indications of Pregnancy

Probable indications of pregnancy are objective findings that can be documented by an examiner. They are primarily related to physical changes in the reproductive organs. Although these signs are stronger indicators of pregnancy, a positive diagnosis of pregnancy cannot be based on these findings.

ABDOMINAL ENLARGEMENT

Enlargement of the abdomen during the childbearing years is a fairly reliable indication of pregnancy, particularly if it corresponds to a slow, gradual increase in uterine growth. Evidence of pregnancy is even more reliable when uterine growth is accompanied by amenorrhea.

CHANGES IN THE CERVIX

Color. The cervix changes from pink to a dark bluish violet. The color change, called Chadwick's sign, extends to the vagina and labia as well as the cervix. The bluish color is due to increased vascularity of the pelvic organs and is one of the earliest signs of pregnancy.

Consistency. Softening of the cervix (Goodell's sign) is noted by the examiner during pelvic examination. At about the sixth week of pregnancy, the lower uterine segment is so soft that it can be compressed to the thinness of paper. This is called Hegar's sign (Fig. 13–7). Because of the softening, the uterus can be easily flexed against the cervix (leading to McDonald's sign).

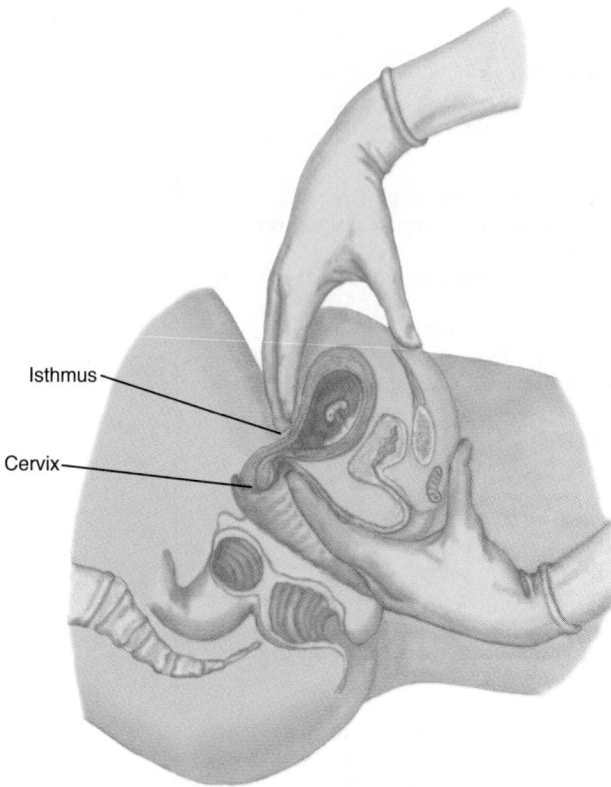

FIGURE 13–7

Hegar's sign—compressibility of the lower uterus—reflects softening of the isthmus of the cervix.

CHANGES IN THE UTERUS

Ballottement.   Near midpregnancy, a sudden tap on the cervix during vaginal examination may cause the fetus to rise in the amniotic fluid and then rebound to its original position (Fig. 13–8). Ballottement is a strong indication of pregnancy, but the same sensation may be caused by other factors such as uterine or cervical polyps.

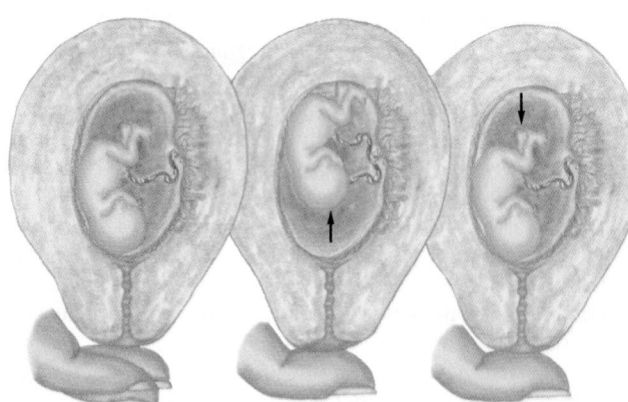

Ballottement

FIGURE 13–8

When the cervix is tapped, the fetus floats upward in the amniotic fluid. A rebound is felt by the examiner when the fetus falls back.

Braxton Hicks Contractions.   Irregular, painless contractions occur throughout pregnancy, although many expectant mothers do not notice them until the third trimester. Braxton Hicks contractions are not positive signs of pregnancy because similar contractions may occur with other conditions.

Palpation of the Fetal Outline.   An experienced practitioner is able to palpate the outlines of the fetal body by the second half of pregnancy. Palpating the fetal outline becomes easier as the pregnancy progresses and the uterine walls thin to accommodate the growing fetus.

Uterine Souffle.   A soft, blowing sound may be auscultated over the uterus. This sound is due to blood circulating through the placenta, and it corresponds to the maternal pulse. Therefore, to identify uterine souffle, the rate of the maternal pulse must be checked simultaneously. Uterine souffle differs from *funic souffle*, the soft, purring sound heard over the umbilical cord and corresponding to the fetal heart rate.

PREGNANCY TESTS

Home Pregnancy Tests.   Pregnancy tests are based on the presence of hCG in maternal urine and may be useful as early as 3 days after a missed menstrual period. They are available for purchase over the counter and are uncomplicated and convenient. Home test kits are capable of greater than 97% accuracy, but test kit instructions must be followed precisely to obtain accurate results (Cunningham et al., 1997).

When pregnancy test results are reported as negative and the woman is in fact pregnant, the results are called false negative. False-negative results may occur when the instructions are not followed properly or the woman has an ectopic pregnancy or impending spontaneous abortion. False-positive tests are due to errors in performing or reading the test or to the use of drugs such as marijuana, methadone, phenothiazine, or aspirin in large quantities.

Radioimmunoassay.   Because radioimmunoassays use radioactively labeled markers to detect antibodies against beta-subunit hCG in blood or urine, they must be performed in a laboratory. They are the most sensitive pregnancy tests available and are accurate as early as 1 week after ovulation.

Positive Indications of Pregnancy

Positive signs of pregnancy are those caused only by pregnancy.

AUSCULTATION OF FETAL HEART SOUNDS

Fetal heart sounds can be heard with a fetoscope by 18 to 20 weeks of gestation. The electronic Doppler scan amplifies fetal heart sounds so that they are audible by 10 to 12 weeks.

It is necessary to distinguish the fetal heartbeat from the maternal pulse. The fetal heart rate is in the range of 160 to 170 BPM in the first trimester (DuBose, 1996). As the fetus grows, the rate becomes slower, and it declines to between 110 and 160 BPM during the third trimester. It should be auscultated while the radial pulse of the expectant mother is being palpated. The fetal heart rate is muffled by amniotic fluid, and the location changes because the fetus moves freely in the amniotic fluid.

FETAL MOVEMENTS FELT BY EXAMINER

Fetal movements are considered a positive sign of pregnancy when felt by an experienced examiner who is not likely to be deceived by similar sensations produced by peristalsis in the large intestine.

VISUALIZATION OF THE FETUS

Transabdominal ultrasound examination is frequently used to confirm pregnancy at 5 to 6 weeks of gestation. The gestational sac and movements of the fetal heart are readily identifiable in the maternal pelvis. Positive confirmation of pregnancy is possible by transvaginal ultrasonography as early as 16 days after ovulation (Cunningham et al., 1997).

Antepartum Assessment and Care

Inadequate antepartum care is associated with low birth weight and an increased incidence of prematurity in neonates. A strong correlation has been found between these two complications and increased infant mortality. Antepartum care is considered adequate when it begins in the first trimester and continues on a regular basis thereafter. In addition to collecting and evaluating laboratory values and physical measurements, prenatal care should also provide health education, counseling, and social support.

Initial Visit

The initial visit is a time to establish rapport with the family and to perform a thorough assessment of the physiologic and psychosocial needs of the family. The nurse practitioner, certified nurse-midwife, or physician must complete a thorough history and physical examination.

HISTORY

Obstetric History. The obstetric history provides essential information about prior pregnancies that may alert the physician or nurse-midwife to possible problems in the present pregnancy. Calculation of gravida and para is essential. Gravida refers to the number of pregnancies, regardless of the duration of the pregnancy. Para refers to the number of pregnancies that end after 20 weeks. The number of fetuses in a pregnancy does not change the para. Thus, a woman who gives birth to twins after her first pregnancy will be a gravida 1, para 1 if birth occurred after 20 weeks of pregnancy.

Use of the TPAL acronym allows a more complete description of pregnancy outcomes than use of gravida and para alone. TPAL stands for term (T), preterm (P), abortions (A), and live (L) births. The TPAL method obtains complete information.

> Nurses must exercise caution when discussing obstetric history with the expectant mother in the presence of her family or significant other. Although the antepartum record may indicate a previous pregnancy or childbirth, she may not have shared this information with her family, and her right to privacy could be jeopardized by probing questions. The confidentiality of the pregnant woman must always be protected.

Calculation of Gravida and Para

A useful method for calculating gravida and para is to use the acronym TPAL to divide pregnancy outcome into the number of term pregnancies (T), preterm pregnancies (P), abortions (A), and live births (L).

To illustrate: Sally Elam is pregnant for the fifth time. She underwent two elective abortions in the first trimester. She has a son who was born at 40 weeks' gestation and a daughter who was born at 36 weeks' gestation. She is gravida 5, para 2. T = 1 (the son born at 40 weeks); P = 1 (the daughter born at 36 weeks); A = 2; L = 2. The two abortions are counted in the gravida but are not included in the para because they occurred before 20 weeks.

Other components of this history include

- Weight of infants at birth, length of gestation
- Labor experience, type of delivery, location of birth, name of caregiver
- Type of anesthesia and any difficulties
- Maternal complications, such as hypertension, diabetes, infection, bleeding
- Complications with the infant
- Method of infant feeding planned (breast or formula)
- Special concerns

Menstrual History. A complete menstrual history is necessary to establish the EDD (or EDB). It is common practice to estimate the EDD on the basis of the first day of the last menstrual cycle, although ovulation and conception occur approximately 2 weeks after the beginning of menstruation in a regular 28-day cycle. The average duration of pregnancy from the first day of the last normal menstrual period is 40 weeks, or 280 days. Nagele's rule is often used to establish EDD. To use this method, subtract 3 months, add 7 days to the first day of the last normal menstrual period (LNMP), and correct the year.

> For example: LNMP June 30, 1999
> Subtract 3 months = March 30, 1999
> Add 7 days and change the year = April 6, 2000

Many health care providers also use a gestational calculator or wheel to calculate EDD quickly, although some wheels are prone to error (Cunningham et al., 1997).

CRITICAL THINKING EXERCISE 13–1

Wilma Turner gave birth to twin girls at 38 weeks of gestation 3 years ago. She had a spontaneous abortion last year at 12 weeks of gestation and thinks she may be pregnant now because she has missed a menstrual period and is experiencing morning sickness. Wilma's last normal menstrual period began June 22.

1. If Wilma is pregnant now, what would be the gravida and para?
2. Explain to Wilma why amenorrhea and morning sickness are not positive indications of pregnancy.
3. Use Nagele's rule to compute the EDD.

Contraceptive History. A detailed history of contraceptive methods is important. Use of oral contraceptives just before pregnancy or continued use during early unrecognized pregnancy remains a source of concern because of the effect of estrogens and some synthetic progestins on the the fetus (Briggs, Freeman, & Sumner, 1998). Some physicians advise women to stop oral contraception and to use alternative methods (condoms, diaphragm) to prevent conception for 3 months before conceiving.

Intrauterine devices can cause complications if pregnancy occurs with an intrauterine device in place. Risks include abortion, premature delivery, and puncture of the uterus.

Medical and Surgical History. Chronic conditions, such as diabetes mellitus, hypertension, and renal disease, can affect the outcome of the pregnancy and must be investigated. Infections such as hepatitis or pyelonephritis, as well as surgical procedures and trauma that may complicate the pregnancy or childbirth, must be documented. The history includes the following:

- Age, race, ethnic background (risk for specific genetic problems, such as sickle cell disease, thalassemia, and Tay-Sachs disease)
- Childhood diseases and immunizations
- Chronic illnesses, such as asthma and heart disease
- Previous illnesses, surgical procedures, injuries
- Previous infections: hepatitis, sexually transmissible diseases, or tuberculosis
- History of anemia and the way it was treated
- Bladder, bowel function (problems or changes)
- Amount of caffeine and alcohol consumed each day
- Tobacco use (number of years and number of packs per day)
- Prescription or other drugs
- General nutrition, history of eating disorders
- Contact with pets, particularly cats (increased risk of infections such as toxoplasmosis)
- Allergies and drug sensitivities
- Occupation and related risk factors

Family Health History. A family history for the woman and her partner provides valuable information about the general health of the family, including chronic diseases such as diabetes and heart disease, and infections such as tuberculosis and hepatitis. Moreover, information about patterns of genetic or congenital anomalies may be revealed.

The use of drugs such as cocaine or alcohol may affect the family's ability to cope with pregnancy and childbirth. Tobacco use by the father poses a risk to both the mother and infant for upper respiratory tract complications as a result of passive smoking. In addition, the father's blood type and Rh factor are important if the mother is Rh negative and there is the possibility of a blood incompatibility between the mother and the fetus.

Psychosocial History. The psychosocial history, which should be completed at the same time, is discussed in Chapter 14.

PHYSICAL EXAMINATION

A thorough evaluation of all body systems is necessary to detect previously undiagnosed physical problems that may affect the pregnancy outcome. It also allows the examiner to establish baseline levels that will guide the treatment of the expectant mother and fetus throughout pregnancy.

Vital Signs

Blood Pressure. Position affects blood pressure in the pregnant woman. Blood pressure should be obtained with the woman seated and her arm supported in a horizontal position at the level of the heart (Knuppel & Drukker, 1993). Documentation should include the position, the arm used, and the pressures obtained.

Pulse. The normal pulse rate is 60 to 90 BPM. Tachycardia is associated with anxiety, hyperthyroidism, and infection and should be investigated. The apical pulse should be assessed for at least 1 minute to determine the amplitude and regularity of the heartbeat.

Respiratory Effort. Respiratory rate during pregnancy is in the range of 16 to 24 BPM. Tachypnea may indicate respiratory infection or cardiac disease. Breath sounds should be equal bilaterally, chest expansion should be symmetric, and lung fields should be free of all abnormal breath sounds.

Temperature. Normal temperature during pregnancy is 36.2° to 37.6°C (98° to 99.6°F). Increased temperature suggests infection that may require medical management.

Cardiovascular System

Venous Congestion. Additional assessment of the cardiovascular system includes observation for venous congestion, which can develop into varicosities. Venous congestion is most commonly noted in the legs, vulva, or rectum.

Edema. Edema of the legs may be a benign condition that reflects pooling of blood in the extremities, which results in a shift of intravascular fluid into interstitial spaces. When pressure exerted by a finger or thumb leaves a persistent depression, the condition is termed pitting edema.

Musculoskeletal System

Posture and Gait. Body mechanics, as well as changes in posture and gait, should be addressed. Body mechanics during pregnancy may place strain on the muscles of the lower back and legs.

Height and Weight. An initial weight is needed to establish a baseline for weight gain throughout pregnancy. Weight should be compared with the ideal-weight-for-height charts. A preconception weight of less than 45 kg (100 lb) or height under 150 cm (60 inches) is associated with preterm labor and low-birth-weight infants. A preconception weight greater than 90 kg (200 lb) is associated with an increased incidence of pregnancy-induced glucose intolerance (gestational diabetes) and hypertension.

Pelvic Measurements. Early in pregnancy, the bony pelvis is evaluated to determine whether the diameters are adequate to permit vaginal delivery (see Chapter 17).

Abdomen. The contour, size, and muscle tone of the abdomen should be assessed. Fundal height should be measured if the fundus is palpable above the symphysis pubis. For the measurement to be accurate, the bladder must be empty before the measurement is taken. With the MacDonald method of measurement, the woman lies on her back with the knees slightly flexed. The top of the fundus is pal-

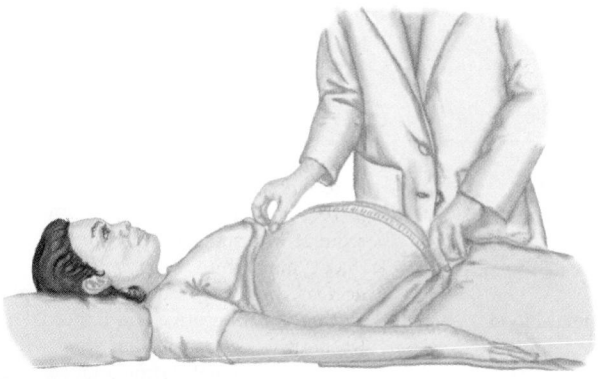

FIGURE 13-9

Measuring the uterus entails measuring from the upper border of the symphysis pubis to the top of the fundus.

pated, and a tape is stretched from the top of the symphysis pubis, over the abdominal curve, to the top of the fundus (Fig. 13–9).

From 22 weeks until term, the fundal height, measured in centimeters, is roughly equal (±2 cm) to the gestational age of the fetus in weeks (Hobel, 1998). If there is a discrepancy between fundal height and weeks of gestation, additional assessment is necessary. The EDD may be incorrect and the pregnancy more or less advanced than thought. The number of fetuses present and fetal growth should also be evaluated.

Fetal heart rate should be measured and recorded if the pregnancy is advanced enough to hear fetal heart tones.

Neurologic System. A complete neurologic assessment is not necessary for young women who are free of signs or symptoms that indicate a problem. Deep tendon reflexes should be assessed, however, because hyperreflexia is associated with complications of pregnancy. (See Procedure 26–1 for assessment of deep tendon reflexes.)

Integumentary System. Skin color should be consistent with racial background. Pallor may indicate anemia. Jaundice may indicate hepatic disease. Lesions, bruising, or areas of hyperpigmentation (chloasma, linea nigra) related to pregnancy, as well as stretch marks (striae), should be noted. Nail beds should be pink, with instant capillary return.

Endocrine System. The thyroid enlarges slightly during the second trimester. Gross enlargement or tenderness, however, may indicate hyperthyroidism and requires further medical evaluation.

Gastrointestinal System
Mouth. Mucous membranes should be pink, smooth, glistening, and uniform. The lips should be free of ulcerations. The gums may be red, tender, and edematous as a result of increased estrogen, which produces hyperplasia.
Intestine. Bowel sounds may be diminished because of the effects of progesterone on smooth muscle. Bowel sounds are often increased if a meal is overdue or if diarrhea is present.

Urinary System. Urine collected for testing should always be a clean-catch midstream sample. Urine is tested to detect signs of urinary tract infection and substances in the urine that may indicate a problem.
Protein. Protein should not be present in urine. Its presence may indicate contamination by vaginal secretions. It may also indicate kidney disease or pregnancy-induced hypertension.
Glucose. Small amounts of glucose may indicate physiologic "spilling" that occurs during normal pregnancy. Larger amounts require glucose screening of the blood.
Ketones. Ketones may be found in the urine after heavy exercise or as a result of inadequate intake of food and fluid.
Bacteria. Increased bacteria in the urine is associated with urinary tract infection, which is common during pregnancy.

Reproductive System
Breasts. Breast size and symmetry, the condition of the nipples, and the presence of colostrum should be noted. Any lumps, dimpling of the skin, or asymmetry of the nipples requires further evaluation.
External Reproductive Organs. The skin and mucous membranes of the perineum, vulva, and anus are inspected for excoriations, growths, ulcerations, lesions, varicosities, warts, chancres, and perineal scars. Enlargement, tenderness, redness, or discharge from Bartholin's glands or Skene's glands may indicate gonorrheal or chlamydial infection. The examiner should obtain a specimen for culture of any discharge from lesions or inflamed glands to determine the causative organisms and to provide effective care.
Internal Reproductive Organs. A speculum inserted into the vagina permits the examiner to see the walls of the vagina and the cervix. Chadwick's sign and Goodell's sign are seen during pregnancy. The external cervical os is closed in primigravidas, but one fingertip may be admitted in multiparas. Routine cervical cultures for gonorrhea and chlamydial infection are standard practice during the initial pregnancy examination at most agencies. The examiner also collects a specimen for a Papanicolaou (Pap) smear, a screening test for cervical cancer.

A bimanual examination involves using both hands to palpate the internal genitalia. The examiner palpates the uterus for size, contour, tenderness, and position. The uterus should be movable between the two examining hands and should feel smooth. The ovaries, if palpable, should be about the shape and size of almonds and should not be tender.

Laboratory Data. Table 13–2 lists laboratory examinations that are commonly performed during pregnancy. The table briefly describes their purpose and the significance of each test.

Risk Assessment. Risk assessment begins at the initial visit, when the health care team identifies factors that put the expectant mother or the fetus at risk for complications and thus in need of specialized care. Many women identified as high risk give birth to healthy term infants. Furthermore, risk factors change as pregnancy progresses, and risk assessment must be updated throughout pregnancy.

TABLE 13-2

. . . .

Common Laboratory Tests

Test	Purpose	Significance
Blood grouping	To determine blood type	Blood replacement may become necessary.
Hemoglobin (Hgb) or hematocrit (Hct)	To detect anemia	Hgb 10.5 g/dl or less or Hct < 33% requires iron supplementation.
Complete blood cell (CBC) count	To detect infection or cell abnormalities	$\geq$15,000/mm^3 white blood cells or decreased platelets requires follow-up.
Rh factor and antibody screen	For possible maternal-fetal blood incompatibility	If mother is Rh-negative and father is Rh-positive or if antibodies are present, additional testing and treatment are required.
VDRL or rapid plasma reagin (RPR) test	Syphilis screen	Treat if positive. Retest at 36 weeks.
Rubella titer	To determine immunity	If titer is <1:8, mother is not immune. Immunize postpartum if not immune.
Skin test	To screen for tuberculosis	If positive, refer for additional testing or therapy.
Hemoglobin electrophoresis	To screen for sickle cell trait if client is African-American	If mother is positive, check partner. Infant is at risk only if both parents are positive.
Hepatitis B screen	To detect presence of antigens in maternal blood	If present, infants should be given hepatitis immune globulin and vaccine soon after birth.
Human immunodeficiency virus (HIV) screen	Offered at first visit to detect HIV antibodies	Positive results require retesting, counseling, and treatment.
Urinalysis	To detect infection, renal disease, or diabetes	Positive for protein, glucose, ketones, or bacteria.
Papanicolaou (Pap) test	To screen for cervical neoplasia	Treat and refer if abnormal cells are present.
Cervical culture	To detect sexually transmissible diseases, such as gonorrhea, group B streptococci	Treat and retest as necessary.
Maternal serum alpha-fetoprotein	To screen for fetal anomalies	Either low or high levels should be investigated.
Maternal blood glucose	To screen for gestational diabetes	If elevated, a 3-hr glucose tolerance test is recommended.

Table 13–3 lists the major risk factors and identifies maternal and fetal-neonatal implications.

Subsequent Assessments

Ongoing antepartum care is important to the successful outcome of pregnancy. The recommended schedule for prenatal assessment in an uncomplicated pregnancy is as follows:

Conception to 28 weeks: every 4 weeks
29 to 36 weeks: every 2 to 3 weeks
37 weeks to birth: weekly

VITAL SIGNS

To be accurate, the blood pressure must be measured in the same arm with the mother in the same position each time. Deviations from baseline values in blood pressure, pulse, or respiratory rate indicate the need for further assessment. The temperature should remain within normal limits.

WEIGHT

Weight should be plotted to document that the expected pattern of weight gain is occurring. Inadequate weight gain may signify that the pregnancy is not as advanced as first thought or that the fetus is not growing as expected. A sudden, rapid weight gain may indicate fluid retention, and further assessment for pregnancy-induced hypertension is indicated. (See Chapter 15 for a thorough discussion of the desired pattern of weight gain.)

URINALYSIS

Urine is tested for protein, glucose, and ketones. A screen for bacteria may be repeated later in the pregnancy if the woman has a history of previous urinary tract infections.

GLUCOSE SCREEN

Blood glucose is often screened between 24 and 28 weeks, using a 50-g glucose load followed by a 1-hour plasma glucose determination. Additional testing is indicated if the result is 140 mg/dl or higher (American College of Obstetricians and Gynecologists, 1994a).

FUNDAL HEIGHT

Measuring fundal height is an inexpensive and noninvasive method for evaluating fetal growth and confirming gestational age.

TABLE 13-3
• • • • • • • • • • •

Summary of High-Risk Factors in Pregnancy

Factors	*Implications*
Demographic Factors	
Age < 16 yr or > 35 yr	Increased risk for preterm labor, pregnancy-induced hypertension, congenital anomalies
Low socioeconomic status or dependent on public assistance	Increased risk for preterm labor, low-birth-weight infants
Nonwhite race	Incidence of infant and maternal death twice that of whites
Multiparity: >4 pregnancies	Increasing parity increases risk of pregnancy loss, antepartum or postpartum hemorrhage, and cesarean birth
Social-Personal Factors	
Weight < 45 kg (100 lb)	Associated with low-birth-weight infant
Weight > 90 kg (200 lb)	Increased risk for pregnancy-induced hypertension, difficult labor, large-for-gestational-age infant, and cesarean birth
Height < 154 cm (5 feet)	Increased incidence of cesarean birth due to cephalopelvic disproportion
Smoking	Associated with low-birth-weight infant, preterm birth
Use of alcohol or addicting drugs	Increased risk of congenital anomalies, neonatal withdrawal syndrome, and fetal alcohol syndrome
Obstetric Factors	
Birth of previous infant weighing > 4,000 g (8.5 lb)	Increased need for cesarean birth; increased risk for infant birth injury, neonatal hypoglycemia, and maternal gestational diabetes
Previous stillborn infant	Maternal psychological distress
Rh sensitization	Fetal anemia, erythroblastosis fetalis, kernicterus
Existing Medical Conditions	
Diabetes mellitus	Increased risk of pregnancy-induced hypertension, cesarean birth, infant either small or large for gestational age, neonatal hypoglycemia, fetal or neonatal death, congenital anomalies
Thyroid disorder	
Hypothyroidism	Increased incidence of spontaneous abortion, congenital anomalies, congenital hypothyroidism
Hyperthyroidism	Maternal risk of pregnancy-induced hypertension, thyroid storm, or postpartum hemorrhage; neonatal risk of thyrotoxicosis
Cardiac disease	Maternal risk for cardiac decompensation and increased death rate, increased risk for fetal and neonatal death
Renal disease	Maternal risk for renal failure and preterm delivery, fetal risk for intrauterine growth retardation
Concurrent Infections	
	Severe fetal implications (heart disease, blindness, deafness, bone lesions) if maternal disease occurred in the first trimester
	Increased incidence of spontaneous abortion or congenital anomalies is associated with some infections

LEOPOLD'S MANEUVERS

Leopold's maneuvers provide a systematic method for palpating the fetus through the abdominal wall during the later part of pregnancy. These maneuvers provide valuable information about the location and presentation of the fetus (see Chapter 17).

FETAL HEART RATE

The fetal heart rate may be heard in early pregnancy with a Doppler transducer or, in later pregnancy, with a fetoscope. The site provides information that may help determine in what position the fetus is entering the pelvis. For instance, fetal heart tones heard in an upper quadrant of the abdomen suggest that the fetus is in a breech presentation.

FETAL ACTIVITY

Usually first noticed by the expectant mother at 16 to 20 weeks of gestation, fetal movements (quickening) gradually increase in both frequency and strength. In the last trimester, the woman may be asked to count fetal body movements. These are commonly called "kick counts." In general, fetal activity indicates that the fetus is physically healthy.

Figure 13–10 is an example of a clinical pathway for prenatal care. Such pathways provide guidelines and a time sequence for specific assessments and interventions. Note that the most common family problems and risk factors are listed at the top of the page and alert the team that additional assessments or care may be needed.

Multifetal Pregnancy

A multifetal pregnancy is a pregnancy in which two or more embryos or fetuses exist simultaneously. (See Chapter 12 for information about development of multifetal gestations.)

DIAGNOSIS

Women with multifetal pregnancies often feel larger than with previous pregnancies, have more fetal movements, and gain more weight. The fundal height is often 4 cm larger than expected on the basis of gestational age computed from the last menstrual period.

The maternal history may be of some help in making the diagnosis. A maternal family history that includes fraternal twins slightly increases the chance of twins. Recent administration of fertility drugs such as clomiphene greatly increases the chance of multifetal pregnancy.

When more than one fetus is thought to exist, the diagnosis should be confirmed by sonography. Separate gestational sacs may be seen as early as 6 weeks of gestation. Multiple fetal parts may be visible by the 10th week.

MATERNAL ADAPTATION TO MULTIFETAL PREGNANCY

Maternal physiologic change is greater with multiple fetuses than with a single fetus. There is a 500-ml increase in blood volume over that needed for a single fetus. This increase heightens the workload of the heart and may contribute to fatigue and activity intolerance. The uterus may achieve a volume of 10 liters or more and weigh more than 20 lb (Cunningham et al., 1997). The weight increases respiratory difficulty because the overdistended uterus causes greater elevation of the diaphragm.

The uterus may also cause more compression of the large vessels, resulting in more pronounced and earlier supine hypotension. Greater compression of the ureters can occur, and maternal edema and proteinuria are common. Compression of the bowel makes constipation a persistent problem.

ANTEPARTUM CARE IN MULTIFETAL PREGNANCY

Many physicians increase the number of times women with a multifetal pregnancy are seen during the antepartum period. More frequent visits permit extra vigilance in the detection of common complications such as anemia, hypertension, premature labor, and congenital anomalies.

Diet must also be considered. The need for calories, iron, vitamins, and folate increases. Women carrying twins are advised to gain 16 to 20.5 kg (35 to 45 lb).

Common Discomforts of Pregnancy

Many women experience discomforts of pregnancy that are not serious in themselves but detract from the woman's feeling of comfort and well-being.

NAUSEA AND VOMITING

Nausea and vomiting of pregnancy are frequently called morning sickness because these symptoms are more acute on arising. They may, however, occur at any time of the day. Women need reassurance that nausea and vomiting, however distressing, are common and that the condition is temporary. Morning sickness must be distinguished from hyperemesis gravidarum, severe vomiting accompanied by weight loss, dehydration, electrolyte imbalance, and ketosis (see Chapter 26).

Although the cause of nausea and vomiting is unknown, these symptoms are believed to be related to increased levels of hCG and estrogen, as well as periodic hypoglycemia. Symptoms may be aggravated by cooking odors, fatigue, and emotional stress.

HEARTBURN

Heartburn is described as an acute burning sensation in the epigastric and sternal regions. It occurs when reverse peristaltic waves cause regurgitation of acidic stomach contents into the esophagus. The underlying causes are diminished gastric motility and displacement of the stomach by the enlarging uterus. Improper diet and nervous tension may be precipitating factors.

BACKACHE

Backache is a common complaint during the third trimester. A primary focus is to prevent backache by teaching correct posture (Fig. 13–11) and body mechanics (Fig. 13–12). Figure 13–13 suggests exercises that relax the shoulders and thighs and help prevent backache.

URINARY FREQUENCY

Although urinary frequency is a common complaint of women during the first trimester and near term, the condition is temporary and is managed by most women without undue distress. Kegel exercises are sometimes recommended to help maintain bladder control.

Text continued on page 285

How to Overcome the Common Discomforts of Pregnancy

Nausea and Vomiting
- Eat dry crackers or toast before arising in the morning; then get out of bed slowly.
- Eat small amounts of carbohydrate foods frequently during the day to prevent an empty stomach and keep meals small.
- Drink fluids separately from meals.
- Avoid greasy or spicy foods or ones with strong odors.

Heartburn
- Eat several small meals daily and avoid fatty foods.
- Curtail smoking and coffee drinking, which stimulate acid formation in the stomach.
- Sit upright to reduce reflux and relieve symptoms.
- Sleep with an extra pillow.
- Sip water to help relieve the burning sensation.
- Use antacids but avoid those that are high in sodium (AlkaSeltzer, baking soda), which cause fluid retention. Antacids high in calcium (Tums, Alkamints) provide relief but may cause rebound hyperacidity.

Backache
- Maintain correct posture: head up, shoulders back.
- To pick up objects, squat rather than bend at the waist.
- When sitting, use foot supports, arm rests, and pillows behind your back.
- Exercise. Tailor sitting, shoulder circling, and pelvic rocking strengthen your back and prepare you for labor.

Urinary Frequency
Performing Kegel's exercises helps to maintain bladder control:

- Identify the muscles to be exercised when you stop the flow of urine midstream. Do not, however, perform the exercise while urinating because urinary retention increases the risk of urinary tract infection.
- Slowly contract the muscles around the vagina and hold for 10 seconds. Relax at least 10 seconds.
- Repeat the contraction-relaxation cycle 30 times per day (Sampselle et al., 1997).

Varicosities
- Avoid constricting clothing and refrain from crossing your legs at the knees because this position impedes blood return from the legs.
- Take frequent rest periods with your legs elevated above the level of your hips.
- Wear support hose or elastic stockings that reach above the varicosities. Apply them before you get out of bed each morning.
- If you work in one position for prolonged periods, walk around for a few minutes at least every 2 hours.

Hemorrhoids
- To prevent hemorrhoids, try to establish a regular pattern of bowel elimination that does not require straining. Drink plenty of water, eat foods rich in fiber, and exercise regularly.
- To relieve existing hemorrhoids, take frequent, tepid sitz baths or warm soaks. Apply cool witch hazel compresses or anesthetic ointments. Lie (on your side) with your hips elevated on a pillow.
- Gently push the hemorrhoids back into the rectum.

To do so, put on a glove and lubricate your index finger. Maintain pressure for 1 to 2 minutes.
- If you have persistent pain or bleeding, call your physician or midwife.

Constipation
Self-care measures generally are as effective as using laxatives, but they do not interfere with absorption of nutrients or lead to laxative dependency.

- Drink at least eight glasses of water each day. These should not include coffee, tea, or carbonated drinks because of their diuretic effect. If you do drink one of these beverages, add a glass of water.
- Add foods high in fiber such as unpeeled fresh fruits and vegetables, whole-grain cereals, bran muffins, oatmeal, baked potatoes with skins, and fruit juices. Four pieces of fruit plus a large salad provide enough fiber for 1 day.
- Restrict cheese consumption, which causes constipation.
- Curtail your intake of sweets, which increase bacterial growth in the intestine and can lead to flatulence.
- Do not discontinue taking iron supplements if they have been prescribed. If constipation persists, consult your health care provider for advice about bulk-forming laxatives or fecal-wetting agents.
- A brisk walk of at least 1 mile per day stimulates peristalsis and improves muscle tone. Swimming and riding a stationary bicycle are also helpful.
- Establish a regular pattern by allowing a consistent time each day for elimination. One hour after meals is ideal to take advantage of the gastrocolic reflex (the peristaltic wave in the colon that is induced by taking food into the fasting stomach). Using a footrest during elimination provides comfort and decreases straining.

Leg Cramps

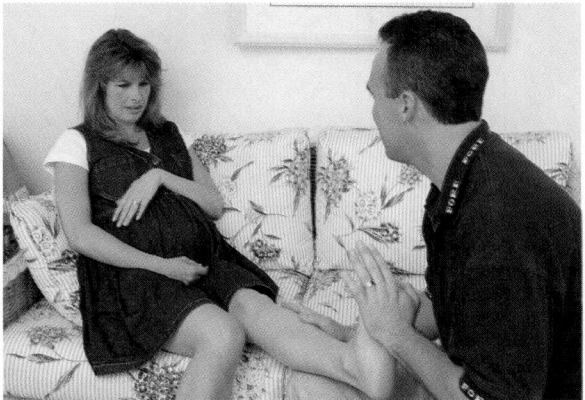

- To relieve cramps, extend the affected leg, keeping the knee straight. Bend your foot toward you, or ask someone to help you flex the foot. If you are alone, stand and apply pressure on the affected leg.
- To prevent cramps, elevate your legs often during the day to improve circulation.
- For frequent leg cramps, your physician or nurse-midwife may suggest aluminum hydroxide gel capsules. These absorb phosphorus and thus raise the level of calcium in the blood.

YORK HEALTH SYSTEM
YORK, PENNSYLVANIA
PRENATAL CARE
CLINICAL PATHWAY

DEMOGRAPHIC LABEL

EDC _____

PRETERM LABOR RISK

1. ☐ Substance abuse
2. ☐ Prior preterm delivery
3. ☐ >2 abortions
4. ☐ <90 lb. pre-pregnancy weight
5. ☐ Placental anomaly
6. ☐ STD current pregnancy
7. ☐ Multiple gestation
8. ☐ Persistent bleeding
9. ☐ Incompetent cervix

DOCUMENTATION CODES

Initialed Box=Meets Standard   ★=Exception on pathway identified   N=Not applicable

STANDARD OF CARE FOR PRENATAL PATIENTS INCLUDES:

• Activity ad lib
• Diet to meet needs of pregnancy.
• Prenatal Vitamins
• FeSO4, if needed

CONSULTS/PROBLEM MANAGEMENT FOR PATIENTS INCLUDE:

• Social Service prn
• Perinatologist prn
• Genetic Counseling prn
• Nutritionist prn
• WIC prn
• Pastoral Care prn
• Lactation Consultant prn (3rd Trimester)

CLINICAL PATH VISITS →	EXPECTED PATIENT/ FAMILY OUTCOMES	MULTIDISCIPLINARY ASSESSMENT (REFER TO STD-0011)	TESTS	EDUCATION & DC PLANNING (REFER TO STD-0011)
NURSE INTERVIEW DATE _____	☐ Referrals made as indicated following Prenatal Standard of Care ☐ Verbalizes understanding of normal vs. abnormal signs and symptoms of pregnancy ☐ Verbalizes agreement to complete Labs, obtain prenatal vitamins and keep scheduled appointments ☐ Verbalizes signs and symptoms of preterm labor ☐ No risk factors PTL identified ☐	• Refer to Standard 0011-Nurse Interview • Weight, Height • Physical, psych/social, behavioral, nutritional risk factors • Knowledge of normal vs. abnormal Signs and Symptoms of pregnancy • Premature labor risk assessment	• CCMS-UA, for nitr/leuk/glucose C and S if applicable. • Prenatal Group • HIV • Sickle cell if applicable • Dating Ultrasound Schedule	☐ Childbirth Ed., Baby Care and Postpartum classes. Exercise during pregnancy. Effects of risk factors on pregnancy. Sexuality during pregnancy. Nutrition education. Normal effects of pregnancy on the body. Fetal Growth/Development. S and S of complications/pre-term labor. Pre-admission Form. Contraceptives/STD Prevention/HIV counseling. Schedule Return-to-Clinic Appointment. Orient to Clinic hours/physical setup, emergency protocol.
RN NAME				
1ST OB Exam	☐ Prenatal group tests within normal limits. ☐ Demonstrates measures to relieve normal complaints of pregnancy. ☐ No change in Preterm Labor risk factors ☐	• Signs and symptoms of normal physical changes, complications • Behavioral Risks • BP, Weight • Urine dipstick for Sugar/Ketone/Protein • Fetal Heart Sounds • Fundal Height • Pelvimetry	• Pap • GC • Chlamydia (if indicated) • Wet smear bacterial/trich./vaginosis Vaginal ph and Whiff Test	
RN NAME				

CLINICAL PATH VISITS →	EXPECTED PATIENT/ FAMILY OUTCOMES	MULTIDISCIPLINARY ASSESSMENT (REFER TO STD-0011)	TESTS	EDUCATION & DC PLANNING (REFER TO STD-0011)
(1-14 WEEKS) DATE _____ _____ _____ RN NAME	□ Demonstrates measures to relieve the normal complaints of pregnancy during 1st Trimester □ Established exercise routine □ Exhibits minimum weight loss/gain □ 1st Trimester test results within normal limits □ Avoids or demonstrates decrease in risk associated behavior (ie. smoking) □ No change in Preterm Labor risk factors □ Takes Prenatal Vitamins □	• Signs and Symptoms of normal physical changes, complications • Behavioral Risks • BP, Weight • Urine Dipstick for Sugar, Ketone, Protein • Fetal Heart Sounds • Fundal Height		□ Reinforce (STD-0011) (Prenatal Standard of Care) Importance of Compliance _____
(15-28 WEEKS) _____ _____ _____ RN NAME	□ Demonstrates measures to relieve the normal complaints of pregnancy during 2nd Trimester. □ Exhibits normal weight gain. □ 2nd Trimester test results within normal limits. □ Continues exercise routine. □ Avoids risk associated behavior. □ Demonstrates self palpation technique and verbalizes signs and symptoms of preterm labor. □ No change in Preterm Labor risk factors. □	• Signs and symptoms of normal physical changes, complications including: • Behavioral Risks • BP, Weight • Urine dipstick for Sugar/Ketone/Protein • Fetal Heart Sounds, Fundal Height • Fetal Movement at 16-20 Weeks • Premature Labor	• Triple Screen (16-19 weeks) • Ultrasound, as needed • Fibronectin (24-26 weeks) **ORDER AT 26 WEEKS:** • Trutol • Antibody Screen (Rh Neg) • Repeat WCBC • RhoGAM at 28 weeks, if indicated _____	□ Fetal Growth/Development for 2nd Tri. Encourage Childbirth, Baby Care and Postpartum classes Reinforce (STD-0011) (Prenatal Standard of Care) Review S and S of preterm labor at 24 week appointment Importance of compliance Home visit _____
(29-42 WEEKS) _____ _____ _____ RN NAME	□ Demonstrates measures to relieve the normal complaints of pregnancy during 3rd Trimester. □ Exhibits normal weight gain. □ Continues exercise routine. □ Normal physical changes of pregnancy w/o complications. □ Avoids risk associated behaviors. □ Attends Childbirth, Baby Care and Postpartum classes □ Responds appropriately to Signs and Symptoms of preterm labor or other complications when indicated. □ Performing nipple preparation, if needed. □ No change in Preterm Labor risk factors. □	• Signs and symptoms of normal physical changes, complications including: • Behavioral Risks • BP, Weight • Urine dipstick for Sugar/Ketone/Protein • Fetal Heart Sounds, Fundal Height • Fetal Movement • Planned method of infant feeding • Nipple exam, if planning to breast feed • Premature Labor	• Ultrasound as needed **ORDER AT 36 WEEKS:** • Recto Vaginal Cultures for GBS **ORDER AT 41 WEEKS:** • NST and AFI Bi-weekly (Amniotic Fluid Index)	□ Fetal Growth/Development for 3rd Trimester Review Signs and Symptoms and Admission procedures for normal labor at 36 weeks. Reinforce (STD-)11) (Prenatal Standard of Care) Review S and S of preterm labor Importance of compliance Update Perinatal Risk Assessment Childbirth Education, Baby Care and Postpartum classes Tubal forms, if indicated by 34 weeks Treatment for inverted nipples if indicated Home visit

F I G U R E 1 3 – 1 0

Prenatal clinical pathway that identifies outcomes, assessments, interventions, and consultations performed during pregnancy. (Courtesy of Women and Children Services of the York Health System, York, Pennsylvania. Reprinted with modifications.)

NURSING CARE PLAN 13–1

· · · · · · · · · · · ·

Discomfort During Early Pregnancy

Assessment	Maria Gomez, a thin, 18-year-old primigravida 8 weeks pregnant, states that she is experiencing nausea with occasional vomiting throughout the day. She reports that the nausea is intensified by the odor of cooking food and that she has little appetite. Although she is always thirsty, she restricts fluids because "they make me sicker." She has no signs of dehydration.
Nursing Diagnosis	Risk for Altered Nutrition: Less than Body Requirements related to nausea, vomiting, and anorexia
Goals/Expected Outcomes	Maria will

Maria will

- Maintain adequate intake of calories and nutrients to meet her needs, as evidenced by continuous weight gain during pregnancy.
- Report less nausea and a decrease in the episodes of vomiting within 2 weeks.
- Demonstrate no signs or symptoms of dehydration.

Intervention	Rationale
1. Recommend that Maria eat two dry crackers half an hour before arising in the morning and that she get out of bed slowly.	1. Food counteracts the hypoglycemia resulting from nightlong fasting and prevents an initial episode of nausea that may become difficult to control.
2. Suggest that Maria consume a high-protein bedtime snack, such as cottage cheese or a turkey sandwich.	2. Proteins are metabolized at a slower rate, which helps prevent morning hypoglycemia.
3. Instruct Maria to eat small, dry meals five to six times a day rather than three large ones.	3. Frequent dry meals prevent the stomach from becoming empty, which increases the feeling of nausea.
4. Recommend that Maria eat a dry cracker, unbuttered popcorn, or dry toast every 2 hours.	4. Nausea is more intense when the stomach is empty.
5. Suggest that Maria avoid fried or greasy foods, foods that are highly seasoned, and foods that have strong odors.	5. Odors and greasy textures are associated with nausea and increased episodes of vomiting.
6. Teach Maria to keep a record of daily intake of food and fluids, episodes of vomiting, and measures that reduce nausea.	6. A record is essential to determine whether adequate nutrients and fluids are being retained and to identify the most helpful measures to control nausea.
7. Suggest that fluids be taken separately from meals.	7. Fluids stretch the stomach and may cause vomiting.
8. Recommend frequent small amounts of ice chips, water, and clear liquids like Jell-O or popsicles. Suggest that Maria avoid coffee or tea.	8. Clear fluids may be tolerated better during periods of nausea. Coffee and tea act as diuretics.
9. Suggest that Maria try ice cream, pudding, watermelon, soups, eggnogs, and vegetable drinks.	9. These foods have more nutrients and are often tolerated well when taken separately.
10. Reassure Maria that nausea and vomiting usually disappear by the second trimester and do not indicate a problem with the pregnancy.	10. Reassurance reduces anxiety, so that the woman knows the condition is self-limiting and does not threaten the fetus.
11. Assess Maria's weight at each prenatal visit and compare her weight gain with that expected for the weeks of gestation.	11. If weight gain is adequate, the focus remains on relieving the discomfort of nausea and vomiting. If weight gain is less than adequate or if signs of dehydration are present, refer her for medical management.
12. Tell Maria to call if she is unable to retain recommended amounts of fluid or has signs of dehydration such as dry, cracked lips, elevated pulse, fever, and concentrated urine.	12. Dehydration should be treated promptly.

Evaluation	Periodic nausea and vomiting continued throughout the first trimester but ceased during the second trimester. Maria did not become dehydrated and gained 4.5 kg (approximately 10 lb) by 20 weeks.

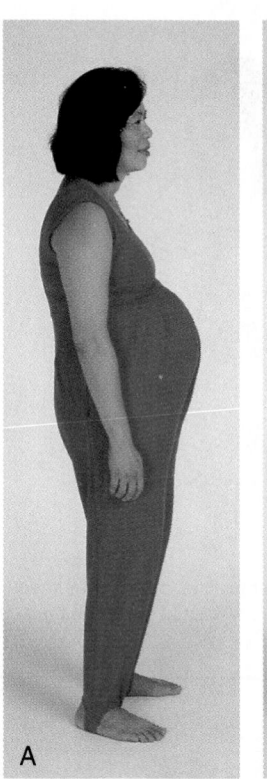
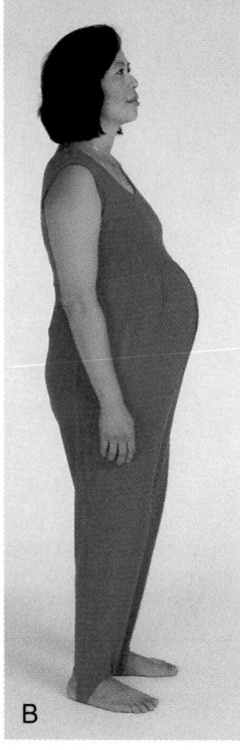

FIGURE 13–11
. . . .
Posture during pregnancy may cause or alleviate backache. *A,* Incorrect posture. The neck is jutting forward, the shoulders are slumping, and the back is sharply curved, creating back pain and discomfort. *B,* Correct posture. The neck and shoulders are straight, the back is flattened, and the pelvis is tucked under and slightly upward.

VARICOSITIES

Varicosities are usually confined to the legs but may involve the veins of the vulva or rectum (hemorrhoids). Varicosities occur most often in women with a family history of varicose veins and are more likely to be a problem in women who are obese or who are multiparas. There may be minimal discomfort at the end of the day or large, tortuous veins that produce severe discomfort with any activity.

Varicosities are common in pregnancy because the weight of the uterus partially compresses the veins that return blood from the legs. This process causes the vessels to dilate, and they may become engorged, inflamed, and painful. Varicose veins are exacerbated by prolonged standing, when the force of gravity makes blood return more difficult.

HEMORRHOIDS

Hemorrhoids are varicosities of the rectum that may be external (outside the anal sphincter) or internal (above the sphincter). Some of the most common causes of hemorrhoids are vascular engorgement of the pelvis, constipation, straining at stool, and prolonged sitting or standing. Pushing during the second stage of labor exacerbates the problem, which may continue into the postpartum period.

CONSTIPATION

Intestinal motility is reduced during pregnancy as a result of progesterone. This change may cause hard, dry stools and decreased frequency of bowel movements. Iron supplementation also causes constipation in some women.

LEG CRAMPS

Painful contraction of the muscles of the lower legs occurs most often during sleep, when the muscles are relaxed. Cramps are also likely to occur when the woman stretches and extends her foot. Leg cramps are believed to be caused by an imbalance of serum calcium and phosphorus. A 1-to-1 ratio of calcium to phosphorus is desired, but this ratio is difficult to achieve in pregnancy, when many women consume large amounts of dairy products high in calcium. Venous congestion in the legs during the third trimester also contributes to leg cramps.

NURSING CARE
. . . .
Family Responses to Physical Changes of Pregnancy

The nursing process focuses on identifying each family's unique responses to the physiologic changes of pregnancy, determining factors that might interfere with the ability to

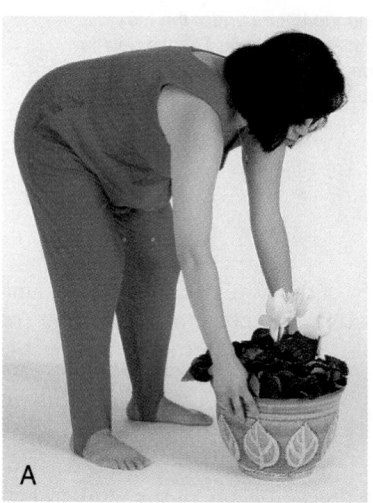
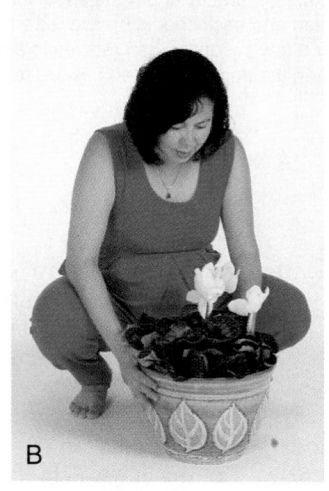

FIGURE 13–12
. . . .
Techniques for lifting. Squatting places less strain on the back. *A,* Incorrect technique. Stooping or bending places a great deal of strain on muscles of the lower body. *B,* Correct technique. Squatting and moving the object close permits the stronger muscles of the legs to do the lifting.

Shoulder circling

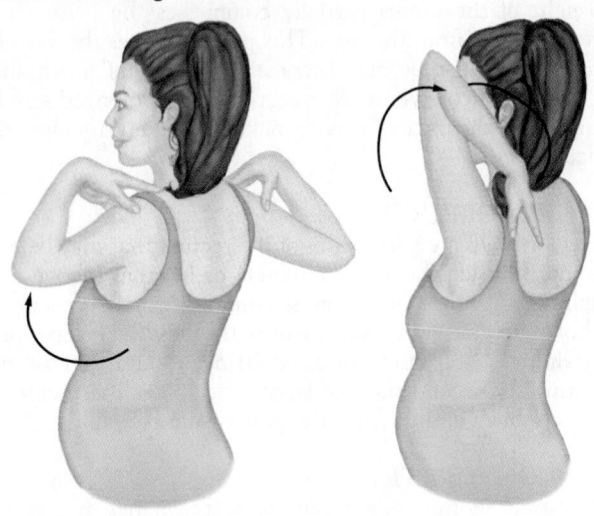

The fingertips are placed on the shoulders, then the elbows are brought forward and up during inhalation, back and down during exhalation. Repeat five times.

Tailor sitting

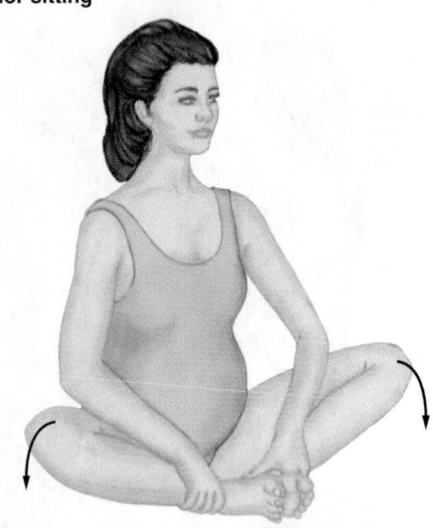

The woman uses her thigh muscles to press her knees to the floor. Keeping her back straight, she should remain in the position for 5 to 15 minutes.

Pelvic tilt or pelvic rocking

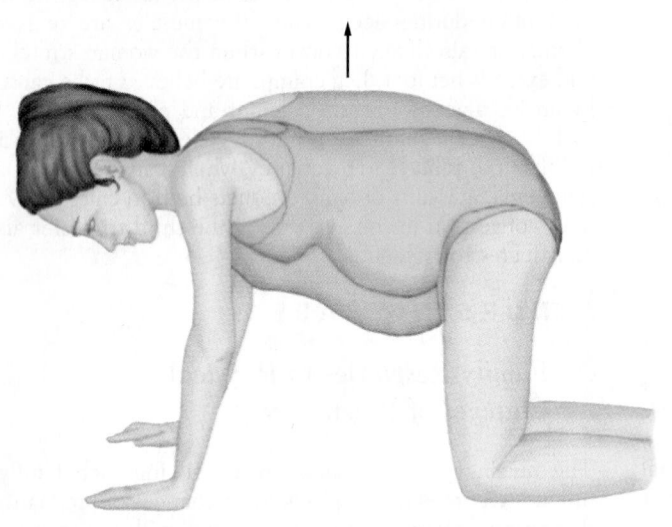

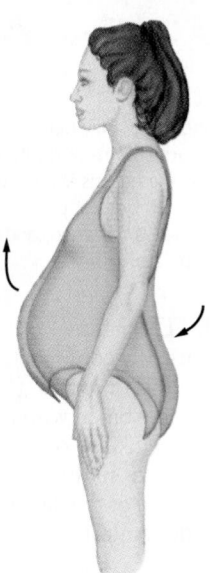

This exercise can be performed on hands and knees, with the hands directly under the shoulders and the knees under the hips. The back should be in a neutral position, not hollowed. The head and neck should be aligned with the straight back. The woman then presses up with the lower back and holds this position for a few seconds, then relaxes to a neutral position. Repeat 5 times. The exercise may also be performed in a standing position when the pelvis is rotated forward to flatten the lower back.

FIGURE 13–13
• • • • • • • • •
Exercises for pregnancy.

adapt to changes that occur, and finding solutions to identified problems.

Assessment

Assess the family's responses to the physiologic processes of pregnancy and the family's preparation for the birth. Include structured interviews, planned teaching-learning sessions, and informal discussions. Significant information may be obtained from a review of the history and physical examination findings. Information may come not only from the expectant mother but also from the partner and other significant family members.

Nursing Diagnosis and Planning

Most families express an intense desire to protect the health of the unborn child and the well-being of the mother. Perhaps the most encompassing nursing diagnosis for the prenatal period is

■ Health-Seeking Behaviors: prenatal care and health practices that provide optimum benefit to the fetus and mother.

Expected Outcomes: The family will demonstrate knowledge of practices that promote the safety and well-being of the mother and fetus throughout pregnancy and will describe measures that provide relief from the common discomforts of pregnancy. The family will describe a realistic plan during the first trimester to modify behaviors or habits that do not promote the health of the mother and fetus.

Interventions

Following the initial assessment, the woman is usually not seen by the health care provider for 4 weeks. Instruct her and her family about signs and symptoms that indicate a serious danger and should be reported immediately.

Teaching Health Behaviors

Bathing.   Bathing protects pregnant women from potential infection and promotes comfort by dissipating heat produced by increased metabolism. During the last trimester, when balance is altered by a changing center of gravity, the woman should be cautioned to use nonskid pads in the tub or shower.

Hot Tubs and Saunas.   Instruct the woman to avoid saunas and hot tubs because they may produce maternal hyperthermia. Maternal hyperthermia, particularly during the first trimester, has been associated with fetal anomalies such as central nervous system defects (Rogers & Davis, 1995).

Douching.   Despite increased vaginal discharge, there is no need for douching before, during, or after pregnancy. The only exception is an order by a physician or nurse-midwife to treat a specific problem. Bulb-type syringes have been associated with deaths caused by air embolism and therefore should never be used. To prevent excessive force of the fluid, douche bags should not be elevated more than 2 feet above the hips. The nozzle should not be inserted

---

CRITICAL TO REMEMBER

Danger Signs During Pregnancy

- Vaginal bleeding, with or without discomfort
- Rupture of membranes (escape of fluid from the vagina)
- Swelling of the fingers (rings become tight) or puffiness of the face or around the eyes
- Continuous, pounding headache
- Visual disturbances (blurred vision, dimness, spots before the eyes)
- Persistent or severe abdominal pain
- Chills or fever
- Painful urination
- Persistent vomiting
- Change in frequency or strength of fetal movements

---

more than 3 inches into the vagina (Cunningham et al., 1997).

Breast Care.   The expectant mother should avoid soap on her nipples, as it removes the natural lubricant that forms there. A supportive bra helps prevent loss of muscle tone as the breasts become heavier during pregnancy. Wide bra straps distribute the weight evenly across the shoulders and provide greater comfort. Breast stimulation, which increases oxytocin secretion and thus initiates uterine contractions, is unsafe if there has been a history of preterm labor or if signs of preterm labor exist.

Clothing.   Clothing should be comfortable and non-constricting. Tight jeans or pantyhose that may constrict venous circulation should be worn only for short periods. Low heels do not interfere with balance, but high heels increase the curvature of the lower spine (lordosis) that is prevalent during the last trimester.

Exercise.   The amount and type of exercise recommended depends on the physical condition of the woman and the stage of pregnancy. Walking is an ideal exercise because it stimulates muscular activity of the entire body, gently increases respiratory and cardiovascular effort, and does not result in fatigue or strain.

Vigorous exercise may divert blood supply from the placenta to maternal muscles and thus deprive the fetus of needed oxygen. It also increases levels of circulating catecholamines, which cause visceral vasoconstriction and decreased placental circulation.

Women should not *begin* strenuous exercise programs or intensify training during pregnancy. Women who have been exercising strenuously should consult the health care provider but may be able to continue much of their usual routine. Sports that require balance or may cause injury, and exercise in the supine position are not safe. As pregnancy progresses, it may be necessary to reduce the level of exercise to prevent physiologic stress. The woman can take her pulse every 10 to 15 minutes and should not exceed a heart rate that has been determined in consultation with the physician or midwife.

Pregnant women must avoid becoming overheated because heat is transmitted to the fetus. They should allow a cool-down period of mild activity after exercising. It is important to take liquids frequently while exercising to prevent dehydration.

Sleep and Rest.   Finding a comfortable position for rest becomes a problem in the third trimester. Pillows can be used to support the abdomen and back and to provide the best opportunity for sleep (Fig. 13–14).

Employment.   Most women of childbearing age in the United States are employed outside the home, and most continue to work during pregnancy.

Maternal Safety.   Work should not lead to undue fatigue. Frequent rest periods are essential. For jobs that require constant standing or sitting, suggest that the woman change positions frequently or walk briefly to stimulate circulation and reduce fatigue. Tasks that require balance may be hazardous because the uterus enlarges and the center of gravity shifts.

Exposure to Teratogens.   Intrauterine exposure to toxic substances is of particular concern during the first trimester, the period of organogenesis. Women should investigate their own occupational hazards. For example, hairdressers

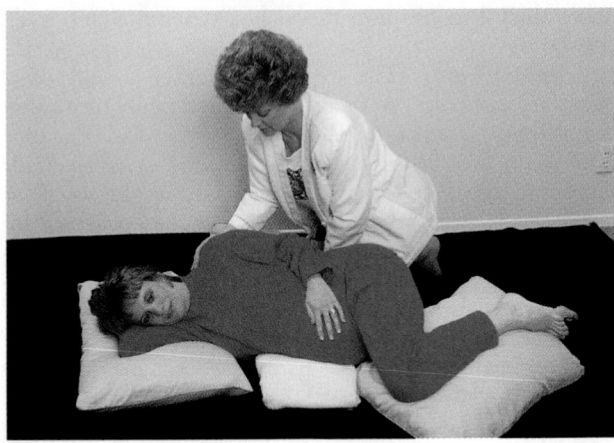

FIGURE 13-14

During the third trimester, pillows supporting the abdomen and back provide a comfortable position for rest.

are exposed to toxic substances in hair dyes and aerosol sprays; nurses and hospital personnel may be exposed to radiation, anesthetic gases, and hexachlorophene; and laundry and dry cleaning workers may be exposed to fetotoxic compounds. In addition, passive smoking is harmful to both mother and fetus.

Travel.   Although travel by car is generally safe, advise frequent stops to allow the expectant mother to empty her bladder and walk around. She must fasten the seat belt snugly, with the lap belt under the abdomen. This position is uncomfortable for some women, and it causes concern about internal injuries should a collision occur. It is much safer to wear the belt, however, than to leave it off and risk being ejected from the car during an accident.

Travel by plane and train is generally safe, although some physicians discourage air travel after 26 weeks. If travel is necessary, women should be advised to walk frequently to maintain adequate peripheral circulation. During travel to remote locations, a major concern is that adequate medical care be available at the destination.

Immunizations.   In general, immunizations that use live virus vaccines are contraindicated during pregnancy because of teratogenic effects on the fetus. These vaccines include measles, mumps, rubella, and oral polio vaccines.

Teaching Necessary Lifestyle Changes

Many expectant parents are willing to make lifestyle changes to avoid adversely affecting the fetus.

Over-the-Counter Drugs.   Advise the pregnant woman to consult with her health care provider before taking any drugs. This precaution is important for over-the-counter drugs as well as for prescription drugs.

Tobacco.   Make every effort to motivate the expectant mother to stop smoking and to avoid contact with others who smoke. It is well documented that pregnant women who smoke have smaller infants and a higher rate of preterm births than women who do not smoke. Moreover, developmental problems, such as short attention span and lower cognitive skills, are also more common in children when the mother continues to smoke during pregnancy.

Alcohol.   Alcohol is a known teratogen, and maternal alcohol use is one of the leading causes of mental retardation in the United States. Alcohol produces a characteristic cluster of developmental anomalies known as fetal alcohol syndrome (see Chapter 25). Conclusive data about the effects of social or moderate drinking on the fetus are not available. Therefore, women who are pregnant or who plan to become pregnant should abstain from all alcohol use.

Illegal Drugs.   Use of so-called street drugs, such as cocaine, heroin, and methamphetamines, is harmful to the fetus. Advise the pregnant woman to discontinue all illicit drug use (see Chapter 25).

Evaluation

- Does the woman practice self-care practices as she was taught?
- Does she develop a plan early in pregnancy to modify habits that do not promote health?
- Can she discuss ways to obtain relief from the common discomforts of pregnancy?

KEY CONCEPTS

- Pregnancy causes a predictable pattern of uterine growth. In general, the uterus can be palpated at the level of the umbilicus at 20 weeks of gestation and at the xiphoid process by 36 weeks.
- Thick mucus fills the cervical canal and protects the fetus from infection caused by bacteria ascending from the vagina.
- The plasma volume expands faster and to a greater extent than red blood cell volume, resulting in a dilution of hemoglobin concentration called physiologic (pseudo) anemia.

- Increased renal plasma flow results in an increased glomerular filtration rate, which often results in "spilling" of glucose and other nutrients in the urine. Increased blood flow to the skin helps reduce the heat generated by the fetus and by the increased maternal metabolic rate.
- The gravid uterus partially occludes the vena cava and the descending aorta when the mother is supine. The occlusion causes supine hypotensive syndrome, which can be prevented or corrected by assuming a lateral position.

- During the last trimester, the uterus pushes the diaphragm upward, decreasing lung capacity. To compensate, the ribs flare, the substernal angle widens, and the circumference of the chest increases.
- Increased hCG and estrogen levels may cause nausea in early pregnancy. Increased progesterone causes relaxation of all smooth muscles, resulting in stasis of urine and the risk of urinary tract infections and constipation.
- Alterations in hormones are also responsible for cutaneous changes, such as hyperpigmentation.

■ The expanding uterus plus the hormone relaxin result in progressive changes that can lead to muscle strain and backache during the last trimester.

■ Progesterone, the hormone of pregnancy, maintains the uterine lining, prevents uterine contractions, and helps to prepare the breasts for lactation.

■ Presumptive and probable signs of pregnancy may be caused by conditions other than pregnancy and thus cannot be considered positive or diagnostic signs. Positive signs can have no other cause.

■ A complete history and physical examination are necessary at the initial antepartum visit to determine the potential risks to the mother and fetus and to obtain baseline data so that a plan of care can be developed.

■ Multifetal pregnancies impose greater physiologic changes than a single-fetus pregnancy and require extra vigilance to detect possible complications.

■ Families need information on self-care and health promotion during pregnancy as well as information on ways to deal with the common discomforts of pregnancy that do not need or respond to medical management.

ANSWERS TO CRITICAL THINKING EXERCISE 13–1

1. If pregnant now, Wilma is gravida 3, para 1 (the twin birth counts as one parous experience). If the acronym TPAL is used, T = 1 (twin infants born at term but counted as 1 parous experience); P = 0 (no preterm infants); A = 1 (one pregnancy ended before 20 weeks' gestation); L = 2 (living twins).

2. Amenorrhea and nausea and vomiting are only presumptive (subjective) indications of pregnancy because they can be caused by conditions other than pregnancy.

3. Count back 3 months to March 22, and add 7 days. This brings the date to March 29. Wilma's EDD is March 29, 2000.

REFERENCES AND READINGS

American Academy of Pediatrics and American College of Obstetricians and Gynecologists. (1997). *Guidelines for perinatal care* (4th ed.). Elk Grove Village, IL, and Washington, DC: Author.

American College of Obstetricians and Gynecologists. (1994a). *Diabetes and pregnancy* (Technical Bulletin No. 200). Washington, DC: Author.

American College of Obstetricians and Gynecologists. (1994b). *Exercise during pregnancy and the postnatal period* (Technical Bulletin No. 189). Washington, DC: Author.

American College of Obstetricians and Gynecologists. (1996). *Guidelines for women's health care*. Washington, DC: Author.

Aminoff, M. J. (1999). Neurologic disorders. In R. K. Creasy & R. Resnik (Eds.), *Maternal-fetal medicine: Principles and practice* (4th ed., pp. 1091–1119). Philadelphia: Saunders.

Andres, R. L. (1999). Social and illicit drug use in pregnancy. In R. K. Creasy & R. Resnik (Eds.), *Maternal-fetal medicine: Principles and practice* (4th ed., pp. 143–164). Philadelphia: Saunders.

Association of Women's Health, Obstetric, and Neonatal Nurses. (1994). *Didactic content and clinical skills verification for professional nurse providers of perinatal home care*. Washington, DC: Author.

Association of Women's Health, Obstetric, and Neonatal Nurses. (1998). *Standards and guidelines for professional nursing practice in the care of women and newborns* (5th ed.). Washington, DC: Author.

Baker, E. R. (1995). Physiologic adaptations to pregnancy. In P. L. Carr, K. M. Freund, & S. Somani (Eds.), *The medical care of women* (pp. 294–303). Philadelphia: Saunders.

Blackburn, S. T., & Loper, D. L. (1992). *Maternal, fetal, and neonatal physiology*. Philadelphia: Saunders.

Briggs, G. G., Freeman, R. K., & Sumner, J. Y. (1998). *Drugs in pregnancy and lactation* (5th ed.). Baltimore: Williams & Wilkins.

Cunningham, F. G., MacDonald, P. C., Gant, N. F., Leveno, K. J., Gilstrap, L. C., Hankins, G. D. V., & Clark, S. L. (1997). *Williams obstetrics* (20th ed.). Norwalk, CT: Appleton & Lange.

Driscoll, J. W. (1996). Psychosocial adaptation to pregnancy and postpartum. In K. R. Simpson & P. A. Creehan (Eds.), *AWHONN perinatal nursing* (pp. 61–71). Philadelphia: Lippincott-Raven.

DuBose, T. J. (1996). First trimester. *Fetal sonography* (pp. 389–425). Philadelphia: Saunders.

Duffy, T. P. (1999). Hematologic aspects of pregnancy. In G. N. Burrow & T. P. Duffy (Eds.), *Medical complications during pregnancy* (5th ed., pp. 79–95). Philadelphia: Saunders.

Ellings, J. M., Newman, R. B., & Bowers, N. A. (1998). Prenatal care and multiple pregnancy. *Journal of Obstetric, Gynecologic, and Neonatal Nursing*, *27*(4), 457–465.

Enkin, M. W., Keirse, M. J., Renfrew, M. J., & Neilson, J. P. (1995). Effective care in pregnancy and childbirth: A synopsis. *Birth*, *22*(2), 101–111.

Fallon, M. K. (1996). Physiologic changes of pregnancy. In K. R. Simpson & P. A. Creehan (Eds.), *AWHONN perinatal nursing* (pp. 43–59). Philadelphia: Lippincott-Raven.

Groff, J. Y., Mullen, P. D., Mongoven, M., & Burau, K. (1997). Prenatal weight gain patterns and infant birth-weight associated with maternal smoking. *Birth*, *24*(4), 234–239.

Hobel, C. J. (1998). Prenatal care. In N. F. Hacker & J. G. Moore (Eds.), *Essentials of obstetrics and gynecology* (3rd ed., pp. 111–122). Philadelphia: Saunders.

Kendig, S., & Barron, M. L. (1996). Antenatal care and risk assessment strategies. In K. R. Simpson & P. A. Creehan (Eds.), *AWHONN perinatal nursing* (pp. 73–103). Philadelphia: Lippincott-Raven.

MacLennan, A. H. (1994). Multiple gestation: Clinical characteristics and management. In R. K. Creasy & R. Resnik (Eds.), *Maternal-fetal medicine: Principles and practice* (3rd ed.). Philadelphia: Saunders.

Mattson, S., & Smith, J. E. (Eds.). (1993). *Core curriculum for maternal-newborn nursing*. Philadelphia: Saunders.

Monga, M. (1999). Maternal cardiovascular and renal adaptation to pregnancy. In R. K. Creasy & R. Resnik (Eds.), *Maternal-fetal medicine: Principles and practice* (4th ed., pp. 783–792). Philadelphia: Saunders.

Newman, R. B., & Ellings, J. M. (1995). Antepartum management of the multiple gestation: The case for specialized care. *Seminars in Perinatology*, *19*(5), 387–402.

Nuwayhid, B., Nguyen, T., & Khalife, S. (1998a). Maternal physiology. In N. F. Hacker & J. G. Moore (Eds.), *Essentials of obstetrics and gynecology* (3rd ed., pp. 85–99). Philadelphia: Saunders.

Nuwayhid, B., Nguyen, T., & Khalife, S. (1998b). Medical complications of pregnancy. In N. F. Hacker & J. G. Moore (Eds.), *Essentials of obstetrics and gynecology* (3rd ed., pp. 234–262). Philadelphia: Saunders.

O'Brien, B., & Zhou, Q. (1995). Variables related to nausea and vomiting during pregnancy. *Birth*, *22*(2), 93–100.

Rapini, R. P. (1999). The skin and pregnancy. In R. K. Creasy & R. Resnik (Eds.),

Although each couple adapts to pregnancy in a unique manner, the psychological responses of prospective parents change as the pregnancy progresses. By the time the infant is born, the woman and her partner have completed developmental tasks that make it possible for them to become parents in the true sense of the word. Both social and cultural factors influence the way the woman adjusts to pregnancy.

■ Maternal Psychological Responses

A woman's psychological response to pregnancy changes over time. Initially she may be uncertain or ambivalent about the pregnancy, and her primary focus is on herself. Gradually her focus shifts, and she becomes increasingly concerned about how she can protect and provide for the fetus she is carrying.

First Trimester

UNCERTAINTY
During the early weeks, the woman is unsure whether she is pregnant and tries to confirm it. She observes her body carefully for changes indicating pregnancy. She may use an over-the-counter pregnancy test kit for validation.

Reaction to the uncertainty of pregnancy depends on the individual. A woman may be eager to find confirming signs, or she may dread the possibility. Usually, she seeks confirmation from a physician, certified nurse-midwife, or nurse practitioner within 12 weeks of the first missed menstrual period.

AMBIVALENCE
Once the pregnancy is confirmed, almost all women have conflicting feelings, or ambivalence, about being pregnant. Many feel that this is not the right time, even if the pregnancy is wanted and planned. Women who had planned to become pregnant often say they thought it would take longer and that they feel unprepared for it. Many pregnancies are desired but unplanned, and these women may wish they had not become pregnant until some specific goals were met.

Many women examine changes to be made in their lives as a result of the pregnancy. If it is a first pregnancy, the woman may worry about the added responsibility and feel unsure of her ability to be a good parent. Some women worry about how this pregnancy will affect their relationship with other children or with the father.

THE SELF AS PRIMARY FOCUS
Throughout the first trimester, the woman's primary focus is on herself, not the fetus. Early physical responses to pregnancy confirm that something is happening to her, but the fetus remains vague and unreal. She may say, "I am pregnant," rather than, "I am going to have a baby."

Physical changes and increased hormone levels may cause emotional lability (unstable moods). Her mood can change quickly from contentment to irritation or from optimistic planning to an overwhelming need for sleep. These changes may be confusing to her partner, who is accustomed to a more stable relationship. The nurse should tell the couple that mood changes are normal and that they do not necessarily indicate unresolved problems.

Second Trimester

PHYSICAL EVIDENCE OF PREGNANCY
During the second trimester, physical changes occur in the expectant mother and make the fetus "real." The uterus can be palpated in the abdomen; weight increases; and breast changes are obvious. Most importantly, she feels the fetus move ("quickening"). This experience is important because it confirms that a life is developing within the uterus. As a result, she no longer thinks of the fetus as simply a part of her body but now perceives it as separate, although entirely dependent on her. Now she might say, "I am going to have a baby" (Fig. 14–1).

THE FETUS AS PRIMARY FOCUS
The woman's major focus during the second trimester becomes the fetus. The pregnant woman generally feels well because the discomforts of the first trimester have usually abated. She is now concerned about how she can produce a healthy infant. She often seeks information about diet and about how the fetus grows and develops. She experiences a feeling of creative energy and satisfaction.

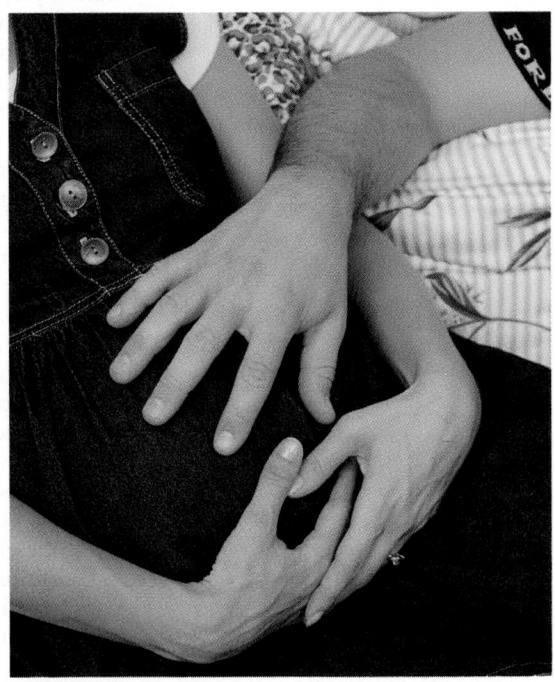

FIGURE 14–1
Fetal movement, "quickening," confirms that a separate life is developing.

NARCISSISM AND INTROVERSION

During this time many women become increasingly concerned about their ability to protect and provide for the fetus. This concern is often manifested as narcissism and introversion. Selecting exactly the right foods to eat or the right clothes to wear may assume more importance than ever before. Some women may lose interest in their jobs because the work seems alien to the events taking place in their bodies. They may be less interested in current events as they concentrate on their pregnancy, or they may become fearful that world events threaten them and therefore present a danger to the fetus.

If she is a primigravida, the expectant mother wonders what the infant is like. She looks at baby pictures of herself and her mate and wants to hear stories about them as infants. Multiparas have concerns about how this child will be accepted by siblings and grandparents.

BODY IMAGE

Rapid and profound changes take place in the body during the second trimester. Changes in body size and contour are noticeable, with obvious bulging of the abdomen, thickening of the waist, and enlargement of the breasts. The changes may be welcomed because they signify growth of the fetus, and this growth creates pride in the woman and her partner. For some women, however, the change in body size and shape, coupled with hyperpigmentation of the skin and striae gravidarum (stretch marks), may contribute to a negative body image. Moreover, changes in body function, such as altered balance, less physical endurance, and discomfort in the pelvis and lower back areas, may also contribute to a negative body image (Nursing Care Plan 14–1).

CHANGES IN SEXUALITY

Sexual interest and activity of pregnant women and their partners are unpredictable: they may increase, decline, or remain unchanged. During the first trimester nausea, fatigue, and breast tenderness may interfere with erotic feelings. Fear of miscarriage may cause couples to avoid intercourse, particularly if the woman has previously lost a pregnancy. Nurses can help reassure the couple that there is no evidence that intercourse is related to early pregnancy loss when no other complications are present.

As a result of pelvic vasocongestion, women experience increased sensitivity of the labia and clitoris and increased vaginal lubrication during the second trimester. These changes, coupled with not having to worry about getting pregnant, may increase the sexual responsiveness of many women.

During the third trimester, the "missionary position" (male on top) may cause discomfort from abdominal pressure. Heartburn, indigestion, and supine hypotensive syndrome may also occur in this position. Alternate positions include side-lying, female-superior, and rear-entry. Fatigue, ligament pain, urinary frequency, and shortness of breath may also interfere with vaginal intercourse. Hugging, kissing, mutual massage, and cuddling are expressions of affection that do not always lead to intercourse.

As they become larger, some women believe that their bodies are ugly, and they may worry about how their partners react to their increased size. Sexual response varies widely among males. Some report heightened feelings of sexual interest, but some men perceive the woman's body in late pregnancy as unattractive. Moreover, for some men, fear of harming the fetus or causing discomfort interferes with sexual activity.

The expectant couple should be made aware of the normal changes in sexual desire that occur during pregnancy and the importance of communicating their feelings openly with each other. Despite the need for information, most women are reluctant to initiate a discussion about sexual activity.

> It may be helpful to use a broad opening statement to initiate discussion about sexual activity. For example, "Sometimes couples are concerned about having sex during pregnancy." Broad opening statements provide a method of introducing the subject in such a way that the woman feels comfortable to pursue it or to let it drop.

The nurse should advise the couple to curtail all sexual activity if the client is at risk for preterm labor because uterine contractions may be initiated by orgasm. The nurse also emphasizes that if membranes have ruptured or if bleeding occurs, they should not have intercourse.

Third Trimester

VULNERABILITY

During the third trimester, particularly in the seventh month of pregnancy, pregnant women have increasing feelings of vulnerability. They often feel that the precious baby may be lost or harmed if not protected at all times (Fig. 14–2). Many mothers have fantasies or nightmares

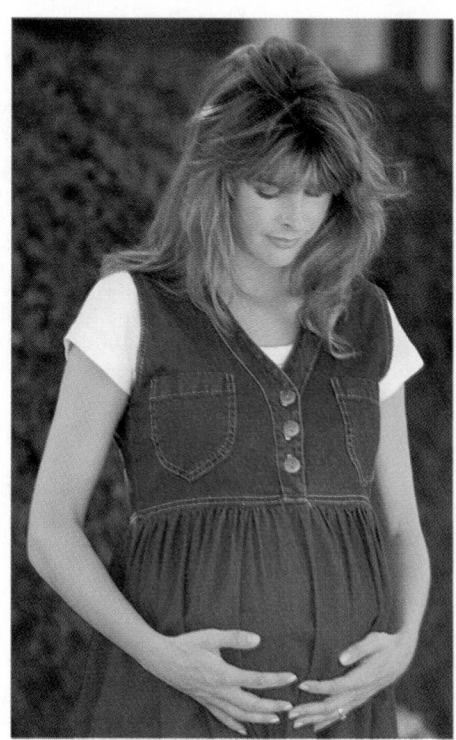

FIGURE 14–2
. . . .
During the third trimester, the mother feels increasingly vulnerable; she cradles her fetus to signify her protectiveness.

NURSING CARE PLAN 14–1

. . . .

Body Image During Pregnancy

Assessment

Dolores White is a 34-year-old primigravida in the 26th week of pregnancy. Both she and her husband have been runners for several years. Dolores stopped running 6 months ago and reports that she now walks "like other old ladies." She verbalizes concern about how much bigger she will get and says she feels "awkward and ugly." She states, "I hate the way I look; I can't wait to get back into shape."

Nursing Diagnosis

Body Image Disturbance related to changes in body size, contour, and function.

Goals/Expected Outcomes

The client will

- Make statements that indicate acceptance of expected body changes during pregnancy.
- Express her feelings about body changes to her husband as well as to the health care team by (date).
- Set realistic goals for weight loss and the resumption of a running program after childbirth.

Intervention

1. Acknowledge Dolores's feelings. "I can see you are disappointed at not being able to run, and I sense you are concerned about how your body has changed as a result of pregnancy."
2. Clarify Dolores's concerns. "You have always been an athlete. You may be wondering how much permanent change will result from pregnancy."

3. Suggest that Dolores share her feelings with her husband and seek his support.

4. Demonstrate the expected pattern of weight gain from 26 weeks to term gestation and correlate this change with the growth and development of the fetus.
5. Help Dolores make realistic plans to lose weight and regain strength after childbirth.
   a. Discuss the expected pattern of weight loss after birth. There is an initial weight loss of 10 to 12 pounds. An additional 5.5 pounds may be lost in the first few postpartum days. By the end of 8 weeks, many women are near their pre-pregnancy weight.
   b. Demonstrate graduated exercises that increase muscle tone and strength.
   c. Explain the purpose of adipose tissue gained during pregnancy. Discuss a diet that provides sufficient calories to meet needs during breast-feeding.

Rationale

1. Feelings must be acknowledged, reflected, and dealt with before the underlying cause can be addressed.

2. An underlying, unvoiced concern may be that pregnancy and childbirth will change the woman from athlete to mother. This altered perception of herself causes fear and/or grief.
3. Although one may assume that the partner observes and understands when negative feelings exist, this response may not be true.
4. Many women are reassured to know that weight gain shows growth of the fetus. Knowledge of expected weight gain may allay unexpressed fears of excessive weight gain.
5. Adipose tissue provides a needed source of energy during birth and lactation. Many women are relieved to know that there is a purpose and that the added weight will be lost gradually. Breast-feeding requires at least 500 additional calories per day.

Evaluation

Dolores makes statements that show more acceptance of body changes during pregnancy. She reports she has discussed her feelings with her husband and that he is very supportive. She discusses her plans for diet and exercise after birth. This area may need more follow-up after the baby is born.

Additional Nursing Diagnoses to Consider

Risk for Situational Low Self-Esteem
Altered Family Processes

about harm coming to the infant and become very cautious as a result. They may avoid crowds because they feel unable to protect the infant from infectious diseases or physical dangers that may be present.

INCREASING DEPENDENCE

The expectant mother often becomes increasingly dependent on her partner in the last weeks of pregnancy. She may insist that he carry a beeper, or she may call his place of work several times during the day just to be sure that he is available. Her need for love and attention from her partner is even more pronounced in late pregnancy. When she is assured of his concern and willingness to provide assistance, she feels more secure and able to cope.

Although the woman may not be able to explain the increasing dependence, she expects her partner to understand the feeling and may become angry if he is not sympathetic. The nurse can encourage couples to discuss their fears and feelings openly so that misunderstandings can be avoided.

PREPARATION FOR BIRTH

Gradually, the feelings of vulnerability decrease as the woman comes to terms with her situation. The fetus continues to grow, and fetal movements are no longer gentle. The woman's relationship with the fetus changes as she acknowledges that although she and the fetus are interrelated, the baby is not a part of herself. Although she may not consciously acknowledge the increasing feelings of separateness, she longs to *see* the baby and to become acquainted with her child.

Most pregnant women are concerned with their ability to determine when they are in labor. They review the signs of labor taught in childbirth education classes and question friends and family members who have given birth. Many couples worry that they will not get to the hospital or clinic in time for the birth, and they may be concerned about how they will cope with labor.

During the last several weeks, the woman becomes increasingly concerned with her expected date of delivery (EDD) and with the experience of labor and delivery. Some women fear labor and dread the EDD, whereas some are so uncomfortable that they look forward to that day, anticipating that it will be the *exact* day the birth will occur.

During the third trimester, an expectant mother may say, "I am going to be a mother" as she prepares for the infant. Obtaining clothing, arranging a place for the infant to sleep, and negotiating how household tasks will be shared with her partner are among the plans made during this period. In addition, many couples complete childbirth education classes.

Table 14–1 summarizes the progressive changes in maternal responses during pregnancy.

▌ *Maternal Role Transition*

The transition into mothering begins during pregnancy and increases with gestational age. An early task of pregnancy is to accept the intrusion of the fetus, then move to developing love for the child as an independent being (Mercer & Ferketich, 1994a). The greatest increase in maternal–fetal attachment seems to occur after quickening, when the mother begins to differentiate herself from the fetus (Bloom, 1995). A pregnant woman prepares for becoming a mother by contemplating her life as a woman with this child. She thinks about what characteristics she wishes to have as a mother and anticipates life changes that will be necessary.

Steps in Maternal Role Taking

Rubin (1984) observed specific steps that provide a framework for understanding the process of maternal role taking: mimicry, role play, fantasy, looking for a role fit, and grief work.

TABLE 14–1

Progressive Changes in Maternal Responses to Pregnancy

First Trimester	Second Trimester	Third Trimester
Emotional Response		
Uncertainty, ambivalence, focus on self	Wonder, increased narcissism, introversion, concern about body and changes in sexuality	Vulnerability Increased dependence Acceptance that fetus is separate but totally dependent
Physical Validation		
No obvious signs of fetal growth	Quickening	Obvious fetal growth Discomfort Decreased maternal activity
Role		
May begin to seek safe passage for self and fetus	Seeks acceptance of fetus and her role as mother	Prepares for birth
"Self" Statement		
"I am pregnant."	"I am going to have a baby."	"I am going to be a mother."

MIMICRY

Mimicry involves observing and copying the behavior of other women who are pregnant or already mothers. It is an attempt to discover what the role is like. Mimicry often begins early, when the woman may wear maternity clothes before they are needed to see how women in more advanced pregnancy feel and to see how people react to her.

ROLE PLAY

Role play consists of acting out some aspects of what mothers actually do. The pregnant woman searches for opportunities to hold or provide care for infants in the presence of another person. Role playing gives her an opportunity to practice the expected role and to receive validation from an observer that she has functioned well. She is particularly sensitive to the responses of her partner and her own mother.

FANTASY

Fantasies allow the woman to try a variety of possibilities and to daydream or to "try on" a variety of behaviors. Fantasies often have to do with how the infant will look and what characteristics he or she will have. The woman may daydream about taking her daughter to the park or about holding the child and reading or playing music.

At times, fantasies are fearful. What happens if something is wrong with the infant? What if the baby cries and won't stop? Fearful fantasies often provoke a pregnant woman to respond by seeking information or reassurance.

LOOKING FOR A ROLE FIT

Looking for a role fit is a process that occurs once the woman has built a set of role expectations for herself and has internalized a view of a "good" mother's behavior. She then observes the behaviors of mothers and compares them with her own expectations of herself. She imagines herself acting in the same way and either rejects or accepts the behaviors, depending on how well they fit her sense of what is right. This process implies that the woman has explored the role of mother long enough to have developed a sense of herself in the role and to be able to select behaviors that reaffirm her sense of herself fulfilling the role.

GRIEF WORK

Grief work may seem incongruous with maternal role taking, but women often experience a sense of sadness when they realize that they must permanently give up certain aspects of their previous selves. A new mother will never again be a carefree girl without a child. She must relinquish some of her old patterns of behavior so that she can move into the new identity of mother. Even simple things such as going shopping or going to the movies will require planning to include the infant or to find alternative care. Changes may be particularly difficult for the adolescent who is not used to planning and who may have to give up or change school plans as well.

Maternal Tasks of Pregnancy

The psychological work of pregnancy has been grouped into four maternal tasks (Rubin, 1984): (1) seeking safe passage for herself and the baby through pregnancy, labor, and childbirth, (2) securing acceptance of the baby and herself by her partner and family, (3) learning to give of herself, and (4) developing attachment and interconnection with the unknown child.

SEEKING SAFE PASSAGE

Seeking safe passage for herself and her baby is the woman's priority task. If she cannot be assured of that safety, she cannot move on to the other tasks. Behaviors that ensure safe passage include seeking the care of a physician or certified nurse-midwife and following recommendations about diet, vitamins, rest, and subsequent visits to the office or clinic.

In addition to following the advice of health care professionals, the pregnant woman must adhere to cultural practices that ensure the safety of herself and the infant. For instance, some Southeast Asian women avoid contact with scissors and knives because they fear sharp instruments may cause cleft lip or abortion (Mattson & Lew, 1995).

SECURING ACCEPTANCE

Securing acceptance is a process that continues throughout pregnancy. It involves reworking relationships so that the important persons in the family accept the woman in the role of mother and welcome the baby into the family. For example, she and the father of the baby must give up an exclusive relationship and make a place in their lives for a child. When the partner expresses pride and joy in the pregnancy, the woman feels valued and comforted. This feeling is so important that many women retain a memory of the partner's reaction to the announcement of pregnancy for many years.

Women's childhood relationships with their own mothers have been shown to be particularly important to the development of maternal attachment (Mercer & Ferketich, 1994a). The pregnant woman gains energy and contentment when her mother freely offers acceptance and support.

Problems may occur if the family strongly desires a child with particular characteristics and the woman believes that the family may reject an infant who does not meet the criteria. For example, if family members wish for a boy, will they accept a girl?

LEARNING TO GIVE OF SELF

Giving is one of the most idealized components of motherhood but one that must be learned. Learning to give begins in pregnancy when the woman allows her body to give space to the fetus. She tests her ability to derive pleasure from giving, often by providing food or care for her family. Their acceptance and enjoyment of the "gift" enhance her pleasure, so the role is strengthened. She may explore further by making and giving small gifts to friends, especially those who are pregnant.

Pregnant women also learn to give by receiving. Gifts received at baby showers are more than needed items: they also confirm continued interest and commitment from friends and family and enhance the woman's ability to give. Intangible gifts from others, such as companionship, attention, and support, help to increase her energy and affirm the importance of giving.

COMMITTING HERSELF TO THE UNKNOWN CHILD

Developing attachment to the unborn baby does not end in pregnancy but continues throughout the neonatal period (Mercer & Ferketich, 1994b). The process begins in early pregnancy when the woman accepts or "binds in" to the idea that she is pregnant, although the baby is not yet real to her. During the second trimester, the baby becomes real, and feelings of love and attachment surge. Mothers report feedback from their unborn infants during the third trimester and describe unique characteristics of the fetus with regard to sleep–wake cycles, temperament, and communication. Love of the infant becomes possessive and leads to feelings of vulnerability. The woman integrates the role of mother into her image of herself. She becomes comfortable with the idea of herself as mother and finds pleasure in contemplating the new role.

Paternal Adaptation

Expectant fathers must also make major psychosocial changes to adapt to their new role. Moreover, the changes may be more difficult because the male partner is often neglected by the health care team as well as by his peer group as attention is focused on the woman.

Variations in Paternal Adaptation

Wide variations exist in how men respond to pregnancy. Some are emotionally invested and explore every aspect of pregnancy, childbirth, and parenting. Others are more task-oriented and see themselves as managers. They may direct the woman's diet and act as coaches during childbirth but remain detached from the emotional aspects of the experience. Other men are more comfortable as observers and prefer not to participate. Some men are culturally conditioned to see pregnancy and childbirth as "women's work," and they may not be able to express their true feelings about pregnancy and fatherhood.

Research indicates that a stable relationship between the partners, financial security, and a sense of closure to the childless part of the couple's relationship contribute to readiness for fatherhood (Tiller, 1995). Additional factors include the man's relationship with his own father, his previous experience with children, and his confidence in his ability to care for the infant.

Developmental Processes

Jordan (1990) described the developmental processes that an expectant father must work through as he deals with the reality of pregnancy and the new child, works to be recognized as a parent, and makes an effort to be seen as relevant to childbearing.

GRAPPLING WITH THE REALITY OF PREGNANCY AND THE CHILD

The pregnancy and the child must become real before a man can take on the identity of father. Initially, changes in the expectant woman's behavior, such as nausea and fatigue, are perceived as symptoms of illness that have little to do with having a baby.

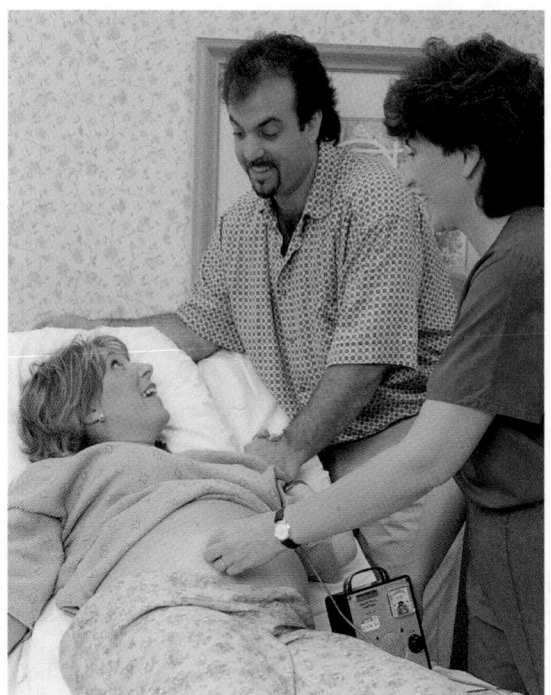

FIGURE 14–3

Reality booster: The existence of the fetus becomes real for the father when he hears the fetal heart beat through the transducer.

A man's initial reaction to the announcement of pregnancy may be pride and joy, but he often experiences the same ambivalence that his partner does, particularly if he is unprepared for the added responsibility or commitment. Various experiences act as catalysts or "reality boosters" that make the child more real (Fig. 14–3). These include hearing the baby's heartbeat, feeling the infant move, and seeing the fetus on a sonogram. Once they can feel the fetus move, many expectant fathers invent a nickname and talk to the fetus (Ferketich & Mercer, 1995).

Preparing the nursery and accumulating supplies for the new addition also reinforce the reality of the forthcoming child. These tasks often represent the first time that the expectant father has the opportunity to do something for the child directly. The birth itself is the most powerful "reality booster," and the infant becomes real to the father when he has an opportunity to see and hold the infant.

STRUGGLING FOR RECOGNITION AS A PARENT

Men tend not to be perceived as parents in their own right by their mates, coworkers, friends, or family. They are often viewed as helpmates but not as coparents. Many men find it upsetting that there is often little validation of their feelings or recognition that they want to be considered a parent as well as a helper.

Expectant mothers play an important role in helping their partners gain recognition as parents. Women who openly share the physical sensations and emotions that they experience help the expectant father to feel that he is part of the process. These women often refer to it as "our" pregnancy and insist that the man be included in all discussions and decisions.

Nurses must learn to view the mother, father, and child as the client and not focus exclusively on the mother and fetus. The nurse should encourage the man to ask questions about his partner's pregnancy. These men are entitled to as much advice and reassurance as expectant women.

CREATING THE ROLE OF INVOLVED FATHER

Men use various means to create a parenting role that is comfortable for them. They may seek closer ties with their fathers to reminisce about their own childhood. They also observe men who are already fathers and "try on" fathering behaviors to determine whether they are comfortable and fit their own concept of the father role. Many men assertively seek information about infant care and growth and development so that they will be prepared.

Parenting Information. Studies indicate that fathers believe they receive inadequate parenting information in prenatal classes (Tiller, 1995). Although adequate information is usually presented, fathers may not be ready for the information at the time it is provided. As a result, they may be unprepared to care for their infants and have unrealistic expectations of the newborn. Nurses must review information about infant care and growth and development after the infant is born, when the information is immediately relevant.

Couvade. The term *couvade* refers to pregnancy-related symptoms and behavior in expectant fathers. In primitive cultures, couvade took the form of rituals involving special dress, confinement, limitations of physical work, avoidance of certain foods, sexual restraint, and in some instances performance of "mock labor."

In modern practice, expectant fathers sometimes experience a cluster of physical symptoms similar to those experienced by women during pregnancy: loss of appetite, nausea and vomiting, headache, fatigue, and weight gain. Couvade symptoms are more likely to occur in early pregnancy and diminish as the pregnancy progresses. Symptoms may be caused by stress, anxiety, or empathy for the pregnant partner. They are usually harmless but may persist and result in nervousness, insomnia, restlessness, and irritability. Although the symptoms are almost always unobserved by the health care team, anticipatory guidance is believed to be beneficial for both partners.

▌ Adaptation of Grandparents

The initial reaction of grandparents depends on a number of different factors.

Age

Age is a major factor in determining the emotional responses of prospective grandparents. Older grandparents have usually dealt with their feelings about aging and react with joy when they find that they are to become grandparents. Younger grandparents may feel conflict and must resolve their self-image with the stereotype of grandparents as old persons. They often have career responsibilities and

may not be accessible because of the continuing demands of their own lives.

Number and Spacing of Other Grandchildren

The number and spacing of other grandchildren also determine how grandparents feel. A first grandchild may be an exciting event that creates great joy. If there are several other grandchildren, however, the birth of another may cause less excitement than with the first grandchild. The subdued reaction may be disappointing to the couple.

Perceptions of the Role of Grandparents

Many grandparents see their relationship with the grandchild as second in importance only to the parent–child relationship. They want to be involved in the pregnancy and look forward to being intimately involved in child care. They offer to care for older children while the mother gives birth, and they assist during the first weeks after childbirth.

In the past, grandparents were often looked to for advice about childbearing and childrearing. Health care workers have now become the "experts," and many grandparents have difficulty adjusting to this change. Special classes are available for grandparents to bring them up to date with current childbearing practices and to help them deal with the changes in their role.

On the other hand, some contemporary grandparents hold different beliefs about the role of grandparents and plan much less participation in pregnancy or child care. This expectation often results in conflict with the parents, who may feel hurt by such an attitude. Parents and grandparents may need to negotiate how the grandparents can be involved without feeling that they must assume care of the child.

▌ Adaptation of Siblings

Toddlers

How siblings adapt to the birth of an infant depends largely on their age and developmental level. Children 2 years or younger are unaware of the maternal changes that occur during pregnancy and are unable to understand that a new brother or sister is going to be born. Because toddlers have little perception of time, many parents delay telling them that a baby is expected until shortly before the birth.

The nurse can make suggestions about helping prepare young children for the birth. Changes in sleeping arrangements should be made several weeks before the birth so that the child does not feel displaced by the new baby. Parents need to realize that toddlers may have feelings of jealousy and resentment when they must share attention with a baby.

Until children feel that their place in the affection of their parents is secure, it is not realistic to expect the 2-year-old to welcome the new "stranger." Frequent reassurances of parental love and affection are of primary importance.

Older Children

Older children, from 3 to 12 years, are more aware of changes in the mother's body and may be aware that a baby is to be born. They enjoy listening to the heart beat and may have questions about how the fetus develops, how it started, and how it will get out of the abdomen. Younger children may expect that the infant will be a full-fledged playmate, however, and are shocked when the infant is small and helpless.

School-age children benefit from being included in preparations for the new baby. They are interested in preparing space and supplies for the infant. These children should be encouraged to feel the fetus move, and many come close to the mother's abdomen and talk to the fetus.

Children as young as 3 years benefit from sibling classes. The classes also provide an opportunity for them to discuss what newborns are like and what changes the new baby will mean for the family.

In some settings, siblings are permitted to be with the mother during childbirth. When they are to be present, children should attend a class that prepares them for the event. A familiar person who has no other role than to provide support and care to a younger child should be present at the birth.

Adolescents

The response of adolescents also depends on their developmental level. Some may be embarrassed because the pregnancy confirms the continued sexuality of their parents. Others may be indifferent to the pregnancy unless it directly affects them or their activities. Some adolescents, on the other hand, become very involved and want to help with preparations for the baby.

▌ Factors That Influence Psychosocial Adaptations

Age

Pregnancy presents a challenge for teenagers, who must cope with the conflicting developmental tasks of pregnancy and adolescence at the same time. The major developmental task of adolescence is to form and become comfortable with a sense of self. On the other hand, one of the major tasks of pregnancy involves learning to give of self, a process that includes sacrificing personal desires for the benefit of the fetus. Giving is particularly difficult for young adolescents, who may not be able to perceive the fetus as real (Bloom, 1995).

Nurses who work with pregnant teenagers should help them tune in to their changing body and the developing fetus. Adolescents also need prompting to follow a lifestyle that promotes the best outcomes for them and for their infants (see also Chapter 25).

Absence of a Partner

The proportion of single women who become pregnant is increasing. Although some unmarried women have the fi-

nancial and emotional support of a partner, many do not. These women often experience more stress about how to tell their family and friends about the pregnancy. They may have to enlist more social support to substitute for that of a partner. They may have legal concerns regarding the father's rights.

Single women without partners often live below the poverty level. They are more likely to delay prenatal care until the second or third trimester and are at increased risk for pregnancy complications and delivery of a low-birth-weight infant. Nurses must be prepared to offer special supportive care for single mothers. Needed social services may include Medicaid, food stamps, and transportation to the prenatal clinic.

Multiparity

Pregnancy tasks are much more complex for the multipara than for the primigravida (Mercer, 1990). The multipara does not have time to take special care of herself as she did during the first pregnancy. Multiparas report more fatigue, and significantly fewer report feeling very well or excellent. They report having serious worries about other children and about finding time and energy for additional responsibilities. When seeking acceptance of the new baby, the multipara may find family members less excited than they were for the first child.

The woman spends a great deal of time working out a new relationship with the first child, who often becomes demanding. This behavior may foster feelings of guilt as she tries to expand her love to include the second child. Developing attachment for the coming baby is hampered by feelings of loss between herself and the first child. She senses that the child is growing up and away from her, and she may grieve for the loss of their special relationship (Fig. 14–4).

Nurses must remember that multiparas may need information about labor, breastfeeding, and infant care. They also need special assistance in integrating an additional infant into the family structure.

Socioeconomic Status

One of the greatest influences on childbearing practices is the socioeconomic status of the family. Socioeconomic sta-

---

CRITICAL THINKING EXERCISE 14–1
• • • • • • • • • •

Emma H., a 24-year-old multipara of 32 weeks' gestation, appears apathetic and tired when she arrives at the prenatal clinic. She states that she is concerned about how her 2-year-old son will accept the new baby and sometimes feels guilty that she is having this baby so soon.

1. How does multiparity affect the maternal tasks of pregnancy?
2. How should the nurse respond to her concerns?
3. What measures can the client take to prepare the 2-year-old before the new baby arrives? After the infant is born?

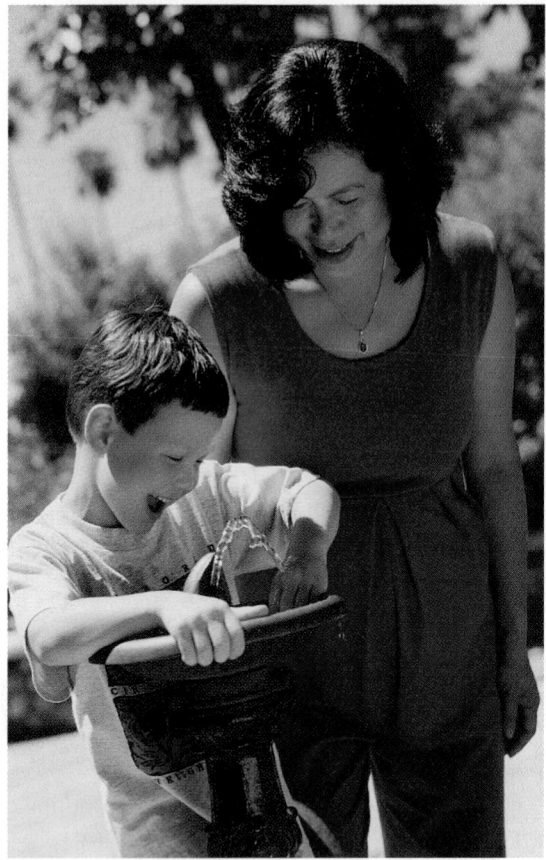

FIGURE 14-4
. . . .
A pregnant multipara seeks to rework her relationship with other children.

tus refers to the resources that the family has to meet the needs for food, shelter, and health care. Socioeconomic status can be divided into the affluent, middle class, working poor, and new poor. Table 14–2 summarizes the impact of socioeconomic status on the family's response to pregnancy.

Barriers to Prenatal Care

The value of prenatal care has been extensively documented. Women who receive inadequate prenatal care are likely to have poor pregnancy outcomes, including higher rates of low-birth-weight babies and increased infant mortality rates. Women's access to prenatal care, however, is limited by financial, systemic, and attitudinal barriers.

Financial barriers are one of the most important factors that limit prenatal care. Many women have no insurance or not enough insurance to cover maternity care. Although Medicaid finances prenatal care for indigent women, the enrollment process is so burdensome that some women do not register (Maloni et al., 1996).

Systemic barriers include institutional practices that interfere with consistent care. For instance, women must often wait 6 to 8 weeks before being seen for their first visit. Prenatal visits are usually scheduled during daytime hours, when some working women cannot attend. Moreover, child care is rarely available, and some woman are unable to find

it. Lack of transportation and inability to take time off from work also prevent women from getting prenatal care.

An important barrier to health care results from the unsympathetic attitude of some health care workers toward those who are unable to pay for prenatal care. Poor families often experience long delays, hurried examinations, rudeness, and arrogance from members of the health care team who work in public clinics. Women may wait 3 to 4 hours for an examination that lasts only a few minutes. Many never see the same health care provider more than once. Women often fail to keep clinic appointments because they do not see the importance of the hurried examinations.

Nurses must understand the importance of treating each family with respect and consideration, and they must insist that poor families who are unable to pay receive the same standard of care as that received by families who can pay.

In addition to unsympathetic attitudes of health professionals, other attitudinal reasons for not seeking early prenatal care include the following:

- Fear of discovering pregnancy
- Advice received from family or friends
- Lack of problems
- Thinking that prenatal care is unimportant
- Consideration of an abortion
- Not wanting anyone to know about the pregnancy (Meikle et al., 1995)

Cultural Influences on Childbearing

More distinct cultural groups live in the United States than anywhere else in the world. Each culture has its own health and healing belief system about major life events such as pregnancy and childbirth. The success of health care depends on how well it fits in with the beliefs of those being served. Therefore, ignorance of culturally divergent beliefs may lead to failure in health care delivery. Groups with beliefs that differ significantly from those of the dominant culture include Native Americans, Hindus (largely from India), Muslims, and Filipinos.

Differences Within Cultures

Wide variations of beliefs and practices exist within each culture, and nurses must recognize that not everyone who shares a culture has identical beliefs. Those who have lived in Western societies for years or even for generations often do not exhibit behaviors prescribed by their culture of origin. Nurses must be careful not to stereotype families or to expect a certain set of behaviors from every family in a particular cultural group. Individual differences are as important as cultural variations.

Cultural Differences That Can Cause Conflict

Cultural differences that cause conflict between health care workers and families during pregnancy are observed most often in the areas of health care beliefs, communication, and time orientation.

TABLE 14-2

Impact of Socioeconomic Factors on Family's Response to Pregnancy

Affluent	*Middle Class*	*Working Poor and Unemployed*	*New Poor*
Resources			
Confident of ability. Financial reserves protect family from economic fluctuations. Own or rent home in safe neighborhood. Have health insurance or can pay for health care. Able to provide enriched environment for their children.	Relative security, but fewer reserves and more debt. Own or rent home in relatively safe neighborhood. Health insurance depends on employment.	Lack skills, bargaining power. Most vulnerable to economic fluctuations. Often live below poverty level and struggle for basic needs.	Previously self-sufficient, but have lost prior resources. May have recently lost job and insurance. Unused to public assistance.
Value Placed on Health Care			
Value preventive care. Expect good health care.	Value health care but must rely on health insurance related to employment.	May value health care but often do not see a way to improve situation.	Value health care but may no longer have finances to access it.
Time Orientation			
Future-oriented; seek prenatal care early.	Future-oriented and seek early prenatal care. Make plans to provide best possible care and education for children.	Priority is to meet needs of present. Often seek prenatal care late. Uncertain future.	Have middle-class time orientation but must meet present needs. May obtain late prenatal care.

HEALTH BELIEFS

For many cultures, health is the balance of mind, body, and spirit. Health-promoting behaviors are the actions used in each of these dimensions to maintain health, prevent illness, or restore health (Spector, 1995).

Health Maintenance. Practices that maintain health include wearing proper clothing, which is believed by some Latinas to ensure a safe birth. The Korean woman may follow *taekyo,* or prenatal care of the fetus through rituals and taboos. This practice includes avoidance of unclean things because they might result in difficult childbirth (Howard & Berbiglia, 1997). Guatemalan women believe that strong emotions, like anger, will affect the fetus (Callister & Vega, 1998). Many groups also believe that concentration, silence, prayer, and meditation maintain mental and spiritual health.

Belief in Fate. Some cultures (Southeast Asian, Middle Eastern) promote a strong belief in fate. Women often believe that the only way in which they can affect the outcome of pregnancy is by eating correctly and observing the taboos of their culture. Because of this belief, it is sometimes difficult to get women to seek early and regular prenatal care.

Preventing Illness. Practices that prevent illness include the use of protective religious objects or charms, such as amulets and talismans. Some women also believe that the type of food one eats can prevent illness or provide a good pregnancy outcome. For instance, those from many backgrounds eat raw garlic or onion or adhere to numerous food taboos and prescribed combinations of foods. Strict adherence to religious codes, morals, and practices is also believed to prevent illness.

Modesty. Fear, modesty, and a desire to avoid examination by men may keep some women from seeking health care during pregnancy. In many cultures (Muslim, Hindu, Latino), exposure of the genitals to men is considered demeaning. Nurses must remember that the reputations of women from these cultures depend on their demonstrated modesty. If necessary, female physicians or female nurse practitioners can perform examinations. If this is not possible, the woman should be carefully draped, with the legs completely covered. A female nurse needs to remain with the woman at all times. It may be necessary to obtain permission from the husband before any examination or treatment can be performed.

Infibulation. Female circumcision (also called female genital mutilation) involves removal of part or all of the clitoris, labia minora, and labia majora and suturing together the lacerations to reduce the size of the introitus. The procedure is widely practiced in parts of northern Africa, Indonesia, Malaysia, and the Mideast (Gibeau, 1998; Shorten, 1995). The practice has been associated with premarital chastity, and in some cultures it is a prerequisite for marriage.

Women who have been infibulated and are now living in the United States need care from physicians and nurses who are knowledgeable about the custom and prepared for the appearance of the women's genitals. Pelvic examination provokes two major concerns: (1) exposure of the genitals, and (2) pain because the introitus is so small, and inelastic scar tissue makes the area especially sensitive.

Nurses must make sure that pelvic examinations are as comfortable as possible by maintaining utmost privacy, draping the woman to provide maximum coverage, and assisting her in locating a health care provider with whom she is comfortable. The infibulated woman may not give any verbal or nonverbal sign of pain, but this lack of response does not indicate an absence of pain.

Restoring Health. Traditional ways to restore health include natural folk medicine such as herbs and plants. Charms, holy words, and holy actions as well as traditional healers are often used before other medical advice is sought. Latinas, for instance, often consult *curanderas* (faith healers), who work with women to keep a balance between hot and cold and to relieve them of their sins, which may be the basis for illness. Some (Africans, Haitians) rely on folk medicine that includes witchcraft, voodoo, and magic.

> To be certain that all essential information about folk medicine is obtained, nurses should inquire whether the client is taking folk remedies. "What do pregnant women take to protect themselves and the baby?" "How often and how much of this do you take?" "Tell me about special foods and drinks that are important."

COMMUNICATION TECHNIQUES

Language. Language is a major barrier to health care. The ideal is to have trained interpreters, preferably women. Sometimes others may be used, but considerations of confidentiality, use of medical jargon, and the possible need to discuss sensitive issues indicate the need for professional interpreters. Adults who came to the United States as children may speak English well and can interpret for their parents and grandparents. Other family members or friends, as well as coworkers in the clinic or hospital, may be helpful, but many are not fluent and can misunderstand instructions, particularly if medical jargon is used (Nursing Care Plan 14–2).

English is spoken by most African-Americans, but variations in pronunciation, grammar, and sentence structure hinder communication. The dialect spoken by African-Americans is sometimes labeled "black English." Nurses who work with African-Americans should realize that "black English" is not just a poor form of English and must avoid labeling and stereotyping those who speak a different dialect.

Communication Style. Styles in communication differ among cultures. For example, among Asians, nodding and smiling do not necessarily show agreement or even understanding but simply, "Yes, I hear you." When presenting information, the nurse should validate how much the person understands by requesting the listener to repeat the information: "Tell me what you understood, and show me what you learned."

Latinas are traditionally diplomatic and tactful. They frequently engage in small talk before bringing up questions they may have about their care. Nurses can use small talk to establish rapport and help accomplish the goals of care.

Eye Contact. Southeast Asians believe that eye contact shows disrespect (Mattson & Lew, 1995). Latinas believe in *mal ojo* (evil eye), a sudden unexplained illness that may occur when an individual with special powers admires a child too openly. Eye contact between unmarried men and women is considered taboo by Hindus, who may view prolonged eye contact as seductive.

Touch. Touch is also an important component of communication. Some Native Americans avoid shaking hands but lightly touch the hand of the person they are greeting. In some cultures (Hindu, Muslim), touch by a woman other than the wife is offensive. In contrast, women from Haiti find touch supportive and reassuring, and gentle touch is particularly important during labor and birth. Nurses must remain sensitive to the response of the person being touched and should refrain from touching if the person indicates that touch is not welcomed.

TIME ORIENTATION

Time orientation varies among cultures. Middle Eastern women, Latinas, and African-American women tend to emphasize the moment rather than the future. This attitude causes conflicts in a health care setting, where tests or appointments are scheduled at particular times. If a woman does not place the same importance on keeping appointments, she may encounter anger and frustration in the health care setting that leaves her bewildered and ashamed.

Culturally Appropriate Nursing Care

To prevent conflict and provide culturally appropriate nursing care, nurses must understand how culture influences individual families in their care during pregnancy.

CULTURAL ASSESSMENT

Cultures are so diverse that nurses cannot know all the specific aspects of each. Some specific questions may elicit information that helps the nurse understand the family's beliefs about appropriate care during pregnancy:

- How will you and your family prepare for the baby?
- What concerns do you have about the pregnancy?
- What would provide the greatest assistance?
- Where do you obtain most health care information?
- What foods are encouraged? Curtailed?
- Who will be with you during labor and birth?

CULTURAL NEGOTIATION

Cultural negotiation involves providing information while acknowledging that the family may hold different views. If the family indicates that the information would be helpful, it can be incorporated into the teaching plan.

> If family members indicate that the information is not helpful or is harmful in their opinion, the conflict must be acknowledged openly and clarified. "I sense that you are unsure of this." "Help me understand your reluctance to try it." The nurse then explains why the recommendation was made and allows family members to continue to express their beliefs until a compromise is worked out.

Language Barrier During Pregnancy

Assessment

Thuy Nguyen, a young Vietnamese primigravida of 26 weeks' gestation, speaks very little English. She listens quietly to the nurse's health care instructions, and although she appears confused, she asks no questions. Her husband has difficulty responding to questions about his wife's health, although he frequently nods and smiles.

Nursing Diagnosis

Impaired Verbal Communication related to foreign language barriers

Goals/Expected Outcomes

The family will

- Keep scheduled appointments, demonstrate ability to follow health care instructions, and verbalize basic needs and concerns.
- Verbalize feelings of support from the health care team throughout prenatal care and childbirth.

Intervention

1. Assess the couple's ability to speak, read, and write in English and determine the languages in which each is fluent.
2. Obtain the assistance of a fluent interpreter.
   a. Establish a list of bilingual staff members in all areas of the facility (business office, housekeeping) who are willing to be educated about the importance of confidentiality and exactness.
   b. Enlist family members or friends who can accompany the client to interpret, if a professional interpreter is not available.
   c. Engage a translator to develop written material, such as colorful cards that have common questions and answers printed in languages that are most frequently spoken.
   d. Develop printed instructions in the most commonly spoken languages.
3. Speak quietly, and use the same interpreter whenever possible.

4. Consider nonverbal factors when communicating.
   a. Speak slowly and softly; smile.
   b. Keep an open posture. Avoid crossing the arms over the chest or turning away from the family.
   c. Determine Mrs. Nguyen's response to light touch on the arm, and either use or avoid touch, depending on her response.
   d. Attend carefully to what the family says by nodding, leaning forward, or encouraging continued talk with frequent "uh-huhs."
   e. Avoid foot shuffling or fidgeting.
   f. Do not expect prolonged eye contact.
5. Determine the availability of prenatal classes in Vietnamese. Explain what is included in such classes and suggest that the couple attend.

Rationale

1. Clients who are not fluent in speaking a language may be more adept at reading it. Many Vietnamese also speak Chinese or French.
2. A fluent interpreter is essential because Vietnamese do not always reveal when they do not understand instructions, and it is essential that follow-up questions can be asked. Communication cards convey interest in communicating and provide a means of eliciting basic information. Printed instructions reinforce information that was given verbally and may answer unasked questions.

3. Soft speech protects the privacy and modesty of the patient. A natural response when people do not understand is to raise the voice. This does not facilitate understanding but may convey impatience or anger.
4. Even subtle body language can indicate interest and empathy or impatience, annoyance, or a desire to escape. Touch and eye contact are sensitive cultural variables, and nurses must be aware that they are not always welcomed.

5. Information is more easily learned in one's own language. Appropriate cultural concerns are likely to be discussed in classes taught in Vietnamese.

Evaluation

Mrs. Nguyen kept all prenatal appointments throughout her pregnancy. She verbalized (through an interpreter) that she was willing to follow instructions and that she was pleased with the support she received from the health care staff.

Additional Nursing Diagnoses to Consider

Knowledge Deficit
Risk for Altered Health Maintenance

Cultural negotiation also involves being sensitive to specific concerns. For example, when caring for childbearing Muslim women, nurses must be aware of Islamic laws governing modesty. The woman must keep her hair, body, arms to the wrist, and legs to the ankles covered at all times when in the presence of a man. Moreover, a Muslim woman is not to be alone in the presence of a man other than her husband or a male relative.

Muslim women prefer female health care providers and should be informed of the availability of female caregivers. Adequate drapes and covers should be available to allow covering all areas of the body except those that must be exposed for examination. Moreover, the woman's husband, a female friend, or male relative should be allowed to be present during examinations.

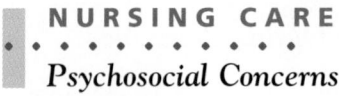

NURSING CARE
Psychosocial Concerns

Assessment

The purpose of a psychosocial assessment is to monitor the adaptation of the family to pregnancy, which has been termed a maturational crisis that requires a major transition in role function and relationships. Some data required for a psychosocial assessment can be obtained from the physical assessment. For example, age, gravida, para, and general health status provide important information in both areas. Table 14–3 identifies areas for assessment, provides sample questions, and indicates nursing implications.

TABLE 14–3

Psychosocial Assessment

Findings (Normal and Unusual)*	Sample Questions	Nursing Implications
Psychological Response		
First trimester: Uncertainty, ambivalence, mood changes, self as primary focus Second trimester: Wonder, joy, focus on fetus Third trimester: Vulnerability, preparing for birth (fear, anger, apathy, lack of preparation)	"How do you/partner feel about being pregnant?" "How will your lives change as a result of being pregnant?" "How do you feel about the changes in your body?" "What preparations have you made for the baby?"	Use active listening and reflection to establish a sense of trust; re-evaluate negative responses (fear, apathy, anger) in subsequent assessments.
Availability of Resources		
Financial concerns (lack of funds, or insurance) Response and availability of grandparents, friends, family (family geographically or emotionally unavailable)	"What are your plans for prenatal care and birth?" "How do your parents feel about being grandparents?" "Whom else can you depend on besides the family?"	Determine if there are adequate funds or if family needs help to find a public clinic that will provide care. Help the couple discover alternative resources if the family is unavailable.
Changes in Sexual Practices		
Mutual satisfaction with changes (concern with comfort or safety)	"How have sexual patterns or satisfaction changed?" "What concerns you most?"	Offer reassurance that intercourse is usually safe; suggest alternative positions and open communication.
Educational Needs		
Many questions about pregnancy, childbirth, and infant care (no questions, absence of interest in educational programs)	"How do you feel about caring for an infant?" "What are your major concerns?" "Whom do you count on for information?"	Respond to priority needs that are expressed; refer couple to appropriate child and parenting classes.
Cultural Influences		
Either the woman or her family is able to speak English or fluent interpreters are available; cultural influences support a healthy pregnancy and infant (unable to communicate verbally, harmful beliefs or health practices).	"What foods are recommended during pregnancy?" "What practices are recommended?" "What is forbidden?" "How can we provide the best care?" "How do your religious beliefs affect pregnancy?"	Locate fluent interpreters if necessary; avoid labeling beliefs as superstitions; reinforce beliefs that promote a good pregnancy outcome; elicit help from accepted source of information to overcome harmful practices.

*Findings that require additional assessment or intervention are shown in parentheses.

Nursing Diagnosis and Planning

Most families strive to maintain the health of the expectant mother and fetus and to complete developmental tasks needed for parenting. The most encompassing nursing diagnosis is probably

- Family Coping: Potential for Growth related to readiness and desire to meet added family needs and to assume parenting roles.
  Expected Outcomes: The family will verbalize emotional responses appropriate to each trimester and will verbalize methods that assist the expectant parents to complete the developmental processes of pregnancy. The family will identify cultural factors that may produce conflicts and collaborate to reduce those conflicts.

Interventions

Providing Information

Provide family members with information and anticipatory guidance about the emotional changes that occur during pregnancy, the developmental tasks of the mother and father, and role transition. Guidance is necessary to prepare prospective parents for the progressive changes that occur during pregnancy and to reassure them that their feelings and behaviors are normal. It also gives them an opportunity to ask questions and explore their feelings.

Discussing Resources

Help couples who have no financial resources or insurance coverage to find the most convenient location to obtain prenatal care and to determine where the woman will give birth. This concern is particularly important for the new poor, who have little idea of how to gain access to government-sponsored care.

Emotional resources include those that assist the new family to adjust to the demands of pregnancy and parenting. If family members who traditionally offer support in times of stress are unavailable, refer the prospective parents to community resources, such as childbirth education classes, support groups, and sibling classes, and later to breastfeeding and new parenting classes.

Helping the Family Prepare for the Birth

During the last trimester, discuss lifestyle changes that will occur when the infant is born. Unanticipated changes that accompany this dramatic life event may add stress and disrupt family processes. Help the prospective parents make practical plans for the infant, such as obtaining clothing and choosing the method of feeding. Siblings should be prepared several weeks or months before the birth, depending on their ages. Older children often benefit from participating in planning for the baby.

Suggest that parents consider how they will work out the division of household and parenting tasks, as well as child care if the mother must return to work after childbirth. If these issues are not addressed, the couple can experience frustration and anger as one parent, usually the mother, assumes total care of the infant and attempts to complete all household tasks. Moreover, exhaustion and frustration can overwhelm the joys of parenting when one parent must provide all care.

Modeling Communication Techniques

When disagreements are evident, it is often helpful to discuss and model therapeutic communication techniques that include all significant family members as the family prepares for the birth. Techniques that clarify, summarize, and reflect feelings can defuse negative feelings that might result in family disruption.

Identifying Cultural Factors That Could Cause Conflict

Possible areas of conflict related to cultural beliefs and health practices that affect pregnancy should be explored.

> It is reassuring to expectant mothers when nurses support health beliefs that are beneficial before confronting them with health care beliefs that cause concern. For example, "It is so good for you and the baby when you eat so many vegetables, but I am worried because you missed your last appointment."

If there is conflict as a result of differences in time orientation, acknowledge the problem, convey understanding of the differences, and emphasize the importance of calling when appointments cannot be kept. Many families do not realize that when they miss their appointment, another family misses the opportunity for health care.

Evaluation

- Does the family verbalize concerns and emotions at each visit?
- Do the partner and significant family members appear interested and involved?
- Do the family members discuss compromises when cultural health practices are harmful?

Perinatal Education

Perinatal education has become increasingly important in helping couples learn about pregnancy, birth, and parenting. With shorter birth facility stays, classes that once focused solely on preparing for childbirth are now expanding to include information formerly received in the birth facility, after the birth.

The goals of perinatal education are to help parents become knowledgeable consumers, take an active role in maintaining health during pregnancy and birth, and learn coping techniques to deal with pregnancy, childbirth, and parenting.

Providers of Education

Most perinatal education classes are taught by registered nurses. Many instructors are certified by organizations such as the American Society for Psychoprophylaxis in Obstetrics (ASPO) or the International Childbirth Education Association (ICEA). Certification ensures that the instructors have received special preparation to provide sound education that adheres to the certifying organization's general philosophy. The Association of Women's Health, Obstetric, and Neonatal Nurses (1993) has published guidelines for educator competencies and class curricula.

Class Participants

Participants in classes about childbearing have traditionally been middle-income couples who are older and better educated than those who do not take classes. Low-income women may not have money to pay for classes. Although inexpensive or free classes are available in some areas, women with little or no prenatal care may not know about this form of education. Classes in languages other than English have become more readily available in areas where they are needed.

People take classes for a variety of reasons. Many have a strong desire to participate actively in all aspects of childbearing. Others are looking for coping strategies to deal with their fear of childbirth or pain. When women feel informed and believe that they have some control over what happens to them, they are more likely to expect birth to be satisfying and fulfilling and to experience it as such.

Choices for Childbearing

One purpose of any perinatal education program is to help parents learn what options are available so that they can make appropriate choices. Parents learn that there are many ways of birthing and that no one "right" method exists. Knowledgeable parents can communicate assertively with their health care providers about their needs and desires. They may make a birth plan that lists their desires about various aspects of their care.

Setting

The woman and her partner must choose a birth setting and select a care provider who practices in that setting. Hospitals are the most frequent setting for birth in North America. They may have birthing suites that provide a homelike atmosphere, or traditional labor and delivery rooms. A freestanding birth center provides an atmosphere

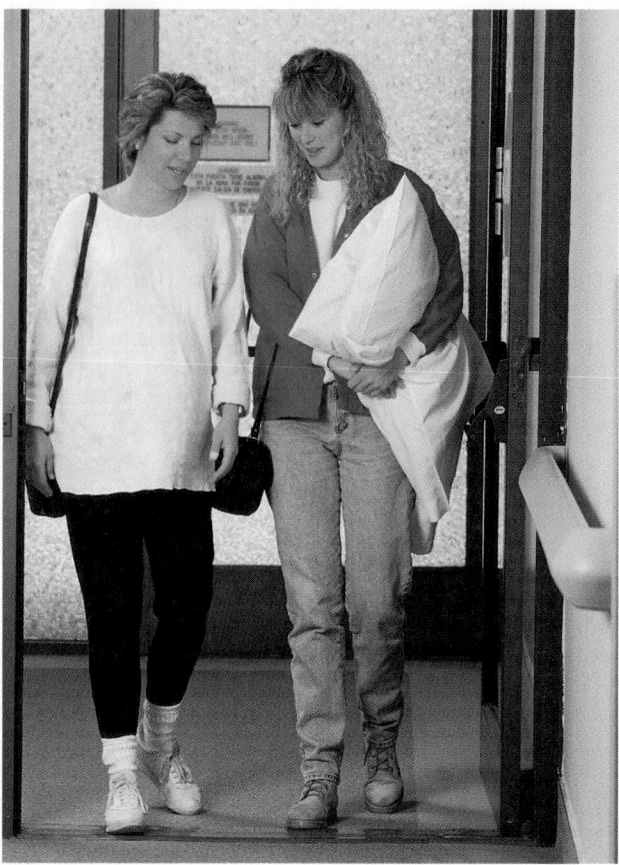

FIGURE 14–5

Often an expectant mother will ask a sister or close female friend to be her labor partner and to attend classes with her.

that is less institutional than that of the hospital. Home birth allows the woman to give birth in her own surroundings, with delivery managed by a midwife.

Support Person

During labor, the woman needs to have someone with her to help her through the experience. The support person is most often the father of her baby, but a relative or friend may also take this role (Fig. 14–5). Some women wish to share the birth experience with several relatives or close friends. Some women hire a support person, such as a doula, to provide support during labor.

Education

Expectant mothers must also decide on prenatal education classes. Their decisions are based on the classes available in the area, the costs, and the kinds of information they need. Some areas have a vast array of classes from which to choose. In others, the selection is limited to childbirth preparation classes only.

Prepared childbirth classes based in birth facilities include detailed information on what to expect in that particular setting but may not cover options that are unavailable at that agency. Hospital classes have sometimes been criti-

---

Birth Plan Considerations

Use of electronic fetal monitoring, continuously or intermittently
Intravenous fluids: use, avoidance, saline lock
Food and oral fluids allowed in labor
Shaving, enemas
Position for labor and delivery
Use of tubs, showers
Episiotomy
Methods of pain relief
Support person(s) present during labor
Breastfeeding, use of formula
Participation of siblings during/after birth
Mother/baby couplet care
Time of discharge
Follow-up care

cized for teaching clients to be "good," or compliant, patients. A woman may wish to talk to the instructor before taking a class to ask about class size and the teacher's philosophy, background, and teaching methods.

Types of Classes Available

PRECONCEPTION CLASSES
Classes for couples who are thinking about having a baby are designed to help them have a healthy pregnancy from the beginning. Information about nutrition before conception, signs of pregnancy, healthy lifestyle, and choosing a caregiver are presented. Preconception classes emphasize early and regular prenatal care and ways to reduce risk factors for poor pregnancy outcome.

EARLY PREGNANCY CLASSES
Early pregnancy classes focus on the first two trimesters. First-trimester classes are sometimes called "earlybird" or "right start" classes. They cover information on adapting to pregnancy, dealing with early discomforts such as morning sickness and fatigue, and understanding what to expect in the months ahead. Emphasis is placed on obtaining prenatal care and avoiding hazards to the fetus.

Second-trimester classes focus on changes that occur during middle pregnancy and on preparing for birth. Information on body mechanics, working during pregnancy, and what to expect during the third trimester is included. Teachers discuss childbirth choices and information to help students become more knowledgeable consumers.

In these classes, parents may begin to learn about the needs of the mother and infant after birth, or they may attend other classes to meet this need. This information is especially important because of the short period they stay in the birth facility.

EXERCISE CLASSES
Exercise classes help women keep fit and healthy during pregnancy. Exercises should be low impact and preceded by warm-up routines. To prevent diversion of blood away from the uterus, women should avoid excessive heart rate elevation. An added benefit of the classes is the opportunity for women to meet others with similar concerns.

CHILDBIRTH PREPARATION CLASSES
In childbirth preparation classes, women and their support persons learn self-help measures and what to expect during labor and birth. Couples learn coping methods that help them approach childbirth in a positive manner. Teachers do not promise prevention of all pain in labor. The increased confidence gained in prepared childbirth classes is, however, associated with a decreased perception and increased tolerance of pain during labor and decreased use of drugs for labor pain (Lowe, 1996).

Classes include information about labor, pharmacologic and nonpharmacologic methods of pain relief, and a tour of the birth setting. Supervised practice of relaxation, breathing techniques, and coping strategies in "labor rehearsals" are part of every class (Fig. 14–6) (see Chapter

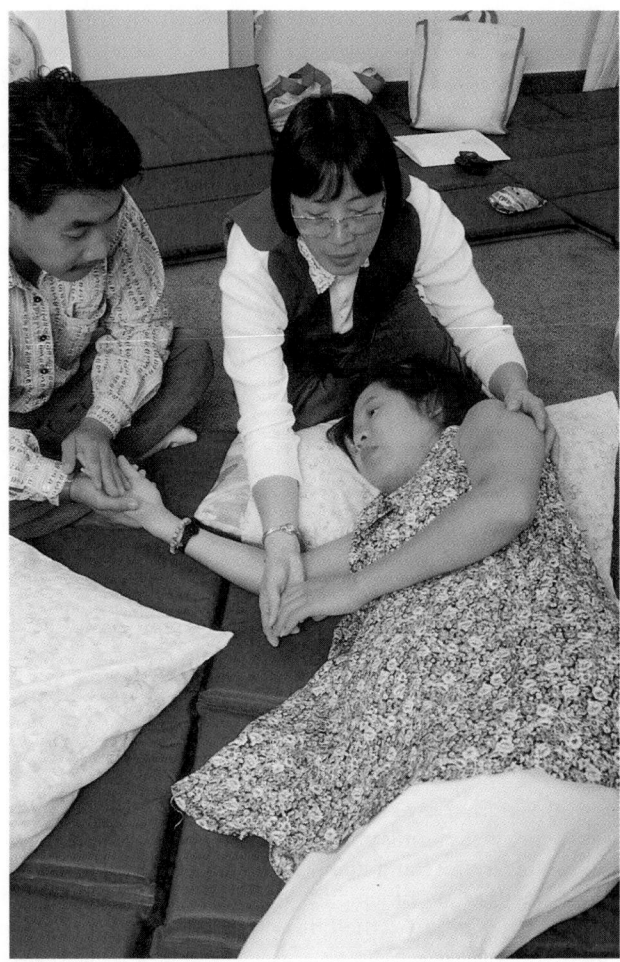

FIGURE 14–6

The nurse teaches the support person how to check for relaxation.

19). Films assist women to develop a realistic picture of the birth process.

Class series range from a 1-day class to four to nine meetings, depending on the content included. Women who have taken classes for a previous birth often take a refresher class for an update of current practices and review of techniques. Classes consist of supervised practice and discussion of role changes in the family and sibling adjustment.

CESAREAN BIRTH PREPARATION CLASSES
Education about cesarean birth may take place in general childbirth classes or may be conducted separately for those expecting a cesarean birth. Topics include indications, options, surgical procedure, and postoperative course. Women who know they will have a cesarean birth may attend planned cesarean birth classes. For those who had a cesarean birth previously, the class offers an opportunity to share experiences and feelings and to clarify misconceptions. Class discussion helps couples feel that they have some control over what happens and provides a basis for discussion with caregivers.

VAGINAL BIRTH AFTER CESAREAN BIRTH

Women who plan to have a vaginal birth after cesarean (VBAC) may take a class to meet their special needs. Content includes explanations of conditions in which a VBAC is possible, the extra precautions taken and their reasons, what to expect during labor and birth, and coping techniques. Although the focus is on positive expectations, situations that might make another cesarean birth necessary are also covered. Discussion includes the emotional aspects of a "failed VBAC" as well.

BREAST-FEEDING CLASSES

Prenatal breast-feeding classes help increase a woman's confidence in her ability to breast-feed successfully and provide her with sources of help if she encounters difficulties. Women who attend prenatal classes that include breast-feeding information are more likely to breast-feed their infants and to do so for longer than 6 months compared with women who do not attend classes (Piper & Parks, 1996).

Breast-feeding classes include information on physiol-ogy of lactation, feeding techniques, establishing a milk supply, and dealing with common problems. Partners who attend learn methods of providing support during breast-feeding.

PARENTING CLASSES

Instruction on parenting and newborn care may be included in prepared childbirth classes or provided separately. Content typically includes general care and common concerns, such as the crying infant and advantages and disadvantages of circumcision. Baby equipment, such as various types of infant car seats, is often displayed. Practice with dolls may also be included. Classes may continue after the birth of the infant.

POSTPARTUM CLASSES

Although the postpartum period is covered in childbirth preparation classes, the mother can also attend classes after birth. Content includes the physiologic and psychological changes of the postpartum period, role transition, sexuality, and nutrition. Some classes focus on exercise for the postpartum period.

KEY CONCEPTS

- Maternal psychological responses progress during pregnancy from uncertainty and ambivalence to feelings of vulnerability and preparation for the birth of the infant.
- As the fetus becomes real, usually in the second trimester, maternal focus shifts from self to the fetus, and the woman turns inward to concentrate on the processes going on in her body.
- Changes in the maternal body during pregnancy may result in a negative body image that affects sexual responses. This change may be especially troubling if the couple does not discuss emotions and concerns related to the changes in sexuality.
- It takes time for a woman to make the transition to the role of mother, and the process involves mimicking the behavior of other mothers, fantasizing about the baby, grieving for the loss of previous roles, and developing a sense of self as mother.
- To complete the maternal tasks of pregnancy, the woman must take steps to seek safe passage for herself and the infant, gain acceptance of significant persons, and form an interconnection and attachment to the unknown child.
- Paternal responses change throughout pregnancy and depend on the ability to perceive the fetus as real, to gain recognition for the role of parent, and to create a role as involved father.
- The most powerful reality boosters for the expectant father during pregnancy are hearing the fetal heart beat, feeling the fetus move, and viewing the infant on a sonogram.
- In primitive cultures, couvade refers to pregnancy-related rituals performed by the man; in modern society, it often refers to a cluster of pregnancy-related signs and symptoms experienced by the man.
- The response of grandparents to the announcement of pregnancy depends on their age, the number and ages of other grandchildren, and their perception of the role of grandparents.
- The response of siblings to pregnancy depends on their ages and developmental levels. Toddlers may feel displaced in their parents' affection unless measures are taken to reassure them.
- It is more difficult for multiparas to complete the developmental tasks of pregnancy because they have less time, experience more fatigue, and must negotiate a new relationship with the older child or children.
- Socioeconomic status is a major factor in determining health practices during pregnancy. Poor families have competing priorities for food and shelter and seek prenatal care late in pregnancy.
- Cultural differences can create major conflicts between expectant families and health care workers. Language, time orientation, and health beliefs are the areas in which conflicts are most likely to occur.
- Education for childbearing helps couples become knowledgeable consumers and active participants in pregnancy and childbirth.
- Many classes are available for pregnant women and their support persons. Early pregnancy classes emphasize having a healthy pregnancy. Those conducted in later pregnancy focus on preparing for childbirth, breast-feeding, and early parenting.

ANSWERS TO CRITICAL THINKING EXERCISE 14 – 1

1. The tasks of pregnancy are more complex for the multipara than for a primigravida. Multiparas have less time and are more likely to be fatigued. They are often very concerned about the effect of the pregnancy on other children and about their ability to handle the added responsibilities of another child.
2. Respond by acknowledging her concerns and reflecting her feelings so that she can fully express how she feels. "You worry that your son will be upset when the new baby is born." Or "You feel guilty that your son will have to share your time and energy with the baby."
3. Suggest that Emma make any changes in sleeping arrangements now so that her son will not feel displaced by the infant. Recommend that she plan ways to have time alone with the older child when the baby arrives, and review measures to reduce sibling rivalry. The mother can tell her 2-year-old how much she loves him, hug and cuddle him frequently, and arrange time together for favorite activities without the newborn. The mother can remind others to pay attention to him as well as to the baby.

REFERENCES AND READINGS

Alteneder, R. R., & Hartzell, D. (1997). Addressing couples' sexuality concerns during the childbearing period: Use of the PLISSIT model. *Journal of Obstetric, Gynecologic, and Neonatal Nursing, 26*(6), 651–658.

American Academy of Pediatrics, Committee on Bioethics. (1998). Female genital mutilation. *Pediatrics, 102*(1), 153–156.

Association of Women's Health, Obstetric, & Neonatal Nurses (AWHONN). (1993). *Competencies and program guidelines for nurse providers of perinatal education.* Washington, DC: Author.

Bloom, K. C. (1995). The development of attachment behaviors in pregnant adolescents. *Nursing Research, 44*(5), 284–289.

Bridgwater, N., & Wiman, B. (1998). Childbirth education options: Exploring one-day classes. *Lifelines, 2*(2), 49–52.

Broude, G. J. (1988). Rethinking the couvade: Crosscultural evidence. *American Anthropologist, 90*(6), 902–911.

Callister, L. C. (1995). Cultural meanings of childbirth. *Journal of Obstetric, Gynecologic, and Neonatal Nursing, 24*(4), 327–331.

Callister, L. C., & Vega, R. (1998). Giving birth: Guatemalan women's voices. *Journal of Obstetric, Gynecologic, and Neonatal Nursing, 27*(3), 289–295.

Choudhry, U. K. (1997). Traditional practices of women from India: Pregnancy, childbirth, and newborn care. *Journal of Obstetric, Gynecologic, and Neonatal Nursing, 26*(5), 533–539.

Ferketich, S. L., & Mercer, R. T. (1995). Paternal–infant attachment of experienced and inexperienced fathers during infancy. *Nursing Research, 44*(1), 31–37.

Fraser, A. M., Brockert, J. E., & Ward, R. H. (1995). Association of young maternal age with adverse reproductive outcomes. *New England Journal of Medicine, 332*(17), 1113–1117.

Galanti, G. (1997). *Caring for patients from different cultures* (2nd ed.). Philadelphia: University of Pennsylvania Press.

Gibeau, A. M. (1998). Female genital mutilation: When a cultural practice generates clinical and ethical dilemmas. *Journal of Obstetric, Gynecologic, and Neonatal Nursing, 27*(1), 85–91.

Howard, J. Y., & Berbiglia, V. A. (1997). Caring for childbearing Korean women. *Journal of Obstetric, Gynecologic, and Neonatal Nursing, 26*(6), 665–671.

Hutchinson, M. K., & BaqiAziz, M. (1994). Nursing care of the childbearing Muslim family. *Journal of Obstetric, Gynecologic, and Neonatal Nursing, 23*(9), 767–771.

Jordan, P. L. (1990). Laboring for relevance: Expectant and new fatherhood. *Nursing Research, 39*(1), 11–16.

Lalonde, A. (1995). Clinical management of female genital mutilation must be handled with understanding, compassion. *Canadian Medical Association Journal, 152*(6), 949–946.

Lowe, N. K. (1996). The pain and discomfort of labor and birth. *Journal of Obstetric, Gynecologic, and Neonatal Nursing, 25*(1), 82–92.

Maloni, J. A., Cheng, C. Y., Liebl, C. P., & Maier, J. S. (1996). Transforming prenatal care: Reflections on the past and present with implications for the future. *Journal of Obstetric, Gynecologic, and Neonatal Nursing, 25*(1), 17–23.

Mattson, S., & Lew, L. (1995). Culturally sensitive perinatal care for Southeast Asians. *Journal of Obstetric, Gynecologic, and Neonatal Nursing, 24*(4), 335–341.

Meikle, S. F., Orleans, M., Leff, M., Shain, R., & Gibbs, R. S. (1995). Women's reasons for not seeking prenatal care: Racial and ethnic factors. *Birth, 22*(2), 81–86.

Mercer, R. T. (1990). *Parents at risk.* New York: Springer.

Mercer, R. T., & Ferketich, S. L. (1994a). Maternal-infant attachment of experienced and inexperienced mothers during infancy. *Nursing Research, 43*(6), 344–351.

Mercer, R. T., & Ferketich, S. L. (1994b). Predictors of maternal role competence by risk status. *Nursing Research, 43*(1), 38–43.

Monto, M. A. (1996). Lamaze and Bradley childbirth classes: Contrasting perspectives toward the medical model of birth. *Birth, 23*(4), 193–201.

Moore, M., & Hopper, U. (1995). Do birth plans empower women? Evaluation of a hospital birth plan. *Birth, 22*(1), 29–36.

Nance, T. A. (1995). Intercultural communication: Finding common ground. *Journal of Obstetric, Gynecologic, and Neonatal Nursing, 24*(3), 249–255.

Piper, S., & Parks, P. (1996). Predicting the duration of lactation: Evidence from a national survey. *Birth, 23*(1), 7–12.

Reichert, G. A. (1998). Female circumcision: What you need to know about genital mutilation. *AWHONN Lifelines, 2*(3), 29–34.

Rubin, R. (1975). Maternal tasks in pregnancy. *Maternal-Child Nursing Journal, 4*(3), 143–153.

Rubin, R. (1984). *Maternal identity and the maternal experience.* New York: Springer.

Shorten, A. (1995). Female circumcision: Understanding special needs. *Holistic Nurse Practitioner, 9*(2), 66–73.

Spector, R. E. (1995). Cultural concepts of women's health and health-promoting behaviors. *Journal of Obstetric, Gynecologic, and Neonatal Nursing, 24*(3), 241–245.

Thorpe, K., Greenwood, R., & Goodenough, T. (1995). Does a twin pregnancy have a greater impact on physical and emotional well-being than a singleton pregnancy? *Birth, 22*(3), 148–152.

Tiller, C. M. (1995). Father's parenting attitudes during a child's first year. *Journal of Obstetric, Gynecologic, and Neonatal Nursing, 24*(6), 508–514.

Walker, L. O., & Montgomery, E. (1994). Maternal identity and role attainment: Long-term relations to children's development. *Nursing Research, 43*(2), 105–110.

Zwelling, E. (1996). Childbirth education in the 1990's and beyond. *Journal of Obstetric, Gynecologic, and Neonatal Nursing, 25*(5), 425–432.

15

Nutrition for Childbearing

LEARNING OBJECTIVES

After studying this chapter, you should be able to:

- Explain the importance of adequate nutrition and weight gain during pregnancy.
- Compare the nutrient needs of pregnant and nonpregnant women.
- Describe common factors that influence a woman's nutritional status and choices.
- Describe how common nutritional risk factors affect nutritional requirements during pregnancy.
- Compare the nutritional needs of the postpartum woman who is breast-feeding with those of one who is not breast-feeding.
- Apply the nursing process to nutrition during pregnancy, the postpartum period, and lactation.

DEFINITIONS

anorexia nervosa Refusal to eat because of a distorted body image and a feeling of obesity.

bulimia Eating disorder characterized by ingestion of large amounts of food, followed by purging behavior such as induced vomiting or laxative abuse.

complete protein food Food containing all the essential amino acids.

essential amino acids Amino acids that cannot be synthesized by the body and must be obtained from foods.

gynecologic age Number of years since menarche (first menstrual period).

heme iron Iron obtained from meat, poultry, or fish sources; the form most usable by the body.

incomplete protein food Food that does not contain all the essential amino acids.

kilocalorie A unit of heat used to show the energy value in foods, commonly called a calorie.

lacto-ovovegetarian A vegetarian whose diet includes milk products and eggs.

lactose intolerance Inability to digest most dairy products owing to a deficiency in the enzyme lactase.

lactovegetarian A vegetarian whose diet includes milk products.

nonheme iron Iron obtained from plant sources.

nutrient density Quantity and quality of protein, vitamins, and minerals per 100 calories in foods.

ovovegetarian A vegetarian whose diet includes eggs.

pica Ingestion of a nonfood substance, such as laundry starch, dirt, or ice.

recommended dietary allowance (RDA) Level of intake of a nutrient that is considered to meet the needs of healthy individuals.

vegan A complete vegetarian who does not eat any animal products.

vegetarian An individual whose diet consists wholly or mostly of plant foods and who avoids animal food sources.

At no time in a woman's life is nutrition as important as it is during pregnancy and lactation. The nurse has ongoing contact with women throughout this period and can provide education about nutritional needs on a continuing basis.

Weight Gain During Pregnancy

Weight gain during pregnancy, especially after the first trimester, is an important determinant of fetal growth. Low birth weight (less than 2,500 g or 5.5 lb), preterm labor, and an increased risk of fetal and newborn mortality and morbidity have been associated with insufficient weight gain during pregnancy. Poor maternal weight gain indicates not only lower caloric intake but also low intake of other important nutrients. Excessive weight gain is another problem. It is associated with a higher risk for macrosomia (large babies), labor abnormalities, meconium staining, and cesarean birth (Kolasa & Weismiller, 1995).

Recommendations for Total Weight Gain

The recommended weight gain during pregnancy is 25 to 35 lb (11.5 to 16 kg) for women who begin pregnancy at normal weight for height. This amount of weight gain is believed to reduce intrauterine growth restriction caused by inadequate maternal intake.

Suggested gains vary according to the woman's weight before pregnancy, as shown in Table 15–1. Women who are 10% below normal weight for their height should gain more during pregnancy to meet the needs of pregnancy and bring their weight up to normal. Overweight women (those 20% over normal weight for height) can gain somewhat less. Obese women (those more than 35% over normal

weight for height) should gain at least 15 lb, which is equivalent to the weight of the products of conception (i.e., fetus and placenta).

Infants of a multifetal pregnancy are often born before term and tend to weigh less than infants born of single pregnancies. A greater weight gain in the mother may help prevent low birth weight. Women who are shorter than 62 inches (157 cm) may not need to gain as much as taller women and should gain only to the lower limits of the recommended range. Young adolescents need to gain to the upper end of the range to provide for their own growth during pregnancy as well as growth of the fetus.

Pattern of Weight Gain

The pattern of weight gain is as important as the total increase. Inadequate early weight gain may be associated with small-for-gestational-age infants, whereas poor gain late in pregnancy is associated with preterm labor. These trends appear even when total weight gain is within normal range (Scholl & Hediger, 1995). The general recommendation is for an increment of about 3.5 lb (1.6 kg) during the first trimester, when the mother may be nauseated and the fetus needs fewer nutrients for growth. During the rest of the pregnancy, the expected weight gain is just under 1 lb (0.44 kg) a week.

Maternal and Fetal Distribution

Women often wonder why they should gain so much weight when the fetus weighs only 7 to 8 lb (3 to 3.6 kg). Explaining the distribution of weight helps them understand this need (Fig. 15–1).

Factors That Influence Weight Gain

Women at risk for inadequate weight gain include those who are young, unmarried, of low income, poorly educated, of short stature, in poor general health, or receiving insufficient prenatal care. African-American, Southeast Asian, and Latino women are more at risk for low weight gain during pregnancy than are white women. Adequate weight gain is especially important for African-Americans and teenagers, who tend to have smaller infants even when they

TABLE 15–1

Recommended Weight Gain During Pregnancy

Weight Before Pregnancy	Total Gain	Total Gain (First Trimester)	Weekly Gain (Second and Third Trimesters)
Normal weight	25–35 lb (11.5–16 kg)	3.5 lb (1.6 kg)	0.97 lb (0.44 kg)
Underweight (10% below normal for height)	28–40 lb (12.5–18 kg)	5 lb (2.3 kg)	1.07 lb (0.49 kg)
Overweight (20% over normal for height)	15–25 lb (7–11.5 kg)	2 lb (0.9 kg)	0.67 lb (0.3 kg)
Twin pregnancies	35–45 lb (16–20.5 kg)	3.5 lb (1.6 kg)	1.5 lb (0.75 kg)

Based on data from *Nutrition during pregnancy*. Part I. *Weight gain*. © 1990 by the National Academy of Sciences. Courtesy of National Academy Press, Washington, DC.

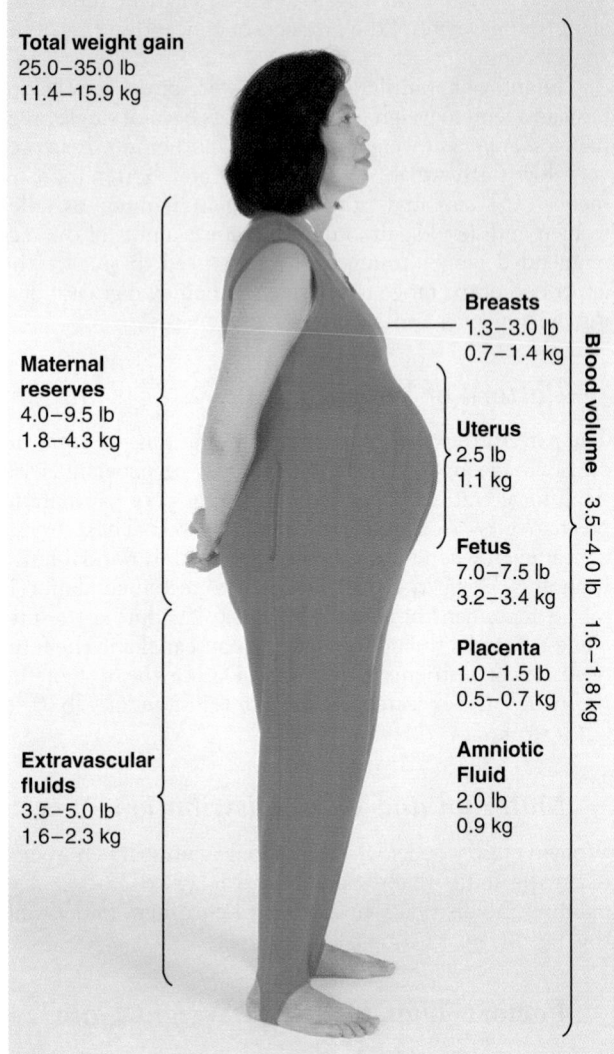

Total weight gain
25.0–35.0 lb
11.4–15.9 kg

Maternal reserves
4.0–9.5 lb
1.8–4.3 kg

Extravascular fluids
3.5–5.0 lb
1.6–2.3 kg

Breasts
1.3–3.0 lb
0.7–1.4 kg

Uterus
2.5 lb
1.1 kg

Fetus
7.0–7.5 lb
3.2–3.4 kg

Placenta
1.0–1.5 lb
0.5–0.7 kg

Amniotic Fluid
2.0 lb
0.9 kg

Blood volume 3.5–4.0 lb 1.6–1.8 kg

FIGURE 15–1

Distribution of weight gain in pregnancy. The numbers represent a general distribution, because there is a great deal of variation among women. The component with the greatest fluctuation is the amount of weight increase attributed to extravascular fluids (edema) and maternal reserves of fat.

gain weight in the same amount as whites or older mothers. The reasons for this difference are not fully understood. Multiparas are at higher risk for low weight gain than women in their first pregnancy. Smoking or substance abuse may interfere with food intake and weight gain.

Nutritional Requirements During Pregnancy

Nutrient needs during pregnancy increase to meet the demands of the mother and fetus. Usually the increases are not large and are relatively easy to obtain through the diet.

Recommended Dietary Allowances

In the United States, the Food and Nutrition Board of the National Research Council sets recommended dietary al-

lowances (RDAs). RDAs refer to the intake of major nutrients necessary for healthy individuals to meet daily nutrient needs. The actual needs of individuals (particularly for calories and protein) may vary according to body size, previous nutritional status, and usual activity level. Table 15–2 shows the current RDAs.

Energy

The energy provided by foods for body processes is calculated in kilocalories. Kilocalories (often used interchangeably with the term *calories*) are obtained from carbohydrates and proteins, which provide 4 calories in each gram, and fats, which provide 9 calories in each gram.

CARBOHYDRATES

Carbohydrates may be simple or complex. Simple carbohydrates include sucrose (table sugar) and those found in fruits and vegetables. Complex carbohydrates are present in starches, such as cereals, and supply vitamins, minerals, and fiber. Because of their value in providing other nutrients, they should be the major source of carbohydrates in the diet.

Another type of carbohydrate is fiber, the nondigestible product of plant foods that produces bulk in the diet. Fiber absorbs water and stimulates peristalsis to help prevent constipation. It also slows gastric emptying, causing a sensation of fullness.

FATS

Fats provide energy as well as fat-soluble vitamins. When reduction of calories is necessary, it is important to reduce but not eliminate carbohydrates and fats. If carbohydrate and fat intake provides insufficient calories, the body uses protein to meet energy needs. This use decreases the amount of protein available for building and repairing tissue.

CALORIES

Approximately 85,000 additional calories are needed during pregnancy (Worthington-Roberts, 1997a). These extra calories furnish energy for the production and maintenance of the fetus, placenta, added maternal tissues, and increased basal metabolic rate. The caloric RDA for women of childbearing age is approximately 2,200 calories per day. Although there is little need for additional calories during the early weeks of pregnancy, caloric intake should increase by another 300 calories per day after that time. A 300-calorie increase can be achieved relatively easily with a variety of foods. For example, a banana, a carrot, a piece of whole-wheat toast, and a glass of low-fat milk consumed over 1 day would provide the extra calories along with other important nutrients.

Nutrient density, the quantity and quality of the various nutrients in each 100 calories of food, is an important consideration. Foods of high nutrient density have large amounts of good-quality nutrients per serving. During pregnancy, the increased need for most nutrients may not be met unless calories are selected carefully. The term *empty calories* refers to foods that are high in calories but low in other nutrients. Many snack foods not only contain excessive calories and low nutrient density but also are high in

TABLE 15-2

Recommended Dietary Allowances

	Nonpregnant (15–18 Years)	Nonpregnant (19–24 Years)	Nonpregnant (25–50 Years)	Pregnant	Lactating (1st 6 Months)	Lactating (2nd 6 Months)
Protein (g)	44	46	50	60	65	62
Vitamin A (μg RE)*	800	800	800	800	1,300	1,200
Vitamin D (μg)†	10	10	5	10	10	10
Vitamin E (mg)‡	8	8	8	10	12	11
Vitamin K (μg)	55	60	65	65	65	65
Vitamin B_6 (mg)	1.5	1.6	1.6	2.2	2.1	2.1
Vitamin B_{12} (μg)	2.0	2.0	2.0	2.2	2.6	2.6
Folate (μg)	180	180	180	400	280	260
Thiamine (mg)	1.1	1.1	1.1	1.5	1.6	1.6
Riboflavin (mg)	1.3	1.3	1.3	1.6	1.8	1.7
Niacin (mg NE)§	15	15	15	17	20	20
Vitamin C (mg)	60	60	60	70	95	90
Iron (mg)	15	15	15	30	15	15
Calcium (mg)	1,200	1,200	800	1,200	1,200	1,200
Phosphorus (mg)	1,200	1,200	800	1,200	1,200	1,200
Zinc (mg)	12	12	12	15	19	16
Magnesium (mg)	300	280	280	300	355	340
Iodine (μg)	150	150	150	175	200	200

* Retinol equivalents. 1 retinol equivalent = 1 μg retinol or 6 μg beta-carotene.

† As cholecalciferol. 10 μg of cholecalciferol = 400 IU of vitamin D.

‡ Alpha-tocopherol equivalents. 1 mg, d-alpha tocopherol = 1 alphaTE.

§ 1 NE (niacin equivalent) = 1 mg of niacin or 60 mg of dietary tryptophan.

Reprinted with permission from *Recommended dietary allowances* (10th ed.). © 1989 by the National Academy of Sciences. Courtesy of the National Academy Press, Washington, DC.

fat and sodium. Increased calories should be "spent" on foods that provide the nutrients needed in increased amounts during pregnancy.

Protein

Protein is necessary for metabolism, tissue synthesis, and tissue repair. The RDA for adults is 0.75 g of protein per 1 kg of body weight daily. This RDA averages to a daily need of 44 to 50 g for females, depending on their age and size. During pregnancy, a protein intake of 60 g/day is recommended to expand the blood volume and support the growth of maternal and fetal tissues.

Protein is generally abundant in diets in most industrialized nations, but diets low in caloric intake may also be low in protein. If calories are low and protein is used to provide energy, fetal growth may be impaired.

The nurse should counsel women at risk for poor-protein diets about determining protein intake and ways to increase food sources of protein. When a woman needs to increase her protein intake, she should eat more high-protein foods rather than use high-protein powders or drinks. Protein substitutes increase protein but do not have the other nutrients provided by foods.

High-Sodium Foods

Products that contain the word "salt" or "sodium," such as table salt, onion salt, monosodium glutamate, bicarbonate of soda (baking soda)

Foods that taste salty, including snack foods like popcorn, potato chips, pretzels, crackers

Condiments and relishes, such as ketchup, horseradish, mustard, soy sauce, bouillon cubes, pickles, green and black olives

Smoked, dried, or processed foods, such as ham, bacon, lunch meats, corned beef

Canned soups, meats, and vegetables unless label states low in sodium

Packaged mixes for sauces, gravies, cakes, and other baked foods

Note: During pregnancy, foods high in sodium should be consumed in moderation. Expectant mothers should be taught to read labels and to avoid products in which sodium is listed among the first ingredients.

Vitamins

Although most people do not eat as much of every vitamin each day as they should, true deficiency states are uncommon in North America. Pregnant women, however, may not eat enough foods high in vitamins B_6, D, or E and folic acid to obtain the recommended levels.

The fat-soluble vitamins include A, D, E, and K. These vitamins can be stored in the liver, so deficiency states are not as likely to occur as with the water-soluble vitamins (B_6, B_{12}, and C, and folic acid, thiamine, riboflavin, and niacin). In excessive amounts, however, fat-soluble vitamins can be toxic. For example, excess vitamin A can cause fetal defects. Further information about the major vitamins is summarized in Table 15–3.

TABLE 15–3

• • • • • • • • • •

Vitamins and Minerals

Sources	Purpose	Importance in Pregnancy
Fat-Soluble Vitamins		
Vitamin A		
Green leafy vegetables, dark yellow vegetables, liver, whole or fortified low-fat or skim milk, egg yolk, butter and fortified margarine.	Important for vision and cell reproduction, growth, and functioning in skin and mucous membranes.	Fetal growth and cell differentiation. Stored in liver, so no increase in RDA in pregnancy. Excessive intake causes spontaneous abortions or serious fetal defects. Women taking isotretinoin (Accutane), a vitamin A derivative, for acne should not take it during pregnancy because it causes fetal defects.
Vitamin D		
Fortified milk, margarine, and soy products, butter, egg yolks. Synthesized in skin when exposed to sunlight. Vegans who are not exposed to sun and who do not eat fortified foods need supplements.	Necessary for metabolism of calcium and prevention of rickets.	Inadequate amounts may result in neonatal hypocalcemia, hypoplasia of tooth enamel, and maternal osteomalacia (softening of the bones). Excessive amounts can cause hypercalcemia and possible fetal deformities. Therefore, supplementary vitamin D should be taken cautiously.
Vitamin E		
Vegetable oils, whole grains, nuts, and green leafy vegetables.	Antioxidant, important for tissue growth and integrity of cells, particularly red blood cell membranes.	Deficiency is rare in pregnant women but can cause anemia in mother and fetus.
Vitamin K		
Green leafy vegetables. Also produced by normal bacterial flora in small intestine.	Necessary for clotting.	No increased RDA in pregnancy. Newborns are temporarily deficient in vitamin K and receive one dose by injection at birth to prevent hemorrhage.
Water-Soluble Vitamins		
Vitamin B$_6$ (Pyridoxine)		
Chicken, fish, liver, pork, eggs, peanuts, whole grains. Vegans at risk for low intake should take supplements.	Important in amino acid metabolism; also in blood, hormone, and immune system function.	Increased metabolism of amino acids during pregnancy.
Vitamin B$_{12}$		
Meat, fish, eggs, milk, fortified soy and cereal products.	Cell division and protein synthesis. Prevents megaloblastic anemia.	Increased formation of red blood cells and protein synthesis.
Folic Acid		
Raw green leafy vegetables, oranges, whole grains and fortified cereals, liver, dried peas and beans, yeast. May be lost in cooking.	Important for cell replication and metabolism and to prevent megaloblastic anemia.	Expanded blood volume and tissue growth. Deficiency in first 6 weeks of pregnancy may cause spontaneous abortion and neural tube defects.
Thiamine		
Pork, whole or enriched grain products, milk, legumes, organ meats, corn, seeds, nuts.	Forms coenzymes necessary to release energy.	Increased due to intake of calories.

TABLE 15–3
• • • • • • • • • • • •

Vitamins and Minerals Continued

Sources	Purpose	Importance in Pregnancy
Riboflavin		
Milk, pork, beef, enriched grain products, deep green vegetables.	Forms coenzymes necessary to release energy.	Increased due to intake of calories.
Niacin		
Meats, legumes, fish, poultry, enriched grains.	Forms coenzymes necessary to release energy.	Increased due to intake of calories.
Vitamin C		
Citrus fruits, peppers, strawberries, cantaloupe, green leafy vegetables, tomatoes, potatoes. Destroyed by heat and oxidation.	Important in collagen formation, tissue integrity, healing, immune response, and metabolism. Severe deficiency causes scurvy.	Necessary for formation of fetal tissue. Need is increased with smoking, drug or alcohol abuse, or aspirin use.

Minerals

Sources	Purpose	Importance in Pregnancy
Iron		
Meats, green leafy vegetables, eggs, grain products, tofu, legumes, nuts.	Formation of hemoglobin, enzymes for metabolism.	Expanded maternal blood volume, formation of fetal red blood cells, and storage in the fetal liver for use after birth.
Calcium		
Dairy products, salmon or sardines with bones, legumes, nuts, dried fruits, dark green leafy vegetables, tofu, broccoli.	Needed in bone formation, cell membrane permeability, coagulation, and neuromuscular function.	Mineralization of fetal bones and teeth.
Phosphorus		
Dairy products, lean meat. High in processed foods, snacks, carbonated drinks.	Needed in 1:1 ratio with calcium for bone formation and cell metabolism.	Mineralization of fetal bones and teeth. Excessive intake causes binding of calcium in intestines and prevents calcium absorption.
Zinc		
Meat, poultry, seafood, eggs, nuts, seeds, legumes, wheat germ, whole grains, yogurt.	Used in cell differentiation and reproduction, DNA and RNA synthesis, metabolism, acid-base balance.	Fetal and maternal tissue growth.
Magnesium		
Whole grains, nuts, legumes, dark green vegetables, scallops, oysters; small amounts in many foods.	Important in cell growth and neuromuscular function; activates enzymes for metabolism of protein and energy.	Same as for nonpregnancy state. Excessive intake may interfere with absorption of iron.
Iodine		
Seafood, iodized salt.	Important in thyroid function.	Deficiency may cause abortion, stillbirth, fetal congenital hypothyroidism, neurologic conditions.
Sodium		
See page 313.	Important for fluid and electrolyte balance.	Needed for expanded fluid volume of pregnancy.

Water-soluble vitamins are easily transferred from food to water in cooking, so foods should be steamed, microwaved, or prepared in only small amounts of water. The remaining water can be used in other dishes, such as soups. Water-soluble vitamins are not stored in the body as well as fat-soluble vitamins. Therefore, they should be included in the daily diet. Excess amounts are excreted in the urine, so there is less chance of toxicity from ingestion of excessive amounts.

Folic Acid

Folic acid (also called folate) can decrease the occurrence of neural tube defects in newborns. Adequate intake of folic acid is especially important just before conception and during the first 6 weeks after conception, when the neural tube is closing. Many pregnancies are unplanned, so all women of childbearing age should consume at least 0.4 mg of folic acid each day. This practice can decrease the incidence of neural tube defects by 50% (Rose & Mennuti, 1995). Women who have given birth to an infant with a neural tube defect should take higher doses of folic acid. A national goal is to reduce the incidence of neural tube defects to 3 per 10,000 live births from 6 per 10,000 in 1990 (U.S. Department of Health and Human Services, 1995). Since 1998, folic acid has been added to flour in an effort to meet this goal.

Minerals

Although most minerals (see Table 15–3) are supplied in adequate amounts in normal diets, the intake of iron, calcium, zinc, and magnesium may drop below recommended levels for pregnancy (Institute of Medicine, 1990).

IRON

During pregnancy, added iron is needed for the 20% to 30% increase in maternal red blood cells and for transfer to the fetus for storage and production of red blood cells. Infants use stored iron during the first 4 to 6 months, when their intake of iron is low. Iron is probably the only nutrient that cannot be supplied completely and easily from the diet dur-

---

**PREGNANT WOMEN
WANT TO KNOW**

About Vitamins and Minerals

- Take only vitamin and mineral supplements prescribed by a physician, nurse practitioner, or certified nurse-midwife. Over-the-counter supplements may not be formulated to meet your individual needs and could be harmful to you and your baby.
- Take iron on an empty stomach, if possible. If you have nausea, heartburn, constipation, or diarrhea, try taking your iron at different times of the day, such as at bedtime or 1 to 2 hours after meals. Taking it with orange juice or another source of vitamin C may increase absorption. Do not take iron with calcium supplements, milk, tea, or coffee because these substances decrease absorption.

TABLE 15–4

Foods High in Iron Content

Food and Amount	Average Amounts of Iron Supplied (mg)
Meats (3 oz)	
Liver	5.3
Red meats (avg.)	2.5
Poultry	
Chicken	0.9
Turkey	1.4
Legumes (1 c)	
Kidney beans	4.6
Lentils	4.2
Peanuts	2.8
Sunflower seeds	15.2
Chickpeas (garbanzo beans)	4.9
Black-eyed peas	3.6
Lima beans, baby	3.5
Peas	2.5
Eggs	
Eggs (each)	1.0
Grains (1 c)	
Rice	1.8
Bran flakes	6.8
with raisins	9.0
Oatmeal	1.6
Bread (slice)	0.9
Fruits	
⅓ c raisins	1.0
4 prunes	1.2
½ c dried apricots	3.0
Vegetables (1 c)	
Asparagus (frozen)	1.2
Broccoli	1.8
Collards	1.9
Spinach	
Raw	1.5
Cooked (frozen)	2.9
Other	
Tofu (2.5 × 2.75 × 1 inch)	2.3

Note: The recommended dietary allowance for iron during pregnancy is 30 mg/day. Although many women do not eat enough iron-containing foods to meet this need and take supplements, iron in foods is often better absorbed. Therefore, the nurse should suggest ways a woman can increase her dietary iron intake.

Data from Mahan, L. K., & Escott-Stump, S. (1996). *Krause's food, nutrition, and diet therapy* (9th ed.). Philadelphia: Saunders.

---

ing pregnancy. Eighty percent of women who do not take iron during pregnancy will have deficient iron stores at term (Niebyl, 1996). Table 15–4 lists common foods high in iron.

Iron is present in many foods, but in small amounts. The average American diet contains only about 6 mg of iron for each 1,000 calories of food. The nonpregnant woman would have to eat approximately 2,500 calories daily and the pregnant woman would need as much as 5,000 calories to meet her iron needs (Worthington-Roberts, 1997b). Thus, many adult women do not meet their daily nonpregnancy requirement for iron and begin pregnancy already anemic or with low iron stores. (Anemia during pregnancy is discussed in Chapter 26.)

Absorption of iron is affected by many other substances. Calcium and phosphorus in milk and tannin in tea decrease iron absorption from plant sources (called nonheme iron) if consumed during the same meal. Coffee binds iron (prevents it from being fully absorbed). Foods cooked in iron pans contain more iron. Foods containing ascorbic acid and meats eaten with other iron-containing foods may increase absorption. Iron from meat (called heme iron) is more readily absorbed than iron from plants and is less affected by other foods.

Because of the difficulty of obtaining enough iron in the diet, physicians and nurse practitioners often prescribe iron supplements of 30 mg/day during pregnancy. Supplementation should begin during the second trimester, when the need increases and morning sickness has usually ended.

Iron taken on an empty stomach is absorbed more completely, but many women find iron difficult to tolerate without some food. Taking it at bedtime may make it easier to tolerate. Side effects occur more often with higher doses and include nausea, vomiting, heartburn, epigastric pain, constipation, and diarrhea.

CALCIUM

Calcium is necessary for bone formation, maintenance of cell membrane permeability, coagulation, and neuromuscular function. It is transferred to the fetus, especially in the last trimester, and is important for mineralization of fetal bones and teeth. Calcium absorption increases during the second trimester. Calcium from the mother's bones may be used to meet the needs of pregnancy, but changes are reversed after pregnancy. A common myth is that calcium is removed from the teeth during pregnancy, leading to excessive decay. Actually, calcium in the teeth is stable and is not affected by pregnancy.

The best source of calcium is dairy products. Whole, low-fat, and skim milk all contain the same amount of calcium and may be used interchangeably to increase or reduce calorie intake. However, women with lactose intolerance (lactase deficiency resulting in gastrointestinal problems when dairy products are consumed) need other sources of calcium.

Calcium is also present in legumes, nuts, dried fruits, dark green leafy vegetables, and broccoli. Although spinach contains calcium, it also contains oxalates, which decrease calcium availability; thus, spinach is not a good source of calcium. Caffeine increases the excretion of calcium.

Women who do not eat dairy products for cultural reasons, because of lactose intolerance, to avoid ingesting animal products, or for any other reason should take calcium supplements. Women younger than 25 years with diets low in calcium may need supplements during pregnancy because their bone density is not complete; lack of available calcium may interfere with adequate bone formation in the mother. To ensure absorption of calcium, women should take sup-

---

• • • • • • • • • •
Calcium Sources Approximately Equivalent to 1 Cup of Milk

1 c yogurt
1½ oz hard cheese
2 c low-fat cottage cheese
1¾ c ice cream or ice milk
3 c sherbet
2½ c peanuts
1 c almonds
9 oz sunflower seeds
2 c refried beans
3 pieces (2.5 × 2.75 × 1 inch) tofu (soybean curd)
1¾ c broccoli
1½ c cooked kale
1 c cooked collard greens
1⅓ c oysters
4 oz salmon with bones
2½ oz sardines with bones
7 corn tortillas
5 tsp. blackstrap molasses

Note: This list can be used to counsel women who are vegans or lactose intolerant. Lactose-intolerant women can often tolerate yogurt and cheese without distress. Although the amounts of some foods listed are more than would be likely to be eaten in the course of a day, they serve for comparison.

Data from Mahan, L. K., & Escott-Stump, S. (1996). *Krause's food, nutrition, and diet therapy* (9th ed.). Philadelphia: Saunders.

---

plements with meals, separately from the time they take iron supplements.

Nutritional Supplementation

PURPOSE

Food is the best source for nutrients. According to the Institute of Medicine Subcommittee on Nutritional Status and Weight Gain During Pregnancy (Institute of Medicine, 1990), women do not routinely need to take vitamin and mineral supplements during pregnancy unless there is reason to believe that the diet is inadequate. The exception is iron, which is unlikely to be obtained in adequate amounts through normal food intake. Expectant mothers who are vegetarians or lactose intolerant or who have special problems in obtaining nutrients through diet alone may need vitamin and mineral supplements. Assessment of each woman's individual needs determines whether supplementation is appropriate.

DISADVANTAGES AND DANGERS OF NUTRITIONAL SUPPLEMENTATION

Because many people think supplements are a harmless way to improve their diets, some women take them without consulting a physician. The use of supplements may increase the intake of some nutrients to doses much higher than the recommended amounts. Excessive amounts of some vitamins and minerals may be toxic to the fetus. Vitamin A can cause craniofacial, central nervous system, and cardiac defects in the fetus when taken in large amounts (Worthington-Roberts, 1997a). Large amounts of vitamin A are taken by women using the drug isotretinoin (Accutane) for acne. Other nutrients that may cause harm in excessive amounts include vitamins B_6, C, and D and the minerals iron and zinc.

Water

Water is important during pregnancy for the expanded blood volume and as a part of the increased maternal and fetal tissues. Women should drink approximately eight to ten 8-ounce glasses of fluids each day, with water constituting most of the fluid intake. Fluids low in nutrients should be limited because they are filling and replace other more nutritional foods and drinks.

Food Guide Pyramid

The U.S. Department of Agriculture's (USDA) food pyramid (Fig. 15–2) provides a guide for healthy eating for adults and children. It can be adapted to serve as a guide

during pregnancy as well. Table 15–5 lists the minimum number of servings of each food pyramid group needed during pregnancy.

WHOLE GRAINS

At the base of the pyramid are breads, cereals, rice, and pastas. They provide complex carbohydrates and fiber as well as vitamins and minerals. Whole grains provide more nutrients than processed grain products. The USDA recommends six to 11 servings of this group for healthy adults over age 25. Pregnant women should have at least seven servings.

VEGETABLES AND FRUITS

Vegetables and fruits form the next two groups of the pyramid and are important sources of vitamins, minerals, and fiber. At least one food that provides vitamin C and one that provides vitamin A should be selected from the fruit and vegetable group each day. Healthy adults should have at least five servings of fruits and vegetables, with a range

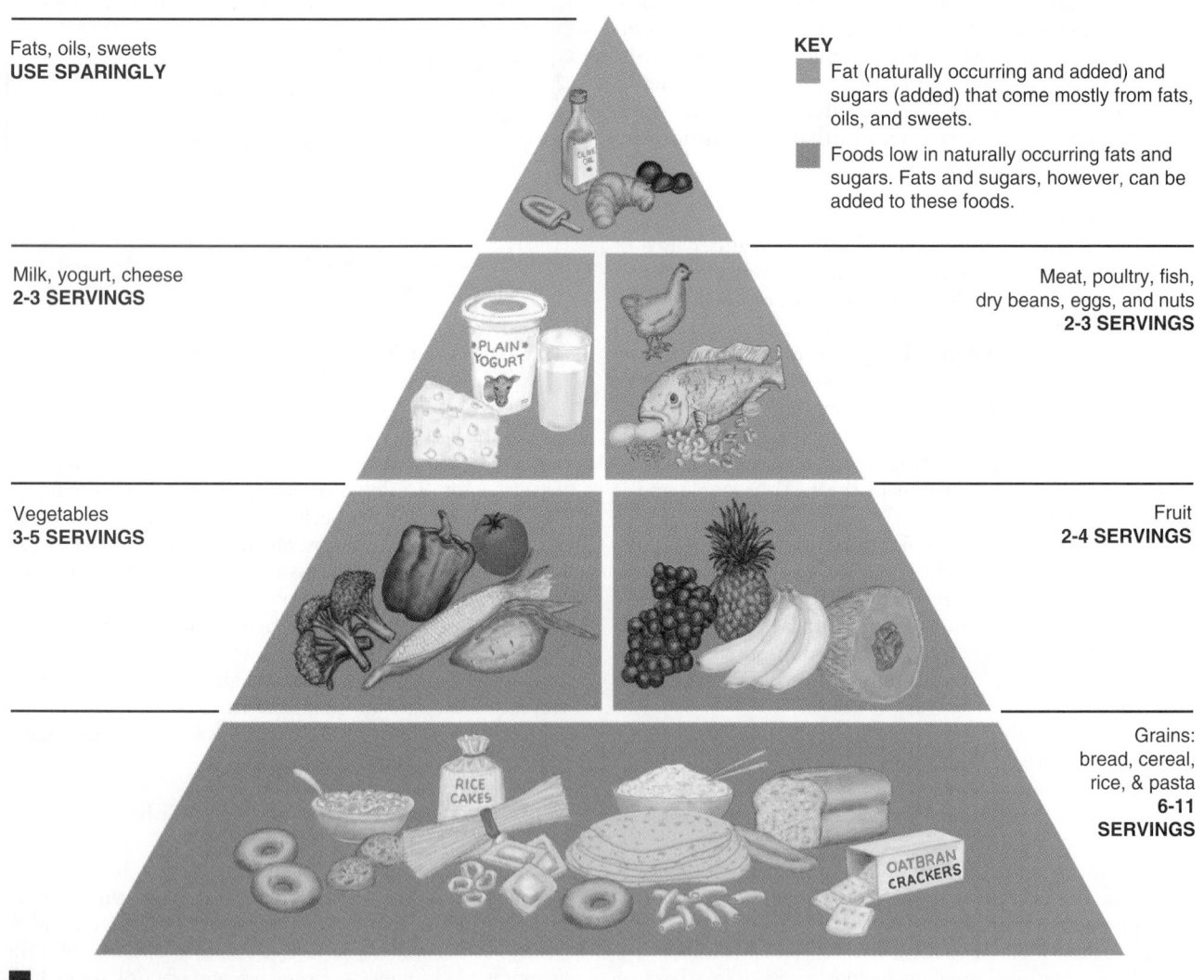

FIGURE 15–2

The food guide pyramid. (Adapted from U.S. Department of Agriculture [1992, April]. USDA's food guide pyramid. *Home and Garden Bulletin,* No. 249.)

TABLE 15-5

Daily Food Plan

Food Guide Pyramid Group	Typical Food Amounts for One Serving	Number of Servings	
		Nonpregnant Women	Pregnant and Lactating Women
Unsaturated fats	1 tsp.	3 tsp.	3 tsp.
Dairy products	1 c milk or yogurt, 1½ oz or ⅓ c grated hard cheese, 2 c cottage cheese	Age <25: 3 or more Age >25: 2 or more	3 or more
Protein sources	1 oz or ¼ c chopped meat, poultry, fish, ½ c cooked legumes, 1 egg, 3 oz tofu, 2 tbsp. peanut butter	5 oz	7 oz
Vegetables and fruits	1 medium piece or ½ c cooked or chopped raw, ¾ c juice, 1 lettuce leaf		
Total servings		5 or more	5 or more
Vitamin C source		1	1
Deep yellow or dark green leafy (vitamin A)		1	1
Other fruits and vegetables		3	3
Whole grains	Breads (1 slice), cereals (½–¾ c), rice and pastas (½ c)	6–11 Age <25: 7 or more Age >25: 6 or more	7 or more

Nurses can use this table as a guide to counsel women about nutrient needs during pregnancy and lactation. Eating *at least* the number of servings listed meets the minimum nutrient need for pregnancy. Additional calories may be necessary to meet individual requirements.

Modified from California Department of Health Services, Maternal and Child Health (1990): *Nutrition during pregnancy and the postpartum period: A manual for health care professionals* (summary). Sacramento, CA: Author.

of three to five servings of vegetables and two to four servings of fruits. The pregnant or lactating woman needs the same amount.

DAIRY FOODS

Dairy foods include foods like milk, yogurt, and cheese. They contain approximately the same nutrient values whether they are whole (4% fat), low fat (2% fat), or nonfat (skim), but the calories and fat are less in the latter two forms. Dairy products are especially good sources of calcium. Adults older than age 25 need two to three servings from this group each day. Younger women and those who are pregnant or lactating need at least three servings.

In the past, calcium supplements and decreased milk intake were recommended to prevent leg cramps by improving the balance of calcium and phosphorus. Both occur in high amounts in milk. The effectiveness of this treatment has not, however, been proved. Because milk provides a large number of nutrients, women generally should not limit it during pregnancy (Neuhouser, 1996; Worthington-Roberts, 1997b).

PROTEIN

Many adults think of meat, poultry, fish, and eggs as the only sources of protein, but legumes (dried beans and peas), nuts, and soybean products such as tofu are also good sources. Adults should consume 5 to 6 ounces of protein foods each day; pregnant or lactating women need 7 or more ounces. A typical serving of meat, fish, or poultry is approximately 3 ounces. Three ounces is about the size of a deck of playing cards.

OTHER ELEMENTS

The tip of the USDA's food guide pyramid represents fats, oils, and concentrated sugars, which should be ingested sparingly. They provide calories for energy but few other nutrients. Three teaspoons of unsaturated fats per day are adequate for this group.

Factors That Influence Nutrition

The nurse must consider cultural background, age, and knowledge about nutrition when counseling women about their diets.

Culture

Food may have special cultural meaning during pregnancy or childbirth. Nurses need knowledge about the habits of a variety of cultures so that they can provide culturally appropriate nutritional counseling. Before making assumptions about the influence of a woman's culture on her diet, the nurse must assess each woman individually. Not all women follow food practices considered typical for their culture.

The nurse should assess the woman's age, her length of time in America, and whether she has adopted prevalent American eating habits. Some women who follow an American diet may return to some aspects of their culture's traditional diet during pregnancy to "be sure" they do not harm the fetus.

Nurses often use pamphlets as a part of teaching and may be able to obtain them in various languages.

The nurse should be certain that the woman can read her own language before giving her written materials. People who cannot read may not readily admit it. In addition, the translation may be too complicated for the woman with little education to understand. Having an interpreter discuss the material with the woman helps to discover whether she can read and aids in other teaching.

Many cultures believe that certain foods, conditions, and medicines are "hot" or "cold" and that they must maintain a balance to preserve health. In Asian cultures, this is referred to as "yin" (cold) and "yang" (hot) and may influence what the mother eats during pregnancy and the postpartum period. Table 15–6 lists common "hot" and "cold" foods.

Food taboos also influence what some women eat during the childbearing period. For example, Korean women may avoid chicken, pork, and blemished fruits during pregnancy. These foods are thought to have a harmful effect on the infant's physical appearance.

Great variety exists in cultural preferences for foods. For instance, some African-Americans may follow a diet that is similar to that of people living in the southeastern United States. Common foods include okra, collards, mustard greens, ham hocks, black-eyed peas, and hominy or grits. The diets of other African-Americans, however, vary according to the geographic area in which they live. Many eat a diet deficient in iron and fresh fruits and vegetables, especially if they have low incomes. Lactose intolerance is common, resulting in lack of calcium if other sources are not present in the diet. Intake of high-sodium and fried foods may present health problems.

Some Jewish women follow a strictly kosher diet. This diet includes meat only from animals with cloven hooves and processed to remove all blood, and avoidance of milk and meat in the same meal. Muslim women do not eat pork and may fast on certain days. The religion, however, exempts pregnant and nursing women from obligatory fasting.

The diet of Native American women may contain corn, beans, and squash but lack fresh fruits and vegetables. Lactose intolerance is common, and meat intake is low. Fat, carbohydrate, sodium, and sugar intake are often high. Low-income Native Americans living on reservations may receive foods such as white flour, corn meal, white rice, and processed meats from federal programs. Some of these families, however, take in less than two thirds of the RDA for calories, calcium, iron, iodine, riboflavin, and vitamins A and C (Davis & Sherer, 1994).

Food preferences for two cultures, Southeast Asian and Latino, show the influence of culture on diet. Immigrants and refugees from Southeast Asia are the newest large group of people to come into the United States. They are likely to continue following diets similar to those in their homelands. Latinos are a large minority group in the United States, and nurses throughout the United States need information about Latino food preferences.

SOUTHEAST ASIAN DIETARY PRACTICES

Southeast Asians come from Cambodia, Laos, and Vietnam. Traditional cooking in these countries includes searing fresh vegetables quickly with a small portion of meat, poultry, or fish in a little oil over high heat. Meals cooked in this manner are low in fat and retain vitamins. Most meals are accompanied by rice, which increases the intake of complex carbohydrates. A salty fish sauce called *nuoc mam* and fresh vegetables are part of most meals.

Effect of Southeast Asian Culture on Diet During Childbearing. In Southeast Asian cultures, pregnancy, especially the third trimester, is considered "hot," and women eat "cold" foods to maintain a balance of hot and cold. Their diet includes sour foods, fruits, noodles, and sweets and avoids fish, excessively salty or spicy foods, alcohol, and rice. The woman also avoids unfamiliar foods for fear that they may harm her or her fetus.

The postpartum period is considered "cold," partly because of the loss of blood, which is "hot." Mothers avoid losing more heat, which would have ill effects on their health. They stay warm physically and choose "hot" foods to eat, including rice with fish sauce, broth, salty meats, fish, chicken, and eggs. They may refuse cold drinks but welcome hot fluids, requesting tea or even plain hot water. Families frequently bring food to the mother while she is in the hospital because hospital food may not meet her preferences.

The diet of Southeast Asians, especially those with low incomes, may be below recommended levels for energy, calcium, iron, zinc, magnesium, and vitamins B_6 and D, but high in sodium. These deficiencies may be of special concern during pregnancy. The woman can often increase her intake of needed nutrients without deviating greatly from her usual diet.

TABLE 15–6

. . . .

Common "Hot" and "Cold" Foods: Southeast Asian and Latino Diets

"Hot" (Yang) Foods	"Cold" (Yin) Foods
Southeast Asian	
Peppers, onions	Most fruits and juices
Meat and poultry	Flour
Fish and fish sauce	Cold fluids
Broth	Sour foods
Eggs	
Spices, sweets	

"Hot" Foods	"Cold" Foods
Latino	
Potatoes, peas, onions, chili peppers	Most fruits and vegetables
Cheese, evaporated milk	Milk
Chicken, lamb	Fish
Flour tortillas	Corn tortillas
Chickpeas and kidney beans	Green and red beans

Note: Although there are variations within cultural groups, foods considered "hot" are used for conditions thought to be "cold," and vice versa. This distinction influences what women are willing to eat during pregnancy or illness, and these customs must be respected as part of nursing care.

Increasing Nutrients with Traditional Foods. Milk products are not part of the traditional Southeast Asian diet, and lactose intolerance is common. Increasing the intake of commonly used dark green leafy vegetables, such as mustard greens, bok choy, and broccoli, however, increases levels of calcium, iron, magnesium, and folic acid. Tofu contains good amounts of calcium and iron. A broth made from pork or chicken bones soaked in vinegar (which removes calcium from the bones) is frequently taken. If the mother avoids fortified milk, she may need vitamin D supplementation. Increasing the intake of meats or poultry elevates levels of vitamin B_6 and zinc.

LATINO DIETARY PRACTICES
Spanish-speaking people, such as Mexican-Americans, Puerto Ricans, and Cuban-Americans, are often referred to as Latinos or Hispanics. Like Asians, Latinos follow the theories of "hot" and "cold" foods and conditions. They also consider pregnancy to be "hot" and the postpartum period to be "cold" and adjust the diet accordingly.

Dried beans (especially pinto beans) are a staple of the Mexican-American diet and are part of most meals, either eaten alone, as refried beans, or mixed with other foods, such as rice. Corn or flour tortillas are eaten with most meals. Corn tortillas are a good source of calcium. Rice is also an important grain.

Although milk is not commonly drunk except by infants, cheese is part of many dishes. Chili peppers and tomatoes are the most common vegetables used. Green leafy and yellow vegetables are seldom included.

Latino foods are often hot and spicy and frequently fried. The diet is high in fiber and complex carbohydrates but also high in calories and fat. The diet may be low in iron, calcium, and vitamins A and D, which should be increased through foods or supplements during pregnancy.

Puerto Ricans and Cubans may add tropical fruits and vegetables from the homeland, when available. Viandas (starchy fruits and vegetables like plantain, green bananas, sweet potatoes, yams, and breadfruit) are common. They may be cooked with codfish and onion. Guava, papaya, mango, and eggplant are also used when available.

Age

The nurse needs to consider age. The adolescent who is not fully mature needs nutritional support for her own growth. Older women who are in good health, however, have the same nutritional requirements as younger pregnant women.

Nutritional Knowledge

Once pregnancy is confirmed, women often become interested in the relationship between what they eat and the effect on the fetus. Some lack basic understanding about nutrition and have misconceptions based on common food myths. These expectant mothers need help from nurses in learning about nutrition.

Nutritional Risk Factors

The nurse must identify risk factors that may interfere with a woman's ability to meet the nutritional needs of pregnancy.

Socioeconomic Status

POVERTY
Low-income women may have deficient diets because of lack of financial resources and nutritional education. Carbohydrate foods are often less expensive than other foods. Therefore, the diet may be high in calories but low in vitamins and minerals. A referral to Temporary Assistance for Needy Families (TANF) or the Special Supplemental Food Program for Women, Infants, and Children (WIC) may be helpful. Vitamin and mineral supplementation may be important for the woman, especially if her diet is inconsistent.

FOOD SUPPLEMENT PROGRAMS
The WIC program is administered by the USDA to provide nutritional assessment, counseling, and education to low-income women and children up to age 5 years who are at nutritional risk. The program also provides food vouchers or foods and formula to qualified women and their children. Eligibility is based on an income below 185% of the federal poverty level. Women are eligible throughout pregnancy and for 6 months after birth if bottle-feeding or 1 year if breast-feeding.

Adolescence

Adolescent pregnancies are associated with higher risk for complications for both the expectant mother and the fetus. Adolescents at greatest risk are the youngest in terms of gynecologic age (number of years since menarche) and those who are still growing. Girls who become pregnant less than 2 years after menstruation begins are not anatomically and physiologically mature, and they need more nutrients to meet their needs than do older adolescents. Those with a gynecologic age of 4 years are usually physically mature and have nutritional demands similar to those of older women (Worthington-Roberts & Rees, 1997) (see also Chapter 25).

Whether the adolescent is still growing, however, is even more important than her age, because some adolescents may continue to grow as long as 6 years after menarche (Scholl et al., 1994). Growing adolescents continue to add fat to their own bodies in late pregnancy rather than use it for support of the fetus. As a result, they tend to have smaller infants even with good weight gains.

To determine the appropriate gain for an individual teenager, the nurse should consider how much weight the adolescent would gain in the next 9 months if she were not pregnant (see growth charts in Appendix H). This amount is added to the recommended weight gain for pregnancy.

NUTRIENT NEEDS
In the past, it was usual to add the RDA for pregnancy to the nutritional requirements for the adolescent. The 1989

Vegetarianism

Although the vegetarian may eat a very nutritional diet, she is at higher risk during pregnancy. If she is new to vegetarian food practices, uninformed about pregnancy needs, or careless with her diet, she could fail to meet her nutrient needs. Plant food combinations that provide complete proteins are listed in Table 15–7. Table 15–8 presents guidelines on vegetarian foods during pregnancy. This scheme is similar to the food pyramid groups followed by nonvegetarians and is easy to remember when planning the daily diet.

TYPES OF VEGETARIANISM

Vegetarianism occurs in a variety of forms. Vegans avoid all animal products and may have the most difficulty meeting their nutrient needs. Their diet may be lacking in adequate iodine, calcium, iron, zinc, riboflavin, and vitamins D and B_{12} (Peckenpaugh & Poleman, 1999). It is easier for

TABLE 15–7

Plant Food Combinations to Provide Complete Proteins

Food	Served With
Grains	
Wheat	Beans
	Soybeans and rice
	Soybeans, rice, and peanuts
	Soybeans and sesame
Rice	Beans (other types)
	Peas
	Sesame
	Soybeans
	Soybeans, peanuts, and wheat
	Soybeans and wheat
Corn	Beans
Legumes	
Soybeans	Peanuts and sesame
	Peanuts, wheat, and rice
	Rice and wheat
	Wheat and sesame
Beans (other types such as garbanzo, navy, peas)	Rice
Nuts and Seeds	
Peanuts	Soybeans and sesame
	Soybeans, wheat, and rice
	Sunflower seeds
Sesame	Beans
	Broccoli
	Cauliflower
	Lima beans
	Rice
	Soybeans and peanuts
	Soybeans and wheat
	Sprouts
Sunflower	Peanuts

Based on data from Lappé, F. M. (1991). *Diet for a small planet.* New York: Ballantine.

TABLE 15–8

Food Plan for Pregnant Vegetarians

Food	No. of Servings
Whole and enriched grains	7
Green and yellow vegetables	3–5
Fruits, including vitamin C	3
Dairy products	3
Legumes, soy products, meat substitutes	2–3

Vitamin and mineral supplements may be necessary according to individual needs. Women who do not consume dairy products need to increase their sources of calcium and may need to take supplements.

lactovegetarians (whose diet includes milk), ovovegetarians (whose diet includes eggs), and lacto-ovovegetarians (whose diet includes milk and eggs) to meet their nutrient needs.

MEETING THE NUTRITIONAL REQUIREMENTS OF THE PREGNANT VEGETARIAN

Energy. Vegetarian diets are low in calories and fat and may not meet the energy needs of pregnancy. The diets are high in fiber and may cause a feeling of fullness before enough calories are eaten. A pregnant woman can increase caloric intake by eating between-meal snacks and foods. If carbohydrate and fat intake are too low, her body may use protein for energy, making it unavailable for other purposes.

Protein. Protein intake is a concern in all vegetarian diets. "Complete" proteins contain all the essential amino acids the body cannot synthesize from other sources. Animal proteins are complete, but vegetable proteins lack one or more of the essential amino acids. Combining incomplete plant proteins with other plant foods that have complementary amino acids allows intake of all essential amino acids. Knowledge of how to mix foods appropriately is needed to ensure adequate intake of essential amino acids. Dishes that combine beans or tofu with rice are examples. Table 15–7 lists combinations of foods that provide complete proteins.

Incomplete proteins can also be combined with small amounts of complete protein foods like cheese to provide all amino acids. Therefore, women who include even small amounts of animal products have less difficulty meeting their protein needs.

Calcium. Vegetarians who include milk products in their diet may meet their pregnancy needs for calcium. Vegans obtain calcium from vegetables, but their high-fiber diet may interfere with calcium absorption. Calcium-fortified soy products, such as soy milk or tofu, may meet the requirements, or calcium supplements may be necessary. Vitamin D supplementation is especially important if the woman drinks no milk and has little exposure to sunlight. Soy milks may be enriched with vitamin D.

Iron. Iron in the vegetarian diet is poorly absorbed because of the lack of heme iron (from meats), which improves absorption. Iron supplementation is particularly important for vegetarian women during pregnancy.

Zinc. The best sources of zinc are meat and fish. Vegans may be deficient in this mineral and need supplements to meet their needs.

Vitamin B$_{12}$. Vitamin B$_{12}$ is obtained only from animal products. Because vegetarian diets contain large amounts of folic acid, anemia due to inadequate intake of vitamin B$_{12}$ may not be apparent at first. Vegans may eat fortified foods such as soy products or may take supplements.

Vitamin A. Vitamin A is abundant in vegetarian diets. If the woman takes a daily multiple vitamin-mineral supplement, she may ingest excessive amounts of vitamin A and may experience toxic effects, such as anorexia, irritability, hair loss, dry skin, and damage to the fetus. Supplementation should be individualized for each woman, based on her diet and her needs.

Lactose Intolerance

Intolerance of lactose is caused by deficiency of the small intestine enzyme lactase, necessary for absorption of the milk sugar lactose. Some degree of lactose intolerance is normal for most of the world's population after early childhood. Groups with a high incidence of lactose intolerance include many African-American, Latina, Asian, Native American, and Middle Eastern women. Although women with lactose intolerance may tolerate cultured or fermented milk products, such as aged cheese, buttermilk, and yogurt, symptoms may occur after drinking as little as a cup of milk. Symptoms include nausea, bloating, flatulence, diarrhea, and intestinal cramping.

Although the ability to tolerate lactose may increase during pregnancy, women who avoid dairy foods may not consume the recommended amounts of calcium. Most women can tolerate small amounts of milk, and they should increase their intake of other foods that provide calcium. Low-lactose milk is available, or the enzyme lactase (Lact-Aid) can be added to milk. See page 317 for additional sources of calcium.

Nausea and Vomiting of Pregnancy

Morning sickness usually ends with the first trimester, but some women experience nausea at other times of the day and for longer than 12 weeks. These women are often able to manage frequent, small meals better than three large meals. Protein and complex carbohydrates are tolerated best, but fatty foods increase nausea. Drinking liquids between meals instead of with meals often helps. At bedtime, a protein snack such as cheese helps to maintain glucose levels through the night. Eating a carbohydrate food like dry toast or crackers before getting out of bed in the morning helps prevent nausea.

Anemia

Anemia is a common concern during pregnancy. Although the normal hemoglobin level for nonpregnant women is 13.5 g/dl, hemoglobin values during the second trimester of pregnancy average 11.6 g/dl as a result of the dilution of the blood caused by plasma increases. This is often called *physiologic anemia* because it is normal (see Chapter 13). One large nutritional survey among low-income women showed that more than 37% of women had hemoglobin levels below 11.0 g/dl (Perry, Yip, & Zyrkowski, 1995).

During the third trimester, hemoglobin levels generally rise to 12.5 g/dl because of increased absorption of iron from the gastrointestinal tract, even though iron is transferred to the fetus primarily during this time. Fetal iron stores during the third trimester are sufficient to prevent anemia in the newborn for the first 4 to 6 months after birth.

Iron stores may be measured by determining the serum ferritin level in the blood. A ferritin level less than 12 micrograms per liter (μg/L) indicates that the anemia is caused by iron deficiency. Pregnant women are considered anemic if the hemoglobin level drops below 10.5 g/dl (Duffy, 1999).

Anemic women need iron supplements and help in choosing foods high in iron (see Table 15–4). Iron supplements are better absorbed if taken between meals with a dietary source of vitamin C to increase absorption. Because high intakes of iron inhibit the body's use of zinc and copper, anemic women may also need to take these minerals.

Abnormal Prepregnancy Weight

In addition to teaching about dietary changes, the nurse should be alert for other problems associated with abnormal prepregnancy weight. The woman who is below normal weight may not have enough money for food or may have an eating disorder. An obese woman may have other health problems, such as hypertension or gestational diabetes, that may affect the nurse's nutritional counseling plan.

Eating Disorders

Eating disorders include anorexia nervosa (refusal to eat because of a distorted body image and feelings of obesity) and bulimia (overeating, sometimes followed by induced vomiting). These women need a great deal of individual counseling to be sure that they meet the increased nutrient needs of pregnancy and understand normal postpartum weight loss.

Pica

The practice of eating substances not normally considered food is called pica. Clay or dirt and solid laundry starch are the most common materials involved, but other items, such as chalk, crushed ice, freezer frost, baking soda, burnt matches, or ashes, may be included. Pica is more common in the southeastern United States but is not limited to any one socioeconomic or geographic area.

The cause of pica is unknown, although cultural values

> **CRITICAL THINKING EXERCISE 15–1**
>
> A pregnant woman very hesitantly confides that the reason she is not gaining much weight is that she eats large amounts of ice. She buys bags of crushed ice or eats the frost that forms in her freezer. "I know I should be gaining more weight, but I'm just not hungry for anything besides ice," she says.
>
> How should the nurse handle this situation?

cause problems include the cabbage family, onions, foods that are highly allergenic (wheat, eggs, cow's milk) or acidic (orange juice), spicy foods, garlic, nuts, chocolate, or large amounts of fresh fruits. Eliminating the suspected food from the mother's diet and then trying it again can often pinpoint whether it was the cause of the problem.

Nutrition for the Nonlactating Mother

The postpartum woman who is not breast-feeding can return to her prepregnancy diet, provided that it meets the RDAs for the adult woman. Her diet should contain protein and vitamin C foods to promote healing. She may continue to take her prenatal vitamin-mineral supplements until her supply is finished. This supplementation ensures adequate intake during the early weeks and helps renew nutrient stores.

The nurse should assess the mother's understanding of the number of servings she needs from each food group. A review of important nutrient sources for calcium and iron may be relevant. If a woman was anemic during pregnancy, an iron supplement is important until the hemoglobin value returns to normal.

When her baby is born, a woman can expect to lose about 12 lb immediately. She loses approximately another 8 lb during the early weeks and probably all but about 2 lb by the end of the first year if she follows a well-balanced diet. To avoid retaining weight, she should take in 300 calories per day less than she did during pregnancy.

Some women are impatient with slow weight loss. Because they need energy to meet the demands of infant care, new mothers should wait at least 3 weeks to start dieting to lose weight. Suggestions for sensible calorie reduction combined with exercise are appropriate. Women who gain excess weight during pregnancy may have more difficulty losing it after birth and may need help from a dietitian in planning a weight loss program.

Mothers may snack instead of planning meals for themselves, especially during the early weeks. The nurse should remind them that snacking often involves high caloric intake without meeting nutritional needs. Meals and snacks should be high in nutrient content.

NURSING CARE

Nutrition for Childbearing

Assessment

Interview

The interview provides an opportunity to develop rapport and to determine whether any specific problems are present that affect dietary intake.

Appetite. Begin the interview by discussing the woman's appetite. Morning sickness may decrease food intake during the first trimester. Determine the severity and duration of nausea and vomiting. Hyperemesis gravidarum is the most serious form of this problem, often requiring intravenous correction of fluid and electrolyte imbalance (see Chapter 26).

Eating Habits. Assess the usual pattern of meals to discover poor food habits, such as skipping breakfast or eating only snack foods for lunch. Determine who does the cooking for the family. If someone else does the cooking, discuss nutritional needs during pregnancy with that person.

Food Preferences. Ask about the woman's food preferences and dislikes. During pregnancy, some women experience an aversion to certain foods, such as meats, that they do not have at other times. Determine whether she has food cravings or eats large amounts of any one particular food or group of foods. Discuss pica in a matter-of-fact way to avoid giving an impression of disapproval. Food items such as ice are sometimes included in pica, so ask about them as well.

> In assessing for pica, you might say, "Have you had any cravings for special things to eat during your pregnancy?" This can be followed by "Women sometimes eat things like clay or starch during pregnancy. Are you fond of those?" Some women are willing to substitute foods such as nonfat dry milk powder for nonfood items like laundry starch.

Psychosocial Influences. Ascertain whether cultural or religious considerations affect the woman's diet. Determine the effect of these on her nutrient intake.

The interview may reveal other factors that interfere with adequate nutrition. Women with low incomes may not know about sources of help. Question the vegetarian to determine how long she has followed the practice and her awareness of changes necessary during pregnancy. A woman's smoking habits, alcohol intake, and substance abuse may become obvious during the interview. Ask about prescription drugs, and determine whether she takes medications that interfere with nutrient absorption.

Ask the woman if she has any special diet concerns. This question may bring out fears about weight gain, concerns that specific foods could hurt the fetus, or other issues not yet addressed.

Diet History

Diet histories provide information about a woman's usual intake of nutrients. They form a basis for counseling about any changes required to meet pregnancy needs.

Twenty-Four-Hour Diet History. Ask the woman to recall what she ate at each meal and snack during the previous 24 hours. Use specific questions about the size of portions and ingredients used. Inquire about beverages as well as food snacks. Determine whether this sample is typical of her usual daily food intake; if not, ask which foods are more representative. Analyze the 24-hour diet history to determine whether the woman has met the recommendations for specific food groups, calories, and protein. Detailed analysis for individual nutrients is unnecessary.

Food Intake Records. Food intake records are used to report foods eaten over one or more days. Ask the woman to list everything she eats throughout the day. The list is more accurate if she writes down each food immediately after eating.

Food-Frequency Questionnaires. Use of food-frequency questionnaires may provide information about diet over a longer period. Ask the woman how often she eats each of the common foods listed. Analyze the list to determine whether foods from each food group are eaten in adequate amounts to meet pregnancy needs.

Physical Assessment

Information about nutritional status includes measurement of weight and examination for signs of nutritional deficiency.

Weight at Initial Visit. To get a baseline value for future comparison, weigh the woman at the first prenatal visit. Ask if this is her usual weight or if she has gained or lost weight. Measure her height without shoes. If her weight is low for height, nutritional reserves are marginal. If it is high, she may be overweight or obese.

Weight at Subsequent Visits. Weigh the woman at each visit on the same scale with approximately the same amount of clothing. Record the weight on a weight grid at each visit throughout the pregnancy. This grid allows

examination of the pattern as well as the total gain to date. It also helps keep track of the amount of gain between individual visits. Figure 15–3 is an example of a weight gain grid.

> Be careful to avoid overemphasizing weight gain. In some instances, a woman may be afraid that caregivers will be disapproving if she gains weight, and consequently she may diet or fast a day or two before her prenatal visit.

Signs of Nutrient Deficiency. Other indications of nutritional status include any signs of deficiency. For example, bleeding gums may indicate inadequate intake of vitamin C. Actual deficiency states, however, are not likely to occur in women in most industrialized countries. The exception is iron deficiency anemia, which is common in a mild form. Signs and symptoms include pallor, low hemoglobin level, fatigue, and increased susceptibility to infection.

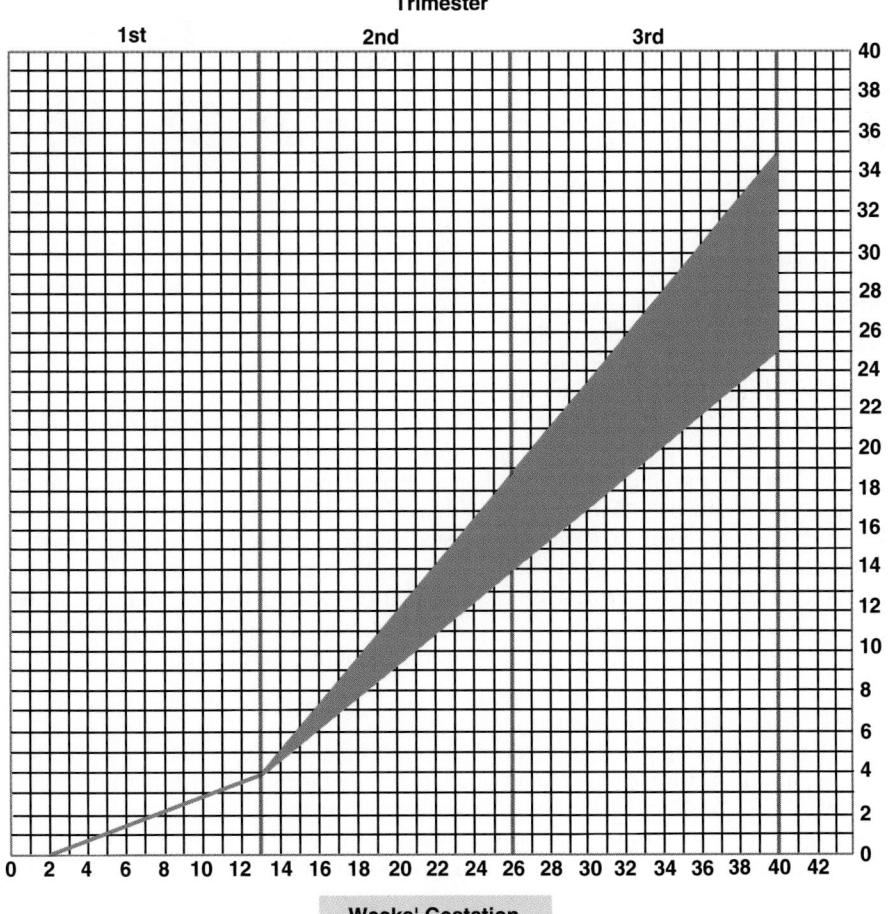

FIGURE 15–3

Weight gain grid for pregnancy. The normal range for weight gain is 25 to 35 lb. Adolescents often need to gain in the higher end of the range. Women who are shorter than 62 inches should gain in the lower portion.

Laboratory Tests

Laboratory tests for in-depth analysis of nutrient intake are generally impractical. Hemoglobin, hematocrit, and in some cases serum ferritin levels are the determinations most often made to detect anemia, particularly iron deficiency anemia.

Nursing Diagnosis and Planning

Although some women consume more calories than they need during pregnancy, the most important nursing diagnosis concerning nutrition is

■ Altered Nutrition: Less Than Body Requirements related to lack of understanding about the nutrient needs of pregnancy.
  Expected Outcomes: The woman will consume a diet meeting the RDAs for nutrients throughout her pregnancy. The woman (of normal weight for height before pregnancy) will gain approximately 3 to 4 lb during the first trimester. She will gain 1 lb per week during the second and third trimesters, for a total gain of 25 to 35 lb.

Interventions

Identifying Problems

Identify any obvious areas of potential deficiency. For example, the woman might eat little meat, avoid vegetables, be lactose intolerant, or follow a vegetarian diet. Also determine the woman's knowledge about nutritional needs during pregnancy.

Explaining Nutrient Needs

Use the woman's diet history as a basis to introduce information about nutrition during pregnancy. Help the woman analyze her own diet so that she understands the process and its importance. Explain which important nutrients are provided in each food group and why they are necessary for her and for the fetus.

Make a rough estimate of calories, protein, iron, and calcium in the diet. To help her determine whether she eats enough of these foods on a regular basis, compare the usual sources of these major nutrients with her diet history and favorite foods. Suggest ways she can increase her intake of nutrients that she is lacking.

Providing Reinforcement

Give frequent positive reinforcement when the woman is eating appropriately. Assist her in evaluating where changes in her diet may be necessary, and plan ways to overcome weaknesses in her present diet (Fig. 15–4).

If the woman can read, give her written materials on nutrition during pregnancy and review them with her. A small pamphlet with pictures might be placed on the refrigerator to help her remember what foods she needs each day.

Evaluating Weight Gain

Compare the woman's weight to a weight gain grid to ascertain whether she has gained the appropriate amount of weight for this point in her pregnancy. Discuss the importance of weight gain and the expected pattern of weight

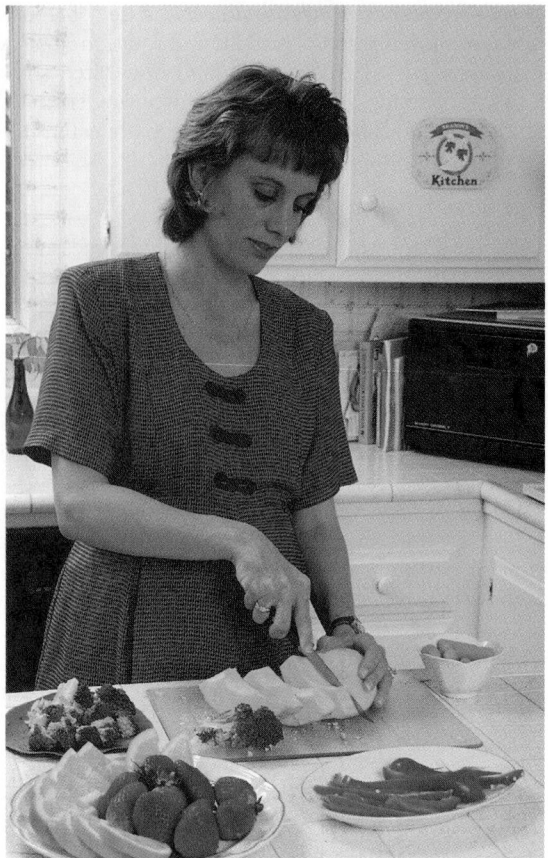

FIGURE 15–4

Women often make changes in their diets for the sake of their unborn child that they would not consider for themselves alone.

gain for her. Explain the importance of eating foods high in nutrient density when she is increasing calories.

For women of normal weight, a monthly gain of less than 2 lb (1 kg) should lead to a discussion of diet and possible problems in food intake. A gain of more than 6.5 lb (3 kg) per month may signify a serious problem such as pregnancy-induced hypertension (see Chapter 26). Errors in calculation of gestation may, however, also reflect a pattern of weight gain different from that expected.

Reassessing Nutritional Status at Each Visit

At each office or clinic visit for prenatal care, reassess the woman's dietary status. Ask her how she is doing with the diet and if she has had any difficulty. Check her weight gain to see if she is within the expected pattern. Evaluate her hemoglobin and hematocrit levels to detect anemia. If the woman is taking vitamin-mineral supplements, determine whether she is taking them regularly. Suggest ways to avoid forgetting the tablets, if that is a problem. Explain side effects, such as constipation with iron supplements.

Making Referrals

Women with health problems such as diabetes, celiac disease, or extreme weight problems may need an initial consultation with a dietitian and follow-up with the nurse. Women with inadequate financial resources to buy food can be referred to public assistance programs such as Temporary Assistance to Needy Families (TANF) or the WIC program. At the next visit, determine whether the woman obtained the help needed and whether other assistance is necessary.

Evaluation

- Does the woman gain 3 to 4 lb during the first trimester and 1 lb per week during the second and third trimesters?
- Is her total pregnancy weight gain between 25 and 35 lb?

KEY CONCEPTS

- Weight gain during pregnancy is an important determinant of fetal growth. Poor weight gain in pregnant women is associated with low birth weight in infants. Excessive weight gain may lead to macrosomia and labor complications.
- The recommended weight gain during pregnancy is 25 to 35 lb. The amount is greater for women who are underweight or who carry more than one fetus, and it is less for obese women.
- The pattern of weight gain is as important as the total increase in weight. The average should be 3 to 4 lb during the first trimester and 1 lb per week thereafter.
- The recommended increase in energy intake during pregnancy is 300 calories per day. Calorie increases should be attained by choosing foods high in nutrient density to meet the other needs of pregnancy.
- Protein should be increased to 60 g/day during pregnancy, an increase of 10 to 16 g/day over nonpregnancy needs.
- Women may not eat enough foods high in vitamins B_6, D, and E and folic acid to meet recommendations.
- Fat-soluble vitamins (A, D, E, and K) are stored in the liver. Excess consumption may result in toxic effects.
- Daily intake of water-soluble vitamins (B and C) is necessary because excesses are not stored but excreted.
- Minerals most likely to be consumed in less than recommended

amounts during pregnancy are iron, calcium, zinc, and magnesium. Iron is often added as a supplement, whereas calcium is added for women with low intake. The nurse can suggest foods high in iron and calcium.
- The routine use of vitamin-mineral supplements is unnecessary and may lead to excessive intake and toxic effects. Increased intake of some nutrients interferes with the use of others and may result in deficiencies.
- Pregnant women should drink eight to ten 8-ounce glasses of fluids each day. They should eat at least seven servings of whole grains, five servings of fruits and vegetables, three servings of dairy products, and seven ounces of protein foods daily.
- Culture can influence diet during pregnancy. The nurse should learn whether a woman follows traditional dietary practices and whether her food practices are consistent with good nutrition.
- Southeast Asian and Latino dietary practices include balancing yin and yang or "cold" and "hot" foods. The nurse must know which foods are acceptable at what times.
- Low-income women may not have enough money or knowledge to meet the nutrient needs of pregnancy. The nurse should refer them for financial assistance and nutritional counseling.
- Adolescents may skip meals and eat snacks and fast foods of low nutrient density. They are sub-

jected to peer pressure that may decrease their nutritional intake.
- Pregnant vegetarians may need help in choosing an adequate diet that includes nonanimal sources of energy, protein, iron, calcium, vitamin B_{12}, and other nutrients. Vegetarians may need vitamin-mineral supplements during pregnancy.
- Lactose-intolerant women should increase calcium intake from foods other than milk, such as calcium-rich vegetables.
- Abnormal prepregnancy weight, anemia, eating disorders, pica, grand multiparity, substance abuse, closely spaced pregnancies, and multifetal pregnancies are all nutritional risk factors that warrant adaptations of diet during pregnancy.
- Lactating women need more of almost every nutrient than women who are not lactating. The increased calories needed for milk production can be met by an added daily intake of 500 calories, and the rest can come from maternal fat stores.
- During lactation, mothers should avoid alcohol, caffeine, and foods that seem to cause distress in the infant.
- The postpartum woman who does not breast-feed should decrease her daily calorie intake by 300 calories but should eat a well-balanced diet to enhance recovery from childbirth. Weight loss should be accomplished slowly and sensibly.

ANSWER TO CRITICAL THINKING EXERCISE 15–1

It is important to be accepting and nonjudgmental in responding to this woman. It is unlikely that she will

discontinue her pica, and she may withdraw and continue to practice it in secret if she feels that the nurse is

disapproving. Therapeutic communication techniques are important to explore the woman's feelings about her cravings. A discussion of her feelings can then lead to teaching about nutrition. The nurse should determine how much ice the woman eats each day and whether she has other crav-

ings. A 24-hour diet history assists in identifying deficient areas in the diet. The nurse can work with the woman to find ways to modify the diet to include more of the food groups that

are lacking. She should be referred to a dietitian for further counseling, but the nurse should also discuss the diet at each prenatal visit.

REFERENCES AND READINGS

Abrams, B., & Pickett, K. E. (1999). Maternal nutrition. In R. K. Creasy & R. Resnik (Eds.), *Maternal-fetal medicine: Principles and practice* (4th ed., pp. 122–131). Philadelphia: Saunders.

American Academy of Pediatrics & American College of Obstetricians and Gynecologists. (1997). *Guidelines for perinatal care.* (4th ed.). Elk Grove Village, IL, and Washington, DC: Author.

American Dietetic Association. (1994). Position of the American Dietetic Association: Nutrition care for pregnant adolescents. *Journal of the American Dietetic Association, 94*(4), 449–450.

Andrews, M. M., & Boyle, J. S. (1995). *Transcultural concepts in nursing care* (2nd ed.). Philadelphia: Lippincott.

Berry, A. (1998). Focusing on folic acid. *Journal of Obstetric, Gynecologic, and Neonatal Nursing, 2*(4), 19–20.

Bronner, Y. L., & Auerbach, K. G. (1999). Maternal nutrition during lactation. In J. Riordan & K. G. Auerbach (Eds.), *Breastfeeding and human lactation* (2nd ed., pp. 515–539). Sudbury, MA: Jones & Bartlett.

Brown, H. L., Watkins, K., & Hiett, A. K. (1996). The impact of the Women, Infants and Children Food Supplement Program on birth outcome. *American Journal of Obstetrics and Gynecology, 174*(4), 1279–1283.

Cooksey, N. R. (1995). Pica and olfactory craving of pregnancy: How deep are the secrets? *Birth, 23*(1), 129–137.

Cunningham, F. G., MacDonald, P. C., Gant, N. F., Leveno, K. J., Gilstrap, L. C., Hankins, G. D. V., & Clark, S. L. (1997). *Williams obstetrics* (20th ed.). Norwalk, CT: Appleton & Lange.

Davis, J., & Sherer, K. (1994). *Applied nutrition and diet therapy for nurses* (2nd ed.). Philadelphia: Saunders.

Duffy, T. P. (1999). Hematologic aspects of pregnancy. In G. N. Burrow & T. F. Ferris (Eds.), *Medical complications during pregnancy* (5th ed., pp. 79–96). Philadelphia: Saunders.

Galanti, G. (1997). *Caring for patients from different cultures* (2nd ed.). Philadelphia: University of Pennsylvania Press.

Godfrey, K. M., Barker, D. J. P., Robinson, S., & Osmond, C. (1997, June). Maternal birthweight and diet in pregnancy in relation to the infant's thinness at birth. *British Journal of Obstetrics and Gynaecology, 104*, 663–667.

Groff, J. Y., Mullen, P. D., Mongoven, M., & Burau, K. (1997). Prenatal weight gain patterns and infant birth-weight associated with maternal smoking. *Birth, 24*(4), 234–239.

Hickey, C. A., McNeal, S. F., Menefee, L., & Ivey, S. (1997). Prenatal weight gain within upper and lower recommended ranges: Effect on birth weight of black and white infants. *Obstetrics and Gynecology, 90*(4, pt. 1), 489–494.

Hutchinson, M. K., & Baziaziz, M. (1994). Nursing care of the childbearing Muslim family. *Journal of Obstetric, Gynecologic, and Neonatal Nursing, 23*(9), 767–771.

Institute of Medicine, National Academy of Sciences, Food and Nutrition Board. (1990). *Nutrition during pregnancy.* Part I: Weight gain. Part II: Nutrient supplements. Washington, DC: National Academy Press.

Institute of Medicine, National Academy of Sciences, Food and Nutrition Board. (1991). *Nutrition during lactation.* Washington, DC: National Academy Press.

Institute of Medicine, National Academy of Sciences, Subcommittee for a Clinical Application Guide. (1992). *Nutrition during pregnancy and lactation: An implementation guide.* Washington, DC: National Academy Press.

Kendig, S., & Barron, M. L. (1996). Antenatal care and risk assessment strategies. In K. R. Simpson & P. A. Creehan (Eds.), *AWHONN perinatal nursing* (pp. 73–108). Philadelphia: Lippincott–Raven.

Kolasa, K. M., & Weismiller, D. G. (1995). Nutrition during pregnancy. *American Family Physician 56*(1), 205–212.

LaLeche League International. (1997). *The breastfeeding answer book* (rev. ed.). Schaumburg, IL: Author.

Lawrence, R. A., & Lawrence, R. M. (1999). *Breastfeeding: A guide for the medical profession* (5th ed.). St. Louis: Mosby.

Lipson, J. G., Dibble, S. L., & Minarik, P. A. (1996). *Culture and nursing care: A pocket guide.* San Francisco: University of California, San Francisco, Nursing Press.

Lust, K. D., Brown, J. E., & Thomas, W. (1996). Maternal intake of cruciferous vegetables and other foods and colic symptoms in exclusively breastfed infants. *Journal of the American Dietetic Association, 96*(1), 46–48.

Mahan, L. K., & Escott-Stump, S. (1996). Nutrition during adolescence. In L. K. Mahan & S. Escott-Stump (Eds.), *Krause's food, nutrition, and diet therapy* (9th ed., pp. 275–286). Philadelphia: Saunders.

Mattson, S. (1995). Culturally sensitive perinatal care for Southeast Asians. *Journal of Obstetric, Gynecologic, and Neonatal Nursing, 24*(4), 335–341.

Mitchell, M. K. (1997). *Nutrition across the life span.* Philadelphia: Saunders.

Morin, K. H. (1998). Perinatal outcomes of obese women: A review of the literature.

Journal of Obstetric, Gynecologic, and Neonatal Nursing, 27(4), 431–440.

Neuhouser, M. L. S. (1996). Nutrition during pregnancy and lactation. In L. K. Mahan & S. Escott-Stump (Eds.), *Krause's food, nutrition, and diet therapy* (9th ed., pp. 181–212). Philadelphia: Saunders.

Niebyl, J. R. (1996). Iron therapy in pregnancy. *Contemporary OB/GYN, 41*(3), 146–150.

Peckenpaugh, N. J., & Poleman, C. M. (1999). *Nutrition essentials and diet therapy* (8th ed.). Philadelphia: Saunders.

Perry, G. S., Yip, R., & Zyrkowski, C. (1995). Nutritional risk factors among low-income pregnant U.S. women: The Centers for Disease Control and Prevention (CDC) pregnancy nutrition surveillance system 1979 through 1993. *Seminars in Perinatology, 19*(3), 211–221.

Purfield, P., & Morin, K. (1995). Excessive weight gain in primigravidas with low-risk pregnancy: Selected obstetric consequences. *Journal of Obstetric, Gynecologic, and Neonatal Nursing, 24*(5), 434–439.

Rose, N. C., & Mennuti, M. T. (1995). Periconceptional folic acid supplementation as a social intervention. *Seminars in Perinatology, 19*(4), 243–254.

Scholl, T. O., & Hediger, M. L. (1995). Weight gain, nutrition, and pregnancy outcome: Findings from the Camden study of teenage and minority gravidas. *Seminars in Perinatology, 19*(3), 171–181.

Scholl, T. O., Hediger, M. L., Schall, J. I., Khoo, C., & Fischer, R. L. (1994). Maternal growth during pregnancy and the competition for nutrients. *American Journal of Clinical Nutrition, 60*, 183–188.

Seidman, R. Y., Jacobson, S., Primeaux, M., Burns, P., & Weatherby, F. (1996). Assessing American Indian families. *MCN: American Journal of Maternal/Child Nursing, 21*(6), 274–279.

Tinkle, M. B., & Sterling, B. S. (1997). Neural tube defects: A primary prevention role for nurses. *Journal of Obstetric, Gynecologic, and Neonatal Nursing, 26*(5), 503–512.

U.S. Department of Health and Human Services, Public Health Service. (1995). *Healthy people 2000: Midcourse review and 1995 revisions.* Washington, DC: Author.

Williams, S. R. (1997). *Nutrition and diet therapy* (8th ed.). St. Louis: Times Mirror/Mosby.

Williams, S. R. (1997). Nutrition assessment and guidance in prenatal care. In B. Worthington-Roberts & S. R. Williams (Eds.), *Nutrition in pregnancy and lactation* (6th ed., pp. 220–253). St. Louis: Times Mirror/Mosby.

Worthington-Roberts, B. S. (1997a). Energy and vitamin needs during pregnancy. In B. Worthington-Roberts & S. R. Williams (Eds.), *Nutrition in pregnancy and lactation* (6th ed., pp. 128–166). St. Louis: Times Mirror/Mosby.

Worthington-Roberts, B. S. (1997b). Mineral needs during pregnancy. In B. Worthing-ton-Roberts & S. R. Williams (Eds.), *Nutrition in pregnancy and lactation* (6th ed., pp. 167–192). St. Louis: Times Mirror/Mosby.

Worthington-Roberts, B. S. (1997c). Nutrition, fertility, and family planning. In B. Worthington-Roberts & S. R. Williams (Eds.), *Nutrition in pregnancy and lactation* (6th ed., pp. 31–57). St. Louis: Times Mirror/Mosby.

Worthington-Roberts, B. S., & Rees, J. M. (1997). The pregnant adolescent: Special concerns. In B. Worthington-Roberts & S. R. Williams (Eds.), *Nutrition in pregnancy and lactation* (6th ed., pp. 292–318). St. Louis: Times Mirror/Mosby.

16

Prenatal Diagnostic Tests

LEARNING OBJECTIVES

After studying this chapter, you should be able to:

- Identify indications for fetal diagnostic procedures.
- Discuss the purpose, procedure, advantages, and risks of each diagnostic procedure presented in the chapter.
- Provide information in response to common questions parents have about procedures.

DEFINITIONS

alpha-fetoprotein Plasma protein produced by the fetus.

amniocentesis Transabdominal puncture of the amniotic sac to obtain a sample of amniotic fluid that contains fetal cells and biochemical substances for laboratory examination.

biophysical profile Method for evaluating fetal status during the antepartum period based on five fetal variables: fetal heart rate, breathing movements, gross movements, muscle tone, and amniotic fluid volume.

chorionic villus sampling Transcervical or transabdominal sampling of chorionic villi (projections of the outer fetal membrane) for analysis of fetal cells.

contraction stress test Method for evaluating fetal status during the antepartum period by observing the response of the fetal heart to the stress of uterine contractions, which may induce recurrent episodes of fetal hypoxia.

late deceleration Slowing of the fetal heart rate after the onset of a uterine contraction that persists after the contraction ends.

lecithin/sphingomyelin ratio (L/S ratio) Ratio of two phospholipids in amniotic fluid that is used to determine fetal lung maturity.

neural tube defect A congenital defect in the closure of the bony encasement of the spinal cord or of the skull.

nonstress test A method for evaluating fetal status during the antepartum period by observing for accelerations of the fetal heart rate.

percutaneous umbilical blood sampling (cordocentesis) Procedure for obtaining fetal blood through ultrasound-guided puncture of an umbilical cord vessel to detect fetal problems such as inherited blood disorders, acidosis, or infection.

phosphatidylglycerol A phospholipid component of surfactant; its presence in amniotic fluid indicates fetal lung maturity.

phosphatidylinositol A phospholipid component of surfactant that is produced and secreted in increasing amounts as the fetal lungs mature.

placenta previa Abnormal implantation of the placenta in the lower uterus, at or near the cervical os.

surfactant A mixture of lipoproteins produced by the lungs of the mature fetus that reduces surface tension in the alveoli, thus promoting lung expansion after birth.

triple-marker screening Analysis of maternal serum for abnormal levels of alpha-fetoprotein, human chorionic gonadotropin, and estriols that may predict chromosomal abnormalities of the fetus.

ultrasonography Technique for visualizing deep structures of the body by recording the reflections (echoes) of sound waves directed into the tissue.

uteroplacental insufficiency Decreased ability of the placenta to exchange oxygen, carbon dioxide, nutrients, and waste products properly between the maternal and fetal circulations.

vibroacoustic stimulation test Use of sound stimulation to elicit acceleration of the fetal heart rate.

Until recently, only nonspecific methods were available to assess the condition of the fetus. Fundal height was measured to estimate fetal growth; the fetal heart rate was auscultated; and the mother's perception of fetal movements was noted. In recent years, however, the development of a variety of sophisticated methods has made it possible to detect physical abnormalities in the fetus and to monitor the fetal condition with greater accuracy.

The ability to predict fetal outcome offers reassurance for some parents but not all. If the fetus is free of anomalies and is determined to be in good condition, the parents are relieved. If fetal health is uncertain and the tests must be repeated, however, the parents may experience anxiety throughout the pregnancy. If fetal anomalies are identified, the parents must then decide whether to continue or terminate the pregnancy. This decision can create emotional conflict and raise ethical dilemmas that impose a great deal of stress on the family.

Indications for Prenatal Diagnostic Tests

In general, two reasons exist for performing fetal diagnostic procedures: to detect congenital anomalies and to evaluate the condition of the fetus. Some procedures, such as amniocentesis and ultrasonography, are used for both purposes.

Many of these procedures are done only if there is reason to believe the fetus may have a problem. Physicians often offer some tests, such as ultrasonography or maternal serum screening, to all pregnant women. Various risk factors increase the likelihood that a fetus will have a problem that can be detected prenatally. Table 16–1 lists some risk factors for which prenatal diagnostic procedures are often recommended.

Ultrasonography

When high-frequency sound waves are aimed in a specific direction, they are deflected by objects in their path and return as echoes. The amount of energy returned as an echo depends on the density of the object that deflected the ultrasonic wave. In obstetrics, when ultrasonic waves are directed through the maternal abdomen, they are deflected by tissue; the returning sound waves are converted to two-dimensional images showing structures of different densities (Fig. 16–1).

Almost all ultrasound procedures in obstetrics now use real-time scanning in which a rapid sequence of fixed images is displayed on the screen, showing movement as it happens. This technique allows the observer to detect fetal heartbeat, fetal breathing activity, and fetal body movement.

Emotional Responses

Some expectant mothers are excited and pleased and report feelings of love and protectiveness when they view the fetus. Others, however, report increased feelings of vulnerability and anxiety about the fetus. Some mothers state that they fear something will be found wrong, and they dread the procedure.

Expectant fathers are often fascinated by fetal movement and insist that the fetus "waved" at them or that they could see the facial expression as the fetus looked directly at them. Some couples wish to be told whether the fetus is male or female and are either disappointed or pleased with

---

TABLE 16–1

Indications for Fetal Diagnostic Procedures

Medical Conditions

Preexisting diabetes mellitus or gestational diabetes
Hypertension (chronic or pregnancy-induced)
Chronic infections (such as pyelonephritis)
Sexually transmissible diseases
Anemia
Parents carry or express a genetic disorder (such as sickle cell anemia or cystic fibrosis)

Demographic Factors

Maternal age <16 or >35 years
Poverty
Nonwhite (twice the risk of neonatal or infant death)
Inadequate prenatal care (initial visit after 20 weeks' gestation or fewer than five prenatal visits to physician or nurse-midwife)

Obstetric Factors

History of low-birth-weight infant (<2,500 g)
Multifetal pregnancy
Malpresentation (breech, shoulder)
Previous fetal loss or birth of infant with congenital anomaly
Previous infant >4,000 g at birth
Hydramnios (>2,000 ml at term)
Oligohydramnios (<500 ml at term)
Decrease or absence in fetal movements
Uncertainty about gestational age
Suspected intrauterine growth restriction
Postmaturity (>42 weeks)
Preterm labor (>20 weeks and <38 weeks of gestation)
Grand multiparity (>5 pregnancies)

Concurrent Maternal Factors

Less than ideal weight for height at conception
More than 20% above ideal weight for height at conception
Inadequate weight gain or poor pattern of weight gain
Excessive weight gain
Use of drugs, alcohol, tobacco

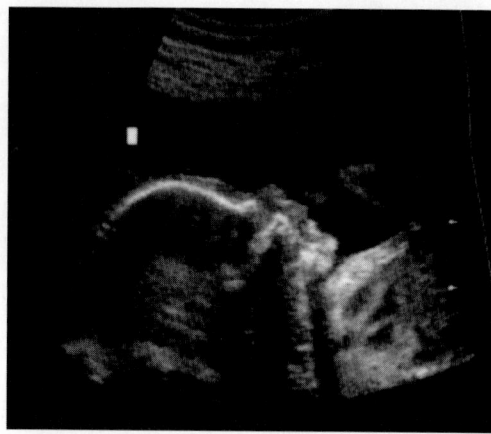

FIGURE 16-1

Sonogram showing profile of fetal facial structures. (Courtesy of Karin Buxton.)

the news. Others do not want to know the sex of the child, even if it is obvious, and prefer to wait and "be surprised."

Although ultrasonography is not yet a standard of care for all women, it is widely used because a great deal of information can be obtained with minimum risk to mother or fetus. Ultrasonography may be used during any trimester, but the procedure and the reasons for its use vary for each trimester.

First Trimester

Transvaginal ultrasonography is often used during the first trimester because the uterus, gestational sac, embryo, and deep pelvic structures, such as the ovaries and fallopian tubes, are clearly visible with this technique.

PROCEDURE

The woman is placed in a lithotomy position for transvaginal ultrasonography. A transvaginal probe that is encased in a disposable cover and coated with a gel that provides lubrication and promotes conductivity is inserted into the vagina. The woman may feel more comfortable if she inserts the probe herself. The procedure takes about 10 to 15 minutes.

PURPOSES

During the first trimester, ultrasonography is most frequently used to do the following:

- Confirm pregnancy
- Verify the location of the pregnancy (uterine or ectopic)
- Detect multifetal gestation
- Determine gestational age
- Confirm fetal viability
- Determine the position of the uterus, cervix, and area of placental formation for transcervical chorionic villus sampling
- Guide the needle insertion for transabdominal chorionic villus sampling

During the first trimester, gestational age is based on the appearance of the gestational sac, which can be seen as

early as 4 weeks after the last menstrual period (Berman, 1996). During the sixth week the embryo and adjacent yolk sac are visible. At this time, the crown-to-rump length of the embryo is the most reliable indicator of gestational age (DuBose, 1996a) (Fig. 16–2).

Fetal viability is confirmed by observing the fetal heartbeat, which is visible by the eighth week following the last menstrual period. The heartbeat averages 168 beats per minute (BPM) at this gestational age. In addition, embryonic organs can be studied for normal growth and appearance (Berman, 1996). Maternal abnormalities, such as bicornuate uterus, uterine fibroids, and ovarian cysts, are also visible.

Second and Third Trimesters

During the second and third trimesters the uterus moves higher out of the pelvis, allowing clear views of the fetus and placenta, which are no longer obstructed by pelvic bones. As a result, transabdominal ultrasonography is most often used.

PROCEDURE

The expectant mother is positioned on her back with her head and knees supported by pillows. If she desires, a display panel can be positioned so that she (and the father) can see the images on the screen. Her head should be elevated, and she should be turned slightly to one side to prevent supine hypotension, which may be caused by compression of the vena cava and aorta by the gravid uterus. A wedge or rolled blanket is placed under one hip to help her maintain this position comfortably. Warm mineral oil or transmission gel is spread over her abdomen, and the sonographer (nurse, physician, or ultrasound technician) slowly moves a transducer over the abdomen to obtain a picture (Fig. 16–3).

The procedure takes 10 to 30 minutes. The sonographer can "freeze" a picture and copy it for permanent records or for the parents if they wish. Many new ultrasound systems offer videotaping of the evaluation, and some facilities provide a small section of videotape for the parents.

During the second trimester a urine-filled bladder displaces the gas-filled intestines and elevates the uterus for better visibility. If a full bladder is necessary, the woman should be instructed to drink 1 to 2 quarts of clear fluid an hour before the time of the examination, and she should be instructed not to void until the examination is completed. Some discomfort may be felt as the transducer is moved over the distended bladder.

PURPOSES

Ultrasonography is used during the second and third trimesters to do the following:

- Confirm gestational age
- Locate the placenta when placenta previa is suspected
- Determine fetal presentation
- Evaluate amniotic fluid volume (p. 337)
- Monitor and document fetal movements
- Guide needle placement when amniocentesis or percutaneous umbilical blood sampling is necessary

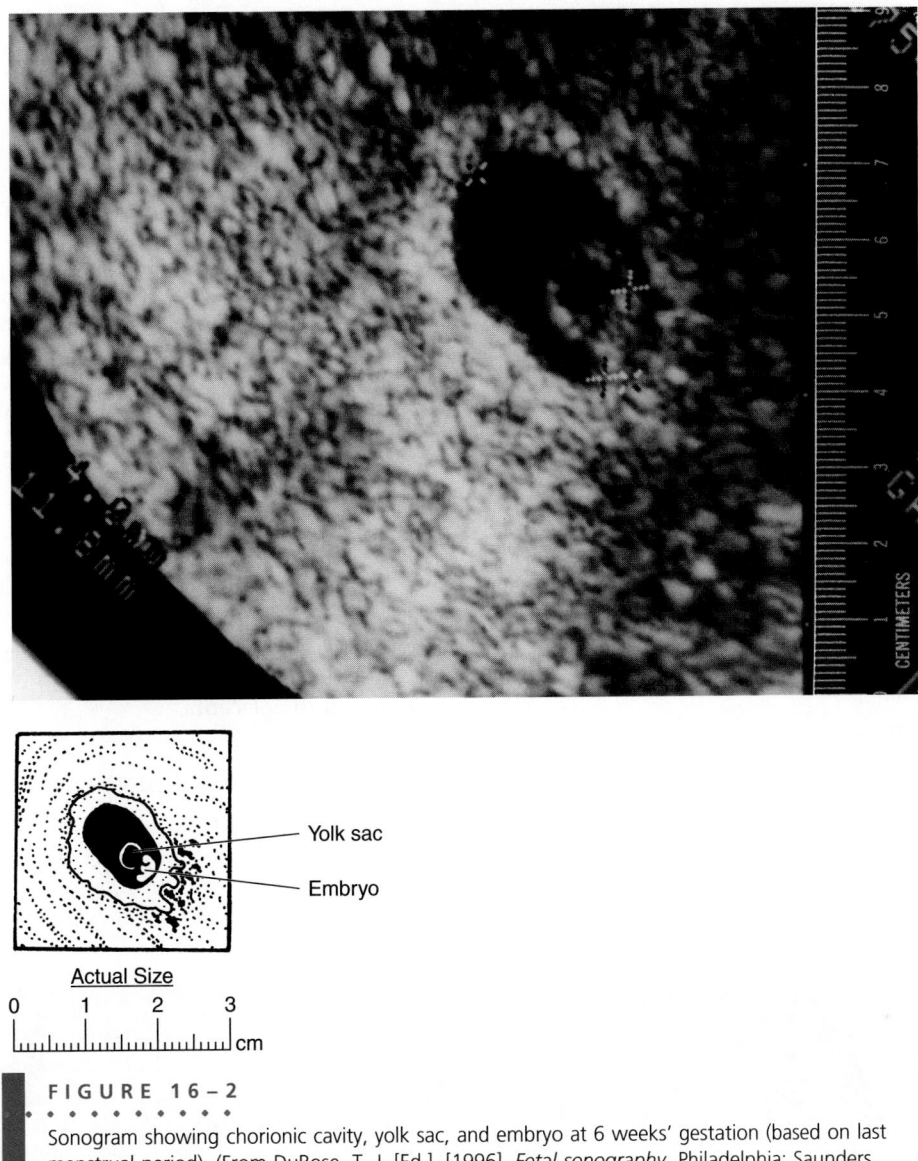

FIGURE 16–2

Sonogram showing chorionic cavity, yolk sac, and embryo at 6 weeks' gestation (based on last menstrual period). (From DuBose, T. J. [Ed.]. [1996]. *Fetal sonography.* Philadelphia: Saunders. Sonogram by T. J. DuBose, MS, RDMS.)

Several measurements help estimate gestational age during the last half of pregnancy, such as biparietal diameter, femur length, and abdominal circumference. Measurements have different reliability at different gestational ages. Multiple measurements will help date the pregnancy more accurately than a single measurement.

Gestational age must be determined accurately when screening for maternal serum alpha-fetoprotein (AFP), which is altered by fetal age. Accurate gestational age is also important if intrauterine growth restriction is suspected or if there is a question about the expected date of delivery.

Assessment of fetal movements is important because coordination of whole-body movement requires complex neurologic control, which indicates that the nervous system is functioning well. Less body movement than expected may indicate fetal compromise, especially if placental perfusion is suspected to be inadequate, with resulting fetal hypoxia and acidosis.

In the second trimester, ultrasound may be targeted toward specific evaluation of fetal anatomy and physiology. Targeted ultrasonography is indicated when an increased risk exists for fetal anomalies. Risk factors include prior birth of an infant with anomalies or abnormal clinical findings, such as *hydramnios* (excessive amniotic fluid), *oligohydramnios* (insufficient amniotic fluid), or abnormal levels of AFP. The fetal anatomy is carefully and systematically examined to identify major system and organ anomalies. Anomalies that can be detected with targeted ultrasonography include neural tube defects, protrusion of intestine through the intestinal wall (gastroschisis), malformed kidneys, hydrocephalus, obstruction in the fetal bowel or urinary system, and cleft lip and palate.

Ultrasonography may be also used to evaluate placental maturity on the basis of the distribution of calcium deposits within the placenta and the increasing delineations that occur as the placenta matures.

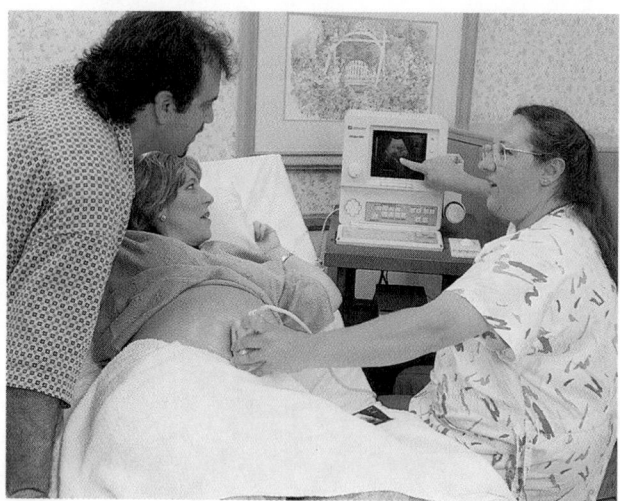

FIGURE 16–3

The nurse provides information as she moves an ultrasound transducer over the mother's abdomen to obtain an image.

Advantages

Ultrasonography allows clear visualization of the fetus and surrounding structures, and it is safe. No clinically significant adverse effects have been reported (Anthony, 1996; Berman, 1996). Ultrasonography is noninvasive and relatively comfortable, and the results are obtained immediately. It is widely available and the scanner is portable, so that it can be moved to the area of need.

Disadvantages

The cost of ultrasonography can be a problem for a woman who does not have insurance or who does not have access to prenatal care in the first trimester of pregnancy.

Doppler Ultrasound Blood Flow Assessment

When an ultrasound wave is directed at an acute angle to a moving target, such as blood flowing through a vessel, the frequency of the echoes changes as the cardiac cycle goes through systole and diastole. This change, referred to as the *Doppler shift*, indicates forward movement of blood within a vessel.

Purpose

The primary indication for Doppler ultrasonography is to detect or confirm intrauterine growth restriction, which is recognizable because of characteristic blood flow abnormalities (Cartier, 1996). Doppler ultrasonography has been used most extensively to study blood flow through the umbilical vessels and the placenta.

Color Doppler Imaging

The location of any Doppler shift can be imaged as either red or blue, depending on whether the direction of the flow is toward the transducer or away from the transducer, respectively. Figure 16–4 illustrates the use of color Doppler

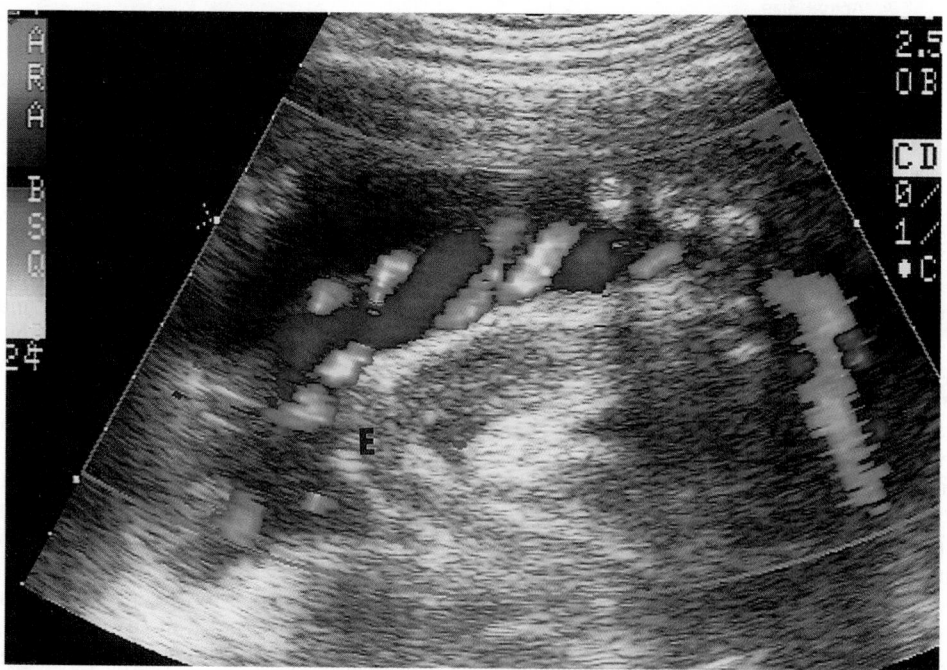

FIGURE 16–4

Color Doppler imaging of the umbilical vein and two arteries. Blood flow toward the transducer is shown in blue and the flow away is shown in red. Three fetal fingers can be seen to grasp and press the cord against the other wrist. (From DuBose, T. J. [Ed.]. [1996]. *Fetal sonography.* Philadelphia: Saunders. Sonogram by T. J. DuBose, MS, RDMS.)

imaging to measure blood flow and velocity in umbilical vessels. Doppler imaging is also useful in assessing fetal blood flow in other areas, such as the brain and aorta.

Alpha-Fetoprotein Screening

Alpha-fetoprotein is the predominant protein in fetal plasma. It diffuses from fetal plasma into fetal urine and is excreted into the amniotic fluid. Some AFP crosses placental membranes into the maternal circulation. Therefore, AFP can be measured in both maternal serum (MSAFP) and in amniotic fluid (AFAFP). Abnormal concentrations of AFP are associated with serious fetal anomalies, requiring additional testing to rule out an abnormality or verify it.

The AFP concentration increases with advancing gestational age of the fetus. It is also higher in multifetal gestations because more than one fetus is producing the protein. Maternal weight influences the maternal serum value because AFP diffuses into a larger maternal compartment in heavier women.

Purpose

Low levels of MSAFP are associated with chromosomal anomalies, such as trisomy 21 (Down syndrome). The most common cause of elevated AFP is failure of the embryonic neural tube to close properly. In this condition, neural tissue is totally exposed or covered with only a very thin layer of tissue, allowing high concentrations of AFP to seep into amniotic fluid and enter maternal serum.

The most common open neural tube defects are anencephaly, in which the cranial vault is absent and most of the brain is undeveloped, and spina bifida, which has a wide range of severity (see p. 1479). See Table 16–2 for other conditions that are associated with abnormal MSAFP.

TABLE 16–2
• • • • • • • • • • •

Conditions Associated with Abnormal Maternal Serum Alpha-Fetoprotein (AFP) Levels

---

Elevated Levels of AFP

Open neural tube defects
Esophageal obstruction
Abdominal wall defects (omphalocele, gastroschisis)
Increased amount leaked by fetal kidney
    (hydronephrosis)
Threatened abortion
Fetal demise
Normal fetus in conjunction with one or more of the
    following:
    Amniotic fluid contaminated with fetal blood
    Underestimation of fetal age
    Multifetal gestation
    Decreased maternal weight
    Maternal insulin-dependent diabetes

Low Levels of AFP

Chromosomal trisomies (e.g., Down syndrome)
Gestational trophoblastic disease
Normal fetuses in conjunction with:
    Overestimation of gestational age
    Increased maternal weight

Procedure

Women should be offered MSAFP screening, ideally between 15 and 18 weeks of gestation (American Academy of Pediatrics [AAP] & American College of Obstetricians and Gynecologists [ACOG], 1997). The mother is informed that MSAFP is a screening test and that further tests will be necessary to investigate abnormal concentrations. If MSAFP levels are abnormal, basic ultrasonography is recommended to determine whether the abnormal concentration is due to multifetal gestation, inaccurate gestational age, or fetal demise.

If ultrasonography fails to explain the abnormal levels of AFP, amniocentesis is the next step offered. Amniotic fluid is analyzed for elevated levels of AFP and for acetylcholinesterase (AChE). Elevations of AChE have been noted in association with open neural tube defects. Amniotic fluid can also be analyzed for chromosome makeup if MSAFP values are lower than expected.

Advantages

Maternal serum AFP evaluation has several advantages:

- It is a simple procedure that requires only a sample of maternal blood.
- It is the least invasive and most economic procedure to screen for an open neural tube defect or chromosome abnormality.
- Prenatal diagnosis allows parents time to examine their options or to prepare for the birth of an infant who will need special care.

Limitations

Some major limitations of MSAFP evaluation are the following:

- It is a screening test only and must be viewed as the first step in a series of diagnostic procedures that are necessary if abnormal concentrations are found.
- Because other benign conditions, such as inaccurate estimation of gestational age, can result in apparently abnormal levels, the parents may experience a great deal of anxiety and expense when follow-up tests are necessary.
- Timing also imposes some limits. Maternal serum AFP evaluation is best performed between 15 and 18 weeks of pregnancy, but many women do not seek prenatal care until after the 18th week and therefore miss the opportunity for MSAFP screening.
- If the maternal weight is inaccurate, interpretation of MSAFP values may be inaccurate as well. For example, if the woman's reported weight is 20 lb lighter than her actual weight, a MSAFP value reported in the normal range may be high for the actual weight.
- Because closed neural tube defects do not produce elevated levels of AFP, normal levels of AFP do not guarantee that the baby will be free of anomalies.

Triple-Marker Screening

Two other markers, human chorionic gonadotropin (hCG) and unconjugated estriol, have been added to MSAFP evaluation to screen for chromosomal abnormalities. This triple-marker screening has been found to increase the detection of trisomy 18 and trisomy 21 (Kellner et al., 1995). Maternal serum samples are taken between 15 and 22 weeks' gestation (based on the last menstrual period), and the results are considered positive if all three markers are low. In that case, the woman should be offered additional testing, such as amniocentesis for karyotyping.

Chorionic Villus Sampling

Chorionic villi are microscopic projections from the outer membrane (chorion) that develop and burrow into endometrial tissue as the placenta is formed. The villi are composed of rapidly dividing cells of fetal origin that reflect the chromosomal and genetic makeup of the fetus. Chorionic villus sampling is used to obtain cells from the chorionic villi for diagnosis of abnormalities that can be identified by studying these cells.

Purpose

Chorionic villus sampling is most often used to diagnose fetal chromosome abnormalities. It cannot be used to diagnose anomalies for which amniotic fluid is essential, such as open neural tube defects, which require measuring AFP levels.

Indications

Chorionic villus sampling is recommended only for women who are at high risk for giving birth to an infant with genetic anomalies that can be diagnosed from the fetal cells. Its use is restricted because of reported complications, such as spotting or bleeding, uterine cramping, and fetal loss. Women past the age of 35 years, those with a history of a previous fetus with anomalies that can be detected with fetal cells, or couples who are carriers or who exhibit genetic defects are at the greatest risk for giving birth to an infant with genetic anomalies. For these women, chorionic villus sampling may be an option to consider.

Procedure

Chorionic villus sampling can be performed under aseptic conditions by two techniques. Both techniques use ultrasonography to guide the sampling. A full bladder is required to push the uterus up and out of the pelvic cavity.

In the transcervical technique, a flexible catheter is inserted through the cervix and a sample of chorionic villi is aspirated (Fig. 16–5). In the transabdominal technique, a needle is inserted through the abdominal and uterine walls and chorionic tissue is aspirated.

Advantages

Chorionic villus sampling offers several advantages over second-trimester procedures for the prenatal diagnosis of genetic defects.

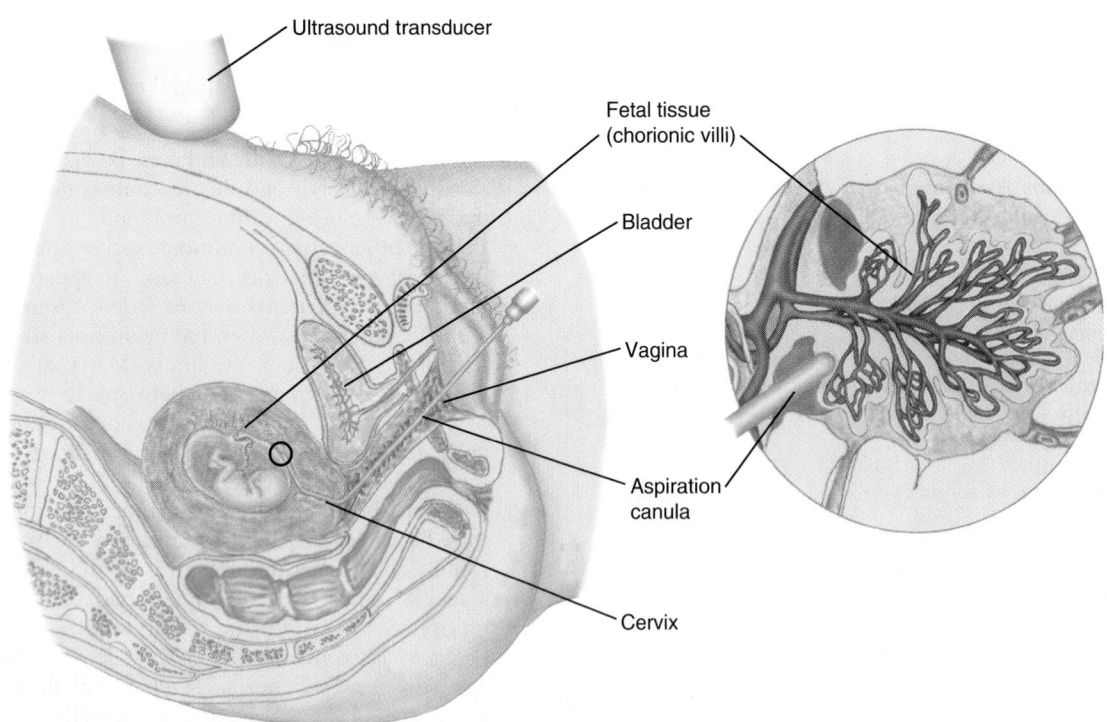

Ultrasound transducer

Fetal tissue (chorionic villi)

Bladder

Vagina

Aspiration canula

Cervix

FIGURE 16–5

Transcervical chorionic villus sampling. Tissue is aspirated to detect the presence of genetic defects in the fetus. A transcervical technique is shown; transabdominal aspiration is an alternative method.

- The results are available quickly, often within 24 to 48 hours.
- The technique allows prenatal diagnosis as early as 10 weeks for women who find second-trimester procedures unacceptable.
- It may save women carrying affected fetuses from the physical and emotional trauma of a second-trimester abortion.

Risks

Although chorionic villus sampling is now considered a safe and effective technique for first-trimester prenatal diagnosis, there are risks.

- The pregnancy loss rate is slightly higher than with amniocentesis. Factors that decrease the risk of pregnancy loss include an experienced team, an anterior placenta, and the ease with which the sample is obtained.
- The are some reports of a higher than expected rate of limb reduction defects when the procedure was performed at 6 to 8 weeks. However, most experienced centers that perform chorionic villus sampling after 10 weeks of gestation have not seen an increase in the rate of limb reduction defects (Wapner, 1997). Still, families should be informed about the possible added risk until definitive studies have been completed.
- The risk for Rh sensitization is increased. Rh_o (D) immune globulin should be administered to all unsensitized Rh-negative women following the procedure (see p. 656).

Infection has not been a major problem with chorionic villus sampling. However, the procedure is contraindicated if endocervicitis, active genital herpes, pelvic inflammatory process, or a positive culture for *Neisseria gonorrhoeae* has been documented.

The family should receive genetic counseling before the test is performed. The risks and benefits of the procedure should be carefully explained and signed consent obtained. The woman should be informed that the actual procedure takes about half an hour, but up to 2 hours should be allotted in case of delays.

After the procedure, maternal vital signs are assessed, and the woman is allowed to void. A small amount of vaginal spotting may appear, but heavy bleeding or the passage of amniotic fluid, clots, or tissue should be reported. The woman needs to rest at home for several hours after the procedure.

Amniocentesis

Amniocentesis is aspiration of amniotic fluid from the amniotic sac for examination (Fig. 16–6). Amniocentesis may be performed during the midtrimester or the last trimester of pregnancy, depending on the purpose. Midtrimester amniocentesis is best performed between 15 and 18 weeks because amniotic fluid volume is adequate and there are many viable fetal cells in the fluid.

Early amniocentesis is possible between 11 and 14 weeks, and may be an option if the woman does not live near a center that offers chorionic villus sampling (Reece, 1997) or if the relatively late test results from later amnio-

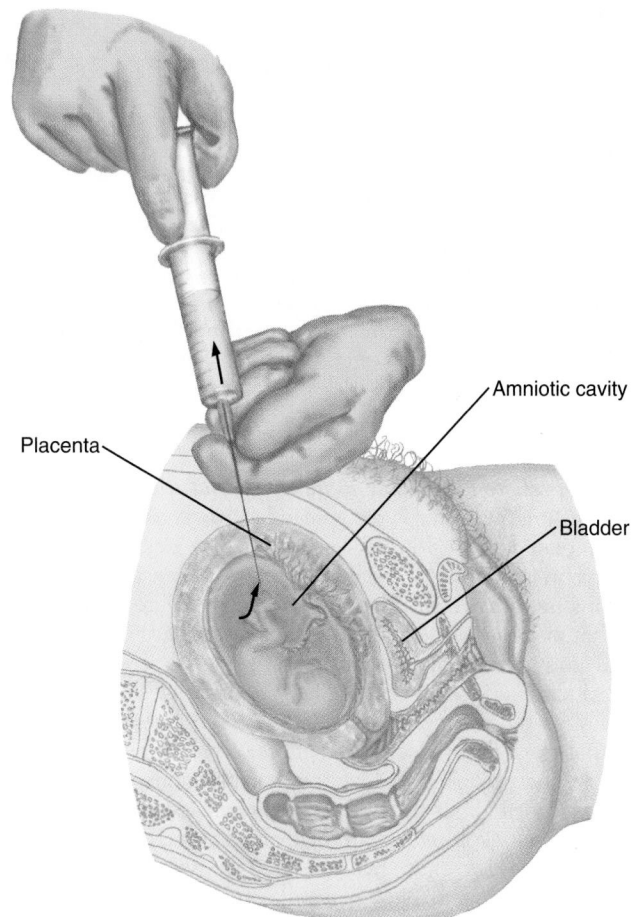

FIGURE 16–6

In amniocentesis, a needle is inserted through the expectant mother's abdomen to aspirate fluid from the amniotic sac. The fluid can then be tested to detect chromosomal abnormalities or other problems and to determine fetal lung maturity.

centesis are unacceptable. Early amniocentesis is associated with a higher fetal loss rate than later amniocentesis (Cunningham, et al., 1997).

Purposes

MIDTRIMESTER

The primary purpose for midtrimester amniocentesis is to examine fetal cells present in amniotic fluid to identify chromosomal abnormalities. Amniocentesis is also used to evaluate the fetal condition when the woman is sensitized to Rh-positive blood, to diagnose amnionitis, and to test the amniotic fluid AFP when MSAFP is abnormal and a cause for the abnormal levels cannot be determined by other tests.

THIRD TRIMESTER

During the third trimester, amniocentesis is usually performed to determine fetal maturity or to diagnose fetal hemolytic disease, most often caused by Rh incompatibility.

Indications for Second-Trimester Amniocentesis

Maternal age > 35 years

Chromosomal abnormality in close family member

Sex determination for maternal carrier of X-linked disorder (such as hemophilia or Duchenne's muscular dystrophy)

Birth of previous infant with chromosomal abnormalities or neural tube defect

Pregnancy after three or more spontaneous abortions

Elevated levels of maternal serum alpha-fetoprotein

Maternal Rh sensitization

Tests to Determine Fetal Lung Maturity. A test for fetal lung maturity is recommended when delivery is contemplated before 38 weeks' gestation. The lecithin/sphingomyelin (L/S) ratio is the best-known test for estimating fetal lung maturity. Lecithin and sphingomyelin are lipoproteins that make up surfactant, which is present in the pulmonary alveoli in term infants. Surfactant keeps the alveoli open by reducing surface tension on their inner walls. The decreased surface tension prevents collapse of the alveoli when the infant exhales, reducing the effort of breathing.

The proportion of lecithin to sphingomyelin is about equal until about the 30th week of gestation. At this time the level of sphingomyelin plateaus, but lecithin continues to rise. An L/S ratio greater than 2:1 (twice as much lecithin as sphingomyelin) generally indicates that surfactant is adequate and the fetal lungs are mature. An L/S ratio of 2:1 does not ensure fetal lung maturity in all women, however, particularly women who have diabetes. Amniotic fluid is therefore also tested for the presence of phosphatidylglycerol (PG) and phosphatidylinositol (PI), which are other phospholipids that boost the properties of lecithin.

Test for Fetal Hemolytic Disease. Amniocentesis is also performed to determine fetal bilirubin concentration if the mother is Rh-negative and is sensitized (that is, has been exposed to the Rh antigen and has developed antibodies against Rh-positive erythrocytes). The level of bilirubin in amniotic fluid reflects the amount of fetal red blood cell destruction that occurs when maternal antibodies destroy Rh-positive fetal red blood cells, leaving the fetus vulnerable to erythroblastosis fetalis and hydrops fetalis (see Chapter 30).

Procedure

The woman is placed in a supine position and is draped with her abdomen exposed. A rolled towel is placed under one buttock to shift the weight of the uterus off the vena cava and aorta. Maternal blood pressure and fetal heart tones are assessed to establish baseline levels.

Ultrasonography is used to locate the fetus and placenta, to identify the largest pockets of amniotic fluid that can safely be sampled, and to guide needle insertion. The skin is prepared with antiseptic solution. A small amount of local anesthetic may be injected into the skin. This step causes the only pain the woman experiences, although she may experience the sensation of pressure as the needle is inserted and mild cramping as the needle enters the myometrium.

A 3- to 4-inch, 20- or 21-gauge needle is inserted into the pocket of fluid. Approximately 20 ml of fluid is removed for analysis. The woman rests quietly for 30 to 60 minutes afterward with electronic monitoring of fetal heart rate. She may resume normal activities after 24 hours (Reece, 1997). She should report persistent uterine contractions, vaginal bleeding, leakage of amniotic fluid, or fever.

As with chorionic villus sampling, Rh_o (D) immune globulin is administered to unsensitized Rh-negative women following amniocentesis to prevent sensitization.

Advantages

Amniocentesis has several advantages:

- It is a simple, relatively safe procedure that permits the diagnosis of many fetal anomalies and confirms fetal maturity.
- It is a brief and relatively painless procedure.
- It has been done for many years, with few reported complications.

Disadvantages

The major disadvantage of midtrimester amniocentesis for genetic prenatal diagnosis is timing. It is done between 15 and 18 weeks of gestation, and test results may take 2 to 3 weeks to be reported. By this time, the pregnancy is obvious, the woman has felt fetal movement, and the woman may face an even more difficult decision about continuing the pregnancy if the results are abnormal.

Early amniocentesis avoids some of the timing disadvantages associated with later amniocentesis for prenatal diagnosis. Early amniocentesis does, however, carry a higher fetal loss rate after the procedure.

Risks

Amniocentesis is a relatively safe prenatal diagnostic procedure. The risk of injury to the fetus or umbilical cord is minimal when ultrasound is used to guide needle insertion. The risk of infection is also minimal, because aseptic technique is used throughout the procedure. The risk of spontaneous abortion associated with amniocentesis is 0.5% or less (Cunningham et al., 1997).

As with all fetal diagnostic procedures, amniocentesis cannot guarantee the birth of a perfect infant. Parents need to be counseled that not all defects are detectable by amniocentesis.

Antepartum Fetal Surveillance

Antepartum fetal surveillance has three goals: to prevent perinatal morbidity and mortality, to determine fetal health or compromise as accurately as possible, and to guide intervention by the obstetric team. The three most common methods of fetal surveillance are the nonstress test, the contraction stress test, and the biophysical profile.

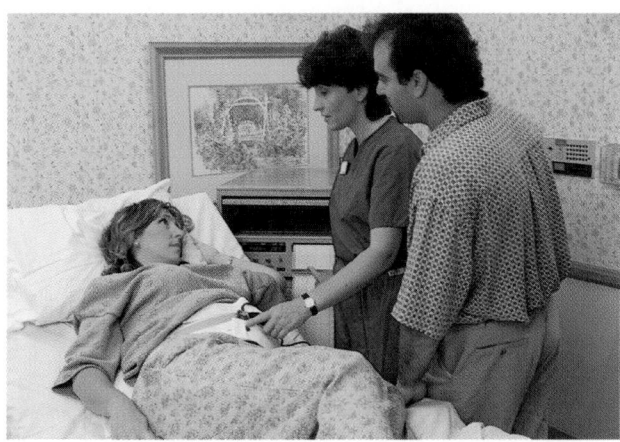

A nonstress test is a noninvasive test that measures the ability of the fetal heart to respond to fetal movements. Here the nurse reassures the parents by pointing to fetal heart rate accelerations detected by the external fetal monitor.

Nonstress Test

PURPOSE

One way to assess fetal well-being is to evaluate the ability of the fetal heart to accelerate, usually in association with fetal movement. Accelerations of the fetal heart rate indicate adequate oxygenation, a healthy neural pathway from the fetal central nervous system to the fetal heart, and the ability of the fetal heart to respond to stimuli. If the fetal heart does not accelerate, an additional test, such as the contraction stress test or the biophysical profile, is necessary to better ascertain the metabolic condition of the fetus.

PROCEDURE

The nonstress test is performed by a nurse with training in fetal monitoring. The nurse instructs the woman about the test and explains why it is recommended. The test is termed "nonstress" because it consists of monitoring only; the fetus is not challenged or stressed by uterine contractions to obtain the necessary data.

The woman usually sits in a reclining chair or in bed in a semi-Fowler's position to prevent supine hypotension. Her blood pressure is checked before the test and every 10 to 15 minutes throughout the test. If hypotension occurs, her position is changed to maintain the baseline pressure.

The nurse applies external electronic monitoring equipment to the woman's abdomen to detect the fetal heart rate and any contractions or fetal movement (Fig. 16–7). The woman may also be given a remote event marker to press each time she senses movement. (See Chapter 18 for more information about fetal monitoring.)

INTERPRETATION

Physicians must review and interpret nonstress test results. Results are judged to be reactive (reassuring) or nonreactive (nonreassuring) (AAP & ACOG, 1997).

- *Reactive:* At least two fetal heart rate accelerations, with or without fetal movement, occurring within a 20-minute period and peaking at least 15 BPM above the baseline and lasting 15 seconds from baseline to baseline (Fig. 16–8). Acoustic stimulation of 1 second that elicits similar fetal heart rate accelerations is also reassuring.
- *Nonreactive:* Tracing does not demonstrate the required characteristics of a reactive tracing within a 40-minute period.

Fetal heart reactivity occurs with maturation of the fetal autonomic nervous system. False-positive nonreactive results are more likely to occur before 28 weeks of gestation (AAP & ACOG, 1997).

ADVANTAGES

The nonstress test is noninvasive and painless and is believed to be without risk to mother or fetus. For these reasons it is the primary means of fetal surveillance in pregnancies that are at increased risk for uteroplacental insufficiency and consequent fetal hypoxia and acidosis. The nonstress test is easy to administer and may be repeated weekly or even daily if necessary. In addition, results are available immediately.

DISADVANTAGES

False-positive results are one disadvantage that may occur with nonstress testing. A common reason for false-positive results is fetal sleep. Forty minutes gives most sleeping fetuses time to awaken.

Awaiting accelerations can prolong the nonstress test. Various methods have been used to stimulate the fetus to elicit accelerations in the fetal heart rate. Some of these methods include having the mother drink orange juice to raise her glucose level, manipulating the woman's abdomen, and fetal sound stimulation. Of these, only vibroacoustic stimulation of the fetus through the maternal abdomen has been shown to be both safe and effective.

Vibroacoustic Stimulation Test

PURPOSE AND PROCEDURE

In recent years, the vibroacoustic stimulation test has been used to confirm nonreactive nonstress test findings or to shorten the time needed to obtain nonstress test data of good quality. The procedure for the vibroacoustic stimulation test is similar to that for the nonstress test. Electronic fetal monitoring equipment is used to obtain a baseline fetal heart rate. Then an artificial larynx is applied to the maternal abdomen over the area of the fetal head for 1 second. The fetus is stimulated by the sound emitted as well as by the vibration created.

POTENTIAL RISKS

Although no known risks exist, there is speculation that repeated use of the artificial larynx may cause fetal hearing loss. Preliminary information, however, suggests that the increased intrauterine sound level is unlikely to lead to significant fetal injury (Smith, 1994).

In addition, prolonged fetal tachycardia has been noted in some instances, but its significance is not known. Moreover, if the test is used frequently, the fetus may become habituated to the stimulus and not respond, making the test results unclear.

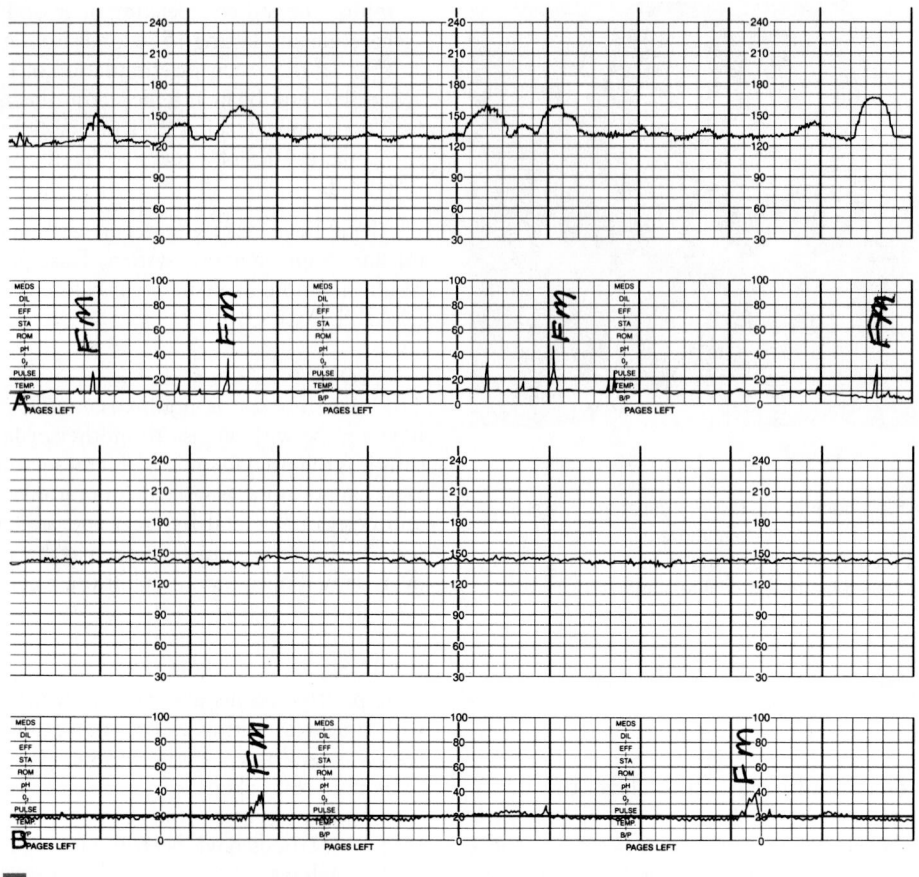

Contraction Stress Test

PURPOSE

A contraction stress test is indicated if nonstress test findings are nonreactive. The concern is that if fetal oxygenation is only marginally adequate when the uterus is at rest, it may be decreased further during uterine contractions. As the name implies, a contraction stress test involves recording the response of the fetal heart rate to stress that is induced by uterine contractions. Uterine contractions compress the arteries supplying the placenta with oxygenated maternal blood; therefore, uterine contractions routinely cause a recurrent decrease in fetal oxygen levels.

The fetus with adequate oxygen reserves can tolerate the temporary hypoxia induced by uterine contractions, so that the fetal heart rate pattern remains reassuring. If the fetus has inadequate reserves, however, and if hypoxia has led to anaerobic metabolism, fetal acidosis may result. This condition leads to myocardial depression that is evidenced by late decelerations in the fetal heart rate. If fetal heart rate variability is also decreased in the presence of persistent late decelerations, the correlation with fetal compromise is increased. (Chapter 18 reviews fetal heart rate monitoring and nonreassuring fetal heart rate patterns.)

PROCEDURE

The nurse is responsible for administering the test and for protecting the safety of the mother and fetus throughout the testing period. In many ways the procedure is similar to that of the nonstress test. The woman is positioned in the same manner, sitting in a reclining chair in a semi-Fowler's position. External electronic fetal monitoring devices are applied to record both uterine activity and fetal heart rate. The major difference between the nonstress test and the contraction stress test is that, in the contraction stress test, the fetal heart rate and patterns must be evaluated in relation to uterine contractions. Three contractions of at least 40 seconds each and occurring within a 10-minute period are required to interpret the contraction stress test. Two methods may be used to initiate uterine contractions if they are not present spontaneously.

Use of *nipple stimulation* is based on the knowledge that stimulation of the nipples causes the release of oxytocin from the posterior pituitary and that oxytocin causes uterine contractions. The woman brushes her palm across one nipple through her clothing for 2 minutes, stopping if a contraction begins. The nipple stimulation is repeated after a 5-minute rest period if no contractions occur.

If nipple stimulation does not result in adequate contractions, *intravenous infusion of low-dose oxytocin* is used to stimulate uterine contractions. The nurse conducting the test inserts a primary intravenous line plus a "piggyback" line to administer the oxytocin solution.

INTERPRETATION

Contraction stress test results may be interpreted as negative (reassuring), positive (nonreassuring), suspicious (equivocal), or unsatisfactory (AAP & ACOG, 1997).

- *Negative:* No late decelerations.
- *Positive:* Late decelerations follow 50% or more of contractions, even if the frequency of contractions is less than three in 10 minutes.
- *Suspicious (equivocal):* Intermittent late or variable decelerations.

- *Unsatisfactory:* Fewer than three contractions within 10 minutes or a poor-quality tracing.

See Figure 16–9 for a summary of contraction stress test interpretations.

Uterine hyperstimulation may occur, resulting in contractions that occur more frequently than every 2 minutes or exceed 90 seconds in duration. If nonreassuring fetal heart rate patterns such as late decelerations occur with hyperstimulation, retesting is appropriate (AAP & ACOG, 1997).

ADVANTAGES

Contraction stress testing has several advantages:

- The test allows follow-up of a nonreactive nonstress test result.

Negative	No late decelerations	Reassuring that the fetus can tolerate labor

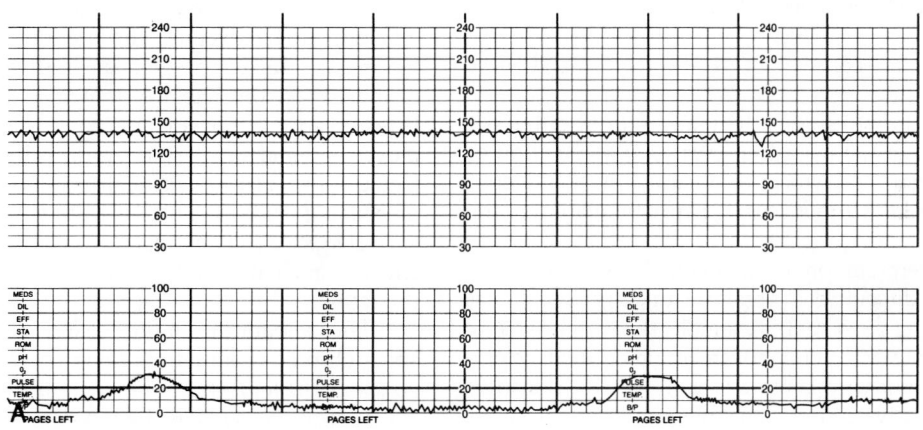

Positive	Consistent late decelerations in ≥ 50% of the contractions, even if contraction frequency is less than 3 in 10 minutes	Indicates UPI and fetal compromise during contractions

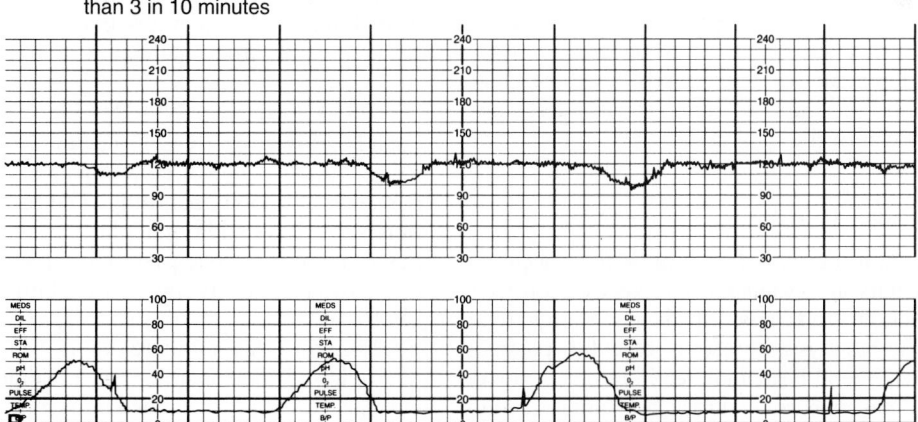

Equivocal	Intermittent late or variable decelerations	A second CST should be repeated within 24 hours
Hyperstimulation	Late decelerations with excessive uterine activity (contractions closer than every 2 minutes or lasting longer than 90 seconds)	Repeat CST within 24 hours with careful monitoring of the situation
Unsatisfactory	Test cannot be interpreted; either not enough data or unsatisfactory tracing; fewer than 3 contactions in 10 minutes	Repeat CST with careful attention to maternal position, oxytocin infusion, and placement of toco-transducer

FIGURE 16–9

Interpretation of contraction stress test (CST). UPI, uteroplacental insufficiency. (Courtesy of Graphic Controls, Buffalo, New York.)

- If the findings are negative, a contraction stress test offers reassurance that the uteroplacental unit will continue to support life for at least a week longer (Cunningham et al., 1997; Murray, 1997). A negative contraction stress test does not reassure that other causes of fetal death will not occur, such as cord accidents or placental abruption (see pp. 640 and 707).
- A positive contraction stress test result allows the physician to analyze available options and to make plans for the birth of an infant who may be compromised because of decreased placental functioning before or during labor.

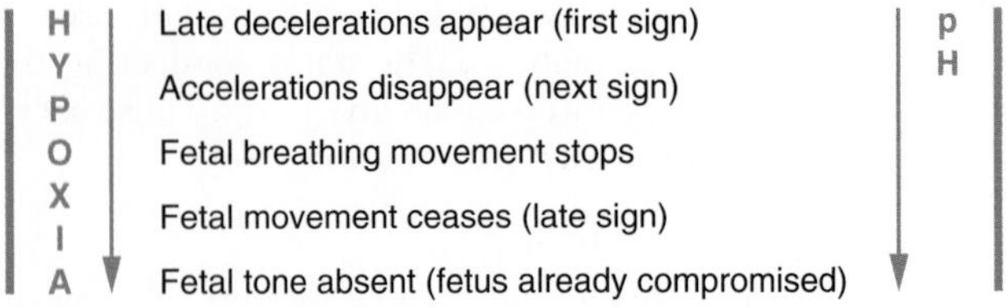

DISADVANTAGES

The contraction stress test is associated with four major disadvantages:

- A contraction stress test cannot be done if uterine contractions are contraindicated. Examples of these conditions include placenta previa (see Chapter 26) or a vertical uterine scar.
- The test is time-consuming, usually requiring about 2 hours.
- The contraction stress test is tedious, requiring either the participation of the woman in breast self-stimulation or careful infusion of oxytocin to obtain an adequate contraction pattern without causing hyperstimulation of the uterus.
- Errors in interpretation are common. These may be due to technical difficulties in obtaining tracings or problems in interpreting the data. For example, the fetal heart rate may accelerate with fetal movement, and late decelerations may occur with contractions (a reactive nonstress test but a positive contraction stress test). Such an interpretation requires further testing, such as a biophysical profile, to confirm the well-being of the fetus.
- The cost is high. A contraction stress test is usually done in a hospital setting, where there is a per-hour charge; equipment and supplies, such as intravenous lines, oxytocin, and infusion pumps, add to the cost. The time spent by a nurse who is educated to administer the test must also be factored into the total cost.

Biophysical Profile

Predicting the condition of the fetus can be most accurate if several parameters are evaluated. Unlike the nonstress test and contraction stress test, which assess only fetal heart activity, the biophysical profile assesses five parameters of fetal activity: fetal heart rate, fetal breathing movements, gross fetal movements, fetal tone, and amniotic fluid volume.

PURPOSE

The individual components of the examination are a combination of both acute and chronic markers of fetal well-being. The acute markers are the fetal heart rate reactivity, fetal breathing movements, gross fetal movements, and fetal tone. The major chronic marker is the amount of amniotic fluid.

The acute markers are controlled by different central nervous system control centers that develop at different stages in gestation. Fetal tone is the earliest to develop, fol-

FIGURE 16-10

Cascade effect of gradual hypoxia.

lowed by fetal movements and then regular breathing movements. Fetal heart rate reactivity is last to develop, occurring at the end of the second or the beginning of the third trimester.

The fetal central nervous system centers that control each individual parameter of the biophysical profile react differently to hypoxemia. The later-developing control centers require higher oxygen levels than earlier-developing centers. Therefore, fetal heart rate reactivity disappears first. Fetal breathing movements are affected next, with fetal movement and finally fetal tone being the last areas affected. Thus, absence of fetal tone indicates advanced asphyxia and acidosis. This progression has been termed the *gradual hypoxia concept*. Figure 16-10 illustrates the cascade effect of gradual hypoxia on the central nervous system of the fetus.

The amount of amniotic fluid provides information about chronic or long-term hypoxia. During periods of hypoxemia, the fetus shunts blood from areas that are not critical to fetal life, such as the kidneys and lungs, toward the vital organs (heart, brain, and placenta). If the hypoxemia is prolonged, blood flow to the fetal kidneys and lungs, which help produce amniotic fluid, may virtually cease. Therefore, oligohydramnios indicates prolonged fetal hypoxia and is a strong indication of fetal compromise.

PROCEDURE AND INTERPRETATION

Fetal heart rate reactivity is measured and interpreted from a nonstress test. The other four parameters are measured by real-time ultrasound scanning. The test is administered by nurses who have additional preparation in ultrasonography. A scoring technique is used to interpret the data, with each of the five parameters contributing either 2 or 0 points (Table 16-3). A score of 10 is perfect; a score of 0 is the worst possible score. A total score of 8 to 10 is reassuring; a score of 4 or less is nonreassuring. Oligohydramnios may indicate chronic fetal hypoxia and warrants more frequent biophysical profile testing or consideration of delivery (AAP & ACOG, 1997).

Modified Biophysical Profile

Some physicians elect to assess the fetus only by ultrasonography and to omit the nonstress test if all parameters are normal. In other medical centers, the test is modified to include only two parameters: an amniotic fluid index (sum of the fluid depths in four quadrants) and a nonstress test. Some physicians, however, now add a sixth parameter: placental grading.

TABLE 16-3

Scoring the Biophysical Profile

Criterion	Points	
	Not present	Present
Reactive nonstress test	0	2
Fetal breathing movements (at least 1 episode of 30 sec in 30 min)	0	2
Gross body movements (at least 3 body or limb movements in 30 min)	0	2
Fetal tone (at least 1 episode of extension with return to flexion)	0	2
Amniotic fluid volume (at least 1 pocket of fluid that measures at least 1 cm in 2 perpendicular planes)	0	2

Interpretation: Normal = 8 to 10 points (if amniotic fluid volume is adequate); equivocal = 6; abnormal = ≤4 and delivery may be considered.

Data from Manning, F. A. (1995). Dynamic ultrasound-based fetal assessment: The fetal biophysical profile score. *Clinical Obstetrics and Gynecology, 38*(1), 26–43.

ADVANTAGES

The biophysical profile is noninvasive and is less costly than some tests because it can be done on an outpatient basis. Results are immediately available, and it may decrease the number of false-positive nonreactive nonstress test findings. The biophysical profile allows conservative treatment of high-risk patients because delivery can be delayed if fetal well-being is indicated.

DISADVANTAGES

Additional research is needed to refine interpretation of the test. For example, each variable is given equal weight, although some variables are more important. At present, not enough research has been done to determine the meaning of low scores to long-term development of the child.

Percutaneous Umbilical Blood Sampling

Percutaneous umbilical blood sampling (PUBS), also called cordocentesis, involves the aspiration of fetal blood from the umbilical cord for prenatal diagnosis or therapy (Fig. 16–11). Major indications for percutaneous umbilical blood sampling include the diagnosis and intrauterine management of Rh disease, genetic studies, diagnosis of abnormal blood-clotting factors, and acid-base status of the fetus.

Procedure

High-resolution ultrasonography is used to locate the fetus, placenta, and umbilical cord. A needle is inserted through the abdomen and into the uterine cavity. The puncture is made into the umbilical cord near the site at which the cord meets the placenta because the cord is almost always stable at this site. The umbilical vein is targeted more commonly than the umbilical arteries because it is larger and is less likely to constrict during the procedure. It is not important to know which vessel (vein or artery) was used when sampling fetal blood for genetic or coagulation studies, but it is very important to know which was used when testing fetal

acid-base parameters. Blood from the umbilical vein contains oxygenated blood and has a lower carbon dioxide content (and thus a higher pH) than blood from an umbilical artery, which comes directly from the fetus after circulation throughout the body.

Risks

It is predicted that percutaneous umbilical blood sampling will become a widely used procedure in the future, but it is

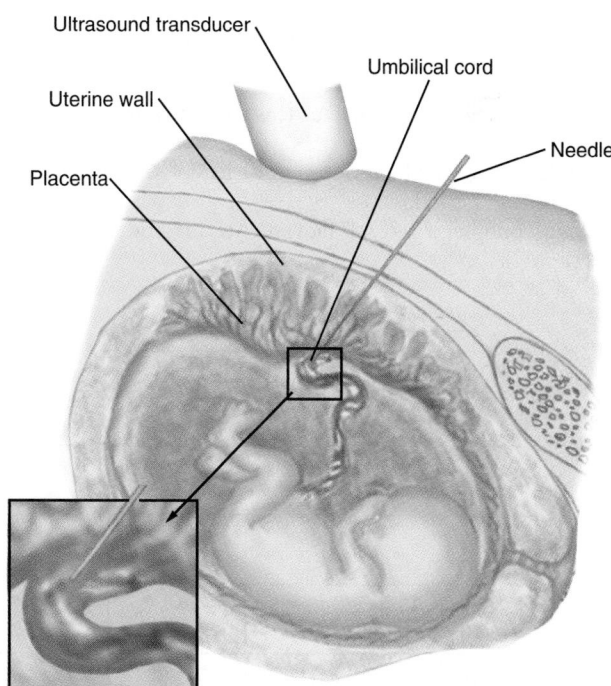

FIGURE 16–11

In percutaneous umbilical blood sampling (cordocentesis) a needle is inserted through the expectant mother's abdomen and into an umbilical vessel (vein or artery) to withdraw a sample of fetal blood.

not risk free. Complications that can occur include infection, fetal bradycardia, cord laceration, cord hematoma, thrombosis, thromboembolism, premature labor, and premature rupture of membranes. After needle withdrawal, the duration of bleeding from the umbilical cord is usually short and can be monitored by ultrasound examination. In addition, the fetal heart can be monitored electronically to identify reassuring or nonreassuring patterns.

Maternal Assessment of Fetal Movement

Movements by the fetus, as assessed by the mother, are sometimes referred to as "kick counts." Fetal movement is associated with fetal condition, and daily evaluation of these movements provides a way of evaluating the fetus.

Procedure

Protocols for assessing the mother's perception of fetal movement vary. The woman lies on her side. She places her hands on the largest part of her abdomen and concentrates on fetal movements. She uses a clock or timer and records the number of movements felt.

The ideal number of movements and the ideal duration for movement counting have not been defined. Ten movements in a period of up to 2 hours is considered reassuring. After ten movements have been perceived, the woman can discontinue the count for that day (AAP & ACOG, 1997). Another approach uses three counting periods of 1 hour each (Fig. 16–12) for maternal evaluation of fetal movement.

Women should notify their health care provider if they experience the following:

* They do not experience at least ten movements in a 2-hour period, or
* They do not feel a movement at least four times in any counting period.
* The number of total movements for the day is less than 12.

* There is any change in the type or character of the movements.

If another protocol for fetal movement evaluation is used, the physician may give slightly different guidelines for notification.

Advantages

Counting fetal movements is one of the oldest methods for evaluating the condition of the fetus. There are some obvious advantages:

* It is inexpensive.
* It is noninvasive.
* It is convenient for the client.

Disadvantages

Many variables make interpretation of fetal movement counts difficult:

* Fetal resting state decreases movements.
* Maternal perception of movement may vary.
* Time of day may affect fetal movement (less in the morning, greater in the evening).
* Maternal use of drugs (methadone, heroin, cocaine, alcohol, tobacco) may affect fetal activity.

NURSING CARE
The Client Who Has Diagnostic Testing

Assessment

Nurses collect information that is important to conducting the diagnostic tests or that is helpful to the physician interpreting the results. Necessary information includes the following:

* Gravida, para, living children, gestation.
* Maternal health problems (hypertension, diabetes, heart disease).
* Current obstetric problems (vaginal bleeding, decreased fetal movement, multifetal gestation, intrauterine growth restriction, malpresentation, hydramnios, oligohydramnios).

Dates: 11/14/98 to 11/20/98

Time of day	Sunday	Monday	Tuesday	Wednesday	Thursday	Friday	Saturday
Morning 8-9 a.m.	卌 卌	卌 ‖	卌 ‖‖				
Afternoon 1-2 p.m.	卌 ∣	卌 ∕∕∕	卌				
Evening 9-10 p.m.	卌 卌 ∕∕	卌 ∕∕∕∣					
Total	28	24					

FIGURE 16–12

Daily fetal movement record in use. The mother counts the number of fetal movements, or "kicks," within a specified period several times a day and indicates each movement on a chart. She reports any abnormality to her health care provider.

- Prior obstetric problems (birth of stillborn infant or infant with congenital anomalies, birth of low-birth-weight infant or large-for-gestational-age infant).
- History of substance abuse, including alcohol and tobacco.
- Client knowledge of reasons for the test and the procedure to be performed. The nurse may ask, "What questions can I answer before we start the test?"
- Client knowledge of surveillance regimen if additional testing is necessary: "Will you tell me what you understand about the need to repeat the test every week?"
- The woman's emotional response to the tests: "What are your major concerns?" "What can we do to make the tests easier for you?"
- The woman's or couple's expectations of the diagnostic tests. Many couples think that the tests can guarantee a perfect baby. They must be told what the test actually reveals.

Nursing Diagnosis and Planning

The following diagnosis is likely to be relevant when a woman requires fetal diagnostic testing.

- Anxiety related to lack of knowledge of diagnostic procedures and the uncertain condition of the fetus.
  Expected Outcomes: The woman and her family will verbalize knowledge of how, when, and why she is to be tested before testing procedures are initiated. The woman and her family will verbalize concerns and seek knowledge about the fetus.

Interventions

Providing Information

Provide the woman and her family simple, clear explanations of what the test assesses and the purpose and frequency of any tests. Tell them how long the test takes and describe the testing procedure to reduce anxiety caused by lack of knowledge. Some tests require teaching about follow-up care and events that should be reported to the health care team.

Providing Support

It is critical that the nurse identify and respond to feelings expressed by prospective parents when antepartum testing procedures are recommended or when fetal problems are confirmed. The woman often experiences frustration with the discomfort, limitations, and time-consuming demands of the pregnancy and the regimen of fetal testing. Skill in therapeutic communication is never more important than when counseling about fetal diagnostic tests.

- Active listening conveys interest and concern.
- Paraphrasing allows for interpretation because it expresses in different words what concerns the family.
- Reflecting what is expressed about feelings helps the family "hear" what their feelings are.
- Clarifying helps prospective parents "see" what the issues are and what options are available.
- Comforting measures such as touch convey empathic concern and are especially important during difficult procedures.

Although nurses offer caring concern and careful reflection of feelings, they do not offer advice. The decisions must be made by the family, but nurses frequently help the family contact persons to whom they turn in troubled times, such as a member of the clergy or a close relative.

Women benefit from knowing that compliance with the testing regimen is beneficial for the fetus. Each day in the uterus allows time for growth and development and increases the chance that the infant will be strong and healthy. The fetus has an improved chance of surviving as long as the test results remain reassuring.

Nurses must examine their own ethical beliefs before they become involved in fetal diagnostic testing. They must be prepared to support whatever decision a woman and her family make, even if it is not one they would make. For example, whether a woman decides to continue or terminate a pregnancy, she is entitled to compassionate care regardless of the nurse's personal views about the decision.

Evaluation

- Did the woman (and her family) verbalize knowledge of why tests are recommended and express an idea of how and when they will be performed?
- Does she actively seek information about the fetal condition to relieve her anxiety?

KEY CONCEPTS

- Ultrasonography is widely used during pregnancy to determine a variety of fetal and placental conditions and to aid in the performance of other tests, such as amniocentesis.
- Alpha-fetoprotein assessment, a screening test performed on maternal serum or amniotic fluid, is used primarily to detect open neural tube defects and chromosomal abnormalities. Additional tests are required if AFP levels are abnormal. Two other markers, human chorionic gonadotropin and estriol, are

assessed along with AFP to screen for chromosomal anomalies.
- Chorionic villus sampling can be performed as early as 10 weeks of gestation to provide parents with information about many chromosomal defects in the first trimester of pregnancy. The risk for pregnancy loss is somewhat higher than it is for amniocentesis, and there may be a risk for limb reduction defects.
- Amniocentesis is usually performed in the second trimester to

identify fetal genetic anomalies or open defects such as neural tube defects. It is done during the third trimester to evaluate fetal lung maturity or Rh incompatibility problems. Early amniocentesis (12 to 14 weeks) is becoming more common for identification of genetic or neural tube defects.
- The nonstress test determines whether the fetal heart rate accelerates. Such acceleration is a reassuring sign associated with adequate fetal oxygenation and an

intact neural pathway from the fetal brain to the heart.
■ Contraction stress tests are used to determine how the fetal heart responds to uterine contractions that temporarily decrease placental blood flow. A positive test result suggests that the placental function has deteriorated.

■ Percutaneous umbilical blood sampling or cordocentesis involves aspirating blood from umbilical vessels to detect blood disorders, acid-base imbalance, infection, or fetal genetic disease.
■ Maternal assessment of fetal movement ("kick counts") is an inex-

pensive and noninvasive method of evaluating the placental function.
■ All perinatal nurses must be prepared to offer clear explanations of diagnostic procedures and to provide support for the family requiring fetal diagnostic tests.

REFERENCES AND READINGS

Alteneder, R. R., Kenner, C., Greene, D., Pohorecki, S. (1998). The lived experience of women who undergo prenatal diagnostic testing due to elevated maternal serum alpha-fetoprotein screening. MCN: American Journal of Maternal/Child Nursing, 23(4), 180–186.

American Academy of Pediatrics & American College of Obstetricians and Gynecologists. (1997). Guidelines for perinatal care (4th ed.). Elk Grove Village, IL, and Washington, DC: Author.

American College of Obstetricians and Gynecologists. (1994). Antepartum fetal surveillance (Technical Bulletin No. 188). Washington, DC: Author.

American College of Obstetricians and Gynecologists. (1995). Chorionic villus sampling (Committee Opinion No. 160). Washington, DC: Author.

Anthony, A. (1996). Biological effects and safety. In T. J. DuBose (Ed.), Fetal sonography (pp. 27–44). Philadelphia: Saunders.

Berman, M. (1996). History of fetal sonography. In T. J. DuBose (Ed.), Fetal sonography (pp. 11–26). Philadelphia: Saunders.

Cartier, M. S. (1996). Fetal Doppler. In T. J. DuBose (Ed.), Fetal sonography (pp. 275–303). Philadelphia: Saunders.

Covington, C., Gielghem, P., Board, F., Madison, K., Nedd, D., & Miller, L. (1996). Family care related to alpha-fetoprotein screening. Journal of Obstetric, Gynecologic, and Neonatal Nursing, 25(2), 125–130.

Cunningham, F. G., MacDonald, P. C., Gant, N. F., Leveno, K. J., Gilstrap, L. C., Hankins, G. D. V., et al. (1997). Williams obstetrics (20th ed.). Norwalk, CT: Appleton & Lange.

DuBose, T. J. (1996a). First trimester. In T. J. DuBose (Ed.), Fetal sonography (pp. 389–425). Philadelphia: Saunders.

DuBose, T. J. (1996b). Second and third trimester. In T. J. DuBose (Ed.), Fetal sonography (pp. 427–471). Philadelphia: Saunders.

Harman, C. R. (1999). Percutaneous fetal blood sampling. In R. K. Creasy & R. Resnik (Eds.), Maternal-fetal medicine (4th ed., pp. 341–363). Philadelphia: Saunders.

Kellner, L. H., Weiss, R. R., Weiner, Z., et al. (1995). The advantages of using triple-marker screening for chromosomal abnormalities. American Journal of Obstetrics and Gynecology, 172(3), 831–836.

Manning, F. A. (1995). Dynamic ultrasound-based fetal assessment: The fetal biophysical profile score. Clinical Obstetrics and Gynecology, 38(1), 26–43.

Manning, F. A. (1999). Fetal assessment by evaluation of biophysical variables: Fetal biophysical profile score. In R. K. Creasy & R. Resnik (Eds.), Maternal-fetal medicine (4th ed., pp. 319–330). Philadelphia: Saunders.

McCarthy, K. E., & Narrigan, D. (1995). Is there scientific support for the use of juice to facilitate the nonstress test? Journal of Obstetric, Gynecologic, and Neonatal Nursing, 24(4), 303–306.

Miller, D. A., Rabello, Y., & Paul, R. H. (1996). The modified biophysical profile: Antepartum testing in the 1990s. American Journal of Obstetrics and Gynecology, 174(3), 812–817.

Moffatt, F. W., Van den Hof, M. (1997). Semi-Fowler's positioning, lateral tilts, and their effects on nonstress tests. Journal of Obstetric, Gynecologic, and Neonatal Nursing, 26(5), 551–557.

Murray, M. (1997). Antepartal and intrapartal fetal monitoring. Albuquerque, NM: Learning Resources International.

Paul, R., & Miller, D. A. (1995). Nonstress test. Clinical Obstetrics and Gynecology, 38(1), 3–9.

Raines, D. A. (1996). Fetal surveillance: Issues and implications. Journal of Obstetric, Gynecologic, and Neonatal Nursing, 25(7), 559–564.

Rayburn, W. F. (1995). Fetal movement monitoring. Clinical Obstetrics and Gynecology, 38(1), 59–67.

Reece, E. A. (1997). Early and midtrimester genetic amniocentesis. Obstetrics and Gynecology Clinics of North America, 24(1), 71–81.

Richardson, B. S., & Gagnon, R. (1999). Fetal breathing and body movements. In R. K. Creasy & R. Resnik (Eds.), Maternal-fetal medicine (4th ed., pp. 231–247). Philadelphia: Saunders.

Santalahti, P., Latikka, A. M., Ryynänen, M., & Hemminki, E. (1996). Women's experiences of perinatal serum screening. Birth, 23(2), 101–107.

Sciosa, A. L. (1999). Prenatal genetic diagnosis. In R. K. Creasy & R. Resnik (Eds.), Maternal-fetal medicine (4th ed., pp. 40–62). Philadelphia: Saunders.

Smith, C. N. (1994). Vibroacoustic stimulation for risk assessment. Clinics in Perinatology, 12(4), 797–809.

Treanor, C. (1998). Exploring nurses' roles in limited ultrasound. AWHONN Lifelines, 2(2), 13–14.

Trudinger, B. (1999). Doppler ultrasound assessment of blood flow. In R. K. Creasy & R. Resnik (Eds.), Maternal-fetal medicine (4th ed., pp. 216–229). Philadelphia: Saunders.

Wapner, R. J. (1997). Chorionic villus sampling. Obstetrics and Gynecology Clinics of North America, 24(1), 83–110.

Wenstrom, K. D., Owen, J., Boots, L., & Ethier, M. (1995). The influence of maternal weight on human chorionic gonadotropin in the multiple-marker screening test for fetal Down syndrome. American Journal of Obstetrics and Gynecology, 173(4), 1297–1300.

17

Giving Birth

DEFINITIONS

abortion   A pregnancy that ends before 20 weeks' gestation, either spontaneously or electively. *Miscarriage* is a lay term for a spontaneous abortion.

amniotomy   Artificial rupture of the amniotic sac (fetal membranes).

attitude   Relationship of fetal body parts to one another.

bloody show   Mixture of cervical mucus and blood from ruptured capillaries in the cervix. Bloody show often precedes labor and increases with cervical dilation.

Braxton Hicks contractions   Irregular, mild uterine contractions that occur throughout pregnancy. These contractions become stronger in the last trimester.

caput succedaneum   Area of edema over the presenting part of the fetus or newborn, resulting from pressure against the cervix. Usually called simply caput.

crowning   Appearance of the fetal scalp or presenting part at the vaginal opening.

EDD   Abbreviation for estimated date of delivery. This date may also be abbreviated EDB (estimated date of birth).

engagement   Descent of the widest diameter of the fetal presenting part to at least a zero station (the level of the ischial spines in the maternal pelvis).

episiotomy   Surgical incision of the perineum to enlarge the vaginal opening.

ferning (or fern test)   Microscopic appearance of amniotic fluid that resembles fern leaves when the fluid is allowed to dry on a microscope slide.

fontanel   Space at the intersection of sutures connecting fetal or infant skull bones.

gravida   A pregnant woman. Also refers to a woman's total number of pregnancies, including the one in progress, if applicable.

lie   Relationship of the long axis of the fetus to the long axis of the mother.

lightening   Descent of the fetus toward the pelvic inlet before labor.

lochia   Vaginal drainage after birth.

molding   Shaping of the fetal head during movement through the birth canal.

multipara   A woman who has given birth after two or more pregnancies of at least 20 weeks' gestation. Also informally used to describe a pregnant woman before the birth of her second or later child.

Nitrazine paper   Paper to determine pH. Nitrazine paper helps to determine whether the amniotic sac has ruptured.

nuchal cord   Umbilical cord around the fetal neck.

nullipara   A woman who has not completed a pregnancy to at least 20 weeks' gestation.

para   A woman who has given birth after a pregnancy of at least 20 weeks' gestation. Para also designates the number of pregnancies that end after at least 20 weeks of gestation. (A multifetal gestation, such as twins, is considered one birth when calculating parity.)

position   Relation of a fixed reference point on the fetus to the quadrants of the maternal pelvis.

presentation   Fetal part that first enters the pelvic inlet; also, the presenting part.

primipara   A woman who has given birth after a pregnancy of at least 20 weeks of gestation. The term is also used informally to describe a pregnant woman before the birth of her first child.

station   Measurement of fetal descent in relation to the ischial spines of the maternal pelvis. See also *engagement*.

sutures   Narrow areas of flexible tissue that connect the fetal skull bones, permitting slight movement during labor.

VBAC   Abbreviation for vaginal birth after cesarean birth.

Care of the woman and her family during labor and birth is a rewarding field of nursing. The birth of a baby is more than a physical event; it has deep personal and social significance for the family. Their roles and relationships are forever altered by this event.

Issues for New Nurses

New nurses and nursing students face several common issues when caring for families during birth.

Pain Associated with Birth

Working with people in pain is difficult, and most nurses feel compelled to relieve pain promptly. Yet pain is an expected part of labor and cannot be eliminated. Helping the woman to manage the pain of birth is a crucial part of nursing care.

Inexperience or Negative Experiences

The nurse who has never given birth may feel inadequate to care for laboring women, although she or he rarely feels it necessary to experience a fracture to care for someone with that problem. Nursing skills needed by the intrapartum nurse are basic: observation, critical thinking, problem solving, therapeutic communication, comfort promotion, empathy, and common sense.

Nurses also may be anxious because of their own difficult experiences during birth. They must be careful not to convey negative attitudes to the laboring woman and her partner.

Unpredictability

Labor is a natural process that follows its own timetable. Some occurrences simply are not easily predicted or explained. Some nurses find the uncertain nature of intrapartum care troubling, whereas others find it exciting.

Intimacy

The intimate nature of intrapartum care and its sexual overtones also make some nurses uncomfortable. They may feel that they are intruding on a private time.

The male nurse often finds this aspect of intrapartum care most anxiety provoking. Although he may have cared for other female clients, his care has not been this focused on the reproductive system. He often wonders how a woman's male partner will accept him as a care provider.

The best approach for both male and female nurses is to maintain professional conduct and take cues from the couple. If they want privacy, the nurse should intervene only as needed to assess the woman and fetus. In more advanced labor, both partners often welcome the presence of a competent, caring nurse of either sex.

Physiologic Effects of the Birth Process

Labor and birth affect the physiologic systems of both the pregnant woman and her fetus. These effects are most striking in the maternal reproductive system and in relation to fetal and neonatal oxygenation.

Maternal Response

Significant changes during labor occur in the woman's cardiovascular, respiratory, gastrointestinal, urinary, and hematopoietic systems as well as in her reproductive system.

REPRODUCTIVE SYSTEM

Characteristics of Contractions. Normal labor contractions are coordinated, involuntary, and intermittent.

Coordinated Contractions. The uterus can contract and relax in a coordinated way, as can other smooth muscles such as the heart. As the woman approaches full term, contractions become organized and gradually assume a regular pattern of increasing frequency, duration, and intensity during labor. Coordinated labor contractions begin in the uterine fundus and spread downward toward the cervix to propel the fetus through the pelvis.

Involuntary Contractions. Uterine contractions are involuntary in that they are not under conscious control, as are skeletal muscles. The mother cannot cause labor to start or stop by conscious effort. Walking or other activity, however, may stimulate existing labor contractions. Anxiety and excessive stress can diminish them.

Intermittent Contractions. Labor contractions are intermittent rather than sustained, allowing relaxation of the uterine muscle and resumption of blood flow to and from the placenta to permit gas, nutrient, and waste exchange for the fetus.

Contraction Cycle. Each contraction consists of three phases (Fig. 17–1). The *increment* occurs as the contraction begins in the fundus and spreads throughout the uterus. The *peak*, or *acme*, is the period during which the contraction is most intense. The *decrement* is the period of decreasing intensity as the uterus relaxes.

The contraction cycle and the overall pattern of contractions are also described in terms of frequency, duration, and intensity. *Frequency* is the period from the beginning of one uterine contraction to the beginning of the next; it is usually expressed in minutes and fractions of minutes. For example, "Contractions are 3½ to 4 minutes apart."

Duration is the length of each contraction from beginning to end; it is usually expressed in seconds. For example, "Her contractions last 55 to 65 seconds."

Intensity is the strength of the contractions. The terms "mild," "moderate," and "strong" are used to describe contraction intensity as palpated by the nurse. Mild contractions are often described as feeling like the tip of the nose, moderate contractions like the chin, and firm contractions

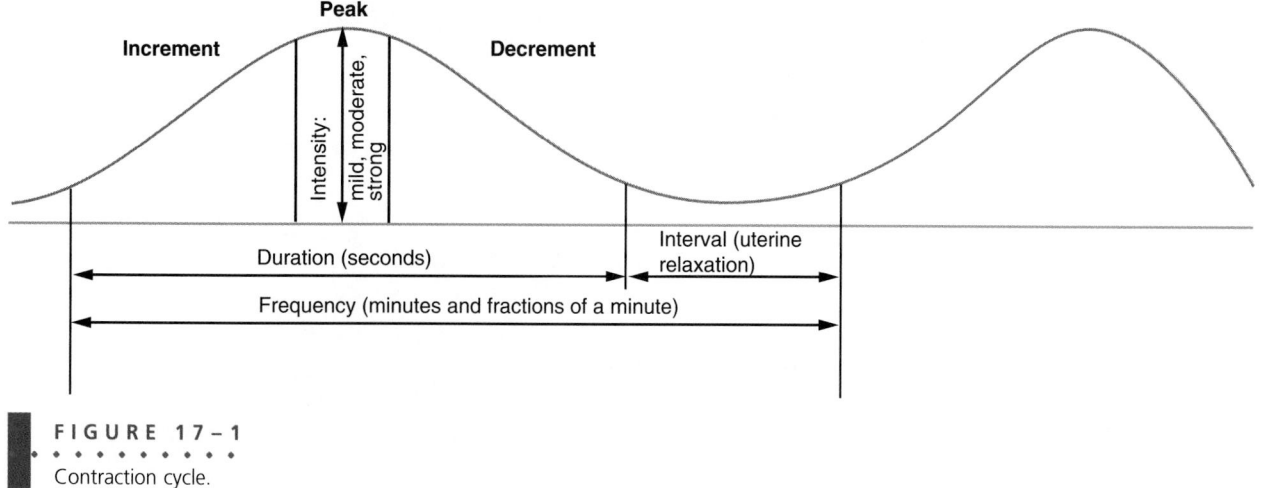

Peak

Increment   **Decrement**

Intensity: mild, moderate, strong

Duration (seconds)

Interval (uterine relaxation)

Frequency (minutes and fractions of a minute)

FIGURE 17–1

Contraction cycle.

like the forehead. Different descriptions of intensity may apply when the electronic fetal monitor is used to record contractions (see Chapter 18).

The *interval* is the period between the end of one contraction and the beginning of the next. The interval is the time when most fetal exchange of oxygen, nutrients, and waste products occurs.

Uterine Body.   Uterine activity during labor is characterized by opposing features. The upper two thirds of the uterus contracts actively to push the fetus down. The lower one third of the uterus remains less active, promoting downward passage of the fetus. The cervix is similar to the lower uterine segment in that it is also passive. The net effect of labor contractions is enhanced because the downward push from the upper uterus is accompanied by reduced resistance to fetal descent in the lower uterus.

Myometrial (uterine muscle) cells in the upper uterus remain shorter at the end of each contraction rather than returning to their original length. In contrast, myometrial cells in the lower uterus become longer with each contraction. These two characteristics enable the upper uterus to maintain tension between contractions to preserve the cervical changes and downward fetal progress made with each contraction.

The opposing characteristics of myometrial contraction in the upper and lower uterine segments cause changes in the thickness of the uterine wall during labor. The upper uterus becomes thicker while the lower uterus becomes thinner and pulled upward during labor. The physiologic retraction ring marks the division between the upper and lower segments of the uterus (Fig. 17–2).

The opposing characteristics of contractions in the upper and lower uterine segments change the shape of the uterine cavity, which becomes more elongated and narrower as labor progresses. This change in uterine shape straightens the fetal body and efficiently directs it downward in the pelvis.

Cervical Changes.   *Effacement* (thinning and shortening) and *dilation* (opening) are the major cervical changes during labor. Effacement and dilation occur together during

labor but at different rates. The nullipara completes most cervical effacement early in the process of cervical dilation. In contrast, the parous woman's cervix is usually thicker than a nullipara's cervix at any point during labor.

Effacement.   Before labor, the cervix is a cylindrical structure, about 2 cm long, at the lower end of the uterus. Labor contractions push the fetus downward against the cervix as they pull the cervix upward. The cervix becomes shorter and thinner as it is drawn over the fetus and amniotic sac (Fig. 17–3). The cervix merges with the thinning lower uterus rather than remaining a distinct cylindrical structure. Effacement is estimated as a percentage of the amount the cervix has thinned, so that a fully thinned cervix is 100% effaced. Effacement also may be recorded as cervical length estimated during vaginal examination.

Dilation.   As the cervix is pulled upward and the fetus is pushed downward, the cervix dilates. Dilation is expressed in centimeters, with approximately 10 cm being full dilation, large enough to allow passage of the average-sized term fetus. The action during effacement and dilation can be likened to pushing a ball out the cuff of a sock.

CARDIOVASCULAR SYSTEM

During each uterine contraction, blood flow to the placenta gradually decreases, causing a relative increase in the woman's blood volume. This temporary change increases her blood pressure slightly and slows her pulse. Therefore, the mother's vital signs are best assessed during the interval between contractions.

Although it is more likely to occur during the antepartum period, supine hypotension also may occur during labor if the mother lies on her back (see Fig. 13–4). *The mother should be encouraged to rest in positions other than the supine to promote blood return to her heart and therefore enhance blood flow to the placenta and promote fetal oxygenation.*

RESPIRATORY SYSTEM

The depth and rate of respirations increase, especially if the woman is anxious or in pain. A woman who breathes rapidly and deeply may experience symptoms of hyperventilation if she exhales too much carbon dioxide. She may also feel tingling in her hands and feet, numbness, and dizziness.

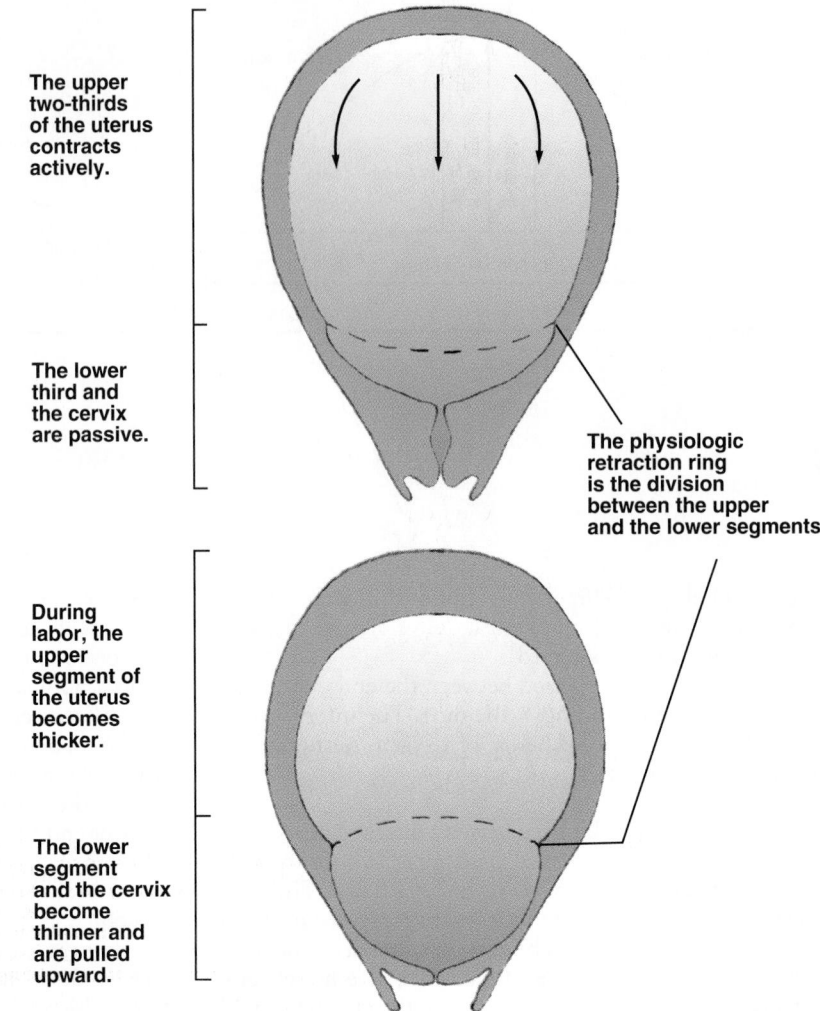

The upper two-thirds of the uterus contracts actively.

The lower third and the cervix are passive.

The physiologic retraction ring is the division between the upper and the lower segments.

During labor, the upper segment of the uterus becomes thicker.

The lower segment and the cervix become thinner and are pulled upward.

FIGURE 17–2

Opposing characteristics of uterine contraction in the upper and lower segments of the uterus.

Helping her to slow her breathing and to breathe into a paper bag or her cupped hands can restore normal blood levels of carbon dioxide and relieve these symptoms.

GASTROINTESTINAL SYSTEM

Gastric motility is reduced to varying degrees during labor. Most women are not actually hungry but are often thirsty and have a dry mouth. General anesthesia is rarely needed for birth, but it is occasionally required. Food and large volumes of liquids are therefore usually withheld to reduce the risk of vomiting and aspiration. Ice chips are commonly provided, and small amounts of other clear liquids or juices, Popsicles, or hard candy on a stick also may be permitted.

URINARY SYSTEM

The most common change in the urinary system during labor is reduced sensation of a full bladder. Because of intense contractions or the effects of regional anesthesia, the woman may be unaware that her bladder is full. Yet a full bladder may contribute to discomfort, especially that which persists after regional anesthesia. A full bladder can also inhibit fetal descent because it occupies space in the pelvis.

After birth, the fluid retention that is normal during pregnancy is quickly reversed, and urine is excreted in large quantities. The bladder may fill rapidly during the first few days after birth.

HEMATOPOIETIC SYSTEM

Most authorities recognize 500 ml as the maximum normal blood loss during vaginal birth. Women usually tolerate this loss well because the blood volume increases during pregnancy by 1 to 2 liters (Guyton & Hall, 1996). A hemoglobin of 11 g/dl and a hematocrit of 33% or higher give most women an adequate margin of safety for blood loss associated with normal birth. The leukocyte count averages 14,000 to 16,000 per cubic millimeter (mm^3) but may be as high as 25,000/mm^3 or higher during labor, a level that might otherwise suggest infection (Cunningham et al., 1997).

Levels of several clotting factors, especially fibrinogen, are elevated during pregnancy and continue to be higher during labor and after delivery. Although the increase in clotting factors provides protection from hemorrhage, it also increases the mother's risk for venous thrombosis during pregnancy and after birth.

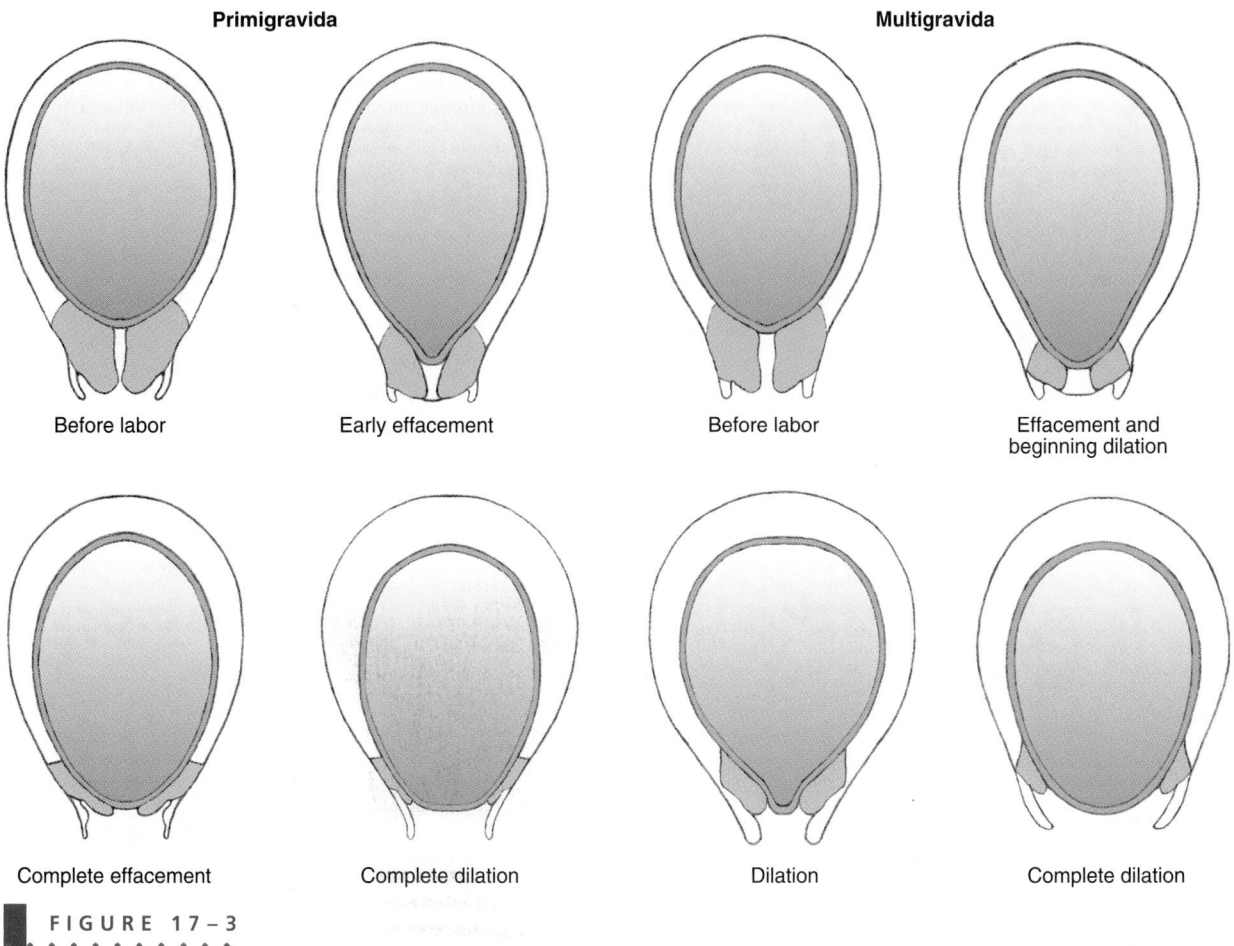

Primigravida

Before labor   Early effacement

Complete effacement   Complete dilation

Multigravida

Before labor   Effacement and beginning dilation

Dilation   Complete dilation

FIGURE 17–3

Cervical dilation and effacement. During labor, the multigravida's cervix remains thicker than the nullipara's.

Fetal Response

Fetal responses are most notable in the placental circulation, the cardiovascular system, and the pulmonary system.

PLACENTAL CIRCULATION

Exchange of oxygen, nutrients, and waste products between mother and fetus occurs in the intervillous spaces without mixing of maternal and fetal blood (see Chapter 12). During strong labor contractions, the maternal blood supply to the placenta stops intermittently as the spiral arteries supplying the intervillous spaces are compressed by the uterine muscle. Therefore, most placental exchange occurs during the interval between contractions.

The placental circulation usually has enough reserve over fetal basal needs to tolerate the intermittent interruption of blood flow. The fetus has protective mechanisms, such as fetal hemoglobin (which more readily takes on oxygen and releases carbon dioxide), a high hematocrit, and a high cardiac output. The fetus may not tolerate labor contractions well in conditions associated with reduced placental function, such as maternal diabetes or hypertension, or in conditions associated with reduced fetal oxygen-carrying capacity, such as fetal anemia.

CARDIOVASCULAR SYSTEM

The fetal cardiovascular system reacts quickly to events during labor. The fetal heart rate is rapid, ranging from 110 to 160 beats per minute (BPM) at term (Menihan, 1996). In general, the preterm fetus has a higher heart rate than the term fetus.

PULMONARY SYSTEM

Before birth, the fetal lungs are filled with fluid to allow normal development of the airways. This fluid must be cleared to allow normal air breathing. As term approaches, production of fetal lung fluid decreases, and its absorption into the interstitium of the lungs increases. Labor intensifies the absorption of lung fluid. Some fluid is expelled from the upper airways as the fetal head and thorax are compressed during passage through the birth canal. The remaining fluid is absorbed into the newborn's pulmonary and lymphatic circulations after birth.

Catecholamines, primarily epinephrine and norepinephrine, produced by the fetal adrenal glands in response to the stress of labor, appear to contribute to the infant's adaptation to extrauterine life. They stimulate cardiac contraction and breathing, speed clearance of remaining lung fluid, and aid in temperature regulation.

Inlet

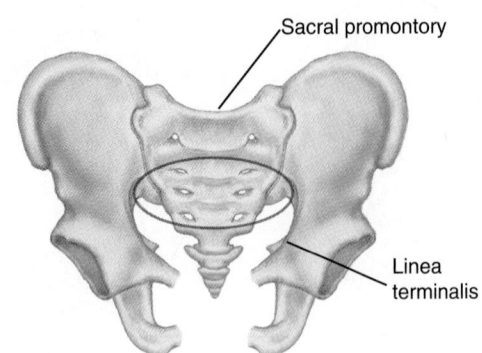

Frontal view, cutaway

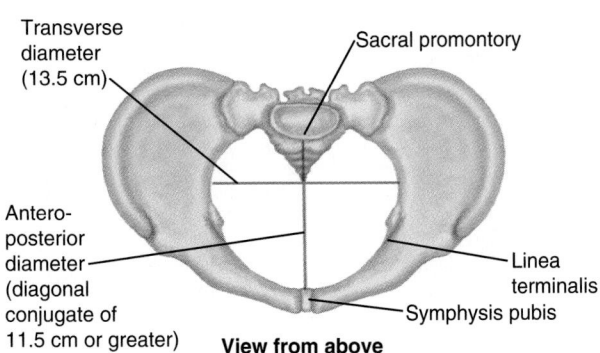

Transverse diameter (13.5 cm)

Sacral promontory

Antero-posterior diameter (diagonal conjugate of 11.5 cm or greater)

Linea terminalis

Symphysis pubis

View from above

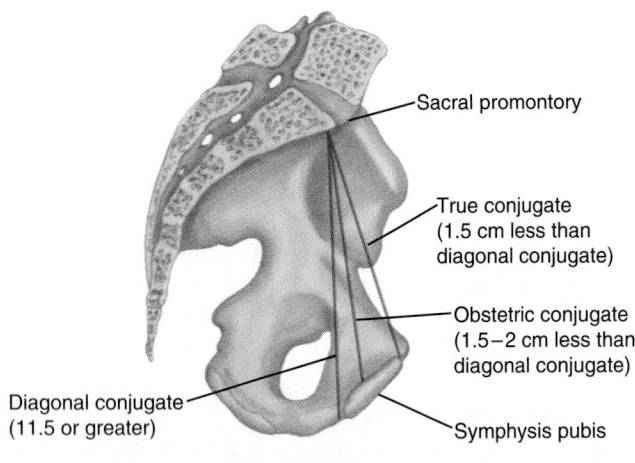

Sacral promontory

True conjugate (1.5 cm less than diagonal conjugate)

Obstetric conjugate (1.5–2 cm less than diagonal conjugate)

Diagonal conjugate (11.5 or greater)

Symphysis pubis

Side view, cutaway

The boundaries of the inlet are the symphysis pubis anteriorly, the sacral promontory posteriorly, and the linea terminalis on the sides. The inlet is slightly wider in its transverse diameter (13.5 cm) than in its anteroposterior (diagonal conjugate) diameter (11.5 cm or greater).

The diagonal conjugate is slightly larger than both the obstetric and true conjugates. The obstetric conjugate is the narrowest of the three conjugate diameters but cannot be measured directly. The obstetric conjugate is estimated by first measuring the diagonal conjugate and then subtracting 1.5 to 2 cm.

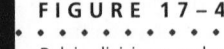

FIGURE 17–4
• • • • • • • • •
Pelvic divisions and measurements.

If the inlet is small, the fetal head may not be able to enter it. Because it is almost entirely surrounded by bone, except for cartilage at the sacroiliac joint and symphysis pubis, the inlet cannot enlarge much to accommodate the fetus. The bony measurements are essentially fixed.

Midpelvis

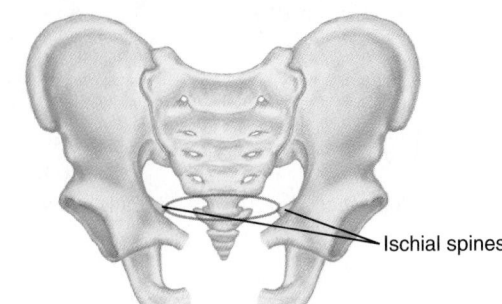

Ischial spines

Frontal view, cutaway

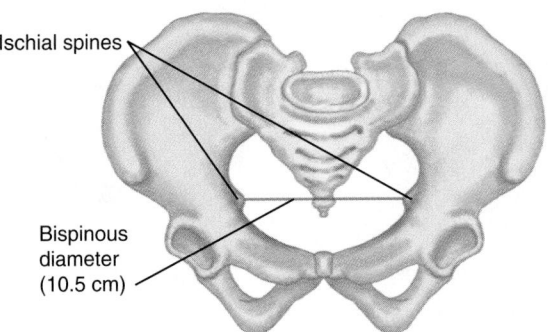

Ischial spines

Bispinous diameter (10.5 cm)

View from above, with pelvis tilted anteriorly

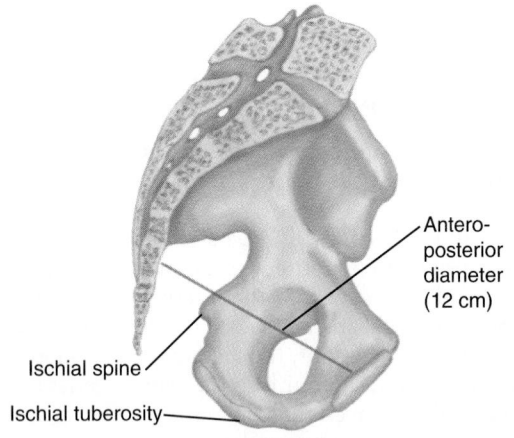

Antero-posterior diameter (12 cm)

Ischial spine

Ischial tuberosity

Side view, cutaway

The midpelvis, or pelvic cavity, is the narrowest part of the pelvis through which the fetus must pass during birth. Mid-pelvic diameters are measured at the level of the ischial spines. The anteroposterior diameter averages 12 cm.

The transverse diameter (bispinous or interspinous) averages 10.5 cm. Prominent ischial spines that project into the midpelvis can reduce the bispinous diameter.

Outlet

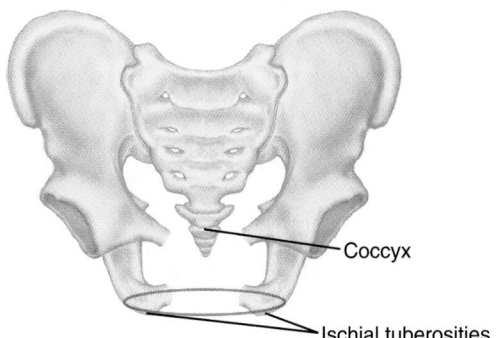

Frontal view, cutaway

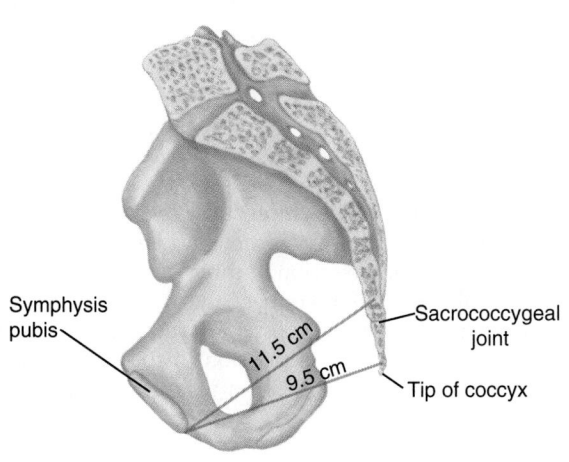

Side view, cutaway

Three important diameters of the pelvic outlet are (1) the anteroposterior, (2) the transverse (bi-ischial or intertuberous), and (3) the posterior sagittal. The angle of the pubic arch is also an important pelvic outlet measure.

The anteroposterior diameter ranges from 9.5 to 11.5 cm, varying with the curve between the sacrococcygeal joint and the tip of the coccyx. The anteroposterior diameter can increase if the coccyx is easily movable.

The transverse diameter is the bi-ischial, or intertuberous, diameter. This is the distance between the ischial tuberosities ("sit bones"). It averages 11 cm.

The posterior sagittal diameter is normally at least 7.5 cm. It is a measure of the posterior pelvis. The posterior sagittal diameter measures the distance from the sacrococcygeal joint to the middle of the transverse (bi-ischial) diameter.

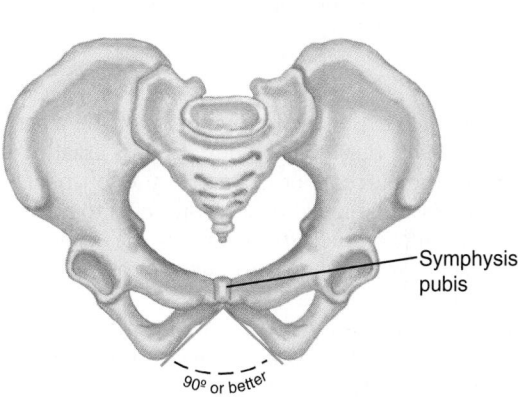

Frontal view, with pelvis tilted anteriorly

The angle of the pubic arch is important because it must be wide enough for the fetus to pass under it. The angle of the pubic arch should be at least 90 degrees. A narrow pubic arch displaces the fetus posteriorly toward the coccyx as it tries to pass under the arch.

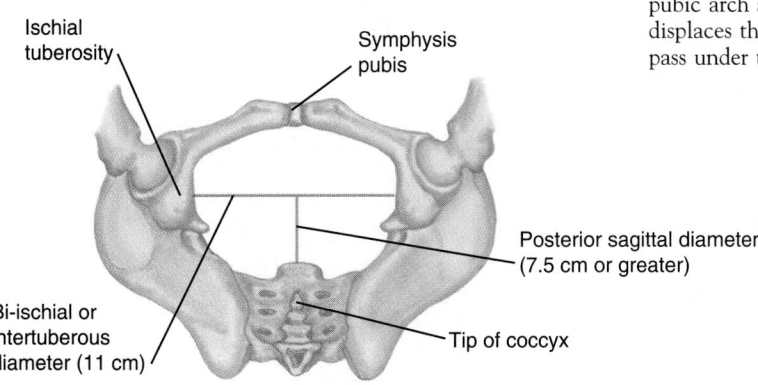

View from below (woman is in lithotomy position)

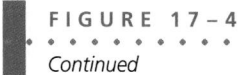

FIGURE 17-4
· · · · · · · · · · · ·
Continued

Components of the Birth Process

Four major factors, often called the "four P's," interact during normal childbirth. They are the powers, the passage, the passenger, and the psyche.

Powers

The two powers of labor are uterine contractions and maternal pushing efforts.

Uterine Contractions.   During the first stage of labor (onset through full cervical dilation), uterine contractions are the primary force moving the fetus through the maternal pelvis.

Maternal Pushing Efforts.   During the second stage of labor (full cervical dilation through birth of the baby), the woman adds her voluntary pushing efforts to the force of uterine contractions to propel the fetus through the pelvis.

Passage

The passage for birth of the fetus consists of the maternal pelvis and the soft tissues. The bony pelvis is usually more important to the outcome of labor than the soft tissue because the bones and joints do not readily yield to the forces of labor. Softening of the cartilage linking the pelvic bones, however, occurs at term because of an increase in the hormone relaxin.

The bony pelvis is divided by the linea terminalis (or pelvic brim) into the false pelvis above and the true pelvis below (see Chapter 11). The true pelvis is most important in childbirth. The true pelvis has three subdivisions: (1) the *inlet*, or upper pelvic opening, (2) the *midpelvis*, or pelvic cavity, and (3) the *outlet*, or lower pelvic opening. The true pelvis is like a curved cylinder with different dimensions at different levels. Figure 17–4 illustrates important pelvic measurements.

Passenger

The passenger is the fetus plus the membranes and placenta.

FETAL HEAD

The fetus enters the birth canal in the cephalic presentation 96% of the time. The fetal shoulders are important because of their width, but they are usually movable and adapt to the pelvis.

Bones, Sutures, and Fontanels.   The bones of the fetal head involved in the birth process are the two frontal bones on the forehead, the two parietal bones at the crown of the head, and the occipital bone at the back of the head (Fig. 17–5). The five major bones are not fused but are connected by sutures composed of strong but flexible fibrous tissue. The fontanels are wider spaces at the intersections of the sutures.

The *anterior fontanel* is diamond shaped and formed by the intersection of four sutures: the two coronal, the frontal, and the sagittal, which connect the two frontal and the two parietal bones. The *posterior fontanel* has a triangular shape formed by the intersection of three sutures, one sagittal and two lambdoid, which connect the two parietal bones and the occipital bone. The posterior fontanel is very small, often more like a slight depression in the skull. The sutures and fontanels allow the bones to move slightly, changing

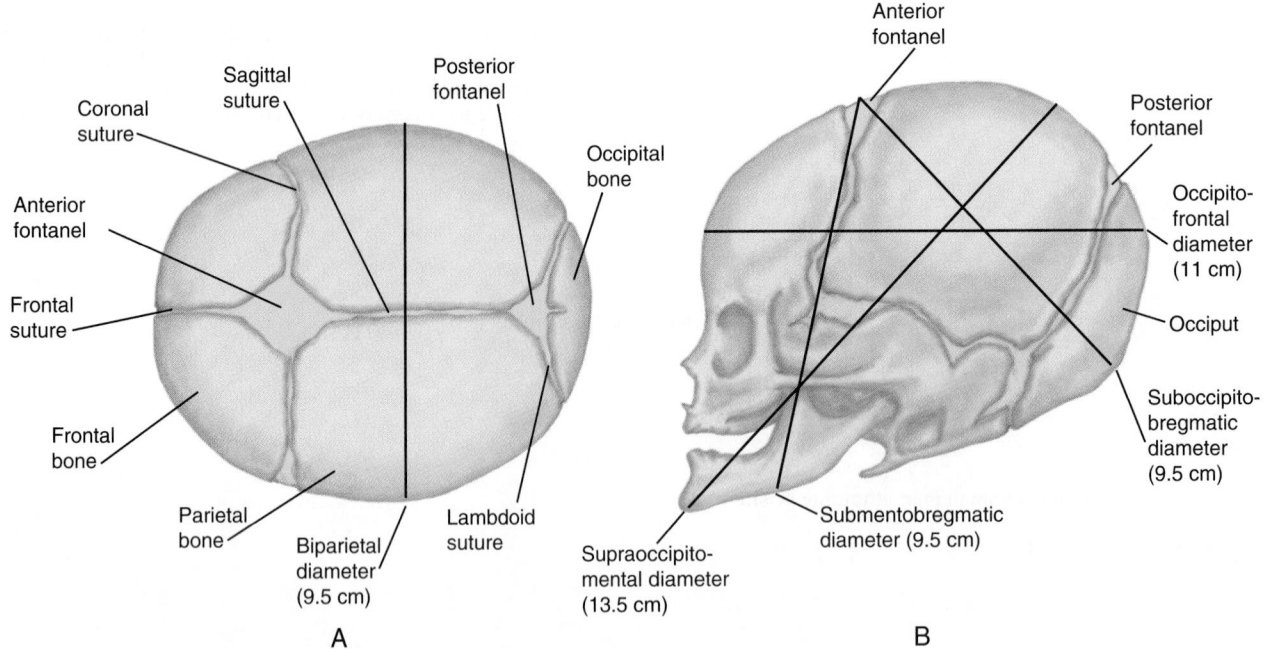

FIGURE 17–5

A, Bones, sutures, and fontanels of the fetal head. Note that the anterior fontanel has a diamond shape, whereas the posterior fontanel is triangular. *B,* Lateral view of the fetal head. Anteroposterior diameters vary with the amount of flexion or extension.

the shape of the fetal head so that it can adapt to the size and shape of the pelvis by molding. The sutures and the different shapes of the fontanels provide landmarks to determine fetal position and head flexion during vaginal examination.

Fetal Head Diameters.   Although most fetuses enter the pelvis in the cephalic presentation, several variations are possible. The major transverse diameter of the fetal head is the biparietal, measured between the two parietal bones. The biparietal diameter averages 9.5 cm in a term fetus.

The anteroposterior diameter of the head varies with the degree of flexion. In the most favorable situation, the head becomes fully flexed during labor, and the anteroposterior diameter is the suboccipitobregmatic, averaging 9.5 cm. See Figure 17–5B for anteroposterior head diameters in different degrees of head flexion and extension.

VARIATIONS IN THE PASSENGER

Fetal Lie.   The orientation of the long axis of the fetus to the long axis of the woman is the fetal lie (Fig. 17–6). In more than 99% of pregnancies, the lie is longitudinal, or parallel to the long axis of the woman. In the *longitudinal lie*, either the head or buttocks of the fetus enter the pelvis first. A *transverse lie* exists when the long axis of the fetus is at right angles to the woman's long axis; it occurs in fewer than 1% of pregnancies. An *oblique lie* is one at some angle between the longitudinal lie and the transverse lie.

Attitude.   The relation of fetal body parts to each other is the attitude of the fetus (Fig. 17–7). The normal fetal attitude is one of flexion, with the head flexed toward the chest and the arms and legs flexed over the thorax. The back is curved in a convex C shape.

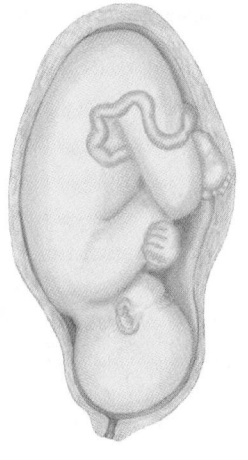 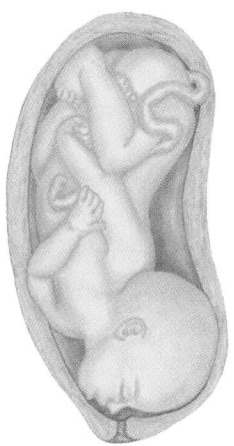

Flexion	Extension
A	B

FIGURE 17–7

Attitude. *A,* The fetus is in the normal attitude of flexion, with the head, arms, and legs flexed tightly against the trunk. *B,* The fetus is in an abnormal attitude of extension. The head is extended and the right arm is extended. A face presentation is illustrated.

Presentation.   The fetal part that enters the pelvis first is the presenting part. Presentation falls into three categories: (1) cephalic, (2) breech, and (3) shoulder. The cephalic presentation with the fetal head flexed is the most common (Fig. 17–8). Other presentations are associated with prolonged labor or other problems and are more likely to require cesarean birth.

Cephalic Presentation.   The cephalic presentation is more favorable than others, for several reasons:

- The fetal head is the largest single fetal part. After the head is born, the smaller parts follow easily as the extremities unfold.
- During labor, the fetal head can gradually change shape to adapt to the size and shape of the maternal pelvis.
- The fetal head is smooth, round, and hard, making it an effective part to dilate the cervix, which is also round.

Cephalic presentation has four variations (see Fig. 17–8).

Vertex.   The vertex presentation is the most common type of cephalic presentation. The fetal head is fully flexed. This presentation is the most favorable for normal progress of labor because the smallest suboccipitobregmatic diameter is presenting.

Military.   In a military presentation, the head is in a neutral position, neither flexed nor extended. The occipitofrontal diameter is presenting.

Brow.   In a brow presentation, the fetal head is partly extended. The longest supraoccipitomental diameter is presenting.

Face.   In a face presentation, the head is fully extended, and the fetal occiput is near the fetal spine. The submentobregmatic diameter is presenting.

Breech Presentation.   A breech presentation occurs when the fetal buttocks or feet enter the pelvis first. Breech presentations are associated with several disadvantages:

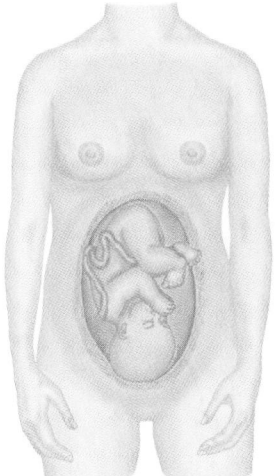

Longitudinal lie	Transverse lie
A	B

FIGURE 17–6

Lie. *A,* In a longitudinal lie, the long axis of the fetus is parallel to the long axis of the woman. *B,* In a transverse lie, the long axis of the fetus is at right angles to the long axis of the mother. The woman's abdomen has a wide, short appearance.

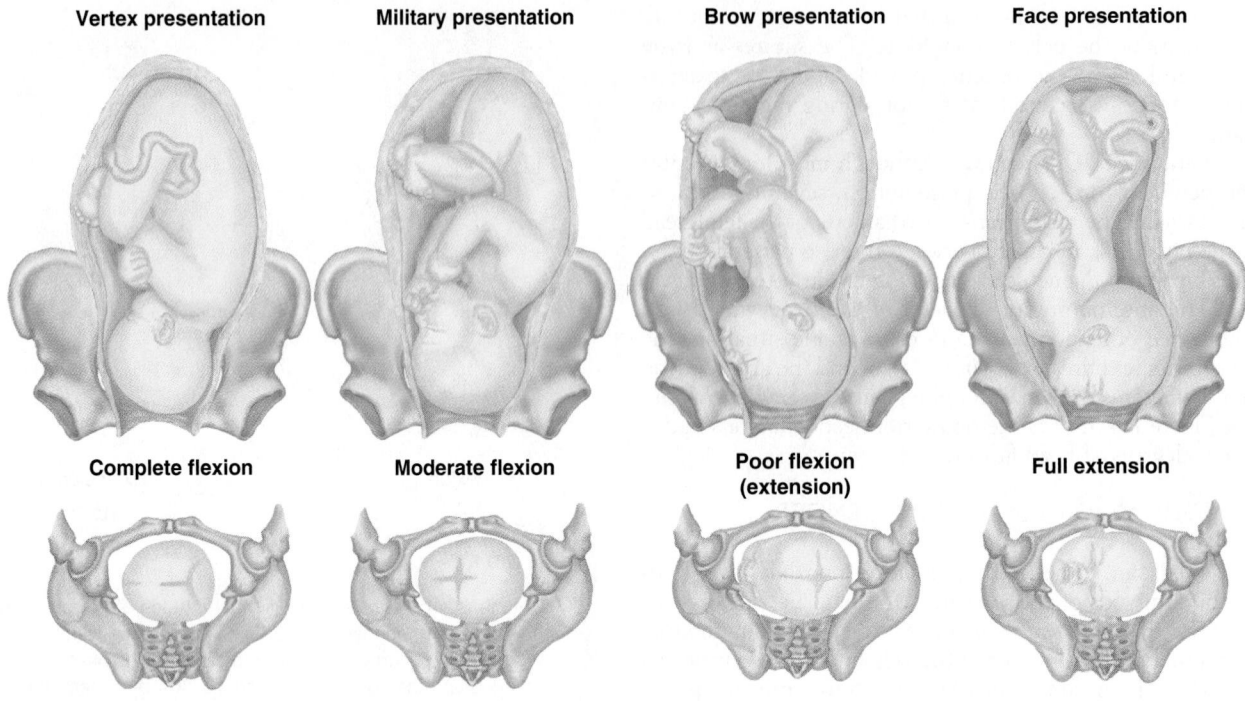

Vertex presentation   **Military presentation**   **Brow presentation**   **Face presentation**

Complete flexion   **Moderate flexion**   **Poor flexion (extension)**   **Full extension**

FIGURE 17–8

Four types of cephalic presentation. The vertex presentation is normal. Note positional changes of the anterior and posterior fontanels in relation to the maternal pelvis.

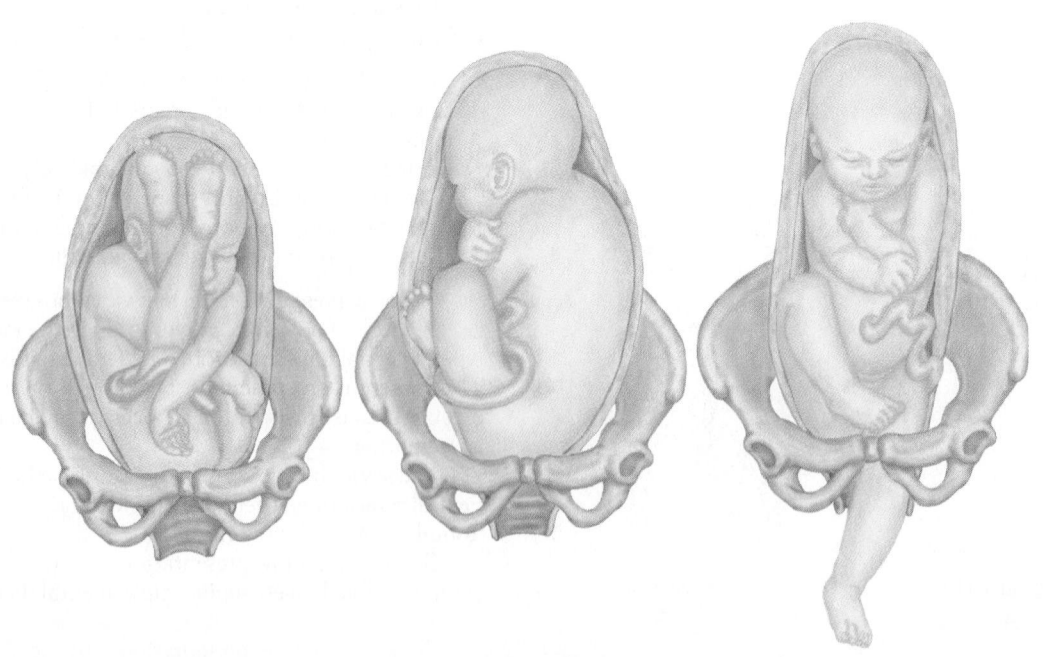

Frank breech   Full breech   Single footling breech

FIGURE 17–9

Three variations of a breech presentation. Frank breech is the most common variation. Footling breeches may be single or double.

- The buttocks are not smooth and firm like the head and are less effective at dilating the cervix.
- The fetal head is the last part to be born. By the time the fetal head is deep in the pelvis, the umbilical cord is outside the mother's body and is subject to compression between the baby's head and the maternal pelvis.
- Because the umbilical cord can be compressed after the fetal chest is born, the head must be delivered quickly to allow the infant to breathe. This necessary speed does not permit gradual molding of the fetal head as it passes through the pelvis.

The breech presentation has three variations, depending on the relationship of the legs to the body (Fig. 17–9).

Frank Breech. The frank breech is the most common variation. In a frank breech presentation the fetal legs are extended across the abdomen toward the shoulders.

Full (or Complete) Breech. The full breech is a reversal of the usual cephalic presentation. The head is flexed, and the knees and hips are also flexed, but the buttocks are presenting.

Footling Breech. The footling breech occurs when one or both feet are presenting.

Shoulder. The shoulder presentation is a transverse lie and accounts for only 0.2% of births (Cunningham et al., 1997). A cesarean birth is almost always necessary.

Position. Fetal position describes the location of a fixed reference point on the presenting part in relation to the four quadrants of the maternal pelvis (Fig. 17–10): right and left anterior and right and left posterior. The fetal position is not fixed but rather changes during labor as the fetus moves downward and adapts to the pelvic contours. Abbre-

viations indicate the relationship between the fetal presenting part and the maternal pelvis.

Right (R) or Left (L). The first letter of the abbreviation describes whether the fetal reference point is in the right or left of the mother's pelvis. If the fetal point is neither to the right nor to the left of the pelvis, this letter is omitted.

Occiput (O), Mentum (M), or Sacrum (S). The second letter of the abbreviation refers to the fixed fetal reference point, which varies with the presentation. The occiput is used in a vertex presentation. The chin, or mentum, is the reference point in a face presentation. The sacrum is used for breech presentations. Letters may also designate the less common brow (F for fronto) and shoulder (Sc for scapula) presentations.

Anterior (A), Posterior (P), or Transverse (T). The third letter describes whether the fetal reference point is in the anterior or posterior quadrant of the mother's pelvis. If the fetal reference point is in neither the anterior nor the posterior quadrant, it is described as transverse.

If the fetal occiput is located in the left anterior quadrant of the mother's pelvis, the position is described as left occiput anterior (LOA). If the occiput is in the mother's anterior pelvis, neither to the right nor to the left, it is described as occiput anterior (OA). If the fetal sacrum is located in the mother's right posterior pelvis, the description is R (right) S (sacrum) P (posterior). See Figure 17–11 for different fetal presentations and positions.

Psyche

The psyche is a crucial part of childbirth. Marked anxiety or fear decreases a woman's ability to cope with pain in labor. Maternal catecholamines secreted in response to anxiety or fear can inhibit uterine contractility and placental blood flow. Relaxation, however, augments the natural process of labor.

Interrelationships of the Components of Birth

The four P's—the powers, passage, passenger, and psyche—are actually an interrelated whole. For instance, a woman with a small pelvis (passage) and a large fetus (passenger) can have a normal labor and birth if the fetus is ideally positioned and the uterine contractions and maternal bearing down efforts (powers) are vigorous. The nurse's supportive attitude strengthens positive psychological elements (psyche) and enhances the processes of birth. The nurse can act as an advocate for the laboring woman and her family or partners to increase their sense of control and mastery of labor, often reducing anxiety and fear.

INDIVIDUAL AND CULTURAL VALUES

A family's culture affects its members' views of birth and the practices that surround it. Culture shapes the values that people hold, their expectations of the birth experience, and their responses to birth. A woman's culture gives her cues about how she should behave and react to labor and how she should interact with her newborn. If the woman, her family, and caregivers have similar views, little conflict in

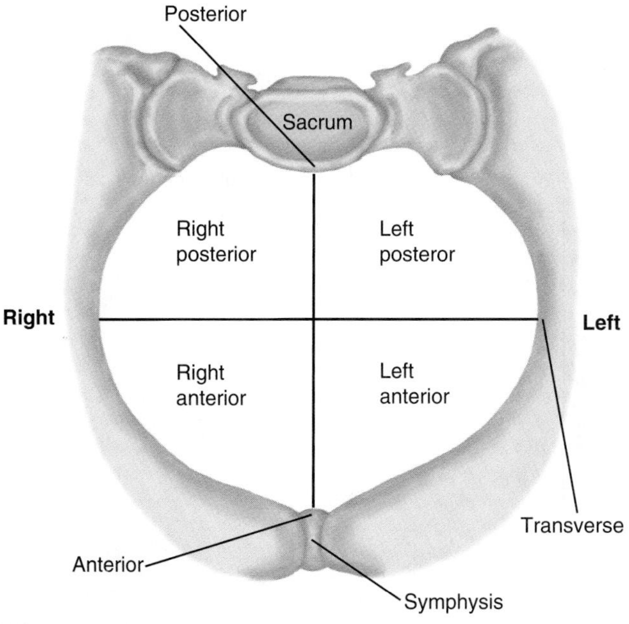

FIGURE 17–10

Four quadrants of the maternal pelvis, used to describe fetal position.

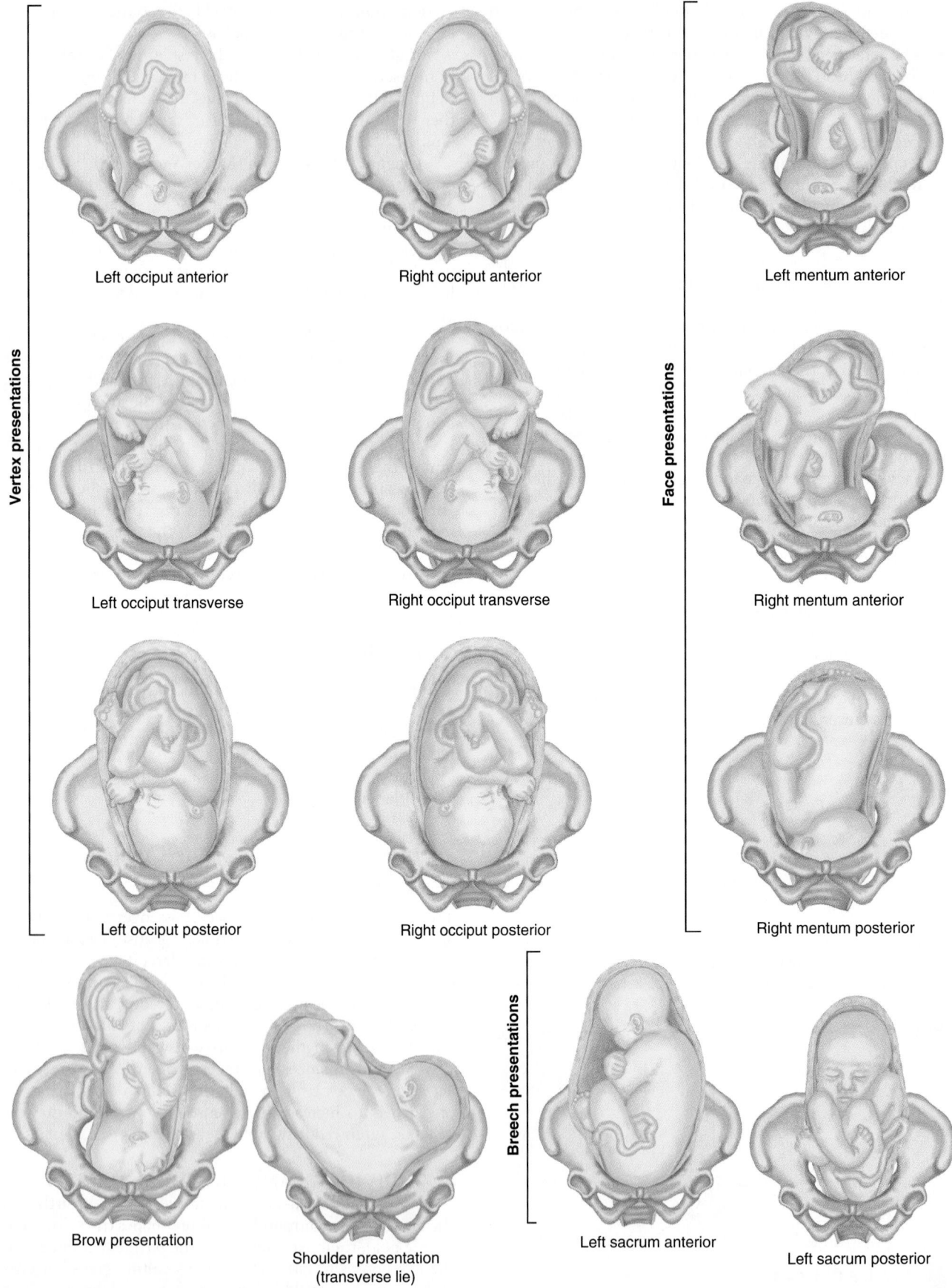

Vertex presentations

Left occiput anterior

Right occiput anterior

Left occiput transverse

Right occiput transverse

Left occiput posterior

Right occiput posterior

Face presentations

Left mentum anterior

Right mentum anterior

Right mentum posterior

Brow presentation

Shoulder presentation
(transverse lie)

Breech presentations

Left sacrum anterior

Left sacrum posterior

FIGURE 17–11

Fetal presentations and positions.

their values and expectations is likely. If these individuals hold markedly different views, however, they may be confused because each expects something different of the other.

Knowledge of the values and practices of cultural groups that the nurse encounters provides a framework to assess and care for the woman and her family, but within a culture, people are individuals. The nurse must assess the personal expectations and birth-related values of each woman and her family within this general framework. Aspects of cultural assessment for the intrapartum period might include the following:

- How long has the family been in the area? Are they recent immigrants, or have their relatives and friends lived in the area for generations?
- What is the family's primary language? Are they comfortable communicating in the nurse's language if the two are different? If an interpreter is needed, are there people the family considers unacceptable?
- Who is the woman's primary support person for labor? What is that person's role? How extensively will that support person interact with the laboring woman?
- If the woman's primary support is to be the baby's father, how does the couple view his role? Will he actively support the woman (e.g., by coaching her breathing), or will he take a less active role?
- Is a caregiver of the same sex and cultural group essential?
- What are the woman's feelings about touch? Is she comfortable telling the nurse when she does or does not welcome touch?
- Are specific symbols, practices, or ceremonies used during the birth period? Who will conduct any ceremonies?

BIRTH AS AN EXPERIENCE

Childbirth is a physical and emotional experience. It is also an irrevocable event that changes a woman forever. Families describe the births of their children as they describe other pivotal events in life: marriages, anniversaries, religious events, and even deaths. With the prevalence of smaller families, parents have greater expectations about the experience of childbirth than in the past. The more realistic a woman's expectations about the birth are, the more likely she is to have a positive experience.

Nursing measures that increase a sense of control and mastery during birth help families perceive the birth as a positive event. Nursing measures to empower families include teaching them about their choices in childbirth in an unbiased way and supporting the choices they make.

Normal Labor

Theories of Onset

The factors that initiate labor remain unknown despite much research on the subject. Labor begins when forces favoring continuation of pregnancy are overcome by forces favoring its end. Factors that have a role in starting labor are the following:

- Increased fetal adrenal gland production of glucocorticoids and androgens, which reduces placental progesterone secretion and increases prostaglandin production. When progesterone levels decline, the uterus becomes more easily stimulated to contract.
- A change in the ratio of maternal estrogen to progesterone so that estrogen levels are higher than progesterone levels. Progesterone promotes uterine muscle relaxation during most of pregnancy. Relatively higher estrogen levels enhance uterine sensitivity to substances that stimulate uterine contractions: prostaglandins from the fetal membranes and oxytocin from the maternal posterior pituitary gland.
- Stretching, pressure, or irritation of the uterus and cervix.

Premonitory Signs

Before labor begins, women usually notice one or more premonitory, or warning, signs that labor is about to begin.

- Braxton Hicks contractions, which occur throughout pregnancy, increase in frequency and are sometimes painful. They may become regular at times, only to decrease spontaneously.
- Lightening ("dropping") occurs as the fetus descends toward the pelvic inlet. Lightening is most noticeable in nulliparas, occurring about 2 to 3 weeks before the onset of labor.
- Increased clear and nonirritating vaginal secretions occur as fetal pressure causes congestion of the vaginal mucosa.
- "Bloody show," a mixture of thick mucus and pink or dark brown blood, may occur as the cervix begins to soften, dilate, and efface slightly ("ripening").
- Some women have an energy spurt ("nesting").
- A small weight loss of about 1 to 3 lb may occur because changing levels of estrogen and progesterone cause excretion of some of the extra fluid that accumulates during pregnancy.

True Labor and False Labor

False labor, also called prodromal labor, is common because the exact time of labor's onset is rarely known and the onset is usually gradual. False labor often causes women to go to the birth center, thinking that labor has started, only to be disappointed when it has not. The term *false labor* is discouraging to women, because they do not realize that these "false" contractions are simply preparation for the main event of true labor, rather than true labor itself.

Several characteristics distinguish true labor from false labor: contractions, discomfort, and cervical change. The best distinction between the two is that the contractions of true labor cause *progressive changes in the cervix*. Effacement and dilation occur with true labor contractions.

Mechanisms of Labor

The mechanisms (cardinal movements) of labor occur as the fetus is moved through the pelvis during birth. The fetus undergoes several positional changes to adapt to the size and shape of the mother's pelvis at different levels (Fig. 17–12). Although the mechanisms of labor are described

How to Know Whether Labor Is "Real"

True labor differs from false labor in three categories.

FALSE LABOR	TRUE LABOR
Contractions	
Inconsistent in frequency, duration, and intensity.	A consistent pattern of increasing frequency, duration, and intensity usually develops.
A change in activity, such as walking, does not alter contractions, or activity may decrease them.	Walking tends to increase contractions.
Discomfort	
Felt in the abdomen and groin.	Begins in lower back and gradually sweeps around to the lower abdomen like a girdle.
May be more annoying than truly painful.	Back pain may persist in some women.
	Early labor often feels like menstrual cramps.
Cervix	
No significant change in effacement or dilation of the cervix.	Effacement and/or dilation of cervix occurs.
	Progressive effacement and dilation of cervix are most important characteristics.

separately in Figure 17–12, some occur concurrently. In a vertex presentation, the mechanisms are the following:

- *Descent* of the fetal presenting part through the true pelvis.
- *Engagement* of the fetal presenting part as its widest diameter reaches the level of the ischial spines of the mother's pelvis.
- *Flexion* of the fetal head so that the smallest head diameters pass through the pelvis.
- *Internal rotation* to allow the largest fetal head diameters to match the largest maternal pelvic diameters.
- *Extension* of the fetal head as it passes beneath the mother's symphysis pubis.
- *External rotation* of the fetal head to allow the shoulders to rotate internally to fit the mother's pelvis as well as possible.
- *Expulsion* of the fetal shoulders and fetal body.

The mechanisms of labor are different in presentations other than the vertex, but the reason is the same: effective use of available space in the maternal pelvis.

Stages and Phases of Labor

Each stage and phase of labor has qualities that set it apart from the others. These descriptions are approximate. Individual women vary in their labor patterns and responses to labor. Use of regional anesthetics, such as the epidural block, is likely to modify the typical maternal behaviors. Table 17–1 provides details of the characteristics of each stage of labor.

FIRST STAGE OF LABOR

Cervical effacement and dilation occur in the first stage of labor, or *stage of dilation*. It begins with the onset of true labor contractions and ends with complete dilation (10 cm) and effacement (100%) of the cervix. The first stage of labor is the longest for both nulliparous and parous women. Labor progress may be plotted on a graph, often called a Friedman curve (Fig. 17–13).

First-stage labor differs from the other stages because it has three phases: latent (early), active, and transition. Each phase is characterized by typical maternal behaviors. These behaviors vary with the woman's preparation, use of coping skills, and use of medication.

Latent Phase. The latent, or early, phase lasts from the beginning of labor until about 3 cm of cervical dilation. Its length is quite variable among women. Despite being called latent, much cervical effacement and fetal position change occur during this phase, preparing for more rapid changes during active labor. The woman is usually sociable and excited during this early phase of labor.

Active Phase. The active phase of labor is aptly named because the pace of labor increases. The cervix dilates from 4 to 7 cm and dilates at a more rapid rate than in the latent phase. Effacement of the cervix is completed. The fetus descends in the pelvis, and internal rotation begins. Discomfort usually increases as the pace of labor picks up.

The woman becomes more anxious and may feel helpless as the contractions intensify. The sociability that characterized early labor is gone, replaced with a serious, inward focus.

Transition Phase. The cervix dilates from 8 to 10 cm, and the fetus descends further into the pelvis. Bloody show often increases with completion of cervical dilation. Transition is a short but intense phase, with very strong contractions. The woman may have an urge to push or bear down during contractions. Leg tremors, nausea, and vomiting are common.

The woman may be irritable and lose control. Her partner may be confused because actions that were helpful just a short time before now bother her.

SECOND STAGE OF LABOR

The second stage (*expulsion*) begins with complete (10 cm) dilation and full (100%) effacement of the cervix and ends with the birth of the baby. As the fetus descends, pressure of the presenting part on the rectum and the pelvic floor causes the mother to have an involuntary pushing response. She may say that she needs to have a bowel movement or "The baby's coming" or "I have to push." Her voluntary pushing efforts augment involuntary uterine contractions. As the fetus descends low in the pelvis and the vulva distends with crowning of the fetal head, she may feel a sensation of stretching or splitting even if no trauma occurs.

The woman often regains a sense of control during the second stage of labor. Contractions are strong, but she may feel more in control because she is doing something to complete the process by pushing with them. "Labor" is a fitting word to describe the second stage. The woman exerts intense effort to push her baby out. Between contractions, she may be oblivious to her surroundings and may appear asleep. She feels tremendous relief and excitement as the second stage ends with the birth of the baby.

THIRD STAGE OF LABOR

The third (*placental*) stage begins with the birth of the baby and ends with the expulsion of the placenta (Fig. 17–14). When the infant is born, the uterine cavity becomes much smaller. The reduced size decreases the size of the placental site, causing the placenta to separate from the uterine wall. Four signs suggest placenta separation:

- The uterus has a spherical shape.
- The uterus rises upward in the abdomen as the placenta descends into the vagina and pushes the fundus upward.
- The cord descends further from the vagina.
- A gush of blood appears as blood trapped behind the placenta is released.

The placenta may be expelled in one of two ways. In the more common *Schultze* mechanism, the placenta is expelled with the shiny, fetal side first (see Fig. 17–14B). The *Duncan* mechanism is less common, with the rough maternal side presenting (see Fig. 17–14A).

The uterus must contract firmly and remain contracted after the placenta is expelled to compress open vessels at the implantation site. Inadequate uterine contraction after birth may result in hemorrhage.

Pain during the third stage of labor results from uterine contractions and brief stretching of the cervix as the placenta passes through it.

FOURTH STAGE OF LABOR

The fourth stage of labor is the *stage of physical recovery* for the mother and infant. It lasts from the delivery of the placenta through the first 1 to 4 hours after birth.

Immediately after birth, the firmly contracted uterus can be palpated through the abdominal wall as a firm, rounded mass about 10 to 15 cm (4 to 6 inches) in diameter at or below the level of the umbilicus. Uterine size varies with the size of the infant and the parity of the mother.

The uterus is larger when the infant is large or the mother is a multipara.

The vaginal drainage during the fourth stage is *lochia rubra,* which consists mostly of blood. See Chapter 21 for more information about lochia.

Many women have a chill after birth. The chill lasts for about 20 minutes and subsides spontaneously. A warm blanket, hot drink, or soup may help shorten the chill and make the woman more comfortable.

Discomfort during the fourth stage usually results from birth trauma or afterpains. Ice packs on the perineum limit discomfort and hematoma formation.

Afterpains are uterine contractions similar to menstrual cramps that occur after birth as the uterus begins its return to the prepregnancy state. The discomfort is similar to that of menstrual cramps. Afterpains are more intense in multiparas, in women who breast-feed, in women who have large babies or other causes of uterine overdistension during pregnancy, or when something interferes with uterine contraction, such as a full bladder or a blood clot that remains in the uterus.

The mother is simultaneously excited and tired after birth. She may be exhausted but too full of nervous energy to rest. The fourth stage of labor is an ideal time for bonding of the new family because the interest of both parents and newborn is high. It is also the best time to initiate breastfeeding if no maternal or infant problems are present. The baby is alert and seeks to make eye contact with the new parents, giving powerful reinforcement for the parents' attachment to their newborn.

Duration of Labor

The total duration of labor is significantly different for women who have never given birth and for those who have previously given birth vaginally. The parous woman usually delivers more quickly than does the nulliparous woman. Women, however, are individuals. Some nulliparas progress through labor quickly, whereas labor for some parous women resembles that of women who have never given birth. A woman who experienced a long labor with her first child may not have a long labor with every baby. If she has a history of rapid labor, however, later births are often rapid as well.

Because vaginal birth after cesarean (VBAC) is common, a parous woman may have had no vaginal births. In this situation, the woman is likely to have a labor more like that of the nullipara, particularly if she did not labor before her previous cesarean birth.

■ Nursing Care During Labor and Birth

Admission to the Birth Center

During the last trimester, the woman needs to know when she should go to the hospital or birth center. Nurses teach women differences between false labor and true labor and offer guidelines for going to the birth center. Not everyone has a typical labor, so a woman should be encouraged to go to the birth center if she is uncertain or has other concerns.

Text continued on page 370

Descent, Engagement, and Flexion

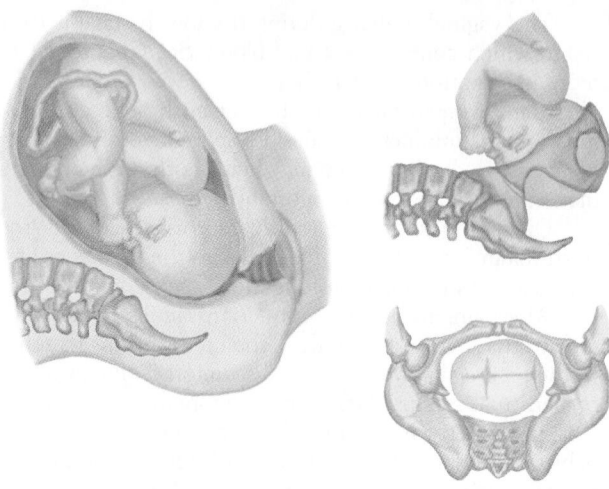

Descent of the fetus is a mechanism of labor that accompanies all the others. Without descent, none of the mechanisms will occur.

Station

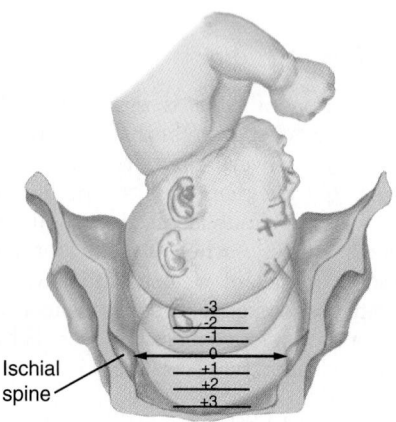

Ischial
spine

Station describes the descent of the fetal presenting part in relation to the level of the ischial spines. The level of the ischial spines is a zero station. Other stations are described with numbers representing the approximate number of centimeters above (negative numbers) or below (positive numbers) the ischial spines. As the fetus descends through the pelvis, the station changes from higher negative numbers (−3, −2, −1) to zero to higher positive numbers (+1, +2, +3, etc.) Sometimes the terms *floating* or *ballottable* may describe a fetal presenting part that is so high that it is easily displaced upward during abdominal or vaginal examination, similar to tossing a ball upward.

FIGURE 17–12
. . . .
Mechanisms (cardinal movements) of labor.

Engagement

Engagement occurs when the largest diameter of the fetal presenting part (normally the head) has passed the pelvic inlet and entered the pelvic cavity. Engagement is presumed to have occurred when the station of the presenting part is zero or lower. Engagement often takes place before onset of labor in nulliparous women. In many parous women and in some nulliparas, it does not occur until after labor begins.

Flexion

As the fetus descends, the fetal head is flexed further as it meets resistance from the soft tissues of the pelvis. Head flexion presents the smallest anteroposterior diameter (suboccipitobregmatic) to the pelvis.

Internal Rotation

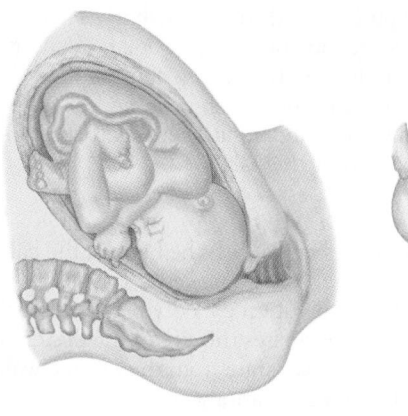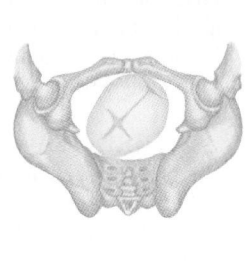

The fetus enters the pelvic inlet with the sagittal suture in a transverse or oblique orientation to the maternal pelvis because that is the widest inlet diameter. Internal rotation allows the longest fetal head diameter (the anteroposterior) to conform to the longest diameter of the maternal pelvis.

The longest pelvic outlet diameter is the anteroposterior. As the head descends to the level of the ischial spines, it gradually turns so that the fetal occiput is in the anterior of the pelvis (OA position, directly under the maternal symphysis pubis). When internal rotation is complete, the sagittal suture is oriented in the anteroposterior pelvic diameter (OA). Less commonly, the head may turn posteriorly so that the occiput is directed toward the mother's sacrum (OP).

Extension

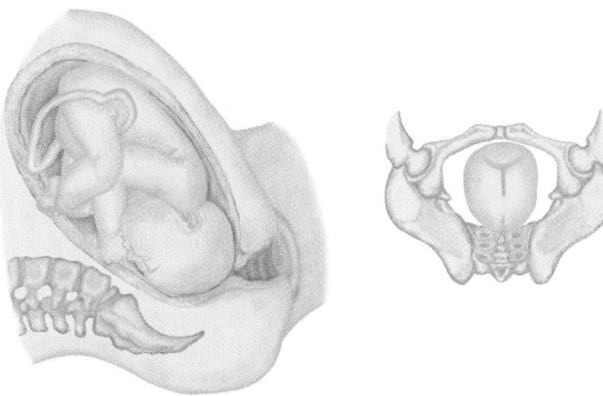

Extension beginning (internal rotation complete)

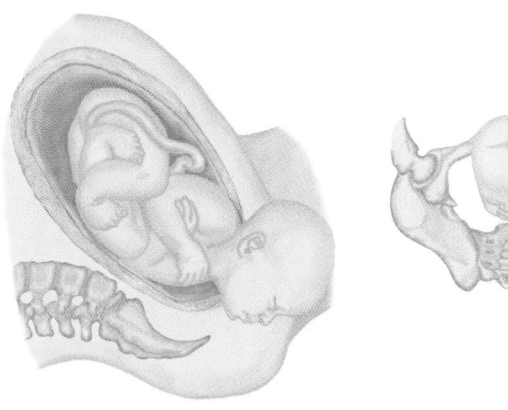

Extension complete

Because the true pelvis is shaped like a curved cylinder, the fetal head is directed posteriorly toward the rectum as it begins its descent. To negotiate the curve of the pelvis, the fetal head must change from an attitude of flexion to one of extension.

While still in flexion, the fetal head meets resistance from the tissues of the pelvic floor. At the same time, the fetal neck stops under the symphysis, which acts as a pivot. The combination of resistance from the pelvic floor and the pivoting action of the symphysis causes the fetal head to swing anteriorly, or extend, with each maternal pushing effort. The head is born in extension, with the occiput sliding under the symphysis and the face directed toward the rectum. The fetal brow, nose, and chin slide over the perineum as the head is born.

External Rotation

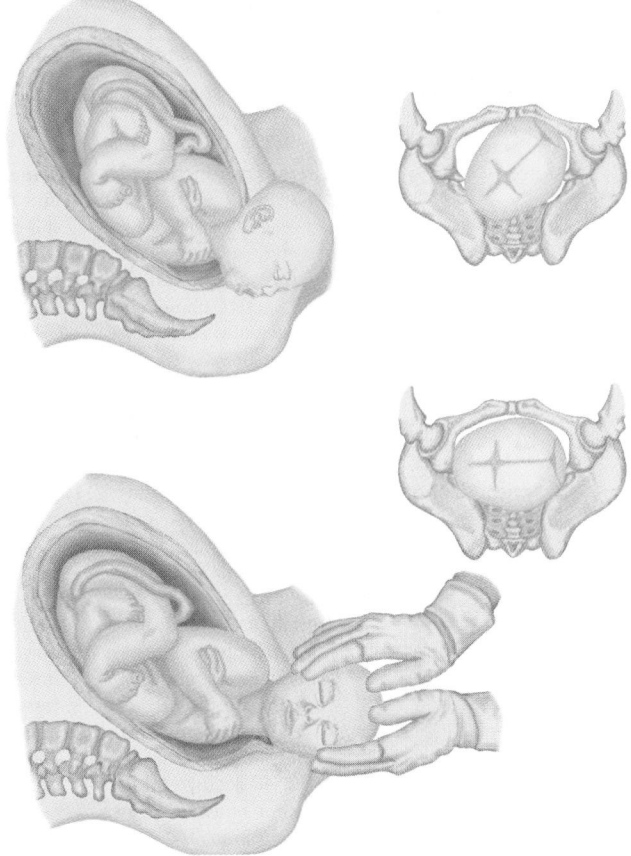

When the head is born with the occiput directed anteriorly, the shoulders must rotate internally so that they align with the anteroposterior diameter of the pelvis.

After the head is born, it spontaneously turns to the same side as it was in utero as it realigns with the shoulders and back (through a process called restitution). The head then turns further to that side in external rotation as the shoulders internally rotate and are positioned with their transverse diameter in the anteroposterior diameter of the pelvic outlet. External rotation of the head accompanies internal rotation of the shoulders.

Expulsion

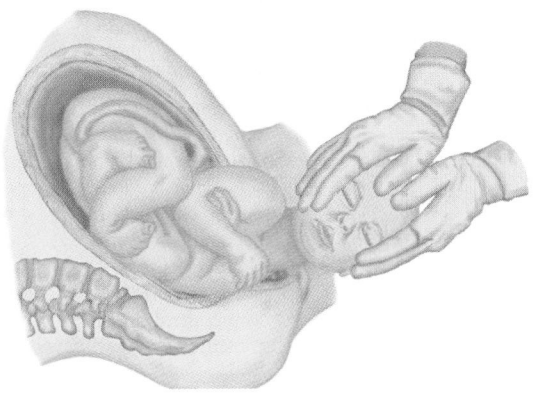

Expulsion occurs first as the anterior, then the posterior, shoulder passes under the symphysis. After the shoulders are born, the rest of the body follows.

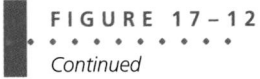

FIGURE 17–12
· · · · · · · · · ·
Continued

TABLE 17-1
• • • • • • • • • • •

Characteristics of Normal Labor

	First Stage	Second Stage	Third Stage	Fourth Stage
Work accomplished	Effacement and dilation of cervix	Expulsion of fetus	Separation of placenta	Physical recovery and bonding with newborn
Forces	Uterine contractions	Uterine contractions and voluntary bearing-down efforts	Uterine contractions	Uterine contraction to control bleeding from placental site
Average duration				
Nullipara	8–10 hr after reaching active phase; dilation averages 1 cm/hr	Average 50 min (range, 30 min–3 hr)	5–10 min; up to 30 min is normal for unassisted placental separation	1–4 hr after birth
Multipara	6–7 hr (range, 2–10 hr) after reaching active phase; dilation averages 1.2 cm/hr	Average 20 min (range, 5–30 min)	Same as for nullipara	Same as for nullipara
Cervical dilation	Latent phase: 0–3 cm Active phase: 4–7 cm Transition phase: 8–10 cm	10 cm (complete dilation)	Not applicable	Not applicable
Uterine contractions	*Latent phase* Initially mild and infrequent; progress to moderate strength, every 5 min with a regular pattern; duration increases to 30–40 sec by end of latent phase *Active phase* Increase in frequency, duration, and intensity until every 2–5 min, 40–60 sec, and moderate to strong intensity *Transition phase* Strong, every 1½ to 2 min, 60 sec	Strong, every 2–3 min, lasting 40–60 sec; may be slightly less intense than during transition phase of first stage; may pause briefly as second stage begins	Firmly contracted	Firmly contracted
Discomfort	Often begins with a low backache and sensations similar to those of menstrual cramps; back discomfort gradually sweeps to the lower abdomen in a girdle-like fashion, discomfort intensifies as labor progresses	Urge to push or bear down with contractions, which becomes stronger as fetus descends; distension of vagina and vulva may cause a stretching or splitting sensation	Little discomfort; sometimes slight cramp is felt as placenta is passed	Discomfort varies; some women have afterpains, more common in multigravidas or those who have had a large baby; as anesthesia wears off, perineal discomfort may become noticeable
Maternal behaviors	Sociable, excited, and somewhat anxious during early labor; becomes more inwardly focused as labor intensifies; may lose control during transition	Intense concentration on pushing with contractions; often oblivious to surroundings and appears to doze between contractions	Excited and relieved after baby's birth; usually very tired; often cries	Tired, but may find it difficult to rest because of excitement; eager to become acquainted with her newborn

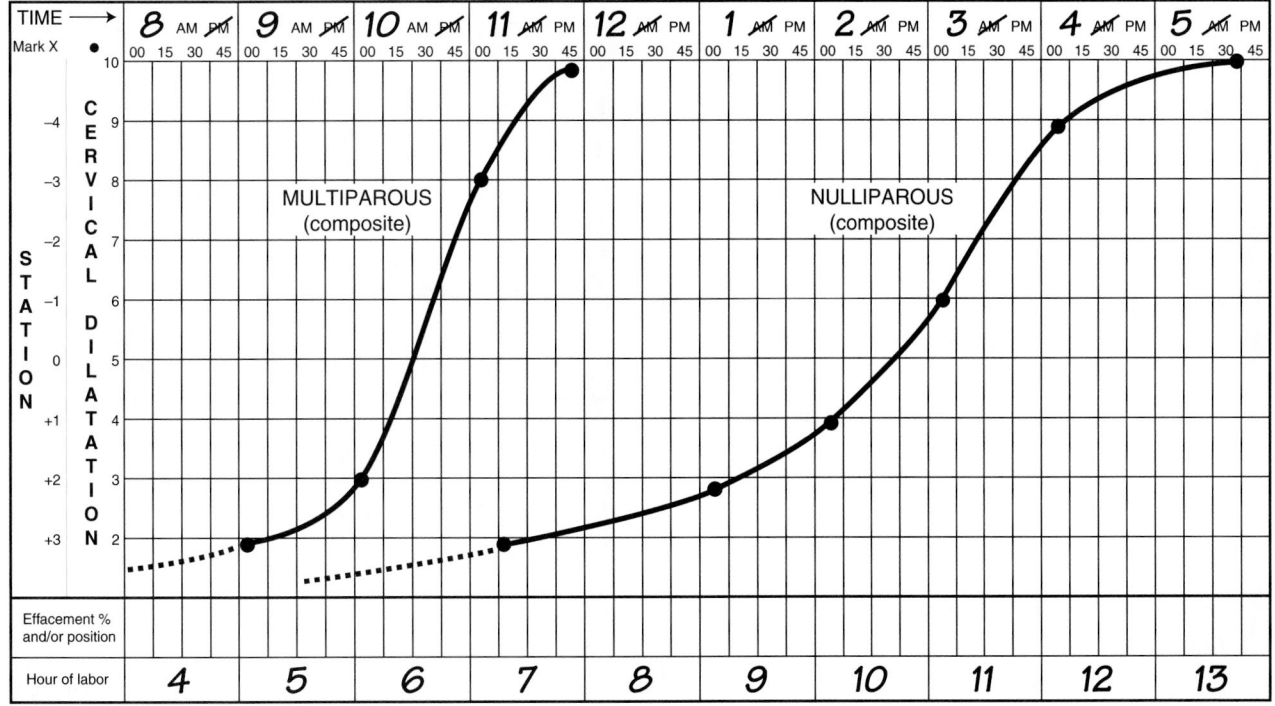

Composite Normal Dilation Curves

FIGURE 17–13

A labor curve, often called a Friedman curve, may be used to identify whether a woman's cervical dilation is progressing at the expected rate.

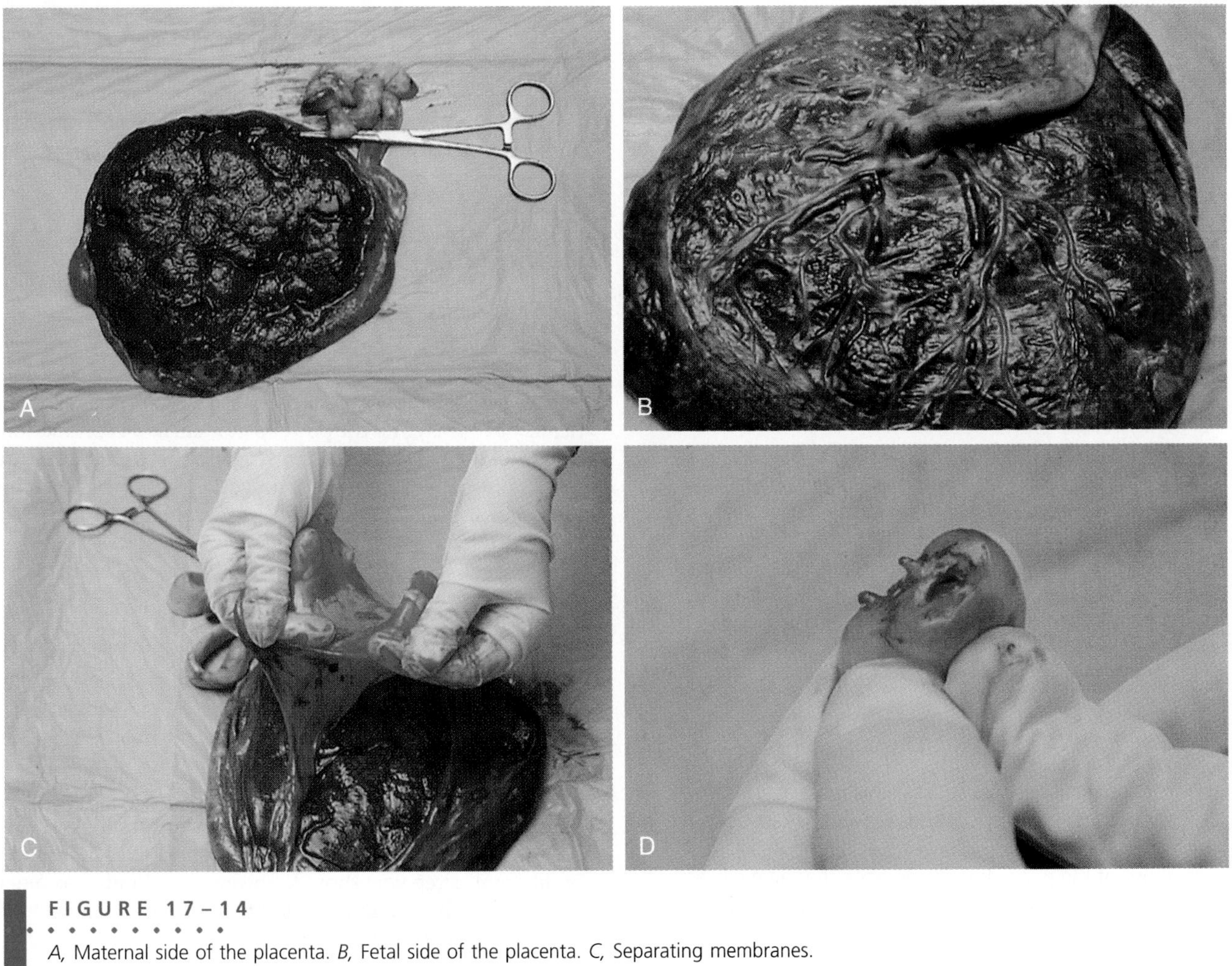

FIGURE 17–14

A, Maternal side of the placenta. *B,* Fetal side of the placenta. *C,* Separating membranes.
D, Umbilical cord vessels—two arteries and one vein.

WOMEN WANT TO KNOW

When to Go to the Hospital or Birth Center

These are guidelines for providing individualized instruction to women about when to enter the hospital or birth center.

Contractions

A pattern of increasing regularity, frequency, duration, and intensity:

- *Nullipara:* Regular contractions, 5 minutes apart, for 1 hour.
- *Multipara:* Regular contractions, 10 minutes apart, for 1 hour.

Ruptured Membranes

A gush or trickle of fluid from the vagina should be evaluated, whether or not you have contractions.

Bleeding

Bright red bleeding that is not mixed with mucus should be evaluated promptly. Normal bloody show is thicker, pink or dark red, and mixed with mucus.

Decreased Fetal Movement

If you notice a decrease in the baby's movement, notify your physician or nurse-midwife or come to the labor unit.

Other Concerns

These guidelines cannot cover all situations. Therefore, please go to the hospital for evaluation of any concerns or feelings that something may be wrong.

Nursing Responsibilities During Admission

The nurse has two priorities when the woman arrives at the birth center: (1) establishing a therapeutic relationship and (2) assessing the condition of the mother and fetus.

ESTABLISHING A THERAPEUTIC RELATIONSHIP

Making the Family Feel Welcome.   A family's first impression influences how family members feel about the quality of the birth experience. Even if the unit is busy, the nurse should communicate interest, friendliness, caring, and competence. Families understand if the nurse is busy; they do not understand rudeness or insensitivity to their needs.

When caring for the woman who has not had prenatal care or childbirth classes, behaviors most nurses value, avoid being judgmental in either words or actions. The woman's priorities and values may not be the same as those of the nurse, but she deserves the same respect, support, and care as the woman who made every preparation for her baby's birth.

CRITICAL THINKING EXERCISE 17–1

Alan Lindsey phones you as you are working in the birth unit of your hospital one night. He says, "My wife's baby is due. She's been having some contractions off and on all day, and they are keeping her awake now. Should we come to the hospital?"

1. Do you need any other information? If so, what information do you need?

You next speak to Heather Lindsey about her symptoms. You find out that her first baby is due the following week and that she has had no leaking of fluid from her vagina. She says, "My contractions are coming every 2 to 10 minutes, and most of them last about 30 seconds. They didn't bother me much until I tried to go to sleep, but now they are keeping me awake. I'm so tired of all this!"

2. What should you tell Heather about her symptoms? What advice should you give her?

Nurses often encounter women who speak a language other than English. Arranging for a culturally acceptable interpreter who is fluent in the woman's language makes the woman and family feel more welcome and promotes safety because it enhances understanding among the woman, her family, and the nurse.

Determining Family Expectations About Birth.   Regardless of how many children they have, women and their partners have expectations about the birth experience. The partners have often studied their options extensively and have planned a birth that best fits their ideals. Some may have a written birth plan filed with their prenatal records. Those who have not made specific plans also have expectations shaped by contact with relatives and friends or by previous birth experiences.

Conveying Confidence.   From the first encounter, the nurse should convey confidence in the woman's ability to give birth and her partner's ability to support her. Contractions and discomfort intensify as labor progresses. A woman having her first baby may find the power of normal labor contractions overwhelming. The nurse can reassure the woman that intense contractions are normal in active labor while helping her deal with them and watching for problems.

Consider the different perspective implied by the phrases "give birth" and "be delivered." The woman who gives birth is an active and able participant; she is the principal action figure. When her baby is "delivered," however, the language implies that she is passive. The nurse might ask, "Who will attend you as you give birth?" rather than, "Who will deliver your baby?"

Assigning a Primary Nurse.   Having one nurse give care during all of labor is usually unrealistic. The number of different caregivers should, however, be limited as much as possible. The woman should know who each caregiver is and what to expect from each.

Using Touch for Comfort. Touch can communicate acceptance and reassurance and can provide physical and emotional comfort to many laboring women. Women who do not usually welcome touch may appreciate it during labor. Cultural norms and personal history influence whether a woman is comfortable with touch from a stranger such as a nurse. One should not assume that the woman desires touch but should ask her if she wants it or benefits from it. As labor progresses, her desire for touch may change; during late labor, it may become an irritant rather than a comfort measure.

Respecting Cultural Values. Cultural beliefs and practices give structure and meaning to the birth experience. The nurse should incorporate a family's cultural practices into care as much as possible if they are beneficial or neutral.

ASSESSMENTS AT THE TIME OF ADMISSION

A record of prenatal care is sent to the center where the woman plans to give birth and is added to her chart when she is admitted. The information can be verified or updated as needed on admission. Women who have not had prenatal care need a more extensive assessment by the nurse and physician. Table 17–2 lists intrapartum assessments, usual findings, significant findings, and appropriate nursing actions.

Focus Assessment. In the intrapartum unit, a focus assessment is done before the broader database assessment, opposite of the usual order. Assessment priorities are to determine the condition of the mother and fetus and whether birth is imminent.

Fetal Heart Rate. Use Leopold's maneuvers (Procedure 17–1) to locate the best place to assess the fetal heart rate. (Procedure 17–2 explains assessment of the fetal heart rate with the fetoscope or Doppler transducer. Chapter 18 presents the procedure for using the electronic fetal monitor.) For a term fetus, these fetal heart rate guidelines are considered reassuring (American College of Obstetricians

Text continued on page 377

TABLE 17–2

. . . .

Intrapartum Assessment Guide

Women who have had prenatal care have much of this information available on their prenatal record. The nurse need only verify it or update it as needed.

Assessment, Method (Selected Rationales)	Common Findings	Significant Findings, Nursing Action
Interview		
Purpose: To obtain information about the woman's pregnancy, labor, and conditions that may affect her care. The interview is curtailed if she seems to be in late labor.		
Introduction: Introduce yourself and ask the woman how she wants to be addressed. Ask her if she wants her partner and/or family to remain during the interview and assessment. (Shows respect for the woman and gives her control over those she wants to remain with her.)	Many women prefer to be addressed by their first names during labor.	The surname (family name) precedes the given name in some cultures. Clarify which name is used to properly address the woman and to properly identify both mother and newborn.
Culture/language: If she is from another culture, ask what her preferred language is and what language(s) she speaks, reads, or verbally understands. (Enables the most accurate data collection.)	Common non-English languages of women in the United States are Spanish or one of the Asian dialects. The most common non-English language varies with location.	Try to secure an interpreter fluent in the woman's primary language. Ask her if there are people who are not acceptable to her as interpreters (e.g., males or one from a group in conflict with her culture). Family members may not be the best interpreters because they may interpret selectively, adding or subtracting information as they see fit.
Communication: Ask the woman to tell you when she has a contraction, and pause during the interview and physical assessment. (Shows that the nurse is sensitive to her comfort and allows her to concentrate more fully on the information the nurse requests.)	Women in active labor have difficulty answering questions or cooperating with a physical examination while they are having a contraction.	If contractions are very frequent, assess the woman's labor status promptly rather than continuing the interview. Ask only the most critical questions.

Table continued on following page

TABLE 17–2

. . . .

Intrapartum Assessment Guide Continued

Women who have had prenatal care have much of this information available on their prenatal record. The nurse need only verify it or update it as needed.

Assessment, Method (Selected Rationales)	Common Findings	Significant Findings, Nursing Action
Nonverbal cues: Observe the woman's behaviors and interactions with her family and the nurse. (Permits estimation of her level of anxiety. Identifies behaviors indicating that she should have a vaginal examination to determine whether birth is imminent.)	*Latent phase:* Sociable and mildly anxious. *Active phase:* Concentrating intently with contractions; often uses prepared childbirth techniques.	The unprepared or extremely anxious woman may breathe deeply and rapidly, displaying a tense facial and body posture during and between contractions. These behaviors suggest that birth is imminent: 1. Her statement that the baby is coming. 2. Grunting sounds (low-pitched, guttural sounds). 3. Bearing down with abdominal muscles. 4. Sitting on one buttock. Euphoria, combativeness, or sedation suggest recent illicit drug ingestion.
Reason for admission: "What brings you to the hospital/birth center today?" (Open-ended question promotes more complete answer.)	Labor contractions at term are the usual reason. Observation for false labor is another common reason for admission.	Bleeding, preterm labor, pain other than labor contractions. Report these findings to the physician or nurse-midwife promptly.
Prenatal care: "Did you see a doctor or nurse-midwife during your pregnancy?" "Who is your doctor or nurse-midwife?" "How far along were you in your pregnancy when you saw the physician or nurse-midwife?" (Enables location of prenatal record.)	Early and regular prenatal care promotes maternal and fetal health.	No prenatal care or care that was irregular or begun in late pregnancy means that complications may not have been identified.
Estimated date of delivery (EDD): "When is your baby due?" (Determines if gestation is term.) "When did your last menstrual period begin?" (For estimation of EDD if woman did not have prenatal care.)	*Term gestation:* 38–42 wk. The woman's gestation may have been confirmed or adjusted during pregnancy with an ultrasound or other clinical examination.	Gestations earlier than 38 wk (preterm) or later than the end of the 42nd wk (postterm) are associated with more fetal or neonatal problems.
Gravidity, parity, abortions: "How many times have you been pregnant?" "How many babies have you had? Were they full-term or premature?" "How many children are now living?" "Have you had any miscarriages or abortions?" "Were there any problems with your babies after they were born?" (Helps estimate probable speed of labor and anticipate neonatal problems.)	Labor may be faster for the woman who has given birth before than for the nullipara. Miscarriage is used to describe a spontaneous abortion because many lay people associate the term "abortion" with only induced abortions.	Parity of 5 or more (grand multiparity) may be associated with placenta previa (see Chapter 26) or post-partum hemorrhage (see Chapter 28). Women who have had several spontaneous abortions or who have given birth to infants with abnormalities may face a higher risk for an infant with a birth defect.
Pregnancy history (Identifies problems that may affect this birth.)		
Present pregnancy: "Have you had any problems during this pregnancy, such as high blood pressure, diabetes, or bleeding?"	Complications are not expected.	Women having diabetes or hypertension may have poor placental blood flow, possibly resulting in fetal compromise. Some complications of past pregnancies, such as diabetes, may recur in another pregnancy. The woman who plans a VBAC may need more support and reassurance to give birth vaginally.

TABLE 17–2

. . . .

Intrapartum Assessment Guide Continued

Women who have had prenatal care have much of this information available on their prenatal record. The nurse need only verify it or update it as needed.

Assessment, Method (Selected Rationales)	Common Findings	Significant Findings, Nursing Action
Past pregnancies: "Were there any problems with your other pregnancy(ies)?" "Were your other babies born vaginally or by cesarean birth?"	Women who had previous cesarean birth(s) often have a trial of labor and vaginal birth (VBAC). A woman who previously had a difficult labor may be more anxious than one who had an uncomplicated labor and birth.	
Other: "Is there anything else you think we should know so that we can better care for you?"	This open-ended question gives the woman a chance to share information that may not be elicited by other questions.	
Labor status: "When did your contractions become regular?" "What time did you begin to think you might really be in labor?" (Facilitates a more accurate estimation of the time labor began.)	Varies among women. Many women go to the birth facility when contractions first begin. Others wait until they are reasonably sure that they are really in labor.	Women who say they have been "in labor" for an unusual length of time (for example, "for 2 days") have probably had false labor. These women may be very tired from the annoying, nonproductive contractions.
Contractions: "How often are your contractions coming?" "How long do they last?" "Are they getting stronger?" "Tell me if you have a contraction while we are talking." (Obtains the woman's subjective evaluation of her contractions. Alerts the nurse to palpate contractions that occur during the interview.)	Varies according to her stage and phase of labor. Labor contractions are usually regular and show a pattern of increasing frequency, duration, and intensity.	Irregular contractions or those that do not increase in frequency, duration, or intensity are more likely to represent false labor. Contractions with a duration of longer than 90 sec or intervals of full uterine relaxation shorter than 60 sec can reduce placental blood flow.
Membrane status: "Has your water broken?" "What time did it break?" "What did the fluid look like?" "About how much fluid did you lose—was it a big gush or a trickle?" (Alerts the nurse of the need to verify whether the membranes have ruptured if it is not obvious. Identifies possible prolonged rupture of membranes.)	Most women go to the birth facility for evaluation soon after their membranes rupture. If a woman is not already in labor, contractions usually begin within a few hours after the membranes rupture at term.	If the woman's membranes have ruptured and she is not in labor or if she is not at term, a vaginal examination is often deferred. Labor may be induced if she is at term with ruptured membranes.
Allergies: "Are you allergic to any foods or medicines?" "What kind of reaction do you have?" "Have you ever had a problem with anesthesia when you had dental work?" (Determines possible sensitivity to drugs that may be used.)	Record any known allergies to food and medication. As needed, describe how they affected the woman.	Allergy to seafood, iodized salt, or x-ray contrast media may indicate iodine allergy. Because iodine is used in many "prep" solutions, alternative ones should be used. Allergy to dental anesthetics may indicate possible allergy to the drugs used for local or regional anesthetics. These drugs usually end in the suffix -caine.
Food intake: "When was the last time you had something to eat or drink?" "What did you have?" (Helps evaluate risk for regurgitation and aspiration of stomach contents during general anesthesia.)	Record the time of the woman's last food intake and what she ate. Include both liquids and solids.	If the woman says she has not had any intake for an unusual length of time, question her more closely: "Is there any food you may have forgotten, such as a snack or a drink of water?"
Recent illness: "Have you been ill recently?" "What was the problem?" "What did you do for it?" "Have you been around anyone with a contagious illness recently?"	Most pregnant women are healthy. An occasional woman may have had a minor illness such as an upper respiratory tract infection.	Untreated urinary tract infections are associated with preterm labor. The woman who has had contact with someone having a communicable disease may become ill and possibly infect others in the facility.

Table continued on following page

TABLE 17–2
. . . .

Intrapartum Assessment Guide Continued

Women who have had prenatal care have much of this information available on their prenatal record. The nurse need only verify it or update it as needed.

Assessment, Method (Selected Rationales)	Common Findings	Significant Findings, Nursing Action
Medications: "What drugs do you take that your doctor or nurse-midwife has prescribed?" "Are there any over-the-counter drugs that you use?" "I know this may be uncomfortable to discuss, but we need to know about any illegal substances that you use to more safely care for you and your baby." (Permits evaluation of the woman's drug intake and encourages her to disclose nonprescribed use.)	Prenatal vitamins and iron are commonly prescribed. Record all drugs the woman takes, including time and amount of last ingestion. Women who use illegal substances often conceal or diminish the extent of their use because they fear reprisals.	Drugs may interact with other medications given during labor, especially analgesics and anesthetics. Substance abuse is associated with complications for the mother and infant (see Chapter 25). If the woman discloses that she uses illegal drugs, ask her what kind and the last time she ingested them (often referred to as a "hit"). A nonjudgmental approach is more likely to result in honest information.
Tobacco or alcohol: "Do you smoke or use tobacco in any other form? About how many cigarettes a day?" "Do you use alcohol? About how many drinks do you have each day (or week)?" (Evaluates use of these legal substances.)	As in substance abuse, women may underreport the extent of their use of tobacco or alcohol.	Infants of heavy smokers are often smaller and may have reduced placental blood flow during labor. Infants of women who use alcohol may show fetal alcohol effects (see Chapter 30).
Birth plans (Shows respect for the woman and her family as individuals and promotes achievement of their expectations. Enables more culturally appropriate care):		
Coach or primary support person: "Who is the main person you want to be with you during labor?" Ask that person how he or she wants to be addressed, such as "Mr. Smith" or "Bob."	This is usually the woman's husband or the baby's father, but it may be her mother, sister, or a friend, especially if she is single.	The woman who has little or no support from significant others probably needs more intense nursing support during labor and after the birth. These clients are more likely to have problems with parent-infant attachment.
Other support: "Is there anyone else you would like to be present during labor?"	Women often want another support person present.	
Preparation for childbirth: "Did you attend prepared childbirth classes?" "Did someone go with you?"	Ideally, the woman and a partner have had some preparation in classes or self-study. Women who attended classes during previous pregnancies do not always repeat the classes during subsequent pregnancies.	The unprepared woman may need more support with simple relaxation and breathing techniques during labor. Her partner may need to learn techniques to assist her.
Preferences: "Are there any special plans you have for this birth?" "Is there anything you want to avoid?" "Did you plan to record the birth with pictures or video?"	Some women or couples have strong feelings regarding certain interventions. Common ones are: (1) analgesia or anesthesia; (2) intravenous lines; (3) fetal monitoring; (4) shave prep or enema; or (5) use of episiotomy or forceps.	Conflict may arise if the woman has not previously discussed her preferences with her physician or nurse-midwife or if she is unaware of what services are available where she gives birth.
Cultural needs: "Are there any special cultural practices that you plan when you have your baby?" "How can we best help you to fulfill these practices?"	Women from Asian and Hispanic cultures often subscribe to the "hot/cold" theory of illness and want specific foods after birth, such as soft-boiled eggs. They may not want their water iced.	Try to incorporate all positive or neutral cultural practices. If a practice is harmful, explain why and try to find a way to work around it if the family does not want to give it up.

TABLE 17-2
· · · · · · · · · · · ·

Intrapartum Assessment Guide Continued

Women who have had prenatal care have much of this information available on their prenatal record. The nurse need only verify it or update it as needed.

Assessment, Method (Selected Rationales)	Common Findings	Significant Findings, Nursing Action
Fetal Evaluation		
Purpose: To determine if the fetus seems to be healthy and tolerating labor well.		
Fetal heart rate (FHR): Assess by intermittent auscultation, or apply an external fetal monitor if that is the facility's policy (most common in the United States). Document fetal heart rate at least this often for the fetus at low risk for complications: 1. Every 30 min during active first-stage labor 2. Every 15 min during second stage	Average at term is a lower limit of 110–120 BPM and an upper limit of 150–160 BPM. Rate should increase when the fetus moves.	These signs may indicate fetal stress and should be reported to the physician or nurse-midwife: 1. Rate outside the normal limits 2. Slowing of the rate that persists after the contraction ends 3. No increase in rate when the fetus moves More frequent assessments should be made of the fetal heart rate.
Labor Status		
Purpose: To identify whether the woman is in labor and if birth is imminent. If she displays signs of imminent birth, this assessment is done as soon as she is admitted.		
Contractions (Yields objective information about labor status): In addition to asking the woman about her contraction pattern, assess the contractions by palpation with the fingertips of one hand. A guideline for women with no risk factors is to assess: 1. At least hourly during the latent phase 2. At least every 30 min during the active phase 3. At least every 15 min during transition and second stage	See interview section earlier in table.	See interview section earlier in table. Women who have intense contractions or who are making rapid progress need to be assessed more frequently.
Vaginal examination (Determines cervical dilation and effacement; fetal presentation, position, and station; bloody show; and status of the membranes.)	Varies according to the stage and phase of labor. It may not be possible to determine the fetal position by vaginal examination when membranes are intact and bulging over the presenting part.	A vaginal examination is not performed if the woman reports or has evidence of active bleeding (not bloody show). Report reasons for omitting a vaginal examination to the physician or nurse-midwife.
Status of membranes: During a vaginal examination a flow of fluid suggests ruptured membranes. A Nitrazine test and/or fern test may be done. (Test needed only if it is not obvious that the membranes have ruptured.)	Amniotic fluid should be clear, possibly containing flecks of white vernix. Its odor is distinctive but not offensive. The Nitrazine test with a color change of blue-green to dark blue (pH > 6.5) suggests true rupture of the membranes but is not conclusive. The fern test is more diagnostic of true rupture of membranes.	A greenish color indicates meconium staining, which may be associated with fetal compromise or postterm gestation. Thick meconium with heavy particulate matter ("pea soup") is most significant (see Chapter 30). Thick green-black meconium may be passed by the fetus in a breech presentation and is not necessarily associated with fetal compromise. Cloudy, yellowish, strong-, or foul-smelling fluid suggests infection. Bloody fluid may indicate partial placental separation (see Chapter 27).

Table continued on following page

TABLE 17–2
• • • • • • • • • • •

Intrapartum Assessment Guide Continued

Women who have had prenatal care have much of this information available on their prenatal record. The nurse need only verify it or update it as needed.

Assessment, Method (Selected Rationales)	Common Findings	Significant Findings, Nursing Action
Leopold's maneuvers: Often done before assessing the fetal heart rate because they help locate the best place to assess the fetal heart rate. (Identifies fetal presentation and position. Most accurate when combined with information from vaginal examination.)	A cephalic presentation with the head well flexed (vertex) is normal. The fetal head is often easily displaced upward ("floating") if the woman is not in labor. When the head is engaged, it cannot be displaced upward with Leopold's maneuvers.	A hard, round, freely movable object in the fundus suggests a fetal head, meaning the fetus is in a breech presentation. Less commonly, the fetus may be crosswise in the uterus: a transverse lie.
Pain: Note discomfort during and between contractions. Note tenderness when palpating contractions. (Distinguishes between normal labor pain and abnormal pain that may be associated with a complication.)	There may be verbal or nonverbal evidence of pain with contractions, but the woman should be relatively comfortable between contractions. The skin around the umbilicus is often sensitive.	Constant pain or a tender, rigid uterus suggests a complication, such as abruptio placentae (separated placenta) (see Chapter 26) or, less commonly, uterine rupture (see Chapter 27).

Physical Examination

Purpose: To evaluate the woman's general health and identify conditions that may affect her intrapartum and postpartum care.		
General appearance: Observe skin color and texture, nutritional state, and appearance of rest or fatigue. Examine the woman's face, fingers, and lower extremities for edema. Ask her if she can take her rings off and on.	Women are often fatigued if their sleep has been interrupted by Braxton Hicks contractions, fetal activity, or frequent urination. Mild edema of the lower extremities is common in late pregnancy.	Pallor suggests anemia. Edema of the face and fingers or extreme (pitting) edema of the lower extremities is associated with pregnancy-induced hypertension (see Chapter 26).
Vital signs: Take the woman's temperature, pulse, respirations, and blood pressure. Reassess the temperature every 4 hr (every 2 hr after membranes rupture or if elevated); repeat blood pressure, pulse, and respirations every hour.	*Temperature:* 35.8°–37.3°C (96.4°–99.1°F). *Pulse:* 60–100/min *Respirations:* 12–20/min, even and unlabored. Blood pressure near baseline levels established during pregnancy. Transient elevations of blood pressure are common when the woman is first admitted, but they return to baseline levels within about ½ hour.	Report abnormalities to physician or nurse-midwife. Temperature of 38°C (100.4°F) or higher suggests infection. Pulse and respirations may also be elevated. Pulse and blood pressure may be elevated if the woman is extremely anxious or in pain. A blood pressure of 140/90 mm Hg or higher is considered hypertensive. For women who did not have prenatal care, there is no baseline to compare.
Heart and lung sounds: Auscultate all areas with a stethoscope.	Heart sounds should be clear with a distinct S_1 and S_2. A physiologic murmur is common because of the increased blood volume and cardiac output. Breath sounds should be clear, with respirations even and unlabored.	The woman who is breathing rapidly and deeply may have symptoms of hyperventilation: tingling and spasm of the fingers, numbness around the lips.
Breasts: Palpate for a dominant mass.	Breasts are full and nodular. Areola is darker, especially in dark-skinned women. Breasts may leak colostrum (clear, sticky, straw-colored fluid) during labor.	Report a dominant mass to the physician or nurse-midwife.
Abdomen: Observe for scars at the same time Leopold's maneuvers and the fetal heart rate are assessed. It is usually sufficient to assess the fundal height by observing its relation to the xiphoid process.	Striae (stretch marks) are common. If scars are noted, ask the woman what surgery she had. The fundus at term is usually slightly below the xiphoid process.	Report a previous cesarean birth to the physician or nurse-midwife. Transverse uterine scars are least likely to rupture if the woman is in labor (see Chapter 27). Measure the fundal height (see p. 277) if the fetus seems small or if the gestation is questionable.

TABLE 17-2

Intrapartum Assessment Guide Continued

Women who have had prenatal care have much of this information available on their prenatal record. The nurse need only verify it or update it as needed.

Assessment, Method (Selected Rationales)	Common Findings	Significant Findings, Nursing Action
Deep tendon reflexes: Assess patellar reflex (see Chapter 26). Upper extremity deep tendon reflexes should be used after epidural block analgesia.	Brisk knee jerk without spasm or sustained muscle contraction is normal. Some women normally have hypoactive reflexes.	Report absent (uncommon unless the woman is receiving magnesium sulfate) or hyperactive reflexes. Hyperactive reflexes and clonus (repeated tapping when the foot is dorsiflexed) are associated with pregnancy-induced hypertension and often precede a seizure (see Chapter 26).
Midstream urine specimen: Assess protein and glucose levels with a dipstick. Follow instructions on the package for waiting times. Send for urinalysis if ordered.	Negative or trace of protein; negative glucose.	Proteinuria is associated with pregnancy-induced hypertension but may also be associated with urinary tract infections or a specimen that is contaminated with vaginal secretions. Glucosuria is associated with diabetes.
Laboratory tests: Women who have had prenatal care may not need additional tests. Common tests include:		
1. Complete blood cell count (or hematocrit done on unit).	1. Hemoglobin at least 11 g/dl; hematocrit at least 33%.	1. Values lower than these reduce maternal reserve for normal blood loss at birth.
2. Blood type and Rh factor.	2. The woman who is Rh-negative usually has received Rh immune globulin at about 28 weeks' gestation to prevent formation of anti-Rh antibodies.	2. Rh-negative mothers need Rh immune globulin if their infant is Rh-positive.
3. Serologic tests for syphilis.	3. Negative.	3. A positive test may indicate that the baby is infected and needs treatment after birth. The mother should be treated if she has not been treated already.

and Gynecologists [ACOG], 1995b; Menihan, 1996; Murray, 1997):

- A lower limit of 110 to 120 BPM and an upper limit of 150 to 160 BPM. (Some sources state that 120 BPM is the lower limit of normal.)
- The presence of variability in the electronically monitored fetal heart rate.
- The presence of accelerations, usually associated with fetal movement, in the fetal heart rate of at least 15 BPM above the baseline rate and lasting for at least 15 seconds.
- An absence of decelerations following contractions.

See Chapter 18 for more information about electronic fetal monitor patterns.

Maternal Vital Signs. Assess maternal vital signs primarily for signs of hypertension or infection. Hypertension during pregnancy is defined as a sustained blood pressure increase to 140 mm Hg systolic or 90 mm Hg diastolic. An elevation of 30 mm Hg systolic or 15 mm Hg diastolic from second-trimester levels is no longer considered diagnostic of hypertension (ACOG, 1996). A temperature of 38°C (100.4°F) or higher suggests infection.

Impending Birth. Occasionally a woman enters the intrapartum unit almost ready to give birth. Grunting sounds, bearing down, sitting on one buttock, or saying urgently something like "The baby's coming" all suggest imminent birth. The nurse then abbreviates the initial assessment and collects other information after birth.

Vital information to obtain if birth is imminent includes the following:

- Mother's name
- Support person's name
- Whether the woman had prenatal care
- Physician's or nurse-midwife's name
- Number of pregnancies and prior births, including whether vaginal or cesarean birth
- Status of membranes
- Estimated date of delivery
- Any problems during this pregnancy
- Allergies to medications
- Time and type of last oral intake
- Maternal vital signs and fetal heart rate

PROCEDURE 17–1

• • • • • • • • • • •

Leopold's Maneuvers

PURPOSE: To determine the presentation and position of the fetus. To aid in location of the fetal heart sounds.

1. Explain the procedure to the woman, the rationale for each step, and what is found at each step to teach her and reassure her when the assessment findings are normal.

2. Ask the woman to empty her bladder if she has not done so recently to reduce discomfort during palpation and make fetal parts easier to feel. Have her lie on her back with her knees flexed slightly to help her relax her abdominal muscles. Place a small pillow or folded towel under one hip to prevent supine hypotension.

3. Wash your hands with warm water to prevent transmission of microorganisms and to make your hands more comfortable when touching the woman. Wear gloves to avoid contact with the woman's secretions if that is likely.

4. Stand beside the woman, facing her head, with your dominant hand nearest her because the first three maneuvers are most easily performed in this position.

First Maneuver

5. Palpate the uterine fundus to distinguish between a cephalic and breech presentation. The breech (buttocks) is softer and more irregular in shape than the head. Moving the breech also moves the fetal trunk. The head is harder, with a round, uniform shape. The head can move without the entire fetal trunk moving.

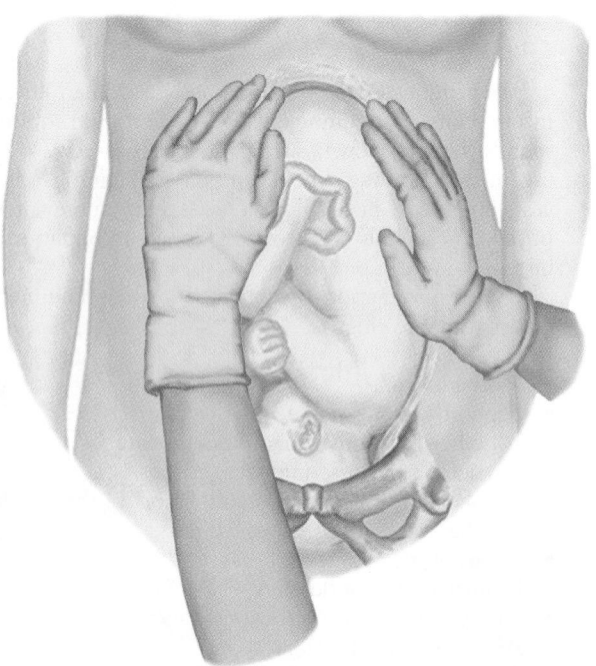

Second Maneuver

6. Hold your left hand steady on one side of the uterus while palpating the opposite side of the uterus with your right hand to determine which side the fetal back is on and which side the arms and legs ("small parts") are on. Then hold your right hand steady while palpating the opposite side of the uterus with your left hand. The fetal back is a smooth, convex surface. The fetal arms and legs feel nodular, and the fetus often moves them during palpation.

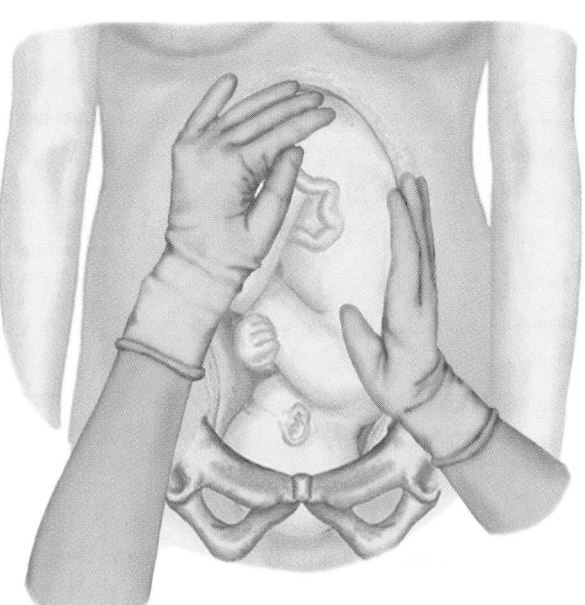

Third Maneuver

7. Palpate the suprapubic area to confirm the presentation felt in the first maneuver and to determine if the presenting part is engaged. If a breech was palpated in the fundus, expect a hard, rounded head in this area. Grasp the presenting part gently between the thumb and fingers. If the presenting part is not engaged, grasping with the fingers moves it upward in the uterus.

PROCEDURE 17–1 *Continued*

Leopold's Maneuvers

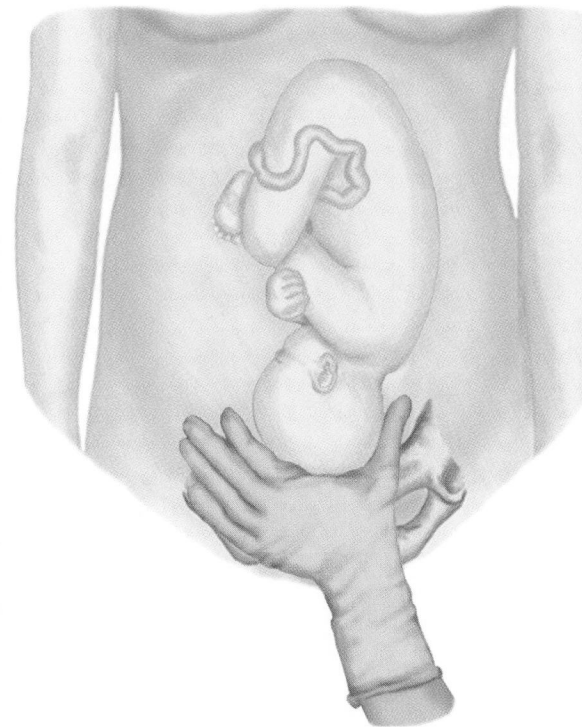

8. Omit the fourth maneuver if the fetus is in a breech presentation because this maneuver is done only in cephalic presentations to determine if the fetal head is flexed.

Fourth Maneuver

9. To perform this maneuver most easily, turn so that you face the woman's feet.

10. Place your hands on each side of the uterus with your fingers pointed toward the pelvic inlet to determine whether the head is flexed (vertex) or extended (face). Slide your hands downward on each side of the uterus. On one side, your fingers easily slide to the upper edge of the symphysis. On the other side, your fingers meet an obstruction, the cephalic prominence. If the head is flexed, the cephalic prominence (the forehead in this case) is felt on the opposite side from the fetal back. If the head is extended, the cephalic prominence (the occiput in this case) is felt on the same side as the fetal back.

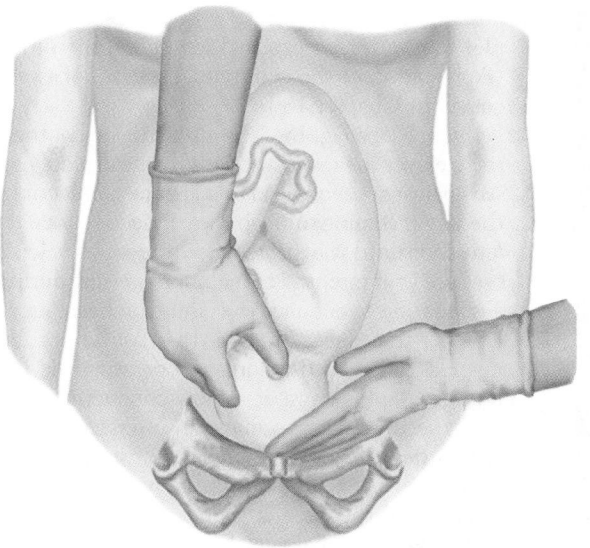

If focus assessments of mother and fetus are normal and birth is not imminent, complete the admission assessment. If the initial assessments are not normal or birth is near, notify the physician or nurse-midwife promptly.

Database Assessment. In addition to the focus assessment, assess the mother and fetus and available maternal support.

Basic Information. Most intrapartum admission forms guide the nurse to ask for essential information. Typical information includes the following:

- The woman's reason for coming to the hospital or birth center (e.g., contractions or rupture of membranes)
- Prenatal care
- Her estimated date of delivery
- Number of pregnancies, births, and abortions
- Medical, surgical, and pregnancy history
- Allergies
- Food intake: what food and when it was eaten
- Recent illness, including treatment
- Medications, including prescription and over-the-counter drugs, tobacco, alcohol, and substances of abuse

- Her subjective evaluation of her labor
- Birth plans, including expected pain management methods
- Support persons: who they are and the role of each
- Screening for domestic abuse (see Chapter 25)

> Be careful when asking about prior pregnancies and births when a woman's family is present. She may have had an abortion or relinquished a baby for adoption, and her family may not know about it. Even if her partner knows about previous pregnancies, her family and friends may not.

Fetal Assessments. Assess the fetal presentation and position and the fetal heart rate. Note the color of the amniotic fluid and the time of rupture if the membranes have ruptured.

Labor Status. Determine the woman's labor status by

- Assessing her contraction pattern
- Determining cervical dilation and effacement, and fetal station, presentation, and position
- Determining if her membranes have ruptured

PROCEDURE 17–2

. . . .

Auscultating the Fetal Heart Rate

PURPOSE: To evaluate the fetal condition and tolerance of labor.

1. Explain the procedure to give information to the woman and her partner. Wash your hands with warm water to reduce the transmission of microorganisms and to make your hands more comfortable when touching the woman's abdomen.

2. Use Leopold's maneuvers to identify the fetal back (Procedure 17–1) because it usually is closest to the surface of the maternal abdomen, where fetal heart sounds are clearest. Illustrations show approximate locations of the fetal heart rate in different presentations and positions.

3. Assess the fetal heart rate with a fetoscope, Doppler transducer, or external fetal heart monitor. (Application of the external fetal monitor is discussed in Chapter 18.)

4. Fetoscope (see Fig. 18–1A): Place the bell of the fetoscope over the fetal back with the head plate pressed against your forehead to add bone conduction to the sound coming through the earpieces. Move the fetoscope until you locate where the sound is loudest. Use your forehead to maintain pressure during auscultation to enhance the faint fetal heart sounds.

5. Doppler transducer (see Fig. 18–1B): Review the manufacturer's instructions for operating the Doppler device. Place water-soluble conducting gel over the transducer to make an interface for clear signal transmission, and turn it on. Place the transducer over the fetal back and move it until you clearly hear the distinct sounds of the fetal heart.

6. With one hand, palpate the mother's radial pulse to be sure that the fetal heart rate is what is actually heard. If her pulse is synchronized with the sounds from the fetoscope or Doppler transducer, try another location for the fetal heart. Other sounds that may be heard are the funic souffle (blood flowing through the umbilical cord) or uterine souffle (blood flowing through the uterine vessels). The funic souffle is synchronized with the fetal heart; the uterine souffle is synchronized with the mother's pulse.

Auscultating the Fetal Heart Rate

7. Assess the fetal heart rate before, during, and after a contraction to allow fetal assessment through a contraction cycle, when blood flow to the placenta is temporarily reduced. Count the baseline fetal heart rate for 30 to 60 seconds between contractions. Note accelerations and slowing of the rate.

8. Note reassuring signs that indicate the fetus seems to be tolerating labor well:
   a. An average rate of 110 to 120 BPM at the lower limit and 150 to 160 BPM at the upper limit for a term fetus.
   b. Accelerations of at least 15 BPM for 15 seconds, usually with fetal movement.

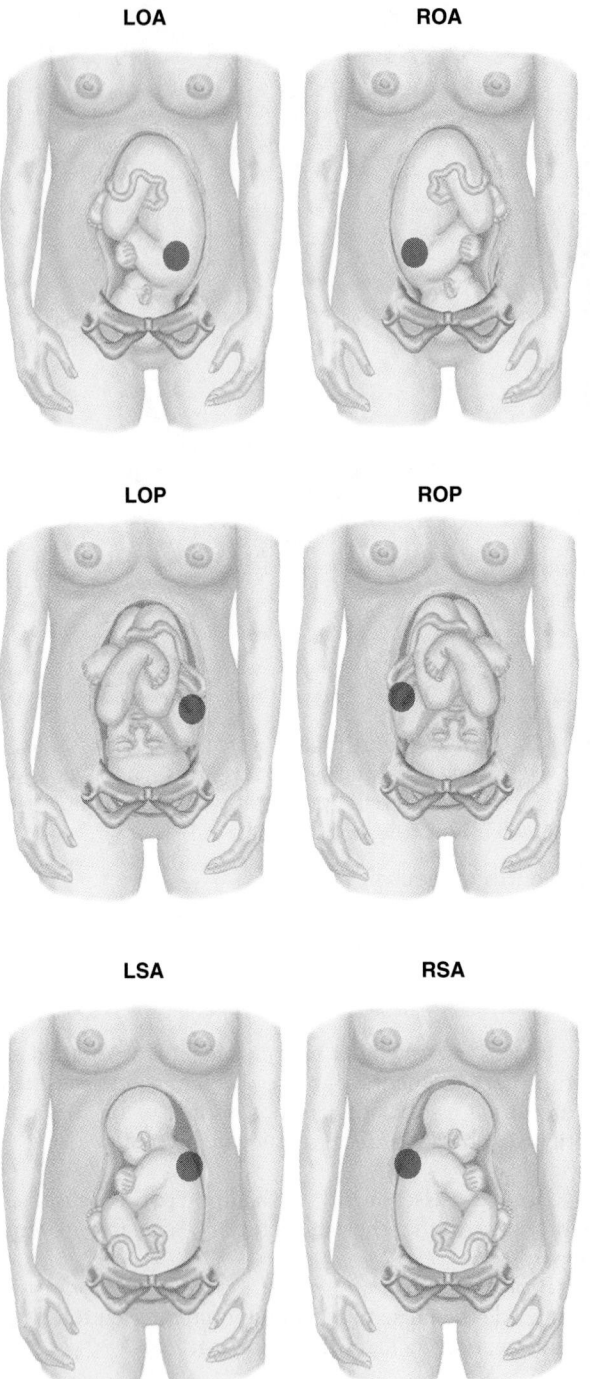

LOA   ROA

LOP   ROP

LSA   RSA

c. The presence of variability (determined by electronic monitoring).

9. Note nonreassuring signs and make more frequent assessments. Notify the physician or nurse-midwife for further evaluation.
   a. Heart rate outside normal limits.
   b. Slowing of the fetal heart rate after the contraction ends.

During a labor admission assessment, a woman quickly denies using drugs other than her prescribed prenatal vitamins. She becomes quiet, answering each of the nurse's questions tersely.

1. What might explain the woman's change in behavior?
2. Should the nurse alter the assessment interview? If so, why?

Physical Examination. If birth is not imminent, perform a brief physical examination to evaluate the woman's overall health. Important general observations that relate to birth include the presence and location of edema, abdominal scars, and the height of the fundus.

ADMISSION PROCEDURES

Notifying the Birth Attendant. After assessment, contact the woman's birth attendant to report on her status and obtain orders. Include the following data in the report:

- Gravidity, parity, and abortions
- Estimated date of delivery
- Contraction pattern
- Fetal presentation and position
- Cervical dilation and effacement, station of the presenting part
- Fetal heart rate
- Maternal vital signs
- Any identified abnormalities or concerns about the maternal or fetal condition
- Pain, anxiety, or other reactions to labor

If the birth attendant admits the woman, any of several procedures may be done.

Consent Forms. The woman signs consent for care during labor, anesthesia, vaginal birth, and possible cesarean birth. Consent for newborn care is often completed as well.

Laboratory Tests. Women who have had regular prenatal care usually need laboratory tests only for specific indications. Simple tests often done on the unit include the following:

- Hematocrit
- Midstream urine specimen for measurement of protein and glucose levels, usually obtained before notifying the birth attendant

Intravenous Access. If used, intravenous access is started with at least an 18-gauge catheter. A saline lock may be used, or the woman may receive continuous infusion of fluids. The lock eases walking during early labor and is less associated with illness, but it still provides quick access if fluids or drugs are needed. Continuous fluid infusion helps prevent or relieve dehydration and is needed if epidural block analgesia is used. Intravenous solutions containing electrolytes, such as lactated Ringer's solution, are common. Glucose-containing fluids are avoided during labor except for specific indications because they may cause neonatal hypoglycemia.

Perineal Preparation. If necessary, hair in the immediate area of an episiotomy is removed by shaving or by clipping the hair near the skin with a shaver or disposable scissors.

Enema. Small-volume enemas (such as Fleet enemas) may be given if the woman has stool in her rectum that causes discomfort or would interfere with fetal descent. Extra lubricant on the enema tip reduces discomfort from hemorrhoids.

ASSESSMENTS AFTER ADMISSION

The woman is usually observed if it is unclear after the initial assessment whether she is in true labor. After 1 or 2 hours, progressive cervical changes (effacement, dilation, or both) strongly suggest true labor. Assess the woman and fetus during the observation period as if she were in early labor.

After the admission assessment, the woman and her fetus need regular assessments based on their risk status and on whether interventions such as epidural analgesia are needed. General guidelines for continuing assessments are listed here.

Fetal Assessments. Fetal assessments are done to identify signs of well-being and signs that suggest compromise. The principal fetal assessments include the fetal heart rate (Procedure 17–2) and patterns and the character of the amniotic fluid. Abnormalities revealed in these assessments may be associated with impaired fetal gas exchange or infection.

Fetal Heart Rate. The fetal heart rate is assessed using either intermittent auscultation or electronic fetal monitoring. Intermittent auscultation is done with a Doppler transducer or a fetoscope. For the fetus at low risk for complications, guidelines for assessment (by either intermittent auscultation or electronic monitoring) and documentation are presented in Table 17–3.

Amniotic Fluid. The membranes may rupture spontaneously (SROM, or spontaneous rupture of membranes), or the birth attendant may perform an amniotomy (AROM, or artificial rupture of membranes). Assess the fetal heart rate for at least 1 minute after the membranes rupture. The umbilical cord could be displaced in a large fluid gush, resulting in compression and interruption of blood flow through it. Charting related to membrane rupture includes the time, fetal heart rate, and character of the fluid.

Amniotic fluid should be clear and may include bits of vernix, the creamy fetal skin lubricant. Cloudy, yellow, or foul-smelling amniotic fluid suggests infection. Green fluid indicates that the fetus has passed meconium before birth. Meconium passage may have been a response to transient hypoxia, although the cause may remain unknown.

Describe quantity in approximate terms; for example, at term, a "large" amount is more than 1,000 ml; a "moderate" amount is about 500 to 1,000 ml; and "scant" amniotic fluid is only a trickle, barely enough to detect. If the fetus is well down into the pelvis when the membranes rupture, a small amount of fluid in front of the fetal head may be discharged (forewaters), with the rest lost at birth.

TABLE 17-3

• • • • • • • • • • •

Guidelines for Assessment and Documentation of Fetal Heart Rate

Women Without Risk Factors	Women with Risk Factors Present on Admission or That Develop During Labor
Active First-Stage Labor	*Active First-Stage Labor*
At least every 30 min, just after a contraction	At least every 15 min, just after a contraction
Second-Stage Labor	*Second-Stage Labor*
At least every 15 min	At least every 5 min

Other Times to Document Fetal Heart Rate

- Before artificial rupture of the membranes; after rupture of the membranes, either artificially or spontaneously
- Before and after ambulation
- Before procedures such as a vaginal examination or catheterization
- If contractions become too frequent, last too long, or if there is an inadequate interval between them
- Before administration of oxytocin and when evaluating the dose for increase, maintenance, or decrease
- Before administration of medications and at time of peak action
- Before epidural analgesia is started and when evaluating it for increase, maintenance, or decrease in dose

Maternal Assessments. Several maternal assessments, such as vital signs and contractions, also relate to the health of the fetus.

Vital Signs. Guidelines for maternal vital signs assessment are listed in Table 17-2. Hypotension, hypertension, elevated pulse and respiratory rates, and elevated temperature should be reported, and assessments should be made more frequently.

Contractions. Contractions can be assessed by palpation (Procedure 17-3) or with the electronic fetal monitor, using the guidelines in Table 17-2.

Progress of Labor. The nurse does a periodic vaginal examination to determine cervical dilation and effacement and fetal descent. The frequency of vaginal examinations depends on the woman's parity, the status of her membranes, and the overall speed of her labor. Vaginal examinations are limited to avoid introducing microorganisms from the perineal area into the uterus.

Intake and Output. Oral and intravenous intake is recorded. Each voiding is recorded. Labor or regional anesthesia may reduce a woman's urge to void, so check her suprapubic area every 2 hours to identify bladder distension.

Pressure of the fetal head on the rectum in late labor makes many women feel the need to defecate. Look at the woman's perineum for crowning of the fetal head if she abruptly expresses a need to defecate or says "something feels different down there" or a comparable remark.

Response to Labor. The woman's behavioral responses change as labor intensifies. She withdraws from interactions but needs more nursing presence and reassurance. She may become more anxious because of pain and fear of bodily injury, unknown outcome, loss of control, unresolved psychological issues that influence her readiness to give birth (such as sexual abuse or previous birth experiences), or unexpected occurrences during labor.

Women vary in the way they handle the pain of labor. The nurse must constantly assess whether added pain control measures are needed. Behaviors that suggest the woman needs help with pain management include the following:

- Expressing that nonpharmacologic measures are ineffective.
- Tensing her muscles or arching her back during contractions.
- Persistence of muscle tension between contractions.
- A tense facial expression.
- Expressions such as "I can't take it anymore."
- Specific requests for medication or other pain control.

The Support Person's Response. Labor is stressful for the woman's support person, often the baby's father. He may become anxious, fearful, or tired. He feels a responsibility to protect and support the woman but may have limited resources for doing so. It is difficult for him to watch the woman he loves in pain, even if the pain is normal. He may respond to stress in many ways: by becoming quiet, suffering silently, pacing, or expressing anger. Some fathers respond by leaving the room frequently or for long periods, whereas others resist taking even short breaks.

Nurses encourage and value the father's presence during labor and birth. This attitude, however, may conflict with a couple's cultural norms, which may dictate that birth is a strictly female activity. The father may be pulled in two directions, wanting to be included but hesitant because it is not customary in his culture to be part of the birth. The nurse should respect the values of each couple and their wishes about the father's involvement.

The support person also may be a parent or other relative, a friend of either sex, or a homosexual partner. The nurse must remember that anyone who assists the woman during labor may feel anxious or helpless at times. Reassurance and care for the labor partner strengthen that person's

PROCEDURE 17–3

. . . .

Palpating Contractions

PURPOSE: To determine whether a contraction pattern is typical of true labor. To identify abnormal contractions that may jeopardize the health of the mother or fetus.

1. Assess at least three contractions in a row to get an idea of the true nature of the contractions. Palpate contractions periodically when an external fetal monitor is used because it is less accurate for intensity as a result of variations in the thickness of the abdominal fat pad, maternal position, and fetal position. Guidelines for minimum frequency of assessments are
   a. Hourly during latent phase.
   b. Every 30 minutes during active phase and transition.
   c. Every 15 minutes during second stage.
2. Place the fingertips of one hand on the uterine fundus because this is where the contractions begin, although the mother usually feels them in her lower abdomen and back. Use light pressure and keep your fingertips relatively still rather than moving them over the uterus because moving your hand over the uterus may stimulate contractions and give an artificial idea of their true pattern. The fingertips are more sensitive to the first tightening of the uterus.
3. Note the time when each contraction begins and ends.
   a. Determine the frequency by noting the average time that elapses from the beginning of

one contraction to the beginning of the next one.
   b. Determine the duration of contractions by noting the average time in seconds from beginning to end of each contraction.
   c. Determine the interval between contractions by noting the average time between the end of one contraction and the beginning of the next one.
4. Estimate the average intensity of contractions by noting how easily the uterus can be indented during the peak of the contraction.
   a. Mild contractions are easily indented with the fingertips. They feel similar to the tip of the nose.
   b. Moderate contractions can be indented with more difficulty. They feel similar to the chin.
   c. Firm contractions feel "woody" and cannot be readily indented. They feel similar to the forehead.
5. Report hypertonic contractions that can reduce placental blood flow:
   a. Durations longer than 90 seconds
   b. Intervals shorter than 60 seconds
   c. Contractions closer than 2 minutes apart
   d. Incomplete relaxation of the uterus between contractions.

---

ability to support the woman and increase the likelihood that both will view the birth experience as positive.

NURSING CARE

. . . .

The Woman with False or Early Labor

Assessment

After assessment, it may be apparent that the woman is not in true labor. If findings are normal and her membranes are intact, she is usually discharged home. The woman who is in very early labor may be discharged to await active labor, especially if she is a nullipara and lives nearby.

Nursing Diagnosis and Planning

The woman may be frustrated because she cannot tell whether labor is real. She may resist returning to the birth center, possibly delaying care needlessly. A nursing diagnosis that applies to many women with false labor contractions is

■ Knowledge Deficit: characteristics of true labor.
   Expected Outcome: The woman and her support person will describe reasons for returning to the birth center for evaluation.

Interventions

Providing Reassurance

A woman sent home after observation often feels foolish and frustrated. Reassure her that even professionals cannot

always identify true labor and that false labor and early true labor have similar characteristics. Tell her that important preparation occurs during late pregnancy, such as softening of her cervix, even if objective progress like cervical dilation has not yet occurred.

Teaching

Review guidelines for returning to the birth center with her: regular contractions, leaking of amniotic fluid, bleeding other than bloody show, and decreased fetal movement. Explain that these are only guidelines and that she should call or return if she has any concerns. It is better for her to return with another false alarm than to arrive at the birth center in advanced labor or to develop complications at home.

Evaluation

• Can the woman and her support person describe guidelines for returning to the birth center?

NURSING CARE

. . . .

The Woman in True Labor

The admission assessment may confirm that the woman is in true labor, or true labor may be evident after observation. Nursing diagnoses and collaborative problems change during labor because the intrapartum period is an evolving process. Those covered in this chapter relate to fetal oxygenation, maternal discomfort, and maternal injury.

Nursing diagnoses are often interrelated during labor. For example, anxiety or fear can affect pain relief measures. A fluid volume deficit can alter fetal oxygenation because less blood is available to circulate to the placenta.

FETAL OXYGENATION

Assessment

Refer to assessments listed in Tables 17–2 and 17–3 for intrapartum assessments. The main assessments related to fetal well-being are the following:

- Fetal heart rate
- Character of amniotic fluid and time of rupture
- Maternal vital signs
- Contractions: frequency, duration, intensity, resting tone, interval

Nursing Diagnosis and Planning

A collaborative problem is appropriate for nursing care related to fetal well-being during labor. Most fetuses tolerate labor well, but conditions such as maternal hypotension or hypertension, maternal fever, excessive (*tetanic*) contractions, or compression of the umbilical cord can compromise fetal oxygenation. Client-centered goals are not made for collaborative problems as they are for nursing diagnoses. Planning includes nursing responsibilities to (1) promote normal placental function and (2) observe for and report problems to the physician or nurse-midwife.

Interventions

Promoting Placental Function

Maternal positioning is the primary measure to promote placental function during normal labor. The woman can choose any position other than the supine to avoid aortocaval compression that would reduce blood flow to the placenta. If she must be in the supine position for a procedure such as catheterization, a small pillow or rolled towel placed under one hip shifts her uterus to maintain good placental blood flow.

Observing for Conditions Associated with Fetal Compromise

Determine whether any conditions associated with fetal compromise exist. If any are identified, assess the fetus more frequently and notify the birth attendant.

Evaluation

Evaluation of client goals or expected outcomes does not apply to a collaborative problem. Throughout labor, the nurse compares actual data with the norms for the mother and fetus.

DISCOMFORT

Assessment

See Table 17–2 for continuing assessments of the laboring woman.

Nursing Diagnosis and Planning

Labor is painful. Women vary in their responses to pain and in the pain management methods they choose. Providing choices for pain management and supporting the woman's choice increase her sense of control over her birth experi-

---

CRITICAL TO REMEMBER

Conditions Associated with Fetal Compromise

- A fetal heart rate outside the normal range for a term fetus: lower limit of 110 to 120 BPM and upper limit of 150 to 160 BPM.
- Little or no variability in the electronically monitored fetal heart rate.
- Slowing of the fetal heart rate that persists after a contraction ends.
- Meconium-stained (greenish) amniotic fluid.
- Cloudy, yellowish, or foul odor to the amniotic fluid (suggests infection).
- Contractions lasting longer than 90 seconds.
- Incomplete uterine relaxation or intervals shorter than 60 seconds between contractions.
- Maternal hypotension (may divert blood flow away from the placenta to ensure adequate perfusion of the maternal brain and heart).
- Maternal hypertension (may be associated with vasospasm in spiral arteries, which supply the intervillous spaces of the placenta).
- Maternal fever (38°C [100.4°F] or higher).

---

ence. The woman who successfully masters the pain and other physical demands of labor is more likely to view her experience as positive. Her support person is likely to feel more satisfaction with the experience as well.

Pain and anxiety are often related nursing diagnoses. Excess anxiety intensifies pain perception, and pain worsens anxiety. The nurse clusters assessment data to determine whether pain or anxiety is the primary client problem. For example, several cues suggest that anxiety is the primary problem: a previous poor experience during birth or expressions of worry and concern. If contractions are intense and labor is progressing quickly, however, pain is the primary concern. The nursing diagnosis is therefore

- Pain related to effects of uterine contractions.
  Expected Outcomes: The woman will state that she is able to tolerate the pain satisfactorily and will use breathing and relaxation techniques. The woman's partner will express satisfaction with his or her ability to support her.

Interventions

Providing Comfort Measures

Ordinary measures reduce irritating surroundings that impair a woman's ability to relax and use coping skills. Nurses must be creative when providing comfort to the laboring woman.

Lighting. Soft, indirect lighting is soothing, whereas a bright overhead light is an irritant. Bright lights imply a hospital ("sick") atmosphere rather than the normal life event that birth is. Use the overhead light only when needed. A small flashlight is handy if the woman wants her room dark.

Temperature. Labor is work. Women in labor are often hot and perspiring. Cool, damp washcloths on the woman's face and neck promote comfort. Keep an ample supply of damp washcloths available, and change them often to keep them cool. An electric fan circulates air in the labor room and directs a breeze on the woman. Be sure that the fan does not blow on the infant after birth, as cool air might cause hypothermia.

Have the woman wear socks if her feet are cold.

Cleanliness. Bloody show and amniotic fluid leak from the woman's vagina during labor. Change the sheets and gown as needed to keep her dry and comfortable. Let her preferences be the guide because she may not want to be disturbed during late labor. Change the disposable underpad regularly to reduce microorganisms that may ascend into the vagina. A folded towel absorbs larger quantities of amniotic fluid than the pad alone.

Mouth Care. Ice chips, Popsicles, or hard candy on a stick reduce the discomfort of a dry mouth. If oral intake is contraindicated, brushing the teeth (without swallowing water) or simply rinsing the mouth helps. Many women appreciate a moist washcloth applied to their lips.

Bladder. A full bladder intensifies pain during labor and can delay fetal descent. Remind the woman to empty her bladder at least every 2 hours.

Positioning. Occasionally, a specific maternal position is recommended to reduce discomfort or to assist the labor process. Otherwise, encourage the woman to assume any position (other than the supine) that she finds comfortable. Frequent changes reduce discomfort from constant pressure, help the fetus adapt to the pelvic contours, and promote fetal descent. Figure 17–15 illustrates various maternal positions for labor.

The woman may have "back labor" if her fetus is in the occiput posterior position and the fetal occiput presses on the mother's sacral promontory with each contraction. The discomfort of back labor is difficult to relieve with medication. Positions that encourage the fetus to fall away from the sacral promontory, such as those in which the mother leans forward or uses the hands-and-knees position, promote her comfort and enhance internal rotation to an occiput anterior position.

Water. Water in the form of a shower, tub, or whirlpool is relaxing and helps many women tolerate contractions. Nipple stimulation by water currents causes release of oxytocin by the posterior pituitary gland, which increases contractions and promotes labor progress. If contractions become too strong, she simply removes her breasts from the water stream.

Teaching

Teaching the woman in labor is a constant and changing task.

First Stage of Labor. Many women become discouraged because several hours are needed to reach 4 or 5 cm of cervical dilation. They believe that the last 5 cm will take as long as the first 5 cm. They may need to know that 5 cm is more like two thirds of the way to full dilation rather than half the way because the rate of dilation increases during the active phase.

The urge to push usually occurs when the woman's cervix is fully dilated and effaced and when the fetus descends deep into the pelvis and internally rotates. As she nears the second stage, however, her baby may descend enough to give her an urge to push before full cervical dilation. If her cervix, which is usually 8 or 9 cm dilated at this time, yields easily to downward pressure, pushing in response to her spontaneous urge rarely causes problems.

Either of two problems may occur if she pushes against a cervix that does not easily yield to pressure from the fetal presenting part:

- The cervix may become edematous, which can block progress.
- The cervix may be lacerated.

Teach the woman to blow out in short breaths if she should not yet push.

Second Stage of Labor. The woman may need help to trust the sensations from her body and to push most effectively during second-stage labor.

Time Limit. Two hours was once considered the upper limit for the duration of the second stage. It is now recognized that a second stage longer than 2 hours is safe as long as the mother and fetus show no signs of compromise.

Women push most effectively when they feel the reflex urge to do so. Many women do not immediately feel the urge to push when the cervix is fully dilated. If maternal and fetal assessments are reassuring, the woman does not need to push before she feels the urge. Pushing vigorously sooner than this time may contribute to birth canal injury because her vaginal tissues are stretched more forcefully and rapidly than they would be if she pushed spontaneously and in response to her body's signals. She does not have to push with every contraction.

Positions. The mother can push in any position she prefers. Position changes promote her natural pushing efforts. Many women prefer semisitting and side-lying positions. Squatting enlarges the pelvic outlet slightly and adds the force of gravity to the mother's efforts; this is an advantage if she has a small pelvis or the fetus is large. Some women push most effectively while sitting on the toilet because that is where they are accustomed to giving in to that sensation. The woman can also turn backward while sitting on the toilet, letting the tank (with a pillow on top) support her upper body.

When the mother pushes, teach her to curve her body around her uterus in a C shape rather than arching her back. For most effectiveness, teach her to pull on her knees, handholds, or a squatting bar while pushing. Women often find that pulling on something from above is efficient.

Method and Breathing Pattern. If she is pushing effectively and safely, do not interfere, but support the woman's spontaneous techniques. She should push with her abdominal muscles while relaxing her perineum. Teach her to take a breath and exhale to begin. Have her take another breath and exhale while pushing strongly for about 4 to 6 seconds at a time. Sustained pushing while breath-holding (the Valsalva maneuver) reduces blood flow to the placenta and is fatiguing. Another deep breath helps her relax at the end of the contraction.

Standing

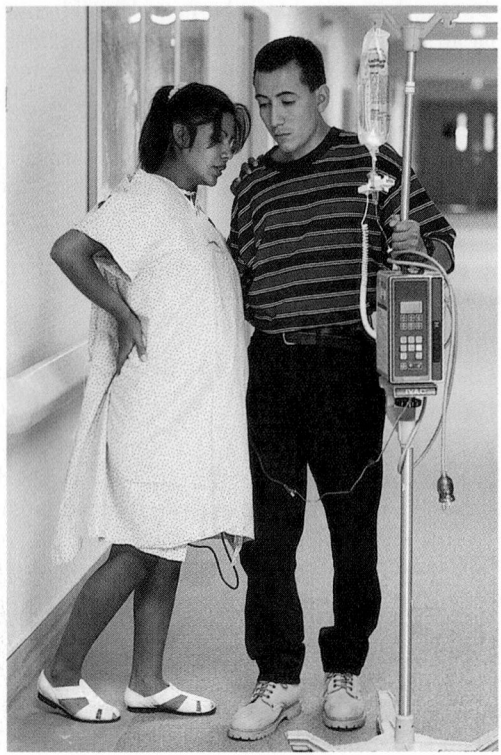

Sitting Upright

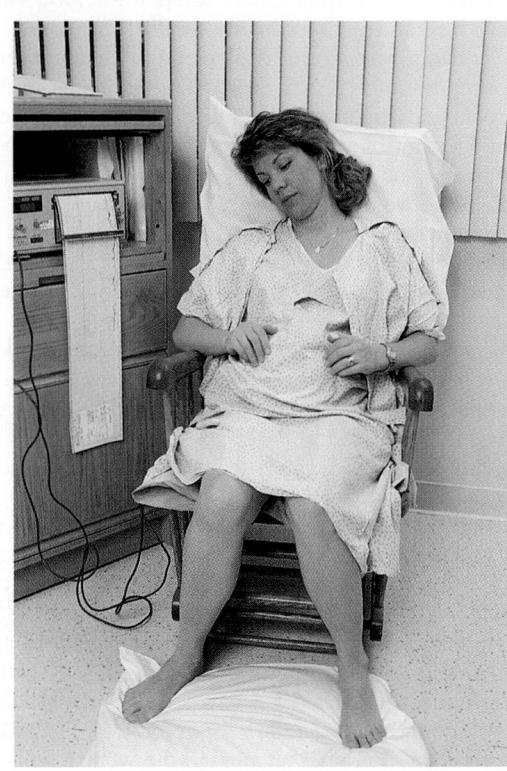

Advantages

Adds gravity to force of contractions to promote fetal descent.
Contractions are less uncomfortable and more efficient.
Variation: Standing, leaning forward with support reduces back pain because fetus falls forward, away from the sacral promontory.

Disadvantages

Tiring over long periods.
Continuous electronic fetal monitoring is not possible without telemetry if woman is walking in the hall.

Nursing Implications

If the woman has intravenous fluid running, give her a rolling pole. Encourage her to alternate walking with other positions whenever she tires or desires to do so.
Remind the woman and her partner when she should return to the labor area for evaluation of the fetal heart rate and her labor status.

Advantages

Uses gravity to aid fetal descent.
Can be done when sitting on side of bed, in a chair, or on the toilet.
Can be used with continuous fetal monitoring.
Avoids supine hypotension.

Disadvantages

May increase suprapubic discomfort.
Contractions are the most efficient when the woman alternates sitting with other positions.

Nursing Implications

A rocking chair is soothing.
Place a pillow on a chair with a disposable underpad over the pillow to absorb secretions.
Use pillows or a footstool to keep the short woman's legs from dangling.
Encourage the woman to alternate positions periodically; for example, she can alternate walking with sitting or sitting with side-lying.

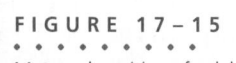

FIGURE 17–15
· · · · · · · · · · ·
Maternal positions for labor.

A woman who is modest or fears losing control may inhibit her best pushing efforts if she is instructed to push as if she were having a bowel movement, particularly if she is in a bed or chair. A more anatomically correct image is to teach the woman to push down and out under her symphysis ("pubic bone"), following the pelvic curve. Seeing a diagram of the pelvis helps her to visualize the curve.

Providing Encouragement

Success breeds success. Tell the woman when her labor is progressing. If she can see that her efforts are effective, she has more courage to continue. Help her touch or see the baby's head with a mirror as crowning occurs.

Praise the woman and her labor partner when they use breathing or other coping techniques effectively. This encouragement reinforces their actions, gives them a sense of control, and conveys the respect and support of the nurse.

Sitting, Leaning Forward with Support

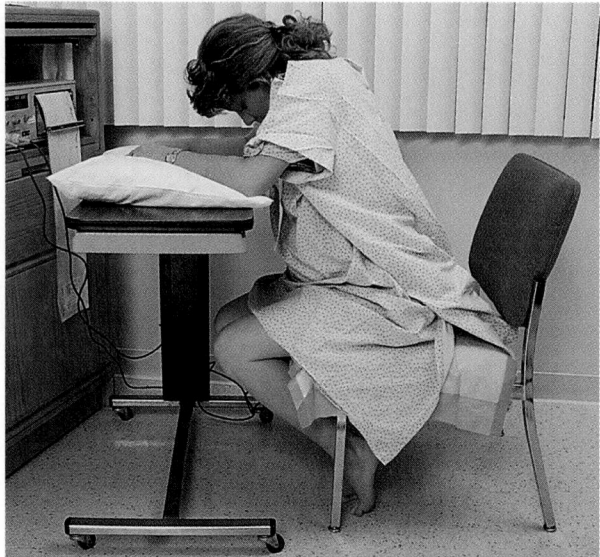

Advantages

Same as for sitting.
Reduces back pain because fetus falls forward, away from sacral promontory.
Partner or nurse can rub back or provide sacral pressure to relieve back pain.

Disadvantages

Same as for sitting.

Nursing Implications

Same as for sitting.

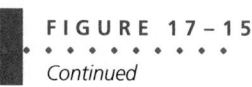

FIGURE 17–15
• • • • • • • • • •
Continued

Semi-sitting

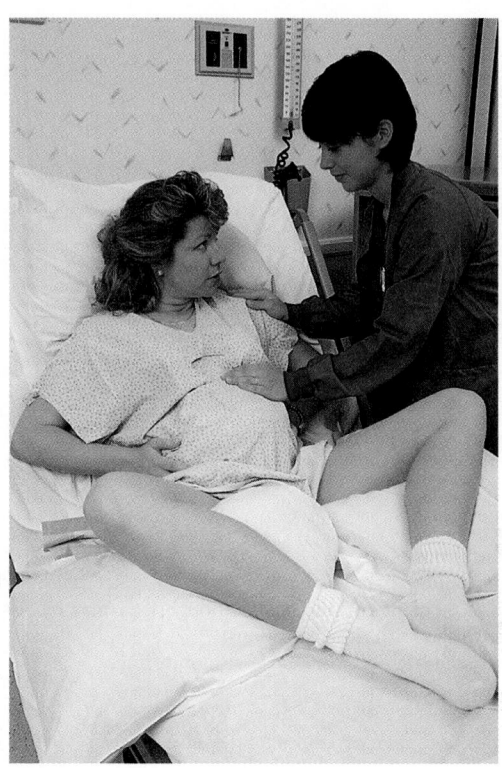

Advantages

Same as for sitting.
Aligns long axis of uterus with pelvic inlet, which applies contraction force in the most efficient direction through pelvis.

Disadvantages

Same as for sitting.
Does not reduce pain as well as the forward-leaning positions.

Nursing Implications

Same as for sitting.
Raise bed to about a 30- to 45-degree angle.
Encourage the woman to use sitting (leaning forward) or side-lying position if she has back pain so that the caregiver can rub her back or apply sacral pressure.

Illustration continued on following page

If one technique is not helpful after a reasonable trial (at least three to five contractions), encourage them to try other techniques.

Giving of Self

The nurse's caring presence is a crucial element in labor support. Even women who are very independent may become dependent during labor and need human contact. Many times the woman simply needs reassurance that all is going well and that the nurse is there for her. The nurse's presence helps to allay her fears of abandonment and conveys safety, acceptance, support, and comfort.

Although the woman and her support person may have prepared for childbirth, they often welcome suggestions and affirmation from the nurse. The nurse who is familiar with the techniques they are using can better support them and avoid contradicting what they have learned and practiced. The nurse's presence, gentle coaching, and encouragement help the laboring woman have confidence in her own body and her fitness to give birth.

Offering Pharmacologic Measures

Some women do not need pharmacologic pain relief during labor. Birth is usually a normal process, and the prepared woman and labor partner can deliver their infant without medication. Many, however, do choose to have pharmacologic pain management. Inform the woman about medications available to her without pressuring her to take them. See Chapter 19 for additional information about pharmacologic measures.

Side-Lying

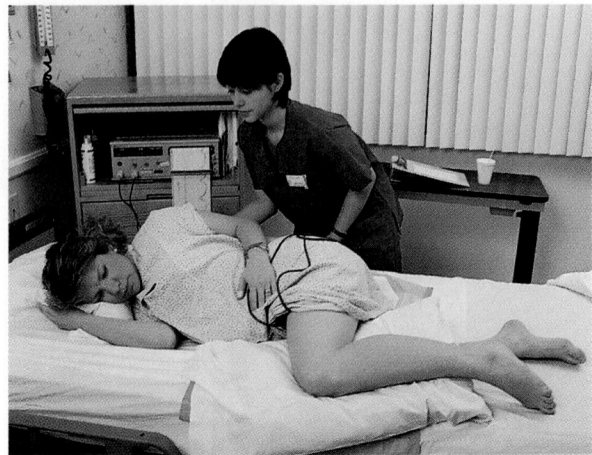

Advantages

Is a restful position.
Prevents supine hypotension and promotes placental blood flow.
Promotes efficient contractions, although they may be less frequent than with other positions.
Can be used with continuous fetal monitoring.

Disadvantages

Does not use gravity to aid fetal descent.

Nursing Implications

Teach the woman and her partner that although the contractions are less frequent, they are more effective.
This position offers a break from more tiring positions.
Use pillows for support and to prevent pressure: at her back, under her superior arm, and between her knees.
Use disposable underpads to protect the pillow between the woman's knees from secretions.
Some women like to put their superior leg on the bed rail. If the woman wants this variation, pad the bed rail with a blanket to prevent pressure.
If she wants to remain recumbent, she should use this position to promote placental blood flow.

Kneeling, Leaning Forward with Support

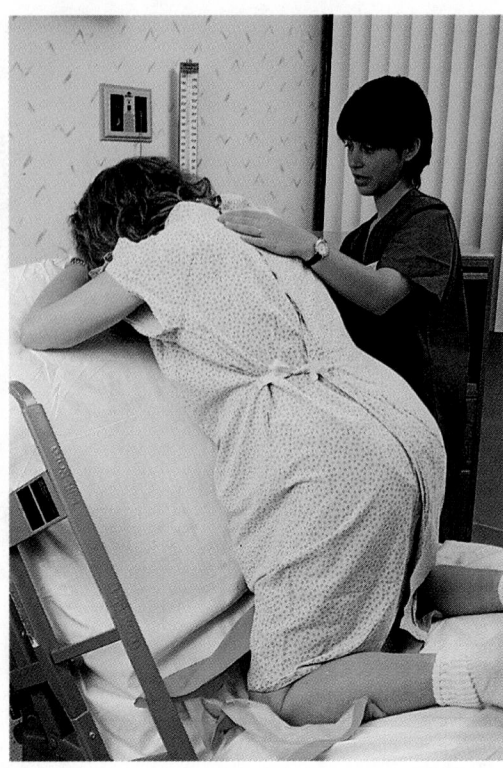

Advantages

Reduces back pain because fetus falls forward, away from sacral promontory.
Adds gravity to force of contractions to promote fetal descent.
Can be used with continuous fetal monitoring.
Caregivers can rub her back or apply sacral pressure.
Promotes normal mechanisms of birth.

Disadvantages

Knees may become tired or uncomfortable.
Tiring if used for long periods.

Nursing Implications

Raise the head of the bed, and have the woman face the head of the bed while she is on her knees.
Another method is for the partner to sit in a chair, with the woman kneeling in front, facing her partner, and leaning forward on him or her for support.
Use pillow under the knees and in front of the woman's chest, as needed, for comfort.
Encourage her to change positions if she becomes tired.

FIGURE 17-15
• • • • • • • • •
Continued

Most women have open minds about using analgesia or anesthesia, but some may have a firm goal of avoiding all pain medication during labor. These women may then feel let down or guilty if they need medication. Other women may plan to use a specific pain relief method, such as epidural analgesia. If something prevents use of their chosen method, they may be upset about this unexpected development in their birth experience. In either case, allow the woman to ventilate her feelings about her experience. Although this development may not be what she wanted, expressing her feelings helps her put it into perspective.

Caring for the Birth Partner

The woman's support person is an integral part of her labor care. Her labor partner can provide care and comfort, which support the woman's ability to give birth. Do not expect too much of the partner, however, or make assumptions about the type and amount of involvement desired.

Hands and Knees

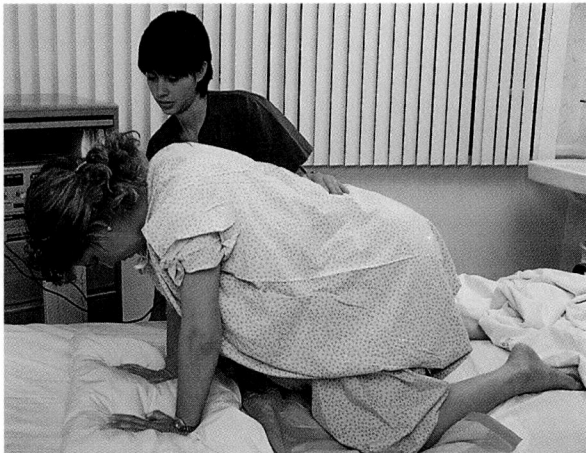

Squatting

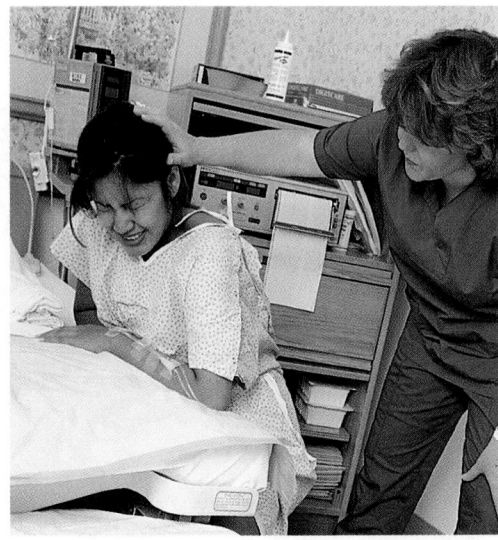

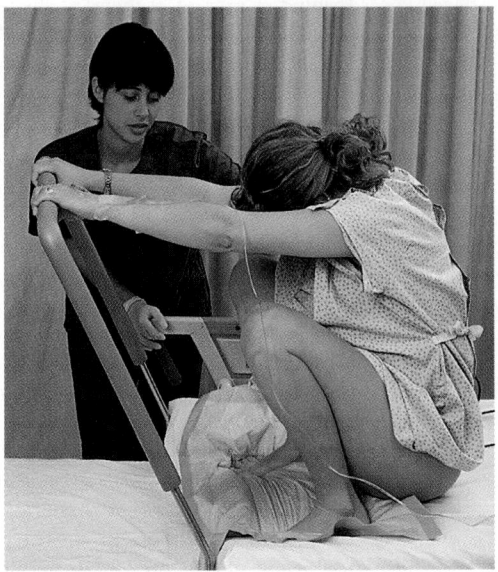

Advantages

Reduces back pain because the fetus falls forward, away from the sacral promontory.
Promotes normal mechanisms of birth.
The woman can use pelvic rocking to decrease back pain.
Caregivers can rub the woman's back or apply sacral pressure easily.

Disadvantages

The woman's hands (especially wrists) and knees can become uncomfortable.
Tiring when used for a long time.
Some women are embarrassed to use this position.

Nursing Implications

Encourage the woman to change to less tiring positions occasionally.
Ensure privacy when encouraging the reluctant woman to try this position if she has back pain.
A second hospital gown with the opening in front covers her back and hips but may be too warm.

Positions for Pushing in Second Stage

Standing

This position may be tiring, and access to the woman's perineum is difficult. Because the infant could fall to the ground if birth occurs rapidly, provide padding under the mother's feet. Gravity aids fetal descent.

Hands and Knees

Advantages and disadvantages are similar to those during first-stage labor. In addition, caregivers must reorient themselves because the landmarks are upside down from their usual perspective.
A variation is for the mother to kneel and lean forward against a beanbag or the side of the bed. This variation reduces some of the strain on her wrists and hands.

Advantages

Adds gravity to force of contractions to promote fetal descent.
Straightens the pelvic curve slightly for more direct fetal descent.
Increases dimensions of pelvis slightly.
Promotes effective pushing efforts in the second stage.
Caregivers can rub back or provide sacral pressure.

Disadvantages

Knees and hips may become uncomfortable because of prolonged flexion.
Tiring over a long time.

Nursing Implications

Provide support with a squat bar attached to the bed or by two people standing on each side of the woman.
If she becomes tired, or between contractions, she can lean back into the sitting position.
Variation: Have the woman squat beside the bed as she pushes.

FIGURE 17–15
. . . .
Continued

Illustration continued on following page

Semi-sitting

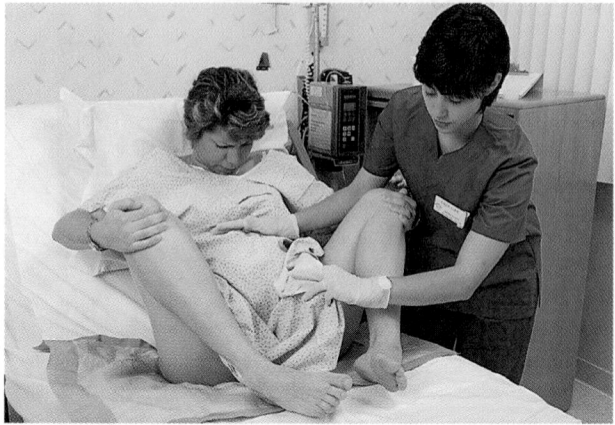

Many women prefer this because they have the security of a back rest; it is also familiar to caregivers and allows easy observation of the perineum. Elevate the woman's back at least 30 to 45 degrees so that gravity aids fetal descent. The woman pulls on her flexed knees (behind or in front of them) as she pushes. She should keep her head flexed and her sacrum flat on the bed to straighten the pelvic curve.

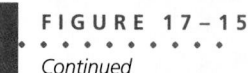

FIGURE 17–15
· · · · · · · · · ·
Continued

Side-Lying

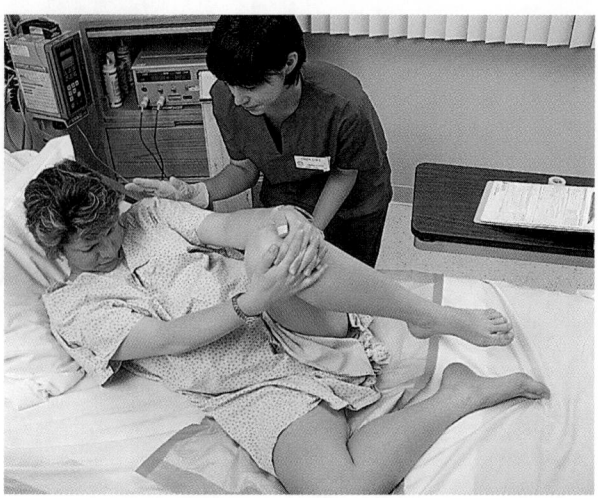

The woman flexes her chin on her chest and curls around her uterus as she pushes. She pulls on her flexed knees or the knee of the superior leg as she pushes.

Some partners are coaches in the true sense of the word, actively assisting the woman through labor. Others want the woman and nurse to lead them and tell them how to help. They are eager to do what they can but expect instructions about how and when to do it. Many couples see the partner's role as one of encouragement, moral support, and just being there for the woman.

To impose unrealistic expectations of leadership, care, and comfort on the partner makes the birth experience unnecessarily stressful. To ensure a positive experience for both people, accept whatever pattern of support the partner is able and willing to provide and whatever the couple finds comfortable. Without taking over or diminishing this role, provide support that the partner cannot.

Encourage the partner to conserve physical strength. The partner may have missed sleep during the hours of early labor or may need a break. The nurse may need to encourage the partner to eat or bring a snack. Remind the partner that support will be more effective if the partner's own needs are met. Support persons who do not eat for a long time are more likely to faint during the birth.

Evaluation

* Does the woman indicate that she is able to tolerate the pain of labor satisfactorily?
* Does the woman use the breathing and relaxation techniques that she was taught?
* Does her partner express satisfaction with his support during labor?

As a nursing diagnosis, pain and related goals for pain management are constantly re-evaluated during labor.

PREVENTING INJURY

Assessment

Nursing assessments of the mother and fetus continue as the woman nears birth. During the second stage of labor, observe the woman's perineum to determine when to make final birth preparations.

The exact time for final birth preparations varies according to the woman's parity, the overall speed of labor, and the fetal station. Preparations are usually completed when crowning in the nullipara reaches a diameter of about 3 to 4 cm. The multipara is prepared sooner, usually when her cervix is fully dilated and the fetal head is well down in the pelvis but before much crowning has occurred.

Nursing Diagnosis and Planning

The woman is vulnerable to injury immediately before and after birth for several reasons: (1) altered physical sensations, such as responses to intense pressure or medication, (2) positional changes for birth, and (3) unexpectedly rapid progress. The nursing diagnosis selected for the laboring woman near the time of birth is therefore

■ Risk for Injury (maternal) related to altered sensations and positional or physical changes.
Expected Outcome: The woman does not have an avoidable injury, such as muscle strains, thrombosis, or lacerations, during birth.

Interventions

Transferring the woman to the delivery site or positioning her in the birthing bed is the first step in the sequence of events that culminates in birth of the baby. During the period surrounding birth, the nurse reduces factors that contribute to maternal injuries.

Transfer to a Delivery Room

Most births occur in a combination labor, delivery, and recovery room. In some facilities or with some client conditions, the woman must be transferred to a separate room for birth. Transfer her early enough to avoid rushed, last-minute preparations, which are stressful for all.

Positioning for Birth

To promote effective pushing and take advantage of gravity, raise the woman's back, shoulders, and head.

Stirrups or foot rests support the woman's legs and feet and make her perineum more accessible. To reduce strain on muscles and ligaments, raise and lower her legs together (if anesthesia limits her movement) and do not separate them too widely. Pad the surfaces that contact the popliteal space behind the knee because veins are near the surface there and pressure on them could lead to thrombus formation. Do not leave her legs in the stirrups for a prolonged time.

Observing the Perineum

The exact time at which a woman is ready to give birth is an educated guess. A woman who has been having a slow labor may suddenly make rapid progress. Birth is near when the fetal head swings anteriorly in extension as the occiput slips under the symphysis pubis. Observe the woman's perineum, especially during late second-stage labor.

A *classic sign of imminent birth is the mother's urgent cry, "The baby's coming!" Look at her perineum, and if the baby will be born before the physician or nurse-midwife arrives, remain calm and support the infant's head and body with gloved hands as it emerges* (Table 17–4).

Evaluation

- During the postpartum period, does the woman show evidence of muscle strains or thrombus formation?

Nursing Care During the Late Intrapartum Period

Responsibilities During Birth

The nurse has added responsibilities during the birth. These may include the following:

- Preparation of a sterile delivery table with gowns, gloves, drapes, solutions, and instruments (see Fig. 17–16)
- Perineal cleansing preparation
- Initial care and assessment of the newborn
- Administration of medications, usually oxytocin, to contract the uterus and control blood loss (see p. 458)

An anesthesiologist or nurse anesthetist may give maternal medications. A nurse from the nursery and often a pediatrician are usually present if the newborn is at risk for problems such as respiratory depression. Nursery nurses may routinely attend deliveries as well (Fig. 17–17).

Eye shields should be worn to protect the nurse from fluid splashing or blood spurting as the cord is cut. At birth, the newborn is covered with blood, amniotic fluid, vernix,

TABLE 17–4

Assisting with an Emergency Birth

The inexperienced nurse rarely must deliver a baby in the hospital or birth center but occasionally helps the more experienced nurse do so. Unplanned out-of-hospital births are not common, but they do occasionally occur.

Nursing Priorities for an Emergency Birth in Any Setting

Prevent or reduce injury to the mother and infant.
Maintain the infant's airway and temperature after birth.

Preparing for an Emergency Birth

Study the delivery sequence in Figures 17–17 and 17–18.
Locate the emergency delivery tray ("precip" tray) on the unit.

During the Birth

Remain with the woman to assist her in giving birth. Use the call bell, or ask her partner to call for help. Stay calm to reduce the couple's anxiety.
Put on gloves, preferably sterile, to prevent contamination with blood and other secretions. Sterile gloves reduce transmission of environmental organisms to the mother and infant. The nurse will be "catching" the infant in this situation. No invasive procedure is done.

After the Birth

Observe the infant's color and respirations for distress. Suction excess secretions with a bulb syringe.
Dry the infant, and place skin-to-skin with the mother or cover with warmed blankets to maintain warmth.
Put the infant to the mother's breast, and encourage suckling to promote uterine contraction, facilitating expulsion of the placenta and controlling bleeding.

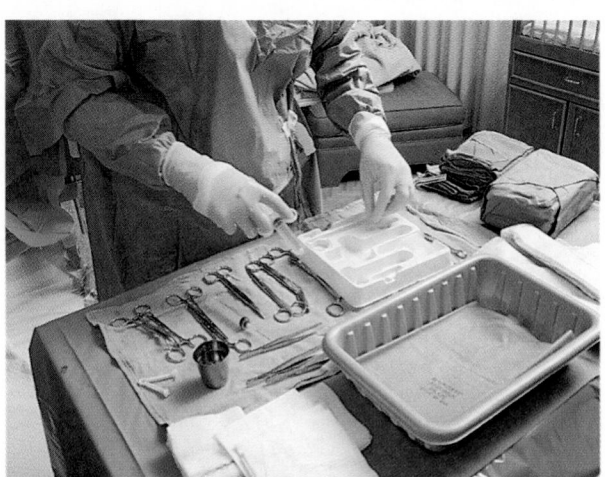

FIGURE 17–16

The nurse makes final preparations for birth. Included on the sterile table are anesthesia trays (if needed), instruments for birth and repair of maternal injury or episiotomy, and infant care materials.

Transfer and Positioning for Birth

Action: When the woman is almost ready to give birth, transfer her to the delivery room or position the birthing bed. The exact time varies with several factors (such as overall speed of labor and rate of fetal descent). *Rationale:* Rushed, last-moment preparations are anxiety-producing for the woman, her partner, and the nurse. Remaining in the birth position for a long time can be tiring.

Action: Continue observing her perineum while making final preparations for birth. *Rationale:* Birth may occur unexpectedly, and the nurse should be prepared to "catch" the infant if the attendant (physician or nurse-midwife) is not in the room.

Action: Continue observing the fetal heart rate (FHR) with continuous monitoring or intermittent auscultation. *Rationale:* Detects changes in fetal condition that may require interventions by the attendant to speed birth.

Action: Elevate the woman's back, shoulders, and head with a wedge (on a delivery table) or by raising the head of the birthing bed. *Rationale:* Allows more effective maternal pushing and uses gravity to aid fetal descent.

Action: Stirrups or foot rests to support the woman's legs and feet may be used on a birthing bed. Pad the surface. *Rationale:* Padding reduces pressure, preventing venous stasis and possible thrombus formation.

Action: When placing the woman's legs in stirrups, elevate them and remove them simultaneously. Do not separate her legs widely. *Rationale:* Reduces strain on muscles and ligaments.

Prepping and Draping

Action: After the woman is in position, cleanse the perineal area with a sterile iodophor and water preparation unless she is allergic. Use warm water to dilute the iodophor scrub. *Rationale:* Removes secretions and feces from perineal area.

Action: After hand washing, apply sterile gloves for the prep procedure. Take a fresh sponge to begin each new area, and do not return to a clean area with a used sponge. Six sponges are needed. The proper order and motions are as follows:

1. Use a zig-zag motion from clitoris to lower abdomen just above the pubic hairline.

2, 3. Use a zig-zag motion on the inner thigh from the labia majora to about halfway between the hip and knee. Repeat for the other inner thigh.

4, 5. Apply a single stroke on one side from clitoris over labia, perineum, and anus. Repeat for the other side.

6. Use a single stroke in the middle from the clitoris over the vulva and perineum.

Rationale: Prevents cross-contamination or recontamination of an area that is already clean.

Action: The attendant may apply sterile drapes if desired. *Rationale:* A vaginal birth is a clean procedure rather than a sterile one because the vagina is not sterile. Sterile drapes are unnecessary, but some attendants may prefer to use them.

Birth of the Head

Action: If an episiotomy is needed, the attendant will perform it when the head is well crowned (see Chapter 20). *Rationale:* Minimizes blood loss from the episiotomy.

Action: As the vaginal orifice encircles the fetal head, the attendant applies gentle pressure to the woman's perineum with one hand while applying counterpressure to the fetal head with the other hand (Ritgen's maneuver). The attendant may ask the mother to blow so that she avoids pushing, or to push gently. *Rationale:* Controls the exit of the fetal head so that it is born gradually rather than popping out; this minimizes trauma to the maternal tissues.

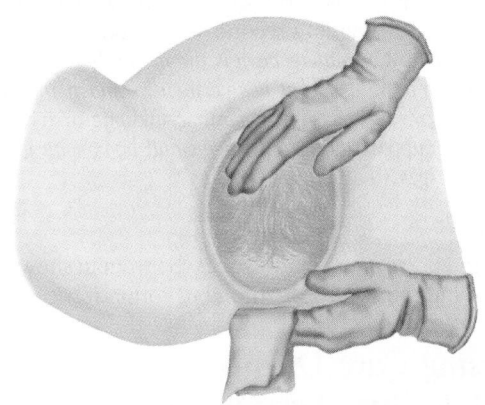

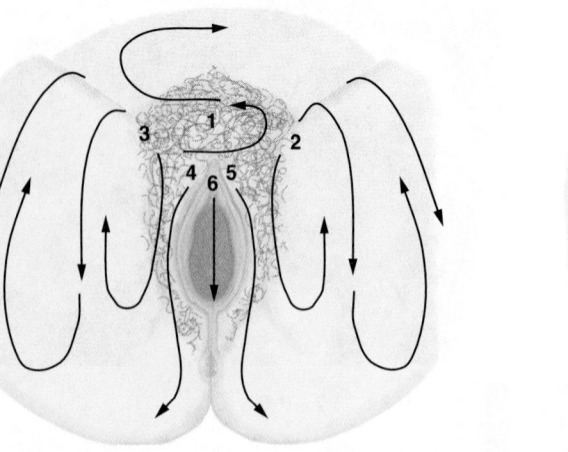

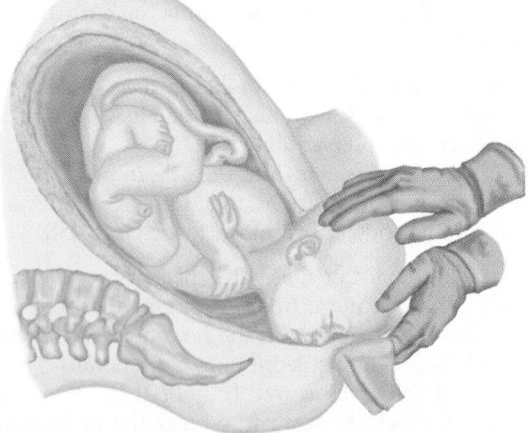

FIGURE 17–17

Sequence of delivery.

Action: The attendant wipes secretions from the infant's face and suctions the nose and mouth with a bulb syringe. *Rationale:* Removes blood and secretions, preventing the infant from aspirating them with the first breaths.

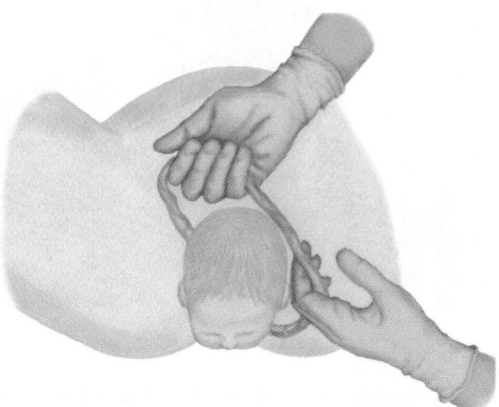

Action: The attendant feels for a cord around the fetal neck (nuchal cord). If it is loose, it is slipped over the head. If tight, it is clamped and cut between two clamps before the rest of the baby is born. *Rationale:* Allows the rest of the birth to occur and prevents stretching or tearing the cord.

Birth of the Shoulders

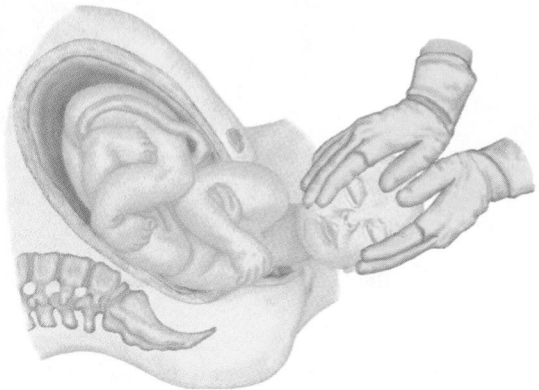

Action: After external rotation, the attendant applies gentle traction on the fetal head in the direction of the mother's perineum. *Rationale:* External rotation allows the shoulders to rotate internally and aligns their transverse diameter with the anteroposterior diameter of the mother's pelvic outlet. Traction on the head in the direction of her perineum allows the anterior fetal shoulder to slip under the symphysis pubis.

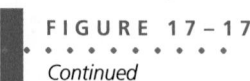
FIGURE 17–17
Continued

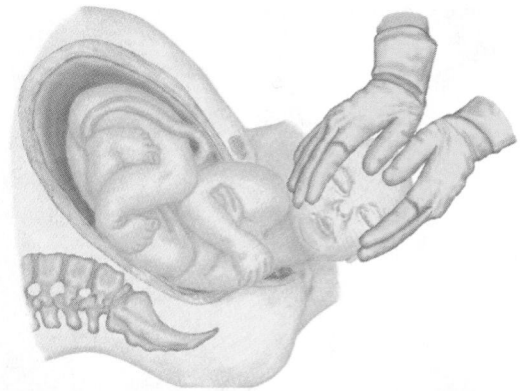

Action: The attendant then lifts the head toward the mother's symphysis pubis. *Rationale:* Permits the posterior fetal shoulder to be eased over the perineum, minimizing trauma to the maternal tissues.

Clearing the Infant's Airway and Cutting the Cord

Action: The rest of the infant's body is born quickly after the shoulders are born. The attendant maintains the infant in a slightly head-dependent position while suctioning excess secretions with a bulb syringe. The infant is often placed on the mother's abdomen. *Rationale:* Gravity aids spontaneous drainage of secretions and prevents aspiration of oral mucus and secretions.

Action: The attendant clamps the cord. Either the father or the attendant cuts the cord above the clamp. *Rationale:* Allows parents to interact more freely with their infant. Prevents flow of blood between placenta and infant, which might result in anemia (if infant is higher than placenta) or polycythemia (if infant is below the placenta).

Delivery of the Placenta

Action: After the placenta separates, it can usually be delivered if the mother bears down. The attendant may pull gently on the cord. *Rationale:* Excess traction on the cord may cause it to break, making the placenta harder to deliver.

Action: The attendant inspects both sides of the placenta. *Rationale:* Ensures that no fragments remain inside the uterus that might cause hemorrhage and infection.

After the infant and placenta are born, the attendant inspects the birth canal for injuries. If needed, any injuries and the episiotomy (if one was done) are repaired.

and other body substances (Fig. 17–18). To avoid contact with potentially infectious secretions, all personnel involved in infant care should wear gloves and other protective equipment until after the first bath. (Nursing Care Plan 17–1 illustrates a normal labor and birth experience.)

Responsibilities After Birth

Intrapartum nursing care extends through the fourth stage of labor and includes care of the infant, the mother, and the family unit. See Chapters 21 through 24 for discussion of later postpartum care of the mother and infant.

CARE OF THE INFANT
Immediate nursing care of the newborn includes supporting cardiopulmonary and thermoregulatory function and placing an identifying band on the infant. In addition, the nurse assesses the infant for approximate gestational age (see p. 550) and examines for obvious anomalies or birth injuries.

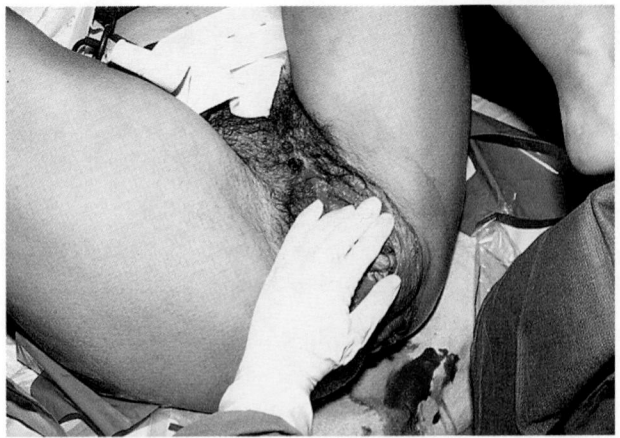

A. *Crowning*

The fetal head distends the labial and perineal tissues. The anus is stretched wide, and it is not unusual to see the woman's anterior rectal wall at this time. Any feces expelled are wiped posteriorly to avoid contaminating the vulva. The attendant (physician or nurse-midwife) is not holding the fetal head back but rather controlling its exit by using gentle pressure on the fetal occiput.

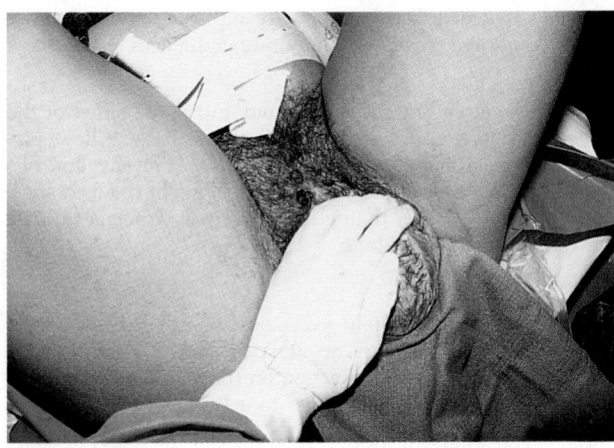

B. *Ritgen Maneuver*

Pressure is applied to the fetal chin through the perineum at the same time pressure is applied to the occiput of the fetal head. This action aids the mechanism of extension as the fetal head comes under the symphysis.

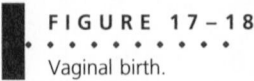

FIGURE 17–18
• • • • • • • •
Vaginal birth.

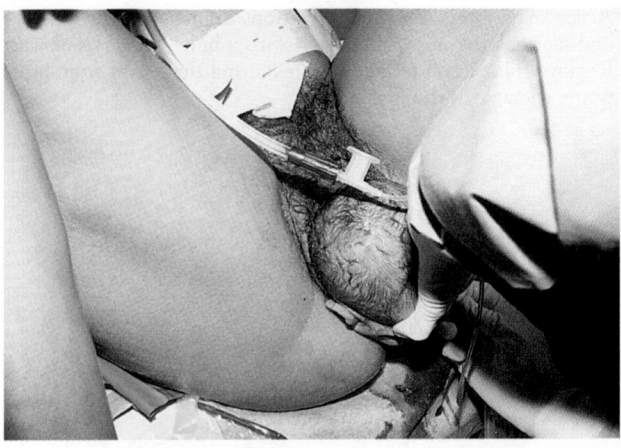

C. *Birth of the Head*

As the head emerges, the attendant prepares to suction the nose and mouth to avoid aspiration of secretions when the infant takes the first breath.

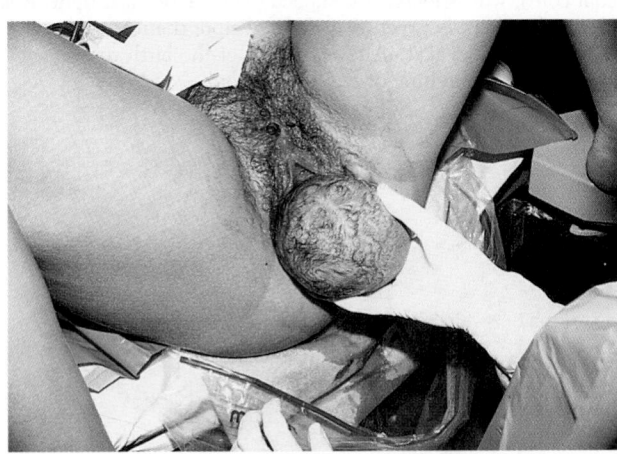

D. *Restitution and External Rotation*

After the head emerges, it realigns with the shoulders (restitution). External rotation occurs as the fetal shoulders internally rotate, aligning their transverse diameter with the anteroposterior diameter of the pelvic outlet.

Maintaining Cardiopulmonary Function. Assess the infant's Apgar score (Table 17–5) at 1 and 5 minutes after birth for rapid evaluation of early cardiopulmonary adaptation. If the Apgar score is 8 or higher, no intervention is needed, other than promoting normal respiratory efforts. If the infant is obviously in distress (i.e., no or low heart rate and/or respirations, limp muscle tone, lack of response to stimulation, blue or pale color), interventions to correct the problem are instituted immediately rather than awaiting the 1-minute Apgar score.

Keep the infant in a flat or slightly head-dependent position briefly while secretions drain. After the infant has a vigorous cry and minimal secretions, tilt the baby to one side with the head flat or slightly elevated. Keeping the infant in a head-dependent position longer than needed limits diaphragm movement because of pressure from the intestines. Suction secretions from the infant's mouth and nose with a bulb syringe as needed, and teach parents how to use the bulb syringe (see p. 569).

Supporting Thermoregulation. To reduce evaporative heat loss, dry the infant. Dry the head well because substantial heat loss can occur from the head, which is

Text continued on page 400

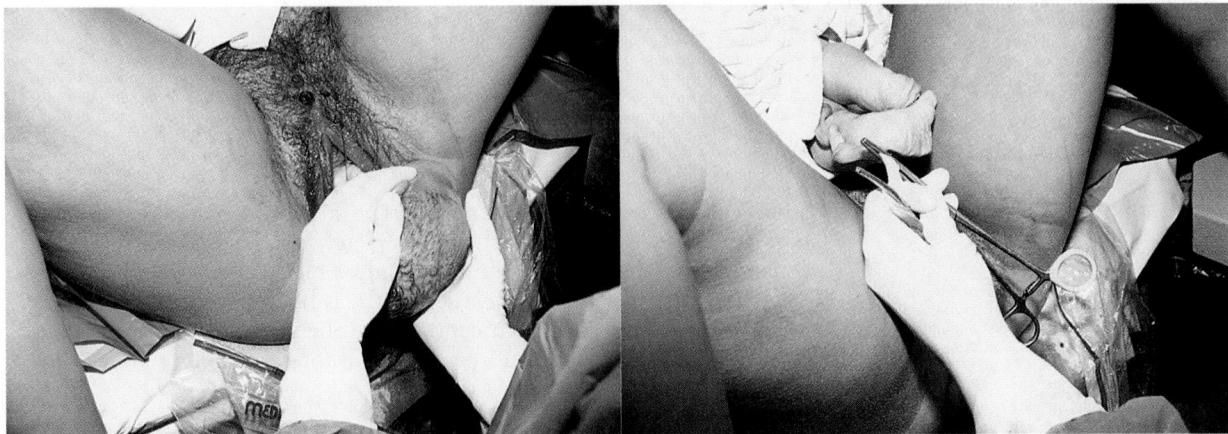

E. Birth of the Anterior Shoulder

The attendant gently pushes the fetal head toward the woman's perineum to allow the anterior shoulder to slip under her symphysis. The bluish skin color of the fetus is normal at this point; it becomes pink as the infant begins air breathing.

H. Cord Clamping

While the infant is in skin-to-skin contact on the mother's abdomen, the attendant doubly clamps the umbilical cord. The cord is then cut between the two clamps. Samples of cord blood are collected after it is cut.

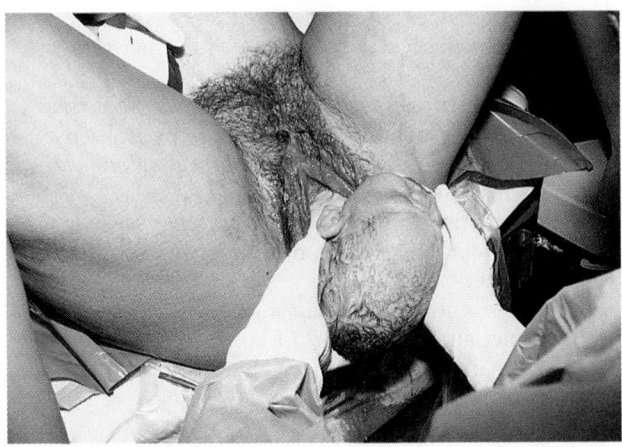

F. Birth of the Posterior Shoulder

The attendant now pushes the fetal head upward toward the woman's symphysis to allow the posterior shoulder to slip over her perineum.

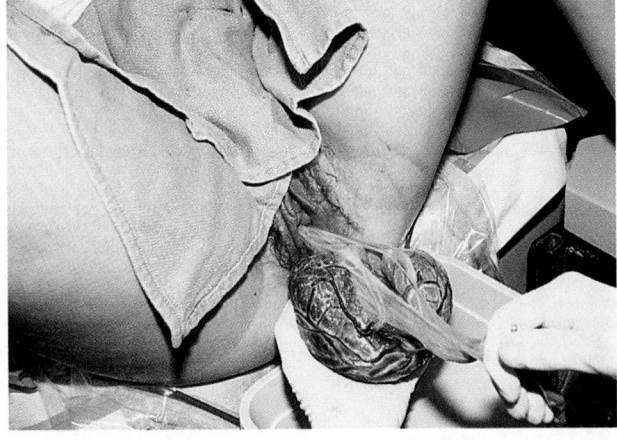

I. Birth of the Placenta

The attendant applies gentle traction on the cord to aid expulsion of the placenta. This placenta is expelled in the more common Schultze mechanism, with the shiny fetal surface and membranes emerging. Note the fetal membranes that surrounded the fetus and amniotic fluid during pregnancy. The chorionic vessels that branch from the umbilical cord are readily visible on the fetal surface of the placenta.

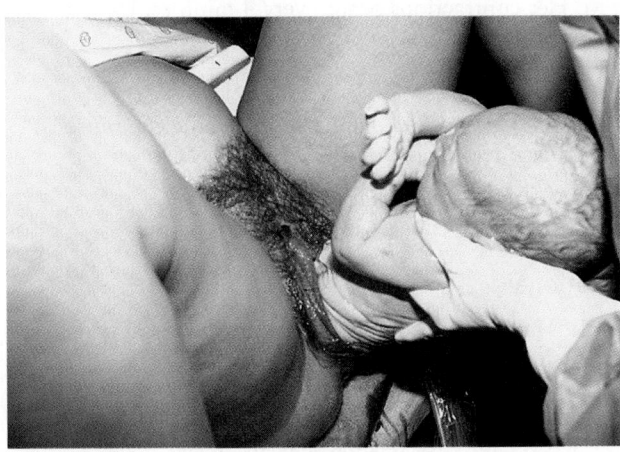

G. Completion of the Birth

The attendant supports the fetus during expulsion. Note that the fetus has excellent muscle tone, as evidenced by facial grimacing and flexion of the arms and hands.

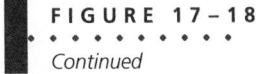

FIGURE 17–18
• • • • • • • • •
Continued

NURSING CARE PLAN 17–1
. . . .

Normal Labor and Birth

Assessment

Cathy Taggart, 17 years old, is a gravida 1, para 0, who is admitted in early labor. Her cervix is 3 cm dilated and completely effaced, and the fetus is at a 0 station. Her membranes are intact. Cathy's husband, Tim, is with her. They did not attend childbirth classes. Cathy is holding Tim's hand tightly and breathing rapidly with each contraction. She says in a shaky voice, "I'm so scared. I've never been in a hospital before. I just don't know if I can do this."

Nursing Diagnosis

Anxiety related to unfamiliar environment and lack of birth preparation.

Goals/Expected Outcomes

- Cathy will express a reduction in her anxiety after admission procedures are completed.
- Cathy will have a relaxed facial expression and body posture between contractions.

Intervention	**Rationale**
1. Maintain a calm and confident manner when caring for Cathy. Express confidence in her ability to give birth.	1. Calm provides reassurance that labor is normal and that she has the resources within her to manage it.
2. Use therapeutic communication when talking with Cathy. Adapt communication to the situation, simplifying explanations and directions as labor intensifies.	2. Clarity identifies dominant concerns so that they can be properly addressed. Intense physical sensations reduce the ability to comprehend complex information.
3. Determine the couple's plans for birth and work within them as much as possible.	3. Determining their plan enhances their sense of control and helps them have a satisfying birth experience.
4. Stay with Cathy as much as possible during labor.	4. A nurse can provide reassurance through human contact and reduce fears of abandonment.
5. Orient Cathy to the labor room and explain procedures and equipment she will encounter.	5. Information reduces fear of the unknown.

Evaluation

Cathy relaxes a bit after talking with the nurse and slows her breathing. Cathy says, "I feel a little better now. I hope I can have my baby before you go home."

Assessment

Cathy's admission vital signs are all normal: temperature, 98.8°F; pulse, 88; respirations, 20; and blood pressure, 112/70 mm Hg. The fetal heart rate averages 140 to 150 BPM. Her contractions occur every 4 minutes, last 50 seconds, and are of moderate intensity.

Potential Complication

Fetal compromise.

Goals/Expected Outcomes

Goals are not formulated for a potential complication because the nurse cannot independently manage fetal compromise. The nurse will

- Take actions to promote normal placental function.
- Observe for and report signs associated with fetal compromise.

Intervention	**Rationale**
1. Encourage Cathy to use any position she desires except the supine.	1. The supine position can cause aortocaval compression, reducing blood flow to the placenta.
2. Assess and document the fetal heart rate using the guidelines in Table 17–3. Report rates outside the normal 110 to 160 BPM, or slowing that persists after contractions. Assess the fetal heart rate more frequently if deviations from normal are identified.	2. Observation allows prompt identification of changes in the rate or of abnormal rates. Fetal heart rate assessments that are outside expected limits should be reported for possible medical intervention.

NURSING CARE PLAN 17–1 *Continued*

Normal Labor and Birth

3. When the membranes rupture, observe the color, odor, and approximate amount of fluid, and note the time of rupture.

4. Assess contractions using the guidelines listed in Table 17–1. Report contractions lasting longer than 90 seconds or occurring at intervals of less than 60 seconds, or incomplete uterine relaxation between contractions.

5. Assess Cathy's blood pressure, pulse, and respirations every hour. Assess her temperature every 4 hours until her membranes rupture, then every 2 hours.

6. See Nursing Care Plan 18–1 for additional interventions if signs of fetal compromise occur.

3. Meconium-stained fluid may be associated with fetal compromise and should be reported. Cloudy, yellow, or foul-smelling fluid suggests infection. Prolonged rupture of membranes increases the risk of infection.

4. Most placental exchange occurs during the interval between contractions. Contractions that are too long or have an inadequate interval between them decrease the time available for the intervillous spaces of the placenta to eliminate wastes and refill with oxygenated blood and nutrients.

5. Maternal hypotension or hypertension can decrease blood flow to the placenta. Maternal fever can increase the fetus's demand for oxygen beyond the mother's ability to supply it. A rising maternal pulse or fetal heart rate may precede the temperature elevation.

6. This nursing care plan addresses basic actions to promote fetal oxygenation and identify possible problems.

Evaluation

Because no client goal is established for a potential complication, evaluation is not done. The fetal heart rate remains approximately the same, and there are no signs of fetal compromise. Cathy finds that sitting in a rocking chair is most comfortable.

Assessment

In 1½ hours, Cathy's cervical dilation progresses to 5 cm, and the fetus descends to a +1 station. Her contractions occur every 3 minutes, last 60 seconds, and are of strong intensity. The fetal heart rate remains near its admission level. Cathy is having difficulty relaxing between contractions and is complaining of back pain. She is relieved that her labor is progressing normally.

Nursing Diagnosis

Pain related to effects of uterine contractions.

Goal/Expected Outcome

• Cathy will express assurance that she can manage labor pain satisfactorily.

Intervention

1. Encourage Cathy to try positions such as standing/sitting and leaning forward, side-lying, leaning over the back of the bed, or on her hands and knees. Remind her to change positions about every half hour or when she feels the need for a change.
2. Teach Tim to rub or apply firm pressure to Cathy's back. Ask her where the best place is and how hard to press. Apply powder to the area rubbed.
3. Offer thermal pain management options:
   a. A warm blanket or hot pack applied to her back.
   b. Cold packs applied to her back.
   c. Alternating warm and cold packs, or use of them for 20 minutes on and 20 minutes off.
   d. Warm water in a shower or whirlpool.

Rationale

1. These positions shift the weight of the fetus away from the sacral promontory, reducing back pain. Alternating positions relieves strain and constant pressure and also helps the fetus adapt to the pelvis.

2. Back rubs or firm pressure counteract some of the back pain. Powder decreases friction and promotes skin comfort.

3. Thermal stimulation interferes with transmission of pain impulses. Changing the thermal stimulation prevents habituation. Nipple stimulation in a shower or whirlpool causes release of oxytocin from the posterior pituitary and enhances contractions.

(continued)

NURSING CARE PLAN 17–1 *Continued*

Normal Labor and Birth

4. Teach Cathy simple breathing and relaxation techniques (see Chapter 19).

5. Observe Cathy's suprapubic area and palpate for a full bladder every 2 hours. Remind her to void if she has not done so recently.

6. Tell Cathy about her progress in labor. Explain that she will probably begin to dilate faster now that she has entered active labor.

7. Tell Cathy what pharmacologic pain relief measures are available to her.

4. Breathing techniques provide distraction from pain and give her a sense of control. Relaxation enhances a woman's ability to manage pain and enhances normal labor processes.

5. A full bladder contributes to discomfort and can prolong labor by obstructing fetal descent.

6. Encouragement and the knowledge that her efforts are having the desired results increase a woman's willingness to continue.

7. Knowing available options gives the woman a sense of control because she can choose whether she wants these measures. (This action may be done during early labor to give a woman more time to consider her options.)

Evaluation

Cathy continues to have back pain but says that she is more comfortable sitting on the side of the bed with her head on a pillow on the overbed table. Tim rubs her back during contractions. She says she is able to manage the pain and does not want medication yet.

Assessment

After another 2 hours, Cathy is quite uncomfortable and requests pain medication. She is occasionally feeling an urge to push. Cathy cries and says she is "losing it" and "can't take it anymore." Tim asks anxiously, "What's wrong? Is Cathy OK? Why is she acting this way?" The fetal heart rate remains near the admission range and shows no signs suggesting fetal compromise. Contractions occur every 2 minutes, last 70 seconds, and are strong.

Cathy's cervix is now 8 cm dilated and the station is +1. Butorphanol (Stadol), 0.5 mg IV, helps her regain control and work with her contractions. She avoids pushing by blowing out at the peak of each contraction.

Cathy is fully dilated in 45 minutes, and the fetal station is +2. She pushes spontaneously several times with each contraction, but tends to stiffen her back and push on the bed with her arms with each push. She pushes for about 10 to 15 seconds at a time, holding her breath each time. She prefers a semi-sitting position.

Nursing Diagnosis

Knowledge Deficit: effective pushing techniques.

Goal/Expected Outcome

• After instruction in more effective pushing techniques, Cathy will use the techniques until the birth occurs.

Intervention

1. Observe Cathy's perineum for fetal crowning with each push.

2. Encourage Cathy to exhale as she pushes strongly for about 4 to 6 seconds at a time.

Rationale

1. A woman having her first baby can still give birth rapidly. Observation permits the nurse to maintain her safety and that of the baby should rapid birth occur.

2. Prolonged pushing against a closed glottis reduces blood return to the heart and maternal oxygen saturation and decreases placental blood flow, especially if it is done with every contraction.

NURSING CARE PLAN 17–1 *Continued*

Normal Labor and Birth

3. Teach Cathy techniques to make each push more effective:
   a. Instruct her to flex her head slightly with each push.
   b. Instruct her to pull against her flexed knees (or hand-holds on the bed) as she pushes, curving her body around her uterus. Encourage upright positions, including squatting.
   c. Have her push toward the vaginal outlet.
   d. Help her relax her perineum as she pushes down.
   e. Keep her sacrum flattened against the bed when she pushes in a semi-sitting position.
4. Do not talk to Cathy unnecessarily between contractions.

3.
   a. Flexing her head directs each push downward into the pelvic cavity.
   b. Pulling provides leverage to gain a more effective push from the abdominal muscles. Upright positions take advantage of gravity, and squatting enlarges the pelvic outlet slightly.
   c. The vagina is the anatomically correct direction.
   d. Relaxation reduces soft tissue resistance to fetal descent.
   e. A flat sacrum straightens the pelvic curve somewhat (and is similar to squatting).
4. Silence allows her to conserve her energy for pushing efforts.

Evaluation

Cathy pushes more effectively with the nurse coaching her during each contraction. In another hour she gives birth to a 7-pound, 6-ounce (3,346-g) boy. The baby's Apgar scores are 9 at both 1 and 5 minutes. Cathy has a small first-degree laceration that is sutured with a local anesthetic. The new family gets acquainted during the recovery period.

TABLE 17–5

APGAR Score*

Assessment	Points 0	1	2
Heart rate	Absent	Below 100/min	100/min or higher
Respiratory effort	No spontaneous respirations	Slow respirations or weak cry	Spontaneous respirations with a strong, lusty cry
Muscle tone	Limp	Minimal flexion of extremities; sluggish movement	Flexed body posture; spontaneous and vigorous movement
Reflex response	No response to suction or gentle slap on soles	Minimal response (grimace) to suction or gentle slap on soles	Responds promptly to suction or a gentle slap to the sole with cry or active movement
Color	Pallor or cyanosis	Bluish hands and feet	Pink (light-skinned) or absence of cyanosis (dark-skinned)

* The Apgar score is a method of rapid evaluation of the infant's cardiorespiratory adaptation after birth. The nurse scores the infant at 1 minute and 5 minutes in each of five areas. The assessments are arranged from most important (heart rate) to least important (color). The infant is assigned a score of 0 to 2 in each of the five areas and the scores are totaled. General guidelines for the infant's care are based on three ranges of 1 minute scores:

0	1	2	3	4	5	6	7	8	9	10

Infant needs resuscitation.	Gently stimulate by rubbing the infant's back while administering oxygen. Determine whether mother received narcotics, which may have depressed infant's respirations. Have naloxone (Narcan) available for administration.	Provide no action other than support of the infant's spontaneous efforts and continued observation.

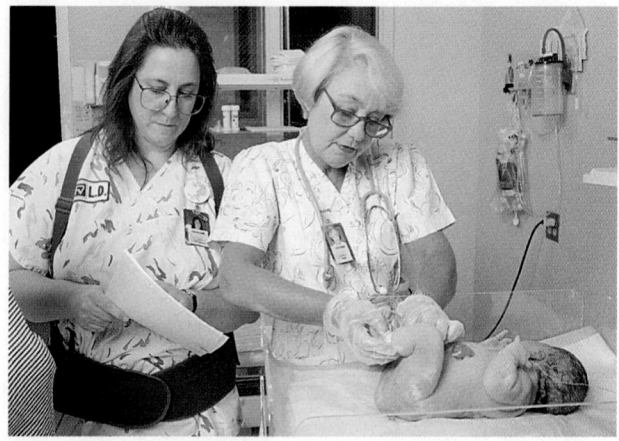

FIGURE 17-19
• • • • • • • • • •
When the birthing room nurse turns care of the newborn over to the nursery nurse, both check the identification bands and record for the same information.

about one fourth of the neonate's body surface area. Discard damp linens.

Place the infant in a prewarmed radiant warmer to limit heat loss while giving initial care. Skin-to-skin contact with a parent has the same effect and also promotes bonding.

Avoid coming between the infant and the heat source. Wrap the infant in warm blankets when he or she is not in the warmer or making skin-to-skin contact. A stockinette cap further reduces heat loss if placed on the baby's *dry* head. A cap is not worn in the radiant warmer because the cap slows transfer of heat to the baby.

Identifying the Infant. Bands having matching imprinted numbers and identifying information are the primary means to ensure that the right baby goes to the right mother after any separation (Fig. 17–19). Apply two bands on the infant, one on an arm and another on an ankle or one on each ankle to prevent facial scratching. Infant bands are applied more snugly than they would be if worn by an adult: leave about one adult fingerwidth of slack in the bands. Apply the longer band to the mother's wrist. A fourth band is usually worn by the father or other primary support person. Check that imprinted numbers and names are identical on each set of bands. A set is needed for each baby in a multiple birth.

CARE OF THE MOTHER

Nursing care of the mother during the fourth stage of labor focuses on observing for hemorrhage and relieving discomfort. Table 17–6 summarizes possible problems during the fourth stage of labor.

TABLE 17-6
• • • • • • • • • • •

Problems During the Fourth Stage of Labor

Sign	Potential Problem	Immediate Nursing Action
Rising pulse rate and/or falling blood pressure	An early sign of hypovolemia due to excessive blood loss (visible or concealed).	Identify the probable cause of the blood loss, usually a poorly contracted uterus. Take steps to correct it (see below).
Soft (boggy) uterus	A poorly contracted uterus does not adequately compress large open vessels at the placental site, resulting in hemorrhage.	With one hand securing the uterus just above the symphysis and the other on the fundus, massage the uterus until firm. Push downward on the *firm* uterus to expel any clots. Empty the woman's bladder (by voiding or catheterization) if that is contributing to the uterine atony.
High uterine fundus, often displaced to one side	Suggests a full bladder, which can interfere with uterine contraction and result in hemorrhage.	Massage the uterus if it is not firm. Help the woman urinate in the bathroom or on the bedpan. If she cannot void, catheterize her.
Lochia exceeding 1 *saturated* perineal pad per hour during the fourth stage	Suggests hemorrhage; however, perineal pads vary in their absorbency, and this must be considered.	Identify cause of hemorrhage, usually uterine atony, which is manifested by a soft uterus. Correct the cause. If lacerations are the suspected cause (excess bleeding with a firm fundus), notify the birth attendant. Keep the woman NPO until the birth attendant evaluates her.
Intense perineal or vaginal pain, poorly relieved with analgesics	Hematoma, usually of vaginal wall or perineum; signs of hypovolemia may occur with substantial blood loss into tissues.	If the hematoma is visible, apply cold packs to the area to slow bleeding into tissues. Notify the birth attendant, and anticipate possible surgical drainage. Keep the woman NPO.

Observing for Hemorrhage. Important assessments related to hemorrhage are the woman's vital signs, uterine fundus, bladder, and lochia. For detailed information about these assessments, see Chapter 21.

Vital Signs. Assess the woman's temperature when recovery care begins. Assess her blood pressure, pulse, and respirations every 15 minutes during the first hour. A rising pulse is an early sign of excessive blood loss because the heart pumps faster to compensate for reduced blood volume. The blood pressure may fall much later as the blood volume is severely reduced.

Fundus. The most common reason for excessive postpartum bleeding is that the uterus does not firmly contract and compress open vessels at the placental site. Assess the firmness, height, and positioning of the uterine fundus with each vital sign assessment. The fundus should be firm, in the midline, and below the umbilicus (about the size of a large grapefruit). If the fundus is firm, no massage is needed; if it is soft (boggy), massage it until it is firm. Nipple stimulation from the infant's suckling releases natural oxytocin from the mother's posterior pituitary gland to maintain firm uterine contraction. Oxytocin in the intravenous solution or given intramuscularly has the same effect.

Bladder. A full bladder interferes with contraction of the uterus and may lead to hemorrhage. Suspect a full bladder if the fundus is above the umbilicus or is displaced to one side, usually the right. If there is no contraindication, such as altered sensation, the mother can walk to the bathroom (with assistance the first few times). The first two voidings are often measured until it is evident that the woman voids without difficulty and empties her bladder completely. Each voiding is usually at least 300 to 400 ml if she is emptying her bladder.

Lochia. Assess lochia with each vital sign and fundal assessment. The amount of lochia seems large to the inexperienced nurse and the new mother. Perineal pads vary in their absorbency, but *saturation* of one pad within the first hour is a guideline for the maximum normal lochia flow. Observe for lochia that pools under the mother's buttocks and back. Small clots may be present, but the presence of large clots is not normal, and the physician or nurse-midwife should be notified. A continuous trickle of bright red blood when the fundus is firm suggests a laceration in the birth canal. A hematoma causes bleeding into the tissues, but excess visible bleeding is unusual.

Relieving Discomfort. Uterine contractions (afterpains) and perineal trauma are common causes of pain after birth. A postpartum chill often adds to discomfort. Pain is usually mild and readily relieved by simple measures. Notify the birth attendant if pain is intense or does not respond to common relief measures.

Ice Packs. To reduce edema and limit hematoma formation, apply an ice pack to the perineum promptly after birth. Small hematomas are common, but a rapidly enlarging hematoma causes significant concealed blood loss and pain. Some perineal pads contain chemical cold packs. These pads absorb less lochia than ordinary pads, so the type of pad should be considered when estimating pad saturation.

Analgesics. Afterpains and perineal pain respond well to mild oral analgesics such as ibuprofen. Regular urination reduces the severity of afterpains because the uterus contracts more effectively.

Warmth. A warm blanket is soothing and can shorten the chill that is common after birth. A portable radiant warmer provides warmth to both the mother and infant. The mother may enjoy warm drinks.

PROMOTING EARLY FAMILY ATTACHMENT

The first hour after birth is an ideal time for parent-infant attachment because the healthy neonate is alert and responsive. Provide privacy while unobtrusively observing the parents and infant. The infant can remain in the parent's arms while you take vital signs, suction small amounts of secretions, and perform many initial assessments.

Assist the mother to breast-feed during the recovery period, if she desires. The infant is usually attentive and nurses briefly. Early nipple stimulation helps initiate milk production.

When the parents are ready, allow siblings, other family members, and friends to visit. Help siblings to see and touch their new brother or sister by putting a stool at the bedside or letting them sit on the bed.

Observe for signs of early parent-infant attachment. Parent behaviors are tentative at first, progressing from fingertip touch to palm touch to enfolding of the infant. Expect parents to make eye contact with the infant and talk to a baby in higher-pitched, affectionate tones.

Cultural variations should be considered when assessing early attachment. The nurse should be knowledgeable about the typical practices of the populations commonly served. In some cultures, great attention to the newborn is considered unlucky (sometimes because of an "evil eye").

KEY CONCEPTS

- Labor contractions are intermittent, allowing placental blood flow and exchange of oxygen, nutrients, and waste products between maternal and fetal circulations during the interval.
- The upper uterus contracts actively during labor, maintaining tension to pull the more passive lower uterus and cervix over the fetal presenting part. These actions bring about cervical effacement and dilation.
- Several occurrences during late pregnancy and labor aid the newborn in making adaptations to extrauterine life: reduced production of fetal lung fluid and increased absorption of lung fluid into the interstitium of the fetal lungs, expulsion of fluid from upper airways

during the compressive forces of labor, and increased catecholamine secretion by the fetal adrenals to stimulate cardiac contraction and breathing speed clearance of remaining lung fluid and aid in temperature regulation.

■ Four interrelated components affecting the process of birth are the powers, the passage, the passenger, and the psyche. Presentation and position further describe the relation of the fetus (passenger) to the maternal pelvis.

■ The mechanisms of labor favor the most efficient passage of the fetus through the mother's pelvis.

■ As labor approaches, the woman may notice one or more premonitory signs that precede its onset: an increase in the frequency and intensity of Braxton Hicks contractions, lightening, increased vaginal secretions, bloody show, a spurt of energy, and weight loss.

■ The conclusive difference between true labor and false labor is progressive effacement and dilation of the cervix.

■ Some women do not have symptoms typical of true labor. They should enter the birth center for evaluation if they are uncertain or have concerns other than those listed in the guidelines.

■ The four stages and phases of labor are characterized by different physiologic events and maternal behaviors. In the first stage, these are cervical dilation and effacement; in the second stage, expulsion of the fetus; in the third stage, expulsion of the placenta; in the fourth stage, maternal physiologic stabilization and parent-infant bonding.

■ Normal labor is characterized by consistent progression of uterine contractions, cervical dilation and effacement, and fetal descent.

■ The initial intrapartum assessments are quick assessments of maternal and fetal health and labor status.

■ Because of complete dependence on the mother's physiologic systems; the fetus is the more vulnerable of the maternal-fetal pair.

■ The normal fetal heart rate at term averages 110 to 120 BPM at the lower limit and 150 to 160 BPM at the upper limit. Other reassuring findings include the presence of variability in the electronically monitored fetus, accelerations of at least 15 BPM for 15 seconds, and absence of decelerations following contractions.

■ Persistent contractions lasting longer than 90 seconds or occurring at intervals of less than 60 seconds may reduce placental blood flow and fetal oxygen, nutrient, and waste exchange.

■ A maternal supine position can reduce placental blood flow because the uterus compresses the aorta and inferior vena cava.

■ General comfort measures promote the woman's ability to relax and cope with labor.

■ Regular changes in position during labor promote maternal comfort and help the fetus adapt to the pelvis.

■ The nurse must be alert for signs of impending birth. The woman may urgently state, "The baby's coming," or she may make grunting sounds or bear down.

■ The priority nursing care of the newborn immediately after birth is to promote normal respirations, maintain normal body temperature, and promote attachment.

■ The priority nursing care of the mother after birth is to assess for hemorrhage, promote firm uterine contraction, and promote parent-infant attachment.

ANSWERS TO CRITICAL THINKING EXERCISES

Exercise 17–1

1. First, you need to speak directly to the woman who is having the contractions. You need some additional information as well: Which baby this is for her? What is her due date? Have her membranes ruptured? What are the characteristics of her contractions (frequency, duration, intensity, effect of activity)?

2. Heather's symptoms sound like those typical of false labor: irregular contractions that are mild, fairly short, and more annoying than truly painful. Although not harmful, these frequent contractions in late pregnancy interrupt the woman's rest. You should tell Heather that these contractions do not

sound like true labor, then review with her the typical signs and symptoms of true labor. Advise her to come to the hospital if her contractions intensify and become more consistent, if her "water breaks," if the baby seems to move much less, or if she has bleeding. And because it is impossible to diagnose labor over the phone, tell her to come to the hospital for assessment if she has any continuing concern.

Exercise 17–2

1. The woman's behavior may have changed for any of several reasons, so the nurse must not make assumptions. For example, she may have felt insulted that the nurse found it necessary to ask her questions

about illicit drug use. Or she may use other drugs (licit or illicit) but prefer not to admit it. She may, however, simply have been surprised by the question about drug use. Women often want their family to remain during the admission assessment but may not admit substance or domestic abuse in their presence. Nonverbal cues, such as a too-quick denial, avoidance of eye contact, or vague responses, are clues that the woman may not be answering these questions truthfully.

2. The nurse should follow up on maternal behaviors privately to clarify the facts that underlie them.

REFERENCES AND READINGS

Albers, L. L., Schiff, M., & Gorwoda, J. G. (1996). The length of active labor in normal pregnancies. *Obstetrics and Gynecology, 87*(3), 355–359.

American Academy of Pediatrics & American College of Obstetricians and Gynecologists. (1997). *Guidelines for perinatal care* (4th ed.). Elk Grove Village, IL, and Washington, DC: Authors.

American College of Obstetricians and Gynecologists. (1995a). *Fetal heart rate patterns: Monitoring, interpretation, and management* (ACOG Technical Bulletin No. 207). Washington, DC: Author.

American College of Obstetricians and Gynecologists. (1995b). *Vaginal delivery after previous cesarean birth* (ACOG Practice Patterns). Washington, DC: Author.

American College of Obstetricians and Gynecologists. (1996). *Hypertension in pregnancy* (ACOG Technical Bulletin No. 219). Washington, DC: Author.

Arrabal, P. P., & Nagey, D. A. (1996). Is manual palpation of uterine contractions accurate? *American Journal of Obstetrics and Gynecology, 174*(1, pt. 1), 217–219.

Association of Women's Health, Obstetric, & Neonatal Nurses (AWHONN). (1998). *Clinical competencies and education guide.* Washington, DC: Author.

Bachman, J., & Kendrick, J. M. (1996). Childbirth. In K. R. Rice & P. A. Creehan (Eds.), *Perinatal nursing* (pp. 151–186). Philadelphia: Lippincott.

Bowes, W. A. (1999). Clinical aspects of normal and abnormal labor. In R. Creasy & R. Resnik (Eds.), *Maternal-fetal medicine: Principles and practice* (4th ed., pp. 541–568). Philadelphia: Saunders.

Chapman, L. L. (1992). Expectant fathers' roles during labor and birth. *Journal of Obstetric, Gynecologic, and Neonatal Nursing, 21*(2), 114–120.

Creehan, P. A. (1996). Pain relief and comfort measures during labor. In K. R. Rice & P. A. Creehan (Eds.), *Perinatal nursing* (pp. 227–245). Philadelphia: Lippincott.

Cunningham, F. G., MacDonald, P. C., Gant, N. F., Leveno, K. J., Gilstrap, L. C., Hankins, G. D. V., et al. (1997). *Williams obstetrics* (20th ed.). Norwalk, CT: Appleton & Lange.

Enkin, M. W., Keirse, M. J., Renfrew, M. J., & Neilson, J. P. (1995). Effective care in pregnancy and childbirth: A synopsis. *Birth, 22*(2), 101–110.

Evans, S., & Jeffrey, J. (1995). Maternal learning needs during labor and delivery. *Journal of Obstetric, Gynecologic, and Neonatal Nursing, 24*(3), 235–240.

Gagnon, A. J., & Waghorn, K. (1996). Supportive care by maternity nurses: A work sampling study in an intrapartum unit. *Birth 23*(1), 1–6.

Guyton, A. C., & Hall, J. C. (1996). *Textbook of medical physiology* (9th ed.). Philadelphia: Saunders.

Haddad, G. G., & Pérez Fontán, J. J. (1996). Development of the respiratory system. In W. E. Nelson, R. E. Behrman, R. M. Kliegman, & A. M. Arvin (Eds.), *Nelson textbook of pediatrics* (15th ed., pp. 1165–1167). Philadelphia: Saunders.

Hodnett, E. (1996). Nursing support of the laboring woman. *Journal of Obstetric, Gynecologic, and Neonatal Nursing, 25*(3), 257–264.

Hutchinson, M. K., & BaqiAziz, M. (1994). Nursing care of the childbearing Muslim family. *Journal of Obstetric, Gynecologic, and Neonatal Nursing, 23*(9), 767–771.

Jackson, M. M., & Rymer, T. E. (1995). Nurses: At special risk. *Journal of Obstetric, Gynecologic, and Neonatal Nursing, 24*(6), 533–540.

Khazoyan, C. M., & Anderson, N. L. R. (1994). Latinas' expectations for their partners during childbirth. *American Journal of Maternal-Child Nursing, 19*(4), 226–229.

Letko, M. D. (1996). Understanding the Apgar score. *Journal of Obstetric, Gynecologic, and Neonatal Nursing, 25*(4), 299–303.

Lowe, N. K., & Reiss, R. (1996). Parturition and fetal adaptation. *Journal of Obstetric, Gynecologic, and Neonatal Nursing, 25*(4), 339–349.

Mattson, S. (1995). Culturally sensitive perinatal care for Southeast Asians. *Journal of Obstetric, Gynecologic, and Neonatal Nursing, 24*(4), 335–341.

Menihan, C. A. (1996). Intrapartum fetal monitoring. In K. R. Rice & P. A. Creehan (Eds.), *Perinatal nursing* (pp. 187–225). Philadelphia: Lippincott.

Murray, M. (1997). *Antepartal and intrapartal fetal monitoring* (2nd ed.). Albuquerque, NM: Learning Resources International.

Roberts, J., & Woolley, D. (1996). A second look at the second stage of labor. *Journal of Obstetric, Gynecologic, and Neonatal Nursing, 25*(5), 415–423.

Rothman, B. K. (1996). Women, providers, & control. *Journal of Obstetric, Gynecologic, and Neonatal Nursing, 25*(3), 253–256.

Rush, J., Burlock, S., Lambert, K., Loosley-Millman, M., Hutchison, B., & Enkin, M. (1996). The effects of whirlpool baths in labor: A randomized controlled trial. *Birth, 23*(3), 136–143.

Simkin, P. (1996). The experience of maternity in a woman's life. *Journal of Obstetric, Gynecologic, and Neonatal Nursing, 25*(3), 247–252.

Supplee, R. B., & Vezeau, T. M. (1996). Continuous electronic fetal monitoring: Does it belong in low-risk births? *American Journal of Maternal and Child Nursing, 21*(6), 301–306.

Tomlinson, P. S., & Mattson Bryan, A. A. (1996). Family centered intrapartum care: Revisiting an old concept. *Journal of Obstetric, Gynecologic, and Neonatal Nursing, 25*(4), 331–337.

Waymire, V. (1997). A triggering time: Childbirth may recall sexual abuse memories. *Lifelines, 1*(2), 47–50.

18

Intrapartum Fetal Monitoring

DEFINITIONS

acidosis A condition resulting from the accumulation of acid (hydrogen ions) or the depletion of base (bicarbonate) in the blood or body tissues. The pH measures acid-base balance.

amnioinfusion Infusion of lactated Ringer's solution or isotonic saline into the uterine cavity during labor to reduce umbilical cord compression; also done to dilute meconium in amniotic fluid, reducing the risk that the infant will aspirate thick meconium at birth.

asphyxia Insufficient oxygen and excess carbon dioxide in the blood and tissues.

baroreceptors Cells that are sensitive to blood pressure changes.

chemoreceptors Cells that are sensitive to chemical changes in the blood, specifically changes in oxygen and carbon dioxide levels and in acid-base balance.

hypercapnia Excess carbon dioxide in the blood, evidenced by an elevated P_{CO_2}.

hypertonic contractions Uterine contractions that are too long or too frequent, have too short a resting interval, or have an inadequate relaxation period to allow optimal uteroplacental exchange.

hypoxemia Reduced oxygenation of the blood, evidenced by a low P_{O_2}.

hypoxia Reduced availability of oxygen to the body tissues.

intermittent monitoring A variation of electronic fetal monitoring in which an initial strip is obtained on admission. If patterns are reassuring, the woman is remonitored for periods of 15 minutes at regular intervals (about every 30 to 60 minutes).

nuchal cord Umbilical cord around the fetal neck.

telemetry Transmission of electronic fetal monitoring data to the bedside monitor unit with radio signals.

tocolytic A drug that inhibits uterine contractions.

transducer A device that translates one physical quantity into another, such as fetal heart motion into an electrical signal for rate calculation or the generation of sound or of a written record.

uterine resting tone Degree of uterine muscle tension when the woman is not in labor or during the interval between labor contractions.

Intrapartum fetal monitoring is the process of fetal surveillance to identify signs associated with well-being and with compromise. Accurate assessment of these signs permits appropriate and timely care to reduce hazards to the fetus. During labor there are two clients: the expectant mother and her fetus. The purposes of intrapartum fetal monitoring are to evaluate how the fetus tolerates labor and to identify hypoxic insult to the fetus during labor. Fetal monitoring cannot identify every compromised fetus.

Two basic approaches are taken to intrapartum fetal monitoring, a low-technology approach and electronic fetal monitoring. Each has advantages and limitations. The low-technology approach uses auscultation of the fetal heart rate and palpation of uterine activity. Electronic fetal monitoring is the second approach to intrapartum fetal surveillance. Although electronic fetal monitoring is used more commonly in U.S. hospital births, its routine use remains controversial because its benefits to the fetus are not always clear.

Fetal Oxygenation

Adequate fetal oxygenation requires five related factors:

- Normal maternal blood flow and volume to the placenta
- Normal oxygen saturation in maternal blood
- Adequate exchange of oxygen and carbon dioxide in the placenta
- An open circulatory path between the placenta and the fetus through vessels in the umbilical cord
- Normal fetal circulatory and oxygen-carrying functions

Labor is stressful for a fetus, but several mechanisms exist to compensate for these stresses. One must understand the dynamics of uteroplacental exchange and fetal circulation to understand fetal responses to labor. (See also Chapter 12 for a discussion of fetal circulation and placental functions.)

Uteroplacental Exchange

Oxygen-rich and nutrient-rich blood from the mother enters the intervillous spaces of the placenta via the spiral arteries (see Fig. 12–7). Oxygen and nutrients in the maternal blood pass into the fetal blood that circulates in capillaries in the intervillous spaces. Carbon dioxide and other waste products pass from the fetal blood into the maternal blood at the same time. Maternal blood carrying fetal waste products drains from the intervillous spaces through endometrial veins and returns to the mother's circulation for elimination by her body. Substances pass back and forth between mother and fetus without mixing of maternal and fetal blood.

During labor, contractions gradually compress the spiral arteries, temporarily stopping maternal blood flow into the intervillous spaces. During contractions, the fetus depends on the oxygen supply already present in body cells, fetal erythrocytes, and the intervillous spaces. The oxygen supply in these areas is enough for about 1 to 2 minutes. As each contraction relaxes, freshly oxygenated maternal blood re-enters the intervillous spaces and waste-laden blood drains out.

Fetal Circulation

The fetal heart circulates oxygenated blood from the placenta throughout the body and returns deoxygenated blood to the placenta. The umbilical vein carries oxygenated blood to the fetus, and the two umbilical arteries carry deoxygenated blood from the fetus to the placenta (see Fig. 12–7).

Regulation of Fetal Heart Rate

Mechanisms that regulate the fetal heart rate are balanced to maintain cardiac output at a level that keeps the fetal heart and brain oxygenated. Fetal cardiac output increase is primarily accomplished by an increase in the heart rate. Conversely, a marked decrease in fetal heart rate decreases the cardiac output.

Five fetal factors interact to regulate the fetal heart rate:

1. the autonomic nervous system
2. the baroreceptors
3. the chemoreceptors
4. the adrenal glands
5. the central nervous system

The balance among forces that increase and those that slow the heart rate result in the characteristic fluctuations in fetal heart rate during the final trimester of pregnancy.

AUTONOMIC NERVOUS SYSTEM

The sympathetic and parasympathetic branches of the autonomic nervous system are balanced forces that regulate the fetal heart rate. Sympathetic stimulation increases the heart rate and strengthens myocardial contractions through release of epinephrine and norepinephrine. The net result of sympathetic stimulation is an increase in cardiac output.

The parasympathetic nervous system, through stimulation of the vagus nerve, reduces the fetal heart rate and maintains short-term variability. The parasympathetic branch gradually exerts greater influence as the fetus matures, beginning between 28 and 32 weeks of gestation. Therefore, the average fetal heart rate in the term fetus is lower than in the preterm fetus.

BARORECEPTORS

Cells in the carotid arch and major arteries respond to stretching when the fetal blood pressure increases. The baroreceptors stimulate the vagus nerve to slow the fetal heart rate and decrease the blood pressure, thus lowering cardiac output.

CHEMORECEPTORS

Cells that respond to changes in oxygen, carbon dioxide, and pH are found in the medulla oblongata and in the aortic and carotid bodies. Decreased oxygen content, increased carbon dioxide content, or a lower pH in the blood or cerebrospinal fluid triggers an increase in the heart rate. However, prolonged hypoxia, hypercapnia, and acidosis depress the fetal heart rate.

ADRENAL GLANDS

The adrenal medulla secretes epinephrine and norepinephrine in response to stress, causing a sympathetic response that accelerates the fetal heart rate. The adrenal cortex responds to a fall in the fetal blood pressure with release of aldosterone and retention of sodium and water, resulting in an increase in the circulating fetal blood volume.

CENTRAL NERVOUS SYSTEM

The fetal cerebral cortex causes the heart rate to increase during fetal movement and decrease when the fetus sleeps. The hypothalamus coordinates the two branches of the autonomic nervous system. The medulla oblongata maintains the balance between stimuli that speed and stimuli that slow the heart rate.

Pathologic Influences on Fetal Oxygenation

Fetal oxygenation may be compromised by alterations in any of the placental or fetal factors or those of the pregnant woman.

MATERNAL CARDIOPULMONARY ALTERATIONS

Actual or relative reductions in the mother's circulating blood volume impair perfusion of the intervillous spaces with oxygenated maternal blood. Hemorrhage causes an actual decrease in her blood volume. Relative reductions in maternal circulating volume involve altered distribution of the blood volume without blood loss. For example, epidural block analgesia may result in vasodilation, which increases the capacity of the maternal vascular bed. However, the amount of blood available to fill the vessels is unchanged. Hypotension then results, with a reduction of placental blood flow.

Maternal hypertension may reduce blood flow to the placenta because of vasospasm and narrowing of the spiral arteries.

A lowered oxygen level in the mother's blood reduces the amount available to the fetus. Maternal acid-base alterations, which often accompany respiratory abnormalities, may also compromise exchange in the placenta. A lower maternal oxygen tension may result from respiratory disorders such as asthma or from smoking.

UTERINE ACTIVITY

Hypertonic uterine activity can reduce the time available for exchange of oxygen and waste products in the placenta. Contractions may be too long (over 90 seconds) or too frequent (closer than every 2 minutes) or have too short an interval (less than 60 seconds). The uterus may not fully relax between contractions, applying continuous compression to the spiral arteries and reducing maternal-fetal exchange in the intervillous spaces. Hypertonic uterine activity may occur spontaneously or with oxytocin administration.

PLACENTAL DISRUPTIONS

Conditions such as abruptio placentae (partial separation of the placenta before birth) and infarcts reduce the placental surface area available for exchange. The amount and location of placental disruption relate to the degree of impairment in uteroplacental exchange.

INTERRUPTIONS IN UMBILICAL FLOW

The usual cause of interrupted blood flow through the umbilical cord is compression. Blood flow through the umbilical cord may be reduced by compression between the fetal presenting part and the pelvis, a nuchal cord or one that is wrapped around the fetal body, or a knot in the cord. It may occur with oligohydramnios because the amount of amniotic fluid is inadequate to cushion the cord. The umbilical cord also may become entangled between fetal body parts.

The thin-walled umbilical vein is compressed initially, resulting in a reduced inflow of more highly oxygenated blood to the fetus. This results in initial hypoxia with hypotension. Baroreceptors and chemoreceptors respond by accelerating the fetal heart rate. Flow through the firmer-walled umbilical arteries is reduced as cord compression continues, resulting in hypertension. Baroreceptors respond to hypertension by stimulating the vagus nerve, thus reducing blood pressure and slowing the fetal heart. The fetal heart rate again accelerates as pressure on the arteries is relieved, and then pressure on the vein.

FETAL ALTERATIONS

Fetal cells may be hypoxic despite an adequate oxygen supply from the mother and adequate exchange within the placenta. A low circulating fetal blood volume, fetal hypotension, or fetal anemia may result in cellular hypoxia. Central nervous system or cardiac abnormalities may cause an abnormal rate or rhythm. For example, a fetus with complete heart block may not respond to stimuli that would normally cause a rate increase.

A prolonged rate lower than 50 beats per minute (BPM) may reduce fetal cardiac output enough to impair brain and heart perfusion. A persistent heart rate faster than 200 BPM, however, also decreases cardiac output because the ventricles do not have time to fill with oxygenated blood during diastole.

Risk Factors for Fetal Compromise

When conditions associated with reduced fetal oxygenation exist (Table 18–1), assessments by either intermittent auscultation and palpation or electronic fetal monitoring are done more often. No absolute indications, including the presence of risk factors, demand the use of electronic fetal monitoring during labor. Properly performed intermittent auscultation is equivalent to continuous electronic monitoring in assessing fetal condition (American College of Obstetricians and Gynecologists, 1995a).

TABLE 18–1

• • • • • • • • • • •

Conditions Associated with Decreased Fetal Oxygenation

Antepartum Period

Maternal History

Prior stillbirth
Prior cesarean birth
Chronic diseases, such as cardiac disease, hypertension, and diabetes
Drug abuse

Problems Identified During Pregnancy

Fetal growth restriction
Gestation > 42 weeks
Marked decrease in fetal movement
Multifetal gestation
Pregnancy-induced hypertension
Gestational diabetes
Placenta previa
Maternal severe anemia
Maternal infection

Intrapartum Period

Maternal Problems

Hypotension
Hypertonic uterine contractions
Abnormal labor: preterm or dysfunctional
Prolonged rupture of membranes
Chorioamnionitis
Fever

Fetal or Placental Problems

Abnormal fetal heart rate or pattern
Meconium-stained amniotic fluid
Abnormal presentation or position
Prolapsed cord
Abruptio placentae

Auscultation and Palpation

The nurse may use intermittent auscultation of the fetal heart rate and palpation of uterine activity for intrapartum fetal surveillance. This approach allows the woman greater freedom to move around during labor than electronic fetal monitoring allows. Intermittent auscultation of the fetal heart rate can be done using either the fetoscope or Doppler ultrasound transducer (Fig. 18–1).

Advantages

Mobility is the primary advantage of auscultation and palpation for intrapartum fetal monitoring. The woman is free to change position and walk around, which is especially helpful during early labor. She can use water-based methods of pain management, such as whirlpool baths or showers. The atmosphere is more natural than technological, which is important to some families during their birth experience.

Limitations

One disadvantage of auscultation and palpation as the primary method of fetal assessment is that fetal heart rate and uterine activity are assessed for a small percentage of the total labor. The fetus is most stressed during contractions because of the normal reduction of blood flow to the placenta at that time. Although the fetal heart rate is assessed during some contractions, it is not recorded during every contraction. Moreover, no continuous printed record is available to show the fetal response throughout labor or to identify subtle trends in the response.

Some women find that interruptions for auscultation are distracting. The pressure of the instrument on the abdomen is uncomfortable for some, and it may require several moves to locate the best place for auscultation.

Intermittent auscultation can be more staff-intensive than electronic monitoring. When many clients are present for the number of nurses, auscultation may not be a realistic option as the primary method of intrapartum fetal surveillance.

Electronic Fetal Monitoring

Electronic fetal monitoring may be continuous, starting shortly after the woman is admitted, or intermittent, with a short recording made at regular intervals during labor.

Advantages

The electronic monitor supplies more data about the fetus than auscultation and prints a permanent record. Gradual trends that suggest problems may be identified because the strip provides a graphic record for review. Continuous electronic fetal monitoring shows how the fetus responds before, during, and after each contraction rather than only occasional contractions.

Many women in the United States expect electronic monitoring and find the constant sound of the fetal heartbeat comforting. The coach can use the tracing of contractions on the monitor strip to help the woman anticipate the beginning and end of each contraction.

Electronic monitoring allows one nurse to observe two laboring women, primarily during uncomplicated early labor. A 1-to-1 nurse-client ratio is needed during the second stage of labor, regardless of the monitoring method used. Electronic monitoring can give the nurse more time for teaching and supporting the laboring woman with breathing and relaxation techniques if the nurse maintains the primary focus on the woman, not on the monitor.

Limitations

Reduced mobility is a limitation of electronic fetal monitoring. Telemetry or intermittent monitoring gives the woman more freedom of movement than continuous electronic monitoring without telemetry.

Frequent maternal position changes or an active fetus may require constant adjustment of equipment. The belts or stockinette used to keep sensors positioned properly for external monitoring are uncomfortable for some women.

The electronic fetal monitor imparts a more technical air to the surroundings and may be objectionable to a woman and her partner.

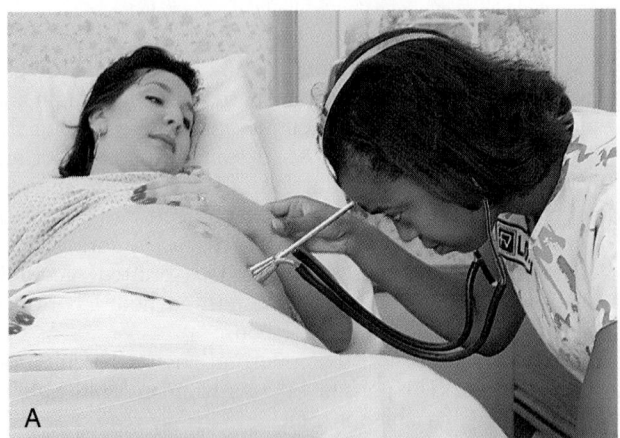

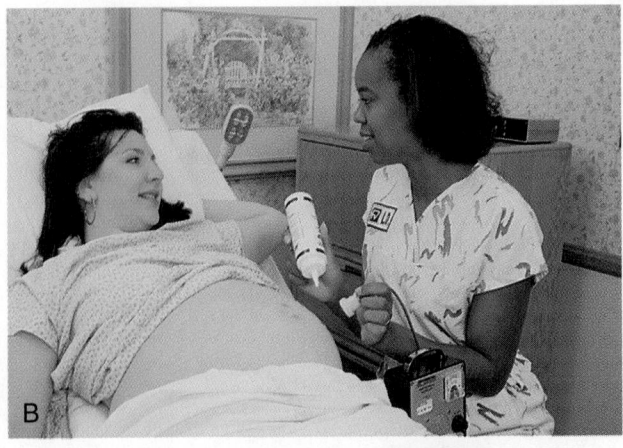

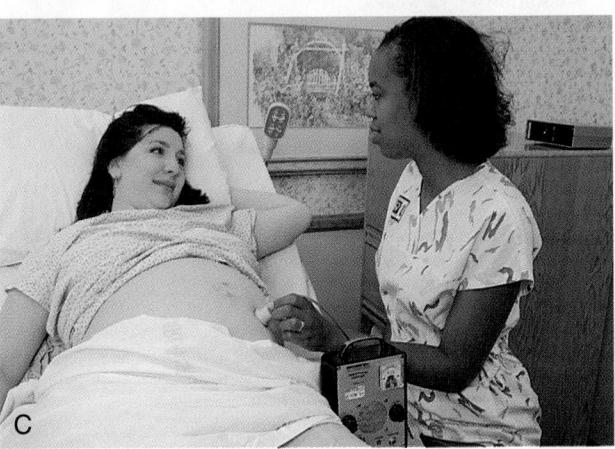

FIGURE 18-1

Low-intervention methods for evaluating the fetal heart rate during labor. *A,* Fetoscope, with head attachment to enhance conduction of faint fetal heart sounds. *B,* Transmission gel improves the clarity of the fetal heart movement sensed by the Doppler ultrasound transducer. *C,* The nurse moves the transducer until the fetal heart sounds are heard clearly. This location is usually over the fetus's back, which is most likely to be located in the woman's right or left lower abdomen.

Electronic Fetal Monitoring Equipment

Electronic fetal monitoring equipment consists of the bedside monitor unit and sensors for fetal heart rate and uterine activity. Sensors for each function may be either internal or external. Additional equipment may include data entry devices, remote units, and computer interfaces.

Bedside Monitor Unit

The bedside monitor unit receives information about the fetal heart rate and uterine activity from the sensors. It processes the information and provides output in the form of a numeric display and a printed strip. Most units can record rates for both fetuses in a twin pregnancy.

Paper Strip

Data about the fetal heart rate and uterine activity are printed on a paper strip having a horizontal grid for the fetal heart rate and another for the uterine activity (Fig. 18–2). Each segment of paper between perforations is numbered for identification and reassembly of a multipart strip. The fetal heart rate is recorded on the upper strip. The range of recorded rates is from 30 to 240 BPM.

Uterine activity is recorded on the lower grid as bell-shaped curves. Contraction intensity and uterine resting tone (from 0 to 100 mm Hg) are recorded on the lower grid.

Vertical lines on both upper and lower grids are time divisions. At a paper speed of 3 cm per minute, dark vertical lines are 1 minute apart. Lighter lines subdivide the 1-minute divisions into six 10-second segments. The vertical lines are used to time the frequency and duration of contractions and to identify the fetal response to the contractions.

Data Entry Devices

Monitors print some notations automatically, such as the date, time, paper speed, and devices being used to detect the fetal heart rate and uterine activity. Most also have data entry devices to enter and print data such as vital signs, vaginal examinations, or other information.

It is essential that times on all clocks in the birth unit, including those on fetal monitors and other machines and on wall clocks, be synchronized. In legal proceedings, the amount of time required to accomplish interventions can make the difference in the defense of a lawsuit.

Remote Surveillance

Many facilities have display units at the nursing station or other locations to allow surveillance when the nurse is not at the bedside. These units display the tracing on a screen

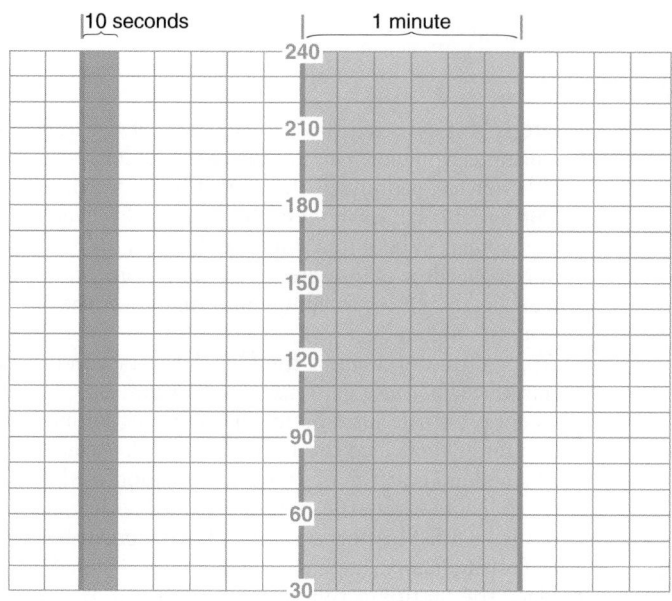

10 seconds

1 minute

Upper grid for recording fetal heart rate. Vertically scaled in beats per minute (BPM)

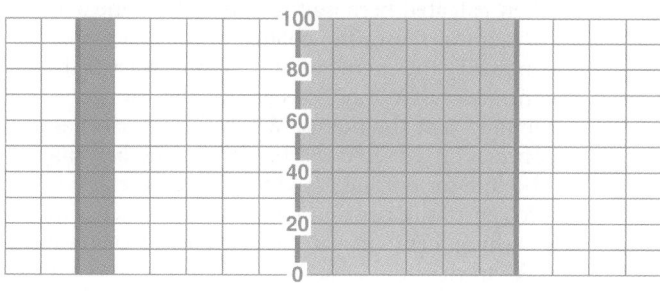

Lower grid for recording uterine activity. Vertically scaled in millimeters of mercury (mmHg)

FIGURE 18–2

Paper strip for recording electronic fetal monitoring data. Each dark vertical line represents 1 minute, and each lighter vertical line represents 10 seconds.

and have settings for alerts, such as range of the heart rate, decelerations, and end of the paper.

Computer Interface

Computers are used increasingly with electronic fetal monitoring to help nurses manage the large amount of data generated during birth. Computer systems can help alert the nurse to suspicious patterns and can store recordings. Systems are available that store all data electronically; a paper strip is not generated unless it is specifically requested.

Devices for External Fetal Monitoring

Both the fetal heart rate and uterine activity can be monitored by external sensors, or transducers. External devices are secured on the mother's abdomen by elastic straps, a tube of wide stockinette, or an adhesive ring (Fig. 18–3). External devices are somewhat less accurate than internal ones but are noninvasive; they do not require ruptured membranes or cervical dilation. Procedure 18–1 contains instructions for using the external electronic fetal monitor.

FETAL HEART RATE MONITORING WITH AN ULTRASOUND TRANSDUCER

A Doppler ultrasound transducer detects fetal heart movement for rate calculation. The transducer sends high-frequency sound waves into the uterus. The sound waves

are reflected, and the monitor's computer calculates the fetal heart rate based on the movement sensed.

Fetal heart motion does not always correlate with electrical heart activity. Other movements, such as fetal or maternal activity or blood flow through the umbilical cord and

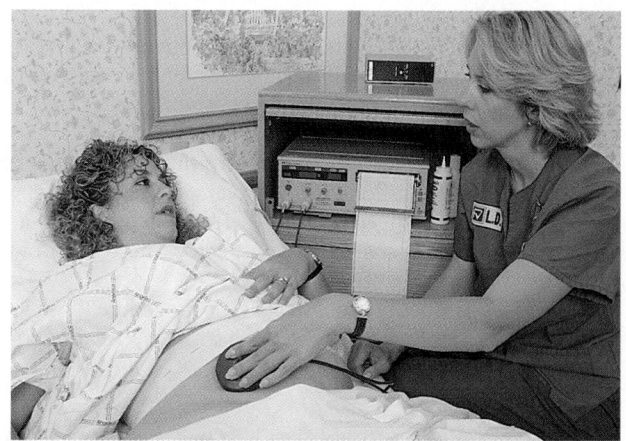

FIGURE 18–3

The nurse applies the uterine activity transducer to the woman's upper abdomen, in the fundal area. The Doppler transducer for sensing the fetal heart rate is usually placed on her lower abdomen when the fetus is in the cephalic presentation.

PROCEDURE 18–1

• • • • • • • • • • •

External Fetal Monitor

PURPOSE: To apply the electronic fetal monitor properly. To perform a basic evaluation of the fetal heart rate (FHR) and uterine activity patterns to identify data needing further assessment by the experienced nurse, physician, or nurse-midwife.

1. Read instruction manual for the equipment to become familiar with proper operation of the equipment and to be able to identify the equipment.

2. Perform a function test, following the manufacturer's instructions, to ensure that the bedside monitor unit is calibrated properly to give accurate data. Each manufacturer sets standards for indicators of proper function. Press the TEST button and observe for result. Common correct test results are
   a. Fetal heart rate: The monitor prints a line at 120, 150, or 200 BPM, depending on the model.
   b. Uterine activity: The monitor adds 50 to uterine activity display.

3. To decrease the woman's fear of the unknown, explain the basic procedure of electronic fetal monitoring to the woman and her partner or family. Teaching her that she can move with the monitor in place enhances her comfort and promotes normal labor. Vary instructions according to equipment used and hospital protocols. A sample is
   a. Using the electronic fetal monitor does not mean that you or the baby have a problem. It is the way we normally assess the baby's response to labor contractions.
   b. Two belts go around your abdomen, one for the fetal heart rate sensor and one for contractions.
   c. Feel free to move with the monitor on. If the tracing is poor, we can adjust the sensors.

4. Apply belts or stockinette if an adhesive ring is not used:
   a. Slide both belts under the woman's back without the sensors attached. To enhance comfort, be sure to keep the belts smooth under her back.
   b. Cut a length of stockinette tubing about 15 to 18 inches long for the average-sized woman. Cut a longer length of wide stockinette for a heavier woman. Slide the stockinette up from her feet to her abdomen.

5. Use Leopold's maneuvers (see Procedure 17–1) to locate the fetus's back because the fetal heart rate is best detected through the back of the fetus. During early labor, this is usually in the left or right lower quadrant of the woman's abdomen. During later labor, the fetal back is usually nearer the woman's abdominal midline. If the fetus is not engaged or is in a breech presentation, the fetal heart rate is probably found higher on the woman's abdomen.

6. Apply ultrasound gel to the Doppler ultrasound transducer because gel improves transmission and reception of the ultrasound waves to provide more accurate data. Place the transducer on the woman's abdomen at the approximate location of the fetus's back. Move the transducer until a clear signal is heard. Most bedside units have a green light or flashing heart shape to indicate a good signal.

7. Place the uterine activity sensor in the fundal area or the area where contractions feel the strongest when palpated because the external uterine activity monitor senses the change in the abdominal contour as the uterus rotates forward with each contraction. Contractions are usually strongest in the fundus of the uterus. When the woman has a contraction, observe the tracing for the bell shape. The line for uterine activity is jagged because it also senses the rise and fall of the abdomen with breathing. Fetal or maternal movement causes a spike in the line. Observe through several contractions to verify correct placement and identify needed position changes.

8. Observe the strip for baseline fetal heart rate, presence of long-term variability, periodic changes, and uterine activity (contraction duration and frequency). Palpate contractions for intensity and relaxation between contractions to identify reassuring and nonreassuring fetal heart rate patterns (see Table 18–2). Contractions having a frequency greater than every 2 minutes, duration longer than 90 seconds, or incomplete uterine relaxation between contractions may reduce maternal blood flow into the intervillous spaces and impair exchange of oxygen and waste products. The external uterine activity sensor is useful only for assessing contraction frequency and duration. It is not accurate for determining actual intensity or uterine resting tone.

9. Notify the physician or nurse-midwife of nonreassuring patterns.

the woman's aorta, can also be detected. Monitors today ignore most of these extraneous sounds to provide a clean tracing.

The Doppler transducer produces a two-part muffled sound resembling galloping horses. Fetal or maternal activity produces a rough, erratic sound rather than the crisp, rhythmic sound characteristic of the fetal heart.

UTERINE ACTIVITY MONITORING WITH A TOCOTRANSDUCER

A tocotransducer (also called a tocodynamometer, or simply a "toco") with a pressure-sensitive area detects changes in abdominal contour to measure uterine activity. The uterus pushes outward against the mother's anterior abdominal wall with each contraction. The monitor calculates changes in this signal and prints them as bell shapes on the lower grid of the strip.

Movement other than uterine activity also registers on the monitor. For example, maternal respirations cause the uterine activity line to have a zig-zag appearance. Other fetal or maternal movements appear as spikes on the uterine activity tracing.

Because uterine activity is sensed through the woman's abdomen, a tocotransducer is useful for observing the frequency and duration of contractions. It does not reliably measure actual contraction intensity and uterine resting tone. Several factors affect apparent intensity as printed on the strip:

- *Fetal size.* A small fetus prevents the uterus from pushing firmly against the abdominal wall with each contraction, making contractions appear less intense.
- *Abdominal fat thickness.* A thick layer of abdominal fat absorbs energy from uterine contractions, reducing the apparent intensity on the printed strip. On the other hand, the uterine activity recording of a thin woman whose uterus rotates sharply forward with each contraction may appear to be more intense than it actually is.
- *Maternal position.* Different maternal positions may increase or decrease the pressure against the transducer.
- *Location of the transducer.* Uterine activity is best de-

tected where it is strongest and where the fetus lies close to the uterine wall. This location is usually over the fundus. Uterine contractions may not be detectable if the transducer is located elsewhere.

Devices for Internal Fetal Monitoring

Accuracy is the main advantage of using internal devices for electronic fetal monitoring. However, their use requires ruptured membranes and about 2 cm of cervical dilation. The devices are invasive, and the risk of infection is slightly increased. As with external devices, the fetal heart rate is printed on the upper grid and the uterine activity is printed on the lower grid of the monitor paper.

FETAL HEART RATE MONITORING WITH A SCALP ELECTRODE

The fetal scalp electrode (or spiral electrode) detects electrical signals from the fetal heart (Fig. 18–4). Fetal or maternal movement does not interfere with accuracy because the rate is calculated from electrical events in the fetal heart. The monitor unit generates a beeping sound with each fetal heartbeat, but this sound can be silenced.

Although called a fetal scalp electrode, the device may be applied to the buttocks in a breech presentation. Areas

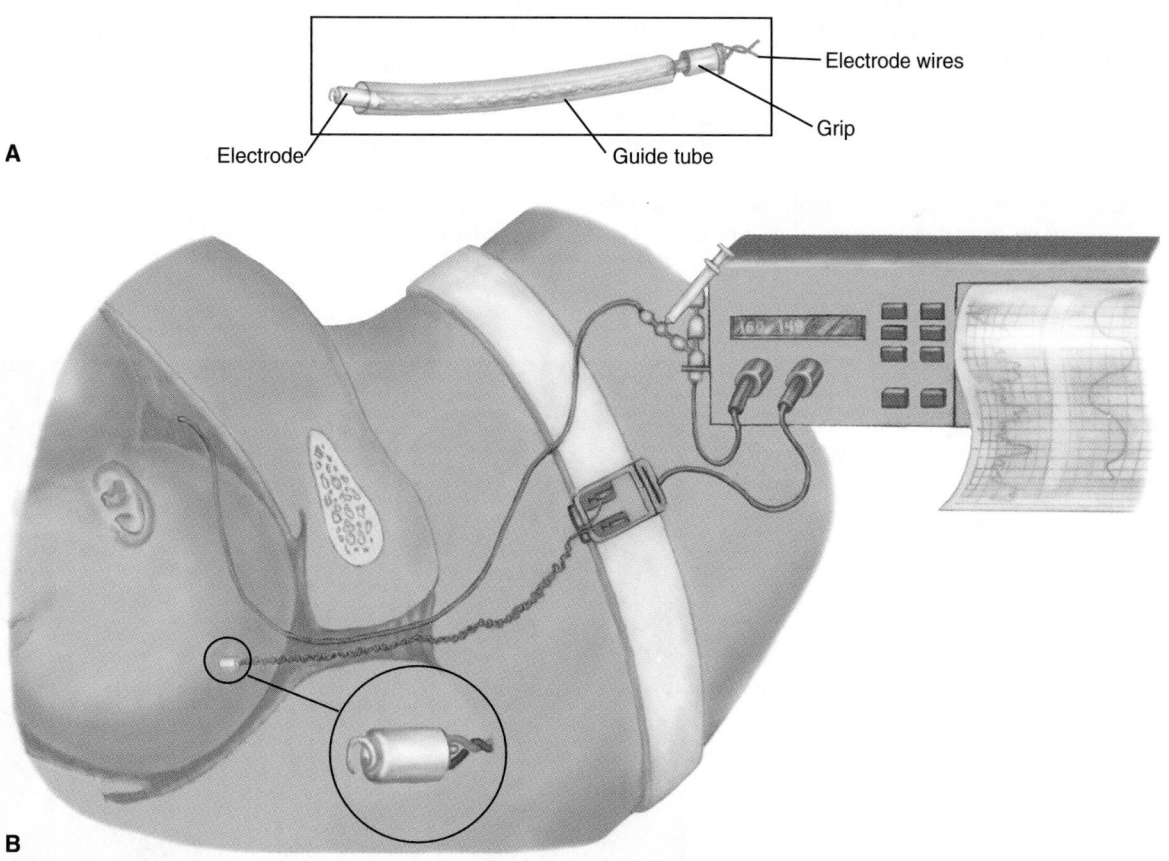

A Electrode   Guide tube   Electrode wires   Grip

B

FIGURE 18–4
• • • • • • • • •
Internal spiral electrode and intrauterine pressure catheter. *A,* Parts of the fetal scalp electrode before it is applied. *B,* Fetal scalp electrode and intrauterine pressure catheter in place and connected to the bedside monitor unit.

to avoid for electrode application are the fetal face, fontanels, and genitals. The wire from the electrode protrudes from the mother's vagina and is attached to a leg plate.

Because it barely penetrates the fetal skin (about 1 mm), the electrode is easily displaced. The tracing then becomes erratic or stops if the electrode is fully detached. Secure attachment of the electrode is often difficult if the fetus has thick hair. The electrode is removed by turning it counterclockwise about one and one-half turns until it detaches.

UTERINE ACTIVITY MONITORING WITH AN INTRAUTERINE PRESSURE CATHETER

Two kinds of intrauterine pressure catheters can be used to measure uterine activity, including contraction intensity and resting tone. These are

- A solid catheter with a pressure transducer in its tip (Fig. 18–5). This catheter may have an additional lumen for amnioinfusion.
- A hollow, fluid-filled catheter that connects to a pressure transducer on the bedside monitor unit.

Both types sense intrauterine pressure and increases in intra-abdominal pressure, such as with coughing or vomiting.

The solid catheter is not affected by height because its transducer is in the catheter. However, the sensor in its tip measures hydrostatic pressure from the amniotic fluid above the fetal presenting part as well as the pressure from uterine activity. Therefore, recorded intrauterine pressures from the solid catheter are higher than those from the fluid-filled catheter, and the nurse must consider this fact when assessing whether uterine activity is normal or hypertonic.

The tip of the fluid-filled catheter in the uterus should be at the level of the transducer on the outside for best accuracy. If the tip is lower than the transducer, the re-corded pressure is lower than the actual intrauterine pressure. If the tip is higher, the recorded pressure may be artificially high. Changes in the mother's position may alter the height of the catheter tip, requiring adjustment of the transducer's height.

▌ Evaluating Electronic Fetal Monitoring Strips

A consistent, organized approach to analyzing fetal monitor patterns ensures completeness. The nurse evaluates the fetal heart rate tracing for baseline rate, variability, and the presence of periodic changes. Uterine activity is evaluated by determining the frequency, duration, and intensity of contractions and by assessing uterine resting tone. Fetal heart rate and uterine activity patterns must be evaluated together.

Other data relevant to strip interpretation are maternal vital signs, maternal position, drug or oxygen administration, character of the amniotic fluid, labor status, and procedures performed. These are recorded on the strip as well as in the labor record.

Baseline Fetal Heart Rate

The baseline fetal heart rate is the most consistent heart rate when the uterus is at rest (Fig. 18–6). The baseline excludes periodic (temporary and recurrent) changes. It is composed of rate and variability. The baseline rate is classified as follows (Menihan, 1996; Murray, 1997):

- *Normal:* For the term fetus, a lower limit of 110 to 120 BPM and an upper limit of 150 to 160 BPM (some sources say that 120 BPM is the lower limit of normal)
- *Bradycardia:* Less than 110 to 120 BPM, persisting for at least 10 minutes

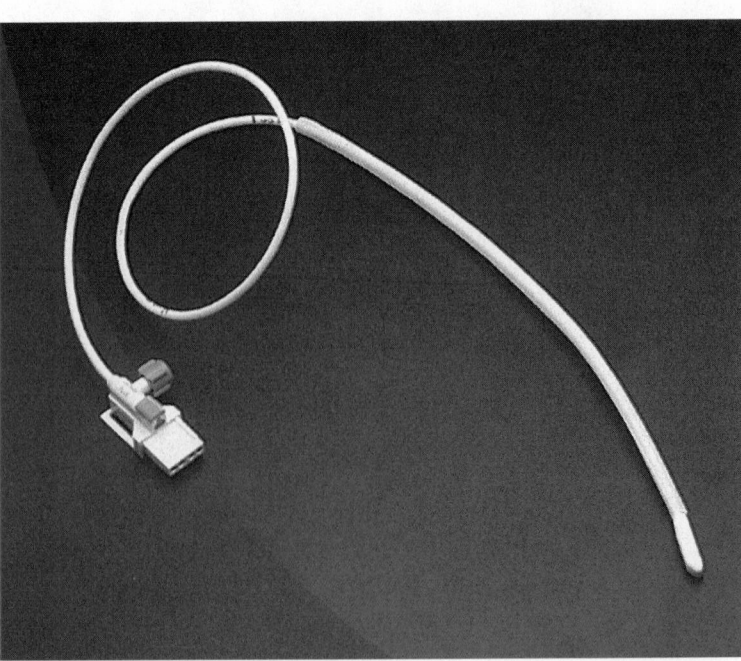

FIGURE 18–5
· · · · · · · · · ·
Solid intrauterine pressure catheter with transducer in its tip. This model also has a lumen for amnioinfusion and is shown with its introducer over the catheter. (Courtesy of Utah Medical Products, Midvale, UT.)

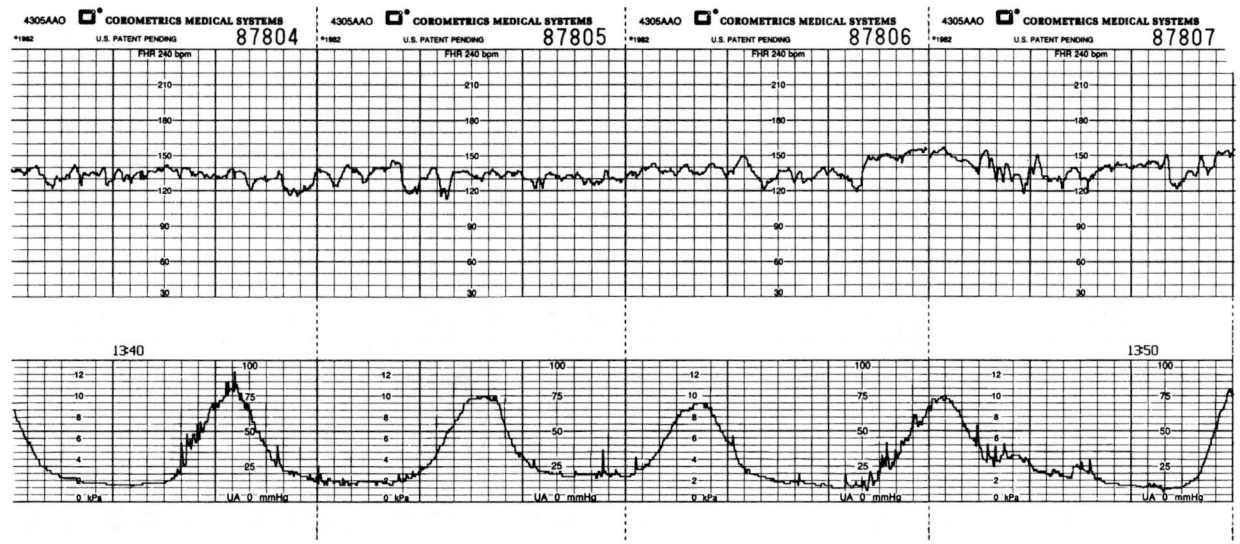

FIGURE 18-6

Electronic fetal monitor strip showing a reassuring pattern of fetal heart rate and uterine activity. The baseline fetal heart rate is 130 to 140 beats per minute (BPM), with a variability of about 10 BPM. There are no periodic changes in this strip. The contraction frequency is approximately every 2 to 3 minutes, duration is about 50 to 60 seconds, intensity is 75 to 90 mm Hg (measured with the internal spiral electrode), and uterine resting tone is approximately 10 mm Hg. (Courtesy of Corometrics Medical Systems, Inc., Wallingford, CT. Redrawn with permission.)

- *Tachycardia:* Greater than 150 to 160 BPM, persisting for at least 10 minutes

Some healthy term fetuses have bradycardia between 100 and 110 BPM with no other signs of compromise. A normal preterm fetus may have a baseline rate slightly higher than that of a term fetus (about 130 to 170 BPM) because the parasympathetic nervous system is immature.

Baseline Fetal Heart Rate Variability

Variability denotes the fluctuations in the baseline fetal heart rate that cause the printed line to have an irregular rather than a smooth appearance (Fig. 18–7). Two types of variability are evaluated together:

- Short-term variability: changes in the fetal heart rate from one beat to the next (beat-to-beat). This variability is most accurately assessed with an internal spiral electrode.
- Long-term variability: broader fluctuations that are apparent over 1-minute intervals. About three to six of these cycles occur each minute.

Both types of variability may be decreased by several nonpathologic and pathologic factors, such as the following:

- Narcotics or other sedative drugs given to the woman, including those given with epidural analgesia
- Fetal sleep (usually lasting 40 minutes or less, but sometimes as long as 80 to 90 minutes [Feinstein & McCartney, 1997])
- Tachycardia
- Prematurity

- Decreased oxygenation of the central nervous system
- Abnormalities of the central nervous system, heart, or both

Both kinds of variability occur because multiple factors constantly speed and slow the fetal heart in a push-and-pull manner. Evaluation of variability helps to clarify how a fetus is tolerating the stress of labor, including factors that cause hypoxia. Variability is a significant component of the fetal heart rate tracing on the electronic monitor, for two reasons:

- Adequate oxygenation promotes normal function of the autonomic nervous system and helps the fetus adapt to the stress of labor.
- Variability evaluates the function of the fetal autonomic nervous system, especially the parasympathetic branch.

No consensus exists on terms to describe variability. Some sources describe short-term and long-term variability separately, whereas others describe the two as a unit. The National Institute of Child Health and Human Development Research Planning Workshop (1997) recommended that no distinction be made between short-term and long-term variability because the two are evaluated visually as a unit. Some use two levels (absent or present), whereas others use as many as five.

Variability of 6 to 25 BPM is considered reassuring by most authorities. For short-term variability, this means that the beat-to-beat rate changes that occur over 1 minute of *baseline* fetal heart rate monitoring are at least 6 BPM but less than 25 BPM. For long-term variability, it means that there are three to six broad cycles of rate changes within the 6 to 25 BPM range.

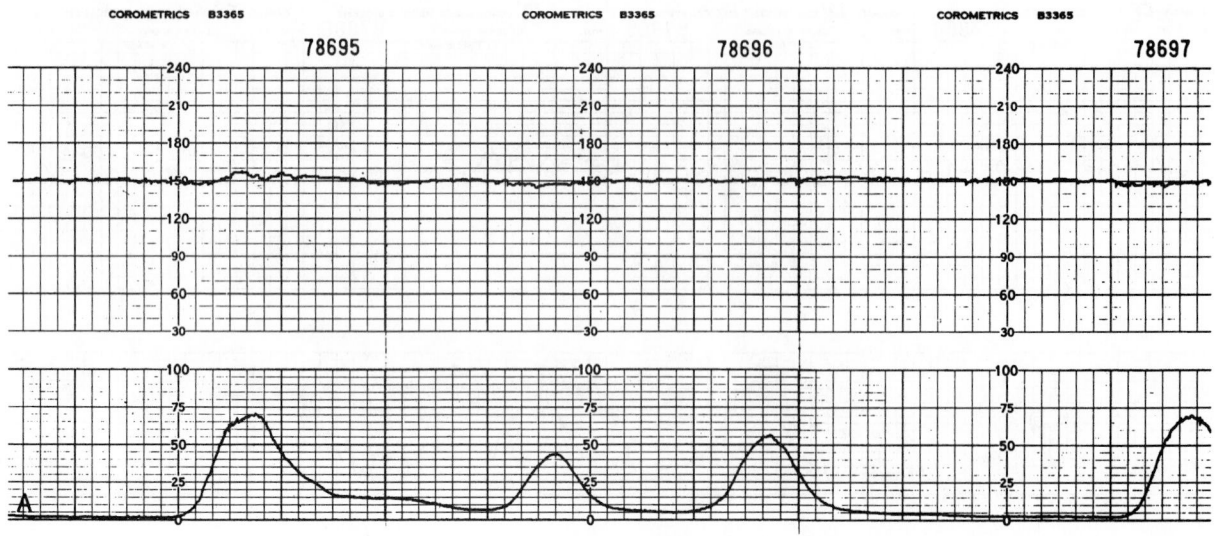

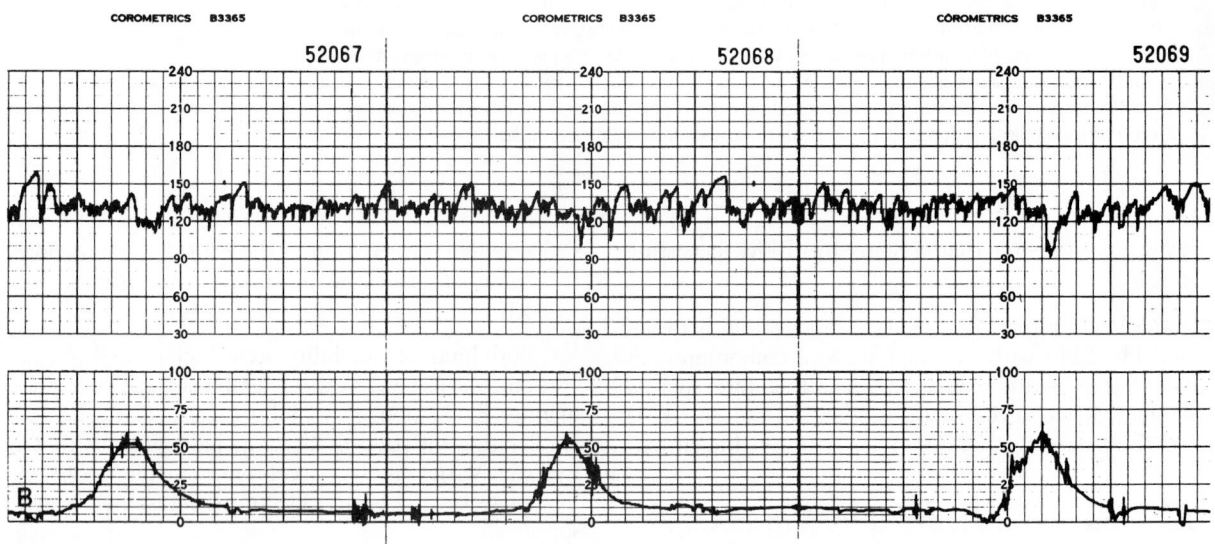

FIGURE 18-7

Contrasts in fetal heart rate variability. A fetal scalp electrode is being used. *A,* Minimal to absent variability (less than 3 BPM). Note the smooth, flat line in the fetal heart rate channel. *B,* Increased variability (about 20 BPM). Note the marked zig-zag appearance of the fetal heart rate line. (Courtesy of Corometrics Medical Systems, Inc., Wallingford, CT. Redrawn with permission.)

Periodic Patterns in the Fetal Heart Rate

Periodic patterns are transient, recurrent changes from the baseline rate that are associated with uterine contractions. They include accelerations and decelerations. Periodic patterns are evaluated with baseline characteristics (rate and variability).

ACCELERATIONS

An acceleration is a brief, temporary increase in the fetal heart rate of at least 15 beats above the baseline that lasts at least 15 seconds (Fig. 18-8). Accelerations may be nonperiodic (having no relation to contractions) or periodic. They may occur with fetal movement, vaginal examina-

tions, uterine contractions, mild cord compression, and when the fetus is in a breech presentation. Accelerations are usually a reassuring sign, reflecting a responsive, nonacidotic fetus.

Accelerations may be briefer and of less amplitude in the fetus younger than 32 weeks of gestation. Accelerations of at least 10 BPM for at least 10 seconds are acceptable for the fetus younger than 32 weeks.

DECELERATIONS

Periodic decelerations are classified into three types, based on their shape and relationship to uterine contractions.

Early Decelerations. Fetal head compression briefly increases intracranial pressure, causing the vagus nerve to slow the heart rate. Early decelerations are not associated

Differences Between Early and Late Decelerations

Early Decelerations

- Occur only during contractions as the fetal head is compressed.
- Return to the baseline fetal heart rate by the end of the contraction.
- Are mirror images of the contraction (fetal heart rate line goes down as contraction line goes up).
- Are not associated with fetal compromise and require no added interventions.

Late Decelerations

- Look similar to early decelerations but begin well after the contraction begins (often near the peak).
- Return to baseline after the contraction ends.
- Reflect impaired placental exchange or uteroplacental insufficiency.
- The degree of fall in rate from baseline is not related to the amount of uteroplacental insufficiency.
- Should be addressed by nursing interventions to improve placental blood flow and fetal oxygen supply.

set and returning to the baseline by the end of the contraction (Fig. 18–9). The rate at the lowest point of the deceleration usually remains above 100 BPM.

Late Decelerations. Deficient exchange of oxygen and waste products in the placenta (uteroplacental insufficiency) may result in a pattern of late (delayed) decelerations. This nonreassuring pattern suggests that the fetus has reduced reserve to tolerate the recurrent reductions in oxygen supply that normally occur with contractions. The cause of uteroplacental insufficiency may be acute, such as maternal hypotension. It may also occur with chronic conditions that impair placental exchange, such as maternal hypertension or diabetes.

Late decelerations look similar to early decelerations but are shifted to the right in relation to the contraction. They often begin after the peak of the contraction. The rate returns to baseline *after* the contraction ends (Fig. 18–10). They have a consistent appearance. The fetal heart rate may remain in the normal range and may not fall much below its baseline level. The amount of rate decrease from the baseline does not indicate how much uteroplacental insufficiency exists.

Variable Decelerations. Conditions that reduce flow through the umbilical cord may result in variable decelerations. These decelerations do not have the uniform appearance of early and late decelerations. Their shape, duration, and degree of fall below baseline rate are variable. They fall and rise abruptly with the onset and relief of cord compression, unlike the gradual fall and rise of early and late decelerations (Fig. 18–11). Variable decelerations also may be nonperiodic, occurring at times unrelated to contractions.

Uterine Activity

Assessment of uterine activity has four components: frequency, duration, and intensity of the contractions, and uterine resting tone.

with fetal compromise and require no intervention. They occur *during* contractions as the fetal head is pressed against the woman's pelvis or soft tissues, such as the cervix.

Early decelerations are consistent in appearance; they are uniform in that one early deceleration looks similar to others. They mirror the contraction, beginning near its on-

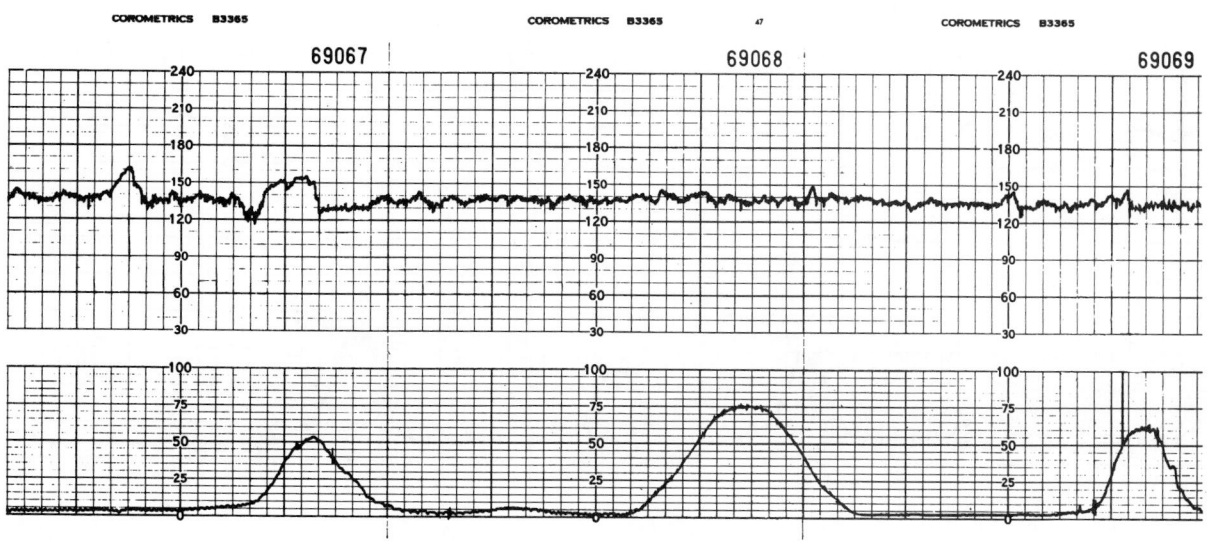

FIGURE 18–8
• • • • • • • • •

Accelerations in the fetal heart rate. (Courtesy of Corometrics Medical Systems, Inc., Wallingford, CT. Redrawn with permission.)

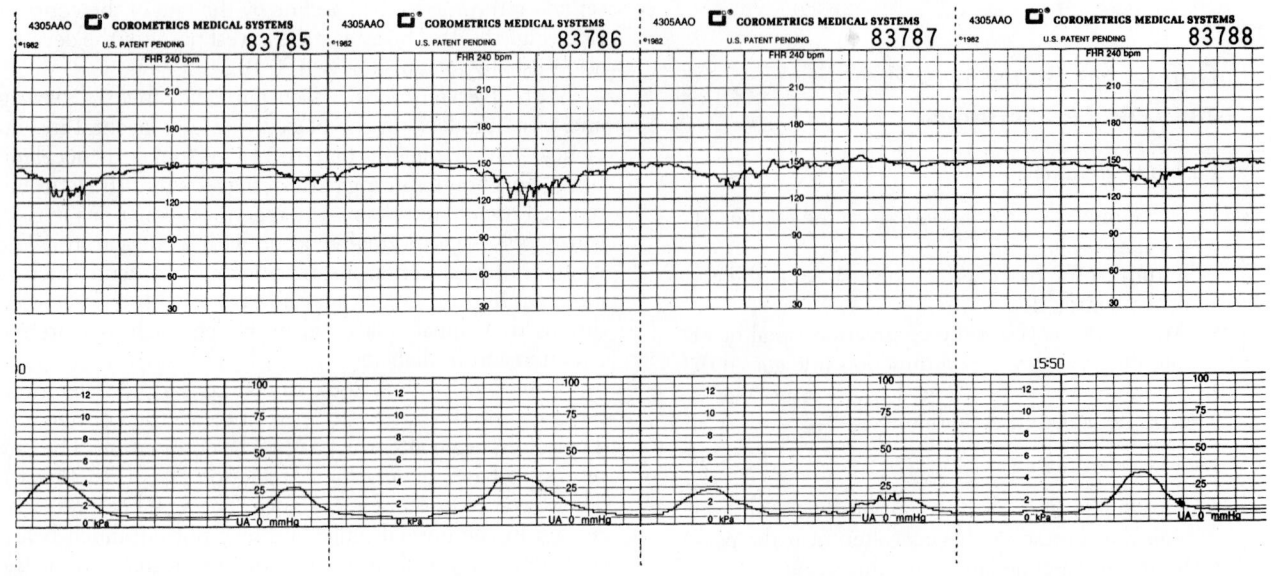

FIGURE 18–9

Early decelerations. Note that the slowing of the fetal heart rate mirrors the contraction. It begins near the beginning of the contraction and returns to the baseline by the end of the contraction. Cause: fetal head compression. (Courtesy of Corometrics Medical Systems, Inc., Wallingford, CT. Redrawn with permission.)

Palpation is used to estimate contraction intensity and uterine resting tone when an external uterine activity monitor is used (see Procedure 17–3). Contraction intensity is described as mild, moderate, or strong. The uterus should relax between contractions for at least 60 seconds.

With the intrauterine pressure catheter, the scale on the paper is used to describe intensity and resting tone. Intensity increases as labor progresses. Uterine contraction intensity with the intrauterine pressure catheter is about 50

to 75 mm Hg during labor, although it may reach 110 mm Hg with pushing during the second stage. Average resting tone is 5 to 15 mm Hg.

Significance of Fetal Heart Rate Patterns

Fetal heart rate patterns on the electronic monitor are classified as either "reassuring" or "nonreassuring." Between

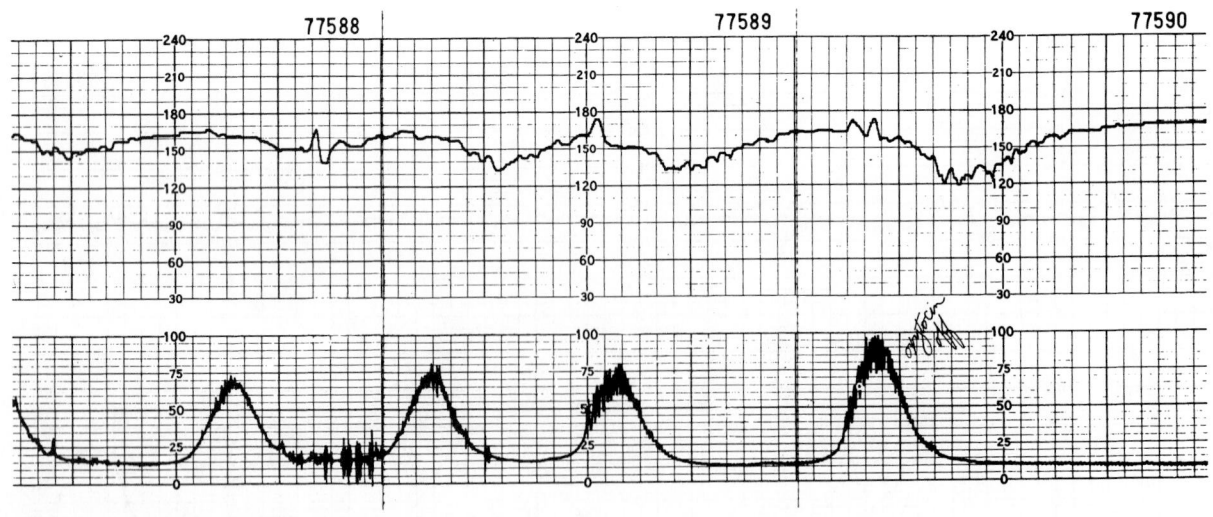

FIGURE 18–10

Late decelerations. Note that the decelerations look similar to early decelerations but are offset to the right. They begin at about the peak of the contraction and do not return to baseline until after the contraction ends. Cause: uteroplacental insufficiency. (Courtesy of Corometrics Medical Systems, Inc., Wallingford, CT. Redrawn with permission.)

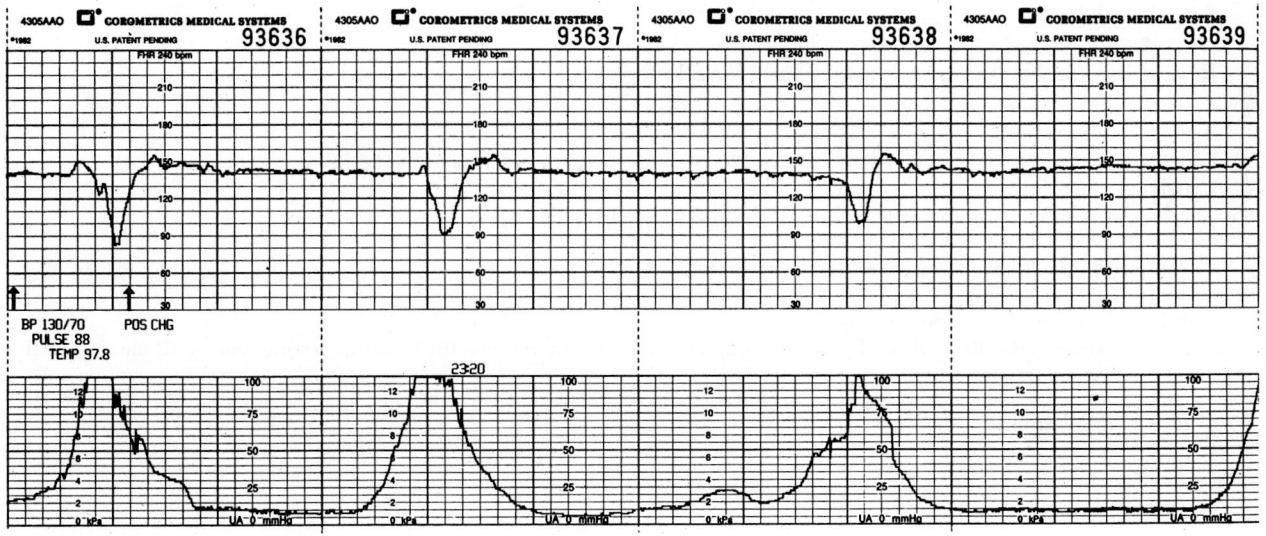

FIGURE 18-11

Variable decelerations. The decelerations are sharp in onset and offset. Note slight rate accelerations (shoulders) after each variable deceleration. Cause: umbilical cord compression. (Courtesy of Corometrics Medical Systems, Inc., Wallingford, CT. Redrawn with permission.)

these two classifications are patterns that are "equivocal"— neither clearly reassuring nor clearly nonreassuring. For equivocal (ambiguous) patterns, several methods may be used to further evaluate the fetal condition. Table 18–2 summarizes reassuring and nonreassuring patterns.

Reassuring Patterns

Reassuring patterns, such as accelerations with fetal movement, are associated with fetal well-being. No intervention is required because the pattern suggests that the fetus is tolerating intrapartum stressors.

Nonreassuring Patterns

Nonreassuring patterns occur if favorable signs are absent or if signs that are associated with fetal hypoxia or acidosis are present. Nonreassuring patterns do not necessarily indicate that fetal hypoxia or acidosis has occurred. Electronic fetal monitoring best identifies the well-oxygenated fetus; it less reliably identifies the compromised fetus. Thus, electronic fetal monitoring is a screening rather than a diagnostic tool.

Nonreassuring patterns are more significant if they occur together and are persistent. For example, bradycardia with short-term variability of less than 3 BPM and late decelerations suggests greater fetal stress than bradycardia with normal variability. The healthy fetus may demonstrate an occasional late deceleration, but a persistent pattern of late decelerations is more likely to represent compromise in a fetus. Nonreassuring patterns include but are not limited to the following:

- Tachycardia
- Bradycardia
- Decreased or absent variability
- Late decelerations
- Variable decelerations falling to less than 70 BPM for longer than 60 seconds
- Prolonged decelerations
- Hypertonic uterine activity

Nonreassuring patterns do not always indicate that labor should end immediately. Several interventions may be used to clarify the fetal condition and to determine the best course of action. Other interventions can increase fetal oxygenation.

CLARIFICATION OF DATA

Any of four methods may clarify data to better understand the fetal condition. Three methods are used during the intrapartum period: fetal scalp stimulation, vibroacoustic stimulation, and fetal scalp blood sampling. A fourth method, analysis of umbilical cord blood gases and pH, is used immediately after birth.

Fetal Scalp Stimulation. Scalp stimulation evaluates the fetus's response to tactile stimulation (Fig. 18–12). This procedure may be performed by the nurse, physician, or nurse-midwife. The examiner applies pressure to the scalp (or other presenting part) with a gloved finger or fingers and sweeps the fingers in a circular motion. An acceleration in the fetal heart rate of 15 BPM for at least 15 seconds is a reassuring response, suggesting a fetus in normal oxygen and acid-base balance. The acceleration may be delayed rather than immediate.

Fetal scalp stimulation is not done in some cases. These situations are essentially those in which vaginal examination would be restricted:

- Preterm fetus (may cause contractions)
- Prolonged rupture of membranes (higher risk of infection)

TABLE 18-2
. . . .

Reassuring and Nonreassuring Fetal Heart Rate Patterns

Reassuring Patterns

Baseline FHR: Stable, with a lower limit of 110–120 BPM and an upper limit of 150–160 BPM at term
Variability of 6–25 BPM
Accelerations with fetal movement: At least 15 BPM above the baseline for at least 15 sec
Uterine activity:
    Contraction frequency: no more frequent than every 2 min
    Contraction duration: no longer than 90 sec
    Interval between contractions: at least 60 sec
    Uterine resting tone: uterus relaxed between contractions (with external monitor); uterine resting tone < 20 mm Hg (with
        intrauterine pressure catheter)

Nonreassuring Patterns

Pattern and Description	Possible Cause
Tachycardia	

Baseline FHR > 160 BPM for at least 10 min
    Mild: 161–180 BPM
    Severe: >181 BPM
	Maternal fever (fetal tachycardia may be the first sign of an
	    intrauterine infection)
	Maternal dehydration
	Maternal or fetal hypoxia
	Fetal acidosis
	Maternal or fetal hypovolemia
	Fetal cardiac arrhythmias
	Maternal severe anemia
	Maternal hyperthyroidism
	Drugs administered to mother (such as terbutaline)

Bradycardia	

Baseline FHR < 110 BPM for at least 10 min
Baseline rates between 100 and 110 BPM are usually not
    associated with fetal compromise if there are no non-
    reassuring patterns
	Fetal head compression
	Fetal hypoxia
	Fetal acidosis
	Fetal heart block
	Umbilical cord compression
	Second-stage labor with maternal pushing

Decreased or Absent Variability	

FHR baseline has a smooth, flat appearance	Fetal sleep (usually lasts no longer than 40 min at a time)
	Fetal hypoxia with acidosis
	Drug effects:
	    CNS depressants
	    Local anesthetic agents

Late Decelerations	

Recurrent decelerations with a uniform appearance and a
    consistent relation to the contraction; begin after the
    contraction starts (usually at the peak) and do not return
    to baseline until after the contraction ends
	Uteroplacental insufficiency, which may be secondary to
	    Maternal hypotension
	    Excess uterine activity
	    Placental interruption, such as abruptio placentae or
	        placenta previa
	    Pregnancy-induced or chronic hypertension
	    Maternal diabetes
	    Maternal severe anemia
	    Maternal cardiac disease

Variable Decelerations	

Sharp in onset and offset
Appearance and relationship to contractions are not
    consistent; may occur as a nonperiodic pattern (randomly)
	Umbilical cord compression, which may be secondary to:
	    Prolapsed cord
	    Nuchal cord (around fetal neck)
	    Oligohydramnios (abnormally small amount of amniotic
	        fluid)
	    Cord between fetus and mother's uterus or pelvis, without
	        obvious prolapse
	    Cord between fetal body parts
	    Knot in cord

Abbreviations: BPM, beats per minute; FHR, fetal heart rate.

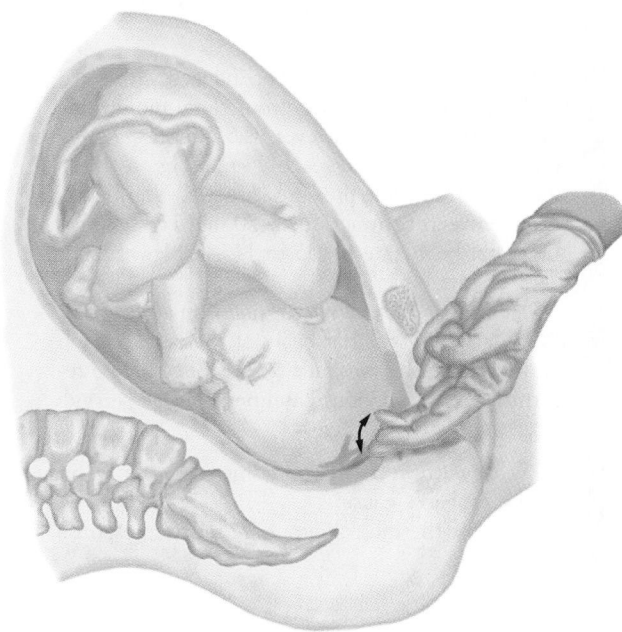

FIGURE 18–12

Fetal scalp stimulation helps identify whether the fetus responds to gentle massage. An acceleration in the fetal heart rate of 15 BPM for 15 seconds suggests that the fetus is in normal oxygen and acid-base balance.

- Chorioamnionitis (intrauterine infection)
- Placenta previa (may cause hemorrhage)
- Maternal fever of unknown origin (with the possibility of introducing microorganisms into the uterus)

Vibroacoustic Stimulation.   Acoustic, or vibroacoustic, stimulation may be used by the nurse, physician, or nurse-midwife to supplement fetal scalp stimulation or if scalp stimulation is contraindicated.

An artificial larynx is applied to the mother's lower abdomen, and it is turned on for up to 3 seconds. The reassuring response is the same as with fetal scalp stimulation: an acceleration in the fetal heart rate of 15 BPM for 15 seconds or more. An absent response, however, does not necessarily mean that the fetus is hypoxic or acidotic.

Fetal Scalp Blood Sampling.   Occasionally, the physician may obtain a sample of fetal scalp blood to evaluate the pH. This procedure is more complex than scalp stimulation or vibroacoustic stimulation. It requires rupture of membranes. Normal scalp pH is 7.25 to 7.35. Acidosis is present if the pH is less than 7.20, and the clinician may hasten the birth by using forceps or cesarean delivery. The scalp sample may be repeated for a borderline pH of 7.20 to 7.24.

Cord Blood Gases and pH.   Umbilical cord blood analysis is used to assess the infant's status immediately after birth for oxygenation and acid-base balance. The samples are analyzed for pH, P_{CO_2}, P_{O_2}, and bicarbonate and for base deficit. This information helps identify whether acidosis exists and whether it is respiratory (short-term), metabolic (prolonged), or mixed. Normal cord blood gases and pH can confirm that the fetus was adjusting normally to the stresses of labor, although the fetal monitoring pattern may have been nonreassuring.

The cord is promptly double clamped (within 20 to 30 seconds of birth) and cut to isolate a 10- to 20-cm (4- to 8-inch) segment. Blood samples from an umbilical artery provide the most accurate information about the newborn's acid-base status because this blood is that which left the fetus for the placenta. Blood is drawn into heparinized syringes to prevent coagulation, and the syringes are capped to avoid altering values by exposure to room air (Fig. 18–13). Samples kept at room temperature are reliable for 30 to 60 minutes (ACOG, 1995b). Samples should be kept in ice if there is a delay beyond this time.

INTERVENTIONS FOR NONREASSURING PATTERNS

Any of several nursing or medical interventions, or both, may be indicated if a nonreassuring fetal heart rate pattern is present. All are directed toward identifying the cause of the nonreassuring pattern and improving fetal oxygenation.

Identifying the Cause of a Nonreassuring Pattern.   Careful examination of the strip may suggest a cause for the nonreassuring fetal heart rate pattern and direct the most appropriate interventions. For example, a pattern of late decelerations suggests uteroplacental insufficiency. Uteroplacental insufficiency however, may be secondary to a variety of causes, such as maternal hypotension and excessive uterine activity. Different causes require different corrective interventions. Checking the mother's vital signs may disclose hypotension, hypertension, and fever. Maternal medications such as narcotics may alter variability.

A vaginal examination may reveal a prolapsed cord, which may cause variable decelerations, bradycardia, or both as it is compressed. A vaginal examination also evaluates the woman's labor status, which helps the birth attendant decide if labor should continue or be ended with a cesarean birth.

Internal monitoring is needed for greater accuracy if a nonreassuring pattern develops when external devices are

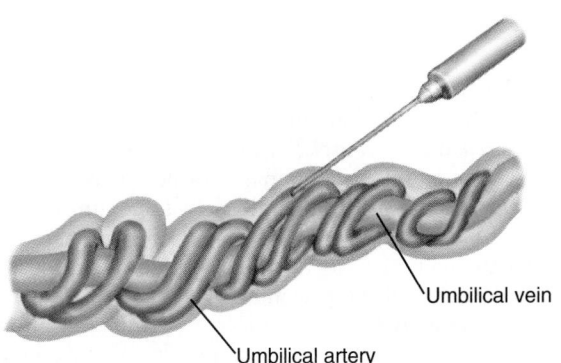

FIGURE 18–13

Obtaining a blood sample to determine umbilical cord blood gas values and pH. Samples are drawn from the umbilical artery, vein, or both. The samples in capped syringes may be kept for up to 60 minutes at room temperature and 3 hours on ice.

CRITICAL TO REMEMBER

Nursing Responses to Nonreassuring Fetal Heart Rate Patterns

1. Identify the cause of the nonreassuring pattern to plan the best interventions:
   • Evaluate the pattern for probable cause (late or variable decelerations, bradycardia or tachycardia, absent variability).
   • Evaluate maternal vital signs to identify hypotension, hypertension, or fever.
   • If not contraindicated, perform vaginal examination to identify a prolapsed umbilical cord.
2. Stop oxytocin infusion if the drug is being administered.
3. Reposition the woman, avoiding the supine position, for patterns associated with cord compression. Repositioning may improve other nonreassuring patterns as well.
4. Increase the rate of infusion of a nonadditive intravenous fluid to expand the mother's blood volume and improve placental perfusion.
5. Administer oxygen by face mask at 8 to 10 L/min to increase her blood oxygen saturation, making more oxygen available to the fetus.
6. Initiate continuous electronic fetal monitoring with internal devices if no contraindication exists.
7. Notify the physician or nurse-midwife as soon as possible. Report and document the following:
   • The pattern that was identified.
   • Nursing interventions taken in response to the pattern.
   • The fetal response after nursing interventions.
   • The response of the physician or nurse-midwife (orders, other response).
8. If the nonreassuring pattern is severe, other staff members should begin preparing for immediate delivery (usually cesarean birth, unless a vaginal birth is imminent).

used. The fetal scalp electrode gives a true picture of variability, which is a strong indicator of fetal condition.

Increasing Placental Perfusion. The woman is positioned on her side to eliminate aortocaval compression, which can reduce placental blood flow. Increasing nonadditive intravenous fluids such as lactated Ringer's solution increases the maternal blood volume, which in turn leads to better perfusion of the placenta.

Uterine activity reduces blood flow into the intervillous spaces, and a fetus with little reserve for stress may be unable to tolerate even normal contractions. Persistent hypertonic uterine activity may compromise a fetus with normal reserves. If a woman is receiving oxytocin, it is discontinued so that uterine activity is not stimulated. A tocolytic drug such as terbutaline (0.125 to 0.25 mg intravenously or 0.25 mg subcutaneously) may be given to reduce uterine activity.

CRITICAL THINKING EXERCISE 18–1

Nancy Joe is having her labor induced with oxytocin and is having internal electronic fetal monitoring. Her contractions occur every 2.5 minutes, are 90 seconds in duration, and reach 75 mm Hg on the scale for the intrauterine pressure catheter. Uterine resting tone between contractions is 20 mm Hg. The baseline fetal heart rate is 135 to 145 BPM with about 7 BPM variability.

Her nurse, Jackie Brown, notes a pattern of uniform decelerations that begin at the peak of each contraction. The rate falls to 125 BPM before returning to the previous baseline about 30 seconds after the contraction ends.

1. What pattern do these findings describe? What is the probable cause?
2. What is the most appropriate nursing response? Why?

Increasing Maternal Blood Oxygen Saturation. Administration of 100% oxygen through a snug face mask makes more oxygen available for transfer to the fetus. A commonly suggested rate is 8 to 10 L/min.

Reducing Cord Compression. If cord compression is suspected, the woman is repositioned. She may be turned from side to side, or her hips may be elevated to shift the fetal presenting part toward her diaphragm. Several position changes may be required before the pattern improves or resolves. The fetal presenting part may be pushed upward slightly.

Amnioinfusion increases the fluid around the fetus and cushions the cord. Lactated Ringer's solution or normal saline is infused into the uterus through an intrauterine pressure catheter. The underpads must be changed regularly because fluid leaks out constantly. Possible complications include overdistension of the uterus and increased uterine resting tone. These complications are relieved by releasing some of the fluid. Amnioinfusion also may be used to wash out and dilute fluid that is stained heavily with meconium so that the infant does not aspirate it at birth.

NURSING CARE

The Woman Having Electronic Fetal Monitoring

The nurse may identify any of several problems if a woman has electronic fetal monitoring. The woman or couple who prefer a nontechnical environment for birth may encounter a decision conflict if electronic fetal monitoring is recommended. Anxiety is likely if the woman does not understand the electronic monitor or if complications develop. Pain may be increased if mobility is restricted during labor.

Two nursing care needs related to intrapartum fetal monitoring are the woman's (or couple's) learning needs and an expansion of nursing care related to fetal oxygenation. Care related to fetal monitoring by either electronic means or auscultation should be combined with that for normal or complicated intrapartum nursing as needed.

CRITICAL THINKING EXERCISE 18-2

LaShonda Blair is in active labor and is having external electronic fetal monitoring for fetal assessment. LaShonda has not had medication, and her labor has been normal so far. Her membranes ruptured about 1 hour ago, and the amniotic fluid was clear. Contractions occur every 3 minutes, are 60 seconds in duration, and are moderately intense. Her uterus fully relaxes between each contraction.

The nursing student who is supporting LaShonda notes abrupt slowing of the fetal heart rate to 90 BPM during the next two contractions, each time lasting about 30 seconds.

Are any nursing actions needed? Why? If nursing actions are needed, what are they? In what order should they be done?

LEARNING NEEDS

Assessment

Determine what the woman and her partner already know about the electronic fetal monitor (Fig. 18–14). If the woman is not familiar with electronic fetal monitoring, assess her perception of it. For example, does she believe that use of the monitor indicates the development of a complication, or does she expect its use? Is the woman comfortable with intermittent auscultation for fetal assessment?

Lack of knowledge contributes to anxiety. Note the anxiety level of the woman and her partner when the monitor is used. For example, is the woman afraid to move because the fetal heart sounds and tracing skip at that time? Does she place the monitor's data above her own comfort? Note questions about the monitor and its data. Reassess after teaching to identify information that is still unclear or causing anxiety.

NURSING CARE PLAN 18-1

Intrapartum Fetal Compromise

Assessment	Glenda Brown is a 30-year-old African-American woman who is accompanied by her husband Paul. She is a gravida 4, para 1, who has had two spontaneous abortions. Glenda has been an insulin-dependent diabetic for 15 years. Her labor is being induced with oxytocin (Pitocin) at 39 weeks' gestation because she had a blood pressure elevation at today's antepartum care appointment. Her blood pressure was 146/94 mm Hg on admission, and repeat assessments have shown little change. Glenda will have electronic fetal monitoring during labor.
Nursing Diagnosis	Knowledge Deficit: Electronic fetal monitoring.
Goals/Expected Outcomes	• Glenda and Paul will state that they understand the reason for electronic monitoring, related equipment and procedures, and the data that are expected.

Intervention

1. Evaluate the parents' present knowledge about electronic fetal monitoring.

2. Provide information about the monitor to Glenda and Paul.

   a. *Purposes:* To provide an audible and written record of the fetal response to labor and to guide caregivers in appropriate interventions if nonreassuring patterns are identified.

   b. *Safety:* The monitoring sensors are electrically isolated from the wall current. The fetal scalp electrode (if used) penetrates the outer layer of skin to about a dime's thickness. The intrauterine pressure catheter lies between the baby and the wall of the uterus.

   c. *Misleading data:* Encourage Glenda to call for assistance if she cannot hear the fetal heartbeat or if she notices that her contractions do not seem to be evident on the strip.

Rationale

1. This evaluation allows the nurse to build on existing accurate knowledge and to correct misunderstandings.

2. Reassure Glenda and Paul that use of the electronic fetal monitor does not mean that something is wrong with Glenda or the baby.

   a. Information tells the parents how the monitor is used.

   b. Information alleviates safety concerns that parents often have.

   c. Sensors, especially external devices, can easily be displaced and stop picking up data. Preparing Glenda and Paul for this possibility reduces their fears if they should stop hearing the fetal heartbeat.

(continued)

Intrapartum Fetal Compromise

d. Encourage Glenda to move about freely. Tell her that a nurse will readjust her monitor if it stops recording properly. Explain that she should urinate about every 2 hours and that the nurse can help her roll the monitor to the bathroom door or temporarily disconnect the sensor.

d. Maternal movement and regular urination enhance normal labor processes. A woman is likely to become anxious and uncomfortable if she concentrates more on maintaining data from the monitor than on coping with labor.

Evaluation

Glenda and Paul say that they expected electronic fetal monitoring during labor. Glenda is familiar with the external monitor because it was used for the biophysical profile. She agrees to have internal monitoring if needed, saying that she understands that greater accuracy is important because of her higher risk status.

Assessment

The nurse applies the external fetal monitor because Glenda's membranes are intact. She is having irregular spontaneous contractions. The fetal heart rate baseline averages 125 to 135 BPM and accelerates when the fetus moves. The nurse begins an oxytocin infusion to induce labor. Glenda's blood pressure is 154/94.

Potential Complication

Fetal compromise.

Goals/Expected Outcomes

Client goals for the fetus are inappropriate because nurses cannot independently manage fetal compromise. Planning for Glenda should reflect the need to

- Compare fetal heart rate and uterine activity data with baseline levels before oxytocin induction.
- Promote normal fetal oxygenation.
- Take corrective actions for nonreassuring patterns.
- Notify Glenda's physician if nonreassuring patterns develop.

Intervention

1. Identify relevant risk factors for fetal compromise.

2. Encourage Glenda to assume any comfortable position other than the supine position.

3. Evaluate the tracing at the following times, signing or initialing the strip each time. Summarize the evaluation on the labor record.
   a. Every 15 minutes during the first stage and every 5 minutes during the second stage.

   b. Before and after procedures such as amniotomy, medications, and epidural anesthesia induction.
   c. With changes of activity, such as urination and repositioning.

4. Use a four-step approach to evaluate the strip:

   a. Baseline fetal heart rate

   b. Variability (with scalp electrode)

   c. Periodic changes: Accelerations, decelerations. Note relationship of periodic changes to fetal movement, contractions, and the woman's status and activity. Note nonperiodic (random) accelerations or variable decelerations.

Rationale

1. Women who have risk factors that could reduce fetal oxygenation should have fetal assessments done more frequently.

2. Compression of the aorta reduces blood return to the heart and reduces cardiac output and placental perfusion.

3. Documentation creates a record that assessment was done. Documenting on both strip and the labor record allows each to stand alone.
   a. Regular documentation provides a framework for regular assessment of the fetal response to labor in the high-risk pregnancy.

   b. These procedures may alter fetal heart rate patterns.
   c. Changes in activity or position could alter the uterine or umbilical cord blood flow. External sensors may need adjustment.

4. The four-step approach provides a systematic framework to evaluate the fetal response to labor.
   a. Tachycardia may be an early response to hypoxia. Bradycardia may occur in response to vagal stimulation or prolonged hypoxia.
   b. Normal variability (6 to 25 BPM) suggests that the fetus is well oxygenated and not in acidosis.

   c. Accelerations are a reassuring sign. Early decelerations are a normal response to head compression. Late (uteroplacental insufficiency) and variable (umbilical cord compression) decelerations are nonreassuring.

Intrapartum Fetal Compromise

d. Uterine activity: Evaluate frequency and duration using either external or internal devices. Estimate their intensity with an external device by palpating three or more contractions. Note whether the uterus relaxes between contractions for at least 60 seconds. If an intrauterine pressure catheter is used, read the contraction intensity and uterine resting tone from a scale on the strip.

5. If nonreassuring patterns develop, take appropriate corrective actions such as discontinuing the oxytocin, increasing the rate of the nonadditive intravenous solution, positioning Glenda on her side, and administering oxygen. Notify the birth attendant of nonreassuring patterns, corrective actions taken, and the fetal response. Document the birth attendant's response and any orders.

d. Contractions that are too long (more than 90 seconds in duration) or too frequent (closer than every 2 minutes), a resting interval of less than 60 seconds, or intrauterine resting pressure of more than 20 mm Hg can reduce placental exchange.

5. The first priority is to identify the cause of the nonreassuring pattern and increase fetal oxygenation. The physician should be notified to remain current with the maternal-fetal status for needed medical orders or interventions.

Evaluation

Goals are not established for collaborative problems. The nurse should have compared data from the fetal monitor and other nursing evaluations with the baseline data before Glenda started having oxytocin or contractions.

For the first 4 hours of the oxytocin induction, the fetal heart rate continued near its baseline of 125 to 135 BPM, with variability averaging 10 BPM. Fetal heart rate accelerations with fetal movement continued. No nonreassuring patterns were noted.

Assessment

The physician ruptures Glenda's membranes and inserts internal devices for assessing the fetal heart rate and uterine activity. Glenda's blood pressure remains near 145/90, and her oxytocin infusion continues. A pattern of repeated late decelerations with baseline variability of 3 BPM develops 1 hour after the membranes are ruptured. The nurse stops the oxytocin infusion and increases the rate of nonadditive intravenous fluid, positions Glenda on her left side, and administers oxygen at 10 L/min with a snug face mask. The physician is notified. Glenda is holding Paul's hand tightly and breathing rapidly. Her vital signs are now blood pressure, 145/90; pulse, 90; and respirations, 32. Uterine activity is normal.

Nursing Diagnosis

Anxiety related to unexpected development of complications.

Goals/Expected Outcomes

- Glenda will have a reduced respiratory rate (14 to 22 breaths per minute) after interventions.
- Glenda will have a more relaxed face and body posture after interventions.

Intervention

1. Maintain calm behavior while performing corrective actions and notifying the physician.

2. Use simple, concise language for all explanations.

3. Explain the following to Glenda and Paul:
   a. The problem that was identified
   b. The usual cause of the problem
   c. Reasons for corrective actions
   d. Expected results
   e. That Glenda can talk with the oxygen mask on
4. Inform Glenda and Paul if the pattern improves or resolves.

Rationale

1. Calm behavior communicates to Glenda and Paul that mother and fetus are receiving competent care. Anxious behavior on the part of caregivers will increase the parents' anxiety.
2. High anxiety or intense physical sensations impair one's ability to comprehend explanations.
3. If Glenda and Paul understand what is happening and why the corrective actions are taken, they are more likely to comply with the care. Knowledge decreases fear of the unknown. Assuring Glenda that she can talk with the oxygen mask on allows her to ask questions and ventilate feelings to reduce anxiety and fear.
4. Knowledge that the nonreassuring pattern has improved or resolved reassures parents about the fetus's condition.

Evaluation

Over the next hour, the fetal heart rate pattern gradually improves. Glenda gradually relaxes her grip on Paul's hand and her body relaxes. Her respiratory rate slows to 22 breaths per minute.

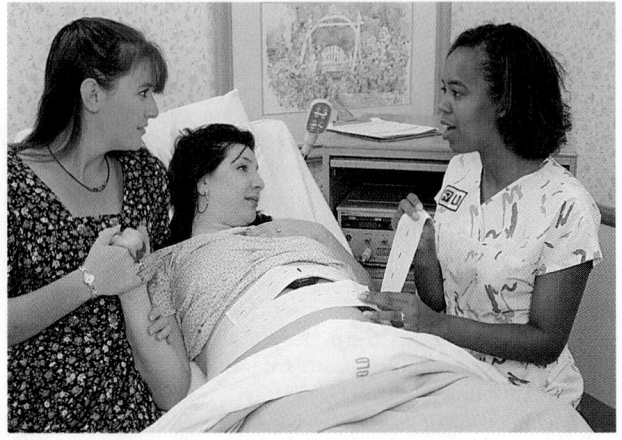

FIGURE 18–14
. . . .
The nurse teaches the woman and her partner about electronic fetal monitoring to limit the woman's anxiety and promote her comfort during labor. Electronic fetal monitoring is only one method used to evaluate fetal well-being during labor.

Nursing Diagnosis and Planning

Many women expect to have continuous electronic fetal monitoring during labor, and they have often been introduced to it during prepared childbirth classes. Most women have additional questions, however, and some women know little about this mode of fetal surveillance. The nursing diagnosis selected is

■ Knowledge Deficit: fetal monitoring.
   Expected Outcome: After being taught about the fetal monitor, the woman and her partner will express understanding of the equipment, procedures, and expected data.

Interventions

Explaining the Electronic Fetal Monitor

Teaching is continuous as circumstances change. Explain the purposes of the monitor and the equipment to be used. A simple explanation entails telling the parents that the monitor is a tool to assess how the fetus reacts to labor, especially during contractions. If true, assure the woman that its use does not mean that something is wrong with her baby. Explain why changes in the monitoring mode (external to internal) are done. It may be helpful to explain

---

PARENTS WANT TO KNOW
• • • • • • • • • • •
About Electronic Fetal Monitoring

When women have electronic fetal monitoring during labor, they often have questions that the nurse may answer. Here are some commonly asked questions and answers the nurse might use.

Can I move around with the monitor?
You can move freely with the monitor. If you notice that the machine isn't picking up the fetal heart sounds or contractions as well, call me and I'll readjust it. Make yourself comfortable; then we'll adjust the machine if necessary.

What if I need to go to the bathroom?
If you need to go to the bathroom, we'll unplug the cords from the machine and you can walk in there, or we can roll the monitor to the door of the bathroom.

Will the monitor shock me? I don't know if I want to be hooked to an electrical outlet, especially since my water has broken.
The part of the monitor that is attached to you and your baby only transmits information into the machine for processing. The sensors on your body are isolated from electrical parts in the monitor.

Why is the baby's heart beating so fast?
A baby's heart normally beats faster than an adult's, both before and after birth. The normal rate is about 110 to 160 beats per minute. A higher or lower rate does not necessarily mean that the baby has a problem, but we do look at the monitor strip closely to see how the baby is doing.

Why do those numbers for the baby's heart rate change so much?
The heart rate of a healthy baby who is awake changes constantly. When the baby moves, the heart often speeds up, just as yours does.

What do those numbers for contractions (external monitor) mean? They change all the time.
The numbers reflect a change in the pressure that the monitor senses. The monitor senses many changes in pressure other than those from contractions, such as changes from breathing, coughing, or movement of you or the baby.

My contractions don't look very strong, but they sure seem strong to me! (External uterine activity monitor is being used.)
The external monitor senses contractions indirectly, rather than sensing the actual pressure within the uterus. Their appearance on the tracing varies because of many factors, such as your position, the position of the sensor on your abdomen, and the thickness of your abdominal wall.

Will the internal monitor hurt my baby?
The spiral electrode attaches only to the outer layer of skin on the baby's head. We are careful to avoid sensitive areas on the head, such as the fontanels (soft spots) or the face. The uterine catheter slides up beside the baby.

that the physician or nurse-midwife evaluates many factors during labor and that the monitor strip is only one of those factors.

Addressing Parents' Safety Concerns

Explain how the equipment functions. Some women are afraid of being attached to an electrical device, especially because cords and electrodes are wet with amniotic fluid and vaginal secretions. Reassure the woman that the connections to her and those to the wall current are isolated from each other.

Parents may be concerned about attachment of the scalp electrode to the fetal presenting part. Show them that the electrode is a very fine wire that penetrates the outer layer of skin only (about 1 mm, or the thickness of a dime). If she is concerned about the intrauterine pressure catheter, tell her that it lies beside the fetus, next to the inner wall of the uterus.

Coping with Misleading Data

Teach the woman that the monitor sometimes gives data that suggest a problem when no problem exists. For example, the fetal heart rate may suddenly fall to zero and the audible tone stop if the sensor (external or scalp electrode) is displaced. Tell her to call the nurse for adjustment or replacement of the sensor.

The woman may be discouraged because the curves representing contractions do not look as strong on the strip as they feel to her. This situation is more likely if an external transducer is used. Explain the many factors that may cause the contraction curves to appear stronger or weaker than they really are. When an external tocotransducer is used, tell her that the strip is used mainly to assess the timing of contractions and the fetus's reaction. Explain that an intrauterine pressure catheter may be recommended if knowledge of intrauterine pressure is crucial.

Reassure the woman that her perception of her contractions and discomfort is important. Value the woman-generated data as well as the machine-generated data. Palpate contractions at intervals as well as evaluating their appearance on the monitor strip.

It is natural for the nurse's attention to be drawn to the electronic fetal monitor when entering the room. Stay focused on the woman and her family rather than devoting excessive attention to the monitoring equipment. The woman is having the baby, not the monitor.

Including the Labor Partner

Tell the partner how to identify the onset and peak of contractions. During active labor, some women discover that contractions become intense before they can prepare for them. If this is the case, have the coach tell the woman when each contraction begins. The coach also can tell her when the peak has passed to encourage her.

Enhancing Comfort

Some women feel tied to the electronic fetal monitor and are reluctant to make themselves more comfortable. Nursing care involves finding ways to make the mother comfortable and the monitor as nonintrusive as possible. Teach her ways to improve comfort while still obtaining an adequate tracing.

Explain that staying in one position is uncomfortable and does not promote normal labor. The woman may assume any position other than supine unless a specific position is needed. Encourage her to find the position in which she is most comfortable; then adjust the external devices to best detect contractions and the fetal heartbeat. Internal devices may be an option if external devices cannot be adjusted to provide useful data.

If the woman finds the sound produced by the electronic fetal monitor distracting or inconsistent with the atmosphere she desires, turn the sound off. Remember that the auditory cues for rate accelerations and decelerations are absent.

If no other contraindications to walking exist, the woman may go to the bathroom to urinate or defecate. Unplug the sensors at the machine and let her walk to the bathroom. Reconnect and adjust them when she returns. Alternatively, you may roll the machine to the door of the bathroom; the cords are usually long enough to remain connected. Document ambulation and any interruption in monitoring on the strip. If the fetus has a nonreassuring pattern, it is preferable not to interrupt the recording.

Evaluation

The evaluation of parental knowledge is continuous because most parents think of questions after initial explanations and as conditions change. Do the partners indicate their understanding after each explanation? Their understanding may be accompanied by a decrease in anxiety as well.

FETAL OXYGENATION

Assessment

Use a systematic approach to evaluate a fetal monitoring strip. Assess the fetal heart rate for baseline, variability, and periodic changes. Assess uterine activity for frequency, duration, and intensity of contractions and for uterine resting tone. Intervals for assessment and documentation should be at least as frequent as those recommended for intermittent auscultation:

- Women without risk factors: every 30 minutes during active first-stage labor and every 15 minutes during the second stage
- Women with risk factors: every 15 minutes during active first-stage labor and every 5 minutes during the second stage

See Table 17–3 for additional guidelines for evaluating and documenting the fetal heart rate.

Take the woman's temperature at least every 4 hours. Maternal fever increases the fetal temperature and fetal oxygen requirements. Assess the woman's pulse, respirations, and blood pressure hourly. Hypotension or hypertension may reduce maternal blood flow to the intervillous spaces.

Assessment of mother and fetus is continuous during the dynamic process of labor. Compare data about fetal heart rate patterns, uterine activity, and maternal vital signs with baseline data and normal ranges. Observe for subtle trends in the data. Distinguish between patterns having similar appearances, such as early and late decelerations.

Vaginal examination may be performed to evaluate specific fetal heart rate patterns—for example, to check for a prolapsed cord if a pattern of variable decelerations occurs (see Chapter 17).

Nursing Diagnosis and Planning

The collaborative problem potential complication: fetal compromise is selected for nursing care related to fetal oxygenation when electronic fetal monitoring is used.

Because the nurse cannot manage fetal distress independently, client (fetal) goals are not made. The nurse's responsibility includes planning to do the following:

- Promote adequate fetal oxygenation.
- Take corrective actions to increase fetal oxygenation if nonreassuring patterns are identified.
- Report nonreassuring patterns to the physician or nurse-midwife.
- Support the woman and her partner if a complication develops.
- Document assessments and care.

Interventions

Measures to promote fetal oxygenation are discussed with the care of the woman in normal labor (see Chapter 17) and of the woman having an epidural or subarachnoid block (see Chapter 19).

Taking Corrective Actions

If a nonreassuring pattern is noted, take actions to identify its cause and improve fetal oxygenation. Birth facilities should have protocols to give nurses a framework for interventions if nonreassuring patterns develop. Nursing interventions may include both independent and delegated actions.

Reassuring Parents

Parents understandably become anxious when a nonreassuring pattern occurs. Remain at the bedside and use a calm manner to avoid increasing their anxiety. Use the call bell to summon other nurses to help with corrective actions and to notify the physician or nurse-midwife.

Explain the problem that was identified and the reason for corrective actions in simple, concise language. Severe anxiety reduces the parents' ability to understand information. Inform them if the fetal heart rate returns to a reassuring pattern. Some corrective actions, such as oxygen administration and positioning, may continue after a reassuring pattern returns. Tell the woman that she may talk with the oxygen mask on.

Reporting Nonreassuring Patterns

Notify the birth attendant of nonreassuring patterns as soon as possible after taking corrective actions. The priority of nursing care is to improve fetal oxygenation. Document the time and content of all consultations with the physician or nurse-midwife about the mother or fetus and the birth attendant's response.

Documenting Assessments and Care

Record data related to fetal well-being in the labor record and on the paper monitor strip. Both are permanent records

---

TABLE 18-3

Documenting Electronic Fetal Monitoring

Documentation When Monitoring Is Initiated

Monitor Strip

Woman's name
Physician's or nurse-midwife's name
Date and time of admission
Date and time electronic monitoring is begun (verify date and time if this information is automatically printed by monitor)
Gravidity, parity, abortions, living children
Gestation in weeks
Presence of identified risk factors
Character of amniotic fluid (if membranes are ruptured)
Function test of monitor accuracy
Initial mode of monitoring (external or internal devices)

Labor Record

Same information as on monitor strip
First panel number when strip is begun

Continuing Documentation

Monitor Strip

Maternal vital signs
Vaginal examinations, including cervical dilation and effacement and fetal station
Rupture of membranes (spontaneously or artificially)
Color, quantity, and character (such as foul odor or cloudiness) of amniotic fluid
Maternal position changes
Maternal or fetal movement
Maternal vomiting, coughing, or other movement that affects tracing
Adjustment of equipment
Medication and anesthesia, including related interventions
Changes of equipment mode (such as external to internal device)
Interventions for nonreassuring patterns
Temporary interruptions in strip, such as woman walking

Labor Record

Same information as on monitor strip
Periodic summary of the baseline rate, variability, periodic changes, and uterine activity (frequency, duration, and intensity of contractions and uterine resting tone)

---

and should be complete and able to document care independently of the other. Table 18-3 shows guidelines for documentation on the monitor strip and labor record. Documentation can demonstrate good nursing care and show that the standard of care has been met.

Write the woman's name, the date, and the time on the strip when electronic fetal monitoring begins. If a break in the strip occurs, such as to change paper, label the new strip with the woman's name, the date, and the time. Record the last panel number of the previous strip on the new strip so that the entire record can be reassembled sequentially.

Continue documenting the heart rate and maternal observations until vaginal birth occurs. If a cesarean birth is needed, continue monitoring by auscultation or electronic means as long as is practical while preparing the woman for surgery. Remove internal devices before securing her legs to the operating table with a strap. Document the time at which monitoring was stopped and the time of abdominal incision.

Evaluation

Client-centered goals are not formulated for a collaborative problem. The nurse compares data with established standards to determine whether they are within normal limits. If nonreassuring patterns are identified, the nurse does the following:

- Takes measures to increase fetal oxygenation
- Notifies the physician or nurse-midwife
- Documents all relevant data

KEY CONCEPTS

- The purpose of intrapartum fetal surveillance is to identify fetal well-being and to identify the fetus who may be having hypoxic stress beyond the ability to compensate for it.
- The two approaches to intrapartum fetal monitoring are intermittent auscultation with palpation of uterine activity and electronic fetal monitoring. Because each type has distinct advantages and limitations, neither approach is superior to the other.
- Fetal oxygenation depends on a normal flow of oxygenated maternal blood into the placenta, normal exchange within the placenta, patent umbilical cord vessels, and normal fetal circulatory and oxygen-carrying function.
- Stimulation of the sympathetic nervous system increases the fetal heart rate and strengthens the heart contraction. Stimulation of the parasympathetic nervous system slows the heart rate and maintains short-term variability.
- External electronic fetal monitoring is less accurate for fetal heart rate and uterine activity patterns than internal monitoring, but it is noninvasive.
- Greater accuracy is the main advantage of internal electronic fetal monitoring devices.
- Nursing responsibilities related to intrapartum fetal monitoring include promoting fetal oxygenation, identifying and reporting nonreassuring findings, supporting parents, communicating with the physician or nurse-midwife, and documenting all care.

ANSWERS TO CRITICAL THINKING EXERCISES

Exercise 18–1

1. The pattern described is one of late decelerations, probably caused by excess uterine activity secondary to the use of oxytocin.
2. Jackie's initial action should be to stop the oxytocin infusion to reduce stimulation of uterine activity and increase the rate of Nancy's nonadditive intravenous fluid. Oxygen should be given through a snug face mask at about 8 to 10 L/min. Nancy should be placed on her side, if she is not already in this position, to increase placental blood flow. After the immediate corrective actions are completed, Jackie should contact Nancy's physician or nurse-midwife, documenting her interventions and the content of the call.

Exercise 18–2

The pattern described is one of variable decelerations, usually associated with cord compression. The novice nurse should use the call bell to summon a more experienced nurse.

At the same time, LaShonda should be asked to change her position. If she is on her left side, she should turn to the right. Changing position may relieve pressure on the cord. The experienced nurse will further evaluate LaShonda and her baby and may perform other interventions.

The physician should be contacted, but attempting to correct the cause of the variable decelerations is the priority.

REFERENCES AND READINGS

American Academy of Pediatrics & American College of Obstetricians and Gynecologists. (1997). *Guidelines for perinatal care* (4th ed.). Elk Grove Village, IL, and Washington, DC: Author.

American College of Obstetricians and Gynecologists. (1995a). *Fetal heart rate patterns: Monitoring, interpretation, and management* (ACOG Technical Bulletin No. 207). Washington, DC: Author.

American College of Obstetricians and Gynecologists. (1995b). *Umbilical artery blood acid-base analysis* (ACOG Technical Bulletin No. 216). Washington, DC: Author.

Association of Women's Health, Obstetric, and Neonatal Nurses (AWHONN). (1998). *Clinical competencies and education guide: Antepartum and intrapartum fetal heart rate monitoring.* Washington, DC: Author.

Barnes, J. (1996). Fetal communication: Calling the placenta (Cassette Recording No. OGN 619). Anaheim, CA: AWHONN, and Philadelphia: Saunders.

Committee on Obstetric Practice, & A.P. Committee on Fetus and Newborn. (1996). Use and abuse of the Apgar score (ACOG Committee Opinion No. 174). *International Journal of Gynecology and Obstetrics, 54,* 303–305.

Cunningham, F. G., MacDonald, P. C., Gant, N. F., Leveno, K. J., Gilstrap, L. C., Hankins, G. D. V., et al. (1997). *Williams obstetrics* (20th ed.). Norwalk, CT: Appleton & Lange.

Cusick, W., Smulian, J. C., & Ventzileos, A. M. (1995). Intrapartum use of fetal heart rate monitoring, contraction monitoring, and amnioinfusion. *Clinics in Perinatology, 22*(4), 875–906.

Feinstein, N., & McCartney, P. (Eds.). (1997). *Association of Women's Health, Obstetric, and Neonatal Nurses' fetal heart monitoring: Principles and practices* (2nd ed.). Dubuque, IA: Kendall/Hunt.

Folsom, M. S. (1997). Amnioinfusion for meconium: Does it help? MCN: *American Journal of Maternal/Child Nursing, 22*(2), 74–79.

Guyton, A. C., & Hall, J. E. (1996). *Textbook of medical physiology*. Philadelphia: Saunders.

Harvey, C. J. (1997). Electronic fetal monitoring update: A look at the new terms. *Lifelines 2*(6), 49–51.

Helwig, J. T., Parer, J. T., Kilpatrick, S. J., & Laros, R. K. (1996). Umbilical cord blood acid-base state: What is normal? *American Journal of Obstetrics and Gynecology, 174*(6), 1807–1814.

Inturrisi, M. (1996). Amnioinfusion (Cassette Recording No. OGN 631). Anaheim, CA: AWHONN.

Low, J. A., Simpson, L. L., Tonni, G., & Chamberlain, S. (1995). Limitations in the clinical prediction of intrapartum fetal asphyxia. *American Journal of Obstetrics and Gynecology, 172*(3), 801–804.

Menihan, C. A. (1996). Intrapartum fetal monitoring. In K. R. Simpson & P. A. Creehan (Eds.), *AWHONN perinatal nursing* (pp. 187–225). Philadelphia: Lippincott.

Murray, M. (1997). *Antepartal and intrapartal fetal monitoring* (2nd ed.). Albuquerque, NM: Learning Resources International.

National Institute of Child Health and Human Development Research Planning Workshop. (1997). Electronic fetal heart rate monitoring: Research guidelines for interpretation. *Journal of Obstetric, Gynecologic, and Neonatal Nursing, 26*(6), 635–640.

Parer, J. (1999). Fetal heart rate. In R. Creasy & R. Resnik (Eds.), *Maternal-fetal medicine: Principles and practice* (pp. 270–299). Philadelphia: Saunders.

Schifrin, B. S. (1995). Medicolegal ramifications of electronic fetal monitoring during labor. *Clinics in Perinatology, 22*(4), 837–854.

Supplee, R. B., & Vezeau, T. M. (1996). Continuous electronic fetal monitoring: Does it belong in low-risk births? MCN: *American Journal of Maternal/Child Nursing, 21*(6), 301–306.

19

◆ ◆ ◆ ◆ ◆ ◆ ◆ ◆ ◆ ◆ ◆ ◆

Pain Management for Childbirth

DEFINITIONS

agonist   A substance that causes a physiologic effect.

analgesic   A systemic agent that relieves pain without loss of consciousness.

anesthesia   Loss of sensation, especially pain sensation, with or without loss of consciousness.

anesthesiologist   A physician who specializes in the administration of anesthesia.

antagonist   A drug that blocks the action of another drug or of body secretions.

aspiration pneumonitis   A chemical injury to the lungs that may occur with regurgitation and aspiration of acidic gastric secretions.

cleansing breath   A deep breath taken at the beginning and end of each labor contraction.

effleurage   Massage of the abdomen or other body part performed during labor contractions.

endorphins   Morphine-like substances that occur naturally in the central nervous system and modify pain sensations.

epidural space   The area outside the dura, between the dura mater and the vertebral canal.

general anesthesia   Systemic loss of sensation with loss of consciousness.

motor block   Loss of voluntary movement caused by regional anesthesia.

nurse anesthetist   A registered nurse who has advanced education and certification in administration of anesthetics. Also called a certified registered nurse anesthetist (CRNA).

pain threshold (or pain perception)   The lowest level of stimulus one perceives as painful. Pain threshold is relatively constant under different conditions.

pain tolerance   Maximum pain one is willing to endure. Pain tolerance may increase or decrease under different conditions.

regional anesthesia   Anesthesia that blocks pain impulses in a localized area without loss of consciousness.

sensory block   Loss of sensation caused by regional anesthesia.

subarachnoid space   Space between the arachnoid mater and the pia mater that contains the cerebrospinal fluid.

Each woman has unique expectations about birth, including expectations about pain and her ability to manage it. The woman who successfully handles the pain of labor is more likely to view her experience as a positive life event. A woman's experience with labor pain varies with several physical and psychological elements, and each woman responds differently. Nonpharmacologic and pharmacologic methods give the nurse and laboring woman a selection of pain management techniques to choose from.

Unique Nature of Pain During Birth

Pain involves two components:

- A physiologic component, which includes reception by sensory nerves and transmission to the central nervous system
- A psychological component, which involves recognizing the sensation, interpreting it as painful, and reacting to the interpretation

Pain is subjective and personal; no one can feel another's pain. One must simply believe what another person says about his or her pain experience.

Childbirth pain, however, differs from other pain in several important respects:

- Childbirth pain is part of a normal process, whereas other types of pain usually indicate an injury or illness. Pain may cause a woman to assume different positions in labor, favoring descent of the fetus through her pelvis.
- The pregnant woman has several months to prepare for labor, including acquiring skills to help manage pain. Realistic preparation and knowledge about the birth process help her develop skills to cope with labor pain.
- Labor pain has a foreseeable end. A woman can expect her labor to end in hours, rather than days, weeks, or months. Other kinds of pain may also be brief, but the baby's birth brings a rapid decrease in pain.
- Labor pain is not constant but intermittent. A woman may describe little discomfort with contractions during early labor. Even during late labor, a woman may be relatively comfortable during the short rest periods between contractions.
- Labor ends with the birth of a baby. The emotional significance of her child's birth cannot be ignored when trying to understand a woman's response to pain. Concern about her fetus often motivates a woman to tolerate more pain during labor than she otherwise might be willing to endure.

Adverse Effects of Excessive Pain

Although expected during labor, pain that exceeds a woman's tolerance can have harmful effects on her and the fetus.

Physiologic Effects

A woman reacts to pain with fear and anxiety, which increase sympathetic nervous system activity and result in increased secretion of catecholamines (epinephrine and norepinephrine). Catecholamines stimulate alpha and beta receptors.

Stimulation of the alpha receptors causes uterine and generalized vasoconstriction and an increase in the uterine muscle tone. These effects reduce uterine blood flow as they increase the maternal blood flow and maternal blood pressure.

Stimulation of the beta receptors relaxes the uterine muscle and causes vasodilation. However, uterine vessels are already dilated, so dilation of other maternal vessels allows a woman's blood to pool in the vessels. The pooling of blood reduces the amount of blood available to perfuse the placenta.

The combined effects of excessive catecholamine secretion are therefore the following:

- Reduced blood flow to and from the placenta, restricting fetal oxygen supply and waste removal
- Reduced effectiveness of uterine contractions, slowing the progress of labor

Labor increases a woman's metabolic rate and her demand for oxygen. Pain and anxiety escalate her already high metabolic rate. She breathes fast to obtain more oxygen, exhaling too much carbon dioxide in the process. Significant changes, more than those expected during labor, can occur in the woman's Pao_2 and $Paco_2$ and in her arterial pH. These maternal respiratory and metabolic changes alter placental exchange. The fetus may have less oxygen available for uptake and be less able to unload carbon dioxide to the mother. The net result is that the fetus shifts to anaerobic metabolism, with the buildup of hydrogen ions (acidosis). This type of acidosis is metabolic and does not resolve as quickly after birth as respiratory acidosis.

Psychological Effects

Poorly relieved pain lessens the pleasure of this extraordinary life event for both partners. The mother may find it difficult to interact with her infant because she is depleted from a painful labor. Unpleasant memories of the birth may affect her response to sexual activity or another labor. Her partner may feel inadequate as a support person during birth.

Variables in Childbirth Pain

Physical and psychosocial factors contribute to a woman's response to the pain of labor.

Physical Factors

Childbirth pain is of two types, visceral and somatic. Visceral pain is a slow, deep pain that is poorly localized. It is often described as dull or aching. Visceral pain dominates during first-stage labor as the uterus contracts and the cervix dilates.

Somatic pain is a faster, sharp pain. It can be precisely

localized. Somatic pain is most prominent during late first-stage labor and during second-stage labor as the descending fetus puts direct pressure on maternal tissues.

SOURCES OF PAIN

Four potential sources of labor pain exist in most labors. Other physical factors may modify labor pain, increasing or decreasing it.

Tissue Ischemia.   The blood supply to the uterus decreases during contractions, leading to tissue hypoxia and anaerobic metabolism. Ischemic uterine pain has been likened to ischemic heart pain.

Cervical Dilation.   Dilation and stretching of the cervix and lower uterus are a major source of pain. Pain stimuli from cervical dilation travel through the hypogastric plexus, entering the spinal cord at the T10, T11, T12, and L1 levels (Fig. 19–1).

Pressure and Pulling on Pelvic Structures.   Some pain results from pressure and pulling on pelvic structures such as ligaments, fallopian tubes, ovaries, bladder, and peritoneum. The pain is a visceral pain; a woman may feel it as referred pain in her back and legs.

Distension of the Vagina and Perineum.   Marked distension of the vagina and perineum occurs with fetal descent, especially during the second stage. The woman may describe a sensation of burning, tearing, or splitting (somatic pain). Pain from vaginal and perineal distension and pressure and pulling on adjacent structures enters the spinal cord at the S2, S3, and S4 levels (see Fig. 19–1).

FACTORS INFLUENCING THE PERCEPTION OR TOLERANCE OF PAIN

Although physiologic processes cause labor pain, a woman's tolerance of pain may be affected by other physical influences.

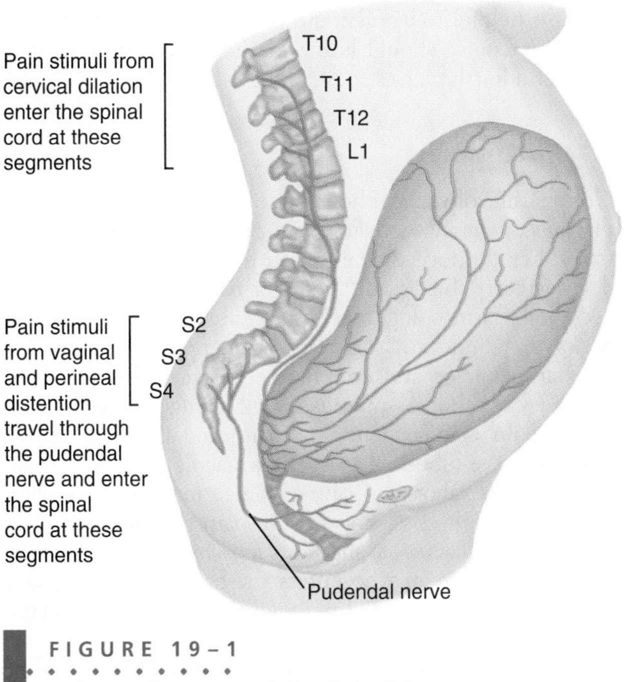

Pain stimuli from cervical dilation enter the spinal cord at these segments

T10
T11
T12
L1

Pain stimuli from vaginal and perineal distention travel through the pudendal nerve and enter the spinal cord at these segments

S2
S3
S4

Pudendal nerve

FIGURE 19–1

Pathways of pain transmission during labor.

Intensity of Labor.   The woman who has a short, intense labor often complains of severe pain because each contraction does so much work (effacement, dilation, and fetal descent). A rapid labor may limit her options for pharmacologic pain relief as well.

Cervical Readiness.   If prelabor cervical changes (softening, with some dilation and effacement) are incomplete, the cervix does not open as easily. More contractions are needed to achieve dilation and effacement, resulting in a longer labor and greater fatigue in the laboring woman.

Fetal Position.   Labor is likely to be longer and more uncomfortable when the fetus is in an unfavorable position. An occiput posterior position is a common variant seen in otherwise normal labors. In this position, each contraction pushes the fetal occiput against the woman's sacrum. She experiences intense back discomfort (*back labor*) that persists between contractions. Often a woman cannot deliver her infant in the occiput posterior position. The fetal head must therefore rotate in a wider arc before the mechanisms of extension and expulsion occur, so labor is often longer (see Chapter 17). Back pain may decrease dramatically when a fetus rotates into the more favorable occiput anterior position. The rate at which labor progresses usually speeds up as well.

Characteristics of the Pelvis.   The size and shape of a woman's pelvis influence the course and length of her labor. Abnormalities may cause a difficult and longer labor and may contribute to fetal malpresentation or malposition.

Fatigue.   Fatigue reduces a woman's ability to tolerate pain and to use coping skills she has learned. She may be unable to focus on relaxation and breathing techniques that would otherwise help her tolerate labor.

Many women sleep poorly during the last weeks of pregnancy. Shortness of breath when lying down, frequent urination, and fetal activity interrupt sleep so that a woman often begins labor with a sleep deficit. If labor begins late in the evening, she may have been awake well over 24 hours by the time she gives birth. Even if a woman begins labor well rested, slow progress may exhaust her.

Intervention of Caregivers.   Although they may be appropriate for the well-being of a woman and fetus, some interventions add discomfort to the natural pain of labor. Intravenous lines cause pain when they are inserted and remain noticeable to many women during labor. Fetal monitoring equipment is uncomfortable to some women. Both may hamper a woman's mobility, which she might use to assume a more comfortable position.

A woman whose labor is induced or augmented often reports more pain and increased difficulty coping with it because contractions reach peak intensity quickly. Vaginal examinations and amniotomy also increase a woman's discomfort briefly because of vaginal and cervical stretching.

Psychosocial Factors

Several psychosocial variables influence a woman's experience of pain.

CULTURE

A woman's sociocultural roots influence how she perceives, interprets, and responds to pain during childbirth. Some cultures encourage loud and vigorous expression of pain, whereas others value self-control. Women are individuals within their cultural groups, however. The experience of pain is personal, and one should not make assumptions about how a woman from a specific cultural or ethnic group will behave during labor.

Women should be encouraged to express themselves in any way they find comforting, and the diversity of their expressions must be respected. Accepting a woman's individual response to labor and pain promotes a therapeutic relationship.

The nurse should avoid praising some behaviors (such as stoicism) while belittling others (such as noisy expression). This restraint is difficult because noisy women are challenging to work with and may disturb others.

The unique nature of childbirth pain and women's diverse responses to it make nursing management complex. The nurse can miss important cues if the woman is either stoic, having little outward expression of pain, or expresses herself loudly and constantly. With either extreme, the nurse may not readily identify critical information such as impending birth or the symptoms of a complication.

ANXIETY AND FEAR

Extreme anxiety and fear magnify sensitivity to pain and impair a woman's ability to tolerate it. They consume energy she needs to cope with the birth process, including its painful aspects.

Anxiety and fear increase muscle tension, diverting oxygenated blood to the brain and skeletal muscles. Tension in pelvic muscles counters the expulsive forces of uterine contractions and the laboring woman's pushing efforts during the second stage. Prolonged tension results in general fatigue, increased pain perception, and reduced ability to use skills to cope with pain.

PREVIOUS EXPERIENCES WITH PAIN

Early in life a child learns that pain is a symptom of bodily injury. Consequently, fear and withdrawal are a woman's natural reactions to pain during labor. Learning about the normal sensations of labor, including pain, helps a woman suppress her natural reactions of fear and withdrawal, allowing her body to do the work of birth.

A woman who has given birth previously has a different perspective. If she has had a vaginal delivery, she is probably aware of normal labor sensations and is less likely to associate them with injury or abnormality. Also, time has a way of blunting the memory of painful experiences.

A woman who had a child by caesarean birth and has never experienced labor may be particularly anxious. The experience of cesarean birth is known to her, whereas labor is unknown. A repeat cesarean birth may seem like the quicker and less painful option. She may have difficulty yielding to the normal forces of birth.

A woman who has previously had a long and difficult labor is more likely to be anxious about the outcome of the present one. If she had a cesarean birth following the difficult labor, she may doubt her ability to give birth vaginally. Her anxiety often intensifies when she reaches the point at which her prior labor ended with the cesarean birth.

Previous experiences do not always adversely affect a woman's ability to deal with pain. She may have learned ways to cope with pain during other episodes of pain or during other births and may use these skills adaptively during labor.

PREPARATION FOR CHILDBIRTH

Preparation for childbirth does not ensure a pain-free labor. A woman should be prepared for pain realistically, including reasonable expectations about analgesia and anesthesia. She may feel that her entire preparation is invalid if what she expects does not happen when she is in labor.

Preparation reduces anxiety and fear of the unknown. It allows a woman to rehearse for labor and learn a variety of skills to master pain as labor progresses. She and her partner learn about expected behavioral changes during labor, and their knowledge decreases their anxiety when those changes occur.

SUPPORT SYSTEM

An anxious partner is less able to provide the support and reassurance that the woman needs during labor. In addition, anxiety in others can be contagious, and an anxious partner can increase her anxiety. She may assume that if others are worried, something is probably wrong.

The birth experiences of a woman's family and friends cannot be ignored. Those individuals can be an important source of support if they convey realistic information about labor pain and its control. If they describe labor as intolerable, however, she may have needless distress. It is equally detrimental for a woman to hear that labor is painless. No two labors are alike, even for the same woman.

◼ Nonpharmacologic Pain Management

The nurse who cares for women in labor and birth can offer nonpharmacologic and pharmacologic pain management methods. Education about nonpharmacologic pain management is the foundation of prepared childbirth classes. To be most helpful to women and their labor partners, the intrapartum nurse should know methods that are taught in local childbirth classes.

Advantages

Nonpharmacologic methods have several advantages over pharmacologic methods if they produce adequate pain control. They do not slow labor and have no side effects, nor do they carry the risk of allergy or neonatal sedation.

Nonpharmacologic techniques are both an alternative to and an adjunct to drugs. Most women use a combination of pharmacologic and nonpharmacologic techniques. The woman who chooses pharmacologic analgesia needs alternative pain management until the drug is given, usually after labor is established. Also, pharmacologic methods may not eliminate labor pain, and a woman may need nonpharmacologic methods to control the pain that remains.

Nonpharmacologic methods may be the only realistic option for a woman who enters the hospital in advanced, rapid labor. In this case, drugs might not have enough time to take effect. Also, the newborn might have respiratory depression if a systemic opioid narcotic reaches its peak action about the time of birth.

Limitations

Nonpharmacologic methods of pain control have limitations, especially if they are used as the sole method of pain control. Women do not always achieve their desired level of pain control using these methods alone. Because of the many variables in labor, even a well-prepared and highly motivated woman may have a difficult labor and need pharmacologic analgesia or anesthesia.

Preparation for Pain Management

The ideal time to learn nonpharmacologic pain control is before labor. During the last few weeks of pregnancy, the woman learns about labor, including its painful aspects, in childbirth classes. She can prepare to confront the pain, learning a variety of skills to use during labor. Her support person learns specific methods to encourage and support her. After admission, the nurse can review and reinforce what the partners learned in class.

The nurse can teach the unprepared woman and her support person nonpharmacologic techniques. The latent phase of labor is the best time for intrapartum teaching because the woman is usually anxious enough to be attentive and interested, yet comfortable enough to understand.

Many methods may become less effective after prolonged use, a process called habituation. Changing techniques counters habituation. The nurse who knows a variety of methods can select those that are most helpful to an individual woman.

Application of Nonpharmacologic Techniques

Four techniques can be applied to intrapartum care: relaxation, cutaneous stimulation, mental stimulation, and breathing.

RELAXATION
Promoting relaxation provides a base for all other methods, both nonpharmacologic and pharmacologic, because it does the following:

- Promotes uterine blood flow, thus improving fetal oxygenation
- Promotes efficient uterine contractions
- Reduces tension that increases pain perception and decreases pain tolerance
- Reduces tension that can inhibit fetal descent

Environmental Comfort. Comfortable surroundings support relaxation. The nurse can reduce irritants such as bright lights and can adjust the room temperature.

Music masks outside noise and provides a background for use of imagery and breathing techniques. It is a distraction that shifts the woman's attention from bodily sensations. Television may have the same effect for some women.

General Comfort. Promoting the woman's personal comfort helps her focus on pain management techniques during labor (Fig. 19–2). This includes actions to increase comfort and reduce the effect of irritants.

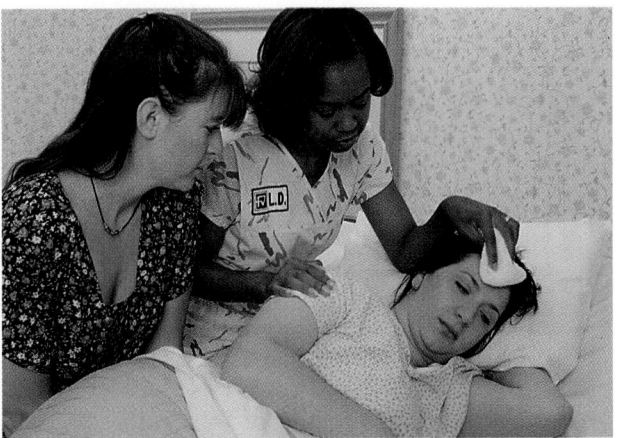

FIGURE 19–2
General comfort measures such as the nurse's reassuring presence or a cool, damp cloth applied to the face supplement other methods of nonpharmacologic and pharmacologic pain control.

Reducing Anxiety and Fear. The nurse may reduce a woman's anxiety and increase her self-control by providing accurate information and focusing on the normality of birth. Hospitals are typically associated with illness or injury, situations that are anxiety provoking. Yet hospitals are the most common site for the normal event of birth.

Simple nursing actions keep the focus on the normality of childbirth, regardless of the setting. For example, referring to a woman as a patient reinforces the atmosphere of illness associated with being in a hospital, whereas calling her by name helps her to see birth as a normal process. Empowerment of the woman and her partner by giving them choices whenever possible helps them to see themselves as competent people who can accomplish the task of giving birth.

Implementing Specific Relaxation Techniques. Relaxation techniques work best if they are learned and practiced before labor. During practice sessions at home, couples may practice *progressive relaxation,* in which the woman contracts and then releases specific muscle groups until all muscles are relaxed. *Neuromuscular dissociation* helps the woman learn to relax all muscles except those that are working (the uterus or the abdominal muscles when pushing). The woman can learn *touch relaxation* in response to her partner's touch, and *relaxation against pain* as the partner deliberately causes mild pain and the woman learns to relax despite the pain.

Even if the woman did not practice these relaxation techniques at home, the nurse can teach her how to consciously relax as labor goes by. The partner can learn to watch for signs of tension, touch that area, and direct the woman to relax.

CUTANEOUS STIMULATION
Cutaneous stimulation has several variations that are often combined with each other or with other techniques.

Self-Massage. The woman may rub her abdomen, legs, or back in a self-massage called *effleurage* to counteract discomfort. Some women find abdominal touch irritating,

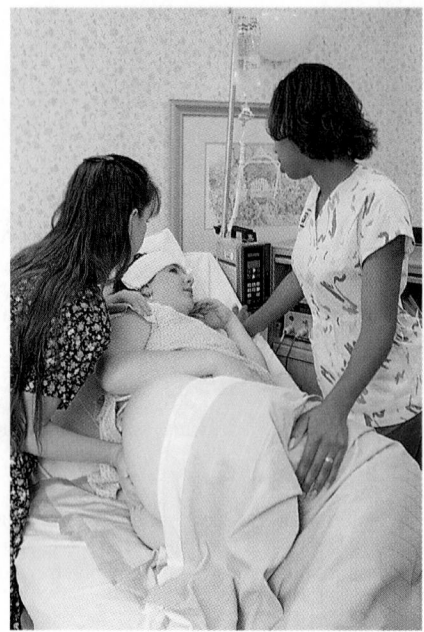

FIGURE 19–3
. . . .
The coach applies sacral pressure to counter the back pain that is common during labor.

especially near the umbilicus. Women in labor may find firm stroking more helpful than very light stroking. They can trace figure-8s or circles on the bed if touch irritates them.

Some women benefit from firm palm or sole stimulation during labor. They may like to have their palms rubbed vigorously by another, rub their hands or feet together, or bang their palms on, or grip, a cool surface. They may hold another person's hand tightly during a contraction. The nurse should determine if these actions indicate excess pain or if they are a woman's way of countering pain and therefore useful.

Massage by Others. The partner or the nurse can rub the woman's back, shoulders, legs, or any area where she finds massage helpful. Sacral pressure is a variation that may help when the woman has back pain, which is usually most intense when the fetus is in an occiput posterior position. Sacral pressure may be applied using the palm of the hand, the fist or fists, or a firm object such as two tennis balls in a sock (Fig. 19–3).

Nonclinical touch by the nurse is a powerful tool if the woman does not object to it. Holding her hand, stroking her hair, or similar actions convey caring, comfort, affirmation, and reassurance at this vulnerable time.

Thermal Stimulation. Many women like to have warmth applied to their back, abdomen, or perineum during labor. A warm shower, tub bath, or whirlpool bath is relaxing and provides thermal stimulation. A sock filled with dry rice and microwaved provides gentle warmth and can be used to apply pressure to the sacral area.

Cool, damp washcloths may be comforting, especially if a woman is hot. She may put them on her head, throat, abdomen, or any place she wants. She also may want to put them in or over her mouth to relieve dryness.

MENTAL STIMULATION
Mental techniques occupy the woman's mind and compete with pain stimuli. They also aid relaxation by providing a tranquil imaginary atmosphere.

Imagery. If the woman has not practiced a specific imagery technique, the nurse can help her create a relaxing mental scene. Most women find images of warmth, softness, security, and total relaxation most comforting.

Imagery can help the woman dissociate herself from the painful aspects of labor. For example, the nurse can help her visualize the work of labor: the cervix opening with each contraction or the fetus moving down toward the outlet each time she pushes. This technique is like visualizing success or movement toward a goal with each contraction.

Focal Point. When using nonpharmacologic techniques, a woman may prefer to close her eyes or may want to concentrate on an external focal point. She may bring a picture of a relaxing scene or an object to use as a focal point and to aid in the use of imagery. She can use any point in the room as a focal point.

BREATHING
Breathing techniques give a woman a different focus during contractions, interfering with pain sensory transmission (Fig. 19–4). Breathing techniques begin with simple patterns and progress to more complex ones as needed. There is no single right time to change patterns during labor. Complex patterns, however, are fatiguing to use for a prolonged time.

First-Stage Breathing. Breathing in the first stage of labor consists of a cleansing breath and various breathing techniques known as *paced breathing*. The method begins with a very simple technique that is used as long as possible. When it is no longer effective, breathing that requires more concentration is added.

Cleansing Breath. Each contraction begins and ends with a deep inspiration and expiration known as the cleansing breath. Like a sigh, a cleansing breath helps the woman

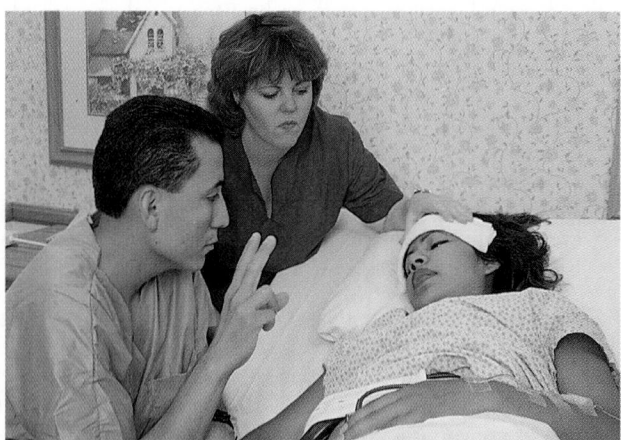

FIGURE 19–4
. . . .
A woman and her partner who are prepared for labor have learned a variety of skills to master pain as labor progresses. The coach uses hand signals to tell the woman how to change her pattern of paced breathing.

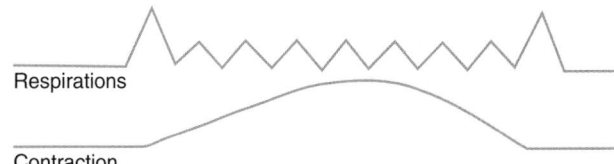

FIGURE 19–5

Slow-paced breathing. Although a specific rate may or may not be taught, slow-paced breathing should be *no slower than half* the woman's usual respiratory rate to ensure adequate oxygenation. This pace is generally about six to nine breaths per minute.

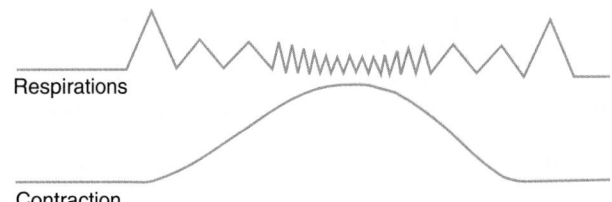

FIGURE 19–7

Combining breathing techniques during a contraction. Slow- and modified-paced breathing can be combined by using the slower breathing at the beginning and end of the contraction and the more rapid breathing over the peak of the contraction.

release tension. It provides oxygen to help prevent myometrial hypoxia, one cause of pain in labor. The cleansing breath also helps the woman clear her mind to focus on relaxing and signals her labor partner that the contraction is beginning or ending. The woman may inhale through the nose and exhale through the mouth or take her cleansing breath in any way comfortable for her.

Slow-Paced Breathing. The first breathing is slow-paced breathing, a slow, deep breathing that increases relaxation (Fig. 19–5). The woman should concentrate on relaxing her body rather than on regulating the rate of her breathing. Relaxation naturally brings about slower breathing, similar to that which occurs during sleep. She can use nose, mouth, or combination breathing, depending on which is most comfortable.

The woman uses slow-paced breathing as long as possible during labor because it promotes relaxation and sufficient oxygenation. Slow-paced breathing is easy for the unprepared woman to learn between contractions and, with the support of the nurse, helps even a frightened woman become calm and able to work with her contractions.

Modified-Paced Breathing. When the woman finds that slow-paced breathing is no longer effective, she begins modified-paced breathing (Fig. 19–6). This chest breathing at a faster rate matches the natural tendency to use more rapid breathing during stress or physical work, such as labor. Although modified-paced breathing is more shallow than slow-paced breathing, the faster rate allows oxygen intake to remain about the same. As with slow-paced breathing, the focus is on release of tension rather than on the actual number of breaths taken.

Women can combine slow- and modified-paced breath-

ing during the course of a contraction (Fig. 19–7). They begin slowly and use shallow, faster breathing at the peak of the contraction. The breathing should not interfere with relaxation but enhance it.

Pattern-Paced Breathing. Pattern-paced breathing (sometimes called "pant blow," "hee hoo," or "hee blow" breathing) involves focusing on the pattern of breathing (Fig. 19–8). It is similar to modified-paced breathing. It differs in that after a certain number of breaths the woman exhales with a slight emphasis or blow, and then begins the modified-paced breathing again. The addition of a blow causes her to focus more on her breathing and reduces habituation. Some educators teach women to make a sound such as "hee" during this breathing and to blow through pursed lips with a "hoo" sound. Others avoid special sounds, which tighten the vocal cords and may decrease relaxation.

The number of breaths before the blow may remain constant (usually between two and six) or may change in a pattern. Variations include a set pattern such as 3-1, 5-1, 3-1 or a stair-step pattern such as 6-1, 5-1, 4-1, 3-1. Some couples use a random pattern determined by the coach, who uses hand signals to show the number of breaths the woman should take before each blow.

Breathing to Prevent Pushing. If a woman pushes strenuously before the cervix is completely dilated, she risks injury to the cervix and the fetal head. Blowing prevents closure of the glottis and breath holding, which are a part of strenuous pushing. The woman blows repeatedly using short puffs when the urge to push is strong. The support person may learn to blow along with her to help the woman

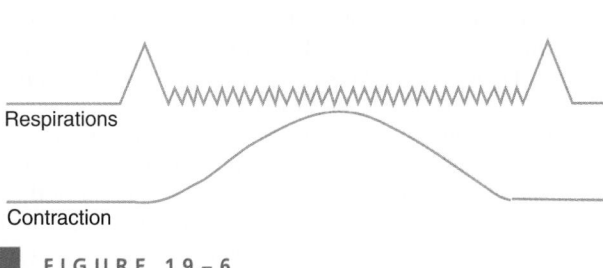

FIGURE 19–6

Modified-paced breathing. The pattern for modified-paced breathing should be comfortable to the woman and *no faster than twice* her normal respiratory rate to prevent hyperventilation or interference with relaxation.

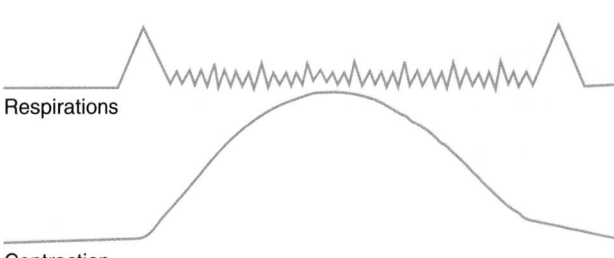

FIGURE 19–8

Pattern-paced breathing. Pattern-paced breathing adds a slight emphasis or "blow" on the exhalation in a pattern. The diagram shows the emphasis after every third inhalation.

concentrate. Some women vary the blowing by using one short breath and one blow.

Common Problems. Hyperventilation and mouth dryness may occur during breathing techniques. Hyperventilation is due to rapid deep breathing that causes excessive loss of carbon dioxide, eventually resulting in respiratory alkalosis. The woman may feel dizzy or lightheaded and have impaired thinking. Vasoconstriction leads to tingling and numbness in fingers and lips. If hyperventilation continues, tetany due to decreased calcium in tissues and blood may result in stiffness of the face and lips and carpopedal spasm.

The woman can blow into a paper bag or her own cupped hands if she feels dizzy. This kind of blowing increases blood carbon dioxide levels.

Dryness of the mouth occurs when the woman uses prolonged mouth breathing. To avoid dryness, she can place her tongue gently against the roof of her mouth to moisturize entering air. The support person can offer ice, mouthwash, sour suckers, or liquids if they are allowed.

Second-Stage Breathing. Breathing in the second stage of labor includes the traditional method of pushing, as well as methods that involve less breath holding.

Traditional Pushing. In traditional pushing, the woman takes one or more cleansing breaths at the beginning of the contraction and then holds her breath, pushing as hard as she can for as long as possible. Generally, the coach counts slowly to 10 while the woman holds her breath. She then quickly exhales, takes another breath, and pushes again, repeating the process until the contraction is over. The concern of those who oppose this method is that pushing against a closed glottis, Valsalva's maneuver, results in an increase in intrathoracic pressure and a decrease in blood pressure and blood return to the heart. The final result may be impaired blood flow to the uterus. Proponents believe that breath holding is important to complete the second stage as quickly as possible, because this may be a time of danger for the fetus.

Other Pushing Methods. Other methods of pushing involve exhalation of small amounts of air through an open glottis during pushing. The woman may push in short bursts only when the urge is very strong instead of using prolonged expulsive efforts. If she holds her breath at all, it is for very short intervals (5 to 6 seconds) only. Proponents believe that this method allows better oxygenation of both expectant mother and fetus.

Pharmacologic Pain Management

Pharmacologic methods for pain management include systemic drugs, regional pain management techniques, and general anesthesia.

Special Considerations When Medicating a Pregnant Woman

Medicating a woman when she is pregnant is not as straightforward as when she is not pregnant, for several reasons:

- Any drug taken by the woman may affect her fetus.
- Drugs may have unusual effects in pregnancy.

- Drugs can affect the course and length of labor.
- Complications may limit the choice of pharmacologic pain management methods.
- Women who need other therapeutic drugs or who practice substance abuse may have fewer safe choices for pain relief.

EFFECTS ON THE FETUS

The effects on the fetus of drugs given to the mother may be direct or indirect. Direct effects result from passage of the drug or its metabolites across the placenta to the fetus. An example of a direct effect on the fetus is decreased fetal heart rate variability following administration of an analgesic to the woman. Indirect effects are secondary to drug effects on the mother. For example, if a drug causes maternal hypotension, blood flow to the placenta is reduced. Fetal hypoxia and acidosis may result.

MATERNAL PHYSIOLOGIC ALTERATIONS

Normal pregnancy changes in four body systems have the greatest implications for pharmacologic pain management methods.

Cardiovascular Changes. Compression of the aorta and inferior vena cava (aortocaval compression) by the uterus can occur when a woman lies in the supine position. Some anesthetics require that she assume the supine position temporarily. In such a case, the uterus is displaced to one side with the hands or with a small wedge placed under one hip.

Respiratory Changes. A pregnant woman's full uterus reduces her respiratory capacity. To compensate, she breathes more rapidly and deeply. As a result, she is more vulnerable to reduced arterial oxygenation during induction of general anesthesia and is more sensitive to inhalational anesthetic agents.

Gastrointestinal Changes. A pregnant woman's stomach is displaced upward by her large uterus; the stomach's interior also has a higher pressure. Progesterone slows peristalsis and reduces the tone of the sphincter at the junction of the stomach and esophagus. These changes make a pregnant woman more vulnerable to regurgitation and aspiration of acidic gastric contents during general anesthesia.

Nervous System Changes. During pregnancy and labor, circulating levels of endorphins are high. Endorphins modify pain perception and reduce requirements for analgesia and anesthesia.

The epidural and subarachnoid spaces are smaller during pregnancy, enhancing the spread of anesthetic agents used for epidural or subarachnoid blocks. Cerebrospinal fluid pressure is higher, reaching a peak during the second stage of labor. Nerve fibers are more sensitive to local anesthetic agents, probably because of acid-base or hormonal alterations. High intra-abdominal pressure causes engorgement of the epidural veins, increasing the risk for intravascular injection of anesthetic agents. The net result of these changes is that a smaller volume of local anesthetic is needed to achieve satisfactory epidural or subarachnoid block.

EFFECTS ON THE COURSE OF LABOR

Most analgesics are not given until labor is well established because they may slow progress if given too early. Caregivers, however, must consider the adverse effects of excessive pain on labor's progress when helping a woman choose methods of pain relief. Regional anesthetics, primarily the epidural block, can slow progress during the second stage if they impair the laboring woman's natural urge to push.

EFFECTS OF COMPLICATIONS

Complications during pregnancy may limit the choices of analgesia or anesthesia. For example, large volumes of intravenous fluids may be infused to prevent hypotension with regional anesthesia. If a pregnant woman has heart disease, this fluid load could be detrimental. Yet without it, she is vulnerable to hypotension.

INTERACTIONS WITH OTHER SUBSTANCES

A woman who ingests drugs (therapeutic, over-the-counter, or illicit) or other substances may have fewer options because of interactions between these substances and analgesics or anesthetics.

Systemic Drugs for Labor

Systemic drugs are those that have effects on multiple systems because they are distributed throughout the body. These intrapartum drugs include opioid analgesics and adjunctive drugs. Although agents used to induce general anesthesia are also systemic, they are discussed separately because they are used only at birth.

OPIOID ANALGESICS

Opioid analgesics reduce the perception of pain without loss of consciousness. Injectable opioid analgesics are the systemic drugs of choice in labor. Common analgesics for intrapartum use are meperidine (Demerol), butorphanol (Stadol), and nalbuphine (Nubain). Table 19–1 summarizes common drugs used for intrapartum pain relief.

Meperidine is a pure opioid agonist, but butorphanol and nalbuphine have mixed opioid agonist and antagonist effects. These agonist-antagonist drugs should not be given

---

TABLE 19-1

Drugs Commonly Used for Intrapartum Pain Management

Drug/Dose	Comments
Opioid Analgesics	
Meperidine (Demerol) 12.5–50 mg every 2–4 hr IV	Respiratory depression (primarily in the neonate) is the main side effect.
Butorphanol (Stadol) 1 mg every 3–4 hr (range, 0.5–2 mg IV)	Has some narcotic antagonist effects. Should not be given to the opiate-dependent woman (may precipitate withdrawal) or after other narcotics such as meperidine (may reverse their analgesic effects). Is a respiratory depressant.
Nalbuphine (Nubain) 10 mg every 3–6 hr IV	Same as butorphanol.
Adjunctive Drugs	
Promethazine (Phenergan) 12.5–25 mg every 4–6 hr IV	Duration of action is longer than that of most narcotics. Enhances respiratory depressant effects of narcotics.
Diphenhydramine (Benadryl) 10–50 mg every 4–6 hr IV	Given to relieve pruritus from epidural narcotics.
Hydroxyzine (Atarax, Vistaril) 25–100 mg IM Z-track only	See promethazine.
Narcotic Antagonists	
Naloxone (Narcan) Adult: 0.4–2 mg IV To reverse pruritus from epidural opioids: 0.04–0.2 mg IV or IV infusion 5–10 µg/kg/hr	Action shorter than that of most narcotics it reverses. Nurse must observe for recurrent respiratory depression and be prepared to give additional doses.
Neonate: 0.1 mg/kg IV (umbilical vein) or intratracheal	For neonatal resuscitation; see also comments for adult dose.
Naltrexone (Trexan) 3–6 mg PO (1 dose)	Long-acting drug to relieve pruritus from epidural narcotics (investigational when used for this purpose).

Abbreviations: IV, intravenously; PO, orally; IM, intramuscularly.

to a woman who is opiate dependent (on a drug such as heroin) to avoid withdrawal effects. These drugs also should not be given if she has already received a pure opioid agonist such as meperidine, because some analgesic effect of the first drug will be reversed.

The primary side effect of opioid analgesics is respiratory depression, which is more likely to occur in the newborn than in the mother. Administration must be timed carefully to reduce neonatal respiratory depression. An infant born at the peak of the drug's action is more likely to have respiratory depression than if born earlier or later. Drugs such as meperidine have metabolites that are active for a long time in the newborn and can cause delayed or prolonged respiratory depression.

During labor, opioid analgesics are usually given intravenously in small, frequent doses to provide a rapid onset of analgesia and a predictable duration of action. A woman benefits from rapid pain control, and there is less likelihood of neonatal respiratory depression. Starting the injection at the beginning of the contraction, when blood flow to the placenta is normally reduced, limits transfer to the fetus. When placental blood flow resumes, much of the drug is in maternal tissues.

OPIOID ANTAGONISTS
Naloxone (Narcan) reverses opioid-induced respiratory depression. Naloxone does not reverse respiratory depression from other causes, such as barbiturates, anesthetics, nonopioid drugs, or pathologic conditions. Naloxone has a shorter duration of action than most of the opioids it reverses. In an opiate-dependent woman or newborn, naloxone may induce withdrawal symptoms. Naloxone is used with other measures as needed to support cardiopulmonary function. (See Chapter 30 for discussion of neonatal resuscitation.)

Naloxone is most often given to the neonate. The recommended neonatal route for administration is intravenous or intratracheal for the most reliable absorption. The neonatal and pediatric resuscitation dose is 0.1 mg/kg by the intravenous or intratracheal route (American Academy of Pediatrics & American College of Obstetricians and Gynecologists, 1997). Intravenous naloxone is given to the neonate through the umbilical vein. The adult dose is 0.4 to 2 mg.

Naltrexone (Trexan) is an opioid antagonist that is usually prescribed for opioid dependence. In the intrapartum setting, naltrexone may be given orally to relieve the pruritus that often occurs when intrathecal or epidural opioid analgesics are used.

ADJUNCTIVE DRUGS
Adjunctive drugs during the intrapartum period include those with antiemetic and tranquilizing effects and sedatives. These drugs are given to reduce nausea and anxiety and to promote rest (see Table 19–1).

Promethazine (Phenergan) relieves the nausea and vomiting that may occur when opioid drugs are given. Promethazine may be given by either the intramuscular or the intravenous route. Use of promethazine allows a lower total dose of opioid to be given, but it does not potentiate the opioid's effects.

SEDATIVES
Sedatives such as barbiturates are not routinely given because they have prolonged depressant effects on the neonate. However, a small dose of a short-acting barbiturate may be given to promote rest if a woman is fatigued from false labor or a prolonged latent phase.

Regional Pain Management Techniques
Regional pain control methods may be used for intrapartum analgesia, anesthesia, or both. These methods provide pain relief without loss of consciousness.

Epidural block analgesia or anesthesia provides pain control during much of labor and for the birth itself. Intrathecal opioids are used for pain control during labor; additional measures are needed during late labor and for the birth. Regional anesthetics that are used only during the birth include the local, pudendal, and subarachnoid blocks.

The major advantage of regional pain management methods is that the woman can participate in birth yet still have good pain control. The woman usually feels some pressure and discomfort, although these sensations are greatly reduced. She can interact with her infant and partner and does not lose her protective airway reflexes, as can happen with general anesthesia. The disadvantages of regional pain control techniques depend on the specific technique used. The effects on the fetus depend on how the woman responds rather than on direct drug effects.

EPIDURAL BLOCK
The lumbar epidural block is a popular regional block that provides pain relief for labor and birth without sedation of the woman and fetus. It is used for both vaginal and cesarean births.

The epidural space is outside the dura mater, between the dura and the spinal canal. It is loosely filled with fat, connective tissue, and epidural veins that are dilated during pregnancy (Fig. 19–9).

The epidural block is done by injecting local anesthetic into the tiny epidural space. It provides substantial relief of pain from contractions and birth canal distension. The level of the epidural block can be extended upward to provide anesthesia for a cesarean birth or tubal ligation after birth. The woman usually retains motor function and some sensation when lower concentrations of anesthetic are used. Higher concentrations of the anesthetic agent that are used for abdominal surgery result in loss of both motor and sensory functions.

Technique. The epidural block is started after labor is established or just before a scheduled cesarean birth. The epidural space is entered at about the L3–L4 interspace (below the end of the spinal cord), and a catheter is passed through the needle into the epidural space (Fig. 19–10). The catheter allows continuous infusion or intermittent injection of medication to maintain pain relief during labor and vaginal or cesarean birth.

Epidural anesthesia requires a larger amount of anesthetic agent than the subarachnoid block because it is outside the meninges. A small (3-ml) test dose of local anesthetic is injected before the full dose is given and before

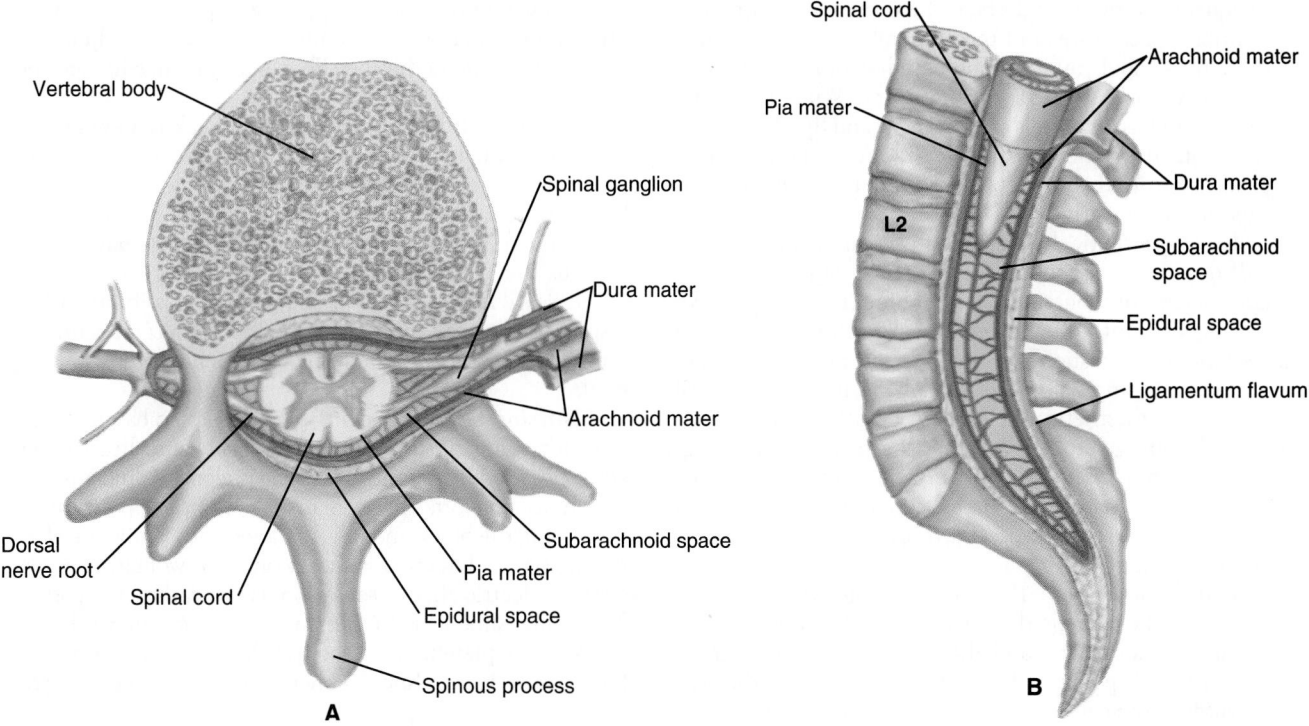

FIGURE 19–9

A, Cross section of spinal cord, meninges, and protective vertebra. The dura and arachnoid lie close together. The pia mater is the innermost of the meninges and covers the brain and spinal cord. The subarachnoid space is between the arachnoid and pia mater. *B,* Sagittal section of spinal cord, meninges, and vertebrae. The epidural and subarachnoid spaces are illustrated. Note that the spinal cord ends at the L2 vertebra.

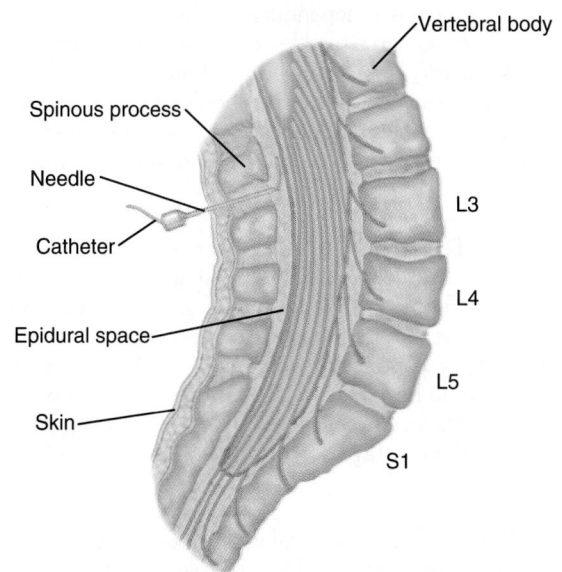

The epidural space is entered with a needle below where the spinal cord ends. A fine catheter is threaded through the needle.

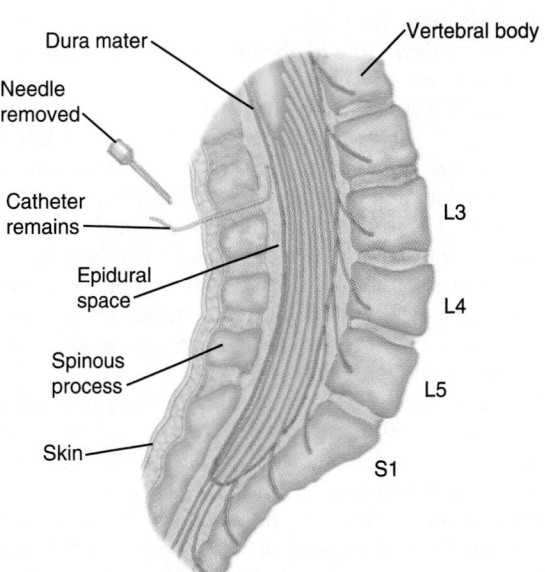

After the catheter is threaded into the epidural space, the needle is removed. Medication can then be injected into the epidural space intermittently or by continuous infusion for pain relief during labor and birth.

FIGURE 19–10

Technique for epidural block.

subsequent intermittent doses. If the catheter is in the sub-arachnoid space instead of the epidural space, the woman experiences rapid, intense motor and sensory block. The test dose also can detect accidental intravascular injection. The woman has numbness of the tongue and lips, lighthead-edness, dizziness, and tinnitus with intravascular injection. Epinephrine in the test dose produces tachycardia if in-jected intravascularly.

Local anesthetic drugs are usually combined with a very small dose of an opioid analgesic such as fentanyl (Subli-maze), sufentanyl (Sufenta), or morphine (Duramorph). All drugs injected into the epidural or subarachnoid spaces are preservative-free. The drug combination provides quicker and longer-lasting pain relief for labor with a lower total dose of local anesthetic and less motor block. Epidural anal-gesics also are given after cesarean birth to provide long-acting pain relief with a low dose. The mother is comfort-able enough to have good interaction with her infant and family. She may require no added analgesics, or oral ones may be sufficient.

Dural Puncture. Because the tough dura and the fragile web-like arachnoid membranes lie close together, du-ral puncture also punctures the arachnoid. If the dura is unintentionally punctured with the large-gauge needle used to introduce the catheter, substantial leakage of cerebrospi-nal fluid can occur, which may result in a spinal headache. Dural puncture and spinal headache also can occur without obvious cerebrospinal fluid leakage.

Contraindications and Precautions. An epidural block is not suitable for all laboring women. Contraindica-tions include the woman's refusal, coagulation defects, un-corrected hypovolemia, an infection in the area of insertion or a severe systemic infection, allergy, or a fetal condition that demands immediate birth.

Adverse Effects of Epidural Block. An epidural block can have adverse effects.

Maternal Hypotension. Sympathetic nerves are blocked along with pain nerves, which may result in vasodilation and hypotension. Rapid infusion of warmed intravenous so-lution such as lactated Ringer's solution before initiation of the block offsets vasodilation by filling the vascular system. The amounts infused are large compared with those given in other settings: often 500 to 1,000 ml or more is rapidly infused (Creehan, 1996). If hypotension occurs, intrave-nous ephedrine in 5- to 10-mg increments promotes vaso-constriction to raise the blood pressure.

Bladder Distension. A woman's bladder may fill quickly because of the large quantity of intravenous solution, yet her sensation to void is reduced. Bladder distention may cause pain that remains after initiation of the block.

Prolonged Second Stage. The urge to push is often less intense than if a woman does not have an epidural block. Forceps- or vacuum extractor–assisted births are more likely because of the reduced urge to push.

Catheter Migration. After accurate placement, the catheter may move. A woman may then have symptoms of intravascular injection, an intense block or one that is too high, absence of anesthesia, or a unilateral block.

Adverse Effects of Epidural Opioids. Adverse mater-nal effects associated with epidural opioids may include nau-sea and vomiting, pruritus, and delayed respiratory depres-sion.

Nausea and Vomiting. As when opioids are given by other routes, nausea and vomiting may occur. Adjunctive drugs such as promethazine (Phenergan) reduce nausea and vomiting.

Pruritus. Itching of the face and neck is an annoying side effect of many epidural opioids. Although she may not specifically complain of itching, a woman may rub or scratch her face and neck frequently. Diphenhydramine (Benadryl), naloxone (Narcan), or naltrexone (Trexan) may relieve pruritus (see Table 19–1).

Delayed Respiratory Depression. The possibility of late respiratory depression exists for up to 24 hours after the ad-ministration of an epidural opioid, depending on the drug used.

Nursing Care. The nurse should record baseline vital signs for comparison after the block is begun. Intravenous access is ensured, and the prescribed preload of fluid is given. The nurse supports the woman in the correct position for instituting the block and tells the anesthesia clinician when the woman is having a contraction. The woman may feel a brief "electric shock" sensation as the catheter is passed. The nurse should assist her in remaining still while the block is completed. After the test dose, the nurse observes for signs of subarachnoid puncture or intravascular injec-tion.

There are currently no national standards for the fre-quency of monitoring of maternal vital signs after an epi-dural block is begun, and standards for fetal assessment are based on risk status (see Chapters 17 and 18). Facility proto-cols and the maternal-fetal status should guide the fre-quency of vital sign measurements and fetal assessments. Pulse oximetry is often used to observe blood oxygenation. Maternal respiratory monitoring may continue for up to 24 hours after birth, depending on the drugs given.

The woman's bladder must be assessed frequently be-cause of the large intravenous fluid load and her reduced sensation to void. The nurse should observe for signs associ-ated with catheter migration from the epidural space and for adverse effects, such as nausea and vomiting and pruritus.

INTRATHECAL OPIOID ANALGESICS

Intrathecal injection of an opioid analgesic is an option for labor pain management that is gaining acceptance. The drug is injected into the subarachnoid space, where it binds to opiate receptors, allowing much smaller doses to be used than would be adequate if the drug were given systemically. The woman can feel her contractions but not the pain.

The advantages of intrathecal analgesics include the following:

- Rapid onset of pain relief without sedation
- No motor block, enabling the woman to ambulate during labor
- No sympathetic block, with its hypotensive effects

The disadvantages may include the following:

- Limited duration of action, possibly requiring another procedure for continued pain relief
- Inadequate pain relief for late labor and the birth itself, requiring added measures to manage pain at that time

Technique. The subarachnoid space is entered with a spinal needle, as in the subarachnoid block. A preservative-free opioid analgesic is then injected.

The drug chosen depends on the expected duration of labor at the time it is given. Drugs that may be used by this route include fentanyl, sufentanyl, and morphine. Fentanyl and sufentanyl have a rapid onset of action and the effect lasts for up to 3 hours. Morphine has a slightly longer onset but its effect lasts longer.

Adverse Effects of Intrathecal Opioids. As with epidural opioids, nausea, vomiting, and pruritus may occur. Delayed respiratory depression may occur, depending on the drug used.

Nursing Care. Vital signs and fetal heart rate are taken at the usual intervals for the woman's stage of labor. Side effects, such as nausea and vomiting or pruritus, are reported and managed similarly to those occurring with the epidural block. Reduced effectiveness suggests that the drug's duration of action is ending or that the woman is in late labor. Other pain management methods may be needed for the remainder of labor and for birth.

LOCAL INFILTRATION ANESTHESIA

Infiltration of the perineum with a local anesthetic is done by the physician or nurse-midwife just before performing an episiotomy or suturing a laceration (Fig. 19–11). Local infiltration does not alter pain from uterine contractions or distention of the vagina. The local agent provides anesthesia in the immediate area of the episiotomy or laceration. There is a short delay between anesthetic injection and the onset of numbness, and the drug burns before its anesthetic action begins. Local infiltration rarely has adverse effects on either mother or infant.

PUDENDAL BLOCK

A pudendal block anesthetizes the lower vagina and part of the perineum to provide anesthesia for an episiotomy and vaginal birth, using low forceps if needed. A pudendal block does not block pain from uterine contractions, and the mother feels pressure.

The physician or nurse-midwife injects the pudendal nerves near each ischial spine with about 10 ml of local anesthetic (Fig. 19–12). The perineum is infiltrated with local anesthetic because the pudendal block does not fully anesthetize this area. As in local infiltration, a delay occurs between injection and the onset of numbness. Possible maternal complications include a toxic reaction to the anesthetic, rectal puncture, hematoma, and sciatic nerve block. If maternal toxicity is avoided, the fetus is usually not affected.

SUBARACHNOID (SPINAL) BLOCK

A subarachnoid block is a simpler procedure than the epidural block and may be done when a quick cesarean birth is necessary and an epidural catheter is not in place. It is similar to local infiltration and pudendal block in that it is done just before birth and so provides no pain relief during most of labor.

The physician or nurse anesthetist injects local anesthetic into the subarachnoid space in a single dose. The woman loses both sensory and motor function below the

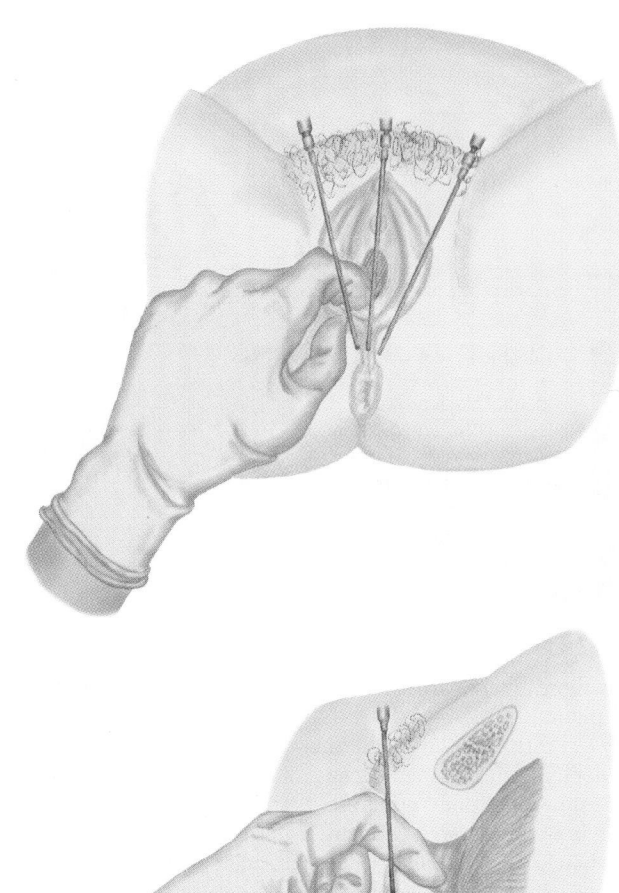

FIGURE 19–11

Local infiltration anesthesia numbs the perineum just before birth for an episiotomy or after birth for suturing of a laceration. The birth attendant protects the fetal head by placing a finger inside the vagina while injecting the perineum in a fan-like pattern.

level of the subarachnoid block, with complete relief of pain from contractions.

Technique. A 25- to 27-gauge spinal needle is placed in the subarachnoid space. Appearance of cerebrospinal fluid at the needle hub assures correct placement, and the local anesthetic is injected (Fig. 19–13).

The level of anesthesia for both epidural and subarachnoid blocks is determined by the volume, concentration, and density of the drug (Fig. 19–14).

Contraindications and Precautions. Contraindications and precautions are similar to those for epidural block: the woman's refusal, coagulation defects, uncorrected hypovolemia, infection in the area of insertion, systemic infection, and allergy.

Adverse Effects of a Subarachnoid Block. Three adverse effects of a subarachnoid block are maternal hypotension, bladder distension, and spinal headache. Hypotension

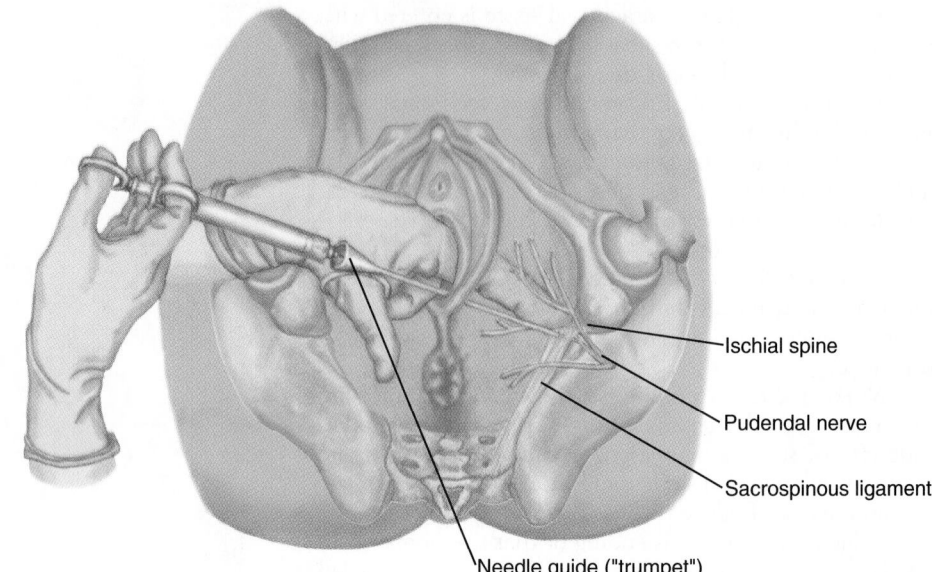

Pudendal block provides anesthesia for an episiotomy and the use of low forceps. A needle guide ("trumpet") protects the maternal and fetal tissues from the long needle needed to reach the pudendal nerve.

Ischial spine

Pudendal nerve

Sacrospinous ligament

Needle guide ("trumpet")

is more likely with the subarachnoid block than with the epidural block.

Postspinal headache may occur after subarachnoid block in some women because of cerebrospinal fluid leakage at the site of dural puncture. A spinal headache is postural; it is worse when a woman is upright and may disappear when she is lying flat. The incidence of spinal headache is lower if a small-gauge needle is used.

Bed rest with oral or intravenous hydration helps relieve the postspinal headache. A blood patch often gives dramatic, definitive relief. The blood patch is done by injecting 10 to 15 ml of the woman's blood (obtained with sterile technique) into the epidural space. The blood forms a gelatinous seal over the hole in the dura, stopping spinal fluid leakage (Fig. 19–15). The blood patch can be repeated if needed.

GENERAL ANESTHESIA
General anesthesia is systemic pain control that involves loss of consciousness. It is rarely used for vaginal births, but

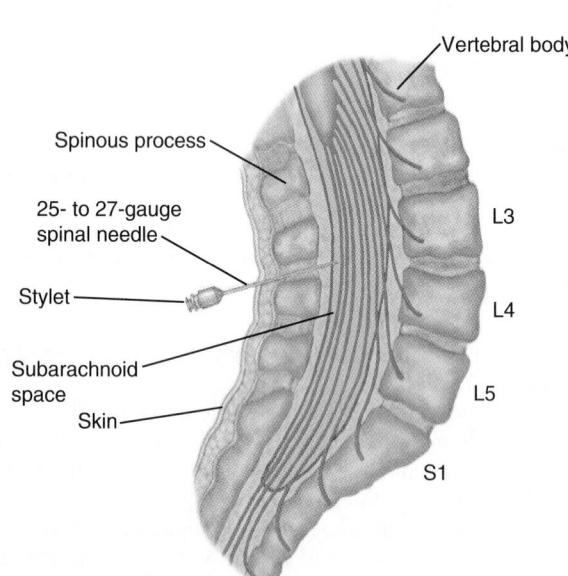

Vertebral body

Spinous process

25- to 27-gauge spinal needle

Stylet

Subarachnoid space

Skin

L3

L4

L5

S1

A 25- to 27-gauge spinal needle with a stylet occluding its lumen is passed into the subarachnoid space below where the spinal cord ends.

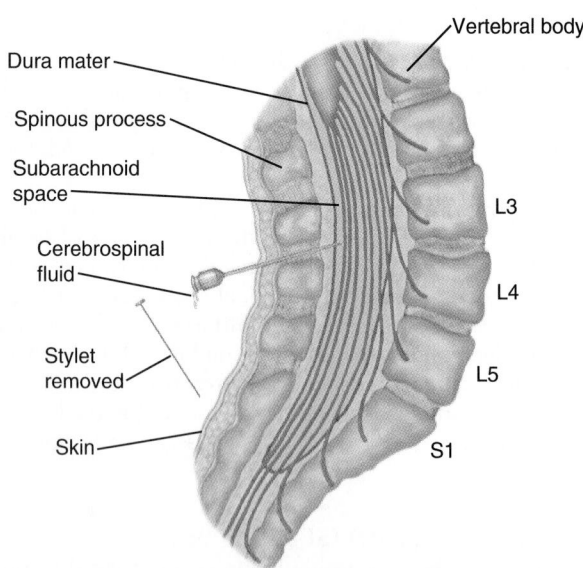

Dura mater

Spinous process

Subarachnoid space

Vertebral body

Cerebrospinal fluid

Stylet removed

Skin

L3

L4

L5

S1

The stylet is removed, and one or more drops of clear cerebrospinal fluid at needle hub confirm correct needle placement. Medication is then injected, and the needle is removed.

Technique for subarachnoid block.

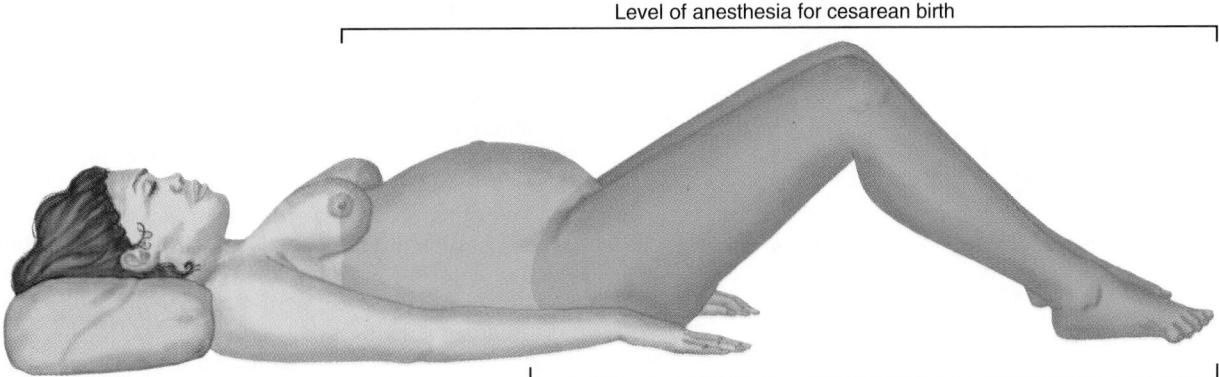

Level of anesthesia for cesarean birth

Level of anesthesia for vaginal birth

FIGURE 19-14

Levels of anesthesia for epidural and subarachnoid blocks. A level of T10 through S5 is adequate for vaginal birth. A higher level, to T4–T6, is needed for cesarean birth.

it still has a place in cesarean birth. Some women either refuse or are not good candidates for epidural or subarachnoid block. In other cases, it may be necessary to perform a cesarean birth so quickly that no time is available to establish either type of regional block.

Technique. Before induction of anesthesia, a woman breathes oxygen for 3 to 5 minutes, or at least four deep breaths, to increase her oxygen stores and those of her fetus for the short period of apnea during anesthesia induction. A wedge is placed under the woman's right side (or the operating table is tilted toward her left side) to reduce aortocaval compression and increase placental blood flow.

Adverse Effects of General Anesthesia. Major adverse effects are possible with the use of general anesthesia.

Maternal Aspiration of Gastric Contents. Regurgitation with aspiration of acidic gastric contents is a potentially fatal complication of general anesthesia. Aspiration of food

particles may result in airway obstruction. Aspiration of acidic secretions results in chemical injury to the airways (aspiration pneumonitis). Infection often occurs after the initial lung injury.

Respiratory Depression. Respiratory depression may occur in either the mother or the infant but is more likely in the baby.

Uterine Relaxation. Some inhalational anesthetics may cause uterine relaxation. This characteristic is desirable for some complications, such as replacing an inverted uterus (see Chapter 27). However, postpartum hemorrhage may occur if the uterus relaxes after birth.

Methods to Minimize Adverse Effects. Measures to reduce the risk of maternal aspiration (or of lung injury, if aspiration occurs) include the following:

- Restricting intake to clear fluids or nothing by mouth if surgery is anticipated.
- Administering drugs to raise the gastric pH and make secretions less acidic, such as sodium citrate and citric acid (Bicitra), ranitidine (Zantac), cimetidine (Tagamet), or famotidine (Pepcid).
- Administering drugs to reduce secretions, such as glycopyrrolate (Robinul).
- Administering drugs to speed gastric emptying, such as metoclopramide (Reglan).
- Using cricoid pressure (Sellick's maneuver) to block the esophagus by pressing the rigid trachea against it (Fig. 19–16).

Neonatal respiratory depression may be averted by doing the following:

- Reducing the time from induction of anesthesia until the umbilical cord is clamped.
- Keeping the anesthesia level as light as possible until the cord is clamped.

To reduce the time from induction of anesthesia to cord clamping, the woman is prepared and draped and the physicians are ready before anesthesia is begun. Before cord clamping, the anesthesia is so light that it is more accurately described as amnesia with profound analgesia. The woman may move on the operating table as the incision is made,

Vertebral body

Spinous process

Dura

Needle

10 to 15 ml of maternal blood

Epidural space

L3

L4

L5

S1

FIGURE 19-15

Blood patch for relief of spinal headache. Ten to 15 ml of the woman's blood is injected into the epidural space to seal a dural puncture.

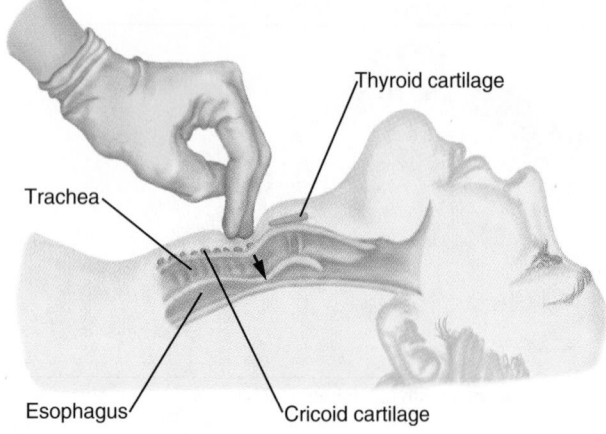

Thyroid cartilage

Trachea

Esophagus

Cricoid cartilage

FIGURE 19–16
• • • • • • • • • •
Sellick's maneuver to prevent vomitus from entering the woman's trachea while she is being intubated for general anesthesia. An assistant applies pressure to the cricoid cartilage to obstruct the esophagus. Once the woman is successfully intubated with a cuffed endotracheal tube, gastric secretions cannot enter the trachea.

but she rarely remembers the experience. If a hazy memory remains, she does not usually remember the experience as painful. The anesthesia level is deepened after the cord is clamped.

NURSING CARE
• • • • • • • • • • • •
Pain Management

The nurse assists laboring women with both nonpharmacologic and pharmacologic methods of pain control as needed (see Nursing Care Plan 19–1). Nursing care related to pain management should be combined with that for normal labor and any complications that arise. Two problems that commonly affect the woman are pain and her potential for respiratory compromise if she needs general anesthesia.

PAIN

Assessment

Pain assessment begins at admission and continues throughout labor. The assessments discussed in Table 17–1 guide the nurse in obtaining data related to pain management. Pain-related assessments include the following:

- Preferences for pain management
- Maternal vital signs
- Fetal heart rate and monitor patterns
- Allergies, focusing especially on allergy to opioid analgesics, dental anesthetics, and iodine (used in most prep solutions)
- Oral intake time and type of intake
- Evidence of pain: verbal evidence: verbal statement, requests for pain relief measures, crying, moaning; and nonverbal evidence: tense, guarded posture or facial expression
- Labor status

In addition to these routine assessments, ask the woman if she needs help with pain management. A stoic woman may give little outward evidence of pain yet may say she wants medication or other pain control if asked.

When assessing pain, clarify the words a woman uses. When asked if she has "pain," the woman may deny it. Changing the word used to "discomfort," "aching," "pulling," "pressure," or other words that may describe labor pain may bring a different response. Do not assume that everyone uses the same words to describe their pain. Just as pain is an individual experience, so also is the expression of pain, including verbal expression.

Asking a woman to rate her pain on a scale of 0 to 10 or a similar scale helps clarify her pain's intensity. Zero represents no pain, whereas 10 is the worst possible pain. Ask the woman to rate her pain on this scale before and after pain relief measures to evaluate their effectiveness.

The woman who remains tense between contractions may be having difficulty coping with pain. Moaning, crying, thrashing, and an inability to use nonpharmacologic techniques suggest that she needs pharmacologic pain relief.

Assess the woman's labor status to help her choose the most appropriate method of pain control. If she has reached a point in labor at which she needs to decide for or against a specific pharmacologic method, inform her. This point does not occur at an exact time or with an exact amount of cervical dilation but is estimated according to when she is likely to give birth, the time needed to establish a specific method, and the pharmacology of the drug or drugs.

Avoid making assumptions about the amount of pain a woman is having on the basis of her rate of labor progress, cervical dilation, or apparent intensity of contractions. It is tempting to assume that a woman whose cervix is 2 cm dilated has little pain and that a woman whose cervix is dilated 8 cm has intense pain. An obese woman's contractions may be strong, but they may appear to be mild if they are assessed by palpation or an external monitor because of her thick abdominal fat pad. *Labor progress or contraction intensity cannot be equated with a woman's pain perception or tolerance.*

A woman's need for pain relief should not be based on her outward expression alone. A quiet woman may need medication but may be reluctant to ask, whereas an expressive woman may be quite satisfied with only nonpharmacologic measures. Because women who do not speak the prevailing language may not know what is available, seek an interpreter to communicate accurately.

Observe for pain that is not typical of labor. Although labor pain is often intense, it should not be constant but should come and go with each contraction. The uterus should not be tender or board-like between contractions. Report atypical pain to the physician or nurse-midwife.

Nursing Diagnosis and Planning

Because pain is an expected part of normal childbirth, a common nursing diagnosis is

■ Pain related to effects of uterine contractions and fetal descent.
  Expected Outcomes: The woman will describe the pain relief measures as satisfactory during labor and will use learned breathing and relaxation techniques during labor.

These two goals are realistic for the unique pain of labor.

Intrapartum Pain Management

Assessment

Beth Anderson is a 28-year-old gravida I, para 0, who was admitted 1 hour ago. Beth's cervix is 3 cm dilated and 100% effaced, the station is −2, and her membranes are intact. Contractions occur every 3 minutes, last 40 to 50 seconds, and are of moderate intensity. The fetal heart rate averages 135 to 145 BPM and has no nonreassuring patterns on the monitor. Beth says that back pain is most troubling. Beth and her husband, Sam, attended prepared childbirth classes and are using breathing techniques they learned.

Nursing Diagnosis

Pain related to effects of uterine contractions and pressure on pelvic structures

Goals/Expected Outcomes

During labor, Beth will

- Continue to use techniques she learned in prepared childbirth classes.
- Have a relaxed facial and body posture between contractions.

Intervention

1. Adjust the environment for comfort.
   a. Adjust room thermostat.
   b. Add warm blankets and socks for warmth.
   c. Offer small electric fan or hand fan if Beth is hot.
2. Reduce distractions.
   a. Close door to reduce outside noise.
   b. Play music of Beth's choice to mask external noise.
   c. Do not stand in front of her focal point.
   d. Try to delay assessments or questions until after a contraction is over.
3. Reduce irritating stimulants.
   a. Keep sheets and underpads dry.
   b. Dim the lights as Beth desires. Use bright lights only when necessary.
   c. Do all procedures and nursing interventions as gently as possible.
   d. Avoid bumping the bed.
4. Encourage Beth to assume positions she finds most comfortable and to change positions regularly (about every 30 to 60 minutes). If there is no contraindication, she may walk around or sit in a chair at the bedside. She should avoid the supine position.

5. Check for bladder distension hourly and encourage Beth to void at least every 2 hours. With an order, catheterize her if her bladder is full and she cannot void.
6. If permitted, give Beth small amounts of clear fluids such as ice chips. If oral intake is prohibited, moisten her mouth with a damp washcloth or have her rinse her mouth with water.

7. Offer a back rub or firm, constant sacral pressure. Ask Beth where and how firm pressure should be applied. Use baby powder when rubbing her back. Have her tell caregivers if this technique becomes uncomfortable or if the location on her back needs to be changed. If Sam is rubbing her back, offer to relieve him occasionally and encourage him to take a break.

Rationale

1. A comfortable environment is conducive to relaxation. Relaxation underlies all other interventions because it increases a woman's ability to use her coping skills to tolerate discomfort.

2. Distractions interfere with use of the skills for pain management taught in prepared childbirth classes.

3. Irritating stimulants are distractions that decrease the woman's ability to use learned childbirth skills and add to her discomfort.

4. Frequent position changes favor fetal descent by encouraging the fetal head to adapt to the pelvic diameters most efficiently. Position changes also reduce muscle tension and unrelieved pressure:
   a. Upright positions enhance descent with gravity.
   b. The supine position is uncomfortable to most women and may cause aortocaval compression with decreased placental perfusion.
5. The sensation to void may be decreased during labor. A full bladder contributes to overall discomfort and may impede fetal descent and prolong labor.
6. Women often use rapid mouth breating during labor, resulting in a dry mouth. These methods may relieve some of the discomfort associated with a dry mouth. Clear liquids limit the risk of aspiration if general anesthesia is needed.
7. Back rubs may reduce discomfort associated with back labor somewhat by stimulating large-diameter fibers and interfering with transmission of the pain impulse to the brain. As labor continues, back rubs may become less effective or even uncomfortable. Powder reduces friction, which could be another source of discomfort. The partner needs a break to conserve energy and better help the woman in later labor.

(continued)

Intrapartum Pain Management

8. Keep Beth and Sam informed about the progress of labor and their baby's condition.

8. Information reduces anxiety and fear of the unknown. Anxiety and fear increase pain perception and reduce pain tolerance.

Evaluation

Beth concentrates on her breathing techniques with each contraction but has a relaxed body posture between them. She continues to use learned skills effectively for about 2 hours, when she begins to have more difficulty coping with her contractions.

Assessment

Three hours after admission, Beth's cervix is 4 cm dilated and 100% effaced, and the fetal station is −1. Membranes have ruptured and the amniotic fluid is clear. Contractions occur every 2 to 3 minutes, last 50 seconds, and are firm. Fetal heart rate and monitor patterns are essentially unchanged. Back discomfort persists, and she is having difficulty relaxing between contractions and is discouraged that labor is not progressing as quickly as she expected. She is no longer able to use prepared childbirth techniques effectively. Beth reluctantly requests an epidural block, which will be given by continuous infusion.

The nurse gives Beth 500 ml or more of ordered intravenous solution before the block begins, which offsets its hypotensive effects. Fetal monitoring, usually by continuous electronic means, helps identify nonreassuring patterns that may occur.

Nursing Diagnosis

Risk for Injury related to altered sensation in her lower extremities

Goals/Expected Outcomes

- Beth will not fall or suffer other injury while experiencing the effects of epidural block.
- The fetus will not be born in an uncontrolled manner.

Intervention

1. Assist Beth to change positions regularly. Keep Beth in bed as long as she has any motor block.

2. Observe for signs of labor progress:
   a. Contractions increasing in frequency, duration, and intensity.
   b. Increase in bloody show.
   c. Statement reflecting urge to push (may *not* be present).
3. If Beth cannot feel a strong urge to push during the second stage, tell her when to push during each contraction.
4. After birth, do not allow Beth to ambulate until sensation and movement have returned to her lower extremities. Ask another nurse to assist when she first ambulates.

Rationale

1. Changing positions reduces constant pressure on one area and helps prevent muscle strain. The epidural block causes a varying degree of motor block, so ambulation is generally contraindicated.
2. Sensation is altered, and rectal pressure associated with fetal descent may not be felt. The fetus could be born unattended because of reduced sensation.

3. Epidural block may alter the reflex urge to push. Coaching about when to push aids fetal descent.

4. Assessing for return of sensation prevents falls due to weakness and inability to sense where her feet are. Having assistance prevents injury if a woman is unexpectedly weak when she ambulates.

Evaluation

Beth is satisfied with her pain relief after the epidural block. She has little motor block. Her blood pressure and the fetal heart rate remain within expected limits. Vaginal dilation progresses to 10 cm (complete) without injury to Beth or her fetus. However, despite her vigorous pushing efforts, the fetal station remains at 0. Beth has a cesarean birth, delivering an 8-pound, 10-ounce girl.

Additional Nursing Diagnoses and Collaborative Problems to Consider

Anxiety	Situational Low Self-Esteem
Risk for Aspiration	Urinary Retention
Powerlessness	Potential Complication: Fetal compromise

Truc Pham is a Vietnamese-American in labor with her first baby. Her cervix is dilated 6 cm, effacement is 100%, and the fetus is at a +1 station. Truc's contractions occur every 3 minutes, last 50 to 60 seconds, and are of strong intensity. She smiles at the nurse each time the nurse talks to her but does not talk much herself. Truc stiffens her body during contractions and interacts little with her husband or the nurse at those times.

1. How should the nurse interpret these data?
2. Does the nurse need additional data?
3. What nursing actions are appropriate?

Interventions

The main points of nursing care related to intrapartum pain management are to reduce factors that hinder the woman's pain control and to enhance those that benefit it. Refer to Chapter 17 for nursing measures that should be included in the care of all laboring women, such as positioning, teaching, encouragement, and care of the partner.

Promoting Relaxation

Simple attention to details helps the woman relax. Adjust her environment so that it is more comfortable. If noise is a problem, suggest music or television to mask it.

A warm blanket or a cool cloth provides tangible comfort and conveys the nurse's caring attitude. Change the linens or underpads as needed to keep the woman reasonably clean and dry.

Offer the woman a warm shower or bath, especially if she is tense and if no contraindications exist (Table 19–2). In general, walking is good during early labor, and water therapy is better during active labor. The mild nipple stimulation that occurs in a whirlpool or shower may intensify contractions in a woman whose labor has slowed because it causes her posterior pituitary gland to secrete oxytocin.

Reduce intrusions as much as possible. For example, wait until a contraction is over before asking questions or doing a procedure. Longer assessments and procedures may span several contractions, but try to stop during each contraction.

Reducing Outside Sources of Discomfort

Anesthetize the intravenous site with 0.1 ml of 1% lidocaine (Xylocaine) before inserting the line if the woman is not allergic and if facility policy permits. Remind her to change position regularly to reduce tension and discomfort from constant pressure. Support her with pillows.

Observe the woman's bladder for distension hourly, and encourage her to void every 2 hours or more often if she has received a large quantity of intravenous fluids. Obtain an order to catheterize her if she cannot void and her bladder is full.

Reducing Anxiety and Fear

Accurate information reduces the negative psychological impact of the unknown. Tell the woman about her labor

TABLE 19–2
· · · · · · · · · ·

Use of Water Therapy During Labor

Use of water therapy has accompanied trends toward a low-intervention approach to intrapartum care. Water therapy can be delivered in several ways:

Shower
Standard tub
Whirlpool

Benefits

Associated with a more natural, home-like atmosphere.
Gives a woman greater control over her labor.
Upright position facilitates progress of labor.
Faster labor progress if contractions are frequent when woman enters the tub.
Buoyancy relieves tired muscles.
Facilitates fetal rotation from occiput posterior or transverse positions to the occiput anterior position. The woman can also assume different positions to aid rotation.
Many women report a perception of less pain.
Reduction in the mean arterial pressure, edema, and increased diuresis. This is especially helpful if the woman has pregnancy-induced hypertension.

Disadvantages

May reduce frequency of contractions and dilation during the latent phase of labor.
Fetus must be assessed with intermittent auscultation rather than electronic fetal monitoring.

Contraindications and Precautions

No specific contraindications if the woman can safely be out of bed.
Thick meconium in the amniotic fluid is an indication for continuous electronic fetal monitoring in most birth facilities and would preclude use of water therapy.
Bleeding.
Oxytocin induction or augmentation. The use of both oxytocin and water therapy could cause excess uterine activity.

and its progress. It is impossible to predict when she will give birth, but tell her if her labor progress is or is not on course. Sometimes she needs only the reassurance from an experienced nurse that her intense contractions are indeed normal. The woman may be willing to endure more discomfort than she otherwise would if she is making progress.

Be honest if problems do occur. A woman usually knows if there is a problem and is more anxious if she does not know what it is. Explain all measures taken to correct the problem, and keep her informed about the results.

Helping the Woman Use Nonpharmacologic Techniques

If the nonpharmacologic method is safe for the woman and fetus and if it is effective, do not interfere with its use. Try not to distract the woman from whatever technique she is using.

Massage. Fetal monitor belts hinder abdominal effleurage. Encourage the woman to do effleurage on uncovered areas of her abdomen or to stroke her thighs. Consider using intermittent fetal monitoring if this method is appropriate.

During massage, baby powder reduces friction and skin irritation. The woman needs to tell the person who is providing sacral pressure or other massage how much pressure helps and the best location for it. Because this information may change during labor or massage may become uncomfortable rather than helpful, seek the woman's feedback regularly.

Mental Stimulation. Use a low, soothing voice when helping a woman use imagery. It is often helpful to speak close to her ear when trying to create a tranquil imaginary scene or to calm her. Music can enhance mental stimulation techniques.

Breathing. Women learn a variety of breathing techniques in prepared childbirth classes and often modify them or invent some of their own during labor. Encourage the woman to change techniques when she needs to, avoiding the complex ones during early labor. If she has trouble maintaining her concentration, the nurse or her partner can make eye contact (if culturally appropriate) and breathe the pattern with her.

Symptoms of hyperventilation (dizziness, tingling and numbness of the fingers and lips, carpopedal spasm) are likely if a woman breathes fast and deep, whether or not she is using patterned breathing techniques. If she hyperventilates, have her breathe into her cupped hands, a paper bag, or a washcloth placed over her nose and mouth.

Teach breathing techniques to the unprepared woman when she is admitted. Review them when she seems to need a different method. Many women make up their own breathing techniques.

When teaching the woman who is in advanced labor nonpharmacologic pain management techniques, follow these guidelines:

- Teach one method at a time.
- Demonstrate the method between contractions.
- Use breathing techniques with the woman while maintaining eye contact.
- Allow her control over her labor: who is present, what technique she will use, and the like.

Incorporating Pharmacologic Methods

All pharmacologic methods require collaboration with medical personnel for orders. Tell the woman soon after admission what medication is available if she needs it. This is not done to undermine her self-confidence but so that she can better understand when she needs to make a choice about medication. Also, analgesia is most effective if it is given before pain is severe.

Tell her that her preferences about pain relief methods will be honored if possible, but it is impossible to predict the course of her labor. Her preferred method of pain management may be inappropriate if labor has unexpected developments. Assure her that no pharmacologic method will be given without her understanding and consent.

If a woman finds some nonpharmacologic methods inadequate, try other nonpharmacologic methods, or offer her available medication. When contacting the birth attendant for medication orders, report the fetal and maternal status

and vital signs, labor status, and the woman's request for medication. If she has a continuous epidural block, contact the person who inserted it if problems occur. Observe special nursing considerations associated with the method used (Table 19–3).

Evaluation

- Is the woman is satisfied with her ability to manage her pain?
- Is she using coping skills somewhat consistently during labor?

RESPIRATORY COMPROMISE

Assessment

General anesthesia may be needed any time during birth, most often for cesarean birth. Document the type (solids or liquids) and time of the woman's last food intake. Question her closely if she reports an unusually long interval since her last oral intake. Anesthesia clinicians can anticipate and prevent problems better if they know the actual oral intake.

Nursing Diagnosis and Planning

Nursing care of laboring women includes monitoring for the short-term risk of aspiration, because it is impossible to pre-

---

PARENTS WANT TO KNOW

How Will This Medicine Affect Our Baby?

Women and their partners often ask whether pain medication or anesthesia will harm their baby. The nurse can help parents choose wisely from available options by providing honest information.

- Pain that is beyond your ability to tolerate is not good for you or your baby, and it reduces the joy of this special event.
- Some risk is associated with every type of pain medication or anesthesia, but careful selection and the use of preventive measures minimize this risk. If complications occur, corrective measures can reduce the risk to you and your baby.
- Pain relievers can cause your baby to be slow to breathe at birth, but carefully controlling the timing and dose of the medication reduces the likelihood that this will occur. We can use another medication to reverse this effect if needed.
- Epidural or spinal anesthesia can cause your blood pressure to fall, which can reduce the blood flow to your baby. However, we give you lots of intravenous fluids to reduce this effect. We have other medications to increase your blood pressure if the fluids are not enough.
- General anesthesia can cause your baby to be slow to breathe at birth. To reduce this risk, the anesthesia will not be started until everything is ready for the surgery, and the doctors will clamp the baby's umbilical cord as quickly as possible.

TABLE 19–3
• • • • • • • • • • • •

Pharmacologic Methods of Intrapartum Pain Management

Method and Uses	*Nursing Considerations*
Opioid Analgesics	
Systemic analgesia during labor and for postoperative pain after cesarean birth. May be combined with an adjunctive drug such as promethazine to reduce the nausea and vomiting that sometimes occur with narcotic use.	1. Assess the woman for drug use at admission. Women who are opiate dependent should not receive analgesics having mixed agonist and antagonist actions (butorphanol and nalbuphine). 2. Observe neonate for respiratory depression, especially if the mother had narcotics within 4 hr of birth: • Delay in initiating or sustaining respirations • Rate < 30/min • Poor muscle tone: limp, floppy 3. The use of adjunctive drugs, such as promethazine, enhances respiratory depressant effects. 4. Have naloxone available. Observe for recurrent respiratory depression after administration of naloxone. Repeat at 20- to 60-min intervals as needed.
Epidural Opioids	
Labor: Mixed with a local anesthetic agent to give better pain relief with less motor block. *Postoperatively:* Gives long-acting analgesia without sedation, allowing the mother and infant to interact more easily.	1. Observe the same nursing implications as with epidural block. 2. Do not give additional opioids or other CNS depressants except as ordered by the anesthesia clinician. 3. Respiratory depression may be delayed for up to 24 hr. Observe respiratory rate, depth, and arousability hourly for 24 hr. Notify anesthesia clinician for rate of <12/min, oxygen saturation of <95% on pulse oximetry, reduced respiratory effort, or difficulty arousing. Cyanosis is a late sign of respiratory depression. 4. Have naloxone, 0.4 mg, readily available. 5. Observe for pruritus or rubbing of the face and neck. Notify anesthesia clinician for relief measures. 6. Urinary retention may occur if the woman does not have a catheter in place. 7. Notify anesthesia clinician for relief of nausea or vomiting. 8. Assess sensation and mobility before allowing ambulation.
Intrathecal Opioid Analgesics	
Provides analgesia for most of first-stage labor without maternal sedation. A very small dose of the drug is needed because it is injected very near the spinal cord where sensory fibers enter. Usually not adequate for late labor or the birth itself.	1. Observe for the common side effects of nausea, vomiting, and pruritus. Notify the anesthesia clinician if these effects occur, and have an antagonist such as naloxone or naltrexone available. 2. Observe for delayed respiratory depression, depending on the drug given. Use a pulse oximeter as indicated.
Local Infiltration Anesthesia	
Numbs perineum for episiotomy or repair of laceration at vaginal birth. No relief of labor pain. Not adequate for forceps-assisted birth.	1. Assess for drug allergies, especially to dental anesthetics because they are related to those used in maternity care. 2. Apply ice to perineum to reduce edema and hematoma formation and to increase comfort.
Pudendal Block	
Numbs the lower vagina and perineum for vaginal birth. No relief of labor pain because it is done just before birth. Provides adequate anesthesia for many forceps-assisted births.	1. Use the same interventions as for local infiltration. A woman may be alarmed by the long needle (about 6 inches [15 cm]). Teach her that it must be long to reach the pudendal nerve and that it will be inserted only about 0.5 inch (1.25 cm) into her tissue. Tell her that a guide ("trumpet") will be used to avoid damaging her or her fetus's tissue.

Table continued on following page

TABLE 19–3
• • • • • • • • • • •

Pharmacologic Methods of Intrapartum Pain Management Continued

Method and Uses	*Nursing Considerations*
Epidural Block	
Labor: Insertion of catheter provides pain relief for labor and vaginal birth (T10–S5 levels). *Cesarean birth:* If epidural was used during labor, level of block can be extended upward (T4–T6 level). Also used for planned cesarean birth and postbirth tubal ligation.	1. Prehydrate the woman with warmed nonglucose crystalloid solution such as Ringer's lactate solution. Common amounts: 500–1,000 ml for labor and vaginal birth; 1,500–2,000 ml for cesarean birth. 2. Displace uterus to left manually or with a wedge placed under the woman's right side to enhance placental perfusion. 3. Assess for hypotension at least every 5 min after block is begun and with each new dose until vital signs are stable. Report to anesthesia clinician: systolic BP of <110 mm Hg or a fall of 20% or more from baseline levels, pallor, or diaphoresis. 4. Assess fetal heart rate for signs of impaired placental perfusion and report to anesthesia clinician and nurse-midwife: tachycardia (>150–160/min), bradycardia (<110–120/min), late decelerations (see Table 18–2). 5. If hypotension or signs of impaired placental perfusion occur, increase the rate of infusion of nonadditive IV fluid, turn woman to her left side and administer oxygen by face mask (8–10 L/min). Have ephedrine available (usually included in epidural tray). 6. Observe for a full bladder and catheterize as ordered. 7. Transfer with help to avoid muscle strains to nurse or client. 8. Ambulate only after sensation and movement have returned. Have another nurse's assistance with the first ambulation.
Subarachnoid Block	

Cesarean birth: Is simpler and can be established more quickly than epidural block.
May rarely be used for complicated vaginal birth.
Does not provide pain relief for labor because it is done just before birth.
	1. See Epidural Block for these interventions:
	  a. IV prehydration
	  b. Uterine displacement
	  c. Observation of blood pressure and fetal heart rate
	  d. Care for hypotension or signs of impaired placental perfusion
	  e. Observation for bladder distension
	  f. Transfer and ambulation precautions
	2. Observe for postspinal headache: a headache that is worse when the woman is upright and that may disappear when she is lying flat. Notify anesthesia clinician if it occurs (a blood patch may be done).
	3. Nursing interventions for postspinal headache: encourage bed rest, increase oral fluids if not contraindicated, give oral caffeine, and give analgesics as ordered.

General Anesthesia	
Cesarean birth if epidural or spinal block is not possible or if the woman refuses regional anesthesia. May be required for emergency procedures such as replacement of inverted uterus.	1. Determine type and time of last food intake on admission. 2. Restrict oral intake to clear liquids or as ordered. Consult with physician or nurse-midwife if surgical intervention is likely. 3. Report to anesthesia clinician: oral intake before and during labor, vomiting. 4. Displace uterus (see Epidural Block). 5. Give ordered drugs such as sodium citrate and citric acid (Bicitra). 6. Maintain cricoid pressure (Sellick's maneuver) during intubation. 7. Maintain woman in a side-lying position (after surgery) until protective (gag) reflexes have returned. 8. Interventions for postoperative respiratory depression: give oxygen by face mask; observe oxygen saturation with pulse oximetry until woman is awake and alert; have woman take several deep breaths if oxygen saturation falls below 95%.

Abbreviations: CNS, central nervous system; BP, blood pressure; IV, intravenous.

dict every woman who will require general anesthesia. The nursing diagnosis is

■ Risk for Aspiration related to impaired protective laryngeal reflexes.
Expected Outcome: The woman will not aspirate gastric contents during the perioperative period.

Interventions

Nursing interventions relate to identifying factors that increase a woman's risk for aspiration, and collaborative and nursing measures to reduce the risk of aspiration or lung injury.

Identifying Risk Factors

Report oral intake both before and after admission to the anesthesia clinician. In general, oral intake during labor is restricted to medications, clear liquids (usually ice chips), Popsicles, or hard candies. Chart all oral intake during labor.

Vomiting is a common discomfort during normal labor, regardless of the mother's oral intake. If vomiting occurs, chart the time, quantity, and character (amount, color, presence of undigested food).

Reducing Risk of Aspiration or Lung Injury

Nursing and medical personnel collaborate to reduce a woman's risk for pulmonary complications.

Perioperative Care. Discontinue the woman's oral intake until after consulting the physician or nurse-midwife if surgical intervention seems likely because the woman may need general anesthesia. Give ordered medications such as sodium citrate and citric acid (Bicitra). Either the nurse or

anesthesia clinician may give parenteral drugs, such as glycopyrrolate (Robinul), depending on when they are administered.

An experienced nurse or a trained anesthesia assistant provides cricoid pressure (Sellick's maneuver) to block the esophagus until the woman is intubated and the cuff of the endotracheal tube is inflated. Successful intubation with the cuffed endotracheal tube blocks passage of any gastric contents into the trachea.

Postoperative Care. Following general anesthesia, the woman is extubated after her protective laryngeal reflexes have returned. Position her on her side until she is awake to allow gravity to drain her secretions or emesis.

Birth facility protocols guide postoperative care. Administer oxygen by mask or face tent until the woman is awake and alert because the agents used for general anesthesia are respiratory depressants. Monitor oxygen saturation with a pulse oximeter. If her oxygen saturation falls below 95%, have her take several deep breaths. Deep breathing also helps her eliminate inhalational anesthetics and reduces stasis of pulmonary secretions.

Assess the woman's pulse, respiration, and blood pressure every 15 minutes for 1 hour or until stable, then continue according to policy. Observe her color for pallor or cyanosis, which suggest shock or hypoventilation.

Evaluation

Interventions for this nursing diagnosis are preventive and short-term because it is a temporary high-risk situation. The goal is met if the woman does not aspirate gastric contents during the perioperative period.

KEY CONCEPTS

■ Childbirth pain is unique because it is normal and self-limiting, can be prepared for, and ends with a baby's birth.
■ Excess or poorly relieved pain can be harmful to the mother and fetus.
■ Pain is a complex physical and psychological experience. It is subjective and personal.
■ Four sources of pain are present in most labors, but other physical and psychological factors may increase or decrease the pain felt from these sources. These sources are cervical dilation, uterine ischemia, pressure and pulling on pelvic structures, and distension of the vagina and perineum.
■ Relaxation enhances other pain management techniques.
■ Any drug that the expectant mother takes, whether therapeutic

or abused, also may affect the fetus. Fetal effects may be direct or indirect.
■ Cutaneous and mental stimulation techniques reduce pain perception. Techniques should be varied to prevent habituation.
■ The purpose of breathing techniques is to increase relaxation. Lamaze breathing should be no slower than half the woman's normal respiratory rate and no faster than twice her normal rate.
■ The physiologic alterations of pregnancy may affect a woman's response to medications.
■ The nurse should observe for respiratory depression, primarily in the newborn, when the mother has received opioid analgesics during labor.
■ The major advantages of regional pain management methods are

that the woman can participate in the birth and that she retains her protective airway reflexes.
■ The nurse should observe for and take actions to prevent maternal hypotension with an epidural or subarachnoid block.
■ The nurse should observe for fetal heart rate changes associated with impaired placental perfusion if the woman is at risk for hypotension, such as with epidural or subarachnoid blocks.
■ The main nursing observations for the woman who receives epidural or intrathecal opioids are for nausea and vomiting, pruritus, and delayed respiratory depression.
■ Regurgitation with aspiration of acidic gastric contents is the greatest risk for a woman who receives general anesthesia.

ANSWERS TO CRITICAL THINKING EXERCISE 19-1

1. Truc's labor progress and pattern of contractions plus her tension suggest that she may need medication. However, the nurse should not assume that she needs or wants medication. Breathing techniques or other nonpharmacologic measures may be adequate for Truc.

   The nurse must not assume that Truc does not need pain relief because she smiles and has not requested pain medication. Asian women often value stoicism and are concerned with harmonious relationships. Truc may be smiling to please the nurse rather than because she is comfortable.

2. The nurse needs additional data about Truc's needs and plans for pain relief.

3. The nurse can share observations about Truc's body posture during contractions. If Truc does not speak English well, an interpreter may improve assessment of her need for pain relief. The nurse can demonstrate nonpharmacologic actions, such as breathing techniques, for Truc to use with or without medication.

REFERENCES AND READINGS

American Academy of Pediatrics & American College of Obstetricians and Gynecologists. (1997). *Guidelines for perinatal care* (4th ed.). Elk Grove Village, IL, and Washington, DC: Author.

American College of Obstetricians and Gynecologists. (1996). *Obstetric analgesia and anesthesia* (ACOG Technical Bulletin No. 225). *International Journal of Gynecology and Obstetrics, 54,* 281–292.

Association of Women's Health, Obstetric, and Neonatal Nurses. (1996a). Clinical commentary: Obstetric epidural analgesia and the role of the professional registered nurse. *AWHONN Voice, 4*(8).

Association of Women's Health, Obstetric, and Neonatal Nurses. (1996b). *Position statement: Role of the registered nurse (RN) in the management of the patient receiving analgesia by catheter techniques (epidural, intrathecal, intrapleural, or peripheral nerve catheters).* Washington, DC: Author.

Creehan, P. A. (1996). Pain relief and comfort measures during labor. In K. R. Simpson & P. A. Creehan (Eds.), *AWHONN's perinatal nursing* (pp. 227–245). Philadelphia: Lippincott.

Cunningham, F. G., MacDonald, P. C., Gant, N. F., Leveno, K. J., Gilstrap, L. C., Hankins, G. D. V., et al. (1997). *Williams obstetrics* (20th ed.). Norwalk, CT: Appleton & Lange.

Dewan, D. M., & Hood, D. D. (1997). *Practical obstetric anesthesia.* Philadelphia: Saunders.

Dick, M. J. (1995). Assessment and measurement of acute pain. *Journal of Obstetric, Gynecologic, and Neonatal Nursing, 24*(9), 843–848.

Goer, H. (1995). *Obstetric myths versus research realities: A guide to the medical literature.* Westport, CT: Bergin & Garvey.

Kendrick, J. (1996). *Controversies in decision-making for pain control in L & D* (Cassette Recording M1). Anaheim, CA: MCN Convention.

Lowe, N. K. (1996). The pain and discomfort of labor and birth. *Journal of Obstetric, Gynecologic, and Neonatal Nursing, 25*(1), 82–92.

Manning, J. (1996). Intrathecal narcotics: New approach for labor analgesia. *Journal of Obstetric, Gynecologic, and Neonatal Nursing, 25*(3), 221–224.

Pasero, C. L., & Britt, R. (1998). Managing pain during childbirth. *American Journal of Nursing, 98*(8), 10–11.

Simkin, P. (1995). Reducing pain and enhancing progress in labor: A guide to nonpharmacologic methods for maternity caregivers. *Birth, 22*(3), 161–171.

Thorp, J., & Breedlove, G. (1996). Epidural analgesia in labor: An evaluation of risks and benefits. *Birth, 23*(2), 63–83.

Weber, S. E. (1996). Cultural aspects of pain in childbearing women. *Journal of Obstetric, Gynecologic, and Neonatal Nursing, 25*(1), 67–72.

Youngstrom, P. C., Baker, S. W., & Miller, J. L. (1996). Epidurals redefined in analgesia and anesthesia: A distinction with a difference. *Journal of Obstetric, Gynecologic, and Neonatal Nursing, 25*(4), 350–354.

## 20

Nursing Care During Obstetric Procedures

LEARNING OBJECTIVES

After studying this chapter, you should be able to:

- Identify clinical situations in which specific obstetric procedures are appropriate.
- Explain risks, precautions, and contraindications for each procedure.
- Identify nursing considerations for each procedure.
- Identify methods to provide effective emotional support to the woman having an obstetric procedure.
- Apply the nursing process to plan care for the woman having a cesarean birth.

DEFINITIONS

abruptio placentae Premature separation of a normally implanted placenta.

amniotomy Artificial rupture of the amniotic sac (fetal membranes).

augmentation of labor Artificial stimulation of uterine contractions that have become ineffective.

cephalopelvic disproportion Fetal head size that is too large to fit through the maternal pelvis at birth. Also called fetopelvic disproportion.

cesarean birth Surgical birth of the fetus through an incision in the abdominal wall and uterus.

chignon Newborn scalp edema created by a vacuum extractor.

chorioamnionitis Inflammation of the amniotic sac (fetal membranes), usually caused by bacterial or viral infections. Also called amnionitis.

dystocia Difficult or prolonged labor, often associated with abnormal uterine activity and cephalopelvic disproportion.

episiotomy Surgical incision of the perineum to enlarge the vaginal opening.

hydramnios Excessive volume of amniotic fluid (more than 2,000 ml at term). Also called polyhydramnios.

iatrogenic An adverse condition resulting from treatment.

induction of labor Artificial initiation of labor.

nuchal cord Umbilical cord around the fetal neck.

oligohydramnios Abnormally small quantity of amniotic fluid (less than 500 ml at term).

placenta previa Abnormal implantation of the placenta in the lower uterus.

premature rupture of the membranes Spontaneous rupture of the membranes before the onset of labor. The gestation may be term, preterm, or postterm.

version Turning the fetus from one presentation to another before birth, usually from breech to cephalic.

Although labor is a normal process, special procedures are sometimes needed to help the mother or fetus. A physician or nurse-midwife performs these procedures; nursing considerations for each are addressed.

▪ Amniotomy

Indications

Amniotomy may be performed to induce labor, augment labor, or allow internal electronic fetal monitoring and fetal scalp blood sampling (see Chapter 18). Although amniotomy is often used for induction or stimulation of labor, its actual effectiveness for these purposes is not always supported by research (Busowski & Parsons, 1995).

Risks

Amniotomy is performed by the physician or nurse-midwife. The nurse must observe for three risks associated with amniotomy and assist in emergency procedures.

PROLAPSE OF THE UMBILICAL CORD
The primary risk is that the umbilical cord will slip down in the gush of fluid. The cord can be compressed between the fetal presenting part and the woman's pelvis, obstructing blood flow to and from the placenta and reducing fetal gas exchange.

INFECTION
With interruption of the membrane barrier, vaginal organisms have free access to the uterine cavity and may cause chorioamnionitis. The risk is low at first but increases as the interval between membrane rupture and birth increases. Birth within 24 hours of amniotomy is desirable, although there is no absolute time when infection occurs.

ABRUPTIO PLACENTAE
Abruptio placentae may occur if the uterus is distended with excessive amniotic fluid when the membranes rupture. As the uterus collapses with discharge of the amniotic fluid, the area of placental attachment shrinks. The placenta then no longer fits its implantation site and partially separates. A large area of placental disruption reduces fetal oxygenation, nutrition, and waste disposal.

Technique

A disposable plastic hook (Amnihook) is commonly used to perforate the amniotic sac (Fig. 20–1). The birth attendant does a vaginal examination to determine cervical dilation and effacement, fetal station, and fetal presenting part.

Amniotomy is deferred if the fetal presenting part is high or if the presentation is not cephalic. The risk of a prolapsed cord is higher in these situations because more room is available for the cord to slip down.

The hook is passed through the cervix and the membranes are snagged. The hole is enlarged with the finger, allowing fluid to drain.

Nursing Considerations

OBTAINING BASELINE INFORMATION
The fetal heart rate is assessed with auscultation or electronic monitoring to identify a reassuring rate and pattern before amniotomy is done. The initial fetal assessment provides a baseline to compare later assessments with. A minimum of 20 to 30 minutes is needed for adequate baseline fetal evaluation.

ASSISTING WITH AMNIOTOMY
Before amniotomy, place two or three underpads under the woman's buttocks to absorb the fluid. A folded bath towel under the buttocks absorbs a large quantity of amniotic fluid. Other supplies needed are a disposable plastic hook, a sterile glove, and a packet of sterile lubricant.

PROVIDING CARE AFTER AMNIOTOMY
Nursing care after amniotomy is the same as that following spontaneous membrane rupture.

Identifying Complications. Assess the fetal heart rate for at least 1 full minute after amniotomy. Nonreassuring monitor patterns or significant changes from previous assessments are reported promptly to the birth attendant. Cord compression is usually accompanied by a rate of less than 100 beats per minute (BPM), which worsens during contractions.

Chart the quantity, color, and odor of the amniotic fluid. Refer to Chapter 17 for expected findings and signs of abnormality in the amniotic fluid.

Assess the woman's temperature every 2 to 4 hours after the membranes rupture. Report elevations above 38°C (100.4°F). Fetal tachycardia (above 160 BPM) may precede maternal fever.

CRITICAL THINKING EXERCISE 20–1

A physician performs an amniotomy on a laboring woman whose cervix is dilated to 5 cm. The amniotic fluid is pale yellow and moderate in amount and has a strong odor. The fetal heart rate is 164 BPM and accelerates when the fetus moves. Maternal vital signs are temperature, 37.6°C (99.7°F); pulse, 92; respirations, 22; and blood pressure, 116/80 mm Hg. Contractions are moderate to firm in intensity and occur every 3 to 4 minutes with a duration of 50 to 60 seconds and complete uterine relaxation between contractions.

1. Which of these observations should the nurse regard as normal? Which observations are abnormal?
2. Should the nurse modify routine labor care based on the postamniotomy assessments?

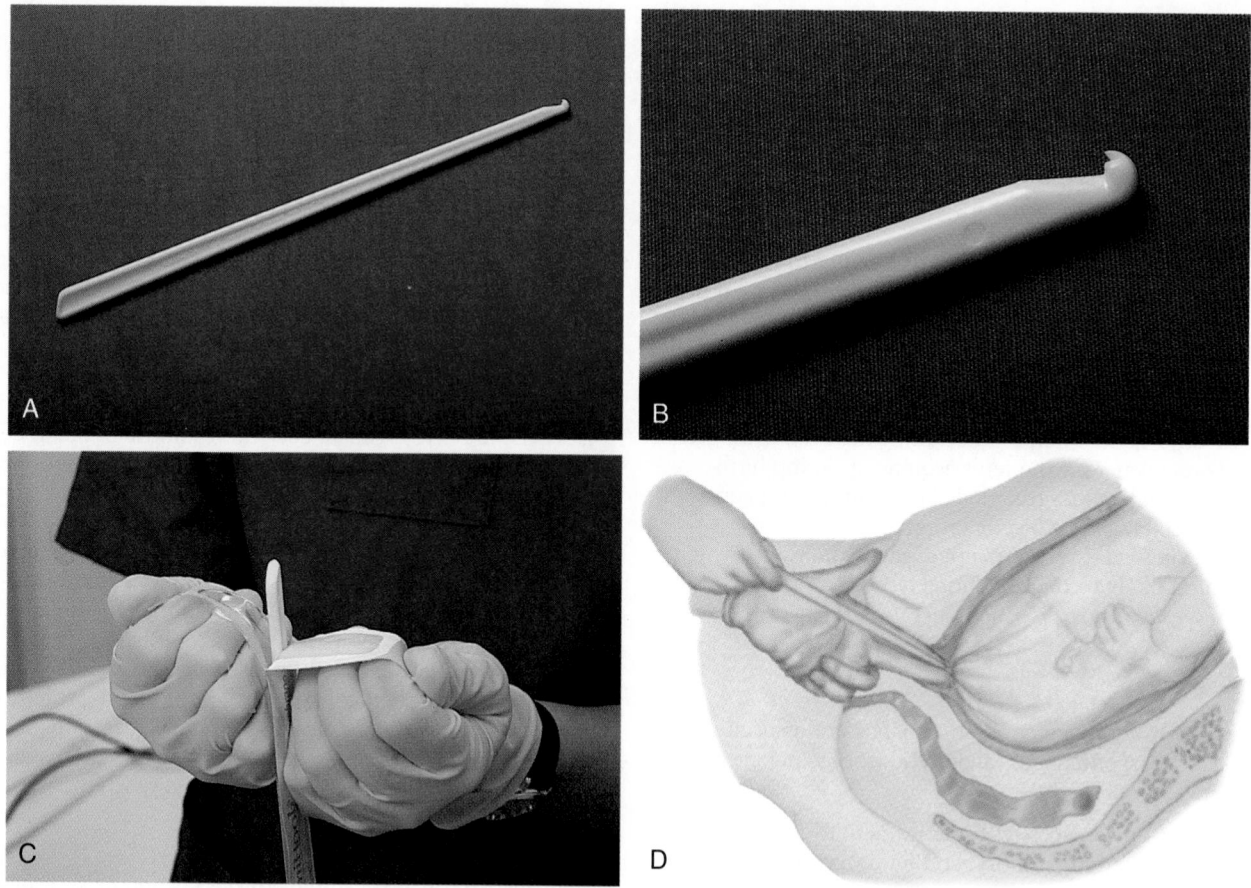

FIGURE 20–1

A, Disposable plastic membrane perforator. *B,* Close-up view of hook end of plastic membrane perforator. *C,* Correct method of opening the package. *D,* Technique for artificial rupture of membranes.

Promoting Comfort. Amniotic fluid continues to leak from the woman's vagina. Change the underpads regularly to keep her drier and reduce the moist environment, which favors bacterial growth.

Induction and Augmentation of Labor

Induction and augmentation of labor use artificial methods to stimulate uterine contractions. Techniques and nursing care are similar for both induction and augmentation.

Indications

Induction of labor is considered when continuing the pregnancy may jeopardize the health of the woman or fetus and when labor and vaginal birth are considered safe. Labor induction is not done if the fetus must be delivered more quickly than the process permits; a cesarean birth would be performed instead. Induction may be done for these specific conditions:

- Pregnancy-induced hypertension, which is associated with reduced placental blood flow

- Spontaneous rupture of the membranes at or near term without onset of labor
- Chorioamnionitis (inflammation of the amniotic sac)
- Maternal medical conditions that are worsening with continuation of the pregnancy (e.g., diabetes, renal disease, pulmonary disease)
- Conditions in which the intrauterine environment is hostile to fetal well-being (such as intrauterine fetal growth restriction, post-term gestation, maternal-fetal blood incompatibility)
- Fetal death

Induction solely for convenience is not recommended. However, factors such as a history of rapid labors or living a long distance from the hospital are valid reasons to induce labor because of the real possibility that the baby would otherwise be born in uncontrolled circumstances.

Prenatal testing sometimes reveals a fetal anomaly for which specialized neonatal care at a distant facility will be needed. The mother may be transported to that facility for labor induction, with the necessary equipment and specialists assembled there to care for the newborn.

Augmentation of labor with oxytocin is considered when labor has begun spontaneously but progress has slowed or stopped because of poor contractions.

Contraindications

Any contraindication to labor and vaginal birth is a contraindication to induction or augmentation of labor. These conditions may include the following:

- Placenta previa, which may result in hemorrhage during labor
- Umbilical cord prolapse
- Abnormal fetal presentation (vaginal birth is often more hazardous; also, the fetus may turn to a normal position by the time spontaneous labor occurs)
- Fetal presenting part above the pelvic inlet, which may be associated with cephalopelvic disproportion or a preterm fetus
- Active genital herpes infection, which can cause serious consequences if the fetus acquires it during birth
- Maternal pelvic structural abnormalities that contribute to cephalopelvic disproportion
- Previous classic (vertical) cesarean incision, which is more likely to rupture during labor than the more common low transverse incision

Risks

Induction and augmentation of labor are associated with risks, as is spontaneous labor. These risks include the following:

- Hypertonic (excessive) uterine activity, which can reduce placental perfusion and fetal oxygenation
- Uterine rupture
- Maternal water intoxication, which is more likely if a dextrose and water intravenous solution is used to dilute the oxytocin and with rates greater than 20 mU/min (Cunningham et al., 1997).

Technique

Surgical and medical methods may be used for labor induction or augmentation. Amniotomy is the method of surgical induction and augmentation because rupturing membranes stimulates uterine contractions if the cervix is favorable.

Medical methods for induction or augmentation use drugs such as prostaglandin or intravenous oxytocin (Pitocin), or both, to stimulate contractions.

DETERMINING WHETHER INDUCTION IS INDICATED

The birth attendant evaluates whether labor and birth are safer for the woman or fetus than continuing the pregnancy. Labor is not induced if the fetus is younger than 39 weeks' gestational age unless there is a compelling reason. Also, induction is more likely to be successful at term because prelabor cervical changes favor dilation.

Cervical assessment estimates how favorable the cervix is for induction. The Bishop scoring system (Table 20–1) uses five factors to estimate cervical readiness for labor: cervical dilation, effacement, consistency, position, and fetal station. Induction is likely to be successful with a Bishop score higher than 6.

Because the Bishop score is subjective and its accuracy depends on the experience of the examiner, more objective methods for evaluating a woman's readiness for induction of labor are being explored. One method being studied is assessment of fetal fibronectin in the cervical and vaginal secretions. Studies have noted that this fetal protein is rarely present in the cervical and vaginal secretions from 21 weeks until 37 weeks, but it is present and increases as labor nears (Blanch, Oláh, & Walkinshaw, 1996).

CERVICAL RIPENING

Procedures to ripen (or soften) the cervix and make it more likely to dilate with the forces of labor are a common adjunct to induction. Most are done the day before the scheduled induction. If there are no complications, the woman may go home afterward and return for induction the following morning.

Chemical Methods. Preparations containing prostaglandin E₂ (PGE₂) may be used to facilitate cervical ripening. PGE₂ may be given as an intravaginal gel, an intracervical gel, or a timed-release vaginal insert (Table 20–2). It is administered in a setting in which fetal monitoring and emergency care are immediately available.

TABLE 20–1

Bishop Scoring System to Evaluate the Cervix

Factor	Score			
	0	1	2	3
Dilation	0 cm	1–2 cm	3–4 cm	5–6 cm
Effacement	0%–30%	40%–50%	60%–70%	≥80%
Station	3	2	1 or 0	+1 or +2
Cervical consistency	Firm	Medium	Soft	
Cervical position	Posterior	Middle	Anterior	

Note: This system is used to estimate how easily a woman's labor can be induced. Higher scores are associated with a greater likelihood of successful induction because her cervix has undergone prelabor changes, often called ripening. A woman who has given birth before usually has a successful induction when her Bishop score is 5 or higher. Delivery in a woman who is having her first baby is most successfully induced if her score is 7 or higher.

Adapted from Bishop, E. H. (1964). Pelvic scoring for elective induction. *Obstetrics and Gynecology, 24*(2), 266–268.

TABLE 20-2

Prostaglandin E₂ Preparations for Cervical Ripening

Hospital-Prepared Gel	Commercially Prepared Gel	Commercially Prepared Vaginal Insert
Dosage		
For vaginal application: up to 5 mg. For intracervical application: 0.5 mg. Repeat up to 3 times in 24 hr at 4- to 6-hr intervals.	For intracervical application: 0.5 mg. Repeat up to 3 times in 24 hr at 6-hr intervals.	10 mg in a timed-release vaginal insert. Rate of release is 0.3 mg/hr. Remove at onset of active labor or 12 hr after insertion.
Actions for Uterine Hyperstimulation		
Place woman in side-lying position. Provide oxygen by face mask at 8–10 L/min. Administer tocolytic drug such as terbutaline or magnesium sulfate.	Same as for hospital-prepared gel.	Remove insert. Implement actions as for hospital-prepared gel if necessary.
When Oxytocin for Induction May Begin		
4 hr after last dose.	6–12 hr after last dose.	30 min after removal of insert.

The major adverse reaction to PGE₂ is hypertonic uterine contractions, which can reduce placental blood flow and oxygen exchange. Prostaglandin should be given cautiously to women who have asthma, glaucoma, or pulmonary, hepatic, or renal disease. The woman should lie flat for 15 to 20 minutes after the gel is inserted to reduce leakage. The fetal heart rate should be monitored for at least 30 minutes for changes, and the uterus should be assessed for excessive contractions.

Misoprostol (Cytotec) is becoming popular for preinduction cervical ripening because of its low cost, stability, and ease of use. Misoprostol is a synthetic prostaglandin tablet that is primarily used for prevention of gastric ulcers. Its use for cervical ripening is currently an unlabeled one. The dose range is 25 to 50 μg, inserted in the vagina. Uterine hyperstimulation is more likely if the 50-μg dose is used.

Mechanical Methods. The most common mechanical method for cervical ripening involves placement of hydrophilic (moisture-attracting) inserts into the cervical canal, where they absorb water and swell, gradually dilating the cervix. Examples of these dilators are the following:

- Dilapan, a synthetic material
- Lamicel, a synthetic sponge containing 450 mg of magnesium sulfate
- Laminaria tents, sterile cone-shaped preparations of dried seaweed

The woman usually goes home overnight, and oxytocin induction of labor begins the following morning.

OXYTOCIN ADMINISTRATION

Oxytocin is a powerful drug, and it is impossible to predict a woman's response to it. Several precautions reduce the chance of adverse reactions in the mother and fetus.

- Oxytocin is diluted in a physiologic electrolyte-containing fluid and given as a secondary (piggyback) infusion so that it can be stopped quickly if complications develop (Fig. 20–2).

- The oxytocin line is inserted into the primary (nonadditive, or maintenance) intravenous line as close as possible to the venipuncture site (the proximal port) to limit the amount of drug infused after changing to the nonadditive fluid.

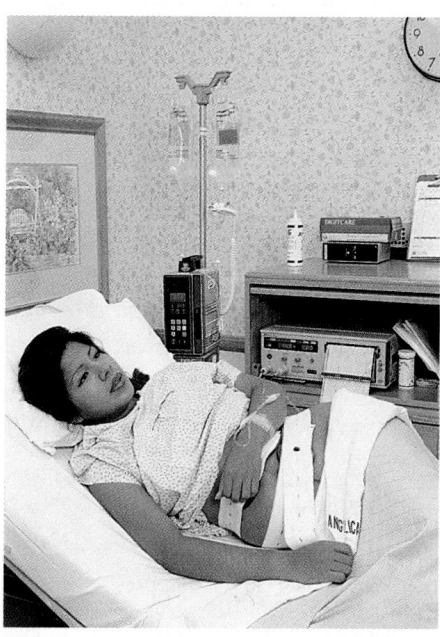

FIGURE 20-2

Intravenous oxytocin setup for induction or augmentation of labor. The primary line (nonadditive, or maintenance line) on the left side of the pole contains no medication. The secondary line with the orange "medication added" label contains oxytocin. The secondary oxytocin line is regulated by the infusion pump and is inserted into the lowest port in the primary fluid line. An external fetal monitor is used to assess the fetal response to oxytocin-stimulated contractions. The woman lies on her side to promote uterine blood flow.

DRUG GUIDE

Oxytocin (Pitocin)

Classification: Oxytocic.

Action: Synthetic compound identical to the natural hormone from the posterior pituitary. Stimulates uterine smooth muscle, resulting in increased strength, duration, and frequency of uterine contractions. Uterine sensitivity to oxytocin increases gradually during gestation. Oxytocin has vasoactive and antidiuretic properties.

Indications: Induction or augmentation of labor at or near term. Maintenance of firm uterine contraction after birth to control postpartum bleeding. Management of inevitable or incomplete abortion.

Dosage and Route *Induction or Augmentation of Labor*

1. *Intravenous infusion* via a secondary (piggyback) line. Dilute 10 units (1 ml) of oxytocin in 1,000 ml of a balanced electrolyte solution such as lactated Ringer's solution, resulting in a concentration of 10 milliunits (mU) of oxytocin per milliliter. Other mixtures of oxytocin and solution may be used, such as 15 units of oxytocin (1.5 ml) plus 250 ml of intravenous solution, resulting in a concentration of 60 mU/ml. Oxytocin infusion is controlled with a pump. The drug may also be given in 10-minute pulsed infusions rather than continuously.
2. Administration protocols vary, but guidelines from the American College of Obstetricians and Gynecologists (1995) suggest (1) starting dosages of 0.5 to 2 mU/min, and (2) increasing dosage by 1 to 2 mU/min increments every 30 to 60 minutes. The actual oxytocin dose is based on uterine response and absence of adverse effects. Shorter intervals between dose increases may result in uterine hyperstimulation. A lower starting dose is usually required to augment labor.
3. After an adequate contraction pattern is established and the cervix is dilated 5 to 6 cm, the oxytocin may be reduced by similar increments.

Control of Postpartum Bleeding
Intravenous infusion: Dilute 10 to 40 units in 1,000 ml of intravenous solution. The rate of infusion must control uterine atony. Begin at a rate of 20 to 40 mU/min, increasing or decreasing the rate according to uterine response and the rate of postpartum bleeding. *Intramuscular injection:* Inject 10 units after delivery of the placenta.

Inevitable or Incomplete Abortion
Dilute 10 units in 500 ml of intravenous solution and infuse at a rate of 10 to 20 mU/min.

Absorption: Intravenous, immediate; intramuscular, 3 to 5 minutes.

Excretion: Liver and urine.

Contraindications and Precautions: Include, but are not limited to, placenta previa, vasa previa, nonreassuring fetal heart rate patterns, abnormal fetal presentation, prolapsed umbilical cord, presenting part above the pelvic inlet, previous classic uterine incision, active genital herpes infection, pelvic structural deformities, invasive cervical carcinoma.

Adverse Reactions: Most result from hypersensitivity to drug or excessive dosage. Adverse reactions include hypertonic uterine activity, impaired uterine blood flow, uterine rupture, and abruptio placentae. Uterine hypertonicity may result in fetal bradycardia, tachycardia, reduced fetal heart rate variability, and late decelerations. Fetal asphyxia may occur with diminished uterine blood flow. Fetal or maternal trauma, or both, may occur from rapid birth. Prolonged administration may cause maternal fluid retention, leading to water intoxication. Hypotension (seen with rapid intravenous injection), tachycardia, cardiac dysrhythmias, and subarachnoid hemorrhage are rare adverse reactions.

Nursing Considerations

Intrapartum: Assess the fetal heart rate for at least 20 minutes before induction to identify reassuring or nonreassuring patterns. Perform Leopold's maneuvers,

a vaginal examination, or both to identify fetal presentation. If nonreassuring fetal heart rate patterns are identified or if fetal presentation is other than cephalic, notify the physician and do not begin induction.

Observe uterine activity for establishment of effective labor pattern: contraction frequency every 2 to 3 minutes, duration of 40 to 90 seconds, intensity of 50 to 80 mm Hg (measured with an intrauterine pressure catheter). Observe for hypertonic uterine activity: contractions less than 2 minutes apart, rest interval shorter than 60 seconds, duration longer than 90 seconds, or an elevated resting tone greater than 20 mm Hg (measured with an intrauterine pressure catheter). Observe fetal heart rate for nonreassuring patterns such as tachycardia, bradycardia, decreased variability, and late decelerations.

If uterine hypertonicity or a nonreassuring fetal heart rate pattern occurs, intervene to reduce uterine activity and increase fetal oxygenation: stop the oxytocin infusion; increase the rate of nonadditive solution; position the woman in a side-lying position; and administer oxygen by snug face mask at 8 to 10 L/min. Notify the physician of adverse reactions, nursing interventions, and response to interventions. Record the maternal blood pressure every 30 to 60 minutes or with each dosage increase. Record intake and output.

Postpartum: Observe uterus for firmness, height, and deviation. Massage until firm if uterus is soft ("boggy"). Observe lochia for color, quantity, and presence of clots. Notify birth attendant if uterus fails to remain contracted or if lochia is bright red or contains large clots. Assess for cramping. Assess vital signs every 15 minutes or according to protocol. Monitor intake and output to identify fluid retention or bladder distension.

Inevitable or Incomplete Abortion: Observe for cramping, vaginal bleeding, clots, and passage of products of conception. Observe maternal vital signs, intake, and output as noted under postpartum nursing implications.

- Oxytocin is started slowly, increased gradually, and regulated with an infusion pump.
- Uterine activity and fetal heart rate and patterns are monitored when oxytocin is given and throughout labor.

The woman's uterus becomes more sensitive to oxytocin as labor progresses. Therefore, the rate of oxytocin infusion may be gradually reduced when she is in the active phase of labor, about 5 to 6 cm of cervical dilation. It may be stopped or reduced after her membranes rupture. When labor is augmented with oxytocin, a lower total dose is usually needed to achieve adequate contractions.

Nursing Considerations

In addition to basic intrapartum care, the nurse observes the woman and fetus for complications and takes corrective actions if abnormalities are noted. If a woman has a cervical ripening procedure, the same nursing care applies until she is discharged home.

The nurse has a great responsibility when administering oxytocin to a pregnant woman. The nurse must decide, within the facility's protocols and medical orders, when to start, change, or stop the oxytocin infusion. This responsibility requires additional education and refinement of the nurse's critical thinking skills.

OBSERVING THE FETAL RESPONSE

Oxytocin stimulates uterine contractions, and they may become too strong (hypertonic). Hypertonic contractions can reduce placental blood flow and therefore reduce exchange of fetal oxygen and waste products. Before induction or augmentation of labor, the nurse determines whether the fetal heart rate and patterns are reassuring. The fetal heart rate is charted in the labor record every 15 minutes during first-stage labor and every 5 minutes during the second stage (Menihan, 1996).

The nurse remains alert for fetal heart rate patterns that suggest reduced placental exchange secondary to hypertonic contractions. Examples of these patterns are fetal bradycardia (rate less than 110 to 120 BPM at term), tachycardia (rate more than 150 to 160 BPM at term), late decelerations (slowing after the peak of the contraction), and decreased fetal heart rate variability (reduced rate fluctuations). Reduced placental exchange also may have causes other than excess uterine activity, such as maternal hypotension. The nurse must assess the woman and fetus carefully to identify the most likely cause of the problem and the indicated corrective actions.

If nonreassuring patterns occur or if contractions are hypertonic, the nurse takes steps to reduce uterine activity and increase fetal oxygenation. These steps include:

1. Reducing or stopping the oxytocin infusion and increasing the rate of the primary nonadditive infusion.
2. Keeping the woman on her side to prevent aortocaval compression and increase placental blood flow.
3. Giving 100% oxygen by snug face mask at a rate of 8 to 10 L/min to increase the woman's oxygen saturation, making more oxygen available for the fetus.

CRITICAL THINKING EXERCISE 20–2
• • • • • • • • • •

A woman is having labor induced with oxytocin. Her cervix is 4 cm dilated and fully effaced, and the fetal head is at station 0. The nurse notes that the fetal heart rate (internal monitor) is near its baseline of 120 to 130 BPM, with variability of 10 BPM. Contractions are firm (100 mm Hg with intrauterine pressure catheter), occur every 2 to 2.5 minutes, and typically last 95 to 100 seconds.

1. What is the correct interpretation of these assessments?
2. What are appropriate nursing actions in this situation, and why are they done?

CRITICAL TO REMEMBER
• • • • • • • • • •

Signs of Hypertonic Uterine Activity

- Contraction duration longer than 90 seconds.
- Contractions occurring less than 2 minutes apart or relaxation of less than 60 seconds between contractions.
- Uterine resting tone above 20 mm Hg (with intrauterine pressure catheter).
- Peak pressure higher than 90 mm Hg during first-stage labor (with intrauterine pressure catheter).
- A fetal heart rate pattern of late decelerations may accompany hypertonic uterine activity.

Nursing Actions for Hypertonic Uterine Activity

- Reduce or stop the oxytocin infusion.
- Increase the rate of the primary nonadditive infusion.
- Keep the laboring woman in a lateral position.
- Give oxygen by snug face mask, 8 to 10 mL/min.
- Notify the physician or nurse-midwife.

The physician may order a drug to reduce uterine activity, such as terbutaline (Brethine) or magnesium sulfate.

OBSERVING THE MOTHER'S RESPONSE

The woman who has a cervical ripening procedure may begin labor before her scheduled induction. The signs of labor's onset should be reviewed (see Chapter 17), and she should be instructed to return to the birth facility if these signs occur.

Uterine activity must be assessed for hypertonus, which can reduce fetal oxygenation and contribute to uterine rupture. Contractions are assessed for frequency, duration, and intensity, and uterine resting tone is assessed for relaxation of at least 60 seconds between contractions. Uterine activity observations are charted at the same intervals as the fetal heart rate. Corrective actions for hypertonic uterine activity are the same as those listed in the discussion of the fetal response. Additionally, a tocolytic drug such as terbutaline may be given.

The woman's blood pressure and pulse are taken every 30 to 60 minutes, or with each increase in the oxytocin dose, to identify changes from her baseline. Her temperature is checked every 2 to 4 hours to identify infection, which can occur with ruptured membranes.

Recording intake and output identifies fluid retention, which may precede water intoxication. Signs and symptoms of water intoxication include headache, blurred vision, behavioral changes, increased blood pressure and respirations, decreased pulse, rales, wheezing, and coughing.

After birth, observe for postpartum hemorrhage caused by uterine relaxation. Postpartum uterine atony is more likely if the woman has received oxytocin for a long time because the uterine muscle becomes fatigued and does not contract effectively to compress vessels at the placental site. It is manifested by a soft uterine fundus and excess amounts of lochia, usually with large clots. Hypovolemic shock may occur with hemorrhage.

Version

Either of two methods may be used to change fetal presentation: external or internal version. Each has different indications and a different technique. External version is much more common.

Indications

EXTERNAL VERSION
The fetus may be changed from a breech, shoulder (transverse lie), or oblique presentation to a cephalic presentation using external version. Successful version may allow the woman to avoid a cesarean birth. One study found that version was successful in 51% of the women in whom it was attempted but that more of these women than expected (31%) eventually had a cesarean birth (Laros, Flanagan, & Kilpatrick, 1995). The reasons for cesarean birth in the version group were primarily induction failure and abnormal labor progress.

INTERNAL VERSION
Malpresentation in twin gestations is usually managed by cesarean birth, but internal version is sometimes used for the vaginal birth of the second twin.

Contraindications

Version is not done if a woman is unlikely to deliver vaginally because that is the goal of the procedure. Contraindications are similar for both internal and external version. Maternal conditions that may contraindicate external version or reduce its success include the following:

- Uterine malformations that limit the room available to perform the version and may be the reason for the abnormal fetal presentation.
- Previous cesarean birth with a vertical uterine incision. Manipulation of the fetus within the uterus may strain and rupture the old incision and a vertical incision is most likely to rupture.
- Disproportion between fetal size and maternal pelvic size.

  Fetal conditions also may contraindicate the use of version:

- Placenta previa. Manipulation of the fetus within the uterus may cause hemorrhage, endangering both mother and fetus. Placenta previa other than marginal is an indication itself for cesarean birth.
- Multifetal gestation, which reduces available room to turn the fetus or fetuses. External version may be done after the first twin is born.
- Oligohydramnios, ruptured membranes, or a cord around the fetal body or neck (nuchal cord). These conditions limit the room in which to turn the fetus and may lead to cord compression and fetal hypoxia.
- Uteroplacental insufficiency. Uterine contractions occurring during the version or during labor may worsen the insufficiency and cause fetal compromise.
- Engagement of the fetal presenting part into the pelvis.

Risks

There are few risks to the woman. The principal risk is that the fetus may become entangled in the umbilical cord, com-

pressing its vessels and resulting in hypoxia. Abruptio placentae also may occur if fetal manipulation disrupts the placental site. Fetal and maternal blood could become mixed because of small breaks in placental vessels, possibly resulting in maternal sensitization to the fetal blood type. Cesarean birth may be needed for fetal compromise at the time of version or later if the fetus returns to an abnormal presentation.

Technique

EXTERNAL VERSION
A nonstress test (see Chapter 16) is done before external version to evaluate fetal health and placental function. If the test is nonreactive or other nonreassuring signs are present, the version is not done. Version would add stress to the fetus already functioning with reduced physiologic reserve. An ultrasound examination confirms fetal gestational age and fetal presentation and demonstrates adequacy of amniotic fluid.

External version is usually attempted after 37 weeks of gestation but before the woman is in labor, for the following reasons:

- As term nears, the fetus may spontaneously turn to a cephalic presentation.
- The fetus is more likely to return to an abnormal presentation if version is attempted before 37 weeks.
- If fetal compromise or onset of labor occurs, a fetus born

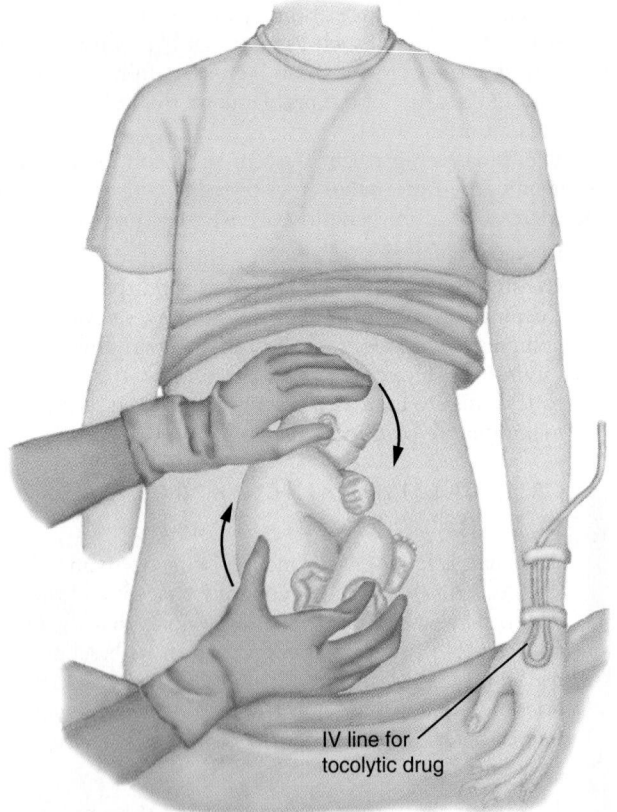

IV line for tocolytic drug

FIGURE 20–3

External version.

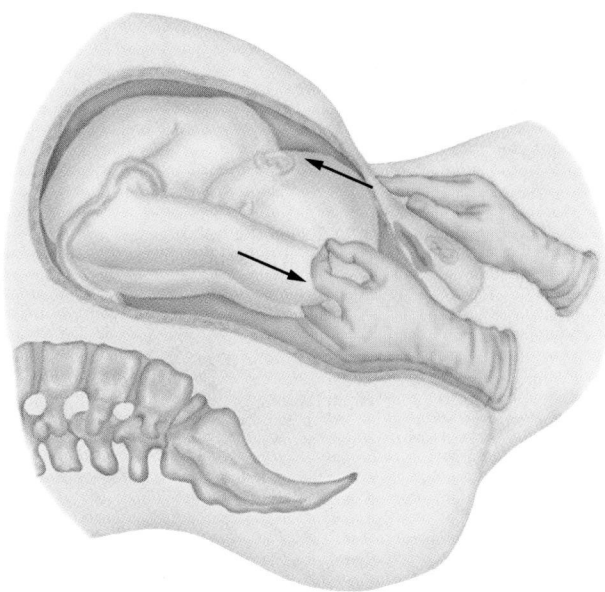

FIGURE 20–4

Internal version for vaginal birth of a second twin.

after 37 weeks is unlikely to have major problems associated with preterm birth, such as respiratory distress syndrome.

The woman is usually given a tocolytic drug such as terbutaline to relax the uterus while the version is performed.

Ultrasonography guides fetal manipulations during external version and helps monitor the fetal heart rate. The physician gently pushes the breech out of the pelvis in a forward or backward roll (Fig. 20–3).

If indicated, Rh immune globulin is given to the Rh-negative woman after external version to prevent Rh sensitization.

INTERNAL VERSION

Internal version is an unexpected and urgent procedure. The physician reaches into the uterus with one hand and, with the other hand on the maternal abdomen, maneuvers the fetus into a longitudinal lie (cephalic or breech) (Fig. 20–4) to allow delivery.

Nursing Considerations

When caring for the woman having external version, the nurse provides information, assesses the woman and fetus, and helps to reduce her anxiety.

PROVIDING INFORMATION

The birth attendant explains the indications and risks for external version to the woman before she signs an informed consent form. The nurse verifies the woman's understanding of the purposes, risks, and limitations of version.

The purposes and side effects of any planned tocolytic drug are reviewed. Tachycardia and tremors are common side effects of tocolytics such as terbutaline and stop shortly after the medication is discontinued at the end of the procedure.

PROMOTING MATERNAL AND FETAL HEALTH

Admission information is collected as if the woman were in labor or having a cesarean birth because the need for operative intervention may arise suddenly. The woman should have nothing by mouth during this short procedure.

Maternal vital signs are assessed, and fetal monitoring is begun to obtain baseline values and to evaluate the initial nonstress test. Abnormalities and nonreassuring fetal heart rate patterns should be reported promptly.

The nurse administers the tocolytic drug. The blood pressure and pulse are checked every 5 minutes, with Doppler or real-time ultrasonography used to guide the version. Fetal bradycardia may occur during the procedure, but the fetal heart rate usually returns to normal when manipulation ends.

After the version, the tocolytic drug is discontinued. The mother and fetus are observed for at least 1 hour after the version for a return of their vital signs to baseline values. Reassuring fetal signs are a heart rate in about the same range as on admission, resolution of bradycardia, and the presence of rate accelerations with fetal movement.

Maternal vital signs are measured every 15 minutes until they return to their baseline level. The presence of regular contractions suggests the onset of labor. Spontaneous rupture of membranes sometimes occurs. Rh immune globulin is given if indicated.

The woman usually has some discomfort during the version, but it should diminish quickly afterward. Persistent or continuous pain suggests a complication such as abruptio placentae.

Because the woman undergoing external version is near term, the nurse should review the signs of true labor with her and explain guidelines for returning to the hospital (see Chapter 17).

REDUCING ANXIETY

The woman may be anxious before version because its success is not certain, and complications may require rapid cesarean delivery. After version, she may still be anxious because the fetus can return to its previous position. The nurse should keep her informed about what is occurring during the version to reduce the woman's fear of the unknown.

The expectant mother is probably concerned about the fetal condition. Pointing out reassuring fetal monitor patterns, such as a normal heart rate and rate accelerations, can help reduce her anxiety about her baby. If problems such as bradycardia develop, the nurse should explain what has happened, what steps are being done to relieve it, and the result of these interventions.

Forceps and Vacuum Extraction

The physician may use forceps or vacuum extraction to apply traction to the fetal head during birth, aiding the woman's expulsive efforts. Both techniques assist descent only or descent and rotation of the fetal head from an occiput posterior or occiput transverse position to the occiput anterior position.

Forceps are metal instruments having two curved blades that can be locked in the center. Many styles are available for different needs. The blades may be closed or open and are

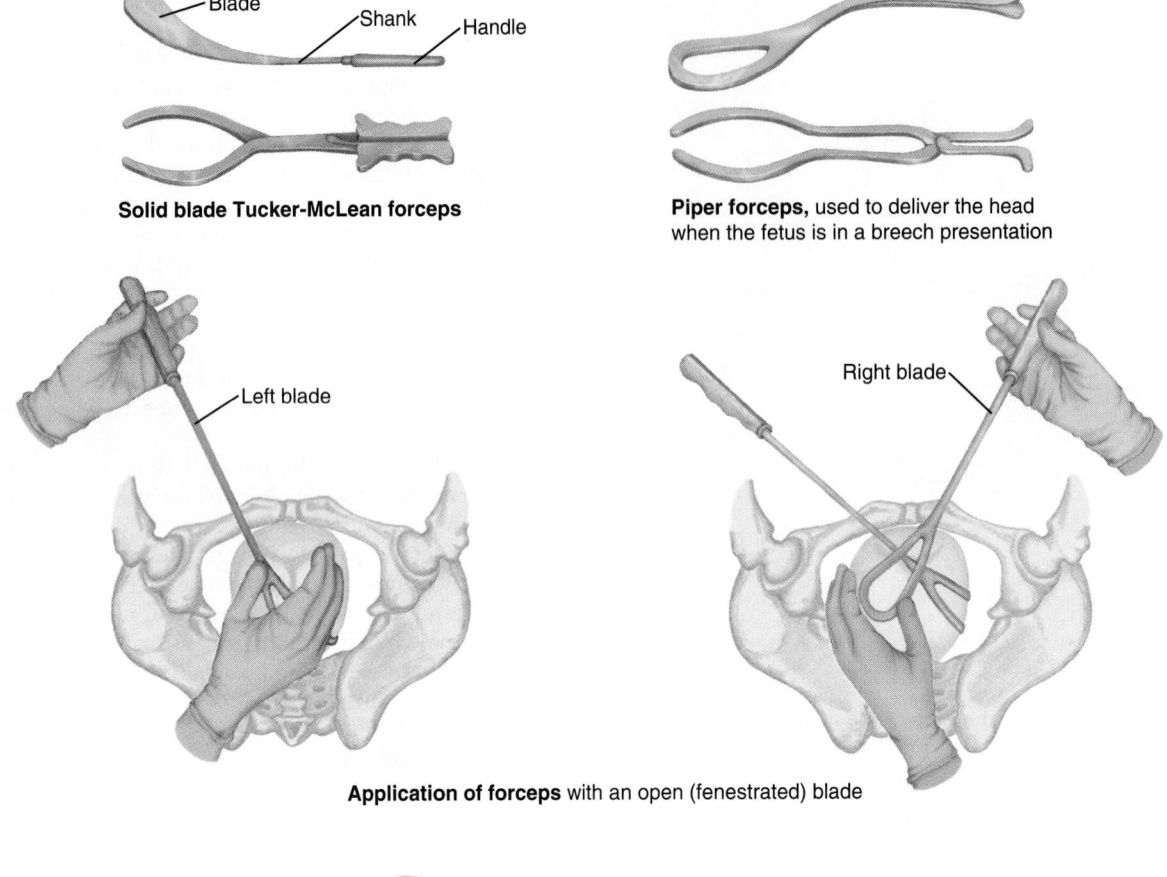

Solid blade Tucker-McLean forceps

Piper forceps, used to deliver the head when the fetus is in a breech presentation

Application of forceps with an open (fenestrated) blade

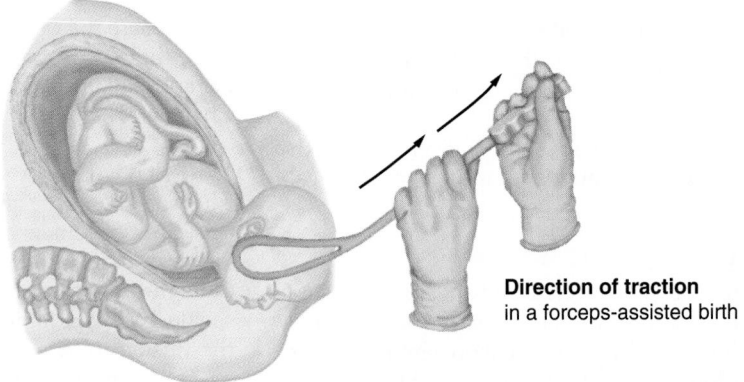

Direction of traction in a forceps-assisted birth

FIGURE 20–5

Obstetric forceps and their application.

shaped to grasp the fetal head (Fig. 20–5). Disposable foam pads are available to cushion the fetal head from the blades. Piper forceps are a special type used to assist birth of the head as it is born last in a vaginal breech birth. Forceps or a vacuum extractor also may be used during a cesarean birth.

A vacuum extractor uses suction to grasp the fetal head while traction is applied (Fig. 20–6). It is not used to deliver the fetus in a nonvertex presentation, such as breech or face; otherwise, its use is similar to that for forceps.

Indications

Forceps or vacuum extraction is considered if the second stage should be shortened for the well-being of the woman,

fetus, or both, and if a vaginal birth can be accomplished quickly without undue trauma. Maternal indications may include exhaustion, inability to push effectively, cardiac or pulmonary disease, and intrapartum infection. Fetal indications may include a prolapsed cord, premature separation of the placenta, and nonreassuring fetal heart rate patterns.

Contraindications

A cesarean birth is preferable if the maternal or fetal condition mandates a more rapid birth than can be accomplished with forceps or a vacuum extractor or if the procedure would

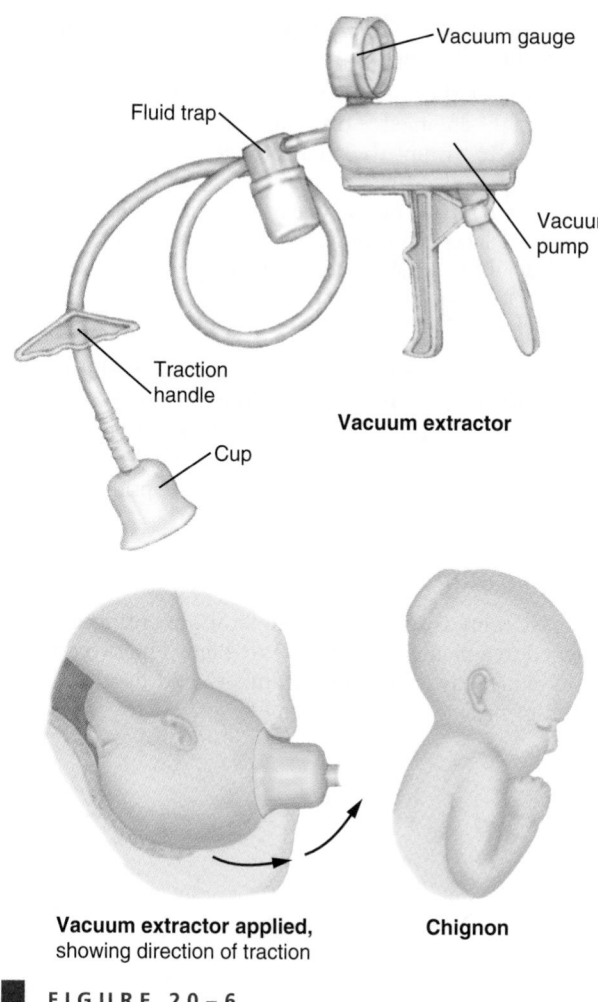

Vacuum extractor

Vacuum gauge

Fluid trap

Vacuum pump

Traction handle

Cup

Vacuum extractor applied,
showing direction of traction

Chignon

FIGURE 20–6
. . . .
Birth assisted with a vacuum extractor. The chignon is scalp edema that often forms under the suction cup when the vacuum extractor is used.

be too traumatic. Examples of these conditions are severe fetal compromise, acute maternal conditions such as congestive heart failure and pulmonary edema, a high fetal station, and disproportion between the size of the fetus and the maternal pelvis.

Risks

The main risk of forceps or vacuum extraction is trauma to maternal or fetal tissues. Because of the relative safety of cesarean birth, the attempt at an instrumental birth is usually abandoned if the fetal head does not descend easily.

Maternal risks include laceration or hematoma of the vagina. The infant may have ecchymoses, facial and scalp lacerations or abrasions, facial nerve injury, cephalhematoma, subgaleal hemorrhage, and other intracranial hemorrhage. A vacuum extractor may create scalp edema called a *chignon* at the application area (see Fig. 20–6). The chignon resolves quickly after birth.

Technique

Preparation for forceps or vacuum extraction is the same as for any vaginal birth. In addition, the woman is often catheterized to provide more room in the pelvis and limit bladder trauma. Membranes must be ruptured and the cervix completely dilated for forceps or vacuum extraction birth. The woman needs adequate anesthesia, usually with a regional block such as a pudendal or epidural block. An episiotomy is often done.

Forceps- and vacuum extractor–assisted births are classified according to how far the fetal head has descended into the pelvis when these instruments are applied (American Academy of Pediatrics & American College of Obstetricians and Gynecologists [AAP & ACOG], 1997). The three classifications are outlet, low, and midforceps.

Outlet. The fetal head is on the perineum, with the scalp visible at the vaginal opening without separating the labia. The position is OA, ROA, LOA, or OP.

Low. The leading edge of the fetal skull is at station +2 (about 2 cm below the level of the mother's ischial spines) or lower.

Midforceps. The leading edge of the fetal skull is between a 0 (at the level of the ischial spines) and a +2 station.

The physician determines the presentation, position, and station of the fetal head and the amount of cervical dilation. When the forceps is correctly applied, the long axis of the blades lies over the fetal cheeks and parietal bones. After checking for proper application, the physician locks the two blades in the center and pulls gently, following the curve of the pelvis. An episiotomy is often done, as the fetal head distends the perineum. The physician may keep the forceps on until the head is born or may remove the blades just before expulsion. The rest of the fetus is born in the usual way.

For vacuum extraction, the cup is connected to a machine that creates a vacuum to hold the cup on the fetal head in the midline of the occiput. The physician applies traction intermittently, as in a forceps-assisted birth.

Nursing Considerations

When a forceps or vacuum extraction birth is anticipated, a catheter is added to the instrument table for the birth. The physician specifies the type of forceps or vacuum cup. The fetal heart rate should be assessed, and any rate lower than 100 BPM should be reported.

After birth, the mother and infant are observed for trauma. The mother may have vaginal wall lacerations or hematoma (see Chapter 28). Cold applications for the first 12 hours reduce pain by numbing the area and limit bruising and edema of the tissues. Heat applications after 12 hours aid resolution of the edema and bruising. The fundus is usually firm unless uterine atony is also present.

The infant often has reddening and mild bruising of the skin where the forceps were applied. These areas do not need treatment. Cold treatment is not done for an infant because of possible hypothermia. Observe for skin breaks that allow entry of microorganisms; keep skin breaks clean. Facial asymmetry, most obvious when the infant cries, suggests facial nerve injury.

After a forceps-assisted birth, a parent may ask why the baby's cheeks are reddened or bruised. A good response is to explain that the pressure of the forceps on the baby's delicate skin may cause minor bruising that usually resolves without treatment. Parents of an infant born with assistance of a vacuum extractor may likewise be concerned about the edema (chignon) on their baby's head. Reassure them that this edema will soon resolve. Point out improvement in the baby's cheeks or scalp during the postpartum stay.

Episiotomy

The routine performance of an episiotomy remains controversial, despite several research studies. The decision about whether an episiotomy is needed must be made just before birth, however, and indications are not always clear.

Indications

Fetal indications for episiotomy are similar to those for forceps or vacuum extraction. An episiotomy may be done to reduce pressure on the fetal head when a small, preterm infant is born.

Maternal indications are also similar to those for forceps or vacuum extraction. Other maternal indications may include the following:

• Control of the direction and extent that the vaginal opening is enlarged. This is an advantage if a laceration is likely to disrupt the anal sphincter.
• A straight, clean-edged incision is created that can be simpler to repair than a large perineal laceration. A small perineal laceration, however, would be easier to repair and would heal better than a larger episiotomy.

Risks

Infection is the primary risk of episiotomy. Perineal pain occurs with both episiotomy and spontaneous tears. However, perineal pain may last longer with episiotomy, mainly because the incision tends to extend into deeper lacerations. Prolonged perineal pain impairs resumption of sexual intercourse.

Technique

An episiotomy is done when the fetal presenting part has crowned to a diameter of about 3 to 4 cm. The two types of episiotomies have different advantages and disadvantages: *median* or *midline* and *mediolateral* (Fig. 20–7).

Median or Midline

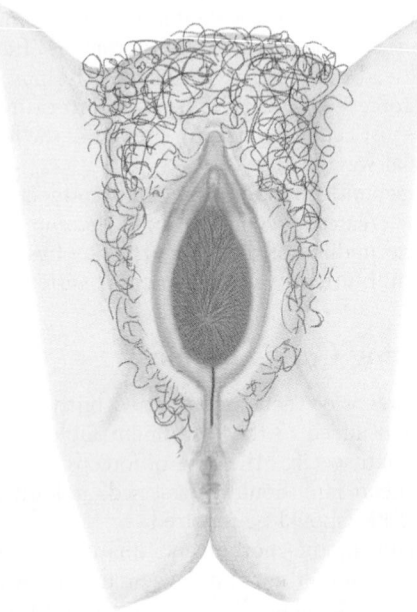

Mediolateral

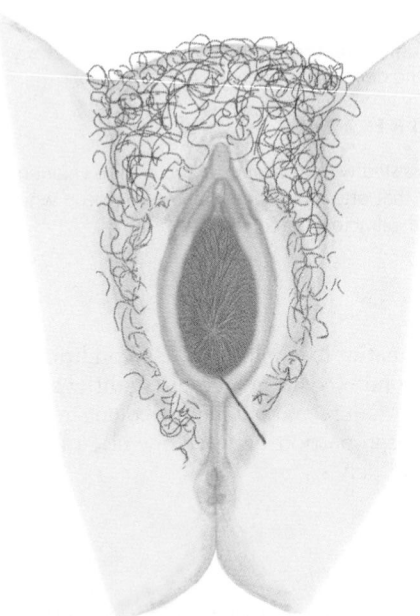

Advantages	**Disadvantages**
Minimal blood loss	An added laceration may extend the median episiotomy into the anal sphincter
Neat healing with little scarring	
Less postpartum pain than the mediolateral episiotomy	Limited enlargement of the vaginal opening because perineal length is limited by the anal sphincter

Advantages	**Disadvantages**
More enlargement of the vaginal opening	More blood loss
Little risk that the episiotomy will extend into the anus	Increased postpartum pain
	More scarring and irregularity in the healed scar
	Prolonged dyspareunia (painful intercourse)

FIGURE 20–7
Types of episiotomies.

Nursing Considerations

An episiotomy can sometimes be avoided (or its length limited) with nursing measures. Assuming an upright position while pushing gently promotes gradual stretching of the woman's perineum. Warm perineal compresses and perineal massage may relax perineal muscles so that the birth canal more readily accommodates the fetal head as it emerges. Further research needs to be done to clarify whether warm compresses, perineal massage, or other techniques are truly effective in reducing the need for episiotomy.

Nursing interventions during the recovery and postpartum periods are similar for episiotomy and perineal laceration. Observe the perineum for hematoma and edema. As with forceps use, perineal cold applications are done for the first 12 hours, followed by perineal heat applications after 12 hours.

▌ Cesarean Birth

In 1965, the cesarean birth rate in the United States was 4.5% of all births, rising to 24% in the late 1980s. The 1994 rate was 22% of all births. Of 1994 births, 15.8% were primary (first) cesareans and 6.2% were repeat cesareans (Clarke & Taffel, 1996).

Several factors led to the high U.S. cesarean birth rate. Paul and Miller (1995) describe several:

- Greater safety of the surgery for the woman makes the surgery a reasonable option in more circumstances.
- Improved survival of very small preterm infants makes the use of cesarean birth reasonable.
- High consumer expectations of a good fetal outcome cause physicians to intervene with a surgical birth quickly.
- A greater threat of litigation if outcomes are not good causes physicians to opt for surgery quickly if the maternal or fetal condition, or both, seems to be at risk.

A national goal for the Healthy People 2000 initiative is to reduce the rate of cesarean births to no more than 15%, with the rate of primary cesarean births being no more than 12% of total births. These goals may be revised when the updated Healthy People 2010 initiative is released. Efforts to accomplish the goal include (1) promoting vaginal birth after cesarean (VBAC) when appropriate, (2) careful evaluation of dystocia, and (3) selection of some women to deliver their infants in the breech presentation. Because previous cesarean birth and dystocia contribute substantially to the current rate, promotion of VBAC and critical evaluation of dystocia can reduce the total rate.

The American College of Obstetricians and Gynecologists (1998) has affirmed their support for VBAC (see accompanying box), but has urged caution in approaching a trial of labor because VBAC is associated with a small but significant risk of uterine rupture. Global mandates to attempt VBAC, such as by third-party payers, are not appropriate because the risks and benefits of VBAC for each woman must be considered by her and her physician. For example, the risk of uterine rupture increases as the number of prior uterine incisions increases, and a woman who has had two prior cesarean deliveries might be reluctant to attempt VBAC for her third birth because of this added risk.

• • • • • • • • • •
Vaginal Birth After Cesarean Birth (VBAC)

- Approximately 60% to 80% of women with one low transverse uterine incision from a previous cesarean birth have successful vaginal births.
- Women whose previous cesarean birth was done for breech presentation or a nonreassuring fetal heart rate pattern appear to have more success with VBAC than if the primary cesarean birth was for cephalopelvic disproportion or failure to progress in labor.
- About 40% to 50% of women who are candidates for a trial of labor refuse it and undergo a repeat cesarean birth.
- Candidates for VBAC include the following:
  - A woman who has one previous low transverse uterine incision. She should be encouraged to attempt labor in her current pregnancy.
  - A woman who has two or more low transverse uterine incisions. She should not be discouraged from laboring in her current pregnancy.
- Estimated fetal weight greater than 4,000 grams by itself is not a contraindication if the woman is not diabetic.
- VBAC is contraindicated if a woman has a previous classic uterine incision.
- Insufficient data are available about the risks and benefits of a trial of labor in a multifetal gestation or with a fetus in breech presentation.
- Normal activity should be encouraged during latent labor.
- Epidural analgesia and anesthesia may be used.
- Induction and augmentation of labor with oxytocin may be done. The risks and benefits of prostaglandin gel have not been thoroughly researched, although there are reports of success using this drug.

Data from American College of Obstetricians and Gynecologists & American Academy of Pediatrics. (1995). *Vaginal delivery after previous cesarean birth* (ACOG Practice Patterns No. 1). Washington, DC: American College of Obstetricians and Gynecologists.

Additionally, the woman who tries VBAC and still requires a repeat cesarean birth may incur double costs because she has both labor and surgical expenses. She and her infant are more likely to have infections that further complicate their recovery and increase costs. The ability of a hospital to respond to an emergency such as uterine rupture must also be considered. Small rural hospitals may be less suitable for the woman attempting VBAC because they do not have the capacity for the rapid response that a larger urban hospital may have.

Experience with electronic fetal monitoring has improved knowledge of normal fetal responses to labor, promoting interventions for fetal benefit that may avoid cesarean delivery. Nurses and birth attendants increasingly recognize that simple interventions, such as walking or squatting during the second stage, may promote normal labor progress. Interventions, both nursing and medical, that reduce the primary (first) cesarean birth rate will also reduce the need for repeat (secondary) cesareans.

Indications

Cesarean birth is performed when waiting for a vaginal birth would compromise the mother, the fetus, or both. Possible indications for cesarean birth include, but are not limited to, the following:

- Dystocia
- Cephalopelvic (fetopelvic) disproportion
- Pregnancy-induced hypertension, if prompt delivery is necessary
- Maternal diseases such as diabetes, heart disease, or cervical cancer, if labor is not advisable
- Active genital herpes
- Some previous uterine surgical procedures, such as a classic cesarean incision
- Persistent nonreassuring fetal heart rate patterns
- A prolapsed umbilical cord
- Fetal malpresentations, such as breech or transverse lie
- Hemorrhagic conditions, such as abruptio placentae or placenta previa

A prior cesarean birth alone is not an indication for another cesarean birth for most women. Women who have had one cesarean birth with a lower-segment uterine incision should be counseled and encouraged to attempt labor and vaginal birth. Women who have had two or more previous cesarean births with low transverse incisions can also be permitted to attempt vaginal birth if there are no contraindications (AAP & ACOG, 1997).

Contraindications

There are few absolute contraindications to cesarean birth, but there are conditions in which it is not desirable because the risks to the woman are too great when compared with the potential benefit to mother or fetus. These conditions include fetal death, a fetus that is too immature to survive, and maternal coagulation defects.

Risks

Cesarean birth is one of the safest major surgical procedures; however, it poses greater risk for the mother than does vaginal birth. Maternal risks include the following:

- Infection
- Hemorrhage
- Urinary tract trauma
- Thrombophlebitis
- Paralytic ileus
- Atelectasis
- Anesthesia complications, such as aspiration of gastric contents

Cesarean delivery poses added risks for the infant, which may include the following:

- Inadvertent preterm birth
- Transient tachypnea of the newborn caused by delayed absorption of lung fluid (see Chapter 30)
- Persistent pulmonary hypertension of the newborn (see Chapter 30)
- Injury, such as laceration, bruising, or other trauma

Diagnostic studies are often done to ensure that the fetal lungs are mature when a cesarean birth is planned (see Chapter 16). These studies include determining the amniotic fluid lecithin/sphingomyelin (L/S) ratio and assessing for the presence of phosphatidylglycerol (PG) and phosphatidylinositol (PI).

Technique

PREPARATION

Regional anesthesia, such as epidural block, is commonly used for cesarean birth. The woman receives nothing by mouth, however, because general anesthesia, with its risk for vomiting and aspiration, may be required. A drug such as famotidine (Pepcid) or sodium citrate with citric acid (Bicitra) is given to reduce gastric acidity before surgery. The woman does not have routine premedication other than drugs to control gastric and respiratory secretions.

Fetal monitoring continues until just before the sterile abdominal skin prep (intermittent auscultation or external monitor) or just after the prep (internal monitor) (AAP & ACOG, 1997). A wedge placed under one hip prevents aortocaval compression and promotes placental blood flow.

Routine laboratory studies vary with the mother's condition and type of anesthesia but often include a complete blood count, clotting studies such as prothrombin and partial thromboplastin times, and blood typing and screening. The physician may order 1 or more units of blood typed and crossmatched to have available for transfusion if the woman's hemoglobin and hematocrit values are low or if she is at increased risk for hemorrhage, such as grand multiparity (five or more births).

A single intravenous dose of a prophylactic antibiotic such as ampicillin or a cephalosporin is often ordered. Additional antibiotic doses are given to a woman who has an increased risk for infection, such as one who has had prolonged rupture of membranes.

If a Pfannenstiel (transverse or "bikini") skin incision is planned, the woman's abdomen is shaved from about 3 inches above the pubic hairline to the mons pubis, about where her legs come together. For a vertical skin incision, the upper border of the shave is just above the umbilicus.

An indwelling catheter inserted before the surgery keeps the bladder away from the operative area, reducing the risk for injury. The catheter allows accurate observation of urine output during and after surgery, which helps evaluate circulatory status.

Preoperative preparations are completed before a general anesthetic is begun to reduce neonatal exposure to anesthesia. The team scrubs, dons gowns and gloves, and drapes the woman before general anesthesia is induced.

A sterile abdominal skin prep is done just before sterile draping. As in other surgical skin preparations, the direction of the scrub is circular, from the center of the operative area outward.

INCISIONS

Two incisions are made: one in the abdominal wall (skin incision) and the other in the uterine wall. Either of two skin incisions is used: a midline vertical incision between the umbilicus and the symphysis or a Pfannenstiel incision just above the symphysis (Fig. 20-8).

Three types of uterine incisions are possible (Fig. 20-9): (1) low transverse, (2) low vertical, and (3) classic, a vertical incision into the upper uterus. The low transverse uterine incision is preferred unless a very large fetus or pla-

Vertical

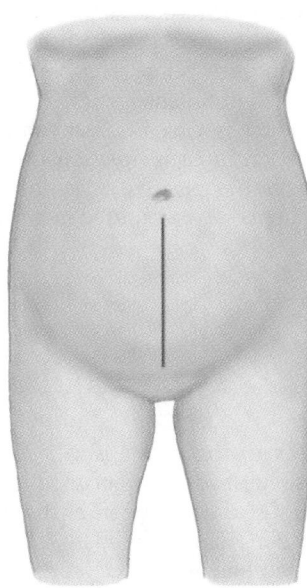

Advantages
Quicker to perform
Better visualization of the uterus
Can quickly extend upward for greater visualization if needed
Often more appropriate for obese women

Disadvantages
Easily visible when healed
Greater chance of dehiscence and hernia formation

Pfannenstiel

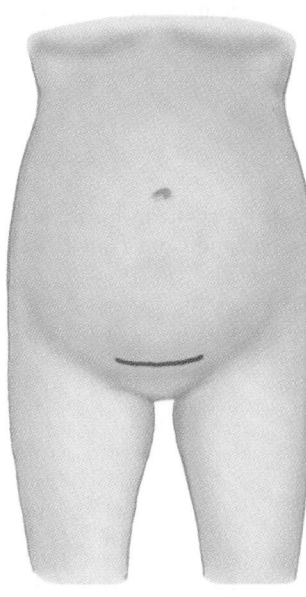

Advantages
Less visibility when healed and the pubic hair grows back
Less chance of dehiscence or formation of a hernia

Disadvantages
Less visualization of the uterus
Cannot be done as quickly, which may be important in an emergency cesarean birth
Cannot easily be extended to give greater operative exposure
Re-entry at a subsequent cesarean birth may require more time

FIGURE 20–8
Skin (abdominal wall) incisions for cesarean birth.

Low Transverse

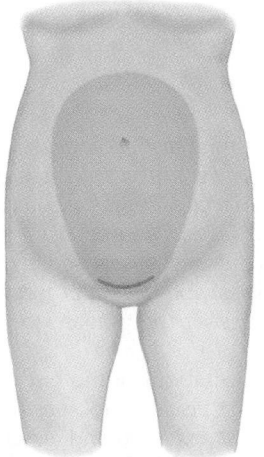

Advantages
Unlikely to rupture during a subsequent birth
Makes VBAC possible for subsequent pregnancy
Less blood loss
Easier to repair
Less adhesion formation

Disadvantage
Limited ability to extend laterally to enlarge the incision

Low Vertical

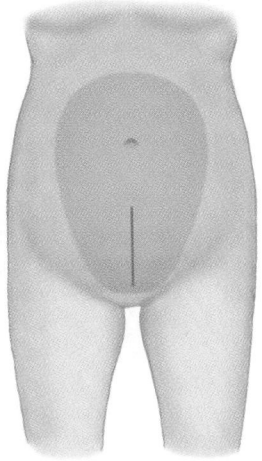

Advantage
Can be extended upward to make a larger incision if needed

Disadvantages
Slightly more likely to rupture during a subsequent birth
A tear may extend the incision downward into the cervix

Classic

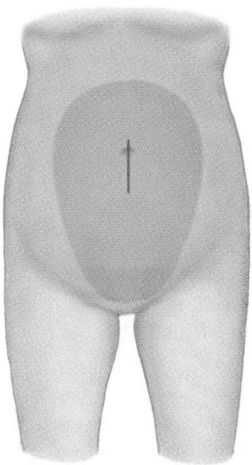

Advantage
May be the only choice in these situations:

Implantation of a placenta previa on the lower anterior uterine wall
Presence of dense adhesions from previous surgery
Transverse lie of a large fetus with the shoulder impacted in the mother's pelvis

Disadvantages
Most likely of the uterine incisions to rupture during a subsequent birth
Eliminates VBAC as an option for birth of a subsequent infant

FIGURE 20–9
Uterine incisions for cesarean birth. The abdominal and uterine incisions do not always match.
VBAC, vaginal birth after cesarean.

centa previa in the lower uterus prevents its use. The uterine incision does not always match the skin incision. For example, a woman may have a vertical skin incision and a low transverse uterine incision.

Nursing Considerations

Nursing care for a woman who has a cesarean birth varies according to the situation (see Nursing Care Plan 20–1).

She may be planning a cesarean birth, or a surgical birth may be unexpected. A planned cesarean may be her first, or she may have had a cesarean birth before. Her previous cesarean may have been planned or an emergency.

Nursing care for all women having cesarean childbirth is similar, but the approach in each situation is different. For example, although preoperative teaching is important, it must be abbreviated or even omitted in a true emergency.

NURSING CARE PLAN 20–1

Cesarean Birth

Assessment

Christina Cole is 22 years old and is expecting her first baby. She is in early labor and expecting a cesarean birth because her baby has remained in a breech presentation. Although her physician discussed cesarean birth with her, Christina is anxious and has many questions about what will happen to her and her baby. Christina's mother and husband Bruce are with her.

Nursing Diagnosis

Anxiety related to unfamiliarity with the setting and procedures for cesarean birth.

Goals/Expected Outcomes

After interventions, Christina will

- State that she feels less apprehensive.
- Verbalize understanding of preoperative and postoperative care.
- Demonstrate postoperative techniques for coughing and deep breathing.

Intervention	Rationale
1. Assess Christina's level of anxiety. Mild to moderate anxiety is expected.	1. Assessment enables the nurse to approach preoperative care of the woman in the most appropriate manner. Mild to moderate anxiety facilitates learning, but high levels impair learning.
2. Remain with Christina as much as possible. Allow her to express her fears. Encourage her mother and Bruce to remain with her.	2. The presence of significant others and a caring nurse provides support. Expression of her fears enables the nurse to answer the woman's concerns specifically.
3. Elicit Christina's feelings about surgery by using broad leads, such as, "What were your thoughts when you found out you might have your baby by cesarean?"	3. Identification of expectations of the birth experience allows actions to be taken to make it a positive one. If a woman's expected and actual experience closely match, she is likely to be more satisfied with it. Misunderstandings and possible feelings of inadequacy or anger are identified.
4. Explain preoperative preparations using simple language, verifying Christina's understanding and giving her the opportunity to ask questions.	4. Knowledge decreases anxiety and fear of the unknown. Simple language facilitates understanding when a woman's attention is narrowed from anxiety. Explanations and the chance to ask questions show respect and give the woman a greater sense of control.
5. Explain what to expect postoperatively, demonstrating as needed.	5. Knowledge reduces anxiety and fear of the unknown. The explanation promotes understanding and acceptance of care that will be painful while providing reassurance of pain control. Return demonstration verifies learning and identifies the need for additional teaching.
6. Reduce unnecessary stimulation.	6. Unnecessary stimulation can add to the woman's anxiety. Its reduction emphasizes that a cesarean delivery is a birth, not just a surgical procedure.

Cesarean Birth

Evaluation

Christina believes that a cesarean birth is best for her baby. She asks a few other questions, then states that she understands preoperative and postoperative care. She demonstrates effective coughing and deep breathing techniques.

Assessment

Christina will have epidural anesthesia for her birth. Her vital signs are temperature, 37.2°C (99°F); pulse, 90 BPM; respirations, 22 breaths per minute; and blood pressure, 122/70 mm Hg. The fetal heart rate is 130 to 140 BPM and accelerates with fetal movement.

Assessment

Christina is transferred to the operating room, and epidural anesthesia is begun.

Nursing Diagnosis

Risk for Injury related to altered sensation from epidural anesthesia and the use of electrical equipment during surgery.

Goals/Expected Outcomes

• Christina will not have injury, such as pressure areas, muscle strains, and electrical injury, during the perioperative period.

Intervention

1. Pad the operating table carefully, particularly under Christina's bony prominences. Avoid obstructing her popliteal area.

2. Transfer Christina to and from the operating table carefully, using enough staff members to keep her body in alignment. Brace the bed and operating table to keep them from separating.
3. After anesthesia is begun, position Christina on the operating table and secure her legs with a safety strap. She should have a wedge under one hip, or the table should be tilted.

4. Apply a grounding pad if electrocautery is to be used.

Rationale

1. Padding reduces potential for tissue damage caused by pressure. An unobstructed popliteal area reduces venous stasis with possible thrombus formation.
2. Having adequate staff reduces the risk of a fall or muscle strains in both Christina and the staff.

3. The safety strap prevents falls or displacement of the woman's legs, which have lost sensation. A hip wedge or tilting the table reduces aortocaval compression, which might reduce placental blood flow.
4. A grounding pad prevents electrical shock or burn.

Evaluation

During surgery, Christina's body was secured in proper alignment, with proper padding of all her bony prominences. The grounding pad ensured electrical safety when the electrocautery was used. She gave birth to an 8-pound, 8-ounce (3,856-g) baby. Christina was transferred to the recovery room without incident. During the recovery period she showed no signs of pressure, electrical, or musculoskeletal injury.

Additional Nursing Diagnoses to Consider

Risk for Aspiration
Pain
Risk for Altered Respiratory Function
Hypothermia
Family Coping: Potential for Growth

Note: Only nursing diagnoses related to the preoperative and intraoperative care of the woman are discussed here. See Chapter 18 for nursing care related to fetal oxygenation. See Chapter 19 for care related to anesthesia. See Chapters 17 and 21 for nursing care of the mother during the recovery and postpartum periods.

. . . .
Nursing Care for a Woman Having Cesarean Birth

BEFORE THE CESAREAN BIRTH

1. Assess the time of last oral intake and what was eaten.
2. Assess for allergies.
3. Have the woman sign an informed consent form.
4. Obtain ordered laboratory work.
5. Do preoperative teaching: what the woman can expect in the operating and recovery rooms.
6. Start ordered intravenous infusion.
7. Do abdominal shave.
8. Insert an indwelling catheter.
9. Administer ordered medication to control gastric secretions.
10. Assist woman to operating table, positioning her with a wedge under her hip (or tilt table).
11. Apply grounding pad for electrocautery.
12. Do cleansing prep of abdomen.

DURING THE RECOVERY PERIOD

1. Begin anesthesia-related interventions: pulse oximeter, oxygen administration, cardiac monitor.
   a. Assess for return of sensation and movement if regional anesthesia was used.
   b. Assess level of consciousness if general anesthesia was used.
2. Do routine assessments every 15 minutes for the first hour, every 30 minutes during the second hour, and hourly thereafter until the woman is transferred to the postpartum unit. Assess the following:
   a. Vital signs
   b. Uterine fundus for firmness, height, and deviation (massage if poorly contracted)
   c. Lochia for color, quantity, and presence of large clots
   d. Urine output for color, quantity, and patency of the catheter and tubing
   e. Abdominal dressing for drainage
3. Assess need for analgesia and administer as ordered.
4. Change position hourly if no contraindication exists. Have her breathe deeply and cough at each routine assessment time. Provide a small pillow to support her incision when coughing or turning.

PROVIDING EMOTIONAL SUPPORT

Emotional support begins well before the birth and extends well after it. A mother who has had a previous cesarean birth may harbor unresolved feelings of grief, guilt, or inadequacy because she perceives that she somehow failed in her expected birth experience.

> The nurse in the prenatal setting can open the subject of a woman's previous cesarean birth with a broad lead, such as, "Tell me about when you had your other baby."

The staff's behavior can either reduce or increase the woman's anxiety. A calm and confident manner helps her feel that she is being cared for by competent professionals. A quiet, low voice is calming. There is little reason to shout, even in an emergency.

The nurse and the woman's significant others are important sources of emotional support. Therapeutic communication with a caring nurse helps clarify her concerns, so explanations to reduce her fear of the unknown can be most effective.

The father or other support person should be encouraged to remain with her during surgery if she has regional anesthesia. In some hospitals, the support person may come into the operating room after the woman is intubated for general anesthesia to foster attachment with the infant and help the mother integrate her birth experience.

Nurses also support a woman's partner and significant others during the cesarean birth. The partner may be as anxious as the woman but may be afraid to express it because the woman needs so much support. The partner may be physically exhausted after hours of labor coaching. The staff should not expect more support from the partner than he or she can provide.

> Although cesarean births are routine in the intrapartum unit, they are not routine to women who undergo them or to their families. Avoid belittling their fears by telling women and their families not to worry or that everything will be all right.

After birth, visiting the mother and her family allows the nurse to answer questions about the surgery and fill in any gaps in their understanding. This helps them understand the experience and promotes a positive perception of the birth.

TEACHING

Knowledge helps to reduce fear of the unknown and increases a woman's sense of control over her infant's birth. The nurse cannot assume that a woman who had a previous cesarean birth already knows what will happen and why. If her previous surgery was done after a long labor or in an emergency, she may recall only part of it and may not understand what she does remember. Teaching should be done in simple language and should include her partner.

The nurse explains preoperative procedures and their purposes, such as the abdominal shave, indwelling catheter, intravenous lines, and dressings. The catheter and intravenous lines usually remain in place no longer than 24 hours after birth. The nurse may need to reinforce anesthetic information provided by the anesthesia clinician.

Women who have regional anesthesia, such as an epidural or subarachnoid block, often fear that they will feel pain during surgery. They do feel pressure and pulling, but these sensations do not mean that the anesthesia is wearing off. The nurse reassures her that her anesthesia clinician will regularly assess her needs for pain management.

If a woman is having general anesthesia, the nurse explains why operative preparations are completed before the woman is anesthetized. She should be reassured that her surgery will not begin until she is asleep and that she will not wake up during the procedure.

The nurse describes the operating room and everyone who will be present to make it less intimidating to her. The operating room is very cool, and the surgery table is narrow. Her labor nurse is often the circulating nurse during surgery, reassuring her with a familiar face and voice.

The support person should be told when he or she can expect to come into the operating room. If it is not already in place, an epidural block is often established after the woman goes to the operating room. Bringing the partner in may be delayed until the regional block and other preparations, such as placement of the indwelling catheter, are complete. These preparations may take 30 to 45 minutes if there is no rush. The support person should be told that he or she will not be forgotten and that the apparent delay does not indicate a problem.

The nurse explains the recovery room and any equipment that will be used, such as a pulse oximeter and automatic blood pressure cuff. The need for routine assessments and interventions such as fundus and lochia checks, coughing, and deep breathing are explained. The woman is taught simple exercises to promote normal circulation in her legs. The nurse reassures her that every effort will be made to promote her comfort with medication, positioning, and other interventions.

PROMOTING SAFETY

Although the need for general anesthesia occurs infrequently, the nurse must assume that it will be needed. The woman's food intake is assessed for type and time on admission. Oral intake and emesis during labor are recorded and reported to the anesthesia clinician. Oral intake other than ordered medications should be discontinued if a cesarean birth becomes very likely. Anesthesia-related drugs to control gastric and respiratory secretions are administered as ordered.

The woman is transferred and positioned carefully to prevent injury, especially if she has received regional anesthesia that reduces motor control and sensation. Her bony prominences are well padded. A safety strap placed across her thighs secures her on the narrow operating table. A wedge placed under one hip or tilting the operating table avoids aortocaval compression and reduced placental blood flow. During positioning, the drain tube of the indwelling catheter should be routed under her leg to promote drainage and keep the tube away from the operative area. The catheter bag is placed near the head of the table so that the anesthesia clinician can monitor urine output.

The nurse verifies proper function of machines such as suction devices, monitors, and electrocautery. Leads for the cardiac monitor and pulse oximeter are placed to observe heart and respiratory functions. A grounding pad permits safe use of the electrocautery.

After the surgery, the incision area is cleansed with sterile water and a sterile dressing is applied. Blood and amniotic fluid are cleaned from the woman's abdomen, buttocks, and back before she is transferred to a bed. Smooth transfers reduce pain and hypotension.

PROVIDING POSTOPERATIVE CARE

Postoperative care for the mother who has had a cesarean birth is similar to that for one who has had a vaginal birth, with added interventions. Her temperature is assessed on admission and according to protocol thereafter. If her condition is stable, other assessments are done every 15 minutes during the first 1 to 2 hours, progressing to every 30 minutes to 1 hour until transfer to her postpartum room. In addition to temperature, routine postoperative assessments include the following:

- Return of motion and sensation (if a regional block was given)
- Level of consciousness (particularly if general anesthesia or sedating drugs were given)
- Vital signs and character of respirations
- Abdominal dressing
- Uterine firmness and position (midline or deviated)
- Lochia
- Urine output (quantity, color, other characteristics)
- Intravenous infusion
- Pain relief needs

The nurse observes for return of motion and sensation if the woman had epidural or subarachnoid block anesthesia. The level of consciousness and respiratory status (skin or mucous membrane color; rate and quality of respirations) are important observations if she had general anesthesia. Respiratory observations are also important if the woman received epidural opioid narcotics, which can cause delayed respiratory depression. Have naloxone (Narcan) available to reverse opioid-induced respiratory depression. (See Chapter 19 for more information about anesthesia and analgesia for cesarean birth.)

The pulse, respirations, and blood pressure provide important clues to the woman's circulatory and respiratory status. If oxygen saturation falls below 95%, having her take several deep breaths usually raises it. A respiratory rate of less than 12 breaths per minute suggests respiratory depression. Deep breathing and coughing move secretions out of the lungs and promote full expansion. A small pillow to support her incision reduces pain when she coughs. Position changes every 2 hours improve ventilation and decrease discomfort from constant pressure.

As with a vaginal birth, the fundus is assessed for height, firmness, and position. To relax her abdominal muscles, thus reducing pain from fundus checks, she should flex her knees and take slow deep breaths. The nurse's fingers are gently "walked" toward her fundus to determine uterine firmness. The woman who has a Pfannenstiel skin incision usually has less pain with fundus checks than the woman with a vertical skin incision. A firm fundus does not need massage. The dressing is checked for drainage with each fundus check.

The nurse assesses the lochia and urine output with other assessments. Lochia may pool under the mother's buttocks and lower back. Urine may be bloody temporarily if the cesarean delivery was done after a long labor or an attempted forceps delivery. The urine drain tubing should be observed for gradual clearing of the blood. Urine should drain freely to prevent bladder distension, which worsens pain and increases the risk for postpartum hemorrhage. The nurse must remember that a falling urine output is an early sign of hypovolemia.

The woman's needs for pain relief should be regularly assessed. The woman who received an epidural analgesic may not need other analgesia during the early postpartum period. If she needs added pain relief while the epidural analgesic is still in effect, the dose ordered is often lower than if she had not had that form of analgesia. Early analgesia is usually given by a patient-controlled analgesia pump or intermittent injections. Oral analgesics usually replace parenteral ones the day after surgery.

PRESENTING VAGINAL BIRTH AFTER CESAREAN

Teaching the woman about VBAC presents a challenge to nurses. Women have often heard the outdated saying, "once a cesarean, always a cesarean," and are anxious about attempting vaginal birth in a later pregnancy. They may know the facts about VBAC but find it impossible to disregard what they have heard for years. Scheduling a repeat cesarean often seems simpler and something the woman can count on. The prospect of laboring and perhaps still needing a cesarean birth is unattractive as well. Also, the nurse cannot promise the woman that she will not ultimately need a cesarean birth after hours of labor.

The physician discusses VBAC during prenatal care, and the nurse reinforces these explanations and identifies misunderstandings. If the woman is planning VBAC, the nurse should reinforce the appropriateness of attempting it and the advantages of a vaginal birth, such as fewer overall complications. Vaginal birth after cesarean should be presented in a positive way, at the same time acknowledging that a cesarean delivery may be needed.

KEY CONCEPTS
. . . .

■ Prolapse and compression of the umbilical cord are the primary risks of amniotomy. As the fluid gushes out, the cord can become compressed between the fetal presenting part and the expectant woman's pelvis.
■ Infection is more likely to occur when membranes have been ruptured for a long time, usually thought to be after about 24 hours.
■ Labor may be induced if continuing the pregnancy is more hazardous to the maternal or fetal health than is the induction. Induction is not done if a maternal or fetal contraindication exists to labor or vaginal birth.
■ Oxytocin-stimulated uterine contractions may be hypertonic, decreasing placental perfusion.

■ External version is done to promote vaginal birth by changing the fetal presentation from a breech or transverse lie to a cephalic lie. Internal version is sometimes used to change the presentation of the second twin after the birth of the first twin.
■ The median episiotomy is less painful but more likely to extend into the rectum. The mediolateral episiotomy is more painful but is not likely to extend into the rectum.
■ Trauma to maternal and fetal tissue is the primary risk associated with use of forceps or a vacuum extractor. Possible trauma to the mother includes vaginal wall laceration and hematoma. Trauma to

the infant may include ecchymoses, lacerations, abrasions, facial nerve injury, and intracranial hemorrhage.
■ The preferred uterine incision for cesarean birth is the low transverse incision because it is least likely to rupture in a subsequent pregnancy. The skin incision does not always match the uterine incision and is unrelated to the risk of later uterine rupture.
■ Some women have feelings of guilt or inadequacy if they have a cesarean birth. Therapeutic communication and sensitive, family-centered care are essential to help them achieve a positive perception of their birth experience.

ANSWERS TO CRITICAL THINKING EXERCISES
. . . .

Exercise 20–1
1. The amount of amniotic fluid is normal, but the pale yellow color and strong odor suggest chorioamnionitis, or infection of the amniotic sac. The risk for chorioamnionitis increases as the duration of ruptured membranes increases, but it can be apparent at any time, including at initial rupture. The fetal heart rate is slightly elevated from the normal maximum rate at term

of 160 BPM. Accelerations with fetal movement are a reassuring sign. The maternal temperature, pulse, and respirations are slightly elevated. It is difficult to accurately interpret these values because the baseline values are not stated. These contractions are typical for a woman entering the active phase of first-stage labor.
2. The nurse should continue to assess the fetus for tachycardia,

which often precedes maternal fever. Assess the woman's temperature at least every 2 hours for a temperature of 38°C (100.4°F) or higher. Report abnormalities to the physician. Observe also for fetal tachycardia and signs of fetal compromise that may occur with maternal infection.

Exercise 20–2
1. The woman is having hypertonic uterine activity because the dura-

tion of contractions is longer than 90 seconds and the rest interval is no longer than 55 seconds. Her peak intrauterine pressure during contractions is 10 mm Hg higher than expected for first-stage labor. Oxytocin stimulation is the probable cause of the excessive contractions. The reassuring fetal heart rate suggests that the fetus is now tolerating the excessive contractions.

2. Fetal oxygenation may be compromised if the excessive contractions continue. Reduce or stop the oxytocin infusion to decrease uterine stimulation. Increase the primary (nonadditive) intravenous infusion as needed to maintain adequate circulating volume and ensure maximum uterine blood flow. Keep the woman in a lateral position to re-

duce aortocaval compression and increase placental blood flow. Oxygen given at 8 to 10 L/min with a snug face mask increases her blood oxygen saturation, making more available to the fetus. (See Chapter 18 for further information about fetal responses to reduced placental perfusion.)

REFERENCES AND READINGS

Ahner, R., Egarter, C., Kiss, H., et al. (1995). Fetal fibronectin as a selection criterion for induction of term labor. *American Journal of Obstetrics and Gynecology* 170(2), 1513–1517.

American Academy of Pediatrics & American College of Obstetricians and Gynecologists. (1997). *Guidelines for perinatal care* (4th ed.). Elk Grove Village, IL, and Washington, DC: Author.

American College of Obstetricians and Gynecologists. (1994). *Operative vaginal delivery* (ACOG Technical Bulletin No. 196). Washington, DC: Author.

American College of Obstetricians and Gynecologists. (1995a). *ACOG practice patterns: Vaginal delivery after previous cesarean birth* (ACOG Technical Bulletin No. 217). Washington, DC: Author.

American College of Obstetricians and Gynecologists. (1995b). *Dystocia and the augmentation of labor* (ACOG Technical Bulletin No. 217). Washington, DC: Author.

American College of Obstetricians and Gynecologists. (1995c). *Induction of labor* (ACOG Technical Bulletin No. 218). Washington, DC: Author.

American College of Obstetricians and Gynecologists. (1998). *Vaginal birth after previous cesarean delivery* (ACOG Practice Bulletin No. 2). Washington, DC: Author.

Annibale, D. J., Hulsey, T. C., Wagner, C. L., & Southgate, W. M. (1995). Comparative neonatal morbidity of abdominal and vaginal deliveries after uncomplicated pregnancies. *Archives of Pediatric and Adolescent Medicine*, 149(8), 862–867.

Bachman, J., & Kendrick, J. M. (1996). Childbirth. In K. R. Simpson & P. A. Creehan (Eds.), *AWHONN's perinatal nursing* (pp. 151–245). Philadelphia: Lippincott.

Bishop, E. H. (1964). Pelvic scoring. *Obstetrics and Gynecology*, 24(2), 266–268.

Blanch, G., Oláh, K. S. J., & Walkinshaw, S. (1996). The presence of fetal fibronectin in the cervicovaginal secretions of women at term: Its role in the assessment of women before labor induction and in the investigation of the physiologic mechanisms of labor. *American Journal of Obstetrics and Gynecology*, 174(1), Pt. 1, 262–266.

Bowes, W. A. (1999). Clinical aspects of normal and abnormal labor. In R. Creasy & R. Resnik (Eds.), *Maternal-fetal medicine:*

Principles and practice (4th ed., pp. 541–568). Philadelphia: Saunders.

Brisson-Carroll, G., Fraser, W., Bréart, G., Krauss, I., & Thornton, J. (1996). The effect of routine early amniotomy on spontaneous labor: A metaanalysis. *Obstetrics and Gynecology*, 87(5), Pt. 2, 891–896.

Busowski, J. D., & Parsons, M. T. (1995). Amniotomy to induce labor. *Clinical Obstetrics and Gynecology*, 38(2), 246–258.

Centers for Disease Control and Prevention. (1995). Rates of cesarean delivery—United States, 1993. *Morbidity and Mortality Weekly Report*, 44(15), 303–307.

Clarke, S. C., & Taffel, S. M. (1996). Rates of cesarean and VBAC delivery, United States, 1994. *Birth*, 22(3), 166–168.

Cunningham, F. G., MacDonald, P. C., Gant, N. F., Leveno, K. J., Gilstrap, L. C., Hankins, G. D. V., et al. (1997). *Williams obstetrics* (20th ed.). Norwalk, CT: Appleton & Lange.

Flamm, B. L., Berwick, D. M., & Kabcenell, A. (1998). Reducing cesarean section rates safely: Lessons from a "breakthrough series" collaborative. *Birth*, 25(2), 117–124.

Fuentes, A., & Williams, M. (1995). Cervical assessment. *Clinical Obstetrics and Gynecology*, 38(2), 224–231.

Hannah, M. E., Huh, C., Hewson, S. A., & Hannah, W. J. (1996). Postterm pregnancy: Putting the merits of a policy of induction of labor into perspective. *Birth*, 23(1), 13–19.

Kaczorowski, J., Levitt, C., Hanvey, L., Avard, D., & Chance, G. (1998). A national survey of use of obstetric procedures and technologies in Canadian hospitals: Routine or based on existing evidence? *Birth*, 25(1), 11–18.

Krammer, J., Williams, M. C., Sawai, S. K., & O'Brien, W. F. (1995). Preinduction cervical ripening: A randomized comparison of two methods. *Obstetrics and Gynecology*, 85(4), 614–618.

Laros, R. K., Flanagan, T. A., & Kilpatrick, S. J. (1995). Management of term breech presentation: A protocol of external cephalic version and selective trial of labor. *American Journal of Obstetrics and Gynecology*, 172(6), 1916–1925.

Lydon-Rochelle, M. (1995). Cesarean delivery rates in women cared for by certified nurse-midwives in the United States: A review. *Birth*, 22(4), 211–219.

Lydon-Rochelle, M. T., Albers, L., & Teaf, D. (1995). Perineal outcomes and nurse-midwifery management. *Journal of Nurse-Midwifery*, 40(1), 13–18.

Maier, J. S., & Maloni, J. A. (1997). Nurse advocacy for selective versus routine episiotomy. *Journal of Obstetric, Gynecologic, and Neonatal Nursing*, 26(2), 155–161.

Menihan, C. A. (1996). Intrapartum fetal monitoring. In K. R. Simpson & P. A. Creehan (Eds.), *AWHONN's perinatal nursing* (pp. 187–225). Philadelphia: Lippincott.

Naef, R. W., Ray, M. A., Chauhan, S. P., Roach, H., Blake, P. G., & Martin, J. N. (1995). Trial of labor after cesarean delivery with a lower-segment, vertical uterine incision: Is it safe? *American Journal of Obstetrics and Gynecology*, 172(6), 1666–1675.

O'Brien, W. F. (1995). The role of prostaglandins in labor and delivery. *Clinics in Perinatology*, 22(4), 973–984.

Paul, R. H., & Miller, D. A. (1995). Cesarean birth: How to reduce the rate. *American Journal of Obstetrics and Gynecology*, 172(6), 1903–1911.

Porreco, R. P., & Thorp, J. A. (1996). The cesarean birth epidemic: Trends, causes, and solutions. *American Journal of Obstetrics and Gynecology*, 175(2), 369–374.

Shyken, J. M., & Petrie, R. H. (1995). Oxytocin to induce labor. *Clinical Obstetrics and Gynecology*, 38(2), 232–245.

Summers, L. (1997). Methods of cervical ripening and labor induction. *Journal of Nurse-Midwifery*, 42(2), 71–85.

Thompson, J. P. Forceps deliveries. (1995). *Clinics in Perinatology*, 22(4), 953–972.

Torgersen, K. (1996). Ask the experts: Please compare prostaglandin E_2 preparations used to ripen the cervix in preparation for induction. *AWHONN Voice*, 4(3), 4.

U.S. Department of Health and Human Services, Public Health Service. (1995). *Healthy people 2000: Mid-course review and 1995 revisions*. Washington, DC: Author.

Williams, M. C. (1995). Vacuum-assisted delivery. *Clinics in Perinatology*, 22(4), 907–931.

Xenakis, E. M. J., Langer, O., Piper, J. M., Conway, D., & Berkus, M. D. (1995). Low-dose versus high-dose oxytocin augmentation of labor: A randomized trial. *American Journal of Obstetrics and Gynecology*, 173(6), 1874–1878.

21

Postpartum Adaptations

LEARNING OBJECTIVES

After studying this chapter, you should be able to:

- Explain the physiologic changes that occur during the postpartum period.
- Describe nursing assessments and nursing care during the postpartum period.
- Discuss the role of the nurse in health education and identify important areas of teaching.
- Describe postpartum home care in terms of criteria for discharge, common problems, and available health care services.
- Compare nursing assessments and care for women who have undergone cesarean birth and vaginal birth.
- Explain the process of bonding and attachment, including the role of maternal touch and verbal interactions.
- Describe the progressive phases of maternal adaptation to childbirth and the stages of maternal role attainment.
- Identify maternal concerns and how they change over time.
- Discuss the cause, manifestations, and interventions related to postpartum blues.
- Describe the processes of family adaptation to the birth of a baby.
- Discuss factors that affect family adaptation.
- Discuss cultural influences on family adaptation.
- Describe assessments and interventions related to postpartum psychosocial adaptations.
- Discuss the need for additional care following discharge of the mother and infant from the birth facility.

DEFINITIONS

afterpain Cramping pain following childbirth, caused by alternating relaxation and contraction of uterine muscles.

atony Absence or lack of usual muscle tone.

attachment Development of strong affectional ties as a result of interaction between an infant and a significant other (mother, father, sibling, caretaker).

bonding Development of a strong emotional tie of a parent to a newborn. Also called claiming or binding in.

catabolism A destructive process that converts living cells into simpler compounds. Process involved in involution (changes) of the uterus after childbirth.

decidua Term referring to the endometrium during pregnancy. All except the deepest layer is shed after childbirth.

diastasis recti Separation of the longitudinal muscles of the abdomen (rectus abdominis) during pregnancy.

dyspareunia Difficult or painful coitus in women.

en face Position that allows eye-to-eye contact between the newborn and a parent. Optimal distance is 20 to 22 cm (8 to 9 inches).

engorgement Swelling of the breasts resulting from increased blood flow and the presence of milk.

engrossment Intense fascination and close face-to-face observation between father and newborn.

entrainment Newborn movement in rhythm with adult speech, particularly high-pitched tones, which are more easily heard.

episiotomy Surgical incision of the perineum to enlarge the vaginal opening.

fingertipping First tactile (touch) experience between mother and newborn. The mother explores the infant's body with her fingertips only.

fourth trimester First 12 weeks following birth, a time of transition for parents and siblings.

fundus Part of the uterus that is farthest from the cervix, above the openings of the fallopian tubes.

involution Retrogressive changes that return the reproductive organs, particularly the uterus, to their nonpregnant size and condition.

Kegel exercises Alternate contracting and relaxing of the pelvic muscles. These movements strengthen the pubococcygeal muscle, which surrounds the urinary meatus and vagina.

lactation Secretion of milk from the breasts. Also describes the period of time of breast-feeding.

letting go A phase of maternal adaptation that involves relinquishing previous roles and assuming a new role as a parent.

lochia alba Whitish or clear vaginal discharge that follows lochia serosa. Occurs when the amount of blood is decreased and the number of leukocytes is increased.

lochia rubra Reddish vaginal discharge that occurs immediately after childbirth; composed mostly of blood.

lochia serosa Pinkish or brown-tinged vaginal discharge that follows lochia rubra; composed largely of serous exudate, blood, and leukocytes.

milk-ejection reflex Release of milk from the alveoli into the ducts. Also known as the letdown reflex.

oxytocin Posterior pituitary hormone that stimulates uterine contractions and the milk-ejection reflex. Also prepared synthetically.

postpartum blues Temporary, self-limiting period of weepiness experienced by many new mothers within the first few days following childbirth.

prolactin Anterior pituitary hormone that promotes growth of breast tissue and stimulates production of milk.

puerperium Period from the end of childbirth until involution of the uterus is complete, approximately 6 weeks.

reciprocal bonding behaviors Repertoire of infant behaviors that promotes attachment between parent and newborn.

REEDA Acronym for redness, ecchymosis, edema, discharge, and approximation. Useful for assessing wound healing or the presence of inflammation or infection.

sibling rivalry Feelings of jealousy and fear of replacement when a young child must share parental attention with a newborn infant.

taking hold Second phase of maternal adaptation, during which the mother assumes control of her own care and initiates care of the infant.

taking in First phase of maternal adaptation, during which the mother passively accepts care and comfort and details about the newborn.

The first 6 weeks following the birth of an infant are known as the postpartum period, or puerperium. During this time, mothers experience numerous physiologic and psychosocial changes. Many postpartum physiologic changes are retrogressive—that is, changes that occurred in body systems during pregnancy are reversed as the body returns to the nonpregnant state. Progressive changes also occur. Most obvious are the initiation of lactation and the return of normal menstrual cycles.

Reproductive System

Involution of the Uterus

Involution refers to the changes that the reproductive organs, particularly the uterus, undergo after childbirth as they return to their nonpregnant size and condition. Uterine involution entails three processes: (1) contraction of muscle fibers, (2) catabolism, and (3) regeneration of uterine epithelium. Uterine involution begins immediately after delivery of the placenta, when uterine muscle fibers contract firmly around maternal blood vessels at the area where the placenta was attached. This contraction controls bleeding from the area left denuded when the placenta separated. Moreover, the uterus becomes smaller as the muscle fibers, which have been stretched for many months, contract and gradually regain their former contour and size.

The enlarged uterine muscle cells are affected by catabolic changes in protein cytoplasm, which cause a reduction in individual cell size. The products of this catabolic process are absorbed by the bloodstream and excreted in the urine as nitrogenous waste.

Regeneration of the uterine epithelial lining begins soon after childbirth. The outer portion of the endometrial layer is expelled with the placenta. Within 2 to 3 days, the remaining decidua separates into two layers. The first layer is superficial and is shed in lochia. The basal layer remains intact and is the source of new endometrium. Regeneration of the endometrium, except at the site of placental attachment, occurs by 2 to 3 weeks.

The placental site, which is about 7 cm (2.7 inches) in diameter, heals by a process of *exfoliation* (scaling off of dead tissue). New endometrium is generated at the site from glands and tissue that remain in the lower layer of the decidua after separation of the placenta (Cunningham et al., 1997). This process leaves the uterine lining free of scar tissue, which would interfere with implantation of future pregnancies. Healing at the placental site takes approximately 6 to 7 weeks.

DESCENT OF THE UTERINE FUNDUS

The location of the uterine fundus helps determine whether involution is progressing normally. Immediately after delivery, the uterus is about the size of a large grapefruit and weighs approximately 1,000 g (2.2 lb). The fundus can be palpated midway between the symphysis pubis and umbilicus. Within a few hours, the fundus rises to the level of the umbilicus and should remain at this level for about 24 hours.

After 24 hours, the fundus begins to descend by approximately 1 cm, or one fingerbreadth, per day, so that by the tenth day it is in the pelvic cavity and cannot be palpated abdominally. Descent is documented in relation to the umbilicus. For instance, U − 1 indicates that the fundus is palpable one fingerbreadth below the umbilicus. Within a week, the weight of the uterus decreases to about 500 g (1 lb); at 6 weeks, the uterus weighs 60 g (2 ounces), which is roughly the prepregnancy weight. Figure 21–1 illustrates normal descent of the uterine fundus as involution occurs.

AFTERPAINS

Etiology. Intermittent contractions, known as afterpains, are a source of discomfort for many women. The discomfort is more acute for multiparas because repeated stretching of muscle fibers leads to loss of the muscle tone that enables alternate contraction and relaxation of the uterus. The uterus of a primipara tends to remain contracted, but she may also experience severe afterpains if the uterus has been overdistended by twins, a large infant, hydramnios (excess of amniotic fluid), or retained blood clots. Oxytocin released from the posterior pituitary during breastfeeding may also cause strong contractions of the uterine muscles.

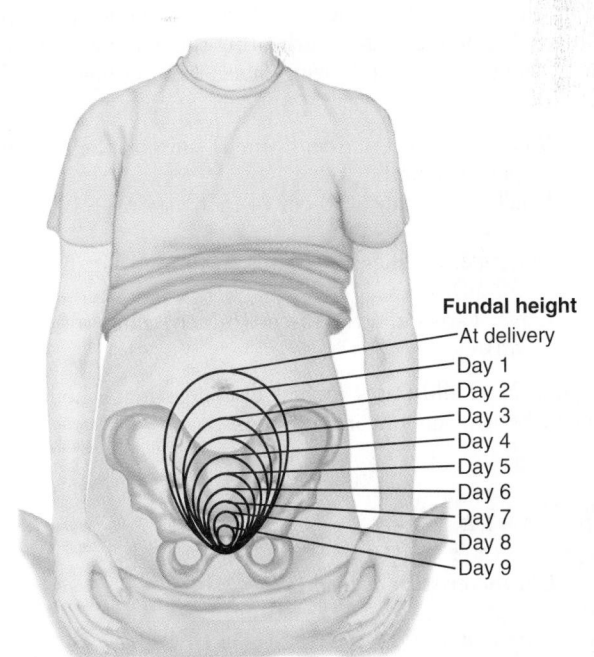

Fundal height
- At delivery
- Day 1
- Day 2
- Day 3
- Day 4
- Day 5
- Day 6
- Day 7
- Day 8
- Day 9

FIGURE 21–1

Involution of the uterus. Height of the uterine fundus decreases by approximately 1 cm/day.

Nursing Considerations. Analgesics are frequently used to lessen the discomfort of afterpains. If the mother is breast-feeding, she achieves maximum relief by taking the medication at least 30 minutes before nursing the infant. There is general agreement that analgesics may be used for short-term pain relief without harm to the infant. The benefits of pain relief, such as comfort and relaxation, which facilitate the milk-ejection reflex, usually outweigh the negligible effects of the medication on the infant.

Some mothers also find that lying in a prone position with a small pillow or folded blanket under the abdomen helps keep the uterus contracted and provides relief. Afterpains are self-limiting and decrease rapidly after 48 hours.

LOCHIA

Changes in the color and amount of lochia also provide information about whether involution is progressing normally.

Changes in Color. For the first 3 days after childbirth, lochia consists almost entirely of blood, with small particles of decidua and mucus. Because of its red color it is termed *lochia rubra*. The amount of blood decreases by about the fourth day. The color of lochia then changes from red to pinkish (*lochia serosa*). Lochia serosa is composed of serous exudate, erythrocytes, leukocytes, and cervical mucus. By about the 11th day, the erythrocyte component decreases. The discharge becomes white or a cream color (*lochia alba*). Lochia alba contains leukocytes, decidual cells, epithelial cells, fat, cervical mucus, and bacteria. It is present in most women until the third week after childbirth but may persist for 6 weeks.

Amount. Because estimating the amount of lochia is difficult, nurses frequently record lochia in terms that are difficult to quantify, such as "scant," "moderate," and "heavy." One method for estimating the amount of lochia in 1 hour uses the following labels (Luegenbiehl et al., 1990):

> *Scant:* Less than a 5-cm (2-inch) stain on the perineal pad (~10 ml).
> *Small:* Less than a 10-cm (4-inch) stain (~10 to 25 ml).
> *Moderate:* Smaller than a 15-cm (6-inch) stain (25 to 50 ml).
> *Large:* Larger than a 15-cm (6-inch) stain (50 to 80 ml).

Figure 21–2 illustrates lochial discharge for 1 hour and quantifies the amount in milliliters.

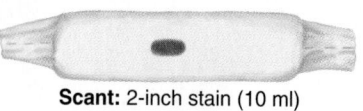
Scant: 2-inch stain (10 ml)

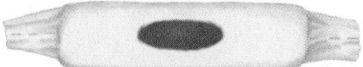
Small: 4-inch stain (10 to 25 ml)

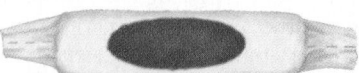
Moderate: 6-inch stain (25 to 50 ml)

Large: >6-inch stain (50 to 80 ml)

FIGURE 21–2

Guidelines for assessing the volume of lochia based on the amount of stain on the perineal pad.

Lochia is often heavier when the new mother first gets out of bed because gravity allows blood that has pooled in the vagina during the hours of rest to flow freely when she stands. Table 21–1 summarizes the characteristics of normal and abnormal lochial discharge.

Cervix

Immediately after childbirth, the cervix is formless, flabby, and open wide. Small tears or lacerations may be present, and the cervix is often edematous. Healing occurs rapidly, and by the end of the first week the cervix feels firm, and the external os is the width of a pencil. The internal os closes as before pregnancy, but the shape of the external os is permanently changed. It remains slightly open and appears slit-like rather than round, as in the nulliparous woman (Fig. 21–3).

Vagina

Soon after childbirth, the vaginal walls appear edematous, and multiple small lacerations may be present. Very few vaginal rugae (folds) are present. The hymen is permanently torn and heals with small, irregular tags of tissue visible at the vaginal introitus.

Although the vaginal mucosa heals and rugae are re-

TABLE 21–1

Characteristics of Lochia

Time and Type	Normal Discharge	Abnormal Discharge
Days 1–3: lochia rubra	Bloody; small clots; fleshy, earthy odor	Large clots; saturated perineal pads; foul odor
Days 4–10: lochia serosa	Decreased amount; serosanguineous; pink or brown	Excessive amount; foul smell; continued or recurrent reddish color
Days 11–21: lochia alba	White or cream color; decreasing amounts	Persistent lochia serosa; return to lochia rubra, foul odor; discharge continuing

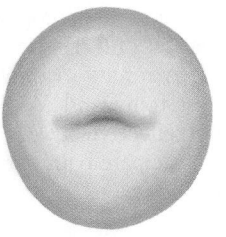 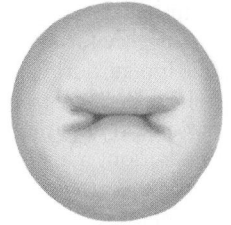

**Nulliparous cervix
with round os**

**Parous cervix
with slit os**

FIGURE 21–3
. . . .
A permanent change occurs in the cervical os after childbirth.

gained by 3 weeks, it takes the entire postpartum period (6 weeks) for the vagina to complete involution and to gain approximately the same size and contour it had before pregnancy. The vagina does not, however, entirely regain the nulliparous size.

During the postpartum period, vaginal mucosa becomes atrophic, and vaginal walls do not regain their thickness until estrogen production by the ovaries is re-established. Because ovarian function, and therefore estrogen production, is not well established during lactation, breast-feeding mothers are likely to experience vaginal dryness and may experience dyspareunia, or discomfort during intercourse, for 4 to 6 months (Blackburn & Loper, 1992).

. . . .
Lacerations of the Birth Canal

PERINEUM

Perineal lacerations are classified in degrees to describe the amount of tissue involved. Some physicians or nurse-midwives also describe the extent of median episiotomies by degree of tissue involvement.

First-degree: Involves the superficial vaginal mucosa or perineal skin.
Second-degree: Involves the vaginal mucosa, perineal skin, and deeper tissues, which may include muscles of the perineum.
Third-degree: Same as second-degree laceration but involves the anal sphincter.
Fourth-degree: Extends through the anal sphincter into the rectal mucosa.

PERIURETHRAL AREA

A laceration in the area of the urethra. Women with periurethral lacerations may have difficulty urinating after birth. They may need an indwelling catheter for a day or two.

VAGINAL WALL

A laceration involving the mucosa of the vaginal wall.

CERVIX

Tears in the cervix may be a source of significant bleeding after birth.

Perineum

Because of pressure from the fetal head, the muscles of the pelvic floor stretch and thin greatly during the second stage of labor. After childbirth, the perineum may be edematous and bruised. In the United States, many women who give birth also have a surgical incision (episiotomy) of the perineal area.

Lacerations of the perineum may also occur during delivery. Lacerations and episiotomies are classified according to tissue involved. (See discussion of episiotomy in Chapter 20.)

DISCOMFORT

Although the episiotomy is relatively small, the muscles of the perineum are involved in many activities (walking, sitting, stooping, squatting, bending, defecating). An incision in this area can cause a great deal of discomfort. In addition, many pregnant women are affected by hemorrhoids (distended rectal veins), which are pushed out of the rectum during the second stage of labor.

NURSING CONSIDERATIONS

Hemorrhoids, as well as perineal trauma, episiotomy, or lacerations, can make physical activity or bowel elimination difficult during the postpartum period. Relief of perineal discomfort is a nursing priority and includes teaching self-care measures, such as sitz baths, perineal care, and the use of topical anesthetics.

Cardiovascular System

Hypervolemia, which produces a 50% increase in blood volume at term, allows the woman to tolerate a substantial blood loss during childbirth without ill effect. On the average, 500 ml of blood is lost in vaginal deliveries and 1,000 ml is lost in cesarean births (Cunningham et al., 1997).

Cardiac Output

Despite the blood loss, a transient increase in maternal cardiac output occurs after childbirth. This increase is caused by (1) an increased flow of blood back to the heart when blood from the uteroplacental unit returns to the central circulation and (2) the mobilization of excess extracellular fluid into the vascular compartment.

The rise in cardiac output, which persists for about 48 hours after childbirth, is probably caused by an increase in stroke volume because bradycardia is often noted during the postpartum period. Bradycardia is defined as a pulse rate of 50 to 60 beats per minute. Gradually, cardiac output decreases and returns to normal levels by 12 weeks after childbirth (Resnik, 1999).

Plasma Volume

The body rids itself of excess plasma volume by diuresis and diaphoresis.

- *Diuresis* (increased excretion of urine) is facilitated by a decline in the levels of the adrenal hormone aldosterone, which increase during pregnancy to counteract the salt-wasting effect of progesterone. As aldosterone production decreases, sodium retention declines, and fluid excretion accelerates. A decrease in oxytocin, which promotes reabsorption of fluid, also contributes to diuresis. A urinary output of 3,000 ml/day is not uncommon for the first few days of the postpartum period.

- *Diaphoresis* (profuse perspiration) also rids the body of excess fluid. Although it is not clinically significant, diaphoresis can be uncomfortable and unsettling for the mother who is not prepared for it. Explanations of the cause and provision of comfort measures, such as showers and dry clothing, are generally sufficient.

Coagulation

During pregnancy, plasma fibrinogen (necessary for coagulation) increases. As a result, the mother's body has a greater ability to form clots and thus prevent excessive bleeding. Plasminogen (necessary for lysis of clots), however, does not rise during pregnancy. The result is that during pregnancy and the postpartum period she is at risk for thrombus (clot) formation.

Although the incidence of thrombophlebitis has declined greatly in recent years, probably as a result of early postpartum ambulation, new mothers are still at increased risk for thrombus formation. Women who have varicose veins, a history of thrombophlebitis, or a cesarean birth are at further risk, and the lower extremities should be monitored closely. Antiembolism hosiery is often applied before a cesarean birth or if the mother is at particular risk because of a history of previous phlebitis or the presence of varicosities. (See discussion of thromboembolic disorders in Chapter 28.)

Blood Values

Several components of the blood change during the postpartum period. Marked leukocytosis occurs, with the white blood cell count increasing from the nonpregnancy normal range of 5,000 to 10,000/mm³ up to 20,000 or even 30,000/mm³ (Cunningham et al., 1997). Neutrophils, which increase in response to inflammation, pain, and stress, account for the major increase in white blood cells.

Maternal hemoglobin and hematocrit values are difficult to interpret during the first few days after birth because of the remobilization and rapid excretion of excess body fluid. The hematocrit is low when plasma (the liquid part of blood) increases and dilutes the concentration of blood cells and other substances carried by the plasma. As excess fluid is excreted, the dilution is gradually reduced. The hematocrit should return to normal values within 3 to 7 days unless excessive blood loss has occurred.

Gastrointestinal System

Soon after childbirth, digestion begins to be active, and the new mother is usually hungry because of the energy expended in labor. Moreover, she is usually thirsty because of the long period of fluid restriction during labor, the fluid loss from exertion, and early diaphoresis. Nurses anticipate the mother's needs and provide food and fluids soon after childbirth.

Constipation is a common problem during the postpartum period, for a variety of reasons. First, bowel tone, which was diminished during pregnancy as a result of progesterone, remains sluggish for several days. Second, restricted food and fluid intake during labor often results in small, hard stools. Third, perineal trauma, episiotomy, and hemorrhoids cause discomfort and interfere with effective bowel elimination. In addition, many women anticipate pain when they attempt to defecate and are unwilling to exert pressure on the perineum.

Temporary constipation is not harmful, although it can cause a feeling of abdominal fullness and flatulence. Stool softeners and laxatives are frequently prescribed to prevent or treat constipation.

Urinary System

Physical Changes

As a result of many changes that occur during pregnancy, the bladder of the postpartum woman has an increased capacity and has lost some of its muscle tone. Moreover, during childbirth the urethra, bladder, and tissue around the urinary meatus may become edematous and traumatized as the fetal head passes beneath the bladder. This condition often results in diminished sensitivity to fluid pressure, and many new mothers have no sensation of needing to void even when the bladder is distended.

The bladder fills rapidly because of the diuresis that follows childbirth. As a consequence, the mother is at risk for overdistension of the bladder, incomplete emptying of the bladder, and retention of residual urine. Women who have received regional anesthesia are at particular risk for bladder distension and for difficulty voiding until feeling returns.

Urinary retention and overdistension of the bladder may cause urinary tract infection and postpartum hemorrhage. Urinary tract infection occurs when urinary stasis allows time for bacteria to multiply. Risk of postpartum hemorrhage increases because uterine ligaments, which were stretched during pregnancy, allow the uterus to be displaced upward and laterally by the full bladder. The displacement results in an inability of the uterine muscles to contract (uterine atony), a primary cause of excessive bleeding (Fig. 21–4).

Chemical Changes

Both protein and acetone may be present in the urine in the first few postpartum days. Acetone suggests dehydration, which often occurs during the exertion of labor. Mild proteinuria is usually the result of the catabolic processes involved in uterine involution.

Musculoskeletal System

Muscles and Joints

In the first 1 to 2 days after childbirth, many women experience muscle fatigue and aches, particularly of the shoulders, neck, and arms, because of exertion during labor. Warmth and gentle massage increase circulation to the area and provide comfort and relaxation.

During the first few days, levels of the hormone relaxin

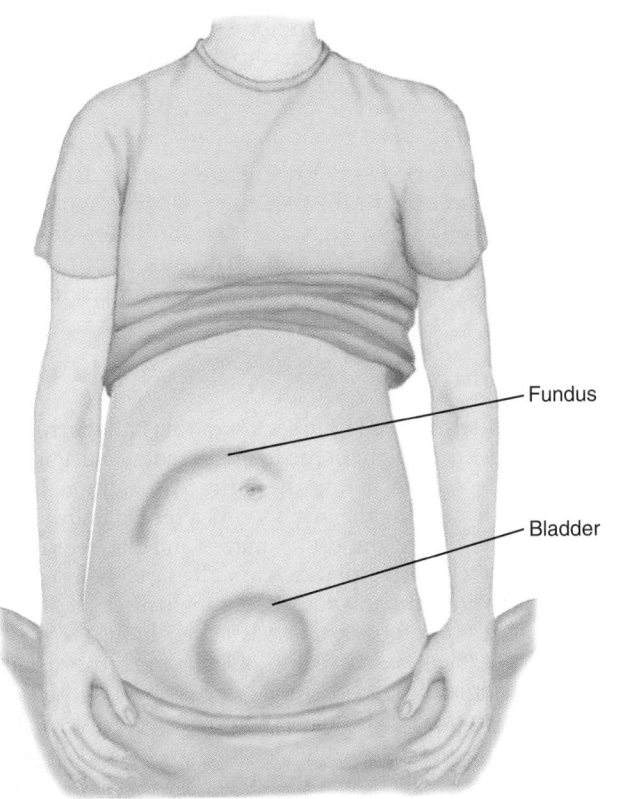

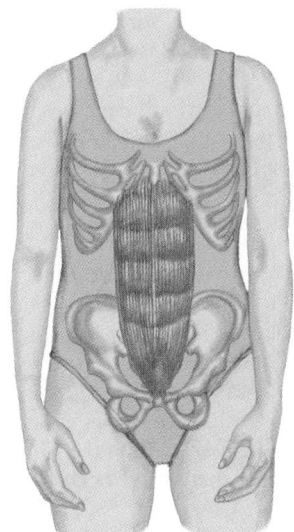
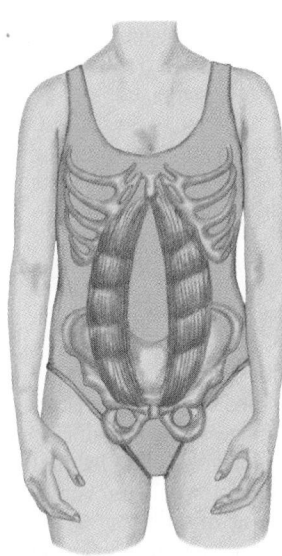

Normal location of rectus muscles of the abdomen

Diastasis recti: separation of the rectus muscles

FIGURE 21–5
• • • • • • • •
Diastasis recti occurs when the longitudinal muscles of the abdomen separate during pregnancy.

FIGURE 21–4
• • • • • • • •
A full bladder displaces and prevents contraction of the uterus.

gradually subside, and the ligaments and cartilage of the pelvis begin to return to their prepregnancy position. These changes can cause hip or joint pain that interferes with ambulation and exercise. It is helpful if the mother understands that the discomfort is temporary and does not indicate a medical problem. Good body mechanics and correct posture are extremely important during this time and should prevent low back pain and injury to the joints. (See Figs. 13–11 and 13–12 for correct and incorrect posture and body mechanics.)

Abdominal Wall

During pregnancy, the abdominal walls stretch to accommodate the growing fetus, and muscle tone is diminished.

Many women, expecting that the abdominal muscles will return to the prepregnancy condition immediately after childbirth, are dismayed to find the abdominal muscles weak, soft, and flabby.

The longitudinal muscles of the abdomen may also separate (diastasis recti) during pregnancy (Fig. 21–5). The separation may be minimal or severe. The mother may benefit from special exercises to strengthen the abdominal wall. Figure 21–6 illustrates exercises that help to correct diastasis recti.

Integumentary System

Many skin changes that occur during pregnancy are caused by an increase in hormones. When the hormone levels decline after childbirth, the skin gradually reverts to the prepregnancy state. For example, levels of melanocyte-stimulating hormone, which caused hyperpigmentation during pregnancy, decrease rapidly after childbirth, and pig-

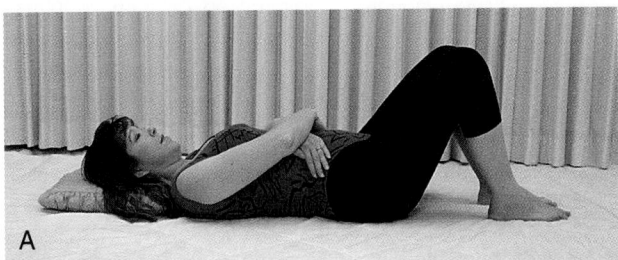
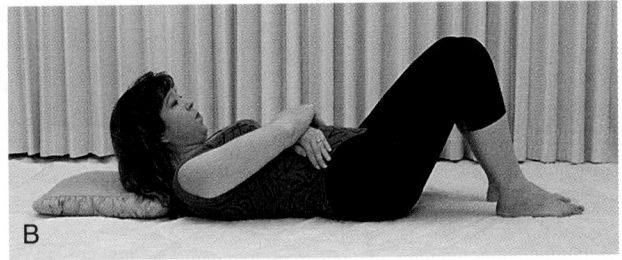

FIGURE 21–6
• • • • • • • •
Abdominal exercises for diastasis recti. *A,* The woman inhales and supports the abdominal wall firmly with her hands. *B,* Exhaling, the woman raises her head as she pulls the abdominal muscles together.

mentation begins to recede. This change is particularly noticeable when the "mask of pregnancy" (*chloasma*) and linea nigra disappear.

Striae gravidarum (stretch marks), which develop during pregnancy when connective tissue in the abdomen and breasts is stretched, gradually fade to silvery lines but do not disappear.

Neurologic System

Many women experience discomfort and fatigue after childbirth. Afterpains, discomfort from episiotomy or incisions, muscle aches, and breast engorgement may contribute to a woman's discomfort and inability to sleep. Anesthesia or analgesia may produce temporary neurologic changes such as lack of feeling in the legs and dizziness. During this time, the priority is prevention of injury that could occur as a result of falling.

Complaints of headache need careful assessment. Although they are uncommon, postpuncture headaches following regional anesthesia may occur. They may be most severe when the woman is in an upright position and are relieved by a supine position. They should be reported to the appropriate health care provider, usually an anesthesiologist. Headache, along with blurred vision, photophobia, and abdominal pain, may also indicate development or worsening of pregnancy-induced hypertension (see Chapter 26).

Endocrine System

Following expulsion of the placenta, a fairly rapid decline occurs in placental hormones such as estrogen, progesterone, human placental lactogen, and human chorionic gonadotropin. Adrenal hormones, such as aldosterone, return to prepregnancy levels. If the mother is not breast-feeding, the pituitary hormone prolactin, which stimulates milk secretion, disappears in about 2 weeks.

Resumption of Ovulation and Menstruation

Most nonnursing mothers resume menstruation within 7 to 9 weeks after childbirth, although times vary widely (Resnik, 1999). Breast-feeding delays the return of both ovulation and menstruation. The length of the delay depends on the duration of lactation and the frequency of breast-feeding. Women who breast-feed for less than 28 days ovulate at approximately the same time as nonnursing mothers. The longer the period of lactation lasts, the longer the average time to the first menstrual period. Women who breast-feed six or more times daily are also likely to ovulate and menstruate later than women who breast-feed less often.

Most lactating women resume menstruation within 12 weeks, although a few do not menstruate for the entire lactation period. Breast-feeding is not an effective form of contraception, however, because ovulation may occur before menstrual cycles are established.

Lactation

During pregnancy, estrogen and progesterone prepare the breasts for lactation. Although prolactin levels also rise during pregnancy, lactation is inhibited at this time by the high levels of estrogen and progesterone. Following expulsion of the placenta, levels of estrogen and progesterone decline rapidly, and prolactin initiates milk production within 2 to 3 days after childbirth. Once milk production is established, it continues because of frequent removal of milk from the breast.

Oxytocin is necessary for milk ejection, or "let down." A hormone secreted by the posterior pituitary gland, oxytocin, causes milk to be expressed from the alveoli into the lactiferous ducts during suckling. The process of lactation and measures to aid in breast-feeding are described in detail in Chapter 24.

Weight Loss

Approximately 5.5 kg (12 lb) is lost during childbirth. This loss includes the weight of the fetus, placenta, and amniotic fluid and blood lost during the birth. An additional 4 kg (8.8 lb) is lost during the first 2 weeks after childbirth. This loss includes the weight lost by diuresis and diaphoresis during the first few postpartum days as well as weight lost as the reproductive organs involute (Cunningham et al., 1997).

Adipose (fatty) tissue that was gained during pregnancy to meet the energy requirements of labor and breast-feeding is not lost initially, and the usual rate of loss is quite slow. Most women approach their prepregnancy weight about 6 months after childbirth, but a year may elapse before all weight is lost. This period may be frustrating for mothers who desire an immediate return to prepregnancy weight. Nurses can provide information about diet and exercise that will produce an acceptable weight loss but does not deplete energy or impair the mother's health. See Chapter 15 for additional information about weight loss and dietary recommendations.

Postpartum Assessments

Providing essential, cost-effective postpartum care to new families is a challenge for maternity nurses. Legislation now mandates that a longer length of stay be allowed than the 24-hour stay that was previously allowed by many insurance companies. The trend toward early discharge, however, continues. Women with an uncomplicated vaginal birth generally leave the birth facility within 48 hours. Those who gave birth by cesarean section may remain in the facility for 96 hours.

Although the length of stay is short, the family's need for care and information remains the same. This need causes nurses a great deal of concern for families who are discharged without adequate preparation or support. Nurses are actively involved in developing ways to provide continuing care in the home.

Clinical Pathways

Many institutions use clinical pathways (also called critical pathways, care maps, or multidisciplinary action plans) to provide necessary care while reducing the length of stay. Clinical pathways identify expected outcomes and establish time frames for specific assessments and interventions that prepare the mother and infant for discharge. The clinical pathway is a guideline and documentation tool. Figure 21–7 shows an example of a clinical pathway for normal spontaneous vaginal birth.

DRUG GUIDE

Rubella Vaccine

Classification: Attenuated live virus vaccine.

Action: Produces a modified rubella infection that is not communicable. This process causes the formation of antibodies.

Indications: Administered after childbirth or abortion to women whose antibody screen shows they are not immune to rubella (German measles). This vaccine prevents rubella infection and possible severe congenital defects in the fetus during a subsequent pregnancy.

Dosage and Route: 0.5 ml of reconstituted vaccine injected subcutaneously into the upper outer aspect of the arm.

Absorption: Well absorbed.

Contraindications and Precautions: Contraindicated in women who have a respiratory or febrile infection or who are immunosuppressed, pregnant, or sensitive to neomycin or eggs. The attenuated virus may appear in breast milk, but this is not a contraindication to vaccination of lactating women.

Adverse Reactions: Lymphadenopathy, rash, urticaria, fever, malaise, sore throat, headache, dizziness, nausea, vomiting, arthralgia, arthritis.

Nursing Implications: The mother and her partner must be warned to avoid pregnancy for at least 3 months after vaccination because of the possibility that a fetus might be affected by the live virus in the vaccine.

Initial Assessments

When caring for postpartum patients, the nurse faces a high risk for contact with body fluids (colostrum, breast milk, amniotic fluid, and lochia from the mother as well as urine, stool, and blood from the infant). Therefore, the recommendations of the Centers for Disease Control and Prevention for standard blood and body fluid precautions must be followed diligently (see Appendix B).

Postpartum assessments begin during the fourth stage of labor (1 to 2 hours after childbirth). During this time the mother is examined to determine whether she is physically stable. Initial assessments include the following:

- Vital signs
- Skin color
- Location and firmness of the fundus
- Amount and color of lochia
- Presence and location of pain
- Intravenous infusions (type of fluid, rate)
- Added medications (type and amount)
- Patency of intravenous line
- Intravenous site for redness, pain, or edema
- Time and amount of last voiding
- Presence of urinary catheter
- Level of feeling and ability to move if regional anesthesia was administered

Chart Review

When the initial assessments confirm that the mother's physical condition is stable, nurses should review the chart to obtain pertinent information and to determine whether there are factors that increase the risk of complications during the postpartum period. Relevant information includes the following:

- Gravida, parity
- Time and type of delivery (use of forceps, vacuum extractor)
- Anesthesia or medications administered during labor
- Significant medical and surgical history, such as diabetes, hypertension, or heart disease

- Medications routinely taken and reasons why they are needed
- Food and drug allergies
- Chosen method of infant feeding
- Condition of the baby
- Perineum for episiotomy or lacerations

Laboratory data are also examined. Of particular interest are the prenatal hemoglobin and hematocrit values, the blood type and Rh factor, hepatitis B surface antigen, and a syphilis screen.

NEED FOR $Rh_o(D)$ IMMUNE GLOBULIN

Prenatal and neonatal records are checked to determine whether $Rh_o(D)$ immune globulin should be administered. $Rh_o(D)$ immune globulin may be necessary if the mother is Rh-negative and the newborn is Rh-positive. To prevent the development of maternal antibodies that would affect subsequent pregnancies, $Rh_o(D)$ immune globulin should be administered within 72 hours after childbirth (see Chapter 26).

NEED FOR RUBELLA VACCINE

A prenatal rubella antibody screen is performed on each pregnant woman to determine if she is immune to rubella. If she is not immune, rubella vaccine is offered after childbirth to prevent her from acquiring rubella during subsequent pregnancies, when it can cause serious fetal anomalies. Rubella vaccine is a live virus that can produce serious consequences for the fetus if the mother becomes pregnant soon after it is administered. Before administration, some agencies require that she sign a statement indicating that she understands the risks of becoming pregnant again within 3 months following the injection. If this statement is not required, the nurse should record in the chart that the risk has been explained and the parents have verbalized their understanding.

RISK FACTORS FOR HEMORRHAGE AND INFECTION

Nurses must be aware of conditions that increase the risk of *hemorrhage* and *infection*, the two most common complications of the puerperium.

Text continued on page 486

YORK HEALTH SYSTEM
YORK, PENNSYLVANIA
CLINICAL PATHWAY
VAGINAL DELIVERY

CLINICAL PATH DAY		EXPECTED PATIENT/ FAMILY OUTCOMES	INTERDISCIPLINARY ASSESSMENT	TESTS	CONSULT
Pre-Natal	DATE	☐ Prenatal test results available [4] ☐ 8 or more prenatal visits complete [4] ☐ Attended baby care and post-partum classes [3] ☐ Risk assessment complete and referral(s) to appropriate agency made as needed.[5] ☐ Low risk pregnancy or monitored high risk pregnancy [4] ☐ _____ ☐ _____	Each visit-maternal weight; BP; urine dipstick-sugar, protein ketones; FHT S/S of pregnancy complication Perinatal risk assessment Social support Knowledge of self and newborn care Knowledge of warning signs of complications Knowledge of signs of labor	Type and Rh Antibody Screen H and H Sickle cell Rubella RPR HBSAG Trutol or 3h GTT GC, Chlamydia Triple Screen Group B Strep	☐ Perinatologist ☐ Diabetic Educator ☐ Behavioral Health ☐ Social Service ☐ _____ ☐ _____ ☐ _____
Admission		☐ Demonstrates knowledge of pain management options [1, 2, 3] ☐ Support person present [2] ☐ Referral made for identified risk factors ☐ Admission procedures completed [4] ☐ _____	Admission assessment Patient needs/desires for pain relief in labor Support system _____ _____	WCBC Type and Rh prn Tube to hold US scan prn _____	☐ Perinatologist ☐ Behavioral Health ☐ Social Service ☐ Neonatology ☐ _____
Labor First Stage		☐☐☐ Achieves desired level of pain relief [1, 2, 3] ☐☐☐ Support person present [2] ☐☐☐ Referral made for identified maternal/fetal risk during labor ☐☐☐ Mother demonstrates normal physiologic parameters [4] ☐☐☐ Fetus demonstrates normal physiologic parameters [4] ☐☐☐ _____	FHR q 30 min UC q 30-60 min P, R, BP q 2h T q 4° (q2 if ROM) Support system Progress of labor Level of comfort _____	_____ _____	☐ Neonatology ☐ _____
Labor Second Stage		☐ Pushing effectively [4] ☐ Support person present {2} ☐ Referral made for identified maternal/fetal risk during labor [4] ☐ Mother demonstrates normal physiological parameters [4] ☐ Fetus demonstrates normal physiological parameters [4] ☐ _____	FHR q 5 min BP q 30 min Vaginal exam prn _____	_____ _____	☐ Neonatology ☐ _____

NAME	INITIALS	NAME	INITIALS

FIGURE 21–7
· · · · · · · · · · ·

Clinical pathway for uncomplicated vaginal birth. (Courtesy of Women and Children's Services of the York Health System, York, Pennsylvania.)

DOCUMENTATION CODES
Initial=Meets Standard
★=Exception on pathway identified
C=Chronic problems
N=Not applicable

PARENT/FAMILY PROBLEMS
1. Pain r/t childbirth
2. Anxiety r/t childbirth and/or parenting
3. Knowledge deficit r/t childbirth and/or parenting
4. Potential alteration maternal/fetal homeostasis

5. Potential for ineffective parenting
6. _____
7. _____

INTERVENTIONS/ACTIVITIES	MEDS	NUTRITION	EDUCATION AND DC PLANNING
_____ _____	Prenatal vitamin, Fe as per order _____	Regular diet _____	Childbirth preparation class Baby care class Breastfeeding class when appropriate Prenatal education
Bed rest with fetal monitor x 30 minutes _____	IV/mini cath _____	NPO with ice chips _____	□ Orient pt/SO/family to L and D area □ Reinforce breathing and relaxation techniques □ _____

Insertion of scalp electrode and IUPC
   as appropriate
Warm/cold compress, massage,
   position change, ambulates and warm
   showers prn
Encourage to void q 1-2°
EFM as ordered
Vaginal exam prn
Catheterize prn
 	
_____
_____
	IV as ordered
	Analgesia prn as ordered
	Epidural as ordered
	Induction/augmentation
	   of labor as ordered
	
	_____
	_____
		NPO with ice chips
		
		_____
			☐☐☐ Reinforce breathing and relaxation
			      technique
			☐☐☐ Review options for pain
			      management
			☐☐☐ Encourage support person
			      involvement
			☐☐☐ Provide explanation of labor
			      progress prn

Position for comfort
Catheterize prn
Warm/cold compress, massage,
   position change and void prn
 	
_____
	IV as ordered
	Continue epidural as
	   ordered
	Augmentation of labor
	   as ordered
	
	_____
	_____
		NPO with ice chips
		
		_____
			□ Assist with pushing
			□ Encourage support person
			   involvement
			□ _____
			□ _____

NAME	INITIALS	NAME	INITIALS

FIGURE 21–7
• • • • • • • • • •
Continued

Ilustration continued on following page

CLINICAL PATH DAY		EXPECTED PATIENT/ FAMILY OUTCOMES	INTERDISCIPLINARY ASSESSMENT	TESTS	CONSULT
Delivery	DATE	☐ Deliver live newborn vaginally [4] ☐ Support person present [2] ☐ Mother demonstrates normal physiologic parameters	Fundus, bleeding _____ _____	Cord blood Rh studies when indicated Placenta to pathology as ordered	_____
	TIME	☐ _____			
Early Recovery	DATE	☐ Postpartum parameters stable [4] ☐ Achieves desired level of pain relief [1] ☐ _____ ☐ _____	Temp X 1 P, R, BP, fundus, lochia, bladder, episiotomy q 15 min x 4, and q 30 min x 2 Level of comfort	_____ _____	_____
2-24 Hours	DATE	☐☐☐ Achieves desired level of pain relief [1] ☐☐☐ Cares for self and infant [3] ☐☐☐ Postpartum parameters stable ☐☐☐ Voiding qs [4] ☐☐☐ Adequate home support system identified [5] ☐☐☐ _____ ☐☐☐ _____	T, P, R, BP, Breasts, fundus, lochia, bladder, episiotomy q 4h Readiness to learn Knowledge of self and newborn care Level of comfort Home support system	_____ _____	_____
24-48 Hours	DATE	☐☐☐ Achieves desired level of pain relief [1] ☐☐☐ Postpartum parameters stable [4] ☐☐☐ Referral made for potential or identified risk (physical/psychosocial) ☐ Cares for self and infant [3] ☐☐☐ _____	T, P, R, BP, bid Breasts, fundus, lochia, bladder, episiotomy q shift WA Level of comfort Readiness to learn Knowledge of self and newborn care	WCBC _____	_____
Day of Discharge	DATE	☐☐☐ Achieves desired level of pain relief [1] ☐☐☐ Postpartum physiological parameters within D/C guidelines [4] ☐ Patient/SO/family verbalization of D/C instructions [3] ☐ Postpartum Home Visit not needed based on Interqual Criteria ☐ Discharge within 2 days after delivery ☐ _____ ☐ _____	T, P, R, BP, bid Breasts, fundus, lochia, bladder, episiotomy bid Level of comfort Readiness to learn Pt/SO/family knowledge of self and newborn care _____ _____	_____ _____	_____

NAME	INITIALS		NAME	INITIALS

NOTE: EACH PATIENT REQUIRES AN INDIVIDUAL ASSESSMENT AND TREATMENT PLAN. THIS CLINICAL PATH IS A RECOMMENDATION FOR THE AVERAGE PATIENT WHICH REQUIRES MODIFICATION WHEN NECESSARY BY THE PROFESSIONAL STAFF.

FIGURE 21–7
· · · · · · · · ·
Continued

INTERVENTIONS/ACTIVITIES	MEDS	NUTRITION	EDUCATION AND DC PLANNING
Catheterize prn Continue IV Continue epidural or local anesthetic _____ _____	Oxytocin after placenta delivered as ordered ☐ _____ ☐ _____	NPO _____ _____	☐ Support parent/infant bonding ☐ _____ ☐ _____
OOB with assist first time Perineal ice pack q 30 min prn Cath prn Shower _____ _____	Analgesia prn Continue epidural if PPTL Continue IV oxytocin as ordered D/C IV or cap IV ☐ _____ ☐ _____	Reg diet as tolerated _____ _____	☐ Support parent/infant bonding ☐ Teach pericare ☐ _____ ☐ _____
OOB with assist first time, then OOB ad lib Catheterize per protocol Epifoam, Tucks prn Ice pack prn Sitz bath 12° after delivery prn _____ _____	Analgesia prn _____ _____	Adv to reg diet as tolerated _____ _____	☐☐☐ Initiate and continue maternal/newborn education record, D/C instructions ☐☐☐ _____ ☐☐☐ _____ _____
OOB ad lib Epifoam, Tucks prn Sitz bath prn _____	Analgesia prn _____ _____	Regular diet _____ _____	☐☐☐ Continue maternal newborn education record ☐☐☐ _____ ☐☐☐ _____ _____

OOB ad lib
Epifoam, Tucks prn
Sitz bath prn
 	
_____
	Analgesia prn
	☐ RhoGAM, when indicated
	☐ Rubella, when indicated
	_____
		Regular diet
		_____
		_____
			☐ Completion of maternal newborn education record
			☐ Physician discharge instructions
			☐ Support services in community:
			  ☐ Breastfeeding Support Services
			  ☐ Perinatal Coaching
			  ☐ City/State Health
			  ☐ Other
			☐ D/C after Pt./family review instructions

DISCHARGE DATE	DISCHARGE TIME	DISCHARGED TO	ACCOMPANIED BY ☐ W/C ☐ AMBULATE

FIGURE 21–7
. . . .
Continued

Postpartum High-Risk Factors

Hemorrhage

- Multiparity (more than three)
- Overdistension of the uterus (e.g., due to a large baby, twins, hydramnios)
- Precipitous labor (less than 3 hours)
- Prolonged labor
- Retained placenta
- Placenta previa or abruptio placentae
- Induction or augmentation of labor
- Administration of tocolytics to stop uterine contractions
- Operative procedures (vacuum extraction, forceps, cesarean birth)

Infection

- Operative procedures (cesarean birth, forceps, vacuum extraction)
- Multiple cervical examinations
- Prolonged labor (more than 24 hours)
- Manual extraction of placenta
- Diabetes
- Indwelling catheter
- Anemia (hemoglobin less than 10 mg/dl)

Focus Assessments Following Vaginal Birth

Nurses perform postpartum assessments according to facility protocol. For example, a protocol might require assessment every 15 minutes for the first hour, every half hour for the next hour, every 4 hours for the first 24 hours, and every 8 hours thereafter. Of course, assessments are performed more frequently if findings are abnormal.

Although assessments vary according to particular problems presented, a focus assessment for a vaginal delivery generally includes the fundus, lochia, bladder elimination, perineum, vital signs, breasts, and lower extremities. The assessment for postcesarean mothers is more complete (see p. 492).

FUNDUS

The fundus should be assessed for consistency and location. It should be firmly contracted and at or near the level of the umbilicus. If the uterus is above the expected level or is shifted from the midline position (usually to the right), the bladder may be distended. The location of the fundus should be rechecked after the woman has emptied her bladder. Procedure 21–1 illustrates how to locate and palpate the fundus. If the fundus is difficult to locate or is soft or "boggy," the nurse stimulates the uterine muscle to contract by gently massaging the uterus.

The nondominant hand must support and anchor the lower uterine segment if it is necessary to massage an uncontracted uterus. Uterine massage is not necessary if the uterus is firmly contracted.

The uterus can contract only if it is free of intrauterine clots. To expel clots, the nurse must support the lower uterine segment, as illustrated in Procedure 21–1. This support prevents inversion of the uterus (turning inside out) when the nurse applies firm pressure downward toward the vagina to express clots that have collected in the uterus. Nurses should observe the perineum for the number and size of clots expelled. Table 21–2 describes normal and abnormal findings of the uterine fundus and includes follow-up nursing actions for abnormal findings.

Drugs are sometimes needed to maintain contraction of the uterus and thus to prevent postpartum hemorrhage. The most commonly used drugs are methylergonovine (Methergine) and oxytocin (Pitocin). Drug Guides for methylergonovine are presented on p. 717 and for oxytocin on p. 458.

LOCHIA

Important assessments include the amount, color, and odor of lochia. Nurses observe the amount and color of lochia

---

Observations of the Uterine Fundus Requiring Nursing Actions

Normal Findings	Abnormal Findings	Nursing Actions
Fundus is firmly contracted.	Fundus is soft, "boggy," uncontracted, or difficult to locate.	Support lower uterine segment and massage until firm.
Fundus remains contracted when massage is discontinued.	Fundus becomes soft and uncontracted when massage is stopped.	Continue to support lower uterine segment; massage until firm and apply pressure to fundus to express clots that may be accumulating in uterus. Notify health care provider and begin oxytocin administration, as prescribed, to maintain a firm fundus.
Fundus is located at level of umbilicus and midline.	Fundus is above umbilicus and/or displaced from midline.	Assess bladder elimination. Assist mother in urinating or catheterize, if necessary, to empty bladder.

PROCEDURE 21-1
· · · · · · · · · ·
Assessing the Uterine Fundus

PURPOSE: To determine the location and firmness of the uterus.

1. To reduce anxiety and elicit cooperation, explain the procedure and rationale for each step before beginning the procedure.
2. Have the mother empty her bladder if she has not voided recently because a distended bladder lifts and displaces the uterus.
3. Place the mother in a supine position with her knees slightly flexed to relax the abdominal muscles and to permit accurate location of the fundus.
4. Put on clean gloves because there may be contact with body fluids. Lower the perineal pads to observe lochia as the fundus is palpated.
5. Place your nondominant hand above the woman's symphysis pubis to support and anchor the lower uterine segment during palpation or massage of the fundus.
6. Use the flat part of your fingers (not the fingertips) for palpation (see illustration) because the larger surface provides more comfort.
7. Begin palpation at the umbilicus, and palpate gently until the fundus is located. Notice how the hand "cups" the uterus to determine firmness and location of the fundus. The fundus should be firm, in the midline, and approximately at the level of the umbilicus. Bladder distension may lift and displace the fundus.
8. If the fundus is difficult to locate or is soft or "boggy," keep your nondominant hand above the woman's symphysis pubis and massage the fundus with your dominant hand until the fundus is firm. The nondominant hand anchors the lower segment of the uterus and prevents trauma while the uterus is massaged. The uterus contracts in response to tactile stimulation.

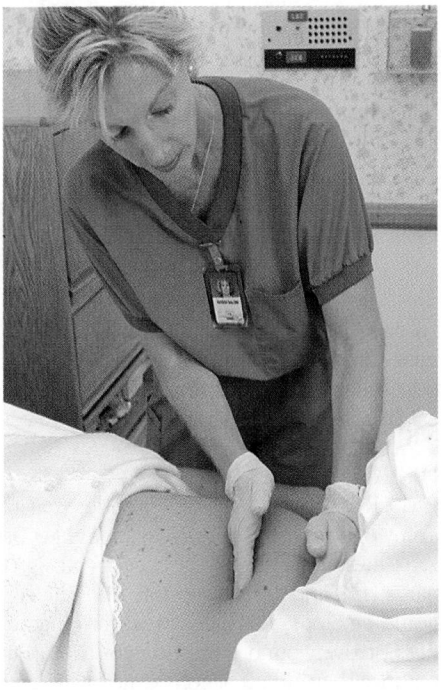

9. Document the consistency and location of the fundus to promote accurate communication and identify deviations from expected findings. Record consistency as "fundus firm," "firm with massage," or "boggy." Record fundal height in fingerbreadths above or below the umbilicus. For example, "fundus firm, midline, U − 2" (two fingerbreadths below umbilicus) or "fundus firm with light massage, U + 2, displaced to right."

on perineal pads and while checking the perineum. They also watch vaginal discharge while palpating or massaging the fundus so that the amount of lochia as well as the number and size of any clots expressed during these procedures can be observed. Refer to Figure 21-2 for criteria to determine the amount of lochia and to Table 21-1 for the normal characteristics of lochia as well as abnormal observations that must be reported. Note these important guidelines:

- A constant trickle of lochia indicates excessive bleeding and requires immediate attention.
- Excessive lochia in the presence of a contracted uterus suggests lacerations of the birth canal, and the health care provider must be notified so that the laceration can be located and repaired.

The odor of lochia is usually described as "fleshy," "earthy," or "musty." A foul odor suggests endometrial infection, and assessments should be made for additional signs of infection. These signs include maternal fever, tachycardia, and uterine tenderness and pain.

Absence of lochia, like the presence of a foul odor, may also indicate infection. If the birth was cesarean, lochia may be scant because the cavity of the uterus was wiped by sponges, removing some of the endometrial lining. Lochia should not, however, be entirely absent.

BLADDER ELIMINATION
Because the mother may not experience the urge to void even if the bladder is full, nurses must rely on physical assessment to determine whether the bladder is distended. Bladder distension often produces an obvious or palpable bulge that feels like a soft, movable mass above the symphysis pubis. Other signs include an upward and lateral displacement of the uterine fundus and increased lochia. Frequent voidings of less than 150 ml suggest urinary retention with overflow. Signs of an empty bladder include a firm fundus in the midline and a nonpalpable bladder.

Some facilities measure the first two voidings to determine whether normal bladder function has returned. When the mother can void at least 300 to 400 ml, the bladder is usually empty. Regardless of the amount voided, however, the fundus must be assessed to confirm that the bladder is empty. Subjective symptoms of urgency, frequency, or dysuria suggest urinary tract infection and should be reported to the health care provider.

PERINEUM

The acronym REEDA is used as a reminder that the site of an episiotomy or a perineal laceration should be assessed for five signs: redness (R), edema (E), ecchymosis (bruising) (E), discharge (D), and approximation (A) (the edges of the wound should be close, as though stuck or glued together).

Redness of the wound may indicate the usual inflammatory response to injury. If accompanied by excessive pain or tenderness, however, it may indicate the beginning of localized infection. Ecchymosis or edema indicates soft tissue damage that can delay healing. There should be no discharge from the wound. Rapid healing necessitates that the edges of the wound be closely approximated. Procedure 21–2 describes the perineal examination.

VITAL SIGNS

Blood Pressure.   Blood pressure varies with position. To obtain accurate results, it should be measured with the mother in the same position each time. Therefore, nurses must record both the mother's position when taking blood pressure and the pressure obtained. Postpartum blood pressure should be compared with that of the predelivery period so that deviations from the parameters that are normal for the mother can be quickly identified. An increase from the baseline suggests pregnancy-induced hypertension. A decrease may indicate dehydration or hypovolemia resulting from excessive bleeding.

Orthostatic Hypotension.   After birth, a rapid decrease in intra-abdominal pressure results in dilation of blood vessels supplying the viscera. The resulting engorgement of abdominal blood vessels contributes to a rapid fall in blood pressure of 15 to 20 mm Hg when the woman moves from a recumbent to a sitting position. This change causes mothers to feel dizzy or lightheaded or to faint when they stand. The nursing diagnosis Risk for Injury applies to women with orthostatic hypotension. (See Nursing Care Plan 21–1 for application of this nursing diagnosis.)

Hypotension may also indicate hypovolemia. Careful assessments for hemorrhage (location and firmness of the fundus, amount of lochia, pulse rate for tachycardia) should be made if the postpartum blood pressure is significantly less than the prenatal baseline blood pressure.

PROCEDURE 21–2

Assessing the Perineum

PURPOSE: To observe perineal trauma and the state of healing.

1. Provide privacy, and explain the purpose of the procedure to elicit cooperation and reduce anxiety.
2. Put on clean gloves to implement standard precautions.
3. Ask the mother to assume a Sims position and flex her upper leg. Lower the perineal pads and lift her superior buttocks to provide an unobstructed view of the perineum. If necessary, use a flashlight for better visibility during inspection of the perineal area.
4. Note the extent and location of edema or bruising. Extensive bruising or asymmetric edema may indicate formation of a hematoma.
5. Examine the episiotomy or laceration for redness, ecchymosis, edema, discharge, and approximation (REEDA), which may indicate infection or problems with healing.
6. Note the number and size of hemorrhoids. Swollen hemorrhoids interfere with activity and bowel elimination.

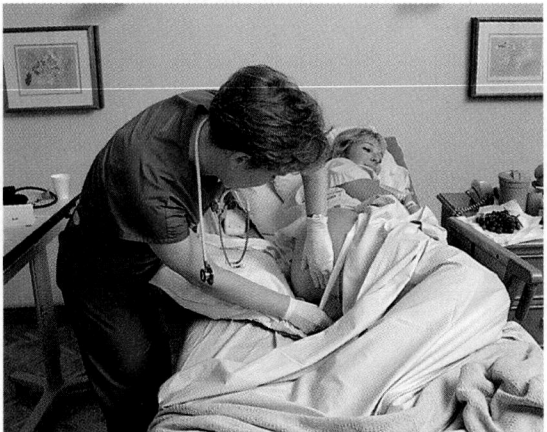

Pulse.   Bradycardia, defined as a pulse rate of 50 to 60 beats per minute, is expected and reflects the large amount of blood that returns to the central circulation following delivery of the placenta. The increase in central circulation results in increased stroke volume and allows a slower heart rate to provide adequate maternal circulation.

Tachycardia may indicate excitement, fatigue, pain, dehydration, hypovolemia, or infection. If tachycardia is noted, additional assessments should include blood pressure, location and firmness of the uterus, amount of lochia, estimated blood loss at delivery, and hemoglobin and hematocrit values. The objective of the additional assessments is to rule out excessive bleeding and to intervene at once if hemorrhage is suspected.

Respirations.   A normal respiratory rate of 16 to 20 breaths per minute should be maintained. It is not necessary to assess breath sounds if the mother has had a normal vagi-

NURSING CARE PLAN 21–1
. . . .

Postpartum Hypotension, Fatigue, and Pain

Assessment	Four hours after giving birth, Jacqueline Tilden became weak and dizzy when she attempted to ambulate the first time. Her gait was unsteady, and the nurse had to lower her back to bed to prevent her fainting. Her color was pale and her pulse was rapid.
Nursing Diagnosis	Risk for Injury related to physiologic effects of orthostatic hypotension.
Goal/Expected Outcome	• Jacqueline will remain free of injury caused by fainting and falling during the postpartum period.

Intervention	Rationale
1. Check the mother's blood pressure while she is in a supine position and in a sitting position; check her blood pressure in the same arm.	1. A decrease of 20 mm Hg in systolic pressure in the upright position indicates orthostatic hypotension. Measuring from the same arm provides more accurate information because the reading may differ slightly in each arm.
2. Assist the mother to elevate the head of the bed for a few minutes and then to sit on the side of the bed for several minutes before standing. Help her to stand slowly.	2. Sitting and dangling the legs allows time for blood pressure to stabilize before she is fully upright, thus maintaining circulation to the brain.
3. Instruct the mother to move her feet constantly when she first stands.	3. Moving the feet increases venous return from the lower extremities, which maintains cardiac output and increases cerebral circulation.
4. Suggest that Jacqueline take brief, tepid (not hot) showers and that she bend her knees and "march" during the shower.	4. Hot water dilates peripheral blood vessels, allowing additional blood to remain in the vessels of the legs. Moving the feet and legs increases blood return from the legs and increases blood to the brain.

5. Initiate measures to prevent injuries that could be sustained if Jacqueline were to faint:
  a. Stay with the mother when she ambulates, and be prepared to assist her in sitting down or in lowering her gently to the floor if she becomes faint.
  b. Call for assistance before attempting to return her to bed.
  c. Remind her to call for assistance before trying to ambulate. Check to see that the call light is conveniently located.
	5. Gravity increases blood flow to the brain when the head is lowered and thus prevents fainting. Adequate assistance prevents falling and possible injury during a fainting episode.

Evaluation	Jacqueline has participated in self-care and has sustained no injury during her hospital stay.
Assessment	On the second day after delivery Jacqueline expresses concern about her third-degree episiotomy and asks what she can do to prevent the pain she experienced during intercourse for several months after the birth of her first child, who is now 18 months old.
Nursing Diagnosis	Altered Sexuality Patterns related to fatigue and pain.
Goals/Expected Outcomes	The couple will • Verbalize measures to promote comfort during sexual activity by (date). • Verbalize a plan to reduce fatigue, which interferes with interest in and energy for sexual activity by (date).

(continued)

Postpartum Hypotension, Fatigue, and Pain

Intervention	Rationale
1. Recommend that the parents postpone vaginal intercourse until the perineum is well healed, usually about 3 weeks. Suggest that the mother continue perineal care, sitz baths, and the use of topical agents until the perineum is healed.	1. These measures promote rapid healing and reduce pain or fear of pain when sexual activity is resumed.
2. Suggest that the infant be breast-fed just before the parents initiate sexual activity.	2. Breast-feeding reduces the chance of leaking milk, which interferes with sexual pleasure for some couples. Feeding the infant may also allow uninterrupted time while the infant sleeps.
3. Suggest the use of a water-soluble vaginal lubricant (Lubrin, Replens, KY Jelly) if the mother is planning to breast-feed for longer than 6 weeks.	3. Breast-feeding delays the return of ovarian hormones to nonpregnant levels, including estrogen, which may result in vaginal dryness that is most noticeable after 6 weeks of breast-feeding.
4. Prior to vaginal intercourse, as part of foreplay, suggest that one finger be inserted into the vaginal introitus to determine areas of tenderness or pain.	4. A finger locates areas of discomfort and stretches the perineal scar gently.
5. Remind parents that sexual arousal may be slower because of decreased hormone levels and fatigue. More stimulation may be necessary before the mother is sexually aroused.	5. Knowledge of postpartum physiologic changes reduces the anxiety and tension that occur if the parents are unprepared for them.
6. Suggest that the woman assume the superior position during intercourse.	6. In this position the woman controls the depth and location of penetration, which can help reduce her discomfort.
7. Remind the mother to perform Kegel exercises until she can comfortably do 30 each day.	7. Kegel exercises strengthen the muscles around the vagina and promote increased sexual satisfaction.
8. Suggest measures that may lessen fatigue: a. Recommend that each partner nap for 30 minutes sometime during the day or evening. b. Suggest that sexual activity occur in the morning or afternoon rather than at the end of a tiring day. c. Suggest that parents rest when the infant has long periods of sleep and that they postpone additional home projects that will increase fatigue until the infant is older and is sleeping through the night.	8. Napping lessens fatigue, which is cited by both mothers and fathers as one of the major causes of decreased interest in sexual activity following childbirth.
9. Discuss the need for frank communication between partners about measures that reduce discomfort as well as specific concerns and needs.	9. Communication facilitates understanding and fosters a feeling of closeness that can enhance sexual interest.

Evaluation

The couple expresses interest in trying various measures to reduce fatigue and discomfort. They verbalize a plan to use the instructions provided.

Additional Nursing Diagnoses to Consider

Altered Family Processes
Risk for Altered Health Maintenance
Risk for Altered Parenting
Health-Seeking Behaviors
Sleep Pattern Disturbance

nal delivery, is ambulatory, and is without signs of respiratory distress. Breath sounds should always be auscultated if the birth has been cesarean, if the mother is a smoker, if she has a history of frequent or recent upper respiratory infections, or if she has a history of asthma.

Temperature. A temperature of up to 38°C (100.4°F) is common during the first 24 hours after childbirth and may be caused by dehydration or normal postpartum leukocytosis. If the elevated temperature persists for longer than 24 hours or if it exceeds 38°C, infection should be suspected and the fever reported to the physician or nurse-midwife.

BREASTS

For the first day or two after delivery, the breasts should be soft and nontender. After that, breast changes depend largely on whether the mother is breast-feeding or is taking measures to prevent lactation. The breasts should be examined even if she chooses formula feeding because the breasts may become engorged despite preventive measures. The size, symmetry, and shape of the breasts should be observed. The skin should be inspected for dimpling or thickening, which, although rare, can indicate breast tumor.

The areola and nipple should be carefully examined for potential problems such as flat or retracted nipples; these problems sometimes make breast-feeding more difficult. Signs of nipple trauma (redness, blisters, or fissures) are often noted during the first days of breast-feeding, especially if the mother needs assistance in positioning the infant correctly. (For full details, see Chapter 24.)

The breasts should be palpated for firmness and tenderness, which indicate increased vascular and lymphatic circulation that may precede milk production. The breasts may feel "lumpy" as various lobes begin to produce milk.

The breast assessment is an excellent opportunity to provide information or reassurance about breast care and breast-feeding techniques.

LOWER EXTREMITIES

The legs are examined for signs or symptoms of thrombophlebitis. These indications include localized areas of redness, heat, edema, and tenderness. Pedal pulses may be obstructed by thrombophlebitis and should be palpated with each assessment.

HOMANS'S SIGN

Discomfort in the calf with sharp dorsiflexion of the foot may indicate deep vein thrombosis. Although the sign is of limited value (Cunningham et al., 1997), it continues to be part of the assessment of the lower extremities in the postpartum period. A negative Homans's sign is indicated by absence of discomfort. A positive Homans's sign is indicated by the presence of discomfort and should be reported to the physician or nurse-midwife.

EDEMA AND DEEP TENDON REFLEXES

Pedal or pretibial edema may be present for the first day or two, until excess interstitial fluid is remobilized and excreted.

Deep tendon reflexes should be 1+ to 2+. Report brisker than average and hyperactive reflexes (3+ to 4+), which suggest pregnancy-induced hypertension. (See Procedure 26–1 for an explanation of assessing deep tendon reflexes.)

COMFORT LEVEL

Nurses must remain alert to signs of afterpains, perineal discomfort, and breast tenderness. Covert signs of discomfort include an inability to relax or sleep, a change in vital signs, restlessness, irritability, and facial grimaces.

Analgesics, such as acetaminophen (Tylenol, Panadol), and nonsteroidal anti-inflammatory drugs, such as ibuprofen (Motrin, Advil), are frequently prescribed for relief of mild to moderate discomfort. Tylenol No. 3 and Percocet are often prescribed for more severe discomfort.

Adequate fluids help restore the balance altered by fluid loss during labor and the birth process. Women should be encouraged to drink approximately 2,500 ml of fluids each day. New mothers generally have a hearty appetite, and nurses should encourage healthy food choices, with respect for ethnic background. Meals and snacks should be available at all times, not only at regular mealtimes.

Care in the Immediate Postpartum Period

The postpartum period is often divided into three periods. The first 24 hours is called the immediate postpartum period; the first week is referred to as the early postpartum period; and the second week to the sixth week is the late postpartum period. Care of the mother during the immediate postpartum period focuses on the following:

- Maintaining the mother's physiologic safety through frequent assessments
- Providing comfort measures
- Establishing bladder elimination
- Providing health education

Providing Comfort Measures

ICE PACKS

Both cold and warmth are used to alleviate perineal pain after childbirth. Ice causes vasoconstriction and is most effective if applied soon after the birth to prevent edema and to numb the area. Chemical ice packs or a glove filled with ice and tied at the cuff is often used during the first 12 hours following a vaginal birth. The ice pack is wrapped in disposable paper before it is applied to the perineum. It should be left in place until the ice melts. It is then removed for 10 minutes before a fresh pack is applied. Some perineal pads have cold packs incorporated in them, but they do not absorb as much lochia as other perineal pads.

PERINEAL CARE

Perineal care consists of squirting warm water over the perineum after each voiding or bowel movement. Perineal care cleanses, provides comfort, and prevents infection. The perineum is gently patted rather than wiped dry.

TOPICAL MEDICATIONS

Anesthetic sprays decrease surface discomfort and allow more comfortable ambulation. The mother is instructed to hold the nozzle of a benzocaine spray, such as Americaine or Dermoplast, 6 to 12 inches from her body and direct it toward the perineum. The spray should be used following perineal care and before clean pads are applied.

SITTING

The mother should be advised to squeeze her buttocks together before sitting and to lower her weight slowly onto her buttocks. This measure prevents stretching of the perineal tissue and avoids sharp impact on the traumatized area. An air cushion ("doughnut") may relieve pressure on the perineum when sitting.

SITZ BATHS

Sitz baths, which provide continuous circulation of water, cleanse and comfort the traumatized perineum. Cool water reduces pain caused by edema and may be most effective within the first 24 hours. Warm water increases circulation and promotes healing and may be most effective after 24 hours. Nurses must be sure that the emergency bell is within easy reach in case the mother feels faint during the sitz bath.

ORAL AND PARENTERAL MEDICATIONS

Mothers should be encouraged to take prescribed medications for afterpains and perineal discomfort.

Promoting Bladder Elimination

Many new mothers have difficulty voiding because of edema and trauma of the perineum as well as diminished sensitivity to fluid pressure in the bladder. As soon as they are able to ambulate safely, mothers should be assisted to the bathroom. It is important to provide privacy and to allow adequate time for the first voiding. Some common measures to promote relaxation of the perineal muscles and to stimulate the sensation of needing to void include the following:

- Running water, placing the mother's hands in water, and pouring water over the vulva.
- Asking the mother to blow bubbles through a straw.
- Encouraging urination in the shower or sitz bath.
- Providing hot tea or fluids of choice. The recommended fluid intake is about 2,500 ml/day.

A distended bladder lifts and displaces the uterus, making it difficult for the uterus to remain contracted. Thus, urinary retention is a major cause of uterine atony (loss of tone), which permits excessive bleeding. Moreover, stasis of

CRITICAL THINKING EXERCISE 21–1

Linda Welker, a 22-year-old multipara, was admitted from the labor, delivery, and recovery unit 2 hours after the birth of an 8-lb (3,600-g) baby boy. An hour later her fundus is firm, located three fingerbreadths above the umbilicus, and displaced to the right. Her perineal pads, which were changed just before transfer, are saturated.

1. What do these data suggest? Why?
2. What nursing action should be taken first? What follow-up assessments are necessary?
3. Why is it necessary to remind Linda to void?

urine in the bladder predisposes the woman to urinary tract infection. Therefore, the mother must be catheterized if

- She is unable to void.
- The amount voided is less than 150 ml.
- The fundus is elevated or displaced from the midline.

Repeated catheterizations increase the chance of urinary tract infection because bacteria may be pushed into the bladder despite scrupulous aseptic technique. To decrease the risk of infection, an indwelling catheter is usually inserted for 24 hours if catheterization is necessary more than once or twice.

◼ Nursing Care After Cesarean Birth

The length of stay for mothers after a cesarean birth has decreased. Most now leave the hospital within 72 to 96 hours following surgery. Many facilities have developed clinical pathways or care maps that are similar to those used for uncomplicated vaginal births. The clinical pathway identifies outcomes and establishes a time frame for assessments and interventions for postcesarean mothers and their infants. Clinical pathways, however, are guidelines only. If a problem arises, sometimes called a variance, additional assessments and interventions are necessary.

Assessment

In addition to the usual postpartum assessments, the postcesarean mother must be assessed as any other postoperative patient.

RESPIRATIONS

Many mothers receive epidural narcotics for postoperative pain relief. The analgesic effect lasts for approximately 24 hours. During this time respirations must be assessed frequently because narcotics depress the respiratory center. In some facilities an apnea monitor is used for 24 hours to detect a decreased respiratory rate. In others, a pulse oximeter is used for this purpose. If these devices are not used, the respiratory rate and depth should be checked every 15 minutes for the first hour, every 30 minutes for 3 to 6 hours, and every 30 minutes to 1 hour for the remainder of the first 24 hours.

If the respiratory rate begins to decline or if the respiratory rate is less than 12 breaths per minute, the nurse should do the following:

- Notify the anesthesiologist immediately.
- Elevate the head of the bed to facilitate lung expansion.
- Administer oxygen and apply a pulse oximeter to measure oxygen saturation.
- Follow facility protocol to administer narcotic antagonists, such as naloxone hydrochloride (Narcan).
- Be aware that the duration of effect of naloxone is approximately 30 minutes and that respiratory depression may recur.
- Recognize that naloxone reduces the level of pain relief.

In addition to observing respiratory rate and depth, the mother's breath sounds should be auscultated because depressed respirations as well as a longer period of immobility allow secretions to pool in the bronchioles. To counteract this risk, the mother must be assisted to turn, cough, and expand the lungs by breathing deeply. Incentive spirometers are also used to expand the lungs and thus to prevent the hypostatic pneumonia that can result from immobility and shallow, slow respirations.

ABDOMEN

Nurses assess gastrointestinal function by auscultating for bowel sounds until normal peristalsis is noted in all abdominal quadrants. Although paralytic ileus (lack of movement in the bowel) is rare following cesarean birth, nurses must be aware of the signs, which include abdominal distension, absent or decreased bowel sounds, and no excretion of flatus or stool.

The surgical dressing should be observed for intactness and discharge. When the dressing is removed, nurses observe the incision, which should be approximated, and use the acronym REEDA to assess for signs of infection, such as redness and edema.

The fundus must be palpated gently because of increased discomfort caused by the uterine incision.

INTAKE AND OUTPUT

The intravenous infusion should be monitored for the rate of flow and the condition of the intravenous site. Any signs of infiltration, such as edema or coolness at the site, as well as signs of infection, such as edema, redness, and pain, should be reported. Ice chips and fluids are usually allowed soon after cesarean birth. The amount as well as the color and clarity of urine should be monitored.

Interventions

THE FIRST 24 HOURS

The mother who gave birth by cesarean section is cared for as one would care for other postoperative clients.

Overcoming the Effects of Immobility. The new mother is on bed rest for the first 8 to 12 hours. To prevent pooling of secretions in the airway, she must be helped every 2 hours to turn, cough, and breathe deeply. Splinting the abdomen with a small pillow reduces incisional discomfort when she coughs. She should be encouraged to flex her legs and to move her feet and legs frequently to improve peripheral circulation. She needs assistance to sit and dangle her feet for the first few times.

Providing Comfort. Placing a pillow behind her back and one between her knees when the mother is in a side-lying position prevents strain and discomfort. Excellent physical care (oral hygiene, perineal care, a sponge bath, and clean linen) comforts and refreshes her.

Postcesarean clients differ from typical postoperative clients in three important ways. First, they typically wish to be alert so that they can interact with their newborn infants. Second, they are concerned about the type and quantity of analgesics they receive and that they could potentially pass them on in their breast milk. Third, compared with other postoperative patients, postcesarean clients tend to want more input into and control over their care.

Although intramuscular injection of narcotics for postcesarean pain was once common, it has been replaced in many institutions by patient-controlled analgesia, administered by continuous intravenous infusion of a low-concentration narcotic solution using a pump specifically designed for that purpose. If the analgesia is insufficient, the woman can self-administer intermittent small doses of narcotic from the infusion pump.

A single dose of narcotic (usually morphine) may be injected into the epidural or subarachnoid space immediately after the surgery to provide 18 to 24 hours of postcesarean analgesia. Side effects of both patient-controlled analgesia and epidural narcotics include respiratory depression, itching (pruritus), nausea and vomiting, and urine retention.

AFTER 24 HOURS

Reinstating Normal Activities. After 24 hours, several normal functions return as postcesarean women are able to participate more actively in their own care:

- Both the indwelling catheter and intravenous infusion are usually discontinued.
- The dressing is usually removed, and often staples or clamps are removed also. Steri-Strips or a small nonsticking dressing may be used to cover the incision.
- Mothers are usually helped to ambulate by the first postpartum day and are comfortable sitting in a chair for brief periods.
- Clear liquids may be changed to a soft diet once bowel sounds are audible. If abdominal distension is minimal, the diet then progresses to a regular regimen.

Nurses must encourage the mother to increase her activity and ambulation each postpartum day. By the second day, she is usually allowed to shower.

Assisting the Mother with Infant Feeding. It is important to help the mother find a comfortable position for holding and feeding her infant. A side-lying position may be most comfortable, but some mothers prefer sitting with a pillow on the lap to protect the incisional area. The football hold is often the most comfortable position for breast-feeding because the infant is not on the lap and thus does not cause incisional discomfort. (Chapter 24 discusses breast-feeding in detail.)

Preventing Abdominal Distension. Abdominal distension is a major source of discomfort, and measures should be taken to prevent or minimize it. Early, frequent ambulation is perhaps the best method. Additional measures include

- Pelvic lifts. Lying supine with her knees bent, the woman lifts her pelvis from the bed. These exercises may be repeated up to 10 times, several times each day.
- Tightening and relaxing the abdominal muscles. These exercises may also be helpful.
- Avoiding carbonated beverages. Both carbonated beverages and the use of straws, which increase the accumulation of intestinal gas, should be restricted.
- Simethecone. This agent may disperse upper gastrointestinal flatulence.
- Rectal suppositories. These suppositories stimulate peristalsis and the passage of flatus.

▮ NURSING CARE
Teaching After Birth

Nurses are responsible for providing health education about a long list of subjects before the family is discharged from the birth facility. This task causes a great deal of concern because so much must be taught during a short time and because it is not the best time to teach mothers, who have not fully recovered from the birth process.

Before beginning teaching, determine the learning needs and the major concerns of each family. For example, multiparas may remember some aspects of self-care but would benefit from a review. On the other hand, primiparas may be anxious about self-care measures and all aspects of infant care. They may need more thorough teaching and more practice. Be aware of the most common barriers to learning: age and developmental level, cultural factors, and difficulty understanding the language.

Nursing Diagnosis and Planning

In general, mothers adapt to the physiologic changes after childbirth, and most nursing care is wellness oriented. Some new mothers, however, lack knowledge of self-care and thus are at risk for a disruption in health. A nursing diagnosis that applies to these women is

■ Risk for Altered Health Maintenance related to insufficient knowledge of self-care, signs of complications, and preventive measures.
Expected Outcomes: The mother will verbalize or demonstrate understanding of self-care instructions by the hour of discharge and verbalize understanding of practices that promote maternal health by a specified date. The mother will describe plans for follow-up care and the signs and symptoms that should be reported to the physician, nurse-midwife, or nurse practitioner by the day of discharge.

Additional diagnoses include Risk for Injury and Altered Sexuality Patterns. These appear in Nursing Care Plan 21–1.

Interventions

Teaching the Process of Involution

Provide the mother with basic information about involution, including how to assess lochia and how to locate and palpate the fundus. This information allows her to recognize abnormal signs, such as prolonged lochia or uterine tenderness, which should be reported to the health care provider. If the mother is a young teenager, another family member may also need to be given the information.

Teaching Self-Care

Hand Washing. Emphasize the importance of thorough hand washing before touching the breasts, after diaper changes, after bladder and bowel elimination, and always before handling the infant.

Breast Care for Lactating Mothers. Instruct the breast-feeding mother to wash her nipples with clear water and to avoid soaps that remove the natural lubrication secreted by Montgomery's glands. Keeping the nipples dry between feedings helps prevent tissue damage, and wearing a good bra provides necessary support as breast size increases.

Measures to Suppress Lactation. If the mother chooses not to breast-feed, initiate measures to suppress lactation. The safest method is to prevent breast distension either by binding the breasts or by having the mother wear a tight-fitting bra 24 hours a day until the breasts become

soft. Discomfort can usually be managed by applying ice, which reduces vasocongestion, and with analgesics. Advise the woman to refrain from stimulating milk production by allowing warm water to fall directly on the breasts during showers or by pumping or massaging the breasts.

Perineal Care. Nurses are responsible for teaching perineal cleansing as soon as possible after childbirth. The most common method is to fill a squeeze bottle with warm water and spray the perineal area from the front toward the back. In some facilities, a small amount of cleansing solution is added; in others, only clear warm water is used. Remind the new mother not to separate the labia during this procedure so that water does not enter the vagina. If a commercial product that includes a nozzle attached to the faucet is used, teach the mother that the nozzle should not touch the perineum during use.

Moist antiseptic towelettes or toilet paper is used in a patting motion to dry the perineum. Teach the mother to dry from front to back to prevent fecal contamination from the anal area to the vaginal introitus. She should perform perineal cleansing and change perineal pads (peripads) after each voiding or defecation.

Many women do not use peripads for menstrual protection and must be taught how to use them correctly. Mesh panties and adhering pads are used in most facilities. Careful handling of the pads is important to prevent localized perineal infection.

• Thorough hand washing is a must before and after changing the pads.
• Unused pads should be stored inside their package.
• Pads should be applied without touching the side that comes into contact with the perineum.
• The pads should be applied and removed in a front-to-back direction to prevent contamination of the vagina and perineum.
• Used pads must be disposed of properly.

Kegel Exercises. All mothers should become familiar with Kegel exercises. These movements strengthen the pubococcygeal muscle, which surrounds the vagina and urinary meatus. This exercise helps prevent the loss of muscle tone that can occur after childbirth.

The Kegel exercise involves contracting muscles around the vagina (as though stopping the flow of urine), holding tightly for 10 seconds, and then relaxing for 10 seconds. The woman should work up to 30 contraction-relaxation cycles each day.

Promoting Rest and Sleep

The mother who is fatigued appears worn out and lethargic, with slumping posture, and often verbalizes a generalized decrease in energy and strength. The extreme fatigue that mothers experience in the puerperium has several causes. Women are tired when they begin the postpartum period because they often did not sleep well during the third trimester and are exhausted by the exertion of labor. New mothers commonly experience feelings of excitement and euphoria for some time after childbirth and are unable to rest. Numerous visitors interfere with periods of rest. Hospital routines, an unfamiliar environment, and physical discomfort also make it difficult for the new mother to rest.

Most mothers are discharged from the facility within

24 to 48 hours after childbirth, and most go home with a tremendous deficit in sleep and energy. Yet new parents may be unprepared for the conflict between their need for sleep and the infant's need for care and attention. The joys of parenting can easily be overshadowed by the exhaustion and frustration that result.

Rest at the Birth Facility. Hospital routines continue around the clock, making uninterrupted rest difficult and increasing the probability that the mother is fatigued when she is discharged. Group assessments and care, and provide time for napping to help the mother obtain needed rest. Suggest that she restrict phone calls and visitors during these times.

Rest at Home. Help the mother understand the impact that her physical discomfort and the demands of the newborn will have on her energy during the first few weeks. Emphasize measures that conserve energy, such as the following:

- Maintaining a flexible routine that focuses on care of the mother and infant
- Planning simple meals and flexible mealtimes
- Accepting assistance with food shopping, meal preparation, and housework
- Postponing major household projects
- Involving friends and family to provide care for other children

Explain to the mother that she should delay her return to employment, if possible, until the infant sleeps through the night (usually by 4 months). Advise all mothers to restrict coffee, tea, colas, and chocolate (which all contain the stimulant caffeine) or to use decaffeinated versions for the first few weeks. The mother should also rest whenever the infant sleeps rather than use the time to catch up on housecleaning tasks.

Relaxation Exercises. Total relaxation exercises (lying quietly, alternately tightening and relaxing the muscles of the neck, shoulders, arms, legs, and feet) are helpful when a nap is not possible. Emphasize to the mother the importance of asking for help when she begins to feel exhausted or overwhelmed. Encourage her to share these feelings with family, friends, and other new mothers.

Providing Nutrition Counseling

Food Supply. Families of low socioeconomic status may benefit from referral to government-sponsored programs, such as food stamps or the Women, Infants, and Children (Food Supplement Program) to help them obtain adequate food. It may also be necessary to determine what facilities are available for cooking and storing food. Sometimes the new family must be referred to a social worker for solutions for their unique problems.

Diet. Although many women are not satisfied with the slow rate of weight loss, they should avoid severe restriction of caloric intake. Explain the need to select foods that provide adequate calories to meet energy needs, taking into account the time and energy needed to care for a newborn. Strict dieting can leave the mother feeling tired, lower her immunity, and interfere with the lactating mother's ability to synthesize milk. A balanced, low-fat diet with adequate protein, complex carbohydrates, fruits, and vegetables provides the nutrients needed. (See discussion of nutrition for breast-feeding in Chapter 15.)

Promoting Regular Bowel Elimination

Explain the role of progressive exercise, adequate fluid, and dietary fiber in preventing constipation. Walking is perhaps the best exercise, and the distance can be increased as strength and endurance increase. Drinking at least eight glasses of water daily will help maintain normal bowel elimination. Dietary fiber is present in fruits and vegetables, particularly when they are unpeeled. Prunes act as a natural laxative. Additional fiber is found in whole-grain cereals, bread, and pasta.

A regular schedule of bowel elimination is also important in overcoming constipation. For instance, bowel elimination following breakfast allows the mother to take advantage of the gastrocolic reflex (stimulation of peristalsis induced in the colon when food is consumed on an empty stomach). Moreover, measures that reduce perineal and hemorrhoidal pain, such as sitz baths, prepackaged witch hazel astringent compresses, and ointments, facilitate bowel elimination.

Promoting Good Body Mechanics

Exercise. Teach exercises in the early postpartum period to strengthen the abdominal muscles and firm the waist. The exercises can be started soon after childbirth and repeated up to five times twice a day, at first. The number of exercises is gradually increased as the mother gains strength. Figure 21–8 illustrates recommended postpartum exercises that the mother may begin with the approval of the physician, nurse-midwife, or nurse practitioner.

Instruct postcesarean mothers to follow the instructions of their health care provider. Generally they should not begin an exercise program for at least 4 to 6 weeks.

Preventing Back Strain. Back strain often can be prevented if the mother and father find a location for infant care, such as a kitchen table or bathroom counter, that does not require bending or leaning forward. For lifting objects, teach parents to hold the back straight as they squat and use the legs rather than bending at the waist (see Fig. 13–12).

Counseling About Sexual Activity

The couple may have concerns about resuming sexual intercourse and contraceptive choices. Cultural or religious convictions may restrict the choice of method for some couples, whereas the availability of health care or limited finances may dictate the choice for others. Discuss previous experience with contraceptives and the satisfaction with those methods.

Many new parents are reluctant to ask about when to resume sexual activity and about potential alterations in sexuality resulting from pregnancy and childbirth. If couples do not indicate such concerns, introduce the topic in a general, nonspecific manner, such as by saying, "You have an episiotomy, which may cause some discomfort with intercourse until it has completely healed," or "Sometimes couples are not aware that some vaginal dryness occurs as a result of breast-feeding." Such broad opening statements permit the family to pursue the topic as they desire.

ABDOMINAL BREATHING

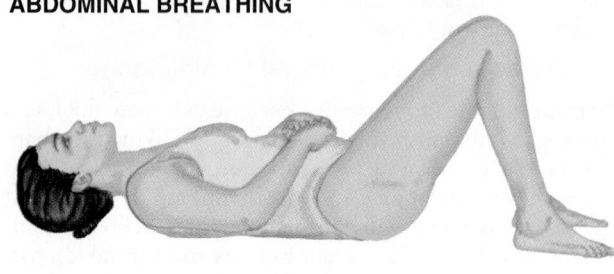

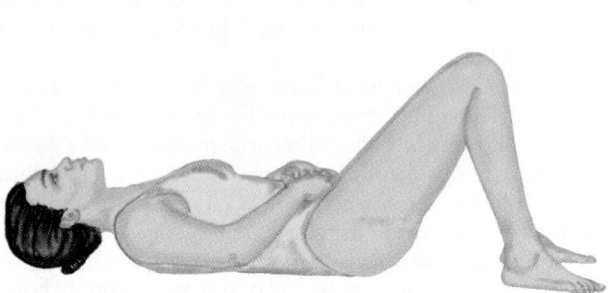

This is one of the simplest exercises and can be started on the first postpartum day. The woman assumes a supine position with knees bent. She inhales through the nose, keeps the rib cage as stationary as possible, and allows the abdomen to expand. She then contracts the abdominal muscles as she exhales slowly through the mouth.

HEAD LIFT

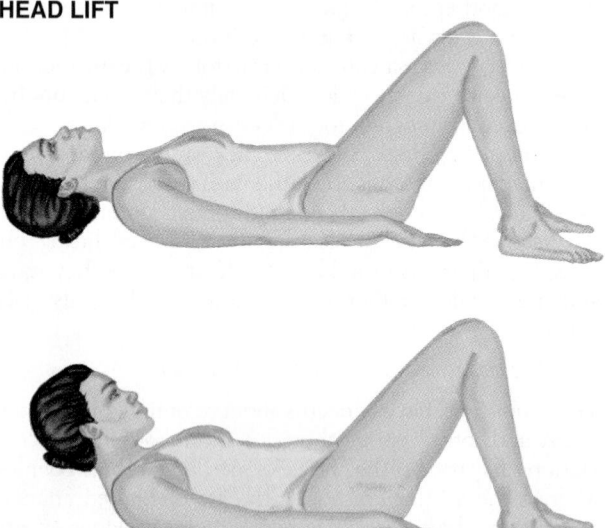

This exercise can be started within a few days after childbirth. The mother is supine with knees bent and arms outstretched at her side. She inhales deeply to begin, then exhales while lifting the head slowly; she holds the position for a few seconds and relaxes.

MODIFIED SIT-UPS

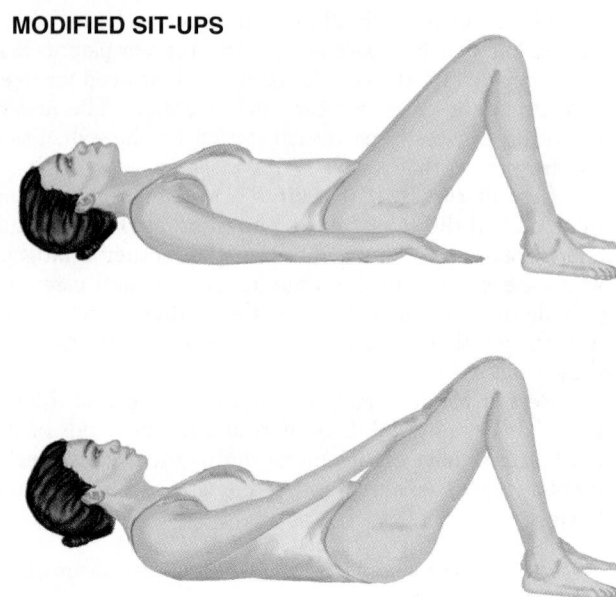

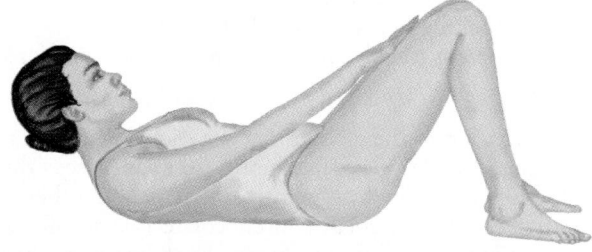

Head lifts may progress to modified sit-ups with the approval of the health care provider; the mother should follow the advice of the health care provider about the number of repetitions.

The exercise begins with the mother supine with arms outstretched and the knees bent. She raises her head and shoulders as her hands reach for her knees. She raises the shoulders only as far as the back will bend; her waist remains on the floor.

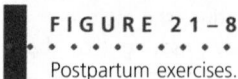

FIGURE 21-8
. . . .
Postpartum exercises.

KNEE AND LEG ROLLS

CHEST EXERCISES

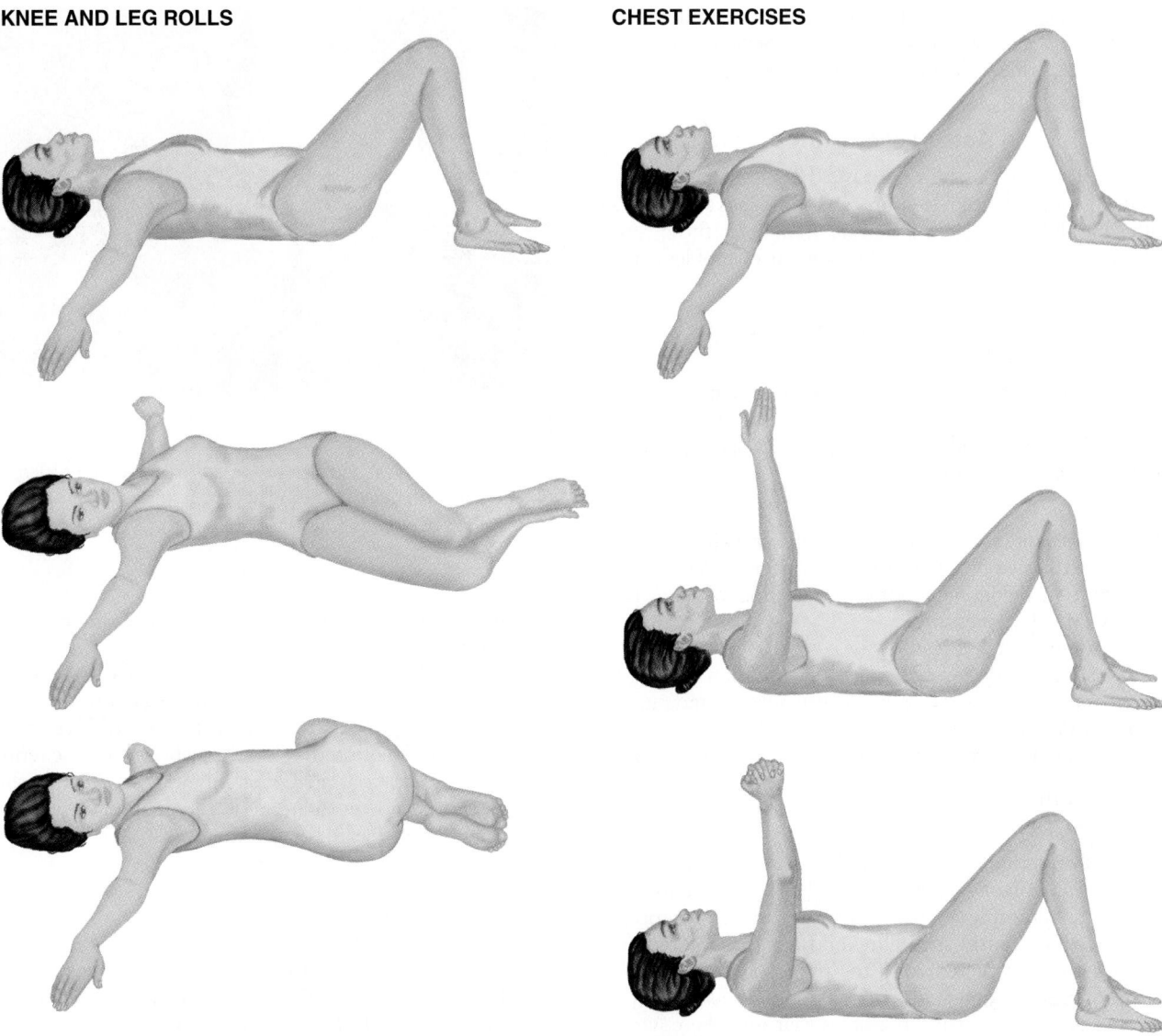

This is an excellent exercise to begin firming the waist. The mother lies flat on her back with knees bent and feet flat on the floor or bed; she keeps the shoulders and feet stationary and rolls the knees to touch first one side of the bed, then the other. She maintains a smooth motion as the exercise is repeated five times. Later, as flexibility increases, the exercise can be varied by the rolling of one knee only. The mother rolls her left knee to touch the right side of the bed, returns to center, and rolls the right knee to touch the left side of the bed.

This is an excellent exercise to strengthen the chest muscles. The mother lies at with arms extended straight out to the side; she brings the hands together above the chest while keeping the arms straight; she holds for a few seconds and returns to the starting position. She repeats the exercise five times initially and follows the advice of the health care provider for increasing the number of repetitions.

Isometric exercises also increase strength and tone; the mother bends her elbows, clasps her hands together above her chest, and presses her hands together for a few seconds. This is repeated at least five times.

FIGURE 21 – 8

. . . .

Continued

Nursing Care Plan 21–1 describes interventions for the nursing diagnosis Risk for Altered Sexuality Patterns related to perineal discomfort, dryness of vaginal mucosa, or fatigue.

Instructing About Follow-up Appointments

The new mother generally returns to her physician or nurse-midwife for postpartum examination at 2 weeks and 6 weeks after childbirth. Explain that examination at those times allows early identification and treatment of problems that may be developing.

Teaching About Signs and Symptoms That Should Be Reported

Teach new mothers and at least one other family member which physical signs and symptoms should be reported to the health care provider right away. These signs and symptoms include the following:

- Fever
- Localized area of redness, swelling, or pain in either breast that is not relieved by support or analgesics
- Persistent abdominal tenderness or feelings of pelvic fullness or pelvic pressure
- Persistent perineal pain
- Frequency, urgency, or burning on urination
- Change in character of lochia (increased amount, resumption of bright red color, passage of clots, foul odor)
- Localized tenderness, redness, or warmth of the legs

Ensuring That All Elements Have Been Taught

Group instruction and hospital classes, such as those that demonstrate infant care and provide breast-feeding instructions, are returning to the postpartum environment. In these settings, nurses streamline and organize information so that it can be presented in the time available.

To prevent omissions, many hospitals use teaching "check-off" sheets listing the areas that must be covered. For example, care of the umbilical cord and circumcision site, using a bulb syringe, and taking a temperature are part of the infant care teaching that must take place before the mother leaves the hospital.

Evaluation

- Does the mother demonstrate correct breast and perineal hygiene?
- Can the mother verbalize her plan to manage diet, rest, and exercise after discharge?
- Can she describe her plan for follow-up care and signs that indicate the need for immediate treatment?

The Process of Becoming Acquainted

Perhaps no other event requires such rapid change in family structure and function as the birth of a baby. The addition of a new baby requires that all family members adjust their roles.

The role of maternity nurses includes not only the care of the mother-infant dyad but also the well-being of the entire family. Nurses are concerned about the family's adjustment to childbearing, not only during the hospital stay

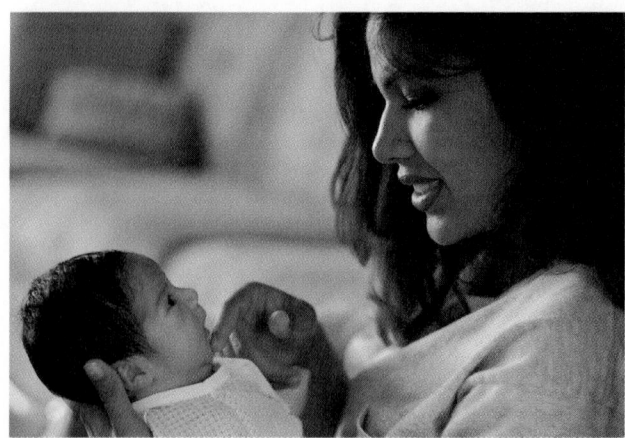

FIGURE 21–9

The infant is quiet and alert during the initial sensitive period. The newborn gazes at the mother and responds to her voice and touch.

but also during the early weeks at home as new parents make the transition to parenthood.

A great deal of information has appeared in nursing literature that describes how parents and newborns become acquainted and progress to develop feelings of love, concern, and deep devotion that last throughout life. The terms *bonding* and *attachment* are commonly used to describe the initial steps. Although the terms are sometimes used interchangeably, their meanings do differ.

Bonding

Bonding describes the initial attraction felt by parents. It is unidirectional, from parent to child, and is enhanced when parent and infant are permitted to touch and interact during a so-called *sensitive period* that extends through the first 30 to 60 minutes following birth. During this time the infant is in a quiet, alert stage. The eyes are open, and the infant seems to gaze directly at the parents (Fig. 21–9). Nurses frequently delay procedures such as instillation of prophylactic eye medications that can interfere with this time between parents and newborns.

Attachment

Attachment is the process by which an enduring bond to a child is developed through pleasurable, satisfying parent-child interaction. The process begins in pregnancy and extends for many months after childbirth. The infant receives warmth, food, and security from the parent. The parent (usually the mother) places the child's needs above her own for years to come. In return, she receives enjoyment and establishes her identity as a mother. Both benefit from the formation of irreplaceable links that continue long after the child ceases to be dependent.

Three important concepts regarding attachment are the following:

- Attachment is a process that follows a progressive, or developmental, course that changes over time. It is rarely

Carol, a 35-year-old primipara, had a cesarean birth after failure to progress in labor. She is very tired, although she is relatively comfortable. Her husband, Bill, is excited about being a father but expresses concern because neither he nor Carol has experience with infants and his job requires almost constant travel.

The day of delivery, Carol readily accepts attention and assistance with hygiene. She recounts the details of her labor to friends on the telephone. She examines her baby girl closely and touches the infant's face and hands gently with her fingertips. She remarks that she plans to breast-feed and is surprised that the infant sleeps so much.

1. What are Carol's priority needs at this time?
2. What phase of recovery is she manifesting? Why does she "fingertip" the infant?

On the first postoperative day, Carol's indwelling catheter is removed, and intravenous fluids are discontinued. She ambulates with minimal assistance and is pleased that she is able to urinate without difficulty. She asks about bowel function and requests the prescribed stool softener. She spends a great deal of time getting the baby to breast-feed. She is very frustrated that the infant does not breast-feed well and asks for assistance from the lactation educator.

3. What are Carol's priority needs now?
4. How have her behaviors changed?

Before discharge, Carol is breast-feeding well. The infant latches on and nurses for 10 to 15 minutes on each side, and Carol's nipples are free of tenderness or signs of trauma. Carol has no relatives in the area, and her husband is home for the weekend only. She states that she will just have to get along by herself after that.

5. What anticipatory guidance should Carol receive about her own care? About the infant's care?
6. What further nursing interventions would be most helpful to her and the baby?

instantaneous. Attachment behaviors of inexperienced or first-time mothers do not differ significantly from those of experienced mothers (Mercer & Ferketich, 1994b).

- Attachment is facilitated by positive feedback, either real or perceived. For example, an infant's grasp reflex around a parent's finger means "I love you" to the parent.
- Attachment occurs through mutually satisfying experiences. Therefore, if the new mother is in severe pain or is exhausted, she needs pain relief and assistance for her to enjoy the early experiences with the baby.

Unlike bonding, attachment is reciprocal—that is, it goes in both directions between parent and infant. For attachment to occur, there must be some response from the infant to parental signals. Alert infants have a whole repertoire of responses called *reciprocal attachment behaviors*. They are the infant's part in the process of early attachment that progresses to lifelong mutual devotion.

Reciprocal Attachment Behaviors

Newborn infants have the ability to do the following:

- Make eye contact and engage in prolonged, intense, mutual gazing.
- Move their eyes and attempt to "track" the parent's face.
- Grasp the parent's finger and hold on.
- Move synchronously in response to rhythms and patterns of the parent's voice. This is called *entrainment*.
- Root, suckle, and finally latch on to the breast.
- Be comforted by the parent's voice or touch.

Maternal Touch

Maternal behavior, particularly maternal touch, changes rapidly as the mother progresses through a discovery phase with her infant. Initially the mother may not reach for the infant, but if the infant is placed in her arms, she holds the baby in an *en face* position, with the infant's face in the same vertical plane as her own. When the infant is awake, the two engage in prolonged mutual gazing, as illustrated in Figure 21–9.

Fingertipping is common during the early minutes as the mother gets acquainted with the tiny stranger. She may gently explore the infant's face, fingers, and toes with her fingertips only (Fig. 21–10).

After "fingertipping," mothers begin to stroke the baby's chest and legs with the palm. Next, the mother uses her entire hand to enfold the infant and to bring the child close to her body. She strokes the baby's hair, presses her cheek against the infant's cheek, and finally feels comfort-

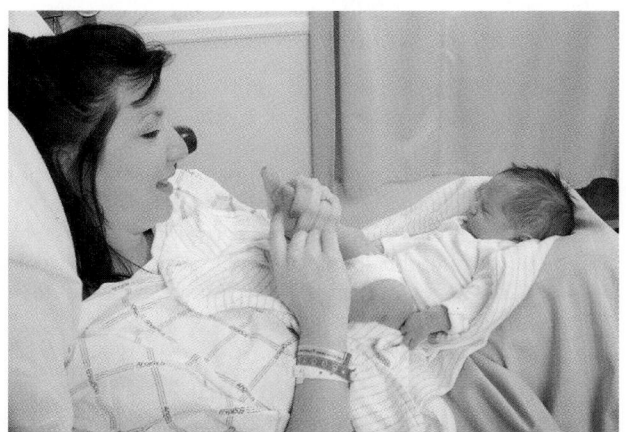

FIGURE 21–10

The mother's initial touch includes *fingertipping,* whereby she becomes acquainted with her infant by touching only with her fingertips.

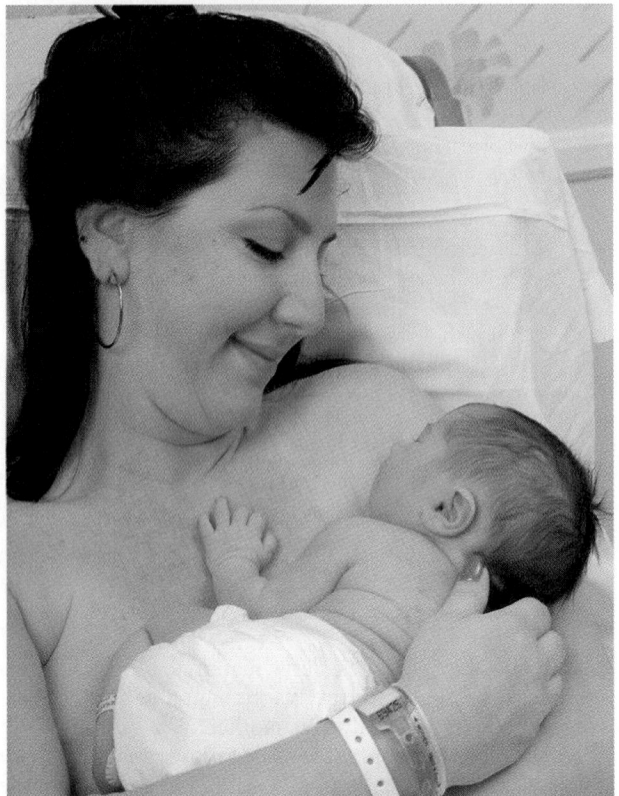

FIGURE 21–11

Mothers progress from exploratory touching to enfolding the infant. Their pleasure is enhanced by skin-to-skin contact.

able enough to engage in a full range of consoling behaviors (Fig. 21–11).

The mother next begins to identify specific features of the newborn. "Look at his little pink mouth." Then she begins to relate features to family members. "He has his father's chin and nose (Fig. 21–12)." This identification process has been termed *claiming* or *binding in* (Rubin, 1977).

Verbal Behaviors

Verbal behaviors are also important indicators of maternal attachment. Most mothers speak to the infant in a high-pitched voice and progress from calling the baby "it" to "he or she" and then to using the given name. Verbal behaviors may provide clues to a mother's early psychological relationship with her infant. Nurses are in a position to observe the interactions of mothers and their infants and, if necessary, to teach and model interactions that foster early attachment between them.

The Process of Maternal Role Adaptation

Puerperal Phases

In the early 1960s, Rubin identified restorative phases that the mother must go through to replenish the energy lost

during labor and to attain comfort in the role of mother. The puerperal phases are called *taking in, taking hold,* and *letting go.* The three phases may provide a useful method to observe progressive change in maternal behavior but should not be used as strict guidelines for maternal assessment. They can, however, be used to anticipate maternal needs and to intervene to meet those needs.

TAKING-IN PHASE

During the taking-in phase, the mother is focused primarily on her own need for fluid, food, and deep restorative sleep. Inexperienced nurses may be puzzled by the mother's passive behavior as she takes in or receives attention and physical care. She also takes in or absorbs every detail of the neonate, but she seems content to allow others to make decisions.

A major task for the mother during this time is to integrate her birth experience into reality. To do this she recounts the details of her labor and delivery over and over. She may spend a great deal of time on the telephone describing her labor and the birth of this child. She repeats her experiences for visitors and attempts to piece together all the details from those who were involved. This process helps the mother realize that the pregnancy is over; the infant is born, and the child is now an individual separate from her.

Although Rubin believed that the taking-in phase lasted for approximately 2 days, it is now believed to last a day or less. The taking-in phase may be prolonged when a cesarean birth, especially an emergency cesarean delivery,

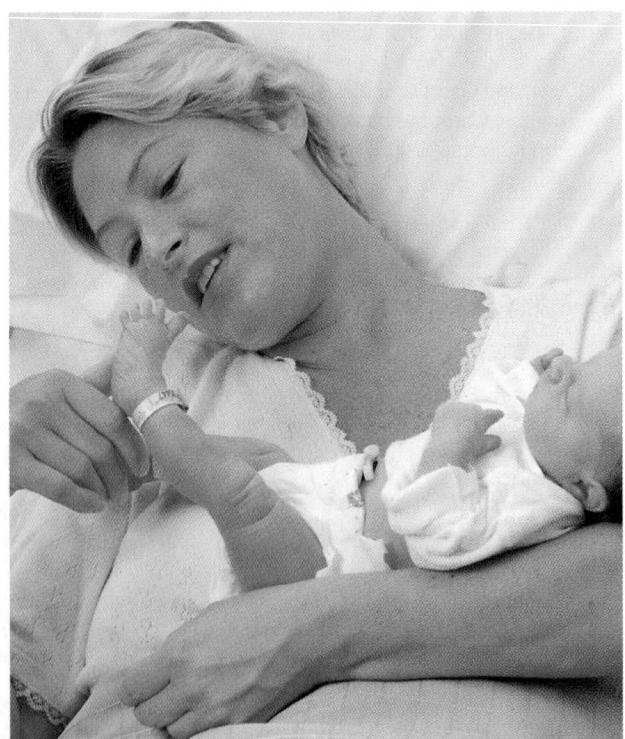

FIGURE 21–12

The *binding-in,* or *claiming,* process includes the mother's identification of her baby's specific features, relating them to other family members. This mother states, "His long toes are exactly like mine."

has been necessary. Many women have difficulty assimilating the unfamiliar and intrusive procedures that occurred very rapidly, and they may express negative perceptions of the birth experience. These women require attention and sensitive care that takes into account their special needs for pain relief and sustained contact with their newborn.

TAKING-HOLD PHASE
The mother becomes more independent in the taking-hold phase. She exhibits concern about managing her own body functions and assumes responsibility for her own self-care. When she feels more comfortable and in control of her body, she shifts her attention from her own needs to the performance of the infant. She welcomes information about the wide variety of behaviors exhibited by newborns.

During the taking-hold phase, the mother may verbalize anxiety about her competence as a mother. She may compare her caretaking skills unfavorably with those of the nurse.

Nurses must be careful not to assume the mothering role but instead to allow the mother to perform as much of the caretaking as possible and to praise each attempt, even if the mother's early care is awkwardly performed.

The taking-hold phase, which extends over several days, has been called the "teachable, reachable, referable moment." Nurses who provide home care can take advantage of this ideal time to review previously taught material and to provide additional instructions and demonstrations.

LETTING-GO PHASE
The letting-go phase is a time of relinquishment for the mother and often for the father. If this is a first child, the couple must give up their previous role as a childless couple and acknowledge the loss of a more carefree lifestyle. Many mothers must also give up idealized expectations of the birth experience. For example, they may have planned to have a vaginal birth with minimal or no anesthesia, but instead they required a cesarean birth or regional anesthesia.

In addition, some mothers (and fathers) are disappointed by the size, sex, or characteristics of the infant who does not "match up" with the fantasy baby of pregnancy.

They must relinquish the infant of their fantasies and accept the real infant. These losses often provoke feelings of grief that may be so subtle that they are unexamined or unacknowledged. Both parents may benefit, however, if given the opportunity to verbalize unexpected feelings and to realize that these feelings are common. If the mother is very young or the pregnancy was unplanned, the feelings of loss and grief may be acute.

Maternal Role Attainment
Role attainment is a process in which the mother achieves confidence in her ability to care for her infant and becomes comfortable with her identity as a mother. The process begins during pregnancy and continues for several months after childbirth. The transition to the maternal or paternal role follows four stages (Mercer, 1985):

1. The *anticipatory stage* begins during the pregnancy when pregnant women choose a physician or nurse-midwife. Many attend childbirth classes to prepare for the birth experience. They seek out role models to learn the role of mother.
2. The *formal stage* begins with the birth of the infant and continues for approximately 6 to 8 weeks (Mercer, 1990). During this stage, behaviors are largely guided by others: health professionals, close friends, or parents. A major task for parents during this stage is to become acquainted with their infant so that they can mesh their caregiving with cues from the infant.
3. The *informal stage* begins once the parents have learned appropriate responses to their infant's cues or signals. They begin to respond according to the unique needs of the infant rather than following textbook or health professionals' directives.
4. The *personal stage* is attained when parents feel a sense of harmony in their role, see the infant as a central person in their lives, and have internalized the parental role. The parents accept and feel comfortable with the role of parent.

REDEFINING ROLES
The mother is particularly concerned about redefining roles and focuses on maintaining a strong, adaptive relationship with her partner. She observes him carefully for any change in behavior and is acutely sensitive to his interaction with the infant. From the father's perspective, anxieties about succeeding in his new role put added pressure on the family. Conflicting demands between work and home, feelings of exclusion, and concerns about his relationship with his partner present additional challenges.

It may be essential for the new parents to agree on a division of tasks and responsibilities that was not necessary before the birth of the infant. This process is accomplished quickly and with very little discord in some families. Role assignment in other families is much less flexible, and any change can be a source of tension and frustration.

Although nurses are not actively involved in redefining family roles, they can use their skills in communication to assist the family in expressing their feelings and concerns so that the changes can be accomplished with minimum stress.

ROLE CONFLICT

Role conflict occurs when one's perception of role responsibilities differs significantly from reality. For example, if the mother perceives that her responsibility is to provide most of the care and comfort for the infant, but reality dictates that she must return to full-time employment, role conflict may occur. Nearly 2 million women in the United States face this conflict each year. Many report feelings of guilt for leaving the infant and experience intense "separation grief" when they first leave the infant with a caregiver. Some report feeling jealous of the caregiver and fear that the caregiver will supplant the mother in the infant's affection.

Acknowledging these feelings and reassuring the mother that her emotions are normal may be helpful. The mother also needs time to reestablish feelings of closeness when she comes home from work, and she needs to develop a schedule that allows maximum time with the infant when she is at home. She may have to negotiate with another family member to take over some of the household tasks until she feels more comfortable with the situation. Nursing Care Plan 21–2 describes additional interventions.

Major Maternal Concerns

After childbirth, mothers have major concerns that change over time. During the first month concerns about feeding, infant behavior, and physical care of the infant predominate. Maternal concerns related to the self include discomfort and fatigue. Concerns about family relationships include having less time with older children and not being interested in sex (Sheil et al., 1995). Mothers who had a cesarean birth may also express concerns about limited activity and incisional healing.

BODY IMAGE

As women gain confidence in their ability to care for the infant and as their physical discomfort decreases, emotional concerns related to the self become more intense. In particular, women express concern about regaining their normal figure. Some mothers have unrealistic expectations about weight loss and the time it takes for the body to regain its prepregnancy shape.

Nurses must emphasize that weight loss should be gradual and that about 6 months is usually required to lose the weight gained during pregnancy. Rigid restriction of calories can lead to depleted energy, decreased immunity, and decreased production of milk.

Moreover, nurses should teach the importance of safe activities such as walking and the importance of graduated exercises to regain muscle tone. Mothers should seek the advice of a health care professional before initiating a rigorous exercise program. See Figure 21–8 for postpartum exercises.

POSTPARTUM BLUES

Mild depression, also known as postpartum blues or maternity blues, is a frequently expressed concern. This transient condition affects 75% to 80% of American women who have given birth. The condition has an early onset (1 to 10 days after a woman has given birth) and usually lasts no longer than 2 weeks (Ugarriza, 1992). It is characterized by fatigue, weeping, mood instability, and anxiety. The symptoms are usually unrelated to events, and the condition does not seriously affect the mother's ability to care for the infant. Typically, the mother says, "I don't know why I am crying; I don't feel sad." Although the direct cause is unknown, it is generally accepted that postpartum blues is related to the wide hormonal fluctuations that occur during labor, delivery, and the immediate postpartum period. Although postpartum blues is self-limiting, mothers benefit greatly when empathy and support are freely given by the family and the health care team.

Postpartum blues must be distinguished from *postpartum depression* and *postpartum psychosis*. These separate entities

---

NURSING CARE PLAN 21–2

• • • • • • • • • • •

Adaptation of the Working Mother

Assessment	Rebecca Sanders, a 30-year-old single mother, gave birth to a baby boy by cesarean delivery 4 days ago. She cares for herself with minimal assistance and demonstrates confidence in breast-feeding. Rebecca must return to work in 6 weeks. She states that she does not want to leave the baby with someone else while she works: "My mother was always there for me and I want to be with Derrek, but it is just impossible. How can I be a mother and work full time?"
Nursing Diagnosis	Anticipatory Grieving related to inability to perform the role of mother as she wishes because of the need to place the infant with another care provider and return to full-time employment.
Goals/Expected Outcomes	Rebecca will • Describe her concerns and feelings about leaving her infant with a caregiver by (specific date). • Verbalize plans to achieve maximum satisfaction in her role as mother by the time she returns to work.

Adaptation of the Working Mother

Intervention	Rationale
1. Allow Rebecca to describe her perception of her role as mother and to express concerns about how employment will interfere with her ability to fulfill this role.	1. Role conflict, stress, and grief can result when a mother must leave the infant with another caregiver and return to her job.
2. Recommend free expression of feelings to significant others and to the care provider who is selected.	2. Candid expression of feelings helps to resolve them and opens the way for a discussion of measures that will help to overcome feelings of conflict.
3. Acknowledge the feelings Rebecca expresses, and reassure her that the feelings are common.	3. Knowledge that the feelings are not trivial and that they are common reinforces their validity and importance.

4. Help Rebecca develop a schedule that allows her maximum time with the infant:
  a. Make a list of errands and supplies needed, to avoid frequent stops that delay getting home from work.
  b. Double the recipe when cooking, and freeze half for future use.
  c. Pick up nutritious take-out meals to avoid cooking each evening.
  d. Work out plans that include the baby in daily walks, exercise, or social visits.
	4. Feelings of frustration and stress can be alleviated if the mother has a plan that allows her long periods of uninterrupted time with the infant.

5. Recommend that Rebecca allow 30 to 45 minutes to hold the infant when she first gets home. Delay all other activities until this need is met.	5. Time is needed to reestablish feelings of closeness, comfort, and attachment.
6. Suggest that Rebecca delay her return to employment, if possible, until the infant is at least 16 weeks old.	6. By 16 weeks most infants are able to sleep through the night. This development reduces the chance that sleep deprivation will add to other stressors.
7. Recommend that Rebecca investigate several day care providers. She should check references, make unannounced visits, insist on seeing required licenses and certification, discuss the number and ages of children cared for, request a schedule of planned care, determine the provider's philosophy of infant care, determine whether the care provider is trained in cardiopulmonary resuscitation (CPR), and know what plans are in place if a fire or disaster occurs.	7. A great deal of stress is eliminated if parents feel confident that a competent and nurturing day care provider has been found.
8. Suggest that Rebecca leave the infant with the chosen day care provider for 2 to 3 days before resuming full-time employment.	8. Allowing both mother and infant to "practice separating" while there is still some flexibility in their schedules makes the first day back at work less traumatic.
9. Recommend that Rebecca pump her breasts and feed the infant by bottle at least once a day before returning to work.	9. Becoming proficient at pumping the breasts and introducing the infant to bottle-feeding prepares both the mother and infant for all-day separation.

Evaluation

Rebecca freely expresses her feelings of guilt, anxiety, and concern about leaving her infant. She has organized a plan to investigate day care in her area and verbalized plans to reorganize her work and social schedule so that she can spend as much time as possible with her son.

Additional Nursing Diagnoses to Consider

Diversional Activity Deficit
Parental Role Conflict
Altered Role Performance

are disabling and require therapeutic management for full recovery. (Chapter 28 provides a discussion of these conditions.)

The Process of Family Adaptation

The birth of an infant requires that roles and relationships within the family be reorganized. Each family member is affected.

Fathers

The father's developing bond to his newborn has been called *engrossment*. It is characterized by intense interest in how the infant looks and responds and a desire to touch and hold the baby. Many fathers comment on the baby's distinctive features. They experience strong attraction to the infant and express elation described as a "high" following the baby's birth. The father's attachment behaviors increase when the infant is awake, makes eye contact, and responds to the father's voice (Fig. 21–13).

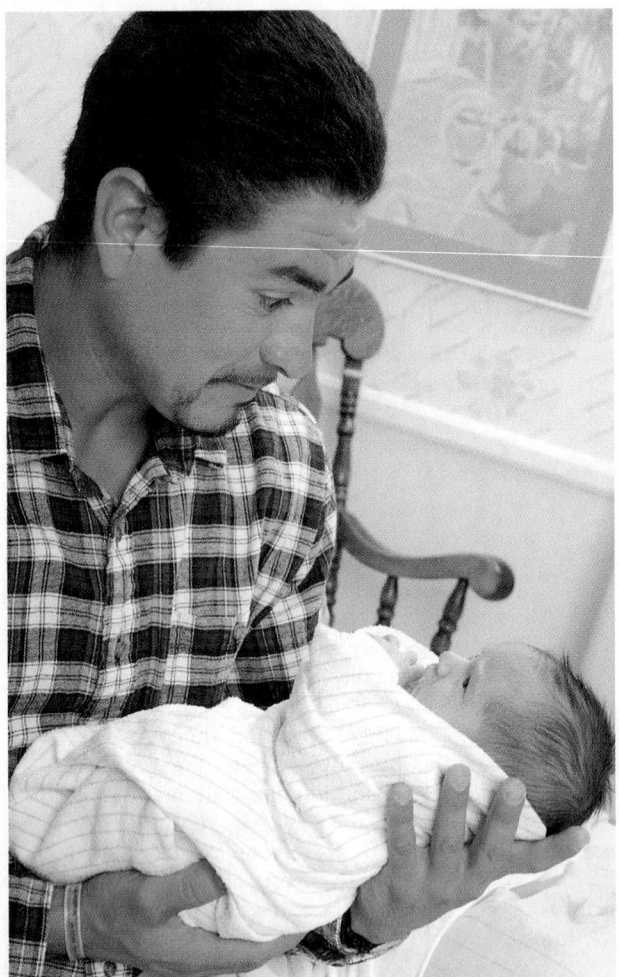

FIGURE 21–13

Fathers' behaviors at initial contact with their infants often correspond to maternal behaviors. The intense fascination that fathers exhibit is called *engrossment*. Note the eye-to-eye contact between father and infant.

Many fathers eagerly look forward to coparenting with their mate. They may, however, lack confidence in providing infant care and are sensitive to being left out of instructions and demonstrations of infant care. They may feel that others expect them only to provide support to the mother. Research indicates that fathers need more parenting information than that provided in prenatal classes. Fathers often do not know what to expect from infants during the first 3 months of life. They would benefit from additional information about normal growth and development during infancy. Moreover, information about child care, presented in the prenatal period, should be reviewed after the child is born (Tiller, 1995).

Siblings

Sibling response to the birth of a new brother or sister depends on age and developmental level. Toddlers are usually not completely aware of the impending birth. They may view the infant as competition or fear that they will be replaced in the parents' affection. Negative behaviors such as sleep problems, an increase in attention-seeking efforts, and regression to more infantile behaviors like renewed bedwetting or thumb sucking may surface. Some may exhibit hostile behaviors toward the mother, particularly when she holds or feeds the newborn. Parents must find opportunities to affirm their continued love and affection for the very vulnerable sibling.

Preschool siblings engage in more looking than touching. Most spend at least some time in proximity to the infant and talk to the mother about the infant (Fig. 21–14). A relaxed, natural setting, without time constraints, may make it easier for young children to interact with the infant. Special care must be taken by the parents, visitors, and nurses to pay as much attention to the sibling as to the new baby.

Grandparents

The involvement of grandparents with grandchildren depends on many factors. One of the most important factors is proximity. Grandparents who live near the child frequently develop strong attachment that evolves into unconditional love and a special relationship that brings joy to the grandparents and an added sense of security to the grandchildren (Fig. 21–15). Grandparents who live many miles from grandchildren must try to devise ways to foster a relationship with grandchildren they seldom see.

Expectations of the role of grandparents are also a factor in how the grandparents adapt to the birth of a grandchild. Many grandparents strive to be fully involved in the care and upbringing of the child. Others desire less involvement.

Grandparents are often a major part of the support system that new parents need. Grandmothers in particular provide assistance with household tasks and infant care, which allows the mother to recover from childbirth and make the transition to parenthood.

Factors Affecting Family Adaptation

Numerous factors influence the family's adjustment. Some, such as discomfort and fatigue, can be anticipated because

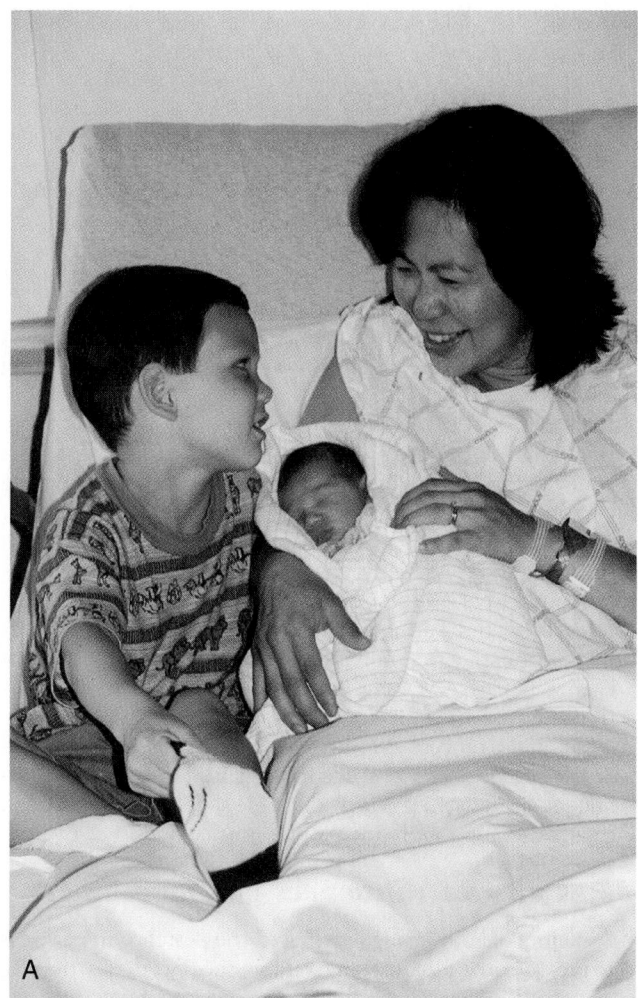
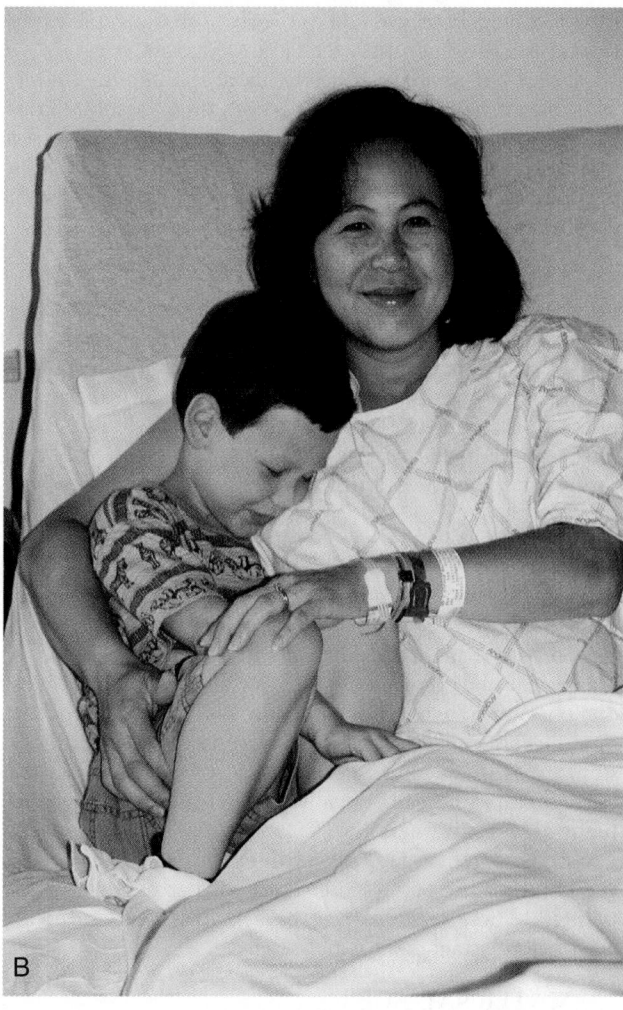

FIGURE 21–14
· · · · · · · · · · ·

A, Although they may hesitate to touch the infant, children often want to be close. *B,* This boy's relief and joy are obvious as he reclaims a favorite spot.

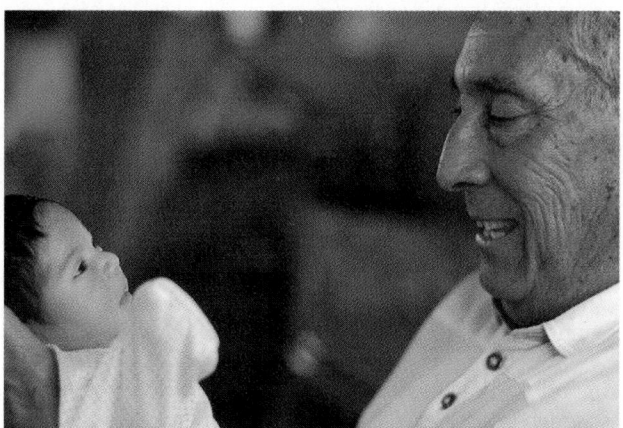

FIGURE 21–15
· · · · · · · · · ·

Grandparents may develop strong bonds with grandchildren.

they are so common. Unanticipated events, such as cesarean birth, birth of a preterm or ill infant, or the birth of twins, also affect the ease and speed with which the family adjusts.

DISCOMFORT AND FATIGUE
Normally, discomfort associated with childbirth resolves within the first days following birth. Discomfort may make it difficult to focus on the needs of the newborn. Fatigue often continues during the first few weeks, when the infant's schedule is erratic and uninterrupted sleep is minimal. When the infant begins to sleep through the night (at about 16 weeks), fatigue becomes less of a factor.

KNOWLEDGE OF INFANT NEEDS
First-time parents are often unsure of how to care for the newborn and become very anxious if they are unable to console a crying infant. Moreover, many are concerned about specific procedures, such as care of the umbilical cord or the circumcision. They want to know if the infant is receiving adequate nutrition. Breast-feeding benefits both mother and

infant. It may, however, add to the stress that parents experience initially when they lack knowledge about it.

Some parents have concerns about spoiling the infant. They may believe that responding each time the infant cries causes the infant to cry to get his or her way. It may be necessary to remind parents that infants cry to indicate a need and to reassure the parents that responding to crying does not spoil the child.

PREVIOUS EXPERIENCE
Previous experience with newborns may also affect family adjustment. Multiparas are more comfortable with infants and exhibit attachment behaviors earlier than do primiparas, who may spend many more hours in the early discovery phase of attachment. Mothers who have previously given birth to infants with anomalies or to infants who did not survive may need more time to feel comfortable with this infant.

EXPECTATIONS OF THE NEWBORN
Unrealistic expectations of the infant may also influence adjustment. Many parents have very little experience with newborns and are disappointed at the way a newborn looks. Nurses must be prepared to teach normal growth and development and to assist the parents in working through their misconceptions. For instance, the capacity of an infant's stomach is small, and the infant must be fed frequently. Also, infants are neurologically unable to sleep through the night for several weeks.

Some parents may be very disappointed in the sex of the child, or they may sense that their partners are disappointed. These feelings must be acknowledged and dealt with before attachment can take place.

MATERNAL AGE
Adjustment to parenthood is a challenge for teenagers who have not achieved a strong sense of their own identity. In general, teenagers tend to talk less, respond less, appear more passive, and sometimes appear less affectionate with their children than do adult parents. They need special assistance to develop necessary parenting skills that promote optimal development of the infant. (See discussion of teenage parenting in Chapter 25.)

MATERNAL TEMPERAMENT
Maternal personality traits are a major influence on attachment. Mothers who are calm and secure in their ability to learn adjust more easily to the demands of motherhood. Conversely, mothers who are excitable, insecure, and anxious have more difficulty.

TEMPERAMENT OF THE INFANT
The infant also affects maternal adjustment. Infants who are calm, easily consoled, and enjoy cuddling increase parental confidence and feelings of competence. In contrast, irritable infants who are difficult to console and who do not respond to cuddling interfere with attachment.

AVAILABILITY OF A STRONG SUPPORT SYSTEM
A strong, consistent support system is a major factor in the adjustment of the new mother. She needs assistance with household tasks such as meal preparation, laundry, and shopping. In addition, she needs encouragement, praise, and reassurance that she is a good mother.

UNANTICIPATED EVENTS
Cesarean Birth. Unanticipated events can make parental adjustment more difficult. For example, an unplanned cesarean birth may result in financial strain, a longer recovery time for the mother, additional discomfort, and increased stress for the family. Birth of a preterm or ill infant results in additional concern about the condition of the infant and may necessitate prolonged separation of parents and child. This separation may delay the process of attachment and create stress on the normally functioning family.

Birth of Twins. Even if expected, the birth of more than one infant may present problems of attachment. It is believed the process of attachment is structured so that the parents become attached to only one infant at a time. Therefore, parents should be encouraged to interact with each child individually, especially in the early getting-acquainted period. Nurses must help the parents to relate to each infant as an individual rather than as part of a unit by pointing out the individual responses and uniqueness of each infant. Early, frequent contacts or rooming-in helps the parents gain confidence in caretaking and facilitates the attachment process. Mothers are sometimes overwhelmed at the prospect of breast-feeding twins. They need reassurance that they will produce an ample supply of milk for each infant because supply increases with demand.

▌ *Cultural Influences on Adaptation*

A major goal of nursing practice in the postpartum period is to provide nursing care that is culture specific; that is, nursing care needs to fit the health beliefs, values, and practices of a particular culture. This effort can be difficult because of the increasing ethnic diversity in countries such as the United States and Canada. A major challenge for nurses is to be aware of cultural beliefs and to acknowledge their importance in family adaptation. Many cultural factors that are relevant to the postpartum period can be grouped into communicative practices, dietary practices, and health beliefs.

Communication

Verbal communication may be difficult because of the numerous dialects and languages spoken. An interpreter should be fluent in the language, of the same religion, and of the same country of origin if possible. This compatibility is particularly important for Middle Eastern families, whose religious orientation may vary widely and who come from countries with long histories of social and religious conflict.

Respecting the privacy and modesty of all families is important, but modesty is especially important to Latinas (women of Mexican, Central American, and South American extraction) and to Middle Eastern and Asian women. Laws of modesty require that Muslim women keep their hair, body, arms to the wrist, and legs to the ankles covered.

Health care workers must remember that tactfulness and warmth are important. Direct communication can be distressing, particularly for Latinas and Native Americans, who approach a subject only after polite and gracious comments have been exchanged.

When the nurse and the family speak different primary languages, it is important to verify that the family has understood what is being said. Nodding or saying "Yes" may be a sign of courtesy rather than of understanding or agreement. To be certain the message has been received, the nurse should ask family members to repeat in their own words what they have been told.

Dietary Practices

Some dietary practices that must be considered center on the hot-cold theory of health and diet. Hot-cold has nothing to do with temperature but with intrinsic properties of certain foods. For example, Southeast Asians (Cambodians, Vietnamese, Hmong, and Laotians) believe that after childbirth the woman should eat only "hot" foods such as eggs, chicken, and rice. They believe "hot" foods help to replace blood lost during childbirth (Mattson, 1995). Women from India also eat special foods to regain a state of balance after childbirth. Dried ginger is often eaten to control postpartum bleeding (Choudhry, 1997).

Some Chinese believe that a combination of yin and yang maintains balance. Yin foods include bean sprouts, broccoli, carrots, and cauliflower. Yang foods include broiled meat, chicken, soup, and eggs.

Health Beliefs

Cultural beliefs and practices provide a sense of security for new mothers. For example, Muslims believe that the first sounds a child hears should be from the Koran in praise and supplication to God (Allah), and parents want to say a prayer in the newly born child's ears at the time of birth. Facilitating this practice goes a long way toward building the family's trust in the relationship with the nurse.

Many Middle Eastern families believe that compliments should be directed to Allah rather than to the newborn. The compliment thus is converted into a blessing so that mistrust or jealousy does not occur. Some Southeast Asians believe the spirit resides in the head and are troubled if someone pats or rubs the head of the newborn.

Health beliefs having to do with hygiene and breastfeeding cause the most conflict in the postpartum period. Southeast Asians and Latinas believe that the mother should be kept warm to avoid upsetting the balance of hot and cold. Some women do not wish to take baths or wash their hair during the postpartum period. This practice is upsetting for nurses who are concerned about hygiene. Tact and sensitivity are needed to find a compromise. Many Southeast Asian women believe that colostrum is "unclean" and that they should not breast-feed until the milk comes in. This belief conflicts with the theory that breast-feeding should start as soon after birth as possible.

Specific religious practices should be accepted and supported. For instance, Muslim mothers are exempted from their obligation to pray while they are bleeding. The father and other family members, however, kneel, place their heads on the floor, and pray five times a day. If possible, provide a clean, quiet room where this obligation can be fulfilled without having to leave the birth facility.

Home Care

Because many mothers and infants are discharged from the birth facility soon after childbirth, most of the assessments and interventions described in this chapter occur in the home. Many mothers leave the birth facility before they have fully recovered from the childbirth experience. Consequently, most psychosocial concerns, such as family adaptation and postpartum blues, surface later, when support from health care professionals is less available.

A variety of methods is currently being tried to provide care for mothers and infants who leave the birth facility within hours after childbirth. These methods include telephone calls, nurse-managed postpartum clinics, home visits, and "baby lines" staffed by nurses who provide information and guidance for families who call. All methods have advantages and disadvantages.

■ NURSING CARE
Maternal Adaptation

Assessment

Several factors, such as how the mother progresses through the puerperal phases, her mood, interaction with the infant, and unanticipated events, affect maternal adaptation to the birth. Table 21–3 summarizes the psychosocial assessment of the mother and nursing considerations related to each assessment.

Nursing Diagnosis and Planning

Parenting involves the parents' ability to create an environment that nurtures the growth and development of the infant. Parenting may be difficult when factors such as maternal discomfort, fatigue, and lack of knowledge or confidence in infant care come into play. Therefore, a common nursing diagnosis is

■ Risk for Altered Parenting related to multiple factors, such as fatigue, discomfort, and lack of knowledge of infant care.
  Expected Outcomes: The mother will verbalize feelings of comfort and support as she progresses through the phases of recovery and will demonstrate progressive attachment behaviors by (specific date) and participate in care of the newborn by (date) or by the first home visit.

Interventions

Assisting the Mother Through Recovery Phases

"Mother" the Mother. The early taking-in phase is a time to mother the mother so that she can move on to more complex tasks of maternal adjustment. During the first few hours after childbirth, she has a great need for physical care and comfort. Provide ample fluids and favorite foods. Keep linens dry, tuck warm blankets around her until chilling has stopped, and use warm water for perineal care.

Monitor and Protect. The new mother depends on nurses to monitor and protect her. Remind her of the need

TABLE 21-3

• • • • • • • • • •

Assessing Maternal Adaptation

Assessments	Nursing Considerations
Progression Through Puerperal Phases	
Taking in (passive, dependent) Taking hold (autonomous, seeks information) Letting go (relinquishes fantasy baby, begins to see self as mother)	Behaviors that should be noted include the mother's need to rest, her need to recount the details of her labor and childbirth, and her readiness to learn infant care and assume control of her own care.
Maternal Mood	
Mood and energy level, eye contact, posture, comfort	Tense body posture, crying, or anxiety may indicate discomfort, fatigue, or the beginning of postpartum blues.
Factors That Affect Maternal Adaptation	
Age of mother	May need additional support if less than 18 years old.
Previous experience	Primiparas often progress through puerperal phases at a slower pace and may need additional assistance. Multiparas often have more experience with infant care. Previous birth of a child with anomalies or death of an infant may delay adaptation.
Maternal/infant temperament	Mothers who are calm, secure in their ability to learn, and free from anxiety adjust more easily to the demands of motherhood. Infants who are easily consoled and enjoy cuddling increase parental confidence. Infants who are difficult to console increase parental frustration.
Unanticipated events	Cesarean birth may result in increased discomfort and longer recovery. The birth of more than one infant can create problems with attachment.
Interaction with Infant	
Maternal touch	Mother progresses from "fingertipping" to enfolding and a full range of comforting behaviors.
Verbal interaction	Mother may call infant "it" initially but progresses quickly to using given name and identifying specific characteristics.
Response to infant cues or signals	Prompt, gentle, consistent response indicates progressive adaptation to parenting role.
Preparation for Parenting	
Classes in breast-feeding, parenting, or infant care	Many mothers feel more prepared after completing classes and participate in care sooner.

to void and assist her to ambulate. Offer pain medication before discomfort is severe, and analgesia is less effective. At the first signs of fatigue, encourage the mother to sleep.

Listen to the Birth Experience. Be prepared to listen to details of the birth experience and to offer sincere praise for her efforts during labor.

Many mothers spend so much time on the telephone that it is difficult to complete assessments and care. It is often helpful to offer a choice. "Excuse me for a moment. I need to check you soon. I can do it now or come back in 5 minutes."

Fostering Independence

As the mother becomes more independent, allow her to schedule her care as much as possible. Collaborate with her to plan when procedures, such as sitz baths, will be done. Encourage her to assume responsibility for self-care, and emphasize that the nurse's role at this point is to assist and to teach.

Promoting Bonding and Attachment

Early, unlimited contact between parents and infants is of primary importance to facilitate the attachment process (Fig. 21–16). In many hospitals and birth centers infants remain in the room with the parents unless complications intervene. This arrangement may be called mother-baby nursing, couplet care, or dyad care. One nurse cares for both the mother and the baby and is able to provide teaching and help with bonding as a part of ongoing nursing care.

Prolonged contact between mothers and infants leads to more touching and caring for the infant. Specific nursing measures to promote bonding and attachment are the following:

- Assist the parents in unwrapping the baby to inspect the toes, fingers, and body. This process allows the parents to become acquainted with the "real" baby that must replace the fantasy baby that many parents imagined during the pregnancy.
- Position the infant in an *en face* position because eye-to-eye contact is a first step in establishing mutual interaction between the infant and the parent.
- Point out the reciprocal bonding activities of the infant: "Look how she holds your finger"; "He has not taken his eyes off you."
- Allow the infant to remain with the parents as long as they wish so that they can progress at their own speed through the discovery or getting-acquainted phase.
- Assist the mother in feeding the infant and answer her questions about feeding.
- Model behaviors by holding the infant close and speaking in high-pitched, soothing tones.

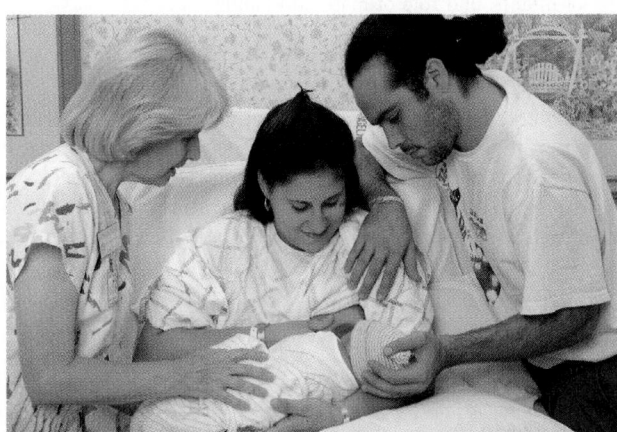

FIGURE 21–16

By teaching about the newborn and family, the nurse helps parents develop confidence in their ability to provide care for the infant.

- Refer to the infant's characteristics positively: "She has the tiniest pink ears and such a lot of dark hair."

Involving Parents in Infant Care

Providing care for the infant fosters feelings of responsibility and nurturing and is an important component of attachment. Moreover, it allows parents to develop confidence in their ability to care for an infant before they go home.

Although teaching begins during pregnancy, review information and repeat demonstrations if time allows. (See Chapter 23 for teaching about infant care.) It is important for the entire staff to agree on how basic care is to be taught. Mothers seek confirmation of information, and they become confused and lose faith in the credibility of the staff if information varies.

Offer parents repeated praise and encouragement because they become easily discouraged if they think they have failed at some attempt to care for their infants.

> Suggestions for care must be tactfully phrased to avoid the implication that the parents are inept: "You burped that baby like a professional. There are a couple of little hints I can share about diapering."

Evaluation

- Does the mother verbalize feelings of comfort as she cares for her infant?
- Does she demonstrate attachment behaviors such as enfolding the infant, using the infant's name, and responding gently when the infant cries?
- Does she participate in infant care (diapering, feeding, and care of the umbilical cord and circumcision)?

NURSING CARE
. . . .
Family Adaptation

Assessment

Fathers

The father's emotional status and interaction with the infant are particularly important because he usually serves as the mother's primary support person. The nurse should assess the father's interaction with the mother and the infant and his knowledge about infants. Unrealistic expectations of the infant may lead to problems. Moreover, if the father expects the mother to recover her energy and libido rapidly, he may become resentful if her recovery takes longer than anticipated.

Siblings

It is important to note the ages of siblings and how they react to the newborn. The nurse should also assess the parents' reaction to sibling behaviors.

Support System

Family members often provide a powerful support system, and their involvement is important to the adaptation of the family. Asking about who will assist the mother when she returns home helps the nurse assess the support system.

TABLE 21–4

Assessing Family Adaptation

Assessments	Nursing Considerations
Characteristics of Infant That May Affect Family Adaptation	
Sex and size of infant	Disappointment in the sex or concern about the small size may interfere with bonding.
Unexpected characteristics (cephalhematoma, jaundice, cranial molding, newborn rash)	Be prepared to explain unexpected appearance or behavior in words parents can comprehend.
Infant behavior (irritable, easily consoled, cuddles)	An easily consoled, cuddly infant increases bonding and attachment.
Paternal Adaptation	
Response to mother and to infant	Mate often provides the most important support for the mother, and his involvement with the infant indicates his acceptance of his parenting role.
Knowledge of infant care	Useful in planning teaching that includes the father.
Response to infant cues or signals (crying, fussing)	Many fathers feel awkward handling the infant but want to become proficient in infant care.
Ages and Developmental Levels of Siblings	
Reaction of siblings	Young children often fear that the newborn will replace them in the affection of parents. Anticipatory guidance for the parents about sibling rivalry may be needed.
Support System	
Interest and availability of family or friends to assist during early weeks	Family may need assistance in identifying available support.
Plans for first few days at home	Review plans for care, support, and rest.
Follow-up plans	Appointments should be scheduled at 2 weeks and 6 weeks with clinic or health care provider.
Cultural Factors	
Cultural beliefs and practices that may affect nursing care	Culture-specific care can be planned for hygiene, dietary preferences, usual care of infants, and role of mate and family.
Expectations of the health care team	

Nonverbal Behavior

Nonverbal behavior is equally important. Are the parents' words congruent with what they do? For example, does the mother verbalize satisfaction with her infant's characteristics but respond slowly to infant signals? Table 21–4 summarizes the family assessment and briefly indicates nursing considerations.

Nursing Diagnosis and Planning

Sometimes a family that usually functions effectively is unable to cope because of a specific event, such as the birth of a baby. A common nursing diagnosis is

■ Altered Family Processes related to lack of knowledge of infant needs and behaviors, stress during the early weeks at home, and sibling rivalry.

Expected Outcomes: The family will verbalize understanding of infant needs and behaviors and identify methods for reducing stress during the early weeks at home. The family will describe measures to reduce sibling rivalry and identify external resources and support system.

Expected outcomes often cannot be evaluated before discharge from the birth facility and overlap with home care. The expected outcome should therefore specify a date.

Interventions

Teaching the Family About the Newborn

Infant Needs. Some new parents have unrealistic expectations of the newborn, and nurses are in the best position to provide information about what the infant is capable of doing and what the infant needs to thrive. Provide them with information about the infant's capabilities as well as the emotional and physical needs.

Infant Signals.   Discuss the importance of responding promptly and gently to cues such as crying or fussing, which indicate that the infant needs attention. Reassure parents that responding to cues does not "spoil" their child but helps the infant learn to trust that the world is a safe, secure place.

Help parents recognize signals that indicate when their infant has had enough and wants to avoid further stimulation. The so-called avoidance cues, such as looking away, splaying the fingers, arching the back, and fussiness, indicate that the infant needs a quiet time.

Helping the Family Adapt

Providing Anticipatory Guidance About Stress Reduction.   Help the family plan for the first weeks at home, when the family must adjust to the demands of a newborn. This is a time when the need for rest is great but the opportunity for uninterrupted sleep is minimal. As a result, fatigue is a common problem.

Emphasize that the priority during the first 4 to 6 weeks should be caring for the mother and baby. The mother should sleep when the infant sleeps and delay visits and phone calls until she is rested. She can reduce family tension by establishing a relaxed home atmosphere and a flexible meal schedule. Enlisting the aid of grandparents, other relatives, and friends to help with meal preparation, shopping, and care of the other children will provide the mother more time for rest.

Teach mothers breathing exercises and progressive relaxation techniques to reduce stress and to energize, especially when a nap is not possible. To help them cope with stress, encourage parents to discuss their feelings openly. Remind them of the need for healthy nutrition and for favorite recreation. It is easy for fatigue and tension to overwhelm the anticipated joys of parenting if no respite is available from constant care.

Providing Ways to Reduce Sibling Rivalry.   Suggest that parents plan time alone with the older child and that they offer frequent expressions of love and affection. It is also helpful if visitors and family do not focus exclusively on the infant but also include the older child in their gift giving and exclamations about the newborn.

Emphasize the importance of responding calmly and with understanding when the child regresses to more infantile behaviors or expresses hostility toward the infant. Acknowledging the child's feelings and offering prompt reassurance of continued love are most valuable.

Identifying Resources.   In many homes, women assume the major responsibilities of day-to-day homemaking. With the birth of an infant, this task becomes more difficult. A division of labor must be negotiated to prevent undue stress and fatigue. This division of labor is particularly important if there are other children whose needs for time, attention, and comfort must also be met.

The mother's primary support is often the father of the baby. Members of the extended family, particularly grandmothers and sisters, or friends also provide valuable support. Community resources such as day care centers, parenting classes, and breast-feeding support groups are available in many areas. Remind the mother that resources are available when she begins to feel isolated and exhausted.

Evaluation

- Do the parents respond to the infant's crying promptly and gently?
- Do the parents have a plan to reduce family stress and sibling anxiety?
- Are they able to describe resources for support?

Postpartum Home Care

Criteria for Discharge

Most women leave the hospital when they are just beginning to recover from giving birth and beginning to learn how to care for themselves and their infants. The following criteria for discharge of mothers were developed by the American Academy of Pediatrics and the American College of Obstetricians and Gynecologists (1997):

- The mother has no complications, and assessments are normal (including vital signs, lochia, fundus, urinary output, incisions, ambulation, ability to eat and drink, and emotional status).
- Pertinent laboratory data have been reviewed, and immune globulin has been administered, if necessary.
- The mother has received instructions on self-care, deviations from normal, and the proper response to danger signs and symptoms.
- The mother demonstrates readiness to care for herself and her baby.
- The mother has received instructions on postpartum activity, exercises, and relief measures for common postpartum discomforts.
- Arrangements have been made for postpartum care.
- Family members or other support persons are available to the mother for the first few days following discharge.

Common Problems of the Postpartum Period

Common problems encountered by new mothers are discomfort, such as perineal, incisional, and nipple pain and uterine cramping. Additional problems include fatigue, constipation, and difficulties with breast-feeding. Women who had a cesarean birth are also concerned about the need for assistance with chores and infant care (Eakes & Brown, 1998). Infants who leave the birth facility within the first 24 hours are at risk for a variety of problems, including feeding difficulties, jaundice, significant weight loss or inadequate weight gain, rashes, and conjunctivitis (Keppler, 1995).

Home Care Services

New parents must be made aware of the services offered for home care. These services include information lines, follow-up telephone calls, home visits, and nurse-managed postpartum outpatient clinics. In addition, some facilities offer breast-feeding and parenting classes, "baby and me" walks or exercise sessions, and postpartum support groups.

INFORMATION LINES

Ideally, information lines should be open 24 hours a day, 7 days a week. They should be staffed by qualified nurses who use agency protocols to respond to the family's questions. Moreover, these nurses must be prepared to triage. That is, they must be skilled at soliciting information to identify problems and determining the priority of the problems identified.

Legal liability is a concern for all agencies and personnel who identify problems, set priorities, and provide information by telephone. Not only must the staff be educated and evaluated for the task, but protocols must also be devised, a documentation system developed, and adequate consultation or "backup" support made available.

A major disadvantage of information lines is that they rely on families to initiate a request for assistance. Not all families recognize a problem as it begins to develop and, as a result, may delay in seeking information.

TELEPHONE CALLS

Some facilities initiate telephone interviews to assess new families and to provide information to families at home. The calls are usually made 1 to 3 days following discharge. As with information lines, a qualified nurse, following the facility protocol, conducts a systematic assessment of the mother and infant. The nurse solicits questions and reinforces important information. Telephone calls are relatively inexpensive. Their major disadvantage, however, is that the nurse cannot confirm the data but must rely on observations made by the family.

HOME VISITS

Home visits allow physical examination of the mother and infant and assessment of family adaptation as well as the home environment. Maternal assessment should include the breasts, fundus, lochia, and psychosocial status (Fig. 21–17). Postpartum visits can provide opportunities for further teaching. If possible, nurses should allow time to observe breast-feeding and to provide encouragement and reassur-

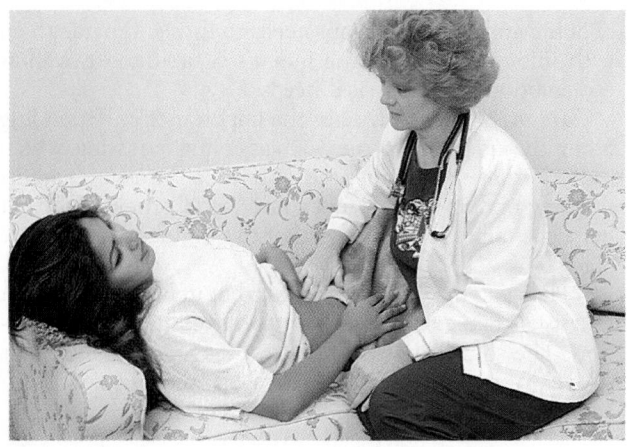

FIGURE 21–17

Postpartum home visits include assessments and health education. Here the nurse evaluates involution while teaching the mother how to palpate her fundus.

ance that is badly needed during the first days before lactation is well established.

The newborn's weight, color, and elimination pattern are important parts of the home visit. Ample time should be allowed to reinforce previous learning, to answer questions, and to introduce new topics. Although home visits are expensive, some agencies believe that they are less expensive than readmissions of the mother or infant to the hospital for problems that could be prevented by follow-up care.

OUTPATIENT CLINICS

Nurse-managed outpatient clinics offer another option for postpartum care. Although transportation is a problem for some families, clinic visits are less costly for the agency than home visits. Like home care, clinic visits include an examination of the mother and infant. There should be time to answer questions about maternal self-care, to provide assistance with infant feeding, and to deal with special concerns, such as care of the umbilical cord or circumcision and postpartum blues (Keppler, 1995).

KEY CONCEPTS

- After childbirth, the uterus returns to its nonpregnant size and condition by involution, which involves contraction of muscle fibers, catabolic processes, and regeneration of uterine epithelium.
- The site of placental attachment heals by a process of exfoliation, which leaves the endometrium smooth and without scars.
- Involution can be evaluated by measuring the descent of the fundus (about 1 cm/day). By the tenth day after childbirth, the fundus should no longer be palpable abdominally.
- Afterpains, or intermittent uterine contractions, cause discomfort for many women, particularly multiparas who breast-feed.
- Vaginal discharge (lochia) progresses from lochia rubra, to lochia serosa, to lochia alba in a predictable time frame. Lochia should be assessed for volume, type, and odor. Foul odor suggests endometrial infection.
- Although vaginal mucosa heals within 3 weeks, it takes 6 weeks for the vagina to regain the same size and contour.
- Perineal trauma and hemorrhoids cause discomfort and can interfere with bladder and bowel elimination.
- As blood from the uteroplacental unit returns to central circulation and extracellular fluid is mobilized into the vascular compartment, the cardiac output increases, and excess fluid is excreted by diuresis and diaphoresis.

- Increased clotting factors predispose the postpartum woman to thrombus formation. Early ambulation helps prevent thrombophlebitis.
- Constipation may occur from inadequate fluid intake during labor, reduced activity, decreased muscle tone, or fear of pain during defecation.
- Increased bladder capacity and decreased sensitivity to fluid pressure may result in urinary retention. Stasis of urine allows time for bacteria to grow and can lead to urinary tract infection.
- A distended bladder lifts and displaces the uterus. This condition can interfere with uterine contraction and result in excessive bleeding.
- Exercises to strengthen the abdominal muscles as well as good posture and body mechanics may reduce musculoskeletal discomfort.
- As hormone levels decline, the skin gradually reverts to its prepregnancy state.
- Breast-feeding may delay the return of ovulation and menstruation, but it is not a reliable method of contraception. All mothers need information about family planning.
- Breast-feeding mothers are more likely to experience dyspareunia as a result of vaginal dryness that results from inadequate estrogen.
- Lactation may be suppressed by wearing a snug bra, by binding the breasts, and by avoiding stimulation of the breasts.
- The postpartum woman should be afebrile. Because of exertion, dehydration, and leukocytosis, however, her temperature may be higher during the first 24 hours after delivery.
- Bradycardia is expected. Tachycardia may be caused by excitement, dehydration, hypovolemia, or infection. Additional assessments are required to determine if excessive bleeding is the cause.
- Orthostatic hypotension occurs when the mother goes from a supine to a standing position quickly.
- The common practice of early discharge challenges nurses to develop a plan for teaching self-care and infant care in a short period.
- The postcesarean woman requires postoperative as well as postpartum assessments and care. She is at increased risk for problems associated with immobility and discomfort.
- Bonding and attachment are gradual processes that begin before childbirth and progress to feelings of love and deep devotion that last throughout life.
- Nurses foster bonding and attachment by providing early, unlimited contact between the parents and infant and by modeling attachment behaviors.
- Maternal touch changes over time as many mothers progress from exploratory "fingertipping" to enfolding and finally to demonstrating a full range of comforting behaviors.
- Verbal behaviors are important indicators of maternal attachment. Nurses often model how to speak to the infant and point out the infant's response to verbal stimulation.
- Maternal adjustment to parenthood is a gradual process that involves restorative phases. Nurses play a valuable role in the process by "mothering the mother" and fostering her independence.
- Postpartum blues, a temporary, self-limiting period of weepiness, is often ignored by the health care team. Explanations and support can assist the mother through this distressing episode.
- Parents usually progress through four stages of role attainment (anticipatory, formal, informal, and personal) as they learn to structure their parenting behaviors to mesh with the infant's needs.
- Many women experience role conflict when they must leave the infant with a caregiver and return to work. Nurses can offer anticipatory guidance that makes the conflict less difficult.
- The birth of a baby necessitates reorganization of family structure and renegotiation of family responsibilities. Nurses can assist the father in coparenting the infant and help the new parents identify family resources.
- Siblings feel jealousy and fear that they will be replaced by the newborn in the affection of the parents. Nurses can help by providing information about how to reduce sibling rivalry.
- Nursing care in the birth facility overlaps with follow-up care that is provided after discharge to meet family needs.

ANSWERS TO CRITICAL THINKING EXERCISES

Exercise 21–1
1. The birth of a large infant increases the risk of postpartum hemorrhage. Saturation of pads in a short time suggests excessive bleeding. The location of the fundus above the umbilicus and displaced to the side indicates that the cause of excessive bleeding might be a distended bladder.
2. Assisting the mother to void is the most appropriate nursing action. If, after voiding, the fundus is located at the level of the umbilicus and firmly contracted, the cause of the bleeding was probably a distended bladder, which made it difficult for the uterus to contract firmly. The location and consistency of the uterus, amount of lochia, blood pressure, and pulse should be assessed frequently so that further excessive bleeding can be controlled.
3. Linda does not experience the urge to void because the bladder has not regained the muscle tone lost during pregnancy and the sensitivity to pressure is decreased.

Exercise 21–2
1. Carol's priority needs are for physical care and comfort. She also needs to make the experience of childbirth part of her reality by recounting the details of her birth experience to anyone who will listen and by trying to fill in the missing pieces about the cesarean birth.
2. Carol is in the taking-in phase. She is getting acquainted with her

"real" baby by exploring with her fingertips. This is usually the first maternal touch observed.

3. Carol's priorities are to assume control of her own body functions and to manage her care so that she can "take hold" and assume care of the baby.

4. Carol has become more independent and demonstrates readiness to learn by requesting the assistance of the lactation educator.

5. Anticipatory guidance should focus on how Carol can manage the care of the infant while still getting adequate rest and nutrition. A flexible schedule, resting while the infant rests, and preparing simple meals are some of the most important items to emphasize.

6. It would be helpful to assist her in identifying a friend or neighbor who could provide some support while her husband is away. She should have telephone numbers for community resources, such as the hospital "baby line." A follow-up telephone call or a home visit by a perinatal nurse would be most helpful. The nurse could assess both the mother and the infant, reinforce teaching, and provide encouragement.

REFERENCES AND READINGS

Affonso, D. D., Mayberry, L., Inaba, A., Matsuno, R., & Robinson, E. (1996). Hawaiian-style "talkstory": Psychosocial assessment and intervention during and after pregnancy. *Journal of Obstetric, Gynecologic, and Neonatal Nursing, 25*(9), 737–742.

Affonso, D. D., Mayberry, L. J., Lovett, S. M., & Paul, S. (1994). Cognitive adaptation to stressful events during pregnancy and postpartum: Development and testing of CASE instrument. *Nursing Research, 43*(6), 338–343.

Alteneder, R. R., & Hartzell, D. (1997). Addressing couples' sexuality concerns during the childbearing period: Use of the PLISSIT model. *Journal of Obstetric, Gynecologic, and Neonatal Nursing, 26*(6), 651–658.

American Academy of Pediatrics & American College of Obstetricians and Gynecologists. (1997). *Guidelines for perinatal care* (4th ed.). Elk Grove Village, IL, and Washington, DC: Author.

Association of Women's Health, Obstetric and Neonatal Nurses. (1998). *Standards and guidelines for professional nursing practice in the care of women and newborns* (5th ed.). Washington, DC: Author.

Berger, D., & Cook, C. A. L. (1998). Postpartum teaching priorities: The viewpoints of nurses and mothers. *Journal of Obstetric, Gynecologic, and Neonatal Nursing, 27*(2), 161–168.

Blackburn, S. T., & Loper, D. L. (1992). *Maternal, fetal, and neonatal physiology: A clinical perspective.* Philadelphia: Saunders.

Brooten, D., Knapp, H., Jacobsen, B., & Arnold, L. (1996). Early discharge after unplanned cesarean birth: Nursing care time. *Journal of Obstetric, Gynecologic, and Neonatal Nursing, 25*(7), 595–600.

Brown, S. G., & Johnson, B. T. (1998). Enhancing early discharge with home follow-up: A pilot project. *Journal of Obstetric, Gynecologic, and Neonatal Nursing, 27*(1), 33–38.

Callister, L. C. (1995). Cultural meanings of childbirth. *Journal of Obstetric, Gynecologic, and Neonatal Nursing, 24*(4), 327–334.

Carpenter, J. A. (1998). Shortening the short stay. *AWHONN Lifelines, 2*(1), 29–34.

Choudhry, U. K. (1997). Traditional practices of women from India: Pregnancy, childbirth, and newborn care. *Journal of Obstetric, Gynecologic, and Neonatal Nursing, 26*(5), 533–539.

Clark, R. A. (1995). Infections during the postpartum period. *Journal of Obstetric, Gynecologic, and Neonatal Nursing, 24*(6), 542–549.

Cunningham, F. G., MacDonald, P. C., Gant, N. F., Leveno, K. J., Gilstrap, L. C., Hankins, G. D. V., et al. (1997). *Williams obstetrics* (20th ed.). Norwalk, CT: Appleton & Lange.

Eakes, M., & Brown, H. (1998). Home alone: Meeting the needs of mothers after cesarean birth. *AWHONN Lifelines, 2*(1), 37–40.

Evans, C. J. (1995). Postpartum home care in the United States. *Journal of Obstetric, Gynecologic, and Neonatal Nursing, 24*(2), 180–186.

Ferketich, S. L., & Mercer, R. T. (1995a). Paternal-infant attachment of experienced and inexperienced fathers during infancy. *Nursing Research, 44*(1), 31–37.

Ferketich, S. L., & Mercer, R. T. (1995b). Predictors of role competence for experienced and inexperienced fathers. *Nursing Research, 44*(2), 89–95.

Fishbein, E. G., & Burggraf, E. (1998). Early postpartum discharge: How are mothers managing? *Journal of Obstetric, Gynecologic, and Neonatal Nursing, 27*(2), 142–148.

Gennaro, S., Fehder, W., York, R., & Douglas, S. D. (1997). Weight, nutrition, and immune status in postpartal women. *Nursing Research, 46*(1), 20–25.

Grohar, J. (1996). Pospartum care. In K. R. Simpson & P. A. Creehan (Eds.), *AWHONN perinatal nursing* (pp. 249–270). Philadelphia: Lippincott-Raven.

Gupton, A., & McKay, M. (1995). The Canadian perspective on postpartum home care. *Journal of Obstetric, Gynecologic, and Neonatal Nursing, 24*(2), 173–179.

Higley, A. M., & Miller, M. A. (1996). The development of parenting: Nursing resources. *Journal of Obstetric, Gynecologic, and Neonatal Nursing, 25*(9), 707–713.

Hutchinson, M. K., & BaqiAziz, M. (1994). Nursing care of the childbearing Muslim family. *Journal of Obstetric, Gynecologic, and Neonatal Nursing, 23*(9), 767–771.

Keppler, A. B. (1995). Postpartum care center: Follow-up care in a hospital-based clinic. *Journal of Obstetric, Gynecologic, and Neonatal Nursing, 24*(1), 17–21.

Klaus, M., & Kennell, J. (1982). *Maternal-infant bonding.* St. Louis: Mosby.

Kramer, R. L., Van Someren, J. K., Qualls, C. R., & Curet, L. B. (1996). Postoperative management of cesarean patients: The effect of immediate feeding on the incidence of ileus. *Obstetrics and Gynecology, 88*(1), 29–32.

Lawrence, R., & Lawrence, R. M. (1999). *Breastfeeding: A guide for the medical profession* (5th ed.). St. Louis: Mosby.

Luegenbiehl, D., Brophy, G., Artigue, G., Phillips, K., & Flack, R. (1990). Standardized assessment of blood loss. *MCN: American Journal of Maternal/Child Nursing, 15*(4), 241–244.

Martell, L. K. (1995). Response to change: Maternity nursing after World War II. *MCN: American Journal of Maternal/Child Nursing, 20*(3), 131–134.

Martell, L. K., & Mitchell, S. K. (1984). Rubin's puerperal change reconsidered. *Journal of Obstetric, Gynecologic, and Neonatal Nursing, 13*(3), 145–148.

Mattson, S. (1995). Culturally sensitive perinatal care for Southeast Asians. *Journal of Obstetric, Gynecologic, and Neonatal Nursing, 24*(4), 335–341.

Mercer, R. T. (1985). The process of maternal role attainment. *Nursing Research, 34*(4), 198–204.

Mercer, R. T. (1990). *Parents at risk.* New York: Springer.

Mercer, R. T. (1995). *Becoming a mother: Research on maternal identity from Rubin to the present.* New York: Springer.

Mercer, R. T., & Ferketich, S. L. (1994a). Predictors of maternal role competence by risk status. *Nursing Research, 43*(1), 38–43.

Mercer, R. T., & Ferketich, S. L. (1994b). Maternal-infant attachment of experienced and inexperienced mothers during infancy. *Nursing Research, 43*(6), 344–351.

Nance, T. A. (1995). Intercultural communication: Finding common ground. *Journal of Obstetric, Gynecologic, and Neonatal Nursing, 24*(3), 249–255.

Phillips, C. R. (1997). *Mother-baby nursing.* Washington, DC: Association of Women's Health, Obstetric and Neonatal Nurses.

Prodromidis, M., Field, T., Arendt, R., Singer, L., Yando, R., & Bendell, D. (1995). Mothers touching newborns: A comparison of rooming-in versus minimal contact. *Birth, 22*(4), 196–200.

Resnik, R. (1999). The puerperium. In R. K. Creasy & R. Resnik (Eds.), *Maternal-fetal medicine: Principles and practice* (4th ed., pp. 102–105). Philadelphia: Saunders.

Rubin, R. (1961). Puerperal change. *Nursing Outlook, 9*(12), 743–755.

Rubin, R. (1977). Binding-in in the postpartum period. *Maternal-Child Nursing Journal, 6*(1), 65–75.

Rubin, R. (1984). *Maternal identity and the maternal experience.* New York: Springer.

Sampselle, C. M., Burns, P. A., Dougherty, M. C., Newman, D. K., Thomas, K. K., & Wyman, J. F. (1997). Continence for women: Evidence-based practice. *Journal of Obstetric, Gynecologic, and Neonatal Nursing, 26*(4), 375–385.

Schneiderman, J. U. (1996). Postpartum nursing for Korean mothers. *MCN: American Journal of Maternal/Child Nursing, 21*(3), 155–158.

Sheil, E. P., Bull, M. J., Moxon, B. E., et al. (1995). Concerns of childbearing women: A maternal concerns questionnaire as an assessment tool. *Journal of Obstetric, Gynecologic, and Neonatal Nursing, 24*(2), 149–155.

Stover, A. M., & Marnejon, J. G. (1995). Postpartum care. *American Family Physician, 52*(5), 1465–1472.

Thorpe, K., Greenwood, R., & Goodenough, T. (1995). Does a twin pregnancy have greater impact on physical and emotional wellbeing than a singleton pregnancy? *Birth, 22*(3), 148–152.

Tiller, C. M. (1995). Fathers' parenting attitudes during a child's first year. *Journal of Obstetric, Gynecologic, and Neonatal Nursing, 24*(6), 508–514.

Troy, N. W., & Dalgas-Pelish, P. (1997). The natural evolution of postpartum fatigue among a group of primiparous women. *Clinical Nursing Research, 6*(2), 126–141.

Ugarriza, D. N. (1992). Postpartum affective disorders: Incidence and treatment. *Journal of Psychosocial Nursing, 30*(5), 29–32.

Valaitis, R., Tuff, K., & Swanson, L. (1996). Meeting parents' postpartal needs with a telephone information line. MCN: *American Journal of Maternal/Child Nursing, 21*(2), 90–95.

Waldenström, U., Borg, I. M., Olsson, B., Sköld, M., & Wall, S. (1996). The childbirth experience: A study of 295 new mothers. *Birth, 23*(3), 144–153.

Weber, S. E. (1996). Cultural aspects of pain in childbearing women. *Journal of Obstetric, Gynecologic, and Neonatal Nursing, 25*(1), 67–72.

Williams, L. R., & Cooper, M. K. (1996). A new paradigm for postpartum care. *Journal of Obstetric, Gynecologic, and Neonatal Nursing, 25*(9), 745–749.

22

• • • • • • • • • • •

The Normal
Newborn:
Adaptation
and Assessment

LEARNING OBJECTIVES

After studying this chapter, you should be able to:

■ Explain the physiologic changes that occur in the respiratory and cardiovascular systems during the transition from fetal to neonatal life.

■ Describe thermoregulation in the newborn.

■ Compare gastrointestinal functioning in the newborn and adult.

■ Explain the causes and effects of hypoglycemia.

■ Describe the steps in normal bilirubin excretion and the development of physiologic, pathologic, and breast milk jaundice.

■ Describe kidney functioning in the newborn.

■ Explain the functioning of the newborn's immune system.

■ Describe the periods of reactivity and the six behavioral states of the newborn.

■ Describe nursing assessments of the newborn.

■ Explain the importance and the components of gestational age assessment.

DEFINITIONS

acrocyanosis Bluish discoloration of the hands and feet due to reduced peripheral circulation.

asphyxia Insufficient oxygen and excess carbon dioxide in the blood and tissues.

bilirubin Unusable component of hemolyzed erythrocytes.

brown fat (or brown adipose tissue) Highly vascular specialized fat found in the newborn that provides more heat than other fat when metabolized.

café au lait spots Light brown birthmarks.

caput succedaneum Area of edema over the presenting part of the fetus or newborn, resulting from pressure against the cervix. Often called simply "caput."

cephalhematoma Bleeding between the periosteum and skull from pressure during birth. It does not cross suture lines.

choanal atresia Abnormality of the nasal septum that obstructs one or both nasal passages.

craniosynostosis Premature closure of the sutures of the infant's head.

cryptorchidism Failure of one or both testes to descend into the scrotum.

epispadias Abnormal placement of the urinary meatus on the dorsal side of the penis.

erythema toxicum Benign rash of unknown cause in newborns, with blotchy red areas that may have white or yellow papules in the center.

fetal lung fluid Fluid that fills the fetal lungs, expanding the alveoli and promoting lung development.

first period of reactivity Period beginning at birth in which newborns are active and alert. It ends when the infant first falls asleep.

hyperbilirubinemia Excessive amount of bilirubin in the blood.

hypospadias Abnormal placement of the urinary meatus on the ventral side of the penis.

jaundice Yellow discoloration of the skin and sclera caused by excessive bilirubin in the blood.

lanugo Fine, soft hair covering the fetus.

milia White cysts, 1 to 2 mm in size, from distended sebaceous glands.

molding Shaping of the fetal head during movement through the birth canal.

mongolian spots Bruise-like marks that occur mostly in newborns with dark skin tones.

neutral thermal environment Environment in which body temperature is maintained without an increase in metabolic rate or oxygen use.

nevus flammeus Permanent purple birthmark. Also called port wine stain.

nevus vasculosus Rough, red collection of capillaries with a raised surface that disappears with time.

nonshivering thermogenesis Process of heat production, without shivering, by oxidation of brown fat.

periodic breathing Cessation of breathing lasting no more than 10 seconds without changes in color or heart rate.

point of maximum impulse Area of the chest in which the heart sounds are loudest when auscultated.

polycythemia Abnormally high number of erythrocytes.

polydactyly More than ten digits on the hands or feet.

pseudomenstruation Vaginal bleeding in the newborn, resulting from withdrawal of placental hormones.

second period of reactivity Period of 4 to 6 hours after the first sleep following birth when the newborn may have an elevated pulse and respiratory rate and excessive mucus.

strabismus A turning inward ("crossing") or outward of the eyes due to poor muscle tone.

surfactant Combination of lipoproteins produced by the lungs of the mature fetus to reduce surface tension in the alveoli, thus promoting lung expansion after birth.

syndactyly Webbing between fingers or toes.

tachypnea Respiratory rate above 60 breaths per minute in the newborn after the first hour of life.

telangiectatic nevi (stork bites, nevus simplex) Flat, pink areas on the nape of the neck and over the eyelids resulting from dilation of the capillaries.

thermogenesis Heat production.

thermoregulation Maintenance of body temperature.

vernix caseosa Thick, white substance that protects the skin of the fetus.

At birth, neonates must make profound physiologic changes to adapt to extrauterine life to meet their own respiratory, digestive, and regulatory needs. During nursing assessments, nurses must be aware of those changes so that they can identify behaviors signifying problems or abnormalities.

▐ Initiation of Respirations

The first vital task in newborn adaptation is the initiation of respirations. Forces occurring throughout pregnancy and during birth bring about this change.

Development of the Lungs

During fetal life, the respiratory tract produces fetal lung fluid that expands the alveoli. As the fetus nears term, the lung fluid begins to move into the interstitial spaces. The fluid shift continues during normal labor and after birth. This shift helps reduce the pulmonary resistance to blood flow that was present before birth and enhances the advent of air breathing (Lowe & Reiss, 1996).

As the lungs mature, they begin to produce surfactant, a slippery, detergent-like lipoprotein that reduces surface tension within the alveoli. Without surfactant, the alveoli collapse as the infant exhales. They must be reopened with each breath, greatly increasing the work of breathing. Sufficient surfactant is usually produced beginning at 34 to 36 weeks of gestation.

Causes of Respirations

Because the alveoli are collapsed, the infant's first breath requires a much larger negative pressure (suction) than subsequent breathing. Breathing is initiated by chemical, thermal, and mechanical factors that stimulate the respiratory center in the medulla of the brain and trigger respirations (Fig. 22–1).

CHEMICAL FACTORS
Chemoreceptors in the carotid arteries and the aorta respond to changes in blood chemistry brought about by the hypoxia that occurs with normal birth. A decrease in blood oxygen (P_{O_2}) and pH and an increase in blood carbon dioxide (P_{CO_2}) stimulate the respiratory center in the medulla. A forceful contraction of the diaphragm results, causing air to enter the lungs.

THERMAL FACTORS
The temperature change that occurs with birth is an important stimulus to the initiation of respirations. Sensors in the skin respond to this sudden change in temperature by send-ing impulses that stimulate the respiratory center and breathing.

MECHANICAL FACTORS
During a vaginal birth, the fetal chest is compressed by the narrow birth canal. A small amount of the fetal lung fluid is forced out of the lungs into the upper air passages and expelled during birth. When the pressure against the chest is released, it recoils, drawing a small amount of air into the lungs. Tactile stimuli and the stimulation of the sounds and lights at delivery may also aid in initiating respirations.

Continuation of Respirations

Once the alveoli expand, surfactant acts to keep them partially open between respirations. Approximately half of the air from the first breath remains in the lungs to become the functional residual capacity.

The remaining fetal lung fluid moves into the interstitial spaces, where it is absorbed by the circulatory and lymphatic systems. Absorption is accelerated by the process of labor and may be delayed after cesarean birth. Although most fluid is absorbed within a few hours, complete absorption may take as long as 24 hours. This process explains why the lungs may sound moist when first auscultated but become clear a short time later.

▐ Cardiovascular Adaptation: Transition from Fetal to Neonatal Circulation

During fetal life, the *ductus arteriosus, foramen ovale,* and *ductus venosus* shunt most of the blood away from the lungs and liver. High pressures within the lungs permit only a small amount of blood flow into the pulmonary vessels (see Chapter 12).

At birth, the shunts close and the pulmonary vessels dilate. These changes occur in response to increases in blood oxygen, shifts in pressure within the heart and pulmonary and systemic circulations, and the clamping of the umbilical cord. The changes necessary for transition from fetal to neonatal circulation occur simultaneously within the first few minutes after birth.

Ductus Arteriosus

In the fetus, the ductus arteriosus connects the pulmonary artery and the aorta. Most of the blood that enters the pulmonary artery passes into the aorta and bypasses the nonfunctioning lungs.

As the newborn takes the first breaths of air at birth, the rise in oxygen causes the ductus arteriosus to constrict. At the same time, resistance in the pulmonary circulation decreases and resistance throughout the systemic circulation increases. These responses cause blood to flow from the pulmonary artery into the lungs for oxygenation.

The ductus arteriosus closes gradually as oxygenation improves. Functional closure occurs within 15 to 24 hours. Until closure is complete, the blood that does flow through the vessel reverses, moving from the aorta to the pulmonary

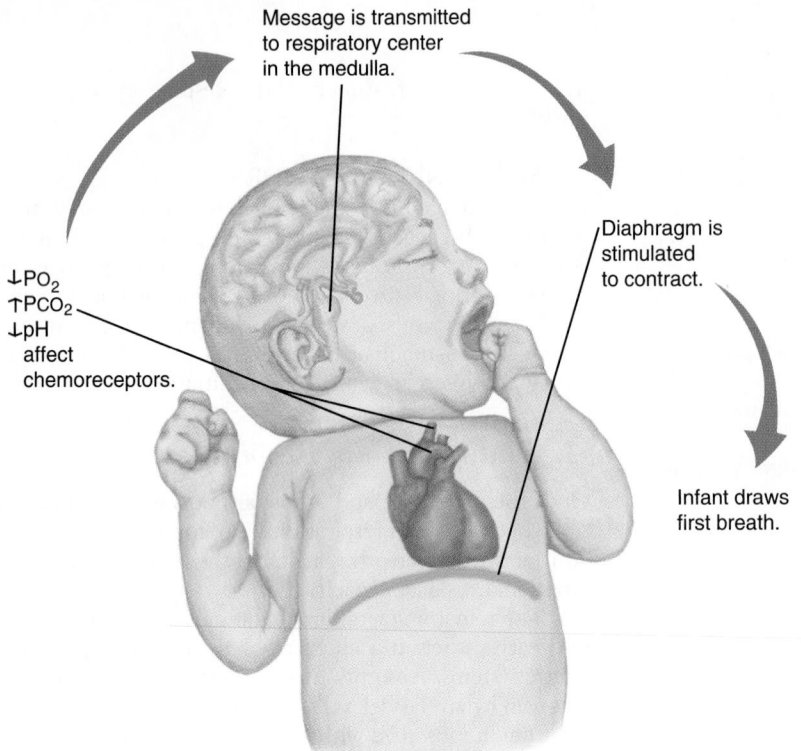

Message is transmitted to respiratory center in the medulla.

Diaphragm is stimulated to contract.

$\downarrow PO_2$
$\uparrow PCO_2$
$\downarrow pH$
affect chemoreceptors.

Infant draws first breath.

Internal stimuli

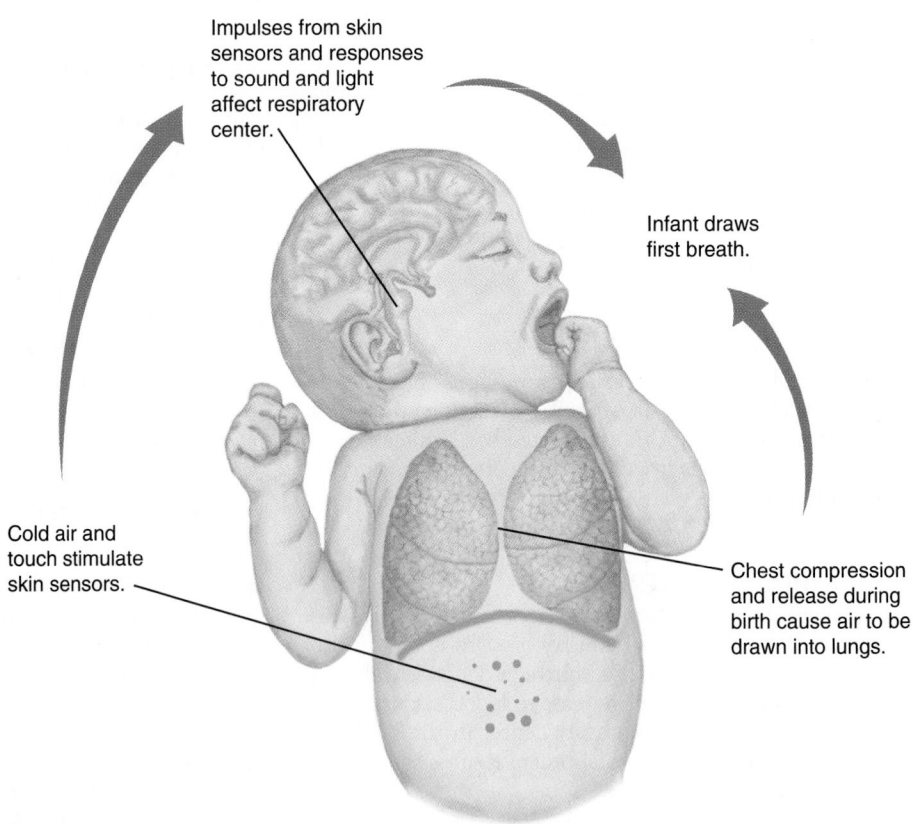

Impulses from skin sensors and responses to sound and light affect respiratory center.

Infant draws first breath.

Cold air and touch stimulate skin sensors.

Chest compression and release during birth cause air to be drawn into lungs.

External stimuli

FIGURE 22–1
. . . .
Internal causes of the initiation of respirations are the chemical changes that take place at birth.
External causes of respirations include thermal and mechanical factors.

artery and increasing blood flow to the lungs. This sequence occurs because pressure in the aorta is now higher than that in the pulmonary artery. A murmur may be heard as a result of blood flow through the partially open vessel.

The ductus arteriosus closes permanently by 3 to 4 weeks and is then called the ligamentum arteriosum (Lott, 1998). Until permanent closure occurs, low levels of oxygen in the blood may cause the ductus arteriosus to dilate and the pulmonary vessels to constrict. These processes may cause a return to fetal blood flow patterns, a serious complication. A patent ductus arteriosus may occur in the infant who experiences asphyxia at birth, becomes hypoxic, or is preterm (see Chapter 46).

Pulmonary Blood Vessels

The pulmonary blood vessels dilate in response to the increased oxygenation that occurs at birth. At the same time, fetal lung fluid shifts into the interstitial spaces and is removed by the blood and lymph system. These changes allow more room for dilation of the pulmonary blood vessels and decrease pulmonary vascular resistance. As a result, the vessels can expand to hold the suddenly increased blood flow from the pulmonary artery.

Foramen Ovale

The foramen ovale is a flap in the septum between the right and the left atria of the fetal heart. It allows oxygenated blood from the inferior vena cava to move from the right atrium and to the left side of the heart. Little mixing occurs with the less oxygenated blood that enters from the superior vena cava and continues to the right ventricle. Thus, most of the better oxygenated blood travels away from the nonfunctioning fetal lungs.

The foramen ovale opens only from right to left. The higher pressure in the right side of the heart from the restricted flow of blood to the lungs causes this right-to-left shunting. The pressure in the right side of the heart decreases at birth, when the umbilical vessels are occluded and blood flows easily into the pulmonary circulation.

Pressure in the left side of the heart builds as blood enters the left atrium from the pulmonary veins and systemic resistance increases because of the lack of blood flow to the placenta. Because the foramen ovale opens only from right to left, it closes when the pressure in the left heart is higher than that in the right heart. This difference increases blood flow from the right ventricle into the lungs. Thus, blood flow through the heart and lungs changes from fetal to neonatal circulation and is similar to that in the normal adult (see Fig. 12–9).

CRITICAL THINKING EXERCISE 22–1

. . . .

Understanding the changes that occur during the transition from fetal to neonatal circulation helps in predicting the effect on blood flow of various defects in the heart. What would be the effect on blood flow of an opening in the septum of the atria of the heart?

The foramen ovale is functionally closed soon after birth because pressure changes in the heart prevent it from opening. Conditions such as asphyxia, however, may reverse the pressures in the heart and cause the foramen ovale to reopen. It is permanently closed several months after birth and is called the fossa ovale.

Ductus Venosus

During fetal life, it is not necessary for the liver to filter the blood. The ductus venosus directs approximately half of the blood flow from the umbilical vein away from the liver and directly to the inferior vena cava. After birth, very little blood enters the ductus venosus. Fibrosis of the ductus venosus occurs by the end of the first week of life, and it is then called the ligamentum venosum.

▌ Neurologic Adaptation: Thermoregulation

Although the fetus produces heat in utero, the consistently warm temperature of the amniotic fluid makes thermoregulation, the maintenance of body temperature, unnecessary. The neonate, however, must produce and maintain heat to prevent cold stress, which can have serious and even fatal effects.

Newborn Characteristics Leading to Heat Loss

Some characteristics of newborns predispose them to lose heat. The skin is thin, blood vessels are close to the surface, and there is little subcutaneous fat. Heat is readily transferred from the internal areas of the body to the cooler skin surfaces and then to the surrounding air. Newborns have three times more surface area to body mass than the adult and lose heat at a rate four times greater than adults do (Behrman, Kliegman, & Arvin, 1996).

The flexed position of the healthy, full-term infant reduces the amount of skin surface exposed to the surrounding temperatures and decreases heat loss. Because of decreased muscle tone, the sick or preterm infant does not maintain a flexed position.

Methods of Heat Loss

There are four methods of heat loss in the neonate (Fig. 22–2):

- *Evaporation:* Drying of the skin that results in cooling. Insensible water loss from the skin and respiratory tract increases heat loss by evaporation.
- *Conduction:* Movement of heat away from the body occurs when newborns come in direct contact with objects that are cooler than their skin.
- *Convection:* Transfer of heat to the air surrounding the infant.
- *Radiation:* Heat transfer to cooler objects that are not in direct contact with the infant.

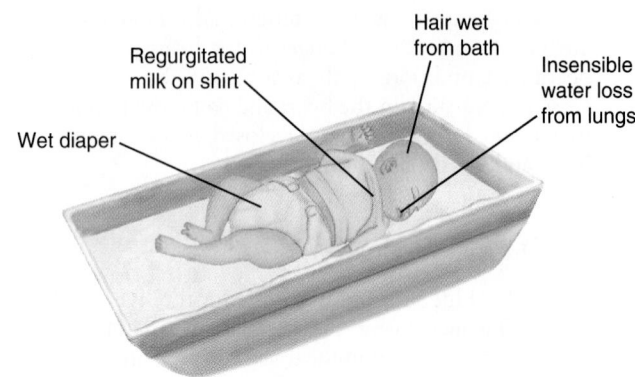

Evaporation can occur during birth or bathing from moisture on skin, as a result of wet linens or clothes, and from insensible loss.

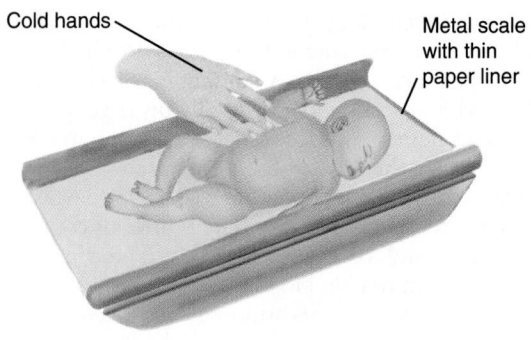

Conduction occurs when the infant comes in contact with cold objects or surfaces such as a scale, a circumcision restraint board, cold hands, or a stethoscope.

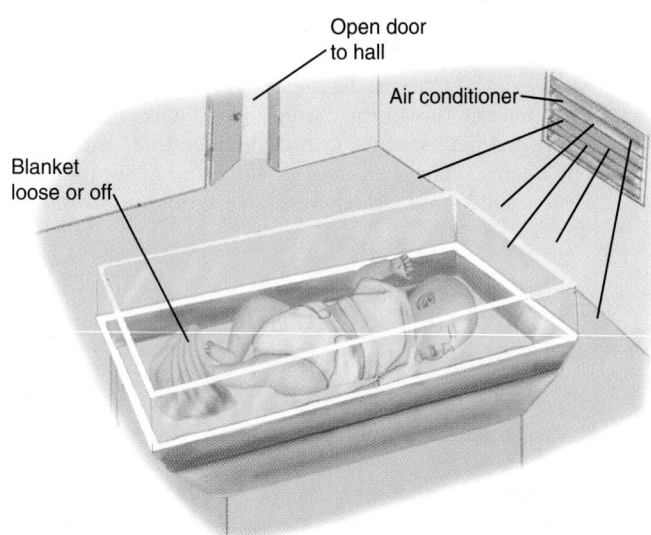

Convection occurs when drafts come from open doors, air conditioning, or even air currents created by people moving about.

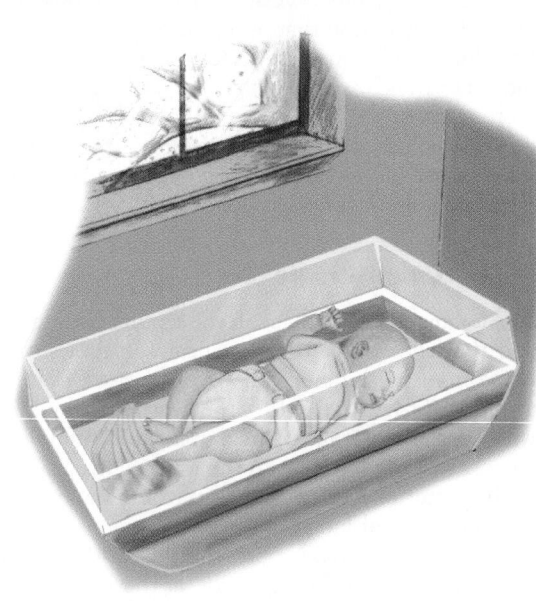

Heat is lost by radiation when the infant is near cold surfaces. Thus, heat is lost from the infant's body to the sides of the crib or incubator and to the outside walls and windows.

FIGURE 22–2
Methods of heat loss.

Nonshivering Thermogenesis

Shivering is not an effective method of heat production for newborns and rarely occurs (Bruck, 1998). Instead, nonshivering thermogenesis is used when the infant becomes cold. Nonshivering thermogenesis is the oxidation of brown fat (also called brown adipose tissue) to produce heat. This highly vascular fat is found only in newborns. It is located primarily around the back of the neck; in the axillae; around the kidneys, adrenals, and sternum; between the scapula; and along the abdominal aorta (Fig. 22–3). As brown fat is metabolized, it generates more heat than other fats. Blood passing through brown fat is warmed and carries heat to the rest of the body.

Preterm infants and those with intrauterine growth restriction may have inadequate brown fat stores. These infants are not able to raise their body temperature if they are subjected to cold stress. They may therefore have serious complications. Brown fat is used up during the early weeks after birth and is not present in the older infant.

Nonshivering thermogenesis begins when thermal receptors in the skin detect a drop in skin temperature. The process goes into effect even before a change occurs in core or interior body temperature, as measured with a rectal thermometer. Therefore, nonshivering thermogenesis may begin in an infant when skin temperature is cool, even though a temperature taken rectally shows a normal reading.

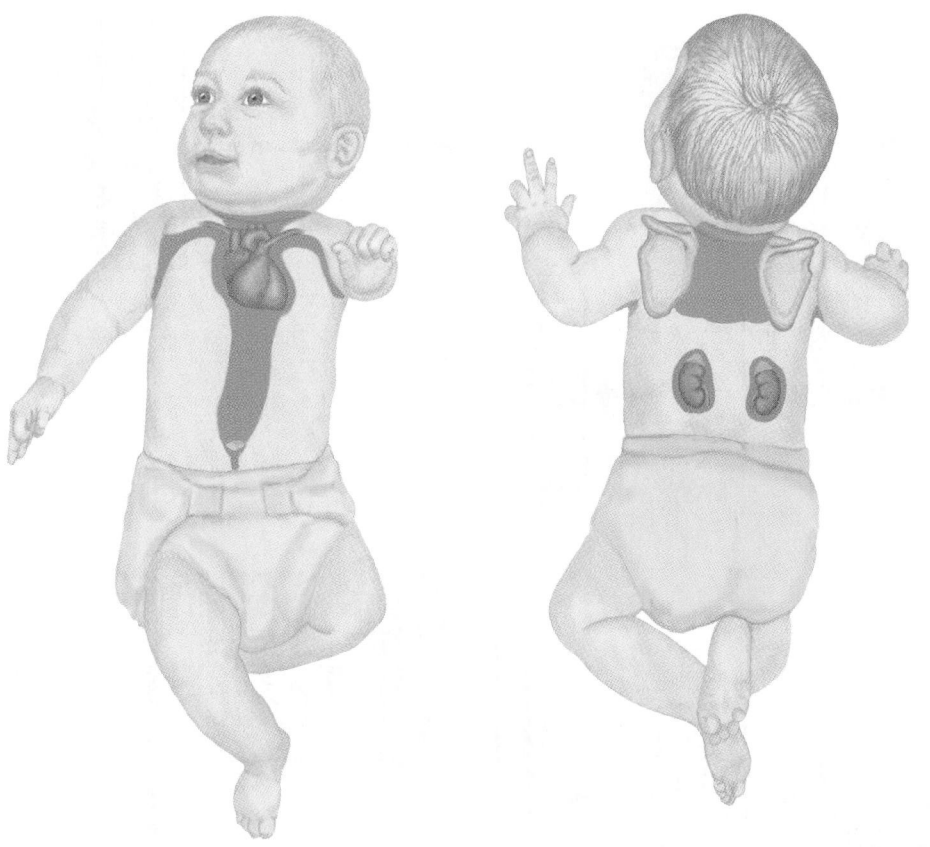

FIGURE 22–3
· · · · · · · · ·
Sites of brown fat in the neonate.

Effects of Cold Stress

Cold stress causes many body changes (Fig. 22–4). It results in the need for more oxygen and glucose because the increase in metabolic rate can lead to a significant rise in the need for oxygen. Even during mild respiratory distress, the infant may experience severe hypoxia as oxygen is used for heat production. The infant may not have sufficient oxygen for the metabolic rate to increase. Cold stress also causes diminished production of surfactant, impeding lung expansion and leading to more respiratory distress.

Glucose is necessary in larger amounts when the metabolic rate rises to produce heat. When the infant's temperature drops, glycogen stores are converted to glucose. The stores may be quickly depleted, causing hypoglycemia. Metabolism of glucose in the presence of insufficient oxygen causes increased production of acids.

Metabolism of brown fat also releases fatty acids. This release can cause metabolic acidosis, which can be a life-threatening condition. Elevated fatty acids in the blood can also interfere with transport of bilirubin to the liver, increasing the risk of jaundice.

As the infant's body attempts to conserve heat, vasoconstriction of the peripheral blood vessels occurs. Vasoconstriction helps reduce heat loss from the skin's surface. Decreased oxygen levels in the blood, however, may also cause vasoconstriction of the pulmonary vessels and a return to fetal circulation patterns, further increasing respiratory distress.

Neutral Thermal Environment

A neutral thermal environment is one in which the infant can maintain a stable body temperature without an increase in oxygen consumption or metabolic rate. The range of environmental temperature that allows this maintenance is called the thermoneutral zone. In healthy, unclothed, full-term newborns, an environmental temperature of 32° to 35°C (89.6° to 95°F) provides a thermoneutral zone (Bruck, 1998).

Hyperthermia

Infants also respond poorly to hyperthermia. With an elevated temperature, the metabolic rate rises, causing an increased need for oxygen and glucose. In addition, vasodilation leads to increased insensible fluid losses. Sweating may occur but is often delayed because sweat glands are immature.

Newborns may be overheated by poorly regulated equipment designed to keep them warm. When infants are under radiant warmers, warming lights, or in warmed incubators, the temperature mechanism must be set to vary the heat according to the infant's skin temperature and thus prevent heat that is too high or too low. Alarms to signal that the infant's temperature is too high or too low should be functioning properly.

Hematologic Adaptation

Factors Affecting the Blood

The average blood volume of the newborn is 80 to 85 ml/kg. If the cord remains unclamped for a few minutes after

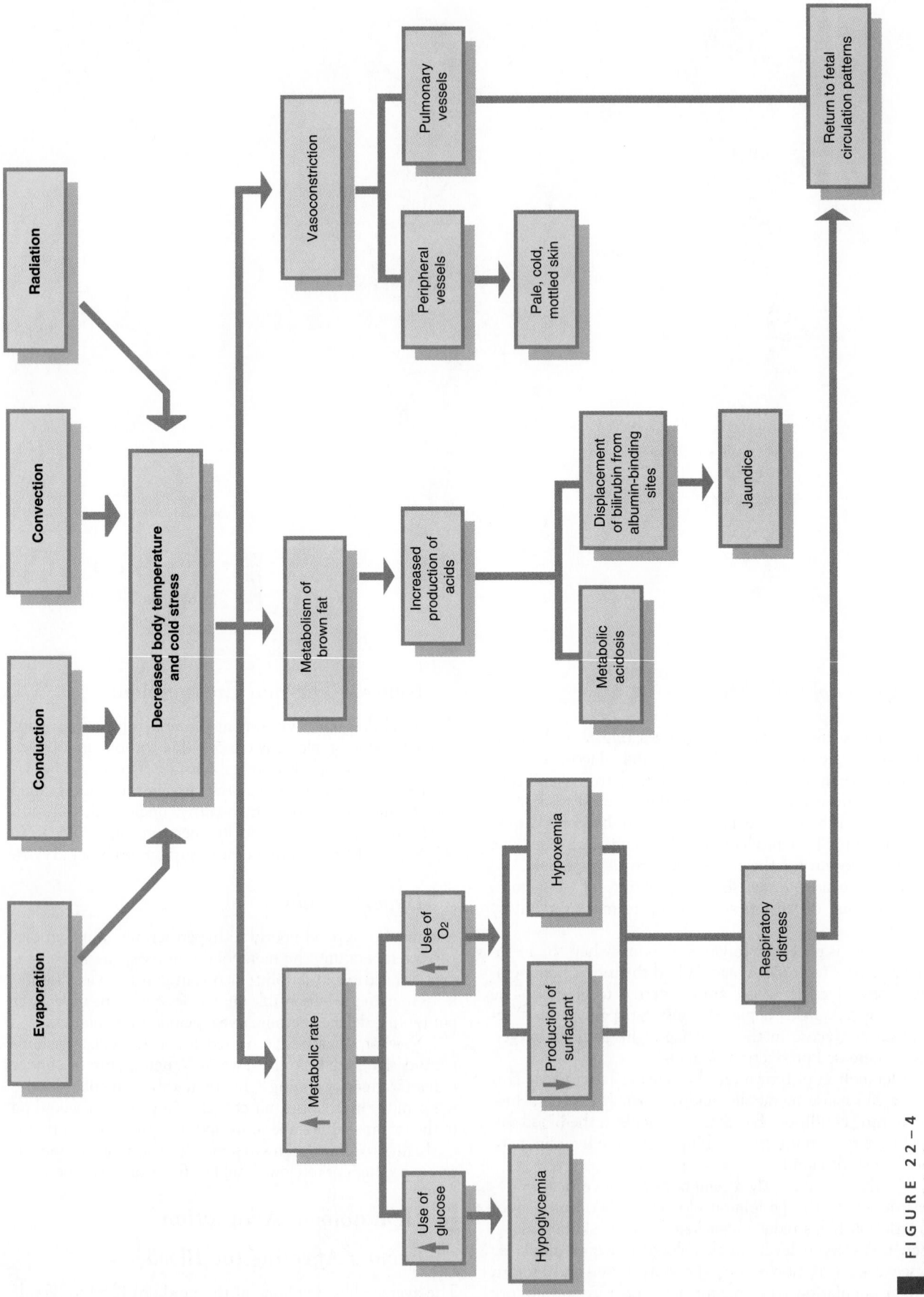

522

FIGURE 22-4
Effects of cold stress.

CRITICAL TO REMEMBER

Hazards of Cold Stress

- Increased oxygen need
- Respiratory distress
- Decreased surfactant production
- Hypoglycemia
- Metabolic acidosis
- Jaundice

---

birth, the infant may have a 75-ml increase in blood volume from the placenta (Guyton & Hall, 1996). The extra blood volume increases the workload of the heart. In addition, as the added red blood cells break down, bilirubin is released, increasing the risk of jaundice.

Blood samples drawn from the heel, where the circulation is sluggish, indicate higher levels of hemoglobin and hematocrit than samples taken from central areas. Venous blood samples are more accurate and are taken when precise measurement is essential. (Newborn laboratory values are listed in Appendix D.)

Blood Values

ERYTHROCYTES AND HEMOGLOBIN

At birth, the infant has comparatively more erythrocytes (red blood cells) and higher hemoglobin and hematocrit levels than the adult. This difference is necessary because the partial pressure of oxygen of fetal blood is much lower than the normal adult level. The large number of erythrocytes and higher hemoglobin level enable the fetal cells to receive enough oxygen. Adequate oxygenation to the cells is also possible because fetal hemoglobin (hemoglobin F) carries 20% to 50% more oxygen than adult hemoglobin (Guyton & Hall, 1996).

Erythrocytes in the newborn have a shorter life span than those of the adult. Excess bilirubin due to the breakdown of large numbers of red blood cells may lead to jaundice.

HEMATOCRIT

The hematocrit level in the normal infant is 48% to 69% from peripheral sites (Nicholson & Pesce, 1996). A level above 65% from a central site indicates polycythemia, an abnormally high erythrocyte count. Polycythemia increases the risk of jaundice and damage to the brain and other organs as a result of blood stasis. Respiratory distress and hypoglycemia are more common in these infants.

LEUKOCYTES

In newborns, an elevated white blood cell (leukocyte) count does not necessarily indicate infection. In fact, the white blood cell count may decrease in infections. Increased numbers of immature leukocytes are a sign of infection or sepsis in the neonate. Platelets (thrombocytes) may also decrease as a result of infections.

Risk of Clotting Deficiency

Newborns are at risk for clotting deficiency during the first few days of life because they lack vitamin K, which is necessary to activate several of the clotting factors (factors II, VII, IX, and X.) Vitamin K is synthesized in the intestines, but food and normal intestinal flora are necessary for this process. To decrease the risk of hemorrhagic disease of the newborn, vitamin K is administered intramuscularly to most newborns. Drugs such as phenytoin (Dilantin), phenobarbital, and aspirin taken by the mother during pregnancy interfere with clotting ability in the infant after birth.

■ Gastrointestinal System

Stomach

The newborn's stomach capacity is approximately 6 ml/kg at birth (Blackburn & Loper, 1992), but expands to approximately 90 ml within the first few days of life. The stomach begins to empty during feeding and is completely empty within 2 to 4 hours. The gastrocolic reflex is stimulated when the stomach fills, causing increased intestinal peristalsis. Infants frequently pass a stool during or after a feeding. The cardiac sphincter between the esophagus and the stomach is relaxed, which explains the newborn's tendency to regurgitate feedings easily.

Intestines

The newborn's intestines are long in proportion to the infant's size and compared with those of the adult. The added length allows more surface area for absorption, but it also makes infants more prone to water loss should diarrhea develop. Air enters the gastrointestinal tract soon after birth, and bowel sounds are present within the first hour.

The digestive tract is sterile at birth. Once the infant is exposed to the external environment and begins to take in fluids, however, bacteria enter the gastrointestinal tract. Normal intestinal flora is established within the first few days of life.

Digestive Enzymes

The newborn can digest simple carbohydrates but is deficient in pancreatic amylase and lipase. Amylase is needed to digest complex carbohydrates such as those in cereal. Sufficient amylase is present at 3 to 6 months of age. Lipase, needed for fat digestion, is present in breast milk and may make it more digestible for the newborn than formula. Protein and lactose, the major carbohydrate in the infant's milk diet, are both well digested.

Stools

Meconium is the first stool excreted by the newborn. It consists of particles from amniotic fluid such as skin cells and hair, along with cells shed from the intestinal tract, bile, and other intestinal secretions. Meconium is greenish-black with a thick, sticky, tar-like consistency. The first meconium stool is usually passed within the first 24 hours of life.

If meconium is not passed within 36 to 48 hours, obstruction is suspected.

Meconium stools are followed by transitional stools, which are greenish-brown and of a looser consistency than meconium. They are followed by the stool that is characteristic of the type of feeding that the infant receives.

The stools of infants fed with breast milk are seedy and have the color and consistency of mustard with a sweet-sour smell. The breast-fed infant in general has more frequent stools than the infant who is formula-fed. Breast-fed newborns excrete as many as ten small stools each day, although some older infants pass only one stool every 2 to 3 days. The normal breast-fed newborn should have at least three stools daily.

The formula-fed infant excretes pale yellow to light brown stools. They are firmer in consistency than those of the breast-fed infant. The infant may excrete several stools daily, or only one or two. The stools have the characteristic odor of feces.

▎ *Hepatic System*

Liver functions include maintenance of blood glucose levels, conjugation of bilirubin, production of factors necessary for blood coagulation, storage of iron, and metabolism of drugs.

Blood Glucose Maintenance

During the last 4 to 8 weeks of pregnancy, glucose is stored in the fetal liver as glycogen for use after birth. Glucose is used rapidly in the newborn for energy during the stress of delivery and for breathing, heat production, movement against gravity, and activation of all the functions that the neonate must take on at birth. The brain requires a constant supply of glucose or damage can result.

Until newborn feedings are adequate to meet energy requirements, stored glycogen is converted by the liver to glucose for use. In the term infant, glucose levels should be 40 to 60 mg/dl (Nicholson & Pesce, 1996). A blood glucose level below 40 mg/dl in the term infant indicates hypoglycemia (Behrman, Kliegman, & Arvin, 1996).

Many newborns are at increased risk for hypoglycemia. In the preterm and small-for-gestational-age infant, adequate stores of glycogen or even fat for metabolism may not have accumulated. Stores of glycogen may be used up before birth in the post-term infant because of poor intrauterine nourishment from a deteriorating placenta.

Large-for-gestational-age newborns may produce excessive insulin that consumes available glucose quickly. This condition is particularly acute if the mother is diabetic. During pregnancy, infants of diabetic mothers produce more insulin in response to large amounts of glucose from the mother. Infants may produce excessive insulin after birth, resulting in hypoglycemia (see Chapter 30).

Almost any stress can predispose a newborn to hypoglycemia. When infants are exposed to such stressors as asphyxia or infection, the glycogen in the liver may quickly be exhausted, and signs of hypoglycemia appear. In newborns who are not kept warm, all available glucose may be depleted to increase metabolism and raise body temperature.

Conjugation of Bilirubin

A major function of the liver is the conjugation of bilirubin (Fig. 22–5). The newborn's liver may not be mature enough to prevent the development of jaundice during the first week of life. Jaundice occurs in 60% of term newborns and 80% of preterm infants (Behrman, Kliegman, & Arvin, 1996).

SOURCE AND EFFECT OF BILIRUBIN

The principal source of bilirubin is the hemolysis of erythrocytes. This is a normal occurrence after birth, when fewer erythrocytes are needed than during fetal life. Bilirubin is toxic to the body and must be excreted.

Bilirubin is released in an unconjugated form. Unconjugated bilirubin, also called indirect bilirubin, is not soluble in water. Before excretion can occur, the liver must change it to a water-soluble form by a process called conjugation. The bilirubin is then known as conjugated or direct bilirubin.

Because unconjugated bilirubin is fat soluble, it may be absorbed by the subcutaneous fat, causing the yellowish discoloration of the skin called jaundice. If enough unconjugated bilirubin accumulates in the blood, staining of the tissues in the brain may occur. This condition is known as kernicterus and may result in bilirubin encephalopathy, which may cause severe brain damage.

NORMAL CONJUGATION

When unconjugated bilirubin is released into the bloodstream, it attaches to binding sites on albumin in the plasma and is carried to the liver. There, the enzyme glucuronyl transferase changes the bilirubin to the conjugated form. Conjugated bilirubin is excreted into the bile and then into the duodenum. In the intestines, the normal flora acts on bilirubin to reduce it to urobilinogen, which is excreted in the stool.

A small percentage of conjugated bilirubin may be converted back to the unconjugated state by the intestinal enzyme beta-glucuronidase. The deconjugated bilirubin is reabsorbed into the bloodstream and carried back to the liver, where it once again undergoes the conjugation process. This recirculation of bilirubin is called the enterohepatic circuit.

FACTORS IN INCREASED BILIRUBIN

Factors that result in an increased incidence of jaundice in the first week of life include

- *Excess production:* Bilirubin is produced in infants during the first 2 weeks of life at a rate twice that in adults (Maisels, 1999).
- *Red blood cell life:* Fetal red blood cells break down more quickly than do adult erythrocytes.
- *Liver immaturity:* The newborn's immature liver may not produce adequate amounts of glucuronyl transferase during the first few days of life. Lack of glucuronyl transferase limits the amount of bilirubin that can be conjugated.
- *Intestinal factors:* Conjugated bilirubin cannot be reduced to urobilinogen for excretion until intestinal flora are established. Large amounts of the enzyme beta-glucuronidase change bilirubin back to the unconjugated state.
- *Delayed feeding:* When feedings are delayed or taken

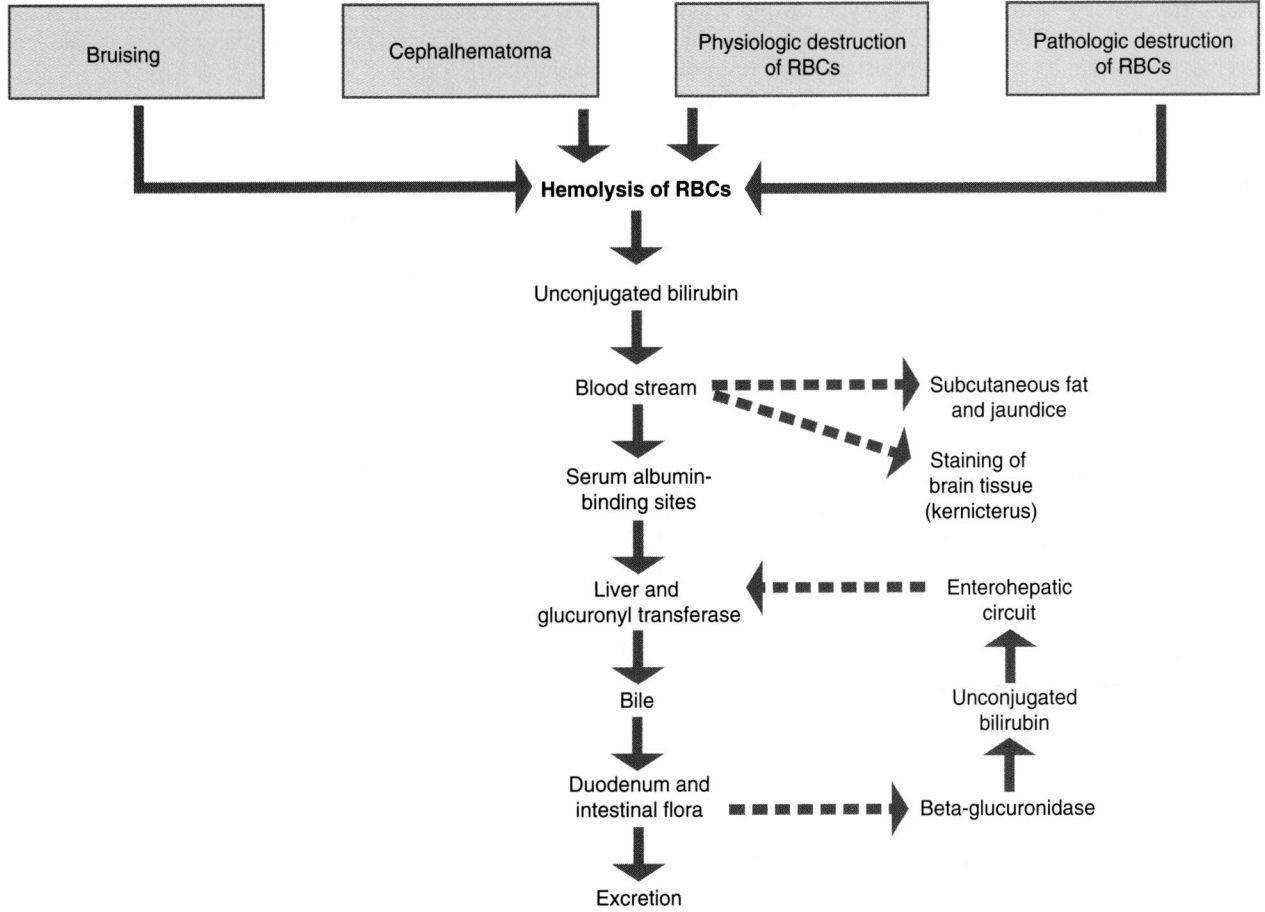

FIGURE 22-5

Sources of bilirubin and how it is removed from the body.

poorly, normal intestinal flora is not established, and passage of meconium, which is high in bilirubin, is delayed. Delayed feedings may therefore increase the time for conjugated bilirubin to be deconjugated.

- *Trauma:* Trauma during birth (bruising, cephalhematoma) causes increased hemolysis of red blood cells.
- *Fatty acids:* Fatty acids have a greater affinity than bilirubin for the binding sites on albumin and bind to albumin in place of bilirubin. Cold stress or asphyxia may increase circulating fatty acids.

CRITICAL TO REMEMBER

Factors that Increase Hyperbilirubinemia

- Hemolysis of excessive erythrocytes
- Short red blood cell life
- Liver immaturity
- Lack of intestinal flora
- Delayed feeding
- Trauma resulting in bruising or cephalhematoma
- Fatty acids from cold stress or asphyxia

Hyperbilirubinemia

PHYSIOLOGIC JAUNDICE

Physiologic jaundice is due to transient hyperbilirubinemia and is considered normal. It is not present during the first 24 hours of life but appears on the second or third day after birth. Jaundice becomes visible when the serum bilirubin reaches 5 to 7 mg/dl. In physiologic jaundice, the serum bilirubin peaks at 5 to 6 mg/dl between the second and fourth day of life. The bilirubin then begins to fall, declining below 2 mg/dl by the end of the first week (Behrman, Kliegman, & Arvin, 1996).

Physiologic jaundice may be treated with phototherapy when the bilirubin levels rise faster or to higher levels than expected. Because preterm and low-birth-weight infants are more susceptible to kernicterus at lower bilirubin levels, phototherapy may be used earlier than in the full-term infant.

PATHOLOGIC JAUNDICE

Physiologic jaundice must be differentiated from pathologic jaundice, which is abnormal and requires further investigation. One of the most important differences is the time at which the jaundice appears. Pathologic jaundice may occur during the first 24 hours after birth, whereas physiologic jaundice begins after the first 24 hours. A direct bilirubin level above 1 mg/dl or a total bilirubin concentration that increases by more than 5 mg/dl per day, is higher than 12 mg/dl in a full-term infant or 10 to 14 mg/dl in a preterm infant, or persists after the second week of life is considered pathologic (Behrman, Kliegman, & Arvin, 1996).

Pathologic jaundice is due to abnormalities causing excessive destruction of red blood cells (erythrocytes). These include incompatibilities between the mother's and infant's blood types (see Chapter 26), infection, and metabolic disorders. Pathologic jaundice is discussed in Chapter 30.

BREAST MILK JAUNDICE
Approximately one of every three normal, breast-fed infants has jaundice at 2 weeks of age (Maisels, 1995).

Early-Onset Breast Milk Jaundice. The most common cause of jaundice in breast-fed infants is insufficient intake, often called early-onset jaundice or breast-feeding jaundice. Jaundice begins within the first week of life, and serum bilirubin may rise above 12 mg/dl.

Infants who are sleepy, have a poor suck, or nurse infrequently may not receive enough colostrum, the substance that precedes true breast milk, to take advantage of its normal laxative effect in eliminating meconium. Lack of adequate suckling also depresses production of breast milk and increases the problem further. Helping the mother with breast-feeding to increase intake and stimulate milk production are the most important treatments.

True Breast Milk Jaundice. True breast milk jaundice, also called late-onset breast milk jaundice, occurs after the first 3 to 5 days of life. The serum bilirubin usually peaks at 5 to 10 mg/dl at approximately 2 weeks, although some infants may have levels over 20 mg/dl. Serum bilirubin falls gradually over several months (Halamek & Stevenson, 1997). The exact cause of breast milk jaundice is unknown. Substances in the breast milk have been suspected to interfere with conjugation or to increase absorption of bilirubin from the intestine, but the exact cause is unknown.

Treatment of breast milk jaundice includes close monitoring of serum bilirubin in the blood and at least eight to ten feedings each 24 hours. Although the levels are higher and last longer than in physiologic jaundice, reported cases of bilirubin encephalopathy from this type of jaundice are very rare (Maisels & Newman, 1995). If bilirubin levels become too high, treatment includes phototherapy, discontinuation of breast-feeding for 24 to 48 hours, or both. These measures cause a rapid drop in bilirubin. The level may rise again when breast-feeding is resumed but usually not high enough to interfere with further breast-feeding.

Blood Coagulation

Prothrombin and coagulation factors II, VII, IX, and X are produced by the liver and activated by vitamin K, which is deficient in the newborn (see p. 523).

Iron Storage

Iron is stored in the liver during the last weeks of pregnancy. Full-term infants whose mothers had adequate diets usually do not need added iron until 4 to 6 months of age. At that time, they should begin iron-containing foods or iron supplements. Infants with poor prenatal iron stores should have iron-fortified formula.

Metabolism of Drugs

The liver metabolizes drugs inefficiently in the newborn. Breast-feeding mothers should alert their primary caregiver before taking medications because harmful amounts may be transferred to the infant through the breast milk.

Urinary System

Kidney Development

The kidneys are completely developed at 35 weeks of gestation. Full kidney function, however, does not occur until after birth. Blood flow to the kidneys increases after birth because of decreased resistance in the renal vessels. The improved perfusion results in a steady improvement in kidney function during the first few days of life.

Kidney Function

The infant's kidney function is immature compared with that of the adult. The ability of the glomeruli to filter and the renal tubules to reabsorb is considerably less than in adults. The glomerular filtration rate doubles during the first weeks of life but does not reach adult levels until 1 to 2 years of age (Bonilla-Felix, Brannan, & Portman, 1998). Therefore, infants have a decreased ability to filter waste products from the blood.

Substances such as glucose and protein may escape into the urine of the neonate. They disappear within the first 3 days of life as kidney function improves. Urate crystals may give a pink color to the urine that is sometimes mistaken for blood.

The first voiding occurs within 24 hours of birth in most newborns. The newborn who does not void within 48 hours may have an inadequate intake of fluids. Absence of kidneys or anomalies that interfere with excretion of urine are usually discovered before birth because it causes low amniotic fluid volume. Only two to six voidings may occur during the first 2 days of life. Then the infant voids at least once after every feeding (Brion, Bernstein, & Spitzer, 1997).

Fluid Balance

Newborns have a lower tolerance for changes in total volume of body fluid than do older infants. In addition, the fluid turnover rate is greater than that in adults. To maintain fluid balance, newborns need 65 ml/kg (30 ml/lb) daily during the first 2 days of life and then 100 to 150 ml/kg (45 to 68 ml/lb) a day (Tsang, DeMarini, & Rath, 1998). For example, an infant who weighs 3.4 kg (7.5 lb) on the third day of life needs 340 to 510 ml of fluid each day.

WATER DISTRIBUTION
Seventy-eight percent of the newborn's body is composed of water, which is distributed differently from the distribu-

---

CRITICAL TO REMEMBER

Intake and Output in the Newborn

First 2 days of life

- Intake: 65 ml/kg (30 ml/lb) a day
- Output: 2 to 6 voids

After the first 2 days

- Intake: 100 to 150 ml/kg (45 to 68 ml/lb) a day
- Output: 5 to 25 voids

---

tion in the adult. The percentage of extracellular water in newborns is more than twice as high as in adults. Because infants have more fluid for their size than adults, and because a larger proportion of it is located outside the cells, total body water is easily depleted. Conditions such as vomiting and diarrhea can quickly result in life-threatening dehydration.

INSENSIBLE WATER LOSS

Water lost from the skin and respiratory tract contributes to insensible water loss. The newborn's large body surface area and rapid respiratory rate cause increased insensible water loss. Fluid losses increase greatly when infants are placed under radiant heaters, which accelerate evaporation from the skin. An elevated respiratory rate or low humidity in the air surrounding the infant raises insensible water losses even further.

URINE DILUTION AND CONCENTRATION

The ability of a newborn's kidneys to dilute urine is relatively good, to a specific gravity of 1.001 to 1.005 (Bonilla-Felix, Brannan, & Portman, 1998). A newborn's kidneys, however, cannot handle large increases in fluids, which result in fluid overload. This is most likely to happen when infants receive too much intravenous fluid. Normal urine output is 1 to 3 ml/kg/hr (Brion, Bernstein, & Spitzer, 1997).

Because they have only half the adult's ability to excrete concentrated urine, newborns have more difficulty preventing loss of fluid in the urine than do adults (Guyton & Hall, 1996). Neonates can concentrate urine only to a specific gravity of 1.015 to 1.020 (Bonilla-Felix, Brannan, & Portman, 1998), compared with the adult level of 1.040. It takes 3 to 6 months for urine concentrations to reach adult levels. The newborn's limited ability to conserve water may result in dehydration more quickly than in the older infant or child.

Acid-Base and Electrolyte Balance

The maintenance of acid-base and electrolyte balance is a primary function of the kidneys and may be precarious in neonates. Newborns tend to lose bicarbonate at lower levels than adults, increasing their risk for acidosis. The excretion of solutes is less efficient in newborns as well. Although newborns conserve needed sodium well, they are less able to excrete sodium efficiently if they receive excessive amounts.

Immune System

The neonate is less effective in fighting off infection than the older infant or child. Leukocytes are delayed in moving to the site of invasion and are not efficient in destroying the invader. Fever and leukocytosis, which occur during infection of the older child, are often not present in the newborn with infection. This lack of response is due to immaturity of the hypothalamus and the inflammatory response.

Because of their immature immune system, infants are susceptible to pathogens such as *Staphylococcus epidermidis* and *Escherichia coli* that do not usually affect older children. Full-term newborns received antibodies from the mother during the last trimester of pregnancy. If the mother breastfeeds, the infant continues to receive antibodies in breast milk. Breast-feeding transfers passive immunity to the infant. Immunoglobulins (serum globulins with antibody activity) help protect the newborn from infection. The major immunoglobulins are IgG, IgM, and IgA.

IgG

IgG crosses the placenta readily and provides the fetus with passive temporary immunity to bacteria and viruses to which the mother has immunity. IgG also protects the fetus from bacterial toxins. Most of the transfer occurs in the third trimester.

Although the fetus begins to make IgG at 20 weeks of gestation, very little is produced until 3 to 4 weeks after birth. The passive immunity lasts for varying amounts of time. Although much of the passive immunity is gone by approximately 3 months of age, the antibodies to measles (rubeola) may last much longer.

IgM

IgM helps protect against gram-negative bacteria. It is rapidly produced beginning a few days after birth. IgM cannot cross the placenta because the molecules are too large. If IgM is found in larger-than-normal amounts in the neonate, exposure to infection in utero is probable.

IgA

IgA does not cross the placenta and must be produced by the infant. It is not produced in adequate amounts until 6 to 12 weeks after birth. Because IgA is important in protection of the gastrointestinal and respiratory systems, newborns are particularly susceptible to infections of those systems. A form of IgA is included in colostrum and breast milk. Therefore, breast-fed infants receive protection that formula-fed infants do not.

Psychosocial Adaptation

Periods of Reactivity

In the early hours after birth, the infant goes through changes called periods of reactivity. There are two periods of reactivity, separated by a period of sleep.

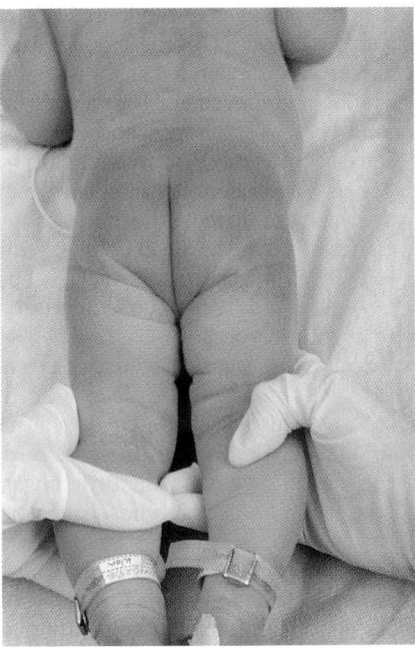

FIGURE 22-10
* * * * * * * *
Note the symmetry of gluteal and thigh creases.

The legs are extended to determine if they are equal in length and if thigh and gluteal creases are symmetric (Fig. 22–10). If the hip is dislocated, the leg on the affected side is shorter, and the creases are asymmetric. When the infant's legs are bent, the knee on the affected side is lower if the hip is dislocated. Because the hip may be unstable but not yet dislocated, these signs are not always present at birth. Treatment of developmental dysplasia of the hip involves immobilizing the leg in a flexed, abducted position, usually with a harness.

VERTEBRAL COLUMN

The nurse palpates the newborn's vertebral column to discover any defects in the vertebrae (see Chapter 52). An indentation, especially with a tuft of hair over it, is a sign of spina bifida occulta, failure of a vertebra to close. Other, more obvious neural tube defects include a meningocele or myelomeningocele. These are protrusions of spinal fluid and meninges or the spinal cord, or both, through the defect in the vertebrae. They appear as a sac on the back and may be covered by skin or only the meninges.

A pilonidal dimple may be present at the base of the spine. It should be examined for a sinus and the depth noted.

Measurements

Measurements provide information about the infant's growth in utero. The weight, length, and head and chest circumference are compared with the norms for the infant's gestational age.

WEIGHT

The newborn's weight ranges between 2,500 and 4,000 g (5 lb, 8 oz and 8 lb, 13 oz) (Glenn, 1993). The average weight of a full-term newborn is 3,400 g (7.5 lb). Factors affecting weight include gestational age, placental functioning, genetic factors, and maternal diabetes, substance abuse, or hypertension.

Infants are weighed each day they are in the birth facility and at follow-up visits. They can be expected to lose 5% to 10% of their birth weight during the first few days of life (Bell & Oh, 1999). This weight loss is due to excretion of meconium from the bowel and normal loss of extracellular fluid. Newborns usually do not take in enough calories to maintain their weight during this period, so that low caloric intake also contributes to early weight loss. Infants normally regain birth weight by the 10th day of life. Thereafter, they gain approximately 20 g (2/3 oz) a day until the middle of the first year (Bowden, Dickey, & Greenberg, 1998).

LENGTH

The infant's length is measured from the top of the head to the end of the outstretched leg (Fig. 22–11). The average length of a full-term newborn is 48 to 53 cm (19 to 21 in.) (Glenn, 1993).

HEAD AND CHEST CIRCUMFERENCE

The diameter of the head is measured around the occiput, just above the eyebrows. The average head circumference of the term newborn is 33 to 35.5 cm (13 to 14 in.) (Glenn, 1993). The measurement may be affected by molding of the skull during the birth process. If a large amount of molding occurred, the head is remeasured when it regains its normal shape. An abnormally small head may indicate poor brain growth and microcephaly. A very large head may be a sign of hydrocephalus.

The chest is measured at the level of the nipples. It is usually 2 to 3 cm smaller than the head. The average circumference of the chest is 30.5 to 33 cm (12 to 13 in.) (Glenn, 1993). If molding of the head is present, the head and chest measurement may be equal at birth.

Assessment of Cardiorespiratory Status

Assessments of respiratory and cardiovascular status are performed together because transitional changes take place in both systems at birth.

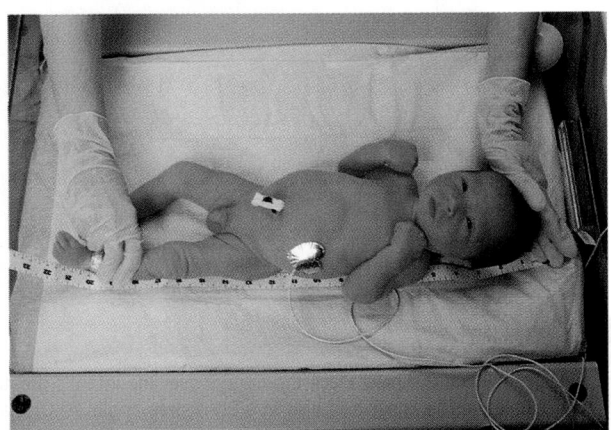

FIGURE 22-11
* * * * * * * *
Measuring length.

History

Information about the pregnancy, labor, and delivery is important in assessing the infant's cardiovascular and respiratory status and the likelihood of problems at birth.

Airway

During birth, some fetal lung fluid is forced into the upper airway. Excessive fluid or mucus in the infant's respiratory passages may cause respiratory difficulty for several hours after birth.

RESPIRATORY RATE

The nurse assesses respirations at least once every 30 minutes until the infant has been stable for 2 hours after birth (American Academy of Pediatrics & American College of Obstetricians and Gynecologists, 1997). If abnormalities are noted, respirations are assessed more often. The normal respiratory rate is 30 to 60 breaths per minute, with an average rate of 30 to 40. The infant may breathe faster immediately after birth, during crying, and during the first and second periods of reactivity. Respirations should not be labored, and the chest movements should be symmetric. Because the pattern and depth of respirations are irregular, they must be counted for a full minute for accuracy (Procedure 22–1).

Periodic breathing, pauses in breathing lasting up to 10 seconds without other changes, may occur is some full-term infants during the first few days, but is more common in preterm infants. Apnea lasting longer than 20 seconds, or accompanied by cyanosis, heart rate changes, or other signs of difficult breathing, is abnormal (Hagedorn, Gardner, & Abman, 1998).

BREATH SOUNDS

The anterior and posterior lung fields are auscultated for breath sounds, which should be present equally throughout. Breath sounds should be clear over most areas. It is not unusual, however, to hear sounds of moisture in the lungs during the first hour or two after birth because fetal lung fluid has not been completely absorbed. Abnormal or diminished sounds should always be reported to the primary care provider if they continue.

CHOANAL ATRESIA

Assessment for choanal atresia is important because newborns are obligate nose breathers for approximately the first 3 weeks of life and so breathe mostly through the nose, except when crying. In choanal atresia, one or both nasal passages are blocked by an abnormality of the septum.

The nurse can assess for choanal atresia by closing the

CRITICAL TO REMEMBER

Normal Vital Signs in the Newborn

- Temperature: 36.5° to 37.5°C (97.7° to 99.5°F) axillary, 36.5° to 37.6°C (97.7° to 99.7°F) rectal
- Apical pulse: 120 to 160 beats/min (100 sleeping, 180 crying)
- Respirations: 30 to 60 breaths/min (average, 30 to 40)

---

infant's mouth and occluding one nostril at a time. The infant is observed for breathing, and breath sounds are auscultated while each nostril is occluded. Another method of assessment is to pass a catheter (nos. 5 to 8 French) through each nostril to check for patency. Infants with choanal atresia may become cyanotic when quiet but pink when crying.

Bilateral choanal atresia causes severe respiratory distress and requires surgery. Blockage of one side puts the infant at risk for respiratory distress if the other side becomes occluded by mucus or edema.

SIGNS OF RESPIRATORY DISTRESS

The nurse must be alert for signs of respiratory distress, which may be present at birth or develop later.

Tachypnea. Tachypnea, a respiratory rate above 60 breaths per minute, is the most common sign of respiratory distress. It is not unusual during the first hour after birth and during the second period of reactivity. Continued tachypnea, however, is abnormal.

Retractions. Retractions result when the soft tissue around the bones of the chest is drawn in with the effort of pulling air into the lungs. Substernal or xiphoid retractions occur when the area under the sternum retracts each time the infant inhales. When the muscles between the ribs are pulled in so that each rib is outlined, intercostal retractions are present. The muscles above the sternum and around the clavicles may also be used to aid in respirations (supraclavicular retractions). Occasional mild retractions are common immediately after birth but should not continue after the first hour.

Flaring of the Nares. A reflex widening of the nostrils occurs when the infant is receiving insufficient oxygen. Flaring of the nares helps to decrease airway resistance and increase the amount of air entering the lungs. Intermittent flaring may occur in the first hour after birth. Continued flaring indicates a more serious respiratory problem.

Cyanosis. Cyanosis is a purplish-blue discoloration that indicates that the infant is not getting enough oxygen. It may be preceded by a dusky or gray hue to the skin. Central cyanosis involves the lips, tongue, and trunk and shows true hypoxia. It indicates that not enough oxygen is reaching the vital organs and requires immediate attention. Acrocyanosis, which involves just the extremities, is normal in the first few hours after birth or if the infant becomes cold. It is due to poor perfusion of blood to the periphery of the body (Fig. 22–12).

Grunting. Grunting describes a noise made on expiration when pressure is increased within the alveoli to help keep them open. Grunting may be very mild and heard only with a stethoscope, or it may be loud enough to hear unaided in an infant having severe respiratory difficulty. Grunting is a common sign of respiratory distress syndrome and necessitates expanded assessment and referral for treatment.

Seesaw Respirations. If the infant's chest falls when the abdomen rises and the chest rises when the abdomen falls during respirations, seesaw respirations are present. These respirations are a sign of severe respiratory difficulty.

Asymmetry. Chest expansion should be equal on both sides. Asymmetry or decreased movement on one side may indicate the collapse of a lung (pneumothorax).

Color

In addition to cyanosis, the nurse assesses for pallor and ruddiness.

PROCEDURE 22-1

Assessing Vital Signs in the Newborn

PURPOSE: To obtain an accurate measurement of newborn vital signs.

Respirations

1. Assess respirations when the infant is quiet or sleeping, if possible, so that lung sounds can be heard more clearly. Count the respirations (and apical pulse) before disturbing the infant for other assessments.
2. Observe, palpate, or auscultate the chest and abdomen. Using more than one method increases accuracy and helps differentiate rapid, irregular respirations from other movements.
3. Lift the infant's blanket and shirt to see the chest and abdomen. Observation of the pattern of respirations before beginning to count makes it easier to count the rate.
4. If desired, place a hand lightly over the infant's chest or abdomen to feel the movement and palpate the rate.
5. To auscultate respirations, place a stethoscope on the right side of the infant's chest to decrease the sounds of the heart.
6. Count for a full minute to increase accuracy because respirations are normally irregular in the newborn.
7. A crying infant may become quiet if allowed to suck on a pacifier or gloved finger. If the infant continues to cry, make a note in the chart because the rate may be faster than when the infant is quiet. Recheck later when the infant is calm.
8. Expect the respiratory rate to be 30 to 60 breaths/min when the infant is at rest. Report signs of respiratory distress (tachypnea, retractions, flaring, cyanosis, grunting, seesawing, apneic periods, and asymmetry of chest movements) to ensure follow-up care.

Pulse

1. If possible, listen to the apical pulse on a quiet or sleeping infant so the sounds can be heard more clearly.
2. If possible, use a pediatric head on the stethoscope to listen. A pediatric head allows better contact between the stethoscope and the chest wall and eliminates some of the sounds from the lungs and intestines.
3. If the infant is crying, insert a pacifier or a gloved finger into the mouth to quiet the infant.
4. If the infant cannot be quieted, increase concentration and time spent listening. This increase helps to separate the sounds heard and to focus in on the heart beat.

5. To get used to the rapid beat, listen briefly before beginning to count. Then count for a full minute. Tapping a finger in rhythm with the beat may be helpful. Expect the heart rate to be 120 to 160 beats/min at rest.
6. Move the stethoscope over the entire heart area to listen to all sounds. Refer any abnormal sounds (arrhythmias, murmurs) for follow-up. Listening over the entire area increases chances of hearing abnormal sounds.

Temperature

AXILLARY

1. Place the thermometer vertically along the chest wall in the center of the axillary space with the infant's arm firmly over it. This placement keeps the thermometer positioned properly and avoids injury to the infant. If the thermometer is held horizontally, it may protrude behind the axilla and give an inaccurate reading.
2. Read thermometer at the proper time: glass, 5 minutes; plastic strip, 1 to 1.5 minutes (with a 10-second wait before reading); electronic, when indicator sounds. Normal range: 36.5° to 37.5°C (97.7° to 99.5°F).

RECTAL

1. Take a rectal temperature only when necessary. Use the axillary method whenever possible to avoid the risk of perforation of the rectum.
2. Lubricate the tip of the thermometer with water-soluble lubricant to ease insertion.
3. Place the infant in a supine position and hold the ankles firmly in one hand. Bend the infant's knees against the abdomen and raise the legs to expose the anus, or place the infant prone or on the side and separate the buttocks. This provides visibility and prevents excessive movement that might cause injury.
4. Insert the thermometer carefully and gently no more than 0.5 in. into the rectum. The rectum turns to the right 1 in. from the sphincter. Inserting the thermometer farther may cause perforation.
5. Do not force the thermometer if it does not insert easily. An obstruction may be preventing insertion of the thermometer.
6. To maintain control and avoid injury to the infant, hold the thermometer securely throughout the time it remains in the rectum.
7. Read the thermometer at the proper time: glass, 5 minutes; electronic, when indicator sounds. Normal range: 36.5° to 37.6°C (97.7° to 99.7°F).

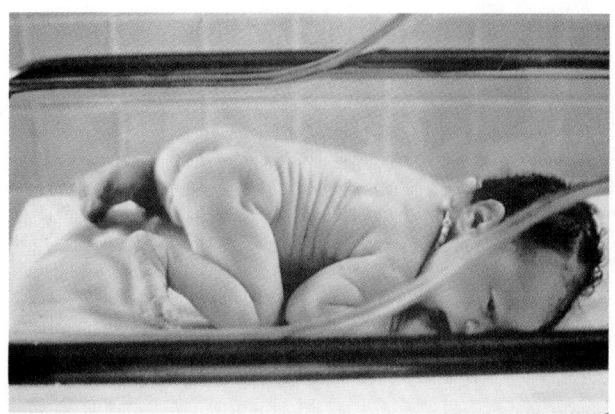

FIGURE 22–12
• • • • • • • • • •
Acrocyanosis. (Courtesy of Jane Deacon, M.S., R.N., N.N.P., The Children's Hospital, Denver, Colorado.)

PALLOR

Pallor can indicate that the infant is slightly hypoxic or anemic. A laboratory examination of hemoglobin and hematocrit or a complete blood count may be ordered by the physician.

RUDDY COLOR

A ruddy or reddish color of the skin may indicate polycythemia, an excessive number of red blood cells. A hematocrit determination confirms polycythemia. Infants with elevated hematocrits are at increased risk for jaundice from the normal destruction of excessive red blood cells that occurs after birth. Jaundice may occur in infants with hematocrits above 65%.

Heart Sounds

The heart is auscultated for rate, rhythm, and the presence of murmurs or abnormal sounds. The nurse should count the apical pulse for a full minute for accuracy and listen for abnormalities. The rate should range between 120 and 160 BPM with normal activity. It may elevate to 180 BPM when infants are crying or drop as low as 100 BPM when they are in a deep sleep.

If no problems are present at birth, the heart rate should be recorded at least once every 30 minutes until the infant has been stable for 2 hours after birth (American Academy of Pediatrics & American College of Obstetrics and Gynecologists, 1997). Monitoring is more frequent if there are abnormalities. Once stable, the heart rate is checked once every 8 hours unless a reason exists to assess it more frequently.

POSITION

The apex of the heart is located at the point of maximum impulse, where the pulse is most easily felt and the sound is loudest. This is at the third or fourth intercostal space, slightly left of the midclavicular line (a line drawn from the middle of the left clavicle). It may be slightly lower in some newborns and at the fifth intercostal space (Vargo, 1996). Conditions that affect the position of the heart include pneumothorax and dextrocardia (in which the heart position is reversed from normal).

RHYTHM AND MURMURS

The rhythm of the heart should be regular, and the first and second sounds should be heard clearly. Abnormalities in rhythm or sounds such as murmurs should be noted. Murmurs are sounds of abnormal blood flow through the heart and may indicate openings in the septum of the heart or problems with blood flow through the valves. Most murmurs in the newborn are normal functional murmurs due to incomplete transition from fetal to neonatal circulation. A murmur is not uncommon until the ductus arteriosus is functionally closed. Any abnormal sounds of the heart are investigated further because they may be signs of cardiac defects.

Brachial and Femoral Pulses

The brachial and femoral pulses should be present and equal bilaterally. The brachial pulse is located over the antecubital space, and the femoral pulse is located at the groin. Pulses should be equal bilaterally and the brachial and femoral pulses should be the same. Differences between the brachial and femoral pulses may be due to impaired blood flow in coarctation of the aorta, a congenital heart defect (see Chapter 46).

Blood Pressure

Measurement of blood pressure is not a necessary part of a routine assessment of the newborn according to the American Academy of Pediatrics and American College of Obstetricians and Gynecologists (1997). The blood pressure is taken on all extremities, however, if the infant shows signs such as unequal pulses or murmurs. Doppler ultrasonography or other electronic measurement makes it easier to obtain an accurate blood pressure. To ensure accurate measurement, the infant should be quiet when the blood pressure is taken because crying elevates it. The width of the blood pressure cuff should be 20% greater than the diameter of the extremity, and the bladder of the cuff should cover two thirds of the upper arm or thigh (Smith et al., 1996).

Blood pressure varies according the infant's age, weight, and gestational age. (See Appendix J for normal blood pressure readings.) Hypotension may occur in the sick infant. The blood pressure of the lower extremities should be the same as or slightly higher than that of the upper extremities. If there is a difference of as much as 20 mm Hg, coarctation of the aorta may be present.

Assessment of Thermoregulation

The neonate's temperature is taken soon after birth while the infant is being held by the mother or is in a radiant warmer with a skin probe attached to the abdomen. The probe allows the warmer to measure and display the infant's temperature continuously. The temperature control is set to regulate the amount of heat produced according to the infant's skin temperature. The temperature should be assessed at least once every 30 minutes until the infant has been stable for 2 hours after birth (American Academy of Pediatrics & American College of Obstetricians and Gynecologists, 1997). It is often checked again at 4 hours and then once every 8 hours as long as it remains stable.

Taking axillary temperatures is safer than taking rectal temperatures because it avoids the possibility of damaging the rectum (Procedure 22–1, Fig. 22–13). Axillary tempera-

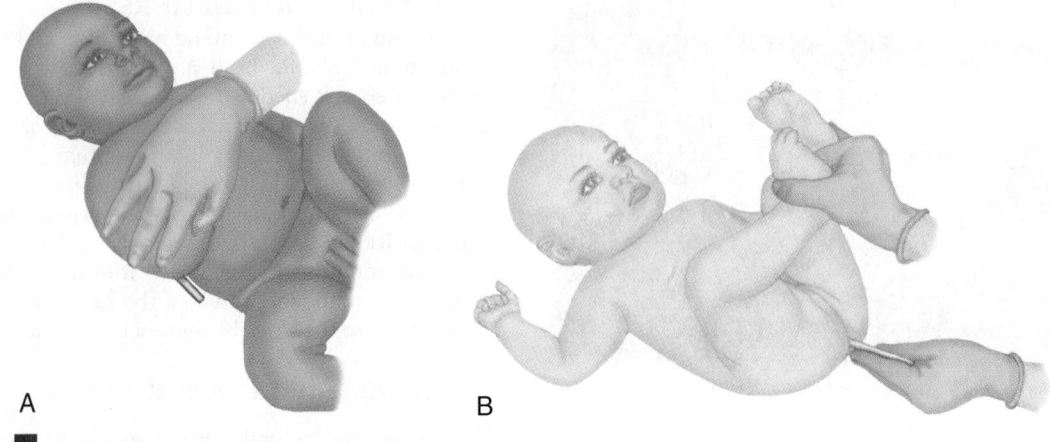

FIGURE 22-13

An axillary (*A*) or rectal (*B*) temperature may be taken. The infant is held securely to prevent injury and obtain an accurate reading.

tures provide a reading very close to rectal measurements. The normal range for axillary temperature is 36.5° to 37.5°C (97.7° to 99.5°F) (Blake & Murray, 1998).

If a rectal temperature is necessary, the nurse should insert the thermometer no more than 0.5 in. into the anus. The colon turns at a sharp right angle approximately 1 inch from the anal sphincter. Inserting the thermometer farther might result in potentially fatal perforation of the intestinal wall. A thermometer should never be forced into the rectum because there could be an imperforate (closed) anus. The normal range of rectal temperature is 36.5° to 37.6°C (97.7° to 99.7°F).

Temperatures can be measured with an electronic or glass thermometer or a disposable plastic strip. Disposable plastic strips change color to indicate temperature change. Tympanic thermometers usually are not used because they are less accurate in newborns.

Assessment of Hepatic Function

The major early assessments of the hepatic system are related to blood glucose and bilirubin conjugation.

Blood Glucose

Observing for signs of hypoglycemia is necessary throughout routine assessment and care.

CRITICAL TO REMEMBER

Risk Factors for Hypoglycemia

- Prematurity
- Postmaturity
- Intrauterine growth restriction
- Asphyxia
- Cold stress
- Large for gestational age
- Small for gestational age
- Maternal diabetes
- Maternal intake of ritodrine or terbutaline

CRITICAL TO REMEMBER

Signs of Hypoglycemia

- Jitteriness
- Poor muscle tone
- Sweating
- Tachypnea
- Dyspnea
- Apnea
- Cyanosis
- Low temperature
- Poor suck
- High-pitched cry
- Lethargy
- Seizures, coma
- Note: Some infants may be asymptomatic.

The American Academy of Pediatrics and American College of Obstetricians and Gynecologists (1997) state that screening for the blood glucose level is necessary only for infants in risk categories. Normal blood glucose during the first day of life is 40 to 60 mg/dl (Nicholson & Pesce, 1996). Because capillary blood is used in screening tests, these tests are less accurate than laboratory tests using venous blood. Therefore, a laboratory analysis (per agency policy) is often used to verify readings below 45 mg/dl on glucometers or glucose strips.

It is important to avoid injuring the infant's foot when taking blood from the heel. If the lancet goes into the calcaneus bone, osteomyelitis may result. To avoid piercing the bone, the skin should be punctured to a depth of less than 2 mm (Meehan, 1998). The site chosen must avoid the major nerves and arteries in the area (Procedure 22-2).

Bilirubin

The nurse identifies infants at increased risk for hyperbilirubinemia. Jaundice is identified by pressing the infant's skin over a firm surface, such as the end of the nose or the

PROCEDURE 22–2

. . . .

Assessing Blood Glucose in the Newborn

P U R P O S E : To measure the infant's blood glucose accurately by heel puncture using the AccuChek or One Touch glucometer or Dextrostix or Chemstrip reagent strips.

1. Wash hands and gather supplies needed: (a) gloves, (b) alcohol wipe, (c) 2 × 2-in. gauze, (d) lancet, (e) adhesive bandage, (f) diaper or commercial warming pack to warm heel, (g) glucometer or glucose screening reagent strips. When using Chemstrip and AccuChek, add a cotton ball. When using One Touch, add a pipette. Having all supplies ready allows efficient performance of procedure.

2. To ensure proper functioning of the machine, calibrate the glucometer and use quality-control measures according to manufacturer's guidelines.

3. If the infant's mother has a blood-borne disease such as hepatitis B or human immunodeficiency virus infection, bathe the infant before puncturing the skin to avoid contamination of the puncture site with maternal blood on the infant's skin.

4. Warm the infant's foot for a few minutes if it is cold or if blood is needed for several tests. Dampen a diaper with warm water and fasten it over the heel, or use a heel-warming pack according to directions. Warming causes vasodilation and allows blood to flow more easily.

5. Apply gloves as part of standard precautions to prevent contamination of hands with blood.

6. Locate the site. Palpate the bone of the heel to avoid puncturing the calcaneus bone, which could result in infection. Place the thumb or finger over the walking surface to avoid damage to nerves and arteries of this area. Choose the puncture site on the lateral heel.

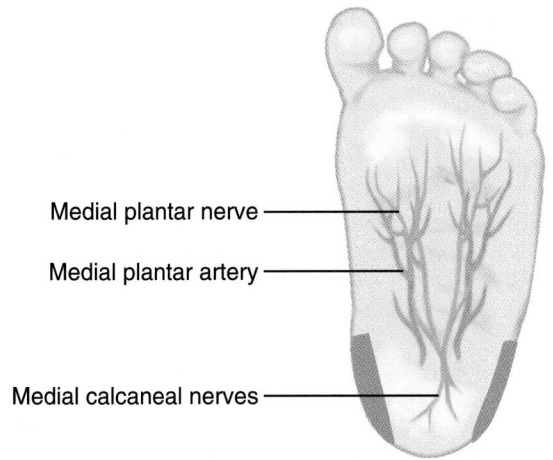

Medial plantar nerve

Medial plantar artery

Medial calcaneal nerves

7. Clean the area with alcohol and dry with sterile gauze or allow to air dry to prevent diluting the specimen with alcohol.

8. Puncture the side of the heel with a lancet to a depth of less than 2 mm to avoid piercing the bone. Place the lancet in sharps container to prevent injury to the infant and injury or unnecessary exposure of others to the infant's blood.

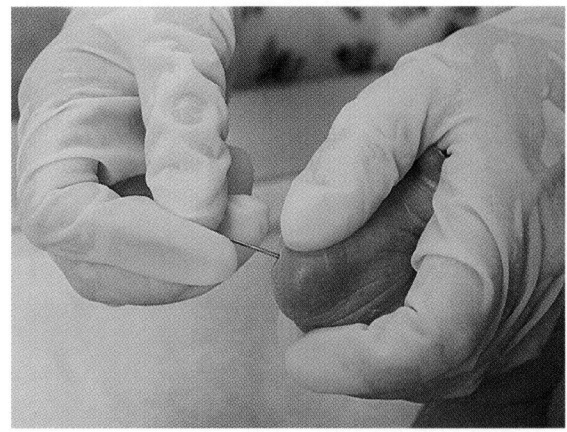

9. If an automatic puncture device is used, place it over the site and activate according to manufacturer's directions.

10. Wipe away the first drop of blood with gauze to avoid dilution with fluid from the area of the puncture (if directed by manufacturer).

11. Collect a large "standup" drop of blood at the puncture site. Avoid excessive squeezing of the foot because it dilutes the sample with tissue fluid. If using AccuChek, Dextrostix, or Chemstrip, place the drop of blood on the treated area of the reagent strip. To ensure accuracy, cover the entire treated area of the strip and do not smear it. If using One Touch, draw blood into the pipette and place it on the reagent strip that has been placed in glucometer.

12. If using AccuChek, Dextrostix, or Chemstrip, remove blood from the strip at the exact time recommended by manufacturer. More or less time affects accuracy of reading.

13. Remove blood by the method appropriate for the type of reagent strip used. For Dextrostix, run cold water slowly over the end of the strip to wash away the blood. Water flowing with too much force can wash away color change. Warm water may affect the color. For AccuChek and Chemstrip, wipe blood completely away with a cotton ball.

14. Obtain results. If using a glucometer, read the glucometer when the sound indicates the results are ready. For Dextrostix and Chemstrip, compare reagent strips with the color chart on the bottle. For Dextrostix, read immediately. For Chemstrip, read after 60 seconds.

15. Apply adhesive bandage to prevent bleeding. Remove it as soon as the bleeding has stopped.

16. Record results. Have laboratory draw blood for verification of abnormal results according to agency policy. To provide calories needed for metabolism and prevent further decrease in glucose levels, feed the infant according to agency policy or for readings below 45 mg/dl.

CRITICAL TO REMEMBER

Common Risk Factors for Hyperbilirubinemia

- Prematurity
- Cephalhematoma
- Bruising
- Delayed or poor intake
- Cold stress
- Asphyxia
- Rh incompatibility
- ABO incompatibility
- Sepsis
- Sibling with jaundice
- Breast-feeding

sternum. Because jaundice begins at the head and moves down the body, the nurse can make a rough estimate of the problem's severity. Jaundice of the face and neck occurs at levels up to 8 mg/dl; jaundice of the upper trunk occurs up to 12 mg/dl (Philip, 1996).

Jaundice becomes visible when serum bilirubin reaches 5 to 7 mg/dl. If it appears before the second day of life, the bilirubin level may not be physiologic. The physician or nurse practitioner may order laboratory determinations of the bilirubin level on the basis of the nurse's assessment.

Assessment of Body Systems

Neurologic System

REFLEXES
The nurse notes the presence and strength of the reflexes and whether both sides of the body respond symmetrically (Fig. 22–14). A diminished overall response occurs in preterm or ill infants. Absence of reflexes may indicate a serious neurologic problem. Asymmetric responses may indicate that trauma during birth caused nerve damage, paralysis, or fracture. Some of the newborn reflexes gradually weaken and disappear during the early months (Table 22–2).

SENSORY ASSESSMENT
Ears. The ears are assessed for placement, overall appearance, and maturity. An imaginary line drawn from the inner to the outer canthus of the eye should be even with the area where the upper ear joins the head (Fig. 22–15). Low-set ears may indicate chromosomal abnormalities.

The nurse examines the ears for skin tags and preauricular sinuses or dimples. If abnormalities of the ear are present, the newborn may have chromosomal abnormalities, mental retardation, or kidney defects. The stiffness of the cartilage and the degree of incurving of the pinna are checked as part of the gestational age assessment.

Hearing is assessed by noting the infant's reaction to sudden loud noises, which should cause a startle response. The infant should respond to the sound of voices, particu-

larly if it is a high-pitched tone of voice or the sound of the mother's voice. Many birth facilities screen for risk factors for hearing loss and refer or perform further testing if necessary.

Eyes. The eyes should be symmetric and equal in size. The usual slate gray-blue color gradually changes to the true color by 3 to 12 months of age. Infants with dark skin may have brown eyes. The eyes are examined for abnormalities and signs of inflammation. A slant of the epicanthal fold in a non-Asian infant may indicate Down syndrome. Edema of the eyelids or subconjunctival hemorrhages (reddened areas of the sclera) result from pressure on the head during birth. The sclera should be white or bluish-white.

Conjunctivitis may result from infection or a chemical reaction to medications. *Staphylococcus, Chlamydia,* and *Neisseria gonorrhoeae* are common organisms that cause infection. Maternal gonorrhea can infect the infant's eyes (ophthalmia neonatorum) and lead to blindness. All infants are treated prophylactically with antibiotics to the eyes to prevent this condition. Any discharge from the eyes is reported for possible culture and treatment.

Transient strabismus ("crossed eyes") is common for the first 3 to 4 months after birth because infants have poor control of their eye muscles. The doll's-eye sign is a normal finding in the newborn: when the head is turned quickly to one side, the eyes move toward the other side. The setting-sun sign (the iris appears low in the eye, and part of the sclera can be seen above the iris) may be an indication of hydrocephalus.

The pupils should be equal in size and react to light. Cataracts (opacities of the lens) appear as white areas over the pupils. They may develop in infants of mothers who had rubella or other infections during the pregnancy. When a light is directed into the eyes, the normal red reflex may not be seen if large cataracts are present. Tears are scant or absent for the first 2 to 4 weeks of life. Excessive tearing may indicate a plugged lacrimal duct, which is treated with massage or surgery.

Although visual acuity is not well developed and the eyes cannot accommodate for distance, newborns should show a visual response to the environment. They should make eye contact when held in a cradle position during a period of alertness and focus on objects that are 8 to 9 inches away. Newborns can follow interesting objects horizontally 180 degrees and vertically 30 degrees. They should respond well to human faces and geometric patterns of black and white or medium-bright colors, but show little interest in pastel colors.

Newborns should blink or close their eyes in response to bright lights. Any infant who does not respond to visual stimuli should be reported to the physician or nurse practitioner for further investigation.

OTHER NEUROLOGIC SIGNS
The newborn is assessed for jitteriness or tremors, usually caused by hypoglycemia, low calcium levels, or prenatal exposure to drugs. Tremors increase each time the infant is touched or moved but stop briefly if the extremity is flexed and held firmly.

Seizures indicate central nervous system abnormality. To differentiate jitteriness from seizures, the infant's ex-

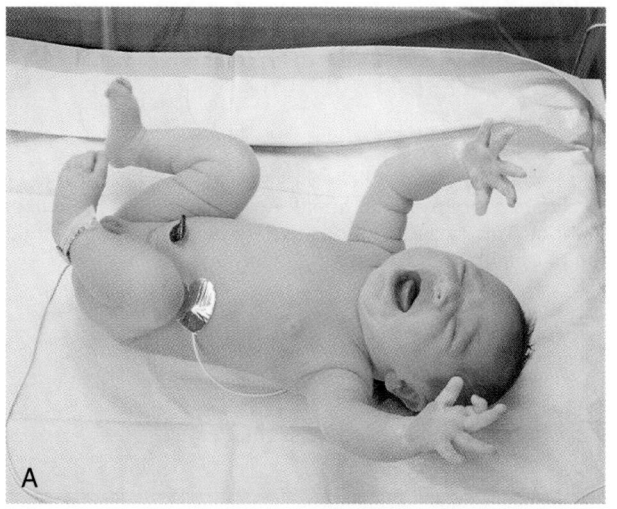

A. **Moro Reflex.**
The Moro reflex is the most dramatic reflex. It occurs when the infant's head and trunk are allowed to drop back 30 degrees when the infant is in a slightly raised position. The infant's arms and legs extend and abduct, with the fingers fanning open and thumbs and forefingers forming a C position. The arms then return to their normally flexed state with an embracing motion. The legs may also extend and then flex.

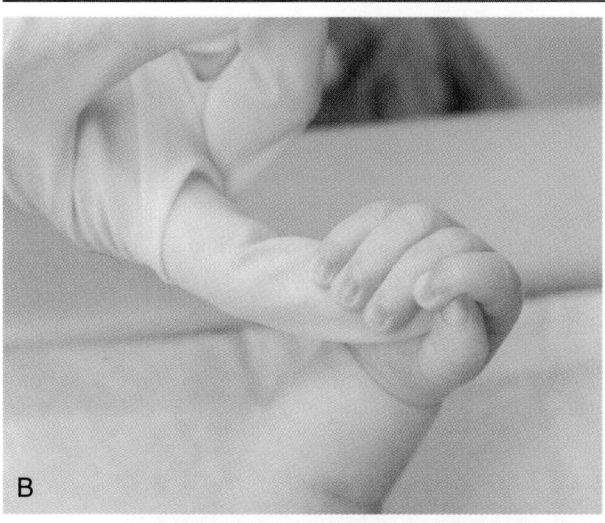

B. **Palmar grasp reflex.**
The palmar grasp reflex occurs when the infant's palm is touched near the base of the fingers. The hand closes into a tight fist. The grasp reflex may be weak or absent if the infant has damage to the nerves of the arms.

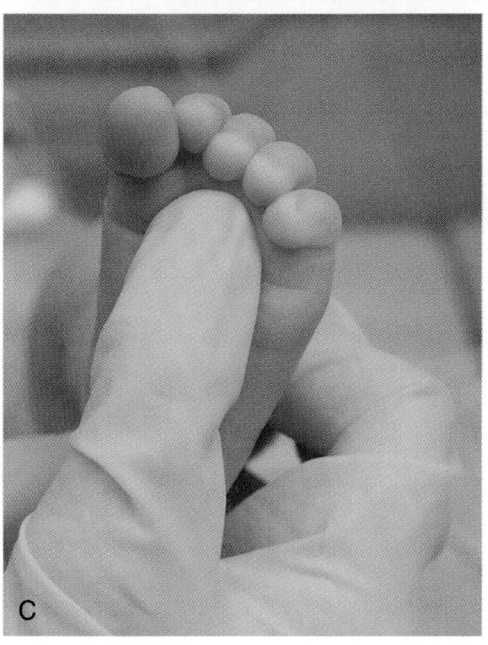

C. **Plantar grasp reflex.**
The plantar grasp reflex is similar to the palmar grasp reflex. When the area below the toes is touched, the infant's toes curl over the nurse's finger.

FIGURE 22–14

Reflexes

Illustration continued on following page

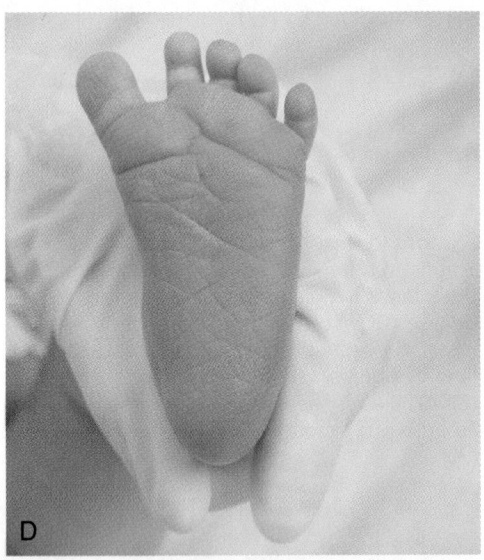

D. **Babinski reflex.**
The Babinski reflex is elicited by stroking the lateral sole of the infant's foot from the heel forward and across the ball of the foot. This causes the toes to flare outward and the big toe to dorsiflex.

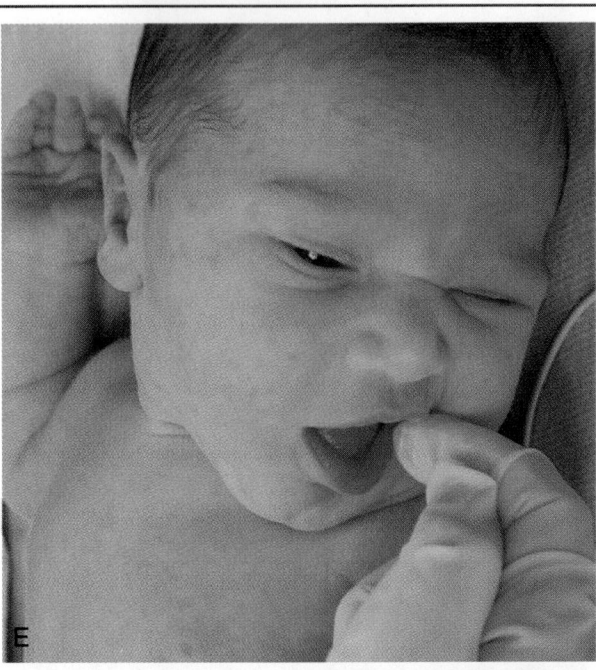

E. **Rooting reflex.**
The rooting reflex is important in feeding and is most often demonstrated when the infant is hungry. When the infant's cheek is touched near the mouth, the head turns toward the side that has been stroked. This response helps the infant find the nipple for feeding. The reflex occurs when either side of the mouth is touched. Touching the cheeks on both sides at the same time confuses the infant.

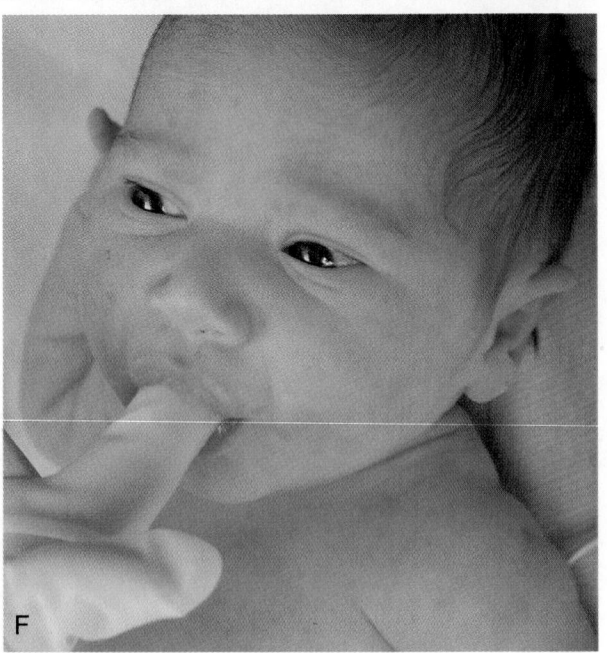

F. **Sucking reflex.**
The sucking reflex is essential to normal life. When the mouth or palate is touched by the nipple or a finger, the infant begins to suck. The sucking reflex is assessed for its presence and strength. Feeding difficulties may be related to problems in the infant's ability to suck and to coordinate sucking with swallowing.

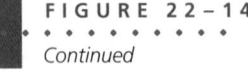

FIGURE 22–14
. . . .
Continued

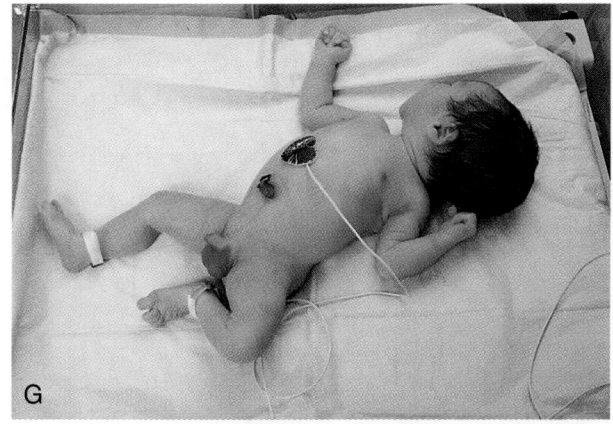

G. Tonic neck reflex.
The tonic neck reflex refers to the posture assumed by newborns when in a supine position. The infant extends the arm and leg on the side to which the head is turned and flexes the extremities on the other side. This response is sometimes referred to as the "fencing reflex" because the infant's position is similar to that of a person engaged in a fencing match.

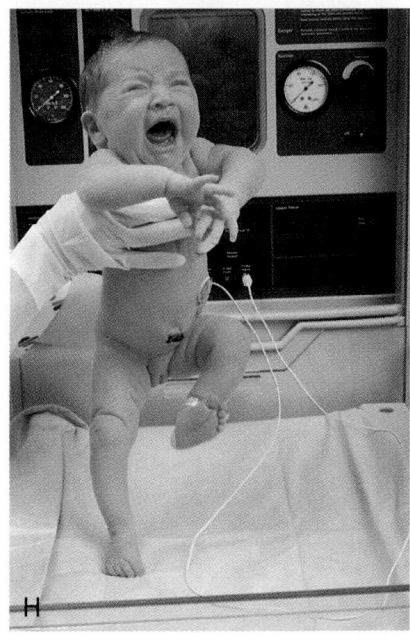

H. Stepping reflex.
The stepping reflex occurs when infants are held upright with their feet touching a solid surface. They lift one foot and then the other, giving the appearance that they are trying to walk.

FIGURE 22–14
. . . .
Continued

tremities are held in a flexed position. This position causes tremors to stop, but a seizure continues. Seizure activity may also include abnormal movements of the eyes or mouth and other subtle signs. Any infant thought to be having seizures is referred for further assessment and treatment.

The pitch of the cry is important. A shrill or high-pitched cry, a cat-like "mewing," or a hoarse cry is abnormal. These cries may indicate a neurologic disorder or other problem.

Normal infants respond to holding and appear content when their needs are met. Rocking motions are often effective in quieting an irritable infant. Most infants "mold" their bodies to that of the people holding them, making them easy to hold and cuddle. The neonate who stiffens the body, pulls away from contact, or arches the back when held is showing signs of central nervous system damage. Infants should react to painful stimuli with crying and an increase in vital signs. Excessive irritability may also be a sign of damage to the nervous system. All such abnormal signs are reported for further neurologic assessment.

Gastrointestinal System

The initial assessment of the gastrointestinal tract occurs during the first hours after birth, as the nurse observes the parts that can be seen and the infant takes the initial feeding.

MOUTH

The mouth is inspected visually and by palpation. Some infants are born with precocious teeth, usually incisors. If the teeth are loose, the physician usually removes them to prevent aspiration. Epstein's pearls are small, white, hard cysts on the hard palate that disappear without treatment.

The nurse examines the tongue for size and movement. A large, protruding tongue is present in hypothyroidism and chromosomal disorders such as Down syndrome. Paralysis of the facial nerve causes drooping of the mouth and affects the movement of the tongue.

Although candidiasis (thrush) is not apparent in the mouth immediately after birth, it may appear a day or two later. The lesions resemble milk curds on the tongue and cheeks that

TABLE 22-2

Summary of Neonatal Reflexes

Reflex	Method of Testing	Expected Response	Abnormal Response/ Possible Cause	Time Reflex Disappears
Babinski	Stroke lateral sole of foot from heel to across base of toes.	Toes flare with dorsiflexion of the big toe.	No response. Bilateral: CNS deficit. Unilateral: local nerve damage.	12 mo
Gallant (trunk incurvation)	Lightly stroke the back lateral to the vertebral column.	Entire trunk flexes toward side stimulated.	No response: CNS deficit.	1 mo
Grasp reflex (palmar and plantar)	Press finger against base of fingers or toes.	Fingers curl tightly; toes curl forward.	Weak or absent: neurologic deficit or muscle damage.	Palmar grasp lessens 3–4 mo, disappears by 5–6 mo. Plantar grasp disappears by 8–9 mo.
Moro	Let infant's head drop back approximately 30 degrees.	Sharp extension and abduction of arms with thumbs and forefingers in "C" position. Followed by flexion and adduction to "embrace" position. Legs follow similar pattern.	Absent: CNS dysfunction. Asymmetry: brachial plexus injury, paralysis, or fractured clavicle or bone of extremity. Exaggerated: maternal drug use.	6 mo
Rooting	Touch or stroke side of cheek near mouth.	Infant turns to side touched. Difficult to elicit if infant sleeping or just fed.	Weak or absent; prematurity, neurologic deficit, depression from maternal drug use.	3–4 mo
Startle	Make a loud noise.	Similar to Moro, but hands remain clenched.	Weak or absent: neurologic damage, deafness.	4 mo
Stepping	Hold infant so feet touch solid surface.	Infant lifts alternate feet as if walking.	Asymmetry: fracture of extremity, neurologic deficit.	4–7 mo
Sucking	Place nipple or finger in mouth, rub against palate.	Infant begins to suck. May be weak if recently fed.	Weak or absent: prematurity, neurologic deficit, maternal drug use.	Well coordinated with swallow by 34–36 wk of gestation. Disappears by 1 yr.
Swallowing	Place fluid on the back of the tongue.	Infant swallows fluid. Should be coordinated with sucking.	Coughing, gagging, choking, cyanosis: tracheoesophageal fistula, esophageal atresia, neurologic deficit.	Present throughout life.
Tonic neck reflex	Gently turn head to one side while infant is supine.	Exension of extremities on side to which head turned, with flexion on opposite side.	Prolonged period in position: neurologic deficit.	May be weak at birth and increase to 1 mo, then disappears by 4 mo.

CNS = central nervous system.

What might be the effect on normal development if reflexes are retained beyond the age when they should disappear?

bleed if attempts are made to wipe them away. Newborns may become infected with *Candida albicans* during passage through the birth canal if the mother has a candidal vaginal infection. The infant is treated with nystatin suspension.

A cleft lip or palate results if the lip or palate fails to close (see Chapter 43). Cleft palate may involve the hard or the soft palate or both, and the condition may appear

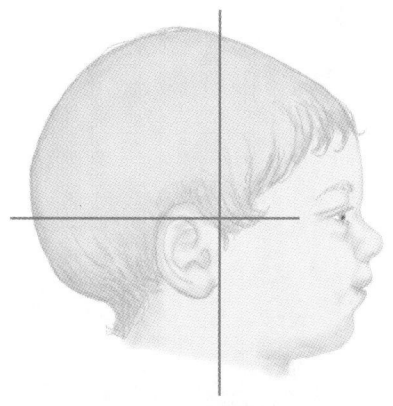

Normal ear location

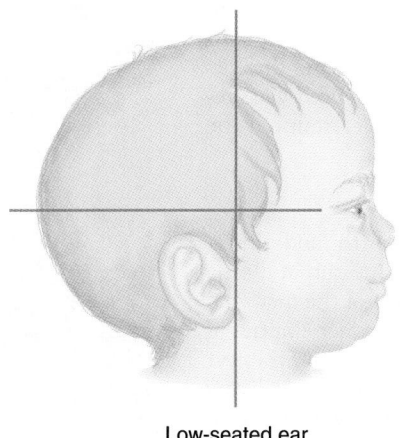

Low-seated ear

FIGURE 22-15
· · · · · · · · · ·
An imaginary line is drawn from the inner to the outer canthus of the eye and then to the ear. The line should intersect with the area where the upper ear joins the head.

alone or with a cleft lip. The palate is inspected when the infant cries. A gloved finger is inserted into the mouth to palpate both the hard and the soft palate. A very small cleft of the soft palate may be missed if only a visual examination is done.

SUCK

The normal full-term infant should have a strong suck reflex, which is elicited when the lips or palate are stimulated. The reflex is weaker in the neonate who is preterm, ill, or has just been fed. The newborn's cheeks have well-developed muscles and sucking pads that enhance the ability to suck.

ABDOMEN

The abdomen should be rounded and protrude slightly but should not be distended. A distended abdomen with stretched, shiny skin may indicate obstruction. Loops of bowel should not be visible through the abdominal wall. Visible bowel could indicate that air and meconium are not passing through the intestines normally.

A sunken or scaphoid appearance of the abdomen occurs in diaphragmatic hernia, in which the intestines are located in the chest cavity instead of the abdomen (see Chapter 43). The nurse listens over the abdomen for bowel sounds, which usually appear within the first hour after birth. Bowel sounds heard in the chest may indicate diaphragmatic hernia.

An umbilical hernia occurs when the intestinal muscles fail to close around the umbilicus, allowing the intestines to protrude through the weak area. The condition is more common in African-American infants. It often disappears when the infant is walking well, although some hernias require surgical repair.

Palpating the abdomen is easiest when the infant is relaxed and quiet. The abdomen should feel soft because the muscles are not yet well developed. Masses may indicate tumors of the kidneys. Palpation of the liver is usually not part of the routine nursing assessment of the abdomen. When palpated, it is normally felt no more than 1 to 3 cm below the right costal margin. If the organ seems large, it should be reported to the physician or nurse practitioner because it may be a sign of congestive heart failure or congenital infection.

INITIAL FEEDING

The initial feeding is an opportunity to assess the newborn further. The nurse observes for choking, coughing, and cyanosis, indicating a connection between the trachea and the esophagus, such as tracheoesophageal fistula. If the mother is breast-feeding, the nurse can observe the infant's response unobtrusively while assisting the mother to position the infant. To decrease regurgitation from overdistension of the stomach, a formula feeding should be no more than 1 ounce.

The infant's ability to suck, swallow, and breathe in a coordinated manner is evaluated. Some newborns choke or gag during the first feeding. Others may become dusky or cyanotic because they become apneic while they are feeding. In either case, the nurse should stop the feeding immediately, suction if necessary, and stimulate the infant to cry by rubbing the back.

Most infants learn to coordinate sucking, swallowing, and breathing by the time the first feeding is finished. Neonates who continue to have difficulty may have a cardiac anomaly (see Chapter 46), tracheoesophageal fistula, or esophageal atresia (see Chapter 43). Infants with tracheoesophageal fistula or esophageal atresia may also drool excessively. Further assessment and referral are necessary.

STOOLS

Stools should be assessed for normal color and consistency. There should never be a "water ring" around the solid part of any stool. This indicates diarrhea, with the watery part absorbed into the diaper.

The nurse should be aware of the time that the infant's last stool occurred and whether any stools have been passed since birth. Most newborns pass the first meconium stool within 24 hours of birth.

Genitourinary System

KIDNEY PALPATION

Palpation of the kidneys is not usually part of the routine nursing assessment of the newborn. The kidneys may be felt, however, just above the level of the umbilicus on each side of the abdomen during the first hours after birth. Abdominal masses may indicate enlargement or tumors of the kidneys. Anomalies of the kidney may accompany other defects because an insult early in fetal development often affects all organs being formed at that time. For example, an infant with only one umbilical artery or defects involving the ears may have renal anomalies. The nurse should observe carefully for urinary output in these infants to determine if the kidneys are functioning.

URINE

Most newborns void within 24 hours of birth, and almost all void by 48 hours. Because absence of urine output during this time may indicate anomalies, the time of the first void is recorded on the chart. The newborn's bladder empties as little as two to six times during the first 2 days, and the first void may be missed. Sometimes it occurs in the delivery room but goes unnoticed because attention is focused on the infant's overall condition. If there is no void in the expected time, the physician or nurse practitioner is alerted.

After the first 2 days of life, the newborn's bladder empties 5 to 25 times each day. Each void is recorded in the infant's chart, including diapers the mother changes. The total number is correlated with what is appropriate for the age of the infant. Mothers should be taught that approximately six to ten wet diapers, after the first 2 days, indicate the infant is taking adequate fluid.

The newborn's urine may contain urate crystals that cause a reddish or pink stain on the diaper. This is known as "brick dust staining" and may be frightening to parents, who may think the infant is bleeding. It does not continue beyond the first few days as the kidneys mature.

GENITALIA

Female. In the full-term female infant, the labia majora should be large and completely cover the clitoris and labia minora. The labia may be darker than the surrounding skin from exposure to the mother's hormones before birth. Edema of the labia and white mucous vaginal discharge are normal. A small amount of vaginal bleeding, known as pseudomenstruation, may occur from the sudden withdrawal of the mother's hormones at birth. Hymenal or vaginal tags are small pieces of tissue at the vaginal orifice. These are normal and disappear in a few weeks. The urinary meatus and vagina should be present.

Male. The scrotum should be pendulous at term and may be dark brown from maternal hormones. Pressure during a breech delivery may cause it to be edematous. Rugae (creases in the scrotum) are deep and cover the entire scrotum in the full-term infant. Enlargement of one or both sides of the scrotum may be due to a hydrocele, a collection of fluid around the testes.

Palpation of the scrotum determines if the testes have descended (Fig. 22–16). Testes feel like small, round, movable objects that "slip" between the fingers. If the testes are not present in the scrotal sac, they may be felt in the inguinal canal. Undescended testis (cryptorchidism) occurs on one or both sides. An empty scrotal sac appears smaller than one with testes (see Chapter 44).

The meatus should be at the tip of the glans penis. It may be abnormally located on the underside of the penis (hypospadias), on the upper side (epispadias), or on the perineum. The prepuce, or foreskin, of the penis covers the glans and is adherent to it. Attempts to retract it in the newborn are unnecessary and can cause damage. Abnormal

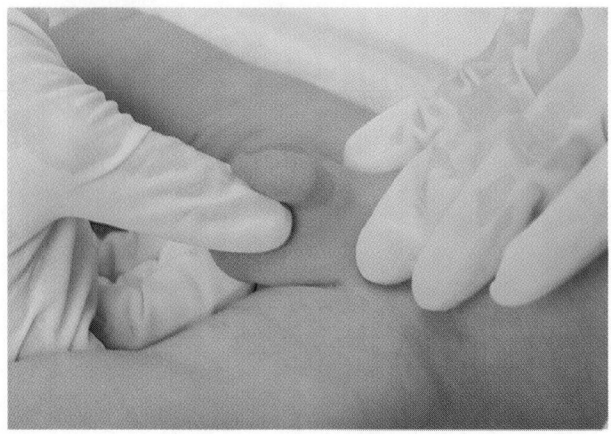

FIGURE 22–16

The testes are palpated from front to back with the thumb and forefinger. Placing a finger over the inguinal canal holds the testes in place for palpation.

placement of the meatus may not be visible because it is covered by the prepuce, but often the prepuce in these infants is incompletely formed. Hypospadias may be accompanied by chordee, a condition in which fibrotic tissue causes the penis to curve downward (see Chapter 44).

Parents are very concerned about any abnormalities of the genitalia. If the meatus is abnormally positioned, they need an explanation of the condition and why the infant may not be circumcised. The foreskin may be needed for later plastic surgery to repair the defect.

Integumentary System

SKIN

The skin of the newborn is fragile, and reddened areas or rashes may develop during the early days of life. The nurse must examine every inch of skin surface carefully during the initial assessment and at the beginning of each shift.

Color. The newborn's skin should be pink or tan. Red, thin skin occurs in preterm infants. Redness (ruddy color) in the full-term infant may indicate polycythemia. Acrocyanosis is common during the first day or two as a result of poor peripheral circulation. The infant's mouth and central body areas should not be cyanotic at any time. Blanching the skin over the nose or chest shows the presence of jaundice. Jaundice is abnormal during the first day of life but common during the first week.

A greenish-brown discoloration of the skin, nails, and cord results if meconium was passed before birth. This discoloration may indicate that the infant was compromised at some time before birth, and it is more common in the post-term infant. These infants must be watched for other complications, such as respiratory difficulty.

Vernix Caseosa. Vernix, a thick, white substance, resembles cream cheese and provides a protective covering for the fetal skin in utero. The full-term infant has little vernix left on the body except small amounts in the creases. A thick covering of vernix may indicate a preterm infant. Yellow-tinged vernix may indicate elevated bilirubin levels

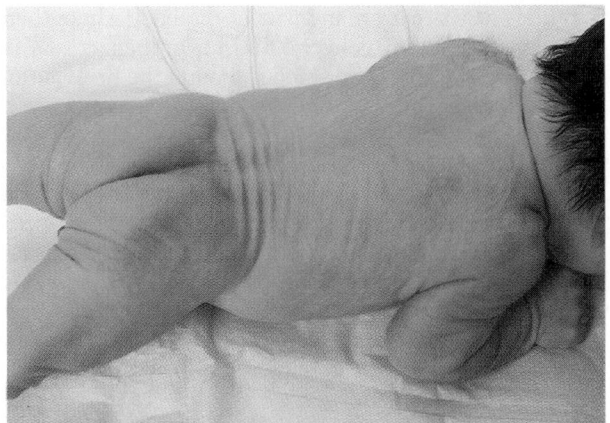

FIGURE 22–17
Lanugo is abundant on this slightly preterm infant.

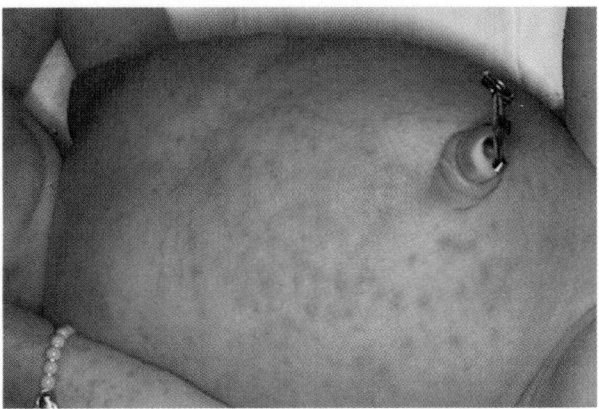

FIGURE 22–19
Erythema toxicum. (From Hurwitz, S. [1993]. *Clinical pediatric dermatology* (2nd ed., p. 13). Philadelphia: Saunders.)

in utero, and green-tinged vernix is due to meconium staining.

Lanugo. Lanugo is fine hair that covers the fetus during intrauterine life (Fig. 22–17). It is assessed with the gestational age assessment.

Milia. Milia are white cysts, 1 to 2 mm in size, due to distension of sebaceous glands (oil glands) that are not yet functioning properly. They occur on the face over the forehead, nose, and chin and disappear within 2 months without treatment (Fig. 22–18).

Erythema Toxicum. The nurse notes the presence of erythema toxicum, red, blotchy areas that may have white or yellow papules in the center (Fig. 22–19). It is commonly called "flea bite" rash or newborn rash and resembles small bites or acne. The rash appears during the first 24 to 48

hours after birth, although occasionally not until 1 to 2 weeks. It is most common over the back, shoulders, and chest. The cause of erythema toxicum is unknown, and it disappears within hours or up to 10 days.

Birthmarks. The size, location, color, elevation, and texture of all birthmarks should be carefully documented. Marks should be explained to parents, who are often concerned.

- Mongolian spots are bluish-black marks that resemble bruises on the sacrum, buttocks, arms, shoulders, or other areas (Fig. 22–20). They occur most frequently in newborns with dark skin and usually disappear after the first few years of life. Some continue into adulthood.
- A telangiectatic nevus is sometimes called nevus simplex or a "stork bite" (Fig. 22–21). It is a flat pink or reddish discoloration from dilated capillaries that occurs on the eyelids, bridge of the nose, or nape of the neck. The color blanches when pressed and is more prominent during crying. Stork bites disappear by age 2 years, although those at the nape of the neck may persist.
- Nevus flammeus (port wine stain) is a permanent, flat, dark reddish-purple mark (Fig. 22–22). It varies in size

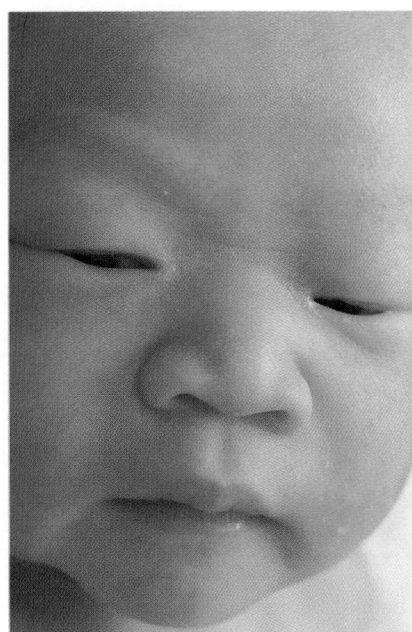

FIGURE 22–18
Milia.

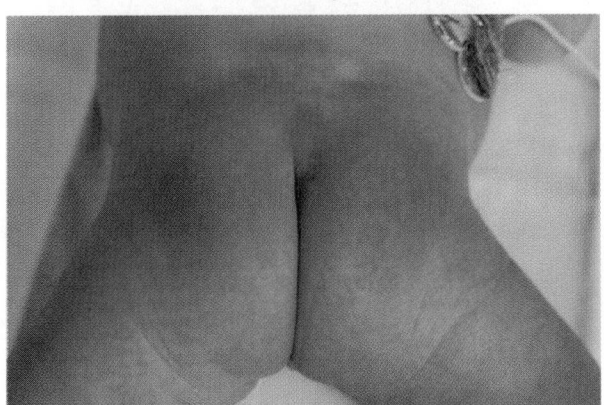

FIGURE 22–20
Mongolian spots.

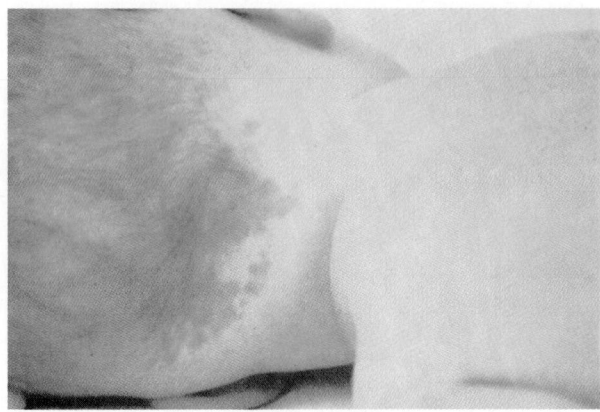

and location and does not blanch with pressure. It can be removed by laser surgery.

- Nevus vasculosus (strawberry hemangioma) consists of enlarged capillaries in the outer layers of skin. It is dark red and raised with a rough surface, giving a strawberry-like appearance. The hemangioma is usually located on the head. It may grow larger for 5 to 6 months but usually disappears by the early school years. No treatment is necessary.
- Café au lait spots are permanent, light brown areas that may occur anywhere on the body. Although they are harmless, the number and size are important. More than six spots or spots larger than 1.5 cm are associated with neurofibromatosis, a genetic condition of neural tissue.

Marks from Delivery. The nurse inspects the infant for marks that may have occurred from injury or pressure during labor or delivery.

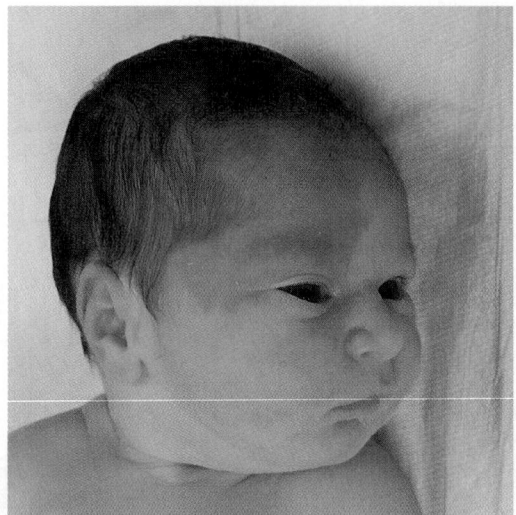

FIGURE 22–22

Port wine stain.

- Bruises may occur on any part of the body where there was pressure during delivery. Bruising of the face may be present if the cord was wrapped around the neck during birth. Bruising on the head may occur from use of a vacuum extractor.
- Petechiae, pinpoint bruises that resemble a rash, may appear over areas such as the back or face. They are due to pressure during the birth process. Widespread petechiae or continued formation of petechiae may indicate infection or a low platelet count.
- A small puncture mark is present on the newborn's head if a fetal monitor scalp electrode was attached. The area should scab and heal normally but should be observed for signs of infection.
- Forceps marks occur over the cheeks and ears where the instruments were applied. They are carefully documented as to size, color, and location. Lack of movement or symmetry of the face may indicate damage to the facial nerve.

Other Aspects of Skin Assessment. The nurse notes other aspects of the skin that may indicate abnormalities. Localized edema may be due to trauma of delivery. Generalized edema indicates more serious conditions, such as heart failure. Peeling of the skin is normal in full-term newborns. Excessive amounts of peeling may indicate a post-term infant.

BREASTS

The nurse notes the placement of the nipples and looks for extra (or supernumerary) nipples, which may appear on the chest or in the axilla. Occasionally, the breasts become engorged and secrete a small amount of white fluid (sometimes called "witch's milk"). This condition is due to hormones from the mother. It resolves within a few weeks without treatment.

HAIR AND NAILS

The hair on the full-term infant should be silky and soft, whereas that on the preterm infant is woolly or fuzzy. The nails come to the end of the fingers or beyond. Very long nails may indicate a post-term infant.

Assessment of Gestational Age

The gestational age assessment is an examination of the newborn to determine the number of weeks from conception to birth. The determination is based on physical and neurologic characteristics. It is important because neonates born before or after term and those whose size is not appropriate for gestational age are at increased risk for complications.

Assessment Tools

The New Ballard Score (Fig. 22–23) is frequently used to determine gestational age based on neuromuscular and physical characteristics. A score is given to each assessment, and the total score is used to determine the gestational age of the infant.

NEWBORN MATURITY RATING & CLASSIFICATION

ESTIMATION OF GESTATIONAL AGE BY MATURITY RATING
Symbols: X - 1st Exam   O - 2nd Exam

Gestation by Dates _____ wks

Birth Date _____ Hour _____ am/pm

APGAR _____ 1 min _____ 5 min

NEUROMUSCULAR MATURITY

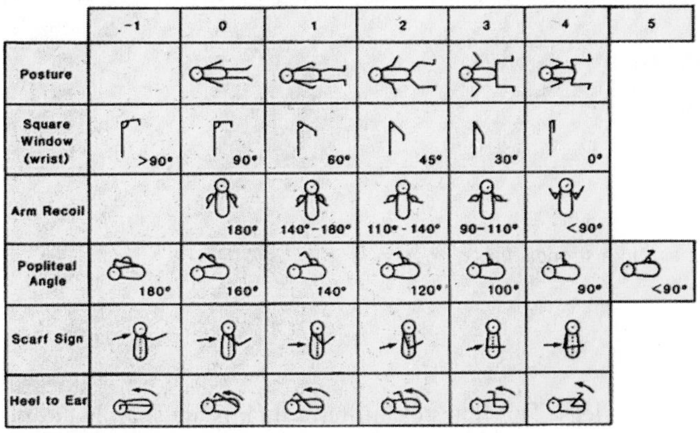

	-1	0	1	2	3	4	5
Posture							
Square Window (wrist)	>90°	90°	60°	45°	30°	0°	
Arm Recoil		180°	140°-180°	110°-140°	90°-110°	<90°	
Popliteal Angle	180°	160°	140°	120°	100°	90°	<90°
Scarf Sign							
Heel to Ear							

PHYSICAL MATURITY

Skin	sticky friable transparent	gelatinous red, translucent	smooth pink, visible veins	superficial peeling &/or rash. few veins	cracking pale areas rare veins	parchment deep cracking no vessels	leathery cracked wrinkled
Lanugo	none	sparse	abundant	thinning	bald areas	mostly bald	
Plantar Surface	heel-toe 40-50mm:-1 <40 mm:-2	>50mm no crease	faint red marks	anterior transverse crease only	creases ant. 2/3	creases over entire sole	
Breast	imperceptible	barely perceptible	flat areola no bud	stippled areola 1-2mm bud	raised areola 3-4mm bud	full areola 5-10mm bud	
Eye/Ear	lids fused loosely:-1 tightly:-2	lids open pinna flat stays folded	sl. curved pinna; soft; slow recoil	well-curved pinna; soft but ready recoil	formed &firm instant recoil	thick cartilage ear stiff	
Genitals male	scrotum flat, smooth	scrotum empty faint rugae	testes in upper canal rare rugae	testes descending few rugae	testes down good rugae	testes pendulous deep rugae	
Genitals female	clitoris prominent labia flat	prominent clitoris small labia minora	prominent clitoris enlarging minora	majora & minora equally prominent	majora large minora small	majora cover clitoris & minora	

MATURITY RATING

score	weeks
-10	20
-5	22
0	24
5	26
10	28
15	30
20	32
25	34
30	36
35	38
40	40
45	42
50	44

SCORING SECTION

	1st Exam=X	2nd Exam=O
Estimating Gest Age by Maturity Rating	_____ Weeks	_____ Weeks
Time of Exam	Date_____ Hour_____ am/pm	Date_____ Hour_____ am/pm
Age at Exam	_____ Hours	_____ Hours
Signature of Examiner	_____ M.D.	_____ M.D.

FIGURE 22-23

New Ballard Score. (Courtesy of Bristol-Myers Company, Evansville, Indiana. From Ballard, J. L., Khoury, J. C., Wedig, K., Wang, L., Eilers-Walsman, B. L., & Lipp, R. [1991]. New Ballard Score, expanded to include extremely premature infants. *Journal of Pediatrics, 19*(3), 417–423.)

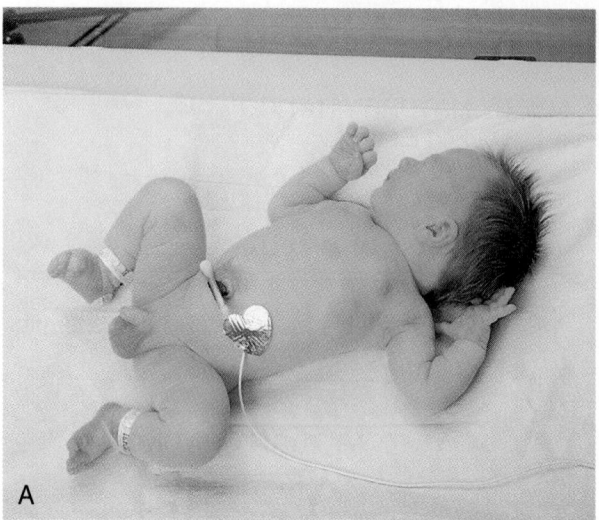
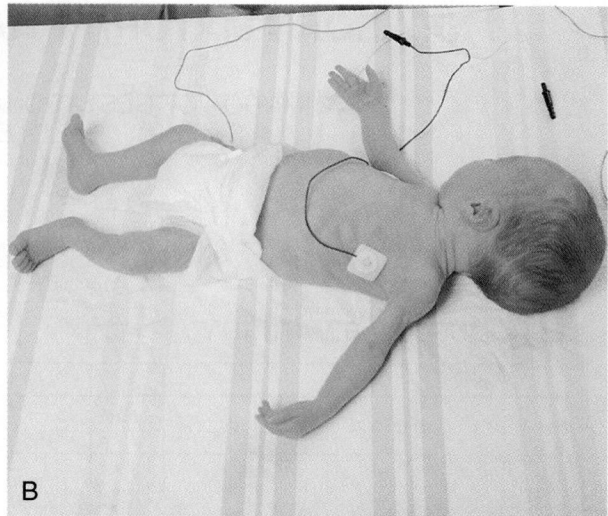

FIGURE 22-24

Posture in newborns. *A,* The healthy, full-term infant remains in a strongly flexed position. *B,* The preterm infant's extremities are extended.

Neuromuscular Characteristics

POSTURE

The posture and degree of flexion of the extremities are scored before disturbing the quiet infant to perform the remainder of the examination (Fig. 22–24). Preterm neonates with immature flexor muscles have extended, limp arms and legs. The limbs of full-term infants are sharply flexed. The legs should be flexed at the hips, knees, and ankles.

SQUARE WINDOW

The square window sign is elicited by bending the hand at the wrist until the palm is as flat against the forearm as possible with gentle pressure (Fig. 22–25). The angle be-

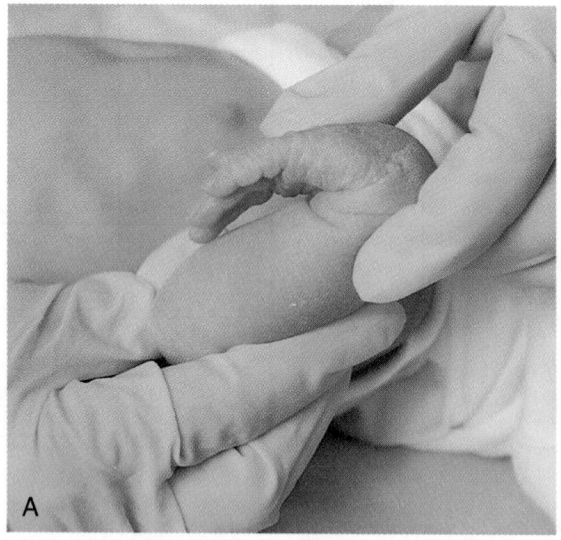
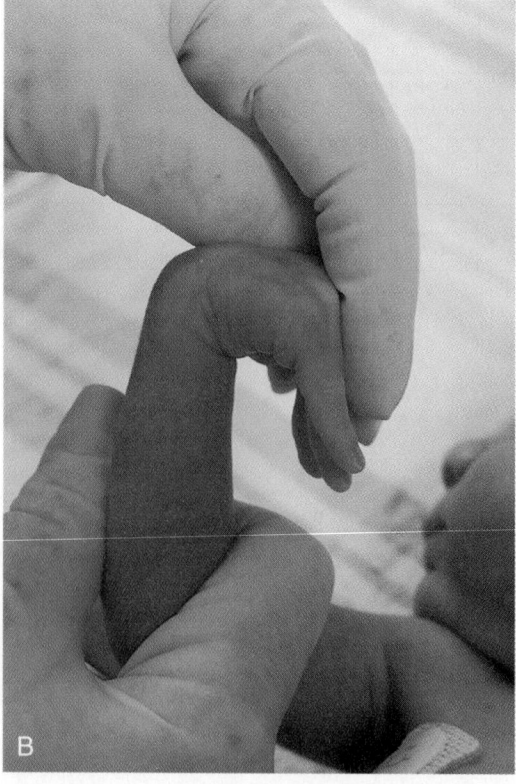

FIGURE 22-25

The square window sign is performed on the arm without the identification bracelet. The nurse bends the wrist and measures the angle. *A,* Infant near full term. *B,* Preterm infant.

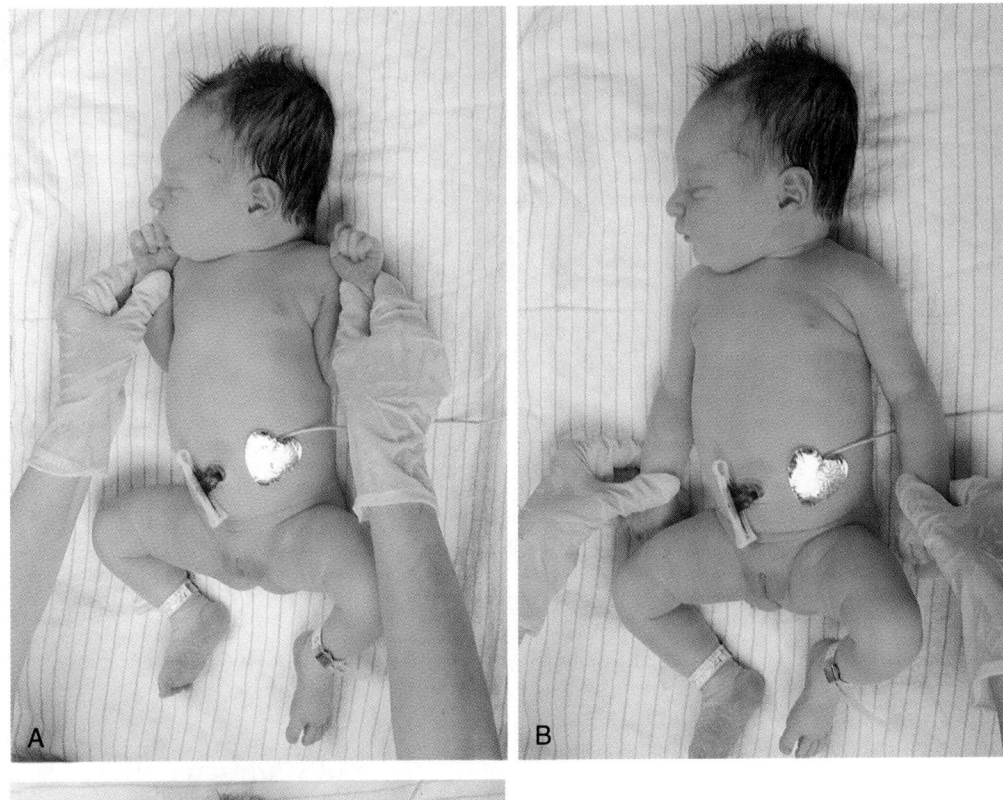

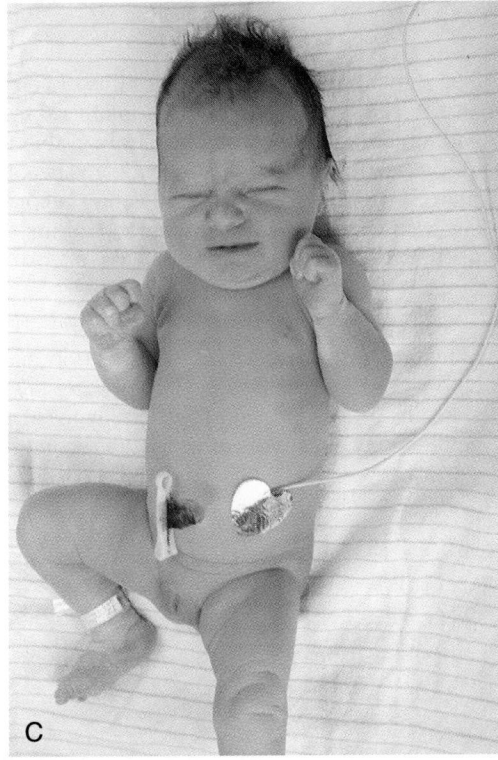

FIGURE 22–26
• • • • • • • •
Arm recoil. *A*, Arms flexed. *B*, Arms extended.
C, Recoil for the full-term infant.

tween the palm and the forearm is measured. The more mature the neonate, the smaller the angle, until the palm folds flat against the forearm at term.

ARM RECOIL
To test for arm recoil, the nurse holds the neonate's arms fully flexed at the elbows for 5 seconds, then pulls the hands straight down to the sides (Fig. 22–26). The hands are

quickly released and the degree of flexion is measured as the arms return to their normally flexed position. Preterm infants may not move the arms at all, whereas the full-term infant has a quick return to flexion.

POPLITEAL ANGLE
To measure the popliteal angle, the newborn's lower leg is folded against the thigh, with the thigh on the abdomen

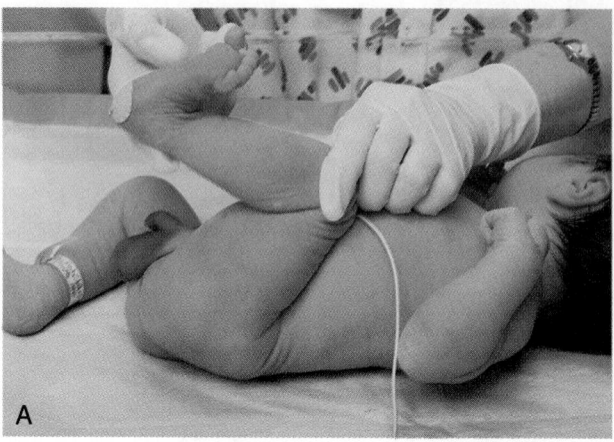
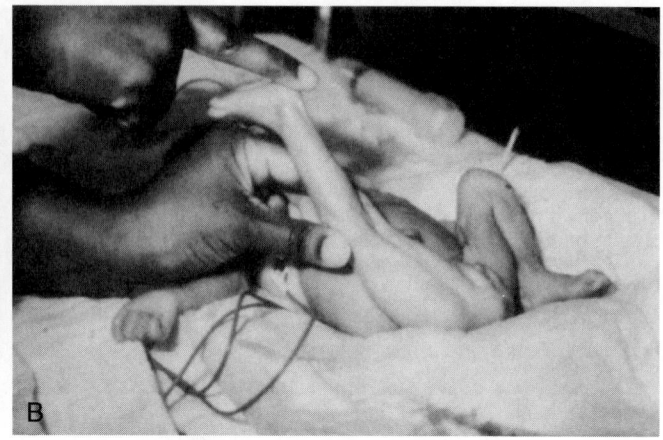

FIGURE 22-27

The popliteal angle is measured by flexing the thigh against the abdomen and extending the lower leg to the point of resistance. *A*, Full-term infant. *B*, Preterm infant.

(Fig. 22–27). Then the lower leg is straightened just until resistance is met. Continued pressure causes the infant to extend the leg further and results in an inaccurate score. The angle at the popliteal space is scored when resistance is first felt.

SCARF SIGN

For the scarf sign, the nurse grasps the infant's hand and brings the arm across the body to the opposite side, keeping the shoulder flat on the bed (Fig. 22–28). The position of the elbow in relation to the midline of the infant's body is noted.

HEEL TO EAR

For the heel-to-ear assessment, the nurse grasps the infant's foot and pulls it straight up toward the ears while the hips remain flat on the surface of the bed (Fig. 22–29). When resistance is first felt, the position of the foot in relation to the head and the amount of flexion of the leg are compared with the diagrams. The more resistance and flexion, the more mature the infant.

Physical Characteristics

SKIN

The skin is assessed for color, visibility of veins, and peeling and cracking. The very preterm infant's skin is red, sticky, and fragile, with veins that are easily visible. In the mature newborn, the skin color is paler; few veins are visible; and there is peeling and cracking. Peeling becomes even more apparent in the post-term infant and during the hours after birth as the skin loses moisture (Fig. 22–30).

LANUGO

Lanugo appears at 20 weeks of gestation and increases in amount until 28 to 30 weeks (see Fig. 22–17). At that time, it begins to disappear until little remains at term. A small amount may remain over the upper back and shoulders, over

FIGURE 22-28

Scarf sign. The nurse determines how far the arm will move across the chest and observes the position of the elbow when resistance is felt. *A*, Full-term infant. *B*, Preterm infant. (Note the many visible veins in the preterm infant and the absence of visible veins in the full-term infant.)

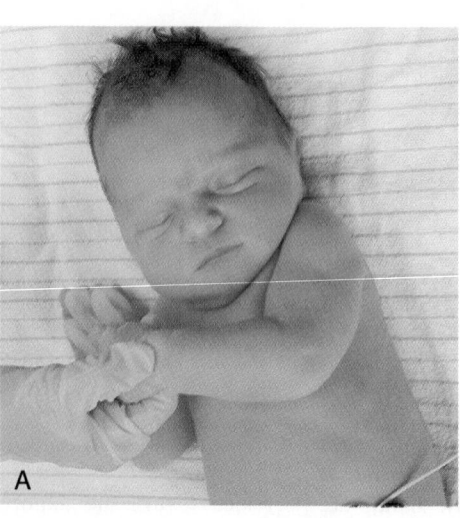
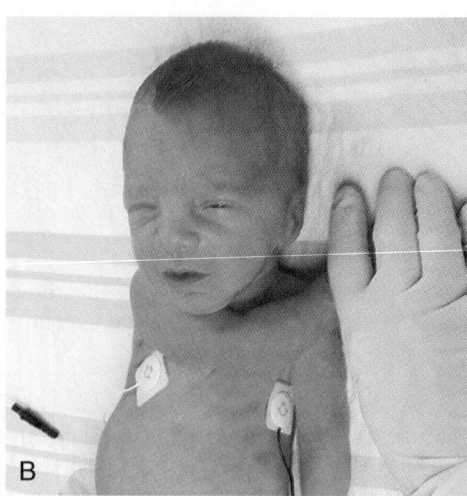

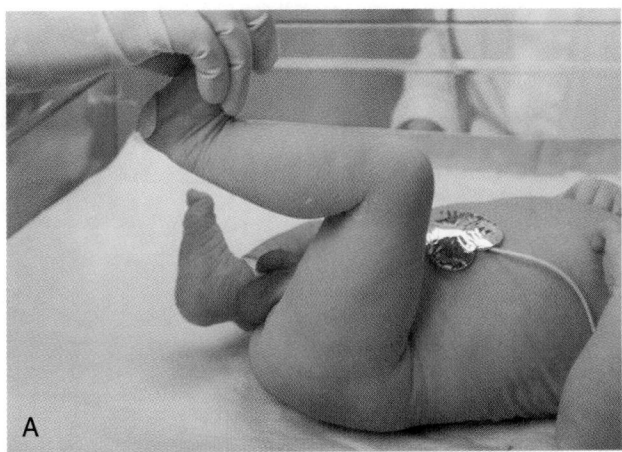
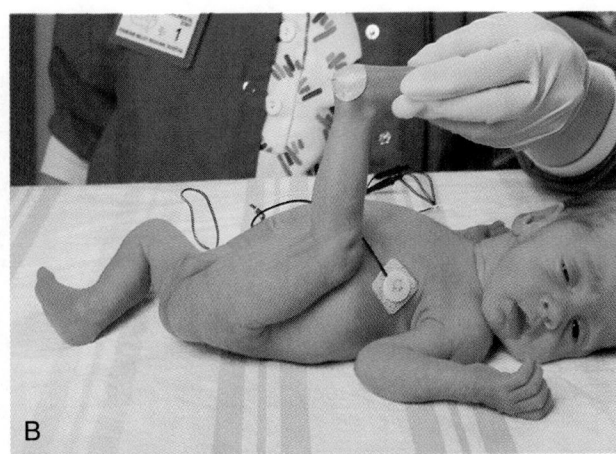

A   **B**

FIGURE 22–29

· · · · · · · · · ·

Heel to ear. The nurse grasps the foot and brings it up toward the ear, keeping the hips flat. The score is recorded when resistance is felt. *A*, Full-term infant. *B*, Preterm infant.

the ears, or on the sides of the forehead. Newborns with dark coloring may have more lanugo (which is dark and more easily noticed) than infants with fair skin and very light hair even though they are the same gestational age. The infant receives a score based on the amount of lanugo present.

PLANTAR SURFACE

Plantar creases begin to appear at 32 weeks of gestation and gradually spread down toward the heel and become deeper

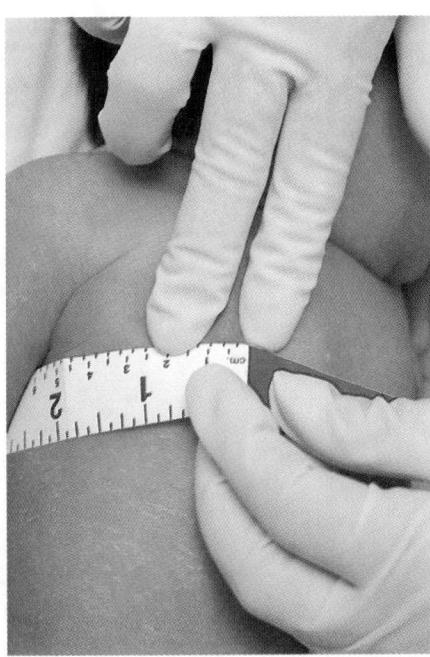

FIGURE 22–30

· · · · · · · · · ·

The nurse places a finger on either side of the breast bud tissue and measures the size. In the full-term infant, breast tissue is raised and the nipple is easily distinguished from surrounding skin. (Note the peeling skin.)

(Fig. 22–31). The plantar creases must be assessed during the early hours after birth because, as the infant's skin begins to dry, the creases appear more prominent.

BREASTS

The formation of the nipples and areolae and size of the subcutaneous fat pads (or breast buds) are assessed and scored. To determine the size of the fat pads, the nurse places a finger on each side and measures the diameter (see Fig. 22–30). Use of the thumb and forefinger may cause excess tissue to be drawn together, resulting in an inaccurate score.

EYES AND EARS

The eyelids are fused until 26 to 28 weeks. The incurving of the upper pinnae begins at the top and continues around the ear. In assessing the ear, the incurving and thickness of each pinna are rated (Fig. 22–32). The ear is folded to assess the resistance and how fast the ear returns to its original state. In infants younger than 32 weeks of gestational age, the ear has little cartilage to keep it stiff. In the term neonate, the ear springs back to its original position immediately.

GENITALS

In the female infant, the relationship in size of the clitoris, labia minora, and labia majora is noted (Fig. 22–33). As the infant nears term, the labia majora enlarge until the clitoris and labia minora are completely covered.

In the male infant, the location of the testes and the rugae on the scrotum are assessed (Fig. 22–34). The testes originate in the abdominal cavity but have moved through the inguinal canal into the scrotum by term. Rugae form on the surface of the scrotum beginning at approximately 36 weeks and cover the sac by 40 weeks. Once the testes are completely down into the scrotum, it appears large and pendulous.

Scoring

As each part of the assessment is performed, the infant's response is matched with the diagrams and explanations on

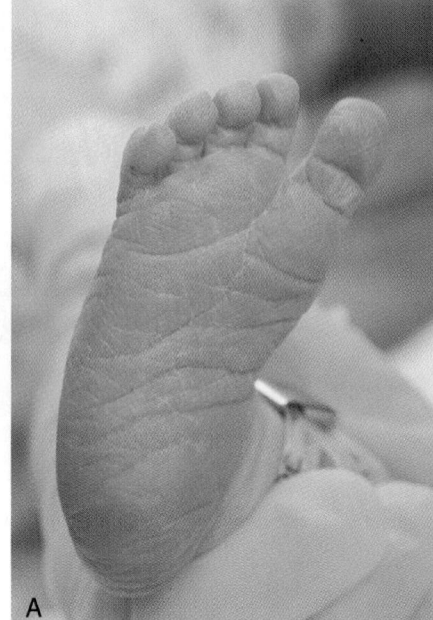
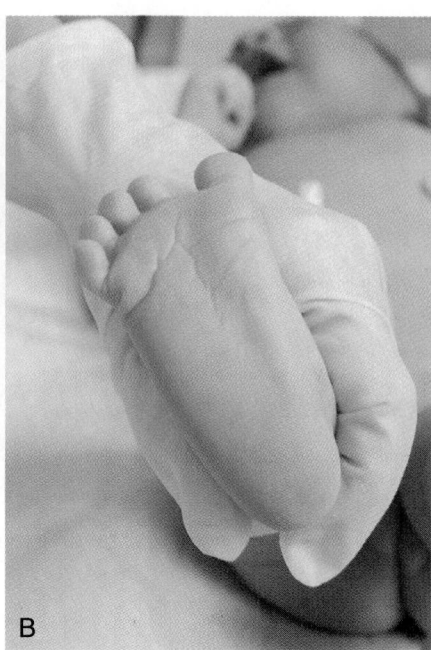

FIGURE 22-31

Plantar creases begin to develop at the base of the toes and extend to the heel. *A,* The post-term infant has deep creases. *B,* The preterm infant has few creases on the entire foot.

the assessment tool (Fig. 22–35). The total score is compared with the corresponding gestational age. It is important to understand that it is the total score of all assessed characteristics that determines the gestational age. One or two characteristics alone cannot be used to assign a gestational age.

Gestational Age and Infant Size

The appropriateness of the neonate's size for gestational age is determined by plotting the gestational age, weight, length, and head circumference on a graph of intrauterine development (see Fig. 22–35). This score determines how

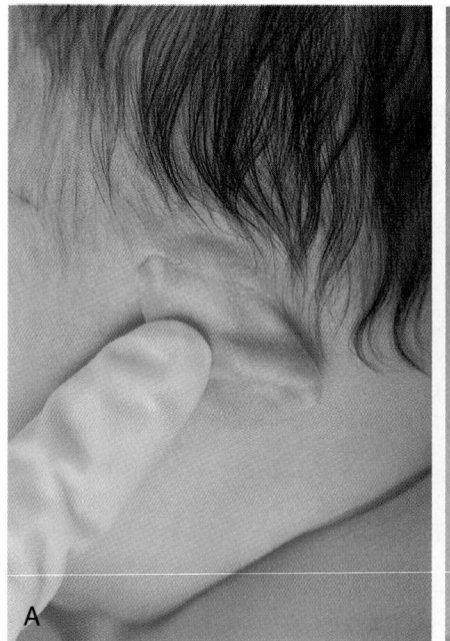
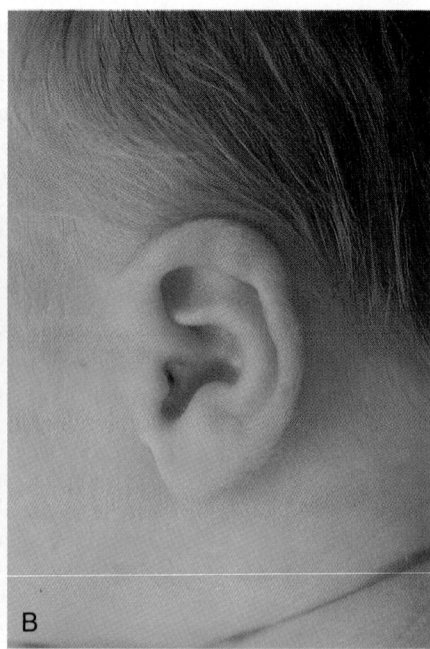
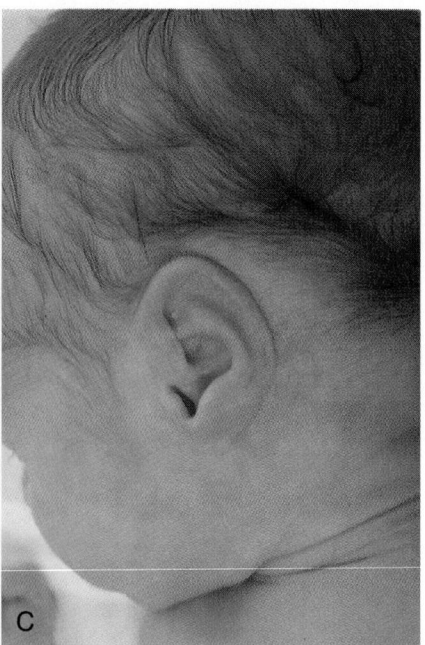

FIGURE 22-32

Ear maturation. *A,* The nurse folds the ears and notes how quickly they return to position. *B,* Ears in the full-term infant are well formed and have instant recoil. *C,* In the preterm infant, ears show less curving of the pinna and recoil slowly or not at all.

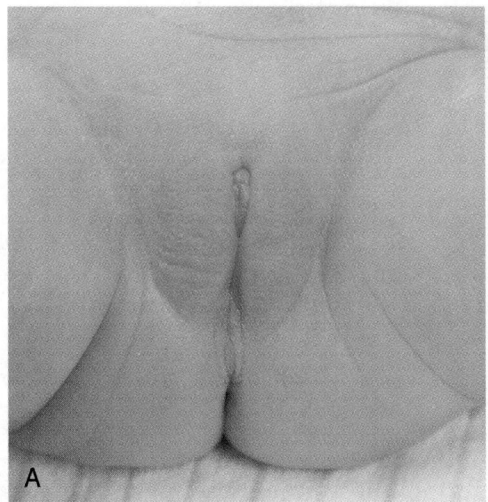 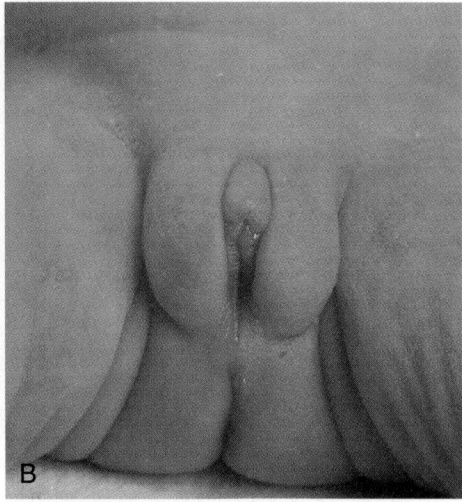

FIGURE 22-33

Female genitals. As the female fetus matures, the labia majora cover the labia minora and clitoris completely; in the preterm infant, these structures are not covered. *A*, Near-term infant. *B*, Preterm infant.

well the infant has grown for the amount of time spent in the uterus. The infant who is appropriate for gestational age falls between the 10th and the 90th percentiles on the graph. The large-for-gestational-age (LGA) infant is above the 90th percentile, whereas the small-for-gestational-age (SGA) infant is below the 10th percentile.

When an infant's gestational age or measurements fall outside the range expected, the nurse monitors for complications specific to the preterm, post-term, SGA, and LGA infant (see Chapter 29).

Assessment of Behavior

Assessment of the infant's behavior helps determine intactness of the central nervous system and provides information about ability to respond to caretaking activities.

Periods of Reactivity

During the first and second periods of reactivity (see p. 527–528), newborns may have elevated pulse and respiratory rates, low temperatures, and excessive respiratory secretions. It is important to observe infants carefully during this time. During the sleep period between the first and second periods of reactivity, newborns cannot be awakened easily and are not interested in feeding.

Behavioral Changes

Nurses assess the infant's behavior and alert the physician to abnormalities. Assessment includes the six different behavioral states: deep sleep, active sleep, drowsy, quiet alert, active alert, and crying. Movement between states should

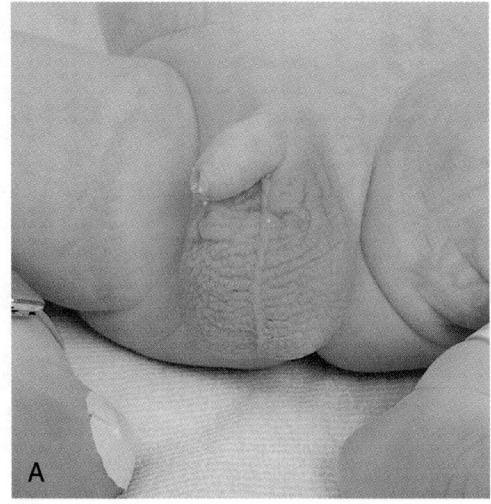 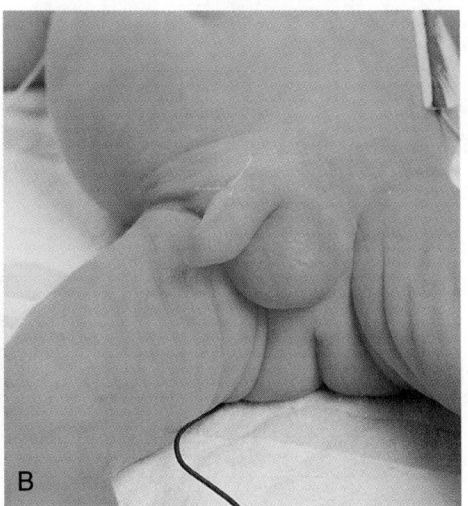

FIGURE 22-34

Male genitals. *A*, The full-term infant has a pendulous scrotum with deep rugae. *B*, In the preterm infant, the testes may not be descended and rugae are few.

CLASSIFICATION OF NEWBORNS –
BASED ON MATURITY AND INTRAUTERINE GROWTH
Symbols: X-1st Exam O-2nd Exam

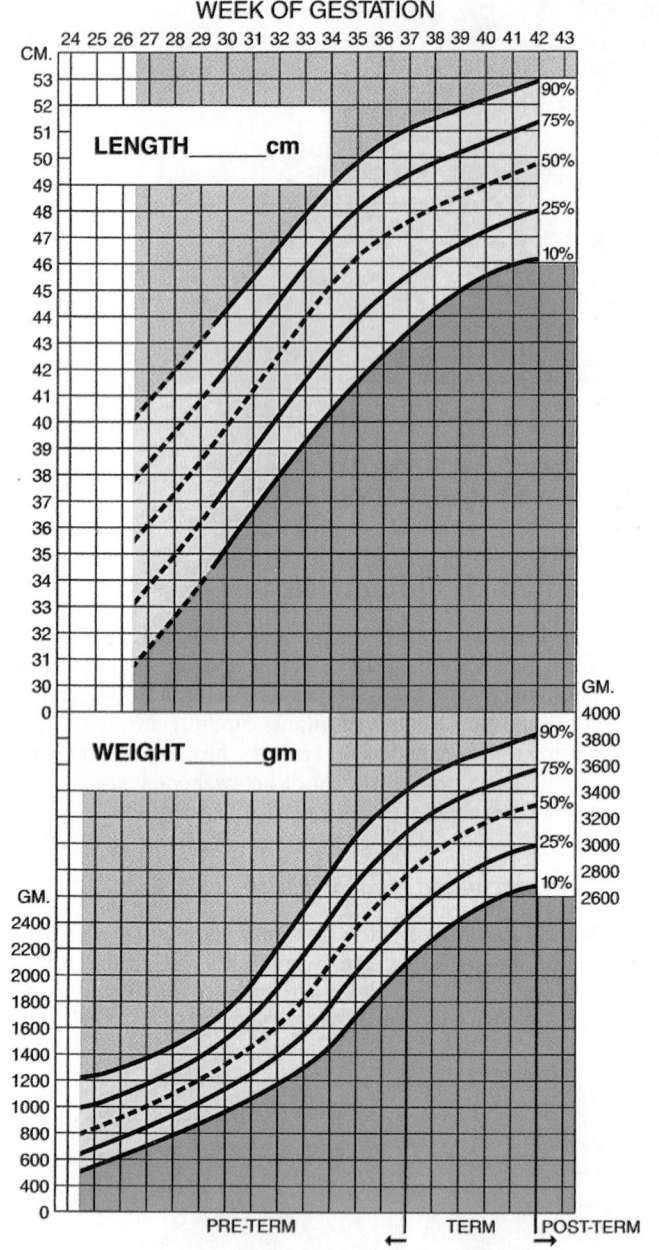

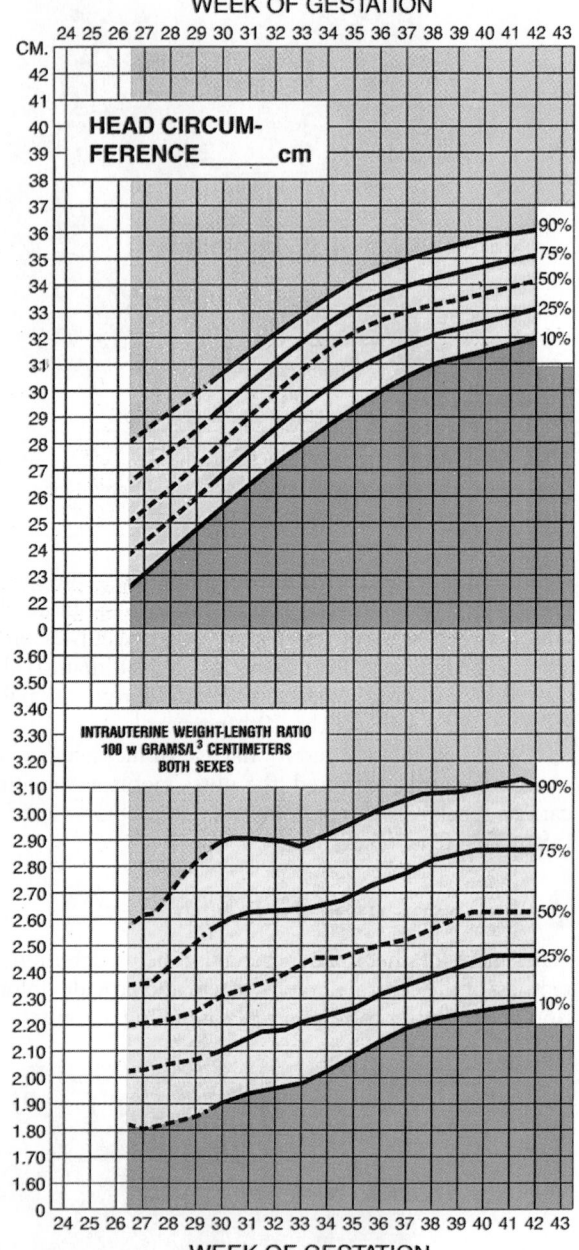

	1st Exam (X)	2nd Exam (O)
LARGE FOR GESTATIONAL AGE **(LGA)**		
APPROPRIATE FOR GESTATIONAL AGE **(AGA)**		
SMALL FOR GESTATIONAL AGE **(SGA)**		
Age at Exam	hrs	hrs
Signature of Examiner	M.D.	M.D.

FIGURE 22–35

Intrauterine growth grids. (Courtesy of Bristol-Myers Company, Evansville, Indiana. Adapted from Lubchenko, L. C., Hansman, C, & Boyd, E. [1966]. *Pediatrics, 37,* 403. Adapted by permission of Pediatrics, Vol. 37, p. 403, 1966; and from Battaglia, F. C., & Lubchenko, L. C. [1967]. *Journal of Pediatrics, 71,* 159.)

be smooth and not abrupt. The Brazelton Neonatal Behavioral Assessment Scale is often used when detailed knowledge about the infant is needed. In addition to assessing behavioral states, the scale analyzes other aspects of the newborn's behavior, such as orientation, habituation, self-consoling behaviors, and social behaviors.

ORIENTATION

The nurse notes the infant's orientation (ability to pay attention) to interesting visual or auditory stimuli. It is most prominent during the quiet alert state. Infants focus their eyes and turn their heads toward a stimulus in an attempt to prolong contact with it.

HABITUATION

The infant's response to a visual, auditory, or tactile stimulus is assessed. Usually, the first response of a healthy newborn to an interesting stimulus, such as a brightly colored object or a bell, is a period of alertness. If the stimulus is disturbing, like a bright light flashed in the eyes, the infant startles and attempts to escape by averting the eyes.

Infants gradually stop responding to continued noxious stimuli. This gradual habituation allows them to ignore the stimuli and save energy for physiologic needs. Newborns may go into a dull drowsy state or fall into a deep sleep. Those who seem unresponsive in a bright, noisy nursery may be in a state of habituation. The preterm infant or one with damage to the central nervous system may not be able to habituate.

SELF-CONSOLING ACTIVITIES

Normal newborns are able to console themselves for short periods. Self-consoling activities include attempting to bring their hands to the mouth and sucking on their fists. Infants who are ill, preterm, or exposed to drugs prenatally have less ability to console themselves.

PARENTS' RESPONSE

The parents' growing ability to respond to the infant's behavioral cues should be noted. To facilitate bonding and help the parents learn how to interpret the infant's cues, the nurse can point out the infant's behavioral changes.

KEY CONCEPTS

- Chemical, thermal, and mechanical factors combine to stimulate the respiratory center in the brain and initiate respirations at birth.
- Surfactant lines the alveoli and reduces surface tension to keep the alveoli open. Fetal lung fluid moves into the interstitial spaces before, during, and after birth and is absorbed by the lymphatic and vascular systems.
- Increases in blood oxygen levels, shifts in pressure in the heart and lungs, and closing of the umbilical vessels cause closure of the ductus arteriosus, foramen ovale, and ductus venosus at birth.
- Infants are predisposed to heat loss because they have thin skin with little subcutaneous fat, blood vessels close to the surface, and a large skin surface area. They lose heat by evaporation, conduction, convection, and radiation.
- Heat is produced in newborns by nonshivering thermogenesis, vasoconstriction, and an increase in metabolism. These factors increase oxygen and glucose consumption and may cause respiratory distress, hypoglycemia, acidosis, and jaundice.
- Laboratory values for erythrocytes, hemoglobin, and hematocrit are higher for newborns than for

adults because oxygen available to them in fetal life was less than after birth.
- The stools progress from thick, greenish-black meconium to loose, greenish-brown transitional stools to milk stools. Stools of breast-fed infants are frequent, soft, seedy, and mustard-colored, whereas those of formula-fed infants are pale yellow to light brown, firmer, and less frequent.
- The brain needs a constant supply of glucose and may be damaged without it.
- Physiologic jaundice occurs in normal newborns after the first 24 hours of life as a result of hemolysis of red blood cells and immaturity of the liver. Pathologic jaundice is abnormal, may begin within the first 24 hours, and often requires treatment with phototherapy. Breast milk jaundice begins later than physiologic jaundice and may be due to substances in the milk.
- The ability of the newborn's kidneys to filter, reabsorb, and maintain fluid and electrolyte balance is less than that of the adult's kidneys. The newborn's body is composed of a greater percentage of water, and fluid is more easily lost.

- Newborns receive passive immunity when IgG crosses the placenta in utero. After birth, IgM and IgA are produced to protect against infection.
- During the first and second periods of reactivity, newborns are active and alert and may be interested in feeding. They may have a low temperature, elevated pulse and respirations, and excessive respiratory secretions. Between these periods, the infant is in a deep sleep with relaxed muscle tone and no interest in feeding.
- Newborns progress through six behavioral states: quiet sleep, active sleep, drowsy, quiet alert, active alert, and crying.
- Nurses assess newborns immediately after birth to detect serious abnormalities. If no problems are detected with a quick assessment, a more comprehensive examination is performed.
- Molding of the head is normal during birth and may cause the head to appear misshapen. Caput succedaneum or a cephalhematoma may be present.
- Measurements are an important way to learn about growth before birth. Abnormal measurements alert the nurse that complications may occur.

- Assessment of cardiorespiratory status includes history, airway, color, heart sounds, pulses, and blood pressure.
- Axillary temperatures are preferred over rectal temperatures because they are safer and provide accurate measurement.
- Hypoglycemia can cause damage to the brain. Early signs of hypoglycemia include jitteriness, poor muscle tone, respiratory distress, sweating, low temperature, and poor suck.
- In performing heel sticks for blood glucose, the nurse must choose the site carefully to avoid damage to the bone, nerves, or blood vessels of the heel.
- Reflexes are an indication of the health of the central nervous system. Asymmetry or retention of reflexes beyond the time when they should disappear is abnormal.
- The initial feeding provides information about the neonate's ability to coordinate sucking, swallowing, breathing, and tolerance to feeding.
- Newborns usually pass the first stool within 24 hours of birth. Absence of stool for 48 hours may signify an obstruction.
- The newborn's first void occurs within 24 to 48 hours. Infants void 2 to 6 times the first 2 days and 5 to 25 times daily thereafter.
- Marks on the skin should be documented, including location, size, and a general description. Explain marks to parents, and offer emotional support if they are upset.
- The gestational age assessment provides an estimate of the infant's age from conception. It alerts the nurse to possible complications of age and development.

ANSWERS TO CRITICAL THINKING EXERCISES

Exercise 22–1

If there were an opening between the right and left atria after birth, blood would flow from the left atrium, where pressures are high, into the right atrium, where pressures are low. This process is the reverse of the blood flow through the foramen ovale during fetal life. The blood would then flow to the right ventricle, the pulmonary artery, and the lungs. This sequence would cause an increased workload on the lungs and could lead to serious complications.

Exercise 22–2

Failure of the reflexes to fade on schedule may interfere with normal development. For example, the palmar grasp reflex must disappear so that the infant can learn to grasp voluntarily and later to release objects at will. Persistence of the plantar reflex would interfere with walking. Retention of reflexes beyond the age when they should disappear indicates a pathologic process and should prompt further investigation.

REFERENCES AND READINGS

American Academy of Pediatrics & American College of Obstetricians and Gynecologists. (1997). *Guidelines for perinatal care* (4th ed.). Elk Grove Village, IL, and Washington, DC: Author.

Association of Women's Health, Obstetric, and Neonatal Nurses (AWHONN). (1996). *Physiologic assessment of the healthy newborn*. Washington, DC: Author.

Ballard, J. L., Khoury, J. C., Wedig, K., Wang, L., Eilers-Walsman, B. L., & Lipp, R. (1991). New Ballard Score, expanded to include extremely premature infants. *Journal of Pediatrics, 19*(3), 417–423.

Behrman, R. E., Kliegman, R. M., & Arvin, A. M. (Eds.). (1996). *Nelson textbook of pediatrics* (15th ed.). Philadelphia: Saunders.

Bell, E. F., & Oh, W. (1999). Fluid and electrolyte management. In G. B. Avery, M. A. Fletcher, & M. G. MacDonald (Eds.), *Neonatology: Pathophysiology and management of the newborn* (5th ed., pp. 345–361). Philadelphia: Lippincott.

Berkowitz, C. D. (1996). *Pediatrics: A primary care approach*. Philadelphia: Saunders.

Blackburn, S. (1995). Hyperbilirubinemia and neonatal jaundice. *Neonatal Network, 14*(7), 15–25.

Blackburn, S. T. (1998). Assessment and management of neonatal neurobehavioral development. In C. Kenner, J. W. Lott, & A. A. Flandermeyer (Eds.), *Comprehensive neonatal nursing: A physiologic perspective* (2nd ed., pp. 564–607). Philadelphia: Saunders.

Blackburn, S. T., & Loper, D. L. (1992). *Maternal, fetal, and neonatal physiology: A clinical perspective*. Philadelphia: Saunders.

Blake, W. W., & Murray, J. A. (1998). Heat balance. In G. B. Merenstein & S. L. Gardner (Eds.), *Handbook of neonatal intensive care* (4th ed., pp. 100–115). St. Louis: Mosby.

Bonilla-Felix, M., Brannan, P., & Portman, R. (1998). Neonatal nephrology. In G. B. Merenstein & S. L. Gardner (Eds.), *Handbook of neonatal intensive care* (4th ed., pp. 535–570). St. Louis: Mosby.

Bowden, V. R., Dickey, S. B., & Greenberg, C. S. (1998). *Children and their families: The continuum of care*. Philadelphia: Saunders.

Brazelton, T. B. (1999). Behavioral competence. In G. B. Avery, M. A. Fletcher, & M. G. MacDonald (Eds.), *Neonatology: Pathophysiology and management of the newborn* (5th ed., pp. 321–332). Philadelphia: Lippincott.

Brion, L. P., Bernstein, J., & Spitzer, A. (1997). Kidney and urinary tract. In R. A. Polin & W. W. Fox (Eds.), *Fetal and neonatal physiology* (Vol. 2, 2nd ed., pp. 1564–1636). Philadelphia: Saunders.

Brooks, C. (1997). Neonatal hypoglycemia. *Neonatal Network, 16*(2), 15–21.

Bruck, K. (1998). Neonatal thermal regulation. In R. A. Polin & W. W. Fox (Eds.), *Fetal and neonatal physiology* (Vol. 1, 2nd ed., pp. 676–702). Philadelphia: Saunders.

Crockett, M. (1995). Physiology of the neonatal immune system. *Journal of Obstetric, Gynecologic, and Neonatal Nursing, 24*(7), 627–634.

Dodd, V. (1996). Gestational age assessment. *Neonatal Network, 15*(1), 27–36.

Fanaroff, A. A., & Martin, R. J. (1997). *Neonatal-perinatal medicine* (Vols. 1 and 2, 6th ed.). St. Louis: Mosby–Year Book.

Fletcher, M. A. (1999). Physical assessment and classification. In G. B. Avery, M. A. Fletcher, & M. G. MacDonald (Eds.), *Neonatology: Pathophysiology and management of the newborn* (5th ed., pp. 301–320). Philadelphia: Lippincott.

Glenn, L. H. (1993). Biological and behavioral characteristics. In S. Mattson & J. E. Smith (Eds.), *NAACOG core curriculum for maternal–newborn nursing* (pp. 375–385). Philadelphia: Saunders.

Gomella, T. L., Cunningham, M. D., Eyal, F. G., & Zenk, K. E. (Eds.). (1999). *Neonatology* (4th ed.). Norwalk, CT: Appleton & Lange.

Guyton, A. C., & Hall, J. E. (1996). *Textbook of medical physiology* (9th ed.). Philadelphia: Saunders.

Hagedorn, M. I., Gardner, S. L., & Abman, S. H. (1998). Respiratory diseases. In G. B. Merenstein & S. L. Gardner (Eds.), *Handbook of neonatal intensive care* (4th ed., pp. 437–497). St. Louis: Mosby.

Halamek, L. P., & Stevenson, D. K. (1997). Neonatal jaundice and liver disease. In A. A. Fanaroff & R. J. Martin (Eds.), *Neonatal–perinatal medicine* (Vol. 2, 6th ed., pp. 1345–1389). St. Louis: Mosby.

Ince, Z., Coban, A., Peker, I., & Can, G. (1995). Breast milk beta-glucuronidase and prolonged jaundice in the neonate. *Acta Paediatrica, 84,* 3237–3239.

Johnson, C. B. (1996). Head, eyes, ears, nose, mouth, and neck assessment. In E. P. Tappero & M. E. Honeyfield (Eds.), *Physical assessment of the newborn* (2nd ed., pp. 53–66). Petaluma, CA: NICU Ink.

Kenner, C., Lott, J. W., & Flandermeyer, A. A. (1998). *Comprehensive neonatal nursing: A physiologic perspective* (2nd ed.). Philadelphia: Saunders.

Leick-Rude, M. K., & Bloom, L. F. (1998). A comparison of temperature-taking methods in neonates. *Neonatal Network, 17*(5), 21–37.

Lepley, C. J., Gardner, S. L., & Lubchenco, L. O. (1998). Initial nursery care. In G. B. Merenstein & S. L. Gardner (Eds.), *Handbook of neonatal intensive care* (4th ed., pp. 70–99). St. Louis: Mosby.

Lott, J. W. (1998). Assessment and management of cardiovascular dysfunction. In C. Kenner, J. W. Lott, & A. A. Flandermeyer (Eds.), *Comprehensive neonatal nursing: A physiologic perspective* (2nd ed., pp. 306–335). Philadelphia: Saunders.

Lowe, N. K., & Reiss, R. (1996). Parturition and fetal adaptation. *Journal of Obstetric, Gynecologic, and Neonatal Nursing, 25*(4), 339–349.

Maisels, M. J. (1999). Jaundice. In G. B. Avery, M. A. Fletcher, & M. G. MacDonald (Eds.), *Neonatology: Pathophysiology and management of the newborn* (5th ed., pp. 765–819). Philadelphia: Lippincott.

Maisels, M. J. (1995). Clinical rounds in the well-baby nursery: Treating jaundiced newborns. *Pediatric Annals, 25*(10), 548–552.

Maisels, M. J., & Newman, T. B. (1995). Kernicterus in otherwise healthy, breastfed term newborns. *Pediatrics, 96*(4), 730–733.

Mattson, S., & Smith, J. E. (1993). *NAACOG core curriculum for maternal-newborn nursing.* Philadelphia: Saunders.

Meehan, R. M. (1998). Heelsticks in neonates for capillary blood sampling. *Neonatal Network, 17*(1), 17–24.

Miklos, A. B., & Creehan, P. A. (1996). Newborn physical assessment. In K. R. Simpson & P. A. Creehan (Eds.), *AWHONN's perinatal nursing* (pp. 307–335). Philadelphia: Lippincott.

National Association of Neonatal Nurses. (1997). *Neonatal thermoregulation: Guidelines for practice.* Petaluma, CA: Author.

Nelson, N. (1999). The onset of respirations. In G. B. Avery, M. A. Fletcher, & M. G. MacDonald (Eds.), *Neonatology: Pathophysiology and management of the newborn* (5th ed., pp. 257–278). Philadelphia: Lippincott.

Nicholson, J. F., & Pesce, M. A. (1996). Laboratory medicine and reference tables. In R. E. Behrman, R. M. Kliegman, & A. M. Arvin (Eds.), *Nelson textbook of pediatrics* (15th ed., pp. 2031–2084). Philadelphia: Saunders.

Philip, A. (1996). *Neonatology: A practical guide* (4th ed.). Philadelphia: Saunders.

Pressler, J. L., & Hepworth, J. T. (1997). Newborn neurologic screening using NBAS reflexes. *Neonatal Network, 16*(6), 33–46.

Reimann, D., & Coughlin, M. (1996). Newborn adaptation to extrauterine life. In K. R. Simpson & P. A. Creehan (Eds.), *AWHONN's perinatal nursing* (pp. 289–306). Philadelphia: Lippincott–Raven.

Sansoucie, D. A., & Cavaliere, T. A. (1997). Transition from fetal to extrauterine circulation. *Neonatal Network, 16*(2), 5–12.

Smith, J. B., Ley, S. J., Curley, M. A. Q., Elixson, E. M., & Dodds, K. M. (1996). Tissue perfusion. In M. A. Q. Curley, J. B. Smith, & P. A. Moloney-Harmon (Eds.), *Critical care of infants and children* (pp. 155–248). Philadelphia: Saunders.

Taeusch, H. W., & Sniderman, S. (1998). Initial evaluation: History and physical examination. In H. W. Taeusch & R. A. Ballard (Eds.), *Avery's diseases of the newborn* (7th ed., pp. 334–353). Philadelphia: Saunders.

Tappero, E. P., & Honeyfield, M. E. (Eds.). (1996). *Physical assessment of the newborn* (2nd ed.). Petaluma, CA: NICU Ink.

Tsang, R. C., DeMarini, S., & Rath, L. L. (1998). Fluids, electrolytes, vitamins, and trace minerals: Basis of ingestion, digestion, elimination, and metabolism. In C. Kenner, J. W. Lott, & A. A. Flandermeyer (Eds.), *Comprehensive neonatal nursing: A physiologic perspective* (2nd ed., pp. 336–353). Philadelphia:p Saunders.

Vargo, L. (1996). Cardiovascular assessment of the newborn. In E. P. Tappero & M. E. Honeyfield (Eds.), *Physical assessment of the newborn* (2nd ed., pp. 77–92). Petaluma, CA: NICU Ink.

23

The Normal Newborn: Nursing Care

The nurse's role in ongoing assessments and care of the newborn is to identify changes in the newborn's condition as the infant adapts to life outside the uterus. Nurses also intervene to keep infants safe and teach parents to provide care.

Clinical Pathways

Birth facilities use clinical pathways to see that all the necessary tasks involved in helping infants and mothers prepare for discharge are accomplished in the time available. Clinical pathways are also used to see that mothers and infants meet the criteria for discharge. Figure 23–1 provides one example of a clinical pathway for newborns. Pathways are individualized by each institution and based on protocols to meet the needs of their clients.

Early Care

Early care after birth involves the assignment of Apgar scores, assessment, and stabilization of the infant as necessary. Immediate care is discussed in Chapter 17, and infant resuscitation is discussed in Chapter 30. Assessment is discussed in Chapter 22. Once the infant is stable, prophylactic medications are given.

Administering Vitamin K

Vitamin K is given to the neonate within the first hour after birth (p. 997) to prevent hemorrhagic disease of the newborn (American Academy of Pediatrics & American College of Obstetricians and Gynecologists, 1997). Because infants cannot synthesize vitamin K in the intestines without bacterial flora, they are deficient in clotting factors. One dose of vitamin K, given intramuscularly, prevents bleeding problems until the infant is able to produce the vitamin independently.

Providing Eye Treatment

Infants also receive erythromycin eye ointment (Fig. 23–2) to prevent ophthalmia neonatorum in case the mother is infected with gonorrhea or *Chlamydia*. Because the ointment may temporarily blur the infant's vision, the treatment may be given near the end of the first hour to allow for bonding with the parents.

In some infants, a mild inflammation develops a few hours after prophylactic treatment. Any discharge from the eyes, however, especially if it is purulent, should alert the nurse to the possibility of infection. Drainage should be removed with sterile saline and cotton. If the mother is infected, the infant needs additional antibiotics because routine prophylactic treatment may not completely prevent infection.

NURSING CARE
Cardiorespiratory Status

In the early newborn period, problems of transition may include temporary problems in cardiorespiratory status.

Assessment

Assess the infant for signs of difficult transition to newborn life. Note the rate and character of the heart rate, respirations, and breath sounds. Look for signs of respiratory distress, including tachypnea, retractions, flaring of the nares, pallor or cyanosis, grunting, seesaw respirations, and asymmetry. Check pulses and blood pressure.

Text continued on page 568

DRUG GUIDE

Vitamin K₁ (Phytonadione)

Classification: Fat-soluble vitamin

Other Names: AquaMEPHYTON, Konakion

Action: Promotes the formation of factors II (prothrombin), VII, IX, and X by the liver for clotting. Provides vitamin K, which is not synthesized in the intestines for the first 5 to 8 days after birth because the newborn lacks intestinal flora necessary for vitamin K production.

Indication: Prevention or treatment of hemorrhagic disease of the newborn.

Neonatal Dosage and Route: 0.5 to 1 mg (0.25 to 0.5 ml) given once intramuscularly within 1 hour of birth for prophylaxis. (The lower dose may be used for small infants weighing less than 2,500 g.) May be repeated or higher doses used if the mother took anticonvulsants during pregnancy. May be repeated if the infant shows bleeding tendencies.

Absorption: Readily absorbed after intramuscular injection. Effective within 1 to 2 hours.

Adverse Reactions: Pain and edema at site of administration. Hemolysis or hyperbilirubinemia, especially in a preterm infant or when large doses are used.

Nursing Considerations: Protect the drug from light until just before administration because it decomposes and loses potency on exposure to light. Incompatible with other drugs. Observe all infants for signs of vitamin K deficiency: ecchymoses or bleeding from any site.

YORK HOSPITAL
YORK, PENNSYLVANIA
CLINICAL PATHWAY

NEWBORN

CLINICAL PATH DAY		EXPECTED PATIENT/ FAMILY OUTCOMES	MULTIDISCIPLINARY ASSESSMENT	TESTS	CONSULT
Immediate Newborn Care	Date & Time	☐ Apgar score >7 at 5 min. [4] ☐ Maintains axillary temp of 36.5C to 37.2C while in radiant warmer or in double blankets [1] ☐ Physiologic parameters WNL [4} ☐ Demonstrates proper latch when breastfeeding [2]	☐ Apgar score 1 & 5 min. ☐ Transitional newborn assessment q 30 min. ☐ Suck reflex	☐ Hypoglycemia protocol when indicated	☐ ________
Newborn Admission	Date & Time	☐ Maintains axillary temp of 36.5C to 37.2C while in radiant warmer or in double blankets [1] ☐ Physiologic parameters WNL [4] ☐ Tolerates initial feeding [2] ☐ ________	☐ Weight ☐ V/S q 30 min x 4 ☐ Multisystem admission assessment ☐ Suck reflex ☐ ________	☐ Hypoglycemia protocol when indicated ☐ ________	☐ ________ ☐ ________
Day of Birth	Date	N D E ☐☐☐ Maintains axillary temp of 36.5C to 37.2C independent of external heat source [1] ☐☐☐ Parents/family verbalize understanding of safety & security measures [6] ☐☐☐ Physiologic parameters WNL [4] ☐☐☐ Parent(s)/family & infant demonstrate attachment behaviors [3] ☐☐☐ Feeding [2] ☐☐☐ Latch score is 7 or greater for breastfed newborn [2] ☐☐☐ No jaundice [4] ☐☐☐ Infant seen by physician within 12 hours [6]	N D E ☐☐☐ Temp, apical pulse, neuro, cardiac, resp., GI, GU, integ. q shift ☐☐☐ Parent/infant attachment ☐☐☐ Positioning and LATCH score of breastfed newborn ☐☐☐ Freq. and amount of bottlefeeding ☐☐☐ ________	N D E ☐☐☐ Hypoglycemia protocol when indicated ☐☐☐ ________	N D E ☐☐☐ ________ ☐ Social service consult if indicated

NAME	INITIALS	NAME	INITIALS

FIGURE 23–1

An example of a clinical pathway for the newborn from birth through the second day and discharge. This form is printed on both sides and is used by all caregivers to plan and document care. (Courtesy of Women and Children Services of the York Health System, York, Pennsylvania. Modified with permission.)

DOCUMENTATION CODES
Initial = Meets Standard
★ = Exception on pathway identified
C = Chronic problems
N/A = Not applicable

PATIENT/FAMILY PROBLEMS
1. Thermoregulation
2. Nutrition
3. Parent-Infant attachment
4. Potential alteration in newborn metabolism
5. Risk for infection
6. Infant safety
7. ____
8. ____

TREATMENTS	MEDS	NUTR.	EDUC & DC PLANNING
☐ Clamp cord ☐ Dry newborn ☐ Radiant warmer or double blanket while being held until temp stable ☐ ID bands	☐ Neonatal eye prophylaxis & Aquamephyton ☐ HBIG if indicated	☐ Determine if bottlefeeding or breastfeeding ☐ Assist with initial breastfeeding	☐ Initiate safety & security measures with parents/ family ☐ Teach breastfeeding mother proper latch
☐ Cord care ☐ Admission bath	☐ ____	Initial feeding: ☐ ____	
N D E ☐☐☐ Cord care ☐☐☐ ____	N D E ☐☐☐ ____	N D E ☐☐☐ Breast/bottle feed on demand (breast: q 2–3 hrs, bottle: q 3–4 hrs)	N D E ☐☐☐ Reinforce safety and security measures w/ parents/family ☐☐☐ Observe & reinforce proper latch and instruct breastfeeding mother/family in alternative positioning ☐☐☐ Give and review new pamphlets: -Message to mothers -Newborn screening -Car seat -Health insurance for newborns -Preparing formula -Breastfeeding, A Guide for Success

NAME	INITIALS	NAME	INITIALS

FIGURE 23–1

Continued

CLINICAL PATH DAY	EXPECTED PATIENT/ FAMILY OUTCOMES	MULTIDISCIPLINARY ASSESSMENT	TESTS	CONSULT
Day 1	Date N D E ☐☐☐ Maintains axillary temp of 36.5C to 37.2C independent of external heat source [1] ☐☐☐ Parent(s)/family & newborn demonstrate attachment behaviors [3] ☐☐☐ Physiologic parameters WNL [4] ☐☐☐ Feeding [2] ☐☐☐ LATCH score 7 or greater for breastfed newborn [2] ☐☐☐ No jaundice [4] ☐☐☐ No signs of infection [5] ☐☐☐ _____	N D E ☐☐☐ Temp, apical pulse, cardiac, resp., neuro, GI, GU, integ. q 8 hr. N/A N/A N/A Weight ☐☐☐ Parent(s)/family & infant attachment behaviors ☐☐☐ LATCH score of breastfed newborn ☐☐☐ Frequency & amt. of bottle feeding ☐☐☐ _____	N D E ☐☐☐ _____	N D E ☐☐☐ Referral made to lactation consultant for LATCH score <7 ☐☐☐ _____
Day 2	Date ☐☐☐ Maintains axillary temp of 36.5C to 37.2C independent of external heat source [1] ☐☐☐ Parent(s)/family & newborn demonstrate attachment behaviors [3] ☐☐☐ Physiologic parameters WNL [4] ☐☐☐ Feeding [2] ☐☐☐ LATCH score 7 or greater for breastfed newborn [2] ☐☐☐ No jaundice [4] ☐☐☐ No signs of infection [5] ☐☐☐ _____	☐☐☐ Temp, apical pulse, cardiac, resp., neuro, GI, GU, integ. q 8 hr. N/A N/A N/A Weight ☐☐☐ Parent(s)/family & infant attachment behaviors ☐☐☐ LATCH score of breastfed newborn ☐☐☐ Frequency & amt. of bottle feeding ☐☐☐ _____	☐☐☐ _____	☐☐☐ Referral made to lactation consultant for LATCH score <7 ☐☐☐ _____
Discharge	☐ Maintains axillary temp of 36.5C to 37.2C independent of external heat source [1] ☐ Parent(s)/family & newborn demonstrate attachment behaviors and appropriate care of newborn [3] ☐ Physiologic parameters WNL [4] ☐ Circumcision w/o bleeding [5] ☐ Voided at least x 1 [4] ☐ Stooled at least x 1 [4] ☐ Feeding [2] ☐ LATCH score 7 or greater for breastfed newborn [2] ☐ Parent(s)/family verbalize newborn D/C instruction [6] ☐ No jaundice [4] ☐ Physician aware of Coombs results ☐ Discharge Day 2 ☐ No signs of infection	☐ Temp, apical pulse, cardiac, resp., neuro, GI, GU, integ. q 8 hr. ☐ Discharge weight ☐ Parent(s)/family & infant attachment behaviors ☐ LATCH score of breastfed newborn ☐ Frequency & amt. of bottle feeding ☐ _____	☐ Newborn screening tests prior to D/C ☐ _____	☐ Referral made to lactation consultant for LATCH score <7 ☐ _____

NAME	INITIALS		NAME	INITIALS

NOTE: EACH PATIENT REQUIRES AN INDIVIDUAL ASSESSMENT & TREATMENT PLAN. THIS CLINICAL PATH IS A RECOMMENDATION FOR THE AVERAGE PATIENT WHICH REQUIRES MODIFICATION WHEN NECESSARY BY THE PROFESSIONAL STAFF.

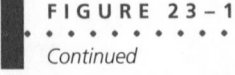

F I G U R E 2 3 – 1
· · · · · · · · · ·
Continued

TREATMENTS	MEDS	NUTR.	EDUC & DC PLANNING
N D E [N/A] [N/A] Cord care [ ][ ][ ] _____	N D E [ ][ ][ ] _____	N D E [ ][ ][ ] Breast/bottle feed on demand (breast: q 2–3 hrs, bottle: q 3–4 hrs)	N D E [ ][ ][ ] Observe return demonst. of breast-feeding mother's use of alternative positioning [ ][ ][ ] Observe parent(s) providing appropriate newborn care; reinforce. [ ][ ][ ] _____
[N/A] [N/A] Cord care [ ][ ][ ] _____	[ ][ ][ ] _____	[ ][ ][ ] Breast/bottle feed on demand (breast: q 2–3 hrs, bottle: q 3–4 hrs)	[ ][ ][ ] Observe return demonst. of breast-feeding mother's use of alternative positioning [ ][ ][ ] Observe parent(s) providing appropriate newborn care; reinforce. [ ][ ][ ] _____
[ ] Cord care [ ] Circumcision care when indicated [ ] Cord clamp removed prior to D/C [ ] _____	[ ] Hepatitis B vaccine per order [ ] _____	[ ] NPO for circumcision when indicated [ ] Breast/bottle feed on demand (breast: q 2–3 hrs, bottle: q 3–4 hrs)	[ ] Review D/C instructions with parent(s)/family [ ] Discuss plan for follow-up care [ ] D/C to mother's care

NAME	INITIALS	NAME	INITIALS

FIGURE 23–1
• • • • • • • • • •
Continued

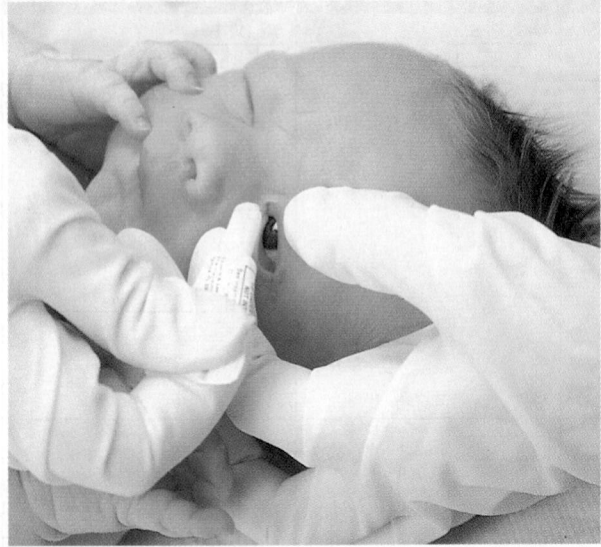

FIGURE 23–2

Administration of ophthalmic ointment. The nurse gently cleans the eyes of blood or vernix using sterile saline. Then, placing a finger and thumb near the edge of each lid, the nurse gently presses against the periorbital ridges to open the eyes, avoiding pressing on the eye itself. A ribbon of ointment is squeezed into each conjunctival sac.

Nursing Diagnosis and Planning

Fluid from the lungs must be removed by absorption or drainage from the respiratory passages after birth. This does not happen immediately and may cause a temporary problem during the early hours after birth. One of the most common nursing diagnoses for the newborn is

■ Ineffective Airway Clearance related to excessive secretions in the respiratory passages.
Expected Outcomes: The newborn will maintain a patent airway with a respiratory rate within the normal range of 30 to 60 breaths per minute and will show no signs of respiratory distress.

Interventions

Positioning the Infant

To aid in draining fluid from the respiratory passages immediately after birth, position the infant with the head slightly lower than the extremities. Use this position briefly whenever the infant is having difficulty clearing the airways, such as during regurgitation. Do not leave the infant in a head-dependent position longer than necessary because pressure from the intestines may interfere with movement of the diaphragm.

Suctioning Secretions

Use the bulb syringe frequently to suction secretions as they drain into the infant's mouth or nose (Procedure 23–1). Keep the bulb syringe in the crib near the infant's head, where it is available if needed quickly. Teach both parents how to use the bulb syringe correctly. Send the syringe home with the infant so that the parents can use it if the infant experiences a problem.

If mechanical suctioning is necessary to remove deeper secretions, choose a small catheter to avoid damaging the tissues of the respiratory tract. Suction for no more than 5 seconds at a time using minimal negative pressure to avoid trauma, laryngospasm, and bradycardia.

Providing Continuing Care

Continue monitoring the infant for problems throughout the stay at the birth facility. By the time of the second period of reactivity, the infant may be alone with the mother without constant attendance by the nurse. Although nurses know that regurgitation, gagging, and episodes of cyanosis are normal during the first and second periods of reactivity, these may be very frightening to the mother. Check frequently with her to see if the infant is having difficulty.

Evaluation

- Is the respiratory rate between 30 and 60 breaths per minute?
- Is the infant free of signs of respiratory distress?

DRUG GUIDE

Erythromycin Ophthalmic Ointment

Classification: Antibiotic

Action: Inhibits cell wall replication in bacteria

Indications: Prophylaxis against the organisms *Neisseria gonorrhoeae* and *Chlamydia trachomatis.* Prevents ophthalmia neonatorum in infants of mothers with gonorrhea and conjunctivitis in infants of mothers with chlamydial infection. Prophylaxis against gonorrhea is required by law for all infants, regardless of whether the mother is known to be infected.

Neonatal Dosage and Route: A "ribbon" of 0.5% erythromycin ointment, 1 to 2 cm (0.5 to 1 in.) long, is applied to the lower conjunctival sac of each eye within 1 hour after birth. May also be used in drop form.

Adverse Reaction: Irritation may result in chemical conjunctivitis, lasting 24 to 48 hours. Ointment may cause temporary blurred vision.

Nursing Considerations: Cleanse the infant's eyes before application, as needed. Hold the tube in a horizontal rather than a vertical position to prevent injury to the eye from sudden movement. Administer from the inner canthus to the outer canthus. Do not touch the tip of the tube to any part of the eye because this may spread infectious material from one eye to the other. Do not rinse. Ointment may be wiped from the outer eye after 1 minute. Observe for irritation. Use a new tube for each infant to prevent spread of infection. Other medications used for prevention of gonorrhea include tetracycline and silver nitrate solution.

PROCEDURE 23–1

Using a Bulb Syringe

PURPOSE: To provide an open airway by removing secretions or regurgitated feeding from the infant's mouth and nose.

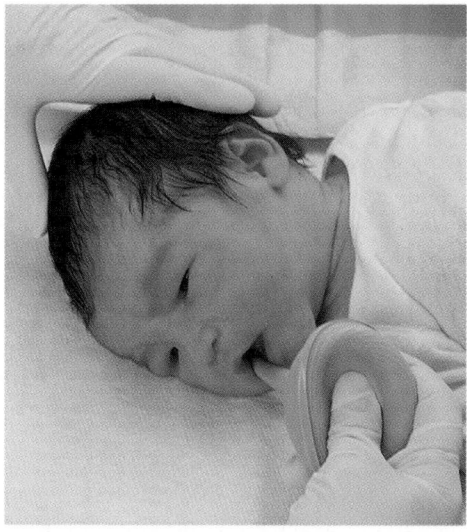

1. To allow drainage from the mouth, position the infant's head to the side or hold the infant with the head slightly lower than the rest of the body.
2. Compress the bulb before inserting it into the mouth. Do not compress the bulb while it is in the infant's mouth, or secretions in the bulb will be expelled back into the mouth.
3. Insert the bulb into the side of the infant's mouth. Do not insert it straight to the back of the throat because this maneuver could stimulate a vagal response, resulting in bradycardia or even apnea.
4. Release the bulb slowly while it is in the mouth to draw in the secretions. Remove and empty it by compressing several times before using again to remove secretions.
5. Suction the nose, if necessary, after the mouth is suctioned. Infants often gasp when the nose is suctioned and might aspirate secretions in the mouth if it is not cleared first.
6. Suction the nose gently because trauma could cause edema and obstruction of nasal passages.

NURSING CARE

Thermoregulation

Because any neonate may have difficulty with thermoregulation, the nurse must identify problems and intervene to prevent complications.

Assessment

Assess the newborn's temperature shortly after birth and then according to agency policy. In general, the temperature is assessed every half hour until it has been stable for 2 hours. It is checked again at 4 hours and then once a shift (every 8 hours). Assess the newborn more often if the temperature is abnormal.

Nursing Diagnosis and Planning

A common diagnosis is

■ Risk for Ineffective Thermoregulation related to immature compensation for changes in environmental temperature.
  Expected Outcome: The infant will maintain body temperature within the normal ranges: axillary, 36.5° to 37.5°C (97.7° to 99.5°F); rectal, 36.5° to 37.6°C (97.7° to 99.7°F).

Interventions

Preventing Heat Loss

Preparing the Environment Before Birth. Begin preventive measures before the infant is born. Prepare a neutral thermal environment with a radiant warmer to use during initial assessments (Fig. 23–3). Check the radiant warmer to be sure it is functioning properly before the delivery. Turn it on early enough to warm the bed before the birth. Set the servocontrol between 36.0° and 36.5°C (96.8° and 97.7°F). This setting regulates the amount of heat produced

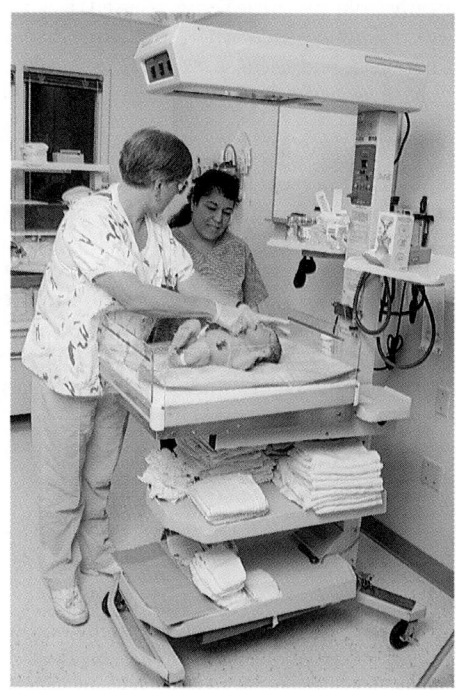

FIGURE 23–3

Radiant warmers allow easy access to the infant without increasing heat loss due to exposure. The nurse should be careful not to come between the infant and the overhead source of heat when giving care.

by the warmer to maintain the infant's skin temperature at the normal level.

Providing Immediate Care. Immediately after birth, place the infant on the mother's abdomen or under the radiant warmer to counteract the cool temperature of the delivery room. Dry the wet infant quickly with warm towels to prevent heat loss by evaporation. Pay particular attention to drying the hair because the head is a large surface area and hair that remains damp increases heat loss. Remove towels or blankets as soon as they become wet and replace them with dry, warmed linens. Cover the infant's head with a cap when the infant is not under a radiant warmer.

Providing Ongoing Prevention. To avoid conduction of heat away from the body, warm anything that comes in contact with the infant. Pad cool surfaces such as scales before placing infants on them. Warm stethoscopes and clothing before using them. Before touching the infant, run warm water over your hands if they are cold.

To prevent heat loss by radiation, position the newborn's crib or incubator away from walls or windows that are part of the outside of the building. It is easy to overlook this source of heat loss when the objects and air around the infant seem warm, but infants may lose heat to objects not in close contact with them. Keep this possibility in mind when positioning cribs in mothers' rooms, which are often short of space. Place the crib at the end of the mother's bed or between the beds (in a two-bed room) rather than next to the windows. Avoid areas with drafts. Keep traffic low around radiant warmers because movement increases air currents.

When assessing or caring for newborns, avoid exposing more of their bodies than necessary. Remove clothing and blankets only from the areas being assessed. Keep the upper part of the infant covered when changing diapers. Wrap them in blankets, and use a stockinette or insulated hat to prevent heat loss from the large surface area of the head.

Restoring Thermoregulation

If an infant has a decreased temperature after initial care, immediately institute nursing measures to assist thermoregulation. If the axillary temperature is low, some nurses check the rectal temperature to determine core temperature; do not wait for the rectal temperature to drop, however. The process of nonshivering thermogenesis begins in the infant before the core temperature becomes abnormal. Core temperature changes indicate that the infant's thermoregulatory resources are exhausted.

Correct obvious causes first. The infant may be un-

wrapped or wearing wet clothing. The mother's room may be cold, or the crib may be placed near the air conditioner.

A slight drop in temperature may require only the addition of extra clothing. Put a shirt on the infant upside down by placing the infant's legs in the sleeves for added warmth. Use two blankets, each wrapped separately around the infant, to increase insulation of heat by trapping air between the layers. Place another blanket over the infant in the crib, and be sure that a hat is on the infant's head. Place linens in a warmer prior to use if added warmth is desired.

A greater drop in temperature requires additional measures. Place the infant under a radiant warmer for a short time. For an infant with a markedly decreased temperature, set the temperature control on the warmer to warm the infant slowly. Too rapid warming can cause complications, including apnea.

Performing Expanded Assessments

Expanded assessments are necessary whenever temperature is decreased in a newborn. Observe for signs of respiratory distress brought on by the additional oxygen requirement of nonshivering thermogenesis.

Because the cold infant uses more glucose to produce heat, test the blood glucose level when the temperature is abnormal. If the glucose is low, have the mother breast-feed or use heated formula. Warm milk helps warm the infant.

Notify the physician or nurse practitioner if the infant does not respond to these measures. Place the infant in an incubator for close observation until the temperature stabilizes. Because low temperature is a common sign of infection, observe for signs of infection.

Evaluation

- Is the temperature within normal range?
- Are there signs of complications from cold stress?

NURSING CARE
Hepatic Function

The major early assessments and care of the hepatic system are related to blood glucose levels and bilirubin conjugation.

BLOOD GLUCOSE

Assessment

Assess all infants for risk factors and signs of hypoglycemia (see p. 540). Perform screening tests for blood glucose according to signs exhibited and agency policy.

Nursing Diagnosis and Planning

For infants who have glucose levels of 40 mg/dl by laboratory analysis or 45 mg/dl by screening tests (or value used by agency), the collaborative problem potential complication: hypoglycemia is appropriate. Client-centered goals for hypoglycemia are inappropriate because this problem requires collaboration between the nurse and the physician. Planning revolves around the nurse's role in the following:

- Assessing for signs of hypoglycemia
- Notifying the physician about signs of hypoglycemia or

CRITICAL THINKING EXERCISE 23–1

You are caring for Nancy Belinsky and her son, Andy, who have both been doing well since Andy was born early this morning. As you enter the room after lunch, Nancy says, "Andy's hands and feet are so cold! And his hands are so shaky. Is he all right?"

1. What are the nursing priorities in this situation?
2. What expanded assessments are necessary?
3. What interventions are necessary?
4. How will you respond to Nancy?

following routine orders left by the physician for infants with hypoglycemia
• Intervening to minimize hypoglycemia

Interventions

Maintaining Safe Glucose Levels

If glucose is not constantly available to the brain, permanent damage may occur. To prevent this development, follow agency policy and physician orders regarding feeding infants with low glucose levels. If this is the infant's first feeding, provide breast milk or formula. Glucose water is not recommended because although it raises the blood glucose, insulin production also increases, causing a drop in blood glucose again. Because of the other nutrients included, milk provides a longer-lasting supply of glucose.

Assist the breast-feeding mother with the first feeding. If she is unable to nurse the infant immediately (because of pain or exhaustion from delivery), feed the infant formula and help her breast-feed at the next feeding. Assist formula-feeding mothers to give the bottle.

Repeating Glucose Tests

Until glucose levels are stable, closely observe newborns who have shown signs of hypoglycemia. Repeat glucose screenings may be performed. Keep the physician or nurse practitioner aware of the newborn's status. If the blood glucose does not remain at an adequate level, other causative factors are investigated. The infant may be transferred to a nursery for more intensive treatment, including intravenous feedings, until blood glucose is regulated with oral feedings.

Providing Other Care

Watch for signs of other complications. If infants do not have enough glucose, they may experience a drop in temperature that could lead to respiratory distress as oxygen is used for nonshivering thermogenesis. Explain the situation to parents. They will be distressed over the multiple heel sticks their infant must endure. Explain the importance of maintaining adequate blood glucose levels and why the tests and frequent feedings are necessary. Encourage parents to feed the newborn as instructed so that enough glucose is available to meet the infant's needs.

Evaluation

Evaluate the collaborative interventions for hypoglycemia by noting the infant's response to interventions and the presence or absence of continued signs of hypoglycemia.

BILIRUBIN

Elevated bilirubin levels are common in newborns. Infants who need treatment for hyperbilirubinemia are discussed in Chapter 30. Prevention, however, is an important aspect of care.

Assessment

Assess for jaundice by blanching the infant's skin on the nose or sternum. Determine how far down the body the jaundice extends. When serum bilirubin tests are ordered, compare the results with what is expected for the infant's age and with previous results.

Nursing Diagnosis and Planning

When infants are discharged early after birth, hyperbilirubinemia may not occur until after they are at home. A nursing diagnosis for this situation is

■ Risk for Injury related to lack of parental knowledge about hyperbilirubinemia.
  Expected Outcomes: Infants with jaundice will be identified early in the birth facility or at home. Parents will identify methods of preventing or reducing jaundice when at home.

Interventions

Determine which infants are at increased risk for hyperbilirubinemia (see p. 542). By using extra vigilance in caring for infants at higher risk, nurses can detect jaundice earlier and take measures to decrease it.

Explain to parents the importance of adequate feedings to stimulate passage of stools and help prevent high levels of bilirubin in the infant. When a newborn is feeding poorly, determine the reasons and intervene appropriately. Help mothers wake sleepy infants to feed and encourage them to spend extra time with an infant with a poor suck. Instruct breast-feeding mothers to nurse every 2 to 3 hours. Avoid giving water to jaundiced infants because water does not stimulate stool excretion.

Before discharge, show parents how to check for jaundice. Instruct them to contact their care provider if they see jaundice or if the infant is not eating every 3 to 4 hours, voiding six to ten times a day, and producing stools appropriately (at least once daily for formula-fed infants, at least three stools daily for breast-fed infants).

Continue to check the infant for jaundice during the early home or clinic visits. Use a transcutaneous bilirubinometer (jaundice meter), if available, to verify the level of bilirubin. The meter is placed on the infant's skin to measure the intensity of the skin color, which is correlated with bilirubin levels (Ruchala, Seibold, & Stremsterfer, 1996). Reinforce teaching about identification of jaundice and importance of feedings and stooling. Answer questions parents may have developed since discharge from the birth facility.

If an infant contracts true breast milk jaundice, explain it to the parents. The mother who must discontinue breast-feeding for a day or two will be very concerned. Reassure her that her milk is adequate and not harmful to the infant. Help her maintain her milk supply by using a breast pump during the time the infant is taking formula.

Evaluation

• Can parents discuss what they will look for regarding jaundice?
• Are parents able to verbalize methods to prevent or reduce jaundice?

■ Ongoing Assessments and Care

A complete assessment is necessary every 8 hours, according to the birth facility's routine, but the nurse must always watch for signs of change in the newborn's condition (see Nursing Care Plan 23–1). Vital signs are assessed once every 8 hours or more often if they are abnormal. The infant is weighed once daily, and weight loss or gain noted.

NURSING CARE PLAN 23-1
. . . .
Normal Newborn

Assessment	Nicholas, a full-term newborn, weighs 7 lb, 8 oz, and is 20 in. long. He is the first baby for his mother, Vicki. Nicholas receives Apgar scores of 8 at 1 minute and 9 at 5 minutes. During the initial assessment, he has an excessive amount of mucus. His respiratory rate is 62, apical pulse is 156, and breath sounds are slightly moist. He has mild substernal retractions. His color is pink with acrocyanosis.
Nursing Diagnosis	Ineffective Airway Clearance related to excessive secretions in airways
Goal/Expected Outcome	• Nicholas will maintain a patent airway and have no signs of respiratory distress throughout the birth facility stay as demonstrated by respiratory rate of 30 to 60 breaths per minute, clear breath sounds, and no cyanosis, retractions, flaring, or grunting.

Intervention	Rationale
1. Place Nicholas in a side-lying position with his head slightly lower than the rest of his body just until drainage has occurred.	1. A head-down position uses gravity to facilitate drainage of secretions from the airways.
2. Suction as needed with a bulb syringe. If the nose also requires suctioning, suction it after suctioning the mouth.	2. Suctioning the mouth first prevents aspiration of oral secretions should Nicholas gasp when his nose is suctioned.
3. Change the infant's position frequently.	3. Position changes promote expansion and drainage of all parts of the lungs.
4. Provide reassurance for Vicki, who may be concerned.	4. The close attention to the infant may make the parents feel that something is wrong.
5. Demonstrate and explain use of the bulb syringe to Vicki. Assess her ability and make suggestions as needed during a return demonstration.	5. Demonstration and return demonstration help ensure that parents learn correct techniques.
6. Continue to observe Nicholas for signs of respiratory distress. Count pulse and respirations every 30 minutes until they have been stable for 2 hours. Increase frequency of assessment if there is any sign of abnormality. Continue to assess for other signs of ineffective airway clearance and respiratory difficulty, such as cyanosis, retractions, flaring, and grunting.	6. Monitoring should be based on history of excessive mucus, ability to cope with mucus, and other signs of respiratory difficulty and changes in the infant's condition.

Evaluation	Nicholas has clear breath sounds within 3 hours of birth, and his respiratory rate stays within normal limits. He has no further signs of respiratory difficulty. Vicki uses the bulb syringe to suction Nicholas appropriately.
Assessment	Nicholas's axillary temperature ranges from 36.2° to 36.8°C (97.2° to 98.2°F). His mother frequently unwraps him to look at him.
Nursing Diagnosis	Risk for Ineffective Thermoregulation related to parental lack of knowledge of newborn thermoregulation abilities and needs
Goals/Expected Outcomes	• Nicholas will maintain a temperature within the normal range of 36.5° to 37.5°C (97.7° to 99.5°F) axillary throughout his birth facility stay. • Vicki will verbalize and practice methods of preventing heat loss by the end of the first day.

Intervention	Rationale
1. Explain the reasons why newborns have problems with thermoregulation.	1. When parents understand the reasons behind precautions given them, they are more likely to practice them.
2. Teach Vicki to dry Nicholas promptly whenever he is wet, such as during bathing and when changing wet diapers or clothing.	2. Heat loss from evaporation occurs when the infant's skin is wet.

NURSING CARE PLAN 23-1 *Continued*

Normal Newborn

3. Instruct Vicki to keep Nicholas's crib away from cold walls, windows, or drafts from air conditioners and open doors or windows.
4. Point out common objects that may be cold when they touch Nicholas. Explain the effect of this contact, and suggest methods to warm them before use.
5. Assess the infant's axillary temperature every 30 minutes until it has been stable for 2 hours.
6. If Nicholas becomes jittery or lethargic, check blood sugar according to birth facility routine. Help Vicki breast-feed him if it is low.
7. Monitor for tachypnea or other signs of respiratory distress. Suction and apply oxygen if needed.

8. If Nicholas is slow to warm or has repeated episodes of low temperature, place him under the radiant warmer. Alert the physician or nurse practitioner.
9. When Nicholas is ready to go into an open crib, dress him in warmed clothes and blankets.
10. Remove extra blankets according to the infant's temperature.
11. Apply a stockinette or insulated hat to the infant's head.
12. After transfer to an open crib, monitor the infant's temperature every 30 to 60 minutes until it is stable.
13. Teach Vicki how to take her son's axillary temperature at home.

3. Heat loss by radiation and convection occurs from exposure to cold objects or air drafts.

4. Heat can be gained or lost by conduction.

5. Continued assessment shows response to interventions.
6. Nonshivering thermogenesis may cause hypoglycemia. Feeding provides calories for heat production.
7. Nonshivering thermogenesis requires use of large amounts of oxygen, increases the work of the respiratory system, and may lead to hypoxia.
8. Radiant heat warms infants and can be adjusted according to their needs. Temperature instability is one sign of infection in newborns.
9. Warming clothing and blankets warms infants by conduction.
10. Overheating increases oxygen and glucose consumption.
11. Covering the head decreases heat loss.

12. Continued monitoring provides prompt identification of problems that develop.

13. Teaching increases parents' competence in infant care.

Evaluation

Nicholas's axillary temperature at 3 hours after delivery is 37°C (98.6°F). He has no further problems with temperature instability during his birth facility stay. Vicki is conscientious in using correct measures to keep Nicholas warm.

Additional Nursing Diagnoses to Consider

Risk for Altered Parenting
Risk for Infection
Health-Seeking Behaviors

Providing Skin Care

The skin is checked for new marks or changes in old ones. To assess skin turgor, the nurse pinches up a small area of skin over the chest or abdomen and notes how quickly it returns to its normal position. The return should be immediate in the normal newborn, with no "tenting." Skin that remains tented is an indication of dehydration.

Bathing

The infant receives a bath to remove blood and excessive vernix as soon after birth as the temperature is stable. Early bathing decreases exposure to maternal blood and possible

blood-borne organisms on the infant's skin. In one study, infants were bathed as soon as the rectal temperature reached 36.5°C (97.7°F), approximately 1 hour after birth. They had no significant drop in temperature compared with infants bathed at 4 hours after birth (Penny-MacGillivray, 1996).

While shampooing the hair, the nurse combs through it to remove dried blood. The infant must be returned to the radiant warmer quickly and dried well to minimize heat loss. Combing the hair out hastens drying.

The nurse wears gloves during all contact with the infant until the bath is completed because of the blood on the infant's skin from birth. After the bath, gloves are necessary only when contact with body fluids will occur.

After the initial bath, the infant may not receive another full bath during the birth facility stay. The skin, however, is cleansed at diaper changes and to remove regurgitated milk. Clear water or a mild soap solution is used according to agency policy.

Providing Cord Care

The cord should be checked for bleeding or oozing during the early hours after birth. The cord clamp must be securely fastened with no skin caught in it. Purulent drainage or redness or edema at the base indicates infection. The cord becomes brownish-black within 2 to 3 days and falls off within approximately 10 to 14 days.

The cord may be treated with a bactericidal substance such as triple-dye solution, an antibiotic ointment, or alcohol. Parents should continue to clean the cord with alcohol at least three times a day at home until the cord falls off. The diaper is folded below the cord to keep it dry and free from contamination by urine.

The cord clamp is removed about 24 hours after birth if the end of the cord is dry (Fig. 23–4). The base of the cord is still moist, but there is no danger of bleeding if the end is dry and crisp.

Cleansing the Diaper Area

Because contact with body fluids is likely while changing diapers, it is important to wear clean gloves. Meconium is very thick and sticky and can be difficult to remove from the skin. Plain water or special soap solutions may be used for cleaning the diaper area.

Assisting with Feedings

The nurse must ensure that infants are eating well and that parents understand their chosen feeding method. Position-ing infants on the side after feedings promotes emptying of the stomach and decreases chances of aspiration. The head of the bed may be elevated for a short time after the feeding. This position helps keep stomach contents from flowing into the esophagus through the relaxed cardiac sphincter.

Protecting the Infant

Safeguarding the infant is a major role of the nurse. Primary ways nurses protect newborns are by (1) ensuring that infants always go to the correct parents, (2) taking precautions to prevent infant abductions, and (3) preventing or recognizing early signs of infection.

IDENTIFYING THE INFANT

Identification bands are placed on the mother, the infant, and the father or other support person at the infant's birth to ensure that the wrong infant is never given to a mother. This type of mistake could result in interference with bonding, lack of confidence in the reliability of the staff, and lawsuits.

Information on each band is identical and includes a number imprinted on the plastic band. The imprinted number is used to identify the mother and the infant every time the infant is brought to the mother (or significant other) after a period of separation, however brief (Fig. 23–5).

Other methods to identify infants include taking footprints of the infant and a fingerprint of the mother or photographs of the infant. A notation of birthmarks or other distinguishing features is made on the nurses' notes.

PREVENTING INFANT ABDUCTION

An unfortunate but essential role of the nurse is protection of the infant from infant abduction (kidnapping). Precautions include teaching parents how to recognize birth facility personnel, whether by a picture identification badge or

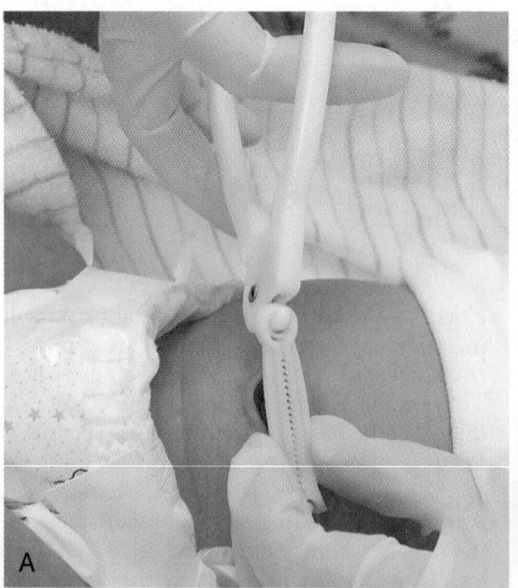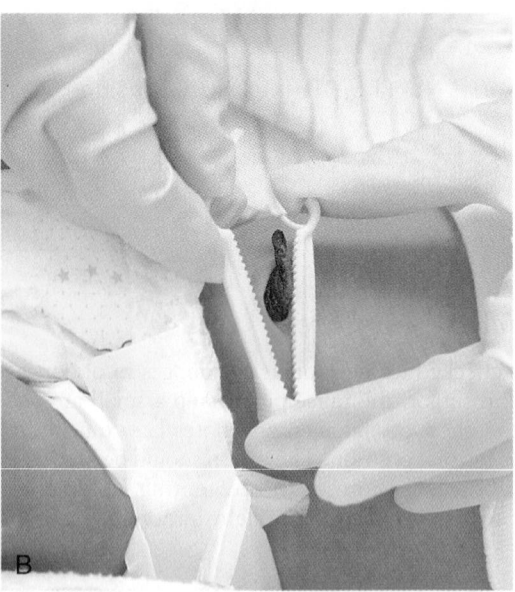

FIGURE 23–4

The cord clamp is removed when the end of the cord is dry and crisp. The clamp is cut *(A)* and separated *(B)*.

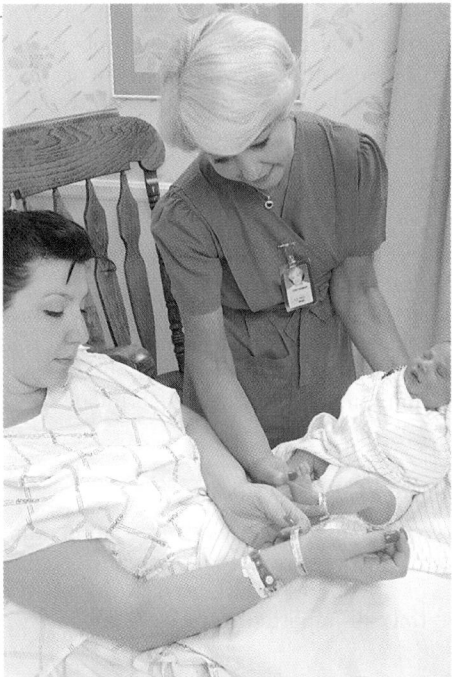

FIGURE 23–5

The nurse unwraps the infant to compare the infant's identification band with the mother's band. The mother may be asked to read the identification number on her band as the nurse checks the infant's band.

by other means. Parents receive written and oral information, including a picture of the special identification badge worn by staff. They should be cautioned never to give their infant to anyone who does not have proper identification.

Staff who are working temporarily on the unit are assigned special identification badges to be worn for the shift. Badges are carefully monitored so that none can be removed from the premises without alerting the staff. In some agencies, an electronic device is attached to each infant's wrist, ankle, or clothing. The maternity unit exits are wired so that an alarm is triggered when the device is near.

Entrances to the maternity unit should be in areas where staff can watch people entering and leaving. Unit doors may be locked at all times. Entrance requires knocking on the door or use of a card-key or a code on the lock (Fig. 23–6). Visitors to maternity units may be required to check in with security guards and wear special visitor identification tags.

Remote exits are often locked and equipped with video cameras and alarms. Staff must respond quickly whenever a door alarm sounds. Although alarms are usually triggered accidentally, it is always possible that a kidnapper is using a remote exit for a quick getaway.

Newborns are usually abducted by women who are familiar with the birth facility and its routines. They are often married and living near the birth facility. They usually visit several times to learn the routines so that they can impersonate birth facility staff to gain access to a newborn. They often know the layout of the facility and the locations of exits well. The woman may have had a previous pregnancy loss or has been unable to have a child of her own. She may

Precautions to Prevent Infant Abductions

1. All personnel must wear appropriate identification at all times. No one without appropriate identification should handle or transport infants.
2. Enlist parents' help in preventing kidnapping. Teach them to allow only hospital staff with proper identification to take their infants from them.
3. Teach parents and staff to transport infants only in their cribs and never by carrying them. Question anyone walking in the hallway carrying an infant.
4. Investigate anyone with a newborn near an exit or in an unusual part of the facility.
5. Be suspicious of anyone who does not seem to be visiting a specific mother or who asks detailed questions about nursery or discharge routines.
6. Be suspicious of unknown people carrying large bags or packages that could contain an infant.
7. Respond immediately when an alarm sounds signaling that a remote entrance has been opened or an infant has been taken into an unauthorized area.
8. Never leave infants unattended at any time. Teach parents that infants must be observed at all times. Suggest that they talk to the nurse if they or a family member cannot watch the infant.
9. Take infants to mothers one at a time. Never leave an infant in the hall unsupervised.
10. When infants are left in mothers' rooms, place them away from the doorways.
11. If entrances to the maternity unit or nurseries are equipped with locks that open to codes, protect the code from others.
12. When a parent or family member comes to the nursery to take an infant, always match the infant and adult identification bracelet numbers. Never give an infant to anyone without an identification bracelet or other proper identification.
13. Alert hospital security immediately of any suspect activity.

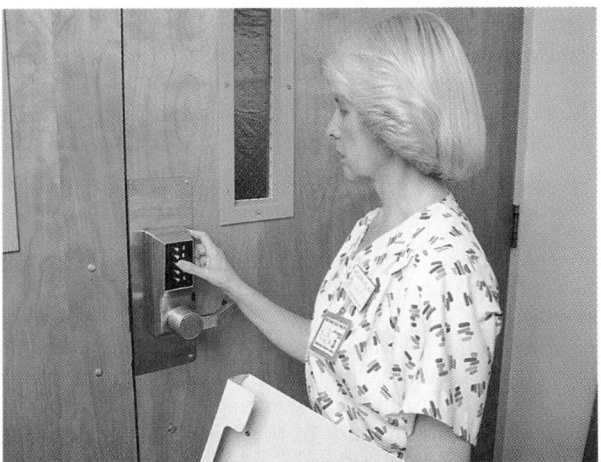

FIGURE 23–6

The nurse uses a code to open the door to the nursery.

want an infant to solidify a relationship with her boyfriend. Although the woman plans the kidnapping, she waits for an appropriate opportunity to take any infant.

PREVENTING INFECTION

Because the newborn has a limited ability to respond to infection, prevention is of utmost importance throughout the birth facility stay and constitutes a major part of parent teaching.

Many nursing actions help prevent infection. At the beginning of their shift, nurses in many agencies perform a scrub of their hands and arms. Hand washing is important before and after touching any infant. It is essential not to handle one neonate and then go to another without again washing one's hands. An infection that develops in one infant could quickly spread to others without these precautions.

The nurse should encourage parents and visitors to wash their hands before handling infants. Parents should be instructed to discourage visitors with colds or other infections from coming in contact with the mother or newborn at the birth facility or during the early days at home.

To avoid cross-contamination, each infant's supplies should be kept separate from those used for other infants. Supplies in drawers or cupboards of each crib unit should be used only for that infant. Using them for another neonate could result in the transfer of infectious organisms.

When the mother has an infection, the physician or nurse practitioner decides whether it is safe for the newborn to remain with her. Although mothers and infants may well share the same organisms, the infant of a mother who is acutely ill may need to stay in the nursery until the mother is no longer contagious and feels able to perform infant care. Often the degree of the mother's fever is one of the determining factors. Nurses must be vigilant for signs of infection during assessment and care of the infant (see Chapter 30). Instead of a fever, there may be a decrease in temperature. The infant may feed poorly or be lethargic. Periods of apnea sometimes occur without obvious cause. Any change in behavior that is unexplained should be recorded and investigated.

NURSING CARE
Parents' Knowledge of Newborn Care

The nurse must use every contact with the parents as an opportunity for further teaching.

Assessment

Assess parents' changing learning needs throughout the birth facility stay. Consider the mother's and infant's physical conditions and any special concerns that the mother may have.

Determine learning needs for experienced mothers. They may be unaware of information that has changed since the birth of the last infant. For example, mothers who have always placed their infants in the prone position for sleep need to know that this position is no longer recommended because it may be associated with sudden infant death syndrome. Mothers should be taught to use the back or side position (American Academy of Pediatrics & American

College of Obstetricians and Gynecologists, 1997). Also assess the father's learning needs and his plans for involvement with infant care. Determine if there are cultural dictates about the father's involvement with the infant.

Nursing Diagnosis and Planning

A common nursing diagnosis for the family with learning needs is

- Health-Seeking Behaviors related to the desire for information about infant care.
  Expected Outcomes: The parents will seek assistance from nurses to meet their information needs, will correctly demonstrate infant care before discharge, and will express confidence in their ability to meet their infant's needs.

Interventions

Determining Who Teaches

Because several different nurses care for mothers and infants during each 24-hour period, coordinate the teaching so that all concerns are addressed. Many facilities use a checklist to ensure that all important topics are covered with every parent.

Setting Priorities

With only a short time available for teaching, it is important to set priorities in determining what to teach. Make a teaching plan with the parents. Use a topic list to help them point out major concerns regarding infant care to ensure effective use of time. Begin by discussing their most pressing concerns to decrease anxiety. Then, as time allows, go on to other subjects.

Using Various Teaching Methods

Use a variety of teaching methods to increase effectiveness. Use oral and written methods, as well as demonstrations. Parents often learn best by seeing skills performed correctly and then practicing them under supervision while the nurse gives suggestions. To increase the likelihood that parents will follow the nurse's instructions, explain the rationale for each point made during teaching sessions.

Discuss information with the mother alone or with her family members, roommate, or a group of mothers. Group teaching is a more efficient use of nursing time, but some mothers learn better with one-to-one teaching. Use audiovisual materials, including pamphlets, magazines, videos, and television programs. Highlight the most important areas and clarify information as necessary to reinforce learning.

Modeling Behavior

Modeling by the nurse is an important teaching tool. Mothers watch closely when nurses handle infants. The nurse demonstrates mothering behavior by the way the infant is held and care is given and by talking to the infant. This guidance is particularly important for the mother with no experience in infant care.

Teaching Intermittently

Plan teaching in small segments that are interspersed with infant care. Check the parents' understanding often. Encourage them to take over until they are performing all of the infant's routine care.

Including the Father

Identify fathers who would like to participate in care of their infants but hesitate. Offer them the same teaching given the inexperienced mother. Give praise liberally when mothers and fathers practice their new infant care skills. Praise increases their confidence and skill.

Documenting Teaching

Document all teaching performed and the parent's abilities to carry out infant care. This information helps other nurses to know what teaching is still needed. It also provides legal proof that teaching was completed before discharge.

Providing for Follow-up Care

Provide information about unmet learning needs to the home or clinic nurse who will see the mother and infant, especially if they are discharged early. Reinforcement can then be provided during out-patient care.

Provide as much information as possible in written form. The parents can then refer to areas where they have concerns. Also provide telephone numbers that they can call for further help. Offer written information in the parents' primary language, if possible. Even if they speak English, parents may prefer to read in their own language.

Incorporating Cultural Considerations

When teaching, consider the family's cultural beliefs about childcare. For example, some Southeast Asian and Latino women are hesitant to breast-feed in the birth facility and wish to wait until the milk comes in when they are home. Asian parents may be uneasy when caregivers are too complimentary about the baby or casually touch the infant's head. Latino parents, however, may prefer that a person who compliments the infant touch the infant to ward off *mal ojo* or the "evil eye." A woman from India who is concerned about the evil eye, or *najar*, places a black dot on the newborn's forehead to ward it off (Choudhry, 1998).

Teaching should include family members who will be caring for the infant. The people involved may vary according to the culture and the availability of the traditional caregiver. The woman's mother is often a major support person. In the Korean culture, however, the husband's mother is the primary caregiver for the infant and the mother in the early weeks. If the mother will not be the primary infant caregiver, she may appear uninterested in the nurse's teachings. Asking the parents who will be helping them care for the infant helps determine family members to be included in the teaching.

Evaluation

- Do the parents ask questions about the infant's care?
- Can they demonstrate correct infant care?
- Do they verbalize growing confidence in their caregiving abilities?

Circumcision

Circumcision is the most common surgical procedure of the neonate. It is the removal of the prepuce (foreskin), a fold of skin that covers the glans penis. Although it can be retracted easily for cleaning in the older child, the prepuce is not usually fully retractable until age 3 years or older. The prepuce should never be forcibly retracted in any infant because trauma and adhesions can result.

Reasons for Choosing Circumcision

Circumcision may reduce urinary tract infections, which occur in approximately 1% of uncircumcised infants (Roberts, 1996). Inflammation of the glans or prepuce and cancer of the penis are uncommon but occur more often in uncircumcised male patients. Uncircumcised men may be more likely to have syphilis and gonorrhea, but circumcised men are more likely to have genital warts (Cook, Koutsky, & Holmes, 1994). These conditions, however, may be related more to poor hygiene than circumcision (Zderic, 1998).

Some parents choose circumcision for religious, cultural, or social reasons. Jewish parents may have their infants circumcised on the eighth day after birth as part of a special ceremony. Muslim culture also includes circumcision. Some parents want their son to look like his circumcised father or peers. Others feel circumcision is an expected part of newborn care, and some do not realize that they have a choice in the matter.

Parents may be concerned that when older, the child might acquire phimosis, a tightening of the prepuce that prevents its retraction and requires circumcision. Although the number of such cases is very small, surgery after the newborn period involves hospitalization and anesthesia and can be psychologically disturbing to the young child.

Lack of knowledge about the care of the prepuce leads to some circumcisions. Poor hygiene may increase the risk of infections and other problems. Teaching the parents and child the proper care of the uncircumcised penis can prevent surgery and complications related to inadequate cleanliness.

Reasons for Rejecting Circumcision

Reasons why parents decide against circumcision are varied. Some parents believe that the incidence of conditions more common in uncircumcised males is still too uncommon to warrant surgery. Others believe that having the infant circumcised to look like the father or peers is cosmetic surgery and therefore unnecessary. These parents especially object to subjecting their sons to pain during and after surgery. Circumcision is uncommon in many countries and less frequent among families from Asian, Latino, and Native American cultures.

Parents may be concerned about removing the prepuce, which serves to protect the glans. When unprotected by the prepuce, the glans is more prone to irritation from constant exposure to urine and rubbing against diapers. Many believe that circumcision decreases sexual pleasure later in life because the glans becomes less sensitive.

Complications are unusual but most often include hemorrhage and infection. Other complications include the removal of too much or too little of the prepuce, stenosis or fistulas of the urethra, adhesions, necrosis, or other damage to the glans.

Only healthy newborns should undergo circumcision. The preterm or sick infant should not be circumcised until he is healthy enough to tolerate the procedure. Infants with blood dyscrasias may have excessive bleeding if circumcised. For the repair of anatomic abnormalities of the penis, such as hypospadias or epispadias, an intact prepuce may be needed for use in plastic surgery.

Pain Relief

Some circumcisions are performed without anesthesia. Although it was once commonly thought that newborns do not feel pain, it is now known that the fetus can perceive pain by the third trimester. During circumcision, newborns show changes in vital signs, oxygen saturation levels, and responses by the adrenals, indicating that they feel pain. Infants may show irritability, altered sleep-wake states, and abnormal feeding patterns for up to 22 hours after being circumcised without pain medication (Agarwal, Hagedorn, & Gardner, 1998). Later in infancy, boys circumcised without pain relief may show more pain responses than uncircumcised boys when undergoing painful procedures such as vaccinations (Taddio, Katz, Illersich, & Koren, 1997).

Injection of the dorsal penile nerves with an anesthetic such as lidocaine is a safe method to eliminate pain during circumcision. Complications are uncommon but include hematomas, local skin necrosis, and absorption of the medication into the bloodstream. Anesthetic cream applied before the procedure may also be used but is less effective and requires a longer waiting period before it is effective.

Nonpharmacologic pain relief methods include pacifiers, oral sucrose, soothing music, recordings of intrauterine sounds, and talking softly to the infant. All have shown some success in reducing an infant's pain responses to circumcision. The effect of these measures is distraction from rather than actual elimination of pain.

Methods

The Gomco (Yellen) clamp (Fig. 23–7) and the Plastibell (Fig. 23–8) are two commonly used devices for performing circumcisions. In each method, the prepuce is first separated from the glans with a probe and incised to expose the glans. A Mogan clamp may also be used for circumcisions, especially for ritual circumcisions for Jewish families.

Nursing Considerations

ASSISTING IN DECISION MAKING
Ideally, parents decide about circumcision early in pregnancy on the basis of careful consideration of the risks and benefits. This ideal, however, is not always the case. Nurses may be called on to answer parents' questions or clarify misconceptions.

Nurses must be certain that their own biases about circumcision do not interfere with their ability to give objective information to parents. Once the parents come to a decision, the nurse should support it.

PREPARING FOR THE PROCEDURE AND PROVIDING CARE DURING CIRCUMCISION
As with any surgical procedure, informed consent is necessary from the parents before a circumcision is performed.

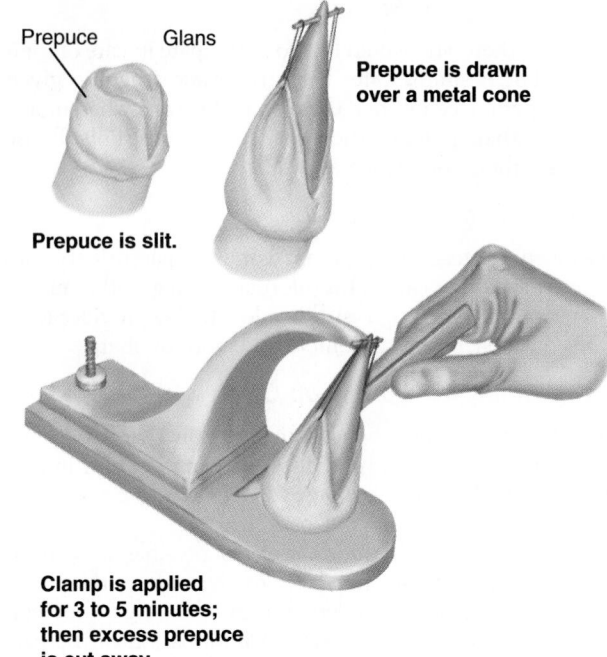

Prepuce   Glans

Prepuce is slit.

Prepuce is drawn over a metal cone

Clamp is applied for 3 to 5 minutes; then excess prepuce is cut away.

FIGURE 23–7
Circumcision using the Gomco (Yellen) clamp. The physician pulls the prepuce over a cone-shaped device that rests against the glans. A clamp is placed around the cone and prepuce and is tightened to provide enough pressure to crush the blood vessels. This procedure prevents bleeding when the prepuce is removed after 3 to 5 minutes.

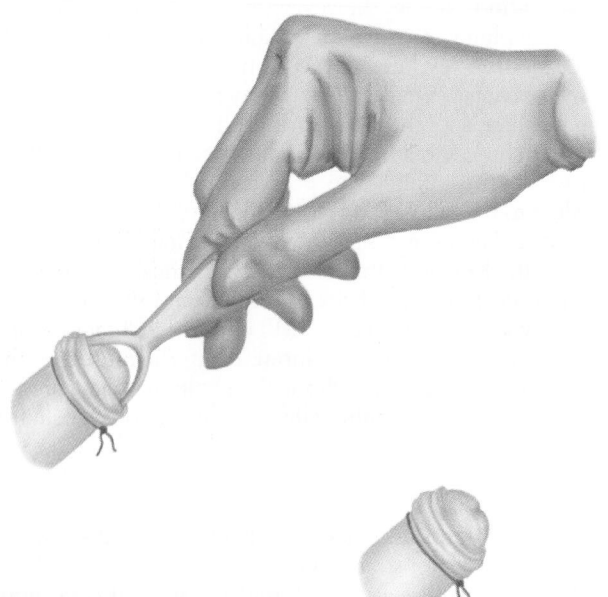

FIGURE 23–8
Circumcision using the Plastibell. The physician places the Plastibell, a plastic ring, over the glans, draws the prepuce over it, and ties a suture around the prepuce and Plastibell. This procedure prevents bleeding when the excess prepuce is removed. The handle is removed, leaving only the ring in place over the glans. The Plastibell falls off in 5 to 8 days.

Caring for the Uncircumcised Penis

Wash your son's penis daily and when soiled diapers are changed. Do not retract the foreskin because it is does not separate from the glans or end of the penis for 3 or more years after birth.

Occasionally, gently pull back on the foreskin to see how much separation has occurred. *Never,* however, force the foreskin to retract. This effort is painful and may cause bleeding, infections, and adhesions. As your son gets older and takes over his own care, teach him to wash under the foreskin by gently pulling it back as far as it retracts each day.

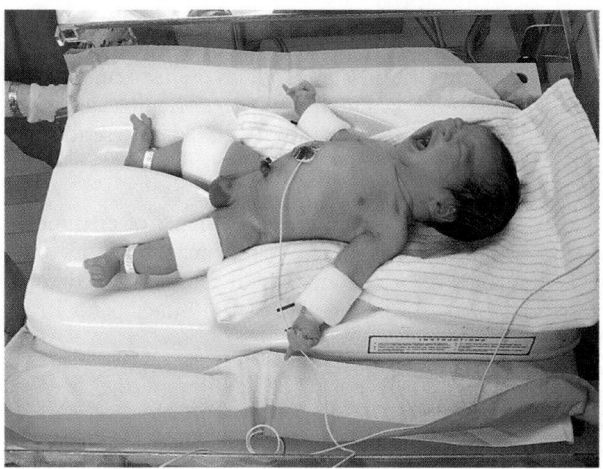

FIGURE 23–9

The infant is placed on the circumcision board just before the procedure is begun.

The nurse sees that the consent has been signed and informs the physician of problems that might impair the infant's ability to withstand circumcision. The infant should be at least 12 hours old and stable.

The nurse gathers equipment and supplies before the procedure. To prevent regurgitation while the infant is restrained in a supine position, feedings may be withheld for 2 to 4 hours before the procedure. A bulb syringe should be placed nearby in case suction is necessary.

When the physician and equipment are ready, the infant is placed on a circumcision board and restrained (Fig. 23–9). A blanket is placed under the infant, and a drape provides warmth and maintains sterility. A heat lamp or radiant warmer helps prevent cold stress. During the procedure, the nurse provides comfort measures.

PROVIDING POSTPROCEDURE CARE

The infant should be removed from the restraints immediately after the circumcision is completed. If a Gomco clamp

was used, the nurse squeezes petroleum jelly or antibiotic ointment over the circumcision site to prevent the diaper from sticking to it. Gauze may be placed over the area. Petroleum jelly should not be used with a Plastibell. The diaper is attached loosely to prevent pressure. The infant should be comforted and returned to his mother, who may be anxious about her son.

The nurse watches carefully for signs of complications after the circumcision. The wound is checked frequently for bleeding during the first few hours after the procedure. If the infant is to be discharged after the circumcision, he should be observed for at least 1 hour before release.

If excessive bleeding occurs, pressure is applied to the site and the physician is notified. A small amount of blood loss may be significant in an infant, who has a small total blood volume. The physician may apply Gelfoam or epinephrine, or may suture the site.

Noting the first urination after circumcision is important because edema could cause an obstruction. If the infant goes home before voiding, the mother is instructed to call the physician if there is no urinary output within 6 to 8 hours.

How to Care for the Circumcision Site

Observe the circumcision site at each diaper change. Call the physician if there are more than a few drops of blood with diaper changes during the first day or any bleeding thereafter. Continue to apply petroleum jelly to the penis with each diaper change for the first 24 to 48 hours. If a Plastibell was used, petroleum jelly should not be applied.

Squeeze warm water from a clean washcloth over the penis to wash it. Fasten the diaper loosely to prevent rubbing or pressure on the incision site.

A yellow crust over the area is normal and should not be removed. Watch for signs of infection such as fever or drainage that smells bad or has pus in it. *Call your physician if you suspect any abnormalities.* The area should be fully healed in approximately 10 days. If a Plastibell was used, the plastic rim will fall off in 5 to 8 days. If it does not fall off by that time, notify your physician.

Signs of Complications After Circumcision

- Bleeding more than a few drops with first diaper changes
- Failure to urinate
- Signs of infection: fever or low temperature, purulent or foul-smelling drainage
- Displacement of the Plastibell
- Scarring (after healing)

TEACHING PARENTS

Each time the site is checked for bleeding, the nurse should show the parents the amount of blood on the diaper to help them understand how much to expect. The normal yellowish exudate that forms over the site should be described and differentiated from purulent drainage. Signs of complications should be discussed fully.

Although nurses usually teach parents of circumcised infants how to care for the penis, they may not think about providing teaching for parents who decide against circumcision. They should include care of the intact penis in the teaching plan for these parents.

Immunization

Hepatitis B is a growing problem in the United States. Immunization for this disease is now included with other routine childhood vaccinations (see Appendix F). Newborns of mothers with acute or chronic hepatitis B infection (hepatitis B surface antigen [HbsAg] positive) may become infected from exposure to the mother's blood at birth. They have a very high chance for development of a chronic infection, which may cause later cancer or other serious liver damage.

These infants should receive both the vaccine and hepatitis B immune globulin (HBIG). The immune globulin provides passive immunity to hepatitis to protect infants until they develop their own antibodies and should be given within 12 hours of birth. The vaccine promotes antibody formation to protect infants from further exposure to the disease.

Newborn-Screening Tests

Most states require that newborns have certain screening tests to detect conditions that result from inborn errors of metabolism or other genetic conditions. Without early treatment, the disorders may cause mental retardation or other serious problems. The tests are easy and inexpensive. More thorough testing is necessary to confirm any abnormal test results.

Although each state determines which conditions must be tested, those most commonly included are phenylketonuria (see Chapter 30), hypothyroidism (see Chapter 51), galactosemia (absence of the enzyme necessary to use the milk sugar, galactose), and hemoglobinopathies such as sickle cell disease and thalassemia (see Chapter 47). Screening may also be performed for maple syrup urine disease, homocystinuria, and other conditions.

Many agencies also include screening for hearing loss. This process may include an interview to determine risk factors with subsequent testing of high-risk infants, or testing of all infants before discharge. Infants who demonstrate a problem are referred for further testing.

Discharge and Newborn Follow-up Care

Discharge

Although state and federal legislation allows women and infants to stay in the birth facility for 48 hours after vaginal birth and 96 hours after cesarean birth, some women choose to go home earlier. The time of discharge varies according to the mother's and newborn's needs and wishes and the primary caregivers' assessment of their conditions.

Early discharge may be considered for term newborns who are appropriate for gestational age and have normal physical examination results. Infants discharged early should have vital signs within normal limits, have fed successfully, and show that they are making the transition from fetal to neonatal life without difficulty. The mother should show adequate knowledge, ability, and confidence to provide adequate care of the newborn (AAP, 1995).

Follow-up Care

Care after discharge from the birth facility is very important. The AAP recommends that follow-up by a health care professional be provided to all newborns who go home from the birth facility less than 48 hours after birth. This should occur within 48 hours of discharge and can be provided in the home, clinic, or office (AAP & ACOG, 1997).

Nursing follow-up care can be provided in a number of ways. These include home visits, clinic visits, and telephone counseling.

HOME VISITS

The home visit is ideally scheduled during the first 24 to 72 hours after discharge. This timing allows early assessment and intervention for problems in nutrition, jaundice, newborn adaptation, and maternal-infant interaction. Visits usually are 60 to 90 minutes to allow enough time for assessment and teaching (Fig. 23–10). Home visits can be cost effective and can reduce health care expenditures (Brown & Johnson, 1998).

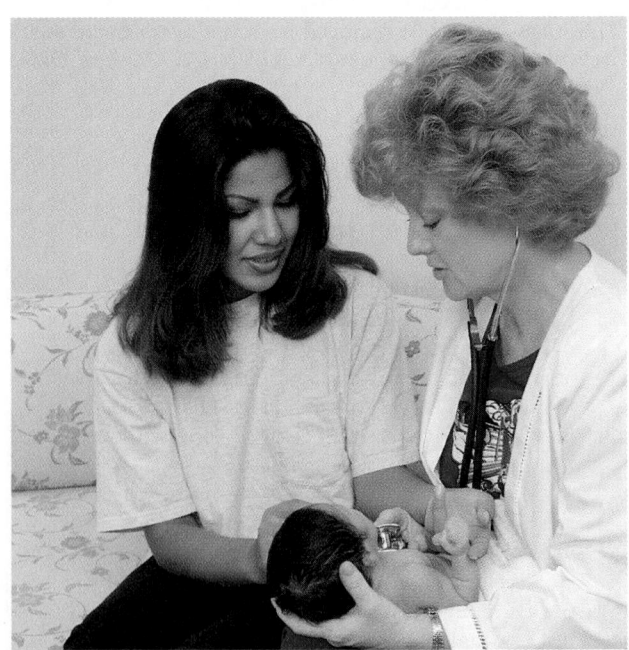

FIGURE 23–10
During the home visit, the nurse performs a complete assessment of the infant. Here a nurse is checking the apical pulse and listening to breath sounds.

Techniques for Infant Care

This guide is written in language that the nurse might use when teaching parents about infant care. Adapt the subjects to meet the needs of individual parents.

Handling the Infant

Head Support

An infant cannot support the heavy head when held in an upright position for the first few months of life. To help support the head, place your hand behind the baby's head whenever you hold the body.

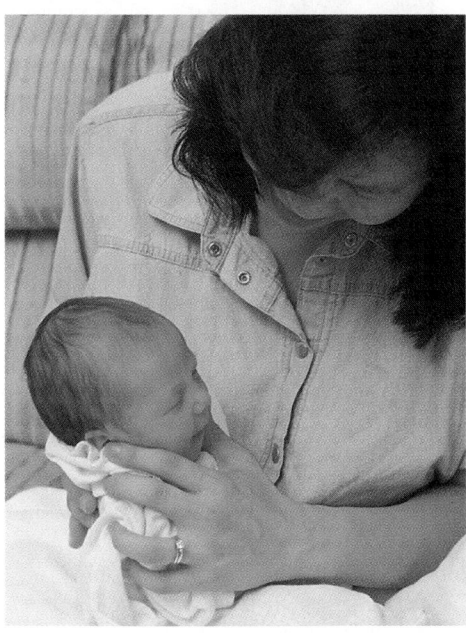

Positions

Most mothers hold the infant in the cradle position. For the "football" position, support the baby's head in the palm of your hand with the body along your arm, supported against your side. This position allows one hand to be free when washing the baby's hair or breast-feeding.

The shoulder hold is good for burping the baby. You can also sit the baby on your lap and support the head and chest with one hand while gently patting or rubbing the infant's back with the other hand. This position allows you to see the baby's face in case of "spit ups."

Always place your baby on the back for sleep. This position helps prevent sudden infant death syndrome (SIDS), the sudden, unexplained death of an infant. The baby may also sleep on the side if the lower arm is brought forward so the baby cannot roll onto the abdomen. The baby should sleep on a firm mattress.

Wrapping

Young infants feel secure when wrapped firmly in a blanket. To swaddle the infant, turn down one corner of a blanket and position the baby's head over the edge. Fold one side of the blanket over the body and arm. Bring the lower corner up and fold it over the chest. Then bring the other side around the infant and tuck it underneath.

Normal Body Processes

Breathing

Newborns normally breathe about 30 to 60 times a minute. Their breathing is irregular and may vary from loud to very soft. Sneezing is usually a normal response to lint from new baby clothes rather than a sign of a cold.

Using a Bulb Syringe

Use the bulb syringe when the infant has excessive mucus in the mouth or nose or spits up milk. Squeeze the bulb before you insert it into the mouth and aim it to the side of the mouth rather than to the back. Extra mucus is common in the first days of life but is usually not a problem thereafter unless a cold develops. Clean the bulb with soap and water and dry well before using again. Call your physician if the baby's skin becomes blue or if the baby stops breathing for more than 15 seconds, has difficulty breathing, or has yellow or green drainage from the nose.

Temperature

When newborns become cold, they need more calories and oxygen than they have available, which can be dangerous to them. Dress your baby as you would like to be dressed. Add a light receiving blanket, except in very hot weather.

Using a Thermometer

Check your baby's temperature under the arm during illness. Hold the arm firmly over the thermometer and be sure the bulb does not protrude behind the arm. Read it at 5 minutes. If you do not know how to read a glass thermometer, a nurse will teach you. Call your physician if the baby has a temperature higher than 100°F or lower than 97.7°F.

Urine Output

Your baby will have at least two to six wet diapers a day during the first day or two and six to ten wet diapers a day thereafter. Counting the number of wet diapers helps you know if the baby is getting enough milk. *Call your baby's doctor if the baby has no wet diapers for more than 12 hours.*

Stool Output

Formula-fed infants pass one to several stools each day. Stools are pale yellow to light brown and formed. Breast-fed infants pass at least three very soft, seedy stools that have a sweet-sour odor and are mustard yellow. Babies are not constipated when they turn red when passing a stool. Constipated infants pass small, hard stools. There are often fewer stools per day than usual.

Diarrhea

Babies with diarrhea pass more frequent stools that are greener and more liquid than usual. There may be a water ring—an area in the diaper where the liquid has absorbed, sometimes around an area of more solid stool. Call your physician if your baby has more than two diarrhea stools.

(continued)

Skin Care

A number of normal marks occur on the newborn's skin. The normal newborn rash resembles small insect bites. Small whiteheads disappear without treatment. Do not squeeze them or they may become infected. Newborns have very dry, peeling skin that will be soft after peeling. It is not necessary to use lotions or creams because they may cause irritation.

Cord

Use a cotton swab dipped in alcohol to clean the cord and the crevices at the base of the cord about three times a day. *Notify your physician if you see bleeding or signs of infection, such as redness, drainage, or a foul odor.*

Keep the cord dry by folding the diaper below it so that it is not wet by urine. The cord usually falls off in about 10 to 14 days. Do not start tub baths until the cord is off and the area is well healed.

Diaper Area

Clean the diaper area with each diaper change. For girls, separate the labia (folds) and remove all stool. For boys, wash under the scrotum to help prevent rashes. If the diaper area becomes red, change the diaper more often. Leaving the diaper off to expose the area to air is also helpful. If an ointment is needed, petroleum jelly or a barrier-type ointment may be used. *If redness persists, ask your baby's doctor for suggestions.*

Bathing

Give your baby a sponge bath until the cord and circumcision areas are healed. Then begin tub baths. Because infants are washed as needed after regurgitation and with diaper changes, it is not necessary to give them a bath every day.

Sponge Baths

Before the bath, gather all the supplies. You need a container or sink for the warm water, washcloth, towel, baby shampoo, alcohol, cotton-tipped swabs, and clean clothes. Soap is not necessary for the young infant, but if it is used, it should be gentle and nonalkaline.

Give the bath in a room that is warm and free of drafts. Bathe the baby on a surface that is comfortable and safe. If you use a counter, pad it with blankets or towels.

Never leave the infant alone on an unprotected surface, even for a minute. Keep one hand on the infant at all times to prevent falls. Taking the phone off the hook during the bath prevents distractions. If you must leave the room, take the baby along or place the baby in the crib.

Keep the baby warm by uncovering only the area you are washing. Wash the face with clear water. Use a separate clean area of the washcloth to wipe each eye. Clean in and around the ears, where regurgitated milk may accumulate. Do not use cotton-tipped swabs in the infant's ears or nose because injury may occur.

To clean the neck folds, put one hand under the baby's shoulders and lift slightly. This maneuver causes the head to drop back enough that the creases in the neck can be washed.

Clean the diaper area last. For baby girls, wipe the diaper area from front to back. This procedure avoids infections that may occur if stool gets into the vagina or urethra.

Shampoo the head while holding the baby in a football position. The fontanel, or "soft spot," is covered with a tough membrane and is not injured by washing. Pulse movements in the fontanel are normal. Dry the hair well to prevent heat loss.

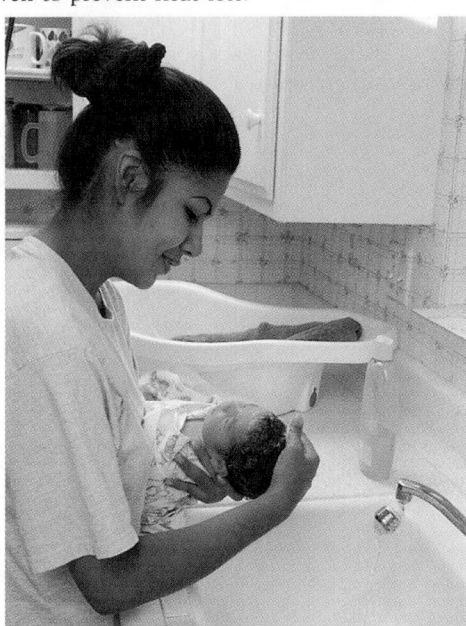

Tub Bath

For a tub bath, use a small plastic tub or a clean sink. Pad the bottom with a towel or foam pad. Place about 3 inches of warm water in the tub. Wash the face and hair before placing the baby in the tub. Keeping the baby dressed until after the hair is washed helps prevent chilling.

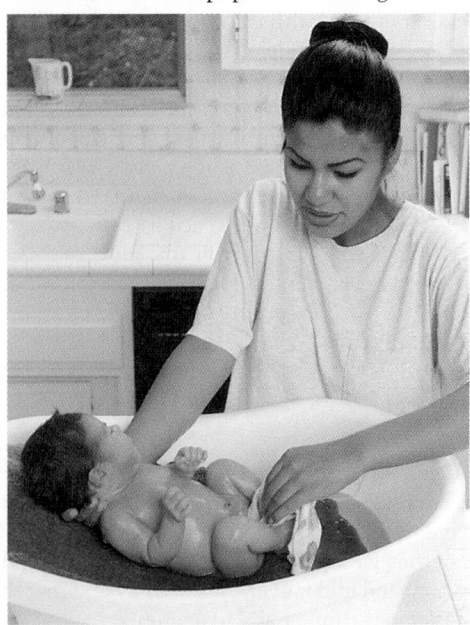

It may be easier, at first, to lather the infant's body and then immerse the baby in the tub for rinsing. It is not unusual for young infants to be frightened when they are first put in water. To help the baby adjust, talk softly and calmly while holding your baby securely.

Behavior
Knowing infants' different behavioral states helps you learn about your baby's individual characteristics.

Sleep Phases. During quiet sleep, the infant sleeps soundly with quiet breathing and little movement. Your baby will not be disturbed by noises from appliances or other children at this time. In active sleep, the baby moves or fusses while still asleep. During the drowsy state, the baby is beginning to wake but may go back to sleep if not disturbed. If it is time for feeding or other activities, however, talk softly to help the baby awaken.

Awake Phases. The quiet alert state is a good time for infant stimulation because the infant seems interested in objects and people. In the active alert, or "fussy," phase infants signal hunger or discomfort. If you do not intervene, the baby soon moves to the crying state. The baby who cries too long may not respond at first to care activities. A few minutes of rocking and holding close may be necessary before the infant settles down.

Socialization
Infants enjoy contact with people. Use an infant seat or an infant carrier to keep the baby near you and the rest of the family. Talking and holding the baby close provide social stimulation. Infants enjoy music that is not too loud. Because they focus their eyes best at a distance of 7 to 12 inches, items such as mobiles should be placed within this range. Infants especially like black-and-white geometric figures. Babies respond best to gentle stimulation during the quiet alert state. Too much stimulation can cause the baby to be irritable and have difficulty going to sleep.

Content of the Home Visit. During the home visit, the nurse performs a physical examination of the mother and infant. Family adaptation to the addition of a new member and the adequacy of the mother's support system are assessed. The nurse reinforces and continues the teaching about self- and infant care that was begun at the birth facility, and parents have an opportunity to ask questions. A feeding session should be assessed, especially if the mother is breast-feeding. Blood may be obtained for metabolic screening if the infant went home too early for reliable testing in the birth facility (Fig. 23–11).

Home visits provide reassurance for parents and may increase a woman's confidence and competence in caring for herself and her infant. Early return to her own environment, coupled with the knowledge that she can receive needed assistance from nurses, helps the woman to feel more in control of her experience.

Identification of Jaundice. Home visits are especially valuable in recognizing jaundice and intervening before bilirubin levels become dangerously high (Fig. 23–12). When jaundice is found, the nurse can discuss the implications and draw blood for testing bilirubin levels. Appropriate care is discussed, as necessary, including hydration and phototherapy (see Chapter 30).

Feeding Concerns. Feeding is a subject about which mothers often have questions, especially when they are breast-feeding. Breast-feeding problems were found in one study in almost a third of infants (Williams & Cooper, 1996). When the nurse observes a feeding and helps a woman deal with problems, the infant's intake may increase. Increased intake helps to prevent dehydration and possible hospital readmission. It also leads to increased excretion of bilirubin, which may prevent a need for phototherapy at home or in the hospital.

General Considerations in Home Visits. The nurse making a home visit is a guest of the family and must adapt nursing care usually given in the birth facility to the home

setting. The needs of other family members may make care in the home quite different from care given in the hospital. For example, the examination of the infant may need to wait for a short time while the mother meets the needs of her other small children.

Careful planning before the visit is essential to make the most of the limited time available. A telephone call allows the nurse to schedule the visit at a time convenient for the family and obtain directions to the home. It is important to set priorities very carefully based on the needs identified by the nurse and the family, especially when only one visit is planned. After the home visit, the nurse may schedule additional visits or provide the family with a telephone number where they may receive further help if needed.

Communication skills are particularly important when the setting is the home and the client is the family. The nurse must develop rapport with family members quickly and work with them to meet shared goals for the visit. A brief social interaction may be beneficial at the beginning of the visit to develop a trusting relationship. The purpose of the visit should be explained and the family's expectations and desires discussed. Open-ended questions and therapeutic communication techniques help the nurse identify and address the family's needs. It is important to make suggestions in a positive manner.

The nurse should be aware of any cultural practices affecting the family's view of care. For example, many Asians find direct eye contact, pointing a finger, or showing the bottom of the shoe offensive. In patriarchal cultures, the father is the head of the family, and teaching should be performed through him. The elder members of the family may also play a large role in determining what health care is essential. In some cultures, the mother-in-law is a very important influence in the care of the mother and infant.

Documentation of the visit is essential. The results of the assessments, teaching, nursing care, referrals, and plans

EXPECTED NEWBORN/FAMILY OUTCOMES	ASSESSMENTS	INTERVENTIONS	RESPONSE
Physical assessment: The newborn assessment is within normal limits.	Vital signs, weight Respiratory status (color, retractions, etc.) Skin (rash, jaundice, cord, circumcision) Fontanelles Activity, sleep, behavior, crying Elimination (number of voids and stools in 24 hours)	Complete systematic assessment.	Outcomes met. Outcome not met (requires further documentation).
Nutrition: Infant's intake is adequate.	Infant's and mother's behaviors during a feeding	Discuss frequency, length of feedings, and amount (in oz. or time at breast). Discuss breastfeeding or other problems. Provide written educational materials.	Outcome met. Outcome not met (requires further documentation). Referral made
Caregiving: Parents correctly describe infant characteristics and needs and demonstrate care.	Parent's knowledge and performance of infant care	Teach and clarify as necessary. Provide written educational materials.	Outcome met. Outcome not met (requires further documentation).
Infant/family relationships: The family demonstrates attachment behaviors.	Interaction of parents and family members with infant	Discuss emotional adjustment of all family members, sibling rivalry, postpartum blues. Provide written educational materials.	Outcome met. Outcome not met (requires further documentation).
Support system: Parents have an adequate support system.	Interaction of family members, sources of support within and outside the immediate family	Discuss availability and need for support, resources. Provide written educational materials.	Outcome met. Outcome not met (requires further documentation). Referral made.
Environment: The home is safe and has adequate facilities and baby equipment and supplies are safe.	Safety and potential hazards in the home; availability of heat, electricity, telephone, sanitation, sleeping arrangements	Provide written educational materials.	Outcome met. Outcome not met (requires further documentation).
Need for care: The parents verbalize understanding of need for well-baby care. They recognize signs of infant illness and how to get help.	Knowledge about well baby checkups and immunizations, signs of illness, how to take a temperature, where to get care	Discuss areas in which there is need; demonstrate temperature taking. Provide written educational materials.	Outcome met. Outcome not met (requires further documentation).

FIGURE 23–11

An example of a clinical pathway for a home visit by a nurse to the family of a normal newborn.

EXPECTED NEWBORN/FAMILY OUTCOMES	ASSESSMENTS	INTERVENTIONS	RESPONSE
Other care: Metabolic screening or other care is received, as ordered.	Need for specimen collection or other care	Collect blood specimens for newborn metabolic screening; give other care (phototherapy, etc.) as ordered. Provide written educational materials.	Outcome met. Outcome not met (requires further documentation).
Referrals: Parents verbalize understanding of referrals.	Need for referrals	Refer to physician, lactation consultant, WIC, community resources, etc. Provide written educational materials.	Outcome met (document to whom referral made). Outcome not met (requires further documentation).

FIGURE 23–11
• • • • • • • • • •
Continued

for follow-up should be recorded. Copies of the record are usually sent to the primary caregiver.

CLINIC VISITS

Clinic visits may be provided by the pediatrician or by the birth facility in clinics managed by nurses. In nurse-

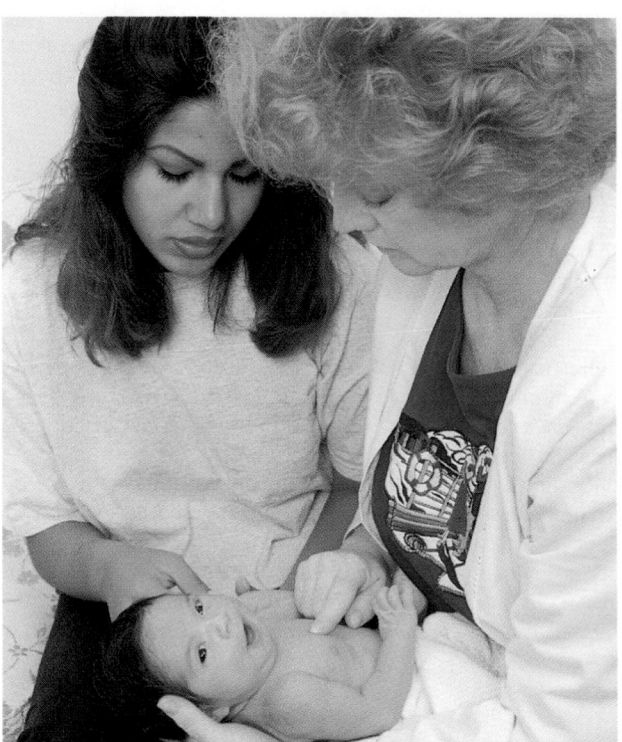

FIGURE 23–12
• • • • • • • • • •
Jaundice is of particular concern when infants are discharged early after birth. The nurse shows the mother how to blanch the skin to check for jaundice and discusses what the mother should do if she sees it.

managed clinics, mothers and infants are seen by a nurse within the first 48 to 72 hours after discharge. The charge is often included in the maternity care package. Assessment and care are essentially the same as those provided for home visits. The advantage of outpatient visits is that the nurse does not have to travel to the home and can see more clients each day, thereby reducing the cost of the service. The disadvantage is that the nurse does not have the opportunity to assess the home setting and the family interaction there. Clinic visits usually last 30 to 45 minutes. Clinic appointments may be made during the discharge procedure from the birth facility.

TELEPHONE COUNSELING

Telephone counseling can occur during follow-up calls to discharged clients or when parents call "warm lines" for help with problems or questions. Telephone calls have the advantage of being much less expensive than home or clinic visits. The major disadvantage is that the nurse cannot perform an in-person assessment of the mother, infant, or home environment and must rely on the caller to present an accurate picture of the situation.

Follow-up Calls.   Follow-up calls are placed by nurses in the first few days after discharge. The nurse asks a series of questions to assess the physical condition of the mother and infant and to identify any needs or problems. All mothers may receive calls or only those considered at risk for problems. In some facilities, the nurse who cared for the woman makes the calls. In others, certain nurses are assigned to make all calls. The nurse may schedule another call or a home visit, if available, or refer the woman to her primary care provider if problems are discovered.

Warm Lines.   Warm lines, also called help lines, provide parents with an opportunity to ask a nurse the questions that often arise after they have faced the reality of parenting. Warm lines are used for situations that cause parents concern but are not emergencies. The service should be available 24 hours each day to best meet the needs of the callers. Parents often call about infant feeding, breast-feeding concerns, and basic care of the mother and infant. Calls last about 15 to 20 minutes. The nurse answers the caller's questions and assesses for other problems. The nurse may call back later to see if the situation has resolved.

Telephone Techniques. It is important that nurses caring for clients by telephone understand telephone counseling techniques. They need special training in telephone communication and triage. Open-ended questions such as "How have you been getting along since you left the hospital?" or "Have there been situations where you weren't sure what to do?" help the mother describe any problems in her own terms.

Telephone triage involves determining whether a serious problem exists and what needs to be done about it. The nurse should help the mother (or caller) describe the major concerns, which may not be those discussed first. "What worries you most?" may help focus on the most important problems. Although most problems discussed are concerns about normal infants, the nurse must be alert for serious situations needing immediate referral.

The nurse should determine if the parents know where and when to obtain more care if the problem is not resolved. They should be told approximately how long it is appropriate to wait before calling the primary care provider or telephone warm line if the situation does not improve.

Nurses often call parents back to check on the progress of the problem.

Guidelines and Documentation. When nurses are giving care by telephone, it is important that they have written protocols and policies that provide guidelines for care. This procedure helps ensure that all who perform this service provide clients with similar information. A list of common questions can be compiled to help nurses obtain appropriate information when parents call about a problem.

Parents should always be told when and how to seek more care if problems are not resolved. If the infant appears ill, referral to the pediatrician or hospital emergency department is most appropriate. The nurse's judgment, based on education, expertise, and experience, is the most important factor in how helpful the service is to clients.

All calls should be documented so that accurate, legal records are available for future reference. The nurse may use a check-off form or a simple written description of the call. Documentation should include identifying information for the caller, including address and phone number. The reason for the call, problems described, advice given, and any referrals should also be recorded. In some agencies, all calls are audiotaped. A copy of the information is sent to the primary caregiver to provide continuity of care.

KEY CONCEPTS

- Prophylaxis against hemorrhagic disease of the newborn and ophthalmia neonatorum is necessary shortly after birth. It is provided by an injection of vitamin K and use of erythromycin ophthalmic ointment.
- Newborns may need help in clearing the airway. Positioning, suction, and close observation may be necessary.
- Nurses can prevent heat loss in newborns by keeping them dry and covered, avoiding contact between them and cold objects or surfaces, and keeping them away from drafts and outside windows and walls.
- The nurse must identify actual or potential hypoglycemia and intervene appropriately.
- Important interventions for jaundice are to monitor for its occurrence, to be sure that the infant is

feeding well, and to explain the condition to the parents.
- Reasons parents choose circumcision include decreased incidence of urinary tract infections and inflammation of the glans, prepuce, or meatus; religious dictates; parent preference; and lack of knowledge about care of the foreskin.
- Risks of circumcision include hemorrhage, infection, over-removal, urethral stenosis or fistula, adhesions, damage to the glans, and pain during and after the surgery.
- Parents may reject circumcision because of cultural practices, the belief that surgery is unnecessary, and concern about pain.
- Parents with uncircumcised sons should be taught not to retract the foreskin until it becomes separate from the glans later in childhood.
- Parents of circumcised infants should be taught signs of com-

plications and how to care for the area.
- The nurse must prevent mistaken identification of infants by checking the mother and infant identification bands whenever they have been separated.
- Parents and nurses must work together to prevent infant abductions. Parents must know how to identify hospital staff. Nurses should be alert for suspect behavior.
- Infection can best be prevented by scrupulous hand washing by staff and all who come in contact with newborns.
- Every nursing contact with parents should be used as an opportunity to teach.
- Screening tests are commonly performed to rule out phenylketonuria, hypothyroidism, galactosemia, and hemoglobinopathies.

ANSWERS TO CRITICAL THINKING EXERCISE 23-1

1. Determine whether Andy is showing signs of hypothermia, hypoglycemia, or both. Reassure and teach Nancy about her son's condition.

2. While taking the infant's temperature, assess for skin temperature, jitteriness, and general behavior. Check the blood glucose level if indicated.

3. If Andy's temperature is slightly low, change any wet linens, double wrap him, and apply a hat. Have Nancy feed him if it is near feeding

time. Recheck the temperature in 30 minutes and place Andy in a radiant warmer if necessary. Notify the physician if the problem continues. (See Nursing Care Plan 23–1 for other interventions.)

4. Praise Nancy for being so observant of her son. Explain that peripheral circulation is sluggish in newborns and causes cool hands and feet. If "shakiness" is the Moro reflex or normal newborn behavior, discuss this. Explain all interventions.

REFERENCES AND READINGS

Agarwal, R., Hagedorn, M. I. E., & Gardner, S. L. (1998). Pain and pain relief. In G. B. Merenstein & S. L. Gardner (Eds.), *Handbook of neonatal intensive care* (4th ed., pp. 173–196). St. Louis: Mosby.

American Academy of Pediatrics (AAP). (1995). Hospital stay for healthy term newborns. *Pediatrics, 96*(4), 788–789.

American Academy of Pediatrics & American College of Obstetricians and Gynecologists. (1997). *Guidelines for perinatal care* (4th ed.). Elk Grove Village, IL, and Washington, DC: Author.

American Academy of Pediatrics Task Force on Infant Positioning and SIDS. (1996). Positioning and sudden infant death syndrome (SIDS): Update. *Pediatrics, 98*(6), 1216–1218.

Association of Women's Health, Obstetric, and Neonatal Nurses (AWHONN). (1995). New data on infant abductions released. *AWHONN Voice, 3*(3), 11.

Association of Women's Health, Obstetric, and Neonatal Nurses (AWHONN). (1996). *Physiologic assessment of the healthy newborn*. Washington, DC: Author.

Association of Women's Health, Obstetric, and Neonatal Nurses (AWHONN). (1998). *Standards and guidelines for professional nursing practice in the care of women and newborns* (5th ed.). Washington, DC: Author.

Avery, G. B., Fletcher, M. A., & MacDonald, M. G. (Eds.). (1994). *Neonatology: Pathophysiology and management of the newborn* (4th ed.). Philadelphia: Lippincott.

Bajo, K., Hager, J., & Smith, J. (1998). Clinical focus: Keeping moms and babies together. *AWHONN Lifelines, 2*(2), 44–48.

Barnes, L. P. (1995). Using the telephone in patient and family teaching. *MCN: American Journal of Maternal/Child Nursing, 20*(6), 341.

Berger, D., & Cook, C. A. L. (1998). Postpartum teaching priorities: The viewpoints of nurses and mothers. *Journal of Obstetric, Gynecologic, and Neonatal Nursing, 27*(2), 161–168.

Brown, S. G., & Johnson, B. T. (1998). Enhancing early discharge with home follow-up: A pilot project. *Journal of Obstetric, Gynecologic, and Neonatal Nursing, 27*(1), 33–38.

Carpenter, J. A. (1998). Shortening the short stay. *AWHONN Lifelines, 2*(1), 29–34.

Choi, E. C. (1995). A contrast of mothering behaviors in women from Korea and the United States. *Journal of Obstetric, Gynecologic, and Neonatal Nursing, 24*(4), 363–369.

Choudhry, U. K. (1997). Traditional practices of women from India: Pregnancy, childbirth, and newborn care. *Journal of Obstetric, Gynecologic, and Neonatal Nursing, 26*(5), 533–539.

Cook, L. S., Koutsky, L. A., & Holmes, K. K. (1994). Circumcision and sexually transmitted diseases. *American Journal of Public Health, 84*(2), 197–201.

Evans, C. J. (1995). Postpartum home care in the United States. *Journal of Obstetric, Gynecologic, and Neonatal Nursing, 24*(2), 180–186.

Freitag-Koontz, M. J. (1997). Prevention of hepatitis B and C transmission during pregnancy and the first year of life. *Journal of Perinatal and Neonatal Nursing, 10*(2), 40–55.

Fuentes-Afflick, E. (1996). Circumcision. In H. W. Taeusch, R. O. Christiansen, & E. S. Buescher (Eds.), *Pediatric and neonatal tests and procedures* (pp. 372–379). Philadelphia: Saunders.

Lowe, M., Millea, D., & Simpson, K. R. (1996). Discharge planning. In K. R. Simpson & P. A. Creehan (Eds.), *AWHONN's perinatal nursing* (pp. 379–399). Philadelphia: Lippincott.

Maisels, M. J. (1998). Length of stay, jaundice, and hospital readmission. *Pediatrics, 10*(6), 995–998.

Mattson, S. (1995). Culturally sensitive perinatal care for Southeast Asians. *Journal of Obstetric, Gynecologic, and Neonatal Nursing, 24*(4), 335–341.

Mattson, S., & Smith, J. E. (1993). *NAACOG core curriculum for maternal-newborn nursing*. Philadelphia: Saunders.

McGregor, L. A. (1996). Short, shorter, shortest: Continuing to improve the hospital stay for mothers and newborns. *MCN: American Journal of Maternal/Child Nursing, 21*(4), 191–196.

National Association of Neonatal Nurses. (1997). *Neonatal thermoregulation: Guidelines for practice*. Petaluma, CA: Author.

Penny-MacGillivray, T. (1996). A newborn's first bath: When? *Journal of Obstetric, Gynecologic, and Neonatal Nursing, 25*(6), 481–487.

Philip, A. (1996). *Neonatology: A practical guide* (4th ed.). Philadelphia: Saunders.

Phillips, C. R. (1997). *Mother–baby nursing.* Washington, DC: Association of Women's Health, Obstetric, and Neonatal Nurses.

Rabinowitz, R., & Hulbert, W. C. (1995). Newborn circumcision should not be performed without anesthesia. *Birth, 22*(1), 45–46.

Roberts, J. A. (1996). Neonatal circumcision: An end to the controversy? *Southern Medical Journal, 89*(2), 167–171.

Ruchala, P., Seibold, L., & Stremsterfer, K. (1996). Validating assessment of neonatal jaundice with transcutaneous bilirubin measurement. *Neonatal Network, 15*(4), 33–37.

Schneiderman, J. U. (1996). Postpartum nursing for Korean mothers. *MCN: American Journal of Maternal/Child Nursing, 21*(3), 155–158.

Simpson, K. R., & Creehan, P. A. (Eds.). (1996). *AWHONN's perinatal nursing*. Philadelphia: Lippincott–Raven.

Smith, C. M. (1995). The home visit: Opening doors for family health. In C. M. Smith & F. A. Maurer (Eds.), *Community health practice: Theory and practice* (pp. 179–204). Philadelphia: Saunders.

Snellman, L. W., & Stang, H. J. (1995). Prospective evaluation of complications of dorsal penile nerve block for neonatal circumcision. *Pediatrics, 95*(5), 705–708.

Stock, C. M. (1995). Standardization of telephone triage: Is it time? *Journal of Nursing Law, 2*(2), 10–25.

Taddio, A., Katz, J., Illersich, A. L., & Koren, G. (1997). Effect of neonatal circumcision on pain response during subsequent routine vaccination. *Lancet, 349,* 599–603.

Tappero, E. P., & Honeyfield, M. E. (Eds.). (1996). *Physical assessment of the newborn* (2nd ed.). Petaluma, CA: NICU Ink.

Valaitis, R., Tuff, K., & Swanson, L. (1996). Meeting parents' postpartal needs with a telephone information line. *MCN: American Journal of Maternal/Child Nursing, 21*(2), 90–95.

Weekly, S. J., & Neumann, M. L. (1997). Speaking up for baby: The case for individualized neonatal discharge plans. *AWHONN Lifelines, 1*(1), 24–29.

Williams, L. R., & Cooper, M. K. (1996). A new paradigm for postpartum care. *Journal of Obstetric, Gynecologic, and Neonatal Nursing, 25*(9), 745–749.

Zderic, S. A. (1998). Developmental abnormalities of the genitourinary system. In H. W. Taeusch & R. A. Ballard (Eds.), *Avery's diseases of the newborn* (7th ed., pp. 1144–1157). Philadelphia: Saunders.

24

Newborn Feeding

LEARNING OBJECTIVES

After studying this chapter, you should be able to:

- Identify the nutritional and fluid needs of the infant.
- Compare the composition of breast milk with that of formula.
- Explain important factors in choosing a method of infant feeding.
- Explain the physiology of lactation.
- Describe nursing management of initial and continued breast-feeding.
- Describe nursing assessments and interventions for common problems in breast-feeding.
- Describe nursing assessments and interventions in formula feeding.

DEFINITIONS

colostrum Breast fluid secreted during pregnancy and the first 2 to 3 days after childbirth.

engorgement Swelling of the breasts resulting from feedings that are delayed, too short, or not frequent enough.

foremilk First breast milk received in a feeding.

hindmilk Breast milk received near the end of a feeding; contains higher fat content than foremilk.

latch-on Attachment of the infant to the breast.

let-down reflex See *milk-ejection reflex*.

mastitis Inflammation of the breast, usually caused by stasis of milk in the ducts or by infection.

mature milk Breast milk that appears after the first 2 weeks of lactation.

milk-ejection reflex Release of milk from the alveoli into the ducts; also known as the let-down reflex.

nonnutritive sucking Sucking during which no milk flow is obtained.

nutritive suckling or sucking Steady rhythmic suckling at the breast or sucking at a bottle to obtain milk.

oxytocin Hormone produced by the posterior pituitary gland that stimulates uterine contractions and the milk-ejection reflex; also prepared synthetically.

prolactin Anterior pituitary hormone that promotes growth of breast tissue and stimulates production of milk.

suckling Giving or taking nourishment from the breast. Sometimes used interchangeably with sucking, which refers only to drawing into the mouth with a partial vacuum, as with a bottle or pacifier.

transitional milk Breast milk that appears between secretion of colostrum and mature milk.

Helping women choose a feeding method and become comfortable using it are important nursing contributions that require knowledge of the infant's nutritional needs and the techniques to meet those needs.

Nutritional Needs of the Newborn

Calories

The full-term newborn needs 110 to 120 kcal/kg (50 to 55 kcal/lb) of body weight each day. Breast milk and formulas used for the normal newborn contain 20 kcal/ounce. The average newborn weighing 3.4 kg (7.5 lb) requires approximately 19 to 21 ounces of breast milk or formula each day to meet caloric requirements.

During the early days after birth, many infants lose 5% to 10% of their birth weight. This loss is due to normal loss of extracellular water and the consumption of fewer calories than needed. Newborns may fall asleep before feeding adequately and have a small stomach capacity at birth. Capacity increases rapidly so that many infants take 2 to 3 ounces by the end of the first week. Infants usually regain the lost weight by age 10 days. This information should be explained to parents.

Other Nutrients

The calories needed by the newborn are provided by carbohydrates, proteins, and fat in breast milk or formula. Full-term neonates digest simple carbohydrates and proteins well. Fats are less well digested because of the lack of pancreatic lipase in the newborn. Vitamins and minerals are provided by both breast milk and formula.

Water

Because newborns lose water easily from the skin, kidneys, and intestines, they must have adequate fluid intake each day. The normal newborn needs approximately 100 to 150 ml/kg (45 to 68 ml/lb) a day after the first 2 days of life (Tsang, DeMarini, & Rath, 1998). Breast milk or formula

supplies the infant's fluid needs. Additional water is unnecessary.

Breast Milk and Formula Composition

Breast Milk

Breast milk is species-specific for human infants and offers many advantages over formula. The nutrients in breast milk are proportioned appropriately for the neonate and change to meet the newborn's changing needs. Breast milk provides protection against infection and is easily digested.

CHANGES IN COMPOSITION
The composition of breast milk changes in three phases: colostrum, transitional milk, and mature milk.

Colostrum. The major secretion of the breasts during the first week of lactation is colostrum, a thick, yellow substance. Colostrum is higher in protein, fat-soluble vitamins, and minerals than mature milk but lower in calories, fat, and lactose. It is rich in immunoglobulins, especially secretory IgA, which helps protect the infant's gastrointestinal tract from infection. Colostrum helps establish the normal flora in the intestines, and its laxative effect speeds the passage of meconium.

Transitional Milk. Transitional milk appears by 7 to 10 days after lactation begins, as the milk changes from colostrum to mature milk. Immunoglobulins and proteins decrease while lactose, fat, and calories increase. The vitamin content is approximately the same as that of mature milk.

Mature Milk. After the first 2 weeks of lactation, mature milk replaces transitional milk. Because breast milk is bluish and not as thick as colostrum, some mothers think their milk is not "rich" enough for the infant. Nurses should explain the normal appearance of breast milk. Mature milk contains approximately 20 kcal/ounce and nutrients sufficient to meet the infant's needs. In general, discussions of breast milk and its contents refer to mature milk unless otherwise stated.

NUTRIENTS
Protein. The concentrations of amino acids in breast milk are suited to the infant's needs and ability to metabolize them. Breast milk is high in taurine, which is important for bile conjugation and brain development. Tyrosine and phenylalanine are low in breast milk, corresponding to the infant's low levels of enzymes to digest them. The proteins produce a low solute load for the infant's immature kidneys.

Casein and whey are the proteins in milk. Casein forms a large, insoluble curd that is harder to digest than the curd from whey, which is very soft. Breast milk is easily digested because it has a high ratio of whey to casein. Commercial formulas must be adapted to increase the amount of whey so that the curd is more digestible.

The protein in cow's milk causes allergies in approximately 3% to 5% of infants fed cow's milk formulas (Schepers, 1996). Because breast milk is made for the human infant, it does not cause allergies (Lawrence, 1999). Long-term follow-up studies have shown a significant de-

---

CRITICAL TO REMEMBER
· · · · · · · · · · · ·
Daily Calorie and Fluid Needs of the Newborn

Calories: 110 to 120 kcal/kg (50 to 55 kcal/lb)
Fluid: 100 to 150 ml/kg (after first 2 days of life)

crease in allergic conditions when infants are breast-fed exclusively for at least 1 month (Saarinen & Kajosaari, 1995).

Carbohydrate. Lactose is the carbohydrate in breast milk. Its higher level in breast milk may improve absorption of calcium (Lawrence, 1999). Lactose also promotes growth of the normal bacterial flora in the intestines.

Fat. Thirty percent to 55% of the calories in breast milk are from fat. The high level of cholesterol may aid in the development of the central nervous system. The fat in breast milk is more easily digested by the newborn than that in cow's milk.

The amount of fat in breast milk varies during the feeding and according to the time of day. More fat is present in the hindmilk, the milk produced at the end of the feeding (Mohrbacher & Stock, 1997).

Vitamins. Vitamin C must be added to commercial formulas to match the levels in human milk, which meet the infant's needs if the mother has an adequate intake. The infant may need added vitamin D if the mother's diet is poor and she or the infant is not exposed to the sun. The infant of a vegan mother may need supplementation with vitamin B_{12}.

Minerals. Although iron in breast milk is lower than in formula, approximately 49% is absorbed, compared with only 4% of that in iron-fortified formula (Lawrence, 1999). The full-term infant who is breast-fed exclusively maintains iron stores for the first 6 months of life. The addition of formula or other foods, however, may decrease the absorption of iron, making supplementation necessary. Preterm infants need iron supplements.

Sodium, calcium, and phosphorus are higher in cow's milk than in human milk. This difference could cause an excessively high renal solute load if formula is not diluted properly.

ENZYMES
Breast milk contains enzymes that aid in digestion. Pancreatic amylase, necessary to digest carbohydrates, is low in the newborn, but the enzyme is present in breast milk. Breast milk also contains lipase to increase fat digestion.

INFECTION-PREVENTING COMPONENTS
Substances in breast milk such as *bifidus factor, lysozymes,* and *lactoferrin* help to prevent infection in the infant. *Immunoglobulins* are present in highest amounts in colostrum but are present throughout lactation. Lymphocytes in the milk produce secretory IgA, which helps prevent intestinal and respiratory infections. Infants who are breast-fed, even partially, have a significantly decreased incidence not only of respiratory and gastrointestinal infections but also of ear infections and hospitalization (Beaudry, Dufour, & Marcoux, 1995).

EFFECT OF MATERNAL DIET
Although the fatty acid content of breast milk is influenced by the mother's diet, malnourished mothers have about the same proportions of protein, carbohydrates, and most minerals as those who are well nourished. Levels of vitamins in breast milk, however, are affected by the mother's intake and stores. It is important that breast-feeding women eat a well-balanced diet to maintain their own health and energy levels. (See Nutrition for Lactation in Chapter 15.)

Formulas

Commercial formulas are produced to replace or supplement breast milk. Manufacturers adapt commercial formulas to correspond to the components in breast milk as much as possible, although an exact match is not possible. A variety of formulas that differ in price and ingredients is available.

COW'S MILK
Unmodified cow's milk is not recommended for infants younger than 12 months old. Modified cow's milk is the source of approximately 80% of commercial formulas. Manufacturers specifically formulate it for infants by reducing protein to decrease renal solute load. Saturated fat is removed and replaced with vegetable fats. Vitamins and other nutrients are added to simulate the contents of breast milk. Examples of formulas are Enfamil and Similac.

FORMULAS FOR ALLERGIC INFANTS
Infants who have formula intolerance or allergies or come from families in which allergies are prevalent are given soy or protein hydrolysate formulas. Examples of soy formulas are ProSobee and Isomil. Many infants with cow's milk allergy are also allergic to soy formulas. Protein hydrolysate formulas, such as Nutramigen, are more universally tolerated by infants with allergies. The protein in these cow's milk–based formulas is treated so that they are hypoallergenic. The formulas are also used for infants with fat malabsorption.

SPECIAL FORMULAS
Some formulas are designed to meet the needs of infants with special problems. The preterm infant may require a more concentrated formula with more calories in less liquid, such as Enfamil Premature and Similac Special Care. Human milk fortifiers, such as Similac Natural Care, can be added to human milk to adapt it to the needs of preterm infants. Formulas such as Pregestimil are produced for infants with gastrointestinal problems. Lactofree formula is modified for infants who do not tolerate lactose. Lofenalac is low in the amino acid phenylalanine for infants with phenylketonuria, a deficiency in the enzyme to digest phenylalanine found in standard formulas.

▮ Considerations in Choosing a Feeding Method

Many women decide on a feeding method well ahead of birth, but some wait until late in their pregnancy. Nurses can help mothers decide on a method and gain confidence in feeding their infants. It is very important for nurses to be sensitive to mothers' feelings about feeding. Although nurses should encourage breast-feeding as the best method of feeding in most circumstances, they should be supportive of the mother's chosen method once the decision is made.

Breast-Feeding

Breast-feeding offers many advantages, summarized in Table 24–1. Both the American Academy of Pediatrics (AAP) and the U.S. Surgeon General recommend breast-feeding.

TABLE 24-1

. . . .

Benefits of Breast-Feeding

For the Infant

No allergic reaction to breast milk

Immunologic properties help prevent infections. May have fewer respiratory, ear, and gastrointestinal infections and less risk for hospitalization

Composition meets infant's specific nutritional needs

Nutritional and immunologic properties change according to infant's needs

Breast milk easily digested

Protein, fat, and carbohydrate in most suitable proportions

No possibility of improper (and potentially dangerous) dilution

Breast milk unlikely to be contaminated, not affected by water supply

Less likely to result in overfeeding

Unlikely to have constipation

For the Mother

Oxytocin release enhances involution of uterus

Mother more likely to rest while feeding

Mother likely to eat balanced diet that improves healing

May help with postpartum weight loss

Frequent, close contact may enhance bonding

Convenient: always available, no bottles to prepare, no formula to buy or heat

Economical: eliminates cost of formula and bottles

Traveling easier: no bottles to prepare, carry, refrigerate, or warm

---

The AAP suggests breast-feeding only for the first 6 months after birth and continuation of breast-feeding after the addition of solids until the infant is at least 12 months old (AAP, 1997) . Only 62.4% of mothers, however, are breast-feeding at the time of discharge. Of mothers who breast-feed, 41.7% are still breast-feeding at 6 months. These statistics show a gradual increase in recent years (Ross Products Division, 1997).

In an effort to promote breast-feeding, the United Nations Children's Fund (UNICEF) and the World Health Organization (WHO) advocate that birth facilities become certified as "baby-friendly" hospitals, where policies are initiated to encourage breast-feeding actively. Guidelines to becoming certified as a baby-friendly hospital emphasize education of staff and parents about breast-feeding, early initiation of breast-feeding, demand feedings, avoidance of formula and pacifiers, and rooming-in.

Formula-Feeding

Mothers choose formula-feeding for many reasons. Some women have medical conditions that interfere with breast-feeding. They may require medications that enter breast milk and are harmful to the infant. Other women are embarrassed by breast-feeding. Many mothers have little experience with family or friends who have had positive breast-feeding experiences. A frequent reason that mothers choose formula-feeding instead of breast-feeding is a lack of adequate knowledge about the two methods.

Combination Feeding

Some parents prefer a combination of breast-feeding and bottle-feeding. If possible, it is best to delay this combination until lactation has been well established at 3 to 4 weeks. Either breast milk or formula may be given in the bottle.

Factors Influencing Choice

Many factors influence a woman's choice of feeding method. These factors must be considered when educating women about their choices.

CULTURE

Cultural influences may dictate decisions about how a mother feeds her infant. For example, many Mormon women believe that breast-feeding is an important part of motherhood. Muslim women often breast-feed for the first 2 years. Some immigrants from countries where breast-feeding is the norm may breast-feed for shorter durations or not at all because they lack the support system they had in their own country. In addition, formula-feeding may be seen as a symbol of the new way of life. For example, Cambodian women rarely bottle-fed infants before coming to the United States but rarely breast-feed infants born in the United States (Rasbridge & Kulig, 1995). In one study, 58% of Hmong women who had previously given birth in Laos or Thailand had breast-fed there, but almost all chose to formula-feed when they gave birth in the United States (Jambunathan & Stewart, 1995). Nurses should be particularly watchful for ways to help mothers from other cultures who might wish to breast-feed but fail to do so because of lack of support.

Some Asian and Latino mothers give their infants formula while in the birth facility and do not begin to breast-feed until at home. This practice may be due to modesty about nursing in front of others in the birth facility, as well as lack of understanding about the value of colostrum. Some believe that breast-feeding before the milk comes in may drain heat and fluids from the mother (Mattson, 1995). Women in some cultures believe that colostrum may be "spoiled" because it has been in the breasts for a long time. They may express colostrum and discard it before they begin to breast-feed the infant.

EMPLOYMENT

The need to return to employment soon after birth may cause concern about feeding methods. The mother may choose formula from the beginning, plan a short period of breast-feeding before weaning the infant to formula, or use a combination of breast-feeding and bottle-feeding. Nurses provide information about breast-feeding and working.

SUPPORT FROM OTHERS

The mother with little support or with active discouragement from her family will probably have a difficult time nursing. Educating family members about the advantages of breast-feeding and how to deal with problems may lead to their encouragement of the breast-feeding mother.

The support the mother receives from the nursing staff plays a significant part in whether she feels comfortable with the feeding method she chooses. Those who do not feel confident in their ability to breast-feed before they leave the birth facility are less likely to continue breast-feeding if they encounter difficulties at home.

■ Normal Breast-Feeding

Breast Changes During Pregnancy

Breast changes begin early in pregnancy (see Chapter 9 and Figures 11–8 and 13–3). The ducts, lobules, and alveoli develop in response to estrogen, progesterone, placental lactogen, prolactin, and chorionic gonadotropin. Prolactin levels are high but milk production is prevented by estrogen, progesterone, and placental lactogen, which inhibit breast response to prolactin.

Milk Production

Milk is produced in the alveoli of the breasts through a complex process by which materials are removed from the mother's bloodstream and reformulated into breast milk. Most milk is synthesized when the infant is suckling.

The milk is ejected from the secretory cells of the alveoli into the alveolar lumen by contraction of the myoepithelial cells. It travels through the lactiferous ducts to the lactiferous sinuses (or ampullae), which the infant compresses during nursing to eject a stream of milk through pores in the nipple.

Hormonal Changes at Birth

PROLACTIN

At birth, loss of progesterone, estrogen, and placental lactogen from the placenta results in increasing levels and effectiveness of prolactin and causes milk production. Suckling and the removal of colostrum or milk causes continued increased levels of prolactin.

OXYTOCIN

Oxytocin increases in response to nipple stimulation. Oxytocin causes the milk-ejection reflex, commonly known as the let-down reflex. When mothers see, hear, or think about their infants, they often have an increase in oxytocin level, bringing about a let-down of milk. Pain or lack of relaxation can inhibit oxytocin release. Oxytocin also causes the uterine contractions mothers may feel at the beginning of nursing sessions (Fig. 24–1).

Continued Milk Production

The amount of milk produced depends primarily on adequate stimulation of the breast and removal of the milk. This "supply and demand" effect continues throughout lactation—that is, increased demand with more frequent and longer nursing results in more milk available for the infant. If milk (or colostrum) is not removed from the breasts, the milk in the ducts is eventually absorbed, the alveoli become smaller, the secretory cells return to a resting state, and milk production ends.

Preparation of Breasts for Breast-Feeding

Little preparation is needed during pregnancy for breast-feeding. The mother should avoid soap on her nipples to prevent removal of the natural protective oils from the Montgomery tubercles of the breasts. The use of creams, nipple rolling, pulling, and rubbing to "toughen" nipples is

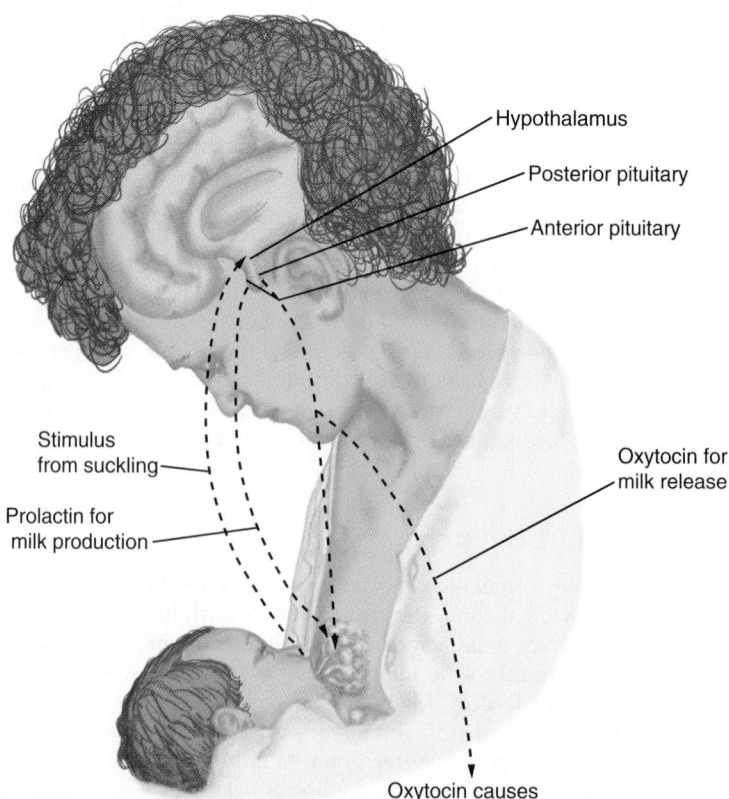

Hypothalamus

Posterior pituitary

Anterior pituitary

Stimulus from suckling

Prolactin for milk production

Oxytocin for milk release

Oxytocin causes uterine contraction.

FIGURE 24–1

Effect of prolactin and oxytocin on milk production. When the infant begins to suckle at the breast, nerve impulses travel to the hypothalamus, which causes the anterior pituitary to secrete prolactin to increase milk production. Suckling also causes the posterior pituitary to secrete oxytocin, producing the let-down reflex, which releases milk from the breast. Oxytocin also causes the uterus to contract, which aids in involution.

unnecessary and may cause irritation or uterine contractions from release of oxytocin.

The breasts should be assessed during pregnancy to identify flat or inverted nipples (Fig. 24–2). Normal nipples protrude. Flat nipples appear soft, like the areola, and do not stand erect unless stimulated by rolling them between the fingers. Inverted nipples are drawn into the breast tissue. Both conditions make it difficult for infants to draw the nipples into the mouth. Some nipples appear normal but draw inward when the areola is compressed in the infant's mouth. Compressing the areola between the thumb and the forefinger determines whether the nipple projects normally or becomes inverted.

Women with flat or inverted nipples sometimes use breast shells during the last weeks of pregnancy and after birth. The shells (also called breast cups) are worn in the bra with the opening over the nipple. They exert slight pressure against the areola and help the nipples protrude.

NURSING CARE
Breast-Feeding

Assessment

Assess both the mother and the infant during the breast-feeding process.

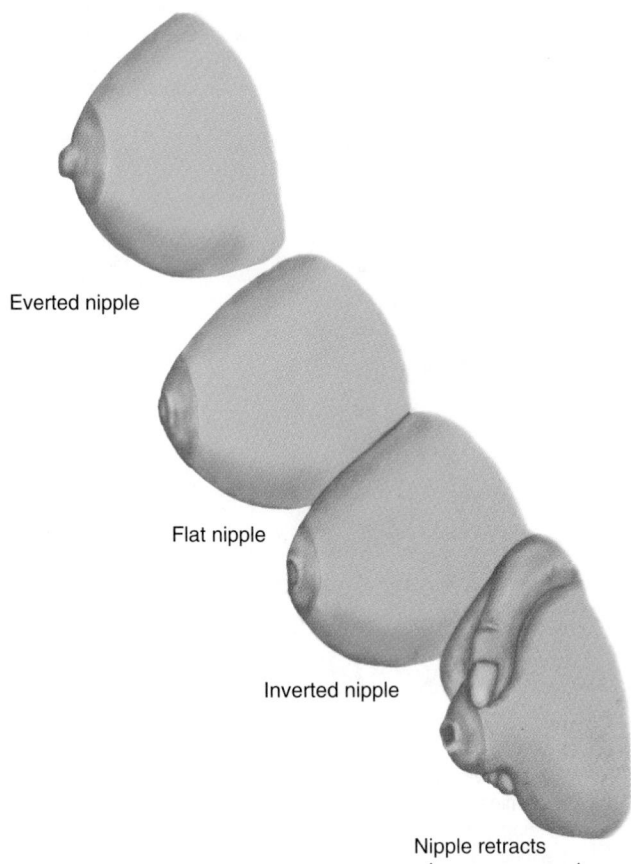

Everted nipple

Flat nipple

Inverted nipple

Nipple retracts when compressed.

FIGURE 24–2

Normal everted nipple and other types of nipples that may cause the infant difficulty in latching-on. Nipples shown after stimulation.

Maternal Assessment

Breasts and Nipples. Examine the breasts and nipples during pregnancy to identify problems that might interfere with feeding. Palpate the breasts to see if they are soft, filling, or engorged. Soft breasts feel like a cheek. If milk is beginning to come in, the breasts may be slightly firmer, which is charted as "filling." Engorged breasts are hard and tender, with taut, shiny skin. Redness, tenderness, or lumps within the breasts are also noted. The nipples may be red, bruised, blistered, fissured, bleeding, or tender.

Knowledge. The mother breast-feeding for the first time may have many questions and may need substantial guidance during her first attempts. If she has nursed before, she may have a better understanding of breast-feeding but may have questions or have forgotten some aspects.

Infant Feeding Behaviors

Before initiating a breast-feeding session, assess the infant's readiness for feeding. The infant should be awake and hungry. Sucking on the hands, rooting when the cheek or side of the mouth is touched, smacking of the lips, and slight fussiness are common hunger cues. Crying is a late sign of hunger. Continue to assess for signs of infant problems throughout the feeding.

Nursing Diagnosis and Planning

Women with and without experience often need information to have a successful breast-feeding experience. Therefore, a common nursing diagnosis for the breast-feeding mother is

■ Risk for Ineffective Breast-Feeding related to lack of knowledge of breast-feeding techniques.
   Expected Outcomes: The infant will breast-feed using nutritive suckling for an average of 15 minutes per feeding before discharge. The mother will demonstrate breast-feeding techniques as taught before discharge and will verbalize satisfaction and confidence with the breast-feeding process before discharge.

Interventions

Interventions are centered on teaching that nurses should provide to all inexperienced breast-feeding mothers. These techniques should be adapted as appropriate for mothers who have some knowledge of breast-feeding but need review or clarification.

Assisting with the First Feeding

The first feeding should take place within the first 1 to 2 hours after birth if both mother and infant are stable. The mother may need assistance in positioning herself and the infant and a demonstration of how to hold the breast.

Teaching Feeding Techniques

Position of the Mother and Infant. Breast-feeding mothers most often use the cradle and football holds and the side-lying position (Figs. 24–3, 24–4, 24–5). To increase her comfort, position pillows behind the mother's back or over an abdominal incision. Use pillows to elevate the infant to the level of the nipple and prevent pulling and tension on the nipple. The infant's head and body should directly face the breast, with the infant's nose and

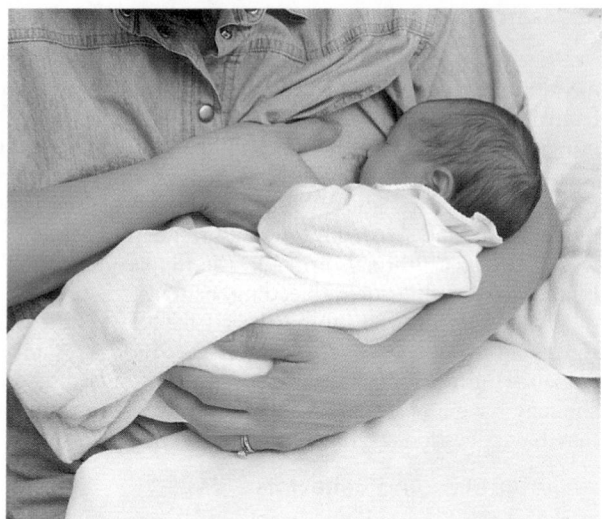

FIGURE 24–3

For the cradle hold, the mother positions the infant's head at or near the antecubital space and level with her nipple with her arm supporting the infant's body. Her other hand is free to hold the breast. Once the infant is positioned, pillows or blankets can be used to support the mother's arm, which may tire from holding the baby.

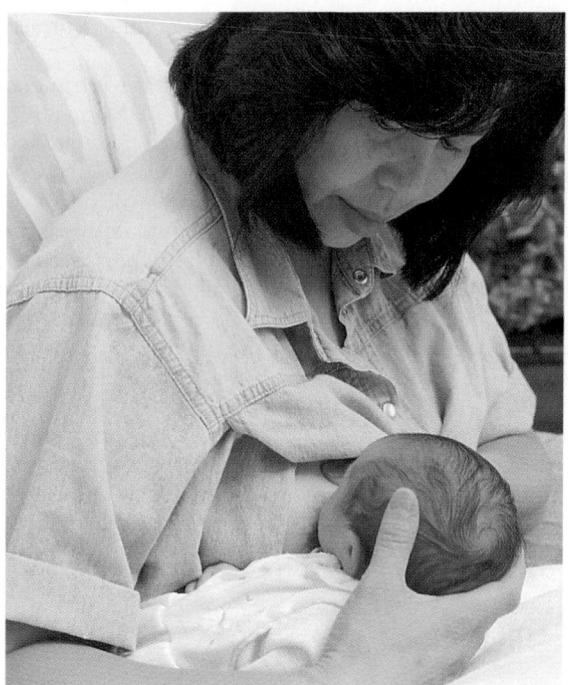

FIGURE 24–4

For the football hold, the mother supports the infant's head in her hand, with the infant's body resting on pillows alongside her hip. This method allows the mother to see the position of the infant's mouth on the breast, helps her control the infant's head, and is especially helpful for mothers with heavy breasts. This hold also avoids pressure against an abdominal incision.

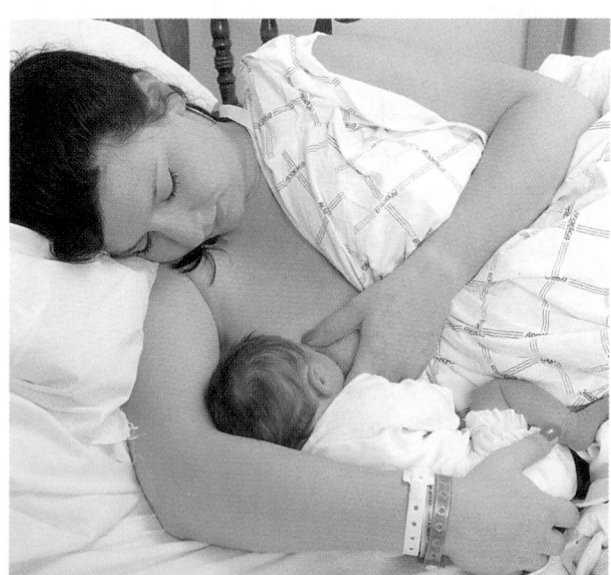

FIGURE 24–5

The side-lying position avoids pressure on episiotomy or abdominal incisions and allows the mother to rest while feeding. She lies on her side, with her lower arm supporting her head or placed around the infant. A pillow behind her back and between her legs provides comfort. Her upper hand and arm are used to position the infant on the side at nipple level and hold the breast. When the infant's mouth opens to nurse, the mother leans slightly forward or draws the infant to her to insert the nipple into the mouth.

chin lightly touching the breast. If the infant must turn the head to reach the breast, swallowing is difficult.

Position of the Mother's Hands. The mother's hand position is also important. In the C position, the mother holds her breast with her thumb on top and the fingers against the chest wall and supporting the underside of the breast (Fig. 24–6). Her fingers should be behind the areola. In the scissors hold, the woman uses her forefinger and middle finger to support the breast. This hold increases the risk that her fingers will slip down the wet areola and interfere with the placement of the infant's mouth.

Although mothers worry about the infant's ability to breathe while nursing, it is unnecessary to indent the breast tissue near the infant's nostrils. This procedure might cause improper positioning of the nipple in the infant's mouth, interfere with the grasp of the nipple, or interfere with milk flow.

Latch-On Techniques. Teach the mother techniques to help the infant latch on to the breast. The infant should be awake and hungry.

Eliciting Latch-On. After positioning the infant to face the breast, instruct the mother to hold her breast so that the nipple brushes against the center of the infant's lower lip. The infant will respond by opening the mouth, although up to a minute of stroking may be necessary. The breast should not be inserted until the infant's mouth is opened wide, or the infant will compress the end of the nipple, causing pain and little milk flow. When the mouth opens wide, the mother should quickly bring the infant close to her so that the infant can latch on to the areola.

Position of the Mouth. The position of the infant's mouth on the breast is important (Fig. 24–7). As much of the areola as possible should be in the infant's mouth to

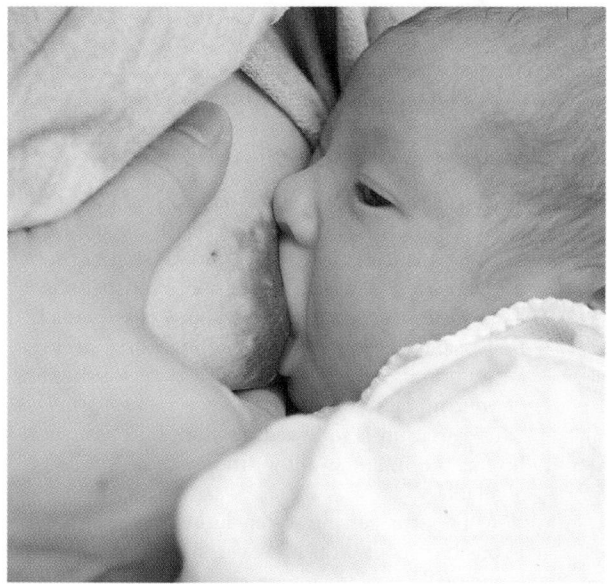

FIGURE 24-6
. . . .
C position of hand on breast. The hand is positioned so the thumb is on top of the breast while the fingers support the breast from below. Note the flaring of the infant's lips.

allow the nipple to be drawn toward the back of the mouth. This position prevents the infant from sucking on the nipple only, which leads to sore nipples and insufficient milk production. The infant's lips should be about 1 to 1.5 inches from the base of the nipple (Lawrence, 1999).

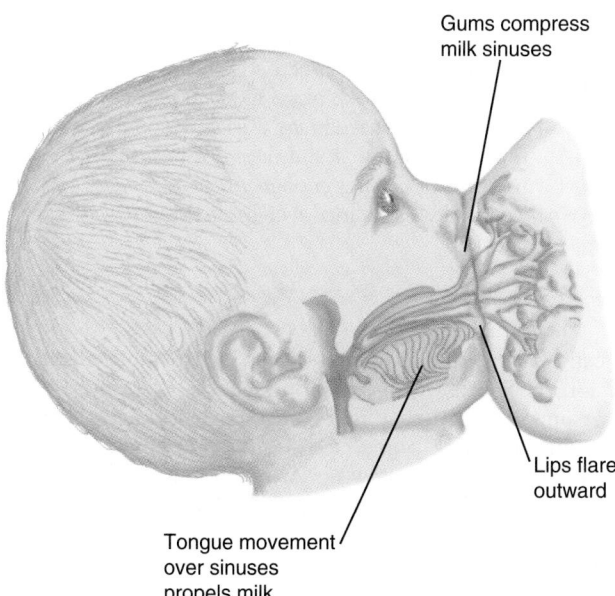

Gums compress
milk sinuses

Lips flare
outward

Tongue movement
over sinuses
propels milk

FIGURE 24-7
. . . .
Position of infant's mouth while suckling. When the nipple and areola are properly positioned in the infant's mouth, the gums compress the milk sinuses behind the areola. The tongue is between the lower gum and the breast. The tongue moves over the sinuses like a peristaltic wave to bring the milk forward into the infant's mouth. The infant's lips are flared outward.

Suckling Pattern. Teach the mother about the infant's suckling pattern. During nutritive suckling, the infant sucks with smooth, continuous movements with only occasional pauses to rest. Each suck may be followed by a swallow, or there may be two or three sucks before the swallow. Nonnutritive sucking often occurs when the infant is falling asleep. There may be a fluttery or choppy motion of the jaw that is not accompanied by the sound of swallowing. When this occurs, the mother should remove the infant from the breast because her nipples may become sore.

Mothers often wonder whether their infants are actually receiving milk from the breast. Point out to them the sound of swallowing when it occurs. A soft "ka" or "ah" sound indicates that the infant is swallowing colostrum or milk.

Short pauses are normal during nursing. Caution mothers not to jiggle the breast in the infant's mouth in an effort to start the suckling again. This process may cause the infant to lose the grasp on the nipple and areola, resulting in "chewing" on the nipple and soreness. If necessary, she should take the infant off the breast to awaken the baby, then start again.

Removal from the Breast. Demonstrate how to avoid trauma to the breast when removing the infant. To break the suction, the mother inserts her finger into the corner of the infant's mouth between the gums. She then removes the breast quickly before the infant begins to suck again.

Frequency of Feedings. Because breast milk moves through the stomach within 1.5 to 2 hours, infants usually feed every 2 to 3 hours. Frequent feedings are especially important in the early days after birth, while lactation is being established and stomach capacity is small. Explaining that the hormone prolactin, which is responsible for milk production, is released in increased amounts while the infant is suckling helps mothers understand the relationship of frequent feeding to milk supply.

During the early weeks of life, however, the infant should usually not be allowed to sleep more than 5 hours without a feeding. Long periods between feedings increase the likelihood of breast engorgement. Generally, the mother should nurse 8 to 12 times in each 24-hour period.

Some infants cluster their feedings and vary the length of feeding and time between each feeding. Several feedings close together (sometimes called "cluster feedings") may be followed by a longer interval between feedings (Mulford, 1995). Strict scheduling of infant feedings is unnecessary and leads to frustration for both mother and infant. A mother should take her cues from her infant.

Length of Feedings. Although early feedings were once limited to only a few minutes per breast to prevent sore nipples, improper positioning, rather than time at breast, is the usual cause of nipple trauma. When feedings are too short, the infant receives little or no colostrum or milk. It may take as long as 5 minutes for the milk-ejection (letdown) reflex to occur at first.

Mothers who are uneasy without a specific length of time for feedings can be instructed to start with feedings lasting approximately 10 minutes on each side, or longer if the infant continues to nurse vigorously. After burping, the feeding continues on the second breast until the infant falls asleep or begins nonnutritive suckling, generally about 10 to 15 minutes. Although variations in the length of feedings occur, early feedings should last no less than a total of 15 minutes on the average (Auerbach & Riordan, 1999). Feeding time increases as needed by the infant over the next few days.

Teach the mother about the differences between foremilk, the watery first milk that quenches the infant's thirst, and hindmilk, which is richer in fat, is more satisfying, and leads to weight gain. Feeding for too short a period prevents the infant from getting the hindmilk and decreases weight gain.

Switching back and forth between breasts several times during a feeding increases the amount of foremilk the infant receives but decreases the amount of hindmilk. Therefore, the mother should continue feeding on the first side as long as the infant nurses vigorously before burping and continuing on the other breast.

Preventing Problems

Frequent checking on the woman as she feeds her infant allows the nurse to answer questions as the woman thinks of them. Intensive teaching during the short stay in the birth facility helps prevent problems after discharge. Include suggestions about common problems and their solutions, as well as how to improve positioning and techniques. Pamphlets and videos provide another means of providing education. Review them before use, however, to ensure that the information is correct and they contain no advertisements for formula.

One of the major reasons for early weaning to formula is mothers' perception of an insufficient milk supply. Therefore, mothers should learn how to assess whether the infant is receiving enough milk. Intake can also be gauged when the physician or nurse practitioner weighs the infant at well-baby checkups. After the initial weight loss after birth, infants generally gain approximately 15 to 30 g (0.5 to 1 oz) each day during the early months of life. Weight gain generally begins by the fifth day of life.

Teach mothers who need to increase milk supply to feed more often and use a breast pump after feedings to increase milk production. Common causes of decreased milk supply include formula use, inadequate rest or diet, smoking, and use of caffeine, alcohol, or some medications.

Evaluation

- Does the infant nurse for an average of 15 minutes per feeding, with good latch-on and nutritive suckling?
- Does the mother use correct techniques for latch-on and positioning?
- Does the mother say she feels confident about the process?

▌ Breast-Feeding Concerns

Because mothers may be discharged from the birth facility before problems arise, nurses should teach them how to prevent and treat common problems.

After discharge, guidance for breast-feeding problems

MOTHERS WANT TO KNOW

Is My Baby Getting Enough Milk?

Your baby is probably getting enough milk if

- You hear the baby swallow frequently during feedings. It sounds like a soft "ka" or "ah" sound.
- You see nutritive suckling, a smooth series of sucking and swallowing with occasional rest periods. This pattern is different from short, choppy sucks that occur when the baby is falling asleep and not getting milk. After pauses, you may feel a tingling of your nipples as a new let-down reflex occurs. This sensation is followed by more nutritive suckling as the infant swallows the increased milk available.
- Your breast is getting softer during the feeding. (Your breasts do not, however, have to be hard [engorged] for you to have enough milk.)
- You can see milk in the baby's mouth or dripping from your breast occasionally.
- You feed your baby 8 to 12 times every 24 hours. When you nurse often, you produce more milk.
- Your baby has at least two to six wet diapers a day for the first 2 days after birth and at least six to eight wet diapers a day by the fifth day. If you are unsure if the diaper is wet, place a tissue or cotton ball inside it to show small amounts of urine. Urine should be light, not dark, yellow.
- Your baby passes at least three bowel movements—and often more—every day during the first month. The bowel movements are yellow by the end of the first week.
- Your baby seems satisfied after feedings. Babies remain quietly awake or go to sleep for at least an hour after most feedings. (An occasional fussy time is not unusual and does not mean that the baby is not getting enough to eat.)
- Your baby has gained weight at the first well-baby checkup.

---

can be continued at home by referring the mother to lactation specialists or organizations such as La Leche League, a support group that gives ongoing assistance to breastfeeding mothers. Some facilities provide home visits (Fig. 24–8), telephone follow-up, or outpatient clinics. Women with more serious breast-feeding problems need referral to a lactation consultant, a professional educated to deal with more complex situations.

Infant Problems

Infant problems require prompt attention to ensure successful breast-feeding.

SLEEPY INFANT

During the first few days after birth, infants often sleep longer than expected or fall asleep at the breast after feeding for only a short time. The nurse should show mothers how

Solutions to Common Breast-Feeding Problems

Problem:
Infant is sleepy at feeding time or falls asleep shortly after beginning feeding.

Prevention

- Gently awaken your baby at feeding time. Talk, gently move the infant's arms and legs, and play with the infant for a short time before beginning the feeding.
- Unwrap the baby's blankets and change the diaper. Leave the blanket off as you begin the feeding. Your body and a blanket added later will provide adequate warmth.

Solutions

If your baby goes to sleep during the feeding and has fed less than 5 minutes, try the following:

- Rub the baby's hair or cheeks gently, stroke around the infant's mouth, or shift the baby's position slightly to see if the infant will wake up.
- Remove the baby from the breast. Rub the infant's back to bring up bubbles of air and help awaken the baby.
- Express a few drops of colostrum onto the nipple. The baby tastes the colostrum when the nipple is offered and often begins renewed suckling.
- Wash the baby's face with a lukewarm washcloth to help the infant wake up.
- If your baby cannot be aroused with a few of the above gentle techniques, a longer sleep period may be needed. Let the infant sleep another half hour, then begin again.

Problem:
Infant who has taken bottles pushes the nipple out of the mouth and sucks poorly during breast-feeding. Infant has become confused about how to suck from the breast.

Prevention

- Avoid all bottles and pacifiers unless necessary. If they are necessary, stop as soon as possible.
- Do not give the baby formula during the night.
- Avoid giving formula at the end of a breast-feeding session, as it is unnecessary for healthy newborns. Adding formula may cause the infant's stomach to become distended, resulting in more "spitting up." If the infant waits longer before nursing again, milk production will decrease.

Solution

- Stop all bottle-feeding and pacifier use so that the baby gets used to suckling from the breast instead of the bottle. Nurse more often to stimulate milk production and help the baby learn what to do.

Problem:
Infant sucks on the end of the nipple or fails to open the mouth widely enough.

Prevention

- Be sure that the baby has the nipple at the back of the mouth and 1 to 1.5 inches of the areola in the mouth.
- Do not insert the breast into the infant's mouth until the infant opens the mouth wide.
- Pull down gently on the infant's chin to help the infant open the mouth if necessary.

Solutions

- Stop the feeding and start again if the infant is sucking on the end of the nipple or you see dimples in the infant's cheeks or hear "smacking" or clicking sounds.

Problem:
Breasts are hard and tender from engorgement.

Prevention

- Breast-feed the infant every 2 to 3 hours day and night.
- Do not give a bottle during the night, as bottle-feeding increases the risk of engorgement.

Solutions

- To reduce edema and pain, apply cold packs to the breasts between feedings. Make inexpensive cold packs from clean rubber gloves or plastic bags filled with crushed ice or frozen washcloths. Cover with a washcloth before applying to the skin.
- Before feedings, apply heat with compresses or a shower to stimulate milk flow. Use warm, wet disposable diapers applied over each breast. Fasten the tabs to keep the diapers in place and prevent dripping.
- To stimulate the let-down reflex so that the baby can nurse more easily, massage the breasts before and during feedings.
- If the breasts are very hard and your baby cannot latch on, express a little milk by hand or with a breast pump.
- Feed more often—every 1.5 to 2 hours.
- Wear a well-fitting bra for support day and night.
- To help you feel more comfortable, take prescribed pain medication 15 to 30 minutes before feedings.

Problem:
Nipples are sore, cracked, blistered, or bleeding.

Prevention

- Position the baby at the breast with enough of the areola in the mouth that the nipple is not compressed between the baby's gums during nursing.
- Avoid engorgement by nursing frequently. Express enough milk to soften the areola if engorgement occurs.
- Do not use soap on the nipples because it removes the protective oils and causes drying.

(continued)

- If you use breast pads for leaking milk, remove them when they become wet to prevent irritation of the skin. Avoid pads with plastic linings that retain moisture.
- Breast creams are unnecessary and may cause sensitivity and irritation. Creams that must be removed before each feeding may increase soreness.

Solutions

- To start the let-down reflex, begin each feeding with the less-sore side first, causing milk to flow more quickly on the second breast.
- Do not use nipple shields (latex nipples that fit over your own nipples). They decrease milk flow so that the baby does not get enough milk and milk production is decreased.
- Vary the position of the infant during nursing. The area of the nipple directly in line with the infant's nose and chin is most stressed during the feeding.
- Apply colostrum or breast milk to the nipples after feedings, as it has healing properties. Or try warm water or warm, wet tea bag compresses to the nipples.
- Expose the nipples to air between feedings by lowering the flaps of your nursing bra. Use a hair dryer held 6 to 8 inches from the breast to apply heat and dry the nipples.

- If you have burning, itching, or stabbing pain throughout your breast, look in the baby's mouth for the white patches of thrush, a yeast infection that can infect the nipples. Call the health care provider for medication to treat both you and your baby.

Problem:
Flat or inverted nipples that the baby has difficulty drawing into the mouth.

Prevention

- None.

Solutions

- Wear breast shells in your bra to help make the nipples protrude.
- Just before beginning breast-feeding, roll the nipple between your thumb and forefinger to help it protrude (see Fig. 24–11).
- To draw out inverted nipples, use a breast pump just before feedings. Put the baby to your breast immediately after the pump causes the nipple to become erect. The normal suckling process usually causes the nipple to stay erect.

to arouse sleepy infants for breast-feeding. When infants fall asleep during feedings, the nurse should evaluate whether the infant has fed adequately, should be awakened to feed longer, or should be fed again sooner than usual. Infants who continue to be excessively sleepy or to nurse poorly need further evaluation. Poor feeding may be an early sign of a complication such as sepsis (see Chapter 30).

NIPPLE CONFUSION
Nipple confusion (or nipple preference) may occur when an infant who has received bottle-feedings confuses the tongue movements necessary for bottle-feeding with the suckling of breast-feeding. The infant may refuse to breast-feed or may use tongue movements that push the breast out of the mouth. Some infants develop a preference for the bottle, from which milk flows freely without effort.

Movement of the mouth and tongue are different in breast-feeding and bottle-feeding. In bottle-feeding, infants must push their tongue over the latex nipple of a bottle to slow the flow of milk and prevent choking (Fig. 24–9). If the infant uses the same thrusting tongue motion while

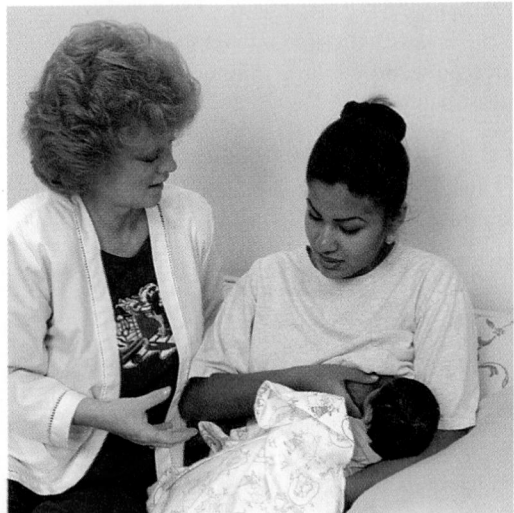

FIGURE 24–8
The nurse offers suggestions on hand position during the home visit.

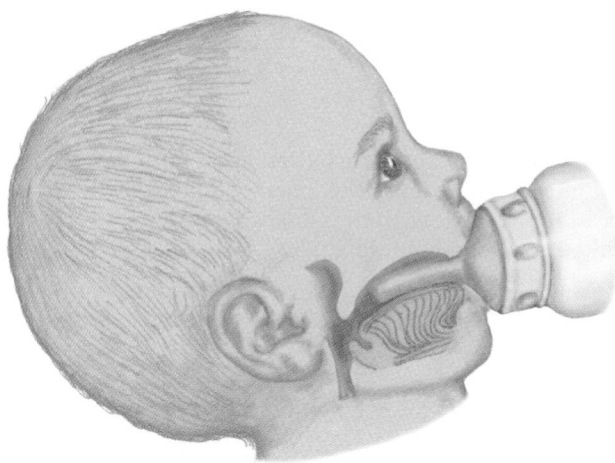

**Tongue thrusts forward
to control milk flow.**

FIGURE 24–9
. . . .
During bottle feeding, infants must thrust the tongue forward
to slow the rapid flow of milk.

nursing, the breast may be pushed out of the mouth. During breast-feeding, the tongue cups around the nipple and areola and presses against the breast like a peristaltic wave to bring milk from the sinuses into the infant's mouth.

Nurses should discourage use of formula in normal breast-feeding infants. It reduces breast-feeding time and decreases production of prolactin and, therefore, milk supply. Formula takes longer to digest, and the infant is not hungry again for about 4 hours. Formula-feeding further limits breast stimulation and milk supply and may lead to engorgement. Women who avoid using bottles during the first month are more likely to continue breast-feeding over 6 months (Piper & Parks, 1996).

SUCKLING PROBLEMS
Suckling problems may occur when the nipple is poorly positioned in the mouth. Dimpling of the cheeks and smacking or clicking sounds may indicate that the infant is sucking on the nipple only. Some infants do not open their mouths widely and suck on the end of the nipple.

Inserting a gloved finger into the infant's mouth helps assess suckling. The peristaltic motion of the tongue should be felt as the infant sucks. The infant who is thrusting the tongue may have become confused by the use of latex nipples, which should be avoided until the problem is resolved. If the infant tends to place the tongue on top of the nipple, placing a finger in the mouth and pressing the infant's tongue down just before latch-on may be effective. More complicated suckling problems may require assistance from a lactation consultant.

INFANT COMPLICATIONS
Infant complications may be minor and cause minimal interference with breast-feeding. The very preterm or ill infant, however, may be unable to breast-feed for a long period (see Nursing Care Plan 24–1).

JAUNDICE
Jaundice (hyperbilirubinemia) need not interfere with breast-feeding. Even when infants receive phototherapy, they can usually be removed from the lights for feedings. Concern over adequate intake may be more prevalent in caring for the infant with jaundice. Infants receiving phototherapy should not be given extra water because it may decrease the intake of breast milk. Frequent breast-feeding is necessary to provide adequate intake of protein and fluid and stimulate production of milk. In addition, breast-feeding increases the number of stools and aids in excretion of bilirubin. Jaundice is discussed in detail in Chapters 22 and 30.

PREMATURITY
If the preterm infant cannot breast-feed immediately after birth, the mother needs encouragement and instruction on how to use a breast pump to establish and maintain her milk supply. Breast milk offers immunologic and nutritional benefits and is adapted to preterm needs. It may help prevent necrotizing enterocolitis, a serious complication of preterm infants. It also helps the mother feel she is providing care for her infant even if she cannot take the infant home with her. The woman can pump her milk and take it to the nursery for the infant's feedings. Feeding the preterm infant is discussed in detail in Chapter 29.

ILLNESS AND CONGENITAL DEFECTS
Illness in the infant and congenital defects such as a cleft palate may cause breast-feeding problems. Parents of these infants need the same type of assistance as parents with preterm infants. The focus is on helping the mother maintain lactation until she is able to nurse the infant. Referral to support groups can be particularly helpful.

Maternal Concerns

COMMON BREAST PROBLEMS
Early nursing intervention can help the mother overcome common breast problems.

Engorgement. Engorgement is likely to occur if breast-feeding is delayed or infrequent. The breasts are edematous, hard, and tender, making feeding or even movement painful. The areola may become hard and the nipples flat, making it difficult for the infant to nurse. The condition may lead to nipple trauma, mastitis, and even the discontinuation of breast-feeding. See p. 597 for prevention and treatment of engorgement.

Nipple Trauma. Nipple pain lasting a minute or less at the beginning of feedings may occur during early breast-feeding as the infant stretches the tissue. Nipple trauma causes more sustained pain. Nipple pain tends to be greatest on the third or fourth day after birth and then to improve.

Traumatized nipples appear red, cracked, blistered, or bleeding (Fig. 24–10). Minor nipple trauma can be treated by independent nursing interventions. Redness of breast tissue, purulent drainage, and fever indicate mastitis or breast abscess and require antibiotic treatment (see Chapter 28). See p. 597 for prevention and treatment of nipple trauma.

Flat and Inverted Nipples. Nipple abnormalities should be treated during pregnancy, if possible, but interventions can begin after birth. Use of breast shells can be

NURSING CARE PLAN 24–1

Breast-feeding an Infant Who Has Complications

Assessment

Ruth James's son John develops respiratory complications at birth and is admitted to the neonatal intensive-care unit. The infant will probably not be able to feed at the breast for a few days. Ruth is disappointed and worried about whether she will be able to breast-feed at all.

Nursing Diagnosis

Interrupted Breast-Feeding related to separation from infant secondary to illness

Goals/Expected Outcomes

Within 2 days, Ruth will

- Verbalize the importance of breast-feeding her infant and her desire to maintain lactation.
- Pump her breasts as taught.
- Breast-feed John successfully (when it becomes possible).

Intervention

1. Explore Ruth's perception of the problem and her understanding of the cause for separation and the effect on breast-feeding.
2. Use therapeutic communication to help Ruth express her feelings of disappointment with the unexpected change in plans.
3. Explain to Ruth how valuable breast milk is for her infant and that she can use a breast pump to maintain lactation until John can breast-feed.
4. Teach Ruth to use a breast pump and store her milk. Instruct her to pump her breasts for 15 to 20 minutes every 3 hours during the day and at least once at night.
5. Explain prevention and treatment of engorgement.

6. Feed John breast milk if possible, whether by bottle or gavage. Teach Ruth how to store her milk and how to prepare it for use for her infant.
7. Arrange for Ruth to spend as much time with John as possible. To answer her questions and provide support, accompany her during the early visits and when she begins to breast-feed.
8. When Ruth begins to breast-feed, offer the same teaching that mothers of well infants receive. In addition, provide continued support if she has concerns.
9. Offer praise and realistic encouragement frequently.

10. If Ruth must go home before John is ready for discharge, provide her with information about purchase or rental of breast pumps. Give her containers to bring her milk into the nursery.

Rationale

1. Discussion of the problem identifies misconceptions and determines the type of teaching and support required.
2. Helping the mother express her feelings and accepting them helps her cope with the situation.

3. Reinforcing the value of breast-feeding and offering encouragement increase the chance of success.

4. Frequent use of a breast pump helps establish lactation by causing release of prolactin and oxytocin so that milk is produced and released from the breasts.
5. Frequent pumping should prevent engorgement. If it does not, the mother will need assistance in treating it.
6. Breast milk has properties that are especially valuable for the sick infant.

7. Bonding occurs more easily if a mother can be with her baby. Accompanying a mother during visits allows the nurse an opportunity to offer support as needed.
8. Women who must delay breast-feeding may be more anxious about the process.

9. A mother needs reinforcement of her abilities to increase self-esteem as a mother. Encouragement must be suited to actual circumstances.
10. The mother who must pump her breasts for a longer period may find that an electric pump is more efficient.

Evaluation

Ruth verbalizes her determination to provide breast milk for John. She maintains lactation and brings breast milk at each visit. At 5 days of age, John is ready to begin breast-feeding. Ruth is very patient in helping John learn to breast-feed with the nurses' help. John is able to nurse well at each feeding by discharge.

taught at this time. Nipple rolling just before feeding helps flat nipples become more erect so that the infant can grasp them more readily (Fig. 24–11). A breast pump may help draw out inverted nipples.

Plugged Ducts.　Engorgement, missed feedings, or a constricting bra may cause occlusion of a lactiferous duct. Localized edema and tenderness are present, and a hard area may be palpated. There may be a tiny white area on the nipple. Massage of the area (Fig. 24–12) followed by heat and continued breast-feeding using varied positions cause the duct to open. A plugged duct may progress to mastitis if not treated promptly. Mastitis involves localized pain accompanied by fever, generalized aching, and malaise. The mother with mastitis is discussed in Chapter 28.

ILLNESS IN THE MOTHER

When the mother is ill, breast-feeding may have to be postponed temporarily because of the mother's condition or the drugs she receives. Abrupt weaning, however, may lead to mastitis as well as maternal depression from decreased prolactin, which has been associated with feelings of well-being (Lawrence, 1999). The nurse should assist the mother in using a breast pump until she resumes breast-feeding.

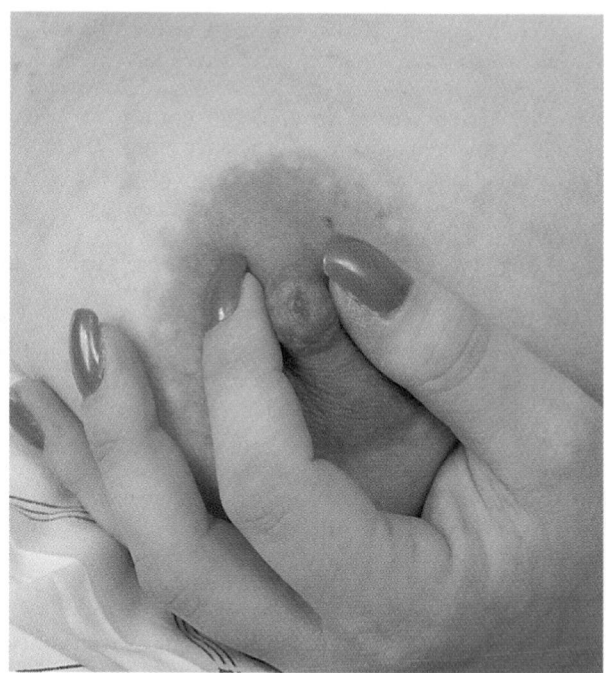

FIGURE 24–11
. . . .
Rolling helps flat nipples become erect in preparation for latch-on.

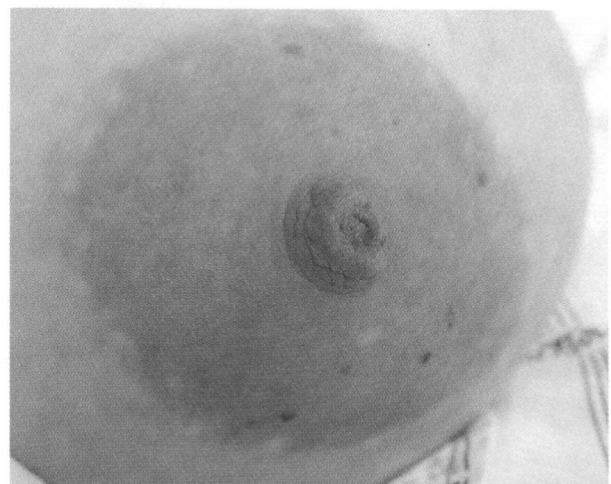

FIGURE 24–10
. . . .
Note the cracked area on this nipple.

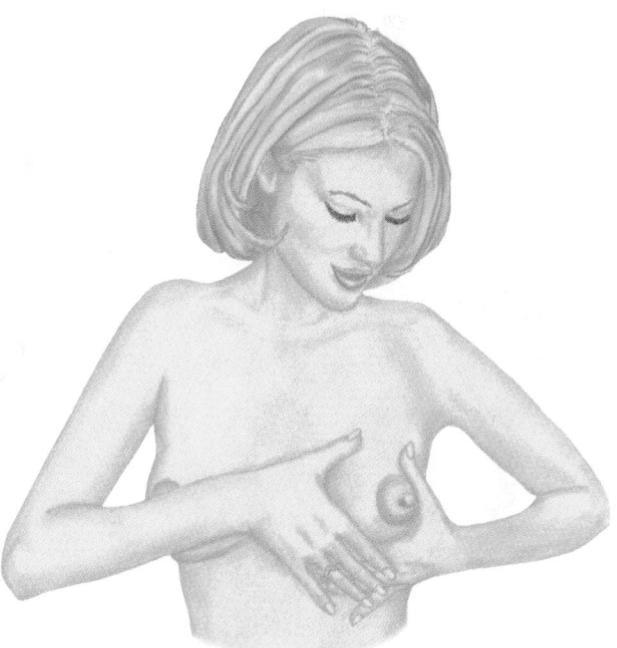

FIGURE 24–12
. . . .
To massage the breasts, the mother places her hands against the chest wall with her fingers encircling the breasts. She gently slides her hands forward until the fingers overlap. The position of the hands is rotated to cover all breast tissue.

Conditions in Which Breast-Feeding Should Be Avoided. In some situations, breast-feeding is contraindicated, often because the mother's serious illness can be transmitted to the infant. Examples are untreated active tuberculosis and human immunodeficiency virus (HIV) infection. Conditions such as cancer may become worse because of hormonal changes of lactation. Maternal drug abuse is also a contraindication.

Drug Transfer to Breast Milk. Most medications taken by the mother cross into the breast milk to some degree. Some interfere with milk production. Therefore, use of both prescription and over-the-counter drugs should be approved by a physician. Another drug can often be substituted for one that affects the infant. If a mother must take a drug that will be harmful to her infant, she should pump her breasts while she is taking the medication. Once the drug clears her bloodstream, she may resume breast-feeding (see Appendix C for information about drug effects during breast-feeding).

MILK EXPRESSION

When there is a need for milk expression, the nurse helps the mother use hand expression (Fig. 24–13) or a breast pump (Fig. 24–14). (The nurse should always wear gloves when contact with breast milk may occur.) Hand expression can be done without other equipment but is not as effective as a breast pump. Hand expression or manual pumps are useful for the mother who wants to save breast milk for another feeding or whose areola is so engorged that the infant cannot grasp it.

The mother who needs to pump her milk for a prolonged period may prefer using a battery-operated or electric breast pump. Battery-operated pumps are small, port-

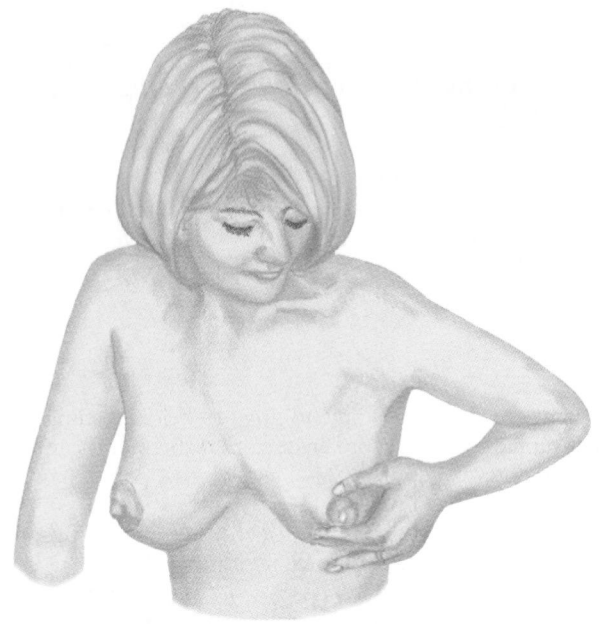

FIGURE 24–13

To express milk from the breast, the mother places her hand just behind the areola, with the thumb on top and the fingers supporting the breast. The tissue is pressed back against the chest wall; then the fingers and thumb are brought together and toward the nipple. This procedure compresses the milk sinuses and causes milk to flow. The action is repeated to simulate the suckling of the infant. Moving the hands around the areola allows compression of all sinuses and complete removal of milk from the breast. Compression should be gentle to avoid trauma.

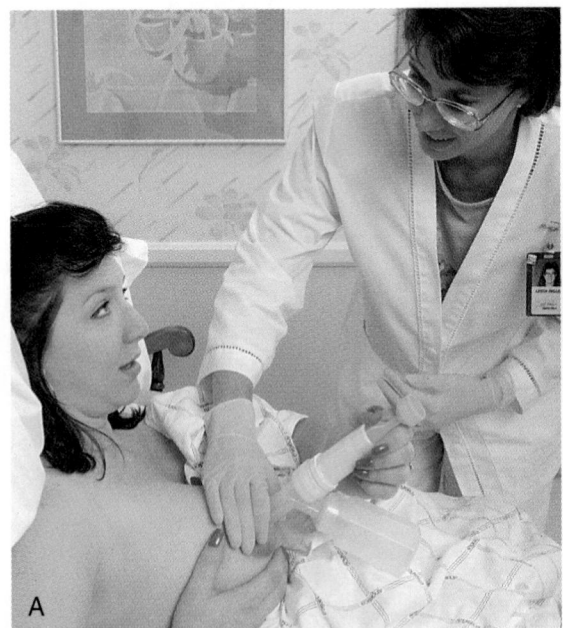

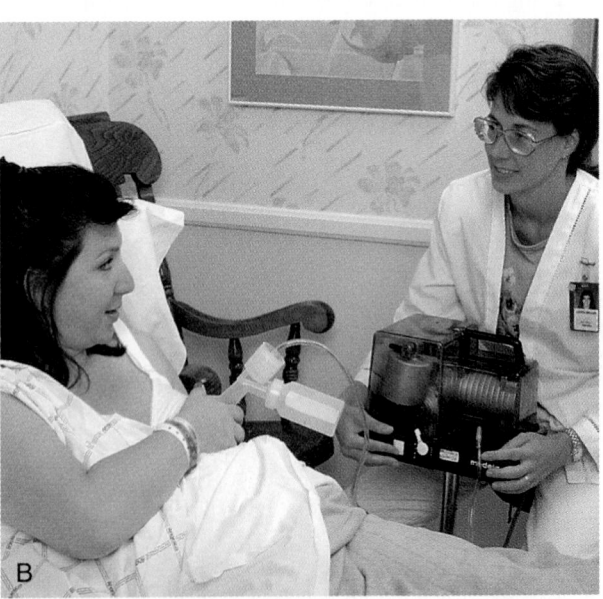

FIGURE 24–14

The nurse demonstrates methods of pumping breast milk. *A,* Manual breast pump. *B,* Electric breast pump.

able, and relatively inexpensive. Large electric pumps can often be rented for home use. They are more efficient than hand or battery pumps and are indicated when the mother must pump to maintain her milk supply for a long period.

Use of the breast pump should begin within the first 24 hours after birth for the woman who cannot breast-feed her infant. She should pump her breasts approximately every 3 hours during the day and at least once at night when prolactin levels are elevated. Sessions should last approximately 15 to 20 minutes. A total of eight or more sessions in each 24 hours is best to maintain milk supply.

Use of massage and heat before pumping helps initiate the flow of milk. Massage during pumping may increase the volume of milk obtained at each session. The amount of suction should be set at a low level in the beginning and gradually increased, if necessary. Too much negative pressure traumatizes the breast. If the woman needs to increase her milk supply, pumping more often rather than for longer periods is more effective.

BREAST-FEEDING AFTER MULTIPLE BIRTHS

To be successful, mothers who have more than one newborn need help and support from nurses and family members. It is important for these mothers to nurse every 2 to 3 hours to build up the milk supply. If the infants cannot breast-feed, the woman will need help to use a breast pump.

If the woman decides to feed two infants simultaneously, she will need help positioning them using the football hold, cradle hold, or a combination of both. She should be encouraged to eat well, get enough rest, and ask for help from family and friends.

EMPLOYMENT

Although some mothers remain at home for 6 weeks or more after birth, others must return to work earlier. Working and breast-feeding can be combined very well with some planning. A week or two before she returns to work, the mother can begin using a breast pump once or twice a day to practice pumping her breasts and to build up a small supply of frozen breast milk.

Milk should be stored in rigid polypropylene plastic containers because antibodies in the milk adhere to glass. The rigid plastic containers maintain the stability of the milk components and are easier to use than plastic bottle liners, which spill easily. The milk can be kept in a refrigerator for 48 hours, a refrigerator freezer for a month, or a deep freeze at 0°F for 6 months. Leukocytes are destroyed by freezing, but most of the other immunologic properties are preserved. Breast milk should be thawed in a refrigerator or by holding the container under running water rather than by heating it. It should not be refrozen or heated in a microwave. Refrigerated milk should be used as much as possible so that the leukocytes are available for the infant.

Most working mothers use a battery-operated or electric pump once or twice a day during lunch or coffee breaks. The milk should be refrigerated or placed in an insulated container with ice and can be used for the next day's feeding.

WEANING

There is no one "right" time to wean the infant. Mothers choose to wean their infants for a variety of reasons. The nurse should provide information so that the mother can make an informed decision about weaning and should support the woman once her decision is made. Explaining that even a short period of breast-feeding offers her infant many advantages is reassuring. Mothers may need help in planning a gradual weaning process. Gradual weaning allows them to avoid engorgement, and infants can get used to a bottle or cup over a longer period.

FORMULA-FEEDING

Although formula-feeding may require less knowledge and skill than breast-feeding, the inexperienced mother often has many questions and may need assistance in learning to use formula correctly.

NURSING CARE
Formula-Feeding

Assessment

To identify areas that need teaching, the nurse assesses the mother's method of positioning the infant and bottle and burping during the initial and subsequent feedings. The mother should know how to prepare formula when she goes home.

Nursing Diagnosis and Planning

Because improper formula preparation and feeding techniques could harm the infant, an appropriate nursing diagnosis for the mother using formula-feeding is

■ Risk for Altered Health Maintenance related to lack of understanding of formula preparation and feeding techniques.

Expected Outcomes: The mother will demonstrate correct techniques in holding the infant and bottle during feedings and will describe how to prepare formula and the frequency of feedings.

Interventions

Teaching about Formula

Teach the mother how to prepare formula correctly. Infection may occur if the milk or water used for preparation is contaminated. It is essential that she follow directions in mixing the formula. Improper dilution of the formula may cause undernutrition or imbalances of sodium, which can be dangerous to the infant.

Types of Formula. Formula may be purchased in three different forms.
Ready-to-Use Preparations. Ready-to-use formula is available in bottles to which a nipple is added or in cans to be poured directly into a bottle. Although expensive, it is practical when there is difficulty mixing the formula or the water supply is in question. An open can should be refrigerated and used within 24 hours.

Concentrated Liquid. Explain to the mother how to dilute concentrated liquid formula. Equal parts of formula and water are mixed together in a bottle to provide the amount desired for each feeding.

Powdered Formula. Powdered formula is more economical and is particularly useful when a breast-feeding mother plans to give an occasional bottle of formula. Usually one scoop of powder is added to each 2 ounces of warm water in a bottle. Formula should be well mixed to dissolve the powder and make the solution uniform.

Equipment. Many different types of bottles and nipples are available. Bottles may be glass or plastic, or a plastic liner that fits into a rigid container is used. Some nipples are designed to simulate the human nipple to promote jaw development. Selection of the type of bottles and nipples depends on individual preference.

Preparation. The mother can prepare a single bottle or a 24-hour supply. If the water supply is safe, sterilization is not necessary. Bottles and nipples can be washed in hot, sudsy water, rinsed well, and allowed to air dry. Bottles may be washed in a dishwasher, but nipples tend to deteriorate quickly unless washed by hand. Instruct the mother to wash her hands as well as the top of the can and the can opener. The formula and water are poured into the bottles, which are then capped. Emphasize that the proportion of water and liquid or powdered formula must be adhered to exactly to prevent illness in the infant.

Explain that if safety of the water supply is questionable, sterilization, by aseptic or terminal method, is required. In both methods, all equipment is washed and rinsed well before beginning. In the aseptic method, equipment needed for the procedure is boiled for 5 minutes in a sterilizer or deep pan. Water for diluting the formula is boiled separately. The bottles are then assembled, using sterilized tongs to avoid contamination by the hands. The formula and boiled water are added, and the bottles are capped and refrigerated until needed.

In the terminal sterilization method, the formula is placed in clean, loosely capped bottles. The bottles are then placed in the sterilizer or pan of water and boiled for 25 minutes. After the bottles cool, the caps are tightened and the bottles refrigerated.

Explaining Feeding Techniques

Positioning. Show the mother how to position the infant in a semi-upright position such as the cradle hold. This position allows the mother to hold the infant close with face-to-face contact. The bottle is held so that the nipple is kept full of formula to prevent excessive swallowing of air (Fig. 24–15).

Burping. Burping or "bubbling" the infant after every half-ounce is needed for the first few days. The infant gradually can take more milk before burping. Show the mother how to place the infant over her shoulder or in a sitting position with the head supported while she pats and rubs the infant's back.

Frequency and Amount. Tell the mother to feed the infant every 3 to 4 hours. The infant takes only 0.5 to 1 ounce per feeding during the first day of life but gradually increases to 2 to 3 ounces per feeding by the third day. Both

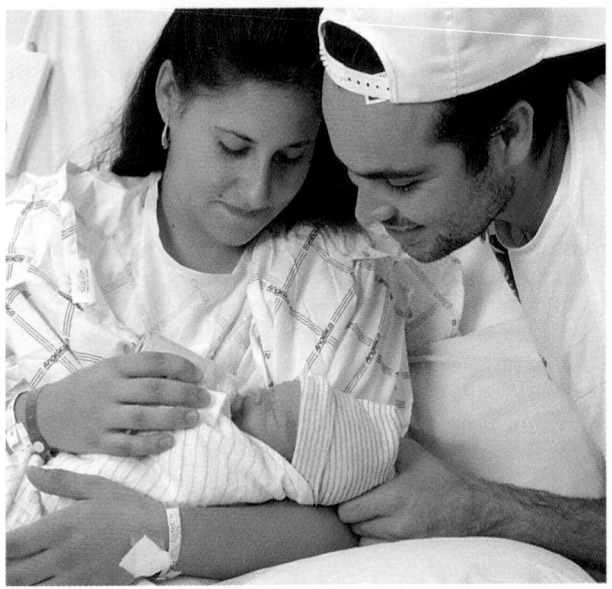

FIGURE 24–15

This mother holds her infant close during bottle feeding. The bottle is positioned so the nipple is filled with milk at all times. The father offers encouragement.

the frequency and amount, however, should be adapted to the infant's needs. An infant who is satisfied often goes to sleep.

Cautions. Caution mothers not to prop the bottle. Propping increases the likelihood of choking if regurgitation occurs and eliminates the holding and cuddling that should accompany feeding. Infants who go to sleep with a bottle propped are at risk for aspiration. Pooled milk in the mouth leads to cavities once the teeth are in. Ear infections are more common in infants who sleep with a bottle.

The mother should not try to coax the infant to finish the bottle at each feeding. This action could result in regurgitation and excessive weight gain.

Discarding unused formula within an hour prevents feeding the infant formula contaminated by rapidly growing bacteria.

Formula should not be heated in a microwave oven because the heating is uneven and may result in some parts of the liquid being very hot, even when the outside of the bottle feels only warm. Formula can be heated by placing it in a container of hot water until it is warm. Suggest that the mother test the formula temperature by allowing a few drops from the bottle to fall on her inner arm.

Infant Variations. Although formula is usually given at room temperature, some infants take heated formula better. The mother of a sleepy infant needs to use the same wake-up techniques discussed for the breast-feeding mother. Angling the tip of the nipple so that it rubs the palate triggers the suck reflex in most infants.

Evaluation

- Does the mother position the infant and the bottle correctly?
- Does she feed the infant the right amount of formula?
- Can she explain how to prepare formula properly?

KEY CONCEPTS

- The newborn may lose weight in the first few days after birth as a result of insufficient intake and normal loss of extracellular fluid.
- Colostrum is rich in protein, vitamins, minerals, and immunoglobulins. Transitional milk appears between colostrum and mature milk. Mature milk is present after the first 2 weeks of lactation.
- Breast milk has nutrients in proportions that the newborn requires and in an easily digested form. Most commercial formulas are cow's milk adapted to simulate human milk.
- Breast milk contains factors that help establish the normal intestinal flora and prevent infection. These include *bifidus* factor, leukocytes, lysozymes, and immunoglobulins.
- A variety of commercial formulas is available. They include modified cow's milk formula, soy-based or protein hydrolysate formulas, and formulas for preterm infants or those with special problems.
- Factors that influence the mother's choice of feeding method include knowledge about each method, support from family and friends, cultural influences, and employment.
- Suckling at the breast causes the mother's posterior pituitary to release oxytocin, which triggers the let-down reflex. It also causes the anterior pituitary to release prolactin, which increases milk production.
- The principle of "supply and demand" applies to breast-feeding. Milk production increases when the infant feeds frequently. When breast-feeding ceases, prolactin is decreased, and eventually the alveoli of the breasts atrophy and stop producing milk.
- Flat and inverted nipples should be identified during pregnancy. Creams and methods to toughen the nipples are not necessary.
- The nurse can help the mother establish breast-feeding by initiating early feeding, assisting her to position the infant at the breast, and showing her how to position her hands. The nurse should teach the mother how to help the infant latch on to the breast, assess the position of the mouth on the breast, and remove the infant from the breast.
- The mother should feed the infant 8 to 12 times each day for an average of at least 15 minutes per feeding, nursing until the infant is satisfied at the second breast.
- Wake-up techniques for sleepy infants include unwrapping the blankets, talking to the infant, changing the diaper, rubbing the infant's back, and expressing colostrum onto the breast.
- When infants suck from a bottle, they must push the tongue against the nipple to slow the flow of milk. When they suckle at the breast, they position the nipple far into the mouth so that the gums compress the areola as the tongue moves over the milk sinuses in a wave-like motion.
- The nurse can help the woman with engorged breasts by encouraging her to nurse frequently, apply heat and cold, and massage and express milk to soften the areola if necessary.
- The nurse should help the mother with sore nipples to check the positioning of the infant at the breast. The mother should vary the position of the infant at the breast, apply breast milk, warm-water compresses, or warm, wet tea bags to the nipples. She should also expose the nipples to air.
- Teaching for the mother who plans to work and breast-feed includes expression of breast milk by hand or pump and proper storage of the milk.
- Mothers who use formula need information about the types of formula available, preparing them correctly, and feeding techniques.

REFERENCES AND READINGS

American Academy of Pediatrics & American College of Obstetricians and Gynecologists. (1997). *Guidelines for perinatal care* (4th ed.). Elk Grove Village, IL, and Washington, DC: Author.

American Academy of Pediatrics Work Group on Breastfeeding. (1997). Breastfeeding and the use of human milk. *Pediatrics, 100*(6), 1035–1039.

Association of Women's Health, Obstetric, and Neonatal Nurses (AWHONN). (1998). *Standards and guidelines for professional nursing practice in the care of women and newborns* (5th ed.). Washington, DC: Author.

Auerbach, K. D. (1999). Maternal employment and breastfeeding. In J. Riordan & K. C. Auerbach (Eds.), *Breastfeeding and human lactation* (2nd ed., pp. 577–636). Boston: Jones & Bartlett.

Auerbach, K. D., & Riordan, J. (1999). The breastfeeding process: The perinatal and intrapartum period. In J. Riordan & K. C.

Auerbach (Eds.), *Breastfeeding and human lactation* (2nd ed., pp. 279–309). Boston: Jones & Bartlett.

Barger, J. (1998). The ten steps to successful breastfeeding: Principles, practicalities, and practices, part I. *Mother Baby Journal, 3*(6), 41–44.

Beaudry, M., Dufour, R., & Marcoux, S. (1995). Relation between infant feeding and infections during the first six months of life. *Journal of Pediatrics, 126*(2), 191–197.

Behrman, R. E., Kliegman, R. M., Arvin, A. M., & Nelson, W. E. (Eds.). (1996). *Nelson textbook of pediatrics* (15th ed.). Philadelphia: Saunders.

Biancuzzo, M. (1997). Breastfeeding education for early discharge: A three-tiered approach. *Journal of Perinatal Neonatal Nursing, 11*(2), 10–22.

Bronner, Y. L., & Auerbach, K. G. (1999). Maternal nutrition during lactation. In J. Riordan & K. G. Auerbach (Eds.),

Breastfeeding and human lactation (2nd ed., pp. 515–539). Boston: Jones & Bartlett.

Buescher, E. S. (1995). Host defense mechanisms of human milk and their relations to enteric infections and necrotizing enterocolitis. *Clinics in Perinatology, 21*(2), 247–262.

Chezem, J., Friesen, C., Montgomery, P., Fortman, T., & Clark, H. (1998). Lactation duration: Influences of human milk replacements and formula samples on women planning postpartum employment. *Journal of Obstetric, Gynecologic, and Neonatal Nursing, 27*(6), 646–651.

Choudhry, U. K. (1997). Traditional practices of women from India: Pregnancy, childbirth, and newborn care. *Journal of Obstetric, Gynecologic, and Neonatal Nursing, 26*(5), 533–539.

Darby, M. K., & Loughead, J. L. (1996). Neonatal nutritional requirements and formula composition: A review. *Journal of Obstetric, Gynecologic, and Neonatal Nursing, 25*(3), 209–217.

Furman, L. (1995). A developmental approach to weaning. *MCN: American Journal of Maternal/Child Nursing, 20*(6), 322–325.

Gigliotti, E. (1995). When women decide not to breastfeed. *MCN: American Journal of Maternal/Child Nursing, 20*(6), 315–321.

Gromada, K. K., & Spangler, A. K. (1998). Breastfeeding twins and higher-order multiples. *Journal of Obstetric, Gynecologic, and Neonatal Nursing, 27*(4), 441–449.

Henly, S. J., Anderson, C. M., Avery, M. D., Hills-Bonczyk, S. G., Potter, S., & Duckett, L. J. (1995). Anemia and insufficient milk in first-time mothers. *Birth, 22*(2), 87–92.

Huggins, K. (1995). *The nursing mother's companion* (3rd ed.). Boston: Harvard Common Press.

Institute of Medicine, National Academy of Sciences, Food and Nutrition Board. (1989). *Recommended dietary allowances* (19th ed.). Washington, DC: National Academy Press.

Jacobi, A. M., & Levin, M. (1997). Promotion and support of breastfeeding. In B. Worthington-Roberts & S. R. Williams (Eds.), *Nutrition in pregnancy and lactation* (6th ed., pp. 393–445). St. Louis: Times Mirror/Mosby.

Jambunathan, J., & Stewart, S. (1995). Hmong women in Wisconsin: What are their concerns in pregnancy and childbirth? *Birth, 22*(4), 204–210.

Kovach, A. C. (1996). An assessment tool for evaluating hospital breastfeeding policies and practices. *Journal of Human Lactation, 12*(1), 41–45.

Lavergne, N. A. (1997). Does application of tea bags to sore nipples while breastfeeding provide effective relief? *Journal of Obstetric, Gynecologic, and Neonatal Nursing, 26*(1), 53–58.

Lawrence, R. A. (1995). The clinician's role in teaching proper infant feeding techniques. *Journal of Pediatrics, 126*(6), S112–117.

Lawrence, R. A., & Lawrence, R. M. (1999). *Breastfeeding: A guide for the medical profession* (5th ed.). St. Louis: Mosby.

Losch, M., Dungy, C. I., Russell, D., & Dusdieker, L. B. (1995). Impact of attitudes on maternal decisions regarding infant feeding. *Journal of Pediatrics, 126*(4), 507–514.

Mahlmeister, L. (1996). Breastfeeding [letter]. *Journal of Obstetric, Gynecologic, and Neonatal Nursing, 25*(1), 15.

Mattson, S. (1995). Culturally sensitive perinatal care for southeast Asians. *Journal of Obstetric, Gynecologic, and Neonatal Nursing, 24*(41), 335–341.

Mohrbacher, N., & Stock, J. (1997). *The breastfeeding answer book* (2nd ed.). Schaumburg, IL: La Leche League International.

Moore, K., & Chute, G. (1996). Newborn nutrition. In D. R. Simpson & P. A. Creehan (Eds.), *AWHONN's perinatal nursing* (pp. 337–354). Philadelphia: Lippincott.

Moore, K., Zale, M., & Moramarco, M. L. (1998). New guidelines for breastfeeding. *RN, 61*(8), 36–39.

Mulford, C. (1995). Swimming upstream: Breastfeeding care in a nonbreastfeeding culture. *Journal of Obstetric, Gynecologic, and Neonatal Nursing, 24*(5), 464–474.

Orlando, S. (1995). The immunologic significance of breast milk. *Journal of Obstetric, Gynecologic, and Neonatal Nursing, 24*(7), 678–683.

Pascale, J. A., Brittian, L., Lenfestey, C. C., & Jarrett-Pulliam, C. (1996). Breastfeeding, dehydration, and shorter maternity stays. *Neonatal Network, 15*(7), 37–43.

Piper, S., & Parks, P. (1996). Predicting the duration of lactation: Evidence from a national survey. *Birth, 23*(1), 7–12.

Pipes, P. L. (1996). Nutrition in infancy. In L. K. Mahan & S. Escott-Stump (Eds.), *Krause's food, nutrition, and diet therapy* (9th ed., pp. 213–230). Philadelphia: Saunders.

Pugh, L. C., Buchko, B. L., Bishop, B. A., Cochran, J. F., Smith, L. R., & Lerew, D. J. (1996). A comparison of topical agents to relieve nipple pain and enhance breastfeeding. *Birth, 23*(2), 88–93.

Rasbridge, L. A., & Kulig, J. C. (1995). Infant feeding among Cambodian refugees. *MCN: American Journal of Maternal/Child Nursing, 20*(4), 213–218.

Righard, L. (1998). Are breastfeeding problems related to incorrect breastfeeding technique and the use of pacifiers and bottles? *Birth, 25*(1), 40–44.

Riordan, J. (1999a). The biologic specificity of breastmilk. In J. Riordan & K. C. Auerbach (Eds.), *Breastfeeding and human lactation* (2nd ed., pp. 121–161). Boston: Jones & Bartlett.

Riordan, J. (1999b). The cultural context of breastfeeding. In J. Riordan & K. C. Auerbach (Eds.), *Breastfeeding and human lactation* (2nd ed., pp. 29–52). Boston: Jones & Bartlett.

Riordan, J. M., & Koehn, M. (1997). Reliability and validity testing of three breastfeeding assessment tools. *Journal of Obstetric, Gynecologic, and Neonatal Nursing, 26*(2), 181–187.

Ross Products Division. (1997). *Updated breastfeeding trend through 1997. Mothers' survey.* Columbus, OH: Ross Products Division, Abbott Laboratories, Inc.

Saadeh, R., & Akre, J. (1996). Ten steps to successful breastfeeding: A summary of the rationale and scientific evidence. *Birth, 23*(3), 154–160.

Saarinen, U. M., & Kajosaari, M. (1995). Breastfeeding as prophylaxis against atopic disease: Prospective follow-up study until 17 years old. *Lancet, 346,* 1065–1069.

Schepers, A. (1996). Nutritional care in food allergy and food intolerance. In L. K. Mahan & S. Escott-Stump (Eds.), *Krause's food, nutrition, and diet therapy* (9th ed., pp. 843–863). Philadelphia: Saunders.

Timbo, B., Altekruse, S., Headrick, M., & Klontz, K. (1996). Breastfeeding among black mothers: Evidence supporting the need for prenatal intervention. *Journal of the Society of Pediatric Nurses, 1*(1), 35–40.

Tsang, R. C., DeMarini, S., & Rath, L. L. (1998). Fluids, electrolytes, vitamins, and trace minerals: Basis of ingestion, digestion, elimination, and metabolism. In C. Kenner, J. W. Lott, & A. A. Flandermeyer (Eds.), *Comprehensive neonatal nursing, a physiologic perspective* (2nd ed., pp. 336–353). Philadelphia: Saunders.

U.S. Department of Health and Human Services (USDHHS). (1991). *Healthy children 2000.* Washington, DC: Author.

Walker, M. (1997). Breastfeeding the sleepy baby. *Journal of Human Lactation, 13*(2), 151–153.

Williamson, M. T., & Murti, P. K. (1996). Effects of storage, time, temperature, and composition of containers on biologic components of human milk. *Journal of Human Lactation, 12*(1), 31–35.

Worthington-Roberts, B. (1997). Human milk composition and infant growth and development. In B. Worthington-Roberts & S. R. Williams (Eds.), *Nutrition in pregnancy and lactation* (6th ed., pp. 345–391). St. Louis: Times Mirror/Mosby.

Worthington-Roberts, B. (1997). Lactation: Basic considerations. In B. Worthington-Roberts & S. R. Williams (Eds.), *Nutrition in pregnancy and lactation* (6th ed., pp. 319–344). St. Louis: Times Mirror/Mosby.

25

The Childbearing Family with Special Needs

LEARNING OBJECTIVES

After studying this chapter, you should be able to:

- Discuss the incidence of and identify the factors that contribute to teenage pregnancy.
- Identify the effects of pregnancy on the adolescent mother, her infant, and the family.
- Describe the role of the nurse in the prevention and management of teenage pregnancy.
- Relate the major implications of delayed childbearing to maternal and fetal health.
- Describe the effects of substance abuse on the mother and the infant.
- Identify nursing interventions to reduce or minimize the effects of substance abuse in the antepartum, intrapartum, and postpartum periods.
- Discuss parental responses when an infant is born with congenital anomalies, and identify nursing interventions to assist the parents.
- Describe parental responses to pregnancy loss, and identify nursing interventions to assist parents through the grieving process.
- Examine the role of the nurse when the mother relinquishes the infant for adoption.
- Identify the factors that promote violence against women, and describe the role of the nurse in assessment, prevention, and interventions.

DEFINITIONS

abstinence syndrome A group of symptoms that occurs when a person who is addicted to a specific drug withdraws or abstains from taking that drug.

addiction Physical or psychological dependence on a substance such as alcohol, tobacco, or drugs, either legal or illicit.

alcoholism A chronic, progressive, and potentially fatal disease characterized by tolerance for and physical dependency on alcohol or by pathologic organ changes due to alcohol abuse or both.

amphetamines Central nervous system stimulants that create a perception of pleasure unrelated to external stimuli.

crack A highly addictive form of cocaine that has been processed to be smoked.

egocentrism Interest centered on the self rather than on the needs of others.

fetal alcohol syndrome A group of physical and mental disorders of the offspring associated with maternal use of alcohol during pregnancy.

methadone A synthetic compound with opiate properties. Used as an oral substitute for heroin and morphine in the opiate-addicted person.

neonatal abstinence syndrome A cluster of physical signs exhibited by the newborn exposed in utero to maternal use of substances such as cocaine or heroin. See also *abstinence syndrome*.

opiate Any narcotic containing opium or a derivative of opium.

prune-belly syndrome An absence of abdominal muscles that results in a flabby, distended, and creased abdomen; may occur in the infant exposed to cocaine in utero.

withdrawal syndrome See *abstinence syndrome*.

All families must make major changes as they adapt to pregnancy and childbirth. For some families, however, the changes are particularly difficult. Those families have special needs related to the parents' age, substance abuse, the birth of an infant with congenital abnormalities, loss of a pregnancy, or family violence. Perinatal nurses can make a difference in the lives of these families.

Adolescent Pregnancy

Incidence of Teenage Pregnancy

Since 1991 there has been a trend toward fewer births to teenagers in the United States, with an overall decrease of 12%. Still, however, approximately 1 million teenage girls become pregnant each year. In 1996, 55 of every 1,000 adolescent girls (almost 500,000) gave birth (Ventura, Curtin, & Matthews, 1998). Most of these pregnancies are unplanned and unwanted. Moreover, adolescents who become pregnant are likely to become pregnant again within 2 years (Fig. 25–1).

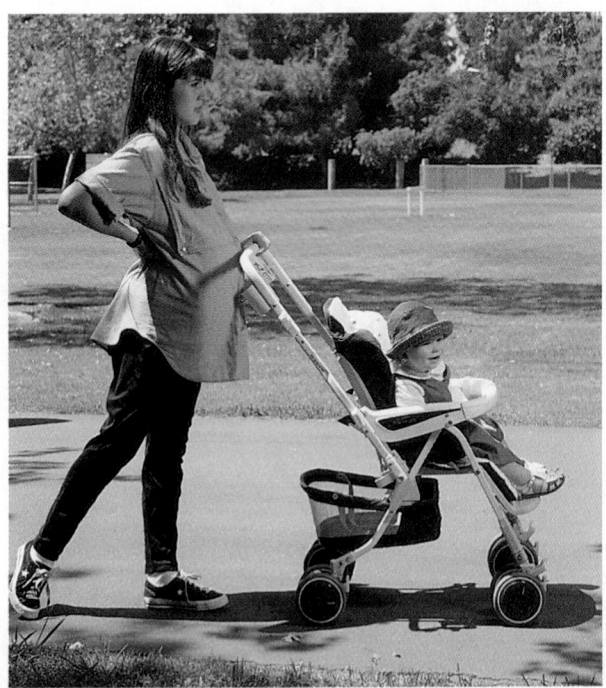

FIGURE 25–1

Pregnant adolescent. Thirty-eight percent of teenage girls who become pregnant will be pregnant again within 24 months.

Factors Associated with Teenage Pregnancy

The high level of sexual activity and low incidence of contraceptive use among adolescents are directly related to the incidence of teenage pregnancies in the United States. More than 50% of adolescents in grades 9 to 12 have had sexual intercourse. Nearly half of sexually active teens report they did not use a condom at last intercourse (Warren et al., 1998).

Moreover, many adolescents fail to understand their vulnerability to pregnancy as a result of their sexual activity. Many subscribe to the "personal fable" that they are immune to pregnancy. Some risk pregnancy and parenthood as a means of gaining a love relationship. Others see it as a means to gain independence.

Sex Education

Sex education is provided in many schools. Most educators emphasize that two major strategies should be employed. First, teenagers should be helped to understand how to set limits on sexual activity. Second, they must be instructed in effective measures to prevent pregnancy and sexually transmissible diseases (STDs).

Learning how to set limits on sexual behavior is particularly important for younger teenagers, who may be pressured to become sexually active before they have developed the maturity to deal responsibly with intercourse, contraception, or unplanned pregnancy. They need advice about how to handle pressure so they can postpone sexual intercourse until they are emotionally and physically ready.

When providing sex education, nurses must keep in mind that adolescent males and females mature at different rates and may be more comfortable learning in separate groups. In talking with teenagers, nurses should use simple but correct language such as uterus, testicles, penis, and vagina. Once the meanings of the terms are understood, most teenagers prefer to use them in their discussions. (See Chapter 10 for information about contraception.)

Factors Contributing to Teenage Pregnancy

Lack of accurate information about how to use contraceptives
Limited access to contraceptive devices
Fear of reporting sexual activity to parents
Ambivalence toward sexuality; intercourse not "planned"
Feelings of invulnerability
Peer pressure to begin sexual activity
Low self-esteem and consequent inability to set limits on sexual activity
Means to attain love or to escape present situation
Lack of appropriate role models
Low level of education correlated with incorrect use of contraceptives

Options When Pregnancy Occurs

An adolescent who becomes pregnant must choose one of three options: (1) to terminate the pregnancy, (2) to continue the pregnancy and place the infant for adoption, or (3) to continue the pregnancy and keep the infant. Although many pregnant teens choose abortion, this is not an acceptable option for some. Moreover, many teenagers do not acknowledge the pregnancy until it is too late for abortion.

Few teenagers choose to continue the pregnancy and place the infant for adoption. Those who do may have complicated feelings of grief, relief that a "bad" experience is over, and anger at parents who were unwilling to provide assistance and thus made adoption the only realistic option. The autonomous decision to relinquish the child "for the child's good," however, may be an important step toward maturity.

Adolescents who choose abortion or adoption receive less assistance in dealing with their experience than those who keep their infants. They need help in coping with their feelings about their decision. (See p. 624 for information about relinquishment by adoption.)

Socioeconomic Implications of Teenage Pregnancy

The financial cost of teenage pregnancy in the United States is high. It includes funds for Temporary Assistance for Needy Families (TANF), Medicaid, food stamps, direct payment to care providers, and administrative costs. Teenage mothers are more likely than older mothers to be nonwhite, poor, less educated, and unmarried. Moreover, teenage mothers are more likely to have larger families at an earlier age, resulting in more children to feed and clothe on an already inadequate income.

Although the financial cost of teenage pregnancy is enormous, the cost in human terms is often tragic. The developmental tasks of adolescence, such as achieving independence from parents and establishing a lifestyle that is personally satisfying, are interrupted. Educational goals are often curtailed, limiting employment opportunities and resulting in reliance on the welfare system. Research has found that in adolescent girls, lack of contraceptive use and having a child are associated with depression, low self-esteem, and little feeling of control over their lives (Kowaleski-Jones & Mott, 1998).

Children born into this situation do not escape unscathed. They show a higher incidence of impaired intellectual functioning and poor school adjustment. The negative cycle is often repeated: a large percentage of teenage parents were children of teenage parents. As a result, children of adolescent parents are often among the poorest people in the United States.

Implications of Teenage Pregnancy for Maternal Health

Pregnancy presents significant problems for the health of adolescent females. They are at increased risk for pregnancy-induced hypertension, anemia, and nutritional deficiencies. (Cunningham et al., 1997). Moreover, the maternal mortality rate is higher for adolescents than for older women.

The high incidence of STDs among pregnant teenagers is another concern. Gonorrhea and chlamydial infection are particularly prevalent during these years.

The reason for the high incidence of complications among teenagers is unclear. It may be due to delayed prenatal care rather than to age. Some pregnant adolescents do not start prenatal care until the third trimester, and others receive none at all. Early prenatal care that includes counseling about nutritional needs and close observation for complications is important.

Implications of Teenage Pregnancy for Fetal-Neonatal Health

The pregnant adolescent is more likely to smoke and less likely to gain adequate weight. Her infant is at high risk for prematurity and low birth weight (less than 2,500 g). These conditions are particularly likely when the mother is 13 to 17 years old (Fraser, Brockert, & Ward, 1995). Infants of teenage mothers have an increased risk of long-term serious disabilities and of dying during the first year of life (Ventura, Curtin, & Matthews, 1998).

The cause of low birth weight may be intrauterine growth restriction, which means that the fetus does not grow as expected. This condition may be due to a variety of causes, such as poor placental perfusion, which occurs during pregnancy-induced hypertension, or the underdeveloped vasculature of the uterus in young primigravidas. Prematurity is also a major cause of low-birth-weight infants. When the infant is born before 38 weeks of gestation, the baby is likely to weigh less than 2,500 g and has the added risks associated with immature organs.

The Teenage Expectant Father

Many adolescent mothers become pregnant by men who are not teenagers but are in their early to middle twenties. These men may accept responsibility for the child, or they may become "phantom fathers," which means that they are absent and rarely involved in raising the child.

Almost all adolescent expectant fathers indicate that they are not ready for fatherhood. Many are depressed as they grapple with the conflicting roles of adolescence and fatherhood. Although some express interest in learning about childbirth and child care, those who do not want to be fathers are less likely to be supportive. Some do not wish to interact with the infant, leaving the pregnant girl to seek support elsewhere.

A disproportionate number of teenage expectant fathers are from environments of poverty and lack job skills or educational preparation. Many need job training before they can earn enough money to contribute to the support of their children.

Impact of Teenage Pregnancy on Parenting

Research indicates that adolescent mothers are at risk to become nonnurturing parents (Thompson et al., 1995). Whether this risk is due to adolescence per se, the higher incidence of premature births, the lower socioeconomic status, or the particular home environment is difficult to determine. Teenage mothers do tend to be less sensitive to infant cues. They display fewer instances of mutual gazing, verbal interaction, and touching than do older mothers. They may have inappropriate parental behaviors, such as pinching, poking, or picking at the infant; these behaviors are rare in older mothers.

The mother's relationship with the father of the baby may affect her parenting abilities. A close and satisfying relationship with the baby's father may increase attachment behaviors in the mother. Thus, the father should be included, when appropriate, in care of the mother and baby (Bloom, 1998).

Adolescent parents may have little understanding of the expected growth and development of infants. They may expect too much too soon from their children. For instance, they may expect that the infant will sleep through the night, smile, or be toilet-trained before it is possible for infants to do these things.

It also appears that family functioning decreases as the infant of the adolescent mother grows. The period of time immediately after the infant is brought home has been termed a honeymoon phase. That phase seems to pass as time elapses and child care difficulties arise (Records, 1994). When family support begins to deteriorate, the teenage mother is likely to experience a great deal of stress.

The ability to deal with stress plays an important part in mothering skills. Young adolescents have immature coping mechanisms, and they may be unable to separate the stress of other life events from the stress that occurs when the infant cries and cannot be consoled. They may respond with immature or punitive measures toward the infant when the source of stress is other factors, such as social isolation or inadequate financial resources.

NURSING CARE
The Pregnant Teenager

Assessment

Physical Assessment

Assessment of pregnant teenagers is similar to that of older women in many respects. At the initial visit, obtain a thorough health and family history to determine whether conditions, such as diabetes or infectious diseases, increase the risk for the mother and fetus. Monitor closely for signs of iron deficiency anemia, pregnancy-induced hypertension, or STDs. Attempt to identify lifestyle behaviors, such as poor nutrition, smoking, or alcohol or drug use, that could harm the mother or fetus.

Structure the interview so that questions can be interspersed in a more general conversation that explores the teenager's likes and concerns. This approach helps to establish rapport and gain a better understanding of the teenager.

Knowledge of Infant Needs

Assess knowledge of infant needs and parenting skills. How does the teenager plan to feed the infant? What will she do when the infant cries? How will she know when the infant is ill and should be taken to a pediatrician? Does she know how much the infant should sleep? What plans have been made to provide for the hygiene and safety needs of the infant?

Cognitive Development

Determine the teenager's cognitive development and ability to absorb health counseling. The three most important areas of cognitive development are

1. *Egocentrism*, which involves the ability to defer personal satisfaction to respond to the needs of the infant: "What would you do if the baby were sick?" "How would you make the baby better?"
2. *Present-future orientation*, which involves the ability to make long-term plans: "What are your plans for finishing high school?"
3. *Abstract thinking*, which involves identifying cause and effect: "Why is it important to keep clinic appointments?" "Why should condoms be used during sexual intercourse?"

Family Assessment

Begin assessment of the family unit by determining the degree of participation by the infant's father. Fathers may plan to marry the expectant mother, participate in the pregnancy and rearing of the child without marriage, or be totally uninvolved.

It is important to assess the adolescent without the presence of her parents, but it is also crucial to determine the availability and amount of family support. Families respond in a variety of ways. A family member (usually the adolescent's mother) may take over the mothering role, or all infant care may be performed by the teenager. In some families, care and responsibilities are shared. This arrangement allows the adolescent to complete the developmental tasks of adolescence as well as learning the mother role.

The pregnant teenager's mother is particularly important when assessing the family. She may feel that she has "failed" as a mother, or she may resent the new cycle of child care in which the pregnancy involves her. If the family is unable or unwilling to provide care for an adolescent with an infant, what other social support can be located?

Nursing Diagnosis and Planning

Many adolescents wait until the second or third trimester to seek prenatal care because they either do not realize that they are pregnant or continue to deny that they are pregnant. Moreover, many teenagers have little information about the physiologic demands that pregnancy imposes on their bodies, such as the increased need for nutrients. As a result, they may have a pattern of sporadic prenatal care and missed appointments (Nursing Care Plan 25–1). One of the most relevant nursing diagnoses is

■ Risk for Altered Health Maintenance related to lack of knowledge of measures to promote health during pregnancy and increased family stress.
  Expected Outcomes: The expectant mother will keep scheduled prenatal appointments. She will communicate concerns and seek knowledge of measures that promote her health and the health of the fetus throughout the pregnancy. She will express knowledge of infant needs and the expected pattern of infant growth and development before the end of the third trimester. The family will verbalize emotions and concerns and maintain functional support of the expectant mother and her infant.

NURSING CARE PLAN 25-1
. . . .

Adolescents' Responses to Pregnancy and Birth

Assessment	Ann Killian, a 16-year-old white female, presented at the prenatal clinic during the 20th week of her pregnancy. She lives with her mother and father, who both work, and a younger sister. Ann remains in school but verbalizes concern about how she looks and feels: "How much bigger am I going to get?" "Why is my face so blotchy?"
Nursing Diagnosis	Body Image Disturbance related to perceived negative effects of pregnancy as evidenced by verbalized concern about appearance
Goals/Expected Outcomes	Ann will

- Verbalize her feelings about pregnancy and her perception of herself during each antepartum visit.
- Make two positive statements about herself during the next antepartum visit.

Intervention	Rationale
1. Allow time at each prenatal visit for Ann to express concerns about weight gain and other physiologic changes of pregnancy, such as hyperpigmentation and stretch marks.	1. The adolescent is often ashamed and uncomfortable with her pregnant body. She feels more comfortable if she is allowed to share these feelings and be reassured that they are a normal part of pregnancy.
2. Initiate interaction about body changes by asking open-ended questions such as, "How do you feel about needing to wear maternity clothes?"	2. Adolescents are often intimidated by health care professionals and may think that their own feelings are not important enough to discuss.
3. Provide anticipatory guidance about normal changes during pregnancy, such as the pattern of weight gain during pregnancy and weight loss after childbirth.	3. Most adolescents do not know what to expect during pregnancy. Anticipatory guidance reduces fear and provides information about expected changes.
4. Explain the reason for changes that are most troublesome at each prenatal visit (weight gain, hyperpigmentation, stretch marks, breast changes).	4. It is often helpful for the adolescent to know that some changes are temporary and that increasing weight indicates that the fetus is growing and developing. This often becomes a source of pride for the young teenager as well as for the older woman.
5. Promote positive self-image by praising grooming, posture, and responsible behavior such as keeping prenatal appointments and following recommendations: "You have never missed an appointment, and your baby is growing so well."	5. Positive reinforcement is particularly important to help the adolescent meet the developmental tasks of developing a sense of identity and self-worth.

Evaluation	Ann discusses her concerns about how she looks and feels about herself. She begins to make positive statements about herself at each prenatal visit.
Assessment	Ann reveals that her father has said that she has "shamed the family," and she is worried that her friends will reject her when they learn that she is pregnant. Ann states that she will have to "drop out of everything." She confides, in a trembling voice, that she feels guilty for "putting my family through this."
Nursing Diagnosis	Anxiety related to feelings of rejection by family and friends as manifested by statements indicating uncertainty about future support for self and infant
Goals/Expected Outcomes	Ann will

- Identify at least two new measures to cope with her anxiety by the end of the current antepartum visit.
- Demonstrate ability to implement these measures during subsequent antepartum visits.

(continued)

NURSING CARE PLAN 25–1 *Continued*

Adolescents' Responses to Pregnancy and Birth

Intervention	Rationale
1. Help Ann identify what she can do to overcome anxiety about rejection from her family and friends before the next prenatal appointment.	1. Planning to approach family and friends reduces anxiety.
a. Role-play how Ann can initiate a conversation with her friends to discuss activities that they can continue to share.	a. Acceptance by the peer group in peer group activities is a primary concern of the adolescent. A change of status within the group is a threat to self-concept that precipitates acute anxiety.
b. Suggest that she talk to family members about her feelings (guilty for the unhappiness she is causing them and fearful they will not assist her through the pregnancy and birth).	b. Although adolescents strive for independence, family values continue to be a significant influence. Rejection by the family at this time would leave her vulnerable to great stress.
c. Recommend that she share her feelings with the father of the infant if she continues to see him.	c. Expectant fathers may be a source of emotional and financial support.
2. Encourage Ann to discuss her economic needs as well as her plans for continuing school when the infant is born.	2. Planning provides some sense of control and increases feelings of competency.
3. Assist Ann in locating and joining the school-age mothers' program if available through her school.	3. This peer group (teenagers who are either mothers or expectant mothers) often replaces the pregnant teenager's previous peer group. The shared concerns and activities provide an opportunity for growth.

Evaluation Ann talks with her family and reports relationships are somewhat improved. She enters a school-aged mothers' program and is very pleased.

Assessment Ann has given birth to a 6-lb, 3-oz girl at 38 weeks' gestation. She has decided not to breast-feed because she plans to go back to school as soon as possible. Ann will live at home, and her mother has agreed to care for the infant while Ann is in school. Ann is very concerned about caring for the newborn. She seems unsure how to respond when the infant cries and handles her only during feedings.

Nursing Diagnosis Risk for Altered Parenting related to knowledge deficit of infant needs and lack of confidence in her ability to care for the infant, as evidenced by uncertain responses to the infant

Goals/Expected Outcomes Ann will

- Demonstrate basic infant care (cord care, bathing, burping, feeding, swaddling) by discharge.
- Verbalize infant needs for gentle, prompt response to crying on the first postpartum day.
- Demonstrate attachment behaviors (eye contact, gazing, holding, verbal stimulation, and positive comments about the infant) before discharge.

Intervention	Rationale
1. Demonstrate infant care on the first postpartum day, and obtain a return demonstration on the second postpartum day before discharge. (See Chapter 23.)	1. Confidence is increased by returning the demonstration of infant care.
2. Role-play for Ann how to respond when the infant cries, and emphasize the importance of promptness and gentleness.	2. Observing nurses respond to the infant increases the likelihood that adolescents will respond in the same manner. Prompt response helps the infant develop trust.

NURSING CARE PLAN 25–1 *Continued*

Adolescents' Responses to Pregnancy and Birth

3. Emphasize the importance of touch and verbal stimulation, and point out the reciprocal bonding behaviors that the infant exhibits.

3. Many teenaged parents do not provide adequate tactile and verbal stimulation for their infants, which may decrease the infant's ability to learn and respond to the environment. The infant has a repertoire of behaviors that stimulates attachment between parent and child.

4. Include the grandmother and the father of the infant in as many demonstrations as possible.

4. When all primary caregivers are included, family cohesiveness and consistency of care are enhanced.

5. Instruct Ann in early growth and development of the infant (how often infants need to eat, how much they sleep, what to do when they cry).

5. Some teenage parents expect "too much, too soon" from infants and become frustrated when the infant does not respond as expected. Anticipatory guidance helps them have realistic perceptions of the infant.

Evaluation

Ann shows a prompt and gentle response when her infant cries. She gives basic care as taught and discusses what to expect in early growth and development of her baby.

Additional Nursing Diagnoses to Consider

Risk for Altered Family Processes
Risk for Altered Health Maintenance
Risk for Altered Growth and Development

Interventions

Eliminating Barriers to Health Care

The two major barriers to health care are scheduling conflicts and negative attitudes of health care workers. Determine the most convenient location and time for appointments. It may be necessary to help the adolescent locate the clinic closest to her and to provide information about public transportation to that location. Moreover, appointments must be available when the girl (and her partner, if he wishes) are not in school.

Pregnant women of all ages state that the attitude of health care workers can discourage them from obtaining prenatal care. Some health care workers, including nurses, physicians, and social workers, are described as rude, insensitive, patronizing, judgmental, hostile, and condescending. This attitude is particularly unfortunate because it discourages families that would benefit most from early, consistent prenatal care. Nurses can be instrumental in finding ways to overcome these negative attitudes, thus encouraging pregnant women, including teenagers, to return for needed follow-up care.

Applying Teaching/Learning Principles

Because peers are important to adolescents, they benefit from participating in small groups with common concerns. Specific needs that might be addressed are the benefits of prenatal care or education to eliminate unhealthful habits such as smoking, drug use, or alcohol consumption. Near the end of pregnancy, preparation for labor and delivery and infant care become the priorities.

Repetition is an important method of teaching and clarifying misinformation. Allow ample time for questions and discussions. Although teenagers do not read or benefit from printed materials to the same degree that older parents do, many learn well from audiovisual aids.

It is particularly important to avoid sounding like a parent when working with adolescents. Avoid using the word "should" or "ought," offering unwanted advice, or making decisions for the teenagers.

Counseling

Allow time to counsel teenagers about their specific problems, such as nutrition, stress reduction, and infant care.

Nutrition. Nutrition counseling is one means of reducing the incidence of low-birth-weight infants. Tailor information to the individual adolescent's likes and peer group habits. Nutrition education must be socially and culturally appropriate. (See Chapter 15 for suggestions on nutrition for adolescents.)

Referrals to food stamp providers, the Special Supplemental Food Program for Women, Infants, and Children (WIC), surplus food distributors, food banks, and food preparation equipment may be necessary because many teenagers have limited access to food and lack the ability to store or prepare food.

Stress Reduction. Teenagers are vulnerable to many sources of stress. Stress may be related to basic needs such as food, shelter, and health care. Fear of labor and delivery and fear of being single, alone, and unsupported all create stress. A major source of stress for teenagers occurs when they attempt to meet the developmental tasks of adolescence while working on the developmental tasks of pregnancy (overcoming ambivalence, attaining the role of parent).

A variety of measures may be used to reduce stress, depending on the teenager's age, situation, and available support. Adolescents with chronic life stress may require the concentrated efforts of a social worker to achieve stabilization. The pregnant teenager often experiences stress because she has not told her parents or the father of the infant about the pregnancy. It may be helpful to role-play the encounter so that she can work out a plan for breaking the news. If the girl is very young or if the pregnancy occurred as a result of rape or incest, social service and law enforcement agencies must become involved to provide protection and assistance.

Infant Care. The priorities for teaching gradually change from maternal to infant needs. Explain and demonstrate infant cues (using behaviors of the infants in videos or in the group as examples). Describe how infants use these behaviors to "talk" without words and how parents can adjust their position, distance, face, voice, and touch to correspond to their infant's cues. Emphasize that eye contact, holding, cuddling, and verbal stimulation are important for the child's development.

Because adolescents tend to have a more rigid and punitive approach to child care, emphasize that infants develop a sense of trust when their needs are met promptly and gently. Moreover, their future development depends on attaining a sense of trust during infancy. Emphasize that crying does not indicate that the infant is spoiled but simply that the infant has a need for food, warmth, or comfort and love.

Emphasize normal growth and development. Explain that development proceeds from the head downward. This information helps the young mother understand that the infant must learn to sit before walking and must walk before toilet training is possible.

Promoting Family Support

The pregnant teenager needs encouragement to include her family in her decision making and problem solving. Topics that should be discussed include who will care for the infant, whether the teenager will return to school, and what financial assistance is available from the family and from the infant's father. Adolescent mothers who have adequate emotional support, are enrolled in school, want to avoid pregnancy for at least 2 years, and believe pregnancy will occur without adequate contraception are more likely to use contraceptives reliably (Berenson & Wiemann, 1997).

If, however, the family has multiple problems that include substance abuse or domestic violence, involving family members may be inappropriate. The teenager should be encouraged instead to communicate with a family friend or other trusted adult.

Providing Referrals

Make referrals to national and community resources for pregnant adolescents that are in convenient locations. These include well-baby clinics, programs for school-age mothers offered by many high schools, TANF offered by state social service agencies, and WIC. Church and community organizations may also provide needed assistance.

Evaluation

- Does the pregnant adolescent keep prenatal appointments?
- Does she ask questions and follow the recommended plan of care?
- Can she explain care and growth and development of the infant?
- Is the family supportive, or have appropriate referrals been made?

Delayed Pregnancy

An increasing number of women become pregnant relatively late in their reproductive life. Although a 35-year-old woman can hardly be considered elderly, she is often referred to as an "elderly primigravida" or "older mother." The term *mature primigravida* is preferred by some.

Maternal and Fetal Implications of Delayed Pregnancy

When the mature woman decides to conceive, she may experience a delay in becoming pregnant. This problem is particularly likely after the age of 35 years because of the normal aging of the ovaries and the increased incidence of reproductive tract disorders. (See Chapter 10 for infertility.)

Once the mature woman conceives, she is at increased risk for complications associated with pregnancy. The risks may be considered in three categories: genetic, preexisting medical conditions, and obstetric complications. The increased risk of fetal chromosomal abnormalities with advancing maternal age is well documented. Trisomy 21 (Down syndrome) is the most common example. The likelihood of a 20-year-old woman having an affected child is approximately 1 in 1,400, compared with a 1 in 100 risk for a 40-year-old woman (Cunningham et al., 1997).

The most common examples of preexisting diseases that can cause maternal or fetal jeopardy are hypertension and diabetes mellitus. Uterine myomas (fibroids) occur with greater frequency in women older than 35 years and may be associated with postpartum hemorrhage. The older primigravida is also at increased risk for obstetric complications, such as multiple gestation, preterm labor, dysfunctional labor, and cesarean birth. Moreover, the risk of a small-for-gestational-age infant increases with maternal age.

Advantages of Delayed Childbirth

Mature primigravidas come to the parenting role with a range of personal resources: psychosocial maturity, self-confidence, and a sense of control over their lives. In addition, they are capable of solving complex problems and are often adept at maintaining interpersonal relationships. Because they are more likely to be financially secure, these women can afford good care for their infants. They are experienced at setting priorities and developing plans. Moreover,

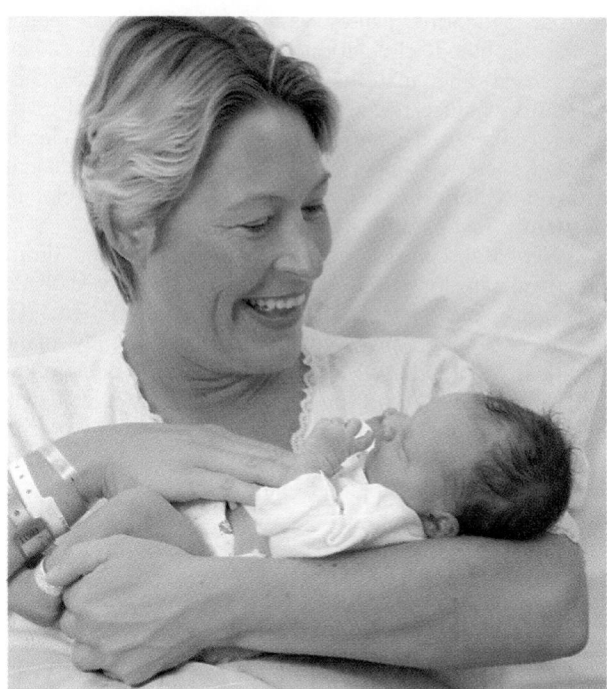

FIGURE 25-2

Older primigravidas bring maturity and problem-solving skills to the maternal role, but they are at somewhat increased risk for physiologic problems related to pregnancy and birth.

they are usually able to manage stress and will independently seek support and assistance (Fig. 25-2).

Disadvantages of Delayed Childbirth

Mature primiparas need more time to recover from childbirth, and they have less energy than their younger counterparts. They may find child care an exhausting experience for the first few weeks, particularly if they had a cesarean birth or other complications of pregnancy.

Peer support may be less available for mature primigravidas. Many of their friends have teenage children and do not relate to the concerns of a new mother. Younger mothers have some of the same concerns, but they often do not share the perspective of older mothers.

Family support may also be lacking for the older woman. Her parents are usually in their 60s or 70s and may not be able to assist with child care to the extent that younger grandparents can.

Nursing Considerations

REINFORCING AND CLARIFYING INFORMATION

Because the fetus of a mature woman is at increased risk for chromosomal anomalies, the woman will be informed about diagnostic tests that are available (see Chapter 16). The tests most often recommended are alpha-fetoprotein screening, chorionic villus sampling, amniocentesis, and ultrasonography. The family's beliefs and attitudes about abortion often determine whether to have the recommended tests.

The woman who would not consider abortion regardless of the condition of the fetus may refuse diagnostic studies. Nurses must respect the decision and acknowledge that it may have been a difficult one to make.

FACILITATING EXPRESSION OF EMOTIONS

Several days or weeks may pass between the performance of diagnostic studies and the time results of the tests are known. This is a particularly difficult time for many expectant parents, and nurses often assist the couple to express their concerns and emotions.

> A broad statement such as, "Many couples find it difficult to wait for the results" will often elicit free expression of how the partners feel. Follow-up questions such as, "What concerns you most?" may reveal worry about the procedure itself or about the possible effects of the procedure on the fetus. Simply acknowledging that it is a stressful time helps the couple to cope with their emotions.

PROVIDING PARENTING INFORMATION

Nurses often help the mature primipara prepare for effective parenting. Anticipatory guidance about measures that will help conserve energy after childbirth is very useful. Such measures may include meal planning and setting realistic housekeeping goals. In addition, many older mothers need to mobilize all available support so that they can reserve their energy for infant care. During the first weeks after childbirth, the mother may experience feelings of social isolation, particularly if her friends have children who are a great deal older. If she is accustomed to a great deal of mental stimulation, she may miss this while staying at home. If she elects to return to work, she is likely to experience guilt and grief because she must leave her infant.

First-time mothers older than age 35 are especially receptive to prenatal classes. These include classes in childbirth education, preparation for cesarean birth, breastfeeding, and early parenting. Older couples are particularly interested in learning how the infant grows and develops and what they can do to provide nurturing care for the infant. They generally comprehend printed materials that can be used to reinforce teaching.

◼ Substance Abuse

The use of legal substances, such as alcohol and tobacco, as well as illicit drugs, such as cocaine and marijuana, increases the risk of medical complications in the mother and poor birth outcomes in the infant.

Incidence of Substance Abuse

More than 4.4 million women use illicit drugs (Lieberman, 1998). Approximately 1 in 10 infants is exposed to one or more mood-altering drugs during pregnancy (American Academy of Pediatrics [AAP], 1997). Although tobacco, alcohol, and marijuana are the most commonly abused drugs, the use of cocaine and heroin has had a major impact on health care for pregnant women and their offspring.

Maternal and Fetal Effects of Substance Abuse

When the pregnant woman takes a substance, the fetus experiences the same systemic effects as the expectant mother but often more severely. For instance, cocaine raises the blood pressure of the woman and the fetus and puts both at risk for intracranial bleeding. A drug that causes intoxication in the woman causes it for prolonged periods in the fetus. This prolonged effect occurs because the fetus cannot metabolize drugs efficiently and will experience the effects long after they have abated in the woman. For a summary of the maternal, fetal, and neonatal effects of commonly abused substances, see Table 25–1.

TOBACCO

The active ingredients of cigarette smoke are nicotine, tar, and harmful gases, such as carbon monoxide and cyanide. Nicotine causes vasoconstriction and reduces placental blood circulation. Carbon monoxide inactivates fetal and maternal hemoglobin. Together these substances reduce the amount of oxygen delivered to the fetus. Indirect effects of cigarette smoking include decreased maternal appetite, which results in inadequate intake of calories as well as decreased absorption of some nutrients.

Neonatal consequences of smoking tobacco during pregnancy are low birth weight and prematurity. Tobacco exposure reduces birth weight an average of 100 to 320 g (Lambers & Clark, 1996). Infants are symmetrically smaller in all areas, including head circumference (Bell & Lau, 1995). Smoking during pregnancy is also associated with delayed neurologic and intellectual development of children. Problems include hyperactivity, shorter attention span, and lower reading and spelling scores during the primary grades.

TABLE 25–1

. . . .

Maternal and Fetal or Neonatal Effects of Commonly Abused Substances

Substance	Maternal Effects	Fetal or Neonatal Effects
Caffeine (coffee, tea, cola, chocolate, cold remedies, analgesics)	Stimulates CNS and cardiac function, causes vasoconstriction and mild diuresis; half-life triples during pregnancy	Crosses placental barrier and stimulates fetus; teratogenic effects are undocumented
Tobacco	Decreased placental perfusion, anemia, PROM, preterm labor, spontaneous abortion	Prematurity, LBW, fetal demise, developmental delays, increased incidence of SIDS, pneumonia
Alcohol (beer, wine, mixed drinks, after-dinner drinks)	Spontaneous abortion	Fetal demise, IUGR, FAS (facial and cranial anomalies, developmental delay, mental retardation, short attention span), fetal alcohol effects (milder form of FAS)
Narcotics (heroin, methadone, morphine)	Spontaneous abortion, PROM, preterm labor, increased incidence of STDs, HIV exposure, hepatitis, malnutrition	IUGR, perinatal asphyxia, intellectual impairment, neonatal abstinence syndrome, neonatal infections, neonatal death (SIDS, child abuse and neglect)
Sedatives (barbiturates, tranquilizers)	Lethargy, drowsiness, CNS depression	Neonatal abstinence syndrome, seizures, delayed lung maturity, possible teratogenic effects
Cocaine ("crack")	Hyperarousal state, generalized vasoconstriction, hypertension, increased incidence of spontaneous abortion, abruptio placentae, preterm labor, cardiovascular complications (stroke, heart attack), seizures, increased STDs	Stillbirth, prematurity, IUGR, irritability, decreased ability to interact with environmental stimuli, poor feeding reflexes, nausea, vomiting, diarrhea, decreased intellectual development; distended, flabby, creased abdomen (prune-belly syndrome) due to absence of abdominal muscles
Amphetamines ("speed" or "ice" when processed in crystals to smoke)	Malnutrition, tachycardia, withdrawal symptoms (lethargy, depression)	Increased risk for cardiac anomalies and cleft palate, IUGR, withdrawal symptoms
	Often used with other drugs: alcohol, cocaine, tobacco; increased incidence of anemia and inadequate weight gain	Unclear, more study needed, believed related to prematurity, IUGR, neonatal tremors, sensitivity to light

Abbreviations: CNS, central nervous system; PROM, premature rupture of membranes; LBW, low birth weight; SIDS, sudden infant death syndrome; IUGR, intrauterine growth restriction; FAS, fetal alcohol syndrome; STDs, sexually transmissible diseases; HIV, human immunodeficiency virus.

ALCOHOL

Researchers are unsure how alcohol causes damage to the fetus. During the first trimester, alcohol is believed to affect cell membranes and alter the organization of tissue. Throughout pregnancy, alcohol interferes with the metabolism of carbohydrates, lipids, and proteins and thus retards cell growth and division.

The teratogenic effects of alcohol include fetal alcohol syndrome (FAS). This syndrome is characterized by three clinical features: prenatal and postnatal growth restriction, central nervous system impairment, and a recognizable combination of facial features. Common facial anomalies associated with FAS include short palpebral fissures (the openings between the eyelids), flat midface, indistinct philtrum (median groove on the external surface of the upper lip), and a thin upper lip (Fig. 25–3). Growth restriction is noted in length, weight, and head circumference.

Manifestations of central nervous system impairment include mental retardation, high activity level, short attention span, and poor short-term memory. Although the range is broad, the average intelligence quotient (IQ) of individuals with FAS is about 70 (Hankin & Sokol, 1995).

Fetal alcohol effects is a term used to describe infants who exhibit mild or partial manifestations of FAS, such as low birth weight, developmental delay that may not be obvious for 1 to 2 years, and hyperactivity. Not all fetuses exposed to alcohol in utero develop FAS, but no safe level of alcohol consumption during pregnancy has been estab-

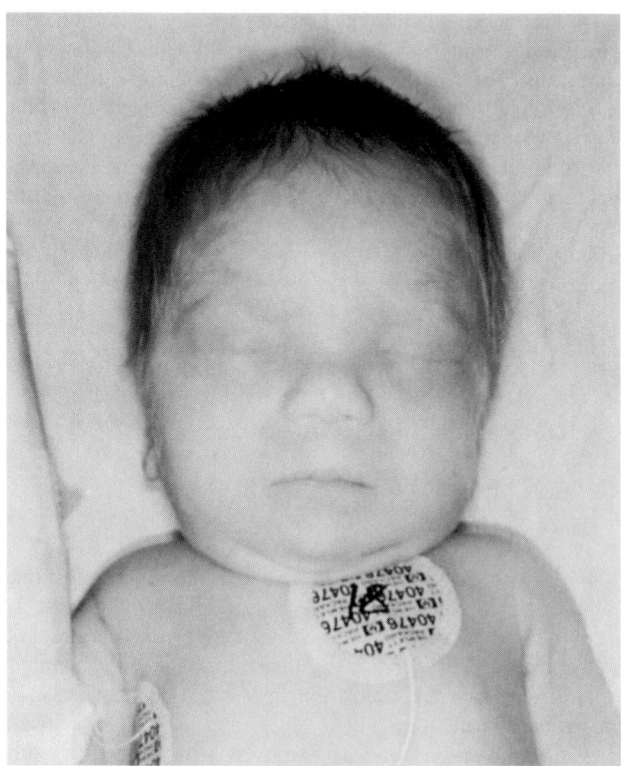

FIGURE 25–3

Infant with fetal alcohol syndrome. Subtle indicators are flat midface, indistinct philtrum, and low-set ears. (Courtesy of Trish Beachy, M.S., R.N., Perinatal Program Coordinator. University of Colorado Health Sciences, Denver.)

CRITICAL TO REMEMBER

Signs and Symptoms of Recent Cocaine Use

Diaphoresis, high blood pressure, irregular respirations

Dilated pupils, increased body temperature

Sudden onset of severely painful contractions

Fetal tachycardia, excessive fetal activity

Angry, caustic, abusive reactions and paranoia

---

lished. It is therefore recommended that women abstain from drinking alcohol throughout their pregnancies.

COCAINE

How Cocaine Works. Cocaine is a powerful, short-acting stimulant of the central nervous system. Cocaine blocks the presynaptic reuptake of the neurotransmitters norepinephrine and dopamine, producing a hyperarousal state that results in euphoria, physical excitement, reduced fatigue, and a heightened sense of well-being and power. Anorexia, hyperglycemia, hyperthermia, and tachypnea are among the array of side effects of cocaine use.

When the initial euphoria wears off, a period of irritability, fatigue, lethargy, depression, and impatience occurs. This state elicits a strong desire for additional cocaine so that the initial feelings can be recaptured.

Physical effects of cocaine use are related to cardiovascular stimulation and vasoconstriction. The heart rate, systolic blood pressure, and demand for oxygen all increase. Complications of generalized vasoconstriction include myocardial ischemia, myocardial infarction, or cardiac arrhythmias. In addition, cocaine has been associated with stroke, subarachnoid hemorrhage, and temporal lobe seizures.

Maternal and Fetal Effects of Cocaine. Because many women who use cocaine also use additional drugs, such as alcohol or marijuana, to "come down" from the superarousal state that cocaine produces, it is difficult to define the precise effects of cocaine use on the fetus. In addition, women who abuse cocaine are less likely to seek prenatal care or to eat a diet that contains adequate nutrition. Moreover, sex is often exchanged for drugs, so that the woman is at increased risk for STDs.

Cocaine stimulates uterine contractions, and premature delivery is common (Bell & Lau, 1995). Because of the vasoconstriction of placental vessels, the incidence of spontaneous abortion and abruptio placentae also increases. Additional complications include premature rupture of membranes, precipitous delivery, and stillbirth.

Clearance of the drug takes a prolonged period in the fetus. Fetal effects include tachycardia, decreased beat-to-beat variability of the fetal heart rate baseline, fetal overactivity, and intrauterine growth restriction.

Neonatal Effects of Cocaine. Clinical symptoms observed in neonates exposed to cocaine in utero include tremors, tachycardia, marked irritability, muscular rigidity, hypertension, and exaggerated startle reflex. These infants are difficult to console and respond poorly to voices or environmental stimuli. They are often poor feeders and have frequent episodes of diarrhea.

Infants may continue to be irritable and have limited interaction with people and objects in their environment. There may be lifelong disabilities, such as learning problems, slower intellectual development, and delayed language and motor development.

MARIJUANA

The active constituent of marijuana is delta-9-tetrahydrocannabinol (THC), which crosses the placenta and accumulates in the fetus. Although marijuana is one of the most commonly used drugs, very little research has been conducted on the effects of marijuana on the pregnant woman or fetus. Because marijuana is often paired with other drugs such as cocaine and alcohol, its precise effects are difficult to determine.

Repeated use of marijuana appears to increase the incidence of maternal anemia and inadequate maternal weight gain. Clinically, the neonate may exhibit hyperirritability, tremors, and unusual sensitivity to light. Long-term effects of marijuana on the development of the child are unknown.

HEROIN

Heroin, an illegal opiate derived from morphine, produces severe physical addiction. Like all opiates, heroin is a central nervous system depressant. It produces a feeling of mental dullness, drowsiness, and finally stupor ("on the nod"). Addiction is present when discontinuance causes withdrawal symptoms (abstinence syndrome) that are quickly relieved by a dose of the drug.

Women who abuse heroin have poor general health with multiple medical problems associated with their drug abuse and addicted lifestyle. Heroin is an appetite suppressant that also interferes with the absorption of nutrients ingested, and many women start pregnancy malnourished and anemic. Additional problems include a high incidence of STDs. Infections such as hepatitis and exposure to HIV occur frequently as a result of sharing unclean needles.

Fetal Effects of Heroin.   Because the street supply of heroin is usually not steady, the fetus suffers frequent episodes of maternal overdose alternating with periods of withdrawal from the drug. These episodes expose the fetus to intermittent hypoxia, which increases the risk of prematurity, growth restriction, and stillbirth. Indirect effects are due to maternal malnutrition and fetal exposure to STDs.

Neonatal Effects of Heroin.   Infants born to mothers addicted to opiates, including heroin, methadone, meperidine, or morphine, exhibit a neonatal abstinence (withdrawal) syndrome. This syndrome affects all body systems. The most consistent symptoms are neurologic: tremors, jitteriness, restlessness, and on occasion seizures. Other manifestations include hypertonicity and prolonged continuous crying.

Additional symptoms of newborn abstinence syndrome include poorly coordinated sucking and swallowing reflexes, vomiting, and diarrhea, which may result in dehydration and failure to gain weight normally. Long-term developmental and learning problems are common. Moreover, the lifestyle of parents who are substance abusers is strongly associated with child neglect and abuse, which are major causes of infant death in this population.

Initial management of the addicted neonate includes decreased environmental stimulation, swaddling, and small, frequent feedings. Caretakers often become frustrated because the infant's body is stiff and extended and the newborn does not respond to cuddling or soothing behaviors that usually console a crying infant. (See Chapter 30.)

Diagnosis and Management of Substance Abuse

In addition to toxicology screening, the pregnant woman who uses illicit drugs must be tested throughout pregnancy for STDs, hepatitis, and exposure to HIV. Fetal diagnostic tests such as nonstress tests are used to identify problems with the fetus. Nurses monitor weight and provide guidance in nutrition to prevent maternal anemia and inadequate weight gain.

Therapeutic management depends on the type of drug used. In the case of opiates, such as heroin, withdrawal during pregnancy has been associated with significant fetal stress and even fetal death due to the effects of abstinence syndrome. One approach to treatment of the pregnant woman who uses heroin is to place her on an alternative drug such as methadone. Methadone is useful because it can be taken orally and is long acting. The woman on methadone can maintain fairly consistent blood levels to decrease adverse fetal effects of wide swings in blood level. The newborn, however, must withdraw from methadone after birth. In addition, women using methadone often use other illicit drugs such as cocaine or marijuana (Brown et al., 1998).

Treatment of substance abuse is aimed at establishing abstinence and preventing relapse. Women may receive outpatient or residential treatment. Education, individual and group therapy sessions, and peer support groups (Narcotics Anonymous, Alcoholics Anonymous, or Cocaine Anonymous) are combined. Because women have extremely positive memories associated with cocaine use, relapse is common. Written contracts that focus on abstinence for one day at a time are often used to help the patient who has relapsed and experiences severe feelings of guilt and self-blame.

▌ NURSING CARE
· · · · · · · · · ·
Maternal Substance Abuse

ANTEPARTUM PERIOD

Assessment

Polydrug abuse appears to be the most common substance abuse problem among women, and all women must be screened at the first prenatal visit for nicotine, alcohol, and other drugs. *Because substance abuse occurs in all populations, the nurse must not make assumptions based on class, race, or economic status.*

Certain behaviors are strongly associated with substance abuse: seeking prenatal care late in the pregnancy, failing to keep appointments, and following recommended regimens inconsistently. Poor grooming, inadequate weight gain, or a poor pattern of weight gain may be signs of a lifestyle that includes substance abuse.

Defensive or hostile behaviors may be overt signs of

substance abuse. Women who use drugs have low self-esteem. They must deal with conflicting issues: the physical or psychological need for the substance, guilt that they may be responsible for harming the fetus, and fear of prosecution for use of illegal drugs.

Many women with substance abuse problems face discrimination and resentment from health care professionals who direct their frustration at the woman rather than at the problem. The nurse taking the health history must exhibit patience, empathy, and tolerance and must use a blend of approaches that reinforce concern for the woman and her infant.

Medical and Obstetric History

Determine whether the woman has medical conditions such as hepatitis or STDs that are prevalent among women who use drugs. Evaluate for past and current complications of pregnancy. Spontaneous abortions, premature deliveries, abruptio placentae, and stillbirths are associated with substance abuse, although they also occur in the population that has never used drugs. Current complications may include vaginal bleeding, an inactive or hyperactive fetus, or intrauterine growth restriction.

Investigate emotional responses, such as anger or apathy, regarding the pregnancy. These feelings are particularly significant during the latter half of the pregnancy, when one would expect the normal feelings of ambivalence to be resolved. Negative feelings toward the pregnancy may interfere with prenatal compliance with follow-up care.

History of Substance Abuse

Obtaining an accurate history of substance abuse is difficult and depends in large part on the way the health care worker approaches the woman. A sincere, nonjudgmental, empathic approach promotes an open exchange of information.

Investigate all forms of drug use, including cigarettes, over-the-counter drugs, prescribed medications, alcohol, and illicit drugs such as cocaine, marijuana, and heroin. Examine patterns of drug use, which can range from occasional recreational use to weekly binges to daily dependence on a particular drug or group of drugs.

Urine toxicology screening is used to validate drug use. Screening is particularly important when the woman denies current use but has a group of signs and symptoms that suggest she is using one or more drugs.

> ### CRITICAL TO REMEMBER
> • • • • • • • • • •
> ### *Behaviors Associated with Substance Abuse*
>
> Seeking prenatal care late in pregnancy
> Failure to keep prenatal appointments
> Inconsistent follow-through with recommended care
> Poor grooming, inadequate weight gain
> Needle punctures, thrombosed veins, cellulitis
> Defensive or hostile reactions
> Anger or apathy regarding pregnancy

Nursing Diagnosis and Planning

Some women do not realize the adverse effects of the drugs they are using, whereas others may be unable to stop using the substances. A nursing diagnosis that addresses both these factors is

■ Risk for Altered Health Maintenance related to lack of knowledge of the effects of substance abuse on self and fetus and inability to manage stress without the use of drugs.

Expected Outcomes: The woman will identify harmful effects of substance on herself and her infant, will verbalize feelings related to continued use of harmful substances, and will identify personal strengths and accept support offered by the health care delivery system to stop using drugs.

Interventions

Effective interventions for substance abuse require that nurses realize that progress is slow and frustrating. The major priority is to protect the fetus and the expectant mother from the harmful effects of drugs.

Examining Attitudes

When working with substance-abusing pregnant women, nurses must identify and acknowledge their own knowledge level, feelings, and prejudices. They may have limited knowledge about perinatal substance abuse and may have negative attitudes toward mothers who abuse substances (Selleck & Redding, 1998). Nurses may find it difficult to maintain feelings of empathy or concern without becoming judgmental or even unknowingly punitive to the pregnant woman. Nurses may also feel angry, helpless, and discouraged when the pregnant woman continues to abuse drugs despite the best efforts of the health care team. In-service education, professional consultation, and peer support are all helpful when working with pregnant women who abuse drugs.

Communicating with the Woman

If possible, allow time to get acquainted with the expectant mother. This effort often involves asking questions about various aspects of her life to obtain a better picture of what other stressors may be contributing to the pattern of substance abuse. Additional stressors may include inadequate housing, economic predicaments, family discord, and emotional or physical illness.

Be honest at all times while displaying a patient, nonjudgmental attitude as well as genuine interest and concern. This approach is especially important when the woman relapses into substance-abusing patterns. Allow her to express guilt and reassure her that abstinence is possible and that she must simply begin again.

Helping the Woman Identify Strengths

Because she generally has a poor self-image, assist the substance-abusing pregnant woman in identifying personal strengths. Acknowledge her actions when she abstains from drugs or alcohol for even a short time. Praise for maintaining an adequate weight gain and attending prenatal classes may increase self-esteem and compliance with the recommended regimen of care.

Providing Ongoing Care

At each antepartum visit, consider the current status of substance use, social service needs, education needs, and compliance with treatment referrals. In particular, address current drug use, because women may change their pattern of drug use during pregnancy. For instance, they may stop using cocaine but increase their use of marijuana or alcohol.

Verify compliance with recommended treatment regimens, such as antepartum clinics and chemical-dependence referral programs. Coordinate care among various service providers with such measures as group therapy and prenatal classes.

Provide continuing prenatal education classes that include the anatomy and physiology of pregnancy and consequences of prenatal substance abuse. Describe how the newborn benefits when the mother abstains from drugs, including tobacco and alcohol. Praise any attempts at abstinence and encourage the expectant mother to try again if she relapses.

Evaluation

- Can the expectant mother identify the effects of substance abuse on herself and her infant?
- Does she discuss her feelings about continued substance abuse?
- Does she identify her own strengths and work with the health care team to stop using drugs?

INTRAPARTUM PERIOD

Assessment

Nurses who work in labor and delivery units must become skilled at identifying drug-induced signs and symptoms.

Cocaine

Behaviors associated with frequent or recent use of crack include profuse sweating, high blood pressure, and irregular respirations, combined with a lethargic response to labor and lack of interest in the necessary interventions. Additional signs include dilated pupils, increased body temperature, and sudden onset of severely painful contractions. Fetal signs often include tachycardia and excessive activity.

Emotional signs of recent cocaine use may include angry, caustic, or abusive reactions to those attempting to provide care. Emotional lability and paranoia are signs of cocaine intoxication.

Heroin

Typically, the pregnant woman addicted to heroin comes to the labor and delivery unit intoxicated from a recent drug administration. When the effects of the drug begin to wear off, withdrawal symptoms may be observed. These include yawning, diaphoresis, rhinorrhea, restlessness, and excessive tearing of the eyes.

Nursing Diagnosis and Planning

One of the most relevant nursing diagnoses during the intrapartal period is
- Risk for Injury related to physiologic and psychological effects of recent drug use.
    Expected Outcome: The woman and the fetus will remain free from injury during labor and childbirth.

Interventions

Preventing Injury

When a laboring woman has recently used a substance such as cocaine, her life and the life of the fetus depend heavily on the nurse, who must intervene to meet the needs for safety, oxygen, and comfort.

Admitting Procedure. Two nurses may be needed to admit the woman into the labor unit. One nurse helps the woman assume a safe position, initiates electronic fetal monitoring, and begins administration of oxygen, as needed. The other nurse acts as communicator.

Because the woman who has recently used a drug often has difficulty following directions, only one nurse should tell her what to do. This nurse states firmly what is happening and exactly what the woman must do: "Lie on your left side." "This helps us watch how the baby is doing." "This gives you more oxygen." This nurse maintains eye contact with the woman while giving her instructions.

Setting Limits. It is critical to realize the importance of setting limits to protect the safety of the mother and the fetus. For instance, the mother cannot smoke when oxygen is in use. If she must remain in bed, she may become agitated. The nurse may say, "I know it is hard to stay in bed, but we can't take good care of the baby when you walk." If it is safe for the woman to walk, the nurse must set limits about where she can walk.

Initiating Seizure Precautions. The laboring woman who recently used cocaine is at risk for hypertensive crisis and must be protected from injury in case of seizures. Seizure precautions should be taken. Keep the bed in a low, locked position. Pad the side rails and keep them up at all times. To prevent aspiration, make sure suction equipment functions properly. Reduce environmental stimuli (lights, noise) as much as possible.

Maintaining Effective Communication

Establishing a therapeutic pattern of communication is one of the primary methods of providing care for the patient who has recently used cocaine. Avoid confrontation; instead, acknowledge feelings: "I know you hurt and you are frightened. I will do everything I can to make you comfortable." When the woman is abusive, be careful not to take the abuse personally or react in a nontherapeutic manner.

Examine your own feelings when women are abusive, and acknowledge when anger is getting in the way of providing care. To allow some relief from unrelenting abusive comments, another nurse may need to assume care of the woman for a time.

Providing Pain Control

Pain control for women who are substance abusers poses a difficult problem because it is often impossible to determine the type or combination of drugs that were used before admission. If the woman has used heroin, medications such as morphine, hydromorphone, and meperidine must be used with caution. Avoid narcotic agonists-antagonists, such as butorphanol (Stadol), because they may cause acute withdrawal symptoms in the woman and the fetus.

Comfort measures may require nonpharmacologic nursing interventions, such as sacral pressure, back rubs, a cool cloth on the head, and continual support and encouragement. If medications can be administered safely, do not withhold them under the false assumption that their use will contribute to addiction.

Preventing Heroin Withdrawal

To prevent or stabilize heroin withdrawal during labor, administer methadone intramuscularly as ordered if the woman is nauseated or vomiting. Give methadone to the woman who usually takes methadone at chemical-dependence centers if she did not receive her daily dose.

Evaluation

• Are the woman and her fetus free of injury during labor and childbirth?

POSTPARTUM PERIOD

During the postpartum period, nursing care is focused on helping the mother with bonding, infant care, and planning to provide for the care of herself and the infant after discharge. These topics are discussed in Chapter 30.

▌ *Birth of an Infant with Congenital Anomalies*

Even when everything goes according to plan, childbirth is a time of stress for parents. When the infant is born with anomalies, the parents are often overwhelmed with shock and grief. Because nurses are with the parents more than other members of the perinatal team, they have an opportunity to help the family adjust and to cope with their feelings.

Factors Influencing Emotional Responses of Parents

TIMING AND MANNER OF BEING TOLD

It was common practice at one time to remove the infant from the delivery area before parents could see a congenital anomaly. This practice changed, however, when it was realized that parents experienced less stress if they were told at once and were permitted to hold the newborn if the physical status of the infant allowed (Fig. 25–4). Physicians and nurses also became aware of the importance of helping the parents accept and bond with the newborn.

PRIOR KNOWLEDGE OF THE DEFECT

In this age of sophisticated prenatal examinations, parents may be aware of the congenital anomaly before the infant is born. These parents may not experience the shock and disbelief that parents who are unprepared do. Their reactions, however, should not be interpreted to mean that they do not experience grief. Instead, they have completed some of the early stages of grieving before the birth.

TYPE OF DEFECT

Although any defect in a newborn produces extreme concern and anxiety, certain defects are associated with long-term parenting problems. It is particularly difficult for the family and the community to accept an infant with facial or genital anomalies. The face is visible to everyone, and parents are fearful about whether the child will be accepted.

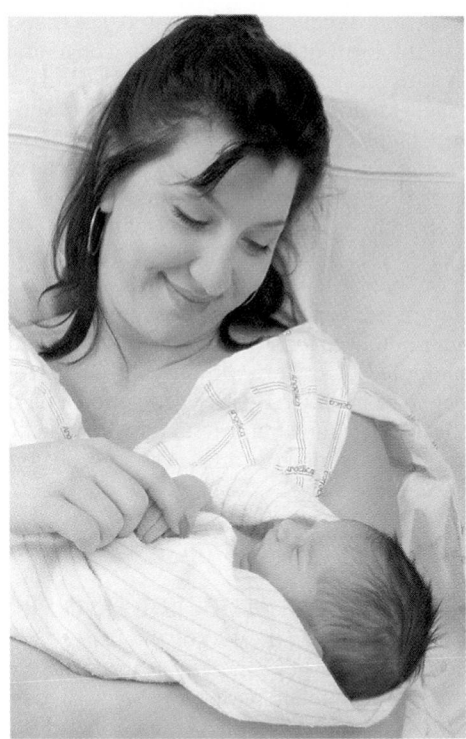

FIGURE 25–4

Touching and cuddling between parents and the infant with a congenital anomaly foster attachment and help resolve the grieving process.

If the defect is cleft lip and palate, the parents are extremely concerned about surgical repair. Parents are often anxious about how grandparents and siblings will accept the child.

Gender is at the core of a person's identity, and any defect of the genitals arouses deep concern in both parents. Some anomalies, such as hypospadias (opening of the urethra on the underside of the penis), are repaired in early childhood. Other genital anomalies, such as ambiguous genitalia, when assignment of gender is in doubt, cause extreme concern in the family and affect such basic issues as what to name the infant, how to dress the infant, and how to respond to questions about the infant's sex.

IRREPARABLE DEFECT

Although the initial impact of any defect is profound disappointment and concern, when the defect is irreparable, the parents have no time limit to their endeavors. Eventually, they must grapple with the knowledge that the infant will have a lifelong disability. Examples of irreparable defects include Down syndrome, microcephaly, and amelia (absence of an entire extremity).

Grief and Mourning

Grief describes the emotional response to loss. *Mourning* is the process of going through the phases of grief until one can accept and resolve the loss. Birth of an infant with an anomaly evokes a grief response, and the family must mourn the loss of the perfect infant they fantasized about during pregnancy. Early emotions include denial, anger, and guilt.

Denial and disbelief are the initial reactions of most parents to the birth of an infant with a congenital defect. Anger is often a pervasive response, and it may take the form of fault-finding or resentment. Anger may be directed toward the family, the medical personnel, or the self, but it is seldom directed toward the infant. Guilt may be expressed as a question of responsibility for the defect: "I shouldn't have taken that trip while I was pregnant."

Other emotions include fear, which may be expressed as concern about what must be done in the immediate or distant future (surgical procedures, complicated health care, the infant's potential for a normal life). Sadness and depression, manifested by crying, withdrawal from relationships, lack of energy, inability to sleep, and decreased appetite, may precede acceptance and resolution. Gradually, often after a prolonged period, feelings of sadness abate, and the family can accept and resolve grief.

Nursing Considerations

ASSISTING WITH THE GRIEVING PROCESS

Parents must grieve for the loss of the perfect infant that they expected before they can form an attachment with this newborn. It is helpful if nurses remain with the parents through the initial phase of shock and disbelief and maintain an atmosphere that encourages them to express their feelings.

Nurses must recognize that grief responses vary with individuals. Moreover, cultural and religious beliefs affect the expression of grief. Some groups express grief openly by crying, becoming angry, or seeking comfort from a support group. Other cultures (such as Chinese, Japanese, or Native Americans) do not. They may appear stoic and may not reveal the depths of their grief. In some cultures (such as Latino), it is acceptable for women, but not for men, to grieve publicly.

PROMOTING BONDING AND ATTACHMENT

A priority nursing intervention is to promote bonding and attachment, which may be disrupted when parents who expected a perfect infant give birth to an infant with an abnormality. The process often begins when the nurse communicates acceptance of the infant.

To do this, the nurse handles the newborn gently and presents the infant as something precious. Parents are particularly sensitive to facial expressions of shock or distress. Many nurses emphasize the normal aspects of the infant's body: "She is so alert and she has beautiful eyes." Perhaps it is most important to help the parents hold their infant as soon as possible. Touching and cuddling are essential to caring.

PROVIDING ACCURATE INFORMATION

Nurses who work in perinatal settings are responsible for becoming informed about follow-up treatment and timing of surgical procedures so that they can clarify and reinforce information provided by the physician. This process involves discussing the plan of care with the physician as well as researching the nursing care that will be required. Parents develop trust in the health care team when consistent information is presented clearly and explained fully.

One primary nurse or team should work with the family throughout the hospital stay. Nurses should expect to repeat information frequently because it may be difficult for the grieving parents to retain it.

FACILITATING COMMUNICATION

Nurses are sometimes fearful of being asked questions that they cannot answer, or they fear that they will say the wrong thing.

The most helpful course of action is to answer questions as honestly as possible. If unsure of information, say so: "I am not sure about that, but I will find out about it for you." In addition to answers, parents need kindness, support, and genuine concern.

It is crucial that family members communicate with one another as well as with the health professionals. Fathers should be included in all discussions, demonstrations, and care of the infant. Information and empathy should be offered consistently to both parents. Without this attention, the father cannot be expected to support his partner, explain the infant's condition to relatives and friends, or begin to deal with his own shock and sadness.

PLANNING FOR DISCHARGE

Often the parents need to learn the special feeding, holding, and positioning techniques that their infant needs. Early participation in infant care fosters feelings of attachment and responsibility for the infant.

Anticipatory guidance may help prevent problems when the infant is discharged. The reaction and behavior of siblings depend on their age and ability to understand the needs of the infant. Young children, who are often jealous of the attention and care that the infant requires, may regress to infantile behaviors, such as bed-wetting or thumb-sucking. Parents should be reminded that this response indicates a need for attention rather than naughtiness.

Although grandparents can be a great source of strength and support, they may also have difficulty adjusting to the infant with an abnormality. When appropriate, include grandparents when teaching special care that the infant will need.

PROVIDING REFERRALS

Finally, nurses often initiate referrals to national and community resources. Besides a referral to the social worker in the hospital, parents may also benefit from information about the National Easter Seal Society for Crippled Children, the March of Dimes Birth Defects Foundation, or the disabled children's services of the public health department. In addition, organizations such as the Shriners provide funds for the care of children.

Pregnancy Loss

Perinatal death can occur at any time. Early spontaneous abortion, fetal demise during the latter half of pregnancy, stillbirth, or neonatal death when the infant survives for a few days or weeks can be equally devastating for the parents.

Parents experiencing perinatal death often feel alone in their grief, because many people do not consider perinatal loss to be on the same level as the loss of an older child or adult. Moreover, friends and family members are often hesitant to discuss the loss for fear of saying the wrong thing.

Fathers often feel a need to appear strong so that they can support their partners. As a result, fathers often hold back their own feelings of grief and pain and are sometimes perceived as needing less support than the mother.

A perinatal loss may affect the woman during a subsequent pregnancy. She may have more anxiety about the pregnancy and may have decreased attachment to the fetus during the pregnancy (Armstrong & Hutti, 1998).

Early Pregnancy Loss

Early pregnancy loss, because of either spontaneous abortion or ectopic pregnancy, may precipitate intense grief by the parents. Many people, however, minimize the grief that occurs at this time. Comments such as, "You shouldn't have any problems getting pregnant again" discount the feelings of mothers and fathers. When ectopic pregnancy is the reason for the loss, the woman must deal with the loss of the pregnancy as well as with the possible loss of one fallopian tube.

Concurrent Death and Survival in Multifetal Pregnancy

Parents experience conflicting and complex feelings of joy and grief when one or more infants in a multifetal pregnancy live and one or more infants in the same gestation die. Contrary to common belief, parents do not grieve less for the dead infant because of the joy that they experience in the surviving infant.

For parents experiencing both survival and death of an infant, the grieving process may be more complicated. They may have fears about the health of the surviving infant, especially if the infant is preterm or ill. They may be unable to grieve for the dead child because of their concerns for the surviving child. They may also have problems with attachment to the surviving infant because of grieving. Moreover, they may receive less support than parents who have lost the only child in a single gestation.

NURSING CARE

Pregnancy Loss

Assessment

Nursing assessment of the family that has experienced the loss of a fetus or infant requires a great deal of sensitivity. In the case of infant death, collect as much information as possible before meeting the woman and her family for the first time so that hurtful mistakes can be avoided. Knowing the child's sex, weight, length, gestational age, and whether any abnormalities were noted will help in communicating effectively.

Many perinatal units design a sticker to place on the door, chart, and Kardex so that all staff who come in contact with the family, including auxiliary, housekeeping, laboratory, and radiology personnel, will be alerted that the infant

has not survived. Designs include a fallen leaf, a teardrop, or a rainbow. This visual symbol diminishes the chance that an uninformed person will make inadvertent comments that cause the family pain.

> Nurses are often unsure how to interact with a family that has experienced the loss of an infant. It is helpful to acknowledge the situation and to clarify the nurse's role at once: "I am Bette Turner. I will be your nurse for the next 8 hours. I am so sorry for your loss. Let me know if there is any way I can be of help." This is not an appropriate time for self-disclosure or for false reassurance. Keep the focus on the family's response and their ability to support one another.

Nurses who provide home care or who make follow-up telephone calls must be aware of subtle cues of grief, such as sighing, excessive sleeping, apathy, poor hygiene, or loss of appetite. These are especially important when assessing members of cultural groups that do not display grief publicly.

Evaluate also the availability of a support system that includes family members or clergy. It may be necessary to ask whether a spiritual adviser would help the family cope with grief. Include the father in assessment, as he may not receive the support he needs.

Nursing Diagnosis and Planning

Grief reactions are unique to each person, and it is inappropriate to assign a time frame in which parents will acknowledge or share their grief. The most obvious nursing diagnosis for anyone who experiences perinatal death is

- Grieving related to newborn (or fetal) death.
  Expected Outcomes: The parents will acknowledge their grief and express the meaning of the loss and will share their grief with significant others.

Interventions

Acknowledging the Infant

It was once believed that, when an infant was stillborn or died shortly after birth, the parents would grieve less if the newborn were quickly taken away before the parents saw the infant. Relatives often disposed of the clothes and the bassinet of the expected infant before the mother returned home, and the parents were left with very few memories of the infant's birth.

The response to perinatal death changed as nurses discovered that the most helpful interventions for grieving parents were those that acknowledged the rights of the baby. These include the right

To be recognized as a person who was born and died
To be named
To be seen, touched, and held by the family
To have life-ending acknowledged
To be put to rest with dignity (Primeau & Lamb, 1995)

Presenting the Infant to the Parents.   The infant's presentation to the parents is extremely important because these are the memories that they will retain. If necessary, wash the infant and apply baby lotion or powder. Wrap the infant in a soft, warm blanket. If possible, bring parents and infant together while the infant is still warm and soft. It may be necessary to keep the infant in a warmed incubator if some time elapses before the parents have contact with the infant. If this is not possible, tell the parents that the skin may feel cool. Allow parents to keep the infant as long as they wish, and make them feel free to unwrap the infant if they wish.

When the stillborn infant has severe deformities, explain the defect briefly and gently. Wrap the infant to expose the most normal aspect. Use diapers to cover genital defects, and use booties and mittens to cover abnormalities of the hands and feet. It is not advisable, however, to try to hide the defects completely. Allow parents to progress at their own speed in inspecting the infant. Clinical experience shows that many parents never unwrap the infant but instead quietly discuss the positive features of the infant.

Allow as much privacy and time as the parents and other family members need to be together. Remain sensitive to cues that members of the family want to talk or prefer not to. A sympathetic smile, and a promise to return in a specific time and then returning at that time are equally important. It is all right to ask, "Do you want to talk?" Then, listening quietly and reflecting the mother or father's feelings are all that is required.

Preparing a Memory Packet. Mourning requires memories. Nurses have explored measures that help the family create memories of the infant so that the existence of the child is confirmed and the parents can complete the grieving process.

Most parents treasure a memory packet that includes a photograph; footprints; the crib card with the infant's name, weight, and length; and, if possible, a lock of hair. Some parents and grandparents want pictures taken of themselves with the infant. The memory packet should be kept on file if the parents do not wish to take it home; they may change their minds later.

Providing Referrals

Parents may find that friends and relatives expect them to recover quickly from perinatal loss and cannot understand their continued grief. The greatest help often comes from contact with persons who have experienced a similar loss, and a variety of support groups have been formed. These include Resolve Through Sharing, AMEND (Aiding a Mother Experiencing Neonatal Death), SHARE (Source of Help in Airing and Resolving Experiences), and HAND (Helping After Neonatal Death).

Evaluation
- Have the parents acknowledged their grief and the meaning of the loss?
- Have they shared their grief with significant others?

Relinquishment by Adoption

Some women carry the pregnancy to term and then relinquish the newborn to the care of another family for adoption. The decision to place the infant for adoption is a painful one that can produce long-lasting feelings of ambivalence. On the one hand, the expectant mother may be satisfied that the infant is going into a stable home where a child is wanted and will receive excellent care; on the

other hand, the social pressures against giving up one's child are often intense.

The relationship between the birth mother and the adoptive parents varies greatly. The adoptive parents may be unknown to the birth mother, or she may know and even choose them. Some adoptive mothers participate in the birth.

Nurses are sometimes unsure of how to communicate with the woman who is relinquishing her infant. First, the nursing staff that comes into contact with the woman must be informed of her decision to place the infant for adoption. Information prevents inadvertent comments that could cause distress. Second, nurses must remember that adoption is *an act of love, not one of abandonment*, as the woman relinquishes the newborn to a family that is better able to provide financial and emotional support.

Nurses must also be prepared to respect any special wishes that the mother may have about the birth. For instance, most birth mothers want to know all about the infant. They may want to see and hold the newborn. Some wish to name the infant or to give it a gift. Many take photographs or save mementos such as the birth bracelet or the crib card. Such actions provide memories of the infant and help the mother through the grieving process that may accompany relinquishment of the child.

> The nurse should try to establish rapport and a trusting relationship with the mother. It is helpful to acknowledge the situation at the initial contact with the woman: "Hello, my name is Denise, and I will be your nurse today. I understand the adoptive family is coming this morning. What can I do to help you get ready?" This communication is more helpful than providing care without reference to an event that is of utmost concern to the mother. It also provides an opening for her to express feelings that may include attachment to the infant, ambivalence about her decision, and profound sadness.

Nurses also teach adoptive families how to care for the newborn and what to expect in growth and development. Teaching requires adequate time and a private place. This family benefits from all the teaching provided to other new parents. They may be anxious, and demonstrations as well as return demonstrations are appropriate.

Violence Against Women

Physical abuse may start or become worse during pregnancy; it has been recognized as a risk to the health of both mothers and infants. The incidence during pregnancy is reported to be 16% (1 in 6) (McFarlane, Parker, & Soeken, 1996a). Physical abuse is recurrent, with 60% of abused women reporting two or more episodes of violence. Although all ethnic groups report similar rates of abuse, major ethnic differences exist, with white women experiencing more frequent and more severe abuse (McFarlane, Parker, & Soeken, 1996a).

Physical abuse may involve threats, slapping, or pushing. It may also escalate to punching, kicking, and beating that results in internal injury or to wounds from weapons. It may end in death. Sexual abuse, including rape, is often part of physical abuse, with almost half the abused women reporting being forced into sex by their male partner.

Physical violence occurs within the context of continuous mental abuse, threats, and coercion. Women go through a process of shame, loss of self-respect, diminished ability to cope as a free adult, and a distancing between self and sources of help and support (Smith, Tessaro, & Earp, 1995). Moreover, physical abuse of the mother may be an indication of what life holds for the unborn child. Most men who batter women also batter their children, and some women who are battered physically abuse their children.

Factors That Promote Violence

Family violence occurs in cultures where male and female roles are based on gender and little value is placed on the woman's role. Men hold power, and women are viewed as less worthy of respect than men.

In many cultures, women earn less than men in the job market, and they are often victimized by marriage. For example, women who hold full-time jobs still carry the major responsibilities for housekeeping and child care. They often remain in unhealthy relationships because they are financially dependent on men. If they divorce, most women become single parents with a standard of living much lower than that of their former husbands.

Stereotyping males as powerful and females as weak and without value has a profound effect on the self-esteem of women. Many women internalize the messages and come to believe that they are less worthy than their partners and that they are the cause of their own punishment. They accept the message from society that when women are battered or raped, "they got what they deserved."

Although alcohol is often stated as a cause of violence against women, chemical dependence and domestic violence are two separate problems. Violence, however, may become more severe or bizarre when alcohol or drugs are involved. See Table 25-2 for a summary of the myths and realities of violence against women.

Characteristics of the Abuser

Physical abuse concerns power, and it is only one of many tactics that abusive men use to control their partners. Other tactics include isolation, intimidation, and threats. Extreme jealousy and possessiveness are typical of the abuser. An abusive man often attempts to control all aspects of the woman's life, such as where she goes and what she wears. He controls access to money and transportation and may force the woman to account for every moment spent away from him.

The abusive man often has a low tolerance for frustration and poor impulse control. He does not perceive his violent behavior as a problem and often blames the woman. Most abusive men come from homes where they witnessed the abuse of their mothers or were themselves abused as children.

TABLE 25-2

Myths and Realities of Violence Against Women

Myths	Realities
The battered woman syndrome affects only a small percentage of the population.	Battering is the single major cause of injury to women; 3 to 4 million women are battered each year by their partners.
Battering of women occurs only in lower socioeconomic classes and in minority groups.	Violence occurs in families from all social, economic, educational, racial, and religious backgrounds.
The problem is really "spouse abuse," couples who assault each other.	Ninety-five percent of serious assaults are male against female; violence against women is about control and power.
Alcohol and drugs cause abusive behavior.	Substance abuse and violence against women are two separate problems. Substance abuse is a disease; violence is a learned behavior that can be unlearned.
The abuser is "out of control."	He is not out of control; he is making a decision, because he chooses who, when, and where he abuses.
The woman "got what she deserved."	No one deserves to be beaten. No one has the right to beat another person. Violent behavior is the responsibility of the violent person.
Women "like" it or they would leave.	Women are threatened with severe punishment or death if they attempt to leave; many have no resources and are isolated, and they and their children depend on the abuser.
Couples counseling is a good recommendation for abusive relationships.	Couples counseling is ineffective for the couple. It can also be dangerous for the abused woman.

Cycle of Violence

Violence occurs in a cycle that consists of three phases: a tension-building phase, a battering incident, and a "honeymoon phase." Being aware of the behaviors that accompany each phase will enable the nurse to counsel the woman. Figure 25–5 depicts these behaviors.

Effects of Battering During Pregnancy

Abuse during pregnancy is correlated with health problems for the mother and the infant. Women battered during pregnancy are more likely to have multiple injury sites, particularly of the abdomen as well as the face and breasts. Abused women tend to enter prenatal care late in the pregnancy, with up to one-fourth starting prenatal care in the third trimester. They are at increased risk for low maternal weight gain and anemia, and a higher percentage report the use of alcohol and illicit drugs (McFarlane, Parker, & Soeken, 1996b). Pregnant women in battering relationships face an increased risk of prematurity and bearing low-birth-weight infants.

Nurse's Role in Prevention of Abuse

Nurses can do a great deal to prevent physical abuse. First, they must examine their beliefs to determine whether they accept the prevailing attitude that blames the victim: "Why does she stay with him?"

Second, nurses can consciously practice in ways that empower women. They should make it clear that the woman owns her body and has the right to decide how it should be treated. Nurses must use language that indicates that the woman is an active partner in her care: "You understand your body: what do you think?"

During examinations, nurses can introduce aspects of care that increase the woman's control over the situation. For example, make sure that the woman meets the physician or nurse practitioner who is to examine her while seated and clothed rather than while unclothed and in a lithotomy position.

School nurses are in an excellent position to influence how teenagers define gender roles: "Real men don't beat up women." "Girls don't have to put up with verbal or physical abuse from anyone."

NURSING CARE
The Battered Woman

Assessment

Because of the prevalence of physical abuse during pregnancy, it is recommended that all women be screened for

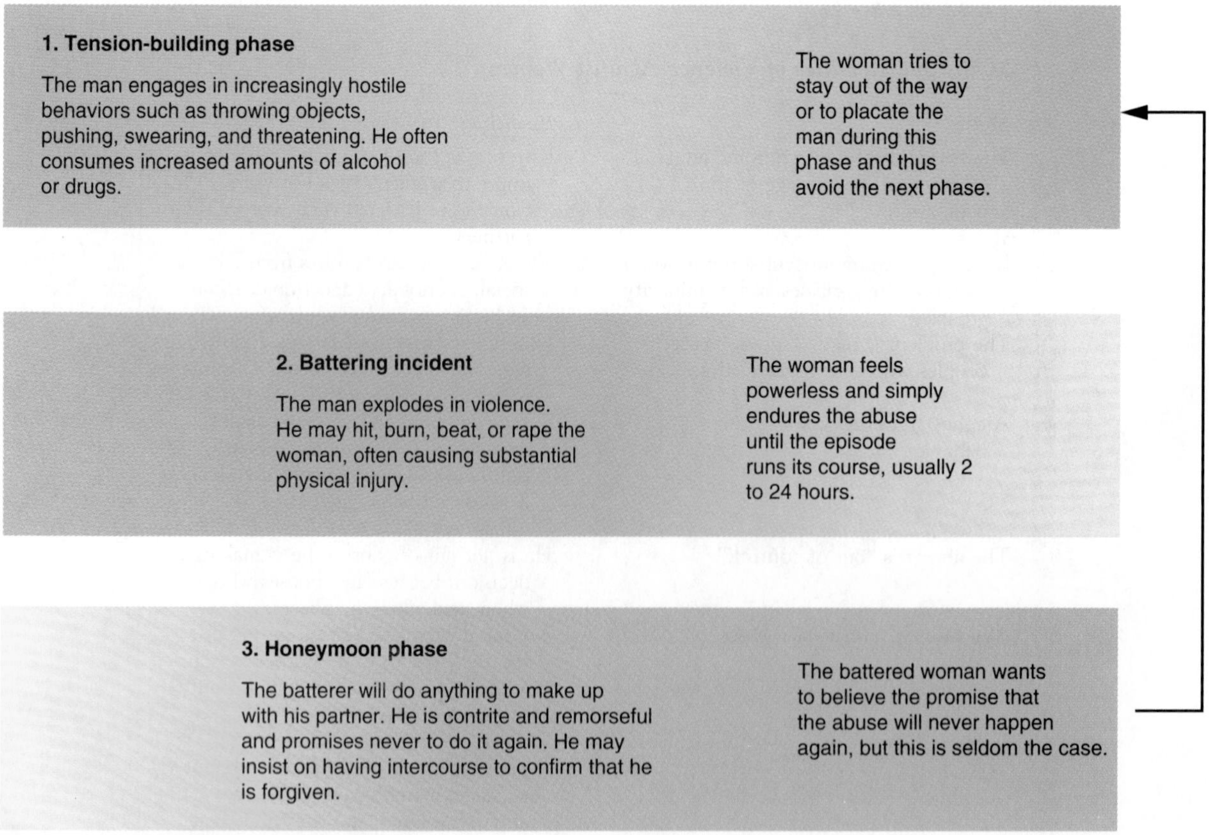

1. Tension-building phase

The man engages in increasingly hostile behaviors such as throwing objects, pushing, swearing, and threatening. He often consumes increased amounts of alcohol or drugs.

The woman tries to stay out of the way or to placate the man during this phase and thus avoid the next phase.

2. Battering incident

The man explodes in violence. He may hit, burn, beat, or rape the woman, often causing substantial physical injury.

The woman feels powerless and simply endures the abuse until the episode runs its course, usually 2 to 24 hours.

3. Honeymoon phase

The batterer will do anything to make up with his partner. He is contrite and remorseful and promises never to do it again. He may insist on having intercourse to confirm that he is forgiven.

The battered woman wants to believe the promise that the abuse will never happen again, but this is seldom the case.

FIGURE 25–5
Types of behaviors evident in each step of the cycle of violence.

physical abuse at each contact. When they are first approached, women may deny that abuse has occurred. Asking or asking more than once, however, may lead the woman to seek help at a later time. Leaving written information in women's restrooms also implies that discussion of violence with the nurse is encouraged and safe.

Nurses are often unsure how to approach the issue of suspected abuse. Women often seek care and are assessed in the "honeymoon phase" of the violence cycle. It is during this phase that the man is often overly solicitous ("hovering husband syndrome") and eager to explain any injuries that the woman exhibits. *Introducing the subject of violence in the presence of the man who may be responsible for it places the woman in danger. It is essential to separate the woman from the man for the interview.*

When a private, secure place has been found, reassure the woman that her privacy will be protected and that confidentiality will be absolute. Ask questions directly. If there is trauma, appropriate questions are, "Did someone hurt you?" "Did you receive these injuries from being hit?" The abused woman often appears hesitant, embarrassed, or evasive. She may be unable to look the nurse in the eye and appears guilty, ashamed, jumpy, or frightened.

Evaluate and document all signs of injury, both past and present. This includes areas of welts, bruising, swelling, lacerations, burns, and scars. Injuries are most commonly noted on the face, breasts, abdomen, and genitalia. Many women have new or old fractures. These are usually frac-

---

> ### CRITICAL TO REMEMBER
> #### Cues Indicating Violence Against Women
>
> *Nonverbal:* Facial grimacing, slow and unsteady gait, vomiting, abdominal tenderness, absence of facial response
> *Injuries:* Welts, bruises, swelling, lacerations, burns, vaginal or rectal bleeding; evidence of old or new fractures of the nose, face, ribs, or arms
> *Vague somatic complaints:* Anxiety, depression, panic attacks, sleeplessness, anorexia
> *Discrepancy between history and type of injuries:* Wounds that do not match the woman's story, multiple bruises in various stages of healing, bruising on the arms (which she may have raised to protect herself), old, untreated wounds

---

tures of the face, nose, ribs, or arms. If there has been sexual abuse, a gynecologic examination is necessary because there is often trauma to the labia, vagina, or cervix.

Be particularly alert for nonverbal cues that indicate that abuse has occurred. Facial grimacing or a slow, unsteady gait may indicate pain. Vomiting or abdominal tenderness may indicate internal injury. A flat affect—that is, absence of facial response—is indicative of women who mentally withdraw from the situation to protect themselves from the horror and humiliation they experience. Keep in mind that the woman may fear for her life because abusive episodes tend to escalate.

Nursing Diagnosis and Planning

Nursing diagnosis depends on the data collected during the assessment. The most meaningful diagnosis for perinatal nurses to make may be

- Fear related to possibility of severe injury to self and/or children during unpredictable cycle of violence.
  Expected Outcomes: The woman will acknowledge the physical assaults, will develop a specific plan of action to implement when the abusive cycle begins, and will identify community resources that provide protection for herself and her children.

The abused woman is often unwilling to leave the abusive situation, and nurses often must work with the woman to plan realistic short-term goals that will protect her from injury.

Interventions

Developing a Personal Safety Plan

Help the woman make concrete plans to protect the safety of herself and her children. For example, describe the cycle of behavior that culminates in physical abuse and instruct her in factors that precipitate a violent episode. These

---

> ### CRITICAL THINKING EXERCISE 25-1
>
> Joan Piszarek, a 28-year-old primigravida, is admitted to the labor, delivery, and recovery unit in active labor. The right side of her face is swollen, evidence of old bruises looks like fingerprints on her upper arms, and a large bruised area is evident on her abdomen. She is accompanied by her husband, who is very solicitous. He verbalizes concern about her labor status and remains close beside her at all times. Joan appears lethargic and avoids eye contact with the nurse who is admitting her. She states that she fainted at home and hurt herself when she fell against the bathtub. The nurse accepts the explanation and asks no further questions.
>
> 1. What assumptions has the nurse made?
> 2. What should make the nurse examine her conclusion that the injuries resulted from falling?
>
> When the relief nurse arrives, she waits for time alone with Joan and asks, "Did you get these injuries from being hit?" Joan appears extremely anxious and says, "Don't say anything! He got so mad when I was late getting home from shopping. It was my fault."
>
> 3. Why did the nurse wait for time alone before asking questions?
> 4. How should the nurse respond? What bias must she guard against?
> 5. How can Joan be protected?

include the use of alcohol or other drugs and behaviors that indicate that the level of frustration and anger is increasing.

Discussing specific safety behaviors with abused women often results in their adopting many of the behaviors (McFarlane et al., 1998). The woman should

- Locate the nearest shelter or safe house and make specific plans to go there once the cycle of violence begins.
- Identify the safest, quickest routes out of the home.
- Obtain and hide extra keys to the car and house.
- Hide money and copies of important papers (birth certificates, social security numbers).
- Devise a code word, and prearrange with someone to call the police when the word is used.
- Memorize the telephone number of the shelter or hotline, because time is often a crucial element in the decision to leave.
- Review the safety plan frequently, because leaving the batterer is one of the most dangerous times.

Affirming She Is Not to Blame

The abused woman often believes that she is responsible for the abuse. Let her know that no one deserves to be hit for any reason. The one who hit her is the person responsible; she did not provoke it, and she did not cause it. Nurses are often responsible for teaching her that violence is not normal and it is usually repeated and usually escalates. She

needs help to understand that battered women have alternatives.

Providing Referrals

Many interventions are outside the scope of nursing practice. Refer the family to community agencies such as the police department, legal services, community shelters, counseling services, and social service agencies.

It is essential to accept the decisions of the battered woman and acknowledge that she is on her own timetable. She may not take any actions at the time that they are recommended. Therefore, listening to her and providing information about resources may be the only help the nurse can provide.

Do not become negative or pass judgment on the partner of an abused woman. She is often tied to the man by both economic and emotional bonds and may become defensive if her partner is criticized. Tell her that resources are available for her partner but that it is necessary for him to admit abuse and seek assistance before help can be offered. Initiating referrals for the partner before he asks for help will increase the danger to the woman if he feels that he has been betrayed.

Evaluation

- Does the woman acknowledge the violence?
- Has she made concrete plans to protect herself and her children from future injury?
- Does she use the community resources available to her?

KEY CONCEPTS

- Teenage pregnancy is a major health problem in the United States. Adolescents need to receive accurate information not only about contraceptives but also about setting limits on sexual behavior.
- Pregnancy poses serious physiologic risks for the adolescent and the fetus. These result in a higher incidence of pregnancy-induced hypertension, anemia, and nutritional deficiencies for the expectant mother as well as prematurity and low birth weight for the infant.
- Teenage pregnancy interrupts the developmental tasks of adolescence and may result in childbirth before the parents are capable of providing a nurturing home for the infant without a great deal of assistance.
- The mature primigravida often has financial and emotional resources that younger women do not have. She may experience

anxiety about recommended antepartum testing, however, and about her ability to be an effective parent.
- Polydrug abuse is a widespread problem that can have devastating fetal and neonatal effects. These may become long-term developmental problems for the child.
- The lifestyle associated with illicit drug abuse includes inadequate nutrition, inadequate prenatal care, and an increased incidence of STDs. It necessitates interdisciplinary interventions to prevent injury to the expectant mother and to the fetus.
- The birth of an infant with congenital anomalies produces strong emotions of shock and grief in the family. It calls for a sensitive response from the health care team to help the family grieve for the loss of the perfect or "fantasy" infant and to form an attachment to the newborn.

- Pregnancy loss at any stage of pregnancy produces grief that must be acknowledged and expressed before it can be resolved. Nurses realize that mourning requires memories, and they intervene to arrange unlimited contact between the family and the stillborn infant and to prepare a packet of mementos for the family.
- Nursing care for the mother who is placing her infant for adoption is based on the knowledge that relinquishment (adoption) is an act of love, not abandonment.
- Multiple factors are associated with violence against women. It is deliberate, severe, and generally repeated in a predictable cycle that often causes severe physical harm (or death) to the woman.
- All perinatal nurses come into contact with abused women who require assistance to protect themselves and their children from serious injury.

ANSWERS TO CRITICAL THINKING EXERCISE 25-1

1. The nurse assumed that the husband's behavior showed concern for his wife. Instead, it may have been a "hovering husband syndrome" that occurs in the honeymoon phase of the cycle of violence.
2. Facial injury, signs of previous bruising that resemble "grab marks," and abdominal bruising. Joan's story of falling and hurting herself is not congruent with the location of abdominal injury and injuries on her arms. Joan's lethargy and avoidance of eye contact also suggest that she is afraid.
3. The nurse should not question Joan's explanation of the injury in her husband's presence because this action increases the danger of escalating violence when the mother and infant are discharged.
4. The nurse should respond, "No one deserves to be hurt. It's not your fault. How can I help you?" Nurses must examine their own thinking to be certain that they do not accept a common bias that physical abuse is deserved by the victim.
5. Joan needs information about protecting herself and the coming infant from future harm. This is not, however, the appropriate time to give her this information. The nurse must inform the physician and the postpartum staff of the problem and must make the necessary referrals to the hospital's social service department for follow-up.

REFERENCES AND READINGS

American Academy of Pediatrics (AAP) & American College of Obstetricians and Gynecologists (ACOG). (1997). *Guidelines for perinatal care* (4th ed.). Elk Grove Village, IL, and Washington, DC: Author.

American College of Obstetricians and Gynecologists (ACOG). (1996). *Guidelines for women's health care.* Washington, DC: Author.

Armstrong, D., & Hutti, M. (1998). Pregnancy after perinatal loss: The relationship between anxiety and prenatal attachment. *Journal of Obstetric, Gynecologic, and Neonatal Nursing, 27*(2), 183–189.

Association of Women's Health, Obstetric, and Neonatal Nursing (AWHONN). (1998). *Standards and guidelines for professional nursing practice in the care of women and newborns* (5th ed.). Washington, DC: Author.

Barnet, B., Duggan, A. K., Wilson, M. D., & Joffe, A. (1995). Association between postpartum substance abuse and depressive symptoms, stress, and social support in adolescent mothers. *Pediatrics, 96*(4), 659–666.

Bell, G. L., & Lau, K. (1995). Perinatal and neonatal issues of substance abuse. *Pediatric Clinics of North America, 42*(2), 261–279.

Berenson, A. B., & Wiemann, C. M. (1997). Contraceptive use among adolescent mothers at 6 months postpartum. *Obstetrics and Gynecology, 89*(6), 999–1005.

Berns, S. M., & Brown, L. A. (1998). The changing family unit. In C. Kenner, J. W. Lott, & A. A. Flandermeyer (Eds.), *Comprehensive neonatal nursing: A physiologic perspective* (2nd ed., pp. 61–68). Philadelphia: Saunders.

Bloom, K. C. (1995). The development of attachment behaviors in pregnant adolescents. *Nursing Research, 44*(5), 284–289.

Bloom, K. C. (1998). Perceived relationship with the father of the baby and maternal attachment in adolescents. *Journal of Obstetric, Gynecologic, and Neonatal Nursing, 27*(4), 420–430.

Bragg, E. J. (1997). Pregnant adolescents with addictions. *Journal of Obstetric, Gynecologic, and Neonatal Nursing, 26*(5), 577–584.

Brown, H. L., Britton, K. A., Mahaffey, D., Brizendine, E., Hiett, A. K., & Turnquest, M. A. (1998). Methadone maintenance in pregnancy: A reappraisal. *Obstetrics and Gynecology, 179*(2), 459–463.

Chazotte, C., Youchah, J., & Freda, M. C. (1995). Cocaine use during pregnancy and low birth weight: The impact of prenatal care and drug treatment. *Seminars in Perinatology, 19*(4), 293–299.

Chez, R. A., & Jones, R. F. (1995). The battered woman. *American Journal of Obstetrics and Gynecology, 173*(3), 677–679.

Christian, A. (1995). Home care of the battered pregnant woman: One battered woman's pregnancy. *Journal of Obstetric, Gynecologic, and Neonatal Nursing, 24*(9), 836–842.

Cockey, C. D. (1998). Preventing teen pregnancy. *Lifelines, 1*(3), 32–40.

Cornelius, M. D., Taylor, P. M., Geva, D., & Day, N. L. (1995). Prenatal tobacco and marijuana use among adolescents: Effects on offspring, gestational age, growth, and morphology. *Pediatrics, 95*(5), 738–743.

Covington, D. L., Dalton, V. K., Diehl, S. J., Wright, B. D., & Piner, M. H. (1997). Improving detection of violence among pregnant adolescents. *Journal of Adolescent Health, 21*(1), 18–24.

Cunningham, F. G., MacDonald, P. C., Gant, N. F., Leveno, K. J., Gilstrap, L. C., Hankins, G. D. U., et al. (1997). *Williams obstetrics* (20th ed.). Stamford, CT: Appleton & Lange.

Fishwick, N. J. (1998). Assessment of women for partner abuse. *Journal of Obstetric, Gynecologic, and Neonatal Nursing, 27*(6), 661–670.

Flandermeyer, A. A. (1998). The drug-exposed neonate. In C. Kenner, J. W. Lott, & A. A. Flandermeyer (Eds.), *Comprehensive neonatal nursing: A physiologic perspective* (2nd ed., pp. 864–892). Philadelphia: Saunders.

Fraser, A. M., Brockert, J. E., & Ward, R. H. (1995). Association of young maternal age with adverse reproductive outcomes. *New England Journal of Medicine, 332*(17), 1113–1117.

Fretts, R. C., Schmittdiel, J., McLean, F. H., Usher, R. H., & Goldman, M. B. (1995). Increased maternal age and the risk of fetal death. *New England Journal of Medicine, 333*(15), 953–957.

Gaines, K. A. (1997). Abuse and pregnancy: What every childbirth educator/nurse should know. *Journal of Perinatal Education, 6*(4), 28–34.

Gazmararian, J. A., Lazorick, S., Spitz, A. M., Ballard, T. J., Salzman, L. E., Marks, J. S. (1996). Prevalence of violence against pregnant women. *Journal of the American Medical Association, 275*(24), 1915–1920.

Hadley, S. M., Short, L. M., Lezin, N., & Zook, E. (1995). Womankind: An innovative model of health care response to domestic abuse. *Women's Health Issues, 5*(4), 189–198.

Hankin, J. R., & Sokol, R. J. (1995). Identification and care of problems associated with alcohol ingestion in pregnancy. *Seminars in Perinatology, 19*(4), 286–291.

Hoffman, S. D. (1998). Teenage childbearing is not so bad after all . . . Or is it? A review of the new literature. *Family Planning Perspectives, 30*(5), 236–239.

Kenner, C., & D'Apolito, K. (1997). Outcomes for children exposed to drugs in utero. *Journal of Obstetric, Gynecologic, and Neonatal Nursing, 26*(5), 595–603.

Kowaleski-Jones, L., & Mott, F. L. (1998). Sex, contraception and childbearing among high-risk youth: Do different factors influence males and females? *Family Planning Perspectives, 30*(4), 163–169.

Kowalski, K. (1996). Loss and bereavement: Psychological, sociological, spiritual, and ontological perspectives. In K. R. Simpson & P. A. Creehan (Eds.), *AWHONN's perinatal nursing* (pp. 271–286). Philadelphia: Lippincott.

Laken, M. P., & Hutchins, E. (1996). *Recruitment and retention of substance-using pregnant and parenting women: Lessons learned.* Arlington, VA: National Center for Education in Maternal and Child Health.

Lambers, D. S., & Clark, K. E. (1996). The maternal and fetal physiologic effects of nicotine. *Seminars in Perinatology, 20*(2), 115–126.

Landry, S. H., & Whitney, J. A. (1996). The impact of prenatal cocaine exposure: Studies of the developing infant. *Seminars in Perinatology, 20*(2), 99–106.

Lee, R. V. (1999). Substance abuse. In G. N. Burrow & T. F. Ferris (Eds.), *Medical complications during pregnancy* (5th ed., pp. 495–513). Philadelphia: Saunders.

Lieberman, L. D. (1998). Overview of substance abuse prevention and treatment approaches in urban, multicultural settings: The Center for Substance Abuse Prevention programs for pregnant and postpartum women and their infants. *Women's Health Issues, 8*(4), 208 – 217.

Leoni, L. C., Woods, J. R., & Woods, J. E. (1998). Caring for patients after pregnancy loss. *Lifelines, 2*(1), 56–58.

Mackay, M. C., & Tiller, C. M. (1998). Adolescents' description and management of pregnancy and preterm labor. *Journal of Obstetric, Gynecology, and Neonatal Nursing, 27*(4), 410–419.

McFarlane, J., & Gondolf, E. (1998). Preventing abuse during pregnancy: A clinical protocol. *MCN: American Journal of Maternal/Child Nursing, 23*(1), 22–26.

McFarlane, J., Parker, B., & Soeken, K. (1996a). Abuse during pregnancy: Associations with maternal health and infant birth weight. *Nursing Research, 45*(1), 37–42.

McFarlane, J., Parker, B., & Soeken, K. (1996b). Physical abuse, smoking, and substance use during pregnancy: Prevalence, interrelationships, and effects on birth weight. *Journal of Obstetric, Gynecologic, and Neonatal Nursing, 25*(4), 313–320.

McFarlane, J., Parker, B., Soeken, K., Silva, C., & Reel, S. (1998). Safety behaviors of abused women after an intervention during pregnancy. *Journal of Obstetric, Gynecologic, and Neonatal Nursing, 27*(1), 64–69.

National Center for Health Statistics. (1998). *Health, United States, 1998, with socioeconomic status & health chartbook.* Hyattsville, MD: Author.

Nichols, J. A. (1998). Bereavement: The state of having suffered a loss. In C. Kenner, J. W. Lott, & A. A. Flandermeyer (Eds.), *Comprehensive neonatal nursing: A physiologic perspective* (2nd ed., pp. 73–84). Philadelphia: Saunders.

Poland, L. M., & Hutchins, E. (1995). *Building and sustaining systems of care for substance-using women and their infants: Lessons learned.* Arlington, VA: National Center for Education in Maternal and Child Health.

Primeau, M. R., & Lamb, J. M. (1995). When a baby dies: Rights of the baby and parents. *Journal of Obstetric, Gynecologic, and Neonatal Nursing, 24*(3), 206–208.

Prysak, M., Lorenz, R. P., & Kisly, A. (1995). Pregnancy outcome in nulliparous women 35 years and older. *Obstetrics and Gynecology, 85*(1), 65–70.

Records, K. A. (1994). Adolescent mothers: Caregiving, approval, and family functioning. *Journal of Obstetric, Gynecologic, and Neonatal Nursing, 23*(9), 792–797.

Robertson, P. A., & Kavanaugh, K. (1998). Supporting parents during and after a pregnancy subsequent to a perinatal loss. *Journal of Perinatal and Neonatal Nursing, 12*(2), 63–71.

Roye, C. F., & Balk, S. J. (1996). Evaluation of an intergenerational program for pregnant and parenting adolescents. *Maternal-Child Nursing Journal, 24*(1), 32–40.

Ryan, J., & King, M. C. (1998). Scanning for violence: Educational strategies for helping abused women. *Lifelines, 2*(3), 36–41.

Selleck, C. S., & Redding, B. A. (1998). Knowledge and attitudes of registered nurses toward perinatal substance abuse. *Journal of Obstetric, Gynecologic, and Neonatal Nursing, 27*(1), 70–77.

Smith, P. H., Tessaro, I., & Earp, J. A. (1995). Women's experiences with battering: A conceptualization from qualitative research. *Women's Health Issues, 5*(4), 173–182.

Stark, M. A. (1997). Psychosocial adjustment during pregnancy: The experience of mature gravidas. *Journal of Obstetric, Gynecologic, and Neonatal Nursing, 26*(2), 206–211.

Thompson, P. J., Powell, M. J., Patterson, R. J., & Ellerbee, S. M. (1995). Adolescent parenting: Outcomes and maternal perceptions. *Journal of Obstetric, Gynecologic, and Neonatal Nursing, 24*(8), 713–717.

U.S. Department of Health and Human Services. (1995). *Healthy people 2000: Midcourse review and 1995 revisions.* Washington, DC: Author.

Ventura, S. J., Curtin, S. C., & Mathews, T. J. (1998). *Teenage birth in the United States: National and state trends, 1990–1996.* National Vital Statistics System, Hyattsville, MD: National Center for Health Statistics.

Warren, C. W., Santelli, J. S., Everett, S. A., Kann, L., Collins, J. L., Cassell, C., et al. (1998). Sexual behavior among U.S. high school students, 1990–1995. *Family Planning Perspectives, 30*(4), 170–172.

Wescott, C. S. (1997). The pain of grief. *Childbirth Instructor Magazine, 7*(5), 38–41.

Wilkerson, N. N. (1997). Screening and assessment for substance abuse in the childbearing population. *Journal of Perinatal Education, 6*(3), 10–19.

26

◆ ◆ ◆ ◆ ◆ ◆ ◆ ◆ ◆ ◆ ◆ ◆ ◆

The Pregnant Woman with Complications

DEFINITIONS

abortion Spontaneous or elective ending of a pregnancy before 20 weeks' gestation. Miscarriage is a lay term for a spontaneous abortion.

antiphospholipid antibodies Autoimmune antibodies directed against phospholipids in cell membranes, associated with recurrent spontaneous abortion, fetal loss, and severe pregnancy-induced hypertension.

bicornuate (bicornate) uterus Malformed uterus having two horns.

caudal regression syndrome Malformation that results when the sacrum, lumbar spine, and lower extremities fail to develop.

cerclage Encircling of the cervix with suture to prevent recurrent spontaneous abortion caused by early cervical dilation.

congestive heart failure Condition resulting from failure of the heart to maintain adequate circulation, characterized by weakness, dyspnea, and edema in body parts lower than the heart.

culdocentesis Needle puncture through the upper posterior vaginal wall (cul-de-sac of Douglas) to aspirate blood or fluid from the pelvic cavity.

diabetogenic Producing the effects of diabetes mellitus. Diabetogenic conditions include pregnancy.

dilation and curettage (D&C) Stretching the cervical os to permit suctioning or scraping of the walls of the uterus. The procedure is performed in abortion, to obtain samples of uterine lining tissue for laboratory examination, and during the postpartum period to remove retained fragments of placenta.

dystocia Difficult or prolonged labor, often associated with abnormal uterine activity and cephalopelvic disproportion.

eclampsia Convulsive form of pregnancy-induced hypertension.

erythroblastosis fetalis Agglutination and hemolysis of fetal erythrocytes due to incompatibility between maternal and fetal blood. In most cases the fetus is Rh-positive and the mother is Rh-negative.

gestational trophoblastic disease A spectrum of diseases that includes benign hydatidiform mole and gestational trophoblastic tumors, such as invasive moles and choriocarcinoma.

gluconeogenesis Formation of glycogen by the liver from noncarbohydrate sources, such as amino acids or fatty acids.

hydramnios Excess volume of amniotic fluid (more than 2,000 ml at term). Also called polyhydramnios.

hypovolemic shock Acute peripheral circulatory failure due to loss of circulating blood volume.

kernicterus Staining of brain tissue caused by accumulation of unconjugated bilirubin in the brain. Also called bilirubin encephalopathy.

ketosis Accumulation of ketone bodies (metabolic products) in the blood; frequently associated with acidosis.

laparoscopy Insertion of an illuminated tube (laparoscope) into the abdominal cavity to observe contents, locate bleeding, and perform surgical procedures.

lipogenic substance Substance, such as insulin, that stimulates the production of fat.

maceration Discoloration and softening of tissues and eventual disintegration of a fetus retained in the uterus after its death.

Marfan syndrome A hereditary condition that involves weakness in connective tissue, bones, and muscles. The vascular system is affected, particularly the aorta.

osmotic diuresis Secretion and passage of large amounts of urine as a result of increased osmotic pressure that can result from hyperglycemia.

perinatologist A physician who specializes in the care of the mother, fetus, and infant during the perinatal period (from the 20th week of pregnancy to 4 weeks following childbirth).

seroconversion Change in a blood test result from negative to positive, indicating the development of antibodies in response to infection or immunization.

toxemia An old term occasionally used to denote pregnancy-induced hypertension, pre-eclampsia, and eclampsia.

vacuum curettage (vacuum aspiration) Removal of the uterine contents by application of a vacuum through a hollow curet or cannula introduced into the uterus.

vasoconstriction Narrowing of the lumen of blood vessels.

Complications during pregnancy occasionally threaten the well-being of the expectant mother, the fetus, or both. These complications fall into two broad categories: complications of pregnancy, when problems develop in the normal processes, and complications related to other disorders that adversely affect the pregnancy or are adversely affected by the pregnancy.

Pregnancy-Related Complications

The most common pregnancy-related complications are hemorrhagic conditions that occur in early pregnancy, hemorrhagic complications of the placenta in late pregnancy, hyperemesis gravidarum, hypertensive disorders of pregnancy, and blood incompatibilities between the mother and fetus.

Hemorrhagic Conditions of Early Pregnancy

The three most common causes of hemorrhage during the first half of pregnancy are abortion, ectopic pregnancy, and hydatidiform mole.

Spontaneous Abortion

Abortion is the loss of pregnancy before the fetus is viable, that is, capable of living outside the uterus. The medical consensus today is that a fetus of less than 20 weeks' gestation or one weighing less than 500 g is not viable. Abortion may be either spontaneous or induced. Lay people often use the term *miscarriage* to denote an abortion that has occurred spontaneously as opposed to one that has been induced. Induced abortion is described in Chapter 31. Spontaneous abortion denotes termination of a pregnancy without action taken by the woman or any other person.

Determining the exact incidence of spontaneous abortion is difficult because many unrecognized losses occur in early pregnancy. The incidence of spontaneous abortion increases with parental age (Cunningham et al., 1997). The incidence is 12% for women less than 20 years old, rising to 26% for women over age 40. Paternal age under 20 years is associated with a spontaneous abortion rate of 12%, rising to 20% for fathers over 40. Most spontaneous abortions occur in the first 12 weeks of pregnancy, with the rate declining rapidly thereafter.

The most common cause of spontaneous abortion is severe congenital abnormalities that are often incompatible with life. Additional causes include maternal infections such as syphilis, listeriosis, toxoplasmosis, brucellosis, rubella, and cytomegalic inclusion disease. Maternal endocrine disorders such as hypothyroidism and abnormalities

of the reproductive organs have also been implicated. In addition, immune factors such as antiphospholipid antibodies are currently being investigated.

Spontaneous abortion is divided into six subgroups: threatened, inevitable, incomplete, complete, missed, and recurrent. Figure 26–1 illustrates threatened, inevitable, and incomplete abortion.

THREATENED ABORTION

Manifestations. The first sign of threatened abortion is vaginal bleeding. Up to 25% of all women experience "spotting," or light bleeding, in early pregnancy, and about half of these pregnancies will not survive (Cunningham et al., 1997).

Vaginal bleeding may be followed by rhythmic uterine cramping, persistent backache, or feelings of pelvic pressure. These symptoms increase the chance that the threatened abortion will progress to inevitable abortion.

Therapeutic Management. Bleeding in the first half of pregnancy must be considered a threatened abortion, and women should be advised to notify their physician or nurse-midwife if they note vaginal bleeding. The nurse obtains a detailed history that includes length of gestation or time of last menstrual period and the onset, duration, and amount of vaginal bleeding. Any accompanying discomfort, such as cramping, backache, or sharp abdominal pain, is also evaluated.

Ultrasound examination is often performed to determine whether the fetus is present and, if so, whether it is alive. Although bed rest may be recommended after each bleeding episode, many physicians now believe that there is no valid basis for advising bed rest (Enkin et al., 1995).

The woman is advised to curtail sexual activity until bleeding has ceased and for at least 2 weeks following the last evidence of bleeding. The woman is instructed to count the number of perineal pads used and to note the quantity and color of blood on the pads. She should also look for tissue passage.

The woman often wonders whether her actions may have contributed to the situation and is anxious about her own condition and that of the fetus. The nurse should offer accurate information and avoid false reassurance, because the woman may lose the fetus despite every precaution.

INEVITABLE ABORTION

Manifestations. Abortion is usually inevitable (that is, it cannot be stopped) when the membranes rupture and the cervix dilates. Excessive bleeding or infection can occur if the products of conception are not completely evacuated.

Therapeutic Management. Initial treatment of inevitable abortion involves allowing natural expulsion of the uterine contents. If tissue remains or if bleeding is excessive, the physician performs a dilation and vacuum curettage (D&C) while the woman is under anesthesia.

INCOMPLETE ABORTION

Manifestations. Incomplete abortion occurs when some but not all of the products of conception are expelled from the uterus. The major manifestations are uterine bleeding and severe abdominal cramping. The cervix is open, and there is passage of fetal and placental tissue.

Threatened abortion

Incomplete abortion

Inevitable abortion

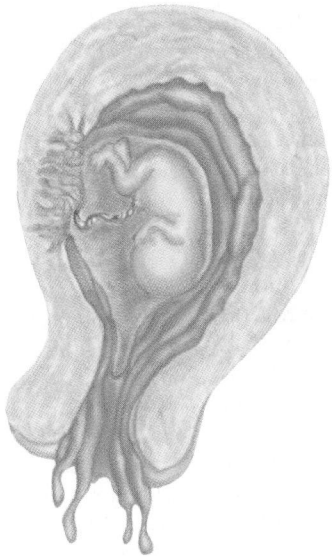
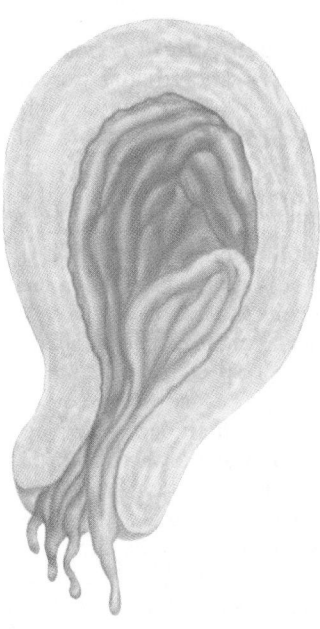

Vaginal bleeding occurs.

Some products of conception have been expelled, but some remain.

Membranes rupture, and cervix dilates.

FIGURE 26–1

Three types of spontaneous abortion.

Therapeutic Management. The retained tissue prevents the uterus from contracting firmly, thus allowing profuse bleeding from uterine blood vessels. Initial treatment should focus on the woman's cardiovascular stabilization. A blood specimen is drawn for crossmatching and blood typing, and an intravenous line is inserted for fluid replacement. When the woman's condition is stable, curettage is usually performed to remove the remaining tissue. This procedure may be followed by intravenous administration of oxytocin (Pitocin) or intramuscular administration of methylergonovine (Methergine) to contract the uterus and control bleeding.

Because of the danger of excessive bleeding, curettage may not be performed if the pregnancy has advanced beyond 14 weeks. In this case, oxytocin or prostaglandin is administered to stimulate uterine contractions until all products of conception (fetus, membranes, placenta, and amniotic fluid) are expelled.

COMPLETE ABORTION

Manifestations. Complete abortion occurs when all products of conception are expelled from the uterus. Uterine contractions and bleeding abate, and the cervix closes after all products of conception are passed.

Therapeutic Management. Once complete abortion is confirmed, no additional intervention is required unless excessive bleeding or infection develops. The woman should be advised to rest and watch for further bleeding, pain, or fever. She should abstain from intercourse until after a follow-up visit with her health care provider. Contraception will be discussed at this visit if she wishes to avoid pregnancy.

MISSED ABORTION

Manifestations. Missed abortion occurs when the fetus dies during the first half of pregnancy but is retained in the uterus. When the fetus dies, the early symptoms of pregnancy (nausea, breast tenderness, urinary frequency) disappear. The uterus stops growing and often decreases in size, reflecting the absorption of amniotic fluid and maceration of the fetus.

Therapeutic Management. In most cases, the pregnancy ends spontaneously after fetal death (Cunningham et al., 1997). If the fetus is not expelled, fetal death is confirmed by ultrasound examination. In addition, serial pregnancy tests should indicate a decline in placental hormone production. When fetal death is confirmed, the uterus may be evacuated by D&C. Prostaglandin compounds may be necessary to induce contractions and empty the uterus if the cervix does not dilate easily.

Two major complications of missed abortion are infection and disseminated intravascular coagulation (DIC). If there are signs of uterine infection, such as an elevated temperature, vaginal discharge with a foul odor, or abdominal pain, evacuation of the uterus is delayed until antibiotic therapy is initiated.

Disseminated Intravascular Coagulation. DIC is a defect in coagulation that may occur if the fetus is retained for a prolonged period. Coagulation defects do not usually occur unless fetal death occurs after the first trimester. DIC is also associated with abruptio placentae and with pregnancy-induced hypertension.

With DIC, anticoagulation and procoagulation factors are activated simultaneously. DIC develops when the clotting factor thromboplastin is released into the maternal bloodstream as a result of placental bleeding and consequent clot formation. The circulating thromboplastin activates widespread clotting in small vessels throughout the body. This process consumes, or "uses up," other clotting factors such as fibrinogen and platelets. The condition is further complicated by activation of the fibrinolytic system to lyse, or destroy, clots. The result is a simultaneous decrease in clotting factors and increase in circulating anticoagulants, which leaves the circulating blood unable to clot. This situation allows bleeding to occur from any area, such as intravenous sites, incisions, or the gums or nose, as well as from expected sites such as the site of placental attachment during the postpartum period.

In DIC, fibrinogen and platelets are usually decreased, prothrombin and partial thromboplastin times may be prolonged, and fibrin degradation products, the most sensitive measurement, are increased.

The priority in treating DIC is delivery of the fetus and placenta to stop the production of thromboplastin, which is fueling the process. In addition, blood replacement products, such as whole blood, packed red blood cells, and cryoprecipitate, are administered to maintain the circulating volume and to transport oxygen to body cells.

RECURRENT SPONTANEOUS ABORTION

Manifestations. Recurrent spontaneous abortion is sometimes referred to as "habitual" abortion; the current definition is three or more consecutive spontaneous abortions. The primary causes of recurrent abortion are believed to be genetic or chromosomal abnormalities and anomalies of the woman's reproductive tract, such as bicornuate uterus or incompetent cervix.

Additional causes include an inadequate luteal phase with insufficient secretion of progesterone and immunologic factors that involve increased sharing of human leukocyte antigens by the sperm and ovum of the man and woman who conceived. The theory is that, because of this sharing, the woman's immunologic system is not stimulated to produce blocking antibodies that protect the embryo from maternal immune cells or other damaging antibodies. Systemic diseases such as lupus erythematosus and diabetes mellitus have been implicated in recurrent abortions. Reproductive infections and some sexually transmissible diseases are also associated with recurrent abortions.

Therapeutic Management. The first step in managing recurrent spontaneous abortion is a thorough examination of the woman's reproductive organs to determine whether anatomic defects are the cause. If her reproductive organs are normal, the woman is usually referred for genetic screening to identify genetic factors that would increase the possibility of recurrent abortions. Additional therapeutic

management of recurrent pregnancy loss depends on the cause. For example, antibiotics are prescribed for the woman with infection.

Recurrent spontaneous abortion may be due to cervical incompetence, an anatomic defect that results in painless dilation of the cervix in the second trimester. In this instance, the cervix may be sutured to keep it from opening (i.e., cerclage). Sutures may be removed near term if vaginal delivery is expected, or they may be left in place if a cesarean birth is planned. Prophylactic antibiotics may be necessary if the woman is judged to be at high risk for infection.

NURSING CONSIDERATIONS

Abortion may be accompanied by various amounts of bleeding. Prevention or identification of hypovolemic shock is the nursing priority when a woman is bleeding heavily. The nurse should observe for tachycardia (often the earliest sign), a falling blood pressure, pale skin and mucous membranes, confusion, restlessness, and cool, clammy skin. The nurse manages fluid and blood replacement as ordered.

Vaginal bleeding of any amount during pregnancy is frightening, and waiting and watching are difficult, although often the only reasonable treatment. Moreover, many families feel an acute sense of loss and grief with spontaneous abortion. Grief often includes feelings of guilt, which may be expressed as wondering if the woman could have done something to prevent the loss. Nurses can help by emphasizing that spontaneous abortions usually occur because of factors or abnormalities that could not be avoided.

Anger, disappointment, and sadness are commonly experienced emotions, although the intensity of the feelings may vary. For many couples the fetus has not yet taken on specific physical characteristics, but they grieve for their fantasies of the lost child. The couple may want to express their sadness but may feel that family, friends, and often health personnel are uncomfortable or unable to provide emotional support after early pregnancy loss.

To recognize the meaning of the loss to each family, nurses must listen carefully to what the couple says and observe how the partners behave. Nurses must attempt to convey unconditional acceptance of the feelings expressed or demonstrated. The couple should be permitted to remain together as much as possible. Providing information and simple, brief explanations of what has occurred and what will be done facilitates the family's ability to grieve.

It is helpful for the family to realize that grief may last from 6 months to a year, or even longer. Family support, knowledge of the grief process, spiritual counselors, and the support of other bereaved couples may provide needed assistance during this time.

Ectopic Pregnancy

Ectopic pregnancy refers to implantation of a fertilized ovum in an area outside the uterine cavity. Ninety percent of ectopic pregnancies are in the ampulla of the fallopian tube. Figure 26–2 shows common sites of tubal implantation.

Ectopic pregnancy has been called "a disaster of reproduction" for two reasons:

- It remains a leading cause of maternal death from hemorrhage.

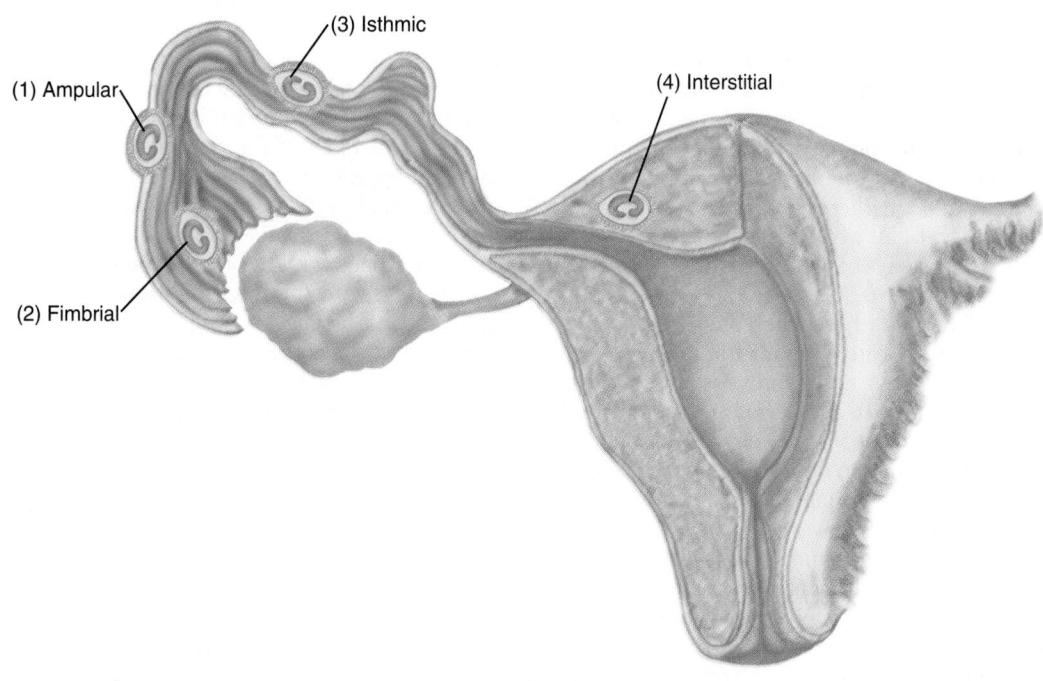

FIGURE 26-2

Sites of ectopic pregnancy. Numbers indicate the order of prevalence.

• It sharply reduces the woman's chance of subsequent pregnancies because of damage to or destruction of a fallopian tube.

INCIDENCE AND ETIOLOGY

The incidence of ectopic pregnancy has increased dramatically throughout the world in the past 20 years. In the United States, the rate has more than quadrupled, to 14 in every 1,000 reported pregnancies. The highest rate is seen in nonwhite women older than 35 (Cunningham et al., 1997). The rapid increase in incidence is attributed to the growing number of women of childbearing age who experience scarring of the fallopian tubes due to pelvic infection, inflammation, or surgery. Pelvic infection is often due to *Chlamydia* or *Neisseria gonorrhoeae*.

Anything that slows the transport of the fertilized ovum through the tube or causes it to implant too early increases the risk that implantation will occur in the tube rather than the uterus.

MANIFESTATIONS

Early signs and symptoms of ectopic pregnancy are the following:

• Missed menstrual period
• Abdominal and pelvic pain
• Vaginal "spotting" or light bleeding

More subtle signs and symptoms depend on the site of implantation. If implantation occurs in the distal end of the fallopian tube, which can accommodate the growing embryo longer, the woman may at first exhibit the usual early signs of pregnancy. Several weeks into the pregnancy, intermittent abdominal pain and small amounts of vaginal bleeding occur. These manifestations initially can be mistaken for those of threatened abortion.

If implantation has occurred in the proximal end of the fallopian tube, rupture of the tube may occur within 2 to 3 weeks of the missed period. Symptoms include sudden, severe pain in one of the lower quadrants of the abdomen as the tube tears open and the embryo is expelled into the pelvic cavity. Pain is often accompanied by profuse hemorrhage. Irritation of the diaphragm, manifested by shoulder or neck pain that is worse on inspiration, occurs in about half of women (Cunningham et al., 1997). Signs of hypovolemic shock (rapid pulse, lightheadedness, syncope, falling blood pressure) may develop without external bleeding.

Risk Factors for Ectopic Pregnancy

• History of sexually transmissible diseases (gonorrhea, chlamydial infection)
• History of pelvic inflammatory disease
• History of previous ectopic pregnancies
• Failed tubal ligation
• Intrauterine device
• Multiple induced abortions
• Maternal age older than 35 years

DIAGNOSTIC EVALUATION

Ectopic pregnancy can usually be diagnosed before rupture occurs. Transvaginal ultrasound can confirm or rule out an intrauterine pregnancy. When used in combination with serum hormone levels of progesterone and the beta-subunit of human chorionic gonadotropin (β-hCG), the physician can make a judgment about whether the pregnancy is intrauterine or ectopic and whether the conceptus is living.

Progesterone levels fall when pregnancy fails, whether it is an intrauterine or an ectopic pregnancy. Women on ovulation induction agents, however, are an exception (Minnick-Smith & Cook, 1997). Their progesterone levels may remain high despite ectopic implantation.

β-hCG normally rises during early gestation to cause the corpus luteum to persist and secrete progesterone. β-hCG then decreases at about 50 to 70 days' gestation as the placenta takes over production of progesterone to maintain the pregnancy. Lower than normal levels of β-hCG suggest an abnormal pregnancy.

The use of sensitive pregnancy tests and high-resolution ultrasound has largely eliminated invasive tests for ectopic pregnancy. Aspiration of blood from the cul-de-sac in a culdocentesis suggests bleeding into the peritoneal cavity from rupture of a fallopian tube. Laparoscopy (examination of the peritoneal cavity by means of a laparoscope) may reveal a characteristic bluish swelling within the tube.

THERAPEUTIC MANAGEMENT

The management of tubal pregnancy depends on whether the tube is intact or ruptured. Medical management may be possible if the tube is unruptured, the pregnancy is early, the pregnancy mass is 3.5 cm or smaller, and cardiac activity is absent (Cunningham et al., 1997; Minnick-Smith & Cook, 1997). The chemotherapeutic agent methotrexate (a folic acid antagonist that interferes with cell reproduction) inhibits cell division in the embryo. The primary impetus for medical management is preserving the tube and improving the chance of future fertility.

Surgical management of a tubal pregnancy that is unruptured may involve a *linear salpingostomy* to salvage the tube for future pregnancies. The tube is opened with a linear incision, the products of conception are removed, and to reduce scarring, the tubal incision is left to heal without suturing. Linear salpingostomy may also be attempted if the tube is ruptured but damage to the tube is minimal.

When ectopic pregnancy results in rupture of the fallopian tube, the goal of therapeutic management is to control the bleeding and prevent hypovolemic shock. When the woman's cardiovascular status is stable, a salpingectomy is performed to remove the affected tube and ligate bleeding vessels. Future pregnancies can still occur when only one tube is present, although the likelihood of fertility decreases. In addition, the same conditions that caused the ectopic pregnancy in the tube that was removed may exist in the other tube.

NURSING CONSIDERATIONS

Nursing care focuses on preventing or identifying hypovolemic shock, controlling pain, and providing psychological support for the woman who experiences an ectopic pregnancy. If methotrexate is used, the nurse must explain adverse side effects, such as nausea and vomiting, and the im-portance of communicating any physical changes to the health care team. The woman must be instructed to refrain from drinking alcohol or ingesting vitamins that contain folic acid, which would decrease the drug's effectiveness. She should not have sexual intercourse until β-hCG levels are not detectable. If the treatment is successful, this hormone disappears from plasma within 2 to 4 weeks (Cunningham et al., 1997). Moreover, the importance of keeping follow-up appointments should be emphasized.

The woman and her family often need emotional support to resolve emotions, which may include anger, grief, guilt, and self-blame. The woman may also be anxious about her ability to become pregnant in the future. Nurses may need to clarify the physician's explanation and to use therapeutic communication techniques that assist the woman to deal with her anxiety.

Gestational Trophoblastic Disease (Hydatidiform Mole)

Hydatidiform mole is a form of gestational trophoblastic disease that occurs when the trophoblasts (peripheral cells that attach the fertilized ovum to the uterine wall) develop abnormally. As a result of the abnormal growth, the placenta, but not the fetus, develops. The condition is characterized by proliferation and edema of the chorionic villi. The fluid-filled villi form grape-like clusters that may grow large enough to fill the uterus to the size of an advanced pregnancy (Fig. 26–3). The mole may be *complete*, with no fetus

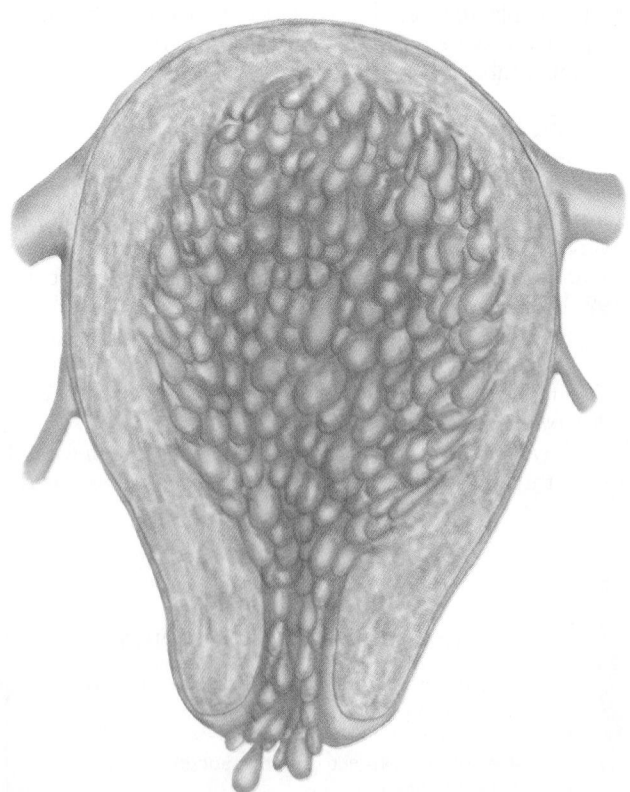

FIGURE 26–3
• • • • • • • • •
Hydatidiform mole.

present, or *partial*, in which fetal tissue or membranes are present. Malignant change of the trophoblastic tissue (choriocarcinoma) is one complication of hydatidiform mole.

INCIDENCE AND ETIOLOGY

In the United States and Europe, the incidence of hydatidiform mole is 1 in every 1,000 pregnancies (Cunningham et al., 1997). Hydatidiform mole is more likely to occur in very young or older mothers. Women who have had one molar pregnancy are at increased risk to have another.

A *complete mole* is believed to occur when the ovum is fertilized by a sperm that duplicates its own chromosomes while the chromosomes of the ovum are inactivated. In a *partial mole*, the maternal contribution is usually present but the paternal contribution is double, and thus the karyotype is triploid (69,XXY or 69,XYY).

MANIFESTATIONS

The signs and symptoms of a complete molar pregnancy include the following:

- Elevated levels of β-hCG
- Vaginal bleeding, which varies from dark brown spotting to profuse hemorrhage
- A uterus larger than expected for the duration of the pregnancy
- No fetal heart activity detected even with sensitive instruments
- Excessive nausea and vomiting, which may be related to excessive β-hCG from the proliferating trophoblasts
- Unusually early development of pregnancy-induced hypertension, which is rarely diagnosed before 24 weeks

DIAGNOSTIC EVALUATION

Ultrasound examination allows a differential diagnosis to be made between two types of molar pregnancies. A complete mole shows multiple small cystic structures but no fetus.

THERAPEUTIC MANAGEMENT

Medical management includes two phases: (1) immediate evacuation of the mole and (2) follow-up to detect any malignant changes in the remaining trophoblastic tissue. Before evacuation, chest radiography, computed tomography, or magnetic resonance imaging may be performed to detect metastatic disease. A complete blood count, laboratory assessment of clotting factors, and blood typing and crossmatching are done in case a transfusion is needed.

Most often, vacuum aspiration is used to extract the mole. After tissue has been removed, intravenous oxytocin is used to contract the uterus. It is important to avoid uterine stimulation with oxytocin before evacuation. Uterine contractions can cause trophoblastic tissue to be drawn into the venous circulation, resulting in pulmonary embolism. Curettage with a sharp curet follows the evacuation to remove all molar tissue, and the tissue obtained is sent for laboratory evaluation to identify malignant changes.

Follow-up is critical to detect choriocarcinoma. The follow-up protocol involves evaluation of serum β-hCG levels every 1 to 2 weeks until normal prepregnancy levels are attained. The test is repeated every 1 to 2 months for a year.

Pregnancy must be avoided during the first year of follow-up because it would obscure the evidence of choriocarcinoma. Oral contraceptives are safe to use, but intrauterine devices may cause irregular bleeding and should not be used.

NURSING CONSIDERATIONS

Women who have had a hydatidiform mole experience many of the same emotions as those who have had any other type of pregnancy loss. In addition, they may be anxious about the possibility of malignancy and the need to delay pregnancy for at least a year.

NURSING CARE
The Woman with a Hemorrhagic Condition of Early Pregnancy

Nurses play a vital role in the management of early pregnancy bleeding, regardless of its cause. Nurses monitor the condition of the pregnant woman and collaborate with the physician to provide treatment.

Assessment

Confirmation of pregnancy and length of gestation is an important initial step. Physical assessment priorities are to determine the amount and character of bleeding and the description, location, and severity of pain. Estimate the amount of vaginal bleeding by examining linen and peripads. If necessary, make a more accurate estimation by weighing the linen and peripads (1 g weight equals 1 ml volume). When asking a woman how much blood she lost at home, ask her to compare the amount lost with a common measure, such as a tablespoon or a cup. Ask how long the bleeding episode lasted and what she has done to control the bleeding.

Bleeding may be accompanied by pain. Uterine cramping usually accompanies spontaneous abortion; deep, severe pelvic pain is associated with ectopic pregnancy. Remember that in ruptured ectopic pregnancy, bleeding may be concealed within the abdomen, and pain is the only symptom.

Assess the woman's vital signs to determine her cardiovascular status. Check laboratory values for hemoglobin and hematocrit and report abnormal values to the physician. Determine the Rh factor so that all women who are Rh-negative can receive $Rh_o(D)$ immune globulin (see p. 658).

Moreover, because abortion may be associated with infections, assess the woman for fever, malaise, and prolonged or malodorous vaginal discharge.

Determine the family's knowledge of needed follow-up care and how to prevent complications such as infection.

Nursing Diagnosis and Planning

Risk for Hypovolemic Shock and Infection are a collaborative problem and nursing diagnosis that can be considered in the woman who has a hemorrhagic complication of early pregnancy. The more complete nursing diagnosis, however, is

- Knowledge Deficit of diagnostic and therapeutic procedures, signs and symptoms of infection, dietary measures to prevent infection, and recommended follow-up care. *Expected Outcomes:* The woman will verbalize understanding of diagnostic and therapeutic procedures, measures to reduce the risk for infection, and signs of infection that should be reported to the health care provider. The woman will develop a plan for obtaining follow-up care.

Interventions

Providing Information About Tests and Procedures

Women and their families experience less anxiety if they understand what is happening. Explain necessary diagnostic procedures, such as transvaginal or abdominal ultrasonography. Include the purpose of the tests, their duration, and whether the procedures cause discomfort. If surgical intervention is necessary, reinforce the explanations of the physicians who will perform the surgery and administer anesthesia. Briefly describe the reasons for blood tests, such as those for determining hCG, hemoglobin, or hematocrit values. Explain that diagnostic and therapeutic measures are performed quickly at times to prevent excessive bleeding.

Teaching Measures to Prevent Infection

The risk for infection is greatest during the first 72 hours following spontaneous abortion or operative procedures, but most women are discharged within a few hours of uterine evacuation. To prevent infection, perineal pads should be used instead of tampons until bleeding has stopped. Teach the woman to wash her hands before and after changing perineal pads. She should consult with the health care provider before resuming sexual intercourse.

Providing Dietary Information

Nutrition and adequate fluid intake help maintain the body's defense against infection and correct anemia. The woman needs foods high in iron to increase hemoglobin and hematocrit values. These foods include liver, red meat, spinach, egg yolks, carrots, and raisins. In addition, she needs foods high in vitamin C, which may increase the utilization of iron (Mahan & Escott-Stump, 1996). These foods include citrus fruits, broccoli, strawberries, cantaloupe, cabbage, and green peppers.

Iron supplements may be prescribed. Gastric upset is less severe when iron is taken with meals, and a diet that is high in fiber and fluid (2,500 ml/day) helps reduce the constipation experienced by many women who take iron supplements.

Teaching Signs of Infection to Report

Ensure that the woman knows how to use a thermometer, and instruct her to take her temperature every 8 hours for the first 3 days at home. Tell her to seek medical help if her temperature goes above 37.8°C (100°F). She should also report to the health care provider additional signs of infection, such as vaginal discharge with foul odor, pelvic tenderness, or general malaise.

Recommending Follow-up Care

A variety of follow-up procedures such as repeat ultrasonic examinations or repeated determinations of serum β-hCG levels may be necessary. The couple that experiences recurrent abortions may become involved in complex investigations of immunologic or genetic abnormalities.

The nurse should help couples that experience a pregnancy loss by answering questions about the cause of the pregnancy loss and the chances of later reproductive success. Acknowledge the couple's grief, which often manifests as anger. Many women have guilt feelings that must be recognized. They often need repeated reassurance that the loss was not due to anything they did or to anything they neglected.

Evaluation

- Did the woman verbalize comprehension of diagnostic and therapeutic procedures, hygienic and dietary measures that reduce the risk of infection, and signs of infection that should be reported?
- Did the woman develop and comply with a follow-up plan of care?

Hemorrhagic Conditions of Late Pregnancy

After 20 weeks of pregnancy, the two major causes of hemorrhage are disorders of the placenta called placenta previa and abruptio placentae. Abruptio placentae may be further complicated by DIC.

Placenta Previa

Placenta previa is implantation of the placenta in the lower uterine segment. Three classifications of placenta previa (total, partial, and marginal) are typically recognized. They depend on how much of the cervical os is covered by the placenta (Fig. 26–4). Improved precision of ultrasound diagnostics, however, may eventually render these three classifications obsolete. Current ultrasonography usually allows precise measurement of the distance between the lowest edge of the placenta and the internal cervical os (Clark, 1999).

Marginal or low-lying placentas (implanted in the lower uterine segment but not extending to the cervical os) that are found on early ultrasound examinations frequently appear to move upward and away from the internal cervical os as the uterus grows to accommodate the pregnancy. Follow-up ultrasonography is performed to determine placental location in relation to the cervical os during the last weeks of pregnancy.

INCIDENCE AND ETIOLOGY

Placenta previa occurs in about 1 in 200 pregnancies in the United States. It is more common in older women, multiparas, women who have had cesarean births, and women who have had prior suction curettage for induced or spontaneous abortion. It is also more likely to recur if a woman had a previous placenta previa. Women of Asian or African ethnicity have an increased risk. Smoking and cocaine use are also associated with placenta previa (Clark, 1999).

MANIFESTATIONS

The classic sign of placenta previa is the sudden onset of painless uterine bleeding in the latter half of pregnancy.

Marginal

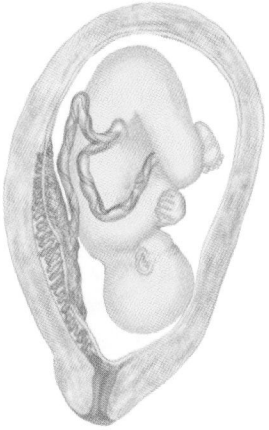

Placenta barely extends to cervical os.

Partial

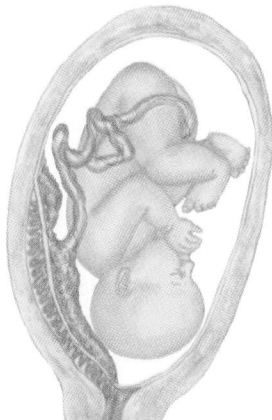

Placenta partially covers cervical os.

Total

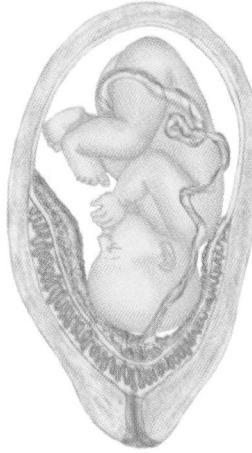

Placenta completely covers cervical os.

FIGURE 26–4

The three classifications of placenta previa.

Many cases of placenta previa, however, are diagnosed by ultrasound examination before the onset of bleeding. Bleeding occurs when the placental villi are torn from the uterine wall, resulting in hemorrhage from the uterine vessels. Bleeding is typically painless because it does not occur in a closed cavity and therefore does not cause pressure on adjacent tissue. Bleeding may be scanty or profuse, and it may cease spontaneously, only to recur later.

Bleeding may not occur until labor starts, when cervical changes disrupt placental attachment. The admitting nurse may be unsure whether the bleeding represents heavy "bloody show" or is a sign of a placenta previa. The laboring woman may have pain associated with the bleeding because of active labor contractions.

Digital examination of the cervical os when placenta previa is present can cause additional placental separation or can tear the placenta itself, causing severe maternal and fetal bleeding. *Until the location and position of the placenta are verified by ultrasonography, no manual examinations should be performed, and administration of oxytocin should be postponed to prevent strong contractions that could result in sudden placental separation and hemorrhage.*

THERAPEUTIC MANAGEMENT

When the diagnosis of placenta previa is confirmed, medical interventions are based on the condition of the mother and fetus. The woman is evaluated carefully to determine the amount of hemorrhage, and electronic fetal monitoring is initiated to determine the condition of the fetus. A third consideration is the fetal gestational age.

Options for management include conservative management if the mother's cardiovascular status is stable and the fetus is immature and without signs of distress. Conservative management may take place in the home or in the hospital.

Home Care. Criteria for outpatient management include the following:

- The client is clinically stable, with no evidence of active bleeding.
- The client can remain on bed rest at home.
- Home is within a reasonable distance from the hospital.
- Emergency transportation is available 24 hours a day (Clark, 1999).

Nurses should help the family develop a plan of care that includes strict bed rest, the presence of a responsible adult at all times, and ready transportation to the hospital. Nurses must teach the mother and the family what to monitor and emphasize the importance of (1) assessing vaginal discharge or bleeding after each urination or bowel movement, or more often as needed, (2) counting fetal movements daily, (3) assessing uterine activity daily, and (4) omitting sexual intercourse to prevent disruption of the placenta. Nurses often make daily phone contact for assessments of uterine activity (cramping, regular or sporadic contractions), bleeding, fetal activity, and adherence to the prescribed treatment plan. In addition, nurses make regular home visits for comprehensive maternal-fetal assessments, including nonstress tests. The family is instructed to report decreased fetal movements, uterine contractions, or vaginal bleeding at once.

Nurses should also provide specific, accurate information about the condition of the fetus. For example, parents are reassured when they hear that the fetal heart rate is within the expected range and daily "kick counts" are reassuring of fetal well-being. Moreover, it may be necessary for nurses to help the family understand the physician's plan of care, such as a cesarean delivery.

Inpatient Care. Hospitalization will be needed if the woman does not meet the criteria for home care. Nursing assessments in the hospital are similar to those done at home and are focused on determining the presence and character of bleeding and looking for signs of preterm labor. Periodic electronic fetal monitoring identifies changes in fetal heart activity that suggest fetal compromise. A significant change in fetal heart activity, an episode of vaginal bleeding, or signs of preterm labor should be reported immediately to the physician.

At times conservative management is not an option. For instance, delivery by cesarean birth is scheduled if the fetus is older than 36 weeks' gestation and the lungs are mature. Immediate delivery of an immature fetus may be necessary if bleeding is excessive, the woman's cardiovascular status is unstable, or there are signs of fetal compromise.

Nurses prepare the woman for surgery whenever cesarean birth becomes necessary. Preparation includes inserting an indwelling urinary catheter, confirming that appropriate preoperative permission forms are signed, validating that blood typing and crossmatching have been done, and starting intravenous fluids as directed by the physician. The preoperative procedures are often performed quickly, and the family and mother are often anxious.

Abruptio Placentae

Separation of a normally implanted placenta before the fetus is born (called abruptio placentae, placental abruption, or premature separation of the placenta) occurs when there is bleeding and formation of a hematoma on the maternal side of the placenta. As the clot expands, further separation occurs. The severity of the complication depends on the amount of bleeding and the size of the hematoma. The hematoma can expand and thus obliterate intervillous spaces where fetal gas and nutrient exchange occurs. Moreover, fetal vessels will be disrupted as placental separation occurs, and there is fetal as well as maternal bleeding.

The major danger for the woman is hemorrhage and consequent hypovolemic shock and clotting abnormalities. The major dangers for the fetus are related to anoxia, blood loss, and preterm birth.

INCIDENCE AND ETIOLOGY

The published incidence of abruptio placentae varies widely but probably averages about 1 in 200 deliveries. Placental abruption extensive enough to cause the death of the fetus has declined to about 1 in 830 deliveries (Cunningham et al., 1997).

The cause of abruptio placentae is unknown, but several factors that increase the risk have been identified. The risk factors include maternal hypertension, maternal cigarette smoking, multigravida status, short umbilical cord, abdominal trauma, and a history of a previous premature separation of the placenta. Maternal use of cocaine, which causes vasoconstriction in the endometrial arteries, is a leading cause of abruptio placentae.

MANIFESTATIONS

The four classic signs and symptoms of abruptio placentae are the following:

- Vaginal bleeding
- Abdominal pain
- Uterine hyperactivity with poor relaxation between contractions
- Uterine tenderness

Additional signs include back pain, nonreassuring fetal heart rate patterns, signs of hypovolemic shock, and fetal death.

Hemorrhage from abruptio placentae may be concealed or apparent. In either type, the placental abruption may be complete or partial. Concealed hemorrhage is bleeding that occurs behind the placenta while the margins remain intact.

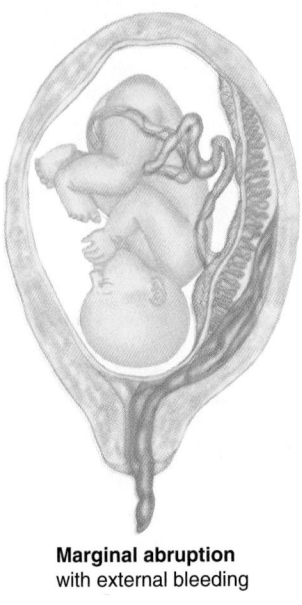

Marginal abruption
with external bleeding

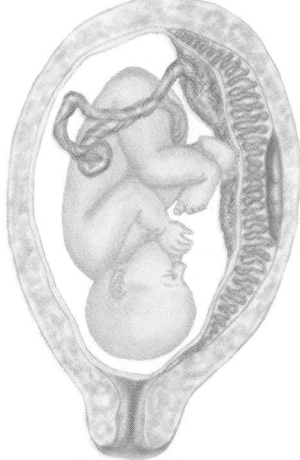

Partial abruption
with concealed bleeding

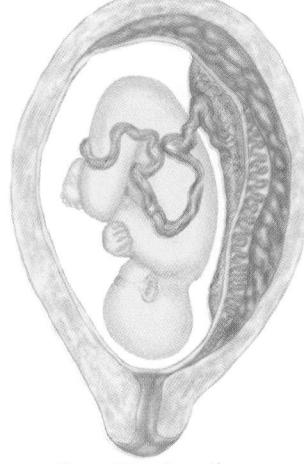

Complete abruption
with concealed bleeding

FIGURE 26–5

Types of abruptio placentae.

The hemorrhage is apparent when bleeding separates or dissects the membranes from the endometrium and blood flows out through the vagina. Figure 26–5 illustrates variations of abruptio placentae with external and concealed bleeding. The actual amount of blood lost may be greater than the visible bleeding. Signs of maternal hypovolemia may be present when there is little or no external bleeding.

Abdominal pain is also related to the type of separation. It may be sudden and severe when there is bleeding into the myometrium (uterine muscle) or intermittent and difficult to distinguish from labor contractions. The abdomen may become exceedingly firm (board-like) and tender, making palpation of the fetus difficult. Ultrasound examination is helpful to rule out placenta previa as the cause of bleeding, but it cannot be used to diagnose abruptio placentae because the separation and bleeding may not be obvious on ultrasonography.

THERAPEUTIC MANAGEMENT

Any woman who exhibits signs of abruptio placentae should be hospitalized and evaluated at once. Evaluation focuses on the condition of the fetus and the cardiovascular status of the expectant mother. If the abruption is mild and the fetus is immature and shows no signs of distress, conservative management may be initiated. Measures include bed rest and may include administration of tocolytic medications to decrease uterine activity (Clark, 1999).

If there are signs of fetal compromise or if the expectant mother exhibits signs of excessive bleeding, either obvious or concealed, immediate delivery of the fetus is necessary. Intensive monitoring of both the woman and the fetus is essential because rapid deterioration of either can occur. Blood products for replacement should be available, and two large-bore intravenous lines should be secured for replacement of fluid and blood.

NURSING CONSIDERATIONS

If immediate cesarean delivery is necessary, the woman may feel powerless as the health care team hurriedly prepares her for surgery. If at all possible, nurses should explain anticipated procedures to the woman and her family to reduce their feelings of fear and anxiety.

Excessive bleeding and fetal hypoxia are always major concerns with abruptio placentae, and nurses are responsible for continuous monitoring of both the expectant mother and the fetus so that problems can be detected early, before the condition of the woman or the fetus deteriorates.

NURSING CARE

The Woman with a Hemorrhagic Condition of Late Pregnancy

Assessment

For hemorrhagic conditions of late pregnancy, some nursing assessments should be performed immediately, and others

---

CRITICAL TO REMEMBER

Signs of Concealed Hemorrhage in Abruptio Placentae

- Increase in fundal height
- Hard, board-like abdomen
- High uterine baseline tone on electronic monitoring strip
- Persistent abdominal pain
- Systemic signs of early hemorrhage (tachycardia [maternal and fetal], falling blood pressure, restlessness)
- Persistent late deceleration in fetal heart rate or decreasing baseline variability
- Vaginal bleeding that may be slight or absent

CRITICAL THINKING EXERCISE 26-1

All women who have experienced prenatal bleeding and invasive procedures are at increased risk for infection.

What common assumptions do nurses make about those who are at risk for developing infections?

---

can be deferred until initial measures have been taken to stabilize the woman's cardiovascular status. The priority nursing assessments are the following:

- *Amount and nature of bleeding:* Time of onset, estimated blood loss before admission to hospital, and description of tissue or clots passed. Peripads and linen savers should be saved so that blood loss can be estimated accurately.
- *Pain:* Type (constant, intermittent, sharp, dull, severe), onset (sudden, gradual), and location (generalized over abdomen, localized). Is the uterus tender on gentle palpation?
- *Maternal vital signs:* To identify hypertension or hypotension and tachycardia that occur with hypovolemia. A normal blood pressure can be misleading in a woman with abruptio placentae because she may have been hypertensive before the blood loss made her blood pressure fall to normal or hypotensive levels.
- *Condition of the fetus:* Application of an electronic monitor to identify fetal heart rate, baseline variability, and fetal response to uterine activity (late decelerations or loss of baseline variability are of particular concern).
- *Uterine contractions:* Application of a monitor to determine uterine resting tone and the frequency and duration of contractions. A uterus that does not relax between contractions and frequent, long contractions are associated with abruptio placentae.
- *Obstetric history:* Gravida, para, previous abortions, preterm infants, previous pregnancy outcomes.
- *Length of gestation:* Date of last menstrual period, fundal height, correlation of fundal height with estimated gestation, results of ultrasound examinations performed during pregnancy. With bleeding into the myometrium, the fundus enlarges rapidly as bleeding progresses. A piece of tape can be used to mark the top of the fundus at a given time and then to observe and report increasing fundal size, which indicates that bleeding into uterine muscles is occurring.
- *Laboratory data:* Hemoglobin, hematocrit, clotting factors, blood type, partial thromboplastin time, and clotting time. Laboratory data are obtained to prepare for transfusions, should they become necessary, and to determine whether signs of DIC are developing.

Despite the emphasis on physical assessment, the emotional response of the expectant mother and her partner must also be addressed (see Nursing Care Plan 26-1). They will most likely be anxious, fearful, confused, and overwhelmed by the activity. They may have very little knowledge of expected medical management and may not realize that the fetus must be delivered as quickly as possible and that a surgical procedure is necessary. Moreover, they may fear for the life of the woman and the fetus.

NURSING CARE PLAN 26-1
· · · · · · · · · · ·
Antepartum Bleeding

Assessment	Beth Dixon, a 28-year-old gravida 2, para 1, is admitted at 34 weeks' gestation following an episode of vaginal bleeding due to total placenta previa. Vital signs are stable, and the fetal heart rate is 140 beats per minute with no nonreassuring signs. Beth and her husband, Bob, appear anxious about the condition of the fetus and the plan of care. Beth is particularly worried about her 5-year-old son, who is at home with a neighbor.
Nursing Diagnosis	Anxiety related to unknown effects of bleeding and lack of knowledge of predicted course of management.
Goals/Expected Outcomes	• The couple will verbalize expected routines and projected management by the end of the first day following admission. • The couple will express less anxiety following teaching.

Intervention	**Rationale**
1. Remain with the couple and acknowledge the emotions that they exhibit: "I know this is unexpected, and you must have many questions. Perhaps I can answer some of them."	1. The nurse's presence and empathic understanding prepare the family to cope with the unexpected situation.
2. Determine the couple's level of understanding of the situation and the projected management: "Tell me what you've been told to expect."	2. Assessing understanding allows the nurse to reinforce the physician's explanations and to notify the physician if additional explanations are necessary.
3. Provide the couple with factual information about projected management. Examples of teaching may include these topics:	3. Client education has proved effective in preventing and reducing anxiety.
a. Hospitalization, which may be necessary so that Beth's condition and the condition of the fetus can be watched closely.	
b. The possible necessity for a cesarean birth this time even though Beth delivered vaginally before.	
c. Information about hospital routines (meals, visiting hours) and monitoring techniques that will be used (electronic fetal monitoring, nonstress tests).	
4. Allow Beth and her family to participate in the routine as much as possible. Family involvement may mean scheduling procedures around times when Tom and their son can visit.	4. Reduces the sense of powerlessness that women often feel when they are confined to bed and a course of treatment is prescribed without consultation.

Evaluation	The interventions are judged to be successful if the couple demonstrates knowledge of the projected management and the reasons it is necessary and reduced anxiety.
Assessment	Although Beth has no more episodes of vaginal bleeding, she cries frequently. She tells the nurse, "I miss my son so much. He just started kindergarten, and he is so shy. I feel useless, and he really needs me now. It's hard on Bob too; he has to do everything."
Nursing Diagnosis	Situational Low Self-Esteem related to temporary inability to provide care for family.
Goals/Expected Outcomes	Beth will • Identify positive aspects of self during hospitalization. • Identify ways of providing comfort and affection for her son during the hospital stay.

NURSING CARE PLAN 26-1 *Continued*

Antepartum Bleeding

Intervention	Rationale
1. Encourage Beth to express her concerns about the need for hospitalization: "What bothers you most about being away from home?"	1. Major concerns may not be identified or may be misunderstood unless the woman clarifies them.
2. After acknowledging Beth's feelings, encourage examination of the need for hospitalization and its consequences: it provides time for the fetus to mature.	2. Careful consideration identifies positive aspects of Beth's important role in maturing her fetus.
3. Explore reality of Beth's self-appraisal ("I feel useless") by assisting her to investigate ways to provide nurturing care for her son while she is hospitalized: a. Keep in close touch by telephone (wake-up, goodnight, and after-school calls). b. Make small handmade items such as bookmarks. c. Explain to him in simple, nonfrightening terms why she must stay in the hospital. d. Offer reassurances of continued love.	3. Daily involvement in the life of the older child helps reduce feelings of isolation and inability to meet needs of her family.
4. Assist Beth to involve her son in plans for the newborn. He might benefit from sibling classes or play time with his mother that involves caring for dolls.	4. Involving siblings provides goals for combined family interaction that increase feeling of self-worth.

Evaluation   Beth is able to make positive comments about the importance of bed rest to the health of the fetus, and she initiates numerous activities that permit her to continue close, comforting contact with her child during the period of hospitalization.

Additional Nursing Diagnoses to Consider

Risk for Altered Family Processes
Diversional Activity Deficit
Fear

Nursing Diagnosis and Planning

The most dangerous potential complication is *hypovolemic shock*, which jeopardizes the life of the mother as well as the fetus. The nurse cannot independently manage the collaborative problem of hypovolemic shock but must confer with physicians for medical orders for treatment. Planning should therefore reflect the nurse's responsibility to do the following:

- Monitor for signs of hypovolemic shock.
- Consult the physician if signs of hypovolemic shock are observed.
- Perform actions to minimize the effects of hypovolemic shock.

Interventions

Monitoring for Signs of Hypovolemic Shock

Observe for any sign of developing hypovolemic shock. The body attempts to compensate for decreased blood volume and to maintain oxygenation of essential organs by increasing the rate and effort of the heart and lungs and by shunting blood from less essential organs. This compensatory mechanism results in the early signs and symptoms of hypovolemic shock:

- Fetal tachycardia (often the first sign)
- Tachycardia, diminished peripheral pulses
- Normal or slightly decreased blood pressure

CRITICAL TO REMEMBER

Signs and Symptoms of Impending Hypovolemic Shock Due to Blood Loss

- Increased pulse rate, falling blood pressure, increased respiratory rate
- Weak, diminished, or "thready" peripheral pulses
- Cool, moist skin, pallor, or cyanosis (late sign)
- Decreased urinary output (<30 ml/hr)
- Decreased hemoglobin, hematocrit levels
- Change in mental status (restlessness, agitation, difficulty concentrating)

- Increased respiratory rate
- Cool, pale skin and mucous membranes

The compensatory mechanism fails if hypovolemic shock progresses and blood volume is insufficient to perfuse the brain, heart, and kidneys. Later signs of hypovolemic shock include the following:

- Falling blood pressure
- Pallor of skin and mucous membranes; skin cold and clammy
- Urine output less than 30 ml/hr
- Restlessness, agitation, decreased mentation

Monitoring the Fetus

Initiate continuous electronic fetal monitoring to identify signs associated with reduced placental blood flow, such as decreasing baseline variability or late decelerations (see Chapter 18). If nonreassuring patterns are noted, contact the physician at once because these fetal signs may be noted before maternal signs of hemorrhage or hypovolemia are obvious.

Promoting Tissue Oxygenation

To promote oxygenation of tissues,

- Place the woman in a lateral position, with the head of the bed flat to increase cardiac return and thus to increase circulation and oxygenation of the placenta and other vital organs.
- Restrict maternal movements and activity to decrease the tissue demand for oxygen.
- Provide simple explanations, reassurance, and emotional support to the woman to help reduce anxiety, which increases the metabolic demand for oxygen.

Collaborating with the Physician for Fluid Replacement

To replace fluids,

- Obtain an order for blood typing and crossmatching so that blood is available for replacement if necessary.
- Insert intravenous lines, usually two lines, using large-bore catheters to allow rapid blood replacement.
- Administer fluids for replacement as directed by the physician to maintain a urinary output of at least 30 ml/hr.

Providing Emotional Support

Explain to the woman what is causing her discomfort, and reassure her that pain relief measures will be initiated as soon as possible without causing harm to the fetus. Although it is unwise to offer false reassurance about the condition of the fetus, provide accurate and timely information to the woman and her family.

Care Related to Surgery

It may be necessary to prepare the woman quickly for cesarean birth. (Care for the woman having a cesarean birth is discussed fully in Chapter 20.) Remain with the woman and her family as much as possible to provide information.

After birth, assess bleeding from the vagina as well as from any surgical sites or puncture wounds (epidural or intravenous sites). Report uncontrolled bleeding or bleeding from unexpected sites, which may indicate DIC. Perform all routine postpartum assessments as well as those related to surgery and to the hemorrhagic complication.

Evaluation

Although client-centered goals are not developed for collaborative problems, the nurse collects and compares data with established norms and judges whether the data are within normal limits. The desired outcome is that the maternal vital signs remain within normal limits and the fetal heart rate demonstrates no signs of compromise, such as late decelerations or decreasing baseline variability.

▋ *Hyperemesis Gravidarum*

Hyperemesis gravidarum is persistent, uncontrollable vomiting that begins in the first weeks of pregnancy and may continue throughout pregnancy. Hyperemesis is associated with weight loss, dehydration, acidosis from starvation, alkalosis from loss of hydrochloric acid in the gastric fluids, and hypokalemia.

Etiology

The cause of hyperemesis gravidarum is not known, but the condition is more common among unmarried white women, during first pregnancies, and in multifetal pregnancies. Theories include endocrine or allergic origins. Elevated hormone levels, such as estrogen and hCG, are considered a possible cause, as is thyroid dysfunction. Psychological factors, such as ambivalence toward the pregnancy and family-related stress, may also play causal roles.

Therapeutic Management

Treatment often occurs in the home, where the woman attempts to control the nausea by methods used for morning sickness (see Chapter 13). In addition, some physicians prescribe vitamins, such as pyridoxine (vitamin B_6), which may provide some relief. The use of antiemetic medications is controversial because reported fetal anomalies associated with them have been widely circulated. A daily vitamin and mineral supplement may be recommended.

The physician will exclude other causes for persistent nausea and vomiting, such as cholecystitis, before diagnosing and treating hyperemesis. Laboratory studies include determining the hemoglobin and hematocrit, which may be elevated as a result of dehydration, which results in hemoconcentration. Electrolyte studies may reveal reduced sodium, potassium, and chloride.

If methods to relieve nausea and vomiting are unsuccessful and weight loss or electrolyte imbalance persists, intravenous fluid and electrolyte replacement or total parenteral nutrition may be necessary. Enteral nutrition via a feeding tube has also been used successfully (Cunningham et al., 1997).

Nursing Considerations

Physical assessment begins with determining the woman's intake and output. Intake includes intravenous fluids and parenteral nutrition as well as oral nutrition, which is allowed once vomiting is controlled. A description of the output includes the amount and character of emesis and urinary output. As a rule of thumb, the normal urinary output is about 1 ml/kg (2.2 lb)/hr. A record of bowel elimination also provides significant information about oral nutrition because bowel movements will be decreased and hard with dehydration. Findings associated with dehydration include decreased fluid intake (less than 2,000 ml/day), decreased urinary output, increased urine specific gravity (above 1.025), dry skin or dry mucous membranes, and nonelastic skin turgor.

The woman should be weighed daily and her urine tested for ketones. Weight loss and the presence of ketones in the urine suggest that fat stores and protein are being metabolized to meet energy needs.

Nursing interventions focus on reducing nausea and vomiting, maintaining nutrition and fluid balance, and providing emotional support.

REDUCING NAUSEA AND VOMITING
Food portions should be small so that the amount does not appear overwhelming. Present foods attractively and eliminate foods with strong odors, because nausea is often associated with food smells. Low-fat foods and easily digested carbohydrates, such as fruit, breads, cereals, rice, and pasta, provide important nutrients and help prevent low blood sugar, which can cause nausea. Soups and other liquids should be taken between meals so as not to overly distend the stomach and trigger vomiting. Sitting upright after meals reduces the frequency of gastric reflux.

MAINTAINING NUTRITION AND FLUID BALANCE
Intravenous fluids and total parenteral nutrition are administered as directed by the physician. Small oral feedings of clear liquids are started when nausea and vomiting begin to subside. When oral fluids are tolerated, parenteral fluids and nutrition are gradually discontinued. Any inability to tolerate oral feedings or continued episodes of vomiting should be reported to the physician so that continued parenteral fluids and nutrition can be prescribed.

Women with nausea and vomiting should eat every 2 to 3 hours. Salting food helps replace chloride lost when hydrochloric acid is vomited. Potassium- and magnesium-rich foods should be encouraged because these nutrients are likely to be depleted and magnesium deficiency can exacerbate nausea.

PROVIDING EMOTIONAL SUPPORT
The woman with hyperemesis gravidarum needs the opportunity to express how it feels to be pregnant and to live with ever-present nausea, but these women often experience a curious lack of sympathy and support. This attitude may stem from reports that hyperemesis gravidarum is psychogenic. Whatever the cause, nurses must use critical thinking to examine their own beliefs and biases so that they can provide comfort and support. Case conferences and educational programs help nurses overcome preset beliefs and meet the woman's needs.

Hypertensive Disorders of Pregnancy
Hypertension in Pregnancy

The terminology used to describe hypertension in pregnancy is often nonuniform and confusing. Several overlapping terms are commonly applied to different clinical manifestations of the same disease process. Two distinct entities, however, are commonly encountered in clinical practice: pregnancy-induced hypertension and chronic hypertension. Furthermore, these two conditions can coexist.

Pregnancy-Induced Hypertension

Pregnancy-induced hypertension (PIH) is a multiorgan disease process that develops during pregnancy and regresses in the postpartum period. Several clinical subsets have been given distinct labels, depending on end-organ effects (Table 26–1). In clinical practice, the terms PIH and pre-eclampsia are often used interchangeably. Eclampsia is the term reserved for PIH that has progressed to involve one or more seizures.

Pre-eclampsia

Pre-eclampsia is a condition in which hypertension develops during the last half of pregnancy in a woman who previ-

TABLE 26–1

Classification of Hypertensive Disorders of Pregnancy

Disorder	Comments
Pregnancy-induced hypertension	Development of hypertension (BP > 140/90) during second half of pregnancy; occurs in previously normotensive woman.
Pre-eclampsia	Renal involvement leads to proteinuria.
Eclampsia	Central nervous system involvement leads to seizures.
HELLP	Clinical picture is dominated by hematologic and hepatic signs and symptoms.
Chronic hypertension	Elevation of blood pressure occurs before 20 weeks' gestation.

Adapted from American College of Obstetricians and Gynecologists. (1996). *Hypertension in pregnancy*. (ACOG Technical Bulletin No. 219). Washington, DC: Author. © ACOG, January 1996.

ously had a normal blood pressure. In addition to hypertension, renal involvement leads to proteinuria. Many women also experience generalized edema. In most women, the manifestations of pre-eclampsia usually decrease rapidly after birth, although they are occasionally first identified in a postpartum woman.

INCIDENCE AND RISK FACTORS

Seven percent of all pregnancies that progress to the second trimester are affected by pre-eclampsia (Magann & Martin, 1995). It is a major cause of perinatal death and is often associated with intrauterine fetal growth restriction (IUGR, also known as intrauterine growth retardation).

Although the cause of pre-eclampsia is unknown, several factors increase a woman's risk that the condition will develop. For example, it is most likely to occur in a first pregnancy, in women older than 40 years of age, in African-Americans, and in those with chronic hypertension or renal disease. A family history of PIH also increases the risk. Although low socioeconomic status and young maternal age have been identified as risk factors, the actual independent contribution of these factors to the risk for PIH is questionable (American College of Obstetricians and Gynecologists [ACOG], 1996). Women having diabetes or multifetal gestations are also more likely to have PIH.

Less well-known risk factors include both genetic and immunologic factors. The presence of the angiotensinogen gene *T235* greatly increases the woman's sensitivity to angiotensin, a powerful vasoconstrictor that could lead to hypertension. Antiphospholipid syndrome (APS) is also strongly associated with the development of PIH (see p. 673).

PATHOPHYSIOLOGY

Pre-eclampsia is due to generalized vasospasm. The underlying cause of the vasospasm remains a mystery, but some of the physiologic processes are known. In a normal pregnancy, there is a significant increase in vascular volume as well as increased cardiac output. Despite these factors, blood pressure does not rise in a normal pregnancy, probably because pregnant women develop resistance to the effects of vasoconstrictors such as angiotensin II. Moreover, a decrease in peripheral vascular resistance occurs due to the effects of certain vasodilators, such as prostacyclin (PGI_2), prostaglandin E (PGE), and endothelium-derived relaxing factor (EDRF).

In pre-eclampsia, however, peripheral vascular resistance increases because of the sensitivity of some women to angiotensin II and a decrease in vasodilators. For instance, there is an increase in the ratio of thromboxane A_2(TXA_2) to PGI_2. Thromboxane, produced by kidney and trophoblastic tissue, causes vasoconstriction and platelet aggregation (clumping). Prostacyclin, produced by placental tissue and endothelial cells, causes vasodilation and inhibits platelet aggregation.

Vasospasm decreases the diameter of blood vessels, which results in endothelial cell damage and decreased EDRF. Vasoconstriction also results in impeded blood flow and elevated blood pressure. As a result, circulation to all body organs, including the kidneys, liver, brain, and pla-

centa, is decreased. The following changes are most significant:

- Decreased renal perfusion reduces the glomerular filtration rate. Consequently, blood urea nitrogen, creatinine, and uric acid levels begin to rise.
- Reduced blood flow to the kidneys results in glomerular damage, allowing protein to leak across the glomerular membrane, which is normally impermeable to large protein molecules.
- Loss of protein from the kidneys reduces colloid osmotic pressure and allows fluid to shift to interstitial spaces. This fluid shift may result in edema and relative hypovolemia, which causes increased viscosity of the blood and a rise in hematocrit.
- In response to hypovolemia, additional angiotensin II and aldosterone are secreted to trigger the retention of both sodium and water. The pathologic processes spiral: additional angiotensin II results in further vasospasm and hypertension; aldosterone increases fluid retention, and edema is worsened.
- Decreased circulation to the liver leads to impaired liver function as well as to hepatic edema and subcapsular hemorrhage, which can result in hemorrhagic necrosis. This process is manifested by elevated liver enzyme levels in maternal serum.
- Vasoconstriction of cerebral vessels leads to pressure-induced rupture of thin-walled capillaries, resulting in small cerebral hemorrhages. Signs and symptoms of arterial vasospasm include headache and visual disturbances, such as blurred vision and "spots" before the eyes, as well as hyperreflexia.
- Decreased colloid oncotic pressure can lead to pulmonary capillary leak that results in pulmonary edema. Dyspnea is the primary symptom.
- Decreased placental circulation results in infarctions that increase the risk of abruptio placentae and DIC. In addition, when maternal blood flow through the placenta is decreased, the fetus is likely to experience IUGR and persistent fetal hypoxemia, which can result in fetal acidosis, mental retardation, or death.

PREVENTIVE MEASURES

Prenatal Care. Proper prenatal care with attention to the pattern of weight gain as well as careful monitoring of blood pressure and urinary protein may minimize maternal and fetal morbidity and mortality.

Low-Dose Aspirin. In recent years, low doses of aspirin (60 to 80 mg/day) have been administered to women at high risk for developing pre-eclampsia. Low-dose aspirin helps to prevent injury to endothelial cells that line the blood vessels by reducing the aggregation of platelets and allowing increased production of EDRF. In addition, aspirin suppresses the synthesis of TXA_2. Aspirin is not, however, recommended for PIH prophylaxis in women with normal blood pressure who are not at risk for developing PIH (ACOG, 1996).

Calcium Supplementation. Some evidence suggests that women who receive calcium supplementation are less sensitive to the pressor effects of angiotensin II and have a lower overall incidence of hypertension (Ferris, 1995).

MANIFESTATIONS

Classic Signs. Hypertension, generalized edema, and proteinuria are the three classic signs of pre-eclampsia. The first indication of pre-eclampsia is usually hypertension. The first sign of edema that the pregnant woman may notice is a rapid weight gain, which is due to fluid retention and consequent generalized edema. Edema may be present in the lower legs, which is common in pregnancy, but also in the hands and face (Fig. 26–6). Edema may not, however, be present in all women who develop pre-eclampsia.

Hypertension is defined as a sustained blood pressure of 140/90 or higher. Earlier data suggested that an increase of 30 mm Hg in systolic pressure or 15 mm Hg in diastolic pressure from baseline was also of diagnostic value, but this concept is no longer considered valid (ACOG, 1996). Because young women often have relatively low blood pressure, however, using a criterion of 140/90 for hypertension may not identify many who develop hypertension during pregnancy (Leicht & Harvey, 1999).

Blood pressure measurements vary with the woman's position, so the blood pressure should be measured uniformly at each office visit. Blood pressure should be measured with the woman seated and her arm supported, and the cuff size should be appropriate for the size of her arm.

Proteinuria usually develops later than hypertension and edema, and the combination of proteinuria and hypertension increases the possibility of fetal jeopardy. A clean-catch specimen prevents contamination of the specimen by vaginal secretions, allowing accurate recognition of proteinuria.

Additional Signs. When the retina is examined, vascular constriction and narrowing of the small arteries are obvious in most women with pre-eclampsia. The vasoconstriction that can be seen in the retina is occurring throughout the body. Deep tendon reflexes may be very brisk (hyperreflexia), suggesting cerebral irritability secondary to decreased circulation and edema.

Symptoms. Pre-eclampsia is dangerous for the expectant mother and fetus for two reasons: (1) it develops and progresses rapidly and (2) the early symptoms are not often noticed by the woman. By the time she experiences symptoms, the disease has often progressed to an advanced state, and valuable treatment time has been lost.

Certain symptoms, such as continuous headache, drowsiness, or mental confusion, indicate poor cerebral perfusion and may be precursors of convulsions. Visual disturbances, such as blurred or double vision or spots before the eyes, indicate arterial spasms and edema in the retina. Numbness or tingling of the hands or feet occurs when nerves are compressed by retained fluid. Some symptoms, such as epigastric pain or "upset stomach," are particularly ominous because they indicate distension of the hepatic capsule and often warn that a convulsion is imminent. Decreased urinary output indicates poor perfusion of the kidneys and may precede acute renal failure.

THERAPEUTIC MANAGEMENT

Pre-eclampsia continues to be categorized as either mild or severe, depending on the frequency and intensity of presenting signs and symptoms (Table 26–2). Because the disease may progress rapidly, however, an apparently mild condition can become severe in a very short time.

Delivery is the only definitive treatment but may not be practical if pre-eclampsia is mild and the fetus is immature. Delivery must be accomplished by induction of labor or ce-

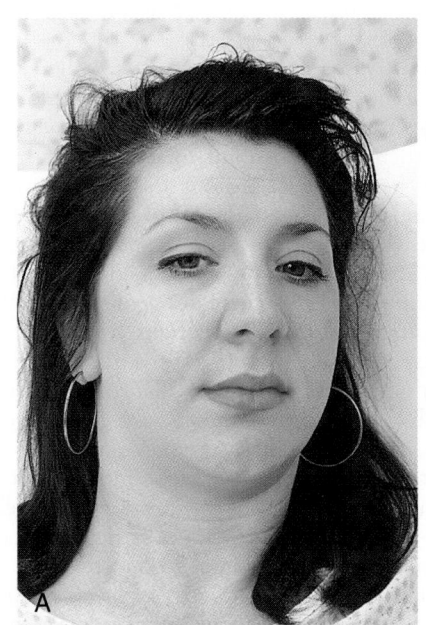
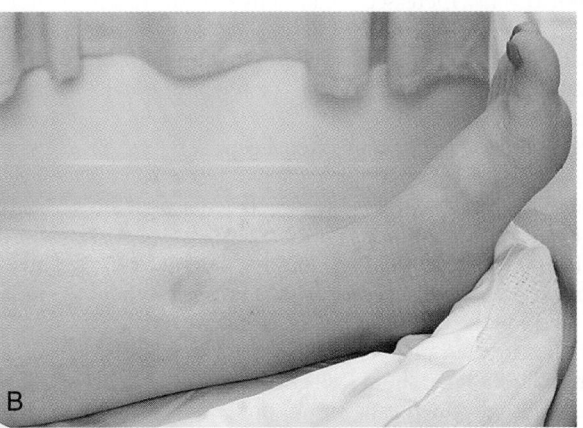

FIGURE 26–6

Generalized edema is a classic sign of pre-eclampsia. *A,* Facial edema may be subtle. *B,* Pitting edema of the lower leg.

TABLE 26–2

Mild versus Severe Pre-eclampsia

Parameter Evaluated	Mild	Severe
Systolic blood pressure	<160	>160
Diastolic blood pressure	<100	>110
Proteinuria	Trace	>5 g/24 hr
Creatinine	Normal	Elevated
Thrombocytopenia	Absent	Present
Oliguria	Absent	<500 ml/24 hr
Liver enzyme elevation	Minimal	Marked
Fetal growth restriction	Absent	Present
Headache, visual disturbances, abdominal pain	Absent	Present

sarean birth, however, if the maternal or fetal conditions deteriorate, regardless of fetal age.

Home Care for Mild Pre-eclampsia. Home management is appropriate if pre-eclampsia is mild, if the woman and fetus are in stable condition, and if she can adhere to the treatment plan. A home care nurse often makes one or more visits daily for assessment of signs and symptoms, review of blood pressure, urinalysis, assessment of fetal movement, and assessment of the woman's weight, activity level, and adherence to treatment plan. Indications of disease progression or fetal deterioration require admission to the hospital.

Activity Restrictions. Bed rest or sedentary activity for most of the day is prescribed (Cunningham et al., 1997; Roberts, 1999). Resting on the left side as much as possible decreases pressure on the vena cava, thereby increasing cardiac return and circulatory volume and thus improving perfusion of vital organs. Increased renal perfusion decreases angiotensin II levels, promotes diuresis, and lowers the blood pressure. The woman is advised to remain quiet and calm. She may need to restrict visitors or telephone calls that cause agitation.

Fetal Activity. The woman often keeps a record of fetal movements, also called a "kick count" (see Chapter 16). She should report a decrease in movements or if no movement is felt during a 4-hour period.

Blood Pressure. The family must be taught to use electronic blood pressure equipment. Blood pressure should be checked two to four times per day in the same arm and with the woman in the same position.

Weight. The woman should weigh herself at the same time each day, usually in the morning, preferably on the same scale and in clothing of similar weight.

Urinalysis. A urine dipstick test for protein, using the first voided midstream specimen, should be performed daily.

Diet. A regular diet without salt or fluid restriction is usually prescribed. Moderate salt restriction may be prescribed for the woman with significant edema, not to alter the course of the disease but to increase her comfort (Roberts, 1999).

Fetal Assessment. Additional fetal surveillance is often recommended and may include serial sonography, weekly nonstress testing, and a contraction stress test or bio-physical profile if the nonstress test indicates possible fetal compromise.

Inpatient Management for Severe Pre-eclampsia. Pre-eclampsia is considered severe when blood pressure is higher than 160/110 mm Hg, proteinuria is greater than 5 g/24 hr (3+ or more), and oliguria is present (500 ml or less in 24 hours). If symptoms occur that were absent in the mild form of the disease or if laboratory findings indicate liver involvement (elevated enzymes or hyperbilirubinemia) or kidney damage (elevated creatinine), the disease is judged to be severe (ACOG, 1996).

Antepartum Management. The woman will be hospitalized for assessment and management. The goals of management are to prevent convulsions and to maintain the pregnancy until it is safe to deliver the fetus.

Bed Rest. The hospitalized woman is kept on bed rest and her environment is kept quiet. External stimuli (lights, noise) that might precipitate a convulsion should be reduced.

Antihypertensive Medications. Blood pressure control does not improve fetal oxygenation, and thus the use of antihypertensives is usually reserved for severe hypertension when there is the possibility of maternal intracranial bleeding (Roberts, 1999). Various antihypertensive agents such as hydralazine may be used (ACOG, 1996). Other antihypertensive medications, such as nifedipine (a calcium channel blocker) or labetalol (a beta-adrenergic blocker), may be administered in some cases (August, 1999).

Anticonvulsant Medications. In the United States, magnesium sulfate ($MgSO_4$) is the drug of choice to prevent convulsions, but phenytoin (Dilantin, Diphenylan) is occasionally used. Magnesium acts as a central nervous system depressant by blocking neuromuscular transmission and decreasing the amount of acetylcholine liberated. Magnesium is not an antihypertensive medication, but it relaxes smooth muscle and thus reduces vasoconstriction. Decreased vasoconstriction promotes circulation to the vital organs of the expectant mother and increases placental circulation. Increased circulation to the maternal kidneys leads to diuresis, as interstitial fluid is shifted into the vascular compartment and excreted.

Magnesium is usually administered by intravenous infusion, which allows for immediate onset of action and does not cause the discomfort associated with intramuscular ad-

DRUG GUIDE
Magnesium Sulfate

Classification: Miscellaneous anticonvulsant.

Action: Decreases acetylcholine released by motor nerve impulses, thereby blocking neuromuscular transmission. Depresses the central nervous system to act as an anticonvulsant, also decreases frequency and intensity of uterine contractions. Produces flushing and sweating due to decreased peripheral blood pressure.

Indications: Prevention and control of seizures in severe pre-eclampsia. Prevention of uterine contractions in preterm labor.

Dosage and Route
An intravenous loading bolus (4 to 6 g given over 20 minutes) is given and followed by continuous infusion (1 to 3 g/hr) via a controlled infusion device (ACOG, 1996; Leicht & Harvey, 1999). Therapeutic range for magnesium is generally considered to be 4 to 8 mg/dl (ACOG, 1996). Deep intramuscular injection is acceptable but is painful.

Absorption
Immediate onset following intravenous administration. Duration of action is 3 to 4 hours.

Excretion
Excreted by the kidneys.

Contraindications and Precautions:
Contraindicated in persons with myocardial damage, heart block, myasthenia gravis, or impaired renal function.

Adverse Reactions: Result from magnesium overdose and include flushing, sweating, hypotension, depressed deep tendon reflexes, and central nervous system depression, including respiratory depression.

Nursing Implications: Monitor blood pressure closely during administration. Assess client for respiratory rate above 12 breaths per minute, presence of deep tendon reflexes, and urinary output greater than 30 ml/hr before administering magnesium. Place resuscitation equipment (suction, oxygen) in the room. Keep calcium gluconate, which acts as an antidote to magnesium, in the room along with syringes and needles.

---

ministration. Intravenous magnesium is administered via a secondary ("piggyback") line so that the medication can be discontinued at any time while the primary line remains functional.

One of the major advantages of magnesium is that it is safe for the fetus or neonate while preventing maternal convulsions (Roberts, 1999). Fetal magnesium levels are nearly identical with those of the expectant mother. As a result, the fetal monitor tracing may show decreased fetal heart rate variability. No cumulative effect occurs, however, because the fetal kidneys excrete magnesium effectively.

Significant adverse reactions and side effects are associated with parenteral administration of magnesium. The most important is central nervous system depression, including depression of the respiratory center. Magnesium is excreted solely by the kidneys, and the reduced urine output that often occurs in pre-eclampsia allows magnesium to accumulate to toxic levels in the woman.

Intrapartum Management. Most seizures occur during labor and the postpartum period. During labor, the woman must be monitored continuously to detect signs of imminent convulsions. She should be kept in a lateral position to promote circulation through the placenta, and pain that may cause agitation and precipitate seizures should be controlled. Narcotic analgesics or epidural analgesia may be administered to reduce pain that could precipitate a convulsion.

Induction of labor by intravenous oxytocin is done if the maternal or fetal conditions deteriorate. Oxytocin to stimulate uterine contractions and magnesium sulfate to prevent convulsions are often administered simultaneously during labor. The woman will have two secondary infusions: one for oxytocin and one for magnesium.

Continuous electronic fetal monitoring identifies fetal heart rate patterns that suggest compromise. If nonreassuring patterns occur, the corrective actions depend on the pattern identified (see Chapter 18). Late decelerations, associated with reduced placental perfusion, or decreased variability are more likely to occur because of vasospasm, but any other nonreassuring pattern may occur as well.

A pediatrician, neonatologist, or neonatal nurse practitioner must be available to care for the newborn at birth.

Postpartum Management. Following birth, careful assessment of the mother's blood loss and signs of shock are essential because the hypovolemia caused by pre-eclampsia may be aggravated by blood loss during the delivery. Assessments for signs and symptoms of pre-eclampsia must be continued for at least 48 hours, and magnesium may be continued to prevent seizures.

Signs that the woman is recovering from pre-eclampsia are the following:

- Urinary output of 4 to 6 L/day, which causes a rapid reduction in edema and rapid weight loss
- Decreased protein in the urine
- Return of blood pressure to normal, usually within 2 weeks

Management of Eclampsia. Eclampsia is marked by convulsions that typically begin with twitching about the mouth. The body then becomes rigid in a state of tonic muscular contractions that last 15 to 20 seconds. Suddenly the facial muscles and then all body muscles alternately contract and relax in rapid succession. This clonic phase of the convulsion may last about 1 minute. Respiration is halted during the convulsion because the diaphragm remains fixed. Breathing usually resumes shortly after the convulsion and is most often rapid and deep (Usta & Sibai, 1995).

Magnesium may be given intravenously to control the convulsions. Sedatives such as phenobarbital or diazepam are used only if magnesium fails to bring the seizures under control. Sedatives should not be given if birth is expected within an hour or two because of their depressant effects on the fetus.

Pulmonary edema, circulatory or renal failure, and cerebral hemorrhage are complications that may occur with eclampsia. The woman's lungs should be auscultated frequently. Furosemide (Lasix) may be administered if pulmonary edema develops. Digitalis may be needed to strengthen contraction of the heart if circulatory failure results. Urine output should be assessed hourly; if output drops below 30 ml/hr, renal failure should be suspected.

Because eclampsia stimulates uterine irritability, the woman should be monitored carefully for ruptured membranes, signs of labor, or abruptio placentae. While the woman is unresponsive, she should be kept on her side to prevent aspiration and to improve placental circulation. The side rails should be kept up to prevent a fall and possible injury. When vital signs have stabilized, delivery of the fetus should be considered.

Aspiration is a leading cause of maternal morbidity following an eclamptic seizure. After initial stabilization, the nurse should anticipate orders for chest radiography and arterial blood gas determination to identify aspiration.

NURSING CARE
The Woman with Pre-eclampsia

Assessment

Weigh the woman on admission and then daily. Check vital signs, and auscultate the chest for moist breath sounds that suggest pulmonary edema. Assess the location and severity of edema at least every 4 hours. Table 26–3 describes a useful method for describing edema. Measure urine output hourly. An indwelling catheter is often ordered. Check the urine for protein every 4 hours. Apply an electronic fetal monitor to identify changes in fetal heart rate or variability that suggest poor placental perfusion or other problems.

Check brachial and patellar reflexes for hyperreflexia that indicates cerebral irritability. Determine whether clonus is present by dorsiflexing the woman's foot sharply while her knee is held in a flexed position. If oscillations or "jerking" motions occur as the foot drops, clonus is present and

TABLE 26–3

Assessment of Edema

Characteristics	Grade
Minimal edema of lower extremities	+1
Marked edema of lower extremities	+2
Edema of lower extremities, face, hands, and sacral area	+3
Generalized massive edema that includes ascites (accumulation of fluid in peritoneal cavity)	+4

should be reported to the physician. Procedure 26–1 details how to assess and rate deep tendon reflexes.

Question the woman carefully about symptoms she may be experiencing, such as headache, visual disturbances, epigastric pain, or increased edema.

> An open-ended question such as "How do you feel?" may not be adequate. Ask targeted questions, such as "Do you have a headache? Describe it for me." "Do you have any pain in the abdomen? Show me where it is and describe it." "Do you see spots before your eyes? Flashes of light? Double vision?" "Is your vision blurred?" "I see you have removed your rings. Did you do that because your hands were swollen? When did that happen?"

Assessments for Magnesium Toxicity

Adverse side effects of magnesium include central nervous system depression, including depression of the respiratory center. Hypotonic reflexes indicate central nervous system depression that precedes respiratory depression. Determine the respiratory rate hourly. Assess the woman's level of consciousness (alert, drowsy, confused, oriented). Table 26–4 summarizes nursing assessments and their implications.

Psychosocial Assessment

The development of pre-eclampsia places a great deal of stress on the childbearing family. The woman may be on bed rest at home or hospitalized for some time. This situation creates anxiety about the condition of the fetus as well as that of the expectant mother. Moreover, many families do not understand the seriousness of the disease; after all, the woman feels well initially.

Investigate how the family will function while the expectant mother is hospitalized or on bed rest at home. Determine how the woman is adapting to the "sick role" and the necessity of being dependent on others instead of functioning in her primary role. Ask how much support is available and who is willing to participate. Finally, determine the major concerns of the family.

Nursing Diagnosis and Planning

Analysis of the data collected can lead to both nursing diagnoses (see Nursing Care Plan 26–2) and collaborative problems or potential complications. Potential complications require nurses to monitor for the onset of new problems or changes in status. Both physician-prescribed and nurse-prescribed interventions are used to minimize the complication. Potential complications for the woman with pre-eclampsia are eclamptic seizures and magnesium toxicity.

Client-centered goals are inappropriate for the potential complications of eclamptic seizures and magnesium toxicity because the nurse cannot independently manage these conditions but must confer with physicians for medical orders for treatment. For seizures, planning should reflect the nurse's responsibility to do the following:

- Perform actions that will minimize the risk of seizures occurring and prevent maternal or fetal injury if seizures do occur.

PROCEDURE 26–1

* * * * * * * * * *

Assessing Deep Tendon Reflexes

PURPOSE: To identify any exaggerated reflexes (hyperreflexia) or diminished reflexes (hyporeflexia).

1. To assess both the brachial and the patellar reflex, plus clonus, you will need a reflex hammer.
2. To assess the brachial reflex, support the woman's arm and instruct her to let it go limp while it is being held so that the arm is totally relaxed and flexed.
3. Place your thumb over the woman's tendon, as illustrated, to allow you to feel as well as see the tendon response when it is tapped. Strike the thumb with the small end of the reflex hammer. The normal response is slight flexion of the forearm.

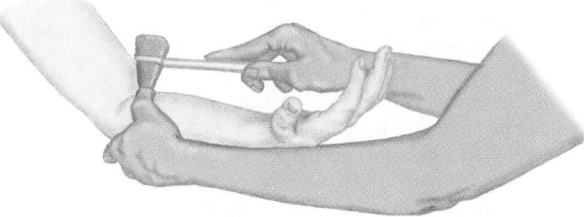

4. The patellar reflex can be assessed with the woman in two positions, sitting or lying. When the woman is sitting, allow her lower legs to dangle freely to flex the knee and stretch the tendons. Strike the tendon with the reflex hammer just below the patella. The patellar reflex is unreliable if the woman has had epidural analgesia.

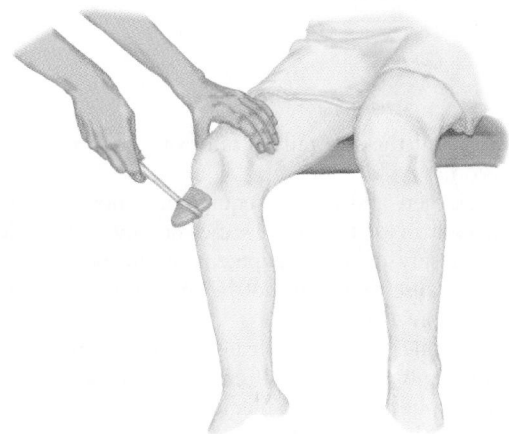

5. When the woman is supine, the weight of her leg must be supported to flex the knee and stretch the tendons because an adequate response requires that the limb be relaxed and the tendon partially stretched. Strike the partially stretched tendons just below the patella. Extension of the leg is the expected response.

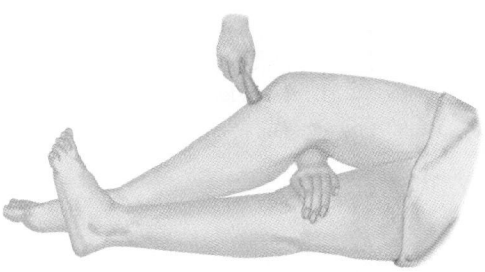

6. Clonus should be tested, particularly when the reflexes are hyperactive. The woman's lower leg should be supported, as illustrated, and the foot sharply dorsiflexed to stretch the tendon. Hold the stretch. With a normal response, no movement will be felt. When clonus (indicating hyperreflexia) is present, rapid rhythmic jerking motions of the foot are obvious.

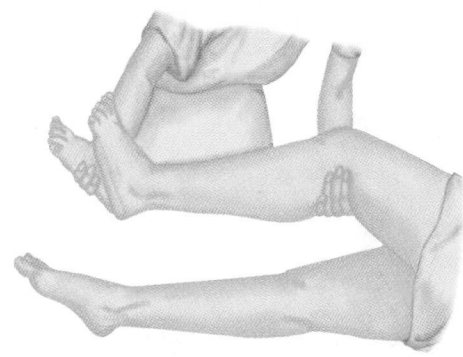

Deep Tendon Reflex Rating Scale

0	Reflex absent
+1	Reflex present, hypoactive
+2	Normal reflex
+3	Brisker than average reflex
+4	Hyperactive reflex with clonus present

* Monitor for signs of impending seizures.
* Support the family of the woman with eclampsia.

For magnesium toxicity, planning should reflect these nursing responsibilities:

* Monitor for signs of magnesium toxicity.
* Consult with the physician if signs of magnesium toxicity are observed.
* Perform actions that will minimize the possibility of magnesium toxicity.

Interventions

Interventions for Seizures

Initiating Preventive Measures. In the presence of cerebral irritability, seizures may be precipitated by excessive visual or auditory stimuli. Nurses should reduce external stimuli by doing the following:

* Admitting the woman to a private room in the quietest section of the unit and keeping the door to the room closed.

TABLE 26–4

Nursing Assessments for Pre-eclampsia and Magnesium Toxicity

Assessment	Implications
Daily weight	Provides estimate of fluid retention.
Blood pressure	To determine response to treatment.
Respiratory rate	Drug therapy ($MgSO_4$) causes respiratory depression, and drug should be withheld and the physician notified if respiratory rate is <12/min.
Breath sounds	To detect onset of pulmonary edema.
Deep tendon reflexes	Hyperreflexia indicates increased cerebral edema; hyporeflexia indicates magnesium excess.
Edema	For estimation of interstitial fluid.
Urinary output	Output of at least 30 ml/hr indicates adequate perfusion of the kidneys.
Level of consciousness	Drowsiness, dulled sensorium indicate therapeutic effects of magnesium; nonresponsive behavior or muscle weakness indicates magnesium excess.
Headache, epigastric pain, visual problems	These findings indicate increasing severity of the condition and the possible development of eclampsia.
Fetal heart rate and baseline variability	Rate should be between 110 and 160 in a term fetus. Decreasing baseline variability may be due to magnesium or to continuous fetal hypoxemia and fetal distress.
Laboratory data	Elevated serum creatinine, elevated liver enzymes, or decreased platelets (thrombocytopenia) are significant signs of increasing severity of disease. Serum magnesium levels should be in the therapeutic range designated by the physician.

- Padding the door to reduce noise when the door must be opened and closed.
- Keeping lights low and noise to a minimum; this may include blocking incoming telephone calls.
- Grouping nursing assessments and care to allow the woman long periods of undisturbed quiet.
- Moving carefully and calmly around the room and avoiding bumping into the bed or startling the woman.
- Collaborating with the woman and her family to restrict visitors.

Monitoring for Signs of Impending Seizures. Signs of impending seizures include the following:

- Hyperreflexia, the presence of clonus, or both
- Increasing signs of cerebral irritability (headache, visual disturbances)
- Epigastric pain

None of these signs is an absolutely reliable predictor of imminent seizure. Nurses must be alert for subtle changes and prepared for seizures in all women with pre-eclampsia.

Preventing Seizure-Related Injury. The bed's side rails should be padded and the bed kept in the lowest position with the wheels locked to prevent trauma should the woman hit the side rails or fall from the bed during a convulsion.

Oxygen and suction equipment should be assembled and ready to use to remove secretions and to provide oxygen as necessary. Check equipment at the beginning of each shift because there will not be time to set up equipment if convulsions occur.

Supplies specific for care in pre-eclampsia should be immediately available, often in a separate box or tray. The supplies include a medium plastic airway, an Ambu bag with mask, an ophthalmoscope, a tourniquet, a reflex hammer, syringes, and needles. Medications that should be on hand include magnesium sulfate, sodium bicarbonate, heparin sodium, epinephrine, phenytoin, and calcium gluconate.

Protecting the Woman and Fetus During a Convulsion. Nurses must protect the woman and the fetus during a convulsion. The nurse's primary responsibilities are the following:

- Remain with the woman and press the emergency bell for assistance.
- Attempt to turn the woman on her side when the tonic phase begins. A side-lying position permits greater circu-

NURSING CARE PLAN 26–2
. . . .
Pre-eclampsia

Assessment

Julie Frost, a 16-year-old primigravida, is seen in the prenatal clinic at 30 weeks of gestation. Her blood pressure is 136/90, and there is some edema of the lower legs and trace proteinuria. She is given instructions about home care for pregnancy-induced hypertension. The regimen includes bed rest; frequent monitoring of blood pressure, weight, and urine; and doing fetal "kick counts." Julie is told she must return to the clinic in a week. She states that she feels fine and doesn't want to miss school. She says that she doesn't see the reason for bed rest.

Nursing Diagnosis

Impaired Adjustment related to lack of knowledge of health status and the need for a change in lifestyle.

Goals/Expected Outcomes

Julie will

- Verbalize the benefits of the recommended regimen by the end of the first prenatal appointment.
- Comply with the recommended care for the next week.
- Keep prenatal appointments.

Intervention	Rationale
1. Allow Julie to verbalize her feelings about the recommended regimen: "What concerns you most about missing school?" Acknowledge her feelings as important: "It must be difficult to think of falling behind in your schoolwork. It isn't any fun to miss all the after-school activities."	1. When feelings are identified and acknowledged as important, anxiety decreases, and teaching and learning can begin.
2. Identify family support that will permit compliance with the recommended regimen of bed rest and home care.	2. Compliance with the regimen is impossible without family assistance, which includes assistance with activities of daily living and necessary assessments.
3. Describe in general terms the pathophysiologic processes that affect Julie and the fetus.	3. Expectant mothers are usually motivated to comply with a therapeutic management that will benefit the fetus.
4. Explain that Julie may feel well even when the condition worsens and that she must be observed for signs and symptoms at home and at the clinic.	4. The expectant mother does not notice hypertension and proteinuria. Many clients consider edema normal, and they may not identify edema above the waist as more significant than dependent edema.
5. Instruct Julie to call the clinic if she notices headache, double vision, or spots before her eyes.	5. These signs indicate rapid progression of the disease and that additional management is needed.
6. Collaborate with Julie to arrange for contact with her boyfriend or selected friends and to arrange for ongoing home-bound classes.	6. Such an agreement will allow a schedule to provide peer support but allow for prolonged periods of quiet. Home-bound classes alleviate the concern that she is falling behind with schoolwork.

Evaluation

Despite maintaining the recommended regimen of bed rest with the help of her mother and sister, Julie's condition worsened with a rise in blood pressure and a rapid gain in weight, indicating generalized edema.

Assessment

Julie is admitted to the hospital at 32 weeks of gestation with a blood pressure of 160/110, heart rate of 92, and respiratory rate of 22 per minute. There is 2+ proteinuria and marked edema of the hands and face. Fetal heart rate is 136 with average variability. An intravenous infusion of magnesium sulfate ($MgSO_4$) is started, seizure precautions are initiated, and environmental stimuli are carefully reduced. Julie is agitated and verbalizes concern that the procedures are going to hurt her or the fetus. She frequently asks, "How sick am I?" "Is the baby going to be okay?" Her hands are perspiring, and they shake when she reaches for a tissue.

(continued)

NURSING CARE PLAN 26-2 *Continued*
• • • • • • • • • • • •

Pre-eclampsia

Nursing Diagnosis	Anxiety related to hospitalization and concern about her health and the health of the fetus.
Goals/Expected Outcomes	Julie will

- Verbalize her concerns and describe the benefits of the treatment while her family is present.
- Manifest less anxiety (agitation, physiologic signs such as tremors, tachycardia, and perspiration).

Intervention

1. Initiate measures to reduce anxiety.
   a. Provide positive reassurance that a solution to anxiety can be found: "I can see you are really worried, and I will try to answer all your questions."
   b. Allow Julie to cry, get angry, or express any feeling that is present.
   c. Encourage a discussion of feelings: "Tell me more about how you feel."
   d. Reflect observations: "I see you wringing your hands; do you want to talk about it?"
   e. Convey empathy and positive regard; use nonverbal behavior, including touch, when appropriate.
2. Provide information about hospital routines and procedures when Julie's anxiety has diminished enough for learning to take place.
   a. Be very specific about procedures, such as fetal monitoring, assessment of deep tendon reflexes, and vital signs. Explain the reasons for these procedures, who will do them, and how long they will be maintained.
   b. Focus on Julie's present concerns; she is not able to be future oriented at this time.
   c. Speak slowly and calmly, give very short directions, and do not ask Julie to make decisions: "Turn on your side." "Breathe slowly."
   d. Allow a friend or family member to remain with Julie and instruct the person on the need for a low-stimulus environment.

Rationale

1. Anxiety is an ominous feeling of tension resulting from a physical or emotional threat to the self. It is a global, often unnamed sense of doom, a feeling of helplessness, isolation, and insecurity. Anxiety needs to be ventilated and then addressed by conveying that the person is not alone and will be protected.

2. Knowledge of procedures to be performed and the purpose of these procedures provides a sense of control that reduces anxiety. Perception is somewhat narrowed when anxiety is high; therefore, short, brief instructions are easier for the anxious person to understand than long explanations.

Evaluation

Julie discusses her feelings with the nurse and with her sister. She feels in control of anxiety, as manifested by fewer signs of agitation and fewer physiologic signs (tachycardia, tachypnea) and by the ability to use relaxation techniques.

Potential Complications to Consider

Magnesium toxicity
Seizures

---

lation through the placenta, and it may also help prevent aspiration.
- Note the time and sequence of the convulsion.
- Insert an airway following the convulsion, and suction the woman's mouth and nose to prevent aspiration. Administer oxygen by mask to increase oxygenation of the placenta and all maternal body organs.

- Observe fetal monitor patterns for signs suggestive of hypoxia, such as bradycardia, tachycardia, or decreased variability.
- Notify the physician that a convulsion has occurred. A seizure is associated with cerebral hemorrhage, premature separation of the placenta, severe fetal hypoxia, and death.

- Administer medications and prepare for additional medical interventions as directed by the physician.

Providing Information and Support for the Family. Explain to the family what has happened without minimizing the seriousness of the situation. A convulsion is frightening for anyone who witnesses it, and the family is often reassured when the nurse explains that the convulsion lasts only a few minutes and that the woman will probably not be conscious for some time afterward. Acknowledge that the convulsion indicates worsening of the condition and that it will be necessary for the physician to determine future management, which may include delivery of the infant as soon as possible.

Interventions for Magnesium Toxicity

Monitoring for Signs of Magnesium Toxicity. Magnesium excess depresses the entire central nervous system, including the brain stem, which controls respirations and cardiac function, and the cerebrum, which controls memory, mental processes, and speech. Carbon dioxide accumulates if the respiratory rate is reduced, leading to respiratory acidosis and further central nervous system depression, which could end in respiratory arrest.

Signs of magnesium toxicity include the following:

- Respiratory rate less than 12 breaths per minute
- Absence of deep tendon reflexes
- Sweating, flushing
- Altered sensorium (confusion, lethargy, slurring of speech, drowsiness, disorientation)
- Hypotension
- A serum magnesium concentration above the therapeutic range of 4 to 8 mg/dl (ACOG, 1996)

Responding to Signs of Magnesium Toxicity. Discontinue magnesium if the respiratory rate is less than 12 breaths per minute or if deep tendon reflexes are absent. Notify the physician. Magnesium is excreted by the kidneys, and if the urinary output falls below 30 ml/hr, the physician should be notified before magnesium is administered.

Calcium gluconate antagonizes the effects of magnesium at the neuromuscular junction. Magnesium toxicity can be reversed by intravenous administration of 1 g (10 ml of 10%) calcium gluconate over 2 minutes (ACOG, 1996).

Evaluation

Collect and compare data with established norms and then judge whether the data are within normal limits. For seizures, interventions are judged to be successful if

- Deep tendon reflexes remain within normal limits (+1 to +3).
- Clonus is absent.
- The woman is free of visual disturbances, headache, and epigastric pain.
- The woman remains free of seizures or free of preventable injury if a seizure occurs.

For magnesium toxicity, determine whether respiratory rates remain above 12 breaths per minute, deep tendon reflexes are present, and maternal plasma levels of magnesium do not exceed the therapeutic dose.

■ *Hemolysis, Elevated Liver Enzymes, and Low Platelets Syndrome*

The acronym HELLP (hemolysis, elevated liver enzymes, low platelets) describes a potentially life-threatening variation of pre-eclampsia. Hemolysis is believed to occur as a result of the fragmentation and distortion of erythrocytes during passage through small damaged blood vessels. Liver enzyme levels increase when hepatic blood flow is obstructed by fibrin deposits. Hyperbilirubinemia and jaundice may also be observed as a result of liver impairment. Low platelet levels are due to vascular damage resulting from vasospasm; platelets aggregate at sites of damage, resulting in thrombocytopenia.

The prominent symptom of the HELLP syndrome is pain in the right upper quadrant, the lower chest, or epigastric area. There may also be tenderness due to liver distension. Additional signs and symptoms include nausea, vomiting, and severe edema. Laboratory data include irregular, damaged red blood cells, thrombocytopenia, and elevated liver enzyme levels (Riely & Fallon, 1999).

It is important to avoid traumatizing the liver by abdominal palpation and to use care in transporting the woman. A sudden increase in intra-abdominal pressure could lead to rupture of the subcapsular hematoma, which is most likely to occur during convulsions (Usta & Sibai, 1995).

Women with the HELLP syndrome should be managed in a setting with full intensive care facilities. Treatment includes administration of magnesium sulfate and hydralazine, followed by cesarean delivery if the fetus is mature (Fagan, 1999). After delivery, most mothers have an uneventful recovery. The platelet count generally returns to normal within 7 days (Fallon & Riely, 1995).

■ *Chronic Hypertension*

A diagnosis of chronic hypertension is made whenever evidence suggests that hypertension preceded the pregnancy or when a woman is hypertensive before 20 weeks' gestation. Chronic hypertension is seen most often in older women, in those who are obese, and in those with diabetes. Heredity, including race, plays a role in the development of chronic hypertension, which is common in African-Americans (Cunningham et al., 1997).

The most common hazard faced by pregnant women with chronic hypertension is the development of pre-eclampsia. The diagnosis of pre-eclampsia is made on the basis of a rise in blood pressure, sustained proteinuria, and generalized edema (Roberts, 1999). Treatment of superimposed pre-eclampsia often requires hospitalization and measures to prevent the development of eclampsia.

A high-protein diet with adequate but not excessive salt is recommended, and the woman is advised to weigh herself every 3 days to detect abnormal weight gain. Antihypertensive medication should be continued if already in use. If not in use, antihypertensive medication should be initiated if the diastolic pressure is consistently higher than 90 mm Hg in early pregnancy (Roberts, 1999). The choice of antihypertensive medication is of great concern because of the possible teratogenic effects of these medications. Methyldopa (Aldomet) is one of the most commonly prescribed antihypertensives during pregnancy, and long-term follow-up evaluations of children whose mothers took methyldopa indicate no signs of teratogenic effects (Roberts, 1999).

Incompatibility Between Maternal and Fetal Blood

Rh Incompatibility

Rhesus (Rh) factor incompatibility during pregnancy is possible only when two specific circumstances coexist: (1) the expectant mother is Rh-negative and (2) the fetus is Rh-positive. For such a circumstance to occur, the father of the fetus must be Rh-positive. Rh incompatibility is a problem that affects the fetus; it causes no harm to the expectant mother during pregnancy.

Rh-negative blood is a recessive trait; therefore, a person must inherit the same gene from both parents to be Rh-negative. Approximately 15% of the white population in the United States is Rh-negative. The incidence is lower in African-Americans and Asians.

PATHOPHYSIOLOGY

People who are Rh-positive have the Rh antigen on their red blood cells, whereas people who are Rh-negative do not have the antigen. When blood from a person who is Rh-positive enters the bloodstream of a person who is Rh-negative, the body reacts as it would to any foreign substance: it develops antibodies to destroy the invading antigen. To destroy the Rh antigen, which exists as part of the red blood cell, the entire red blood cell must be destroyed.

Theoretically, no mixing of fetal and maternal blood occurs during pregnancy. In reality, however, small placental accidents may allow a drop or two of fetal blood to enter the maternal circulation and initiate the production of antibodies to destroy the Rh-positive blood. Sensitization can also occur during a spontaneous or elective abortion or during antepartal procedures such as amniocentesis and chorionic villus sampling. Figure 26–7 illustrates the process of maternal sensitization.

Most exposure of maternal blood to fetal blood occurs during the third stage of labor, when active exchange of fetal and maternal blood can occur as the placenta separates. The woman's first child is usually unaffected because antibodies are formed following the birth of the infant. Subsequent Rh-positive fetuses may be affected, however, unless the mother receives $Rh_o(D)$ immune globulin (RhoGAM) to prevent antibody formation after the birth of each Rh-positive infant.

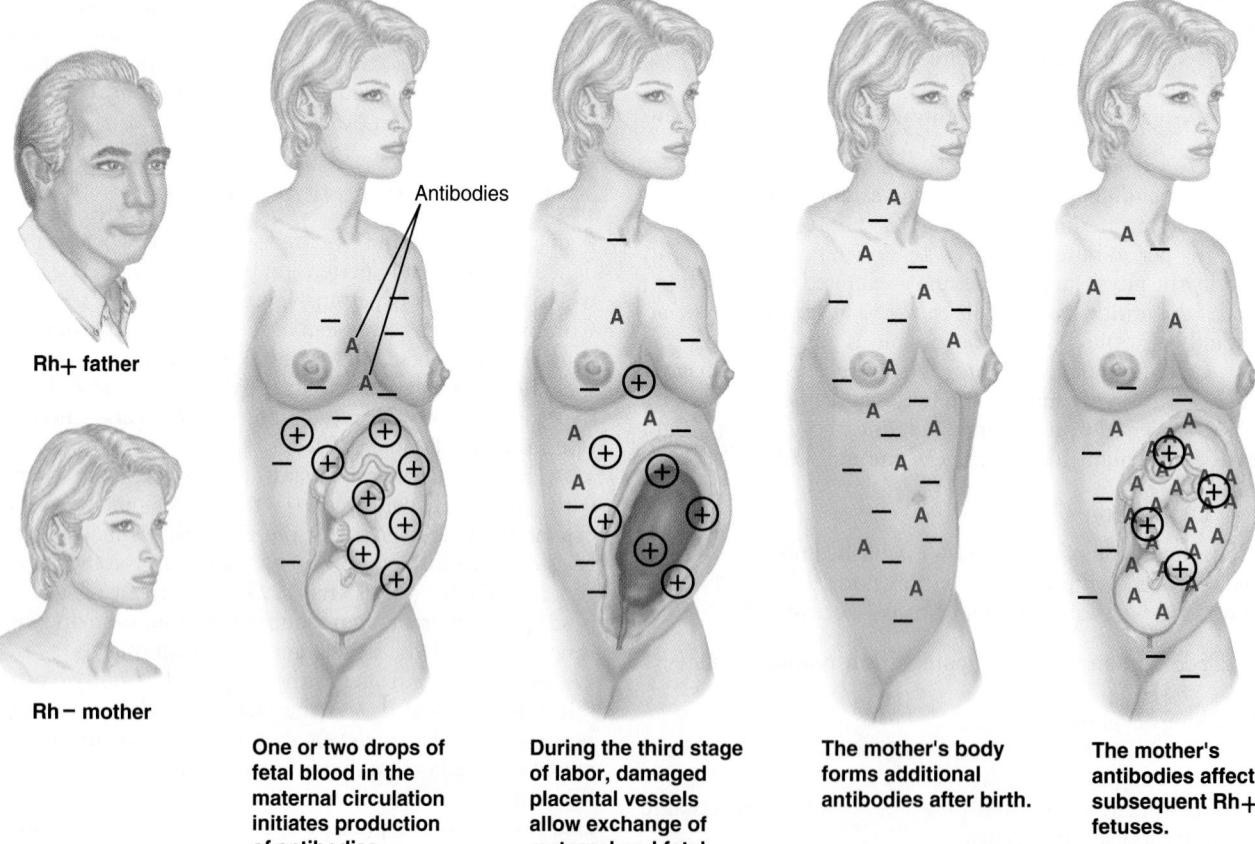

Rh+ father

Rh− mother

Antibodies

One or two drops of fetal blood in the maternal circulation initiates production of antibodies.

During the third stage of labor, damaged placental vessels allow exchange of maternal and fetal blood.

The mother's body forms additional antibodies after birth.

The mother's antibodies affect subsequent Rh+ fetuses.

FIGURE 26–7

The process of maternal sensitization to the Rh factor.

About Rh Incompatibility

What does it mean to be Rh-negative?
Those who are Rh-negative lack a substance that is present in the red blood cells of those who are Rh-positive.

How can the expectant mother be Rh-negative and the fetus be Rh-positive?
The fetus can inherit the Rh-positive factor from the father.

What does sensitization mean?
Sensitization means that the expectant mother has been exposed to Rh-positive blood and has developed antibodies against the Rh factor.

Do the antibodies harm the expectant mother?
No. The mother is unaffected because she does not have the Rh factor.

Do Rh-positive men always father Rh-positive children?
No. Rh-positive men who have an Rh-positive gene and an Rh-negative gene can also father Rh-negative children.

Why is RhoGAM necessary during pregnancy and following childbirth?
RhoGAM prevents the development of Rh antibodies, which might be harmful to subsequent fetuses.

Why will the next fetus be jeopardized if RhoGAM is not administered?
If RhoGAM is not administered when the fetus is Rh-positive, the mother may develop antibodies to fetal Rh-positive blood that crosses the placental barrier. These antibodies may destroy the erythrocytes of the next Rh-positive fetus.

FETAL AND NEONATAL IMPLICATIONS

If antibodies to the Rh factor are present in the expectant mother's blood, they cross the placental barrier and destroy fetal red blood cells. The fetus becomes deficient in red blood cells, which are needed to transport oxygen to fetal tissue. As fetal red blood cells are destroyed, fetal bilirubin levels increase (*icterus gravis*), which can lead to severe neurologic disease (*bilirubin encephalopathy*). This hemolytic process results in rapid production of erythroblasts (immature red blood cells), which cannot carry oxygen. The entire syndrome is termed *erythroblastosis fetalis*. The fetus may become so anemic that generalized fetal edema (*hydrops fetalis*) results and can terminate in fetal congestive heart failure. Management of the infant born with erythroblastosis fetalis is discussed in Chapter 30.

PRENATAL ASSESSMENT AND MANAGEMENT

All pregnant women should have a blood test to determine blood type and Rh factor at the initial prenatal visit. Rh-negative women should have an antibody titer (indirect Coombs test) to determine whether they are sensitized (have developed antibodies) as a result of previous exposure to Rh-positive blood. If the indirect Coombs test is negative, it is repeated at 28 weeks of gestation to identify cases of later sensitization. A negative indirect Coombs test result accurately identifies the fetus as not at risk for hemolytic disease of the newborn.

As a preventive measure, an $Rh_o(D)$ immune globulin (such as RhoGAM) is administered to the unsensitized, Rh-negative woman at 28 weeks of gestation. RhoGAM is a commercial preparation of passive antibodies against Rh factor. It effectively prevents the formation of active antibodies if fetal Rh-positive blood is accidentally transported into the circulation of an Rh-negative mother during the remainder of the pregnancy.

If the indirect Coombs test result is positive—that is, if it indicates maternal sensitization and the presence of antibodies—it is repeated at frequent intervals throughout the pregnancy to determine whether the antibody titer is rising. An increase in titer indicates that the process is continuing and that the fetus will be in jeopardy.

Amniocentesis may be performed to evaluate change in the optical density (ΔOD) of amniotic fluid. This measure reflects the amount of bilirubin (residue of red blood cell destruction) present in the amniotic fluid. If the fluid optical density remains low, it may indicate that the fetus is Rh-positive but in no jeopardy or, more likely, that the fetus is Rh-negative. If the optical density is elevated, indicating fetal jeopardy in a hostile environment, intrauterine transfusion may be planned. If the fetal age is more than 32 weeks, early delivery may provide the best opportunity for survival.

Ultrasound examination is also used to evaluate the condition of the fetus. Generalized fetal edema, ascites, an enlarged heart, or hydramnios indicate serious fetal compromise.

POSTPARTUM MANAGEMENT

If the mother is Rh-negative, umbilical cord blood is taken at delivery to determine blood type, Rh factor, and antibody titer (direct Coombs test) of the newborn. Rh-negative, unsensitized mothers who give birth to Rh-positive infants are given an intramuscular injection of RhoGAM within 72 hours following delivery. If RhoGAM is given to the mother in the first 72 hours following delivery of an Rh-positive infant, any Rh antigens present are destroyed, and therefore the mother does not form natural, permanent antibodies.

If the infant is Rh-negative, there is no possibility of antibody formation, and RhoGAM is not necessary. RhoGAM is also administered following abortion, chorionic villus sampling, and amniocentesis when fetal-to-maternal transfusion is possible, and at 28 weeks of gestation if the mother is Rh-negative and unsensitized.

Families are often very concerned about the fetus. Nurses must be sensitive to cues and signals that indicate that the family is anxious, and must be able to offer honest reassurance. This is especially important if the expectant mother is sensitized and fetal testing is necessary throughout pregnancy.

At birth, the physician or nurse should collect cord blood to determine the blood type and Rh factor of the

Rh₀(D) Immune Globulin (RhoGAM, HypRhoD, Gamulin Rh)

Classification: Concentrated immuno-globulins directed toward the red blood cell antigen Rh₀(D).

Action: Prevents production of anti-Rh₀(D) antibodies in Rh-negative women who have been exposed to Rh-positive blood by suppressing the immune reaction of the Rh-negative woman to the antigen in Rh-positive blood. Prevents antibody response and subsequently prevents hemolytic disease of the newborn in future pregnancies of women who have conceived an Rh-positive fetus.

Indications: Administered to Rh-negative women who have been exposed to Rh-positive blood by

- Delivering an Rh-positive infant
- Aborting an Rh-positive fetus
- Having chorionic villus sampling, amniocentesis, or intra-abdominal trauma while carrying an Rh-positive fetus

- Accidental transfusion of Rh-positive blood to an Rh-negative woman

Dosage and Route
One *standard dose* administered intramuscularly:

- At 28 weeks of pregnancy and within 72 hours of delivery
- Within 72 hours following the termination of a pregnancy of 13 weeks or more of gestation

One *microdose* within 72 hours following the termination of a pregnancy of less than 13 weeks' gestation.

After accidental transfusion, dosage is calculated based on the volume of blood erroneously administered.

Absorption
Well absorbed from intramuscular sites.

Excretion
Metabolism and excretion unknown.

Contraindications and Precautions: Women who are Rh-positive or women previously sensitized to Rh₀(D) should not receive Rh₀(D) immune globulin. Used cautiously for women with previous hypersensitivity reactions to immune globulins.

Adverse Reactions: Local pain at intramuscular site, fever, or both.

Nursing Implications: Type and cross-match of mother's blood and cord blood of the newborn must be performed to determine the need for the medication. The mother must be Rh-negative and negative for Rh antibodies; the newborn must be Rh-positive. If there is doubt regarding the fetus's blood type following termination of pregnancy, the medication should be administered. The drug is administered to the mother, not the infant. The deltoid muscle is recommended for intramuscular administration.

---

newborn. During the postpartum period, nurses are responsible for follow-up to determine whether RhoGAM is necessary and to administer the injection within the prescribed time.

ABO Incompatibility

ABO incompatibility occurs when the expectant mother is blood type O and the fetus is blood type A, B, or AB. Blood types A, B, and AB contain a protein component (antigen) that is not present in type O blood.

People with type O blood develop anti-A or anti-B antibodies naturally as a result of exposure to antigens in the foods that they eat or to infection by gram-negative bacteria. As a result, some women with type O blood have developed high serum anti-A and anti-B antibody titers before pregnancy. The antibodies may be either IgG or IgM. When the woman becomes pregnant, the IgG antibodies cross the placental barrier and cause hemolysis of fetal red blood cells. Although the first fetus can be affected, ABO incompatibility is less severe than Rh incompatibility because the primary antibodies of the ABO system are IgM, which do not cross the placenta.

No specific prenatal care is needed, but the nurse must be aware of the possibility of ABO incompatibility. At birth, cord blood is taken to determine the blood type of the newborn and the antibody titer (direct Coombs test). The newborn is carefully screened for jaundice, which indicates hyperbilirubinemia. See Chapter 30 for medical and nursing management of hyperbilirubinemia in newborns.

▮ Concurrent Disorders During Pregnancy

Pregnancy may alter the course of a concurrent disease, or a disease and its treatment may have unwanted effects on the pregnancy. As a result, the usual antepartum care must be adapted to include increased surveillance of the mother and the fetus. Moreover, some disorders that are mild or even subclinical in the pregnant woman can cause massive damage to a fetus.

▮ Diabetes Mellitus

Pathophysiology

ETIOLOGY

Diabetes mellitus is a complex disorder of carbohydrate metabolism caused primarily by a partial or complete lack of insulin secretion by the beta cells of the pancreas. Some cells, such as those in skeletal and cardiac muscles and in adipose tissue, require insulin to carry glucose across the cell membranes. Without insulin, glucose accumulates in the blood, resulting in hyperglycemia. The body attempts to dilute the glucose load by any means possible. The first strategy is to increase thirst (*polydipsia*), one of the classic symptoms of diabetes mellitus. Next, fluid from the intracellular spaces is drawn into the vascular bed, resulting in dehydration at the cellular level but fluid volume excess in the vascular compartment. The kidneys attempt to excrete large volumes of this fluid plus the heavy solute load of glucose (osmotic diuresis). This excretion produces the second sign of diabetes, *polyuria*, as well as *glycosuria* (glucose in the urine). Without glucose, the cells starve, so weight loss occurs even though the person ingests large amounts of food (*polyphagia*).

Because the body is unable to metabolize glucose, it begins to metabolize protein and fat to meet energy needs. Metabolism of protein produces a negative nitrogen balance, and the metabolism of fat results in the buildup of ketone bodies (such as acetone, acetoacetic acid, or beta-hydroxybutyric acid) or ketosis (accumulation of acids in the body).

If the disease is not well controlled, serious complications may occur. Hypoglycemia or hyperglycemia can result if the amount of insulin does not match the diet. Moreover, fluctuating periods of hyperglycemia and hypoglycemia damage small blood vessels throughout the body. This damage can cause serious impairment, especially in the kidneys, eyes, and heart.

EFFECT OF PREGNANCY ON FUEL METABOLISM

To comprehend the relationship of diabetes mellitus and pregnancy, it is necessary to understand how pregnancy and diabetes alter the metabolism of food.

Early Pregnancy. Metabolic changes can be divided into those that occur early in pregnancy (from 1 to 20 weeks) and those that occur late in pregnancy (from 20 to 40 weeks). During early pregnancy, maternal metabolic rates and energy needs change little. During this time, however, insulin release in response to serum glucose levels increases. As a result, significant hypoglycemia may occur, particularly in women who experience the nausea, vomiting, and anorexia that often occur during the first weeks of pregnancy.

In an uncomplicated pregnancy, the availability of glucose and insulin favors the development and storage of fat during the first half of pregnancy. Accumulation of fat prepares the mother for the rise in energy use by the growing fetus during the second half of pregnancy.

Late Pregnancy. During the second half of pregnancy, when fetal growth accelerates, levels of placental hormones rise sharply. These hormones, particularly estrogen, progesterone, and human placental lactogen, create resistance to insulin in maternal cells to provide an abundant supply of glucose for the fetus. The hormones have a diabetogenic effect, however, in that they may leave the woman with insufficient insulin and episodes of hyperglycemia.

For most women, insulin resistance is not a problem. The pancreas responds by simply increasing the production of insulin. If the pancreas is unable to respond, however, the woman will experience periods of hyperglycemia.

During late pregnancy, the fetus continuously withdraws nutrients, such as glucose and amino acids, from maternal blood. The result is an earlier than normal switch from carbohydrate metabolism to gluconeogenesis (formation of glycogen from noncarbohydrate sources such as proteins and fat). Because the fetus uses many of the amino acids, the process becomes predominantly one of fat utilization. This process produces high levels of free fatty acids that further inhibit the uptake and oxidation of glucose and thus preserve glucose for use by the central nervous system

and the fetus. These metabolic changes are similar to those that occur during "accelerated starvation," when fat is metabolized to meet the body's energy needs.

Classification

Diabetes is classified as type 1 (insulin dependent) or type 2 (non-insulin dependent) according to whether the client requires the administration of insulin to prevent ketoacidosis. The onset of glucose intolerance during pregnancy is *gestational diabetes*. About 90% of the cases of diabetes during pregnancy are gestational diabetes.

Incidence

One of every 200 pregnant women has preexisting diabetes (type 1 or type 2). Five of every 200 pregnant women will develop gestational diabetes (Reece, 1996).

Preexisting Diabetes Mellitus

MATERNAL EFFECTS

The risk of pregnancy-induced hypertension is four times greater in the woman with diabetes than in the normal population, even in the absence of vascular or renal complications (Cunningham et al., 1997). The development of ketoacidosis is a threat to women with insulin-dependent diabetes and is most often precipitated by infection or missed insulin doses. Moreover, ketoacidosis may develop during pregnancy at lower thresholds of hyperglycemia than those seen in nonpregnant individuals. Untreated ketoacidosis can progress to fetal and maternal death.

Urinary tract infections are more common, possibly because glucose-rich urine provides a good medium for bacterial growth. Other effects include hydramnios, which may result from fetal hyperglycemia and consequent fetal diuresis, and premature rupture of membranes, which may be caused by overdistension of the uterus by hydramnios or a large fetus. A difficult labor, shoulder dystocia (delayed or difficult birth of fetal shoulders after the head is born), and injury to the birth canal are more likely if the fetus is large. Large fetal size also increases the likelihood that a cesarean birth will be necessary and increases the risk of postpartum hemorrhage.

• • • • • • • • • • •

Classification of Diabetes Mellitus

Type 1, Insulin Dependent. Onset in childhood or young adulthood. Involves autoimmune destruction of pancreatic beta cells. Prone to ketosis.

Type 2, Non-Insulin Dependent. Usual onset after 40 years. Associated with obesity. Insulin resistance usually sufficient to prevent ketosis.

Gestational. Onset of glucose intolerance first diagnosed during pregnancy. Exogenous insulin may or may not be needed.

Data from American Diabetes Association. (1999). American Diabetes Association: Clinical practice recommendations 1999. *Diabetes Care, 22*(Suppl. 1).

FETAL EFFECTS

Fetal and neonatal effects of preexisting diabetes depend on the timing and severity of maternal hyperglycemia and the degree of maternal vascular impairment. During the first trimester, when major fetal organ development is occurring, the effects of the abnormal metabolic environment, such as hypoglycemia, hyperglycemia, and ketosis, may lead to an increased incidence of spontaneous abortion or major fetal malformations.

Congenital Malformation. The most common major congenital malformations associated with preexisting diabetes are neural tube defects, caudal regression syndrome, and cardiac defects. Major malformations have been reported in 4% to 11% of infants born to mothers with type 1 diabetes, compared with only 1.2% to 2.1% of infants of nondiabetic mothers (Healy, Jovanovic-Peterson, & Peterson, 1995). Fewer malformations occur if the woman maintains a normal and stable blood glucose level before conception and throughout early pregnancy.

Variations in Fetal Size. Fetal growth is related to maternal vascular integrity. In women without vascular impairment, glucose and oxygen are easily transported to the fetus; if the woman is hyperglycemic, so is the fetus. Although maternal insulin does not cross the placental barrier, the fetus produces insulin by the tenth week of gestation. Fetal macrosomia results when elevated levels of blood glucose stimulate excessive production of fetal insulin, which acts as a powerful growth hormone. Macrosomia increases the likelihood of cesarean birth or birth injury from shoulder dystocia.

Conversely, placental perfusion may be decreased with vascular impairment. Vascular impairment may be caused by complications of the diabetes or by vasoconstriction that occurs in pregnancy-induced hypertension, a common added complication for the woman with diabetes. When placental perfusion is impaired, the supply of glucose as well as oxygen will be decreased. As a result, the infant is likely to be small for gestational age (intrauterine fetal growth restriction).

NEONATAL EFFECTS

The four major neonatal complications of preexisting diabetes are hypoglycemia, hypocalcemia, hyperbilirubinemia, and respiratory distress syndrome.

Hypoglycemia. The neonate is at higher risk for hypoglycemia because fetal insulin production was accelerated during pregnancy to metabolize excessive glucose received from the expectant mother. The constant stimulation of hyperglycemia leads to hyperplasia and hypertrophy of the islets of Langerhans in the pancreas. At birth, when the maternal glucose supply is withdrawn, the level of neonatal insulin exceeds the available glucose, and hypoglycemia develops rapidly.

Hypocalcemia. During the last half of pregnancy, large amounts of calcium are transported across the placenta from the mother to the fetus. At the time of birth, this transfer is abruptly stopped, leading to a dramatic decrease in total and ionized calcium. Hypocalcemia, defined as a calcium concentration of 7 mg/dl or less, most often occurs between 24 and 36 hours after birth (Tyrala, 1996). It is associated with preterm birth, birth trauma, and perinatal asphyxia, all common problems of the infant born to a mother with diabetes mellitus. Reduced fetal parathyroid function may also play a role (Moore, 1999).

Hyperbilirubinemia. The fetus who experiences recurrent hypoxia due to maternal vascular impairment compensates by producing additional erythrocytes to carry oxygen supplied by the mother. After birth, the excess in erythrocytes is broken down, releasing large amounts of bilirubin into the neonate's circulation.

Respiratory Distress Syndrome. Fetal hyperinsulinemia retards cortisol production, which is necessary for synthesis of surfactant (lipoproteins that prevent collapse of alveoli), and the inadequate production of surfactant increases the risk that the newborn will experience respiratory distress syndrome. (See Chapters 29 and 30 for additional information about neonatal complications.)

The occurrence of maternal and fetal-neonatal complications can be greatly diminished if the mother maintains normal and stable blood glucose levels throughout pregnancy. The objective of the team providing treatment is to devise a plan that allows the woman to maintain a blood glucose level as close to normal as possible (see Nursing Care Plan 26–3).

MATERNAL ASSESSMENT

The initial prenatal assessment for the woman with preexisting diabetes includes a history, physical examination, and laboratory tests.

History. A detailed history should include the onset and management of the diabetic condition. How long has she had the disease? How does she maintain normal blood glucose levels? Can she monitor her blood glucose level and self-administer insulin? The degree of glycemic control before pregnancy is of particular interest. Effective management depends on her adherence to a plan of care. Therefore, her knowledge of how diabetes and pregnancy interact must be determined. Her support person's knowledge also must be assessed, and specific learning needs should be identified. In addition, the woman's emotional status should be assessed to determine how she is coping with pregnancy superimposed on preexisting diabetes.

All women with diabetes should be seen by a qualified nurse educator for an individualized assessment to ensure that they can monitor blood glucose accurately. Accurate readings depend on performing the test correctly and as often as recommended by the health care team. In addition to home monitoring of blood glucose levels, the nurse must observe the woman's skill in mixing and administering insulin.

Physical Examination. In addition to routine prenatal examination (see Chapter 13), specific efforts should be made to assess the effects of diabetes. A baseline electrocardiogram (ECG) determines cardiovascular status. Evaluation for retinopathy should be performed, with referral to an ophthalmologist if necessary. The woman's weight and blood pressure must be monitored carefully because of the increased risk for the development of pregnancy-induced hypertension. Fundal height should be measured, noting any abnormal increase in size that may indicate macrosomia or hydramnios. Reduced growth in fundal height suggests intrauterine growth restriction associated with maternal vascular impairment.

NURSING CARE PLAN 26-3

Pregnancy and Diabetes Mellitus

Assessment	Kathy Ringold is a 24-year-old primigravida carrying a fetus of 9 weeks' gestation; she was diagnosed with type 1 diabetes mellitus 6 years ago. She has been on a daily regimen of insulin and is comfortable with insulin administration and blood glucose monitoring. She is experiencing daily nausea and vomiting. Kathy states that she is concerned because she is not eating as much as before becoming pregnant. She also reveals that she had sometimes "binged" on food before becoming pregnant and didn't always monitor blood glucose as often as directed. She does not see why her blood glucose has to be watched so carefully.
Nursing Diagnosis	Risk for Altered Health Maintenance related to knowledge deficit of the effects of pregnancy on diabetes control.
Goals/Expected Outcomes	Kathy will

Kathy will

- Describe predicted changes in insulin needs throughout pregnancy.
- Follow prescribed schedule of blood glucose monitoring, insulin administration, diet, and exercise.
- Describe the importance of frequent fetal surveillance and follow the prescribed schedule.

Intervention	Rationale

1. Reduce barriers to learning
  a. Allow Kathy to express emotions and concerns before teaching.
  b. Examine her beliefs and past experiences related to diabetes.
  c. Assess readiness to learn, based on interest, attention, and participation in scheduled learning sessions.
	1. Motivation and readiness to learn are essential for permanent learning to occur. Kathy will learn only if she sees the value of the information.

2. Instruct Kathy about the predicted changes in diabetes management during pregnancy.
  a. Explain the importance of blood glucose testing; Kathy will need less insulin because of the nausea and vomiting occurring in the first trimester.
  b. Emphasize that she will probably need more insulin during the second and third trimesters because of the effects of the placental hormones.
  c. Describe the importance of following the prescribed diet and exercise regimen to maintain normal blood glucose levels.
	2. Behaviors change when learning occurs. Understanding how insulin needs change throughout pregnancy, labor, and the postpartum period increases the likelihood that Kathy will follow the recommended regimen.

3. Inform Kathy about specific fetal surveillance techniques recommended during pregnancy (serial nonstress tests, contraction stress tests, biophysical profiles) and explain the importance of the tests.	3. Some frequently ordered tests are time-consuming and expensive. The woman is more likely to comply if she understands the importance of monitoring the fetal condition at frequent intervals.
4. Allow time for Kathy to focus on her feelings and concerns at each teaching session; offer praise and encouragement for her adherence to the prescribed regimen.	4. Motivation to comply with the regimen is strengthened by praise and the awareness that the woman's feelings are important.
5. Explain in simple, positive terms the advantages to the fetus of maintaining a normal maternal blood glucose level. These advantages include an optimal pattern of growth, the increased likelihood that the baby will be born near term, and fewer complications associated with prematurity.	5. Understanding that the fetus benefits when maternal glucose levels are normal reduces anxiety and increases the likelihood that the mother will comply with recommended treatment.
6. Review the recommended plan for diet and exercise during pregnancy and determine whether Kathy knows the importance of these factors in her care.	6. Maintenance of normal blood glucose depends on coordinating the amount of food, insulin, and exercise. If any of these factors is altered, the others must also be altered to prevent hypoglycemia or hyperglycemia.

(continued)

NURSING CARE PLAN 26-3 *Continued*

Pregnancy and Diabetes Mellitus

Evaluation	Kathy verbalizes her understanding of changing insulin needs and the importance of glucose monitoring. She states that she feels in better control of the diabetes and plans to comply with the recommended schedule of fetal surveillance, diet, and exercise.
Assessment	At 32 weeks' gestation, Kathy's blood glucose is consistently above the desired level, and daily nonstress tests are prescribed. The tests are reactive, indicating no present fetal compromise. Kathy, however, verbalizes anxiety about the condition of the fetus and asks when it will be safe for the baby to be born.
Nursing Diagnosis	Anxiety related to perceived threat to the health of the fetus and lack of knowledge about the timing of the delivery.
Goals/Expected Outcomes	Kathy will

- Relate her perception of the condition of the fetus and the significance of the reactive nonstress test as the tests are performed.
- Describe her concerns about the timing of the delivery at the conclusion of the next nonstress test.

Intervention	**Rationale**
1. Ask Kathy to describe her concern about the fetus and to clarify her feelings.	1. Kathy's concerns must be identified and clarified so that misconceptions do not occur.
2. Explain that a reactive nonstress test indicates that the fetal heart rate accelerates whenever the fetus moves; this is a good sign that the fetus is not in immediate jeopardy.	2. Reassurance that the fetus is not in jeopardy and that the daily tests will detect early signs if a problem develops reduces anxiety about the fetal condition.
3. Ask Kathy how she feels about the labor and delivery; determine whether she is taking childbirth education classes and whether she has selected her coach.	3. It is normal for women to become concerned about the birth process and how they will cope with labor during the last few weeks of pregnancy. Medical professionals sometimes neglect the need for normal pregnancy care for women with high-risk pregnancies.
4. Assist Kathy in investigating a childbirth education class if she has not done so previously, and suggest that she and her coach begin classes.	4. Knowledge learned at childbirth classes may reduce the anxiety about the birth processes.
5. Acknowledge that the prospect of labor and delivery causes many women some anxiety, even when the condition of the infant is not in question.	5. Knowledge that her feelings are common to most women may provide some relief from anxiety.

Evaluation	Kathy says she is reassured by explanations regarding the reactive nonstress test but is concerned about how she will do in labor. She initiates plans to attend a childbirth education class with her sister as the coach.

Additional Nursing Diagnoses to Consider

Risk for Altered Family Processes
Risk for Altered Parenting
Risk for Injury

Laboratory Tests. In addition to routine prenatal laboratory examinations, baseline renal function should be assessed with a 24-hour urine collection for total protein excretion and creatinine clearance. The urine should be checked at each prenatal visit for possible urinary tract infections and for the presence of glucose and ketones. Thyroid function tests should be performed because of the risk for coexisting thyroid disease.

Glycemic control should be evaluated on the basis of *glycosylated hemoglobin*. With prolonged hyperglycemia, a percentage of hemoglobin will remain saturated with glucose for the life of the red blood cell. The glycosylated hemoglobin assay (HbA$_{1c}$) is an accurate measurement of the average glucose concentrations during the preceding 4 to 8 weeks (Homko & Khandelwal, 1996). Unlike other tests, which reflect the amount of glucose in the plasma at that moment, the HbA$_{1c}$ assay result is not affected by recent intake or restriction of food.

FETAL SURVEILLANCE

Because of the increased risk for congenital anomalies, fetal surveillance should begin early for women with preexisting diabetes mellitus. Testing for anomalies includes determining the maternal serum alpha-fetoprotein concentration at 16 weeks to identify possible neural tube or other open defects, and performing ultrasonography and fetal echocardiography at 20 to 22 weeks to determine the integrity of the fetal body and cardiac structure (Moore, 1999).

During the third trimester, fetal surveillance includes maternal assessment of fetal movement ("kick counts"), nonstress tests, contraction stress tests, and biophysical profiles. Ultrasonography is also used to document fetal growth rates. Doppler velocimetry may be recommended if vascular complications exist or if hypertension develops. See Chapter 16 for a complete description of fetal diagnostic procedures.

THERAPEUTIC MANAGEMENT

The goals of therapeutic management for a pregnant woman with diabetes are (1) to maintain normal and stable maternal blood glucose levels, (2) to increase the likelihood that the baby will be born healthy, and (3) to avoid accelerated impairment of blood vessels and other major organs. Pregnant women with diabetes are cared for by a team, which may include a diabetologist, who assists in regulation of maternal blood glucose, a perinatologist, who monitors the mother and fetus and determines the optimal time for birth, a dietitian, who provides a balanced meal plan that considers the woman's individual needs, and a nurse, who provides ongoing education and support. The team is completed by a neonatologist, who will care for the newborn, and by the family physician and the pediatrician, who will provide ongoing care for the infant and mother after birth.

Preconception Care. Ideally, care should begin before conception. Both prospective parents should participate in care sessions to learn more about the following issues:

- Establishing the optimal time for pregnancy, based on maintenance of normal maternal blood glucose levels, to reduce the risk of major fetal malformations
- Evaluating the degree of maternal vascular complications
- Understanding the importance of maintaining normal blood glucose levels throughout the pregnancy
- Correctly performing home glucose monitoring techniques

Diet. The average daily intake for the pregnant woman with diabetes ranges from 2,200 to 2,400 calories per day. Approximately 50% to 60% of the calories should be from carbohydrates, 12% to 20% from protein, and the remaining calories from fat (ACOG, 1994). Caloric intake should be distributed among three meals and two to four snacks. Women who are less active or who gain excessive weight need fewer calories.

Self-Monitoring of Blood Glucose. A typical glucose monitoring schedule consists of six checks: on rising, 2 hours after breakfast, before and after lunch, before dinner, and at bedtime (Moore, 1999). In addition to regular monitoring, the woman should also perform a glucose test whenever she experiences symptoms of hypoglycemia. The woman should record all test results on a log sheet for review by the health care provider at each visit.

Insulin Therapy. The need to maintain rigorous control of maternal metabolism during pregnancy requires more frequent doses of insulin than usual. Most treatment regimens rely on three daily injections, with a combination of short-acting (regular or lispro [Humalog]) insulin and intermediate-acting (NPH) insulin given before breakfast, regular insulin before dinner, and NPH insulin at bedtime. Lispro acts more quickly than regular insulin and should be injected just before a meal. Lispro reduces postprandial hyperglycemia but is less likely to cause between-meals hypoglycemia (Moore, 1999). Because placental hormones cause insulin needs to change throughout pregnancy, insulin coverage will need to be adjusted as pregnancy progresses.

First Trimester. Insulin needs generally decline during the first trimester because the secretion of placental hormones that are antagonistic to insulin remains low during this time. The woman may also experience nausea, vomiting, and anorexia, resulting in decreased intake of food, and thus may need less insulin. Moreover, the fetus receives its share of glucose, which reduces maternal plasma glucose levels and decreases the need for maternal insulin.

Second and Third Trimesters. Insulin needs increase markedly during the second and third trimesters, when placental hormones, which initiate maternal resistance to the effects of insulin, reach their peak. The nausea of early pregnancy usually resolves, and the woman needs 300 additional calories per day to meet the increased metabolic demands of pregnancy.

During Labor. Insulin needs during labor are based on the blood glucose level. The vigorous muscular exertion and lack of oral intake should decrease the amount of insulin needed. Intravenous glucose, however, is sometimes given, making it necessary to administer insulin. Hourly glucose monitoring allows adjustment of the insulin dosage and intravenous infusion to maintain the blood glucose level between 70 and 100 mg/dl (Kitzmiller & Davidson, 1998). Tight glucose control during labor is needed to reduce neonatal hypoglycemia.

Postpartum. Insulin needs should decline rapidly after delivery of the placenta and the abrupt cessation of placental hormones. Blood glucose levels should be monitored at least four times daily, however, so that the insulin dose can be adjusted to meet individual needs.

Timing of Delivery. The pregnancy should be allowed to progress to term, if possible, so that the fetal lungs can mature, reducing the risk of neonatal respiratory distress syndrome. With evidence of fetal compromise, such as nonreactive nonstress tests or late decelerations on a contraction stress test, amniocentesis may be done to evaluate fetal lung maturity by a lecithin/sphingomyelin (LS) ratio and presence of phosphatidylglycerol (PG) in the amniotic fluid (ACOG, 1994; Moore, 1999).

Gestational Diabetes Mellitus

RISK FACTORS

Gestational diabetes is a carbohydrate intolerance of variable severity that develops or is first recognized during pregnancy. Factors known to increase the risk for gestational diabetes include the following:

- Obesity (more than 90 kg or 198 lb)
- Chronic hypertension
- Maternal age older than 25 years
- Family history of diabetes
- Previous birth of a large infant (more than 4,000 g)
- Previous birth of an infant with unexplained congenital anomalies
- Previous unexplained fetal death
- Gestational diabetes in previous pregnancy

IDENTIFYING GESTATIONAL DIABETES MELLITUS

Glucose Challenge Test. Depending on the setting, all pregnant women may be screened with a 50-g, 1-hour glucose challenge test (GCT) between 24 and 28 weeks of pregnancy, or only those having risk factors may be screened (AAP & ACOG, 1997). The woman does not need to fast, and the test does not follow a meal. The woman should ingest 50 g of oral glucose solution; 1 hour later a blood sample should be taken. If the blood glucose concentration is 140 mg/dl or greater, a 3-hour oral glucose tolerance test (OGTT) is recommended (ACOG, 1994). Some practitioners use a lower cutoff of 130 mg/dl (Kendrick, 1999). A result of 200 mg/dl on the GCT is diagnostic for gestational diabetes and does not require further testing (Kendrick, 1999).

Oral Glucose Tolerance Test. The OGTT is diagnostic for diabetes mellitus. Although it is the gold standard for diagnosing diabetes, it is a more complicated test. The woman must ingest a high-carbohydrate diet for 2 days before the scheduled test and must fast from midnight before the day of the test. After a fasting plasma glucose level is determined, the woman should ingest 100 g of oral glucose solution. Plasma glucose levels should be determined at 1, 2, and 3 hours. Gestational diabetes is the diagnosis if the fasting blood glucose level is abnormal or if two or more of the following values occur on the OGTT (ACOG, 1994):

- Fasting, greater than 105 mg/dl
- 1 hour, greater than 190 mg/dl
- 2 hours, greater than 165 mg/dl
- 3 hours, greater than 145 mg/dl

MATERNAL, FETAL, AND NEONATAL EFFECTS

With a few important exceptions, the effects of gestational diabetes are similar to those associated with preexisting diabetes. The differences are that gestational diabetes is not associated with an increased risk for ketoacidosis or spontaneous abortion. Because gestational diabetes develops after the first trimester, which is the critical period of major fetal organ development (organogenesis), it is not usually associated with an increase in the incidence of major congenital malformations. Nevertheless, gestational diabetes, characterized by maternal hyperglycemia during the third trimester, is associated with increased neonatal morbidity and mortality. The major fetal complications are macrosomia, leading to birth injuries or making cesarean birth necessary, and neonatal hypoglycemia. Other problems, such as hypocalcemia, hyperbilirubinemia, and respiratory distress, may also occur. Table 26–5 summarizes maternal, fetal, and neonatal effects of diabetes mellitus and their probable causes.

THERAPEUTIC MANAGEMENT

Diet. The diet should provide the calories and nutrients needed for maternal and fetal health, result in euglycemia, and prevent ketosis due to inadequate carbohydrate intake. Calories should be distributed in a way similar to that for preexisting diabetes. Simple sugars found in concentrated sweets should be eliminated from the diet. Calories should be divided among three meals and at least three snacks (Kitzmiller & Davidson, 1998).

Exercise. Exercise plays a significant role in managing blood glucose levels in women who develop gestational diabetes and in women with type 2 diabetes who become pregnant. A contracting skeletal muscle increases its glucose uptake and helps regulate glucose transport. Moderate exercise for active women and regular activity for sedentary women help normalize blood glucose levels (Artal, 1996). The exercise regimen should be recommended by a physician who takes into account each woman's risk factors and risks to the fetus.

Glucose Level Monitoring. Blood glucose levels should be evaluated to determine if glucose levels are normal. The most common methods are *fasting blood sugar* (no food for the previous 4 hours) and *postprandial blood sugar* (2 hours after a meal). The American College of Obstetricians and Gynecologists (1994) recommends that fasting blood glucose be maintained below 105 mg/dl and that postprandial levels be less than 120 mg/dl. Insulin is recommended if levels repeatedly exceed these thresholds (Buchanan & Coustan, 1995).

Fetal Surveillance. Women with diet-controlled gestational diabetes who maintain normal fasting and postprandial glucose values are at low risk for fetal death (Landon & Gabbe, 1996). Maternal assessment of fetal activity, or "kick counts," however, is often initiated during the last trimester. In addition, antepartum fetal testing is usually initiated if (1) the mother needs insulin, (2) hypertension develops, or (3) there is a history of a previous stillbirth. The most common fetal surveillance techniques used during the third trimester include "kick counts," the nonstress test, the amniotic fluid index, and a biophysical profile (see Chapter 16).

NURSING CONSIDERATIONS

The care of a pregnant woman with diabetes mellitus focuses primarily on helping her maintain normal blood glucose levels. Some women respond calmly to the intense medical supervision; others respond with anxiety, fear, denial, or anger and feel inadequate or unable to control the diabetes to the degree expected by the health care team.

TABLE 26–5

Major Effects of Diabetes Mellitus on Pregnancy

Increased Maternal Risks	Probable Cause
Pregnancy-induced hypertension	Unknown but increased even without renal or vascular impairment
Urinary tract infections	Increased bacterial growth in nutrient-rich urine
Hydramnios	Fetal osmotic diuresis caused by hyperglycemia
Ketoacidosis	Uncontrolled hyperglycemia or infection
Preterm labor and premature rupture of membranes	Overdistension of uterus caused by hydramnios and fetal macrosomia
Difficult labor, injury to birth canal, cesarean birth, and postpartum hemorrhage	Fetal macrosomia and overdistension of uterus

Increased Fetal and Neonatal Risks	Probable Cause
Perinatal death	Poor placental perfusion because of maternal vascular impairment
Congenital anomalies	Maternal hyperglycemia in first trimester
Macrosomia (>4,000 g)	Fetal hyperglycemia stimulating production of insulin to metabolize carbohydrates; excess nutrients transported to fetus
Birth injury	Large fetal size
Intrauterine fetal growth restriction	Maternal vascular impairment
Polycythemia	Fetal hypoxemia stimulating erythrocyte production
Hyperbilirubinemia	Breakdown of excessive red blood cells after birth
Hypoglycemia	Neonatal hyperinsulinemia after birth when maternal glucose is no longer available (but insulin production remains high)
Hypocalcemia	Transfer of calcium abruptly stopped at birth, reduced fetal parathyroid function
Respiratory distress syndrome	Inadequate production of pulmonary surfactant

Increasing Effective Communication.   Nurses must ask specifically about the feelings and concerns the woman and her family have about the pregnancy.

> Broad opening questions, such as "What are your major concerns?" and "How do you feel about the plan of care?" are helpful. These should be followed with more specific questions, such as "How do you feel about the fetal testing?" and "What would you like to change about your diet?"

The nurse must be an active listener and allow time for the woman and her family to express concerns and feelings. The nurse must convey acceptance of feelings that are expressed, whether they are negative or positive. Sharing of emotions will help the woman avoid unnecessary guilt, anxiety, or frustration and thus promote positive feelings about her ability to participate successfully in her plan of care.

Most women benefit from praise when diabetic control is well maintained. They feel competent and trusted by the health care team and are motivated to continue their efforts.

Providing Opportunities for Control.   Allowing the woman to make as many decisions as possible increases her sense of being in control. For instance, she can select foods from the exchange list that provide the necessary nutrients but still allow her some choice. She may also develop a regular schedule of exercise and sleep that helps to keep the blood glucose level under control. Nurses should allow as much flexibility as possible when scheduling stressful events, such as fetal monitoring tests and amniocentesis.

Providing Normal Pregnancy Care.   The nurse caring for a woman with diabetes should provide education and counseling regarding normal pregnancy changes and discomforts. Also, because women with diabetes are concerned about how they will manage during labor and delivery, nurses should offer childbirth preparation classes and discuss with them the experiences common to all pregnant women.

CRITICAL THINKING EXERCISE 26-2

Marcia Mahoney, a 28-year-old primigravida, is diagnosed with gestational diabetes in her 30th week of pregnancy. The health care team provides her with a diet and exercise regimen and tells her that she will need weekly tests to monitor her condition and that of the fetus. Although Marcia accepts the information without comment, she does not keep the next scheduled appointment.

1. What assumptions has the health care team made?
2. What could the team have done to ensure Marcia's compliance with the recommendations?

Marcia is located and agrees to return to the clinic for follow-up care. She states she does not "see what all the fuss is about." She understands she may have a large baby but states that her mother had a 10-lb baby who did just fine. She wonders if the weekly tests are necessary and if they could harm the baby.

3. How can the nurse respond to Marcia's comments about having a large baby without frightening her?
4. How can the nurse explain the necessity for weekly nonstress tests?

NURSING CARE

The Pregnant Woman with Diabetes Mellitus

Assessment

Determine how well the woman understands the prescribed management and how the family plans to carry out the recommended regimen. She may be newly diagnosed and may have no experience in the necessary skills and procedures. On the other hand, she may be skilled in monitoring glucose levels and administering insulin but may have no knowledge of the effects of diabetes on pregnancy or the effects of pregnancy on diabetes management.

To determine whether her techniques are accurate, ask the expectant mother to demonstrate how she monitors her blood glucose level and observe how she mixes and injects insulins. Verify that she and her family are aware of the need to select appropriate sites and injection techniques.

Although diet is prescribed by a dietitian, it is necessary to assess how well the family understands the diet. Identify any special problems with food preferences or the availability of recommended foods. It may be necessary to review the exchange list and ask the woman how she plans to substitute and exchange foods.

Identify the woman's knowledge of potential complications, such as hypoglycemia and hyperglycemia, so that she and her family can be provided with pertinent information.

Determine her knowledge of fetal surveillance techniques and her response to the need for frequent tests. Some women are highly motivated to continue the treatment regimen when test results indicate the fetus is thriving. Other women dread the tests and are puzzled by the need for such frequent testing.

Nursing Diagnosis and Planning

One of the most common nursing diagnoses is

■ Risk for Altered Health Maintenance related to knowledge deficit of specific measures to maintain normal blood glucose levels; signs, symptoms, and management of hypoglycemia and hyperglycemia; and recommended fetal surveillance procedures.

Expected Outcomes: The woman and her family will demonstrate competence in home glucose monitoring and administration of insulin before home management is initiated and will describe a plan for meeting dietary recommendations. The woman and her family will identify signs and symptoms of hypoglycemia and hyperglycemia and the management required for each and will verbalize knowledge of fetal surveillance procedures and keep scheduled appointments for testing.

Interventions

Although management of diabetes mellitus during pregnancy is a team effort, the nurse's major responsibility is to provide accurate information about the recommended therapeutic regimen and to offer consistent support for the woman's efforts to comply with the recommendations. It may be necessary to demonstrate specific skills that the woman and her family must master, and to review and reinforce information that comes from other members of the health care team.

Teaching Self-Care Skills

Demonstration and return demonstration are effective ways to teach and evaluate psychomotor skills. The woman (and her family) must learn to obtain a small sample of blood to test for glucose determination and to mix and inject insulin. Both procedures are invasive and cause mild discomfort, which may make the woman reluctant to start. Acknowledge these feelings before teaching begins.

Home Blood Glucose Monitoring. Spring devices, available for sticking the finger, make home blood glucose monitoring easier. Recommend that the expectant mother use the side of the fingertip, which is less sensitive than the pad. Teach her to cleanse the area with warm water to prevent infection before obtaining a sample. Each home monitoring kit contains specific instructions for timing and washing or blotting the blood from the reagent strip, and these directions must be followed exactly to obtain an accurate reading.

Insulin Administration. Two types of insulin are usually prescribed: intermediate-acting (NPH) and short-acting (regular or lispro) insulin. Teach the expectant mother the difference in onset, peak, and duration of action of each type of insulin. She also needs to learn how to mix the two insulins in the same syringe.

Insulin is administered subcutaneously. Common sites include the upper thighs, abdomen, and upper arms. Because the pregnant woman is injecting insulin frequently, emphasize these precautions:

• To prevent hypoglycemia, a meal should be taken 30 minutes after regular insulin is injected. Because of its 10-minute onset of action, lispro insulin may be injected just before eating.

- Unless the woman is very thin, insulin should be injected with the needle inserted at a 90-degree angle so that the tip of the needle reaches the fatty tissue layer.
- The needle should be inserted quickly to minimize discomfort.
- The tissue pinch, if used, is released after inserting the needle and before injecting insulin because pressure from the pinch can promote insulin leakage from the subcutaneous tissue.
- It is not necessary to aspirate when injecting into subcutaneous tissue.
- Insulin is injected slowly (over 2 to 4 seconds) to allow tissue expansion and to minimize pressure, which can cause insulin leakage.
- The needle is withdrawn quickly to minimize the formation of a track, which might permit insulin to leak out.

Emphasize the importance of administering the correct dosage at the correct time. Teach the woman and her family the function of insulin and the importance of following the directions of her physician in regard to coordinating meals with the administration of insulin.

Continuous Subcutaneous Insulin Infusion. The use of programmable insulin infusion pumps allows tailoring of insulin administration to the woman's individual lifestyle. Prompt emergency counseling and assistance must be available 24 hours a day to deal with unexpected problems such as pump malfunction.

Teaching Dietary Management

Although a dietitian prescribes the recommended diet, the nurse must be aware of the general requirements and must be sensitive to the expectant mother's dietary habits and preferences. There is often a need to review and clarify how the exchange lists are used to plan meals and snacks. Teach the woman to avoid simple sugars (candy, cake, cookies, juice), which raise the blood glucose levels quickly, and to include foods high in fiber, which are believed to help reduce glucose levels.

It may be necessary to help the woman select foods high in nutrients but low in cost. Animal protein is especially expensive, and alternative sources of protein (beans, peas, corn, grains) can be substituted to meet some of the protein needs.

Recognizing and Correcting Hypoglycemia and Hyperglycemia

Every woman and her family must be aware of the signs and symptoms that indicate abnormal blood glucose levels. If they are not identified and corrected quickly, hypoglycemia and hyperglycemia pose a threat to mother and fetus.

Hypoglycemia. Treat hypoglycemia at once to prevent damage to the brain, which depends on glucose. If the woman is able to swallow, have her drink 8 ounces of milk and eat two crackers. Repeat the snack in 15 minutes if symptoms persist or her blood glucose level is between 40 and 80 mg/dl. Glucose tablets are often recommended to treat hypoglycemia because of their consistent glucose content. Sucrose or unrefined sugar should not be ingested during hypoglycemic episodes. They can result in high blood glucose levels that disturb glycemic control for many hours (Moore, 1999).

CRITICAL TO REMEMBER

Signs and Symptoms of Maternal Hypoglycemia

- Shakiness (tremors)
- Sweating
- Pallor; cold, clammy skin
- Disorientation, irritability
- Headache
- Hunger
- Blurred vision

Teach family members how to inject glucagon in the event that the woman cannot swallow or retain food. Notify the physician at once. Intravenous glucose will be administered if she is hospitalized. If untreated, hypoglycemia can progress to convulsions and death.

To prevent episodes of hypoglycemia, instruct the woman to have meals at a fixed time each day and to plan snacks at the recommended times. Suggest that she carry glucose tablets or a container of milk and some dry crackers whenever possible.

Hyperglycemia. Because infection is the most common cause of hyperglycemia, pregnant women must be instructed to notify the physician whenever they have an infection of any type.

If untreated, hyperglycemia can lead to ketoacidosis, coma, and maternal and fetal death. If signs and symptoms occur, notify the physician at once so that treatment can be initiated. Hospitalization is often necessary for monitoring blood glucose levels and intravenous administration of insulin.

Explaining Procedures, Tests, and Plan of Care

Explain the schedule and the reasons for frequent checkups and tests. Encourage the woman and her family to ask questions if any part of the schedule is confusing. Pregnant women and their families need to know why frequent nonstress tests or other tests are necessary. They need to know that their diabetic care will take more time and effort than

---

CRITICAL TO REMEMBER

Signs and Symptoms of Maternal Hyperglycemia

- Fatigue
- Flushed, hot skin
- Dry mouth, excessive thirst
- Frequent urination
- Rapid, deep respirations; odor of acetone on the breath
- Drowsiness, headache
- Depressed reflexes

it did before pregnancy but that this care greatly improves the likelihood that they will have healthy infants.

Evaluation

After the procedures, tests, and plan of care have been explained, the family should be evaluated.

- Can the expectant mother and one family member demonstrate competence in blood glucose monitoring and administration of insulin?
- Can the family describe a plan for meeting dietary requirements?
- Can the woman and her family list the signs and symptoms of hypoglycemia and hyperglycemia?
- Can the woman and her family describe the initial management of these conditions?
- Can the woman verbalize knowledge of the reason for fetal surveillance procedures and keep appointments for tests?

Heart Disease

In every pregnancy, cardiovascular function changes to meet additional maternal metabolic demands and the needs of the fetus. Plasma volume, venous return, and cardiac output all increase. Heart rate and stroke volume, the two components of cardiac output, increase during pregnancy. The heart rate gradually rises above baseline during the third trimester, but an increase in stroke volume is primarily responsible for the overall rise in cardiac output during early pregnancy.

A normal heart adapts to the changes so that the woman tolerates pregnancy and birth without difficulty. With preexisting or underlying heart disease, however, the changes can impose an additional burden on an already compromised heart, and cardiac decompensation and congestive heart failure can result.

Incidence and Classification

Heart disease complicates about 1% of pregnancies (Cunningham et al., 1997). Pregnancy may unmask a previously asymptomatic heart condition or may aggravate known heart disease.

The two major categories of heart disease are rheumatic heart disease and congenital heart disease. Although rheumatic fever is uncommon in the United States, it is prevalent in less-developed countries. The incidence of pregnancy complicated by congenital heart disease is increasing because more women with congenital heart disease now survive to reproductive age. A third category, mitral valve prolapse, is a benign condition that usually does not complicate pregnancy.

RHEUMATIC HEART DISEASE

A remarkable decline in rheumatic heart disease has occurred in North America and western Europe as a result of early treatment of streptococcal pharyngitis (strep throat), which often precedes the onset of rheumatic fever. Even one bout of rheumatic fever may cause scarring of the heart valves, resulting in stenosis (narrowing) of the openings between the chambers of the heart.

The mitral valve is the most common site of stenosis. Mitral stenosis obstructs free flow of blood from the left atrium to the left ventricle. The left atrium becomes dilated. As a result, pressure in the left atrium, the pulmonary veins, and pulmonary capillaries is chronically elevated. This elevation may lead to pulmonary hypertension, pulmonary edema, or congestive heart failure. The first warnings of heart failure include persistent rales at the base of the lungs, dyspnea on exertion, cough, and hemoptysis. Progressive edema and tachycardia are additional signs of heart failure.

CONGENITAL HEART DISEASE

Congenital heart defects can be grouped into those that cause a left-to-right shunt and those that result in a right-to-left shunt. Those defects that produce left-to-right shunting include atrial and ventricular septal defects and patent ductus arteriosus. Right-to-left shunting occurs with a cyanotic heart defect, such as tetralogy of Fallot. Right-to-left shunting may also occur through a septal defect or a patent ductus arteriosus when pulmonary vascular resistance exceeds peripheral vascular resistance, and pulmonary hypertension (Eisenmenger syndrome) occurs.

Left-to-Right Shunt

Atrial Septal Defect.   Atrial septal defect is often first discovered in women of childbearing age because symptoms are absent or vague. This defect produces a left-to-right shunt because pressure in the left side of the heart is higher than it is in the right side. Pregnancy is well tolerated by patients with no complications (Caulin-Glaser & Setaro, 1999). Bacterial endocarditis is rare, and prophylactic antibiotics are not required. Atrial septal defects are not associated with heart failure; therefore, digitalis, diuretics, and extreme limitation of intravenous infusions are not warranted (Shabetai, 1999). Left-to-right shunting, however, may increase the chance of pulmonary hypertension because the additional blood that moves to the right side of the heart is transported to the lungs via the pulmonary artery.

Ventricular Septal Defect.   Although ventricular septal defects are more common at birth than atrial septal defects, ventricular septal defects are usually detected and corrected before females reach childbearing age. Most women with these defects who become pregnant are asymptomatic, but occasionally fatigue or symptoms of pulmonary congestion occur.

Pregnancy is well tolerated with small to moderate left-to-right shunts (Cunningham et al., 1997). Pregnancy, however, occasionally precipitates heart failure or an arrhythmia, either of which is managed as in nonpregnant patients. Bacterial endocarditis is common with unrepaired defects, and antibacterial prophylaxis is recommended.

Patent Ductus Arteriosus.   The communicating shunt between the pulmonary artery and aorta is usually discovered and treated in childhood. If untreated, the physiologic effects are related to size. If small, this lesion, like septal defects, may be well tolerated during pregnancy unless complicated by pulmonary hypertension. The patent ductus arteriosus tends to become infected, so antibiotic prophylaxis is recommended, particularly during labor.

Right-to-Left Shunt

Tetralogy of Fallot. The primary cause of right-to-left shunting is tetralogy of Fallot, a combination of four defects (ventricular septal defect, pulmonary valve stenosis, right ventricular hypertrophy, and rightward displacement of the aorta). Untreated patients with tetralogy of Fallot have obvious symptoms of heart disease that include (1) cyanosis, (2) clubbing of the fingers, indicating proliferation of capillaries to transport blood to the extremities, and (3) inability to tolerate activity.

Women who have undergone repair, and in whom cyanosis did not reappear, may do well during pregnancy. With uncorrected tetralogy of Fallot, maternal mortality approaches 10% (Cunningham et al., 1997).

Eisenmenger Syndrome. Eisenmenger syndrome develops when pulmonary resistance exceeds systemic resistance to blood flow and a right-to-left shunt develops in a patient with a previous left-to-right shunt. In this case, pregnancy should be avoided (Caulin-Glaser & Setaro, 1999).

MITRAL VALVE PROLAPSE

Mitral valve prolapse is one of the most common cardiac conditions among the general population. The incidence among otherwise healthy young women is 5% (Cunningham et al., 1997). Although the condition appears to be inherited, mitral valve prolapse is associated with a variety of other cardiac disorders, such as atrial septal defects and Marfan syndrome.

The leaflets of the mitral valve prolapse into the left atrium during ventricular contraction. Mitral valve prolapse is considered a benign condition, and most women with mitral valve prolapse are asymptomatic. Some women experience arrhythmias or chest pain, but most women with mitral valve prolapse tolerate pregnancy well. The condition is considered by some to be a significant risk factor for bacterial endocarditis, and some physicians administer prophylactic antibiotics before and during labor and delivery. If arrhythmia or chest pain occurs, beta-blockers, such as propranolol hydrochloride (Inderal), are administered to prevent stimulation of myocardial, vascular, and pulmonary receptor sites.

Diagnostic Evaluation

Early recognition of underlying heart disease is essential, and careful assessment for specific signs and symptoms of heart disease is part of every initial prenatal visit. Signs and symptoms include dyspnea, syncope (fainting) with exertion, hemoptysis, paroxysmal nocturnal dyspnea, and chest pain with exertion. Additional signs that confirm the diagnosis are (1) diastolic, presystolic, or continuous heart murmur, (2) cardiac enlargement, (3) a loud, harsh systolic murmur associated with a thrill, or (4) serious arrhythmias.

The diagnosis of heart disease may be made from clinical signs and symptoms and physical examination. It is often confirmed by chest radiography, electrocardiography, or echocardiography.

Once the diagnosis is made, the severity of the disease can be determined by the woman's ability to endure physical activity. A clinical classification based on the effect of exercise on the heart has been developed by the New York Heart Association.

New York Heart Association Functional Classification of Heart Disease

Class I. Uncompromised. No limitation of physical activity. Asymptomatic with ordinary activity.

Class II. Slightly compromised, requiring slight limitation of physical activity. Comfortable at rest, but ordinary physical activity causes fatigue, dyspnea, palpitations, or anginal pain.

Class III. Marked limitation of physical activity. Comfortable at rest, but less than ordinary activity causes excessive fatigue, palpitation, dyspnea, or anginal pain. Markedly compromised.

Class IV. Inability to perform any physical activity without discomfort. Symptoms of cardiac insufficiency even at rest.

In general, maternal and fetal risks with classes I and II disease are small but are greatly increased with classes III and IV.

Therapeutic Management

CLASS I AND CLASS II HEART DISEASE

All pregnant women with heart disease should do the following:

- Limit physical activity so that cardiac demand does not exceed the functional capacity of the heart. In other words, the woman should remain free of symptoms of cardiac stress, such as dyspnea, chest pain, or tachycardia.
- Avoid excessive weight gain, which places extra demands on the heart. A diet adequate in protein, calories, and sodium is necessary. A low-sodium diet prevents excessive expansion of blood volume and may be needed for some women with cardiac disease (McAnulty, Metcalfe, & Ueland, 1995).
- Prevent anemia, which decreases the oxygen-carrying capacity of the blood and results in a compensatory increase in heart rate. Most anemia is prevented by administration of iron and folic acid.
- Prevent infection. Prevention may include administration of prophylactic antibiotics.
- Undergo careful assessment for the development of congestive heart failure, pulmonary edema, or cardiac arrhythmias.

CLASS III AND CLASS IV HEART DISEASE

The primary goal of management is to prevent cardiac decompensation and the development of congestive heart failure. Moreover, every effort is also made to protect the fetus from hypoxia and IUGR, which can occur if placental perfusion is inadequate.

DRUG THERAPY

Anticoagulants. During pregnancy, clotting factors normally increase and thrombolytic activity decreases. These changes may predispose the pregnant woman to thrombus formation. Superimposed cardiac problems, such as mitral valve stenosis, may require anticoagulant therapy during pregnancy. Warfarin is associated with fetal malformations and should be restricted throughout pregnancy. Heparin, which does not cross the placental barrier, is an effective alternative anticoagulant for most women. Heparin should be administered subcutaneously to decrease the likelihood of maternal and placental bleeding. Careful monitoring of the partial thromboplastin time, activated partial thromboplastin time, and platelet count is essential to achieve effective, safe anticoagulation.

Antiarrhythmics. When medication to control arrhythmias is necessary during pregnancy, the effect on the fetus must be considered. Digoxin, quinidine, and procainamide are not harmful to the fetus. Beta-blockers have been associated with neonatal respiratory depression, sustained bradycardia, and hypoglycemia when administered late in pregnancy or just before delivery (Moore, 1999).

Anti-infectives. Anti-infective agents, such as ampicillin and gentamicin, may be administered as prophylaxis against bacterial endocarditis.

Diuretics. When congestive heart failure is uncontrolled by restriction of activity and sodium intake, diuretics should be instituted, with careful monitoring of electrolytes and water balance. Experience is greatest with thiazides and furosemide. Fetal growth retardation has been associated with furosemide, and neonatal jaundice, thrombocytopenia, anemia, and hypoglycemia have been associated with thiazide diuretics (Moore, 1999).

INTRAPARTUM MANAGEMENT

Every effort is made to minimize the effects of labor on the cardiovascular system. For example, with every contraction, 300 to 500 ml of blood is shifted from the uterus and placenta into the central circulation. This extra fluid causes a sharp rise in cardiac workload. Therefore, careful management of intravenous fluid administration is essential to prevent fluid overload. The woman should be positioned on her side, with her head and shoulders elevated. Oxygen is administered to increase the blood oxygen saturation. Sedation and epidural anesthesia are recommended early in labor to reduce discomfort. The environment is kept as quiet and calm as possible to decrease anxiety, which can cause tachycardia.

The fetus is monitored electronically, and signs of fetal compromise as well as maternal signs of cardiac decompensation (tachycardia, rapid respirations, moist rales, exhaustion) should be reported immediately to the physician.

A vaginal delivery produces less trauma and is recommended for a woman with heart disease unless there are specific indications for cesarean birth. Outlet forceps are often used to shorten the second stage of labor.

The fourth stage of labor is associated with special risks. After delivery of the placenta, about 500 ml of blood is added to the intravascular volume. To minimize the risks of overloading the circulation, the woman's legs are kept level with the body by avoiding the use of stirrups or by lowering them during the third stage of labor. Moreover, the uterus should not be massaged to expedite separation of the placenta. Careful assessment for signs of circulatory overload, such as a bounding pulse, distended neck and peripheral veins, and moist rales in the lungs, is performed during the third and fourth stages of labor.

POSTPARTUM MANAGEMENT

Women who have shown no evidence of distress during pregnancy, labor, or childbirth may still decompensate during the postpartum period. They must be observed closely for signs of infection, hemorrhage, or thromboembolism. These conditions can act together to precipitate postpartum heart failure in women with underlying heart disease.

Nursing Considerations

To plan care better, the nurse should determine what functional classification the physician has assigned the woman. Assess for changes in vital signs such as tachycardia. Note increasing fatigue or other signs of congestive heart failure. Review the chart to identify the presence of other factors that can increase the woman's cardiac workload, such as anemia, infections, anxiety, or inadequate support to manage the activities of daily living.

During pregnancy, nursing care focuses on helping the woman and her family understand factors that increase the workload of the heart and measures they can adopt to help the woman maintain any needed activity restrictions. Explain how gaining excessive weight during pregnancy or any other time increases the burden on the heart. Anemia causes the heart to pump faster to circulate available erythrocytes to the tissues. A well-balanced diet that yields approximately 2,200 calories/day is recommended, with adequate high-quality protein. Emphasize the importance of taking iron and folic acid supplements to prevent anemia.

Simple modifications can allow the woman to live within her cardiac reserve. Explain how she can take rest periods during the day and for an hour after meals. Instruct her to sit rather than stand, if possible, when performing activities. If she performs an activity that increases her heart rate, teach her to rest every few minutes to allow the heart to recover. She should stop the activity if she experiences dyspnea, chest pain, or tachycardia. Chapter 27 contains suggestions for coping with bed rest if it is required.

The woman should avoid extremes of temperature when possible. Instruct her to dress for the cold in layers and to avoid exertion during hot and humid weather.

Emotional stress also increases cardiac demand. Discuss methods for stress management, such as meditation, progressive relaxation, and biofeedback. Teach that cigarette smoking and the use of illicit drugs, such as cocaine and amphetamines, greatly increase stress to her heart.

The woman is vulnerable post partum, as interstitial fluid is mobilized into the vascular space for elimination. Continue to observe for signs of congestive heart failure. The mother may not be able to assume the care of her infant, but nurses should make every effort to promote contact between the mother and infant. Include the father and other family members in the infant's care if possible. Breastfeeding may not be recommended because of its added demands on the mother's heart. Encourage her to feed the baby anytime she feels able.

The mother and new family may need help at home. Consult physicians and make any needed referrals for follow-up care, which may include home visits by a nurse or nursing assistant. Before the woman is discharged, review the signs and symptoms of cardiac complications and note the times when she should contact the physician.

Anemias

Anemia is a condition in which a decline in circulating red blood cell mass reduces the capacity to carry oxygen to the vital organs of the mother or fetus. During pregnancy and the puerperium, anemia is defined as a hemoglobin concentration of less than 10.5 to 11.0 g/dl (Cunningham et al., 1997; Kilpatrick & Laros, 1999).

Anemia is one of the most common problems of pregnancy. The incidence varies according to geographic location and socioeconomic group. Anemia may be caused by a variety of factors, including nutrition, hemolysis, or blood loss. The most common types of anemia observed during pregnancy include iron deficiency anemia, folic acid deficiency anemia, the anemia associated with sickle cell disease, and thalassemia.

Iron Deficiency Anemia

It is difficult to meet pregnancy needs for iron through the diet alone, although iron is present in many foods. The primary sources of iron are meat, fish, chicken, liver, and green leafy vegetables.

MATERNAL EFFECTS
Signs and symptoms of iron deficiency anemia are often minimal but may include pallor, fatigue, lethargy, and headache. Clinical findings may also include inflammation of the lips and tongue. Pica (consuming nonfood substances such as clay, dirt, ice, or starch) is also a sign of iron deficiency anemia (Kilpatrick & Laros, 1999). Laboratory findings include red blood cells that are *microcytic* (small) and *hypochromic* (pale). The plasma iron and serum ferritin concentrations are low, whereas the total iron-binding capacity is higher than normal.

FETAL AND NEONATAL EFFECTS
The effects of maternal iron deficiency anemia on the fetus and neonate are unclear. In general, even with significant maternal iron deficiency, the fetus will receive adequate stores at a cost to the mother. If the mother is severely anemic, the fetus may have reduced red cell volume, hemoglobin, and iron stores.

THERAPEUTIC MANAGEMENT
Iron replacement is easily achieved in most women with administration of ferrous sulfate, gluconate, or fumarate tablets. The daily dosage should equal about 200 mg of *elemental iron*. Many women experience less gastrointestinal discomfort if iron is taken with meals. Therapy is often continued for about 3 months after the anemia has been corrected. Parenteral therapy may be necessary if the woman cannot take oral preparations.

Folic Acid Deficiency (Megaloblastic) Anemia

Folic acid is essential for cell duplication and for fetal and placental growth. It is also an essential nutrient for the formation of red blood cells.

MATERNAL EFFECTS
Maternal needs for folic acid double during pregnancy in response to the demand for greater production of erythrocytes and for fetal and placental growth. A deficiency in folic acid results in a reduction in the rate of DNA synthesis and mitotic activity of individual cells, resulting in the presence of *large, immature erythrocytes* (*megaloblasts*). Folate deficiency is the primary cause of megaloblastic anemia during pregnancy.

Nonnutritional factors that contribute to folic acid deficiency include hemolytic anemias with increased red blood cell turnover; some medications, such as phenytoin (Dilantin); and malabsorption entities. Folic acid deficiency is often present in association with iron deficiency anemia.

FETAL AND NEONATAL EFFECTS
Folate deficiency is associated with an increased risk of spontaneous abortion, abruptio placentae, and fetal anomalies. There is particular interest in the relation between folic acid deficiency anemia and fetal neural tube defects.

THERAPEUTIC MANAGEMENT
The recommended daily allowance for folic acid doubles during pregnancy, and some women have difficulty ingesting the amount needed, even though folic acid occurs widely in foods. The best sources of folic acid are liver, kidney beans, lima beans, and fresh, dark green leafy vegetables. As a result of the increased demands for this vitamin during pregnancy, supplementation with folic acid, 400 µg (0.4 mg)/day, has become a standard component of care.

Sickle Cell Disease

Sickle cell disease is an autosomal recessive genetic disorder. It occurs when the gene for the production of S hemoglobin is inherited from both parents. The defect in the hemoglobin causes erythrocytes to respond to hypoxia, acidosis, or dehydration by changing their shape to form a sickle, or crescent. Because of their distorted shape, the erythrocytes have difficulty passing through small arteries and capillaries and tend to clump together and occlude the blood vessel.

The disease is characterized by chronic anemia, increased susceptibility to infection, and periodic crises when the abnormally shaped erythrocytes obstruct blood vessels. Sickle cell disease occurs most often in people of African-American or Mediterranean ancestry. The incidence is 1 in 400 African-Americans, and 70,000 Americans are affected by sickle cell disease (Emory University School of Medicine, Department of Pediatrics, 1997).

MATERNAL EFFECTS

Pregnancy may worsen sickle cell disease and bring on *sickle cell crisis*. This broad term encompasses several different conditions, particularly temporary cessation of bone marrow function, hemolytic crisis with massive erythrocyte destruction resulting in jaundice, and severe pain caused by infarctions in the joints and all the major organs. In addition, expectant mothers with sickle cell disease are prone to pyelonephritis, bone infection, and heart disease.

FETAL AND NEONATAL EFFECTS

The fetus is prone to serious complications, including prematurity and IUGR. The incidence of fetal death is particularly high in the presence of sickle cell crisis.

THERAPEUTIC MANAGEMENT

Women with sickle cell disease should seek early prenatal care and should be informed of the maternal and fetal risks associated with the pregnancy. Frequent evaluations of hemoglobin, complete blood count, serum iron, total iron-binding capacity, and serum folate are necessary to determine the degree of anemia and iron and folic acid stores. Fetal surveillance studies (ultrasonography, nonstress tests, biophysical profiles) assess fetal growth and development and placental function.

The goal of nursing management is to help the pregnant woman maintain a healthy status and avoid hospitalization. Women must be encouraged to keep all prenatal care appointments, usually every other week. Topics in prenatal education include (1) the need to maintain adequate hydration to prevent sickling, (2) the need for adequate nutrition to meet metabolic needs, (3) the need for folic acid supplementation for erythrocyte production, (4) the need for rest periods throughout the day as well as good hygiene practices and the avoidance of persons with infectious illnesses, and (5) the need for prompt treatment of fever or other signs of infection.

Nurses must be alert for signs of sickle cell crisis. The most common indications are pain in the abdomen, chest, vertebrae, joints, or extremities; pallor; and signs of cardiac failure. Nurses must also provide comfort measures, such as repositioning, good skin care, assisting with ambulation and movement in bed, and assisting the woman to splint the abdomen with a pillow when she must cough or breathe deeply.

Intrapartum care focuses on preventing the development of sickle cell crisis. Oxygen is administered continuously, and fluids should be administered to prevent dehydration because hypoxemia and dehydration as well as exertion, infection, and acidosis stimulate the sickling process.

Thalassemia

Like sickle cell disease, thalassemia is a genetic disorder that involves the abnormal synthesis of alpha or beta chains of hemoglobin. This leads to alterations in the red blood cell membrane and a decreased life span of red blood cells. Thalassemia is named and classified by the type of chain that is inadequately produced. Beta-thalassemia is most frequently encountered in the United States. Beta-thalassemia minor refers to the heterozygous form that results from the inheritance of one abnormal gene from either parent. Beta-thalassemia major refers to inheritance of the gene from both parents. Females with beta-thalassemia major (Cooley's anemia) usually die in childhood or adolescence. Those who survive are often sterile (Cunningham et al., 1997). Beta-thalassemia is most often found in those of Mediterranean or Asian (particularly Chinese) origin.

MATERNAL EFFECTS

Women with beta-thalassemia minor are often mildly anemic but healthy otherwise. Laboratory values normally associated with beta-thalassemia minor indicate a mild hypochromic and microcytic anemia. This can lead to the diagnosis of iron deficiency anemia and iron supplementation therapy. This treatment is potentially dangerous because beta-thalassemia is associated with increased iron absorption and storage and a susceptibility to iron overload (Duffy, 1999).

FETAL AND NEONATAL EFFECTS

Controversy regarding whether thalassemia is associated with increased fetal or neonatal morbidity remains unresolved. There appears to be no increase in the rate of prematurity, low-birth-weight infants, or abnormal size for gestation. The fetus may inherit the serious problem of beta-thalassemia major if both parents have beta-thalassemia minor.

THERAPEUTIC MANAGEMENT

There is no specific therapy for beta-thalassemia minor during pregnancy. Most often the outcomes for the mother and fetus are satisfactory (Cunningham et al., 1997). Infections, which depress production of red blood cells and accelerate erythrocyte destruction, should be identified and treated promptly.

■ Immune Complex Diseases

Systemic Lupus Erythematosus

Systemic lupus erythematosus (SLE) is a chronic, inflammatory, autoimmune disease that can affect any organ or system in the body. Although the cause is unknown, an imbalance appears to develop between immune response and tolerance of specific antigens, so that the body produces antibodies to its own cells and tissue. Signs and symptoms result from inflammation of multiple organ systems, especially the joints, skin, kidneys, and nervous system. The most common symptoms are joint pain, photosensitivity, and a "butterfly" rash on the face.

The disease tends to affect young women, but it may occur in any age group. The incidence is believed to be approximately 1 per 1,000 persons. It is more common in African-Americans and persons of Latin descent.

SLE is associated with an increased incidence of abortion and fetal death during the first trimester. There is an increased risk for later pregnancy loss or premature birth due to hypertension, renal complications, and preterm rupture of membranes.

The newborn may have a congenital heart block, which may be detected prenatally. Skin lesions resembling those of the adult with SLE may be present for most of the first year.

Because pregnancy can exacerbate SLE, the woman must be carefully observed during pregnancy for signs that the disease has worsened. Renal complications pose a special risk. Women with a history of kidney problems should be advised to seek the advice of a physician before becoming pregnant. Pregnancy is most likely to have a favorable outcome in the woman whose disease is under good control at the beginning.

Antiphospholipid Syndrome

Antiphospholipid syndrome (APS) is an autoimmune condition characterized by the production of antiphospholipid antibodies, combined with certain clinical features. The most specific clinical features include thrombosis, decreased platelets, and pregnancy loss. Stroke may occur as a consequence of arterial thrombosis. An unusually high rate of pre-eclampsia has been noted in women with APS. Pre-eclampsia and uteroplacental insufficiency contributes to the high rate of preterm births and fetal loss with APS.

Although the syndrome occurs most often in women with other underlying autoimmune diseases, such as SLE, it is also diagnosed in women with no other recognizable autoimmune disease.

Women with APS should be informed of the potential maternal and obstetric problems, ideally before conception. They should be assessed for evidence of anemia, thrombocytopenia, and underlying renal disease. Heparin and low-dose aspirin are now recommended for pregnant women with APS (Silver & Branch, 1999).

▮ Neurologic Disorders: Epilepsy

Convulsive seizures are the most common form of epilepsy, which is a recurrent disorder of cerebral function. Epilepsy occurs in 0.3% to 0.6% of pregnant women (Aminoff, 1999). Pregnancy may affect management of seizure disorders, and the seizure disorder may affect the course of pregnancy.

The effect of pregnancy on the course of epilepsy is variable and unpredictable. The frequency of seizures may increase, decrease, or remain the same. In general, the longer the woman has been seizure-free before pregnancy, the less likely she is to develop seizures during pregnancy. Women with epilepsy have a higher than normal incidence of stillbirth and may have a higher incidence of preterm labor. Maternal bleeding may occur as a result of a deficiency of clotting factors associated with anticonvulsant drugs such as diphenylhydantoin (Dilantin) or phenobarbital. Anticonvulsant drugs also compete with folate for absorption, which may result in folate deficiency.

A major concern is the teratogenic effects of anticonvulsant drugs. One specific syndrome is *fetal hydantoin syndrome*, which includes craniofacial abnormalities, limb re-

duction defects, growth restriction, mental retardation, and cardiac anomalies. Other anticonvulsants, such as trimethadione, paramethadione, and carbamazepine, are also associated with malformation syndromes. The teratogenic effects of phenobarbital are difficult to assess because it is often combined with other drugs.

Health professionals should recommend that the pregnant woman consult a neurologist before conception. The goals of treatment are to prevent grand mal seizures and to reduce the adverse effects of anticonvulsant medications on the fetus. The woman and her family must be made aware of the risks involved when anticonvulsant drugs must be used during pregnancy. They also should realize that treatment cannot be stopped during pregnancy unless the woman has been free of seizures for a prolonged time. Grand mal seizures result in fetal hypoxia and acidosis and thus pose a serious problem for the fetus.

▮ Trauma in Pregnancy

Blunt Force Injuries

Automobile accidents cause most cases of blunt force injuries to the pregnant woman, followed by violent assault and suicide (Gonik, 1999). Maternal deaths are most often caused by head injury or intra-abdominal hemorrhage, which may follow sudden premature separation of the placenta or rupture of the uterus. Pelvic fracture is also a commonly reported injury in automobile accidents or as a result of falls.

During the first trimester, the fetus is protected from external forces by the bony pelvis, the amniotic fluid, and soft tissue surrounding the pelvis. Later in pregnancy, the fetal compartment extends beyond the bony pelvis, and as a result the fetus is more vulnerable to blunt force injury. Fetal injury may include skull fracture and intracranial hemorrhage. Moreover, disruption of uteroplacental blood flow due to premature separation of the placenta can result in fetal anoxia.

The use of seat belt restraints improves maternal and fetal outcomes in automobile accidents significantly. Current recommendations are that the pregnant woman wear three-point restraint seat belts during automobile travel. The lower part of the belt should be over the lap and not placed over the protruding uterus.

Penetrating Injuries

Gunshot and knife wounds are the most common penetrating injuries and are associated with assaults or suicide attempts. Because the uterus acts as a shield for the abdominal structures (Gonik, 1999), mortality rates from penetrating wounds in the pregnant woman are less than those in nonpregnant women. The fetus fares less well, with high injury and mortality rates.

Therapeutic Management

The initial management of trauma in pregnant women is similar to that in the nonpregnant person. Primary goals are

- Maintenance of maternal cardiopulmonary function
- Evaluation and stabilization of maternal injuries

Basic rules are applied to resuscitation: establishing ventilation and supporting cardiac function. To minimize compression of the large blood vessels by the heavy uterus, prolonged supine positioning should be avoided during resuscitation and other treatment. Lateral displacement of the uterus can be accomplished by placing a wedge along the right or left side of the woman. The need for large amounts of blood and fluid replacement should be anticipated.

After resuscitation, evaluation continues for fractures, bleeding sites, and internal injuries. Exploratory abdominal surgery may be necessary to identify and control internal bleeding. The uterus and fetus must also be evaluated for injuries.

Electronic fetal monitoring may reflect the condition of the mother as well as that of the fetus. For example, although the mother is stable, electronic monitoring may detect signs of premature separation of the placenta, such as uterine contractions, fetal tachycardia, and late decelerations. Fetal tachycardia often precedes changes in maternal vital signs due to hemorrhage.

The necessity for a cesarean birth to deliver a live fetus depends on several factors, including the age of the fetus, the fetal condition, and the extent of uterine injury. Because placental abruption usually develops soon after trauma, electronic monitoring is begun as soon as the mother is stabilized. It is continued as long as there are signs of uterine contractions, vaginal bleeding, uterine tenderness, or ruptured membranes.

Infections During Pregnancy

Infections may cause harm to the woman, the fetus, or both. A mild infection in the adult may have devastating effects on the developing fetus. Table 26–6 presents nursing considerations in relation to sexually transmissible diseases and vaginal infections. Table 26–7 summarizes urinary tract infections and their effect on pregnancy.

Viral Infections

Viral infections are often mild or even asymptomatic in adults, but they may have catastrophic fetal or neonatal consequences. Maternal infections with cytomegalovirus, rubella, varicella-zoster virus, herpes simplex, hepatitis B, and human immunodeficiency virus have the greatest potential for harming the fetus or neonate.

CYTOMEGALOVIRUS

Cytomegalovirus (CMV), a member of the herpesvirus group, is widespread and eventually infects most humans. Although CMV is widespread, it produces serious effects only in the fetus, immunodeficient persons, or those receiving immunosuppressant therapy. CMV has been isolated from urine, saliva, blood, cervical mucus, semen, breast milk, and feces. The highest rate of infection occurs in persons ages 15 to 35 years; thus, the possibility of CMV infection occurring during pregnancy is high.

After primary infection, the virus becomes latent, but, like other herpesviruses, CMV may produce periodic reacti-

---

TABLE 26–6

• • • • • • • • • • •

*Sexually Transmissible Diseases and Vaginal Infections:
Their Impact on Pregnancy*

Maternal, Fetal, and Neonatal Effects	Nursing Considerations
Sexually Transmissible Diseases	

Syphilis (Causative Organism: Spirochete Treponema pallidum)

If untreated, the infection may cross the placenta to the fetus and result in spontaneous abortion, a stillborn infant, premature labor and birth, or congenital syphilis. Major signs of congenital syphilis are enlarged liver and spleen, skin lesions, rashes, osteitis, pneumonia, and hepatitis.	Penicillin is the only treatment that will cure the disease in both the woman and fetus. Women who are allergic are desensitized and then treated (CDC, 1998c; Hollier & Cox, 1998).

Gonorrhea (Causative Organism: Bacterium Neisseria gonorrhoeae)

Not transmitted via the placenta; vertical transmission from mother to newborn during birth may cause ophthalmia neonatorium. Endocervicitis and weakness of the fetal membranes increase the risk of premature rupture of membranes and preterm labor.	Ceftriaxone or cefixime plus amoxicillin or erythromycin are now recommended for penicillin-resistant organisms because 20%–50% of women with gonorrhea will also have chlamydial infection (CDC, 1998c; Gibbs & Sweet, 1999). The partner must also be treated to prevent reinfection. All infants are treated with an ophthalmic antibiotic at birth to prevent serious eye infections.

TABLE 26–6
· · · · · · · · · · ·

Sexually Transmissible Diseases and Vaginal Infections:
Their Impact on Pregnancy Continued

Maternal, Fetal, and Neonatal Effects	*Nursing Considerations*

Chlamydial Infection (Causative Organism: Bacterium Chlamydia trachomatis)

The fetus may be infected during birth and suffer neonatal conjunctivitis or pneumonitis, which manifests within 4–6 weeks. Conjunctivitis is prevented by erythromycin ophthalmic ointment. *Chlamydia* may also be responsible for premature rupture of membranes, premature labor, and chorioamnionitis.	Education is particularly important because *Chlamydia* infection is the most common sexually transmissible disease in the United States, and infection is usually asymptomatic. Both partners should be treated to prevent recurrent infection. As with all sexually transmissible diseases, the use of condoms decreases the risk of infection. Erythromycin or amoxicillin is the recommended treatment (CDC, 1998c).

Trichomoniasis (Causative Organism: Protozoan Trichomonas vaginalis)

Not transmitted across the placental barrier; the organism cannot survive in the infantile, nonestrogenized vagina. Associated with premature rupture of membranes and postpartum endometritis.	Because of teratogenicity, metronidazole (Flagyl) can be used safely only during the second and third trimesters. Clotrimazole may provide relief of symptoms during first trimester.

Condyloma Acuminatum (Causative Organism: Human Papillomavirus)

Transmission of condyloma acuminatum, also called venereal warts, may occur during vaginal birth and is associated with the development of epithelial tumors of the mucous membranes of the larynx in children. Pregnancy can cause proliferation of lesions, which are associated with cervical dysplasia and cancer.	Podophyllin is contraindicated as treatment during pregnancy because of the possible teratogenic effects. Applications of trichloracetic acid or cryotherapy are often recommended instead (CDC, 1998c; Youngkin, 1995).

Vaginal Infections

Candidiasis (Causative Organism: Yeast Candida albicans)

Oral candidiasis (thrush) may develop in newborns if infection is present at birth. Thrush is treated with application of nystatin (Mycostatin) over the surfaces of the oral cavity four times a day for several days. Characteristic "cottage cheese" vaginal discharge with vulvar pruritus, burning, and dyspareunia. Vulva may be red, tender, and edematous.	Candidiasis (previously called *Monilia* infection) is a persistent problem for many women during pregnancy. Effective treatment may be obtained with miconazole nitrate (Monistat) or clotrimazole (Gyne-Lotrimin), both available over the counter.

Bacterial Vaginosis* (Causative Organism: Gardnerella vaginalis)

No known fetal effects. May be associated with postpartum endometritis; has been associated with preterm birth. Marked by a major shift in vaginal flora from the normal predominance of lactobacilli to a predominance of anaerobic bacteria. Causes profuse, malodorous, "fishy" vaginal discharge, itching, and burning.	The causative organism is sensitive to metronidazole, which may be used during the second and third trimesters without concern about teratogenic effect (Lee, 1995).

*Formerly called nonspecific vaginitis or *Gardnerella* vaginitis.

TABLE 26–7

Urinary Tract Infections and Their Effect on Pregnancy

Maternal, Fetal, and Neonatal Effects	Nursing Considerations
Asymptomatic Bacteriuria (Causative Organisms: Escherichia coli, Klebsiella, Proteus)	
Ascending bacterial infection can result in cystitis or pyelonephritis in later pregnancy if condition remains untreated.	Defined as recovery of the same pathogen from two consecutive urine samples (midstream, clean-catch specimens) of 100,000 colony-forming units per milliliter of urine. Treated with oral sulfonamides or ampicillin in early pregnancy; sulfonamides displace bilirubin from albumin in fetal circulation in late pregnancy and can result in neonatal jaundice.
Cystitis (Causative Organisms: E. coli, Klebsiella, Proteus)	
Emphasize importance of reporting signs of urinary tract infection. Stress the importance of taking all the medication prescribed even if the symptoms abate. Provide information about hygiene measures.	Signs and symptoms include dysuria, frequency, urgency, and suprapubic tenderness. Ascending infection may lead to pyelonephritis.
Acute Pyelonephritis (Causative Organisms: E. coli, Klebsiella, Proteus)	
Increased risk of preterm labor and premature delivery. Maternal complications include septic shock and adult respiratory distress syndrome.	Inform women with asymptomatic bacteriuria or cystitis of signs and symptoms, such as sudden onset of fever, chills, flank pain or tenderness, nausea, and vomiting, so that treatment can begin promptly. Woman may be hospitalized for intravenous administration of antibiotics.

vation and shedding of the virus. Primary CMV infection is the most dangerous to the fetus. The best way to establish the presence of CMV is by isolating the virus (Gibbs & Sweet, 1999). Most infections are asymptomatic, so they may not be suspected or diagnosed.

Fetal and Neonatal Effects. Two percent of all live neonates are infected with the virus; about 90% of these are asymptomatic and appear normal (Landry, 1999). The most serious complications in infected infants are deafness, mental retardation, seizures, blindness, and dental abnormalities. Some of these conditions may not be obvious for several months or even years.

Therapeutic Management. No effective therapy is currently available for the treatment of congenital infection. Antiviral agents, such as adenosine arabinoside, have been used for severe infections, but these drugs are toxic and only temporarily suppress shedding of the virus (Gibbs & Sweet, 1999). If a primary infection is diagnosed during the first 20 weeks of gestation, therapeutic termination of the pregnancy may be considered.

RUBELLA
Rubella is caused by a virus that is transmitted by droplets or through direct contact with articles contaminated with nasopharyngeal secretions. Rubella is a mild disease; major symptoms are fever, general malaise, and a characteristic maculopapular rash that begins on the face and spreads over the body. Although the overall incidence has declined since rubella vaccine became available, many young adults remain at risk. Recent outbreaks of rubella have tended to occur where young adults congregate and in Latinos, who are more likely to remain unvaccinated (Gibbs & Sweet, 1999).

Fetal and Neonatal Effects. Rubella remains a serious concern because the virus crosses the placental barrier and can infect the fetus. The greatest risk to the fetus occurs during the first trimester, when fetal organs are developing. If maternal infection occurs during this time, approximately one third of these cases will result in spontaneous abortions, and the surviving fetuses may be seriously compromised. Deafness, mental retardation, cataracts, cardiac defects, IUGR, and microcephaly are the most common fetal complications. Moreover, infants born to mothers who had rubella during pregnancy shed the virus for many months and thus pose a threat to other infants as well as to susceptible adults who come in contact with them.

Therapeutic Management. Prevention is the only effective protection for the fetus. Women who are immune do not become infected, so it is critical to determine the immune status of all women of childbearing age. A rubella titer of 1:8 or greater provides evidence of immunity. Women who are not immune should be vaccinated before they become pregnant, and they should be advised not to become pregnant for 3 months after vaccination because the live-virus vaccine poses a possible risk to the fetus. Many nonimmune women are vaccinated during the postpartum period so that they will be immune before becoming pregnant again.

VARICELLA-ZOSTER VIRUS

Varicella infection (chickenpox) is caused by varicella-zoster virus, a herpesvirus that is transmitted by direct contact or via the respiratory tract. The varicella virus can become latent in nerve ganglia. When the virus is reactivated, herpes zoster (shingles) results. Potential maternal complications of acute varicella infection may include preterm labor, encephalitis, and varicella pneumonia, which is the most serious complication associated with varicella-zoster virus.

Fetal and Neonatal Effects.   Fetal and neonatal effects depend on the time of maternal infection. If the infection occurs during the first trimester, the fetus has a small risk for congenital varicella syndrome; clinical findings include limb hypoplasia, cutaneous scars, chorioretinitis, cataracts, microcephaly, and symmetric IUGR. In later pregnancy, transplacental passage of maternal antibodies usually protects the fetus. If the fetus is exposed to the virus in utero and is born before the development of maternal antibodies, however, the infant is at risk for the development of life-threatening neonatal varicella infection (Gibbs & Sweet, 1999).

Therapeutic Management.   Immune testing may be recommended for pregnant women presumed to be susceptible. Varicella-zoster immune globulin should be administered to women who have been exposed and are susceptible (Rouse et al., 1996). Women who contract chickenpox during pregnancy should be instructed to report pulmonary symptoms immediately. Hospitalization, fetal surveillance, full respiratory support, and hemodynamic monitoring should be available for women diagnosed with varicella pneumonia.

For infants born to mothers with varicella, authorities recommend immunization with varicella-zoster immune globulin within 72 hours of birth. Women and infants with varicella are highly contagious and should be placed in strict isolation. Only staff members known to be immune to varicella should come in contact with these clients.

HERPESVIRUS SEROTYPES 1 AND 2

Genital herpes is one of the most common sexually transmissible diseases. It may be caused by herpesvirus serotype 1 or serotype 2, but 90% of episodes of genital herpes are caused by type 2. Infection occurs as a result of direct contact of the skin or mucous membrane with an active lesion. Lesions form at the site of contact and begin as a group of painful papules that progress rapidly to become vesicles, shallow ulcers, pustules, and crusts. The woman sheds the virus until the lesions are completely healed. The virus then migrates along the sensory nerves to reside in the sensory ganglion, and the disease enters a latent phase. It can be reactivated later as a recurrent infection.

Vertical transmission (from mother to infant) generally occurs in two ways: (1) after rupture of membranes, when the virus ascends from active lesions, and (2) during birth, when the fetus comes in contact with infectious genital secretions.

The diagnosis is usually based on clinical signs and symptoms. A definitive diagnosis, however, involves isolation of the virus from a lesion.

Fetal and Neonatal Effects.   Complications of pregnancy from a recurrent infection are rare. If primary infection occurs during the first 20 weeks, however, an increase occurs in the rate of spontaneous abortions, IUGR, and preterm labor (Riley, 1998). Neonatal herpes infection is a major perinatal problem. About 1,000 cases of neonatal herpes occur in the United States each year. Symptoms usually appear within 2 to 3 days of birth, and the disease progresses rapidly. The mortality in infants with disseminated herpes infection is approximately 60%. Long-term morbidity, such as mental retardation, spasticity, blindness, and learning disability, is significant in survivors of disseminated neonatal herpes infection (Riley, 1998).

Therapeutic Management.   To reduce symptoms and shorten the duration of lesions, acyclovir may be administered in pregnancy. The ability of acyclovir to prevent maternal-fetal transmission of the infection has not been proved. According to the U.S. Food and Drug Administration, however, acyclovir is in pregnancy risk category C and should be used with caution.

For women with a history of genital herpes, vaginal delivery is allowed if there are no genital lesions at the time of labor. For women with active lesions, either recurrent or primary, at the time of labor, cesarean birth is often recommended. Use of fetal scalp electrodes, which cause a break in the skin, should be limited in the infected woman.

After delivery, isolation of the mother from her infant is not necessary as long as direct contact with lesions is avoided and mothers use careful hand-washing techniques. Mothers may breast-feed if there are no lesions on the breasts. The infant is observed carefully for signs of infection, including temperature instability, lethargy, poor sucking reflex, jaundice, seizures, and herpetic lesions.

Expectant mothers need information about effective ways to deal with the emotional as well as the physical effects of herpes. Many women are concerned about privacy and do not want family members to know why cesarean birth is necessary. Such women must be assured that their wishes will be respected. Many women need an opportunity to discuss their feelings of shame, anger, or anxiety about the disease.

PARVOVIRUS B19

Erythema infectiosum, also called *fifth disease,* is caused by human parvovirus B19. It is an acute, communicable disease that is characterized by a highly distinctive rash. The rash starts on the face with a "slapped-cheeks" appearance, followed by a generalized maculopapular rash. Other symptoms include fever, malaise, and joint pain. Erythema infectiosum is more common among children and often occurs in community epidemics. The prognosis is usually excellent. If the disease occurs in pregnancy, however, there are potential fetal and neonatal effects.

Fetal and Neonatal Effects.   When infection occurs during pregnancy, fetal death can result, usually from failure of fetal red blood cell production, followed by severe fetal anemia, hydrops (generalized edema), and heart failure.

Some association has been noted between elevated levels of maternal serum alpha-fetoprotein (MSAFP) and poor pregnancy outcomes for women infected with parvovirus, but an elevated MSAFP level does not appear to be a strong predictor of fetal risk (Markenson & Yancey, 1998). Serial ultrasonography can also be performed to detect hydrops.

At delivery, the umbilical cord blood should be examined for virus or IgM antibody, which reveals whether or not the virus has crossed the placenta and infected the fetus. If the fetus has been infected, the infant is examined for any defect, and the child is assessed regularly for several years to exclude the possibility of delayed complications.

Therapeutic Management.   Infection with parvovirus B19 has no specific treatment. Starch baths may help reduce pruritus, and analgesics may be necessary to relieve mild joint pain.

HEPATITIS B

Six types of hepatitis virus have currently been identified: A, B, C, D, E, and G. Hepatitis B can be transmitted perinatally; maternal-fetal transmission of hepatitis C also may occur in women with very high antibody titers. Hepatitis C has no immunoprophylaxis, although it is available for hepatitis B. Hepatitis G is related to hepatitis C, but its clinical significance is not yet known. Hepatitis B is responsible for about 35% of hepatitis cases in the United States (Duff, 1998).

Hepatitis B, formerly known as serum hepatitis, is caused by a virus that is transmitted via blood, saliva, vaginal secretions, semen, or breast milk and across the placental barrier. The disease is prevalent in certain population groups, such as Africans, Asians, Southeast Asian immigrants, Native Americans, Eskimos, and intravenous drug users. Symptoms may include vomiting, abdominal pain, jaundice, fever, rash, and painful joints. Fortunately, most infected adolescents and adults recover within 6 months and acquire long-lasting immunity.

Fetal and Neonatal Effects.   Hepatitis B infection in pregnancy is associated with an increased incidence of prematurity, low birth weight, and neonatal death. Infants born to mothers who had hepatitis B during pregnancy or who are chronic carriers of hepatitis B surface antigen (HBsAg) are at risk for the development of acute infection at birth. Newborns as well as children infected with hepatitis B virus before the age of 5 years will become chronic carriers of the virus.

Therapeutic Management.   Hepatitis B infection is completely preventable. Simple hygiene measures such as safe sex and the use of standard precautions with body fluids provide primary prevention. Highly effective hepatitis B vaccines have been available for more than a decade in the United States. A series of three intramuscular injections given during a 6- to 12-month period produces a protective antibody response for most infants, children, and adults. Vaccination is recommended for any population at risk, including nurses who frequently come in contact with blood.

All pregnant women should be screened for HBsAg. Women at high risk for hepatitis should be rescreened in the third trimester if the initial test is negative. Household members and sexual contacts should be tested and offered vaccination if they are susceptible. No specific treatment exists for hepatitis. Recommended supportive treatment includes bed rest and a high-protein, low-fat diet.

Infection of a newborn whose mother is known to be HBsAg positive can usually be prevented by administration of hepatitis B immune globulin (HBIG, Hep-B-Gammagee), followed by hepatitis B vaccine (Recombivax-HB or Engerix-B) soon after birth. To prevent infections from skin surface contamination, the newborn must be carefully bathed before any injections are given. The vaccine should be repeated at 1 month and 6 months of age.

Infants born to mothers who were not screened for HBsAg should receive the vaccine soon after birth. If the mother is found to be HBsAg positive, HBIG should be administered, followed by a second and third dose of vaccine. Breast-feeding is considered safe as long as the newborn has been vaccinated.

HUMAN IMMUNODEFICIENCY VIRUS

Acquired immunodeficiency syndrome (AIDS) is caused by a retrovirus known as human immunodeficiency virus (HIV). HIV infection is transmitted predominantly through three modes: (1) sexual exposure to genital secretions of an infected person, (2) parenteral exposure to infected blood or tissue, and (3) from an infected mother to an infant (vertical transmission) perinatally. It is also probable that the virus can be transmitted through breast milk (Minkoff, 1998).

In the past, the populations at highest risk for HIV exposure were homosexual and bisexual men, intravenous drug users (who often share contaminated needles), and inhabitants of West Africa and Haiti. Women who acquire HIV infection heterosexually or through intravenous drug abuse now constitute a major part of the infected population. The rate of HIV infection has increased much faster in women than in men. Approximately 107,000 to 150,000 women in the United States are now infected with HIV, and most of them are of childbearing age. In 1985, women accounted for only 7% of the known AIDS cases, but that figure had increased to 22% by 1997. Between 1995 and 1996, a 3% increase in initial HIV diagnoses occurred among women, while HIV diagnoses declined 3% among men (Centers for Disease Control and Prevention [CDC], 1998a).

The ethnic distribution of female AIDS cases is unequal. Seventy-nine percent of AIDS cases reported among women in 1996 occurred among African-American and Latino women, whereas these two groups make up only 21% of the female population in the United States. In 1996 HIV infection was the fourth leading cause of death among women ages 25 to 44 and the leading cause of death among African-American women in this age group (CDC, 1998a; Minkoff, 1998).

Pathophysiology.   Like other retroviruses, HIV can integrate its viral genetic makeup into the genetic makeup of the cell when infecting it. This process produces a cell that cannot perform its functions properly. At the same time, this abnormal cell replicates and produces more viruses that invade more cells. The disease worsens as more and more cells cease to function, and at the same time, a greater number of viruses are produced. The principal mechanism whereby HIV leads to immunodeficiency is through its effect on helper (CD4) lymphocytes. These cells play a key role in organizing the body's immune response.

As the number of CD4 cells declines, the immune response becomes inadequate, and opportunistic infections are able to overwhelm the person who is HIV positive. A CD4 count of less than 200 cells/mm^3 confirms the diagnosis of AIDS.

The clinical course of HIV infection follows four fairly predictable stages:

- An early, or acute, stage that occurs several weeks after HIV exposure. Flu-like symptoms may develop and last a few weeks. Antibodies to HIV (seroconversion) generally appear within a few months but may occasionally be delayed for more than a year.
- A middle, or asymptomatic, period of minor or no clinical problems. This period is characterized by continuous low-level viral replication and CD4 cell loss. The latent period from infection to AIDS is approximately 11 years (Minkoff, 1999).
- A transitional period of symptomatic disease, characterized by immune dysfunction.
- A late, or crisis, period of symptomatic disease that lasts months or years. This period is characterized by infections and cancers that occur principally in persons with immune system compromise.

During stages 1 and 2, the infected person is said to be HIV positive; during stages 3 and 4, the immune system no longer offers adequate protection, and opportunistic diseases occur. The person is then said to have AIDS. (For a more complete discussion of adult HIV infection and AIDS, consult a medical-surgical nursing text.)

Fetal and Neonatal Effects.   Because of new antiretroviral drugs, the prognosis for HIV-infected women and their infants has considerably improved in the past few years. Maternal-infant transmission of HIV was 25% to 35% of infants born to infected mothers during the early 1990s. With appropriate drug intervention during pregnancy, up to 95% of these infants can now be born uninfected (Minkoff, 1998). A 1995 analysis of data found, however, that only 53% of infants received the full benefit of drug treatment, primarily because over one fourth of their mothers did not have prenatal care.

The infected newborn is typically asymptomatic at birth, but signs and symptoms usually become obvious during the first year of life. The most common early signs are enlargement of the liver and spleen, lymphadenopathy, failure to thrive, persistent thrush, and extensive seborrheic dermatitis (cradle cap). Infants frequently experience chronic bacterial infections, such as meningitis, pneumonia, osteomyelitis, septic arthritis, and septicemia. The progression from HIV infection to AIDS occurs more quickly in the infant than in the adult. See Chapter 41 for more information about HIV infection and its treatment in infants and children.

Prevention.   Prevention remains the only way to avoid HIV infection. Sexual transmission can be avoided by several methods. Abstinence would render a person safe from all sexually transmissible diseases, including HIV, but for many people sexual expression adds to the quality of life, and many are not willing to practice total abstinence. Sexual transmission of HIV can also be prevented if infected persons do not have intercourse with susceptible persons. If intercourse does occur, the use of barrier methods of contra-

ception, such as latex condoms in conjunction with spermicidal jellies containing nonoxynol 9, has been demonstrated to be effective. A rubber dam or a condom offers protection from transmission of the virus during cunnilingus or fellatio (oral sex).

Intravenous drug users who refuse rehabilitative treatment should be taught to wash the equipment with water, soap, and bleach before each use to prevent transmission of the virus from one person to another via a soiled needle.

Therapeutic Management.   Although the long-term outlook for persons infected with HIV remains poor, powerful new drugs have substantially slowed the progression of the infection, greatly improving the short-term outlook. Of particular interest is a regimen of zidovudine (ZVD) given during pregnancy and labor and to the newborn for 6 weeks, which has dramatically reduced the rate of transmission from mother to infant (CDC, 1994; Minkoff, 1999). Zidovudine (previously called azidothymidine [AZT]) is thought to inhibit replication of the virus and thus to prolong the mother's life. Currently, zidovudine is recommended for pregnant women who are HIV positive to reduce vertical transmission of the virus (CDC, 1994).

Women with HIV are treated with a combination of drugs to prevent the development of drug resistance, which can occur when a single drug is used. Protease inhibitors are a new class of drugs that reduce the amount of virus in the blood. Saquinavir (Invirase) is the first protease inhibitor approved by the U.S. Food and Drug Administration. Several antiretroviral drugs and protease inhibitors are available to treat people with HIV infection or AIDS. One concern is that zidovudine is the only drug that has been shown to benefit the infant by preventing maternal-fetal transmission, while the effects of other drugs used for combination maternal therapy have unknown effects on the fetus. For this reason, zidovudine treatment is delayed until after the first trimester for a woman who is not taking any antiretroviral therapy. If the woman is already taking one or more of these drugs, however, the effects of stopping or continuing therapy until after the first trimester are unknown

---

Recommendations for Zidovudine Prophylaxis for the Prevention of Perinatal HIV Transmission

- *Pregnancy:* Zidovudine, 100 mg orally 5 times per day, 200 mg 3 times per day, or 300 mg twice daily, initiated between 14 and 34 weeks of gestation.
- *Labor:* Intravenous zidovudine with a 1-hour loading dose of 2 mg/kg, followed by continuous infusion of 1 mg/kg/hr.
- *Newborn:* Oral zidovudine syrup, dose of 2 mg/kg every 6 hours for 6 weeks, beginning 8 to 12 hours after birth.

From Centers of Disease Control and Prevention. (1994). Recommendations for the use of zidovudine to reduce perinatal transmission of human immunodeficiency virus. *Morbidity and Mortality Weekly Report, 43*(RR-11), 2–4; Minkoff, H. L. (1998). HIV and pregnancy. *Seminars in Perinatology, 22*(4), 302.

(Newshan & Hoyt, 1998). Several clinical trials are currently under way to evaluate the benefits and risks of drug combinations when taken by pregnant women.

Nursing Considerations. Learning of HIV infection during pregnancy can have a devastating and immobilizing effect on the entire family. A nursing diagnosis of Anticipatory Grieving related to multiple losses, including probable loss of the woman's life and possible death of the infant, should be considered. Crisis intervention may be necessary initially to help the family cope.

Nurses must frequently determine what the family perceives as the most pressing needs and worries. Some of the most common fears are loss of control, loss of support and love, social isolation, and loss of privacy. The nurse's response may involve finding ways for the woman to retain control while she is physically able and to assist her in selecting those in her family who will provide continued love and emotional support. Above all, it is necessary to reassure the woman that her right to privacy will not be violated.

Nurses can help the woman maintain the highest level of wellness possible. Adequate, high-quality nutrition decreases the risk of opportunistic infections and promotes vitality. A daily regimen should include sufficient rest and activity. It is important to avoid large crowds, travel to areas with poor sanitation, or exposure to infected individuals. Meticulous skin care is essential, especially during recurrent herpes infections.

The woman will need to know that breast-feeding is contraindicated but that she can provide all other care for her infant. She will almost certainly experience a great deal of anxiety about whether the infant will be HIV positive. Nurses need to respond honestly that testing will be required but that many infants do not get the virus. Moreover,

nurses must reinforce information about medications such as zidovudine that reduce the rate of vertical transmission.

Nonviral Infections

TOXOPLASMOSIS
Toxoplasmosis is a protozoal infection caused by *Toxoplasma gondii*. Infection is transmitted through organisms in raw or undercooked meat, through contact with infected cat feces, or across the placental barrier to the fetus if the expectant mother acquires the infection during pregnancy.

Toxoplasmosis is often subclinical; the woman may experience a few days of fatigue, muscle pains, and swollen glands but may be unaware of the disease. If the infection is suspected, diagnosis can be confirmed by positive serologic test results, which include indirect fluorescent antibody tests for IgG and IgM.

Fetal and Neonatal Effects. Toxoplasmosis may cause abortion or result in the birth of a live infant with the disease. About 50% of infants born to mothers infected during pregnancy have congenital toxoplasmosis. Affected infants may be asymptomatic at birth or may have low birth weight, enlarged liver and spleen, jaundice, and anemia. Complications, usually chorioretinitis or signs of neurologic damage, may develop several years later.

Therapeutic Management. All pregnant women should be advised to do the following:

- Cook meat thoroughly, particularly pork, beef, and lamb.
- Avoid touching mucous membranes of the mouth or eyes while handling raw meat.
- Wash all kitchen surfaces that come in contact with uncooked meat.
- Wash the hands thoroughly after handling raw meat.
- Avoid uncooked eggs and unpasteurized milk.
- Wash fruits and vegetables before eating.
- Avoid contact with materials that are possibly contaminated with cat feces (cat litter boxes, sandboxes, or garden soil).

Toxoplasmosis is usually self-limiting, and treatment for mothers is controversial in the United States. Some physicians recommend a combination of pyrimethamine and sulfadiazine, accompanied by folinic acid to reduce the toxicity of the other two drugs. All authorities agree, however, that this combination should be administered to symptomatic infants with congenital toxoplasmosis (Gibbs & Sweet, 1999). The most serious consequences occur if the disease is contracted during the first 20 weeks of pregnancy, so abortion may be presented as an option for the parents to consider.

GROUP B STREPTOCOCCUS INFECTION
Group B streptococcus (GBS) is a leading cause of life-threatening perinatal infections in the United States. The gram-positive bacterium colonizes the rectum, vagina, cervix, and urethra of pregnant and nonpregnant women. Approximately 10% to 30% of pregnant women are colonized with GBS in the vaginal or rectal area (CDC, 1996). Often, these women are asymptomatic, although symptomatic maternal infections can occur. These infections include uri-

nary tract infection, chorioamnionitis, and endometritis. Most women respond quickly to antimicrobial therapy, but potentially fatal complications, such as meningitis, fasciitis, or intra-abdominal abscess, can occur.

Fetal and Neonatal Effects.   Early-onset GBS disease occurs within 7 days of birth and accounts for approximately 80% of all GBS cases in newborns (ACOG, 1996). In these newborns, the mortality rate ranges from 5% to 20% (ACOG, 1996; CDC, 1996). Sepsis, pneumonia, and meningitis are the primary infections. Late-onset disease occurs after the first week of life, and meningitis is the most common clinical manifestation. Permanent neurologic consequences may be seen in 15% to 30% of those who survive meningeal infections. See Chapter 30 for additional information about manifestations and recommended management of neonatal sepsis.

Therapeutic Management.   Health care providers have difficulty identifying women who are asymptomatic GBS carriers during pregnancy because the duration of carrier status is unpredictable. Prenatal screening cultures may not identify the woman who will be a GBS carrier at the time of membrane rupture or onset of labor (CDC, 1996). Optimal identification of the GBS carrier depends on culture timing and technique. Material for culture should be obtained from the rectum and vagina (not the cervix) between 35 and 37 weeks' gestation, and if GBS is present, the woman should be offered intrapartum penicillin to prevent neonatal infection (CDC, 1996).

The CDC (1996) also recommends that intrapartum penicillin be administered in specific high-risk situations:

- If the mother previously gave birth to an infant with GBS disease
- If GBS is present in the urine during the current pregnancy
- If the infant is born before 37 weeks' gestation
- If the mother has a fever (temperature ≥38°C [≥100.4°F]) during labor
- If the membranes ruptured 18 or more hours before childbirth

Research is under way to develop a vaccine to prevent GBS disease. Guidelines for administration and timing of any future vaccine have not been worked out (Mitchell et al., 1997).

TUBERCULOSIS

Tuberculosis results from infection by *Mycobacterium tuberculosis*. It is transmitted by aerosolized droplets of liquid containing the bacterium, which are inhaled by a noninfected individual and taken into the lung. Initially, most individuals are asymptomatic. Women obtaining prenatal care should be screened for tuberculosis. This screening involves an intradermal injection of mycobacterial protein (purified protein derivative). If the reaction is positive, the woman's abdomen should be protected by a lead shield while a radiograph is taken of her chest. The diagnosis is confirmed by isolating and identifying the bacterium in the sputum.

Symptomatic persons have general malaise, fatigue, loss of appetite, weight loss, and fever. These symptoms occur in the late afternoon and evening and are accompanied by night sweats. As the disease progresses, a chronic cough develops and a mucopurulent sputum is produced.

Tuberculosis is associated with poverty, malnutrition, and HIV infection. Worldwide, it is responsible for more deaths than any other communicable disease. Moreover, the incidence is increasing in inner-city areas and among homeless persons. It is also prevalent among immigrants from Southeast Asia and Central and South America.

Fetal and Neonatal Effects.   Although perinatal infection is rare, it may be acquired as the fetus swallows infected amniotic fluid or is exposed through the umbilical vein. The diagnosis is made by finding the bacilli in a gastric aspirate of the neonate or in placental tissue. Signs of congenital tuberculosis include failure to thrive, lethargy, respiratory distress, fever, and enlargement of the spleen, liver, and lymph nodes. If the mother remains untreated, the newborn is at high risk for acquiring tuberculosis by inhalation of infectious respiratory droplets from the mother.

Therapeutic Management.   The treatment of tuberculosis is based on two principles. First, more than one drug must be used to prevent the growth of resistant organisms. Second, treatment must continue for a prolonged period. Isoniazid is the principal drug for treating tuberculosis in pregnancy and is usually given with ethambutol. Pyridoxine (vitamin B_6) should be administered with isoniazid to prevent fetal neurotoxicity (AAP & ACOG, 1997). Pyrazinamide is increasingly used instead of ethambutol because it quickly clears the sputum of the organism and because 6-month rather than 9-month treatment is effective. The information about the safety of pyrazinamide for the fetus is inadequate, but neither is there a body of adverse experience (de Swiet, 1999).

Management of the infant born to a mother with tuberculosis involves preventing the disease or treating early infection. Prevention focuses on teaching family members how the disease is transmitted so that they can protect the infant from airborne organisms. The infant should be skin tested at birth and may be started on preventive isoniazid therapy. Skin testing should be repeated at 3 months, and isoniazid may be stopped if the skin test result remains negative. If the skin test result converts to positive, a full course of drug therapy should be given.

Nursing Considerations.   When the pregnant woman has tuberculosis, a potential nursing diagnosis is Ineffective Management of Therapeutic Regimen. The woman with tuberculosis must adhere to a prolonged treatment regimen that has significant side effects. Added socioeconomic stressors such as poverty, malnutrition, and sometimes language barriers may add to the risks associated with infection and make it more difficult for her to follow the prescribed treatment regimen.

The nurse must determine whether the woman knows how the disease is transmitted and how important it is to complete the prescribed course of medications. Does she know the major side effects of medications?

Providing information about the transmission of tuberculosis to others helps the woman and her family understand the needed precautions. For example, infants should be isolated from those who have bacteria in their sputum. Covering the mouth when coughing, sneezing, or laughing helps prevent bacteria from entering the air. Washing the hands carefully after any contact with body substances or soiled tissues decreases exposure of others, as it does for any infection.

The nurse can also furnish reassuring information about pregnancy and tuberculosis. It is rare for the infant to be infected at birth. No adverse fetal effects are associated with maternal skin testing, and several effective antitubercular drugs have not shown adverse fetal effects. The good news is that tuberculosis may be cured or arrested if medication is taken as prescribed.

The nurse should teach the woman about the correct administration of prescribed medications, interactions with other medications or substances such as alcohol, expected side effects, and adverse effects that she should report. Em-

phasize the necessity of continuing medication to eradicate the infection even though the symptoms may have disappeared. Emphasize the importance of keeping follow-up appointments.

An occasional new mother still has organisms in her sputum when she delivers, and she must be placed in respiratory isolation, separated from her newborn. The nursing staff must provide emotional support and counseling so that the mother can deal with the anxiety and frustration she may feel at not being allowed to care for her infant. Language barriers and cultural implications should also be addressed. A referral to social services may be needed to arrange temporary care of the newborn outside the home until the infant and mother have received adequate treatment.

KEY CONCEPTS

- Spontaneous abortion is a leading cause of pregnancy loss. Treatment focuses on preventing complications, such as hypovolemic shock and infection, and providing emotional support for grieving.
- The incidence of ectopic pregnancy in the United States is increasing as a result of pelvic inflammation associated with sexually transmissible diseases. The goals of therapeutic management are to prevent severe hemorrhage and to preserve the fallopian tube so that future fertility is retained.
- Management of hydatidiform mole involves two phases: (1) evacuation of the molar pregnancy and (2) regular follow-up for 1 year to detect malignant changes.
- A woman with placenta previa typically presents with painless vaginal bleeding during the last half of pregnancy. Bleeding from abruptio placentae may be visible or concealed and is likely to be accompanied by pain, uterine tenderness, and uterine hyperactivity.
- Disseminated intravascular coagulation is a life-threatening complication of missed abortion, abruptio placentae, and pre-eclampsia, in which procoagulation and anticoagulation factors are simultaneously activated.
- The goals of management for hyperemesis gravidarum are to prevent dehydration, malnutrition,

and electrolyte imbalance. Emotional support is a most important therapy and a responsibility of nurses.
- Generalized vasospasm, which occurs with pregnancy-induced hypertension, decreases circulation to all organs of the body, including the placenta. Major maternal organs affected include the liver, kidneys, and brain.
- The treatment of pre-eclampsia includes bed rest, reducing environmental stimuli, and administering anticonvulsants.
- Magnesium sulfate is used to prevent convulsions in pregnancy-induced hypertension. Its most serious adverse effect is central nervous system depression, which includes depression of the respiratory center. Hyporeflexia precedes respiratory depression.
- Nurses monitor the woman with pre-eclampsia to determine the effectiveness of medical therapy and to identify signs that the condition is worsening, such as increasing hyperreflexia. Nurses also control external stimuli and initiate measures to protect the woman in case of eclamptic seizures.
- Women who have chronic hypertension are at increased risk for pre-eclampsia and should be monitored closely for proteinuria or generalized edema. Antihypertensive medication should be continued or initiated if diastolic blood pressure is consistently higher than 90 mm Hg.

- Rh incompatibility can occur when an Rh-negative woman conceives a child who is Rh-positive. As a result of exposure to the Rh-positive antigen, maternal antibodies may develop and cause hemolysis of fetal Rh-positive red blood cells in subsequent pregnancies. Administration of RhoGAM prevents production of anti-Rh antibodies, thus preventing destruction of Rh-positive red blood cells in subsequent pregnancies.
- ABO incompatibility usually occurs when the mother has type O blood and has naturally occurring anti-A and anti-B antibodies, which cause hemolysis if the fetal blood is not type O. ABO incompatibility may result in hyperbilirubinemia of the infant, but it usually is a mild condition.
- During early pregnancy, the release of insulin accelerates and may result in episodes of hypoglycemia. Placental hormones, which reach their peak during the second and third trimesters, create resistance to insulin in maternal cells and cause changes in insulin needs throughout pregnancy.
- Women with type 1 diabetes mellitus have a greater risk for pregnancy-induced hypertension, urinary tract infections, and ketosis.
- Because maternal hyperglycemia during the first trimester increases the risk for congenital anomalies in the fetus, a major goal of management is to establish normal blood glucose levels before pregnancy occurs.

- Fetal growth depends on the condition of maternal blood vessels and the blood glucose levels. With no vascular impairment and adequate placental perfusion, the infant is likely to be of normal size (if maternal glucose levels are normal) or large (i.e., having macrosomia). With high maternal glucose levels and vascular impairment, placental perfusion may be compromised, and the fetus may be growth restricted (IUGR).
- In addition to congenital anomalies, the infant of a diabetic mother is at increased risk for hypoglycemia, hypocalcemia, hyperbilirubinemia, and respiratory distress syndrome.
- The maternal effects of gestational diabetes include increased risks for urinary tract infections, hydramnios, premature rupture of membranes, and the development of pregnancy-induced hypertension.
- Gestational diabetes is responsible for two major complications for the fetus or neonate, fetal macrosomia and neonatal hypoglycemia.
- Gestational diabetes can usually be treated by diet and exercise. Insulin, however, may be administered if blood glucose remains high.
- Cardiovascular changes that occur in normal pregnancy impose an additional burden that may result in cardiac decompensation if the expectant mother has preexisting heart disease.
- The primary goal of management of the pregnant woman with heart disease is to prevent the development of congestive heart failure by restricting activity, limiting weight gain, and preventing anemia and infection, so that cardiac demand does not exceed cardiac reserves.
- Intrapartum and postpartum management of heart disease focuses on preventing fluid overload, which can cause a sharp rise in cardiac effort.
- Iron supplementation is needed during pregnancy because most women do not have sufficient iron stores to meet the demands of pregnancy.
- Folic acid deficiency is associated with an increased risk of spontaneous abortion, abruptio placentae, and fetal anomalies, such as neural tube defects. A folic acid supplement may be necessary to prevent maternal and fetal effects.
- Sickle cell disease is exacerbated by pregnancy, and a primary goal is to prevent sickle cell crisis during pregnancy.
- Laboratory values for thalassemia are similar to those of iron deficiency, but administration of iron is risky because increased iron absorption and storage make the woman susceptible to iron overload.
- Although women with systemic lupus erythematosus can have a normal pregnancy and give birth to a normal newborn, the pregnancy must be treated as high risk because of the increased incidence of abortion, fetal death during the first trimester, and possible exacerbation of the disease.
- Antiphospholipid syndrome (an autoimmune disorder) is a cluster of clinical entities and is associated with an increased risk for thrombosis, fetal loss, and the presence of antiphospholipid antibodies.
- The management of epilepsy is complicated by the teratogenic effects of anticonvulsant medications.
- Automobile accidents are the major cause of blunt force trauma that may result in premature separation of the placenta, hemorrhage, fractures, and internal injuries. Penetrating injuries caused by knives or bullets are particularly dangerous for the fetus.
- The treatment of trauma during pregnancy is similar to that in a nonpregnant person. Providing cardiopulmonary support and controlling bleeding are the priorities. Careful evaluation of the uterus and fetus is also essential.
- Viral infections that occur during pregnancy can be transmitted to the fetus in two ways: across the placenta or by exposure to organisms during birth. Although they are mild or even subclinical in the mother, viral infections can have serious effects for the fetus.
- Human immunodeficiency virus is a retrovirus that invades the CD4 subset of lymphocytes and destroys them, producing AIDS, which allows opportunistic infections to overwhelm the immune system.
- Pregnant women who are HIV positive experience anxiety, fear, and grief as they contemplate the losses they will experience as a result of the disease. Nurses must provide emotional support, information, and counseling, which will help the woman cope with her emotions and retain control of her care for as long as possible.
- Nonviral infections such as toxoplasmosis, group B streptococcus infection, and tuberculosis can be prevented or treated.

ANSWERS TO CRITICAL THINKING EXERCISES

Exercise 26–1
Nurses often assume that clients know how to use a thermometer and that they know the signs of infection. Moreover, many nurses assume that clients recognize the connection between blood loss and the tendency to develop infection. As a result, nurses may not emphasize the need for a diet high in nutrients that increase hemoglobin and hematocrit.

Exercise 26–2
1. The team may have assumed that Marcia knew the maternal and fetal effects of gestational diabetes and the importance of following the plan of care.

2. The team could have explained the reasons for the recommended plan and allowed adequate time to answer all questions. It is particularly important to emphasize why it is necessary to monitor the condition of the fetus, because mothers are usually motivated to do whatever they can to ensure the health of the fetus.

3. The nurse should acknowledge Marcia's belief. "I realize that we haven't made our concerns clear to you. Let me explain why it is important for you and for your baby to be watched carefully during these last weeks." The nurse must then provide clear, simple explanations and allow time to answer questions.

4. The nurse must acknowledge that weekly tests are time-consuming but that they provide valuable information about the well-being of the baby. Usually the information is reassuring, but additional tests can be performed if there are questions.

REFERENCES AND READINGS

American Academy of Pediatrics & American College of Obstetricians and Gynecologists. (1997). *Guidelines for perinatal care* (4th ed.). Elk Grove Village, IL, and Washington, DC: Author.

American College of Obstetricians and Gynecologists. (1991). *Fetal macrosomia* (ACOG Technical Bulletin No. 159). Washington, DC: Author.

American College of Obstetricians and Gynecologists. (1994). *Diabetes and pregnancy* (ACOG Technical Bulletin No. 200). Washington, DC: Author.

American College of Obstetricians and Gynecologists. (1996). *Hypertension in pregnancy* (ACOG Technical Bulletin No. 219). Washington, DC: Author.

American Diabetes Association. (1999). American Diabetes Association: Clinical practice recommendations 1999. *Diabetes Care, 22*, suppl. 1.

Aminoff, M. J. (1999). Neurologic disorders. In R. K. Creasy & R. Resnik (Eds.), *Maternal-fetal medicine: Principles and practice* (4th ed., pp. 1091–1119). Philadelphia: Saunders.

Artal, P. (1996). Exercise: An alternative therapy for gestational diabetes. *The Physician and Sports Medicine, 24*(3), 54–66.

Atterbury, J. L., Groome, L. J., Hoff, C., & Yarnell, J. A. (1998). Clinical presentation of women readmitted with postpartum severe preeclampsia or eclampsia. *Journal of Obstetric, Gynecologic, and Neonatal Nursing, 27*(2), 134–141.

Atterbury, J. L., Munn, M. B., Groome, L. J., & Yarnell, J. A. (1997). The antiphospholipid antibody syndrome: An overview. *Journal of Obstetric, Gynecologic, and Neonatal Nursing, 26*(5), 522–530.

August, P. (1999). Hypertensive disorders in pregnancy. In G. N. Burrow & T. P. Duffy (Eds.), *Medical complications during pregnancy* (5th ed., pp. 53–77). Philadelphia: Saunders.

Beazley, D. M., & Egerman, R. S. (1998). Toxoplasmosis. *Seminars in Perinatology, 22*(4), 332–338.

Berman, M. L., DiSaia, P. J., & Brewster, W. R. (1999). Pelvic malignancies, gestational trophoblastic neoplasia, and nonpelvic malignancies. In R. K. Creasy & R. Resnik (Eds.), *Maternal-fetal medicine: Principles and practice* (4th ed., pp. 1128–1150). Philadelphia: Saunders.

Bevier, W. C., Jovanovic-Peterson, L., & Peterson, C. M. (1995). Pancreatic disorders of pregnancy: Diagnosis, management, and outcome of gestational diabetes. *Endo-*

crinology and Metabolism Clinics of North America, 24(1), 103–138.

Boden, G. (1996). Fuel metabolism in pregnancy and in gestational diabetes mellitus. *Obstetrics and Gynecology Clinics of North America, 23*(1), 1–10.

Bowman, J. M. (1999). Hemolytic disease (erythroblastosis fetalis). In R. K. Creasy & R. Resnik (Eds.), *Maternal-fetal medicine: Principles and practice* (4th ed., pp. 736–767). Philadelphia: Saunders.

Brown, H. L., & Abernathy, M. P. (1998). Cytomegalovirus infection. *Seminars in Perinatology, 22*(4), 260–266.

Carpenito, L. J. (1997). *Handbook of nursing diagnosis* (7th ed.). Philadelphia: Lippincott.

Caulin-Glaser, T., & Setaro, J. (1999). Pregnancy and cardiovascular disease. In G. N. Burrow & T. P. Duffy (Eds.), *Medical complications during pregnancy* (5th ed., pp. 111–133). Philadelphia: Saunders.

Centers for Disease Control and Prevention. (1994). Recommendations for the use of zidovudine to reduce perinatal transmission of human immunodeficiency virus. *Morbidity and Mortality Weekly Report, 43*(RR-11), 1–20.

Centers for Disease Control and Prevention. (1996). Prevention of perinatal group B streptococcal disease: A public health prospective. *Morbidity and Mortality Weekly Report, 45*(RR-7), 1–24.

Centers for Disease Control and Prevention. (1998a, July 24). Critical need to pay attention to HIV prevention for women: Minority and young women bear greatest burden. *CDC Update* [On-line]. Available: http://www.cdc.gov/nchstp/hiv_aids/pubs/facts/women.htm

Centers for Disease Control and Prevention. (1998b, July 24). Status of perinatal HIV prevention: U.S. declines continue: Hope for extending success to developing world. *CDC Update* [On-line]. Available: http://www.cdc.gov/nchstp/hiv_aids/pubs/facts/perinatal.htm

Centers for Disease Control and Prevention. (1998c). 1998 guidelines for treatment of sexually transmitted diseases. *Morbidity and Mortality Weekly Report, 47*(RR-1), 1–118.

Chapman, S. J. (1998). Varicella in pregnancy. *Seminars in Perinatology, 22*(4), 339–346.

Clark, S. L. (1999). Placenta previa and abruptio placentae. In R. K. Creasy & R. Resnik (Eds.), *Maternal-fetal medicine: Principles and practice* (4th ed., pp. 616–631). Philadelphia: Saunders.

Classen, S. R., Paulson, P. R., & Zacharias,

S. R. (1998). Systemic lupus erythematosus: Perinatal and neonatal implications. *Journal of Obstetric, Gynecologic, and Neonatal Nursing, 227*(5), 493–500.

Comport, K. A., & Seng, J. K. (1997). Aortic stenosis in pregnancy: A case report. *Journal of Obstetric, Gynecologic, and Neonatal Nursing, 26*(1), 67–77.

Corrarino, J. E. (1998). Perinatal hepatitis B: Update and recommendations. *MCN: American Journal of Maternal/Child Nursing, 23*(5), 246–252.

Coustan, D. R. (1996). Screening and testing for gestational diabetes mellitus. *Obstetrics and Gynecology Clinics of North America, 23*(1), 125–136.

Cunningham, F. G., MacDonald, P. C., Gant, N. F., Leveno, K. J., Gilstrap, L. C., Hankins, G. D. V., & Clark, S. L. (1997). *Williams obstetrics* (20th ed.). Norwalk, CT: Appleton & Lange.

de Swiet, M. (1999). Rheumatologic and connective tissue disorders. In R. K. Creasy & R. Resnik (Eds.), *Maternal-newborn medicine: Principles and practice* (4th ed., pp. 1082–1090). Philadelphia: Saunders.

Doshier, S. (1995). What happens to the offspring of diabetic pregnancies? *MCN: American Journal of Maternal/Child Nursing, 20*(1), 25–28.

Duff, P. (1998). Hepatitis in pregnancy. *Seminars in Perinatology, 22*(4), 277–283.

Duffy, T. P. (1999). Hematologic aspects of pregnancy. In G. N. Burrow & T. P. Duffy (Eds.), *Medical complications during pregnancy* (5th ed., pp. 79–85). Philadelphia: Saunders.

Emory University School of Medicine, Department of Pediatrics. (1997). Sickle cell information center. [On-line]. Available: http://www.emory.edu.PEDS/SICKLE

Enkin, M., Keirse, M. J., Renfrew, M., & Neilson, J. (1995). *A guide to effective care in pregnancy and childbirth* (2nd ed.). Oxford & New York: Oxford University Press.

Fagan, E. A. (1999). Diseases of liver, biliary system, and pancreas. In R. K. Creasy & R. Resnik (Eds.), *Maternal-fetal medicine: Principles and practice* (4th ed., pp. 1064–1081). Philadelphia: Saunders.

Finch, C. M. (1995). Human parvovirus B19 in pregnancy. *Journal of Obstetric, Gynecologic, and Neonatal Nursing, 24*(6), 495–498.

Flemming, D. R. (1999). Challenging traditional insulin injection practices. *American Journal of Nursing, 99*(2), 72–74.

Freeman, S. B. (1995). Common genitourinary infections. *Journal of Obstetric, Gynecologic, and Neonatal Nursing, 24*(8), 735–741.

Gibbs, R. S., & Sweet, R. L. (1999). Maternal and fetal infectious diseases. In R. K. Creasy & R. Resnik (Eds.), *Maternal-fetal medicine: Principles and practice* (4th ed., pp. 659–725). Philadelphia: Saunders.

Gonik, B. (1999). Intensive care monitoring of the critically ill pregnant patient. In R. K. Creasy & R. Resnik (Eds.), *Maternal-fetal medicine: Principles and practice* (4th ed., pp. 895–920). Philadelphia: Saunders.

Healy, K., Jovanovic-Peterson, L., & Peterson, C. M. (1995). Pancreatic disorders of pregnancy. *Endocrinology and Metabolism Clinics of North America, 24*(1), 73–101.

Hewell, S. W., & Hammer, R. H. (1997). Antiphospholipid antibodies: A threat throughout pregnancy. *Journal of Obstetric, Gynecologic, and Neonatal Nursing, 26*(2), 162–168.

Hill, J. A. (1999). Recurrent pregnancy loss. In R. K. Creasy & R. Resnik (Eds.), *Maternal-fetal medicine* (4th ed., pp. 423–443). Philadelphia: Saunders.

Hollier, L. M., & Cox, S. M. (1998). Syphilis. *Seminars in Perinatology, 22*(4), pp. 323–331.

Homko, C. J., & Khandelwal, M. (1996). Glucose monitoring and insulin therapy during pregnancy. *Obstetrics and Gynecology Clinics of North America, 23*(1), 47–74.

Inzucchi, S. E. (1999). Diabetes in pregnancy. In G. N. Burrow & T. P. Duffy (Eds.), *Medical complications during pregnancy* (5th ed., pp. 25–51). Philadelphia: Saunders.

Kendrick, J. M. (1999). Diabetes mellitus in pregnancy. In L. K. Mandeville & N. H. Troiano (Eds.), *AWHONN's high-risk and critical care intrapartum nursing* (2nd ed., pp. 224–255). Philadelphia: Lippincott.

Kilpatrick, S. J., & Laros, R. K. (1999). Maternal hematologic disorders. In R. K. Creasy & R. Resnik (Eds.), *Maternal-fetal medicine: Principles and practice* (4th ed., pp. 935–963). Philadelphia: Saunders.

Kitzmiller, J. L., & Davidson, M. B. (1998). Diabetes and pregnancy. In M. B. Davidson (Ed.), *Diabetes mellitus: Diagnosis and treatment* (4th ed., pp. 313–343). Philadelphia: Saunders.

Landon, M. B., & Gabbe, S. G. (1996). Fetal surveillance and timing of delivery in pregnancy complicated by diabetes mellitus. *Obstetrics and Gynecology Clinics of North America, 23*(1), 109–124.

Landry, M. L. (1999). Viral infections. In G. N. Burrow & T. P. Duffy (Eds.), *Medical complications during pregnancy* (5th ed., pp. 337–362). Philadelphia: Saunders.

Langer, O., & Hod, M. (1996). Management of gestational diabetes mellitus. *Obstetrics and Gynecology Clinics of North America, 23*(1), 137–160.

Larrabee, K., & Cowan, M. (1995). Clinical nursing management of sickle cell disease and trait during pregnancy. *Journal of Perinatal Neonatal Nursing, 9*(2), 29–41.

Leicht, T. L., & Harvey, C. J. (1999). Hypertensive disorders in pregnancy. In L. K. Mandeville & N. H. Troiano (Eds.), *AWHONN's high-risk and critical care intrapartum nursing* (2nd ed., pp. 159–172). Philadelphia: Lippincott.

Lucas, L. S., & Jordan, E. T. (1997). Phenytoin as an alternative treatment for preeclampsia. *Journal of Obstetric, Gynecologic, and Neonatal Nursing, 26*(3), 263–269.

Magann, E. F., & Martin, J. N. (1995). Complicated postpartum preeclampsia-eclampsia. *Obstetrics and Gynecology Clinics of North America, 22*(2), 337–357.

Mahan, I. K., & Escott-Stump, S. (1996). *Krause's food, nutrition, and diet therapy* (9th ed.). Philadelphia: Saunders.

Maiolatesi, C. R., & Peddicord, K. (1996). Methotrexate for nonsurgical treatment of ectopic pregnancy: Nursing implications. *Journal of Obstetric, Gynecologic, and Neonatal Nursing, 25*(3), 205–208.

Markenson, G. R., & Yancey, M. K. (1998). Parvovirus B19 infections in pregnancy. *Seminars in Perinatology, 22*(4), 309–317.

McKenna, D. S., & Iams, J. D. (1998). Group B streptococcal infections. *Seminars in Perinatology, 22*(4), 267–276.

Minkoff, H. L. (1998). Human immunodeficiency virus infection in pregnancy. *Seminars in Perinatology, 22*(4), 293–308.

Minkoff, H. L. (1999). Human immunodeficiency virus. In R. K. Creasy & R. Resnik (Eds.), *Maternal-fetal medicine: Principles and practice* (4th ed., pp. 725–735). Philadelphia: Saunders.

Minnick-Smith, K., & Cook, F. (1997). Current treatment options for ectopic pregnancy. *MCN: American Journal of Maternal/Child Nursing, 22*(1), 21–25.

Mitchell, A., Steffenson, N., Hogan, H., & Brooks, S. (1997). Group B streptococcus and pregnancy: Update and recommendations. *MCN: American Journal of Maternal/Child Nursing, 22*(5), 242–248.

Monga, M. (1999). Maternal cardiovascular and renal adaptation to pregnancy. In R. K. Creasy & R. Resnik (Eds.), *Maternal-fetal medicine: Principles and practice* (4th ed., pp. 783–792). Philadelphia: Saunders.

Montgomery, K. S. (1996). Caring for the pregnant woman with sickle cell disease. *MCN: American Journal of Maternal/Child Nursing, 21*(5), 224–228.

Moore, T. R. (1999). Diabetes in pregnancy. In R. K. Creasy & R. Resnik (Eds.), *Maternal-fetal medicine: Principles and practice* (4th ed., pp. 964–995). Philadelphia: Saunders.

Nathan, L., & Huddleston, J. F. (1995). Acute abdominal pain in pregnancy. *Obstetrics and Gynecology Clinics of North America, 22*(1), 55–68.

Newshan, G., & Hoyt, M. J. (1998). Use of combination antiretroviral therapy in pregnant women with HIV disease. *MCN: American Journal of Maternal/Child Nursing, 23*(6), 307–312.

Reece, E. A. (1996). Preface. *Obstetrics and Gynecology Clinics of North America, 23*(1), xi–xii.

Reece, E. A., & Eriksson, U. J. (1996). The pathogenesis of diabetes-associated congenital malformations. *Obstetrics and Gynecology Clinics of North America, 23*(1), 29–46.

Reece, E. A., Homko, C. J., & Hagay, Z. (1996). Prenatal diagnosis and prevention of diabetic embryopathy. *Obstetrics and Gynecology Clinics of North America, 23*(1), 11–28.

Riely, C. A., & Fallon, H. J. (1999). Liver diseases. In G. N. Burrow & T. P. Duffy (Eds.), *Medical complications during pregnancy* (5th ed., pp. 269–294). Philadelphia: Saunders.

Riley, L. E. (1998). Herpes simplex virus. *Seminars in Perinatology, 22*(4), 284–292.

Roberts, J. M. (1999). Pregnancy-related hypertension. In R. K. Creasy & R. Resnik (Eds.), *Maternal-fetal medicine: Principles and practice* (4th ed., pp. 833–872). Philadelphia: Saunders.

Rosa, C. (1998). Rubella and rubeola. *Seminars in Perinatology, 22*(4), 318–322.

Rouse, D. J., Gardner, M., Allen, S. J., & Goldenberg, R. L. (1996). Management of presumed susceptible varicella (chickenpox)-exposed gravida: A cost-effectiveness/cost-benefit analysis. *Obstetrics and Gynecology, 87*(6), 932–936.

Savoia, M. C. (1999). Bacterial, fungal, and parasitic disease. In G. N. Burrow & T. P. Duffy (Eds.), *Medical complications during pregnancy* (5th ed., pp. 295–335). Philadelphia: Saunders.

Scott, L. D. (1999). Gastrointestinal disease in pregnancy. In R. K. Creasy & R. Resnik (Eds.), *Maternal-fetal medicine: Principles and practice* (4th ed., pp. 1038–1053). Philadelphia: Saunders.

Shabetai, R. (1999). Cardiac diseases. In R. K. Creasy & R. Resnik (Eds.), *Maternal-fetal medicine: Principles and practice* (4th ed., pp. 793–819). Philadelphia: Saunders.

Shermer, R. H. (1995). Group B streptococcus during the perinatal period. *Journal of Obstetric, Gynecologic, and Neonatal Nursing, 24*(6), 562–566.

Silver, R. M., & Branch, D. W. (1999). Immunologic disorders. In R. K. Creasy & R. Resnik (Eds.), *Maternal-fetal medicine: Principles and practice* (4th ed., pp. 465–483). Philadelphia: Saunders.

Snell, L. H., Haughey, B. P., Buck, G., & Marecki, M. A. (1998). Metabolic crisis: Hyperemesis gravidarum. *Journal of Perinatal-Neonatal Nursing, 12*(2), 26–37.

Tyrala, E. E. (1996). The infant of the diabetic mother. *Obstetrics and Gynecology Clinics of North America, 23*(1), 221–241.

Urbanski, T. K., Higgins, P. G., Murray, M. L., & Joffe, G. (1996). Caring for a woman with a hydatidiform mole and coexisting pregnancy. *MCN: American Journal of Maternal/Child Nursing, 21*(2), 85–89.

Usta, I. M., & Sibai, B. M. (1995). Emergent management of puerperal eclampsia. *Obstetrics and Gynecology Clinics of North America, 22*(2), 315–335.

van Stuijvenberg, M. E., Schabort, I., Labadarios, D., & Nel, J. T. (1995). The nutritional status and treatment of patients with hyperemesis gravidarum. *American Journal of Obstetrics and Gynecology, 172*(5), 1585–1591.

Weinberger, S. E., & Weiss, S. T. (1999). Pulmonary disease. In G. N. Burrow & T. P. Duffy (Eds.), *Medical complications during pregnancy* (5th ed., pp. 363–400). Philadelphia: Saunders.

Yero, T., Mayer, J., Parsons, A., & Maroulis, G. (1995). A prospective of unruptured ectopic pregnancies treated by tubal injection with hyperosmolar glucose. *Obstetrics and Gynecology, 85*(2), 265–268.

Youngkin, E. Q. (1995). Sexually transmitted diseases: Current and emerging concerns. *Journal of Obstetric, Gynecologic, and Neonatal Nursing, 24*(8), 743–758.

27

The Woman with an Intrapartum Complication

DEFINITIONS

abruptio placentae Premature separation of a normally implanted placenta.

amniotic fluid embolism An embolism in which amniotic fluid with its particulate matter is drawn into the pregnant woman's circulation, lodging in her lungs.

cephalopelvic disproportion (CPD) Fetal head size that is too large to fit through the maternal pelvis at birth. Also called fetopelvic disproportion.

chorioamnionitis Inflammation of the amniotic sac (fetal membranes); usually caused by bacterial or viral infection. Also called amnionitis.

dystocia Difficult or prolonged labor; often associated with abnormal uterine activity and cephalopelvic disproportion.

hydramnios Excessive volume of amniotic fluid (more than 2,000 ml at term). Also called polyhydramnios.

hypertonic labor dysfunction Ineffective labor characterized by erratic and poorly coordinated contractions. Uterine resting tone is higher than normal.

hypotonic labor dysfunction Ineffective labor characterized by weak, infrequent, and brief but coordinated uterine contractions. Uterine resting tone is normal.

macrosomia Unusually large fetal size; infant birth weight more than 4,000 g (8.8 lb).

multifetal pregnancy A pregnancy in which the woman is carrying two or more fetuses. Also called multiple gestation.

occult prolapse See *prolapsed cord*.

oligohydramnios Abnormally small volume of amniotic fluid (less than 500 ml at term).

placenta accreta A placenta that is abnormally adherent to the uterine muscle. If the condition is more advanced, it is called placenta increta (the placenta extends into the uterine muscle) or placenta percreta (the placenta extends through the uterine muscle).

placenta previa Abnormal implantation of the placenta in the lower uterus, at or very near the cervical os.

precipitate birth A birth that occurs without a trained attendant present.

precipitate labor An intense, unusually short labor (less than 3 hours).

preterm labor Onset of labor after 20 weeks and before the beginning of the 38th week of gestation.

prolapsed cord Displacement of the umbilical cord in front of or beside the fetal presenting part. An occult prolapse is one that is suspected on the basis of fetal heart rate patterns; the umbilical cord cannot be palpated or seen.

shoulder dystocia Delayed or difficult birth of the fetal shoulders after the head is born.

tocolytic A drug that inhibits uterine contractions.

uterine inversion Turning of the uterus inside out after birth of the fetus.

uterine resting tone Degree of uterine muscle tension when the woman is not in labor or during the interval between labor contractions.

uterine rupture A tear in the wall of the uterus.

Birth is usually free of major complications. Sometimes, however, complications make childbearing hazardous for the woman or her baby. The nurse's challenge is to identify and manage the complications promptly and to provide effective care for these mothers while supporting the entire family at this significant time in their lives.

■ *Dysfunctional Labor*

Normal labor is characterized by progress. Dysfunctional labor is one that does not result in normal progress of cervical effacement, dilation, and fetal descent. *Dystocia* is a general term that describes any difficult labor or birth. A dysfunctional labor may result from problems with the powers of labor, the passenger, the passage, the psyche, or a combination of these. Dysfunctional labor is often prolonged but may be unusually short and intense.

An operative birth (vacuum extractor– or forceps-assisted or cesarean) may be needed if dysfunctional labor does not resolve or if fetal or maternal compromise occurs. Signs that indicate the need for an operative birth include persistent nonreassuring fetal heart rate (FHR) patterns (see Chapter 18), fetal acidosis, and meconium passage. Maternal exhaustion or infection may occur, especially with long labors.

Problems of the Powers

The powers of labor may not be adequate to expel the fetus because of ineffective contractions or ineffective maternal pushing efforts.

INEFFECTIVE CONTRACTIONS

Effective uterine activity is characterized by coordinated contractions that are strong and numerous enough to propel the fetus past the resistance of the woman's bony pelvis and soft tissues. It is not possible to say how frequent, long, or strong labor contractions must be. One woman's labor may progress with contractions that would be inadequate for another woman. Possible causes of ineffective contractions include

- Maternal fatigue
- Maternal inactivity
- Fluid and electrolyte imbalance
- Hypoglycemia
- Excessive analgesia or anesthesia
- Maternal catecholamines secreted in response to stress or pain
- Disproportion between the maternal pelvis and the fetal presenting part
- Uterine overdistention, such as with multiple gestation or hydramnios

Two patterns of ineffective uterine contractions are hypotonic and hypertonic dysfunction (Table 27–1). Hypotonic dysfunction is more common than hypertonic. Characteristics and management of each are different, but the result—poor labor progress—is the same if they persist.

Hypotonic Dysfunction. Hypotonic contractions are coordinated but are too weak to be effective. They are infrequent and brief and can be easily indented with fingertip pressure at the peak.

Hypotonic dysfunction usually occurs during the active phase of labor, when progress normally quickens. Uterine overdistention is associated with hypotonic dysfunction because the stretched uterine muscle contracts poorly.

The woman may be fairly comfortable because her contractions are weak. Persistent hypotonic dysfunction is fatiguing and frustrating for the mother. Fetal hypoxia is not usually seen with hypotonic labor.

Management depends on the cause. Providing intravenous or oral fluids corrects maternal fluid and electrolyte imbalances or hypoglycemia. Maternal position changes, particularly upright positions, favor fetal descent and promote effective contractions. The woman who moves about actively typically has better labor progress and is more comfortable than one who remains in one position.

The nurse should use therapeutic communication to help the woman identify anxieties or beliefs about labor and its progress. Helping her to get her anxieties in the open is the first step to managing them effectively so that the stress response does not slow her labor.

Some women need measures such as amniotomy or oxytocin infusion to promote labor progress. The birth attendant evaluates the woman's labor to confirm that she is having hypotonic active labor rather than a long latent phase (the first 3 cm of dilation) of labor. The maternal pelvis and fetal presentation and position are assessed to identify abnormalities.

Amniotomy or oxytocin augmentation (see Chapter 20) may be used to stimulate a labor that slows after it is established. Reduced placental perfusion due to excessive uterine contractions is the most common risk of oxytocin labor augmentation.

Hypertonic Dysfunction. Hypertonic dysfunction of labor is less common than hypotonic. Contractions are uncoordinated and are erratic in their frequency, duration, and intensity. The contractions are painful but ineffective. Hypertonic dysfunction usually occurs during the latent phase of labor.

The uterine resting tone between contractions is high, reducing uterine blood flow. This ischemia decreases fetal oxygen supply and causes the woman to have almost constant cramping pain. Because high resting tone and constant pain are also seen in abruptio placentae, this complication should be considered as well.

The mother becomes very tired because of nearly constant discomfort. She may lose confidence in her ability to give birth and to cope with labor. Frustration and anxiety further reduce her pain tolerance and interfere with the normal processes of labor. The nurse should accept her frustration and discomfort. It is important not to equate cervical

TABLE 27–1

• • • • • • • • • • •

Patterns of Labor Dysfunction

Hypotonic Dysfunction	*Hypertonic Dysfunction*
Contractions	
Coordinated but weak	Uncoordinated, irregular
Become less frequent and shorter in duration	Short and poor intensity, but painful and cramp-like
Easily indented at peak	
Woman may have minimal discomfort because the contractions are weak.	
Uterine Resting Tone	
Not elevated	Higher than normal. Important to distinguish from abruptio placentae, which has similar characteristics (p. 640).
Phase of Labor	
Active. Typically occurs after 4 cm dilation	Latent. Usually occurs before 4 cm dilation
More common than hypertonic dysfunction	Less common than hypotonic dysfunction
Therapeutic Management	
Amniotomy (may increase the risk of infection)	Correct cause if it can be identified.
Oxytocin augmentation	Sedation
Cesarean birth if no progress	Hydration
	Tocolytics to reduce high uterine tone and promote placental perfusion
Nursing Care	
Interventions related to amniotomy and oxytocin augmentation	Promote uterine blood flow: side-lying position.
Encourage position changes. An abdominal binder may help direct the fetus toward the mother's pelvis if her abdominal wall is very lax.	Promote rest, general comfort, and relaxation.
Ambulation if no contraindication and if acceptable to the woman	Pain relief
Emotional support: Allow her to ventilate feelings of discouragement. Explain measures taken to increase effectiveness of contractions. Include her partner/ family in emotional support measures as they may have anxiety that will heighten the woman's anxiety.	Emotional support: Accept the reality of the woman's pain and frustration. Reassure her that she is not being childish. Explain reason for measures to break abnormal labor patterns and their expected results. Allow her to ventilate her feelings during and after labor. Include partner/family (see hypotonic labor).

dilation with the amount of pain a woman "should" experience.

Management of hypertonic labor depends on the cause. Relief of pain is the primary intervention to promote a normal labor pattern. Warm showers or baths promote relaxation and rest, often allowing a normal labor pattern to ensue. Systemic analgesics or occasionally epidural analgesia may be required to achieve this purpose.

Oxytocin is not usually given because it can intensify the already high uterine resting tone. Very low doses of oxytocin, however, are sometimes given to promote coordinated uterine contractions. Tocolytic drugs may be ordered to reduce uterine resting tone and improve placental blood flow.

INEFFECTIVE MATERNAL PUSHING

A reflex urge to push with contractions usually occurs as the fetal presenting part reaches the pelvic floor during second-stage labor. Ineffective pushing may result from

- Use of incorrect pushing techniques or inappropriate pushing positions
- Fear of injury because of pain and tearing sensations felt by the mother when she pushes
- Decreased or absent urge to push
- Maternal exhaustion
- Analgesia or anesthesia that suppresses the woman's urge to push
- Psychological unreadiness to "let go" of her baby

Management focuses on correcting the causes contributing to ineffective pushing. If maternal and fetal vital signs are normal, there is no maximum allowable duration for the second stage. Each woman is evaluated individually by her birth attendant to determine whether labor should be ended with an operative delivery or can continue safely. For most women, this occurs after about 2 to 3 hours of *vigorous* pushing efforts that do not result in fetal descent to the pelvic floor.

Nursing care to promote effective pushing helps the mother make each effort more productive. Upright positions such as squatting add the force of gravity to her efforts. Semi-sitting, side-lying, and pushing while sitting on the toilet are other options (see Chapter 17).

The woman who fears injury because of the sensations she feels when she pushes may respond to accurate information about the process of fetal descent. If she understands that sensations of tearing often accompany fetal descent but that her tissues can expand to accommodate the baby, she may be more willing to push with contractions. Warm perineal compresses and massage may increase perineal distensibility and reduce the chance of tearing, although this is unproven.

A reduced urge to push may occur when epidural block analgesia is given. If a woman cannot feel the urge to push or cannot feel it strongly, she can be coached to push as each contraction begins.

The woman who is exhausted may push more effectively if she is encouraged to rest and to push only when she feels the urge, or she may push with every other contraction. Oral or intravenous fluids provide energy for the strenuous work of second-stage labor. Reassuring her about fetal well-being and the fact that she has no deadline to meet help her work with her body's efforts most effectively. This reassurance also helps the woman who may be emotionally readying herself to "let go" of her fetus in exchange for a newborn as she labors.

Problems with the Passenger

Fetal problems associated with dysfunctional labor are those related to

- Fetal size
- Fetal presentation or position
- Multifetal pregnancy
- Fetal anomalies

These variations may cause mechanical problems and contribute to ineffective contractions.

FETAL SIZE
Macrosomia.   The macrosomic infant weighs more than 4,000 g (8.8 lb) at birth. The head or shoulders may not be able to adapt to the pelvis. In addition, distention of the uterus by the large fetus reduces the strength of contractions both during and after birth.

Size is relative, however. The woman with a small pelvis or one that is abnormally shaped may not be able to deliver an average-sized or small infant. A woman with a large pelvis may easily give birth to a larger infant.

Shoulder Dystocia.   Delayed or difficult birth of the shoulders may occur as they become impacted above the maternal symphysis pubis. As soon as the head is born, it retracts against the perineum, much like a turtle's head drawing into its shell (sometimes referred to as the "turtle sign").

Shoulder dystocia is an urgent situation because the umbilical cord is compressed but chest compression within the vagina prevents respirations. Any of several methods may be used to relieve the impacted fetal shoulders quickly (Fig. 27–1). The infant's clavicles should be checked for crepitus, deformity, or bruising, each of which suggests fracture.

ABNORMAL FETAL PRESENTATION OR POSITION
An unfavorable fetal presentation or position may interfere with cervical dilation or fetal descent.

Rotation Abnormalities.   Persistence of the fetus in the occiput posterior (OP) or occiput transverse (OT) position can contribute to dysfunctional labor. These positions delay fetal descent and other mechanisms of labor (cardinal movements). Most fetuses that begin labor in an OP position rotate spontaneously to an occiput anterior position, promoting normal extension and expulsion of the head. Although many women cannot readily deliver their fetus in the OP position, the woman with a large pelvis compared with the fetal size may be able to do so.

Labor is usually longer and more uncomfortable when the fetus remains in the OP or OT position. Intense back or leg pain that is poorly relieved with analgesia makes it difficult for the woman to cope with labor. "Back labor" aptly describes the sensations a woman feels when her fetus is in an OP position.

Maternal position changes promote fetal head rotation to an occiput anterior position and descent (see Chapter 17). Examples are as follows:

- Hands and knees. Rocking the pelvis back and forth while on hands and knees encourages rotation.
- Side-lying (on her left side if the fetus is in a right OP position and on her right side for a left OP position)
- The lunge (Simkin, 1995), in which the mother places one foot on a chair with her foot and knee pointed to that side. She lunges sideways repeatedly during a contraction for 5 seconds at a time. This action can also be performed in a kneeling position. The nurse or her partner must secure the chair and help her balance.
- Squatting (for second-stage labor)
- Sitting, kneeling, or standing while leaning forward

Using a birthing ball, a large plastic ball capable of supporting an adult's weight, helps support the woman when in the hands-and-knees position. She can also sit on it, providing many of the benefits of squatting. Additionally, the woman tends to move her hips back and forth, favoring fetal descent.

Upright maternal positions promote descent, which is usually accompanied by fetal head rotation. The hands and knees and the side-lying positions promote rotation because the mother's abdomen is dependent in relation to her spine. The convex surface of the fetal back tends to rotate toward the convex anterior uterus, similar to nesting two spoons together (Fig. 27–2). Moreover, these positions decrease the mother's discomfort by reducing fetal head pressure on her sacrum. A side-lying position has a similar effect.

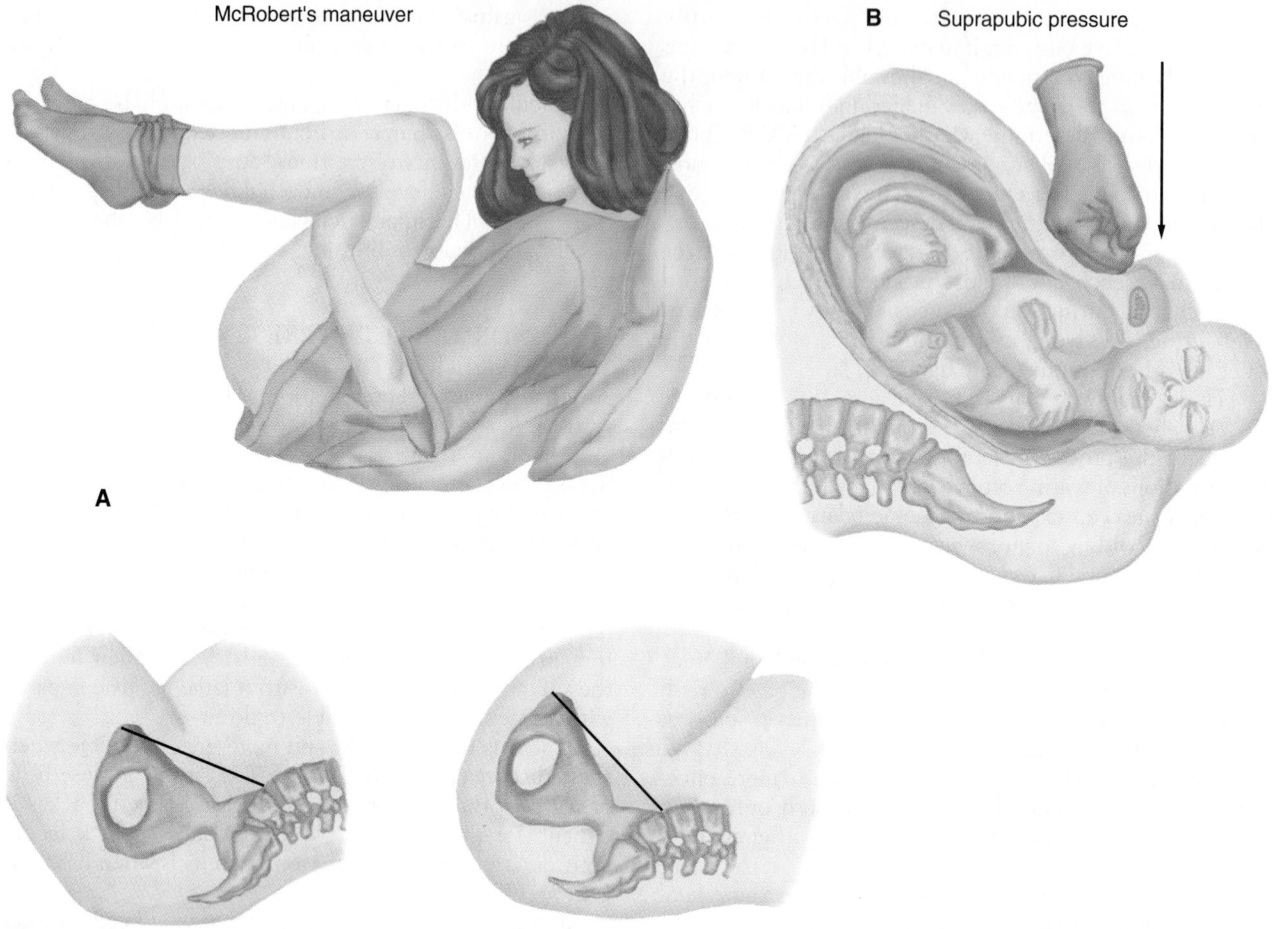

McRobert's maneuver

B Suprapubic pressure

A

FIGURE 27-1

Methods that may be used to relieve shoulder dystocia. *A,* McRobert's maneuver. The woman flexes her thighs sharply against her abdomen, which straightens the pelvic curve. A supported squat has a similar effect and adds gravity to her pushing efforts. *B,* Suprapubic pressure by an assistant pushes the fetal anterior shoulder downward to displace it from above the mother's symphysis pubis. Fundal pressure should not be used, as it will push the anterior shoulder more firmly against the mother's symphysis.

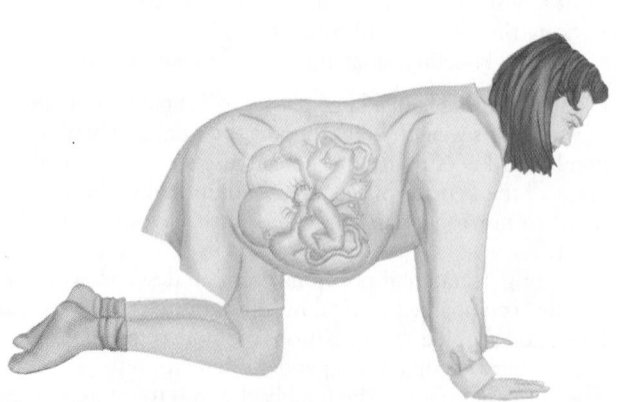

FIGURE 27-2

A "hands-and-knees" position helps the fetus rotate from a left occiput posterior (LOP) position to an occiput anterior position.

The lunge widens the side of the pelvis toward which the woman lunges. If the fetal position is known, she lunges toward the side where the occiput is located (Fig. 27–3). If the fetal position is not known, the woman can lunge toward the side that gives her greater comfort.

All variations of the squatting position aid rotation and fetal descent by straightening the pelvic curve and by enlarging the pelvic outlet. They also add gravity to the force of maternal pushing.

If spontaneous rotation does not occur, the physician may assist rotation and descent of the head with forceps. The vacuum extractor cannot usually be applied to the fetal head when it remains in an OP position. Cesarean birth may be needed if forceps use is not successful.

Deflexion Abnormalities. The poorly flexed fetal head presents a larger diameter to the pelvis than if flexed with the chin on the chest (see Fig. 17–8). In the *face presentation,* the head diameter is similar to that of the vertex presentation, but the maternal pelvis can be traversed only if the fetal chin (mentum) is anterior.

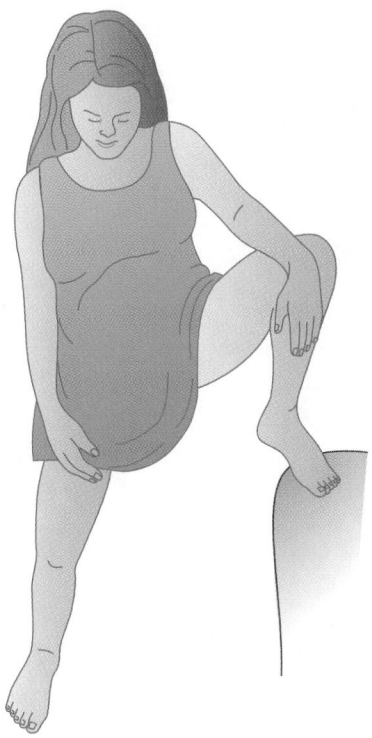

FIGURE 27-3

The "lunge" to one side promotes rotation of the fetal occiput from a posterior position to an anterior one.

Breech Presentation. Cervical dilation and effacement are often slower when the fetus is in a breech presentation because the buttocks or feet do not form a smooth, round dilating wedge like the head. The greatest fetal risk is that the head—the largest fetal part—is last to be born. By the time the lower body is born, the umbilical cord is well into the pelvis and may be compressed. The shoulders, arms, and head must be delivered quickly so that the infant can breathe.

A breech presentation is common well before term, but only 3% to 4% of term fetuses remain in this presentation. Adverse outcomes that are associated with breech birth may include

- Fetal injury with a difficult vaginal birth
- Prolapsed umbilical cord

CRITICAL THINKING EXERCISE 27-1

A woman having her first baby has been in labor for several hours. Her nurse-midwife performs a vaginal examination and says that the cervix is 6 cm dilated and completely effaced, with the fetus in right occiput posterior position. The mother is having persistent back pain that worsens during contractions.

1. How should the nurse interpret this information?
2. Should the nurse take any specific action based on the examination?

- Low birth weight due to preterm gestation, multifetal pregnancy, or intrauterine growth restriction
- Fetal anomalies, such as hydrocephalus
- Complications secondary to placenta previa or cesarean birth

External version may be attempted to change the fetus in a breech presentation or transverse lie to a cephalic presentation (see Chapter 20). If the fetus remains in the abnormal presentation, cesarean birth is usually performed to avoid complications of a difficult vaginal birth. Birth for the nulliparous woman with a fetus in a breech presentation is almost always cesarean. The fetus remaining in a transverse lie is delivered by cesarean.

The physician may recommend that vaginal birth be attempted when the fetus is in a breech presentation if

- The maternal pelvis is of normal size and shape
- The estimated fetal weight is less than 3,600 g (8 lb)
- Other complications, such as placenta previa and prolapsed cord, are not present

MULTIFETAL PREGNANCY

Multifetal pregnancy may result in dysfunctional labor because of uterine overdistention, which contributes to hypotonic dysfunction, and abnormal presentation of one or both fetuses (Fig. 27–4). In addition, the potential for fetal hypoxia during labor is greater. The risk for postpartum hemorrhage resulting from uterine atony because of uterine overdistention is greater.

Because of these problems, birth for a woman with a multifetal pregnancy is often cesarean. The physician considers fetal presentations, maternal pelvic size, and the presence of other complications, such as pregnancy-induced hypertension.

During labor, each twin's FHR is monitored separately. When in bed, the woman should remain in a lateral position to promote adequate placental blood flow. After vaginal birth of the first twin, assessment of the second twin's FHR continues until birth. The nurse observes for signs of hypotonic dysfunction throughout labor.

Whether the birth is vaginal or cesarean, the intrapartum staff must be prepared for the care and possible resuscitation of multiple infants. Cord clamps, bulb syringes, radiant warmers, and resuscitation equipment must be prepared for each infant. One or more neonatal nurses, a neonatal nurse practitioner, a pediatrician, or a neonatologist should be available to care for each infant. One nurse should be free to care for the mother.

FETAL ANOMALIES

Fetal anomalies such as hydrocephalus or a large fetal tumor may prevent normal descent of the fetus. Abnormal presentations, such as breech or transverse lie, are also associated with fetal anomalies. These abnormalities may be discovered by ultrasound examination before labor. A cesarean birth is scheduled if vaginal birth is not possible or if it is inadvisable.

Problems of the Passage

Dysfunctional labor may occur because of variations in the maternal bony pelvis or because of soft tissue problems that inhibit fetal descent.

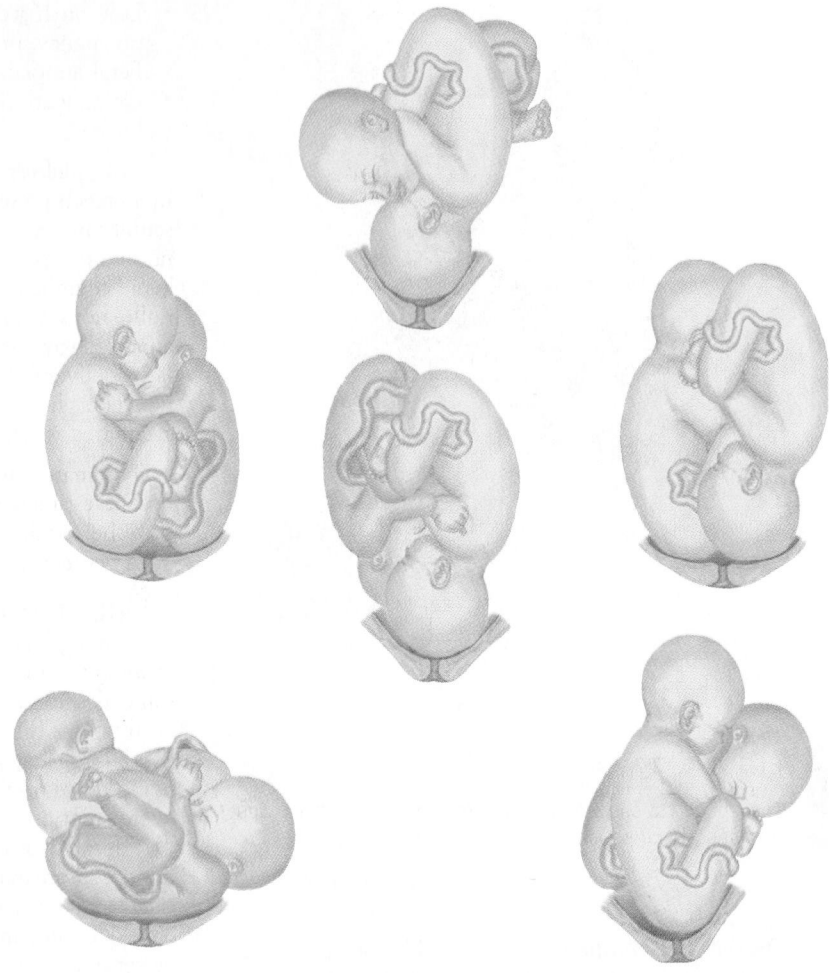

FIGURE 27–4
• • • • • • • • •
Twins can present in any combination.

PELVIS

A small (contracted) or abnormally shaped pelvis may retard labor and obstruct fetal passage. The woman may experience poor contractions, slow dilation, slow fetal descent, and a long labor. The danger of uterine rupture is greater with thinning of the lower uterine segment, especially if contractions remain strong.

There are four basic pelvic shapes, each with different implications for labor and birth (Fig. 27–5). Most women have mixed characteristics from two or more types.

MATERNAL SOFT TISSUE OBSTRUCTIONS

During labor, a full bladder is a common soft tissue obstruction. Bladder distention reduces available space in the pelvis and intensifies maternal discomfort. The woman should be assessed for bladder distention regularly and encouraged to void every 1 to 2 hours. Catheterization may be needed if she cannot urinate.

Problems of the Psyche

A perceived threat caused by pain, fear, nonsupport, or one's personal situation can result in excessive maternal stress and interfere with normal labor progress. The woman's perception of stress more than the actual existence of a threat is important.

The body responds to stress, preparing itself for fight or flight. Responses to excessive or prolonged stress, however, interfere with labor in several ways:

- Increased glucose consumption reduces the energy supply available to the contracting uterus.
- Secretion of catecholamines (epinephrine and norepinephrine) by the adrenal glands stimulates uterine beta-receptors, which inhibit uterine contractions (an action similar to that of tocolytic drugs, such as terbutaline).
- Adrenal secretion of catecholamines diverts blood supply from the uterus and placenta to skeletal muscle.
- Labor contractions and maternal pushing efforts are less effective because these powers are working against the resistance of tense abdominal and pelvic muscles.
- Pain perception is increased and pain tolerance is decreased, which further increase maternal anxiety and stress.

Helping the woman relax helps her body work more effectively with the forces of labor and promotes normal progress. General nursing measures involve

- Establishing a trusting relationship with the woman and her family
- Making the environment comfortable by adjusting temperature and light
- Promoting physical comfort, such as cleanliness

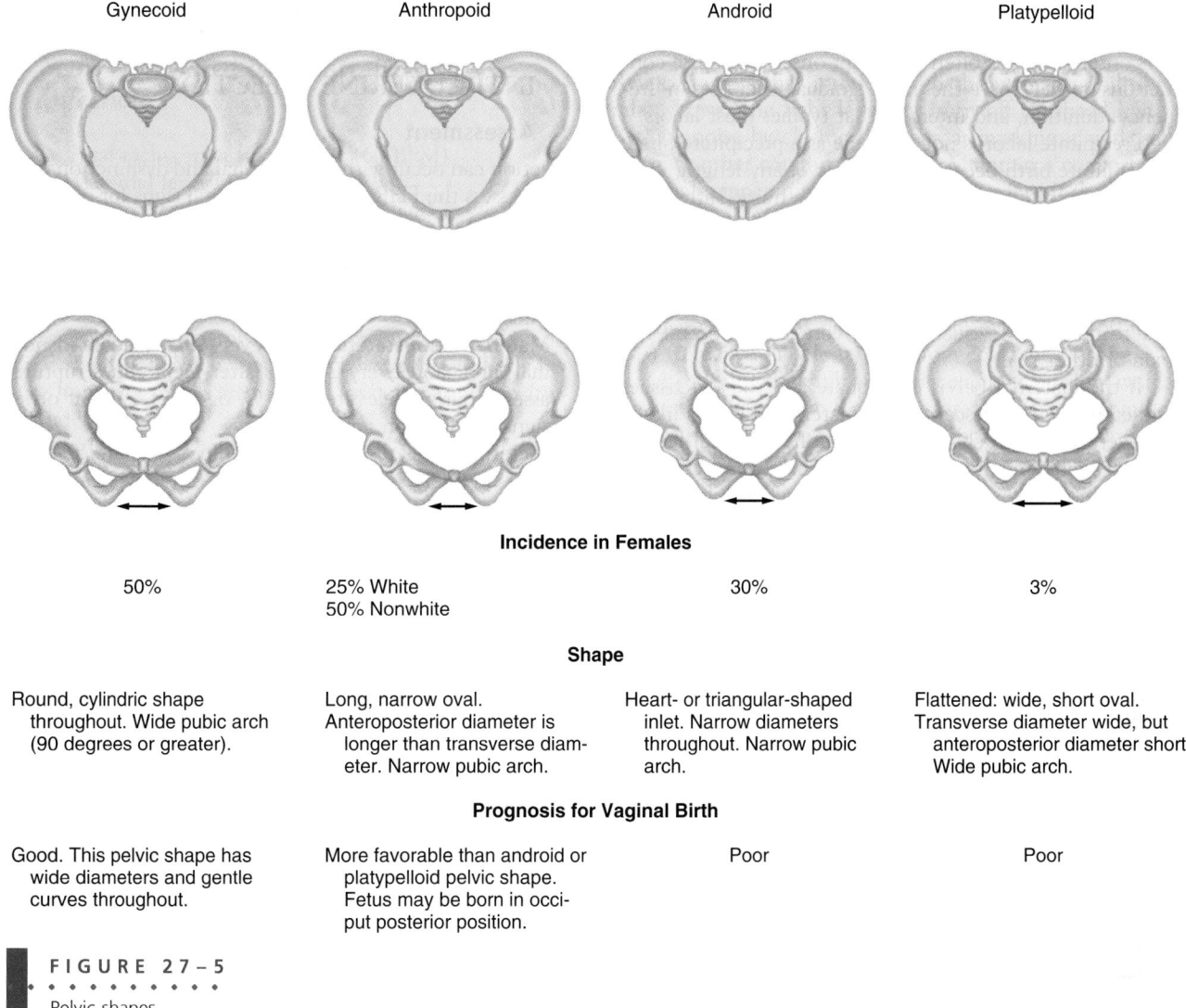

Gynecoid	Anthropoid	Android	Platypelloid

Incidence in Females

50%	25% White 50% Nonwhite	30%	3%

Shape

Round, cylindric shape throughout. Wide pubic arch (90 degrees or greater).	Long, narrow oval. Anteroposterior diameter is longer than transverse diameter. Narrow pubic arch.	Heart- or triangular-shaped inlet. Narrow diameters throughout. Narrow pubic arch.	Flattened: wide, short oval. Transverse diameter wide, but anteroposterior diameter short. Wide pubic arch.

Prognosis for Vaginal Birth

Good. This pelvic shape has wide diameters and gentle curves throughout.	More favorable than android or platypelloid pelvic shape. Fetus may be born in occiput posterior position.	Poor	Poor

FIGURE 27–5
• • • • • • • • • •
Pelvic shapes.

• Providing accurate information
• Implementing nonpharmacologic and pharmacologic pain management

Chapters 17 and 19 describe specific methods to encourage relaxation and promote comfort.

Abnormal Labor Duration

An unusually long or short labor may result in maternal, fetal, or neonatal problems.

PROLONGED LABOR

Prolonged labor is a type of dysfunctional labor that results from problems with any of the factors in the birth process. After the woman reaches the active phase of labor, cervical dilation should proceed at a minimum rate of 1.2 cm per hour in the nullipara and 1.5 cm per hour in the parous woman. Descent of the fetal presenting part is expected to occur at a minimum rate of 1.0 cm per hour in the nullipara and 2.0 cm per hour in the parous woman (American College of Obstetrics & Gynecology [ACOG], 1995b). If all

previous births were by cesarean before much cervical dilation occurred, the criteria that apply to a nullipara may be applied to a multipara.

Potential maternal and fetal problems in prolonged labor include

• Maternal infection, intrapartum or postpartum
• Neonatal infection, which may be severe or fatal
• Maternal exhaustion
• Higher levels of anxiety and fear during a subsequent labor

Maternal and neonatal infections are more likely if the membranes have been ruptured for a prolonged time because organisms ascend from the vagina. The mother is more likely to have an intrapartum or a postpartum infection, or both.

Nursing measures for the woman who has prolonged labor include promotion of comfort, conservation of energy, emotional support, position changes that favor normal progress, and assessments for infection. Nursing care for the fetus includes observation for signs of intrauterine infection and for compromised fetal oxygenation (see Chapter 18).

in smooth muscles such as the uterus, so blocking calcium reduces the muscular contraction. Flushing of the skin, headache, and a transient increase in the maternal and fetal heart rates are common side effects. Because nifedipine is a vasodilator, the woman may have postural hypotension.

The nurse should observe for side effects of nifedipine and report a maternal pulse rate greater than 110. The woman should be assisted when sitting or standing and should do so gradually to reduce the effects of postural hypotension.

ACCELERATING FETAL LUNG MATURITY

The physician may order corticosteroids to speed fetal lung maturation if preterm birth seems inevitable. Steroid therapy may reduce the incidence and severity of respiratory distress syndrome (RDS) in the preterm infant. Evidence also suggests that steroids given before preterm birth reduce the mortality rate and decrease the incidence of intraventricular hemorrhage and necrotizing enterocolitis. Betamethasone and dexamethasone are common drugs for this purpose.

Corticosteroids are indicated if the woman is between 24 and 34 weeks' gestation because of the high incidence of RDS at this age. For greatest benefit in reducing RDS, birth must occur no sooner than 24 hours after beginning the drug but within 7 days. Evidence shows that steroids received within 24 hours of birth offer some benefits to the infant, so steroids are recommended unless birth is imminent. Although the National Institutes of Health concluded that steroids are beneficial for women with ruptured membranes between 24 and 32 weeks, ACOG (1995c) recommends further study of this issue. Repeated steroid doses may be given if birth does not occur within 7 days (up to 34 weeks' gestation), although further study is needed to determine if repeated dosing is safe and effective.

The nurse should observe for and teach the woman

signs of pulmonary edema, because corticosteroids can cause sodium retention with accompanying fluid retention. The nurse assesses lung sounds with other vital signs. The woman is taught to report any chest pain or heaviness or any difficulty breathing.

■ NURSING CARE
· · · · · · · · · ·
The Woman in Preterm Labor

Nursing care for the woman with preterm labor may include interventions related to tocolytic, corticosteroid, or antibiotic drug therapy. If labor cannot be halted, care is similar to that for other laboring women, with additional care to prepare for a preterm infant's needs at birth. Support for anticipatory grieving may be needed if the infant is very immature and is expected to die.

Care for the family when an extremely preterm infant (20 to 25 weeks' gestation) is expected to be born can be heavily laden with ethical and legal issues. For example, if labor cannot be halted, should fetal monitoring be used if fetal survival is unlikely? If no intervention is done for a nonreassuring pattern, it can distress parents and caregivers alike. On the other hand, knowledge of the fetal response to labor helps the neonatologist make better decisions about how to treat the infant. In addition, ultrasound estimates of gestational age have considerable variation at this time. A fetus presumed to be 24 weeks of gestation before birth may be assessed to be 26 weeks after birth and thus suited to more aggressive treatment than was planned.

Much of the general nursing care for a woman having preterm labor also applies to women with other high-risk pregnancies. Women may need multiple hospitalizations, and these may occur in the middle of the night, disrupting sleep and family routines. These women often have some activity restriction and may have to stop working. There-

---

DRUG GUIDE
· · · · · · · · · ·
Betamethasone, Dexamethasone

Classification: Corticosteroids

Indications: Acceleration of fetal lung maturity to reduce the incidence and severity of respiratory distress syndrome. Studies suggest that antenatal steroids can also reduce the incidence of intraventricular hemorrhage and necrotizing enterocolitis in the preterm infant. Greatest benefits accrue if at least 24 hours elapse between the initial dose and birth of the preterm infant, but the drug is indicated if birth is not imminent.

Dosage and Route: Betamethasone: 12 mg IM for two doses, 24 hr apart
Dexamethasone: 6 mg IM every 12 hr for four doses
The doses may be repeated if birth has not occurred within 7 days.

Absorption: Rapid and complete after IM administration

Excretion: Metabolized in the liver. Excreted in urine.

Contraindications: Active infection, such as chorioamnionitis, is a relative contraindication, although further study is needed. The National Institutes of Health recommend use of corticosteroids for the woman who has preterm rupture of the membranes (24 to 32 weeks' gestation), but the American College of Obstetrics and Gynecology has not yet endorsed this recommendation.

Precautions: Possible infection. Pregnancies complicated by diabetes.

Adverse Reactions: Few, owing to the short-term use of the drug. Pulmonary edema is possible secondary to sodium and fluid retention.

Nursing Considerations: Explain the potential benefits of corticosteroid administration to the preterm neonate. Explain that the drug cannot prevent or lessen the severity of all complications of prematurity. If the woman is diabetic, explain that more frequent blood glucose determinations are common because these levels are often slightly higher. Assess lung sounds. Report chest pain or heaviness or dyspnea.

fore, this section focuses on the family's psychosocial concerns, management of home care, and the woman's boredom.

PSYCHOSOCIAL CONCERNS

Assessment

The entire family is affected by stressors associated with a complicated pregnancy. Assess how the woman and her family usually cope with crisis situations and how they are coping with this one. To prioritize care, identify their greatest concerns.

The woman or her family may have physical, emotional, and cognitive impairments because of the unexpected problems. Physical signs of emotional distress, such as trembling, palpitations, and restlessness, are also side effects of β-adrenergic drugs. The woman may express fear, helplessness, or disbelief. She may be irritable and tearful. Her ability to concentrate may be impaired at a time when she needs to absorb new information.

Her partner often feels at loose ends. He struggles to keep the household running if she must be inactive. Young children pick up on their parents' anxiety and may misbehave or regress.

The family may be under financial strain. The woman must often curtail or stop working. If she does not have sick time or other benefits, the family suffers an abrupt drop in income at a time when medical expenses are mounting.

Overlaid on the sudden change in lifestyle is the family's concern for fetal well-being. A woman may feel pulled in opposite directions by the needs of all her children—those already born and the fetus she is trying to mature. She may be concerned about the effects of drug therapy on the fetus and on her own body.

Nursing Diagnosis and Planning

The outcome of any pregnancy is never certain, and this is especially true when the pregnancy is a high-risk one for any reason. The unexpected development of complications during pregnancy can prevent a woman and her family from using their normal coping mechanisms. Goals focus on the family's ability to cope with the crisis of preterm labor. The nursing diagnosis is

■ Anxiety related to uncertain outcome of the pregnancy, disruption of family relationships, and financial concerns.
Expected Outcome: The family will identify methods to cope with the temporary disruption in their lives.

Interventions

Providing Information

Knowledge decreases anxiety and fear related to the unknown. Include appropriate family members so that they are more likely to be supportive. Determine what the woman knows about preterm birth and about the specific therapy that is recommended. Determine what information the parents need about the problems that a preterm infant may face. Use this opportunity to correct misinformation and reinforce accurate information.

Initially, the woman for whom activity restriction is prescribed may be highly motivated to maintain the recommended level of activity. Because she usually feels well, however, she may begin to feel lazy and unproductive. Continue to explain how limiting her activity benefits her baby and to affirm that she is indeed doing an important job.

Promoting Expression of Concerns

Encourage the woman and her family to express their concerns. Begin by exploring common concerns of women with problem pregnancies. For example, say, "Most women are worried when they have to stop working. How has this affected your family?" An open question gives them a chance to ventilate their feelings so that they can take the next step: identifying constructive methods to cope with the situation. Collaboration with a social worker may identify financial or other community resources available.

Teaching What May Occur During a Preterm Birth

Because preterm birth may occur despite all interventions, a pregnant woman and her partner should be prepared for that possibility. If the hospital has a neonatal intensive care unit, a nurse often visits the parents to explain what might occur there if their baby is born early. One or both parents tour the unit to see the equipment and care infants receive there. A tour of the intensive care nursery may motivate the woman to maintain the recommended therapy to prevent preterm birth.

In hospitals with neonatal intensive care units, one or more neonatal nurses, a neonatal nurse practitioner, a neonatologist, or a combination of these is present at birth to care for the infant. The woman who planned to give birth in a hospital without a neonatal intensive care unit may be transferred to a facility with this type of unit before the birth to allow immediate care and stabilization of her newborn. The infant may also be transferred after birth if there is no time to transfer the woman before birth or if the infant has more problems than anticipated. Hospitalization of the mother or infant, or both, at a distant location adds to the stress on the family.

Evaluation

• Can the woman and her family identify constructive methods to deal with their anxiety?

If a high-risk pregnancy situation is prolonged, or if the family has difficulty adapting constructively to the situation, a nursing diagnosis of Altered Family Processes may be more appropriate.

MANAGEMENT OF HOME CARE

Assessment

Part of the care of women with high-risk pregnancies, including a risk for preterm birth, often occurs in their homes. Many daily household activities are managed by the woman. When she is disabled, even briefly, the usual roles of family members are disrupted.

Determine the level of activity prescribed by the physician, and identify the role of each family member. A good way to do this is to have the woman describe a usual day

NURSING CARE PLAN 27-1

Preterm Labor

| Assessment | Rhonda Ellis is a 28-year-old gravida IV, para III. Her children were born at 40 weeks, 28 weeks, and 32 weeks of gestation. Her children are 7 and 4 years, and 18 months old. She has mild cramping and pelvic pressure at 28 weeks and comes to the hospital right away. Her cervix is dilated 1 to 2 cm and is beginning to efface. She responds to intravenous magnesium sulfate to stop her contractions. The physician also orders betamethasone 12 mg IM for two doses, 24 hours apart. After her contractions stop, Rhonda is started on oral terbutaline to maintain tocolysis and will be discharged home in 48 hours if no recurrent symptoms develop. |

Nursing Diagnosis   Impaired Home Maintenance Management related to activity restrictions and family demands

Goal/Expected Outcome
- By hospital discharge, Rhonda will relate ways that she can maintain prescribed activity restrictions.

Intervention

1. Assess what support systems are available and financially feasible to help Rhonda with child care and transportation, such as day care, mother's day out programs at churches, family, and friends.
2. Encourage Rhonda to lower her standards for home management temporarily.
   a. Eat nourishing take-out or fast food.
   b. Prioritize household tasks that must be done.
   c. Let her children do tasks that are within their abilities.
   d. Make lists of tasks for different people who ask to help her.
3. Encourage Rhonda to accept help from others. Remind her that this situation is temporary and that she may be able to help someone else at another time.

Rationale

1. Responsibilities for other children may impede a woman's ability to maintain activity limits. Coordination among several resources helps provide all-day coverage for child care.
2. Many usual roles must be reallocated during this time. Having alternative arrangements increases the chance that the woman can maintain therapy.

3. If a woman feels that she can help others at another time, she may be more willing to accept help when she needs it.

Evaluation   Rhonda identifies three friends in addition to her mother-in-law who may be able to help with child care. She says she cannot afford to continue sending her children to their day care center if she is not working. She feels that if her children are cared for, her husband can handle the other home management needs.

Assessment   At 31 weeks' gestation, Rhonda again experiences preterm labor and goes to the hospital. Her cervix is dilated 2 to 3 cm and is 75% effaced (about 0.5 cm long). Her contractions occur every 6 to 7 minutes, and last about 20 to 30 seconds each. The physician again orders a magnesium sulfate infusion and betamethasone injections. The physician explains that preterm birth may be delayed but will probably occur within the next 24 to 48 hours. Rhonda begins crying and says, "I did what I was supposed to do and now I'm still going to have another preemie! It will be weeks before I can be a real mother!"

Nursing Diagnosis   Anticipatory Grieving related to loss of expected birth experience

Goal/Expected Outcome
- Rhonda will express her feelings about the loss of her expected birth at term.

Intervention

1. Sit down and spend time with Rhonda. Use therapeutic communication to encourage her to express her feelings.

Rationale

1. Unhurried time allows expression of feelings, which is the first step in dealing with the anticipated loss.

NURSING CARE PLAN 27–1 *Continued*

Preterm Labor

2. When she has expressed her frustration about this development in her pregnancy, explain that much remains unknown about why labor begins, whether at term, preterm, or post-term.

3. Explain that Rhonda's efforts have paid off because she has gained 3 valuable weeks of gestation for her baby.

2. If a woman knows that professionals do not have all the answers but must make recommendations based on what is known or appears to work for an individual woman, she may be more accepting of the inevitability of preterm birth.

3. Knowing that her self-care has benefits, although not the hoped-for term birth, reduces the sense of failure that she may feel.

Evaluation

Rhonda cries and expresses her frustration about the developments in her pregnancy. She says that she knew she was more likely to have another preterm infant but hoped that this time would be different. As the day goes by, Rhonda gradually begins expressing feelings that she did do something positive for this baby. She begins making specific plans to deal with the probable preterm birth.

Additional Nursing Diagnoses to Consider

Health-Seeking Behaviors
Altered Family Processes
Altered Health Maintenance
Ineffective Individual or Family Coping

---

before she had any limitations. Determine the number and ages of children in the home.

Evaluate the home itself, either by visual inspection or by questioning the family. Does the home or apartment have more than one level? Determine if a telephone is available for emergency contact.

Evaluate the family's resources and their willingness to use them. Ask whether family members and friends in the area are available to help. Explore local support groups, such as churches or mother-to-mother networks, that the family might contact for assistance. Determine whether insurance covers assistance such as homemaker services.

Nursing Diagnosis and Planning

The nursing diagnosis is

■ Impaired Home Maintenance Management related to change in usual roles and responsibilities.
  Expected Outcomes:
  Short-term: The family will identify methods for managing daily household routines.
  Long-term: The woman will be able to maintain the prescribed level of activity and drug therapy.

Interventions

The pregnancy threatened by preterm labor or other complications is a self-limiting situation, making temporary adjustments somewhat easier. Needed changes in home routines may be brief but sometimes extend over several weeks.

Caring for Children

The woman who has children has different concerns than the woman who does not. Knowledge of growth and devel-

opment helps the nurse identify the most appropriate way to ensure adequate care for the children and strengthen family relationships.

Toddlers and preschoolers rarely understand why their mother does not play with them as usual. If they are already in day care, this may continue if the family can afford it. They may live with a relative or friend temporarily. Toddlers may feel that their parents have abandoned them if they are sent away, although this may be the only realistic solution if no one besides the mother is available to supervise them.

School-age children usually understand the situation better and are often quite helpful. They may assist with care of other children, but they should not be put into the role of an adult. They may resent responsibility that is excessive for their age.

Adolescents may welcome the trust their parents have in them, but they also may resent the intrusion on independent activities with their peers. Teenagers who drive can be very helpful in taking younger siblings to school and other activities. They may be enlisted for grocery shopping and meal preparation. If resentment flares, the parents and nurse can remind teenagers that the situation is temporary and that they are making valuable contributions to the health of the new baby.

Maintaining the Household

The first step to home maintenance during this time may be for the woman to lower her standards of housekeeping. Things may not be as clean or organized as she would like. The partner may take over many household tasks, but these compete with his responsibilities outside the home.

Advise the woman to have a list of tasks ready when friends and family ask, "Can I do anything to help?" If they offer to bring a meal or do laundry, encourage her to accept. Remind her that people who offer to help mean it and that she may be able to return the favor to someone else. Homemaker services may be an option to help the family deal with the woman's temporary disability.

Transportation of school-age children may be a concern. If no family or friends are available, the school nurse or parent-teacher association (PTA) may help find someone willing to take the children to school each day.

Evaluation

- Short-term goal: Does the family identify how to manage minimal household care?
- Long-term goal: Can the woman maintain the prescribed therapy until birth?

BOREDOM

Assessment

If activity is to be restricted, determine what skills the woman has for coping with boredom. Although the benefit of bed rest in prolonging gestation is questionable, often at least some reduction in activity is prescribed. At first, a prescription for rest may sound wonderful, but after a short while it can become trying.

To identify activities that are still appropriate within the restrictions prescribed, ask about a usual day. Ask about hobbies, present and past. What type of leisure activities does the woman enjoy? Which activities are available or possible? Does she have good alternative places to maintain rest and still give her a change of scenery?

Assess her personality. Is she calm and composed, taking whatever comes with serenity, or does she need to be busy most of the time? No matter how motivated, the woman who finds inactivity tiresome will find even limited activity restrictions difficult to maintain.

Nursing Diagnosis and Planning

The nursing diagnosis is

- Diversional Activity Deficit related to lack of knowledge about alternative activities.
  Expected Outcomes: The woman will identify activities that are appropriate for her level of activity restriction and will pursue (with the help of others) activities to relieve boredom.

Interventions

Identifying Appropriate Activities

Determine the woman's understanding about needed activity restrictions to identify misunderstandings and reinforce correct information. Help her identify which usual activities are permitted and which ones should not be done and why. If she understands the rationale, she may be more willing to comply with restrictions.

Some women continue work activities, such as paperwork or phone calls, that can be accomplished while at rest. Workplace deadlines can increase stress, even if she works at home. The feeling of usefulness gained by such activities, however, may be beneficial if it means she is willing to maintain activity restrictions. Moreover, work-related activities can help reduce some of the family's financial concerns.

Suggest activities to help the woman keep busy and productive. These may include household activities that can be done at rest, volunteering for activities such as phone calls, and leisure activities such as puzzles, games, and needlework. Help her identify someone who can obtain the necessary supplies for her. This might be a good time to reactivate an old (quiet) hobby.

The woman can participate in some activities with her children while she is in bed. She can read to them and play board or card games. Encourage her to help the children with their homework and stimulate their development with thought-provoking discussions.

Changing the Physical Surroundings

Encourage the woman to identify at least two areas where she can maintain her prescribed rest. This gives her a change of scene and helps her feel more a part of the family activities. Each area should include pillows, blankets, and a clipboard with writing materials. An adjustable ironing board can provide a movable table for her things, and a shoe bag helps keep supplies organized and at hand. Ideally, the telephone is within reach or is cordless, and she has a television with a remote-control unit in both areas.

Evaluation

- Can the woman accurately discriminate between appropriate and inappropriate activities?
- Does the woman actually pursue only appropriate activities?

Prolonged Pregnancy

A prolonged pregnancy is one that lasts longer than 42 weeks. Many apparent cases of prolonged pregnancy are only miscalculation of the estimated date of delivery (EDD) because the woman has had irregular menstrual periods or has forgotten the date of her last normal one. Late prenatal care limits the use of clinical methods such as ultrasonography, which might otherwise be used to pinpoint her EDD.

Complications

The main physical risk in prolonged pregnancy is to the fetus or newborn. Insufficiency of the placental function secondary to aging and infarction reduces transfer of oxygen and nutrients to the fetus and removal of waste. Because the fetus with placental insufficiency has less reserve to tolerate uterine contractions, signs of fetal compromise, such as late decelerations and decreased variability, may develop during labor. In addition, the reduced amniotic fluid volume (oligohydramnios) that often accompanies placental insufficiency can result in umbilical cord compression. Meconium in the amniotic fluid may cause respiratory distress in the newborn if it is aspirated before or during birth. The infant may have growth restriction and may appear to have lost weight.

Many post-term fetuses do not suffer from placental insufficiency and may continue growing. The woman and fetus then may have complications related to dysfunctional labor, inadequate postpartum uterine contraction to control bleeding, and injury if the birth is traumatic.

Psychologically, the woman often feels as if her pregnancy will never end. She may fear induction of labor, a possible cesarean birth, and problems with her baby. The added fatigue imposed by prolonged pregnancy diminishes her resources for tolerating the added stress and anxiety.

Therapeutic Management

Therapeutic management begins with determination of the true gestation with the greatest accuracy possible. If a woman did not have early prenatal care, several markers used to pinpoint gestation, such as ultrasonography, fundal height measurements, and dates of quickening and first auscultation of the fetal heart tones with a nonamplified fetoscope, may be lost. Also, the woman may have forgotten the date of her last menstrual period.

Another factor in management decisions is whether the fetus is thriving in the uterus. If antepartum tests such as a biophysical profile indicate that the fetus is doing well, the birth attendant can take a more conservative approach than if the fetus is suffering from reduced placental function.

If the gestation appears to be truly post-term and there is no fetal urgency to deliver quickly, management depends on whether the cervix is favorable for induction of labor. If the cervix is favorable, induction is usually begun. If the cervix is not favorable, the physician may take a "wait-and-see" approach, repeating fetal surveillance tests as needed. The woman may undergo a cervical ripening procedure (see Chapter 20) to make the cervix more favorable for induction.

Nursing Considerations

Nursing care for the woman with a prolonged pregnancy is tied to the management chosen. The nurse's role may include

- Teaching about procedures, such as antepartum testing or induction of labor
- Support for the woman's psychological and physical fatigue
- Nursing care related to specific procedures, such as induction of labor

Intrapartum Emergencies

Placental Abnormalities

Women with placental abnormalities (see Chapter 26) may experience hemorrhage during the antepartum or intrapartum period. Placenta previa is sometimes associated with an abnormally adherent placenta (placenta accreta). Placenta accreta may cause immediate or delayed hemorrhage immediately after birth because the placenta does not separate cleanly, often leaving small fragments that prevent full uterine contraction. More extreme degrees of abnormal adherence occur when the placenta penetrates the uterine muscle

itself (placenta increta) or even all the way through the uterus (placenta percreta). All or only part of the placenta may be involved. A hysterectomy is often required if a large portion of the placenta is abnormally adherent.

Prolapsed Umbilical Cord

A prolapsed umbilical cord slips down after the membranes rupture, subjecting it to compression between the fetus and pelvis (Fig. 27–6). It may slip down immediately with the fluid gush or long after the membranes rupture. Interruption in blood flow through the cord interferes with fetal oxygenation and is potentially fatal.

ETIOLOGY
Prolapse of the umbilical cord is more likely when the fit is poor between the fetal presenting part and the maternal pelvis. When the fit is good, the fetus fills up the pelvis, leaving little room for the cord to slip down. Although prolapse of the cord is possible during any labor, it is more likely if the following conditions are present:

- A fetus that remains at a high station
- A very small fetus
- Breech presentations (the footling breech is more likely to be complicated by a prolapsed cord because the feet and legs are small and do not fill the pelvis well)
- Transverse lie
- Hydramnios (often associated with abnormal presentations; also, the unusually large amount of fluid exerts more pressure to push the cord out)

MANIFESTATIONS
Prolapse may be complete, with the cord visible at the vaginal opening. A prolapsed cord may not be visible but may be palpated on vaginal examination as it pulsates synchronously with the fetal heart. An occult prolapse of the cord is one in which the cord slips alongside the fetal head or shoulders. The prolapse cannot be palpated or seen but is suspected because of changes in the FHR, such as bradycardia or variable decelerations.

THERAPEUTIC MANAGEMENT
Medical and nursing management often overlap, as they do in many emergency situations. The nurse or the birth attendant may be the first to discover cord prolapse. Birth is almost always cesarean unless vaginal delivery can be accomplished more quickly and less traumatically.

CRITICAL TO REMEMBER

· · · · · · · · · · · ·

Factors That Increase a Woman's Risk for a Prolapsed Umbilical Cord

Ruptured membranes *and*

- The fetal presenting part at a high station
- A fetus that poorly fits the pelvic inlet because of small size or abnormal presentation
- Excessive volume of amniotic fluid (hydramnios)

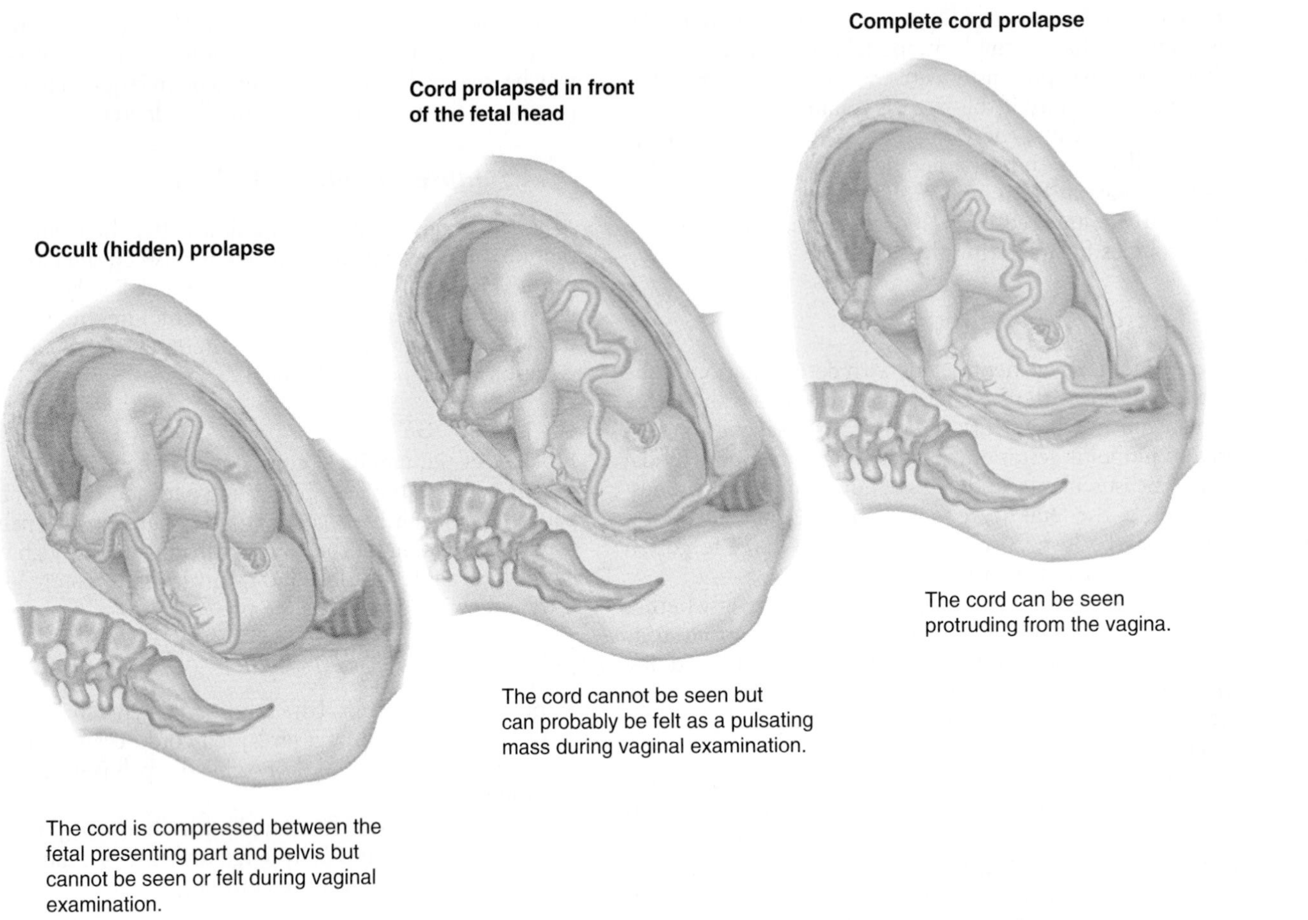

Complete cord prolapse

Cord prolapsed in front of the fetal head

Occult (hidden) prolapse

The cord can be seen protruding from the vagina.

The cord cannot be seen but can probably be felt as a pulsating mass during vaginal examination.

The cord is compressed between the fetal presenting part and pelvis but cannot be seen or felt during vaginal examination.

FIGURE 27–6

Variations of prolapsed umbilical cord.

When cord prolapse occurs, the priority is to relieve pressure on the cord to restore blood flow through it until delivery. None of these interventions should delay the promptest possible delivery. Push the call light to summon help. Others should call the physician and prepare for birth. Notify the neonatal nurses and pediatrician and prepare for possible neonatal resuscitation.

Prompt actions are taken to relieve cord compression and increase fetal oxygenation:

1. Position the woman's hips higher than her head to shift the fetal presenting part toward her diaphragm. Any of these methods (Fig. 27–7) may be used:
   a. Knee-chest position
   b. Trendelenburg position
   c. Hips elevated with pillows, with side-lying position maintained
2. With a gloved hand, push the fetal presenting part upward. Maintain this position until the physician orders it stopped, which may not be until a cesarean incision is made.

Give oxygen at 8 to 10 liters per minute by face mask to increase maternal blood oxygen saturation, making more oxygen available for the fetus.

Other actions may enhance fetal oxygenation, but prompt delivery is the priority and often no time remains for these measures. A tocolytic drug, such as terbutaline, may be ordered to inhibit contractions, increasing placental blood flow and reducing intermittent pressure of the fetus against the pelvis and cord. Warm saline-moistened towels retard cooling and drying of the cord. Cooling causes vasospasm within the cord, further reducing blood flow to and from the placenta. If the cord is protruding from the vagina, no attempt should be made to replace it because to do so could traumatize it and further reduce blood flow through it.

Prognosis for the woman is good because the only additional risks are those associated with cesarean birth. Prognosis for the infant depends on how long and how severely blood flow through the cord has been impaired. With prompt recognition and corrective actions, the infant usually does well.

NURSING CONSIDERATIONS

In addition to prompt corrective actions, the nurse must consider the woman's anxiety. The nurse must remain calm during this time and acknowledge the woman's anxiety. Explanations must be simple because anxiety interferes with the woman's ability to comprehend them. Her partner and family should be included as much as possible.

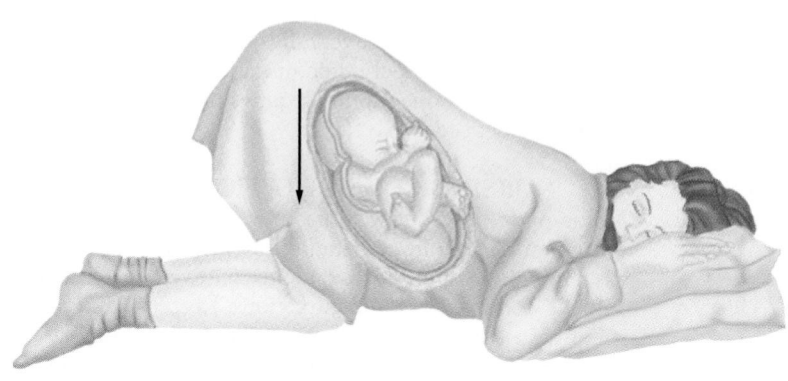

A gloved hand in the vagina pushes the fetus upward and off the cord.

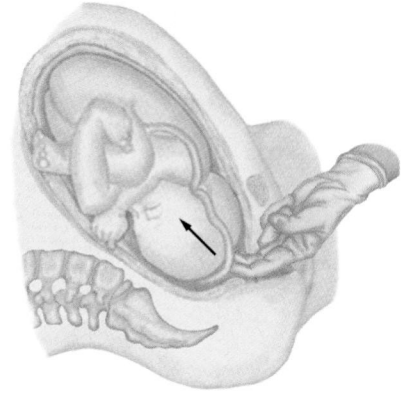

Knee-chest position uses gravity to shift the fetus out of the pelvis. The woman's thighs should be at right angles to the bed and her chest flat on the bed.

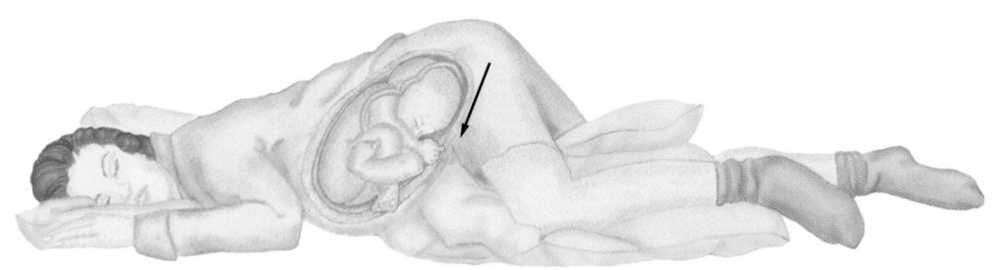

The woman's hips are elevated with two pillows; this is often combined with the Trendelenburg (head down) position.

FIGURE 27–7

Measures that may be used to relieve pressure on a prolapsed umbilical cord until delivery can take place.

Uterine Rupture

Sometimes a tear in the wall of the uterus occurs because the uterus cannot withstand the pressure against it (Fig. 27–8). There are three variations of uterine rupture:

- *Complete rupture* is a direct communication between the uterine and peritoneal cavities.
- *Incomplete rupture* is rupture into the peritoneum covering the uterus or into the broad ligament but not into the peritoneal cavity.
- *Dehiscence* is a partial separation of an old uterine scar. There may be little or no bleeding. There may be no signs or symptoms, and the rupture ("window") may be found incidentally during a subsequent cesarean birth or other abdominal surgery.

ETIOLOGY

Although uterine rupture is rare, dehiscence is not unusual. Uterine rupture is associated with previous uterine surgery, such as cesarean birth or surgery to remove fibroids. The risk for rupture in a woman who has had a prior cesarean

birth depends on the type of uterine incision. The risk for rupture is greater in women with a classic incision (vertical into the upper uterine segment) than in women with a low transverse incision. For this reason, vaginal birth after cesarean is not recommended for women who have had a previous classic cesarean birth.

Rupture of the unscarred uterus is more likely for women of high parity with a thin uterine wall, women sustaining blunt abdominal trauma, and women with intense contractions, especially if fetopelvic disproportion is present. Excessively strong (hypertonic) contractions may cause the intrauterine pressure to exceed the tensile strength of the uterine wall. If the fetus cannot be expelled downward through the pelvis, contractions may push it through the lower uterine segment. Intense contractions are more likely to occur when oxytocin is administered for induction or augmentation of labor, but they also may occur spontaneously.

MANIFESTATIONS

Dehiscence does not produce symptoms initially and may not interfere with labor or vaginal delivery if the area is

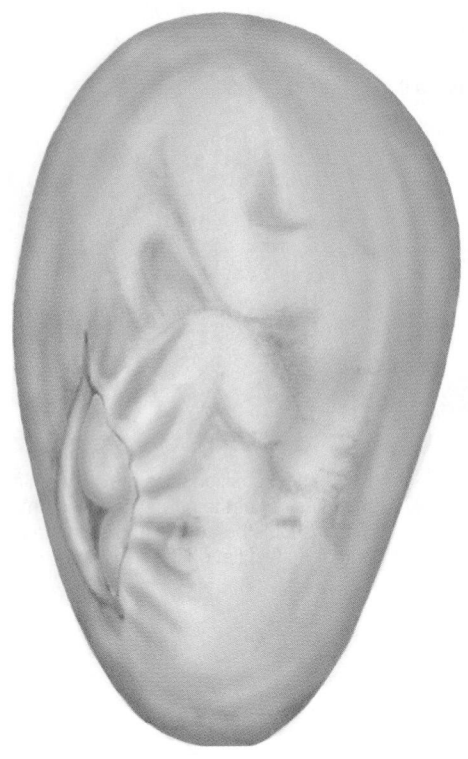

FIGURE 27–8

Uterine rupture in the lower uterine segment.

small. However, labor progress may stop because the open area prevents efficient expulsion of the fetus. Intrauterine pressures may have little change during contractions. A larger area of dehiscence may cause abdominal pain that persists despite analgesia.

Manifestations of uterine rupture vary with the degree of rupture and may mimic other complications. Possible signs and symptoms of uterine rupture include

- Abdominal pain and tenderness. The pain may not be severe; it may occur suddenly at the peak of a contraction. The woman may describe a feeling that something "ripped."
- Chest pain, pain between the scapulae, or pain on inspiration. Pain occurs because of the irritation of blood below the woman's diaphragm.
- Hypovolemic shock caused by hemorrhage: falling blood pressure, tachycardia, tachypnea, pallor, cool and clammy skin, anxiety. Signs of shock may not occur until after birth.
- Signs associated with impaired fetal oxygenation, such as late decelerations, reduced variability, tachycardia, and bradycardia
- Absent fetal heart tones with a large disruption of the placenta
- Cessation of uterine contractions
- Palpation of the fetus outside the uterus (usually occurs only with a large, complete rupture). The fetus is often dead if the placenta is involved.

If the rupture is incomplete, blood loss is slower and signs of shock, chest pain, or intrascapular pain may be de-

layed. Complete rupture results in massive blood loss. Signs of shock and pain develop quickly. External bleeding may not be impressive, because most of the blood is lost into the peritoneal cavity.

THERAPEUTIC MANAGEMENT

Initial management is to stabilize the woman and fetus and to perform cesarean delivery. If the rupture is small and the woman wants other children, it may be repaired. A woman with a large uterine rupture requires hysterectomy. Blood is replaced if needed.

NURSING CONSIDERATIONS

The nurse must be aware if the woman is at increased risk for uterine rupture and must stay alert for the signs and symptoms. Administer oxytocin cautiously to reduce the likelihood of excessive contractions. Keep in mind that hypertonic contractions can occur in either a stimulated or an unstimulated labor, and monitor for their presence. Notify the birth attendant if hypertonic contractions occur.

Uterine rupture may not be detected before birth. If postpartum bleeding is excessive and the fundus is firm, injury to the birth canal, including uterine rupture, is possible. Bleeding may be concealed if the ruptured area bleeds into the broad ligament. In this case, signs of hypovolemic shock are likely to develop quickly.

Uterine Inversion

An inversion occurs when the uterus completely or partly turns inside out, usually during the third stage of labor. Such an event is uncommon but potentially fatal.

ETIOLOGY

Often no single cause is identified. Predisposing factors are

- Pulling on the umbilical cord before the placenta detaches from the uterine wall
- Fundal pressure during birth
- Fundal pressure on an incompletely contracted uterus after birth
- Increased intra-abdominal pressure
- An abnormally adherent placenta
- Congenital weakness of the uterine wall
- Fundal placenta implantation

MANIFESTATIONS

The birth attendant notes that the uterus is either absent from the abdomen or a depression in the fundal area is present. The interior of the uterus may be seen through the cervix or protruding into the vagina. Massive hemorrhage, shock, and pain quickly become evident. The woman has severe pelvic pain.

THERAPEUTIC MANAGEMENT

Quick action by nursing and medical personnel is required to reduce maternal morbidity and mortality rates. The physician tries to replace the uterus through the vagina into a normal position. If that is not possible, laparotomy with replacement is done. Hysterectomy may be required.

Two intravenous lines are established to allow rapid fluid and blood replacement. General anesthesia or a tocolytic drug is often needed to relax the uterus enough to re-place it. After the uterus is replaced, oxytocin is given to contract the uterus and control blood loss. *Oxytocin is not given until the uterus is repositioned to avoid trapping the inverted fundus in the cervix.*

NURSING CONSIDERATIONS

Nursing care during the emergency supplements that of other staff members. Postpartum nursing care is directed toward observing and maintaining maternal blood volume and correcting shock. The woman may be transferred to the intensive care unit.

Assess the uterine fundus for firmness, height, and deviation from the midline. Assess vital signs every 15 minutes or more frequently until stable, then according to recovery room routine. Observe for tachycardia and a falling blood pressure, which are associated with shock. A cardiac monitor identifies dysrhythmias, which may occur with shock. Invasive hemodynamic monitoring is commonly used.

An indwelling catheter is often inserted to observe fluid balance and to keep the bladder empty so that the uterus can contract well. Assess the catheter for patency, and record intake and output. Urine output should be at least 30 ml per hour. A fall in urine output may indicate hypovolemia or an obstructed catheter.

The woman is allowed nothing by mouth until her condition is stable. She can usually receive fluids and progress to solid foods quickly because uterine inversion does not usually recur. It may recur in a future pregnancy, however, if conditions favor its development.

Amniotic Fluid Embolism

Amniotic fluid embolism occurs when amniotic fluid is drawn into the maternal circulation and carried to the woman's lungs. Fetal particulate matter (skin cells, vernix, hair, meconium) in the fluid obstructs pulmonary vessels. Abrupt respiratory distress, heart failure, and circulatory collapse occur. Disseminated intravascular coagulation (see Chapter 26) is likely because thromboplastin-rich amniotic fluid interferes with normal blood clotting. This infrequent disorder is often fatal. Survivors may have neurologic deficits.

Amniotic fluid embolism is more likely when the labor is very strong. High intrauterine pressure forces amniotic fluid into open uterine or cervical veins. The meconium that often accompanies a stressed fetus in such a labor adds to the particulate matter forced into the woman's circulation and increases the likelihood of death from this embolism.

Therapeutic management of amniotic fluid embolism is primarily medical and includes

- Cardiopulmonary resuscitation
- Oxygen with mechanical ventilation
- Blood transfusion
- Correction of coagulation deficits with platelets or fibrinogen

Trauma

Most trauma during pregnancy occurs because of accidents, assault, or suicide. Battering is a significant cause of maternal-fetal trauma during pregnancy. (The social and emotional issues of battering are addressed in Chapter 25.) Trauma may be blunt, such as that sustained in an automobile accident, or penetrating, such as gunshot and knife wounds. Burns and electrical injuries also may occur.

Although fetal injury may not be fatal, later neurologic deficits are sometimes found. Direct fetal trauma, such as skull fracture or intracranial hemorrhage, may occur from pelvic fracture, penetrating wounds, or blunt trauma. Indirect causes of fetal injury or death include abruptio placentae and disruption of the placental blood flow secondary to maternal hypovolemia or uterine rupture. The most common cause of fetal death is death of the mother.

The anatomic and physiologic changes of pregnancy make trauma care unique. During early pregnancy, the uterus is surrounded by the pelvis and is well protected from direct damage. As the uterus grows, it protrudes and becomes a large target for trauma. At the same time, it acts as a shield for other maternal organs such as the kidneys, often protecting them from direct trauma.

Normal alterations of pregnancy can affect the maternal and fetal outcomes after traumatic injury and can affect the interpretation of diagnostic studies that may be done. Pregnant women have a greater blood volume than nonpregnant women, which gives them a cushion against blood loss. However, the fetus may suffer if the woman hemorrhages because maternal blood is diverted from the placenta. This can lead to fetal hypoxia, acidosis, and death.

Maternal fibrinogen levels are higher during pregnancy (300 to 600 mg/dl). A decrease to lower levels is associated with abruptio placentae and may indicate that disseminated intravascular coagulation is developing.

THERAPEUTIC MANAGEMENT

Care of the pregnant trauma victim first focuses on injuries that threaten her life. Management of the fetus depends on whether the fetus is living and on the gestational age. The fetus may be delivered by cesarean birth if it is mature enough to survive and if the maternal or fetal condition is likely to be improved by prompt delivery. The fetus that is dead or too immature to survive is not usually delivered unless birth can improve the outcome for the mother.

NURSING CONSIDERATIONS

Nursing care of the pregnant trauma victim also focuses first on maternal and then on fetal stabilization. A wedge is placed under one side to prevent supine hypotension and further hemodynamic instability and to improve placental blood flow. Vital signs are taken as needed, based on the woman's condition. Vital signs and urine output (at least 30 ml per hour) provide information about the adequacy of her blood volume. Bloody urine suggests bladder or renal damage. Other nursing care is directed toward specific injuries and implementation of medical care.

Signs suggesting abruptio placentae (vaginal bleeding with uterine pain and tenderness) should be reported because this complication may occur with abdominal trauma. The uterine height may also increase as the uterus fills with blood.

Once the woman's condition is stable, nursing care intensifies for the fetus. External monitoring is appropriate if the fetus has reached a viable gestational age. Preterm labor may occur but may not be recognized if the woman is unconscious or if pain from injuries overshadows discomfort from contractions. Recurrent restlessness or moaning may accompany contractions. *The nurse should palpate the woman's uterus for contractions periodically because they may not be evident on the fetal monitoring strip, especially if the fetus is small.*

Although the nurse is usually anxious in an emergency situation too, it is important to keep a calm attitude. The woman and her family quickly pick up on the staff's anxiety, and consequently theirs escalates. To reduce fears of abandonment, the nurse should remain with the woman and, if possible, hold her hand. The nurse should speak in a low, calm voice.

KEY CONCEPTS

■ Dysfunctional labor may occur because of abnormalities in the powers, the passenger, the passage, or the psyche. Combinations of abnormalities are common.

■ Nursing care in dysfunctional labor focuses on prevention or prompt identification and action to correct additional complications: fetal hypoxia, infection, injury to the mother or fetus, and postpartum hemorrhage.

■ Premature rupture of the membranes is associated with infection as both a cause and an effect.

■ The early indications of preterm labor are often vague. Prompt identification of preterm labor enables the most effective therapy to delay preterm birth.

■ Nursing care for the woman at risk for a very early preterm birth focuses on helping her delay birth long enough to provide time for fetal lung maturation with corticosteroids, allow transfer to a facility with neonatal intensive care, or reach a gestation at which the infant's problems with immaturity are minimal.

■ The main risk in prolonged pregnancy is reduced placental function. This may compromise the fetus during labor and may result in meconium aspiration in the neonate. Dysfunctional labor may occur as a fetus continues growing during the prolonged pregnancy.

■ The key intervention for umbilical cord prolapse is to relieve pressure on it and to expedite delivery.

■ Be aware of women at risk for uterine rupture, and observe for signs and symptoms: signs of shock, abdominal pain, a sense of tearing, chest pain, pain between the scapulae, abnormal FHR patterns, cessation of contractions, and palpation of the fetus outside the uterus.

■ Uterine inversion is often accompanied by massive blood loss and shock. Recovery care promotes uterine contraction and maintenance of adequate circulating volume.

■ Amniotic fluid embolism is more likely to occur when labor is intense and the membranes have ruptured.

■ Medical and nursing care of the pregnant trauma victim focuses on stabilization of the mother first. Management of the fetus depends on gestational age and whether the fetus is alive. Abruptio placentae and uterine rupture are obstetric complications that may occur with direct abdominal trauma.

ANSWERS TO CRITICAL THINKING EXERCISE 27–1

1. When the fetus is in an occiput posterior position, back pain is usually persistent because the fetal head presses on the mother's sacrum with each contraction. This is often called "back labor." Additionally, the fetal head has to rotate internally through a wider arc to reach an occiput anterior position for birth; this process prolongs labor in most women.

2. The nurse should take actions to make the woman more comfortable and to promote rotation of the fetal head to an occiput anterior position. The nurse should encourage the woman to change positions regularly. Positions that cause her uterus to fall forward reduce pressure on her sacrum and straighten the pelvic curve somewhat to encourage fetal rotation. Examples of these are leaning forward while sitting, kneeling, standing, and a hands-and-knees position. Lunging toward her right side provides slightly more room on that side of her pelvis. If she wants to lie in bed, a left side-lying position favors fetal rotation toward an occiput anterior position. Consult with the nurse-midwife if the woman wants analgesia or anesthesia.

REFERENCES AND READINGS

Abbott, J. T. (1999). Emergency management of the obstetric patient. In G. N. Burrow & T. P. Duffy (Eds.), *Medical complications during pregnancy* (5th ed., pp. 225–236). Philadelphia: Saunders.

American Academy of Pediatrics (AAP) &

American College of Obstetricians and Gynecologists (ACOG). (1997). *Guidelines for perinatal care* (4th ed.). Elk Grove Village, IL, and Washington, DC: Author.

American College of Obstetricians and Gynecologists (ACOG). (1995a). *Technical bulletin no. 196: Operative vaginal delivery.* Washington, DC: Author.

American College of Obstetricians and Gynecologists (ACOG). (1995b). *Technical bulletin no. 218: Dystocia and the augmentation of labor.* Washington, DC: Author.

American College of Obstetricians and Gynecologists (ACOG). (1995c). *Technical bulletin no. 206: Preterm labor*. Washington, DC: Author.

Bachman, J., & Kendrick, J. M. (1996). Childbirth. In K. R. Simpson & P. A. Creehan (Eds.), *AWHONN's perinatal nursing* (pp. 151–186). Philadelphia: Lippincott.

Bowes, W. A. (1999). Clinical aspects of normal and abnormal labor. In R. K. Creasy & R. Resnick (Eds.), *Maternal-fetal medicine: Principles and practice* (4th ed., pp. 541–568). Philadelphia: Saunders.

Boyle, J. G. (1995). Beta-adrenergic agonists. *Clinical Obstetrics and Gynecology, 38*(4), 688–696.

Burke, M. E., & Poole, J. (1996). Common perinatal complications. In K. R. Simpson & P. A. Creehan (Eds.), *AWHONN's perinatal nursing* (pp. 109–148). Philadelphia: Lippincott.

Creasy, R. K., & Iams, J. D. (1999). Preterm labor and delivery. In R. K. Creasy & R. Resnick (Eds.), *Maternal-fetal medicine: Principles and practice* (4th ed., pp. 498–531). Philadelphia: Saunders.

Crowther, C. A. (1995). Commentary: Bed rest for women with pregnancy problems: Evidence for efficacy is lacking. *Birth, 22*(1), 13–14.

Cunningham, F. G., MacDonald, P. C., Gant, N. F., et al. (1997). *Williams obstetrics* (20th ed.). Norwalk, CT: Appleton & Lange.

de Veciana, M., Porto, M., Major, C. A., & Barke, J. I. (1995). Tocolysis in advanced preterm labor: Impact on neonatal outcome. *American Journal of Perinatology, 12*(4), 294–298.

Escher-Davis, L. (1996). Fetal fibronectin: A biochemical marker for preterm labor. *AWHONN Voice, 4*(3), 1, 6–7.

Freda, M. C. (1995). Arrest, trial, and failure. *Journal of Obstetric, Gynecologic, and Neonatal Nursing, 24*(5), 393–394.

Gardner, M. O., & Goldenberg, R. I. (1995). The clinical use of antenatal corticosteroids. *Clinical Obstetrics and Gynecology, 38*(4), 746–754.

Garite, T. J. (1999). Premature rupture of the membranes. In R. K. Creasy & R. Resnick (Eds.), *Maternal-fetal medicine: Principles and practice* (4th ed., pp. 644–658). Philadelphia: Saunders.

Geary, M., & Lamont, R. F. (1997). Prediction of preterm birth. In M. G. Elder, R. Romero, & R. Lamont (Eds.), *Preterm labor* (pp. 51–63). New York: Churchill-Livingstone.

Goodwin, T. M., Valenzuela, G., Silver, H., Hayashi, R., Creasy, G., & Lane, R. (1996). Treatment of preterm labor with the oxytocin antagonist atosiban. *American Journal of Perinatology, 13*(3), 143–146.

Gordon, M. C., & Iams, J. D. (1995). Magnesium sulfate. *Clinical Obstetrics and Gynecology, 38*(4), 706–712.

Gordon, M. C., & Samuels, P. (1995). Indomethacin. *Clinical Obstetrics and Gynecology, 38*(4), 697–705.

Hall, S. P. (1997). The nurse's role in the identification of risks and treatment of shoulder dystocia. *Journal of Obstetric, Gynecologic, and Neonatal Nursing, 26*(1), 25–32.

Hodnett, E. (1996). Nursing support of the laboring woman. *Journal of Obstetric, Gynecologic, and Neonatal Nursing, 22*(4), 311–315.

Huzel, P. A., & Remsburg-Bell, E. A. (1995). Fetal complications related to minor maternal trauma. *Journal of Obstetric, Gynecologic, and Neonatal Nursing, 25*(2), 121–124.

Iams, J. D. (1997). Uterine contraction monitoring and preterm birth. In M. G. Elder, R. Romero, & R. Lamont (Eds.), *Preterm labor* (pp. 185–193). New York: Churchill-Livingstone.

Joffe, G. M., Symonds, R., Alverson, D., & Childton, L. (1995). The effect of a comprehensive prematurity prevention program on the number of admissions to the neonatal intensive care unit. *Journal of Perinatology, 15*(4), 305–309.

Jones, D. P., & Collins, B. A. (1996). The nursing management of women experiencing preterm labor: Clinical guidelines and why they are needed. *Journal of Obstetric, Gynecologic, and Neonatal Nursing, 25*(7), 569–592.

Josten, L. E., Savik, K., Mullett, S. E., Campbell, R., & Vincent, P. (1995). Bed rest compliance for women with pregnancy problems. *Birth, 22*(1), 1–12.

Lewis, R., & Mercer, B. M. (1995). Adjunctive care of preterm labor: The use of antibiotics. *Clinical Obstetrics and Gynecology, 38*(4), 755–770.

Luke, B., Mamelle, N., Keith, L., et al. (1995). The association between occupational factors and preterm birth: A United States nurses' study. *American Journal of Obstetrics and Gynecology, 173*(3), Part I, 849–862.

Malone, F. D., & D'Alton, M. E. (1999). Multiple gestation: Clinical characteristics and management. In R. K. Creasy & R. Resnick (Eds.), *Maternal-fetal medicine: Principles and practice* (4th ed., pp. 598–615). Philadelphia: Saunders.

Maloni, J. A. (1996). Bed rest and high-risk pregnancy: Differentiating the effects of diagnosis, setting, and treatment. *Nursing Clinics of North America, 31*(2), 313–325.

McGregor, J. A., French, J. I., Parker, R., et al. (1995a). Prevention of premature birth by screening and treatment for common genital tract infections: Results of a prospective controlled evaluation. *American Journal of Obstetrics and Gynecology, 173*(1), 158–167.

McGregor, J. A., Jackson, G. M., Lachelin, G. C. L., et al. (1995b). Salivary estriol as risk assessment for preterm labor: A prospective trial. *American Journal of Obstetrics and Gynecology, 173*(4), 1337–1342.

Poole, G. V., Martin, J. N., Perry, K. G., Griswold, J. A., Lambert, C. J., & Rhodes, R. S. (1996). Trauma in pregnancy: The role of interpersonal violence. *American Journal of Obstetrics and Gynecology, 174*(6), 1873–1876.

Potter, J. (1996). *Controversies in preventing and managing preterm labor*. (Cassette recording no. T6). New Orleans: MCN Convention.

Ray, D., & Dyson, D. (1995). Calcium channel blockers. *Clinical Obstetrics and Gynecology, 38*(4), 713–721.

Resnik, R., & Calder, A. (1999). Post-term pregnancy. In R. K. Creasy & R. Resnick (Eds.), *Maternal-fetal medicine: Principles and practice* (4th ed., pp. 532–539). Philadelphia: Saunders.

Ruiz, R. J. (1998). Mechanisms of full-term and preterm labor: Factors influencing uterine activity. *Journal of Obstetric, Gynecologic, and Neonatal Nursing, 27*(6), 652–660.

Sauve, R. S. (1996). Tocolytics: The neonatal perspective. *Birth, 23*(1), 43–45.

Schroeder, C. A. (1996). Women's experience of bed rest in high-risk pregnancy. *Image: Journal of Nursing Scholarship, 28*(3), 253–258.

Simkin, P. (1995). Reducing pain and enhancing progress in labor: A guide to nonpharmacologic methods for maternity caregivers. *Birth, 22*(3), 161–171.

Simpson, K. R., & Pode, J. H. (1998). *Cervical ripening and induction and augmentation of labor*. Washington, DC: Association of Women's Health, Obstetric, and Neonatal Nurses.

Sisson, M. C. (1997). Preventing preterm labor: Is terbutaline our best option? *Lifelines, 1*(2), 42–46.

Wright, L. L., Horbar, J. D., Gunkel, H., et al. (1995). Evidence from multicenter networks on the current use and effectiveness of antenatal corticosteroids in low birth weight infants. *American Journal of Obstetrics and Gynecology, 173*(4), 263–269.

28

The Woman with a Postpartum Complication

LEARNING OBJECTIVES

After studying this chapter, you should be able to:

- Describe the predisposing factors, causes, manifestations, and therapeutic management of postpartum hemorrhage.
- Explain major causes, manifestations, and therapeutic management of subinvolution.
- Describe three major thromboembolic disorders (superficial venous thrombosis, deep vein thrombosis, pulmonary embolism), together with their predisposing factors, causes, manifestations, and therapeutic management.
- Discuss the location, predisposing factors, causes, manifestations, and therapeutic management of puerperal infection.
- Describe two major affective disorders (postpartum depression and psychosis).
- Describe the role of the nurse in the management of women with postpartum complications.

DEFINITIONS

atony Absence or lack of usual muscle tone.

dilation and curettage (D&C) Stretching of the cervical os to permit suctioning or scraping of the walls of the uterus. The procedure is performed in abortion, to obtain samples of uterine lining tissue for laboratory examination, and during the postpartum period to remove retained fragments of placenta.

embolus Clot, usually part or all of a thrombus, brought by the blood from another vessel and forced into a smaller one, thus obstructing circulation.

hematoma Localized collection of blood in a space or tissue.

hydramnios Excess volume of amniotic fluid (more than 2,000 ml at term). Also called polyhydramnios.

hypovolemia Abnormally decreased volume of circulating fluid in the body.

hypovolemic shock Acute peripheral circulatory failure due to loss of circulating blood volume.

placenta accreta Placenta that is abnormally adherent to the uterine muscle. If the condition is more advanced, it is called placenta increta (the placenta extends into the uterine muscle) or placenta percreta (the placenta extends through the uterine muscle).

psychosis Mental state in which a person's ability to recognize reality, communicate, and relate to others is impaired.

thrombus Collection of blood factors, primarily platelets and fibrin, that may cause vascular obstruction at the point of formation.

Pregnancy and childbirth are natural functions from which most women recover without complication. Nurses, however, must be aware of problems that may occur and their effect on the family. The most common physiologic complications are hemorrhage, thromboembolic disorders, and infection. Psychogenic complications include postpartum depression and postpartum psychosis.

Postpartum Hemorrhage

Postpartum hemorrhage is defined as blood loss that exceeds 500 ml after vaginal childbirth or 1,000 ml after cesarean birth. Blood loss to this extent in the first 24 hours after childbirth is termed early postpartum hemorrhage. When it occurs after 24 hours, it is called late postpartum hemorrhage.

Estimating blood loss is difficult, especially when bleeding is brisk or hemorrhage is concealed. Furthermore, blood loss during childbirth is frequently underestimated and constitutes only approximately half the actual loss (Cunningham et al., 1997). This is important to remember when excessive bleeding occurs later.

Postpartum hemorrhage complicates approximately 4% of deliveries (Hayashi, 1998). Hemorrhage, along with infection and hypertensive disorders, is one of the leading causes of maternal morbidity and mortality.

Early Postpartum Hemorrhage

The two major causes of early postpartum hemorrhage are uterine atony and trauma to the birth canal during labor and delivery. Abnormalities of the third stage of labor, such as placenta accreta (abnormal adherence of the placenta to the uterine wall) and inversion of the uterus, are described in Chapter 27.

UTERINE ATONY

Seventy-five to 80% of cases of early hemorrhage are caused by uterine atony (Hayashi, 1998). *Atony* refers to lack of muscle tone that results in failure of the uterine muscle fibers to contract firmly around blood vessels when the placenta separates. The relaxed muscles allow rapid bleeding from the endometrial arteries at the placental site. Bleeding continues until the uterine muscle fibers contract to stop the flow of blood. Figure 28–1 illustrates the effect of uterine contraction on the size of the placental site and the amount of bleeding that occurs.

Predisposing Factors. Knowledge of factors that increase the risk of uterine atony can be used to anticipate and thus reduce excessive bleeding. Overdistension of the uterus from any cause (multiple gestation, a large infant, hydramnios) makes it more difficult for the uterus to contract with enough firmness to prevent excessive bleeding.

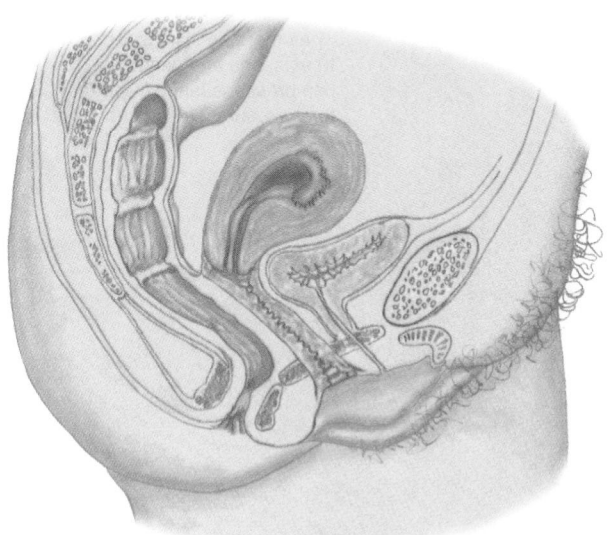

A Contracted uterus

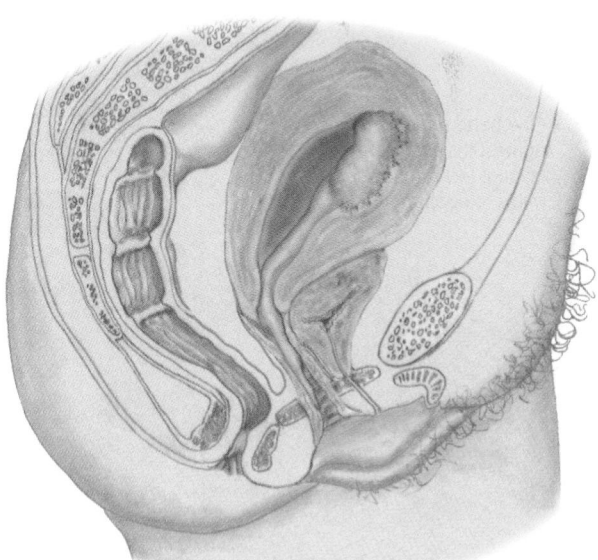

B Uterine atony
Uterus remains uncontracted.

FIGURE 28–1

A, When the uterus remains contracted, the placental site is smaller, so bleeding is minimal. *B*, If uterine muscles fail to contract around the endometrial arteries at the placental site, hemorrhage occurs.

• • • • • • • • • •
Common Predisposing Factors for Postpartum Hemorrhage

Overdistension of the uterus (multiple gestation, large infant, hydramnios)
Multiparity (>5)
Use of tocolytic drugs
Precipitate labor or delivery
Prolonged labor
Use of forceps or vacuum extractor
Cesarean birth
Manual removal of the placenta
Previous postpartum hemorrhage
General anesthesia
Low implantation of placenta
Administration of magnesium sulfate
Clotting disorders
Previous uterine surgery

Multiparity results in muscle fibers that have been stretched repeatedly, and these flaccid muscle fibers may not remain contracted after birth. Intrapartum factors include contractions that were barely effective, resulting in prolonged labor, or contractions that were excessively vigorous, resulting in precipitate labor. Labor that was induced or augmented with oxytocin is more likely to be followed by postdelivery uterine atony and hemorrhage. Retention of a large segment of the placenta does not allow the uterus to contract firmly and can result in uterine atony.

Manifestations. Major signs of uterine atony include

• A uterine fundus that is difficult to locate
• A soft, or "boggy," feel when the fundus is located
• A uterus that becomes firm as it is massaged but loses its tone when massage is stopped
• A uterine fundus that is located above the expected level
• Excessive lochia

For the first 24 hours after birth, the uterus should feel like a firmly contracted ball roughly the size of a large grapefruit. It should be easily located at about the level of the umbilicus. Lochia should be dark red and moderate in amount. Saturation of more than one peripad per hour is considered excessive. The nurse must realize that although bleeding may be profuse and dramatic, a constant steady trickle is just as dangerous (see Chapter 21 for assessment of the uterus and lochia).

Therapeutic Management. Nurses are with the mother during the hours after childbirth and are responsible for assessments and initial management of uterine atony. If the uterus is not firmly contracted, the first intervention is to massage the fundus until it is firm and to express clots that may have accumulated in the uterus. One hand is placed just above the symphysis pubis to support the lower uterine segment while the fundus is gently but firmly massaged in a circular motion. Clots that may have accumulated in the uterine cavity are expressed by applying firm but gentle pressure on the fundus in the direction of the vagina. It is critical not to attempt to express clots until

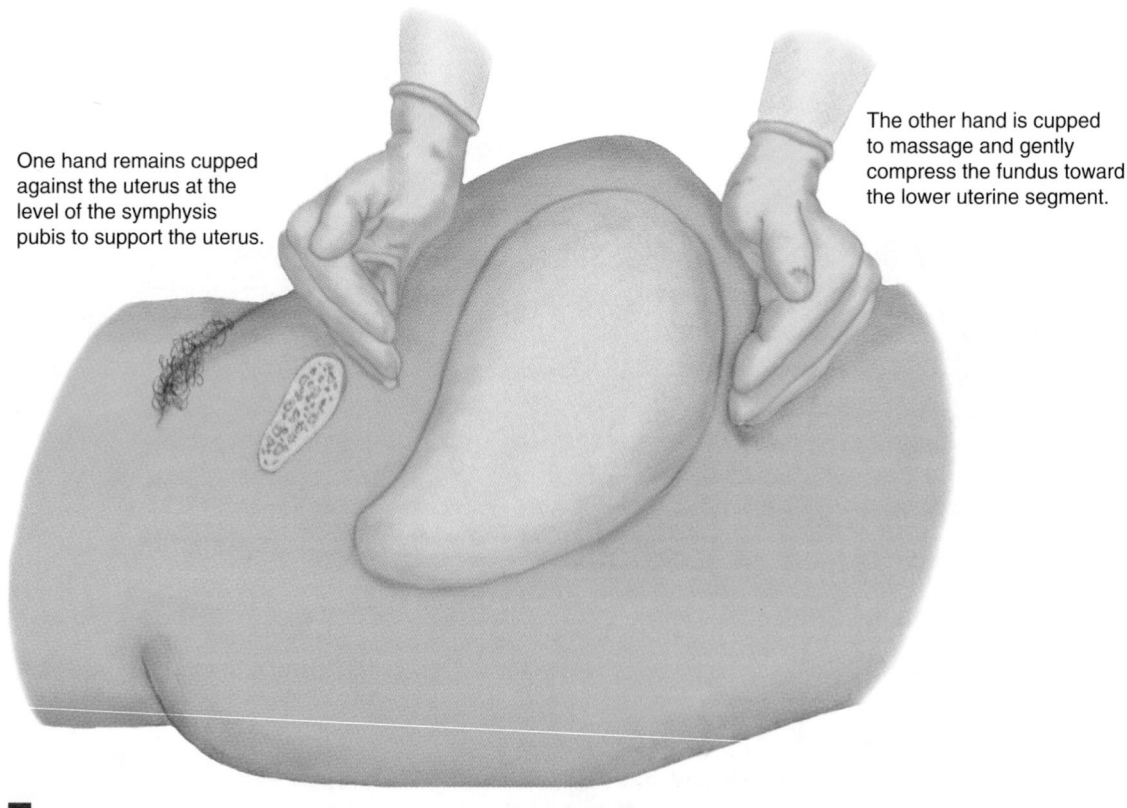

One hand remains cupped against the uterus at the level of the symphysis pubis to support the uterus.

The other hand is cupped to massage and gently compress the fundus toward the lower uterine segment.

FIGURE 28-2
• • • • • • • •
Technique for fundal massage.

DRUG GUIDE

Methylergonovine (Methergine)

Classification: Oxytocic.

Action: Directly stimulates contraction of the uterus.

Indications: Used for the prevention and treatment of postpartum or post-abortion hemorrhage caused by uterine atony or subinvolution.

Dosage and Route: Usual dosage is 0.2 mg intramuscularly (IM) every 2 to 4 hours for up to five doses. Change to oral route 0.2 mg every 6 to 12 hours for 2 to 7 days.

Absorption: Well absorbed after oral or IM route.

Excretion: Metabolized by the liver and primarily excreted in urine.

Contraindications and Precautions: Do not use to induce labor. Do not use IM if the mother is hypersensitive to phenol. Contraindicated for hypertensive women; those with hepatic, renal, or coronary artery disease; and during the third stage of labor.

Adverse Reactions: Nausea and vomiting, dizziness, headache, dyspnea, palpitations, hypertension, peripheral ischemia, and uterine and gastrointestinal cramping.

Nursing Considerations: Before administering medication, assess blood pressure. Follow facility protocol if medication must be withheld (usually a reading of 136/90). Caution the mother to avoid smoking because nicotine constricts blood vessels. Remind her to report any adverse reactions.

---

the uterus is firmly contracted. Pushing on an uncontracted uterus could invert the uterus and cause massive hemorrhage. Figure 28–2 illustrates correct hand placement for fundal massage.

If the uterus does not remain contracted as a result of uterine massage, the problem may be a distended bladder. A full bladder lifts and displaces the uterus and prevents effective contraction of the uterine muscles. Nurses should assist the mother to urinate or catheterize her, if necessary, to correct uterine atony caused by bladder distension.

Pharmacologic measures may also be necessary to maintain firm contraction of the uterus. A rapid intravenous infusion of dilute oxytocin (Pitocin) often increases uterine tone and controls bleeding. Twenty units in 1,000 ml of lactated Ringer's or normal saline at a rate of 600 ml/hr is often recommended (Cunningham et al., 1997). If the uterus remains atonic and bleeding continues, methylergonovine (Methergine) may be given intramuscularly (Cunningham et al., 1997). Methylergonovine has the side effect of elevating blood pressure and should not be given to a woman who is hypertensive. Analogues of prostaglandin $F_{2\alpha}$ (carboprost tromethamine; Hemabate, Prostin) given intramuscularly are sometimes effective in controlling postpartum hemorrhage caused by uterine atony.

If uterine massage and pharmacologic measures are ineffective in stopping uterine bleeding, the physician or nurse-midwife may use bimanual compression of the uterus to stop the bleeding. In this procedure, one hand is inserted in the vagina and the other compresses the uterus through the abdominal wall (Fig. 28–3). It may also be necessary to return the woman to the delivery area to explore the uterine cavity and to remove placental fragments that interfere with uterine contraction.

Hemorrhage requires prompt replacement of intravascular fluid volume. Lactated Ringer's solution and whole blood as well as other plasma extenders may be used. Enough fluid should be given to maintain urine flow of at least 30 ml/hr (Cunningham et al., 1997). The nurse is often responsible for obtaining properly typed and cross-matched blood and for inserting large-bore intravenous lines that are capable of carrying whole blood.

Operative procedures are the last resort. A hysterec-tomy may be necessary to save the life of a woman with uncontrollable postpartum hemorrhage.

TRAUMA

Trauma to the birth canal is the second most common cause of early postpartum hemorrhage. Trauma can include vaginal, cervical, or perineal lacerations as well as hematomas.

Predisposing Factors. Many of the same factors that increase the risk of uterine atony also increase the risk of soft-tissue trauma during childbirth. For example, trauma to the birth canal is more likely to occur if the infant is large or if labor and delivery occur rapidly. Induction and augmentation of labor increase the risk of tissue trauma, as does the use of assistive devices (see p. 716 for predisposing factors).

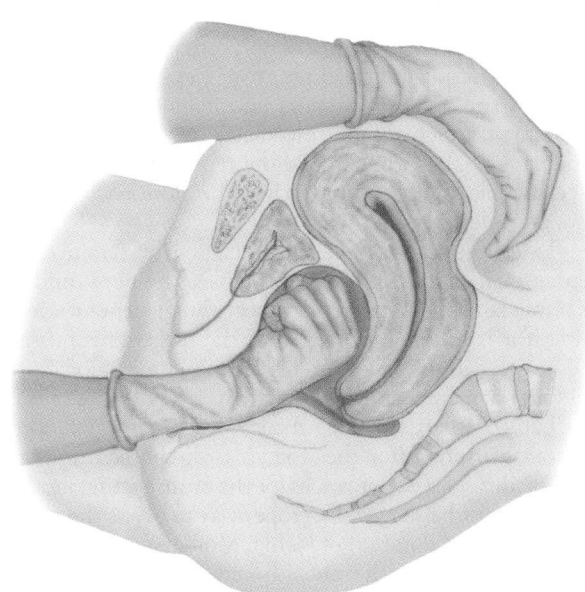

FIGURE 28–3

Bimanual compression. One hand is inserted in the vagina, and the other compresses the uterus through the abdominal wall.

Lacerations. The perineum, vagina, cervix, or the area around the urethral meatus are the most common sites for lacerations. Cervical lacerations occur frequently when the cervix dilates rapidly during the first stage of labor. Lacerations of the vagina, perineum, and periurethral area usually occur during the second stage of labor, when the fetal head descends rapidly or when assistive devices, such as forceps or a vacuum extractor, are used to assist in delivery of the fetal head.

Lacerations of the birth canal should always be suspected if excessive uterine bleeding continues when the fundus is contracted firmly and is at the expected location. Bleeding from lacerations of the genital tract is often bright red, in contrast to the darker red color of lochia.

Hematomas. Hematomas occur when bleeding into loose connective tissue occurs while overlying tissue remains intact. Hematomas develop as a result of injury to soft tissue in spontaneous deliveries as well as in deliveries in which forceps or vacuum extractors are used. Hematomas may be found in vulvar, vaginal, or retroperitoneal areas.

Visible vulvar hematomas appear as discolored, bulging masses. Hematomas produce deep, severe, unrelieved pain and feelings of pressure. Formation of a hematoma should also be suspected if the mother demonstrates systemic signs of concealed blood loss, such as falling blood pressure or tachycardia, when the fundus is firm and lochia is within normal limits.

Therapeutic Management. When postpartum hemorrhage is caused by trauma to the birth canal, surgical repair is often necessary. The mother is returned to the delivery area, where surgical lights enhance visibility, and the laceration is repaired.

Small hematomas usually reabsorb naturally. Large hematomas, however, may require incision, evacuation of the clots, and location of the bleeding vessel so that it can be ligated.

Late Postpartum Hemorrhage

The most common causes of late postpartum hemorrhage are subinvolution (delayed return of the uterus to its prepregnant size and consistency) and fragments of placenta that remain attached to the myometrium when the placenta is delivered. Clots form around the retained fragments, and excessive bleeding can occur when the clots slough several days after delivery.

Late postpartum hemorrhage caused by retained placental fragments usually is preventable. The nurse-midwife or physician should carefully inspect the placenta to determine if it is intact. If a portion of the placenta is missing, the health care provider can explore the uterus, locate the missing fragments, and remove them.

Late postpartum hemorrhage, which typically occurs without warning after the woman is discharged from the birth facility, can be dangerous for the unsuspecting mother. Families must be taught the proper way to assess the fundus and the normal duration of lochia. Moreover, they must be instructed to notify their health care provider if bleeding persists or becomes unusually heavy.

PREDISPOSING FACTORS
Attempts to deliver the placenta before it separates from the uterine wall, manual removal of the placenta, and placenta accreta are the primary predisposing factors for retention of placental fragments.

THERAPEUTIC MANAGEMENT
Initial treatment for late postpartum hemorrhage is directed toward control of the excessive bleeding. Oxytocin, methylergonovine, or prostaglandins are the most commonly used pharmacologic measures. Placental fragments are often dislodged and swept out of the uterus by the bleeding, and if the bleeding subsides when oxytocin is administered, no other treatment is required. Sonography can exclude placental fragments as the cause of delayed postpartum hemorrhage (Cunningham et al., 1997). If bleeding continues or recurs, curettage may be necessary. This treatment should be performed only when other treatment has failed, because curettage may cause trauma and additional bleeding. Broad-spectrum antibiotics may also be given if postpartum infection is suspected because of uterine tenderness, foul-smelling lochia, or fever.

▌ NURSING CARE
The Woman with Excessive Bleeding

Assessment

The initial postpartum assessment includes a chart review to determine whether factors such as prolonged labor or birth of a large infant have increased the risk for the woman to bleed excessively (see p. 716).

Uterine Atony

Priority assessments for uterine atony include the fundus, bladder, lochia, vital signs, skin temperature, and color. Assess the consistency and the location of the uterine fundus. The fundus should be firmly contracted, at or near the level of the umbilicus and midline. If the uterus is not firmly contracted, the fundus feels soft (boggy), and bleeding from the placental site is rapid and continuous. If the fundus is above the level of the umbilicus and displaced, a full bladder may be the cause of excessive bleeding. A full bladder lifts the uterus and impedes contraction, which allows excessive bleeding. The accumulation of clots also expands the uterus, making contraction difficult and resulting in continued bleeding.

It is difficult to estimate the volume of lochia by visual examination of peripads. More accurate information is obtained by weighing peripads and bed liners before and after use and subtracting the difference. One gram (weight)

CRITICAL TO REMEMBER
Early Signs of Postpartum Hemorrhage

- An uncontracted uterus
- Large gush or slow, steady trickle of blood from the vagina
- Saturation of more than one peripad per hour
- Severe, unrelieved perineal or rectal pain
- Tachycardia

equals 1 ml (volume). When inspecting for blood loss, always ask the woman to turn on her side to be certain that large amounts of blood are not pooling undetected underneath her. Although bleeding may be profuse and dramatic, a constant, steady trickle may lead to significant blood loss that becomes increasingly life-threatening.

Measure vital signs at least every 15 minutes to detect trends, such as tachycardia or a decrease in pulse pressure, that may reveal a deteriorating status in a woman with significant blood loss. Initially, the body compensates for excessive bleeding by constricting the blood vessels and shunting blood to vital organs. Therefore, vital signs may remain normal although the woman is becoming hypovolemic.

The skin should be warm and dry; mucous membranes of the lips and mouth should be pink; and there should be prompt capillary return when the nails are blanched. These signs confirm adequate circulating volume to perfuse the peripheral tissue.

Trauma

If the fundus is firm but bleeding is excessive, the cause may be lacerations of the cervix or birth canal. Inspect the perineum to determine whether a laceration is visible in that area. Lacerations of the cervix or vagina are not visible, but bleeding in the presence of a contracted uterus suggests a laceration. This sign warrants examination of the vaginal walls and the cervix by the health care provider.

If the mother complains of deep, severe pelvic or rectal pain or if vital signs or skin changes suggest hemorrhage but excessive bleeding is not obvious, the cause may be concealed bleeding and the formation of a hematoma. Examine the vulva for bulging masses or discoloration of the skin. A hematoma may be developing in the vagina or in the retroperitoneal area, however, and will not be obvious when the vulva is examined. Table 28–1 summarizes

assessments, abnormal signs and symptoms, and nursing implications.

Nursing Diagnosis and Planning

Postpartum hemorrhage is a potential complication that requires the efforts of the health care team to control the hemorrhage and prevent further complications, such as hypovolemic shock. Client-centered goals are inappropriate for this potential complication because the nurse cannot manage postpartum hemorrhage independently but must

---

CRITICAL THINKING EXERCISE 28–1

Dolores Navarra, a 26-year-old multipara, is admitted to the postpartum unit after rapid labor and the birth of her fourth infant 2 hours ago. The baby weighed 4,000 g (8 pounds, 12 ounces). At the initial assessment, Dolores's fundus is firm, at the level of the umbilicus. Lochia is heavy, with occasional small clots expressed. Vital signs are unchanged from prenatal norms.

1. What are the "red flags" that suggest a potential problem or complication? What actions should the nurse take as a result?
2. The nurse observes that the fundus is soft and that lochia is excessive. What are the priority interventions? Why?
3. Within an hour, the fundus becomes boggy again and is located 3 cm above the umbilicus and displaced to the right. What is the priority nursing action? Why?
4. Dolores voids 500 ml. The fundus is difficult to locate, however, and lochia is excessive. What is the next nursing action? Why?

TABLE 28–1

Nursing Assessments for Postpartum Hemorrhage

Assessments	Abnormal Signs/Symptoms	Nursing Implications
Chart review	Presence of predisposing factors	More frequent evaluations are necessary.
Fundus	Soft, boggy, displaced	Massage, express clots, assist to empty bladder, notify primary health care provider if measures are ineffective.
Lochia	Excessive bleeding (saturation of more than 1 pad/hr, steady trickle or profuse flow)	Assess for trauma, save and weigh pads and bed liner so estimation of blood loss will be more accurate. Notify physician or nurse-midwife.
Vital signs	Tachycardia, decreasing pulse pressure	Signs of excessive blood loss should be reported.
Comfort level	Severe pelvic or rectal pain	Signs of hematoma, usually perineal or vaginal; examine vulva for masses or discoloration.
Skin	Cool, damp, pale	Vigilant assessment for signs of hemorrhage and hypovolemia is necessary.

PART II: MATERNITY NURSING CARE

confer with the physicians or nurse-midwife for medical orders to treat the condition. Planning should reflect the nurse's responsibility to do the following:

- Monitor for signs of postpartum hemorrhage.
- Consult with the health care provider if signs of postpartum hemorrhage are observed.
- Perform actions that minimize postpartum hemorrhage and prevent hypovolemic shock.

Interventions

Preventing Hemorrhage

Every nurse should be aware of factors that put the new mother at risk for postpartum hemorrhage. This knowledge alerts the nurse to be particularly vigilant in monitoring these women so that excessive bleeding can be anticipated and minimized.

When predisposing factors are present, frequent assessments are necessary. Many hospitals and birth centers have a standard of care that calls for assessments every 15 minutes during the first hour after delivery, every 30 minutes for the next 2 hours, and hourly for the next 4 hours. This protocol, however, may not be adequate for the woman at known risk for postpartum hemorrhage because bleeding occurs rapidly. A delay in assessment may result in a great deal of blood loss.

Collaborating with the Health Care Provider

Notify the physician or nurse-midwife when excessive bleeding is suspected. Weighing the blood-soaked pads and linens allows the nurse to report the amount of blood lost in a certain period.

Begin uterine massage to control bleeding. In some hospitals or birth centers, protocols permit nurses to initiate specific laboratory studies, such as hemoglobin and hematocrit levels and typing and cross-matching of blood, so that blood is available should transfusions be necessary. Many protocols also allow the nurse to start intravenous fluids while the health care provider is being informed of the mother's condition. These actions do not substitute for notifying the health care provider, but they do allow nurses to make initial interventions quickly.

Keep the woman on bed rest to increase venous return and maintain cardiac output. The Trendelenburg position may interfere with cardiac function and is not advised. Continue assessments, call for assistance, and save all pads, linen savers, and linen so that an accurate estimation of blood loss can be made. Assistance is necessary because one nurse must continue to massage the uncontracted uterus and perform and record assessments while the other notifies the health care provider of the mother's condition.

Document the time and content of each communication when the health care provider is notified, for example, "1300: Dr. X notified of difficulty maintaining uterine contraction and continued excessive bleeding. Requested Dr. X to see client. Orders received."

Administer medications and fluids ordered by the health care provider. Note the effects and relay the information to the health care provider. If measures fail to control bleeding, notify the health care provider so that additional procedures can be initiated. These may include preparation for operative intervention (surgical preparation, consent signed for operative procedure, or confirmation that blood replacement is available).

Providing Support for the Family

The unusual activity of the hospital staff may make the mother and her family anxious.

> Acknowledge their anxiety, and provide simple, appropriate explanations of the activity. "I know all this activity must be frightening. She is bleeding a little more than we would like, and we are doing several things at once." Keeping family informed is one of the most effective ways of reducing anxiety.

Evaluation

- Does the fundus remain firm?
- Is lochia moderate?
- Do vital signs remain near predelivery levels?

Hypovolemic Shock

The pregnant woman can tolerate blood loss that approaches the volume of blood added during pregnancy (approximately 1.5 L; Knuppel & Hatangadi, 1995). When more than this reserve is lost, hypovolemic shock can ensue. Hypovolemia endangers vital organs by depriving them of oxygen. The brain, heart, and kidneys are especially vulnerable to hypoxia and may sustain damage in a brief period.

Pathophysiology

During hypovolemic shock, the body compensates by constriction of peripheral blood vessels and release of catecholamines to cause vasoconstriction and increase the heart rate and blood pressure. As shock worsens, the compensatory mechanisms fail. Inadequate organ perfusion and decreased cellular oxygen for metabolism result in a buildup of lactic acid and the development of metabolic acidosis. Decreased serum pH (acidosis) results in vasodilation, which further increases bleeding. If circulating volume becomes insufficient to perfuse cardiac and brain tissue, the mother dies.

Manifestations

Tachycardia is one of the earliest signs of hypovolemic shock, and even gradual increases in the pulse rate should be noted. A decrease in blood pressure and narrowing of pulse pressure (difference between systolic and diastolic blood pressure) occurs when the circulating volume of blood is sufficiently decreased. The respiratory rate increases as the woman becomes more anxious and attempts to take in more oxygen.

Skin changes also provide early cues. Vasoconstriction in the skin causes it to become pale and cool to the touch. As hemorrhage worsens, pallor increases, and the skin becomes cold and clammy.

As shock progresses, changes also occur in the central nervous system. The mother becomes anxious, then confused, and finally lethargic when blood loss totals 30% to

40% of the total blood volume. Urine output also decreases from more than 30 ml/hr in early shock to less than 5 ml/hr when more than 40% of the blood is lost.

Therapeutic Management

The goals of therapy are to control bleeding and to prevent hypovolemic shock from becoming irreversible. A second intravenous line should be inserted with a large-bore (16-gauge) catheter capable of carrying whole blood. Sufficient fluid volume is infused to produce a urinary output of at least 30 ml/hr. The health care team makes every effort to locate the source of bleeding and to stop the loss of blood. Interventions may include uterine packing; ligation of the uterine, ovarian, or hypogastric artery; or hysterectomy.

Nursing Considerations

IMMEDIATE CARE

One person should be assigned to evaluate and record vital signs, location and consistency of the fundus, amount of lochia, skin temperature and color, and capillary return every 3 to 5 minutes. Nurses often follow facility protocols that allow them to draw blood for hemoglobin, hematocrit, clotting studies, type, and cross-match. In addition, a pulse oximeter should be applied to determine oxygen saturation of the blood. A urinary catheter is inserted so that hourly urinary output can be measured. The catheter is also necessary if a surgical procedure to control the hemorrhage is required. Oxygen may be needed to increase the saturation of fewer red blood cells. It should be administered by tight face mask at 6 L/min or as directed by the health care provider.

Nurses are also responsible for administering fluids, whole blood, and medications as directed and for reporting on their effectiveness. Moreover, nurses must make every effort to provide information and emotional support for the woman and her family.

HOME CARE

Nurses who work in home care or nurse-managed postpartum clinics must be aware that women who have had postpartum hemorrhage are subject to a variety of complications. In general, they are exhausted, and it may take weeks for them to feel well again. Anemia often results and a course of iron therapy may be prescribed to restore hemoglobin level. Some women need extra assistance with housework and care of the new infant. Exhaustion may interfere with bonding and attachment. Moreover, extensive blood loss increases the risk of postpartum infection, and the woman must be taught to observe for specific signs and symptoms.

Subinvolution of the Uterus

Subinvolution refers to a slower-than-expected return of the uterus to its prepregnancy size after childbirth. Normally, the uterus descends at the rate of approximately 1 cm or one fingerbreadth per day. By 2 weeks, it is no longer palpable above the symphysis pubis. The endometrial lining

has sloughed off as part of the lochia, and the site of placental attachment is well healed by 6 weeks after birth.

The most common causes of subinvolution are retained placental fragments and pelvic infection. Signs of subinvolution include prolonged lochial discharge, irregular or excessive uterine bleeding, and sometimes profuse hemorrhage (Cunningham et al., 1997). Many women report pelvic pain or feelings of pelvic heaviness, backache, fatigue, and persistent malaise. On bimanual examination, the uterus feels larger and softer than normal for the particular period of the puerperium.

Therapeutic Management

Treatment is tailored to correct the cause of subinvolution. Oral methylergonovine maleate (Methergine), 0.2 mg every 3 to 4 hours for 24 to 48 hours, provides sustained contraction of the uterus (see p. 717). Infection responds to antimicrobial therapy.

Nursing Considerations

In most cases, subinvolution is not obvious until the mother has returned home after childbirth. For this reason, nurses must teach the mother and her family how to assess for the condition and how to recognize its occurrence.

The nurse should demonstrate how to palpate the fundus and how to estimate fundal height in relation to the umbilicus. The uterus should become smaller each day (by approximately one fingerbreadth). The nurse also explains the progressive changes from lochia rubra, to lochia serosa, and then to lochia alba (see Chapter 21).

The mother is instructed to report any deviation from the expected pattern or duration of lochia. A foul odor often indicates uterine infection. Additional signs include pelvic or fundal pain, backache, or feelings of pelvic pressure or fullness.

■ Thromboembolic Disorders

The three most common thromboembolic disorders encountered during pregnancy and the postpartum period are superficial venous thrombosis, deep venous thrombosis, and pulmonary embolism. Superficial venous thrombosis usually involves the saphenous venous system and is confined to the lower leg. Deep venous thrombosis can involve veins from the foot to the iliofemoral region. It is a major concern because it predisposes to pulmonary embolism. Pulmonary embolism is a dangerous and potentially fatal complication that occurs when the pulmonary artery is obstructed by a blood clot that was swept into circulation from a vein.

Incidence

The incidence of thromboembolic disease in pregnancy and the puerperium is five times higher than that in nonpregnant women of a similar age. It remains a major cause of maternal death in the United States. Deep venous thrombosis occurs in 1 in 2,000 women during pregnancy and 1 in 700 women after birth (Nuwayhid, Nguyen, & Khalife, 1998). There has been a decrease in the frequency of deep venous thrombosis and pulmonary embolism in the puerperium. This is a result of early ambulation after childbirth. Ambulation prevents stasis of blood in the legs and decreases the likelihood of thrombus formation.

Etiology

A *thrombus* is a collection of blood factors, primarily platelets and fibrin, on a vessel wall. Once started, the thrombus can enlarge with successive layering of platelets, fibrin, and blood cells as the blood flows past the clot. Thrombus formation is often associated with an inflammatory process in the vessel wall, which is termed *thrombophlebitis*.

The three major causes of thrombosis are venous stasis, hypercoagulable blood, and injury to the intima (the innermost layer) of the blood vessel. Venous stasis and hypercoagulable blood are present in all pregnancies.

VENOUS STASIS
During pregnancy, venous stasis occurs from compression of the large vessels of the pelvis and legs by the enlarging uterus. Stasis is most pronounced when the pregnant woman stands for prolonged periods. It results in dilated vessels and the potential for continued pooling of blood postpartum. Prolonged time in stirrups for delivery and repair of the episiotomy may also promote venous stasis and increase the risk of thrombus formation.

HYPERCOAGULATION
Pregnancy also causes changes in the coagulation and fibrinolytic systems that persist in the postpartum period. During pregnancy, the levels of most coagulation factors (particularly fibrinogen and factors III, X, and VIII) are elevated. In addition, the fibrinolytic system (plasminogen activator and antithrombin III) is suppressed, which hinders clot disintegration (lysis). The net result is that factors that promote clot formation are increased to prevent maternal hemorrhage and factors that prevent clot formation are decreased, resulting in a higher risk for thrombus formation.

BLOOD VESSEL INJURY
Injury to the intima of the blood vessel usually does not occur, except possibly during cesarean births, which could trigger a pelvic vein thrombosis. Thrombosis is three times more likely to occur if the birth was cesarean (Laros, 1999).

ADDITIONAL PREDISPOSING FACTORS
Factors that create additional risk include varicose veins, obesity, a history of thrombophlebitis, and smoking.

Factors That Increase the Risk of Thrombosis
Inactivity
Obesity
Cesarean birth
Smoking
History of previous thrombosis
Varicose veins
Diabetes mellitus
Prolonged time in stirrups in second stage of labor
Maternal age older than 35 years
Parity greater than 3

Women older than 35 years or who have had more than three pregnancies are also at increased risk.

Superficial Venous Thrombosis

MANIFESTATIONS
Superficial venous thrombosis is often seen in association with varicose veins. It is usually limited to the calf area. Signs and symptoms include swelling of the involved extremity as well as redness, tenderness, and warmth. It may be possible to palpate the enlarged, hardened vein. Patients sometimes experience pain when they walk.

THERAPEUTIC MANAGEMENT
Treatment includes analgesics, rest, and elastic support. Elevation of the lower extremity improves venous return. Warm packs may be applied to promote healing. There is no need for anticoagulants unless the condition persists. After 5 to 7 days of bed rest, the woman may ambulate gradually if symptoms have disappeared. She should avoid standing for long periods and continue to wear support hose to help prevent venous stasis and a subsequent episode of superficial thrombosis. There is little chance of pulmonary embolism if the thrombosis remains in the superficial veins of the lower leg.

Deep Venous Thrombosis

Signs and symptoms of deep venous thrombosis are often absent or diffuse. If they are present, they are caused by an inflammatory process and obstruction of venous return. Calf swelling, erythema, heat and tenderness, and pedal edema are the most common signs.

It is a common belief that a positive Homans' sign (presence of pain behind the knee when the foot is dorsiflexed) is an indicator of deep venous thrombosis in postpartum women, but Homans' sign has proved to be of little value in the diagnosis because pain may also be caused by a strained muscle or contusion.

Reflex arterial spasms may cause the leg to become pale and cool to the touch with decreased peripheral pulses. At one time, this condition was called *milk-leg*. Additional symptoms may include pain on ambulation, chills, general malaise, and stiffness of the affected leg.

DIAGNOSTIC EVALUATION
Doppler ultrasonography of the deep veins of the upper legs is often used to detect alterations in blood flow to diagnose deep venous thrombosis. Impedance plethysmography, which measures changes in venous blood volume and flow, may also be used. Venography is an accurate method for diagnosing deep venous thrombosis, but the radiographic dye may cause chemical phlebitis.

THERAPEUTIC MANAGEMENT
Preventing Thrombus Formation. To prevent thrombus formation, the mother should ambulate frequently and as early as possible. If she is unable to ambulate, range-of-motion and gentle leg exercises, such as flexing and straightening the knee and raising one leg at a time, should begin

WOMEN WANT TO KNOW

How Do I Prevent Thrombosis?

Methods to improve peripheral circulation help prevent the occurrence of thrombophlebitis. Especially important are these measures:

- Improve your circulation with a regular schedule of activity, preferably walking.
- Avoid prolonged standing or sitting in one position.
- When sitting, elevate your legs and avoid crossing them. This position increases the return of venous blood from the legs.
- Maintain a daily fluid intake of at least 2,500 ml (approximately 2.5 quarts) to prevent dehydration and consequent sluggish circulation.
- Stop smoking.

within 8 hours after childbirth. In addition, the mother should avoid using pillows or the knee gatch because sharp flexion at the knees and pressure on the popliteal space cause pooling of blood in the lower extremities.

Antiemboli stockings are used for mothers with varicose veins, a history of thrombosis, or cesarean birth. To prevent venous congestion when she stands, the stockings should be applied before the mother gets out of bed. It is important that she understand the correct way to put on the antiemboli stockings because they can roll or bunch, slowing venous return from the legs if improperly applied.

Stirrups should be padded during childbirth to prevent prolonged pressure against the popliteal angle during the second stage of labor. It may also be possible to decrease the time in stirrups to no more than 1 hour.

Before discharge from the birth facility, the mother should be taught about lifestyle changes that can improve peripheral circulation.

Initial Treatment. The mother is placed on bed rest, with the affected leg elevated to decrease interstitial swelling and to promote venous return from that leg. She is allowed to ambulate gradually when symptoms have disappeared. Anticoagulant therapy is begun with continuous infusion of intravenous heparin to delay the clotting time of the blood and prevent extension of the thrombus. Activated partial thromboplastin time should be monitored, and the heparin dose should be adjusted to maintain a therapeutic level of 1.5 to 2.5 times control (Laros, 1999). The mother receives analgesics to control pain and antibiotic therapy, as necessary.

Subsequent Treatment. The long-term management of deep venous thrombosis depends on whether the woman is pregnant or in the postpartum period. After several days of treatment with heparin, the postpartum woman is started on warfarin (Coumadin), which is often continued for 4 to 6 months (Laros, 1999). The usual anticoagulating dose of warfarin is 10 to 15 mg daily until a therapeutic level is reached. Prothrombin time and the international normalized ratio (INR) are used to monitor coagulation time when warfarin is used. The INR corrects for variations in the po-

tency of the thromboplastins used by different laboratories. An appropriate ratio for treatment of deep venous thrombosis is 2.0 to 3.0 (Laros, 1999).

Warfarin is contraindicated during pregnancy because of teratogenic effects and the risk of fetal hemorrhage. Therefore, pregnant women are given heparin, which is administered by continuous infusion or subcutaneously. Heparin does not cross the placenta.

NURSING CARE

The Mother with Deep Venous Thrombosis

Assessment

Assessment focuses on determining the status of the venous thrombosis. Palpate the pedal pulses in each foot to determine presence, equality, and strength. Inspect the leg for unusual warmth or redness, which indicates inflammation, and for unusual coolness or cyanosis, which indicates venous obstruction. Compare the affected and unaffected leg for size and color and measure the circumference to obtain an accurate estimation of the edema. Ask the woman about discomfort. Pain is caused by tissue hypoxia, and increasing pain indicates progressive obstruction.

Evaluate the laboratory reports of clotting studies. In addition to activated partial thromboplastin time, whole-blood partial thromboplastin time and platelets may be evaluated when heparin is used. Thrombocytopenia is a concern when heparin is administered for a prolonged period (Laros, 1999). Prothrombin time and INR are evaluated when the anticoagulant for the postpartum woman is changed to warfarin.

Nursing Diagnosis and Planning

The treatment of deep venous thrombosis includes the administration of anticoagulants for a prolonged period. As a result, a collaborative problem, hemorrhage secondary to anticoagulation therapy, is one of the most troubling potential complications. Planning should reflect the nurse's responsibility to do the following:

- Monitor for signs of hemorrhage.
- Consult with the physician if signs of hemorrhage are observed.
- Perform actions that will minimize the risk of hemorrhage.

Interventions

Monitoring for Signs of Bleeding

At least twice a day, assess the mother for the appearance of bruising or petechiae. Instruct her to report the appearance of any bleeding: bloody nose, blood in urine, bleeding gums, or increased vaginal bleeding. The nurse must be alert to signs of hemorrhage, such as tachycardia, falling blood pressure, or other signs of shock that may indicate internal bleeding.

Unless frank hemorrhage is present, the usual treatment for excessive anticoagulation is temporary discontinuance of the anticoagulant. Protamine sulfate, the antidote for heparin, should, however, be available. The antidote for warfarin is vitamin K.

Explaining Continued Therapy

Carefully explain the treatment regimen, including the schedule of medication and possible side effects, such as unexplained fever, unusual fatigue, or sore throat (signs of agranulocytosis or diminished number of neutrophils). It is important to caution the mother not to "double up" if a dose is missed. The mother and another family member should learn how to inject heparin, if necessary.

Emphasize the importance of keeping the health care provider informed about any medications the mother takes, because oral anticoagulants are associated with many clinically significant drug interactions. Common over-the-counter medications, such as aspirin and nonsteroidal anti-inflammatory drugs, increase the risk of hemorrhage. The woman should understand that any unusual bleeding should be reported.

Suggest that the mother use a soft toothbrush and floss her teeth gently to prevent bleeding from the gums. She should postpone dental appointments until the therapy is completed. A depilatory to remove unwanted hair is safer than a razor during anticoagulant therapy. Remind the mother to avoid activities that may cause injury, and caution her about using alcohol, which inhibits the metabolism of oral anticoagulants.

Helping the Family Adapt to Home Care

Nurses often assist the family to adapt to home care. The first step is to assess family structure and function to determine how prepared the family is to cope with the mother's illness. Determine the ages of the children and availability of family members or friends to help while the mother is confined to bed or on limited activity. Although the health of the mother is of primary importance, care must be taken that the attachment process between her and the infant progresses normally.

Evaluation

- Does the woman maintain therapeutic levels of her anticoagulant?
- Is she free from signs of unusual bleeding or other side effects of the medication?

Pulmonary Embolism

Pathophysiology

Pulmonary embolism is a rare but dreaded complication of deep venous thrombosis. It occurs when fragments of a blood clot are carried to the lungs. The embolus occludes a vessel and obstructs the flow of blood into the lungs, either entirely or partially. If pulmonary circulation is severely compromised, death may occur within a few minutes. If the embolus is small, adequate pulmonary circulation may be maintained until treatment can be initiated.

Manifestations

Sudden, sharp chest pain, tachycardia, syncope, tachypnea, pulmonary rales, cough, and hemoptysis are the most common signs of pulmonary embolus. Arterial blood gas determinations show decreased partial pressure of oxygen, and chest radiography reveals areas of atelectasis and pleural effusion.

Therapeutic Management

Treatment of pulmonary embolism is aimed at dissolving the clot and maintaining pulmonary circulation. Heparin therapy is initiated and may be continued for many months to prevent further emboli. Oxygen is used to decrease hypoxia, and narcotic analgesics are used to reduce pain and apprehension. The woman is kept at bed rest, with the head of the bed slightly elevated to reduce dyspnea. Intensive care, support of ventilation, and other measures depend on her pulmonary status. Pulse oximetry should be initiated, and arterial blood gases should be evaluated. Thrombolytic drugs, such as streptokinase or urokinase, may be used for massive pulmonary emboli. Embolectomy (surgical removal of the embolus) may be necessary.

Nursing Considerations

MONITORING FOR SIGNS
When caring for a woman with deep venous thrombosis, nurses look for early signs and symptoms of pulmonary embolism. Observation includes frequent assessment of respiratory rate and auscultation of breath sounds. Abnormalities, such as diminished or unequal breath sounds or coughing, should be reported immediately to the health care provider. Additional signs that require immediate attention include air hunger, dyspnea, tachycardia, pallor, and cyanosis.

FACILITATING OXYGENATION
Oxygen should be administered at 8 to 10 L/min by tight face mask (Grohar, 1996). The nurse should remain with the mother to allay fear and apprehension. The head of the bed should be raised to facilitate breathing. Narcotic analgesics, such as morphine, may be used to relieve pain.

SEEKING ASSISTANCE
The woman's condition is precarious until the clot is lysed or until it adheres to the pulmonary artery wall and is reabsorbed. The primary nurse should call for assistance to initiate interventions. These include intravenous administration of heparin, continuous assessment of vital signs, and administration of any emergency drugs that may be needed. The woman who has pulmonary embolism requires critical care nursing skills and is usually transferred to an intensive care unit.

Puerperal Infection

Puerperal infection is a term used to describe bacterial infections after childbirth. Infection occurs in 3% of all women who have had vaginal births and in 15% to 20% of those who have had cesarean births (Gibbs & Sweet, 1999). Until the advent of antibiotics, puerperal infection often resulted in death. Even today, it is one of the leading causes of maternal deaths.

The most common postpartum infections are metritis, wound infections, urinary tract infections, mastitis, and septic pelvic thrombophlebitis.

Definition

The definition of puerperal infection, according to the Joint Committee on Maternal Welfare, is a fever of 38°C (100.4°F) or higher after the first 24 hours after childbirth, occurring on at least 2 of the first 10 days after the first 24 hours. Although a slight elevation of temperature may occur during the first 24 hours because of dehydration or the exertion of labor, any mother with fever should be assessed for other signs of infection.

Pathophysiology

Every part of the reproductive tract is connected to every other part, and organisms can move from the vagina, through the cervix, into the uterus, and out the fallopian tubes to infect the ovaries and the peritoneal cavity. Moreover, the entire reproductive tract is particularly well supplied with blood vessels during pregnancy and after childbirth. Blood vessels or lymphatics can carry the infection to the rest of the body, which can result in life-threatening septicemia.

The normal physiologic changes of childbirth increase the risk of infection. During labor, the acidity of the vagina is reduced by the amniotic fluid, blood, and lochia, which are alkaline. An alkaline environment encourages growth of bacteria.

Necrosis of the endometrial lining and the presence of lochia provide a favorable environment for the growth of anaerobic bacteria. Many small lacerations, some microscopic in size, occur in the endometrium, cervix, and vagina during birth and allow bacteria to enter the tissue. Although the uterine interior is not sterile until 3 to 4 weeks after delivery, infection does not develop in most women, partly because granulocytes in the lochia and endometrium prevent infection.

Etiology

Other factors may predispose a woman to infection. Cesarean birth, the major predisposing factor, increases the risk 5 to 30 times above that for vaginal delivery (Gibbs & Sweet, 1999). The risk is higher because of the trauma to the tissues that occurs in surgery: the incision provides an entrance for bacteria; contamination is possible during surgery; and foreign bodies, such as sutures, can promote infection. In addition, women who must have a surgical delivery because of a problem that develops during labor may have other risk factors, such as prolonged labor, that raise the chances of infection. Colonization of the vagina with organisms, such as group B streptococci, *Chlamydia trachomatis*, *Mycoplasma hominis*, and *Gardnerella vaginalis*, also predisposes to the development of infection after childbirth.

Any trauma to maternal tissues increases the hazard of infection. Trauma may occur with rapid delivery, birth of a large infant, use of forceps or a vacuum extractor, or the need for manual delivery of the placenta, as well as lacerations and episiotomies. Catheterization during labor increases the chance of introduction of organisms into the bladder and adds to the urinary tract trauma that occurs during normal childbirth.

With prolonged rupture of membranes during labor, organisms from the vagina are more likely to ascend into the uterine cavity, especially if more than 24 hours pass before delivery. A long labor or many vaginal examinations during labor increases the danger of infection. Each vaginal examination increases the possibility of contamination from gloves or from organisms in the vagina being pushed through the open cervix. If part of the placenta remains inside the uterus after delivery, the tissue becomes necrotic and provides a good place for bacteria to grow.

Additional factors include postpartum hemorrhage, which causes loss of some of the infection-fighting components of the blood, such as leukocytes, and leaves the mother in a weakened condition. Prenatal conditions (poor nutrition, anemia) interfere with the mother's ability to resist infection. Lack of knowledge of hygiene or lack of access to facilities that permit adequate hygiene increases the risk of postpartum infection. Table 28–2 includes other risk factors for infection.

Specific Infections

METRITIS

Infections of the uterus have been called endometritis, endomyometritis, and endoparametritis. The preferred term is *metritis with pelvic cellulitis* because infection involves the decidua, myometrium, and parametrial tissues (Cunningham et al., 1997).

Etiology.   Metritis is usually caused by organisms that are normal inhabitants of the vagina and cervix. Several organisms are responsible for most infections. Organisms most often involved include gram-negative coliform bacteria, such as *Escherichia coli*, *Bacteroides*, *Staphylococcus*, and anaerobic nonhemolytic *Streptococcus*. Group B streptococci are often involved and are a major cause of sepsis in the newborn as well.

Manifestations.   The major signs and symptoms of metritis are fever, chills, malaise, anorexia, abdominal pain and cramping, uterine tenderness, and purulent, foul-smelling lochia. Additional signs include tachycardia and subinvolution. In most cases, the signs and symptoms occur within the first 2 to 7 days (Gibbs & Sweet, 1999). When the causative organisms are group A or group B streptococci, however, the woman may exhibit no signs except fever.

Laboratory data may confirm the diagnosis. The results of a complete blood count may show an elevation of leukocytes, although leukocytes are normally elevated to 20,000 or as high as 30,000 during labor and for a short time afterward. Elevations in the upper ranges of normal should cause suspicion. Specimens may be taken from the blood, endocervix, and uterine cavity for cultures. A catheterized urine specimen should also be obtained.

Therapeutic Management.   Intravenous administration of antibiotics is the initial treatment for metritis. Broad-spectrum antibiotics, such as ampicillin and cephalosporins, are rapidly effective for mild to moderate infection after vaginal birth. Response to antibiotics after cesarean birth is less dramatic, and a combination of clindamycin plus gentamicin may be necessary (Gibbs & Sweet, 1999).

Improvement in clinical signs usually follows within 48 to 72 hours. Oral antibiotics may be used after completion of an intravenous course of treatment. Some physicians give

TABLE 28–2

Risk Factors for Puerperal Infection

Risk Factor	Reason
History of previous infections (urinary tract infection, mastitis, thrombophlebitis)	May be more vulnerable to infectious process
Colonization of lower genital tract with pathogenic organisms such as group B streptococci, *Chlamydia trachomatis, Staphylococcus aureus, Escherichia coli,* and *Gardnerella vaginalis*	Infections usually caused by several microbes that have ascended to the uterus from the lower genital tract
Cesarean birth	Increased portals of infection
Trauma	Provides entrance for bacteria and makes tissues more susceptible
Prolonged rupture of membranes	Allows access for organisms to interior of uterus
Prolonged labor	Increases number of vaginal examinations and allows time for bacteria to multiply
Catheterization	Could introduce organisms into bladder
Excessive number of vaginal examinations	Increases chance that organisms from vagina or outside source are carried into the uterus
Retained placental fragments	Provide growth medium for bacteria and may interfere with flow of lochia
Hemorrhage	Loss of infection-fighting components of blood
Poor general health (excessive fatigue, anemia, frequent minor illnesses)	Increases vulnerability to infections and complications of labor
Poor nutrition (decreased protein, vitamin C)	Less able to repair tissue and defend against infection
Poor hygiene	Excessive exposure to pathogens
Medical conditions, such as diabetes mellitus	Decreases ability to defend against infections of any kind
Low socioeconomic status	More likely to have poor nutrition and inadequate prenatal care

prophylactic antibiotics intravenously, orally, or both for any woman who is having a cesarean birth or who is particularly at risk for infection. Other drugs include antipyretics for fever and oxytocics, such as methylergonovine, to increase drainage of lochia and promote involution.

Complications. If the infection spreads outside the uterine cavity, there may be infection of the fallopian tubes (*salpingitis*) or the ovaries (*oophoritis*), which could result in sterility. *Peritonitis* (inflammation of the membrane lining the walls of the abdominal and pelvic cavities) may occur and lead to formation of a pelvic abscess. In addition, the risk of pelvic thrombophlebitis is increased when pathogenic bacteria enter the bloodstream during episodes of metritis. Figure 28–4 illustrates complications of metritis.

Signs and symptoms that the infection is spreading may be similar to those of metritis, but more severe. Fever and abdominal pain will be particularly pronounced. Peritonitis may result in paralytic ileus and a distended, board-like abdomen with absent bowel sounds.

Nursing Considerations. The mother with metritis should be placed in a Fowler's position to promote drainage of lochia. She may be medicated as needed for abdominal pain or cramping, which may be severe. The nurse should give the medications as directed and observe the mother for signs of improvement or new symptoms, such as nausea and vomiting, abdominal distension, absent bowel sounds, and severe abdominal pain. Comfort measures include warm blankets, cool compresses, cold or warm drinks, or use of a heating pad.

Teaching incorporates signs and symptoms of worsening condition, side effects of therapy, and the importance of adhering to the treatment plan and follow-up care. If the woman must be isolated from her infant, a nursing diagnosis of Risk for Altered Parenting related to separation from infant should be considered. If the mother is breast-feeding, she will need help to pump her breasts to establish and maintain lactation.

WOUND INFECTION

Wound infections are common types of puerperal infection because any break in the skin or mucous membrane provides a portal for bacteria. The most common sites are cesarean surgical incisions; the perineum, where episiotomies and lacerations are common; and the vagina.

Manifestations. Signs of wound infection are edema, warmth, redness, tenderness, and pain. The edges of the wound may pull apart, and there may be seropurulent drainage from the wound. If the wound remains untreated, gener-

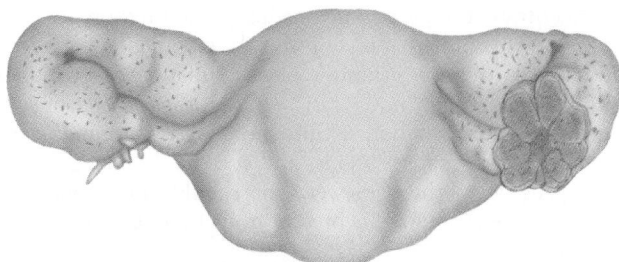

Salpingitis: Infection in fallopian tubes causes them to become enlarged, hyperemic, and tender.

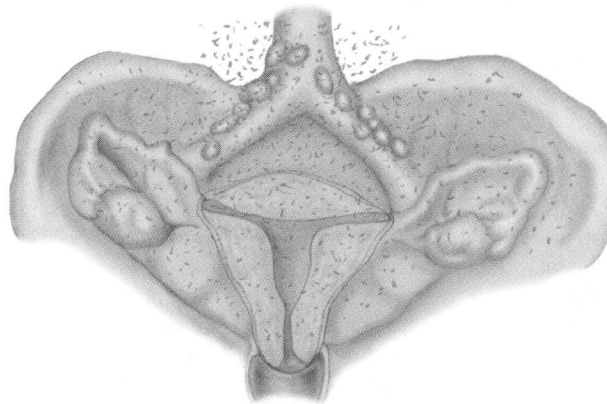

Peritonitis: Infection spreads through the lymphatics to the peritoneum; a pelvic abscess may form.

FIGURE 28–4
Areas of spread of uterine infection.

alized signs of infection, such as fever and malaise, may develop as well. As with other puerperal infections, cultures may reveal mixed aerobic and anaerobic bacteria.

Therapeutic Management. The physician or nurse-midwife may decide to remove some sutures to open the area and allow for drainage. Packing, such as iodoform gauze, may be placed in the open lesion to keep it open and to facilitate drainage. Broad-spectrum antibiotics are ordered until a report of the organism is returned. Analgesics are often necessary, and warm compresses or sitz baths may be used to provide comfort and to promote healing by increasing circulation to the area.

Nursing Considerations. Wound infections are painful and annoying to the mother out of proportion to their size. Perineal infections cause discomfort during many activities, such as walking, sitting, or defecating.

Wound infections may require readmittance to the hospital or home health care visits. The woman requires reassurance and supportive care. Comfort measures might include sitz baths, warm compresses, and frequent perineal care. The woman is taught to wipe from front to back and to change perineal pads frequently. Good hand washing techniques are emphasized. Adequate fluid intake and diet are important. Activity may be modified depending on the site, severity, and treatment of the wound infection.

The infant is not routinely isolated from the mother with a wound infection, but she must be advised to protect her infant from contact with contaminated articles. Anticipatory guidance should include teaching side effects of medication, signs of worsening condition, and any self-care measures that will be needed.

URINARY TRACT INFECTIONS

Etiology. During childbirth, the bladder and urethra are traumatized by the pressure from the descending fetus. Insertion of a catheter, with its risk of infection, occurs at least once during many labors. After birth, the bladder and urethra are hypotonic, with urinary stasis and retention common problems. Moreover, there may be residual urine and reflux of urine during voiding. Women who had bacteria in the urine during pregnancy are at increased risk for postpartum urinary tract infections, which are usually caused by coliform bacteria such as *E. coli.*

Manifestations. Symptoms typically begin on the first or second postpartum day. They include dysuria (a burning pain on urination), urgency, and frequency of urination. A low-grade fever is sometimes the only symptom. In some women, an upper urinary tract infection, such as pyelonephritis, may develop the third or fourth day, with chills, spiking fever, costovertebral angle tenderness, flank pain, and nausea and vomiting. If not promptly treated, this infection of the kidney pelvis may result in permanent damage to the kidney.

Therapeutic Management. With the exception of pyelonephritis, most urinary tract infections can be treated on an outpatient basis. If the mother is breast-feeding, the most commonly prescribed medication is ampicillin, which can be taken safely during pregnancy and lactation (Hodgson & Kizior, 1998). Sulfonamides, nitrofurantoin, or cephalosporins should be used cautiously during lactation.

Pyelonephritis warrants intravenous hydration and intravenous administration of broad-spectrum antibiotics until the causative organism and its sensitivity are known. The antibiotic therapy can then be adjusted.

Nursing Considerations. The woman with a urinary tract infection must be instructed to take the medication for the entire time it is prescribed and not to stop when symptoms abate. In addition, she must drink at least 3,000 ml of fluid each day to help dilute the bacterial burden and flush the infection from the bladder. Acidification of the urine inhibits multiplication of bacteria, and drinks that acidify urine, such as apricot, plum, prune, or cranberry juices, are frequently recommended. Carbonated drinks should be avoided because they increase urine alkalinity.

Teaching should also include measures to prevent urinary tract infections, such as proper perineal care, increasing fluid intake, and urinating frequently.

MASTITIS

Mastitis, an infection of the lactating breast, occurs most often during the second and third weeks after birth, although it may develop at any time during breast-feeding. It is more common in mothers nursing for the first time and usually affects only one breast.

Etiology. Mastitis usually is caused by *Staphylococcus aureus* or *E. coli.* The bacteria are most often carried on the hands of the mother or agency staff or in the mouth of the newborn. The organism may enter through an injured area of the nipple, such as a crack or blister, although there may be no obvious signs of injury. Soreness of a nipple may result in insufficient emptying of the breast resulting from pain during breast-feeding. Engorgement and stasis of milk frequently precede mastitis, often when a feeding is skipped, when the infant begins to sleep through the night, or when breast-feeding is suddenly stopped. Constriction of the breasts from a bra that is too tight may interfere with emptying of all the ducts and may lead to infection. The mother who is fatigued or stressed or who has other health problems that might lower her immune system is also at increased risk for mastitis.

Manifestations. Initial symptoms may be flu-like with fatigue and aching muscles. Symptoms progress to include fever of 38.4°C (101.1°F) or higher, chills, malaise, and headache. Mastitis is characterized by a localized area of redness and inflammation. Although rare, purulent drainage may be present. Untreated mastitis may progress to breast abscess. Figure 28–5 illustrates mastitis.

Therapeutic Management. Antibiotic therapy and continued decompression of the breast by breast-feeding or breast pump constitute the first line of treatment. With early antibiotic treatment, mastitis usually resolves within 24 to 48 hours, and abscess formation is unusual. Supportive measures include application of heat or ice packs, breast support, and analgesics (Lawrence & Lawrence, 1999). The mother should continue to breast-feed from both breasts. If the affected breast is too sore, a breast pump can be used. Regular emptying of the breast is important in preventing abscess formation. If an abscess forms and ruptures into the breast ducts, breast-feeding on that side should be discontinued and a breast pump used to empty the breast temporarily. Milk obtained should be discarded.

Nursing Considerations. Because mastitis rarely occurs before discharge from the birth facility, the nurse must concentrate on providing adequate information for the family. Measures to prevent the development of mastitis include correct positioning of the infant and avoiding nipple trauma and milk stasis. The mother should breast-feed every 2 to 3 hours. She should avoid formula supplements and nipple shields, and she should change nursing pads when they are wet. She should also avoid continuous pressure on the breasts from tight bras or infant carriers.

Once mastitis occurs, nursing measures are aimed at increasing comfort and helping the mother maintain lactation. Moist heat promotes comfort and increases circulation. A shower or hot packs should be used before feeding or pumping the breasts.

The breast should be completely emptied at each feeding to prevent stasis of milk, which can result in an abscess. If the mother is too sore to breast-feed on the affected side or if she is taking antibiotics that are contraindicated during lactation, she should be instructed to express the milk or use a mechanical pump to empty the breasts. Breast-feeding or pumping every 1.5 to 2 hours makes the mother more comfortable and prevents stasis. Starting the feeding on the unaffected side causes the milk-ejection reflex to occur in the painful breast and makes the process more efficient. Massage over the affected area before and during the feeding helps to ensure complete emptying. The mother should stay in bed during the acute phase of her illness. Her fluid intake should be at least 3,000 ml/day. Analgesics may be required to relieve discomfort.

The mother with mastitis is likely to be very discouraged and may need much encouragement. Some mothers decide to stop breast-feeding because of the discomfort involved. Weaning during an episode of mastitis may increase engorgement and stasis, leading to abscess formation or recurrent infection. Therefore, the nurse should encourage the mother to continue breast-feeding.

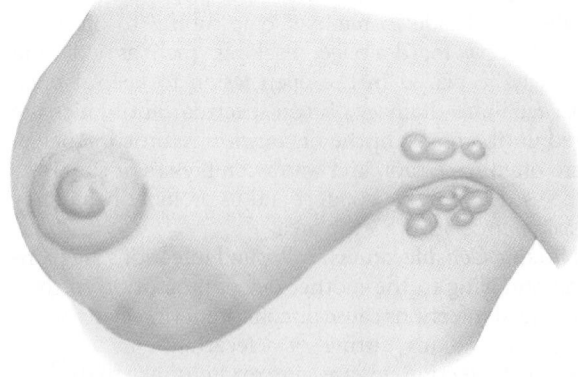

Early mastitis

Enlarged, tender axillary lymph nodes
Tender "flush" without swelling

Acute mastitis

Enlarged, tender axillary lymph nodes
Area of inflammation is red, swollen, hot, and tender

FIGURE 28–5

Mastitis is an infection that usually occurs 2 to 3 weeks after birth in the breast of a woman who breast-feeds.

SEPTIC PELVIC THROMBOPHLEBITIS

Septic pelvic thrombophlebitis is the least common of the puerperal infections. It usually is not seen until 2 to 4 days after childbirth. It occurs when infection spreads along the venous system and thrombophlebitis develops. It is seen more often in women with wound infection and usually involves the ovarian, uterine, or hypogastric veins.

Manifestations. The primary symptom is pain in the groin, abdomen, or flank. There may be fever, tachycardia, gastrointestinal distress, and decreased bowel sounds. Laboratory data may be used to exclude other diagnoses and usually include complete blood count with differential, blood chemistries, coagulation studies, and cultures. The only signs may be fever that does not respond to antibiotic therapy.

Therapeutic Management. Readmittance to the hospital is usually necessary. Treatment includes anticoagulation therapy with intravenous heparin and usually causes reduction of fever within 36 hours (Laros, 1999). Intravenous antibiotics are also given. Supportive care is similar to that for deep venous thrombosis and includes monitoring for safe levels of anticoagulation therapy and for signs and symptoms of pulmonary embolism.

▌ NURSING CARE
The Woman with an Infection

Assessment

Although all women are observed for indications of infection as part of routine nursing assessments, the nurse must practice increased vigilance for mothers who are at increased risk of infection (see Nursing Care Plan 28–1).

Assessment focuses on signs that may be expected in infection, such as fever, tachycardia, pain, or unusual amount, color, or odor of lochia. Generalized symptoms of malaise and muscle aching may also be significant. Examine all wounds each shift for signs of localized infection, such as redness, edema, tenderness, discharge, or pulling apart

---

CRITICAL TO REMEMBER
Signs and Symptoms of Postpartum Infection

- Fever, chills
- Pain or redness of wounds
- Purulent wound drainage or wound edges not approximated
- Tachycardia
- Uterine subinvolution
- Abnormal duration of lochia, foul odor
- Elevated white blood cell count
- Frequency or urgency of urination, dysuria, or hematuria
- Suprapubic pain
- Localized area of warmth, redness, or tenderness in the breasts
- Body aches, general malaise

---

of incisions or sutured lacerations. Ask the mother about difficulty emptying her bladder or discomfort related to urination.

Evaluate the mother's knowledge of hygiene practices that prevent infections, such as proper hand washing, perineal care, and handling of perineal pads. Also important are her knowledge of breast-feeding and the presence of problems that might result in breast engorgement and stasis of milk in the ducts. Examine the nipples for signs of injury that might provide a portal of entry for organisms.

Nursing Diagnosis and Planning

Because all women are at risk for infection after childbirth, most facilities have developed standards of practice that protect postpartum women from infection, and individual nursing care plans are usually not necessary. When predisposing factors increase the likelihood of infection, however, routine assessments and care may need to be modified and preventive measures intensified. In this case, the most relevant nursing diagnosis is

- Risk for Infection related to the presence of significant risk factors.

Nursing Care Plan 28–1 develops goals and interventions for this nursing diagnosis.

▌ *Affective Disorders*

Affective (mood) disorders are disturbances in function, affect, or thought processes that can affect the family after childbirth as severely as physiologic problems. They include postpartum psychosis, postpartum depression, and postpartum blues. Postpartum blues is a transient, self-limiting mood disorder that is discussed in Chapter 21. Postpartum psychosis and postpartum depression are more serious disorders that disrupt the family and require intervention to resolve.

Postpartum Psychosis

Postpartum psychosis is a rare condition that affects approximately 1 in 1,000 postpartum women. It usually surfaces within 3 weeks of delivery. It may occur as bipolar disorder with manic and depressive episodes or as major depression consisting of depression without manic episodes. Women who have had one episode of postpartum psychosis have a 50% risk of having another episode (Pearlstein et al., 1998).

Women with bipolar disorder suffer from irritability, hyperactivity, euphoria, and grandiosity. They exhibit little need for sleep and are seldom aware they have a problem. The poor judgment and confusion they experience make self-care and infant care impossible and can be life-threatening for the mother and infant.

The depressions of the bipolar disorder and major depression are similar and are characterized by tearfulness, preoccupations of guilt, feelings of worthlessness, sleep and appetite disturbances, and an inordinate concern with the baby's health. Delusions about the infant being dead or defective are common.

Assessment and management of postpartum psychosis are beyond the scope of maternity nurses, and mothers who

Postpartum Infection

Assessment

Lisa Pyle, a thin, pale, 16-year-old primipara, is admitted to the postpartum unit after a cesarean birth. Her membranes were ruptured for 14 hours, and she was in labor for 16 hours before the birth. She was catheterized twice during labor and now has an indwelling catheter. She plans to breast-feed her infant.

Nursing Diagnosis

Risk for Infection related to presence of favorable conditions for infections

Goals/Expected Outcomes

Lisa will

- Remain free of signs of infection during the postpartum period.
- Verbalize methods of prevention of infection and signs that infection may be present by discharge.

Intervention

1. Assess vital signs every 4 hours.

2. Observe the surgical incision for redness, tenderness, or edema and note odor of lochia every 4 hours. Ask Lisa if she experiences frequency, urgency, or pain with urination when the catheter is removed.
3. Instruct Lisa in hygienic practices to prevent infection:
   a. Careful hand washing before and after perineal care
   b. Perineal cleansing after elimination
   c. Changing peripads frequently
   d. Wiping the perineum from front to back
4. Initiate measures to reduce the risk of urinary tract infection.
   a. Provide fluids of Lisa's choice when she is able to take them and emphasize the importance of drinking 2,500 to 3,000 ml/day.
   b. Monitor bladder distention to prevent overfilling. Teach Lisa the importance of emptying her bladder every 2 to 3 hours during the first days after childbirth.
   c. Use methods to promote bladder emptying, such as running water in the shower or sink, running warm water over the perineum, and providing pain medication as needed.
5. Assist Lisa in breast-feeding. Explain the reasons for proper positioning and frequent feedings.
6. Offer and encourage Lisa to eat well balanced meals when she progresses to a regular diet. Emphasize the importance of a diet high in protein and vitamin C.
7. Teach Lisa signs of infection that she should report to her health care provider. Include fever, chills, dysuria, increased incisional tenderness or drainage, and foul odor of the lochia.

Rationale

1. Temperature above 38°C (100.4°F) or tachycardia suggests an infectious process and should be reported.
2. Redness, pain, or swelling of the incision suggests wound infection. Foul odor of lochia suggests endometrial infection. Frequency, urgency, or painful urination may indicate urinary tract infection.
3. Hand washing is the most important defense against infection and its spread. Perineal cleansing helps prevent growth of bacteria. Frequent pad changes remove accumulated lochia, which provides an excellent culture for bacteria. Wiping from front to back prevents fecal contamination of the vagina.
4. Adequate hydration and frequent emptying of the bladder help prevent stasis of urine, which increases the risk of urinary tract infection. Relief of pain may allow the mother to relax enough to void. The sound of running water may stimulate the urge to void.

5. Poor positioning and infrequent feedings may cause nipple trauma and engorgement and lead to mastitis.
6. Adequate protein and vitamin C are necessary for healing damaged tissues.

7. Prompt recognition and reporting of signs of infection ensures early treatment and reduces further complications.

Evaluation

Lisa remains free of the signs and symptoms of infection throughout her hospital stay. She discusses measures that she will use to reduce the risk of infection when she is discharged from the hospital.

Additional Nursing Diagnoses to Consider

Activity Intolerance
Pain
Fatigue
Risk for Altered Parenting

experience these conditions must be referred to specialists for comprehensive therapy.

Hospitalization is usually necessary to treat women with postpartum psychosis. Women who have manic symptoms are usually treated with the standard medications (lithium, antidepressants, antipsychotics). Lithium is not recommended during pregnancy, but it may be resumed in the postpartum period if the mother is not breast-feeding. Women who have depressive symptoms must be assessed for suicidal potential and treated according to the severity of the threat. Antipsychotics and antidepressants are used for treatment, and careful monitoring is required because of the effect of hormonal imbalances on the mother's reaction to the prescribed medication.

Postpartum Depression

INCIDENCE
Depression is the most common affective disorder of the postpartum period. It occurs in 10% and 15% of women during pregnancy and after birth, respectively (Pearlstein et al., 1998). The incidence may be as high as 25% in women after multifetal pregnancy (Leonard, 1998). Moreover, many investigators believe that postpartum depression is underdiagnosed and underreported.

MANIFESTATIONS
The woman experiencing postpartum depression shows less interest in her surroundings and a loss of her usual emotional response toward her family. Although she cares for the infant in a loving manner, she is unable to feel pleasure or love. She sees the infant as demanding and feels she is inept at mothering. The woman may have intense feelings of unworthiness, guilt, and shame. Generalized fatigue, complaints of ill health, and difficulty in concentrating are also present. She often has little interest in food and experiences sleep disturbances. She may describe panic attacks and relentless obsessive thinking. Most of the symptoms are intensely and consistently present for at least a 2-week period.

IMPACT ON THE FAMILY
Postpartum depression creates strain on each family member's usual methods of coping and often causes difficulties in relationships. Stressors tend to be magnified and, as a result, family members may decrease their interactions with the depressed mother when she needs support the most. Communication is impaired because she gradually withdraws from contact with others. Moreover, the decreased libido commonly associated with depression may also affect her relationship with her significant other.

Depressed mothers interact differently with their infants than do women who are not depressed. They appear tense, are more irritable, and feel less competent as mothers. They may not pick up on their infants' cues or smiles, thus failing to meet the infants' needs and to enjoy their positive feedback (Beck, 1995). Infants of depressed mothers tend to be fussier and more discontented, and they make fewer positive facial expressions.

ETIOLOGY
The cause of postpartum depression is unknown. Factors believed to increase the risk of its occurrence include

- Hormonal fluctuations that follow childbirth
- Medical problems during pregnancy, such as pregnancy-induced hypertension, pre-existing diabetes mellitus, or thyroid dysfunction
- History of depression, mental illness, or alcoholism, either in the woman or in her family
- Personality characteristics, such as immaturity and low self-esteem
- Marital dysfunction or difficult relationship with the significant other, resulting in lack of support
- Anger at the pregnancy
- Feelings of isolation
- Fatigue, lack of sleep, financial worries, and birth of an infant who is ill or has anomalies
- Multifetal pregnancy

THERAPEUTIC MANAGEMENT
Depression responds best to a combination of psychotherapy, social support, and medication, such as antidepressants. The woman's partner and immediate family must be included in counseling sessions so they can develop an understanding of what the woman feels and needs.

NURSING CARE
The Woman with Postpartum Depression

Assessment
Observe for subjective symptoms, such as apathy, lack of interest or energy, anorexia, or sleeplessness. The mother's verbalizations of failure, sadness, loneliness, anxiety, or vague confusion are also important cues. Assess for objective data, such as crying, poor personal hygiene, or inability to follow directions or to concentrate.

Assessment includes availability of family support. Single mothers or mothers with an absent or unavailable support system may feel increasingly isolated, leading to stress that they are unable to manage. Inappropriate expressions of blame or anger toward the partner and unmet expectations of the baby or the parenting role are sometimes present.

Nursing Diagnosis and Planning
A likely nursing diagnosis is

- Risk for Ineffective Individual Coping related to depression secondary to stressors associated with childbirth and parenting.
  Expected Outcomes: The new mother will verbalize feelings with the health care provider and the significant other throughout the postpartum period and will identify strengths and resources that are available during the postpartum period.

Interventions

Demonstrating Caring
Conveying a caring attitude is one nursing strategy to help mothers decrease their emotional distress and to guide them

Aricella Nunez, a 23-year-old multipara, gave birth several days ago to her second baby. She is crying when the nurse makes a telephone follow-up call after discharge. Aricella says, "I feel so stupid. I can barely get out of bed in the morning, and I am worn out just trying to take care of the kids." The nurse responds, "Oh, that is just the 'baby blues.' Just look at those beautiful babies and you will feel better."

1. What assumption has the nurse made?
2. Is her response helpful for Aricella? Why or why not?
3. What would be a more therapeutic response?
4. What additional action should the nurse take?

in regaining their well-being during the postpartum period. Acknowledge that the woman feels depressed. Reassure the woman that the condition is not her fault. Postpartum depression is an illness that can be treated and will end. It is particularly important for nurses to reinforce that it is an illness and is not the woman's fault.

Providing Anticipatory Guidance

Provide all new mothers with anticipatory guidance about the early weeks at home. Emphasize the need for frequent contact with other adults so that the mother does not become isolated. Continued communication with the partner or with a close friend who is available to provide support when loneliness or anxiety becomes a problem is important. Explain the importance of adequate rest and nutrition for maintaining energy and a feeling of health and well-being.

Helping the Mother Verbalize Feelings

Many women and their families minimize depression because they cannot find the exact cause. Moreover, many in the health care delivery system also trivialize the problem by making comments such as "You'll get over it. After all, you have a beautiful baby."

Recommend that although some of her feelings may seem "unreasonable" (e.g., anger, guilt, shame), the woman should acknowledge the feelings to herself and insist that others acknowledge them as well. It may be helpful to rehearse some situations that may occur, such as a fussy baby or being home alone and feeling lonely, as a means to develop perspective and to find solutions before the situation occurs.

Enhancing Sensitivity to Infant Cues

Help the mother to plan measures that enhance her sensitivity to infant cues. Music, relaxation therapy, and massage techniques just before mother-infant interactions have been used to alter the mother's depressed mood at least temporarily and thus increase the mutual response between the mother and infant (Beck, 1995).

Discussing Options and Resources

Assist the new mother in identifying people who are available to provide support. Suggest that she explain her anticipated needs to those people before the development of symptoms. In addition, give the mother telephone numbers for support groups in the area.

Evaluation

- Can the mother identify stressors in her life that contribute to postpartum depression?
- Can she verbalize her feelings and insist that others acknowledge the feelings and their impact on her?
- Does she identify sources that will provide support during this time?

KEY CONCEPTS

- Postpartum hemorrhage can sometimes be prevented by careful examination of factors that predispose to excessive bleeding.
- Overstretching of the muscle fibers during pregnancy or repeated stretching during past pregnancies predisposes to uterine atony and excessive uterine bleeding.
- Initial management of uterine atony focuses on measures to contract the uterus and provide fluid replacement.
- Soft-tissue trauma (lacerations, hematomas) can cause rapid loss of blood even when the uterus is firmly contracted. Management involves repairing the trauma before excessive blood loss occurs.

- Compensatory mechanisms maintain the blood pressure so that vital organs receive adequate oxygen. When these mechanisms fail, hypovolemic shock follows.
- The process of uterine involution is delayed (causing subinvolution) when placental fragments are retained or when the inner lining of the uterus is infected (causing metritis).
- Subinvolution of the uterus develops after the mother goes home. The nurse teaches the family the process of normal involution and the signs and symptoms that should be reported to the health care provider.
- Venous stasis that occurs during

pregnancy, increased levels of coagulation factors, and decreased thrombolytic factors that persist into the postpartum period increase the risk of thrombus formation during the puerperium.
- Treatment for deep venous thrombosis includes anticoagulants, analgesics, and bed rest, with the affected leg elevated to decrease interstitial edema and improve venous return.
- Nurses who administer anticoagulant therapy assess the mother to determine whether her clotting time is within the recommended therapeutic range so that overmedication with anticoagulants does not result in bleeding.

■ Pulmonary embolism is a complication of deep venous thrombosis that occurs when a clot is dislodged from the vein and carried by the blood to a pulmonary vessel, which may become completely or partially occluded.

■ The risk of infection is increased with childbearing because there is open access to bacteria from the vagina through the fallopian tubes and into the peritoneal cavity. Increased blood supply to the pelvis and the alkalinization of the va-

gina by the amniotic fluid further increase the risk of metritis.

■ Any break in the skin or mucous membranes during childbirth provides a portal of entry for pathogenic organisms and increases the risk of puerperal infection. Nurses must assess women for any signs of infections.

■ Urinary stasis and urinary tract trauma increase the risk of urinary tract infection. Nurses must initiate measures to prevent urinary stasis.

■ Nurses must provide information about the importance of completely emptying the breasts at each feeding and about measures to prevent nipple trauma to prevent mastitis.

■ Postpartum depression is a disabling affective disorder that affects the entire family. Nurses help the woman acknowledge her feelings and assist her in identifying measures that will help her cope with the condition.

ANSWERS TO CRITICAL THINKING EXERCISES

Exercise 28–1

1. Her history of multiparity, birth of a large infant, and rapid labor and delivery indicate that Dolores is at risk for postpartal hemorrhage. The nurse should assess the fundus, lochia, vital signs, and skin temperature and color more frequently.

2. Massage the fundus and express clots that may have accumulated in the uterus. Massage stimulates uterine contractions that compress myometrial blood vessels and stop excessive bleeding. Continued assessment of the fundus and lochia is imperative.

3. Assist Dolores to void because a distended bladder lifts the uterus, making contraction more difficult and resulting in excessive bleeding.

4. Notify the physician or the nurse-midwife because excessive bleeding requires the combined efforts of primary health care providers and nurses to prevent postpartum hemorrhage.

Exercise 28–2

1. The nurse assumed that Aricella has the transient, self-limiting moods of depression that come and go in most women who give birth. She fails to obtain additional data that may indicate whether Aricella is experiencing postpartum depression that requires additional therapy.

2. Her response is not helpful because it minimizes the feelings Aricella has expressed and it offers no measures for dealing with the feelings.

3. The nurse should acknowledge Aricella's feelings and ask questions that allow her to express those feelings fully.

4. The nurse must convey her genuine interest and caring. She can do this best by
   a. Indicating that she is aware that something may be wrong
   b. Sharing as much time as Aricella needs to express her feelings
   c. Providing hope by reassuring Aricella that her feelings are not her fault and that the condition can be cured
   d. Making appropriate referrals that try to provide as much continuity of care as possible

REFERENCES AND READINGS

American Academy of Pediatrics & American College of Obstetricians and Gynecologists. (1997). *Guidelines for perinatal care* (4th ed.). Elk Grove Village, IL, and Washington, DC: Author.

Beck, C. T. (1995). The effects of postpartum depression on maternal-infant interaction: A meta-analysis. *Nursing Research, 44*(5), 298–304.

Beck, C. T. (1998). A checklist to identify women at risk for developing postpartum depression. *Journal of Obstetric, Gynecologic, and Neonatal Nursing, 27*(5), 39–46.

Clark, R. A. (1995). Infections during the postpartum period. *Journal of Obstetric, Gynecologic, and Neonatal Nursing, 24*(6), 542–548.

Cunningham, F. G., MacDonald, P. C., Gant, N. F., Leveno, K. J., Gilstrap, L. C., Hankins, G. D. V., & Clark, S. L. (1997). *Williams obstetrics* (20th ed.). Norwalk, CT: Appleton & Lange.

Ely, J. W., Rijhsinghani, A., Bowdler, N. C., & Dawson, J. D. (1995). The association between manual removal of the placenta and postpartum endometritis following vaginal delivery. *Obstetrics and Gynecology, 86*(6), 1002–1006.

Gibbs, R. S., & Sweet, R. L. (1999). Maternal and fetal infectious disorders. In R. K. Creasy & R. Resnik (Eds.), *Maternal-fetal medicine: Principles and practice* (4th ed., pp. 659–724). Philadelphia: Saunders.

Grohar, J. (1996). Postpartum care. In K. R. Simpson & P. A. Creehan (Eds.), *AWHONN perinatal nursing* (pp. 249–270). Philadelphia: Lippincott–Raven.

Hager, W. D. (1998). Puerperal mastitis. *Contemporary Obstetrics and Gynecology, 43*(4), 27–33.

Hayashi, R. H. (1998) Postpartum hemorrhage and puerperal sepsis. In N. F. Hacker & J. G. Moore (Eds.), *Essentials of obstetrics and gynecology* (3rd ed., pp. 333–342). Philadelphia: Saunders.

Hodgson, B. B., & Kizior, R. J. (1998). *Saunders nurse's drug handbook 1998.* Philadelphia: Saunders.

Knuppel, R. A., & Hatangadi, S. B. (1995). Acute hypotension related to hemorrhage in the obstetric patient. *Obstetrics and Gynecology Clinics of North America 22*(1), 111–130.

Laros, R. K. (1999). Thromboembolic disease. In R. K. Creasy & R. Resnik (Eds.), *Maternal-fetal medicine: Principles and practice* (4th ed., pp. 821–831). Philadelphia: Saunders.

Lawrence, R. A., & Lawrence, R. M. (1999). *Breastfeeding: A guide for the medical profession* (5th ed.). St. Louis: Mosby.

Leonard, L. G. (1998). Depression and anxiety disorders during multiple pregnancy and parenthood. *Journal of Obstetric, Gynecologic, and Neonatal Nursing, 27*(3), 329–337.

Luegenbiehl, D. L. (1997). Improving visual estimation of blood volume on peripads. *MCN: The American Journal of Maternal/Child Nursing, 22*(6), 294–298.

Nuwayhid, B., Nguyen, T., & Khalife, S. (1998). Medical complications of pregnancy. In N. F. Hacker & J. G. Moore (Eds.), *Essentials of obstetrics and gynecology* (3rd ed., pp. 234–262). Philadelphia: Saunders.

Pearlstein, T., Diaz, S., Howard, M., Zlotnick, C., & Jain, N. (1998). Dysphoric disorders in women: A case of perinatal depression. *Medscape Women's Health* [On-line serial], 3(4). Available: http://www.medscape/womenshealth/1998/v03.n04/wh3067.pear/wh3067.pear-01.html.

Savoia, M. C. (1999). Bacterial, fungal, and parasitic disease during pregnancy. In G. N. Burrow & T. F. Ferris (Eds.), *Medical complications during pregnancy* (5th ed., pp. 295–335). Philadelphia: Saunders.

Scott-Conner, C. E. H. (1997). Diagnosing and managing breast disease during pregnancy and lactation. *Medscape Women's Health* [On-line serial], 2(5). Available: http://www.medscape/womenshealth/journal/1997/v02.n05/wh3148.scott-conner/wh3148scottconner.html.

Straub, H., Cross, J., Curtis, S., Iverson, S., Jacobsmeyer, M., Anderson, C., & Sorenson, M. (1998). Proactive nursing: The evolution of a task force to help women with postpartum depression. MCN: *The American Journal of Maternal/Child Nursing, 23*(5), 262–265.

Williams-Judge, S. (1998). Managing postpartum hemorrhage. *Mother Baby Journal, 3*(6), 5–12.

Wood, A. F., Thomas, S. P., Droppleman, P. G., & Meighan, M. (1997). The downward spiral of postpartum depression. MCN: *The American Journal of Maternal/Child Nursing, 22*(6), 308–316.

29

The High-Risk Newborn: Problems Related to Gestational Age and Development

After studying this chapter, you should be able to:

- Explain the special problems of the preterm infant.
- Identify common nursing diagnoses for preterm infants, and explain the nursing care for each.
- Describe the complications that may result from premature birth.
- Describe the characteristics and problems of the infant with postmaturity syndrome.
- Explain the effects of intrauterine growth restriction.
- Compare the problems of the large-for-gestational-age infant with those of the small-for-gestational-age infant.

DEFINITIONS

apneic spells Cessation of breathing for more than 15 seconds, accompanied by cyanosis or bradycardia.

bronchopulmonary dysplasia Chronic pulmonary condition in which damage to the infant's lungs requires prolonged dependence on supplemental oxygen.

compliance Stretchability or elasticity of the lungs and thorax, which allows distension without resistance during respirations.

containment A method of increasing comfort in infants by swaddling or other methods to keep the extremities in a flexed position near the body.

corrected gestational age Gestational age that a preterm infant would be if still in utero. May also be called developmental age.

enteral feeding Nutrients supplied to the gastrointestinal tract orally or by feeding tube.

intrauterine growth restriction Failure of a fetus to grow as expected for gestational age. May also be called intrauterine growth retardation.

large-for-gestational-age infant An infant whose size is above the 90th percentile for gestational age.

low-birth-weight infant An infant weighing less than 2,500 g at birth.

macrosomia Unusually large fetal size; infant birth weight more than 4,000 g.

necrotizing enterocolitis Condition of injury, invasion by bacteria, and possible necrosis of the intestines.

noncompliance Resistance of the lungs and thorax to distension with air during respirations.

parenteral nutrition Intravenous infusion of all nutrients needed for metabolism and growth.

periventricular-intraventricular hemorrhage Bleeding into and around the ventricles of the brain.

postmaturity syndrome Condition in which a post-term infant shows characteristics indicative of poor placental functioning before birth.

post-term infant An infant born after 42 weeks of gestation.

preterm infant An infant born before the beginning of the 38th week of gestation. Also called premature infant.

pulse oximetry Method of determining the level of blood oxygen saturation by sensors attached to the skin.

respiratory distress syndrome Condition caused by insufficient production of surfactant in the lungs; results in atelectasis (collapse of the lung alveoli), hypoxemia, and hypercapnia.

retinopathy of prematurity Condition in which interference with blood supply to the retina may cause decreased vision or blindness.

small-for-gestational-age infant An infant whose size is below the 10th percentile for gestational age.

transcutaneous oxygen/carbon dioxide monitoring Method of continuous noninvasive measurement of oxygen and carbon dioxide levels in the blood by transducers attached to the skin.

very-low-birth-weight infant An infant weighing 1,500 g or less at birth.

Nurses identify and care for the immediate needs of neonates with gestational complications until they are transferred to the neonatal intensive care unit (NICU). Nurses also provide information and emotional care for parents. Neonatal intensive care, however, is a nursing specialty requiring further study. Nurses who work in NICU nurseries have additional education and experience to prepare them for this role.

Care of High-Risk Newborns

Approximately 9% of all newborns are sick enough at birth to require intensive care (Behrman, Kliegman, & Arvin, 1996). Nurses care for minor illness in the normal newborn nursery, but more serious problems require care in specialized nurseries designed for that purpose (Fig. 29–1).

Preterm Infants

Preterm infants (also called premature infants) are born before the beginning of the 38th week of gestation. The word preterm is sometimes confused with the term *low birth weight* (LBW), which refers to infants weighing 2,500 g (5 lb, 8 oz) or less at birth. *Very-low-birth-weight* (VLBW) infants weigh 1,500 g (3 lb, 5 oz) or less at birth. Although most of these infants are preterm, others are full-term and have failed to grow normally while in the uterus, a condition called *intrauterine growth restriction* (IUGR).

Incidence and Etiology

SCOPE OF THE PROBLEM
Advances in technology have resulted in survival at much lower birth weights than ever before. The number of early births, however, is not decreasing. In fact, 7.5% of newborns weighed less than 2,500 g in 1996. Prematurity and low birth weight are the second leading cause of infant death (Guyer et al., 1998). In medical expense, lost potential, and suffering of infants and their parents, preterm birth is extremely costly.

CAUSES
The exact causes of preterm birth are not known, but all risk factors in pregnancy are potential causes of complications for the newborn as well (see Chapter 13).

PREVENTION
Prevention of preterm birth is best accomplished by provision of adequate prenatal care for every pregnant woman to identify and treat risk factors as early as possible. Teaching women signs of preterm labor will help them seek care when halting the labor is still a possibility (see Chapter 27).

Characteristics of Preterm Infants

Preterm infants vary by gestational age. For example, the appearance and problems of infants born at 34 weeks' gestation are different from those of infants born at 26 weeks' gestation. Some characteristics, however, are common to all preterm infants.

APPEARANCE
Preterm infants appear frail and weak, and they have underdeveloped flexor muscles and muscle tone. Their extremities are limp, and they typically lie in an extended position (Fig. 22–24).

Preterm infants lack subcutaneous fat, which makes their thin skin appear red and almost transparent, with blood vessels clearly visible. The nipples and areola may be barely perceptible, whereas vernix caseosa and lanugo may be abundant. Plantar creases are absent in infants of less than 32 weeks' gestation (Fig. 22–31).

The pinna of the ear is soft and flat, lacking the rolled-over look of full-term ears (Fig. 22–32). In the female infant, the clitoris and labia minora appear large and are not covered by the small, separated labia majora. The male infant may have undescended testes, with a small, smooth scrotal sac (Figs. 22–33 and 22–34).

BEHAVIOR
Preterm infants have little excess energy for maintaining muscle tone. They are easily exhausted from noise and rou-

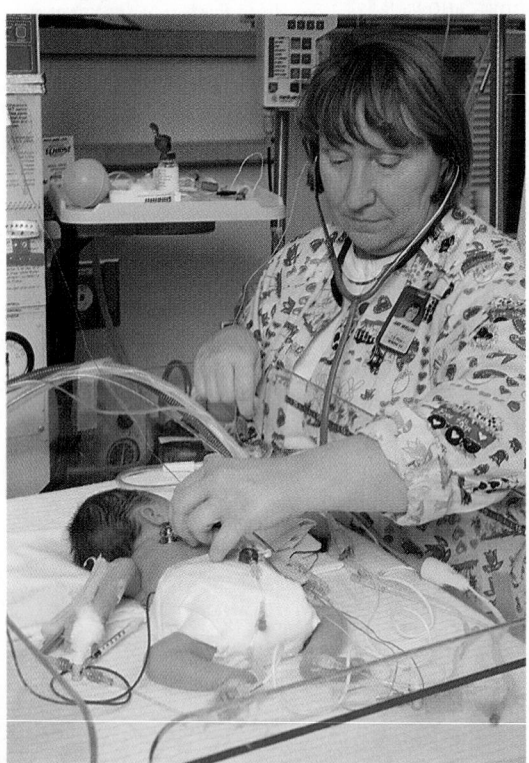

FIGURE 29–1
The infant in an NICU nursery is cared for by nurses with highly specialized skills.

tine activities. Their response is varied, including lowered oxygenation levels and behavior changes. The cry is feeble and seldom heard because the infant is too weak to cry.

Assessment and Care of Common Problems

Preterm infants are prone to problems that affect all systems and body processes.

PROBLEMS WITH RESPIRATION
Problems of the respiratory system are a major concern because preterm newborns have immature lungs. The presence of surfactant in adequate amounts is of primary importance. Surfactant reduces surface tension in the alveoli and prevents their collapse with expiration. Infants born before surfactant production is adequate develop respiratory distress syndrome (p. 752).

Assessment. The infant's respiratory status must be observed constantly. The lungs are assessed for adventitious breath sounds or areas of absent breath sounds. The Silverman-Andersen index is a useful tool for evaluating the degree of respiratory distress (Fig. 29–2).

The nurse differentiates periodic breathing from apneic spells. Periodic breathing is the cessation of breathing for 5 to 10 seconds without other changes. Apneic spells generally last more than 15 seconds or are accompanied by cyanosis and bradycardia, or both. They are common in preterm infants, increasing in incidence with lower gestational age. Apnea without an identified cause in a preterm infant is called apnea of prematurity and generally improves as the infant matures. The infant may require gentle stimulation or bag-and-mask ventilation.

The weak or absent cough reflex and the very small air passages make the preterm infant susceptible to obstruction by mucus. Because newborns are nose breathers, obstruction of the nasal passages may cause respiratory distress.

The nurse observes the effort required for breathing and the location and severity of retractions. Retractions are particularly noticeable in the preterm infant, whose weak chest wall is drawn in with each inspiration. The excessive compliance (elasticity) of the chest cage during retractions may interfere with full expansion of the lungs.

Grunting may be an early sign of respiratory distress syndrome. It closes the glottis and increases the pressure within the alveoli. This process keeps the alveoli partially open between breaths and increases the amount of oxygen absorbed.

Nursing Interventions. Interventions focus on collaborating with other team members, such as the respiratory therapist, to manage technical equipment and facilitate removal of secretions.

Working with Respiratory Equipment. The infant may need an endotracheal tube and mechanical ventilation. Continuous positive airway pressure may be necessary to keep the alveoli open and improve expansion of the lungs. It can be delivered with nasal prongs or an endotracheal tube. High-frequency ventilation may be used to provide very fast, frequent respirations with less pressure than other methods. Inhaled nitric oxide and partial liquid ventilation are newer methods used for infants with respiratory difficulty.

An oxygen hood is often used for infants who can breathe alone but who need extra oxygen. The hood is a plastic box-like device that fits over the infant's head. The infant breathes the higher levels of oxygen surrounding the head, and the device does not interfere with access to the rest of the infant's body for care (Fig. 29–3).

Oxygen may also be given by nasal cannula to the infant who breathes well alone. After discharge, many preterm infants continue to receive oxygen via nasal cannula at home. Oxygen must be humidified to prevent insensible water loss and drying of the delicate mucous membranes. It is warmed to maintain body temperature.

When oxygen is administered, the level of oxygen in the infant's blood must be monitored. Arterial blood may be drawn for testing arterial oxygen levels. Pulse oximetry or transcutaneous monitoring may also be used. They are less invasive and provide continuous information about oxygen partial pressure (Po_2) levels through sensors attached to the skin.

The nurse must observe the infant's increasing or decreasing dependence on breathing assistance and need for oxygen. The infant's response to activity that may increase oxygen need, such as handling, feeding, and linen changes, may require changes in settings on equipment to meet the infant's needs.

Positioning the Infant. The infant should be placed in a side-lying or prone position to facilitate drainage of respiratory secretions and regurgitated feedings. The prone position is not recommended for normal newborn infants because it is associated with an increased incidence of sudden infant death syndrome (SIDS). In the preterm infant, however, the prone position allows more efficient use of the respiratory muscles, decreases respiratory effort, and results in better oxygenation and lung compliance (Lefrak-Okikawa & Lund, 1993).

If the infant must be in a supine position, the nurse can elevate the head of the bed and turn the infant's head to the side. Rolled blankets by the head can prevent movement, if necessary. A small roll under the shoulders will straighten the airway. Frequent position changes will help air passages drain and prevent stasis of secretions.

Suctioning Secretions. Suction equipment must be available at all times. The nurse checks equipment at the beginning of each shift to ensure that it is functioning properly. A bulb syringe is less likely to be traumatic than wall suction, but it may not reach mucus deep in the respiratory tract.

The infant is suctioned as mucus becomes apparent. Suction should always be gentle to avoid traumatizing the delicate mucous membranes. Trauma could cause edema, which could further decrease the size of the air passages and lead to more respiratory difficulty.

Performing Chest Physiotherapy. Chest physiotherapy (postural drainage, percussion, and vibration) and suctioning are used in some hospitals to help keep the airway clear. Postural drainage helps the affected areas of the lung drain into the major bronchi. Percussion helps loosen secretions and bring them into the bronchi, where they can be removed by suction. Percussion is not used on small infants, however, because the stimulation causes stress and may increase intracranial pressure.

| Grade | 0 | 1 | 2 |

CHEST/ABDOMINAL MOVEMENT

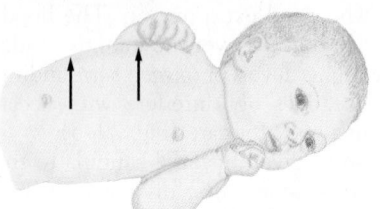 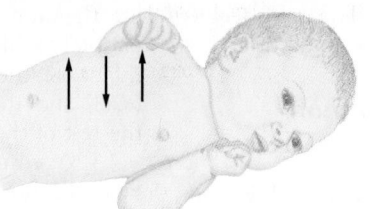 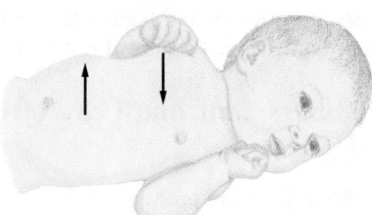

Synchronized respirations   Lag in inspiration   Seesaw respirations

INTERCOSTAL SPACES

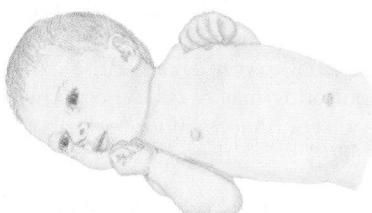 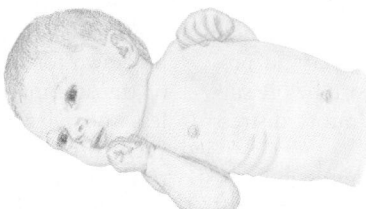 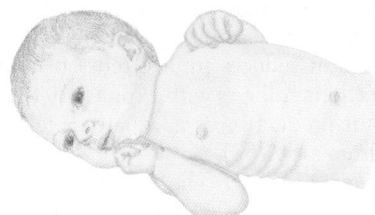

No retraction   Retraction just visible   Marked retraction

XIPHOID AREA

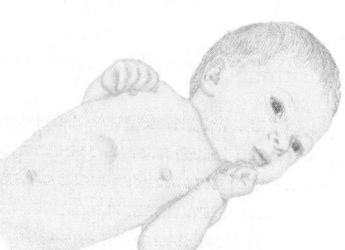 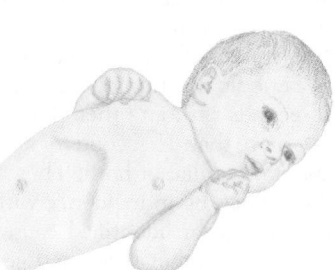

No retraction   Retraction just visible   Marked retraction

NARES

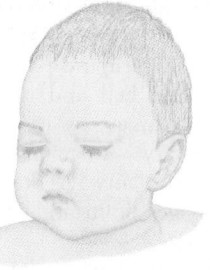 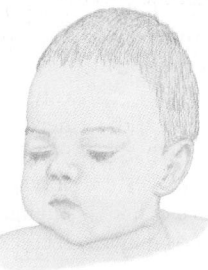 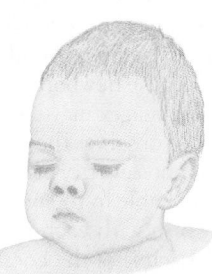

No dilation   Minimal dilation   Marked dilation

EXPIRATORY SOUND

 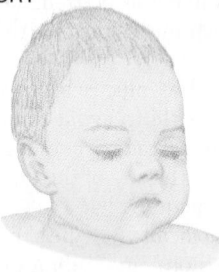 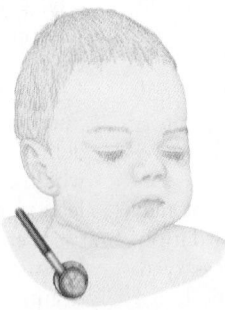 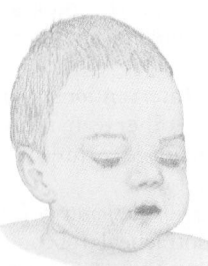

No expiratory grunting   Expiratory grunting audible by stethoscope   Expiratory grunting audible to unaided ear

FIGURE 29–2

Assessment of respiratory distress. The Silverman-Andersen index is used to score the infant's degree of respiratory difficulty. The score for individual criteria matches the grade, with a total possible score of 10 indicating severe distress. (Modified with permission from Silverman, W., & Andersen, D. [1956]. A cold clinical trial of effects of water mist on obstructive respiratory signs, death rate, and necropsy findings among premature infants. *Pediatrics, 17*(4), 1–9).

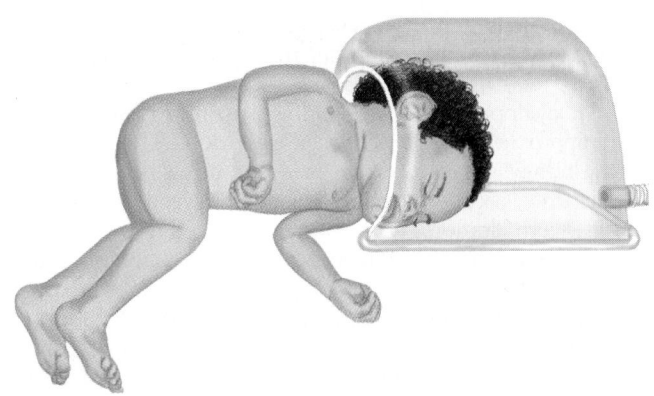

FIGURE 29–3

The oxygen hood is one way of delivering oxygen to an infant who can breathe unassisted.

CRITICAL TO REMEMBER

Signs of Inadequate Thermoregulation

Axillary temperature <36.3°C or >36.9°C
Abdominal skin temperature <36°C or >36.5°C
Change in feeding behavior
Lethargy
Irritability
Decreased muscle tone
Cool skin temperature
Mottled skin
Signs of hypoglycemia
Signs of respiratory difficulty

Maintaining Hydration. Adequate hydration is essential to keep secretions thin so that they can be removed by drainage or suction. If infants become dehydrated, secretions will become thick and viscous and could obstruct tiny air passages. Fluid intake should be increased, within the limits of the overall treatment plan, if secretions seem to indicate even minimal dehydration. Small amounts of saline may be administered through endotracheal tubes just before suctioning to thin secretions.

PROBLEMS WITH THERMOREGULATION

Although heat loss can be a problem for full-term infants, it is even more significant in preterm infants. They have thin skin and little subcutaneous fat for insulation. There is less brown fat for nonshivering thermogenesis. Their body surface area is proportionately larger than full-term infants' and their extended extremities increase exposure. The temperature control center of the brain of preterm infants is less mature and may be further impaired by asphyxia. These conditions all contribute to heat loss.

Complications of heat loss are more likely in the preterm infant than the full-term infant. They include hypoglycemia, metabolic acidosis, pulmonary vasoconstriction, and impaired surfactant production.

Assessment. The infant's temperature is monitored continuously by a skin probe, which is attached to the heat control mechanism of the radiant warmer or incubator. The infant's temperature as shown on the monitor should be recorded every 30 to 60 minutes initially and every 3 to 4 hours when the infant is stable. The nurse should assess the axillary temperature every 4 to 8 hours and compare it with the heat control reading to ensure that the machinery is functioning properly.

The axillary temperature for a preterm infant should remain between 36.3° and 36.9°C (97.3° and 98.6°F) (Blake & Murray, 1998). If the infant has accumulated brown fat, a normal axillary temperature when the monitor shows a decreased skin temperature may indicate that brown fat in the axillary space is being used to maintain the infant's core temperature.

Indications of inadequate thermoregulation include poor feeding or intolerance to feedings in an infant who previously had little difficulty, lethargy, irritability, poor muscle tone, cool skin temperature, and mottled skin (Fig. 29–4). Hypoglycemia and respiratory distress may be the first signs that the infant's temperature is low. Because temperature instability may be an early sign of infection, the nurse should assess for other evidence that infection may be present.

Nursing Interventions. Maintenance of heat in preterm infants involves the same basic nursing care principles as for the full-term infant (see Chapter 23). These principles, however, must be adapted to meet the needs of the preterm infant.

Maintaining a Neutral Thermal Environment. A neutral thermal environment is especially important to prevent the need for increased oxygen to maintain body temperature. Radiant warmers or incubators are used until infants can maintain normal body temperature alone. Because they lose more heat and produce less, smaller, less mature infants need more warmth to maintain body heat than larger or older preterm infants.

Infants needing many procedures are usually placed under the open radiant warmer to make it easier to see them and work with equipment. Air currents around an un-

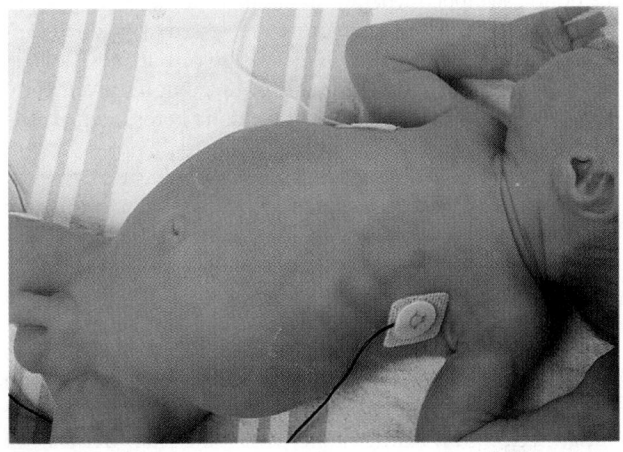

FIGURE 29–4

This preterm infant has mildly mottled skin and slight abdominal distension and retractions.

clothed infant can, however, cause heat loss by convection despite the heat generated by the warmer. Doors near the warmer should be closed and traffic kept to a minimum to decrease convective heat loss further. The infant should receive only warmed oxygen, because thermal receptors in the face are very sensitive to cold. Cold oxygen could quickly lead to cold stress.

Equipment or caregivers should not come between the infant and the heat source, preventing heat from reaching the infant. A transparent plastic blanket over the infant allows heat from the warmer to pass across to the infant and decreases insensible water loss while maintaining visibility of the infant's body parts.

When infants are in incubators, nurses should keep portholes and doors closed as much as possible. A significant amount of heat is lost every time the incubator is opened, and it takes time to build up again. On removal from the incubator for procedures or holding, the infant should be placed in heated blankets, and head coverings should be used. To retain heat inside, the incubator doors should be closed while the infant is out of it.

Although temperature loss is the most common concern, overheating is also a problem for preterm infants. Overheating may occur when heating devices such as radiant warmers are set too high. Overheating leads to an increase in the metabolic rate, with increased oxygen and glucose needs, and insensible water losses.

Weaning to an Open Crib. Preparation of infants for moving to open cribs should begin early. When stable, an infant can be dressed in a shirt, diaper, and hat while in the incubator. Clothing conserves heat and helps infants adjust to a different temperature on the face than the rest of the body. Infants who are about 1,500 g and have a consistent weight gain for 5 days can begin gradual weaning from external heat (Medoff-Cooper, 1994).

Each NICU has its own protocol for the weaning process. The incubator temperature is usually decreased 1° to 1.5°C each day. It is raised if the infant's temperature falls below the desired range. If the temperature remains stable, the process can continue the next day.

An infant who can tolerate the incubator setting at 28°C is ready for transfer to an open crib. The infant should be double-wrapped with warm blankets at first to help insulate body heat. The temperature is assessed at gradually increasing intervals until the infant is on a routine schedule. A blanket is added for a low temperature, but if the temperature does not rise to normal, the infant is returned to the incubator.

Nurses should observe the infant carefully during the first few days after transfer to an open crib. Signs that may indicate inadequate thermoregulation include decreased weight gain, poor feeding, or increased requirement for oxygen.

PROBLEMS WITH FLUID AND ELECTROLYTE BALANCE

Preterm infants lose fluid very easily. The rapid respiratory rate and the use of oxygen can increase fluid loss from the lungs. Their thin skin is more permeable than the skin of term infants. The large surface area, in proportion to body weight, and lack of flexion further increase insensible water losses. Radiant warmers and the heat from phototherapy lights cause even more fluid loss through the skin. Radiant warmers heighten insensible water losses by 40% to 50%, compared to water loss in an incubator (Blake & Murray, 1998).

Development of the kidneys is not complete until approximately 35 weeks of gestation. The ability of the kidneys to concentrate or dilute urine is poor before that time, causing a fragile balance between dehydration and overhydration. With variation according to size and gestational age, the fluid needs of preterm infants range from 90 to 150 ml/kg per day on the second and third days of life (Adcock, Consolvo, & Berry, 1998). Monitoring intake and output of fluids is important in determining fluid balance. Normal urinary output is 1 to 3 ml/kg per hour.

The kidneys' regulation of electrolytes is also a problem. Preterm infants need higher intakes of sodium because the kidneys do not reabsorb it well. If they receive sodium, however, they may be unable to increase sodium excretion adequately and are susceptible to sodium and water overload as a result.

Assessment. The nurse must be alert for fluid overload or deficit. The infant's intake and output by all routes are carefully calculated. Parenteral, feeding tube, or oral fluids are included when measuring intake. Output from drainage tubes and urine should be measured. A urine output of less than 1 ml/kg per hour may indicate inadequate fluid intake, whereas more than 3 ml/kg per hour is a sign of overhydration (Gomella et al., 1999). The nurse must also keep track of the amount of blood taken for laboratory tests; the amount can be substantial.

Urinary Output. There are several methods of measuring urinary output. Plastic bags that adhere to the perineum are often not suitable for the preterm infant because they may damage the fragile skin. Weighing diapers is less invasive to the infant. The weight of dry diapers is subtracted from the weight of wet diapers to determine the amount of urine excreted. One gram is equivalent to 1 ml of urine. Humidification, however, may add moisture to the diaper, and a radiant warmer may cause evaporation of urine on the diaper. When precise measurement is essential, diapers can be fastened instead of placing them open under the infant.

Specific gravity should be checked to determine if urine is more concentrated or dilute than expected. Urine is collected by placing cotton balls at the perineum. The specific gravity should range between 1.005 and 1.015.

Weight. Changes in the infant's weight can give an indication of fluid gain or loss, especially if the changes are sudden and greater than would be expected from feeding changes. The undressed infant should be weighed daily at the same time with the same scale. Very small infants are often placed in a bed that has a scale on it so that they do not have to be disturbed for daily weighing. They may be weighed twice a day to monitor their fluid status more closely.

Signs of Dehydration or Overhydration. The nurse should observe for signs that indicate that the infant has received too little or too much fluid. Early signs of dehydration include decreased urine output and increased specific gravity. Weight loss may exceed that expected for the infant's age and general condition. Dry skin or mucous membranes, sunken anterior fontanel, and poor tissue turgor are late signs. Changes in the blood include increased sodium, protein, and hematocrit levels resulting from decreased plasma volume.

Signs of overhydration include increased output of urine with a below-normal specific gravity. Edema and weight gain occur from retention of fluids. Bulging fontanels and decreased blood sodium, protein, and hematocrit levels are also present. Complications of excess fluid may include patent ductus arteriosus and congestive heart failure.

Nursing Interventions. The nurse must carefully regulate intravenous fluids and use infusion control devices to help prevent fluid volume overload. Intravenous medications should be diluted in as little fluid as is consistent with safe administration of the drug and should be included when measuring intake. Starting intravenous lines on infants with poor veins is a lengthy, difficult procedure. Infants must be restrained as necessary to prevent infiltration. If they infiltrate, some fluids cause extensive damage as a result of tissue sloughing.

PROBLEMS WITH INFECTION
The incidence of infection in preterm infants is three to ten times greater than that in full-term newborns (Behrman, Kliegman, & Arvin, 1996). Many preterm infants have one or more episodes of sepsis during their hospital stays. Factors contributing to the high rate of infection include exposure to maternal infection, lack of transfer of immunoglobulin G from the mother during the third trimester, and immature immune response to infection.

Preterm infants are often exposed to situations that may cause infection. Their skin is fragile, permeable, and easily damaged. They are subject to many invasive procedures such as insertion of intravenous lines and drawing of blood specimens.

Assessment. The nurse should be alert for signs of infection at all times (see Chapter 30).

Nursing Interventions. Nursing care involves scrupulous cleanliness and maintaining the infant's skin integrity. Even the normal flora on the hands of caretakers may cause sepsis. Therefore, parents and staff members should scrub their hands and arms before handling infants. Exposure to family members or staff members who have contagious diseases should be prevented.

The nurse should avoid the use of chemicals on the infant's skin, as they can injure it or may be absorbed through it. If alcohol or providone-iodine is used on the skin, a sterile water rinse minimizes damage. Tape should be used as little as possible. Tape that is specially prepared to be less traumatic on removal helps protect the skin. Easily removed pectin-based products are available for skin probes and monitor leads.

Infants and their equipment should be positioned to avoid undue pressure on the skin. Frequent position changes are important but should be based on the infant's ability to tolerate changes.

PROBLEMS WITH PAIN
Infants in the NICU undergo many painful procedures each day. Caregivers once thought that newborns, particularly preterm infants, were neurologically too immature to feel pain. It is now recognized that pain stimuli cause physiologic and behavioral changes in infants. Preterm infants may be even more sensitive to pain than older infants (Evans et al., 1997). The long-term effects of pain in the neonate are not yet fully understood.

Assessment. The nurse must assess the infant's response to painful stimuli. Physiologic changes include changes in heart rate and respirations, increased blood pressure and intracranial pressure, and decreased oxygen saturation. Hormonal and metabolic changes occur as well. Physiologic changes may be unpredictable and cannot be used alone to assess pain.

Behavioral changes include high-pitched, intense, harsh crying. In infants who are intubated or too weak to cry, a "cry face" is seen, a crying facial expression without the sound of a cry.

Nursing Interventions. Nurses should prepare infants for potentially painful procedures by waking them slowly and gently and using containment. Containment simulates the enclosed space of the uterus and is comforting to infants. It involves keeping the extremities in a flexed position near the body by swaddling, blanket rolls, or the nurse's hands. At least one hand should be near the mouth for sucking.

Comfort measures help the infant cope with short-term, mild pain and reduce agitation. They include nonnutritive sucking, talking softly, restraining the extremities to prevent flailing, and holding and rocking. Measures should be adapted according to infants' responses.

The nurse should discuss the infant's pain with the primary care provider to ensure that medications are available for long-term and more severe pain. Morphine and general anesthesia can be tolerated by preterm infants. Ordered medications are given before painful procedures and when the infant demonstrates signs of pain. To determine the need to increase or decrease the dosage, the nurse should carefully note the infant's response.

Case Management and Clinical Pathways

Preterm infants may remain in the NICU for many days, at a cost of thousands of dollars. Case management and clinical pathways are methods to reduce the length of stay to return infants to their parents at home more quickly.

The case manager is a nurse who follows infants from admission to discharge to identify or prevent situations that would interfere with progression toward discharge. Clinical pathways list the care infants will need along a time line and the expected outcomes of that care. Different pathways are created to meet the needs of different types of infants, such as infants with various complications of prematurity.

NURSING CARE
The Preterm Infant

Preterm infants commonly have difficulty with stress from the NICU environment and obtaining adequate nutrition. Their parents may have difficulty with bonding.

ENVIRONMENTALLY CAUSED STRESS
Preterm infants are exposed constantly to a bright, loud environment. The sounds of alarms, ventilators, doors, and people create a noise level above that of loud traffic. Noise and routine nursing interventions are often accompanied by changes in heart rate, oxygen saturation levels, and behavior states.

Preterm infants undergo multiple assessments and treatments that often cause frequent interruptions of sleep and may interfere with the development of normal sleep-wake cycles. Energy is used coping with an overstimulating and stressful environment and may be unavailable for normal growth and development.

Assessment
Assess the amount of noise to which the infant is exposed. Determine how often interruptions occur and how the infant responds to different types of care.

CRITICAL TO REMEMBER

Signs of Overstimulation in Preterm Infants

Oxygenation Changes
Increase or decrease in pulse and respiratory rate
Cyanosis, pallor, or mottling
Flaring nares
Decreased oxygen saturation levels
Coughing
Yawning

Behavior Changes
Stiff, extended arms and legs
Fisting of the hands or splaying of the fingers
Alert, worried expression
Turning away from eye contact
Hiccuping
Regurgitation
Fatigue

Assess the infant's ability to tolerate activity and noise. Overstimulation results in changes in oxygenation and behavior.

Nursing Diagnosis and Planning
A nursing diagnosis appropriate for preterm infants having difficulty enduring the multiple stimuli in their environment is

■ Risk for Altered Growth and Development related to stress from an overstimulating environment.
Expected Outcomes: The infant will conserve energy for growth and development by showing decreasing signs of overstimulation during routine activity and will gradually show an ability to withstand more activity before signs of overstimulation occur.

Interventions
Interventions are focused on providing developmentally supportive nursing care that meets the preterm infant's ability to tolerate stimulation. Developmental care keeps stressors in the environment to a minimum based on the infant's physiologic and behavioral responses.

Scheduling Care
Schedule periods of undisturbed rest to allow the infant to recover from treatments. Avoid disturbing rest by arranging routine care to correspond with the infant's awake periods. Plan care so that several tasks are performed at one time. Be alert, however, to the infant's signs of stress. Too many activities may be more than the infant can tolerate. If the infant shows signs of overstimulation, allow short rest periods within grouped activities or during long or painful procedures.

Decrease the frequency of taking vital signs and providing other routine care as soon as possible. Even the handling involved in routine sponge bathing may cause changes in heart rate and oxygenation saturation levels in small infants

(Peters, 1996a). If the procedure causes stress responses in an infant, it should be limited to necessary cleaning only.

Reducing Stimuli

Keep noise around the infant as low as possible. Place incubators away from traffic and congestion of people and avoid talking near the incubator. Set alarm volumes on low and respond quickly when they sound. Open and close doors on incubators and cupboards gently. Do not place objects on top of the incubator or use it as a writing surface, because this activity increases the noise inside.

The lights that are on 24 hours a day in the nursery may interfere with the development of sleep cycles. Position the incubator so that the infant is not facing bright lights, and drape blankets over the back and ends to decrease light further. Use a dimmer switch to vary the intensity of lights as needed. Place infants in a prone position to help them avoid looking at ceiling lights.

Promoting Rest

When possible, schedule "quiet periods" when lights and noise in the unit are kept to a minimum to promote rest. Scheduled naps when infants are disturbed as little as possible help increase sleep, decrease waking, and lead to longer uninterrupted sleep (Holditch-Davis et al., 1995). They may be associated with decreased periods of apnea and increased weight gain for some infants. A daytime and evening nap and two during the night will help the infant begin to differentiate day and night sleeping patterns.

Contain the infant's arms and legs to promote flexion and reduce energy loss from flailing extremities. Provide a "nest" with rolled blankets placed around the infant for boundaries. Use the prone position to increase quiet sleep periods. In the side or supine position, arrange the infant's arms and legs in a flexed position, with the hands near midline.

Promoting Motor Development

Preterm infants may have musculoskeletal and developmental problems from prolonged immobilization and the effects of gravity on their immature neuromuscular system. Because the extensor muscles mature before the flexor muscles, the infant tends to remain in an extended, "frog-leg" position. Shoulder retraction, abduction of the lower extremities, and lateral flexion of the arms may result. When possible, swaddle the infant with the extremities flexed and the hands positioned near the mouth to allow the infant to suck the hands for comfort. Turn the infant every 2 hours, avoiding the supine position, and use blankets and rolls to maintain flexion.

Individualizing Care

The ability to tolerate stress varies with each infant. Adapt general care according to the infant's ability to tolerate it. Even positive stimuli, such as soft music or soft talking, can overstimulate the infant. Use these measures judiciously according to the infant's tolerance level.

Infants often require extra energy to adjust to changes in care. Observe how well an infant tolerates changes such as moving from assisted to more independent breathing or introduction of new feeding methods. Increase rest periods during these times.

Communicating Infants' Needs

Use the nursing care plan, Kardex, and shift reports to inform other caregivers of techniques that are especially effective for certain infants. Explain all techniques to parents.

Evaluation

- Does the infant display signs of overstimulation less often?
- Does the infant show increasing tolerance to activity before signs appear?

NUTRITION

Preterm infants are born before full accumulation of nutrient stores has occurred. Full-term newborns have reservoirs of calcium, iron, and other substances, but these are lacking in preterm infants. Fat stores are minimal or absent, and glucose reserves are used up soon after birth. Low blood glucose levels develop very quickly and must be prevented or treated quickly because the brain needs a steady supply of glucose.

Preterm infants need approximately 120 kcal/kg per day, but this amount varies according to activity, illness, and other factors. These infants also need increased amounts of nutrients such as protein, iron, calcium, and phosphorus.

The gastrointestinal tract of preterm infants does not absorb nutrients as well as full-term infants'. Although they digest protein fairly well, preterm infants have insufficient bile acids and pancreatic lipase to absorb fat adequately. They have some lactase deficiency but digest glucose and sucrose adequately. Although their smaller stomach capacity limits the volume that they can tolerate at each feeding, preterm infants need more of many nutrients per kilogram than do full-term infants and require supplementation.

Coordination of sucking and swallowing occurs as early as 32 weeks of gestation but may be delayed because of other problems in the infant (Lefrak & Dowling, 1998). Infants of less than 34 weeks' gestation or those who weigh less than 1,500 g generally have difficulty coordinating sucking, swallowing, and breathing. The gag reflex, which helps prevent aspiration, may function poorly. Oral feeding may cause the very weak infant to expend too much oxygen and glucose. When sucking is uncoordinated or takes too much energy, the infant must receive intravenous or gavage feedings.

Assessment

Readiness for Nipple-Feeding

Preterm infants are often fed parenterally or by gavage initially to conserve energy for growth and basic functioning. During feedings, watch for signs that nipple-feeding may soon be possible, such as rooting; sucking on the gavage tube, a finger, or a pacifier; and an increasing ability to tolerate holding and handling. Note whether the infant gags on the tube or a gloved finger inserted into the mouth. Infants who do not have a gag reflex are more likely to aspirate feedings.

When the infant begins to feed by nipple, assess coordination of suck and swallow and observe for aspiration. Frequent choking, gagging, or cyanosis during feedings may indicate that the infant cannot coordinate sucking, swallowing, and breathing well enough for nipple-feeding. Some infants are so weak that the usual signs of aspiration are minimal or absent.

Assess the respiratory rate before and during feedings. When the respiratory rate is more than 60 to 70 breaths per minute before feedings, gavage-feed to prevent aspiration. Observe for signs that the effort of nipple-feeding requires too much energy and oxygen for the infant.

Feeding Tolerance

Assess how well the infant tolerates feedings, whether by feeding tube or nipple. Before beginning a gavage feeding, withdraw the gastric contents to measure the amount left from the previous feeding. This procedure helps determine whether the stomach is emptying and prevents overdistension. Excessive residuals may indicate that the amount or type of formula needs changing or may be an early sign of a complication.

Observe for other signs of intestinal complications. Obtain objective data about abdominal distension by using a tape to measure abdominal girth at the level of the umbilicus. Test stools for reducing substance by dissolving stool in water and mixing with a Clinitest tablet. The presence of reducing substance indicates malabsorption of carbohydrates. Also check for occult blood.

Vomiting or frequent regurgitation may indicate that the feedings are too large. Vomitus containing bile may be a sign of intestinal obstruction and may require surgery. Diarrhea may be caused by rapid advancement of the feeding or intolerance to the type of formula. Report signs of feeding intolerance to the physician or nurse practitioner because they may be early indications of complications, such as il-

eus, sepsis, obstruction of the gastrointestinal tract, or necrotizing enterocolitis.

Nursing Diagnosis and Planning

The nursing diagnosis that addresses the nutritional problems of the preterm infant is

■ Risk for Altered Nutrition: Less Than Body Requirements related to uncoordinated suck and swallow and fatigue during feedings
Expected Outcomes: The infant will take in adequate amounts of breast milk or formula to meet nutrient needs for age and weight and will gain weight as appropriate for age.

The actual amount of feedings and weight gain vary according to the infant's gestational age and other conditions. What is appropriate for a particular infant can be discussed with the physician or nurse practitioner.

Interventions

Administering Parenteral Feedings

The nurse manages the administration of parenteral nutrition, which may be necessary for very immature infants because of respiratory problems, limited gastric capacity, and reduced peristalsis. Parenteral nutrition is the intravenous infusion of solutions containing the major nutrients needed for metabolism and growth. It provides calories, amino acids, fatty acids, vitamins, and minerals in amounts adapted to the needs of infants.

Administering Gavage Feedings

Enteral feedings (feeding into the gastrointestinal tract, orally or by feeding tube) are started as soon as possible because they may help promote intestinal growth and maturity. Infants of less than 34 weeks' gestation or those who weigh less than 1,800 g (4 lb) may need special formulas or fortified breast milk. Special formulas are adapted to meet the need for easily digestible, concentrated nutrients in a smaller volume of fluid. Preterm infants may need 24 kcal/oz (instead of 20 kcal/oz used for the full-term infant) to meet their requirements. Preterm formulas contain added calcium, phosphorus, and vitamins needed by the preterm infant. Breast milk fortifiers add needed nutrients to breast milk to make it more concentrated.

Gavage feedings are usually started before oral feedings for preterm infants (see Procedures 37–11 and 37–12). A small, soft catheter is inserted through the mouth at each feeding for intermittent (bolus) feedings, or a nasogastric catheter may be inserted and left in place for a period of time to provide for continuous feedings. Leaving the catheter in place decreases the vagal stimulation that causes apnea and bradycardia during multiple insertions, but it may interfere with air flow through the infant's small nasal passages. In addition, bacteria counts in the milk or formula may become too high, and fats tend to adhere to the tubing during continuous feeding.

Gavage feedings are begun in small amounts, with gradual increases as tolerated by the infant. Only a few milliliters of feeding are given at first. Very small feedings may help increase later feeding tolerance (Pereira, 1995). Carefully observe the infant's tolerance at each feeding to determine when the feeding type or amount can be changed.

If the infant can suck, use a pacifier during feedings to help associate the comfortable feeling of fullness with sucking. Nonnutritive sucking also helps prepare the infant for nippling, improves weight gain, and decreases oxygen consumption. It may help quiet a fussy infant as well.

Administering Oral Feedings

Oral feedings are often begun when the infant reaches what would be 32 to 34 weeks' corrected gestational age and weighs at least 1,500 g (Pickler, Mauck, & Geldmaker, 1997). At this time, most healthy preterm infants can coordinate sucking with swallowing and breathing, have a functional gag reflex, and have enough energy to feed orally without compromising oxygenation (Fig. 29–5). The first nipple-feedings may be only a few milliliters once a day, completed by gavage. Placing the gavage tube before beginning oral feedings helps prevent regurgitation stimulated by passing the catheter. Gradually increase the amount and frequency of oral feedings until the infant feeds by breast or bottle once a shift, then every second or third feeding, and eventually every feeding.

Preparing for Feedings. Provide for heat maintenance during feeding times. When infants have stable temperature maintenance, wrap them in warm blankets and hold for feedings.

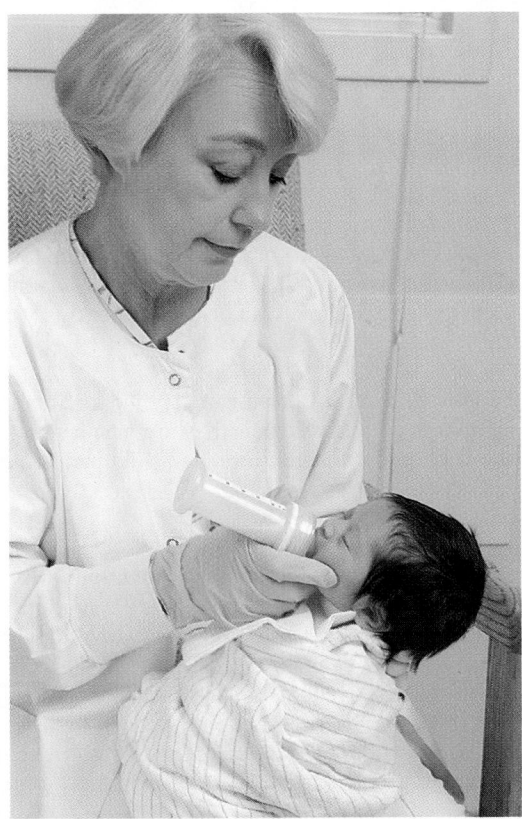

FIGURE 29–5
. . . .
The nurse positions her hands to provide cheek and jaw support for feeding this preterm infant.

Nipple-feedings involve a greater expenditure of energy by the infant than gavage-feedings. Allow a period of rest before and after feedings. Use of a pacifier before feedings may enhance oral feeding success. Infants may be fed according to a feeding schedule or at times when they demonstrate cues that they are ready.

Giving Bottle Feedings. Nursing interventions for bottle-feeding the preterm infant are presented in Nursing Care Plan 29–1.

Facilitating Breast-Feeding

Encourage mothers who would like to breast-feed. Contributing her milk helps the mother feel that she has something important to offer at a time when she may feel there is little she can do to help her baby. The immunologic benefits of breast milk are particularly important to the preterm infant who did not receive passive immunity during fetal life. Nutrients in breast milk are more easily digested, and enzymes, hormones, and growth factors important for the preterm infant are provided. Although milk from mothers of preterm infants is higher in protein, fat, and electrolytes during the early weeks, it may be necessary to add fortifiers to meet total nutrient needs.

Breast milk may increase feeding tolerance, reduce later allergies, improve retinal function, enhance neurologic development, and help prevent necrotizing enterocolitis (Meier & Brown, 1996). Breast-feeding may be less stressful than bottle-feeding for preterm infants. Oxygenation levels are often higher during breast-feeding because the infant can regulate breathing and suckling better than with bottle-feeding. In addition, the mother's body temperature helps keep the infant warm.

When the mother plans to breast-feed, she will need help in maintaining lactation until the infant is mature enough to nurse. Teach her how to use a breast pump and give her sterile containers to store her milk. Tell her to place it in a refrigerator or freezer until she brings it to the NICU for the infant. If fortifiers will be added to the milk, explain the higher needs of the preterm infant so the mother does not believe that her milk is inadequate.

Support the mother in her efforts in feeding, which may be difficult at first. Provide as much privacy as possible, using a separate room or screens. Help the mother feel comfortable holding the tiny infant and any attached equipment, such as monitor leads.

Adapt breast-feeding teaching to the needs of a very small infant. Show the mother how to use the cross-cradle hold, which is very effective for small infants. She should hold her breast with the hand on the same side and press slightly back and downward behind the areola to make the nipple prominent. The other hand holds the infant's head and brings it to the breast. This position allows the mother to see the infant well during latching-on and throughout the feeding.

Make the same observations of the infant during breast-feeding as during bottle-feeding. Signs of fatigue, bradycar-

CRITICAL THINKING EXERCISE 29–1
. . . .

What are the major differences between formula-feeding a preterm infant and a full-term infant?

NURSING CARE PLAN 29-1

The Preterm Infant

Assessment

John was born at 33 weeks' gestation and now weighs 1,800 g (4 lb). He breathes on his own with oxygen by hood. John needs many treatments throughout the day. He demonstrates pallor and increased respiratory rate when tired. Noises often cause a drop in oxygen saturation. When held or disturbed for care, John may stiffen and extend his arms with the fingers splayed. He sleeps most of the time when he is undisturbed.

Nursing Diagnosis

Activity Intolerance related to weakness, fatigue, and possible overstimulation

Goals/Expected Outcomes

- John will not show signs of overstimulation (increased respirations, pallor, decreased oxygen saturation level, stiffening of arms and legs, or splaying of fingers) as a result of normal activity.
- John will increase tolerance to activity gradually, as demonstrated by fewer signs of fatigue or stress.

Intervention	Rationale
1. Whenever possible, arrange to provide routine care to correspond with John's natural awake periods.	1. Preterm infants need undisturbed sleep to promote growth.
2. Schedule periods of uninterrupted rest, especially before and after energy-draining activities.	2. Infants tolerate activities best when they begin in a rested state and are allowed to recover from them before other activities are necessary.
3. Experiment with grouping care to determine the number and combination of care activities that John tolerates best.	3. Grouping accomplishes more tasks at once so that longer rest periods are possible between tasks. Too many activities, however, may cause too much fatigue.
4. Assess carefully to determine what activities bring about signs of overstimulation and fatigue. Stop activities and allow short periods of rest, if possible.	4. Careful observation allows the nurse to be sensitive to the infant's ability to tolerate care.
5. Reduce the noise level around John. Avoid talking unnecessarily; open and close doors softly; keep alarm volumes low.	5. Noise may be overstimulating and result in increased oxygen need.
6. Place John prone and facing away from bright lights. Partially cover the incubator to keep out light but allow visibility of infant.	6. Continuous lighting interferes with the infant's sleep. Reducing light in the infant's face will increase rest.
7. Use blanket rolls to form "boundaries" around John and keep the extremities flexed.	7. Because it is similar to the small space of the uterus, enclosed space promotes rest and comfort.
8. Collaborate with other nurses to determine what works best to decrease John's fatigue. Tape signs on the bed to provide this information to parents and others.	8. All caregivers should have information available to help meet the infant's needs consistently.
9. Explain to the parents John's needs for rest and low stimulation. Suggest ways that they can interact appropriately to meet John's needs, and point out signs that he is receiving too much stimulation. Ask for their input.	9. Parents who are informed can care for the infant appropriately and feel that they are members of the team and are parenting their child by learning his needs.

Evaluation

John gradually shows increased ability to tolerate progressive activity with fewer episodes of overstimulation. His respirations and oxygen saturation levels remain stable, and he rarely stiffens his arms and legs during activity.

Assessment

Two or three times a day, John receives feedings by nipple supplemented by gavage when he becomes too tired. He has occasional episodes of increased respirations or short cyanotic spells when fed. He sometimes takes only half the feeding before falling asleep and must receive the rest by gavage. John's mother has decided to formula-feed.

Nursing Diagnosis

Risk for Altered Nutrition: Less Than Body Requirements related to fatigue during feedings

746

The Preterm Infant

Goals/Expected Outcomes   John will

- Take 216 kcal/day to meet his needs at a weight of 1,800 g.
- Gain 27 to 36 g daily.
- Complete nipple-feedings without signs of excessive fatigue (such as increased respiratory rate or falling asleep during feeding).

Intervention	Rationale
1. Schedule nursing care to provide a rest period before and after nipple-feedings.	1. Nippling consumes a great deal of energy. Rest helps prevent excessive fatigue that might prevent the infant from completing the feeding.
2. Use a feeding container (such as a Volutrol) on which each milliliter is marked. Place the container in warm water to warm milk to room temperature or slightly warmer. Do not use a microwave oven to warm.	2. Exact measurement of the amount taken is important to ensure that infants receive required nutrients. Some infants take slightly warmed milk better. Microwaving provides uneven heating of formula and may cause the infant to be burned.
3. Determine the type of nipple that works best for John. Choose between various sizes and consistencies.	3. A "preemie" nipple is more pliable than regular nipples and requires less energy for sucking. Some infants need firmer nipples because soft nipples allow milk to flow too fast, cause choking, and interfere with breathing between sucking bursts. Infants with very small mouths require smaller nipples.
4. Wrap John in warmed blankets and place a hat on his head. Feed him in the incubator or under the warmer if needed.	4. A hat and blankets help maintain the temperature. If infants have difficulty with temperature maintenance, an incubator or warmer provides warmth during feedings.
5. Position John at a 45° to 60° angle facing the nurse. Position the head slightly forward and the chin slightly down. Place a finger on each cheek and one under the jaw at the base of the tongue midway between the chin and the throat. Provide gentle pressure.	5. This position allows the nurse to observe the infant's suck response to feeding, and any regurgitation. The finger position increases sucking strength and helps support the tongue.
6. Feed slowly, with frequent stops to burp and allow the infant to rest. Do not force the preterm infant to resume feeding before he or she is ready.	6. Slow feeding is necessary because of the infant's decreased energy. Preterm infants may swallow more air than full-term infants because sucking is less efficient. Preterm infants need rest periods during feedings because they have difficulty regulating their breathing while feeding.
7. Observe for coughing, gagging, cyanosis, changes in heart rate or respirations, and apnea. Evaluate the infant's ability to continue.	7. These signs show difficulty coordinating sucking, swallowing, and breathing, and possible aspiration.
8. Assess for signs of overfatigue: falling asleep during feedings, feedings lasting more than 25 to 30 minutes, increased respirations.	8. Feedings may require more energy than the infant has available. Infants who are overfatigued are more likely to aspirate.
9. Finish feeding by gavage if necessary.	9. Completing the feeding by gavage conserves energy and prevents aspiration.
10. After feeding, position John on the right side or prone with his head elevated approximately 30°.	10. If regurgitation occurs, fluid will run out of the mouth easily so that the infant will not aspirate it. The right-side position and elevation of the head allow gravity to help empty the stomach.
11. Include parents in the feedings. Teach them to assess the infant's response to feedings.	11. Feeding allows parents to participate in the infant's care. Their comfort with feedings and learning about the infant's responses will help them prepare for discharge.

(continued)

NURSING CARE PLAN 29–1 *Continued*

The Preterm Infant

Evaluation

John consumes an average of 220 calories and gains an average of 31 g daily. He gradually takes more of his feeding by nipple and rarely needs gavage feeding to finish. His respiratory rate remains less than 60 breaths/minute, and he stays awake for the entire feeding.

Additional Nursing Diagnoses to Consider

Ineffective Thermoregulation
Ineffective Airway Clearance
Altered Family Processes
Risk for Caregiver Role Strain
Risk for Altered Parenting
Risk for Infection
Pain

dia, tachypnea, or apnea may show lack of readiness for breast-feeding. Be sure that the infant stays warm. The mother's body heat will help maintain the infant's temperature during feedings. Kangaroo care (p. 750) can often be combined with breast-feeding.

Making Ongoing Assessments

Continuously assess the infant's responses to all feeding methods. Record the amount of breast milk or formula that the infant takes by gavage- or bottle-feeding and compare it with the amount needed to meet nutrient needs for the infant's age and weight. Because it is difficult to estimate milk intake accurately, infants may be weighed on an electronic scale before and after breast-feedings. This sequence allows gavage-feeding amounts to be calculated based on the infant's oral intake.

Weigh the infant daily at the same time with the same scale. Record the length and head circumference each week. Plot measurements on a growth chart for preterm infants to see if changes are within expected ranges. Weight increase not accompanied by increased length may be caused by edema and may be a sign of a complication such as congestive heart failure.

Observe changes in the infant's ability to take feedings. As the infant becomes more mature, less energy should be expended during the feeding sessions. The infant will take the feedings more quickly and show fewer signs of fatigue, such as falling asleep during feedings.

Evaluation

- Does the infant consume adequate amounts of formula or breast milk to meet nutrient needs for age and weight?
- Is the pattern of weight gain appropriate for the infant's age?

PARENTING

The extended hospitalization of the preterm infant causes separation of the parents from their newborn, produces emotional trauma, and disrupts family life. Some parents feel they play such a small part in the preterm infant's life that the infant almost belongs to the hospital.

Parents need help to understand the infant's condition and what is expected to occur throughout the hospital stay. Parents perceive nurses as being among the most helpful in helping them to cope with these stresses (Miles, Carlson, & Funk, 1996). Nurses must evaluate the progress of bonding and assist parents to feel important in caring for their infant.

Assessment

Assess for signs of parental attachment on the first and subsequent visits to the NICU nursery. Expect parents to be fearful at first but more able to focus on the infant as they get over the initial shock of preterm birth. Assess for common behaviors that show normal progression of attachment. These include talking about the infant in positive terms, making eye contact, pointing out physical characteristics, naming the infant, and calling the infant by name. When they can hold and participate in the care of the infant, observe for gradual increase in comfort and skill. The parents should smile and talk to the infant and verbalize increasing confidence in their caretaking abilities.

Watch for signs that bonding is not occurring as expected. Determine if there are other stressors in the parents' lives that may interfere with their ability to visit and attach to the infant.

After the critical period in the early days after birth, healthy preterm infants become more stable. They still require specialized nursing care and hospitalization but gradually need fewer technological interventions. They are sometimes called "growers" at this time. This is a time when parental participation in the infant's care should increase in preparation for discharge.

Nursing Diagnosis and Planning

For most parents of infants with problems at birth, the nursing diagnosis is

■ Risk for Altered Parenting related to separation of parents from infant and lack of understanding about the preterm infant's condition and characteristics.
Expected Outcomes: The parents will demonstrate bonding behaviors, including visiting frequently and

CRITICAL TO REMEMBER

Signs That Bonding May Be Delayed

Using negative terms to describe the infant

Discussing the infant in impersonal or technical terms

Failing to give the infant a name or to use the name

Visiting or calling infrequently or not at all

Decreasing the number and length of visits

Showing interest in other infants equal to that in their own infant

Refusing offers to hold and learn to care for the infant

Showing a decrease in or lack of eye contact and in time spent talking to or smiling at the infant

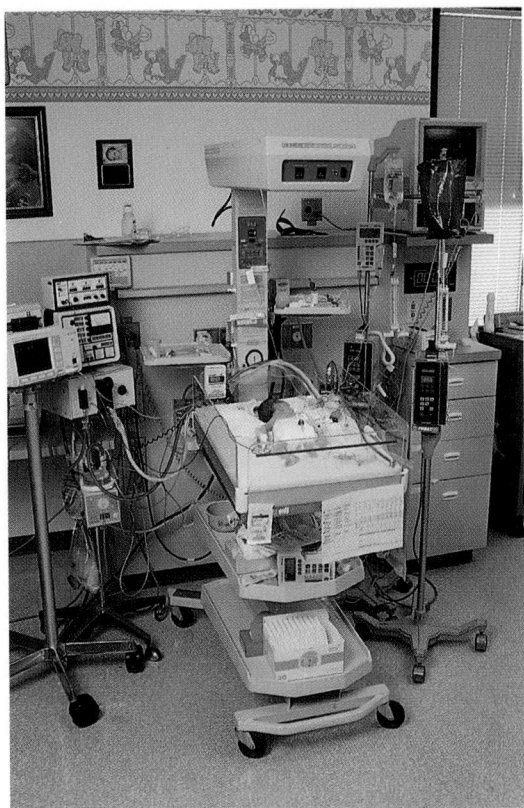

FIGURE 29-6

An infant in the NICU is surrounded by highly technological equipment. This can be very frightening to parents at first. Preparation of parents before they visit is an important nursing responsibility.

interacting as appropriate for the infant's condition throughout the hospital stay. The parents will verbalize understanding of the preterm infant's condition and characteristics within 2 days and will express increasing comfort in participating in infant care within 1 week (as appropriate).

Interventions

Making Advance Preparations

Preparing for threatening situations such as preterm birth helps parents cope with the actual event. Parents expected to have a preterm birth should visit the NICU nursery before delivery. If the mother is confined to bed, arrange for a nurse from the NICU to visit her. The father or another support person should tour the nursery so that he can discuss the nursery environment with the mother.

Assisting Parents at Birth

After the birth, allow the mother to see the newborn in the delivery room so that she has a realistic idea of the infant's appearance and condition. If possible, allow the father to watch the initial care in the NICU. Explain what is happening and why. This attention allows him to see the intensive efforts made on behalf of his infant, increases his confidence in the staff, and enables him to give the mother a full description later. Support the father as well as the mother.

If the infant must be transported to another facility, ask the transport team to visit the mother before leaving, if possible. The visit helps the mother feel connected to her infant and to the staff providing care. Leaving photographs with the mother is one way of helping her bond with the infant.

Supporting Parents During Early Visits

Take the mother to the NICU nursery as soon as she is able. If she is too sick to be with her infant, bring her photographs. Prepare parents before the first visit. Describe the equipment and its purposes, the various attachments to the infant, and the sounds of alarms (Fig. 29–6). Explain how the infant will look and behave. Table 29–1 provides specific steps that the nurse can follow to help parents become familiar with the NICU setting.

At first, stay with the parents during visits. When they are comfortable, allow them time alone with the infant so that they can interact in private. Answer questions and explain changes in the infant's condition and treatment. Use therapeutic communication as the parents cope with their grief, guilt, and emotional turmoil.

Parents should touch the infant as soon as possible because touching helps promote the development of attachment. They may be hesitant initially because of fear that they will interfere with equipment. Show them how to touch in ways appropriate for the infant, such as holding the infant's hand through the portholes of the incubator. Some parents may hesitate to touch because they are afraid of becoming attached to an infant whom they may lose. They need sensitive support from the nurse until they are ready to progress in their relationship with the infant.

Providing Information

Explain all nursing care, its purpose, and the expected response. To help parents develop a realistic understanding of the infant's capabilities, point out how preterm infants are similar to and different from full-term infants.

TABLE 29-1

Introducing Parents to the Neonatal Intensive Care Unit Setting

Before Parents Visit the NICU

Describe the NICU environment. Include the noise of alarms, the busyness of the staff, the number of people and sick infants.

Show parents photographs of the infant. These help prepare the parents, but are not as overwhelming as seeing the infant in person.

Describe the infant. Include the size, the lack of fat, the breathing, the weak cry. Explain that no sound of crying can be heard if the infant is intubated. Include some personal aspects: "He's a real fighter" or "She makes the funniest faces during her feedings."

Describe the equipment. Include ventilators, intravenous lines, and monitors. Explain how they look and how they are attached to the infant. Keep the explanations simple, without technical details.

When Parents Visit the NICU

Help parents perform scrubbing and gowning procedures while explaining the purpose.

Stay with the parents during their visit. Having a familiar person nearby will help them feel more comfortable while they adjust to this unfamiliar environment.

Introduce them to the NICU nurse. Ask the nurse to explain some of the things being done for the infant.

Provide parents with written information about the NICU so that they can take it home to read later.

Tell the parents that they will receive instruction on how to care for their infant in time. Encourage them to visit the infant as much as they can. Emphasize how important they are to their infant.

Offer realistic encouragement based on the infant's condition.

Provide an opportunity for the parents to express their concerns and feelings and to ask questions.

Offer realistic reassurance about the infant's condition, emphasizing positive aspects while being truthful. If parents have misconceptions or did not understand a physician's explanations, clarify or ask the physician to go over specific information again. Translate medical terms into words that the parents can understand. Use an interpreter if the parents do not understand English.

Repeat explanations, especially at first. Because of their emotional distress, parents are often unable to comprehend fully or remember what is said to them.

Offer written information in the parents' language about NICU policies and procedures. Explanations about visiting hours, who can visit, routines for scrubbing, and the role of parents can be reinforced in writing and be available for later reading by parents who are overwhelmed.

Instituting Kangaroo Care

Begin kangaroo care (KC) as soon as possible. KC is a method of providing skin-to-skin contact between preterm infants and their parents. Explain the advantages of KC to parents and elicit their participation. This method of care has been found safe for stable infants, even if intubated. It provides an opportunity for parents to participate in the infant's care, and it increases attachment. The infant, wearing only a diaper and hat, is placed under the mother's clothes between her breasts. Mothers may breast-feed if they wish and the infant is able. Fathers may also participate in KC.

In a study comparing KC with traditional holding (cradle position with the infant wrapped in blankets), infants having KC could maintain their temperature better than those without KC. They had stable heart rates and oxygen saturation levels. Mothers generally were pleased with the care and preferred the kangaroo method of holding (Legault & Goulet, 1995).

KC provides the developmental care so important for the preterm infant and helps with parental attachment. The upright position of the infant against the parent's chest makes breathing easier. The containment of the extremities decreases purposeless movements that use up oxygen and calories. In addition, parents are often gratified when infants fall into a quiet sleep during KC, and feelings of confidence and closeness to the infant are increased (Ludington-Hoe & Swinth, 1996).

Facilitating Interaction

Parents may feel rejected by the infant's lack of response during interactions. Explain to them that infants born at less than 34 weeks' gestation may not be able to cope with socialization. Interaction effective with full-term infants may be too stimulating for very young or sick preterm infants. Suggest forms of touch and interaction based on the individual infant's capacity. Quiet holding or gentle stroking may be better until the infant can tolerate more.

Teach parents signs of overstimulation. Discuss methods to avoid too much stimulation and ways to calm the infant. If several types of stimulation (such as rocking, eye contact, and talking) cause signs of distress, suggest they stop one or more activities until the infant has had a rest period. Show them how to position the infant with the hands near the mouth so the infant can suck on them as a self-comforting measure. When the infant is ready for more interaction, suggest appropriate types of stimulation.

Point out small signs of improvement and even minor strengths. Talk about individual characteristics that make this infant different from all others. The way the infant eats, reacts to sounds, or seems to get tangled in the monitor leads may help parents feel closer to their newborn.

Involve the parents in care of the infant as soon as possible to help them feel a sense of control (Fig. 29-7). At first, plan to change the linens in the incubator or radiant warmer when the parents are there so that they can hold their infant. As the infant's condition improves, parents can develop skill in caring for the tiny infant by changing diapers, feeding, and bathing.

Increasing Parental Decision Making

Give parents the information they need to take an active part in decisions made about the infant's treatment plan. This knowledge will increase their feelings of control over a situation in which many parents feel they have little power.

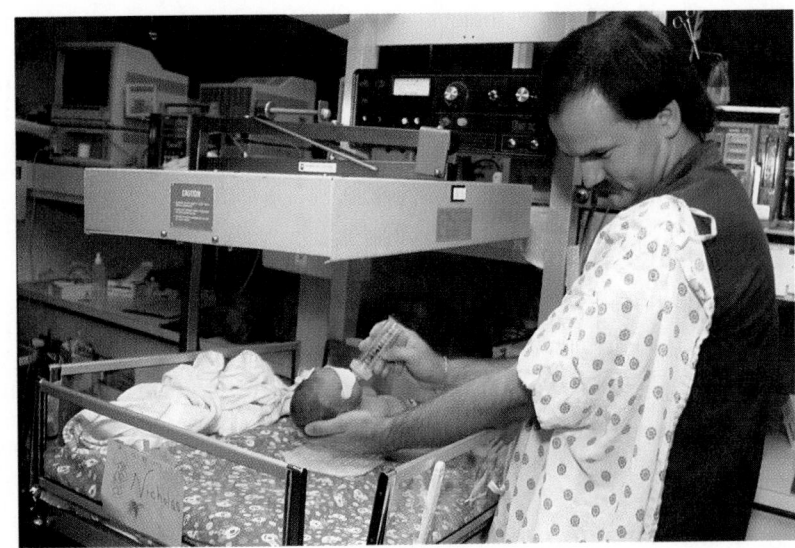

FIGURE 29–7
• • • • • • • • • •
To promote family bonding with the infant, parents are involved as much as possible in the care of their infant. This father bottle-feeds his infant in a radiant warmer.

Alleviating Concerns

Invite parents to call the NICU at any time for information about their infant. Phone calls are beneficial for parents who cannot visit the infant because of distance or other reasons. Put them in touch with other parents who have had preterm infants and refer them to parent groups. Talking with those who have faced the same problems can be very comforting. They can compare notes and get down-to-earth suggestions from an experienced parent's point of view.

Helping with Ongoing Problems

Parents may be unprepared for the inconsistent progress infants often make after surviving the risks of the early days. They expect steady progress once the infant can eat and breathe alone. Complications such as necrotizing enterocolitis, however, can cause major setbacks at this time. To cope with a new crisis, parents need extensive support from the nurse. Use therapeutic communication techniques to help them express and cope with their extreme disappointment. Give information about the infant's changing condition and what to expect in the days ahead.

Preparing for Discharge

Because infants go home very early, it is important that the parents understand the expected hospital course. If a clinical pathway is being used for the infant, give them a copy. They can chart the infant's achievement of major milestones in development and changes in care as the infant moves toward discharge. This information helps them prepare themselves and their home to provide the special care that their infant may need after discharge.

Begin early to teach parents and other caregivers any special procedures, treatments, and medications that the infant will need after discharge (Fig. 29–8). Observe the parents performing care until they are comfortable and can do it safely. Help them learn what is normal for their infant and how to recognize and respond to abnormal signs. Some hospitals have parents spend a night in a special "parent room," where they take over full 24-hour care of the infant.

Help the parents determine what adaptations they will need to make at home for discharge. Utility companies

should be notified if the infant is considered medically fragile. This notice ensures the family receives priority service in cases of power failure. Arrange home nursing services and delivery of special equipment before discharge.

Discuss what to expect in care of the infant after discharge. Many infants need feedings every 3 hours, day and night, to help them gain the 20 to 40 g a day expected (Sifuentes, 1996). Feedings may be time consuming, and parental fatigue resulting from sleep interruptions may be more than they expected.

Help parents to have realistic expectations of the infant. For example, they should know that the infant will accomplish developmental tasks, such as crawling and walking, later than full-term infants. Parents should base expectations on the infant's developmental rather than chronologic age. Developmental age is the chronologic age minus the number of weeks the infant was born early. Many in-

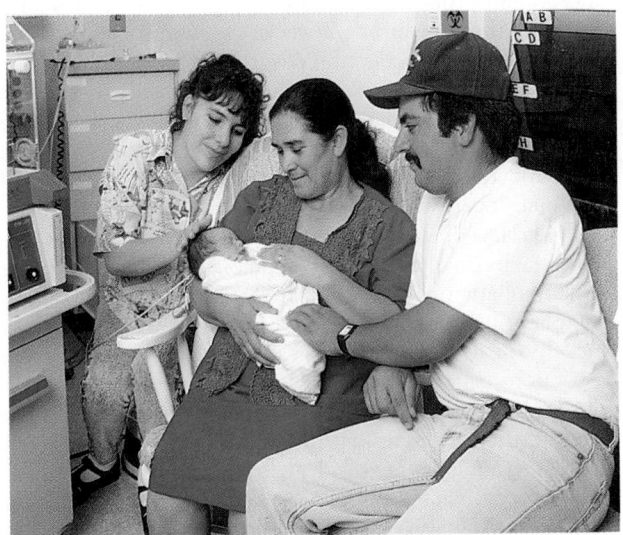

FIGURE 29–8
• • • • • • • • • •
The parents look on while the grandmother holds the infant in the NICU.

fants catch up to their chronologic age when they are approximately 2.5 years old (Sifuentes, 1996).

Assist the parents in planning for integrating the new infant into the family. Meeting the needs of their other children, in addition to the new responsibilities of caring for the preterm infant, is a major source of worry. Listen to their concerns about other children and encourage siblings to visit, if possible. Siblings should touch or hold the infant, if possible, to help them bond.

Evaluation

- Do the parents demonstrate common bonding behaviors?
- Do they verbalize understanding of the preterm infant's special needs and treatments?
- How active are the parents in caring for the infant?

▌ Common Complications of Preterm Infants

Complications of prematurity increase as the infant's gestational age and birth weight decrease. Those common to full-term and preterm infants, such as hyperbilirubinemia, are discussed in Chapter 30.

Respiratory Distress Syndrome

The frequency of respiratory distress syndrome (RDS), also called hyaline membrane disease, increases as gestational age decreases. It is also seen in birth by cesarean and infants of diabetic mothers because these conditions interfere with surfactant production. It is less frequent, however, when chronic fetal stress, such as in heroin addiction and pregnancy-induced hypertension, causes the lungs to mature more quickly (Hansen & Corbet, 1998b).

PATHOPHYSIOLOGY

RDS is caused by insufficient production of surfactant, a phospholipid that lines the alveoli. Surfactant is first produced in the alveoli at 22 weeks' gestation. By 34 to 36 weeks' gestation, production of surfactant is usually mature enough to enable the infant to breathe normally outside the uterus (Hagedorn, Gardner, & Abman, 1998). Immature cell and vascular development in the lungs also plays a part.

Surfactant decreases surface tension to allow the alveoli to remain open when air is exhaled and must be continuously produced. With too little surfactant, the alveoli collapse each time the infant exhales. The lungs become noncompliant or "stiff," and they resist expansion. Noncompliant lungs require a much higher negative pressure for the alveoli to open each time the infant inhales. Severe retractions occur with each breath, drawing the weak muscles of the chest wall inward. The resulting pressure on the lungs further interferes with expansion.

As fewer alveoli expand, atelectasis and hypoxia occur. This process causes pulmonary vasoconstriction and decreased blood flow to the lungs. Persistent pulmonary hypertension can result in a return to fetal circulation patterns, with opening of the ductus arteriosus. Acidosis and alveolar necrosis complicate the condition by interfering with surfactant synthesis. Hyaline membranes, consisting of debris from necrotic cells in a proteinaceous material, are an added problem.

Lecithin, sphingomyelin, and phosphatidylglycerol are components of surfactant that can be detected by tests of amniotic fluid. These tests can predict whether the fetal lungs are mature enough for survival outside of the uterus (see Chapter 16). The incidence and severity of RDS may be reduced by giving the mother corticosteroids at least 24 hours before birth (Chapter 27).

MANIFESTATIONS

Signs of RDS begin during the first hours after birth and include tachypnea, nasal flaring, retractions, and cyanosis. Grunting on expiration is characteristic and signifies physiologic efforts to maintain lung expansion. Breath sounds may be decreased or wet. Acidosis develops as a result of hypoxemia. Chest radiographs show the "ground glass" appearance of the lungs that is characteristic of RDS. Areas of atelectasis are present.

THERAPEUTIC MANAGEMENT

Surfactant replacement therapy is now common. Surfactant is instilled into the infant's trachea immediately after birth or as soon as signs of RDS become apparent. Improvement in breathing occurs in minutes. Infants treated with surfactant have higher survival rates and fewer of some complications of RDS, although they may have other complications resulting from their prematurity.

Other supportive treatment includes mechanical ventilation, correction of the acidosis, intravenous feedings, and care of developing complications.

NURSING CONSIDERATIONS

The nurse observes for signs of developing RDS at birth and during the early hours after delivery. Changes in the infant's condition are constantly assessed. For example, diuresis may occur with improvement in the disease. Changes in ventilator settings may be necessary as the infant's ability to oxygenate increases. Observation for common complications, such as patent ductus arteriosus and bronchopulmonary dysplasia, is important. The nurse must monitor the results of laboratory tests for abnormalities in blood gases and acid-base balance. Early signs of sepsis must be identified and reported. Other care is similar to general care for the preterm infant.

Bronchopulmonary Dysplasia

Bronchopulmonary dysplasia (BPD) is a chronic condition occurring in as many as 40% of infants weighing less than 1,500 g at birth (Hagedorn, Gardner, & Abman, 1998). It is discussed in detail in Chapter 45.

Periventricular-Intraventricular Hemorrhage

Periventricular-intraventricular hemorrhage (PIVH) occurs in 20% to 30% of infants of less than 32 weeks' gestation or those who weigh less than 1,500 g (Moe & Paige, 1998).

PATHOPHYSIOLOGY

PIVH results from rupture of the fragile blood vessels in the germinal matrix, located around the ventricles of the brain. It is most often associated with hypoxic injury to the vessels, increased blood pressure, and increased or fluctuating cerebral blood flow. Rapid volume expansion, hypercarbia, anemia, and hypoglycemia are other causes.

Hemorrhage is graded 1 through 4, according to the amount of bleeding. Grade 1 is a very small bleed outside ventricle walls, producing few if any clinical changes. Grade 2 hemorrhage extends into the lateral ventricles, and grade 3 distends at least one ventricle. Grade 4 hemorrhage causes ventricular dilation and damage to brain tissue.

Infants with grade 3 and 4 hemorrhages are likely to have neurologic abnormalities and developmental delays. Those with grade 4 hemorrhage have a poor survival rate. The mortality rate is 5% to 20% for infants with moderate hemorrhage and 50% for those with severe hemorrhage (Blackburn, 1998).

MANIFESTATIONS

Signs of PIVH are determined by the severity of the hemorrhage. They may include lethargy, poor muscle tone, deterioration of respiratory status with cyanosis or apnea, drop in hematocrit level, decreased reflexes, full or bulging fontanel, and seizures. Subtle aberrations of eye position or movement may occur. Because some infants show no signs, early and repeated screening by ultrasonography is performed on preterm infants younger than 32 weeks' gestation.

THERAPEUTIC MANAGEMENT

Treatment is supportive and focuses on maintaining respiratory function and dealing with other complications. Hydrocephalus may develop from blockage of cerebrospinal fluid flow. Lumbar taps or a ventriculoperitoneal shunt may be necessary to drain the fluid.

NURSING CONSIDERATIONS

Many aspects of care may increase cerebral blood flow. These include mechanical ventilation, suctioning, and exchange transfusions. Therefore, the nurse must be alert for early signs of PIVH. Nursing care includes measurement of the head circumference daily and observation for changes in neurologic status, which may be subtle. Increases in blood pressure from excessive handling or crying and suctioning should be avoided. Developmental care has been found helpful in preventing or minimizing the problem.

Parents need assistance to cope with the diagnosis and their concerns regarding long-term implications. They should learn to assess for signs of hydrocephalus and understand that follow-up care may include periodic ultrasound examinations.

Retinopathy of Prematurity

Retinopathy of prematurity (ROP), once called retrolental fibroplasia, may result in visual impairment or blindness in preterm infants. It occurs more often in infants weighing less than 1,500 g.

PATHOPHYSIOLOGY

ROP is caused by damage to immature blood vessels in the retina. Although the exact cause of the damage is unknown, it is thought to result partly from high arterial blood oxygen levels. It is the level of oxygen in the blood rather than the amount of oxygen the infant receives that is important. Because ROP has developed in some infants who have not received oxygen, other causative factors may also be involved.

In ROP, immature blood vessels in the retina constrict and become permanently occluded. New vessels proliferate to reestablish circulation. If the vessels extend into the vitreous humor, fluid leakage and hemorrhage occur. The result may be scarring, traction on the retina, and retinal detachment.

THERAPEUTIC MANAGEMENT

LBW infants are screened 4 to 6 weeks after birth or at 31 to 33 weeks' corrected age to detect changes of the eye (American Academy of Pediatrics & American College of Obstetricians and Gynecologists, 1997). Cryotherapy and laser surgery have been used to destroy the proliferating blood vessels. Reattachment of the retina may also be necessary. Many infants have spontaneous regression with little or no impairment of vision.

NURSING CONSIDERATIONS

The nurse should check the pulse oximetry equipment and readings frequently for any infant receiving oxygen. Parents should be informed about ophthalmology tests and the results should be explained. Mydriatic eye drops may be given to dilate the eyes; the nurse should watch for feeding intolerance when they are used. If surgery is performed, the eye is assessed for drainage. Ice packs may be used for edema, and pain medication should be given.

Necrotizing Enterocolitis

Necrotizing enterocolitis (NEC) is a serious condition of the intestinal tract, with necrotic lesions of the mucosa of the intestines. There is a 25% to 30% mortality rate (Berseth & Abrums, 1998).

PATHOPHYSIOLOGY

Although the exact causes are unknown, NEC may be due to interference with blood supply to the intestinal mucosa. This condition occurs during asphyxia, sepsis, polycythemia, and maternal cocaine use. The resulting ischemia may make the mucosa more susceptible to invasion with bacteria. When infants are fed, bacteria proliferate, and gas-forming organisms may invade the intestinal wall. Eventually, necrosis, perforation, and peritonitis may occur.

MANIFESTATIONS

Signs include increased abdominal girth caused by distension, increased gastric residuals, decreased or absent bowel sounds, loops of bowel seen through the abdominal wall, vomiting, bile-stained residuals or emesis, blood in the stools, and signs of infection. Apnea, bradycardia, temperature instability, and lethargy are less specific signs also seen in sepsis. On radiographs, loops of bowel dilated with air and layers of gas in the intestinal wall are present. Free air in the peritoneum indicates perforation.

THERAPEUTIC MANAGEMENT

Treatment includes antibiotics, nasogastric suction, discontinuation of oral feedings, and use of parenteral nutrition to rest the intestines. Surgery may be necessary if there is perforation or continued lack of improvement. The necrotic area is removed, and an ostomy may be performed. Breast milk may have a preventive effect on the development of NEC. Other preventive strategies include corticosteroids given to the mother, slow advancement of feedings, and oral immunoglobulin A (Parker, 1995).

NURSING CONSIDERATIONS

Early recognition of signs of NEC is essential to decrease the mortality rate. Because nurses are constantly observing infants, they often can note the early, subtle signs that lead to prompt diagnosis. Noting one or more signs will prompt the nurse to withhold the next feeding and notify the physician. The infant should be positioned on the side to minimize the effects of pressure on the diaphragm from the distended intestines. During recovery, the nurse must observe for signs for feeding intolerance when feedings are resumed. Scar tissue may cause partial or complete bowel obstruction.

▌ Post-Term Infants

Post-term infants are those who are born after the 42nd week of gestation. Their longer-than-normal gestation places them at risk for a number of complications.

Scope of the Problem

Approximately 6% to 12% of all pregnancies are considered post-term. Post-term infants have a two to three times higher perinatal mortality rate than infants born at term. The major concern is how well the placenta functions during the last weeks of pregnancy. In 20% to 30% of post-term pregnancies, placental function deteriorates, causing interference with oxygen and nutrient supply (Ogundipe & Hamilton, 1998). This condition results in hypoxia and malnourishment in the fetus and is called *postmaturity syndrome* or *dysmaturity syndrome*.

In most cases, however, the fetus continues to be well supported by the placenta. Some may grow to more than 4,000 g (8 lb, 13 oz) and are at risk for birth injuries or need a cesarean birth.

Assessment

Signs of postmaturity syndrome may occur during pregnancy, during labor, or after birth. Diminished fetal growth or oligohydramnios may cause decreased uterine size during the last weeks of pregnancy. When labor begins, poor oxygen reserves may cause fetal compromise. The fetus may pass meconium as a result of hypoxia before or during labor, increasing the risk of meconium aspiration at delivery (Chapter 30).

At birth, the cord, skin, and nails may be stained, indicating that meconium was present for some time. The hyperalert, wide-eyed, worried look common to these in-

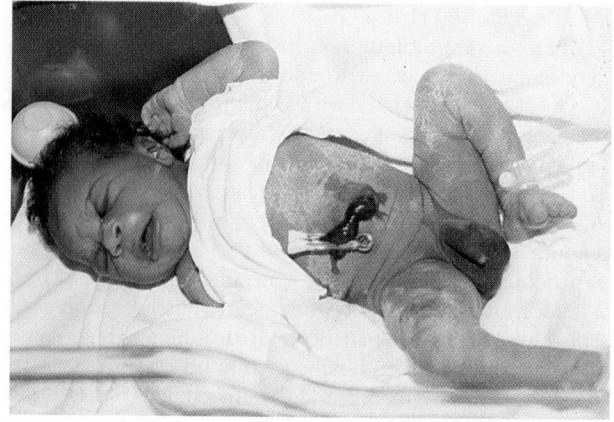

FIGURE 29–9
. . . .
The postmature infant has no vernix and dry, cracked, peeling skin.

fants is a sign of chronic intrauterine hypoxia. Inadequate oxygen in utero may cause the infant to have polycythemia (Chapter 30, pp. 770–771).

A poorly nourished fetus has wasting and growth restriction. The infant is thin and has loose skin with little subcutaneous fat. There is little or no lanugo and vernix caseosa but abundant hair on the head and long nails. The skin is cracked and peeling (Fig. 29–9).

Therapeutic Management

Therapeutic management focuses on prevention and symptomatic treatment. Labor is induced if there are signs of placental deterioration. Apgar scores less than 7 are more likely in post-term infants. In cases of asphyxia or meconium aspiration, respiratory support is needed at birth (Chapter 30).

Nursing Considerations

Signs of postmaturity syndrome in infants are noted during the initial assessment. Respiratory problems may necessitate continued assessment and care. Infants with any indications of postmaturity should be tested for blood glucose level soon after birth and again an hour later. They need early and more frequent feedings to help compensate for the period of poor nutrition in utero.

Temperature regulation may be poor because fat stores were used for nourishment in utero. Extra blankets, frequent temperature assessment, and teaching parents about prevention of cold stress may be necessary throughout the hospital stay. Polycythemia increases the risk of hyperbilirubinemia.

▌ Small-for-Gestational-Age Infants

Small-for-gestational-age (SGA) infants are those who fall below the 10th percentile in size on growth charts. They have had intrauterine growth restriction (IUGR). The terms SGA and IUGR are often used interchangeably.

SGA infants may be preterm, full-term, or post-term but have failed to grow at the rate expected for the time spent in utero. Approximately one third of all LBW infants are full-term but SGA (Behrman, Kliegman, & Arvin, 1996).

Etiology

Many risk factors may cause an infant to be SGA. Congenital malformations, chromosomal anomalies, and fetal infections may cause IUGR. Poor placental function resulting from aging, small size, separation, or malformation may interfere with fetal growth. Illness in the expectant mother, including pregnancy-induced hypertension or severe diabetes, restricts uteroplacental blood flow and decreases fetal growth. Smoking, drug or alcohol abuse, and severe maternal malnutrition also impair fetal growth.

Scope of the Problem

Infants affected with IUGR have higher perinatal morbidity and mortality rates than infants who are not growth restricted. Death may occur from asphyxia before or during labor because of poor placental functioning.

SGA infants are subject to many of the same complications as those who are preterm or post-term, depending on the cause and degree of growth restriction. Problems tend to be greatest in infants who are preterm in addition to being SGA.

Low Apgar scores, meconium aspiration, and polycythemia are increased in incidence in SGA infants. Hypoglycemia is common because of little storage of glycogen in the liver. Infants are prone to inadequate thermoregulation because subcutaneous and brown fat stores have been used to survive in utero.

Characteristics of Small-for-Gestational-Age Infants

The appearance of the SGA infant varies according to whether the cause of growth restriction began early or late in the pregnancy. Variation occurs because growth restriction affects the weight first. If it continues, the length and then the head size will eventually be affected.

Symmetric growth restriction may be caused by congenital anomalies or exposure to infections or drugs early in pregnancy. Although the infant is small, the body is proportionate and appears normally developed for size. There is a decrease in the total number of cells, and the infant may have long-term complications. These infants are often small throughout their lives.

Asymmetric restriction is caused by complications that begin after the first half of pregnancy. In asymmetric restriction, the head is normal in size but seems large for the rest of the body. The length is normal, but the weight is less than that expected for gestational age. The infant appears long and thin. The loose skin has longitudinal thigh creases from loss of subcutaneous fat. The infant has sparse hair, a thin cord, dry skin, and the wide-eyed look associated with intrauterine hypoxia. These infants generally catch up in growth if they are adequately nourished after birth.

Therapeutic Management

Therapeutic management focuses on prevention with good prenatal care to identify and treat problems early. When growth restriction cannot be prevented, ultrasound examination may permit early discovery of the condition so that the infant can be delivered early, if necessary, and preparation can be made for the expected complications at birth. Problems after birth are treated as they occur.

Nursing Considerations

Because the causes of growth restriction are so varied, care of the SGA infant must be adapted to meet the specific problems of the infant. When signs of growth restriction are present, the nurse must observe for the complications that commonly accompany it. The general appearance and measurements give an indication of the type of growth restriction that has occurred. Measurements of the head, chest, length, and weight are less than normal in the infant with symmetric growth restriction. If the restriction is asymmetric, the head circumference and length are normal and the chest circumference and weight are low.

The nurse should assess for hypoglycemia, especially in asymmetric growth-restricted infants. The brain of the infant is normal and needs large amounts of glucose, but the liver is small and has inadequate stores of glycogen. Calorie needs are greater than for a normal infant, making early and more frequent feedings important. Temperature regulation and respiratory support are added nursing concerns.

■ Large-for-Gestational-Age Infants

Large-for-gestational-age (LGA) infants are those who are above the 90th percentile on intrauterine growth charts. They may weigh more than 4,000 g (8 lb, 13 oz) and are usually born at term, although they may be preterm or post-term. The preterm LGA infant may be mistaken for full-term but has the same problems as other preterm infants.

Etiology

LGA infants may be born to multiparas, large parents, and members of certain ethnic groups known to have large infants. Diabetes in the mother may also cause increased size, as may erythroblastosis fetalis (Chapter 30).

Scope of the Problem

The LGA infant is more likely to go through a longer labor, have injury during birth, or need a cesarean birth. Shoulder dystocia may occur because the shoulders are too large to fit through the pelvis. Fractures of the clavicle, damage to the brachial plexus or facial nerve, cephalhematoma, and bruising occur more often in these infants than in those of normal size. Congenital heart defects are more common and the mortality rate is greater (Behrman, Kliegman, & Arvin, 1996).

Therapeutic Management

Therapeutic management is based on identification of macrosomia (large size) during pregnancy by measurements of fundal height and ultrasound examination. Delivery problems may lead to the use of vacuum extraction, forceps, or cesarean birth. Specific treatment involves identification and treatment of birth injuries and complications as they arise.

Nursing Considerations

The nurse assists in a difficult delivery or cesarean birth resulting from dystocias when the infant is LGA. After birth, the infant is carefully assessed for injuries or other complications such as hypoglycemia or polycythemia (see pp. 540 and 770–771). Nursing care is geared to problems presented.

KEY CONCEPTS

- Preterm infants differ in appearance from full-term infants. Some differences include small size, limp posture, red skin, abundant vernix and lanugo, and immature ears and genitals.
- The lungs of preterm infants may lack adequate surfactant, which may cause the lungs to be noncompliant, increasing the amount of energy necessary for breathing and leading to atelectasis.
- Other factors that may increase respiratory problems are poor cough reflex, narrow respiratory passages, and weak muscles.
- Preterm infants should be positioned on the side or prone to increase drainage of respiratory secretions. Prone position decreases breathing effort because respiratory muscles are used efficiently. In the supine position, a small roll should be placed under the shoulders to straighten the airway.
- Preterm infants are prone to cold stress because they have thin skin with blood vessels near the surface, little subcutaneous or brown fat, a large surface area, a limp position, and an immature temperature control center.
- It is important to maintain a neutral thermal environment at all times for infants. The nurse should prevent drafts, use warmed oxygen, and keep incubator doors and portholes closed. When taken out of heating devices, the infant should be wrapped in warmed blankets and wear a hat.
- Preterm infants are subject to increased insensible water losses and have difficulty maintaining fluid balance. Their kidneys do not concentrate or dilute urine as well as those of full-term infants. Intake and output must be carefully measured.
- Preterm infants are subject to infections because they lack passive antibodies from the mother, have an immature immune system, have fragile skin, and are subjected to many invasive procedures.
- The nurse must watch carefully for signs of pain and use comfort measures and medications to alleviate it.
- Infants demonstrate that they are receiving too much stimulation by changes in oxygenation and behavior. The nurse should schedule care to allow rest periods, keep noise to a minimum, and teach parents to interact with the infant appropriately.
- Preterm infants lack nutrient stores and need more nutrients but do not absorb them well. They lack coordination in sucking and swallowing and fatigue easily.
- Signs indicating that an infant may be ready for nipple-feeding include rooting, sucking on a gavage tube or pacifier, presence of gag reflex, and respiratory rate less than 60 breaths per minute.
- The nurse can help the mother who wishes to breast-feed her preterm infant by teaching her to use a breast pump and store her milk until the infant is ready to breast-feed. The nurse can provide privacy, give support and encouragement, explain the infant's behavior, and answer general questions about breast-feeding.
- Nurses can increase parents' comfort with their preterm infant by providing information about the NICU environment, the infant's condition and characteristics, and the equipment and care. Spending time with parents during visits, offering therapeutic communication and realistic encouragement, and involving parents in care of the infant will also help with bonding.
- Preparation for discharge should be started early in the infant's hospital stay. Preparation allows parents to learn gradually about and take on increasing responsibility in the care of the infant until they are comfortable with complete care.
- Common complications of preterm birth are RDS, BPD, PIVH, ROP, and NEC.
- Infants with postmaturity syndrome may appear thin, with loose skin folds, cracked peeling skin, and meconium staining. They appear hyperalert and worried. They may have respiratory difficulties at birth and suffer hypoglycemia and inadequate temperature regulation.
- Infants with IUGR may be SGA at birth. In symmetric growth restriction, the infant is proportionately small; in asymmetric growth restriction, the head and length are normal and the body is thin.
- LGA infants may have birth injuries such as fractures, nerve damage, or bruising as a result of their size. They may have hypoglycemia or polycythemia.

ANSWER TO CRITICAL THINKING EXERCISE 29–1

The preterm infant may need a special formula and smaller amounts. The preterm infant will take longer to feed, might need gavage feedings before introduction of a bottle, and would be more prone to complications in feeding. See Nursing Care Plan 29–1 for interventions appropriate for bottle-feeding the preterm infant.

REFERENCES AND READINGS

Adcock, E. W., Consolvo, C. A., & Berry, D. D. (1998). Fluid and electrolyte management. In G. B. Merenstein & S. L. Gardner (Eds.), *Handbook of neonatal intensive care* (4th ed., pp. 243–258). St. Louis: Mosby.

Als, H., & Gilkerson, L. (1997). The role of relationship-based developmentally supportive newborn intensive care in strengthening outcome of preterm infants. *Seminars in Perinatology, 21*(3), 178–189.

American Academy of Pediatrics & American College of Obstetricians and Gynecologists. (1997). *Guidelines for perinatal care* (4th ed.). Elk Grove Village, IL, and Washington, DC: Author.

Andrews, J. D., & Krowchuk, H. V. (1997). Stool patterns of infants diagnosed with necrotizing enterocolitis. *Neonatal Network, 16*(6), 51–57.

Association of Women's Health, Obstetric, and Neonatal Nurses. (1995). *Clinical commentary: Pain in neonates.* Washington, DC: Author.

Behrman, R. E., Kliegman, R. M., & Arvin, A. M. (Eds.). (1996). *Nelson textbook of pediatrics* (15th ed.). Philadelphia: Saunders.

Bell, E. H., Geyer, J., & Jones, L. (1995). A structured intervention improves breastfeeding success for ill or preterm infants. *MCN: American Journal of Maternal/Child Nursing, 20*(6), 309–414.

Bell, R. P., & McGrath, J. M. (1996). Implementing a research-based kangaroo care program in the NICU. *Nursing Clinics of North America, 31*(2), 387–403.

Berseth, C. L., & Abrams, S. A. (1998). Special gastrointestinal concerns. In H. W. Taeusch & R. A. Ballard (Eds.), *Avery's diseases of the newborn* (7th ed., pp. 965–978). Philadelphia: Saunders.

Blackburn, S. (1995). Problems of preterm infants after discharge. *Journal of Obstetric, Gynecologic, and Neonatal Nursing, 24*(1), 43–49.

Blackburn, S. T. (1998). Assessment and management of neurologic dysfunction. In C. Kenner, J. W. Lott, & A. A. Flandermeyer (Eds.), *Comprehensive neonatal nursing: A physiologic perspective* (2nd ed., pp. 564–607). Philadelphia: Saunders.

Blake, W. W., & Murray, J. A. (1998). Heat balance. In G. B. Merenstein & S. L. Gardner (Eds.), *Handbook of neonatal intensive care* (4th ed., pp. 100–115). St. Louis: Mosby.

Bosque, E. M., Brady, J. P., Affonso, D. D., & Wahlberg, V. (1995). Physiologic measures of kangaroo versus incubator care in a tertiary-level nursery. *Journal of Obstetric,* *Gynecologic, and Neonatal Nursing, 24*(3), 219–226.

Boyle, K. M., Baker, V. L., & Cassaday, C. J. (1995). Neonatal pulmonary disorders. In S. L. Barnhart & M. P. Czervinske (Eds.), *Perinatal and pediatric respiratory care* (pp. 445–479). Philadelphia: Saunders.

Bracht, M., Ardal, F., Bot, A., & Cheng, C. M. (1998). Initiation and maintenance of a hospital-based parent group for parents of premature infants: Key factors for success. *Neonatal Network, 17*(3), 33–37.

Bruno, J. P. (1995). Systematic neonatal assessment and intervention. *MCN: American Journal of Maternal/Child Nursing, 20*(1), 21–28.

Corbett, J. V., & Omlin, K. L. (1995). Prenatal and postnatal use of corticosteroids. *MCN: American Journal of Maternal/Child Nursing, 20*(6), 346.

Cox, C. A., Wolfson, M. R., & Shaffer, T. H. (1996). Liquid ventilation: A comprehensive overview. *Neonatal Network, 15*(3), 31–43.

Darby, M. K., & Loughead, J. L. (1996). Neonatal nutritional requirements and formula composition: A review. *Journal of Obstetric, Gynecologic, and Neonatal Nursing, 25*(3), 209–217.

Dodd, V. (1996). Gestational age assessment. *Neonatal Network, 15*(1), 27–36.

Evans, J. C., Vogelpohl, D. G., Bourguignon, C. M., & Morcott, C. S. (1997). Pain behaviors in LBW infants accompany some "nonpainful" caregiving procedures. *Neonatal Network, 16*(3), 33–40.

Fanaroff, A. A., & Martin, R. J. (1997). *Neonatal-perinatal medicine* (6th ed.). St. Louis: Mosby.

Gomella, T. L., Cunningham, M. D., Eyal, F. G., & Zenk, K. E. (Eds.). (1999). *Neonatology: Management, procedures, on-call problems, diseases, drugs* (4th ed.). Norwalk, CT: Appleton & Lange.

Gomez, M., Hansen, T., & Corbet, A. (1998). Principles of respiratory monitoring and therapy. In H. W. Taeusch & R. A. Ballard (Eds.), *Avery's diseases of the newborn* (7th ed., pp. 576–594). Philadelphia: Saunders.

Gordin, P. (1997). Issues in nursing care of the newborn. In H. W. Taeusch & R. A. Ballard (Eds.), *Avery's diseases of the newborn* (7th ed., pp. 576–594). Philadelphia: Saunders.

Gordon, M., & Montgomery, L. A. (1996). Minimizing epidermal stripping in the very low birth weight infant: Integrating research and practice to affect infant outcome. *Neonatal Network, 15*(1), 37–44.

Gray, K., Dostal, S., Ternullo-Retta, C., & Armstrong, M. A. (1998). Developmentally supportive care in a neonatal intensive care unit: A research utilization project. *Neonatal Network, 17*(2), pp. 33–38.

Griffin, T. (1998). Nurses and families in the NICU: The visitation policy. *Neonatal Network, 17*(2), 75–76.

Guyer, B., Martin, J. A., MacDorman, M. F., Martin, J. A., Peters, K. D., & Strobino, D. M. (1998). Annual summary of vital statistics—1997. *Pediatrics, 102*(6), 1333–1349.

Hagedorn, M. I., Gardner, S. L., & Abman, S. H. (1998). Respiratory diseases. In G. B. Merenstein & S. L. Gardner (Eds.), *Handbook of neonatal intensive care* (4th ed., pp. 437–499). St. Louis: Mosby.

Hansen, T., & Corbet, A. (1998a). Chronic lung disease. In H. W. Taeusch & R. A. Ballard (Eds.), *Avery's diseases of the newborn* (7th ed., pp. 634–647). Philadelphia: Saunders.

Hansen, T., & Corbet, A. (1998b). Disorders of the transition. In H. W. Taeusch & R. A. Ballard (Eds.), *Avery's diseases of the newborn* (7th ed., pp. 602–629). Philadelphia: Saunders.

Hicks, M. A. (1995). A systematic approach to neonatal pathophysiology: Understanding respiratory distress syndrome. *Neonatal Network, 14*(1), 29–35.

Higley, A. M., & Miller, M. A. (1996). The development of parenting: Nursing resources. *Journal of Obstetric, Gynecologic, and Neonatal Nursing, 25*(9), 707–713.

Holditch-Davis, D., Barham, L. N., O'Hale, A., & Tucker, B. (1995). Effect of standard rest periods on convalescent preterm infants. *Journal of Obstetric, Gynecologic, and Neonatal Nursing, 24*(5), 424–432.

Ikuta, L. M. (1998). An exemplary service: Neonatal individualized developmental care and assessment program in the NICU. *Journal of Perinatal Education, 7*(1), 27–31.

Kirkpatrick, J. M., Alesander, J., & Cain, R. M. (1997). Recovering urine from diapers: Are test results accurate? *MCN: American Journal of Maternal/Child Nursing, 22*(2), 96–102.

Lefrak, L., & Dowling, D. A. (1998). Nutrition: Physiologic basis of metabolism and management of enteral and parenteral nutrition. In C. Kenner, J. W. Lott, & A. A. Flandermeyer (Eds.), *Comprehensive neonatal nursing, a physiologic perspective* (2nd ed., pp. 354–370). Philadelphia: Saunders.

Lefrak-Okikawa, L., & Lund, C. H. (1993). Nursing practice in the neonatal intensive care unit. In M. H. Klaus & A. A. Fanaroff (Eds.), *Care of the high-risk neonate* (pp. 212–227). Philadelphia: Saunders.

Legault, M., & Goulet, C. (1995). Comparison of kangaroo and traditional methods of removing preterm infants from incubators. *Journal of Obstetric, Gynecologic, and Neonatal Nursing, 24*(6), 501–506.

Ludington-Hoe, S. M., & Swinth, J. Y. (1996). Developmental aspects of kangaroo care. *Journal of Obstetric, Gynecologic, and Neonatal Nursing, 25*(8), 691–703.

McGrath, J. M., & Conliffe-Torres, S. (1996). Integrating family-centered developmental assessment and intervention into routine care in the neonatal intensive care unit. *Nursing Clinics of North America, 31*(2), 367–386.

Medoff-Cooper, B. (1994). Transition of the preterm infant to an open crib. *Journal of Obstetric, Gynecologic, and Neonatal Nursing, 23*(4), 329–335.

Medoff-Cooper, B., & Ray, W. (1995). Neonatal sucking behaviors. *IMAGE: Journal of Nursing Scholarship, 27*(3), 195–200.

Meier, P., & Brown, L. P. (1996). State of the science: Breastfeeding for mothers and low birth weight infants. *Nursing Clinics of North America, 31*(2), 351–365.

Meier, P. P., Brown, L. P., & Hurst, N. M. (1999). Breastfeeding the preterm infant. In J. Riordan & K. Auerbach (Eds.), *Breastfeeding and human lactation* (2nd ed., pp. 449–481). Boston: Jones & Bartlett.

Meier, P., Engstrom, J. L., Fleming, B. A., Streeter, P. L., & Lawrence, P. B. (1996). Estimating milk intake of hospitalized preterm infants who breastfeed. *Journal of Human Lactation, 12*(1), 21–26.

Miles, M. S., Carlson, J., & Funk, S. G. (1996). Sources of support reported by mothers and fathers of infants hospitalized in a neonatal intensive care unit. *Neonatal Network, 15*(3), 45–51.

Miles, M. S., & Holditch-Davis, D. (1997). Parenting the prematurely born child: Pathways of influence. *Seminars in Perinatology, 21*(3), 254–266.

Militello, L., & Lim, L. (1995). Patient assessment skills: Assessing early cues of necrotizing enterocolitis. *Journal of Perinatal Neonatal Nursing, 9*(2), 42–52.

Moe, P., & Paige, P. L. (1998). Neurologic disorders. In G. B. Merenstein & S. L. Gardner (Eds.), *Handbook of neonatal intensive care* (4th ed., pp. 571–603). St. Louis: Mosby.

Nash, P. (1996). Common neonatal complications. In K. R. Simpson & P. A. Creehan (Eds.), *AWHONN's perinatal nursing*. Philadelphia: Lippincott–Raven.

Ogundipe, O. A., & Hamilton, L. A. (1998). Intrauterine growth restriction, postterm pregnancy, and intrauterine fetal demise. In N. F. Hacker & J. G. Moore (Eds.), *Essentials of obstetrics and gynecology* (3d ed.) (pp. 324–332). Philadelphia: Saunders.

Palmer, M. M., & VandenBerg, K. A. (1998). A closer look at neonatal sucking. *Neonatal Network, 17*(2), 77–79.

Parker, L. A. (1995). Necrotizing enterocolitis. *Neonatal Network, 14*(6), 17–26.

Pereira, G. R. (1995). Nutritional care of the extremely premature infant. *Clinics in Perinatology, 22*(1), 61–75.

Peters, K. L. (1996a). Research update: Dinosaurs in the bath. *Neonatal Network, 15*(1), 71–73.

Peters, K. L. (1996b). Selected physiologic and behavioral responses of the critically ill premature neonate to a routine nursing intervention. *Neonatal Network, 15*(1), 74.

Philip, A. (1996). *Neonatology: A practical guide* (4th ed.). Philadelphia: Saunders.

Pickler, R. H., Mauck, A. G., & Geldmaker, B. (1997). Bottle-feeding histories of preterm infants. *Journal of Obstetric, Gynecologic, and Neonatal Nursing, 26*(4), 414–420.

Premji, S. S. (1998). Ontogeny of the gastrointestinal system and its impact on feeding the preterm infant. *Neonatal Network, 17*(2), 17–24.

Raines, D. A. (1998). Values of mothers of low birth weight infants in the NICU. *Neonatal Network, 17*(4), 41–46.

Schanler, R. J., Berseth, C. L., & Abrams, S. A. (1998). Parenteral and enteral nutrition. In H. W. Taeusch & R. A. Ballard (Eds.), *Avery's diseases of the newborn* (7th ed., pp. 944–964). Philadelphia: Saunders.

Short, M. A. (1998). A comparison of temperature in VLBW infants swaddled versus unswaddled in a double-walled incubator in skin control mode. *Neonatal Network, 17*(3), 25–31.

Short, M. A., Brooks-Brunn, J. A., Reeves, D. S., Yeager, J., & Thorpe, J. A. (1996). The effects of swaddling versus standard positioning on neuromuscular development in very low birth weight infants. *Neonatal Network, 15*(4), 25–31.

Sifuentes, M. (1996). Well child care for preterm infants. In C. D. Berkowitz (Ed.), *Pediatrics: A primary care approach* (pp. 76–80). Philadelphia: Saunders.

Stevens, B. J., Johnston, C. C., & Grunau, R. V. E. (1995). Issues of assessment of pain and discomfort in neonates. *Journal of Obstetric, Gynecologic, and Neonatal Nursing, 24*(9), 849–855.

Symington, A., Ballantyne, M., & Stevens, B. (1995). Indwelling versus intermittent feeding tubes in premature neonates. *Journal of Obstetric, Gynecologic, and Neonatal Nursing, 24*(4), 321–328.

Thompson, D. G., & Maringer, M. (1995). Using case management to improve care delivery in the NICU. *MCN: Maternal/Child Nursing Journal, 20*(5), 257–260.

Townsend, S. F., Johnson, C. B., & Hay Jr., W. W. (1998). Enteral nutrition. In G. B. Merenstein & S. L. Gardner (Eds.), *Handbook of neonatal intensive care* (4th ed., pp. 275–299). St. Louis: Mosby.

Tsang, R. C., DeMarini, S., & Rath, L. L. (1998). Fluids, electrolytes, vitamins, and trace minerals: Basis of ingestion, digestion, elimination, and metabolism. In C. Kenner, J. W. Lott, & A. A. Flandermeyer (Eds.), *Comprehensive neonatal nursing, a physiologic perspective* (2nd ed., pp. 336–353). Philadelphia: Saunders.

Vecchi, C. J., Vasquez, L., Tadin, T., & Johnson, P. (1996). Neonatal individualized predictive pathway (NIPP): A discharge planning tool for parents. *Neonatal Network, 15*(4), 7–13.

Wereszczak, J., Miles, M. S., & Holditch-Davis, D. (1997). Maternal recall of the neonatal intensive care unit. *Neonatal Network, 16*(4), 33–40.

Wilson, S. K. (1998). Incubator to open crib: a three-phase process. *Mother Baby Journal, 3*(3), 7–13.

Zahr, L. K. (1998). Two contrasting NICU environments. *MCN: American Journal of Maternal/Child Nursing, 23*(1), 28–36.

The High-Risk Newborn: Acquired and Congenital Conditions

LEARNING OBJECTIVES

After studying this chapter, you should be able to:

- Describe the steps involved in neonatal resuscitation.
- Explain the common respiratory problems in the newborn.
- Explain the causes and significance of pathologic jaundice.
- Describe the nursing care of the infant with pathologic jaundice.
- Describe causes of neonatal infections and nursing care for infants with infections.
- Explain the effect of maternal diabetes on the newborn.
- Describe the effect of maternal substance abuse on the newborn.

DEFINITIONS

asphyxia Insufficient oxygen and excess carbon dioxide in the blood and tissues.

bilirubin encephalopathy Brain damage resulting from deposits of unconjugated bilirubin in the brain tissue.

erythroblastosis fetalis Agglutination and hemolysis of fetal erythrocytes due to incompatibility between the maternal and fetal blood types. In most cases, the fetus is Rh positive and the mother is Rh negative.

hydrops fetalis Heart failure and generalized edema in the fetus secondary to severe anemia resulting from destruction of erythrocytes.

kernicterus Staining of brain tissue caused by accumulation of unconjugated bilirubin in the brain.

meconium aspiration syndrome Obstruction and air trapping due to meconium in the infant's lungs, which may cause severe respiratory distress.

neonatal abstinence syndrome A cluster of physical signs exhibited by the newborn exposed in utero to maternal use of substances such as heroin or cocaine.

persistent pulmonary hypertension Vasoconstriction of the infant's pulmonary vessels after birth; may result in right-to-left shunting of blood flow through the ductus arteriosus, the foramen ovale, or both.

transient tachypnea of the newborn Condition of rapid respirations due to inadequate absorption of fetal lung fluid.

In addition to the high-risk conditions related to gestational age discussed in Chapter 29, the newborn at risk may have acquired or congenital complications. Acquired conditions may be associated with prenatal complications or may occur at birth or shortly thereafter.

■ Respiratory Complications

Respiratory distress is one of the most common problems of the neonate. It may be caused by asphyxia before or during birth, disease of the respiratory system, or other conditions that affect the infant's ability to breathe. The nurse is responsible for the identification and evaluation of respiratory status at birth and throughout the hospital stay.

Asphyxia

Asphyxia is a lack of oxygen and an increase of carbon dioxide in the blood. It may occur in utero, at birth, or later. When asphyxia occurs at birth, it may be a continuation of asphyxia that began in utero, or it may be the result of other factors, such as preterm lungs with insufficient surfactant to function adequately.

Apnea may be primary or secondary. In primary apnea, a few gasping breaths at birth are followed by cessation of respirations and a rapid fall in heart rate. Stimulation alone or with oxygen may restart respirations. If asphyxia continues, gasping respirations may resume weakly until the infant enters a period of secondary apnea. In secondary apnea, the blood oxygen level continues to decrease, the infant loses consciousness, and stimulation is ineffective. Resuscitative measures must be initiated immediately to prevent permanent damage to the brain or death.

Lack of oxygen to the cells leads to anaerobic metabolism and the production of lactic acid. Metabolic acidosis develops when available bicarbonate can no longer buffer the accumulating acids. The partial pressure of carbon dioxide in arterial blood ($Paco_2$) is high and the partial pressure of oxygen (Po_2), pH, and bicarbonate level are low. Vasoconstriction decreases blood flow to all organs except the brain, myocardium, and adrenal glands. The ductus arteriosus and foramen ovale may remain open because of the low oxygen level in the blood, the high resistance to blood flow through constricted pulmonary vessels, and the elevated pressure on the right side of the heart. Thus, even circulating blood remains low in oxygen. Progress toward brain damage and death is rapid unless intervention is prompt.

INFANTS AT RISK

Complications during pregnancy, labor, or birth increase the risk for asphyxia. In addition, if the expectant mother receives narcotics for analgesia shortly before delivery, the infant may be too depressed at birth to breathe spontaneously. Naloxone (Narcan) is given to these infants.

NEONATAL RESUSCITATION

All personnel involved in deliveries should know how to perform resuscitative measures. Neonatal resuscitation is presented in Procedure 30–1.

Nurses must be prepared for situations in which asphyxia may develop. Equipment should be readily available and functioning properly at all times so that there is no delay in starting resuscitation. Nurses begin resuscitation measures and assist the physician as necessary.

Once the infant is stabilized, the nurse assesses for further change. Infants with asphyxia often have other complications as well. Communication with the parents is a vital nursing function. Parents need explanations, realistic reassurance, and continued support after the crisis.

DRUG GUIDE
Naloxone Hydrochloride (Narcan)

Classification: Narcotic antagonist.

Action: Reverses central nervous system and respiratory depression caused by narcotics (opiates). Competes with narcotics at receptor sites.

Indications: Severe respiratory depression when the mother has received narcotics within 4 hours of delivery.

Dosage and Route: Available in 0.4 mg/ml and 1 mg/ml. Dosage is 0.1 mg/kg. Given intravenously, intramuscularly, subcutaneously, or into an endotracheal tube. Intravenous and endotracheal routes are preferred during resuscitation.

Absorption: Well absorbed by all routes. Onset of action is 1 to 2 minutes if given intravenously.

Excretion: Metabolized by the liver and excreted by kidneys.

Contraindications and Precautions: Duration of effect is 1 to 4 hours. The dose may need to be repeated because the narcotic may have a longer half-life than naloxone. If given to an infant of a mother addicted to drugs, it will cause withdrawal and may cause seizures. Resuscitative measures should be used as necessary.

Nursing Considerations: Note the strength of the medication available when calculating the dose. Prepare the syringe before birth with 1 ml of the drug. After birth, the excess is removed from the syringe, and the amount is given according to the estimate of the infant's weight. Inject rapidly. Monitor for response, and be prepared to give repeated doses if necessary.

PROCEDURE 30-1

• • • • • • • • • • •

Performing Resuscitation in Newborns

PURPOSE: To ensure adequate oxygenation of the neonate with asphyxia.

1. Before *every* birth, check all equipment and supplies and preheat the warmer to ensure all is ready, should resuscitation be necessary.

2. Place the infant under a preheated radiant warmer immediately. Dry thoroughly and determine if resuscitation is necessary. Remove wet linens. Drying prevents cold stress and increased oxygen need.

3. Position the infant with the neck only slightly extended, in a "sniffing" position, so that the airway is open. Avoid hyperextension or flexion of the neck. Place a small blanket under the shoulders. Proper positioning helps maintain an open airway. Hyperextension or flexion may obstruct the airway.

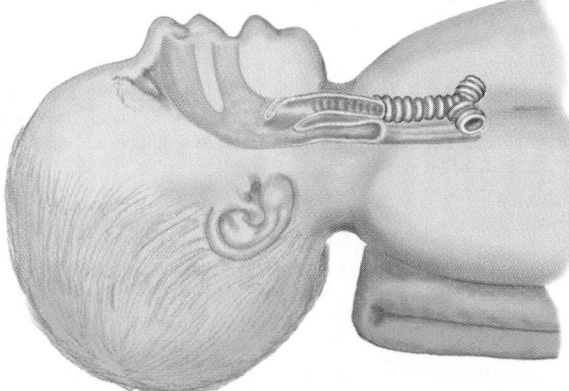

4. Suction the mouth and then the nose to remove mucus from the airways. Infants often gasp when the nose is suctioned and may aspirate secretions from the mouth into the lungs.

5. Evaluate respiratory effort, heart rate, and color. Use stimulation and positive-pressure ventilation (PPV) for apnea or gasping. Use PPV for heart rate less than 100 beats per minute. Give free-flow oxygen for central cyanosis. A quick evaluation determines the steps to take next.

6. Stimulate the infant if necessary. Rub the infant's back or slap the soles of the feet if additional stimulation is needed. Spontaneous respirations should begin within the first 30 to 45 seconds after birth. Drying and suctioning may be sufficient stimulation to cause spontaneous respirations. If not, additional stimulation may be needed.

7. If there is no response after stimulating once or twice, stop and initiate immediate resuscitation. Do not delay resuscitation until the Apgar scores are given. Drying, clearing the airway, and stimulation should take no more than 20 seconds. Resuscitation becomes more difficult the longer it is delayed.

8. Begin PPV with a bag and mask if the infant fails to breathe spontaneously with initial stimulation or the heart rate is less than 100 beats per minute when respirations have begun. This effort ensures oxygen entry into the lungs.

9. Attach the bag to oxygen so that the infant will receive 90% to 100% oxygen. Place the mask snugly over the infant's nose and mouth. Squeeze the bag gently to force air into the infant's lungs with a pressure that will deliver 20 to 30 ml of air. If possible, use a bag with a gauge, to show the amount of pressure being used, and a "pop-off" valve, which releases if the pressure is high enough to cause lung damage. Great care must be taken to use a pressure that will deliver the 20 to 30 ml of air necessary to inflate the lungs without causing damage from overinflation.

10. Observe the rise and fall of the chest during ventilation. If the chest does not move, suction secretions and reposition the head and the mask. Ventilate the infant at a rate of 40 to 60 breaths per minute until the infant is breathing spontaneously and the heart rate is more than 100 beats per minute. The airway must not be occluded by positioning or secretions.

11. Pause after 15 to 30 seconds of ventilation to check the heart rate. Use a stethoscope or feel the pulsations at the base of the cord. If the rate is less than 60 beats per minute, or between 60 and 80 beats per minute and not increasing, a second person should begin chest compressions while the first continues to ventilate the infant. Adequate ventilation causes improvement of bradycardia in most infants. Evaluation of the infant's status determines whether ventilation can be discontinued or chest compressions must be added.

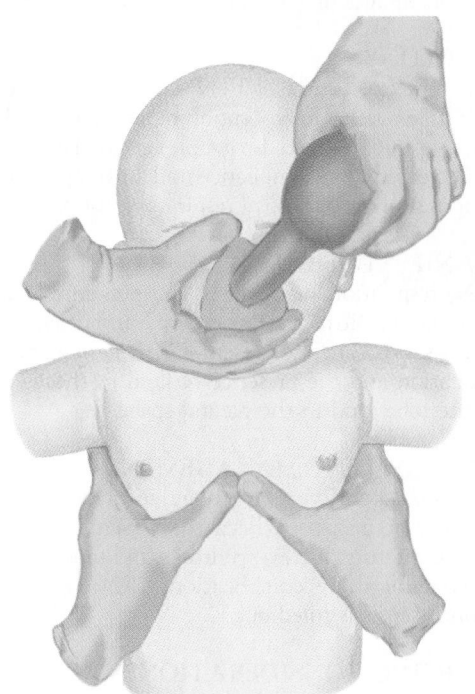

Procedure continued on following page

PROCEDURE 30-1 *Continued*

Performing Resuscitation in Newborns

12. Compress the chest by placing the hands around the infant's chest with the fingers under the back for support and the thumbs over the sternum. Position the thumbs over the lower third of the sternum and above the xiphoid. Correct hand position compresses the heart but avoids or minimizes injury to the liver or spleen, fractures of the ribs, or pneumothorax.

13. Compress the sternum ½ to ¾ inch, with three compressions followed by one ventilation, at a rate of 90 compressions and 30 ventilations each minute. Pause for ½ second after every third compression for ventilation. Simultaneous compression and ventilation may interfere with adequate ventilation. The short pause allows air to enter the lungs.

14. Stop compressions after 30 seconds to check the heart rate for 6 seconds. If it is 80 beats per minute or more, discontinue compressions but continue ventilation until spontaneous breathing begins. If the heart rate is less than 80 beats per minute, continue compressions with periodic re-

checks of the heart rate. Periodic evaluation is necessary to ensure that treatment is appropriate to the infant's status.

15. Prepare medications if the heart rate is less than 80 after 30 seconds of compression. They may include epinephrine given through an umbilical vein catheter or through an endotracheal tube to stimulate the heart. Volume expanders, naloxone, or a 10% dextrose solution may also be given. Sodium bicarbonate is given only after prolonged arrest and only with effective ventilation. Volume expanders may be used for bleeding. Naloxone counteracts the effects of narcotics given to the mother in labor. Dextrose prevents or treats hypoglycemia. Sodium bicarbonate corrects acidosis after prolonged asphyxia that does not respond to other treatment.

Data from Bloom, R. S., Cropley, C., & AHA/AAP Neonatal Resuscitation Program Steering Committee. (1996). *Textbook of neonatal resuscitation.* Dallas: American Heart Association and American Academy of Pediatrics.

Transient Tachypnea of the Newborn

Infants with transient tachypnea of the newborn (TTN) develop rapid respirations soon after birth. This condition resolves within a few days. Risk factors include maternal analgesia, bleeding, or diabetes; cesarean birth; and asphyxia. Mild immaturity of surfactant production may also be a factor. Infants may be term or preterm.

ETIOLOGY

Although the exact cause of TTN is unknown, it is thought to result from a delay in absorption of fetal lung fluid by the pulmonary capillaries and the lymph vessels. This condition causes decreased lung compliance and air trapping and produces signs similar to those of respiratory distress syndrome.

MANIFESTATIONS

In TTN, respirations as high as 150 per minute develop within hours of birth. Retractions, nasal flaring, grunting, and mild cyanosis are also present. Chest radiography shows hyperinflation and the presence of fluid in the fissures between the lobes and in the pleural space.

THERAPEUTIC MANAGEMENT

Treatment is supportive. Oxygen and intravenous or gavage feeding may be necessary. Because the signs are similar to those of respiratory distress syndrome and sepsis, the infant is observed for those complications. Antibiotics may be given until sepsis is ruled out.

NURSING CONSIDERATIONS

After identifying signs, the nurse notifies the appropriate caregiver and carries out treatment. General nursing care is similar to that of the respiratory care of the preterm infant (see Chapter 29).

Meconium Aspiration Syndrome

Meconium aspiration syndrome (MAS) occurs most often in post-term infants, but it also occurs in term infants who have suffered intrauterine asphyxia. It causes obstruction of the airways, pneumonitis, and air trapping. It may also lead to persistent pulmonary hypertension of the newborn.

ETIOLOGY

Although the normal fetus may pass meconium, MAS most often occurs when hypoxia causes relaxation of the anal sphincter before or during labor. MAS develops when meconium enters the lungs during fetal life or at birth. It may be drawn into the lungs if gasping movements occur in utero as a result of asphyxia and acidosis, or the meconium in the upper airways may be pulled deep into the respiratory passages when the infant takes the first breaths after birth.

Obstruction of the airways may be complete or partial. In partial obstruction, air can enter but not escape from the alveoli. During inhalation, the bronchioles expand slightly as air flows into them past the meconium. During exhalation, the passages constrict, and meconium blocks movement of air out of the lungs.

This ball-valve mechanism results in air trapping. The overdistended alveoli may develop an air leak, with escape of air into the pleural cavity (pneumothorax) or mediastinum (pneumomediastinum). In addition, meconium is irritating to lung tissue and causes an inflammatory reaction and chemical pneumonitis. Persistent pulmonary hypertension may result.

Severe MAS develops in only a small number of newborns with meconium below the vocal cords. The addition of meconium to a lung damaged by asphyxia may increase the severity of the condition. Damage from asphyxia interferes with clearing of lung fluid and production of surfactant, and it causes pulmonary vasoconstriction that can result in a return to fetal circulation.

MANIFESTATIONS

If meconium in the amniotic fluid is light, respiratory problems usually do not develop. Thick meconium, however, may cause serious respiratory pathology. Signs of mild to severe respiratory distress are present at birth, with tachypnea, cyanosis, retractions, nasal flaring, grunting, and coarse breath sounds. Radiography shows atelectasis, consolidation, and hyperexpansion from air trapping.

THERAPEUTIC MANAGEMENT

At birth, the airway must be cleared, especially if meconium is thick. The infant's mouth and pharynx are suctioned as soon as the head is delivered and before delivery of the rest of the body. This procedure helps prevent drawing the meconium from the upper air passages deep into the lungs during the infant's first breath.

Immediately after birth and before the infant takes the first breath, a laryngoscope is inserted and the trachea is suctioned. An endotracheal tube is inserted to allow deep suction of meconium and ventilation, if necessary. If the meconium is thin and the infant is vigorous and showing no respiratory difficulty, intubation may not be necessary.

Infants may need only warmed, humidified oxygen, or extensive respiratory support with a ventilator may be required. High-frequency ventilation may be used. Supportive care to meet the problems presented makes up ongoing management.

Infants with severe MAS who do not respond to conventional treatment may benefit from extracorporeal membrane oxygenation (ECMO). This is a method to oxygenate the blood while bypassing the lungs to allow the infant's lungs to rest temporarily and recover.

NURSING CONSIDERATIONS

When meconium is noted in the amniotic fluid during labor, the nurse notifies the primary caregiver so that delivery care can be adapted as necessary. The nurse ensures that equipment is available and functioning and assists with care at delivery. After the infant's birth, nursing care is adapted to the problems presented. Although meconium is sterile, lung damage promotes the growth of bacteria, and infants should be closely observed for infection.

Persistent Pulmonary Hypertension of the Newborn

Persistent pulmonary hypertension of the newborn (PPHN) is a condition in which the vascular resistance of the lungs does not decrease after birth and normal changes to neonatal circulation are impaired. For this reason, the condition is also called *persistent fetal circulation*.

ETIOLOGY

The cause of PPHN may be abnormal lung development, maternal use of nonsteroidal anti-inflammatory agents or aspirin, and hypoxemia and acidosis from conditions such as asphyxia, meconium aspiration, sepsis, or respiratory distress syndrome.

Delayed relaxation of the pulmonary vessels produces increased resistance in the lungs. The elevated pulmonary vascular resistance causes a rise in pressure on the right side of the heart. This development may result in a right-to-left shunt of blood through the foramen ovale and patent ductus arteriosus, as occurs during fetal circulation.

MANIFESTATIONS

Infants with PPHN are usually term or post-term and develop signs of PPHN within the first 24 hours after birth. Tachypnea, respiratory distress, and progressive cyanosis often worsen with handling. Oxygen saturation and partial pressure of oxygen in arterial blood (Pao_2) are decreased. Other signs may result from associated conditions.

THERAPEUTIC MANAGEMENT

Management involves treating the underlying cause and relieving pulmonary vasoconstriction. Arterial pH may be increased with respiratory and drug therapy to cause pulmonary vasodilation. High-frequency ventilation, surfactant therapy, and ECMO therapy may all be necessary. Inhalation of nitric oxide, which dilates pulmonary vessels, is being investigated. Nursing care is similar to care of other infants with severe respiratory disease. Because infants become hypoxic with activity and other stimuli, handling and noise are kept to a minimum.

Hyperbilirubinemia (Pathologic Jaundice)

When the bilirubin level reaches 5 to 7 mg/dl, jaundice is visible in the newborn's skin (MacMahon, Stevenson, & Oski, 1998b). (Conjugation of bilirubin and physiologic jaundice are discussed in Chapter 22.) Jaundice is considered pathologic in the following circumstances:

It appears in the first 24 hours after birth.
The total bilirubin rises to more than 12 mg/dl in a full-term infant or 10 to 14 mg/dl in a preterm infant, or more than 5 mg/dl in 24 hours.
The direct bilirubin level is more than 1 mg/dl.
Jaundice continues beyond the second week of life (Behrman, Kliegman, & Arvin, 1996).

Pathologic jaundice is a concern because it may lead to kernicterus. In kernicterus, bilirubin deposits cause yellowish staining of the brain, especially the basal ganglia, cerebellum, and hippocampus. It is more likely to occur in infants who have suffered sepsis, hypoxia, or respiratory acidosis, which impairs the blood-brain barrier and allows unconjugated bilirubin to enter the brain. Kernicterus causes bilirubin encephalopathy.

Although bilirubin encephalopathy is rare today because of improved treatment measures, the mortality rate of affected infants is high. Those who survive may suffer cerebral palsy, mental retardation, hearing loss, or more subtle long-term neurologic and developmental problems. The exact level at which these conditions begin to develop is not known, but they may occur when total bilirubin levels are more than 20 mg/dl in full-term infants and when lower levels are reached in preterms or neonates with other complications.

Etiology

The most common cause of pathologic jaundice is hemolytic disease of the newborn from incompatibility between the blood of the mother and that of the fetus. The best known cause is Rh incompatibility, in which the Rh-negative mother forms antibodies when Rh-positive blood from the fetus enters her circulation (see Chapter 26). The antibodies cross the placenta and destroy fetal red blood cells, causing erythroblastosis fetalis.

Infants with erythroblastosis fetalis are anemic from destruction of red blood cells. Severely affected infants may have hydrops fetalis, a severe anemia that results in heart failure and generalized edema. Use of $Rh_o(D)$ immune globulin (RhIG), such as RhoGAM, to prevent the mother from forming antibodies against Rh-positive blood has greatly decreased the incidence of erythroblastosis fetalis.

ABO incompatibility also causes pathologic jaundice. Mothers with type O blood have natural antibodies to type A or B blood. The antibodies cross the placenta and cause hemolysis of fetal red blood cells. The destruction, however, is much less severe than with Rh incompatibility and causes milder signs.

Other causes of pathologic jaundice include infection, hypothyroidism, glucuronyl transferase or other enzyme deficiency, polycythemia, and biliary atresia. Any condition that causes destruction of erythrocytes or impairment of the liver may result in pathologic bilirubin levels.

Therapeutic Management

The focus of therapeutic management is prevention of kernicterus. The cause is determined by history and diagnostic tests to identify infections or blood abnormalities. During pregnancy, a positive Coombs' test result of the expectant mother's blood shows the presence of antibodies against fetal blood. Amniocentesis may be performed to determine the degree of hyperbilirubinemia.

At birth, a direct Coombs' test is performed on the cord blood. A positive result indicates that antibodies from the mother have attached to the infant's red blood cells. Bilirubin levels are followed closely for changes that indicate that treatment should be initiated or changed.

PHOTOTHERAPY

The most common treatment of jaundice is phototherapy or "bili" lights, special fluorescent lamps placed over the infant. A fiberoptic phototherapy blanket that is placed against the infant's skin is another option. The infant can be swaddled and does not require patches over the eyes when the blanket is used. Double phototherapy lights or a combination of blanket and lights may be used if the bilirubin level is high. Another option is a bilibed, a device containing phototherapy lights that fits into a crib and on which the infant lies. Although the infant must remain in the bed during therapy, the bed can be moved into the mother's room, and eye shields are not necessary.

During phototherapy, bilirubin in the skin absorbs the light and changes into water-soluble products (photobilirubin and lumirubin). These do not require conjugation by the liver and can be excreted in the bile and urine.

Side effects of phototherapy include frequent, loose green stools, resulting from increased bile flow and peristal-

Home Care for the Infant Receiving Phototherapy

Position the phototherapy or "bili" light at the proper distance from your baby according to the manufacturer's directions. Placing it too close to the infant could result in fever or burns. Placing it too far away will make the treatment ineffective.

Close the baby's eyes and place patches over the eyes before placing the infant under the lights. Check at least every hour to see that the patches remain in place. They must cover the eyes but not press on the nose because they can interfere with breathing.

The infant may be removed from the lights for feedings, diaper changes, and other general care but should receive phototherapy for 18 hours every day (or the number of hours ordered by the physician). Hold and cuddle your infant during the time that the baby is out of the lights. When the infant is under the lights, you can talk to your baby. The sound of your voice will be comforting.

If you are using a fiberoptic blanket, keep it next to the baby's skin at all times. Be sure the baby does not roll off the blanket. You may wrap the baby with a receiving blanket over the "bili" blanket and hold the baby for feedings and other care. It is not necessary to cover the infant's eyes if the blanket alone is used.

Check your baby's temperature under the arm before every feeding. The temperature should remain between 97.7° and 99.5°F. If it is abnormal, see if the heat in the room is too low or high or if the "bili" light is out of position. Use warm blankets when you remove the baby from the warmth of the light. Call your physician if the baby has a temperature less than 97.7° or more than 100°F.

Change your baby's position about every 2 hours so that the light reaches all areas of the body. Dress the baby in only a diaper to expose as much skin as possible to the lights.

Feed your baby every 2 to 3 hours because the lights cause the baby to lose fluid from the skin and have loose stools. This process could cause dehydration. The infant needs protein, which helps eliminate the bilirubin that causes the jaundice.

Keep a list of your baby's wet diapers and stools. Increase the feedings if the baby has less than six wet diapers a day or if the urine appears dark.

Call the physician or home care nurse if you have questions about care, if the baby has a fever or appears sick to you, if the mouth seems dry, or if the urine is dark or less than normal.

sis. African-American infants may experience a tanning effect from the light. Bronze baby syndrome, a grayish-brown discoloration of the skin, occurs in infants with cholestatic jaundice, in whom liver function and production or flow of bile are impaired. A skin rash similar to erythema toxicum may also occur. The color changes and rash disappear when phototherapy is ended. Some infants experience a temporary lactose intolerance during therapy and need formula without lactose.

Home phototherapy allows the infant to go home yet continue treatment. Parents need extensive teaching on managing the equipment and caring for the infant. Home visits by nurses are important to help ensure that the infant is making adequate progress and that the parents understand how to provide care.

EXCHANGE TRANSFUSIONS

Exchange transfusions are necessary when phototherapy does not reduce dangerously high bilirubin levels quickly enough. This treatment removes sensitized red blood cells, antibodies, and unconjugated bilirubin in the blood. It also corrects severe anemia.

Procedure. During the exchange transfusion, 5- to 10-ml portions of blood are removed and replaced with an equal amount of donor blood. Because the donor blood mixes with the infant's blood, it is necessary to administer approximately twice the infant's blood volume. At the end of the transfusion, approximately 85% of the infant's red blood cells have been replaced.

When the level in the blood decreases, bilirubin from the tissues moves into the plasma. This rebound elevation of bilirubin may necessitate repeat transfusions, but phototherapy is generally adequate to resolve it.

Complications. Complications of exchange transfusions include infection, hypervolemia or hypovolemia, cardiac dysrhythmias, and air embolism. Hypocalcemia is also a problem because preservatives in the blood lower the infant's blood calcium level. Signs of hypocalcemia are jitteriness, irritability, tachycardia, and electrocardiographic changes.

Role of the Nurse. The nurse's role during exchange transfusion is to prepare equipment, assess the infant during and after the procedure, and keep accurate records. A cardiac monitor is attached to the infant, and adequate warmth is provided by a radiant heater. The nurse must also clarify any misunderstandings that the parents may have about the treatment and help allay their anxiety.

NURSING CARE
The Infant with Hyperbilirubinemia

Although collaborative care of the infant with jaundice is an important part of the nurse's role, several nursing diagnoses are appropriate. Risk for Injury is one common finding. Risk for Fluid Volume Deficit is discussed in Nursing Care Plan 30–1.

Assessment

Assess the level of jaundice at the initial assessment each shift. Determine the areas of the body affected by the jaundice, and document carefully for comparison during future assessment. Jaundice begins at the head and moves down the body as the bilirubin levels rise. Monitor laboratory bilirubin levels for change.

Assess for risk factors that might further increase bilirubin levels. Note temperature fluctuations, hypoglycemia, or infection. Determine the infant's oral intake and number of stools.

Diagnosis and Planning

Nurses can do many things to prevent situations that might cause further rises in bilirubin. They must also protect the infant from injury from the light during phototherapy. The nursing diagnosis is

■ Risk for Injury related to preventable causes of further elevation of bilirubin and damage to the eyes or gonads secondary to phototherapy.
  Expected Outcomes: The infant will avoid injury resulting from increased bilirubin and will avoid injury of the skin, eyes, or gonads from the phototherapy lights.

Interventions

Maintaining a Neutral Thermal Environment

Prevent situations, such as cold stress or hypoglycemia, that could result in increased levels of fatty acids in the blood caused by acidosis, thereby decreasing the availability of albumin-binding sites for unconjugated bilirubin. Prevent cold stress at birth and during all care by maintaining the infant in a neutral thermal environment. Check the infant's axillary temperature every 2 to 4 hours to identify an early decrease before it becomes a problem. Use warmed clothes and blankets when removing the infant from phototherapy lights.

Prevent elevation of the infant's temperature from exposure to the heat of the "bili" lights. To maintain the environmental temperature appropriately, use a skin probe if the infant is in an incubator. Position the lights according to the manufacturer's guidelines to prevent overheating or burning the skin.

Providing Optimal Nutrition

Ensure that the infant receives feedings every 2 to 3 hours, whether by breast or bottle. Feedings prevent hypoglycemia, provide protein to maintain the albumin level in the blood, and promotes gastrointestinal motility and prompt emptying of bilirubin from the bowel. Avoid offering water because the infant may take less milk, which is more effective in removing bilirubin from the intestines. If breast-feeding must be supplemented, use formula instead of water.

Protecting the Eyes

Provide patches to protect the eyes from retinal damage from the phototherapy lights (Fig. 30–1). To avoid abrasions to the cornea, close the infant's eyes before placing the patches. Check the position of the patches at least every hour. Poorly positioned patches can dig into the eyes or compress the nose and interfere with breathing.

Enhancing Response to Therapy

Expose as much skin as possible to the light. Turn the infant frequently to expose all areas evenly. Remove all clothing except a diaper to cover the testes or ovaries. Turn the light

---

CRITICAL THINKING EXERCISE 30–1

Why is it important to remove the patches from the eyes each time the infant is taken from the phototherapy lights for feeding?

NURSING CARE PLAN 30-1
• • • • • • • • • • •
The Infant with Jaundice

Assessment

Holly, a 2-day-old, full-term infant, is jaundiced secondary to ABO incompatibility and is receiving phototherapy. She weighs 3.2 kg (7 lb, 1 oz), and her mucous membranes appear slightly dry. Skin turgor is good with quick recoil, and the anterior fontanel is flat. Urine appears slightly dark. Holly had three loose green stools with no water ring on this shift. She is a sleepy infant who takes formula poorly. Holly's mother, Valerie, had a cesarean birth and appears tired and frustrated with Holly's slow eating behavior.

Nursing Diagnosis

Fluid Volume Deficit related to inadequate oral intake to meet needs of increased insensible water loss and frequent loose stools

Goals/Expected Outcomes

Holly will

- Take at least 320 to 480 ml of fluid per day (100 to 150 ml/kg/day) to meet normal needs.
- Show no signs of dehydration (dry mucous membranes, inelastic skin turgor, sunken fontanels, inadequate urine output, urine specific gravity >1.020).

Intervention

1. Instruct Valerie to feed Holly every 2 to 3 hours. Feed Holly in the nursery at night or when Valerie needs rest, if she prefers.
2. Explain to Valerie why Holly needs frequent feedings.

3. Observe Valerie feeding Holly and offer suggestions as needed. Show Valerie how to waken the infant by unwrapping and gentle stimulation. Try warming the formula slightly. Stroke around Holly's mouth, and insert a gloved finger to elicit the suck reflex before feedings.
4. Tell the parents about the need for frequent feeding to provide added fluid, protein, and other nutrients.

5. Avoid offering water or dextrose water. Use formula instead.

6. If water loss appears excessive, check the specific gravity of the urine and weigh all diapers. Urine output should be 1 to 3 ml/kg/hr. Specific gravity should be 1.001 to 1.020 for full-term infants.

7. Use therapeutic communication techniques to help Valerie vent her frustrations. Offer praise for her attempts to feed Holly.

Rationale

1. Adequate intake is necessary to meet the infant's nutrient and fluid needs and ensure excretion of bilirubin in the stools.
2. The mother's understanding of the need and the reasons will increase her willingness to work with the infant.
3. Observation of feedings may identify problems and interventions that work for this situation. A wide-awake infant is more likely to feed well. Some infants prefer warm milk. Oral exercises may help infant suck effectively.

4. Infants receiving phototherapy have a greater-than-normal insensible water loss. Albumin (protein) is necessary to carry bilirubin to the liver for conjugation. Heightened intestinal motility decreases absorption of nutrients.
5. Water supplements may decrease intake of formula. Formula increases excretion of bilirubin in stools, but water does not.
6. Weighing the diapers and checking specific gravity will identify inadequate output and dehydration early. The wet diaper weight in grams minus the weight of a dry diaper equals the milliliters of urine.

7. Helping the mother deal with her feelings helps her meet the infant's needs. Praise increases her concept of herself as a "good mother."

Evaluation

Holly drinks a total of 450 ml (15 oz) of formula during 24 hours. Valerie is able to wake Holly, who begins to suck more vigorously. Holly's mucous membranes are moist, and there are 12 wet diapers during the 24 hours.

Additional Nursing Diagnoses to Consider

Altered Skin Integrity
Anxiety
Altered Parenting
Ineffective Thermoregulation

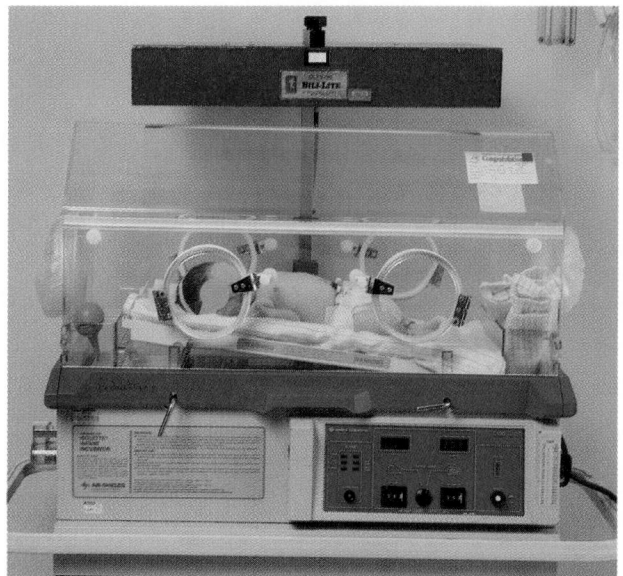

FIGURE 30-1

The infant receiving phototherapy is wearing eye patches to protect the eyes and a diaper to protect the gonads.

off when changing diapers because there is a possibility that damage to DNA may occur from exposure of the gonads to phototherapy.

If a fiberoptic blanket is used, check its position frequently. Infants sometimes need to be repositioned so that the blanket remains in contact with the skin.

Use a light meter to check the level of irradiance to be sure the apparatus is functioning appropriately.

Observe for other complications. Although bilirubin encephalopathy is rare today, monitor for signs that indicate its presence. These include lethargy, poor muscle tone, decreased or absent Moro reflex, high-pitched cry, opisthotonos, and seizures. Note the presence of rashes or changes in the color of the skin, and inform parents that they are not harmful and will disappear when phototherapy is discontinued.

Evaluation

- Is the infant free of signs of injury?
- Are the skin, eyes, and gonads protected from injury from the phototherapy lights?

Infection

Neonatal infection is responsible for approximately 30% of all neonatal deaths (Lott et al., 1998). The nurse must be constantly alert for this condition.

Transmission of Infection

Newborns acquire infections in several ways:

- In utero by passage of organisms across the placenta. These infections may cause long-term consequences. Examples are rubella, cytomegalovirus, syphilis, and toxoplasmosis.
- During labor and birth as bacteria ascend the vagina. Examples are group B streptococci, hepatitis B, and herpes.

- After birth from infected mothers, family members, or caregivers, and from contaminated equipment. Examples include staphylococcal infections.

Some of the most common infections and their effects on the neonate are listed in Table 30–1. Infections acquired during pregnancy are also discussed in Chapter 26.

Sepsis Neonatorum

Infection that occurs during or after birth may result in sepsis neonatorum, systemic infection with bacteria in the bloodstream. Bacterial sepsis occurs in one to eight infants per 1,000 live births (Klein & Remington, 1995).

Newborns are particularly susceptible to sepsis because their immune systems are immature and they react more

---

CRITICAL TO REMEMBER

Signs of Sepsis in the Newborn

General Signs
Temperature instability (usually low)
Nurse's feeling that infant is not doing well
Rash

Respiratory Signs
Tachypnea
Apnea
Respiratory distress—nasal flaring, retractions, grunting

Cardiovascular Signs
Color changes: cyanosis, pallor, mottling
Tachycardia
Hypotension
Decreased peripheral perfusion

Gastrointestinal Signs
Decreased oral intake
Vomiting
Gastric residuals measuring more than half of previous feeding
Diarrhea
Abdominal distension
Hypoglycemia or hyperglycemia

Central Nervous System Signs
Decreased muscle tone
Lethargy
Irritability
Bulging fontanel

Signs That May Indicate Advanced Infection
Jaundice
Evidence of hemorrhage (petechiae, purpura, pulmonary bleeding)
Anemia
Enlarged liver and spleen
Respiratory failure
Shock
Seizures

TABLE 30–1
. . . .

Common Infections in the Newborn

Transmission	Effect on Newborn	Nursing Considerations
Viral Infections		
Cytomegalovirus		
Transplacental	Most infants asymptomatic at birth. LBW, IUGR, enlarged liver and spleen, jaundice, mental retardation, hearing loss, blindness, epilepsy. May have no signs for months or years.	Most common perinatal infection. A major cause of mental retardation. Diagnosed by urine culture. May shed virus in saliva and urine for months. Antiviral drug therapy.
Hepatitis B		
Usually during birth through contact with maternal blood. Also transplacental, breast milk.	Asymptomatic at birth. LBW, prematurity. Most of those infected become chronic carriers. Risk of later liver cancer.	Wash well to remove all blood before skin is punctured for any reason. After cleaning, administer hepatitis B immune globulin and hepatitis B vaccine to prevent infection.
Herpes		
Usually during birth through infected vagina or ascending infection after rupture of membranes. Transplacental rarely.	Clusters of vesicles, temperature instability, lethargy, poor suck, seizures, encephalitis, jaundice, purpura. Death or severe neurologic impairment is very likely with disseminated infection.	Contact precautions. Obtain lesion specimens for culture. Antiviral drugs.
Human Immunodeficiency Virus/Acquired Immunodeficiency Syndrome		
Transplacental, during birth from infected blood and secretions, from breast milk. Transmission rate lower if mother takes antiretroviral drugs during pregnancy.	Asymptomatic at birth, signs usually apparent at 4 to 12 months. Enlarged liver and spleen, lymphadenopathy, failure to thrive, pneumonia, persistent candidal and bacterial infections.	Diagnosed from symptoms or at 6 to 18 months when antibodies from mother gone. Wash early and before skin is punctured to remove blood. Treat with antiretroviral drugs and prophylaxis against other infections.
Rubella		
Transplacental	Asymptomatic or IUGR, cataracts, cardiac defects, deafness, mental retardation. Damage greatest in first trimester.	Contact precautions. Infant may shed virus for months after birth. Diagnosed by presence of antibody. No treatment.
Varicella Zoster Virus (Chickenpox)		
Transplacental	Skin scarring, limb hypoplasia, eye and brain damage, IUGR, death. Damage greatest before the 20th week of gestation.	Immune globulin for infants of mothers infected just before delivery. Acyclovir. Airborne isolation of infants with lesions.
Other Infections		
Group B Streptococcal Infection		
During birth or ascending after rupture of membranes	Sudden onset of respiratory distress in infant usually well at birth, pneumonia, shock, meningitis. May have early or late onset.	Early identification essential to prevent death. Treated with IV antibiotics to mother in labor or to infant after birth.
Gonorrhea		
Usually during birth	Conjunctivitis (ophthalmia neonatorum), with red, edematous lids and purulent eye drainage. May result in blindness if untreated.	All infants receive erythromycin or tetracycline eye ointment for prevention. Silver nitrate previously used. Treated with antibiotics.
Chlamydial Infection		
During birth	Conjunctivitis, pneumonia, otitis media.	Erythromycin or tetracycline eye ointment for prevention of conjunctivitis. Infection treated with erythromycin.

TABLE 30-1

Common Infections in the Newborn Continued

Transmission	Effect on Newborn	Nursing Considerations
Candidiasis		
During birth	White patches in mouth (thrush) that bleed if removed. Rash on perineum. May be systemic.	Administer nystatin drops or cream and teach parents how to administer them. Assess mother for vaginal or breast infection.
Toxoplasmosis		
Transplacental	Asymptomatic, or LBW, thrombocytopenia, enlarged liver and spleen, jaundice, anemia, seizures, microcephaly, hydrocephalus, chorioretinitis. Signs may not develop for years.	Consider in infants with IUGR. Confirmed by serum tests. Treatment: pyrimethamine, sulfadiazine, and folinic acid.
Syphilis		
Transplacental	Asymptomatic or enlarged liver and spleen, jaundice, lymphadenopathy, anemia, rhinitis, pink or copper-colored peeling rash, pneumonitis, osteochondritis, CNS involvement.	Diagnosed by blood and cerebrospinal fluid testing. Administer penicillin as ordered.

Note: Standard precautions for infection control apply to all patients and are not listed above. They include precautions for contact with blood; all body fluids, secretions, and excretions except sweat; nonintact skin; and mucous membranes. Contact precautions are used when transmission of the disease may occur from direct contact with the patient's dry skin or articles in the patient's environment. See Appendix B for more information about infection control.

Abbreviations: LBW, low birth weight; IUGR, intrauterine growth restriction; IV, intravenous; CNS, central nervous system.

slowly to invasion by organisms. They fail to localize infection as well as older children, and this inability allows the infection to spread easily from one organ to another. The blood-brain barrier is less effective in keeping out organisms, and central nervous system infection may result. Preterm and low-birth-weight infants are especially susceptible to infection.

ETIOLOGY

The most common causative agents of neonatal sepsis are group B β-hemolytic streptococci and *Escherichia coli*. Other common causes include *Staphylococcus epidermidis* (most often in very small preterm infants), *Staphylococcus aureus* (usually hospital acquired), *Hemophilus influenzae*, and *Listeria monocytogenes*. Sepsis may be divided into early onset and late onset, according to when signs of disease begin.

Early-onset sepsis is often caused by complications of labor such as prolonged rupture of membranes, prolonged labor, or chorioamnionitis. It usually begins in the first 24 hours after birth and has a more rapid progression than late-onset sepsis. The mortality rate is 15% to 50% (Klein & Marcy, 1995). It often involves the respiratory system or causes meningitis.

Late-onset sepsis generally develops after the first week of life from exposure to organisms during or after birth and usually involves the central nervous system. The mortality rate is 10% to 20% (Klein & Marcy, 1995), and serious long-term effects can be common.

THERAPEUTIC MANAGEMENT

Diagnostic testing helps identify sepsis and the organism responsible. A complete blood count with differential may show decreased neutrophils, increased bands (immature neutrophils), and decreased platelets. Presence of elevated immunoglobulin M levels in cord blood or shortly after birth indicates that infection was acquired in utero, because this immunoglobulin does not cross the placenta. It often indicates transplacental infection.

Cultures of the blood, cerebrospinal fluid, urine, trachea, and gastric aspirate may be obtained. Chest radiography helps differentiate between respiratory distress syndrome and sepsis. Blood glucose levels should be checked because they may be unstable (high or low) in sepsis.

Broad-spectrum antibiotics are given intravenously until culture and sensitivity results are available. Continued antibiotic therapy is based on culture results. Commonly used antibiotics include ampicillin, penicillin G, gentamicin, and cefotaxime. Intravenous immunoglobulins may also be used in prevention and treatment of sepsis in some preterm infants. Other care is supportive to meet the infant's specific needs. The infant may require oxygen or even intubation and mechanical ventilation. Fluid balance maintenance, monitoring of the blood pressure, and hourly urine output measurements are important.

NURSING CONSIDERATIONS

Assessment

Risk Factors. The nurse should identify infants at risk for infection. The mother who had a prolonged or precipitous labor, prolonged rupture of membranes, signs of infection, or foul-smelling or meconium-stained amniotic fluid may have an infant with sepsis. Preterm or low-birth-weight infants and those with other complications are also at risk. Invasive procedures, such as use of intravenous catheters and endotracheal tubes, are another source of infection.

Signs of Infection. In the newborn, signs of infection are often subtle and could indicate other conditions. There may be temperature instability (with a low temperature most common), respiratory problems, and changes in feeding habits or behavior. Experienced nurses may have a feeling that the infant is not doing well even before specific signs of infection are present. When suspecting infection, the nurse expands the assessment and watches carefully for the development of other signs. Early identification and treatment are important because infants can deteriorate rapidly from normal to fulminant septic shock with little warning, especially if the causative agent is group B streptococci.

Nursing Interventions

Providing Antibiotics. The nurse must be knowledgeable about the specific antibiotics used and possible side effects. The nurse starts the intravenous fluids and ensures that medications are administered on time. If more than one antibiotic is ordered, the timing of administration must be coordinated to increase effectiveness. Laboratory analysis of peak and trough levels may be ordered to measure blood levels of the medications at times when they are expected to be at the highest and lowest points. Changes in dosage are based on the results of the laboratory tests. Antibiotics are usually continued for 10 days or longer.

Providing Other Supportive Care. Oxygen or other respiratory support is used if needed. The infant may need treatment for shock, hypoglycemia or hyperglycemia, electrolyte imbalances, and problems in temperature regulation. Gavage feeding may be necessary if the infant cannot take oral feedings. Signs of disseminated intravascular coagulopathy are noted.

Preventing Spread of Infection. Transmission of infection to other infants in the nursery is prevented by hand washing, separation of infants' supplies, and standard precautions for infection control. Placing the infant in an incubator provides a physical separation between infected and well infants, similar to placing adults in isolation in private rooms.

Supporting Parents. The infant with sepsis often appears healthy at birth but suddenly becomes critically ill. Parents experience shock, fear, and disappointment when their apparently healthy newborn is suddenly moved to the intensive-care nursery. They benefit from a chance to talk about their feelings. Keeping the parents informed of the infant's changes in condition and involving them in care are essential.

Infant of a Diabetic Mother

Scope of the Problem

The infant of a diabetic mother (IDM) faces a number of risks. Infants of mothers with long-term diabetes and vascular changes may be small for gestational age because decreased placental blood flow causes intrauterine growth restriction. Hypertension occurs more often in diabetic women and further compromises uteroplacental blood flow.

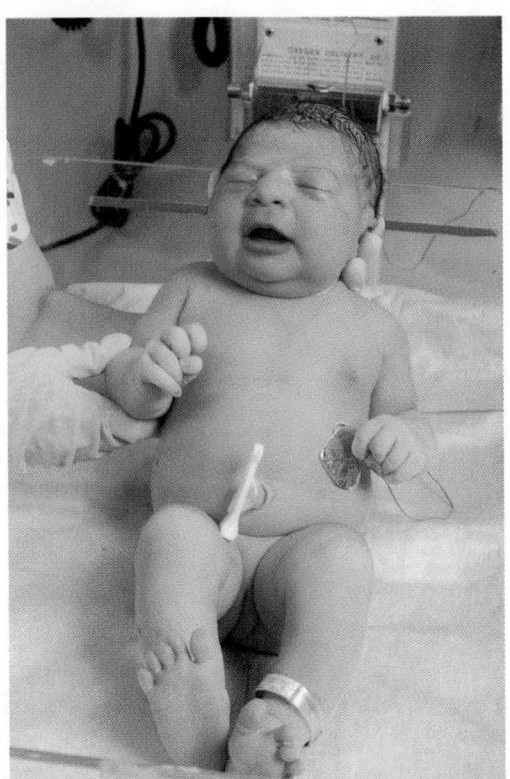

FIGURE 30–2

Macrosomia is common in infants of diabetic mothers.

Infants born to women with gestational diabetes or diabetes without vascular changes may be large for gestational age, particularly if the diabetes is not well controlled (Fig. 30–2).

When the mother is hyperglycemic, large amounts of amino acids, free fatty acids, and glucose are transferred to the fetus, but maternal insulin is not. This condition causes hypertrophy of the islet cells of the fetal pancreas. The islet cells produce large amounts of insulin, which acts as a growth hormone. The accelerated protein synthesis and the deposition of fat and glycogen in fetal tissues result in macrosomia. Macrosomic infants are at risk for trauma during birth, including fractures or nerve damage.

Congenital anomalies are more likely in IDMs. Caudal regression syndrome and anomalies of the neural tube, heart, and kidney are most common. The incidence of anomalies is lower if blood glucose levels remain within normal limits, especially before conception and in the early weeks of gestation, when organs are forming.

Other complications for which the IDM is at risk include respiratory distress syndrome because high levels of insulin interfere with the production of surfactant. Hypoglycemia may occur after birth, when the maternal supply of glucose ends but the infant's high level of insulin produc-

CRITICAL THINKING EXERCISE 30–2

Why is breast milk or formula usually given instead of 10% glucose when an infant's glucose level is low?

tion continues. Hypocalcemia may result from decreased parathyroid hormone production, especially when the mother's diabetes was poorly controlled.

Polycythemia (hematocrit level more than 65%) occurs when infants produce more erythrocytes than normal because of poor oxygenation during fetal life. Organ damage from decreased blood flow, renal vein thrombosis, and necrotizing enterocolitis are possible effects of polycythemia. Polycythemia also results in hyperbilirubinemia as the excessive red blood cells break down after birth.

Characteristics of Infants of Diabetic Mothers

The small-for-gestational-age IDM is similar to small-for-gestational-age infants from other causes but is more likely to have congenital anomalies. The macrosomic IDM has hypertrophy of the liver, adrenals, and heart. All organs except the brain are larger than normal. The length and head size are generally within the normal range for gestational age. Infants of diabetic mothers have a characteristic appearance. The face is round and red, and the body is obese. There is poor muscle tone at rest, but the infant becomes irritable and may have tremors when disturbed.

Therapeutic Management

Therapeutic management includes controlling the mother's diabetes to decrease complications in the fetus (see Chapter 26). If the infant is large, a cesarean birth may be required. Immediate care of respiratory problems and continued observation for complications determine treatment.

Nursing Considerations

ASSESSMENT
The IDM is assessed for signs of complications, trauma, and congenital anomalies at delivery and during the early hours after birth. Hypoglycemia may be present without observable signs. The blood glucose level is screened according to hospital protocol. An example is screening every hour for 4 to 6 hours after birth and every 4 hours until the results are normal (Philip, 1996).

The most frequent sign of low glucose is jitteriness or tremors. Diaphoresis is uncommon in newborns but may occur with hypoglycemia. Rapid respirations, low temperature, and poor muscle tone are also common (see Chapter 22, p. 540). If jitteriness occurs and the glucose levels are normal, the infant may have hypocalcemia.

NURSING INTERVENTIONS
Feeding. If hypoglycemia develops, infants must be fed early to correct it. Gavage feeding may be used if the infant does not suck well or if the respirations are high. Some infants need intravenous glucose to maintain balance and prevent damage to the brain.

Other Complications. The nurse must be alert for signs of other complications. Signs of respiratory distress syndrome or other respiratory complications may occur. Cold stress increases the need for oxygen and glucose. A check of the hematocrit level will identify polycythemia. These infants must be hydrated adequately to prevent slug-

gish blood flow and ischemia to vital organs. Monitoring of bilirubin levels is important if jaundice occurs.

Support. Providing support to parents is important. They may not understand why their infant, who appears fat and healthy to them, needs close observation and frequent blood tests. The mother may have had a difficult pregnancy and may feel guilty, even if she followed a program of good diabetic control. Ample opportunity for discussion of feelings as well as information about the care of the infant is important.

█ Prenatal Drug Exposure

Substance abuse affects the fetus at any time during pregnancy. The effects of substance abuse on pregnancy, the fetus, and the neonate are discussed in Chapter 25. Neonatal abstinence syndrome is a disorder in which neonates demonstrate signs of drug withdrawal.

Identification of Drug-Exposed Infants

Maternal substance abuse may be identified before an infant is born, or it may be unknown to health professionals. A history of no prenatal care or behaviors during birth that indicate substance abuse may raise suspicion. When there is any cause to suspect drug use, the infant is observed closely for signs of prenatal drug exposure.

Neonatal abstinence syndrome occurs in infants who have suffered prenatal drug exposure sufficient to cause withdrawal signs after birth. It usually begins during the first 48 to 72 hours after birth, depending on the time of the

---

CRITICAL TO REMEMBER
• • • • • • • • • • • • • •

Signs of Intrauterine Drug Exposure

Behavioral Signs
Irritability
Jitteriness, tremors
Muscular rigidity, increased muscle tone
Restless, excessive activity
Exaggerated startle reflex
Prolonged high-pitched cry
Difficult to console

Signs Relating to Feeding
Uncoordinated sucking and swallowing
Frequent regurgitation or vomiting
Diarrhea

Other Signs
Poor sleeping patterns
Yawning
Nasal stuffiness, sneezing
Tachypnea
Apnea
Seizures
Diaphoresis

Note: Some infants with prenatal drug exposure have no abnormal signs at all, or signs may be delayed.

NURSING CARE PLAN 30-2 *Continued*
· · · · · · · · · · · ·
The Drug-Exposed Infant

2. Assist Gloria to hold and feed Tracy. Explain nursing actions such as placing the crib in a secluded area.

3. Demonstrate comfort measures such as swaddling and rocking. Show her how to place a rolled blanket around the infant to provide a feeling of security.

4. Explain that Tracy's behavior is normal for drug-exposed infants. Point out signs that Tracy is overstimulated. Such signs include gaze aversion and increase in irritability.

5. Model ways of interacting with Tracy and calming her. Point out signs that Tracy is ready to interact. Suggest only one stimulus at a time, such as talking softly without rocking.

6. Point out positive points about Tracy, such as her long eyelashes or delicate fingers. Point out signs that show that Tracy is making progress.

7. Explain the routine care of a newborn. Spread teaching out over Gloria's visits.

8. Give praise and encouragement frequently as Gloria works with Tracy.

9. Use therapeutic communication techniques to help Gloria discuss her feelings as she cares for Tracy.

10. Discuss sources of support from family members or friends. Refer her to support groups in the community.

11. If Gloria will have custody of Tracy, help her make plans for discharge. Discuss ongoing problems and concerns such as sudden infant death syndrome (SIDS).

2. Encouraging the mother to participate in care of the infant helps her get to know her infant and how to care for the infant.

3. When the mother learns ways to comfort her infant, the positive response from the infant may increase bonding.

4. The mother needs to learn that the infant's behavior is part of the infant's problem and is not caused by the mother's handling of her.

5. The mother learns appropriate interaction when she sees it performed by the nurse. Infants may need short time-outs before they are ready for more stimulation.

6. The mother needs help to focus on positive aspects of the infant as well as the problems.

7. The mother needs to learn the usual care of any newborn as well as the infant's special needs.

8. The mother needs positive reinforcement and help to feel that she is capable of mothering her infant.

9. Mothers often find it frustrating to care for the drug-exposed infant. Helping them vent their feelings may increase their ability to cope with the infant's needs.

10. Ongoing support is necessary for the woman with addiction problems. Support for the mother will help her care more effectively for her infant.

11. Infants will have ongoing problems that will continue in the home setting. Infants exposed to heroin have an increased incidence of SIDS.

Evaluation

Gloria begins to visit more often, coming three or four times a week. She participates in care, begins to talk about her "pretty little girl," and discusses her plans for taking Tracy home with her.

Additional Nursing Diagnoses to Consider

Altered Nutrition
Altered Family Processes
Ineffective Individual Coping
Impaired Skin Integrity
Disorganized Infant Behavior

The mother's participation also provides a chance to assess the mother's infant care skills and areas in which further discussion of the newborn's needs will be helpful. In addition, it gives the nurse an opportunity to demonstrate parenting skills. Many mothers who use drugs have not had good parenting role models and do not know what to do. Frequent positive feedback about the mother's participation is also important.

The mother needs the same teaching given to all new parents, plus special techniques necessary to meet the needs of drug-exposed infants. The nurse should teach her about her newborn's special characteristics and help her take on more of the infant's care as she demonstrates readiness.

Signs of overstimulation in drug-exposed infants have some similarities with those for the preterm infant. In addition, these infants cannot tolerate more than brief periods of interaction. They may not make eye contact, or they may avert their eyes after 30 to 60 seconds of social interaction.

The nurse should teach the mother that the infant responds poorly to everyone so that she does not think that only she is being rejected.

The nurse can provide information and referral to any special programs available to help parents learn special stimulation techniques appropriate for drug-exposed infants. If the mother cannot care for the newborn, the same interventions can be used to help the person who will take over care of the infant on hospital discharge.

Cocaine, amphetamines, and other drugs pass into breast milk. Trying to breast-feed an infant with poorly developed feeding skills may be too much stress for the mother who is trying to recover from addiction. Therefore, mothers likely to continue drug use after delivery should be discouraged from breast-feeding. In some situations, however, breast-feeding may be acceptable. If the woman has a strong desire to breast-feed, the nurse should consult the health care provider.

Hypocalcemia

Hypocalcemia is a total serum calcium concentration of less than 7.0 mg/dl. It is divided into early onset (less than 48 hours of age) and late onset (at about 1 week of age).

Etiology

Early-onset hypocalcemia occurs most often in IDMs and in infants with asphyxia, prematurity, and low birth weight. Late hypocalcemia is due to maternal hyperparathyroidism or vitamin D deficiency, high-phosphate formula, low magnesium levels, and congenital hypoparathyroidism. Other causes of hypocalcemia include alkalosis, administration of bicarbonate or citrate-preserved blood, furosemide therapy, and renal disease.

Therapeutic Management

Laboratory testing of the serum calcium level determines the presence of the problem. Oral or intravenous calcium gluconate is given if feeding alone does not raise the calcium level. A cardiac monitor is necessary when intravenous calcium is given, as bradycardia can occur.

Nursing Considerations

ASSESSMENT

The nurse must be alert for signs of hypocalcemia. These include irritability, tremors, poor feeding, high-pitched cry, tachycardia, apnea, muscle twitching, seizures, and electrocardiographic changes. The condition is often asymptomatic.

NURSING INTERVENTIONS

Oral calcium should be given with feedings because it may cause gastric irritation. Intravenous calcium should be administered slowly and stopped immediately if bradycardia or dysrhythmia develops. The intravenous site should be assessed frequently because infiltration can cause necrosis and ulceration.

Phenylketonuria

Phenylketonuria (PKU) is a genetic disorder that causes central nervous system damage from toxic levels of the amino acid phenylalanine in the blood. All newborns are screened for this condition before or shortly after discharge from the birth facility. Mental retardation occurs in untreated infants and children.

Etiology

PKU is due to a deficiency of the enzyme phenylalanine hydroxylase, which is necessary to convert phenylalanine to tyrosine for use. It is an autosomal recessive disorder (see Chapter 12).

Therapeutic Management

Positive screening tests are followed by other testing. Treatment is a low-phenylalanine diet. Small amounts of phenylalanine are allowed, as it is a necessary amino acid. Early and continued treatment are necessary to prevent mental retardation.

Nursing Considerations

ASSESSMENT

The nurse should determine if the newborn was screened for PKU. Signs of the disease include digestive problems, vomiting, seizures, musty or mousy odor of the urine, and mental retardation. Older children have eczema, hypertonia, hyperactive behavior, and hypopigmentation of the hair, skin, and irises.

NURSING INTERVENTIONS

Screening performed before 24 to 48 hours of age should be repeated, as the infant must have taken in enough protein for the test to be accurate. The nurse assists parents in regulating the diet to meet the infant's changing phenylalanine needs. Parents can be reassured that good control should allow normal infant growth and development.

KEY CONCEPTS

- Asphyxia before or during birth causes apnea, acidosis, pulmonary hypertension, and possible death. Neonatal resuscitation must be initiated immediately.
- Nurses must identify conditions that increase the risk of asphyxia, begin resuscitation promptly, and assist other members of the team during treatment. Continued follow-up of the infant and parental support are important.
- In transient tachypnea of the newborn, respiratory difficulty in full-term or preterm infants is caused by failure of fetal lung fluid to be absorbed completely. It usually resolves spontaneously with supportive care.

- In meconium aspiration syndrome, meconium enters the lungs before birth or during the first breaths after birth. It causes inflammation and blocks air flow.
- The nurse's role in meconium aspiration syndrome is to prepare for care at birth, assist with care, and continue aftercare.
- Pathologic jaundice appears in the first 24 hours of life, rises faster and to higher levels than physiologic jaundice, or both. It may result in damage to the brain from kernicterus.
- The nurse's role in phototherapy includes decreasing situations such as cold stress or hypoglycemia

that might further elevate bilirubin levels, seeing that lights are used properly, observing for excessive fluid loss or skin impairment, ensuring adequate oral intake, and teaching parents.
- Infection can be transmitted to the neonate from the mother during pregnancy or birth or from the mother, family members, or agency staff after birth. Infections may have serious consequences.
- The IDM may have congenital anomalies, may be large or small for gestational age, and may have respiratory distress syndrome, hypoglycemia, hypocalcemia, and polycythemia.

- Nursing responsibilities in caring for IDMs include early identification and follow-up of complications, monitoring blood glucose levels, ensuring early and adequate feedings, and supporting parents.
- Infants with prenatal exposure to drugs may have congenital defects and behavioral and feeding abnormalities. They may have difficulty relating to others and fail to gain weight.
- Nursing care for infants with neonatal abstinence syndrome includes decreasing stimuli from lights, noise, or handling; increasing feeding abilities; and fostering the mother's attachment to and ability to care for her infant.

ANSWERS TO CRITICAL THINKING EXERCISES

Exercise 30–1
Patches hide the eye area, and an infection might not be noticed immediately. Removal of the patches at feedings allows inspection for signs of infection such as redness, edema, and drainage. Removal also allows a time

of visual stimulation for the infant. If parents give the feeding, being able to see the infant's eyes enhances attachment.
Exercise 30–2
Giving infants fluids with high levels of glucose will correct the immediate

problem of hypoglycemia, but will stimulate the production of additional insulin. This causes a rebound hypoglycemia. Giving glucose in a form that will be metabolized more slowly provides longer levels of normal glucose.

REFERENCES AND READINGS

American Academy of Pediatrics. (1998). Policy statement: Neonatal drug withdrawal. *Pediatrics, 101*(6), 1079–1088.

American Academy of Pediatrics & American College of Obstetrics and Gynecology. (1997). *Guidelines for perinatal care* (4th ed.). Elk Grove Village, IL, and Washington, DC: Author.

American Academy of Pediatrics, Provisional Committee for Quality Improvement and Subcommittee on Hyperbilirubinemia. (1994). Practice parameter: management of hyperbilirubinemia in the healthy term newborn. *Pediatrics, 94*(4), 558–565.

Askin, D. F. (1995). Bacterial and fungal infections in the neonate. *Journal of Obstetric, Gynecologic, and Neonatal Nursing, 24*(7), 635–643.

Association of Women's Health, Obstetric, and Neonatal Nurses. (1995). *Clinical commentary: Perinatal group B streptococcal disease.* Washington, DC: Author.

Association of Women's Health, Obstetric, and Neonatal Nurses. (1998). *Standards and guidelines for professional nursing practice in the care of women and newborns* (5th ed.). Washington, DC: Author.

Behrman, R. E., Kliegman, R. M., & Arvin, A. M. (Eds.). (1996). *Nelson textbook of pediatrics* (15th ed.). Philadelphia: Saunders.

Bell, G. L., & Lau, K. (1995). Perinatal and neonatal issues of substance abuse. *Pediatric Clinics of North America, 42*(2), 261–281.

Berkowitz, C. D. (1996). Infants of substance abusing mothers. In C. D. Berkowitz, *Pediatrics: A primary care approach.* Philadelphia: Saunders.

Blackburn, S. (1995). Hyperbilirubinemia and neonatal jaundice. *Neonatal Network, 14*(7), 15–25.

Bloom, R. S., Cropley, C., & AHA/AAP Neonatal Resuscitation Program Steering Committee. (1996). *Textbook of neonatal resuscitation.* Dallas: American Heart Association and American Academy of Pediatrics.

Boyle, K. M., Baker, V. L., & Cassaday, C. J. (1995). Neonatal pulmonary disorders. In S. L. Barnhart & M. P. Czervinske (Eds.), *Perinatal and pediatric respiratory care* (pp. 445–479). Philadelphia: Saunders.

Cordero, L., Treuer, S. H., Landon, M. B., & Gabbe, S. G. (1998). Management of infants of diabetic mothers. *Archives of Pediatric Adolescent Medicine, 152,* 249–253.

D'Apolito, K., & McRorie, T. I. (1996). Pharmacologic management of neonatal abstinence syndrome. *Journal of Perinatal and Neonatal Nursing, 9*(4), 70–80.

DeBoer, S. L., & Stephens, D. (1997). Persistent pulmonary hypertension of the newborn: Case study and pathophysiology review. *Neonatal Network, 16*(1), 7–13.

Doshier, S. (1995). What happens to the offspring of diabetic pregnancies? *MCN: American Journal of Maternal/Child Nursing, 20*(1), 25–29.

Fanaroff, A. A., Martin, R. J., & Miller, M. J. (1999). Identification and management of problems in the high-risk neonate. In R. K. Creasy & R. Resnik, *Maternal-fetal medicine* (4th ed., pp. 1151–1193). Philadelphia: Saunders.

Flandermeyer, A. A. (1998). The drug-exposed neonate. In C. Kenner, J. W. Lott, & A. A. Flandermeyer (Eds.), *Comprehensive neonatal nursing: A physiologic perspective* (2nd ed., pp. 864–892). Philadelphia: Saunders.

Franck, L., & Vilardi, J. (1995). Assessment and management of opioid withdrawal in ill neonates. *Neonatal Network, 14*(2), 39–48.

Frank, D. G., Cooper, S. C., & Merenstein, G. B. (1998). Jaundice. In G. B. Merenstein & S. L. Gardner (Eds.), *Handbook of neonatal intensive care* (4th ed., pp. 393–412). St. Louis: Mosby.

Hagedorn, M. I., Gardner, S. L., & Abman, S. H. (1998). Respiratory diseases. In G. B. Merenstein & S. L. Gardner (Eds.), *Handbook of neonatal intensive care* (4th ed., pp. 437–499). St. Louis: Mosby.

Halamek, L. P., & Stevenson, D. K. (1997). Neonatal jaundice and liver disease. In A. A. Fanaroff & R. J. Martin, *Neonatal-perinatal medicine* (6th ed., pp. 1345–1389). St. Louis: Mosby.

Healy, K., Jovanovic-Peterson, L., & Peterson, C. M. (1995). Pancreatic disorders of pregnancy: Pregestational diabetes. *Endocrinology and Metabolism Clinics of North America, 24*(1), 73–101.

Kaftan, H., & Kinney, J. S. (1998). Early onset neonatal bacterial infections. *Seminars in Perinatology, 22*(1), 15–24.

Kenner, C., & D'Apolito, K. (1997). Outcomes for children exposed to drugs in utero. *Journal of Obstetric, Gynecologic, and Neonatal Nursing, 26*(5), 595–603.

Klein, J. O., & Marcy, S. M. (1995). Bacterial sepsis and meningitis. In J. S. Remington & J. O. Klein (Eds.), *Infectious diseases of the fetus & newborn infant* (4th ed., pp. 835–890). Philadelphia: Saunders.

Klein, J. O., & Remington, J. S. (1995). Current concepts of infections of the fetus and newborn infant. In J. S. Remington & J. O. Klein (Eds.), *Infectious diseases of the fetus & newborn infant* (4th ed., pp. 1–19). Philadelphia: Saunders.

Lott, J. W., Nelson, K., Fahrner, R., & Kenner, C. (1998). Assessment and management of immunologic dysfunction. In C. Kenner, J. W. Lott, & A. A. Flandermeyer (Eds.), *Comprehensive neonatal nursing, a physiologic perspective* (2nd ed., pp. 496–519). Philadelphia: Saunders.

Ludwig, M. A., Marecki, M., Wooldridge, P. J., & Sheman, L. M. (1996). Neonatal nurses' knowledge of and attitudes toward caring for cocaine-exposed infants and their mothers. *Journal of Perinatal Neonatal Nursing, 9*(4), 81–85.

MacMahon, J. R., Stevenson, D. K., & Oski, F. A. (1998a). Management of neonatal hyperbilirubinemia. In H. W. Taeusch & R. A. Ballard (Eds.), *Avery's diseases of the newborn* (7th ed., pp. 1033–1043). Philadelphia: Saunders.

MacMahon, J. R., Stevenson, D. K., & Oski, F. A. (1998b). Physiologic jaundice. In H. W. Taeusch & R. A. Ballard (Eds.), *Avery's diseases of the newborn* (7th ed., pp. 1003–1007). Philadelphia: Saunders.

Merenstein, G. B., Adams, K., & Weisman, L. E. (1998). Infection in the neonate. In G. B. Merenstein & S. L. Gardner (Eds.), *Handbook of neonatal intensive care* (4th ed., pp. 413–436). St. Louis: Mosby.

Miller, M. J., Fanaroff, A. A., Martin, R. J. (1997). Respiratory disorders in preterm and term infants. In A. A. Fanaroff & R. J. Martin (Eds.), *Neonatal-perinatal medicine* (6th ed., pp. 1040–1065). St. Louis: Mosby.

Mitchell, A., Steffenson, N., Hogan, H., & Brooks, S. (1997). Neonatal group B streptococcal disease. *MCN: American Journal of Maternal/Child Nursing, 22*(5), 249–253.

Nash, P. (1996). Common neonatal complications. In K. R. Simpson & P. A. Creehan (Eds.), *AWHONN's perinatal nursing* (pp. 353–375). Philadelphia: Lippincott–Raven.

National Association of Neonatal Nurses. (1997). *Neonatal thermoregulation: Guidelines for practice.* Petaluma, CA: Author.

Peng, T. C. C., Gutcher, G. R., & Van Dorsten, J. P. (1996). A selective aggressive approach to the neonate exposed to meconium-stained amniotic fluid. *American Journal of Obstetrics and Gynecology, 175*(2), 296–303.

Philip, A. (1996). *Neonatology: A practical guide* (4th ed.). Philadelphia: Saunders.

Shermer, R. H. (1995). Group B streptococcus during the perinatal period. *Journal of Obstetric, Gynecologic, and Neonatal Nursing, 24*(6), 562–566.

Stamos, J. K., & Rowley, A. H. (1995). Timely diagnosis of congenital infections. *Pediatric Clinics of North America, 41*(5), 1017–1033.

Steinhorn, R. H., Millard, L. L., & Morin, F. C. (1995). Persistent pulmonary hypertension of the newborn. *Clinics in Perinatology, 22*(2), 405–428.

Strodtbeck, F. (1995). Viral infections of the newborn. *Journal of Obstetric, Gynecologic, and Neonatal Nursing, 24*(7), 659–667.

Suevo, D. M. (1997). The infant of the diabetic mother. *Neonatal Network, 16*(5), 25–33.

Tan, K. L. (1995). Comparison of the efficacy of fiberoptic and conventional phototherapy for neonatal hyperbilirubinemia. *Journal of Pediatrics, 125*(4), 607–612.

Tsang, R. C., DeMarini, S., & Rath, L. L. (1998). Fluids, electrolytes, vitamins, and trace minerals: Basis of ingestion, digestion, elimination, and metabolism. In C. Kenner, J. W. Lott, & A. A. Flandermeyer (Eds.), *Comprehensive neonatal nursing, a physiologic perspective* (2nd ed., pp. 336–353). Philadelphia: Saunders.

Tyrala, E. E. (1996). The infant of the diabetic mother. *Obstetric Clinics of North America, 23*(1), 221–241.

Wiswell, T. E., & Bent, R. C. (1998). Meconium-stained amniotic fluid and the meconium aspiration syndrome. *Pediatric Clinics of North America, 45*(3), 511–529.

Wolach, B. (1997). Neonatal sepsis: Pathogenesis and supportive therapy. *Seminars in Perinatology, 21*(1), 28–38.

Zahka, K. G., & Patel, C. R. (1997). Cardiovascular problems of the neonate. In A. A. Fanaroff & R. J. Martin, *Neonatal-perinatal medicine* (6th ed., pp. 1158–1167). St. Louis: Mosby.

31

Women's Health Care

LEARNING OBJECTIVES

After studying this chapter, you should be able to:

■ Explain examinations and various screening procedures that are recommended to maintain the health of women.

■ Define four benign disorders of the breast, relate them to expected age of onset, and describe the diagnostic procedures used to rule out cancer of the breast.

■ Describe the incidence, risks, pathophysiology, management, and nursing considerations of malignant tumors of the breast.

■ Discuss the four most common menstrual cycle disorders.

■ Explain nursing considerations for women who experience premenstrual syndrome.

■ Discuss procedures, possible complications, and follow-up care related to induced abortion.

■ Describe the physical and psychological changes associated with menopause and the risks versus benefits of hormone replacement therapy.

■ Discuss preventive measures for osteoporosis.

■ Describe the causes, treatments, and nursing considerations for the major disorders associated with pelvic relaxation.

■ Discuss the signs and symptoms, management, and nursing considerations for the most common benign and malignant disorders of the reproductive tract.

■ Describe care of the woman with an infectious disorder of the reproductive tract, including candidiasis, sexually transmissible diseases, pelvic inflammatory disease, and toxic shock syndrome.

DEFINITIONS

adjuvant therapy Additional treatment that increases or enhances the action of the primary treatment.

adnexa Accessory organs of the uterus, such as the fallopian tubes and ovaries.

amenorrhea Absence of menstruation. Primary amenorrhea is a delay of the first menstruation. Secondary amenorrhea is cessation of menstruation after its initiation.

atrophic vaginitis Inflammation that occurs when the vagina becomes dry and fragile, usually as a result of estrogen deficit after menopause.

autogenous graft Tissue moved from one part of the body to another part of the same person's body.

axillary tail Wedge of tissue extending from the breast into the axilla (also called the tail of Spence).

carcinoma in situ Malignant neoplasm in surface tissue that has not extended into deeper tissue.

climacteric Endocrine, body, and psychic changes occurring at the end of a woman's reproductive cycle. Also informally called *menopause*.

colposcopy Examination of the vaginal and cervical tissue with a colposcope for magnification of cells.

condyloma A wartlike growth of the skin seen on the external genitalia, in the vagina, on the cervix, or near the anus. Condyloma may be caused by human papillomavirus (condyloma acuminatum) or by syphilis (condyloma latum).

cryotherapy Destruction of tissue using extreme cold.

cystocele Prolapse of the urinary bladder through the anterior vaginal wall.

dysmenorrhea Painful menstruation.

dyspareunia Difficult or painful coitus in women.

dysplasia Abnormal development of tissue.

dysuria Painful urination, often associated with urinary tract infection.

endometrial hyperplasia Excessive proliferation of normal cells of the uterine lining; may be due to administration of estrogen during the postmenopausal period.

endometriosis Presence of tissue resembling the endometrium outside the uterine cavity.

laparoscopy Insertion of an illuminated tube into the abdominal cavity to see contents, locate bleeding, and perform surgical procedures.

laparotomy Incision through the abdominal wall to examine the abdominal or pelvic organs.

mammogram Study of breast tissue using very-low-dose radiography; primary tool in the diagnosis of breast tumors.

menarche Onset of menstruation; average age is 12.8 years.

menometrorrhagia Uterine bleeding that is irregular in frequency and excessive in amount.

menopause Permanent cessation of menstruation during the climacteric.

menorrhagia Excessive bleeding at the time of menstruation in duration, amount of blood lost, or both.

metrorrhagia Bleeding from the uterus at any time other than during the menstrual period.

osteoporosis Increased spaces (porosity) in bone; process greatly accelerates following menopause.

peau d'orange Dimpled skin condition that resembles an orange; associated with lymphatic edema and often seen over the area of breast cancer.

rectocele Herniation (protrusion) of the rectum through the posterior vaginal wall.

toxic shock syndrome Rare, potentially fatal disorder caused by toxin produced by *Staphylococcus aureus*; has been associated with improper use of tampons.

Nurses have an important role in primary and preventive care of women as it relates to routine assessments, screening procedures, and management of specific health concerns. The nurse acts as educator and advocate for women. Nurses explain screening and diagnostic procedures, clarify options so that women can make informed decisions about care, and provide support to women when they experience disruptions in their health.

Health Maintenance

Health maintenance refers to measures that can be taken to prevent or to detect specific diseases. Unfortunately, many women do not take advantage of recommended health maintenance procedures. Some seek care only when they have a problem. For others, the only health care they receive comes from a gynecologist or nurse practitioner. Therefore, it is important that those who provide health care for women are familiar with principles of screening and counseling in areas that are not traditionally associated with gynecology, such as assessing risk factors for colon cancer and heart disease.

Health History

The health history is most important in the determination of risk factors for a variety of conditions. The focus of a health history depends on the woman's age, but some topics need to be discussed with all women. Table 31–1 provides a summary of information that should be obtained.

Family history is essential to assess risk profiles. History on hyperlipidemia, heart disease, osteoporosis, and thyroid disease indicates which screening tests and examinations are needed. A list of family members who have had cancer and their ages when it was discovered provides important information about the risk of cancer, particularly breast and colon cancer. A family history of heart disease is especially important when the woman is postmenopausal because estrogen, which protects against coronary artery disease, decreases after menopause.

Physical Assessment

A thorough physical examination is necessary to detect general health problems. Vital signs and weight are measured at each visit. Height is taken at the initial examination and yearly after that. Loss of height and abnormal curvature of the vertebral column (dorsal kyphosis or scoliosis) are important observations in evaluating osteoporosis in the postmenopausal woman.

The heart is auscultated at the initial visit to determine whether the rate and rhythm are normal and to detect heart murmurs. The extremities are observed for varicosities or edema, and pedal pulses are palpated. Palpation of the abdomen for tenderness, masses, or distension is an important part of the physical examination.

Additional assessments are necessary if the woman is in a high-risk group. For instance, if she has a family history of diabetes mellitus, a fasting glucose test may be indicated. If she has a history of multiple sexual partners or a sexual partner with multiple contacts, she may require testing for sexually transmissible diseases.

Preventive Counseling

Physical examination provides an excellent opportunity to counsel women about preventive care. Major preventable problems are obesity, inactivity, and smoking. Approximately one-fifth of the women in the United States are obese (American College of Obstetricians and Gynecolo-

---

TABLE 31–1

Health History

Personal History

Demographic data (name, age, marital status)
Reason for seeking medical care (chief complaint)
Current and past state of health, previous surgeries
Appetite, dietary intake
Exercise pattern
Habits (smoking, use of alcohol, drugs), allergies
Sleep and rest patterns
Patterns of elimination (current or chronic problems)
Degree of stress and stress management techniques

Sexual History

Sexual activity (one partner, multiple partners, age when first sexually active)
Method of contraception (satisfaction with method, adverse reactions)
Knowledge/practice of measures to protect self from sexually transmissible diseases

Menstrual History

Age of menarche
Regularity, duration of menstrual cycle
Menstrual discomfort

Obstetric History

Gravida, para, length of gestation, weight of infant at birth
Labor experience and method of delivery

Family History

Cardiovascular problems (anemia, hypertension, clotting disorders, stroke, heart attacks)
Cancer (breast, uterine, ovarian, bowel, lung)
Osteoporosis

Psychosocial History

Primary language, additional languages spoken or understood
Marital status, employment, occupation, education (relevant to determine financial, social, and emotional support)

gists [ACOG], 1996). Obesity is associated with diabetes and hypertension. Inactivity is associated with osteoporosis, elevated levels of cholesterol, and coronary artery disease. Cigarette smoking is on the rise in young women, and smoking increases the risk for a wide variety of diseases, including cardiovascular problems and cancer. Counseling regarding diet should be offered, and positive behaviors, such as exercise, should be reinforced. Use of latex condoms provides some protection against transmission of viruses, such as human immunodeficiency virus (HIV) and human papillomavirus (HPV), which is strongly implicated as a risk factor for cervical cancer.

The history or physical examination may indicate other areas for which counseling would be beneficial. These include the dangers of malignant melanoma with repeated exposure to ultraviolet rays of the sun. In addition, the health risks associated with alcohol and other substance abuse may be particularly important for some women.

Screening Procedures

Screening procedures are important because early diagnosis allows early treatment while the pathologic process is still treatable. A variety of screening procedures are recom-

---

TABLE 31–2

Screening Procedures

Procedure	Purpose
Breast self-examination	To assess monthly for breast changes or masses that might indicate breast tumors
Clinical breast examination	To detect masses that women might miss
Mammography Every 1–2 y from 40–49 y, every 1 y over 50 y (ACOG, 1996) Annually (American Cancer Society, 1998)	To detect breast lumps before they become palpable, to promote long-term survival
Vulvar self-examination	To detect signs of precancerous conditions or infections
Pelvic examination	To confirm that no disease exists, or for early detection if disease does exist
Papanicolaou test	To detect abnormal cervical cytology as early as possible
Rectal examination	To check for hemorrhoids and lesions and to evaluate sphincter control
Fecal occult blood test	To detect blood in stool, an early sign of colon cancer
Urinalysis	To screen for diabetes and urinary infections

Additional Procedures Based on Risk Factors

Procedure	Risk Factors
STD testing	Multiple sexual partners of the woman or her partner, history of STDs
HIV testing	Seeking treatment for STDs, intravenous drug use, sexual partner who is HIV positive or bisexual or injects drugs, recurrent or persistent episodes of STDs such as candidiasis and herpes
Lipid profile	Diabetes, smoking, no estrogen use after menopause, family history of high cholesterol or coronary artery disease
Fasting glucose test	Obesity, history of gestational diabetes, family history of diabetes
Rubella antibodies	To assess immunity to rubella
Thyroid-stimulating hormone	Signs or strong family history of thyroid disease
Transvaginal ultrasound examination or blood test for CA 125	Family history of ovarian cancer
Sigmoidoscopy or colonoscopy	Family history of bowel cancer or age >50 y

Abbreviations: STD, sexually transmissible disease; HIV, human immunodeficiency virus.

How to Perform Breast Self-Examination

- Observe your breasts in a mirror while your arms are at your sides, then raised above your head; while your hands are pressed against your hips; and while you are bending forward. Look for a change in shape or color, dimpling of the skin, and any nipple changes or discharge.

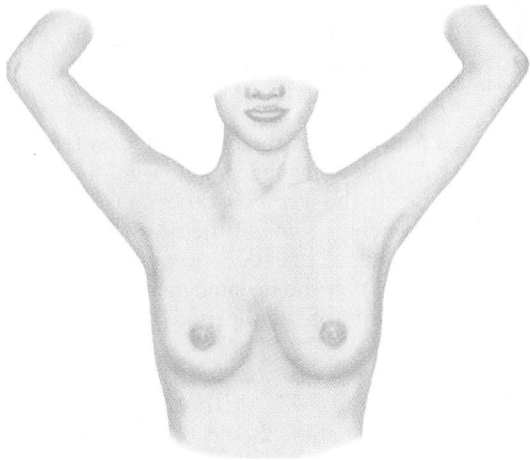

- Lie down. Flatten your right breast by placing a pillow under your right shoulder. If your breasts are large, lie on your left side with the right shoulder rotated back toward the bed while you examine the outer half of your right breast.

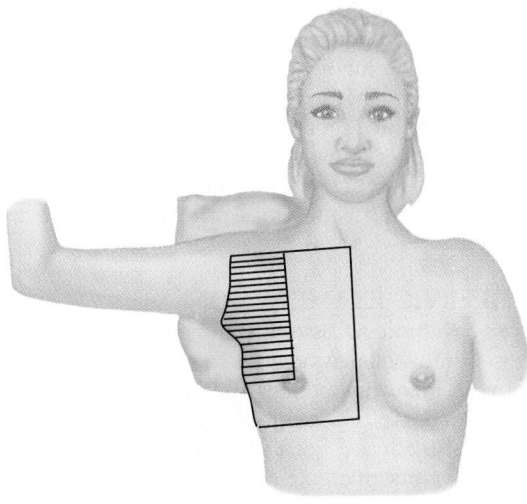

- Use the sensitive pads of the middle three fingers on your left hand and a circular motion to feel for lumps or changes in the breast tissue.
- Press firmly enough to distinguish different breast textures.
- Completely palpate, or feel, all parts of the breast and chest area, as shown. Most breast cancers occur in the upper outer quarter of the breast.

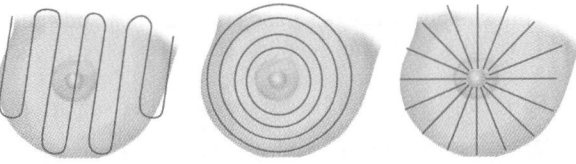

- Examine your breasts by beginning at the middle of the armpit and moving down to below the breast in a vertical strip. Then move your fingers a finger's width toward the center and palpate a vertical strip up to the collar bone. Continue until you have covered all areas of the breast.
- Alternative patterns are to palpate in overlapping circles around the breast or in wedges.
- Examine the area under your armpit with your arm relaxed at your side.
- When you have completely examined your right breast, examine the left breast. Compare what you feel in one breast with the other.
- You may also want to examine your breasts while bathing, when the skin is wet and lumps may be easily palpated.

mended for all women, including three screening procedures for early detection of breast cancer as well as vulvar self-examination and screening for cervical cancer. Table 31–2 provides a summary of screening procedures.

BREAST SELF-EXAMINATION
Most breast cancers are discovered by the woman herself. Yet, only approximately half of all women examine their breasts each month. Breast self-examination (BSE) should be performed monthly by all women older than 20 years of age. Women should perform BSE approximately 1 week

after the onset of menses, when hormonal influences on the breasts are at a low level. If the woman no longer menstruates, she may choose a day that is easy to remember and perform the test on that day every month. An example is the first day of the month.

CLINICAL BREAST EXAMINATION
Clinical breast examination (performed by a health care professional) may detect questionable areas that the woman misses during BSE. It should be performed every 3 years for women aged 20 to 40 years and yearly for those older than

40 years. The examination includes inspection and palpation.

Inspection. Follow these steps for breast inspection:

1. While the woman is in an upright position, the examiner inspects the breasts for size, symmetry, color, and skin changes. The nipples and areola are inspected for differences in size and color, unilateral retraction of a nipple, and asymmetric nipple direction, which may indicate an underlying tumor.
2. The woman raises her hands above her head, and the examiner inspects the sides and underneath portions of the breast for asymmetry and differences in color.
3. The woman places her hands on her hips and presses down to reveal skin dimpling or masses.

Palpation. Follow these steps for breast palpation:

1. With the woman in an upright position and while the arm is at the side and relaxed, each axilla is carefully palpated for enlarged or tender lymph nodes.
2. The woman lies in a supine position for palpation of the breasts. A small pillow or folded towel is placed under the shoulder, and the arm is placed at a 90-degree angle to stretch the tissue and thus flatten the breast. The examiner uses the flat part of the first three fingers to palpate the breast, rotating the fingers against the chest wall. Tissue that extends into the axilla, the tail of Spence, should also be palpated. The procedure is repeated on the opposite side. Normal breast tissue is described as firm, lumpy, nodular, tender, and thickened. Abnormal breast tissue is often likened to a raisin, watermelon seed, or grape. If a suspicious area is found, follow-up by mammography is recommended.
3. The nipples are compressed to detect the presence of discharge. A sample of any discharge should be collected for culture and examination of cells.

MAMMOGRAPHY

Mammography may be used either to screen for cancer or to assist in the diagnosis of a palpable mass in the breast. Mammography is the only screening tool that can detect breast lumps long before they are large enough to be palpated. This procedure allows early diagnosis and treatment and thus increases the chance of long-term survival.

The American Cancer Society (1999) recommends yearly mammography for women older than 40 years of age. Women at high risk for breast cancer may need earlier or more frequent evaluation. Despite the known value of mammography, many women have never had a mammogram. Reasons for this include expense, fear that x-ray exposure will cause cancer, fear of pain, and reluctance to hear "bad news."

Nurses provide information and reassurance to help the woman overcome her objections to the use of this valuable screening tool. Although mammography is relatively expensive, it is often covered by health insurance, and screening mammograms are frequently offered by the community at low cost. It is important to acknowledge that some discomfort occurs when the breast is compressed between two plates while the radiograph is taken. One measure that reduces discomfort is scheduling the mammography after a

- - - - - - - - - - -
Risk Factors for Breast Cancer

Female
Age older than 50 years
History of breast cancer
Family history (mother, sister, daughter)
Previous uterine, ovarian, or colon cancer
Nulliparity or first term pregnancy after 35 years
Early menarche (<12 years), late menopause (>55 years)
Lifestyle factors: high intake of dietary fat, excessive consumption of alcohol, smoking

menstrual period, when the breasts are less tender. Knowledge that the risk of mammography is minimal to nonexistent because of the very-low-dose x-rays used may help women to overcome some of their fear.

No screening test is 100% accurate. Therefore, nurses must emphasize that the mammogram should be performed *along with* monthly BSE and periodic clinical breast examinations.

VULVAR SELF-EXAMINATION

Vulvar self-examination should be performed monthly by all women older than 18 and by those younger than 18 years of age who are sexually active. Vulvar self-examination is visual inspection and palpation of the female external genitalia to detect signs of precancerous conditions or infections.

The woman is instructed to sit in a well-lighted area and to use a hand-held mirror to see the external genitalia. She is taught to examine the vulva in a systematic manner, starting at the mons pubis and progressing to the clitoris, labia minora, labia majora, perineum, and anus. Palpation of the vulvar area should accompany visual inspection. New moles, warts or growths of any kind, ulcers, sores, changes in skin color, or areas of inflammation or itching should be reported to the woman's health care provider as soon as possible.

PELVIC EXAMINATION

Every gynecologic assessment includes a pelvic examination. The woman is advised to schedule the examination between menstrual periods and not to douche or have sexual intercourse for at least 48 hours before the examination. She is also advised not to use vaginal medications, sprays, or deodorants that might interfere with interpretation of cytology specimens that are collected.

Before the examination, the procedure is carefully explained and the woman empties her bladder. She is placed in a lithotomy position, with a pillow under her head. If she wishes, she may assume a semisitting position and use a hand mirror so that she can observe the external genitalia and the examination. She is draped so that only the parts being examined are exposed.

Equipment needed for the examination includes gloves, speculum, slides, cotton swabs, a fixative agent, and a cytobrush and spatula for obtaining material for the Papanicolaou (Pap) smear. A stool specimen may be obtained by the examiner during the rectal examination, and a slide for this specimen should also be available.

External Organs. The pelvic examination is conducted systematically and gently. The external organs are scrutinized for the degree of development or atrophy of the labia, the distribution of hair, and the character of the hymen. Any cysts, tumors, or inflammation of Bartholin's glands are noted. The urinary meatus and Skene's glands are inspected for purulent discharge. Perineal scarring due to childbirth is noted.

Speculum Examination. A bivalve speculum of the appropriate size is used to inspect the vagina and cervix. The speculum is warmed with tap water and then gently inserted into the vagina. No other lubrication is used because it interferes with accurate cytology results. The size, shape, and color of the cervix are noted. A sample is taken for the Pap test. In addition, a sample of any unusual discharge is obtained for microscopic examination or culture.

Bimanual Examination. The bimanual examination provides information about the uterus, fallopian tubes, and ovaries. The labia are separated, and the gloved, lubricated index finger and middle finger of the examiner's nondominant hand are inserted into the vaginal introitus.

The cervix is palpated for consistency, size, and tenderness to motion. The uterus is evaluated by placing the dominant hand on the abdomen with the fingers pressing gently just above the symphysis pubis so that the uterus can be felt between the examining fingers of both hands. The size, configuration, consistency, and motility of the uterus are evaluated (Fig. 31–1).

The ovaries are palpated between the fingers of both hands. Because ovaries atrophy after menopause, it is often impossible to palpate the ovaries of a postmenopausal woman.

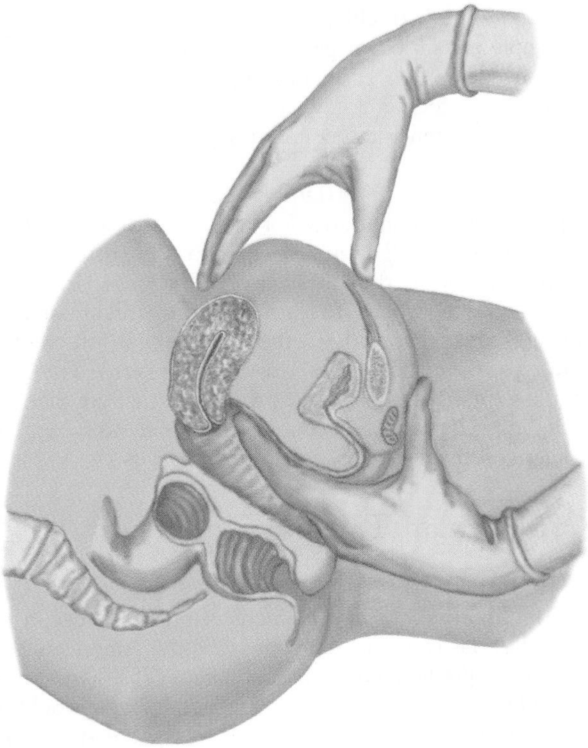

THE PAPANICOLAOU TEST

Purpose. Changes occur in cells of the cervix before cervical cancer develops. Cervical cytology, or the Pap test, is the most useful procedure for detecting precancerous and cancerous cells that may be shed by the cervix. The Pap test (also called Pap smear) prevents at least 70% of cervical cancers by finding premalignant changes that can be treated before they become malignant (Policar, 1998).

Procedure. A speculum is inserted into the vagina and excess cervical mucus is wiped away. Samples of the superficial layers of the cervix and endocervix are obtained with a spatula or a cytobrush.

Most lesions develop at the squamocolumnar junction (the border where developing squamous tissue meets the immature columnar epithelium). The cytobrush is most effective in obtaining an adequate specimen from this site, particularly in postmenopausal women, in whom the squamocolumnar junction recedes into the endocervix. The material is placed on slides that are then sprayed with or immersed in a fixative solution before being sent to the laboratory for analysis.

Classification of Cervical Cytology. Cervical cytology findings are reported using the Bethesda system. It consists of three elements: (1) a statement of specimen adequacy, (2) a general categorization (normal or abnormal), and (3) a descriptive diagnosis regarding abnormal cytology.

The terminology for epithelial cell abnormalities includes the following categories:

- Atypical squamous cells of undetermined significance (ASCUS): An immediate colposcopy may be recommended or follow-up Pap tests may be done every 4 to 6 months until three normal results are obtained or a second ASCUS result requires colposcopy.
- Squamous intraepithelial lesion (SIL), which is subdivided into (1) low-grade SIL (including cellular changes of HPV) and (2) high-grade SIL (previously categorized as carcinoma in situ). Most low-grade SIL regresses or remains the same for long periods, but some slowly progresses to malignancy. Follow-up is the same as for ASCUS results. Women with high-grade SIL should have a colposcopy.
- Squamous cell cancer: Treatment may include colposcopy, biopsy, conization, or hysterectomy, depending on the extent of involvement.

RECTAL EXAMINATION

The anus is inspected for hemorrhoids, inflammation, and lesions. The lubricated index finger is gently inserted, and sphincter tone is noted. A slide may be prepared to test for the presence of occult blood in stool.

Fecal occult blood testing is a useful screening measure for colorectal cancer. Special instructions are necessary to prevent false test results when materials for fecal occult blood testing are sent home with the woman. She should be instructed to do the following:

- Avoid aspirin and nonsteroidal anti-inflammatory drugs (NSAIDs) such as ibuprofen or naproxen for at least 7 days before collecting the specimen.

FIGURE 31–1

Bimanual palpation provides information about the uterus, fallopian tubes, and ovaries.

- Avoid red meat, raw fruits and vegetables, horseradish, and vitamin C for 72 hours before testing.
- Collect a specimen from three consecutive stools.
- Return slides as directed within 4 to 6 days after the specimens are collected.

Breast Disorders

Benign Disorders of the Breast

There are four relatively common benign disorders of the breast. The risk for each disorder is related to a specific age.

FIBROADENOMA

Fibroadenomas are the most common benign tumors of the breast and are most common during the teenage years and the twenties. Fibroadenomas are composed of both fibrous and glandular tissue. They are felt as firm, rubbery, freely mobile nodules that may or may not be tender when palpated. Fibroadenomas do not change during the menstrual cycle. They are usually located in the upper, outer quadrant of the breast, and more than one may be present.

Treatment may involve careful observation for a few months, or the tumor may be excised and the specimen analyzed to rule out malignancy.

FIBROCYSTIC BREAST CHANGES

Fibrocystic breast changes, also called mammary dysplasia, are the most common breast disorders during the reproductive years. Fibrosis, or thickening of the normal breast tissue, occurs in the early stages. Cysts form in the latter stages and are felt as multiple, smooth, well-delineated nodules.

The most common symptoms of fibrocystic changes are pain and tenderness. The pain is often bilateral and particularly noticeable during the premenstrual phase of the normal cycle. Women often improve during pregnancy and lactation because of the hormonal changes.

Fibrocystic breast changes are not a disease but represent the way a woman's breasts respond to normal monthly hormonal fluctuation. Fine-needle aspiration may be performed to study cells in the aspirate. Open biopsy is necessary if the fluid is bloody or if a residual mass remains after aspiration. Medical treatment is rare because side effects of the drugs may be more distressing than the breast discomfort. If drugs are administered, they may include progesterone, tamoxifen (Nolvodex; an antiestrogen), bromocriptine (Parlodel), or, in severe cases, danazol (Danocrine) (Droegemueller, 1997a).

Although controversy exists about whether caffeine contributes to the development of fibrocystic breast changes, some physicians and nurse practitioners recommend limiting consumption of tea, coffee, colas, and chocolate. Some women also benefit from restricting sodium intake to reduce fluid retention the week before menstruation starts, when symptoms are often most acute.

DUCTAL ECTASIA

Ductal ectasia usually occurs as the woman approaches menopause. It is characterized by dilation of the collecting ducts, which become distended and filled with cellular debris. This initiates an inflammatory process resulting in a mass that feels firm and irregular, enlarged axillary nodes, nipple retraction, pain, and discharge that is green, brown, or black. These signs and symptoms are similar to those of breast cancer, and accurate diagnosis is vital. Although ductal ectasia is benign, the ducts may be excised to prevent further discharge.

INTRADUCTAL PAPILLOMA

Intraductal papilloma develops most often just before or during menopause. It occurs when papillomas (small elevations or protuberances) develop in the epithelium of the ducts of the breasts. As the papilloma grows, it causes trauma and erosion within the ducts that result in serous or serosanguineous discharge from the nipple. Treatment consists of excision of the mass and ductal area, plus analysis of nipple discharge to rule out a malignant tumor.

DIAGNOSTIC EVALUATION

When a lesion or lump is discovered in the breast, the physician must determine if it is benign or malignant. Ultrasound examination can be used to differentiate fluid-filled cysts from solid tissue that is potentially malignant. Needle aspiration biopsy can be performed to remove fluid from suspected cysts for analysis of the cells. Surgical biopsy is performed under these conditions:

- Bloody fluid removed from a cyst on aspiration
- Failure of the mass to disappear completely after fluid aspiration
- Recurrence of the cyst after one or two aspirations
- Solid dominant mass not diagnosed as fibroadenoma
- Bloody nipple discharge
- Nipple ulceration or persistent crusting
- Skin edema and erythema suspicious for inflammatory breast carcinoma
- Suspect mammography findings (ACOG, 1996)

NURSING CONSIDERATIONS

It is of primary importance for the nurse to acknowledge the anxiety that all women feel when a breast disorder is discovered and as they await a final diagnosis. It may be helpful for some women to learn that 90% of all breast disorders are benign. For others, the most helpful intervention is to encourage them to express their concerns. The nurse should explain the diagnostic procedures that are planned, including what the procedures entail and how long the woman will have to wait to learn the results.

Malignant Tumors of the Breast

INCIDENCE

The lifetime risk for development of breast cancer in the United States is one in eight. In 1999, the American Cancer Society predicted that approximately 175,000 new cases would be diagnosed that year, and 43,700 deaths would occur from cancer of the breast. Cancer of the breast is second only to lung cancer as a cause of death from cancer among women.

The incidence of breast cancer is approximately five times higher in the United States and northern Europe than in Japan (Prout, 1995). Possible reasons for the high incidence in these areas—high per capita consumption of dietary fat and smoking—are being studied.

PREDISPOSING FACTORS

Although the actual cause of breast cancer remains unknown, several factors are known to increase the risk for the development of breast cancer (see p. 782). In addition, two genes (BRCA1 and BRCA2) thought to be responsible for most cases of familial breast cancer have been identified.

Although risk factors are important, 80% of women with breast cancer have none of the identified risk factors (Marchant, 1997a). Therefore, it is important that all women, not only those at "high risk," take advantage of available screening procedures.

PATHOPHYSIOLOGY

Although the rate of growth varies, the average breast cancer doubles in diameter every 300 days, taking 6 to 8 years to reach 1 cm. In approximately another year, the mass reaches 2 cm, the size most common when a woman discovers the lump during regular BSE (Droegemueller, 1997a).

The woman may have a ductal or lobular carcinoma in situ, a precancerous lesion that may progress to invasive carcinoma if untreated. The most common breast cancer is infiltrating ductal carcinoma. When it penetrates the duct into surrounding tissue, it is classified as invasive. Growth occurs in irregular patterns and invades the lymphatic channels, eventually causing lymphatic edema and the dimpling of the skin that resembles an orange peel (peau d'orange).

Cancer cells are carried by the lymph channels to the lymph nodes, and metastasis occurs when the cells are spread by both blood and lymph systems. The most common sites of metastasis are the lungs, liver, and bones.

MANIFESTATIONS

When breast cancer becomes palpable, the woman or caregiver feels a breast lump, thickening, or distortion. There may be dimpling, nipple retraction, or changes in the skin or shape of the breast. Most breast pain is benign. Changes on the mammogram may occur before the cancer is palpable.

STAGING

Although confirmation of malignancy is the first step in evaluating the woman with cancer, staging is necessary to understand the severity of the cancer. Staging is generally based on the TNM (tumor, node, metastasis) system used to describe the cancer's anatomic extent. Stages of breast cancer progress from stage 1, indicating a small tumor without lymphatic involvement or metastases, to stage 4, which indicates spread to lymph nodes and metastases to other organs. The stages are often used to determine treatment, and they are useful guides to prognosis. The type of cancer cell, the presence of hormone receptors, and the proliferative rate of the breast cancer cells are also important factors in the rate of recurrence.

THERAPEUTIC MANAGEMENT

The woman with breast cancer must choose from a variety of treatments offered. A combination of surgical excision and adjuvant therapy is often recommended.

Surgical Treatment. The surgical procedure depends on the type, stage, and location of the disease. The most common surgeries are the following:

- *Breast conservation treatment,* which involves wide local excision (sometimes called lumpectomy) of the tumor to microscopically clear margins. The excision can be performed without major cosmetic deformity. Some axillary lymph nodes are usually removed to rule out spread of the disease. In most instances, radiation therapy is required to complete the treatment.
- *Simple mastectomy,* which is removal of the entire breast. Axillary dissection is omitted, although some lymph nodes may be removed for staging purposes. Simple mastectomy is recommended for recurrence after partial mastectomy and for selected cases in which prophylactic removal of the opposite breast is considered. It is also performed for elderly women who are poor operative risks and in whom no axillary involvement or distant disease is present (Marchant, 1997b).
- *Modified radical mastectomy,* which involves removal of breast tissue, axillary nodes, and some chest muscles. The pectoralis major and minor muscles, however, are preserved. This surgical procedure is recommended when a large primary lesion is found in a relatively small breast, there are contraindications to radiation therapy, or there is evidence of multifocal disease (ACOG, 1996).

Adjuvant Therapy. Adjuvant therapy is supportive or additional therapy that may be recommended after the surgical procedure. Radiation, chemotherapy, and hormone therapy are the recommended adjuvant therapies. The decision about whether to use adjuvant therapy is based on the woman's age, the stage of the disease, the woman's preference, and the hormone receptor status of the lesion.

Radiation and chemotherapy are known to improve the chance of long-term survival after surgery. Because some tumors are estrogen receptor positive, meaning that their growth is stimulated by estrogen, estrogen blocking medications are administered. Tamoxifen is the hormone therapy most recommended. Tamoxifen blocks estrogen by binding to estrogen receptors, thereby suppressing tumor growth by reducing the effects of estrogen. The drug has been approved as a method of prevention for women who do not have breast cancer but are at very high risk for the disease.

Side effects of tamoxifen vary from woman to woman. The most commonly mentioned side effects are hot flashes, vaginal dryness or increased vaginal discharge, nausea, and anorexia. Women are at increased risk of endometrial cancer, deep vein thrombosis, and pulmonary embolism when taking tamoxifen. All side effects should be discussed with the woman before tamoxifen is administered so she can weigh the risks against the benefits and make an informed decision.

Breast Reconstruction. *Timing.* Breast reconstruction has become an integral part of the treatment of breast cancer, and the timing of reconstruction should be discussed with the woman before surgical treatment. A woman may choose immediate reconstruction because facing breast cancer and the loss of her breast simultaneously is overwhelming. Other women may delay reconstruction to have time to learn about the methods of reconstruction, to heal from the mastectomy, and to consider the extent of the disease and the side effects associated with adjuvant therapy.

Method. A variety of methods of breast reconstruction are available. The *tissue expansion method* is the most popular postmastectomy reconstruction (Versaci, 1997). The method uses an empty silicone prosthesis fitted with a valve that can be accessed by percutaneous needle puncture. The bag is filled with saline in small increments to expand the tissue slowly. When the desired volume is attained, the incision is reopened and the expander exchanged for the appropriate implant. In newer models, only the valve must be removed, and the expander serves as the permanent implant.

Autogenous grafts have been successfully used for reconstruction. They are recommended for women who have received radiation therapy. Implants do not do well in such wounds, whereas tissue transfers work well because the flaps carry their own blood supply. The graft is often taken from the abdomen and includes muscle and cutaneous tissue.

Nipple-Areola Reconstruction. The nipple can be reconstructed from tissue taken from the opposite nipple, from skin that covers the prosthesis mound, or from other body tissue. After the nipple has been reconstructed, many surgeons inject pigment into the area to create an areola.

PSYCHOSOCIAL CONSEQUENCES OF BREAST CANCER

The time from discovery to treatment of breast cancer is the most stressful time for many women. Factors that contribute to presurgery distress include a sense of uncertainty, inadequate information, the need to make difficult treatment decisions, and scheduling problems. Treatment usually involves consultations with one or more specialists, including a surgeon, a radiotherapist, a plastic surgeon, and a medical oncologist. When there are scheduling difficulties or conflicting opinions expressed by the health care team, the woman feels frustrated and confused.

Concerns frequently expressed during treatment for breast cancer include fear of recurrence and death, uncertainty about the quality of life, changes in body image, the effect on sexuality, and side effects of recommended therapy. For many women, the knowledge that they will lose their hair as a result of chemotherapy creates one of the most difficult situations in therapy.

Breast cancer can have psychological consequences not only for women but also for their significant others. Difficulties reported include sleep disturbances, eating disorders, and problems with work responsibilities. There may be strain on the marital relationship, primarily in the areas of sexual relations and communication about matters related to the illness. Women and their partners sometimes differ in regard to how much they want to discuss the illness. Some women have a great need to discuss their diagnosis, treatment, and fears of recurrence. Other women and many men view discussion of such fears as negative thinking that delays adjustment.

NURSING CONSIDERATIONS

The woman who is diagnosed with breast cancer depends on nurses for emotional support and accurate information.

They must allow time for the woman to express her feelings and convey a sense of empathic understanding by quiet presence, touch, and close attention to the woman's concerns. Many women feel that they have lost control and that their lives have been taken over by cancer and the recommended treatment. They may have concerns about family relationships and how their sexual partner will respond. Each woman should be allowed to express her fears and worries. Nurses must provide time and demonstrate genuine interest in the woman's concerns.

The anxiety that most women experience is reduced when procedures and care are clearly understood. Preoperative teaching should include significant others, to increase their ability to support the woman. Teaching should include the length of the hospital stay and what will happen during that time. The nurse should describe the dressings, drainage tubes, and appearance of the incision. Lymphedema of the arm on the same side as the mastectomy is possible because of blocked lymphatic vessels. Specific exercises such as arm lifts and pulley exercises may be necessary.

Discharge teaching focuses on the need for follow-up care and treatment. Some areas of concern include how to minimize the risk of wound infection, side effects of adjuvant therapy, and signs and symptoms that should be reported to the physician. Most women also benefit from information about such groups as Reach to Recovery and Encore, which provide support, information, and guidance after mastectomy.

Using nursing diagnoses to plan and implement care could ensure that care is complete. Relevant diagnoses might include the following:

- Fear related to uncertain outcome
- Body Image Disturbance related to loss of breast and temporary loss of hair during chemotherapy
- Altered Family Processes related to illness of primary caregiver or lack of information about the course of the disease
- Altered Sexuality Patterns related to concern about altered body structure

Menstrual Cycle Disorders

Although most menstrual cycle disorders are benign, all require comprehensive gynecologic assessment. Nurses must be knowledgeable about underlying processes, diagnostic procedures, and expected treatment so they can provide client advocacy, education, and supportive counseling.

Amenorrhea

Amenorrhea is normal before menarche, during pregnancy, during the puerperium and lactation, and after menopause. Amenorrhea at other times is abnormal, and it is called either primary or secondary amenorrhea, depending on when it occurs.

PRIMARY AMENORRHEA

Primary amenorrhea is the failure to menstruate by age 16.5 years in girls after breast development or pubic and axillary hair appear, by age 14 years in girls with no secondary sexual characteristics, or within 2 years of breast or pubic hair development (Nelson, 1998).

Etiology. The most common cause for primary amenorrhea associated with absence of breast or pubic hair development is Turner's syndrome. This syndrome occurs when girls have only one normal X chromosome. When the secondary sex characteristics are present, the cause may be incomplete development of the uterus, ovaries, and fallopian tubes. Intrauterine exposure to diethylstilbesterol is associated with abnormal development of the uterus. Other causes may include hormonal imbalances, systemic disease, and hypothalamic–pituitary abnormalities that result in inadequate secretion of gonadotropins. It may also be due to excessive exercise, malnutrition, or eating disorders, such as anorexia nervosa and bulimia, that cause a decrease in ovarian hormones.

Therapeutic Management. The success of medical management depends on the cause. Counseling for eating disorders and reducing excessive exercise may prove helpful. Hormone therapy may establish normal menses if the cause is hormone imbalance. Some conditions cannot be successfully treated. For example, if the cause is reproductive tract or congenital anomalies, normal menses and fertility may not be possible, and psychological support becomes the most important therapy.

SECONDARY AMENORRHEA

Secondary amenorrhea is the cessation of menstruation for 6 months or more in a woman who has established a pattern of menstruation, or absence of menstruation for 12 months in women with oligomenorrhea (Schlaff & Kletzky, 1998). It may be due to a variety of causes, including systemic diseases such as diabetes mellitus, tuberculosis, hypothyroidism, or central nervous system lesions. Hormonal imbalances, strenuous aerobic exercise, poor nutrition, use of oral contraceptives, and ovarian tumors may also be the cause.

Assessment includes a thorough medical and obstetric history and laboratory testing of hormone levels, as well as questions about eating habits, history of dieting, and current exercise pattern. Women are also questioned about their use of drugs, such as hormonal contraceptives, phenothiazines, and antihypertensives, which can cause secondary amenorrhea.

Medical treatment aims at identifying and correcting the underlying cause. Pregnancy testing is mandatory for any sexually active woman, and medications that are potentially teratogenic must be withheld until pregnancy is ruled out. Hormone replacement therapy, ovulation stimulation, and periodic progesterone withdrawal often result in menstruation.

NURSING CONSIDERATIONS

Amenorrhea causes a great deal of concern for the young woman and her family, who may worry that it indicates a serious disease. Moreover, menstruation is a unique function of women, and absence of menstruation may provoke concerns about femininity and the ability to have children.

Teaching includes the importance of adequate nutrition and discouragement of rigorous dieting. The nurse should explain that, although exercise is beneficial, strenuous workouts or aerobic training can cause amenorrhea. The nurse also provides emotional support and explanation of proposed treatment.

Abnormal Uterine Bleeding

Menstruation is considered normal when bleeding occurs every 24 to 35 days and lasts for 2 to 7 days (Weiss, 1995). Abnormal bleeding can be defined as bleeding that occurs with abnormal frequency (metrorrhagia) or lasts an abnormal length of time or is excessive in amount (menorrhagia).

ETIOLOGY

The most common causes of abnormal bleeding fall into five basic categories:

1. Pregnancy complications, such as spontaneous abortion
2. Anatomic lesions, either benign or malignant, of the vagina, cervix, or uterus
3. Drug-induced bleeding, such as "breakthrough" bleeding that may occur in women who use hormonal contraceptives
4. Systemic disorders, such as diabetes mellitus, clotting disorders, and hypothyroidism
5. Failure to ovulate (dysfunctional uterine bleeding)

THERAPEUTIC MANAGEMENT

Medical treatment for abnormal bleeding depends on the cause. Medications include the use of progestin–estrogen combination oral contraceptives that allow a more stable endometrial lining to form. Prolonged menorrhagia may result in decreased hemoglobin, and the woman may need treatment for iron-deficiency anemia.

Surgical therapy may include dilation and curettage to remove polyps or to diagnose endometrial hyperplasia, which may be treated with progesterone. Hysterectomy is often performed if the uterus is enlarged as a result of fibroids or adenomyosis (benign invasive growth of the endometrium into the muscular layer of the uterus) and if the woman no longer wishes to bear children. Endometrial ablation with laser or electrocautery may be chosen to remove the endometrial lining permanently.

NURSING CONSIDERATIONS

Nurses are often able to encourage women to seek medical attention promptly when abnormal bleeding occurs. Nurses also help the woman keep a menstrual calendar to note when vaginal bleeding occurs, as well as the number of pads and tampons saturated each day. Finally, nurses must provide support for women who fear that irregular bleeding indicates a serious disease, such as cancer. It is unwise to offer false reassurance, but information about diagnostic procedures and treatment options may be helpful.

Pain Associated with the Menstrual Cycle

Cyclic pelvic pain must be distinguished from acute pelvic pain. Acute pelvic pain is sudden in onset, and it is not experienced with each menstrual cycle. It may indicate a serious disorder, such as ectopic pregnancy or appendicitis. On the other hand, cyclic pelvic pain occurs repetitively and predictably in a specific phase of the menstrual cycle.

The most common causes of cyclic pelvic pain are mittelschmerz, primary dysmenorrhea, and endometriosis.

MITTELSCHMERZ

Mittelschmerz ("middle pain") refers to pelvic pain that occurs midway between menstrual periods, or at the time of ovulation. The pain is due to growth of the dominant follicle in the ovary or rupture of the follicle and subsequent spillage of follicular fluid and blood into the peritoneal space. The pain is fairly sharp and is felt on the right or left side of the pelvis. It usually lasts from a few hours to 2 days, and slight vaginal bleeding may accompany the discomfort. Usually, explanation of the discomfort or mild analgesics is sufficient treatment.

PRIMARY DYSMENORRHEA

Primary dysmenorrhea refers to menstrual pain without an identified pathologic process. Commonly called *cramps*, primary dysmenorrhea affects at least half of all women and causes 10% to miss work or school (Somani, 1995).

Manifestations. The pain of dysmenorrhea begins within hours of the onset of menses and is spasmodic or colicky in nature. It is felt in the lower abdomen but often radiates to the lower back or down the legs. Primary dysmenorrhea occurs in ovulatory cycles, and it is most common in young, nulliparous women.

Etiology. One of the most confusing aspects of primary dysmenorrhea has been why it is experienced by some, but not all, women. It is now known that some women produce excessive endometrial prostaglandins during the late luteal phase of the menstrual cycle. The prostaglandins (particularly E_2 and $F_{2\alpha}$) diffuse into endometrial tissue and cause abnormal uterine muscle contractions, uterine ischemia, and hypoxia. This process accounts for the cramping uterine pain as well as symptoms that often accompany it, such as diarrhea, nausea, and vomiting.

Therapeutic Management. Oral contraceptives and NSAIDs provide marked relief for primary dysmenorrhea. Oral or injected contraceptives decrease the endometrial growth that occurs during the menstrual cycle and thus re-duce the production of endometrial prostaglandin. For women who do not wish to take hormonal contraceptives, NSAIDs such as ibuprofen (Motrin, Advil) and naproxen (Naprosyn, Anaprox) act as prostaglandin inhibitors to offer relief. To be effective, these must be taken before menses and the onset of cramps.

ENDOMETRIOSIS

Endometriosis occurs when endometrial tissue is present outside the uterus. It is estimated that over 15% of women have the disease (Moore, 1998).

Etiology. The cause of endometriosis remains unknown. One theory is that retrograde menstruation (reflux of menstrual flow through the fallopian tubes) causes endometrial cells to attach to nearby structures and proliferate, creating spots of endometrial tissue. Endometriosis may also represent an autoimmune process.

Pathophysiology. Endometrial tissue outside the uterus responds to stimulation from estrogen and progesterone in the same manner that tissue inside the uterus responds. That is, it grows and proliferates during the follicular and luteal phases of the cycle and then sloughs during menstruation.

The menstruation from endometriosis lesions, however, occurs in a closed cavity, which causes pressure and pain on adjacent tissue. In addition, prostaglandins secreted by the endometriosis lesions irritate nerve endings and stimulate uterine contractions that further increase pain. Moreover, cyclic bleeding into the pelvic cavity initiates chronic inflammation that may cause scarring and adhesions and make conception and implantation difficult. The most common sites of endometriosis lesions are illustrated in Figure 31–2.

Manifestations. The two major symptoms of endometriosis are cyclic pain and infertility. The pain of endometriosis differs from that of primary dysmenorrhea. Endometriosis pain is deep, unilateral or bilateral, and either sharp or dull. It is constant, as opposed to the spasmodic or colicky pain of primary dysmenorrhea. Dyspareunia (painful intercourse) is typical, particularly with deep penetration. Rectal pain is common, especially during defecation. Diar-

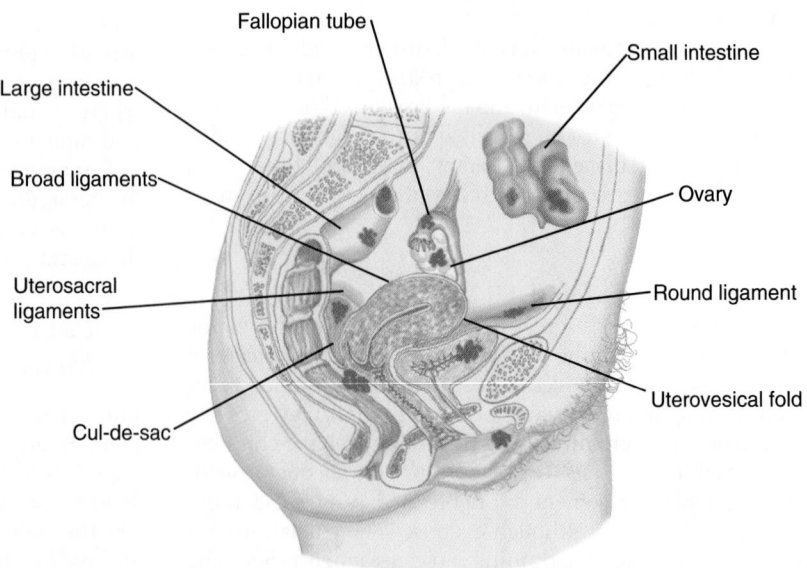

FIGURE 31–2
Common sites of endometriosis.

rhea, constipation, and sensations of rectal pressure or urgency are other symptoms of endometriosis. Although the cause of infertility is not completely understood, pelvic adhesions and tubal disease due to chronic inflammatory changes are certainly contributing factors.

Therapeutic Management. Treatment may be either medical or surgical, and the therapy chosen must weigh the need for relief of pain and the desire to maintain fertility against the side effects that accompany many treatment regimens. Because growth of endometriosis depends on the production of estrogen and progesterone during the menstrual cycle, medical therapy is aimed at interrupting the menstrual cycle. As a result, the woman experiences symptoms associated with estrogen deficit and is at increased risk for postmenopausal conditions, such as adverse serum lipid changes and osteoporosis.

Danazol and analogues of gonadotropin-releasing hormone (GnRH) can be used for 6 to 9 months. Danazol (Danocrine, Cyclomen) is an androgen derivative that has been used for many years. The GnRH agonists include leuprolide acetate (Lupron), goserelin acetate (Zoladex), and nafarelin (Synarel). Both danazol and GnRH agonists interfere with production of gonadotropins (follicle-stimulating hormone and luteinizing hormone) and thus stop the menstrual cycle, creating a "pseudomenopause."

Side effects of danazol include headache, dizziness, irritability, and decreased libido. In addition, danazol often produces masculinizing effects, such as deepening of the voice, facial and body hair, and weight gain. The GnRH drugs have fewer side effects but may produce hot flashes, vaginal dryness, insomnia, decreased libido, and loss of bone mineral density, which is recovered when the drug is discontinued. Add-back therapy, the addition of small amounts of estrogen and progesterone, may be used to decrease the side effects of GnRh agonist drugs and may extend the time they can be used without adverse effects (Kettel & Hummel, 1997).

Pregnancy also interrupts menstruation, and if the woman wishes to conceive, she may be advised not to delay conception. If pregnancy is not an immediate option, continuous noncyclic oral contraceptives or injected contraceptives are sometimes recommended, although they are not as effective as the other drugs.

Surgical treatment can take many forms. Laparoscopy may be performed for lysis of adhesions and laser vaporization of the lesions of endometriosis. This procedure is used especially when infertility is a problem. For women with severe pain who no longer wish to have children, a hysterectomy with bilateral salpingo-oophorectomy (removal of the uterus, both fallopian tubes, and both ovaries) and excision of all lesions offers the greatest chance for cure. This surgery results in early menopause with permanent estrogen deficit. Postoperative hormone replacement therapy may be recommended if all lesions are removed.

NURSING CONSIDERATIONS

Dysmenorrhea varies from mild "menstrual awareness" to incapacitating pain that affects the quality of life for many days of each month. Too often the pain is belittled ("It's just cramps"). One of the most important nursing actions is to acknowledge the pain in a supportive manner.

The nurse should suggest nonpharmacologic pain relief measures, such as frequent rest periods, application of heat to the lower abdomen, moderate exercise, and a well-balanced diet. The woman should avoid scheduling stress-provoking situations during the menstrual period. NSAIDs provide relief for some women. The woman should be counseled to report unusual side effects, such as headache, dizziness, or unusual fluid retention, to the physician or nurse practitioner.

The nurse should allow time for the woman to express her concerns about the therapy. She should be instructed not to use oral contraceptives when medical therapy, such as GnRH or danazol, is used. Some women benefit from information about measures that promote sleep and relaxation, and, most important, from the knowledge that someone is available to provide support and guidance when needed.

Premenstrual Syndrome

Premenstrual syndrome (PMS) is a group of symptoms that occur only during the second half of the menstrual cycle and cause problems in a woman's work and relationships with others. It occurs in approximately 40% of women at one time or another (Stenchever, 1997).

ETIOLOGY
The cause of PMS is unknown. Theories include an imbalance between estrogen and progesterone, low levels of beta-endorphins, low serotonin levels, and abnormal production of prostaglandins.

MANIFESTATIONS
Diagnosis of PMS depends on the following criteria:

- The signs and symptoms must be cyclic and recur in the luteal phase (after ovulation) of the menstrual cycle.
- The woman should have no symptoms during the follicular phase (before ovulation) of the menstrual cycle and at least 7 symptom-free days per cycle.
- Symptoms must be severe enough to have an impact on work, lifestyle, and relationships.
- Diagnosis must be based solely on *prospective* symptom charting by the woman; that is, charting of symptoms as they occur rather than recall of symptoms that occurred in the past (ACOG, 1996).

Figure 31–3 illustrates one type of PMS calendar or diary the woman can use to record her symptoms and their severity.

Premenstrual syndrome puts a consistent strain on family relationships because symptoms recur monthly. Clinical descriptions of severe family disruptions include increased family conflict, disrupted communication, and decreased family cohesion. Of particular concern is the group of women who report symptoms of loss of control, child battering, self-injury, and increased accidents.

THERAPEUTIC MANAGEMENT
Treatment of PMS is based on the symptom profile of each woman. Mild potassium-sparing diuretics may be prescribed for women with fluid retention and weight gain. Vitamin B$_6$

How to Relieve Symptoms of Premenstrual Syndrome

Diet

- Decrease consumption of caffeine (coffee, tea, colas, chocolate), which increases irritability, insomnia, anxiety, and nervousness.
- Avoid simple sugars (cake, candy) to prevent elevations of blood glucose followed by a rapid decline and a period of low blood glucose (hypoglycemia).
- Decrease intake of salty foods to reduce fluid retention.
- Drink at least 2,000 ml (2 quarts) of *water* per day, and do not include other beverages in this total.
- Eat six small meals a day to prevent hypoglycemia. Plan well-balanced meals with emphasis on fresh fruits and vegetables, complex carbohydrates, and nonfat milk products.
- Avoid alcohol, which aggravates depression.

Exercise

Increase physical exercise to relieve tension and to decrease depression. Aerobic activity, such as jogging or walking, several times a week is recommended.

Stress Management

During the time when there are no symptoms of PMS, acknowledge the effect of PMS on daily life and make plans to avoid stressful situations during the premenstrual period when symptoms are acute.

Use guided imagery, conscious relaxation techniques, warm baths, and massage to reduce stress.

Sleep and Rest

To reduce fatigue and combat insomnia:

- Adhere to a regular schedule for sleep.
- Drink a glass of milk, which is high in tryptophan and is known to promote sleep, before bedtime.
- Schedule exercise in the morning or early afternoon rather than late afternoon.
- Engage in relaxing activities, such as reading, before bedtime, and avoid excitement at this time.

Symptoms of Premenstrual Syndrome (PMS)

PHYSICAL SYMPTOMS

Edema
Weight gain
Abdominal bloating
Constipation
Hot flashes
Breast pain
Headache
Acne
Rhinitis
Heart palpitations

BEHAVIORAL SYMPTOMS

Anxiety
Depression
Irritability
Mood swings
Aggressive behavior
Increased appetite
Food cravings
Fatigue
Inability to concentrate
Insomnia

Note: Symptoms listed in approximate order of occurrence.

(pyridoxine) and progesterone supplementation have been tried but have been found ineffective. Antianxiety medications are usually reserved for severe anxiety that does not respond to other therapy. Alternative therapy may be helpful for some women. Measures include acupuncture, biofeedback, hypnosis, psychotherapy, and stress management. Calcium (1,200 mg daily) has been shown to cause significant improvement of most symtoms (Thys-Jacobs et al., 1998).

NURSING CONSIDERATIONS

Many women experience some of the symptoms and diagnose themselves as having PMS. Nurses must discourage this practice because serious systemic disease can be missed if the criteria for diagnosis are ignored. Nurses should recommend that the woman consult with her health care provider so that a complete history and physical examination can be performed to rule out other causes.

Once the diagnosis of PMS is confirmed, nurses can educate the family about lifestyle changes that may help. Nurses should acknowledge that dietary changes are particularly difficult because many women crave salty or sweet foods, which should be restricted. Women also benefit from education about expected cyclic changes. As they learn to predict the pattern of symptoms and gain a sense of control over them, the symptoms often diminish.

Education and support must be expanded to include the family. When the woman exhibits symptoms of PMS, family members often respond by withdrawing or confronting the woman.

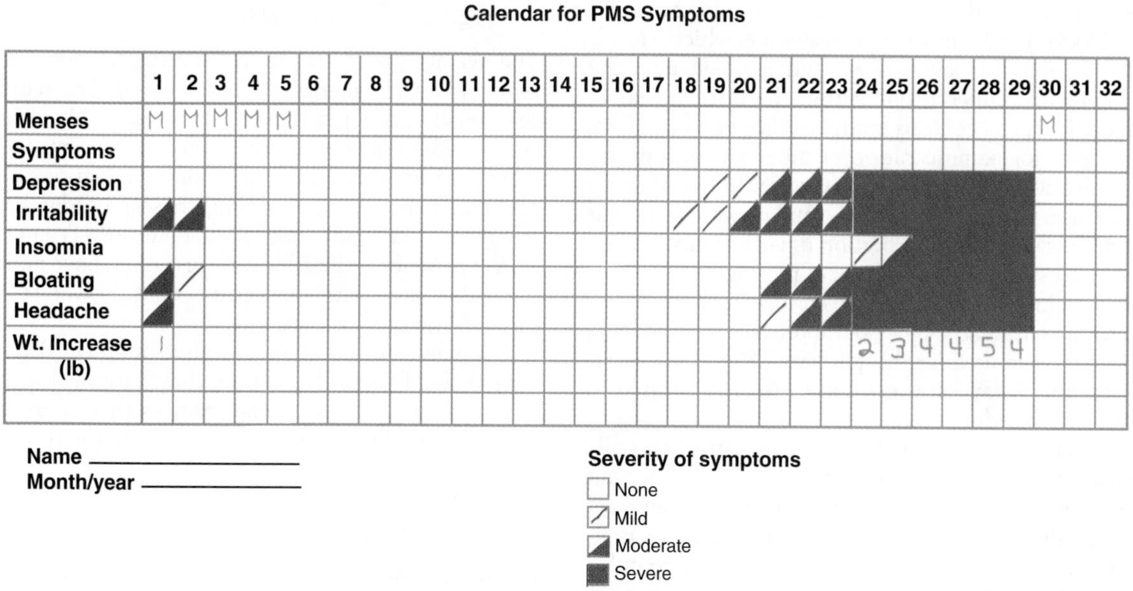

Calendar for PMS Symptoms

	1	2	3	4	5	6	7	8	9	10	11	12	13	14	15	16	17	18	19	20	21	22	23	24	25	26	27	28	29	30	31	32
Menses	M	M	M	M	M																									M		
Symptoms																																
Depression																																
Irritability																																
Insomnia																																
Bloating																																
Headache																																
Wt. Increase (lb)	1																							2	3	4	4	5	4			

Name _____

Month/year _____

Severity of symptoms
☐ None
◨ Mild
◪ Moderate
◼ Severe

FIGURE 31–3

The woman uses a diary to record occurrence and severity of premenstrual symptoms.

It is more helpful if the family acknowledges feelings they believe the woman is experiencing. For instance, saying "It must be disturbing to feel so irritable. What can I do to help?" provokes a different emotional response than confronting or blaming comments.

Family members should also be encouraged to express their feelings so that anger and resentment within the family can be diminished.

Nurses must help the woman make concrete arrangements to obtain relief when she feels she is losing control or when she fears that she may harm herself or a child. A neighbor, friend, or family member should be identified to provide immediate relief, without questions or explanations, when the woman feels she is losing control.

Induced Abortion

Induced abortion is a voluntary method of terminating a pregnancy. It may be performed to preserve the health of the mother, to prevent the birth of an infant with severe genetic defects, or to end a pregnancy caused by rape or incest. A woman may also choose to terminate a pregnancy for economic or social reasons. Abortions involve social and ethical implications (see Chapter 1).

Methods of Abortion

The technique used to induce abortion depends on the length of gestation. Up to 13 weeks' gestation, vacuum aspiration or curettage is the method of choice. General anesthesia or a paracervical block may be used during the procedure. The cervix is dilated and a plastic cannula is inserted into the uterine cavity. The contents are aspirated with negative pressure, and the uterine cavity may be scraped with a curet to ensure that the uterus is empty. Cramping may

last 20 to 30 minutes after the procedure is completed. Complications may include uterine perforation, hemorrhage, cervical lacerations, and adverse reactions to the anesthetic agent.

Mifepristone (RU 486), a pill that induces early abortion, has been used effectively in other countries and may

WOMEN WANT TO KNOW

Self-Care Measures After Induced Abortion

- Normal activities may be resumed, but strenuous work or exercise should be avoided for a few days.
- Bleeding or cramping may occur for a week or two. If either becomes severe, medical advice should be sought. Light "spotting" may occur for approximately a month.
- Sanitary pads should be used instead of tampons for the first week after the abortion to avoid possible infection.
- To prevent infection, douching should be avoided for at least 1 week.
- Intercourse should be curtailed for 1 week after the abortion because of the possibility of infection until the uterine lining heals.
- Birth control measures should be used if sex is resumed before menstruation begins because it is possible to become pregnant during this time. Menstruation usually resumes in 4 to 6 weeks.
- Temperature should be taken twice a day to detect possible infection; a temperature above 37.8°C (100°F) should be reported to the health care provider.
- It is important to keep the follow-up appointment in 2 weeks.

become available in the United States in the future. Mifepristone blocks development of progesterone, which a fertilized ovum needs to develop. To end a pregnancy, the woman must take mifepristone within the first 7 weeks of pregnancy. The protocol calls for three office or clinic visits, including one for administration of mifepristone, one for the administration of misoprostol (Cytotec), a prostaglandin that causes uterine contractions, and one to verify that the abortion was complete. Abortion usually occurs approximately 4 hours after administration of prostaglandin. Complications include heavy or prolonged bleeding.

Methotrexate, although not approved for inducing abortion, has been used for this purpose. Misoprostol is administered 6 to 7 days after methotrexate and repeated in 24 hours if no bleeding occurs.

From 13 to 16 weeks, a dilation and evacuation is usually performed. The procedure is similar to vacuum curettage but requires greater cervical dilation and a larger aspirator because the products of conception are larger. The cervix is dilated with prostaglandin E_1 or laminaria (short, rounded pieces of material that absorb water). When laminaria are inserted into the cervix, they draw fluid from the cervical canal and expand, causing the cervix to dilate. Cervical dilation occurs slowly and is less traumatic to the cervix.

After 16 weeks' gestation, labor induction can be carried out with several agents that produce uterine contractions. Prostaglandin E_1 (misoprostol) or E_2 (dinoprostone), may be given vaginally to stimulate contractions. Side effects of dinoprostone include nausea, vomiting, and fever.

Nursing Considerations Related to Induced Abortion

The nurse's role in caring for women seeking induced abortion is to provide physical and emotional support and information. The nurse may take a history and collect specimens for laboratory testing. Counseling and emotional support are nursing responsibilities unless a designated counselor performs these services. Nurses are also responsible for providing information for self-care after an abortion. They should teach the woman signs of complications such as excessive bleeding or infection.

▌ Menopause

Menopause simply means "the end of menstruation." Many people, however, use the term to indicate all changes that occur at the end of the reproductive period. The entire process, frequently called the *change of life*, is correctly termed the *climacteric*. *Premenopause* refers to the early part of the climacteric, before menstruation ceases but after the woman experiences some of the climacteric symptoms, such as irregular menses. *Perimenopause* includes premenopause, menopause, and at least 1 year after menopause. *Postmenopause* refers to the phase after menopause, when menstrual periods have ceased altogether.

Once a woman is postmenopausal, *unplanned bleeding should always be investigated as soon as possible* because it is highly suggestive of endometrial cancer. Women who take estrogen and progesterone sequentially have planned bleeding when they stop taking the drugs, usually once a month. This allows the uterine lining to be sloughed and prevents endometrial hyperplasia.

Age at Menopause

The average age for naturally occurring menopause is 51.5 years in North America (ACOG, 1996). The natural process usually takes place over 3 to 5 years. Menopause can be created artificially, however, at any age, by surgical removal of the ovaries or destruction by radiation. The most common reason for performing these procedures is treatment of gynecologic cancer or endometriosis. Young women who experience artificial menopause often have more symptoms associated with menopause than do women who go through the process naturally.

Women can now expect to live another 30 years after menopause. During this period, they must deal with physical, psychological, and social changes that often require a reevaluation of their primary roles and restructuring of personal goals.

Physiologic Changes

During the premenopausal period, the ovaries are less responsive to gonadotropins. Although increased amounts of follicle-stimulating hormone are secreted, ovulation is sporadic and menstrual periods are irregular. With progressive aging, the ovaries become unresponsive, even to high levels of gonadotropins, and ovulation, menstruation, and the secretion of ovarian hormones (estrogen and progesterone) cease. Lack of estrogen has a significant effect on the health of women during the postmenopausal years.

When estrogen levels decline, the organs of reproduction undergo regression. The labia become thin and pale. The vaginal mucosa atrophies, and vaginal tissue loses its lubrication and is easily traumatized. Dyspareunia is not uncommon, and bacterial invasion of the epithelium may lead to frequent vaginal infections. This process is called atrophic vaginitis. Breasts become smaller, and atrophy of the uterus occurs. A concurrent benefit is that uterine myomas (fibroids) and endometriosis lesions also atrophy. Estrogen deficit can also result in atrophic changes in the bladder and urethra that may give rise to loss of urethral tone and frequent atrophic cystitis.

In addition, absence of estrogen is associated with an adverse change in serum lipids. Low-density lipoproteins, which carry cholesterol to blood vessels, increase. High-density lipoproteins, which carry cholesterol to the liver and protect against the development of coronary artery disease, decrease.

Most menopausal women experience hot flashes or flushes, which are the result of vasomotor instability. The cause of vasomotor instability is unknown, but it is closely associated with increased secretion of gonadotropins. Hot flashes are characterized by a sudden feeling of heat or burning of the skin, followed by perspiration. They occur more frequently during the night, causing fatigue from interrupted sleep.

Psychological Responses

Psychological and social changes also accompany menopause, and individual responses vary widely. Many women are relieved that their childbearing and childrearing tasks are coming to an end. Other women grieve that the possibility of childbearing is past, especially if they are childless.

DRUG GUIDE
• • • • • • • • • •

Conjugated Estrogens (Premarin, Ogen)

Classification: Hormone estrogen.

Action: Increases synthesis of DNA, RNA, and various proteins in responsive tissues. Reduces release of gonadotropin-releasing hormone, thus reducing follicle-stimulating hormone and luteinizing hormone. Promotes normal growth and maintenance of female genital organs, maintaining genitourinary function and vasomotor stability. Restores hormone balance in deficiency states, reduces blood cholesterol, and restores balance of bone resorption. Decreases serum concentration of testosterone.

Indications: Treatment of vasomotor symptoms of menopause, such as hot flashes; prevention of postmenopausal osteoporosis; management of atrophic vaginitis.

Dosage and Route: Dosage for relief of menopausal symptoms and prevention of osteoporosis, 0.6 to 1.25 mg orally. If the woman has had a hysterectomy, estrogen alone may be administered daily or in a repeating cycle. If the uterus is present, estrogen may be given for 21 days, with progesterone added for the final 10 days. Both medications are then stopped for 7 days and predictable bleeding occurs. An alternative schedule involves the administration of estrogen, 0.625 mg, and progesterone, 2.5 to 5 mg daily. This schedule eliminates episodes of planned bleeding. Vaginal cream applied daily for 21 days, off for 7 days, and then repeated, may be useful for atrophic vaginitis.

Absorption: Well absorbed following oral administration, readily absorbed through skin and mucous membranes.

Excretion: Metabolized largely by the liver. As hepatic recirculation occurs, more absorption occurs from the gastrointestinal tract.

Contraindications and Precautions: Contraindicated in thromboembolic diseases, undiagnosed vaginal bleeding, estrogen-dependent cancers, pregnancy, and lactation. Used cautiously in underlying cardiovascular disease and severe hepatic or renal disease. Unopposed use may increase the risk of endometrial carcinoma.

Adverse Reactions: Headache, dizziness, intolerance to contact lenses, nausea, jaundice.

Nursing Considerations: Assess blood pressure, pulse, and weight gain periodically throughout therapy. Assess frequency and severity of hot flashes. Instruct the woman to report skin changes and to protect skin from excessive exposure to sunlight to prevent hyperpigmentation. Assess for vaginal bleeding, amenorrhea, or changes in menstrual flow, and instruct the woman to report these signs to her health care provider. Caution the woman to avoid use of any medication that has not first been approved by her health care provider.

Some symptoms do not have a physiologic explanation, but they are no less real to women who experience them. Depression, mood swings, irritability, and agitation are common climacteric complaints. Insomnia and fatigue are frequently mentioned as major problems.

One of the most puzzling aspects of menopause is the wide variation in both physical and psychological symptoms that women experience. For some women, the only changes are mild, infrequent hot flashes and amenorrhea. Other women experience severe, debilitating hot flashes, atrophic vaginitis, and multiple psychological symptoms, such as irritability and prolonged depression.

Hormone Replacement Therapy

Hormone replacement therapy is considered the treatment of choice for many of the common discomforts of menopause. The type of hormone replacement, either estrogen

DRUG GUIDE
• • • • • • • • • •

Medroxyprogesterone (Provera, Cycrin, Amen)

Classification: Hormone progestin.

Action: A synthetic form of progesterone that transforms the endometrium from a proliferative to a secretory phase and promotes withdrawal bleeding when estrogen is also present. Promotes relaxation of uterine smooth muscle and growth of mammary alveolar tissue.

Indications: Used to reduce the risk of endometrial carcinoma when estrogen is administered to control postmenopausal symptoms or to prevent osteoporosis. Also used for secondary amenorrhea and abnormal uterine bleeding.

Dosage and Route: For induction of secretory endometrium after estrogen priming, 5 to 10 mg orally for 10 days; or 2.5 to 5 mg daily with exogenous estrogen to prevent endometrial hyperplasia.

Absorption: Unknown, metabolized by the liver.

Excretion: Primarily excreted in the urine.

Contraindications and Precautions: Contraindicated in pregnancy, thromboembolic disease, carcinoma of the breast, and liver disease. Used with caution with cardiovascular disease, seizure disorders, and mental depression.

Adverse Reactions: Depression, thrombophlebitis, edema, weight gain, dizziness, fatigue, headache, insomnia. Fluid retention may complicate other conditions such as asthma, heart disease, and renal disorders.

Nursing Considerations: Assess blood pressure throughout therapy. Monitor weight gain, and emphasize that steady weight gain should be reported to health care provider. Advise women to anticipate withdrawal bleeding 3 to 7 days after discontinuing medication. Emphasize the importance of reporting the following signs and symptoms: visual changes, sudden weakness, headache, leg or calf pain, shortness of breath, jaundice, depression, and skin rash.

alone or estrogen in combination with progestin, depends on whether the woman has had a hysterectomy. Estrogen only is prescribed for the woman who has had a hysterectomy. Estrogen and progestin are prescribed for the woman who retains the uterus and is at risk for endometrial hyperplasia if unopposed estrogen is administered.

BENEFITS

Although hormone replacement therapy is the primary treatment for the symptoms of menopause, the risks as well as the benefits of estrogen must be evaluated for each woman. Estrogen controls hot flashes and alleviates genital atrophy, which is associated with atrophic vaginitis, atrophic cystitis, and urinary incontinence. Either oral or topical estrogen may be administered for atrophic vaginitis.

Estrogen also offers protection from cardiovascular disease, which increases dramatically in postmenopausal women. The cardiovascular benefits of estrogen are believed to be due to its ability to increase high-density lipoprotein and to decrease low-density lipoprotein. Progestins have an opposite effect on lipids, but studies have not shown that this effect negates the cardiovascular protection (ACOG, 1996). Estrogen is also known to protect against bone loss and the development of osteoporosis.

Many women expect more from estrogen than it can deliver. Estrogen does not prevent aging of the skin, and evidence is inconclusive about whether it relieves depression or other psychological symptoms. Clinical experience, however, suggests that estrogen replacement relieves insomnia, promotes increased energy, and improves the overall quality of life.

TREATMENT REGIMENS

Three treatment regimens are used for hormone replacement therapy:

- *Cyclic regimen*, in which estrogen is given at specific intervals (such as 25 days per month) with the addition of progestin for the last 10 to 14 days. (Many women are unhappy with the monthly "period" that occurs when the hormones are stopped for several days each month.)
- *Combined regimen*, in which estrogen and a low dose of progestin are given daily, and planned bleeding is avoided.
- *Estrogen alone*, in which estrogen is given for 25 days per month or daily. This regimen is used for women who have had hysterectomies.

RISKS

Administration of unopposed estrogen has been associated with an increased risk of endometrial cancer. To overcome this risk, small doses of progestin are given with estrogen. The addition of progesterone eliminates the constant stimulation of the endometrium that occurs when estrogen is used alone. Some data suggest a minimally increased risk of breast cancer for women who used estrogen for more than 10 to 20 years, but the risk is unclear and data are confusing (ACOG, 1996).

Estrogen is contraindicated for some women. Growth of existing estrogen receptor–positive breast cancer may be stimulated by estrogen. Estrogen stimulates blood coagulation, and women who have had a thrombosis should not

---

WOMEN WANT TO KNOW
About Hormone Replacement Therapy

- Take the medication with meals to reduce nausea.
- If you miss a dose, take the medication as soon as you remember, but not immediately before the next scheduled dose. *Do not take double doses.*
- Expect withdrawal bleeding (if your uterus is intact) when estrogen and progestin are temporarily discontinued.
- Report unplanned or unanticipated bleeding to your health care provider.
- To reduce the risk of serious thrombotic disorders, such as thrombophlebitis, stop smoking.
- Use sunscreen and protective clothing to prevent increased pigmentation.
- Continue follow-up physical examinations, including blood pressure measurements, Pap tests, and examinations of breasts, abdomen, and pelvis.

---

take it. Because estrogen is metabolized by the liver, it should not be used by women who have hepatitis or liver disease.

Not being able to take estrogen presents a dilemma for some women. Not only is osteoporosis an increased risk, but the atrophic changes of menopause and vasomotor instability remain major problems. When estrogen is contraindicated, women also have increased risk of coronary artery disease because they do not receive the protective effects that estrogen provides. Clonidine hydrochloride (Catapres, Dixarit), an antihypertensive, is sometimes prescribed to decrease the severity and frequency of hot flashes.

Nursing Considerations Related to Menopause

Nursing care focuses on helping women understand the physical changes that occur and the psychological responses that may occur during menopause. Nurses must clarify the individual regimen of hormone replacement therapy as well as the risks and benefits of the therapy. For instance, women should be told that although hormone replacement therapy effectively treats atrophic vaginitis and reduces dyspareunia, it may not correct the loss of libido that some women experience.

If hormone replacement therapy is contraindicated, nurses are often the primary source of information about alternative measures that mitigate symptoms:

- Vitamin E, ginseng, and other herbs can be effective in relieving hot flashes.
- Water-soluble lubricants, such as Lubrin and Replens, provide relief from vaginal dryness and dyspareunia. Oil-based lubricants should not be used because they adhere to the mucous membrane and provide a medium for bacterial growth.
- Kegel exercises increase muscle tone around the vagina and urinary meatus and help counteract the effects of genital atrophy.

- Drinking at least eight glasses of water a day decreases the concentration of urine and reduces bacterial growth, preventing atrophic cystitis.
- Wiping from front to back after urination and defecation reduces the transfer of bacteria from the anus to the urinary meatus and helps prevent cystitis.

Osteoporosis

Osteoporosis is one of the greatest hazards of the postmenopausal years. It is characterized by decreased bone density, leaving the bones porous, fragile, and susceptible to fractures. The vertebrae, wrists, and hips are the most common sites of fractures. In the United States, 1.3 million fractures occur yearly as a result of osteoporosis. Of these, 500,000 vertebral fractures and 250,000 hip fractures occurred in women. Between 12% and 20% of the women who have a hip fracture die as a result of complications, such as pneumonia (Freund, 1995).

PREDISPOSING FACTORS

Small-boned, fair-skinned white women of northern European extraction and Asian women are at greatest risk for osteoporosis. Other risk factors may include a family history of the disease, early menopause, and a sedentary lifestyle. Women who smoke, drink alcohol, or take corticosteroids, as well as those who consume excessive amounts of caffeine, also have an increased risk for osteoporosis (Freund, 1995). Inadequate lifetime intake of calcium is a major risk factor because it results in failure to achieve peak bone mass.

MANIFESTATIONS

Osteoporosis has been called the "silent thief" because it takes place gradually throughout the course of many years without symptoms. The first noticeable signs are loss of height and back pain that occurs when the vertebrae collapse. Later signs include the "dowager's hump," which occurs when the vertebrae can no longer support the upper body in an upright position. Secondary to this, the waistline disappears and the abdomen protrudes because the rib cage moves closer to the pelvis. Depending on the number of fractures, several inches of height may be lost. Figure 31–4 illustrates progressive changes in posture associated with osteoporosis.

Diagnosis of osteoporosis depends on history and physical examination. Bone mineral analysis may be performed if results will influence the decision to use hormone replacement therapy. Conventional radiography is of little help because more than 30% of the bone mass must be lost before changes are apparent. Dual-energy x-ray absorptiometry is a highly accurate, fast method of diagnosis that involves low exposure to radiation.

PREVENTION AND THERAPEUTIC MANAGEMENT

The major goal of treatment is to prevent the development of osteoporosis and to stabilize remaining bone mass. The most effective measures are estrogen replacement, supplemental calcium, and exercise.

Estrogen Replacement.   Estrogen halts bone loss and reduces the incidence of fractures. In women who do not take estrogen, 25% have vertebral fractures by age 60 years

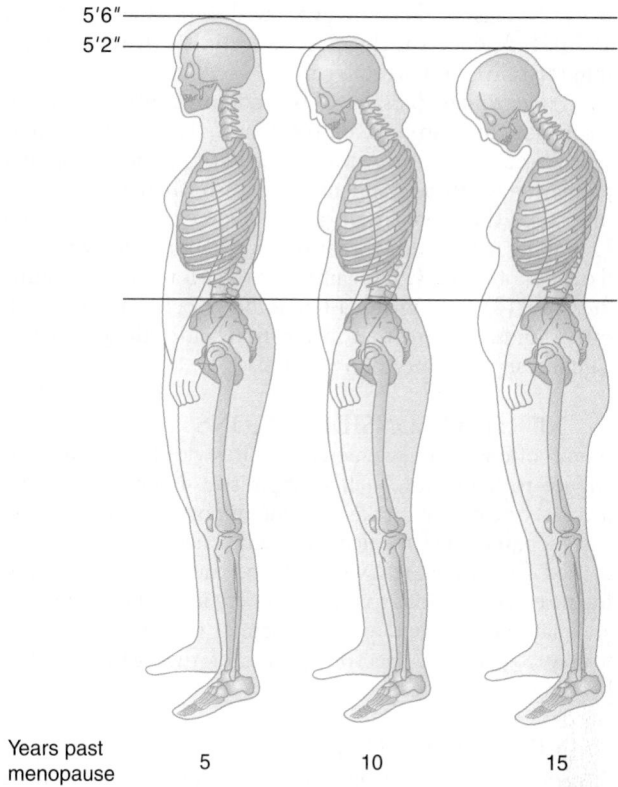

Years past menopause   5   10   15

FIGURE 31–4

With progression of osteoporosis, the vertebral column collapses, causing loss of height and back pain. *Dowager's hump* is the term used for this curvature of the upper back.

(Mishell, 1997c). Estrogen is usually started in the perimenopausal period, and 0.625 mg/d is thought to provide protection from bone loss (ACOG, 1996). When therapy is begun in early menopause, it must be continued for at least 5 to 8 years to protect against the rapid bone loss that occurs during this time (Freund, 1995). Many women continue hormone therapy throughout their lives.

Calcium.   Although calcium does not prevent bone loss, other therapies cannot be effective if calcium is deficient. A postmenopausal woman should receive 1,500 mg/d of calcium. Because it is difficult to ingest this amount daily, the use of supplements is recommended (ACOG, 1996). Vitamin D is necessary for calcium to be absorbed from the intestine. Supplemental vitamin D, 400 to 800 units, is recommended for many women (Gamble, 1995).

Exercise.   Weight-bearing exercise has been shown to increase lumbar spine bone mineral density in postmenopausal women. Walking, hiking, stair climbing, and dancing are examples of weight-bearing exercises. High-impact exercises should be avoided because of the risk to fragile vertebrae.

Alternative Medications.   Women who are especially at risk for osteoporosis, already have bone loss, or who cannot take estrogen need other medications. Calcitonin is available by injection or by nasal spray (Miacalcin). It is indicated for treatment of postmenopausal osteoporosis in women who are 5 years past menopause and demonstrate low bone mass by dual-energy x-ray absorptiometry (Moore, 1996). Side effects include nausea, rhinitis (with nasal administration), and arthralgias.

Alendronate (Fosamax) is a potent inhibitor of bone resorption and can increase bone mass. The most common side effects are nausea, stomach irritation, and abdominal pain. Many of these complaints diminish when women carefully take the medication as directed. Directions include (1) taking it first thing on arising in the morning with 6 to 8 ounces of water, (2) remaining upright for at least 30 minutes, and (3) waiting at least 30 minutes before taking food, other fluids, or any other medications (including antacids, calcium supplements, and vitamins).

NURSING CONSIDERATIONS

Nurses often counsel women about lifestyle factors that contribute to bone loss, such as cigarette smoking, excessive alcohol or caffeine intake, and the importance of following the recommended medical regimen. Nurses are also concerned about how to prevent falls and thus reduce the risk of fractures. Suggestions to increase safety in the home include adequate lighting and avoiding objects that might increase falls such as loose electrical cords or rugs with nonskid backing.

NURSING DIAGNOSES

A variety of nursing diagnoses are important for the woman with osteoporosis. Examples include the following:

- Activity Intolerance related to discomfort and fear of falling
- Body Image Disturbance related to altered posture and functional limitations
- Self-Care Deficit (specify) related to physical limitations and depression

Pelvic Floor Dysfunction

Pelvic floor dysfunction affects at least one third of adult women (Bump & Norton, 1998). It occurs when muscles, ligaments, and fascia that support the pelvic organs become damaged or weakened. This relaxation of pelvic support allows the pelvic organs to prolapse into, and sometimes out of, the vagina. Pelvic disorders usually occur in the perimenopausal period and may be the delayed result of traumatic childbirth.

Vaginal Wall Prolapse

The vagina may prolapse at either the anterior or posterior wall. Anterior wall prolapse involves the bladder and urethra and is called cystocele. Prolapse of the posterior wall produces enterocele or rectocele.

CYSTOCELE

When the weakened upper anterior wall of the vagina is no longer able to support the weight of urine in the bladder, cystocele develops (Fig. 31–5A). The bladder protrudes downward into the vagina, resulting in incomplete emptying of the bladder and consequent cystitis. Urethral displacement may occur when the urethra bulges into the

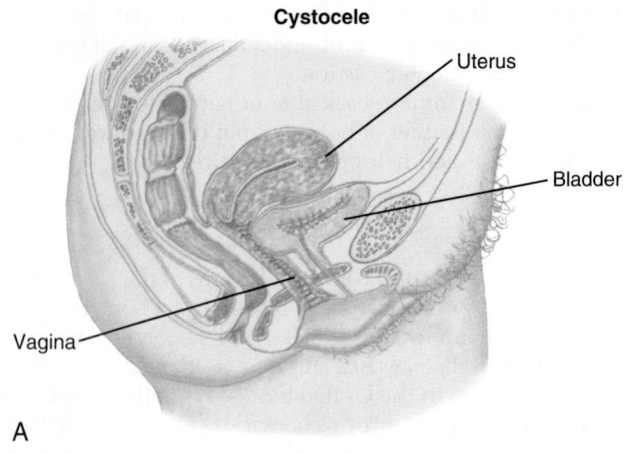

Cystocele

A

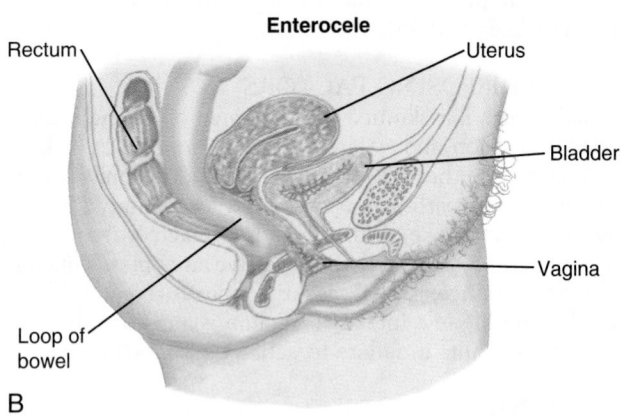

Enterocele

B

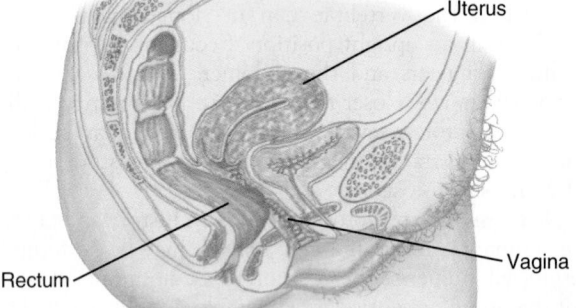

Rectocele

C

FIGURE 31–5

Three types of vaginal wall prolapse. *A*, Note bulging of bladder into the vagina. *B*, Note loop of bowel between rectum and uterus. *C*, Note bulging of rectum into vagina.

lower anterior vaginal wall, producing stress incontinence. Stress incontinence is the loss of urine that occurs with a sudden increase in intra-abdominal pressure from sneezing, coughing, lifting, or other sudden, jarring motions.

ENTEROCELE

Enterocele refers to prolapse of the upper posterior vaginal wall between the vagina and rectum. This condition is almost always associated with herniation of the pouch of Douglas (a fold of peritoneum that dips down between the rectum and the uterus) and may contain loops of bowel (Fig. 31–5B). Enterocele often accompanies uterine prolapse.

RECTOCELE

Rectocele occurs when the posterior wall of the vagina becomes weakened and thin. When the woman strains at defecation, feces are pushed against the thin wall, causing further stretching, until finally the rectum protrudes into the vagina (Fig. 31–5C). Many rectoceles are small and produce few symptoms. If the rectocele is large, the woman may have difficulty emptying the rectum. Some women facilitate bowel elimination by applying digital pressure on the posterior vaginal wall to keep the rectocele from protruding during a bowel movement.

Uterine Prolapse

Uterine prolapse occurs when the cardinal ligaments, which support the uterus and vagina, are unduly stretched during pregnancy and do not return to normal after childbirth. This development allows the uterus to sag backward and downward into the vagina. The condition occurs most often in women who have had many vaginal deliveries or large infants. Figure 31–6 illustrates three degrees of uterine prolapse, from first degree, in which the uterus remains in the vagina, to third degree, in which the cervix protrudes through from the vagina.

MANIFESTATIONS

Symptoms usually become obvious during the menopausal period, when decreased estrogen causes atrophic changes in the supporting structures. Symptoms include feelings of pelvic fullness, a dragging sensation, pelvic pressure, and fatigue. Low backache and a feeling that "everything is falling out" are sometimes described.

Symptoms also relate to the structures involved. For instance, urinary frequency, urgency, and urinary incontinence occur in women with cystocele. Constipation, flatulence, and difficulty defecating are major symptoms of rectocele. Regardless of the structures involved, symptoms become worse after prolonged standing and are relieved by lying down. Symptoms of uterine prolapse are produced by the weight of the descending structures and may include pelvic pressure, backache, and fatigue. Cervical ulceration and bleeding occur if the cervix protrudes from the vaginal introitus.

THERAPEUTIC MANAGEMENT

Treatment of disorders related to pelvic floor dysfunction depends on the woman's age, physical condition, sexual activity, and degree of prolapse. Surgical procedures provide the most satisfactory therapy for women who have significant discomfort. The most common procedures are the anterior and posterior colporrhaphy. The anterior colporrhaphy, performed for a cystocele, involves suturing the pubocervical fascia to support the bladder and urethra. For a rectocele, a posterior colporrhaphy (suturing the fascia and perineal muscles that support the perineum and rectum) is performed.

Surgical treatment for prolapse of the uterus depends on the degree of prolapse. An anterior and posterior colporrhaphy may be effective for a first-degree prolapse. Treatment for more severe prolapse may include vaginal hysterectomy, in which the uterus is removed through the vaginal canal rather than through an abdominal incision. Vaginal hysterectomy may also be combined with anterior and posterior colporrhaphy.

If surgery is contraindicated, a pessary (a device to support pelvic structures) may be inserted into the vagina. The pessary must be inspected and changed frequently by a physician or nurse practitioner to prevent vaginal ulceration or infection.

Medical therapy may include hormone replacement, which is beneficial in reducing the genital atrophy that contributes to pelvic relaxation. It may be provided orally or by vaginal cream.

NURSING CONSIDERATIONS

Pelvic Exercises. Kegel exercises strengthen the pubococcygeus muscle, which surrounds the urethra, vagina, and rectum and provides support for the pelvic floor. Before teaching Kegel exercises, the nurse should ask the woman to try to contract the pubococcygeus muscle while urinating. If she can stop the stream of urine, she is able to perform the exercise. The exercise should be performed at times other than while urinating after the first time.

Kegel exercises involve conscious contracting and relaxing of the pelvic muscles. Only the pelvic muscles should be used; the abdomen, thighs, and buttocks should *not* tighten. Women should be taught to exhale and keep the mouth open to avoid bearing down when contracting the pelvic muscles for 10 seconds, followed by a 10-second period of relaxation. Repeating the exercise approximately 30 times a day should strengthen the muscle tone (Sampselle et al., 1997). The woman must understand that for muscle tone to be maintained, the exercise must be continued for the rest of her life.

Graduated weight cones may be used as an adjunct to

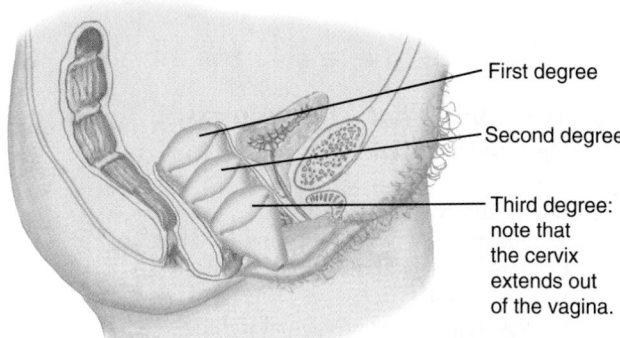

First degree

Second degree

Third degree: note that the cervix extends out of the vagina.

FIGURE 31–6

Three degrees of uterine prolapse.

pelvic muscle exercise. Incrementally weighted cones are inserted into the vagina, and the woman attempts to hold the weights in place. As the weight of the cones increases, the resistance against which the pelvic muscles contract increases, thereby strengthening the pelvic muscles.

Measures that help reduce the symptoms of pelvic relaxation may also prove helpful. These include lying down with the legs elevated or assuming a knee-chest position for a short time several times a day. Additional teaching includes measures to prevent constipation.

Urinary Incontinence.　Nurses must acknowledge the reluctance many women feel about discussing incontinence and help them overcome these feelings and seek medical intervention.

Direct questions, such as "Do you have trouble with your bladder?" or "Do you ever unintentionally lose urine?" may encourage women to discuss urine control problems.

Continence may be enhanced by teaching health promotion activities, such as Kegel exercises and bladder training, which involves adhering to a prescribed schedule for emptying the bladder (Sampselle et al., 1997). Women who cannot execute even a weak pelvic muscle contraction or are unable to implement bladder training may benefit from biofeedback or electrical stimulation. Surgical correction may be necessary.

Women often benefit from knowing about some of the commercial products that protect the skin and prevent odor. These products are made of material that traps urine and prevents constant contact with the skin.

Women often restrict fluids, believing that this will decrease urinary incontinence. Restricting fluids may actually make the condition worse because the bladder does not fill to its normal capacity. Furthermore, decreased fluid intake can lead to highly concentrated urine that can irritate bladder mucous membranes and increase the urge to void. Alcohol and caffeine can also irritate the bladder and worsen incontinence.

Disorders of the Reproductive Tract

Benign Disorders

The most common benign conditions of the reproductive tract include cervical polyps, uterine leiomyomas (fibroids), and ovarian cysts.

CERVICAL POLYPS

Polyps are small tumors, usually only a few millimeters in diameter, that are usually on a pedicle (a stem-like structure). They are caused by proliferation of cervical mucosa, and they often cause intermittent vaginal bleeding.

Cervical polyps are surgically removed in an outpatient setting, and the specimen is sent for pathologic examination to rule out the possibility of malignancy.

UTERINE LEIOMYOMAS

Approximately one third of American women older than 30 years of age have benign tumors called leiomyomas or fibroids (ACOG, 1996). Although the cause is unknown, uterine fibroids develop from smooth muscle cells and are estrogen dependent. As a result, they grow rapidly during the childbearing years. During menopause they begin to atrophy, unless growth is stimulated by estrogen replacement therapy. Fibroids may occur throughout the muscular layer of the uterus.

Uterine fibroids usually produce no symptoms, but increased uterine size, pelvic pain, and excessive menstrual bleeding may occur. Excessive bleeding may result in anemia, weakness, and fatigue. Additional symptoms include feelings of pelvic pressure, bloating, and urinary frequency that occurs when the tumor applies pressure on the bladder.

Treatment depends on the size of the fibroids and the symptoms experienced. In the absence of symptoms, treatment may consist of observation only. If abnormal bleeding is a problem, surgical intervention may be necessary. The two most common surgeries are myomectomy (removal of the tumor only) and hysterectomy. Medical treatment with GnRH agonists may be effective in reducing the size of myomas and lessen the need for surgical removal of the tumor.

OVARIAN CYSTS

An ovarian cyst may be either follicular or luteal. If the ovarian follicle fails to rupture during ovulation, a follicular cyst may develop. These cysts are usually asymptomatic, and they usually regress during the subsequent menstrual cycle. A lutein cyst may develop if the corpus luteum becomes cystic and fails to regress. A lutein cyst is more likely to cause pain and some delay in the next menstrual cycle. Occasionally, an ovarian cyst can rupture or twist on its pedicle and become infarcted, causing pelvic pain and tenderness.

Treatment depends on differentiating a cyst from a solid ovarian tumor that may indicate cancer. If the woman is in her childbearing years, when the risk of ovarian cancer is less, the physician may wait until after the next menstrual cycle and examine the woman again. Transvaginal ultrasound examination is useful to determine if it is a fluid-filled cyst or a solid tumor. Laparoscopy or laparotomy may be performed to remove the cyst from the ovary for examination by a pathologist.

Malignant Disorders

The primary sites for cancer in the female reproductive organs are the cervix, uterus, and ovaries. Although cancer can occur at any age, the incidence increases with age.

CRITICAL TO REMEMBER

Symptoms That Must Always Be Investigated

- Irregular vaginal bleeding
- Unexplained postmenopausal bleeding
- Unusual vaginal discharge
- Dyspareunia
- Persistent vulvar or vaginal itching
- Elevated or discolored lesions of the vulva
- Persistent abdominal bloating or constipation
- Persistent anorexia or vomiting
- Blood in stools

TABLE 31–3
• • • • • • • • • • •

Risk Factors for Cancer of the Reproductive Organs

Uterus

Obesity
Nulliparity
Late menopause
Diabetes mellitus
Hypertension
Gallbladder disease
Breast, colon, or ovarian cancer
Chronic unopposed estrogen stimulation

Cervix

First coitus before 20 y
Multiple sexual partners
Lower socioeconomic status (may be related to
    infrequent gynecologic examinations)
Race (incidence higher in African Americans)
History of sexually transmissible diseases (strong link
    with human papillomavirus)

Ovaries

Race (increased in white women)
Menopause >52 y
Family history of ovarian or uterine cancer
Nulliparity

PREDISPOSING FACTORS

Predisposing factors vary according to the site of the cancer (see Table 31–3 for a summary of risk factors for cancer of the reproductive organs). Risk factors for cervical cancer include a history of multiple sex partners, first intercourse during the teenage years, and infection with HPV. Prolonged use of unopposed estrogen replacement therapy predisposes to overgrowth (hyperplasia) of endometrial tissue and is a significant risk factor for uterine cancer.

Family history is an important risk factor for ovarian cancer. Other factors include nulliparity and late menopause. Use of talcum powder may increase the risk, whereas several pregnancies or use of oral contraceptives decreases the risk.

MANIFESTATIONS

Cancer of the reproductive organs may not be diagnosed until it is advanced because few symptoms are experienced in the early stages. When symptoms occur, they are often nonspecific and could be caused by other conditions. Cancer of the ovaries is particularly difficult to diagnose because the condition may remain "silent" until far advanced, when the chance of long-term survival is greatly reduced.

DIAGNOSTIC EVALUATION

Early diagnosis is strongly associated with long-term survival. A variety of screening and diagnostic procedures are useful in early detection. Screening tests include periodic pelvic examinations, Pap tests, and ultrasonography. Serum tests for tumor markers such as CA 125, which may be increased with ovarian or other cancers, are nonspecific and

are performed when other tests indicate possible malignancy. Diagnostic procedures include endometrial sampling and colposcopy, which can identify patterns of abnormality near the cervical os, where most cancers of the cervix develop.

THERAPEUTIC MANAGEMENT

Treatment of cancer of the reproductive organs is based on location and extent of the disease as well as the age and desire of the woman to have children. Early treatment of cervical cancer may consist of cryosurgery, destruction of abnormal tissue by laser, loop electrodiathermy excision procedure, or surgical conization of the cervix to remove the affected area. After treatment, a surveillance schedule should be established because there is risk of recurrent squamous epithelial lesions (SIL) after treatment.

Treatment for uterine, ovarian, or advanced cervical cancer usually consists of a total abdominal hysterectomy and bilateral salpingo-oophorectomy, and may include adjuvant therapy with radiation or chemotherapy.

■ Infectious Disorders of the Reproductive Tract

Candidiasis

Candidiasis, also known as moniliasis and yeast infection, is the most common form of vaginitis. The cause is believed to be related to a change in vaginal pH that allows accelerated growth of *Candida albicans*, a yeast-like fungus commonly found in the digestive tract and on the skin. Some conditions, such as pregnancy, diabetes mellitus, oral contraceptive use, and systemic antibiotic therapy, result in changes in vaginal pH and flora that favor accelerated growth of *C. albicans*. It is not considered a sexually transmissible disease.

The hallmark presenting symptoms for candidiasis are vaginal and perineal itching. Vulvar and vaginal tissues are inflamed, causing burning on urination. Vaginal discharge is white with a typical "cottage cheese" appearance. Diagnosis is made by identifying the spores of *C. albicans*.

Treatment consists of vaginal application of miconazole nitrate (Monistat), clotrimazole (GyneLotrimin), or nystatin (Mycostatin). These medications are available without prescription. Fluconazole (Diflucan) taken once orally is available by prescription. Women should be advised to seek medical attention with the first infection or if the infection persists or recurs frequently (four or more times in a year). Recurrent yeast infections that resist treatment are associated with HIV infection.

Sexually Transmissible Diseases

Sexually transmissible diseases are transmitted through sexual activity. For some diseases, such as gonorrhea and chlamydial infection, sexual activity is almost the only method of transmission. For other diseases, such as bacterial vaginosis, sexual activity may or may not be the mode of transmission. A woman may have more than one sexually transmissible disease at a time.

INCIDENCE

Sexually transmissible diseases are epidemic today, with the highest incidence among adolescents and young adults. Furthermore, it is believed that the number of untreated infected people with no symptoms is immense, especially because many women do not have symptoms. Because the vagina and microscopic tears in mucosa from intercourse provide favorable conditions for infection, women are twice as likely as men to be infected by a sexually transmissible disease (Sharts-Hopko, 1997).

Methods of contraception have a significant impact on the risk of sexually transmissible diseases. The best protection is the use of condoms. Barrier methods, such as the diaphragm and cervical cap, are less effective than the condom in preventing sexually transmissible diseases, but they provide some protection for the upper genital tract. Other methods may prevent pregnancy but do not prevent exposure to sexually transmissible diseases.

Major concerns include the following:

- The vulnerability of women to sexually transmissible diseases
- The resistance of some organisms to antibiotics
- The relationship between HIV infection and other sexually transmissible diseases
- Failure of asymptomatic people to seek treatment when their sexual partner is infected

See Chapter 26 for the impact of sexually transmissible diseases on pregnancy and the fetus.

TYPES OF SEXUALLY TRANSMISSIBLE DISEASES

Chlamydial Infection.   The most common sexually transmissible disease in Western countries is caused by the gram-negative bacterium *Chlamydia trachomatis.* Approximately 2 to 4 million new cases occur each year. (Cates, 1998). The incidence is particularly high in the teenage population, and it is increased in women using oral contraceptives.

Chlamydial infection is often asymptomatic in women, making diagnosis and control of the disease difficult. It should be suspected when the male sexual partner is treated for nongonococcal urethritis and when the culture results for gonorrhea are negative, yet the woman exhibits symptoms similar to those of gonorrhea, such as a yellowish vaginal discharge and painful urination.

Untreated, chlamydial infection ascends from the cervix to cause pelvic inflammatory disease (PID), and it is one of the chief causes of tubal scarring that results in infertility or ectopic pregnancy. The usual treatment is azithromycin, doxycycline hyclate, or tetracycline, and concurrent treatment of all sexual partners is essential to prevent recurrence.

Gonorrhea.   Gonorrhea is an infection of the genitourinary tract caused by the gonococcus *Neisseria gonorrhoeae.* The woman is often asymptomatic, but she may have purulent discharge, dysuria, and dyspareunia. Diagnosis is based on a positive culture for the gonococcus. Gonorrhea, like chlamydial infection, is associated with PID, which increases the risk of tubal scarring and can result in infertility or ectopic pregnancy.

Because chlamydial infection and gonorrhea frequently occur together, ceftriaxone, cefixime, or ciprofloxacin in combination with doxycycline may be used to treat both infections at once. If possible, all sexual partners should be treated simultaneously.

Herpes Genitalis.   Herpes genitalis is a recurrent sexually transmissible disease caused by the herpes simplex virus (HSV). Two types of HSV have been identified: type I and type II. HSV II usually causes genital lesions. Approximately one in five adults is infected with HSV II (Department of Health and Human Services [DHHS], 1998b). Transmission occurs through direct contact with an infected person.

Within 2 to 20 days after the primary infection, vesicles (blisters) appear in a characteristic cluster on the vulva, perineum, or perianal area. The initial lesions may cause severe vulvar pain and tenderness as well as dyspareunia. Lesions may also occur on the cervix or in the vagina, where the woman cannot see them. The vesicles rupture within 1 to 7 days and form ulcers. Viral shedding lasts for 2 to 3 weeks after the appearance of lesions.

At the initial infection, the woman may also experience flu-like symptoms, including fever, general malaise, and enlarged lymph nodes. When symptoms abate, the virus remains dormant in the nerve ganglia and periodically reactivates, particularly at times of stress, fever, and menses. Recurrent episodes are seldom as extensive or painful as the initial episode, but they are just as contagious. Diagnosis is often based on clinical signs and symptoms and confirmed by viral culture of fluid from the vesicle.

Treatment offers no cure, but acyclovir (Zovirax), an antiviral drug, helps reduce or suppress symptoms, shedding, and recurrent episodes. The safe use of acyclovir in pregnancy has not been established. Women should be advised to abstain from sexual contact until the lesions are completely healed. With an initial infection, the woman should continue to abstain until she becomes culture negative because prolonged viral shedding may occur in such cases.

Condylomata Acuminata.   Condylomata acuminata, also known as venereal or genital warts, are caused by HPV. It is estimated that one half of sexually active adults are infected with HPV (DHHS, 1998b). The dry, wart-like growths may be microscopic, small and discrete, or cauliflower-like clusters. Common sites include the vagina, labia, cervix, and perineal area.

Condylomata acuminata are of particular concern because of the increasing evidence of the association of HPV with precursor states of cervical cancer. Colposcopy is usually recommended to evaluate abnormal cervical tissue and to identify HPV. Women with condylomata acuminata should be advised to have semiannual or annual Pap tests to detect cervical dysplasia.

The goal of treatment is to remove the warts. Applications of 25% trichloroacetic acid, podophyllin, or self-administered podofilox or imiquimod may be used. Podophyllin should not be applied during pregnancy and should be washed off after 1 to 4 hours. Cryotherapy, electrocautery treatment, or laser therapy may also be used to remove the warts.

It is important that the woman understand that none of these treatments eradicates the virus and that she may have recurrences. Furthermore, all sexual partners must be

About Sexually Transmissible Diseases

What are the most common symptoms of sexually transmissible diseases (STDs)?

- Unexpected, nonbloody vaginal discharge (increased amount, unusual color, or odor) or vaginal bleeding
- Vulvar itching or swelling
- Pelvic pain, including painful intercourse, painful urination, and abdominal tenderness
- Skin eruptions or changes (rashes, ulcers, warts, blisters)
- Flu-like symptoms (fever, swollen or painful lymph glands, loss of appetite, nausea or vomiting)
- Presence of symptoms in a sexual partner, even though symptoms are absent in the woman

What are the common methods of diagnosis?

- Culture (vaginal discharge, cervix, lesions) to identify organism
- Blood test (serology) to determine if antibodies for specific diseases are present

How can STDs be prevented?

- Limit number of sexual partners.
- Establish monogamous relationship with uninfected partner.
- Use mechanical and chemical barriers (latex condoms along with nonoxynol 9).
- Remember that one episode of an STD offers no protection from future infection.
- Make sure partner is simultaneously treated to prevent reinfection.

What are the most important things to know about the treatment?

- The entire course of medication must be completed even if symptoms subside.
- It is essential to comply with follow-up care.
- Sexual intercourse should be avoided until free of active infection.
- Partner must be examined and treated before sexual intercourse is resumed.
- Side effects of medications, such as skin rashes, difficulty breathing, or headaches, should be reported.
- Not all STDs can be cured (herpes, AIDS, venereal warts), and treatment is aimed at slowing the disease and preventing complications.

Are there measures that provide comfort and prevent secondary infections?

- Keep the vulva clean but avoid strong soaps, creams, and ointments unless prescribed by health care provider.
- Keep the vulva dry. A hair dryer turned on low may help.
- Wear absorbent cotton underwear and avoid pantyhose and tight pants as much as possible.
- Take analgesics (aspirin or acetaminophen) as directed by health care provider.
- Cool or tepid sitz baths may provide relief from itching.
- Wipe vulva from front to back after urination or defecation and then carefully wash hands.

treated. Sexual contact should be avoided until all lesions are healed, and the use of condoms is recommended to reduce transmission.

Syphilis. Syphilis is caused by the spirochete *Treponema pallidum*, and it is divided into primary, secondary, and tertiary stages. The first sign of primary syphilis is a painless chancre (ulceration) that develops on the genitalia, anus, or lips or oral cavity. Diagnosis is made by identifying the spirochete on dark-field microscopy in material scraped from the base of the chancre. A serologic test usually is negative in the primary stage.

The chancre heals in approximately 6 weeks, if untreated, but the spirochete is carried by the blood to all parts of the body. Approximately 2 months after the initial infection, signs of secondary syphilis appear. These include enlargement of the spleen and liver, headache, anorexia, and a maculopapular skin rash on the palms of the hands and soles of the feet. Skin eruptions, called condylomata lata, may develop on the vulva during this time. They resemble warts and contain numerous spirochetes. Serologic tests usually are positive at this time.

If untreated, the disease enters a latent phase that may last for several years. Tertiary syphilis, which follows the

latent phase, may involve the heart, blood vessels, and central nervous system. General paralysis and psychosis may result.

The usual screening test for syphilis is the Venereal Disease Research Laboratory (VDRL) serum test, which detects antibodies produced in response to the infection. The rapid plasma reagin (RPR) and fluorescent treponemal antibody absorption (FTAABS) tests are more specific and are commonly performed to confirm a positive VDRL.

Treatment of all stages of syphilis is with penicillin. Tetracycline or doxycycline are alternatives if the woman is not pregnant.

Trichomoniasis. Trichomoniasis is caused by *Trichomonas vaginalis*, a protozoon that thrives in an alkaline environment. The presenting symptoms include a profuse, malodorous, greenish-yellow vaginal discharge. Vulvar itching, edema, and redness may also be present. The diagnosis is made by identifying the organism in a wet-mount preparation.

If the woman is not pregnant, the treatment of choice is metronidazole (Flagyl, Protostat). Women should be advised to avoid using alcohol during treatment with metronidazole and for 24 hours thereafter. If the woman is pregnant, clotrimazole (GyneLotrimin) may provide relief of symptoms during the first trimester. Metronidazole may be used after the first trimester. The woman's partner may be asymptomatic but should be treated to prevent reinfection.

Bacterial Vaginosis. This infection, previously referred to as nonspecific vaginitis or *Gardnerella* vaginitis, occurs when anaerobic bacteria such as *Gardnerella vaginalis* proliferate and replace normal vaginal lactobacilli that inhabit the vagina of healthy women.

Chief symptoms are a thin, grayish-white vaginal discharge that typically exudes a fishy odor. The diagnosis is made by preparing a saline wet mount and identifying characteristic clue cells (epithelial cells with numerous bacilli clinging to their surface).

Treatment for bacterial vaginosis is directed toward reestablishing the balance of flora in the vagina. Metronidazole has been shown to relieve symptoms and to improve vaginal flora. Clindamycin cream and metronidazole gel are alternative treatments.

Acquired Immunodeficiency Syndrome. Acquired immunodeficiency syndrome (AIDS), caused by HIV, is the most devastating of the sexually transmissible diseases. The rate of infection is increasing more rapidly in women than in men, and diagnosis in women may not occur until late in the disease (Burdge, 1996). HIV has been isolated from blood, semen, vaginal secretions, urine, saliva, tears, cerebrospinal fluid, amniotic fluid, and breast milk (Goodman, 1998). The primary modes of transmission are intimate contact with infected bodily secretions, exposure to infected blood and blood products, and perinatal transmission from mother to infant.

The treatment of HIV/AIDS is a rapidly developing and changing field. Although there is no cure, new medications show a great deal of promise. In addition to the problems shared with men with HIV/AIDS, infected women may need treatment for genital herpes, vaginal candidal infections, HPV infection, abnormal Pap tests and cervical intraepithelial neoplasia (CIN), or other gynecologic conditions. See Chapter 26 for a discussion of HIV and AIDS in pregnant women and neonates.

NURSING CONSIDERATIONS

In their role as teachers and counselors, nurses can play a major part in preventing the spread of sexually transmissible diseases. To fulfill this role, nurses must be prepared to do the following:

- Teach preventive measures
- Teach the signs and symptoms that require medical attention
- Explain diagnostic or screening tests
- Explain treatments

Pelvic Inflammatory Disease

Pelvic inflammatory disease, infection of the upper genital tract, is a serious health problem in the United States. It is estimated that PID develops in 1 million women each year, and 25% of those have complications such as chronic pelvic pain, infertility, and ectopic pregnancy (Droegemueller, 1997c).

ETIOLOGY AND PATHOPHYSIOLOGY

Although organisms such as *Escherichia coli* may cause PID, the primary sources of infection are *C. trachomatis* and *N. gonorrhoeae*. These organisms invade the endocervical canal and cause cervicitis. Bacteria ascend and infect the endometrium, fallopian tubes, and pelvic cavity. The chronic inflammatory response is responsible for extensive tubal scarring and peritubal adhesions, which interfere with conception and with transport of the fertilized ovum through the obstructed fallopian tubes.

MANIFESTATIONS

Some women with PID are asymptomatic, whereas others experience pelvic pain, fever, purulent vaginal discharge, nausea, anorexia, and irregular vaginal bleeding. Findings during physical examination may include abdominal or adnexal tenderness and tenderness of the uterus and cervix when they are moved during bimanual examination (cervical motion tenderness). Laboratory evaluation may reveal a marked leukocytosis and increased sedimentation rate. A urinalysis is needed to rule out urinary tract infection, and cervical cultures for *N. gonorrhoeae* and *C. trachomatis* help to diagnose the disease.

THERAPEUTIC MANAGEMENT

Women with serious infection, as manifested by fever, abdominal pain, and leukocytosis, may be admitted to a hospital. They are most often treated with intravenous administration of cefoxitin or cefotetan plus doxycycline, or clindamycin and gentamicin. Ambulatory treatment is appropriate for some women who are less ill and are able to comply with the recommended regimen.

NURSING CONSIDERATIONS

Nurses can play an important role in preventing PID by teaching women how to prevent sexually transmissible diseases. Prevention occurs on two levels: primary and secondary. Primary prevention involves avoiding exposure to these diseases or preventing acquisition of infection during exposure. Measures include limiting the number of sexual partners and avoiding intercourse with those who have had multiple partners. Barrier methods (latex condoms with spermicide containing nonoxynol 9) used consistently and correctly during all sexual activity help prevent sexually transmissible diseases.

Secondary prevention involves preventing a lower genital tract infection from ascending to the upper genital tract. Also important is preventing further transmission within the community. Nurses should advise women to seek medical attention promptly after having unprotected sex with someone suspected of having a sexually transmissible disease and when unusual vaginal discharge or genital lesions are apparent. Moreover, periodic medical assessment is necessary if the woman is not in a mutually monogamous relationship, even if she is asymptomatic. Additional measures include taking medication as prescribed and returning for follow-up evaluation.

Toxic Shock Syndrome

Although toxic shock syndrome is rare, it is a potentially fatal condition caused by toxin-producing strains of *Staphy-*

lococcus aureus. The toxin produced alters capillary permeability, which allows intravascular fluid to leak from the blood vessels, leading to hypovolemia, hypotension, and shock. The toxin also causes direct tissue damage to organs and precipitates serious defects in coagulation.

If toxin-producing strains of *S. aureus* inhabit the vagina, certain factors increase the risk that the toxin will gain entry into the bloodstream. These include the use of high-absorbency tampons during menstruation and barrier methods of contraception (cervical cap or diaphragm), both of which may trap and hold bacteria if left in place for a prolonged time.

Symptoms of toxic shock syndrome include a sudden spiking fever and flu-like symptoms (headache, sore throat, vomiting, diarrhea), hypotension, a generalized rash resembling sunburn, and skin peeling from the palms of the hands and the soles of the feet 1 to 2 weeks after the onset of the illness.

Treatment consists of fluid replacement, administration of vasopressor drugs, and antimicrobial therapy. Corticosteroids may be used to treat skin changes.

Nurses are often responsible for providing information that may help to prevent toxic shock syndrome.

TAMPON USE
Nurses should instruct women to do the following:

- Wash the hands thoroughly to remove bacteria before inserting tampons.
- Change tampons at least every 4 hours to prevent excessive bacterial growth on the tampon.
- Do not use super-absorbent tampons at any time because they may be left in the vagina for a prolonged period, allowing bacteria to proliferate.
- Use pads rather than tampons during hours of sleep, which usually exceed the 4-hour segments of tampon use.

DIAPHRAGM USE
Nurses should tell women to do the following:

- Wash the hands thoroughly before inserting the diaphragm.
- Do not use a diaphragm during menstrual periods.
- Remove the diaphragm within the time recommended by the health care provider.

KEY CONCEPTS

- *Health maintenance* refers to examinations and screening procedures that allow early detection of specific conditions, such as breast or cervical cancer, and allow for early treatment that increases the chance of long-term survival.
- A major role of nurses is to explain screening procedures and to encourage women to have them on a regular basis. The most common screening procedures include BSE, clinical breast examination, and mammography for breast cancer; vulvar self-examination to detect precancerous conditions or infections; pelvic examination to detect abnormalities of the uterus or ovaries; Pap test for cervical cancer; and screening for fecal occult blood.
- Disorders of the breast may be benign, such as fibrocystic changes that occur in relation to the menstrual cycle, or malignant. The discovery of any breast disorder creates anxiety in women, and nurses must be prepared to explain diagnostic procedures.
- Breast cancer develops in one in eight women in the United States. Besides gender, the great-

est risk factors are advancing age and prior history of breast cancer. Additional factors include family history of breast cancer and previous uterine, ovarian, or colon cancer. Lifestyle factors such as a high intake of dietary fat, smoking, and consumption of alcohol are also suspected to increase risk.
- Management of breast cancer includes surgical removal of the tumor plus varying amounts of surrounding tissue and lymph glands. Adjuvant therapy includes radiation, chemotherapy, and hormone therapy.
- Breast reconstruction is an integral part of the surgical management of breast cancer. Methods include tissue expansion and autogenous grafts.
- Nursing care for women with cancer of the breast focuses on providing emotional support and accurate information.
- Menstrual cycle disorders include amenorrhea, abnormal uterine bleeding, cyclic pelvic pain, and PMS. Some of the disorders, such as PMS, respond to lifestyle alterations such as changes in diet, exercise habits, and stress management.

- Induced abortion may be performed by medical or surgical methods, and each method is associated with social and ethical conflicts.
- Menopause, more correctly termed the *climacteric*, is a combination of endocrine, somatic, and psychic changes that occur at the end of the reproductive cycle. Women's responses to menopause vary widely. After menopause, all women are in a permanent state of estrogen deficit that can result in bone loss (osteoporosis) and increased incidence of coronary artery disease.
- Hormone replacement therapy is commonly prescribed to manage the symptoms of estrogen deficit, such as hot flashes and atrophic vaginitis, and to decrease osteoporosis and cardiovascular disease.
- Estrogen replacement has risks as well as benefits and is contraindicated for women who have thromboembolic disease, undiagnosed vaginal bleeding, previous episodes of breast cancer or untreated uterine cancer, or chronic liver disease. For these women, alternative measures are needed to control the symptoms of menopause.

■ Relaxation of pelvic support structures occurs as a delayed result of traumatic childbirth and becomes troublesome when a deficiency in estrogen hastens genital atrophy.

■ Benign disorders of the reproductive tract include cervical polyps, uterine leiomyomas (fibroids), and ovarian cysts. Malignant disorders include cancer of the cervix, uterus, and ovaries.

■ Although some infections of the reproductive tract are related to a change in the pH or the flora of the vagina, such as candidiasis, most are transmitted by sexual contact. The incidence of sexually transmissible diseases is reduced by barrier methods of contraception, particularly the condom, which prevents potentially infected ejaculate from entering the lower genital tract.

■ Pelvic inflammatory disease is often a complication of untreated sexually transmissible diseases, particularly chlamydial infection or gonorrhea, which can result in infertility or ectopic pregnancy because of scarring of fallopian tubes resulting from inflammatory processes in the pelvic cavity.

■ Toxic shock syndrome is a life-threatening condition resulting from infection with toxin-producing strains of *S. aureus*. The infection is believed to be related to use of high-absorbency tampons, cervical caps, and diaphragms that trap and hold bacteria in nutrient-rich menstrual blood for an extended time.

REFERENCES AND READINGS

American Cancer Society. (1997). *Breast self-examination.* Atlanta: Author.

American Cancer Society. (1999). *Cancer facts and figures.* Atlanta: Author.

American College of Obstetricians and Gynecologists (ACOG). (1996). *Guidelines for women's health care.* Washington, DC: Author.

Association of Women's Health, Obstetric, and Neonatal Nurses. (1998). Guideline for a nursing health assessment in midlife women. In *Standards and Guidelines for Professional Nursing Practice in the Care of Women and Newborns* (pp. 10–11). Washington, DC: Author.

Brunt, M. J. (1995). Amenorrhea and oligomenorrhea. In P. L. Carr, K. M. Freund, & S. Somani (Eds.), *The medical care of women* (pp. 168–181). Philadelphia: Saunders.

Bump, R. C., & Norton, P. A. (1998). Epidemiology and natural history of pelvic floor dysfunction. *Obstetrics and Gynecology Clinics of North America, 25*(4), 723–746.

Burdge, D. R. (1996). Bridging the gender gap in HIV diagnosis and care. *Medscape Women's Health* [On-line serial], *1*(10). Available: http://www.medscape/womenshealth/journal1996/v01.n10/w83.burdge/w83.burdge.html

Buzby, M. (1996). Viral hepatitis: A sexually transmitted disease? *Nurse Practitioner Forum, 7*(1), 10–15.

Cates, J. R., Alexander, L., & Cates, W. (1998). Prevention of sexually transmitted diseases in an era of managed care: The relevance for women. *Women's Health Issues, 8*(3), 169–186.

Cates, W. (1998). Reproductive tract infections. In R. A. Hatcher, J. Trussell, F. Stewart, W. Cates, G. K. Stewart, F. Guest, & D. Kowal (Eds.), *Contraceptive technology* (17th ed., pp. 179–210.). New York: Ardent Media.

Centers for Disease Control and Prevention. (1998). Guidelines for treatment of sexually transmitted diseases. *Morbidity and Mortality Weekly Reports, 47*(RR-1), 1–118.

Creehan, P. A. (1995). Toxic shock syndrome: An opportunity for nursing intervention. *Journal of Obstetric, Gynecologic, and Neonatal Nursing, 24*(6), 557–561.

Dahlbeck, S. W., Donnelly, J. F., & Theriault, R. L. (1995). Differentiating inflammatory breast cancer from acute mastitis. *American Family Physician, 52*(3), 929–934.

Department of Health and Human Services (DHHS). (1995). *Healthy people 2000: Midcourse review and 1995 revisions.* Washington, DC: U.S. Public Health Service.

Department of Health and Human Services (DHHS). (1998a). *Health, United States, 1998, with socioeconomic status and health chartbook.* Washington, DC: U.S. Public Health Service.

Department of Health and Human Services (DHHS). (1998b). *Healthy people 2000: Progress review.* Washington, DC: U.S. Public Health Service.

Droegemueller, W. (1997a). Breast diseases: Diagnosis and treatment of benign and malignant disease. In D. R. Mishell, M. A. Stenchever, W. Droegemueller, & A. L. Herbst (Eds.), *Comprehensive gynecology* (pp. 353–387). St. Louis: Mosby-Year Book.

Droegemueller, W. (1997b). Infections of the lower genital tract. In D. R. Mishell, M. A. Stenchever, W. Droegemueller, & A. L. Herbst (Eds.), *Comprehensive gynecology* (pp. 601–659). St. Louis: Mosby-Year Book.

Droegemueller, W. (1997c). Infections of the upper genital tract. In D. R. Mishell, M. A. Stenchever, W. Droegemueller, & A. L. Herbst (Eds.), *Comprehensive gynecology* (pp. 661–690). St. Louis: Mosby-Year Book.

El-Rfaey, H., Rajasekar, D., Abdalla, M., Calder, L., & Templeton, A. (1998). Induction of abortion with mifepristone (RU 486) and oral or vaginal misoprostol. *New England Journal of Medicine, 332*(15), 983–987.

Ferreira, N. (1996). Sexually transmitted *Chlamydia trachomatis. Nurse Practitioner Forum, 7*(1), 40–46.

Foulks, M. J. (1998). The Papanicolaou smear: Its impact on the promotion of women's health. *Journal of Obstetric, Gynecologic, and Neonatal Nursing, 27*(4), 367–373.

Freeman, S.B. (1995). Common genitourinary infections. *Journal of Obstetric, Gynecologic, and Neonatal Nursing, 24*(8), 735–741.

Freund, K. M. (1995). Osteoporosis. In P. L. Carr, K. M. Freund, & S. Somani (Eds.), *The medical care of women* (pp. 643–651). Philadelphia: Saunders.

Galsworthy, T. D. (1996). It steals more than bone. *American Journal of Nursing, 96*(6), 27–33.

Gamble, C. L. (1995). Osteoporosis: Drug and nondrug therapies for the patient at risk. *Geriatrics, 50*(8), 39–43.

Gaydos, C. A., Howell, M. R., Pare, B., Clark, K. L., Ellis, D. A., Hendrix, R. M., Gaydos, J. C., McKee, K. T., & Quinn, T. C. (1998). *Chlamydia trachomatis* infections in female military recruits. *New England Journal of Medicine, 339*(11), 739–744.

Goodman, J. R. (1998). AIDS and infectious diseases in pregnancy. In N. F. Hacker & J. G. Moore (Eds.), *Essentials of obstetrics and gynecology* (3rd ed., pp. 208–223). Philadelphia: Saunders.

Grady, D., Gebretsadik, T., Ernster, V., & Petitti, D. (1995). Hormone replacement therapy and endometrial cancer risk: A meta-analysis. *Obstetrics and Gynecology, 85*(2), 304–313.

Hautman, M. A. (1996). Changing womanhood: Perimenopause among Filipina-Americans. *Journal of Obstetric, Gynecologic, and Neonatal Nursing, 25*(8), 667–672.

Hindle, W. H. (1997). The diagnostic evaluation. In D. J. Marchant (Ed.), *Breast disease.* (pp. 69–82). Philadelphia: Saunders.

Huff, B. C. (1996). Prevention, screening and early detection of gynecologic cancers. *AWHONN Voice, 4*(5), 1–13.

Kendig, S. & Sanford, D. G. (1998). *Midlife and menopause: Celebrating women's health.* Washington, DC: Association of Women's Health, Obstetric, & Neonatal Nurses.

Kettel, L. M., & Hummel, W. P. (1997). Modern medical management of endometriosis. *Obstetrics and Gynecology Clinics of North America, 24*(2), 361–373.

Kottmann, L. M. (1995). Pelvic inflammatory disease: Clinical overview. *Journal of Obstetric, Gynecologic, and Neonatal Nursing, 24*(8), 759–767.

Leach, G. & Haab, F. (1998). Impact of female pelvic anatomy on stress urinary incontinence. *Contemporary OB/GYN, 43*(10), 45–58.

LeBoeuf, F. J., & Carter, S. G. (1996). Discomforts of the perimenopause. *Journal of Obstetric, Gynecologic, and Neonatal Nursing, 25*(2), 173–180.

Lebherz, T. B. (1998). Infectious and benign diseases of the vagina, cervix, and vulva. In N. F. Hacker & J. G. Moore (Eds.), *Essentials of obstetrics and gynecology* (3rd ed., pp. 393–411). Philadelphia: Saunders.

Lindheim, S. R. (1998). Treatment options for recurrent endometriosis. *Contemporary OB/GYN, 43*(10), 34–39.

Marchant, D. J. (1997a). Contemporary management of breast cancer. In D. J. Marchant (Ed.), *Breast disease* (pp. 111–113). Philadelphia: Saunders.

Marchant, D. J. (1997b). Invasive breast cancer: Surgical treatment alternatives. In D. J. Marchant (Ed.), *Breast disease* (pp. 179–193). Philadelphia: Saunders.

McHahon, S. (1995). Prevention and early detection of cancer in women. *Seminars in Oncology Nursing, 11*(2), 88–102.

McHugh, D. R. (1996). Syphilis: An old disease with modern health concerns. *Nurse Practitioner Forum, 7*(1), 34–39.

McKeon, V. A. (1998). The breast cancer prevention trial: Should women at risk take tamoxifen? *Lifelines, 2*(5), 20–25.

Mishell, D. R. (1997a). Family planning. In D. R. Mishell, M. A. Stenchever, W. Droegemueller, & A. L. Herbst (Eds.), *Comprehensive gynecology* (pp. 283–352). St. Louis: Mosby-Year Book.

Mishell, D. R. (1997b). Menopause: Endocrinology, consequences of estrogen deficiency, effects of hormonal replacement therapy, treatment regimens. In D. R. Mishell, M. A. Stenchever, W. Droegemueller, & A. L. Herbst (Eds.), *Comprehensive gynecology* (pp. 283–352). St. Louis: Mosby-Year Book.

Mishell, D. R. (1997c). Primary and secondary amenorrhea: Etiology, diagnostic evaluation, management. In D. R. Mishell, M. A. Stenchever, W. Droegemueller, & A. L.

Herbst (Eds.), *Comprehensive gynecology* (pp. 353–387). St. Louis: Mosby-Year Book.

Moore, A. A. (1996). Osteoporosis and the older woman. *AWHONN Voice, 4*(5), 1–14.

Moore, A. A., & Noonan, M. D. (1996). A nurse's guide to hormone replacement therapy. *Journal of Obstetric, Gynecologic, and Neonatal Nursing, 25*(1), 24–31.

Moore, J. G. (1998). Endometriosis and adenomyosis. In N. F. Hacker & J. G. Moore (Eds.), *Essentials of obstetrics and gynecology* (3rd ed., pp. 433–445). Philadelphia: Saunders.

Nelson, A.L. (1998). Menstrual problems and common gynecologic concerns. In R. A. Hatcher, J. Trussell, F. Stewart, W. Cates, G. K. Stewart, F. Guest, & D. Kowal (Eds.), *Contraceptive technology* (17th ed., pp. 95–140). New York: Ardent Media.

Policar, M. S. (1998). Female genital tract cancer screening. In R. A. Hatcher, J. Trussell, F. Stewart, W. Cates, G. K. Stewart, F. Guest, & D. Kowal (Eds.), *Contraceptive technology* (17th ed., pp. 43–67). New York: Ardent Media.

Prout, M. N. (1995). Breast cancer: Epidemiology, screening, and prevention. In P. L. Carr, K. M. Freund, & S. Somani (Eds.), *The medical care of women* (pp. 153–160). Philadelphia: Saunders.

Sampselle, C. M., Burns, P. A., Dougherty, M. C., Newman, D. K., Thomas, K. K., & Wyman, J. F. (1997). Continence for women. *Journal of Obstetric, Gynecologic, and Neonatal Nursing, 26*(4), 375–385.

Schlaff, W. D., & Kletzky, O. A. (1998). Amenorrhea, hyperprolactinemia, and chronic anovulation. In N. F. Hacker & J. G. Moore (Eds.), *Essentials of obstetrics and gynecology* (3rd ed., pp. 580–593). Philadelphia: Saunders.

Scott, M. A. K. (1996). Reducing the risks: Adolescents and sexually transmitted diseases. *Nurse Practitioner Forum, 7*(1), 23–29.

Scura, K. W., & Whipple, B. (1997). How to provide better care for the postmenopausal woman. *American Journal of Nursing, 96*(6), 36–43.

Sharps, P. W. (1997). Reproductive, gynecologic, and urinary tract conditions and disorders. In K. M. Allen & J. M.Phillips (Eds.), *Women's health across the lifespan: A comprehensive perspective* (pp. 168–192). Philadelphia: Lippincott-Raven.

Sharts-Hopko, N. C. (1997). STDs in women: What you need to know. *American Journal of Nursing, 97*(4), 46–54.

Somani, S. (1995). Evaluation and management of pelvic pain. In P. L. Carr, K. M. Freund, & S. Somani (Eds.), *The medical care of women* (pp. 55–66). Philadelphia: Saunders.

Stenchever, M. A. (1997). Primary and secondary dysmenorrhea and premenstrual syndrome. In D. R. Mishell, M. A. Stenchever, W. Droegemueller, & A. L. Herbst (Eds.), *Comprehensive gynecology* (pp. 1011–1023). St. Louis: Mosby-Year Book.

Stewart, F. (1998). Menopause. In R. A. Hatcher, J. Trussell, F. Stewart, W. Cates, G. K. Stewart, F. Guest, & D. Kowal (Eds.), *Contraceptive technology* (17th ed., pp. 77–93). New York: Ardent Media.

Thys-Jacobs, S., Starkey, P., Bernstein, D., & Tian, J. (1998). Calcium carbonate and the premenstrual syndrome: Effects on premenstrual and menstrual symptoms. *American Journal of Obstetrics and Gynecology, 179*, 444–452.

Urso, P., & Jordan, M. L. (1996). Less common dermatological sexually transmitted diseases. *Nurse Practitioner Forum, 7*(1), 30–33.

Versaci, A.D. (1997). Plastic surgery: Breast reconstruction following mastectomy. In D. J. Marchant (Ed.), *Breast disease* (pp. 247–258). Philadelphia: Saunders.

Weiss, R. M. (1995). Abnormal uterine bleeding. In P. L. Carr, K. M. Freund, & S. Somani (Eds.), *The medical care of women* (pp. 113–120). Philadelphia: Saunders.

Wilbur, J., Miller, A. M., Montgomery, A., & Chandler, P. (1998). Women's physical activity patterns: Nursing implications. *Journal of Obstetric, Gynecologic, and Neonatal Nursing, 27*(4), 383–392.

III

Pediatric Nursing Care

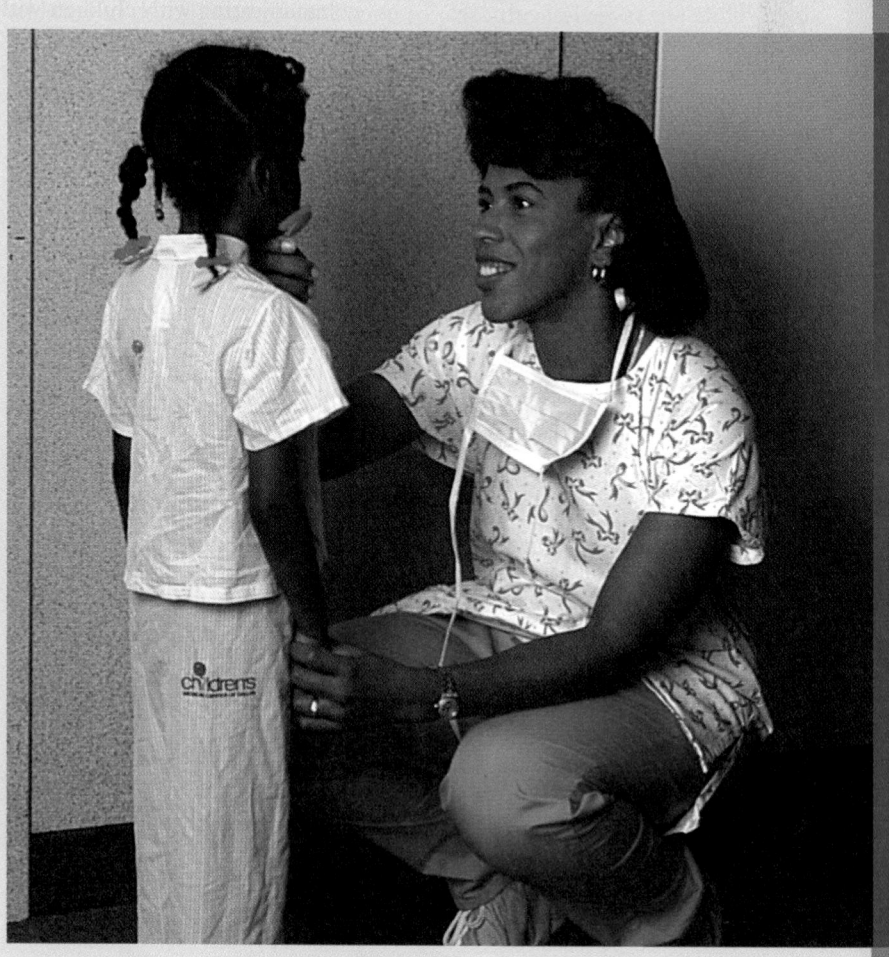

cautiously when meeting new children and families, respecting each individual's personal space. For example, the nurse should pull over a chair from across the room to sit closer to the child and family. This action puts the nurse at eye level. Standing over the child and family can be intimidating. If a chair is not accessible, the nurse may also stoop, squat, or sit on the floor by the child. The important part is to be at eye level while remaining at a comfortable distance for the child and family (see Fig. 32–1).

The nurse should not overlook privacy or underestimate its importance. A room should be available for conducting private conversations away from roommates or family members and visitors. Privacy is particularly critical when working with adolescents, who typically will not discuss sensitive topics with parents present. The nurse's skill and ease with parents of adolescents will increase the adolescents' trust in the nurse. Hallway conversations, particularly outside a child's room, should be avoided because children and parents may hear only some words or phrases and misinterpret their meaning. Overhearing may lead to unnecessary stress and lead to mistrust between the health care providers and the child or family.

Listening

Messages given must be received for communication to be complete. Therefore, listening is an essential component of the communication process. By practicing active listening skills, nurses can be effective listeners. *Active listening* skills include

- *Attentiveness.* The nurse needs to be intentional about giving the speaker undivided attention. Eliminating distractions is important, whenever possible. For example, the nurse should maintain eye contact, close the door, and eliminate potential distractions (television, computer, video games).
- *Clarification Through Reflection.* Using similar words, the nurse should express back to the speaker what was heard and understood about the content of the message. For example, when the child or family member says, "I hate the food that comes on my tray," an appropriate response would be "You are unhappy with the food you've been given?"
- *Empathy.* The nurse should identify and acknowledge feelings expressed in the message. For example, if a child is crying after a procedure, the nurse might say, "I know it is uncomfortable to have this procedure. It is OK to cry. You did a great job holding still."
- *Impartiality.* To understand and avoid prejudicing what is heard with personal bias, the nurse should listen with an open mind. For example, if an adolescent expresses concern that she's having difficulty with relationships at school and that she feels disconnected socially because she's a lesbian, the nurse should remain a supportive listener. The nurse can then help her identify ways to connect with peers and interact with her as with all children, regardless of the nurse's personal values and beliefs.

Children must also learn to be effective listeners. In working with children, the nurse is responsible for ensuring that messages are accurately comprehended. When communicating with children, the nurse should be aware of their level of growth and development, age, sex, health status,

---

CRITICAL TO REMEMBER

Tips to Enhance Listening and Communication Skills

- Children understand better than they can talk.
- To develop conversations with children, ask open-ended questions rather than questions requiring yes/no responses.
- Comprehension is increased when the nurse uses different methods to present and share information.

---

personality, communication behavior, and intellectual abilities. These characteristics can suggest ways a child may respond to various messages. Such insight can be a foundation for selecting the content, structure, and form of the message most likely to achieve the child's comprehension (Haynes & Shulman, 1994).

To enhance the effectiveness of communication and maximize normal language patterns that contribute to language development, the nurse should focus on talking *with* children rather than *to* them. Develop conversations with children.

The nurse must be prepared to listen with the eyes as well as with the ears. Information will not always be audible, so the nurse must be alert to subtle cues in body language and physical closeness. Only then can one fully understand the messages of children. For example, when the nurse enters the room to complete an initial assessment of a 4-year-old child and observes the child turning away and beginning to suck her thumb, the child is communicating about her basic security and comfort level, even though she hasn't said a word.

Visual Communication

Eye contact is a communication connector. Making eye contact helps confirm attention and interest between the individuals communicating.

Clothing, physical appearance and objects being held are visual communicators. Children may react to an individual's presence based on a white lab coat, a bushy beard, a syringe, or a video game in hand. The nurse needs to think ahead and anticipate visual stimuli a child may find startling as well as those that may be pleasing, and make appropriate adjustments when possible. For example, it is a routine practice for nurses to bring a medication in a syringe for insertion into an intravenous line. Unless the purpose of the syringe is immediately explained, children may immediately assume they are about to receive an injection.

Some children, as well as some adults, are visual learners. They learn best when they can see or read instructions, demonstrations, diagrams, or information. Using various methods of presenting and sharing information will increase comprehension.

Concepts can be presented more vividly using photographs, videotapes, dolls, computer programs, charts, or graphs than using written or spoken words alone. The nurse needs to select teaching tools and materials that appropriately match the child's growth and developmental level.

Tone of Voice

The spoken word comes to mind most often when communication is the topic. Communication consists not only of what is said, however, but also the way it is said. The tone and quality of voice often communicate more than the words themselves.

Because infants' cognitive understanding of words is limited, their understanding is based on tone and quality of voice. A soft, smooth voice is more comforting and soothing to infants than a loud, startling, harsh voice. Infants can sense from the tone of voice whether their caregiver is angry or happy, frustrated or calm. The nurse can assess awareness of infants' sensitivities to these messages by observing their body language. Infants are relaxed when they hear a calm, happy caregiver and tense and rigid when they hear an angry, frustrated caregiver.

Children can detect anger, frustration, joy, and other feelings voices convey, even when the accompanying words are incongruent. This incongruity can be very confusing for children. The nurse should strive to make words and their intended meanings match.

Verbal communication extends beyond actual words. All audible sounds convey meaning. An infant's primary mode of audible communication is crying. Crying is a cue to check basic needs, including hunger, pain, discomfort (e.g., wet diaper), or temperature. Cooing and babbling, also heard during the first year of life, generally convey messages of comfort and contentment. As children develop and mature they will have increasing vocabularies to express their ideas, thoughts, and feelings verbally.

The choice of words is critical in verbal communication. The nurse should avoid talking down to children but should not expect them to understand adult words and phrases. Technical health care terms should be used selectively, and jargon should be avoided.

Body Language

From the gentle caress of holding an infant to sitting and listening intently to an adolescent's story, body language is a factor in communication. An open body stance and positioning invite communication and interaction, whereas a closed body stance and positioning impede communication and interaction.

Using an open body posture improves the nurse's understanding of children and the children's understanding of the nurse. Nurses need to learn to read children's body language and should become more aware of their own body language. Table 32–1 compares open and closed body postures.

Timing

Recognizing the appropriate time to communicate information is a developed skill. A distraught child whose parents have just left for work is not ready for a diabetic teaching session. The session will be much more productive and the information better comprehended if the child has a chance to make the transition. The child's needs must be met first rather than the convenience of a schedule.

TABLE 32–1

Open and Closed Body Postures

Open	Closed
Leaning toward other person	Leaning away from other person
Arms loose at the sides	Arms folded across chest
Frequent eye contact	No eye contact
Hands moving freely	Hands on hips
Soft stance, body swaying slightly	Rigid stance
Head up	Head bowed
Calm, slow movements	Constant motion, squirming
Smiling, friendly facial cues	Frowning, negative facial cues
Conversing at eye level	Conversing at diagonal eye level

Family-Centered Communication

Any discussion about effective ways to communicate with children must also include a discussion of effective communication with families. *Family-centered care* emphasizes that the family is intricately involved in the care of the child. Family-centered care is achieved when health care professionals can create partnerships with families, recognizing that the family is essential to the child and that the family has the right to participate fully in planning, implementing, and evaluating the child's plan of care.

Commitment to family-centered care means that the nurse respects the family's cultural, educational, and socioeconomic variations and can use the strengths of these variations. Family-centered care also means that the nurse truly believes that the child's care and recovery are greatly enhanced when the family fully participates in the child's care (Fig. 32–2).

Establishing Rapport

Critical to establishing good rapport with families is the nurse's ability to convey genuine respect and concern during the first encounter. Family members need to know that the nurse is interested in their well-being. A nonjudgmental

CRITICAL TO REMEMBER

Communicating with Families

- Include all involved family members. One of the most essential steps toward achieving a family-centered care environment is to develop open lines of communication with the family.
- Encourage families to write down their questions.
- Remain nonjudgmental.
- Give families both verbal and nonverbal messages that send a message of availability and openness.
- Respect and encourage feedback from families.

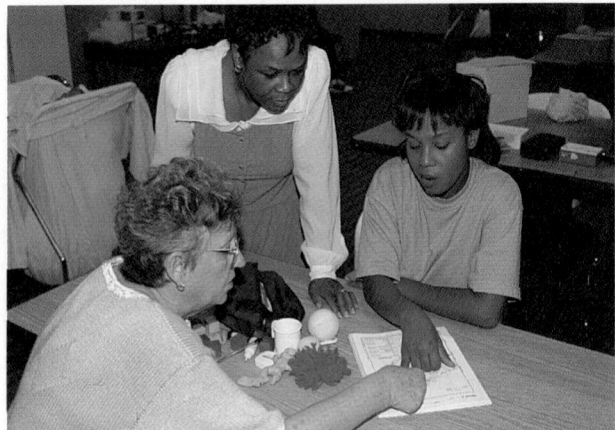

This nurse practitioner has learned Spanish to communicate better with her many Spanish-speaking clients. Speaking with family members in their own language encourages the family to remain in the health care system. The nurse is also using eye contact and has positioned herself at the mother's eye level. (Courtesy of Parkland Health and Hospital System Community Oriented Primary Care Clinic, Dallas, Texas)

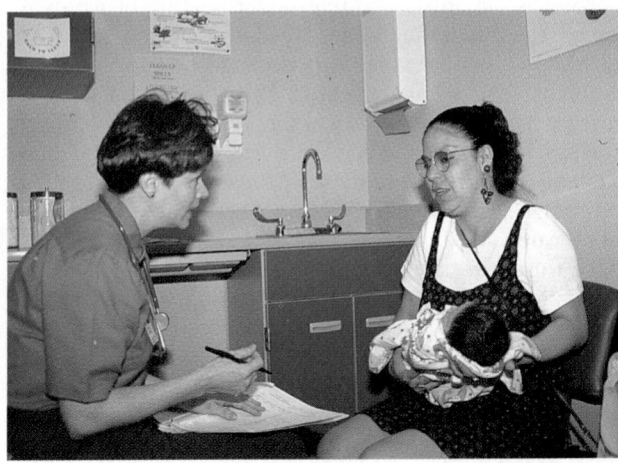

◀ The nurse explains a child's test results to his mother and grandmother. Including all important family members in the child's health care reflects a commitment to family-centered care. (Courtesy of The University of Texas at Arlington School of Nursing, Arlington, Texas)

FIGURE 32–2

The child's ongoing health care, both preventive and during illness, is enhanced by participation of the family.

approach and willingness to assist them in effectively caring for their child establish rapport.

Identifying Needs and Expectations

A thorough needs assessment of the child and family elicits information about problem-solving skills, cultural needs, coping behaviors, and the child's routines. A thorough assessment requires the nurse to obtain information from the child as well as the family. Assessment enables the nurse to develop better insight by gathering information from multiple perspectives and facilitates the development of a more comprehensive plan of care. The nurse should also describe routines and provide information about what the child and family can expect during their visit.

> The nurse might say, "Mrs. Brown, I value your input as well as your child's. Hearing Michael explain his understanding of his diabetic dietary restrictions in his own words will help us gain better insight into how best to manage his care. Let's take a few minutes to hear from Michael, and then we can talk about your perspective."

Availability and Openness to Questions

A nurse who does not take time to see how a child and family are doing—such as a nurse who leaves a room immediately after a treatment or administration of a medication—will not encourage or invite families to ask questions. Families want and need unrushed and uninterrupted time with the nurse. Sometimes this time can be made available only by purposefully scheduling it into the day.

> For example, encouraging families to write down their questions will enable them to take full advantage of their time with the nurse. The nurse might encourage use of time by saying, "I know you have a lot of questions and are very anxious to learn more about your son's condition. I have another patient who has an immediate need, but I will be available in 10 minutes to meet with you. In the meantime, here is a parent handbook that gives general information about seizures. Please feel free to review it and write down any questions that we can discuss when I return."

Family Education and Empowerment

Educating parents about their child's condition, ensuring their continued involvement in planning and evaluating the plan of care, and teaching them the skills to participate empower the family. Families need support as they gain confidence in their skills, and they need guidance to assist them as they navigate through the health care experience. Communication is enhanced when families feel competent and confident in their abilities.

Feedback from Children and Families

The nurse must be alert for verbal as well as nonverbal cues. Routinely checking with family members about their experiences, satisfaction with communications, teaching sessions, and health care goals is an effective way to ensure that health care providers obtain appropriate feedback. To enhance the delivery of care, the nurse should explain how this feedback will be used. The nurse should listen and observe carefully to make sure that what family members are saying is truly what they are feeling.

TABLE 32–2

Choosing Words Carefully

Poor Words	Rationale	Better Words	Rationale
Policies allowed or *not permitted*	Convey attitude that hospital personnel have authority over parents in matters concerning their children	*Guidelines, working together, welcome*	Convey openness and appreciation for position and importance of families
Noncompliant, uncooperative, difficult (when referring to parents and other family members)	Imply that health care providers make the decisions and give instructions that families must follow without input	*Partners, colleagues, joint decision-makers, experts about their child*	Acknowledge that families bring important information and insight and that families and professionals form a team
Dysfunctional, in denial, overprotective, uninvolved, uncaring (labeling families)	Pronounce a judgment that may not incorporate a full understanding of a family's situation, reactions, or perspective	*Coping* (describing family's reactions with care and respect)	Leaves room to build a more complete and appreciative understanding of families over time

For example, while one nurse was teaching the mother of a 2-year-old who was recently diagnosed with diabetes mellitus, the mother reported that although she was the primary caregiver of her child, the child's grandmother frequently cared for the child while the mother was at work. The nurse therefore notified the other team members and altered the teaching plan for diabetes care to include the child's grandmother.

Effective Management of Conflict

When conflict occurs, it should be addressed in an expedient manner to prevent further breakdown in communication. Table 32–2 discusses the importance of choosing words carefully to make families feel welcome and to further facilitate family-centered care.

Transcultural Communication: Bridging the Gap

Conflict can arise when the nurse comes from a different cultural background than the child and family. Such differences could influence the approach to care. As the demographics in the United States continue to change, health care professionals will be challenged to become more cross-cultural in their approach to clients if they want to continue to be effective in their relationships with children and families. Health care professionals need to be aware of their own values and beliefs, and need to recognize how these influence their interactions with others. They also need to be aware of and respect the child's and family's values and beliefs. In working with children and families, the initial assessment should address values, beliefs, and traditions. The nurse can then consider ways in which culture might affect communication style, methods of decision making, and other behaviors related to health care practices.

During the initial interview, the nurse should ascertain the following information related to the child and family:

- *Decision-making practices:* Are decisions made by individuals or collectively as a group?

Strategies for Managing Conflict

- *Understand the parents' perspective (walk in their shoes).* Imagine yourself as the parent of a child in a hospital where your values and beliefs are exposed and scrutinized. Try to understand their perspective better by encouraging them to share it.
- *Determine a common goal and stay focused on it.* Determine the result agreed upon and work toward it. By staying focused on a common goal, the parties involved are more likely to find workable strategies to achieve the identified goal.
- *Seek win-win solutions.* Conflict should not be about who is right and who is wrong. Effective conflict management focuses on finding a solution whereby both "win." By establishing a *common* goal, both parties win when this goal is achieved.
- *Listen actively.* Critical to resolving situations of conflict is the ability to listen and understand what the other person is saying and feeling. In active listening, the receiver actively and empathically listens to gain a better understanding of the actual and the implied message.
- *Openly express your feelings.* Talking about feelings is much more constructive than acting them out.

  For example, the nurse might say, "I am very concerned about Jamie's safety when you leave his side rails down."

- *Avoid blaming.* Each party owns part of the problem. Pointing fingers and blaming others will not solve the problem. Instead, identify the part of the problem that each party owns and work together to resolve it. Seek win-win solutions.
- *Summarize the decision.* At the end of any discussion, summarize what has been decided and identify who is responsible for follow-up. This process ensures that everyone is clear about the decision and facilitates accountability for implementing solutions.

- *Child-rearing practices:* Who are the primary caregivers? What are their disciplinary practices?
- *Family support:* What is the family structure? Whom does the patient and family turn to for support?
- *Communication practices:* How is the information communicated to the rest of the family?
- *Health and illness practices:* Do family members seek professional help or rely on other resources for treatment and advice?

Once this information is obtained, the nurse can use this knowledge to individualize the treatment plan and approach for the child's and family's needs. For example, if the parents of a child with an Orthodox Jewish religious background request a kosher diet, the nurse facilitates the routine delivery of kosher meals and communicates the family's wishes to the rest of the team members so that they can also respect the family's customs. If the family of a child who suffered a severe brain injury requests the services of a healer, the nurse enables the family to arrange the visit. Coordinating the child's daily schedule to provide an uninterrupted visit with the healer is one aspect of family-centered care.

Therapeutic Relationships: Maintaining Professional Boundaries

The nurse needs always to identify and maintain professional boundaries. Because nurses are caring, nurturing people and the profession demands that nurses sometimes become intimately involved in other people's lives, maintaining the balance between relating and professional separation is at times very difficult. The key to establishing a supportive therapeutic relationship, however, lies in the ability to maintain this balance successfully. The nurse who loses sight of this boundary and becomes too emotionally involved loses effectiveness as an objective professional resource (Barnsteiner & Gillis-Donovan, 1990). The erosion of professional boundaries greatly diminishes the nurse's ability to guide families effectively in meeting the health care needs of their children.

Family members may display feelings of incompetence, fear, and loss of control by expressing anger, withdrawal, or dissatisfaction. Most important in working with these families is to promote the parents' feelings of competency through education and empowerment. The nurse should keep parents well informed of the child's care through frequent phone calls and involvement in decision making. The nurse should promote their confidence, enhance their self-esteem, and foster their independence by teaching them the skills necessary to care for their child.

CRITICAL TO REMEMBER
Maintaining a Therapeutic Relationship

Maintaining professional boundaries requires that the nurse constantly be aware of the fine line between empathy and overinvolvement.

Warning Signs of Overinvolvement

- Buying gifts for individual children or families
- Giving out a home phone number
- Competing with other staff for the child/family's affection
- Inviting child/family to social gatherings
- Accepting invitations to family gatherings (e.g., birthday parties, weddings)
- Visiting or spending time with child/family during off-duty time
- Revealing personal information
- Lending or borrowing money
- Making decisions for the family about the child's care

Nurses must be able to recognize their own personal and professional needs. Awareness of the motives for one's own actions will greatly enhance the nurse's ability to understand the needs of children and families and to give families the tools to manage care effectively.

Communication Strategies for Nurses

Determining the Best Communication Approach

Nurses working with children should determine the best communication approach for each child individually, based on the child's age and developmental abilities. This decision requires that the nurse understand developmental milestones and be able to assess the child's comprehension and communication skills. This assessment needs to include an evaluation of the child's cognitive and emotional development as well as language abilities. Table 32–3 presents an overview of developmental milestones related to communication skills in children and some approaches to facilitate successful interactions.

Play

Play can greatly facilitate communicating with children. Approaching children at their developmental level with fa-

CRITICAL THINKING EXERCISE 32–1

The nurse caring for 8-year-old Jimmy observes him lying in his bed with his back facing the door. He is crying, although he quickly wipes his eyes when he sees the nurse at the door. Jimmy has been hospitalized because of leukemia. He lives in a small community 350 miles from the hospital. His parents visit on the weekends.

1. Identify two things that might be upsetting Jimmy.
2. What strategies could you use to encourage Jimmy to talk about his feelings related to the problems you have identified?

TABLE 32-3

Developmental Milestones and Their Relationship to Communication Approaches

Development	Language Development	Emotional Development	Cognitive Development	Suggested Communication Approach
Infants (0–12 Months)				
The infant experiences the world through the senses of hearing, seeing, smelling, tasting, and touching.	Crying, babbling, cooing Single-word production Able to name some simple objects	Dependent on others; high need for cuddling and security Responsive to environment (sounds, visual stimuli, etc.) Distinguish between happy and angry voices as well as between familiar and strange voices Beginning to experience separation anxiety	Interactions largely reflexive Beginning to see repetition of activities and movements Beginning to initiate interactions intentionally Short attention span (1–2 minutes)	Use calm, soft, soothing voice. Be responsive to cries. Engage in turn-taking vocalizations (adult imitates baby sounds). Talk and read regularly to infants. Prepare infant as you are about to perform care. Talk to infant about what you are about to do. Use a slow approach and allow child time to get to know you.
Toddlers (1–2 Years)				
Toddlers experience the world through the senses of hearing, seeing, smelling, tasting, and touching.	Two-word combinations emerge. Participate in turn-taking in communication (speaker/listener) "No" becomes a favorite word. Able to use gestures and verbalize simple wants and needs.	Strong need for security objects Separation/stranger anxiety heightened Participate in parallel play Thrive on routines Beginning development of independence: "Want to do by self" Still very dependent on significant adults	Experiment with objects Participate in active exploration Begin to experiment with variations on activities Begin to identify cause-and-effect relationships Short attention span (3–5 minutes)	Learn the toddler's words for common items and use them in conversations. Describe activities and procedures as they are about to be done. Use picture books. Use play for demonstrations. Be responsive to child's receptivity toward you and approach cautiously. Preparation should occur immediately prior to the event.
Preschool Children (3–5 Years)				
Preschool children use words they do not fully understand, nor do they accurately understand many words used by others.	Further development and expansion of word combination (able to speak in full sentences) Upward growth in correct grammatical usage Use pronouns Clearer articulation of sounds Vocabulary rapidly expanding; may know words without understanding meaning	Like to imitate activities and make choices Strive for independence but need adult support and encouragement Demonstrate purposeful attention-seeking behaviors Learn cooperation and turn-taking in game playing Need clearly set limits and boundaries	Begin developing concepts of time, space, and quantity Magical thinking prominent World seen only from child's perspective Short attention span (5–10 minutes)	Seek opportunities to offer choices. Use play to explain procedures and activities. Speak in simple sentences and explore relative concepts. Use picture and story books, puppets. Describe activities and procedures as they are about to be done. Be concise; limit length of explanations (<5 minutes). Engage in preparatory activities 1–3 hours prior to the event.

Table continued on following page

TABLE 32–3
. . . .

Developmental Milestones and Their Relationship to Communication Approaches Continued

Development	Language Development	Emotional Development	Cognitive Development	Suggested Communication Approach
School-Age Children (6–11 Years)				
Communicate thoughts and appreciate viewpoints of others. Words with multiple meanings and words describing things they have not experienced are not thoroughly understood.	Expanding vocabulary enables child to describe concepts, thoughts, and feelings Development of conversational skills	Interact well with others Understand rules to games Very interested in learning Build close friendships Beginning to accept responsibility for own actions Competition emerges Still dependent on adults to meet needs	Able to grasp concepts of classification, conversation Concrete thinking emerges Become very oriented to "rules" Able to process information in serial format Lengthened attention span (10–30 minutes)	Use photographs, books, diagrams, charts, videos to explain. Make explanations sequential. Engage in conversations that encourage critical thinking. Establish limits and set consequences. Use medical play techniques. Introduce preparatory materials 1–5 days in advance of the event.
Adolescents (12 Years and Older)				
Adolescents are able to create theories and generate many explanations for situations. Beginning of communicating like an adult.	Able to verbalize and comprehend most adult concepts	Beginning to accept responsibility for own actions Perception of "imaginary audiences" Need independence Competitive drive Strong need for group identification Frequently have small group of very close friends Question authority Strong need for privacy	Able to think logically and abstractly Attention span up to 60 minutes	Engage in conversations about adolescent's interests. Use photographs, books, diagrams, charts, and videos to explain. Use collaborative approach and foster/support independence. Introduce preparatory materials up to 1 week in advance of the event. Be respectful of privacy needs.

miliar forms of play increases their comfort and allows the nurse to be seen in a more positive, less threatening role.

Because play is an everyday part of children's lives and a method they use to communicate, they are less likely to be inhibited when participating in play interactions. Through play, children may express thoughts and feelings they may be unable to verbalize.

Storytelling

Storytelling is an innovative and creative communication strategy. It is also a skill that can be acquired and refined through practice. Familiarity with stories and frequent practice in storytelling increase a nurse's confidence and competence as storyteller. Storytelling can be a routine part of a nurse's day. Its purposes range from establishing rapport to approaching uncomfortable topics such as loss, death, fear,

. . . .
Storytelling Strategies

- Capture a story on paper or on videotape as told by a child or group of children.
- Tell a "yarn story" with two or more people. A long piece of yarn with knots tied at varied intervals is slid loosely through the hands of the teller until a knot is felt, at which time the yarn is passed to the next person, who continues the story.
- Initiate a game of sentence completion, either oral or written, with sentences beginning "If I were in charge of the hospital . . . ," "I wish . . . ," "When I get home I will . . . ," or "My family. . . ."
- Read stories with themes related to issues a child is facing. The children's section of the local public library is an excellent resource.

grief, and anger. In storytelling, there is a teller and a listener. In individual situations the child may be the teller or the listener, although in a shared story, adult and child may each take a turn in both roles.

Explaining Procedures and Treatments

Preparation before a procedure, which includes explaining the reasons for the procedure and the expected sequence of events and outcomes, can greatly reduce a child's fears and anxieties. Preparation enables the child to experience some mastery over events, gives the child time to develop effective coping behaviors, and fosters trust in those caring for the child. Adequate preparation is the key to helping a child have a successful, positive health care experience.

In general, the younger the child, the closer to the event preparation should occur. For example, a 3-year-old will generally be very anxious and therefore should be prepared immediately before, whereas a teenager would benefit from a longer preparation time so that he or she can develop

strategies for dealing with the situation. See Table 32–3 for age-related attention span guidelines.

Key elements for communicating complete and accurate information are as follows (Gaynard et al., 1990):

- *Learn the procedure.* To explain a procedure adequately, the nurse must understand what is involved. What pieces of equipment will be used? Where will the procedure take place? Essentially, the nurse needs to learn what the child can expect to happen during the procedure.
- *Determine what information to share with the child and family.* The preparation should include information only about what the child will experience or perceive directly. Consultation with the family will allow the nurse to learn words and terminology used by the child. Table 32–4 offers other concrete suggestions in choosing appropriate language for nurses to use in working with children.
- *Provide sensory information.* Allowing children to see, hear, feel, taste, smell, and experience similar sensations during their preparation will greatly enhance their preparedness and diminish their anxieties. For example, in

---

TABLE 32–4

Considerations in Choosing Language

Potentially Ambiguous	*Concrete Explanation*
"The doctor will give you some dye." *To make me die?*	"The doctor will put some medicine in the tube that will help her see your _____ more clearly."
Dressing, dressing change *Why are they going to undress me?* *Do I have to change my clothes?*	Bandages; clean, new bandages
Stool collection *Why do they want to collect little chairs?*	Use child's familiar term, such as "poop" or "BM" or "doody."
Urine *You're in?*	Use child's familiar term, such as "pee."
Shot *When people get shot, they're really badly hurt.*	Describe giving medicine through a (small, tiny) needle.
CAT scan *Will there be cats?*	Describe in simple terms and explain what the letters of the common name stand for.
PICU *Pick you?*	Explain as above.
ICU *I see you?*	Explain as above.
IV *Ivy?*	Explain as above.
Stretcher *Stretch her? Stretch whom?*	Bed on wheels
Special; funny (words that are usually positive descriptors) *It doesn't look/feel special to me.*	Odd, different, unusual, strange
Gas, sleeping gas *Is someone going to pour gasoline into the mask?*	"A medicine, called anesthesia, is a kind of air you will breathe through a mask like this to help you sleep during your operation so you won't feel anything. It is a different kind of sleep." (Explain differences.)

Table continued on following page

TABLE 32-4
• • • • • • • • • •

Considerations in Choosing Language *Continued*

Potentially Ambiguous	Concrete Explanation
"The doctor will put you to sleep." *Like my cat was put to sleep? It never came back.*	"The doctor will give you medicine that will help you go into a very deep sleep. You won't feel anything until the operation is over. Then the doctor will stop giving you the medicine, so you can wake up."
"Move you to the floor" *Why are they going to put me on the ground?*	Unit, ward (Explain why the child is being transferred, and where.)
OR (or treatment room) table *People aren't supposed to get up on tables.*	A narrow bed
"Take a picture" (x-ray, CT, and MRI machines are far larger than a familiar camera, move differently, and don't yield a familiar end product.)	"A picture of your insides" (Describe appearance, sounds, and movement of the equipment.)
"Flush your IV" *Flush it down the toilet?*	Explain

Words can be experienced as "hard" or "soft" according to how much they increase the perceived threat of a situation. For example, consider the following word choices.

Harder	Softer
"This part will hurt."	"It (you) may feel (or feel very) sore, achy, scratchy, tight, snug, full, or _____ (other manageable, descriptive term)." (Words such as scratch, poke, or sting might be familiar for some children and frightening to others.)
"The medicine will burn."	"Some children say they feel very warm."
"The room will be very cold."	"Some children say they feel very cold."
"The medicine will taste (or smell) bad."	"The medicine may taste (or smell) different from anything you have tasted before. After you take it, will you tell me how it was for you?"
"Cut," "open you up," "slice," "make a hole"	"The doctor will make an opening." (Use concrete comparisons, such as "your little finger" or "a paper clip" *if* the opening will indeed be small.)
"As big as _____" (e.g., size of an incision or of a catheter)	"Smaller than _____."
"As long as _____" (e.g., for duration of a procedure)	"For less time than it takes you to _____."
"As much as _____" (These are open-ended and "extending" expressions.)"	Less than _____." (These expressions help confine, familiarize, and imply the manageability of an event or of equipment.)

The unfamiliar usage or complexity of some common medical words or expressions can be confusing and frightening.

Potentially Ambiguous	Concrete Explanation
"Take your vitals" (or "your vital signs")	"Measure your temperature," "see how warm your body is," "see how fast and strongly your heart is working." (Nothing is "taken" from the child.)

TABLE 32–4

Considerations in Choosing Language Continued

Potentially Ambiguous	Concrete Explanation
Electrodes, leads	"Sticky like a Band-Aid, with a small wet spot in the center, and small strings that attach to the snap (monitor electrodes); paste like wet sand, with strings with tiny metal cups that stick to the paste (EEG electrodes). The paste washes off easily afterward; the strings go into a box that will make a picture of how your heart (or brain) is working." (Show child electrodes and leads before using. Let child handle them and apply them to a doll or to self.)
"Hang your (IV) medication"	"We will bring in a new medicine in a bag and attach it to the little tube already in your arm. The needle goes into the tube, not into your arm, so you won't feel it."
NPO	"Nothing to eat. Your stomach needs to be empty." (Explain why.) "You can eat and drink again as soon as _____." (Explain with concrete descriptions.)
Anesthesia	"The doctor will give you medicine—you may hear it called 'anesthesia.' It will help you go into a very deep sleep. You will not feel anything at all. The doctors know just the right amount of medicine to give you so you will stay asleep through your operation. When the operation is over, the doctor stops giving you that medicine and helps you wake up."

Note: Words or phrases that are helpful to one child may be threatening for another. Health care providers must listen carefully and be sensitive to the child's use of and response to language.

Adapted with permission of the Association for the Care of Children's Health, 7910 Woodmont Ave., Suite 300, Bethesda, MD 20814, from Gaynard, L., Wolfer, J., Goldberger, J., Thompson, R., Redburn, L., & Laidley, L. (1990). *Psychosocial care of children in hospitals: A clinical practice manual from ACCH Child Life Research Project.* Bethesda, MD: The Association for the Care of Children's Health.

preparing a child for an intravenous line insertion, the nurse can show the child the catheter or explain the purpose of the tourniquet and allow the child to put it on or to put it on the arm of a doll, if the child so desires. The nurse should let the child smell an alcohol swab and feel its coolness when applied to the skin. Showing the child the treatment room and allowing the child to sit on the treatment table where the procedure will be performed is an effective way to convey information.

• *Explain the sequence of events.* Preparation includes a description of the sequence in which events will occur. Recognizing the procedure as a series of sequential steps allows children to anticipate appropriately and gives them a sense of control as well as a better understanding of the number of steps to expect before the procedure is over.

• *Explain how long the procedure will last.* Whenever possible, the nurse should allow the child to have simulated play experiences. Allowing the child to perform the procedure on a doll or stuffed animal is often effective and gives children a real sense of time as well as firsthand experience with the sequence of events. If a concrete demonstration is not possible, the nurse should explain the timing in terms that the child can understand; for example, the nurse might say, "The procedure will last as long as it takes to sing your favorite song."

• *Monitor accuracy of information (feedback).* Feedback can be used to modify or reinforce future preparation sessions. Feedback also allows the nurse to correct any misunderstandings the child may have and provides an opportunity for the child to process verbally and express feelings about the experience.

TABLE 32–5

Self-Esteem in Children: Communication Practices

Techniques to Enhance Self-Esteem	Practices That Harm Self-Esteem
Praise efforts and accomplishments.	Criticize efforts and accomplishments.
Use active listening skills.	Be too busy to listen.
Encourage expression of feelings.	Tell children how they should feel.
Acknowledge feelings.	Give no support for dealing with feelings.
Use developmentally based discipline.	Use physical punishment.
Use "I" statements.	Use "you" statements.
Be nonjudgmental.	Judge the child.
Set clearly defined limits and reinforce them.	Set no known limits or boundaries.
Share quality time together.	Give time grudgingly.
Be honest.	Be dishonest.
Describe behaviors observed when praising and disciplining.	Use coercion and power as discipline.
Compliment the child.	Belittle, blame, or shame the child.
Smile.	Use sarcastic, caustic, or cruel "humor"
Touch and hug the child.	Avoid coming near child even when the child is open to touching, holding, or hugging. Touch and hold only when performing a task.
Rock the child.	Avoid comforting through rocking.

Open, honest communication about treatments and procedures and attentiveness to the learning needs of the child will greatly facilitate the achievement of the treatment goals.

Strategies for Enhancing Self-esteem

Stanley Coopersmith (1967) defined self-esteem as a "personal judgement of worthiness that is expressed in the attitudes the individual holds toward himself or herself." Communication practices play an important role in the development of children's self-esteem. Nurses are in an excellent position to model communication practices that enhance self-esteem. Table 32–5 offers comparisons of helpful and harmful communication practices.

The words adults choose, their tone of voice, and the place and timing of message delivery all influence the child's interpretation of the message. The interpretation may be positive, negative, or neutral. To enhance the child's self-esteem, adults should strive for positive language. Active listening, the use of positive language, discarding "labels," and encouraging rather than pressuring are some of the ways to communicate that help build self-esteem (Sifuentes, 1996).

▌Communicating with Children Who Have Special Needs

The opportunity to interact with children who have special communication needs presents an exciting challenge for nurses. To identify successful alternative methods of communication, the nurse needs to learn particular techniques for working with children and families. Alternative methods of communicating are critical. Children need to express

CRITICAL TO REMEMBER

Communicating with Children with Special Needs

In working with children with special needs, the nurse must carefully assess each child's physical, mental, and developmental abilities and determine the most effective methods of communication.

their wants and needs accurately. Through adequate preparation and reassurance, the nurse can offer the child comfort and understanding. Successfully meeting this challenge is a rewarding experience for the nurse and a positive, supportive experience for the child and family.

The Child with a Visual Impairment

For the child with a visual impairment, the nurse can do the following:

- Obtain a thorough assessment of the child's self-help skills and abilities (include toileting, bathing, dressing, feeding, and mobility).
- Orient the child to the surroundings. Walk the child around the room and unit several times, indicating landmarks (such as doors, closets, bedside tables, windows) while guiding the child by the hand. Explain sounds that the child may frequently hear (such as monitors, alarms, nurse call bell).
- Encourage the parents to stay with the child. They can

facilitate communication and greatly enhance the child's comfort in this unfamiliar environment.

- Keep furniture and other items in the same consistent place. Consistency aids in the child's orientation to the room, and fosters independence, and promotes safety.
- Keep the nurse call bell in the same place and within the child's reach.
- Identify yourself when entering the room and tell the child when you are departing.
- Carefully and fully explain all procedures.
- Allow the child to handle equipment while explaining the procedure to enhance understanding.

The Child with a Hearing Impairment

For the child with a hearing impairment, the nurse can do the following:

- Thoroughly assess the child's self-help skills and abilities.
- Identify the family's method of communication and, if possible, adopt it.
- Encourage a family member to stay with the child at all times to decrease the stress of hospitalization and facilitate communication.
- If sign language is used, learn the most frequently used signs and use them whenever able.
- Develop a communication board with pictures of most commonly used items or needs (e.g., television, cup, toothbrush, toilet, shower).
- Determine whether the child uses a hearing aid. If so, make sure the batteries are working and the hearing aid is clean and intact.
- When entering the room, do so cautiously and gently touch the child before speaking.
- Always face the child when speaking. If the child is a lip reader, face-to-face visibility will greatly enhance the child's ability to understand.
- Do not shout or exaggerate speech. This behavior distorts the face and can be very confusing. Rather, speak in a normal tone and at a regular pace.
- Remember that nonverbal communication can speak as loud as, if not louder than, speech (e.g., a frown or worried face can say more than words).
- When performing a procedure that requires standing behind the child, such as when giving an enema or assisting with a spinal tap, have another person stand in front of the child and explain the procedure as it is being performed.
- Whenever possible, use play strategies to help communicate and demonstrate procedures (see pp. 814, 816).

The Child Who Speaks Another Language

For the child who speaks another language, the nurse can do the following:

- Thoroughly assess the child's abilities in speaking and understanding both languages.
- Ask family members if they would like an interpreter, and involve them in the selection. Whenever possible, avoid using children as interpreters because this role can

place psychological stress on a child (Lynch & Hanson, 1992).

- Identify an interpreter, perhaps another adult family member, friend of the family, or other individual with proficiency in both languages.
- Use an interpreter whenever possible but especially when explaining procedures, determining understanding, teaching new skills, and assessing needs.
- Use a communication board with the names of items printed in both languages.
- Learn the words and names of commonly used items in the child's language and use them whenever possible. Using the familiar language not only aids in communication but also demonstrates sincere interest in learning the language and respect for the culture.
- Learn as much about the child's culture as possible and develop plans of care that demonstrate respect for the culture. Sincere attempts to learn to communicate with the child and family demonstrate your concern for their well-being.
- Use play strategies whenever possible. Play seems to be a universal language.

The Aphonic Child

For the aphonic child, the nurse can do the following:

- Thoroughly assess the child's self-help skills and abilities. Determine the child's and family's methods of communicating and adopt these as much as possible.
- Encourage parents to stay with the child to decrease anxiety and foster communication.
- Determine whether the child uses sign language or augmented communication devices.
- Use a communication board.
- Be attentive to and maximize the child's nonverbal communication. Facial grimaces, frowns, smiles, and nods are effective means of communicating responses and expressing likes and dislikes.
- If appropriate, encourage the child to use writing boards (dry erase, chalk, or pads of paper) to write needs, wants, questions, and concerns.

The Child with a Profound Neurologic Impairment

For the child with a profound neurologic impairment, the nurse can do the following:

- Because hearing, vision, and language abilities are often hard to determine in this population, assume the child can hear, see, and comprehend something in what is said. Use a friendly tone of voice that conveys warmth and respect.
- Address the child when entering and exiting the room. Gently touch the child while saying the child's name.
- Speak softly, calmly, and slowly to allow the child time to process what you are saying.
- While in the room with the child, talk to the child. Do not talk as if the child were not there. For example, the nurse might say, "Jenny, I am going to wash your arm now," or "Jenny, now I am going to take your tem-

perature by putting the thermometer under your arm." Identifying an assistant, the nurse might say, "Jenny, Kristi, another nurse, is here to help me lift you into your chair."

- Talk to the child about activities and objects in the room, things that the child might see, hear, smell, touch, taste, or sense. For example, the nurse might say, "It is a sunny day today; can you feel the warm sun shining on you through the window?"
- When asking the child questions, allow the child adequate time to respond. Be careful to ask questions only of children who are capable of responding.
- Ascertain the child's ability to respond to simple ques-

tions. Some children can respond to yes/no questions by squeezing a hand and/or blinking their eyes (once for yes and twice for no).

- Be extremely attentive to any signs or gestures (facial grimaces, smiling, eye movements) that may convey responses to likes or dislikes. Signs or gestures may be the child's only means of communicating.
- As with all children with special communication needs, thoroughly document and communicate to others who interact with them any special techniques that work. Providing information will greatly enhance continuity and more fully facilitate the child's ability to communicate.

KEY CONCEPTS

- Components of effective communication with children involve verbal as well as nonverbal interactions. Essential components include touch, physical proximity, environment, listening, eye contact, visual cues, pace of speech and tone of voice, and overall body language.
- Nurses should determine the best communication approach for an individual child, based on the child's age and developmental abilities. Strategies include play and storytelling, explaining procedures

and treatments, and modeling communication practices that enhance self-esteem.
- Communication pitfalls, such as using jargon, talking down to children or beyond their developmental level, and avoiding or denying a problem, can lead to a breakdown in the relationship between the nurse and the child and family.
- Family-centered communication strategies include establishing rapport, identifying needs, establishing expectations, being available

and open to questions, family education, empowerment, obtaining feedback from children and families, promoting effective conflict management, learning techniques for transcultural communication, and maintaining professional boundaries.
- In working with children with special needs, the nurse should carefully assess each child's physical, mental, and developmental abilities and determine the most effective methods of communication.

ANSWERS TO CRITICAL THINKING EXERCISE 32–1

1. Two areas that the nurse should explore are Jimmy's feelings about separation from his family and issues related to having leukemia, including the discomfort, treatment, and prognosis.
2. School-age children often do not readily discuss their feelings. The nurse needs to build trust with the child. Involving the child in a board game can be a useful strategy

to help the child relax. As the game progresses, the nurse can begin to talk with the child using a lead in such as, "You seem very quiet today" or "You seemed upset when I came into your room." The child can choose to validate or deny the nurse's observation.

Another approach would be to say, "If you could have one wish today, what would it be?" Some chil-

dren will use this as an opportunity to describe what they would like to change. The nurse can cue into this disclosure. It is important to remember that all children are different, and what works for one child may not work for another. Every nurse caring for children needs to understand growth and development and learn related communication techniques.

REFERENCES AND READINGS

Print References

Adams, R. J., & Parrott, R. (1995). Pediatric nurses' communication of role expectations to parents of hospitalized children. *Journal of Applied Communication Research, 22*(1), 36–47.

Almquist, N. L., Bisson, S., & Wynia, A. (1998). Bringing an early pediatric literacy

program to the clinic setting. *Journal of Pediatric Health Care, 12*(5), 276–279.

Anteau, C. M., & Williams, L. A. (1997). The Oklahoma bombing: Lessons learned. *Critical Care Nursing Clinics of North America, 9*(2), 231–236.

Barnsteiner, J. H., & Gillis-Donovan, J. (1990). Being related and separate: A stan-

dard for therapeutic relationships. *MCN: American Journal of Maternal/Child Nursing, 15,* 223–228.

Bob, P. S. S., & Famolare, N. E. (1998). Teaching and communication strategies: Working with the hospitalized adolescent with pelvic inflammatory disease. *Pediatric Nursing, 42*(1), 17–20.

Coopersmith, S. (1967). *The antecedents of self-esteem*. San Francisco: Freeman.

Garbarino, J., Stott, F. M., & Faculty of the Erikson Institute. (1990). *What children can tell us: Eliciting, interpreting and evaluating information from children*. San Francisco: Jossey-Bass.

Gaynard, L., Wolfer, J., Goldberger, J., Thompson, R., Redburn, L., & Laidley, L. (1990). *Psychosocial care of children in hospitals: A clinical practice manual from ACCH Child Life Research Project*. Bethesda, MD: The Association for the Care of Children's Health.

Grover, G. (1996a). Talking to adolescents. In C. D. Berkowitz (Ed.), *Pediatrics: A primary care approach*. Philadelphia: Saunders.

Grover, G. (1996b). Talking to children. In C. D. Berkowitz (Ed.), *Pediatrics: A primary care approach*. Philadelphia: Saunders.

Grover, G. (1996c). Talking to parents. In C. D. Berkowitz (Ed.), *Pediatrics: A primary care approach*. Philadelphia: Saunders.

Haynes, W. O., & Shulman, B. B. (1994). *Communication development: Foundations, processes, and clinical applications*. Englewood Cliffs, NJ: Prentice Hall.

Hobbie, C. (1995). Maximizing healthy communication: Readability of patient educational materials. *Journal of Pediatric Health Care, 9*(2), 92–93.

Horn, J. D., Feldman, H. M., & Ploof, D. L. (1996). Parent and professional perceptions about stress and coping strategies during a child's lengthy hospitalization. *Social Work in Health Care, 21*(1), 107–127.

Jeppson, E. S., & Thomas, J. (1995). *Essential allies: Families as advisors*. Bethesda, MD: Institute for Family-Centered Care.

Lynch, E. W., & Hanson, M. J. (1992). *Developing cross-cultural competence: A guide for working with young children and their families*. Baltimore: Paul H. Brookes.

Manworren, R. C., & Woodring, B. (1998). Evaluating children's literature as a source for patient education. *Pediatric Nursing, 24*(6), 548–553.

McElveen, K. A. (1997). Practical hints: Communicating with children. Could you use some help? MCN: *American Journal of Maternal/Child Nursing, 22*, 108–111.

Shaner, K. H., & Bechtel, N. M. (1997). Bridging the gap: How to communicate with pediatric patients and their families. *Emergency Medical Services, 26*(3), 46.

Sieving, R. E., & Zirbel-Donisch, S. T. (1990). Development and enhancement of self-esteem in children. *Journal of Pediatric Health Care, 4*(6), 290–296.

Sifuentes, M. (1996). Fostering self-esteem. In C. D. Berkowitz (Ed.), *Pediatrics: A primary care approach*. Philadelphia: Saunders.

Stanley, J. M. (1998). The effect of music and multimodal stimulation on responses of premature infants in neonatal intensive care. *Pediatric Nursing, 42*(6), 532–538.

Woodgate, R., & Kristjanson, L. J. (1996). "Getting better from my hurts": Toward a model of the young child's pain experience. *Journal of Pediatric Nursing, 11*(4), 233–242.

Video References

Association for the Care of Children's Health. (1991). *Communicating with children: Supportive interactions in hospitals* [Film]. (7910 Woodmont Ave., Bethesda, MD 20814)

University of Colorado Health Science Center School of Nursing. (1993). *Communication with preverbal infants and young children*. (Available from Learner Managed Designs, Inc., P.O. Box 747, Lawrence, KS 66044).

Hall, J. (Executive Producer), & Atkins, P. (Producer/Director). (1995). *Designing for family-centered care* [Film]. (Available from Institute for Family-Centered Care, Bethesda, MD)

(1976). Having an operation. In *Mr. Rogers*. Family Communications, Inc., 4802 5th Ave., Pittsburgh, PA.

(1986). Going to the doctor. In *Mr. Rogers*. Family Communications, Inc., 4802 5th Ave., Pittsburgh, PA.

University of Colorado Health Science Center School of Nursing. (1993). *The process of communication: Facilitating interactions with young children with severe disabilities in mainstream early childhood programs*. (Available from Learner Managed Designs, Inc., P.O. Box 747, Lawrence, KS 66044)

33

Physical Assessment of Children

LEARNING OBJECTIVES

After studying this chapter, you should be able to:

- Apply principles of anatomy and physiology to the systematic physical assessment of the child.
- Describe the major components of pediatric history taking.
- Identify the principal techniques for doing a physical examination.
- Use a systematic and developmentally appropriate approach for examining a child.
- Describe the general sequence of the physical examination of the infant, the young child, the school-age child, and the adolescent.
- Describe normal findings of a physical examination.
- List common terms used in describing the findings on physical examination.
- Record physical examination findings in a systematic way.

DEFINITIONS

auscultation Elicitation and evaluation of sounds produced by the body, frequently by using a stethoscope to magnify body sounds.

circumduction Circular movement of a limb or an eye.

crepitation A dry, crackling sound or sensation.

development Changes that occur over time in function and psychosocial and cognitive behavior.

fasciculation A small, local, involuntary muscular contraction visible under the skin.

fremitus A vibration perceptible on palpation or auscultation.

growth Measurable physical and physiologic changes that occur over time.

history The aggregate of subjective data that describe past and present health status.

inspection Careful observation to identify physical findings.

obtund To render dull or blunt.

palpation The use of touch to determine such factors as texture, temperature, moisture, and organ location.

percussion Tapping of the body to determine the density, location, and size of organs.

systematic assessment Organized method of collecting data.

Nurses perform physical assessments of infants and children in various settings—the clinic, the hospital, the school, and the home. The physical examination may be part of a well-child assessment, it may be the admission examination when a child enters the hospital, or it may be part of an initial assessment for home health care. The physical examination provides objective and subjective information about the child. It allows health care providers to determine the child's health status and make judgments about the need for nursing care.

General Approaches to Physical Assessment

As when providing any nursing care for infants and children, the nurse applies knowledge of growth and development. Such knowledge assists in preparing the child and performing the examination. Parents should be involved as much as possible, and the child should be encouraged to handle and play with instruments that are safe, such as the stethoscope.

The physical examination is often the first direct contact between the nurse and the child. Establishing a trusting relationship between the child and the examiner is important. Throughout the examination the nurse should be sensitive to the cultural needs of and differences among children. A quiet, private environment should be provided for the history and physical examination. The classic systematic approach to the physical examination is to begin at the head and proceed through the entire body to the toes. When examining a child, however, the physical assessment must be tailored to the child's age and developmental level.

Infants 1 to 6 Months

Infants age 1 to 6 months are responsive to human faces, are increasingly interested in their environment, and do not

---

CRITICAL TO REMEMBER

Adapting the Physical Examination to the Child

The classic systematic approach to the physical examination is to begin at the head and proceed to the toes. For children, the physical examination is tailored to the child's age and developmental level. Painful or frightening procedures should be left to last. Involving parents by asking them to hold or stand by the child can decrease children's anxiety and assist them in relaxing.

---

mind being undressed (see Chapter 5). Their examination should therefore be relatively easy. If the infant is nursing or asleep in the parent's arms, auscultate the heart, lungs, and abdomen without waking the baby. If the baby is awake, lay the baby on the examining table with the parent close by. As body parts are examined, incorporate evaluation of the primitive reflexes—palmar grasp, plantar grasp, placing, stepping, and tonic neck reflexes. Leave all uncomfortable procedures, such as abduction of the hips, speculum examination of the tympanic membranes, and eliciting the Moro reflex, until last. Before beginning the examination, undress the infant, leaving the diaper on a male child. Refocus an unhappy infant by calmly talking in a soft voice, distracting with a rattle, or using a pacifier.

Infants 6 to 12 Months

For an older infant, follow the same procedures used for the infant from birth to 6 months, but keep in mind that infants 6 months and older experience stranger anxiety and so are more difficult to examine. Distracting a child of this age with a toy or object may be useful. It is easier to do as much of the examination as possible with the child held on the parent's lap. Leave ear, oral, and other uncomfortable procedures until last.

Toddlers

Toddlers are the most challenging to examine because they are least likely to "cooperate" (see Chapter 6). To form a supportive relationship with the parent and toddler, the examiner begins by sitting or standing next to the parent. To facilitate relaxation, the examiner can provide a few toys and books and encourage the child to explore. Fears can be decreased by allowing the child to handle objects used during the examination (see pp. 826–828). Communicating with the child, using age-appropriate words to describe what is about to be done, can also help decrease fear.

Portions of the examination can be done before the child is totally undressed. The order of the examination is flexible, and painful or frightening procedures should be left to last. Resistance is common with toddlers. Assure the parent that the child's response to the examination is normal. The parent is the best assistant and can be asked to hold the child's outstretched arms against the child's head or abdomen while the examiner's body immobilizes the lower half of the child's body.

Preschoolers

The preschool child is usually more cooperative, but these children still like to have their parents nearby (see Chapter 6). Preschool children are happy to show nurses that they can undress themselves. They can also be expected to cooperate. The nurse may proceed with the examination from the head to the toes but should still save the more invasive procedures, such as the speculum ear examination and the oral examination, until the end of the examination. The examiner can reinforce the child's interest by allowing the child to participate in the examination and by praising the child for cooperating.

HEALTH SCREENING FOR A 2-YEAR-OLD

◆ ◆ ◆ ◆ ◆ ◆ ◆

Community-based clinics promote optimum health in their clients. Children and their parents can develop an ongoing relationship with a provider, which encourages them to return for needed care in both health and illness. This 2-year-old girl is having a routine checkup at a clinic.

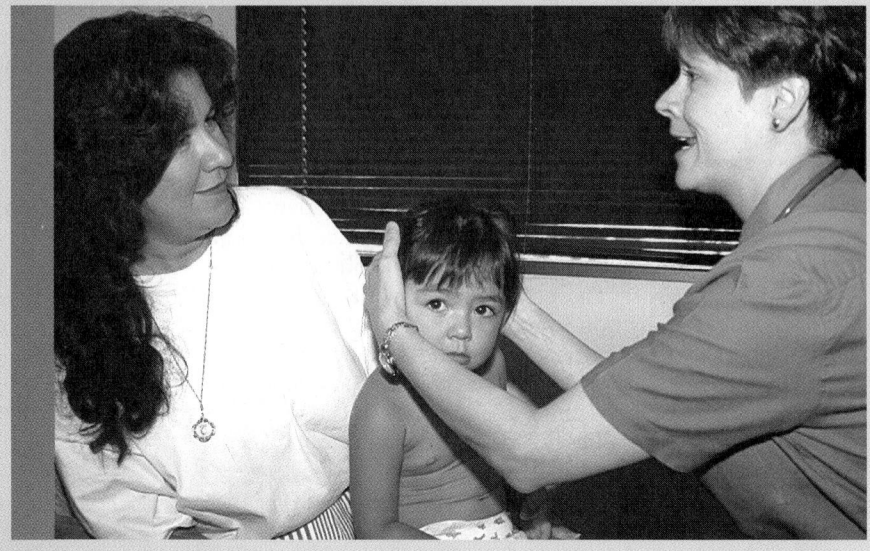

Communicating and enlisting the child's trust are vital elements in a successful physical examination. This girl remains in the security of her mother's arms as the nurse assesses her head. The little girl's anterior fontanel is not quite fully closed. The nurse reassures her mother that, although the fontanel usually closes by 18 months, the child's open fontanel likely represents a normal variation. Note that the nurse is at the mother's eye level and makes eye contact with her, promoting effective communication.

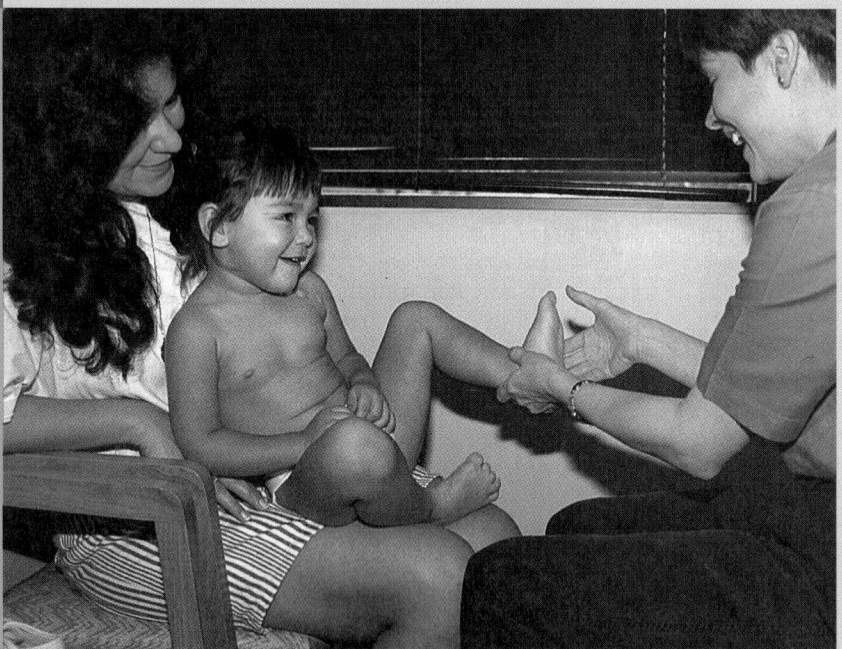

The nurse examines the child's feet for normal or abnormal reflexes and for straightness.

To limit the child's stress, the nurse creates an "examination table" by placing her knees next to the mother's knees. The child then lies across their laps as the nurse examines her thorax and abdomen.

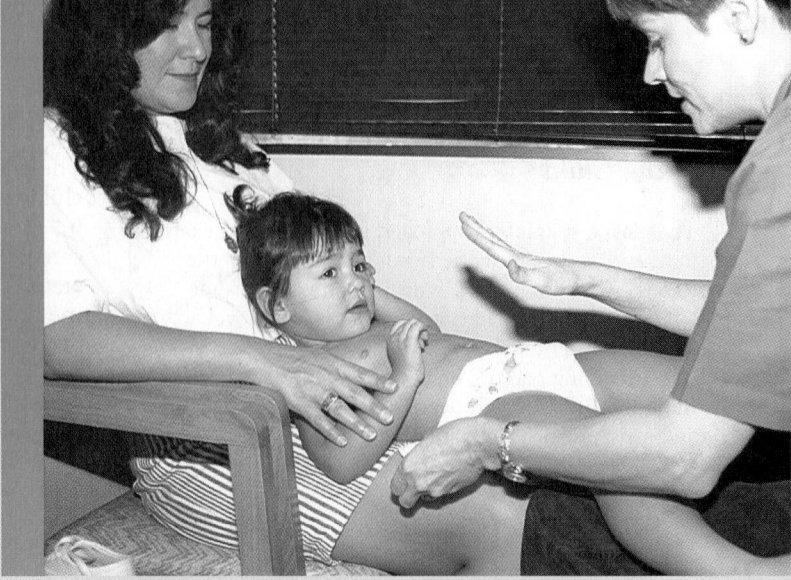

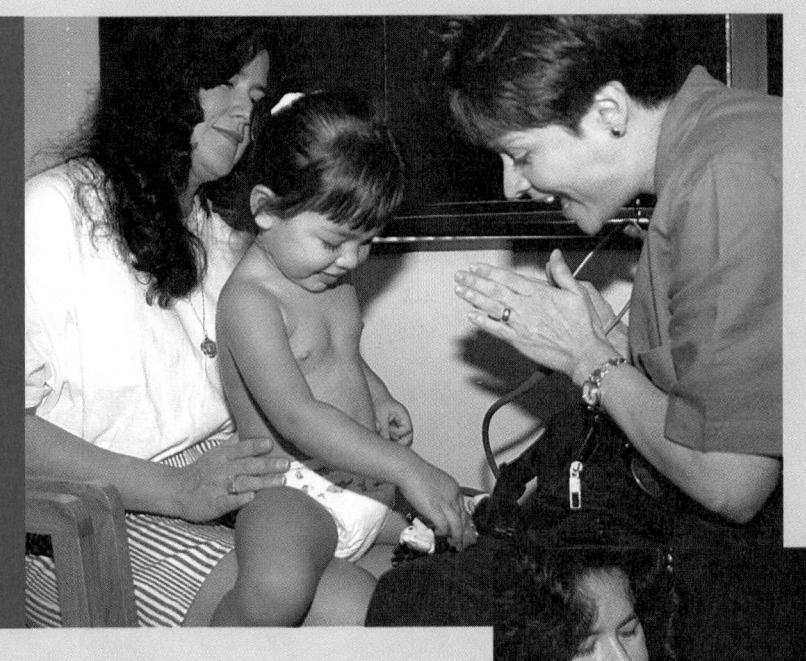

Allowing the child to check Mickey Mouse with a stethoscope before the nurse auscultates her chest enlists the child's cooperation and reduces her stress. This effort is especially important for assessments that are best done when the child is quiet. As the nurse auscultates her chest, the child is distracted by handling Mickey. Toddlers must be prepared for procedures immediately before they occur because a toddler's attention span is so short.

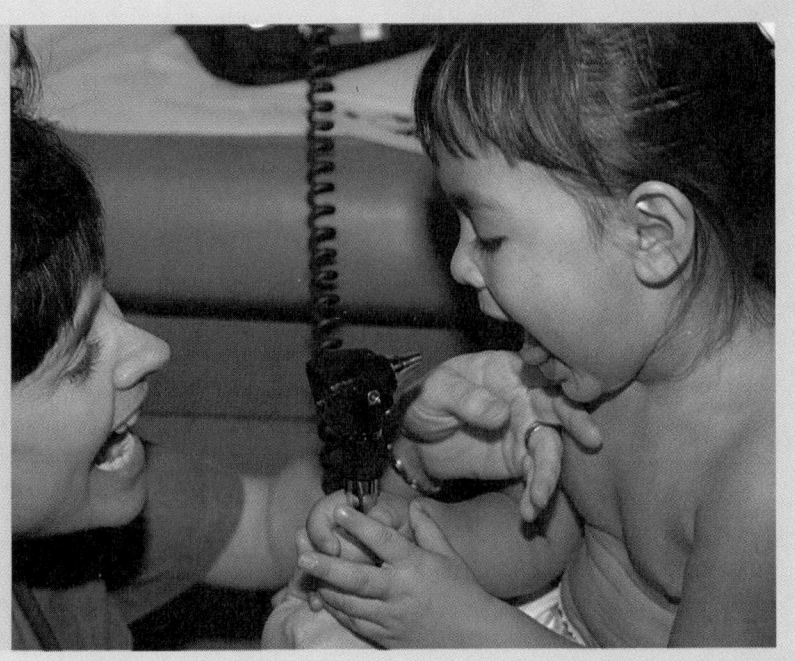

Pant like a puppy!" the nurse tells the child as she examines her mouth and throat. Incorporating play and fun into examinations promotes the child's trust in the nurse as well as enlisting her cooperation.

CONTINUED

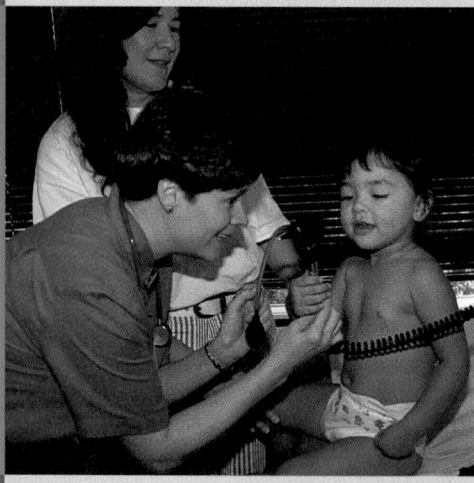

As in other examinations, the nurse helps the child examine the otoscope just before using it to examine her ears.

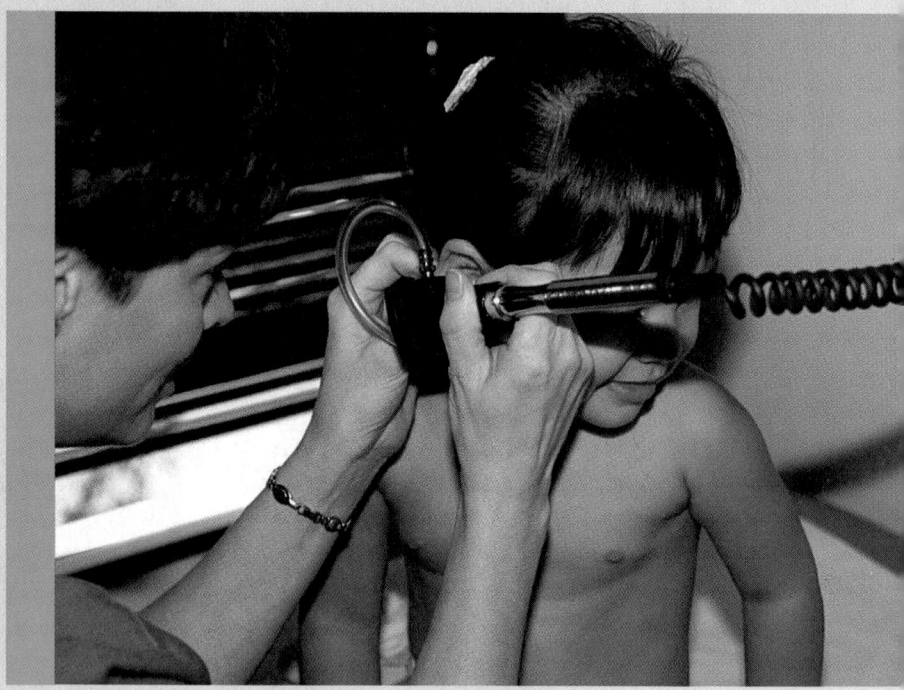

The nurse deftly examines the child's ears, pulling the pinna down and back. Ear examinations are especially important during the toddler years to identify fluid accumulation in the middle ear, which can interfere with hearing and speech development.

The nurse concludes the examination by checking the unclothed child for normal genital development, straightness of her spine and extremities, and evidence of previously undiagnosed hip dysplasia. To identify problems in motor development, the nurse observes the child's gait.

The nurse determines that this little girl's development is appropriate for her age. She is tall, like her mother, so the cherubic toddler appearance is less apparent than it might otherwise be. The nurse shares her findings as she does the examination and summarizes them for the mother at the end. Because the child is developing normally, she does not need to return to the clinic for a checkup until she is 3 years old.

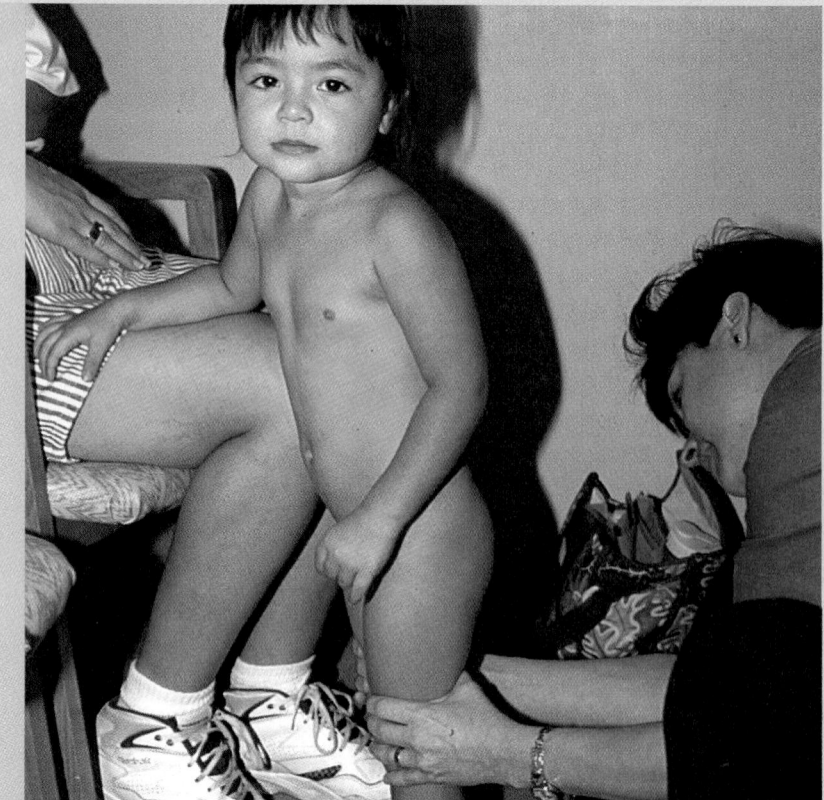

Photos courtesy of Parkland Health and Hospital System Community Oriented Primary Care Clinic.

School-Age Children

To establish trust with the school-age child, the examiner addresses to the child questions the child can answer. Children in elementary school will talk about school, favorite friends, and activities (see Chapter 7). Older school-age children may have to be encouraged to talk about their school performance and activities. The examiner encourages the parent to support and reinforce the child's participation in the examination.

The examination proceeds from head to toe. Children of this age prefer a simple drape over their underpants, and the examiner should be sensitive to the child's modesty. The examination is a wonderful opportunity to teach the child about the body and personal care. The nurse answers questions openly and in simple terms.

Adolescents

Adolescents are most comfortable with a straightforward, uncondescending approach (see Chapter 8). Decisions about who should be present during the examination should be openly discussed with the adolescent. The order of the examination is the same as for the school-age child.

It is best to incorporate the genital examination into the middle of the examination. If possible, proceed from the abdominal examination to the genital examination, to allow ample time for questions and discussions about this part of the examination. The physical examination is a wonderful opportunity to assure the pubertal child about normal developmental stages and to answer concerns children this age frequently have about what is happening to their bodies. The adolescent is expected to undress and wear a gown. The adolescent is draped appropriately during the examination.

▌ Techniques for Physical Examination

When performing the physical assessment, the nurse uses the four basic techniques of inspection, palpation, percussion, and auscultation, in that order. During the abdominal examination the sequence is altered: inspection is performed first, then auscultation, percussion, and palpation. The sequence of the abdominal examination is changed so as not to alter bowel sounds before determining their presence and characteristics, and to determine the size of abdominal organs before palpation.

Inspection

Most information is gathered during the physical examination by systematic and deliberate visual observations. The nurse first surveys an entire area of the body and then focuses on specifics, such as color, shape, size, or movement. Inspection can be both direct and indirect. Direct inspection relies on the examiner's senses of sight and hearing. Indirect inspection is accomplished with the use of special equipment, such as an otoscope, to examine a specific body area.

CRITICAL TO REMEMBER
• • • • • • • • • • • • •
Using the Hands for Palpation

Fingertips are used to palpate the breast, lymph nodes, and pulses.
The back of the hand is used to assess temperature.
The palm of the hand is used to identify vibrations.

Palpation

During palpation the nurse uses the sense of touch to make judgments about pulsations and vibrations and to locate structures and masses. Palpation allows the nurse to determine characteristics such as size, texture, warmth, mobility, and tenderness of various areas of the body.

Different parts of the hands are used to detect different characteristics. The fingertips are used to palpate the breast, lymph nodes, and pulses. The back of the hand is used to assess temperature. The palm of the hand is used to detect vibrations.

The type of palpation used is governed by the structure to be examined and the need to avoid any unnecessary discomfort to the client. Light palpation is accomplished by gently applying fingertip pressure to depress the skin surface approximately $1/2$ to $3/4$ inch and then moving the fingertips in a circular motion.

Deep palpation is used to detect abdominal masses and is performed after light palpation. The surface is depressed approximately $1 1/2$ to 2 inches to detect underlying masses. Bimanual palpation is performed using both hands. The examiner superimposes one hand over the other to increase pressure or places one hand near the other to capture and trap a mass or structure between them, such as the kidneys or spleen.

Percussion

To percuss, the nurse uses quick, sharp tapping of the fingers or hands to produce sounds. Percussion is performed to locate the position, size, and density of underlying structures. The three basic methods are mediate, or indirect percussion, in which the finger of one hand is placed against the body surface and the finger of the other hand acts as the hammer; immediate percussion, performed by striking the finger of one hand directly against the body; and fist percussion, in which the ulnar aspect of the fist is used to deliver a firm blow directly to the area. The method used depends on the area to be percussed. The nurse uses quick, light blows to create vibrations that penetrate approximately 2 inches below the surface. Sounds identified by percussion are classified as flat, dull, resonant, or tympanic.

Auscultation

Auscultation entails eliciting and listening to body sounds created in the lungs, heart, blood vessels, and abdominal viscera. The most common way to auscultate is to use a stethoscope. Most sounds auscultated result from air or fluid movement within the body. The diaphragm of the stethoscope is most effective in assessing high-pitched sounds, such as heart and breath sounds. The bell of the stethoscope

Sounds Identified When Percussing

Flat: High-pitched, soft-intensity sound elicited by percussing over solid masses such as bone or muscle

Dull: Medium-pitched, medium-intensity sound elicited when percussing over high-density structures such as the liver

Resonance: Low-pitched, loud-intensity sound elicited over a hollow organ such as the lungs

Tympany: High-pitched, loud-intensity sound heard over air-filled body parts such as the bowel or stomach

is most effective in hearing low-pitched sounds, such as blood pressure and vascular sounds. Auscultation requires a quiet environment. The nurse places the stethoscope on the skin in the appropriate area. Sounds heard are described according to pitch, intensity, duration, and quality.

Smell

While examining the child, the nurse uses the sense of smell to detect general body odors, common in children who are neglected or dirty. Odor may also indicate infection. Odors from the mouth, urine, or feces can be important. In particular, some diseases are characterized by odors coming from the mouth (Barkauskas et al., 1998).

The Complete History

The content of the complete or initial history includes

1. **Statistical information:** Name, age, address, telephone number, Social Security number, names of parents or guardians, and source of support.
2. **Client profile:** Times the child eats and sleeps, educational level, developmental level, race and nationality, religion, economic status, and health status perception. If an interpreter was used to gather the health history, the person's name is included in the record, usually in this section of the history. Also included is a statement about the reliability of an informant, such as an older sibling who answers questions concerning a younger sibling or an aunt or uncle who answers questions regarding a child visiting them.
3. **Health history:** Birth history, growth and development, common childhood illnesses, immunizations, previous hospitalizations, accidents or injuries, allergies or allergic reactions and exact symptoms the allergy produced. The person taking the history should ask about medications taken daily or for an acute episode of an illness and should list all medications being taken, including dose and frequency. The parent should name both prescription and over-the-counter medications. The examiner also asks if the child has ever had a blood transfusion or has received any blood products. For any hospitalizations, serious illnesses, and injuries, the nurse should obtain the following information:
   a. Reason for admission
   b. Place of admission
   c. Length of stay
   d. Surgical procedures
   e. Outcomes
   f. Other

Problem-Oriented History

Chief complaint: Use the child's own words.

Bodily location: Place the problem somewhere on the body.

Quality: Define what the problem is like for the child.

Quantity: Describe the intensity of the problem for the child.

Chronology: Determine when the problem began, the periodicity and frequency, and the course of symptoms.

Setting: Identify where the problem occurs.

Aggravating and alleviating factors: Find out what makes the problem better or worse.

Associated manifestations: Document other related information.

Sequence of Physical Examination

General Appearance

During the first contact with the child and parent, the examiner forms an initial impression by making a general survey. The nurse determines the child's age, sex, and race and identifies clues concerning the child's behavior and health

4. **Family history:** Information concerning the health status of the child's mother, father, siblings, and specific blood relatives such as aunts, uncles, and grandparents. If any are deceased, the history includes the age and cause of death. The purpose is to determine constitutional and hereditary factors that are likely to affect the child's health.
5. **Lifestyle and life patterns:** The child's interaction with the social, psychological, physical, and cultural environment. Growth and development, use of street drugs and smoking, roles and relationships, and family life information are all important.
6. **Review of systems:** A systematic review of the major anatomic and physiologic parts. A head-to-toe review focusing on the health function and maintenance of each body part should occur in this order:
   a. General appearance
   b. Head
   c. Hair
   d. Face
   e. Eyes
   f. Ears
   g. Nose and sinuses
   h. Mouth
   i. Throat
   j. Neck
   k. Lungs
   l. Heart
   m. Breasts
   n. Abdomen
   o. Kidneys and bladder
   p. Bowels, rectum, and anus
   q. Genitals
   r. Extremities

Potential Indicators of Child Abuse

Dress: Inappropriate for the weather; ragged or excessively dirty; the latest fad

Grooming and personal hygiene: Dirty teeth, broken and dirty fingernails, matted and dirty hair

Posture and movements: Crouching in a corner; slow, concentrated movements

Body image distortion: Being thin but describing self as fat

Speech and communication: Answering questions in words of one syllable, looking to others to respond first, seeking approval for answers

Facial characteristics and expressions: Fearful, anxious, tearful, sad, or angry expressions

Psychological state: Labile, demanding, bizarre, overly dramatic, or condescending

status. Because each child is a unique human being, individual differences in behavior and health status related to growth and development will be evident. During the general survey the examiner continually notes the parent-child interaction and the way the parent responds to the child's needs and behavior. These, together with other indicators of the child's health status, may provide clues to distress or abuse.

History Taking

Taking an accurate history of the child is the single most important component of the physical examination. Practitioners obtain three different types of health histories: the complete, or initial, history; the well, interim history; and the episodic, or problem-oriented, history.

In the *complete, or initial, history*, data are gathered about the child from the time of conception to the child's current status. In the *well, interim history*, data are gathered about the child from the last well visit to the current visit. When doing a well, interim history, the examiner assumes that a database is in place. In a *problem-oriented, or episodic, history*, information is gathered about a current problem. Information about the specific problem is then added to the existing database.

CRITICAL THINKING EXERCISE 33–1

Ann Maloney, a 17-year-old single mother, brings her 6-month-old daughter, Kerrie, to the clinic. This is Kerrie's first visit. Ms. Maloney had made several earlier appointments for Kerrie but was always unable to keep them. She states, "I am very busy trying to work and care for Kerrie. I have had to miss work because Kerrie has had lots of colds. I hate to take time off when she is well. My supervisor at work said that it was important for her to have her immunizations and a physical examination. I guess I messed up."

1. What assumptions could the nurse make about Ms. Maloney?
2. How should the nurse respond to Ms. Maloney's comment?
3. How can the nurse best act as an advocate for both Kerrie and her mother?

Recording of Data

The information gathered during the history is documented concisely to provide all necessary information from pregnancy to the child's current status. Milestones in growth and development, immunizations, and family status are always included in the child's history.

Vital Signs

Vital signs are taken on every child at every visit in ambulatory settings and are monitored throughout the day in a hospitalized child. Assessment of vital signs (temperature, pulse, respirations, and blood pressure) is an important way to measure and monitor vital body functions. Measuring vital signs provides the basis for decisions concerning the child's overall health and illness. In children, changes in vital signs are important signs of changes in health status. Table 33–1 describes normal vital signs by age, and Chapter 37 details the procedure for taking vital signs in children.

TABLE 33–1

Normal Vital Signs by Age

Age	Temperature* Fahrenheit	Temperature* Celsius	Pulse Rate (BPM)	Respiratory Rate (Breaths/min)	Blood Pressure (mm Hg)
Newborn	96.8–99 (axillary)	36–37.2 (axillary)	120–160	30–60	Systolic: 46–92 Diastolic: 38–71
3 Years	97.5–98.6 (axillary)	36.4–37 (axillary)	80–125	20–30	Systolic: 72–110 Diastolic: 40–73
10 Years	97.5–98.6 (oral)	36.4–37 (oral)	70–110†	16–22	Systolic: 83–121 Diastolic: 45–79
16 Years	97.5–98.6 (oral)	36.4–37 (oral)	55–90	15–20	Systolic: 93–131‡ Diastolic: 49–85

* The normal range of the child's temperature will depend on the measuring method used. Temperatures exhibit circadian rhythms at all ages.

† After age 12 years, a boy's pulse is 5 BPM slower than a girl's.

‡ After age 14 years, blood pressure in boys is higher than in girls.

TEMPERATURE

The method for measuring children's temperature may vary from one setting to another. Some parents are comfortable taking a rectal or axillary temperature. Health care providers may use a mercury, a tympanic membrane sensor, an electronic, or a digital thermometer. Currently, parents are encouraged to take axillary rather than rectal temperatures. Reasons for the recommendation are the invasive nature of rectal temperature measurements, the risk of injury, and their questionable accuracy with febrile children, as feces retain body heat for hours after a fever has diminished. Axillary temperatures, when taken correctly, provide accurate information concerning changes in the child's health status.

Tympanic temperature measurements are frequently used in health care agencies because they can be performed quickly and involve less cross-contamination. When recording a tympanic temperature, the nurse notes the side on which the temperature was elicited. Variation can occur from one ear to the other on the same child. An oral thermometer may be used with older children, usually at age 5 or 6. For oral temperature measurements, an electronic thermometer is unbreakable and registers quickly, but it may not be available. (See Chapter 37 for a discussion of various methods of assessing temperature.)

PULSE

Apical pulse rates are taken in children under 2 and in any child who has an irregular heart rate or known congenital heart disease. Radial pulse rates may be taken in children older than 2. To account for normal irregularities, the nurse counts the pulse for a full minute. Chapter 37 details the procedure for measuring pulse.

Arterial pulses are palpated to determine pulse rate and rhythm and to evaluate blood flow, arterial wall elasticity, and vessel patency. To determine the position of the heart in the anterior precordium, the nurse palpates the apical impulse in infants and children under age 6 years. In the acute care setting an apical impulse is always palpated on every child, and the location of the apical impulse is noted. Simultaneously, the examiner palpates and compares femoral, radial, and carotid pulses on children of any age. The nurse may also compare a carotid pulse with a femoral or radial pulse for equality of pulses. In infants the nurse notes the pulsating anterior fontanel. The pulse may be increased significantly above normal in infants and children with anxiety, fever, exercise, inflammatory illnesses, shock, or congestive heart failure. The resting heart rate changes with increasing age.

The rhythm of the heartbeat is assessed for equal spacing between consecutive beats. Irregular cardiac rhythms are not uncommon in children and are often related to changes in rhythm that occur in response to respiratory inspiration and expiration.

RESPIRATIONS

The nurse observes the rate, depth, and ease of respiration in the child. Respirations vary with age. The respiratory rate, like the heart rate, is significantly influenced by emotion and exercise. In infants, the rate may be determined by observing abdominal excursion. In toddlers and older children, the nurse observes thoracic excursion. Because the movements are irregular, the rate should be assessed for 1 minute in infants and young children. Respirations are best counted when the child is not paying attention to the examiner. Respirations should be counted while the examiner continues to keep fingers on a pulse or the stethoscope on the chest, as though checking the pulses. This effort will ensure that the child is unaware that the examiner is counting respirations.

The depth and rhythm of respiration are determined subjectively and compared with norms for a particular age group. The ease or difficulty of respiration is a somewhat subjective observation. Respirations should be quiet and appear effortless. Stridorous respirations—a crowing noise heard on inspiration—are worrisome in a child and may be a sign of croup or epiglottitis.

BLOOD PRESSURE

Blood pressure measurements are taken on all children at every ambulatory visit and at least daily, and often more frequently, depending on the child's condition, in an acute care setting. The appropriate-size cuff must be used to auscultate the blood pressure. Blood pressure measurements in healthy ambulatory children are compared with standard norms. (See Table 33–1 for the effects of age on vital signs.) Blood pressure is monitored more closely on any child suspected of having a condition that affects blood pressure, such as hypertension, cardiovascular disease, kidney diseases, or liver disease.

The size of the cuff is important. Cuffs that are too small will cause falsely elevated values; those that are too large will cause inaccurate low values. The cuff should cover two thirds of the distance between the antecubital fossa and the shoulder. Several determinations may be needed to obtain values unaffected by anxiety. Instructing the child that the balloon will gently squeeze the arm, or give the arm a "hug," will usually decrease anxiety. To alleviate anxiety, the child can also assist with taking a blood pressure on a doll, a stuffed animal, or the parent.

Anthropometric Measurement

Anthropometrics entails measuring the human body and assessing nutritional status as well as growth and development. Weight, height, and head circumference are always measured in children and are compared to averages for age group and sex. Midarm muscle circumference, skin fold thickness, and weight provide information about three body tissues (subcutaneous tissue, muscle, and fat) altered by nutrition. Anthropometric measurements are most valuable when they are evaluated serially so that trends can be monitored.

Measuring height and weight is a routine procedure that provides valuable information about the health of a child. Children grow and develop rapidly, and this growth and development must be constantly evaluated. Physical measurements of a child reflect the rate of growth; a failure in growth, an acceleration in growth, or any change in growth pattern may be the first clue to serious problems. A child's falling off the child's own growth curve is the most significant indicator of changing health status. Measurements must be correct and accurate and are taken at every visit from birth to adulthood.

HEIGHT

The methods of measurement of a child vary with age. Length of infants and toddlers is best measured with the child lying down on a flat measuring board. This method is used until the child is able to stand independently. The child's head is held secure to the headboard, and the movable footboard is stretched to touch the child's heel. If a measuring board is not available for the infant and young child, it is possible to position the child's body on a flat surface, mark the point where the heel touches the surface, and then mark the point where the tip of the head is lying on the surface, taking care to ensure that the child's legs and body are straight on the surface. The examiner then removes the child and measures the distance between the two points with a measuring tape. Measuring the length of the child in this manner is not as accurate as using a measuring board.

When a child is able to cooperate and stand without support, around age 2, the examiner stands the child in stocking feet next to a standard measuring tape that begins at the child's heel and is not displaced by room molding. A flat, hard surface is used to reach from the top of the child's head to the tape so that the examiner does not guess or add height because of the hair.

Once the measurement is taken, it must be plotted on a standardized growth chart (see Appendix H). Height and weight are evaluated by determining whether the child is following a predictable percentile curve on a growth chart. Height and weight are related to hereditary factors and will vary from child to child.

WEIGHT

The method and equipment for weighing vary with the child's age. All scales must be balanced first before weighing. Infants are placed in a lying position on a regular baby scale with all their clothing removed. Older children who are able to stand or walk without support may be weighed on the adult standing scale. On the older child, remove all clothing except underwear. Like height, weight is plotted on a standardized growth chart (see Appendix H).

HEAD CIRCUMFERENCE

Head circumference is measured on all children from birth to age 36 months and plotted on a standard growth chart on all visits. Children over age 3 with any questionable head size—megalocephaly or microcephaly—should have their head circumference measured at every visit. To measure the

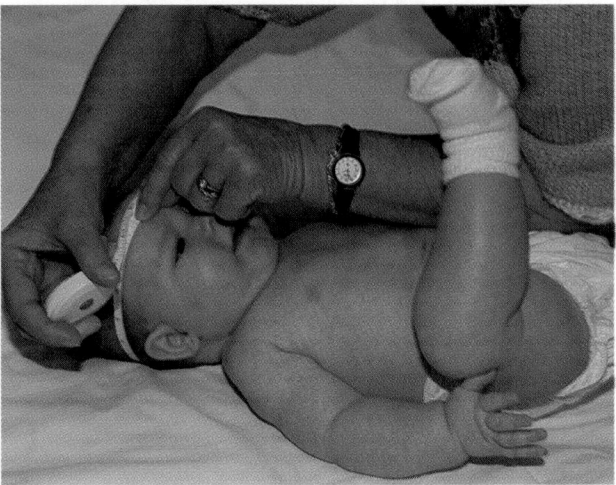

head circumference, a nonstretching measuring tape is wrapped above the supraorbital ridges and over the most prominent part of the occiput (Fig. 33–1).

The head circumference is plotted on a standardized growth chart. During the first 6 months of life the head circumference normally increases by 1.5 cm each month, and it increases by 0.5 cm per month between ages 6 and 12 months. Head circumference can reflect an abnormal rate of development, give some indication of nutritional status, and possibly indicate tumor growth.

CHEST CIRCUMFERENCE

Chest circumference is routinely measured only in the newborn. The newborn's head circumference is larger than the chest circumference. Chest circumference is almost equal to head circumference after age 1 year. To measure chest circumference, the measuring tape is wrapped around the chest at the nipple line. The measurement is taken between inspiration and expiration.

MIDARM CIRCUMFERENCE

Midarm circumference reflects muscle mass and fat. To measure midarm circumference, the midpoint on the arm between the acromial process and the olecranon process is determined. Then, with the arm hanging loosely at the side, the child's arm is measured at the midpoint with a tape measure. The measurement is recorded in centimeters. With a decrease in fat or muscle atrophy, the midarm circumference decreases. It will increase with weight gain.

TRICEPS SKIN FOLD

Triceps skin fold thickness indicates total body fat because at least half of body fat is directly below the skin. Metal calipers are used to obtain this measurement. On the non-dominant arm the midpoint of the arm is determined using the same method as is used for measuring midarm circumference. With the arm hanging loosely at the side, a fold of skin at the midpoint on the posterior aspect of the arm is grasped. To avoid error, the child is asked to flex the arm muscle after the examiner grasps the skin. If contraction is felt, then muscle as well as fat has been grasped. The examiner applies the caliper and takes a reading after waiting 3 seconds. Fat stores decrease with long-term undernutrition and malnutrition.

Use of Growth Charts

An accurate record of an infant's or child's overall pattern of growth is best determined by serial measurements over months or years. The National Center for Health Statistics (NCHS) publishes growth charts (see Appendix H). The charts, currently in revision, provide a single set of references to assess body size and monitor growth in infants, children, and adolescents in the United States. They are intended to serve as a reference rather than as growth standards or clinical ideals to be achieved (Kuczmarski, 1998).

National survey data for all racial/ethnic groups are being combined to develop the revised growth charts. Racial/ethnic differences in growth appear to be attributable primarily to environmental influences. In addition, the national health examination surveys do not have adequate samples to create charts specific to all racial and ethnic groups in the United States (Kuczmarski, 1998).

The revised charts will include these components:

- Infant charts for birth to age 3 relate length, weight, and head circumference to age and relate weight to length.
- Charts for ages 2 through 19 relate stature, weight, and body mass index (BMI) to age. Body mass index has been recommended for evaluating and tracking overweight children and adolescents. The 85th percentile line helps identify children at risk for overweight.
- Separate charts exist for boys and girls.

To plot on a growth chart, the exact age of the child is determined on the chart's horizontal axis. The corresponding measurement is marked on the chart's vertical axis. The chart is marked where the two lines intersect. The percentile lines on these charts indicate the number of children expected to fall above and below the child's measurement.

Skin, Hair, and Nails

SKIN

Assessment of the skin includes inspection and palpation. The entire skin surface is examined. This examination may be combined with assessment of other areas of the body.

Inspection. The nurse observes the color and pigmentation of the skin. Skin color reflects the amount of melanin and can range from pink to black. In dark-skinned infants and children, erythema will appear dusky red or violet; cyanosis will appear black; and jaundice will appear diffusely darker (Hurwitz, 1993). In dark-skinned infants and children it is best to determine the normal skin color and

then compare any color change with the normal color. Color changes to the skin may be related to sun exposure or tattooing.

Palpation. The examiner palpates the skin to assess moisture, temperature, turgor, edema, and lesions. *Moisture* is assessed by lightly stroking the skin surface and body creases. The external skin on exposed areas is normally dryer than unexposed areas of the skin.

Temperature is assessed by using the back of the hand, as it is more sensitive to skin changes. The two sides of the child's body are compared with each other.

Normal *texture* of the skin is described as being smooth and soft. Scars or excessive scar tissue should be noted.

Turgor is assessed by grasping the skin between the thumb and index finger and quickly releasing it (Fig. 33–2). The skin normally returns to place without excessive skin markings. Skin that "tents" when released indicates dehydration. The abdomen and upper arm are the best places to test for tissue turgor on a child.

Edema, the accumulation of excessive salt and water in the interstitial spaces, is identified by pressing the thumb into areas of the body that may appear puffy. The extremi-

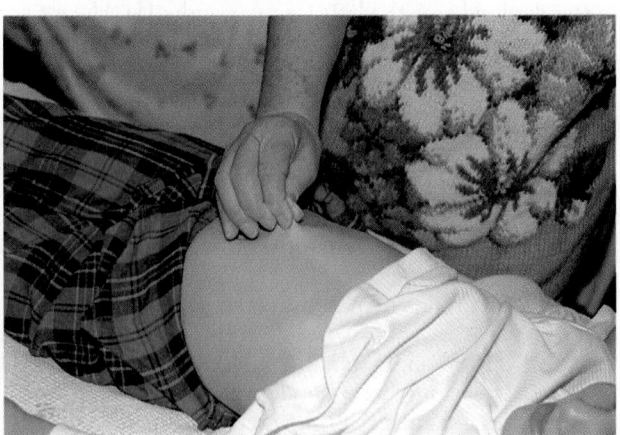

FIGURE 33–2
• • • • • • • • • •
Skin turgor is best tested by grasping the abdominal skin between the thumb and forefinger and quickly releasing it. "Tenting" (persistent elevation of the skin when released) suggests dehydration. (Courtesy of The University of Texas at Arlington School of Nursing, Arlington, Texas.)

ties and buttocks are classic areas to palpate for edema in the child. Periorbital edema is observed on the eyelids.

Lesions are identified, noting configuration, distribution, color, and size. Skin lesions are identified as primary lesions, arising from normal skin, or secondary lesions, resulting from an alteration of a primary lesion. Configuration of a skin lesion refers to the arrangement or position of several lesions in relation to each other or to the arrangement of a single lesion. Distribution refers to the body location and the symmetry or asymmetry of lesions.

HAIR

Hair normally covers the entire body except for the palms, soles, and parts of the genitalia. Hair is examined for texture, changes in color, unusual distribution, and cleanliness.

Scalp hair has a wide range of normal textures, including straight, curly, or kinky. The hair is usually shiny, silky, and strong. The examiner should keep in mind the age and development of the child. Fine downy hair is normal for a newborn, whereas in an older child it would lead the examiner to consider nutrition and endocrine abnormalities. Brittle hair, identified when the hairs break off easily when bent between the fingers, might also indicate endocrine and nutritional abnormalities.

The color of the hair may be anything from pale blond to black. Changes in color may be due to depigmentation, hereditary factors, or chemicals applied to the hair.

The distribution of the hair over the head is identified. In most children the hair begins in a whorl and then is distributed over the head. Some children may have more than one whorl. Scalp hair does not grow beyond the nape of the neck or down to the eyebrows. *Hirsutism* is defined as excessive hair growth; *alopecia* is unusual hair loss.

The hair is separated and examined for cleanliness, signs of trauma, lesions, or scaling. The scalp should be clean and free of any infestations. Most cases of head lice (*pediculosis capitis*) are first detected when one or more children are seen scratching their heads. Closer observation may reveal nits adhering to the hairs. Usually these are the whitish to sand-colored empty shells of eggs that have hatched (Meinking & Taplin, 1995).

NAILS

Nails are inspected and palpated for shape and contour. The nail surface is normally flat or slightly convex. The edges of the nails should be smooth, rounded, and clean. Clubbing of fingernails can be identified by looking at the index finger; the angle at the nail base and the finger should be less than 160°. On palpation, the base of the fingernail should be firm. On touching the index fingernails back to back, a diamond of light below the knuckle and above where the fingernails touch will be present. In early clubbing the diamond shape is decreased or not apparent (see Fig. 45–6).

Capillary refill of the nails is assessed by pressing on the nail edge and releasing; the nail will blanch and color return to the nail within 1 or 2 seconds. A capillary refill time of more than 2 seconds may be due to anemia, peripheral edema, vasoconstriction, or decreased cardiac output due to hypovolemia, shock, or congestive heart failure (Barkauskas et al., 1998).

Lymph Nodes

Lymph nodes are inspected and palpated. Lymph tissue is found all over the body and must be evaluated as the examiner assesses body systems. Always assess for enlarged lymph nodes in the head and neck, the axillary region, the arms, and the inguinal region (Fig. 33–3). Examination of lymph

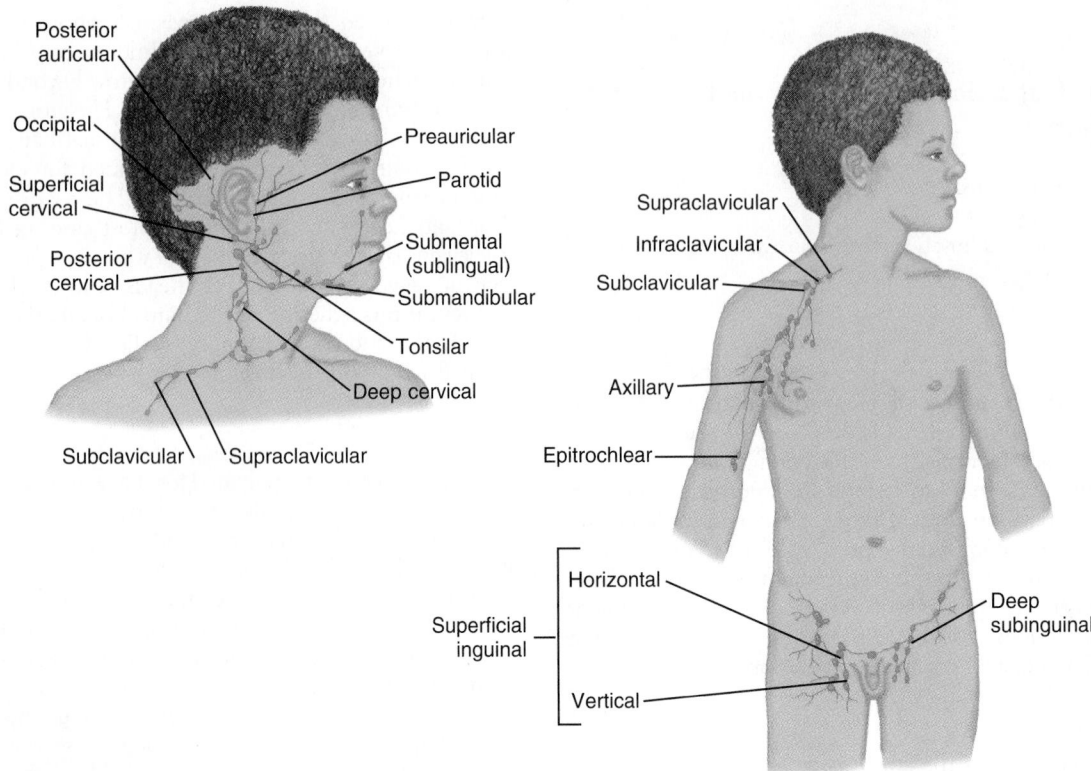

FIGURE 33–3

Location of superficial lymph nodes.

nodes should be incorporated into the examination when that part of the anatomy is being assessed. When an enlarged lymph node or a mass is found during examination, its characteristics should be described.

To palpate for most lymph nodes, the examiner uses the distal portion of the fingers and gently but firmly moves the fingers in a circular motion to determine the node's characteristics.

Lymph nodes that are enlarged, warm, firm, and fluctuant are a sign of infection. Lymph nodes that are small, firm, and shotty (freely palpable and very small) are often palpable in normal infants and children in the cervical, axillary, inguinal, and occipital areas (Green, 1998).

Head, Face, and Neck

HEAD

The head is inspected and palpated. To examine the head, the examiner must see and feel. The head is evaluated from the front, the back, and the sides. The head is examined for symmetry, paralysis, weakness, and movement.

Head Shape Terminology

Normocephalic: Normal-size head
Microcephalic: Head small for body size and age
Macrocephalic: Abnormally large head
Bossing: Frontal enlargement

Symmetry is assessed by looking at and feeling the entire head. If any lumps or bumps are seen or felt, the examiner notes their exact location and size and density. The suture lines in infants should be palpated. Sutures are felt as prominent ridges in the newborn but usually flatten by 6 months.

Paralysis and weakness of the head are directly related to the condition of the neck muscles. That is, paralysis and weakness of the head will occur with paralysis or weakness of the neck muscles.

Head movement is evaluated by observing the child move the head. Head control is observed with the child in a lying position and while the examiner grasps the child's hands and pulls the infant into a sitting position. An infant younger than 4 months may show some head lag, but the infant in an upright position should be able to maintain the head upright for several seconds. Head lag after age 6 months may indicate poor muscle development. The head should be put through a full range of motion by asking the older child to look up, down, and sideways. After age 4 months, inability to move the head or to hold the head in an upright position may be related to paralysis or weakness of the neck muscles.

The *fontanels* are inspected and palpated for size, tenseness, and pulsation (Fig. 33–4). The posterior fontanel is closed by age 6 to 8 weeks. The anterior fontanel should be soft and flat when the child is sitting. Measure the width and length of an open anterior fontanel. The anterior fontanel should be less than 5 cm in length and width after age 12 months and should be completely closed by age 12 to 18 months. A sunken fontanel is associated with dehydra-

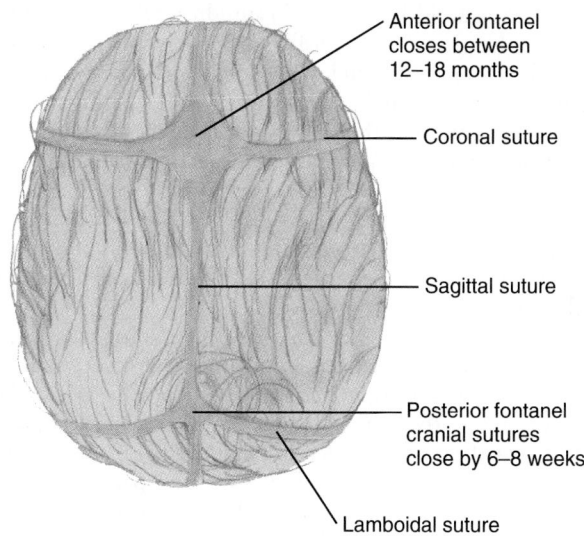

Anterior fontanel
closes between
12–18 months

Coronal suture

Sagittal suture

Posterior fontanel
cranial sutures
close by 6–8 weeks

Lamboidal suture

FIGURE 33–4

Fontanels are inspected and palpated for size, tenseness, and pulsation.

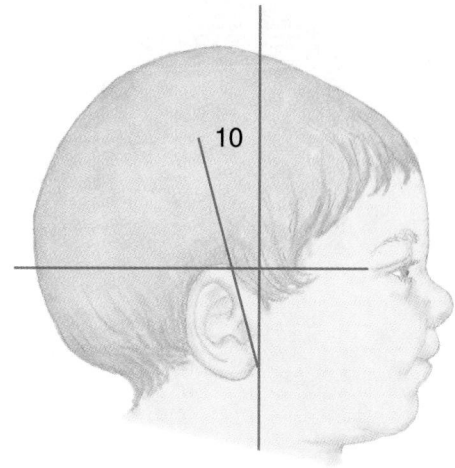

Normal alignment

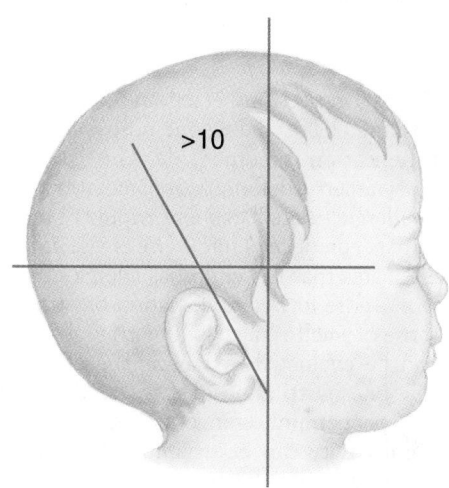

Low-set ears and
deviation in alignment

FIGURE 33–5

The child's ears are inspected for alignment. Low-set ears could indicate mental retardation or renal anomalies.

tion, and a bulging fontanel can be associated with increased intracranial pressure. A bulging fontanel is normally seen when an infant cries, coughs, or vomits (Bates, 1995).

NECK

In the child the neck is inspected and palpated for symmetry, size, and shape, which is directly related to the use or disuse of the neck muscles. The neck should be viewed from the front, the back, and both sides. Webbing of the neck, the presence of an extra fold of skin posteriorly, is associated with some chromosomal abnormalities such as trisomy 21, or Down syndrome.

While palpating the child's neck, the *thyroid gland* is palpated by identifying the isthmus of the thyroid across the trachea. To identify an enlarged thyroid in a child, the examiner gently displaces the thyroid gland laterally and palpates thyroid tissue with the opposite thumb and fingers. The lobe may be more palpable when the child swallows.

FACE

The child's face is inspected and palpated for dysmorphic features. Spacing and symmetry of facial features are noted. The face is observed for any changes in color or the presence of edema such as cellulitis. The eyes are examined for size, position, and configuration. *Hypertelorism* is a condition in which the eyes are unusually widely spaced; in *hypotelorism*, the eyes are unusually close together. The child's nostrils should be oval in shape and equal in size, with no evidence of a hypoplastic philtrum (shallow crease or absence of a crease below the nose). The lips should be equal on either side of the midline. The child's ears are inspected for alignment. Low-set ears are identified when the auricle of the ear does not cross or touch the eye-occiput line. The position of the auricle should be almost vertical, with no more than a 10-degree lateral posterior angle (Fig. 33–5).

The functions of cranial nerve V (trigeminal nerve) and cranial nerve VII (facial nerve) are evaluated while as-

sessing the face. Cranial nerve V is evaluated by observing chewing or sucking, which demonstrates the strength of the temporomandibular joint, and by touching the child's forehead and cheeks with a piece of cotton. The child should move the head or bat the object away. Cranial nerve VII is evaluated by having the child frown, smile, or make a face while the examiner observes for symmetry of movement. Having the child puff out the cheeks or whistle also allows the examiner to evaluate cranial nerve VII (Jarvis, 1996).

Nose, Mouth, and Throat

NOSE

The examiner should wear gloves when doing the nasal examination. Note any drainage coming from the nose. Describe the amount, color, and consistency.

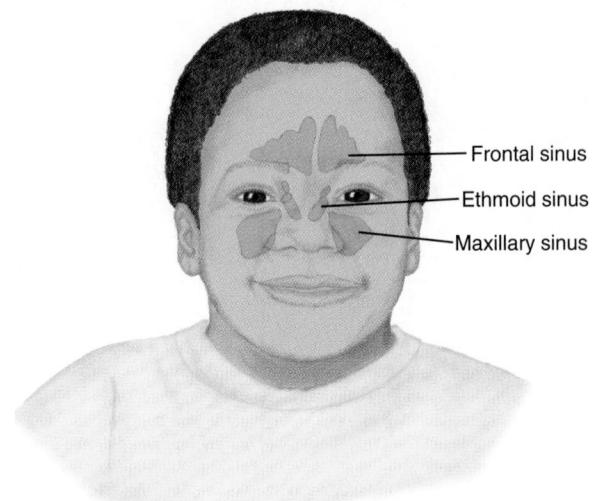

FIGURE 33–6
• • • • • • • • •
The frontal, ethmoid, and maxillary sinuses.

The external nose is inspected and palpated. Patency can be determined by occluding one nostril and having the child sniff. Repeat on the other side. The external nose is observed for symmetry, deformity, inflammation, or skin lesions. The "allergic salute," frequent wiping of the nose because of drainage, produces a transverse crease on the child's nose and indicates that the child has allergies. Palpate the entire external nose for septal deviation or other deformities. The sense of smell is mediated by cranial nerve I. This function can be evaluated by having the child close the eyes, occlude one nostril, and identify familiar odors such as cinnamon, peppermint, orange, or cherry.

The nasal cavity can be examined by using a short, wide-tipped speculum on the otoscope and inserting it into the nasal vestibule, being careful not to put pressure on the nasal septum. The nasal mucosa is inspected for color and moisture. The nasal mucosa is normally smooth, moist, and has a bright pink color. In children with allergies the mucosa is pale and appears boggy. With infectious diseases the mucosa is erythematous and swollen; the nasal drainage may be yellow or green. The nasal septum is examined for intactness and for any deviation.

The *frontal* and *maxillary sinuses* are inspected and palpated (Fig. 33–6). The areas over the sinuses are examined for color and swelling. Puffiness and redness over the sinuses and dark circles under the eyes may indicate an inflammatory process in children. The frontal sinuses are palpated by pressing over the sinuses below the eyebrow. The maxillary sinuses are palpated by pressing upward with the thumbs under the maxillary bones.

MOUTH AND THROAT

Assessment of the mouth in a young child should be performed at the end of the physical examination because it may create anxiety. The examination should proceed from the anterior structures to the internal structures of the mouth.

The *philtrum*, the little notch between the nose and

upper lip, should be intact. In children with dysmorphic features the philtrum is invisible or incompletely "dug out."

The examiner should wear gloves when doing the oral examination. A tongue blade and a good penlight assist with visualization of the oral cavity. The mouth and internal structures are examined using inspection, palpation, and the sense of smell.

Lips are inspected for color, moisture, cracking, or the presence of any lesions. The alveolar frenulum, which attaches the lips to the gums, should be intact. The lips are palpated to identify any masses.

The *buccal mucosa* is examined by holding the cheeks open with a tongue blade and examining for color, nodules, or lesions. Significant mouth odors should be noted. For many children this part of the examination can be unpleasant. To facilitate the child's cooperation, the examiner may want to demonstrate on a doll or on the parent or allow the child to place the tongue blade in the parent's mouth. The buccal mucosa should be pink, smooth, and moist. Dark-skinned children may have patchy areas of hyperpigmentation. The opening of the *parotid gland* is found as a small dimple on the buccal mucosa opposite the upper second molar. The entire surface of the buccal mucosa is palpated for changes in consistency or masses.

Teeth are inspected for number, cavities, tooth formation, and occlusion. The number and characteristics of the teeth will change with growth and development (Fig. 33–7). The eruption of deciduous teeth begins around the sixth month of extrauterine life; all 20 deciduous teeth are present by age 30 months. Have the child close the mouth, and note the position of the teeth. The upper teeth will protrude slightly over the lower teeth. The color and shape of each tooth should be noted. The crown is white, with some variation from person to person. Permanent teeth are larger and have a darker color than deciduous teeth. Brown or black discoloration of the teeth is usually due to dental caries. Chronic use of certain medications (i.e., tetracycline and iron) may stain teeth. With excessive fluoride ingestion, the enamel of the permanent teeth may appear mottled. The shape of the tooth will be determined by age, development, and the amount of wear.

The *gums* (gingiva) are inspected and palpated for color and swelling. The gum surface will have a pink, stippled appearance and will feel firm. Dark-skinned children may have a dark-pigmented line along the gingival margin.

The floor of the mouth can be inspected by asking the child to lift the tongue to the roof of the mouth. Observe the frenulum, sublingual ridge, and Wharton ducts that lie on either side of the frenulum. The color of the floor of the mouth will be pink.

The *tongue* is inspected and palpated. The dorsum of the tongue should appear dull red, moist, and glistening, with a white coat. The anterior portion of the tongue should have a slightly roughened appearance with papillae and small fissures. The tongue is palpated for indurations or ulcerations. While palpating the mouth of a young child, biting can be prevented by holding the child's cheeks.

Cranial nerve XII (hypoglossal nerve) is examined by asking the child to stick out the tongue as though licking a lollipop and observe for any deviation of the tongue to one side. The examiner can determine the strength of the

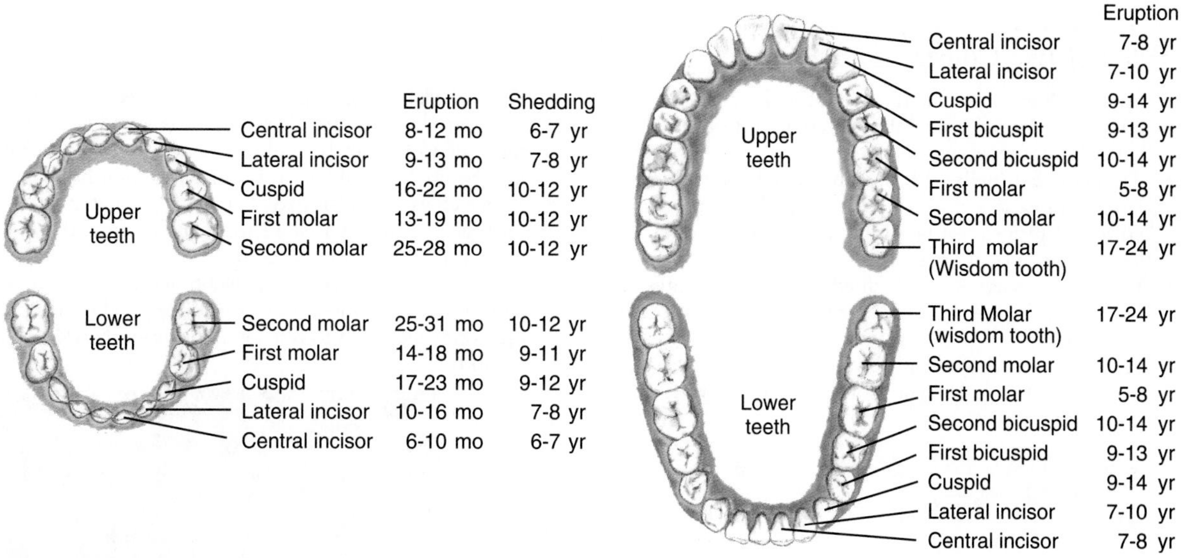

Upper teeth		Eruption	Shedding
	Central incisor	8-12 mo	6-7 yr
	Lateral incisor	9-13 mo	7-8 yr
	Cuspid	16-22 mo	10-12 yr
	First molar	13-19 mo	10-12 yr
	Second molar	25-28 mo	10-12 yr
Lower teeth			
	Second molar	25-31 mo	10-12 yr
	First molar	14-18 mo	9-11 yr
	Cuspid	17-23 mo	9-12 yr
	Lateral incisor	10-16 mo	7-8 yr
	Central incisor	6-10 mo	6-7 yr

Upper teeth		Eruption
	Central incisor	7-8 yr
	Lateral incisor	7-10 yr
	Cuspid	9-14 yr
	First bicuspit	9-13 yr
	Second bicuspid	10-14 yr
	First molar	5-8 yr
	Second molar	10-14 yr
	Third molar (Wisdom tooth)	17-24 yr
Lower teeth		
	Third Molar (wisdom tooth)	17-24 yr
	Second molar	10-14 yr
	First molar	5-8 yr
	Second bicuspid	10-14 yr
	First bicuspid	9-13 yr
	Cuspid	9-14 yr
	Lateral incisor	7-10 yr
	Central incisor	7-8 yr

FIGURE 33-7

Sequence of eruption of primary and secondary teeth.

tongue by placing a finger in the side of the child's cheek and asking the child to press the tongue against the examiner's finger. The tongue should feel equally strong on each side.

The *hard palate, soft palate,* and *uvula* are examined by asking the child to tilt the head back. The examiner inspects the hard palate for shape and color. The hard palate is whitish and convex, with transverse rugae. The examiner palpates the hard palate for the height of the arch and intactness. The examiner can allow the infant to suck on a gloved finger while palpating the hard palate to determine the strength of the sucking reflex. The soft palate is continuous with the hard palate and is concave and pinker in color. The uvula varies in length and thickness and is located in midline as a continuation of the soft palate. Cranial nerves IX (glossopharyngeal nerve) and X (vagus nerve) are evaluated at this time. The child is asked to say "ah"; normally, the soft palate rises symmetrically while the uvula remains in midline.

A tongue blade is used to depress the tongue and observe the *oropharynx.* This action can be unpleasant for the child. To minimize discomfort, the examiner slides the tongue blade along the side of the tongue until reaching the soft palate, then compresses the tongue to elicit the gag reflex (cranial nerve X) and observes the back of the throat. The tonsillar pillars are inspected with particular notation of size and color of tonsils. The tonsils are pink in color.

The size of tonsils will vary; large tonsils are common in young children. Tonsils may have crypts where food particles collect. With inflammatory processes, the crypts may contain exudate. A child whose parents complain of the child's snoring or waking up by snoring may have grossly enlarged tonsils. The posterior wall of the pharynx should be smooth and glistening pink; the wall may have small irregular spots of lymphatic tissue and small blood vessels (Seidel, 1995).

Eyes

The eyes are inspected and palpated as well as evaluated for visual acuity and extraocular muscle function.

VISUAL ACUITY

Visual acuity can be difficult to evaluate in a young child. Acuity develops over time, and evaluation requires the child's cooperation. Items needed for evaluating visual acuity in a child are an eye cover and visual charts. The chart chosen will be determined by the child's age and development. The infant from birth to age 1 or 2 months will gaze at black-and-white contrasting figures and faces. At age 4 weeks or older an infant will fix on a brightly colored object and follow it.

Depending on verbal ability, children age 2 may be able to use Allen cards to identify pictures from a distance of 15 feet. Each eye is tested separately. The child should be able to name three of seven cards in a maximum of five tries.

Preschool children can be tested using the HOTV chart at 10 feet. A card with HOTV is given to the child to hold. One eye is covered, and the child is instructed to keep the eye covered and to match the letters on the chart at 10 feet. The child holds the letters, or they are placed on a table directly in front of the child.

Older children's visual acuity can be tested using the Snellen chart, placed on a wall 20 feet away from the child. The chart should have no glare and should be well illuminated. No other materials should be around or near the chart. Both eyes are tested first, then each eye separately. If the child has corrective lenses, the procedure should be repeated with the corrective lenses on. Unless the child is known to have very poor vision, testing is begun at the distance on the chart for 40 feet. To determine at what level the child cannot see, the examiner finds the distance at

• • • • • • • • • • •
Types of Eye Charts

- **Snellen chart:** A standardized chart with graduated letters for testing far vision of children at 20 feet. Used with children over age 6.
- **Tumbling E (Snellen E):** A standardized chart using the letter E in various directions that is used with preschoolers ages 3 to 6 to test far vision at 20 feet. Also available for a distance of 10 feet.
- **Preliterate chart:** A standardized chart with pictures used with children ages 3 to 6 to test far vision at a distance of 20 feet.
- **HOTV chart:** A standardized chart with letters *HOTV* in graduated sizes. Designed for use at 10 feet with children ages 3 to 6.

- **Allen cards:** Picture cards of familiar objects for testing children 2½ years and older. Vision is tested at a distance of 15 feet. If the child is cooperative, Allen cards may be used in children as young as 24 months.
- **Jaeger chart:** Standardized chart with graduated letters for testing near vision at 12 to 14 inches from the eyes. Used with children over age 6.
- **Ishihara chart:** A series of polychromatic cards with a pattern of dots printed against a background of many colored dots. Designed to test for color vision between ages 4 and 6.

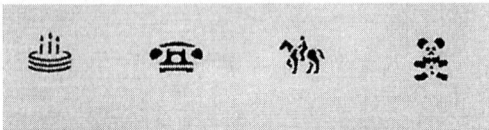

Allen cards, for testing preliterate children. (From Cassin, B. [1995]. *Fundamentals for ophthalmic technical personnel* [p. 160]. Philadelphia: Saunders.)

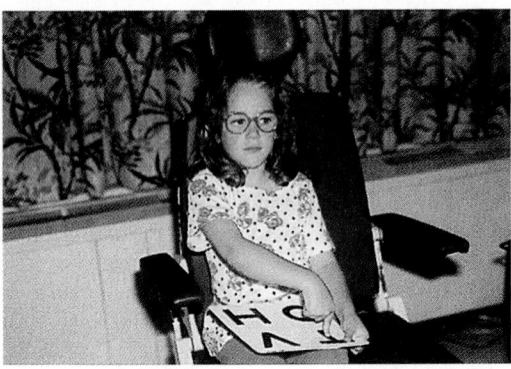

HOTV chart, for children ages 3 to 6 years. The letters *H O T V* are presented at a distance, and the child points to the corresponding letter on the card resting on her lap. (From Albert, D. M., & Jakobiec, F. A. [1994]. *Principles and practice of ophthalmology* [Vol. 4, p. 2722]. Philadelphia: Saunders.)

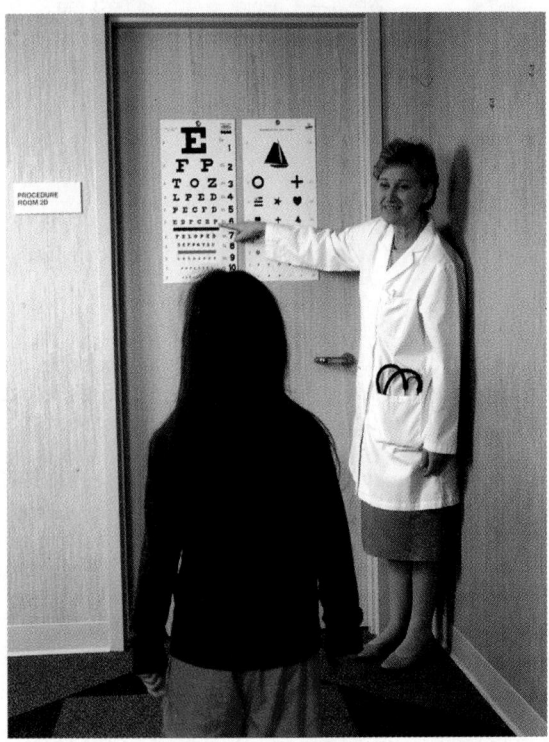

The standard Snellen E chart can be used for an older child who can read letters. The picture chart to the right of the Snellen chart can be used to assess vision in 3- to 6-year-olds. (From Jarvis, C. [1996]. *Physical examination and health assessment* [2nd ed., p. 329]. Philadelphia: Saunders.)

which the child misses half plus one of the symbols on a line of the chart. The visual acuity would then be designated as the smallest line at which the child is able to identify more than half of the symbols on the line. For corrective lenses, the examiner notes the last date the child was examined for a prescription. Findings are recorded by noting the distance of the line correctly read for both eyes (i.e., right eye 20/20 and left eye 20/20). This annotation means that the child has correctly interpreted the letters on the chart for 20 feet at a distance of 20 feet, which matches what the average child can see at that distance. If the child correctly identifies the letters on the line labeled 40 feet, that child can see at 20 feet what the average child can see at 40 feet.

Visual acuity changes with age and varies according to the test used. Normal ranges are

> *Birth:* Fixates on objects (8 to 12 inches), 20/100 to 20/150
> *4 months:* 20/50 to 20/80
> *1 year:* 20/40 to 20/70
> *4 years:* 20/30 to 20/40
> *5 years:* 20/20 to 20/30

COLOR VISION
Color vision deficit, less correctly termed color blindness, is an inherited recessive X-linked trait that, in varying de-

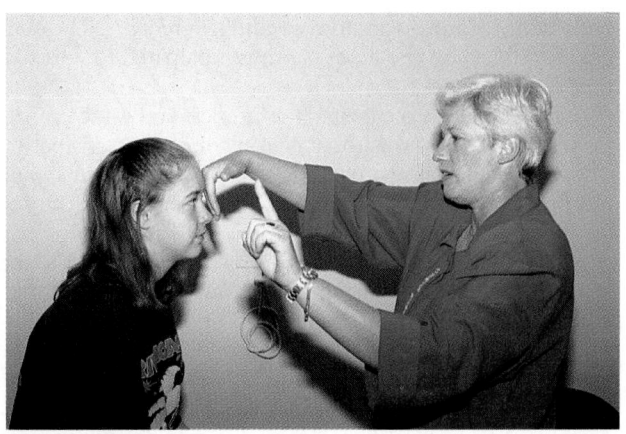

FIGURE 33-8

Visual fields (cranial nerve II) are tested in each eye separately. One eye is covered as the child stares straight ahead. An object is slowly moved from the side of the head into the field of vision. The child says "now" when first seeing the object.

grees, may affect the child's ability to discern traffic lights, brake lights, and color-coordinated clothing. Color vision deficit may affect learning if the learning is color related. The condition is very rare in females but affects 8% to 10% of males.

Color vision is evaluated using Ishihara's charts, a series of polychromatic cards. These cards have a pattern of colored pictures embedded in the charts. Boys between ages 4 and 8 years are tested once and are asked to touch or identify the embedded patterns. A child with this deficit cannot see the patterns against the field of color.

PERIPHERAL VISION

Visual fields are evaluated in older children to identify peripheral vision. The examiner's face is positioned directly in front and on the level of the child, about 2 feet away.

The visual fields should roughly mirror the examiner's. The examiner covers one eye and has the child mimic by covering the opposite eye. Slowly a puppet or some other test object is brought from the periphery into the child's field of vision. The object should come from a position slightly behind the child's head, and the child is asked to say "now" when the object is in view (Fig. 33–8). Testing for visual acuity and visual fields evaluates cranial nerve II, the optic nerve, which mediates vision.

BINOCULAR VISION AND STRABISMUS

Extraocular muscle function is evaluated to test binocular vision and the presence of strabismus. Strabismus, or "crossed eyes," is the abnormal or incomplete development of binocular visual alignment. Three tests are performed: the corneal light reflex (Hirschberg) test, a field-of-vision test, and the cover/uncover (alternate cover) test.

Corneal Light Reflex Test. The corneal light reflex is assessed by shining a light directly onto the irises from a distance of about 40.5 cm (16 inches). The reflection of the light should appear in exactly the same spot on both eyes. If the light falls off center in one eye, then the eyes are malaligned. Children with epicanthal folds (Fig. 33–9) may give a false impression of malalignment (pseudostrabismus).

Field-of-Vision Test. The six cardinal fields of vision are tested by holding the child's chin so that the head does not move and asking the child to follow a puppet or a familiar object held approximately 12 inches away from the face as the object is moved to each of the six cardinal positions. As the object is moved to the margins of each cardinal position, the examiner holds it momentarily in that position before proceeding back to the center. The eyes will track in a parallel fashion to each position. As the eyes are in the margins of each position, the examiner can note *end-stage nystagmus,* a gentle oscillation of the eye, which is considered normal. Young children under age 2 or 3 years may not be able too cooperate with this test.

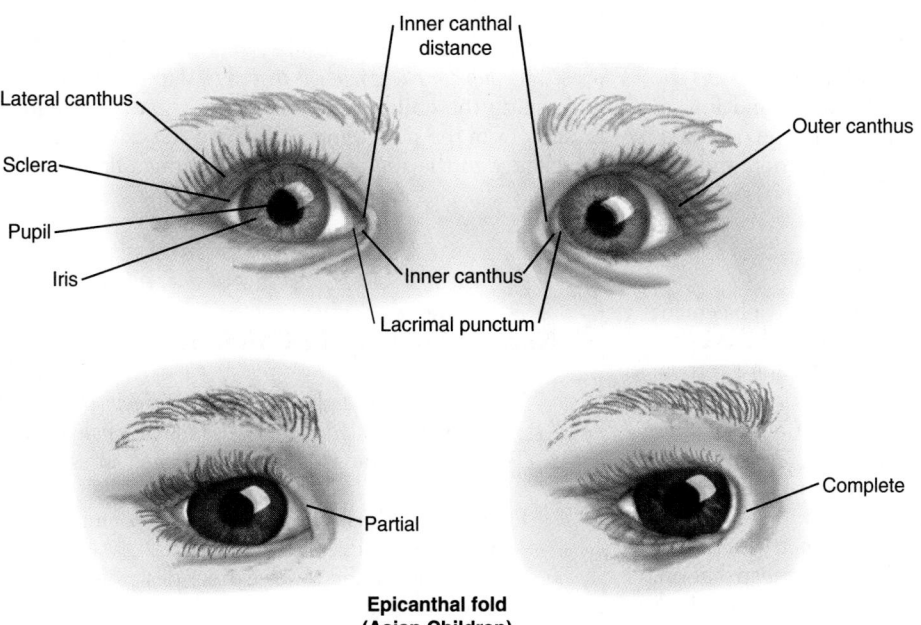

**Epicanthal fold
(Asian Children)**

FIGURE 33-9

External structures of the eye.

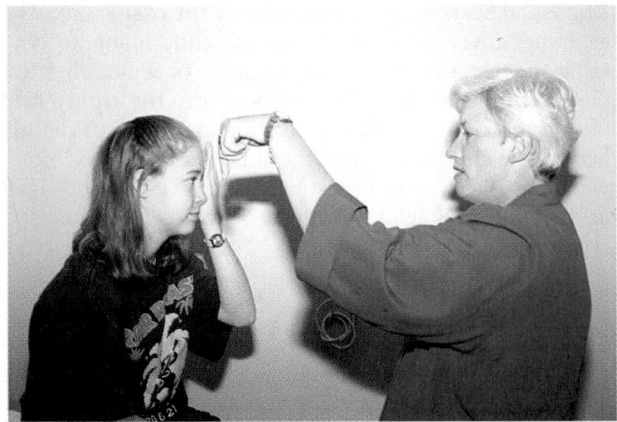

FIGURE 33–10

The cover/uncover test detects small degrees of deviated eye alignment. With one eye covered, the child gazes straight ahead with the uncovered eye. The cover is then removed and the eye should continue to stare straight ahead. Movement in either eye suggests muscle weakness. Extraocular muscle function is controlled by cranial nerves III, IV, and VI.

Cover/Uncover Test. The cover/uncover test is used to detect small degrees of deviated alignment by interrupting fusion of the eyes as they gaze at a fixed object. One eye is covered with an opaque card while the child stares straight ahead, at which time the examiner observes the uncovered eye. A steady fixed gaze is maintained by the uncovered eye. Next the eye is uncovered and observed for any movement; it should continue to stare straight ahead (Fig. 33–10). The procedure is repeated with the opposite eye. Any movement in either eye in the process of covering or uncovering may indicate muscle weakness.

Testing for extraocular muscle function in children under age 5 years is critical to identifying any muscle imbalance, so that it can be corrected at an early age to preserve vision. Extraocular muscle function evaluates three cranial nerves: cranial nerve VI, the abducent, which innervates the lateral rectus muscle (responsible for abducting the eye); cranial nerve IV, the trochlear nerve, which innervates the superior oblique muscle (responsible for down and inward movement of the eye); and cranial nerve III, the oculomotor nerve, which innervates the superior, inferior, and medial rectus and the inferior oblique muscles (Nelson et al., 1998).

EXTERNAL EYE

The external eye is evaluated for position and placement (see Fig. 33–9). The examiner notes whether the eyes are set wide apart or close together. *Epicanthal folds* are vertical folds that partially or completely cover the inner canthi. Epicanthal folds are seen in Asian children and in some non-Asian children as well (see Fig. 33–9). The slant of the eyes is determined by drawing an imaginary line across the inner canthi.

The *eyebrows* are inspected for symmetry and hair growth. The *eyelashes* are inspected for even distribution. The *lacrimal apparatus* is assessed by asking the child to look down. The outer part of the upper lid is palpated along the bony orbit for any discomfort, swelling, or redness. The puncta (tear duct) on the inner canthus is palpated for obstruction in the infant.

The eye globe is palpated for firmness and can be gently pushed into the orbit without causing discomfort. Palpation of the eye may cause anxiety in small children and should not be done unless there is a serious concern about the size of the eye.

Eyelids are inspected for color, swelling, discharge, and lesions. The position of the eyelids on the globe is noted. With the eyelids open, the upper lid normally falls below the superior limbus but does not cover any of the pupil. The lower lids normally fall just at the inferior limbus. The limbus is the point where the sclera of the eye meets the color portion of the iris. When closed, the eyelids approximate each other completely, without tremor, fasciculations, or tics.

The *conjunctiva* has two portions to evaluate. The palpebral portion of the conjunctiva lines the lids. The palpebral conjunctiva is examined by pulling down as the child looks up. It is normally clear, with a pink color, and may have several small blood vessels visible. The upper lid can be inspected by everting the upper eyelid over a cotton-tipped applicator. Eversion of the upper eyelid is not normally done because eye manipulation may cause apprehension in a child. The bulbar portion of the conjunctiva is transparent and lies over the sclera, allowing the white of the sclera to be clearly visible.

The following anterior structures of the eye are inspected: sclerae, cornea and lens, anterior chamber, and irises. The sclerae are white. Dark-skinned children may have small brown macules or a gray-blue or "muddy" color, particularly at the limbus. These variations are normal. The corneas are clear and transparent. Shining a light obliquely across the cornea highlights any abnormal irregularities on the corneal surface. The examiner illuminates the anterior chamber by shining a light across the eye from the temporal side to illuminate the entire iris without producing a shadow. The irises are round, regular-shaped, and clear. The irises are similar in color but may exhibit some variation between them.

Pupils appear round, regular, and of equal size in both eyes. The *pupillary light reflex* is tested by darkening the room and asking the child to gaze into the distance. A light is brought from the side (temporally), and the examiner notes the change in the size of the pupil. Shining a light directly

---

CRITICAL TO REMEMBER

Normal Findings in Children

Small, firm, nontender, and shotty (freely palpable and very small) lymph nodes may be palpable.

Tonsils are of varying sizes, often larger in young children.

Pupils are of equal size, round, and accommodating to light (PERRLA).

Pulses in upper and lower extremities are bilaterally symmetric.

into a pupil will cause the pupil to constrict (direct light reflex). The procedure is repeated while the opposite eye is observed. The opposite eye will constrict (consensual light reflex) in response to the light shone in the other eye. Pupils should constrict at equal speeds.

Pupil size should be the same in both eyes. In some children, pupils of unequal size are normal, but in general, unequal pupils call for a consideration of central nervous system injury. Accommodation can be tested by asking the child to focus on a distant object. The pupils normally dilate. An object such as a puppet or a finger brought into the line of vision about 7 to 8 cm from the nose should cause pupillary constriction and convergence of the axes of the eyes (Nelson et al., 1998).

OPHTHALMOSCOPIC EXAMINATION

The ophthalmoscopic examination requires a cooperative child, practice, and patience. Lights in the room will need to be dim. Most children will enjoy playing with the light of the "flashlight," and watching the light as you move it around the room facilitates cooperation. Minimally all practitioners will view the red reflex, but the procedure requires demonstration and practice. When the ophthalmoscope is placed in front of the pupil and the light hits the lens, a red color is reflected from the retina to the examiner. The retina, choroid, optic disk, macula, fovea centralis, and retinal vessels are also visible with the ophthalmoscope.

Ears

Assessment of the ears includes testing for hearing acuity, inspection and palpation of the external ear, and examination of the internal ear using the otoscope.

HEARING ACUITY

Infant Assessment. In an infant, hearing is assessed by asking the parent to speak to the infant from behind and observing the infant's response to the parent's voice. The examiner can stand behind the infant and ring a bell or make a sound the infant is familiar with and observe the infant turning to locate the sound. A very young infant, younger than 4 months, may demonstrate a startle reflex to loud sounds.

Preschool and School-Age Assessment by Audiometry. In preschool and school-age children the audiometer gives a precise (quantitative) assessment of the child's ability to hear. The child is placed in a soundproof room and is asked to identify tones played at a level the child can hear. With the audiometer, two tests are used to evaluate hearing: the sweep test and the pure tone hearing test. The *sweep test* is used to screen for hearing losses. The *pure tone test* is used to determine the exact extent of the hearing loss.

School-Age and Adolescent Assessment: The Whisper Test. The whisper test is performed on school-age children and adolescents. The child is asked to cover one ear or occlude one ear canal and to repeat what is heard as the examiner stands about 0.3 meter (1 foot) behind or to the side of the child.

For a preschool child the examiner stands in front of the child approximately 0.6 to 0.9 meter (2 to 3 feet) and gives the child a command such as "Please put the toy on the floor."

Conduction Tests (Tuning Fork Hearing Tests). Tuning fork tests are qualitative tests done to determine the ability to hear by air conduction and by bone conduction. In the normal child, air conduction of sound is greater than bone conduction. The *Rinne* hearing test is used to determine if air conduction is greater than bone conduction. The *Weber* hearing test determines the child's ability to hear by bone conduction. Testing the child's hearing evaluates cranial nerve VIII (acoustic nerve).

EXTERNAL EAR

The external ear is inspected and palpated. Ear placement and position are evaluated when assessing the face, but the external ear is also examined for any malformations or unusual markings (Fig. 33–11). Any discharge coming from the auditory meatus is noted, and its amount and characteristics are described. Soft yellow-brown cerumen (ear wax) is normally seen in the external auditory meatus.

The bony prominence of the mastoid process behind the ear is palpated for tenderness. The auricles are gently pulled to determine if discomfort is created.

OTOSCOPIC EXAMINATION

The *tympanic membrane* is examined by using the otoscope (Fig. 33–12). Many children may be apprehensive about this examination. If necessary, a small child is positioned on the parent's lap, and the child's arms are secured. The examiner uses the largest speculum that will fit comfortably into the ear canal. In a child younger than 3 years the ear canal is straightened by pulling the pinna of the ear down and back. If a child is 3 years old or older, the pinna is pulled up and back. As much of the canal as possible should be visible before inserting the speculum into the auditory meatus.

The canal is inspected for any lesions and for cerumen. The tympanic membrane is inspected for landmarks, color, and mobility. A puff of air is injected into the canal with an insufflation bulb, and the tympanic membrane is observed for movement. Normally, the tympanic membrane moves inward with a slight puff and outward with a slight release.

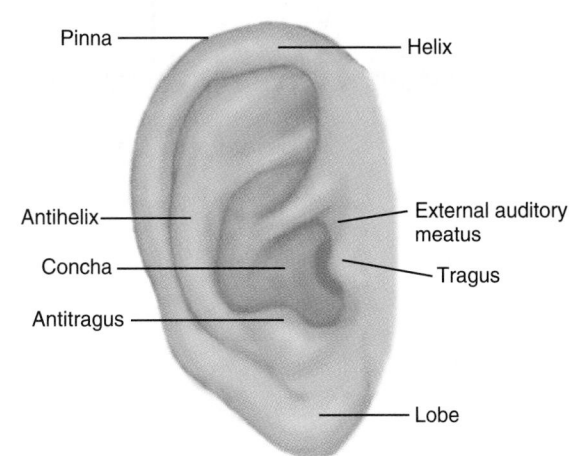

FIGURE 33–11

Landmarks of the external ear.

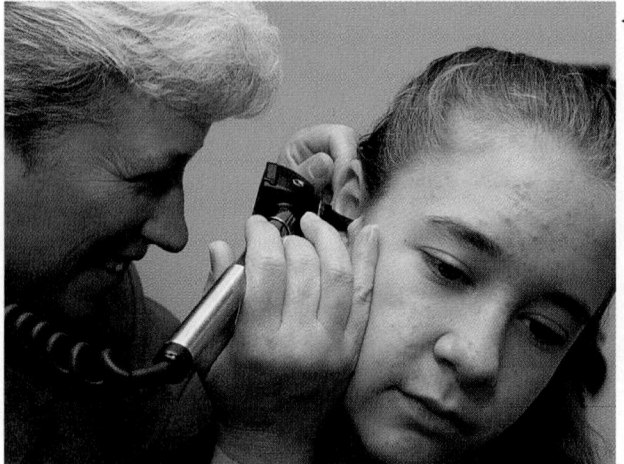

◀ To straighten the ear canal of a child older than age 3, the nurse pulls the child's pinna up and back.

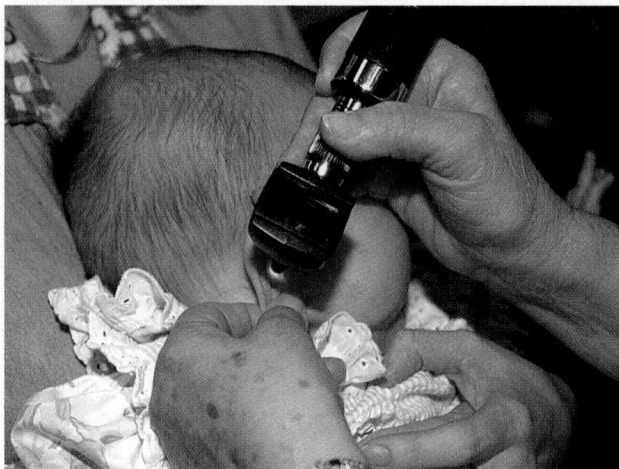

For children under age 3, the pinna is pulled down ▶ and back.

◀ Structures of the ear

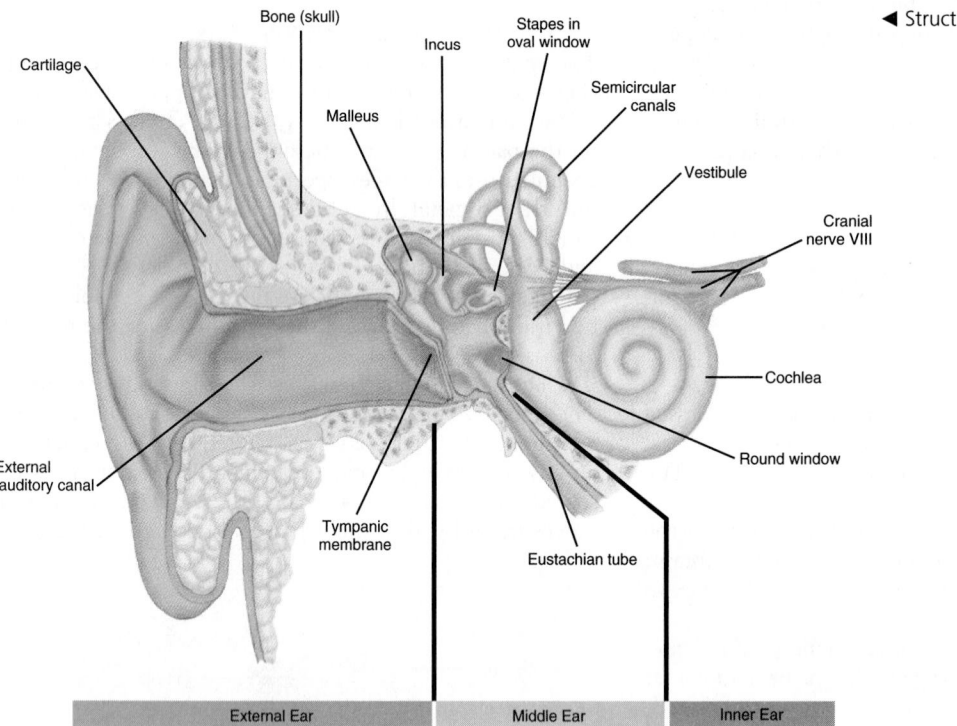

Landmarks of the tympanic membrane ▶

FIGURE 33–12

Inspection of the tympanic membrane using the otoscope. The auditory canal is inspected before inserting the otoscope to see the child's tympanic membrane.

Thorax and Lungs

Assessment of the thorax and lungs consists of inspection, palpation, percussion, and auscultation, in that order. To assist with localizing findings on the thorax, anatomic landmarks such as the ribs and intercostal spaces are identified, and imaginary lines are drawn on the surface (Fig. 33–13).

Location of lung tissue will depend on the age and development of the child. In an infant, lung tissue on the anterior chest can be located from the apex, above the clavicle, to the level of the fifth rib in the midclavicular line. By age 6 years, lung tissue is assessed from the apex to the level of the sixth rib in the midclavicular line. Laterally, lung tissue is assessed from the axilla to the level of the eighth rib. Posteriorly, lungs are assessed from the level of the first thoracic vertebra to the tenth thoracic vertebra.

INSPECTION

The child's shirt or clothing covering the chest is removed. In adolescent females the breasts should be kept covered and exposed only when necessary. Inspection of the chest includes observing the child for any cough, stridor, grunting, hoarseness, snoring, wheezing, and type and amount of any sputum, if present. *Respiratory rate* and *pattern* are observed. In young children and infants, breathing is more diaphragmatic or abdominal. (See Table 33–1 for the effect of age on vital signs.) The chest wall should expand symmetrically during respiration. Respirations should be easy, regular, and without apparent distress.

Thoracic configuration is evaluated by determining the shape and symmetry of the chest from the front, sides, and back (Fig. 33–14). Two common alterations in structure in the anterior chest are *pectus carinatum* (pigeon breast) and *pectus excavatum* (funnel breast).

PALPATION

Palpation of the chest begins with the posterior chest. To alleviate fear in a young child, the examiner should stand in a position that allows the child visibility at all times. The posterior chest is palpated for areas of tenderness, tactile fremitus, and chest excursion.

To palpate for tenderness, the examiner touches the entire thorax with the palmar aspects of the fingers. This process elicits any points of discomfort or pain. The examiner notes any masses or edema (Fig. 33–15).

To evaluate for *tactile fremitus*, the examiner palpates the chest wall while the child says "ninety-nine." Vibrations felt on the chest wall are the result of vibrations produced in the vocal cords and transmitted to the chest wall through the respiratory tract.

Percussion of the chest is performed by advanced practitioners to determine changes in sound produced by the density of the underlying tissues.

AUSCULTATION

Auscultation of the chest is done to determine the characteristics of breath sounds heard with a stethoscope. Breath sounds heard with the stethoscope are made by the flow of air through the respiratory tree and are characterized by intensity, pitch, quality, and duration.

It is best to listen to breath sounds with the child sitting upright, if possible. Infants and toddlers can be held in the parent's lap; have the parent assist with removal of clothing and positioning of the child. The examiner's position is on the side of the child, allowing the child to observe the examiner's movements. Before touching the chest, the examiner allows the young child to hold or play with the stethoscope, and warms the stethoscope before placing it on the child's chest.

An anxious or frightened child may cry during this part of the examination. Distracting the child or having the young child focus on another activity may facilitate listening. For the inconsolable child, the examiner listens to breath sounds between each cry. If the young child is sleeping or comfortable in the parent's arms, the examiner listens to the chest first before proceeding to the rest of the examination.

For listening to the posterior thorax, the child is positioned with the head bent forward and hands folded in front. Having the child raise the arms overhead while sitting erect allows the examiner to listen laterally. To auscultate the anterior chest, have the child sit erect with the shoulders back (Fig. 33–16).

The examiner begins on the posterior thorax and has the child open the mouth and breathe in and out while the examiner listens with the diaphragm of the stethoscope. Having the young child blow bubbles, pretend to blow out birthday candles, or blow a tissue will increase breath sounds. Compressing the hand holding the stethoscope on the chest wall and placing the other hand on the opposite side of the chest accentuates expiration and makes end-expiratory sounds (e.g., wheezes) easier to hear. The sequence for listening to breath sounds is posterior chest, right and left lateral chest, and anterior chest (Fig. 33–17).

ADVENTITIOUS BREATH SOUNDS

In addition to normal breath sounds, adventitious sounds may be audible with the stethoscope. Table 33–2 describes the origin and characteristics of adventitious sounds. Adventitious sounds are additional sounds heard in an abnormal clinical state. They are described by their quality. The examiner notes whether they are continuous or discontinuous and where they occur in the respiratory phase. The effects of coughing are also noted. When adventitious sounds are heard, they are described as to their location, timing, and intensity.

Heart

The techniques for assessing the heart are inspection, palpation, and auscultation. The sequence of this examination depends on the age, growth, and development of the child being examined. For an infant or young child, the examiner may want to listen to the child's heart while the parent is holding the child, before doing other parts of the examination. Infants and children have varying degrees of dependence on parents and may be fearful of the examination. Percussion of the heart primarily indicates the size and shape of the heart and is not routinely done. The heart is assessed with the child in a supine position, a left lateral recumbent position, and in a sitting position while leaning forward slightly.

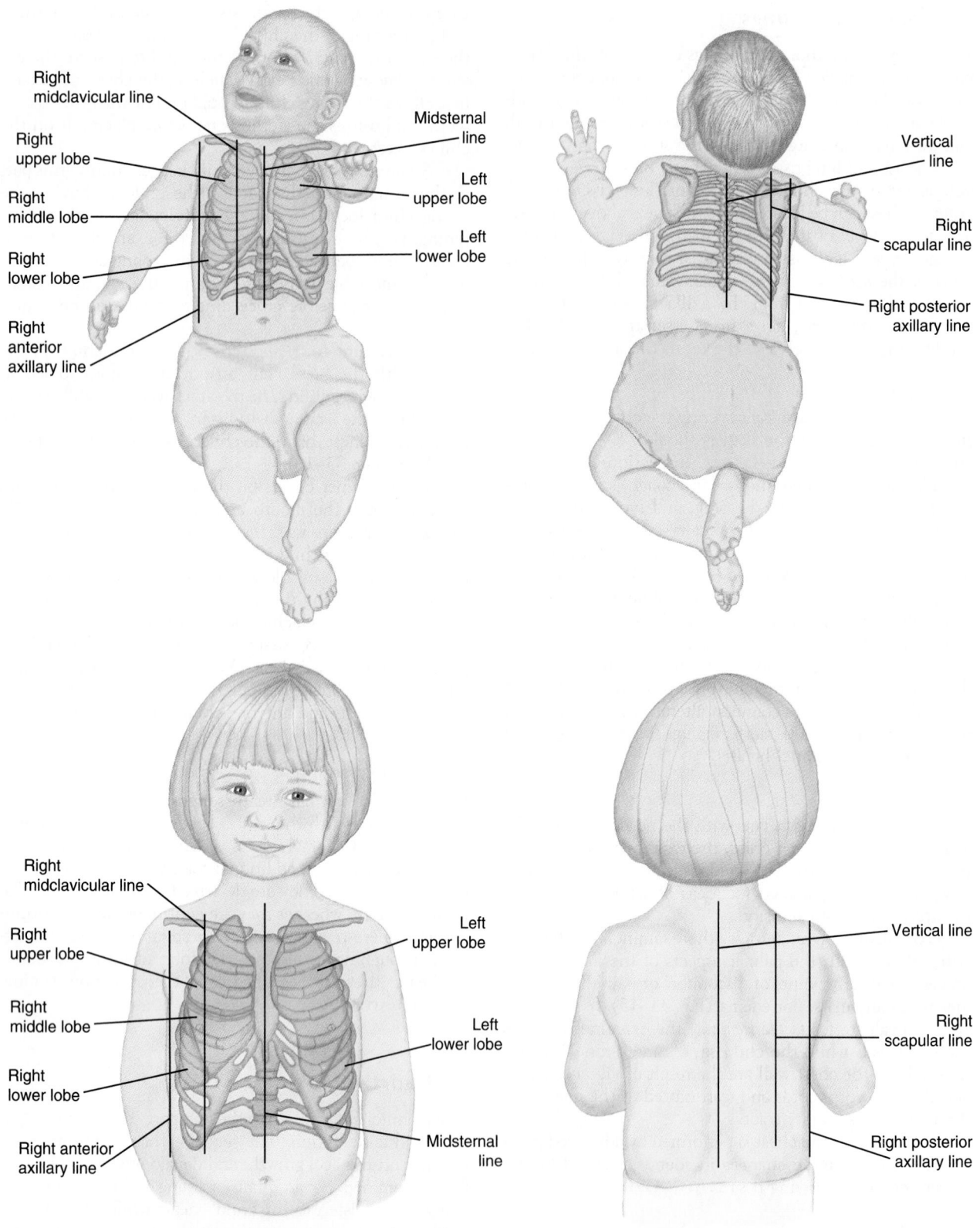

Right
midclavicular line

Right
upper lobe

Right
middle lobe

Right
lower lobe

Right
anterior
axillary line

Midsternal
line

Left
upper lobe

Left
lower lobe

Vertical
line

Right
scapular line

Right posterior
axillary line

Right
midclavicular line

Right
upper lobe

Right
middle lobe

Right
lower lobe

Right anterior
axillary line

Left
upper lobe

Left
lower lobe

Midsternal
line

Vertical line

Right
scapular line

Right posterior
axillary line

FIGURE 33–13

Anatomic landmarks of the thorax in infants and children.

Normal Infant

The chest of the normal infant is approximately round or barrel shaped in cross-section. A barrel chest in a child older than 6 suggests a chronic pulmonary disease such as asthma or cystic fibrosis.

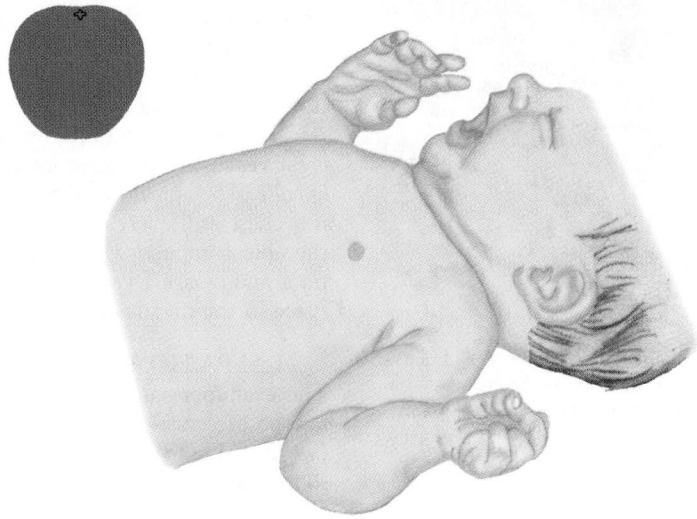

Funnel Chest (Pectus Excavatum)

A funnel chest has a depression in the lower portion of the sternum. Compression of the heart and great vessels may cause murmurs.

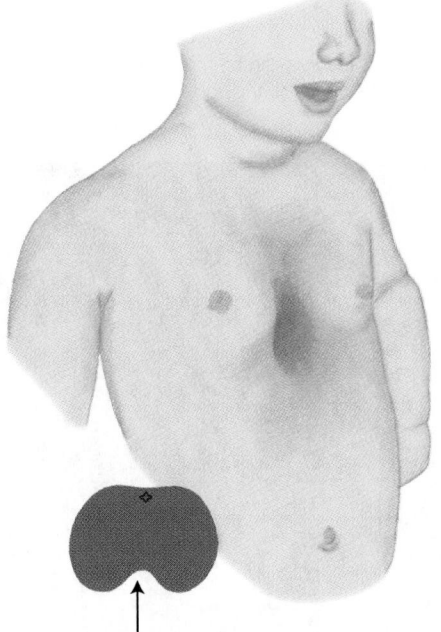

Pigeon Chest (Pectus Carinatum)

In pigeon chest, the sternum is displaced anteriorly, increasing the anteroposterior diameter. Grooves in the chest wall accentuate the deformity.

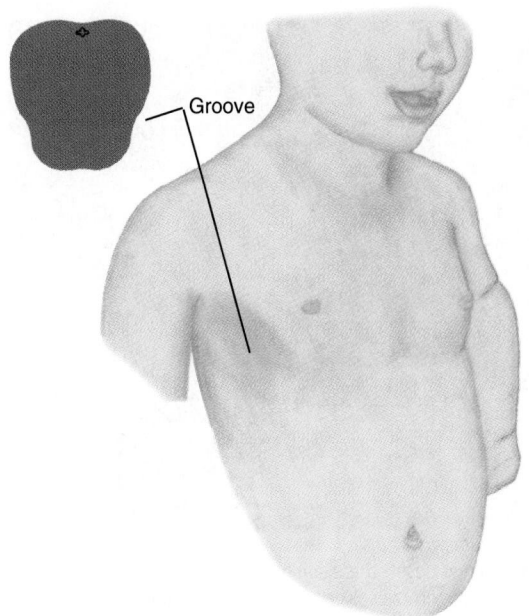

Groove

FIGURE 33–14

Common alterations in chest configuration.

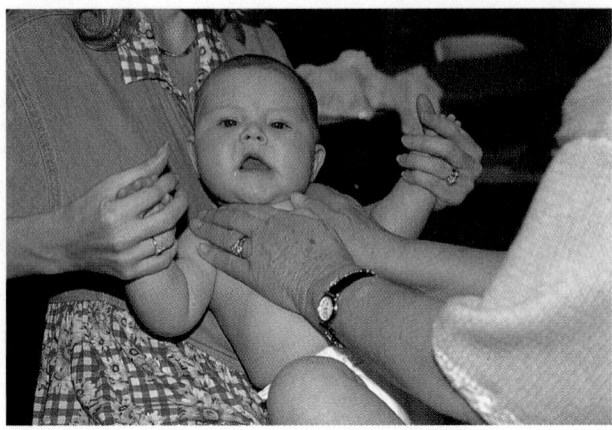

FIGURE 33–15
. . . .
To identify areas of fremitus, tenderness, symmetry, and depth and equality of expansion the nurse palpates the child's posterior and anterior chest. When palpating any area, warm hands increase the child's comfort. (Courtesy of The University of Texas at Arlington School of Nursing, Arlington, Texas.)

INSPECTION

The anterior chest is systematically inspected, with special attention paid to the following five areas: second right intercostal space (aortic area), second left intercostal space (pulmonic area), left sternal border (right ventricular area), fifth left intercostal space in the midclavicular line (apex), and just below the xiphoid process (epigastric area). The areas

will differ at different ages (Fig. 33–18). During infancy the heart is more horizontal in the thorax, and the apex is one or two intercostal spaces above the fifth intercostal space and lateral to the midclavicular line. The second intercostal space is located by identifying the sternal angle. The second rib is attached to the sternum just below or at the sternal angle. The second intercostal space is below the second rib. Other ribs and intercostal spaces are identified by their relationship to the second rib.

The precordium (anterior chest overlying the heart and great vessels) is inspected for *bulges*, *lifts*, *heaves*, and *apical impulse*. The apical impulse is the light tapping of the anterior chest wall every time the heart beats. The location of the apical impulse will change gradually as the child matures and by age 7 years can be seen at the fifth intercostal space in the midclavicular line.

PALPATION

The examiner palpates the precordium with the fingertips for the presence of any pulsations at each individual area (see Fig. 33–18). The examiner locates the apical pulse, sometimes identified as the point of maximal impulse (PMI), or the point where the light tapping of the heart is felt the best. Using the palmar aspect of the hand to feel for *thrills*, the examiner then palpates each individual area of the precordium. Thrills are palpable vibrations of the heart.

AUSCULTATION

Auscultation of the heart is done by listening both with the bell and with the diaphragm of the stethoscope as the child

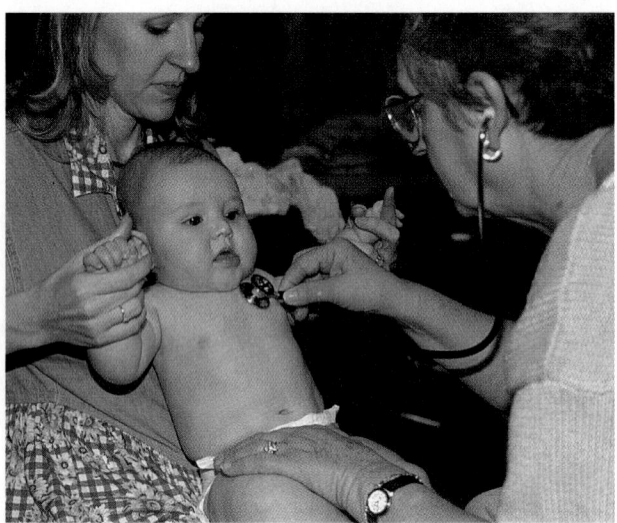

If the child is upset, the examiner may have to listen to breath ▶ sounds between cries. Keeping this child in the comfort of her mother's arms lessens her distress.

◀ Infants and toddlers can be held sitting upright in the parent's lap while the nurse listens to breath sounds.

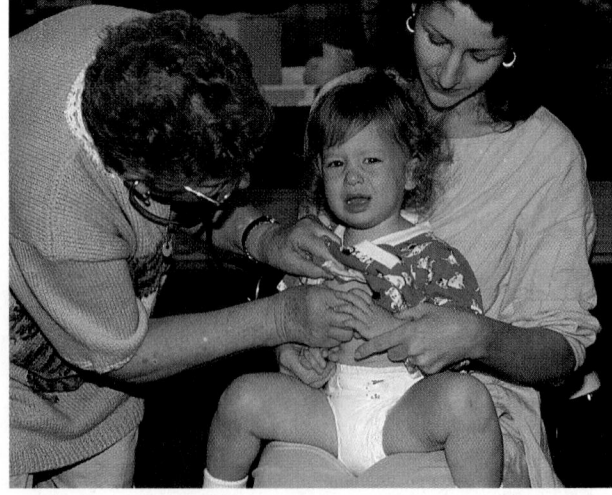

FIGURE 33–16
. . . .
To hear heart and breath sounds, the nurse auscultates the child's chest with a stethoscope in an orderly way. Auscultation is best performed when the child is quiet, so this part of the examination is best performed first if the child is quiet or asleep. To allay fears and make the examination more comfortable, the child can play with the stethoscope first and warm the instrument. The child also can be distracted with a toy while listening. (Photo courtesy of The University of Texas at Arlington School of Nursing, Arlington, Texas.)

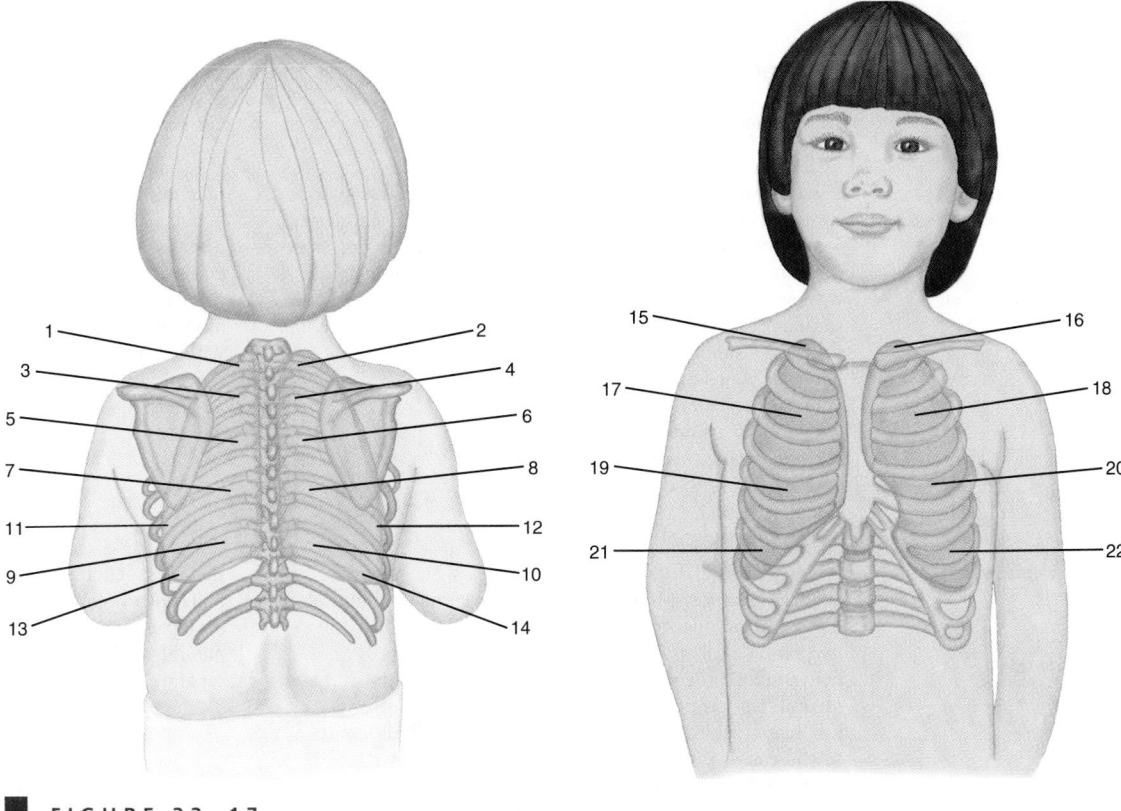

FIGURE 33-17
· · · · · · · · · ·
Sequence for listening to breath sounds.

is lying down, in a left lateral recumbent position, and sitting up. To auscultate heart sounds, the examiner uses a systematic approach. Sounds heard with the stethoscope are predominantly produced with the closing of the heart valves. The four traditional areas for listening to heart sounds are the aortic valve area in the second right intercostal space, the pulmonic valve area in the second left intercostal space, the tricuspid valve area in the left lower sternal border, and the mitral valve area in the fifth intercostal space at the left midclavicular line (see Fig. 33–18). The position for listening to these areas will depend on the age of the child. It is best to listen to heart sounds by inching the stethoscope across the precordium in a Z pattern, from the base of the heart across and down, or from the apex upward. All areas are auscultated with both the bell and the diaphragm of the stethoscope.

Sounds produced by the closing of the valves can be heard all over the precordium, so it will be necessary to concentrate on one heart sound at a time. The heart sounds are divided into two components, the first heart sound (S_1) and the second heart sound (S_2). S_1 is heard best at the apex of the heart, and S_2 is heard best at the base. S_1, phonetically described as *lub*, is produced by the closing of the mitral and tricuspid valves. S_2, phonetically described as *dub*, is produced by the closing of the aortic and pulmonic valves and is heard best at the base of the heart.

The physiologic splitting of S_2, an audible pause between the closing of the aortic and pulmonic valves, is frequently heard in children of all ages and is considered normal. Splitting of S_2 can be heard best at the pulmonic area

because ejection times on the right side of the heart are slightly longer than on the left side. Splitting of S_2 is greatest at the peak of inspiration and decreases or goes away during expiration.

The routine for assessing heart sounds is the following sequence:

1. Identify the rate and rhythm.
2. Identify S_1 and S_2.
3. Assess S_1 and S_2 separately to determine where they are best heard.
4. Listen for extra heart sounds.
5. Identify murmurs.

Normal Rate and Rhythm. The normal rate of a child's heart is different at different ages (see Table 33–1). Children's heart rates often increase with inspiration and slow down during expiration. To decrease the irregular rhythm associated with respirations, the examiner has the child hold the breath as the examiner continues to listen.

Extra Heart Sounds, Including Murmurs. Extra sounds, sounds heard over and above the normal heart sounds, may be described as opening snaps, ejection clicks, mid- to late systolic clicks, and murmurs. Snaps and clicks are short, high-pitched sounds heard with valve disorders and do not vary with respirations. *Murmurs* are blowing, swooshing sounds that occur because of some disruption in the blood flow into, through, or out of the heart. Innocent or functional heart murmurs are frequently heard in children. They do not radiate and change with position change.

TABLE 33-2
• • • • • • • • • • • •

Origin and Characteristics of Adventitious Breath Sounds

Sound	Description	Mechanism	Clinical Example
Discontinuous Sounds			
Crackles—fine (rales, crepitations); heard when fluid is in airways.	Discontinuous, high-pitched, short, crackling, popping sounds heard during inspiration and not cleared by coughing. You can simulate this sound by rolling a strand of hair between your fingers near your ear, or by moistening your thumb and index finger and separating them near your ear. Described as discrete (short), discontinuous.	Inhaled air collides with previously deflated airways; airways suddenly pop open, creating crackling sound as gas pressures between the two compartments equalize.	*Late inspiratory* crackles occur with restrictive disease: pneumonia, congestive heart failure, and interstitial fibrosis. *Early inspiratory* crackles occur with obstructive disease: chronic bronchitis and asthma.
Pleural friction rub.	A very superficial sound that is coarse and low-pitched; it has a grating quality, as if two pieces of leather were being rubbed together. A pleural friction rub sounds just like crackles, but close to the ear. It sounds louder if you push the stethoscope harder into the chest wall.	Caused when pleurae become inflamed and lose their normal lubricating fluid. Their opposing roughened pleural surfaces rub together during respiration. This sound is heard best in the anterolateral wall, where lung mobility is greatest.	Pleuritis, accompanied by pain with breathing. (Rub disappears after a few days if pleural fluid accumulates and separates pleurae.)
Continuous Sounds			
High-pitched wheeze heard with narrowing of the air passages due to fluid, swelling, spasm, and tumors.	High-pitched, musical squeaking sounds that predominate in expiration but may occur in both expiration and inspiration. Coughing frequently will change the character of the sound.	Air squeezed or compressed through passageways narrowed almost to closure by collapsing, swelling, secretions, or tumors. The passageway walls oscillate in apposition between the closed and barely open positions. The resulting sound is similar to that produced by a vibrating reed.	Obstructive lung disease such as asthma.
Low-pitched wheeze (sonorous rhonchi).	Low-pitched, musical snoring, moaning sounds. They are heard throughout the cycle, although they are more prominent on expiration and may clear somewhat by coughing.	Air flow obstruction as described by the vibrating reed mechanism. The pitch of the wheeze does not correlate with the size of the passageway that generates it.	Bronchitis.

Note: Although nothing in clinical practice seems to differ more than the nomenclature of adventitious sounds, most authorities concur on two categories: (1) discontinuous, discrete crackling sounds, and (2) continuous, coarse, or wheezing sounds.

To describe and classify extra heart sounds, the nurse needs advanced training and practice.

Peripheral Vascular System

Arterial pulses are examined for decreased or absent pulses. Pulses are palpated, with the examiner noting the rate, rhythm, elasticity of the vessel wall, and equal force of bilateral pulses. The pulse force should be symmetric and should be the same for upper and lower extremities. Comparing opposite pulses is necessary in children. The examiner compares one femoral pulse with the opposite carotid pulse for equality, and compares one lower extremity pulse with an upper extremity pulse for equality.

Breast

The examiner inspects and palpates breast tissue. Developmental differences occur in response to circulating hormones and affect the appearance of breast tissue. In infants

Cardiac Landmarks

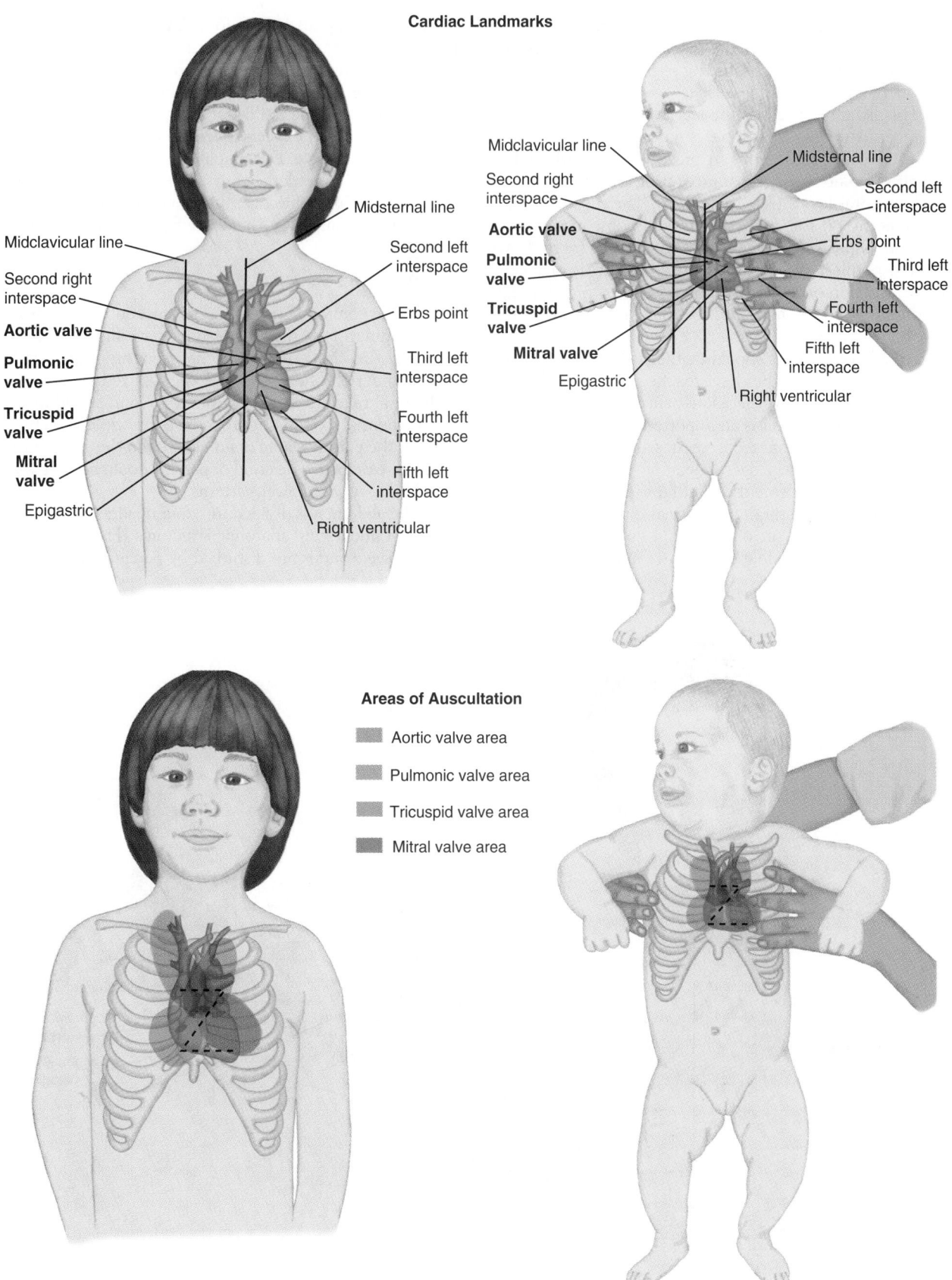

Aortic valve area

Pulmonic valve area

Tricuspid valve area

Mitral valve area

FIGURE 33–18

Location of the heart within the thorax in the infant and the older child, showing landmarks and areas of auscultation.

of both sexes the breasts may appear engorged because of maternal estrogen crossing the placenta. *Thelarche*, breast development, marks the beginning of puberty in preadolescent girls and can occur as early as age 8 years.

The examiner inspects the *nipples* for position and appearance. In infants the nipple is flat and symmetric with darker areola pigmentation. In preadolescent and adolescent girls, Tanner's sexual maturity rating is used to evaluate developmental levels (see Table 8–2). The nipples should be symmetric on the chest, and should point in the same direction. Nipples may appear to be inverted or everted. An inverted nipple is significant if the inversion is of recent origin. The skin of the breast should be smooth and free of any dimpling. It is common to see some asymmetry during growth.

All adolescent girls should be taught how to do breast self-examination once they have reached menarche. Teaching self-examination to the adolescent and reinforcing its importance at every visit is an important role for the nurse. Many adolescents do not do breast self-examinations because of lack of knowledge or fear of finding something wrong. Once the adolescent is familiar with how her breasts look and feel, the natural and normal changes that occur in the breast as a result of hormonal fluctuations can be easily identified. The adolescent girl should be taught to do a breast self-examination 3 to 4 days after menses, as the breasts are least tender and sensitive at that time. Chapter 31 describes the procedure for examining the breasts.

The examiner uses the same technique to palpate the breast tissue and the axillas of the adolescent boy. In the male, the examiner expects to feel a thin layer of fatty tissue overlying the muscle. During puberty some boys experience *gynecomastia*, an enlargement of breast tissue, felt as a smooth, firm, movable disk. It frequently affects only one breast and is temporary (Fuller & Schaller-Ayers, 1994).

Abdomen

The child's comfort should be considered during the abdominal examination. An empty bladder, a warm room, and positioning the child supine on the examining table with a pillow under the head and the knees flexed will enhance abdominal relaxation. For an infant or young child most of the abdominal examination can be done while the child is lying in the parent's lap. For an older child the genitalia and breasts are draped. The child or parent should be questioned about urinary and bowel patterns.

The abdomen is divided into four quadrants that correlate with underlying anatomic structures (Fig. 33–19). Because bowel sounds are disturbed by percussion and palpa-

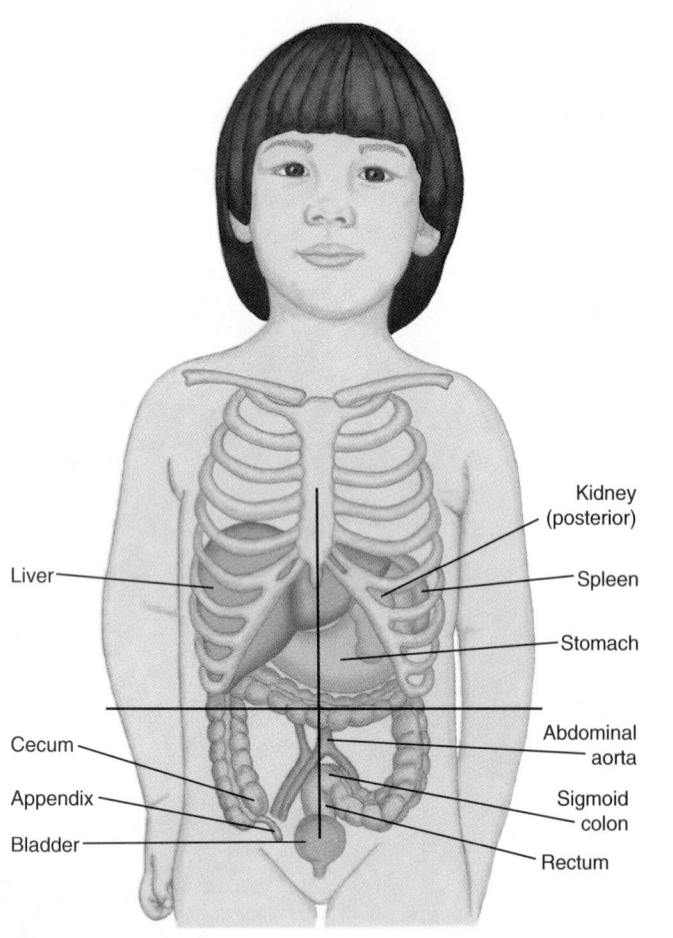
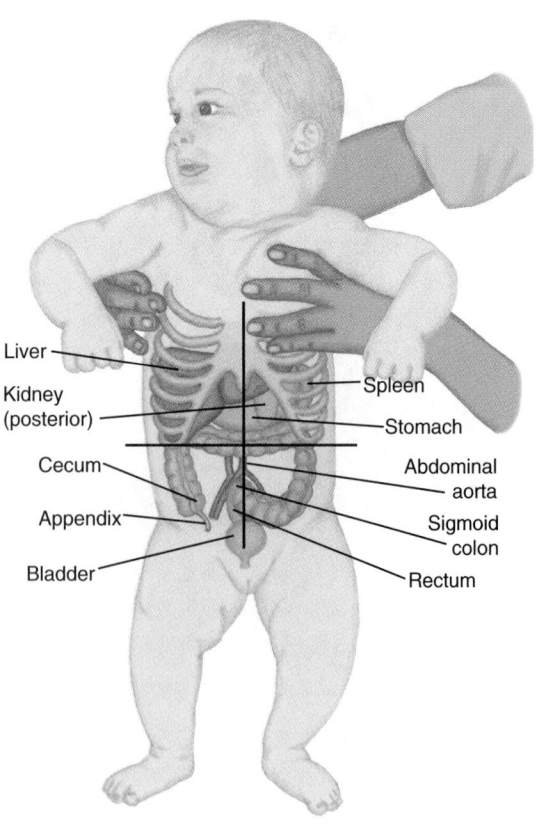

FIGURE 33–19

Abdominal quadrants and structures.

tion, the sequence of techniques differs in abdominal assessment. The abdomen is first inspected, then auscultated, then percussed, and lastly palpated.

INSPECTION

Abdominal inspection is done to determine contour, symmetry, characteristics of the umbilicus and skin, pulsations or movement, and hair distribution. *Contour* is the profile of the abdomen from the rib margin to the pubic bone and is best determined by looking tangentially across the abdomen. The contour is described as flat, scaphoid, rounded, or protuberant (Fig. 33–20). The abdominal contour provides an overall indicator of nutritional state. The abdomen should be *symmetric* bilaterally. The examiner looks for distentions, bulging, visible mass, or asymmetric shape.

The *umbilicus* is normally midline and inverted. There should be no signs of discoloration, inflammation, or hernia. Throughout the neonatal period, the umbilical cord is inspected for signs of infection or bleeding.

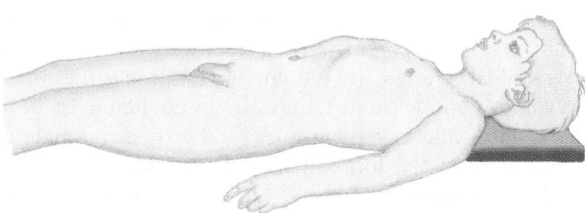

Flat: Thin child

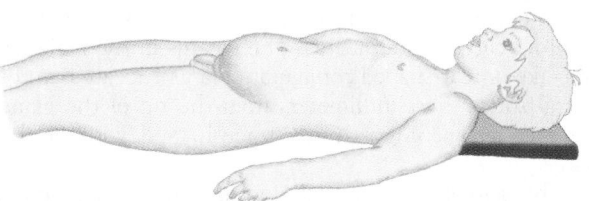

Rounded: Normal appearance of abdomen in a young child

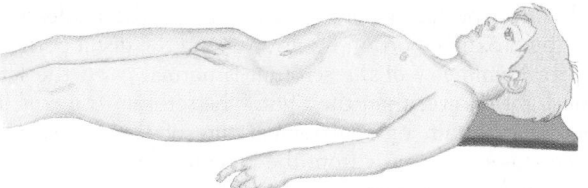

Scaphoid: Emaciated or malnourished child

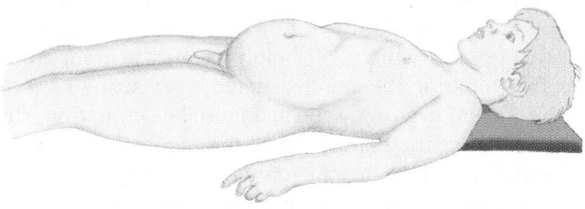

Protuberant: Recent distention with flatus; or extremely obese child. (If adolescent female, may indicate pregnancy.)

FIGURE 33–20
. . . .
Abdominal contours. The contour of the abdomen provides an indication of the child's overall nutritional state.

The skin of the abdomen is inspected for color and the presence of scars, lesions, and striae. A fine venous network may be seen in infants and small children.

The abdomen is inspected for *pulsations* and *movement*. In thin children the examiner may see the pulsations from the aorta beneath the skin in the epigastric area. Most children will have abdominal movement with respirations. Peristalsis of the abdomen should not be visible.

AUSCULTATION

Auscultation of the abdomen follows inspection. The diaphragm of the stethoscope is held lightly against the skin to note the character and frequency of bowel sounds. Bowel sounds are high-pitched, gurgling sounds heard in all four quadrants. They are irregular and can occur from 5 to 34 times a minute. The examiner begins in the lower right quadrant and listens in all four quadrants. To determine that there are no bowel sounds, the examiner must listen for up to 5 minutes in an area where no bowel sounds are heard.

The bell of the stethoscope is used to listen for bruits over the aortic, renal, iliac, and femoral arteries. The examiner also listens in the epigastric region and around the umbilicus for a venous hum—a soft, low-pitched, continuous sound.

PERCUSSION

Advanced practitioners perform abdominal percussion. The technique reveals tympany, liver span, and splenic dullness.

PALPATION

Abdominal palpation is done to identify any mass or tenderness and to determine the size, consistency, and location of certain organs.

The examiner should have warm hands before palpating the abdomen. Palpation of the infant or young child can be done in the parent's lap by laying the child's head and thorax across the parent's legs and extending the child's abdomen and legs across the examiner's legs. The child should be prepared for palpation of the abdomen by flexing the knees.

Fear and anxiety may cause the child to resist when the examiner touches the abdomen. Distracting the young child with a toy or talking is helpful. Beginning with light palpation shows the child that palpation will not "hurt."

Ask an older child who is anxious or ticklish to assist with this part of the examination. The child places a hand on the abdomen and the examiner places a hand, with fingers touching the abdomen, on top of the child's hand and asks the child to push as the examiner pushes. This technique allows the child some control as the examination begins and it reduces the sensation of tickling. To assist with relaxation of the abdominal muscles, the examiner can ask the child to take deep breaths.

The examiner begins with light palpation of all four quadrants using light, even pressure and pressing the palmar surface of the fingers no more than 1 cm into the abdomen. The hand is lifted while moving from area to area. Sudden jabs should be avoided. As the examiner circles around the abdomen, the abdomen should feel soft and smooth. Light palpation is useful in identifying areas of tenderness and muscular resistance. Guarding, resistance, or tenderness should alert the examiner to move cautiously with deeper palpation.

Tenseness can be either voluntary or involuntary. In a child, tenseness and rigidity may be due to fear and anxiety. Distracting the child or waiting for the child to breathe will assist with determining whether the tenseness is voluntary or involuntary. The examiner gently indents the fingers into the abdominal wall during inspiration. With even pressure, the abdomen should feel soft. Rigidity, a constant boardlike hardness of the abdomen, is usually associated with an acute inflammation of the peritoneum.

Using the same techniques, the examiner deeply palpates the abdomen. The examiner pushes down about 5 to 8 cm into the abdominal wall, beginning in the right lower quadrant. The entire abdomen is examined to identify palpable organs and masses.

To palpate the liver's edge, the examiner begins at the level of the umbilicus in the midclavicular line, using the side of the hand to indent into the abdomen about 5 to 8 cm. With deep penetration of the abdominal wall, the hand is gently inverted toward the costal margin. Then the examiner progresses upward with the same maneuver until palpating the border of the liver. The edge of the liver is felt as soft and smooth. The firm border moves downward when the child takes a deep breath. In infants and young children, the examiner can begin at the costal margin and, using the palmar aspects of the fingers, indent into the abdominal wall about 5 to 8 cm. The examiner should move down from the costal margin until the hand falls off the edge of the liver border. In infants and toddlers, the liver edge may be palpated 1 to 3 cm below the costal margin.

Advanced practitioners palpate the spleen and kidneys to determine the presence and size of masses or enlargement.

When areas of tenderness are elicited during palpation, a special procedure for identifying rebound tenderness is used. A site away from the identified tenderness is chosen. The examiner places a hand perpendicular to the abdomen, pushes down slowly and deeply into the abdomen, and then lifts the hand quickly. With peritoneal inflammation, the sudden release of the pressure will cause severe pain and muscle rigidity.

While palpating the abdomen, the examiner checks skin turgor and palpates the femoral pulses and inguinal lymph nodes.

The child is turned over and the buttocks are inspected. The buttocks in children are full, with symmetric folds. No evidence of scars or ecchymosis should appear on the buttocks. The sacrococcygeal area is examined for any dimples or tufts of hair.

Male Genitalia

The approach to examining the male genitals will depend on the child's growth and development. In an infant, toddler, or young child the nurse tells the child what will occur and then concurs with the parent or guardian that the nurse should proceed to examine the child's genitalia.

Adolescent boys are normally apprehensive about the genital examination. Concerns arise from modesty, fear of pain, negative judgment, or a previous uncomfortable experience. A matter-of-fact approach and direct communication will facilitate this part of the physical examination. The genital examination is performed during or immediately after the abdominal examination. In the adolescent the physical examination should not conclude with the genital examination so as to allow further opportunity for communication. A good practice is to conclude the physical examination with the musculoskeletal and neurologic examination after the genital examination has been completed.

Gloves should be worn during every genital examination. The examiner begins by inspecting the *penis*. The size of the penis is directly related to age and to growth and development. In infants and young boys the penis is approximately 2 to 3 cm. Genital hair distribution is noted. The adolescent shows a wide variation in normal development of the genitals. Tanner's stages are used for determining the level of development in the adolescent (see Table 8–2).

The skin on the penis normally appears wrinkled, hairless, and without lesions. In the adolescent a prominent dorsal vein may be apparent. Any indurations on the penile shaft should be noted. In the circumcised male the glans looks smooth and without lesions. In an uncircumcised infant the glans may not be visible. By the time the male is age 5 or 6 years the foreskin should be easily retractable behind the corona of the glans. The adolescent is asked to retract the foreskin himself.

The *meatus* is evaluated by compressing the glans between the thumb and forefinger anteroposteriorly. The adolescent may be requested to compress the glans so that the examiner can see the meatus. The meatus in the male has a slit-like or tear-shaped configuration and is located on the ventral surface just millimeters from the tip of the glans. The meatus opening is pink, smooth, and without discharge.

The *scrotum* is inspected for size and configuration, which will change with growth and development. In the infant or young boy the proximal portion of the scrotum is wider and the distal portion narrower. In the adolescent boy the proximal portion is narrower and the distal portion wider. Asymmetry of the scrotum is normal, with the left half slightly lower than the right. The scrotum is movable and, to maintain optimal temperature of the testes, will move closer to or away from the body in response to environmental temperature.

The contents of the scrotum are palpated. The cremasteric reflex in young boys may cause the testes to withdraw into the inguinal canal, making palpation more difficult. If the boy is old enough, have him sit in a cross-legged, or "tailor," position, which will help prevent the cremasteric reflex by stretching the muscle, thereby preventing its contraction. Before beginning the abdominal examination, the examiner warms the hands, blocks the inguinal canal with one hand, and palpates for the scrotal contents (Fig. 33–21). The examiner uses the thumb and first two fingers to palpate each *testis* and *epididymis*. The testes should be smooth, rubbery, and free of nodules. The size of the testes will change with growth and development. Tanner's growth and development stages are used for appropriate interpretation. Because of the high incidence of testicular tumors in young

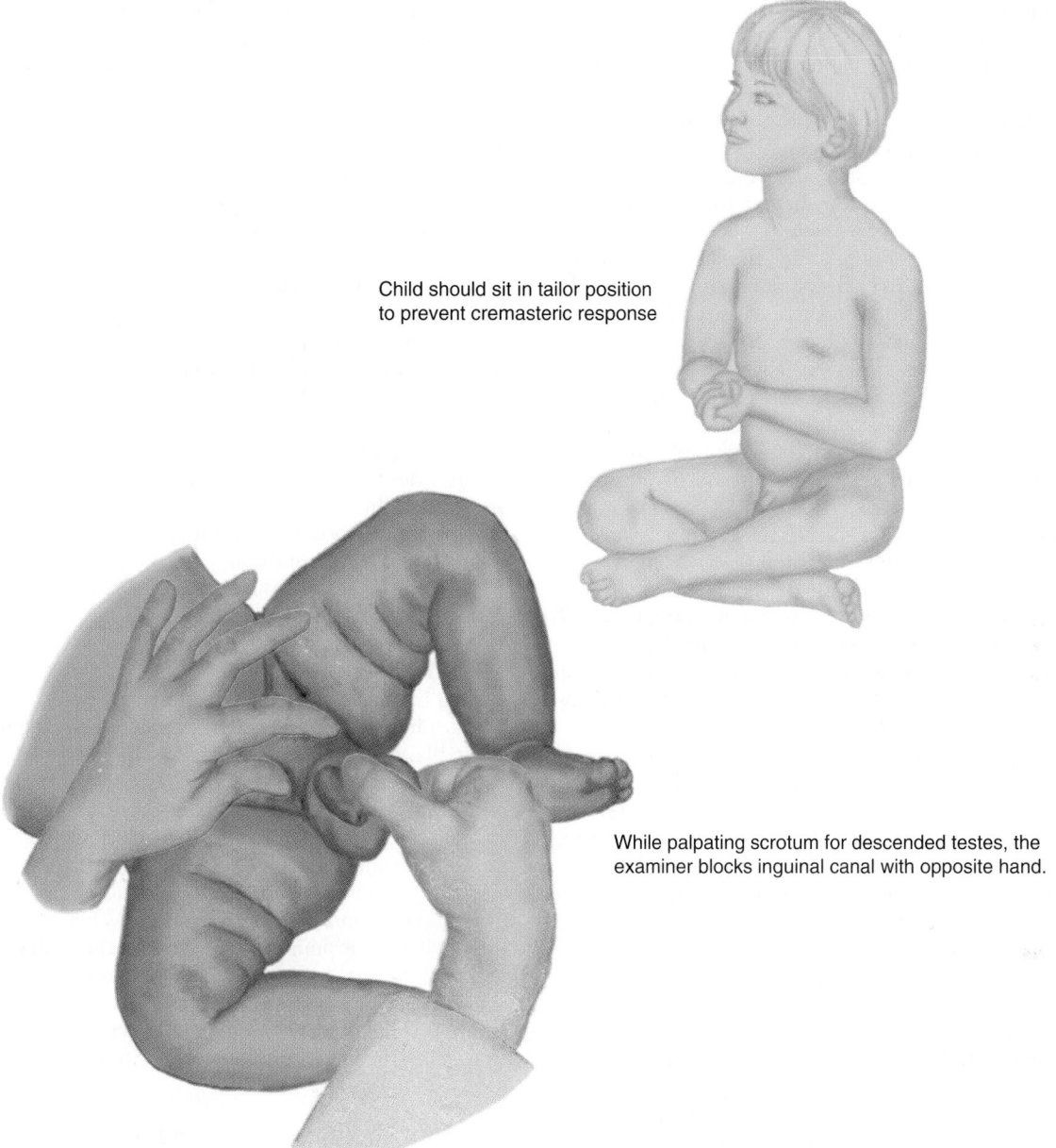

Child should sit in tailor position to prevent cremasteric response

While palpating scrotum for descended testes, the examiner blocks inguinal canal with opposite hand.

FIGURE 33–21
. . . .
When a boy's scrotum is examined, the cremasteric reflex may cause the testes to withdraw into the inguinal canals. To prevent this reflex, the examiner can have the boy sit in a tailor position. The examiner uses one hand to block the inguinal canals and the other to palpate.

men, adolescents should be taught to do testicular self-examination.

Female Genitalia

In general, the anogenital examination in prepubescent girls is limited to visual inspection and gentle palpation of the external area. Internal speculum examinations are not routine in prepubescent children. The appearance of the external genitalia in females varies from child to child and with growth and development. A relaxed, caring attitude will reassure both child and parent.

To safeguard privacy, reinforce modesty, and decrease anxiety, the child is draped appropriately. The examiner should communicate with the child what will be done and concur with the parent or guardian that it is appropriate to examine the genitalia. With the child in different positions, the genitals will differ in tone, relaxation, and appearance. Generally, examination of the genitalia in young girls is performed with the child supine, gently drawing the legs up onto the abdomen to expose the genitalia.

The examiner dons gloves and begins by inspecting the mons pubis and labia majora. The skin should be smooth and clean. The examiner notes the distribution of pubic hair. Tanner's stages are used to determine appropriate growth and development (see Table 8–2).

In the newborn the labia majora and minora may be edematous, with the labia minora often more prominent. In the infant the hymen may protrude and may appear thick and vascular. The clitoris may appear relatively large. The hymen is centrally located and about 0.5 cm in diameter. The examiner determines whether the hymen has an opening.

In the young girl or adolescent, the labia majora may be gaping or closed, shriveled or full, and dry or moist, depending on the age and development of the child. The labia majora are usually symmetric (see Fig. 11–1).

The examiner uses the fingers to gently spread the labia majora and then inspects and palpates the labia minora, the clitoris, the urethral orifice, and the vaginal introitus. The *labia minora* should appear symmetric, dark pink, and moist. On palpation the tissue should be soft and homogeneous with no tenderness.

With the labia majora spread, the examiner can look superiorly and inspect the *clitoris* for size and length. The clitoris will vary with growth and development. Progressing inferiorly, the examiner locates the *urethral meatus*, which may be close to or inside the vaginal introitus. The urethral meatus is usually in the midline. The opening may appear irregular or slit, depending on the characteristics of the hymen. This tissue is usually moist.

The *vaginal introitus* may be a thin vertical slit or a large orifice with irregular edges, depending on the characteristics of the hymen. The hymen may or may not be stretched across the vaginal opening. By menarche the opening should be at least 1 cm wide. The tissue is usually moist. The amount and characteristics of any vaginal discharge will depend on the circulating hormones in the child. A normal vaginal discharge is odorless and may be cloudy or clear, thick or thin.

Normally, *Skene's glands*, located just inferior to the urethral meatus, are not seen or felt and have no discharge. Any discharge from Skene's glands is an indication of an infection. The examiner inspects and palpates *Bartholin's glands*, located in the posterolateral portion of the labia majora. Bartholin's glands should have no swelling or tenderness.

A speculum examination of the internal reproductive organs is not indicated for young girls. The adolescent girl has special needs during the genital examination, which is performed by advanced practitioners.

Musculoskeletal System

The musculoskeletal system is composed of the bones, joints, cartilage, ligaments, and muscles. Joint motions are defined as flexion, extension, abduction, adduction, internal rotation, external rotation, and circumduction. The musculoskeletal examination focuses principally on the upper and lower extremities and the spinal column. Musculoskeletal evaluation begins with observing the child during play or history taking. Observation of the child climbing, jumping, hopping, rising from a sitting position, and manipulating toys and other objects provides evidence of joint function, range of motion, bone stability, and muscle strength. Assessment of fine motor and gross motor ability is accomplished

during the Denver II test for the child less than 5 years old (see Chapter 4 and Appendix J).

General inspection begins with visual scanning of the body using a cephalocaudal (head-to-toe) organization. The child can be examined in shorts or underwear. The examiner compares the two sides of the body for symmetry, contour, size, and involuntary movement. The examiner then inspects the two sides for areas of swelling or edema and for ecchymoses or other discolorations. The structural relationship of the feet to the legs, the hips to the pelvis, the upper extremities, the shoulder girdle, and the upper trunk are evaluated.

Common deformities of the extremities are *varus* and *valgus* deformities. With the reference point of the midline of the body, a varus deformity is a medial adduction or turning inward. A valgus deformity is a medial abduction or turning outward (see Chapter 50).

Injuries to the extremities are common in children and are caused by overexertion and strenuous movements. Sprains are the most common injury, followed by fractures, dislocations, and lacerations.

Deformities of the spine are *scoliosis, kyphosis,* and *lordosis,* which are discussed in Chapter 50.

INFANTS
During infancy, symmetric flexion of the arms and legs is noted. Limbs should be freely movable, with symmetry of the axillary, gluteal, femoral, and popliteal creases. The examiner inspects the hands, noting the shape, number, and position of the fingers and palmar creases. The clavicle should feel smooth, regular, and without crepitus. By age 2 months the infant can lift the head while prone.

The examiner observes range of motion as the infant spontaneously moves the extremities. When the infant is lifted with the examiner's hands under the axillae, the infant with normal muscle strength wedges securely between the hands. The examiner checks the hips for congenital dislocation. The *Ortolani* and *Barlow maneuvers* are performed by a trained examiner on every visit until the infant is 1 year old (see Chapter 22).

TODDLERS, PRESCHOOLERS, AND SCHOOL-AGE CHILDREN
The examiner may want to start with the child's hands and arms by checking for range of motion and the presence of pain while the child is sitting. Children are willing to show their hands, so this is an excellent way to make contact with the child.

The child should stand so that the examiner can observe the posture from behind. The shoulders should be level and the scapulae symmetric. Lordosis is common in young children. Anteriorly, the examiner begins with the feet and observes for adduction and pronation of the foot. Pronation is common between ages 12 and 30 months because of the young child's broad-based stance. Adduction, or toeing in, is demonstrated when the child walks on the lateral side of the foot. Adduction tends to correct itself by age 3, as long as the foot is flexible. *Genu varum* (bowleg) is present when a space of more than 2.5 cm is measured between the knees as the medial malleoli are held together. Genu varum is normal for 1 year after the child has begun to walk. *Genu valgum* means that more than 2.5 cm remains between the medial malleoli when the knees are held together. Genu valgum is present between age 2 and 3½ years (see Fig. 50–3).

The child is instructed to stand on one leg and then the other while the examiner watches from behind. The iliac crest should stay level when the weight is shifted.

ADOLESCENTS

For adolescents, the examiner follows the sequence described for school-age children but with special attention to the spine. Adolescents frequently have kyphosis (Fig. 50–8) due to poor posture. Children ages 9 through 15 should be screened for scoliosis.

RANGE OF MOTION

The examiner notes the child's ability to perform active range-of-motion movements. The equality of movement for each joint and for contralateral joints should be noted. There should be no pain, limitation of movement, spastic movement, joint instability, deformity, or crepitation during movement. Passive range-of-motion movements are performed on joints where limitations are noted. Passive range-of-motion movement is accomplished by the examiner anchoring the joint with one hand while the other hand slowly moves the joint to its limit. Active and passive ranges of motion should be the same.

MUSCLE STRENGTH AND MASS

The examiner assesses the strength of each muscle group. The child is asked to flex the muscle and then resist as opposing force is applied against flexion. Muscle tone should be firm on palpation. When appropriate, the evaluation of muscle strength is integrated with examination of the associated joint for range of motion. The motor segment of cranial nerve V (trigeminal nerve) is evaluated by applying

---

. . . .
Screening Procedure for Scoliosis

To ensure early detection and treatment, children ages 9 through 15 should be screened for scoliosis. At greatest risk are girls from age 10 through adolescence.

The child should be unclothed or wearing underpants only so that the chest, back, and hips can be clearly seen. Have the child stand with her or his weight equally on both feet, legs straight, and arms hanging loosely at the sides. Observe for the following signs of scoliosis:

- Nonpainful lateral curvature of the spine.
- A curve with one turn ("C curve") or two compensating curves ("S curve").
- Lateral deviation and rotation of each vertebra, observed better by looking at the ribs as well as the spinal column itself.
- Unequal shoulder heights.
- Congenital scoliosis visible in the infant lying prone. The condition is sometimes more prominent if the infant is suspended prone.
- Unequal scapular prominences and heights. (Note that the muscle masses may be somewhat unequal, especially if the child uses one shoulder more than the other, as in carrying books. Look for bony, not muscular, prominence.)
- Unequal waist angles.
- Unequal rib prominences and chest asymmetry.
- Unequal rib heights when the child stands in Adam's position (see photograph).

The physical examination should also include

- Observation for equal leg lengths.
- Examination of the skin for hairy patches, nevi, café au lait spots, lipomas, dimples.
- Neurologic examination.
- Cardiac examination for Marfan syndrome.

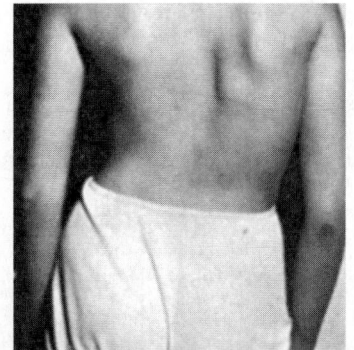

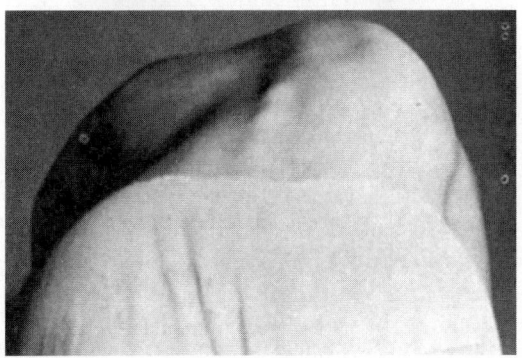

Adam's position with rib hump of structural scoliosis. Lateral curvature of thoracic and lumbar segments of the spine, usually with some rotation of involved vertebral bodies.

Functional scoliosis is flexible; it is apparent with standing and disappears with forward bending. It may be compensatory for other abnormalities such as leg-length discrepancy.

Structural scoliosis is fixed; the curvature is evident both when the individual stands and when the individual bends forward. Note the rib hump with forward flexion. When the child is standing, note unequal shoulder elevation, unequal scapulae, obvious curvature, unequal elbow level, and unequal hip level.

Data from Burns, C. E. (1996). Musculoskeletal disorders. In C. E. Burns, N. Barber, M. A. Brady, & A. M. Dunn (Eds.), *Pediatric primary care: A handbook for nurse practitioners* (p. 778). Philadelphia: Saunders. Photographs from Delp, M. H., & Manning, R. T. (1981). *Major's physical diagnosis: An introduction to the clinical process* (9th ed., p. 450). Philadelphia: Saunders.

opposing force to the temporalis muscle while the child clenches the teeth. Cranial nerve XI (spinal accessory nerve) is tested by assessing the strength of the sternocleidomastoid and trapezius muscles with rotation of the head from side to side and chin to shoulder.

Muscle mass is measured when atrophy or hypertrophy is suspected. Muscles are best measured at their greatest circumference. With the joint used as a landmark, the distance from the joint to a point on the extremity is measured. A comparison with the opposite muscle is made. One measurement is not as significant as a series of measurements to determine changes in size of muscles.

JOINTS

The examiner palpates each joint for temperature, tenderness, swelling, crepitation, or masses. In children, fatigue, stiffness, or weakness, along with heat and redness, are frequently associated with disorders of the joints. Children will usually not move a joint if they are experiencing pain.

GAIT

Assessment of gait and the ability to ambulate is an essential part of both the musculoskeletal and neurologic assessments. The developmental acquisition of the ability to walk follows a prescribed sequence in infants and toddlers (Table 33–3). (See pp. 84–87.)

Gait is assessed in two phases, stance and swing. The stance phase begins when the heel strikes the floor, then the weight is transferred to the ball of the foot and the toes push off the floor. The swing phase consists of acceleration, swingthrough, and deceleration.

Neurologic System

The purpose of the neurologic examination in the child and adolescent is to identify any nervous system malfunction and to ascertain the extent of nervous system development and functioning. In cases of neurologic deficit, the examiner needs to determine the degree, type, and location of nervous system lesions. In the child, the examiner determines the degree to which the nervous system is functioning so that the healthy portion of the nervous system can be used for habilitation or rehabilitation. For the child under age 5, neurologic functioning is best evaluated by using the Denver II test (see Chapter 4 and Appendix I). For the child over age 5, the sequence of the neurologic examination should be adapted to the child's ability to understand and cooperate.

Testing cerebral function, cranial nerves, and cerebellar function gives a picture of nervous system functioning above the spinal cord. The child's age and development will determine the sequence of the neurologic examination. The infant and younger child will not be able to cooperate with neurologic testing. A review of developmental milestones attained will help establish the rate and consistency of development in the infant and younger child. The 3- or 4-year-old will cooperate with testing when it is approached as a game.

TABLE 33–3

Gross Motor Development in the Infant: Progression to Walking

Activity	Age
Raises head and holds position.	2 weeks to 2 months
Moves all extremities, kicking arms and legs when prone.	2 months
Draws up knees and raises abdomen off table. Rocks back and forth while up on hands and knees. Rolls over.	3 to 6 months
Sits alone, using hands for support (tripod fashion).	By 7 months
Lurches forward and pulls legs to chest in "inchworm" fashion, may move backward in same fashion. Creeps and rolls.	By 9th month
Crawls in one-sided manner (moves arm and leg on same side of body, then other side).	6 to 9 months
Crawls in regular fashion, alternating arm and opposite leg.	6 to 9 months
Begins to pull up.	By 11 months
Attempts to walk with support or holding on to something stable.	By 12 months
Momentarily lets go and maintains balance for a few seconds.	Once comfortable standing and holding on
Takes first steps (a broad stance with arms flexed for balance).	Once standing balance accomplished
Sits from a standing posture.	By 12 months
Walks alone.	By 15 months

• • • • • • • • •
Specific Cerebral Function Tests

- **Sound recognition:** Can the child identify familiar sounds with the eyes closed?
- **Auditory/verbal comprehension:** Does the child answer questions and carry out instructions appropriate for age?
- **Recognition of body parts and sidedness:** Does the child recognize the parts of the body? Does the child know right from left?
- **Performance of skilled motor acts:** Can the child drink from a cup, button clothes, use a common tool?
- **Visual object recognition:** Ask the child to identify a familiar toy or object (wristwatch).
- **Visual/verbal comprehension:** Can the child read appropriately and explain the meaning?
- **Motor speech:** Does the child imitate different sounds and phrases?
- **Automatic speech:** Can the child repeat series learned (e.g., nursery rhymes or days of the week)?
- **Volitional speech:** Does the child answer questions relevantly?
- **Writing:** Can the child write his or her name or the name of an object?

CEREBRAL FUNCTION

The evaluation of cognitive function focuses on appearance, behavior, orientation, speech patterns, memory, logic, and affect. The examiner needs to obtain information from the primary caregiver about changes in the child's behavior, personality, appearance, and age-appropriate school performance. Evaluation of cognitive function in the older child and adolescent is based on observation of level of consciousness, awareness, thought processes, and communication.

The level of consciousness in the older child or adolescent is determined by the degree of response to sensory stimuli. The child is described as alert, lethargic, obtunded, stuporous, or comatose.

The older child and adolescent have the ability to understand, think, feel emotions, and appreciate sensory information about the self and surroundings. Awareness is evaluated by observing the older child's or adolescent's level of orientation in relation to person, place, and time. The normally functioning child is oriented to person, place, and time.

Thought processes include abstract thinking, problem solving (simple calculations and concentration), insight, memory (recent and remote), and judgment. The child's school performance may or may not be an accurate indicator of thought processes. Factors that may influence thought processes are attention span, communication, perceptual problems, and emotional withdrawal and depression.

Language ability is evaluated through speech patterns and comprehension. The child is questioned about reading and writing ability. Is the child's speech intelligible? Does the child answer questions appropriately for age and developmental level? The normally functioning child is able to speak fluently, name objects correctly, and write both name and address.

CRANIAL NERVES

Assessment of the cranial nerves (Table 33–4) should be incorporated into the examination of the system each nerve affects. Games, such as making faces or performing tests on a parent or the examiner, will enhance cooperation.

CEREBELLAR FUNCTION

Proprioception, balance, and coordination are tested by having the child perform specific movements. The cerebellum controls balance and coordination. Proprioception evaluates laterality and orientation in space. The techniques used vary with the child's age and development. The child should attempt the technique and show continued improvement with maturation.

MOTOR SYSTEM

Muscle size, muscle tone, involuntary movements, and muscle strength are assessed during the musculoskeletal examination.

Muscles are inspected and palpated while at rest for size, consistency, and possible atrophy. The examiner notes symmetry of posture and of muscle contours and outlines.

Muscle tone is evaluated by palpating the muscles at rest and noting resistance to passive movement. The examiner inspects the muscles for involuntary movements. Muscle strength is tested first without resistance and then against resistance. Corresponding muscles are compared on each side. The examiner then tests the major joints for flexion, extension, and other movements.

SENSORY SYSTEM

Sensory testing depends on the child's perception and interpretation of the stimuli and on the child's age and development. Sensory tests should first be done in an educational practice session before being done in a testing situation. Sensory testing compares both sides of the body, corresponding extremities, and the sensitivity of the distal and proximal parts of each extremity for each form of sensation. Sensory testing is performed to determine if sensory changes involve one entire side of the body, are dermatomal in distribution, or are confined to the peripheral nerves.

REFLEX STATUS

Most brain growth occurs in the first year of life. Primitive reflexes in the newborn are inhibited when more advanced cortical functions and voluntary control take over as the child matures and grows. Commonly elicited reflexes are described and illustrated in Table 33–5.

Motor maturation proceeds in a cephalocaudal direction. The ability to elicit a reflex requires an intact afferent nerve fiber, functional synapses in the spinal cord, intact motor nerve fibers, functional neuromuscular junctions, and competent muscle fibers. The examiner compares the responses on the right and left side, which should be equal. Diminished or hyperreflexic responses are reported for further evaluation.

NEUROLOGIC "SOFT" SIGNS

Neurologic "soft" signs are findings that indicate the child's inability to perform certain activities related to the child's age. They may provide subtle clues to an underlying central nervous system deficit or neurologic maturation delay. Al-

TABLE 33-4
. . . .

Assessing Cranial Nerves

Cranial Nerve	Procedure
Cranial nerves are tested when the system in which they occur is assessed.	
I (olfactory nerve)	The child is asked to identify familiar odors with the eyes closed. Each side of the nose is tested separately.
II (optic nerve)	Visual acuity is tested using the Snellen chart, HOTV chart for young children, or the tumbling E chart for very young children. Each eye is tested separately, and then both eyes together. If corrective lenses are worn, the eyes are tested both with and without correction.
III, IV, and VI (oculomotor, trochlear, abducens nerves)	The child is asked to follow a toy or the examiner's finger as the object moves in all directions of gaze (six cardinal fields of gaze).
V (trigeminal nerve)	The child is asked to identify a wisp of cotton on the face. Corneal reflex is tested by observing for blinking when the examiner approaches the face closely. The masseter and temporal muscles' strength can be evaluated by having the child bite down on a tongue blade as the examiner tries to remove it.
VII (facial nerve)	The child is asked to imitate the examiner's frown, wrinkled forehead, smile, and raised eyebrow. The child tries to keep the eyes closed while the examiner attempts to open them, to test the strength of the eyelid muscles. The sensory portion of the facial nerve can be evaluated by having the child identify the taste of sugar and salt placed on the anterior part of the tongue on each side.
VIII (acoustic nerve)	Cochlear nerve tests are tests for hearing. Audiometric testing is a quantitative evaluation of hearing. The Weber (lateralization) and Rinne (air and bone conduction) tests are qualitative evaluations of hearing.
IX (glossopharyngeal nerve)	The glossopharyngeal and vagus nerves are tested together. With a tongue depressor, the gag reflex is tested by touching the posterior pharyngeal wall. The palatal reflex is tested by stroking each side of the mucous membrane of the uvula. The side touched should rise. Normal function of the vagus nerve is revealed by the child's ability to swallow and to speak clearly.
XI (accessory nerve)	The examiner palpates and notes the strength of the trapezius and sternocleidomastoid muscles against resistance, or the child shrugs the shoulders against resistance.
XII (hypoglossal nerve)	The child is asked to stick out the tongue, and the examiner notes any lateral deviation when it is protruded. The strength of the tongue is assessed by having the child push against the examiner's finger pressed against the cheek with the child's tongue.

Cerebellar Function: Tests of Balance and Coordination

Balance and coordination are tested by having the child perform the following movements:

- **Finger-to-nose test.** Child performs first with one hand, then with the other; first with the eyes open, then with the eyes closed. Ask child first to touch a finger to the child's own nose and then to your finger as you change the position of your finger. Repeat this action with increasing rapidity. The tests are performed with each hand.

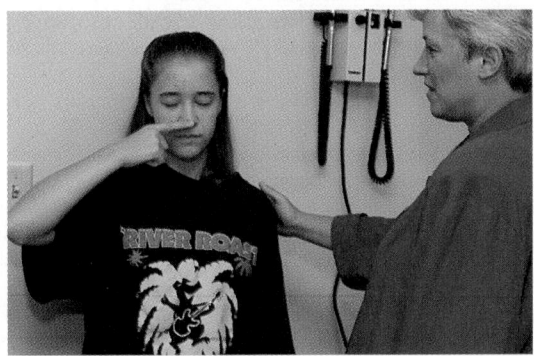

- **Rapid alternating movements.** The child rapidly pats the knee with the palms and backs of the hands by pronating and supinating the hands (demonstrate first). Ask the child to touch the thumb to each of the fingers in rapid succession (demonstrate first).

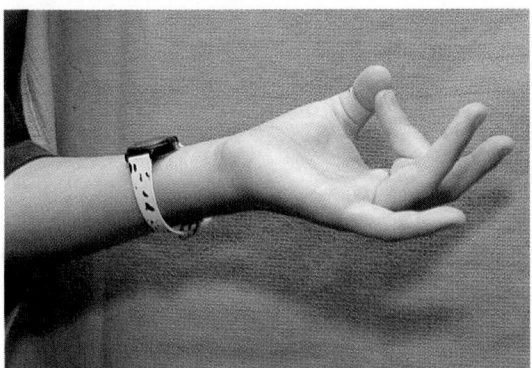

- The child stands erect, first with the eyes open and then with the eyes closed. Stand near the child to prevent injury if the child begins to fall.

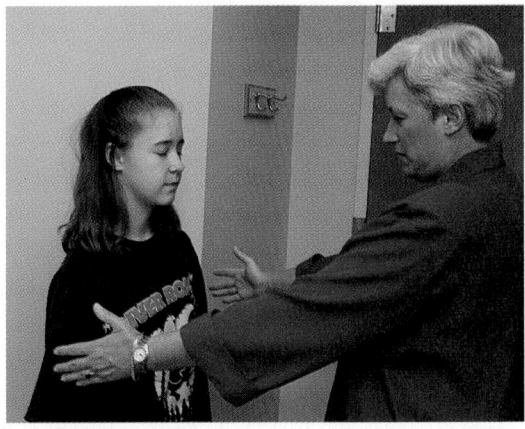

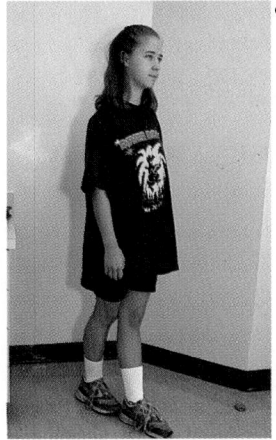

- The child walks in tandem fashion, placing the heel immediately in front of the opposite foot's toe and alternating while walking a straight line.

- Ask the sitting child to run each heel down the opposite shin. With the child lying down, ask the child to point to your hand with each big toe.

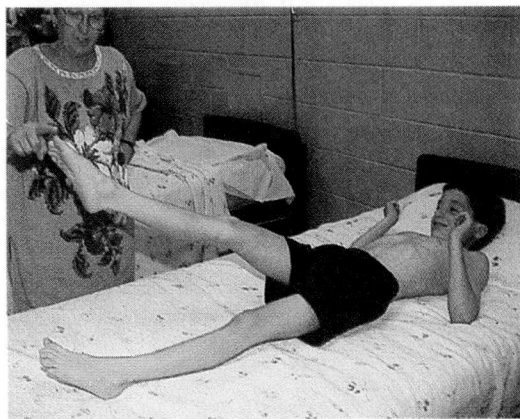

Tests for Evaluating Sensory Function

PRIMARY FORMS OF SENSATION

Check in sequence the hands, forearms, upper arms, trunk, thighs, lower legs, and feet for the following:

- **Superficial tactile sensation:** Touch the child with a wisp of cotton.
- **Superficial pain:** Touch the child with a pin or other sharp object. Be careful not to injure or frighten the child.
- **Sensitivity to temperature:** Touch the various parts of the child's body with test tubes containing warm and cold water. This test is infrequently done with children because of the difficulty of keeping water warm or cold enough for the child to distinguish the difference.
- **Sensitivity to vibration:** Hold a vibrating tuning fork to the bony prominences, noting the child's ability to perceive the vibration and tell you when the vibration stops.
- **Deep pressure pain:** Press the tip of your fingernail against the child's fingernail. The child will feel discomfort. You may also squeeze the Achilles tendons, calf, and forearm muscles, noting sensitivity.
- **Motion and position:** Hold the sides of the toes, thumbs, and fingers by grasping them between your index finger and thumb. Move the fingers and toes passively and ask the child to tell you the final position of the digit.

CORTICAL AND DISCRIMINATORY FORMS OF SENSATION

These forms of sensation are complex somatic sensory impressions that require interpretation by the cerebral cortex. The following sensations can be evaluated, depending on the age and development of the child being tested.

- **Two-point discrimination:** Can the child differentiate between one and two points? With the child's eyes closed, various parts of the body are touched simultaneously with two sharp objects. Alternate touching the child with one point or two points. Different areas of the body differ in the distance by which the child can differentiate one from two points. This test is more appropriate for older children.
- **Point localization:** With the eyes closed, can the child locate the spot where the child was touched?
- **Texture discrimination:** Can the child recognize, with the hands, the difference in the feel of materials such as cotton, wool, and silk?
- **Stereognostic function:** Can the child identify familiar objects placed in each hand? Place several objects in a paper bag and have the child identify them with each hand and show you the object.
- **Graphesthesia:** Can the child identify letters or numbers traced on the palm or back of the hand with a blunt point? Numbers are easier than letters for a young child to recognize.
- **Extinction phenomenon:** With the eyes closed, can the child identify touch on both sides? Touch opposite sides of the body in identical areas simultaneously. This test is used for older children only.

TABLE 33–5

Evaluating Common Reflexes

Deep Tendon Reflexes	*Deep tendon reflexes* are elicited by tapping briskly on a tendon or a bony prominence, evoking a sudden stretching of certain muscles and their resulting contraction. For an adequate response, the limb should be relaxed and the muscle partially stretched. The reflex is stimulated by directing a sharp blow of the reflex hammer onto the muscle's insertion tendon.
Biceps Reflex	The child's arm should be flexed up to 45 degrees at the elbow. The biceps tendon in the antecubital fossa is palpated. The thumb is then placed on the biceps tendon, and a blow is struck on the thumb. The response will be a visible or palpable flexion of the forearm.

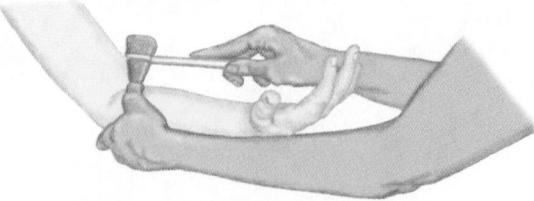

TABLE 33–5

Evaluating Common Reflexes Continued

Triceps Reflex	The arm is suspended by holding the upper arm and instructing the child to just let the arm "go limp." Alternatively, the forearm can be supported on the examiner's arm. The triceps tendon is struck directly just above the elbow. The response will be extension of the forearm.

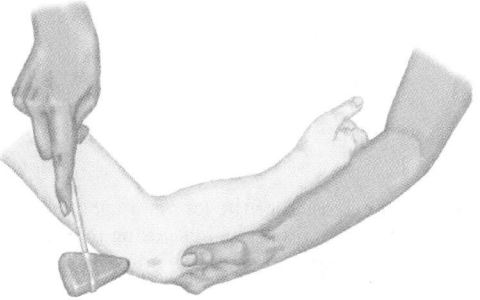

Brachioradialis Reflex	The child's arm is supported on the examiner's arm, and the elbow flexed up to 45 degrees. The brachoradial tendon is struck with the reflex hammer 1–2 inches above the radial styloid process. The response will be pronation and flexion of the elbow.

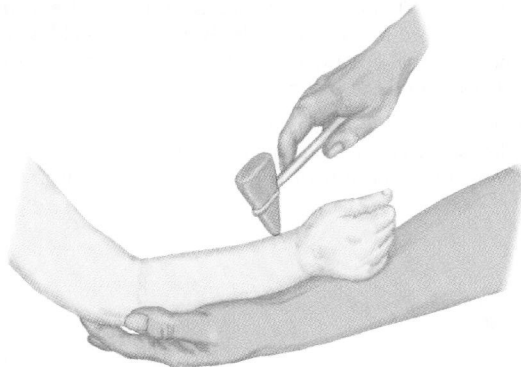

Patellar Reflex	The lower leg is allowed to dangle freely by flexing the child's knee up to 90 degrees. The examiner supports the upper leg with the hand and strikes the patellar tendon just below the patella. The response will be extension of the lower leg.

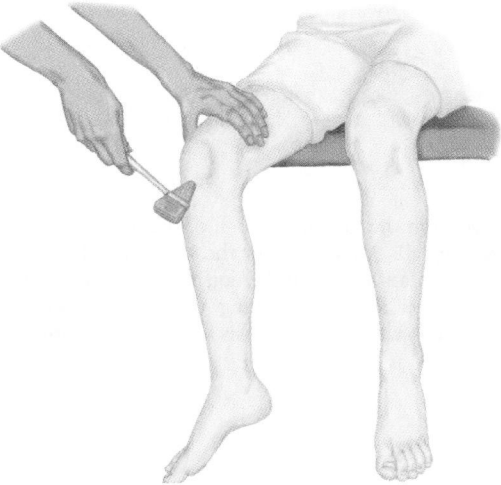

Table continued on following page

TABLE 33–5
• • • • • • • • • • •

Evaluating Common Reflexes Continued

Achilles Reflex

The hip is externally rotated, and the foot is held in dorsiflexion. The Achilles tendon is struck directly. The response will be plantar flexion of the foot. An alternative way to elicit this reflex is to have the child kneel on a chair with the toes pointing toward the floor; the examiner then strikes the Achilles tendon directly.

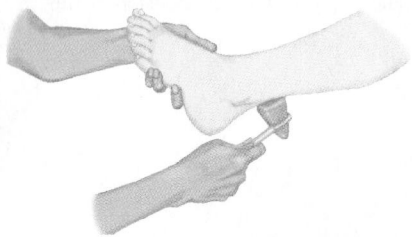

Clonus Reflex

Eliciting a *clonus*, a continued, rapid flexion and extension of the foot and hand, is attempted in children. Clonus is elicited by suddenly and briskly dorsiflexing the foot or hand and applying sustained and moderate pressure. No rhythmic oscillating movements should be palpated.

Superficial Reflexes

Superficial reflexes are tested by stroking the skin with an object that is moderately sharp but not sharp enough to break the skin. The receptors are in the skin rather than the muscles.

Upper and Lower Abdominal Reflexes and Cremasteric Reflex

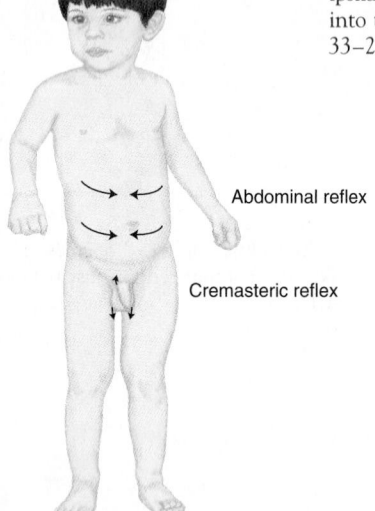

Abdominal reflex

Cremasteric reflex

Upper and lower abdominal reflexes: While the child is in a supine position and with the abdomen exposed and knees slightly bent, the skin of the abdomen is stroked. Movement of stroking is from the side of the abdomen toward the midline at both the upper and lower abdominal levels. The response will be ipsilateral contraction of the abdominal muscle with an observable movement of the umbilicus toward the side being stroked.

Cremasteric reflex: In the male, light stroking of the inner aspect of the thigh causes the ipsilateral testicle to elevate. This reflex may cause a young male to withdraw the testicles into the inguinal canal when the abdomen is touched with very cold hands. (See Fig. 33–21 to prevent this reflex.)

Plantar Reflex (Babinski Reflex)

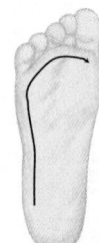

The lateral aspect of the sole of the foot, from the heel to the ball of the foot, is stroked in a movement curving medially across the ball. A fingernail or the wooden end of an applicator stick may be used. The response in an infant will be dorsiflexion, fanning of the toes, and hyperextension of the great toe. Once a child is walking, the response will be plantar flexion of the toes. Some children will withdraw from this stimulus by flexing the hip and the knee.

Gluteal Reflex

When the buttocks are separated, the skin tenses at the gluteal area.

Examples of Neurologic "Soft" Signs

Short attention span
Poor motor coordination
Clumsiness
Frequent falling
Hyperkinesis, voluntary or involuntary
Uneven perceptual development
Incomplete laterality, with no side clearly dominant
Language disturbances: articulation disorders, dyslexia
Motor outflow (movements involving more muscles than intended)
Mirroring movements of the extremities (for example, both hands in motion when only one is performing a function)

though these findings may fall in a gray area, they should be recorded and reported when observed. Children with multiple soft signs are often found to have learning problems (Seidel, 1995).

Conclusion and Documentation

When the physical examination has been completed, the examiner should ask the parents and child, if age appropriate, whether they have any questions concerning the examination. Findings are documented in a complete and concise manner. Deviations from normal and risk factors should be identified and documented. Depending on the setting, referrals may be made.

KEY CONCEPTS

- A systemic approach to the physical examination is to begin at the head and proceed through the entire body to the toes. The physical examination is tailored to the child's age and developmental level.
- The order of the examination should be flexible, and intrusive and frightening procedures should be done at the end of the examination. The examiner should develop creative approaches to complete the physical examination for children of different ages.
- An accurate history is the single most important component of the physical examination. The history and physical examination provide both subjective and objective data for identifying health and illness.
- Vital signs should be assessed on every visit in ambulatory settings and monitored on a routine basis in the hospitalized child.
- Assessment of vital signs is an important way to measure and monitor vital body functions.
- Examination findings are recorded completely and concisely. Deviations from normal and risk factors should be identified, recorded, and, when appropriate, reported for further evaluation.
- Anthropometrics measure the human body and assess nutritional status as well as growth and development. These measures are of

most value when they are evaluated serially so that trends can be evaluated.
- The skin is observed for color and palpated to determine moisture, temperature, turgor, edema, and lesions.
- The general appearance of the child is observed for signs of abuse, both physical and psychological.
- Examination of the lymph nodes is incorporated into the examination when that part of the anatomy is being assessed.
- The head is inspected for symmetry, movement, control, and shape.
- The fontanels are inspected and palpated for size, tenseness, and pulsation.
- The eyelids, eyebrows, palpebral fissures, nasolabial folds, mouth, and nose are inspected for spacing and symmetry.
- The nasal mucosa is inspected for color and moisture.
- Assessment of the mouth in a young child should be performed at the end of the examination because it may cause anxiety.
- The chart chosen to evaluate visual acuity is determined according to the age and development of the child.
- Assessment of the thorax and lungs entails inspection, palpation, percussion, and auscultation.

- Auscultation of the heart is done by listening with both the bell and the diaphragm of the stethoscope with the child lying down, in the left lateral recumbent position, and sitting up.
- An empty bladder, a warm room, and the child supine with a pillow under the head and the knees flexed will enhance abdominal relaxation.
- Examination of the genitalia may evoke concerns regarding modesty, fear of pain, negative judgment, or a previous uncomfortable experience. A matter-of-fact approach and direct communication will help create a positive experience.
- The musculoskeletal examination is predominantly directed toward the upper and lower extremities and the spinal column.
- The neurologic examination is done to identify any nervous system malfunction and to evaluate current nervous system development and functioning.
- When the physical examination has been completed, the examiner should ask the child and the parents if they have any questions concerning the examination.

ANSWERS TO CRITICAL THINKING EXERCISE 33-1

1. The nurse could assume that Ms. Maloney does not provide adequate care for her child. She might also assume that all teenage mothers lack the skills to be good parents. She might also assume that Kerrie has been neglected in other ways. In fact, however, Ms. Maloney may really be trying to meet all of Kerrie's needs but may not know what those needs are or how to meet them.

2. The nurse should display empathy and avoid displays of disapproval, perhaps by stating, "Children take a great deal of time and energy. You must be very busy trying to balance caring for Kerrie and working. Let's take some time today to look at how we can help you."

3. The nurse can take a thorough history and determine Kerrie's health status from conception to the present. A head-to-toe assessment will provide baseline data. Assuming that no abnormalities are present, the nurse will want to focus on anticipatory guidance related to nutrition, immunizations, safety, and any age-related growth and development issues. While doing the assessment, the nurse role models activities that increase Kerrie's language, motor, sensory, and psychological skills. The nurse cannot provide care for Kerrie without meeting the needs of her mother. Support systems should be evaluated and, if weak, should be addressed. If Ms. Maloney understands she needs to bring Kerrie to the clinic for preventive care, she is more likely to give clinic visits a higher priority. Teaching is therefore critical. Because of the history of this case, the nurse should assist Ms. Maloney in making the next appointment while in the clinic and should follow up with a call prior to the visit.

REFERENCES AND READINGS

Albert, D. M., & Jakobiec, F. A. (1994). *Principles and practice of ophthalmology.* Philadelphia: Saunders.

Allwood, J. S. (1995). The primary care management of burns. *Nurse Practitioner Journal, 20*(8), 74–87.

Barkauskas, V. H., Stoltenberg-Allen, K., Baumann, L. C., & Darling-Fisher, C. (1998). *Health and physical assessment* (2nd ed.). St. Louis: Mosby–Year Book.

Bates, B. (1995). *A guide to physical examination* (6th ed.). Philadelphia: Lippincott.

Berkowitz, C. (1996). *Pediatrics: A primary care approach.* Philadelphia: Saunders.

Boisvert, J. T., Reidy, S. J., & Lulu, J. (1995). Overview of pediatric arrhythmias. *Nursing Clinics of North America, 30*(2), 365–379.

Burg, F. D., Ingelfinger, J., Wald, E., & Polin, R. (1999). *Gellis & Kagan's current pediatric therapy.* Philadelphia: Saunders.

Chadwick, D. L., et al. (1989). *Color atlas of child sexual abuse.* Chicago: Year Book.

Coupey, S. (1997). Interviewing adolescents. *Pediatric Clinics of North America, 14*(6),1349–1364.

Dinulos, J., & Graham, E. A. (1998). Influence of culture and pigment on skin conditions in children. *Pediatrics in Review, 19*(8), 268–275.

Fuller, J., & Schaller-Ayers, J. (1994). *Health assessment: A nursing approach* (2nd ed.). Philadelphia: Lippincott.

Gladstein, J., Holden, E. W., Peralta, L., & Raven, M. (1993). Diagnoses and symptom patterns in children presenting to a pediatric headache clinic. *Headache, 33*(9), 497–500.

Goldbloom, R. (1997). *Pediatric clinical skills* (2nd ed.). New York: Churchill Livingstone.

Graham, M. V., & Uphold, C. (1994). *Clinical guidelines in child health.* Gainesville, FL: Barmarrae Books.

Green, M. (1998). *Pediatric diagnosis.* Philadelphia: Saunders.

Greif, J., & Hewitt, W. (1998). The living canvas. Health issues in tattooing, body piercing, and branding. *Advances for Nurse Practitioners, 6*(6), 26–31, 82.

Hayman, L. L., & Ryan, E. A. (1994). The cardiovascular health profile: Implications for health promotion and disease prevention. *Pediatric Nursing, 20*(5), 509–515.

Heffwernam, A. E., & O'Sullivan, A. (1998). Pediatric sun exposure. *Nurse Practitioner, 23*(7), 67–78.

Hurwitz, S. (1993). *Clinical pediatric dermatology* (2nd ed.). Philadelphia: Saunders.

Jarvis, C. (1996). *Physical examination and health assessment.* Philadelphia: Saunders.

Kaleida, P. H., & Stool, S. E. (1992). Assessment of otoscopists' accuracy regarding middle-ear effusion: Otoscopic validation. *American Journal of Diseases of Children, 146*(4), 433–435.

Kuczmarski, R. (1998). Revised growth charts due in late '98. *AAP News, 14*(9).

Meinking, T., & Taplin, D. (1995). Infestations. In L. Schachner & R. Hansen (Eds.), *Pediatric dermatology* (2nd ed.). Philadelphia: Saunders.

Miola, E. S. (1994). The otoscope: An update on assessment skills. *Journal of Pediatric Nursing, 9*(4), 283–286.

Nagengast, S. L., Baun, M. M., Megel, M., & Leibowitz, J. M. (1997). The effects of the presence of a companion animal on the physiological arousal and behavioral distress in children during a physical examination. *Journal of Pediatric Nursing, 12*(6), 323–330.

Nelson, L. B., et al. (1998). *Harley's pediatric ophthalmology* (4th ed.). Philadelphia: Saunders.

Schreiner, B., & Brondum, L. A. (1994). Nutrition in pediatric primary care: Assessment and common problems. *Nursing Practice Forum, 5*(1), 13–23.

Seidel, H. B. (1995). *Mosby's guide to physical examination* (3rd ed.). St. Louis: Mosby–Year Book.

Simon, C., & Janner, M. (1990). *Color atlas of pediatric diseases* (2nd ed.). Philadelphia: Decker.

Smith, D. M., Kovan, J., Rich, B., & Tanner, S. (1997). *Preparticipation physical evaluation* (2nd ed.). Minneapolis: McGraw-Hill Healthcare.

Smith, K. M. (1997). The innocent heart murmur in children. *Journal of Pediatric Health Care, 11*(5), 207–214.

Stone, R. (1996). Primary care diagnosis of acute abdominal pain. *Nurse Practitioner, 21*(22), 19–39.

Thomas, D. (1996). Assessing children: It's different. *RN, 59*(4), 38–45.

van der Net, J., van der Hoeven, H., Esseveld, F., de Wilde, E. J., Kuis, W., & Helders, P. J. (1995). Musculoskeletal disorders in juvenile onset mixed connective tissue disease. *Journal of Rheumatology, 22*(4), 751–757.

Weston, W. L., & Lane, A. T. (1991). *Color textbook of pediatric dermatology.* St. Louis: Mosby–Year Book.

Young, K. T., Davis, K., Schoen, C., & Parker, S. (1998). Listening to parents: A national survey of parents with young children. *Archives of Pediatric and Adolescent Medicine, 152,* 255–262.

34

◆ ◆ ◆ ◆ ◆ ◆ ◆ ◆ ◆ ◆ ◆ ◆ ◆ ◆

Emergency Care of the Child

LEARNING OBJECTIVES

After studying this chapter, you should be able to:

- Describe general principles that encourage cooperation and help to make examination and treatment of children in emergency settings more comfortable for the child and family.
- List the developmental issues that are significant in caring for infants, toddlers, preschool and school-age children, and adolescents.
- Compare the airway anatomy of a child with that of an adult and explain the significance of the differences in managing the pediatric airway.
- Assess the early signs of shock in infants and children, recognizing that changes in heart rate and skin signs are more accurate signs of early shock than decreased blood pressure.
- Define triage and list the most important factors to assess when obtaining an overall impression of an infant's or child's general condition.
- Describe the general guidelines for cardiopulmonary resuscitation in infants and children and discuss what additional precautions and procedures are required for infants and children with traumatic injuries.
- List indications that suggest a child brought into the emergency care setting has been neglected or abused and discuss the nurse's responsibility for reporting possible neglect or abuse.
- Identify several possible roles for nurses in prevention of submersion injuries, traumatic injuries, and poison ingestions.

DEFINITIONS

ABCDEs Airway, Breathing, Circulation, Disability, and Exposure. When assessing children, the nurse should remember each of these areas.

airway management Correct positioning of airway, appropriate interventions used to ensure patency of the airway, and adequate oxygenation and ventilation.

cardiopulmonary resuscitation (CPR) Protocol performed when a patient's respiratory and cardiovascular systems require support, as in the pulseless, nonbreathing patient. Airway management, ventilation, and chest compressions are provided to improve tissue perfusion until the patient can receive definitive care.

dental emergency Injury or infection of a tooth or teeth occurring when the period of time to definitive care is critical for the survival of the tooth or to alleviate pain.

emergency A psychological, medical, or traumatic condition that requires immediate care or care within an hour to prevent further deterioration.

envenomation Injection of venom by an animal (usually snakes, lizards, spiders, scorpions, and the like) into a human body.

extracorporeal membrane oxygenation (ECMO) Mechanical circulatory and pulmonary support for infants and children in severe end-stage cardiogenic shock.

hypothermia Cooling of body temperature to subnormal levels. Temperature levels considered to be dangerous to infants and children are core body temperatures below 35.6°C (96°F).

ingestion Swallowing of a potentially toxic substance, such as a large amount of medication, petroleum products, or toxic plants.

shock Inadequate tissue perfusion, usually caused by illness or injury, that causes respiratory or cardiovascular compromise.

submersion injury Injury resulting from a near-drowning incident. Such an injury may be immediately apparent or may appear up to 48 hours after the submersion incident.

trauma Injury from an external cause, such as a motor vehicle accident, gunshot wound, or stabbing. Trauma may be self-inflicted, may be deliberately inflicted or accidental, and may be physical or psychological.

trauma score A numeric score assessed by health care providers to determine the condition of patients. The score usually results from adding, subtracting, dividing, or multiplying numbers representing physiologic parameters or specific types of injuries. These scores are used for field triage and are assessed serially to determine whether a patient's condition is improving or deteriorating. They are also correlated with survivability.

triage A sorting process used to decide the urgency of a patient's illness or injury and allocate appropriate resources effectively. The purpose of triage is to ensure that the most seriously ill or injured patients receive the appropriate level of care, before patients with less urgent or emergent conditions.

◼ General Guidelines for Emergency Nursing Care

Many factors affect the psychological impact of an emergency on both the child and family. In addition to the expected fears children have at various developmental stages (e.g., separation, pain, and altered body image), an overriding concern expressed by both children and parents in emergency settings is fear of the unknown. The suddenness with which the child and family come in contact with emergency personnel, the necessity for rapid assessment and intervention, and the relative seriousness of the child's condition can intensify a fearful response and overwhelm normal coping mechanisms. In addition, children and families are unfamiliar with the setting, the staff of the health care facility, the equipment, and the procedures. Emergency nurses can use some simple interventions to make examination and treatment of children in the emergency setting more comfortable for the child and for the family and to decrease the adverse psychological effects of the experience.

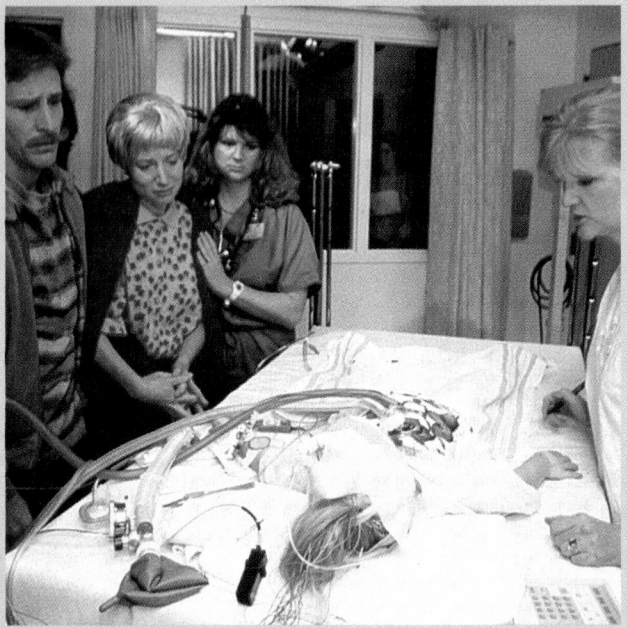

Encouraging parents to remain with their child in the emergency setting can bolster the family's coping. (Courtesy of Cook Children's Medical Center, Fort Worth, Texas.)

Communicate an attitude of calm confidence. This attitude can be difficult to maintain when the situation is critical, but families in crisis look to nurses for reassurance and expect to see competent, professional behavior. Speak quietly and calmly to the child and parents, and remain firmly in charge. Remember to talk to the family often throughout the visit—silence is a form of communication that is easily misinterpreted. Keep the parents informed of any untoward delays. Acknowledge the child's and family's fears (Newberry, 1998).

Establish a trusting relationship with the child and family. Make eye contact with the child and family when you speak to them. To establish a trusting relationship, check back with the family and provide periodic updates if the child and family are separated. When parents are confident that they are being kept informed, they are less likely to make demands for additional attention and information. When speaking to the child and family, use simple, nonmedical terms and remember that children (and sometimes adults) can have inaccurate ideas of how their bodies function and the location of body parts (Kitt et al., 1995). Providing comfort measures to the family members also builds a trusting relationship. Protect their privacy, direct them to a public telephone or cafeteria, and provide space where they can talk quietly.

Try to avoid separating the child and parents. As much as possible, include the parents as partners in their child's treatment. Unless the child does not want a parent in the room (as with some adolescents), a parent can help to calm the child, and many examina-

tions and procedures can be performed with the child on a parent's lap. For parents who do not know exactly how to be of assistance in these situations, it can be helpful to explain how a parent might help, such as "I think he might stay calmer if you hold his hand and tell him a story while I clean this burn" or "Try counting to ten with her while I start this intravenous line." Although having the family remain with the child can be calming and supportive, respect the family's right to leave if the child's condition or the painful nature of a procedure provoke more anxiety than the family member is able to handle.

Whenever possible, designate one staff member as the child's caretaker and liaison to the parents. In the unfamiliar emergency setting the child and family find that having one contact person is less confusing. Consistency is helpful in a crisis because the child and family may feel overwhelmed in the busy and sometimes confusing emergency department environment.

Tell the truth. To establish a trusting relationship, be as honest as possible. If a procedure will be painful, tell the child (usually briefly beforehand). Only then can the child believe health care providers when they say that a procedure will *not* be painful. Keeping a child informed of what will occur by describing sensations ("This will feel cold and wet as I clean your arm") is more helpful than describing the actual procedure.

Provide incentives and rewards. Provide positive feedback when either the child or the parents are being helpful. Children from 3 to 12 years of age especially appreciate concrete rewards for good behavior, such as stickers, fancy bandages, or inexpensive toys (Henderson & Brownstein, 1994). Adults also appreciate being thanked for their patience and for their assistance in the care of their child. All of these techniques help to create as positive an experience as possible.

Assess the child's unspoken thoughts and feelings. Try to determine what the child is thinking or feeling, but not verbalizing. Encourage the child to express thoughts and feelings, because sometimes the child might be misinterpreting a situation, or because the child might need to express emotions (Zink, 1996). Always call the child by name to personalize care and provide individualized support. Treat the child and family kindly and gently.

In some cases, however, the child's and family's coping mechanisms break down, causing inappropriate behavior. If violence or abusive behavior is an issue, you might need to obtain assistance from law enforcement or hospital security officers. For an emotional crisis that does not involve abusive or aggressive behavior, some simple rules apply:

- Encourage the person in crisis to move to a quiet place. Observers and stimuli from other sources tend to aggravate a crisis.
- Encourage the child or parent to talk about feelings rather than the "facts" of the situation. Use reflective statements.
- Avoid defensiveness, explanation, or justification of your own or others' behavior.
- Speak in simple sentences. Use sentences of no more than five words, with words no longer than five letters (e.g., "Let's sit down over here," "Let me help," "Please let go of that.").

Pediatric Emergency Equipment

Airways (oral and nasopharyngeal): infant to adult size
Endotracheal tubes: cuffed sizes 6.5–8
    uncuffed sizes 2.5–7
Laryngoscope with blades: sizes 0–3 straight
    sizes 2–3 curved
Magill forceps
Oxygen equipment: sizes infant to adult masks and cannulas
Bag-valve-mask: infant to adult size
Chest tubes: sizes 10–38 French
Pediatric peripheral intravenous equipment and solutions, including over-the-needle catheters, 14–24 gauge
Intraosseous device: 15–18 gauge
Nasogastric tubes: sizes 5–18
Urinary catheters: sizes 5–18
Suction catheters: sizes 8–14 French
Pediatric tracheostomy tubes
Medication dosage length-based chart or tape
Defibrillator with pediatric paddles

When interacting with families in distress, a good general rule is to try to listen rather than talk. Simply being present for children and families and empathizing with them are useful interventions. Help families identify specific problems and assist them to explore reasonable solutions.

When coping mechanisms break down entirely, however, some direction is necessary. Consulting social services, spiritual counselors (i.e., chaplain), or crisis intervention professionals can be helpful. Early intervention and support for appropriate coping mechanisms are far easier and less time consuming than intervening after a child's or parent's emotional decompensation.

Pediatric Emergency Medications

Medication	Use
Activated charcoal	Reduces drug absorption in toxic ingestions
Adenosine	Treatment for supraventricular tachycardia
Atropine sulfate	Treats symptomatic bradycardia
Bretylium	Treats ventricular tachycardia; ventricular fibrillation prophylaxis
Calcium chloride	Treatment of hypocalcemia, hypomagnesemia, hyperkalemia, and calcium channel blocker overdose
Dopamine	Treats hypotension or poor peripheral perfusion in the child
Dobutamine hydrochloride	Treats hypoperfusion, severe congestive heart failure, or cardiovascular shock
Epinephrine	For bradycardia or asystolic arrest
Lidocaine	Treats recurrent ventricular tachycardia, ventricular fibrillation, or ventricular ectopy
Naloxone	Reverses the effects of some narcotics
Sodium bicarbonate	Treats severe acidosis associated with cardiac arrest, unstable hemodynamic status, or hyperkalemia

Very few experiences are as frightening to a family as a child's sudden illness or injury. Caring for children and families in the emergency setting, therefore, presents special challenges to the health care team. Nurses play an important role in emergency settings because they are most often responsible for the initial contact, triage, and continuing care throughout an emergency visit. The goals of emergency nursing care include not only addressing the physical problems of the child but supporting the child's and family's coping mechanisms and creating an atmosphere where the family is valued and kept as intact as possible.

Growth and Development Issues in Emergency Care

Emergency nursing care of children needs to address both the physiologic and psychological differences in children in terms of age and development. Paying close attention to developmental issues assists in obtaining a more accurate assessment and can affect the course of care (see Chapters 4 to 8 for approaches to children of different ages). The nurse treats each child as an individual. Although children of the same age group are similar, one toddler might be much more mature than another, and one adolescent might lean more toward school-age behaviors than another.

The Infant

An infant experiences the world through the senses; hunger, satiation, cold, warmth, quiet, and noise affect the infant's comfort or discomfort. An infant has not learned patience and has little tolerance for physical or emotional discomfort, including pain (see Chapter 39 for management of pain in infants and children).

Although infants are able to discriminate their parents from others, older infants (9 to 18 months of age) can exhibit signs of both separation and stranger anxiety. The nurse should allow the parent to hold the infant as much as possible for examination and treatment. This might not be possible in a critical situation, but nurses need to remember to reunite parent and child whenever feasible.

The Toddler

Toddlers are just beginning to explore the world and seem to have limitless energy and curiosity. They are also beginning to have a clearer image of themselves as autonomous and distinct human beings. For this reason, they do not respond well to restrictions and tend to push any limits imposed. This tendency can be a problem in the emergency setting because some nursing care might involve securing and restraining the toddler, which makes the toddler feel vulnerable. The nurse should be sure to remove any restriction or restraint as soon as safety permits. Toddlers have little understanding of time, so procedures should be introduced just before they are initiated.

The Preschooler

The preschool child is talking and beginning to be more independent. This outward appearance of organization is somewhat misleading, however, because the preschool period is also the stage of fear and fantasy. Preschool children have nightmares and can have exaggerated ideas and impressions. They are also confused about the concept of responsibility and tend to blame themselves for illnesses and injuries.

The preschool child might be more willing than the toddler to be separated from parents, but the nurse should keep this separation as brief as possible. The nurse can include the parents in treatments and provide them with instruction on calming the child, if they seem unsure. The nurse should never ask a parent to restrain the child because this role may be confusing to the child and difficult for the parent.

The School-Age Child

School-age children are interested in learning and gradually acquire reasoning skills, including some abstract thinking. They are able to understand the cause of illness and injury and are much less likely to fantasize and exaggerate. School-age children have extensive vocabularies and they can understand simple explanations of procedures. They are also able to make decisions about their own care. By this time, they have also developed personal techniques to help them through painful times. The nurse helps them use coping techniques that work for them.

The Adolescent

Although adolescents are at varying stages of puberty, they begin to resemble adults in appearance. They are also beginning to explore the adult world and develop their own unique identities. The nurse needs to remember, however, that even though adolescents might appear physically mature, they might not be emotionally mature and continue to require support. Coping with extraordinary changes in their physical appearance, they are often concerned with whether they are "normal" and whether others have similar thoughts and feelings.

Although this is an age of risk taking, which can make them prone to very serious injury, adolescents can be quite fearful of death. Although they are aware of the possibility of their own death, they avoid thinking about its reality. Adolescents consider themselves invincible, and many experience overwhelmingly emotional feelings when a friend dies unexpectedly.

Adolescence is an age of extremes: teenagers might either exaggerate or underplay the seriousness of a condition. Sometimes it is difficult for the nurse to assess the full extent of an adolescent's illness or injury. Expert care of the adolescent requires sensitivity to both verbal and nonverbal cues.

. . . .
Working with Children in Emergencies: Developmental Guidelines

INFANTS

- Allow the use of a pacifier.
- Use a quiet, soothing voice.
- Touch, rock, or cuddle the infant. Holding the infant securely or swaddling a young infant can also be comforting.
- Keep the infant warm; if the infant must be left undressed, use warming lights to ensure a comfortable temperature.
- As much as possible, allay parents' fears so they will not be communicated to the infant.
- Remember that infants experience pain (see Chapter 39 for pain interventions).

TODDLERS

- Give treatments and perform procedures with the toddler sitting up on the stretcher or examining table or on the parent's lap.
- Perform the most distressing/intrusive parts of the examination last.
- Reassure the family as much as possible—the child will benefit from their confidence.
- Allow the child to have familiar objects (transitional objects) such as a blanket, doll, or toy to help him or her feel safe (Henderson & Brownstein, 1994).
- Keep frightening objects out of the child's line of vision. Also try to keep machines that make loud noises away.

PRESCHOOLERS

- Explain a procedure or treatment a few seconds rather than minutes beforehand because allowing the child time to think about it may result in frightening fantasies or exaggerations.
- Talk to preschool children throughout procedures, describing the sensations they are feeling or will feel and telling them how they can help.
- Distract the child with noises or bright objects. Counting with some preschool children might help to calm them during procedures.
- Avoid criticizing the preschool child for crying, struggling, or fighting during a procedure. Reassuring a child that the child did try the best will help to build a positive self-image.
- Encourage the preschool child to talk about how the illness or injury occurred. If the child is inappropriately taking responsibility for the illness or injury, try to reassure that the child is not to blame for the situation.

- Remember that preschool children can seem to understand more than they actually do. Health care providers often overestimate understanding in a child of this age, so be sure to explain things in words the child understands.
- Use positive terms such as "make better" and "help," and avoid more frightening terms like "shot" and "cut."
- Use adhesive bandages over small wounds and injection sites. Preschool children might imagine their blood leaking out through puncture wounds.

SCHOOL-AGE CHILDREN

- Offer simple choices whenever possible to help the child feel more in control. The school-age child is capable of deciding in which arm to have an injection or in which hand to hold a nebulizer.
- Talk directly to the child, explaining procedures in simple terms. When explaining treatments or care options to the parent, include the child.
- Ask the child about the level of understanding and allow time for questions.
- Address the child's fears or concerns directly, rather than treating them as foolish or inconsequential.
- Give rewards, such as a sticker or inexpensive toy, after a procedure, regardless of the child's behavior. Think of this gesture as a reward for undergoing the procedure, not as a judgment of "good" or "bad" behavior.

ADOLESCENTS

- Preserve the adolescent's modesty; offer adolescents a choice as to whether they want their parents present.
- Consider the legal issues regarding the right to privacy for pregnant adolescents and adolescents with sexually transmissible diseases.
- Provide an opportunity for questions.
- Listen to the adolescent's concerns nonjudgmentally and without belittling the young person. Developing a teasing relationship with an adolescent is often a temptation, but this has potential for harm—the adolescent is easily embarrassed.
- Explain procedures or treatments carefully and allow choices. Adolescents are capable of complex abstract thinking and can make intelligent and reasoned decisions about their own care.

▌ *The Family of a Child in Emergency Care*

Stress on the family results directly and indirectly from the child's illness or injury. The way a child perceives an illness or injury often is related to the parents' attitude, so caring for the child requires assessment of and intervention with the family.

The most common emotions experienced by parents of children cared for in emergencies are fear and anxiety. Parents are afraid that

- Their child might die. This fear is the greatest source of anxiety and can be present even when death is highly unlikely, as in the case of minor illnesses or injuries. This anxiety is often the underlying cause of parents' anger toward health care providers.
- Their child might experience pain. As a rule, parents try very hard to protect children from pain. Even when pain is necessary, it is difficult for parents to understand and accept.
- The child's body may be permanently altered. Parents often fear that their children will have permanent scars or bodily changes.

Parental guilt is another frequently seen emotion. Parents can feel guilty because

- They feel responsible for their child's illness or injury.
- They are submitting their child to a painful experience.
- They do not have enough knowledge to make educated decisions about their child's care.

In addition, parents might have had negative experiences with health care providers in the past or may have other concerns about siblings, financial arrangements, and work schedules.

The particular causes of stress for families in emergencies are unique to the circumstances and to the family involved. All of the stressors combined could stretch parents' coping mechanisms to the limit and result in anger, withdrawal, or tearfulness. Stress also can manifest itself in hyperactivity—making numerous phone calls, repeating questions, and involving a large number of people in decision-making processes.

Including family members in their child's care can reduce feelings of helplessness and promote positive coping mechanisms. It is far easier and less time consuming to intervene early and provide support for appropriate coping mechanisms than it is to intervene after a child's or parent's emotional decompensation.

Emergency Assessment of Infants and Children

In the emergency setting, assessment of the ill or injured child must be rapid and accurate to identify abnormal findings quickly. In children, initial evidence of life-threatening conditions can be very subtle, with few signs of impending respiratory or cardiopulmonary arrest. It is particularly important to make as many initial observations as possible without touching the child, so that assessments can reflect the child's baseline, resting condition. For an infant or young child, most of the examination required for general triage can be performed with the child on the parent's lap. The nurse also observes the relationship between the parents and child during the examination process.

The triage nurse usually performs the initial observation in the emergency setting and decides the level of care needed for the child. Triaging is an important skill that improves with experience. The nurse bases much of the "initial" assessment on an overall sense of how the child looks—sick or well. Because children do not try to cover up either how they feel or how they look, the nurse receives a fairly accurate impression of illness or wellness immediately.

Three essential factors combine to form a first impression: respiratory rate and effort, skin color, and response to the environment. If results of all three of these assessments appear to be normal, the nurse follows the initial assessment with a more thorough and in-depth evaluation. If the general impression is that the child is seriously ill, the nurse must intervene immediately and combine any additional evaluation with intervention.

PRIMARY ASSESSMENT

Primary assessment, which is part of the initial triage assessment, consists of assessing the *ABCDEs*—airway, breath-

ing, circulation, the child's level of consciousness, and exposure. Because the two most common pathways to mortality in children are respiratory failure and shock, interventions would include providing respiratory and circulatory support.

Airway Assessment. Although determining the etiology of respiratory distress or failure in an ill child ultimately will be important, more important is recognizing symptoms and signs of respiratory distress. In the emergency setting, initial treatment is the same regardless of the cause.

Because of some differences in airway anatomy and physiology, children are at greater risk of airway problems than adults (Table 34–1). When assessing children's airways, the nurse pays particular attention to breath sounds (often audible to the naked ear) as well as snoring, stridor, wheezing, and grunting. Snoring is caused by obstruction in the upper airway (often the tongue relaxing against the posterior pharynx) and can be heard in a child with decreased mental status. Stridor is a high-pitched sound, heard on inspiration (laryngeal obstruction) or on both inspiration and expiration (mid-tracheal obstruction). Wheezing, a high-pitched, musical sound heard primarily on expira-

TABLE 34–1
. . . .

Primary Assessment in Pediatric Emergencies

Assessment	Pediatric Differences	Nursing Implications
A—Airway: patency, positioning for air entry, audible sounds, airway obstruction (blood, mucus, edema)	**A** • The child's airway is narrower than an adult's, and more easily obstructed by foreign bodies, small amounts of mucus, or tissue edema. Infants are preferential nasal breathers for the first several months of life; therefore, nasal secretions can cause respiratory compromise. Children are more susceptible to infectious respiratory diseases that contribute to risk of airway obstruction. Edema and mucus in a narrow airway cause incrementally more obstruction than in a wider one (Chameides, 1994). • The tongue is relatively large in relation to the oral cavity and can more easily fall into the airway in the unconscious child. • Cartilage of the larynx is relatively soft, and the trachea is thinner and more flexible than an adult's. The larynx is higher and more anterior, increasing the risk of obstruction and aspiration. • The submandibular area is softer and can be more easily compressed to occlude the airway. • Deciduous teeth are poorly anchored and easily dislodged.	A—Allow the child to maintain a position of comfort or manually position the airway (jaw thrust or head tilt–chin lift); encourage the child to avoid flexing or hyperextending the neck; use spinal immobilization and airway adjuncts as required.
B—Breathing: increased or decreased work of breathing, nasal flaring, use of accessory muscles of respiration (retractions), pattern, quality, oxygen saturation	**B** • The chest wall is thin, softer, and more compliant. Rib alignment is more horizontal. The younger child is more susceptible to respiratory distress and failure. Retractions commonly occur with respiratory distress and can compromise the ability to increase tidal volume. • The diaphragm is the predominant muscle of respiration. Pressure above or below the diaphragm can impede respiratory effort. • Infants and children have a higher metabolic rate and increased oxygen demand. Hypoxia occurs more rapidly.	B—Provide supplemental oxygen; initiate assisted ventilation with bag-valve-mask and prepare for intubation as indicated; provide gastric decompression by use of orogastric or nasogastric tube.
C—Circulation: skin color, temperature, and capillary refill (<2 sec); strength of peripheral and central pulses	**C** • The child's circulating blood volume per body weight is much larger than an adult's, even though actual blood volume is much smaller. Therefore, small-volume losses have more severe circulatory consequences. • A higher percentage of fluid is located in the extracellular compartment, causing more rapid fluid shifts. • A higher metabolic rate and oxygen demand requires an increased heart rate; tachycardia is the first compensatory mechanism for decreased oxygenation, *not* hypotension.	C—Control bleeding through application of direct pressure, obtain vascular access; initiate volume replacement; perform chest compressions; defibrillate or provide synchronized cardioversion; initiate drug therapy.

Table continued on following page

TABLE 34-1
• • • • • • • • • •

Primary Assessment in Pediatric Emergencies Continued

Assessment	Pediatric Differences	Nursing Implications
D—Disability: level of consciousness or activity level; response to the environment; pupillary response	**D** • A larger head/body ratio and weak neck muscles contribute to more serious head injury from shaking or impact. • The anterior fontanel remains open until approximately 18 months. An open fontanel allows for expanded cranial space in response to increased cranial volume, so signs of increased intracranial pressure, which indicate underlying brain injury, might be delayed. • A thinner skull predisposes the child to more severe injury. • Nerve myelinization is incomplete during infancy; unmyelinated tissue is more vulnerable to shearing injury (Bernardo, 1998).	**D**—Treat the underlying cause (e.g., signs of increased intracranial pressure; fluid or blood volume deficit, hypoxia).
E—Expose: to identify underlying injuries or additional signs of illness.	**E** • Bulging fontanel, periorbital edema, unusual rashes, and edema or exudate in the pharynx can indicate a variety of severe childhood communicable diseases. • Bruising, unusual burns, vaginal tearing, rectal bleeding, and discharge suggest child abuse.	**E**—Remove all clothing, including diapers; save any clothing needed for evidence; maintain an appropriately warm environment.

Data from: Bernardo, L. (1998). Multiple trauma. In: M. Slota (Ed.). *Core curriculum for pediatric critical care nursing* (pp. 568–571). Philadelphia: Saunders; and Emergency Nurses Association. (1998). *ENPC provider manual* (2nd ed., pp. 61–67). Park Ridge, IL: Author.

tion, signals obstruction of the lower airway. Crackles or rales are fine, popping noises heard on inspiration; they usually indicate that fluid is in the lungs, as in pneumonia.

Breathing Assessment. The rate and depth of breathing, as well as the respiratory effort made by the child, indicate relative oxygenation. A rapid respiratory rate with shallow breathing indicates respiratory distress. Very slow breathing in an ill child is an ominous sign, indicating respiratory failure. A slowly breathing child might no longer have the energy for adequate ventilation. Abdominal breathing is normal in the infant or young child, so the nurse observes the rise and fall of the abdomen instead of the chest.

The use of accessory muscles for breathing invariably indicates respiratory distress. The chest wall of a child is relatively weak and unstable, so retractions occur with increased work of breathing. Assessment of breathing includes observing the child for intercostal, substernal, suprasternal, supraclavicular, and infraclavicular retractions. As a child becomes exhausted, retractions might diminish, usually indicating respiratory failure. Nasal flaring with inspiration is another form of accessory muscle use. Grunting, a sound made by expiration against partially closed vocal cords, represents the body's effort to improve oxygenation by generating positive end-expiratory pressure, and is a sign of hypoxemia.

The nurse observes the child's preferred body posture.

A child in respiratory distress is upright with the jaw thrust forward, leaning forward on outstretched arms—the "tripod" position. This position helps to maximize airway opening and the use of accessory muscles of respiration.

Once the work of breathing has been carefully observed, listening to the chest provides some useful information. Children have small chests, and breath sounds can be transmitted throughout the chest. The nurse therefore auscultates a child's chest at both sides of the body at the mid-axillary line and over the trachea to confirm equality of breath sounds and to distinguish upper from lower airway noises.

Normal respiratory rates for children vary by age, and are faster than for adults (see Table 33–1). A respiratory rate over 60 breaths per minute, however, is abnormal for any age. Another important adjunct for respiratory assessment is the pulse oximetry reading (see Chapter 37).

Cardiovascular Assessment. Cardiovascular assessment includes observing the child's skin color and temperature, checking capillary refill, determining heart rate, and measuring blood pressure. A child can compensate more effectively for fluid loss, through increased heart rate and peripheral vasoconstriction, than an adult can. Tachycardia and decreased peripheral perfusion are early signs of cardiovascular compromise in a child, and require immediate intervention to prevent decompensation. A systolic blood pressure below 70 mm Hg in an ill or injured child can suggest uncompensated shock, which requires immediate and aggressive intervention (Chameides, 1994). Children can maintain a normal blood pressure until up to 25% of their circulating blood volume is lost, so hypotension is a late sign.

Disability: Neurologic Assessment. The infant's or child's level of consciousness is an essential component of the primary assessment. This assessment can be made only when the child is awake. If the child is sleeping, the nurse asks the parent to awaken the child gently, to establish arousability.

Most methods of assessing level of consciousness in adults include some form of verbal feedback, which is not possible in a preverbal child. One method for assessing neurologic status in preverbal children is AVPU: Alert, Verbal (responds to verbal stimuli), Painful stimuli (responds to painful stimuli), Unresponsive. This method, which is adequate for the emergency setting, provides a global assessment and includes documentation of the type of stimuli used to evoke responses or lack of response. More thorough and sophisticated means of assessment are used later, if needed (see Chapter 52).

Exposure. Primary assessment ends with exposure, or removing the child's clothing to identify additional injuries or indicators of illness. The nurse needs to preserve the child's clothing appropriately if it will be needed for evidence in any potential civil or criminal proceeding. To prevent heat loss, the nurse keeps the child warm.

SECONDARY ASSESSMENT

After the primary assessment is complete and intervention (if necessary) has stabilized the child, the nurse begins the secondary assessment. Components of the secondary assessment include vital signs, history and head-to-toe assessment, and inspection (Table 34–2).

Vital Signs. Vital signs are useful in the triage assessment of the child, but because age variations make their significance more difficult to interpret, they are not as reliable an indicator as in adult assessment. This variation is especially applicable to temperature. For example, an infant has an immature thermoregulatory system and might not have a fever, even in the presence of infection, so the nurse needs to be alert for supporting signs. Infants and young children also have a greater body surface area/weight ratio, which contributes to increased heat loss. The nurse needs to keep young children warm to prevent shivering, which increases metabolic needs. (See Chapter 37 for methods of temperature taking.)

When taking children's vital signs, the nurse observes the respiratory rate first, then obtains the pulse, and obtains the temperature and blood pressure last, because they can be the most upsetting for children. The nurse should be certain to use the right-size blood pressure cuff and take both the respiratory and heart rates for 1 full minute, because subtle differences are important in the child. Normal respiratory and heart rates are faster than an adult's, whereas the blood pressure is lower on average. (See Table 33–1 and Appendix J for normal vital signs by age.) The nurse performs pulse oximetry, if indicated.

History and Head-to-Toe Assessment. A brief history obtains information about prior illness or injury that might affect the emergency care of the child. A format often used for pediatric patients is AMPLE:

A—allergies
M—medications taken and immunization history
P—prior illness and/or injury
L—last meal/eating habits
E—events leading up to this injury or illness (e.g., exposure to other children, mechanism of injury)

This mnemonic gives sufficient information to determine whether the child's medical history will play an important role in assessment and treatment of the current illness or injury. In emergency departments that care for children, a list of immunizations and the appropriate ages should be posted in a convenient location (see Appendix F).

After obtaining an appropriate history, the nurse begins to perform a head-to-toe assessment, documenting any

---

TABLE 34-2

. . . .

Secondary Assessment in Pediatric Emergencies

Assessment	Nursing Implications
F—Full set of vital signs: evaluate the child's vital signs, including temperature, for abnormal findings; obtain weight in kg. Family presence: assess the needs of the family for support and inclusion in care.	**F**—Continuously monitor the child's vital signs, including temperature; weigh child, obtain estimated weight if child's condition prohibits measured weight. Provide family support in a culturally appropriate way.
G—Give comfort measures: discomfort is usually related to the underlying problem; use pain assessment scales for children.	**G**—Frequently monitor pain level and response to pain relief measures; include non-pharmacologic techniques for reducing pain.
H—Head-to-toe assessment: perform a complete head-to-toe assessment and obtain a history; during triage assessment the head-to-toe (secondary) assessment may need to relate to the chief complaint.	**H**—Continuously monitor the child for changes in condition; assess for any unusual odors.
I—Inspect the back and isolate: observe the back for obvious or hidden injuries; assess for communicable illness or susceptibility to illness (immunocompromised patients).	**I**—Reinspect the back as indicated; provide isolation as indicated.

Adapted and reprinted with permission from Emergency Nurses Association. (1998). *ENPC provider manual* (2nd ed., pp. 68–75). Park Ridge, IL: Author.

findings that might affect the child's condition. The nurse inspects all body surfaces, looking for fractures, lacerations, contusions, and penetrating injuries. The nurse also observes the skin for petechiae or rashes. The presence and pattern of any pain is described. The nurse pays particular attention to signs of pneumothorax or hemothorax (e.g., decreased breath sounds on the affected side, signs of hypoxemia, signs of shock). The nurse then palpates the child's abdomen and auscultates for presence of bowel sounds. Any sign of hematuria indicates genitourinary injury. Blood found at the urinary meatus suggests disruptive injury of the lower urinary tract and the need to avoid inserting a urinary catheter.

Diagnostic Tests. Once the child has arrived in the emergency setting and has undergone initial assessment and interventions, many diagnostic tests assist in the evaluation process. Standard protocols for laboratory tests usually comprise a complete blood count (CBC) with differential count, serum electrolytes, and urinalysis. Additional studies might be necessary for the child who has multiple trauma. These include coagulation profiles, blood urea nitrogen (BUN), creatinine, glucose, amylase, lipase, SGOT (serum glutamic oxaloacetic transaminase, also known as AST, or aspartate aminotransferase), SGPT (serum glutamic-pyruvate transaminase, also known as ALT, or alanine aminotransferase), and blood type and crossmatch.

Radiologic films may be obtained, depending on the presenting problem and assessment data. Placement of a nasogastric tube, urinary catheter, or other device might be required.

Weight. Determining the weight of the child is absolutely essential in emergency care because all medication dosages and fluid amounts are calculated according to the child's weight in kilograms. The nurse weighs the child on an appropriate scale, if possible. If not possible, the nurse obtains a weight history from the parent or approximates the weight using standard growth charts.

Another way to determine the child's weight and medication dosages is through the use of a length-based tape, such as the Broselow tape. A length-based tape is placed on a gurney or stretcher next to the child, and the child's length is measured. The length is keyed to emergency medication dosages, usually listed on the tape. The tape also indicates fluid bolus volumes, defibrillation energy levels, and sizes of the pediatric airway, bag-valve-mask, laryngoscope, endotracheal tube, nasogastric tube, urinary catheter, chest tube, and intravenous catheter.

When all else fails, it is sometimes easiest to remember three estimated average weights for children younger than 6 years of age, and estimate the child's weight from there:

2 years	10 kg
4 years	20 kg
6 years	30 kg

Parent-Child Relationship. Rapid triage assessment of the child also includes observation of the child in relation to the parents. If the relationship does not appear to be close, comfortable, and trusting, the nurse might want to explore further. Especially with trauma, the nurse considers possible causes and manifestations of dysfunctional parent-child relationships, such as child abuse or neglect (Henderson & Brownstein, 1994).

Cardiopulmonary Resuscitation of the Child

AIRWAY AND BREATHING
Initial Assessment and Intervention. Early recognition of and intervention for respiratory distress and compensated shock can be life saving for the child. Assistance with ventilation and administration of fluids might prevent further deterioration in the child's condition. Once the child progresses to respiratory failure and shock, cardiopulmonary resuscitation (CPR) becomes an absolute necessity (Fig. 34–1). Resuscitation of children requires attention to the differences between adults and children, as described in Table 34–1.

After appropriately opening the airway, the nurse looks for chest rise and listens and feels for exhaled breath against his or her cheek. When the child is not breathing or ventilation is not adequate after positioning the airway correctly, the nurse gives at least two slow breaths by means of a bag-valve-mask device, watching for the rise and fall of the chest. *The nurse should stop inflating the lungs when the chest just begins to rise and allow enough time for exhalation (longer than inhalation).* Endotracheal intubation is necessary if the child cannot be ventilated adequately with these measures.

A pressure gauge attached to the bag and mask device helps deliver breaths at the correct pressure, especially for infants and young children. Choosing the appropriate-size mask and the correct-volume bag is important. The mask should cover the child's mouth and nose but not place pressure on the eyes. A good fit ensures a seal around the face and under the chin. Gastric decompression by use of an orogastric or nasogastric tube is indicated during assisted ventilation.

Obstructed Airway Management. Inability to inflate the lungs suggests airway obstruction, a life-threatening emergency. When ventilation is not possible, the infant or child will die in a very short time.

> When a child's airway is obstructed and the child is coughing or is able to breathe adequately despite partial obstruction, the child should be allowed to maintain whatever position is comfortable until specialized care is available. The nurse remains with the child and encourages the child to remain calm by reassuring in a soothing manner.

Management of airway obstruction depends on the cause and on the child's age. Definitive treatment depends on diagnosis. Foreign body aspiration, for example, is a problem frequently seen in young children, with a large number of aspirations attributed to small toy parts (Centers for Disease Control and Prevention [CDC], 1997b). When a child is unable to ventilate adequately and aspiration of a foreign body is suspected as the cause, the nurse initiates maneuvers to remove the obstruction.

Although controversy remains about how to clear a foreign body from the airway, for children older than 1 year the American Heart Association recommends using the Heimlich maneuver for a conscious child and abdominal thrusts for the unconscious child (Fig. 34–2). Removal of a foreign

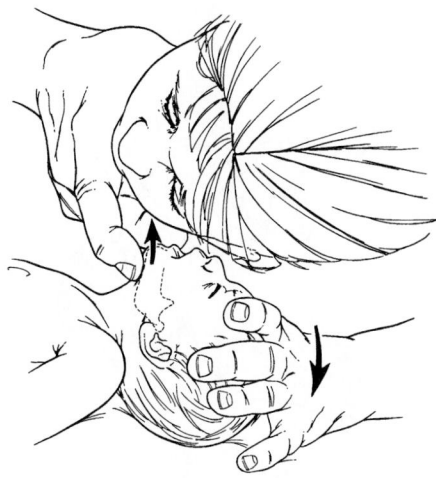

A. Opening the airway with the head tilt-chin lift maneuver. One hand is used to tilt the head, extending the neck. The index finger of the rescuer's other hand lifts the mandible outward by lifting on the chin. Use a jaw-thrust maneuver if cervical spine injury is suspected.

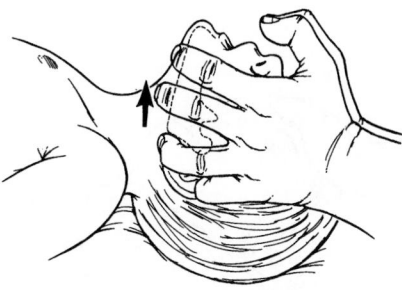

B. Opening the airway with the jaw-thrust maneuver. The airway is opened by lifting the angle of the mandible. The rescuer uses two or three fingers of each hand to lift the jaw while the remaining fingers guide the jaw upward and outward.

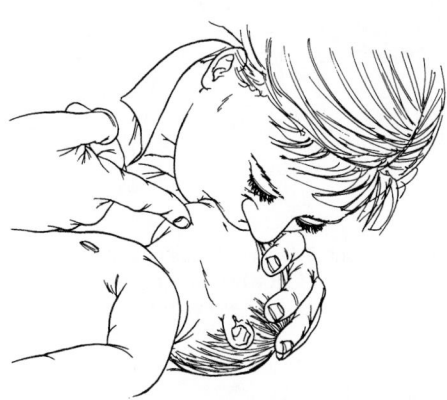

C. Rescue breathing in an infant. The rescuer's mouth covers the infant's nose and mouth, creating a seal. One hand performs head tilt while the other hand lifts the infant's jaw. Avoid head tilt if the infant has suspected head or neck trauma.

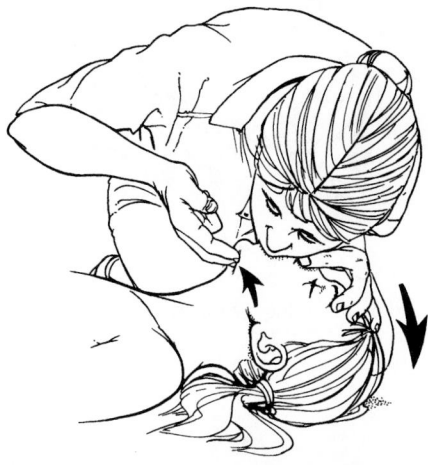

D. Rescue breathing in a child. The rescuer's mouth covers the mouth of the child, creating a mouth-to-mouth seal. One hand maintains head tilt; the thumb and forefinger of the same hand are used to pinch the child's nose. If head or neck trauma is suspected, immobilize the head in neutral position and do not perform head tilt.

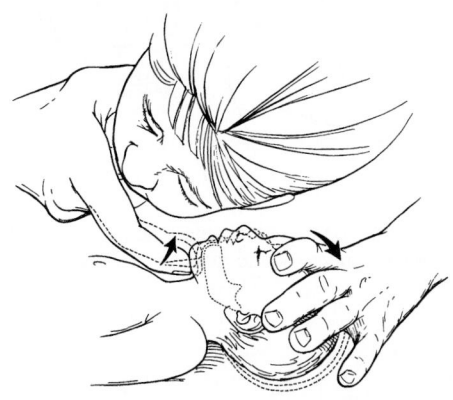

E. Movement of victim's head into positions of progressive neck extension until position of optimum airway patency (and effective ventilation) is achieved. Such manipulation of the head should not be performed if head, neck, or cervical spine injury is suspected.

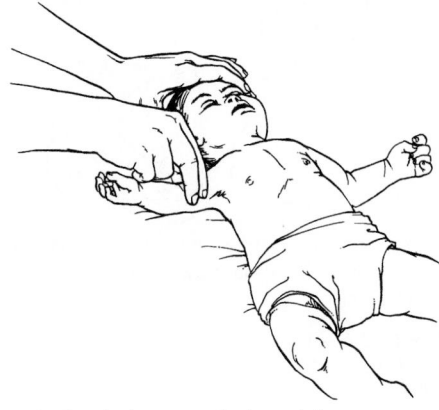

F. Palpating the brachial artery pulse in an infant.

FIGURE 34–1
. . . .

Cardiopulmonary resuscitation for infants and children. (Reproduced with permission from American Heart Association. [1997]. *Basic Life Support for Health Care Providers*. Dallas: Author. Copyright American Heart Association.)

Figure continued on following page

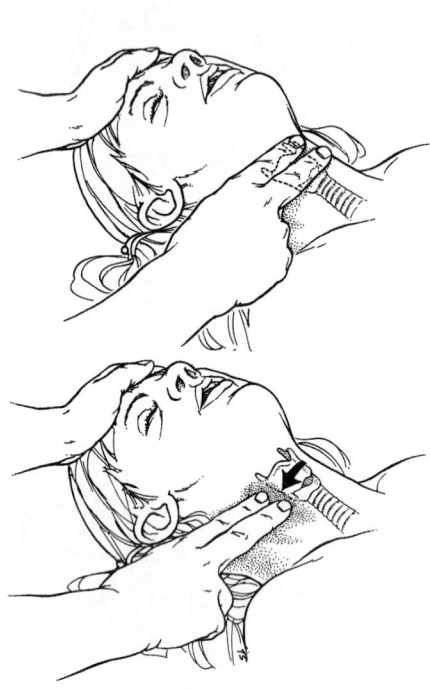

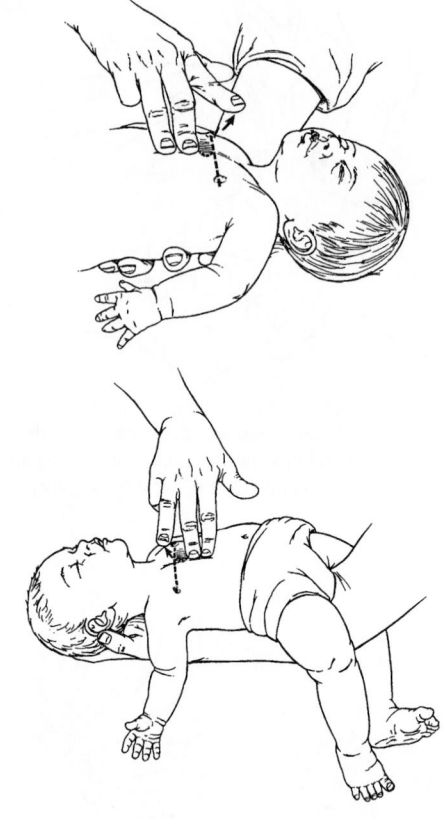

G. Locating and palpating the carotid artery pulse in the child.

H. Cardiac compressions. Top, Infant supine on palm of the rescuer's hand. Bottom, Performing CPR while carrying the infant or small child. Note that the head is kept level with the torso.

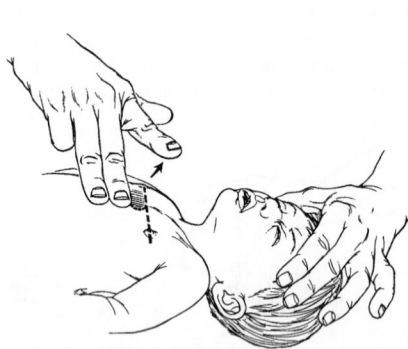

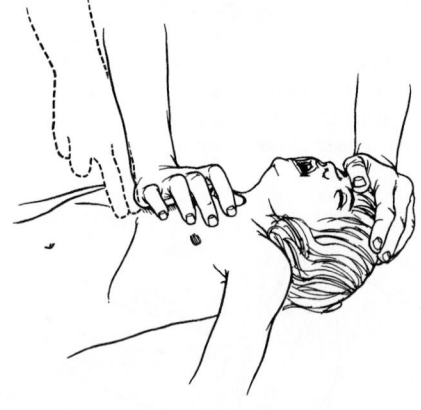

I. Locating proper finger position for chest compression in infant. Note that the rescuer's other hand is used to maintain head position to facilitate ventilation.

J. Locating hand position for chest compression in child. Note that the rescuer's other hand is used to maintain head position to facilitate ventilation.

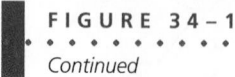

FIGURE 34–1
• • • • • • • • •
Continued

body from an infant involves placing the infant in a downward-slanting position and giving back blows and chest thrusts (see Fig. 34–2). Blind finger sweeps to remove a foreign body are not recommended for infants and children because of the risk of forcing the object further down into the airway. A finger sweep can be used if the object is visible.

If obstruction continues after these maneuvers, subsequent actions can include direct laryngoscopy and use of a Magill forceps to remove the foreign body. Tracheostomy is used as a last resort. When the lower airway is obstructed because of a disease process such as asthma, medication to open the airway might be necessary.

THE INFANT: BACK BLOWS AND CHEST THRUSTS

The following sequence is used to clear a foreign-body obstruction from the airway of an infant. Back blows are delivered while the infant is supported in the prone position (face down) straddling the rescuer's forearm, with the head lower than the trunk. Chest thrusts are delivered while the infant is supine, held on the rescuer's forearm, with the infant's head lower than the body. The rescuer should perform the following steps to relieve airway obstruction in the conscious infant:

1. Hold the infant face down, resting on the forearm. Support the infant's head by firmly holding the jaw. Rest your forearm on your thigh to support the infant. The infant's head should be lower than the trunk.
2. Deliver up to five back blows forcefully between the infant's shoulder blades, using the heel of the hand (Fig. A).

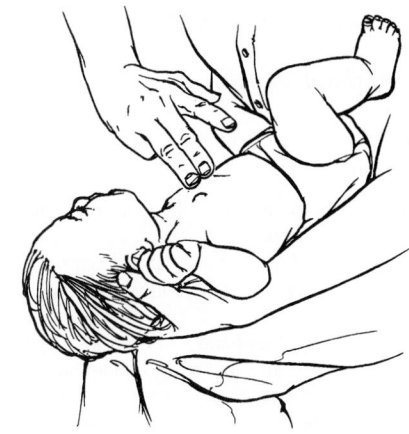

B. Chest thrusts to relieve foreign-body airway obstruction in the infant.

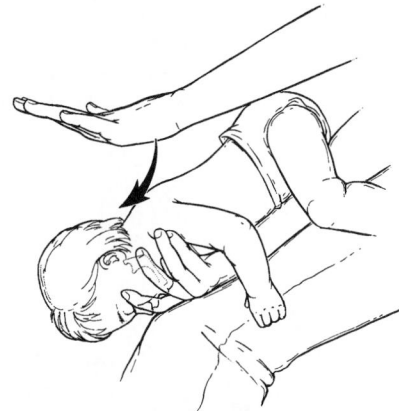

A. Back blows to relieve foreign-body airway obstruction in the infant.

3. After delivering the back blows, place your free hand on the infant's back, holding the infant's head. The infant is effectively sandwiched between your two hands and arms. One hand supports the head and neck, jaw, and chest while the other supports the back.
4. Turn the infant while the head and neck are carefully supported, and hold the infant in the supine position, draped on the thigh. The infant's head should remain lower than the trunk.
5. Give up to five quick downward chest thrusts in the same location and manner as chest compressions—two fingers placed on the lower half of the sternum, approximately one finger's breadth below the nipples (Fig. B). If the rescuer's hands are small or the infant is large, these maneuvers may be hard to perform. If so, place the infant supine on the lap, with the head lower than the trunk and the head firmly supported. After you have given up to five back blows, turn the infant as a unit to the supine position and give up to five chest thrusts.

6. Open the airway by grasping both the tongue and lower jaw and lifting the mandible (tongue-jaw lift). Remove the foreign body if you see it (see below).

Steps 1 through 6 should be repeated until the object is expelled or the infant loses consciousness. If the infant loses consciousness, open the airway using a tongue-jaw lift and remove the foreign object if you see it and attempt to rescue breathing and relief of airway obstruction.

If the victim is or becomes unconscious,

1. Open the infant's airway. If the loss of consciousness is witnessed, and foreign-body obstruction is suspected, lift the chin using a tongue-jaw lift and remove the object with a finger sweep if you see it.
2. Attempt rescue breathing.
3. If the first attempt is unsuccessful, reposition the head and reattempt ventilation.
4. If ventilation is unsuccessful, give five back blows and five chest thrusts.
5. Open the mouth using a tongue-jaw lift and remove the foreign object if you see it.
6. Repeat steps 2 through 4 until ventilation is successful (chest rises).
7. Activate the EMS system after approximately 1 minute, then resume efforts.
8. If the victim resumes effective breathing, place in the recovery position and monitor closely until rescue personnel arrive.

▌ **FIGURE 34–2**
• • • • • • • • • • •
Procedures for clearing airway obstruction in infants and children. (Reproduced with permission from American Heart Association. [1997]. *Basic Life Support for Health Care Providers.* Dallas: Author. Copyright American Heart Association.)

Figure continued on following page

CIRCULATION

The nurse feels for the pulse and in the child older than 1 year of age, palpates the carotid artery. For an infant younger than 1 year of age, the nurse uses the brachial artery because the infant's relatively short, fat, neck makes palpation of the carotid artery difficult. If no pulse is palpated or if the infant's heart rate is less than 60 beats/min, the nurse begins chest compressions (see Fig. 34–1).

The nurse obtains venous access for fluid resuscitation and medication administration. If venous access through a peripheral vein cannot be obtained within 90 seconds or with three attempts, the next consideration is an intraosseous line (placed in the upper tibia). Children should be given 20 ml/kg intravenous (IV) fluid, usually lactated Ringer's or normal saline solution, as an initial bolus for shock. The nurse administers additional boluses as needed after reassessing cardiovascular status and warms the solution before any rapid infusion.

THE CHILD: THE HEIMLICH MANEUVER

Abdominal Thrusts with Victim Conscious (Standing or Sitting)

Perform the following steps to relieve complete airway obstruction in the conscious victim:

1. Stand behind the victim, arms directly under the victim's axillae encircling the victim's torso.
2. Place the thumb side of one fist against the victim's abdomen in the midline slightly above the navel and well below the tip of the xiphoid process.
3. Grasp the fist with the other hand and exert a series of quick upward thrusts (Fig. C). Do not touch the xiphoid process or the lower margins of the rib cage because force applied to these structures can damage internal organs.

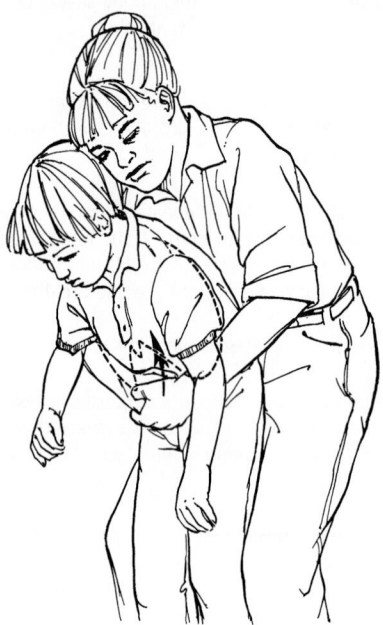

C. Abdominal thrusts with victim standing or sitting (conscious).

4. Each thrust should be a separate, distinct movement, intended to relieve the obstruction. Continue abdominal thrusts until the foreign body is expelled or the patient loses consciousness.
5. If the victim loses consciousness, open the airway using a tongue-jaw lift and remove the obstructing object with a finger sweep if you see it.
6. Attempt rescue breathing. If the chest fails to rise, reposition the head and reattempt rescue breathing again. If the airway remains obstructed in the unconscious victim, repeat the Heimlich maneuver.

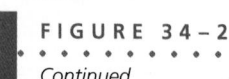

FIGURE 34 – 2
• • • • • • • • •
Continued

Abdominal Thrusts for the Victim Who Is Unconscious or Who Becomes Unconscious

The rescuer should perform the following steps:

1. Place the victim supine.
2. If the loss of consciousness is witnessed and foreign-body airway obstruction is suspected, open the airway using a tongue-jaw lift and remove the object with a finger sweep if you see it.
3. Attempt rescue breathing. If ventilation is unsuccessful, reposition the head and reattempt ventilation. If ventilation is still unsuccessful, continue with steps 4 through 8 below.
4. Kneel beside the victim or straddle the victim's hips.
5. Place the heel of one hand on the child's abdomen in the midline slightly above the navel and well below the rib cage and xiphoid process. Place the other hand on the top of the first.
6. Press both hands into the abdomen with a quick upward thrust (Fig. D). Each thrust is directed upward in the midline and should not be directed to either side of the abdomen. Perform a series of five thrusts. Each thrust should be a separate and distinct movement.

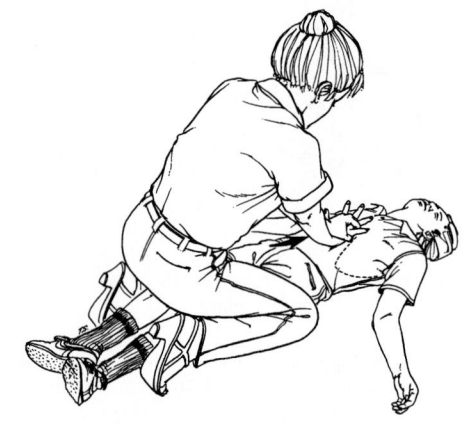

D. Abdominal thrusts with victim lying (conscious or unconscious).

7. Open the airway by grasping both the tongue and lower jaw and lifting the mandible (tongue-jaw lift). If you see the foreign body, remove it using a finger sweep.
8. Repeat steps 3 through 7 until ventilation is successful.

Epinephrine is the drug of choice for management of cardiac arrest. It can be given through the endotracheal tube when necessary. Atropine diminishes vagally mediated bradycardia. Sodium bicarbonate is given on the basis of arterial blood gas results, and dextrose can be used on the basis of blood glucose results or for patients unresponsive to resuscitative efforts.

Although cardiac rhythm disturbances in children are rare, rapid heart rates can occur, including sinus tachycardia, supraventricular tachycardia, and ventricular tachycar-

dia. Cardiac output is a function of stroke volume and heart rate. Because children are unable to increase stroke volume, they can increase cardiac output only by increasing their heart rate. As heart rates increase, cardiac filling time decreases, and cardiac output falls.

Sinus tachycardia usually requires observation and determination of the cause. Cardioversion at 0.5 to 1.0 joules/kg might be necessary for symptomatic supraventricular tachycardia (heart rate 200 beats per minute). Valsalva maneuvers or adenosine would be considered for the stable pa-

---

CRITICAL TO REMEMBER

Basic Life Support Maneuvers in Infants and Children

Maneuver	Infant (< 1 year)	Child (1 to 8 years)
Airway	Head tilt-chin lift (if trauma is present, use jaw-thrust)	Head tilt-chin lift (if trauma is present, use jaw-thrust)
Breathing		
Initial	At least two breaths at 1 to 1.5 seconds/breath	Two breaths at 1 to 1.5 seconds/breath
Subsequent	20 breaths/min (approximate)	20 breaths/min (approximate)
Circulation		
Pulse check	Brachial/femoral	Carotid
Compression area	Lower half of sternum	Lower half of sternum
Compressed width	Two or three fingers	Heel of one hand
Depth	Approximately one third to one half the depth of the chest	Approximately one third to one half the depth of the chest
Rate	At least 100/min	100/min
Compression–ventilation ratio	5:1 (pause for ventilation)	5:1 (pause for ventilation)
Foreign body airway obstruction	Back blows/chest thrusts	Heimlich maneuver

Reproduced with permission from American Heart Association. (1997). *Basic Life Support for Health Care Providers.* Dallas: Author. Copyright American Heart Association.

---

tient. Ventricular tachycardia in a child is usually the result of congenital abnormalities or chronic cardiac disease and requires complex interventions.

Resuscitation of the child requires a team effort; training and rehearsal, such as mock codes, are very helpful, as are national courses now available, such as the Pediatric Advanced Life Support (PALS) program provided by the American Heart Association.

The Child in Shock

Shock is an acute, complex, unstable physiologic state in which decreased circulation to tissues compromises oxygen delivery to vital body organs. Decreased tissue perfusion (circulation of blood through the vascular bed of tissue) leads to tissue hypoxia and ischemia, metabolic acidosis, and multisystem organ failure (Callow, Suddaby, & Slota, 1998). Shock can be more specifically identified according to its etiology, but regardless of precipitating factors, all forms of shock eventually result in cardiogenic shock (Callow, Suddaby, & Slota, 1998).

Etiology

HYPOVOLEMIC SHOCK

Hypovolemic shock is circulatory collapse caused by massive blood or body fluid loss. The result is decreased intravascular fluid volume. Blood loss can be caused by trauma or surgery; fluid and plasma losses can occur with vomiting and diarrhea. All can contribute to hypovolemic shock.

SEPTIC SHOCK

Septic shock occurs when microbial toxins (from bacteria, viruses, fungi, or rickettsiae) are present in the blood. These toxins cause a cascade of metabolic, hemodynamic, and clinical changes, resulting in decreased perfusion and hypotension. Organisms most frequently implicated include *Neisseria meningitidis, Streptococcus pneumoniae, Streptococcus pyogenes,* and *Staphylococcus aureus* (Kaplan & Davis, 1999). Infants and children with debilitating illnesses, patients in the intensive care unit for prolonged periods with many invasive lines, and those who are immunosuppressed are at greatest risk for development of septic shock.

CARDIOGENIC SHOCK

Cardiogenic shock occurs when myocardial function is impaired so that cardiac output is not sufficient to meet the body's metabolic demands. The causes of cardiogenic shock include structural abnormalities related to congenital heart disease, infectious and noninfectious cardiomyopathies, trauma, ischemia, metabolic abnormalities, drug intoxication, and impaired cardiac function after intracardiac surgical repair.

Manifestations

The clinical manifestations of shock are different for each type of shock. Infants and children with septic shock first demonstrate early signs indicating a compensated state and then late signs indicating a decompensated state of shock. Table 34–3 presents the general appearance of a child in shock.

PATHOPHYSIOLOGY
of Shock

HYPOVOLEMIC SHOCK

Hypovolemic shock results from an abnormal decrease in plasma volume. Water constitutes a much greater portion of an infant's or child's body weight than it does an adult's, and because the bulk of fluid volume in young children is primarily located in the extracellular tissue spaces, infants and young children are more susceptible to hypovolemic shock. Infants, with their large body surface area and increased metabolic rate also experience increased insensible fluid loss, thus compounding hypovolemia.

When intravascular volume is reduced, the body initially compensates by increasing the heart rate and redistributing the blood flow to the vital organs (the brain and heart). Decompensation occurs when the total blood and fluid volume is reduced by 20% to 25%. If fluid resuscitation is not initiated within an appropriate time frame, decreased oxygen delivery and cellular ischemia and necrosis result.

SEPTIC SHOCK

Septic shock occurs when an invading organism infects a susceptible host, overwhelms the host's first and second lines of defense, and enters the bloodstream. The presence of toxins or organisms in the blood produces endocrine, metabolic, and immunologic reactions. Endotox-ins, produced by lysis of bacteria, cause maldistributed blood flow, cardiac dysfunction, oxygen supply and demand imbalance, and metabolic alterations (Rosenthal-Dichter, 1998). The early phase of septic shock is marked by adequate tissue perfusion and even increased cardiac output. The late phase is marked by decreased cardiac output, increased systemic vascular resistance, and decreased peripheral tissue perfusion.

CARDIOGENIC SHOCK

Cardiogenic shock is characterized by low cardiac output and hypotension, which results in inadequate tissue perfusion. Unlike hypovolemic shock, the compensatory mechanisms that occur in a child with cardiogenic shock can cause further myocardial dysfunction. These compensatory mechanisms redistribute blood away from the peripheral, splenic, and mesenteric circulation to help maintain the circulation to the vital organs, the heart and brain. Initially, compensatory mechanisms increase the heart rate, myocardial contractility, and vasoconstriction. Subsequent events result in sodium and fluid retention, producing a greater workload on the left ventricle (after-load). The increased workload causes increased oxygen demands of the myocardium in response to a depleted oxygen upply. This process leads to myocardial ischemia, which further depresses cardiac function, thereby establishing a vicious cycle.

Diagnostic Evaluation

The diagnosis of shock in infants and children is established chiefly on the basis of clinical manifestations and medical history. A chest radiograph may help to differentiate cardiogenic shock from hypovolemic and septic shock. In cardiogenic shock, the heart is usually enlarged and may show signs of pulmonary edema. In hypovolemic or septic shock, the chest radiograph is usually normal, and the heart is smaller than normal. In septic shock, chest radiographs may indicate pneumonia, which may be the source of the infection. An echocardiogram can identify underlying structural cardiac disease.

Laboratory studies used in the diagnosis of septic shock include blood cultures and cultures of other sites that may be the source of infection (i.e., urine, sputum, wound drain-

TABLE 34–3

Assessing a Child's General Appearance: "Looks Good" Versus "Looks Bad"

	"Looks Good"	"Looks Bad"
Color	Pink mucous membranes Consistent color over the trunk and extremities	Mottled color
Skin perfusion	Warm Brisk capillary refill (<2 sec)	Cold (peripheral to proximal cooling) Sluggish capillary refill (>2 sec)
Activity	Age-appropriate (may be frightened, unhappy, unwilling to be separated from parents) Will engage in play	Fretful, then lethargic
Responsiveness	Age-appropriate	Irritable (early), then lethargic Decreased response to painful stimulus is worrisome
Infant feeding	Eats well	Weak suck Tires during feeding May have respiratory distress during feedings

Adapted from Hazinski, M. F. (1990). Shock in the pediatric patient. *Critical Care Nursing Clinics of North America, 2*(2), 313.

age, indwelling lines). Other laboratory tests for all types of shock include arterial blood gas values, glucose levels, electrolytes, BUN, creatinine levels, CBC, and coagulation studies.

Therapeutic Management

The therapeutic management of the child in shock includes basic life support: maintaining airway, breathing, and circulation.

Monitoring with pulse oximetry and increasing ambi-

ent oxygen are indicated in most cases. If vascular access cannot be obtained, an intraosseous line can be used until the child is resuscitated, at which time the temporary intraosseous line can be replaced with an intravenous line. Central line access (femoral, subclavian, internal jugular veins) allows rapid administration of large volumes of fluids and is essential for administering some vasoactive drugs (O'Rourke, 1996).

HYPOVOLEMIC SHOCK

Once the airway, breathing, and circulation are established, the next priority is adequate vascular access. A crystalloid infusion of warm normal saline or lactated Ringer's solution should be initiated promptly. If hypovolemic shock is caused by hemorrhage, appropriate blood products should be administered to replace losses after the child has received the crystalloids.

Colloids (albumin) are protein-containing fluids that may be used in volume resuscitation after the initial treatment with crystalloids. Colloids are primarily used for dehydration or body fluid losses other than blood.

SEPTIC SHOCK

The therapeutic management of septic shock involves restoring hemodynamic status with fluid resuscitation and promptly treating infection with antibiotics. Inotropic medications are used to manage the cardiovascular instability. Vasoconstrictors may be used to increase vascular tone and counteract the effects of toxins. Maintaining a secure, patent airway may be necessary if significant respiratory distress occurs. Surgery also might be indicated to eliminate the source of infection (as with an abscess).

CARDIOGENIC SHOCK

The initial management of an infant or child with cardiogenic shock includes adequate oxygenation by maintaining both the airway and proper ventilation. Invasive monitoring of central venous pressure, arterial blood pressure, and pulmonary artery pressure helps to identify hemodynamic changes. Vigilant monitoring, however, may identify subtle clinical signs and symptoms of decreased cardiac output (e.g., cyanosis, decreased skin temperature, and delayed capillary refill), which can indicate the early stages of shock. Early detection allows uncompensated cardiac failure to be avoided.

With an excess of intravascular fluid volume, diuretics may be prescribed. Usually, furosemide (Lasix), 1 mg/kg, provides effective diuresis.

The heart rate must be in the normal range or higher than normal to improve the cardiac output. Children, especially infants younger than 6 months of age, have a decreased ability to increase stroke volume and thus are much more dependent on an increased heart rate to improve cardiac output. Pharmacologic therapy is the mainstay of medical treatment in children with cardiogenic shock. Frequently, a combination of pharmacologic agents is necessary to stabilize the child. Dobutamine or dopamine are the initial drugs of choice for treating cardiogenic shock.

Extracorporeal membrane oxygenation (ECMO) is a means of mechanical circulatory and pulmonary support for infants and children in severe end-stage cardiogenic shock.

ECMO provides the temporary support needed while the child's cardiac function improves.

NURSING CARE
The Child in Shock

Assessment

Nursing assessment of a child in shock should be thorough, with attention focused on the cardiopulmonary system. Early identification of shock in infants and children is crucial to decreasing morbidity and mortality. An assessment of airway, breathing, and circulation is the primary focus. Initial concerns are ensuring a patent airway and monitoring the child's respiratory effort to confirm adequate air exchange with good chest expansion. Central circulation is assessed by checking a brachial, carotid, or femoral pulse.

Hypovolemic Shock

A child in hypovolemic shock may have a history of vomiting and diarrhea or may have anorexia. The parent may report a decrease in wet diapers or explain that the child has not voided recently. With trauma, the child may demonstrate obvious signs of injury or bleeding.

The child in hypovolemic shock requires frequent assessment of vital signs, including blood pressure (every 15 minutes to 1 hour). Skin color, turgor, and temperature should be monitored very closely. The anterior fontanel (if present) should be assessed to determine whether it is depressed or full. A depressed fontanel may be a manifestation of dehydration, whereas a full or level fontanel usually suggests that fluid volume is adequate.

In addition, the child's neurologic status must be assessed and monitored closely. A depressed or deteriorating level of consciousness should be reported promptly. The nurse auscultates heart and lungs and palpates peripheral pulses. Capillary refill time, moistness of mucous membranes, and general muscle tone/strength should be assessed and urine output monitored closely. In very young children, diapers should be weighed to quantify urine output. If the child has diarrhea, a urine bag or Foley catheter should be placed. The abdomen should be palpated and auscultated for the presence of bowel sounds. Abdominal injury must be ruled out, especially if the abdominal girth appears to be increasing, with evidence of abdominal distension. Any abnormal bruising or obvious trauma must be recognized quickly.

Septic Shock

Early signs of septic shock include hyperthermia or hypothermia. The temperature should be monitored every 1 to 2 hours. In early septic shock (the hyperdynamic phase), the skin is typically warm and flushed. In late shock (the hypodynamic phase), skin is ashen and cold. Indeed, shock of any etiology may cause microcirculatory dysfunction leading to abnormal function of coagulation factors and platelets. Therefore, the skin should be observed closely for signs of petechiae, oozing of blood from invasive lines, or purpuric lesions. The presence of petechiae that are spread diffusely over the body may indicate severe sepsis. In children, hypotension is a late sign of all types of shock.

Cardiogenic Shock

A child with cardiogenic shock requires close monitoring of the heart and lungs for adventitious sounds. The liver should be paplated and its size measured. The child's respiratory effort must also be assessed. Retractions, grunting, and nasal flaring may be apparent. Periorbital and peripheral edema may be present. Close monitoring of the peripheral pulses and capillary refill is extremely important.

Nursing Diagnosis and Planning

The following nursing diagnoses and expected outcomes may be appropriate following assessment of the child with shock.

- Altered Tissue Perfusion (cardiopulmonary, cerebral, and peripheral) related to decreased fluid volume (in hypovolemic shock), abnormal distribution of blood flow, metabolic acidosis, or both (in septic shock), or decreased cardiac contractility (in cardiogenic shock).
  Expected Outcome: The child will maintain adequate tissue perfusion as evidenced by strong peripheral pulses, appropriate skin turgor, normal capillary refill time, pink and warm mucous membranes and nail beds, vital signs within normal limits for age, and no evidence of dyspnea.
- Impaired Gas Exchange related to possible decreased pulmonary blood flow, increased interstitial fluid in alveoli, and inflammatory response of alveoli.
  Expected Outcome: The child will have adequate gas exchange as evidenced by oxygen saturation level between 95% and 100% and normal arterial blood gas measurements.
- Risk for Infection related to invasive venous and arterial lines, indwelling catheters, presence of endotracheal tube, and possible incisional wounds.
  Expected Outcome: The child will remain free from signs of infection.
- Anxiety and Fear related to the care of a critically ill child with a possible grave prognosis.
  Expected Outcome: The child and parent will express feelings, verbalize understanding of the condition, and demonstrate adequate coping skills.

Interventions

Interventions for the child experiencing shock are directed toward maintaining tissue perfusion, ensuring adequate oxygenation, preventing infection, and enhancing child and family coping.

Maintaining Tissue Perfusion

Careful and frequent observation of the child's cardiovascular status is essential. Take vital signs and check capillary refill every 1 to 2 hours. After establishing an adequate IV access, administer appropriate fluid replacement. Carefully document intake and output, and report urine output of less than 1 ml/kg/hr or any major discrepancy between intake and output. Weigh the child daily on the same scale. Report any rapid weight gain to the physician.

Because infants have high glucose requirements and low glycogen stores, alterations in glucose metabolism are frequently seen in response to stress. Monitor blood glucose levels every 2 to 4 hours.

Administer ordered medications by IV pump to ensure

appropriate delivery of medication. Because dobutamine and dopamine can cause tissue necrosis if infiltration occurs in peripheral tissues, these agents are preferably administered through a central line.

Ensuring Oxygenation

Observe and record respiratory rate and effort, skin color, chest expansion, and aeration. Note signs of respiratory distress and report them to the physician promptly. Administer oxygen as ordered, making sure the delivery mode is appropriate for the child's age. Monitor oxygen saturation, arterial blood gases, and hemoglobin levels. Maintain a patent airway and have emergency endotracheal intubation and ventilation equipment available.

Preventing Infection

Because children in a compromised state are prone to infection, maintain strict aseptic technique when handling IV lines, invasive tubes, and incisional or puncture sites. Closely monitor the child's temperature and report any rectal temperature greater than 38.5°C or 101.0°F. Observe secretions/body fluids, incisions, and puncture sites for erythema, edema, or purulence. Report positive blood culture results and elevated white blood cell counts promptly. Administer ordered antipyretics and ensure adequate caloric intake. If the child is unable to tolerate oral or nasogastric feedings, discuss alternative methods of feeding with the physician.

Enhancing Coping

Provide concise, accurate information to parents. Determine the child's developmental level and level of comprehension. Provide simple explanations of procedures before initiating them. Provide information in a calm, relaxed, and concerned manner. Answer all questions honestly. Be empathic.

Allow the child and parents to vent their feelings, concerns, and anxieties. Encourage the parents to participate in the child's care as appropriate (e.g., bathing, combing hair). This assistance provides them with some control. Be nonjudgmental in response to parents' actions. Use available resources (e.g., social worker, chaplain, or other family members) to help calm parents who are exhibiting uncontrolled feelings.

Elicit the parents' perceptions of the event and provided reassurance or clarify any misconceptions. Determine the availability of support systems and encourage their use. Help the parents to identify coping mechanisms that have been effective in the past and encourage parents to determine whether these mechanisms may be effective during the current crisis.

Evaluation

- Does the child demonstrate pink mucous membranes, brisk capillary refill, alertness, responsiveness, and normal vital signs for age?
- Is the oxygen saturation at least 95% on room air, and are blood gas values within normal limits?
- Does the child demonstrate a normal breathing rate and pattern?
- Is the child afebrile with negative culture results?

- Can the parents and child vent their feelings to staff or significant others?
- Is the family demonstrating decreased anxiety by using available resources and effective coping mechanisms?

■ Pediatric Trauma

Injury is the leading cause of death for young children between the ages of 1 and 4 years in the United States (Scholer, Mitchel, & Ray, 1997). Motor vehicle injuries are the leading cause of unintentional death in children younger than 19 years of age in the United States, followed by drownings, and fires (CDC, 1997a). The term *injury* is used in preference to *accident* when describing trauma because some trauma is not accidental and much of it is preventable.

Injury prevention and education can decrease the incidence of trauma in the pediatric population. Successful prevention and education steps include motor vehicle safety restraints, firearm education, bicycle helmet programs, safety caps and locked medications, and eliminating potential hazards, such as old refrigerators and unfenced pools. On discharge from the emergency department, the nurse provides injury prevention information to the families of all child victims of trauma. Injury prevention is also discussed at every well-child visit through adolescence (see Chapters 5 through 8).

Mechanism of Injury

Knowing the mechanism of injury helps to identify common injury patterns and predict patient needs and outcomes. Blunt or penetrating force causes tissue trauma. Blunt trauma is responsible for 87% of pediatric trauma (motor vehicle accidents and falls), whereas penetrating trauma (firearms, sharp penetrating objects) constitutes only 10% of injuries. The remaining mechanisms are categorized as submersion and other injuries (Gausche, 1995).

BLUNT TRAUMA
Injuries sustained from blunt trauma are often less apparent but can be more serious than those from penetrating trauma.

Motor Vehicle Trauma. A common cause of blunt trauma is acceleration–deceleration force, often from motor vehicle accidents or falls. Just before a motor vehicle collision, both the occupant and the vehicle are traveling at the same speed. When the vehicle meets an opposing force, the speed of both the occupant and the vehicle rapidly decelerate. When this change occurs, three collisions take place: the moving vehicle collides with the opposing object; the occupant's body collides with the interior portion of the vehicle; and the occupant's internal organs and tissues collide with rigid internal structures (Bernardo, 1998).

Unrestrained occupants in a motor vehicle accident have a higher incidence of injury than restrained occupants because they are tossed around the interior of the vehicle or are ejected at the point of collision. This principle applies also to children riding unrestrained in the back of open pickup trucks; they become missiles ejected out of the vehicle into oncoming traffic or onto the road. Children who are held on an adult's lap during a motor vehicle accident can be instantly crushed between the rigid part of the automobile and the moving adult.

Restraining devices in vehicles offer some protection but also have some consequences for the child. Because of differences in developmental anatomy, children can suffer injuries when placed in adult restraining mechanisms. Children 4 to 9 years of age have a shorter sitting height than adults, and a larger proportion of their bodies is located above the safety belt. This difference can cause more forward motion during impact and increase the potential for head injury from striking the dashboard (if the child is sitting in the front passenger seat). The child also can jackknife over a lap belt during impact, causing abdominal and high spinal cord injuries. An improperly fitting adult shoulder restraint might cross the child's face or neck, leading to potential airway injury.

Recently, childhood injuries and deaths have occurred as a result of air bag deployment. As of the beginning of 1998, 50 deaths had been reported from air bag use in the United States (CDC, 1998). Injury in small children from air bags occurs from impact with the dashboard near the air bag as well as from impact or displacement from the deployed air bag itself. The CDC advises that all children younger than 12 years of age be placed in rear seats in all cars, especially those with passenger air bags.

Pedestrian Injury. Pedestrian injuries in children are also a significant problem, with the largest number of incidences occurring in children 1 to 4 years of age (CDC, 1997a). Most of these injuries occur during the daylight hours as the child darts out into the middle of the street between parked cars or stands unnoticed behind a vehicle backing out of a driveway.

When a child is hit by a motor vehicle, a triad of injuries, referred to as Waddell's triad, occurs (Fig. 34–3). This one traumatic event results in three different types of injuries:

1. After being struck by the bumper and hood of the car, the child sustains abdominal or thoracic injuries.
2. The child is then propelled into the air, lands on the ground, and sustains femur or other leg injury.
3. As the child is propelled like a missile to the ground, the large size and weight of the child' s head results in skull fracture or closed head injury to the contralateral side of the head.

PENETRATING TRAUMA

Penetrating injury is produced when force from a penetrating object (e.g., a knife or bullet) is introduced into body tissue. Damage to the body tissue can result from the penetrating object itself and secondarily from radiating energy forces along the pathway of the penetrating object. The severity of an injury depends on the anatomic area penetrated, the length of the penetrating object, the type of gun and bullet, the distance from bullet to impact, and the angle of penetration (Bernardo & Kelley, 1994). With gunshot wounds, what might seem like a fairly innocuous wound can actually be very severe, depending on the amount of damage occurring after the initial penetration.

Multiple Trauma

A child with multiple trauma incurs injuries to more than one body system. A positive outcome for a child who has sustained multiple trauma depends on rapid assessment and intervention, which begins at the scene of the accident and continues through the trauma center emergency department, the critical care and acute care units, and the rehabilitation phase. Ideally, a critically injured child should be rapidly transported to a trauma facility with the personnel, equipment, and commitment to provide specialized care to children.

At the trauma center, and even in the emergency department of the community hospital, the presence of qualified trauma team members to assess and treat the trauma patient is crucial. A trauma team usually consists of skilled surgeons, physicians, nurses, social workers, and other health professionals, each with a specific role and duties during trauma resuscitation. The team usually assembles after notification of pending arrival by emergency personnel and readies the trauma room with personnel and equipment (e.g., emergency medications, endotracheal tubes, catheters, fluid warmer, and O-negative blood in the blood bank).

All patients with multiple trauma require a rapid, complete, and thorough assessment to determine injuries sustained. Assessment and intervention must proceed at the same time in the patient with trauma—the two cannot be separated. As with the ill child, assessment of a child with multiple trauma includes primary and secondary surveys.

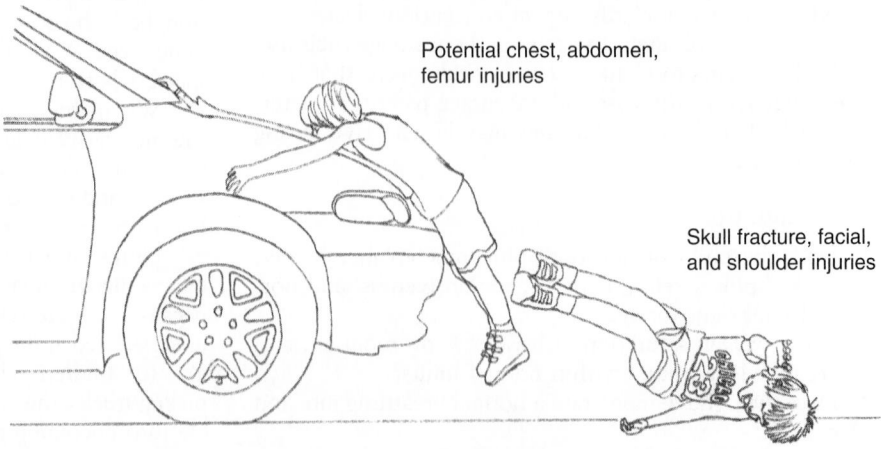

Potential chest, abdomen, femur injuries

Skull fracture, facial, and shoulder injuries

FIGURE 34–3
Waddell's triad of injuries.

PRIMARY SURVEY

The goal of the primary survey is to assess and manage life-threatening injuries. The primary assessment (see p. 876) proceeds with the following additions.

Airway Assessment and Management. The priority is to open and maintain the airway, using the jaw-thrust maneuver to prevent movement of the cervical spine. The nurse inspects for loose teeth or other potential obstruction. Because the child's lower airway is narrow and easily obstructed by edema and mucus, oral suctioning might be required to keep the airway clear (Gausche, 1995). A pediatric immobilization board secures a child when there is concern over spinal cord injury (Fig. 34–4). If a cervical collar is necessary, the correct size for maximum stability is used: the chin must rest securely in the chin holder, with the collar below the ears, and the lower end not extending below the upper part of the sternum. The cervical immobilization device and spinal immobilization device (long backboard) must remain in place until spinal injury has been ruled out.

In instances when a child is brought to the emergency setting in the car seat, the nurse places rolled towels on either side of the child's head and secures these with tape to maintain cervical immobilization without removing the child from the seat. If otherwise stable, the child can remain in the car seat until radiographs have shown there is no injury to the cervical spine.

Breathing Assessment and Management. Pulse oximetry readings are an adjunct to evaluating ventilation and adequate oxygenation. Because there are no contraindications to oxygen use in the child with multiple trauma, the nurse starts supplemental oxygen at a rate of 4 to 6 liters by nasal cannula or 10 to 12 liters by mask. Placing the cannula or mask on the child's face before starting the oxygen flow should avoid startling the child. If the child is alert and does not tolerate the mask, using blow-by oxygen with the tubing only, or using a plastic cup attached to the end of the tubing, might be less threatening to a child.

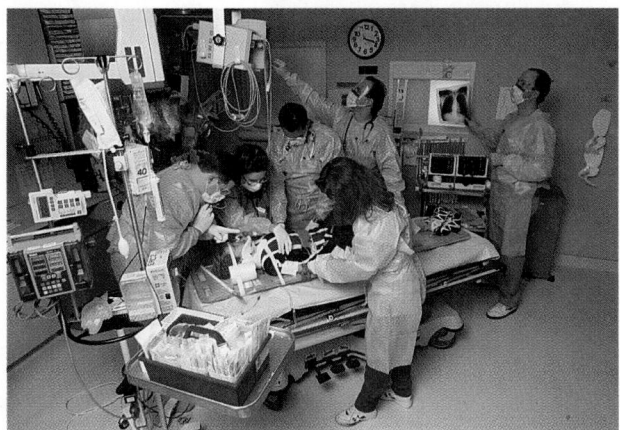

FIGURE 34–4

The child with multiple trauma injuries must remain on an immobilization board (long backboard) with a cervical immobilization device in place until being evaluated for spinal injuries. (Courtesy of Children's Medical Center, Dallas, Texas.)

If ventilation is inadequate or absent, the nurse begins to ventilate the child (as described on p. 877) using a bag-valve-mask with a reservoir and high-flow oxygen. Using an oropharyngeal or nasopharyngeal airway maintains patency in a child with altered consciousness, although airways should be used only for children older than 1 year of age and without signs of facial trauma (Gausche, 1995). When head injury is severe, a nasopharyngeal airway might cause further injury by entering the cranial vault during insertion.

Endotracheal intubation might be needed for airway control and oxygenation in children with altered level of consciousness, lack of spontaneous respirations, or severe head injury. The nurse hyperventilates the child before this procedure.

While observing the child for respiratory difficulty, the nurse checks the neck for jugular vein distension or tracheal deviation (the cervical collar can be opened for this assessment and then closed, keeping the neck in alignment). Because respiratory difficulty can be caused by chest injury, the nurse observes the chest for contusions, penetrations, abrasions, and paradoxical movement. A chest tube insertion or intervention for cardiac tamponade might be indicated for a penetrating chest injury.

Severe facial trauma, although rare in children younger than 5 years of age, can be life threatening, primarily because of the potential to obstruct ventilation—both fractures and soft tissue injury can cause narrowing of the airway. Facial trauma in children is treated as it is in adults. Nursing intervention includes ensuring an adequate airway and breathing, observing for possible progressive obstruction, and keeping the injured areas clean to prevent infection.

Circulation Assessment and Management. Cardiovascular assessment of the child focuses on early recognition and treatment of hypovolemia (Gausche, 1995). Blood loss in children is usually caused by internal abdominal or chest injury or severe injuries to the extremities. The early indicators of shock in children are tachycardia, increased capillary refill time (greater than 2 seconds), mottled skin, apprehension, pallor, and cool extremities. A decrease in blood pressure is a very late and ominous sign, indicating that the child is unable to compensate for the fluid loss. Decreased level of consciousness, dusky skin color, clammy extremities, bradycardia, and hypotension are late signs, indicating that cardiac arrest is imminent.

Cardiac monitoring and frequent cardiovascular assessments are necessary during the acute stage. During this stage, any external hemorrhage is noted and controlled, and intravenous or other access to the circulatory system is obtained.

The nurse assesses extremities for fractures and decreased peripheral circulation and splints any suspected fracture, assessing peripheral circulation after applying any splint. Assessment includes motor (can the child move the extremity? Is there pain?), circulatory (is there a pulse and good capillary refill?), and neural function (is sensation to the area intact? Is there any numbness or tingling in the extremity?). If neurovascular or circulatory compromise is present, immediate intervention is necessary.

Disability. During the primary survey phase a brief neurologic examination is performed, establishing level of consciousness along with pupillary size and reactivity and muscle movement. AVPU can assess mental status. Sudden changes such as agitation or somnolence might indicate hypoxia or decreased cerebral perfusion.

SECONDARY SURVEY

After exposing the child by removing all the child's clothing, the trauma staff carefully inspects and documents any and all signs of injury by performing the head-to-toe assessment and obtaining a history of the injury.

Obtaining a History of the Injury. Determination of the degree and severity of injuries is truly both an art and a science. Diagnosis depends on knowing the mechanism of injury as well as the presenting signs and symptoms. Nurses can obtain a comprehensive history by asking specific questions. Thorough assessment depends on a systematic trauma evaluation, which takes place along with life-saving intervention.

History of Injury Questions

FOR A VICTIM OF A MOTOR VEHICLE ACCIDENT

Was the child wearing a seat belt or in a child's car seat?
What was the type of seat belt (lap or lap and shoulder)?
What was the speed of the motor vehicle?
With what did the motor vehicle collide?
At what point on the motor vehicle was the location of impact?
Where was the victim seated in the motor vehicle?
How much damage was done to the motor vehicle?

FOR A VICTIM OF A FALL

How far did the child fall?
How did the child land (on what part of the body)?
On what type of ground did the child land?
Was the child's fall broken by any objects?

FOR A VICTIM OF A PENETRATING INJURY

How long and how wide was the blade of the knife?
How far away was the gun when it was fired?
What type of gun was used and what was the caliber of the gun?

Trauma Scoring Systems

TRAUMA SCORE (TS)

Adult scoring tool sometimes used with children.
Assesses respiratory rate and effort, blood pressure, and capillary refill.
Includes the Glasgow Coma Scale (GCS).

REVISED TRAUMA SCORE (RTS)

Comprises the GCS, blood pressure, and respiratory rate.

PEDIATRIC TRAUMA SCORE (PTS)

Adapted for the pediatric patient.
Assesses size, airway, central nervous system response, systolic blood pressure, open wounds, and skeletal fractures.

Trauma Scoring. Various kinds of scoring, performed and documented by on-site emergency medical personnel and nursing staff, are used as an objective measure of the severity of the injury caused by a traumatic event and, sometimes, to decide the facility most appropriate for treating the child. Most of the scoring systems are for the assessment of injury to adults and do not take the anatomic differences of children into account.

Assessing for Child Abuse. Child maltreatment can be a cause of injury. (See Chapter 53 for an in-depth discussion of child abuse.) Nurses working in emergency settings play an important role in both the assessment and reporting of child maltreatment. In acute care settings, there is rarely time to assess parent-child interactions or to observe at length the child's behavioral indicators, although these may provide important information. Some of the most important indicators that raise the suspicion of child maltreatment in the emergency setting include

* A history inconsistent with physical findings
* Activity reportedly leading to the trauma that seems inconsistent with the age of the child
* Delay in seeking treatment for the trauma
* A history of other emergency visits

Certain physical findings should also raise the level of suspicion:

* Bruises or fractures in various stages of healing noted on radiography
* Injuries rarely found in children (e.g., long bone or rib fractures) when the history is not appropriate for the injury
* Patterns of injury indicating that a specific object caused injury (e.g., belt marks, cigarette burns)

The nurse carefully assesses these indicators in the context of the injury and in relation to the affect of the child and family. The nurse also observes the family's reaction to the child and staff, keeping in mind that people behave very differently depending on culture, ethnicity, experience, and psychological makeup. Above all, health care providers do not assume an investigative role—that is law enforcement's responsibility. Nurses are required to report suspicion of child maltreatment, however, and so must be careful to document any observations in detail. It might help to remember that over 90% of parents who have abused their children feel ashamed of doing so but are unable to control the impulse. When child maltreatment is suspected, the intervention of child protective services is essential to ensure the safety of the child and to prevent additional injury.

NURSING CONSIDERATIONS

The Child and Family. The most critical aspect of nursing care of the child with traumatic injury is continuous assessment of respiratory and circulatory status. The nurse observes these children for the early signs of shock and intervenes immediately to prevent rapid and irreversible deterioration. Preparing for the many procedures and examinations required and observing the equipment used for monitoring should not interfere with close and continuous observation of the child's signs and symptoms.

Nursing care of the child also requires care of the family. When the family arrives at the hospital, one staff member should become the contact person and should provide regular updates. Family members should be allowed to be with the child as soon as possible, if they so desire. Even when the child is in critical condition, parents should be allowed in, however briefly, attended by a staff member who will be responsible for them. Hospital staff is often uncomfortable about parental presence in a critical situation, but all personnel agree that they would want to be there if it were their child. Remember that consent must be obtained from the families of patients for all procedures, unless the intervention is required to save the child's life.

The Child During Recovery. Regardless of the cause of the injury, most children with traumatic injury do well, unless the injuries are extremely severe. Their cardiovascular systems are strong and their bodies are growing, allowing them to compensate for even the most serious injuries. Even children with severe head injuries have far more favorable chances of recovery than do adults. These children and their families require nursing support to recover from both the physical and psychological effects of trauma; the need for rehabilitation must be considered from the moment the child arrives in the emergency setting.

Submersion Injuries (Near Drowning)

Submersion injury is the second leading cause of accidental death in children. *Drowning* is submersion that results in asphyxia and death within 24 hours. If the child survives longer than 24 hours after submersion, the event is referred to as *near drowning*.

One of the most important nursing responsibilities related to drowning is prevention of injury, including water safety education and training, support of legislative efforts to pass drowning prevention measures, and teaching of CPR. Nurses must emphasize the importance of adequate adult supervision when children are in or around water.

Etiology

Most drownings happen in residential swimming pools, although drownings can occur in any body of water, including hot tubs, spas, bathtubs, toilets, and even buckets. Open-water sites, such as lakes, rivers, and oceans, are more likely to be the site of accidents among teenagers. Alcohol is often a factor in teenage drownings because it alters judgment and increases risk-taking behaviors.

Incidence

Each year, approximately 1,600 children die in the United States from drowning. Near drowning accounts for three to four times as many injuries as drowning. The average age of approximately 40% of drowning victims is under 4 years. Boys are five times more likely than girls to die from drowning. Drowning is more likely to occur in the summertime, on weekends, and between 4 and 6 P.M., when adults are usually distracted by the dinner hour.

Manifestations

The child's condition after near drowning varies with the extent of injury. Five factors contribute to the child's eventual prognosis: (1) age, (2) submersion time, (3) elapsed time before resuscitation efforts are instituted, (4) neuro-

> ### PATHOPHYSIOLOGY
> ### of Submersion Injury
>
> Hypoxia causes the injury to organ systems when drowning occurs. Drowning progresses in a predictable sequence of events. Drowning victims panic, struggle, and attempt to hold their breath. In doing so, they begin to swallow water, which is then vomited and aspirated. This process can cause laryngospasm, which leads to hypoxia, seizures, and death (called *dry drowning* because laryngospasm prevents large amounts of water from entering the respiratory system). If the child becomes unconscious before laryngospasm, hypoxia causes loss of airway reflexes and subsequent aspiration of large amounts of water (leading to wet drowning). As hypoxia and acidosis progress, cardiopulmonary arrest occurs. Swallowing large amounts of fresh water also causes electrolyte shifts into the intracellular spaces, resulting in hyponatremia and cerebral edema.
>
> Submerged children lose body heat quickly in cold water because of their relatively large body surface area. Severe hypothermia offers some protection to the brain through the diving reflex, which is stimulated when the face is submerged in cold water. This neurologic reflex shunts blood away from the periphery, increasing blood flow to the brain and heart. The diving reflex is stronger in young children. Irreversible brain damage usually occurs after 4 to 6 minutes of submersion, but some children have had a complete recovery after lengthy submersion (10 to 40 minutes) in very cold water.

Parents react in many different ways, according to their cultures, religious beliefs, and individual personalities. Remember that denial can be protective initially, and allow the family to accept information gradually. Ask family members if they want other family members or clergy contacted. Religious rites, including baptism, may be very important to families. A list of clergy from a variety of religions should be readily available for use by the nursing staff.

Providing hope for the family is always important. At times, the only hope may be that the child is not suffering or did not suffer. If the child survives the incident, the parents will have ample time to adjust to the worst news, so it is not necessary to insist on their acceptance at this point. There have been many miraculous recoveries after lengthy submersions, although these are usually in very cold water. In the emergency setting, however, it is impossible to predict the ultimate outcome for a child. A realistically positive attitude, while acknowledging the strong possibility of long-term effects for the child, is the most reasonable approach.

Evaluation

- Has the child's neurologic status returned to its predrowning state?
- Does the child demonstrate adequate oxygenation (normal Po_2 and Pco_2) and independent breathing?
- Is the child's urine output greater than 1 to 2 ml/kg/hr?
- Do the parents verbalize their feelings and concerns appropriately?

▌ Ingestions and Poisonings

The combination of curiosity, lack of fear, and evolving motor ability place all children at risk for toxic exposure and ingestion. There are differences, however, in types of incident by age-group. Younger children (1 through 5 years of age) are indiscriminately curious, and can innocently ingest a toxic substance in a matter of seconds. As children grow, they gradually learn from parents to avoid dangerous substances, but accidental ingestions and exposures still can occur. In adolescence, the risk is higher for deliberate ingestion.

Incidence

The most common age for poisoning deaths in young children in the United States is 1 to 4 years of age. The largest number of deaths from poisonings is in the adolescent age group (15 to 19 years of age), with approximately 60% of the incidents deliberately intended (CDC, 1997a). Most poisonings occur as a result of oral ingestion. Ocular or topical exposure, inhalation, or envenomation account for the remainder of poisoning incidents. Young children most often ingest household products, plants, or medications such as acetaminophen (Tylenol), aspirin, vitamins, or minerals. Adolescents have a much higher incidence of ingestion of psychopharmacologic drugs (tranquilizers, sedatives, antidepressants).

Manifestations

Assessment and treatment of toxic exposure and ingestion go hand in hand. Although identification of the type and amount of the exposure is important, the child must initially be treated on the basis of physical signs and symptoms.

An accurate history of the ingestion is useful in planning care for the child. History given by the child, parent, friend, or caretaker might not always be accurate or complete—there are often areas of confusion as well as a reluctance to provide information that might be damaging to themselves or others. It can be helpful to interview all those involved individually if they are available. The information obtained in the history of the ingestion is combined with the child's presenting physical assessment to provide a complete picture of the event and to plan treatment. Laboratory analysis provides definitive diagnosis.

Most ingestions seen in emergency settings occur acutely, and the child is brought in immediately or when parents realize this event has occurred. An exception to this is lead poisoning. Although lead poisoning is relatively common, it is rarely identified in the emergency setting. A child who has unusual neurologic signs or symptoms, neuropathy, or anemia that cannot be attributed to other causes might have lead poisoning. This condition most often occurs when a child ingests or inhales paint chips or powder of lead-based paint. Other common sources of lead include dust or soil contaminated by emissions from lead smelters, some vinyl miniblinds, improperly glazed pottery, and paint from peeling walls or dust from remodeling in older buildings. A careful history can assist in the diagnosis of lead poisoning, but testing serum lead levels provides the only accurate diagnosis. The child usually is admitted to the hospital; chelation therapy, if needed, is administered on an inpatient basis to remove lead from the blood and tissue. When a child is found to have elevated lead levels, other children in the home should be tested as well because of the environmental nature of the ingestion.

Diagnostic Evaluation

Laboratory tests are performed to assess serum levels of the substance and the effect of the toxin on body systems. Regional poison control centers and clinical pharmacists should be included as members of the treatment team. The blood glucose level might be tested initially by means of a reagent strip. Measurement of serum glucose level and toxicologic analysis of urine, serum, and stomach contents are the most common laboratory tests ordered for toxic exposure or ingestion. Blood gases are required if the child is hypoventilating.

Therapeutic Management

The first step in treatment of a toxic exposure or ingestion is to assess ABCs and to stabilize the patient. Oxygen can be given and breathing supported with a bag-valve-mask device if necessary. If the child has an altered level of consciousness, endotracheal intubation may be necessary to protect the airway. When the child has ingested a sufficient amount of a substance to cause rapid deterioration in mental status, an intubation tray should be at the bedside even when the child is awake and alert. If the child is in shock or shows signs of compensated shock, IV fluid resuscitation is initiated. Cardiac rhythm disturbances can result from many ingested substances, so placement of a cardiac monitor and pulse oximeter are also indicated.

Care of the child who has been exposed to or ingested a toxic substance depends on the amount ingested and the toxicity of the ingested substance (Table 34–4). After ini-

TABLE 34-4
. . . .

Common Poisonous Substances

Substance	Pathophysiology	Clinical Manifestations	Treatment
Acetaminophen (Tylenol, many over-the-counter products)			
Toxic dose: Uncertain, do not exceed recommended levels. Seriousness of the ingestion is determined by the amount ingested and the length of time before intervention.	Metabolic byproducts deplete liver glutathione and cause damage to hepatic cells. Children younger than 6 years of age seem to be more resistant to development of hepatotoxicity than older children and adults.	*First stage* (first 24 hr): Malaise, nausea, vomiting, sweating, pallor, weakness. *Second stage* (24–48 hr): Latent period with a rise in liver enzymes (aspartate and alanine aminotransferase) and bilirubin, right upper quadrant pain, prolonged prothrombin time. *Third stage* (3–7 days): Jaundice, liver necrosis, possible death from hepatic failure. *Fourth stage* (5–7 days): Liver functions begin to normalize in the recovering child.	Induce vomiting or gastric lavage within 1 hour of ingestion, depending on amount ingested. Administer activated charcoal or antidote: acetylcysteine (Mucomyst) as ordered. IV fluids. Sodium-restricted, high-calorie, high-protein diet.
Salicylates (Aspirin, many over-the-counter products, oil of wintergreen)			
Toxic dose: Single dose exceeding 200–280 mg/kg. Peak gastric absorption occurs within 2 hr of ingestion.	*First stage:* Stimulation of respiratory center, leading to respiratory alkalosis. *Second stage:* Loss of potassium, increase in metabolic rate, and accumulation of ketones leading to metabolic acidosis, hypokalemia, and dehydration. Inhibition of prothrombin formation, decreased platelet levels and adhesiveness, and capillary fragility (chronic poisoning).	GI effects: Nausea, vomiting, thirst. CNS effects: Hyperventilation, tinnitus, confusion, seizures, coma, respiratory failure, circulatory collapse. Renal effects: Oliguria. Hematopoietic effects: Bleeding tendencies. Metabolic effects: Sweating, dehydration, fever, hyponatremia, hypokalemia, dehydration, hypoglycemia.	Induce vomiting with syrup of ipecac or perform gastric lavage; administer activated charcoal to decrease absorption. IV fluids, sodium bicarbonate (which enhances excretion), potassium replacement; volume expanders as needed to support circulation. Vitamin K for bleeding tendencies (chronic poisoning). Glucose for hypoglycemia. Hemodialysis in severe cases if child unresponsive to therapy.
Corrosives (Toilet and drain cleaners, bleach, ammonia)			
Extent of damage depends on the causticity of the substance and the amount ingested.	Severe chemical burns of mouth, throat, esophagus. Alkali substances can continue to cause damage after initial contact. If damage is severe, long-term care is needed, including repeated esophageal dilatations and surgical repair of esophagus, sometimes with colon tissue transplant (done when child is older).	Whitish burns of mouth and pharynx, color darkens (red, swollen, and oozing as ulcerations form and tissue erodes). Edema, difficulty swallowing, drooling. Respiratory distress, pain. Difficulty swallowing; subsequent healing of burns can produce esophageal strictures. Severe burns causing perforation can lead to vascular collapse and shock.	Do not induce vomiting: do not lavage. Activated charcoal may be given. Dilute with small amounts of water or milk (take care not to stimulate vomiting). Flood external areas with large amount of water. Endoscopy to diagnose esophageal burns. Possible gastrostomy, possible esophageal dilatations to prevent strictures and to maintain patency of esophagus. IV fluids while NPO. Analgesics, steroids, antibiotics, nasogastric tube feedings.

Table continued on following page

TABLE 34–4

. . . .

Common Poisonous Substances Continued

Substance	Pathophysiology	Clinical Manifestations	Treatment
Hydrocarbons (Gasoline, kerosene, paint thinner, lighter fluid, turpentine, furniture polish)			
	Chemical pneumonitis from aspiration of hydrocarbon. Pneumonia and acute hemorrhagic necrotizing disease, usually in 24 hr.	Burning sensation in mouth and pharynx. Characteristic petroleum breath odor. Nausea, vomiting, anorexia, CNS depression, fever.	Do not induce vomiting. Support ventilation; administer oxygen. IV fluids.
Lead (Paint chips, soil contaminated with lead, lead solder used in plumbing, vinyl miniblinds, improperly glazed pottery)			
Diet high in fat and low in iron and calcium increases lead absorption. Serum lead level >10 μg/dl are considered harmful. 10–15 μg/dl: more frequent screening indicated; 15–20 μg/dl: nutritional and educational interventions and environmental investigation; >20 μg/dl: possible removal and treatment.	GI tract is the major route of absorption. Lead is deposited in the blood, bone, and soft tissue. Major toxic effects occur in the bone marrow, nervous system, and kidney. Amount of lead ingested, size of the particle, and repeated ingestion over time contribute to severity of lead poisoning.	Symptoms may be vague with insidious onset. CNS effects: irritability, lethargy, hyperactivity, cognitive and perceptual-motor difficulties, clumsiness, seizures, coma, and death (associated with blood level of 100 μg/dl). Hematopoietic effects: anemia. GI effects: anorexia, nausea, vomiting, constipation, lead line along gums. Skeletal effects: increased density of long bones, lead line in long bones. Renal effects: glycosuria, proteinuria, possible acute or chronic renal failure. Kidney damage is reversible early in the disease, but with continued lead exposure, permanent kidney damage may occur.	>25 μg/dl: remove child from lead source, hospitalize if level is significantly higher. Administer chelating agents: succimer orally for lead level of 35–45 μg/dl; EDTA for level >70 μg/dl given IV over several hours for 5 days (causes lead to be deposited in bone and excreted by kidneys); bronchoalveolar lavage every 4 hours for six doses for level >70 μg/dl. Monitor kidney function because EDTA is nephrotoxic; monitor calcium levels because EDTA enhances excretion of calcium. Provide adequate hydration. Calcium, phosphorus, and vitamins C and D. Anticonvulsants. Oral or intramuscular iron for anemia. Follow-up lead levels to monitor progress (lead is excreted more slowly than it accumulates in the body).
Carbon Monoxide			
Most often from improperly ventilated heaters; also from poorly ventilated vehicles. The cause of the exposure should be determined and eliminated.	An odorless, colorless gas that binds to receptors on hemoglobin more effectively than does oxygen, thereby causing hypoxia.	Headache, visual disturbances. Altered level of consciousness, cherry-red lips and cheeks, nausea, and vomiting.	100% oxygen by rebreathing mask. Serum carboxyhemoglobin levels, hyperbaric chamber treatment may be necessary for patients with high carboxyhemoglobin levels. Other interventions are based on signs and symptoms.

CNS, central nervous system; EDTA, ethylenediaminetetraacetic acid; GI, gastrointestinal; IV, intravenous.

tial stabilization, removing the poison or preventing its absorption is the primary goal. Several methods frequently used to treat toxic ingestions include dilution of the toxin, administration of syrup of ipecac, administration of activated charcoal, and gastric lavage.

DILUTING THE TOXIN

Administering water or milk can dilute the toxic effects of acid or alkali ingestion. These substances, when ingested, can cause burning of tissue along the gastrointestinal tract. Because these caustic substances continue to cause damage until neutralized, inducing emesis is contraindicated.

SYRUP OF IPECAC

There is an ongoing controversy about the value of syrup of ipecac in the treatment of acute poison ingestion. Ipecac produces vomiting and rapid stomach emptying. Emesis occurs approximately 20 to 30 minutes after ipecac is administered and might last for several hours. Because of its potentially prolonged period of gastric emptying, ipecac's effects can delay administration of activated charcoal, which is used to bind chemicals and toxins to its surface (West, 1997; Krenzelok, 1996). Ipecac should be followed with 6 to 12 ounces of clear fluid.

Ipecac is available without prescription and should be cautiously administered to any child younger than 1 year of age. Ipecac is most useful in the home, when a poison ingestion is recognized and treated before enough time has elapsed for significant absorption. Ipecac should not be administered without prior advice from a poison control center. The box on page 123 discusses the usual dosage of ipecac for infants and children. Contraindications to ipecac use include

- Decreased level of consciousness
- Ingestion of corrosive or petroleum-based substance
- Ingestion of drugs that result in rapid deterioration of mental status

GASTRIC LAVAGE

Gastric lavage is used for gastric emptying in the first 1 to 2 hours after the ingestion. This method is selected when the toxic ingestion has potentially serious complications such as seizures, decreased level of consciousness, respiratory depression, and cardiac effects. Because of the danger of esophageal perforation, lavage should not be used after ingestion of corrosive substances. The nurse places the child on the left side, with the head lowered approximately 10 degrees in the Trendelenburg position. Depending on the size of the child, a 24- to 40-French orogastric tube is inserted. In comatose children, endotracheal intubation is recommended before beginning gastric lavage (Krenzelok, 1996). To prevent electrolyte disturbances, younger children are lavaged with normal saline or half normal saline. The nurse observes the returned fluid for any pill fragments or toxic substance, sends a specimen of lavage fluid to the laboratory for analysis, and administers activated charcoal after completion of the lavage process.

ACTIVATED CHARCOAL

Activated charcoal is a charcoal substance with a porous surface that binds to the toxin and passes through the gas-

trointestinal system. Activated charcoal has become the recommended treatment for acute poisonings in the pediatric population, particularly for incidents where identification of the poison is delayed. Activated charcoal can bind to the toxin at any point along the gastrointestinal tract. The longer the time between activated charcoal administration and the time the toxin was ingested, however, the less effective it will be. If the child has received ipecac, ongoing vomiting can delay administration and retention of activated charcoal.

Administering activated charcoal is a nursing challenge because the substance is unpalatable in both taste and appearance to young children. Mixing the activated charcoal with chocolate milk or other flavoring sometimes makes it easier to drink. Placing the charcoal in a covered opaque or decorated container prevents the child from seeing the substance while drinking (West, 1997). Often, children refuse to drink the activated charcoal, and it must be administered by nasogastric tube. Activated charcoal administration might be repeated to prevent reabsorption of the toxin from fluid secreted in the biliary tract. The dosage is usually 1 to 2 g/kg in children.

ANTIDOTES

Specific antidotes can be used to inhibit the absorption of the toxin at the receptor site or reduce the concentration. Examples of commonly used antidotes are acetylcysteine (Mucomyst) for acetaminophen ingestion and naloxone for narcotics (see Table 34–4).

NURSING CARE
· · · · · · · · · ·
The Child Who Has Ingested a Toxic Substance

Assessment

Accurate and rapid assessment of the poisoned child can mean the difference between life and death. Assess ABCs. Take frequent vital signs. Initiate respiratory or circulatory support as needed. Because shock is a result of ingestion of many toxic substances, blood pressure, tissue perfusion, and urine output are carefully monitored. Observe and document the child's mental status frequently to determine any changes in level of consciousness. Assess changes in pupil size or reactivity as well as occurrence of seizures.

The nurse needs to take the responsibility for assessing the cause of poisoning. A poisoning incident is extremely

---

CRITICAL TO REMEMBER
· · · · · · · ·
Assessment of Poison Ingestion

Obtain information about the following:

- Substance ingested, if known
- Amount ingested
- Approximate time of ingestion
- Change in the child's condition
- Treatment administered at home

distressing to parents. Defer detailed questioning until the child's condition is stabilized. If the ingestion was purposeful, psychological consultation and referral should be provided.

Nursing Diagnosis and Planning

The following diagnoses apply to the child and family:

- Risk for Injury related to insufficient parental knowledge about first aid for toxic ingestion and accidental poisonings.
  Expected Outcome: The child will receive appropriate treatment by parents if accidental poisoning occurs.
- Ineffective Breathing Pattern related to effects of toxic substances.
  Expected Outcome: The child will maintain adequate oxygenation and ventilation as evidenced by normal arterial blood gases and serum pH or pulse oximetry.
- Risk for Fluid Volume Deficit related to effects of ingested substances, treatment modalities, or decreased fluid intake.
  Expected Outcome: The child will maintain a urine output of 1 to 2 ml/kg/hr, with age-appropriate specific gravity.
- Ineffective Family Coping related to sudden hospitalization and emergency aspects of illness.
  Expected Outcomes: The family will demonstrate an understanding of the child's condition and treatment, appropriately verbalize feelings and concerns, and remain with the child as much as possible.
- Risk for Poisoning related to insufficient parental knowledge about poisoning prevention.
  Expected Outcomes: The parent makes the necessary changes in the home environment to prevent future poisoning.

Interventions

Stabilizing the child is the nurse's priority in caring for the child who has ingested a poisonous substance. Nursing care also includes reducing the child's and the family's fear and anxiety, providing preventive teaching concerning the storage of poisons and supervision of children, and removal of the poison from the child's skin and mucous membranes to reduce further injury.

Parents usually are overwhelmed by feelings of self-blame, fear, and anger when their child has ingested a poisonous substance. Providing an opportunity for them to express their feelings in a nonjudgmental atmosphere helps parents cope with this experience. Aspects of treatment such as induction of vomiting, placement of a nasogastric tube, or support of ventilation are disturbing and frightening to parents. Offer support by explaining treatment and keeping the parents informed about the status of their child.

Ideally, nurses intervene with parents before a poisoning incident occurs. Discussion of safe storage of medications and other potentially toxic substances as well as age-appropriate supervision of children are essential aspects of poison prevention. Instruct the parent to keep one dose of syrup of ipecac for each child under age 5 years available in the home and to be familiar with its use and proper dosage. Advise the parent to post the poison control phone number clearly and to call the poison center before treating

the child. This and other injury prevention information should be readily available in emergency care settings and should be given to families when a child is discharged. Education through community programs to prevent poisoning and reduce drug abuse should be directed to young children as well as to adolescents, parents, and caretakers.

Evaluation

- Do parents verbalize common household hazards that can result in child poisoning?
- Are preventive measures in place in the home?
- Is the appropriate amount of ipecac available in the home?
- Do parents verbalize the appropriate actions to take when a child has been poisoned?

Animal, Human, and Snake Bites

Etiology

ANIMAL AND HUMAN BITES

Both animal and human bites involve soft tissue damage from crushing, lacerations, and puncture wounds. All animal bites have potential for infection. Although human bites are relatively rare, they carry the greatest risk of infection if they break the skin, particularly if they are on the scalp, face, hands, wrists, or feet. Serious injury can result from any type of bite, but most dog bites are not life threatening.

SNAKE BITES

Envenomations of children on land are usually from snakes, scorpions, and spiders. Envenomation can also result from marine animals such as jellyfish, sea urchins, and stingrays. Fatalities from envenomation are rare; most occur from snakebites.

Incidence

Animal bites in the pediatric age-group are most often from domestic animals and have the highest incidence in school-age male children (Weiss, Friedman, & Coben, 1998; Gershman, Sacks, & Wright, 1994; Sinclair & Zhou, 1995). Most bites are from dogs, usually a dog familiar to the victim (Wiggins, Akelman, & Weiss, 1994). Larger dogs can cause serious damage. Chows, Dobermans, German shepherds, pit bulls, and Rottweilers have all caused serious bite injuries to children (Gershman, Sacks, & Wright, 1994).

Cats are the most common family pets, and although a cat bite is less likely to cause serious injury initially, it is more likely to become infected than a dog bite. Bites from pet birds, rats, ferrets, pigs, hamsters, turtles, fish, alligators, snakes, horses, and many other animals have been seen in emergency settings, as have varieties of wild animals such as raccoons, skunks, coyotes, and others.

In the United States, the two groups of poisonous snakes are pit vipers (Crotalidae)—such as rattlesnakes, water moccasins, and copperheads—and coral snakes (Elapidae). Each year 45,000 snakebites are reported, and fewer than 20% of these are from venomous snakes (Gold & Wingert, 1994). Almost half (45%) of the bites from venomous snakes are dry bites, delivering no venom (Gold & Wingert, 1994). Annually, 9 to 15 fatalities, mostly children and the elderly, occur from snakebites (Gold & Wingert, 1994).

Manifestations

ANIMAL BITES

Because of the risk of infection, human bites are more serious and can be differentiated from dog bites by the distance between the canines; in human bites the distance is generally greater than 3 cm. A human bite is horseshoe shaped and rarely breaks the skin (Kelley, 1994).

SNAKE BITES

To determine the cause of envenomation, medical staff in emergency settings should have some knowledge of the venomous snakes likely to be encountered in the surrounding geographic area.

Regardless of whether the snake can be positively identified, treatment should be based on physical assessment and symptoms. These local signs and symptoms are the most common signs and symptoms suggesting envenomation:

- Bite marks that look like fang marks
- Burning at the site
- Ecchymosis
- Pain or numbness
- Swelling and erythema

These systemic signs and symptoms suggest severe envenomation:

- Nausea and vomiting
- Sweating, chills
- Numbness, paresthesia of the tongue and perioral region
- Hypotension

Systemic signs and symptoms can develop within 15 minutes of severe envenomation. When a substantial amount of venom has been injected and when treatment is delayed, envenomation can progress to disseminated intravascular coagulation, respiratory failure, renal failure, seizures, shock, and death.

Therapeutic Management

ANIMAL BITES

Emergency care for animal bites depends on the type of bite but usually includes thorough irrigation and débridement. Tetanus prophylaxis is given if the child's immunization is not up to date or if documentation is unavailable. Antibiotics are prescribed if there is a high probability of infection. Smaller bite wounds are often left open, rather than sutured, because puncture wounds and wounds closed with sutures have more potential for infection. Treatment of the child for rabies might be necessary, depending on the specifics of the situation.

SNAKE BITES

Three factors influence the severity of bite from a venomous snake:

1. Age, size, and general health of the victim
2. Size of the snake (larger snakes produce more venom)
3. Location of the injury (peripheral injuries account for 90% of the bites and are less severe)

When assessing the patient with a snakebite, identification of the type of snake is helpful, but this is not always possible. In most cases, an expert in the treatment of snake bites should be consulted. Although traditional emergency treatment of envenomation once included use of a tourniquet, incision, and extraction of the venom, these measures are no longer recommended (Gold & Wingert, 1994). First aid now includes immobilization of the extremity in a position below the level of the heart and prompt administration of sufficient quantities of antivenin. Snake venom is absorbed through the lymph system; thus, decreasing the child's activity aids in decreasing the systemic spread of the venom.

An intravenous line should be established if envenomation is suspected, for administration of antivenin and possible fluid resuscitation. When no signs or symptoms of envenomation appear within 4 hours of the bite, it can be considered a dry bite. For mild envenomation (fang marks and local swelling), the child is observed and may or may not be given antivenin. Moderate to severe envenomations will require antivenin. To assess hypersensitivity, a small test dose of antivenin is given intradermally before the full dose. All patients with venomous bites are admitted to the hospital. Laboratory studies include CBC, platelet count, coagulation studies, electrolytes, and renal function.

NURSING CARE
The Child with Animal, Human, or Snake Bite

With severe bites, significant envenomation, or anaphylaxis, nursing interventions for bites and envenomations begin with attention to the ABCs and support of vital functions. With envenomation, nursing care includes keeping the patient as calm as possible to help prevent spread of the toxin or venom. Few hospitals have sufficient antivenin for severe envenomation, so nurses should make sure that available protocols include the location of centers to contact for additional antivenin.

Carefully clean the injury site of all bites and give tetanus prophylaxis if immunizations are not up to date. When the bite or envenomation is located on an extremity, immobilize the extremity. Remove any jewelry on the affected digit or extremity immediately. As swelling occurs, the jewelry might be constricting and have to be cut off or bent during removal.

If antivenin is to be administered, obtain a careful history of allergies because some antivenins are made from horse serum. Document the type and location of the injury, the length of time since the injury, and the signs and symptoms resulting from the injury.

The cause of any bite should be carefully explored. Questions include inadequate supervision or inadequate containment of potentially dangerous animals. When the injury appears to be a human bite, child abuse or neglect should be considered a possibility and reported when necessary.

In most states, notification of the local animal control agency is required for animal bites. Document rabies immunization status of the animal, if available, in nursing notes. Quarantine of the animal responsible for the attack might be necessary if the animal can be found.

Discharge instructions should include observation for signs and symptoms of infection and wound care. Provide injury prevention education to all families. Give parents information about how to teach their children to avoid dog bites.

Dental Emergencies

Incidence and Etiology

Injury to the teeth, particularly the anterior teeth, is common in children. Toddlers, because of their lack of coordination, receive dental injuries from falling from or onto furniture. School-age children are more likely to have their teeth injured on playgrounds and in the course of sports activities. The first teeth begin to erupt at approximately 6 months of age. By approximately 2 years of age, a child has all 20 primary teeth. Permanent teeth come in at approximately 5 or 6 years of age. By adolescence, a child usually has the full complement of 32 permanent teeth, although the eruption of wisdom teeth might be somewhat delayed. Injury to primary and permanent teeth is considered equally serious. Teeth are imbedded in the bones of the maxilla and mandible. Injuries to teeth are usually divided into the following categories:

Concussion	Tooth is not displaced, but pressure may cause pain.
Subluxation	The tooth is moveable within the socket but is displaced less than 2 mm. There is no damage to the socket.
Intrusion	The tooth is pushed into its socket with injury to the underlying structures.
Extrusion	An upper tooth is dislodged downward from the socket, or a lower tooth is dislodged upward.
Luxation	Lateral movement of the tooth with tearing of the periodontal ligament.
Avulsion	The tooth is no longer in the socket, and the socket itself might be damaged.

Therapeutic Management

Dental emergencies require specialized care, which is often difficult to obtain immediately. Survival of the tooth depends on the periodontal ligament attachment, so concussion, subluxation, lateral luxation, and extrusion, in which the periodontal ligament is still attached, have a better prognosis than complete avulsion of a tooth. Intrusion of a tooth might damage underlying structures to a greater extent and diminish chances for tooth survival.

Time is of the essence in caring for dental injuries.

With injury to a child's mouth, the nurse observes for missing teeth. If a missing tooth cannot be found in the oral cavity, possible aspiration should be considered (especially when the child has difficulty breathing); radiographs might be needed to determine the location of the tooth. To determine whether other teeth are loose or malpositioned, the nurse gently palpates (using standard infection precautions) the teeth for movement. If a tooth is loose in the socket, it should not be removed. If the position is not correct, repositioning may be necessary when a specialist is available.

In general, primary teeth are not replanted because damage to the developing tooth bud can occur. Complete avulsion of a permanent tooth requires care of the socket and of the tooth itself. Survival of an avulsed tooth depends to a large extent on the length of time it is out of the mouth. Irreversible damage to the periodontal ligament due to dehydration of the open socket may occur after 60 minutes.

Emergency care by the dentist includes cleaning of the tooth and socket, placement of the tooth in the socket, and splinting of the tooth. Tetanus immunization is given if needed, and an antibiotic may be prescribed.

NURSING CARE
The Child with a Dental Emergency

Parents calling for emergency advice should be instructed to keep the tooth moist in the child's mouth if possible (in front of the lower incisors or under the tongue, for instance). Alternatively, the tooth can be kept in the parent's mouth. If this is not possible, the tooth may be immersed in saline, water, or milk. The teeth should not be cleaned or scrubbed. Although some recommend replacing the tooth in the socket immediately, a parent might replace the tooth backwards, or the tooth or socket may not be clean or free of debris or clots; these problems would decrease the chances of tooth survival. The child should see a dentist, if possible, or should go to an emergency facility for care without delay.

Parents should be given careful discharge instructions and appropriate referrals for continuing care. When appropriate, reassure the family that first teeth are replaced by the second set of teeth and that there are many ways to ensure a good cosmetic outcome, even with loss of a permanent tooth.

KEY CONCEPTS

- Because of children's smaller sizes, the different equipment and dosages needed for their care, and age-related psychological differences, nursing care of ill and injured children may seem more complicated than care of adults.
- Familiarity with the issues related to growth and development of the child, continuing education in pediatric emergency care, and careful organization of pediatric equipment, supplies, referrals, and reference lists can help to decrease anxiety in health care providers and improve the care of children in emergency settings.
- Airway management is the most critical element in pediatric emergency care. Emergency assessment and triage should include airway assessment and intervention. Without adequate oxygenation and ventilation, patients have little hope of survival.
- Shock must be recognized early in the pediatric patient and should always be considered a possibility when the heart rate increases, breathing increases, or changes occur in color, temperature, or moisture of the infant's or child's skin.
- Care of the family and developmental stage of the child should always be considered when providing nursing interventions in the emergency setting. The parents' reactions and the child's developmental factors affect compliance, cooperation, and anxiety levels.
- Trauma assessment of the pediatric patient includes the standard primary and secondary survey and intervention but must also include assessment of skin signs, use of appropriate age-related tools for determining the level of consciousness, and prevention of or intervention for hypothermia.
- Injury prevention plays an important role in the nursing care of children. Motor vehicle injuries, submersion injuries, ingestions, and poisonings are largely preventable. Nurses can play an important role in offering anticipatory guidance and in providing injury prevention materials and instruction to children and their families.

ANSWERS TO CRITICAL THINKING EXERCISE 34–1

1. First assess level of consciousness and ABCs. Initiate appropriate resuscitation if necessary. If the child is conscious and alert, observe her mouth carefully, being sure not to touch it without appropriate barrier protection.
2. If a tooth is missing, ask for help finding it. When it is found, your primary goal is to keep it moist to enhance eventual reimplantation. Asking the child to put the tooth back in her mouth in the space between the bottom lip and lower teeth is appropriate, so long as there is no danger the child will aspirate the tooth. Do not try to replace the tooth in the socket. Alternatively, if there is no source of liquid readily available, wrapping the tooth in a wet handkerchief is also an acceptable way of transporting it. Advise that the child be seen by dental personnel within 2 hours.

REFERENCES AND READINGS

Bartacherer, D. (1997). Syrup of ipecac: Appropriate use in the emergency department. *Journal of Emergency Nursing, 23*(3), 251–253.

Bernardo, L. (1996). Parent-reported injury-associated behaviors and life events among injured, ill, and well preschool children. *Journal of Pediatric Nursing, 11*(2), 100–109.

Bernardo, L. (1998). Multiple trauma. In M. Slota (Ed.), *Core curriculum for pediatric critical care nursing* (pp. 551–594). Philadelphia: Saunders.

Bernardo, L., & Kelley, S. (1994). Care of the multiply injured child. In S. Kelley (Ed.), *Pediatric emergency nursing* Norwalk, CT: Appleton & Lange.

Bernardo, L., & Schenkel, K. (1995). Pediatric medical emergencies. In S. Kitt, J. Selfridge-Thomas, J. Proehl, & J. Kaiser (Eds.), *Emergency nursing: A physiologic and clinical perspective* (2nd ed.). Philadelphia: Saunders.

Bernardo, L., & Trunzo, R. (1995). Pediatric trauma. In S. Kitt, J. Selfridge-Thomas, J. Proehl, & J. Kaiser (Eds.), *Emergency nursing: A physiologic and clinical perspective* (2nd ed.). Philadelphia: Saunders.

Beyda, D. (1998). Childhood submersion injuries. *Journal of Emergency Nursing, 24*(2), 140–143.

Brownstein, D., & Rivara, F. (1996). Emergency medical services for children. In W. Nelson, R. Behrman, R. Kliegman, & A. Arvin (Eds.), *Nelson textbook of pediatrics* (15th ed., pp. 232–239). Philadelphia: Saunders.

Callow, L., Suddaby, E., & Slota, M. (1998). Cardiovascular system. In M. Slota (Ed.), *Core curriculum for pediatric critical care nursing* (pp. 144–196). Philadelphia: Saunders.

Centers for Disease Control and Prevention. (1997a). Recommended framework for presenting injury mortality data. *Morbidity and Mortality Weekly Report*, (RR-14), 11.

Centers for Disease Control and Prevention. (1997b). Toy-related injuries among children and teenagers: U.S., 1996. *Morbidity and Mortality Weekly Report, 46*(50), 1186–1189.

Centers for Disease Control and Prevention. (1998). National child passenger safety week: February 8–14, 1998. *Morbidity and Mortality Weekly Report, 47*(3), 59–60.

Chameides, L. (Ed.). (1994). *Textbook of pediatric advanced life support.* Dallas: American Heart Association.

Coburn, M., & Pfeifer, J. (1995). Nonoperative management of splenic and hepatic trauma in the multiply injured pediatric and adolescent patient. *Archives of Surgery, 130*(3), 328–338.

Coffman, S., Martin, V., & Prill, N. (1998). Perceptions, safety behaviors, and learning needs of parents of children brought to an emergency department. *Journal of Emergency Nursing, 24*(2), 133–138.

Cosby, C. (1998). Pediatric emergencies. In L. Newberry (Ed.), *Sheehy's emergency nursing: Principles and practice* (4th ed.). St. Louis: Mosby.

Emergency Nurses Association. (1995). *Emergency Nurses Association policy statement.* Park Ridge, IL: Author.

Finberg, L. (1998). Poisonings and environmental hazards. In L. Finberg (Ed.), *Saunders manual of pediatric practice* (pp. 1017–1024). Philadelphia, PA: Saunders.

Gausche, M. (1995). Pediatric trauma. In J. Siedel & D. Henderson (Eds.), *Pre-hospital care of pediatric patients*. Boston: Jones & Bartlett.

Gershman, K. A., Sacks, J. J., & Wright, J. C. (1994). Which dogs bite? A case-control study of risk factors. *Pediatrics, 93*(6 Pt), 913–917.

Giguere, J., St-Vil, D., Turmel, A., DiLorenzo, M., Pothel, C., Manseau, S., & Mercier, C. (1998). Airbags and children: A spectrum of C-spine injuries. *Journal of Pediatric Health Care, 12*(3), 130–138.

Gold, B. S., & Wingert, W. A. (1994). Snake venom poisoning in the United States: A review of therapeutic practice [see comments]. *Southern Medical Journal, 87*(6), 579–589.

Haller, J., Papa, P., Drugas, G., & Colombani, P. (1994). Nonoperative management of solid organ injuries in children: Is it safe? *Annals of Surgery, 219*(6), 625–631.

Henderson, D., & Brownstein, D. (1994). *Pediatric emergency nursing manual*. New York: Springer.

Huston, C. (1997). Dental luxation and avulsion. *American Journal of Nursing, 97*(9), 48.

Huston, C. (1998). Cervical spine injury. *American Journal of Nursing, 98*(6), 33.

Kaplan, S., & Davis, S. (1999). Septic shock. In F. Burg, E. Wald, J. Ingelfinger, & R. Polin (Eds.), *Gellis and Kagan's current pediatric therapy* (16th ed.). Philadelphia: Saunders.

Kelley, S. (1994). *Pediatric emergency nursing* (2nd ed.). Norwalk, CT: Appleton & Lange.

Kitt, J., Selfridge-Thomas, J., Proehl, J., & Kaiser, J. (1995). *Emergency nursing: A physiologic and clinical perspective* (2nd ed.). Philadelphia: Saunders.

Klinkhammer, B., & Andreoni, C. (1998). *Quick reference for emergency nursing*. Philadelphia: Saunders.

Krenzelok, E. (1996). Acute poisonings. In F. Burg, E. Wald, J. Ingelfinger, & R. Polin (Eds.), *Gellis and Kagan's current pediatric therapy* (15th ed.). Philadelphia: Saunders.

Lanphear, B., Byrd, R., Auinger, P., & Schaffer, S. (1998). Community characteristics associated with elevated blood lead levels in children. *Pediatrics, 101*(2), 264–270.

Martinez, K., & Moore-Koehler, K. (1997). Poisoning and toxic effects of drugs: A critical pathway for improving outcomes. *Pediatric Nursing, 23*(6), 609–612.

McGrath, N. (1996). Head injury. In J. Seidel & D. Henderson (Eds.), *Prehospital care of the pediatric emergencies*. Boston: Jones & Bartlett.

Nadkarni, V. (1997). ILCOR advisory statements: Pediatric resuscitation. *Circulation, 95*, 2185–2195.

Newberry, L. (Ed.). (1998). *Sheehy's emergency nursing: Principles and practice* (4th ed.). St. Louis: Mosby.

O'Rourke, P. (1996). Shock. In R. Behrman, P. Kliegman, & A. Arvin (Eds.), *Nelson textbook of pediatrics* (15th ed., pp. 263–264). Philadelphia: Saunders.

Roddy, S., et al. (1998). Minimal head trauma in children revisited: Is routine hospitalization required? *Pediatrics, 101*(4), 575–577.

Rosenthal-Dichter, C. (1998). Septic shock. In M. Slota (Ed.), *Core curriculum for pediatric critical care nursing* (pp. 627–651). Philadelphia: Saunders.

Royall, J. (1998). Cardiogenic shock/hypertensive crisis. In L. Finberg (Ed.), *Saunders manual of pediatric practice* (pp. 604–607). Philadelphia: Saunders.

Scholer, S., Mitchel, E., & Ray, W. (1997). Predictors of injury mortality in early childhood. *Pediatrics, 100*(3), 342–347.

Seidel, J., Tittle, S., Hodge, D., et al. (1998). Guidelines for pediatric equipment and supplies for emergency departments. *Journal of Emergency Nursing, 24*(1), 45–48.

Semonin-Holleran, R. (1993). Taking the sting out of summer. *RN, 56*(7), 40–46.

Shah, B. (1998). Child poisoned by unknown substance. In L. Finberg (Ed.), *Saunders manual of pediatric practice* (pp. 1013–1016). Philadelphia: Saunders.

Shah, B. (1998). Child with multisystem trauma. In L. Finberg (Ed.), *Saunders manual of pediatric practice* (pp. 1010–1013). Philadelphia: Saunders.

Shoemaker, B., & Ose, M. (1997). Pediatric lap belt injuries: Care and prevention. *Critical Care Clinics, 13*(3), 611–628.

Sinclair, C. L., & Zhou, C. (1995). Descriptive epidemiology of animal bites in Indiana, 1990–92: A rationale for intervention. *Public Health Reports, 110*(1), 64–67.

Sladky, J. (1996). Near drowning. In F. Burg, E. Wald, J. Ingelfinger, & R. Polin (Eds.), *Gellis and Kagan's current pediatric therapy* (15th ed.). Philadelphia: Saunders.

Solomon, B. (1997). Emergency nursing: There is no typical day. *Nursing in Pediatrics,* Fall/Winter, 4–7.

Soud, T. D., & Rogers, J. S. (1998). *Manual of pediatric emergency nursing*. St Louis: Mosby–Year Book.

Tuggle, D. W., Taylor, D. V., & Stevens, R. J. (1993). Dog bites in children. *Journal of Pediatric Surgery, 28*(7), 912–914.

Walsh, E., & Ioli, J. (1994). Childhood near-drowning: Nursing care and primary prevention. *Pediatric Nursing, 20*(3), 265–269.

Walsh-Kelly, C., & Strait, R. (1998). Impact of violence and the emergency department response to victims and perpetrator. *Pediatric Clinics of North America, 45*(2), 449–457.

Weiss, H., Friedman, D., & Coben, J. (1998). Incidence of dog bite injuries treated in emergency departments. *JAMA, 279*(1), 51–53.

West, L. (1997). Innovative approaches to the administration of activated charcoal in pediatric toxic ingestions. *Pediatric Nursing, 23*(6), 616–619.

Wiggins, M. E., Akelman, E., & Weiss, A. P. (1994). The management of dog bites and dog bite infections to the hand. *Orthopedics, 17*(7), 617–623.

Zink, K. (1996). Emotional support in pediatric trauma: Remembering children like Caleb. *Journal of Pediatric Nursing, 11*(6), 345–347.

35

The Ill Child in the Hospital and Other Care Settings

LEARNING OBJECTIVES

After studying this chapter, you should be able to:

- Discuss the nurse's role in various settings where care is given to ill children.
- List common stressors affecting hospitalized children.
- Describe the child's response to illness.
- Discuss the stages of separation anxiety.
- Describe the factors that affect children's response to hospitalization and treatment.
- Discuss the psychological responses of families to the illness of a child in the family.

DEFINITIONS

denial A defense mechanism in which unpleasant realities are denied and kept out of conscious awareness.

egocentric Preoccupied with one's own interests and needs.

regression Defense mechanism in which conflict or frustration is resolved by returning to a behavior that was successful in an earlier stage of development.

separation anxiety Distress and apprehension caused by being removed from parents, home, or familiar surroundings.

situational crisis Unanticipated event that poses a threat to an individual's psychosocial or psychological well-being.

therapeutic play Guided play that promotes the psychophysiologic well-being of a child.

Because of current trends in health care management, the care of ill children continues to move from the traditional acute hospital setting to community-based settings and the home. Hospitalized children are more acutely ill than in the past, and their stays are shorter. In addition, the hospitalized child is more likely to have a chronic or terminal disease. These changes do not mean that the need for pediatric nurses has diminished; their role is ever-changing and expanding. Pediatric nurses will continue to care for children in hospitals, schools, clinics, and the home.

All children experience some form of illness. The ways in which stressors and developmental needs are addressed are important factors in resolving the immediate crisis and in dealing with future illnesses. The nurse is often the first person the child sees when the child enters the health care system, and the nurse spends more time with an ill child than any other health care worker. The nurse therefore has a unique opportunity to influence that child's physical and emotional health.

Settings of Care

The Hospital

Entering the hospital is somewhat like visiting a foreign country. The language, culture, activities, and expectations may be unfamiliar to the child and the family. The nurse acts as a "tour guide" and provides a safe environment, both physically and emotionally. Being the guide includes activities as diverse as explaining the jargon (NPO, IV, "vitals"), explaining procedures that are often painful, and facilitating the parent's access to hospital resources such as social services, case managers, spiritual counselors, and ethics specialists. Above all, the nurse must educate the child and family about the disease process, its treatment, hospital procedures, and discharge issues.

Hospitalizations can be categorized according to length of stay, planned or unplanned admission, surgical or medical intervention, and outpatient (day) or inpatient status. Even though they overlap, these categories provide a framework for examining the child's experience.

Another variable is the type of facility. Children may be hospitalized in a pediatric hospital, on a pediatric unit within a general hospital, or in a general hospital that occasionally admits children. Pediatric units within a general hospital or hospitals that do not have a specific pediatric unit may not have as many child-oriented services as a pediatric hospital. Special play areas and child-size equipment and fixtures often are not available in general hospitals. Staff who routinely do not care for children may be less comfortable in that role.

The nurse is aware of these challenges and can provide support for the child and the family, for example, by taking extra time when the child is admitted to explain routines and procedures or by placing the child close to the nurse's station. This support might include moving a cot into the room for the parent and ordering special foods for the child. Sometimes it means removing food from a tray that is about to be served so that the child is not overwhelmed by the large servings intended for an adult. Ultimately, it means being sensitive to the needs of the child and the family.

24-HOUR OBSERVATION

Children become ill quickly and recover quickly. For this reason, they may need acute care for a short time. (Children who are dehydrated or are having an episode of acute asthma are examples.) At the end of 24 hours, the child is evaluated to determine whether further hospitalization is needed or whether discharge with home care instructions is appropriate.

The nurse must prepare the child and family for discharge and assess the parents' ability to care for the child at home. Instructions should be written, and the parent should be encouraged to ask questions. The parent should be told when to notify the primary health care provider in the event the child's condition worsens. An awareness of cultural differences enhances the nurse's assessment ability. For example, is the parent smiling because of contentment, or is the parent embarrassed to ask a question? Are parents nodding because they understand or because they are too embarrassed to say they cannot read?

EMERGENCY HOSPITALIZATION

Because of limited time for preparation, an emergency admission can be traumatic. The admission can be the result of trauma or acute sudden illness. The family may arrive at the hospital with little money, clothing, or other resources. Siblings may also be present, competing with the sick child for the parent's attention. In addition to caring for the sick child, the staff may be called on to help meet the family's basic needs for food, clothing, and a place to stay. A social service referral is appropriate in such situations.

Because of the intense level of activity in emergency departments, care of the family is often overlooked. The family may fear that the child will die or be permanently disabled. Although nurses may see many similar situations each day in which children do well, they must be sensitive to the family's fears and keep them informed of the child's condition and care.

Having parents present can affect the way a child reacts to a stressful situation. In most cases, children are more secure and relaxed if at least one parent remains with them. In the past, it was the practice to keep parents out of the room until the child's condition was stabilized. The staff believed that they were protecting the parents, but the parents often wondered if they would ever see their child again. In most situations, the parents can decide whether they want to be with the child. If the parents' behavior impairs the staff's ability to provide care, they are asked to wait outside the room and kept informed.

The time for preparing a child is usually limited in emergencies. Nurses must seize every opportunity to prepare children for the care they will receive. Holding and touching the child, talking softly, distracting the child, and involving the child in the procedure are methods of support used in emergencies. After the child is stable, the nurse returns and uses therapeutic communication to talk about the event. A child life specialist may also help the child express feelings. The use of dolls, puppets, and hospital equipment can aid children in communicating their feelings. (Chapter 34 provides more detailed information about caring for children and their families in an emergency setting.)

For example, one 7-year-old boy was admitted to the medical-surgical unit after spending several hours in the emergency department because of acute asthma. Although his mother brought him to the hospital, she had his younger brother and sister with her and could not remain with him in the room. The boy remained quiet, but the nurse noticed that he watched every move she made.

In such a case, the nurse might say, "Some kids say it's scary to come to the hospital and especially to be in the emergency room, with the bright lights and everyone rushing around. If you'd like, I can spend a little time with you, and we can talk about being in the hospital."

Outpatient and Day Facilities

Outpatient facilities have evolved in an effort to keep children out of the hospital unless absolutely necessary. The outpatient facility may be part of a hospital, or it may be freestanding. The child arrives in the morning, undergoes a procedure, test, or surgery, and goes home by the evening. Common procedures performed during such admissions include tympanostomy tube placement, hernia repair, tonsillectomy, cystoscopy, and bronchoscopy.

This mode of care has three main advantages: (1) it minimizes separation of the child from the family, (2) it decreases the risk of infection, and (3) it decreases cost. A disadvantage is that outpatient facilities that are not connected to a hospital may not be equipped for overnight stays. If complications develop that require continued observation and treatment, the child may have to be transferred to a hospital. This situation can be upsetting to the child and the family.

Although the procedure may be short, teaching the child and the parent is as important as in the acute care setting. When possible, a tour of the facility before the procedure can decrease fear of the unknown. Parents have indicated that although they like the idea of outpatient care, taking a child home afterward can be frightening.

Assessment of the parent can assist the nurse in deciding whether the parent is capable of handling the child's care at home or whether home health care is needed. Written instructions specific to the child and procedure are helpful and reassuring. At the very least, a follow-up phone call to the home should be required. Parents should also be encouraged to call the facility if they have any concerns, and they should be given other resources to contact after the facility closes. Families who live far from the health care facility may want to spend the night at a nearby hotel or consider an overnight admission.

Rehabilitative Care

After a serious illness or trauma, the child's ability to function may change. After the acute situation has resolved, the child may be admitted to a rehabilitation hospital. Staff from nursing, medicine, physical therapy, occupational therapy, and other areas collaborate to develop a treatment plan in which the child, family, and health professionals work to help the child regain previous abilities. Children with neurologic injuries, such as head injuries, or children with serious burns may thrive in this environment, which usually resembles a home environment with facilities available for the child to relearn the activities of daily living.

Nurses in rehabilitative settings must balance nurturing and firm discipline as they help children reclaim independence. Parents often need encouragement and support because they are torn between doing for their child and watching the child struggle to function independently. Overprotection is a common reaction, and parents can be assisted in identifying the child's developmental need to master the environment. The focus should be on what the child can do rather than on the child's limitations.

The Medical-Surgical Unit

Children admitted to the hospital are usually acutely ill or have a chronic disease or disability that requires frequent, often long-term hospitalizations. (Care of the child with a chronic disease is discussed in Chapter 36.) The average length of hospital stay for the acutely ill child has shortened significantly, and the need for teaching has increased in proportion.

Preparation for a planned hospitalization is essential. Some hospitals provide an opportunity for the child to visit the hospital before admission, and many pediatric hospitals host preoperative parties or classes to introduce children to the strange sights and sounds experienced during a surgical experience. Many children's books about the experience of illness and hospitalization are available in public libraries. Some children's hospitals also have libraries. Parents should answer questions honestly and encourage the child to talk about the hospitalization. Videos may also be available for family members to view together and then discuss.

The Intensive Care Unit

When a child is admitted to the intensive care unit (ICU), both the child and the parents experience increased stress because of the seriousness of the admitting diagnosis and the high-tech, unfamiliar environment. In addition, the child often is experiencing pain, uncomfortable procedures, noise, and constant lighting. In many instances the child cannot eat or talk. Meanwhile, the parents are experiencing a parent's worst fear, the possible loss of a child.

The child and family need intense emotional support. All of the normal responses to hospitalization are magnified and need to be assessed. When possible, planned admissions to the ICU (e.g., for cardiac surgery) should be preceded by visits to the unit or special classes that provide information about special procedures and operations at a level the child can understand.

The parent should be encouraged to remain with the

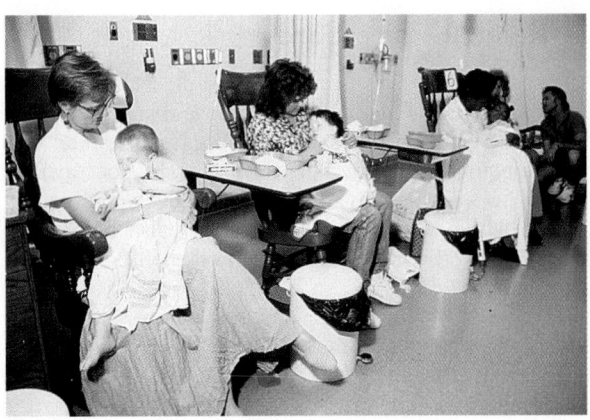

FIGURE 35-1

When nursing care centers on the family, hospital rules must be altered. These parents are holding their children and rocking them in a postanesthesia care unit, normally a place off-limits to those not on the staff. (Courtesy of Cook Children's Medical Center, Fort Worth, Texas.)

child and should be kept informed of the child's condition (Fig. 35–1). Procedures, equipment, and treatments should be explained, in appropriate language, to both the child and the parent. If the parent leaves and the child's condition changes or a new tube or piece of equipment has been added, the nurse should prepare the parent for the change before the parent sees the child. Nurses should encourage parents to provide care and to touch their child as much as possible. The nurse's active listening is essential.

Siblings of the seriously ill hospitalized child can easily be overlooked. Siblings may need to talk, be comforted, or have the hospital experience explained to them. Parents may feel pulled between the ill child and the rest of the family. Often family members want to help but do not know what to do. Suggesting that a grandparent or other relative relieve a parent so that the parent has time with the ill child's sibling can help both the parent and the child. Helping parents by discussing options can relieve stress and may lead to solutions. Inclusion of family members in the provision of care, such as bathing and feeding, is important to both the family members and the child.

School-Based Clinics

School-based clinics have been part of health care for more than 25 years, but with the recent changes in health care delivery, this setting is now a site for expanding primary care. School-based clinics play an important role in providing care for children in remote rural communities and in underserved inner-city areas. Clinics are typically staffed by school nurses, nurse practitioners, physicians, social workers, and other health care providers. This area of practice will continue to grow, and many believe that school-based clinics are the perfect setting for providing primary care for selected groups of children and adolescents because they are well situated to influence the health and well-being of underserved students (Kaplan et al., 1998).

Prevention remains the focus of school-based care as children learn health habits to prevent their developing

acute problems. Nurses identify children who need immunizations and provide immunizations when necessary. Screening that once required referral can often be handled on site. Through school-based clinics, children can receive medical services in a timely manner and avoid expensive emergency visits. For example, a child who is experiencing an earache at school can be seen on site, treated, and sent home if warranted. The child's compliance with treatment can be monitored and a follow-up visit scheduled to determine whether treatment has been effective. One clinic documented that school absences decreased significantly after a school-based clinic was established (Pietrobono, 1994). Funding for school-based clinics is increasing, and they will continue to be a focus of health care delivery in the community.

Nurses in school-based clinics must be sensitive to parental concerns about certain topics in health care, especially areas related to sexuality (e.g., birth control, sexually transmissible diseases, abortion). Community involvement and support can dispel concerns and assist in setting guidelines for such clinics. School-based nurses must also be team members who act in collaboration with other health care workers and have a strong background in preventive health as well as the ability to think critically.

The school-based clinic provides a setting for parental education in preventive health, growth and development, anticipatory guidance, parenting skills, and care of acutely ill children. The nurse respects the rights and wishes of the parents, but respecting parents' wishes can be a challenge when the value systems of the health care provider and the parent are different. The pediatric nurse is a patient advocate but must exercise caution unless the child is being harmed. (Child abuse is discussed in Chapter 53.)

Community Clinics

Community health clinics provide primary care for children and their families. In these settings, nurses, nurse practitioners, and physicians provide case management of illness and health promotion. Because most children enter this setting during illness, preventive care is integrated into the child's acute care. Support services and groups (e.g., social services, a dental clinic, day care) may be available in the same center, and referrals to medical specialists and other health care providers are also available.

Although many children seen at community health clinics are ill, nurses must use the opportunity to take a health history to assess immunization, nutrition, anticipatory guidance, and growth and development. If the child is ill at the time of the visit, the nurse can set an appointment for the child to return for immunizations or other care that cannot be given when the child is ill (see Appendixes F and G).

In some urban areas, nurses are involved in primary prevention and offer information and education about childhood immunization, the signs and symptoms of childhood illnesses, injury prevention, and parenting skills (Fig. 35–2). Demonstration projects have proved that support and education reduce hospitalization and emergency department visits, increase compliance with prescribed medical care, and improve health outcomes for the entire family (Struk, 1994).

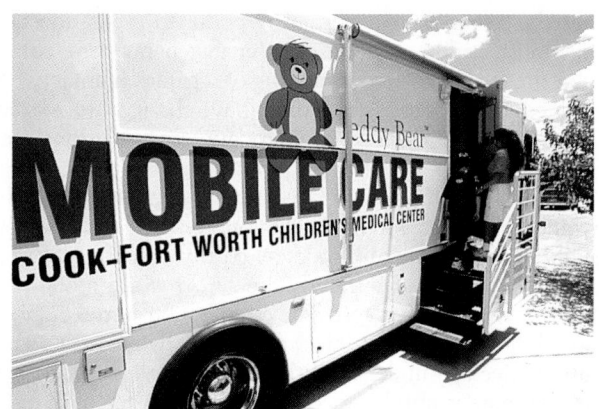

FIGURE 35-2

Nurses today help take health care on the road to provide services to those who otherwise might not obtain them. This mobile van is stationed at a public school, where it offers health screenings and prevention services to children. (Courtesy of Cook Children's Medical Center, Fort Worth, Texas.)

Home Care

Pediatric home care is the provision of skilled care within the child's home. Nurses in this setting are part of a multidisciplinary team that usually includes physicians, physical therapists, speech therapists, occupational therapists, and social workers. Children cared for at home include those receiving respiratory therapy, having dressing changes, receiving total parenteral nutrition, or needing skilled care because of a chronic illness or an injury.

Nurses who work in home care should have previous hospital experience in their practice area. The nurse must be able to make independent decisions and think critically and should have good clinical, documentation, communication, and teaching skills. To meet the needs of each child and family, the nurse must understand various cultures and socioeconomic backgrounds.

Although the separation of child from family is not a problem in home health care, the child may experience many of the other effects of illness, such as fear of the unknown, loss of control, anger, guilt, and regression. In addition, care is taking place in the family's domain, and the nurse is a guest in the home. The family may have to adjust to unfamiliar noises and equipment, such as special beds, ventilators, or intravenous pumps, in their home. They may feel that they have lost their privacy and cannot "be themselves" because someone outside of the family is frequently there. Awareness of siblings' needs is also a nursing goal in this setting.

The nurse's role as a teacher is especially important because many of the tasks that the nurse might perform in the hospital are delegated to the family, with the nurse monitoring the care. Here the nurse acts as a case manager and coordinator of care.

Stressors Associated with Illness and Hospitalization

Age, cognitive development, preparation, coping skills, and culture influence a child's reaction to illness. Previous expe-

CRITICAL TO REMEMBER

Children's Response to Illness

- Fear of the unknown
- Separation anxiety
- Fear of pain or mutilation
- Loss of control
- Anger
- Guilt
- Regression

rience with the health care system and the parent's reaction to the illness also affect the child.

Each child is unique, so that predicting reactions to an illness is often difficult. Much of the research on the effects of hospitalization on children has been based on adult assumptions of the child's experience and on children's self-reports. Several categories have been identified: separation, physical harm or bodily injury, fear of the unknown, uncertainty about limits, and loss of control (Visintainer & Wolfer, 1975). Previous experience may not reduce fear but rather may replace fear of the unknown with fear of the known (Hart & Bossert, 1994).

Although preschoolers and young school-age children experience separation anxiety, it is most significant in infants and toddlers, especially those ages 6 to 30 months. In times of stress, anxiety related to separation increases.

Each age group has its own fears related to pain and injury. The past decade has seen an expansion of knowledge about pain and its treatment, negating many erroneous beliefs about children and pain. Children quickly learn to associate health care activities and professionals with pain and injury. The fear is usually focused on "shots." (Chapter 39 discusses issues related to pain.)

A child's feeling of having control over a situation has been shown to affect distress in reaction to medical events (LaMontagne, 1993). If children believe that they have personal control over a situation, they are more likely to feel confident and master a task, whether it is holding still while a needle is inserted or lying still while tomography is performed.

Although specific fears are related to the child's age, hospitalization puts all children at high risk for fears related to their unfamiliarity with the people, surroundings, and events. The child has not developed trust in the health care provider and therefore does not know what to expect. The child may have real or imagined fears: Will the nurse know when I am hungry or hurting? Will the nurse hurt me?

The Infant and Toddler

SEPARATION ANXIETY

Infants and toddlers, especially those between 6 and 30 months, experience separation anxiety. Separation is this age group's major stressor, and it is traumatic to both the child and the parent. The child experiences several stages in reaction to the separation: *protest, despair,* and *detachment.*

In the initial phase, known as protest, the child demon-

● ● ● ● ● ● ● ● ●
Stages of Separation

Protest: Child is agitated, resists caregivers, cries, and is inconsolable.

Despair: Child experiences hopelessness and becomes quiet, withdrawn, and apathetic.

Detachment: Child becomes interested in the environment, plays, and seems to form relationships with caregivers and other children. If parents reappear, the child may ignore them.

strates distress by crying and rejecting anyone other than the parents (Fig. 35–3). The child appears angry and upset. During the despair phase, the child experiences hopelessness and becomes quiet and withdrawn. Crying decreases, and the child becomes apathetic. If separation from the parent continues, the child enters the detachment phase. During this phase, the child again becomes interested in the environment and begins to play. Nurses may misinterpret this phase as a positive sign that the child has adjusted to the hospitalization. In reality, the child has "given up." If the parents return during this stage, the child may ignore them, and the parents may think that the child does not want to see them. The reaction, however, is a coping mechanism to protect the child from further emotional pain related to the separation.

Nurses in acute care settings see the first two stages of separation—protest and despair—much more frequently than the final stage, detachment, which is more common in long-term separations. Parents may misunderstand their child's behavior. They may even perceive the child's reaction as a behavior problem. Nurses need to reassure parents that this reaction is a normal response to separation and that most children will not suffer any permanent effects from the event. As understanding of separation anxiety has evolved, changes in visiting times have changed from structured hours to more flexible rooming-in situations (see Fig. 35–3).

Most practitioners believe that if separation can be avoided, the child will be much more resilient during a hospitalization. Infants and toddlers go through the stages of separation. The older the children in this age group, the more elaborate the protest. The child not only cries but may also cling to the parent, kick, and generally create a scene. Parents need to understand that this behavior is a sign of healthy parent-child attachment. The toddler may resist bedtime and eating and may have temper tantrums more frequently than normal for this age. Regression may occur in toileting and eating. Nurses need to explain to parents that regression is normal and encourage parents to reinforce appropriate behavior while allowing the regressive behavior to occur.

For example, a parent might ask whether someone needs to be with a hospitalized toddler all of the time and may be especially concerned because the parents work and have other children. The nurse may respond, "We encourage parents to stay with their children when they are in the hospital. If you have to leave, however, we will spend time with your child and check on your child frequently. You may call us at any time, day or night. When you return, perhaps you could bring a favorite toy or stuffed animal and something that reminds the child of you. A picture or a piece of clothing will make your child feel more secure because it is familiar."

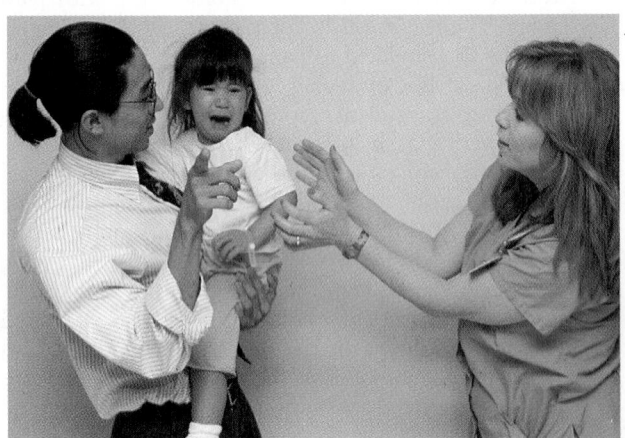

Hospitals try to reduce the stress of hospitalization for both parents and the child by having rooming-in arrangements. Rooming-in promotes parental attachment and provides many opportunities to teach parents how to care for their child's needs.

◄ Between the ages of 6 and 30 months, a child is expected to have separation anxiety. The child initially reacts with protest, as this girl is doing. If separation continues, the child becomes quiet and withdrawn (despair phase). In the final phase, detachment, the child may ignore the parents.

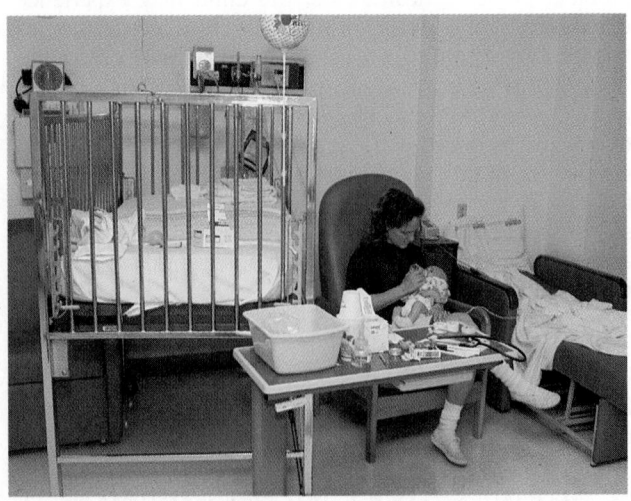

FIGURE 35–3
● ● ● ● ● ● ● ● ●
Separation is one of the stressors of hospitalization that affects both child and parent. (Courtesy of T. C. Thompson, Children's Hospital of Chattanooga, Tennessee.)

FEAR OF INJURY AND PAIN

Previous experiences, separation from parents, restraint, and preparation affect the reaction of infants and toddlers to pain and bodily injury. The young child views injury and pain concretely. Nurses who have worked with toddlers know that most toddlers react to any intrusive procedure, whether it is painful or not. (See Chapter 39 for a more extensive discussion of pain in infants and toddlers.)

LOSS OF CONTROL

According to Erikson, the major task of the toddler period is developing autonomy. Control is a major issue with this age group. The toddler experiences the environment through all of the senses and loves to explore the environment. At the same time, toddlers need sameness (rituals and routines). Because of the changes in growth and development taking place in the toddler, familiar rituals and routines (e.g., those for eating, sleeping, playing) provide reassurance and stability.

Hospitalization, which has its own set of rituals and routines, can severely disrupt the life of a toddler. The child may be confined to a crib, and the crib may have a cover over it. Because of safety issues, the child is not allowed to run in the halls. If the parents are unable to be with the child, the way the child is put to bed or bathed may be unfamiliar. Information obtained from parents about routines for feeding, going to bed, and playing can assist the nurse in maintaining usual and comforting routines. When children are unable to do things themselves, their sense of control and autonomy is weakened. They are frustrated and may have temper tantrums. Choices, even simple ones, can return some control to the child.

This lack of control is often exhibited in behaviors related to feeding, toileting, playing, and bedtime. The nurse should remember that each of these activities may have associated rituals and routines and that the child may also show some regression in these areas.

The Preschooler

SEPARATION ANXIETY

Separation anxiety occurs among preschoolers, but it is generally less obvious and less serious than in the toddler. Although the preschooler may already be spending some time away from parents at a day care center or preschool, illness adds a stressor that makes separation more difficult.

The preschooler expresses the same protest as the toddler but tends to be less direct. The nurse may find a preschooler quietly crying because the parents have told the child to "act like a big boy." Children of this age may refuse to eat or take medications, and they may be generally uncooperative. They may repeatedly ask when their parents will be coming for a visit; with access to a phone, the child may constantly call the parents. All of these behaviors are signs that the child is having difficulty coping with the situation.

FEAR OF INJURY AND PAIN

The preschooler fears mutilation. The child who must have surgery affecting a limb or other body part experiences increased fear. The preschooler generally does not understand body integrity. Children of this age are also afraid of intrusive procedures, and because of their literal interpretation of words, they often imagine treatments to be much worse than they are. Finally, the child's active imagination can go wild during illness. The preschooler may believe that the illness occurred because of some personal deed or thought, or perhaps just because the child touched something or someone. (The preschooler's specific reactions to pain are further discussed in Chapter 39.)

LOSS OF CONTROL

The preschooler has attained a good deal of independence in self-care and has been given more independence at home, preschool, or day care. Some children expect to maintain their independence in the hospital. For example, the preschooler may like to wander about the unit and may not be happy when restricted to the bed or room. Like the toddler, a preschooler likes familiar routines and rituals and may show some regression if not allowed to maintain some areas of control.

> For example, one 5-year-old boy refused to have his dressing changed by the nurse who cared for him during the previous day. She reported that he cried, pulled up the covers, and said that she was "mean." This behavior was unusual for him, and the nurse suspected that he had been told to do too many things and had not been given choices. In response, the nurse might say, "I know there have been many changes for you since you came to the hospital. Today, we are going to decide together what is going to happen. I see you have chosen a video to watch. Would you like me to change your dressing before you watch the video, or after?" This approach gives the preschooler a choice and some control while maintaining boundaries.

GUILT AND SHAME

Because their thinking is egocentric and magical, preschoolers may believe that their illness is somehow related to a thought or deed. This belief can lead to feelings of guilt, shame, and increased stress at a time when the child has to cope with several other stressors. Because the child typically does not share these feelings with adults, parents and caregivers must be aware of the possibility of guilt and shame in this age group.

The nurse's role is to assess the child for this type of thinking and, through therapeutic communication, assist the child in identifying unfounded fears and beliefs. The child may be able to relate perceptions of what is happening. The use of puppets, dolls, and drawings can help children deal with their feelings. A tremendous decrease in anxiety can result when the nurse helps the child identify a perceived punishment and then reassures the child that nothing the child did could cause the illness.

The School-Age Child

SEPARATION

The school-age child is accustomed to periods of separation from parents, but just as in the preschooler, as stressors are added, the separation becomes more difficult. The younger school-age child may already have been experiencing separation anxiety related to starting school.

Older children may be more concerned with missing school and the fear that their friends will forget them. The need to adjust to an unfamiliar environment and the regression seen in ill children, however, increase the likelihood that some separation anxiety will take place.

FEAR OF INJURY AND PAIN

The school-age child is concerned with body disability and death. The child is more relaxed about having a physical examination or having the eyes or an ear examined but is uncomfortable with any type of sexual examination. These children want to know the reasons for procedures and tests, and they ask relevant questions about their illness. Because school-age children can understand cause and effect, they can relate actions to becoming ill. Their parents may tell them that if they do not get enough rest, wear warm clothes, or eat nutritious meals, they will get a cold. If they become ill, they associate their actions with the disease. (For further discussion of pain in the school-age child, see Chapter 39.)

LOSS OF CONTROL

School-age children are movers and shakers. They control their self-care and typically are highly social. They like being involved, and most fill their days with activities. Illness can change all of these patterns. If children of this age have physical limitations, they can feel helpless and dependent (Fig. 35–4).

Friends are important to this age group, and school-age children may think that their friends will forget them while they are ill. They are also accustomed to making choices about meals and activities. By capitalizing on the child's abilities and needs, the nurse can encourage children of this age to become involved in their own care. School-age children can select their own menus, assist with some treatments, keep their rooms neat, and visit with younger children when it is appropriate for both. With these opportunities for independence, children retain a sense of control, enhance their self-esteem, and continue to work toward achieving a sense of industry.

The Adolescent

SEPARATION

Adolescents often are unsure whether they want their parents with them when they are hospitalized. Some enjoy the freedom and the period of independence. Others, in response to the stress of illness, become more dependent and want their parents nearby. A third group cannot decide what they want, and this situation can be frustrating to the parents. All of these responses are consistent with the normal growth and development of an adolescent.

Because of the importance of the peer group, separation from friends is a source of anxiety to the adolescent. Ideally, the peer group will support the ill friend. Some adolescents are reluctant to visit friends in the hospital, either because of their own health fears or because the reality of illness in someone their age is difficult for them to handle. Hospitalized adolescents may be upset if their friends simply go on with their lives, excluding them. Special activity areas and other opportunities for the adolescent to meet and interact with hospitalized adolescents are important (see Fig. 35–4).

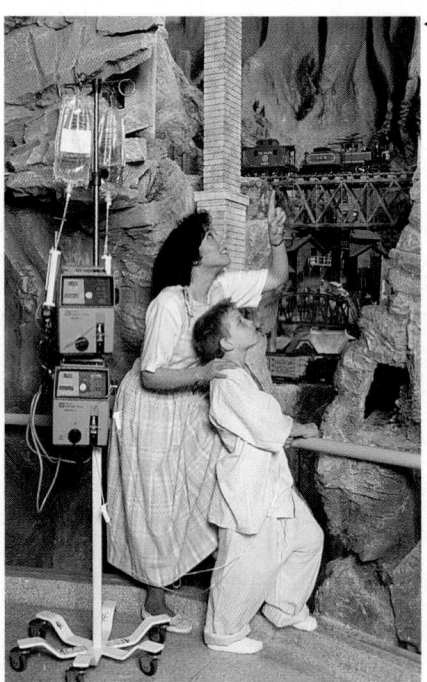

◄ This multilevel trainscape in a children's hospital provides children and adults alike with a welcome respite from real-life stresses. (Courtesy of Children's Medical Center, Dallas, Texas.)

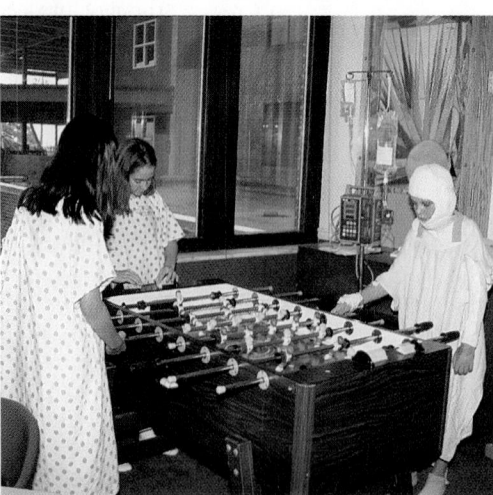

◄ Hospitalized teens need to interact with their peers, as they do when they are well. A lounge area that is separate from the playroom used by younger children fulfills this need.

FIGURE 35–4
• • • • • • • •
Activities for the hospitalized child are important for growth and development, stress relief, socialization, and a sense of control.

FEAR OF INJURY AND PAIN

To the adolescent, appearance is crucial. Therefore, illness or injury that changes adolescents' perceptions of themselves can have a major impact. Even children who have seemingly adjusted to a chronic disease in their earlier years may have difficulty during adolescence simply because they do not want to be different. The diabetic adolescent may not want to eat different foods or take time out from an activity for injections. Adolescents do not want attention drawn to them, so they may eat the wrong foods and skip their medication.

Adolescents may also give the impression that they are not afraid, even though they are terrified. Adolescents may think that being "cool" means being in control. They may question everything, or they may appear overly confident. Because of their concern with their bodies, they are guarded when any areas connected to sexual development are examined. Nurses need to be sensitive to adolescents' concerns and reassure them that they are normal, if in fact they are. Some adolescents also believe that they are invincible and that nothing can hurt them or cause death. This belief can cause them to take risks and to be noncompliant because they may not see the consequences of their behavior. (Pain management is discussed in Chapter 39.)

LOSS OF CONTROL

Control is important to the adolescent. Some of the challenges in caring for an ill adolescent stem from control issues, and understanding this issue is key when caring for adolescents. Giving the adolescent some control avoids endless power struggles. Behaviors exhibited in response to loss of control may include anger, withdrawal, and general uncooperativeness.

Control issues can cause a major conflict between the adolescents and their parents. Parents often feel like Ping-Pong balls as they are bounced back and forth by a child who wants help one minute and rejects it the next. Parents who do not understand growth and development can become frustrated and angry over such behavior. Educating the parents increases understanding and facilitates parent-child communication.

Adolescents may also feel that they are losing control of their social lives as they sit on the sidelines of activities. Time to plan for the separation (e.g., scheduled surgery) allows a greater sense of control than an unplanned hospitalization (e.g., trauma).

Fear of the Unknown

The sights and sounds of the hospital can be frightening and confusing to the child. The child may have many questions: Why are the nurses wearing masks? Why does that alarm keep ringing? Am I dying? Why are they putting tubes in me? Why am I under a plastic tent?

The child's routines and rituals may have been disrupted, and the child may wonder what will happen next. Understanding these fears can assist the nurse in structuring care and teaching in a way that avoids unnecessary anxiety.

Regression

Children may regress in toileting or may cry for a bottle even though they have been weaned for several months.

CRITICAL TO REMEMBER
. . . .
Maintaining a Safe Place

A designated safe area can enhance the child's security. For example, intrusive procedures may cause discomfort or anxiety and should be in the treatment room, not in the child's room. The playroom should also be a place for playing, not treatments and administering medications.

They may want more attention at bedtime or have temper tantrums. The older child may react to separation by clinging or crying or may have fears about shadows on the walls or noises in the halls.

Parents may be overly concerned about regression. They should be told that the child might continue the behavior at home. The child may need more emotional support while the parent slowly returns the child to normal routines. If the child has regressed in toileting, the parent should wait until the child has returned to a daily routine and then begin the toilet training again. Behavior appropriate for the child's age should be reinforced.

> For example, the nurse might explain, "I know that you are concerned because David has been soiling his pants since he has been in the hospital. This soiling is a normal reaction to the stress of being ill and in the hospital. When he returns home and things return to normal for him, he will resume his previous schedule."

Factors Affecting a Child's Response to Illness and Hospitalization

Each child responds to illness or hospitalization differently. The expression "perception is everything" certainly applies to the ill child. How children perceive the incident will affect their response before, during, and after the illness or hospitalization. How a child reacts is often related to the parents' response to the illness and the child's age, level of cognitive development, preparation, previous experiences, and coping skills.

If the child has had a previous illness or hospitalization, how that event unfolded and the child's response to it greatly affect the child's view of future occurrences. Children with chronic diseases who experience multiple hospitalizations have a different perception of illness than those who have an occasional cold (see Chapter 36). A visit to a pediatrician's office will show the wide range of responses children have. Some older children have more negative responses as they begin to associate certain people, colors, and surroundings with what was for them an unpleasant experience.

Age and Cognitive Development

Children's developmental level affects their reactions to illness. These differences need to be taken into consideration

Developmental Approaches to the Hospitalized Child

NEONATE

- Anticipate needs and fulfill them in a timely manner.
- Provide opportunities for nonnutritive (comfort) sucking and oral stimulation, using a pacifier.
- Provide swaddling, with the infant's hands drawn to the midline and close to the face. Use facilitated tucking and soft talking to soothe.
- If the infant is very ill, provide a quiet, soothing environment. Pay close attention to light and sound stimulation.
- When stimulation is appropriate, provide stimulation for each sense (e.g., mobiles, music, smell, soft stuffed animals). Use contrasting colors and textures.
- Watch for cues of overstimulation such as eye avoidance, extension of arms, splaying of fingers, and "zoning-out" behavior.
- Before painful procedures, provide comforting touch and nonnutritive sucking. Follow painful procedures with tucking, holding, and cuddling.
- Model and share appropriate behaviors with family members regarding stimulation, touch, verbalization, and feeding.
- Provide consistency in caregivers when parents are not available.
- Collaborate with parents on ways to provide home care.
- Involve the parents in the care of their infant as much as possible.
- Encourage parents to room-in if possible.

INFANT

- For the younger infant, provide the same care given for neonate.
- The older infant will begin to anticipate painful procedures and fight. Use sheets and blankets to provide swaddling, if necessary. Allow nonnutritive sucking for comfort.
- Expect regressive behavior, and inform parents to expect it and why.
- Limit the number of caregivers to whom the infant must adjust.
- Request that parents bring the infant's security object (e.g., blanket, stuffed animal).
- Encourage parents to be present during procedures.

TODDLER

- Expect regression, and inform parents about behaviors.
- Follow home routines and rituals.
- Involve parents in the care of the toddler.
- Provide for rooming-in if possible.
- Allow opportunities for mobility when it can be done safely.
- Employ all possible methods of pain control when the child must have a painful procedure.
- Anticipate temper tantrums when the child's frustration level is high.
- Maintain a safe environment for toddler's physical acting out and temper tantrums.
- Encourage the child to be independent (e.g., feed self, use potty-chair, put on socks).
- Provide support when the toddler needs to be dependent (e.g., hold after a procedure, comfort if parents leave).
- Approach with a positive attitude ("I am going to give you your medicine").

PRESCHOOLER

- Provide safe ways to act out aggression (e.g., with punching bags, painting, clay).
- Take time for communication. Answer questions with simple, concrete explanations. Explain all procedures honestly. Allow for choices whenever possible.
- Expect egocentric behavior.
- Provide for a safe and secure environment (e.g., with a nightlight, view of others, objects from home).
- Be consistent.
- Ask the parents how the child usually copes in new situations.
- Tell the child that the child did not cause the illness.
- Involve parents in care, and follow home routines.
- Place the child with other children of the same age, if possible.
- Provide for play activities in the playroom and in the room.
- Accept regression if it occurs, and explain it to parents.
- Encourage the child to be independent (e.g., feeding, dressing, toileting).

SCHOOL-AGE CHILD

- Inform the child of limits and enforce them (no water fights, wheelchair races, leaving the unit, etc.).
- Involve the child in planning and implementing care (e.g., allow child to choose from menu and assist with some procedures).
- Explain all procedures, and allow the child time for questions and answers. Use medical and scientific terminology and diagrams, body outlines, or anatomically correct dolls to explain the procedure.
- Accept regression but encourage independence.
- Provide privacy.
- Encourage the child to assist in keeping room and belongings in order.
- Assist the child in contacting friends. Encourage parents to contact the teacher and have school friends send cards and letters.
- If the child's condition supports visits and calls from friends, encourage this contact.
- Provide for the educational needs of the child by encouraging parents to bring in work and scheduling study times. If the child will have a prolonged period of hospital or home care, arrange for a teacher to work with the child. Some hospitals have a hospital-based teacher.

ADOLESCENT

- Provide privacy for care and visiting.
- Encourage the adolescent to wear street clothes and perform normal grooming.
- Encourage questions about appearance and the effects of illness on the adolescent's future.
- Use scientific and medical terminology to prepare the adolescent for procedures.
- Use body outlines and diagrams and give the rationale for the procedure.
- When possible, provide for a special activity area that is limited to adolescent use. Introduce the child to other adolescents on unit.
- Encourage peers to call and visit if the adolescent's condition can tolerate this action.
- Assist parents in communicating, supporting, and guiding their adolescents by providing them with information about growth and development.
- Allow favorite foods to be brought in if the adolescent does not need a special diet.
- Approach the adolescent with caring, understanding, and acceptance.
- Provide for educational needs, as for a school-age child.

when planning nursing care. Preparing a toddler for hospitalization or a procedure differs from preparing a school-age child. The content, the time frame, the setting, and the method of preparation are all based on the child's growth and development. Pediatric nurses must have a clear understanding of the cognitive abilities of each age group.

Parental Response to Illness or Hospitalization

Children have sharp observation skills and know when their parents are anxious and upset. This anxiety is transferred to the child, and the child's anxiety then increases. If the parents talk outside their child's room or within hearing range but in whispers, the child begins to imagine what the parents are saying. All children, but especially preschoolers, who have such active imaginations, can invent elaborate stories to explain what is happening.

The parent who does not answer the child's questions or who does not tell the truth for fear it will frighten the child only confuses and weakens the child's trust in the parent. The child wants to believe that someone is in control and that that person can be trusted. Some parents cannot be honest with their children because of their own fears and insecurities. The nurse must assess all of these issues.

PREPARATION OF THE CHILD AND FAMILY

Stress has been defined as a nonspecific response of the body to any demand made on it. Perceived stressors, the conditioning factors brought to the situation, and the coping mechanisms used to adapt all affect each person's adaptation to a stress-producing situation (Selye, 1974). Preparing for an event, in this case hospitalization, can decrease stress in several ways. During preparation, the child's and the parent's perceptions of the event can be explored. In addition, previous experiences that might affect the impending hospitalization and the use of previous coping strategies can be identified and discussed.

The depth and method of preparation vary among children and are based on an understanding of the child's individual needs. Variables that the nurse should consider include the child's age and developmental level, involvement of the family, timing, the child's physiologic status and psychological status, the setting, sociocultural factors, and the child's experiences with illness and hospitalization (Brown et al., 1997; Manion, 1990).

Preparation sessions should be planned. Teaching is more effective if the nurse and family develop trust. Honesty and language appropriate for the child's age are imperative. When possible, all of the child's senses should be involved. The child should be allowed to see the intensive care area before being admitted, to take the blood pressure of a stuffed animal, or to handle the mask that will be used in surgery. The nurse should avoid using medical terms that children and their parents may not understand. Literal interpretation of some words may be confusing and scary to some children, especially the preschooler (see Chapter 32). Some children assume that certain procedures include pain. Explanation and the opportunity to handle equipment, when possible, can help a child master the fear of hospitalization and treatment.

COPING SKILLS OF THE CHILD AND FAMILY

Coping is the process of contending with difficulties in an effort to overcome or work through them. How the child copes with illness or hospitalization is related to age, perception of the event, previous hospitalizations and encounters with the health care profession, support from significant others, and the child's and parent's coping skills.

The child's coping behaviors include words, descriptions, phrases, and actions that children use to help them through stressful situations (Corbo-Richert, Caty, Barnes, 1993). The child may also cope by ignoring or negating the event. The younger child is more likely to use emotional expression, whereas the older child and adolescent are more likely to withdraw or practice more self-control behaviors. For example, whereas the younger child might scream and kick during a procedure, the older child might remain stoic and say that it did not hurt, even though it did. Some children try to appear brave and meet self-imposed or parental expectations.

Breathing (e.g., blowing bubbles, pinwheels, or party blowers) helps with relaxation and offers a focus for the child. Teaching coping mechanisms and practicing them before a procedure can help a child feel more in control as well as successful. Distraction (e.g., waterwheels, games, books) and imagery (e.g., tapes, scenarios) for older children are effective tools for coping. Parents, nurses, and child life therapists may all serve as facilitators for these techniques.

Psychological Benefits of Hospitalization

Some think that hospitalization causes only negative psychological effects. The stress of illness and hospitalization can actually be growth enhancing by promoting a child's coping skills and bolstering self-esteem. Children can increase their self-confidence as they overcome the anxiety related to hospitalization and perhaps master some self-care skills. They feel good about their recovery or increased ability to cope with any disability they have. In addition, hospitalization offers an opportunity for children to ask questions and obtain new information. Some even become interested in a career in health care while observing professionals caring for them. Hospitalization can also be an opportunity to teach parents about children's growth and development, improve parenting skills, and assess the child's immunization record.

Playrooms in Health Care Settings

Hospitals and clinics often provide playrooms where children may go to play with toys, participate in age-appropriate arts and crafts, and socialize with other children. Children should always see this area as a safe place where procedures and treatments do not take place. Children, when their condition is stable, may be taken to the playroom in their beds and wheelchairs (Fig. 35–5). A separate activity area should be provided, when possible, for adolescents to listen to music, play video games, and visit with their peers.

Therapeutic Play

When a child is hospitalized, one component of the child's plan of care is the use of *therapeutic play*. Therapeutic play

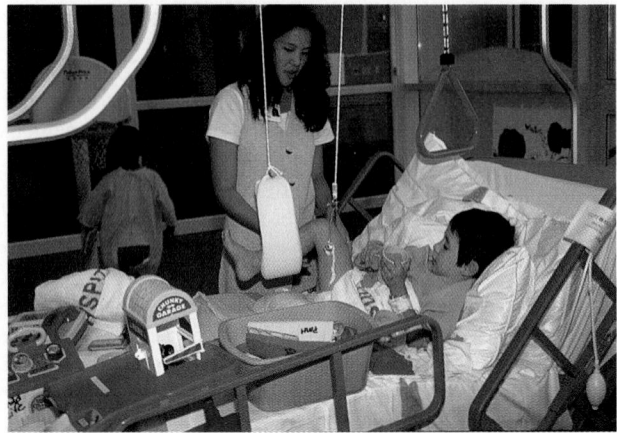

FIGURE 35-5
. . . .
Being in traction is no reason not to enjoy the hospital's play
facilities. To give him a change of surroundings and allow him
to interact with her and with other children, the play therapist
wheels this child in his bed to the playroom. Because his
mobility will be limited for a significant period, providing
diversion is especially important. (Courtesy of Parkland Health
and Hospital System, Dallas, Texas.)

differs from normal play in its design and intent. Members
of the health team guide it, and activities are planned to
meet the physical and psychological needs of the child.
Therapeutic play can provide an emotional outlet, instruct,
or improve physiologic abilities (Vessey & Mahon, 1990).
Supervised play with medical equipment helps reduce fear
and separate reality from fantasy.

Child life specialists or play therapists are available in
many hospitals and share their expertise in child growth
and development and the use of play. Child life programs
have as their goals maintaining normal living patterns, minimizing psychological trauma, and promoting optimal development of the child and family. Nurses should also be
involved in this type of activity, either in conjunction with
the child life specialist or individually when a child life specialist is not available. Interpretations of the child's play
behavior and some types of play therapy require guidance
by a skilled health care worker.

Emotional Outlet Play

Emotional outlet play is often called *dramatic play*. During
this type of play the child acts out or dramatizes real-life
stressors. These might include emotional stressors, such as
abuse or neglect, or a painful physical stressor, such as a
bone marrow aspiration. The hospitalized child who is separated from family and friends might use a wooden hammer
and pegs to express anger over the separation. A child who
has been sexually abused might not be able to communicate
verbally the experience but may be able to use an anatomically correct doll to show what happened.

Many commercially crafted toys are available for dramatic play. Anatomically correct dolls and puppets are
available. Some dolls have removable parts that enable the
child to see the various organs of the body.

Children can express their inner beliefs and perceptions through drawing. A child may draw a very big bed
with a tiny child on it surrounded by large hovering adults,
or a huge syringe with a long needle. Children often express
their thoughts and feelings through the use of paper and
crayons or colored markers (Fig. 35-6).

Supervised needle play is an appropriate intervention
with the child who has to undergo frequent blood work,
injections, intravenous therapy, or any other therapy involving needles. Safety when using needle play is always
important, and the nurse should assess the child's growth
and development level before using this type of directed
play. An adult is always present during needle play. The
child can give a doll an injection and can thereby work
through anger and anxiety. Wooden hammers and peg-
boards, Nerf balls, and boxing gloves are all avenues for release of stress or anger.

Teaching Through Play

Play can also be used to teach. It can be used in preoperative
teaching and teaching before a new, painful, or extensive
procedure (see Fig. 35-6). The nurse assesses the child's
cognitive level before this type of teaching, and the play
should be appropriate to the child's level.

Numerous books are available to assist in teaching.
Hospital equipment is often used in this type of play. The
nurse might demonstrate taking a blood pressure on the
child's stuffed animal before putting the cuff on the child.
A breathing treatment might be "given" to the child's doll
before the child is given the treatment. The nurse might
use drawings and diagrams to explain procedures or surgery.

Some hospitals have preoperative visits during which
children come and meet the people who will be taking care
of them and see the physical surroundings. They may see
the scrub gowns and masks worn by the surgical staff and
visit a typical room. Children and parents can ask questions
and meet other children and parents who are going through
the same experience as they tour the area.

Enhancing Cooperation Through Play

Children with illnesses that require unpleasant or painful
therapies often are uncooperative. Developing a plan that
will stimulate and engage the child in the activity is a challenge. The nurse should include age-appropriate growth and
development activities when planning care. The school-age
child who loves competition and games is more likely to
increase range of motion of an arm if points can be made
each time the Nerf ball is thrown through the hoop.

Deep-breathing exercises can be enhanced by allowing
the child to blow bubbles, a whistle, or a pinwheel or to
simulate blowing out the nurse's penlight. Range of motion
can be accomplished by throwing Nerf balls, beanbags, and
paper balls. The child who needs to increase intake can
sometimes be motivated to drink more fluids if a graph
shows the amount taken in and the child receives a reward
when a selected goal is reached. Including the child in planning and identifying rewards and goals enhances motivation. Colorful stickers, baseball cards, small toys, and special
pencils can be used as awards.

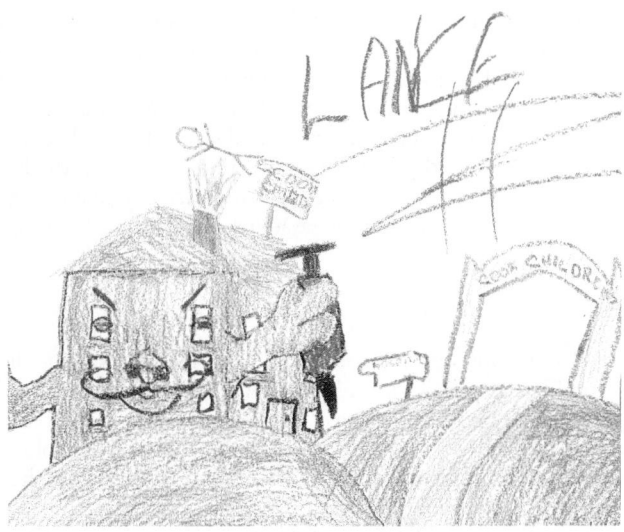

Art materials allow children to express their thoughts and feelings about health care problems.

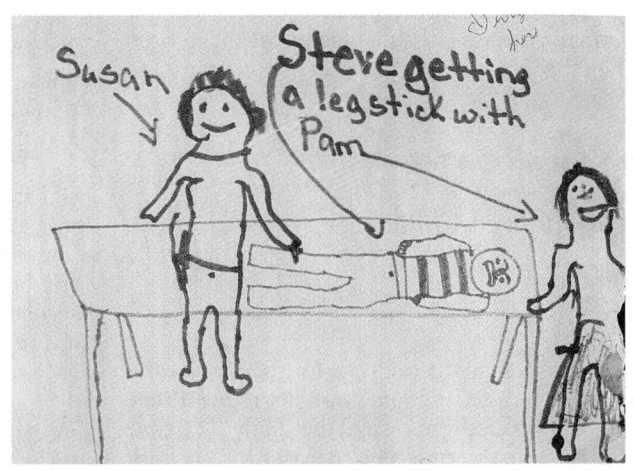

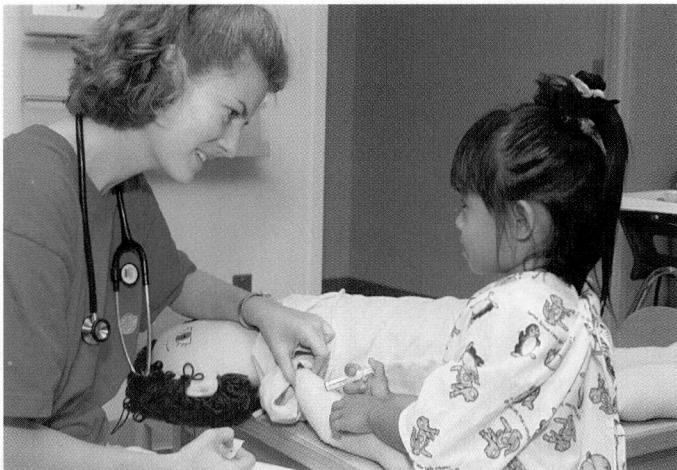

◄ Giving a doll an injection can help a child work through anxiety and anger about injections she may be receiving.

FIGURE 35–6
. . . .

Therapeutic play can be used to teach children about medical procedures or help them work through their feelings about what has happened to them in the health care setting. Child life specialists or play therapists are often members of the team in children's hospitals to provide expert guidance for therapeutic play.

Unstructured Play

In addition to therapeutic play, the nurse encourages unstructured play in the hospital setting. Through unstructured play, children can control events, ideas, and relationships.

Hospitals that do not have a special room set aside for play should be encouraged to provide developmentally appropriate toys, games, and books. These items can be kept in a special box accessible to the nursing staff.

Evaluation of Play

Therapeutic play should be reflected in the child's nursing care plan. During the evaluation step of the nursing process, the nurse looks at the outcome criteria to determine whether the goals have been met. The nurse is asking whether play enhanced the care of the child. Is the child coughing and deep breathing every 2 hours? Is the child relating feelings of fear over the separation from parents? Is the child eating or sleeping? If the client goals have been achieved, then the interventions have been appropriate and effective.

NURSING CARE

The Hospitalized Child

Assessment

Admission

The admission procedure sets the tone for the hospitalization. It should not be a series of questions but rather a time of collaboration between the nurse and the family. The time the family has spent in the emergency department, the seriousness of the illness, and other family needs (e.g., other children with parents or left with neighbors) may affect the interview process.

> The nurse can acknowledge the parent's concerns. For example, the nurse might say, "Mrs. Smith, I know you're concerned about your other children. Would you like to call your neighbor before I ask you some questions about Heidi and her illness?"

Most hospitals provide an admission interview form. Some of the information is essential for providing immediate care, and some can be collected later. By recognizing the family's needs, the nurse can structure each admission to fit that child and family. If the parent has entered the system through the emergency department, some of the questions may have previously been answered. By looking at the forms from other departments, repetition can be avoided, but data about allergies, medications taken at home, the history of the illness, and other relevant details must be repeated.

Although hospitals have policies and procedures for admission, the routine may need to be altered because of the child's condition. For example, a severely dehydrated child should have an intravenous infusion started, and a child in pain should be medicated before any other interventions are performed. On the other hand, the primary needs of the child and family may be emotional. A parent who has just been told that her child may have a terminal disease may have difficulty remembering the dates of the child's immunizations. In this situation, the nurse should provide the parent with support and assistance in mobilizing coping mechanisms and support systems rather than focusing on data gathering.

Physical Assessment

Initial Assessment. The initial assessment determines the need for any immediate or emergency care that must be provided before other information can be obtained. After the child is made comfortable (Fig. 35–7), obtain a more thorough assessment of the body systems and a health and psychosocial history.

Baseline Data. For all types of admissions, perform a complete physical assessment and complete an admission data sheet. The format of the admission data sheet varies from hospital to hospital, but most admission forms ask for much of the same information: history; allergies; nutritional, sleep, elimination, and psychosocial information; and the results of the initial physical assessment.

The physical assessment should be thorough, and special attention should be given to the body system involved in the child's admission. Many admission forms have an outline of the child's body on which the nurse should indicate any bruises, scratches, or other skin markings that provide specific objective data. (The process of interviewing, taking a history, and physical assessment is explained in Chapter 33.)

Nursing Diagnosis and Planning

Data collected at admission are used to formulate nursing diagnoses and the child's plan of care and should be placed in the body of the child's chart, not at the back of the chart, where it can be forgotten.

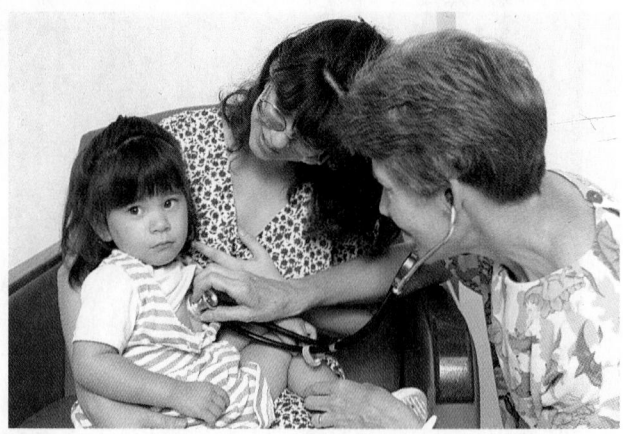

FIGURE 35–7

To reduce the stress of unfamiliar surroundings and people, the nurse assesses this child while the girl remains in the security of her mother's arms. (Courtesy of T. C. Thompson, Children's Hospital, Chattanooga, Tennessee.)

Nursing Diagnosis, Planning, Intervention, and Evaluation

Nursing Diagnosis
- ■ Altered Nutrition: Less Than Body Requirements related to unfamiliar foods, separation from caregiver, strange environment, or disease process.

Expected Outcome
- • The child's nutritional intake will meet the metabolic needs for the age group.

Intervention	Rationale
1. Assess the child's current nutritional intake and identify the normal nutritional requirements for the child's age. Measure height and weight and plot on growth chart.	1. Assessment data form a baseline, and normal nutritional requirements are the foundation for formulating a plan of care.
2. Identify the cause of the child's anorexia.	2. Identifying the cause of anorexia can assist in the elimination of the problem.
3. Obtain a nutritional history, including the child's favorite foods and eating rituals.	3. Identification of normal nutritional habits will aid in providing the child with familiar foods and eating routines; these in turn will reduce anxiety associated with unfamiliar surroundings.
4. Encourage parents to bring foods from home and to be with the child during meals.	4. The parents' presence simulates the home environment and increases the likelihood that the child will eat.
5. Allow the child to select food from the menu.	5. Allowing the child to select foods gives the child control and provides an opportunity to select foods that the child likes and will eat.
6. Offer frequent, nutritious snacks and encourage parents to do the same.	6. Children may eat junk food and then refuse nutritious foods offered at mealtimes.
7. Offer small portions. Use small dishes, cups, and glasses.	7. Children may be overwhelmed by large portions and refuse to eat any of the food.
8. If parents cannot be available during meals, allow the child to eat with other children.	8. Other children may distract the child and decrease separation anxiety.
9. Request a nutritional consultation.	9. Dietitians can assist in planning age-appropriate nutritious meals.
10. Respect the child's cultural and religious dietary requests.	10. Religious and cultural preferences may restrict a child's food choices. Efforts should be made to meet the individual needs of each child.

Evaluation
- • Did the child maintain baseline body weight during hospitalization?
- • Was the child's nutritional intake appropriate for the age and body weight?

Nursing Diagnosis
- ■ Ineffective Individual Coping related to anxiety associated with hospitalization.

Expected Outcome
- • The child will maintain the current level of toilet training.

Intervention	Rationale
1. Follow home routines of elimination.	1. Compliance will increase and anxiety will decrease if the child's normal routines and rituals are maintained.
2. Inquire about the child's terms for elimination.	2. Communication will be enhanced if the nurse and child use the same terms.
3. Do not scold the incontinent child.	3. If the incontinence is caused by anxiety, scolding will only increase the anxiety.
4. Explain to parents that some regression is normal in hospitalized children and that most children resume their normal routines soon after discharge.	4. Parents may be concerned about the child's regression and may increase the child's anxiety by focusing on the child's incontinence.
5. Discourage parents from beginning toilet training during hospitalization.	5. Toilet training can add another stressor at a difficult time.

Evaluation
- • Did the child experience incontinence of urine or stool while hospitalized?

Nursing Diagnosis
- ■ Anxiety related to fear of the unknown and separation from significant others and familiar surroundings.

Expected Outcome
- • The child will display decreased indicators of distress (e.g., crying, withdrawal).

Intervention	Rationale
1. Orient the child and parent to the hospital and the routines of the unit.	1. Familiarity with the environment and its expectations will decrease anxiety related to fear of the unknown.
2. Prepare the child and parent for all procedures.	2. Preparation for an event decreases anxiety and fear.
3. Encourage parents to stay with the child when possible and to be involved in the care of the child.	3. The presence of parents supports the parental role and decreases the child's separation anxiety.
4. Hold, rock, and cuddle the infant or young child.	4. Holding and cuddling children increases feelings of security and trust.
5. If the parents cannot stay with the child, provide for a consistent caregiver.	5. Continuity of care provides the child with a consistent person with whom the child can develop a trusting relationship.
6. Follow home routines and rituals when possible.	6. Familiar routines help the child be able to predict events and reduce anxiety caused by the unfamiliar setting.
7. Encourage the parents to be honest with the child when they leave and to inform the nurse where they can be reached and when they will return. Encourage the parents to call while they are away. Older children can talk on the phone with their parents.	7. Trust is increased when parents and caregivers are honest with the child. If parents just disappear, the child will feel anger, abandonment, and acute anxiety. By keeping open lines of communication, the parent's anxiety is decreased.
8. Encourage parents to bring transitional objects (e.g., blanket, teddy bear) and to provide reminders of themselves (e.g., pictures, scarf, handkerchief) if they cannot be with the child.	8. Transitional objects give the child a feeling of security. Both transitional objects and reminders of the parents comfort the child and help decrease the anxiety related to separation.
9. Take the child to the playroom and introduce to other children when appropriate.	9. Other children provide a form of distraction and assist the child in adapting to the environment.
10. For the older child, arrange for peer contact through visits, phone calls, and letters.	10. The older child may fear being replaced by peers. By maintaining contact and sharing information with peers, the child maintains a sense of importance and security.
11. Offer choices and allow the child to make decisions when appropriate.	11. Choice increases the child's sense of control.
12. Involve the child in his or her own care when appropriate.	12. Involvement increases the child's self-esteem.
13. Encourage the child to wear street clothes and to decorate the room.	13. Normal attire gives the child an opportunity for self-expression and makes the child feel more comfortable in the environment.
14. Provide opportunities for the older child to express feelings about the illness and hospitalization.	14. Fear and anxiety may decrease if the child has an opportunity to communicate feelings, have them validated, and participate in problem-solving techniques.

Evaluation
- Is the child playing and communicating with other children and staff?
- Does the child perform self-care when appropriate?
- Does the child separate from the parents with greater ease?

Nursing Diagnosis
- ■ Diversional Activity Deficit related to separation from normal activities and peers.

Expected Outcome
- The child becomes involved in play activities.

Intervention	Rationale
1. Plan for play activities. Spend time with the child reading, playing board games, drawing, or working on a journal.	1. Play is a normal part of a child's life. Play is a means of communication. It can decrease stress and boredom and act as a means of releasing anger associated with the illness.
2. Plan diversional activities based on the child's age, developmental level, interests, limitations, and safety issues.	2. Play is a part of a child's development. The needs of each age group are different.
3. Have parents bring the child's favorite toys from home.	3. Familiar toys can act as transitional objects for the child and decrease anxiety by giving the child a sense of security.
4. Communicate with a child life specialist about the child's identified needs (e.g., fear, anxiety, anger, boredom, lack of information).	4. Child life specialists can work with the child to identify fears and concerns, provide an avenue for release of feelings, and teach about procedures or surgery.

5. Provide opportunities for the child to meet other children. Assign the child a roommate of the same age, sex, and physical capabilities when possible.
6. Encourage peers to visit, call, and send cards and letters.

7. Document the child's response to play.

8. If the child is too ill, play for the child.

5. Peer activities are especially important to the older child and the adolescent. Children who have more in common are more likely to interact.
6. Spending time with friends and reading cards and letters can provide distraction for the hospitalized child.
7. Observation of play can provide information about the child's developmental level, psychosocial skills, level of anxiety, and adjustment to hospitalization.
8. Children who are too ill to play often benefit from watching someone else play (e.g., parents, siblings, nurse).

Evaluation
- Does the child engage in play with other children in the playroom or in the child's room?

Nursing Diagnosis
- ■ Altered Family Processes related to hospitalization of a child.

Expected Outcome
- The parents will participate in the care of the child and maintain mutual support of each member of the family.

Intervention

1. Assess the physical and emotional needs of the family.

2. Orient the parents to the hospital and provide information related to their physical needs (e.g., food, sleep, bathing).

3. Encourage the family to express their feelings and to ask questions about the child's illness.
4. Provide the family with information about the child's condition, treatment, and support systems.
5. Identify with the family the ways in which they are coping. Support parenting skills.

6. Refer the family to other professionals (e.g., social worker, clinical psychologist, clinical specialist, psychiatrist, clergy) when their problems are not within the scope of nursing.

Rationale

1. Assessment assists in identifying factors that might interfere with an appropriate adjustment to the child's illness.
2. The physical needs of the parents must be met for them to meet the child's needs and their own emotional needs. Meeting these needs indicates support for the parents from the health care giver.
3. Expression decreases anxiety and clarifies misconceptions.
4. Information gives the parents a sense of control and decreases their anxiety.
5. Individuals are not always aware of their coping mechanisms, and the nurse should evaluate the effectiveness of the family's coping mechanisms.
6. Early identification of family problems can decrease the possibility of escalation of the problems. Collaboration with other professionals can bring a holistic approach to the care of the child and family.

Evaluation
- Does the family support each other and seek other resources when necessary? Does the family assist the child in moving from a sick role to a well role?

Nursing Diagnosis
- ■ Self Care Deficit related to physical disability, change in environment, and regression.

Expected Outcome
- The child will participate physically in age-appropriate feeding, dressing, toileting, and bathing activities.

Intervention

1. Assess the child's usual self-care activities.

2. Encourage the child to participate in self-care according to developmental abilities.
3. Teach the child self-care behaviors and provide opportunities for the child to relearn or adapt to an activity.

4. Assist the child when the ability to perform self-care is limited because of fatigue, discomfort, or other factors related to the disease process.
5. Explain to the parents that regression is a re-

Rationale

1. Assessment provides a baseline of the child's actual abilities rather than age-expected criteria, which may be inaccurate if the child has a chronic illness or other factors that have caused delays.
2. Self-care increases the child's self-esteem and feeling of control.
3. Limitations may be placed on the child because of immobility, sensory alterations, or cognitive deficits. The child's sense of self-worth increases when abilities are used to their maximum.
4. The disease process may limit the child's ability, physically or mentally, to perform self-care.

5. Regression may be a defense mechanism in re-

sponse to illness and may affect the child's ability to perform self-care.

6. Provide the necessary equipment for self-care and place it within easy reach.

7. Offer choices and include them in the plan of care.

sponse to a threatening situation (i.e., illness and hospitalization).

6. Accessible equipment decreases the complexity of providing self-care by making the environment easier to manipulate.

7. Choice reduces the child's feelings of powerlessness and promotes self-worth and a feeling of control.

Evaluation

• Is the child able to feed, toilet, and bathe at the same level as before illness?

Nursing Diagnosis

■ Sleep Pattern Disturbance related to unfamiliar environment, separation from caregiver, or discomfort.

Expected Outcome

• The child will maintain a balance of sleep and activity.

Intervention	Rationale
1. Determine the child's usual sleep routine, including time, hygiene practices, and rituals, such as rocking, stories, or snacks.	1. An understanding of the child's normal sleep patterns will assist in planning care. Maintaining a routine decreases anxiety and increases the child's ability to sleep.
2. Decrease the child's level of anxiety or discomfort (see pp. 915–916). (See Chapter 39 for information on relief of pain.)	2. Inability to sleep can be caused by anxiety or discomfort.
3. Plan care to allow time for periods of sleep. Care can be organized so that vital signs can be measured and other procedures performed when medication is given.	3. Planning allows for uninterrupted sleep. Children who are awakened a short time after they have fallen asleep often have difficulty going back to sleep.
4. Post a sign on the door when the child is asleep to prevent other staff and visitors from waking the child. Unplug the phone, turn off the TV, close the door unless the child must be observed, and pull the blinds.	4. Environmental distractions can be major sleep interruptions.
5. If the parents are not with the child, explain that you will be nearby and will check during the night. Provide a nightlight.	5. Feelings of security are increased if the child understands that someone is watching.

Evaluation

• Does the child take naps and sleep an appropriate amount of time based on age requirements?

■ *The Family of an Ill Child*

Parents

A child's illness may cause a situational crisis for the family. If the illness leads to hospitalization, either planned or unplanned, the anxiety in the family increases. Ill children become the central focus of the parents. Four dimensions of support that nurses can provide for parents have been identified (Miles, Carlson, & Brunssen, 1999):

• Supportive communication and provision of information related to the child's illness, treatments, care, and related issues
• Parental support focused on respecting, enhancing, and supporting the parental role
• Emotional support to help the parents cope with their own emotional responses and needs related to the child's illness
• Caregiving support involving the quality of care provided to the child (Fig. 35–8)

Parents may wonder why their family is facing the crisis of a childhood illness or may believe that if they had sought treatment earlier, the child would not be so ill. A parent may have delayed taking a child with a low-grade fever and

vague symptoms to a physician. If the symptoms were a sign of serious illness, the parent may feel guilty for not having sought care earlier.

Parents have varied responses to a child's illness. They may initially deny that their child is ill, especially if the illness is serious. The period of denial may be followed by anger. The anger may be directed at the nurse, another family member, or sometimes at God. When the immediate crisis is over, a period of depression may occur. At this point, the parents are usually exhausted, both physically and psychologically. Often, they have been spending long hours at the hospital while working and trying to care for the other children in the family.

The nurse needs to be aware of parents' feelings and to listen closely to what is said. The nurse can then assist the parents in working through their feelings.

The parental role often changes when the child is admitted to the hospital. The parent who had been in control before the admission is now in an unfamiliar environment. Parents may be confused as to what they can and cannot do. Can they bathe their child? Can they even hold their child, or will they disturb the tubes? When the parent is not given permission to perform some of the care, both the child and the parent suffer.

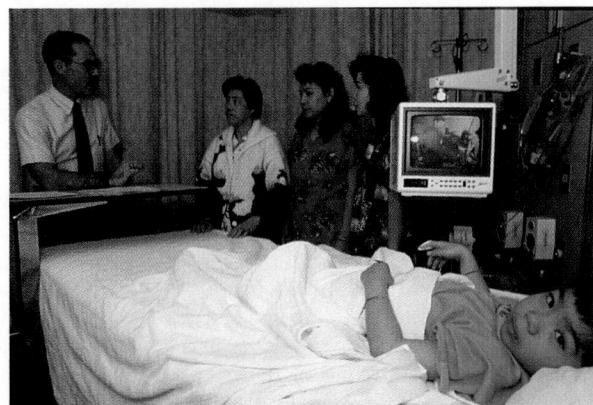

FIGURE 35–8

Sometimes the family of a hospitalized child may not speak the prevailing language. Interpreters on call at many hospitals help such parents communicate with hospital personnel and provide a familiar link to the parents' and child's culture and language. (Courtesy of Cook Children's Medical Center, Fort Worth, Texas.)

The needs of fathers are sometimes forgotten. The father may come to the hospital only after he has spent a day at work and then, after a short visit, may need to go home to be with other children. He may not be there when the primary care physician makes rounds and therefore receives most of his medical information from someone else. The father may think that he needs to be the strong one in the family and not show his fear and anxiety. In some families, the mother works outside the home while the father stays with the child. In either case, an awareness of each parent's role will assist the nurse in identifying the individual needs of the parents.

Because of dual roles, long separations, increased stress, and numerous other factors, the parents' marriage may be strained. This situation is especially likely in marriages that are already at risk. Even when both partners are at the hospital, they may not have any time alone.

Many children have stepmothers and stepfathers. In such cases both sets of parents need recognition, support, and education. How the family copes with the illness of a child depends on its coping strategies. A family that is already in crisis or one without support systems (e.g., family, friends, church) will have more difficulty adjusting to the change than a family that is organized and adjusted. A family that deals successfully with the crisis is strengthened by the experience. (For further discussion of the effects of illness on the family, see Chapter 3. For a discussion of the family with a child with a chronic illness, see Chapter 36.)

Siblings

The illness or hospitalization of a brother or sister can be difficult for children. The siblings of the ill child may experience jealousy, insecurity, resentment, confusion, and anxiety. Children often have difficulty understanding why their ill sibling is getting all of the attention and why their parents seem so preoccupied and have so little time for them. They may worry that if their sibling could get sick, so could

Caring for the Siblings of an Ill or Hospitalized Child

FACTORS THAT ADD TO THE STRESS OF SIBLINGS

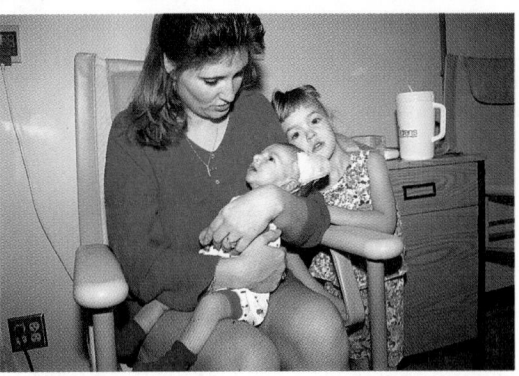

Her brother's repeated hospitalizations for problems associated with a diaphragmatic hernia have been difficult for this girl. Siblings of ill children may experience jealousy, insecurity, resentment, confusion, and anxiety. The nurse can help this child to cope by paying attention to her when she is providing care to the infant. (Courtesy of Children's Medical Center, Dallas, Texas.)

- Age younger than 10 years
- Emotional closeness to the hospitalized child
- Receiving only a limited explanation of the experience
- Fear of getting the illness themselves
- Being cared for outside their own home
- Perceiving that their parents are acting differently toward them
- Having a sibling who is progressively ill

NURSING CARE GUIDELINES FOR MEETING THE NEEDS OF SIBLINGS

- Encourage caregivers to have the ill child retell what happened. This experience may be uncomfortable for the adult, but it helps the sibling to put the illness or accident in perspective.
- If the sibling suggests feelings of guilt, address the child's concerns directly. If the feelings of guilt continue, suggest a consultation with a counselor.
- Give parents educational materials and show them how to use them with the sibling.
- Schedule a time for the sibling to visit. Prepare the sibling for the medical equipment and any changes in the ill child's appearance that may cause concern.
- If the sibling cannot visit, send photographs.
- Encourage the sibling to talk with the child on the telephone.

Adapted from Craft, M., Wyatt, N., & Sandell, B. (1985). Behavior and feeling changes in siblings of hospitalized children. *Clinical Pediatrics, 24*(7), 374–378.

they. Preschool children, who engage in magical thinking, may worry that they somehow caused the illness. All of these thoughts and feelings are compounded by children's difficulty expressing their feelings. Although some are at greater risk than others, many children hold everything inside. The amount of stress the sibling experiences varies according to the type of sibling relationship, the residence of the well sibling during the hospitalization, the frequency of sibling visitation, and the amount of parental behavior change perceived by the sibling (Simon, 1993). (A detailed discussion of siblings can be found in Chapters 3 and 36.)

NURSING CARE

The Family with a Hospitalized Child

Through family-centered care, the nurse considers and treats the child in the context of the family and recognizes the family as the primary and continuing provider of care for the child. Although the nurse sometimes must plan care without involving the family, it is difficult to do so.

Several factors (identified in Chapter 3) affect a family's adjustment to illness and hospitalization. Assess each of these factors, along with the history of the child's admission. Was the admission an emergency? Were there previous admissions, and how did the parents perceive those hospitalizations? How serious is the illness or trauma? Are some factors unknown, such as the cause of the disease or the child's prognosis? Special attention should also be given to any information obtained in the admission interview.

Providing the parents with information that will enable them to care for their child can enhance the transition from hospital to home. A systematic approach should be used to assist the family in their readjustment to the home environment.

- Assess the family's knowledge.
- Provide information about the illness or trauma and expected outcomes. Tell the parents when they should consult the primary care physician or nurse.
- Explain medications to be given at home and provide written information about times, route, side effects, and any special care to be taken when giving the medication.
- Explain any special nutritional needs.
- Identify specific activities in which the child may and sometimes should participate.
- Provide a date when the child may return to school.
- Explain, demonstrate, and request a return demonstration of any treatments or procedures that will be done at home. This teaching should be an ongoing process and not left until the time of discharge, because learning takes place at different rates.
- Provide the parents with a date to bring the child back to the hospital, clinic, or office for follow-up care.
- Provide the parents with information about any referral agency needed for the child or family.

CRITICAL THINKING EXERCISE 35–1

Tommy, age 4, was admitted to the hospital with pneumonia. Tommy has cystic fibrosis. His family has recently moved to the area, and this is his first admission to your hospital. Tommy loves to play with his dinosaur collection and spends much of his day playing and watching his favorite videos. His mother visits for short periods during the lunch hour and his father visits in the evening. Tommy cries when his parents leave. You mention to a colleague that you think Tommy's parents should spend more time with him. She responds, "We don't know what their other responsibilities are."

1. What other responsibilities might the family have?
2. What are some of the nursing interventions that would support a family with a child in the hospital?

KEY CONCEPTS

- Pediatric nurses may care for children in the hospital, school, community, or home. Each setting requires special interventions.
- Common stressors affecting hospitalized children include fear of the unknown, separation anxiety, fear of pain or mutilation, and loss of control.
- Children may experience anger, guilt, and regression in response to illness.
- The stages of separation anxiety are protest, despair, and detachment.
- The more stressed children become, the more difficult it is for them to separate from their parents.
- A child's reaction to pain and fear of injury is related to the child's developmental stage, previous experiences, separation from parents, restraint, and amount of preparation.
- Children who feel that they have control over their illness and hospitalization are more likely to feel confident and be cooperative.
- Regression is a common response to illness and hospitalization. The child returns to an earlier form of behavior.
- How children react to illness and hospitalization is affected by their perception of the event, age, cognitive ability, preparation, previous experiences, coping skills, and the parent's response.
- Nursing care of the ill child is directed toward meeting the child's needs related to self-care, separation anxiety, growth and development, diversion, family, control, and pain.
- Parents may experience guilt, denial, anger, and depression when their child is hospitalized.
- Therapeutic play can provide an emotional outlet, instruct, or improve physiologic abilities.
- Play can be incorporated into nursing care when the nurse is teaching or providing a therapeutic intervention that the child finds unpleasant or painful. Compliance increases when deep breathing and range-of-motion exercises, for example, are made fun activities.

ANSWERS TO CRITICAL THINKING EXERCISE 35–1

1. Families' two most common responsibilities are care of other children and work. A family with a child with cystic fibrosis has the added responsibility of caring for a child with a chronic disease who may or may not have frequent hospitalizations. In addition, family members have the expenses associated with the treatment of the child and, in most cases, cannot afford to miss work. They also risk losing their jobs because of missing work when the child is ill. Families often must balance work, caring for other children, and providing for the needs of the ill child.

2. In most cases, families of ill children are doing the best they can and may not know of available resources that might support them both emotionally and financially. The nurse should review the history obtained on admission to seek additional information about this family. In addition, the nurse should talk with the parents when they visit to determine if they have a support system and if a social service consultation is appropriate. Because the family is new to the area, their needs will probably be greater than the needs of a family surrounded by extended family and friends. If other family members and friends, such as grandparents or church members, are available, the nurse can guide them in identifying ways in which they might assist the family. The staff's awareness that Tommy is often alone can mobilize staff to spend extra time with him. The child life department, if one is available, should also be consulted.

REFERENCES AND READINGS

Agazio, J. G. (1997). Family transition through the termination of private duty home care nursing. *Journal of Pediatric Nursing, 12*(2), 74–84.

Als, H. (1996). *Newborn individualized developmental care & assessment program (NIDCAP) program guide.* Boston: National NIDCAP Center.

Baker, N. (1994). Avoiding collisions with challenging families. *MCN: American Journal of Maternal/Child Nursing, 19*(2), 97–101.

Biester, D. (1994). Schools and health: A partnership for a healthier future. *Journal of Pediatric Nursing, 9*(6), 414–416.

Bossert, E. (1994). Factors influencing the coping of hospitalized school-age children. *Journal of Pediatric Nursing, 9*(5), 299–306.

Boyd, J. R., & Hunsberger, M. (1998). Chronically ill children coping with repeated hospitalizations: Their perceptions and suggested interventions. *Journal of Pediatric Nursing, 13*(6), 330–342.

Brennon, A. (1994). Caring for children during procedures: A review of the literature. *Pediatric Nursing, 20*(5), 451–461.

Brown, R. T., Frank, N., Blount, R. L., & Smith, A. (1997). Hospitalization. In G. G. Bear, K. M. Minke, & A. Thomas (Eds.), *Children's needs II: Development, problems and alternatives.* Bethesda, MD: National Association of School Psychologists.

Burke, S. O., Handley-Derry, M. H., Costello, E. A., Kauffmann, E., & Dillon, M. C. (1997). Stress-point intervention for parents of repeatedly hospitalized children with chronic conditions. *Research in Nursing and Health, 20*(6), 475–485.

Carnevale, F. A. (1997). The experience of critically ill children: Narratives of unmaking. *Intensive and Critical Care Nursing, 13*(1), 49–52.

Clatworthy, S., Simon, K., & Tiedeman, M. E. (1999). Child Drawing: hospital—an instrument designated to measure the emotional status of hospitalized school-aged children. *Journal of Pediatric Nursing, 14*(1), 2–9.

Clatworthy, S., Simon, K., & Tiedeman, M. E. (1999). Child Drawing: hospital manual. *Journal of Pediatric Nursing, 14*(1), 10–18.

Corbo-Richert, B., Caty, S., & Barnes, C. (1993). Coping behaviors of children hospitalized for cardiac surgery: A secondary analysis. *MCN: American Journal of Maternal/Child Nursing, 21*, 27–36.

Craft, M., Wyatt, N., & Sandell, B. (1985). Behavior and feeling changes in siblings of hospitalized children. *Clinical Pediatrics, 24*(7), 374–378.

Dixon, D. M. (1996). Unifying concepts in parents' experiences with health care providers. *Journal of Family Nursing, 2*(2), 111–132.

Dokken, D. L., & Sydnor-Greenberg, N. (1998). Family matters: Helping families mobilize their personal resources. *Pediatric Nursing, 24*(1), 66–69.

Ellerton, M., Ritchie, J., & Caty, S. (1994). Factors influencing young children's coping behaviors during stressful healthcare encounters. *MCN: American Journal of Maternal/Child Nursing, 22*(3), 74–82.

Fisher, M. (1994). Identified needs of parents in a pediatric intensive care unit. *Critical Care Nurse, 14*(3), 82–90.

Grey, M. (1993). Stressors and children's health. *Journal of Pediatric Nursing, 8*(2), 85–99.

Hart, D., & Bossert, E. (1994). Self-reported fears of hospitalized school-age children. *Journal of Pediatric Nursing, 9*(2), 83–89.

Heuer, L. (1993). Parental stressors in a pediatric intensive care unit. *Pediatric Nursing, 19*(2), 128–133.

Horn, J. D., Feldman, H. M., & Ploof, D. L. (1995). Parent and professional perceptions about stress and coping strategies during a child's lengthy hospitalization. *Social Work in Health Care, 21*(1), 107–127.

Johnson, A., & Lindschau, A. (1996). Staff attitudes toward parent participation in the care of children who are hospitalized. *Pediatric Nursing, 22*(2), 99–102.

Jones, D. (1994). Effect of parental participation on hospitalized child behavior. *Issues in Comprehensive Pediatric Nursing, 17*(2), 81–92.

Kaplan, D. W., Brindis, C., Naylor, K. E., Phibbs, S. L., Ahlstrand, K. R., & Melinkovich, P. (1998). Elementary school based center use. *Pediatrics, 101*(6), e12–26.

Kashani, J., Canfield, L., Borduin, C., Soltys, S., & Reid, J. (1994). Perceived family and social support: Impact on children. *Journal of the American Academy of Child and Adolescent Psychiatry, 33*(6), 819–823.

Kristensson-Hallstrom, I., & Elander, G. (1997). Parents' experience of hospitalization: Different strategies for feeling secure. *Pediatric Nursing, 23*(4), 361–367.

LaMontagne, L. (1993). Bolstering personal control in child patients through coping interventions. *Pediatric Nursing, 19*(3), 235–237.

LaMontagne, L. L., Hepworth, J. T., Byington, K. C., & Chang, C. Y. (1997). Child and parent emotional responses during hospitalization for orthopaedic surgery. *MCN: American Journal of Maternal/Child Nursing, 22*, 299.

Lieber, M. (1997). Community-based pediatric experiences: Education for the future. *Journal of Pediatric Nursing, 12*(2), 85–88.

Manion, J. (1990). Preparing children for hospitalization, procedures, or surgery. In M. Craft & J. Denehy (Eds.), *Nursing interventions for infants and children.* Philadelphia: Saunders.

Manworren, R. C., & Woodring, B. (1998). Evaluating children's literature as a source for patient education. *Pediatric Nursing, 24*(6), 548–553.

McClowry, S. G., Galehouse, P., Hartnagle, W., Kaufman, H., Just, B., Moed, R., & Patterson-Dehn, C. (1996). A comprehensive school-based clinic: University and community partnership. *Journal of the Society of Pediatric Nurses, 1*(1), 19–26.

Melnyk, B. (1994). Coping with unplanned childhood hospitalization: Effects of informational interventions on mothers and children. *Nursing Research, 43*(1), 50–55.

Melnyk, B. N., Alpert-Gillis, L. J., Hensel, P. B., Cable-Beiling, R. C., & Rubenstein, J. S. (1997). Helping mothers cope with a critically ill child: A pilot test of the COPE interventions. *Research in Nursing and Health, 20*(1), 3–14.

Meyer, F. C. (1998). Parental perception of stress during a child's health crisis. *Evidence-Based Nursing, 1*(2), 60.

Miles, M. S., Carlson, J., & Brunssen, S. (1999). The nurse patient support tool. *Journal of Pediatric Nursing, 14*(1), 44–50.

Moore, M. L., & Krowchuk, H. (1997). Parent line: Nurse telephone intervention for parents and caregivers of children from birth through age 5. *Journal of Society of Pediatric Nurses, 2*(4), 179–186.

Mu, P., & Tomlinson, P. (1997). Parental experience and meaning construction during a pediatric health crisis. *Western Journal of Nursing Research, 19*(5), 608–636.

Page, N. (1994). Visitation in the pediatric intensive care unit: Controversy and compromise. *AACN Clinical Issues in Critical Care Nursing, 5*(3), 289–295.

Pietrobono, J. (1994). Taking health care where the kids are. *Texas Medicine, 90*(6), 14–23.

Ryan-Wenger, N. A. (1996). Children, coping, and the stress of illness: A synthesis of the research. *Journal of the Society of Pediatric Nursing, 1*(3), 126–138.

Scott, L. D. (1998). Perceived needs of parents of critically ill children. *Journal of the Society of Pediatric Nurses, 3*(1), 4–12.

Selye, H. (1974). *Stress without distress.* New York: Lippincott.

Simon, K. (1993). Perceived stress of nonhospitalized children during the hospitalization of a sibling. *Journal of Pediatric Nursing, 8*(5), 298–304.

Struk, C. (1994). Women and children: Infant mortality, urban programs, and home care. *Nursing Clinics of North America, 29*(3), 395–408.

Vessey, J., & Mahon, M. (1990). Therapeutic play and the hospitalized child. *Journal of Pediatric Nursing, 5*(5), 328–333.

Visintainer, M., & Wolfer, J. (1975). Psychological preparation for surgical pediatric patient: The effect on children's and parents' stress response and adjustment. *Pediatrics, 56*(2), 187–202.

Yoos, H. L., & McMullen, A. (1996). Illness narratives of children with asthma. *Pediatric Nursing, 22*(4), 285–290.

Ziegler, D., & Prior, M. (1994). Preparation for surgery and adjustment to hospitalization. *Nursing Clinics of North America, 29*(4), 655–669.

36

The Child
with a Chronic
Condition
or Terminal
Illness

DEFINITIONS

anticipatory grief   The processes of mourning, coping, interacting, planning, and psychosocial reorganizing that occur as part of the response to the impending death of a loved one.

bereavement   The objective condition or state of loss.

chronic illness/condition   A condition or illness that is long term and either without cure or has residua that limit activities of daily living.

chronic sorrow   Recurrent feelings of grief, loss, and fear related to the child's condition and the loss of the ideal, healthy child.

grief   A psychophysiologic process that occurs in response to a specific loss.

hospice care   A system of specialized and comprehensive care that provides support and assistance to clients and families affected by terminal illness. The purpose of hospice care is to humanize the dying experience while providing the means for living as comfortably and as fully as possible. These goals are accomplished by providing respectful, noninvasive care, pain and symptom control, and emotional, physical, psychological, and spiritual support.

normalization   Responses used to negate an illness or abnormal behavior in order to maintain valued social roles. Normalization is a common response among family members of a chronically ill child.

palliative treatment   Medical treatments or procedures that aim to promote comfort and quality of life, not to cure the underlying disease.

terminal care   A philosophy of care for the dying child in a hospital setting that is based on the tenet that the remaining time is precious for both the child and the family. During terminal care, procedures and treatments deemed necessary for comfort and pain relief are arranged so as not to disrupt the family. Such care is provided on a 24-hour basis and reflects the needs and desires of the family.

R apid advances in medicine have changed the experience of chronic illness in childhood. Children with
chronic illnesses are living longer, and an increasing
number of children are living with illnesses previously considered to be fatal. Both quality of life and longevity have
been enhanced by improvements in early diagnostic testing
and treatment.

Chronic Illness Defined

A *chronic illness* or condition is one that is long term and
either without cure or with residual characteristics that
limit activities of daily living (ADL) and require adaptation
or special assistance. Severity varies among chronic conditions. Many, such as bleeding disorders, diabetes, or sickle
cell disease, although not physically apparent, have a tremendous impact on the child and family. A short-term but
terminal condition may also have serious long-term effects
on the family.

The federal Maternal and Child Health Bureau's Division of Services for Children with Special Health Care
Needs (Westbrook, Silver, & Stein, 1998) developed the
following definition for planning and advocacy purposes:

> Children with special health care needs are those
> who have or are at increased risk for a chronic physi-
> cal, developmental, behavioral, or emotional condi-
> tion and who also require health and related services
> of a type or amount beyond that required for chil-
> dren generally.

Common Chronic Conditions of Childhood

Asthma (reactive airway disease)
Bleeding disorders (e.g., hemophilia)
Bronchopulmonary dysplasia
Cancer
Cerebral palsy
Congenital heart disease
Chronic renal failure
Cystic fibrosis
Diabetes mellitus
Down syndrome
Epilepsy
Human immunodeficiency virus (HIV) infection and
    acquired immunodeficiency syndrome (AIDS)
Hydrocephalus
Juvenile rheumatoid arthritis
Lupus erythematosus
Muscular dystrophy
Neural tube defects
Phenylketonuria
Sickle cell disease

The Family of the Child with Special Health Care Needs

Impact on the Family

Increased technology, insurance provisions, and allocation
of health care have all affected the family's role in caring
for the child with a chronic illness. Children with special
needs can now be safely cared for in the home setting. This
type of care, which includes psychosocial support, is the
most cost-effective and desirable care for both child and
family.

Although improved quality of life, longevity, and increased involvement in physical care are positive developments, they do present certain difficulties. Despite recent
medical advances, the child and family must live with an
ongoing physical problem that requires continued attention
and adaptation.

Chronic illness is stressful and can create situational
crises for families. A *situational crisis* is an unexpected crisis
for which the family's usual problem-solving abilities are not
adequate. However, various studies show that some families
reorganize and actually become stronger in response to a
situational crisis. These families are considered resilient;
that is, they are able to recover from adversity.

Resilient families exhibit many important traits, but
the predominant trait is family cohesiveness (Patterson,
1991). This cohesion is achieved by active efforts to keep
the family intact, not only by sharing the new responsibilities related to the chronic condition but also by sharing
the enjoyable activities of family life. Social integration and
support are important factors in these activities.

Maintaining social integration involves balancing the
needs of the family with the needs imposed by the child's
condition. Resilient families are careful in allocating resources, including money, time, and energy, as they balance
various needs. This balance ensures that the other children
in the family are not neglected or overindulged and that
the condition-related needs of the ill child are balanced
with normal growth and development needs and without
overprotection. In resilient families, the child's condition-
related needs are incorporated into the family's daily life;
they do not become the focus around which the activities
of the entire family revolve. This integration helps to

Traits of the Resilient Family System

- Balancing the illness with other family needs
- Maintaining clear family boundaries
- Developing competence in communicating
- Attributing positive meaning to the experience
- Maintaining family flexibility
- Maintaining a commitment to the family as a unit
- Engaging in active coping efforts
- Maintaining social integration
- Developing collaborative relationships with profes-
  sionals

From Patterson, J. M. (1991). Family resilience to the challenge
of a child's disability. *Pediatric Annals, 20*(9), 491–499.

---

achieve and maintain the new normality imposed by the illness. In such a family setting, baseball practices, school activities, ballet recitals, and other activities do not stop for either the ill child or the well sibling. Rather, as much as possible, medical appointments and treatments are arranged around these activities. When conflicts do arise, parents (or other family members or friends) alternate responsibility for maintaining the activities of the ill child and siblings.

Sharing care giving and encouraging parental involvement with well siblings helps maintain appropriate family boundaries. When one parent becomes primarily involved in meeting the needs of the ill child, both parental and marital relationships suffer. To keep these boundaries intact, resilient families pay specific attention to the marital relationship. They also work to avoid showing favoritism toward the ill child. Boundary problems of a different sort can arise when the need for outside care and assistance increases. External family boundaries can be negatively affected at such times, but difficulties can be minimized if family members adopt an assertive role in managing the child's care and maintain professional relationships with caregivers.

Resilient families work consistently to ensure appropriate communication, which may be more difficult because of new, disorder-related language (medical or otherwise), an increased need for problem-solving communication, and, most important, the need to express emotions. Accepting the validity of all emotions and learning suitable means of expressing them may be difficult. However, many families report that the experience of living with a chronic illness brings about positive life changes, such as increased empathy, increased family unity, and new meanings to life.

Even when positive meaning is attached to a child's chronic illness, much flexibility is required of family members with regard to roles, family rules, and expectations of each other. This flexibility is also required of the health care team, both for the benefit of the family and as a means of achieving a positive, collaborative relationship between the team and the family. The team of health care professionals becomes an integral part of family life, and the quality of the relationship can affect how the entire family adapts to and copes with the child's condition.

For resilient families, coping is an active process that entails learning about their child's illness and the resources available to them. These families do not sit idly by, letting others meet their child's needs. The nurse and other members of the health care team have an important role in helping families learn to meet their child's special health care needs.

At times of extreme stress, such as periods of relapse, unexpected physical setbacks, worsening of the condition, and death, families may slip into less effective patterns. Gentle reminders and encouragement may be all that a resilient family needs to help family members resume the behaviors that foster resiliency, despite the many stressors and uncertainties of a chronic illness.

The Grieving Process

The most important aspect of a chronic illness is that it affects not only the child but also the entire family. This scope of concern necessitates consistent family-centered

---

• • • • • • • • • • • •

Kubler-Ross's Five Stages of Dying

- First stage: Denial and isolation
- Second stage: Anger
- Third stage: Bargaining
- Fourth stage: Depression
- Fifth stage: Acceptance

Reprinted by permission of Simon & Schuster from *On Death and Dying*, by Elisabeth Kubler-Ross. Copyright © 1969 by Elisabeth Kubler-Ross.

---

nursing care (see Chapter 1). All family members respond to chronic illness, but their responses will vary according to the relationship and involvement with the ill child, age, developmental level, and previous experience with a medical problem.

Chronic disorders involve the loss of health and result in *grief*. Common responses to a chronic disorder include the five stages of the grieving process delineated by Elisabeth Kubler-Ross (1969). These are denial and shock, anger and resentment, bargaining, sadness or depression, and acceptance. Individuals need different periods to work through and resolve the feelings of one stage before proceeding to the next stage, and some fluctuation may occur across stages before acceptance is reached.

Acceptance of a chronic illness can occur even in the face of apparent denial, which might appear to be sustained throughout the course of the disease. Because children have less variable protective mechanisms, they may use denial frequently. An individual who has a positive, optimistic outlook and who focuses on concerns and tasks of the day, rather than on fears about the illness, is using adaptive denial as a protective mechanism.

The time frame for denial is important. In the short term, true denial, although often considered maladaptive, can instead be adaptive and is universally experienced at the onset of a chronic illness as a normal stage of grieving. Persistence of such denial over the course of the illness, however, is maladaptive (Walker et al., 1993).

As adjustment to the disorder progresses, many parents experience *chronic sorrow*, or the recurrent feelings of grief, loss, and fear related to the child's disorder and the loss of the ideal, healthy child. As identified and defined by Fraley (1990), chronic sorrow is a normal process and involves grief that may never resolve.

The nurse needs to recognize grief as a normal, healthy mechanism and chronic grief as a normal process, both for the child with a chronic illness and for the family. The first step in supporting families and helping them deal with chronic sorrow is to listen to and recognize their pain. They can then be assisted in recognizing and acknowledging the normality of such pain. Although families should be encouraged to acknowledge and express their feelings of chronic sorrow, they should also be encouraged to verbalize and demonstrate realistic hopes and dreams.

Many organizations, both general and disease-specific, offer family support and assistance, and the nurse should help the family use these services fully. Such support is particularly important when observation and assessment of family behaviors indicate problems that may require professional attention. In caring for children with special health care needs and their families, one factor that is often overlooked is the difficulty of acknowledging that death can occur unexpectedly or sooner than planned. This consider-

ation is important, even when the child's condition is chronic but not terminal. Supporting the family requires understanding the family's knowledge base, coping skills, and personal beliefs, as well as recognition of and attention to actual grief-related problems (see p. 940).

The Illness Experience: The Child and Adolescent

INFANT

Developmental Task: Achievement of awareness of being separate from significant other
Impact of Illness: Potential distortion of differentiation of self from parent/significant others
Cognitive Age/Stage: Sensorimotor (birth to 2 years)
Major Fears: Separation, strangers
Interventions: Provide consistent caretakers. Minimize separation from parents/significant others. Decrease parental anxiety, which is projected to infant. Maintain crib/nursery as "safe place" where no invasive procedures are performed.

TODDLER

Developmental Task: Initiation of autonomy
Impact of Illness: Interference with or loss of developing sense of control, independence
Cognitive Age/Stage: Preoperational (2 to 7 years): egocentric, magical, little concept of body integrity
Major Fears: Separation, loss of control
Concept of Illness: Phenomenism (2 to 7 years): Perceives external, unrelated, concrete phenomena as cause of illness (e.g., "being sick because you don't feel well"). Contagion: Perceives cause of illness as proximity between two events that occurs by "magic" (e.g., "getting a cold because you are near someone who has a cold").
Interventions: Minimize separation from parents/significant others. Keep security objects at hand. Provide simple, brief explanations. Explain and maintain consistent limits. Encourage participation in daily care. Provide opportunities for play.

PRESCHOOLER

Developmental Task: Creation of a sense of initiative
Impact of Illness: Interference with or loss of accomplishments such as walking, talking, controlling basic bodily functions
Cognitive Age/Stage: Preoperational thought: egocentric, magical, tendency to use and repeat words child does not understand, providing own explanations and definitions. Literal translation of words. Inability to abstract.
Major Fears: Bodily injury and mutilation, loss of control, the unknown, the dark, being left alone
Concept of Illness: Phenomenism, contagion
Interventions: Provide simple, concrete explanations. Advance preparation is important: days for major events, hours for minor events. Verbal explanations are usually insufficient, so use pictures, models, actual equipment, and medical play.

SCHOOL-AGE CHILD

Developmental Task: Sense of industry
Impact of Illness: Potential feelings of inadequacy or inferiority if autonomy and independence are compromised

Cognitive Age/Stage: Concrete operational thought (7 to 10 years)
Major Fears: Loss of control, bodily injury and mutilation, failure to live up to expectations of important others, death
Concept of Illness: Contamination: Perceives cause as a person, object, or action external to the child that is "bad" or "harmful" to the body (e.g., "getting a cold because you didn't wear a hat"). Internalization: Perceives illness as having an external cause but being located inside the body (e.g., "getting a cold by breathing in air and bacteria").
Interventions: Provide choices whenever possible to increase the child's sense of control. Stress contact with peer group. Use diagrams, pictures, and models for explanations because thinking is concrete. Emphasize the "normal" things the child can do, as the child does not want to be seen as different. Reassure the child that he or she has done nothing wrong; hospitalization, for example, is not punishment.

ADOLESCENT

Developmental Task: Achieving a sense of identity
Impact of Illness: Potential alteration in or relinquishment of newly acquired roles and responsibilities
Cognitive Age/Stage: Formal operational thought (11+ years): beginning of ability to think abstractly. Existence of some magical thinking (e.g., feeling guilty for illness) and egocentrism
Major Fears: Loss of control, altered body image, separation from peer group
Concept of Illness: Physiologic: Perceives cause as malfunctioning or nonfunctioning organ or process, can explain illness in sequence of events. Psychophysiologic: Realizes that psychological actions and attitudes affect health and illness.
Interventions: Allow adolescent to be an integral part of decision making regarding care. Give information sensitively, as adolescents react both to the content of information and the manner in which it is delivered. Allow as many choices and as much control as possible. Be honest about treatment and its consequences. Stress what the adolescent can personally do and the importance of cooperation and compliance. Assist in maintaining contact with peer group.

Developed by Martha Blechar Gibbons in Gibbons, Psychosocial aspects of serious illness in childhood and adolescence. *Hospice Care for Children* (chap. 3). In A. Armstrong-Dailey & S. Z. Goltzer (Eds.), New York: Oxford University Press, 1993. Based on Bibace, R., & Walsh, M. E. (1980). Development of children's concepts of illness. *Pediatrics,* 66, 912–918.

The Child with Special Health Care Needs

Growth and Development Concerns

Children with chronic disorders have many different concerns and needs related to their conditions, not the least of which is successful navigation of the stages of growth and development. Children's responses to illness are influenced by their age at the onset of the disorder and by distinct growth and development considerations. Nursing care must be planned accordingly. (See Chapter 4 for a more complete discussion of the normal stages of growth and development.)

Often, chronic conditions span several years and developmental stages. Regardless of the growth and developmental stage, however, concerns related to self-esteem, self-reliance, and autonomy are prevalent among children with chronic conditions. Many such children experience altered body awareness and image as a result of physical changes related to the illness or treatment, and these changes frequently have a negative impact on their self-esteem. Control and autonomy may be decreased because of hospitalizations and treatment regimens that offer few decision-making opportunities for the child. Social activities and adjustment may be limited as a result of hospitalization or the effects of the illness or treatment, or both. Such effects may include altered appearance, decreased physical ability, or increased susceptibility to infection. These factors may profoundly affect a child's acquisition of age-appropriate growth and developmental skills, especially in adolescence. To minimize the effects of illness and hospitalization and to maximize the child's potential at any given age, issues concerning self-esteem and autonomy must be understood in relation to each stage of growth and development.

Despite the best efforts and interventions of family and staff, a variety of changes and effects frequently occur in children with a chronic illness. Most are minimal, short-lived, and expected as a part of the "normal" course of a chronic condition. For example, among older infants and toddlers, stranger anxiety may be heightened or may reappear months after previous resolution.

Temporary regression is common from older infancy through the young school-age years. Toddlers use regression frequently and effectively as they attempt to cope with the stress of a serious illness. Despite its frequent occurrence, regression may be extremely unsettling, as it entails the loss of recently acquired skills. Common regressive behaviors include reverting back to the baby bottle or thumb sucking, a decline in toileting skills, an increased incidence of bed-wetting, and an increased use of "baby talk" or communication techniques more appropriate for younger ages.

Another possible difficulty is loss of communication in a child whose communication skills were previously age-appropriate or beyond. Lack of communication often occurs exclusively in the clinic or hospital setting, with regular patterns of communication used at home. Among older preschoolers, a lack of communication may be a form of withdrawal or an expression of stubbornness and a refusal to cooperate. This problem may also be seen in school-age children and adolescents and is related to issues involving independence and self-esteem. (Chapter 35 provides a more in-depth description of the impact of illness on each individual age group.)

Parental Responses to Developmental Issues

Regardless of the developmental stage or the number of years that a chronic illness has existed, the basic tenets of child rearing and development still apply. As with the well child, discipline and consistency are very important. For example, one mother of a 3-year-old with neuroblastoma would frequently remind both the ill child and her sibling that cancer is no excuse for bad manners!

Experiencing a chronic illness is confusing, especially for children whose cognitive ability is not sufficiently developed to allow the comprehension that could ease stress somewhat. When changes in their world begin to affect the only constant they know, their family unit, children's behavior often reflects this change. Negative behavior may result from the stress of the illness or from changes in their family and environment, or both. Previously existing negative behaviors may worsen, making treatment, including a positive relationship and compliance with the medical team, difficult. Future behavior and long-term development may be affected as well. At the time their child is diagnosed, parents should be instructed about the need to maintain any previous rules and expectations. The focus should be on the accomplishment of developmental tasks, not on the disease process (Clawson, 1996).

NURSING CARE
The Child with a Chronic Illness

The goal for any child with a chronic illness is to achieve and maintain the highest level of health and function possible. The aim is similar for the family system, including parents, siblings, and extended family members. This attempt to maintain a normal pattern of living for the family is termed *normalization*. The goals for the family are to remain intact, achieve and maintain normalization, and maximize function throughout the illness. Therefore, all care provided

---

CRITICAL TO REMEMBER

Goals for Chronic Care

Goals for the Child

- To achieve and maintain normalization
- To obtain the highest level of health and function possible, physically, emotionally, and psychosocially

Goals for the Family

- To remain intact
- To achieve and maintain normalization
- To maximize function throughout the course of the illness

by members of the health care team must use a family-centered approach.

The nursing diagnoses and care of the child with a chronic illness may be very complex because the goals are both physical and psychosocial. Care takes place in a psychosocial environment, is provided over a span of years, and must incorporate rapid changes in the child's growth and development. The long time frame means that the nurse must be prepared for a changing assessment, regardless of whether problems are physical or psychosocial. Nursing care includes assisting the child and family to accept, understand, and incorporate the illness appropriately into each stage of growth and development, regardless of the child's age at diagnosis.

Planning and implementation of nursing care are based on several factors. The child's actual condition is the first consideration. The nurse should not generalize across broad illness categories, such as cancer, respiratory conditions, and cardiac problems. Each illness will include specific implications, including subsequent disabilities. The child's and family's needs, coping mechanisms, and available resources are other influencing factors.

Ongoing Care

As with assessment and diagnosis, effective intervention involves the entire family. Evaluation will be an ongoing process, often done on a daily basis because of the chronic condition. Unexpected setbacks, such as a relapse, critical infection, an undesirable response to medication, lack of physical progress, or the need to undergo a medical or surgical procedure unexpectedly or sooner than anticipated, may be a part of the standard course of the illness. Goals may have to be revised frequently. These facts may be stressful and difficult, even for the most "seasoned" ill child and family. Continuous support and reassurance are necessary throughout the illness.

Education

Education is directed toward the child and the family and addresses both psychosocial and clinical issues, such as the physical care of the child. With an illness that continues for several years, the education process will be ongoing and may change frequently with the child's advancing age or with changes in the child's physical condition.

A special consideration is use of a child life specialist (Fig. 36–1). Educational methods used by either nursing or child life specialists include medical play, medical art, therapeutic play, and therapeutic art (see Chapter 4). All are similar in that they present the child with an opportunity for increased self-expression of ideas or situations that may present difficulties.

Communication

Communication with the child is frequently more difficult than the actual physical care (see Chapter 32). Often, communication is the most important factor in determining the success of teaching efforts and in establishing a good relationship, whether the child has a chronic or a terminal illness. Appropriate communication is based on the child's age and development and always involves honesty as well as compassion. Following these principles helps decrease the child's fears and misunderstandings and increase confidence

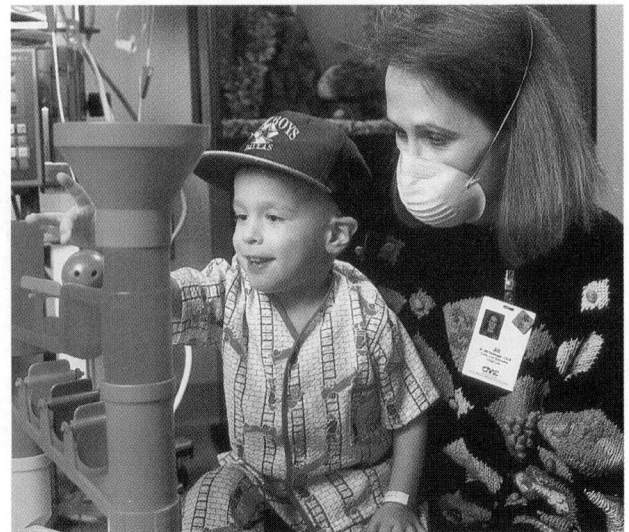

FIGURE 36–1

The nurse or a child life specialist can use therapeutic play, medical play, and therapeutic art to enhance self-expression, education, and growth and development. (Courtesy of Norm Tindell for Cook Children's Medical Center, Fort Worth, Texas.)

in the nurses and other members of the health care team. Increased compliance and cooperation is an additional benefit. If fears and misunderstandings are not ameliorated at the outset and caregivers do not gain the child's trust, establishing trust at a later date can be very difficult especially when the nursing care involves unpleasant or painful medications and treatments.

To prevent misinterpretations and misunderstandings, the nurse can ask children to explain what they know and understand. The nurse or caregiver should also strive to understand what the child is really asking. The classic example of miscommunication is the child who asks where he comes from and hears the entire reproduction story explained, when all he really wanted to know was whether his family is from Texas or Oklahoma! Clarification of the question can help the nurse avoid overinforming children, frightening them unnecessarily, or hindering them from asking future questions.

Honesty and trust must be maintained at all times in the care of the child, and these elements should be encouraged among the family and other members of the health care team. Complete honesty may cause problems for some individuals, family, or staff, especially when they face the difficult questions that often arise when caring for a chronically or terminally ill child. The most difficult and feared questions are, of course, "Am I going to die?" "Why did I get sick?" "Why do I have to die?" These are followed closely by questions concerning the death of others whom the child has known and with whom the child has developed a close relationship. Children are often reluctant even to ask questions of adults at all, much less questions whose answers they fear. Many times the child already knows the answer, so that the question becomes a test and a benchmark in the child's relationship with the adult, whether parent or staff. For children with a chronic or terminal condition, honesty may increase the child's emotional pain, something not always handled well. As with adults, children need honesty in order to establish trust. Children may not understand the use of dishonesty as a means of protecting them against discomfort or unpleasantness. Once aware of dishonesty, children may feel that they cannot and will not trust those who have been deceitful. Dishonesty may therefore have disastrous effects, particularly when one is trying to reassure the child and gain the child's cooperation. Many times, a chronic condition may progress to impending death, at which point the child's trust can be paramount to achieving comfort and peace (see p. 940).

Assessment

Family-centered care mandates assessment of the entire family system. Existing coping mechanisms must be assessed. If they are inappropriate, suggestions and support for changing to healthy, beneficial mechanisms should be offered. Additionally, the nurse should explore the family's response to the child's illness and the family's recognition of the impact of illness on the entire family system. Evaluating perceptions of the illness includes discovering what each individual actually understands about the disease process and the treatment regimen and determining whether any processes have changed as a result of misinformation or misinterpretation. Learning about existing support systems is also necessary. Such support not only helps the family cope but may also shape the family's method of coping, responses, and beliefs. Given the ongoing challenges of a chronic condition and the potentially frequent changes in the child's physical status, education should be viewed as a continual process. This ongoing effort ensures that the family shares an accurate knowledge base if and when family members assume physical care for the child.

The child's level of development and abilities (physical and cognitive) must be assessed jointly by the child, family, and interdisciplinary team. This baseline assessment of skills and abilities helps to ensure consistency of expectations and gauge the level of assistance that will be needed. Psychosocial abilities assessed should include family patterns of communication and behavior, as well as emotional concerns.

Issues of self-esteem, self-reliance, and autonomy are primary concerns for the child with a chronic illness. The child is considered at risk for self-esteem problems related to physical changes, which are frequently the result of the condition, the treatment, or both. Even with apparently minor changes, altered body awareness and body image can lead to a negative impact on self-esteem.

The nurse therefore should always assess the child's perception of physical changes and their effects. This assessment must consider the special concerns of each developmental stage. This assessment, perhaps more than any other, may change with the passing years. A child of 8 may be very comfortable with and well adjusted to a physical change or disability yet may experience difficulties with the same circumstances upon becoming a young adolescent.

Coping and adaptive abilities must also be assessed. This information will guide the health care team to explore any possible sources of difficulties in the family process. As these areas are examined during the course of a chronic illness, the nurse needs to keep in mind the physiologic progression of the disease. As the condition unfolds and the child's condition changes, so will the impact on the family and the work necessary to cope.

Nursing Diagnosis, Planning, Intervention, and Evaluation

Nursing Diagnosis	■ Altered Growth and Development related to chronic illness or disability.
Expected Outcomes	• The child will experience minimal disturbance of normal growth and development (physical, cognitive, and psychological), as evidenced by minimal delays, documented by an age-appropriate developmental screening tool. • The child will experience minimal disturbance of normal growth and development, as evidenced by ability to interact in an age-appropriate manner socially, physically, and cognitively, to the degree allowed by the existing disability. • The child will experience minimal disturbance of normal growth and development, as evidence by ability to perform and usual age-appropriate ADL as allowed by the existing disability

Intervention	Rationale
1. Educate the child and family about the physical conditions, expected physical changes or disabilities, and prescribed treatment. Education should be in a manner appropriate for the child's cognitive abilities rather than chronological age.	1. Education encourages a sense of control and acceptance of the physical changes related to the condition, as well as increased compliance with the prescribed treatment. Many children with a chronic condition are wise beyond their years, with a cognitive ability that does not necessarily correspond to their chronological age. Among such children, even those as young as 6 years may be able to discuss medical matters, such as laboratory values or the results of a diagnostic procedure, knowledgeably.

2. Set reasonable goals for improving and maximizing abilities in relation to any existing disability. Goal setting should be a group effort involving the child, family, and interdisciplinary team.

3. Assist child to develop a sense of pride in existing abilities and to gain the desire to achieve physical abilities.

4. Encourage and provide opportunities for autonomy and situational control by offering as many choices as possible. Include the child in age-appropriate decisions regarding treatment. Control can be offered in the form of choices, such as whether to be admitted to the hospital before or after lunch or whether to reserve the time after a treatment for a family celebration or a special time of sharing between child and parent. Teenagers may be given the option of driving themselves to the clinic, provided this effort is physically possible, for the treatment planned that day.

5. Encourage and provide opportunities for normal, age-appropriate ADL and self-care. Provide assistive devices, and educate the child in their proper use.

6. During hospital stays, provide regular street clothes (when possible) and items from home for grooming, eating, recreation, and so forth.

7. Provide age-appropriate activities and encourage the child to continue regular peer interaction (sports, school clubs or activities, church, social groups, and so forth). Activities should be done both in and out of the hospital, to the degree allowed by the child's physical condition or treatment. When possible, clinic visits, treatments, and hospitalizations should be arranged so as not to interfere with social, school, or church events. During hospitalizations, support and encourage the completion of school work, as well as peer visits and activities (Fig. 36–2). Misunderstandings and fear regarding the child's condition or the medical setting may decrease involvement of the child's well peers. A nurse and child life therapist can offer education through school visits. Include well peers in special events during hospitalizations.

8. Encourage the child to participate in the general or disease-specific support groups found at most pediatric hospitals. It may be appropriate to offer the strongest encouragement when the child is initially diagnosed (i.e., when fears and concerns are likely to be increased). Encourage participation in support groups, but accept the decision not to join if that is the child's choice. Disease-specific camps, where all campers share the same problem, are also available; examples include camps for children with renal, endocrine, neurologic, pulmonary, hematologic, or oncologic conditions.

2. Goal setting assists children and families to increase their abilities and self-esteem through successful accomplishment of tasks. Goal setting may also increase a sense of situational control.

3. Focusing on activities or skills once enjoyed can set achievable goals. For example, the child with a prosthesis can strive toward once more becoming an accomplished skier, but on one leg! Or the child can establish a goal of learning to drive an automatic instead of a standard-shift automobile, receiving a driver's license along with peers.

4. Autonomy and situational control are often lost as a result of limitations imposed by the condition or treatment. The child often cannot have a say in accepting a treatment or determining the type of treatment received but can be made to feel a part of the decision-making process. Situational control and autonomy are positively connected to self-esteem. Choices are not always possible, but when they are, no matter how small, they should be offered. Goal setting and the reasons for achieving the goal will be facilitated if the goal has meaning for the child, not just for the family or staff.

5. Self-care encourages independence and gives the child an opportunity to practice and improve abilities.

6. Personal items promote normalization despite an illness or disability and help to minimize disturbances in the patient's usual routines. Normalization also maintains and maximizes the child's sense of control.

7. Ongoing social connections encourage development and maintenance of age-appropriate activities and developmental skills. Social involvement also contributes positively to the child's self-esteem and autonomy.

8. Tremendous and valuable support can be derived from peers who are experiencing a similar medical situation. Such a setting creates acceptance and understanding not frequently found among those who are well. Because comfort levels and the type of support needed vary, however, such support groups may not be the best or only answer for every child.

Evaluation

- Does the child exhibit minimal developmental delays?
- Does the child exhibit age-appropriate social, physical, and cognitive interactions?
- Does the child perform age-appropriate ADL, as allowed by existing disability?

Nursing Diagnosis

- Body Image Disturbance related to actual or perceived physical differences or disabilities caused by an illness.

Expected Outcomes

- The child will exhibit minimal disturbance of body image and adaptation to the illness and related physical changes or disabilities, as evidenced by expression of all attitudes and feelings (positive and negative) concerning the condition, physical change, or disability.
- The child will express acceptance regarding the condition, physical changes, or disability, will maintain as much independence as possible, as allowed by the physical changes or disability, and will maintain a well-groomed physical appearance.

Intervention	Rationale
1. Encourage and provide opportunities for the child to verbalize all feelings, positive and negative, regarding the illness, physical change, or disability. Emphasize the normality of negative emotions.	1. Negative emotions will occur. To assist the child to progress to a positive accepting attitude, these should be expressed and dealt with by the health care team and family in an accepting, nonjudgmental fashion.
2. Educate child regarding physical changes or disability, expected limitations, or the progression of the disease, its duration, required assistive devices, and newly required self-care skills.	2. Misperceptions concerning physical changes or disability may hamper acquisition of a positive, accepting attitude, compliance with treatment, and the acquisition of new skills.
3. Encourage and assist the child to achieve as much independence as allowed by the physical change or disability.	3. Independence in self-care promotes self-esteem and a sense of control.
4. Provide constant reassurance about the child's self-worth and ability to be autonomous, despite a physical change or disability. Teach the child and family the actual self-care skills necessitated by the physical change or disability.	4. An ongoing physical disability can cause poor self-esteem. It may also cause doubts regarding the child's ability to become and remain self-reliant and autonomous. These skills must be taught, encouraged, and supported.
5. Focus positively on the unchanged physical attributes of the child and the intact physical abilities. Teach and encourage the child and family to do the same.	5. Achieving and maintaining a positive body image (with resulting increased self-esteem) is often difficult when physical changes have resulted from a condition, treatment, or use of an assistive device.
6. Assist the child to use aesthetic devices, such as wigs, special clothing, and makeup. Educate the child and family about more extensive measures, such as prosthetics and reconstructive surgery. Support any decision made about use of such measures.	6. Adults may consider physical changes, such as hair loss or scarring, to be minor when compared to limb loss or salvage, which result in disability. Children, however, often consider physical changes to be severe, resulting in negative emotions and poor self-esteem.
7. Teach and encourage positive, accepting attitudes about physical differences. Foster new ideas regarding what constitutes physical attractiveness. Many programs are available to help children adapt to physical changes. For instance, some offer advice about head coverings and makeup for the cancer patient (Look Good, Feel Better, the American Cancer Society). Some provide fashion alternatives for those with braces or prosthetics. Disease-specific support groups provide information about available programs.	7. Minimizing or disguising physical changes is often necessary to foster a positive self-image. These adaptations may also be necessary to assist others to accept physical differences more easily.
8. Encourage and assist the child to use special support groups and special camps for children with similar health problems or disabilities. Accept and respect the decision of children and families that choose not to participate in such support groups.	8. Support groups help provide peer interaction, possibly on a more comfortable, familiar level. Such programs may also provide activities that foster positive self-esteem. Individual comfort levels will vary, as will the type and amount of support needed by each child. Support groups may not be the best or only answer for every child.

9. Refer the child or family to appropriate personnel to manage coping or adjustment difficulties requiring therapeutic or nonprofessional intervention.

9. Some children experience serious problems, such as depression. Early intervention may lead to acceptance, adjustment, and resolution of such problems.

Evaluation

- Does the child openly express feelings, both negative and positive, regarding the condition, physical changes, or disability?
- Does the child express acceptance of the condition, physical changes, or disability?
- Does the child maintain independence as allowed by the physical change or disability?
- Has the child maintained a well-groomed appearance?

Nursing Diagnosis

■ Altered Family Processes related to care of the child with a chronic illness.

Expected Outcomes

- The child and family will experience minimal disturbance of appropriate family process, as evidenced by positive adjustment to and acceptance of the illness.
- The family will exhibit appropriate parenting and parent-child interactions and will demonstrate effective family coping.

Intervention

1. Educate the family about the child's condition, including expected disease progression, physical changes or disabilities, and treatment options. Assist the family to achieve a positive, realistic view of the child in relation to the condition.
2. Assist the family to identify fears and emotions pertaining to the child's illness. Emphasize that all feelings are normal and that appropriate verbalization is a positive and healthy part of coping.
3. Act as a role model for appropriate, accepting, positive attitudes and behaviors concerning the child.

4. Refer the family or child to additional resources (social worker, clergy, professional counselor) when necessary (i.e., if problems are beyond the nurse's scope or if the family requests referral).

Rationale

1. Education enables and encourages appropriate interaction with the health care team and compliance with treatment, in addition to decreasing fears and misconceptions.

2. Verbalization of feelings, with positive feedback, can help decrease stress and facilitate resolution of negative emotions.

3. Grief over the loss of a healthy child, discomfort with providing medical care, or a physical disability may hamper positive adjustment and acceptance. A positive role model may facilitate adjustment.
4. Situations requiring psychosocial assistance that is beyond the scope of nursing practice are not always indicators of family dysfunction requiring mental health intervention. When such intervention is indicated, however, early referral leads to a greater opportunity for positive outcomes.

Evaluation

- Does the family exhibit a positive adjustment to the illness?
- Does the family exhibit appropriate parenting and parent-child interactions?
- Does the family exhibit effective family coping?

Care of the Parents

Some needs of parents of children with a chronic disease are especially significant (Graves & Hayes, 1996). These include

- Obtaining information about the child's chronic condition and future services
- Receiving support through reading material related to parents with similar children
- More time for self
- Opportunities to meet and talk with parents of similar children
- Help in locating babysitters or respite care providers
- Assistance in paying for food, housing, medical expenses, clothing, and so on
- Help in discussing problems and reaching solutions

Grief Education and Support

Nursing care should include education about the child's condition and treatment as well as education concerning the grieving process. The nurse must assist all family members, including the child, to understand and express the emotional responses of grief. Taking time to provide care and support in this area is as important as physical care. Many adults have not experienced illness or death before a child's diagnosis and are not accustomed to the idea of

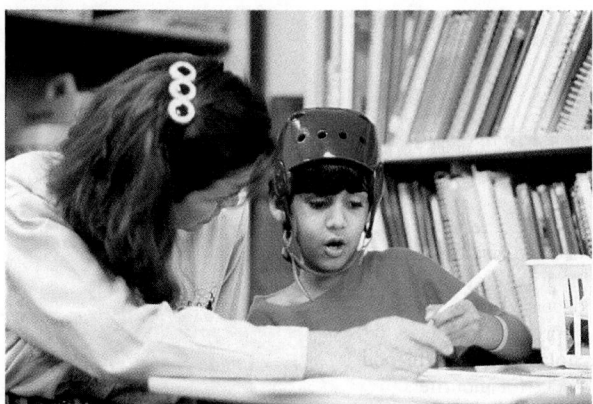

FIGURE 36-2

As more children with chronic conditions are living longer, more attend public school. Because these children are likely to be hospitalized frequently, however, hospitals often provide an area where teachers can help them keep up with their studies. (Courtesy of Cook Children's Medical Center, Fort Worth, Texas.)

grief, much less grief as a normal, healthy process. The nurse must educate the family about the importance of this process and provide opportunities for grieving. This care means conversation, listening, and being present for all family members as the need arises.

Cultural and Religious Beliefs

To provide caring and comprehensive grief support, the nurse must be aware of the impact of culture and religion on the grieving process in both illness and death (Table 36–1). Culture and religion influence the meaning of death and illness and customs observed by the family at such times. The family's explanation of the child's disease is revealing and may well lead to more culturally sensitive interventions (Sterling, Peterson, & Weekes, 1997).

When faced with an unfamiliar culture or religion, nurses must acquaint themselves with standard beliefs and practices, and the health care team must communicate acceptance of these beliefs and practices. Team members cannot assume that an individual or family belongs to a particular religion solely on the basis of cultural background. If in doubt, the nurse should question the family, stressing the need to provide the most comprehensive and appropriate care possible.

Referrals

To the degree possible, the nurse should not only meet the physical, emotional, psychosocial, and intellectual needs and concerns of the child but also meet those of the family. In addition, nursing care means assisting family members to provide for the child's needs themselves. Regardless of culture or religion, in some cases the nurse may not be able to provide the necessary support, usually because of lack of time or expertise. At such times the family should be referred to other personnel, such as a chaplain or social worker. If these individuals cannot provide assistance, they are generally in a better position to refer the family to outside professionals or services. The social service department will also be able to provide information concerning other re-

sources needed by the family. This information may include financial information, such as insurance and public assistance, housing and transportation assistance, as well as assistance with medical care and supplies. (See Appendix L for a list of general and disease-specific support organizations.)

The Nurse as Liaison

The nurse acts as a liaison for the family in many different situations. The most important liaison work, however, links the family with other members of the health care team, particularly the physician. Acting in this capacity, the nurse can ensure that family members receive correct information and have a solid understanding of their child's condition and resulting needs. These efforts facilitate the family's health care planning, help ensure a good relationship and appropriate communication with the health care team, and increase compliance with treatment.

Care of the Siblings

For the sibling as for the client, concerns and needs in relation to the chronic illness vary according to age and development. Fluctuations are common when the condition exists for several years. Siblings experience many of the same anxieties and fears as their parents.

Regardless of whether a child is past the age of magical thinking, siblings frequently have feelings of guilt regarding their role in the ill child's condition. What sibling has not had thoughts as to what life would be like without having to share material possessions and parental love with another child? The well sibling should be reassured about the normality of such feelings and told that the illness is definitely not the result of anything that the child said or did.

Nursing care of the sibling involves education about the ill child's condition, treatment, physical changes or disabilities, and expected disease progression. The hospital setting—rules, equipment, and personnel—must also be explained.

Like the ill child, siblings may also regress in developmental stage and activities. Parents frequently do not expect such behavioral changes from a well sibling and may need to be reminded that regression is a normal coping mechanism for all children, both ill and well, in the face of a stressful event.

Helping the sibling understand that illness creates stress that often results in difficult emotions, such as anger and jealousy, is a nursing goal. Children need to know that these emotions are a normal part of life, although they are often perceived as negative and harmful. Children must be allowed to experience and express each of these feelings (Fig. 36–3). While the physical and emotional needs of the ill child are generally well tended to, health care professionals may too easily exclude siblings and neglect their emotional needs. This oversight can lead to an additional set of stress-producing problems that have to be dealt with by the entire family.

CRITICAL THINKING EXERCISE 36-1

How can the nurse apply the principles of family-centered nursing to the family with a chronically ill child?

TABLE 36–1
• • • • • • • • • •

Cultural and Religious Variations in Grief and Death

Religious Attitudes	Grief Expression	Death Rituals	Resources for Support
Japanese/Chinese			
Very protective of people's feelings. Believe in afterlife. Decedents return to Nirvana. Deceased infants become "little Buddhas."	Not publicly expressive.	Chanting ceremony at bedside after death. Accepting clothes of deceased may not be appropriate. Japanese prepare gift food packs for mourners.	Families
Indochinese			
After death, soul lives in land of *tian*. Deceased baby returns in body of another child. Stillborns are "marked" on soles of the feet. Assign number to baby instead of name for first few days of life.	May weep or wail aloud.	May cover baby's head after death as a sign of respect for soul believed to be housed in the head. Women's mourning attire consists of a white outfit; men wear a black armband.	Families
African-Americans			
Commonly recognized western concept of heaven/hell. Deceased do not watch over earthlings.	Very expressive.	The funeral rite is an informal gathering that may include prayers, scripture reading, songs, and crying or screaming.	Minister, family, friends, church. Strong family kinship
Mexican-Americans			
Illness and death are God's will.	Very expressive.	Dependent on religious beliefs.	Families
Native Americans			
No life after death: return to ancestors. Navajos are fearful of death, will burn decedent's possessions. Beliefs in spirits and need to be in harmony with nature.	May or may not be publicly expressive.	May evoke nature names, monotonous singing over the dead to frighten away evil spirits.	Families, shaman, tribal group
Arabs			
Anticipatory grief work is not acceptable. Children are an integral part of family activities.	Express grief openly. Much touching of decedent's body.	Remain with body until it is transported. Do life review at decedent's bedside.	Family

Developed and used by permission of Roy Martin, D.Min., Professor Emeritus, Cook Children's Medical Center, Fort Worth, Texas.

The nurse and family can include the sibling as much as possible in the life and activities of the ill child, whether the child is hospitalized or receiving outpatient care. The family should be educated regarding the pros and cons of sibling involvement. Many families choose to minimize siblings' time and involvement in the medical setting as a means of keeping their lives as normal and uninterrupted as possible. Spiritual or cultural beliefs may affect this decision. Other families try to maintain the existing degree of closeness and may choose complete involvement, including the presence of the sibling during the day and for overnight visits if allowed by the institution. Regardless of the choice or the reasons behind it, the family's decision must always be supported.

When extensive involvement is chosen, the nurse should ensure that the sibling is appropriately educated in order to decrease misunderstanding and fear. As with the ill child, medical play, therapeutic play, and therapeutic art are excellent means of educating the sibling and allaying

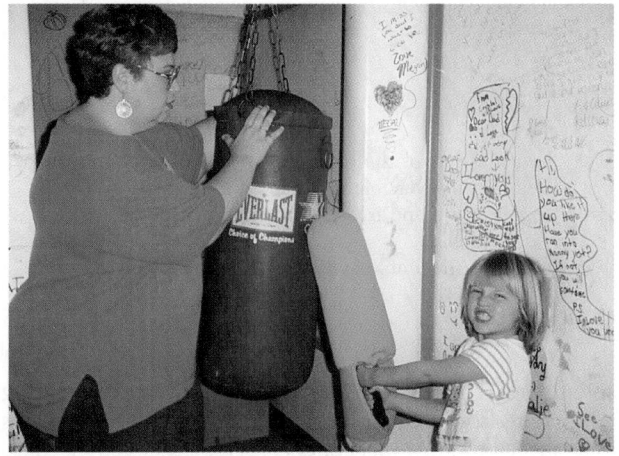

Chronic illness is stressful for the siblings of an ill child. Siblings' emotional needs may be overlooked. Siblings should be given the opportunity to express negative feelings, such as anger and jealousy, through therapeutic art and play and through physical outlets, such as striking a punching bag, as this little girl is doing.

fears and misunderstandings about the ill child's condition and medical treatment. These activities are also an excellent mechanism for support, allowing siblings to gain some understanding of their often intense and confusing emotional responses while venting them in a healthy, appropriate manner. Involvement with the health care team and a sense of connection with the ill child are also provided.

This type of extensive involvement brings with it additional risks. The sibling will frequently be exposed to the ill child's intense physical and emotional experiences, which can certainly have emotional consequences for the sibling. Close attention from staff and family helps to detect problems of this type. If problems do arise, the necessary support and intervention should be provided by appropriate team members (medical, nursing, child life, and family services personnel).

CRITICAL TO REMEMBER

Nursing Care for Children with Chronic Conditions and Their Families

- Caring for a child with a chronic condition means attending to the needs of the family system. Both parents and siblings may need additional support.
- The age and developmental level of the chronically ill child affect both the child's understanding and the family's needs. Goals may need to be revised frequently to meet the child's changing developmental needs.
- The nurse needs to listen carefully to the child's perception of the chronic condition. Children's experience of illness does not always match an adult's understanding of physical limitations and emotional strains.

Nurses striving to teach and include siblings in the hospital life of the child should collaborate with the child life specialist. This interaction can help the entire family discover, explore, and resolve feelings that might otherwise be problematic for both the ill child and the siblings.

The relationship between client and sibling may be altered because of normal but unintentional feelings of resentment, jealousy, and competition as the ill child receives more attention. This change may be accentuated if the sibling spends extended time at the hospital, thus witnessing the extra attention given to the ill child. Siblings may experience guilt and shame about such feelings. The nursing staff or child life specialist can devote individual attention to the sibling, separately from the ill child, as a means of providing sibling support. The opportunity to verbalize emotions and interact with a caring, nonjudgmental individual may help siblings understand and accept the normality of their feelings. Additionally, sibling support groups are a resource available at many hospitals.

The ill child often receives extra attention, including gifts, from family and friends during the course of the illness. Often, siblings associate illness with this extra attention and gifts, subsequently experiencing real or imagined illnesses themselves as a bid for similar attention. An important aspect of sibling support is to also remember the sibling at special times when the ill child is recognized, such as birthdays or graduations.

The Terminally Ill or Dying Child

The Child's Concept of Death

An understanding of death and dying in relation to childhood is necessary when caring for the child approaching death. The established and accepted guidelines concerning children's concepts of death are based on the stages of growth and development. As Waechter (1984) and Wass (1985) explain, these concepts correlate with age and cognition (Table 36-2). A child's concept of death is also affected by intellectual, social, and psychological life experiences (Bowden, 1993).

INFANTS AND TODDLERS
Infants and toddlers view death in relation to the loss of a caretaker and the subsequent emptiness in their lives. They are also affected by the loss of comforting measures, as when they experience pain or cold. Consequently, time with primary caregivers is quite important. As they approach death, they often sense the severity of their condition through their parents' nonverbal communication. Children of this age may react to the dying process on the basis of the sadness, anger, and anxiety conveyed by their parents. Reactions will be expressed through crying, attachment to the primary caregiver, and separation anxiety.

PRESCHOOLERS
Preschoolers view death as a separation or departure and believe it to be only temporary. Death is also seen as reversible. Magical thinking and egocentricity at this age often lead to guilt and shame, as children may believe that their

TABLE 36-2
. . . .

The Child's Concept of Death

Age	Cognitive Stage	Concept
Infant/toddler (0–2 yr)	Sensorimotor	Death as loss of the caretaker
Early childhood (2–7 yr)	Preoperational	Death as a reversible and temporary separation
Middle childhood/school-age (7–11/12 yr)	Concrete operations	Death as sad and irreversible but not necessarily inevitable
Adolescence (12+ years)	Formal operations	Death as inevitable and irreversible but often a distant event

thoughts or actions caused the death. The child's first exposure to death frequently involves a dead animal, such as an insect, bird, or pet.

Preschoolers facing an impending death frequently view their condition as punishment for behaviors or thoughts. They respond with guilt, anger, sadness, and fear. Their self-imposed guilt may cause them to believe that others, including parents, see them as "bad" and are angry with them. Feelings are kept inside, and these children may withdraw from everyone, including those whom they love and on whom they depend. Children may direct their anger at those they care about, and the intensity of their anger frightens them. Great patience and understanding are required of their parents and nurses, particularly when emotions are labile and subject to frequent, acute changes. Indeed, all children feel greater security when adults maintain discipline and suitable, customary limits, especially when the dying child is experiencing multiple changes and discrepancies in daily life.

SCHOOL-AGE CHILDREN
By the school-age years, death begins to be understood as a sad and irreversible event, yet it still may be considered inevitable only for adults. By the age of 10 years or so, children begin to understand that they, too, can die. Some associated feelings of guilt often persist for school-age children. They may continue to believe that thoughts or actions can cause death or that death serves as a punishment for wrongdoing.

The school-age child has increased cognition and other resources necessary to cope with the dying process, but these same abilities may lead to additional questions and fears. School-age children may wonder why they are ill and must die so young. Fear about the process of dying and what follows also may arise. Even in children who have a foundation of faith and spiritual beliefs, this fear may persist because they do not have a concrete knowledge of what heaven or the hereafter is like. They may also fear being without the love and support of the parents they have always known. Moreover, school-age children may feel vulnerable and doubt their ability to cope with the knowledge of their impending death, as well as the experience itself.

ADOLESCENTS
Most adolescents have a fully developed understanding of death as inevitable and irreversible. Because of an increasingly independent frame of reference, however, many adolescents view death as a distant event and may consider themselves resistant to death. Although adolescents may understand death and dying, they do not necessarily have

an emotional acceptance. Adolescents who are attempting to separate from their parents often test and break rules as they stride toward independence. This process may cause guilt for the dying child, especially when contemplating the spiritual aspects of life and death.

Adolescents may become isolated from their peers as a result of an illness. The terminal illness or disability of a peer forces adolescents to abruptly and unwillingly face and question their own mortality and wholeness. Discomfort with this possibility is often the cause of infrequent visits or no visits at all, even from close friends. Adolescents may also become isolated from caring adults, family, and staff because of feeling that adults do not understand them. Consequently, many feel lonesome and become afraid that they will die without the love and support that they need and desire. Realizing that they face death when their lives are just beginning, many adolescents respond with bitterness and sadness, particularly when they consider the adult experiences that will be denied them. Such bitterness and sadness may lead to depression.

Responses to Death and Dying

The process of dying, as well as the actual death of a child, is a unique and complex situation. The responses of all involved—child, family, and staff—will be affected by various factors, such as personal and spiritual beliefs, previous experiences with illness and death, and experiences during the dying process. An individual's progression through the stages of grief and death are also important, as is the relationship with the dying child. At any given time, the child, parents, and siblings may all be experiencing a different stage of grief and expressing that grief in very different ways.

THE CHILD'S RESPONSE
A child who is dying wants to feel safe and does not want to be alone or in pain. These concerns are frequently more intense and problematic with school-age children and adolescents. The child's responses to death and dying will be multiple and varied, not always fully correlating with the child's chronological cognition and development. The often traumatizing experiences of a chronic condition and its treatment tend to make children more mature and wise beyond their years. Additionally, children with a terminal illness may reach a point where they consider their illness and treatment worse than death. Relief is frequently evident as the dying child works through the five stages of grief and dying. The responses and actions of the dying child may also be affected by the behaviors and feelings of those

around them, particularly family and staff. Progression through the five stages is often accomplished rapidly, to achieve the necessary acceptance and closure.

The child's response to dying and the resulting actions are often more precocious than would be expected, particularly among preschool children. Family or staff often consider precocious actions and those of a spiritual nature to be inappropriate or unbelievable and may attribute these responses to physical alterations, such as a low hemoglobin level, altered neurologic status, or medications, such as analgesics or sedatives.

Spiritual beliefs may influence the child and be reflected in conversation and actions. Children may speak of seeing or even interacting with angels or the higher being recognized by their particular faith. They may also speak of going to heaven to be with the angels or other spiritual beings. Moreover, children may speak of going to play or be with a child or relative who has already died. This type of conversation may take place only days or hours before death, with children giving specifics as to when they will see or be with deceased individuals.

Dying children often experience a heightened sense of understanding and awareness, particularly as death nears. Many know when they will die, and death often occurs after they are successful in achieving closure of some type. Closure may be a special event in their life or that of a loved one, such as a graduation, holiday, or birthday. Frequently, closure also entails resolution of unfinished business, such as interacting with a loved one who has been absent or correcting a wrong.

Correspondingly difficult to understand is the concept of "allowing" the child to die. For most children, allowing death means giving the child permission to die. A predominant issue of childhood is that a child should obey the directives of parents. This assumption is based on the knowledge that parents know best and provide guidance so that their children will do what is safe and correct.

Additionally, as noted by Kubler-Ross (1983), children are afraid not of death but of abandonment. Children who are enveloped by hope, joy, and love will maintain their grasp on their precious and fragile lives. Accordingly, most children, particularly those who are younger, need verbal permission to die, as well as reassurance that it is safe to do so. Such reassurance should include a description of what and whom to expect as they die and in the time afterward. Children may also need reassurance that the family, friends, and loved ones who are left behind will be all right and that they will take care of each other. Equally important to children of all ages is the need to be remembered.

THE PARENTS' RESPONSE

When a child is initially diagnosed with any condition that is potentially fatal, every parent faces and begins to cope with the *possibility* of the child's death. When they are informed that nothing more can be done medically, parents face the *reality* of their child's death. The stages of grief worked through in relation to the illness must now be experienced in relation to the death of their child. Acceptance does not always occur. Some parents may find it difficult or unacceptable to discontinue treatment. They may choose to continue treatment of a curative rather than a palliative nature. Such a choice, however, does not always indicate denial. It may simply represent a belief system based on spiritual or personal convictions. Legally, emotionally, and psychosocially, the family's decision must be upheld and supported.

> Parents will exhibit the need to talk about their child and the experience of their child's illness and death. They talk in order to assimilate the experience, but more important, they talk to remember their child.

When a chronic condition has extended over time, the parents' initial reaction to their child's death is often relief that the child is no longer suffering and that the uncertainty of their situation has ended. Many times, this relief and feeling of peace may begin before death, when a definite resolution is known to be imminent. This relief may correlate with numbness, followed by intense sadness and a sense of profound loss and emptiness. The grief of a child's grandparent is similar to that of the parents, yet threefold greater. The grandparent must grieve for their grandchild, for themselves, and for their own child, the parent (Ponzetti, 1992).

THE SIBLINGS' RESPONSE

Like their responses to the illness itself, siblings' responses to death and dying, as well as their progression through the stages of grief, will vary according to age and development. Although children usually experience all five stages of grief and dying, these may not necessarily occur in the given sequence. Frequently, children move between the stages in a seemingly random fashion, often experiencing a stage several times. This process is an appropriate coping mechanism for children's cognitive and developmental needs and abilities. Issues dealt with successfully earlier in the illness, such as concern over having caused the illness or death, may resurface. Without appropriate guidance and assistance, these issues may persist. Siblings may experience other emotions, many of which are the same as those experienced by their parents. Because of their level of cognition and development, however, they may not be as well equipped to understand, to cope, and to work their way through the grieving process successfully.

Unresolved grief contributes to many problems in adult life. Children work through the grieving process differently from adults, and they often need assistance to complete the process. Many centers are now available that provide grief support for the child who has experienced the death of a loved one.

The most important aspect of providing support for the grieving child is to acknowledge that the loss of a sibling is just as significant as the parents' loss of their child. It is common practice for the health care team to send sympathy cards and other correspondence to parents after their child's death. This gesture can be taken an important step further by also addressing cards, phone calls, and other statements of sympathy to siblings individually. Such validation of their grief can be a first and important step in their successful navigation of the grieving process.

NURSING CARE
The Terminally Ill or Dying Child

Despite medical advances and current technology, many chronic disorders ultimately terminate in death. Providing

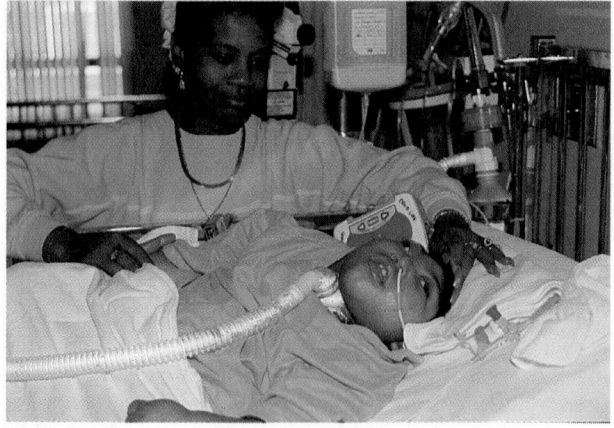

FIGURE 36-4

. . . .

The family of the child with a terminal condition needs compassion and support from the nurse. This child has anencephaly (absence of most of the brain), a birth defect that is usually fatal before birth or in the first few days after birth. His grandmother is his primary caregiver. His nursing care includes not only physical care but also support of the grandmother's care giving and assistance with the grieving process. (Courtesy of Parkland Health and Hospital System, Dallas, Texas.)

nursing care to the child with a fatal illness who is nearing death and to family members requires a heightened level of understanding, compassion, and support. A family's coping abilities are often tested beyond measure. Nursing care includes assisting the family to withstand the tremendous pressures and to meet the emotional demands of the situation (Fig. 36-4).

Professional Boundaries

Nurses must be cognizant of potential stresses, not only for the child and family but also for themselves. Caring for the child who is approaching death can be very rewarding, but it may also severely test the nurse's coping skills. Compassion is a must, but also essential is awareness and maintenance of professional boundaries. These boundaries are necessary for the nurse to provide clinically sound, compassionate care while also maintaining emotional, physical, and spiritual health. To provide professional care and support, nurses must understand and accept their own feelings and beliefs about death. Unresolved difficulties may interfere with nursing care.

Communication

Staff and family must be aware of the communication needs and patterns of the dying child. This awareness requires openness and acceptance on the part of all involved. Nurses and parents should provide assurance that the child will not be abandoned or alone and that loved ones will always be present. Children should emphatically be assured that the illness and approaching death are not the result of anything they have or have not done or said.

Children must also be assured that their emotions and actions are not wrong and that they are loved and accepted, no matter what. Children, parents, and siblings need assistance to understand their often varied, intense emotions,

especially such emotions as anger and guilt, which are often perceived negatively. Parents in particular need opportunities away from the child to express their grief and anger. This opportunity helps to minimize or prevent the child from feeling responsible for the parents' difficult emotions. It also contributes to an environment that is as soothing, comfortable, and stress-free as possible, where parents can have uninterrupted time with their child and the opportunity to provide whatever level of physical care they wish to handle.

Regardless of age, most dying children will follow the rules and patterns of communication set by those closest to them. As death approaches, the essential element of communication between child and family can decline in both extent and effectiveness. The nurse should take into account how communication was handled at particularly stressful times, such as the time of diagnosis, relapse, or periods of disease exacerbation. Generally, what has been effective in the past will continue to be effective. Blanket assumptions should be avoided, however, and each circumstance should be evaluated carefully to ensure the best communication possible for the child and family.

The most common issue that arises in relation to a child's impending death is whether or not to inform the child of the prognosis. The needs of the child, parents, and staff frequently conflict, but the needs of all must be considered. The suggested approach is to adopt a policy that allows the child to maintain open awareness and communication with those who choose to do so. Such open acknowledgment makes it possible to meet the child's need for someone to know and to acknowledge the child's dying while simultaneously allowing mutual pretense and decreased communication with those who prefer that approach. This flexible system has been found to be effective, and is prevalent among dying children and those who care for them.

Despite such flexibility, nurses may be caught between children who wish to talk about their death and parents who would forbid any such conversation. As the caregiver and primary advocate, the nurse should first meet the needs of the child. Any skirting of the issues or dishonesty with the child may destroy the nurse-client relationship, possibly denying the child a much-needed source of comfort and support. Nurses can inform the parents that they will not initiate any discussion with the child but that they need and intend to respond openly and honestly when the child initiates such a discussion. This policy allows nurses both to respect the wishes of the parents and to provide assistance or support when needed by the child.

Words are not always necessary. Presence—simply sitting with the child—or a light touch, such as holding a hand, may be all the child needs. The silence itself may be a therapeutic intervention, or it may help to open the door for desired verbal communication.

The Family's Beliefs and Practices

To support parents appropriately during this difficult time, the death of their child, nursing care must impart consistent respect and acceptance. This effort must occur regardless of any differences between the spiritual or cultural beliefs and practices of the family and those of the nurse.

The nurse will encounter different beliefs and practices surrounding death and the grieving process. These practices may include wearing prayer cloths, applying holy water or oil, viewing religious pictures, icons, or other objects, extemporaneous prayer gatherings, the preparation and serving of certain foods, and so on. Some practices may be troublesome to deal with because of concern over whether they are in the best interest of the child or even safe at all.

Parents' last-ditch attempts may include the use of unproven medications or treatments, such as those used in other countries. Although difficult to justify in our world of FDA-approved medical care, many of these attempts are not physically harmful to the child. Indeed, they may be emotionally beneficial to both parent and child, for such efforts affirm that everything possible was tried, a notion that may be very important to the child and family. These efforts may also instill hope, which under no circumstances should be taken from the child or parents. At times, however, such medication or treatment may be harmful to the child, as with painful intramuscular injections or treatments that may cause bleeding in a child with a low platelet count. In such instances, the staff may decide not to administer the treatment. The decision and the rationale for it must be explained compassionately yet firmly, always noting that the decision was made in the best interest of the child.

Often, parents make treatment decisions that do not offer any hope of increased comfort and quality of life and are not based on cultural or spiritual beliefs. These decisions often do not seem to be in the best interest of the child. For instance, parents may refuse pain medication for their child because they want the child to be alert, or they may request treatments that are traumatic and offer no hope of long-term survival. The issue of pain medication may be more easily resolved than the question as to whether extraordinary means should be used to keep the child alive. These situations may cause emotional, spiritual, and professional distress for the nurse, particularly if the action conflicts with the nurse's beliefs and seems useless for the child. To provide the necessary appropriate care, the nurse must cope with and resolve these situations. If unable to do so, the nurse should be given the option of not participating in the child's care.

Pain Control

For all involved—child, family, and staff—the most pressing and emotional issue relating to the dying child is usually pain control. The nurse should educate the child and family regarding pain control and then provide constant, consistent reassurance that everything will be done to guarantee the child's continued comfort. Families and older children may express concerns about addiction in the same breath as concerns that pain relief will not be adequate. Without belittling the feelings of those involved, the nurse should remind the family of the terminal condition, reassuring them that their concerns regarding addiction are unnecessary and inappropriate under the circumstances.

When there is a physical reason for pain medication, such as with a terminal condition, addiction does not and will not occur. Questions regarding increasing doses of narcotics and addiction may arise just as frequently in the care of a pediatric client as they do in the care of an adult. The child and family should be informed that the pain associated with terminal conditions may escalate acutely and frequently, with a corresponding decrease in the child's response to narcotics. The nurse should also emphasize that any necessary increase in medication dosage or change in

regimen will always occur in response to escalating pain. The child and family must always know and believe that pain will be handled in a manner that provides comfort as well as the optimal environment for meeting their psychosocial and spiritual needs. (For further information and discussion of pain control in children, see Chapter 39.)

Hospice Care

For many terminally ill children and their families, a non-hospital environment, involving either an inpatient or a home hospice program, may be the preferred choice for meeting their various needs during the dying process. *Hospice care* is a specialized, comprehensive system of care that provides support and assistance to the dying (and their families) in the last phase of a terminal illness. This phase is generally the last 6 months of a person's life.

The use of hospice care for children, either in a home setting or in an inpatient setting, is increasing. In part, this increase is due to the wide range of support services offered by hospice programs. Although nursing support is perhaps the primary reason hospice care is feasible, it is only one component of the array of services available through a comprehensive hospice program. For instance, social workers provide a number of services that assist families with a wide range of difficulties. These services include, but are not limited to, identifying sources of financial assistance, locating and bringing home family members who are in the armed services or living at a distance, planning a funeral, and facilitating legal affairs. The accessibility of equipment that can easily be managed by the layperson has also contributed to the increased use in hospice care. Such equipment includes hospital beds, bedside commodes, assistive devices such as walkers and bath chairs, oxygen administration setups, and other respiratory equipment.

In general, death usually occurs peacefully for children, but hospice care and death in the home afford a more natural, relaxed backdrop than the traditional hospital setting. At home, children can have close at hand family, pets, friends, and the comfort of their own rooms.

Just as home hospice care has been increasingly used for children, so too has inpatient hospice care. Inpatient hospice care may be provided in a free-standing setting or as a separate unit within an acute care setting. Families may choose an inpatient hospice for a variety of reasons:

- Physical care requirements and emotional burdens are too great for family caregivers to manage.
- The physical symptoms may require aggressive management, or the child may experience pain requiring intensive and complex medication control (Lombardi, 1993).

Brief periods of inpatient hospice care may also be used to meet a family's respite care needs, providing an environment that is less threatening and more home-like than that available in a regular hospital or medical center.

Hospice care should always be an alternative offered to families, along with the information necessary for making an educated choice. Some families may choose home-based hospice care but later admit the child to a hospital during the final hours or days of life. This choice, which always remains available to families, may be based on fears about pain control, adequate physical care of the child, or concerns over handling the emotional aspect of a death at home. Parents may be particularly anxious as to how successfully siblings will cope with living in their home once a death has occurred there. The health care team and family should discuss these fears early in the hospice experience and then deal with them appropriately. Regardless of such discussions, however, families may still elect hospitalization when death nears. The family's choices must be accepted and supported, regardless of the type or frequency of changes in decision making.

Assessment

Nursing care of the dying child and family is based on a complex set of issues. Circumstances affecting the child, parents, and siblings must be assessed and taken into consideration. Some of these circumstances include the family's relationship to and involvement with the child; the child's cognition, developmental stage, and previous experiences with illness and death; and the family's and child's experiences during the current illness. The nurse also explores the individual's progression through the stages of grief and dying. Children and their families experienced these stages in relation to the grief caused by the chronic illness; now they must experience them in relation to the impending death.

Anxiety can negatively affect the child physically, exacerbating pain or bringing on other physical symptoms such as dyspnea. Negative psychosocial effects may also exist for both the child and the family. Anxiety and concerns exhibited during the current illness should be assessed, particularly during times of increased stress, such as at diagnosis or during disease exacerbations or relapses. The nurse also assesses the coping and adaptive mechanisms of both child and family.

Nursing Diagnosis, Planning, Intervention, and Evaluation

Nursing Diagnosis	■ Anticipatory Grieving related to the impending death of a child.

Expected Outcomes

- The child and family will experience appropriate progression through the five stages of grief, as evidenced by verbalization of an understanding of the five stages of grief, expression of all emotions in an appropriate manner, and expression of feelings by each family member in a communication style most comfortable for the individual.
- The child and family will exhibit behaviors indicating acceptance of the child's impending death and will provide care and support—emotional, physical, and psychosocial—in the manner desired by the child.

Intervention

1. Explain the five stages of grief and their necessity for healthy grieving, including resolution to acceptance.
2. Identify the stage of grief being experienced and provide each family member with the opportunity to verbalize feelings corresponding to that stage. Provide positive feedback for appropriate progression.
3. Educate family about grief stage progression characteristic of children (the client and any siblings). Encourage patience with the extended time frame for a child's grief.
4. Offer all family members the opportunity to verbalize and act out, as necessary, all emotions in an appropriate manner.
5. Exhibit a nonjudgmental attitude toward and acceptance of verbalization and behaviors.

6. Encourage open, honest communication with the child to the degree requested. Demonstrate appropriate communication techniques.
7. Offer family members the opportunity to participate in the patient's physical care, as desired by both parties. Demonstrate care in a gentle, supportive fashion.

Rationale

1. An understanding of the normal grieving process may be lacking. An explanation should facilitate grief progression and guide behaviors in each stage.
2. Verbalization of feelings and receiving positive feedback will guide behaviors and facilitate continuing progression.

3. Understanding the ways in which children's coping mechanisms differ from those of adults will facilitate acceptance and understanding by parents.

4. Venting of emotions helps to decrease stress and to facilitate resolution of anger.

5. An attitude of acceptance will convey care and support. It will also encourage appropriate, needed expression of all emotions, both negative and positive.
6. Appropriate communication with the child will provide comfort and support. It will also ease closure and resolution of problems for the patient.
7. Many individuals fear the atmosphere of dying and the provision of physical care. Learning by example will lessen fears and enhance provision of care.

Evaluation

- Do the child (if cognitively able) and family verbalize an understanding of the five stages of grief and express all emotions in an appropriate manner and in a communication style most comfortable for each individual?
- Do the child and family exhibit behaviors that indicate acceptance of the impending death?
- Does the family provide physical, emotional, and psychosocial care and support in the manner and environment desired by the child?

Nursing Diagnosis	■ Anxiety related to the diagnosis or impending death.
Expected Outcomes	• The child and family will experience minimal fear, as evidenced by open verbalization of all feelings and emotions and questions concerning the diagnosis and prognosis. • The child and family will express physical, emotional, and spiritual comfort.

Intervention	Rationale
1. Educate the child and family about the terminal phase of illness, including what to expect physically, emotionally, and spiritually. Explain how needs will be met. Offer alternatives, such as hospice care.	1. Misconceptions may lead to increased fear and anxiety. Expression of feelings by family members may distress an otherwise comfortable child.
2. Assure the child and family that the child will be safe and comfortable and will not be alone. Provide frequent reassurance as needed.	2. Fears about the child's comfort and security are the most common. Frequent reassurances are often necessary as the disease or symptoms worsen.
3. Provide as much privacy as possible for the child dying in the hospital setting. Allow and encourage parents and siblings to stay with the child, as desired by the family. Regulate visitation by those outside the immediate family and friends as necessary.	3. Families may need extended time for closure. Although visitors may be well-meaning, their increased visits as death nears may interfere with time needed by the family. Because of concerns over hurt feelings, the family may have difficulty regulating visitors. If so, the staff must help by regulating visitors as a means of ensuring the family's privacy.
4. Provide extensive opportunities for the family to care for the child. Teach family members the necessary physical skills. Allow the family to decline provision of care when it is physically distressing or painful.	4. Children are usually most comfortable when cared for by family members. In some instances, however, the child and family may be more comfortable and less anxious if certain care is provided by the staff.

Evaluation	• Do the child and family openly and appropriately verbalize all feelings, emotions, and questions concerning the diagnosis and prognosis? • Do the child and family exhibit physical, emotional, and spiritual comfort?

The Process of Dying and the Time of Death

The care needs of the dying child are much like those of the chronically or seriously ill child. Much of the care is directed by the physical, emotional, and spiritual needs of the child and family. The goal of nursing care is to provide time for the child and family with minimal disruptions. Whether the death is occurring at home, in the hospital, or on an inpatient hospice unit, the child's room should be secluded, comfortable, and quiet. Appropriate surroundings contribute significantly toward creating a meaningful time for the child and family.

Privacy for the Child and Family

Disruptions by staff and even by friends or extended family should be discouraged and minimized to the degree possible. Often, members of the immediate family will request private time with the dying child. Occasionally, this request may cause others, such as grandparents, to become distraught or to insist on spending time with the child. In a hospital or inpatient hospice setting, this response is less difficult to handle. In such an environment, the nurse can more easily treat the matter as a request that the nurse is appropriately responsible for enforcing. In the home environment, the nurse has no such authority yet is still responsible to the child and family. Here, the nurse must attempt to communi-

cate the family's desires to others and must also educate others about the importance of meeting such desires and needs for privacy.

Regardless of whether privacy is required because of emotional or spiritual needs, privacy is needed for physical reasons. The dying child's endurance will be greatly diminished, with increased needs for daytime napping and extended nighttime sleep. The child may also experience difficulties with sleep, such as sleep deprivation, frequent wakefulness, or nightmares. Privacy and careful control of the number and frequency of visitors will help to ensure as much normality and quality in sleep as possible. Also helpful is the knowledge that loved ones are present or close by. In the home or inpatient hospice setting, where privacy may not be as great a problem, open doors or an intercom system (such as a baby monitor) can help to reassure the child that loved ones are always available.

Changes in Family Routines

Because the child requires increasingly frequent and prolonged periods of sleep, the availability of loved ones becomes much more important. Regardless of the duration—moments, minutes, or hours—intervals spent with the child can become treasured memories. The nurse should therefore facilitate family contact as much as possible. Special care must be taken to explain to siblings the reasons for rearranging life around the ill child's wakeful times. Siblings must also be allowed to have their time with the ill child. Most important, their feelings should be explored and emotional support provided.

Family Concerns About Oral Intake

The entire family often needs heightened emotional support with regard to nutrition and oral intake for the dying child. Disinterest in eating and drinking is a normal part of the dying process. Yet diminishing nutritional needs can be one of the most difficult aspects of dying with which families must cope. Parents and siblings may worry that the child will starve to death and that hunger will add to other physical discomforts.

The nurse should remind the family that at a point before death—often days before or (rarely) weeks before—intake will cease as the child loses the ability to swallow. The family needs enhanced emotional support and reminders that lack of oral intake does not cause added discomfort for the dying child, even when it continues for an extended time.

Fluids and Oral Care

A lack of oral intake, however, has some implications for the nurse in the physical care of the child. Any feelings of dry mouth and thirst (usually minimal) should be eased with small amounts of ice chips or fluids, given when desired and requested by the child. In light of decreased swallowing function and the possibility of aspiration, water would appear to be the best choice. Given the terminal situation, however, physical and emotional comfort can be enhanced by meeting the child's requests. Many children continue to drink their favorite fluid, such as milk or root beer, up until the time of death. A lack of strength or coordination may make drinking from a glass or straw difficult. In such cases, fluids can be squirted into the child's mouth easily and tidily with a medicine dropper or syringe. A catheter-tip syringe may be an even better choice, as the child may find it easier to close the mouth around the syringe's wide opening and long tip, although care must be taken with such a wide opening not to deliver too much fluid and cause choking. Many older children also find it easy to drink from the cups used to assist toddlers as they first learn to drink. These cups usually have easy-to-grip handles, a secure lid, and a small spout that requires little strength for sucking out fluids. Drinking out of a cup may also give the child a small sense of independence and control, which are often lost in the process of dying.

If oral discomfort occurs because of lack of fluids, several interventions may prove useful and appropriate. Good oral care will help minimize discomfort, swelling, and infection. Sponge swabs can be used to clean the lips and mouth, but lemon and glycerin swabs should be avoided, as they are drying. Dryness can be further minimized through the use of artificial saliva preparations, which can be swished if the child is able and then swallowed or spit out. These preparations may also be applied with the sponge swabs, along with agents to reduce inflammation or pain. Lip balm or petroleum jelly products can be applied to dry, chapped lips. Good oral care will help minimize odor and unsightliness, which may be distressing to the child and family. Providing oral care may also give the family a feeling of usefulness and an opportunity for much-needed physical

contact with the child. Provision of physical care should therefore be encouraged until the time of death, regardless of whether the child is alert enough to notice or to benefit physically.

Responsiveness and Communication

A child's degree of awareness or wakefulness until the time of death is frequently an overwhelming concern for family members. This aspect of dying varies from person to person, in both children and adults. The child may become unresponsive in the days or hours before death or may be intermittently responsive until the actual moment of death. The nurse should explain the variation to family members and remind them that hearing is the last sense to cease before death. For this reason, verbal communication and physical touch should be encouraged until death occurs, and even after, as desired by the family.

Occasionally, personal fears or beliefs make such actions difficult but may simply reflect a different comfort level in relation to the dying process, a different need for personal space, or different expression of emotions. The absence of either verbal communication or physical touch may not necessarily be emotionally harmful to either child or family. The nurse, however, should investigate the cause and offer assistance only when lack of interaction indicates a negative effect. No matter what the type or level of touch and communication, family members should be reassured that heightened awareness of loved ones is common among the dying, regardless of age. This information may impart an added sense of comfort and security.

Indicators of Imminent Death

Security and comfort may also come from knowing that reliable physical indicators usually signal the time when death is imminent. This phase may last a few hours or a few days. The heart rate increases, with a concomitant decrease in the strength and quality of peripheral pulses, and the blood pressure decreases. Pulses and blood pressure may become nonpalpable, a state that can last for hours. Cardiac changes generally occur before respiratory changes, but not always. Even if mild respiratory changes occur without significant cardiac changes, the nurse should remember how quickly and acutely a cardiac transition can occur. In some cases apparently innocuous respiratory variations, with normal heart rate and blood pressure, have been followed by death in less than 30 minutes.

Respiratory changes, which usually follow a typical pattern and are both visible and audible, are more readily assessed by family members. The effectiveness of the respiratory effort may decline, as evidenced by rapid, shallow respirations. An increased work of breathing, along with apnea, may also be evident. The respiratory picture may fluctuate between the two states. Respirations may cease after rapid, increasingly shallow breaths. Cessation may occur after a continuing increase in the amount and length of apneic episodes, coupled with a tremendous increase in the work of breathing (referred to as Cheyne-Stokes, or agonal, respirations). Respirations may become more audible and may be accompanied by an expiratory sigh, which often resembles moaning and may alarm family members, as the sound seems to signal pain. If the child is otherwise without verbal or physical indications of pain, the family should be reassured that the child's pain level is well controlled. The nurse can reinforce this information by educating the family as to the cause of the sounds and noting their correlation with each breath.

All of these variations in respiratory patterns will result in either hypoxia or hypercapnia. The agitation of hypoxia should be treated with oxygen, which provides physical comfort for the child and emotional comfort for the family. If the nurse is uncertain as to whether the agitation results from hypoxia or pain, the child should be treated for pain as well. A rising carbon dioxide level may actually contribute to a peaceful and comfortable death through its sedative and analgesic qualities. Continuing respiratory and cardiac changes may lead to cool extremities and cyanosis. These effects most often begin in the lower extremities and progress upward to the face. All of these changes, although potentially distressing, are usually well handled by the family with adequate preparation and education.

Perhaps most distressing is the noisy breathing caused by the rattling secretions in the upper airway. This rattling—often called the "death rattle"—occurs when the child has lost the strength and ability to clear airway secretions. Even with preparation, this sound can be extremely difficult for the family. Pharyngeal suctioning can be helpful but may need to be done frequently and can be a source of discomfort for the child. Until a prescribed medication takes effect, the child can be positioned on the side to facilitate drainage of the secretions. A cloth should be placed appropriately and the family prepared to expect secretions draining from the mouth. The child is very rarely aware of this respiratory occurrence, so the focus of care should be symptom management to ensure the emotional comfort of the family.

When respirations have ceased, a short delay may occur before the heart stops beating. There may also be a final gasping noise after the respirations and heartbeat have stopped. Reassure the family that this sound is normal and not painful.

The Family After Death

After death has occurred, family members should have the opportunity to spend as much time with the child as they desire. They might spend time before the body is cleaned, although cleaning is preferably done first because of the drainage, bleeding, and spontaneous elimination of body wastes that often occur at the time of death. Before the body is bathed, the family often appreciates the opportunity to make hand and foot prints or cut a lock of hair as a remembrance of the child. The family should be invited to assist in the bathing if they so desire. This final act of physical care may be a special means of closure.

Frequently, siblings or other children are interested in this procedure. Adults may find this interest distressing, whether or not they wish to assist. Encourage the family to allow sibling participation, noting that it may facilitate closure, as well as correct or prevent fears and misconceptions about death or the deceased child. The nurse should respect whatever decisions are made and offer an explanation as to what the care will involve, even if the family chooses not to participate.

The nurse should inform the family that the child can go to the funeral home either in a hospital gown or in per-

CRITICAL TO REMEMBER

Nursing Care for the Dying Child and the Child's Family

- The nurse should be available to assist both the dying child and family but must not impose personal beliefs and expectations on either the child or the family members.
- The siblings of a dying child need time and attention. They, too, will experience grief and will need to resolve their feelings.
- Most family members need to talk about the experience of illness and death. Open communication maintains family resilience and helps family members remember the child after death.
- Terminal care includes adequate pain control, oral care, ensuring privacy, and providing information on the signs of imminent death and what to expect in the immediate postmortem period.
- After death occurs, family members should have as much time as they desire with the child.

sonal clothes and should reassure the family that the clothes will be returned after the child is dressed for burial. If the family will not be participating in postmortem care, the period just after death is a good time to choose clothing and a personal item, such as a blanket or toy. These items will also be returned. Sibling participation in this process is another good closure mechanism. As family members prepare to hold the deceased child, the nurse informs them that physical changes after death may occur very quickly. Changes include cooling of the body, cyanosis or paleness, and stiffening. The nurse attempts to prevent further drainage of any body fluids, particularly if family members will be holding the child. The nurse prepares the family emotionally and provides towels if preventive measures are not possible or are ineffective.

The nurse should allow privacy for the family, promising to be close by and to return as needed or desired. The nurse always offers the support of clergy, even if there has been no such involvement previously. If no personal clergy has been identified or one is not available, the nurse reminds the family of the availability of hospital or hospice personnel. If a funeral home has not been chosen, clergy or social services personnel are usually good sources for assistance.

The Nurse's Response to the Dying Child

Not all health care providers can deal with the reality of death. This limitation may hold serious implications for the nurse who works in an area where death is common. Caring for dying children and their families can be stressful and emotionally demanding. Even the nurse who works closely and frequently with dying children is not immune to the pressures and responses experienced in such an environment. The demands of chronic or terminal illness may require increased emotional and psychosocial strength, as well as clinical expertise.

The nurse's response to the dying process and death of

a child will correlate to a certain degree with the stages of grief and dying. The nurse who has become more accustomed to the reality and frequency of death may not experience each stage. Length of treatment and personal affinity often cause the nurse to become more involved with or closer to one child or another, a development that can lead to a more intense response or a delay in appropriate resolution of grief. In providing competent and caring nursing care, the nurse may have difficulty maintaining appropriate boundaries between personal involvement and professional care. A nurse who is more detached and professional may be able more easily to provide care on a continuing basis. Regardless of the depth of involvement, level of profession-

alism, or the number of deaths encountered, however, every nurse who cares for dying children will experience loss and grief. Consequently, the nurse will need support through the difficult times. Both staff nurses and management must recognize this need. All must work together to provide mutual support through both active, organized support programs and simple acts of respect, concern, and care among colleagues. To normalize feelings, facilitate self-reflection, and create a supportive environment, the novice nurse may benefit from working with a more experienced nurse (Rashotte, Fothergill-Bourbonnais, & Chamberlain, 1997). Care of the caregiver is also an integral part of caring for the child with a chronic or terminal illness.

KEY CONCEPTS

■ Children with chronic conditions are living longer, and more children are living with conditions that were once considered fatal. Despite improvement in quality of life and longevity, chronic illness is stressful and a situational crisis for families, one that requires ongoing attention and adaptation.

■ The most important aspect of a chronic illness is that it affects the entire family, not just the child.

■ Families dealing with chronic illness have many varied concerns and needs, including meeting the physical and emotional needs of the child, providing care for the rest of the family, and meeting financial burdens. The family must strive to meet the physical, emotional, psychosocial, and spiritual needs of each of its members.

■ The stages of grief, as well as of

death and dying, are applicable to pediatric clients, but with special considerations for both child and family. The child's concepts of death and dying are based on the child's stage of growth and development. These concepts are further affected by age, cognition, and experiences of life—intellectual, social, and psychological. Both ill children and well siblings experience changing understanding of death and dying.

■ The dying child, like the dying adult, desires the comfort, safety, and presence of loved ones.

■ Parents must move from *fearing* the child's death to *acknowledging* the child's impending death. For parents caring for a dying child, pain is the greatest concern.

■ Although the grief of parents is often more intense, siblings' lesser

cognitive abilities and changing developmental needs and capabilities can make the grief of siblings more difficult to address.

■ Grief is similar for all families (adults and children); grief must be processed and the loss integrated. Loved ones must understand that the person who has died is gone, and must experience the resulting emotions. Family members must reinvest in life and go forward with their lives.

■ Nursing care of the terminally ill or dying child can be extremely stressful and demanding. It requires strict attention to one's own physical, emotional, and spiritual health. Care of the caregiver is imperative if the nurse is to provide physical and psychosocial care for families at such a difficult time.

ANSWER TO CRITICAL THINKING EXERCISE 36–1

The nurse can assist family members in using their coping skills and in problem solving. The family should be educated about the medical aspects of the disease and how to care for the child at home. Interpersonal com-

munication among family members and the development of social supports should be encouraged. Siblings should be included in the assessment of the family and incorporated into the plan

of care for the family. Community resources that support both the child and family should be identified and the family assisted in accessing these support systems.

REFERENCES AND READINGS

American Academy of Pediatrics Committee on Bioethics. (1994). Guidelines on forgoing life-sustaining medical treatment. *Pediatric Nursing, 20*(5), 517–521.

American Academy of Pediatrics Committee on Bioethics. (1996). Ethics and the care of critically ill infants and children. *Pediatrics, 98*(1), 149–152.

American Academy of Pediatrics Committee on Children With Disabilities. (1995). Guidelines for home care of infants, children, and adolescents with chronic disease. *Pediatrics, 96*(1), 161–164.

American Academy of Pediatrics Committee on Children With Disabilities. (1997). General principles in the care of children

and adolescents with genetic disorders and other chronic health conditions. *Pediatrics, 99*(4), 643–644.

American Academy of Pediatrics Committee on Pediatric Emergency Medicine. (1994). Death of a child in the emergency department. *Pediatrics, 93*(5), 861–862.

Bakewell-Sachs, S., & Porth, S. (1995). Discharge planning and home care of the technology-dependent infant. *Journal of Obstetric, Gynecologic, and Neonatal Nursing, 24*(1), 77–83.

Bowden, V. R. (1993). Children's literature: The death experience. *Pediatric Nursing, 19*(1), 17–21.

Capen, C., & Dedlow, E. (1998). Discharging ventilator-dependent children: A continuing challenge. *Journal of Pediatric Nursing, 13*(3), 175–184.

Chapman, K. J., & Pepler, C. (1998). Coping, hope, and anticipatory grief in family members in palliative home care. *Cancer Nursing, 21*(4), 226–234.

Clawson, J. (1996). A child with chronic illness and the process of family adaptation. *Journal of Pediatric Nursing, 11*(1), 52–61.

Davies, B., Cook, K., O'Loane, M., Clarke, D., MacKenzie, B., Stutzer, C., Connaughty, S., & McCormick, J. (1996). Caring for dying children: Nurses' experience. *Pediatric Nursing, 22*(6), 500–507.

Diamond, J. (1996). Family-centered care for children with chronic illness. *Journal of Pediatric Health Care, 8*, 196–198.

Doka, K. J. (1995). *Children mourning: Mourning children.* Washington, DC: Hospice Foundation of America.

Fleming, J., Challella, M., Eland, J., Hornick, R., Johnson, P., Martinson, I., Nativio, D., Nokes, K., Riddle, I., Steele, N., Sudela, K., Thomas, R., Turner, Q., Wheeler, B., & Young, A. (1994). Impact on the family of children who are technology dependent and cared for in the home. *Pediatric Nursing, 20*(4), 379–388.

Fraley, A. M. (1990). Chronic sorrow: A parental response. *Journal of Pediatric Nursing, 5*(4), 268–273.

Gallo, A. M., & Knafl, K. (1998). Parents' reports of "tricks of the trade" for managing childhood chronic illness. *Journal of the Society of Pediatric Nurses, 3*(3), 93–100.

Gravelle, A. M. (1997). Caring for a child with a progressive illness during the complex chronic phase: Parents' experience of facing adversity. *Journal of Advanced Nursing, 25*(4), 738–745.

Graves, C., & Hayes, V. (1996). Do nurses and parents of children with chronic conditions agree on parental needs? *Journal of Pediatric Nursing, 11*(5), 288–299.

Hanson, W., Ridder, K., Liebergen, A., Olson, J., Barnard, M., & Tobin-Rommelhart, S. (1997). Outcomes of nursing interventions for siblings of chronically ill children: A pilot study. *Journal of the Society of Pediatric Nurses, 2*, 127–137.

Heffernan, S., & Zanelli, A. S. (1997). Behavior changes exhibited by siblings of pediatric oncology patients: A comparison between maternal and sibling descriptions. *Journal of Pediatric Oncology Nursing, 14*(1), 3–14.

Heiney, S., Ruffin, J., & Goon-Johnson, K. (1995). The effects of a support group on selected psychosocial outcomes of bereaved parents whose child died from cancer. *Journal of Pediatric Oncology Nursing, 12*(2), 51–58.

Heiney, S., Wells, L., & Ruffin, J. (1996). A memorial service for families of children who died from cancer and blood disorders. *Journal of Pediatric Oncology Nursing, 13*(2), 72–79.

Hillman, K. A. (1997). Comparing child-rearing practices in parents of children with cancer and parents of healthy children. *Journal of Pediatric Oncology Nursing, 14*(2), 53–67.

Itano, J., & Taoka, K. (1997). *Core curriculum for oncology nursing.* Philadelphia: Saunders.

Johnson, L. C., Rincon, B., Gober, C., & Rexin, D. (1993). The development of a comprehensive bereavement program to assist families experiencing pediatric loss. *Journal of Pediatrics, 8*(3), 142–146.

Johnston, C. E., & Marder, L. R. (1994). Parenting the child with a chronic condition: An emotional experience. *Pediatric Nursing, 20*(6), 611–614.

Knafl, K., Breitmayer, B., Gallo, A., & Zoeller, L. (1996). Family response to childhood chronic illness: Description of management styles. *Journal of Pediatric Nursing, 11*(5), 315–326.

Komp, D. M. (1994). *Hope springs from mended places: Images of grace in the shadows of life.* Grand Rapids: Zondervan.

Kubler-Ross, E. (1969). *On death and dying.* New York: Macmillan.

Kubler-Ross, E. (1983). *On children and death.* New York: Macmillan.

Kushner, H. S. (1981). *When bad things happen to good people.* New York: Avon Books.

Lehna, C. R. (1998). A childhood cancer sibling's oral history. *Journal of Pediatric Oncology Nursing, 15*(3), 163–171.

Lombardi, N. (1993). Palliative care in an inpatient hospital setting. In A. Armstrong-Dailey & S. Goltzer (Eds.), *Hospice care for children.* New York: Oxford University Press.

Mahon, M. M. (1994). Death of a sibling: Primary care interventions. *Pediatric Nursing, 20*(3), 293.

Menten, T. (1995). *Where is heaven? Children's wisdom on facing death.* Philadelphia: Running Press.

Newacheck, P., Strickland, B., Shonkoff, J., Perrin, J., McPherson, M., McManus, M., Lauver, C., Fox, H., & Arango, P. (1998). An epidemiologic profile of children with special health care needs. *Pediatrics, 102*(1), 117–123.

Patterson, J. M. (1991). Family resilience to the challenge of a child's disability. *Pediatric Annals, 20*(9), 491–499.

Patterson, J. M., Jernell, J., Leonard, B. J., & Titus, J. C. (1994). Caring for medically fragile children at home: The parent-professional relationship. *Journal of Pediatric Nursing, 9*(2), 98–106.

Pearson, L. (1997). Family matters: Family-centered care and the anticipated death of a; newborn. *Pediatric Nursing, 23*(2), 178–182.

Ponzetti, J. J. (1992). Bereaved families: A comparison of parents' and grandparents' reactions to the death of a child. *Omega, 25*(1), 63–71.

Rabin, N. B. (1994). School reentry and the child with a chronic illness: The role of the pediatric nurse practitioner. *Journal of Pediatric Health Care, 8*, 227–232.

Rashotte, J., Fothergill-Bourbonnais, F., & Chamberlain, M. (1997). Pediatric intensive care nurses and their grief experiences: A phenomenological study. *Heart and Lung: The Journal of Acute & Critical Care, 26*(5), 372–386.

Ruden, B. M. (1996). Bereavement follow-up: An opportunity to extend nursing care. *Journal of Pediatric Oncology Nursing, 13*(4), 219–225.

Scott, L. (1998). Perceived needs of parents of critically ill children. *Journal of the Society of Pediatric Nurses, 3*(1), 4–12.

Sokol, M. (1995). Creating a community of caring for families with special needs. *Journal of Obstetric, Gynecologic, and Neonatal Nursing, 24*(1), 64–69.

Sterling, Y., Corson, L., Johnson, D., & Bowen, M. (1996). Parents' resources and home management of the care of chronically ill infants. *Journal of the Society of Pediatric Nurses, 1*(3), 103–109.

Sterling, Y., Peterson, J., & Weekes, D. (1997). African-American families with chronically ill children: Oversights and insights. *Journal of Pediatric Nursing, 12*(5), 292–300.

Waechter, E. H. (1984). Dying children: Patterns of coping. In H. Wass & C. A. Corr (Eds.), *Childhood and death* (pp. 51–68). New York: Hemisphere.

Wagner, T., Higgins, P. G., & Wallerstedt, C. (1997). Perinatal death: How fathers grieve. *Journal of Perinatal Education, 6*(4), 9–16.

Walker, C. L., Wells, L., Heiney, S., Hymovich, D. P., & Weekes, D. P. (1993). Nursing management of psychosocial care needs. In G. V. Foley, D. Fachtman, & K. H. Mooney (Eds.), *Nursing care of the child with cancer.* Philadelphia: Saunders.

Wass, H. (1985). Concepts of death: A developmental perspective. *Issues in Comprehensive Pediatric Nursing, 8*(1–6), 3–25.

Westbrook, L., Silver, E., & Stein, R. (1998). Implications for estimates of disability in children: A comparison of definitional components. *Pediatrics, 101*(6), 1025–1030.

Williams, P., Hanson, S., Karlin, R., Ridder, L, Liebergen, A. Olson, J., Barnard, M., & Tobin-Rommelhart, S. (1997). *Journal of the Society of Pediatric Nurses, 2*(3), 127–137.

Woodgate, R. (1998). Adolescents' perspectives of chronic illness: "It's hard." *Journal of Pediatric Nursing, 13*(4), 210–222.

Yoder, L. (1994). Comfort and consolation: A nursing perspective on parental bereavement. *Pediatric Nursing, 20*(5), 473–477.

37

Principles and Procedures for Nursing Care of Children

LEARNING OBJECTIVES

After studying this chapter, you should be able to

- Describe how to prepare children and families for selected procedures frequently seen in an acute care setting.
- Compare anatomic and physiologic differences in children and adults as they apply to selected procedures.
- Identify psychosocial considerations unique to children undergoing selected procedures.
- Describe techniques useful for eliciting cooperation from the child undergoing selected procedures.
- Describe step-by-step nursing actions and the reasons for performing selected procedures.

DEFINITIONS

antipyretic   An agent that reduces or relieves fever.

apical pulse rate   Heart rate determined by placing the stethoscope over the point of maximum intensity and counting for 1 minute.

auscultate   To listen to body sounds (e.g., heart sounds, breath sounds).

enteral   By way of the alimentary canal (e.g., enteral feeding).

epiglottitis   Inflammation of the epiglottis.

fluorosis   Staining of the teeth due to excessive fluoride ingestion.

hypoxia   Reduced or inadequate cellular oxygenation.

informed consent   A requirement, both legal and ethical, that the child and the parent or guardian completely understand proposed procedures or treatments, including their benefits and risks.

lavage   Wash.

phenylketonuria (PKU)   A protein metabolic condition.

pyrogens   Substances that cause fever.

standard precautions   Infection control guidelines developed by the National Center for Infectious Disease and the Hospital Control Practices Advisory Committee to prevent the spread of infectious organisms from blood, body fluids, secretions and excretions, mucous membranes, and nonintact skin (see Appendix B).

Children need preparation before, and accurate information about, any procedure that is performed. This information is essential. It promotes a sense of security, decreases fear, elicits cooperation, and improves coping skills. Parents also need preparation, as their anxiety may be transferred to the child.

The responsibility of the nurse caring for a child undergoing a procedure is twofold: (1) to help the child and parents through the procedure effectively and (2) to ensure that the procedure is done as efficiently as possible (Brennan, 1994). The nurse can implement strategies to help the child and parents through all phases of a procedure, including the anticipation and preparation for the procedure, the actual procedure, and the period following the procedure. Teaching before performing procedures also helps to increase the knowledge base of the child and family.

Preparing Children for Procedures

Adequately preparing children and families for procedures, especially those that are painful, threatening, or invasive, necessitates a thorough, individualized assessment. This process should include an assessment of the child's age and developmental level, personality, existing level of knowledge, present level of understanding, past experience, coping skills, and family situation. The nurse can then match explanations and teaching to the specific needs of a child and family.

Explaining Procedures

Mentally reviewing the procedure before giving explanations is especially important if the procedure is seldom performed, new, or unfamiliar. Thinking about the procedure in advance provides an opportunity for the nurse to request sedation, gather extra supplies, and obtain assistance, as necessary. Gather all equipment to be used and check that it functions before beginning any procedure.

Explaining procedures includes demonstrating equipment and describing anything the child will feel, see, hear, and smell. Use words the child will understand, and use a developmentally appropriate approach. It helps to relate the experience to an object or situation that the child is familiar with or has an interest in.

Appropriately timing the explanation is critical. Many children respond better to procedures if the explanation is given either just before the procedure or step by step as the procedure unfolds. Some older children and adolescents like to be prepared well in advance, in case they have questions that need answering. Advance preparation allows the child to express feelings about the procedure through role play. Often, parents can inform the nurse about the best timing

for their child. If possible, time should be allowed for questions and for the child to become familiar with the equipment.

Also important for a child's successful coping with an invasive or painful procedure is the presence of someone the child trusts. Time spent establishing a trusting relationship with a child is time well spent. Trust in health care providers can enhance the child's unique coping strategies.

Before procedures, ensure the child's privacy by closing the door to the room and drawing a curtain around the bed or, optimally, by taking the child to a treatment room. The treatment room contains appropriate equipment for invasive procedures and is a private area away from the "safe haven" of a child's room or the playroom (Fig. 37–1). Visitors should be asked to leave, and parents might also choose to leave at this point, although parental participation is supported and encouraged.

CRITICAL TO REMEMBER
Standard Precautions

Always wash your hands and follow standard precautions (see Appendix B) before beginning any procedure.

Telling children or parents what they can do to help gives them control and decreases potential feelings of powerlessness. For example, if the child must hold an extremity still for the placement of an intravenous (IV) catheter, the child must know about this need *before* the procedure is begun. The child should be asked whether he or she will be able to hold still. If not, obtain assistance to help the child remember to do so. Offer children choices, when feasible. For example, let a child choose the type of colorful bandage that will cover an injection site or whether to have a procedure done before or after the next television show.

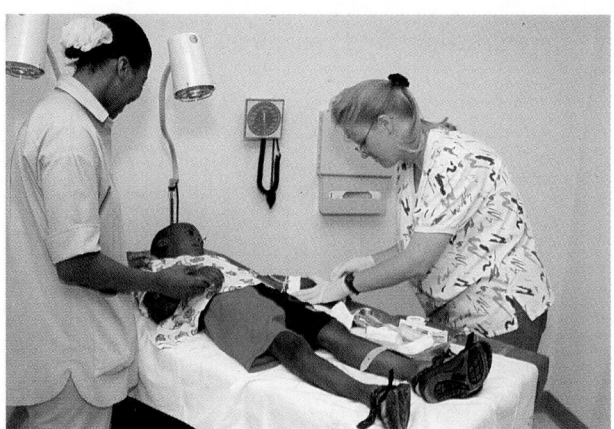

FIGURE 37–1
Because a child should feel that the hospital room is a safe place, a treatment room is used for invasive or painful procedures. The parent is present not to restrain the child but to provide emotional support.

••••••••
Tips for Preparing and Supporting Children Undergoing Procedures

BEFORE THE PROCEDURE

- Offer the child ways of coping with pain or discomfort. For example, some children can use coping strategies, such as guided imagery. Others might listen to a radio, increasing the volume as the discomfort level increases. Give the child permission to cry or yell if necessary.
- Use developmentally appropriate words when discussing the procedure and expectations.
- Give the child as much choice over what will happen as is possible. For example, when possible, the child might be allowed to choose an injection site or a site for IV catheter placement.
- Be sure the consent form has been signed, if applicable.
- Always wash your hands thoroughly before beginning any procedure and follow standard precautions.

DURING THE PROCEDURE

- Talk to the child during the procedure, if the child desires. If the child is using a coping strategy such as guided imagery, however, talking will be a distraction and will decrease the child's ability to cope with what is happening.

- Keep the child informed of the procedure's progress.
- Tell the child when the procedure is nearly completed and the "worst is over."

AFTER THE PROCEDURE

- *Praise* the child for *attempts* at cooperation, even if the child did not do anything you asked. Trying counts! Specifically praise the child for accomplishing an expected task.
- Provide an opportunity for the child to vent feelings about the procedure. Remember that it is OK for feelings of anger to be expressed when appropriate. Tell the child that you understand if the child does not want to talk with you right now and that you will return later.
- If parents were not present during the procedure, reunite the child with the parents and allow them to provide comfort and support.
- Reward the child, using age-appropriate methods such as stickers.
- Record the preparation process and procedure performance, who performed the procedure, the child's tolerance of the procedure, and its outcomes.

Do not threaten children with punishment for not cooperating. Nurses need to have realistic expectations that are based on the child's developmental level and knowledge of the child's capacity for cooperation.

Involve parents as much as they desire, according to what is possible during procedures. For example, a child might be much more cooperative in taking oral medications if the mother administers them. Often, by explaining what the parents will be seeing and what they can do, the nurse helps them feel comfortable staying with and supporting their child. The nurse should recognize, however, that parents might be very uncomfortable remaining with their child during a painful or invasive procedure. Give parents permission to leave, if they so desire, and assure them that they will be called if they are needed or as soon as the procedure is completed.

Consent for Procedures

All surgical or diagnostic invasive procedures, particularly those that involve risk to the child, require *informed consent*. Some examples are lumbar puncture, chest tube insertion, and bone marrow aspiration. There are both legal and ethical requirements to inform the child, if appropriate, and the child's parents of the benefits and risks of the proposed procedure or treatment. Informed consent must be obtained from the parent or legal guardian *before* the procedure is performed.

Other procedures, such as IV line insertions, specimen collection, and medication and oxygen administration, are covered under the general consent to treat that is provided in signed form upon admission. It is now also customary to obtain *assent* from children 7 years old and older. Assent means that the child has been fully informed about the procedure and concurs with those giving the informed consent. Laws on informed consent vary from state to state, so nurses should become familiar with the laws and policies of their institution. (See Chapter 1 for specific information related to legal issues.)

The person performing the procedure should obtain the consent. Nurses need to check that the consent form is signed and witnessed, and need to answer questions relating to the procedure. Occasionally, an emergency or life-threatening situation arises in which it is not possible to contact the parent or legal guardian for consent. In such cases, administrative consent may be obtained to allow physicians to perform the indicated procedures. (Refer to Chapter 1 for legal issues related to informed and emergency consent provisions.)

CRITICAL TO REMEMBER
••••••••••••
Preparation for Procedures

- A treatment room is the preferred location for performing procedures. It is a private area away from the "safe haven" of a child's hospital room, and it usually contains the necessary equipment for a variety of procedures (see Fig. 37–1).
- Ensure that a person the child trusts is there for support.
- Use terminology appropriate for the child's developmental level. Avoid using words or phrases that the child might misinterpret (e.g., dye, put to sleep, stick).
- Offer the child choices, if appropriate.
- Tell the child and family how they can help with the procedure.
- Do not threaten punishment for lack of cooperation.
- Encourage parental participation in the procedure, but do not force an unwilling parent to stay.

Transporting Infants and Children

Infants and children sometimes must be transported to other areas within the hospital unit or even outside the unit. A change in location might be a response to changes in the child's condition or might be done to increase parental involvement in the child's care (e.g., rooming-in). Children might also be transported for specialized care (e.g., rehabilitation) or for diagnostic testing. Children might also be transported to different areas on the same unit (e.g., treatment room, play room).

The method of transportation will depend on the child's age, developmental level, and physical condition, the destination, safety factors, and whether specialized equipment is needed to accompany the child. Any special accommodations should be arranged before the time of the planned transfer.

Infants transported within a unit can be held in several positions (Fig. 37–2). The nurse should hold the infant securely, anticipating sudden movement. Cradle infants up to 2 to 3 months of age by holding them in a horizontal position, supporting the back, and grasping the thigh (Fig. 37–2A). When using the football hold, tuck the infant between your body and elbow, with your arm carrying the infant's body and your hand supporting the head (Fig. 37–2B). When carrying the infant upright, hold the infant erect against your chest (Fig. 37–2C). Rest the infant's buttocks on your forearm and support the infant's head and

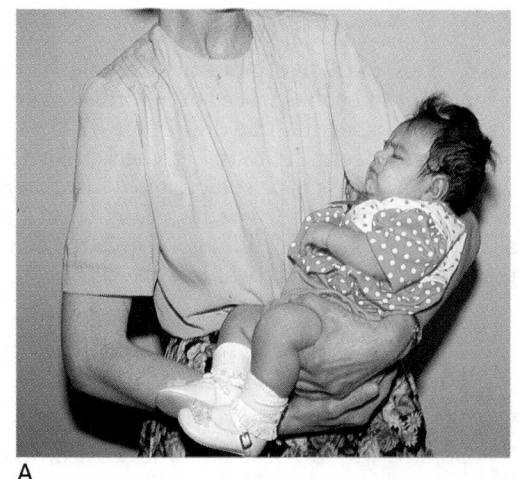

A

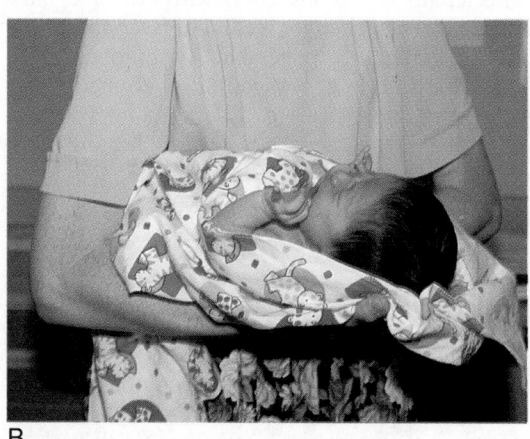

B

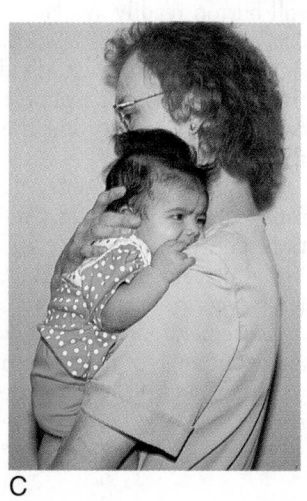

C

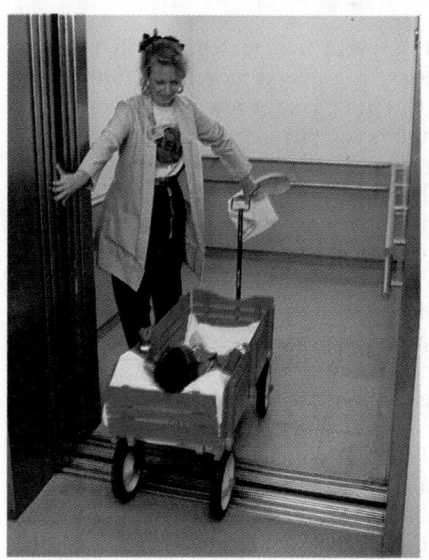

D

FIGURE 37–2

Methods of transporting infants and children. The nurse carries the infant securely, anticipating sudden movement. *A,* Cradle carry. *B,* Football hold. *C,* Over-the-shoulder carry, which can be used until the infant is 6 to 7 months. *D,* Transport can be fun for young children, especially when it is on wheels. (Infant transport photos courtesy of Parkland Health and Hospital System District Community Oriented Primary Care Clinic, Dallas, Texas. Wagon photo courtesy of Cook Children's Medical Center, Fort Worth, Texas.)

shoulders with your other arm. Even for infants with well-developed neck muscles and head control, this extra support prevents the infant from falling backward should the infant make a sudden move.

Infants and toddlers can also be transported in their bassinet or crib. The rails should always be up, and for older infants and toddlers the protective top should be in place. Strollers and wagons can also be used to transfer older infants and toddlers to other areas on the unit (see Fig. 37–2). Use safety belts, and make sure the sides of the wagon are raised. Do not leave the infant or toddler unattended. In all methods of transfer, equipment can be pushed along with the transporting vehicle or, in some cases, stored on a lower shelf of the transport vehicle. Do not place equipment in the transporting unit with infants or young children.

Transport older children in the same manner as adults (e.g., in wheelchairs or on stretchers with the side rails raised). In some cases, such as for a child in traction, transporting the child in the bed is preferable. Alternatively, preschoolers may enjoy a ride in a wagon or other unconventional means of transport (see Fig. 37–2). As for younger children, remember to use safety belts, raised sides, and constant supervision.

■ Using Restraints

Safety is of paramount concern when a child is hospitalized. Nurses need to be especially vigilant about raising side (crib) rails and keeping small objects away from young children. *Always place your hand on an infant's or child's back or abdomen when the sides of the bed are down or when the child is in a high place.*

Occasionally, to prevent trauma, temporarily restraining a child is necessary to suspend movement during certain procedures. In this instance, the restraint is removed as soon as the procedure is complete.

Some children are particularly active and prone to injury. Restraining the child might be the only option for maintaining the child's safety. All possible alternatives to restraint should be considered before applying the restraint. These alternatives might include using a sitter; behavior modification techniques, such as a time-out; or diversional activities such as reading. If restraint is considered for unruly or dangerous behavior, the cause of the behavior should also be examined. Causes can include hypoxia, sedation, adverse drug reactions, and mental illness.

The Omnibus Budget Reconciliation Act of 1987 states that restraints should be used only as a last resort for the protection of the client and others. The legislation further specifies that restraints should not be applied merely for the staff's convenience.

Physical restraints include such items as safety vests (jackets), mitts, and ankle and wrist restraints. Most facilities require a physician's order stating why the restraint is needed and how long it will be in place. The restraint chosen should be the least restrictive device that will prevent

---

CRITICAL TO REMEMBER
....
Using Restraints

- Use the least restrictive restraint.
- Choose the proper device for the child's condition.
- Ensure proper fit of the device.
- Tie knots that can be easily untied for quick access.
- Secure ties to bed frames (not mattresses or side rails) or to the frames of wheelchairs, or other stable device.
- Frequently check and record the child's neurovascular status, behavior, and general condition.

---

injury. Less restrictive protective restraints include such mechanisms as bubbles placed over a crib. Examples of pediatric restraints are illustrated in Figure 37–3.

Before placing the restraint, check the area to be restrained for any sign of compromised circulatory, integumentary, and neurologic systems. Also note any orthopedic alterations. If these conditions exist, extra monitoring of the restrained extremity will be needed.

Preparing the Child and Family

When restraints are applied, the child and family should be informed why the restraint will be used, where it will be applied, what movement it will prevent, and how long it will be in place. Tell the child and family how often a nurse will be coming in to check on the child. Have the call button readily available to older children so that they can call the nurse as needed. If possible, you need to consider and meet the child's developmental needs, such as thumb sucking. For example, an infant's or toddler's arm can be restrained so that the thumb can still be placed in the mouth.

Check the extremity distal to restraints for temperature, pulses, and capillary refill (CSM—circulation, sensation, and motion) every 15 minutes for 1 hour following initial placement. After that, check and record findings at least every hour, and more often if the child is aggressive or extremely active. Remove restraints every 2 hours to allow for range-of-motion movement and repositioning and to offer the child food or the opportunity to use the bathroom.

Documentation

Record findings on hourly neurovascular checks and any other changes in the child's behavior or condition. Every 2 hours, record removal of restraints, range of motion, and position changes. Be particularly alert for skin irritation under the restraints.

Clove hitch restraint

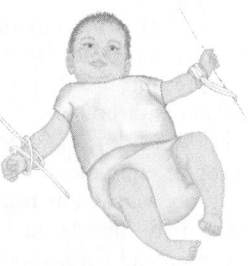

Prevents movement of extremities.
Use on wrists or ankles.

Elbow restraint

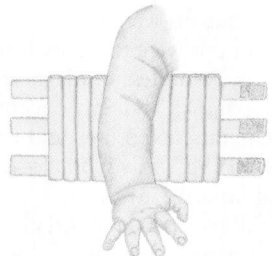

Prevents child from flexing and reaching face,
head, IV and other tubes. Position so that it
does not rub against the axilla.

Mummy restraint (body restraint)

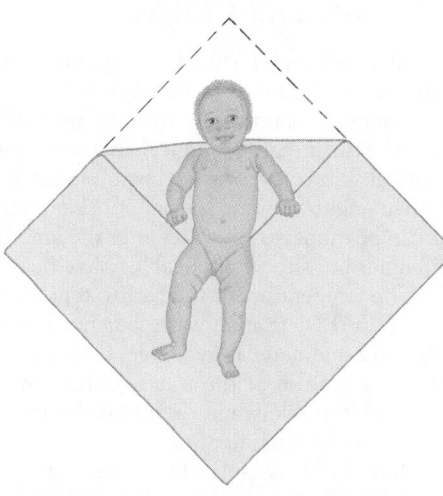

A restraint can be made from a sheet folded
into a square of the appropriate size for the
infant. Start by folding the top corner under the
infant's shoulders and aligning the infant's head
with the folded edge.

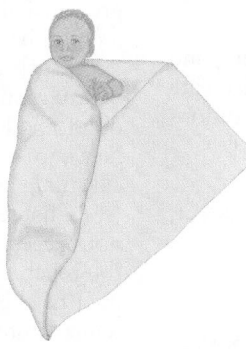

Fold one point of the
sheet across the child
and tuck it firmly behind
the back.

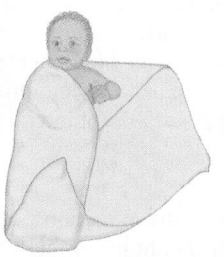

Fold the bottom corner
of the sheet up to cover
and restrain the infant's
feet.

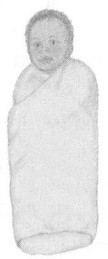

Fold the remaining
corner over the child
and tuck firmly behind
the back.

Jacket restraint

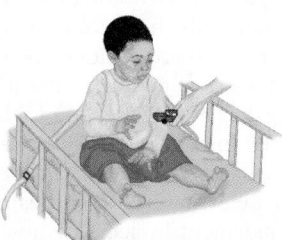

Tied to the back of the child and to the frame
of the bed. Used primarily to keep children
flat in bed after surgery.

Crib top bubble restraint

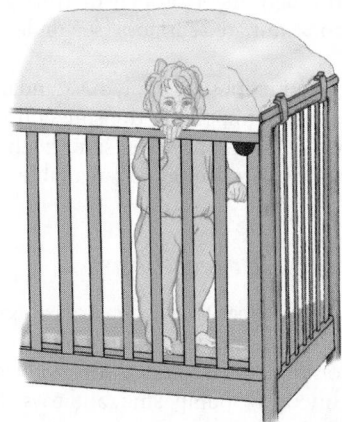

Prevents older infant and younger child
from falling and climbing out of bed.

FIGURE 37–3
• • • • • • • • •
Examples of pediatric restraints.

Isolation

In 1985 *universal precautions* were introduced. These blood and body fluid precautions were to be applied universally in caring for all patients, regardless of diagnosis. The precautions included using masks and eye coverings to protect against mucous membrane exposures and using individual ventilation devices. In 1987 *body substance isolation* was implemented as an alternative to diagnosis-driven isolation recommendations. All moist and potentially infectious body substances (blood, feces, urine, sputum, saliva, wound drainage, and other body fluids) from all patients, regardless of their presumed infection status, were to be considered infectious and handled with gloves. Unfortunately, this system did not adequately address droplet transmission, transmission of microorganisms from dry skin or environmental sources, or airborne transmission. There are both similarities and differences between universal precautions and body substance isolation recommendations. The two systems caused confusion and were subject to individual interpretation.

The confusion pointed to a need for a new system, and the major features of both systems were combined to create *standard precautions* (see Appendix B). Standard precautions apply to

- Blood
- All body fluids, secretions, and excretions, except sweat, regardless of whether they contain visible blood
- Nonintact skin
- Mucous membranes (Garner, 1996)

Under the new system there are two tiers of precautions. Standard precautions, precautions in the first tier, apply in the care of all hospitalized patients without regard for diagnosis or presumed infectious state. Second-tier precautions apply in the care of specific patients and are referred to as transmission-based precautions. They are for patients known or suspected to be infected by pathogens that are transmitted through air or droplet or through contact with dry skin or contaminated surfaces (see table in Appendix B).

The complete guidelines for applying standard precautions, as well as those for applying transmission-based precautions, are quite detailed and extensive. Each facility is responsible for making these guidelines available and implementing the precautions.

Implementing Precautions

It is important to remember that when transmission-based precautions are in effect, the items with which the infected child comes in contact are also contaminated. These items include the bed, linens, IV pump, sink, and toys. Therefore, the nurse who is going into the room to reset an IV pump, pick up soiled linens, and so forth must use whatever protective equipment is mandated by the type of precaution (gown, mask, gloves).

Children placed on transmission-based precautions often need extra attention to avert boredom. They need more diversional activities, such as games or movies, and more psychosocial support. Young children, for example, may think that they are being punished. Finally, visitors might hesitate to enter the child's room and may need additional support or reassurance from the nurse.

Family Teaching

Family education is crucial, and it is important to emphasize to parents, other visitors, and other health care providers that infection control precautions are important and must be followed closely. Parents often state that they are there to visit only their child and do not understand the need to wear special clothing or equipment. The nurse needs to emphasize that some diseases, such as respiratory syncytial virus, can live on inanimate objects, such as clothing, for up to 48 hours and can spread throughout the hospital or to the home if infection control measures are not followed. Encourage family members to visit the child frequently, as visits will decrease the child's sense of isolation.

Bathing Infants and Children

Strictly observing safety principles when bathing a child can prevent falls, burns, or aspiration of water. When bathing a child, be sure to take the opportunity to note any problems, such as altered skin integrity, surgical incisions, loss of sensation, abnormal skin color, bruising, paralysis, or any other condition that might warrant special consideration. Newborn infants can be immersed in water after the umbilical stump and circumcision site (if applicable) have healed (see Chapter 23). The temperature of the bathwater should not exceed 37.8°C (100°F)—that is, warm but not hot to the touch. If a bath thermometer is available, it should be used to check the temperature of the water. Otherwise, a temperature that is comfortable when tested on the inside of your wrist or elbow is appropriate.

Before bathing any child, assess the family's preferences and home practices. Factors to consider include the time of day usually set aside for the bath, bathing rituals, special equipment, any product allergies, and the type of bath preferred. You can also use this time to determine the amount of assistance needed and to address any learning needs related to hygiene. Because bathing is one of the few areas over which parents might be allowed to retain control when a child is hospitalized, it is important to allow them to make as many decisions as possible. Decision making also allows parents to maintain a part of the home routine with their child.

An infant who cannot sit unaided can be given a sponge bath or a tub bath. Support the infant's body and head at all times during the bath (Fig. 37–4). Older infants and toddlers can be bathed in either a bedside tub or a regular bathtub. *Never leave an infant or small child unattended in the bath.* Older children can take showers, if facilities are available. The nurse should use judgment in deciding how much supervision an older child needs while bathing. It is most important to provide privacy for the school-age child or adolescent.

Special Considerations

Bed baths are frequently used for hospitalized infants and children. When bathing a newborn or young infant, soap is not necessary. In fact, soap can be very drying to the skin if used too frequently. If soap is necessary or desired by the parent, use a gentle, nonalkaline soap.

To prevent chilling when giving a sponge bath, be sure to keep the infant covered with a cotton blanket. Cover the entire body except for the body part being washed or

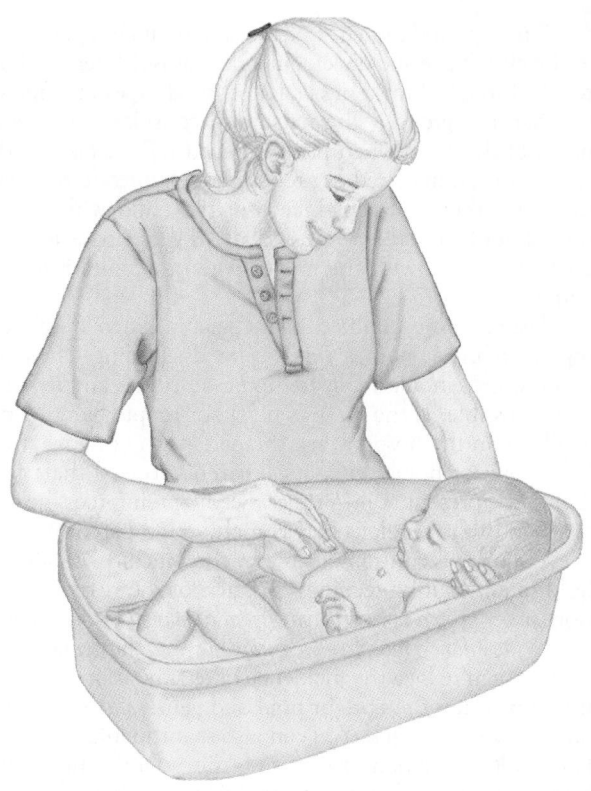

Using hand to support infant's neck and head

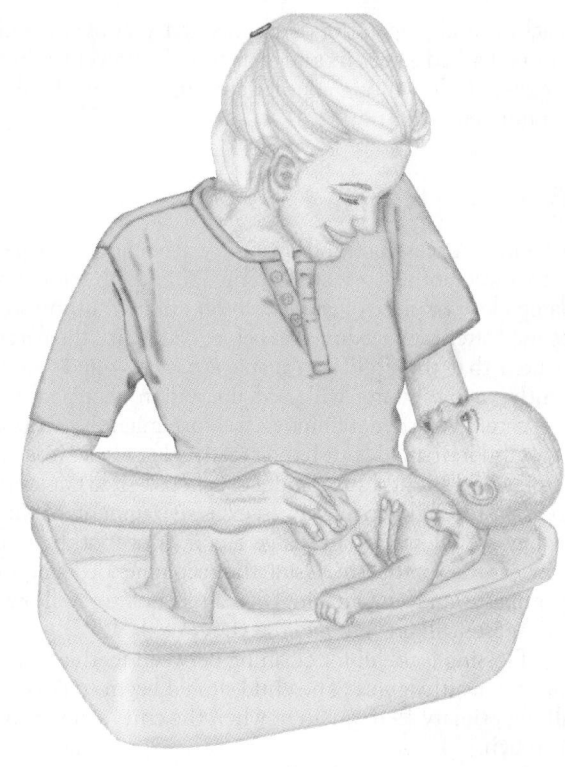

Using arm to support infant's neck and head

FIGURE 37–4

When giving an infant a tub bath, the nurse supports the infant's body at all times.

rinsed. Begin the bath with the face, and clean the diaper area last. Clean any eye discharge using a wet cotton ball and clean from the inner canthus outward. Use a clean cotton ball for each eye. Outer ears can be cleaned with a wet face cloth.

If bathing an infant in a bathtub, line a plastic infant tub with a towel to provide comfort as well as traction to prevent slipping. To prevent accidental drowning should the infant slip out of your grasp, fill the tub with no more than 3 inches of water.

When finished with the infant bath, wrap the infant in a dry towel or cotton blanket. Using the football hold, and holding the infant over the tub, shampoo the infant's head with baby shampoo. Be sure to shampoo over the fontanel. Avoid using talcum powder or corn starch in the infant's diaper area. When these substances get moist, they provide a medium for organism growth. Talcum powder and corn starch, if accidentally inhaled, can also cause severe respiratory consequences (Schmitt, 1992; Silver, Sagy, & Rubin, 1996).

The technique for bathing a child differs little from that used in bathing an adult. The nurse performs the same assessment as with any client and provides assistance as necessary.

Adjust the room temperature to a comfortable setting and draw the curtain around the bed. As with any bed bath, the nurse begins with the face and proceeds in a head-to-toe progression. Obtain fresh water when it is time to rinse the child. As with the infant, drape the child adequately

for privacy and warmth, and to prevent chilling, dry each body section as it is rinsed. The bath can be followed with application of lotion or deodorant if desired.

Some bathing restrictions might apply to patients with surgical incisions, skin traction, IV catheters, casts, urinary catheters, artificial airways, and feeding tubes. Some children are also restricted in position and mobility. For example, children who have undergone orthopedic or neurosurgical procedures often must remain supine. Other children may be intolerant of position changes because of underlying physiologic conditions or injury. It is imperative to assess for these special needs before beginning the bath.

Documentation

Documentation includes the type of bath, child or family participation, procedure tolerance, and any abnormal findings noted, such as bruising, rashes, or excoriation. Any lotions or other skin preparations used should also be recorded.

Parent Teaching

General principles of hygiene and safety might need to be reinforced with some parents. (See Chapter 23 for instructions for care of the newborn infant.) Instruction in the use of special bathing equipment, such as infant bathtubs, safety bars, or tub grips, should be included as part of discharge teaching and preparation. After about 1 year of age, a child can be bathed safely in a regular tub. To prevent injury or accidental drowning, appropriate supervision should be maintained at all times.

▮ Oral Hygiene

To remove excess food and bacteria, wipe infants' gums gently with a wet cloth after each feeding. After teeth erupt, a soft, damp cloth or piece of gauze or a soft child's toothbrush can be used after each feeding and before bed. Until the parent is assured that the child can manage correctly and independently, young children will need supervision when performing oral care. Even then, reminders to brush might be necessary.

Children should brush their teeth at least twice a day with a soft child's toothbrush and a *small* (pea-sized) amount of toothpaste. Children may ingest excessive amounts of fluoride if they are allowed to use large amounts of toothpaste or if they eat the toothpaste. Using the recommended amount of toothpaste and encouraging the child not to swallow the toothpaste will prevent *fluorosis* (Levy et al., 1997).

Flossing is useful for cleaning between teeth and maintaining healthy gums. The child should begin to floss when all the primary teeth are in or when the child's molars begin to touch.

Immunosuppressed children, in particular, need excellent oral hygiene. Soft toothbrushes, sponge-covered toothettes, or moistened gauze sponges can be used for dental care in the child who is at risk for gingival bleeding (see Chapter 48).

Discharge teaching in the area of oral hygiene is very important and often forgotten. Many parents do not realize that infants' gums and teeth can and should be cleaned. Children should have their first visit to a dentist by the time the first teeth erupt and no later than age 2½ years. Thereafter they should be seen on a regular basis (every 6 months) for checkups.

The risk of dental caries is increased if formula, milk, or other liquids remain in a child's mouth overnight. Allowing an infant to fall asleep drinking a bottle of one of these liquids can cause a condition known as "bottle-mouth syndrome," which results in severely decayed primary teeth. Discourage parents from putting a child to bed with a bottle of formula, juice, or sweetened liquid. If the child will not fall asleep without a bottle, advise the parent to use water only.

Good nutrition influences dental health, and vice versa. Dental teaching often provides a means for educating the child and family about proper nutrition and health maintenance.

▮ Feeding

Mealtimes can be difficult for the hospitalized child. Changes in routine, diet, and surroundings, as well as dietary restrictions and illness, affect the child's ability and desire to eat. Refusing to eat might also be the only way the child can control the environment.

Assess the child's preferences and dislikes on admission and before ordering meals. Also note mealtime rituals and routines and cultural food variations. Serving favorite and preferred foods and offering nutritious snacks can ensure appropriate caloric intake.

The type and form of food chosen should be appropriate to the child's age and developmental status. (Refer to Chapters 5 through 8 for a discussion of food types appropriate for each age group.) The nurse also considers any special needs of the child when planning meals. For example, the child with an impaired gag reflex cannot tolerate the same foods as other children. Likewise, the child with nausea should not be offered favorite foods, as these foods may become associated with the nausea when the child is feeling better.

Feeding a hospitalized infant seldom differs from feeding an infant at home. Types of foods, feeding schedules, and routines should replicate home schedules and routines when possible. If the infant's bottle or nipple brand is not available in the hospital, ask the parents to bring what the infant uses at home. Encourage parents to feed their children or be present at mealtimes. Feeding reinforces the special bond that develops between child and parent.

Unless it is contraindicated by their medical condition, hold infants during feedings. Because of the risk of aspiration, *never prop a bottle (leaving it on a pillow or rolled blanket next to the infant's mouth)*. Frequent burping during and after feedings can reduce the incidence of regurgitation. Burp the infant by using the upright hold and gently patting or rubbing the infant's back. You can also seat the infant on your knees with your hand supporting the infant's chin. After feeding, position the infant on the right side to facilitate the flow of the feeding toward the lower end of the stomach and to allow any swallowed air to rise to the esophagus.

Toddlers and preschoolers often use food as a source of control. They might exhibit "food jags," during which they will only eat one or two items for a period of several days. They enjoy finger foods but are beginning to use spoons or forks fairly competently. Use colorful plates and cups to encourage a reluctant child to eat. Also, allow parents to bring the child's own cups or utensils from home to simulate the usual mealtime routines as closely as possible.

Cut foods into pieces appropriate in size and texture to decrease the risk of aspiration. Avoid foods such as hot dogs, popcorn, peanuts, or grapes because, if aspirated, these can occlude the airway. Do not allow young children to eat unsupervised. Secure them appropriately at a table, in a high chair, or in bed using a bedside table during meals. "Roaming" while eating should be discouraged. Allow children to feed themselves, if possible, and restrict the feeding time to 15 to 20 minutes. Discontinue the meal if the child begins to play with the food.

Older children and adolescents seldom have difficulty expressing their dietary preferences. Difficulty may arise, however, when children this age are placed on a restricted or special diet. For example, the diabetic child often has difficulty staying on a restricted diet in the face of peer pressure. Support and setting clear limits are often needed to ensure cooperation.

Special Considerations

Keeping accurate intake and output (I & O) measurements might be necessary for some children. Measure and record all intake, both oral and parenteral. All output, including output from urine and stool, drainage from tubes, stomas, or fistulas, and emesis, is also measured and recorded.

Documentation

Recording the child's nutritional intake assists in determining the child's overall health. It is important to record not only food intake and preferences but also observations about the child's appetite and eating patterns. Particularly note abnormal eating habits in an older child or adolescent, the age at which eating disorders are prevalent.

Different institutions have different forms for recording accurate I & O. Follow institutional procedure for recording, and use volumes as determined by the containers and equipment used by the institution.

Parent Teaching

Parental education is very important, particularly if the hospital admission is related to eating disorders or accidents, such as food aspiration. Carefully instruct parents about any food restrictions or special diets. For example, a child with *phenylketonuria* (PKU) or diabetes is at high risk for injury if the diet is not followed closely.

▌ Vital Signs

The procedure for taking vital signs on an infant is similar to taking vital signs on a newborn (see Procedure 23–2 for specific instructions for taking vital signs in infants). The principles of measuring vital signs in children are similar to those for adults, with some minor modifications. Obtain vital signs when the infant or child is quiet. If this timing is not possible, record any activity that affects accurate measurement (e.g., crying, playing).

Measuring Temperature

Temperature is an objective and reliable indicator of illness, and measuring temperature is an integral part of pediatric assessment. A child's temperature can be measured in a variety of ways. Oral, rectal, axillary, and tympanic temperatures can be measured using glass, electronic, digital, or tympanic membrane thermometers. Whatever method is chosen, the child's temperature should be measured at the same site and with the same temperature-measuring device, to maintain consistency and allow for reliable comparison and tracking of temperatures over time. (See Table 33–1 for normal temperatures in children.)

Axillary temperatures should be measured in infants and children younger than 4 to 6 years of age and in any child who is uncooperative, immunosuppressed, or neurologically impaired or who has had oral surgery (Fig. 37–5). Axillary temperatures are approximately 0.6°C (1°F) lower than the body's core temperature. Because to be accurate, a glass thermometer must remain in the child's axillary area for a full 5 minutes, consider seating the child on your lap and reading a story or singing songs to help pass the time and help the child remain quiet.

Temperatures are measured orally in most children 6 years old or older, including adolescents. It is a challenge

Axillary Temperature

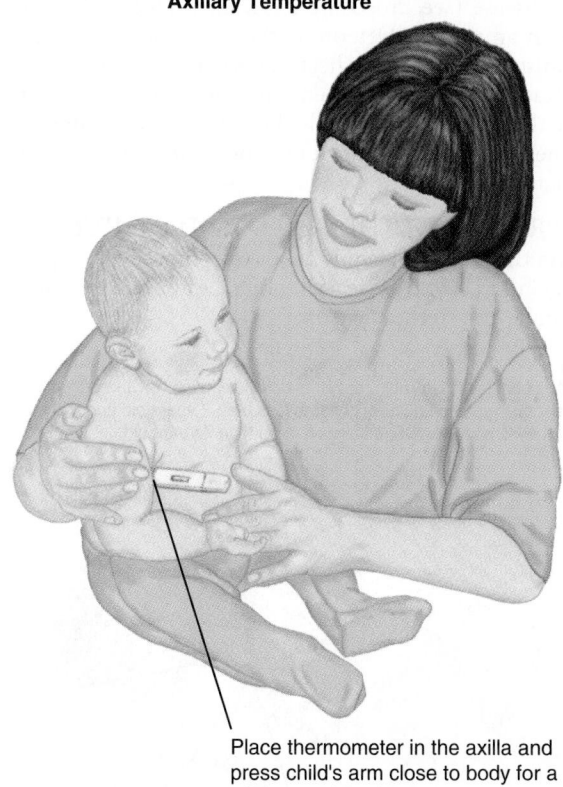

Place thermometer in the axilla and press child's arm close to body for a minimum of 5 minutes.

Tympanic Temperature

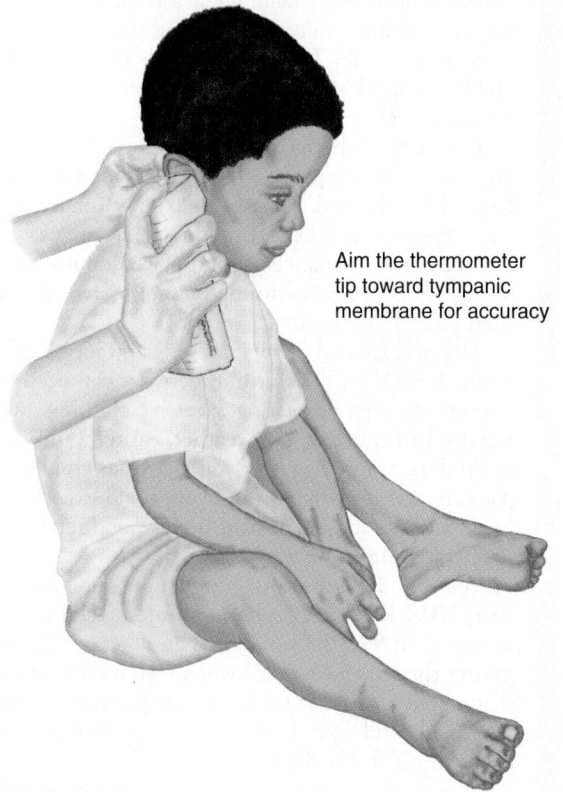

Aim the thermometer tip toward tympanic membrane for accuracy

▌ FIGURE 37–5
⋯⋯⋯⋯⋯⋯
Two methods of temperature measurement.

for the child to keep a glass thermometer in place for a minimum of 3 minutes. Encourage the child to keep the mouth closed around the thermometer (in a "kiss" position), and if a glass thermometer is used, instruct the child not to bite the thermometer. The child should avoid liquids for 30 minutes before the oral temperature measurement. Temperatures measured orally might be inaccurate because of oral intake, oxygen administration, nebulized treatments, or crying (Pontious et al., 1994).

Because of the risk of rectal perforation and the intrusive and upsetting nature of the procedure, temperatures are measured rectally only when no other route can be used (see Procedure 23–2). Because of the injury risk, glass thermometers are not recommended for measuring rectal temperatures.

Digital thermometers, which run on a button battery and measure the temperature quickly, usually in less than 30 seconds, can be used to measure temperatures orally, rectally, or in the axillary area. To prevent cross-contamination, use disposable covers for obtaining temperatures.

PARENTS WANT TO KNOW

Temperature Measurement

Accurately measuring your child's temperature, along with other symptoms, helps your doctor determine whether your child needs to be seen for assessment and treatment. Feeling your child's forehead can give you a clue as to whether the child's temperature should be measured, but does not give accurate information about the child's body temperature. Temperature strips placed on the child's forehead also give only an approximate reading.

A variety of thermometer types is available at the drugstore. An inexpensive digital thermometer can be used to take oral, rectal, and axillary (under the arm) temperatures. Digital thermometers are easy to read because the numbers are displayed on a small screen. They are easier to use but are more expensive than glass thermometers.

The average body temperature, when measured orally, is 98.6°F (37°C). Mild increases can occur as a result of exercise, wearing excessive clothing, taking hot baths, during hot weather, eating warm food, or drinking warm drinks. If you take your child's temperature and it is higher than you would expect it to be, encourage the child to sit quietly, and retake the temperature in ½ hour.

Your child has a fever if the temperature is greater than 100.4°F (38.0°C) when measured rectally, greater than 99.5°F (37.5°C) when taken orally, and greater than 99°F (37.2°C) when measured by the axillary method. If your infant is younger than 6 weeks, you should call your doctor if the baby's temperature is above 100°F (37.8°C).

In general, the height of the fever is not an indication of the seriousness of the illness. What is important is how your child is acting. If your child has a fever and is acting sick, notify your doctor.

Tympanic temperature measurement is now frequently done in pediatric practice (see Fig. 37–5) and can also be done at home. These measurements are quickly obtained, usually within a few seconds, and correlate fairly consistently with core body temperature to within 0.3°C (Worral & Luke, 1998). Tympanic temperature measurement might not be as accurate in toddlers because a child's excessive movement interferes with creating an appropriate seal. Use of the "ear tug"—putting posterior traction on the pinna to expose the tympanic membrane completely—enhances the accuracy of tympanic temperature measurements (Wells et al., 1995).

DOCUMENTATION
Record the method used to measure the temperature in the child's medical record. Include the measurement obtained and any action taken. Record and report core temperatures of less than 36°C (96.8°F) or more than 38°C (100.4°F). Reassess and document as necessary.

PARENT TEACHING
Some parents may need to learn how to take the child's temperature at home. Demonstrate how to take the child's temperature, then observe the parent perform the procedure. Make sure the parent is comfortable with the procedure and is able to read the thermometer accurately.

Measuring Pulse

Apical pulse rate measurements (Fig. 37–6) are recommended in infants and children younger than 2 years old and in any child who has an irregular heart rate or known congenital heart disease (see Procedure 23–2 for assessing the apical pulse in an infant). Determine the apical heart rate before administering certain medications, such as digoxin.

Radial pulse measurements are appropriate for children older than 2 years (see Table 33–1 for normal pulse measurements). The procedure for taking a radial pulse is similar to that for an adult.

PREPARING THE CHILD AND FAMILY
Inform the child and family about the purpose of the procedure. Children who are fearful should be allowed to examine or handle the stethoscope.

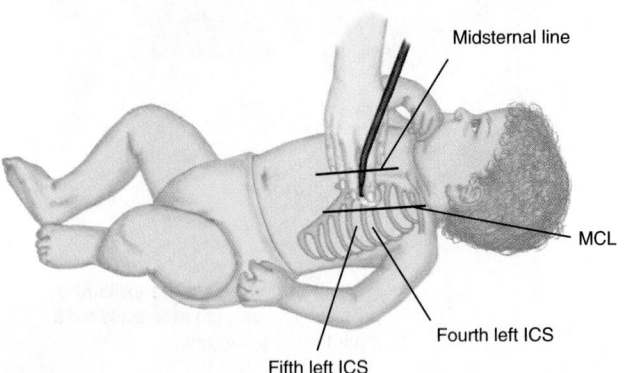

Apical pulse is lateral to the left midclavicular line (MCL) and fourth intercostal space (ICS) in children less than 7 years old and to the left MCL and fifth ICS in children more than 7 years old.

Midsternal line

MCL

Fourth left ICS

Fifth left ICS

FIGURE 37–6

Locating the apical pulse.

DOCUMENTATION

Record the method used to measure the pulse in the child's medical record. Record the measurement obtained and any action taken.

PARENT TEACHING

Some parents might need to be taught how to determine their child's heart rate accurately, as well as the acceptable range for their child. Special considerations relating to parents' notifying the physician may need to be made for children who are taking certain medications, such as digoxin.

Evaluating Respirations

Infants often have irregular respiratory rates that change with stimulation, crying, and feeding. Some infants will initially exhibit a Cheyne-Stokes type of respiratory pattern, but this pattern should disappear by 4 weeks of age. Table 33–1 shows normal rates. (See Procedure 23–2 for measurement of respirations.) Either observe or auscultate respirations in the older child.

DOCUMENTATION

Record and report any deviations from the expected norm, both in the respiratory rate and rhythm and in breath sounds.

PARENT TEACHING

Parents might not be aware that younger children are primarily diaphragmatic breathers, necessitating observation of the rise and fall of the abdomen rather than the chest. Emphasize the importance of diversional activities during the counting, as well as the importance of counting respirations for 1 full minute.

TABLE 37–1

Recommended Blood Pressure Cuff Sizes

Arm Circumference (cm)	Cuff Name	Bladder Width (cm)	Bladder Length (cm)
5–7.5	Newborn	3	5
7.5–13	Infant	5	8
13–20	Child	8	13
24–32	Adult	13	24
32–42	Large adult	17	32
42–50	Thigh	20	42

Measuring Blood Pressure

Blood pressure usually is assessed at least once per shift when a child is hospitalized. Unless a problem is suspected, however, blood pressure may not be assessed more than once per year during routine physical examinations.

Choosing the appropriate cuff size is extremely important (see Table 37–1 for recommendations), because an inappropriate cuff size will yield a blood pressure that is too high or too low. Base the cuff size on a midpoint limb circumference. Blood pressure measurement will differ according to the measuring technique used and the site selected (see Appendix J for normal results).

Blood pressures can be measured in the upper arm, lower arm, thigh, calf, or ankle (Fig. 37–7). To ensure consistency, take measurements in the same limb, in the same

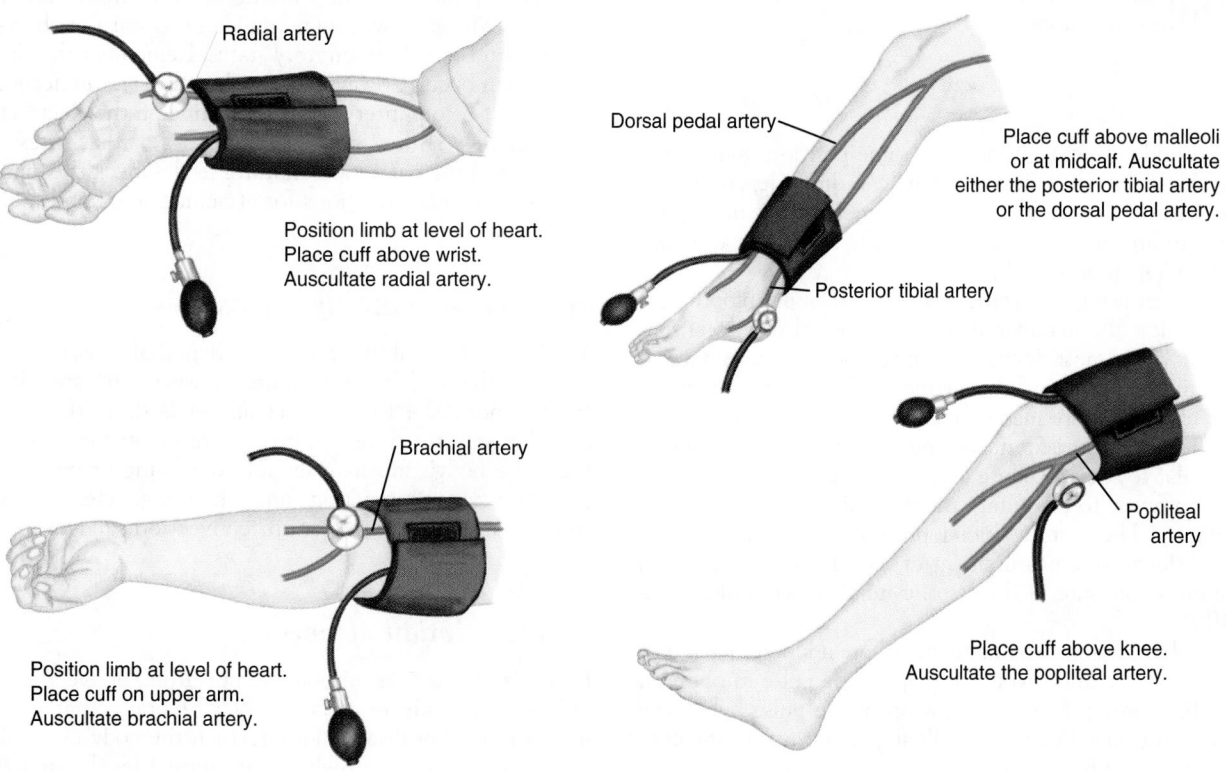

Radial artery — Position limb at level of heart. Place cuff above wrist. Auscultate radial artery.

Dorsal pedal artery / Posterior tibial artery — Place cuff above malleoli or at midcalf. Auscultate either the posterior tibial artery or the dorsal pedal artery.

Brachial artery — Position limb at level of heart. Place cuff on upper arm. Auscultate brachial artery.

Popliteal artery — Place cuff above knee. Auscultate the popliteal artery.

FIGURE 37–7

Blood pressures can be measured in the upper arm, lower arm, thigh, calf, or ankle. It is important that an appropriate-size cuff be used to obtain accurate results (see Table 37–1).

place, and with the child in the same position. Remember that blood pressure measurements can differ depending on the site used. For example, calf measurements are not equivalent to arm measurements, especially in infants and toddlers (Crapanzano et al., 1996).

When using electronic devices to measure blood pressure, follow the manufacturer's guidelines closely to ensure accuracy. For most devices, the first reading is considered a "priming" reading and the second reading is considered the true blood pressure measurement.

The procedure for measuring blood pressure in children is similar to the procedure for adults. It might not be possible, however, to auscultate the diastolic pressure in young children. The systolic blood pressure sometimes can be heard down to a measurement of zero. In this case, record the blood pressure as the systolic number over pulse (e.g., 90/P).

When it is impossible to auscultate a blood pressure in infants and toddlers, you can palpate the pulse to obtain a systolic reading. Find the location of the pulse below the cuff with your index and middle finger and inflate the cuff, as for an auscultated pressure. As the cuff deflates, note the point at which the pulse is first felt. Record this systolic measurement as if you had heard the systolic beat down to zero.

PREPARING THE CHILD AND FAMILY

Inform the child and family of the purpose of the procedure. Allow the child to handle the equipment while you explain how it is used. You can tell young children that the cuff feels like a "hug" or a "squeeze." Many children have pretend cuffs at home and so are familiar with the concept.

DOCUMENTATION

Record blood pressure measurements and note any changes from previous readings. Record palpated pressures as described previously.

PARENT TEACHING

If the child's condition requires home blood pressure monitoring, teach the procedure to the parent. You can provide helpful suggestions about the size of the cuff and methods to involve the child who might resist this procedure. For instance, parents might make a smaller cuff for the child's favorite doll or stuffed animal.

Special Considerations: Cardiorespiratory Monitors

Some children need cardiorespiratory monitoring so that heart rate, respiratory rate, blood pressure, and temperature can be measured continuously. Children who are acutely ill or who are undergoing procedures might be placed on a monitor to help health care providers detect subtle changes in the child's condition.

The procedure and indications for attaching a child to a cardiorespiratory monitor are no different from those for an adult. Monitors will sound an alarm to warn of changes in the child's cardiorespiratory status. Remember that false alarms can occur. Always look at the child and perform an assessment before intervening. A flat line on the electrocardiogram (ECG) does not always signal a cardiac arrest. It may be nothing but a loose monitor lead. Check the manufacturer's recommendations for attaching leads and monitoring selected vital signs.

Fever-Reducing Measures

The body's internal thermostat, the hypothalamus, attempts to keep the body's temperature between 36° and 38°C (96.8° and 100.4°F). This regulation is done through a complex series of interactions that result in heat gain or loss. The body's mechanisms for conserving or producing heat are vasoconstriction and shivering. Heat is lost through radiation, conduction, convection, and evaporation.

Description of Fever

Fever is defined as a body temperature above 38.0°C (100.4°F) rectally or 37.5°C (99.5°F) orally that results from an insult or disease during which the body's set-point temperature rises to a higher than normal level. After the cause of the fever is removed, the body resets its set-point at the normal level.

The body's attempt to defend itself against illness is

manifested by fever, which is triggered by endogenous *pyrogens* produced during the inflammatory response. Because research studies have not conclusively demonstrated whether fever is beneficial or detrimental, practitioners vary in their approach to managing fevers secondary to infections. Mild degrees of fever might or might not require intervention, depending on the underlying cause and the child's response. Most fevers are brief and benign and resolve when the underlying infection resolves. It is generally accepted that children with chronic cardiac or respiratory disease, those with neurologic disease, and those prone to febrile seizures should be treated for fever. Children with fevers of 40°C (104°F) or higher also should be treated.

Fever is uncomfortable, and children might become irritable. For every 1°C of temperature elevation, the body's metabolic rate increases 10% to 12%, resulting in increased insensible fluid loss, increased oxygen consumption, and increased stress on the cardiovascular system (Lorin, 1998). Regardless of the fever's cause, the comfort of the child is the primary reason for treating a fever in a normally healthy child.

Medications and Environmental Management

Treatment can consist of environmental measures, antipyretics, or a combination of interventions. External cooling is one of the oldest and most common forms of fever management, particularly when the elevated temperature is caused by hyperthermia. Removing blankets and clothing and reducing the environmental temperature can reduce fever. Tepid sponge baths and the use of mechanical cooling blankets can reduce a moderate to high fever fairly quickly (see Procedures 37–1 and 37–2). The challenge is to reduce the fever without causing shivering, which produces heat.

In febrile illnesses, the body attempts to resist external cooling, resulting in the need for antipyretics in addition to external cooling interventions. Fevers in children are treated with antipyretics such as acetaminophen and ibuprofen (Tables 37–2 and 37–3). Aspirin is avoided because of its association with Reye syndrome in children with viral illnesses such as influenza and varicella.

Children with elevated temperatures often experience

PROCEDURE 37–1

Giving Sponge Baths

PURPOSE: To reduce fever.

1. Explain the purpose and the reason for selecting the intervention using developmentally appropriate language. If possible, provide toys or some other distraction for the child. The parent can be present to help comfort or play with the child.
2. Gather the following equipment: (a) tepid water (water temperature should be between 29° and 32°C, 85° and 90°F), (b) cotton blankets, (c) washcloths, and (d) toys. The use of rubbing alcohol is contraindicated because of skin irritation, the risk of neurologic depression from the fumes or absorption through the skin, and too rapid cooling, which can result in shivering.
3. Assist the infant or child to sit or lie in a position of comfort in the bed. Place the infant or child on a cotton bath blanket.

When Bathing the Child Outside a Tub

4. Using tepid water, wet the washcloths or towels and place them on the child, exposing one area at a time. Tepid water, and not ice water, is used because it allows the body temperature to drop gradually, thus avoiding heat-producing responses, such as shivering, which are caused by too rapid cooling.

When the Child Is Placed in a Tub

5. Alternatively, the child can be placed in a tub of warm water, with cool water added until the desired temperature is reached. Gently pour or spray water over the child's back and chest. Continue this for 20 to 30 minutes. Use water toys to provide distraction during this nursing intervention.

Remember: An infant or young child should never be left unattended in the tub!
6. Dry the child. Dress the child in lightweight clothing or pajamas, and place in a dry bed.
7. Recheck the child's temperature approximately 30 minutes later to evaluate the effectiveness of the intervention. *If shivering occurs, the procedure should be terminated immediately.*
8. Document in the nurses' notes the child's baseline vital signs, hydration status, general appearance, interventions used for fever reduction, the indications for the interventions, the duration, the child's response, and any problems identified. Also document any family teaching, as well as the degree of understanding the information given.
9. Take the opportunity to teach the parent how to care for a child with an elevated temperature. Provide information about how to take a temperature, how to read a thermometer, normal temperature range, administration of antipyretics, the use of tepid baths, and when to seek professional help. It is important to emphasize in your teaching that ice water and isopropyl alcohol should never be used for sponging or bathing the child with a fever.
10. Additional points to cover with parents include the importance of accuracy in dosing, the timing of doses, methods of administration, and appropriate medication choices when giving antipyretics. Parents need reassurance that fever is a common symptom of illness and rarely poses a threat to the child's well-being.

PROCEDURE 37-2

. . . .

Using a Cooling Blanket

PURPOSE : To reduce hyperthermia.
1. Using developmentally appropriate language, explain the purpose and the reason for using a cooling blanket. Encourage the parent to be present to help comfort or distract the child.
2. You will need the following equipment: (a) a commercial cooling blanket, (b) sheets or small blankets as needed, and (c) a temperature probe.
3. Place the cooling blanket on the bed and cover it with a sheet or thin blanket.
4. Connect the blanket to the cooling unit and set the control mode (manual or automatic) and the desired blanket or body temperature. Temperature parameters should be set according to the manufacturer's recommendations and physician's orders.
5. Check the child's skin condition before, during, and after use of the blanket, and record the findings.

6. Cover the child lightly to maintain privacy and reduce shivering.
7. To prevent too rapid cooling or overcooling, monitor the child's vital signs frequently. A temperature probe can be used to monitor the patient's temperature continually during this cooling method.
8. To reduce shivering, wrap the child's extremities with towels or baby blankets.
9. Keep the child completely dry to reduce the risk of frostbite from dampness.
10. Reposition the child who is on a cooling unit frequently and gently to reduce the risk of skin breakdown.
11. Record the type of unit used, the control mode and temperature settings selected, and the condition of the child's skin before, during, and after use.

loss of appetite. Dehydration can occur from decreased oral intake and increased insensible water loss through the lungs and the skin. Meet the need for adequate hydration by offering the child additional oral fluids. For those who refuse oral hydration or who are unable to take in adequate volume, consider giving fluids intravenously.

It is important to remember that infants who are being

cared for in servocontrolled heating environments must be carefully monitored because of the potential for accidental dislodgment of the skin temperature probe. This problem can cause an increase in the heat production of the unit and a resulting increase in the infant's temperature. In addition, the insensible water loss in infants in these controlled units is greatly increased. These additional fluid

TABLE 37-2

. . . .

Dosage Chart for Children's and Junior Strength Tylenol (Acetaminophen)

Weight and Age	Grape Suspension Drops and Original Fruit Drops (80 mg/0.8 ml*)	Bubble Gum and Cherry Suspension Liquid and Original Grape and Cherry Elixir (160 mg/5 ml*)	Bubble Gum, Grape and Fruit Chewables (80-mg Tabs*)	Junior Strength Caplets and Grape and Fruit Chewables (160 mg*)
6–11 lb/0–3 mo	½ dppr†	‡	‡	‡
12–17 lb/4–11 mo	1 dppr†	½ tsp	‡	‡
18–23 lb/12–23 mo	1½ dppr†	¾ tsp	‡	‡
24–35 lb/2–3 yr	2 dppr†	1 tsp	2 tab	‡
36–47 lb/4–5 yr		1½ tsp	3 tab	‡
48–59 lb/6–8 yr		2 tsp	4 tab	2 cap/tab
60–71 lb/9–10 yr		2½ tsp	5 tab	2½ cap/tab
72–95 lb/11 yr		3 tsp	6 tab	3 cap/tab
≥96 lb/12–14 yr				4 cap/tab

Notes to parents: Consult a physician if your child's age or weight range is within the orange shaded area. Use only under physician's direction. Consult your physician as your child grows to be sure you are giving the most accurate dose based on your child's weight and age.

Consult a physician if fever persists for more than 3 days or if pain continues for more than 5 days. In case of accidental overdosage, contact a physician or poison control center immediately.

A calibrated dropper or dosage cup is included in each liquid package.

Do not use any of the products listed with other products containing acetaminophen.

*Doses should be administered 4 or 5 times daily or as directed by your doctor. Do not exceed 5 doses in 24 hours.

†0.8 ml dropperful (dropper enclosed in package).

‡Do not use this form in this weight/age group unless directed by a physician.

Courtesy of McNeil Consumer Products Company, Division of McNeil-PPC, Inc., Fort Washington, PA 19034.

TABLE 37–3

Dosage Chart for Ibuprofen, by Weight and Age

Weight and Age	5 mg/kg (Temp. $\leq$ 102.5°F)		10 mg/kg (Temp. > 102.5°F)	
	mg	tsp	mg	tsp
13–17 lb/6–11 mo	25	1/4	50	1/2
18–23 lb/12–23 mo	50	1/2	100	1
24–35 lb/2–3 yr	75	3/4	150	1 1/2
36–47 lb/4–5 yr	100	1	200	2
48–59 lb/6–8 yr	125	1 1/4	250	2 1/2
60–71 lb/9–10 yr	150	1 1/2	300	3
72–95 lb/11–12 yr	200	2	400	4

Note: Give every 6–8 hours. Do not exceed 40 mg/kg/day.

losses must be considered when calculating fluid replacement.

Commercial Cooling Blankets

Commercial cooling blankets also can be used to control hyperthermia. These units, which can be controlled manually or automatically, lower the body temperature through cold transfer between the blanket and the child. Cooling unit operation varies among manufacturers. Therefore, it is important to read the operating manual before using this equipment. Some cooling blankets may be reusable, but blankets designed for single patient use are preferred. Shivering, frostbite, and skin breakdown are concerns when using a cooling blanket.

Specimen Collection

Specimens are collected from children for the same reasons they are collected from adults, but children often need more of an explanation of the reasons and procedure for specimen collection. All explanations should be given in age-appropriate language, and children should be prepared for any sensations that they might experience.

Regardless of the type of specimen to be obtained, use standard precautions (see Appendix B). The use of gloves, gowns, masks, eye protection, and hand washing provides protection for individuals coming in contact with potentially infectious materials. The use of equipment for standard precautions will vary according to the degree of "potential splash." *Any time there is a chance for contamination, use standard precautions.* Follow procedures for handling biologic hazards as directed by individual facilities, on the basis of standard precautions.

Urine Specimens

VOIDED SPECIMENS
Older children and adolescents often cooperate in the collection of urine specimens. Most can use a bedpan, urinal, or specimen cup with little difficulty. Younger children and preschoolers often have difficulty voiding on re-

quest. The nurse should take care to use familiar terms, such as "peepee," "tinkle," or "potty" when telling the child what is needed. It is helpful to have a potty chair or collection "hat" that fits in the toilet available for young children. Parents can be very helpful in obtaining a specimen from children this age. Parents might also be successful obtaining specimens from older toddlers who are being toilet trained. Infants and young toddlers, however, are unable to void on request. Because they are not toilet trained, specimen collection devices are needed (Procedure 37–3).

If the specimen must be collected under special conditions (as in the case of a midstream urine sample), the nurse carefully explains to the child what preparation is needed and ensures that the child understands all directions. An adult might need to accompany the child during the collection. A young child might be able to sit on the toilet but be unable to manipulate a specimen cup. The parent or nurse can hold the cup while the child voids. For a boy who wishes to stand while voiding, the cup can be held in the stream as he voids. If the specimen is to be carried to another room or down a hallway, provide a plastic bag or other container for transport.

Although many methods have been used to collect urine from incontinent children (such as placing plastic wrap in a diaper to catch urine), the most reliable is the pediatric urine collection bag or urine "wee bag." This collection device is a plastic bag with an opening lined with adhesive so that it can be attached to the perineum. It is available in two sizes, infant and pediatric, to accommodate almost any child. Twenty-four-hour collection bags are also available. These bags have a tube that extends from the end of the bag, allowing each void to be removed.

Although some facilities use sterile urine collection bags to obtain a specimen for urine culture, this method of collecting urine might be inappropriate to rule out a urinary tract infection. Bags can become contaminated with organisms usually present in the perineal area (Schlager et al., 1995). Many physicians choose to use straight catheterization or suprapubic aspiration to obtain urine for culture from an incontinent child.

A urine specimen can be obtained directly from a disposable diaper. This method has demonstrated good correla-

PROCEDURE 37–3
· · · · · · · · · ·
Urine Specimen Collection from the Incontinent Child

PURPOSE: To monitor urine output accurately or obtain a specimen for testing.

1. Before beginning the procedure, provide adequate privacy. The child may be more relaxed if a parent is present. If both blood and urine specimens need to be obtained from the incontinent child, position the collection bag *before* drawing the blood. Infants and toddlers often void during a painful procedure.

2. Obtain the following equipment: (a) nonsterile gloves, (b) urine collection bag, (c) sterile specimen cup, (d) mild soap, warm water, and a washcloth, (e) diaper and towel, (f) label and requisition form.

3. Clean the perineal area. Cleaning the perineum will remove any lotions or ointments and help the bag to adhere.

   a. *For girls:* Clean from front to back and from the urinary meatus to the labia majora (in to out).

   b. *For boys:* Clean from the tip of the penis in a circular motion. *Do not* retract an infant's or young child's foreskin.

4. After the perineum has been cleansed, dry it thoroughly. The skin must be completely dry for the bag to adhere properly.

5. Remove the backing from the adhesive surface of the bottom half of the collection device.

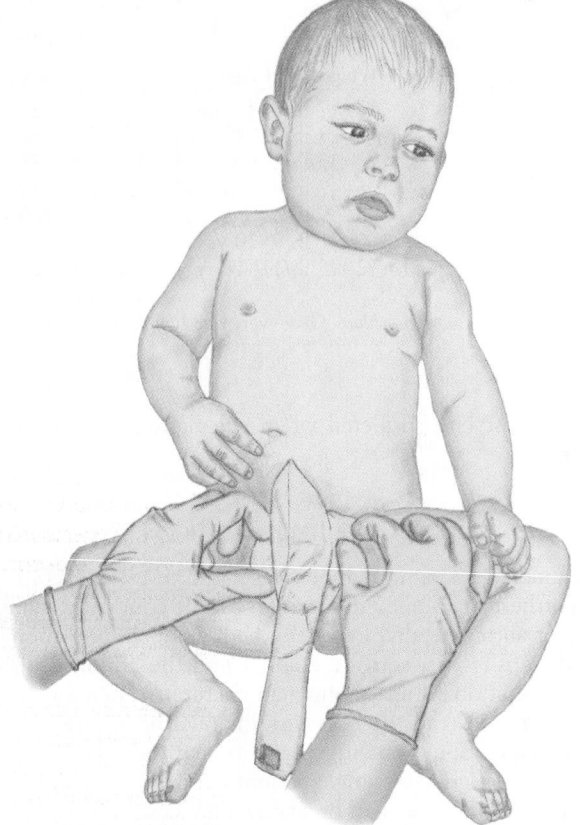

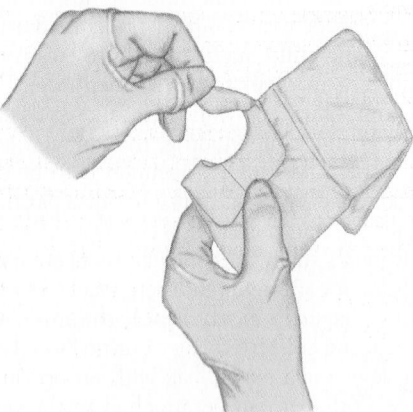

6. Place the child in a frog-leg position to eliminate skin folds that may interfere with bag adherence. Apply the bag.

   a. *With girls:* Hold the perineum taut and apply the adhesive portion of the bag, working outward. To keep the feces from contaminating the specimen, the narrow "bridge" on the adhesive patch must be placed on the tiny area of skin between the anus and the genitals.

b. *With boys:* Place the penis and scrotum (if small enough) inside the bag.

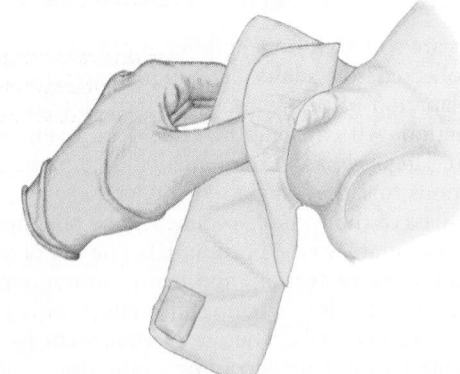

7. After the bag is attached, a diaper can be re-applied. Before replacing the diaper, cut a slit in the diaper and pull the end of the empty bag through the slit so that the bag protrudes from the diaper. This step reduces the chance of leaking, and allows for observation of urine.

8. Check the bag every 30 minutes. Applying slight pressure over the suprapubic area or stroking along the older infant's spine will often induce voiding. As soon as urine is noticed in the bag, remove the bag gently from the perineum.

PROCEDURE 37–3 *Continued*

Urine Specimen Collection from the Incontinent Child

9. Transfer the urine into a sterile specimen cup. Most bags have a small tab that can be removed to allow the urine to be poured. If the bag does not have a tab, clean the outside of the bag with an alcohol pad and withdraw the urine with a needle and syringe for placement in the appropriate container.

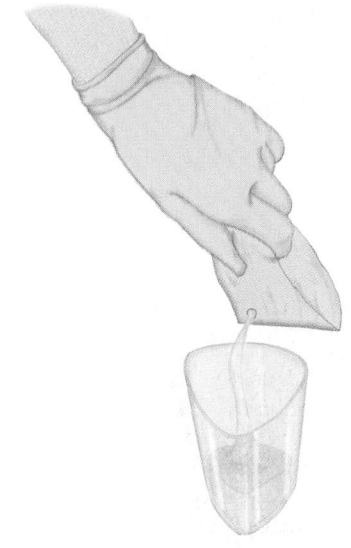

10. Label the urine specimen with the child's name and date and time of collection and deliver it promptly, together with a requisition form, to the laboratory. Urine for culture that cannot be tested within 30 minutes should be refrigerated or placed in a sterile container with a preservative.
11. Record the collection of the specimen in the child's chart. Include the date and time of collection and the amount, color, and appearance of the urine.
12. If a urine specimen is to be obtained at home, give instructions to the parent and provide the appropriate equipment. Parents can keep the urine collected at home in the refrigerator until they are asked to bring it to the laboratory. The specimen should be kept chilled during transport (i.e., placed in a cooler or plastic bag packed with ice).

---

tion with catheterized or aspirated urine for identification of urinary tract infection (Cohen et al., 1997). Take saturated absorbent material from the disposable diaper and place in a 10-ml syringe from which you have removed the plunger. Reinsert the plunger into the barrel of the syringe and express the urine into a specimen container.

URINARY CATHETERIZATION

The basic procedure for urinary catheterization is much the same in children as in adults (Procedure 37–4). Aside from psychological considerations, the major difference is in the size of the catheter. Pediatric catheterization kits often contain a completely closed collection system (with the catheter end already enclosed in the collection tube). The catheter should be small enough so that it can be inserted easily into the urinary meatus but large enough to prevent leakage of urine. Urinary catheters are available in sizes as small as No. 5 French and can be matched to the child's age as follows:

> *Infants up to 1 year old:* No. 5 to 8 French
> *Children 1 to 5 years old:* No. 8 French
> *School-age children:* No. 8 to 14 French
> *Adolescents:* No. 10 to 14 French

Some children, particularly those who undergo multiple urinary tract catheterizations (e.g., children with spina bifida), are at high risk for developing latex sensitivity. These children and other children with known or suspected latex allergy should be identified as early as possible, and latex-free catheters should be used.

Stool Specimens

Stool specimens are obtained to test for the presence of fat, blood, bacteria, parasites, or reducing substances in the stool. If a stool specimen from an incontinent child is needed, it often can be scraped from a diaper and placed in an appropriate container. If the stool is watery, a specimen may be collected by placing a piece of gauze in the diaper to absorb some of the stool or by applying a "wee bag" over the anus.

A bedpan or a specimen collector designed to be placed in the toilet can be used to obtain a specimen from an older child. Because older children may be embarrassed about providing a stool sample, the nurse should use a calm, matter-of-fact manner when explaining why the specimen is needed and the procedure for handling the specimen.

Blood Specimens

Nurses use a variety of techniques to collect blood samples from children. Because blood collection is an invasive procedure, it should be performed in a treatment room, if one is available.

Regardless of the sampling procedure used, most children find blood collection distressing. Some are concerned about the pain involved, while others fear the perceived loss of body fluid. The use of EMLA, a topical anesthetic cream, can reduce the child's discomfort. To be effective, EMLA must remain on the site for at least 45 minutes. (See Chapter 39 for a discussion of EMLA.)

In children who need long-term venous access for nu-

PROCEDURE 37-4
• • • • • • • • • •
Urinary Catheterization

PURPOSE: To obtain a sterile urine sample.

1. Prepare the child for the procedure by using age-appropriate methods. Explain what the child will feel and what the child can do to "help." It may be helpful to demonstrate the procedure on a teaching doll. Teach the child to take slow, deep breaths during the procedure and have the child practice breathing prior to the procedure. Encouraging the child to sing also helps relax the appropriate muscles. The child might feel a need to urinate during the catheter insertion. Reassure the child that the feeling is normal. The assistance of another adult is often necessary with younger children.

2. Make sure the area is well lighted, and gather all necessary equipment. If equipment is not contained in the catheterization kit, bring the appropriate-size catheter, sterile gloves (extra pairs in case of contamination), specimen cup, label, and requisition form. If the child is to have an indwelling catheter, bring a closed drainage bag.

3. When using an indwelling catheter, measure the distance from the catheter tip to the end of the balloon. Once urine is observed, insert the catheter an additional amount equal to this distance before inflating the balloon. Total insertion

length is usually 5 cm (2 inches) for girls and 7–10 cm (3–4 inches) for boys (Smith & Adams, 1998). Before inserting a Foley catheter, inflate and deflate the balloon to check for function and leaks.

4. The procedure is the same as for an adult, with the following additions:
   a. Take extra care to be gentle when cleansing the meatus or glans penis.
   b. Choose the appropriate-size catheter (see p. 963).
   c. In girls, direct the catheter slightly upward and insert it gently through the meatus 1 to 2 inches (2.5–5 cm), or until urine appears. In boys, hold the penis at a 90-degree angle from the boy and gently insert the catheter 2 to 4 inches (5–10 cm) (longer in older boys) or until urine appears. Never force the catheter. The older child can assist in relaxing the external sphincter by bearing down.

5. Record the date and time the procedure was done, as well as the size of catheter used and the amount, color, and appearance of the urine. Note how the infant or child tolerated the procedure. Deliver the labeled specimen promptly, together with the requisition form, to the laboratory.

---

trition or medications and who have a central venous catheter or port in place, the nurse can obtain blood for laboratory studies from the central venous catheter or port. This procedure, however, may be performed *only* by specially trained, licensed personnel.

Venipuncture in children is often performed using a butterfly catheter (Procedure 37–5). The most commonly used sites are the veins of the hand and the antecubital area. Always follow standard precautions when collecting blood specimens or when assisting other personnel in collecting blood.

JUGULAR AND FEMORAL VENIPUNCTURE
Jugular and femoral venipuncture are performed by a physician, with the nurse assisting and monitoring the child. If obtaining blood from one of the large superficial external jugular veins, place the child in a mummy restraint (see Fig. 37–3), allowing enough area at the top edge of the restraint to permit access to the jugular vein. If a restraint is not used, the arms and legs can be held by a second nurse. The child's head is hyperextended to the side opposite the site, over the edge of a table or a small pillow (Fig. 37–8). Apply pressure to the site for 3 to 5 minutes or until bleeding stops. Care should be taken not to overextend the head to the point of causing airway problems.

If performing a femoral venipuncture, place the child supine in the frog-leg position to expose the groin area (see Fig. 37–8). One nurse stands above the child's head, holding the child's arms with the elbows and the legs with the

hands. Place a cloth diaper over the infant's perineal area, tucked under the buttocks with the site exposed. The diaper protects the area in case the child urinates. Apply pressure to the site with a dry, sterile gauze square after the specimen is obtained.

CAPILLARY BLOOD SAMPLING
When a small blood sample is needed, a disposable pediatric lancet (inserted 2.4 mm deep) can be used for a finger or heel puncture (see Procedure 37–6 and Procedure 22–3 for a description of heel stick sampling). For finger punctures, the third (ring) finger of the nondominant hand should be used. Make the puncture just to the side of the fingerpad rather than at the tip. There are fewer nerve endings, and the areas are highly vascular. The heel is used in infants; it is warmed first to increase blood flow. The heel is not used once the infant is walking because calluses make it more difficult to puncture.

Sputum Specimens

Sputum specimens are most frequently obtained to identify or rule out a respiratory infection. When obtaining any specimen, follow standard precautions. If splashing is anticipated, wear masks and goggles or protective eyewear in addition to gloves.

It is easy to obtain sputum in the older child because most older children and adolescents can cough deeply and produce a sputum sample, which can then be placed in the

PROCEDURE 37–5
. . . .
Venipuncture

PURPOSE: To obtain a blood sample for laboratory testing with minimal trauma to the child.

1. As with any procedure, prepare the child using age-appropriate language. Be sure to include what the child will see and feel. Ask the parents whether it is better to prepare their young child in advance or to describe what you are doing as you are performing the procedure. It is often necessary to obtain help to restrain the child during the procedure. Parents might or might not wish to remain in the room.

2. Take the child to the treatment room. Have the following equipment available: (a) 23- or 25-gauge butterfly catheter, (b) gloves, (c) alcohol and/or povidone-iodine (Betadine) swabs or pads, (d) syringe(s), (e) labels, (f) appropriate collection containers, (g) requisition form, and (h) tourniquet. (*Note*: Most tourniquets are composed of rubber tubing that is ½ to 1 inch wide. Although rubber bands have been used as tourniquets in infants, these are not preferred, as they may abrade the skin.)

3. Restrain the child by having one nurse place one hand under the child's arm (usually at the shoulder) and the other hand on the child's hand. The sampling nurse is then able to draw the blood with less likelihood of missing the vein. The vein of the antecubital area is commonly used for venipuncture in children. A butterfly needle is often used; the needle is inserted into the vein with the bevel up. When blood flows and reaches the end of the catheter, the syringe is attached and the sample is gently drawn into the syringe.

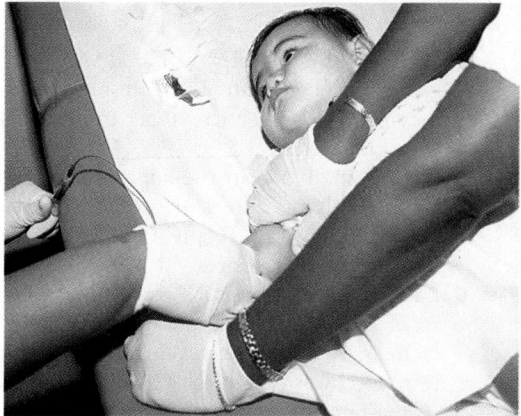

Courtesy of Parkland Health and Hospital System Community Oriented Primary Care Clinic, Dallas, Texas.

4. Apply a tourniquet tight enough to restrict blood flow toward the heart but not so tight as to cause pain or restrict arterial blood flow. Tourniquets are used to slow venous blood return to the heart and cause distension of the veins, thus making them more visible. To facilitate easy removal, the tourniquet should be looped when applied. To prevent hemoconcentration, a tourniquet should be left in place no longer than 2 minutes.

5. Lightly pat or rub the sample site to help the veins become more visible.

6. Using a circular motion, clean the site with alcohol and allow to dry. If the child is immunocompromised, use povidone-iodine (Betadine) to cleanse the skin.

7. Insert the needle of the butterfly catheter into the vein, bevel side up.

8. When blood begins to flow into the catheter, avoid the temptation to place the syringe on the end of the catheter and attempt to speed up the blood flow by pulling back the plunger. Instead, to avoid venospasm wait until the blood reaches the end of the catheter, attach the syringe and slowly draw the appropriate amount of blood into the syringe.

9. After obtaining the required amount of blood, release the tourniquet, withdraw the needle, and apply pressure to the puncture site until the bleeding has stopped. Fill the appropriate specimen tubes or containers. Be sure to dispose of needles and contaminated gauze properly.

10. Comfort the child and offer praise for cooperation. Encourage the parent to provide comfort. Band-Aids are important, as they help to prevent bleeding from the puncture site. Specially colored or cartoon character Band-Aids are available commercially and are appropriate for children's "booboos." The nurse can also give the child a reward, such as a sticker.

11. Label the specimen with the child's name and record the date and time of collection, the amount of blood collected, the site used for puncture, and the reason blood was drawn (e.g., diagnostic test). Note the child's reaction to the procedure and the number of attempts made before a specimen was obtained.

appropriate container. Specimens are easily obtained from children with artificial airways by attaching a mucous or suction trap to a suction catheter and suctioning the airway to obtain the specimen. A cough can be elicited by placing a suction catheter into the back of the throat in an infant or young child.

Because younger children and infants can seldom produce a deep cough on demand and often swallow those secretions, obtaining sputum samples in infants and young children often requires a nasal washing, or *lavage* (Procedure 37–7). Nasal washing is used particularly to obtain a sample for identifying respiratory syncytial virus (RSV) and pertussis.

Infant positioned for jugular venipuncture

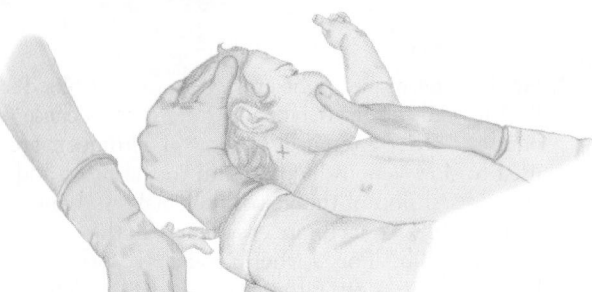

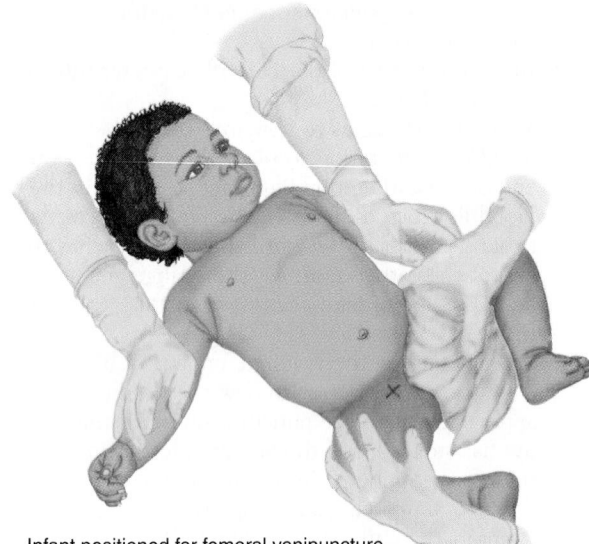

Infant positioned for femoral venipuncture

FIGURE 37-8

Two additional sites for obtaining blood specimens from infants and young children are the large superficial external jugular veins and the femoral veins.

Throat and Nasopharyngeal Specimens

Throat cultures can identify the causative agent of "sore throats" or tonsillitis in children. Nasopharyngeal cultures are mainly used to identify pertussis (Procedure 37–8).

Cerebrospinal Fluid Specimens

Physicians perform lumbar punctures to examine the cerebrospinal fluid (CSF) for bacteria or abnormal cells, to measure pressure within the cerebrospinal cavities, or to inject certain medications (i.e., for pain control, to prevent or eradicate specific diseases, or as contrast agents for scans) (Procedure 37–9). A hollow spinal needle, inserted into the subarachnoid space between the 3rd and 4th lumbar vertebrae, provides for fluid exit and collection. An attached stopcock and manometer are used to measure spinal fluid pressure.

Because a lumbar puncture is frequently performed

PROCEDURE 37-6
* * * * * * * * * * * *
Finger Stick Capillary Blood Sampling

PURPOSE: To obtain a small sample of capillary blood.

1. Prepare the child appropriately for the procedure using developmentally appropriate explanations (finger poke, "owie"). You can warm the site before proceeding or have the older child wash the hands in warm water.
2. Bring the child to the treatment room, where the following equipment should be available: (a) disposable lancets or microlancets, (b) alcohol or povidone-iodine (Betadine) swabs, (c) sterile gauze pads, (d) gloves, (e) warm washcloth, (f) specimen containers, (g) labels and requisition forms.
3. After appropriately cleaning the site, make a puncture with the lancet across the fingerprint halfway between the center of the ball of the finger and its side (Garza & Becan-McBride, 1993). Use the third, or ring, finger of the nondominant hand. Do not use a bruised, edematous, or abraded finger, and avoid old puncture sites.

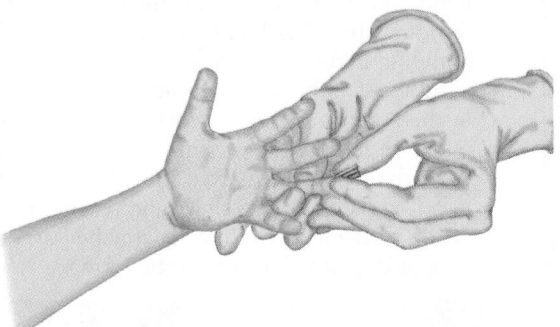

4. Wipe off the first drop of blood with a sterile gauze pad. To ensure adequate blood flow, you may gently massage the finger from its base to the tip.
5. Collect the blood in the appropriate container(s). Apply pressure with sterile gauze until the bleeding stops. Apply a decorative Band-Aid if the child desires.
6. Label the specimen with the child's name and record the date, time, amount of blood collected, site used for the puncture, and reason the blood was drawn. Note the child's reaction to the procedure and whether more than one puncture was necessary.

when a child is acutely ill—with meningitis or leukemia, for example—this stressful procedure becomes even more stressful for the child and family. The nurse must provide a great deal of support and education for the child and family. The physician will explain what is planned and will obtain an informed consent from the parents or guardians. Only a physician or qualified nurse practitioner performs

PROCEDURE 37-7

Nasal Washing

PURPOSE: To obtain a sputum sample from an infant or young child.

1. Prepare the child for the procedure by using developmentally appropriate language and describing any expected sensations (the procedure will make the child sneeze).
2. Gather the following equipment: (a) butterfly catheter, (b) syringe, (c) sterile saline, (d) gloves, (e) sterile specimen container or pertussis kit, (f) labels and requisition form.
3. Ask for assistance restraining the child, or mummy-wrap an infant to restrain the arms and legs.

4. Cut the "butterfly" (needle and wings) off the butterfly catheter and discard.
5. Attach a syringe (without needle) containing 1 to 3 ml of sterile saline to the catheter and fill the catheter.
6. Place the child in a supine position and gently place the catheter into one nostril.
7. Instill the saline into the nostril and immediately withdraw into the syringe, or aspirate secretions after the saline instillation with a small sterile bulb syringe.
8. Place the saline into a sterile, labeled container.
9. Record the amount of saline instilled and the method of collection used. Note the date, time, amount, color, and consistency of secretions.

PROCEDURE 37-8

Throat or Nasopharyngeal Culture

PURPOSE: To obtain a specimen for culture.

1. Explain the procedure to the child in appropriate language. For a throat culture, explain that the child will need to look up toward the ceiling, open the mouth very wide, and might feel like coughing or gagging. Emphasize that the procedure doesn't hurt. For a nasopharyngeal swab, tell the child to look up and explain that you will be inserting the swab into the nose. The child will feel like sneezing. Do not do these procedures immediately after the child has taken medication, eaten, or had something to drink. Assistance may be needed to restrain a younger child.
2. Gather the following equipment: (a) tongue depressor, (b) throat or nasopharyngeal swab (cotton-tipped swab with a flexible wire extension), (c) collection containers and labels (if not included with the swab), (d) gloves, (e) sterile saline.
3. An older child can sit in a chair or sit upright in bed for the culture. A younger child should be placed supine on a bed or examining table.

Throat Culture

4. Have the child open the mouth and say "Ahhh." Eliciting a cry from an infant will give optimal access to the pharyngeal area. Insert a tongue depressor into the mouth with the nondominant hand so that it covers the anterior half of the tongue, and depress the tongue to allow observation of the pharyngeal area. Swab the area quickly, avoiding the tongue, buccal mucosa, and palate. If the child opens the mouth wide enough for adequate visibility, a tongue depressor might not be needed. Only one swab should be used for each culture.

Nasopharyngeal Culture

5. Ask the child to look up. Bend the wire so that, when the swab is inserted, the tip will go beyond the back of the nares and into the pharyngeal area. Dip the swab tip into saline and gently insert it into one nares, down to the posterior nasopharynx. Leave it in place for several seconds, then remove.
6. Place the swabs in the appropriate culture media and transport them to the laboratory.
7. If possible, offer the child cool fluids to drink following the procedure. Assist the parent to support and comfort the child during and after the procedure.
8. Record the date and time, the appearance of the specimen, and the child's response to the procedure.

CRITICAL TO REMEMBER

Throat Cultures

- Never attempt to obtain a throat specimen for culture in a child for whom a diagnosis of *epiglottitis* is suspected because the procedure could precipitate sudden airway obstruction.
- Before obtaining a specimen for throat culture, assess for the presence of high fever of sudden onset, drooling, muffled voice, and erythema or exudate (signs of epiglottitis).

a lumbar puncture. The nurse assists by positioning, restraining, and monitoring the patient.

Bone Marrow Aspirates

Bone marrow aspiration is performed to obtain specimens of marrow for diagnostic testing, for evaluation of response to treatment, or for transplantation (Procedure 37–10). The most common site of bone marrow aspiration in the child is the posterior iliac crest. Other sites include the anterior iliac crest and the tibia.

Because the reasons for a bone marrow aspiration include ruling out serious disease, such as leukemia, or assess-

PROCEDURE 37-9
. . . .
Lumbar Puncture

PURPOSE: To obtain a cerebrospinal fluid sample.

1. Take the child to the treatment room and explain that the child will be lying on the side, curled up into a ball. Tell the child that you will be "hugging" him or her to keep the knees close to the chin and that the child should tell you if you are holding too closely. The child will need to stay very still until the physician is finished. If local anesthesia is to be used, the child might feel a "pinch." If time permits, the child should be allowed to practice the position so as not to feel frightened or suffocated.

2. You will need the following equipment: (a) lumbar puncture tray (usually comes with all equipment needed by the physician), (b) povidone-iodine (Betadine) solution or swabs, (c) extra sterile gloves, (d) additional light source if needed, (e) gloves, (f) requisition forms.

3. Open the lumbar puncture kit if requested. Use sterile gloves and aseptic technique.

4. Place the child in the appropriate position. The two positions used for lumbar puncture are the lateral, or side-lying, position and the sitting position. The intraspinal fluid pressure can be measured only if the child is in the lateral position. Both positions can be used for collecting CSF or injecting medications. Restraint is sometimes better obtained in the side-lying position, but modify the position on the basis of experience.

5. If the child is in a side-lying position, secure the child by holding the child under the thighs and behind the neck. Extreme care should be taken to avoid airway obstruction. The infant placed in a sitting position can be secured by holding the infant along the sides with the nurse's thumbs across the infant's shoulder blades. The older child

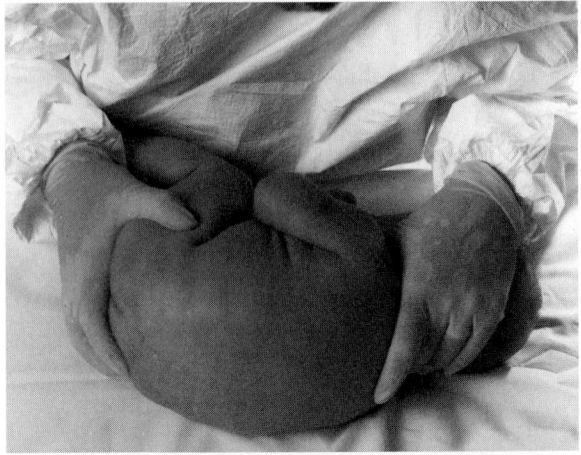

B. For the lumbar puncture: Curl the infant into a tight ball by curving the spinal vertebrae and bringing the baby's knee up to the head. (Note the proximity of the baby's knees to the elbows.) Meanwhile support the head and neck with your other hand.

CHILD (4 MONTHS AND OLDER): LATERAL POSITION

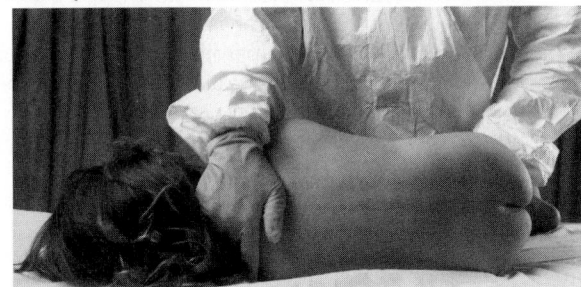

C. Place the child in a side-lying position, placing one hand behind the child's neck and shoulders and the other hand under the child's bent upper thighs.

INFANT (3 MONTHS AND YOUNGER): LATERAL POSITION

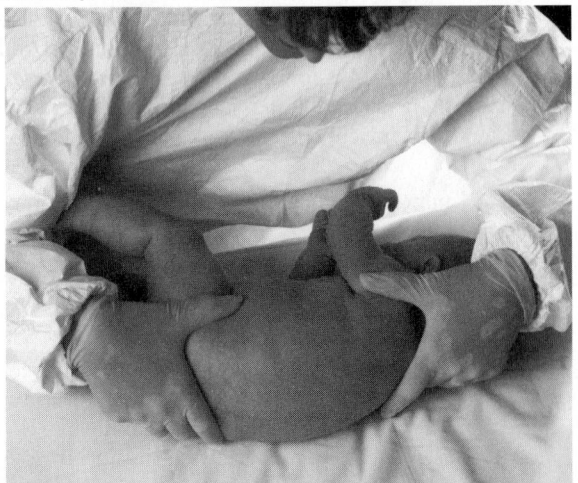

A. Place the infant on one side, placing one hand across the baby's hips and the other hand on the baby's shoulders and back of head.

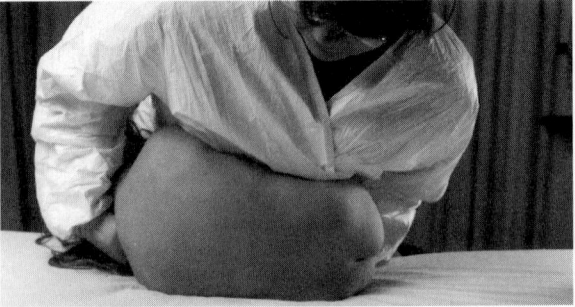

D. For the lumbar puncture: Place a hand farther down, under the child's neck. Your forearm moves behind the child's head to support the neck. Place the other arm farther under the child's upper thighs and curl the body by bringing the knees up to the head. Note that this nurse's weight is supported on the edge of the gurney, and the nurse leans lightly over the child, controlling the arms and legs. Because direct visibility of the child's respiratory status is limited in this position, a cardiorespiratory monitor must be on the child, or another nurse should be at the bedside.

Lumbar Puncture

INFANT (3 MONTHS AND YOUNGER): SITTING POSITION

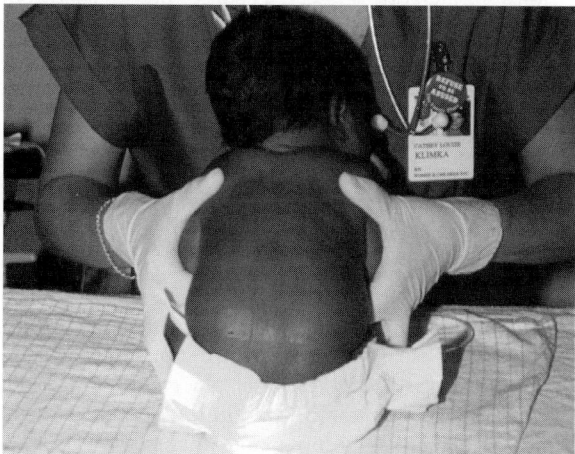

E. Secure the infant in a sitting position with your thumbs across the baby's scapulae.

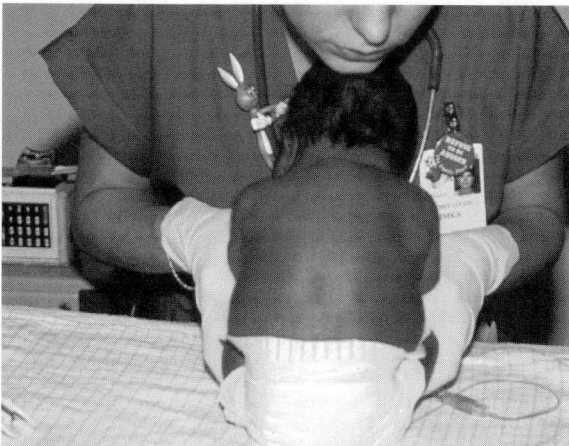

F. An alternative method useful for small infants: Hold the infant in a sitting position. The child's arms are between your thumbs and index fingers and the child's legs are between your index and middle fingers. Note that this nurse steadies the child's head with her chin and so maintains the head in alignment with the child's spine.

CHILD (4 MONTHS AND OLDER): SITTING POSITION

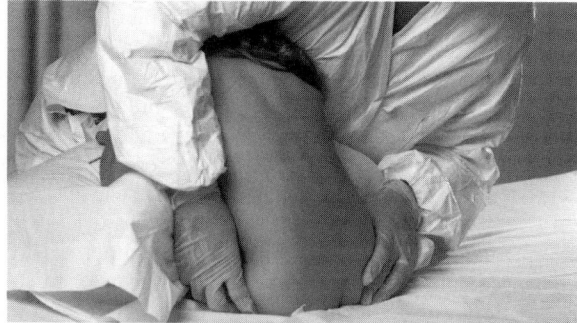

G. Seat the child upright on the stretcher and place a pillow in the child's lap. Allow the child to lean over a pillow while turning the head to the side. The child can sit cross-legged or can dangle the legs straight down. Then place one arm behind the head and around the child's upper shoulders and place a hand on each upper thigh.

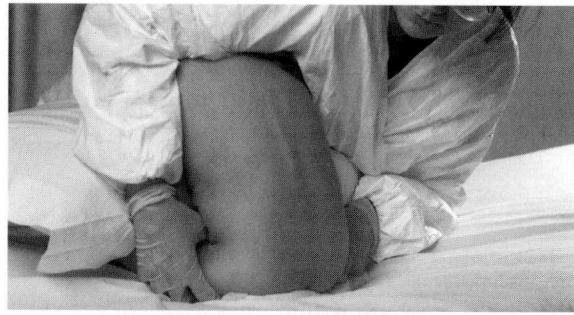

H. For the lumbar puncture: Lean farther down over the child, using your upper body to hold the child still while bending the child back into a convex curve. Both hands hold the hips still.

can lean over a pillow with the nurse placing an arm across the child's back.

6. Explain to the child that he or she will feel something cold as the back is washed and that the child may feel a "sting" when the physician injects local anesthetic. EMLA (see Chapter 39) might be used to eliminate pain.

7. Explain that the child may feel pressure when the spinal needle is inserted and, possibly, some pain in a leg if medication is injected.

8. During the procedure, provide constant verbal reassurance *unless* the child is using guided imagery. (If the child is using guided imagery, your speaking will ruin the child's ability to concentrate.) Monitor the child's cardiorespiratory status either visually or electronically during the procedure.

9. After the needle is inserted into the vertebral space, flexion may be relaxed. If appropriate, encourage the child to relax and take slow breaths. Maintain restraint, however, to prevent the child from moving.

10. The physician will obtain CSF samples and might measure CSF pressure. After completing the sampling and measurement, the needle is removed. Explain that the child will feel light pressure and a Band-Aid being applied.

11. The child might need to remain in bed with the head of the bed flat or elevated no more than 15 degrees for 4 to 6 hours. Monitor the child for complaints of headache, fever, or CSF leakage at the puncture site.

12. Record the date, time, and name of the physician performing the procedure. Monitor the child's vital signs as ordered and observe for changes in responsiveness or motor activity, headache, bradycardia, and condition of the puncture site. Note the color, clarity, and pressure of the CSF.

13. Assist parents to comfort the child during and after the procedure. Inform parents of the child's need for quiet and fluid intake.

Text adapted from Zappa, S. C. (1994). Pediatric practice review: Lumbar punctures. Restraining the pediatric patient. *Nursing in Pediatrics* (Fall), a publication of Cook Children's Medical Center, Fort Worth, Texas, pp. 22–23. Photographs A–D and G–H © Bob Lukeman. Photographs E and F courtesy of Parkland Health and Hospital System, Dallas, Texas.

CRITICAL TO REMEMBER

Lumbar Puncture

- Correct positioning and adequate restraint during the procedure will minimize trauma and ensure an appropriate specimen.
- Observe the child carefully during the procedure for airway obstruction or bradycardia related to neck flexion. Use a cardiorespiratory monitor or pulse oximeter to monitor oxygen saturation.
- If electronic monitoring is not available, ask another nurse to monitor the child's condition.

---

ing the progress of cancer treatment, the child and family need a tremendous amount of support and preparation prior to the procedure.

Gavage and Gastrostomy

Because some infants and children are unable to tolerate adequate oral nutrition, the physician might select an alternative method of feeding. *Enteral feedings* are an option for infants and children who are premature, ill, or injured or who have congenital anomalies, respiratory distress, swallowing disorders, or neurologic impairment or have previously undergone surgery. Feedings are given through an orogastric, nasogastric, or transpyloric tube or through a gastrostomy tube or button.

Tube Route and Placement

Placement of a gastrostomy tube or gastrostomy button is a surgical procedure performed by the surgeon. The nurse usually places an orogastric, nasogastric, or transpyloric tube (Procedures 37–11 and 37–12). Nasogastric tubes are used most frequently because the tube is easier to stabilize with nasal placement than with oral placement (Hill & Rath, 1993). Because of increased mucus production caused by irritation from the tube, nasal placement can potentially interfere with respiratory function. Children with head or nasal anomalies or injuries and infants who are still preferential nose breathers (usually those 4 months old or younger) will need orogastric tube placement.

A transpyloric tube is more difficult to insert than an orogastric or nasogastric tube. A transpyloric tube also requires radiographic confirmation of correct placement. Although various methods may be used to secure the tube, its desired position is often difficult to maintain (Hill & Rath, 1993).

PROCEDURE 37–10

Bone Marrow Aspiration

PURPOSE: To obtain a bone marrow sample for testing or transplantation.

1. Prepare the child in advance for the procedure using developmentally appropriate language and explanations. Explain that the child will need to be positioned on the abdomen (tummy) on top of a small pillow. The child will feel something cold as the hip is washed and might feel a "sting" when the physician injects a local anesthetic.
2. The physician performing the procedure obtains consent, and the child and family need to be given the opportunity to ask questions about the procedure. This procedure is usually performed under sedation in a treatment room.
3. Gather the following equipment: (a) bone marrow aspiration tray, (b) sterile and nonsterile gloves, (c) sterile 2 × 2-inch gauze pads, (d) tape, (e) antiseptic ointment (povidone-iodine [Betadine]), (f) labels and requisition forms.
4. Position the child prone with a small pillow under the hips to facilitate access to the posterior iliac crest. If other sites are to be used, alter the position accordingly. The child can also be positioned sitting up the same as for lumbar punctures.
5. Encourage the parent to stand at the child's head and talk reassuringly to the child throughout the procedure. Because the procedure is painful, the parents might not want to stay. In that circumstance enlist a nurse whom the child trusts to provide support.

6. Restrain the child adequately to prevent movement during the procedure. If adequate sedation has not been given, a second nurse may be needed to help restrain the child.
7. After cleaning the site, the physician inserts a needle into the bone and withdraws the marrow by suction. Prior to the suction, explain that the child might feel a sharp pain and encourage the child to take deep breaths, sing or count, or use other relaxation techniques.
8. The physician examines the marrow for the presence of white marrow spicules. If they are not present, the syringe is reattached to the needle and aspiration is attempted again.
9. After the procedure is complete, the needle is withdrawn, and the nurse applies pressure to the site.
10. Cover the site with a pressure bandage or Band-Aid and return the child to the room. Assess the child's vital signs until stable (this assessment is particularly important if the child has received preprocedural sedation). Monitor the puncture site for signs of bleeding and later for signs of infection. After the child has fully recovered from sedation and if the site shows no signs of complications, the child may resume normal activities.
11. Record the date and time and the name of the physician performing the procedure. Record the child's vital signs, the appearance of the specimen and the sampling site, and the child's response to the procedure.

PROCEDURE 37–11
. . . .
Feeding Tube Insertions

PURPOSE: To provide enteral nutrition.

1. Using developmentally appropriate language, explain the procedure to the child and family and assess their needs and concerns (e.g., previous experience with tube insertion, ability to assist with the procedure, need for restraint). Therapeutic play can be utilized to allay the child's and parents' fears related to the procedure.

2. Gather the following equipment before starting the procedure: (a) feeding tube of appropriate size and type, (b) ¼- or ½-inch hypoallergenic tape, (c) 20-ml syringe, (d) sterile water for oral use, (e) stethoscope, (f) water-soluble lubricating jelly (for nasal insertion only), (g) pH reagent strips, (h) gloves, (i) feeding pump and setup (enteral feeding bag or burette), and (j) the enteral fluid to be administered.

3. Position the child on the back or right side with the head of the bed elevated. To facilitate cooperation and decrease fear, a small child can be held in a parent's arms, with the child's head on the parent's shoulder. An older child may sit up in the bed. Restrain if necessary.

4. Wash your hands and don gloves.

5. Measure the length of the catheter to be inserted and mark with a waterproof marker or with tape.

   a. To place a nasogastric tube in a child, measure the distance from the tip of the nose to the earlobe and then down to the xiphoid process. Mark the total measurement with tape or indelible marker.

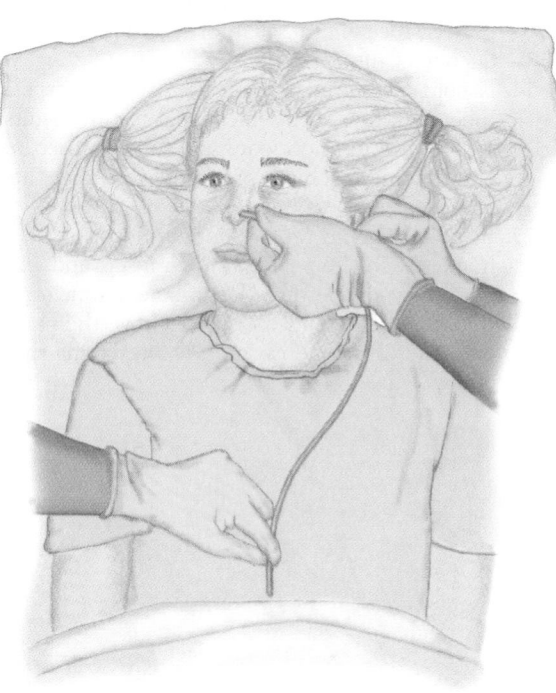

b. To place an orogastric tube in an infant, measure the tube from the tip of the nose to the earlobe and to the midpoint between the end of the xiphoid process and the umbilicus. The total measurement, NEX (nose–ear–xiphoid), should be marked on the tube with tape or indelible marker.

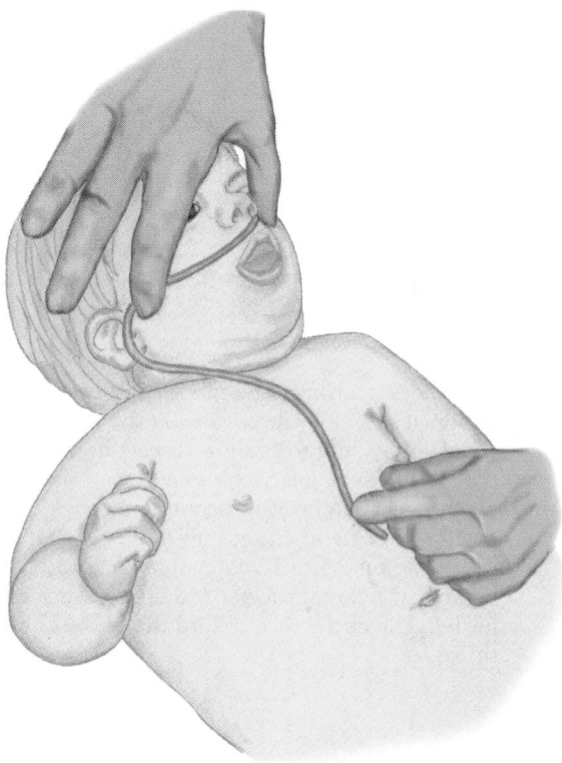

6. To facilitate passage through the nasopharynx, lubricate the tube with water or lubricant. In neonates and for orogastric placement, use water only.

7. Insert the tube gently but firmly through the mouth or nose and down the throat. If you encounter obstruction or if the tube curls in the mouth, remove the tube and repeat this step. If the child gasps, coughs, gags, or turns cyanotic, withdraw the tube and wait for the response to subside before proceeding.

Procedure continued on following page

PROCEDURE 37–11 *Continued*

Feeding Tube Insertions

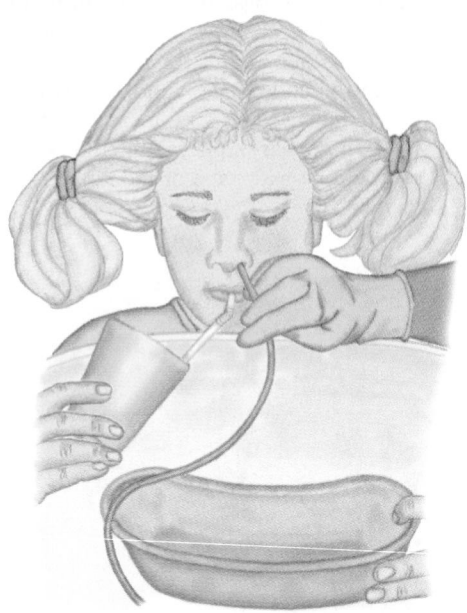

8. Continue to advance the tube gently to the predetermined mark. While advancing the tube, ask the cooperative child to swallow repeatedly when the tube reaches the pharynx, or give small sips of water through a straw, if not contraindicated. Swallowing will ease insertion into the esophagus. Advance the tube 5 to 10 cm with each swallow. Giving an infant a pacifier will encourage swallowing. Direct the tube toward the back of the throat.

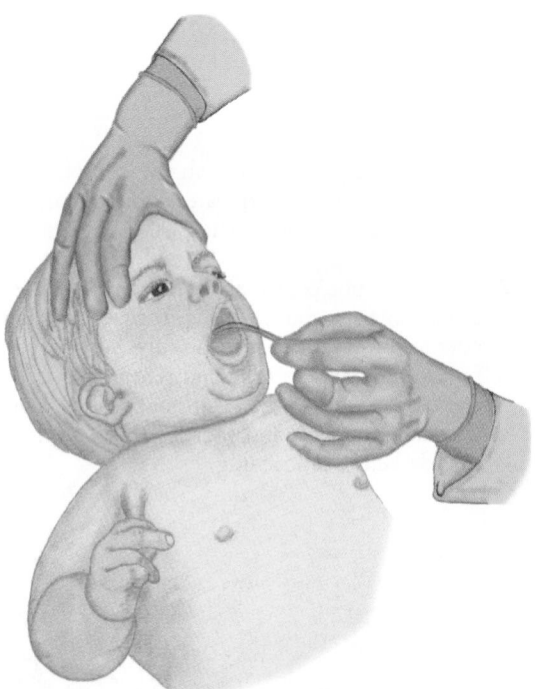

9. Temporarily secure the tube with tape to stabilize it while you check the tube position.

10. Attach the syringe to the end of the tube and insufflate 1 to 5 ml (more for an older child or adolescent) of air while auscultating over the stomach area. Then, after withdrawing the air, attempt to aspirate the gastric contents for pH testing. Choking or soundless coughing may indicate placement in the trachea. Accidental placement of a small-diameter tube into the lungs may not be as apparent as with larger tubes, particularly if the child's cough or gag reflex is absent or suppressed, and radiographic confirmation of small-bore tube placement may be necessary (Metheny et al., 1998).

11. Check the pH of the aspirate to confirm gastric or intestinal placement. (*Note:* Administration of antacid and gastric acid inhibitors will alter the pH of the aspirate to near-neutral levels, thus affecting the reliability of the pH test [Metheny et al., 1998].)

12. If a transpyloric tube (TPT) with a guide wire has been used, remove the guide wire by holding the tube at the child's nostril or the corner of the mouth and slowly removing it. To allow gravity to assist in the advancement of the tube into the duodenum, keep the child on the right side. A plain abdominal film will be ordered by the physician to confirm tube placement in the duodenum.

13. Once tube placement is confirmed, tape the tube securely in place and label the tube with the date and time of insertion. Refer to your facility's policy/procedure manual for recommended frequency of tube change.

14. Record in the nurses' notes the size and type of tube used, route, placement, pH testing results, results of auscultation, date and time of insertion, child/family teaching, procedure tolerance, and any problems encountered.

15. If the child is to receive enteral nutrition at home, teach the parent how to insert and check placement of the tube. Describe comfort measures that may be helpful. Be sure to have the parent give a return demonstration before taking the child home.

PROCEDURE 37-12
. . . .
Administering Enteral Feedings (via the Orogastric, Nasogastric, or Transpyloric Route)

PURPOSE: To provide adequate nutrition in a child who cannot tolerate oral feedings.

1. Using developmentally appropriate language, explain the procedure to the child and family. Assess their needs and concerns related to the procedure, such as previous experience with enteral feedings, ability to assist with the procedure, and need for restraint. Use therapeutic play to allay the child's and parent's fears related to the procedure.

2. The following equipment is needed: (a) stethoscope, (b) irrigation syringe, (c) room temperature formula and water, (d) pacifier for neonates and infants, (e) electronic feeding pump (for continuous tube feedings), (f) gloves.

Intermittent Feedings (Bolus)

3. Technique
   a. Position the child and remove the syringe or cap from the tube.
   b. Check for proper tube placement and aspirate for residual volume from the previous feed. Follow the facility's policy/procedure manual or physician's orders for disposition of residual volume.
   c. Remove the plunger from the syringe and attach the syringe to the tube.
   d. Pour room-temperature formula into the syringe and allow the feeding to flow slowly into the tube (usually over a period of 15 to 30 minutes). Raising or lowering the level of the syringe increases or decreases the flow of formula. Discontinue the feeding if signs of respiratory distress, cyanosis, abdominal distension, or vomiting occur. Notify the physician.
   e. After the prescribed volume has been infused, rinse the tube with sterile water and clear the tube by injecting 1 to 5 ml of air.
   f. Discard the used syringe and close or clamp the tube unless otherwise indicated.
   g. Leave the child lying on the right side with the head of the bed elevated for 30 minutes to 1 hour after the feeding.

Continuous Feedings

4. Technique
   a. Position the child and check tube placement.
   b. Fill the feeding bag, volume control set, or syringe and tubing with the prescribed formula.
   c. Attach infusion tubing to the feeding tube and begin the infusion at the prescribed rate.
   d. Check tube placement and residual volumes every 4 hours.
   e. To reduce the incidence of reflux and aspiration, keep the child positioned on the abdomen or right side.

5. If aspirate was present, record the amount, color, and consistency. Note whether it was re-fed or discarded. Note the type and amount of formula and the child's tolerance of the procedure. Note the position of the child after feeding and whether the tube is clamped or open (an open clamp allows venting of air).

6. Assess the parents' ability to perform enteral feedings. Parents should be encouraged to make this as normal a procedure as possible (e.g., by holding the infant during feedings). Ask the parent to demonstrate the procedure. Assistance with home care can be provided by a home health agency.

There is controversy regarding measurement of the length of the tube to be inserted. The two most common methods of measurement are (1) from the nose to the ear and to the end of the xiphoid process and (2) from the nose to the ear and to a point midway between the xiphoid process and umbilicus. Studies have examined the role that height—and, in low-birth-weight infants, weight—play in gastric insertion distance. Additional research is needed in this area.

Tube Selection

Many types and sizes of tubes are commercially available. Factors influencing the selection of feeding tubes include the child's age and size, the viscosity of the formula, the reason for the enteral feeding, and whether an infusion device will be used. A feeding tube of size 5 to 10 French is used in infants, and the size increases proportionately for older children. Selecting the smallest-bore tube for the infusion and a tube of soft material will decrease the child's discomfort.

SAFETY ISSUES RELATED TO TUBE PLACEMENT

Tube placement must be verified at the time the tube is inserted, any time feeding is interrupted, before each bolus feeding, and every 4 to 8 hours during continuous feeding (Metheny, 1993). Although auscultation is the most frequently used method for checking tube placement, aspiration and pH measurement of the aspirate are considered to be more reliable (Metheny et al., 1998). Insufflation of air (1 to 5 ml in infants and small children; 5 to 20 ml in adolescents) through the tube while auscultating over the epigastrium, stomach, or left upper quadrant for a distinctive "whooshing" or "gurgling" sound might indicate whether the tube is in the stomach. The same sound can be heard, however, if the tube is placed in the respiratory tract. Aspiration of enteral fluid can indicate whether the tube is in the stomach (pH of 6 or lower) or in the intestine (pH of 7 or higher) (Metheny et al., 1998). A pH above 6 that is associated with a decreased level of consciousness, uncooperative or restless behavior, recent intubation or extubation, or decreased cough or gag reflexes suggests respiratory tube placement (Metheny et al., 1998).

Do not assume that a feeding tube has remained in proper position just because the external position has not changed. Tubes can become dislodged with suctioning, retching, or vomiting (Metheny, 1993). Transpyloric tube placement should be confirmed radiographically prior to initiating feedings and any time the tube position is questioned.

CONTRAINDICATIONS TO TUBE PLACEMENT

Determine any preexisting contraindications to the procedure, such as prior operations or trauma or congenital anomalies (e.g., choanal atresia, tracheoesophageal fistula, esophageal strictures) that could interfere with passage of the tube. If any of these findings are present, the physician might use fluoroscopy to guide the insertion. *Do not reinsert a dislodged tube that was placed during or through a surgical repair. Notify the surgeon if the tube becomes dislodged.*

Gastrostomy Feedings

The procedure for gastrostomy feedings is much the same as for orogastric, nasogastric, or transpyloric feedings. As with any tube feeding, hold the infant or young child, when possible, to associate the feeding with pleasant sensations and socialization and to promote normal development and bonding.

Special considerations for patients with gastrostomy tubes or buttons include skin and stoma care. Assess the site for abnormal findings, such as leakage, redness around the site, drainage, bleeding, and skin breakdown. Clean the skin around the tube insertion site with soap and water once or twice daily, depending on the condition, and with each spillage. To facilitate complete cleansing, rotate gastrostomy buttons in a full circle during cleaning.

CRITICAL TO REMEMBER
. . . .
Enteral Feedings

- Begin the feeding *only* after tube placement in the stomach has been properly verified.
- Discontinue feedings and notify the physician if signs of respiratory distress, cyanosis, abdominal distension, or vomiting occur.
- Provide a pacifier to infants so that they can associate sucking with feeding. Encourage older children to sit at a table during meals to promote the normal socialization associated with eating.
- To avoid accidental overfeeding should the infusion pump malfunction, use only an amount of formula appropriate for a 4-hour feeding. Discard any formula that has been opened for more than 4 hours.
- Follow the facility's policy or procedure manual or physician's orders regarding disposing of residual volumes and the prescribed frequency for changing feeding equipment.

Capped gastrostomy tubes extend several inches from the insertion site. Check to be sure that there is no tension on the external tube. If necessary, coil the tube and tape near the exit site. Gastrostomy buttons are placed close to the skin surface. They have a one-way valve that eliminates the need for clamping, and offer the added advantage of allowing children to participate in regular childhood activities. When feeding a child with a gastrostomy button, you might need to place extension tubing between the button and the feeding pump.

Watch for signs that the tube or button might need to be replaced. These signs include leaking, tube occlusion, malfunction of the anti-reflux valve, or abnormal tube position. Report these findings to the physician.

Many children are discharged home with gastrostomy tubes in place. Parents must be able to provide all required care. Parent teaching is a major part of the nursing care of a child with a feeding tube. Parents must know how to check tube position, how to administer feedings, how to care for the tube, what symptoms should be reported, and what to do if the tube becomes dislodged. Booklets are available to assist the family in the care of the child with a gastrostomy tube or button.

▋ Enemas

Enemas are given when stool needs to be removed from the bowel because of severe constipation or in preparation for a diagnostic procedure or surgery. Giving an enema to an infant or child differs very little from the procedure for an adult. The differences are the type and amount of fluid administered and the distance that the enema tip is inserted into the rectum.

Enema Administration

Rectal damage and perforation can occur with improper insertion of the enema tip. Insert a lubricated tip gently 2.5 cm to 7.5 cm, depending on the age and size of the child. Commercially prepared single-use enemas come with a prelubricated tip of appropriate length.

Solutions and Volumes

The amount of the enema solution will vary with the age and size of the child. Unless the physician's orders specify a different amount, the values listed in Table 37–4 for volume and depth of enema insertion into the rectum are recommended. Only isotonic solutions should be used with chil-

---

TABLE 37–4
. . . .

Recommended Volume and Depth for Enema Insertion, by Age

	Volume (ml)	Depth of Insertion
Infants	120–240	1 in. (2.5 cm)
2–4 yr	240–360	2 in. (5.0 cm)
4–10 yr	360–480	3 in. (7.5 cm)
11 yr and older	480–720	4 in. (10.0 cm)

P R

Ch

Cup
air th
throu
secr

Clap
sequ
Elbo
rela:
popp

Post
segr
lowe

Ante
righ

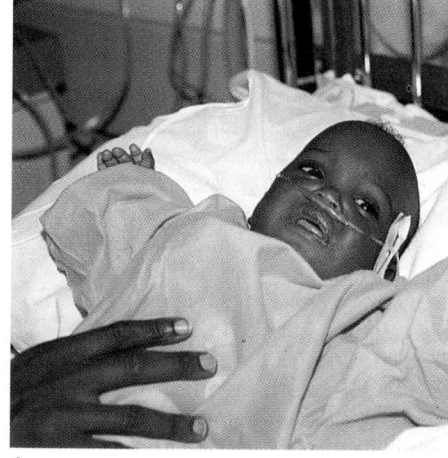

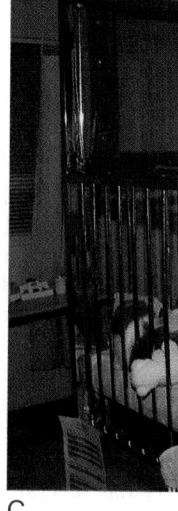

FIGURE 37–9
. . . .

Administering oxygen to children differs from
equipment and in the greater need to educat
cannula. B, Simple face mask. C, Oxygen mis
climbing over the crib rail. (Courtesy of Parkla

nose to the cleft of the chin. Attach the ma:
ified oxygen source and adjust the flow rate t
level. Then place the mask over the child':
the nose clip and head strap.

When humidified oxygen is required to
or to assist the child in mobilizing secretions,
or mist tent is indicated. These devices are pa
in the treatment of croup, epiglottitis, pneum
chiolitis (see Chapter 45). The mist moist:
minimizes fluid loss from the lungs, and prov
ronment, which aids in temperature reducti:
child's temperature frequently to prevent hy
be sure to keep the child in dry clothing and

When a hood or tent is used, it is dif
oxygen concentrations greater than 40%,
is heavier than air and will escape readily
check that the sides and the end of the te
tucked to prevent oxygen leakage. Also,

dren. Plain tap water should never be used because it is hypotonic and can cause a rapid fluid shift and fluid overload.

After completing an enema administration, diaper the infant. Toddlers can use the bedpan or "potty" if possible. Older children and adolescents can use the bedpan or bedside commode or be assisted to the bathroom. Record in the nurses' notes or I & O sheet the date and time the enema was given, the type and amount of solution, the amount and characteristics of stool, any unusual findings (blood, mucus, foreign bodies, worms, etc.), and the child's tolerance of the procedure.

Care of Ostomies

Urinary and fecal diversion may be needed when normal methods of elimination are temporarily or permanently halted. Some conditions requiring the creation of a fecal stoma include imperforate anus, Hirschsprung disease, necrotizing enterocolitis, some cases of intestinal atresia, intussusception, Crohn disease, and ulcerative colitis (see Chapter 43). The anatomic location of the stoma will dictate the consistency of the stool. The higher the stoma, the more liquid is the stool.

Urinary diversion is usually the result of obstructive uropathy, congenital anomalies, or occasionally neurogenic bladder (see Chapter 44). The ureters can be brought out through the abdominal wall (ureterostomy) or connected to a segment of small bowel (ileal conduit).

Nursing care of the child with an ostomy focuses on minimizing the obstacles the child and family face in learning to care for the ostomy, encouraging the child and family to be actively involved in the treatment regimen, providing support and guidance, and making appropriate referrals to an enterostomal therapist or other support system (Procedure 37–13).

The actual management and care of pediatric ostomies differs little from that in adults with ostomies. The major difference is the need to use developmentally appropriate terminology to explain the procedure and care of the ostomy to the child and family. A teaching model, such as a doll with a stoma, can facilitate child and family education.

In many cases, a pediatric ostomy appliance is fitted soon after surgery. The appliance allows for accurate measurement of stoma output from the pouch. If an appliance has not been applied, place a piece of Vaseline gauze and dry dressing over the stoma and measure the output by weighing the wet dressing and comparing it to the dry weight (1 ml = 1 g). Early application of an ostomy appliance also helps prevent excoriation of surrounding skin.

Young children may pull at the stoma pouch in an attempt to remove it. If such pulling occurs, apply a cloth diaper or dressing to cover the area. Older children can participate in the care of the stoma, including skin care, application of the appliance, and identification of potential problems. Evaluate each child individually to determine the child's developmental level and desire to assume partial responsibility for the care of the stoma.

Oxygen Therapy

Hypoxemia, resulting from apnea or inadequate ventilation, occurs more rapidly in children than in adults because of

the child's higher metabolic rate and increased oxygen consumption. Because cardiopulmonary arrest in children can follow progressive respiratory distress, early recognition of subtle signs and symptoms of respiratory distress is a necessary skill for every nurse.

Oxygen is an essential body requirement for any energy-consuming activity or function. For infants and children who are unable to maintain a normal arterial oxygen pressure (Pao_2), supplemental oxygen might be needed. Because oxygen is a drug, a physician's order is needed for administration, except in an emergency situation. Follow your facility's policy for oxygen administration in emergencies.

Oxygen Delivery

Oxygen may be administered to children by nasal cannula, face mask (simple, nonrebreather, partial rebreather, Venturi, or aerosol), an oxygen hood, or an oxygen tent (Fig. 37–9). The method of delivery depends on the concentration needed and the child's ability to cooperate with the chosen method. In most facilities, a respiratory therapist is responsible for the setup, maintenance, and management of oxygen equipment. However, the nurse needs to have a working knowledge of the oxygen delivery system used.

Oxygen administration systems for children differ very little from those used in adults. The primary differences are the size of the equipment and the teaching and emotional support needed for children receiving oxygen and their families. Usually, an oxygen hood is used to provide maximum oxygenation for neonates and infants. Older infants and young toddlers might better tolerate a nasal cannula, blowby oxygen, or face mask. Oxygen delivery by nasal cannula, the blow-by method, or a face mask works well for toddlers and preschoolers. School-age children and adolescents prefer nonrebreather masks to achieve maximum oxygenation.

Children experiencing difficulty breathing might be less than cooperative when an attempt is made to place a mask or cannula on the face. Explain to the child and family in developmentally appropriate language what will happen, why the mask is needed, and how it will feel. Provide assistance, if needed, to keep the oxygen delivery system in place. Check the physician's orders for the percentage of oxygen to be delivered and the method of delivery.

A nasal cannula is a low-flow delivery system that is indicated for infants and children who need modest amounts of supplemental oxygen (up to 40%). Flow rates should not exceed 6 L/min. The loop of the cannula can be enlarged to slip easily over the child's ears. Place the prongs in the nares and tighten the loop. If the child is active, you can tape the cannula to the sides of the child's face to maintain proper position. Be aware, however, that a flow rate exceeding 6 L/min can irritate the nasopharynx and cause gastric distension and regurgitation without appreciably improving the child's oxygenation.

The simple face mask and the Venturi mask are indicated for infants and children who need modest amounts of supplemental oxygen (35% to 60%, or a flow rate of 6 to 10 L/min). The Venturi mask can be adjusted to deliver specific concentrations of oxygen (i.e., 24%, 28%, 35%, 40%, or 50%). You must maintain a minimum flow rate of 6 L/min to prevent rebreathing of exhaled carbon dioxide.

Partial and full nonrebreathing masks are simple face

PROCEDURE 37-13

Ostomy Care

PURPOSE: To assess output, moni
nary function, and preserve skin inte

1. Explain the procedure and its pu
   and family in developmentally a
   guage. Determine their previous
   the procedure and allow the chil
   voice questions and concerns. De
   procedure on a stoma doll, if ava
   them visualize the site and equip
2. Assemble the following equipme
   warm water, (b) a product that a
   adhesive material, (c) mild soap,
   (e) towels and washcloths, (f) sk
   (g) scissors, (h) petroleum gauze,
   (j) gauze, (k) ostomy appliance (
   (l) protective equipment.
3. Assist the child into a position o

Ostomy Without an Appliance

4. Technique
   a. After putting on gloves (and g
      cated), remove the diaper cov
      and place in an appropriate re
   b. Remove peristomal skin barrie
      moving the wafer or paste. Us
      and a mild soap, gently and th
      the skin. If paste is difficult to
      well, dust with powder, and th
   c. Assess the stoma output for vo
      tency, and odor in relation to
      cation of the stoma.
   d. Wipe the peristomal skin with
      Use a tightly rolled piece of ga
      the stoma to act as a wick duri
      ensure adherence to the skin a
      leaks, the skin must be comple
      applying the skin barrier.
   e. Apply a protective barrier (wafe
      der). If using a wafer, use the ter
      to cut a hole that is slightly larg
      stoma. Apply paste/powder in a
      over the peristomal skin and ext
      stoma's edge outward in a 3-incl
   f. Apply a folded cloth diaper ove
      secure it with a regular diaper, t

Ostomy with an Appliance

5. Technique
   a. Remove the pouch and barrier
      and discard in an appropriate r

masks with an attached reservoir that allo
exhaled gas to remain in the bag and mi
These masks supply oxygen concentrations
at a rate of 10 to 12 L/min. A nonrebreat
deliver almost 100% oxygen at a flow rate
min.

CARING FOR AN INFANT WITH A TRACHEOSTOMY

Caring for the child with a tracheostomy can involve several steps, including respiratory therapy treatments, suctioning, and changing the ties that secure the tube. Because many children are discharged from the hospital with tracheostomies, their parents and other home caregivers must be taught these procedures.

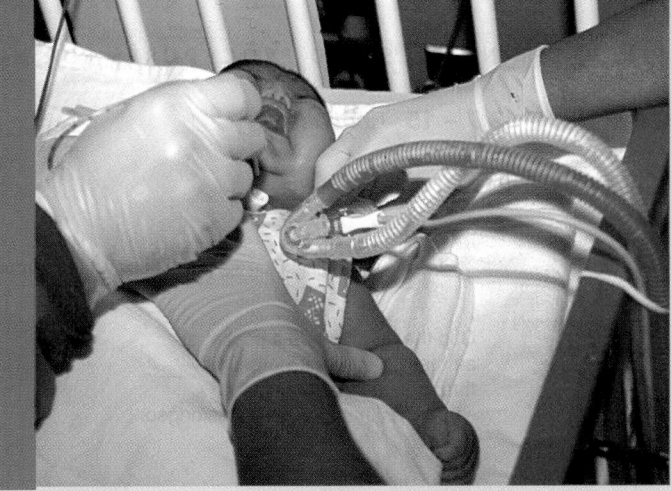

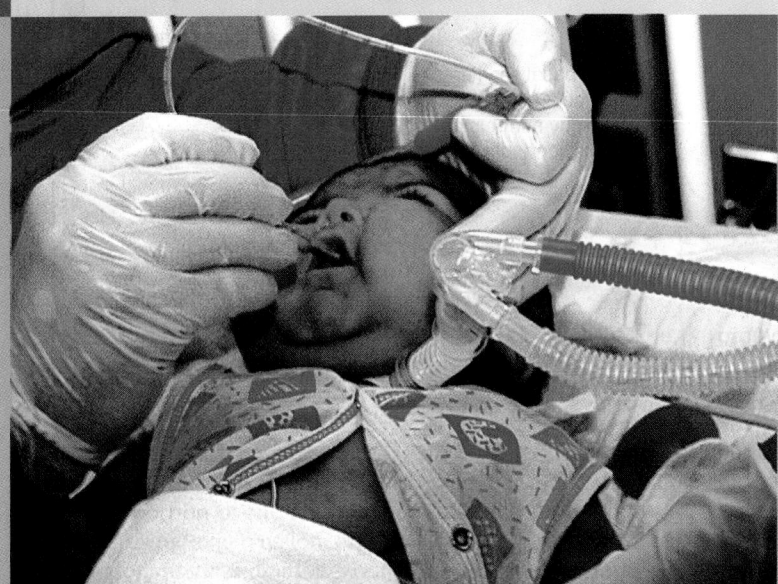

Often the oral cavity requires suctioning as well. The technique is similar to that for suctioning the tracheostomy: the catheter is inserted, then suction is applied while the catheter is withdrawn.

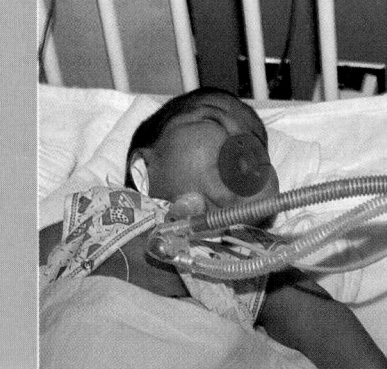

The infant who has a device such as a tracheostomy tube or a gastrostomy feeding tube still needs to suck. A pacifier fulfills this need. Because tracheostomy care is often tiring, the child should be allowed to rest afterwards.

Secretions are removed from this infant's airway with a suction catheter. Appropriate techniques minimize problems with suctioning, such as hypoxia, tissue damage, or infection. The suction catheter is inserted into the tube with the suction turned off. After the appropriate length of tubing is inserted, suction is applied, and the catheter is withdrawn using a twisting motion. Do not suction longer than 5 seconds at a time.

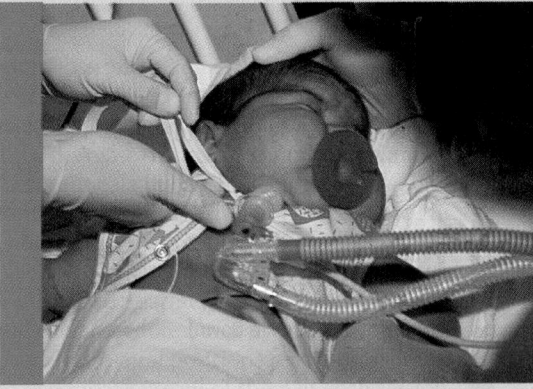

When changing the infant's tracheostomy ties, the nurse has an assistant hold the tube in place to reduce the chance that it will be displaced. The nurse makes sure the ties are snug, but not too tight. When the new ties are in place, the nurse checks their snugness by inserting a finger beneath them.

Photos courtesy of Parkland Health and Hospital System.

PROCEDURE 37–16

Cleaning and Care of the Tracheostomy Site and Inner Cannula

PURPOSE: To maintain a patent airway and prevent infection.

1. Using developmentally appropriate language, explain the procedure, its purpose, and other pertinent information to the child and parent. Some hospital facilities use videotapes and stoma dolls to demonstrate the procedure.

2. If the facility does not have a preassembled tracheostomy care kit, assemble the following: (a) a small tray to hold the cleaning solution, (b) cotton-tipped applicators, (c) pipe cleaners or a brush for cleaning the inner cannula, (d) forceps, (e) tracheostomy ties, (f) sterile dressing (optional), (g) gauze pad, (h) gloves (sterile and nonsterile), (i) towel or blanket roll, (j) hydrogen peroxide, (k) sterile normal saline.

3. To hyperextend the head and neck to expose the site, position child with a towel or blanket under the shoulders.

4. Wash your hands and open the tray, creating a sterile field.

5. Pour equal parts of normal saline and hydrogen peroxide in one small tray and normal saline in the other small tray. Use the large tray for holding cotton-tipped applicators, clean tracheostomy ties, and gauze pad.

6. Don nonsterile gloves and remove the dressing around the tracheostomy, if present. Discard the dressing and gloves according to agency policy. A dressing placed between the skin and the tube can increase the risk for skin breakdown because it will absorb any secretions. For this reason, it may not be used in some facilities. Assess the stoma for redness, drainage or discharge, and skin breakdown.

7. Don sterile gloves and, using cotton-tipped applicators moistened in half-strength solution, clean the child's neck under the tracheostomy tube flanges and tracheostomy tape and allow to dry.

If the child has a tracheostomy without an inner cannula, skip to step 11.

8. Unlock the inner cannula (if using a three-piece tracheostomy system) by rotating it counterclockwise. Using pipe cleaners or a brush, quickly clean it in half-strength hydrogen peroxide solution. (Alternatively, it may be replaced with a new or extra inner cannula, if available.) Rinse the cannula thoroughly in normal saline and inspect it for cleanliness. Repeat the cleaning procedure if necessary.

9. To remove excess moisture, tap the cleaned inner cannula on the edge of the sterile container. Do not dry the outside of the inner cannula because moisture will act as a lubricant during reinsertion.

10. Reinsert the inner cannula into the tracheostomy tube and lock it in place by rotating it clockwise.

Note: Some facilities require two people to change ties, in which case the following procedure is used. While the assistant wearing sterile gloves gently holds the tube in place, remove the existing tape from the flanges. Clean the skin under the ties and inspect the skin for pressure sores from the ties.

11. Loop the new tracheostomy ties through the flange on one side of the tracheostomy (see p. 985). Bring the ties around the back of the child's neck and tie them securely to the opposite flange. Ties are tight enough if only one finger can be inserted between the ties and neck. Tie the ties on the side, not the back, of the neck to prevent confusing the tracheostomy ties with bib ties and to avoid putting pressure on the back of the neck. Use triple knots to prevent accidental untying and dislodging of the tracheostomy. Clean and assess the skin under the ties.

12. Carefully cut and remove the soiled tracheostomy ties and any excess clean tracheostomy tape. Make sure the tracheostomy tube is secure before leaving the bedside.

13. Discard used supplies in appropriate receptacles. Record in the nurses' notes the date, time and type of procedure, the condition of the stoma and skin, any abnormal findings or complications and the nursing action taken, the child's tolerance of the procedure, and any child or family teaching done, as well as their understanding of and involvement in the care.

14. Assess the family's ability to perform the procedure. It might be necessary to engage the assistance of a home health agency if the family needs temporary assistance and support. Begin to teach tracheostomy care early in the child's hospitalization, and teach more than one family member how to do the care. All those caring for the child must also know cardiopulmonary resuscitation (CPR). Write clear instructions, and observe all caregivers perform the procedures. Return demonstrations of the technique are imperative. Advise the caregiver that $1/2$-inch width cotton seam binding, which can be found in fabric stores, makes acceptable tracheostomy ties.

Shiley single-lumen tracheostomy tubes are available in a variety of sizes (up to a No. 8 for an adult-sized patient). Tracheostomy tubes with inner cannulas are available in sizes No. 4 and larger.

Tracheostomy care for the infant or child rarely differs from that appropriate for adult patients (Procedure 37–16). The primary differences include the types and sizes of tubes, the ability of the child to cooperate with procedures, and the parental support and teaching needed to prepare for home care (if indicated).

Routine tracheostomy care includes assessing the stoma area for signs of infection and skin breakdown, changing tracheostomy ties, cleaning the tracheostomy site and inner cannula, changing the tracheostomy tube, and suctioning. Clean the area around the tube at the time the tracheostomy ties are changed or more frequently if needed to keep the site clean and dry. Tracheostomy care can be given at various intervals but should be done at least every 8 hours. The tracheostomy tube is usually changed weekly. The tracheostomy is held in place with ties made of a durable, nonfraying material. These are changed daily or more frequently if they become soiled. *To prevent the tube from being accidentally dislodged, an assistant should always be present when tracheostomy care is performed.*

Keep an extra tracheostomy tube of appropriate size at the bedside (or taped to the head of the bed) for easy access in an emergency. Because of the risk of aspiration and possible occlusion of the trachea, avoid giving the child small toys, toys with small parts, plastic bibs, and plastic bedding. In addition, do not use talcum powders and aerosol products near children with tracheostomies because of the risk of inhalation injury secondary to breathing the particles.

Suctioning

In children with tracheostomies, secretions are removed from the airway by means of a catheter inserted into the airway. Using appropriate techniques and equipment for suctioning can prevent problems sometimes encountered during suctioning, such as hypoxia, tissue damage, and infection. The suctioning procedure for children varies little from that used in adults (Procedure 37–17). Suctioning in infants and children requires the use of a smaller suction catheter and lower suction settings than in the adult. Catheter sizes range from No. 5 French to No. 14 French, with smaller sizes used for smaller tubes. To avoid total airway occlusion, catheter size should be approximately half the inner diameter of the tracheostomy tube. Suction settings for tracheostomy care vary by age, as follows:

Neonates: 60–80 mm/Hg
Infants: 80–100 mm/Hg
Larger children: 100–120 mm/Hg

Assess and record the child's breath sounds, respiratory rate, and character of respirations every 4 hours. Suction the tra-

PROCEDURE 37–17
• • • • • • • • • •
Suctioning a Tracheostomy Tube

PURPOSE: To maintain patency of the tracheostomy tube.

1. After using developmentally appropriate language to explain the procedure, its purpose, and other pertinent information to the child and parent, gather the following equipment: (a) a sterile suction catheter of appropriate size, (b) sterile gloves, (c) normal saline solution, (d) 3-ml syringe without needle for the required amount of normal saline.
2. Adjust the suction vacuum pressure to the prescribed level, then put on the sterile gloves.
3. Using sterile technique, instill normal saline, 0.5 to 2 ml (if being used), to loosen secretions into the trachea.
4. Insert the catheter the length of the tracheostomy tube (measure another tracheostomy tube the same size) *with suction off.* Do not apply suction as the catheter is being inserted.
5. Apply intermittent suction and withdraw the catheter using a twisting motion. Limit insertion and suctioning time to 5 seconds to prevent hypoxia. Holding your own breath during suctioning is a good reminder. If you need a breath, then the child probably does too.
6. Reoxygenate between suction catheter passes and allow a sufficient recovery time after each pass. This time can include allowing the child to rest and take a few breaths, or it may involve "bagging" (giving oxygen by bag and mask).

"Bagging" of children on ventilatory support is imperative.
7. Assess the child to determine whether secretions are still present. Auscultate to listen for air exchange. Repeat the procedure until the airway sounds clear, rinsing the suction catheter with normal saline between each insertion. Normal saline lavage may be used if thick secretions are encountered. Refer to your facility's procedure or policy manual regarding this controversial issue.
8. Assess the child's breath sounds and respiratory rate after suctioning to evaluate the effectiveness of suctioning.
9. Discard the suction tube and gloves in an appropriate container. Record in the nurses' notes the date and time the procedure was performed, the amount and characteristics of the secretions obtained, the character of the breath sounds before and after suctioning, the child's response to the procedure, and any teaching done with the child and family, as well as their level of understanding and their response to the teaching.
10. The family will need much support and encouragement to feel comfortable with suctioning and tracheostomy care. The child can take baths, but care should be taken to prevent water from entering the trachea. Showers are not recommended. To avoid tracheal spasm, the tracheostomy can be covered loosely during cold or windy days.

cheostomy every 2 to 4 hours or as needed. Always use standard precautions.

Surgical Procedures

The child undergoing surgery has increased physical and psychological needs. Although each surgical procedure is unique, a general body of knowledge relates to all children experiencing surgery. Surgery can be a very traumatic event for a child.

With the rising cost of health care, managed-care contracts, and the need for cost containment in health care, many operations are now done on an outpatient basis. Ambulatory, or same-day, surgery uses the same standards of care that apply to all routine hospital admissions, but with the added benefit of lower cost.

Preparation for Surgery

A multidisciplinary approach should be used when preparing a child for surgery. Include the following: parents, nursing staff, child life specialist, physician, and any other specialty area involved in the individual child's care. Preparation for outpatient procedures depends on the type of procedure to be done and the age and developmental level of the child. Psychological preparation for an outpatient experience is just as important as for an inpatient hospital experience. Indeed, much of the preparation is the same, regardless of whether the surgery will be done on an outpatient or an inpatient basis, and a multidisciplinary approach to teaching is appropriate for both settings.

Assess the physical and psychosocial needs of the child and family. Both the child and the family will be anxious, so the nurse needs to be a calming influence. Being aware of the stressors of surgery will guide the nurse in providing family-centered care. These stressors include the following (Holden, 1995; Squires, 1995):

- Separation from significant others
- Pain
- Fear of mutilation
- The presence of strangers
- Disruptions of routine
- Lack of privacy
- Disability
- Disfigurement

Fear of the unknown is another common fear of children. By assessing the presence of these and other stressors, the nurse can develop a plan of care.

Preparing the child and family for surgery establishes a foundation of trust between the nurse and the family. Schedule formal sessions no more than 1 week before admission. Children younger than 4 years of age seem to do best when information is received no more than 3 days before admission (Squires, 1995). Waiting too long to initiate preparation for surgery can give rise to fantasies and increase the child's fear. A short preparation might not provide enough time to answer questions posed by the child or family so that they feel adequately prepared for the surgery.

Although preparation may vary from setting to setting, all teaching should be planned, should use a developmental approach, and should provide information that is simple

and truthful. Many hospitals include a tour of the perioperative area. Conduct a review of the teaching on the day of the surgery. If a child life specialist participates in the preparation, that person should be present on the day of surgery.

The use of therapeutic play is an essential tool, both in preparation and perioperatively. (Therapeutic play is discussed in Chapter 4.) Keeping children busy is especially important if they have a waiting period before their scheduled surgery time. Provide age-appropriate toys in holding areas or in the child's room, if that is the area where the child is waiting.

Parents need to explain to the child as clearly as possible why the child is going to the hospital or surgery center and what will happen during the stay. Nurses can assist the parents in preparing their child. Books on hospitalization or surgery that are geared toward children help prepare them for the experience. Videotapes are also available.

Regardless of the procedure planned, some preoperative activities are routine. These include

- No food or drink after a specified time
- A consent form for the procedure signed by the parent or guardian
- Preoperative medications

Reassure children that they will not be left alone and that they will not feel the procedure as it is done.

. . . .

Sample Preoperative Feeding Instructions

Give the parents the following instructions:

For your child's safety, it is very important that you follow these instructions carefully. If these instructions are not followed, your child's operation or procedure may be canceled or delayed.

1. At 8 P.M.* the evening before surgery, stop all food, including
   Solid food, candy,† and chewing gum
   Milk, milk products, and formulas
   Orange juice and juice containing pulp
2. Breast-feeding may continue until 3 hours‡ before the time you are to arrive at the hospital.
3. Clear fluids may be continued until 2 hours§ before the time you are to arrive at the hospital.
4. Clear fluids include

Water	Clear broth
Apple juice	Pedialyte
Clear juice drinks	Ice Popsicles
Plain Jell-O	

---

*Many hospitals use midnight rather than 8 P.M. for the beginning of the NPO period.

†Hard sucking candy is probably of little concern, and the significance of gum chewing remains controversial.

‡The duration for fasting after formulas is uncertain at present, and shorter intervals may be appropriate.

§It usually takes a minimum of 30 minutes to process a day surgery patient, but parents occasionally make subtraction errors when the instructions are not stated using whole numbers of clock hours.

From Schreiner, M. S. (1994). Preoperative and postoperative fasting in children. *Pediatric Clinics of North America, 41*(1), 118.

Because children are at greater risk for dehydration than adults, the period during which they can have nothing by mouth might be shorter. This period varies according to the protocol of the facility and the anesthesiologist.

Some procedures require preoperative laboratory tests, such as a complete blood cell count or urinalysis, and a chest x-ray. Most hospitals and surgical centers have preoperative checklists (similar to those used in adult care) that assist the nurse in documenting the child's preparation for the procedure. These lists usually include checking the child's identification, obtaining a signed consent form, laboratory results, administering preanesthetic medication, and other documentation. After the preanesthetic medication has been administered, the parent may hold the child or place the child on a stretcher with the side rails raised.

Preoperative Anesthesia

Preoperative medication is used primarily to decrease anxiety in the child. In some settings, premedication is not used if the parents are present. It is becoming increasingly common for parents to be present during the induction of anesthesia. Many safe and painless premedication methods are now available. After parents are asked to leave the child for surgery, the nurse keeps them informed of the anticipated length of the surgery and their child's status throughout the surgery.

Postanesthesia Care

After the surgery, the child is taken to the postanesthesia care unit (PACU) or recovery room. There the nurse performs frequent assessments of the child's cardiorespiratory and circulatory systems until the child is fully awake. When the child awakens from surgery, it is important for the parent(s) to be present to comfort and calm the child. The child might also want a favorite toy or object. Providing warm blankets and a rocking chair as a comfort measure can assist both the child and the parent. Pain medication should be provided as needed (see Chapter 39). Depending on the procedure performed, the child might be discharged from the hospital or admitted to an inpatient unit for the remainder of the hospital stay.

Postoperative Care

Most facilities have a specific protocol that is followed for postoperative care. After a surgical procedure the child's vital signs are monitored frequently until they are stable. The surgical site is checked for drainage, and the child is assessed for pain. The use of patient-controlled analgesia (PCA) and the routine administration of analgesia afford effective pain control. Refer to Chapter 39 for a more detailed discussion of pain management in children.

Atelectasis is a common complication of surgery. The condition is related to the effects of anesthesia in combination with small tidal volume breathing, somnolence, splinting secondary to pain, and cough suppression caused by pain or opioid analgesics (Yaster et al., 1994). Auscultate the lungs to determine any abnormal breath sounds or areas of diminished or absent sounds. In addition, encourage early

---

• • • • • • • • • •
Pediatric Anesthetic Induction Techniques

PREMEDICATIONS—SEDATIVES

Rectal midazolam
Oral benzodiazepine or barbiturate or narcotic
Intranasal benzodiazepine or ketamine
Transmucosal (lollipop) fentanyl

INDUCTION AGENTS—SLEEP-INDUCING

Barbiturates: rectal or intravenous
Ketamine: intramuscular or intravenous
Etomidate: intravenous
Propofol: intravenous
Potent inhalational agents

MODIFICATIONS OF MASK INDUCTION

Give the child the option of sitting up, either in a chair or on a lap.
Let the child hold the mask.
Provide a choice of flavored gases.
Conceal the breathing circuit—"Trojan horse"
    "Halothan Phone"—concealed in play phone
    "Pungent Pacifier"—concealed behind a pacifier
    "Sleepy Bear"—concealed with a stuffed animal

MODIFICATIONS OF INTRAVENOUS INDUCTION

Use EMLA cream to place an intravenous cannula.
Use a 25- or 27-gauge "butterfly" needle.
Allow the child to push a syringe containing the appropriate dose of drug through a preexisting IV access line.
Create diversions (i.e., have the child count backward from 100, or tell jokes or stories).

From Zuckerberg, A. L. (1994). Perioperative approach to children. *Pediatrics Clinics of North America, 41*(1), 25.

---

ambulation, deep breathing, and coughing. Using incentive spirometers can increase respiratory movement. Games such as blowing cotton, a windmill, or bubbles can also facilitate air exchange for children unable or unwilling to use a spirometer.

Children generally recuperate more quickly in a familiar environment; as a result, they are discharged as soon as is safely possible after surgery. Because of decreased lengths of stay, discharge planning begins at the time of admission. Using an organized plan of care, the discharge planner works closely with the child and family to identify needs and resources and then develops an efficient, cost-effective plan for meeting those needs.

Some children will need specialized care in the home following discharge from the hospital. The ability of the family to provide some or all of the care will determine the extent of education provided prior to discharge and the need for involvement of a home health agency after discharge. The family and the nurse must identify the level of knowledge needed and any specific equipment or home modifications required to care for the child adequately at home. It is usually the responsibility of the home health agency to make the necessary arrangements for durable or disposable equipment. It is helpful, when possible, for equipment and supplies to be provided by the same agency that provides assistance with home nursing care. Some agencies also will provide education for the family prior to the child's discharge. To ensure the child and family the smoothest transition possible from hospital to home, these issues and delegation of responsibilities need to be addressed as soon as they are identified.

Nursing diagnoses frequently associated with the child undergoing surgery include the following:

- Anxiety and Fear related to separation from significant other(s), surgery, unfamiliar environment, and personnel
- Pain related to the surgical incision

- Knowledge Deficit about the procedure and expected outcomes
- Altered Family Processes related to the surgical procedure
- Risk for Fluid Volume Deficit related to NPO status before and after surgery, as well as to nausea and vomiting

Additional Information

See Chapter 32 for assistance with communication challenges. Chapter 35 provides information on care related to hospitalization and separation, Chapter 39 discusses pain-related issues, and Chapter 42 presents nursing care as it relates to fluid volume deficits. To deliver quality care, the nurse must identify the child's growth and developmental needs, along with the care needs associated with the disorder for which the operation is being performed.

KEY CONCEPTS

- Whenever possible, perform procedures in the treatment room, away from the child's room.
- Some procedures require informed consent. Children 7 years old and older must give assent to some procedures. Because laws on informed consent vary from state to state, nurses must be familiar with the laws and policies of their institution.
- Use developmentally appropriate and descriptive words when preparing children for procedures.
- Praise children for attempts at co-

operation during a procedure even if they did not follow instructions. Praise them for accomplishing an expected task.
- Documentation of a procedure includes recording the preparation, who performed the procedure, the child's tolerance, the actual procedure, and outcomes.
- Follow standard precautions when collecting all specimens. Standard precautions are used with all hospitalized patients and are not based on diagnosis or presumed infectious state. Transmission-based

precautions are used with clients known or suspected to be infected by pathogens that are conveyed by airborne or droplet transmission or by contact with dry skin or contaminated surfaces.
- Use restraints only as a last resort to protect the child and others.
- Because of children's developmental level and activity, be particularly conscious of safety measures when caring for children in a hospital setting.

REFERENCES AND READINGS

Arvin, A. (1996). Fever. In R. Behrman, R. Kliegman, & A. Arvin (Eds.), *Nelson textbook of pediatrics* (15th ed., pp. 692–694). Philadelphia: Saunders.

Bar-Mor, G. (1997). Preparation of children for surgery and invasive procedures: Milestones on the way to success. *Journal of Pediatric Nursing, 12*(4), 252–255.

Brennan, A. (1994). Caring for children during procedures: A review of the literature. *Pediatric Nursing, 20*(5), 451–458.

Brown, R., & Ioli, J. G. (1993). A pediatric resuscitation poster: Development and multiple uses. *Pediatric Nursing, 19*(1), 56–58.

Bryant, K., Davis, C., & Lagrone, C. (1997). Streamlining discharge planning for the child with a new tracheotomy. *Journal of Pediatric Nursing, 12*(3), 191–192.

Burke, K. (1996). The tympanic membrane thermometer in pediatrics: A review of the literature. *Accident and Emergency Nursing, 4*(4), 190–193.

Burns, C., Barber, N., Brady, M., & Dunn, A. (1996). *Pediatric primary care.* Philadelphia: Saunders.

Carlson, D., & Mowery, D. (1997). Standards to prevent complications of urinary catheterization in children: Should and should-knot. *Journal of the Society of Pediatric Nurses, 2*(1), 37–41.

Carroll, C. (1993). Clinical applications of pulse oximetry. *Pediatric Nursing, 19*(2), 150–151.

Cohen, H., Woloch, B., Linder, N., Vardi, A., & Barzilai, A. (1997). Urine samples from disposable diapers: An accurate method for urine cultures. *Journal of Family Practice, 44*(3), 290–292.

Crapanzano, M., Strong, W., Newman, I., Hixon, R., Casal, D., & Linder, C. (1996). Calf blood pressure: Clinical implications and correlations with arm blood pressure in infants and children. *Pediatrics, 97*(2), 220–224.

Davis, A. (1993). The accuracy of tympanic measurement in children. *Pediatric Nursing, 19*(3), 267–272.

French, J. P. (1995). *Pediatric emergency skills.* St. Louis: Mosby.

Garner, J. (1996). Guidelines for isolation precautions in hospitals. *American Journal of Infection Control, 24*, 24–52.

Garza, D., & Becan-McBride, K. (1993). *Phlebotomy handbook* (3rd ed.). Norwalk, CT: Appleton & Lange.

Hanna, D. (1995). Using pulse oximeters safely. *Nursing '95,* 26.

Hazinski, M. F. (1986). Pediatric home tracheostomy care: A parent's guide. *Pediatric Nursing, 12*(1), 41–48.

Hess, D., & Kacmarek, R. M. (1993). Techniques and devices for monitoring oxygenation. *Respiratory Care, 38*(6), 646–669.

Hill, A. S., & Rath, L. (1993). The care and feeding of the low birthweight infant. *Journal of Perinatal and Neonatal Nursing, 6*(4), 56–68.

Holden, P. (1995). Psychosocial factors affecting a child's capacity to cope with surgery and recovery. *Seminars in Perioperative Nursing, 4*(2), 75–79.

Levy, S., Kiritsy, M., Slager, S., Warren, J., & Kohout, F. (1997). Patterns of fluoride dentifrice use among infants. *Pediatric Dentistry, 19*(1), 50–55.

Lorin, M. (1998). Fever: Pathogenesis and treatment. In R. Feigin & J. Cherry (Eds.), *Textbook of pediatric infectious diseases* (4th ed., pp. 89–94). Philadelphia: Saunders.

Metheny, N. (1993). Minimizing respiratory complications of nasoenteric tube feedings: State of the science. *Heart and Lung, 22*(33), 213–223.

Metheny, N., Wehrle, A., Wiersema, L., & Clark, J. (1998). Testing feeding tube placement: Auscultation vs. pH method. *American Journal of Nursing, 98*(5), 37–42.

Montagne, L. (1993). Bolstering personal control in child patients through coping interventions. *Pediatric Nursing, 19,* 235–237.

Mower, W., Sachs, C., Nicklin, E., & Baraff, L. (1997). Pulse oximetry as a fifth pediatric vital sign. *Pediatrics, 99*(5), 681–685.

Murphy, K. (1992). Acetaminophen and ibuprofen: Fever control and overdose. *Pediatric Nursing, 18*(4), 428.

Pontious, S., Kennedy, A. H., Shelley, S., & Mittrucker, D. (1994). Accuracy and reliability of temperature measurement by instrument and site. *Journal of Pediatric Nursing, 9*(2), 114–123.

Runton, N. (1992). Suctioning artificial airways in children: Appropriate techniques. *Pediatric Nursing, 18*(2), 115–118.

Schlager, T., Hendley, O., Dudley, S., Hayden, G., & Lohr, J. (1995). Explanation for false-positive urine cultures obtained by bag technique. *Archives of Pediatric and Adolescent Medicine, 149,* 170–173.

Schmitt, B. (1992). *Instructions for pediatric patients.* Philadelphia: Saunders.

Selekman, J., & Snyder, B. (1997). Institutional policies on the use of physical restraints on children. *Pediatric Nursing, 23*(5), 531.

Silver, P., Sagy, M., & Rubin, L. (1996). Respiratory failure from corn starch aspiration: A hazard of diaper changing. *Pediatric Emergency Care, 12*(2), 108–110.

Smith, A., & Adams, L. (1998). Insertion of indwelling urethral catheters in infants and children: A survey of current nursing practice. *Pediatric Nursing, 24*(3), 229–234.

Sneed, N. V., & Hollerbach, A. D. (1995). Measurement error in counting heart rate: Potential sources and solutions. *Critical Care Nurse, 15*(1), 36–40.

Soud, T. (1993). Pediatric update: The febrile child in the emergency department. *Journal of Emergency Nursing, 19*(4), 355–358.

Squires, V. L. (1995). Child-focused perioperative education: Helping children understand and cope with surgery. *Seminars in Perioperative Nursing, 4*(2), 80–87.

Taeusch, H. (1996). Blood drawing techniques. In H. Taeusch, R. Christiansen, & S. Buescher, *Pediatric and neonatal tests and procedure* (pp. 599–607). Philadelphia: Saunders.

Thompson, V. (1994). An IV therapy teaching tool for children. *Pediatric Nursing, 20*(4), 351–355.

Thorne, S., Radford, M., & McCormick, J. (1997). The multiple meanings of long-term gastrostomy in children with severe disability. *Journal of Pediatric Nursing, 12*(2), 89–99.

Thornlow, D. K. (1995). Is chest physiotherapy necessary after cardiac surgery? *Critical Care Nurse, 15*(3), 39–46.

Warnock, C., & Porpora, K. (1994). A pediatric trach card: Transforming research into practice. *Pediatric Nursing, 20*(2), 186–188.

Wells, N., King, J., Hedstron, C., & Youngkins, J. (1995). Does tympanic temperature measure up? *Maternal Child Nursing, 20,* 95–100.

Worral, P., & Luke, S. (1998). Tympanic thermometry. *SPN News, 7*(2), 1.

Yaster, M., Sola, J. E., Pegoli, W., & Paidas, C. N. (1994). The night after surgery: Postoperative management of the pediatric outpatient. Surgical and anesthetic aspects. *Pediatric Clinic of North America, 41*(1), 199–219.

38

♦ ♦ ♦ ♦ ♦ ♦ ♦ ♦ ♦ ♦ ♦ ♦ ♦

Medicating Infants and Children

LEARNING OBJECTIVES

After studying this chapter, you should be able to:

■ Describe different methods of administering medications to children.

■ List the advantages and disadvantages of each route of administering medication to children.

■ Describe the physiologic differences between children and adults that affect medicating a child.

■ Describe psychosocial interventions for teaching and successful medication administration for each age group.

DEFINITIONS

blood-brain barrier Selective anatomic or physiologic capillary obstruction that prevents potentially harmful substances, such as certain medications, radioactive ions, and viruses, from entering the parenchyma of the brain.

central venous access device Venous access device in which the catheter is placed centrally rather than peripherally, usually in the superior vena cava or jugular vein; used for long-term intravenous therapy.

eutectic mixture of local anesthetics (EMLA) Cream used to numb the skin at a depth of 0.5 mm; used before needle punctures.

implanted venous access device (IVAD, Infusaport) Surgically implanted port or reservoir in which the catheter tip is placed in the superior vena cava; used for long-term intravenous therapy.

intermittent infusion port Intravenous catheter used to administer intermittent intravenous medications or fluids; remains clamped when not in use.

metered-dose inhaler Hand-held device that delivers "puffs" of medication for inhalation.

peripherally inserted central catheter (PICC) Central line that is inserted peripherally (usually through an antecubital vein) into the superior vena cava.

pharmacodynamics Behavior of medications at the cellular level.

pharmacokinetics The time and movement relationships of medications.

sustained-release medication Medication taken in a single dose but designed to dissolve slowly, releasing medication into the bloodstream over a specified period of time (usually 12 to 24 hours).

tunneled central line A surgically placed central line that is held in place by a Dacron cuff located in a subcutaneous tunnel; most commonly placed in the external jugular vein.

Medicating infants and children is one of the nurse's most important responsibilities. The nurse plays a key role in administering medications, supporting the child and family during the experience, and teaching the child and parents about pharmacologic aspects of the child's care. Although physicians or nurse practitioners prescribe medications, the nurse or caregiver is responsible for their administration. The nurse has a legal responsibility to administer medications safely and accurately. Safe administration of medications to children requires an understanding of the dosages of the medications used in pediatrics as well as the expected actions, possible side effects, and signs of adverse reactions or toxicity. Nurses should use reliable sources of information (e.g., pharmacists, drug handbooks) when administering drugs that are unfamiliar or used infrequently, and should question orders they do not understand before administering the medication.

Giving medications to children requires special skill. To gain the child's cooperation and to administer the medication in the least traumatic manner, the nurse needs to understand the physical characteristics and psychological needs of children at each developmental level. The nurse should use developmentally appropriate strategies to handle children's fears, prevent injury, and enhance coping.

It is vitally important to provide parents with information about medications used in their child's treatment and to encourage parents to support their child during potentially uncomfortable experiences. Involving parents in the task of eliciting their child's cooperation not only makes the job easier but also gives the family a sense of self-management and control. If the parents will be asked to administer medications to their child at home, the nurse ensures that the parents are properly instructed before the child is discharged. Recent research has suggested that, after leaving the health care setting, parents remember only about half of the instructions they were given by health care personnel (Matsui, 1997). Medication administration times that fit into the family routine, medications that are palatable to the child, and clear, written instructions improve compliance (Matsui, 1997).

Pharmacokinetics in Children

An understanding of pharmacokinetics and pharmacodynamics guides appropriate interventions in children. *Pharmacokinetics* refers to the actions of a drug (movement, biotransformation, and so forth) within the human body over time, and *pharmacodynamics* is the behavior of a drug as it interacts with the biochemical and physiologic milieu of the body. The pharmacokinetic actions of absorption, distribution, metabolism, and excretion are influenced by the physiologic environment in which the drug moves, and this environment differs between adults and children (Fig. 38–1). The physiologic differences in body systems are most striking in the neonate.

Absorption

ORAL ROUTE

When a medication is given orally, several factors influence its absorption along the gastrointestinal (GI) tract. Because most medication absorption occurs in the small intestine, the drug must reach that location in a form suitable for maximum absorption. Four factors influence this process:

- Gastric acidity
- Gastric emptying time
- Gastrointestinal motility, or transit time through the GI tract
- Function of the pancreatic enzymes

Gastric Acidity. Infants' gastric secretions are less acidic than older children's or adults'. Secretions slowly increase in acidity during the first 2 years of life. Children, particularly infants, eat more frequently than adults and are more likely to have food and digestive enzymes present in their stomachs. Formula or milk can increase the alkalinity of gastric secretions, decreasing the absorption of medications that require a more acidic environment and enhancing the absorption of medications that require a more alkaline milieu. These factors can greatly affect serum drug levels.

Gastric Emptying. Gastric emptying is intermittent and unpredictable in infants but usually is slower than in older children. This slower pace can prolong the time it takes a medication to reach the intestinal absorption site.

Gastrointestinal Motility. Depending on whether the infant or young child has eaten recently, peristaltic activity in the intestine can be faster or slower than in the older child or adult. Certain adverse health conditions, such as diarrhea, can alter intestinal motility by increasing peristalsis. The longer the transit time in the intestine, the more medication is absorbed. Conversely, a shortened transit time decreases absorption.

Enzyme Activity. Pancreatic enzyme activity also is variable in infants for the first 3 months of life as the GI system matures. Medications that require specific enzymes for dissolution and absorption might not be digested to a form suitable for intestinal action.

OTHER ROUTES

Adequate absorption of medication administered intravenously (IV) depends on adequate peripheral perfusion. Medications given IV are immediately available for absorption into the child's bloodstream. The child's peripheral circulation is less reliable and more responsive to environmental changes than the adult's. As a result, vasoconstriction or dilation can occur and alter the absorption of a parenteral medication. Also, the cardiovascular system is less able to accommodate large or rapid changes in volume, and the child can develop fluid overload if volumes of IV infusions are not carefully monitored.

A child's muscle mass is less than an adult's. The infant's body weight is about 25% muscle, whereas the adult's

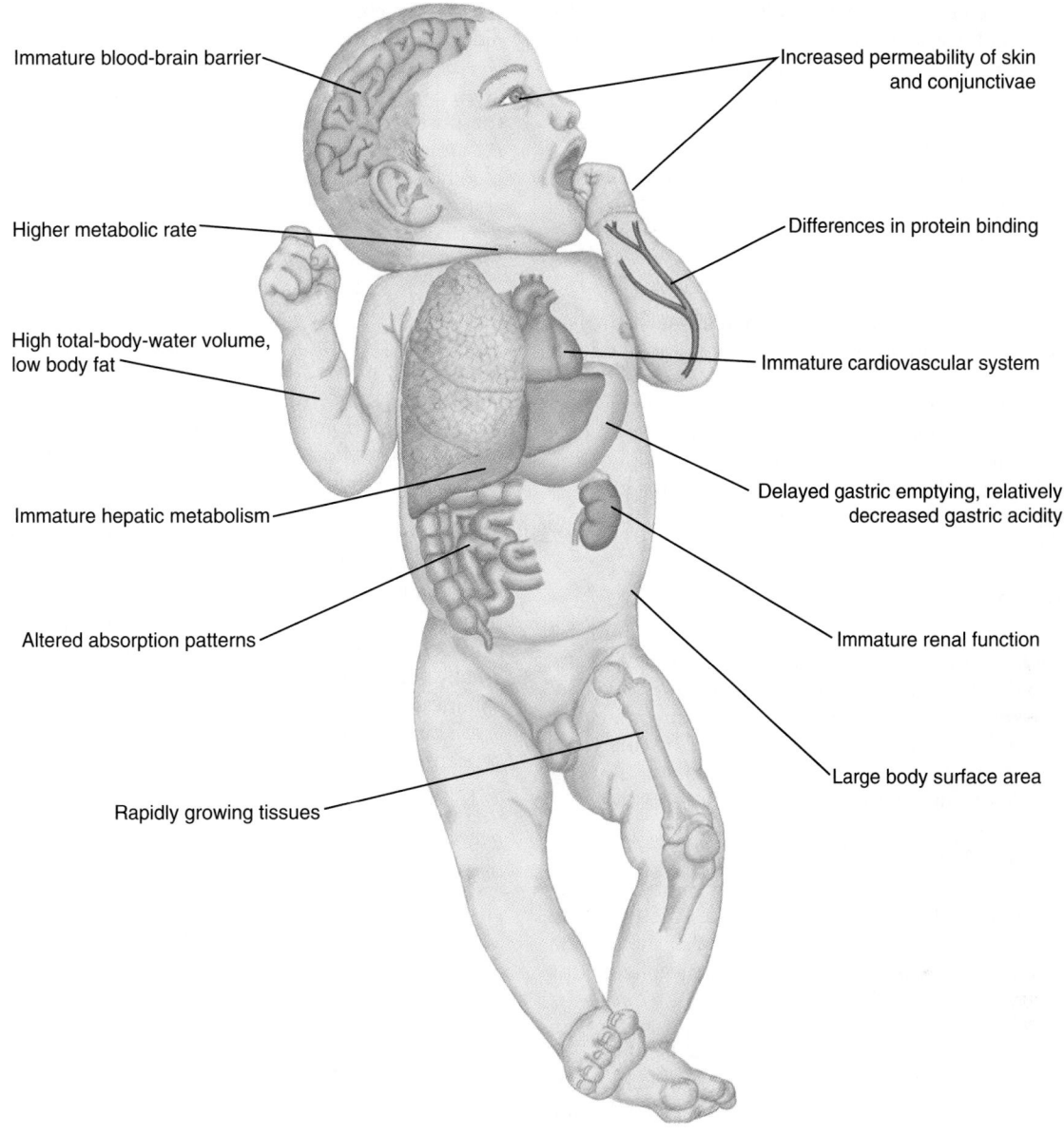

FIGURE 38–1
. . . .
Physiologic differences between children and adults affect drug absorption, metabolism, distribution, and excretion. These differences are most extreme in the neonate.

is about 40%. Because of the smaller muscle mass in infants, fewer sites are available for intramuscular (IM) injections. Blood flow to muscles in the young child is erratic and can affect the absorption of injected medications.

Infants and young children have a thinner outer skin layer (stratum corneum) and a larger body surface area (BSA)/weight ratio. Because the ratio of BSA to weight varies inversely with length, the infant has more surface area relative to weight than the adult. This difference affects the absorption of topical medications. Absorption of a similar dose of a topical medication in an infant and an adult is approximately three times greater in the infant because of the greater BSA and thinner skin layer (Reed, 1996).

Skin pH varies with age. This factor also can affect the absorption of topical medications. A child's skin is also

more prone to irritation, making contact dermatitis and other allergic reactions more common. Irritated or open skin can enhance the absorption of topical medications.

Distribution

Distribution refers to the general and specific concentration of the medication in body fluids and tissues. The medication is distributed to body tissues through blood and body fluids.

DIFFERENCES IN BODY FLUIDS
Dosages of medication must consider fluid differences between children under 2 years of age and older children. The body fluid content in infants and children ranges from 75% to 60% (2 years and older) of body weight. Because of their

greater fluid volume per weight, children need a higher dose per kilogram of a water-soluble medication to achieve the desired distribution effects (see Chapter 42).

A higher percentage of the young child's body fluid is located in the extracellular fluid compartment. During certain illnesses, this extracellular fluid can be lost rapidly, causing fluid depletion. It is important to adjust medication dosages accordingly in the ill infant or young child, to avoid overdosing or underdosing.

DIFFERENCES IN FAT PERCENTAGES
Percentages of fat also change as the child grows. Fat makes up about 16% of an infant's weight, although total body fat varies from child to child. This percentage increases in a 1-year-old but decreases during the preschool years. The percentage of body fat affects the distribution of fat-soluble medications in children. Because the body fat must be saturated with a fat-soluble medication before the drug becomes detectable in the blood, dosages often must be varied to achieve the desired effects.

DIFFERENCES IN PROTEINS
Medications bind to plasma proteins, mainly albumin, for distribution. Only free, unbound medication can be absorbed by the body. Because infants have lower levels of plasma proteins than older children, more unbound drug circulates and is available for absorption. This increased concentration of unbound drug alters the amount of medication needed to maintain a therapeutic drug level.

BLOOD-BRAIN BARRIER
The blood-brain barrier does not fully mature until the child is about 2 years old. This immaturity causes the barrier to be less selective and allows for distribution of medication into the central nervous system. As a result, encephalopathy can occur with some medications.

The relative immaturity of the neurologic system also can lead to paradoxic effects from certain medications. For example, medications that normally cause sedation in adults may have the opposite effect in many children and cause hyperactivity.

Metabolism

Most medications are metabolized in the liver. Because the metabolic enzyme systems are less mature in newborn and premature infants, they might not be able to properly metabolize all the medication in a prescribed dosage. Toddlers and preschoolers can have a much greater metabolizing capacity than adults for certain drugs. For this reason, larger dosages or more frequent administration of certain drugs (such as pain medications) might be needed for young children, to achieve therapeutic results.

Excretion

Most medications are excreted through the renal system. The renal system also is immature at birth. The newborn's glomerular filtration rate is about 30% to 50% that of an adult's, and the renal tubules also function less efficiently. Adult rates are reached after approximately 1 year. Infants

and young children cannot concentrate urine as well as older children or adults.

Because of renal immaturity, medications might not be filtered out of the circulating blood volume and excreted in the urine (the primary method of medication excretion). As a result, medications can circulate longer and reach toxic blood levels. Likewise, loss of fluid may decrease the child's ability to excrete medications. Therefore, dehydration has a serious effect on drug serum levels.

Concentration

To administer appropriately therapeutic medication doses to children, nurses need to be aware of the importance of knowing the concentration of certain medications in serum. Maintaining serum levels within a safe therapeutic range maximizes the effect of a medication while reducing the risk of toxicity. When certain medications are used, the physician will order a peak and a trough serum level to be measured, to monitor medication concentration. The peak concentration is not necessarily the highest concentration but is the concentration of the medication after it has been distributed. The time at which a medication reaches peak concentration differs according to the specific medication but usually occurs a specified time after the medication has been administered.

The medication trough is the level at which the serum concentration is lowest. Trough levels usually are obtained just prior to the next medication dose. Knowing the usual therapeutic peak-and-trough range for a specific medication will assist the nurse in an accurate assessment of the child's response and the potential for toxic medication effects.

Psychological and Developmental Factors

Growth and developmental principles and differences among age groups must always be taken into consideration when medicating a child.

> Always approach children at their developmental level and provide developmentally appropriate explanations about a medication procedure. To decrease feelings of powerlessness, give the child as many choices as possible.

Honesty, reward, and praise are important for gaining trust and cooperation. Give honest explanations, and tell the child when a procedure will be painful or uncomfortable. Also tell the child approximately how long the pain will last and what the child can do to help during that time. Use terms familiar to the child, such as pinching or stinging.

> Praising the child after the procedure for attempts at cooperation is important and helps gain trust and cooperation for future procedures. Do not scold a child for failure to cooperate.

Restraints are seldom necessary for administration of medications. It is appropriate to ask a parent or other staff member to assist with holding a child during an injection, if the child's movements appear to jeopardize safe administration of the medication. Approaches include taking the child to a procedure room where another staff member assists in helping the child to remember to hold still. Physical restraint devices, such as arm boards and mummy restraints are occasionally necessary. It is important to explain that the staff person is helping the child to remember to hold still. Do not threaten a child with restraint.

Rewards for good behavior often help the child feel better about the procedure. Rewards should always be safe and appropriate for the child's age. Stickers are a good choice for younger children. Older children might want a sticker or might choose a small toy or a privilege, such as watching a favorite video.

Infants

Infants are easier to medicate than toddlers but more difficult than children who can follow directions (see Chapter 5). Parents always need to know why the infant is receiving the medication. Because keeping a squirming infant still may be difficult, the nurse should get help in administering the medication, if necessary. Maintaining a routine and cuddling and comforting the infant before and after the procedure are important interventions.

Toddlers and Preschoolers

Older toddlers (2 to 3 years) are prone to magical thinking and might view the administration of medication (especially if painful or intrusive) as punishment for "bad" thoughts (see Chapter 6). Give toddlers age-appropriate explanations, using play, if possible. Allowing older toddlers to examine the equipment before the procedure might enhance cooperation. Because the toddler might react negatively to restraint, use as little restraint as possible and allow the toddler to sit on the parent's lap, if the parent is willing. Praise and cuddling after the procedure are important. Rewards, such as stickers, are useful for this age group.

Preschoolers (3 to 5 years) continue to use magical thinking. They fear the unknown and painful procedures (see Chapter 6). This age group benefits greatly from therapeutic play and participation. Allow as much control over the procedure and offer as much choice as possible (e.g., "Do you want your medication with juice or milk?"). Ask preschoolers if they can hold still for a painful procedure; if they cannot, they usually will say so. Adhesive bandages are important to children in this age group after an invasive procedure, such as an injection. Preschoolers believe that these bandages "make it better"—an example of magical thinking.

School-Age Children

School-age children (6 to 12 years) fear loss of control, pain, and injury. At this age, a child can understand more complex explanations (see Chapter 7). Provide as much choice as possible. School-age children often cooperate fully, even with painful procedures, but might need a source of distraction (e.g., a radio to turn up as pain increases, counting out loud for the length of pain time) and support (see Chapter 39). School-age children still need praise, and rewards (e.g., stickers) are appreciated.

PARENTS WANT TO KNOW

Medication Administration

Parents want to know how they can help their children when a procedure for administering medication is expected to be uncomfortable. They also become concerned if the child refuses to take a medication that is intended to help the child recover from an illness. Nurses should do the following to empower parents:

- Obtain the following information before administering the medication:

  1. Medication allergies or sensitivities
  2. The child's ability to take medications (e.g., can the child swallow pills?)
  3. What method the parent usually uses to administer the medication (e.g., mixing it with certain foods)

- Give the parent a thorough explanation about the medication before administration. Include information about why the child needs the medication, any possible side effects, and how and where you expect to administer the medication.
- Allow the parent to administer certain medications if the child is more comfortable (e.g., oral, otic, ophthalmic). Check the medication "rights" before you allow a parent to administer a medication. Show the parent the most acceptable position for administering the particular medication.
- Encourage the parent to express concern that a medication might not be effective or might be making the child ill. Parents know their children and often are aware of subtle changes long before hospital personnel notice them.
- Help the parent determine the best way to administer the child's medication at home. Recommend the use of positive reinforcements such as rewards or stickers to increase cooperation. Encourage the parent to explain to the child why the medication is needed and to be firm that the child take the medication.

Adolescents

Adolescents (11 to 21 years) fear separation from peers and loss of control (see Chapter 8). Children in this age group understand adult explanations and can assist in making decisions about their care. Often, however, adolescents exhibit a hyperresponse to procedures that can seem inconsistent with their age. It is important to praise their cooperation and find outlets for their frustration (e.g., drawing or writing).

Calculating Dosages

Pediatric medications usually do not have standard dosages. Instead, dosages are calculated based on the child's weight (mg/kg). This practice usually is the most reliable method

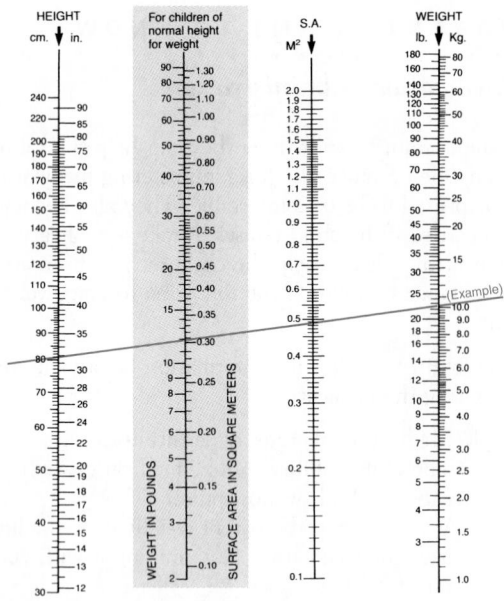

FIGURE 38–2

Nomogram for calculating body surface area, used for determining medication dosages for infants and children. (From Behrman, R. E., Kliegman, R. M., & Arvin, A. M. [1996]. *Nelson textbook of pediatrics* [15th ed., p. 2079]. Philadelphia: Saunders.)

for precisely determining doses. For example, for a child weighing 10 kg, the daily dose of amoxicillin is 20 to 40 mg/kg, or 200 to 400 mg/day.

Dosages can also be calculated based on BSA (body surface area, mg/m²) or according to other standardized methods (Fig. 38–2). To calculate medications on the basis of surface area, the following formula is used:

$$\text{Approximate dose} = \text{BSA of child (m}^2)/1.7 \times \text{adult dose}$$

Administration Procedures

Because the margin of safety is minimal in pediatric patients, accuracy is a prime consideration when administering medications. Inaccurate dosage calculations can result in a tenfold or more dosage error if the decimal point is in the wrong place. Always check medication doses for accuracy in the following areas: (1) recommended dosage in mg/kg/day, (2) number of divided doses recommended (e.g., every 4 hours, t.i.d., every 12 hours, and so forth), and (3) recommended route of administration. To further avoid errors, adhere to the following procedures:

- Adhere to the "six rights" of medication administration: right child, right drug, right dose, right time, right route, and right documentation.
- Always double-check medication calculations before administration.
- Double-check calculations of medications provided by the pharmacy in a unit dose form.
- Ask another nurse to double-check the following medications:
    Insulin
    Narcotics
    Chemotherapy
    Digoxin or other inotropics
    Anticoagulants
    K⁺ and Ca²⁺ salts

Many institutions also require two nurses to check any medication given by continuous infusion or by medication syringe pump.

Administering Oral Medications

The oral route is the most widely used and economical method of administering medications. It is also one of the least reliable methods of administration because absorption is affected greatly by the presence or absence of food in the stomach, gastric emptying time, GI motility, and acidity of the stomach. The oral route can also be less predictable because of medication loss to spillage, leaking, or spitting out.

Oral medications are available in liquid (elixir or suspension), tablet or capsule, chewable tablet, or sprinkle (powder) forms. If the child cannot swallow tablets or capsules, the nurse determines whether the medication is available in a liquid form and, if it is not, determines whether it can be crushed.

Before administering oral medications, the nurse assesses the child's gag reflex and ability to swallow. The oral form used should be tailored to the child's developmental level and ability to successfully take the form prescribed. An assessment of the way the child takes medications at home also helps to determine the proper form. Some older infants and toddlers can successfully take crushed tablets but refuse liquid forms.

MEDICATION PREPARATION

When preparing to administer an elixir or suspension, the nurse first ensures that the correct dose is drawn for administration. Physicians' orders often specify the dosage in milligrams, *not* milliliters, for liquid medications. It is important to calculate the milliliter dose properly, based on the number of milligrams per milliliter in the liquid medication on hand.

Because tableware spoons vary in volume, use a calibrated spoon or dropper designed for medication administration. Calibrated syringes (preferably oral administration syringes) should be used for doses of less than 5 ml or doses that are not in 5-ml increments. Pour larger volumes into calibrated plastic medicine cups. Avoid using paper measuring cups because their volumes tend to vary.

If a tablet is to be crushed and mixed with food, or is available as a sprinkle or powder, mix it with a nonessential food, such as applesauce or pudding, not orange juice or formula. Giving medication with a favorite food can alter the flavor of the food. Avoid using syrup or other high-sugar substances. Never give infants medication or foods mixed with honey, as honey has been known to cause infantile botulism.

Determine a medication's compatibility with food before giving it to the child. Mix any medication with a small amount (5–10 ml) of food or liquid and give to the child before a feeding, if not contraindicated.

Sustained-release tablets or capsules should never be

crushed because their function is to release the medication slowly over a long period. Enteric-coated tablets (tablets covered with a substance that prevents the drug from dissolving until it reaches the intestine) can have an unpleasant taste or odor if crushed. Crushing also interferes with the function of the enteric coating.

MEDICATION ADMINISTRATION

The method of administering oral medications differs according to the child's age and developmental level. Infants usually receive elixir or suspension forms of oral medications. Administer these with an empty nipple or oral syringe. First place the infant in an upright or semi-upright position. The position used for feeding the infant can be used for administering medications. Open the infant's mouth by applying gentle pressure to the chin or both cheeks. If using a nipple, place the nipple in the infant's mouth and add the medication to the empty nipple when the baby begins to suck. Unpleasant-tasting medications should not be given through a nipple because the taste can cause a future aversion reaction to the nipple, thus interfering with feeding.

If using an oral syringe or medicine dropper to administer the medication place the syringe or dropper gently in the infant's mouth along the side of the cheek, and squirt the medication in slowly as the infant sucks (Fig. 38–3). Aiming the medication toward the back of the throat is dangerous because it can cause choking and aspiration.

Toddlers and preschoolers can easily take liquid medi-

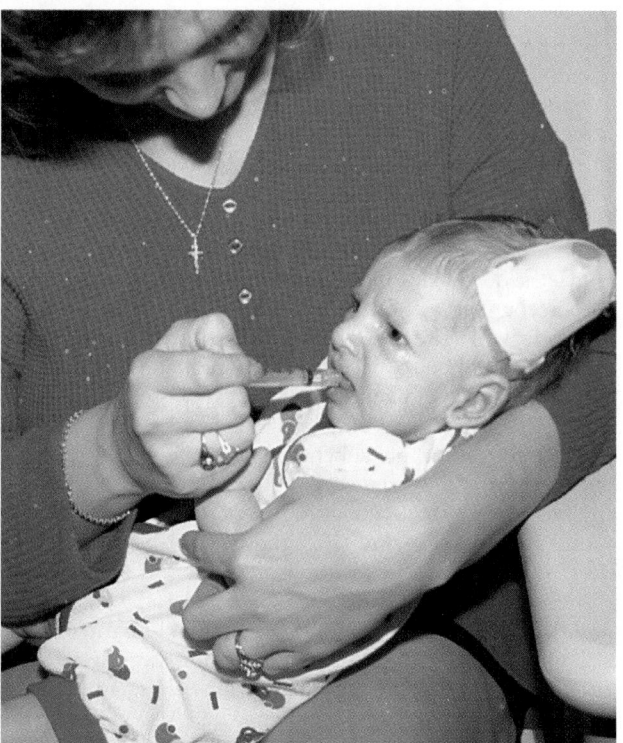

FIGURE 38–3

Administering an oral medication to an infant with an oral syringe. (Courtesy of Parkland Health and Hospital System, Dallas, Texas.)

cations from an oral syringe or medicine cup. If the liquid medication has an unpleasant taste, offer to let the child take it through a straw. If a straw is used, cut the straw in half to avoid a loss of medication. Allowing children to take their own medication, giving rewards as incentives, and providing choices that fit into the medication regimen enhance autonomy.

Preschoolers can usually manage chewable tablets without difficulty. Most older children can swallow tablets or capsules. The nurse, however, should determine whether the child can swallow pills. If not, the nurse should determine whether the medication can be crushed and mixed with food or a small amount of liquid. If the child cannot swallow tablets or capsules and they cannot be crushed, the nurse needs to contact the pharmacy to identify another form for administration (elixir or suspension). If the child can swallow tablets and capsules, ask what the child prefers for the "chaser" (usually water or juice).

Administer oral medications with the child in an upright or slightly recumbent position. The nurse should always use the least amount of force or restraint possible to administer the medication safely and avoid choking and aspiration. If the child is reluctant to take a necessary medication, the child can be positioned in the nurse's lap, as follows:

- Seat the child sideways on your lap, facing your dominant hand.
- Hug the child by bringing the arm closest to your body under your arm and around your waist or back.
- Bring your nondominant arm around behind the child's neck and hold the child's free arm or hand with yours. This position cradles the child's head between your arm and body (see Fig. 38–3).
- If the child is really resistant, secure the child's legs between yours as well.

If the child vomits or spits up after the administration of medication, notify the physician. Another dose may need to be reordered depending on how long it has been since administration, the type of medication, and the amount vomited.

ALTERNATIVE ORAL ROUTES

Oral medications can be administered directly into the GI tract through a feeding tube. If the medication is to be administered through a feeding tube, verify tube placement before administration (see Chapter 37) and, depending on the type of tube (i.e., transpyloric), determine whether the tube is the proper route for the medication. After the medication is administered, flush the tube with water to ensure the medication has reached the GI tract and to prevent blockage in the tube.

Administering Injections

Injected medications are rapidly absorbed by diffusing into either plasma or the lymphatic system. Although injection results in faster and more reliable absorption than the oral route, injections are stressful and threatening to children and are not preferred. Injections are used most often for one-time doses of antibiotics (e.g., ceftriaxone for the initial treatment of severe infection), immunizations, iron admin-

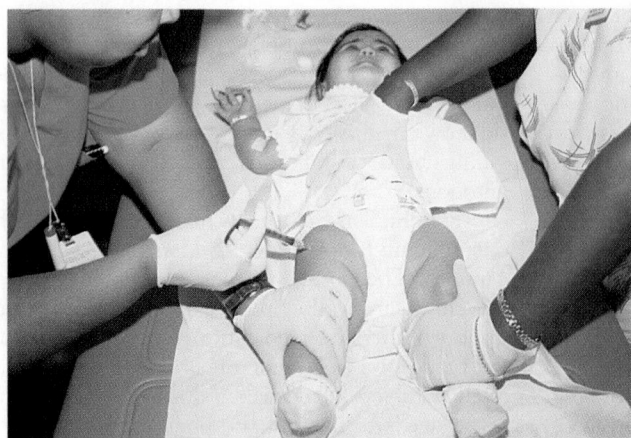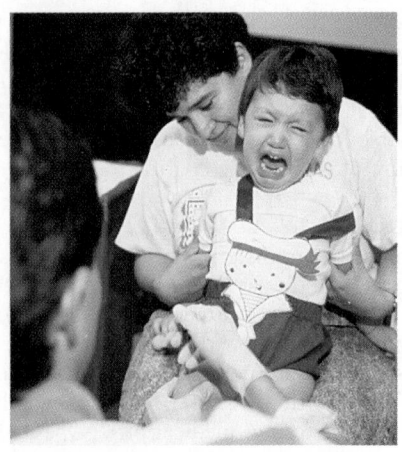

FIGURE 38-4

Two methods of restraint for IM injection at the vastus lateralis site. (Left: Courtesy of Parkland Health and Hospital System Community Oriented Primary Care Clinic, Dallas, Texas. Right: Courtesy of Cook Children's Medical Center, Fort Worth, Texas.)

istration, purified protein derivative (PPD), or allergy skin testing. Injections are potentially more dangerous in infants than in older children because of the infant's decreased muscle mass and variable blood flow to muscles.

Appropriately preparing the child for injections can reduce emotional and anticipatory concerns. Depending on the child's developmental level, explain the reason for the injection, any sensations the child might experience, and the length of time they are anticipated to last. Tell the child that the injection is not a punishment but is needed to make the child better or keep the child healthy. Practice counting, singing, deep breathing, or other distraction techniques with the child in advance.

Offer parents the option to leave if they feel unable to cope with the procedure; inform them when the procedure is completed. Most parents prefer to remain. Some are willing to help reassure the child or hold the child during the procedure.

To reduce the risk of injury, it is sometimes necessary to restrain the child before administering an injected medication. Restraint can be accomplished by swaddling the child or obtaining the assistance of another health care professional. Toddlers and older children often respond better to injections if allowed to be held and comforted by parents during the procedure (Fig. 38–4). The parent, however, must feel confident in the ability to keep the child still enough to prevent injury.

Children perceive injections to be very painful. Even with the best preparation, it is hard for a child to understand that the pain of an injection lasts only seconds. Ice applied to the anticipated injection site for several minutes prior to the injection can numb the pain sensation. Topical anesthetic agents such as EMLA have also been shown to be effective in reducing injection pain. (See p. 1006 and Chapter 39.)

Children can be taught to deal with the pain of an injection using guided imagery, distraction, or other methods, such as taking a deep breath and blowing out the pain, or turning the "pain switch" off (Kachoyeanos & Friedhoff, 1993).

Careful documentation of the injection is also important. Documentation includes recording the amount of medication injected and the site used. If the child will receive several injections, it is important to rotate sites to prevent tissue irritation and possible muscle atrophy and wasting. Federal vaccine regulations now require nurses to record the vaccine manufacturer and lot number for each immunization given, as well as any prior vaccine reaction the child might have incurred.

PREPARING AND ADMINISTERING INTRAMUSCULAR INJECTIONS

When filling a syringe for an injection, it is important to remember that most syringes and needle hubs contain approximately 0.2 ml of dead space. Therefore, to keep the dose accurate, do not flush the needle and hub after injection. On the rare occasion that a Z-track method is used (a method in which a small air bubble locks in the medication), the dead space in the hub of the needle must be taken into account so as not to overdose.

Select the site before the child is given an injection; the site should be soft, well vascularized, and healthy. It is important to avoid puncturing blood vessels, nerves, or bones and also to avoid injecting medications intended for IM administration into subcutaneous tissue. Inadvertent injection into any of these areas can result in accidental IV injection, pain, tissue sloughing, or nerve damage. The preferred IM injection sites in children are shown in Table 38–1, and methods of restraint are shown in Figure 38–4.

Select an appropriate needle size (21 to 25 gauge) and length (0.5 to 1.5 inches) for the injection. Use the smallest size that will *safely and comfortably* administer the medication. For example, a viscous medication is less painful when injected through a larger-gauge needle. Also consider the amount of body fat, the distance to the muscle, the size of the muscle, the volume of medication, and the properties of the medication.

Safe volumes for IM injection range from 0.5 ml to 2.5 ml, depending on the age and size of the child. Wipe the injection site with a skin cleanser and allow to dry. Insert

TABLE 38-1
• • • • • • • • • • • •

Preferred Intramuscular Injection Sites in Children

Site	Key Points	Site	Key Points
Vastus lateralis	Located on the anterior lateral thigh. Well developed at birth. Good choice for all age groups, but usually used in children younger than 3 years. Able to tolerate larger volumes and not located near vital structures, such as nerves and blood vessels.	Dorsogluteal	Located by drawing a diagonal line between the posterior superior iliac spine and the greater tochanter of the femur. The dorsogluteal muscle is found above and lateral to this line. It develops with walking, so it should not be used until the child has been walking for at least 1 year. The child should be asked to "toe in" to avoid tensing the muscle. Can hold 1 to 2.5 ml but has the slowest and poorest absorption of all sites.

Vastus lateralis

Dorsogluteal

Site	Key Points	Site	Key Points
Ventrogluteal	Located by placing the heel of the hand on the greater trochanter with fingers pointed toward the child's head. Place the index finger over the anterior superior iliac spine and the middle finger along the iliac crest posteriorly as far as possible to form a V. The injection is given in the center of the V. Site is safe for IM injection in children older than 18 months because it is free of major blood vessels and nerves. Can generally hold larger volumes (up to 2.5 ml in adolescents). Care should be taken to avoid bone and joint.	Deltoid	Use the part of the muscle located about two fingerwidths below the acromion process. This site is not used for injection in young children because the small muscle mass cannot hold large volumes of medication or medications that must be injected deep into muscle mass. This is the least painful site for injecting smaller volumes.

Ventrogluteal

Deltoid

> **CRITICAL TO REMEMBER**
>
> *Guidelines for Maximum Safe Volumes for IM Injections*
>
> | | | Site | | |
> |---|---|---|---|---|
> | Age | Deltoid | Ventrogluteal | Dorsogluteal | Vastus Lateralis |
> | Premature | — | — | — | 0.5 ml |
> | Neonate | — | — | — | 0.5 ml |
> | Infant | — | — | — | 1 ml |
> | Young child (3–6 yr) | — | 1.5 ml | 1 ml | 1.5 ml |
> | Older child (6–14 yr) | 0.5 ml | 1.5–2.0 ml | 1.5–2.0 ml | 1.5 ml |
> | Adolescent (15 yr– adult) | 1 ml | 2.0–2.5 ml | 2.0–2.5 ml | 1.5–2.0 ml |

the needle at a 90 degree angle with a quick darting motion. Pull back gently on the plunger to aspirate for blood. If blood is noted, withdraw the needle to avoid giving the medication IV. Change the needle and the site. If no blood is noted, give the injection slowly. Unless contraindicated, massage the injection site afterward.

ADMINISTERING SUBCUTANEOUS INJECTIONS

A subcutaneous injection is given into the tissue that lies just below the skin. This type of administration is used for medications that provide a sustained effect (e.g., heparin, insulin). A subcutaneous injection should be given only into healthy tissue. If circulation is impaired—for example because of edema, decreased temperature, or shock—a subcutaneous injection should not be used because absorption will be impaired.

Preferred subcutaneous injection sites are the fat pads located above the iliac crests, hips, lateral upper arms, and anterior thighs (Fig. 38–5). Rotate sites to avoid the development of abscesses and to facilitate drug absorption. Record the site of the subcutaneous injection to avoid using the same site and causing tissue irritation.

Subcutaneous injections are usually given with a small (25 to 27 gauge), short (no more than ½ to ⅝ inch) needle to ensure that the medication is not inadvertently given IM. Volumes for subcutaneous injections are small, usually averaging 0.5 ml. Because the needle is so small and narrow, changing to a new needle after withdrawing medication through the stopper of a vial makes the injection more comfortable for the child.

Clean the site with alcohol and allow it to dry. Pinch the tissue to raise the fatty tissue from the muscle. The angle of needle insertion is usually 45 degrees, although some practitioners insert the ½-inch needle at a 90-degree angle. Unless the child has little subcutaneous tissue, the short needle does not reach the muscle, even if it is inserted at the straight angle. Massage the insertion site after administration unless massage is contraindicated for the injected medication, such as heparin.

If subcutaneous injections are to be ongoing (e.g., insulin administration), pay special attention to client education. Older children and adolescents can usually learn to perform this procedure without difficulty.

INTRADERMAL INJECTIONS

Intradermal injections enter just below the outer layer of skin, the epidermis, and usually on the inner aspect of the forearm, or on the upper back. They are most often used for testing (e.g., allergy, PPD). The needle is small (25 to 27 gauge) and short (½ to ⅝ inch). The volume is also small (usually 0.1 ml). After cleaning the site with alcohol and allowing it to dry, turn the bevel of the needle up and insert gently at a 15-degree angle. The needle will barely penetrate the skin. Inject the medication to form a wheal (similar in appearance to an insect bite) (Fig. 38–6). If the injection does not form a wheal, or if bleeding is noted after the injection, administration was probably too deep and should be repeated. If several intradermal injections are made in the same area, each site should be marked with permanent ink for later identification.

The child who is to receive multiple injections might benefit significantly from supervised needle play. In needle play the child uses a syringe and needle to give shots to a doll. The nurse uses this play to prepare the child for injections and to help the child gain a sense of mastery over the experience of receiving an injection. The nurse offers a brief explanation of what will occur and why the child must receive an injection. Through therapeutic play the child's anxiety is decreased.

Rectal Administration

The rectal route of administration is unreliable and is not used as often as other routes. It is most often reserved for times when a child cannot tolerate the oral route (e.g., because of nausea and vomiting). It has many possible complications, including the Valsalva response, rectal perforation, and other damage to the rectum or anus.

This route should not be used if the rectum is full of stool. Rectal administration is stressful for children because they fear intrusive procedures. Carefully prepare the child and give an explanation about the procedure. Tell the child the reason why the medication is being given in this form and what the child can do to help. The child is also told whether the suppository must be retained or expelled.

Position the child on the left side with the right leg flexed and expose the rectal area sufficiently for visibility. Adequate draping is essential for preschool and older chil-

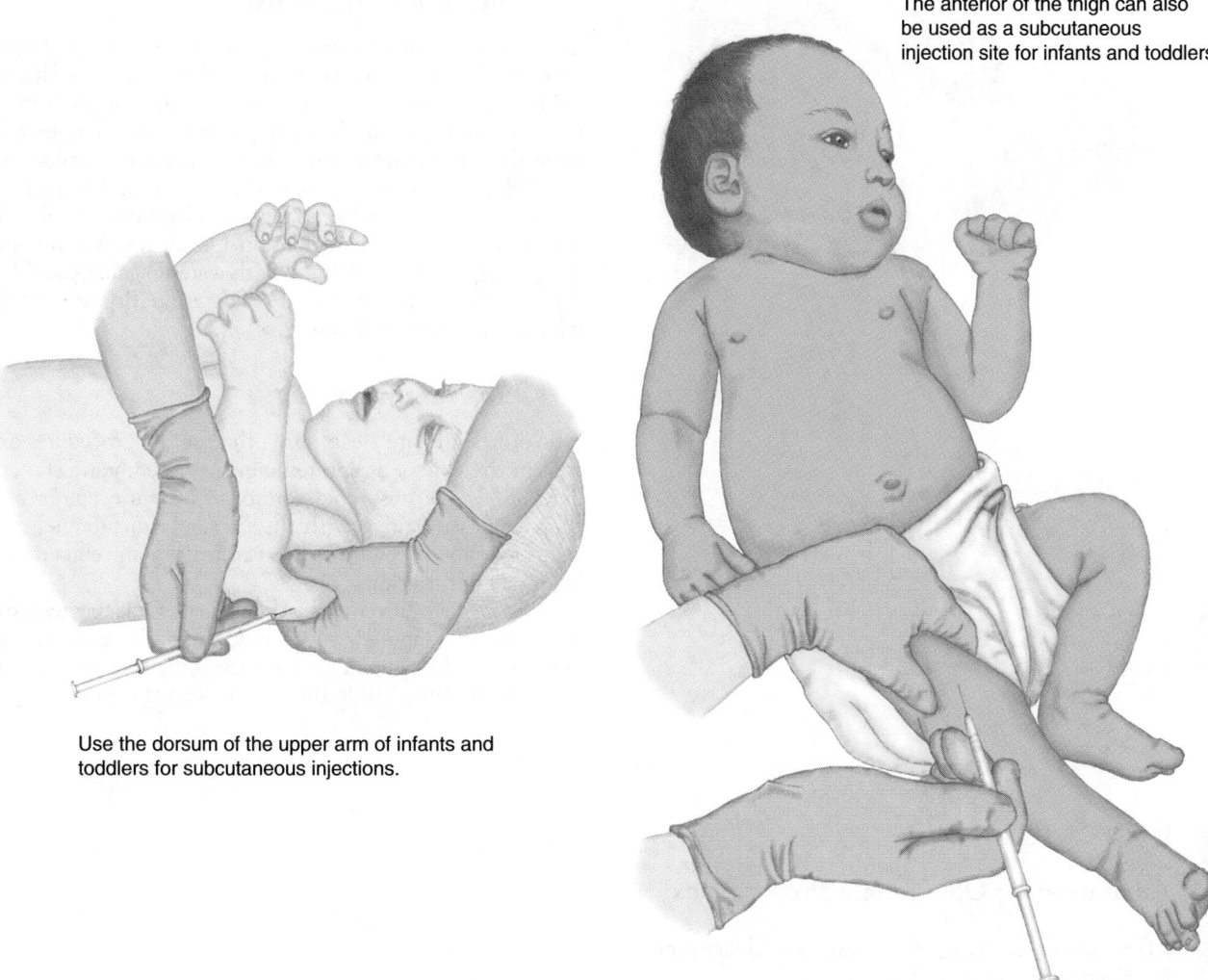

The anterior of the thigh can also be used as a subcutaneous injection site for infants and toddlers.

Use the dorsum of the upper arm of infants and toddlers for subcutaneous injections.

FIGURE 38–5

Two of the preferred subcutaneous injection sites in children. The fat pads above the iliac crests and hips may also be used.

dren. Often the child needs help to relax. Distraction and deep-breathing exercises can help the child relax the external sphincter. Lubricate the suppository well with a water-soluble lubricant before inserting.

Advise the child to take a deep breath or bear down if possible to relax the sphincter further. Then, gently insert past the internal sphincter. The child's rectal vault is not as long as an adult's, and the distance required to place medication is approximately 1 to 2 cm (0.5 to 1 inch). After insertion, hold the child's buttocks together until the urge to expel the suppository has passed.

Vaginal Administration

Although the vaginal route is not often used in infant, toddler, or preschool-age girls, it might be required for school-age or adolescent girls, most often to treat candidal infections or possibly for birth control. It is essential to explain the procedure, why it is indicated, and how the child can help.

Ask the child to void and then assist her into a supine position with the soles of her feet together and her knees resting on the bed (frog-leg position). Remember to drape the child and provide for privacy. Using a gloved hand, gently spread the labia so that the vaginal orifice is visible. If necessary, lubricate the tablet, suppository, or applicator with warm water or a water-soluble lubricant. Have the client take a deep breath, then gently insert the vaginal tablet, suppository, or applicator approximately 9 to 10 cm (3.5 to 4 inches) along the posterior wall of the vagina. To reduce discomfort, the nurse should follow the natural angle of the vagina by pointing the finger or applicator toward the sacrum.

After the procedure is completed, the child might need to remain in a supine position for a period of time. Older school-age children and adolescents can be taught to instill their own vaginal medications. It is important that these girls receive good education and give a return demonstration of the procedure, especially if the instillations are contraceptives.

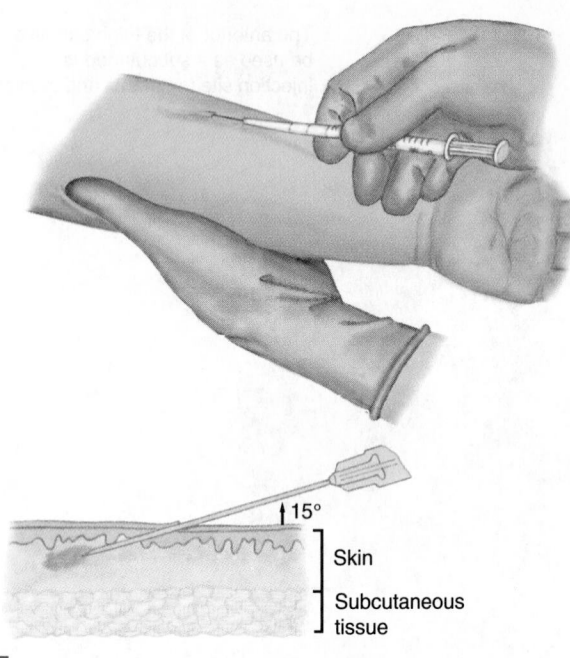

FIGURE 38-6
· · · · · · · · · · ·
Intradermal injection site and technique.

Ophthalmic Administration

Instillation of ophthalmic preparations is a clean rather than sterile procedure (Procedure 38–1). Most pediatric ophthalmic solutions are available as either drops or ophthalmic ointment. If these preparations are refrigerated, allow them to warm to room temperature before instillation.

Before administering, note the expiration date and inspect the drops for color changes or cloudiness. Shake all suspensions well before instillation. Gently remove any exudate by wiping the child's eye with a sterile gauze pad from the inner to outer canthus. If exudates are dry or crusted, wipe with a warm wet compress.

Otic Administration

Otic procedures are clean rather than sterile procedures except in the case of a ruptured tympanic membrane (Procedure 38–2). Because cold eardrops can cause pain when they come in contact with the tympanic membrane, otic solutions should be allowed to warm to room temperature before administration.

Before administering eardrops, gently clean any exudate from the outer ear with sterile gauze. Because the risk of rupturing the tympanic membrane is high, never attempt to place anything inside the ear to clean the canal.

PROCEDURE 38-1
· · · · · · · · · · ·
Administering Ophthalmic Preparations

PURPOSE: To treat an eye infection, dilate pupils for diagnostic testing, or keep eyes moist.

1. Explain the purpose for the medication or lubricating drops. Tell the child how to help with the procedure. Explain that the child might experience blurred vision for a short time afterward.
2. Gather needed equipment: (a) eyedrops or ointment, (b) gauze pads, (c) tissues. Wash your hands before proceeding.
3. Assist the child into a supine position with the neck slightly hyperextended (e.g., by placing a rolled towel or small blanket under the shoulder blades).
4. If the drops are to be instilled into an infant's eyes, obtain assistance in restraining the child's arms and head or use a mummy wrap as necessary.
5. Instruct an older child to look upward and gently pull the lower lid down and away from the eye.
6. Place the drops or a ribbon of ointment into the space between the eye and lower lid, taking care not to contaminate the end of the dropper or tube.
7. If both drops and ointment are ordered, the drops should be administered first. If they are placed after the ointment, they will not be absorbed.
8. Have the child look down as the lower lid is released. Encourage the child to close both eyes and keep them closed for several seconds. Hand the child a tissue to blot any excess medication gently.

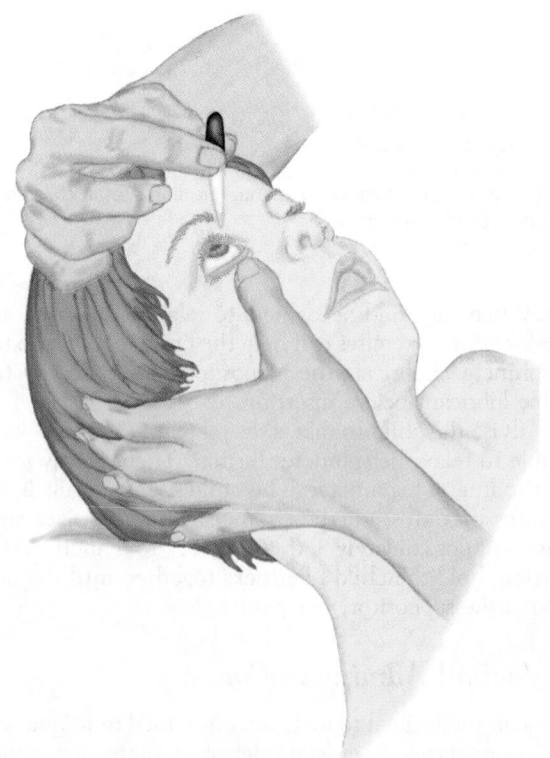

9. As with any procedure, praise the child for cooperation and assistance. Document the medication in the appropriate location.

PROCEDURE 38-2

Administering Otic Drops

PURPOSE: To treat inflammation or infection of the ear canal, relieve pain, or prevent otitis externa.

1. Explain any expected sensations to the child in developmentally appropriate terms (e.g., "It may sound like there is a butterfly flying inside your ear") and describe how the child can help. Assistance in restraining a young child might be necessary.
2. Gather the following equipment: (a) otic drops, (b) cotton pieces. Wash your hands before the procedure.
3. Position the child lying down with the affected ear up or sitting with the head turned so the affected ear is up.
4. Brace the administering hand against the child's head above the ear.

5. If the child is 3 years or younger, pull the pinna of the ear back and down, holding near the lobe. If the child is older than 3 years, pull the pinna back and up.
6. Insert the required number of drops. Then gently massage the tragus (anterior portion) to ensure that the drops reach the tympanic membrane.
7. Pack cotton loosely into the canal, if ordered. Instruct the child not to remove the cotton or place anything inside the ear.
8. Keep the child on the unaffected side for several minutes after the administration. If medication is to be administered in both ears, the procedure should be repeated in the other ear after a wait of at least 1 minute.
9. Document the medication in the appropriate place.

For a child older than 3 years:
pull pinna up and back.

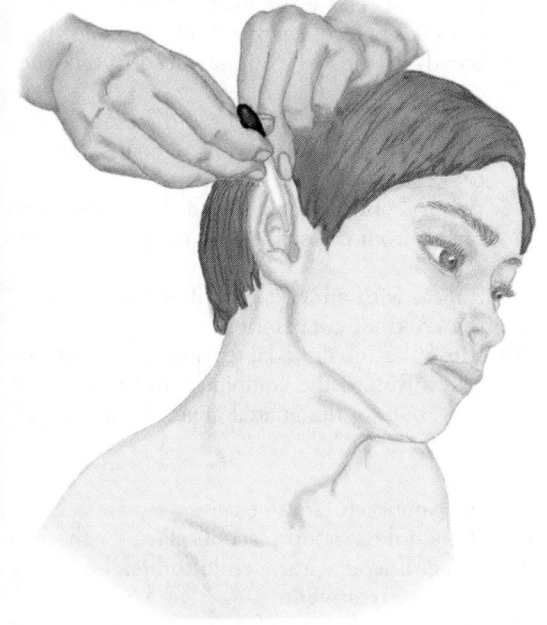

For an infant or a child younger than 3 years:
pull lobe down and back.

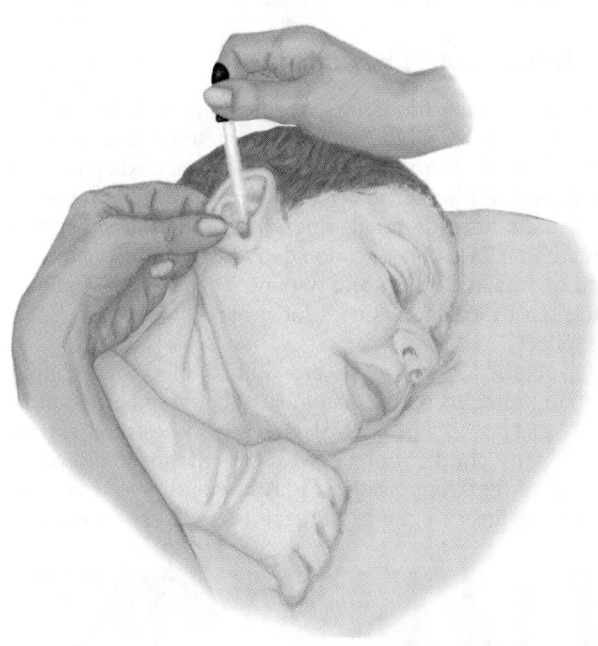

Nasal Administration

Although the mucous membrane route is generally used only for localized treatment, it has fairly rapid systemic absorption and may be used for the administration of certain systemic medications (e.g., antidiuretic hormone).

When administering nose drops to an infant, the nurse removes any excess mucus by gently suctioning before administration. To make eating more comfortable, saline nose drops followed by gentle suction should be given 20 to 30 minutes before feedings.

Receiving nose drops is stressful for young children, who might feel that they are drowning during the instillation. A thorough explanation of what the child will feel, why the medication has been ordered ("to help unstop your

nose"), and what the child needs to do to help is necessary. Assistance with restraint is also necessary with the young child, or mummy restraint or swaddling may be used.

Assist the child into a supine position and hyperextend the neck slightly by placing a rolled towel or small blanket under the shoulder blades. Keeping the head in a midline position, instill the number of drops ordered into each nares. The head is kept in the same position to allow the drops to reach the ethmoid and sphenoid sinuses. Then briefly have the child turn the head slightly in either direction and back to midline to disburse the medication to the maxillary and frontal sinuses.

After the drops have been instilled, the child remains in a supine position for several minutes to allow the medication to be distributed to the sinuses. Instruct the child not to blow the medication out of the nose. Praise all efforts at cooperation.

Topical Administration

Because skin is relatively impermeable when intact and has a large surface area, topical administration of drugs is generally limited to localized treatment. If the medication is applied to abraded skin, over a large area, or over a long period, however, systemic effects can result. Solvents added to the medication to break down skin oils and occlusive dressings also increase absorption. Monitor the child carefully for systemic absorption effects.

As with all other procedures, explain what will be done, why it will be done, and what sensations the child will experience. Clean the skin gently to remove any exudate, scales, or other residue and allow it to dry. To avoid contaminating the container, place the estimated amount of medication on a sterile pad. Wear gloves and apply the ointment or cream as ordered or as recommended by the manufacturer. Cover the site afterward with a sterile pad, if ordered. Encourage the child to avoid touching or scratching the area, and praise the child for cooperation.

Inhalation Therapy

Respiratory medications, used frequently in children, are delivered either by nebulizer or with a metered-dose inhaler, a handheld device that delivers "puffs" of medication for inhalation. Although many inhaled medications have an unpleasant taste or smell, this route is a relatively non-threatening form of medication delivery. Monitoring for desired therapeutic effects and systemic effects is essential because most medications used for inhalation have systemic side effects.

Nebulized medications are diluted in normal saline and administered with a handheld small-volume nebulizer (SVN or HHN). The SVN device aerosolizes the medication for the child to inhale. Medication can be delivered through a mask or through a plastic mouthpiece held between the lips or close to the face (Fig. 38–7). A mask is

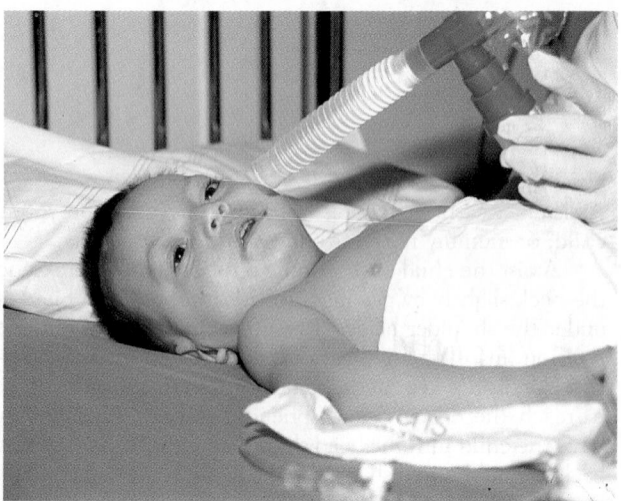

FIGURE 38–7

Administration of nebulized medication in an infant.

PROCEDURE 38-3

Using a Metered-Dose Inhaler

PURPOSE: To deliver medication directly to the respiratory system.

1. Verify the physician's order for medication(s) to be administered and number of puffs.
2. If one of the medications is an inhaled steroid, administer it last.
3. Explain the procedure to the child and parent or caregiver. It is often helpful to demonstrate the use of the inhaler and to explain specifically what the child is expected to do.
4. Place the inhaler in the spacer. Tell the child not to inhale too quickly or the spacer will whistle.
5. Tell the child to exhale (big breath out) and place the spacer mouthpiece in the mouth or the spacer mask over the face. The child might be more comfortable holding the spacer and helping you.
6. Tell the child that you will squeeze the inhaler and release the medication into the spacer. Then direct the child to inhale (big breath in) slowly. You may need to talk the child through this process.
7. Encourage the child to hold the breath for about 10 seconds or until you count slowly to 5.
8. Ask the child to exhale and then take another breath from the spacer and hold it for 10 seconds.
9. Repeat with another puff, if ordered. Praise the child for cooperation.
10. Rinse the inhaler adapter and spacer with cool water. Return the equipment to the medication room or designated area. Document.

---

preferred for young children because they are seldom able to successfully hold a mouthpiece in place for the required length of time. Encourage the child to breathe deeply and slowly during the treatment.

Metered-dose inhalers offer an inexpensive, portable means of delivering inhaled medications. Many people, particularly children, have difficulty using a metered-dose inhaler correctly. The effectiveness of these medications is increased with the use of an inhalation aid such as a spacer device. These aids might be equipped with a mouthpiece or a mask for young children or those who have difficulty using a mouthpiece.

Although both forms of delivering inhaled medications are effective, the nebulized medication offers the advantage of delivery with supplemental oxygen to children in an acute episode of respiratory distress. Nebulized medications can also be delivered to an unconscious or intubated child by inserting the aerosol administration device in-line between the child and a bag-valve mask.

Education of the parent and child is important to ensure the effectiveness of this form of medication delivery. The technique must be demonstrated and a return demonstration given. Use of the metered-dose inhaler should be reviewed at each return visit.

Intravenous Therapy

Intravenous therapy is widely used for children. Fluids and electrolytes, nutrition, blood products, and medications can be delivered by the IV route. When used to administer medications, IV therapy produces a steadier and more therapeutic blood level and is the only acceptable route of administration for some medications that might be irritating. The risks of IV therapy include possible fluid overload and possible complications with administration errors.

Intravenous Catheter Insertion

Typically, children's IVs are infused through an over-the-needle catheter or a butterfly catheter. The type of catheter chosen often depends on hospital policy. Over-the-needle catheters are generally preferred because they are more flexible and stable, thus decreasing the risk of infiltration. Over-the-needle catheters come in even sizes (e.g., 24 and 22 gauge), and butterfly catheters are available in odd sizes (e.g., 23 and 25 gauge).

Venous access sites in children are shown in Figure 38–8. The rate and type of fluid to be infused and the availability of veins often determine site selection in children. The nurse also considers the developmental level of the child. For example, placement of an IV line into the foot of a toddler is often a poor choice because it inhibits walking, a newly learned skill. Avoid inserting an IV into a dominant hand, if possible, because the site will interfere with activities of daily living. The hand, wrist, and antecubital sites are most frequently used in infants and children. Scalp veins are sometimes used in infants. Scalp veins have no valves and can be infused in either direction. IV catheters placed in this area can be adequately secured to allow the infant to move without dislodging the IV line.

Vein size and the kind of fluid to be infused also guide the choice of catheter. Generally, the smallest catheter through which fluids and medications can be safely infused should be used (often a 22- or 24-gauge catheter). For most children, a 20- to 24-gauge catheter provides adequate access.

Before an IV line is started, explain the procedure to the child and parent. Include information about what will happen (what the child will see and feel) during each step of the procedure, why the catheter will be placed, where it will be placed (if possible), how long it will be in place (if known), and what function it will perform. Explain to the parent the purpose of both the IV therapy and any additional equipment (e.g., an infusion pump). Reassure the parent that once the IV catheter is in and stabilized, the child can be held as usual. Bring the child to the treatment room.

Assess the child's ability to hold the affected extremity still during the procedure. Give children suggestions for coping with the discomfort and have them practice coping techniques in advance, if possible. Nonpharmacologic interventions include guided imagery (e.g., putting on an imaginary magic glove that keeps the hand from hurting) and distraction (e.g., music, novelty toys, seek-and-find books). Pharmacologic interventions include ice and topi-

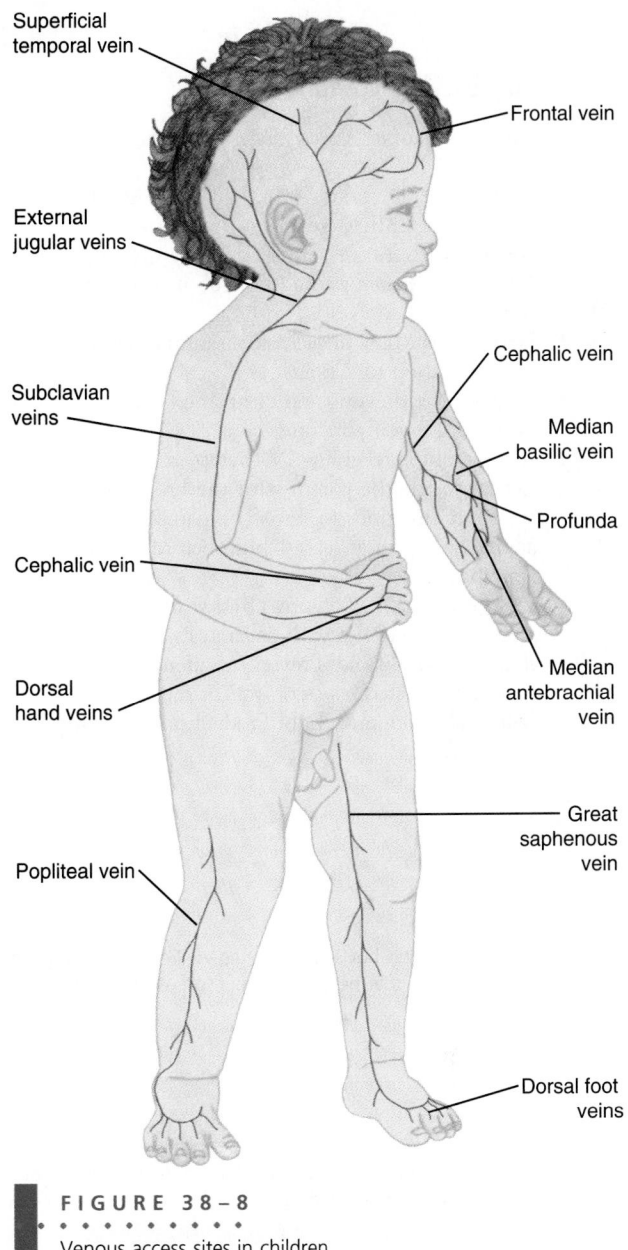

FIGURE 38–8

Venous access sites in children.

cal numbing gels or pastes, such as EMLA. Buffered lidocaine injections, although used in some instances, can be threatening to children because they require a needle puncture of the skin. If the child is not able to hold still, obtain assistance before attempting to start the IV. (See Chapter 39 for further discussion of pain management techniques.)

Have all the needed equipment ready in advance. Equipment includes an IV catheter of appropriate size, ordered IV solution, primed infusion set (most facilities now use needleless sets), extension tubing with a T-connector, tape, occlusive dressing or other sterile dressing, a padded arm board, a tourniquet, alcohol pads, gloves, and blood-sampling tubes (if required). Povidone-iodine preparations might be necessary for immunosuppressed children. Bacteriostatic normal saline, 3 ml, is used to flush the catheter after any required blood samples have been obtained.

Encourage parents to remain with the child if they desire. Parents should not, however, be expected to restrain the child during the procedure. Explain the procedure at each step. The nurse usually selects the IV site, beginning with the veins of the nondominant hand or forearm and moving proximally. As the catheter is inserted and the child experiences a "big sting" or "pinch," it might be helpful to advise the child to take a deep breath and blow out the pain.

Catheter placement is confirmed by a blood return. A normal saline flush verifies that there is no infiltration. After the catheter is placed, secure it in place with tape and a sterile clear occlusive dressing or tape and a small sterile dressing. The dressing allows for adequate visibility of the insertion site. Additionally, secure the catheter extension tubing to the extremity with tape. Be sure to leave the plastic clamp accessible.

After fully stabilizing the IV catheter and tubing, you might need to prevent injury by securing the extremity to a well-padded arm board. This is particularly important for active children. Secure the extremity in an anatomic position to prevent nerve damage. You can further protect the catheter by using a plastic shield. This can be a medicine cup that is cut in half and taped on the edges, or a commercially available device (Fig. 38–9).

Intravenous Monitoring and Maintenance

To prevent fluid overload in children receiving IV therapy, IV fluids or medications are administered through an infu-

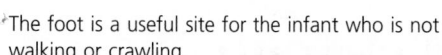

This boy's IV is secured well enough so he can pretend ▶ that he is Magic Johnson as he shoots baskets in the playroom.

The foot is a useful site for the infant who is not walking or crawling.

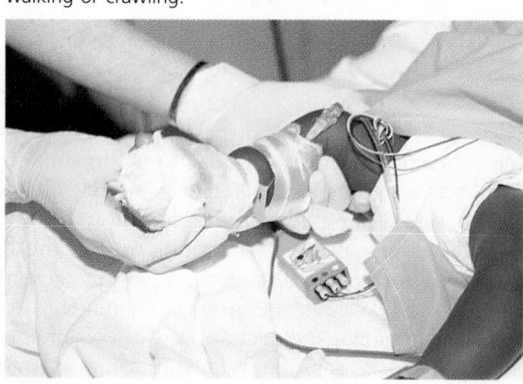

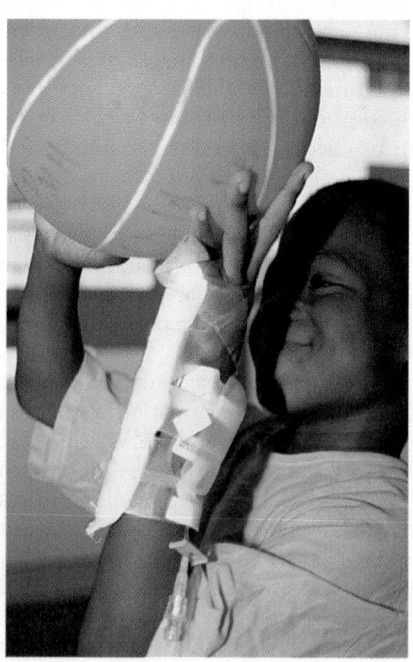

FIGURE 38–9

Because children's veins are fragile and IV lines can be difficult to place, the site must be well protected to prevent the child from removing the catheter and to tolerate the child's activity. Hand veins may be good for preschoolers and older children because IV lines placed here do not limit walking. A padded arm board gently limits movement of the foot or hand, reducing the risk of infiltration of the IV. A plastic shield allows visibility of the site while protecting it. (Courtesy of Parkland Health and Hospital System, Dallas, Texas.)

sion pump that delivers a preset volume at an hourly rate. Most infusion pumps are easily programmable with dose limits to prevent accidental fluid overload. If available, a pump with a tamper-proof design should be used.

An additional safety feature, used in many institutions, is the in-line volume-control set and tubing (burette; Buretrol, Soluset, Metriset), which is used in place of regular IV tubing. A volume-control set usually has a 100- to 150-ml capacity (a 1- to 2-hour supply of fluid). The nurse programs the infusion pump to deliver only the amount in the volume-control set; the clamp between the burette and the IV container remains closed to prevent fluid from inadvertently dropping into the volume-control chamber. Medications can be mixed with an appropriate amount of fluid in the volume-control set by injecting the medication through the available port. The infusion pump is then set at a rate to infuse the amount in the burette over the correct time period.

To precisely administer very low volumes of fluid or medications, a volumetric infusion pump is used (Baxter, Bard). A syringe with the appropriate fluid volume or medication is attached to primed, low-volume tubing and placed in the pump. After connecting the tubing to the child, the nurse programs the pump to deliver the volume of fluid or medication in the syringe over a specified time period (Fig. 38–10). Volumetric infusion pumps are used for both continuous and intermittent therapy.

The nurse assesses an IV site at least every hour (or according to institutional policy, if different) for signs and symptoms of infiltration or phlebitis. Using a transparent dressing over the IV site facilitates assessment. Feel the temperature of the site, observe for any redness or swelling, and assess for pain. One way to assess for infiltration is by observing for symmetry in the size and shape of limbs or scalp. Gently touch the site to determine whether it is soft or taut or whether the scalp site is boggy. If signs of complications (e.g., edema, erythema, pain, blanching, coolness, streaking of the skin above the vein) are noted, discontinue the infusion immediately and notify the physician. Elevating the extremity can decrease edema. Dry heat can be applied if the infused solution or medication is neither a vessicant nor a sclerosing agent.

Unlike the situation with adults, children's IV sites are not changed every 72 hours because of the fragility of children's veins and the difficulty of finding a new site. Change IV fluid containers every 24 hours and tubing according to hospital policy. Most facilities require tubing to be changed every 48 or 72 hours. Many institutions, however, change total parenteral nutrition tubing every 24 hours in an attempt to decrease infection rates.

Infusion Rates and Methods

In most instances the physician orders an hourly IV fluid infusion rate. The rate is based on normal fluid maintenance requirements and additional fluids to replace deficits as needed. At some facilities, nurses can adjust the child's IV rate to infuse fluids in the required time frame. In other facilities a physician's order is needed to adjust the IV infusion rate. Before adjusting the rate, the nurse must know the maintenance rates appropriate for the child's weight, to avoid increasing the rate too much and causing fluid over-

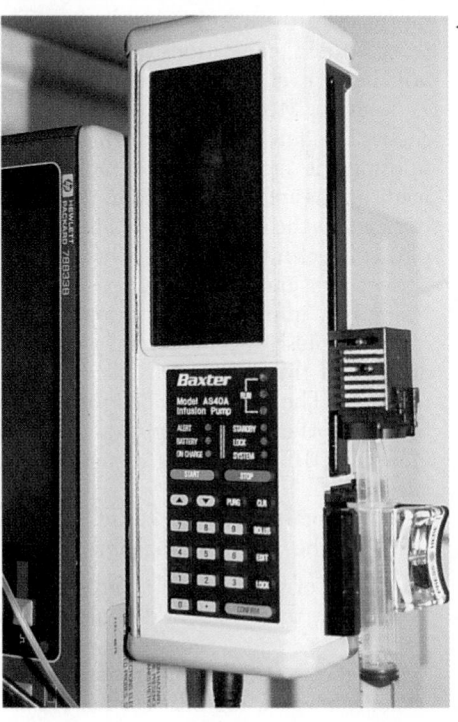

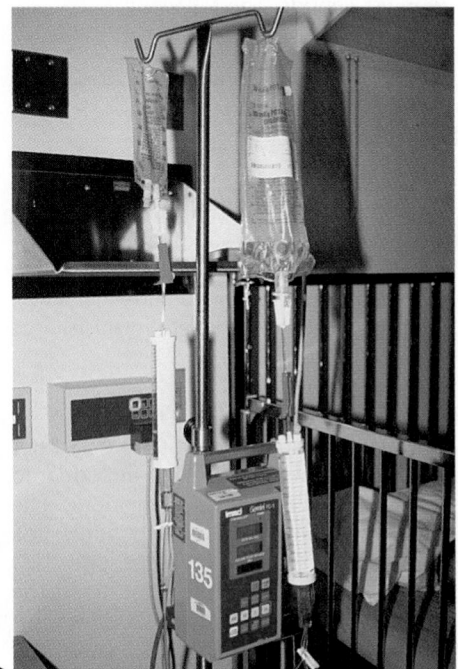

◄ Volumetric infusion pump.

In-line volume-control set. ►

FIGURE 38–10
. . . .
Two types of infusion pumps. (Courtesy of Parkland Health and Hospital System, Dallas, Texas.)

load. The nurse can determine maintenance fluid rates according to the following formula for daily fluid requirements:

0–10 kg	100 ml/kg/day
>10 kg–20 kg	1,000 ml for the first 10 kg of body weight + 50 ml/kg/day for each kg between 10 and 20
>20 kg	1,500 ml for the first 20 kg of body weight + 20 ml/kg/day for each kg in excess of 20

The preceding formulas give the daily fluid requirements. To determine an hourly rate, take the total milliliters per day and divide by 24. For example,

1. A child weighing 15 kg should receive 1,000 ml (1,000 for the first 10 kg) + (50 × 5) (50 ml/kg for each 1 kg between 10 and 20) = 1,250 ml/day.
2. The result is 1,250 ml/24 hr = 52 ml/hr.

It is most important to ensure that the appropriate amount of fluid is absorbing. *Even if the child is receiving fluids through an infusion pump, the nurse checks the fluid absorption at least hourly.* Pumps can malfunction, risking fluid overload if not meticulously checked.

Administering Intravenous Medications

Intravenous medications can be administered as a continuous infusion (e.g., potassium chloride) or intermittently (e.g., antibiotics). Methods of administering IV medications include piggyback, push, and retrograde methods. It is imperative that the appropriate method is chosen to meet the needs of the child and fit any restrictions posed by the medication and fluid volume.

When administering IV solutions and medications to children, the nurse must consider the following:

- Type of IV solution
- Compatibility of the medication and IV solution
- Dilution volume of the medication
- Amount of flush needed
- Administration rate

The administration method, type of IV tubing used, and hospital policies and procedures determine some factors, such as the amount of flush needed. Information about specific medications, their reconstitution, compatible fluids, and rates of infusion can be obtained from pharmacists, drug inserts, or texts.

INTRAVENOUS PUSH ADMINISTRATION

Medications delivered by IV push are reconstituted, but not diluted in additional solution, and are pushed directly into the IV catheter using the port closest to the patient. The volume of medication infused is small (usually <5 ml), and the effects (both desired and adverse) are immediate.

This method is used to give pain medications in the immediate postoperative period, administer sedatives, induce paralytic effects in ventilated patients, and administer other medications. To administer a medication by IV push, the nurse must first ensure that the medication can be administered safely in this way. Verify compatibility with the infusing solution (if there is a running IV line) and deter-

mine the administration rate (usually mg/min). If hospital policy requires, check the medication with another nurse or physician before administering it. In explaining the procedure, reassure the child that the procedure is painless.

Before administering the medication, check the IV site for complications and the running IV line for patency. Clamp the IV tubing above the injection port closest to the child, and clean the port with alcohol. Use Betadine if the line is a central access catheter or the child is immunosuppressed. If the medication is not compatible with the infusing IV fluid or if the medication is going into an intermittent infusion port, flush the tubing with approximately 2 ml of normal saline before and after administering the medication. Attach the medication syringe to the port and administer the medication at the prescribed rate. Medications given by IV push are usually administered slowly and should not be administered faster than the rate the manufacturer suggests. Remove the medication syringe, wipe the port with alcohol, and cover the port if the IV administration system requires a port cover.

Monitor the child carefully for the effects of the medication, including undesired side effects. This evaluation can be done by monitoring the child's vital signs (including blood pressure) and reassessing frequently.

INTRAVENOUS PIGGYBACK ADMINISTRATION

Medications given by piggybacking an IV line frequently are diluted in at least 20 ml of IV solution and administered over at least 15 minutes. These medications might be diluted by the pharmacy and sent to the nursing unit in a separate IV bag, or they can be prepared on the unit with a needleless mixing system, which allows the powdered medication to enter the diluent bag. The nurse can dilute reconstituted medications by injecting them directly into a volume-control set containing a predetermined amount of IV solution. Medications given by IV piggyback to children should be administered through an infusion pump to avoid infusing the medication too rapidly or too slowly. If the medications are to be diluted in the volume-control set, the nurse notes the total amount of fluid (volume of medication plus volume in the burette) when setting the pump for the correct infusion rate.

When infusing medications by piggyback, the nurse must also flush the IV tubing with fluid to complete the delivery of the medication out of the IV tubing and into the child. The volume needed for the flush varies and must be added when accounting for the total volume infused. Generally, 16 to 20 ml is required to flush the IV tubing adequately.

The total volume to be infused should be within safe limits for the child. For example,

- 150 mg of vancomycin is ordered for a 15-kg child. Remember that the child's maintenance hourly rate is 52 ml.
- The recommended concentration for administering vancomycin is 5 mg/ml. To achieve that concentration, 30 ml fluid would be needed (150 ÷ 5).
- Add a 20-ml flush, for a total volume of 50 ml to be administered over the course of 30 to 60 minutes.
- This amount is within the 52 ml hourly volume the child should be receiving.

Determine that the IV line is functioning and that the site is free of complications. Clean the injection port on the volume-control set with alcohol, and add the medication to the required amount of diluent. Agitate the volume-control set gently to mix the medication and diluent. Set the pump to infuse the medication; the rate should be based on the volume actually in the volume-control set. It is important to set the pump to alarm when the volume is infused so that the nurse can return and add the volume needed to complete the flush. Label the volume-control set with the medication added. Document what has infused. All flush and medication volumes must be added to recorded intake and calculated into the total volume limits to avoid fluid overload.

If the child does not have a running IV line but is receiving medication intermittently by piggyback, be sure to flush the IV catheter with saline before attaching the piggyback set. This procedure ensures patency of the line. In some instances, depending on hospital equipment, the medication and the regular IV infusion can be run concurrently, so long as the medication is compatible with the running IV fluid.

INTRAVENOUS RETROGRADE ADMINISTRATION

The IV retrograde method uses smaller volumes of both medication and flush and generally has a slightly shorter administration time than the piggyback method. The nurse clamps the IV tubing below the injection port nearest the child. After wiping the port with an appropriate cleansing solution, the nurse injects the medication into the port in a direction away from the child (retrograde), causing it to flow into the tubing above the injection port. The IV pump is then set to deliver the medication volume plus the amount of flush needed to flush the IV tubing from the injection port to the child.

Some infusion pumps do not allow the pressure created by retrograde infusion. To prevent a problem with back-pressure, low-volume extension tubing, two stopcocks, and two syringes are used for administration of the medication (Fig. 38–11). The syringe containing the medication is attached to the distal stopcock (the stopcock nearest the child), and an empty syringe of equal volume is attached to the proximal stopcock. The distal stopcock is turned off to the child and on to the extension tubing. The IV medication is injected through the distal stopcock into the extension tubing (away from the child). The empty syringe fills with the displaced fluid from the extension tubing as the medication is injected. The displaced fluid is discarded. The syringes are removed, and sterile injection caps are placed into each stopcock side port. The stopcocks are turned to resume the flow of IV fluid. The nurse must take extra care, however, when using the stopcock method to administer retrograde medications. Because the closed system is opened

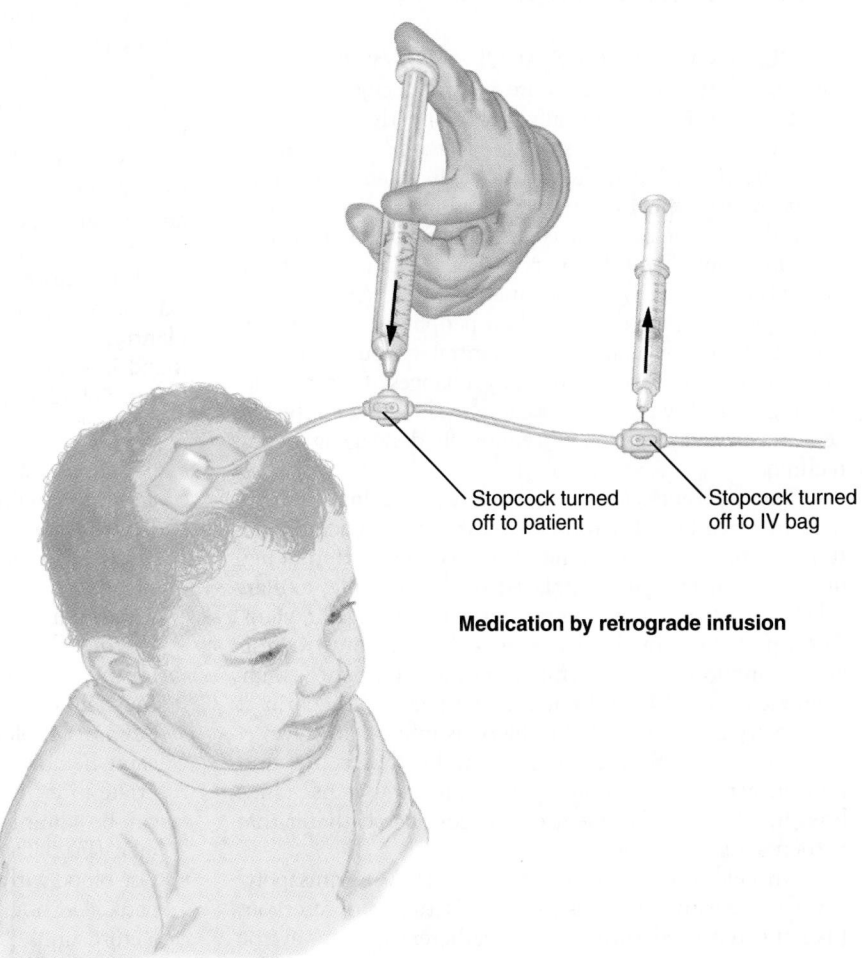

Stopcock turned off to patient

Stopcock turned off to IV bag

Medication by retrograde infusion

FIGURE 38–11

Retrograde infusion method used with an infusion pump that cannot accommodate the pressure created by the retrograde infusion.

each time a medication is to be administered, aseptic technique is particularly important. The nurse must also ensure that stopcocks are secured and kept away from children, who have a tendency to explore and could inadvertently open the system.

Venous Access Devices

INTERMITTENT INFUSION PORTS

Intermittent infusion ports (saline or heparin locks) allow drugs to be administered IV without the need for a running IV line. The intermittent infusion port is an IV catheter that is placed, flushed with normal saline or heparin to maintain patency, and then locked with a male adapter. The port is accessed when needed for fluid or medication infusion. Site observation and site care are the same as for any IV catheter.

The frequency of flushing is controversial and determined by personal preference and hospital policy. Routine flushing to maintain patency is performed every 6 to 12 hours. The device is flushed with saline before and after medication administration and with heparinized saline solution after blood is drawn or infused. The use of heparinized solution to maintain patency has also become controversial. Research has indicated that normal saline is as effective as heparin in maintaining patency in 22-gauge catheters but might not be as effective with smaller-gauge catheters (Beecroft et al., 1997; Mudge, Forcier, Slattery, 1998).

CENTRAL VENOUS ACCESS DEVICES

Central venous access devices are venous access devices in which the catheter is centrally placed directly into a major blood vessel. These devices are most often used to administer medications, blood products, IV fluids, and parenteral nutrition over the long term to chronically ill children. These devices can be tunneled or nontunneled central catheters and implanted infusion ports. *Peripherally inserted central catheters* (PICCs) are also used for children who need IV access for a period longer than peripheral IV catheters can be adequately maintained. Central venous access devices need routine care (dressing changes, flushing) according to facility protocol. Because these devices enter the central venous system, all procedures are done using aseptic technique.

Tunneled central lines are surgically placed lines that are held in place by a Dacron cuff located in a subcutaneous tunnel. They are most commonly placed in an external jugular vein but may also be placed in the cephalic, axillary subclavian, femoral, saphenous, or internal jugular veins. The tip of the tunneled catheter is threaded until it rests at the junction of the superior vena cava and right atrium. Tunneled central lines are usually flushed with heparin at least every 24 hours and after blood is infused or drawn.

Short-term or nontunneled central catheters are most frequently placed in the subclavian or femoral veins. These lines involve the placement of a large-gauge catheter that is then sutured in place.

An *implanted venous access device* (IVAD, Infusaport) consists of a catheter that is connected to a port or reservoir. Like the tunneled catheter, the catheter tip rests at the junction of the superior vena cava and right atrium. The port is under the skin and is accessed with a noncoring needle placed through the skin into the port. The needle is then covered with a bio-occlusive dressing, and an extension set is attached to the end. When the port is no longer needed for infusions or obtaining blood specimens, the port is flushed with heparin and the needle withdrawn. The child with an implanted port can participate in all typical childhood activities, except those with a potential for high-impact contact with the chest (e.g., competitive football).

Peripherally inserted central catheters (PICC lines) are long catheters made of polyurethane or silicone and threaded through an introducer placed in the antecubital vein. They are usually placed by specially trained nurses and are frequently used for home antibiotic therapy. After the catheter is threaded so that the tip is located in the superior vena cava, the introducer is removed. The catheter is then covered with a bio-occlusive dressing, and placement is verified by x-ray. These catheters are usually left in place for several weeks to months. The major complications of this type of line are phlebitis, infection, and thrombosis (Macklin, 1997).

Administration of Blood or Blood Products

Education of the child and parent is essential whenever a transfusion is administered. Children and parents must receive all necessary information honestly, consistently, and at a developmentally appropriate level. Information includes why the transfusion is necessary, how long it will take, what the child will feel and hear, and the types of blood products to be used. Ask the parent or caregiver about the child's transfusion history and whether the child has ever experienced a transfusion reaction. The nurse discusses the risks of receiving versus not receiving the blood product and explains each step as it is to be performed. It is important to use clear, concise, age-appropriate terminology.

Information about the types of blood products, the indications and procedures for their administration, and the identification and treatment of transfusion reactions is found in standard medical-surgical nursing texts. The key features of administration of blood products to children are as follows:

- To prevent circulatory hypervolemia, packed red blood cells are usually administered to infants and children.
- Identify the child and verify blood (type, Rh factor, donor number, expiration date) with another nurse or physician.
- Take vital signs, including blood pressure, before administering blood. Then take vital signs every 15 minutes for the first 2 hours and every 30 minutes thereafter until the infusion is complete.
- Administer blood with normal saline (dextrose solutions cause hemolysis) on a piggyback setup, through an appropriate filter. If a central line is in place, other solutions can be administered concurrently through a different lumen (Fitzpatrick & Fitzpatrick, 1997)
- Use blood within 30 minutes of its arrival from the blood bank. Do not store blood in regular unit refrigeration. Return unused blood to the blood bank. Order only as much blood as can be used in 4 hours.

- The rate of infusion of packed red blood cells is approximately 5 ml/kg/hr over no more than 4 hours (Oakes & Rosenthal-Dichter, 1998). Run the infusion slowly for the first 15 minutes because many transfusion reactions are seen during this brief period. If the child has not displayed any signs of a reaction during this time, increase the rate to the ordered rate for the remainder of the dose.
- Cytomegalovirus-negative blood, blood that has tested negative for cytomegalovirus, is used for cytomegalovirus-negative, immunocompromised children, low-birth-weight neonates, bone marrow transplant recipients, and children younger than 2 years who are receiving chemotherapy.
- Blood that has been irradiated to prevent lymphocyte replication helps to prevent graft-versus-host disease in immunocompromised children, such as bone marrow transplant recipients; it also is used in neonates.
- Although type and crossmatch should be less than 48 hours old, infants younger than 4 months rarely form red cell antibodies and therefore usually undergo a type and crossmatch only once. These results can be used until the infant reaches 4 months of age or is discharged from the hospital (Kevy & Gorlin, 1998).
- During the administration of blood or blood products, the child and parents should notify the nurse immediately if the child feels "bad" or has fever or chills, headache, nausea, pain at the needle site, or difficulty breathing. Children and parents often do not know how they are supposed to feel and will not notify the nurse of the signs and symptoms of a transfusion reaction. The child should not be left alone while receiving blood products.
- In neonates and small infants, auscultate the lungs before and frequently during a transfusion to detect signs of respiratory distress from fluid overload.
- If a reaction is suspected, stop the transfusion immediately and infuse normal saline through new tubing. Notify the physician. Continue to monitor vital signs. Monitor urine output hourly, and send samples of the child's blood and urine to the laboratory.
- If the child's maintenance IV rate was decreased to avoid fluid overload, the blood sugar level must be monitored with reagent strips (Dextrostix) or another form of measurement because reducing the maintenance IV rate decreases the amount of IV glucose received by the child and may lead to hypoglycemia.
- After the transfusion, praise the child and family for their cooperation and help during the procedure.

Child and Family Education

Teaching children and their caregivers about medications is an essential part of therapy. Statistics about compliance suggest that approximately 50% of children taking medications for an acute condition complete their prescribed regimen. Compliance is higher in children taking medication for a chronic health problem (Matsui, 1997). In addition to such factors as forgetting to give a medication, refusal to take the medication because of unpleasant taste, and discontinuing a medication because symptoms have improved, lack of understanding about a medication and its effects is a major reason cited for noncompliance (Matsui, 1997).

Teaching the family about medications begins with a thorough assessment that includes a list of all medications the child is currently taking, including over-the-counter medications. Any history of allergies to medications should be noted to prevent potential drug interactions.

Note as well any special learning needs, such as a hearing or speech disability, language barrier, or illiteracy. The nurse must make provisions to accommodate the child's special needs. For example, information should be presented in a variety of ways (e.g., spoken, written, and illustrated). Written instructions should accompany any oral instruction.

Problem-solve with the family before discharge. This process includes devising acceptable schedules for medication administration, suggesting alternative methods of administering oral medications (e.g., crushing and mixing with food), and identifying foods that might be mixed with the medications.

Emphasize taking the medication as ordered. Particularly highlight finishing the full course of a prescribed antibiotic, not changing dosages without consulting the physician, and returning for follow-up appointments.

Reinforce general safety information, such as keeping medications out of the reach of children and keeping all medications in their original containers. Evaluate your interventions by asking questions (scenarios work well) and providing a demonstration and asking for a return demonstration. Document all teaching and validation of understanding.

KEY CONCEPTS

- Standardized dosage ranges for many medications have not been established for children.
- A child's body proportions and composition are different from those of adults, and a child's response to medications differs accordingly.
- The nurse must incorporate principles of growth and development into medication administration.
- The margin of safety for medication administration is narrow for pediatric patients.
- Oral medications should be administered using developmentally appropriate equipment.
- Injections are stressful to children and are not usually the first

choice of administration route. Take care to choose the appropriate site for the child's size and age, and use the shortest and smallest-gauge needle possible to ensure safe administration of the medication.

- The site selected for venipuncture is often determined by the rate and type of fluid to be infused and the availability and accessibilty of veins.
- Children receiving IV infusions should receive their fluids through a pump that can be set to deliver a predetermined amount of fluid safely. A volume-control set can be used as well to decrease the chance of fluid overload.

- A baseline assessment must be performed before a blood product is administered to a child. This assessment includes auscultating an infant's lungs so that signs of fluid overload during the transfusion are immediately recognized.
- As with any client, the infant or child receiving a transfusion needs to be carefully monitored throughout the procedure to assess effects and adverse reactions.
- Education of the child and parent is important to ensure that medications are administered to achieve therapeutic effects and avoid dangerous side effects.

ANSWERS TO CRITICAL THINKING EXERCISE 38–1

1. The nurse needs to emphasize the following to the father:
   - Even though symptoms have disappeared, it is important for the child to take the entire amount of medication.
   - The medication prescribed is the one best able to treat the child.
   - Some children do react adversely to certain tastes, but

there are methods of disguising the taste.
   - Children of this age will react positively to expectations for compliance.

2. If, after a firm statement of expectation by the father for the child to take the medication, the child still refuses, suggest to the father that

he try mixing the medication in a small (2-teaspoon) amount of a liquid (juice, soda) to disguise the taste. The nurse can also describe how to hold the child properly for administering an oral medication with control. If these methods do not work, the father should call back.

REFERENCES AND READINGS

Anderson, K. C., & Ness, P. M. (1994). *Scientific basis of transfusion medicine.* Philadelphia: Saunders.

Arts, S. E., Abu-Saad, H. H., Champion, G. D., Crawford, M. R., Fisher, R. J., Juniper, K. H., & Ziegler, J. B. (1994). Age related response to lidocaine-prilocaine (EMLA) emulsion and effect of music distraction on the pain of intravenous cannulation. *Pediatrics, 93*(5), 797–801.

Beecroft, P. C., et al. (1997). Intravenous lock patency in children: Dilute heparin versus saline. *Journal of Pediatric Pharmacy Practice, 2*(4), 211–223.

Centers for Disease Control. (1995). *Epidemiology and prevention of vaccine preventable diseases.* Atlanta: Author.

Fitzpatrick, L., & Fitzpatrick, T. (1997, August). Blood transfusion. *Nursing 97,* 34–42.

Ford, D., Leist, E. R., & Phelps, S. J. (1993). *Guidelines for administration of intravenous medication to pediatric patients* (4th ed.). Bethesda, MD: American Society of Hospital Pharmacists.

Gulanick, M., Gradishar, D., Puzas, M. K., & Gettrust, K. V. (1994). *Ambulatory pediatric nursing.* Albany, NY: Delmar.

Hanrahan, K., Kleiber, C., & Fagan, C. A. (1994). Evaluation of saline for IV locks in children. *Pediatric Nursing, 20*(6), 549–552.

Harovas, J., & Anthony, H. (1993). Your guide to trouble-free transfusions. *RN, 56*(11), 26–34.

Heilskov, M. A., Johnson, K., & Miller, J. (1998). A randomized trial of heparin and saline for maintaining intravenous locks in neonates. *Journal of the Society of Pediatric Nurses, 3*(3), 111–115.

Kachoyeanos, M., & Friedhoff, M. (1993). Cognitive and behavioral strategies to reduce children's pain. MCN: *American Journal of Maternal/Child Nursing, 18*(1), 14–19.

Kelley, S. J. (1994). *Pediatric emergency nursing* (2nd ed.). Norwalk, CT: Appleton & Lange.

Kemper, K. J. (1997). A practical approach to chronic asthma management. *Contemporary Pediatrics, 14*(8), 86–95.

Kevy, S., & Gorlin, J. (1998). Red cell transfusion. In D. G. Nathan & S. H. Orkin (Eds.), *Hematology of infancy and childhood* (5th ed.). Philadelphia: Saunders.

Kleiber, C., Hanrahan, K., Fagan, C. A., & Zittergruen, M. (1993). Heparin vs. normal saline for peripheral IVs in children. *Pediatric Nursing, 19*(4), 405–409.

Koss, J. (1997, Fall/Winter). Making medical procedures less stressful. *Nursing in Pediatrics,* 16–17.

LeDuc, K. (1997). Efficacy of normal saline solution versus heparin solution for maintaining patency of peripheral intravenous catheters in children. *Journal of Emergency Nursing, 23*(4), 306–308.

Macklin, D. (1997). How to manage PICCs. *American Journal of Nursing, 97*(9), 27–33.

Matsui, D. (1997). Drug compliance in pediatrics. *Pediatric Clinics of North America, 44*(1), 1–14.

McMullen, A., Fioravanti, I. D., Pollack, V., Rideout, K., & Sciera, M. (1993). Heparinized saline or normal saline as flush solution in intermittent intravenous lines in infants and children. MCN: *American Journal of Maternal/Child Nursing, 18*(2), 78–85.

Medical Economics Data Production Company. (1999). *Physicians' desk reference* (53rd ed.). Montvale, NJ: Author.

Mudge, B., Forcier, D., & Slattery, M. J. (1998). Patency of 24-gauge peripheral intermittent infusion devices: A comparison of heparin and saline flush solutions. *Pediatric Nursing, 24*(2), 142–145.

Niederhauser, V. (1997). Prescribing for children: Issues in pediatric pharmacology. *Nurse Practitioner, 22*(3), 16–28.

Nursing 99 Books. (1999). *Nursing 99 drug handbook.* Springhouse, PA: Springhouse.

Oakes, L., & Rosenthal-Dichter, C. (1998). Hematology and immunology. In M. Slota (Ed.), *Core curriculum for pediatric critical care nursing.* Philadelphia: Saunders.

Rakel, B., Titler, M., Goode, C., Barry-Walker, J., Budreau, G., & Buckwalter, K. (1994). Nasogastric and nasointestinal feeding tube placement: An integrative review of research. *AACN Clinical Issues, 5*(2), 194–206.

Reed, M. (1996). Principles of drug therapy. In W. Nelson, R. Behrman, R. Kliegman, & A. Arvin (Eds.), *Nelson textbook of pediatrics* (15th ed.). Philadelphia: Saunders.

Sansivero, G. E. (1995, July). Why pick a PICC? *Nursing '95,* 35–41.

Taylor, D., et al. (1996). Use of occlusive dressings on central venous catheter sites in hospitalized children. *Journal of Pediatric Nursing, 11*(3), 169–174.

Theroux, M. C., West, D. W., Corddry, D. H., Hyde, P. M., Bachrach, S. J., Cronan, K. M., & Kettrick, R. G. (1993). Efficacy of intranasal midazolam in facilitating suturing lacerations in preschool children in the emergency department. *Pediatrics, 91*(3), 624–627.

U.S. Department of Health and Human Services. (1993). *Transfusion alert* (NIH Publication No. 90-2668). Bethesda, MD: National Heart, Lung and Blood Institute, National Institutes of Health.

Vallino, L. (1998). I.V. HOUSE: Pediatric nurses contribute to refinement of IV protector. *Journal of Pediatric Nursing, 13*(3), 196–198.

Widmer, A. F. (1993). IV related infections. In R. P. Wenzel (Ed.), *Prevention and control of nosocomial infections* (2nd ed., pp. 556–579). Baltimore: Williams & Wilkins.

39

Pain
Management
for Children

After studying this chapter, you
should be able to:

- Define pain.
- Discuss the gate-control theory of
  pain.
- Discuss the myths and realities of
  pain.
- Differentiate between acute and
  chronic pain.
- Explain the assessment of pain in
  children according to children's developmental levels.
- Describe common pain assessment
  tools.
- Discuss nonpharmacologic and
  pharmacologic interventions that
  may be used to relieve pain in children.
- Use the nursing process to describe
  nursing care of the child in pain.

DEFINITIONS

AHCPR   Agency for Health Care
Policy and Research, a federal
agency established in 1989.

conscious sedation   "Light sedation"
during which the child retains airway reflexes and can respond to
verbal stimuli.

epidural   Situated within the spinal
canal, on or outside the dura
mater; synonyms are *extradural* and
peridural.

NSAID   Nonsteroidal anti-inflammatory drug, an aspirin-like drug
that reduces pain and inflammation arising from injured tissue.

pain   An unpleasant sensory and
emotional experience associated
with actual or potential tissue damage or described in terms of such
damage.

pain threshold   Level of intensity at
which pain becomes appreciable or
perceptible.

PCA   Patient-controlled analgesia:
self-administration of an analgesic
by a client instructed in doing so.
PCA usually refers to self-dosing
with an intravenous opioid.

TENS   Transcutaneous electrical
nerve stimulation, a method of producing electroanalgesia through
electrodes applied to the skin.

There is considerable difficulty defining, identifying, and treating pain in children. Infants and children are often unable to communicate the presence of pain or its intensity. In addition, some physicians and nurses have outdated beliefs about pain and pain control in infants and children (Table 39–1).

As a result of increased research on pain in children, the prescription and administration of analgesics in the pediatric population are improving. Newer resources and strategies for pain management, however, are not always implemented, underscoring the need for education. Nurses, who have frequent opportunities to interact with physicians and other health care workers, can make a significant difference in managing pain in infants and children. Individual nurses vary in their assessment of pain. Some of these differences have been linked to the nurse's experience and personal assessment style (Seymour et al., 1997).

Definitions and Theories of Pain

There are many definitions of pain. In a commonly accepted definition, pain is whatever the experiencing person says it is, existing whenever the person says it does (McCaffrey, 1972). The International Association for the Study of Pain defines pain as "an unpleasant sensory and emotional experience associated with actual or potential tissue damage, or described in terms of such damage" (1979). Whatever the definition, pain is subjective and personal. The problem in pediatric care is the infant's or child's inability to communicate the presence and intensity of pain.

Gate-Control Theory

Pain impulses travel between the initial site of injury and the brain, and certain mechanisms affect pain relief. According to the gate-control theory, proposed by Melzack and Wall in 1965, a gating mechanism at the level of the dorsal horn can facilitate or dampen the transmission of pain signals, and stimulation of the larger afferent nerves, which carry benign sensations, can blunt the transmission of pain signals. The gating mechanisms are influenced by the relative activity in the sensory fibers. Input from the large fibers closes the gate, whereas input from the small fibers opens it. For instance, rubbing an injured part activates large-fiber activity, which decreases the ability of small-fiber activity to open the gate. The theory further postulates that cognitive processes such as attention, emotion, and memory influence the gating mechanism and have an impact on the transmission of pain. The gate-control theory lends support for the use of both physiologic and psychological interventions in pain management.

TABLE 39-1

. . . .

Pain and Pain Management in Children: Myths and Realities

Myth	Reality
Neonates do not experience pain because of incomplete myelinization in the peripheral nerves and CNS.	Myelinization is not necessary for pain perception. Pain impulses are carried more slowly in the neonate, but there is a shorter distance for the impulse to travel.
Children have no memory of pain.	Feeding and sleeping differences have been reported in studies of infants who experienced pain, which suggests that the procedure had consequences extending beyond the event (Schechter, 1989).
There is a correct amount of pain for a given injury.	The amount of pain a child experiences cannot be predicted because of cognitive and emotional factors affecting the child (Schechter, 1989).
Children can easily become addicted to narcotic analgesics.	Health care workers often confuse physical dependence with addiction. The actual risk of addiction is very low (Agency for Health Care Policy and Research, Acute Pain Management Guideline Panel, 1992b; Zeltzer et al., 1997).
Narcotic administration can easily cause respiratory depression.	No data support the belief that children are at higher risk for respiratory depression than adults (Eland, 1990).

Acute and Chronic Pain

Children may experience acute as well as chronic pain. Acute pain usually has a sudden onset and continues for a limited time. Acute pain is experienced during and after procedures and after surgery, with fractures, and with other insults to the body. Chronic pain continues for an unpredictable period of time and affects the child's ability to live a normal life. Children with such chronic conditions as juvenile rheumatoid arthritis, sickle cell disease, and cancer experience chronic pain.

Research on Pain in Children

The past two decades have seen a tremendous increase in pediatric pain-related research. Research on pain in the very young, however, is still limited (Maikler, 1998).

In 1989, the Agency for Health Care Policy and Research (AHCPR) was created to focus on the development of scientifically based practice guidelines for selected problems. Pain was a targeted area. The development of guidelines for caring for children in pain were based on retrieval and review of articles related to postoperative, procedural, and trauma pain. The research studies tested pain assessment tools and pharmacologic and nonpharmacologic pain relief. Other studies included the description of pain in children, the development of pain assessment tools, and other issues related to pain in children. This work produced a document titled *Acute Pain Management Guidelines in Infants,*

Children, and Adolescents: Operative and Medical Procedures (AHCPR, 1992a). It is a useful guide for nurses working with children experiencing pain.

Identified needs include educating health care providers about effective pain management, making available information about pain management in neonates and infants, collaboration between nurses and physicians when managing pain in children, and support for nurses to influence pain management (Margolius, Hudson, & Michel, 1995). As new analgesics are introduced, their safety and efficacy in children will need to be tested (Maikler, 1998).

Myths About Pain and Pain Management in Children

Probably the two beliefs that interfere most with the provision of adequate pain relief in infants and children are fear of addiction and fear of respiratory distress. Table 39–1 lists and refutes other prevalent myths about pain and pain management in children.

Assessment of Pain in Children

Pain in children is multidimensional (Schechter, 1988; Wallace, 1989; Zeltzer et al., 1997) and is affected by emotional status, developmental level, culture and ethnicity, previous experience associated with pain, type of pain, temperament, parental response to child's pain, and sex. When

Assessment According to Developmental Levels

NEONATE AND INFANT

- Changes in facial expression, including frowns, grimaces, expressions of surprise, and facial flinching.
- Increases in blood pressure and heart rate and decrease in arterial saturation.
- High-pitched, tense, harsh crying.
- Generalized or total-body response in neonate and young infant that becomes more purposeful as the infant matures.
- Extremities may thrash about. Some infants exhibit tremors.
- Older infants rub painful area, pull away, or guard the involved part.

TODDLER

- Loud crying.
- Verbalizes words that indicate discomfort (ouch, hurt, boo-boo).
- Attempts to delay procedures perceived as painful.
- Generalized restlessness.
- Guards the site.
- Touches painful areas.
- May run from the nurse.

PRESCHOOLER

- May think the pain is punishment for some deed or thought.
- Crying, kicking.

- Describes the location and intensity of pain (e.g., "ear hurts bad").
- Regression to earlier behaviors (loss of bladder and bowel control).
- Withdrawal.
- Denying pain to avoid a possible injection.
- May have been told to "be brave" and deny pain even though it is present.

SCHOOL-AGE CHILD

- Able to describe pain.
- Fears bodily harm.
- Has an awareness of death.
- Stiff body posture.
- Withdrawal.
- Procrastinates or bargains to delay procedure.

ADOLESCENT

- Perceives pain at a physical, emotional, and mental level.
- Understands cause and effect.
- Describes pain.
- Increased muscle tension.
- Withdrawal and decreased motor activity.
- Uses words like sore, ache, pounding to describe pain.

assessing pain in a child, the nurse considers all of these factors. Assessing pain in infants and children is more difficult than in adults. Infants and young children do not have the language and cognitive abilities to communicate their pain, and the nurse must use a combination of behavioral and physiologic signs to assess pain in this age group (Van Keuren & Eland, 1997). Although older children may be able to verbalize their discomfort, they are often afraid of the cure (injections), or they may have been told to "be brave." Studies have shown that children are undermedicated for pain (Kachoyeanos & Zollo, 1995; Sutters & Miaskowski, 1997).

Assessment According to Developmental Level

NEONATES AND INFANTS

Because neonates and young infants have immature central nervous systems, without myelination of pain fibers, clinicians have long believed these children to be incapable of perceiving pain. Increasingly, however, research has challenged this assumption and suggested that very young children do indeed experience pain. (Gardner, 1994; Howard & Thurber, 1998; Phillips, 1995; Van Cleve, Johnson, & Pothier, 1996).

Because infants are preverbal, the nurse's pain assessment should be based on physiologic, biochemical, and behavioral responses. Although biochemical measures indicate hormonal and metabolic changes in infants experiencing pain, such measures are difficult to obtain in the acute care setting. Physiologic changes are more easily assessed. Increases in blood pressure and heart rate and decreases in arterial oxygen saturation have been associated with pain in neonates, although these changes can also be linked to other alterations in the infant's body. Distinguishing between pain and agitation is sometimes difficult. If an infant is treated for pain and the cause is agitation, the intervention will be inappropriate, and the agitation may increase (Gardner, 1994). Crying may affect the infant's physiologic response. Rawlings, Milles, and Engel (1980) reported that oxygenation will decrease in response to pain but may increase after vigorous crying, so that data can be confusing. The nurse should realize that the physiologic changes are just one part of the assessment of pain in the neonate and infant and should suspect that an infant is in pain before physiologic changes occur.

Indicators of infant pain include fussiness, restlessness, grimacing, crying, an increasing heart rate, an increasing respiratory rate, wiggling, rapid state changes, wrinkling of forehead, and clenching of fists (Howard & Thurber, 1998). Some researchers assert that facial expression is the best indicator of pain in infants (Johnston & Strada, 1986). Facial expression, in combination with short latency to onset of cry and a long duration of the first cry cycle, typifies infants' reactions to acute invasive procedures (R. Grunau, Johnston, & Craig, 1990). Cries associated with pain may sound different from those associated with hunger, discomfort, and stress (Anand & Hickey, 1987); these cries are higher-pitched, tense, and harsh. Parents and nurses may therefore be able to differentiate between the usual cries of infants and the cries of pain.

CRITICAL THINKING EXERCISE 39–1

You are about to care for a 3,500-g full-term neonate who is status 24 hours post operative diaphragmatic hernia repair. The nurse who has been caring for Jane reports that Jane has slept for small periods throughout the shift, sucks vigorously on her pacifier, and occasionally cries. The nurse notes that she has not medicated Jane for pain because she does have periods when she sleeps for 15 to 30 minutes. Her blood pressure is 98/74, pulse 170, and respirations 50/min.

1. What would be your first nursing action?
2. What principles related to pediatric pain control would apply to this infant?

Motor movements associated with pain in the neonate and infant progress from a generalized bodily response to more purposeful movements. For example, infants ages 9 to 12 months can use their hands to push the nurse away if they perceive a painful action about to begin (Mills, 1989). The responses of neonates to painful stimuli are sometimes described as total-body responses (Fig. 39–1). The infant's extremities may thrash about, and some infants exhibit tremors. Older infants may rub the painful area, pull away, or guard the involved body part.

TODDLERS

The toddler experiencing pain tends to cry longer than the infant. As verbal abilities become more advanced, the toddler can verbally express displeasure when a painful experience occurs. The toddler asks for parents, verbalizes words that indicate discomfort ("ouch," "hurt"), and may attempt to delay the nurse's attempts to do a procedure perceived as painful. The older toddler can often show the part of the body that hurts.

Generalized restlessness, guarding the site, and touch-

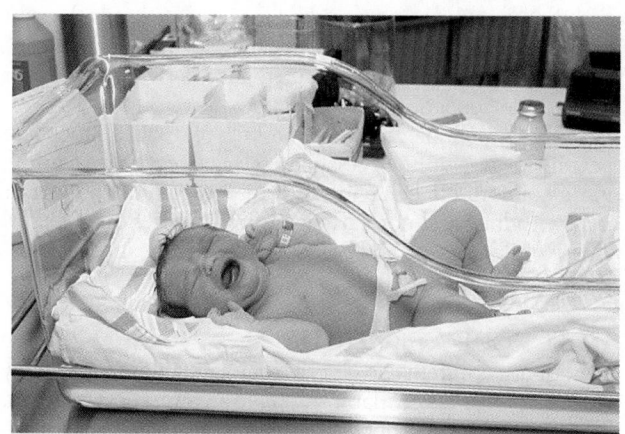

FIGURE 39–1

Neonates and infants have a total-body response to pain. Parents can usually distinguish the infant's cry of pain from other cries because it is tense, high-pitched, and harsh-sounding.

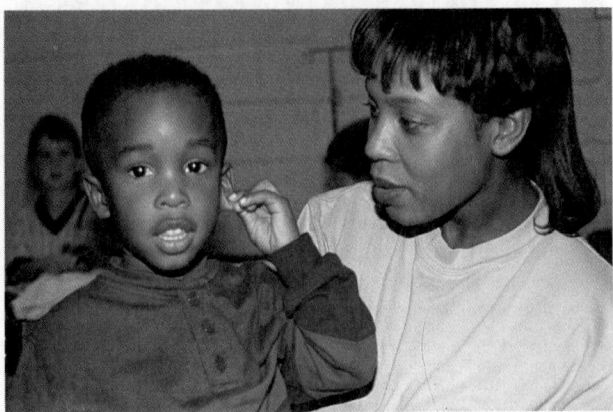

FIGURE 39-2

Toddlers and preschoolers may express pain by guarding or touching the painful area. Pulling on the ear is a characteristic expression of ear pain that accompanies otitis media. (Courtesy of The University of Texas at Arlington School of Nursing, Arlington, Texas.)

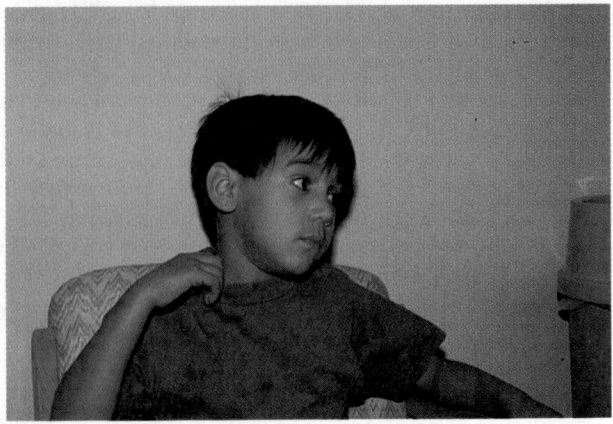

FIGURE 39-3

School-age children may withdraw and become very quiet when they are ill or in pain. Notice how dull this boy appears. Although he has asthma, his mother knew something else was wrong because he was unusually quiet and withdrawn. (Courtesy of Parkland Health and Hospital System Community Oriented Primary Care Clinic, Dallas, Texas.)

ing the painful area are signs of pain in the toddler (Fig. 39–2). The toddler may associate discomfort with a particular procedure, like a dressing change, and may run from the nurse when approached. The toddler's face may show anger and fear. The child may avoid eye contact or look sad.

PRESCHOOLERS

Preschoolers are egocentric. Relating only to the here and now, they cannot relate discomfort to any positive outcome. For example, the preschooler will not understand how debriding a painful burn will ultimately have a positive effect. The child who is unable to understand why an uncomfortable procedure might be positive may find pain disorienting and be affected more profoundly than older children (Schechter, 1988).

Preschoolers tend to think pain will magically go away and that they are being punished for some previous thought or deed. They also fear body mutilation; males in this age group fear castration. Preschoolers may deny pain in order to avoid an injection.

The preschooler may cry and kick to avoid a procedure perceived as painful. Preschoolers may regress to earlier, more comfortable behaviors as a response to discomfort or may withdraw and not participate in activities on the unit. These children can, however, describe the location and intensity of pain.

SCHOOL-AGE CHILDREN

School-age children can describe pain and relate it to a body part. They fear bodily harm and have an awareness of death. Therefore, they may appear to overreact to illness or injury. As in all age groups, the school-age child remembers previous pain experiences, which will affect the child's response. The child's culture, sex, and cognitive abilities will also affect the pain experience.

Nonverbal cues are very important in school-age children. The child may exhibit a stiff body posture, may

withdraw, or may be found quietly sobbing (Fig. 39–3). If the school-age child resists a treatment, cries loudly, or otherwise acts in an aggressive manner, the child may later deny the behavior. School-age children may also make attempts to procrastinate or bargain to delay a painful procedure.

ADOLESCENTS

Adolescents can perceive pain at a physical, emotional, and mental level. They can think abstractly, understand cause and effect, and clearly describe pain, their feelings about pain, and the strategies that help when they experience pain (Savedra, Tesler, & Wegner, 1988). Having these abilities does not mean the adolescent will exercise them. Adolescents are often confused by control issues and are uncertain of their role as they move from childhood to adulthood. Regression may also occur.

CRITICAL TO REMEMBER

Assessing Pain in Children

- Physiologic changes are only one source of information when assessing pain in the infant and neonate and should not be relied on before intervening. Behavioral changes must also be assessed.
- The use of a pain assessment tool is imperative in the assessment of pain in children. The tool is part of the child's chart.
- Fear and anxiety may also cause physiologic changes. Because physiologic changes tend to occur during the acute period and then return to normal, they are not valid indicators of chronic pain.

TABLE 39–2

Pain Assessment Tools

Tool	Description	Age
The Oucher (Beyer, 1984, 1989; Beyer & Aradine, 1986; Beyer, Denyes, & Villarruel, 1992; Beyer & Knott, 1998)	A poster with two scales: one is numeric, for use by children who can count to 100; the other is a photographic scale to be used by children who cannot count to 100. The bottom picture (or 0) is no pain; the top picture (or 100) is the greatest pain (see Fig. 39–4).	3 to 12 years
Poker Chip Tool (Hester, 1979)	Four poker chips are used; each chip represents a piece of hurt. One poker chip represents a little hurt, and four chips represent the most hurt the child could have.	4 to 12 years
The Adolescent and Pediatric Pain Tool: APPT (M. Savedra et al., 1989; M. C. Savedra et al., 1992)	Three-part tool composed of a body outline, an intensity scale, and a pain descriptor word list (see Fig. 39–5).	8 to 17 years
Visual analog scale (VAS)	Usually a 10-cm line with one end representing "no pain" and the opposite end "the worst pain."	Older school-age children and adolescents. May be used by younger school-age children, but less abstract tools are more appropriate.
Numeric rating scale (NRS)	Uses numbers (e.g., 0 to 10 or 0 to 100) to indicate increasing pain.	Child must know numbers.

Because adolescents are egocentric, they tend to think that others also focus on their behavior and so may suppress manifestations of pain or expect the nurse to be aware of it. Adolescents tend to exhibit fewer outward signs of pain than young children. Signs observed in the adolescent include increased muscle tension, withdrawal, and decreased motor activity. Hospitalized adolescents use words such as "sore," "like an ache," "pounding," and "miserable" to describe pain. They complete the statement, "When I have pain, I most often feel . . ." with "sick to my stomach," "scared," "angry," "like crying, but I don't," "like hitting someone," and "like screaming" (Savedra, Tesler, & Wegner, 1988).

Assessment Tools

Several pain assessment tools have been developed so that more objective data on pain assessment can be collected. Self-report and behavioral instruments are available, and validity and reliability have been established for some of them. Children benefit when a pain assessment tool is used because they are given a simple and effective way to communicate the pain they are experiencing. Assessment tools provide more objective data, with less chance that the more discreet signs of pain will be overlooked. Unfortunately, they are not always used in the clinical setting.

An assessment tool should be selected according to the child's age and developmental abilities. Self-report tools are effective in children over age 4 years. The Oucher, the

Poker Chip Tool, and a faces scale are examples of tools for preschoolers and school-age children (Table 39–2). For some children, the African-American or Latino versions of the Oucher pain scale provide more culturally sensitive assessment (Fig. 39–4). The Oucher might also facilitate communication between health care providers and children. Matching the tool to the child's race and ethnicity can provide better information about pain experienced by children from nonwhite populations and so promote better pain control for these children (Beyer & Knott, 1998).

School-age children can understand concepts of order and number and can use numeric rating scales, horizontal word-graphic rating scales, and visual analog scales. Table 39–2 describes pain assessment tools and lists the appropriate age or developmental level for each tool (see Figs. 39–4 and 39–5). To avoid confusing the child and to obtain consistent data, the same scale should be used each time the child is assessed. Ideally, the child should be taught how to use the tool before pain is experienced (e.g., preoperatively). Obviously, in emergencies, such preparation will not be possible. Appropriate use of any tool is essential. Using a tool in a way other than the developer intended may invalidate the information obtained.

In assessing pain, the nurse should also

- Question the child (pain history, word used for pain—"owie," "hurt") (Table 39–3).
- Question the parent (pain history, cultural beliefs, other factors affecting child) (Table 39–3).

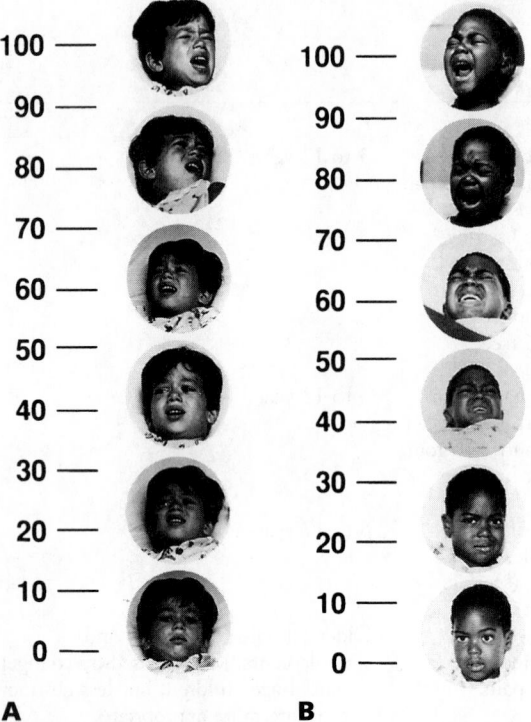

A   **B**

FIGURE 39-4
· · · · · · · ·

A. The Hispanic (Latino) version of the Oucher pain scale. (Developed and copyrighted by Antonia M. Villarruel, R.N., Ph.D., and Mary J. Denyes, R.N., Ph.D., 1991.) *B.* The African-American version. (Developed and copyrighted by Mary J. Denyes, Ph.D., R.N., FAAN [Wayne State University] and Antonia Villarruel, Ph.D., R.N., FAAN [University of Pennsylvania] at the Children's Hospital of Michigan in 1990. Cornelia P. Porter, Ph.D., R.N., and Charlotta Marshall, M.S.N., R.N., contributed to the development of this scale. Reprinted with permission.)

- Observe behavioral changes.
- Note physiologic changes (pulse, blood pressure, and respirations usually increase and then return to normal).

Nonpharmacologic and Pharmacologic Pain Interventions

At times, nonpharmacologic interventions are the only action needed to relieve discomfort. Some nurses prefer to use medication as the first line of action and thus subject the child to unneeded medication. At other times, the only way to break the cycle of pain is to give a pharmacologic agent. The nurse's assessment determines the appropriate intervention.

Nonpharmacologic Interventions

Parents play a very important role in controlling pain in children. They are a resource for determining what methods of pain relief were effective in the past and can aid the nurse in assessing their child's need for intervention. Holding, touching, massage, distraction, and relaxation are all techniques that can be done by the person the child trusts the most, the parent.

The nurse caring for a child in pain can sometimes relieve pain by reducing anxiety and fear of the unknown and by preparing the child for all procedures and treatments (see Chapter 35). The use of therapeutic touch can also soothe the child and reduce anxiety and pain.

DISTRACTION

Distraction is one of the most effective ways to relieve pain (Vessey et al., 1994) (Fig. 39-6). Distraction works by refocusing the child from the discomfort to something else. It does not imply total pain relief, and children experiencing severe pain cannot be distracted. The form of distraction should be appropriate for the child's developmental level. The child's ability to use distraction does not mean that the child is not experiencing pain. Children may distract themselves to "forget" their pain, but the child's watching TV does not mean the child is pain free.

Distraction may be accomplished with music, stories, number games, video games, board games, or even doing multiplication tables or spelling words. If a child has a favorite doll or stuffed animal, it may be used to create a story or a game. Children love to talk about their pets, and the nurse can ask the child to tell a favorite story about the pet. Another distraction technique is to allow the child to help by handing, opening, or holding objects. This technique should be used only when it is safe and there is no danger of contamination of materials or of a site.

For example, a child brought to the emergency department after an accident is invariably frightened. Even if the injury is minor by emergency department standards, the fear and pain are real to the child. Through the use of distraction, the nurse can decrease both anxiety and pain. Although each child is different, cues often indicate whether the nurse should hold the child's hand, touch the child's head, or provide some other intervention.

Once both the child and nurse can communicate personally, the nurse might say, "I see you have a baseball shirt on. Do you play baseball?" If the child expresses an interest in the game, the nurse can continue, "Which team is your favorite? What was the most exciting play you saw this year? Have you been to a game?" The nurse should be comfortable with the topic because the child will sense a lack of genuine interest. The nurse might interject a personal note: "I love baseball also. When I was a child, it was my biggest treat to go with my father to see the St. Louis Cardinals play." This conversation could go on for 10 to 15 minutes, certainly long enough for sutures to be put in or other minor procedures completed. The child will not be focusing on the procedure but rather on baseball. The topic is not important; the important thing is focusing the child on something other than the injury.

CODE _____

DATE _____

Adolescent and Pediatric Pain Tool (APPT)

INSTRUCTIONS:

1. Color in the areas on these drawings to show where you have pain. Make the marks as big or small as the place where the pain is.

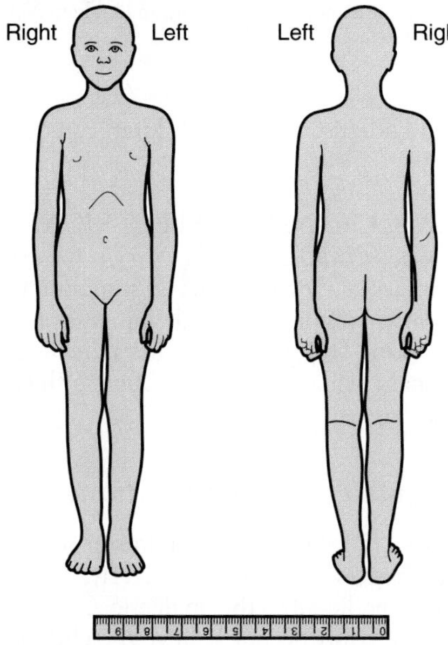

Right   Left   Left   Right

2. Place a straight, up and down mark on this line to show how much pain you have.

| No pain | Little pain | Medium pain | Large pain | Worst possible pain |

3. Point to or circle as many of these words that describe your pain.

1	5	10	15
annoying	blistering	awful	off and on
bad	burning	deadly	once in a while
horrible	hot	dying	sneaks up
miserable	6	killing	sometimes
terrible	cramping	11	steady
uncomfortable	crushing	crying	
2	like a pinch	frightening	If you like,
aching	pinching	screaming	you may add
hurting	pressure	terrifying	other words:
like an ache	7	12	
like a hurt	itching	dizzy	_____
sore	like a scratch	sickening	_____
3	like a sting	suffocating	_____
beating	scratching	13	
hitting	stinging	never goes away	For office use only.
pounding	8	uncontrollable	
punching	shocking	14	BSA: _____
throbbing	shooting	always	IS: _____
4	splitting	comes and goes	
biting	9	comes on all of	#S (2-9) ____ /37=____ %
cutting	numb	a sudden	#A (10-12)____ /11=____ %
like a pin	stiff	constant	#E (1,13) ____ /8= ____ %
like a sharp knife	swollen	continuous	#T (14,15)____ /11=____ %
pin like	tight	forever	
sharp			Total ____ /67=____ %
stabbing			

FIGURE 39–5

Adolescent and Pediatric Pain Tool, appropriate for use with 8-to 17-year-olds. (From Savedra, M. C., Tesler, M. D., Holzemer, W. L., & Ward, J. A. [1992]. *Adolescent and Pediatric Pain Tool: User's manual.* San Francisco: University of California, San Francisco, School of Nursing. Copyright © 1989, 1992. For original tools, write or call 415-476-4040.)

TABLE 39–3

Pain Experience History

Child Form	Parent Form
Tell me what pain is.	What word(s) does your child use in regard to pain?
Tell me about the hurt you've had before.	Describe the pain experiences your child has had before.
Do you tell others when you hurt? If yes, who?	Does your child tell you or others when your child is hurting?
What do you do for yourself when you are hurting?	How do you know when your child is in pain?
What do you want others to do for you when you hurt?	How does your child usually react to pain?
What don't you want others to do for you when you hurt?	What do you do when your child is hurting?
What helps the most to take your hurt away?	What does your child do when hurting?
Is there anything special that you want me to know about you when you hurt? (If yes, have child describe.)	What works best to decrease or take away your child's pain?
	Is there anything special that you would like me to know about your child and pain? (If yes, describe.)

Adapted with permission from Hester, N. O., and Barcus, C. S. (1986). Assessment and management of pain in children. *Pediatrics: Nursing Update, 1,* 2–8.

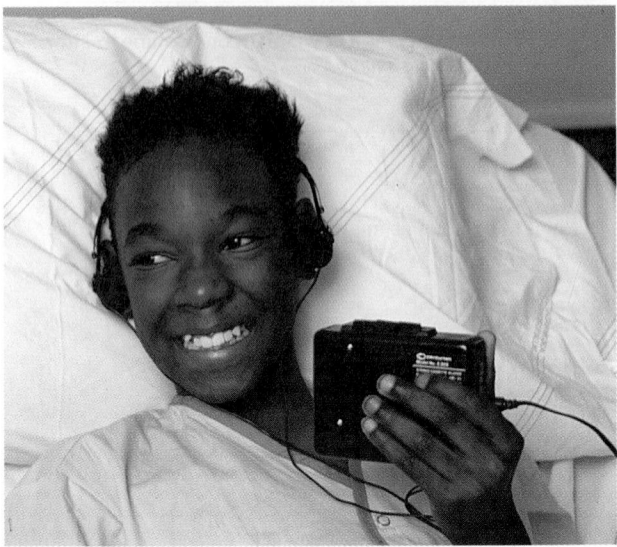

FIGURE 39–6

Distraction effectively reduces pain by helping the child refocus his or her attention. This boy listens to the radio through earphones, allowing him to be distracted without annoying others. (Courtesy of Children's Medical Center, Dallas, Texas.)

RELAXATION IMAGERY

Relaxation imagery is a process involving relaxation and focus on mental images. The child can be encouraged to think of a favorite place and then given permission to go to that place. The nurse, in a quiet, soothing voice, can guide the child on a "make-believe" trip. Breathing techniques can also relax the child. The child is instructed to take several slow, deep breaths while thinking pleasant thoughts. Children often need guidance, and the nurse may suggest remembering a birthday or a special time with family, friends, or a pet.

BIOFEEDBACK

Biofeedback provides visual or auditory evidence that physiologic changes are taking place. Visual feedback involving changes in colors or numbers or involvement in computer games are effective ways to use this technique. Biofeedback gives the child a response that can be seen instantly and can keep the child interested.

HYPNOSIS

Hypnosis is a form of focused attention, an altered state of consciousness, or a trance, often accompanied by relaxation. Hypnosis is effective in relieving pain and symptoms in children undergoing painful procedures associated with cancer, burns, and sickle cell disease. For example, hypnosis can alleviate the nausea and vomiting associated with chemotherapy (Cravero, Manzi, & Rice, 1988; Valente, 1991). Nurses need special training to learn hypnosis. In settings where this is not possible, the child who would benefit from this therapy should be referred to a qualified professional

Disadvantages of Intramuscular Analgesics

Altered tissue absorption leads to peaks and troughs in analgesia.
Children run out of sites quickly.
Intramuscular analgesics have a shorter duration of action than orally administered analgesics.
Intramuscular analgesics are contraindicated in children with low platelet counts.
Children hate them.
Nurses dislike administering them.

Adapted from Eland, J. (1990). Pain in children. *Nursing Clinics of North America, 25*(4), 871–884.

who can provide the service. Children can be taught self-hypnosis.

TRANSCUTANEOUS ELECTRICAL NERVE STIMULATION

In transcutaneous electrical nerve stimulation (TENS) a unit with electrodes delivers small amounts of electrical energy to the skin. The stimulation interferes with the transmission of pain signals and helps suppress the sensation of pain in that area.

Pharmacologic Interventions

Many nurses are reluctant to administer analgesics. Some nurses and physicians believe, incorrectly, that children will easily become addicted to the analgesic. Others fear respiratory distress or really do not believe the child is experiencing enough pain to warrant administration of an analgesic. If a procedure, surgery, or trauma causes pain in an adult,

PARENTS WANT TO KNOW

About Pain Relief for Their Child

- Parents are given a pain assessment tool, together with instructions on its use. They should give a return demonstration.
- The dose, route, and schedule of any pain medication to be given is explained to the parents orally and in writing.
- Nonpharmacologic interventions that are appropriate for the child's particular discomfort (e.g., massage, warm/cold compresses, reposition) are explained and demonstrated.
- Parents are instructed to notify the primary health care provider if pain relief interventions are ineffective or if the child shows behavior or physiologic changes not consistent with the expected outcomes for the child.
- A phone number where parents can contact a nurse if they have any questions about their child's condition is given to the parents.

then it will cause pain in a child. In some cases, however, the analgesia ordered might not be the appropriate dosage for the child, so that lack of adequate analgesia causes needless pain.

ADMINISTRATION OF ANALGESICS

Analgesics can be administered by various routes—oral, rectal, intravenous, intramuscular, epidural, and intranasal. (See Chapter 38 for a discussion of the common routes.)

Patient-Controlled Analgesia. One of the most effective ways of administering analgesia is through the use of a patient-controlled analgesia (PCA) pump. Children as young as age 6 or 7 can effectively and safely use a PCA pump (Houck, 1998). In some institutions parents or nurses activate the PCA pump for children under that age. Further research is needed on the use of PCA in the younger child.

The child receives small intravenous doses of the medication when a button connected to the pump is pushed (Fig. 39–7). After each dose the pump will not release the medication for a period, even if the button is pushed. The pump also delivers a maximum amount of medication over a given period, usually an hour. The child is checked frequently to ensure that pain control is effective and the equipment is functioning correctly.

The child should be monitored carefully for signs of overmedication (especially depressed respiratory rate or inability to rouse) and the side effects that may accompany narcotic administration. Vital signs should be assessed every

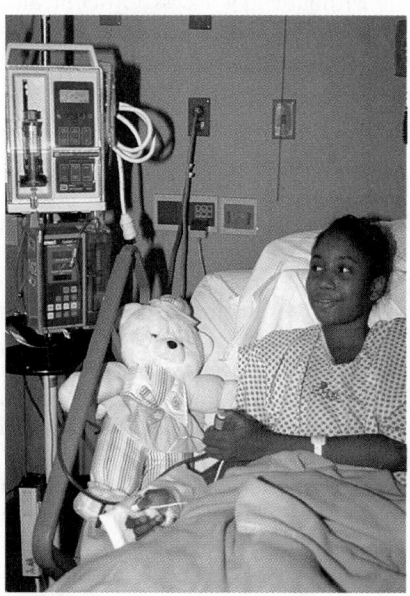

FIGURE 39–7

Patient-controlled analgesia (PCA) gives the older child greater control over pain management. The child presses the button when pain medication is needed and the machine delivers a preprogrammed bolus through the IV line. The child cannot overdose because the controller has a lock-out feature to prevent excess analgesia. (Courtesy of Children's Medical Center, Dallas, Texas.)

15 to 30 minutes when PCA therapy is first initiated and then every 2 to 4 hours thereafter. The policies of many institutions also require that children receiving PCA therapy be placed on continuous pulse oximetry or cardiorespiratory monitoring, or both. Oxygen, a bag and mask, and naloxone should be readily available.

Topical Anesthetic Cream. A topical anesthetic cream, lidocaine-prilocaine 5% cream (EMLA), can be used to reduce the pain associated with selected procedures, such as venipuncture, lumbar puncture, suture removal, immunizations, bone marrow aspiration, and removal of foreign bodies from the skin. Research related to the use of EMLA in the treatment of acute pain in neonates is ongoing (Taddio et al., 1998). The main side effect is skin blanching or redness, which lasts a few hours and actually helps "guide" to the anesthetized area (Zappa, 1994–95, Winter).

EMLA cream is applied liberally to intact skin under an occlusive dressing 60 minutes before anesthesia is needed. The cream is applied in a mound, not rubbed in. The duration of anesthesia is at least 2 hours and not more than 5 hours.

Parents may apply the cream at home before scheduled immunizations and successfully manage pain. EMLA comes with directions in Spanish and English for use by parents. Care should be taken with small children to avoid their removing the dressing and rubbing the cream in their eyes or eating the cream, which looks like cake frosting. Children may still fear needles, and distraction should be used until they realize the "stick" will not hurt.

NONSTEROIDAL ANTI-INFLAMMATORY DRUGS

Because of their ability to inhibit prostaglandin, nonsteroidal anti-inflammatory drugs (NSAIDs) are used primarily for pain associated with inflammation, bone pain, and rheumatic conditions. Aspirin, ibuprofen, and naproxen (Naprosyn) are three of the most common drugs in this category. Because aspirin has been associated with Reye syndrome, it is used cautiously in children.

Acetaminophen lacks the anti-inflammatory effects of the other NSAIDs and does not inhibit prostaglandin. It is the most commonly used analgesic and is the drug of choice for treating fever in children in the United States. It is used in managing mild to moderate pain. The short-term use of this drug is safe, even in neonates. It does not have the gastric side effects of aspirin, and although it can cause hepatic damage, this effect is usually related to overdosage.

OPIOIDS

Opioids are the preferred drugs in the management of most forms of acute severe pain, including postoperative pain, post-traumatic pain, the pain of sickle cell vaso-occlusive crisis, and chronic cancer pain. Some of the more commonly used opioids are morphine, codeine, meperidine, methadone, and fentanyl.

Although opioids may be given by most routes, the oral route should be used when it is effective and appropriate for the child. Elixirs are available for children who cannot effectively swallow tablets. The intravenous (IV) route can be used when the oral route is contraindicated. Intravenous opioids may be given by bolus or continuous infusion.

The nurse needs to remember that opioids produce sedation and respiratory depression in addition to analgesia. Other effects include nausea, vasodilation, cough suppression, urine retention, and constipation. Although these effects must be closely monitored, most children can tolerate these drugs if their dosages are adjusted. Nausea can usually be controlled through the administration of antiemetics.

Morphine is the preferred opioid in children. It reaches its peak effect 20 minutes after IV administration. It produces both sedation and analgesia. Maximum respiratory depression occurs 7 minutes after IV administration. Naloxone (Narcan) should be available to reverse the analgesia, sedation, or respiratory depression if necessary.

Meperidine (Demerol) should be used only for short-term pain control in children who have shown a bold allergy or intolerance to other opioids. The duration of analgesia is shorter with meperidine than with morphine. Some experts believe that meperidine should be given only IV in children (Zajac, 1992). Normeperidine, a metabolite of meperidine, has been associated with convulsions and dysphoria, especially with long-term administration. Meperidine is most often used postoperatively and in combination with other medications for procedural pain.

The use of meperidine (Demerol), promethazine (Phenergan), and chlorpromazine (Thorazine), known as DPT (or "pediatric cocktail"), is discouraged. This combination is thought to be outdated and can cause significant adverse effects, including respiratory arrest, prolonged sedation, and decreased oxygen saturation (American Academy of Pediatrics Committee on Drugs [AAPCD], 1995; Coté, 1994). A combination of opioids and benzodiazepines is much safer.

Fentanyl and its analogues (sufentanil, alfentanil) have a shorter duration of action than morphine and are 50 to 100 times more potent than morphine. Because much less histamine is released, these agents cause less vasodilation and pruritus. The short duration of effect makes these drugs appropriate for use when a short, painful procedure is to be performed (e.g., inserting a chest tube or changing a burn dressing) and when children are critically ill. Fentanyl should be administered in a closely monitored setting.

Methadone is metabolized very slowly and therefore has a prolonged duration of action. It is absorbed well after both oral and IV administration. Because of its long duration, it must be carefully titrated. It is equal in potency to morphine.

Codeine is the most commonly given oral opioid for moderate pain. It is usually given in combination with acetaminophen or aspirin. It can cause constipation and gastrointestinal upset.

Hydromorphone (Dilaudid) is very similar to morphine. It is approximately eight times more potent than morphine. It may be used to control chronic pain in cancer patients.

CRITICAL TO REMEMBER

Administering Analgesics to Children

- The preferred routes of administering analgesics to children are intravenous or oral.
- Infants and children receiving intravenous and epidural opioids should be monitored by pulse oximetry.
- Naloxone hydrochloride should be used to reverse the effects of opioids when oxygen and stimulation of the child are ineffective.

CONSCIOUS SEDATION

Conscious sedation is a medically controlled state of depressed consciousness that allows protective reflexes to be maintained, retains the child's ability to maintain a patent airway independently and continuously, and permits appropriate response to physical stimulation or verbal command (AAPCD, 1992).

Midazolam (Versed) is a short-acting drug that can be given by multiple routes—parenteral, intranasal, rectal, intramuscular, oral, or sublingual. It can be used for conscious sedation and preoperative sedation and as an induction agent for general anesthesia. The intranasal route of administration is used in pediatrics for procedures and as an induction to anesthesia. Advantages to using midazolam include minimal side effects, short duration of sedation, and ability to administer without an IV access. Other medications used for conscious sedation include ketamine, fentanyl, and propofol. After conscious sedation, the child's vital signs, oxygen saturation, and level of consciousness should be closely monitored.

EPIDURAL ANALGESIA

Pain medication (usually fentanyl or bupivacaine) can be administered through an epidural catheter inserted into the epidural space at the lumbar level and secured to the child's back with an occlusive dressing. This form of administration is most useful for children undergoing abdominal, thoracic, and major orthopedic surgeries. Because the medication does not cross the blood-brain barrier, it allows for control of pain without the side effects normally associated with narcotic administration.

Nursing care of the child with an epidural catheter is similar to that for a child receiving PCA therapy. The nurse monitors the child for adequate pain relief and the presence of undesired side effects (particularly decreased respirations), as well as for the complications that might accompany the catheter. "Log rolling" the child is preferable, and bnthe nurse avoids any action that would place pulling stress on the catheter. The nurse also monitors the catheter site frequently for slippage, bleeding, loss of cerebrospinal fluid, or a hematoma at the insertion site—a rare but serious complication that needs to be reported immediately. Other side effects include itching, nausea, and vomiting.

NURSING CARE

The Child in Pain

Nursing Diagnosis	■ Pain related to physical, biologic, or chemical agents (edema, disease process, surgery, infection, trauma).
Expected Outcomes	• The child will express less discomfort on an assessment tool, will display a relaxed body posture, and will exhibit reduced facial grimacing and decreased crying and behavioral change. • The child will return to the activity level he or she experienced before the discomfort began.

Intervention	Rationale
1. Observe and document signs of pain in the child (behavioral and physiologic). Note both verbal and nonverbal responses. Assess vital signs.	1. Assessment of pain in children is based on behavioral and sometimes physiologic changes. Infants and children have difficulty verbalizing pain. Physiologic changes vary in response to pain and should be evaluated together with other data.
2. Assess for factors that might be affecting the child (separation, fear, anxiety, loss of control).	2. The child's perception of pain and ultimate reaction to pain may be influenced by other factors.
3. Assessment of pain should be based on the child's developmental stage.	3. Infants and children at each developmental level have their own way of reacting to and coping with pain.
4. Utilize a developmentally appropriate pain assessment tool (see Table 39–2).	4. Infants and children have difficulty communicating about their pain, and assessment tools provide more objective quantitative information.
5. Note if the child's pain level is different when at rest, ambulating, playing, during procedures, and before and after receiving analgesics.	5. Pain relief measures can be enhanced by an understanding of cause and effect.
6. Implement nonpharmacologic pain reduction strategies: a. Distraction b. Relaxation techniques c. Cutaneous stimulation d. Quiet, calm environment e. Repositioning f. Decrease environmental noise/light g. Comfort measures (holding, rocking, music, books, touch, massage)	6. When appropriate, nonpharmacologic pain reduction strategies should be implemented prior to administering analgesics. a. Distraction interrupts the transmission of pain. b. Relaxation is also thought to interrupt pain. c. Cutaneous stimulation blocks pain transmission. d. A quiet, calm environment is more conducive to rest, which enhances the effects of analgesia. e. A change in position may relieve pressure or provide for a more relaxed, comfortable body. f. A quiet, comfortable environment can have a soothing, relaxing effect on the body. g. Comfort measures decrease anxiety and the skeletal muscle tension that often accompanies pain.
7. Administer the appropriate analgesic. Give by oral or IV route. Avoid injections.	7. Nonnarcotic analgesics are appropriate for mild to moderate pain. Narcotic analgesics should be given for moderate to severe pain. To avoid an injection, children may deny pain.
8. Involve parents in care.	8. The presence of parents may reduce fear and anxiety and thus reduce the amount of pain experienced. Parents also know their child best and can assist in the assessment of pain and its relief.
9. Evaluate and record the response to both pharmacologic and nonpharmacologic pain reduction measures.	9. Documentation aids in determining the effectiveness of pain relief measures.
10. Observe for side effects of medication.	10. Respiratory despression is the most serious side effect of opioids but is rare. Other side effects include nausea and vomiting, constipation, sedation, and personality changes.

11. Record the child's response to both pharmacologic and nonpharmacologic interventions. A copy of the pain assessment tool is part of the child's chart for easy reference.

11. Without documentation, the effectiveness of pain reduction measures cannot be evaluated.

Evaluation

- Does the child have less pain, as shown by a relaxed body position, verbalization of the absence of pain, absence of crying, and a return to normal activities?

KEY CONCEPTS

■ Pain is an unpleasant sensory and emotional experience associated with actual or potential tissue damage or described in terms of such damage.

■ The gate-control theory of pain postulates that gating mechanisms at the level of the dorsal horn can facilitate or inhibit pain transmission. The theory further states that stimulation of the larger afferent nerves, which carry benign sensations, can dull pain.

■ Two of the myths that interfere the most with the provision of adequate pain relief medication to infants and children are the fear of addiction and the fear of increased respiratory depression. Neither belief is supported by research.

■ Pain assessment in infants and children takes a multidimensional approach. The child and parent should be questioned and behavioral and physiologic changes noted.

■ Both pharmacologic and nonpharmacologic measures should be used in the treatment of pain in children. Morphine is the opioid of choice for severe pain and acetaminophen for less severe pain. Nonpharmacologic interventions include distraction, relaxation and imagery techniques, hypnosis, TENS, and biofeedback.

■ To effectively document pain management, a pain assessment tool should be used for each child. The tool should be developmentally correct and must be administered according to instructions, for the results to be valid.

ANSWERS TO CRITICAL THINKING EXERCISE 39–1

1. An assessment to determine objective and subjective data should be performed. You will be looking for both behavioral (crying, facial expression, motor responses) and physiologic cues. When Jane cries, describe the crying and duration. Note whether holding and cuddling can quiet her. If not, her behavior could be an indication of discomfort. Obtain current vital signs and compare them with earlier signs. One clue from the nurse giving the report was that Jane is not having periods of uninterrupted sleep. This information, together with the vital signs, type of surgery, and postoperative day are strong indications that Jane should be medicated for pain. After completing the assessment, a review of the chart will determine patterns, and a nursing judgment can be made. It should also be confirmed through documentation that pain medication was not given during the previous shift.

2. Research has shown that neonates do experience pain. Because they are preverbal, pain assessment is based on physiologic, biochemical, and behavioral responses. Biochemical changes are difficult to obtain. Physiologic and behavioral changes, plus an understanding of the type of surgery and postoperative day, are all valid indicators of pain in infants of this age.

REFERENCES AND READINGS

Agency for Health Care Policy and Research, Acute Pain Management Guideline Panel. (1992a). *Acute pain management in infants, children, and adolescents: Operative and medical procedures. Quick reference guide for clinicians* (AHCPR Pub. No. 92-0020). Rockville, MD: Public Health Service, US Department of Health and Human Services.

Agency for Health Care Policy and Research, Acute Pain Management Guideline Panel. (1992b). *Acute pain management: Operative or medical procedures and trauma. Clinical practice guideline* (AHCPR Pub. No. 92-

0032). Rockville, MD: Public Health Service, US Department of Health and Human Services.

Alfieri, D., & Cagen, D. (1995). Transdermal fentanyl. *Pediatric Nursing, 21*(1), 72–74.

American Academy of Pediatrics Committee on Drugs. (1992). Guidelines for monitoring and management of pediatric patients during and after sedation for diagnostic therapeutic procedures. *Pediatrics, 89*(6), 1110–1115.

American Academy of Pediatrics Committee on Drugs. (1995). Reappraisal of lytic

cocktail/demerol, phenergan and thorazine (DPT) for the sedation of children. *Pediatrics, 95*(4), 598–602.

Anand, K., & Hickey, P. (1987). Pain and its effects in the human neonate and fetus. *New England Journal of Medicine, 317*(21), 1321–1347.

Asprey, J. (1994). Postoperative analgesic prescription and administration in a pediatric population. *Journal of Pediatric Nursing, 9*(3), 150–156.

Beyer, J. (1984). *The Oucher: A user's manual and technical report.* Evanston, IL: Judson Press.

Beyer, J. (1989). *The Oucher: A user's manual and technical report*. Denver: University of Colorado Health Sciences Center.

Beyer, J., & Aradine, C. (1986). Content validity of an instrument to measure young children's perceptions of the intensity of their pain. *Journal of Pediatric Nursing, 1*(6), 386–395.

Beyer, J., Denyes, M., & Villarruel, A (1992). The creation, validation, and continuing development of the Oucher: A measure of pain intensity in children. *Journal of Pediatric Nursing, 7*(5), 335–346.

Beyer, J. E., & Knott, C. B. (1998). Construct validity estimation for the African-American and Hispanic versions of the Oucher Scale. *Journal of Pediatric Nursing, 13*(1), 20–31.

Boughton, K., Blower, C., Chartrand, C., & Dircks, P. (1998). Impact of research on pediatric pain assessment and outcomes. *Pediatric Nursing, 24*(1), 31–35.

Brazy, J. (1988). Effects of crying on cerebral blood flow and cytochrome aa3. *Journal of Pediatrics, 112*(3), 457–461.

Broome, M. E., Rehwaldt, M., & Fogg, L. (1998). Relationships between cognitive behavioral techniques, temperament, observed distress, and pain reports in children and adolescents during lumbar puncture. *Journal of Pediatric Nursing, 13*(1), 48–54.

Carlson, K. L. (1998). Selected resources on pediatric pain. *Journal of Pediatric Nursing, 13*(1), 64–66.

Chambers, C. T., & McGrath, P. J. (1998). Pain measurement in children. In M. A. Ashburn & L. J. Rice (Eds.), *The management of pain* (pp. 625–634). Philadelphia: Saunders.

Colwell, C., Clark, L., & Perkins, R. (1996). Postoperative use of pediatric pain scales: Children's self-report versus nurse assessment of pain intensity and affect. *Journal of Pediatric Nursing, 11*(6), 375–382.

Coté, C. (1994). Sedation for the pediatric patient. *Pediatric Clinics of North America, 41*(1), 31–51.

Cravero, J. P., Manzi, D. J., Rice, L. J. (1998). The management of procedure-related pain in the child. In M. A. Ashburn & L. J. Rice (Eds.), *The management of pain* (pp. 667–681). Philadelphia: Saunders.

Deady, A., & Gorman, D. (1997). Intravenous conscious sedation in children. *Journal of Intravenous Nursing, 20*(5), 245–252.

Eland, J. (1990). Pain in children. *Nursing Clinics of North America, 25*(4), 871–882.

Eland, J. (1991). The use of TENS with children who have cancer pain. *Journal of Pain and Symptom Management, 6*(3), 137.

Fanurik, D., Koh, J., Schmitz, M., & Brown, R. (1997). Pharmacobehavioral intervention: Integrating pharmacologic and behavioral techniques for pediatric medical procedures. *Children's Health Care, 26*(1), 31–46.

Foster, R., & Hester, N. (1990). The relationship between pain ratings and pharmacologic interventions for children in pain. *Advances in Pain Research Therapy, 15*, 31–36.

French, G., Painter, E., & Coury, D. (1994). Blowing away shot pain: A technique for pain management during immunization. *Pediatrics, 93*(3), 384–388.

Gardner, S. (1994). Pain and pain relief in the neonate. *MCN: American Journal of Maternal/Child Nursing, 19*, 85–90.

Gedaly-Duff, V., & Huff-Slankard, J. (1998). Sleep as an indicator for pain relief in an infant: A case study. *Journal of Pediatric Nursing, 13*(1), 32–40.

Gill, K. M., Wilson, J. J., & Edens, J. L. (1997). The stability of pain coping strategies in young children, adolescents, and adults with sickle cell disease over an 18-month period. *The Clinical Journal of Pain, 13*(2), 110–115.

Goodenough, B., Addicoat, L., Champion, C. D., McInerney, M., Young, B., Juniper, K., & Ziegler, J. B. (1997). Pain in 4- to 6-year-old children receiving intramuscular injections: A comparison of the faces pain scale with other self-report and behavioral measures. *The Clinical Journal of Pain, 13*(1), 60–73.

Grunau, R., Johnston, C., & Craig, K. (1990). Neonatal facial and cry responses to invasive and non-invasive procedures. *Pain, 42*, 295–305.

Grunau, R. E., Whitfield, M. F., Petrie, J. (1998). Children's judgement about pain at age 8–10 years: Do extremely low birthweight (<1000g) children differ from full birthweight peers? *Journal of Child Psychology and Psychiatry, 39*(4), 587–594.

Hester, N. (1979). The preoperational child's reaction to immunization. *Nursing Research, 4*(28), 250–254.

Hester, N. O., & Barcus, C. S. (1986). Assessment and management of pain in children. *Pediatrics: Nursing Update, 1*, 2–8.

Howard, V. A., & Thurber, F. W. (1998). The interpretation of infant pain: Physiological and behavioral indicators used by NICU nurses. *Journal of Pediatric Nursing, 13*(3), 164–174.

Houck, C. S. (1998). The management of acute pain in the child. In M. A. Ashburn & L. J. Rice (Eds.), *The management of pain* (pp. 651–666). Philadelphia: Saunders.

Huth, M. M., & Moore, S. M. (1998). Prescriptive theory of acute pain management in infants and children. *Journal of the Society of Pediatric Nurses, 3*(1), 23–32.

International Association for the Study of Pain. (1979). Pain terms: A list with definitions and notes on usage. *Pain, 6*, 249.

Johnston, C., & Strada, M. (1986). Acute pain response in infants: A multidimensional description. *Pain, 24*, 373–382.

Kachoyeanos, M., & Zollo, M. B. (1995). Ethics in pain management of infants and children. *MCN: American Journal of Maternal/Child Nursing, 20*, 142–147.

Keck, J. F., Gerkensmeyer, J. E., Joyce, B. A., & Schade, J. G. (1996). Reliability and validity of the faces and word descriptor scales to measure procedural pain. *Journal of Pediatric Nursing, 11*(6), 368–374.

Kotzer, A. M., Coy, J., & LeClaire, A. D. (1998). The effectiveness of a standardized educational program for children using patient-controlled analgesia. *Journal of the Society of Pediatric Nurses, 3*(3), 117–126.

Lesko, S., & Mitchell, A. (1995). An assessment of the safety of pediatric ibuprofen. *Journal of the American Medical Association, 273*(12), 929–933.

Maikler, V. E. (1998). Pharmacologic pain management in children: A review of intervention research. *Journal of Pediatric Nursing, 13*(1), 3–14.

Margolius, F., Hudson, K., & Michel, Y. (1995). Beliefs and perceptions about children in pain: A survey. *Pediatric Nursing, 21*(2), 111–115.

McCaffrey, M. (1972). *Nursing management of the patient in pain*. Philadelphia: Lippincott.

McCarthy, A. M., Cool, V. A., & Hanrahan, K. (1998). Cognitive behavioral interventions for children during painful procedures: Research challenges and program development. *Journal of Pediatric Nursing, 13*(1), 55–63.

Melzack, R., & Wall, P. (1965). Pain mechanisms: A new theory. *Science, 150*, 971–979.

Mills, N. (1989). Pain behaviors in infants and toddlers. *Journal of Pain and Symptom Management, 4*, 184–190.

Nahata, M., Clotz, M., & Krogg, E. (1985). Adverse effects of meperidine, promethazine and chlorpromazine for sedation in pediatric patients. *Clinical Pediatrics, 24*(10), 558–560.

Palermo, T. M., & Lambert, S. A. (1997). A descriptive study of children's beliefs concerning the use of analgesics in treating postoperative pain. *Children's Health Care, 26*(1), 47–59.

Phillips, P. (1995). Neonatal pain management: A call to action. *Pediatric Nursing, 21*(2), 195–199.

Rayhorn, N. (1998). Sedating and monitoring pediatric patients. *MCN: American Journal of Maternal/Child Nursing, 23*(2), 76–84.

Rawlings, D., Milles, P., & Engel, R. (1980). The effect of transcutaneous Po2 in term infants. *American Journal of Diseases of Children, 134*, 676–678.

Savedra, M., Tesler, M., Holzemer, W., Wilkie, D., & Ward, J. (1989). Pain location: Validity and reliability of body outline markings by hospitalized children and adolescents. *Research in Nursing and Health, 12*, 307–314.

Savedra, M., Tesler, M., & Wegner, C. (1988). How do adolescents describe pain? *Journal of Adolescent Health Care, 9*(4), 315–320.

Savedra, M. C., Tesler, M. D., Holzemer, W. L., & Ward, J. (1992). *Adolescent and Pediatric Pain Tool: User's manual*. San Francisco: University of California, San Francisco, School of Nursing.

Schechter, N. (1988). An approach to the child with pain. *Patient Care, 3*, 116–131.

Schechter, N. (1989). The undertreatment of pain in children: An overview. *Pediatric Clinics of North America, 36*, 781–794.

Schechter, N., Allen, D., & Hanson, K. (1986). Status of pediatric pain control: A comparison of hospital analgesic usage in children and adults. *Pediatrics, 77*, 11–15.

Seymour, E., Fuller, B. F., Pedersen-Gallegos, L., & Schwaninger, J. E. (1997). Modes of thought, feeling, and action in infant pain assessment by pediatric nurses. *Journal of Pediatric Nursing, 12*(1), 32–49

Sutters, K. A., & Miaskowski, C. (1997). Inadequate pain management and associated morbidity in children at home after tonsillectomy. *Journal of Pediatric Nursing, 12*(3), 178–185.

Taddio, A., Nulman, I., Goldbach, M., Ipp, M., & Koren, G. (1994). Use of lidocaine-prilocaine cream for vaccination pain in infants. *Journal of Pediatrics, 124*, 643–648.

Taddio, A., Ohlsson, A., Einarson, T. R., Stevens, B., & Koren, G. (1998). A systematic review of lidocaine-prilocaine cream (EMLA) in the treatment of acute pain in neonates. *Pediatrics, 101*(2), E1.

Tesler, M., Savedra, M., Holzemer, W., Wilkie, D., Ward, J., & Paul, S. (1991). The word-graphic rating scale as a measure of children's and adolescents' pain intensity. *Research in Nursing and Health, 14*, 361–371.

Tesler, M. D., Holzemer, W. L., & Savedra, M. C. (1998). Pain behaviors: Postsurgical responses of children and adolescents. *Journal of Pediatric Nursing, 13*(1), 41–47.

Trentadue, N. O., Kachoyeanos, M. K., Lea G. (1998). A comparison of two regimens of patient-controlled analgesia for children with sickle cell disease. *Journal of Pediatric Nursing, 13*(1), 15–19.

Valente, S. (1991). Using hypnosis with children for pain management. *Oncology Nursing Forum, 18*(4), 699–704.

Van Cleve, L., & Andrews, S. (1995). Pain responses of hospitalized neonates to venipuncture activities. *MCN: American Journal of Maternal/Child Nursing, 20*, 148–152.

Van Cleve, L., Johnson, L., & Pothier, P. (1996). Pain responses of hospitalized infants and children to venipuncture and intravenous cannulation. *Journal of Pediatric Nursing, 11*(3), 161–168.

Van Cleve, L., & Savedra, M. (1993). Pain location: Validity and reliability of body outline markings by 4- to 7-year-old children who are hospitalized. *Pediatric Nursing, 19*(3), 217–220.

Van Keuren, K., & Eland, J. A. (1997). Perioperative pain management in children. *Nursing Clinics of North America, 32*(1), 31–44.

Vesely, C. (1995). Pediatric patient-controlled analgesia: Enhancing the self-care construct. *Pediatric Nursing, 21*(2), 124–128.

Vessey, J., Carlson, K., & McGill, J. (1994). Use of distraction with children during an acute pain experience. *Nursing Research, 43*(6), 369–372.

Wallace, M. (1989). Temperament: A variable in children's pain management. *Pediatric Nursing, 15*(2), 118–121.

Woodgate, R., & Kristjanson, L. J. (1996). "Getting better from my hurt": Toward a model of the young child's pain experience. *Journal of Pediatric Nursing, 11*(4), 233–242.

Zajac, J. (1992). Pediatric pain management. *Critical Care Nursing Quarterly, 15*(2), 35–51.

Zappa, S. (1994, Spring). EMLA cream: A topical anesthetic. *Nursing in Pediatrics*, 28–31.

Zappa, S. (1994–95, Winter). A topical anesthetic and hemophilia care. *Nursing Network/Psychosocial News*, 6.

Zeltzer, L., Bush, J., Chen, E., & Riveral, A. (1997). A psychobiologic approach to pediatric pain: Part II. Prevention and treatment. *Current Problems in Pediatrics, 27*, 264–284.

Zeltzer, L., Jay, S., & Fisher, D. (1989). The management of pain associated with pediatric procedures. *Pediatric Clinics of North America, 36*(4), 941–964.

40

♦ ♦ ♦ ♦ ♦ ♦ ♦ ♦ ♦ ♦

The Child with an Infectious Disease

LEARNING OBJECTIVES

After studying this chapter, you should be able to:

- Describe the infectious process.
- Describe the modes of transmission of infectious diseases.
- Discuss the pathophysiology, clinical manifestations, complications, and nursing management of childhood infectious diseases.
- Discuss the pathophysiology, clinical manifestations, complications, and nursing management of sexually transmissible diseases.
- Use the nursing process to describe the nursing care of a child with an infectious disease.

DEFINITIONS

antitoxin   A particular kind of antibody produced by the body in response to the presence of a toxin.

attenuated vaccine   Vaccine derived from microorganisms or viruses whose virulence has been weakened because of passage through another host.

exanthem   An eruption or rash on the skin.

immunity   Resistance of the body to the effects of a harmful organism or its toxin.

inactivated vaccines   Vaccine that contains killed microorganisms.

infection   Invasion of an organism by pathogenic or nonpathogenic organisms, such as bacteria, viruses, protozoa, helminths, or fungi.

inflammation   A tissue response to injury or destruction of cells.

pathogen   A disease-producing microorganism.

prodrome   The initial stage of a disease; symptoms indicating an approaching disease.

toxin   A poison produced by pathogenic microorganisms.

vector   A carrier that transfers an infective agent from one host to another.

virulence   Strength of effect produced by a pathogenic organism.

Review of Disease Transmission

Microorganisms exist throughout the environment. Most are harmless residents—a normal part of human flora. An organism that invades body tissue, causing tissue damage and disease, however, is a *pathogen*. For pathogens to invade a host, they must breach the normal host defenses, either by attaching to or penetrating the host. The power of these pathogens, known as their *virulence*, depends on their ability to overcome the host defense mechanisms. Thus, a highly virulent organism can cause disease with relative ease.

Microorganisms can have one of several relationships with the host: commensalism, mutualism, or parasitism. Those that cause infectious disease are classified into five types: bacteria, viruses, fungi, protozoa, and helminths.

Exogenous pathogens are transmitted from outside the body. They are transmitted by direct contact, by animal or insect contact, through contaminated food or water, or by contact with a contaminated object. The organisms may be carried by a *vector* from one host to another. The vector may be an insect or an animal. For example, a certain species of mosquito carries the malaria parasite; likewise, certain bats carry the rabies microorganism. Transmission may occur by inhalation, ingestion, injection (insect bites), or direct contact (sexual). Infected breast milk may be the source of the pathogen.

Endogenous transmission of pathogens involves the body's normal flora or microorganisms. Normally, the human flora contains harmless microorganisms. They exist in the skin, nose, mouth, gastrointestinal tract, and urogenital tract. For example, *Staphylococcus epidermidis* inhabits the skin, and *Escherichia coli* is found in the intestines. These microorganisms are beneficial, playing an important role in the body's defenses. They help prevent colonization by virulent pathogens by maintaining an acidic pH environment to discourage pathogen attachment, by taking up epithelial space to prevent growth of pathogens, and by stimulating the immune system. Nevertheless, situations may arise in which these normally benign organisms become virulent.

. . . .
Microorganisms and Host Relationships

Commensalism: Host provides shelter and food for the organism; organism retains the ability to exist independently.
Mutualism: Host provides shelter and food for the organism; both benefit.
Parasitism: Host provides shelter and food; the parasite benefits, but the host may be harmed.

Transmission of Pathogens

For a pathogen to maintain its infectious state, it must be transmitted to another host. Exit transmission occurs through several sources. From the respiratory tract, for example, pathogens are shed through sneezing, coughing, and talking. Because these transmission mechanisms are relatively uncontrollable, infections can easily be spread in crowded conditions; that is, one person can directly spread pathogens to another person's respiratory tract.

Pathogens may also be shed through fecal matter. When personal hygiene is poor and hand washing is not routinely practiced, pathogens have ample opportunities to enter through the mouth. Unclean hands may also contaminate food.

In the urogenital tract, pathogenic transmission does not generally occur through infected urine. Rather, sexual activity involving direct mucosal contact is the most common means of transmission of sexually transmissible diseases (STDs). If the mother's birth canal is infected, newborn infants can be infected by direct contact during birth. Saliva is another avenue of transmission, as is direct contact with infected skin. Pathogens can also be present in breast milk and can infect a nursing infant.

A tick or mite can inject pathogens into the skin and blood of the host. Contamination with the blood of the infected host can then occur through transfusions, blood products, and the use of contaminated needles. Moreover, a pregnant woman can transmit such pathogens through the placenta.

Infection and Host Defenses

The first stage of *infection* begins with *colonization*. Microorganisms invade either by adhering to tissues or by invading cells. When replication of the pathogen first begins, it does not cause tissue damage. Thus, colonization can occur without development of a clinical infection. As the host "recognizes" the invasion, the defense system—the immune response—is activated. The two components of the immune response are the innate, nonspecific immune response and the adaptive, specific immune response: cell mediated and humoral (see Chapter 41).

The first lines of defense in the innate immune system are the skin and intact mucous membranes. The skin serves as a barrier, preventing colonization of most pathogens. The acid secreted in sweat and by sebaceous glands inhibits pathogenic invasion. Smooth muscle contraction and ciliary actions such as those seen in bladder and bowel emptying and coughing and sneezing provide for mechanical removal of pathogens. Physical and chemical barriers are provided by mucus production by goblet cells of mucous

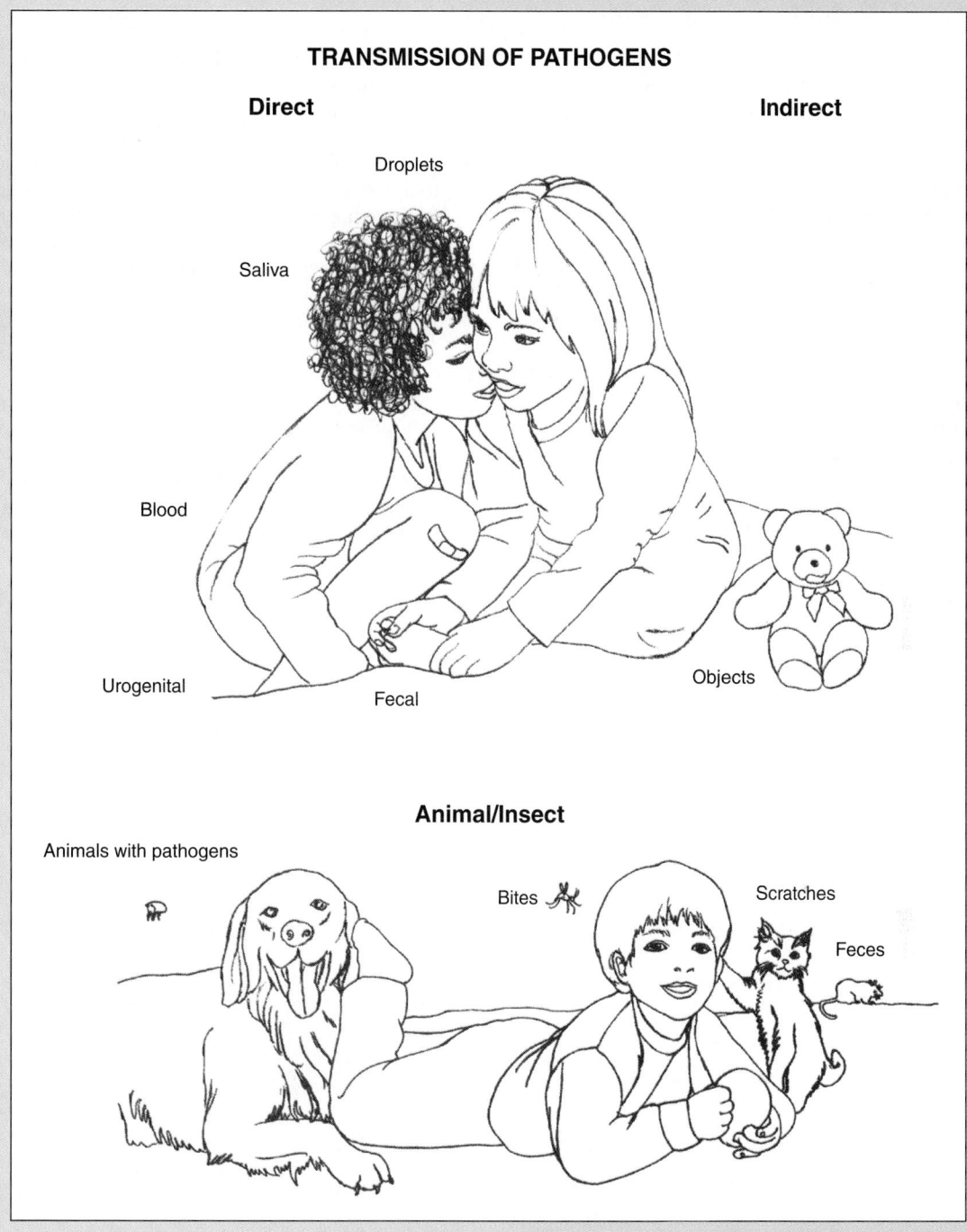

TRANSMISSION OF PATHOGENS

Direct   **Indirect**

Droplets

Saliva

Blood

Urogenital   Fecal   Objects

Animal/Insect

Animals with pathogens   Bites   Scratches   Feces

membranes. Nevertheless, the innate system may be unable to prevent the invasion. Phagocytosis, the process by which phagocytic cells digest and thereby destroy foreign microorganisms, is overwhelmed. Large numbers of pathogens or their *toxins* can inhibit phagocytosis. When this process occurs, the *adaptive immune system* is activated. This system "recognizes" and responds to pathogens and destroys them. The adaptive immune system "imprints" on these pathogens so that if the body encounters them again, the response will be rapid and specific.

▌ *Immunity*

Immunity is the body's resistance to the effects of harmful agents. It occurs as an antigen-antibody reaction that takes place whenever a foreign agent or its toxins enter the bloodstream. Immunity can be either active or passive (Chapter 41).

Some childhood diseases have been reduced and some nearly eliminated through the administration of vaccines.

Types of Vaccines

Artificially active or artificially passive immunity is produced through the administration of a vaccine. Several preparations of vaccines can accomplish immunity. These include the following:

- **Live or attenuated vaccines:** Vaccines that have had their virulence (potency) diminished so as to not produce a full-blown clinical illness. In response to vaccination, the body produces antibodies and causes immunity to be established. An example is the measles vaccine.
- **Killed or inactivated vaccines:** Vaccines that contain pathogens made inactive by either chemicals or heat. These vaccines, which are noninfectious, cause the body to produce antibodies. Their disadvantage is that they elicit a limited immune response from the body; therefore, several doses are required. Examples include the Salk polio, rabies, and pertussis vaccines.
- **Toxoids:** Bacterial toxins that have been made inactive by either chemicals or heat. The toxins cause the body to produce antibodies. Examples include the diphtheria and tetanus vaccines.
- **Human immune globulin:** A vaccine made of human immune globulin, obtained from the pooled blood of many people. This type of vaccine provides antibodies to a variety of diseases, such as measles, rubella, and infectious hepatitis. Its disadvantage is that it offers only temporary passive immunity. Some immune globulin can be disease specific and is derived from individuals with a specific disease.
- **Animal serums (antitoxins):** Vaccines derived from the serum of immunized animals. Animal serums have the disadvantage of being foreign substances, which may cause hypersensitivity reactions. Thus a history and sensitivity testing should precede vaccine administration. The serums derived from this method are used to stimulate production of antibodies for hepatitis, chickenpox, rabies, diphtheria, smallpox, cytomegalovirus (CMV) infection, botulism, snake bites, and spider bites.

The Child with an Infection

Children from infancy to adolescence may experience an infectious disease. Most of these diseases are self-limiting and rarely produce a devastating illness, yet health care is still indicated. Many infectious diseases present with subtle and common symptoms that may be difficult to identify. Because rashes and fever are common symptoms of many diseases, the nurse needs to obtain a complete history, including the earliest signs of the developing disease (*prodrome*), recent exposures, and a description of the rash.

Once the causative organism and disease are identified, nursing care focuses on treating symptoms (e.g., fever, itching), providing comfort measures, and preventing the spread of the disease. In addition, the nurse provides education and emotional support to the family. The family and child may also need assistance in adjusting to the isolation necessitated by the disease. Finally, the nurse must educate the child and parents as to the modes of transmission of infectious diseases and the importance of immunizations.

Assessment

Assessment begins with a history of exposure to an infectious disease and a history of current symptoms. The physical examination includes the following documentation:

- Type, configuration, and distribution of lesions
- Vital signs, especially body temperature
- General wellness
- Any other manifestations (arthralgia, malaise, pain, etc.)

Infectious diseases are a major reason why health care is sought for infants and children. Although most infections are not life-threatening, in some cases complications develop that can be fatal. At increased risk is the infant or child with an immature or compromised immune system. In addition, a child's illness has an impact on the family. Absence from work and the accompanying missed income can be devastating for both single- and two-income families.

Nurses in both community and hospital settings should be able not only to recognize the signs and symptoms of infectious diseases but also to educate parents about them. In the hospital setting, relatively mild diseases, such as chickenpox, may pose potentially fatal problems to the immunosuppressed child. In such cases, the staff nurse must assess and recognize the signs and provide appropriate protection by isolating the infected child. In the community setting, the office or school nurse may be the professional who first recognizes the manifestations of infectious diseases and must take measures to limit the exposure of other children.

Nursing Diagnosis, Planning, Intervention, and Evaluation

Nursing Diagnosis	■ Risk for Infection (cross-contamination of self or others) related to infectious disease.
Expected Outcome	• No other individuals will contract the infection.
	• The child will demonstrate absence of infection, as evidenced by vital signs within normal parameters for the child, resolving lesions with no evidence of redness or swelling, a white blood cell count that is within acceptable limits for the child, and a lack of irritability and lethargy.

Intervention	Rationale
1. Initiate infection control measures as recommended by CDC (see Chapter 37 and Appendix B). Instruct the family as to the need for isolation (gowns, gloves, masks) and the underlying rationale. Instruct the family about proper hand-washing techniques.	1. Infection precautions help prevent transmission of infectious organisms from the child to others.
2. Instruct the family and child about the underlying concepts and the modes of preventing the spread of infectious disease.	2. Understanding promotes compliance with isolation techniques.
3. Instruct the family and child about the sources of infection and the risk of spreading infection.	3. Understanding promotes cooperation with the treatment protocol and other necessary procedures.
4. Teach the family and child reporting methods, signs and symptoms of disease, risks of transmission of disease, and potential complications.	4. Providing information about the causes and treatment of the disease and about preventive measures promotes understanding and reduces others' risk of exposure.

5. Hand washing helps prevent the transmission of pathogens to others.
6. Assess the child for fever, malaise, fatigue, lesions, or other signs of disease. Monitor laboratory values.
7. Administer prescribed medication(s) to control progression of disease or to treat the infection. Instruct the family about the action and side effects of the medication(s) chosen.
8. Provide written instructions for treatment and care upon discharge. Assess the parents' knowledge of the instructions and, if necessary, have them demonstrate procedures or techniques.

5. Instruct the family and child in proper hand-washing techniques and medical asepsis.
6. Recognizing the signs and symptoms of specific infectious diseases helps one differentiate among different diseases.
7. Medication is used to prevent or treat infections. Sharing information with the family promotes compliance with the treatment regimen.
8. Written information assists parents in maintaining compliance in the home setting.

Evaluation
• Have other individuals contracted the disease?
• Is the child free from infection and afebrile?

Nursing Diagnosis
■ Impaired Skin Integrity related to scratching, lesions, inflammation, and/or infection of lesions.

Expected Outcome
• The child will have improved skin integrity, as evidenced by healing of existing lesions, absence of lesion extension, decreased scratching, and decreased discomfort.

Intervention

1. Keep the child's nails short and clean.
2. Use cotton mittens on infants and young children if necessary.
3. Bathe or soak the child in cool water (90° to 100.4°F; 32° to 38°C). Use oatmeal colloid (Aveeno) or baking soda (½ cup in bath water) rather than soap, which can be irritating. Use superfatted soaps or soaps for sensitive skin (Dove, Basis, Neutrogena, Aveeno).
4. Administer antihistamines or antipruritics as prescribed.
5. Dress the child in lightweight clothing that is not irritating. Avoid wool and scratchy materials.
6. Apply soothing lotions, such as calamine, to lesions.
7. Avoid the use of topical corticosteroids unless so ordered by the physician.
8. Apply emollient creams (Lubriderm, Moisturel, Curel, petroleum jelly).

Rationale

1. Secondary infection and scarring are reduced if the child's nails are short and clean.
2. Mittens prevent infants and young children from scratching.
3. Cool baths soothe pruritus and may help prevent scratching. By contrast, hot water may cause vasodilation and increase pruritus. These special soaps are less alkaline and thus less drying.
4. Antihistamines counteract the release of histamine, which causes itching. Antipruritics have a sedative effect.
5. Light clothing provides ventilation and minimizes perspiration that otherwise might intensify itching.
6. The lotions promote drying of lesions and aid in preventing scratching and discomfort. Avoid the use of diphenhydramine-containing calamine, as it can be very sensitizing.
7. Topical steroids can be misused, and they can mask infections. Intermittent rather than continuous use will provide improved results with less risk of side effects.
8. The creams seal in water and hydrate the skin. They can have a soothing effect on the skin.

Evaluation
• Is the skin intact, and are any previously injured areas healing?
• Have the skin lesions remained free of secondary infection?
• Has the child scratched infrequently or not at all?

Nursing Diagnosis
■ Altered Body Temperature related to infection.

Expected Outcome
• The child will be afebrile, as evidenced by a body temperature that is within normal parameters for the child, and will be alert and oriented.

Intervention

1. Administer antipyretics as ordered.
2. Keep the environment cool (in conjunction with antipyretic administration).

Rationale

1. Antipyretics reduce the body temperature to normal parameters (96.8° and 100.4°F [36° and 38°C]).
2. A cool environmental temperature helps to reduce a child's body temperature by promoting evaporation.

3. Keep clothing and bedding minimal (in conjunction with antipyretic administration).
4. Encourage fluid intake (in conjunction with antipyretic administration).

5. Apply a cool, moist compress to the skin (in conjunction with antipyretic administration). Use tepid water to avoid shivering. Do not use alcohol for sponge baths.

3. Minimal clothing and bedding helps to reduce a child's body temperature by promoting evaporation.
4. Increased fluid intake assists in maintaining the child's hydration level. An elevated temperature is associated with increased metabolism and fluid use.
5. Cool compresses assist in heat dissipation. Shivering, however, increases metabolism and causes heat production. Alcohol produces too rapid heat loss, is absorbed through the skin, and has a drying effect on the skin.

Evaluation
- Has the child maintained a body temperature within normal parameters?
- Is the child alert and oriented?

Nursing Diagnosis
■ Fatigue related to fever secondary to infectious disease.
■ Pain related to joint inflammation.

Expected Outcome
- The child will experience an increase in comfort level and energy, as evidenced by verbalization of decreased discomfort, a relaxed body posture, decreased crying and irritability, and maintenance of body temperature at baseline parameters for age.

Intervention	Rationale
1. Perform interventions to decrease disruptions in the skin and causes for discomfort related to impaired skin integrity.	1. Relieving the symptoms will decrease the amount of discomfort from impaired skin integrity.
2. Administer antipyretics as ordered.	2. Antipyretics help to reduce the body temperature to normal parameters (96.8° and 100.4°F [36° and 38°C]).
3. Keep the environment cool and provide light clothing and bedding. Monitor the child's temperature every 4 hours or more frequently if indicated.	3. A cool environment decreases skin irritation. Monitoring temperatures will determine the need for additional nursing measures and help assess the effectiveness of the measures.
4. Administer antihistamines and antipruritics as ordered.	4. Antihistamines and antipruritics reduce itching and discomfort.
5. Apply lotions and provide soaks or baths using oatmeal colloids or baking soda.	5. Lotions and baths decrease the discomfort from skin irritation.
6. Encourage bed rest.	6. Bed rest provides comfort in individuals with joint pain or fever.
7. Provide cool, nonacidic liquids. Provide frequent small feedings of favorite bland foods (pudding, ice cream, Jell-O).	7. Cool liquids provide comfort while encouraging and maintaining adequate intake.
8. Allow the child to gargle.	8. Saline rinses may soothe irritated lesions. Avoid the use of commercial mouthwashes because they can cause drying and irritation.
9. Provide lozenges to relieve irritation of the mouth and throat.	9. Lozenges provide a soothing effect.
10. Provide cool mist.	10. Cool mist keeps mucous membranes moist and decreases the irritation caused by drying.
11. Monitor the status of lesions.	11. Monitoring the child's condition allows the nurse to determine the effectiveness of nursing measures.
12. Provide activities that are age-appropriate and energy-appropriate, depending on the child's level of wellness.	12. Nonpharmacologic techniques such as distraction provide diversion.
13. Keep the child's skin clean and change linens and clothing frequently. Wash clothes and linen in mild detergent and double-rinse.	13. Clean clothing helps to prevent the spread of secondary infections. Double-rinsing reduces the potential irritants in the clothing, thereby minimizing irritation.

Evaluation
- Has the child demonstrated minimal evidence of discomfort?

Nursing Diagnosis
■ Social Isolation related to the communicable disease.

Expected Outcome
- The child and family will demonstrate an understanding of the necessity for isolation while maintaining social contact and will incorporate this isolation into their home management, as evidenced by the child's participating in activities, maintaining appropriate interactions with peers, and verbalizing knowledge of the duration of isolation.

Intervention	Rationale
1. Provide activities involving play with masks, gowns, and gloves.	1. Playing with medical equipment helps the child adjust to personnel required to use the same equipment when caring for the child.
2. Encourage parents to stay with the child.	2. The presence of the family helps the child adjust to activity limitations, reduces boredom, and provides emotional support.
3. Encourage contact with friends and family by telephone or mail.	3. Contact with family and friends promotes social interaction with others and helps to prevent boredom.
4. Provide age-appropriate play activities.	4. Providing play activities prevents boredom and promotes normal growth and development.
5. Explain to the family and child the purpose for and length of the isolation.	5. Understanding promotes compliance with the treatment regimen and isolation requirements.

Evaluation	• Is the child engaging in age-appropriate activities? • Is the family able to maintain isolation and still provide social situations for the child?
Nursing Diagnosis	■ Knowledge Deficit related to lack of information or inexperience with infectious diseases.
Expected Outcome	• Parents will be able to verbalize and/or demonstrate the care necessary to manage their child's health care needs at home, as well as the preventive measures necessary to prevent the spread of the infectious disease.

Intervention	Rationale
1. Instruct parents about the requirements for infection control (gloves, gown, masks).	1. The risk of transmission is decreased when the principles of infection control are practiced.
2. Instruct the parents on measures that can decrease discomfort from lesions and pruritus.	2. The child's level of discomfort will be decreased if parents provide comfort measures.
3. Instruct the parents about the signs and symptoms that would indicate potential complications related to their child's infectious disease.	3. Knowledgeable parents can identify situations requiring medical attention.
4. Instruct parents in the administration of any ordered medications and have parents demonstrate administration. Educate parents about the signs and symptoms of adverse reactions to medications and the actions to take in the event of an adverse reaction.	4. An understanding of the treatment regimen promotes compliance. Parents will then seek medical help when appropriate.
5. Provide parents with information about immunizations. Answer parents' questions about various aspects of immunization.	5. Understanding the relationship between the prevention of infectious diseases and immunizations promotes the use of immunizations.

Evaluation	• Has the family received instruction in the care of the child? • Have the parents verbalized and/or demonstrated appropriate home care? • Have the parents had their child(ren) immunized?

■ *Viral Infections*

Viruses are small parasitic organisms. They have characteristics that cause them to be very different from other organisms. They contain only one type of nucleic acid—either DNA or RNA—which prevents them from reproducing on their own. Instead, a host cell is needed to allow the virus to replicate.

The virus first attaches itself to a host cell. Some of the viruses are selective about the cells to which they attach; for example, the human immunodeficiency virus (HIV) prefers the T cell. After attachment, a virus must invade the interior of the cell. Replication of the virus's nucleic material begins after the envelope and capsule (capsid) are shed and the nucleic material of the virus is released into the cell; the host cell then assists in the formation of the necessary nucleic material. New capsules are then formed and released into the host and new host cells. The infected host cell can respond to the viral invasion by cell death (lysis) and destruction, but infected cells can also remain alive and continue to function while new viral particles are slowly released. This slow release occurs in an asymptomatic person who is a carrier of the virus.

A virus can invade a host, remaining dormant until a

trigger stimulates the virus to begin replicating. Many of the triggering factors are not understood. Some factors, such as stress, however, have been identified as triggers in such viral diseases as herpes simplex, which results in the formation of cold sores.

Nursing Considerations for the Child with a Viral Exanthem Infection

An *exanthem* is an eruption or rash on the skin. Several childhood diseases are characterized by rashes with different characteristics. Indeed, rashes may have more than one characteristic. The nurse needs to obtain a history of the onset and progression of the rash, as well as any associated symptoms. Recent exposures, the child's immunization history, and any prior history of the disease need to be explored and documented. Additionally, the nurse should note any medications taken, any history of upper respiratory tract infection, and any exposure to known infections. The skin and mucous membranes should be examined, and the distribution and type of rash should be recorded. The eyes, nose, ears, and throat should also be examined for signs of inflammation, swelling, and secretions. The temperature of the child should be recorded, as should the child's general state of health. The spleen, liver, and lymph nodes should be examined for any enlargement.

Children with typical uncomplicated viral exanthems are usually cared for at home. Hospitalization is indicated when there are complications. Care of the hospitalized child will be determined by the child's specific needs. The hospitalized child will require respiratory or contact isolation. High-risk children and children with an infectious disease should not be cared for by the same nurse.

Rubeola (Measles)

Causative agent:	RNA virus
Incubation period:	7 to 14 days
Infectious period:	ranges from 1 to 2 days before onset of symptoms to 4 days after appearance of the rash
Transmission:	airborne particles or direct contact with infectious droplets
Immunity:	natural disease or live attenuated vaccine
Season:	winter/spring

MANIFESTATIONS

The measles virus enters the body and slowly spreads. Respiratory symptoms appear after an average of 10 days. The child will have a profuse runny nose (coryza), cough, and fever. Conjunctivitis may be present, along with photophobia. *Koplik spots* appear approximately 2 days before the appearance of the rash (Fig. 40–1). Koplik spots are small, blue-white spots with a red base that occur on the buccal mucosa. These spots last approximately 3 days, after which time they slough off. The measles rash usually begins behind the ears, at the hairline, on the forehead, and on the upper part of the neck. It spreads downward to the feet. The rash is red and maculopapular; it blanches easily with pressure

PARENTS WANT TO KNOW

About Caring for Their Child with a Viral Exanthem

- For elevated temperature, the child's activity should be restricted to quiet activities and bed rest. As the fever decreases, the activity level can be gradually increased to a normal level. Fever can be controlled with acetaminophen, sponge baths, decreased clothing, decreased environmental temperature, and increased fluid intake. Bed linens may need to be changed frequently during periods of high fevers. Parents should be instructed about the possibility of febrile seizures. Seizure precautions should be in effect for any child with a seizure history.

- The amount of skin irritation and discomfort will vary. Lukewarm baths using colloid preparations (Aveeno) or baking soda (1/2 cup in tub of water) may help relieve itching. Creams or emollients may also provide comfort. Soaps should be avoided to prevent drying of irritated skin. Fingernails should be short. If the child continues to scratch, cotton mittens or socks can be applied to the child's hands. It is essential to maintain the integrity of the skin and prevent any secondary infections. Should secondary infections occur, antibiotic therapy might be necessary.

- Coughing can be managed with cool humidification of the room and antitussives.

- For arthralgia, anti-inflammatory medications may be used. Involvement of weight-bearing joints may warrant bed rest.

- Some viral exanthems cause photophobia. In such cases, keeping the room dimly lighted or providing sunglasses for the child may be helpful. If the child has conjunctivitis, secretions or crust should be removed with tepid water and a clean cloth to prevent contamination.

- Fluid intake is important. The parents and child should understand that fluid intake is critical in successfully managing febrile stages of the disease. The child should be encouraged to drink cool liquids frequently. If the child's mucous membranes are involved, soft, bland foods may be beneficial.

- As the child progresses through the stages of illness, it will be necessary to provide diversional activities during the period of isolation. Evaluation of the child's favorite activities will provide ideas. The activities chosen should reflect the child's stage of wellness.

- Parents' understanding of the care necessary for their child is important. Parents need to be educated about immunizations and measures to prevent the spread of infectious diseases. They should also be taught to recognize the signs and symptoms of complications so that they can seek medical treatment when warranted. Providing parents with written instructions that they can refer to at home may prove helpful.

First day   Third day

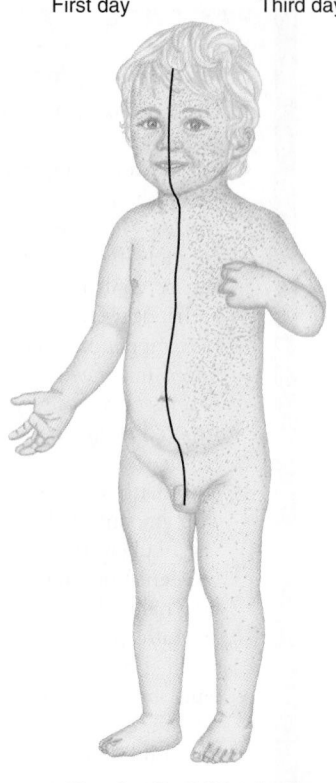

- Preceded by Koplik spots on buccal mucosa

- Begins behind ears, at hairline, and on upper neck and spreads downward toward feet

- Red, maculopapular rash that gradually turns brownish

- Duration: 6–7 days

Measles Rash Distribution

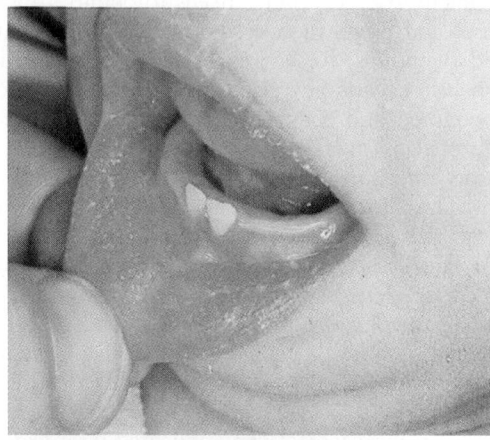

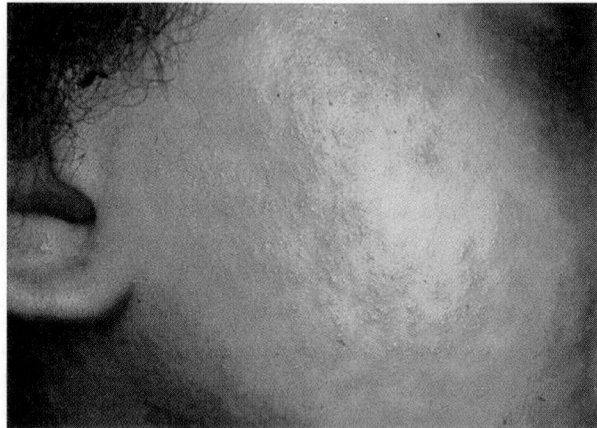

Measles Rash, Dark Skin

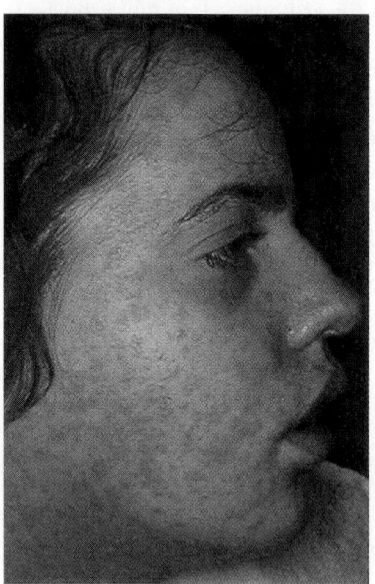

Measles Rash, Light Skin

FIGURE 40–1

Rubeola (measles) lesions and rash distribution. (Photos from Feigin, R. D., & Cherry, J. D. [Eds.]. [1998]. *Textbook of pediatric infectious diseases* [4th ed.]. Philadelphia: Saunders, p. 724, Figs. 67–1 and 67–2; Hurwitz, S. [1993]. *Clinical pediatric dermatology: A textbook of skin disorders of childhood and adolescence* [2nd ed.]. Philadelphia: Saunders, p. 350, Fig. 12–5.)

and will gradually turn a brownish color. The duration of the rash is about 6 to 7 days.

A partially immune child, such as an infant less than 9 months old who has passively acquired maternal antibod-ies or a child given immune gamma-globulin, may contract modified measles. The prodromal period is shorter and the symptoms are minimal, with few to no Koplik spots. The rash progression follows the pattern of regular measles.

COMPLICATIONS

Because of the respiratory involvement, secondary bacterial infections, such as pneumonia and otitis media, can occur. These are the most common complications. Complications may also involve the central nervous system (CNS).

THERAPEUTIC MANAGEMENT

The treatment of measles is symptomatic, whether the child is hospitalized or remains at home. If hospitalized, the child will require airborne precautions. During the febrile period, the child should be restricted to quiet activities and bed rest.

The American Academy of Pediatrics (AAP, 1997) has recommended that vitamin A be considered for the treatment of measles in certain circumstances, including

- Children ages 6 months to 2 years who are hospitalized with complications (pneumonia, croup, diarrhea)
- Children older than 6 months of age who have the following risks: immunodeficiency, evidence of vitamin A deficiency, impaired intestinal absorption, moderate to severe malnutrition, or recent immigration from an area with high mortality from measles

In such children, vitamin A has been found to reduce morbidity and mortality.

Rubella (3-Day Measles, German Measles)

Causative agent:	RNA virus
Incubation period:	14 to 21 days
Infectious period:	ranges from 7 days before onset of symptoms to 14 days after appearance of the rash
Transmission:	airborne particles or direct contact with infectious droplets, transplacental transmission
Immunity:	natural disease or live attenuated vaccine
Season:	winter/spring

MANIFESTATIONS

Rubella is usually a mild disease for children and adults. The virus enters the host, producing a rash after about 14 to 16 days. Young children are often asymptomatic until the appearance of the rash. Older children may complain of profuse nasal drainage, diarrhea, malaise, sore throat, headache, low-grade fever, polyarthritis, eye pain, aches, chills, anorexia, and nausea. Children of all ages usually have lymphadenopathy involving the posterior cervical and posterior, auricular, and suboccipital nodes.

The rash presents as a pinkish rose maculopapular exanthema that begins on the face, scalp, and neck (Fig. 40–2).

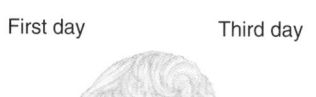

First day   Third day

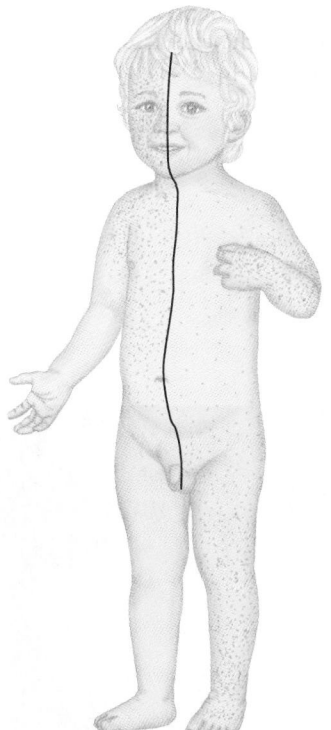

- Begins on face, neck, and scalp and spreads downward to entire body. Fades on face as it spreads to trunk.

- Pinkish, maculopapular

- Reddish, pinpoint petechiae may occur on soft palate (Forscheimer's sign).

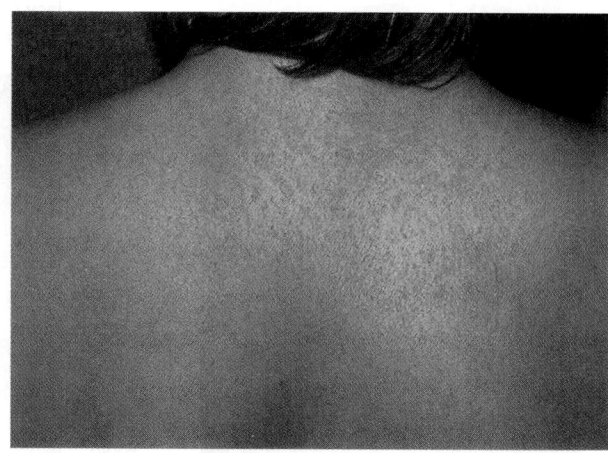

German Measles Rash Distribution

FIGURE 40–2

Rubella (German measles) lesions and rash distribution. (Photo from Hurwitz, S. [1993]. *Clinical pediatric dermatology: A textbook of skin disorders of childhood and adolescence* [2nd ed.]. Philadelphia: Saunders, p. 356, Fig. 12–13.)

trunk and may be surrounded by a whitish ring. Normally, it persists for 24 to 48 hours before fading.

COMPLICATIONS

Complications associated with roseola are uncommon. Convulsions related to the high fever may occur, however, and rare cases of encephalitis, hemiplegia, paresis, and mental retardation have been reported.

THERAPEUTIC MANAGEMENT

The treatment of roseola is supportive.

Mumps

Causative agent: paramyxovirus
Incubation period: usually 16 to 18 days, but may extend to 25 days
Infectious period: from 7 days before swelling to 9 days after onset
Transmission: airborne droplets, salivary secretions, possibly urine
Immunity: natural disease or live attenuated vaccine
Season: late winter/spring

MANIFESTATIONS

Prodromal manifestations may include fever, muscular pain, headache, and malaise. The classic clinical sign of parotid glandular swelling (parotitis) often follows these, although a substantial number of individuals experience no such swelling. When parotid swelling does occur, it may be accompanied by fever.

COMPLICATIONS

Mumps generally affects the salivary glands but can involve multiple organs. The most common complication is aseptic meningitis, with the virus identified in the cerebrospinal fluid (CSF). Common signs include nuchal rigidity, lethargy, and vomiting. Individuals with these manifestations usually recover completely. Meningoencephalomyelitis is another complication that generally has a good prognosis.

The complication of most concern to parents is orchitis (inflammation of a testis), which occurs in males. Unilateral orchitis occurs more frequently than bilateral orchitis. About 1 week after the appearance of parotitis there is an abrupt onset of pain, tenderness, fever, chills, headache, and vomiting. The affected testicle becomes red, swollen, and tender. Atrophy resulting in sterility occurs in only a small number of cases.

Although deafness does not occur frequently, mumps is one of the leading causes of unilateral nerve deafness. The loss can be transient or permanent. Other rare complications include pancreatitis, nephritis, thyroiditis, myocarditis, arthritis, and mastitis.

THERAPEUTIC MANAGEMENT

Uncomplicated mumps may require only symptomatic care. Droplet precautions are indicated until 9 days after the onset of the parotid swelling. Orchitis requires bed rest, intermittent application of ice packs, and emotional support. Meningoencephalomyelitis, which reflects CNS involvement,

---

PARENTS WANT TO KNOW
• • • • • • • • •
About Caring for the Child with Mumps

- Generally, children with mumps are not seriously ill. They will, however, be uncomfortable. Antipyretics and analgesics can be given to control fever and malaise.
- Warm or cold compresses applied to the neck may be of benefit. Intake of food may be painful; soft, bland foods may be preferred. Acidic or spicy foods should be avoided.
- The affected child will need to be isolated while infectious.
- While the child is in isolation, diversional activities should be planned according to the child's interests. Bed rest may be of benefit during the prodromal period.
- In boys with orchitis, ice packs, bed rest, and scrotal support may be indicated.
- Emotional support may be of great importance to the parents. Concern over sterility may be a source of stress.
- Parental education regarding the course of the disease and any potential complications may need to be reinforced. Parents often need additional instruction in preventing the spread of infection and maintaining their child's immunizations.

---

manifests with fever, headache, nausea, vomiting, nuchal rigidity, and changes in sensorium. The affected child is treated symptomatically and generally has an uneventful recovery.

NURSING CONSIDERATIONS

The nurse needs to obtain a history of the onset of symptoms and to examine the child's ears and throat. The characteristics of the lymph nodes in the neck should be documented, as should the child's temperature and general level of wellness. A neurologic evaluation should also be performed. In boys, an examination of the testes should be included in the assessment.

Typically, children with mumps are not hospitalized unless they have complications. Hospitalized children will be placed in isolation according to the facility's policies. Hand washing is of utmost importance. Contaminated articles should be disposed of according to the facility's policies. The family, child, and visitors should be instructed in good hand-washing techniques. Because the mode of transmission is airborne, the child or family should be instructed to cover the child's nose and mouth during sneezing or coughing episodes.

Varicella-Zoster Infections (Chickenpox, Shingles)

Causative agent: varicella-zoster virus
Incubation period: 10 to 21 days
Infectious period: 1 to 2 days before the onset of rash until all lesions are dried, usually 5 to 7 days

Transmission:	direct contact, droplet, airborne particles
Immunity:	natural disease of varicella; same virus causes zoster and may contract zoster at a later time; varicella vaccine
Season:	late winter through early spring

Chickenpox is the result of a primary infection with the varicella-zoster virus. Typically, this is one of the most common childhood diseases seen in children ages 5 to 9 years. Zoster (shingles), which is the reactivation of the latent varicella-zoster virus, occurs most frequently in the elderly. It can also occur in children, however, especially adolescents and young adults. Varicella and zoster in children are not usually life-threatening. In children who are immunosuppressed, however, this relatively mild disease can be serious and may become life-threatening.

MANIFESTATIONS

Varicella. During the 24 to 48 hours before the appearance of the rash, symptoms may include a slightly elevated body temperature, malaise, and anorexia. The macular rash generally first appears on the trunk and scalp (Fig. 40–5). The lesions may be in various stages of development, beginning

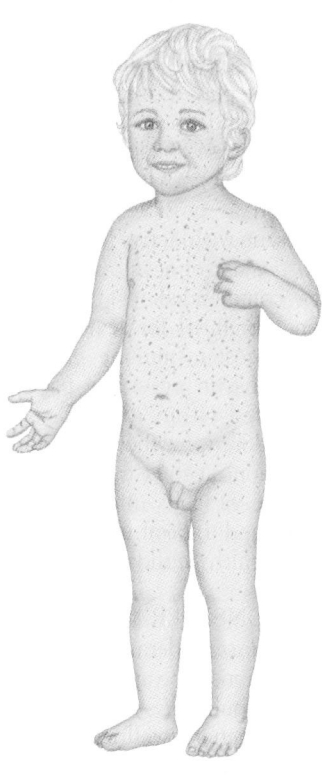

- Macular rash 24–48 hours following slight fever, malaise, anorexia

- Lesions appear in "crops," first on trunk and scalp, then moving sparsely to extremities. May appear in mucous membranes (mouth, genital area, rectum).

- Generally 3 successive eruptions over 3–4 days

- Lesions begin as a macular rash, develop into a red papular rash, then move quickly into teardrop vesicles with erythematous base. Vesicle becomes pustular and begins drying, and a crust develops.

- Rash varies from child to child

Chickenpox Rash Distribution

Chickenpox

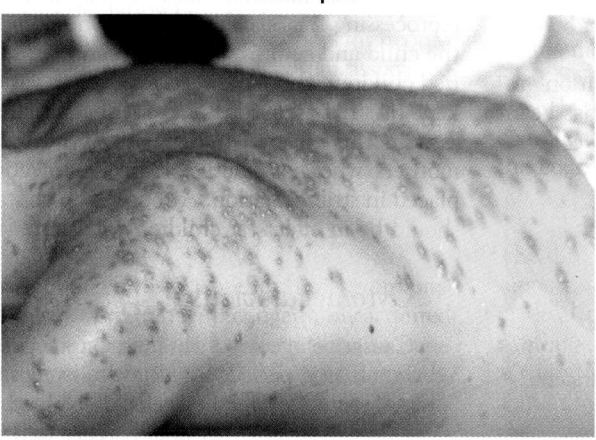

Shingles

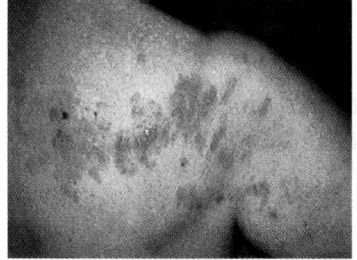

FIGURE 40–5

Chickenpox and shingles lesions, and rash distribution. (Shingles photo from Moschella, S. L., & Hurley, H. J. [1992]. *Dermatology* [3rd ed.]. Philadelphia: Saunders, p. 219, Fig. 8–25D.)

• • • • • • • • • •
Preventive Measures to Avoid Insect Bites

- Children should wear long pants, long-sleeved shirts, long socks, and a hat when in woods and grassy areas. Pants should be tucked into socks. Paths should be followed and dense areas avoided.
- Insect repellents that contain DEET and permethrines should be used. Clothing and exposed skin should be protected every 4 to 8 hours. Care should be taken to avoid contact of repellent with the child's eyes or mouth. The repellent should not be applied to the hands so as to avoid contact with the eyes and mouth.
- Repellents should be used with caution in infants because of the risk of encephalopathy.
- Insect repellent should not be applied to wounds or irritated skin.
- The body should be inspected periodically for ticks, which may resemble small moles or blood blisters.
- Ticks should be removed with tweezers. The tick should be removed as close to the skin as possible.
- Care should be taken to avoid handling the tick with bare hands or crushing the tick's body.
- Ticks may be preserved in alcohol for later identification.
- Pets should be kept free of ticks by dipping and spraying during tick season. Yards should be kept free of brush and undergrowth.

second most common manifestation is arthritis. Other manifestations that accompany the rash are malaise, fatigue, headache, stiff neck, vomiting, nausea, and sore throat. There may be general lymphadenopathy. These symptoms may occur from 1 to 4 months after the bite. The signs and symptoms generally resolve over a few days, but many individuals have a recurrence. Skin lesions may recur but are smaller and more diffuse than the initial ones.

CNS symptoms may include headache with myelitis, aseptic meningitis, Bell's palsy, and cerebral ataxia. Cardiac disease is usually brief and uncommon in children. Large joints are most commonly affected by arthritis. The knee is most often involved. The joints become warm, painful, and swollen. Recurrent attacks of arthritis are common.

THERAPEUTIC MANAGEMENT
Early detection and treatment appear to affect the course of the disease. Disease identified in early stages and treated does not progress to later stages. The characteristic rash of Lyme disease linked to other symptoms should lead to a diagnosis except in cases where the child has atypical manifestations of the disease.

Presently, treatment involves the use of tetracycline or doxycycline for children over 9 years and amoxicillin for children under 9 years. Intravenous cefotaxime is given for rheumatologic or neurologic disease. Most children who are treated early have an uncomplicated course. A vaccine for high-risk groups has been approved, but not for children younger than 15. Safety and efficacy studies in children are currently in progress.

NURSING CONSIDERATIONS
Assessment should include a complete history of rash onset and characteristics, medications taken, recent exposures to infectious diseases, and recent hiking or other activities in wooded areas. The rash should be examined and its distribution and morphology recorded.

Fever, headache, and arthralgia should be treated with antipyretics and analgesics. Antibiotics should be given as ordered. Parents should have an understanding of the course of treatment. Generally, affected children will be treated at home, so home care education is important. Education in the prevention of Lyme disease continues to be an important factor.

Evaluation includes a review of the child's skin integrity, which should be maintained. The child should be free of pain, and both the child and the parents should be able to verbalize an understanding of prevention of Lyme disease.

▌ Helminths

Helminths are worms that live as parasites. The three groups with the greatest impact on humans are tapeworms, flukes, and roundworms (Table 40–1). Children are more commonly infected than adults, primarily as a result of frequent hand-to-mouth activity and the likelihood of fecal contamination. Transmission may occur by oral-fecal ingestion, ingestion of contaminated tissue from another host, skin penetration, or the bite of a blood-sucking insect.

Therapeutic Management

Treatment consists of the administration of oral medications effective against a specific helminth. Treatment is provided to the entire family. Enteric isolation and education of the family regarding personal hygiene and sanitary practices are also necessary.

Nursing Considerations

A thorough history, including the child's general wellness, personal hygiene practices, and nutritional intake, should be obtained. Education focuses on the course of treatment. Parents should be informed of the need and rationale for evaluating and treating the entire family for infection. They need to clearly understand the various modes of transmissions and the methods effective in preventing cross-contamination of family members.

Most parasites are identified in fecal smears obtained from stool specimens. The nurse needs to provide clear instructions regarding the collection of specimens. Sample size and number, as well as proper storage, should be clearly explained. Stool specimens that have not been contaminated with urine are ideal. Obtaining urine-free specimens may be difficult, however, especially in very young children. Older children can be cooperative in obtaining the specimen. At home, clear plastic wrap can be placed over the toilet bowl, or a potty chair can be used. If the child wears diapers, specimens can be collected from the diaper. These specimens do not need to be collected in a sterile manner. The specimen is collected using a clean tongue blade and

TABLE 40–1

Common Helminths

Class and Typical Agent	Transmission	Manifestations	Diagnosis	Treatment
Roundworm (*Ascaris lumbricoides*)	Ingestion of eggs from contaminated soil or food, transfer to mouth from fingers, toys, or other vectors	Abdominal pain or distension, abdominal obstruction, vomiting with bile staining, pneumonitis	Fecal smear	Mebendazole Pyrantel pamoate
Pinworm (*Enterobius vermicularis*)	Ingestion or inhalation of eggs, transfer from hands to mouth	Nocturnal anal itching, sleeplessness	Scotch tape test and microscopic examination	Pyrantel pamoate Mebendazole
Tapeworm (*Taenia saginata*)	Ingestion from handling or eating infected beef or pork	Asymptomatic, segments of worms seen in stool, abdominal pain, nausea, anorexia, weight loss, insomnia	Fecal smear or microscopic examination	Praziquantel (safety under age 4 not established and use is investigational)
Hookworm (*Necator americanus*)	Skin penetration from direct contact with contaminated soil	Dermatitis, anemia, pneumonitis, blood loss, malnutrition	Fecal smear or microscopic examination	Pryantel pamoate

PARENTS WANT TO KNOW

About Preventing Parasitic Infections

- Hand washing (including under the fingernails) with soap and water should be done before eating or handling of food, as well as after toileting.
- Placing hands in the mouth and nail biting should be discouraged.
- Toilets or other appropriate facilities should be used for toileting.
- Clean bathroom facilities, cleaned with agents containing bleach, should be provided.
- Scratching of the anal area with bare hands should be discouraged.
- Dogs and cats should be kept at a distance from play areas and sandboxes, and the latter need to be covered when not in use.
- Shoes should be worn when outside.
- All fruits and vegetables should be washed before being eaten.
- Diapers should be changed frequently and disposed of properly (out of children's reach).
- Swimming facilities that allow diapered children should be avoided.
- Only bottled water should be used during camping outings.

is placed in the specified container. The container should be marked with the child's name and the date and time of collection. It should then be refrigerated until it is delivered to the laboratory.

Teaching the family about prevention is the most important nursing responsibility. Families need to gain a clear understanding of good hygiene and health habits.

Fungal Infections

Fungi are free-living organisms that can be found throughout the environment. Some species of fungi are part of the normal human flora, especially those in the mouth, intestine, vagina, and skin. A fungus is transmitted through inhalation or penetration of tissue as a result of trauma. Fungi grow very slowly, so clinical symptoms may appear only after a prolonged period of time. They are aerobic, can grow in a wide range of temperatures, and are resistant to most antibiotics. They exist in two forms: *molds* and *yeasts*.

Infections caused by fungi are classified into four groups:

- opportunistic—secondary to a defect in host immunity
- systemic—involving deep tissues and organs
- subcutaneous—limited to deep subcutaneous tissue
- superficial—limited to skin, hair, and nails

Common fungal infections include tinea capitis, tinea pedis, and candidal infections. (See Chapter 49 for a discussion).

Sexually Transmissible Diseases

The rates of infection of many sexually transmissible diseases (STDs), or diseases transmitted through sexual activity, are highest among adolescents. Those adolescents at highest risk are male homosexuals, sexually active heterosexuals, younger sexually active adolescents, and intravenous-drug users. Adolescents are at greater risk because they have frequent unprotected intercourse, are biologically more susceptible to infection, and face multiple obstacles to access to health care (Centers for Disease Control and Prevention, 1998a). Often, adolescents lack knowledge of methods for preventing STDs. Moreover, the use of drugs and alcohol makes unsafe, unprotected sex more likely to occur.

Neonates are at risk for transplacental transmission from an infected mother or from direct contamination during the birthing process (see Chapter 55). Children who acquire STDs after the neonatal period should be highly suspect of being sexually abused. These children may present without the typical genital symptoms but with a variety of physical or behavioral complaints. Related changes in behavior may include insomnia, eating disorders, bed wetting, or emotional withdrawal. A careful, complete examination is required. The examination should include inspection of oral, anal, and genital mucosa for any signs of trauma or infection. Because obtaining a complete history may be difficult, children should undergo a complete laboratory evaluation, and all potentially infected areas should be cultured.

Gonorrhea

Causative agent:	*Neisseria gonorrhoeae*
Incubation period:	2 to 7 days
Transmission:	intimate contact (perinatally, through sexual abuse, by sexual intercourse)

Gonorrhea may be transmitted three different ways:

- *Perinatally:* Transmission can occur during birth of a neonate whose mother is infected or with premature rupture of the membranes. The neonate can acquire the disease through aspiration of vaginal secretions, which leads to sepsis; through direct contact through the conjunctiva; or through direct contact through attachment of a fetal scalp electrode.
- *Sexual abuse:* Any child with a positive culture and without a prior history of voluntary sexual behavior should be strongly considered a potential sexual abuse victim. Transmission through sexual play with children has been documented but is rare. Almost all children diagnosed with gonorrhea at the age of 1 year or older have experienced sexual abuse.
- *Voluntary sexual activity:* This route of transmission remains the primary route of infection among adolescents. Sexual abuse should not, however, be excluded as a possibility.

MANIFESTATIONS

Ophthalmia neonatorum is the most common type of gonorrheal infection in the infant, presenting 1 to 4 days after birth. A thick, purulent discharge from the eyes may be present and, if not treated promptly, will progress to corneal ulceration, rupture, and blindness (see Chapter 55). Ophthalmia neonatorum has been controlled through prophylactic treatment with an ophthalmic antibiotic given immediately after birth. In older children, ophthalmic infection can be the result of self-inoculation from the genital site.

Girls with gonorrheal infection may present with a purulent vulvovaginitis, whereas boys often have urethritis. A history of purulent discharge with burning during urination is often elicited. Adolescent girls may present with cervicitis, urethritis, perihepatitis, and salpingitis. Gonorrhea in adolescent and younger females may progress to pelvic inflammatory disease (PID). PID is the most common cause of infertility in young women (Gutman, 1998a).

THERAPEUTIC MANAGEMENT

Because syphilis and chlamydial infection are also often present in individuals with gonorrhea, testing should also take place for those diseases. Penicillin-resistant *N. gonorrhoeae* strains have influenced the choice of therapy. Currently, the drug of choice for gonorrhea is a third-generation cephalosporin, such as ceftriaxone. Ceftriaxone is effective in treating syphilis but not chlamydial infections. It is recommended, therefore, that a course of tetracycline or doxycycline be administered in conjunction with ceftriaxone for those with chlamydial infection. Sexual partners should be treated.

Syphilis

Causative agent:	*Treponema pallidum*
Incubation period:	acquired primary infection—10 to 90 days (average, 21 days)
Transmission:	intimate contact, transplacentally, or sexually

Congenital syphilis may be transmitted transplacentally by an infected mother at any time during pregnancy or birth. Acquired syphilis is contracted through sexual contact. In children, syphilis diagnosed after the neonatal period can almost always be linked to sexual abuse.

MANIFESTATIONS

Infants with congenital syphilis may be asymptomatic or may exhibit signs and symptoms within the first 3 months of life. The classic signs are rhinitis, a maculopapular rash, and hepatosplenomegaly. Diagnostic radiographs may show osteochondritis, periosteitis, or metaphyseal changes, especially in the long bones of the femur and humerus. Late manifestations are a result of the scarring from the systemic disease process. There is involvement of the bones, teeth, eyes, and eighth cranial nerve. The teeth are notched (Hutchinson's teeth), and hearing loss can occur suddenly around the age of 8 to 10 years.

Acquired syphilis has the same clinical course in children as in adults. Primary syphilis presents with a painless chancre at the site of exposure. It is generally a single, rounded ulcer with a rubbery base and defined margins. The lesion may persist for 3 to 6 weeks before healing. Secondary syphilis may occur 3 to 6 weeks after the appearance of the chancre. The primary lesion may still be present, or it may have healed. Symptoms include local or generalized rash, general adenopathy, malaise, fever, headache, and pharyngitis. As a result of the systemic infection, a positive culture of syphilis may be obtained from CSF. The secondary stage may last 3 to 12 weeks before resolving.

The latent stage begins with the resolution of the secondary stage. This stage is a result of the chronic inflammation of bone, teeth, and the CNS. Signs include Hutchinson's teeth, interstitial keratitis, eighth nerve deafness, bone changes, frontal bossing, and saddle nose (Behrman, Kliegman, & Arvin, 1996).

THERAPEUTIC MANAGEMENT
Syphilis responds well to penicillin. Aqueous crystalline penicillin G or procaine penicillin are effective with congenital syphilis. Acquired syphilis can be treated with benzathine penicillin G. Tetracycline or doxycycline can be used for a child with a history of penicillin allergy.

Chlamydial Infection

Causative agent:	*Chlamydia trachomatis, Chlamydia psittaci, Chlamydia pneumoniae*
Incubation period:	7 to 21 days
Transmission:	during birth if mother is infected, through sexual activity

Chlamydial infection has become one of the most prevalent STDs. Infants are infected during the birthing process. Chlamydial infection can cause morbidity in the infant and is responsible for neonatal eye infections and interstitial pneumonia.

MANIFESTATIONS
Neonatal conjunctivitis manifests with a watery discharge that becomes purulent. There is eyelid edema, and the conjunctiva may become inflamed. Mucoid rhinorrhea may be associated with the infection. Many infants with conjunctivitis will develop infection of the nasopharynx, which can progress to pneumonia. These infants may have a history of a cough and congestion. Long-term abnormalities of pulmonary function may result in chronic respiratory problems.

Urethritis with dysuria, urinary frequency, or mucopurulent discharge may indicate chlamydial infection. Any identification of this organism in presexual children indicates possible child abuse.

THERAPEUTIC MANAGEMENT
In infants with conjunctivitis or pneumonia, a 10- to 14-day course of erythromycin is recommended. In children older than 8, doxycycline may also be used.

Trichomoniasis

Causative agent:	*Trichomonas vaginalis*
Transmission:	perinatal contact during delivery, sexual activity

MANIFESTATIONS
Only 25% to 50% of female patients with trichomoniasis will exhibit symptoms. Most male patients are asymptomatic. When symptoms occur, they may include dysuria, vaginal itching and burning (in females), and a foamy, yellowish green, foul-smelling discharge. Infected mothers can infect their newborn infants during birth. Children having a positive culture for *Trichomonas* should be investigated for possible sexual abuse.

THERAPEUTIC MANAGEMENT
The treatment of choice is a single dose of metronidazole (Flagyl, Protostat) for adolescents and adults. For prepubertal girls, the drug is given in three divided doses. Sexual partners should also be treated. Metronidazole should not be used during the first trimester of pregnancy.

Human Papillomavirus

Causative agent:	human papillomavirus (HPV)
Incubation period:	4 weeks to many months
Transmission:	direct sexual contact, perinatal contact during delivery

Human papillomavirus is responsible for the common wart and for venereal warts (condylomata acuminata). These anogenital warts may be contracted through direct sexual contact or perinatally during the delivery process. Children with anogenital warts should be investigated for sexual abuse. Warts can be obtained through autoinoculation from other body sites. A break in skin integrity is necessary for infection to occur.

MANIFESTATIONS
Anogenital warts begin as small papules that grow into soft, clustered lesions. They are found in moist areas, such as the labia minora, vagina, cervix, anus, rectum, and glans penis. Most warts in children resolve within several years.

THERAPEUTIC MANAGEMENT
Treatment can include surgery, cryotherapy, electrocautery, and laser therapy or chemical ablation. For sexually active individuals, transmission can be decreased by the use of condoms.

NURSING CONSIDERATIONS
Prevention and early identification and treatment are the goals of care associated with STDs. The nurse plays a key role in educating young people about STDs. Often, the school nurse is the health care professional whom adolescents feel they can trust, so school nurses may be the care providers in the best position to educate this population. A nonjudgmental approach and reassurance of confidentiality are key. The nurse must be aware of symptoms and assist in identifying those who are at risk for STDs. Encouraging abstinence in those who are not sexually active and condom use in sexually active adolescents are ways of preventing STDs. The nurse may be the one to assume responsibility for helping the adolescent obtain proper medical treatment and gain an understanding of the importance of completing the entire course of medication as well as treatment of partners. (See Chapters 26 and 31 for a discussion of STDs in pregnancy.)

KEY CONCEPTS

■ Microorganisms that cause infectious disease are classified as bacteria, viruses, fungi, protozoa, and helminths.

■ The skin is the first line of defense in the innate immune system.

■ Infectious diseases can be transmitted by direct contact with another infected person, by contact with animal or insect carriers, by ingestion of contaminated food or water containing the pathogens, and by contact with a contaminated object.

■ Exogenous pathogens are transmitted by direct contact, by animal or insect contact, through contaminated water or food, or by contact with a contaminated object.

■ Vaccines can be live or attenuated, killed or inactivated, toxoids, human immune globulin, or animal serums or antitoxins.

■ Assessment of the child with an infectious disease includes recording the type, configuration, and distribution of lesions; the child's temperature; and any other manifestations.

■ Children with infectious diseases usually can and should be cared for at home.

■ Children who acquire an STD after the neonatal period should be evaluated for possible sexual abuse.

■ Gonorrhea can be transmitted during delivery of a neonate or with premature rupture of the membranes, through sexual abuse, and through voluntary sexual activity.

■ Positive findings associated with STDs include discharge from the vagina or penis, itching around the genitals or anus, soreness or swelling in the genital area, pain, body rashes, odors from the genitals, and fever or fatigue.

ANSWER TO CRITICAL THINKING EXERCISE 40-1

The child who develops varicella while hospitalized poses a great risk to immunocompromised children and nonimmune pregnant women. Nursing measures include strict isolation. The nurse who cares for the child may not care for any immunocompromised children. If a female nurse is not immune to varicella, she should not care for this child because of the possibility of acquiring a potentially fatal case of varicella pneumonia. If the child is febrile, administer antipyretics. Provide a cool environment to decrease skin irritation. Administer antihistamines and antipruritics to reduce itching and discomfort. Provide cool liquids and distraction.

REFERENCES AND READINGS

American Academy of Pediatrics Committee on Infectious Diseases. (1993). Vitamin A treatment of measles. *Pediatrics, 91*(5), 1014–1015.

American Academy of Pediatrics Committee on Infectious Diseases. (1995). Recommendations for the use of live attenuated varicella vaccine. *Pediatrics, 95,* 791–796.

American Academy of Pediatrics Committee on Infectious Diseases. (1997). *Report of the Committee on Infectious Diseases: 1997 Red Book* (24th ed.). Washington, DC: Author.

Betz, C. L. (1998). Sexually transmitted disease and adolescents. *Journal of Pediatric Nursing, 13*(3), 139.

Bonny, A. E., & Biro, F. M. (1998). Recognizing and treating STDs in adolescent girls. *Contemporary Pediatrics, 15*(3), 119–143.

Centers for Disease Control and Prevention. (1998a). 1998 guidelines for treatment of sexually transmitted diseases. *Morbidity and Mortality Weekly Report, 47*(RR-1), 1–118.

Centers for Disease Control and Prevention. (1998b). HIV prevention through early detection and treatment of other sexually transmitted diseases—United States. Recommendations of the Advisory Committee for HIV and STD prevention. *Morbidity and Mortality Weekly Report, 47*(RR-12), 1–24.

Cherry, J. D. (1998). Rubella virus. In R. D. Feigin & J. D. Cherry (Eds.), *Textbook of pediatric infectious diseases* (4th ed., pp. 1922–1949). Philadelphia: Saunders.

Feigin, R. D., & Cherry, J. D. (Eds.). (1998). *Textbook of pediatric infectious diseases* (4th ed.). Philadelphia: Saunders.

Fortenberry, J. D. (1997). Health care seeking behaviors related to sexually transmitted diseases among adolescents. *American Journal of Public Health, 87*(3), 417–420.

Gershon, A. A. (1998). Varicella-zoster virus. In R. D. Feigin & J. D. Cherry (Eds.), *Textbook of pediatric infectious diseases* (4th ed., pp. 1769–1777). Philadelphia: Saunders.

Gildea, J. H. (1998). Human parvovirus B19: Flushed in face though healthy (fifth disease and more). *Pediatric Nursing, 24*(4), 325–329.

Gordon, S. L. (1994). Lyme disease in children. *Pediatric Nursing, 20*(4), 415–418.

Gutman, L. T. (1998a). Gonorrhea. In R. D. Feigin & J. D. Cherry (Eds.), *Textbook of pediatric infectious diseases* (4th ed., pp. 1157–1169). Philadelphia: Saunders.

Gutman, L. T. (1998b). Sexually transmitted diseases. In R. D. Feigin & J. D. Cherry (Eds.), *Textbook of pediatric infectious diseases* (4th ed., pp. 548–561). Philadelphia: Saunders.

Haffner, D. W. (1998). Facing facts: Sexual health for American adolescents. *Journal of Adolescent Health, 22*(6), 453–459.

Kenney, J. W. (1996). Ethnic differences in risk factors associated with genital human papillomavirus infections. *Journal of Advanced Nursing, 23*(6), 1221–1227.

Long, S. (1996). Diphtheria. In R. E. Behrman, R. Kliegman, & A. Arvin (Eds.), *Nelson textbook of pediatrics* (15th ed., pp. 776–779). Philadelphia: Saunders.

Overall, J. C. (1998). Viral infections of the fetus and neonate. In R. D. Feigin & J. D. Cherry (Eds.), *Textbook of pediatric infectious diseases* (4th ed., pp. 856–892). Philadelphia: Saunders.

Selekman, J. (1998). Infectious diseases and the immunizations of today and tomorrow. *Pediatric Nursing, 24*(4), 309–315.

Stechenberg, B. W. (1998). Borrelia (Lyme disease). In R. D. Feigin & J. D. Cherry (Eds.), *Textbook of pediatric infectious diseases* (4th ed., pp. 1522–1528). Philadelphia: Saunders.

Stevens-Simon, C. (1997). Reproductive health care for your adolescent female patients. *Contemporary Pediatrics, 14*(2), 35–69.

Taylor, C. A., Keller, M. L., & Egan, J. J. (1997). Advice from affected persons about living with human papillomavirus. *Image—The Journal of Nursing Scholarship, 29*(1), 27–32.

41

The Child with
an Immunologic
Alteration

After studying this chapter, you should be able to:

- Describe how the immune system attempts to maintain homeostasis of the internal and external environment, and what happens when it overfunctions or underfunctions.
- Explain how neonates acquire active and passive immunity.
- Delineate how to prevent the spread of organisms in children with an immunodeficiency.
- Describe how to care for and support HIV-affected children and their families throughout the entire spectrum of illness.
- Outline critical information needed by families with children receiving long-term corticosteroid therapy.
- Describe nursing interventions to help prevent the sudden death of a child having an anaphylactic reaction.

DEFINITIONS

active immunity Protection that forms in response to exposure to natural antigens or vaccines; protection can last months, years, or a lifetime.

allergy A hypersensitivity reaction in various body systems resulting from the immune system's response to exposure to an irritant (allergen).

antibody A protein that the immune system produces to bind to specific antigens and eliminate them from the body.

antigen A substance that possesses unique configurations enabling the immune system to recognize it as foreign.

autoimmune disease Disease that occurs when the immune system produces antibodies—called autoantibodies—against cells of the body.

complement An accessory system to a humoral response that is composed of serum proteins that facilitate enzyme action and antigen death.

immune (lymphoreticular) system The body's internal defense against foreign substances, such as bacteria, viruses, parasites, and fungi.

immunodeficiency A defect in the immune system leading to increased susceptibility to multiple and repeated infections.

leukocytes White blood cells, whose chief function is to protect the body against foreign substances. There are five types: lymphocytes, monocytes, neutrophils, eosinophils, and basophils.

lymphocytes The primary white blood cells of the immune system (e.g., B lymphocytes or B cells and T lymphocytes or T cells).

nonspecific immune functions Protective barriers, such as chemicals, interferon, inflammation, and phagocytosis, which are activated in the presence of an antigen but are not specific to that antigen.

passive immunity Protection that occurs when serum containing an antibody is given or transmitted to a person who does not have that antibody.

specific immune functions Humoral (B-cell and antibody production) and cell-mediated (T-cell) responses that are activated in a highly discriminatory way to antigens that survive in the body.

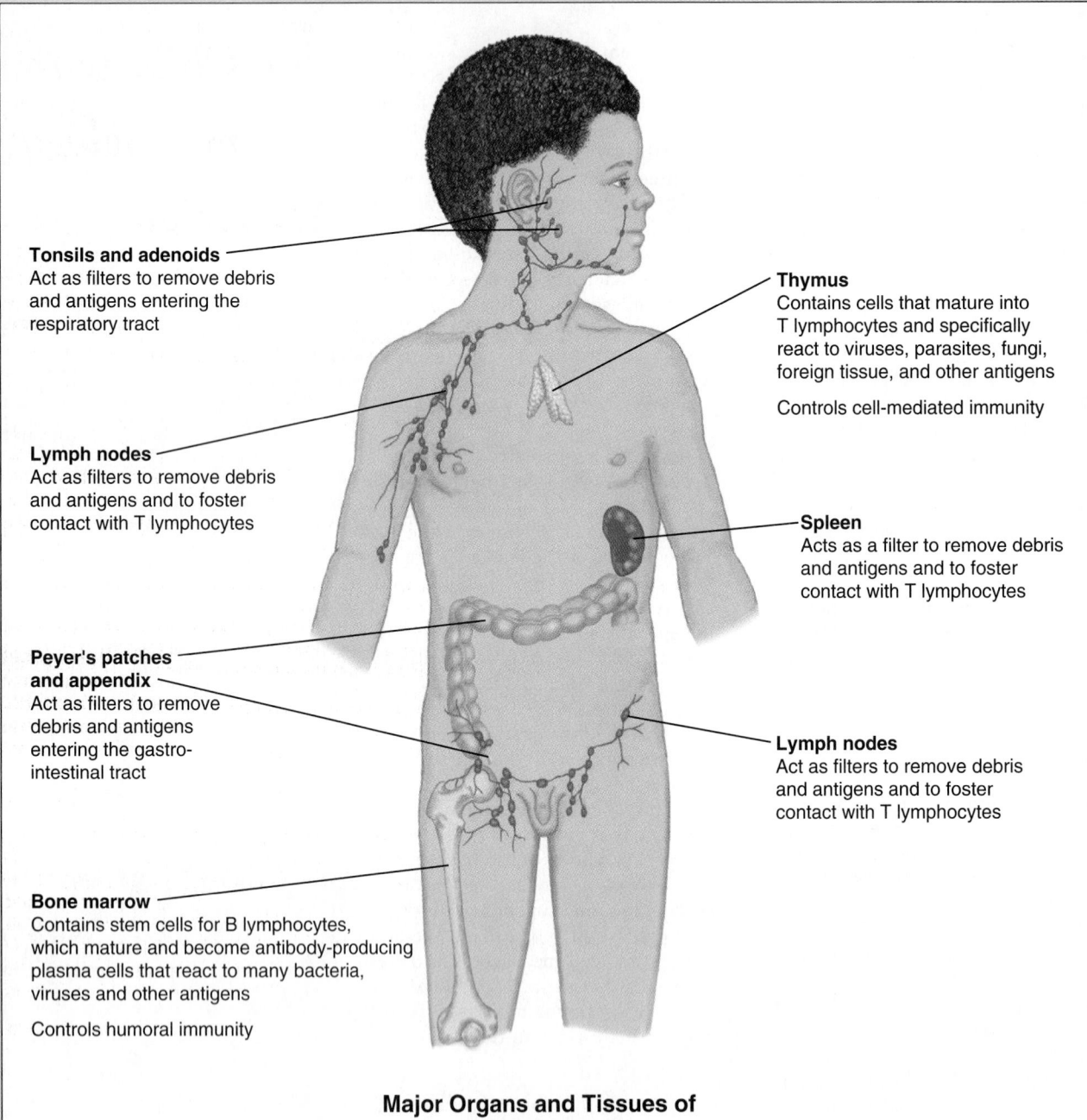

Tonsils and adenoids
Act as filters to remove debris and antigens entering the respiratory tract

Thymus
Contains cells that mature into T lymphocytes and specifically react to viruses, parasites, fungi, foreign tissue, and other antigens

Controls cell-mediated immunity

Lymph nodes
Act as filters to remove debris and antigens and to foster contact with T lymphocytes

Spleen
Acts as a filter to remove debris and antigens and to foster contact with T lymphocytes

Peyer's patches and appendix
Act as filters to remove debris and antigens entering the gastro-intestinal tract

Lymph nodes
Act as filters to remove debris and antigens and to foster contact with T lymphocytes

Bone marrow
Contains stem cells for B lymphocytes, which mature and become antibody-producing plasma cells that react to many bacteria, viruses and other antigens

Controls humoral immunity

Major Organs and Tissues of the Immune System

Review of the Immune System

The body's network of first-line, or external, defenses—intact skin and mucous membranes, and such processes as sneezing, coughing, and tearing—helps keep it free of disease. When a foreign substance penetrates first-line defenses, the immune or internal defense system provides secondary and tertiary protection through nonspecific and specific responses. The immune system is able to distinguish the body's own cells, or self, from foreign substances, or nonself; activate a response to detect and destroy foreign substances; suppress a response against the self; and memorize and store information.

Foreign substances, or antigens, possess unique configurations that mark them as foreign. The immune system first responds to the invader through nonspecific immune functions. If the antigen survives the action of the nonspecific response, the immune system initiates specific immune functions. It begins producing proteins called antibodies or immunoglobulins. Each antibody is specific for a particular antigen, contains sites that are complementary, and can combine with the antigen. This combination of antigen and antibody is called the antigen-antibody complex or immune complex. The immune complex acts to destroy the antigen.

The major organs and tissues of the immune system include the bone marrow, thymus, spleen, lymph nodes, and

Cells Involved in the Immune Response

Cell Type	Nonspecific Immune Response
Granulocytes	
Neutrophils	First leukocytes to respond to tissue damage. Ingest and destroy antigens, especially bacteria, by phagocytosis. Increase in number during acute inflammation, bacterial infection, and necrosis. Immature neutrophils are called bands. Increased bands (shift to the left) indicate infection.
Eosinophils	Neutralize histamine. Increase in number during allergic reactions and infestation with parasitic worms.
Basophils	Secrete histamine, heparin, and serotonin in inflammation and immediate hypersensitivity reactions. Basophils located in tissue rather than in blood are called mast cells.
Agranulocytes	
Monocytes/Macrophages	Monocytes are large phagocytic agranulocytes. In tissue, they are called macrophages. Monocytes ingest and introduce antigens into the circulation. Macrophages engulf bacteria and cellular debris to finish the cleanup process started by the neutrophils.

Cell Type	Specific Immune Response
B lymphocytes	Noncirculating, short-lived cells responsible for humoral immunity. As plasma cells, produce antibodies to bacteria. First responder to viral infection. Some become memory cells for recognition of specific antigens.
T lymphocytes	Responsible for cellular immunity. Interact with specific antigens on cell surfaces and directly attack invading microorganisms. Respond to viruses, fungi, parasites, and foreign tissue. T-cell regulatory functions mobilize or deactivate the other cells in the immune system.
Helper (CD4+) T cells	Recognize antigens that have been processed and presented to them by B cells or macrophages. CD4+ cells secrete lymphokines that stimulate B cells to manufacture antibodies.
Suppressor T cells	Inhibit the actions of helper T cells and B cells. Help keep the immune system cells in check.
Cytotoxic T cells	Phagocytize target cells; make cells more vulnerable to chemical attack via production of lymphokines.

Data from Applegate, E. J. (1995). *The anatomy and physiology learning system: Textbook* (p. 300). Philadelphia: Saunders; Copstead, L. E. (1995). *Perspectives on pathophysiology* (p. 191). Philadelphia: Saunders; Hansen, M. (1998). *Pathophysiology foundations of disease and clinical intervention.* Philadelphia: Saunders.

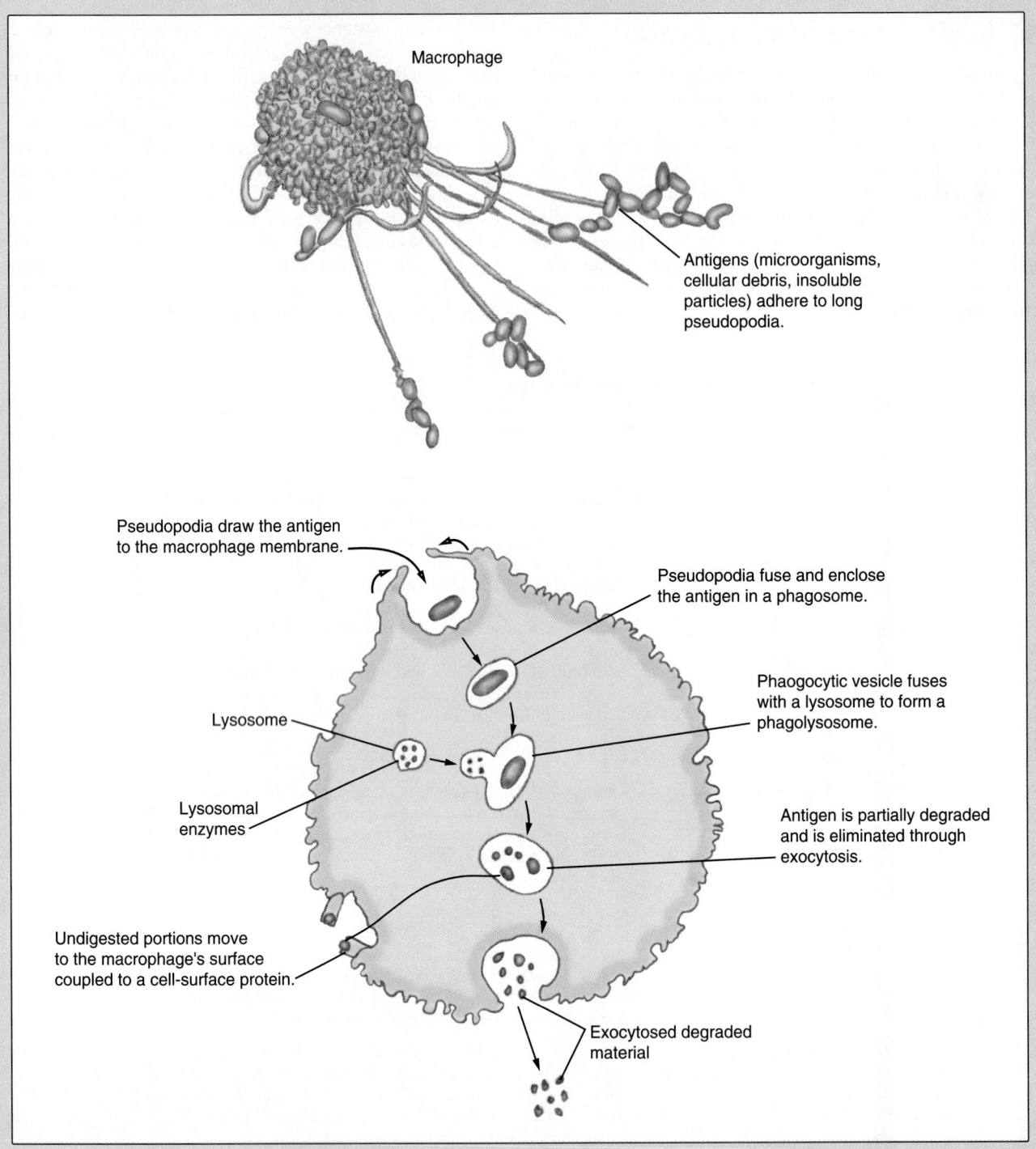

Macrophage

Antigens (microorganisms, cellular debris, insoluble particles) adhere to long pseudopodia.

Pseudopodia draw the antigen to the macrophage membrane.

Pseudopodia fuse and enclose the antigen in a phagosome.

Phaogocytic vesicle fuses with a lysosome to form a phagolysosome.

Lysosome

Lysosomal enzymes

Antigen is partially degraded and is eliminated through exocytosis.

Undigested portions move to the macrophage's surface coupled to a cell-surface protein.

Exocytosed degraded material

lymphoid tissue. Both the circulatory system and the lymphatic system connect these organs and tissues to one another. Specific types of cells are also important to the immune system.

Nonspecific Immune Functions

The body's innate immune system consists of nonspecific immune functions, which are protective barriers activated in the presence of an antigen but not specific to that antigen. Among these nonspecific immune functions are chemical barriers, such as bactericides and fungicides and enzymes in body secretions; interferon, a protein produced in response to viruses; and inflammation, increased capillary permeability, vasodilation, phagocytosis (cell-eating), and elimination of cell products.

Phagocytosis can occur alone or as part of the inflammatory response (see figure). Phagocytes ingest the antigen and either survive or die. In dying, the phagocytes release additional chemicals that draw more phagocytes to the area.

. . . .

Immunoglobulin Function and Pediatric Implications

IG Type	% of Total IG*	Function and Pediatric Significance	Location
IgG	70–80	Contains most antibodies against bacteria, viruses, and fungi in blood and body spaces. Crosses the placenta; provides maternal antibody protection to infants. Responsible for Rh reactions. IgG response is longer and stronger than that of the other immunoglobulins.	Appears in all internal body fluids; present in majority of B cells.
IgM	5–10	Produced 48–72 hours after an antigen enters the body and remains in the blood. First immunoglobulin produced in response to bacterial and viral infections. Responsible for transfusion reactions in the ABO blood typing system. Does not cross placenta, so values are low in newborns. However, IgM is produced early in life, and level increases after 9 months of age. Presence in cord or infant blood may mean infection in utero or newborn period.	Appears mostly in intravascular serum. Attached to B cells; released into plasma during immune response.
IgA	10–15	Prevents infection across mucous membranes (local immunity). Especially important in antiviral protection. Passes to newborn in breast milk. Those having congenital IgA deficiency are prone to autoimmune disease.	Appears in body fluids (nasal and respiratory secretions, saliva, tears, breast milk).
IgE	0.004	Leads to release of histamines producing an allergic response. Elevation may indicate allergy in children. Plays a role in defense against parasites.	Appears in serum. Found on the surface membranes of basophils and mast cells. Produced by plasma cells in mucous membranes and tonsils.
IgD	0.2	Poorly understood. Thought to influence B-cell differentiation.	Appears in small amounts in serum. Attached to B cells.

*Normal immunoglobulin values differ for age.

Data from Applegate, E. J. (1995). *The anatomy and physiology learning system: Textbook* (p. 300). Philadelphia: Saunders; Copstead, L. E. (1995). *Perspectives on pathophysiology* (p. 191). Philadelphia: Saunders; and Sandberg, E., & Shearer, W. (1996). Normal immune responses. In C. W. Bierman, D. Pearlman, G. Shapiro, & W. Busse (Eds.), *Allergy, asthma, and immunology from infancy to adulthood*. Philadelphia: Saunders.

Increased capillary permeability and vasodilation result in redness and edema. The products of phagocyte-antigen death include toxins that give rise to fever, pain, and purulence. As the antigens are destroyed, the toxins are cleared from the lymph nodes, which often become enlarged. If the immune response is effective, the inflammation subsides; if ineffective, fever follows.

Specific Immune Functions

If the antigen survives within the phagocyte, then two types of specific immune functions can recognize and destroy it: humoral and cell-mediated. Both responses are closely related.

Lymphocytes (white blood cells) function in both types of immune response. Lymphocytes circulate in the blood and the lymphatic system. They make up 53% to 57% of white blood cells during the first year of life, when specific immunity develops rapidly, but only 25% to 30% after 12 months of age. Two classes of lymphocytes are involved in the immune response: B lymphocytes (B cells) and T lymphocytes (T cells).

B cells, which promote the humoral response, originate in the bone marrow or liver but mature in the lymphoid tissue, becoming plasma cells. When exposed to antigens, some of the plasma cells produce antibodies while others become memory cells. Antibodies are classified as immunoglobulins G, M, A, D, and E, often abbreviated IgG, IgM, IgA, IgD, and IgE. Immunoglobulins bind to antigens and facilitate their destruction.

T cells, which are responsible for the cell-mediated response, originate in the bone marrow and mature in the thymus, where they react specifically to viruses, fungi, parasites, foreign tissue, and other antigens. There are three types of T cells: suppressor T cells, cytotoxic cells, and helper T cells or CD4+ cells.

Natural killer cells, or large granular lymphocytes, can directly destroy tumor cells and other antigens. They are not antigen specific (Hansen, 1998; Sandberg & Shearer, 1996).

THE HUMORAL RESPONSE

The humoral response chiefly involves B cells, although the cooperation of helper T cells is almost always necessary. Macrophages ingest antigens and introduce them into the circulation. In response, the B cells and helper T cells interact. The helper T cells secrete substances that cause B cells to multiply and differentiate into plasma cells, which produce vast quantities of antibodies specific to the antigen. These antibodies combine with the antigens to form immune complexes. The antibodies either destroy the antigens or activate an accessory system called complement, a series of serum proteins involved in enzyme action and antigen death. Suppressor T cells reduce the production of antibodies after the antigens are eliminated from the body (Hansen, 1998).

THE CELL-MEDIATED RESPONSE

A cell-mediated response is also initiated by macrophages presenting antigens. Once activated, helper T cells secrete substances that spur additional T cells to grow. One set of T cells, called cytotoxic T cells, tracks down and kills viruses, tumor cells, and other pathogens. Suppressor T cells draw the immune response to a close (Hansen, 1998).

Development of Immunity

The normal fetus can produce IgM by 20 to 24 weeks of gestation. The neonate's immune protection comes from prenatal transfer of maternal antibodies (IgG) and breast milk transfer of IgA. Gradually, the normal newborn's own humoral and cell-mediated responses to infections begin; immunity is acquired both actively and passively.

ACTIVE IMMUNITY

When the body reacts to an antigen through either a humoral or a cell-mediated response, it is developing active immunity. Active immunity is long-lived and measured in months, years, or even a lifetime; it follows exposure to environmental antigens or vaccines. Immediately after exposure, there is a latency period when antibody levels are low. When the body recognizes the antigen as foreign, it makes antibodies. The first antibodies produced are predominantly IgM and subsequently IgG. After a second exposure to the antigen, antibodies appear at a faster rate and the latency period is shortened or nonexistent. The antibody

. . . .
Pediatric Differences in the Immune System

The organs of the immune system mature during infancy and childhood.

- Lymphoid tissue increases in mass during infancy and early childhood. It reaches adult size by 6 weeks of age, grows larger during the prepubertal years, and involutes at puberty.
- The thymus reaches its peak mass before puberty and then involutes.
- The spleen reaches its full size during adulthood.
- The number of Peyer's patches increases until the adult mean is exceeded during adolescence.

Immaturity of the immunologic system places the infant and young child at greater risk for infection.

- The infant has a limited capacity to mount an antibody response. The ability to respond to infections develops gradually as the infant acquires immunity actively and passively.
- Because of the immaturity of the inflammatory response in neonates, the more common signs and symptoms of infection (e.g., fever) are less pronounced, making diagnosis more difficult.
- Neonates' diminished nonspecific immune response allows a more rapid spread of infection, leading potentially to sepsis.
- The term newborn receives an adult level of IgG as a result of transplacental transfer from the mother. This level begins to disappear during the first 6 to 8 months, causing a physiologic drop in IgG.
- Premature infants are more susceptible to neonatal infections because of lower levels of transplacental transfer of IgG from the mother and a more severe physiologic drop in IgG.
- IgM, IgE, IgD are normally in low concentration at birth. IgM, IgE, IgA, IgD do not cross the placenta. The immunoglobulins reach adult levels at different ages (Behrman, 1996):

IgM: 1 yr
IgA: 6–7 yr
IgG: 7–8 yr
IgE: 10–15 yr

- Absolute lymphocyte counts reach a peak during the first year. Helper T cells reach adult levels by 6 years of age.
- Passive placental transfer of IgG may affect infants' response to active immunization (i.e., pertussis and/or diphtheria).
- Immature or inexperienced immune cells affect the reliability of delayed hypersensitivity skin reactions. For this reason, allergy skin tests are not routinely used with infants.

Disorders of the immune system present differently in children than in adults.

- Primary immunodeficiencies typically present in the first 6 months of life.
- HIV infection, the major secondary immunodeficiency in children, typically (1) infects an infant through the mother, not sexually; (2) is diagnosed by measuring an aspect of the virus, not antibodies as in adults; and (3) has a shorter latency period in infants, with several different AIDS-defining illnesses.

• • • • • • • • • •

Common Laboratory and Diagnostic Tests of Immune Function

Test	Function	Nursing Considerations
Serum immunoglobulins (IgG, IgM, IgA and IgE)	Tests humoral immunity Measures levels of immunoglobulins by separating them through immunoelectrophoresis.	Immunization and toxoids received in the last 6 months as well as blood transfusions, tetanus antitoxin, and gamma-globulin received in the last 6 weeks can affect results and should be noted on the laboratory requisition. Total immunoglobulins tend to be elevated in early months, then decrease over the first year of life. These also may be unusually high early in HIV infection, then decrease.
Lymphocyte surface antigen	Determines the types and subtypes of lymphocytes present in blood. Names of lymphocyte surface antigens are based on "clusters of differentiation" (CDs). CD antigens on a leukocyte allows its identification. The two most commonly used surface antigens and the cell types they identify are: CD4: helper T cells CD8: suppressor T cells	To determine the number of a particular type of cell, a complete blood cell (CBC) count must also be done.
Serum antibody titer to antigens in vaccines received (e.g., D, T)	Tests humoral immunity.	Tests antibody level to specific antigens.
Skin tests to mumps, tuberculin, tetanus, Candida	Tests cell-mediated immunity.	Measures the immune system's ability to develop antibody to foreign substances.
Differential WBC	Part of the CBC count, composed of five types of WBCs (leukocytes): neutrophils, eosinophils, basophils, monocytes, and lymphocytes. The differential WBC count is expressed in no. per cubic millimeters (mm^3) and as a percent of the total number of WBCs.	These tests measure whether immune cells can ingest and destroy foreign substances.
Allergy skin tests	Upon administration of antigen into the skin to test either immediate or delayed-type hypersensitivity.	Because anaphylactic reactions can occur even in the presence of minimal allergen exposures, emergency equipment and medications should be immediately available.
Radioallergosorbent test (RAST)	Measures the quantity and increase of antigen-specific IgE present in the serum. Exact quantities of antibodies to pollens, foods, etc., can be tested.	More expensive than traditional allergy skin testing, but provides precise information without risk of hypersensitivity reaction.

Refer to Appendix E for normal values.

Data from Corbett, J. V. (1992). *Laboratory tests and diagnostic procedures with nursing diagnoses.* East Norwalk, CT: Appleton & Lange; Kee, J. L. (1991). *Laboratory and diagnostic tests with nursing implications.* East Norwalk, CT: Appleton & Lange; Taeusch, H. W., Christiansen, R. O., & Buescher, E. S. (1996). *Pediatric and neonatal tests and procedures.* Philadelphia: Saunders.

levels remain high and persist for much longer periods of time. The predominant antibody in a secondary response is IgG.

Infants receive specific live or attenuated vaccines on a recommended schedule to induce immunity against the antigens in the vaccine (see Appendix F).

PASSIVE IMMUNITY
Passive immunity results from antibody transfer from one person to another. Transfer of antibodies from a woman to her fetus is an example of passive immunity. The fetus re-ceives maternal IgG antibodies across the placenta and becomes protected against many infections. Most maternal antibodies dissipate in the infant by 6 to 9 months of age, but some persist for up to 18 months. The duration depends on the level of a particular antibody in the maternal plasma. Protection against measles, for example, may last through the second year of life, whereas protection against certain bacterial infections may last only 1 to 2 months. The reason neonates are so susceptible to infections by bacteria such as *Escherichia coli* is because the respective antibodies do not cross the placenta.

• • • • • • • •

Age-Adjusted CD4+ Counts and Percentages

Immunologic Category	<12 Months	1–5 Years	6–12 Years
No evidence of suppression	≥1,500	≥1,000	≥500
	≥25%	≥25%	≥25%
Evidence of moderate suppression	750–1,499	500–999	200–499
	15%–24%	15%–24%	15%–24%
Severe suppression	<750	<500	<200
	<15%	<15%	<15%

From Centers for Disease Control and Prevention. (1998). Guidelines for the use of antiretroviral agents in pediatric HIV infection. *Morbidity and Mortality Weekly Report, 47*(RR-4), Table 1.

Common Laboratory and Diagnostic Tests of Immune Function

IMMUNODEFICIENCIES

A variety of laboratory tests evaluate immune system function. Laboratory evaluation determines intactness of its major functions, B-cell immunity, T-cell immunity, and phagocytosis. Many values vary significantly with age, especially during infancy. Among these are the differ- ential in the complete blood cell count, the amount of various immunoglobulins, the lymphocyte surface anti- gen count (e.g., CD4+ count), and the total lymphocyte count.

ALLERGY

Measurement of eosinophilia and IgE levels, along with a radioallergosorbent test and skin testing, is helpful in diag- nosing allergic reactions.

• • • • • • • •

Laboratory and Clinical Screening Tests for Allergy

Test	Findings Suggestive of Allergy
CBC, differential	Excess eosinophils (>5% of WBCs)
Total eosinophil count	>750 eosinophils
Nasal smear	Excess eosinophils
Serum IgE	Elevated for age
RAST test, antigen-specific IgE	Increase in antigen-specific IgE in the serum
Skin testing	Urticarial wheal appears on skin within ½ hour after administration of selected potential allergens. The reaction can be immediate or delayed and can even include anaphylaxis.

Modified from Centers for Disease Control and Prevention. (September 30, 1994). *Morbidity and Mortality Weekly Report, 43*(RR-12), 1–10.

Immunologic alterations typically are chronic, lasting from months to years and interfering with a child's life. Physical symptoms can range from simple, such as impaired skin integrity, to complex, such as overwhelming infection. Intervals of wellness, relapses, and sometimes a decline in health should be expected. Repeated office visits and hospitalizations, disruptions in family routines, altered social interactions, and emotional and financial strain are often coupled with anxiety about the future.

Initially, the nurse helps the family adjust to a new, often devastating, diagnosis. Care during the acute phase of the illness may be critical in nature, as underlying organisms are diagnosed and treated and fevers and pain are controlled. Once the acute crisis has resolved, the nurse prepares the family for discharge by teaching home management and identifying community resources and referrals for ongoing support. The nurse also teaches the family how to prevent the spread of microorganisms through infection control practices at home and describes parameters for when to call the physician. The nurse discusses ways to maintain the child's skin integrity, the body's first line of protection against microorganisms, and recommends a diet that supports immune cell growth. The nurse must keep abreast of current information because the field of immunology continues to evolve. Nurses also play a vital role in advocating for children with such stigmatized conditions as human immunodeficiency virus (HIV) infection.

Despite all efforts, rehospitalization is often inevitable. The family is an integral part of the multidisciplinary team, keeping the physicians, nurses, and social workers informed of changes in the child's condition, administering medications, providing respiratory care, and often making difficult decisions about continued treatment and comfort.

▌ The Child with an Immunodeficiency

A deficiency in one or more components of the immune system results in immunodeficiency disorders. Immunodeficiency disorders can be inherited, acquired through infection or other illness, or produced as a side effect of certain medications.

Some children are born with defects of their immune system. Children born with defects in the humoral system are unable or only partially able to produce antibodies, thus making them susceptible to bacterial infections. Other children are born with an abnormal thymus, which affects T-cell production. These children are more susceptible to viral and fungal infections as well as to certain cancers. In rare cases, children demonstrate deficiency in both B cells and T cells, a condition termed severe combined immunodeficiency disease (SCID). The most devastating acquired im-

. . . .

Clinical Findings Associated with Immunodeficiency

FREQUENTLY PRESENT, HIGHLY INDICATIVE SIGNS

- Repeated or persistent respiratory tract infection
- Repeated or persistent otitis media or sinusitis
- Severe bacterial infections
- Opportunistic infections, such as *Pneumocystis carinii* pneumonia or cryptosporidiosis
- Poor response to appropriate therapy

FREQUENTLY PRESENT, SOMEWHAT SUGGESTIVE

- Skin lesions
- Failure to thrive or grow
- Chronic diarrhea
- Thrush
- Hepatosplenomegaly
- Anemia, thrombocytopenia, neutropenia
- Small or absent lymph nodes, tonsils, and adenoids

munodeficiency is HIV infection, which destroys helper T, or CD4+, cells.

Medication can also cause acquired immunodeficiency. For example, antibiotics can disrupt normal flora, making the body more susceptible to other microorganisms. Immunosuppressive agents and corticosteroids suppress components of the immune system, resulting in a decrease in the inflammatory response and an increased risk of bacterial invasion.

▌ Human Immunodeficiency Virus Infection

HIV infection is an acquired cell-mediated immunodeficiency disorder that causes a wide spectrum of illness in children ranging from no symptoms to mild and moderate symptoms to severe symptoms. Acquired immunodeficiency syndrome (AIDS) is the most severe manifestation of this illness.

Etiology

HIV, present in an infected individual's blood or body fluids, can enter an uninfected adult's or adolescent's body in several ways, including sharing of needles or syringes, engaging in unprotected sexual intercourse with an infected person, or receiving an infected blood product. Infected women can transmit the virus to a fetus across the placenta during pregnancy, to the infant at delivery, and to the young child through breast-feeding. The potential for such transmission was about 25% before 1994, when the Centers for Disease Control and Prevention (CDC) recommended identifying and treating HIV-positive pregnant women (Mofenson & Read, 1999) (see Chapter 26). The transmission rate has dropped to as low as 8% in infants whose infected mothers received zidovudine (ZDV) during pregnancy and delivery and who themselves received zidovudine for 6 weeks after birth (Mofenson & Read, 1999). A risk of children acquiring HIV infection through sexual abuse exists.

Historically, children, especially those with hemophilia, acquired AIDS through tainted blood products. Most of those children have died, having been infected prior to widespread and accurate screening of donor blood. A small percentage of HIV-positive young adolescents are long-term survivors of perinatally acquired infection.

Incidence

In the United States approximately 7,500 children younger than 13 years of age have been diagnosed with AIDS. Perinatal transmission has been implicated in 90% of the accu-

• • • • • • • • • •
Body Substances Potentially Infectious with Blood-Borne Pathogens

- Human blood, blood products, or blood components such as factor
- All body fluids, secretions, and excretions *except sweat*, regardless of whether they contain visible blood
- Nonintact skin
- Mucous membranes

From Garner, J. S. (1996). Guidelines for isolation precautions in hospitals: Part I. Evaluation of isolation practices. Hospital Infection Control Practices Committee. *American Journal of Infection Control, 24*(1), 24–31. Reproduced with permission.

PATHOPHYSIOLOGY
• • • • • • • • • •
of HIV Infection

HIV is a retrovirus composed of RNA and an enzyme, reverse transcriptase, which plays a key role in viral replication. HIV gains entry into a CD4+ cell by direct fusion of the viral envelope to CD4+ receptors on the cell surface. Within the CD4+ cell, reverse transcriptase causes the synthesis of HIV DNA. This integrates with the CD4+ cell's DNA. The HIV virus then uses the CD4+ cell to make more of itself. The new viruses assemble at the host cell's surface. As they bud through the cell membrane, the viruses mature, are released, and can infect other CD4+ cells. The most critical result of HIV entry into the CD4+ cell is cell incapacitation and death (Hansen, 1998; Schiff & Harville, 1996). Because CD4+ cells primarily enhance cell-mediated immunity, severely infected infants and children will exhibit symptoms of viral or fungal infection. In addition, CD4+ helper cells interact with the humoral immune response. Immunoglobulins become nonfunctional, making the child extremely vulnerable to bacterial infections.

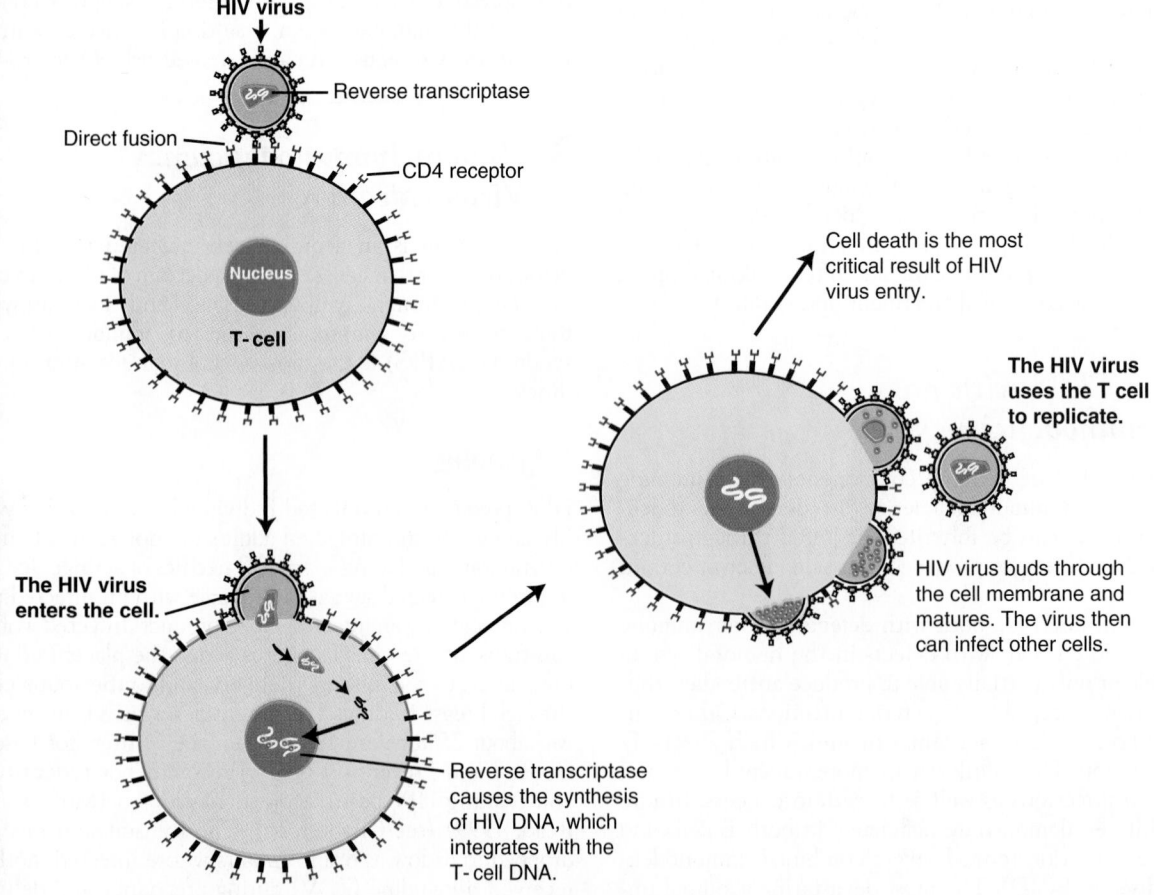

HIV virus

Reverse transcriptase

Direct fusion

CD4 receptor

Nucleus

T-cell

The HIV virus enters the cell.

Reverse transcriptase causes the synthesis of HIV DNA, which integrates with the T-cell DNA.

Cell death is the most critical result of HIV virus entry.

The HIV virus uses the T cell to replicate.

HIV virus buds through the cell membrane and matures. The virus then can infect other cells.

mulated cases; 8% are attributed to contaminated blood transfusions. Between 1988 and 1993, 6,000 to 7,000 infants were born to HIV-infected women; over 1,500 of these infants became infected. The highest incidence occurred in non-Latino black and Latino infants (Centers for Disease Control and Prevention [CDC], 1996). Subsequent to 1994 the infection transmission has decreased by two thirds.

Although only 2,000 teenagers with AIDS have been reported in the United States, ten times that number of 20- to 29-year-olds have been diagnosed with the disease. Insofar as the known median HIV incubation period in adults is 10 years, these young adults probably became infected in their teens (CDC, 1994). HIV infection is the seventh leading cause of death in infants and children under 14 years of age in the United States (CDC, 1998a).

Manifestations

HIV infection in children and adults differs in several ways (Schiff & Harville, 1996):

- The time between infection and AIDS diagnosis is shorter in infants and young children; most untreated infants develop symptoms of AIDS by 1 year of age.
- Symptoms in children include physical and developmental failure to thrive.
- Children experience early opportunistic infections, a greater number of bacterial infections from childhood illnesses, and lymphoid interstitial pneumonitis (LIP), a condition causing parotid gland enlargement, hypoxia, and digital clubbing.

Pneumocystis carinii pneumonia (PCP) in children with perinatally acquired HIV infection can occur as early as 2 months, with the average age at onset being between 3 and 6 months of age (Mofenson & Read, 1999).

The CDC classifies the clinical manifestations of HIV infection as mild, moderate, or severe in children younger than 13 years of age (CDC, 1998b). Mild signs of the illness may be nonspecific and include lymphadenopathy, hepatomegaly, splenomegaly, dermatitis, parotitis, and recurrent or persistent upper respiratory infection, sinusitis or otitis media. In moderate disease, some signs are considered to be important if they persist or recur, particularly anemia, neutropenia, or thrombocytopenia; diarrhea; fever for longer than 1 month; herpes simplex; and oral candidiasis in children more than 6 months old. Other signs of moderate infection include bacterial meningitis, pneumonia, or sepsis (one episode); cardiomyopathy; complicated chickenpox; herpes zoster; hepatitis; nephropathy; LIP; and toxoplasmosis onset before age 1 month. In addition to LIP, the most common indicators of AIDS in children younger than 13 years of age are serious bacterial infections (multiple or recurrent), PCP, cytomegalovirus (CMV), encephalopathy, and wasting syndrome (Moye, 1995).

Diagnostic Evaluation

Because most HIV infections in infants and children occur during perinatal transmission, HIV-positive pregnant women must be identified, educated, and treated. Early identification and treatment reduce the HIV transmission rate and enable early diagnosis for infected infants.

Traditional HIV antibody measurement by enzyme-linked immunosorbent assay (ELISA) or Western blot assay is not accurate in infants less than 18 months old because of the persistence of maternal antibodies. Virologic testing (DNA polymerase chain reaction, viral culture, RNA plasma assay) definitively diagnoses HIV infection by the time an infant is 6 months old, often within the first month (CDC, 1998b). Early diagnosis is essential for appropriate treatment. HIV-exposed infants should have virologic testing done before 48 hours after birth (Table 41–1) and follow-up testing according to the initial results. Because of potential maternal contamination during delivery, umbilical cord blood should not be used for testing.

CD4+ counts and RNA assays are used to assess an infected young child's immune status, risk for disease progression, and need for PCP prophylaxis after 1 year of age. CD4+ counts are measured at ages 1 and 3 months, every 3 months until the age of 2 years, and at least every 6 months thereafter. More frequent monitoring of CD4+ counts is indicated when PCP prophylaxis and antiretroviral therapy is recommended (CDC, 1995).

Therapeutic Management

HIV-EXPOSED INFANTS

Infants of HIV-positive mothers receive zidovudine therapy immediately after birth, to reduce the risk of infection, or as soon as the mother's HIV status is confirmed. Treatment continues for at least 6 weeks. Zidovudine comes in syrup form for easy administration to newborns.

Because PCP can affect an infant as young as 2 months, PCP prophylaxis is initiated when an exposed infant is 4 to 6 weeks old, regardless of HIV status. Treatment with trimethoprim-sulfamethoxazole usually continues until the infant is 1 year old or is determined to be HIV negative.

HIV-INFECTED INFANTS AND CHILDREN

In 1998, the CDC issued new guidelines for the treatment of infants and children infected with HIV. These recommendations were based on the following principles:

- HIV infection causes rapid immune system deterioration in young infants and children.
- Accurate diagnosis early in infancy is now possible.
- Maximally reducing viral replication to below detectable levels reduces organism resistance and preserves immune function.
- Newer and more effective combinations of antiretroviral medications are available in a form and dosage that can be administered to infants and young children.
- Laboratory monitoring in conjunction with therapy has become more precise.

Combination antiretroviral therapy is given to all HIV-infected infants and children who exhibit clinical symptoms of infection or whose immune status is moderately or severely depressed. Combination antiretroviral therapy also is initiated for all HIV-infected infants less than 1 year old as soon as the diagnosis is confirmed.

Two approaches are recommended for children 1 year old or older who are asymptomatic: provide antiretroviral therapy for all asymptomatic children, because most infants

TABLE 41-1

Testing for the Presence of HIV

Infants with Negative Tests	Infants with Positive Tests
Repeat the test as soon as possible after initial testing and again at 14 days.	Repeat the test as soon as possible after initial testing.
Retest at 1–2 months.	CD4+ lymphocyte count at the time of the second virologic test.
Retest at 3–6 months.	Determine sequential CD4+ lymphocyte counts every 2–3 months.
Test for HIV antibody after age 6 months.	
HIV infection can be reasonably excluded in infants with (1) two or more negative virologic tests at or after age 1 month, with one of those tests performed at or after age 4 months, or (2) no symptoms and two separate negative antibody tests performed at least 1 month apart and after the infant is 6 months old. HIV infection can be definitely excluded if the antibody test is negative and the child is asymptomatic at 18 months.	HIV infection is diagnosed from two positive virologic tests performed on separate blood samples.

Data from Centers for Disease Control and Prevention. (1998). Guidelines for the use of antiretroviral agents in pediatric HIV infection. *Morbidity and Mortality Weekly Report, 47*(RR-4), 1–31; Mofenson, L., & Read, J. (1999). Human immunodeficiency virus infection. In F. Burg, E. Wald, J. Ingelfinger, & R. Polin (Eds.), *Gellis & Kagan's current pediatric therapy* (16th ed.). Philadelphia: Saunders.

and children have depressed CD4+ percentages by 1 year of age, or defer treatment for those with normal immune status, a low viral load, and few medication compliance risks, realizing that these children will need frequent and careful monitoring.

Antiretroviral combination regimens usually include two nucleoside analogs, such as zidovudine (ZDV) and didanosine (ddI), which target the virus during its reverse transcription phase. To these is added a protease inhibitor (e.g., ritonavir, nelfinavir). An individual's antiretroviral drug regimen may be changed in response to worsening immune status, medication intolerance or toxicity, or the development of a newer and better regimen. Combination therapy

CRITICAL THINKING EXERCISE 41-1

Some states in the United States have begun considering mandatory HIV antibody testing of newborns. This test is done at the same time as the other mandatory newborn screenings (e.g., for phenylketonuria, sickle cell disease). Because recent HIV medication protocols have produced a marked decrease in the perinatal infection transmission rate, and because very early treatment of HIV-infected infants has been shown to prolong intact immune status, universal HIV testing appears warranted.

What are the major issues, positive and negative, that legislators should consider before approving legislation for mandatory universal HIV testing for infants?

for infected adolescents is similar but, dosages are based on Tanner stage of puberty, not age. Dosages for adolescents in Tanner stage I or II are based on children's dosages, while those for adolescents in Tanner stage V are based on the adult dosage. Those at other Tanner stages need to have dosages monitored and adjusted for effectiveness.

In addition to antiretroviral therapy, aggressive treatment of infections is essential. Ensuring appropriate immunizations, monitoring growth and development, providing nutritional support, and referring for multidisciplinary care are additional therapeutic interventions (Table 41-2).

ADDITIONAL ISSUES RELATED TO HIV

Most important for successful treatment of HIV-infected children and adolescents is meticulous adherence to the medication regimen. Failure to follow the regimen can result in the development of drug resistance and treatment failure. It is most important to educate and reinforce medication compliance at every visit. Palatability of the medication, ability to meld the medication schedule with existing routines, denial, and embarrassment about the diagnosis are all barriers to appropriate adherence to the regimen.

NURSING CARE

The Child with HIV Infection

Assessment

Many children with HIV infection experience normal health. When the immune system becomes more compro-

TABLE 41–2

Recommendations for Routine Immunization of Children with HIV Exposure or Infection

Vaccine	Give to Exposed or Infected Children?
Diphtheria, tetanus, and acellular pertussis (DTaP)	Yes
Oral polio vaccine (OPV)	No
Inactivated polio vaccine (IPV)*	Yes
Mumps, measles, and rubella (MMR)	Yes, except when severely immunosuppressed
Influenza*	Yes, if the child is at least 6 months old
Pneumococcal†	Yes
Hemophilus influenzae type B (Hib)	Yes
Hepatitis B	Yes
Varicella	Not recommended at this time

Note: Always check the most current immunization schedule. Administer immune globulin after measles exposure and varicella-zoster immune globulin after chickenpox exposure, unless administered during the previous 3 weeks. Administer tetanus immune globulin in the management of tetanus-prone wounds.

*Including siblings and other family members.

†At or after 2 years of age.

Data from Barrett, D., & Sleasman, J. (1997). Pediatric AIDS: So now what do we do? *Contemporary Pediatrics, 14*(6), 111–124; Mofenson, L., & Read, J. (1999). Human immunodeficiency virus infection. In F. Burg, E. Wald, J. Ingelfinger, & R. Polin (Eds.), *Gellis & Kagan's current pediatric therapy* (16th ed.). Philadelphia: Saunders.

mised and symptoms develop, hospitalization becomes necessary. Therapeutic management focuses on the treatment of serious bacterial and opportunistic infections that might affect multiple organs and systems. The nurse should engage the family in a helping relationship and put aside biases regarding mode of transmission so that they do not interfere with listening, supporting, and providing care. The nurse should use an interpreter, if needed, to provide culturally sensitive care.

Determine whether an HIV diagnosis has been made and what the family understands about the HIV-related spectrum of illness, including immunologic status. The nurse should assess the child's growth and development according to age-appropriate parameters and ask the caregivers about any fever, nausea, vomiting, diarrhea, ear pulling, or changes in appetite, sleep pattern, or behavior that might suggest secondary infections.

Focus the physical examination on indicators of an infection:

- *Hydration status:* Assess the skin for turgor and the mucous membranes for moistness, drying, or cracking; confirm the absence or presence of tears; determine whether the anterior fontanel is palpable and soft; measure intake, urine output, and specific gravity.
- *Respiratory status:* Listen and observe for nasal flaring, retractions, cough, difficulty breathing, tachypnea, grunting, wheezing, rhonchi, and decreased breath sounds.
- *Mouth lesions:* Observe for white patches on the tongue or inside the cheeks, or blisters on the lips.
- *Skin lesions (especially in the diaper area):* Observe for blotchy, red, flat areas, or blistering or dryness.

Assess pain by obtaining a self-report from the child, using faces, number, or color scales when appropriate; by observing the child's speech, facial expressions, body movements and responses; and by talking with the family.

Unlike other chronic illnesses, pediatric HIV infection is often an intergenerational health problem. Many families affected by the disease have limited financial resources or emotional support systems. As a result, the nurse may consult with a social worker to ensure that basic needs, such as food, housing, and transportation, are met.

Other issues, such as disclosure and do-not-resuscitate (DNR) orders, will need to be explored when the time is right. For example, when trust is established, families may talk about their feelings about disclosure. Some choose to share the diagnosis with a trusted friend. For most, however, keeping the secret is a way of life. Although it is stressful and lonely, there are many legitimate reasons for doing so (Cohen et al., 1995). The nurse can listen as the family talks about its reasons and ask what other family members and friends know, including the child. See Appendix L for a listing of support organizations for families affected by HIV infection.

Because it is currently assumed that all women and children with HIV infection will eventually develop AIDS and die, the nurse, at some point, might ask an infected mother what her plans are for her children's future. This can include exploring the efficacy of standby guardianship, kinship care, or foster and adoptive placement (Merkel-Holguin, 1994). In addition, families have to make difficult decisions about an infected child's ongoing care. Should aggressive treatment continue, or should the goal of treatment be to make the child comfortable? Most of the time, these decisions are made in consultation with a multidisciplinary team. The nurse can help assess when that time is right.

Caring for the Child with an HIV Infection

Review the following information and health practices at the time of initial testing and subsequent visits.

Transmission
HIV can be spread from

- Unprotected sexual intercourse
- Sharing of needles
- An infected mother to her baby
- Open wounds (if there is blood-to-blood contact)

HIV cannot be spread by

- Sharing knives, forks, spoons, or cups
- Using the same toilet seats, bathtubs, or showers
- Coughing or sneezing
- Hugging, holding, or touching people

Prevention
The best way to prevent the spread of HIV is to

- Abstain from sex and from sharing needles, or
- Use latex condoms with nonoxynol 9, and
- Wash needles in a 1:10 bleach solution

The best way to prevent pregnancies is to

- Abstain from sex, or
- Use a latex condom
- Use birth control pills
- Undergo tubal ligation

If infected with HIV,

- Do not breast-feed
- Do not donate blood, sperm, or organs

Testing

- The most common HIV tests used for older children and adults are the ELISA and the Western blot assay, which measure levels of antibodies to the virus.
- The most common HIV tests used for infants and children less than 18 months old are the HIV DNA polymerase chain reaction and HIV RNA assays, which detect the presence of the virus itself.
- CD4+ counts indicate how well the immune system is working.

Illness (AIDS)
Children with HIV infection might initially be asymptomatic. Mild and moderate symptoms include

- Persistent upper respiratory and ear infections
- Thrush
- Skin conditions
- Vomiting and diarrhea
- Enlarged liver, spleen, lymph nodes, and parotid gland
- Growth and development problems
- LIP—a rare lung disease

Some severe symptoms of the illness include

- Opportunistic infections such as PCP and CMV
- Recurrent bacterial infections such as sepsis and meningitis
- Severe developmental delay
- Wasting syndrome

Home Care
Offer a high-calorie, high-protein diet:

- Mix formula as directed.
- Do not add extra water or cereal to formula.
- Give supplemental vitamins and minerals as ordered.

Practice basic infection control measures and follow standard precautions, including the following practices:

- Avoid touching blood.
- Do not share toothbrushes, pierced earrings, razors, or nail clippers.
- Use a barrier when caring for a cut or bloody nose.
- Cover open sores.
- Leave scabs alone.
- Wipe up blood spills with a paper towel, wash the area with soap and water, rinse with bleach and water, and air-dry.
- Wrap disposable materials soiled with blood in newspaper, tie off in a plastic bag, and throw away in a plastic-lined trash can.
- Wash hands with soap and water if you touch blood.
- Rinse blood-soiled clothing with hydrogen peroxide or cold water and then wash as usual.
- Allow blood to air-dry on dry-clean-only clothing.

Keep your child's immunizations up-to-date. Your child should also receive the following

- Pneumococcal vaccine at 2 years of age
- Flu shot each fall
- Immune globulin after measles exposure
- Varicella-zoster immune globulin after chickenpox exposure
- Tetanus immune globulin for tetanus-prone wounds

Call the doctor if any of the following symptoms occur:

- Fever higher than 101°F
- Vomiting and diarrhea
- Decreased appetite, difficulty swallowing, drooling
- Rashes, bumps, lumps, or sores on the skin
- Coughing or chest congestion
- Ear pain, pulling on the ears, or drainage from the ears
- Wounds that will not heal
- Exposure to measles or chickenpox

Give prophylaxis against PCP and antiretroviral drugs as ordered.

Nursing Diagnosis, Planning, Intervention, and Evaluation

Nursing Diagnosis	■ Risk for Infection related to cell-mediated immunodeficiency.
Expected Outcome	• The child will be free of secondary and opportunistic infections and will have up-to-date immunization status.

Intervention	Rationale

1. Follow basic infection control and standard precautions at all times. (See Appendix B for standard precautions.)
2. Administer antimicrobial therapy as ordered; monitor the child for side effects. Monitor for signs and symptoms of infection.

3. Administer antipyretics for fever as ordered; monitor the effects and notify the physician if the fever does not resolve. Offer fluids. Organize care to allow for rest periods.
4. Administer intravenous immune globulin (IVIG) as ordered; monitor the child for side effects. Notify the physician of any reaction and adjust the rate as ordered.
5. Reinforce principles of infection control, appropriate immunization schedules, and indications for contacting a physician (see p. 1070). Teach families how to administer medications and take the child's temperature, as well as when to administer antipyretics at home.

Rationale:

1. Children with HIV are susceptible to infections. Standard precautions protect caregivers from infection.
2. Children with HIV mount a poor antibody response. Common pathogens include *Salmonella*, *Shigella*, *Campylobacter*, *Yersinia*, *Giardia lamblia*, *Isospora belli*, and *Cryptosporidium*.
3. Children with HIV often have fevers. The increased respiratory rate that accompanies increased activity can lead to further fluid loss.
4. IVIG can prevent serious bacterial infections and hospitalizations; however, it does not affect the child's overall survival rate.
5. The best way to prevent the spread of organisms at home is through good hand washing. The child with HIV and the siblings receive inactivated polio vaccine. All household members receive the influenza vaccine. If the child with HIV is exposed to measles or chickenpox, the family must notify the physician immediately.

Evaluation	• Is the child free from signs of infection?
	• Does the child respond well to antimicrobial therapy; is the child free of secondary and opportunistic infections?
	• Is the child afebrile?
	• Are the child's immunizations up to date?
	• Can the family describe signs and symptoms of infection and when to notify the physician?

Nursing Diagnosis	■ Altered Nutrition: Less Than Body Requirements related to inadequate caloric intake and altered gastrointestinal function.
Expected Outcome	• The child will eat foods from the recommended food groups, will take in adequate calories to meet metabolic and growth needs, will be free of painful oral lesions that interfere with eating, will have a regular bowel pattern, and will maintain growth parameters appropriate for age.

Intervention	Rationale

1. Offer foods high in protein and calories; give vitamin and mineral supplements; consult with a nutritionist.
2. Offer milk, nonacidic juice, or water after meals.

3. Offer licks of a Popsicle or ice before meals.
4. Allow older children to use a straw.
5. Offer soft, bland, lightly seasoned foods that are nutritious and easy to eat.

6. Serve food at room temperature.
7. Offer six small meals a day. Increase calories by adding milk, butter, or cheese to potatoes, eggs, casseroles, vegetables, soups, or gravies; by using sauces on rice, noodles, or potatoes; and by offering shakes.

Rationale:

1. Children with HIV are often small in size and stature. Mouth sores and malabsorption can exacerbate problems with weight gain.
2. Children can fill up on liquids before eating and not meet nutrition requirements.
3. Cold may numb the mouth when sores are present.
4. A straw keeps liquids from touching sore spots.
5. Spicy or salty foods can irritate mouth sores. Favorite foods can be mashed, ground, or pureed to facilitate consumption.
6. Hot or cold temperatures can aggravate mouth sores.
7. There may be times when children just do not have an appetite. Allow them to eat the food they want, but attempt to increase calories.

8. Offer bland, low-fiber, nonirritating foods, as ordered, along with Pedialyte, Gatorade, or cranberry juice.
9. Encourage the family to visit at mealtimes, or assign a consistent person to feed the child at a set time.
10. Weigh the child every morning, and review caloric intake every 24 hours. Measure specific gravity at every void; compare consistency of stools; obtain specimens as ordered.
11. Begin tube or parental feedings as ordered.

12. Review with the family how to reconstitute formula at home, give vitamins, increase protein and calories, and adjust intake based on oral lesions and evidence of malabsorption. Teach families how to give alternative feeds as ordered.
13. Administer liquid oral antifungals as ordered.

8. Children with HIV often have stomach cramps and diarrhea because of secondary infections.
9. Children tend to eat better in the presence of family or a familiar trusted person.
10. It is important that the child follow his or her individual growth curve, even if small for age. Children with HIV often experience diarrhea.
11. Alternative feeding techniques are necessary when the child is not gaining weight or is deviating from his or her established growth curve because of mouth or esophageal lesions, malabsorption, or neurologic findings.
12. Proteins and calories are important to immune cell function. Because some families may add water to formula to make it last longer, while others may add cereal to increase calories, it is important to reinforce formula preparations.
13. Eliminates or reduces mouth lesions caused by *Candida*.

Evaluation
- Is the child eating from all recommended food groups?
- Is the child growing according to normal and individual parameters?
- Are the child's stools of normal consistency and frequency?

Nursing Diagnoses
- Impaired Gas Exchange related to secondary or opportunistic infections.
- Ineffective Airway Clearance related to ineffective cough or fatigue.

Expected Outcome
- The child will demonstrate clear breath sounds, will have normal pulse and respiratory rates for age, will breathe comfortably with minimal exertion, and will have an oxygen saturation measurement within normal limits.

Intervention

1. Maintain oxygen therapy as ordered and monitor pulse oximetry values.

2. Administer PCP prophylaxis/treatment as ordered, with a large glass of water or juice; monitor the child for side effects.

3. Administer corticosteroids, as ordered, with food or milk (see p. 1077). Monitor the child for side effects.
4. Perform chest physiotherapy as ordered. Turn and position the child every 2–3 hours; elevate the head of the bed. Encourage the child who is able to get out of bed to do so frequently. Have the child practice coughing and deep breathing using an incentive spirometer. Obtain a sputum sample for culture as ordered.
5. Instruct the parents how to administer trimethoprim-sulfamethoxazole (and steroids as ordered) at home; teach the family chest physiotherapy and coughing and deep breathing exercises for the child, as well as how to administer aerosol treatments at home. Arrange for oxygen tanks and nebulizers as ordered. Nebulizer pieces are cleaned with warm water after each treatment and left to air-dry. They are soaked in white vinegar and water for 30 minutes at the end of the day.

Rationale

1. Changes in the child's pulse oximetry values or clinical condition may indicate a need for a change in oxygen therapy.
2. Specific sulfonamides, such as trimethoprim-sulfamethoxazole, can help prevent or treat PCP. PCP causes dyspnea, tachypnea, cyanosis, and a nonproductive cough.
3. Corticosteroids are used to treat lymphocytic interstitial pneumonia (LIP).

4. Changing position and getting out of bed, even if the child is simply held upright in someone's arms, allows for lung expansion and helps to prevent atelectasis of dependent lung segments.

5. PCP prophylaxis is usually taken twice a day, 3 days a week. Nebulizer treatments help to open the airway before chest physiotherapy.

Evaluation
- Have the child's breath sounds improved on auscultation?
- Is the child's pulse oximetry value greater than 95%?
- Does the child breathe effortlessly when at rest?
- Can the child expectorate upper airway secretions?

Nursing Diagnosis
■ Risk for Impaired Skin Integrity related to cellular immunodeficiency.

Expected Outcome
- The child's skin will be clean, dry, and intact, and the child's throat and mouth will be free of sores or inflammation.

Intervention

1. Use mild soap. Offer liquids throughout the day. Apply baby oil to the scalp. Avoid tight braids or pony tails. Use salve to keep lips moist.
2. Clean open sores with warm water; pat dry or air-dry. Apply antiviral agents as ordered; cover with a nonadherent pad. Monitor the effectiveness of treatment.
3. Clean the child's teeth 2–3 times a day with a soft brush. For infants, clean the mouth with a cotton swab and plain water.
4. Using a cotton swab, clean the mouth and apply an oral antifungal agent. Do not offer food or drink for 30 minutes after application. Monitor the effects of treatment.
5. Use extra care to keep the diaper area smooth and soft. Change diapers as soon as they are wet. Clean the area with mineral oil and warm water, then pat dry or air-dry. Do not use wipes.
6. Leave the diaper area open to the air. Avoid wiping (squeeze a wet cloth over the bottom to wash stool away). Pat dry or air-dry (do not rub). Apply a thin layer of antifungal agent as ordered, and monitor its effectiveness. Handle the child gently. Maalox (applied topically) and colloidal oatmeal baths are effective if skin breakdown is severe.
7. Reinforce techniques to be used at home for meticulous mouth and skin care. Mouth care includes inspecting for white patches, blisters, and sores that recur and persist despite meticulous treatment and care. Skin care of the diaper area is especially important. Teach the family how to apply topical antifungal agents.

Rationale

1. Children with HIV may have very dry skin, scalp, and lips. Oil reduces dryness. Tight hairstyles stress the skin.
2. Children with HIV may develop herpes lesions on the skin or in the mouth. Acyclovir is often ordered.
3. The skin inside the mouth must be kept clean to prevent infections and dental caries. A soft brush decreases injury to gums.
4. Children with HIV often develop a fungal infection due to *Candida albicans,* which causes pain with swallowing and can spread down the esophagus. Nystatin is used initially, followed by ketoconazole.
5. Some brands of disposable diapers and wipes may be irritating to the skin; moistness contributes to skin breakdown.
6. Children with HIV often develop fungal infections in the diaper area. Nystatin powder is used if the rash is wet and weepy. Nystatin cream allows the skin to breathe.

7. The skin and mucous membranes are the body's first line of defense against infecting microorganisms that challenge the immune system.

Evaluation
- Is the child free of further skin breakdown?
- Are the child's skin lesions and open sores healing?

Nursing Diagnosis
■ Altered Growth and Development related to the effects of the virus on the neurologic system, chronicity of the illness, separation from family, and hospitalization.

Expected Outcome
- The child's motor, cognitive, and psychosocial development will be within normal limits.

Intervention

1. Encourage the family to visit the child as often and as long as possible. Supplement family visits with visits from volunteers.
2. Administer antiretroviral drugs as ordered. Monitor the child for side effects.

Rationale

1. Personal interaction is essential to prevent withdrawal and promote language and motor skills.

2. HIV can infect brain cells. Opportunistic organisms, like CMV and *Toxoplasma,* can cause brain infections. Thrombocytopenia can cause internal bleeding. As a result, some children with progressive disease exhibit developmental delay. Many children taking antiretroviral drugs, however, have achieved developmental milestones after a previous delay and gained weight.

3. Interact with the child according to the child's developmental level. Provide safe, age-appropriate toys; integrate physical, occupational, and speech therapy techniques into the child's activities of daily living and play. Assess the child each week for changes in any aspect of development.
4. Reinforce physical and occupational therapy techniques, but not to the point of pain. Encourage the family to follow speech therapy instructions, especially those that enhance receptive language skills.

3. Developmental delay is a manifestation in HIV infected children; motor impairment may become more profound as the disease progresses.

4. As a child begins to lose motor function, the family continues to feel hopeful when general comprehension persists.

Evaluation

- Are all aspects of the child's development within normal limits?
- Is the child's communication appropriate for age?

Nursing Diagnosis

■ Pain related to the physical condition.

Expected Outcome

- The child will be able to communicate where any pain is located, will participate in activities to the maximum extent, and will be comfortable, as evidenced by ability to participate in activities and obtain appropriate rest.

Intervention

1. Continuously anticipate, assess, recognize, and treat pain appropriately. Use developmentally appropriate pain assessment scales and document pain rating every 2 to 4 hours.
2. Offer acetaminophen and nonsteroidal anti-inflammatory drugs (NSAIDs) for mild pain; add codeine for moderate pain and morphine or methadone for severe pain.
3. Plan care so that rest periods are possible and everything that requires touching is done at once. Line the bed with soft blankets or cushions, or a partially inflated mattress. Alternate the child's positions, using the palms of your hands for lifting. Keep the environment calm, speak in gentle tones, play quiet music, dim the lights. Apply mild heat and offer a warm bath.
4. Teach deep-breathing exercises and use distraction techniques (imaging, singing, watching TV, reading a story) to manage pain.
5. Teach the family how to administer analgesics and use nonpharmacologic interventions for managing pain at home. Remind the family to call the doctor if the pain cannot be controlled.

Rationale

1. Pain management requires multidisciplinary input: the caregiver reports pain to the physician, who may order analgesics.

2. A "ladder" approach to analgesia has proved effective in managing pain (Oleske, 1995).

3. Organizing care, environmental control, and distraction are important nonpharmacologic interventions for managing pain.

4. Giving children power to help control pain can help lessen it.

5. Children should not have to be in pain. There is always something that can be done. Families know their children best and are positioned to assess and manage pain at home with lots of support.

Evaluation

- Has the child's pain improved, as evidenced by improved relaxation and ability to sleep, absence of crying and expressed discomfort?
- Is the child able to participate in age-appropriate activities?

Nursing Diagnosis

■ Anxiety (primary caregiver) related to fear of disclosure.

Expected Outcome

- The family will share the diagnosis with health care professionals who need to know. The family will move through the stages of disclosure and will feel comfortable sharing its feelings about the diagnosis with one significant person. The family will answer the child's questions honestly and share the diagnosis when the time is right.

Intervention

1. Listen quietly when the family talks about the diagnosis of HIV. Note their stage of disclosure (secrecy, exploratory, readiness, or full disclosure).

Rationale

1. Sharing the diagnosis occurs on a continuum, with secrecy at one end and full disclosure at the other. Families initially will want to keep their feelings about the diagnosis private. However, there may come a time when they wish to talk; the nurse should develop rapport and gain trust.

2. Encourage the family to share the diagnosis with health care professionals.

3. Help the family decide who else needs to know the child's diagnosis; ask them to name one person they wish to share the diagnosis with. Encourage peer support groups when the family is ready.

4. Encourage the family to be honest with the child and to explain the reason for doctors' visits and procedures.

5. Encourage the family to listen to the questions the child is asking and to answer the questions briefly using words the child can understand. Look for readiness cues that indicate the child wants to know more.

6. Encourage the family to speak with a health care professional when the child asks questions that are difficult to answer. Suggest that the parent seek counseling to help find the appropriate language for answering the child.

7. Promote normal routines at home.

2. Health care professionals who plan and coordinate care need to know the diagnosis.

3. Although many people would like to know the diagnosis, only a handful need to know. Ask families to consider the following when choosing whom to tell: the child's age, clinical condition, and health care requirements; the likelihood that bloody injuries will occur; the use of standard precautions.

4. When to tell the child the diagnosis is a personal choice, but families need to understand that children will worry more if no one talks with them or if they sense dishonesty.

5. It is important for families to understand what their children are asking and to answer their questions, keeping responses short and simple.

6. Role-playing is a useful technique that allows families to practice potential responses to difficult questions. The nurse can offer to accompany them if they decide to share the diagnosis.

7. Children with HIV infection can go to school, church, and parties; play sports and games; and develop or maintain friendships.

Evaluation

- Is the family able to share the diagnosis with all appropriate health care professionals and at least one significant person?
- Does the family appear to be moving through the stages of disclosure and seeking out support from peers?
- Is the family able to seek social and health services for which they qualify based on their HIV/AIDS status?
- Can family members answer the child's questions in a developmentally appropriate way?

Nursing Diagnosis

■ Ineffective Management of Therapeutic Regimen: Noncompliance related to lack of support systems or denial of the illness.

Expected Outcome

- The mother will keep her health care appointments. The family will work toward accepting the diagnosis. Family members will view themselves as valued members of the health care team.

Intervention

1. Use language that shows respect. Offer information in a language that can be understood by the child and family. Use a translator as needed.

2. Encourage the mother to keep her own health care appointments.

3. Accept the parents' use of denial during periods of emotional respite. Refer for counseling to assist with the grieving process.

4. Maintain realistic hope when possible.

Rationale

1. Families affected by HIV do not want their children called innocent victims or AIDs babies, nor do they want to be judged as promiscuous or substance abusers. Labels can create barriers, which can result in noncompliance with health care recommendations.

2. HIV-infected women often neglect their own health care needs as they attend to those of their children.

3. The diagnosis of HIV brings a series of losses, including the loss of the future and all that the future holds for a child. Denial is a coping mechanism.

4. With new prophylaxis for HIV-positive pregnant women and their infants, only 8% of all seropositive babies actually develop HIV infection, and antiretroviral treatments have been successful with preserving immune function.

5. Refer the family to social services for assistance with finances, transportation, food, housing, clothing, medical care, and respite care, as needed.

6. Teach the family how to give antiretroviral agents at home, keep a log, and adjust the schedule to accommodate school schedules. Monitor medication compliance at every visit. Suggest ways to make medications more palatable to children (e.g., by using liquid forms or mixing with foods).

5. Although some women with HIV infection are judged to be uncaring because of missed appointments or because their child fails to gain weight, many simply lack the basic resources for compliance.

6. The antiretroviral regimen may include a combination of three drugs in addition to the other medications a child is taking. A daily log helps families keep track.

Evaluation

- Is the mother able to take care of herself?
- Have the parents or caregivers been able to move from denial to anger to acceptance of the diagnosis?
- Are the primary caregivers active, participatory, and valued members of the health care team?
- Does the child adhere to the medication regimen?

Corticosteroid Therapy

Corticosteroids, given as part of a treatment regimen, act as natural products of the adrenal glands, reducing local and systemic inflammatory symptoms.

Incidence

Topical steroids are applied to the skin or mucous membranes to reduce edema and redness and to counteract itching. They may be used to treat ophthalmic reactions and skin conditions such as eczema. Hydrocortisone cream is one example of a topical steroid. *Systemic steroids* reduce the inflammatory symptoms of generalized allergic reactions (e.g., asthma, hives, severe contact dermatitis). Systemic steroids are also given increasingly to treat malignant or autoimmune disorders. An example of a systemic steroid is prednisone.

Aerosol steroids produce a very strong local action and can control symptoms in children with asthma and allergic

---

PARENTS AND CAREGIVERS WANT TO KNOW

Basic Infection Control for the Child with Immunodeficiency

Review the following basic infection control practices for the child with immunodeficiency.

To prevent contact with germs

- Keep immunizations up to date.
- Keep child home when sick.
- Turn away when someone coughs or sneezes.
- Do not share cups, bottles, plates, utensils, drinks, or pacifiers.
- Do not kiss babies on the mouth.
- Do not use fingers as a pacifier.
- Discard unused refrigerated formula after 24 hours.
- Change diapers—away from food areas—every 2 to 3 hours or sooner if the baby has a stool.
- Dispose of trash daily.

To create a barrier to germs if contact is unavoidable

- Cover your mouth when coughing or sneezing.
- Use a tissue to wipe nose.
- Cover unused food and formula and refrigerate.
- Keep a bowl close by if feeling nauseated.
- Fold soiled disposable diapers inward and tab.
- Discard dirty diapers and used tissues in a tightly covered, plastic-lined container.
- Cover sandboxes when not in use.

To kill germs if contact is made

- Wash hands (using friction) with soap and warm water for 15 seconds before eating and after using the bathroom, wiping noses, changing diapers, cleaning up vomit, or catching a sneeze.
- Provide meticulous skin and mouth care.
- Carefully wash all fruit and vegetables that are to be eaten raw.
- Cook food well, especially meat, fowl, and eggs.
- Wash eating utensils, baby bottles, nipples, and pacifiers with soap and hot water or in the dishwasher.
- Rub the inside of the nipple with salt and rinse well if slimy.
- Clean kitchen and bathroom surfaces, shelves, pails, trash cans, and mops routinely.
- Clean litter boxes, bird cages, and turtle homes frequently and carefully.

Adapted from Ward-Wimmer, D., & Riley, M. W. (1991). *Caring at home: A guide for families.* Washington, DC: The Child Welfare League of America.

rhinitis who are corticosteroid dependent. An example of an aerosol steroid is beclomethasone (see Chapters 45 and 49).

Pathophysiology

Corticosteroids have many different effects but are usually prescribed for their anti-inflammatory or immunosuppressive properties. As anti-inflammatories, they inhibit the process of edema, capillary dilation, phagocytic activity, and the migration of leukocytes into an inflamed area (McDuffie, 1996). As immunosuppressives, they decrease monocyte and macrophage differentiation and lymphokine production, leading to T-cell inhibition (Michaels & Green, 1999).

The side effects of steroids vary widely with the child and the medication. Generally, the higher the dose and the longer the medication is taken, the more serious are the side effects. More knowledge about reactions and a broader selection of steroids and alternatives have significantly reduced untoward reactions in recent years.

Manifestations

Clinical manifestations of excess topically administered steroids include skin atrophy, delayed wound healing, telangiectasis or dilation of the cheek blood vessels, striae, and excess absorption leading to any of the clinical manifestations of systemic use.

Some clinical manifestations of excess steroid administered systemically include

- Edema, particularly in the face
- Gastrointestinal irritation, even bleeding
- Bruising and delayed wound healing
- Susceptibility to infections
- Growth limitations
- Hypertension
- Loss of muscle mass
- Increased appetite and weight gain
- Amenorrhea
- Pancreatitis
- Joint pain and osteoporosis
- Cataracts

Diagnostic Evaluation

The diagnosis of corticosteroid excess is suspected when clinical manifestations appear and is confirmed by administering a bolus of adrenocorticotropic hormone (ACTH) to the child. ACTH challenges the adrenal gland to respond to pituitary stimulation. If serum cortisol levels do not rise after administration of ACTH, adrenal suppression—or cortisone excess—is present.

Therapeutic Management

Every effort is made to prevent corticosteroid excess by observing the following guidelines:

- Institute short-term, high-dose therapy (for 1 week or less) if there is a strong indication for the use of steroids.

- If long-term use is necessary, alternate-day administration may be prescribed.
- At the time of an acute infection or surgery, supplementary steroids are indicated for children who have received them over a long period of time.

Because of immunosuppression, killed-virus vaccines are substituted for live-virus vaccines for children receiving high-dose or long-term steroids.

NURSING CARE
The Child Receiving Corticosteroids

Assessment

Assessment of a child receiving long-term steroid therapy includes measuring height, weight, and blood pressure at each visit. In addition, the nurse observes the child for facial puffiness, abdominal pain, increased appetite, blurred vision, and increased thirst or urination. Families may report recent illnesses, bruising, or delayed wound healing.

Nursing Diagnoses and Planning

The following nursing diagnoses and expected outcomes may be appropriate following assessment of a child receiving corticosteroid therapy:

- Ineffective Management of Therapeutic Regimen: Noncompliance related to associated complications.
  Expected Outcome: The child will take all medications as directed.
- Body Image Disturbance related to changes caused by treatment.
  Expected Outcome: The child will share feelings about any changes in appearance.
- Risk for Infection related to immunosuppression.
  Expected Outcome: The child will not experience secondary infections.
- Risk for Injury related to knowledge deficit.
  Expected Outcome: The child will not experience injuries.
- Risk for Altered Growth and Development related to growth suppression and muscle wasting.
  Expected Outcome: The child will continue to grow according to his or her own height and weight curve.

Interventions

The nurse should provide the family with written instructions that specifically state what to do if a dose is missed and when to decrease dosages. The nurse should emphasize not to discontinue corticosteroid therapy abruptly.

The child needs to take the medication with foods or milk to minimize the risk of gastrointestinal bleeding. Because the child's appetite may be increased, encouraging low-calorie snacks throughout the day is appropriate. (The nurse should remind the family that salt may increase fluid retention.)

Changes in appearance are temporary and reversible. The nurse can compare changes in appearance and weight gain at each visit and encourage expression of the child's feelings. Weight and height monitoring of the child on long-term corticosteroid therapy is important; fluid retention can mask muscle wasting and growth suppression.

Corticosteroids can also mask infections. The family should be instructed to call the doctor in the event of temperature elevation, cough, runny nose, ear tenderness, decreased appetite, nausea, vomiting, diarrhea, behavioral change, or even if the child just doesn't seem right. The child's skin should be checked routinely for bruising and signs of wound infection and lesions that do not resolve as expected should be reported. The family should not treat the child with over-the-counter products without consulting the physician. The child receiving long-term therapy should avoid others who are sick; parents should promptly report any exposure to a communicable disease, such as measles or chickenpox, to the health care provider.

Potential environmental hazards and accident prevention strategies based on the child's developmental age should be emphasized. If the child should get a cut, the parents may hold gentle pressure to the site for 3 to 5 minutes to stop the bleeding and prevent hematoma formation. The child should wear a Medic-Alert bracelet stating the key clinical manifestations of corticosteroid excess or adrenal insufficiency.

Evaluation

• Is the child taking corticosteroids as directed?
• Is the child able to express feelings about any changes in appearance?
• Does the child remain free of infections?
• Is the child's skin intact?

Immune Complex and Autoimmune Disorders

Immune Complex Disorders

Immune complexes are clusters of interlocking antigens and antibodies. Under normal conditions, immune complexes are removed from the blood. In some circumstances, how-

ever, immune complexes continue to circulate. Eventually they become trapped in the tissues of the kidney, lungs, skin, joints, or blood vessels. There they set off reactions that lead to tissue inflammation and damage.

Deposition of immune complexes is considered to be a precipitator for several different conditions in childhood. Kawasaki disease (see Chapter 46) and acute poststreptococcal glomerulonephritis (see Chapter 44) are both thought to be caused by immune complex deposition in tissue.

Autoimmune Disorders

Sometimes the immune system's ability to differentiate self from nonself breaks down and the body begins to make antibodies against its own cells, tissues (particularly connective tissue), and organs. Such antibodies are known as autoantibodies. Autoantibodies are common in such conditions as rheumatic fever (see Chapter 46), juvenile rheumatoid arthritis (see Chapter 50), and systemic lupus erythematosus.

It is still unclear what initiates an autoimmune response. Several theories have been proposed:

• Activation of immature B cells that do not develop antigen-specific receptors
• Alteration of normal tissue cells by infection or other process, which causes them to become antigenic
• Similarity between the structures of some infectious organisms and self-antigens, causing a cross-reaction
• Genetic predisposition of defective immune regulation

The response is exacerbated by a malfunction of helper T and suppressor T cells, when there are too many helper cells and not enough suppressor cells to turn off the immune response. Some autoimmune disorders also manifest with increased tissue deposits of immune complexes.

Systemic Lupus Erythematosus

Systemic lupus erythematosus (SLE) is a chronic, multisystem, autoimmune disease characterized by inflammation of the connective tissue. SLE varies in severity and is marked by remissions and exacerbations.

Etiology

Although the etiology of SLE is not known, genetic, environmental, hormonal, and immune response factors are likely to be responsible. Environmental factors can include exposure to the sun, ultraviolet light, stress, fatigue, viruses, bacteria, certain medications, and some food additives. Exacerbations can occur with the use of birth control pills, menses, pregnancy, and the postpartum period (O'Neil, 1998).

Incidence

The overall incidence of SLE in the United States is 40 cases per 100,000 population (Hansen, 1998). The condition is relatively rare in young children. In young children, the female to male ratio is 3:1; after puberty, this ratio increases to 9:1 (O'Neil, 1998). Onset in girls is most common between the ages of 9 and 15. More African-American,

PATHOPHYSIOLOGY

of Systemic Lupus Erythematosus (SLE)

Many abnormalities in the immune system are associated with SLE. Nonspecific activation of B lymphocytes causes hypergammaglobulinemia, a process that triggers autoantibodies. This response is exacerbated by a reduction in the number of suppressor T cells. These autoantibodies—referred to as antinuclear antibodies, or ANAs—initiate an abnormal immune complex response and deposition, producing inflammation and damaging tissues and organs, including the skin, joints, heart, lungs, kidneys, brain, and circulatory vessels (Hansen, 1998; O'Neil, 1998).

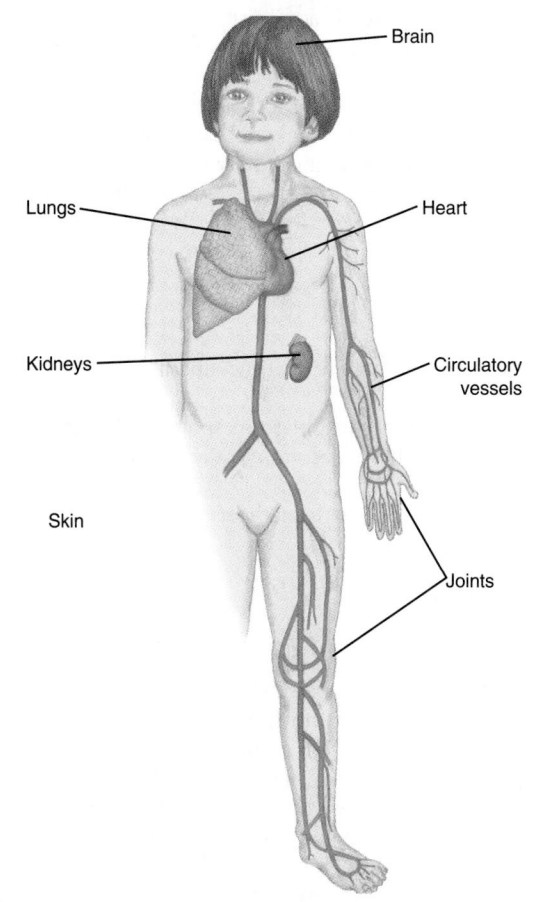

- Photosensitivity—skin rash from sun exposure
- Oral and nasal ulcers—usually painless lesions
- Arthritis—painful, swollen joints with edema
- Pleuritis, pericarditis, or peritonitis
- Nephritis—protein, casts, or red cells in urine
- Neurologic disorders—headaches, personality changes, seizures, or psychosis
- Hematologic disorders—anemia, leukopenia, lymphoma, or thrombocytopenia
- Immunologic disorders
- Positive antinuclear antibody (ANA) assay

A child with SLE also might experience weight loss, growth impairment, headache, and memory problems. Occasionally, children will have Raynaud's phenomenon, in which the digits of the hands and feet suddenly change color (mottled to white to blue) in response to cold. The most serious complications of SLE include renal disease and neurologic problems.

Diagnostic Evaluation

The presence of four or more of the clinical manifestations listed above, whether or not they occur simultaneously, is suggestive of SLE. In addition, a number of tests can be used to diagnose and monitor the progress of SLE. A positive ANA test and the presence of anti-DNA antibody are highly suggestive of SLE but can also occur in other autoimmune disorders. Blood urea nitrogen (BUN) levels, gamma-globulin levels, and the erythrocyte sedimentation rate might be elevated. Complement levels (C3 and C4) can be decreased. Pathologic changes compatible with SLE may be confirmed by electrocardiography, computed tomography, and magnetic resonance imaging and by skin and renal tissue biopsies demonstrating immune complexes.

Therapeutic Management

The treatment of SLE is tailored to the organ system(s) affected and is aimed at preventing exacerbations and

Latino, and Asian children are affected than Caucasian children.

Manifestations

Malaise, arthralgia, and recurrent fever of unknown etiology frequently are among the early manifestations of SLE. The symptoms, however, depend on what organs the immune complexes affect and can include the following (O'Neil, 1998):

- Malar butterfly rash—a fixed red, flat, or raised rash over the cheeks and bridge of nose (Fig. 41–1)
- Discoid rash—red, round, raised patches that spread

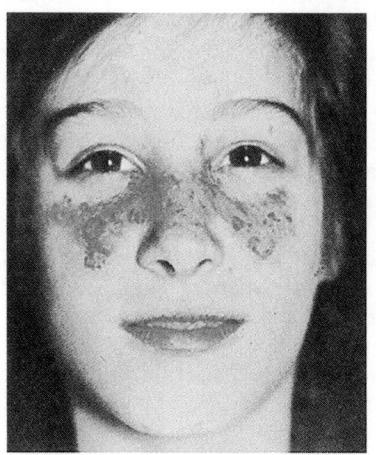

FIGURE 41–1

The butterfly rash of systemic lupus erythematosus. (From Behrman, R. E., Kliegman, R. M., & Arvin, A. M. [1996]. *Nelson textbook of pediatrics* [15th ed.]. Philadelphia: Saunders. Color Plate Fig. 150–1. Reproduced with permission.)

complications. The goal of treatment is to use the least amount of pharmacologic intervention needed. Helping the child and family develop long-term coping strategies is important.

Systemic corticosteroids are most often given to control the inflammatory response. When steroid treatment is not effective or renal progression is rapid, cyclophosphamide (Cytoxan) might be considered. NSAIDs, excluding ibuprofen, are used to treat arthritis, serositis, and febrile attacks. Children with renal and neurologic disorders generally receive anticonvulsant and antihypertensive therapy, whereas those with skin lesions and joint problems take antimalarial drugs, such as hydroxychloroquine (Plaquenil). Killed-virus vaccines rather than live-virus vaccines are used in affected children. A low-salt diet may reduce fluid retention and prevent elevated BUN levels; a low-protein diet helps preserve renal function.

The long-term prognosis for children with SLE is positive; the 10-year survival rate is 90% (O'Neil, 1998).

NURSING CARE
The Child with Systemic Lupus Erythematosus

Assessment

During a period of disease exacerbation, a child can become acutely ill. The nurse should monitor the child's vital signs, mobility, activity level, and pain, and should complete a neurologic examination that assesses for decreased sensation, weakness in the extremities, and changes in behavior. Of equal importance is evaluation of the effect of living with a chronic illness on a young child's self-image and interaction with peers.

Nursing Diagnoses and Planning

The following nursing diagnoses apply to the child with SLE:

- Body Image Disturbance related to changes secondary to the disease process and treatments.
  Expected Outcome: The child will share feelings about appearance.
- Activity Intolerance related to the disease process.
  Expected Outcome: The child will participate in activities to the extent possible.
- Pain related to arthritis and numbness of the hands and feet.
  Expected Outcome: The child will be free of pain.
- Ineffective Management of Therapeutic Regimen: Noncompliance related to associated complications and developmental level.
  Expected Outcome: The child will take all medications as directed.

Interventions

The nurse needs to help the child and family understand the importance of drug therapy and activity restriction during acute exacerbations. Avoiding triggers that cause exacerbations is essential (e.g., avoiding exposure to sun or

avoidable germs). Wearing an appropriate sunscreen is a necessity (SPF above 15, waterproof, PABA free, UVA and UVB protective). Raynaud's phenomenon can be prevented by dressing warmly in cold weather, paying particular attention to hat, gloves, and warm socks.

An adolescent will have difficulty achieving a balance between the need to take risks and be accepted by peers and the realities of a chronic illness (see Chapter 36). The teenager with a chronic illness needs to participate as fully as possible in activities at home and in the community. Documenting episodes of fatigue along with associated activities allows the young person to gain some control. They can then use this information to make sensible decisions about participation in extracurricular activities. The adolescent should be encouraged to plan an appropriate and convenient medication self-administration schedule and should be able to describe the side effects of the prescribed medications.

Anger about the diagnosis and alienation from peers are common. Wearing makeup can mask rashes and improve appearance. Keeping a diary also helps the young person vent anger. An affected peer who is in remission can offer support, as can national SLE organizations (see Appendix L). The Internet is also a source of support and information.

Evaluation

- Does the child share feelings about his or her appearance?
- Does the child participate in sports and extracurricular activities without becoming overly fatigued?
- Is the child free of pain?
- Is the child taking all medications as directed?

Allergic Reactions

Allergy is the immune response to an antigen, called an allergen, which causes a hypersensitive reaction in various body systems. This hypersensitive reaction occurs with a second exposure to an antigen and can be immediate or delayed. The classification of allergic reactions often reflects the pathophysiology of each type (Table 41–3). In most children with allergies, there is a genetic link. Common allergic conditions include allergic rhinitis, hives, eczema, asthma, colic, and migraines (Table 41–4).

Allergic rhinitis is an immediate hypersensitivity reaction to allergens trapped by the hairs and mucus that line the inside of the nose (see Chapter 45). Anaphylaxis is a life-threatening allergic response. Allergic reactions are related to the antibody IgE.

Anaphylaxis

Anaphylaxis, a severe immediate hypersensitivity reaction to an excessive release of chemical mediators, affects the entire body.

Etiology

Penicillin is the major cause of anaphylaxis, although other antibiotics and medications can also cause such a reaction.

TABLE 41–3

Classification of Allergic Reactions

Type		Pathophysiology	Examples
I	Immediate (anaphylactic) hypersensitivity	IgE attaches to mast cells and basophils, causing rupture and release of all contents (i.e., histamines).	Allergic rhinitis, acute anaphylaxis, hives, eczema, asthma
II	Cytotoxic hypersensitivity	An allergen (e.g., a red blood cell) stimulates IgE or IgM to react and mobilize complement to destroy the allergen.	Transfusion reaction after receiving incompatible blood
III	Arthus hypersensitivity (immune complex)	Immune complex is formed and can destroy tissues.	Serum sickness, glomerulonephritis
IV	Delayed cell-mediated hypersensitivity	An allergen reacts with T lymphocytes, and these lead other cells to produce damage.	Contact dermatitis (poison ivy)

In addition, an anaphylactic response can be caused by foods, such as eggs, nuts, or shellfish; by insect stings; by immunizations and allergy immunotherapy; and by diagnostic contrast media, chemotherapeutic agents, and blood products. Anaphylactic reactions to products containing latex have increased in incidence, especially among children with spina bifida (see Chapter 52) and children with abnormalities of the urinary tract.

Incidence

Anaphylaxis is rare in infancy and childhood.

Manifestations

The onset of anaphylaxis is sudden, usually occurring within seconds to minutes after exposure to an allergen. Initial symptoms of impending anaphylaxis include the following:

TABLE 41–4

Common Allergic Conditions in Children

Allergens	Manifestations	Diagnosis
Inhalants		
Pollen, dust, mold, dander	Sneezing; red itchy nose, eyes, pharynx, and palate; edematous nasal passages; tongue clicking; runny or congested nose; mouth breathing; chronic cough; dark circles under eyes; nose wrinkling; pale, boggy nasal mucous membranes	Allergic rhinitis
Applicants		
Heat, cold, wool, cosmetics, hair-permanents, sunscreens, plants, grasses	Well-defined red, raised skin or mucosal lesions	Hives
Foods		
Milk, wheat, eggs, strawberries, tomatoes, oranges, chocolate, nuts, shellfish	Intestinal cramping, nausea, vomiting, and diarrhea Bronchospasm Red patches on cheeks, face, wrists, neck, hands, extremities; swelling; itching; weeping; scales and crust Well-defined red, raised skin or mucosal lesions Vascular headaches	Colic Asthma Eczema Hives Migraines
Medicines		
Penicillin, cephalexin, immunizations, allergy immunotherapy, chemotherapy	Redness, swelling, pain Weakness, restlessness, edema, laryngospasm, and cardiovascular collapse	Local inflammation Anaphylaxis
Insects		
Stings of bees, wasps, hornets	Redness, swelling, pain Weakness, restlessness, edema, laryngospasm, and cardiovascular collapse	Local inflammation Anaphylaxis

- Sneezing
- Tightness or tingling of the mouth or face, with subsequent swelling of the lips and tongue
- Severe flushing, urticaria, and itching of the skin, especially on the head and upper trunk
- Rapid development of erythema
- A sense of impending doom

These symptoms might be followed by gastrointestinal and respiratory symptoms, which include nausea, vomiting, diarrhea, and cramping, as well as rhinorrhea, stridor, wheezing, and hoarseness.

The most serious features of anaphylaxis are laryngospasm, edema, cyanosis, hypotensive shock, vascular collapse, and cardic arrest.

Diagnostic Evaluation

Anaphylaxis occurs suddenly, allowing no time for diagnosis. The etiology is determined later by obtaining the child's history, and the suspected allergen is confirmed by skin or radioallergosorbent (RAST) studies.

Therapeutic Management

Treatment of anaphylaxis must begin immediately, as it may be only a matter of minutes before the child experiences shock. Epinephrine is the first drug of choice in the acute treatment of anaphylaxis. Administration of corticosteroids and antihistamines helps to prevent waves of anaphylaxis several hours later. To manage anaphylactic shock,

- Ensure an adequate airway, possibly by endotracheal intubation.
- Place a tourniquet proximal to the site of injection or insect sting.
- Administer epinephrine in the uninvolved extremity and in the area of reaction, with repeat dosing within 5 to 10 minutes.
- Administer oxygen.
- Start an IV line.
- Administer corticosteroids and antihistamines.
- Keep the child warm and lying flat or with feet slightly elevated.

Children who have experienced life-threatening insect sting anaphylaxis and demonstrate venom-specific IgE antibodies on skin or RAST studies are candidates for venom immunotherapy. All children experiencing episodes of ana-

PATHOPHYSIOLOGY
of Anaphylaxis

Anaphylaxis occurs when an allergen binds with IgE on the mast cells and basophils, accompanied by a release of histamine and other chemical mediators, which affect the magnitude of the response. The reaction is severe and life-threatening and can result in anaphylactic shock and subsequent death. An allergen that has previously evoked a response, or one that has not, can cause anaphylaxis.

phylaxis in the community should be transported by ambulance to an emergency facility (see Chapter 34).

NURSING CARE
The Child with Anaphylaxis

Assessment

The child should be monitored closely for airway obstruction and vascular collapse during the acute phase of anaphylaxis. Assessment includes noting airway patency, respiratory rate and effort, heart rate, peripheral pulses, capillary refill time, oxygen saturation, urine output, and level of consciousness. Following emergency efforts, the nurse can try to determine the cause of the attack by correlating when the symptoms first occurred with foods ingested, medications administered, and the possibility of an insect sting.

Nursing Diagnoses and Planning

The following nursing diagnoses apply to the child with anaphylaxis and family:

- Ineffective Breathing Pattern and Decreased Cardiac Output related to an excessive hypersensitive reaction to an allergen.
  Expected Outcome: The child will maintain a patent airway and adequate cardiac output (short term).
- Knowledge Deficit related to allergens and prevention through risk reduction.
  Expected Outcome: The child and family will avoid known allergens (long term).

Interventions

Initially, the nurse maintains an adequate airway by administering oxygen and assisting with aerosol treatments and intubation as necessary. A laryngoscope, intubation tray, and tracheostomy kit should be available and the code cart should be nearby. In the case of an insect sting or injected medication, a tourniquet applied to the affected extremity just proximal to the site might help to confine the allergen. It is important to have IV access, with a large-bore needle, in at least one site, preferably two, for medication adminis-

CHILDREN WANT TO KNOW
How to Prevent Insect Stings

- Select clothes with white or khaki colors, not dark or decorative ones.
- Wear fitted clothes with long sleeves, pants, and shoes.
- Use unscented soaps, lotions, and deodorants.
- Apply insect skin protection.
- Avoid orchards, flowers, blooming trees, or shrubs.
- Stay away from picnic areas.
- Keep out of the garden.
- Keep car windows closed while driving.
- Place screens on all windows.
- Cover all garbage cans.
- Move away slowly from approaching insects.

tration. The nurse administers IV fluids, epinephrine, corticosteroids, and antihistamines as ordered and informs the physician of the child's improvement or deterioration. Extra fluids (crystalloids or colloids) and plasma expanders should be administered if the child shows signs of vascular collapse (see Chapter 34).

Because epinephrine causes vasoconstriction and an increase in cardiac output, a child receiving the drug might experience heart palpitations and tachycardia. This is frightening and aggravated by the emergency nature of the situation. The nurse should offer gentle reassurance to the child, and provide the family with frequent reports about the childs condition.

Following an initial anaphylactic episode, the nurse should assure the child and family that they were not at fault for the anaphylactic reaction, and discuss how to prevent recurrences. Any child who has experienced anaphylaxis from an insect sting should have and learn to use an insect sting kit. The Epi-Pen Jr. for children delivers 0.15 mg of epinephrine through a spring-loaded injector. Teach the parent or child to hold the injector against the skin of the upper outer region of the child's thigh for 10 seconds after administering the injection to deliver the medication completely. A Medic-Alert bracelet alerts others to the child's allergy.

Evaluation

- Is the child awake and alert with adequate oxygenation and a patent airway?
- Are the child's vital signs within normal limits for age?
- Is the family taking appropriate steps to reduce the risks of another anaphylactic reaction?
- Do the child, family, and other appropriate adults demonstrate the proper use of the insect sting kit?

KEY CONCEPTS

- The immune system maintains homeostasis of the internal and external environment through nonspecific functions (inflammation and phagocytosis) and specific functions (humoral and cell-mediated immunity). Any derangement results in an immunologic imbalance whereby the immune system either underfunctions or overfunctions.
- When the immune system underfunctions, susceptibility to infections is increased (immunodeficiency). When the immune system overfunctions, it produces antibodies against cells of the body in autoimmune disease, or against external sensitizing agents, forming the basis for allergies.
- The immune response is produced either actively or passively. Active immunity means the body has reacted to antigens in nature or vaccines. The effect of active immunity lasts months to a lifetime. Passive immunity results from

antibody transfer from a person with active immunity to a person who does not have that antibody. The effect of passive immunity is transitory.
- Children with acquired or congenital immunodeficiency are vulnerable to bacterial and viral infections. The best way to prevent the spread of organisms is to wash hands routinely and to follow basic infection control practices, based on three principles: (1) prevent contact with organisms, (2) create barriers if contact is unavoidable, and (3) kill organisms if contact is made.
- HIV infection is the best-known acquired immunodeficiency disease. It causes a wide spectrum of illness in children, ranging from no symptoms to mild and moderate symptoms to severe symptoms. AIDS represents the most severe form of the illness.
- Standard treatments for HIV infection include a modified immunization program, antiretroviral therapy, PCP prophylaxis, and the aggressive use of antibiotics.
- For children with HIV, nurses have the challenging tasks of promoting normal growth and development, preventing infections, providing comfort, and respiratory management. In addition, nurses must support families in dealing with a stigmatizing illness that is ultimately terminal.
- Corticosteroids have immunosuppressive and anti-inflammatory properties. Tapering the dose during both long- and short-term therapy regimens allows for the gradual return of adrenal function.
- Emergency treatment takes priority in an anaphylactic reaction, as it is only a matter of minutes before the child will go into shock. Initially, the goal is to maintain an adequate airway, sometimes necessitating endotracheal intubation. This is followed by the administration of epinephrine.

ANSWER TO CRITICAL THINKING EXERCISE 41–1

Negative Considerations: HIV antibody testing in infants less than 18 months old is unreliable because antibodies (indicating infection) are passed from the mother to the child. HIV antibody testing in infants only indicates the HIV infection status of the mother. Several problems are associated with this:
- The mother might not know or suspect she is HIV positive.
- Her denial on learning of her diagnosis might delay her and the baby's treatment.

- Early discharge of mother and infant from the hospital complicates follow-up.
- Some infants are not brought for well-child care and the mother does not receive the information.

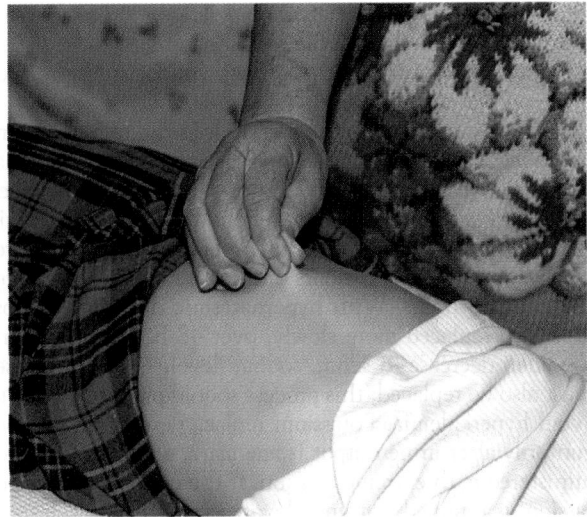

FIGURE 42–1

Testing skin turgor. *Turgor* refers to the elasticity of the skin, which is affected by the extent of hydration. The nurse tests turgor by gently grasping the skin. When the skin is released, it should instantly spring back into place; if it does not, tissue turgor is considered poor. (Courtesy of The University of Texas at Arlington School of Nursing, Arlington, Texas.)

fants indicates dehydration. Suture lines may also become prominent with dehydration.

Vital signs: Fever increases the metabolic rate and fluid requirements. With dehydration, the pulse is rapid, weak, and thready. Metabolic acidosis, which often accompanies dehydration, is compensated for by an increase in the respiratory rate. Blood pressure may be decreased in moderate and severe dehydration, but it is a late sign of hypovolemia.

Behavior: Irritability, lethargy, confusion, or seizures may be present. The child's cry may be high-pitched and weak.

Nursing Diagnosis and Planning

The following nursing diagnosis applies to the dehydrated child:

■ Fluid Volume Deficit related to fluid volume loss through gastrointestinal contents, hemorrhage, burns, other illness, or failure of regulatory mechanisms.

Expected Outcome: The infant or child will display adequate fluid volume, as evidenced by age-appropriate urine output (1 to 2 ml/kg/hr), age-appropriate urine specific gravity, elastic skin turgor and moist mucous membranes, serum pH and electrolyte levels within normal limits, and return to the pre-illness weight.

Interventions

Teach parents how to prevent dehydration. Parents should be taught to give infants and young children extra fluids during hot weather, to avoid overdressing, and to encourage frequent rest periods during high-energy playtimes. During minor illness, providing additional fluids to a child with fever may prevent the development of more serious problems. Teach parents how to identify the early signs and symptoms

About Dehydration

Signs and Symptoms of Dehydration
Parents should be taught to watch for the following signs and symptoms of dehydration:

• Fewer wet diapers (especially no wet diaper for more than 6 to 8 hours)
• No tears when crying
• Irritability; high-pitched cry
• Difficulty in awakening
• Increased respiratory rate or difficulty breathing
• Sunken fontanel, sunken eyes with dark circles
• Abnormal skin color, temperature, or dryness
• Because a young child's condition may worsen faster than an older child's, parents of infants younger than 6 months should seek professional assistance early.

Oral Rehydration Therapy
Parents must understand that giving plain water alone or in large amounts can be extremely dangerous because it does not contain needed electrolytes. Instead, commercially available oral rehydration solutions, such as Rehydralyte, Infalyte, or Pedialyte, should be given.

of dehydration, and instruct them to seek professional help if these signs and symptoms should occur.

Also, teach parents how to replace fluids when the child is mildly dehydrated. Oral rehydration formulations such as Rehydralyte, Infalyte, or Pedialyte contain the appropriate concentration of electrolytes and should be used when fluid is the child's only intake for a prolonged period or in times of decreased intake. Parents need to understand that giving plain water alone or in large amounts can be extremely dangerous, and why.

When caring for the hospitalized child with fluid and electrolyte imbalance, the nurse assumes the responsibility of continuously monitoring the child's condition and administering oral and intravenous fluids safely (see Chapter 38 for a discussion of intravenous therapy). When caring for children with conditions such as fever, burns, diarrhea, vomiting, or trauma, the nurse must continuously assess for signs of dehydration.

Evaluation

• Is urine output appropriate for age (1 to 2 ml/kg/hr) with a specific gravity of 1.005 to 1.020?
• Is the skin elastic and soft?
• Are the mucous membranes moist?
• Are serum pH and electrolyte levels within normal limits?

■ Diarrhea

Diarrhea, one of the most common disorders in childhood, is defined as an increase in the frequency, fluidity, and volume of stools. In the United States, children younger than 5 experience 20 to 35 million episodes of diarrhea, with more than 200,000 hospitalizations per year (Barber &

PATHOPHYSIOLOGY

of Diarrhea

Increased motility and rapid emptying of the intestines result in impaired absorption of nutrients and water, as well as electrolyte imbalance. Water, sodium, potassium, and bicarbonate are drawn from the extracellular space into the stool, resulting in dehydration, electrolyte depletion, and metabolic acidosis.

Diarrhea occurs when there is excess fluid in the small intestine. This condition can result from a number of processes:

- Bacterial toxins stimulating active transport of electrolytes into the small intestine. Cells in the mucosal lining of the intestines are irritated and secrete increased amounts of water and electrolytes.
- Organisms invading and destroying intestinal mucosal cells, decreasing intestinal surface area and impairing the intestine's capacity to absorb fluids and electrolytes.
- Inflammation, which decreases the intestine's ability to absorb fluid, electrolytes, and nutrients. This condition occurs in malabsorption syndromes.
- Increased intestinal motility, resulting in impaired intestinal absorption.

Masiello, 1996). Diarrhea accompanies many childhood disorders. Diarrhea in children may be acute or chronic, inflammatory or noninflammatory. Diarrhea caused by infection is usually called gastroenteritis. Viral gastroenteritis is the cause of approximately 80% of all cases, making it the most common cause of diarrhea in children over age 1.

If not treated, acute diarrhea can lead to dehydration, electrolyte imbalance, and hypovolemic shock. Acute diarrhea can be life-threatening in infants and small children if gastrointestinal fluid losses are not adequately replaced.

Etiology and Incidence

There are many causes of both acute and chronic diarrhea (Table 42–3). Diarrhea with ensuing dehydration is the leading killer of children worldwide and is a major cause of morbidity, as well as a primary sign of many other conditions. In the United States, diarrhea accounts for approximately 10% of all acute care visits by children under age 2 years (Limbos & Lieberman, 1995). It can be either a short- or a long-term condition. In infants and young children, diarrhea can be life-threatening if the losses are not replaced.

Manifestations

Diarrhea may manifest either quickly or insidiously. Its manifestations include the following:

- Integumentary—dry, hot skin; changes in skin texture and turgor; and dry mucous membranes.
- Small intestine—cramps, nausea, and vomiting; large-volume stools, light in color, loose to watery in texture; and stools that tend to be soupy, greasy, or foul-smelling.
- Large intestine—the urge to defecate with insignificant stool present; mushy, jelly-like, or even bloody fecal matter; stool that is usually dark in color; and stool that is rarely foul-smelling.
- Other—increased heart and respiratory rates, decreased tearing, and fever.

Diagnostic Evaluation

Most infectious causes of diarrhea are self-limiting, making comprehensive testing of minor cases of diarrhea impractical. Because of the different possible causes, the diagnostic workup is frequently geared toward ruling out infectious agents as well as anatomic and physiologic reasons, such as allergies, food intolerance, and bowel problems. Tests to be performed after an initial history has assessed for food intolerance, stress, or school- or work-related problems include the following:

Stool: Cultures (for bacteria, ova, parasites, rotavirus), pH, red blood cells, leukocytes, glucose (Clinitest), blood (guaiac test or Hemoccult).

Breath hydrogen test: Checking for carbohydrate malabsorption.

Blood tests: Especially blood cell counts, electrolytes, blood urea nitrogen, glucose, and blood cultures (if an infectious agent is suspected).

X-rays: To check for possible bowel abnormalities.

History: Food or formula intolerance or allergies.

Therapeutic Management

The treatment of diarrhea is aimed at restoring fluid and electrolyte balance and returning the bowel to normal function. Preventing the spread of infection to others is an important component of care. Mild cases of diarrhea can usually be treated at home (American Academy of Pediatrics [AAP] Provisional Committee on Quality Improvement, 1996; O'Loughlin et al., 1995). Parents must be informed of specific fluid intake requirements and signs of dehydration, which would signal a worsening of the child's condition. Treatment includes replacing fluids, providing early feedings, and close monitoring and observation for the treatment of diarrhea and prevention of dehydration. Infants should continue to be given breast milk or regular-strength formula. The early reintroduction of feeding can prevent dehydration, reduce stool frequency and volume, and hasten recovery. It does not prolong diarrhea, and there is evidence that it may reduce the duration of diarrhea by approximately half a day (AAP Provisional Committee, 1996). Early reintroduction of feeding represents a change from the more traditional approach of "resting the bowel" (i.e., placing the child NPO, using intravenous therapy for fluid replacement, and a more gradual introduction of food) (Gremse, 1995; Meyers, 1995).

Oral rehydration therapy is the preferred treatment of fluid and electrolyte losses caused by diarrhea in children with mild to moderate dehydration. Oral rehydration solutions such as Rehydralyte, Infalyte, or Pedialyte may be given. Rice-based oral rehydration solutions increase the absorption of salt, water, and glucose from the intestine and

TABLE 42–3

• • • • • • • • • • •

Causes and Manifestations of Diarrhea in Infants and Children

Causes of Diarrhea	Manifestations
Intestinal infection:	Watery stools containing mucus and possibly blood.
Bacterial (*Campylobacter jejuni,** *Salmonella,** *Shigella,** *E. coli*)	Pain, cramps, nausea, vomiting, and fever (over 101.6°F [38.5°C] with bacterial infection). Risk of dehydration, electrolyte imbalance, and shock.
Viral (rotavirus;* cause of over 50% of cases of acute diarrhea in children; enteric adenovirus)	
Parasitic (*Giardia lamblia,** *Cryptosporidium**—high incidence of both in day care centers)	
Fungal overgrowth	
Food intolerance (lactose intolerance, overfeeding, introduction of new foods)	Diarrhea, increased mucus in stools, flatus, and pain after ingestion of lactose or offending food.
Malabsorption (cystic fibrosis, disaccharide deficiencies, celiac disease)	Diarrhea, cramps, distension, steatorrhea occurring after meals. May experience anorexia, weight loss, and fatigue.
Medications (antibiotics, chemotherapy)	Diarrhea after administration of medications, which usually stops when medications are discontinued.
Colon disease (ulcerative colitis, Crohn's disease, enterocolitis)	Inflammation and ulceration of intestinal walls, increased motility. May have 10–20 stools a day. Abdominal pain, fever, chills, anorexia, and weight loss.
Irritable bowel syndrome	Diarrhea alternating with constipation or normal bowel function. Pain, distension, and nausea may be present.
Intestinal obstruction (including intussusception)	Partial obstruction may result in diarrhea caused by increased intestinal motility. Pain, nausea, and sometimes bloody stools; may note mucus in stools.
Emotional stress (anxiety, fatigue)	Increased motility.
Infectious disease (otitis media, upper respiratory infection, urinary tract infection)	Diarrhea frequently accompanies other infections.

*Most common causative organisms.

may be more beneficial than glucose-based oral rehydration solutions (Misra & Ament, 1998). These solutions are not the same as rice water or commercial products that derive their carbohydrates from glucose polymers purified from rice. Early refeeding can provide similar benefits (AAP Provisional Committee, 1996).

The oral rehydration solutions have changed from the days of homemade recipes (mixtures of water, salt, sugar, and cereals) to today's commercially available, lower-osmolality fluids. Because of their osmotic effect, the high carbohydrate content in fluids such as apple juice, sports drinks, or colas may further aggravate diarrhea and cause additional fluid loss. In addition, Gatorade and other sports drinks do not provide the electrolytes needed to replace the losses in stool during severe diarrhea.

Children and infants who have diarrhea and are not dehydrated should continue to be fed age-appropriate diets. Those needing rehydration should be fed age-appropriate

CRITICAL THINKING EXERCISE 42–1

• • • • • • • • •

Mrs. Peters calls the clinic about 8-month-old David. She states that David has had diarrhea for 2 days and that she doesn't know what to do. She also states that her neighbor said she should stop breast-feeding and give David clear liquids. Mrs. Peters tells you that she is afraid she may have done something to cause David to get sick.

1. What questions should you ask Mrs. Peters about her infant?
2. What teaching can you do to help Mrs. Peters?

diets as soon as they have been rehydrated (AAP Provisional Committee, 1996). If adding milk to the diet increases diarrhea, transient lactose intolerance may be considered, although it is not as common as was once thought. If present, it may be necessary to give the infant a soy formula until the deficiency resolves, usually within several weeks (Limbos & Lieberman, 1995). Common foods that are especially well tolerated during diarrhea are bland but nutritional foods, including complex carbohydrates (e.g., rice, wheat, potatoes, cereals), yogurt, cooked vegetables, and lean meats. Fatty foods and foods high in simple sugars (e.g., tea, juices, soft drinks) should be avoided. This recommendation is a change from the formerly recommended BRAT diet, which consisted of bananas, rice, applesauce, and toast. The BRAT diet can be tolerated but is low in energy, density, fat, and protein.

For infants with mild to moderate diarrhea who have not become dehydrated, oral rehydration therapy is started at home. Breast-feeding should be continued. If an infant or child has become mildly to moderately dehydrated and requires a visit to a clinic or emergency department, oral rehydration solution is recommended. Feeding of solids or formula is started as soon as the child is rehydrated. Children should be encouraged to eat frequently, every 3 to 4 hours. Parents should be instructed that although stool output may increase, feeding will not prolong diarrhea, and the child will be absorbing necessary nutrients and calories. For a child with severe dehydration and ongoing losses, oral rehydration therapy is not recommended. Such children are usually admitted to a hospital for observation and intravenous therapy.

If bacteria, parasites, or fungi cause the diarrhea, other types of medication along with antibiotics may be ordered. The use of antidiarrheal medication is not recommended in children because of the binding nature of these products and the potential for toxicity. Antidiarrheal medications have not been found to shorten the course of the diarrhea, and in cases where the diarrhea is caused by pathogens, they may increase fluid and electrolyte loss by interfering with the body's attempt to rid itself of the organism and allowing the pathogen to remain in the body longer.

Prognosis

Most children experiencing diarrhea and subsequent dehydration usually have a relatively quick recovery, provided that the cause of the diarrhea is determined and therapy is started as soon as possible.

NURSING CARE
The Child with Diarrhea

Assessment

The child's condition and hydration status should be the first area of assessment. The concern about dehydration is the potential for shock. The child and family should be questioned about possible food allergies, intolerance of foods, food eaten over the past 24 hours, and outbreaks of diarrhea in the nuclear or extended family or day care setting. If diarrhea is present, stools should be assessed for amount, color, consistency, and time—abbreviated as ACCT—and odor. When assessing and monitoring for ACCT, note the quantity and quality of the stool, its color (e.g., green, brown, black, clear, blood tinged), consistency (watery, loose), the presence of mucus, and the length of time since the stool's consistency has changed.

Other ongoing assessments include monitoring intake and output; assessing the current weight and comparing it with the last known weight; assessing for thirst, along with skin turgor and texture and mucous membranes; and monitoring the child's level of activity. If diarrhea is severe, it may be necessary to apply a urine bag to measure urine output and to obtain urine to measure specific gravity.

Home Care

Because diarrhea is often treated at home, parents need clear, specific instructions in caring for their sick child. The main goal is to prevent dehydration by giving enough oral fluids to stay abreast of fluid loss through diarrhea. A common myth is that the bowel should be "put to rest" by restricting food and fluids. Limiting fluids, however, can be dangerous, especially in infants and small children. Severe dehydration can develop quickly in a fluid-restricted infant with diarrhea.

Nursing Diagnosis, Planning, Intervention, and Evaluation

Nursing Diagnosis	■ Fluid Volume Deficit related to increased stool output.
Expected Outcome	• The child will maintain fluid balance within normal limits, as evidenced by age-appropriate urine output, capillary refill time less than 2 seconds, elastic skin turgor, moist mucous membranes, and maintenance of pre-illness weight.

Intervention	Rationale
1. Weigh the child carefully on admission and daily on the same scale and at the same time each day.	1. Weight is a useful indicator of fluid status.
2. Monitor and document intake and output hourly. Monitor urine color every 4 hours and specific gravity when appropriate. Weigh diapers after each voiding and stool. (Each gram of diaper weight is equivalent to 1 ml of urine.) Notify physician of signs of dehydration.	2. Urine output should be at least 2 ml/kg/hr for infants and toddlers and 1 ml/kg/hr for school-age children. Older children have lower minimum milliliter per kilogram requirements.
3. Monitor vital signs at least every 4 hours or more frequently as indicated. Temperature should not be taken rectally. Report abnormalities to physician.	3. Dehydration can quickly lead to shock in infants and small children. Using a rectal thermometer can stimulate peristalsis and cause more diarrhea. Fever can be both a cause and a sign of dehydration.

4. Assess for signs of dehydration (dry mucous membranes, decreased tearing, sunken fontanel) frequently. Assess and record the amount, frequency, color, and consistency of stools.
5. Administer oral and intravenous fluids as ordered. Check the intravenous line for patency and infiltration every hour.
6. Administer medications as ordered.

7. Send stools to laboratory for culture and other ordered tests. Perform tests for guaiac, pH, and reducing substance. Monitor laboratory reports (electrolytes, pH, hematocrit, serum albumin, urine specific gravity). Notify physician of abnormal laboratory values or increased frequency of stools.
8. Implement measures to reduce fever (give antipyretics as ordered).

4. Such signs are often the first signs of dehydration.

5. Excessive output without replacement leads to fluid deficit and electrolyte imbalances.
6. Medications may be administered to treat the cause of the diarrhea as well as to assist in minimizing possible sequelae.
7. Laboratory reports are monitored to evaluate response to therapy.

8. See Chapter 37 for a discussion of care of the child with fever.

Evaluation

• Is the infant or child well hydrated, as evidenced by moist mucous membranes, flat fontanel, age-appropriate urine output (1 to 2 ml/kg/hr), and a specific gravity of 1.005 to 1.020?

Nursing Diagnosis

■ Impaired Skin Integrity related to exposure to stool.

Expected Outcome

• The child will have no sign of skin breakdown, as evidenced by intact perineal and perianal skin, and will exhibit signs of healing on affected or excoriated areas.

Intervention

1. Assess the extent of skin breakdown (color, texture, lesions, drainage).
2. Attempt to reduce peristalsis and avoid solutions or foods irritating to mucosal lining.
3. Wash diaper area with water and mild soap after each stool and dry thoroughly. Commercial cleaning wipes often contain alcohol and may cause irritation and pain. Apply medicated ointment or cream as ordered. Do not use plastic pants if hydrocortisone cream is used.
4. Expose affected area to air as much as possible (but not with explosive diarrhea). Keep clothing and linen clean and dry.
5. Use protective moisture barriers, such as creams or ointments.
6. Measure axillary or otic temperatures only. Do *not* take rectal temperatures.

7. Turn the child every 2 hours and protect reddened bony prominences. Use prophylactic pressure-relieving devices in bed and chairs.
8. Teach parents skin care routines.

Rationale

1. Skin breakdown greatly increases the potential for infection.
2. External stimuli aggravate the condition.
3. Thorough and consistent skin care decreases the risk of skin breakdown. Plastic can increase absorption of medication.

4. Exposure of skin to air decreases irritation and promotes healing.

5. Barrier creams are useful for protection from diarrhea stools.
6. Inserting a thermometer in the rectum stimulates peristalsis and may further damage excoriated tissue.
7. Decreasing pressure on irritated skin promotes healing.

8. Parent involvement is necessary to provide ongoing care of the child.

Evaluation

• Have signs of excoriation, redness, blisters, pruritus, and infection been reduced or eliminated?

Nursing Diagnosis

■ Risk for infection (in others) related to lack of knowledge about transmission prevention.

Expected Outcome

• Family members will show no signs of infection and will demonstrate correct precaution technique (contact precautions).

Intervention	Rationale
1. Practice careful hand washing. Wear gloves when caring for the child. Isolate the child according to institution policy.	1. Good hand washing and adherence to isolation guidelines help prevent nosocomial infection.
2. Instruct family and visitors in proper hand washing and observe a return demonstration. Assess parents' understanding of the need for isolation. Discuss the importance of maintaining isolation and explain isolation technique. Teach parents how to contain organisms, and demonstrate techniques to prevent spread. Offer explanations using simple, accurate terminology appropriate to the parents' level of understanding. (See Chapter 37 and Appendix B for a further discussion of isolation technique.)	2. If isolation measures are not maintained, infection may spread to the family and others.
3. Dispose of linen and other soiled items correctly.	3. Proper disposal of contaminated articles decreases the risk of spread of infection.
4. Clean toys, desk, trays, and other equipment after each diaper change and after contact.	4. Proper cleaning of contaminated articles decreases the risk of spread of infection.

Evaluation
- Are family members free of infection?
- Do family members demonstrate an understanding of isolation technique on a consistent basis?

Nursing Diagnosis
- ■ Altered Nutrition: Less Than Body Requirements related to decreased intake and inability of body to absorb fluid.

Expected Outcome
- The child will tolerate diet, as evidenced by weight gain and no recurrence of diarrhea.

Intervention	Rationale
1. Assess the child's weight on admission and daily, using the same scale and after removing the child's clothes. Older children may wear underwear.	1. Weight is a useful indicator of fluid status.
2. Monitor the child's intake and output every 8 hours.	2. Urine output should be at least 2 ml/kg/hr for infants and toddlers and 1 ml/kg/hr for school-age children. Older children have lower minimum requirements.
3. Assess serum electrolyte, calcium, vitamins B_{12} and K^+, folic acid, and zinc levels if ordered.	3. Laboratory values are assessed to determine actual or potential deficiencies.
4. Assess and record bowel sounds and any abdominal distension.	4. Peristalsis (as evidenced by bowel sounds) is necessary for the child to tolerate oral feedings. Hyperactive bowel sounds may indicate excessive peristalsis.
5. When ordered, begin oral rehydration solutions (Rehydralyte, Pedialyte, Infalyte). Discourage the use of Popsicles and other sugary drinks.	5. Fluids high in sugar have high osmotic activity and may increase diarrhea.
6. Offer oral rehydration solution in small, frequent feedings (beginning with 5 to 15 ml every 10 minutes). If tolerated, the volume can be gradually increased.	6. Fluids should be offered in small amounts at first to prevent gastric distension and vomiting.
7. Give liquids at room temperature.	7. Cold liquids stimulate peristalsis.
8. Apple juice, sports beverages, and colas should be avoided during oral rehydration therapy.	8. These beverages have low electrolyte concentrations for oral rehydration therapy and high carbohydrate content.
9. After rehydration, introduce age-appropriate foods that are bland but nutritional and include complex carbohydrates (see p. 1099).	9. Once rehydration has been achieved, an age-appropriate diet provides necessary nutrients.
10. Keep room as odor free as possible. Provide oral hygiene.	10. Minimizing unpleasant stimuli increases intake and feelings of well-being.

Evaluation
- Can the child retain food and fluids?
- Are normal bowel elimination patterns present?
- Has the child maintained or shown an increase in weight?

About Caring for a Child with Diarrhea

Diet
Diet depends on the age of the child and the severity of the diarrhea.

Mild Diarrhea (Mushy Stools) in Children of Any Age
Continue with an age-appropriate diet. Continue breast-feeding, formula, or milk. Encourage an increased intake of fluids and extra water. Avoid fruit juices, as they may worsen diarrhea. Provide bland but nutritious foods. Avoid raw fruits and vegetables and fatty or spicy foods.

Moderate Diarrhea (Watery or Frequent Stools) in Children Younger Than 1 Year
Provide oral rehydration solutions for 6 to 24 hours. Infalyte, Pedialyte, Rehydralyte, or other similar commercially prepared oral rehydration solutions should be given. Juices should be avoided, as they may increase diarrhea.

After the infant has been on clear liquids for 6 to 24 hours, regular formula can be resumed. If the diarrhea was severe or if the diarrhea does not improve after 3 days on regular formula, the infant should be given soy formula (Isomil, ProSobee) instead of cow's milk formula. Soy formula should be continued until the diarrhea is gone for 3 days.

Solids may be given after liquids are fully tolerated. Foods include the ABCs (applesauce, bananas, strained carrots), mashed potatoes, rice cereal, yogurt, and other bland foods.

Breast-feeding should not be discontinued because of diarrhea. Offer more frequent feedings, and if urine decreases, offer oral rehydration solutions in addition to breast-feeding.

Moderate Diarrhea (Watery or Frequent Stools) in Children Over 1 Year
- Give clear liquids (oral rehydration solution) for 6 to 24 hours.
- After clear liquids, provide foods that are appropriate for your child's age and that are nutritional, bland, and high in starch. Suggested foods include breads, crackers, rice, mashed potatoes, noodles, yogurt, cooked vegetables, and lean meats.
- Avoid raw fruits and vegetables, beans, spices, and fatty foods.
- Avoid sports drinks, colas, and apple juice.

Preventing the Spread of Infection
Diarrhea is very contagious. Some of the infectious agents can live on toys, water fountains, and other inanimate objects for several days. Thorough hand washing after diaper changing or using the toilet is crucial to prevent others in the household from getting diarrhea. All family members should be taught the importance of thorough and frequent hand washing. Diapers should be changed on a surface designated for that purpose and *not* on the kitchen counter where food is prepared. Changing areas should be cleaned with disinfectant after each diaper change.

Skin Care
To prevent breakdown of the sensitive skin in the diaper area, diarrhea stools should be completely washed off with mild soap and water after each bowel movement. (Washing the child under running water in the bathtub makes the job easier. The tub should be cleaned with disinfectant before anyone else uses it.) The skin should be patted dry and a layer of A & D ointment or other protective or "barrier" ointment applied.

Changing diapers immediately after bowel movements is important to prevent skin breakdown. The use of commercial baby wipes should be avoided, because they may further irritate and cause additional breakdown of the skin. To prevent overflow of diarrhea from the diaper, diapers should be applied snugly.

When to Call the Doctor
Call the doctor immediately if

- The child does not urinate for longer than 6 hours.
- Crying produces no tears or the mouth becomes dry.
- The infant's fontanel appears sunken.
- Blood appears in the diarrhea or the diarrhea becomes severe (e.g., a bowel movement every hour for more than 8 hours, or more than ten watery bowel movements in one day).
- Severe abdominal cramps occur.
- The child becomes dizzy when standing.
- The child starts acting very sick.
- Fever over 100°F (37.8°C) has been present for more than 72 hours.
- Mild diarrhea lasts more than 1 week.

Adapted from American Academy of Pediatrics Provisional Committee on Quality Improvement, Subcommittee on Acute Gastroenteritis. (1996). The management of acute gastroenteritis in young children. *Pediatrics, 97*(3), 424–435; Schmitt, B. D. (1999). *Instructions for pediatric patients* (pp. 72–73). Philadelphia: Saunders.

Vomiting

Vomiting is the forcible ejection of stomach contents through the mouth. It involves a complex reflex associated with sweating, salivation, and often tachycardia (all symptoms of autonomic nervous stimulation). Other terms that may be used to differentiate vomiting episodes include spitting up (or chalasia, which is a normal process during infancy), regurgitation (associated with gastroesophageal reflux or overfeeding), and, if severe, projectile vomiting (usually indicative of obstruction, tumor, pyloric stenosis, or increasing intracranial pressure). Isolated incidents of vomiting are usually of little concern. The consequences of persistent or prolonged vomiting, however, can be serious.

PATHOPHYSIOLOGY
of Vomiting

Vomiting is under the control of the emetic center, located in the reticular core of the medulla (in the brain stem). The emetic center receives stimuli from one of three sources:

- From the vagal and sympathetic afferent nerves, such as the stimulation of irritation, distension, obstruction, or inflammation.
- Chemically, from drugs (e.g., ipecac and other opioids), cerebral hypoxia, inner ear disturbances, or increased intracranial pressure.
- From the higher cortical centers, with stimuli such as sights, odors, and fright or fear.

The mechanism of vomiting occurs in the presence of several complex reflexes:

- Autonomic nervous system discharge, which causes salivation, sweating, pallor, and an increased heart rate.
- Contraction of the stomach antrum and duodenum.
- Relaxation of the remainder of the stomach, esophagus, and sphincters.
- Closure of the glottis and soft palate.
- Contraction of the diaphragm and abdominal muscles, which increases intra-abdominal pressure and compresses abdominal contents, thus propelling them into the esophagus and out the mouth.

Etiology

Vomiting, which occurs frequently in children, is usually a sign of some other underlying problem or disease. Vomiting has many possible causes. Some of them include infections, obstructions, motion sickness, metabolic alterations, and psychological alterations. If vomiting occurs in association with diarrhea, it may be related to gastroenteritis. Vomiting can also result from allergic reactions, as a side effect of medications (such as chemotherapy), as a toxic effect of medications or ingested substances, and in certain eating disorders.

Manifestations

Sour milk curds without green or brownish color and undigested food from the stomach are manifestations of vomiting. Greenish emesis usually indicates the presence of bile and possible intestinal obstruction below the ampulla of Vater. A fecal odor indicates lower intestinal obstruction or peritonitis. Emesis may be blood tinged, or the color may be bright red or look like coffee grounds. Bright red blood indicates that the blood has not been in contact with gastric juices.

The force of vomiting varies. Regurgitation, a backward flow of undigested food, could be due to overfeeding. Forceful vomiting could indicate some obstruction. Projectile vomiting may indicate obstruction, tumor, or increased intracranial pressure.

CRITICAL TO REMEMBER
Caring for the Child Who Is Vomiting

Nursing care of the child who is vomiting is directed toward

- Observation and reporting of vomiting
- Assessing for associated problems, such as dehydration
- Implementing measures to reduce the vomiting
- Recording accurate intake and output
- Evaluating the effectiveness of therapy
- Preventing aspiration

Diagnostic Evaluation

Vomiting is usually of brief duration and not severe. If vomiting continues and the child starts to look deficient in fluid or electrolytes, however, the following tests may be indicated:

- Complete blood cell counts and electrolyte studies, blood urea nitrogen, glucose levels and urine tests
- Radiographic studies (if an obstructive or neurologic process is suspected)
- Blood cultures (if an infectious disease is suspected)
- Arterial blood gas determinations

Therapeutic Management

The primary focus of managing vomiting is detecting and treating the cause, with the secondary intent of preventing complications. Oral rehydration therapy, as indicated for the treatment of diarrhea, is also appropriate for the vomiting child and may be given in small, frequent amounts. The time intervals and volume depend on the child's weight and age. Even with continued vomiting, most children can maintain hydration with small frequent feedings of an oral rehydration formulation. As the vomiting decreases in frequency, the amount and interval between feedings can increase. If the vomiting is severe or prolonged in neonates and young infants, however, intravenous therapy is initiated. Most children will respond well, but some will need antiemetics.

Once the vomiting has ceased, liquids or foods should be reintroduced gradually, as tolerated. The mouth should be rinsed and the teeth brushed after vomiting, to rid the mouth of the hydrochloric acid as well as to freshen the mouth.

NURSING CARE
The Vomiting Child

Assessment

Determine and describe the type and force of vomiting (i.e., "spitting up" as opposed to regurgitation, forceful vomiting, or projectile vomiting), as well as the character (ACCT) of the vomitus. Because vomiting is often associated with gastric distension, the relationship, if any, with infant feeding should be assessed (e.g., poor feeding techniques, failure to bubble or burp, regurgitation with burp or "wet burp," improper positioning).

Nursing Diagnosis and Planning

The following nursing diagnoses and expected outcomes may be appropriate in the treatment of the vomiting child:

- Fluid Volume Deficit related to increased loss of gastrointestinal contents.
  Expected Outcomes: The child will maintain fluid balance within normal limits, as evidenced by age-appropriate fluid intake, and will have appropriate urine output (1 to 2 ml/kg/hr), a capillary refill time of less than 2 seconds, elastic skin turgor, and moist mucous membranes.
- Altered Nutrition: Less Than Body Requirements related to inability of body to retain gastric contents.
  Expected Outcomes: The child will maintain electrolyte balance within normal limits, as evidenced by serum sodium and potassium levels within normal limits, and a normal level of activity and alertness. The child will tolerate diet, as evidenced by no recurrence of vomiting.

Interventions

The vomiting child should be placed in an upright or side-lying position to prevent aspiration. Because vomiting is often the primary symptom of many different conditions, it is very important to assess and record its occurrence, as well as any other associated manifestations. Nursing interventions are frequently determined by the cause of the vomiting and therefore may be very specific. For example, if the vomiting is found to be due to incorrect feeding techniques or solutions, the nurse's role is to educate the family regarding appropriate feeding techniques (e.g., adequate bubbling and burping as well as positioning after the feeding) and preparation of formulas.

Major concerns with vomiting are dehydration and fluid and electrolyte imbalance; therefore, it is essential that hydration status be carefully assessed, including accurate monitoring of intake and output, weight, fontanels in infants, skin turgor, eyes, skin, and heart and respiratory rates. If the child has repeated vomiting or vomits large volumes, the physician should be notified so that intravenous therapy can be initiated.

Once the cause of vomiting has been determined, nursing interventions are directed toward ensuring a continued reduction in the vomiting. In reintroducing oral fluids and feedings for the child who is vomiting, start with an appropriate electrolyte-containing solution. Offer an oral rehydration solution in small, frequent feedings to avoid gastric distension. If tolerated, the volume can be gradually increased. If oral fluids are well tolerated, solid foods may be added. Another important consideration is education for the child and family about avoidance of certain foods (such as fatty, acidified, or seasoned foods), as well as minimizing stimuli such as stress, anxiety, or unfavorable-smelling foods, which might lead to nausea and subsequent vomiting. Antiemetic medications, decreased stimuli, and avoidance of food or activities that might tend to upset the stomach, either directly or by association, may be helpful in decreasing nausea and vomiting.

Evaluation

- Is the child taking age-appropriate amounts of fluid without vomiting?
- Is the child's urine output 1 to 2 ml/kg/hr?
- Is the child's skin turgor elastic, with a capillary refill time of 2 seconds or less?
- Does the child have moist mucous membranes?
- Are the child's serum sodium and potassium levels within normal limits?
- Is the child tolerating an age-appropriate diet?

KEY CONCEPTS

- Infants and children are at a much greater risk than adults for fluid and electrolyte disturbances.
- The three mechanisms by which acid-base balance is maintained are chemical buffering, respiratory control of carbon dioxide, and renal regulation of bicarbonate and secretion of hydrogen ions.
- The two major forms of acid-base disturbance are acidosis and alkalosis, either of which may be respiratory or metabolic.

- The treatment of metabolic disturbances is directed toward correcting the underlying problem. Interventions for respiratory alterations are implemented toward re-establishing alveolar ventilation.
- Dehydration may be classified as isonatremic (the most common form), hyponatremic, or hypernatremic.
- Monitoring of intake and output, vital signs, and level of activity

(or sensorium) is crucial in appropriately assessing the child with a fluid or electrolyte disturbance.
- Diarrhea can lead to loss of bicarbonate (and subsequently to acidosis).
- Oral rehydration therapy is indicated for the child with diarrhea, dehydration of any degree, and vomiting.

ANSWERS TO CRITICAL THINKING EXERCISE 42-1

1. When taking a history related to diarrhea it is very important that you have accurate information. One person's definition of diarrhea may be very different from the next. David may indeed have severe diarrhea, or he may just have an increase in stools. Ask Mrs. Peters the following questions:

- How long has David had diarrhea?
- How many stools has he had? What is the color, amount, and consistency of the stools?
- How many wet diapers has David had in the last 24 hours?
- Is David playing and acting normally?
- What is David's temperature?
- When David cries, does he have tears?
- Has David been in a day care setting or church nursery?
- Does anyone else in the family have diarrhea?
- What solids does David eat?

2. On the basis of Mrs. Peters's response, you can develop a teaching plan. Three areas need to be addressed: diet, infection control, and emotional support. Although you may think diet and infection control are priorities, until Mrs. Peters is less anxious she will not be able to give full attention to the information you are about to give her. For that reason, you should provide emotional support and assurance.

Emotional Support. Mrs. Peters seems to be blaming herself for David's illness. Provide an environment that encourages her to talk about her feelings. The use of therapeutic communication will build trust and allow her to share her concerns. You can commend her for breast-feeding and point out that breast-feeding provides extra help in fighting infections. Because David is now 8 months old, the antibodies that Mrs. Peters passed to him during her pregnancy are gone, and he is more susceptible to infections. As you talk with Mrs. Peters, you are constantly assessing her emotional needs and responding to her questions.

Diet. Mrs. Peters should continue breast-feeding David. If he shows no signs of dehydration, an age-appropriate diet of solids should be continued. Fruit juices and raw fruits and vegetables should be discontinued because they may increase the diarrhea. If David is mildly dehydrated, Mrs. Peters should be encouraged to breast-feed at more frequent intervals. If urine output is decreased, she can also add an oral rehydration solution for 6 to 24 hours. David can be given a regular diet that is age-appropriate as soon as he is rehydrated. Foods given should be nutritional and include complex carbohydrates. Suggested foods include cereal, mashed potatoes, strained bananas, strained carrots, and applesauce. Mrs. Peters should be given instructions regarding signs of dehydration, as well as when she should notify David's primary health provider if his condition worsens.

Infection Control. Instructions should also cover hand washing and infection control. Instruct Mrs. Peters in the disposal of contaminated linens and other soiled items. Instruct her in the cleaning of areas where diapers are changed and where children play with toys. Instruct her to clean the bathtub after use. Reinforce the importance of not sharing toys among children who have diarrhea.

REFERENCES AND READINGS

Acra, S. A., & Ghishan, F. K. (1996). Electrolyte fluxes in the gut and oral rehydration solutions. *Pediatric Clinics of North America, 43*(2), 433–449.

American Academy of Pediatrics. (1997). *Textbook of pediatric advanced life support.* Dallas: American Heart Association.

American Academy of Pediatrics Provisional Committee on Quality Improvement, Subcommittee on Acute Gastroenteritis. (1996). The management of acute gastroenteritis in young children. *Pediatrics, 97*(3), 424–435.

Barber, C., & Masiello, M. (1996). Oral rehydration therapy. *Topics in Emergency Medicine, 18*(3), 21–26.

Barclay, D. V., Gil-Ramos, J., Mora, J. O., & Dirren, H. (1995). A packaged rice-based oral rehydration solution for acute diarrhea. *Journal of Pediatric Gastroenterology and Nutrition, 20*(4), 408–416.

Behrman, R., & Kliegman, R. (1998). *Nelson essentials of pediatrics* (3rd ed.). Philadelphia: Saunders.

Childhood diarrhea: New solutions. (1996). *Health News, 14*(6), 7–8.

Dabbagh, S., Atiyeh, B., Fleischmann, L. E., & Gruskin, A. B. (1999). Fluid and electrolyte therapy. In F. D. Burg, J. R. Ingelfinger, E. R. Wald, & R. A. Polin (Eds.), *Gellis & Kagan's current pediatric therapy* (16th ed.). Philadelphia: Saunders.

Dimond, R. J. (1995). Nutritional support in pediatric diseases. *Current Opinion in Gastroenterology, 11*(2), 168–173.

Eliason, B. C. (1998). Gastroenteritis in children: Principles of diagnosis and treatment. *American Family Physician, 58*(8), 1769–1776.

Fann, B. D. (1998). Fluid and electrolyte balance in the pediatric patient. *Journal of Intravenous Nursing, 21*(3), 153–159.

Fayad, I. M., Hashem, M., Duggan, C., Refat, M., Bakir, M., Fontaine, O., & Santosham, M. (1993). Comparative efficacy of rice-based and glucose-based oral rehydration salts plus early reintroduction of food. *Lancet, 342*(8874), 772–775.

Finberg, L., Kravath, R., & Hellerstein, S. (1993). *Water and electrolytes in pediatrics* (2nd ed.). Philadelphia: Saunders.

Gorelick, M. H., Shaw, K. N., & Murphy, K. O. (1997). Validity and reliability of clinical signs in the diagnosis of dehydration in children. *Pediatrics, 99*(5), e6.

Gremse, D. A. (1995). Effectiveness of nasogastric rehydration in hospitalized children with acute diarrhea. *Journal of Pediatric Gastroenterology and Nutrition, 21*(2), 145–148.

Harrison, M. S. (1998). Rotavirus: An overview. From discovery to vaccine. *Pediatric Nursing, 24*(4), 317.

Hoekelman, R. A. (Ed.). (1997). *Primary pediatric care.* St. Louis: Mosby–Year Book.

Horne, M., Heitz, U., & Swearingen, P. (1991). *Fluid, electrolyte and acid-base balance: A case study approach.* St. Louis: Mosby–Year Book.

Johnson, K. (Ed.). (1996). *The Harriet Lane handbook.* St. Louis: Mosby–Year Book.

Keller, V. E. (1995). Management of nausea and vomiting in children. *Journal of Pediatric Nursing, 10*(5), 280–286.

Lam, W. H. (1998). Fluids in paediatric patients. *Care of the Critically Ill, 14*(3), 93–96.

Liacouras, C. A., & Baldassano, R. N. (1998). Is it toddler's diarrhea? *Contemporary Pediatrics, 15*(9), 131–144.

Limbos, M. A., & Lieberman, J. M. (1995). Management of acute diarrhea in children. *Contemporary Pediatrics, 12*(12), 68–91.

Meyers, A. (1995). Modern management of acute diarrhea and dehydration in children. *American Family Physician, 51*(5), 1103–1118.

Misra, S., & Ament, M. E. (1998). Gastrointestinal tract infections. In R. D. Feigin & J. D. Cherry (Eds.), *Textbook of pediatric infectious diseases* (4th ed.). Philadelphia: Saunders.

Nordeman, L., & Hamilton, R. (1996). Dehydration and gastroenteritis. *Topics in Emergency Medicine, 18*(3), 11–20.

O'Loughlin, E. V., Notaras, E., McCullough, C., Halliday, J., & Henry, R. L. (1995). Home-based management of children hospitalized with acute gastroenteritis. *Journal of Pediatrics and Child Health, 31*(3), 189–191.

Pizarro, D., Poseda, G., Sandi, L., & Moran, J. (1991). Rice-based oral electrolyte solutions. *New England Journal of Medicine, 324*(8), 517–521.

Schmitt, B. D. (1999). *Instructions for pediatric patients.* Philadelphia: Saunders.

Straughn, A., & English, B. (1996). Oral rehydration therapy: A neglected treatment for pediatric diarrhea. *MCN: American Journal of Maternal/Child Nursing, 21*, 144–147.

ogy, and nursing care. These distinct problems are all abnormal openings in the lip or palate. The defects may occur unilaterally (on either side) or bilaterally.

Incidence

The incidence ranges from 1 in 1,000 births for cleft lip and palate to 1 in 2,500 births for cleft lip. Cleft lip is predominantly seen in males and cleft palate in females. The incidence of cleft is higher in Asians and lowest in African-Americans (Behrman, Kliegman, & Arvin, 1996). Cleft lip and palate accounts for 35% to 40% of these facial malformations.

Manifestations and Diagnostic Evaluation

Cleft lip has the following manifestations: a notched vermilion border, variably sized clefts that involve the alveolar ridge, and dental anomalies (usually deformed, supernumerary, or absent teeth). Cleft palate includes nasal distortion, midline or bilateral cleft with variable extension from the uvula and soft and hard palates, and exposed nasal cavities.

The diagnosis of cleft lip and cleft palate is based on observation at birth and complete examination in the neonatal period. Cleft lip is readily diagnosed through inspection of the lip. The first sign of cleft palate may be formula coming from the nose. A gloved finger placed in the mouth to feel the defect or visual examination with a flashlight will confirm the diagnosis.

Therapeutic Management

Management is based on the severity of the defect. A number of professionals are involved in this process, including surgeons, nurses, geneticists, psychologists or psychiatrists, ear, nose, and throat specialists, audiologists, and occupational and speech therapists. Orthodontists and plastic surgeons become involved in the lengthy management. Pediatricians provide ongoing child health care.

The first intervention involves modifying feeding techniques as needed to allow adequate growth. Use of special feeding techniques, obturators, and unique nipples and feeders can usually accomplish this goal and provide for early discharge with parents (Fig. 43–1).

Cleft lip repair is usually performed by age 4 weeks and at some centers in the first 2 to 3 days of life (Richard, 1994a). Early repair may improve bonding and makes feeding much easier. The surgical technique involves the use of a staggered suture line to minimize scarring. Some cosmetic modifications may be needed again at age 4 to 5 years.

Cleft palate repair is individualized and based on the degree of deformity and size of the child. Closure is completed between ages 6 months and 2 years. Most teams recommend repair by 1 year. Earlier closure facilitates speech development (Richard, 1994a).

Concurrent treatment of altered dentition, recurring otitis media, speech dysfunction, emotional issues, and cosmetic concerns complete the ongoing therapy. Children

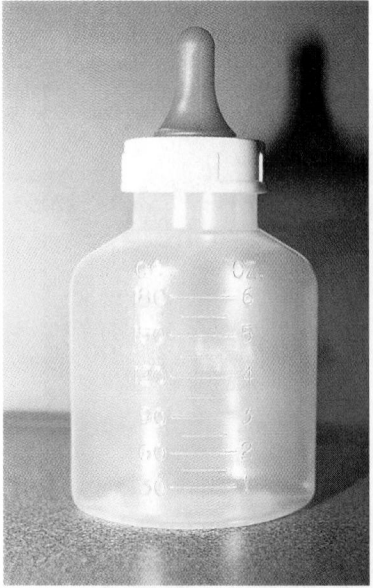

After a cleft lip repair, a syringe with a rubber tip is used for feeding to prevent trauma to the incision.

◀ A feeder with compressible plastic sides allows the person feeding the baby gently to squeeze the sides of the bottle to help eject the breast milk or formula. A slightly longer nipple allows the milk to be swallowed with less chance of entering the nasopharynx and yet is not so long that it stimulates the gag reflex.

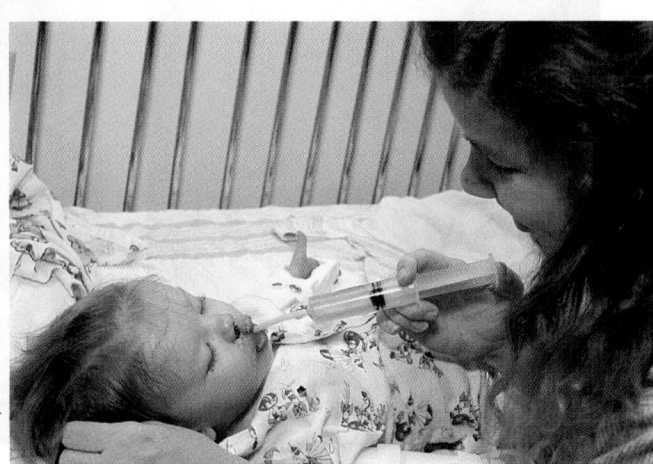

FIGURE 43–1
· · · · · · · · · ·
Before and after repair of a cleft lip or palate, special feeding techniques are essential for adequate nutrition.

Care of the Child with Cleft Lip or Palate

Your infant may require a special feeding method to maximize growth while waiting for surgery, and you may need to practice the feeding method to be used after surgery until the incision heals. The ESSR method is used for infants who are bottle-fed. The ESSR method involves the following steps:

- *Enlarge* the nipple by cross-cutting the hole so that food is delivered to the back of the throat without strong sucking.
- *Stimulate* sucking by rubbing the nipple on the baby's lower lip.
- *Swallow*.
- *Rest* to allow your baby to finish swallowing the breast milk or formula.

After surgery, elbow restraints may be required so that your baby cannot touch the stitches. Follow these recommendations:

- Do not apply the restraints too tightly. They should be loose but still prevent elbow bending.
- Remove restraints at least every 2 hours for 10 to 15 minutes and play games with your child that encourage movement of the elbows. Look for any skin irritation every time you remove the restraints.
- Remove only one restraint at a time.

Do not brush your child's teeth for 1 to 2 weeks after surgery. Feeding a small amount of water after meals will help keep the teeth clean.

with cleft palate are at high risk for developing chronic otitis media. Parents should be aware of this risk so that otitis media can be diagnosed early to decrease the chance of long-term scarring and hearing loss (Resnick & Zarem, 1996).

NURSING CARE

The Child with a Cleft Lip or Palate

Assessment

Cleft lip and cleft palate are readily apparent at birth, and the degree of involvement should be documented during the newborn examination (see Chapter 22). After identifying this condition, assess the infant's ability to suck, swallow, and breathe without distress and handle normal secretions. Because the occurrence of cleft lip and palate is usually unexpected and its appearance can be frightening to parents and families, assess and record parents' reactions as well as their interactions with the neonate.

Parents of an infant with a cleft lip or palate may need help to resolve feelings about their infant's appearance. The parents might need to deal with many questions from family members, stares from strangers, and expressions of pity from other new parents. Providing information about the etiology of the defect and showing them pictures of other children before and after surgical repair can give them some relief from these fears and concerns. In addition, modeling and encouraging bonding through touching, holding, and examining their newborn can be very reassuring. Pointing out the newborn's positive attributes can help decrease the focus on the defect. For example, emphasize how alert the baby is, or the infant's responsiveness or beautiful eyes.

Nursing Diagnosis, Planning, Intervention, and Evaluation

Nursing Diagnoses	■ Altered Nutrition: Less Than Body Requirements related to inability to suck and to the surgical repair. ■ Knowledge Deficit about feeding techniques and surgery related to unfamiliarity with the information.
Expected Outcomes	• The child will drink the desired amount of fluid within 30 minutes and be content during and after feedings and will gain weight and height according to the normal growth curve. • The parent will express satisfaction with progress of feedings and will understand expected preoperative and postoperative care.

Intervention	Rationale
1. Describe the degree of cleft and impairment of sucking.	1. Infants with cleft lip alone or simple cleft dental arch may be successful with breast- or bottle-feeding without modifications.
2. Teach the ESSR (enlarge, stimulate, swallow, rest) method. Some infants may be able to breast-feed with assistance.	2. Infants who are fed using the ESSR method have a better growth rate than children fed by other methods (Richard, 1994b).
3. Keep care and teaching simple and as closely related to normal infant feeding as possible.	3. Nutrition, parent-infant relationship, and compliance may be improved if normal techniques can be utilized.

4. Provide alternative assistive feeding devices as needed and ordered.

5. Burp frequently and hold the infant in a more upright position.
6. Document the feeding program in written form for parents to use at home and provide the plan to other health professionals.
7. Provide emotional support and positive reinforcement to parents as they learn to feed their child.
8. Keep an accurate record of the child's growth by using a growth chart.
9. Explain preoperative and postoperative procedures: oral feedings withheld for 6 hours, placement of intravenous lines, use of arm restraints, appearance of repair in the immediate postoperative period.
10. Postoperatively
    a. Keep straws, pacifiers, spoons, or fingers away from the child's mouth for 7 to 10 days. Do not take temperatures orally.
    b. Advance the child's diet as ordered and tolerated from clear liquids to a normal *soft* diet within 48 hours.
    c. After repair of a cleft lip, resume preoperative feeding techniques.
    d. After repair of a cleft palate, provide short nipples that do not rest on palatal sutures; give baby food or baby food mixed with water (Richard, 1994a).

4. Techniques and equipment vary among institutions. Use what is available and effective for each child.
5. Burping minimizes air swallowing and GI flatus.
6. Documentation provides consistency at home and at other times, when the family is in contact with numerous medical professionals treating the child.
7. Self-care and bonding are improved when parents can assume total care.
8. A chart identifies growth changes early, when intervention can be most effective.
9. Explanation decreases parental anxiety and encourages involvement.

10. For postoperative care
    a. Avoiding contact with the incision site reduces stress on surgical repair and prevents accidental tearing of very fine sutures.
    b. A normal diet minimizes nutritional deficits and stress on the child. No foods that can tear sutures are offered.
    c. Little evidence shows that sucking causes excess suture stress (Richard, 1994a).
    d. Studies indicate that nipples may be used postoperatively without stressing sutures (Richard, 1994a).

Evaluation
- Is the infant following the appropriate growth curve?
- Is the infant happy and content during and after feedings?
- Is the parent satisfied with the feeding technique used and the time required to complete a feeding?
- Can the parent explain and demonstrate expected preoperative and postoperative care?

Nursing Diagnosis
■ Altered Family Processes related to a visible defect.

Expected Outcomes
- The parents will demonstrate positive behaviors toward the infant.
- The parents will access appropriate support.

Intervention

1. Encourage parents to discuss their fears, concerns, and negative emotions.
2. Encourage touching and holding.

3. Make appropriate referral to a cleft lip and palate team of nurses, physicians, and other specialists as soon as possible.
4. Express acceptance of the baby by modeling feeding and close physical contact.
5. Refer parents to community resources and parent groups (see Appendix L).
6. Encourage parents to share concerns about long-term care and emotional and financial stress.

Rationale

1. Grief, anxiety, confusion, guilt, denial, and anger are not uncommon and should be expressed.
2. Contact encourages bonding and prevents a delayed attachment.
3. A health care team can provide accurate information and begin to outline a plan of action.
4. These interventions assist parents with the adaptation process.
5. Acceptance and adaptation are facilitated by sharing with others in similar situations.
6. Long-term concerns require extensive follow-up and can strain many families' resources. Identifying concerns early can increase problem-solving options.

Evaluation
- Can the parents identify their infant's positive characteristics?
- Do the parents hold, cuddle, and make eye contact with the infant?
- Have the parents sought personal, community, or national support?

Nursing Diagnosis

- ■ Impaired Skin Integrity related to the surgical repair.
- ■ Risk for Infection related to the surgical repair.

Expected Outcome

- • The repair site will heal without complications.

Intervention	Rationale
1. Clean the lip repair site according to physician protocol. Many physicians recommend cleaning with sterile water using a cotton swab or saline after feeding and as ordered. Use a rolling motion vertically down the suture line. Have parents demonstrate this cleaning technique.	1. The procedure decreases the medium for bacterial growth, decreases crusting, and minimizes scarring.
2. Apply anti-infective ointment as ordered.	2. Anti-infective ointment prevents infection, crusting, and scarring.
3. Use elbow restraints to keep the child from touching the repair site. Continue for 6 to 8 days. Remove every 2 hours for 10 to 15 minutes. Remove restraint from only one elbow at a time, with a parent or nurse in constant attendance.	3. Elbow restraints prevent accidental rupture or tear of sutures. Periodically removing restraints promotes contact with the child, decreases anxiety, and allows the nurse to assess skin integrity and circulation.
4. Do not brush the child's teeth for 1 to 2 weeks.	4. Avoiding brushing prevents accidental tear of palatal sutures.
5. Keep the child in a supine position or on the side opposite to the repair.	5. Careful positioning prevents contact of suture lines with bed linens.
6. Observe for redness, swelling, excessive bleeding, drainage, respiratory distress, or fever.	6. Signs of infection must be identified early because additional inflammation can increase scarring.
7. To clean the palate repair site, rinse the child's mouth with water after feedings.	7. Rinsing after feeding removes food and residual sugars from suture lines, reducing the risk of infection.
8. Encourage the parents to hold and cuddle the child, as the child desires.	8. Crying puts additional stress on the suture line.
9. Maintain lip protective devices, if ordered.	9. Protective devices prevent separation of lip suture lines.

Evaluation

- • Is the suture site clean, dry, and without redness, heat, or drainage?
- • Is the suture site intact and healing without crusting or excessive scarring?

Nursing Diagnosis

- ■ Pain related to the surgical incision.

Expected Outcome

- • The child will be free from pain.

Intervention	Rationale
1. Describe and document pain using appropriate tools (see Chapter 39).	1. Infants and young children do not react to pain in typical adult ways, and alternative observations are needed to validate assessment findings.
2. Provide comfort measures, especially holding, rocking, and parental voices.	2. Comforting increases parental involvement, relieves discomfort, and reduces stress on sutures caused by crying.
3. Provide analgesics and sedatives on a regular basis as ordered. Pain should decrease significantly after 24 to 48 hours.	3. Medication can prevent peaks of pain that cannot be managed appropriately.
4. Report pain not managed by usual means.	4. Pain may indicate hematoma formation or other complications of the repair.

Evaluation

- • Does the child participate in age-appropriate activities?
- • Is the child responding well to pain medication?
- • Does the child appear relaxed and content at rest?
- • Does the parent describe a child who is not in pain?

Nursing Diagnosis

- ■ Altered Health Maintenance related to the need for long-term care.

Expected Outcome

- • The parents will seek continued follow-up care to evaluate and manage long-term complications.

Intervention	Rationale
1. Make appropriate and early referrals for any problems with speech impairment or language-based learning disabilities.	1. Speech and language-learning impairments are common complications of cleft lip and palate. Early intervention minimizes harm.
2. Monitor for recurrent or chronic otitis media. Schedule frequent hearing tests.	2. Because of craniofacial deformities, otitis media can occur frequently and must be treated to prevent language and learning problems.
3. Encourage early speech attempts. Arrange speech therapy as needed.	3. Cleft palate can make speech difficult to understand, and the child may feel self-conscious about speech errors. Practice improves development.
4. Encourage good dental care.	4. With abnormalities of teeth and the alveolar ridge, malocclusion and dental caries are a major concern.

Evaluation

- Do the parents continue to seek follow-up care (ENT, speech therapy, dental)?
- Does the child demonstrate age-appropriate speech?
- Does the child have normal hearing?
- Does the child have normal dentition?

Upper Gastrointestinal Hernias

A hernia is an abnormal protrusion of part of an organ or tissue through the structures that normally contain it. Hernias can be either congenital or acquired. Some hernias can be reduced, whereas others become incarcerated and cannot be returned by manipulation. A medical emergency occurs when a hernia becomes strangulated and blood supply is cut off. This condition can occur suddenly and requires immediate treatment. The most common hernias of the upper GI tract are discussed in Table 43–1.

Other Developmental Disorders

Table 43–2 discusses other developmental disorders of the upper and lower GI tract.

Gastroesophageal Reflux

Gastroesophageal reflux (GER) is regurgitation of gastric contents back into the esophagus. GER is a normal physiologic phenomenon; all adults and infants experience reflux periodically, especially after meals. Reflux can be divided into three types: physiologic, functional, and pathologic.

Etiology

Many factors contribute to the development of GER. Neurologic impairment such as cerebral palsy, Down syndrome, and head injury may affect the transmission of neural signals to the lower esophageal sphincter (LES). Delayed gastric emptying of a liquid meal due to distension may also contribute. LES relaxations can also be triggered by partial or incomplete swallowing dysfunctions or drugs such as theophylline or caffeine. Increased intra-abdominal pressure incurred while straining, crying, coughing, or

slumping tend to promote increased episodes of GER. These postural effects are most likely primary contributing factors in infants. Obesity and hiatal hernias also promote GER. Finally, during the first 6 months of life, the LES pressure undergoes maturational development. Because infants have a short abdominal LES, they experience GER more often. As the infant grows the LES matures, and the reflux improves.

Types of Gastroesophageal Reflux

PHYSIOLOGIC

- Infrequent emesis
- Parents may not be concerned or may think it is normal

FUNCTIONAL

- Painless, frequent emesis after meals
- No failure to thrive
- 40% asymptomatic by 3 months
- 70% asymptomatic by 18 months
- Medical management very effective

PATHOLOGIC

- Failure to thrive
- Aspiration pneumonia
- Apnea
- Frequent emesis, amount varies
- Often requires surgery

Data from Shannon, R. (1993). Gastroesophageal reflux in infancy: Review and update. *Journal of Pediatric Health Care, 7*(2), 71–75.

TABLE 43-1
. . . .

Upper Gastrointestinal Hernias

Description	Clinical Manifestations	Therapeutic Management	Nursing Management
Hiatal Hernia			
Protrusion of a portion of the stomach through the esophageal hiatus of the diaphragm	• Vomiting • Coughing, wheezing, short periods of apnea • Failure to thrive	Medical management similar to that for the child with reflux Surgical repair of defect	Monitor intake and output, document vomiting, observe for respiratory distress, provide routine postoperative care for GI surgery. Teach parents about surgery and medical treatment of reflux.
Congenital Diaphragmatic Hernia (CDH)			
Opening in the diaphragm through which abdominal contents herniate into the thoracic cavity during prenatal development *and* some degree of pulmonary hypoplasia, determined by the timing and size of the herniation Mortality: 50%–80% Degree of pulmonary hypoplasia determines outcome Incidence: 1 in 2,200–5,000 live births	Clinical findings depend on severity of defect, and may include • Abdominal organs in chest (by fetal ultrasonography) • Diminished or absent breath sounds on affected side • Bowel sounds that may be heard over the chest • Cardiac sounds that may be heard on the right side of the chest • Respiratory distress developing soon after birth: dyspnea, cyanosis, nasal flaring, tachypnea, retractions • Scaphoid abdomen	If diagnosed prenatally mother moved to tertiary care center before delivery *Neonatal emergency* Nasogastric intubation with suction Ventilate with high-frequency ventilation; manage acidosis with bicarbonate and ventilation Extracorporeal membrane oxygenation (EMCO) Manage pulmonary hypertension Surgical reduction of hernia after physiologically stable May wait 6–18 hours after birth Respiratory support, ECMO until lungs functioning after surgery	Identify clinical findings and report immediately. Place child in semi-Fowler's position on affected side with head of bed elevated. Maintain patency of NG tube. Monitor IV fluids. Maintain mechanical ventilation, ECMO, chest tubes, assess oxygenation. Provide minimal stimulation. Provide routine postoperative care. Monitor for signs of infection, respiratory distress, and feeding difficulties and report to physician. Support family mourning, loss of perfect child. Provide clear, truthful information. Encourage the parent to see and touch the infant. Provide referral to support groups. Provide discharge teaching. Use prescribed feeding techniques.

Incidence

Pathologic GER occurs in about 3% of all newborns (Sterling, Jolley, Besser, et al., 1991). Boys are affected three times more than girls, and premature infants are affected more than full-term infants. Almost all infants with GER will have symptoms by age 6 weeks. In the absence of therapy, 2% to 5% will die of respiratory complications and 3% to 5% will develop significant esophageal scarring that will require medical and surgical management.

Manifestations and Diagnostic Evaluation

Vomiting or spitting up after a meal, hiccuping, and recurrent otitis media related to pooled secretions in the nasopharynx during sleep are the hallmarks of all types of GER. In addition, the infant with pathologic GER can experience weight loss, failure to thrive, irritability, discomfort, and abdominal pain. Severe GER can result in hematemisis or melena and anemia. Frequently respiratory illness is associated

Text continued on page 1124

T A B L E 4 3 – 2

Developmental Gastrointestinal Defects

	Esophageal Atresia with Tracheoesophageal Fistula	Imperforate Anus	Gastroschisis	Omphalocele	Umbilical Hernia
Pathophysiology, etiology, and clinical manifestations	Esophageal development terminates before esophagus reaches the stomach, or an unnatural connection exists between the esophagus and the trachea. Most common defect is a blind upper esophageal pouch with a fistula between the distal trachea and the lower esophagus. Feeding causes regurgitation and coughing, constant drooling of saliva, and gastric distension from air passing from the trachea into the stomach. A history of maternal polyhydramnios is a significant prenatal clue. The diagnosis is confirmed if an NG tube cannot be passed 10 to 11 cm beyond the gum line, and by abdominal radiography.	Incomplete development or absence of the anus in its normal position in the perineum. Defect can be high (above the levator ani muscle) or low (below the levator ani muscle). Symptoms include failure to pass meconium stool, absence of anorectal canal, presence of an anal membrane, and external fistula to the perineum. Condition is diagnosed during the newborn examination with radiography, ultrasound, or CT used to determine the level of the lesion.	Embryonal weakness in abdominal wall causes herniation of gut on one side of umbilical cord during early development, most commonly on right side. Viscera are outside the abdominal cavity and are not covered with the sac.	Large herniation of gut into umbilical cord. Viscera are outside the abdominal cavity but inside translucent sac, covered with peritoneum and amniotic membrane.	Imperfect closure of umbilical ring allows gut to push outward at umbilicus during straining and crying. Viscera are inside the abdominal cavity and under the skin. The hernia is usually 1–3 cm and easily reduced.
Incidence	1 in 2,000–4,500 live births	1 in 500–5,000 live births	1 in 20,000 live births More common in males than females	1 in 5,000 to 10,000 live births	Most common in low-birth-weight and African-American infants

Associated anomalies	Cardiac, CNS, and other GI disorders Prematurity and low birth weight	Genitourinary, sacral, or additional GI anomalies	Malrotation of intestines Decreased abdominal capacity Atresia, stenosis rare Higher incidence of Meckel's diverticulum Other anomalies rare	Malrotation of intestines Decreased abdominal capacity Atresia, stenosis common Higher incidence of Meckel's diverticulum Cardiac, genitourinary, or chromosomal anomalies in one third to one half of cases Associated with Beckwith syndrome (hypoglycemia, macrosomia, macroglossia)	Commonly occurs in children with Down syndrome, hypothyroidism, Hurler syndrome
Morbidity and mortality	Prognosis depends on the type of defect.	Prognosis depends on the level of the lesion. Complete continence may be impossible.	Mortality is 10% to 15%.	Mortality is 20% to 30%. Common complications include sepsis and intestinal obstruction.	Minimal
Therapeutic management	An NG tube is placed immediately and aspirated frequently. A one-stage surgical repair is performed that entails repair ligation of the fistula and end-to-side anastomosis of atresia. A temporary gastrostomy may be needed for gastric decompression or stabilization.	Anal stenosis is treated with repeated dilation. All other defects require surgical intervention. High defects may require a colostomy and bowel pull-through procedure.	IV and NG tubes are placed immediately. Total parenteral nutrition is provided. Synthetic material (Silastic) is used to cover the gut in a sac (if the sac has ruptured or the omphalocele is large). If defect is large, the sac is suspended over the child's abdomen, and gravity is used to return the gut slowly to the abdominal cavity over 28 days or longer. The defect is closed surgically after all contents have been returned to the abdominal cavity. Even if the defect is small, immediate surgical repair may be done in several stages. If the condition is diagnosed prenatally, surgical delivery is recommended. Necrotic bowel may need to be removed surgically.		Most umbilical hernias disappear spontaneously by 1 year. No surgical repair is necessary unless the hernia causes symptoms, persists past age 5 years, becomes strangulated, or continues to grow.

Table continued on following page

TABLE 43–2

Developmental Gastrointestinal Defects Continued

	Esophageal Atresia with Tracheoesophageal Fistula	Imperforate Anus	Gastroschisis	Omphalocele	Umbilical Hernia
Nursing care	Assess respiratory status immediately after birth and any associated signs, such as excessive oral secretions, choking, and unexplained cyanosis after feeding. Measure abdominal girth to assess for distension, and monitor for signs of respiratory distress. Place infant in a radiant warmer and administer humidified oxygen. Elevate the infant to a 30-degree angle. Postoperative care involves supporting fluid balance, maintaining thermoregulation, relieving pain, monitoring for infection, and supporting bonding. The infant may have a chest tube initially.	Report any skin dimples or the presence of stool in the urine or vagina. Determine anal patency if meconium is not passed in the first 24 hours after birth. Assess for other GI or GU anomalies. Facilitate bonding. Provide appropriate postoperative care, including care of the colostomy (see Chapter 37).	Thermoregulation is critical because significant heat loss can occur through the exposed intestines. Use warmers, and monitor the child's temperature. Use sterile technique in dealing with the defect. Immediately cover with warm, moist, sterile gauze and wrap with plastic to keep moist. Minimize movement of the infant and handling of the intestines. Assess for circulatory compromise, obstruction, and sepsis: monitor temperature, pulses, capillary refill time, skin color, changes in respiratory patterns, and heart rate. Observe for respiratory distress secondary to high intra-abdominal pressure as the gut returns to the peritoneal cavity. Fluid-volume management is a crucial nursing responsibility: monitor intake and output and daily weights, assess fontanels, monitor electrolytes, and maintain IV line. Postoperatively, monitor and manage ileus, which commonly lasts for 24 weeks: maintain NG tube for decompression, monitor bowel sounds and stools, and measure abdominal girth. Maintain parenteral nutrition to sustain growth. Offer pacifier to meet sucking needs. Provide emotional support for parents as they deal with the loss of the "perfect child." Encourage parents to provide care as they are able, talk to and touch infant and hold the infant, when appropriate.		Binding is not effective in reducing or minimizing the bulge. Monitor for changes in size of hernia. Assess for changing bowel sounds and an irreducible mass, which may indicate strangulation.

Provide skin care at the stoma site if esophagostomy is performed (change gauze frequently, clean with half-strength peroxide daily, use skin barrier).

Initially elevate the gastrostomy tube to allow gastric contents to pass to small intestine and air to escape.

Provide a pacifier to stimulate sucking and swallowing reflexes when the infant tolerates oral secretions (see Chapter 37 for care of the child with a gastrostomy).

Teaching and home care

Teach parents the care of the esophagostomy and gastrostomy.

Demonstrate how to provide oral stimulation, to encourage sucking and swallowing.

Teach assessment criteria for recognizing skin or respiratory problems.

Teach parents colostomy care.

Demonstrate anal dilation (use only prescribed dilator, insert no more than 1 to 2 cm, and use a water-soluble lubricant).

Refer parents for counseling and support.

Provide guidance for toilet training.

Encourage parents to hold, cuddle, and bond with infants as soon as possible.

Provide developmental stimulation for long-term hospitalization.

Assist parents in dealing with feelings of guilt and disappointment.

Use pictures to help parents understand the defect.

Contact national support groups and community resources.

Teach parents signs of bowel obstruction: vomiting, pain, irritability, anorexia, and firm abdomen.

Provide follow-up from nutritional support personnel, as needed.

Teach parents signs of strangulation: vomiting, pain, and irreducible mass at umbilicus.

Contact physician immediately if strangulation is suspected.

PATHOPHYSIOLOGY
of Gastroesophageal Reflux

The lower esophageal sphincter (LES), a zone of tonically contracted smooth muscle surrounding the distal esophagus, is innervated by vagal nerves and receives signals from multiple organs. A defect in this neural control may result in a dysfunctional LES with periods of transitory spontaneous relaxation. These periods of relaxation allow gastric contents to reflux back into the esophagus.

In addition, the esophagus traverses both the abdominal and thoracic cavities, with the LES positioned strategically between the two. Most of the LES is abdominal. The greater the length of intra-abdominal esophagus, the more competent this valve becomes. Any condition that shortens the abdominal segment of the LES will increase the likelihood of reflux.

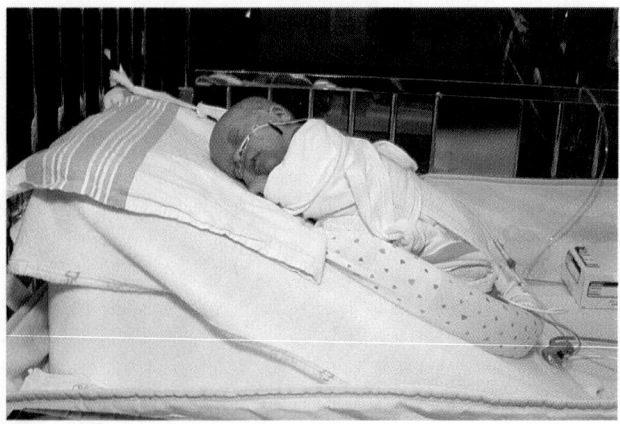

FIGURE 43–2

The infant having gastroesophageal reflux may be positioned prone on a wedge that provides a head-up tilt of 30 degrees. A harness around the torso keeps the baby positioned properly. This child also had liver failure, which caused increased intra-abdominal pressure and accounts for the jaundice.

with GER, and the child may experience coughing, choking, wheezing, pneumonia, apnea, or bradycardia.

A variety of chronic and acute illness have been associated with GER. It is necessary to confirm the presence of GER only after other major conditions have been ruled out. Diagnostic tests include barium swallow examination, upper GI study, fiberoptic endoscopy, esophageal manometry, ambulatory pH studies, and gastroesophageal scintigraphy (radionuclide scan).

Therapeutic Management

Therapy for GER is based on the severity of symptoms and includes dietary alterations, positional changes, medications, and surgery. Many infants suspected of functional GER are treated conservatively, without time-consuming and costly diagnostic testing.

DIET
Small, frequent feedings of predigested formulas such as Nutramigen or Pregestimil will reduce the amount of formula in the stomach, decrease distension, and minimize reflux. These smaller, more frequent feedings with frequent burping are often tried as the first line of treatment. Feedings thickened with rice cereal may reduce episodes of emesis but do not affect reflux time. In fact, thickened feedings actually may increase the risk of GER by delaying gastric emptying time. Concentrated formulas and nasogastric (NG) tube feedings provide nutritional supplementation for the child with failure to thrive. Caffeine and fatty foods lower LES pressure and should be eliminated.

POSITIONING
Much attention has been given to the best positioning for GER. A 30-degree head-elevated prone or right side-lying position (Fig. 43–2) generally results in fewer and shorter episodes of GER. A simple prone position may be equally effective, and infants with GER are excepted from the American Academy of Pediatrics's position statement on the prevention of SIDS (Orenstein, 1999).

MEDICATIONS
Although most medications used in the treatment of GER have not been approved by the Food and Drug Administration (FDA) for children, their use in children is quite common. Antacids for symptom relief, H_2-receptor antagonists (e.g., cimetidine, ranitidine) to decrease acid secretion, and prokinetic agents (e.g., cisapride) to accelerate gastric emptying may be used.

TREATMENT OF ACUTE BLEEDING
Bleeding is a complication of longstanding GER and esophagitis. Stomach lavage (washing) via an NG tube is commonly performed to evacuate blood and blood clots during an episode of upper GI bleeding. The use of iced saline lavage to stop bleeding is no longer advocated. Radiologic procedures or surgery to coagulate bleeding vessels may be needed.

SURGERY
Up to 15% of infants with GER will require fundoplication. A 270-degree to 360-degree wrap to the stomach fundus is made around the distal esophagus. This procedure tightens the LES and prevents gastric reflux. Gas bloat syndrome may develop because of the child's inability to burp, and a gastrostomy tube may be temporarily needed for gastric decompression.

NURSING CARE
The Infant with Gastroesophageal Reflux

Assessment

Nursing assessment begins with a thorough history, including the amount and frequency of feedings, changes in formula, and position during feedings. The frequency and pattern of emesis should be recorded, including documentation of whether it is projectile, painful, or contains blood. A medical history of frequent respiratory problems or pneumonia, apnea, choking, or cyanosis should be gathered. Observing the child during a feeding can provide critical information about choking, gagging, coughing, color change, and comfort during feeding.

Plot the child's length, weight, and head circumference on a growth chart. Assess the infant for *Sandifer movements*, unusual postural habits that may be observed in infants with severe reflux-induced esophagitis. These typically irritable infants may demonstrate head-cocking, arching, and arm thrashing. Drawing the head to one side may relieve pain by keeping gastric secretions from entering the esophagus or mouth. If a history of respiratory symptoms is present, assess the infant for abnormal breath sounds or retractions.

Assessment of the family should not be overlooked. Assessment should include observations of parent-child interactions and feeding styles and a discussion of feelings and concerns about the child who vomits frequently, is difficult to feed, and may have failure to thrive.

Nursing Diagnosis and Planning

The following nursing diagnoses and expected outcomes are appropriate following assessment of the child with GER:

- Risk for Aspiration related to GER.
  Expected Outcome: The infant will maintain a patent airway, without signs of aspiration or respiratory distress.
- Fluid Volume Deficit related to vomiting.
  Expected Outcome: The infant will retain feedings, with regurgitation of less than 10 ml.
- Altered Nutrition: Less Than Body Requirements related to anorexia, vomiting, and dysphagia.
  Expected Outcome: The infant will maintain and gain weight according to growth charts.
- Pain related to esophagitis.
  Expected Outcome: The infant will remain free from the discomfort of esophageal irritation.
- Impaired Swallowing related to esophagitis.
  Expected Outcome: The infant will swallow effectively without choking, coughing, or cyanosis.
- Risk for Infection related to surgical repair.
  Expected Outcome: The infant will have a surgical site that is clean, dry, and free from redness or exudate.
- Knowledge Deficit related to unfamiliarity with the disease process and home care.
  Expected Outcome: The parents will learn infant cardiopulmonary resuscitation (CPR) and will explain GER and the reasons for diagnostic tests, medications, dietary changes, or surgery.
- Impaired Home Maintenance Management related to complex, long-term care.
  Expected Outcome: The parents will demonstrate effective coping mechanisms for dealing with the long-term consequences of GER.

Interventions

Nursing care requires a thorough understanding of therapeutic management as well as postoperative care. It involves dietary modifications, positioning, medication administration, respiratory support, and perioperative care.

Dietary Modifications

Formulas and feeding routines are frequently changed to promote optimal gastric emptying. Parents need to understand the reasons for these changes and may need assistance with developing new feeding techniques or schedules. If thickened formula or thickened breast milk is used, 1 to 3 teaspoons of rice cereal per ounce is most common and may require cross-cutting the nipple. Thickened feedings are only for infants who are not on solid foods. Toddlers are fed their solids first, followed by liquids. Chocolate and caffeine should be eliminated from the diets of older children. Be prepared to offer alternative treats.

Positioning

Proper positioning is one of the mainstays of reflux management. The prone position is appropriate for infants, and this position is maintained until the infant remains asymptomatic for 6 weeks. The use of slings, harnesses, achalasia boards, wedges, and towel rolls is essential for infants who require head elevation. These items are available for home use in a variety of sizes. To decrease the risk of aspiration, avoid excessive handling of the infant immediately after feeding.

Older infants and children with GER achieve better results in an upright position (standing or sitting) while awake. The prone position is advised for sleeping.

Pacifiers can be used to decrease crying, which can increase reflux episodes. Pacifiers can also increase clearance of refluxed stomach contents.

Providing developmental stimulation is essential for the child who may have more limited mobility. Mobiles, activity boxes, mirrors, and musical toys can be useful. Moving the child's crib into areas of activity can also enhance stimulation.

Medications

The nurse administers GER medications as ordered but must be aware of the many drug interactions and side effects associated with the sometimes complicated and long-term regimen. Medications must be scheduled around mealtimes. Determine the child's feeding schedule and assist family members in adjusting their schedule, if necessary.

Respiratory Support

The varying respiratory alterations associated with GER present many challenges. Parents of infants with GER may feel overwhelmed by doubt and anxiety over their ability to adequately care for their child. Repeated instructions, written materials, home health nurse visits, emotional support, and support groups can be very important.

Infants experiencing apnea, bradycardia, or color change will need continuous cardiac and apnea monitoring. This monitoring requires extensive parental training and follow-up. The ability of *all* caretakers to perform infant CPR must be determined. Offer training where it is needed.

Surgical Care

Because surgery is considered the last resort in the treatment of GER, sufficient preoperative preparation time is available to answer questions and prepare the parent for intravenous (IV) lines, NG tube, and possible gastrostomy. Frequently, a gastrostomy tube will be placed at the time of fundoplication. This provides relief from gastric distension and provides a mechanism for enteral tube feedings. The child's ability to burp or vomit will eventually return after a fundoplication. Discuss postoperative problems of retching and difficulty in swallowing with the parents. In addition, parents need to understand that dumping syndrome may develop. Dumping syndrome begins within 30 minutes after a feeding and may include diaphoresis, palpitations, weakness, syncope, abdominal fullness, nausea, or diarrhea. The condition improves with age.

Home Care

Supporting the parents and teaching modifications in positioning and diet and medication administration are essential nursing interventions. Because the plan of care is usually continued for at least 6 weeks after symptoms improve, continued follow-up and support by a nurse are of paramount importance. Be prepared to teach diet, positioning, medications, and respiratory support by demonstrating specific techniques, providing appropriate equipment, and providing written schedules and information.

Evaluation

- Is the child's airway patent, without choking, coughing, cyanosis, or retractions?
- Is the child growing according to the growth chart?
- Can the child retain feedings with regurgitations of less than 10 ml? Is the child able to swallow appropriately?
- Is the child receiving medications as prescribed at the correct times and in the correct dosages?
- Is the child content and comfortable during feedings?
- Have the parents and all caregivers demonstrated infant CPR?
- Can the parents explain GER and the reasons for positioning and dietary modifications?
- Can parents verbalize side effects that require physician notification?
- Can the parents explain the need for a surgical procedure?
- Do the parents demonstrate appropriate care of the NG tube and is the incision site free of redness and signs of infection?
- Have the parents assumed all care responsibilities?

Constipation and Encopresis

Constipation is the infrequent and difficult passage of dry, hard stools. A major concern with constipation is the development of encopresis, or fecal incontinence. With encopresis, children often complain that soiling is involuntary and occurs without warning. Parents find the situation frustrating, and soiling often becomes a major issue between parent and child (Seth & Heyman, 1994). Often encopresis causes children to feel ashamed or embarrassed, and they may avoid situations in which embarrassment might be heightened, such as spending the night with a friend or even going to school. If the condition persists over a long period, it usually affects the child's self-esteem and may impair social relations. Often, the parents experience guilt and shame or revulsion, disgust, or anger, and they may project these feelings onto the child.

PATHOPHYSIOLOGY
of Constipation and Encopresis

When stool passes into the rectum, distension of the walls stimulates mass peristaltic movements in the bowel. This process is called the defecation reflex. If defecation is not desired, the external sphincter contracts, and voluntary retention of stool occurs. As the stool remains in the rectum, the rectum relaxes and the defecation reflex wanes. Water reabsorption from the colon continues, resulting in hard, dry stool that is difficult to pass. The eventual passage of that stool may result in pain or anal fissures. If retention of stool continues, more fissures may develop or become worse, so that eventually even soft stool may produce pain. A cycle of pain develops whereby the stool is retained to avoid pain but the retention leads to even more difficult defecation. Over time, the rectum becomes enlarged. An enlarged rectum can result in failure to control the external sphincter, which in turn results in encopresis.

Etiology and Incidence

Constipation can have many causes, such as changes in diet, dehydration, lack of exercise, emotional stress, certain drugs, pain from anal fissure, or excessive milk intake. If the child has no neurologic or anatomic disorders, encopresis is usually the result of recurrent fecal impaction and an enlarged rectum caused by chronic constipation. Factors predisposing to encopresis include inadequate or inconsistent toilet training or some type of psychological stress, such as starting school or the birth of a sibling.

Constipation can affect any child at any time. Encopresis generally affects the 3- to 7-year-olds (Abi-Hanna & Lake, 1998). Three to six times more boys than girls are affected. The incidence of encopresis is higher in lower socioeconomic classes and among children with learning disabilities.

Manifestations

CONSTIPATION

The principal symptoms of constipation are absence of stool, abdominal pain and cramping without distension, and palpable, movable fecal masses with large amounts of stool in an enlarged rectum. The child may also experience diarrheal overflow; normal or decreased bowel sounds; malaise, anorexia, and headache; nausea and vomiting; or anal fissure.

ENCOPRESIS

Children with encopresis have evidence of soiling clothing and fecal odor without apparent awareness. Anal irritation leads to scratching or rubbing of the anal area. Social withdrawal and avoidance of extended contact with others (such as overnight stays or camp) is common. Children with constipation or encopresis often have a higher incidence of urinary tract infections and urinary incontinence than those without encopresis (Loening-Baucke, 1997).

Diagnostic Evaluation

Abdominal radiographs may demonstrate an enlarged rectum with large amounts of stool and gas. The definitive diagnostic procedure is a rectal examination. This is rarely performed because of its emotional impact on the child and the possibility of pain from anal fissure. A thorough history is usually sufficient for the diagnosis.

Therapeutic Management

The best form of treatment is preventing development of the chronic problem through appropriate diet, exercise, and regular toileting habits. Education about "normal" bowel function can prevent a psychogenic component from compounding the problem. The focus of management is to remove the impaction, retrain the rectum to be aware of when it is full, and help the child overcome the pain-retention cycle.

Treatment usually involves three phases:

1. Disimpaction
   - Enemas until impaction is cleared
   - Stool softener or laxative
2. Maintenance
   - Mineral oil, 2 ml/kg b.i.d., up to 180 to 240 ml/day (not in infants); the dosage is adjusted depending on results achieved
   - Dietary changes, including limiting milk intake, increasing water intake, and increasing residue
3. Changing the retention habit
   - Sitting on the commode for 5 to 10 minutes approximately 20 to 30 minutes after meals
   - Keeping a behavioral chart with positive rewards (daily stars may be helpful)

The goal is for the child to pass two to three soft stools per day without pain within the first month. Medications are weaned slowly over 3 to 6 months after the fear of pain has been lost.

For infant constipation, rectal stimulation is discouraged. For example, rectal thermometers and glycerine suppositories should not be used. Barley cereal can be substituted for rice cereal. Fructose such as prune juice or lactulose can help. High-fiber vegetables will also improve constipation (Staiano & Tozzi, 1998).

NURSING CARE

The Child with Constipation or Encopresis

Assessment

Obtain a thorough history of the soiling events, including frequency, intensity, and duration. Because parent-child relationships are often strained, it is often helpful to interview the parents and child separately to reduce the child's embarrassment. The nurse can explain to parents that a medical history and examination will be performed to rule out organic causes of the chronic constipation such as Hirschsprung disease.

Nursing Diagnosis and Planning

The following nursing diagnoses and expected outcomes may be appropriate after assessing for constipation or encopresis in the child:

- Constipation or Bowel Incontinence related to inconsistent patterns of elimination, anxiety, or pain during elimination.
  Expected Outcome: The child will have normal bowel function, as evidenced by the passage of soft stools without pain or incontinence.
- Ineffective Family Coping related to persistent stress, guilt, and embarrassment about the child's elimination difficulty.
  Expected Outcomes: The family will function effectively as a unit, openly discuss problems, and develop a plan to achieve control over incontinence.
- Social Isolation related to embarrassment, peer teasing, and odor from bowel incontinence.
  Expected Outcomes: The child will verbalize positive, realistic feelings about self and verbalize appropriate ways to achieve control over bowel incontinence.
- Impaired Skin Integrity related to poor hygiene in anal area, bowel incontinence, and lack of knowledge.
  Expected Outcome: The child will maintain skin integrity, as evidenced by clean, intact skin.

Interventions

Because constipation and encopresis represent a continuum of the same problem, a variety of approaches can be tried as needed to deal with the problem. Simple constipation may resolve with only dietary changes or changing a habit of retention. Severe encopresis may require that all interventions be continued for 3 to 6 months.

Overcoming Withholding

Before bowel retraining can begin, the child's bowel must be evacuated of all hard stool and impactions. This goal is best accomplished with the use of appropriate-size Fleet or isotonic enemas every 12 hours until the impaction is cleared, usually within 48 hours. Teach parents to administer enemas at home. During this time, the child should be monitored for hypernatremia or hyperphosphatemia, which could result from repeated use of Fleet enemas (see Chapter 37 for a discussion of enema administration).

After bowel cleansing has been achieved, the child is started on mineral oil (Staiano & Tozzi, 1998). Mineral oil is best tolerated when it is given chilled or mixed with cold drinks. Mixing the oil with ice cream or chocolate milk, blending it with ice cubes and fruit juice, or chilling it help to disguise the taste. It is not unusual for the child to leak oil when dosages are high, and parents and children need to be aware that leakage does not constitute encopresis. At the end of this intervention, the child should be passing soft stool without pain or incontinence.

Dietary Changes

Dietary modifications are used as a part of the treatment. Increasing water and fiber intake by offering granola bars, dried fruits, whole-grain cereals, and fresh vegetables with low-fat dip can increase the bulk in stool and make it easier to pass. Decreasing sugar and milk intake will also help keep stools soft. Advise supplementing with fat-soluble vitamins when mineral oil is being used because the oil can theoretically interfere with vitamin absorption in the small intestine.

Changing the Retention Habit

To help reestablish a normal bowel habit, the child should sit on the toilet for 5 to 10 minutes after breakfast and dinner. This routine will allow the normal gastrocolic reflex to assist with defecation and will eliminate the need to be involved with retraining during school hours. Star charts and small prizes may be helpful in rewarding success. These interventions are continued for at least 3 to 6 months, during which the rectum will resume its normal size and the child will relearn to attend to the defecation reflex. If fecal impaction occurs at any time, enemas are again administered and the dosage of mineral oil is adjusted.

Emotional Support

Allow the child and parents to express their feelings of success and failure with the ongoing program. To minimize the damage to the child's self-esteem, encourage self-care as much as possible. To decrease embarrassment, it is helpful for school-age children to have a complete change of pants and underwear at school, should leakage or an accident occur. Age-appropriate support groups may be available in a center with a large population or encopresis clinic.

> Teaching is a major intervention. Encouraging the child and parents to share feelings of embarrassment is equally important. Allow the child to verbalize any concerns and provide developmentally appropriate anatomic information to assist with understanding the etiology of the problem. Using drawings and books may be an effective way to begin this sharing of feelings and information. Relieving the child of shame and embarrassment may improve cooperation with the plan of care.

Home Care

Because this condition is managed at home, teaching parents is the critical intervention. The parents need to understand the correct way to administer enemas (see Chapter 37). They also need support in implementing and documenting the child's successes and setbacks. The child and parents need encouragement to continue, even when the successes seem few. This problem develops over time and takes time, patience, and perseverance to resolve.

Evaluation

- Is the child passing soft stools without pain?
- Does the food diary indicate a well-balanced, high-fiber diet?
- Is the child experiencing any incontinence?
- Are mineral oil, enemas, or laxatives still needed?
- Are fat-soluble vitamin supplements taken during first phase of treatment?
- Is the child experiencing success with bowel control as a result of implementation of a family-designed plan?
- Does the child more readily participate in age-appropriate activities?
- Is the skin in the anal area clean and intact?

Irritable Bowel Syndrome

Irritable bowel syndrome is the result of increased intestinal motility, which can lead to spasm and pain.

Etiology and Incidence

Stress and emotional factors are thought to be the most common cause of this disorder. Theoretically, an abnormality in the autonomic nervous system accounts for the changes in motility and secretion, but this hypothesis has not been adequately proven (Carlson, 1998). In infants, it may be related to a lactase deficiency. It is not associated with any psychopathology.

Irritable bowel syndrome occurs after infancy and is most common in toddlers (in whom it is sometimes called chronic nonspecific diarrhea of childhood) and adolescents. The condition tends to occur in families with a history of other bowel disturbances or infantile colic (Boyle, 1996). The condition tends to resolve by late adolescence but is sometimes present in adults.

Manifestations and Diagnostic Evaluation

Manifestations of irritable bowel syndrome include diffuse abdominal pain unrelated to meals or activity; alternating constipation and diarrhea, with undigested food and mucus present in the stool; and normal growth.

The diagnosis is based on the elimination of major GI pathology, including Crohn's disease, giardiasis, lactose intolerance, and genitourinary abnormalities. Abdominal ultrasound, stool cultures, abdominal radiography, and a complete gynecologic assessment are often ordered.

Therapeutic Management and Nursing Considerations

There is no definitive treatment for this poorly understood functional bowel problem. Management is aimed at decreasing symptoms. The primary nursing intervention should be reassurance that it is a self-limiting, intermittent problem. Unless lactose intolerance is suspected, no dietary modifications are required other than the maintenance of a healthy, well-balanced, moderate-fiber diet. Encourage the child to eat slowly and not to drink carbonated beverages.

Family and psychosocial assessment may reveal a family

> **PATHOPHYSIOLOGY**
> • • • • • • • • • •
> ### of Irritable Bowel Syndrome
>
> The precipitating factors in irritable bowel syndrome are unknown but result in two distinct problems. The first is disorganized contractility, which causes spasmodic peristaltic rushes and lulls. This disorganization causes alternating diarrhea and constipation with intermittent abdominal pain. The second component is excess mucous production in the lumen of the bowel. This produces maldigestion and the passage of incompletely digested food and nutrients.

that is worried about a serious life-threatening disease and is very focused on the bowel habits of the child. The family may not be reassured by the normal findings on a physical and developmental examination.

The primary nursing interventions are teaching and reassurance. Health promotion activities such as exercise, balanced nutrition, and school activities have the best influence on the disease. Because of the associated psychosocial component, referral to mental health and family counseling services can be effective in cases that are unresponsive to other measures. The child and family will express feelings and concerns that will assist in evaluating the interventions.

Ulcers

A peptic ulcer is an area of sharply circumscribed loss of the mucosa, submucosa, or muscular tissue occurring in areas of the digestive tract exposed to acid and pepsin. Peptic ulcers can be either primary or secondary, gastric or duodenal. Primary, or idiopathic, ulcers occur in the absence of underlying systemic disease. Secondary, or stress, ulcers are acute and are found in conjunction with other illnesses such as shock, respiratory failure, sepsis, hypoglycemia, severe burns, or intracranial lesions.

Gastric ulcers occur in the stomach, particularly the gastric antrum, and are uncommon in childhood. Duodenal ulcers occur in the pylorus or duodenum, are often chronic, frequently lead to complications, and are the most commonly encountered ulcers in children.

Etiology

Known factors that can alter the mucus-bicarbonate barrier in children include the following:

Bile salts—Bile breaks down the adherent mucous structure of the gastric-duodenal lining and exposes the mucosa to acid.

Lack of prostaglandins—Prostaglandins augment both the mucous gel lining and bicarbonate secretion. Deficiencies in mucosal prostaglandins may cause impairment of the mucus-bicarbonate barrier.

Genetic factors—Duodenal ulcers show a familial tendency. This, together with environmental factors, may predispose children to ulcer formation. An association between ulcer activity and type O blood has also been noted.

Bacteria—*Helicobacter pylori* is a gram-negative spiral bacterium that has been identified in the gastric antrum of children with duodenal ulcer. It infects most adults with ulcer disease and acts by weakening the gastric mucosal barrier and allowing acid and peptic digestion of the susceptible mucosa.

Psychological factors—The importance of psychological factors is questionable. They likely influence exacerbations or complications but not initial ulcer activity.

Stress—Stress accounts for at least 80% of secondary ulcers encountered during infancy and early childhood. They tend to be acute and occur in seriously ill children.

PATHOPHYSIOLOGY
of Ulcers

The stomach and duodenum are lined by a thick mucus-bicarbonate barrier, a layer of mucus that provides a buffer zone for acid neutralization. Stomach acids diffuse slowly through this layer toward the gastric wall but are encountered and neutralized by slowly diffusing bicarbonate ions liberated from surface epithelial cells. The establishment of a neutral pH at the gastric epithelial surface provides protection from the combined effects of acid and pepsin. Ulcers result when any imbalance in the process occurs and erosions develop on the surface of the gastric or duodenal mucosa.

Diet—Diet does not seem to influence the development of ulcer disease in children. Although certain foods may cause indigestion, no convincing data show that dietary factors cause, perpetuate, or reactivate ulcers, especially duodenal. Colas, teas, and chocolate do, however, increase acid secretions and may be contributing factors.

Medications—Many medications, such as aspirin, nonsteroidal anti-inflammatory agents, and indomethacin, as well as tobacco and alcohol, are known to adversely affect the gastroduodenal mucosa in adults but appear to have little importance in pediatric ulcer disease.

Incidence

The true incidence of peptic ulcer disease in children is unknown because ulcers often spontaneously heal before a diagnosis is made. The average age for ulcer activity is 11 to 12 years, with boys affected two to three times more than girls. Duodenal ulcers occur more frequently in children over age 6. Children under age 6 frequently develop gastric ulceration. Stress ulcers account for 80% of ulcers occurring during infancy and early childhood, affect both sexes, and are equally distributed between the stomach and duodenum.

Manifestations and Diagnostic Evaluation

Manifestations of ulcer disease in children are burning, cramping pain when the stomach is empty; awakening during the night or early morning complaining of abdominal discomfort; and vomiting in children under age 6 years. Hematemesis and melena are common in infants and young children.

Fiberoptic upper endoscopy is the diagnostic tool of choice for all children, including neonates. Endoscopy not only provides direct visual observation of the lining of the esophagus, stomach, and proximal duodenum, it also is a means for obtaining biopsy or culture material. Ultrasound may be performed to rule out gallstones, tumors, or mechanical obstruction. The fecal occult blood test may be done to check for GI bleeding.

Therapeutic Management

Medical management is the most common treatment for ulcer disease in children. Factors considered in ulcer treatment include drug safety, symptom relief, patient and parent compliance, and the prevention of complications or ulcer recurrence. A bland diet with milk and small, frequent feedings was long thought to be the mainstay of ulcer therapy. It has been shown, however, that the protein and calcium in milk actually stimulate more acid secretions than they buffer. A regular diet low in caffeine is now generally prescribed because caffeine is a potent stimulant of acid secretion and exacerbates GER. A diet high in fiber and polyunsaturated oils may also play a role in ulcer prevention (Andrews, 1994).

Medications are now considered the first line of treatment. They include antacids, H_2-receptor antagonists, mucosa-protective agents, and prokinetic agents.

Surgery is indicated for the management of ulcer complications such as hemorrhage, perforation, or obstruction. Vagotomy, pyloroplasty, ligation of a bleeding vessel, or closure of a perforation may be performed.

If the child is actively bleeding, an NG tube is inserted to remove blood, decompress the stomach, and estimate blood loss. Intravenous fluids, oxygen, blood replacement, and vasoactive drugs like Pitressin (vasopressin) may be given. Balloon tamponade with a Sengstaken-Blakemore tube may be indicated. Blood or clots are removed with room temperature gastric lavage. The use of iced saline lavage to stop GI bleeding is no longer advocated because it increases bleeding and clotting times and prolongs the prothrombin time. It also imposes a risk of hypothermia on an already compromised child.

The long-term prognosis for children diagnosed with peptic ulcer disease remains controversial. Marked improvement in symptoms, however, is noted with the use of H_2-receptor blockers and other medications. Without adequate treatment, peptic ulcer disease frequently persists into adult life.

Nursing Considerations

Nursing assessment of the child with peptic ulcer disease begins with a thorough history, including a family history of ulcer disease, past episodes of abdominal pain, or recent stressful events in the home, school, or community. A complete assessment of pain includes a description of the nature of the pain and its location; its relationship to meals, defecation, or voiding; episodes of nocturnal pain; and medications used to effectively relieve the pain. The child is examined for the presence of epigastric tenderness, nausea, vomiting, abdominal distension, hematemesis, melena, or recent changes in appetite or eating habits.

All stools and emesis fluid should be checked for the presence of blood. Bowel sounds are auscultated for 5 minutes. If vomiting is present, the child is assessed for signs of dehydration. If bleeding is observed, the child is monitored for changes in vital signs, and the physician is notified immediately. Finally, the nurse assesses family members for their understanding of the disease, the presence of a viable support system, and their ability to participate in their child's care.

PROVIDING INFORMATION

The major focus of nursing interventions is teaching. The nurse reviews pathophysiology, medication administration, diet, and assessing for complications.

Preparing the child for diagnostic tests also is an important nursing intervention. Because fiberoptic endoscopy is often performed, the child must be prepared for conscious sedation. Keeping the child NPO for at least 6 hours, maintaining an IV line, and monitoring vital signs and respiratory function during the procedure are nursing responsibilities. Upper GI examinations and ultrasonography may also be performed.

HOME CARE

Ulcers are managed almost exclusively in the home environment, so teaching, follow-up, and home health referral are essential. The correct use of medications and dietary modifications are parental responsibilities that may require educational materials, emotional support, help with time organization, and encouragement to continue even when symptoms are relieved.

Infectious Gastroenteritis

Infectious gastroenteritis is caused by a group of viruses, bacteria, and parasites capable of causing serious communicable diarrhea, massive fluid and electrolyte loss, sepsis, and death (for further discussion of fluid and electrolyte alterations, see Chapter 42).

Etiology

Ingestion of contaminated food or water and person-to-person contamination are the most frequent causes of infectious gastroenteritis in the United States. High-risk groups include children in day care centers, preschools, and long-term care facilities and those infected with the human immunodeficiency virus (HIV). *Giardia* is the most common pathogen seen in children in day care settings, and rotavirus is the most common gastrointestinal pathogen seen in infants and young children (Cohen & Laney, 1999; Wald, 1999). In most cases the pathogen is not identified (Table 43–3).

Incidence

Gastroenteritis is one of the most common outpatient infectious diseases in children. In children under age 5 in the United States, over 20 million cases of diarrhea occur each year. Infections peak in the summer and have an equal sex distribution. Despite the usually self-limiting nature of the condition, each year approximately 300 to 400 children in the United States and greater than 4 million worldwide die from gastrointestinal illness (Cohen & Laney, 1999).

Manifestations

Gastroenteritis will likely manifest with diarrhea of varying amount and consistency, vomiting, and abdominal pain. In addition, the child might experience tenesmus and fever. Dehydration is a severe consequence of gastroenteritis and occurs mainly in children less than 2 years old. A history of travel to other regions of the world can provide clues to the causative organism.

Diagnostic Evaluation

A definitive diagnosis can be made when a rectal or stool culture yields a pathogen, but these cultures are expensive and result in many false negatives. Ova and parasites are more reliably found. Usually only children who appear toxic or have bloody stools, abdominal pain, or tenesmus undergo a diagnostic workup. The presence of white blood cells (WBCs) and blood in the stool can support the presumptive diagnosis based on clinical findings. Blood cultures may also be needed in the acutely ill infant and young child. An unprepared sigmoidoscopy can be useful in the diagnosis of the amount of mucosal involvement and in obtaining more reliable samples for culture, and may be useful in diagnosis.

Therapeutic Management

The priority therapy is to replace water and correct acid-base or fluid and electrolyte disturbances with IV fluids or oral (PO) electrolyte replacement liquids. The rate of replacement may be as high as 50 to 100 ml/kg over 4 to 6 hours (one to two-and-a-half times maintenance requirements). Because diarrheal fluid is high in sodium, potassium, and bicarbonate, oral rehydration solutions should be used to match losses. Hospitalization for treatment is not uncommon, especially in the infant or small child, to allow for continued assessment and management of symptoms or sepsis. Antimicrobial therapy is useful in cases of infection with *Shigella* and *Giardia*, and in some cases of infection with *Salmonella*, *Clostridium difficile*, and *Escherichia coli*, but not for rotavirus infection. Rotavirus immunization is available but is still undergoing study because of complications associated with the vaccine.

NURSING CARE
The Child with Infectious Gastroenteritis

Assessment

Obtain an adequate history of the event, including the length of symptoms, the frequency and consistency of stools, and the presence of blood or mucus in stools. Noting the amount, color, consistency, and time (ACCT) of each stool is a consistent way to document findings. The concurrent appearance of symptoms in other members of the family can be helpful in the diagnosis. Any travel to other countries or wilderness areas should be recorded. Evaluating formula and food preparation at home and in day care facilities as well as examining sanitation and hygiene in these places can provide valuable information.

The child may appear moderately to severely dehydrated with hyperactive bowel sounds and severe diarrhea, which is often bloody. Blood in the stool usually appears after the maximum fluid loss has occurred and can be useful in determining the stage of illness. The presence of abdominal pain, vomiting, tenesmus, and fever should be assessed. Headache, nuchal rigidity, irritability, and seizures are important symptoms of the neurotoxic effects of *Shigella*.

Assessment of hydration status is critical. Poor urine output, high urine specific gravity, poor skin turgor, dry mucous membranes, crying without producing tears, a sunken or depressed fontanel in infants, and skin tenting can occur quickly with the large amount of fluid lost through diarrhea. Loss of bicarbonate from severe diarrhea and dehydration make metabolic acidosis a major concern. The compensatory mechanisms of increased respiratory rate and effort are important to document.

TABLE 43-3

Characteristics of Infectious Diarrhea

Infectious Agent	Characteristics	Clinical Manifestations	Diagnostic Findings	Treatment
Shigella (enteroinvasive with cytotoxin)	Incubation period 1–7 days Most common in summer Fecal-oral spread Remains communicable for 1–3 weeks	Symptoms last 5–10 days Diarrhea begins as watery, progresses to small, bloody, with mucus Severe abdominal pain High fever Neurologic symptoms (headache, nuchal rigidity, convulsions) Risk for sepsis, hemolytic uremic syndrome, rectal prolapse, DIC	Blood, mucus, WBCs in stool Positive culture in some cases	Bactrim, 8–10 mg/kg/day × 5 days, OR Ampicillin, 50–100 mg/kg/day × 5 days Contact precautions Identify source if possible
Salmonella (enteroinvasive)	Incubation 6 hours to 3 days Most common in summer, fall Usually food-borne Infectious for duration of illness and variable period afterward	Symptoms last 2–5 days Rapid onset Secretory diarrhea Abdominal pain, nausea, vomiting common	Blood and polymorphonuclear leukocytes (PMNs) in stool	For infants younger than 12 weeks, same as for Shigella Contact precautions Identify source if possible
Escherichia coli (enteroinvasive with enterotoxin)	Variable incubation Most common in summer Food-borne most common	Green, watery, secretory diarrhea May cause hemorrhagic colitis Fever	Blood and PMNs in stool	Same as for Shigella Contact precautions
Campylobacter	Incubation 1–8 days Most common in infants and adolescents	History of consumption of contaminated shellfish Severe abdominal pain Foul-smelling, watery diarrhea	Blood and PMNs in stool	Possibly treated with erythromycin for 7 days Contact precautions
Giardia lamblia	Most common cause of parasitic diarrhea Spread in water	Afebrile Abdominal distension, flatulence Variable diarrhea	Ova and parasites found in stool, but no blood or PMNs Parasites found on duodenal biopsy	Metronidazole (Flagyl) for 7 days Contact precautions Treat all unknown water sources with chlorine/iodine before drinking.
Rotavirus	Incubation 1–3 days Common in winter months Accounts for 50% of cases of acute diarrhea in children	Symptoms usually last 2–6 days History of preceding or concurrent respiratory illness Fever for 24–48 hours	Virus in stool detected by enzyme immunoassay	No pharmacologic treatment Contact precautions Preventive immunization undergoing testing
Clostridium difficile	Antibiotic-associated Most common nosocomial diarrhea	Diarrhea develops after antibiotic treatment	Blood and PMNs in stool	Cholestyramine used to enhance mucosal recovery and decrease length of diarrhea Possibly treated with vancomycin or metronidazole (Flagyl) for 10 days

Nursing Diagnosis and Planning

The following nursing diagnoses and expected outcomes may be appropriate for the infant or child with gastroenteritis:

- Fluid Volume Deficit related to severe diarrhea.
  Expected Outcomes: The child will be adequately hydrated without electrolyte disturbance, as evidenced by moist mucous membranes, good skin turgor, return to normal weight, and normal serum sodium, potassium, and bicarbonate levels, and the child will have soft, formed stools without diarrhea, blood, or mucus.
- Risk for Infection related to exposure of family members and others to infectious agents.
  Expected Outcome: The child will not transmit pathogens to others.
- Pain related to abdominal cramping.
  Expected Outcome: The child will be free from abdominal pain, as evidenced by a return to normal activity and no complaints of pain.
- Knowledge Deficit related to inadequate information about the disease and its control.
  Expected Outcome: The parents will demonstrate an understanding of the communicability of the condition, as evidenced by the use of standard and contact precautions when handling the child's secretions.
- Altered Nutrition: Less Than Body Requirements related to malabsorption.
  Expected Outcomes: The child will resume a normal diet and will regain weight lost during the acute phase within 1 week after symptoms abate.
- Risk for Impaired Skin Integrity related to skin contact with feces and the necessity for frequent cleansing.
  Expected Outcome: The child will maintain skin integrity, as evidenced by clean, dry intact skin without redness, drainage, or breakdown.

Interventions

Maintaining Fluid Balance

Critical nursing interventions are related to the fluid volume deficit. Oral or parenteral rehydration with correction of acid-base imbalances is essential to establish homeostasis. Accurate intake and output and weight measurements are important. Monitoring skin turgor, urine output, and serum electrolyte levels will provide evaluation criteria in this area (see Chapter 42 for a further discussion of fluid and electrolyte alterations).

Decreasing Risk

Providing safety, assessing neurologic symptoms, and monitoring for seizures are also priorities for the child with *Shigella* infection. Preventing the spread of infection remains a critical nursing intervention. Thorough hand washing is a must. Contact precautions must be strictly enforced for all staff and family members to minimize the risk of infection. These precautions must be maintained at home for up to 2 weeks, fewer if antibiotics are given. Pain and fever may be treated with acetaminophen, but symptomatic treatment with antidiarrheals is not recommended because it tends to increase the length of symptoms. Symptomatic

---

PARENTS WANT TO KNOW

Care of the Child with Infectious Diarrhea

If your child has infectious diarrhea, you must do the following:

- Wash your hands frequently and thoroughly, and insist that your child do so as well. Always wash your hands after changing diapers.
- Allow your child to use a separate bathroom, if available.
- Administer oral fluids using appropriate rehydration solutions (e.g., Rehydralyte) in small, frequent amounts (every 30 minutes). If your child is vomiting, administer one teaspoon of fluid every 5 to 10 minutes.
- Continue to follow these measures for several weeks because bacterial diarrhea may be communicable for several weeks after symptoms disappear.
- When your child is ready to eat, avoid foods containing lactose (milk). Use special formulas (e.g., Isomil DF) and introduce milk products gradually.
- Keep day care providers aware of dietary changes and provide supervision in food or formula preparation as needed.

---

care of the febrile child includes tepid sponging and light dressing.

Parents and children will need to be taught these interventions and given information about the disease process during this period. Depending on the organism causing the gastroenteritis, follow-up by the Public Health Department may be necessary. Organisms like *Salmonella* and *E. coli* can be found in food and present a significant public health concern. A dietary recall for possibly contaminated foods can be important in establishing the cause and minimizing the risk of spread to the public.

Home Care

The most important intervention that can be implemented at home is proper rehydration to prevent the need for hospitalization and IV therapy (see Chapter 42 for a discussion of oral rehydration fluids and care for the child with diarrhea). After rehydration has been successful and symptoms have subsided, feeding should resume.

Clear liquids are recommended for 24 hours after symptoms have subsided. After that time, the normal diet can be resumed slowly. Isomil DF, a lactose-free formula with added fiber, is a good start for the formula-fed infant. Older children and toddlers can gradually resume a soft diet of easily digestible foods such as cereals, cooked vegetables, and lean meats. Infants and children with gastroenteritis may experience temporary lactose intolerance, so milk-based foods should be avoided.

Preventing the spread of infection is also essential for home care. Good hand washing, the disinfection of contaminated linens, clothes, and diapers, and the use of surface disinfectant sprays are important preventive measures.

Evaluation

- Has the child returned to pre-infection weight?
- Does the child have good skin turgor, moist mucous membranes, and a urine specific gravity of less than 1.025?
- Does the child have a serum sodium level of 139 to 145 mmol/L and a serum potassium level of 4.1 to 5.2 mmol/L?
- Is the child passing soft, formed stools without diarrhea, blood, or mucus?
- Can the child tolerate an age-appropriate regular diet and has the child begun to gain weight?
- Are other family members free from infectious diarrhea and is the family following the appropriate precautions to prevent transmission?
- Is the child complaining of abdominal pain?
- Does the child guard the abdomen during palpation?
- Is the day care facility practicing appropriate infection control procedures, if appropriate?
- Is the child's skin intact and free from irritated areas?

▌ *Appendicitis*

Appendicitis is the inflammation and infection of the vermiform appendix, a small lymphoid, tubular, blind sac at the end of the cecum. It is the most common cause of emergency surgery in children and adolescents.

Etiology and Incidence

Common causes of obstruction and subsequent appendicitis include lymphoid swelling related to viral infection, impacted fecal material, foreign bodies, and parasites. In most cases no definitive cause can be identified at the time of surgery.

Appendicitis occurs with equal frequency in both sexes, with most cases occurring during adolescence and early adulthood. Annually, approximately 80,000 children in the United States undergo surgery to remove the appendix (Mattei, Stevenson, & Ziegler, 1999). Appendicitis is uncommon under age 4, but in young children it is associ-

PATHOPHYSIOLOGY

of Appendicitis

Obstruction of the appendix allows normal mucous secretions to accumulate in the appendix, producing distension. Distension eventually causes occlusion of the capillaries and engorgement of the walls of the appendix. Microabscesses form and can progress to abscess and fistulas. Perforation occurs as a result of tissue breakdown and swelling. Bowel contents then contaminate the mesenteric bed and peritoneum, leading to peritonitis and sepsis.

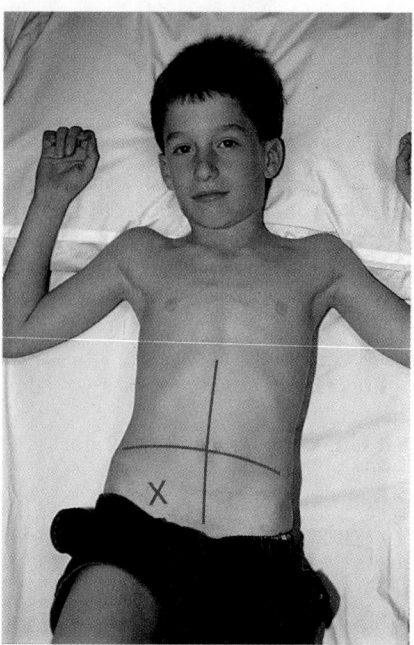

FIGURE 43–3

McBurney's point is midway between the right anterior superior iliac crest and the umbilicus. It is usually the location of greatest pain in the child with appendicitis. (Courtesy of The University of Texas at Arlington School of Nursing.)

ated with a very high frequency of perforation, most likely related to the difficulty in establishing the diagnosis.

Manifestations and Diagnostic Evaluation

The cardinal symptom of appendicitis is pain, progressing in intensity and localizing to the right lower quadrant at McBurney's point (Fig. 43–3). Associated signs and symptoms include nausea and vomiting, anorexia, diarrhea or constipation, and fever and chills. If the appendix perforates, the child will initially experience relief of pain. Other signs and symptoms will worsen, so that the child will appear acutely ill with high fever and signs of dehydration.

The diagnosis is usually based on the classic abdominal findings of pain at McBurney's point: guarding, rebound tenderness, nausea, vomiting, and fever. A WBC count of 15,000 to 20,000 cells/μl can support the clinical findings. A quick, safe, and accurate diagnosis can usually be made with ultrasound, which shows an enlarged, incompressible appendix that may be fluid-filled and locally inflamed. Computed tomography (CT) of the abdomen can increase the accuracy of the diagnosis (Rao, Rhea, Novelline, et al., 1998).

Therapeutic Management

The definitive treatment for appendicitis and suspected appendicitis is appendectomy. Preoperatively the child is managed with fluid therapy, immobilization to control pain, NPO status, and antibiotics. The procedure may be done laparoscopically or through an open abdominal approach if perforation is suspected.

Assessing Appendicitis in the Young Child

Because symptoms of appendicitis can be vague and can develop slowly over approximately a 12-hour period, the condition can be very difficult to assess in young children. The complaint that "my tummy hurts" often is the only initial complaint. Appendicitis should be suspected if pain, anorexia, or nausea and vomiting and fever occur simltaneously. The young child will usually refuse to play, preferring instead to lie down. Often, the child will lie in a knee-chest position to be comfortable. One way of helping the child describe the pain focus is to ask the child to stand on tiptoes and then drop to flat feet. The pain location elicited from this maneuver usually will be in the right lower quadrant.

NURSING CARE

The Child with Appendicitis

Assessment

The nursing assessment will reveal a history of vomiting, pain, fever, and diarrhea or constipation. The physical examination discloses abdominal tenderness and guarding. The child may assume a supine position with the right leg flexed to decrease tension on the abdominal wall. The nurse must be keenly aware of the symptoms of perforation, including a sudden relief from pain followed by an increase in pain, rigid abdomen, and early shock symptoms. Behavioral changes and refusal to eat are important indicators in infants.

Assess anxiety in the child and family members, who are most likely facing unexpected surgery. Because of the pain, the child may be uncooperative with abdominal assessment. The parents may have financial concerns related to the unplanned surgery.

Nursing Diagnosis and Planning

The following nursing diagnoses and expected outcomes may be appropriate after assessing the child with appendicitis:

- Pain related to abdominal inflammation and surgical incision.
  Expected Outcome: The child will be free from pain, as evidenced by resumption of normal activity and movement, with no complaints of pain.
- Risk for Infection related to rupture and surgery.
  Expected Outcomes: The child will have a clean, dry surgical incision that is free from redness, heat, or exudate and will be afebrile with a WBC count of 5,000 to 15,000 cells/μl.
- Fluid Volume Deficit related to vomiting or diarrhea.
  Expected Outcome: The child will be well hydrated, as evidenced by moist mucous membranes, good skin turgor, and urine output of at least 1 to 2 ml/kg/hr.

- Anxiety related to unplanned surgery.
  Expected Outcomes: The parent or child will express feelings about surgery and will verbalize the need for emergency hospitalization.

Interventions

Uncomplicated Appendicitis

On admission, vital signs should be taken to monitor for signs of sepsis or shock. Institute comfort measures, including topical cold application, pain medications, and encouraging positions of comfort. Enemas or laxatives should not be administered. No heat should be applied to the abdomen because it may increase the chance of perforation secondary to vasodilation. IV fluid therapy is started to prepare the child for surgery and correct any existing acid-base disturbance related to vomiting and diarrhea.

If the procedure is performed by laparoscopy, the nurse can expect the child to be discharged within 24 hours. Open surgery may be followed by several days of recovery in the hospital. After either operation, the child will be NPO until bowel function has returned.

Ruptured Appendix

The child with a ruptured appendix needs special care (Fig. 43–4). If perforation is suspected, prepare the child for NG tube insertion. The NG tube provides decompression prior to surgery and allows gastric content drainage postoperatively. The child will need IV antibiotics, which may be started preoperatively. For the child with a perforation, IV antibiotics are continued and hospitalization may last 5 to 14 days. During this time the diet should be advanced gradually as tolerated so that the child can tolerate a normal diet without vomiting or diarrhea.

Depending on the extent of the peritonitis, the child is likely to have postoperative incisional drains. These drains may be attached to suction, and aseptic technique and maintenance of patency are essential. Carefully document the drainage amount each shift. The wound is often left open and treated with sterile wet-to-dry (saline-soaked gauze) dressings and wound irrigation with antibacterial solutions.

Round-the-clock opioid analgesics provide relief from incisional pain and from pain caused by frequent dressing changes (see Chapter 39). Continued reassessment of abdominal pain is essential for evaluating the presence of abscess or fistula.

Monitor vital signs, including temperature, every 2 to 4 hours. NG suction will likely be continued postoperatively until normal bowel sounds return. Positioning the child to facilitate drainage and minimize the spread of infection into the upper abdomen should be done by elevating the head of the bed or having the child lie on the operative side.

Home Care

After surgery and discharge, parents must be prepared to assume responsibility for the child's care. The surgical incision and any drain sites must be assessed for redness, drainage, dehiscence, or suture infections. Report any problems to the physician. The diet should be advanced slowly. Parents should begin with liquids and soft foods and progress

APPENDECTOMY-PERFORATED
(Uncomplicated-without multi-system problems)
ICD-9 Codes 540.0 and 540.1

Expected LOS-5 Days
D#.#=Key interventions for this study.

Examples of appropriate Co-morbidities
Otitis Media
Acute Sinusitis
Pharyngitis
chronic illness not in active stage

Examples of Co-morbidities that are not appropriate:
HIV
Pneumonia
Sickle Cell
Hemophilia
Immuno-compromised patients
cardiac patients
reflux
oncology diagnoses

Refer to Variance Sheet for Recording

	Admission Day	Day 2	Day 3	Day 4	Day 5
Aspect of Care	Date___ Unit ___ ED/OR_____	Date___Unit ___	Date___Unit ___	Date___Unit ___	Date ___Unit ___
DAILY OUTCOME			Ambulating	NG tube out	Afebrile Discharge *(D 7.1 If not d/c by Day 7. record on tracking sheet)*
TESTS	CBC BUN, Cr Sonogram (if ind)	BUN,Cr		CBC (+/-)	CBC (+/-)
CONSULTS	Surgeon		Consider Home Health		
FLUID/ELECTROLYTE MANAGEMENT	Strict I&O	Strict I&O	Routine I&O	Routine I&O	Routine I&O
TREATMENTS/ PROCEDURES	Appendectomy NG Irrigation Wound Care	NG Irrigation Wound Care	NG Irrigation Wound Care	Wound Care	Wound Care
MEDICATIONS	IV (pump, site check) *D1.1 Gentamicin w/ Clindamycin q 8 hrs. +/-Ampicillin q 6 hrs +/- Mefoxin q 6 hrs. Methadone or morphine for pain.*	IV (pump, site check) *D2.1 Gentamicin w/ Clindamycin q 8 hrs. +/-Ampicillin q 6 hrs +/- Mefoxin q 6 hrs. Methadone or morphine for pain.*	IV (pump, site check) *D3.1 Gentamicin w/ Clindamycin q 8 hrs. +/-Ampicillin q 6 hrs +/- Mefoxin q 6 hrs. Methadone or morphine for pain.*	IV (pump, site check) *D4.1 Gentamicin w/ Clindamycin q 8 hrs. +/-Ampicillin q 6 hrs +/- Mefoxin q 6 hrs. Methadone or morphine for pain.*	Hep lock *D5.1 Gentamicin w/ Clindamycin q 8 hrs. +/-Ampicillin q 6 hrs +/- Mefoxin q 6 hrs. Methadone or morphine for pain Analgesics p.o. if tol.*
CLINICAL SUPPORT	NPO Parent Support Bed/Chair Extra Patient Checks Routine Safety	NPO Parent Support Chair Routine Safety	NPO Parent Support Ambulate Routine Safety	NPO/Cl liq (+/-) Parent Support Ambulate Routine Safety	Full liq/Regular Parent Support Ambulate Routine Safety Pain Control Wound Care Activity Follow-up Visit

Original 7/22/1994   Revised 11/2/1995 5/1/97

Disclaimer: This clinical pathway is provided as a general guideline for use by physicians and staff in planning the care and treatment of patients and their families. **It is not intended to be and does not establish a standard of care.** Each patient's care is individualized according to specific needs.

Cook Children's Medical Center
M:\WPFILES\PATHWAYS\APPYPERF.WPD

This pathway is not a permanent part of the patient's medical record.

FIGURE 43–4
. . . .
Clinical pathway for a child undergoing an appendectomy. (Courtesy of Cook Children's Medical Center, Fort Worth, Texas.)

to the child's normal diet if it can be tolerated without nausea or vomiting. Teach parents to watch for vomiting, abdominal pain, or distension as possible signs of bowel obstruction or peritoneal infection.

Evaluation

- Does the child complain of pain?
- Does the child demonstrate guarding on abdominal palpation?
- Has the child returned to normal activity level?
- Is surgical incision clean, dry, and free from redness, heat, purulent drainage, or dehiscence?
- Is the child afebrile, with a WBC count of 5,000 to 15,000 cells/μl?
- Is the child tolerating an age-appropriate regular diet without vomiting, diarrhea, or increased abdominal pain?
- Are the child and parents able to express relief from anxiety?

Inflammatory Bowel Disease

Inflammatory bowel disease is a chronic inflammatory condition of the small or large intestine. It includes two distinct conditions: ulcerative colitis and Crohn's disease. Ulcerative colitis affects only the colon and involves both the mucosal and submucosal layers of the intestine. Crohn's disease can occur anywhere in the GI tract, from the mouth to the anus, and is transmural, involving all layers of the intestine.

Etiology

The exact cause of inflammatory bowel disease is not known. Several triggers have been identified, including viral and other infectious agents, food allergies, vasculitis, increased intestinal permeability, immunologic dysfunction, and genetic factors. Increasing evidence demonstrates a connection between an individual with inflammatory bowel disease in a stressed state generating an immune response that affects the disease outcome (Anton, 1999).

Incidence, Manifestations, and Diagnostic Evaluation

The incidence, manifestations, and diagnostic evaluation for both ulcerative colitis and Crohn's disease are summarized in Table 43–4.

PATHOPHYSIOLOGY
• • • • • • • • • • •
of Inflammatory Bowel Disease

The triggering factor, whether viral, allergic, or immunologic, causes the bowel to "respond" as if to an injury and results in capillary vasoconstriction and histamine release within the bowel. The histamine has two effects on the bowel. The first is vasodilation, which results in swelling that can cause malabsorption by distorting the surface area of the villi. Swelling then produces cell death and ulceration, which can progress to the development of fissures, strictures, fistulas, adhesions, and bowel obstruction. The second effect of histamine release is increased capillary permeability, which results in increased fluid in the intestine and subsequent diarrhea. Crohn's disease affects all the layers of the bowel; ulcerative colitis affects the mucosa and submucosa only.

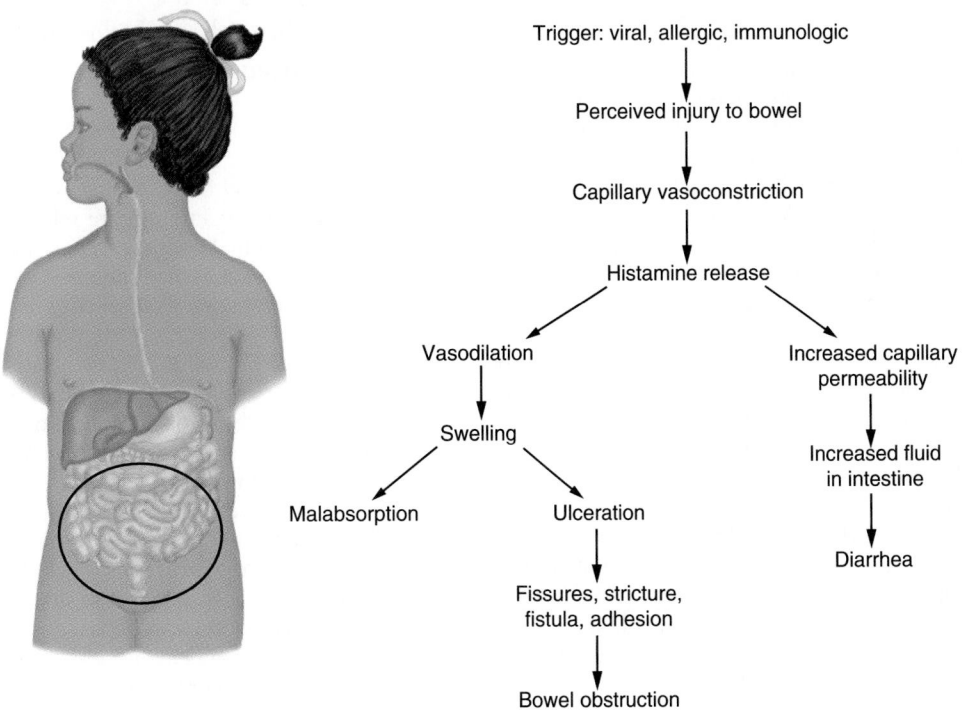

TABLE 43-4

Crohn's Disease and Ulcerative Colitis

	Crohn's Disease	Ulcerative Colitis
Pathophysiology	Affects entire GI tract	Involves only colon, starting at the rectum and moving upward
	Transmural involvement	Mucosa/submucosa only
	Cobblestone appearance of mucosa	Mucosa lacking in most cases
	Fistulas common	Fistulas rare
	Remissions and exacerbations	Remissions uncommon
Diagnostic evaluation:		
Colonoscopy	"Skip" lesions with deep fissures and	Continuous spreading with superficial
Rectoscopy	granulomas	ulceration
Barium enema	Normal	No normal mucous membrane
Incidence	5 per 100,000 and increasing	5 per 100,000
	Equal sex distribution	Equal sex distribution
	Not seen in infants; peaks in teens, early 20s	Peaks between ages 15 and 40 years
	Clusters in families	Clusters in families
	Associated with higher standard of living	Affects whites more than others
Clinical manifestations	Abdominal pain	Abdominal pain unusual
	Diarrhea, nonbloody	Diarrhea, occasionally with hemorrhage and anemia
	Fever	
	Palpable abdominal mass	No masses
	Anorexia and severe weight loss	Moderate weight loss
	Significant growth impairment	Mild growth impairment
	Perianal and anal lesions	Rare
	Fistulas and obstructions	Fistulas and obstructions rare
	Extraintestinal symptoms (arthralgia and arthritis)	Risk of toxic megacolon
Morbidity and mortality	Life expectancy not reduced	12%–15% mortality
	50%–70% will eventually require surgery for obstruction or fistula	10% chance of cancer after 10 years

Therapeutic Management

Management for inflammatory bowel disease is multidimensional and includes medication, dietary and nutritional support, and symptomatic treatment. Pharmacologic treatment includes anti-inflammatory, antibacterial, antibiotic, and immunosuppressive drugs. The principal medications used to treat inflammatory bowel disease include azathioprine (AZA), 6-mercaptopurine (6-MP), methotrexate, and cyclosporin A. AZA and 6-MP are first-line immunosuppressants that allow selected patients with Crohn's disease to avoid steroids and their side effects (Aranda & Horgan, 1998).

For ulcerative colitis, avoidance of milk products and ingestion of a low-fiber, low-residue, high-protein diet can be useful. Total parenteral nutrition (TPN) may be needed during acute flare-ups or surgery to maintain nutritional support. Total colectomy is the only true cure.

Crohn's disease is best managed before permanent structural changes have developed. Malnutrition is a common problem and can involve protein, fat, carbohydrate, and vitamin deficiencies. Nutritional support and teaching are essential. Surgery is not curative but may be necessary to treat abscesses, fistulas, or chronic recurrent obstruction. Bowel resection is the usual procedure.

NURSING CARE

The Child with an Inflammatory Bowel Disease

Assessment

Recurrent or chronic diarrhea is the primary finding in the nursing history of a child with inflammatory bowel disease. The major assessment findings are related to this diarrhea and the associated malabsorption that occurs. Weight loss, dehydration, anorexia, growth failure, vitamin deficiencies, and anemia are common. The severity of the GI symptoms and the amount and length of steroid use will have a significant influence on a child's growth rate. Remissions and exacerbations of symptoms are common. Frank bleeding is possible in ulcerative colitis. Intermittent cramping discomfort exacerbated by eating is common in Crohn's disease. The child with Crohn's disease may complain of oral lesions and perianal skin breakdown.

Inflammatory changes can also occur outside the GI system. Arthralgia and arthritis, especially of the lower extremities, can cause discomfort and mobility problems.

Depression, anxiety, fears about social interactions, and low self-esteem occur and are most likely related to the need to have quick access to restrooms at all times and to be close to home should an accident occur. The chronic nature of this condition and its unknown prognosis can lead to family stress and tax the family financial resources and family support systems. Assessment should include questions about family and peer support, resources, and knowledge about the disease.

Nursing Diagnosis and Planning

The following nursing diagnoses and expected outcomes may apply to the child with inflammatory bowel disease and to the child's family:

- Altered Nutrition: Less Than Body Requirements related to chronic malabsorption.
  Expected Outcomes: The child will have acceptable bowel patterns, as evidenced by passing no more than four stools a day and being free from nocturnal diarrhea, and the child will receive adequate nutrition, as evidenced by normal hemoglobin values and normal growth that follows the growth curve.
- Pain related to cramping.
  Expected Outcome: The child will be free from abdominal pain, as evidenced by resumption of normal activity and no complaints of pain.
- Self-Esteem Disturbance related to chronic diarrhea and colostomy.
  Expected Outcome: The child will have a positive self-concept, as evidenced by leading an active lifestyle without depression.
- Altered Growth and Development related to malnutrition, chronic illness, and steroid use.
  Expected Outcome: The child will meet normal developmental milestones, as evidenced by progress on standard developmental screenings.
- Body Image Disturbance related to weight loss and water retention from steroid therapy.
  Expected Outcome: The child will state reasons for changes in body appearance and will share concerns about changes with family and support personnel.

Interventions

Nursing interventions focus on maintaining pharmacologic interventions, developing long-term nutritional management, educating, and providing emotional support.

Medications

Teaching appropriate administration of medications is an important nursing role. Enemas are used before critical diagnostic tests and as a method of medication administration. Any child who will be taking steroids needs to understand the importance of regular administration. Steroids should be given with food or antacids if GI distress becomes a problem. The steroids, although beneficial in suppressing symptoms, may actually exacerbate the growth delays associated with inflammatory bowel disease.

Nutritional Management

Nutritional support varies with the disease and the child's tolerance of changes. In general, maintaining a low-fiber, low-residue, milk-free diet provides some relief, although strict restrictions do not alleviate symptoms. A balanced, nutritious diet is recommended, as are vitamin, iron, and folate supplements.

During acute flare-ups or surgery, TPN and lipids may be needed to restore a seriously malnourished child. These interventions do not change the course of the inflammation in the bowel but will provide essential nutritional support. Elemental diets, which can be absorbed without significant digestion, may be used during acute episodes of Crohn's disease to allow the bowel to rest. NG or gastrostomy tube feedings during the night may be necessary during puberty to prevent further growth impairment (see Chapter 37).

Continued assessment of nutritional status, growth patterns, and development are important elements of nursing care for children with this chronic problem. Assessing the number of stools, nutritional status, weight, developmental milestones, and pain will help in evaluating the child's response to treatment.

Family Education and Support

Education and support can be provided by appropriate community resources. The Crohn's Colitis Foundation of America will supply educational materials and give the child and family information on local resources and support groups (see Appendix L). Long-term nursing care can be improved by providing consistent caregivers and encouraging the child to form relationships. Self-care and management should be major goals in working with children with inflammatory bowel disease, as with other chronic diseases.

The parents and child will be assuming responsibility for home care. Because Crohn's disease is a long-term health problem with numerous medical, pharmacologic, and surgical interventions required, family support and financial resources can be strained to the limit. National and local support groups may be able to give essential support to the family in these areas. In addition, emotional support for caregivers becomes very important.

Home Care

Home care is a mainstay of treatment. Teaching parents to administer steroids, including providing information on their inherent side effects and the importance of not discontinuing their use abruptly, should be a high priority. Also teach techniques of enema administration and skin care for perianal lesions. Keeping nutrition diaries can provide useful information. TPN may be administered at home, and parents need complete instructions.

In addition, helping children and parents know when to seek care is important. Sudden exacerbations of symptoms, weight loss, blood loss, and severe abdominal pain should be reported to health care professionals. Stress management such as exercise may increase the quality of life and may help modulate the disease (Anton, 1999).

Evaluation

- Is the child free from nocturnal diarrhea?
- Is the child passing more than four stools per day?
- Do the child and family seek help when exacerbations occur?
- Is the child gaining weight appropriately and following the growth chart?
- Is the child's hemoglobin value between 11 and 16?

- Does the child complain of abdominal pain?
- Does the child participate in age-appropriate activities without evidence of depression?
- Has the child or family sought external support through appropriate referral groups?

▌ *Hypertrophic Pyloric Stenosis*

Pyloric stenosis results when the circular area of muscle surrounding the pylorus hypertrophies and obstructs gastric emptying. This condition is one of the most common surgical disorders of early infancy.

Etiology and Incidence

The exact cause of pyloric stenosis remains unknown, but muscular hypertrophy is not present at birth. Pyloric stenosis may be associated with other GI anomalies such as malrotation, short gut syndrome, esophageal and duodenal atresia, anorectal anomalies, hiatal hernia, and GER. Heredity and family predisposition seem to increase the risk of pyloric stenosis.

The incidence of pyloric stenosis is 3 in 1,000 births. First-born children and offspring of affected children are at highest risk. Males are affected five times more often than females, and full-term infants are affected more often than premature infants (Phillips, 1999). The incidence is also higher in white infants than in African-American or Asian infants.

Manifestations

Progressive projectile, nonbilious vomiting in a previously healthy infant is the major manifestation of pyloric stenosis.

PATHOPHYSIOLOGY
• • • • • • • • • • •

of Hypertrophic Pyloric Stenosis

Pyloric spasms cause milk curds to be propelled against a narrowed pyloric channel and subsequently irritate its sensitive mucosal lining. Edema of the pyloric mucosa results. This edema further reduces the size of the pyloric canal and creates resistance to the flow of milk. To promote gastric emptying and compensate for this resistance, the pylorus contracts with more force and gradually enlarges. This enlarged pyloric muscle slowly begins to constrict the pyloric channel, and when the mucosal edema subsides, the resistance to flow still remains. A vicious cycle develops and progresses to a high-level obstruction of the pyloric canal.

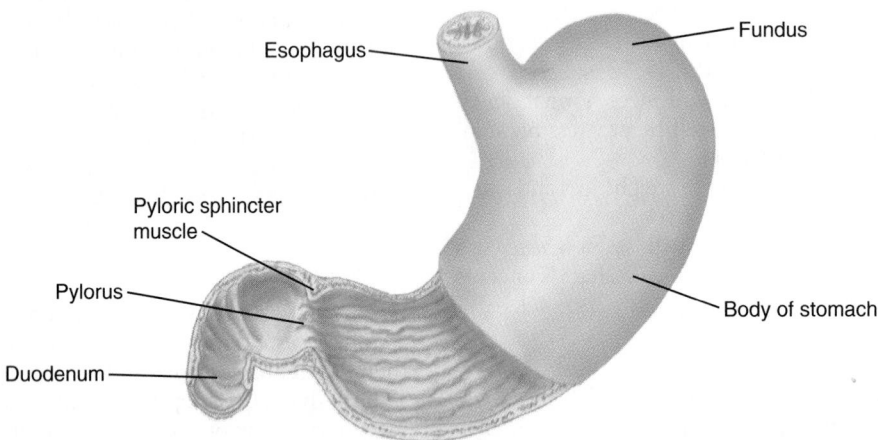

Normal pyloric opening

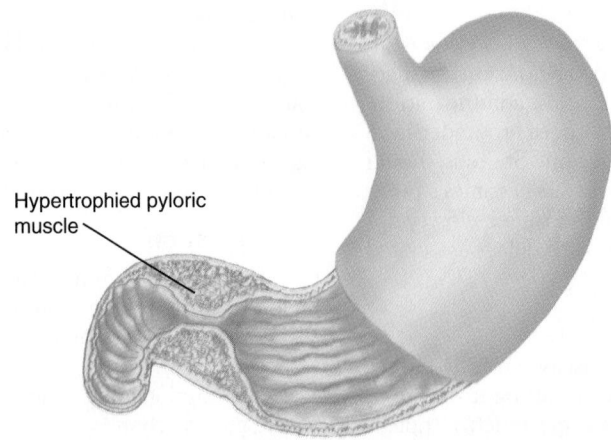

Pyloric stenosis

A movable, palpable, firm, olive-shaped mass is felt in the right upper quadrant. Deep gastric peristaltic waves from left upper quadrant to right upper quadrant may be visible immediately before vomiting. The infant will be irritable and hungry a short time after being fed. If the condition progresses, the infant may become dehydrated and experience metabolic alkalosis.

Diagnostic Evaluation

The diagnosis is based on a history of vomiting, visible peristaltic waves, and a palpable pyloric mass. When the mass cannot be palpated, radiography and ultrasonography are helpful. A flat plate of the abdomen will show a narrow pylorus with a dilated stomach and the absence of gas distal to the pylorus. Ultrasonography can confirm the presence of a pyloric mass. A barium swallow examination will disclose the long, narrow pyloric canal and detect delayed gastric emptying. Laboratory findings may indicate metabolic alkalosis due to vomiting, including decreased serum potassium and sodium levels, increased pH and bicarbonate, and a decreased chloride level. Indirect bilirubin may be elevated.

Therapeutic Management

Because pyloric stenosis is usually diagnosed early, few infants are seen in advanced stages of dehydration, malnutrition, and alkalosis. If present, these conditions must be corrected before surgery. An infant who is slightly dehydrated with a CO_2 of 25 mEq/L or less or an infant who is moderately dehydrated with a CO_2 of 26 to 35 mEq/L is managed with replacement parenteral fluids and electrolytes and an NG tube for stomach decompression. Once the stomach is empty, most infants will stop vomiting. Surgery is usually delayed 24 to 48 hours until fluid and electrolyte deficits and the acid-base balance are corrected. Severely dehydrated and malnourished infants with CO_2 levels above 35 mEq/L may need a 3- to 5-day course of IV fluids, electrolyte replacement, and infusions of plasma or packed red blood cells (RBCs) before surgical repair.

There is universal agreement that a *pyloromyotomy*, an incision of the pyloric muscle to release the obstruction, is the definitive treatment. Pyloromyotomy is not considered an emergency procedure but is usually performed without delay in well-hydrated infants.

NURSING CARE
The Child with Hypertrophic Pyloric Stenosis

Assessment

Hypertrophic pyloric stenosis is suspected in infants who present with a history of projectile vomiting, especially after meals. A thorough nursing history includes the infant's feeding schedule with the type, amount, and frequency of fluid taken. Determine and document the relationship of feedings to vomiting. Vomiting is assessed for frequency, amount, color, and consistency, as well as projection.

Assess for signs of dehydration, such as the absence of

CRITICAL TO REMEMBER

Gathering Information from a Parent About Infant Vomiting

Eliciting a description of the amount and characteristics of vomiting can be difficult as descriptive terms are nonspecific and estimation of amounts is very inconsistent. Useful questions might include

- Could you wipe the vomitus off the child with a diaper or rag?
- Did it require a change of clothes for the infant or caregiver?
- If it was on a bed or sheet, how big a circle did it make?
- If it was on the floor, how big a circle did it make?
- Did it happen after every feeding?
- Did it look like what was just eaten, or was it curdled?
- What color was it?
- Did it appear to be under force and projected away from the child?

Encouraging the parents to keep a written record of answers to these questions can provide essential assessment information.

---

tears, a weak cry, a depressed fontanel, poor skin turgor, and dry mucous membranes. Signs of potassium, sodium, and chloride depletion should be noted. The abdomen is checked for distension, tenderness, bowel sounds, the presence of a pyloric mass, or gastric peristaltic waves. Assess family members for their understanding of the disorder, a viable support system, and the ability to participate in their child's care.

Nursing Diagnosis and Planning

The following nursing diagnoses and expected outcomes are appropriate following assessment of the child with hypertrophic pyloric stenosis:

- Fluid Volume Deficit related to vomiting.
  Expected Outcome: The infant will have a balanced intake and output, be free of signs of dehydration, and have a urine output greater than 1 to 2 ml/kg/hr.
- Altered Nutrition: Less Than Body Requirements related to persistent vomiting.
  Expected Outcome: The infant will tolerate regular feedings, and continue to show growth according to a growth chart.
- Impaired Skin Integrity and Risk for Infection related to a surgical incision.
  Expected Outcome: The infant will have a clean, dry, intact incision without redness or exudate.
- Knowledge Deficit related to the need for surgery or pyloric stenosis.
  Expected Outcome: The parents will describe pyloric stenosis, verbalize an understanding of expected preoper-

Andrew, age 5 weeks, is seen in the outpatient clinic of a large hospital. This is his first visit to the clinic since birth. Andrew's mother states that Andrew is her first child, and that she has been concerned that Andrew "spits up" so much. She states she called the clinic about 2 weeks ago but the nurse told her that all babies spit up and that she could talk with someone when she came in for Andrew's 1-month check-up. She missed the appointment because she could not get a ride to the clinic. She further states that the "spitting up" has increased, and for the past 2 days she hasn't been sure whether Andrew was keeping any of his feedings in his stomach; also, he has been very fussy. After several unsuccessful attempts to speak to someone at the clinic by phone, she decided to bring Andrew in to be seen.

1. What will be your priority nursing action?
2. Identify two issues that you should address with Andrew's mother related to seeking care when health care information is needed.

ative and postoperative care, and assume total care of the infant before discharge.

Interventions

Preoperative Care

Preoperatively, the infant is NPO and is stabilized with IV fluids and electrolytes. Measuring the vital signs, weighing the infant daily, and monitoring laboratory values and intake and output are essential nursing interventions. Intake and output should include all IV and PO fluids, blood products, emesis, urine output, stools, and NG drainage. Keep the dehydrated infant warm and quiet. The nurse should provide oral care and skin massage with lotions and oils because skin and membranes are more susceptible to breakdown in their dehydrated state.

Elevate the head of the bed to reduce the risk of aspiration. The NG tube should be patent and properly positioned. Record the amount, color, and type of drainage. Assess for respiratory distress.

Postoperative Care

Postoperatively, the care varies with each surgeon. Most surgeons remove the NG tube immediately and order feedings within the first 4 to 6 hours after surgery if bowel sounds are normal. Because gastric peristalsis is normally depressed for 12 to 18 hours after the pyloromyotomy, others delay feedings for 24 hours and leave the NG tube in place.

Feeding is started with small amounts of an oral electrolyte solution, such as Pedialyte, and the amount is slowly increased. Formula is offered in half-strength concentrations and advanced to full strength within 48 hours after surgery. If the child is receiving breast milk, dilution is not necessary. Feedings are not advanced until the child can tolerate the previous amount without vomiting. IV fluids

are continued until the infant is taking and retaining sufficient amounts of formula. Many infants experience some vomiting during the early postoperative periods, but vomiting is usually temporary and without complications.

Postoperative nursing care follows the same guidelines as preoperative care, with accurate monitoring of all vital signs, laboratory values, respiratory problems, and hydration. In addition, the nurse assesses the small surgical incision for redness, swelling, or drainage. Encourage parents to participate as much as possible in their infant's care, but they may need emotional support in the unfamiliar environment of the hospital.

Home Care

Because symptoms normally abate in the immediate postoperative period, parents may find taking care of their infant much easier than it had been before repair. They need to be instructed, however, to report any excessive vomiting, abdominal tenderness, fever, incisional redness, or drainage. If the child is discharged before the diet has been advanced to full strength, written instructions for advancing the diet are essential.

Evaluation

- Are intake and output balanced?
- Does the child have a flat fontanel, good skin turgor, moist mucous membranes, a urine specific gravity of less than 1.025, and a sodium level within normal limits?
- Is the child tolerating oral feedings without vomiting?
- Has the child's weight returned to pre-illness level?
- Is the surgical site clean, dry, intact, and without drainage or redness?
- Can the parents explain need for surgery and routine preoperative and postoperative care?
- Have the parents assumed all care responsibilities?

Intussusception

Intussusception is an invagination of a section of the intestine into the distal bowel that results in bowel obstruction. In children, this condition most often occurs as a section of terminal ileum telescopes into the ascending colon through the ileocecal valve. It is the most common cause of bowel obstruction in children under age 2 years (West & Grosfeld, 1999). Although relatively rare, it does represent a pediatric emergency with classic assessment findings.

Etiology and Incidence

In young children, the cause of intussusception is unknown. Contributing factors include a preexisting upper respiratory tract infection or other viral infection. Pathology within the colon, such as a mass or anatomic defect is the most likely cause in children older than 6 years.

Intussusception generally affects infants and young children, with most cases occurring before age 2. This incidence is 1 to 4 per 1,000 births, but the condition is more common in children with celiac disease and cystic fibrosis (West & Grosfeld, 1999; Wyllie, 1996). The male-female ratio is 4:1. There is a risk of recurrence.

PATHOPHYSIOLOGY
of Intussusception

As the bowel telescopes inside itself, obstruction develops. In addition, the mesenteric vessels become trapped between the walls of the two layers, and ischemia occurs. This pressure on the bowel leads to bleeding and "currant jelly" stools. Mesenteric ischemia also causes edema and possible strangulation or infarction of the bowel, which can progress to perforation, peritonitis, sepsis, shock, and death.

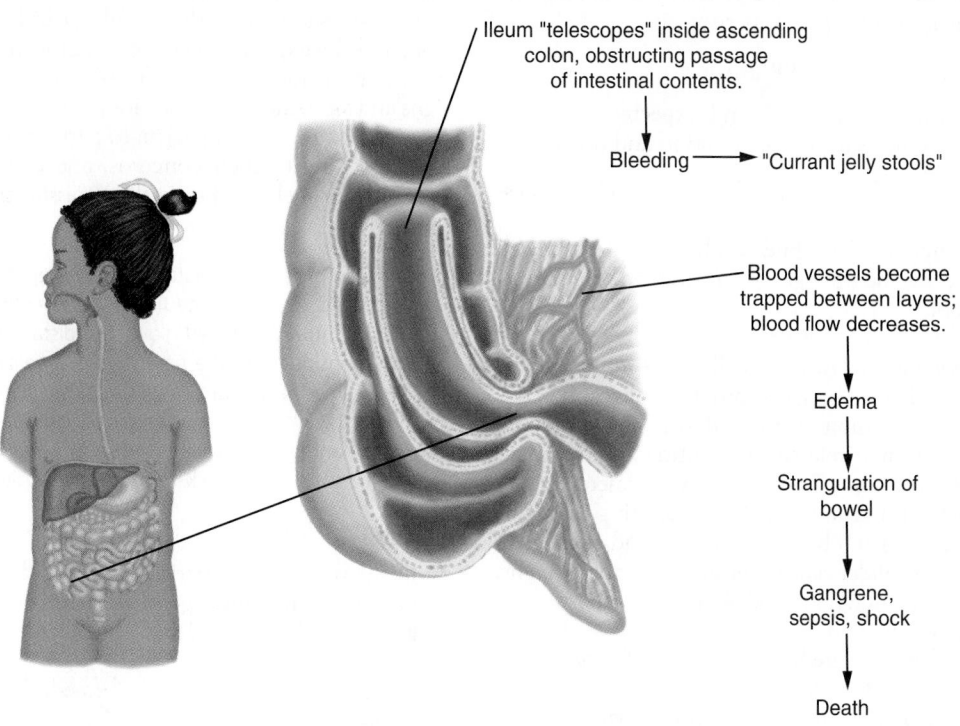

Ileum "telescopes" inside ascending colon, obstructing passage of intestinal contents.

Bleeding ⟶ "Currant jelly stools"

Blood vessels become trapped between layers; blood flow decreases.

Edema

Strangulation of bowel

Gangrene, sepsis, shock

Death

Manifestations and Diagnostic Evaluation

Intussusception occurs in children who are well nourished and without a history of GI problems. Paroxysms of pain occur, subside, and recur during the first several hours, then progress to a more constant severe pain. The child may vomit. The classic signs of intussusception are

- passage of bloody mucus ("currant jelly") stool and diarrhea, which may not occur until the postoperative period
- a sausage-shaped abdominal mass

Symptoms of shock and sepsis are present if obstruction has been present for longer than 12 to 24 hours. The child may be listless. Older children may present with pain without other symptoms.

Abdominal radiographs may show abnormal gas patterns related to the bowel obstruction or a soft tissue mass. Ultrasonography is useful in identifying the location of the intussusception and the amount of edema in the area. A definitive diagnosis can be made and treatment provided simultaneously with a barium enema or air enema examination.

Therapeutic Management

The goal of treatment is to restore the bowel to its normal position and function as quickly as possible. In children who do not show symptoms of shock or sepsis, attempts at hydrostatic reduction are made with a barium or air enema until free flow of barium into the terminal ileum is evident. This procedure can be done in approximately 80% of cases. If reduction fails or findings indicate damage to the bowel, immediate surgery is performed. If the intussusception is detected and reduced within 24 hours, morbidity is minimal. New video laparoscopy equipment can now reduce intussusception, except where bowel necrosis is present (Puddoubnyi, Dronov, Blinnikov, et al., 1998).

NURSING CARE
The Child with Intussusception

Assessment

The nursing history typically reveals a previously healthy infant who suddenly began crying and flexing the legs in severe pain. This problem may resolve, only to recur a short time later and become more constant. Assess any child with these signs for indicators of bowel obstruction: vomiting, nausea, distension, and hypoactive or hyperactive bowel sounds. A palpable abdominal mass and passage of "currant jelly" stools will help confirm the diagnosis. Assess the child's hydration status on admission. Fever, an increased heart rate, changes in level of consciousness or blood pressure, and respiratory distress should be reported immediately as possible indicators of sepsis or peritonitis.

Nursing Diagnosis and Planning

The following nursing diagnoses and expected outcomes may apply to the child with intussusception and the family:

■ Altered Tissue Perfusion (GI) related to bowel compression.
Expected Outcome: The child will have a patent bowel, as evidenced by the passage of soft, formed, Hematest-negative stools.
■ Pain related to bowel obstruction.
Expected Outcomes: The child will be free from abdominal pain, as evidenced by age-appropriate play and activity, and will not exhibit guarding during palpation.
■ Fluid Volume Deficit related to vomiting and diarrhea.
Expected Outcomes: The child will tolerate age-appropriate food and fluids without vomiting or recurrence of symptoms and be free from fluid and electrolyte disturbances, as evidenced by return to normal weight, moist mucous membranes, good skin turgor, and normal serum sodium level and hematocrit.
■ Knowledge Deficit related to possibility of surgery and the need for immediate intervention.
Expected Outcomes: The parents will verbalize an understanding of the need for immediate intervention and will explain the mechanisms of intussusception and hydrostatic reduction.
■ Sleep Pattern Disturbance related to colicky abdominal pain.
Expected Outcome: The child will return to normal sleep patterns.

Interventions

Once the diagnosis is made, immediate plans are made to admit the child to the hospital for hydrostatic reduction. Prompt assessment for dehydration, shock, or sepsis is essential, including documenting mental status, capillary perfusion, and urine output. The child is given IV fluids, and an NG tube is inserted if distension is present. During reduction, pain medications or sedation may be needed to decrease spasm. After reduction, clear liquids are started and advanced gradually as tolerated.

Observe for the passage of barium and note the characteristics of stool. Also note the recurrence of previous symptoms of bowel obstruction; the risk of recurrence following nonsurgical reduction is about 10%. Resumption of a normal diet and normal activity and the passage of stool without blood will indicate a successful outcome. If hydrostatic reduction is unsuccessful, the child must be prepared for abdominal surgery. If hydrostatic reduction is unsuccessful, continue to monitor for return of normal bowel function because spontaneous resolution could occur, eliminating the need for surgery.

Postoperatively, the child is kept NPO until bowel function returns. Nasogastric suction and IV therapy, pain medications, maintenance of respiratory function, frequent assessment, and meeting developmental needs remain nursing responsibilities.

During this difficult time for parents, relieving their anxiety by providing appropriate information is essential. This effort should include a description of the pathophysiology of intussusception, the usefulness of hydrostatic reduction, and the expected recovery care for their child, including the need for IV fluids, NG suction, and frequent vital signs and assessments. In addition, emotional support can be provided by encouraging them to participate in their child's care, listening to their concerns, and encouraging expression of their feelings during this stressful time.

> To help parents understand intussusception, use a hospital glove. As you press one finger (representing the terminal ileum) into the inflated glove (the distal colon) and cause it to go inside itself, the parents can visualize the telescoping. The same mechanism can show how hydrostatic reduction works. As you press on the glove (the distal portion) with your hand, you can see and feel how the telescoped portion is pushed back to its normal position.

Evaluation

• In the preoperative period, does the child achieve moist mucous membranes, good skin turgor, a urine specific gravity of less than 1.025, and a return to pre-illness weight?
• Is the child passing soft, formed, Hematest-negative stools?
• Does the infant guard the abdomen during palpation?
• Is the child demonstrating age-appropriate activity levels, sleep patterns, and play?
• Is the child tolerating age-appropriate food and fluids without vomiting or recurrence of symptoms?
• Can the parents explain the rationale for hydrostatic reduction?
• Are all the parents' questions answered to their satisfaction?

Volvulus

Volvulus is a condition caused by a malrotation or twisting of the bowel that causes a bowel obstruction. It is the result of a defect in fetal development in which the midgut, which normally rotates 270 degrees around the superior mesenteric artery, fails to rotate and fixes itself to the abdominal wall.

Affected infants usually manifest pain, bilious vomiting, and other signs of bowel obstruction. Surgery is essential to prevent bowel ischemia. The nursing care is similar to that for the child with intussusception who has undergone surgery.

Hirschsprung Disease

Also known as congenital aganglionosis or megacolon, Hirschsprung disease is the result of an absence of ganglion cells in the rectum and, to varying degrees, upward in the colon. Seventy-five percent of cases affect the rectosigmoid region; 15% progress to the right colon (Kirschner & Black, 1994).

Etiology and Incidence

The disease is a result of embryonic failure of migration of the hindgut ganglion cells to the most caudal portion of the GI tract, the rectum. The initiating factor in this failure is unknown.

Hirschsprung disease occurs in 1 in 5,000 live births, with a 4:1 male-female ratio (Abi-Hanna & Lake, 1998). It has a strong hereditary component and a higher incidence in children with Down syndrome.

Manifestations and Diagnostic Evaluation

Delayed passage or absence of meconium stool in the neonatal period is the cardinal sign of Hirschsprung disease. Any child who fails to pass meconium within the first 24 hours and who is prone to constipation or stool infrequency in the first month after birth is suspected of having Hirschsprung disease. The neonate may exhibit signs of bowel ob-

struction, abdominal pain and distension, and failure to thrive. Chronic constipation beginning in the first month of life results in pellet-like or ribbon stools that are foul-smelling.

A rectal examination will reveal the absence of stool, followed by an often explosive release of gas and feces related to the sudden but transient increase in rectal size. Barium enema examination will demonstrate an abrupt change in the size of the colon from a very distended ganglionic proximal portion to the contracted, sawtoothed appearance in the aganglionic distal portion, with a transitional zone of tapered bowel between them. Significantly, the child will fail to evacuate barium after the examination. The definitive diagnosis is made by rectal biopsy. During biopsy, a small core or punch sample that contains all layers of the bowel mucosa is removed. Absence of ganglionic cells in the sample confirms the diagnosis of Hirschsprung disease.

Therapeutic Management

Treatment for mild to moderate Hirschsprung disease is based on relieving the chronic constipation with stool

PATHOPHYSIOLOGY
. . . .
of Hirschsprung Disease

Ganglia provide parasympathetic innervation of the colon. In Hirschsprung disease, ganglia are absent from a variable length of colon extending proximally from the anus. Adequate peristalsis cannot occur in the affected colon, leading to a tonic contraction of the lumen. This produces a functional bowel obstruction, chronic consti-

pation, and the passage of ribbon-like stools. It can lead to a complete bowel obstruction. Because of the constriction of the lumen, huge amounts of feces and gas collect proximal to the aganglionic portion, resulting in a gross enlargement of this segment. The enlarged segment of colon is actually normal in its function.

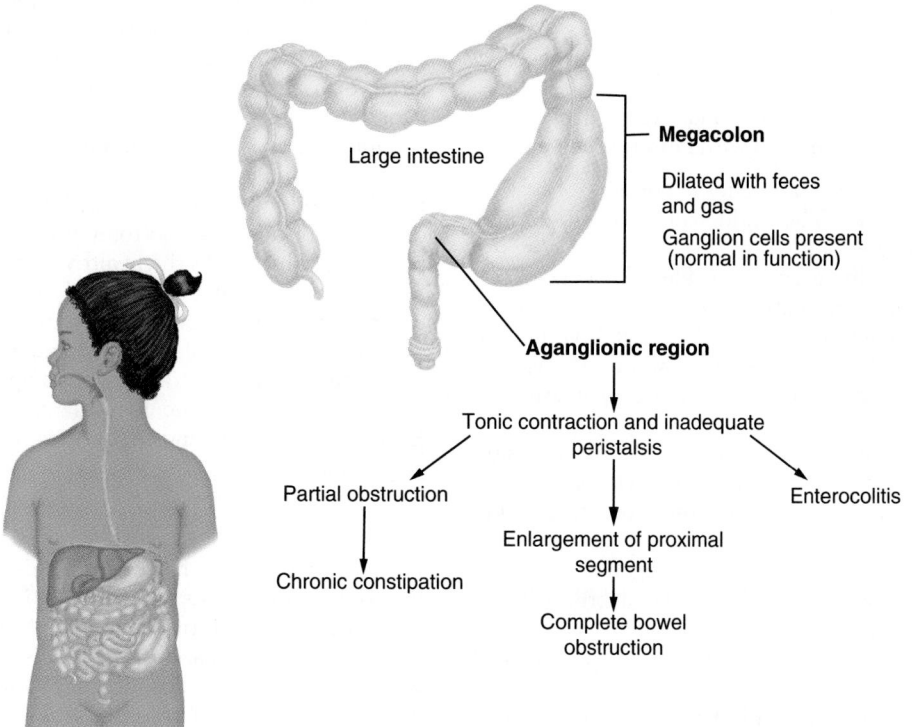

softeners and rectal irrigations. Treatment for moderate to severe Hirschsprung disease involves removing the aganglionic portion of the intestine in a two-step surgical intervention. In the neonatal period, the obstruction is relieved by performing a temporary colostomy with the most distal section of normal bowel. A complete surgical repair is delayed until the child weighs 8 to 10 kg (18 to 20 lb), at which time a pull-through procedure is performed to excise all aganglionic portions of the bowel and re-anastomose the normal bowel to the anal canal. The colostomy is closed during this procedure, and normal bowel function returns shortly thereafter.

NURSING CARE
. . . .
The Child with Hirschsprung Disease

Assessment

The child with Hirschsprung disease will have constipation that has been present since the neonatal period and frequent passage of foul-smelling ribbon-like or pellet stools. Nutritional status should be assessed because malnutrition can develop secondary to extreme distension or enterocolitis. Thin extremities, abdominal distension, and a history of poor feeding should be noted.

If the child is acutely ill on presentation, enterocolitis must be suspected. Document the assessment of bowel sounds and abdominal distension, the frequency of vomiting and diarrhea, and changes in abdominal circumference. Assess temperature using a route other than rectal.

Assess family members' concerns and their methods of dealing with the problem. This disease can drain family and financial resources during the diagnosis and surgical treatment. Mild disease may not be diagnosed until the child is older. Assessing the older child's feelings about chronic constipation and its treatment is important.

Nursing Diagnosis and Planning

The following nursing diagnosis and expected outcomes may be appropriate for the child with Hirschsprung disease:

■ Constipation related to aganglionic bowel.
 Expected Outcome: The child will pass soft, formed stools without retention.
■ Risk for Fluid Volume Deficit or Fluid Volume Excess related to surgical preparation.
 Expected Outcome: The child will be free from fluid or electrolyte disturbances related to bowel cleansing.
■ Impaired Skin Integrity related to colostomy and surgical repair.
 Expected Outcome: The surgical and colostomy sites will be clean and free from exudate, redness, or drainage; the colostomy site will be intact without bleeding or skin irritation.
■ Risk for Infection related to surgical repair.
 Expected Outcome: The child will be afebrile without signs of infection at the site.
■ Altered Nutrition: Less Than Body Requirements related to GI surgery.
 Expected Outcome: The child will have normal bowel sounds, pass stool, and tolerate a regular diet.

■ Pain related to surgical incisions.
 Expected Outcome: The child will be free from pain and able to participate in usual activities of daily living.
■ Knowledge Deficit related to incomplete information about the need for surgery, irrigation, or care of the ostomy.
 Expected Outcome: The parent will state the necessity of rectal irrigations or surgical intervention, and the parent or child will assume responsibility for care of the ostomy.
■ Body Image Disturbance related to colostomy and irrigations.
 Expected Outcome: The child and family will express feelings about irrigations, ostomy care, and the impact the condition has had on the child's body image.

Interventions

Preparing the Child for Surgery

The nurse closely monitors and records the child's bowel elimination pattern. Isotonic saline enemas are administered preoperatively until the return is clear (see Chapter 37). An alternative bowel-cleansing regimen is to administer a polyethylene glycol–electrolyte lavage solution (GoLytely) orally or through the NG tube. This regimen is used only in children older than 5 and is given at a dosage of 25 to 60 ml/kg/hr. After bowel cleansing, keep the child NPO until surgery. Provide IV fluids as needed, and keep strict intake and output records.

Preventing Infection and Maintaining Skin Integrity

Neomycin 1.0% solution given by rectum or stoma is administered preoperatively to sterilize the bowel for surgery. Additional sterilization is provided by IV antibiotics, which also prevent infection at the surgical incision site. Monitor vital signs carefully and measure the child's abdominal circumference with each vital sign measurement. Use tympanic or axillary methods for taking the temperature to avoid traumatizing the rectal mucosa. Monitor the surgical site for redness, swelling, and purulent drainage.

If the child has a colostomy, monitor the stoma site for bleeding and impaired skin integrity (see Chapter 37 for a discussion of care of a colostomy site). After a pull-through procedure, which pulls the healthy bowel to the anal opening, monitor the anal site carefully for redness, discharge, and the presence of stool. To prevent skin breakdown, provide meticulous skin care of abdominal, perineal, and ostomy sites by changing dressings and appliances as needed. Use the appropriate-size hypoallergenic ostomy supplies. Encourage the parent and child to begin ostomy care as soon as possible.

Maintaining Nutritional and Hydration Status

Postoperatively, keep the child NPO until bowel sounds return or the child passes flatus; set the NG tube to intermittent suction until peristalsis returns. Monitor the child for signs of dehydration and acid-base disturbances. Begin advancing the diet from clear liquids to a regular diet. To prevent dehydration, keep the child on IV fluids until the child tolerates oral fluids well.

Relieving Pain

Provide pain medications on a regular basis as ordered. Most school-age children can use patient-controlled analgesia for effective pain control (see Chapter 39). The nurse should encourage the parents to institute nonpharmacologic pain control measures such as repositioning, back rubs, music, holding, rocking, massage, and quiet talking. If pain is not controlled by usual means, the child may be experiencing a bowel obstruction or infection.

Providing Education

Before the time of scheduled surgery, the parents may need to manage rectal irrigations at home. It is necessary to teach not only the procedure but also observing for distension and signs of obstruction. Encourage the parents to express any concerns they may have about the need for irrigations or their ability to perform them. Teach the parents and child about the surgery and recovery process. If the child is to have a colostomy, it is helpful for the child and parents to see and manipulate the equipment.

Postoperatively, encourage preschoolers and young school-age children to draw pictures, use dolls, and play to express concerns about bodily appearance, irrigations, and the colostomy. Teach colostomy care in the immediate postoperative period, and encourage the parents to participate in the child's care as quickly as possible in the supervised setting. Promote self-care as soon as possible for the older child. Referral to an enterostomal therapist can be helpful. The nurse also can refer the family to support groups for children with ostomies.

Evaluation

- Has the child tolerated the bowel-cleansing regimen without signs of fluid and electrolyte imbalance, as evidenced by moist mucous membranes, good skin turgor, and a urine output of 1 to 2 ml/kg/hr?
- Is the child afebrile, and are surgical sites free from redness, purulent drainage, excess heat, and dehiscence?
- Is the colostomy or anal pull-through area free from bleeding and skin breakdown?
- Are bowel sounds active and present in all four quadrants, and is the child tolerating a developmentally appropriate diet without vomiting or diarrhea?
- Does the child pass soft, formed stools without retention following completion of the surgical correction?
- Does the child appear to be free of pain, as evidenced by the ability to sleep comfortably and participate in appropriate play activities when awake?
- Can the parents and child demonstrate all procedures needed for appropriate care?
- Is the child able to express feelings about body changes related to treatments or procedures?

Lactose Intolerance

An inability to tolerate lactose, the sugar found in dairy products, is the result of an absence or deficiency of lactase, an enzyme found in the secretions of the small intestine and needed for the digestion of lactose. The two types of lactose intolerance are congenital and developmental. Congenital lactose intolerance, which is very rare, appears at birth, with

> **PATHOPHYSIOLOGY**
> • • • • • • • • • • •
> *of Lactose Intolerance*
>
> An absence or deficiency of lactase leads to inability to digest lactose and the subsequent accumulation of lactose in the lumen of the small intestine. As a result, water is drawn into the colon, resulting in watery osmotic diarrhea containing undigested lactose. In addition, GI bacteria break down lactose and release hydrogen, which causes excess gas production, bloating, and abdominal pain.

a complete absence of lactase. Developmental lactose intolerance, which is more common, is a deficiency of lactase that appears in early to late childhood.

Etiology and Incidence

Most cases of lactose intolerance are the result of inadequate levels of lactase. The exact reason for this deficiency is unknown. The disease is likely to be more severe during and after other illnesses affecting the GI mucosa, such as viral gastroenteritis or food poisoning.

The condition appears to have an ethnic association, with higher incidence in Asians, Arabs, Jews, African-Americans, and southern Europeans.

Manifestations and Diagnostic Evaluation

Manifestations of lactose intolerance include diarrhea that is frothy but not fatty, abdominal distension, crampy abdominal pain, and excessive flatus. The symptoms are not usually seen until lactase activity begins to decrease after age 3 or during other GI insults. If the child has congenital lactose intolerance, symptoms will be immediate and may be severe.

A history of improvement after a lactose-free diet has been implemented provides a presumptive diagnosis. The diagnosis can be supported by the finding of 1+ or greater sugar values on Clinitest examination of the stool. Breath hydrogen testing may indicate the amount of lactase available by indirectly measuring the amount of undigested carbohydrate.

Therapeutic Management

The treatment for lactose intolerance is removal of lactose from the diet. In most cases, total elimination is unnecessary. Removing milk as the beverage of choice can provide enough relief from symptoms. Additional dietary changes may be necessary to provide adequate sources of calcium and, in the infant, protein and calories. Formulas that do not contain lactose (Isomil, Nursoy, Nutramigen, ProSobee, and other soy-based formulas) may be given to the infant suspected of having lactose intolerance. Breast-feeding mothers are urged to eliminate lactose products from their diet.

These dietary changes can be supplemented with the use of commercial lactase preparations (LactAid, DairyEase,

LacDose) that can be taken with lactose-containing food to provide adequate lactase levels and variable relief from symptoms.

NURSING CARE
The Child with Lactose Intolerance

Assessment

Assessment will reveal a healthy-looking child with episodic abdominal pain and occasional diarrhea without any nutritional deficiencies or other health problems. If the problem is congenital, and thus likely to be more severe, diarrhea may be a major concern. The neonate or infant may appear extremely dehydrated, with severe diarrhea and weight loss. The child and family may or may not be able to correlate symptoms with food intake.

Nursing Diagnosis and Planning

The following nursing diagnoses and expected outcomes may be appropriate for the infant or child with lactose intolerance:

■ Pain related to bloating and flatus.
Expected Outcomes: The child will be free from abdominal pain, as evidenced by developmentally appropriate play and activity, and will have normal bowel sounds with a soft abdomen that is not painful during palpation.
■ Diarrhea related to maldigestion.
Expected Outcome: The child will have soft, formed stools.
■ Knowledge Deficit related to incomplete understanding about needed dietary changes.
Expected Outcomes: The child will take in a minimum of 800 mg of calcium per day, as reported in the dietary history. The family will state foods to be avoided or provided in small amounts and will provide adequate calcium sources in diet and select appropriate lactase products.

Interventions

The principal nursing intervention is teaching. Symptoms are often relieved after a lactose-free diet is followed for a short period. Foods containing small amounts of lactose may be added gradually after this time to assess the child's reaction. If small amounts of milk are tolerated, it is useful to offer food or lactase preparations simultaneously with milk. These simple changes can offer instant relief.

After diagnosis and initial management, this condition is often perceived to be only a minor nuisance. Emotional support for the family, however, may be needed. Referring the family to self-help and information groups and encouraging family members to share successes and concerns are important nursing interventions.

Evaluation

• Is the child happy, content, and free of excess gas and bloating?
• Does the child show adequate growth according to a growth chart?
• Does the food diary indicate an intake of at least 800 mg of calcium daily for a child age 1 to 10 years?

PARENTS WANT TO KNOW
Care of the Child with Lactose Intolerance

• It is necessary for your child to avoid all high-lactose foods (e.g., milk, ice cream). If you are unsure about whether a food contains lactose, examine labels for milk or milk products.
• You can use soy-based, lactose-free formulas as needed for your infant (Isomil, Nursoy, Nutramigen, ProSobee). If you are breast-feeding, limit your own intake of dairy products.
• You or your older child can obtain calcium through other foods besides milk. They include egg yolk, green leafy vegetables, dried beans, cauliflower, and molasses. Calcium supplements are also available.
• Once your child's symptoms have disappeared, you can gradually add yogurt, hard cheeses, and small amounts of milk to assess tolerance.
• If you are having difficulty determining what foods are lactose free or need help finding tasty recipes using lactose-free foods, ask for a dietary consultation.

• Can the parent state what foods it is essential to avoid?
• Does the parent express satisfaction with control of the child's condition?

Celiac Disease

Celiac disease, also known as gluten enteropathy or tropical sprue, results from the inability to digest fully the gliadin or protein part of wheat, barley, rye, and oats. This is a lifelong deficiency requiring dietary modification to prevent chronic maldigestion and malabsorption.

Etiology and Incidence

Celiac disease is considered genetic. From 80% to 90% of children with celiac disease have the genetic marker HLA-B8, a human leukocyte antigen complex located on chromosome 6. This chromosomal variation results in the inability to digest gliadin, causing severe GI mucosal changes that continue on exposure to gluten.

The incidence of celiac disease varies in different regions. In the United States the incidence is about 1 in 1,000 live births. There is a much higher incidence in Europe. Siblings and children of affected individuals are at highest risk for the disease (Troncone & Auricchio, 1999).

Manifestations

The major manifestations in the child with celiac disease include diarrhea and growth failure. The child's growth usually is below the 25th percentile on growth charts.

The child may also experience abdominal distension, vomiting, anemia, irritability and anorexia, muscle wasting,

PATHOPHYSIOLOGY
. . . .
of Celiac Disease

Gluten—the protein found in rye, oats, barley, and wheat—breaks down into gliadin and other by-products. Celiac disease results from an inability to digest gliadin. This results in the accumulation of glutamine in the intestine, which has a toxic effect on the mucosal cells. This leads to atrophy of the villi and a marked de-crease in the absorptive surface. Malabsorption of fats, carbohydrates, and vitamins develops. *Celiac crisis* is a re-sult of sudden accumulation of glutamine and the subse-quent destruction of the mucosal cells, causing severe di-arrhea and dehydration.

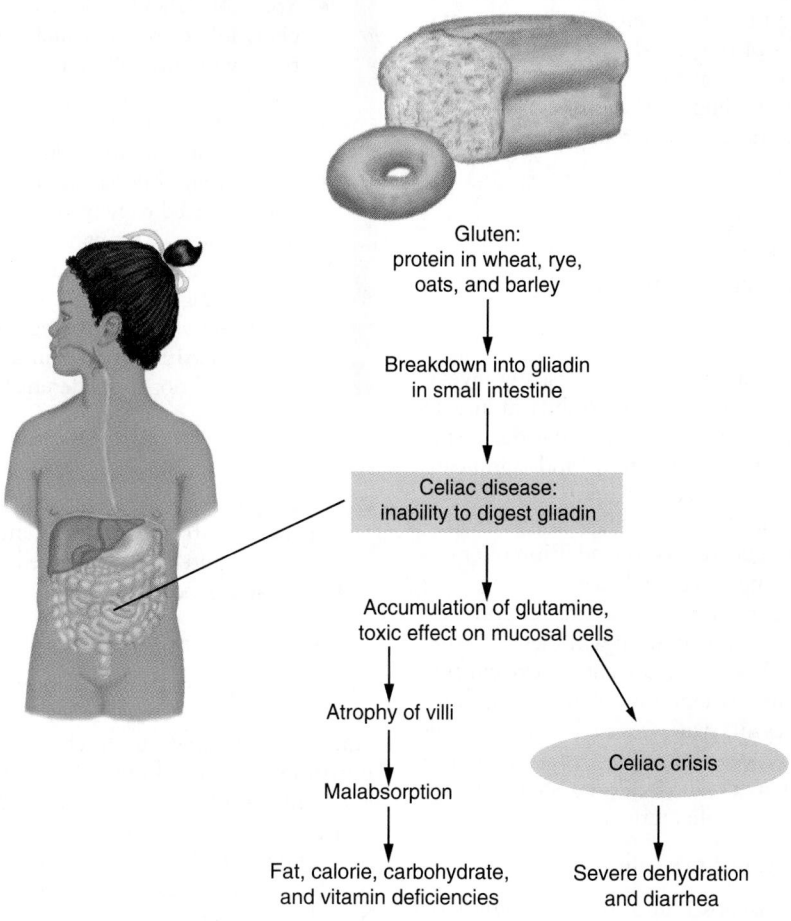

Gluten:
protein in wheat, rye,
oats, and barley

↓

Breakdown into gliadin
in small intestine

↓

Celiac disease:
inability to digest gliadin

↓

Accumulation of glutamine,
toxic effect on mucosal cells

Atrophy of villi → Celiac crisis

↓

Malabsorption

Fat, calorie, carbohydrate,
and vitamin deficiencies

Severe dehydration
and diarrhea

and edema. Symptoms are not seen until 3 to 6 months after the introduction of grains to the diet, usually at age 9 to 12 months. The child in celiac crisis exhibits profuse, watery diarrhea, and vomiting.

Diagnostic Evaluation

The serum antigliadin antibody (AGA) assay is a diagnostic test and allows continued assessment and evaluation of di-etary changes. In the past, this test required specialized labo-ratory equipment. Now, however, a newer method, the strip AGA test, requires only a single drop of blood, and results can be determined quickly and inexpensively. Its ease of use makes the diagnosis of celiac disease simpler and more cost-effective. A newer, more accurate test measures transgluta-mine tTG through enzyme-linked immunosorbent assay (ELISA). The test is also effective in evaluating the ade-quacy of dietary changes (Dieterich, Laag, Schopper, et al.,

1998). Jejunal biopsy will unequivocally identify ulcerations in the GI tract. The diagnosis is supported by monitoring the reaction to a gluten-free diet. Symptoms are often re-lieved in 1 week by removal of gluten from the diet.

Further diagnostic testing may include the breath hy-drogen excretion test to identify the amount of carbohy-drate malabsorption occurring. This test is not specific for sprue. D-xylose testing indicates the amount of mucosal damage; the remaining absorptive surface can be estimated.

Therapeutic Management

Dietary management is the mainstay of treatment. All wheat, rye, barley, and oats should be eliminated from the diet and replaced with corn and rice. To correct deficien-cies, vitamin supplements, especially with fat-soluble vita-mins and folate, may be needed in the early period of treat-ment.

Dietary restrictions are likely to be lifelong, although small amounts of grains may be tolerated after the ulcerations have healed. It is difficult for adolescents to maintain a gluten-free diet without having an unbalanced diet high in protein and fat. An adolescent on a strict gluten-free diet still has a risk for dietary imbalance (Mariani, Viti, Monturo, et al., 1998). Support from dietary services is essential for maintenance.

Occasionally the nurse is the first to see a child in celiac crisis. Celiac crisis causes profuse, watery diarrhea and vomiting and can quickly lead to severe dehydration and metabolic acidosis. The cause of the crisis, usually an infection or a hidden source of gluten, must be identified. The child is given fluids IV to correct fluid and acid-base imbalance, albumin to treat shock, and corticosteroids to decrease severe mucosal inflammation.

NURSING CARE
The Child with Celiac Disease

Assessment

Assessment of the infant with celiac disease usually reveals an irritable, malnourished infant who exhibits failure to thrive by 9 to 12 months. Any child with diarrhea, especially one with foul-smelling, fatty stools and significant growth delays, should be suspected of having this disorder. A noticeable decline in the child's rate of growth as charted on the growth curve, associated with the addition of grains to the diet, is essential supportive evidence.

Abdominal assessment will reveal distension and ascites with an increasing girth; observation will identify other signs of malnutrition such as thin, edematous extremities, pallor, and muscle wasting. Anemia is a common finding.

The child who presents with severe diarrhea, foul-smelling stools, vomiting, poor perfusion, edema, or changes in vital signs (shock or metabolic acidosis) should be referred for emergency care of celiac crisis.

Nursing Diagnosis and Planning

The following nursing diagnoses and expected outcomes may be appropriate for the infant or child with celiac disease:

- Altered Nutrition: Less Than Body Requirements related to malabsorption.
  Expected Outcome: The infant or child will have soft, formed stools without diarrhea.
- Pain related to abdominal distension.
  Expected Outcome: The infant or child will be free from abdominal pain, as evidenced by age-appropriate play and activity.
- Altered Growth and Development related to malnutrition.
  Expected Outcome: The infant or child will return to and follow a normal growth pattern according to a growth chart.
- Knowledge Deficit related to dietary changes.
  Expected Outcomes: The family will offer appropriate foods to the infant or child, as evidenced by a food diary, will state the need for lifelong dietary changes, and will seek emotional and educational support as needed.

PARENTS WANT TO KNOW
Care of the Child with Celiac Disease

- You must eliminate all wheat, rye, barley, oats, and hydrolyzed vegetable protein from your child's diet.
- You can substitute corn, rice, or millet as grains. These can be obtained as flour for baking.
- Your child should take vitamin supplements, especially folate and fat-soluble vitamins, because these vitamins will be hard to provide in your child's diet.
- You will need to read all labels on foods and medications carefully to avoid any unknown additives.
- When your child is old enough to understand, you will need to help your child make appropriate food choices. This can be difficult for an older child or adolescent because popular foods often contain ingredients that will make your child's condition worse. Encourage your child to talk with a nutritionist to plan a diet that is appropriate and not too different from peers'.

- Fluid Volume Deficit related to celiac crisis.
  Expected Outcome: The infant or child will be adequately hydrated, as evidenced by moist mucous membranes and good skin turgor.

Interventions

The most important nursing intervention is teaching parents to modify their child's diet. Pain will likely be relieved quickly by eliminating gluten in the diet. Involvement of nutritionists in teaching and follow-up is helpful. Careful and consistent follow-up will be necessary to ensure the infant resumes a normal growth and development pattern as soon as possible. When the child has normal stools without diarrhea and resumes a normal growth pattern, teaching will have been effective.

Because celiac disease is a lifelong condition, support groups can be useful in managing the problem. The American Celiac Society is an excellent source of information and support (see Appendix L). Referral to this group and other family support organizations is essential. Encourage the parents to share their fears and concerns about the chronic nature of the disease and its impact on family life.

Evaluation

- Does the child have soft, formed stools without diarrhea or signs of dehydration?
- Is the child free of abdominal pain?
- Has the child resumed a normal growth pattern according to a growth chart?
- Does a food diary indicate an intake of approximately 100 kcal/kg for the infant and for the child up to age 3?
- Do the parents use available support and education groups?
- Do the parents express satisfaction with the way they are coping with dietary changes?

Viral Hepatitis

Hepatitis is an acute or chronic inflammation of the liver caused by several different viruses and some toxins or disease states. Although each type of hepatitis is unique, assessment findings and treatment have many similarities.

Etiology

The most common causes and modes of transmission of viral hepatitis are discussed in Table 43–5. Rubella, cytomegalovirus (CMV), herpes simplex virus, and Epstein-Barr virus may also occasionally produce hepatitis in children.

In children, hepatitis A virus (HAV) is highly contagious and spreads readily in households and day care centers. Infection with hepatitis B virus (HBV) can be transmitted perinatally. The incidence of HBV infection transmitted by blood transfusions has decreased in recent years as a result of improved blood product screening procedures. Contaminated body fluids splashed into the mouth or eyes can cause HBV infection. HBV can survive in the dried state for 1 week or longer, and percutaneous contact with contaminated objects can transmit infection.

Incidence

More than 60,000 cases of hepatitis are reported each year. Because the virus may be excreted for 2 to 3 weeks before the appearance of clinical signs and for 2 to 3 weeks afterward, outbreaks are common wherever good hand washing is not practiced.

In the United States and other Western industrialized countries HBV infection occurs most often in adolescents and adults. From 5% to 8% of the U.S. population has been infected with HBV, and 0.2% to 0.9% are chronically infected. In developing countries where sanitation is poor, HBV occurs most often in infants and children younger than 5 years. From 70% to 90% of the adult population of these areas has been infected, and 8% to 15% are chronically infected. HBV infection is the leading cause of acute and chronic liver disease worldwide (Katkov, 1995).

TABLE 43–5

. . . .

Differentiation of Viral Hepatitis

Type/Etiology	Transmission	Incubation	Clinical Manifestations	Recovery Prognosis
Hepatitis A virus (HAV), previously called infectious hepatitis	Fecal-oral Food or water contaminated with HAV	15–50 days (average, 28 days) Most contagious 1–2 weeks before symptoms Onset at 28–30 days	Mild, flu-like symptoms or asymptomatic, no jaundice in children Adolescents: fever, malaise, anorexia, nausea, jaundice	Good prognosis Chronic infections Carriers don't occur Recovery provides life-long immunity
Hepatitis B virus (HBV), previously called serum hepatitis	Blood and blood products Secretions Prenatally, perinatally Sexual contact	15–180 days (average, 90 days)	Same as HAV Severity ranges from asymptomatic to fatal fulminant infection Anicteric or asymptomatic most common in children 90% of infected neonates will develop chronic carrier state	Good prognosis; generally a full recovery except in chronic carriers 40%–90% of infected children <10 years old develop chronic carrier state and are predisposed to cirrhosis and hepatocellular cancer.
Hepatitis C (HCV), non-A, non-B hepatitis	Blood and blood products	14–115 days (average 45 days)	Same as HAV	50% progress to chronic hepatitis and cirrhosis or cancer.
Hepatitis delta virus (HDV), occurs only in patients with acute or chronic HBV infection	Blood and blood products More common in Mediterranean countries, and among IV drug users and hemophiliacs	21–90 days	Occurs with HBV and causes it to be more severe	More likely to develop fulminating hepatitis than other strains
Hepatitis E virus (HEV), enterically transmitted non-A, non-B hepatitis	Fecal-oral More common in adults	15–60 days (average, 40 days)	Epidemic with characteristics of HAV Uncommon in developed countries	High incidence of mortality in pregnant women

Data from Aach, R. (1998). Viral hepatitis due to hepatitis viruses A–E and GB virus. In R. Fagin & J. Cherry (Eds.), *Textbook of pediatric infectious diseases* (4th ed.). Philadelphia: Saunders.

PATHOPHYSIOLOGY

of Viral Hepatitis

Hepatitis viruses cause necrosis of the parenchymal cells of the liver. The inflammatory response causes swelling and blockage of the drainage system in the liver. Biliary stasis and further destruction of the hepatic cells occur. Because the liver cannot excrete bile into the intestine, bile appears in the blood (causing hyperbilirubinemia), urine (as urobilinogen), and skin (causing hepatocellular jaundice).

Hepatitis infection may result in asymptomatic or mild illness, in which complete regeneration of liver cells occurs within 2 to 3 months. More severe forms of hepatitis include fulminant hepatitis, in which hepatic necrosis and death can occur within 1 to 2 weeks, and subacute, or chronic, hepatitis, which can result in permanent scarring of the liver and impaired liver function. Chronically infected persons are carriers of the disease and are at increased risk for developing chronic liver disease (e.g., cirrhosis, chronic persistent hepatitis) or liver carcinoma later in life.

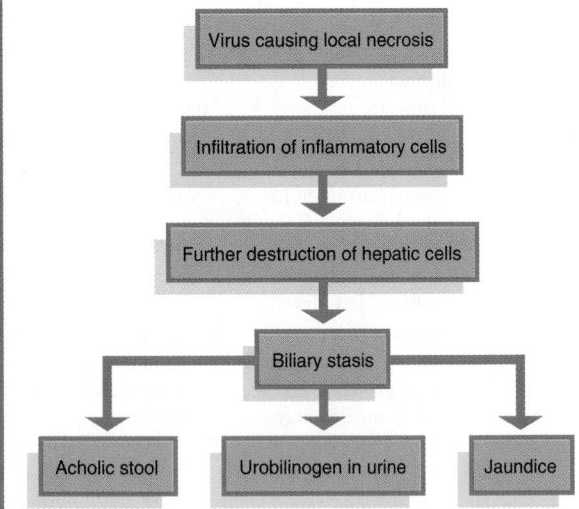

Manifestations

In infants and preschool-age children, HAV infection is usually asymptomatic or causes mild, nonspecific symptoms such as anorexia, malaise, and easy fatigability. In adults, the disease causes the more severe symptoms of nausea, jaundice, and malaise. Because most children with HAV infection are asymptomatic or have mild, nonspecific symptoms, the disease may not be diagnosed until an outbreak of hepatitis occurs. Thus, spread of HAV infection in a day care center often occurs before the initial case is identified.

HBV infection may cause a wide range of clinical manifestations, from asymptomatic infection to fatal acute fulminant hepatitis. Symptomatic acute hepatitis occurs in two stages: the anicteric phase, without jaundice, and the icteric (jaundiced) phase.

During the anicteric phase, manifestations include anorexia, nausea and vomiting, right upper quadrant or epi-

gastric pain, fever, malaise in which the child feels ill, fatigue, depression, and irritability. The anicteric phase lasts approximately 5 to 7 days. During the icteric phase, manifestations include jaundice, urticaria, dark urine, and light-colored stools. The child begins to feel better as jaundice becomes more apparent. Acute fulminating hepatitis is marked by bleeding problems, encephalopathy, ascites, and acute hepatic failure. Fulminant hepatitis is due primarily to hepatitis B and hepatitis C.

The symptoms and clinical changes should return to normal within 3 months of onset. If not, a chronic state should be suspected. Infection with hepatitis B, hepatitis D, and hepatitis C viruses can result in chronic hepatitis and cirrhosis. Chronic HBV infection can also cause hepatic carcinoma.

Diagnostic Evaluation

A history of exposure to jaundiced individuals, confirmed outbreaks in day care centers, or percutaneous exposure to blood or body fluids should raise the suspicion of hepatitis. Although no liver function test is specific for hepatitis, tests of liver function, especially AST, ALT, and bilirubin levels and sedimentation rate, can indicate liver damage caused by hepatitis. Serum bilirubin levels peak 5 to 10 days after jaundice appears. A history and the course of the disease are essential in making the appropriate diagnosis.

Hepatitis is diagnosed by identification of the antigens (HBsAg, HBeAg) responsible for the disease or the antibodies (anti-HAV, anti-HBc, anti-HBe, anti-HBs, or anti-HCV) that develop as a result. IgM anti-HAV antibodies are present at the onset of illness. They usually disappear within 6 months but may persist for 12 months. IgG anti-HAV antibodies develop shortly after IgM anti-HAV antibodies do. The presence of IgG without IgM anti-HAV antibodies indicates past infection (Aach, 1998). HCV serologic assays are used mainly to detect chronic hepatitis C because they remain negative for at least 1 to 3 months after onset of the illness (Aach, 1998).

Liver biopsy may be needed to evaluate the chronic active forms of the disease and to determine the extent of damage in advanced or fulminant cases. Liver fibrosis increases with the duration of HCV infection (Guido, Rugge, Jara, et al., 1998).

Therapeutic Management

Acute viral hepatitis has no specific treatment. In uncomplicated viral hepatitis, treatment is mainly supportive because the disease is self-limiting. Treatment is aimed at maintaining comfort and adequate nutritional balance. A low-fat, balanced diet can be helpful if the child is bothered by nausea and anorexia. Hospitalization is rarely needed.

In fulminant hepatitis, intensive care may be needed to provide hemostasis, nutritional and fluid support, neurologic assessment, and management until the liver has had a chance to recover.

HEPATITIS A

Control of further spread is essential. Because HAV can survive on contaminated objects for weeks, good hand washing and thorough disinfection of diaper-changing surfaces are imperative. Children and adults who have had direct contact with a person infected with HAV should receive immune globulin (IG) as soon as possible after exposure. A vaccine has been developed to prevent HAV infection, and immunization is recommended for day care workers, homosexually active males, military personnel, and travelers to areas of high endemicity. Cases of hepatitis should be promptly reported to local public health officials. Testing for IgM anti-HAV antibodies should be done in suspected cases of infected day care center employees and household contacts of infected persons (American Academy of Pediatrics Committee on Infectious Diseases, 1994).

HEPATITIS B

Children with acute or chronic HBV infection should be cared for with scrupulous standard precautions. The most effective means of preventing HBV infection is immunization with hepatitis B vaccine. Hepatitis B vaccination is recommended beginning in infancy as part of the routine childhood immunization schedule and for all unimmunized children before they reach adolescence. Other persons who should receive hepatitis B immunization include IV drug users, health care and residential facility workers, household contacts and sexual partners of HBV carriers, inmates of correctional facilities, and international travelers. Hepatitis B immune globulin (HBIG) is effective in preventing HBV infection if given within 2 weeks after exposure. It is possible to prevent hepatitis D by preventing hepatitis B.

NURSING CARE
The Child with Viral Hepatitis

Assessment

The nursing history may identify a source of infection. In children, flu-like symptoms of fever, malaise, anorexia, fatigue, and nausea may be the *only* symptoms of viral hepatitis. Abdominal assessment may disclose right upper quadrant tenderness and hepatomegaly. Stools will be pale and clay-colored, and urine may be dark and frothy. Jaundice, if present, is best assessed in sclera, nail beds, and mucous membranes and usually follows a cephalocaudal progression. In HBV infection, arthralgias may be the presenting complaint.

Fulminant hepatitis will likely manifest as acute hepatic failure with associated encephalopathy, bleeding, fluid retention, ascites, and an icteric appearance.

Nursing Diagnosis and Planning

The following nursing diagnoses and expected outcomes may be appropriate after assessing the child with viral hepatitis and the child's family:

- Altered Nutrition: Less Than Body Requirements related to anorexia.
  Expected Outcomes: The child will tolerate age-appropriate diet without weight loss, vomiting, or abdominal pain and will return to a normal activity level.
- Risk for Infection related to exposure of family members to infectious agents.
  Expected Outcomes: The family will practice good hand washing and other necessary isolation procedures and will remain free from infection.

- Risk for Injury related to fulminant hepatitis.
  Expected Outcome: The child will return to pre-illness weight and activity level.
- Knowledge Deficit related to incomplete information about home care and long-term prognosis.
  Expected Outcome: The parents will verbalize a basic understanding of hepatitis and the importance of treatment and prevention.

Interventions

Unless fulminant hepatitis develops, children are usually treated at home, so parental education is crucial. Teaching parents the importance of a nutritious low-fat diet as tolerated by the child, rest, and general supportive care are important. The child with hepatitis is often anorexic. Several small meals and snacks throughout the day are better tolerated than regular portions at mealtimes.

Fatigue and malaise can last for several weeks. Adequate rest and sleep are important for recovery. Because HAV is not infectious within a week after the onset of jaundice, the child may return to school at that time if well enough.

Child and Parent Teaching

Teach the parents the danger signals that could indicate a worsening of the child's condition, specifically changes in neurologic status, bleeding, and fluid retention. Jaundice may worsen before it resolves, and parents should be prepared for this possibility. Also, teach parents not to give their child any over-the-counter medications, because impaired liver function may result in inadequate metabolism and excretion of the medication. Caution adolescents not to drink alcohol during the illness or recovery period.

Preventing the spread of infection is an essential intervention for HAV. Prevention should include the use of contact precautions for at least 1 week after the onset of jaundice and excellent hand washing. Hand washing is the most important preventive measure. Teach family members to institute appropriate precautions and to clean exposed household surfaces with bleach. Diapers should not be changed on or near surfaces used for preparing or serving food. Explain to family members the ways in which HAV (fecal-oral route) and HBV (parenteral route) are spread to others. Provide education about the recommendations concerning hepatitis A and hepatitis B vaccination (see Appendix F).

If the child has HBV infection especially neonatal HBV, prepare the parents for the possibility of a chronic carrier state and the development of cirrhosis and hepatocellular cancer in later years. If a child or adolescent with HBV infection has a history of illicit IV drug use, the nurse has the responsibility of teaching the dangers of such behaviors, including the risk of transmission of hepatitis and other infections. The youth should be assisted to obtain counseling through a drug program.

Home Care

Children with hepatitis are almost always managed at home. Nursing interventions include teaching parents hand-washing skills, the use of gloves, and disinfection of contaminated surfaces and articles. Parents should be taught to monitor for complications, provide a well-balanced, low-fat diet, and monitor other family members for infection.

All children in the family should be immunized against hepatitis.

Evaluation

- Has the child maintained a weight within 5% of the pre-illness weight?
- Is the child free of vomiting?
- Is the child participating in age-appropriate activities and play?
- Do family members practice good hand washing and adhere to procedures?
- Has the spread of hepatitis to other family members been avoided?
- Have all family members been immunized as appropriate?
- Can the parents explain the symptoms to watch for in other family members?

▌ Biliary Atresia

Biliary atresia refers to the obstruction or absence of the extrahepatic bile ducts. At birth, the liver structure itself is normal without inflammation, but the structural problem leads to significant cellular damage and eventual liver failure and death.

Etiology and Incidence

The cause of biliary atresia is unknown. Because the problem originates during the prenatal period, viruses, toxins, and chemicals cannot be ruled out. The condition is unlikely to recur within the same family.

Extrahepatic biliary atresia occurs in 1 in 10,000 to 20,000 births, with a slightly higher incidence in females than in males (C. MacDonald, 1991).

Manifestations

The child is apparently healthy at birth. Developing manifestations, however, include acholic stools (light in color because of the absence of bile pigment), bile-stained urine, and hepatomegaly.

PATHOPHYSIOLOGY
• • • • • • • • • •

of Biliary Atresia

Obstruction of the extrahepatic bile ducts causes obstruction of the normal flow of bile out of the liver and into the gallbladder and small intestine. As a result, bile plugs form, causing bile to back up in the liver. This process causes inflammation, edema, and hepatic degeneration. Eventually the liver becomes fibrotic, and cirrhosis and portal hypertension develop, leading to liver failure. The gradual degeneration of the liver causes jaundice, icterus, and hepatomegaly. Because bile is not present in the intestine, fat and fat-soluble vitamins cannot be absorbed. This condition leads to malnutrition, deficiencies in fat-soluble vitamins, and growth failure.

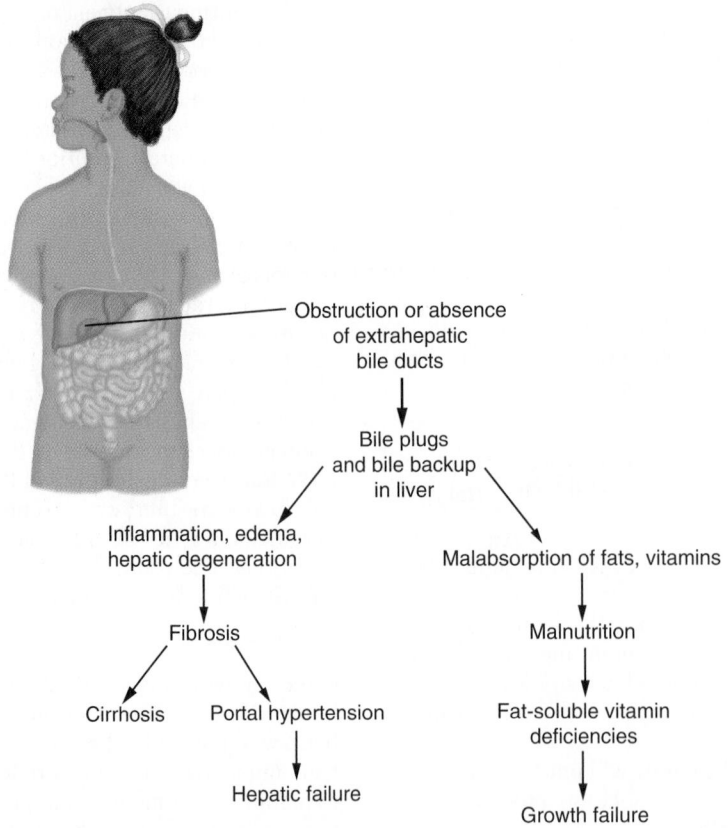

Diagnostic Evaluation

Investigations of liver function (bilirubin, aminotransferases [ALT, AST]) and clotting studies (prothrombin time, partial thromboplastin time) are useful screening tools. To rule out inborn errors of metabolism such as galactosemia and alpha-1-antitrypsin deficiency, which can produce similar initial findings, metabolic screens are essential in these children. Hepatitis and other viral titers are also necessary so that neonatal hepatitis can be eliminated as the source of dysfunction. Urine and stool should be examined and urobilinogen levels determined as an indication of the degree of obstruction.

Liver biopsy can provide a definitive diagnosis if bile plugs, edema, and fibrosis are found in the presence of normal hepatic lobular structure (Behrman et al., 1996). Cholangiography may be used to determine the extent of atresia.

Therapeutic Management

During and after exploratory laparotomy, the size of the lesion can be identified, and drainage can be attempted. If no correctable lesion is found, a hepatic portoenterostomy (Kasai procedure) will be performed to allow bile to drain from the liver. This procedure allows bile to flow directly into the intestine through an anastomosis of the jejunum to the porta hepatis, the point at which the hepatic ducts join to form the common bile duct. The Kasai procedure does provide some long-term benefits, but hepatic dysfunction will persist. The main goal of the procedure is to allow growth and development of the child until liver transplantation can be performed.

The medical management of the child involves managing the malnutrition and providing symptom relief. Medium-chain triglyceride (MCT) oil added to formula to increase calories, or TPN (total parenteral nutrition) provides essential nutrition. Vitamin malabsorption must be treated to prevent night blindness (vitamin A), neuromuscular degeneration (vitamin E), rickets (vitamin D), and hypoprothrombinemia (vitamin K). Assessment for and treatment of portal hypertension with its concomitant problems of ascites and variceal bleeding must be instituted. Controlling bleeding, restricting salt, and using diuretics are important in managing portal hypertension.

Nursing Considerations

During the early phase of disease, in the first months of life, the infant with biliary atresia will appear jaundiced, with mild hepatosplenomegaly and increased abdominal girth. As the disease progresses, the child may appear thin, with failure to thrive, marked jaundice, and evidence of rickets secondary to chronic vitamin D deficiency. Pruritus becomes a major problem; the child may develop skin infections or xanthoma (lipid deposits in the skin) secondary to retention of cholesterol in the skin.

After the Kasai procedure, the child needs to be assessed for evidence of portal hypertension, which may include the development of ascites and GI bleeding. Even after repair, it would not be unusual to find acholic stools and bile-stained urine.

Psychosocial and family assessment should have a high priority. Biliary atresia is a life-threatening, chronic problem that requires surgical intervention, contacts with numerous health care personnel, repeated hospitalization, and eventually an extended wait for a transplant. The nurse gathers information about family and financial resources, emotional support available, and the feelings of the child and family about the progress and management of the disease.

Nursing interventions are directed toward six major areas: nutritional support, skin care, developmental stimulation, continued assessment, education, and emotional support.

NUTRITIONAL SUPPORT
Providing adequate calories, aiding in vitamin supply and absorption, and preventing hepatic encephalopathy are important goals. Calorie counts, daily weights, and abdominal girths are important assessments and will provide the data necessary to improve nutritional support. Concentrating calories with the use of Polycose and providing MCT supplements that do not require the presence of bile salts to digest will significantly change the nutritional status of the child. NG tube feeding or TPN may become necessary at times. Supplements of vitamins A, D, E, and K as well as calcium, phosphate, and zinc are essential for adequate nutrition. Protein may need to be limited to avoid the development of hepatic encephalopathy. Using growth charts and weighing on a monthly basis will provide evaluation criteria.

SKIN CARE
Bile acid binders such as cholestyramine and phenobarbital aid in the excretion of bile salts and decrease pruritus and the development of xanthomas (Behrman et al., 1996). Colloidal oatmeal baths (Aveeno) can relieve severe itching. Preventing skin breakdown from severe scratching is essential. Using gloves during sleep and applying soothing lotions and creams for dry skin may prevent infection.

DEVELOPMENTAL STIMULATION
Teaching parents activities to provide developmental stimulation and using resources available through physical and occupational therapy are essential nursing responsibilities. As the child awaits a transplant, efforts should be made to facilitate as much development as possible by providing stimulation for gross and fine motor skills and social and emotional growth. Routine screening tests can document developmental growth and help evaluate interventions.

CONTINUED ASSESSMENT
Continued assessment for the development of portal hypertension is vital. The parents must be taught to watch for GI bleeding and the development of severe edema and ascites. Should any of these occur, sodium restriction, diuretics, IV albumin, and hospitalization may become necessary.

FAMILY EDUCATION AND SUPPORT
The family has many educational needs, and the nurse needs to help them understand the disease process, deal with nutritional changes, manage skin care, assess for danger signs, and enhance the child's development. National resources are available to help these families. The Children's Liver Foundation can provide programs, educational materials, and referral to support groups as needed (see Appendix L).

The nurse plays a critical role by listening to parental concerns, providing resources and support, and encouraging participation and involvement. Provide information about daily care, and focus the parents' attention on the future liver transplant and its long-term care and treatment. Because transplantation usually occurs within the first 2 years of life, age-appropriate explanations for the toddler are also indicated.

The child and family should be prepared for the eventual need for a liver transplant and the possible death of their child. The life-threatening condition requires numer-

ous hospitalizations, and the many diagnostic tests place immense stress on families. Arranging the educational and emotional support needed by family members so that they can manage their child until liver transplantation becomes possible is a critical nursing intervention.

HOME CARE

The parents must be able to assume all home care responsibilities. They need to be able to monitor growth and nutritional intake, mix special formulas, manage NG feedings, provide skin care, and give medications. Their ability to assess for GI bleeding, ascites, edema, and skin infections is critical so that treatment can begin as soon as possible.

KEY CONCEPTS

- The gastrointestinal (GI) system is formed in the first 4 weeks of embryonic development. Congenital defects can be traced to this period.
- The GI system is anatomically fully developed at birth but physiologically immature, affecting enzymes, sphincter tone, permeability, secretion, and reabsorption.
- Assessment of GI distress is very difficult in small children and must include a thorough history, physical assessment, and general appraisal of the child's distress, as well as the parent's perception of the child's pain.
- Fluid balance is very quickly affected if the child is experiencing vomiting, diarrhea, or anorexia, so the nurse must assess changes quickly and completely.

- Gastroesophageal alterations often place the child at risk for respiratory distress secondary to aspiration and compression of the abdomen into the pulmonary spaces. Assessment of respiratory function and maintaining the airway are critical interventions.
- Medications play a crucial role managing some upper GI alterations, so the nurse must be aware of dosages, indications, side effects, and teaching needs.
- The emotional needs of the parents need to be addressed quickly if the child has a congenital condition.
- Surgery to repair congenital defects and obstructive conditions requires nursing care similar to that for an adult, but with special emphasis on nutrition, fluid status,

pain control, parental involvement, and the developmental level of the child.
- Using appropriate standard precautions is essential to prevent the spread of infection in children with GI disorders.
- Some malabsorptive GI disorders are managed by simple dietary changes.
- Home care and teaching have a high priority because parents must have the necessary information to care for their child during the management of GI alterations.
- Community and home health resources are a critical part of nursing care for the child with GI alterations.

ANSWERS TO CRITICAL THINKING EXERCISE 43–1

1. An accurate history is essential to identify the cause of Andrew's problem and any pathophysiologic process that is occurring. Guide Andrew's mother in carefully describing the frequency, amount, and character of the emesis. Ask about the relationship of feeding to vomiting, and determine whether the vomiting is projectile. A comparison of birth weight and current weight will determine whether Andrew is receiving normal nutrition to support weight gain, and will assist in an assessment for dehydration. Assess the skin turgor, the fontanel, mucous membranes, and alertness appropriate for his age.

2. Parents, especially first-time parents, often are uncertain of when to seek health care advice. The nurse's responsibility is to set a tone that encourages questions and to give guidelines as to when to seek help. Andrew's mother had called the clinic, but either she did not give an accurate description of the problem or the nurse did not ask the questions that would have made that happen.

   Access to health care is often limited because clients do not have transportation and do not live near public transportation. Nurses can assist clients to identify resources

that are more accessible or resources that assist them in other ways (e.g., financial aid, child care). Stories of frustration told by parents seeking access to care should be a red flag for change within the system. Some clinics have hotlines that parents can use. Nurses can also manage caseloads of clients and track both preventive and acute care of those clients assigned to them. This process enables them to identify infants and children who are not receiving preventive care, monitor those receiving acute care, and respond to cues that additional intervention is needed.

REFERENCES AND READINGS

Aach, R. (1998). Viral hepatitis due to hepatitis viruses A–E and GB virus. In R. Fegin & J. Cherry (Eds.), *Textbook of pediatric infectious diseases* (4th ed., pp. 612–640). Philadelphia: Saunders.

Abi-Hanna, A., & Lake, A. (1998). Constipation and encopresis in childhood. *Pediatric Review, 19*(1), 23–30.

Alexander, I. (1998). Viral hepatitis: Primary care, diagnosis and management. *The Nurse Practitioner, 23*(10), 13–40.

American Academy of Pediatrics Committee on Infectious Diseases. (1994). *Report of the Committee on Infectious Diseases: 1994 red book* (23rd ed.). Elk Grove Village, IL: American Academy of Pediatrics.

American Academy of Pediatrics Task Force on Infant Position and SIDS. (1992). Positioning and SIDS. *Pediatrics, 89*, 1120–1126.

Andrews, C. (1994). Ulcer-healing drugs and their actions and side effects. *Nursing Times, 90*(33), 38–40.

Anton, P. (1999). Stress and mind-body impact on the course of inflammatory bowel disease. *Seminars in Gastrointestinal Disease: Problem-Solving Approach for Clinical Diagnosis and Management, 10*(1), 14–19.

Aranda, R., & Horgan, K. (1998). Immunosuppressive drugs in the treatment of inflammatory bowel disease. *Seminars in Gastrointestinal Disease: Problem-Solving Approach for Clinical Diagnosis and Management, 9*(1), 3–9.

Barone, M. (1996). *The Harriet Lane handbook: A manual for pediatric house officers* (12th ed.). St. Louis: Mosby.

Behrman, R., Kliegman, R. M., & Arvin, A. M. (Eds.). (1996). *Nelson textbook of pediatrics* (15th ed.). Philadelphia: Saunders.

Berube, M., & Parrish, R. (1994). Home care of the infant with gastroesophageal reflux and respiratory disease. *Journal of Pediatric Health Care, 8*(4), 173–180.

Borkowski, S. (1994). Common pediatric surgical problems. *Nursing Clinics of North America, 29*(4), 551–562.

Boyle, J. T. (1996). Chronic diarrhea. In R. Behrman, R. Kliegman, & A. Arvin (Eds.), *Nelson textbook of pediatrics* (15th ed.). Philadelphia: Saunders.

Carlson, E. (1998). Irritable bowel syndrome. *The Nurse Practitioner, 23*(1), 82–89.

Cohen, M., & Laney, D. W. (1999). Infectious diarrhea. In R. Wyllie & J. Hyams (Eds.), *Pediatric gastrointestinal disease* (2nd ed., pp. 348–370). Philadelphia: Saunders.

Cooke, D. (1991). Inflammatory bowel disease: Primary health care management of ulcerative colitis and Crohn's disease. *The Nurse Practitioner, 16*(8), 27–39.

Curtin, G. (1990). The infant with cleft lip or palate: More than a surgical problem. *Journal of Perinatal/Neonatal Nursing, 3*(3), 80–89.

Dieterich, W., Ehni, T., Bauer, M., Donner, P., Volta, U., Riecken, E., & Schuppan, D. (1997). Identification of tissue transglutaminase as the autoantigen of celiac disease. *National Medicine, 3*(7), 797–801.

Dieterich, W., Laag, E., Schopper, H., et al. (1998). Autoantibodies to tissue transglu-

taminase as predictors of celiac disease. *Gastroenterology, 115*(6), 1317–1321.

Eliason, M. (1991). Cleft lip and palate: Developmental effects. *Journal of Pediatric Nursing, 6*(2), 107–113.

Evans, K. (1990). Pediatric management problems: Constipation. *Pediatric Nursing, 16*(6), 590–591.

Evans-Storer, N., & Lysen, K. (Eds.). (1997). Clinical nutrition [Special issue]. *Nursing Clinics of North America, 32*(4).

Frost, G. (1992). Hirschsprung's disease in infants and children. *Gastroenterology Nursing, 15*(1), 45–48.

Gauderer, M. W. (1997). When to operate immediately and when to observe. *Seminars in Pediatric Surgery, 6*(2), 65–73.

Griffiths, A., Nguyen, P., Smith, C., MacMillan, J., & Sherman, P. (1993). Growth and clinical course of children with Crohn's disease. *Gut, 34*(7), 939–943.

Guido, M., Rugge, M., Jara, P., Hierro, L., Giacchino, R., Larrauri, J., Zancan, L., Leandro, G., Marino, C., Balli, F., Bagni, A., Timitilli, A., & Bortolotti, F. (1998). Chronic hepatitis C in children: The pathological and clinical spectrum. *Gastroenterology, 115*(6), 1525–1529.

Haas-Beckert, B., & Heyman, M. (1993). Comparison of two skin-level gastrostomy feeding tubes for infants and children. *Pediatric Nursing, 19*(4), 351–354.

Hagelgans, N., & Janusz, B. (1994). Pediatric skin care issues for the home care nurse: Part 2. *Pediatric Nursing, 20*(1), 69–76.

Hillemeier, C. (1996). Gastroesophageal reflux. *Pediatric Clinics of North America, 43*(1), 197–212.

Hubbard, P. (1994). Medication review: Cisapride. *ANNA Journal, 21*(6), 374–380.

Kadia, S., Cassaday, M., & Shaffer, R. (1994). Comparison of Foley catheters as a replacement gastrostomy tube with commercial replacement gastrostomy tube. *Gastrointestinal Endoscopy, 40*(2), 188–193.

Katkov, W. N. (1995). Hepatitis vaccines. *Gastroenterology Clinics of North America, 24*(1), 147–159.

Kenner, C., Brueggemeyer, A., & Gunderson, L. (1993). *Comprehensive neonatal nursing: A physiologic perspective*. Philadelphia: Saunders.

Kent, P., & Curley, M. (1992). Challenges in nursing: Infants with congenital diaphragmatic hernia. *Heart and Lung, 21*(4), 381–389.

Kirschner, B., & Black, D. (1994). *Essentials of Pediatrics* (2nd ed.). Philadelphia: Saunders.

Ladebauche, P. (1992). Intussusception in pediatric patients. *Journal of Emergency Nursing, 18*(3), 275–279.

Litwack-Saleh, K. (1993). Practical points in the care of the patient post-cleft lip and palate repair. *Journal of Post Anesthesia Nursing, 8*(1), 35–37.

Loening-Baucke, V. (1997). Urinary incontinence and urinary tract infection and their resolution with treatment of chronic constipation and urinary symptoms. *Pediatrics 100*, 288–232.

Lord, L. (1997). Enteral access devices. *Nursing Clinics of North America, 32*(4), 685–704.

MacDonald, C. (1991). Biliary atresia. *Journal of Pediatric Nursing, 6*(6), 374–383.

MacDonald, T. (1993). Etiology of Crohn's disease. *Gut, 34*(Suppl. 2), 939–943.

Mariani, P., Viti, M., Monturo, M., Vecchia, A., Cipoletta, E., & Bonamilo, M. (1998). The gluten-free diet: A nutritional risk factor for adolescents with celiac disease. *Journal of Pediatric Gastroenterolgy and Nutrition, 27*(5), 519–523.

Martin, S. (1992). The ABCs of pediatric LFTs. *Pediatric Nursing, 18*(5), 445–449.

Mattei, P., Stevenson, R., & Ziegler, M. (1999). Appendicitis. In R. Wyllie & J. Hyams. (Eds.), *Pediatric gastrointestinal disease* (2nd ed., pp. 466–471). Philadelphia: Saunders.

McCance, K., & Huether, S. (1994). *Pathophysiology: The biologic basis for disease in adults and children*. St. Louis: Mosby.

Moreno, C., & Iovanne, B. (1993a). Congenital diaphragmatic hernia: Part I. *Neonatal Network, 12*(1), 19–27.

Moreno, C., & Iovanne, B. (1993b). Congenital diaphragmatic hernia: Part II. *Neonatal Network, 12*(2), 21–27.

Neal, J., & Slayton, D. (1992). Neonatal and pediatric PEG tubes. *MCN: American Journal of Maternal/Child Nursing, 17*(4), 184-191.

Not, T., Ventura, A., Peticarari, S., Basile, S., Torre, G., & Dragovic, D. (1993). A new, rapid, noninvasive screening test for celiac disease. *The Journal of Pediatrics, 123*(3), 425–427.

Orenstein, S. R. (1999). Gastroesophageal reflux. In R. Wyllie & J. Hyams (Eds.), *Pediatric gastrointestinal disease* (2nd ed., pp. 164–188). Philadelphia: Saunders.

Pappas, S. C. (1995). Fulminant viral hepatitis. *Gastroenterology Clinics of North America, 24*(1), 161–173.

Perucca, R. (1992). Understanding Crohn's disease. *Journal of Intravenous Nursing, 15*(3), 164–169.

Phillips, J. D. (1999). Abdominal surgical emergencies. In R. Wyllie & J. Hyams (Eds.), *Pediatric gastrointestinal disease* (2nd ed., pp. 138–146). Philadelphia: Saunders.

Phillips, S., & Pemberton, J. (1998). Megacolon: Congenital and acquired. In M. Sleisenger & J. Fordtran (Eds.), *GI diseases: Pathophysiology, diagnosis and management*. Philadelphia: Saunders.

Puddoubnyi, I., Dronov, A., Blinnikov, A., Smirnov, I., Darenkov, T., & Dedov, K. (1998). Laparoscopy in the treatment of intussusception in children. *Journal of Pediatric Surgery, 33*(8), 1194–1197.

Ramos-Soriano, A. G., & Schwarz, K. B. (1994). Recent advances in hepatitis: Part I. *Gastroenterology Clinics of North America, 23*(4), 753–767.

Rao, P., Rhea, J., Novelline, R., Mostafavi, A., & McCabe, C. (1998). CT for appendicitis: No more surprises. *Gastroenterology, 115*(6), 1596–1598.

Resnick, J., & Zarem, H. (1996). Diseases and injuries of the oral region. In F. D. Burg, J. R. Ingelfinger, W. R. Wald, & R. A. Polin (Eds.), *Gellis and Kagan's current pediatric therapy* (15th ed., pp. 1029–1032). Philadelphia: Saunders.

Manifestations of Urinary Tract Infection in Infants and Children

Infants	Children	Children with Pyelonephritis
• Nonspecific	• Abdominal or suprapubic pain	• Same symptoms as children with urinary tract infection
• Fever or hypothermia in neonate	• Voiding frequency	• Fever
• Irritability	• Voiding urgency	• Back pain
• Dysuria as evidenced by crying when voiding	• Dysuria	• Costovertebral angle tenderness
• Change in urine odor or color	• New or increased incidence of enuresis	• Nausea and vomiting
• Poor weight gain	• Fever	• Appears sick
• Feeding difficulties		

child and infant are more vague and nonspecific. *Fever (38°C, 100.4°F) without a focus for infection in any boy younger than 6 months of age and any girl younger than 2 years of age suggests a UTI.*

An abdominal mass can suggest hydronephrosis in an infant. Other signs and symptoms of hydronephrosis are similar to those for an infant with a UTI.

Diagnostic Evaluation

Bacteria in the urine establishes a diagnosis of UTI. Symptoms of UTI in the absence of bacteriuria can be caused by perineal inflammation, vaginitis, pinworms, or chemical irritation from bubble baths.

Routine urinalysis that demonstrates hematuria, presence of WBCs, and positive nitrites can suggest a UTI. Urinalysis should be performed on a first morning urine specimen to be most accurate.

Urine culture is the single determining diagnostic study for a UTI. Any bacterial growth of a single strain bacteria exceeding 10^5 colony-forming units/ml of a clean-catch urine establishes a diagnosis of UTI. Obtaining a sterile urine is difficult in children, especially children who are not yet toilet trained. A child who can void on demand can provide a midstream clean-catch urine specimen. In infants and children who are not toilet trained, attaching a sterile pediatric urine collection bag to the perineum can collect a urine specimen (see Chapter 37). Collecting urine by this method is less invasive but not as accurate as by other methods, and the urine specimen must be plated as quickly as possible. If the urine cannot be plated within 10 minutes of collection, it should be refrigerated.

When accurate determination of bacteria is the goal, more intrusive methods of bladder catheterization (see Chapter 37) or suprapubic aspiration are the collection methods of choice. If suprapubic aspiration is necessary, the area above the pubis is cleaned with an antiseptic solution, a needle attached to a syringe is inserted into the bladder,

and urine is aspirated. If catheterization or suprapubic aspiration is used to obtain a urine culture, the growth of any bacteria indicates infection.

More intensive evaluation for underlying structural abnormalities is necessary for certain infants and children with UTIs. Evaluative studies most often include a voiding cystourethrogram (VCUG) or an isotope cystogram, renal ultrasound, and a dimercaptosuccininc acid (DMSA) renal scan.

Therapeutic Management

A 7- to 10-day course of oral antibiotics is the treatment of choice for an uncomplicated UTI without systemic symptoms. The antibiotic chosen should be sensitive to the specific bacteria (identified by culture), easily administered, and have minimal adverse effects. Oral trimethoprim-sulfamethoxazole and cephalosporins are frequently used. A follow-up urine culture evaluates treatment success.

Children with pyelonephritis require initial treatment with parenteral antibiotics followed by oral antibiotic treatment. The older child who does not need hospitalization can receive daily intramuscular ceftriaxone for 1 to 2 days followed by 10 to 14 days of oral antibiotics (Rushton, 1997). Infants and children admitted to the hospital for treatment usually receive an intravenous (IV) ampicillin or cephalosporin and an aminoglycoside (e.g., gentamicin). Oral antibiotics may follow this initial treatment.

CRITICAL TO REMEMBER

• • • • • • • • • •

Evaluation After a Documented Urinary Tract Infection

Radiologic studies are indicated for infants and children who are likely to experience renal damage associated with structural abnormalities. Studies can diagnose underlying abnormalities as well as monitor the extent of potential renal scarring. The following recommendations guide the necessity for follow-up:

• Radiographic imaging studies for at risk infants and children (all boys with UTIs and all girls younger than 5 years of age) after the *first* UTI.

• Evaluation of older girls with recurrent UTIs.

• Renal ultrasound before discharge in all infants and children hospitalized for treatment of a febrile UTI or suspected pyelonephritis.

• VCUG or isotope cystogram for at-risk children when symptoms have disappeared and the urine culture is negative. Some practitioners prefer to wait 4 to 6 weeks after the resolution of the UTI to allow transitory VUR to resolve.

• Renal scan for children diagnosed with VUR and children with suspected pyelonephritis.

• Evaluation of children after the first UTI who have hypertension, a family history of urinary tract abnormalities, or exhibit delayed growth.

When anatomic abnormalities are detected or UTIs re-occur, prophylactic antibiotic therapy might be initiated. Prophylactic antibiotics also are given to children after their initial course of treatment while they are waiting for imaging studies to confirm an underlying structural abnormality.

Because 60% to 80% of children with grades I to III VUR experience spontaneous resolution of the reflux, most physicians choose nonsurgical management of this condition (Belman, 1997). Children are given prophylactic antibiotics and screened for UTI every 2 to 4 months and when febrile. Cystography every 12 to 18 months monitors the progress of resolution.

Surgical intervention, or reimplantation of the ureters into the bladder, is indicated for severe grade IV and V reflux. Other indications for surgical treatment include frequent UTIs, presence of renal scarring, or noncompliance with antibiotic therapy. Nonsurgical treatment of the child with hydronephrosis is similar to the child with VUR. Surgery is required for children with complete obstruction.

NURSING CARE
. . . .
The Child with a Urinary Tract Infection

Assessment

The nurse obtains a history of signs and symptoms of UTI from the child and family, which will vary according to age. Determining bowel elimination patterns is important as well because constipation can increase the risk for UTI in certain children.

Physical assessment includes temperature, blood pressure, abdominal examination for masses, examination for costovertebral angle tenderness, and examination for genital abnormalities. It is important to obtain a urinalysis and urine culture before initiating antibiotics.

Nursing Diagnosis and Planning

The following nursing diagnoses apply to the child with UTI and family:

■ Risk for Injury to the kidney related to complications from the infectious process.
Expected Outcome: The child will be free of recurrent UTIs.
■ Fluid Volume Deficit related to decreased intake and increased fluid loss from fever.
Expected Outcome: The child will maintain adequate intake of fluids and electrolytes for age.
■ Knowledge Deficit related to incomplete understanding of disease process, diagnostic tests, antibiotic administration, and preventive measures for UTI.
Expected Outcome: The parent or child will verbalize an understanding of disease process, diagnostic tests, and preventive measures for UTIs. The child will receive appropriate follow-up care, including antibiotic administration and imaging studies, if recommended.

Interventions

Infants admitted to the hospital with fever of unknown origin often are evaluated to rule out a focal infection or septicemia, even though UTI is one of the most frequent causes of fever in infants. The evaluation includes blood studies and cultures, lumbar puncture, and urinary catheterization or suprapubic aspiration for urine culture. Parents already are anxious about their infant, so it is imperative that the

---

THE CHILD AND FAMILY WANT TO KNOW
. . . .
How to Manage and Prevent Urinary Tract Infections

If your child has been diagnosed with a urinary tract infection, it is most important for you to do the following:

• Give your child the prescribed medication for the full number of days your doctor recommends. Some children need to continue on a lower dose of the antibiotic after the initial treatment is finished.
• Be sure to take a follow-up urine culture to the laboratory if your doctor has requested one. Use a sterile container to collect the urine. If the laboratory has not given you a sterile plastic container, you can use a sterilized glass container with a cover that has been sterilized. Make sure the urine stays refrigerated or in a cooler while you take it to the laboratory.
• If the doctor has ordered some follow-up studies of your child's urinary system, make sure to keep the appointment. These studies can help the doctor diagnose a structural problem with your child's urinary system, or monitor the kidney for any problems.
• If your child has a fever or symptoms that make you think the infection has returned, call your doctor.

Preventing a urinary tract infection from reoccurring is important because repeated infections can cause kidney damage. Some of the following suggestions can help prevent a urinary tract infection.

• Wipe babies and teach young girls to wipe from front to back after going to the bathroom. This takes any germs away from the opening that leads into the urinary system. Be sure to keep the foreskin on uncircumcised baby boys as clean as possible.
• Encourage your toilet-trained child to avoid "holding" urine and to urinate at least four times a day, emptying the bladder completely.
• Give your child lots of fluids throughout the day to help flush out the bladder.
• Avoid dressing your child in tight clothing or diapers. Use cotton underwear, rather than nylon.
• Bubble baths can irritate your child's urinary system and should be avoided.
• If your daughter is sexually active, emphasize proper hygiene and encourage her to urinate immediately after having sexual intercourse.

of Acute Poststreptococcal Glomerulonephritis

Acute glomerulonephritis after a streptococcal infection is thought to occur as a result of an immunologic response. The body responds to the *Streptococcus* bacteria by forming antibodies, which combine with the bacterial antigens to form immune complexes. As these antigen-antibody complexes travel through the circulation, they become trapped in the glomerulus and activate an inflammatory response in the glomerular basement membrane. Products of the inflammatory response damage the glomerular capillaries and reduce the size of the capillary lumen. This process causes a decrease in the glomerular filtration rate, leading to renal insufficiency. Sodium and fluid are retained, and the child exhibits edema and oliguria. In addition, injury to the capillary walls interferes with their permeability so that larger molecules and structures such as red blood cells, casts, and proteins can pass through into the urine.

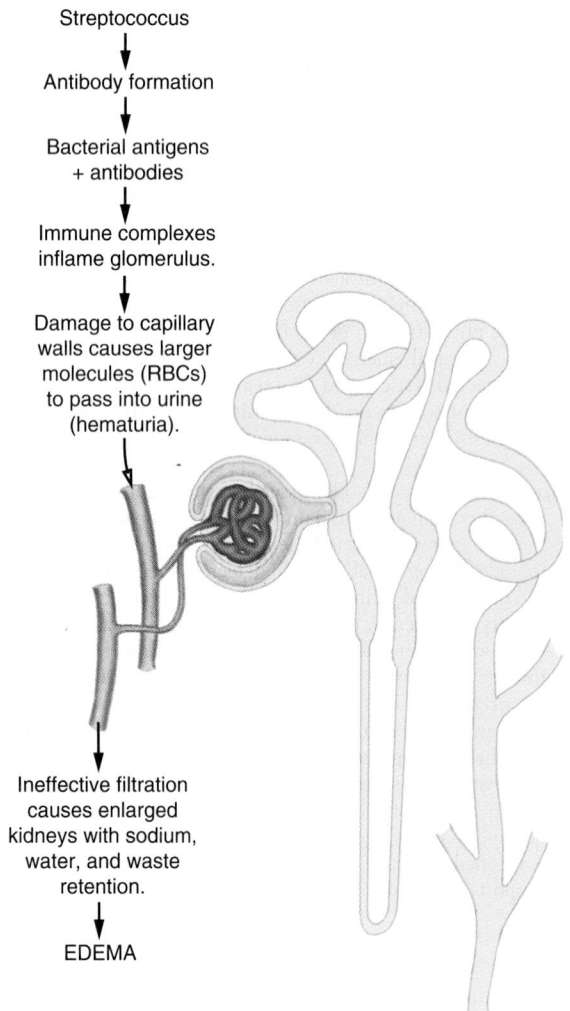

Streptococcus
↓
Antibody formation
↓
Bacterial antigens + antibodies
↓
Immune complexes inflame glomerulus.
↓
Damage to capillary walls causes larger molecules (RBCs) to pass into urine (hematuria).
↓
Ineffective filtration causes enlarged kidneys with sodium, water, and waste retention.
↓
EDEMA

of acute glomerulonephritis usually appear 7 to 10 days after a streptococcal infection (Blowey, 1998).

Manifestations

Hematuria, which is a cardinal sign of poststreptococcal glomerulonephritis, ranges in severity from microscopic to gross, as evidenced by smoky or tea-colored urine. Edema, which is worse in the morning, primarily affects the eyelids and ankles. This can be accompanied by decreased urinary output. Hypertension can be severe. The child may be febrile. Many children experience fatigue. Pulmonary edema can be a life-threatening complication.

Diagnostic Evaluation

History, presenting symptoms, and laboratory results can establish the diagnosis of acute poststreptococcal glomerulonephritis. A urinalysis reveals macroscopic or microscopic hematuria with red cell casts, which indicate glomerular injury. Proteinuria is also present but not severe. Blood chemistry values are usually within the normal range. If renal insufficiency is severe, however, BUN and creatinine levels are elevated. Electrolyte disturbances, such as high serum potassium and low serum bicarbonate, can result from inadequate glomerular filtration.

The complete blood count usually demonstrates normal white blood cells (WBCs) and mild anemia. The lower hemoglobin and hematocrit values reflect the dilutional effect of extra fluid in the blood as a result of decreased glomerular filtration.

Immunologic studies are important in diagnosing acute poststreptococcal glomerulonephritis. Serum complement (C3) may be low because of the fixation of complement in immune complexes. An antistreptolysin (ASO) titer, which indicates the presence of antibodies to streptococcal bacteria, or a Streptozyme test can be elevated. The ASO titer might not be elevated in a streptococcal skin infection. Culture of the throat or skin lesion (if present) may be helpful for isolating the bacteria. Again, this is useful only if the infection is recent and the child has not received antibiotics. A renal biopsy may be indicated for two reasons: (1) for those children whose signs and symptoms are not characteristic of acute poststreptococcal glomerular nephritis, and (2) for those children whose symptoms do not improve as expected.

Therapeutic Management

There is no specific therapy for acute poststreptococcal glomerulonephritis. Supportive care and medical management are directed to the associated signs and symptoms and guided by the degree of renal dysfunction the child experiences. Children with acute renal failure should be hospitalized to allow for fluid and electrolyte management until their renal function has stabilized.

Antihypertensive therapy may be necessary. This can be accomplished by limiting sodium and water intake or by the administration of diuretics or antihypertensive medication. The prognosis for children with acute poststreptococcal glomerulonephritis is excellent. The acute clinical episode is usually self-limiting, with diuresis signaling the beginning of resolution. Laboratory values usually return to baseline in 6 to 12 weeks. Most children experience a complete recovery.

NURSING CARE
The Child with Acute Poststreptococcal Glomerulonephritis

Assessment

Assess the child for presence of periorbital or lower extremity edema. Obtaining vital signs and monitoring daily weight is important for assessing the degree of fluid retention and hypertension. Be sure to use the appropriate size blood pressure cuff for the most accurate blood pressure measurement (see Chapter 37). Monitor the child's level of fatigue and anxiety.

Assess the respiratory system for presence of any respiratory difficulty such as cough, increased respiratory rate, or increased work of breathing. Auscultate the breath sounds for crackles. Monitor laboratory values, especially urinalysis and serum electrolytes.

Determine what the child and family understand about the illness and reason for hospitalization. The parents may be anxious about permanent damage to the child's kidneys as a result of this condition.

Nursing Diagnosis and Planning

The following nursing diagnoses apply to the child with acute poststreptococcal glomerulonephritis and family:

■ Fluid Volume Excess related to retention of sodium and fluid.
  Expected Outcome: The child will maintain normal fluid status, as evidenced by urine output of at least 1 to 2 ml/kg/hr, normal blood pressure, no increase in weight, and no symptoms of respiratory distress.
■ Risk for Activity Intolerance related to fatigue.
  Expected Outcome: The child will be rested, as evidenced by the ability to tolerate daily care and play activities.
■ Risk for Impaired Skin Integrity related to edema and decreased activity.
  Expected Outcome: The child will exhibit no signs of skin breakdown, as evidenced by skin that is intact, normal color for race, and nontender to touch.
■ Altered Nutrition: Less Than Body Requirements related to fluid and diet restrictions.
  Expected Outcome: The child will have adequate hydration and nutrition, as evidenced by moist mucous membranes and maintenance of weight at pre-illness level.
■ Anxiety related to knowledge deficit regarding disease process or hospitalization.
  Expected Outcomes: Anxiety will be decreased in the child, as evidenced by cooperation with daily care and interest in developmentally appropriate play. Parents or caregiver will verbalize understanding of disease process.

Interventions

Preventing the Consequences of Fluid Excess

Frequent, accurate assessment of intake and output is essential for evaluating fluid status. Children with severe renal impairment might require measurement of intake and output every 2 to 4 hours. Fluid intake includes oral intake and intravenous fluids. Report urine output of less than 1 to 2 ml/kg/hr because oliguria suggests impending renal failure.

Accurate daily weights are important for determining fluctuation in fluid status. The nurse obtains daily weights, remembering to weigh the child on the same scale at approximately the same time every day for maximum consistency. Infants and young children should be weighed without diapers and older children should wear only a gown.

Because hypertension from fluid overload and glomerular damage is a severe consequence of this condition, the nurse measures blood pressure with an appropriately sized cuff every shift and documents the results. Report increasing values immediately. More frequent readings might be required if the child has significant hypertension or receives antihypertensive medication.

Auscultate breath sounds every shift and document increased respiratory effort. Rapid respirations, retractions, nasal flaring, or crackles are signs of developing pulmonary edema, which can result from fluid overload.

Limit fluid intake if ordered. Limitation might be difficult if children are old enough to sneak drinks on their own or obtain them from people who are unaware of restrictions. The nurse should inform parents, visitors, and hospital staff of the need to limit fluids. Be sure to record the child's favorite fluids on the nursing care plan, so the child is able to enjoy the fluids given. Encourage the child to consume fluids gradually, rather than large amounts all at once. Provide the child with only the agreed-on amount for the period involved.

Excessive sodium can increase fluid retention. The nurse ensures that a low-sodium diet is followed if ordered. Inform parents and visitors of any diet restrictions.

Providing Adequate Rest

If fatigue is a problem, it is important that the child have ample opportunity to rest. Children with glomerulonephritis may tire easily when first hospitalized, although most children participate in activities according to their level of fatigue. The nurse needs to arrange daily care so that the child has some uninterrupted time for sleep and naps. Encourage parents to bring a favorite sleep toy or blanket for the child, and allow for nap time and bed time to coincide with the child's home schedule as much as possible. Try to follow home rituals. If the child is unable to limit activity, the nurse can limit play time to short periods and extend as the child's condition improves.

Maintaining Skin Integrity

Frequent position changes decrease pressure on bony prominences and help to decrease edema in dependent areas. Encourage the child to change position at least every 2 hours during the day. If the child is experiencing edema of the lower extremities, elevate them with pillows when the child is sitting or lying in bed. Promote activity as the child improves because activity increases the circulation and promotes reabsorption of fluid in edematous areas.

To prevent skin breakdown, the nurse maintains good hygiene by giving baths and cleaning the skin well after

Nursing Diagnosis, Planning, Intervention, and Evaluation

Nursing Diagnosis

■ Risk for Impaired Skin Integrity related to edema and decreased circulation

Expected Outcome

• The child will not exhibit signs of skin breakdown, as evidenced by the absence of redness, tenderness to touch, and ulceration.

Intervention	Rationale
1. Ensure that the child changes position every 2 hours.	1. Frequent position change decreases pressure on body parts and helps relieve edema in dependent areas.
2. Maintain good hygiene by giving daily baths and changing linen daily. Use lotion for dry skin.	2. Body secretions and debris on linens can irritate the skin. Gentle massage when bathing and applying lotion help increase circulation.
3. Support or elevate edematous body parts with pillows while the child is in bed or sitting in a chair.	3. Edema is gravity dependent. Elevation helps move fluid away from dependent body parts.
4. Promote physical activity, as the child is able to tolerate, by providing developmentally appropriate play activities.	4. Increased activity helps promote circulation.

Evaluation

• Is the child's skin intact without redness or tenderness?

Nursing Diagnosis

■ Risk for Infection related to urinary loss of gamma-globulins and immunosuppressive therapy

Expected Outcome

• The child will demonstrate no evidence of an infection, as evidenced by normal WBC count, normal body temperature, and absence of abdominal pain and cough.

Intervention	Rationale
1. Screen visitors for signs of infection such as upper respiratory symptoms, sore throats, or exposure to communicable diseases.	1. Communicable diseases, especially varicella, pose a serious threat because the child on immunosuppressive therapy is not able to respond appropriately to infection.
2. Administer antibiotics as ordered.	2. Antibiotics are usually given for peritonitis prophylaxis during the edematous phase.
3. Use good hand washing techniques and instruct family members to do the same.	3. Hand washing helps decrease transmission of germs.
4. Monitor child for fever, cough, sore throat, or complaints of abdominal pain each shift. Monitor laboratory values.	4. Frequent monitoring ensures early detection of infectious processes. Abdominal pain can be an indication of peritonitis.

Evaluation

• Does the child maintain normal body temperature and exhibit normal laboratory values?
• Is the child free from cough, pain, or other signs of infection?

Nursing Diagnosis

■ Risk for Fluid Volume Deficit (intravascular) related to proteinuria, edema, and effects of diuretics

Expected Outcome

• The child does not experience decreased fluid volume as evidenced by normal blood pressure measurement, adequate urine output, and normal hematocrit and hemoglobin.

Intervention	Rationale
1. Monitor vital signs, including blood pressure and pulse, every shift. Report variance from baseline.	1. Low blood pressure and increased heart rate are signs of hypovolemia. Blood pressure may be elevated due to renin release.
2. Monitor intake and output every shift. Report if child has output of less than 1 to 2 ml/kg/hr of urine.	2. Accurate intake and output measurement is essential for evaluating fluid status.
3. Monitor laboratory values.	3. Increasing values of hemoglobin, hematocrit, and platelets may indicate hemoconcentration or low intravascular volume.

4. Observe for signs of dehydration such as appearance of mucous membranes, capillary refill, and level of activity. (Capillary refill may be altered because of edema; assess in nonedematous area.) Report positive findings.

4. The pathophysiology of nephrotic syndrome may predispose the child to decreased intravascular volume. This condition is compounded by the use of diuretics.

Evaluation

- Are the child's vital signs within normal limits?
- Is the urine output at least 1 to 2 ml/kg/hr?
- Does the child have moist mucous membranes and good skin turgor?

Nursing Diagnosis

■ Fluid Volume Excess related to decreased excretion of sodium and fluid retention

Expected Outcome

- The child will not demonstrate fluid overload as evidenced by stable daily weights and normal respiratory pattern.

Intervention	Rationale
1. Monitor intake and output each shift.	1. Accurate intake and output are essential for evaluating fluid status.
2. Obtain accurate daily weights. Weigh child on same scales, at same time each day, in gown only.	2. Daily weights are necessary to detect changes in fluid status. Clothing or presence of wet diaper can alter weight. Readings of weight can vary from scale to scale and time of day.
3. Adhere to no-added-salt diet.	3. Excessive sodium intake can increase amount of water retention.
4. Measure and record abdominal girth each day. Ensure accuracy by measuring in same area each time.	4. Edema commonly occurs in the abdomen.
5. Monitor blood pressure at least once each shift.	5. Increased total-body fluid volume and concurrent steroid therapy can result in increased blood pressure.
6. Administer diuretics as ordered. Ensure adequate potassium intake.	6. Diuretics may aid in the elimination of excessive fluid. Diuretics can increase excretion of potassium.
7. Monitor pulmonary status by listening to breath sounds for crackles and observing for signs of increased work of breathing and presence of cough.	7. Fluid overload can result in pulmonary edema.

Evaluation

- Does the child maintain a stable weight?
- Is the child free from respiratory distress?

Nursing Diagnosis

■ Anxiety (parental) related to hospitalization of child and caring for a child with chronic disease.
■ Knowledge Deficit about home management related to anxiety or incomplete understanding.

Expected Outcomes

- The parents will demonstrate decreased anxiety as evidenced by participating in the care of their child and verbalizing an understanding of the disease process.
- The parents will be able to explain principles of home management.

Intervention	Rationale
1. Allow parents to verbalize frustration and fears. Encourage them to ask questions and provide them with information about nephrotic syndrome and its treatment.	1. Verbalization of fears is often therapeutic in itself. Information helps decrease anxiety because people often fear the unknown.
2. Incorporate the parents' help in the daily care of the child. Have them practice using Albustix, taking blood pressures, and assessing edema.	2. Nephrotic syndrome can be a chronic condition and is usually managed at home. It is important for the parents to feel comfortable with caring for their child.
3. Arrange for a dietary consult.	3. Steroid therapy stimulates appetite. Children should be informed about low-calorie snacks and portion size. Encourage the parent to cook without salt and remove the salt shaker from the child's access.

4. Teach the parent how to maintain a daily calendar of protein readings, how to do a daily weight, what medications are appropriate for the child, and how to prevent infection. Encourage the parent to report any exposure to communicable disease.

4. Providing appropriate information allows the family to manage the child's care. The child's urine protein results are monitored for signs of relapse. It is important to check with the nephrologist before giving the child any over-the-counter medications because some medications can aggravate hypertension. Children on steroids are unable to respond appropriately to viral or bacterial infections and may require additional treatment.

Evaluation

• Do the parents verbalize understanding of their child's condition and required treatment?
• Do the parents actively participate in the child's care?

Acute Renal Failure

Acute renal failure is defined as the sudden, severe loss of kidney function. In acute renal failure, the kidneys can no longer filter waste products, regulate fluid volume, or maintain chemical balance. Most children with acute renal failure regain renal function.

Etiology and Incidence

Possible causes of prerenal failure are dehydration, perinatal asphyxia, hypotension, septic shock, hemorrhagic shock, and renal artery obstruction. Nephrotoxins such as aminoglycosides and contrast dye, ureterovesical obstruction, he-

molytic uremic syndrome (HUS), glomerulonephritis, and pyelonephritis cause intrarenal acute renal failure. Postrenal acute renal failure is associated with structural abnormalities such as ureteropelvic obstruction, ureterovesical obstruction, posterior urethral valves, neurogenic bladder, and outlet obstruction by stones, tumor, or edema.

Hemolytic uremic syndrome is the most frequent cause of acute renal failure in children. HUS is an acute disorder characterized by anemia, thrombocytopenia, and acute renal failure. Children with HUS become infected by *E. coli* in improperly cooked meat or contaminated dairy products. Acute renal failure in the child is uncommon.

Manifestations

Manifestations of acute renal failure include electrolyte imbalances, fluid imbalances, increased BUN and serum creatinine, acid-base imbalances, and nonspecific manifestations such as poor feeding or decreased appetite, vomiting, lethargy, seizures, and pallor. In children with HUS, gastrointestinal illness characterized by abdominal pain, fever, vomiting, and bloody diarrhea may be present.

Diagnostic Evaluation

Determining the underlying cause of acute renal failure is very important. If the underlying cause can be reversed, renal function usually returns to normal.

HISTORY
The history often gives an indication of the underlying cause of the acute renal failure. Vomiting, diarrhea, and fever may indicate dehydration and prerenal acute renal failure. It is necessary to ascertain any recent history of bloody diarrhea that might suggest HUS.

FLUID STATUS
Acute renal failure is usually associated with dehydration and oliguria (urine output <1 ml/kg/hr). Urine output might be normal or increased.

LABORATORY DATA
Serum creatinine and BUN levels are increased. BUN, an end product of protein catabolism, may reflect the nutritional status of the child. Metabolic acidosis can occur, as indicated by low serum bicarbonate. Serum potassium may be increased. Serum sodium may be increased or decreased

PATHOPHYSIOLOGY
of Acute Renal Failure

Acute renal failure is categorized as prerenal, intrarenal, or postrenal. *Prerenal acute renal failure* is the result of decreased perfusion of the kidney. The kidney must have adequate blood flow for effective functioning. The decreased blood flow and subsequent ischemia cause cellular swelling and injury, and possible cell death. *Intrarenal acute renal failure* is the result of actual ischemic damage to kidney tissue. *Postrenal acute renal failure* is the result of obstruction of urine outflow. The obstruction increases pressure within the kidney, which decreases renal function.

Impaired perfusion markedly decreases the glomerular filtration rate, triggering oliguria (markedly decreased urine output), azotemia (elevated blood levels of urea, creatinine, and uric acid), and associated electrolyte imbalances. Tissue injury further magnifies the damage and the decreased perfusion.

As the underlying problem is treated, recovery of the renal endothelial and tubular cells begins and renal function gradually returns. Because the glomerular filtration rate returns to normal faster than the tubular transport mechanisms, the child begins to diurese large amounts of dilute urine. The danger for dehydration is high at this time (Hansen, 1998). Renal function gradually returns to normal.

PATHOPHYSIOLOGY

of Hemolytic Uremic Syndrome

Most affected children have an associated prodrome of gastrointestinal symptoms, including bloody diarrhea, which suggests that an infectious agent may be the cause of HUS. Studies have shown a strong association between the syndrome and an enteric infection with *E. coli* 0157:H7 (Neumann & Urizar, 1994). Two important characteristics of *E. coli* 0157:H7 contribute to the development of HUS. First, because this bacterium attaches itself to the intestinal mucosa, its clearance through normal intestinal peristalsis is decreased, allowing the bacteria to grow and multiply. Second, the bacteria produce a toxin that damages the endothelial cells of capillary walls, and the subsequent inflammatory response results in occlusion of capillaries. This is especially significant in the renal glomeruli. The occlusion of glomerular vessels decreases filtration and results in acute renal failure. However, it is important to understand that the vascular process seen in HUS can affect *any* organ. Anemia results from fragmentation of red blood cells, which are damaged as they try to pass through the occluded vessels and are removed from circulation by the spleen. Thrombocytopenia occurs because the platelets get trapped within the small vessels.

depending on fluid status. The child with HUS exhibits hemolytic anemia, thrombocytopenia, hematuria, urine casts, proteinuria, and *E. coli* by stool culture.

PHYSICAL EXAMINATION
The child may be hypertensive. Edema secondary to decreased urine output and fluid overload may be present. The child may be in respiratory distress secondary to fluid overload.

IMAGING STUDIES
Renal ultrasound may help with diagnosis of obstruction and postrenal acute renal failure. Renal scan can be helpful in the diagnosis of the cause of renal failure. It can assess blood flow, function, and obstruction.

Therapeutic Management

Many children in acute renal failure are managed without dialysis. Management includes the following principles.

FLUID IMBALANCES
Fluid balance is an important component of the management of a child with acute renal failure. If the child is dehydrated, careful fluid replacement is essential. Fluid restriction is necessary for a child who has decreased or absent urine output and is adequately hydrated or fluid overloaded. Fluid intake is carefully calculated to replace insensible fluid loss and urinary output. Maintaining fluid restriction can be difficult for some children. It is helpful to give small amounts more frequently, rather than a large amount occa-

sionally. Older children can participate in decision making about the kind and frequency of fluids.

ELECTROLYTE IMBALANCES
Potassium. Most children with acute renal failure have a high potassium level, requiring intervention when the serum potassium level is 6 mEq/L. Potassium is restricted from the diet and IV fluids. Interventions to remove potassium include instituting gastric suction; administration of an exchange resin such as Kayexalate; or administration of sodium bicarbonate, glucose, and insulin.

Sodium. The sodium level may be elevated or decreased. It is more common for the level to be decreased because of water overload. Fluid restriction helps improve the serum sodium level. Any replacement sodium is adjusted to maintain a normal sodium level.

Acid-Base. Children with acute renal failure are unable to excrete hydrogen ions and ammonia through the kidney, and develop metabolic acidosis (low serum bicarbonate). Additional sodium bicarbonate can be administered orally or intravenously.

NUTRITION
Children with acute renal failure are at risk for malnutrition because of decreased appetite and restricted intake (Heiliczer, 1999). The underlying principle of nutritional therapy for these children is to provide maximum calories and protein within the fluid restrictions. Foods should be low in sodium and potassium.

DIALYSIS
Dialysis is a process of removing waste products and excess body fluid and regulating electrolytes and minerals. Two types of dialysis are hemodialysis and peritoneal dialysis.

NURSING CARE

The Child with Acute Renal Failure

Most children with acute renal failure are cared for in special care units. Principles of nursing care include (1) monitoring and maintaining fluid, electrolyte, and acid-base balance; (2) preventing infection; (3) providing adequate nutrition; (4) reducing parent and child anxiety; and (5) teaching about dialysis.

CRITICAL TO REMEMBER

Indications for Dialysis in Acute Renal Failure

- Severe fluid overload
- Pulmonary edema or congestive heart failure secondary to fluid overload
- Severe hypertension
- Metabolic acidosis not responsive to medications
- Hyperkalemia not responsive to medications
- Blood urea nitrogen greater than 120 mg/dl

Dialysis

Dialysis is a process of removing waste products and excess body fluids, and regulating electrolytes and minerals. It is sometimes necessary in acute renal failure. When chronic renal failure progresses to end-stage renal disease, dialysis or kidney transplantation is required.

There are two types of dialysis: hemodialysis and peritoneal dialysis.

HEMODIALYSIS

Hemodialysis cleanses the blood by circulating it through a special filter called an *artificial kidney*. Blood is pumped through the artificial kidney and returned to the body. Hemodialysis occurs through a vascular access such as a double-lumen central line or an arteriovenous fistula or shunt. The access is surgically placed. Children who receive chronic dialysis usually receive treatments three times a week for 3 to 4 hours each time.

The major complications of hemodialysis include access infection and access obstruction. In addition, there is a disruption of school, peer, and family life because of the treatment schedule. However, children treated with hemodialysis in a specialized pediatric unit can thrive. In infants and small children, hemodialysis is technically more difficult, and fluid and electrolyte shifts more pronounced.

Hemodialysis is more efficient and requires less time than peritoneal dialysis. In addition, there is less responsibility for the family.

PERITONEAL DIALYSIS

In peritoneal dialysis, fluid enters the peritoneal cavity through a catheter, which may be placed in the child at the bedside or in the operating room. The dialysis fluid remains in the cavity for a prescribed time, during which waste products, chemicals, and fluid pass through the peritoneal membrane into the fluid. The fluid is then drained and the process is repeated.

In children receiving chronic dialysis, the exchanges can be performed overnight with an automated cycler, or manually four to five times per day. The treatments usually are performed at home.

Peritoneal dialysis is technically easier than hemodialysis. Advantages over hemodialysis include more independence for the child and family, and a more stable physiologic state because of frequent dialysis. The disadvantages include the risk of infections (peritonitis and catheter exit site), and family and child fatigue from treatment demands.

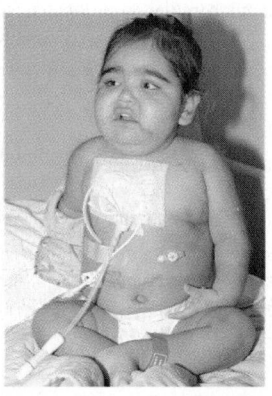

◄ Peritoneal dialysis. Implanted lines allow instillation of the dialyzing fluid into this child's peritoneal cavity. This child has rejected a transplanted kidney and receives peritoneal dialysis until another transplant will be attempted. She was previously on steroids in an attempt to control rejection, which accounts for the characteristics typical of Cushing's syndrome.

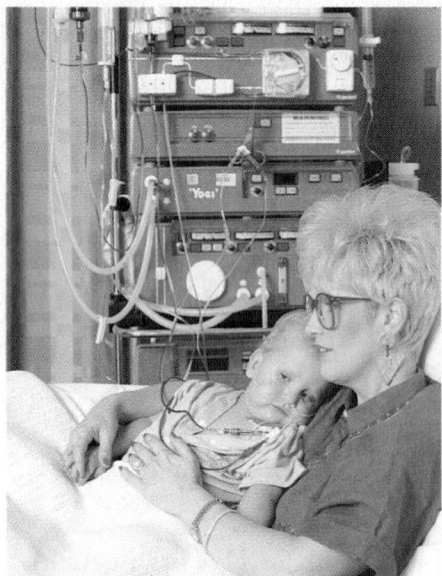

Child receiving hemodialysis. Family members should participate in the child's care as much as possible.

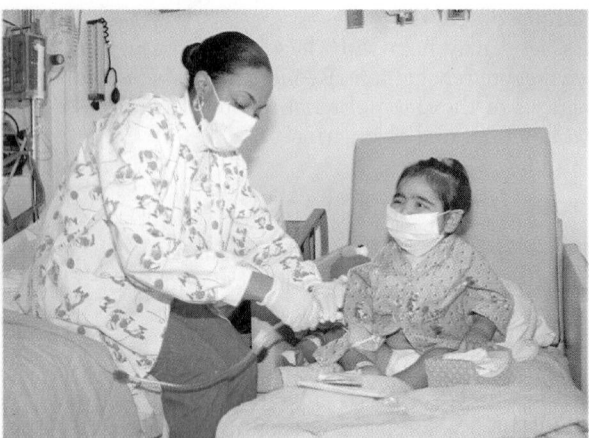

Infection of the peritoneal cavity is the chief hazard of peritoneal dialysis. When the lines are open to begin or end the dialyzing cycle, both adult and child wear masks.

Photos courtesy of Children's Medical Center, Dallas, Texas.

Chronic Renal Failure and End-Stage Renal Disease

Chronic renal failure is an irreversible loss of kidney function that occurs over months to years. It can be managed conservatively with medications and diet restrictions. Chronic renal failure progresses to ESRD, which is the permanent, irreversible loss of kidney function that can no longer be managed conservatively to maintain life and health. Dialysis or transplantation is required to treat ESRD. Treatment usually occurs when only 5% to 10% of kidney function remains.

Pathophysiology

Regardless of the cause of kidney damage, chronic renal failure progresses to ESRD. The exact mechanisms are unclear. The factors that may contribute negatively are ongoing immunologic injury, hyperfiltration (the overwork of the remaining nephrons), high dietary protein and phosphorus intake, persistent proteinuria, and hypertension.

Etiology

The causes of chronic renal failure in children are different from those in adults. The most common cause, especially in younger children, is congenital anomalies such as obstruction, VUR, and renal dysplasia. Chronic renal failure can develop in children from diseases such as glomerulonephritis, pyelonephritis, and HUS. In general, secondary causes of ESRD such as diabetes and high blood pressure are not seen in children. In adults, approximately 35% of people with insulin-dependent diabetes contract ESRD (Foster, 1994).

Incidence

The incidence of chronic renal failure with ESRD among children younger than 19 years of age is approximately 1 in 100,000 (Taylor, 1996). The incidence is higher in adolescents, in boys, and in whites.

Manifestations

Manifestations of chronic renal failure and ESRD include electrolyte imbalance, fluid imbalance (dehydration or fluid overload), acid-base imbalance, renal bone disease (osteodystrophy) and rickets, anemia, poor growth, hypertension, fatigue, decreased appetite or poor feeding, nausea and vomiting, and neurologic symptoms from accumulation of wastes.

Diagnostic Evaluation

Chronic renal failure may present itself nonspecifically. Physical examination may reveal short stature and failure to thrive. The child may be hypertensive. Blood work reveals electrolyte abnormalities (varying according to the underlying disease process), calcium and phosphorus abnormalities (decreased calcium and bone calcium resorption, elevated serum phosphorus), or anemia. Rising creatinine and BUN suggest ESRD. Creatinine clearance testing measures the ability of the renal system to excrete metabolic products. Bone radiographs diagnose renal osteodystrophy. The child may have normal fluid volume, be dehydrated, or have fluid overload.

The history may or may not include known renal disease. Diagnostic tests may be performed to determine etiology and prognosis. These may include VCUG, renal ultrasound, renal scan, and renal biopsy.

Therapeutic Management

CHRONIC RENAL FAILURE

The diet of a child with chronic renal failure is modified secondary to the decreased ability of the kidney to regulate fluids, electrolytes, minerals, and waste products. This might include the following restrictions: salt and fluid to prevent fluid overload and hypertension, protein because of the kidney's inability to remove waste products, phosphorus to help prevent bone disease, and potassium because of the kidney's inability to remove it.

Diuretics also are indicated to control fluid balance, and antihypertensives are given for hypertension. Sodium bicarbonate may be necessary to maintain acid-base balance. Vitamin D and phosphorus-binding medications may be helpful in preventing bone disease.

Advances in the treatment of infants and children with chronic renal failure such as recombinant erythropoietin and recombinant growth hormone have improved the quality of life of these children (Taylor, 1996). Recombinant erythropoietin is used to treat anemia, thus avoiding repeated blood transfusions and improving the energy level. The use of recombinant growth hormone has significantly improved the growth of children with chronic renal failure.

END-STAGE RENAL DISEASE

Once a child reaches ESRD, dialysis or kidney transplantation is required for health and life. The diagnosis of ESRD is made by monitoring serum creatinine, glomerular filtration rate, and the quality of the child's life. ESRD usually is diagnosed when the glomerular filtration rate decreases to about 10%.

KIDNEY TRANSPLANTATION

Transplantation is the goal for most children with ESRD, and offers the best opportunity to have a normal lifestyle. Unfortunately, transplantation is not a cure. Children who have received transplants must continue to take immunosuppressive medication, have blood tests, and keep clinic appointments.

Kidneys come from two types of donors: living donors and cadaveric donors. A living donor is someone in the child's family such as a parent or grandparent. A person who donates must be in good health and have healthy kidneys. A cadaveric donor kidney is a healthy kidney obtained from someone who is brain dead and whose family has consented to the transplantation. The blood and tissue types of the donor and recipient need to be compatible. Transplantations using kidneys from a relative have been more successful in children than those using cadaveric kidneys.

Rejection is the most common complication of kidney transplantation. Immunosuppressive medications, taken to help prevent rejection, include cyclosporine, azathioprine, and prednisone. Newer immunosuppressive drugs include tacrolimus (Prograf), mycophenolate mofetil, and a new form of cyclosporine (Neoral).

As with all medications, immunosuppressive medications have side effects. When the immune system is suppressed, there is an increased risk of infection related to the body's decreased ability to fight infection. Children with renal transplants should be monitored for infection and may take anti-infective medications routinely.

High blood pressure is also a complication of transplantation. Underlying renal disease, the transplanted kidney, or immunosuppressive medication side effects can cause high blood pressure.

NURSING CARE
The Child with Chronic Renal Failure and End-Stage Renal Disease

Assessment

The assessment of the child with chronic renal failure or ESRD is directed toward clinical manifestations of the renal failure and its possible complications. Blood work is monitored for abnormalities and response to interventions. Monitoring hemoglobin and hematocrit assesses for potential anemia and monitors response to therapy in the child receiving recombinant erythropoietin. Serum calcium and phosphorus, alkaline phosphatase, and parathyroid hormone levels, as well as bone radiographs are obtained to monitor for renal osteodystrophy.

The nurse assesses fluid status for fluid overload and dehydration. Monitor fluid status by obtaining weight, monitoring blood pressure and heart rate, and observing and recording edema, skin turgor, mucous membranes, and fontanel.

Obtain accurate weights and height measurements regularly to assess growth and development. Ask the parent about the child's dietary and caloric intake. Information regarding attainment of development tasks, school performance, and peer relationships is helpful.

Nursing Diagnosis and Planning

The following nursing diagnoses apply to the child with chronic renal failure and family:

■ Altered Nutrition: Less Than Body Requirements related to decreased appetite and dietary restrictions.
Expected Outcome: The child will receive adequate nutrition for growth and health as measured by appropriate growth for age.
■ Knowledge Deficit about disease process, treatment, or diet restrictions related to anxiety or incomplete understanding of principles.
Expected Outcome: The child/parents will be able to explain the disease process, its treatment, and dietary restrictions.

■ Fluid Volume Excess/Deficit related to fluid and electrolyte imbalances secondary to renal dysfunction.
Expected Outcome: The child will exhibit no signs of fluid overload or deficit as measured by weight, blood pressure, and absence of edema or signs of dehydration.
■ Altered Growth and Development related to restricted diet, chronic illness, and anemia.
Expected Outcome: The child will attain maximum growth and development.
■ Altered Family Processes related to having a child with chronic and potentially life-threatening disease.
Expected Outcome: The child and family will achieve successful coping strategies, as measured by their ability to care for child.
■ Risk for Impaired Skin Integrity related to edema and poor nutrition.
Expected Outcome: The child's skin will not show signs of break in skin integrity (redness, irritation, breaks).

Interventions

The care of the child with chronic renal failure or ESRD is complex and requires a multidisciplinary team. Maintaining adequate nutritional intake within the dietary restriction parameters is a challenge. The nurse individualizes the diet of the child with chronic renal failure and includes foods the child likes. Small, frequent meals may be helpful. Diet supplements may be necessary to meet caloric needs. Recombinant growth hormone may allow the child to have adequate growth.

Children with chronic renal failure and their families have multifaceted information requirements. The parents need information regarding diet, medications, potential effects of the renal failure, and its treatment. They need to be informed regarding treatment options such as hemodialysis, peritoneal dialysis, and transplantation.

Provide appropriate fluid intake and ongoing assessment of fluid status. Instruct the child and family about fluid restriction and hydration assessment such as weight, blood pressure, and appearance of edema.

Encourage the child to participate in school and age-appropriate activities. Parents may find it difficult to allow the child autonomy and will need support to do so.

The child with chronic renal failure and the family need support. They need opportunities to ask questions, verbalize feelings, and express concerns. Involving children in their own care and decisions regarding treatment is beneficial. Determine the family's prior successful coping strategies and encourage family members to use those. Additional help from social service, psychology, or psychiatry may be helpful.

Evaluation

• Has the child shown normal growth patterns for age?
• Can the parents and the child discuss diet restrictions?
• Is the child free of edema?
• Is the family involved in the care of the child?
• Has the integrity of the child's skin been maintained?
• Has the child verbalized anxiety related to disease?

KEY CONCEPTS

- The kidney reaches near-adult function at 6 to 12 months of age.
- Infants cannot concentrate urine as efficiently as older children and adults.
- Most children eventually outgrow enuresis with therapeutic intervention.
- The clinical manifestations of UTIs vary according to the child's age, underlying anatomic or neurologic abnormalities, and frequency of recurrence.
- Urinary tract infection is the most common clinical manifestation of VUR. Medical management includes low-dose prophylactic antibiotic therapy to prevent renal scarring.
- Nursing care of the child with a UTI includes giving information to the parents and child about peri-

neal hygiene, increased fluid intake, emptying of bladder, and the wearing of cotton underwear.
- Most infants with cryptorchidism have spontaneous descent of their testes during the first year of life.
- The goal of surgery to correct hypospadias is to make urinary and sexual function as normal as possible and to improve the cosmetic appearance of the penis.
- Children with glomerulonephritis should be assessed for hypertension and the presence of any respiratory difficulty such as cough, increased respiratory rate, and difficulty breathing, which may indicate fluid overload.
- Children at risk for fluid volume excess due to decreased urine output should be weighed daily on the same scale, at the same time, wear-

ing only a gown. Infants should have their diapers removed.
- Children with edema should have their position changed at least every 2 hours and their lower extremities elevated when they are sitting or lying in bed.
- Edema related to nephrotic syndrome is first noted in the periorbital spaces and dependent areas of the body. The child may awaken with facial edema; as the day progresses, edema becomes more noticeable. Prednisone usually induces a remission in the child with nephrotic syndrome.
- Most children with acute renal failure regain renal function.
- Children with chronic renal failure and ESRD and their families require multidisciplinary care and extensive nursing support.

ANSWERS TO CRITICAL THINKING EXERCISE 44–1

1. The nurse should first determine whether Thomas has ever been able to be dry at night. This information helps discriminate between primary and secondary nocturnal enuresis. Other information the nurse will need includes (1) whether Thomas has experienced any excessive thirst or weight loss (signs of diabetes mellitus), (2) whether he complains about anal itching (rule out pinworms), and (3) whether he has a fever or other signs of a urinary tract infection. It would also be

helpful to know what approach the parents used during toilet training and whether either parent had enuresis as a child.
2. After underlying problems have been ruled out, the nurse can reassure Mr. Sampson that nighttime wetting is not unusual in children of this age, and the initial approach should be one of benign neglect. Focusing too much on the problem can create anxiety in the child, and decreased self-esteem if the problem persists later into childhood. The nurse can suggest

that the parents encourage Thomas to wear a disposable diaper or waterproof pull-up at night. They can explain to Thomas that lots of children this age need to be in pull-ups for a while, and that it does not mean that he is a baby. When he has stayed dry, he can decide to try going without the pull-up. Putting a plastic draw sheet covered by a regular draw sheet over the middle portion of the bed can reduce the amount of laundry required and preserve the mattress.

REFERENCES AND READINGS

Ahmed, S. (1998). Evaluation and treatment of urinary tract infections in children. *American Family Physician, 57*(7), 1573–1579.

Arant, B. (1999). Vesicoureteral reflux. In F. Burg, E. Wald, J. Ingelfinger, & R. Polin (Eds.), *Gellis and Kagan's current pediatric therapy* (16th ed., pp. 849–851). Philadelphia: Saunders.

Barkin, R., & Rosen, P. (1993). *Emergency pediatrics: A guide to ambulatory care* (3rd ed.). St. Louis: Mosby.

Behrman, R., Kliegman, R. M., & Arvin, A. M. (1996). *Nelson textbook of pediatrics* (15th ed.). Philadelphia: Saunders.

Belman, A. B. (1997). Vesicoureteral reflux.

Pediatric Clinics of North America, 44(5), 1171–1190.

Blowey, D. (1998). Acute glomerulonephritis. In L. Finberg (Ed.), *Saunders manual of pediatric practice* (pp. 688–690). Philadelphia: Saunders.

Borer, J., & Hendren, H. (1999). Disorders of the bladder and urethra. In F. Burg, E. Wald, J. Ingelfinger, & R. Polin (Eds.), *Gellis and Kagan's current pediatric therapy* (16th ed., pp. 843–849). Philadelphia: Saunders.

Bowers, V., Hawnigan, K., & Kushner, K. (1995). Bladder extrophy and epispadias. In K. Karlowicz (Ed.), *Urologic nursing: Principles and practice* (pp. 565–592). Philadelphia: Saunders.

Brouhard, B., & Travis, L. (1992). Acute postinfectious glomerulonephritis. In C. M. Edelmann (Ed.), *Pediatric kidney disease* (2nd ed., pp. 1199–1215). Boston: Little, Brown.

Chandra, M. (1999a). Common voiding disorders. In F. Burg, E. Wald, J. Ingelfinger, & R. Polin (Eds.), *Gellis and Kagan's current pediatric therapy* (16th ed., pp. 837–840). Philadelphia: Saunders.

Chandra, M. (1999b). Neurogenic voiding dysfunction in children. In F. Burg, E. Wald, J. Ingelfinger, & R. Polin (Eds.), *Gellis and Kagan's current pediatric therapy* (16th ed., pp. 840–843). Philadelphia: Saunders.

Clark, G., & Barratt, T. (1993). Minimal change nephrotic syndrome and focal segmental glomerulosclerosis. In M. Holliday, T. Barratt, & E. Avner (Eds.), *Pediatric nephrology* (3rd ed., pp. 767–787). Baltimore: Williams & Wilkins.

Cole, B., & Salinas-Madrigal, L. (1993). Acute proliferative glomerulonephritis and crescentic glomerulonephritis. In M. A. Holliday, T. M. Barratt, & E. D. Avner (Eds.), *Pediatric nephrology* (3rd ed., pp. 697–718). Baltimore: Williams & Wilkins.

Daouk, G., & Ingelfinger, J. (1999). Nephrotic syndrome. In F. Burg, E. Wald, J. Ingelfinger, & R. Polin (Eds.), *Gellis and Kagan's current pediatric therapy* (16th ed., pp. 882–887). Philadelphia: Saunders.

Dwyer, J. (1993). Vegetarian diets for treating nephrotic syndrome. *Nutrition Reviews, 51,* 44–46.

Fogo, A., & Kon, V. (1993). Pathophysiology of progressive renal disease. In M. A. Holliday, T. M. Barratt, & E. D. Avner (Eds.), *Pediatric nephrology* (pp. 1228–1240). Baltimore: Williams & Wilkins.

Foster, D. W. (1994). Diabetes mellitus. In K. J. Isselbacher, E. Braunwald, J. D. Wilson, J. B. Martin, A. S. Fauci, & D. L. Kasper (Eds.), *Harrison's principles of internal medicine* (pp. 1979–2000). New York: McGraw-Hill.

Gill, B., & Kogan, S. (1997). Cryptorchidism: Current concepts. *Pediatric Clinics of North America, 44*(5), 1211–1227.

Goldberg, E. (1997). Physical assessment of children ages 1 to 10 years with renal disease. *ANNA Journal, 24*(2), 222–228.

Gonzalez, R. (1996). Urologic disorders in infants and children. In R. Behrman, R. Kliegman, & A. Arvin (Eds.), *Nelson textbook of pediatrics* (15th ed., p. 1527). Philadelphia: Saunders.

Hansen, M. (1998). *Pathophysiology: Foundations of disease and clinical intervention.* Philadelphia: Saunders.

Heiliczer, J. (1999). Acute renal failure. In F. Burg, E. Wald, J. Ingelfinger, & R. Polin (Eds.), *Gellis and Kagan's current pediatric therapy* (16th ed., pp. 890–894). Philadelphia: Saunders.

Hellerstein, S. (1998). Urinary tract infections in children: Why they occur and how to prevent them. *American Family Physician, 57*(10), 2440–2446.

Hendrix, W. (1992). Dialysis therapies in critically ill children. *Clinical Issues in Critical Care Nursing, 3*(3), 605–613.

Hoberman, A. (1999). Infections of the urinary tract. In F. Burg, E. Wald, J. Ingelfinger, & R. Polin (Eds.), *Gellis and Kagan's current pediatric therapy* (16th ed.). Philadelphia: Saunders.

Kass, E., & Lundak, B. (1997). The acute scrotum. *Pediatric Clinics of North America, 44*(5), 1251–1259.

Kelleher, R. (1997). Daytime and nighttime wetting in children: A review of management. *JSPN, 2*(2), 73–82.

Kelsch, R. C., & Seduran, A. B. (1993). Nephrotic syndrome. *Pediatrics in Review, 14,* 30–37.

Miller, K. (1996). Urinary tract infections: Children are not little adults. *Pediatric Nursing, 22*(6), 473–480, 544.

Montagnino, B., Welch, V., & Hoyler-Grant, C. (1995). Congenital anomalies that affect the kidney, ureter, and bladder. In K. Karlowicz (Ed.), *Urologic nursing: Principles and practice* (pp. 567–592). Philadelphia: Saunders.

Neumann, M., & Urizar, R. (1994). Hemolytic uremic syndrome: Current pathophysiology and management. *ANNA Journal, 21*(2), 137–143.

Reynolds, R. E., & Hoberman, A. (1995). Diagnosis and management of pyelonephritis in infants. *Maternal/Child Nursing, 20,* 78–100.

Ribby, K., & Cox, K. (1997). Organization and development of a pediatric end stage renal disease teaching protocol for peritoneal dialysis. *Pediatric Nursing, 23*(4), 393–399.

Rushton, H. G. (1997). Urinary tract infections in children: Epidemiology, evaluation, and management. *Pediatric Clinics of North America, 44*(5), 1133–1165.

Shaw, K., Gorelick, M., McGowan, K., Yakscoe, N., & Schwartz, J. S. (1998). Prevalence of urinary tract infection in febrile young children in the emergency department. *Pediatrics, 102*(2), e16.

Simckes, A. (1998). Nephrotic syndrome. In L. Finberg (Ed.), *Saunders manual of pediatric practice* (pp. 691–693). Philadelphia: Saunders.

Sugar, E., Firlit, C., & Reisman, M. (1993). Pediatric hypospadias surgery. *Pediatric Nursing, 19*(6), 585–588, 615.

Sugar, E., & Huyler-Grant, C. (1995). Disorders of the external genitalia in children. In K. Karlowicz (Ed.), *Urologic nursing: Principles and Practice* (pp. 498–518). Philadelphia: Saunders.

Taylor, J. (1996). End stage renal disease in children: Diagnosis, management, and interventions. *Pediatric Nursing, 22*(6), 481–487.

Vogt, B. (1997). Identifying kidney disease: Simple steps can make a difference. *Contemporary Pediatrics, 14*(3), 115–127.

Zaontz, M., & Packer, M. (1997). Abnormalities of the external genitalia. *Pediatric Clinics of North America, 44*(5), 1207–1297.

45

The Child
with a
Respiratory
Alteration

After studying this chapter, you should be able to:

- Describe the differences in the anatomy and physiology of the infant's or child's respiratory system that increase the risk for respiratory disease.
- Outline nursing care for a child with allergies to inhalants.
- Discuss and describe the pathophysiology, clinical manifestations, and therapeutic management of common acute and chronic respiratory alterations.
- Identify the nursing care needs of infants and children with acute and chronic respiratory alterations.
- Develop guidelines for the home care of a child with an acute respiratory alteration.
- Identify common triggers of asthma symptoms and measures that can be taken to prevent and treat asthma episodes.
- Identify teaching needs for children with asthma and their families.
- Describe the nursing care of the child with cystic fibrosis.
- Discuss measures to maintain adequate oxygenation and provide appropriate developmental stimulation for the child with bronchopulmonary dysplasia.
- Describe the correct method of administering and evaluating tuberculosis skin tests.
- Identify ways to prevent the transmission of tuberculosis and explain the importance of administering antituberculosis medications as prescribed.

DEFINITIONS

atelectasis A collapsed or airless state of the lung that may involve all or part of the lung.

crackles An abnormal, discontinuous, nonmusical sound heard on auscultation, primarily during inhalation; also called rales.

dyspnea Difficulty breathing.

grunting A sound similar to a grunting noise that can be heard with or without a stethoscope.

hypercapnia Increased levels of carbon dioxide in the blood, as indicated by an elevated $Paco_2$ as determined by blood gas analysis.

hypocapnia Decreased levels of carbon dioxide in the blood.

hypoxemia Decreased levels of oxygen in the blood.

hypoxia Decreased oxygenation of cells and tissues.

nasal flaring A serious sign of air hunger demonstrated by widening of the nares to enable an infant or young child to take in more oxygen.

orthopnea Difficulty breathing except in an upright position.

retractions An abnormal movement of the chest wall during inspiration that may occur intercostally and substernally.

rhonchi Adventitious breath sounds caused by the passage of air through an airway obstructed by thick secretions; sounds do not clear with coughing.

stridor A shrill, harsh sound that can be heard during inspiration, expiration, or both; produced by the flow of air through a narrowed segment of the respiratory tract.

tachypnea Increased respiratory rate.

wheezing High-pitched, musical whistles that can be heard with or without a stethoscope; may be inspiratory or expiratory. Wheezing is caused by bronchial constriction or obstruction of the airway and commonly occurs in asthma.

■ Review of the Respiratory System

The respiratory system consists of the nose, pharynx, trachea, bronchi, and lungs. It is further divided into the *upper respiratory tract* (nose, pharynx, larynx) and the *lower respiratory tract* (trachea, bronchi, and lungs).

The Upper Airway

Air enters the body through the *nares*, or nostrils, two nasal cavities lined with mucous membrane. In older infants and children, air can also enter through the mouth into the pharynx, or throat. The *nasopharynx* is located immediately behind the nasal cavity; the *oropharynx* is located behind the mouth. The *laryngeal pharynx* lies below the oropharynx and opens into the larynx toward the front and into the esophagus toward the back.

The *larynx* is located between the pharynx and the trachea. The vocal cords are at the upper end of the larynx. The proximity of the upper esophagus to the upper respiratory system can put an individual at risk for inhaling food or liquids, but the *epiglottis* covers the larynx during swallowing and helps keep food out of the lower respiratory tract.

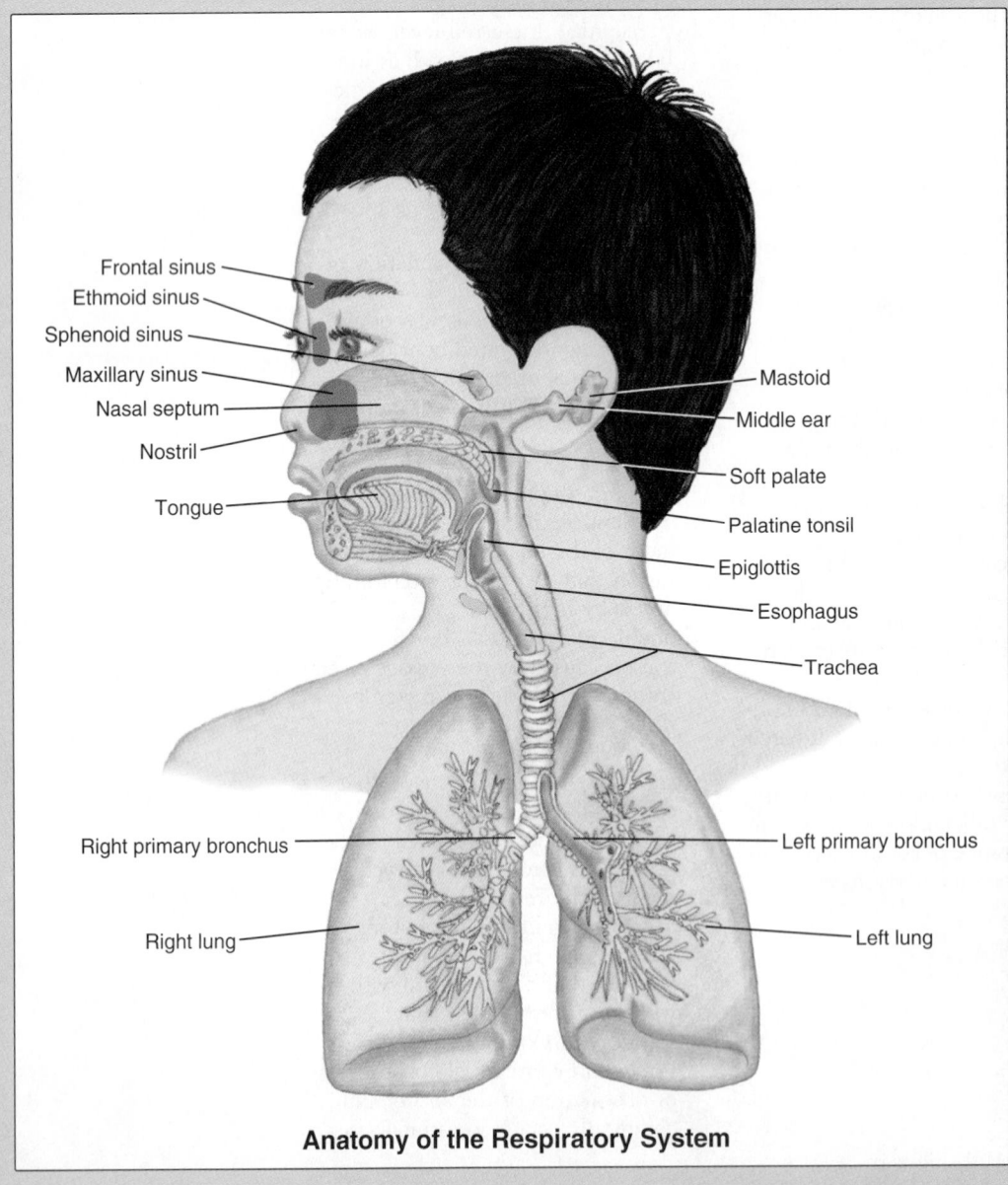

Frontal sinus
Ethmoid sinus
Sphenoid sinus
Maxillary sinus
Nasal septum
Nostril
Tongue

Mastoid
Middle ear
Soft palate
Palatine tonsil
Epiglottis
Esophagus
Trachea

Right primary bronchus
Right lung

Left primary bronchus
Left lung

Anatomy of the Respiratory System

Cilia are hair-like processes that move mucus and fluid. Damage to cilia interferes with the removal of mucus from the respiratory tract. Ciliated mucous membranes line the larynx and filter dust and other particles from the air. The particles are then carried to the pharynx to be removed by sneezing, blowing, or coughing. After being filtered, the air that enters the respiratory system is humidified and warmed before proceeding into the lungs. There are three types of tonsils: the oval *palatine tonsils* are located on either side of the pharynx, the *lingual tonsils* are located below the palatine tonsils at the base of the tongue, and the *pharyngeal tonsils*, or *adenoids*, are located at the nasopharyngeal border. The tonsils are composed mainly of lymphoid tissue. They help filter the circulating lymph of bacteria and other foreign material that enters the body, especially through the mouth and nose.

The Lower Airway

The *trachea* conducts air between the larynx and the lungs. It divides into right and left main *bronchi* at its lower end, the *carina*. The right main bronchus is shorter and wider than the left. The main bronchi divide into *lobar bronchi*, *segmental bronchi*, and *bronchioles* and terminate in *alveoli*. Mucus-secreting goblet cells line the bronchi and protect the lungs from dust and bacteria.

The *lungs* are two conical structures within the thoracic cavity. The right lung has three *lobes* (upper, middle, and lower); the left has two lobes (upper and lower). The *pleura* consists of two layers, the *parietal pleura* and the *visceral pleura*. The parietal pleura lines the entire thoracic cavity; the visceral pleura encases each lung. The pleura helps maintain lung stability. Negative pressure within the intrapleural space prevents the lungs from separating from the thorax. *Diffusion* of gases takes place in the lungs. Terminal bronchioles lack mucus-secreting goblet cells and cilia, and gas exchange does not take place here.

Distal to the terminal bronchioles are the alveoli, where most gas exchange occurs. Thinness of the alveolar walls aids in gas exchange. Within the alveolar walls there is an almost solid sheet of capillaries, so that the alveolar gases are in close proximity to the capillary blood.

Prenatal Respiratory Development

The respiratory system must mature before birth for the neonate to survive. The placenta performs oxygenation in utero, but, to adapt to extrauterine life, the neonate must be able to inflate the lungs, establish continuous breathing, and transfer the gases needed to meet metabolic needs.

Postnatal Respiratory Changes

Postnatal changes in the respiratory system occur as follows:

1. Compression of the thorax during delivery forces out some fetal lung fluid.
2. Respirations are stimulated by hypoxemia, hypercarbia, cold, tactile stimulation, and a possible decrease in the concentration of prostaglandin E_2.
3. Inflation of the normal lung is complete within a few breaths, and most alveoli have expanded within the first hour of life.
4. Surfactant in the lung liquid lowers surface tension and facilitates lung expansion.
5. Pulmonary blood flow increases.
6. Closure of the foramen ovale and the ductus arteriosus (see Chapter 46) establishes the pulmonary and circulatory systems.

Gas Exchange and Transport

Two-way diffusion takes place between the walls of the alveoli. In *diffusion*, molecules move from an area of greater

Pediatric Differences in the Respiratory System

- Surfactant is lacking in premature infants. Infants born before 34 weeks' gestation have a higher risk for respiratory distress syndrome.
- Smaller lower airways and undeveloped supporting cartilage predispose the child to an increased risk of obstruction by mucus, edema, and foreign bodies. The neonate's airway is 50% smaller than that of adults. A premature infant has a more compliant chest wall and weaker respiratory muscles than a term infant.
- Lung size is proportional to body height. Therefore, lung volumes and capacities do not vary from age to age.
- Infants are obligatory nose breathers; they have difficulty breathing through the mouth. If the infant has nasal congestion, breathing becomes more difficult.
- The diaphragm is the neonate's major respiratory muscle. Intercostal muscles are not well developed. Retractions are more common in the infant than in older children and adults.
- Brief periods of apnea (10 to 15 seconds) are common in the neonate. The respiratory pattern may be irregular.
- Children's normal respiratory rate is higher than that of adults.
- An increased metabolic rate increases oxygen needs.
- Alveoli develop from approximately 20 million to 200 million by age 3 years. There is a gradual decrease of alveolar development after age 3 years; few develop after age 8 years.
- The lung surface increases until 5 to 8 years. Actual lung growth continues into the adolescent years.
- Eustachian tubes are relatively horizontal, which increases the risk of bacteria entering the middle ear.
- Tracheal size approximately triples by adulthood.
- Tonsillar tissue is normally enlarged in early-school-age children.
- Infants and children use abdominal muscles to inhale until about age 5 to 6 years.
- The child's flexible larynx is more susceptible to spasm.

concentration to one of lesser concentration. Blood entering the lung capillaries is somewhat low in oxygen. Oxygen will diffuse from the alveoli, where its concentration is higher, into the blood. Similarly, carbon dioxide moves out of the blood and into the alveoli. Most oxygen that diffuses into the capillary blood in the lungs is bound to the hemoglobin of red blood cells. A small percentage is dissolved in plasma. For oxygen to enter the cells, it must separate from hemoglobin. Carbon dioxide diffuses into the blood from the tissues and is transported to the lungs by the blood. In this activity hemoglobin is a buffer that enables blood to take up carbon dioxide without altering the blood pH significantly. The uptake and delivery of gases by the blood is a continuous process.

Ventilation occurs through *inspiration* and *expiration*. In inspiration the diaphragm contracts and flattens, expanding the vertical dimension of the chest; the lung volume increases. In expiration the diaphragm and chest wall relax, decreasing thoracic volume. Intrathoracic pressure increases and gas flows out of the lungs, taking with it the carbon dioxide that was delivered to the lungs by the blood. Ventilation of the lungs is intermittent. Inspired air is 21% oxygen; end-expired air is 16% oxygen and 35% carbon dioxide.

◼ *Diagnostic Tests*

In most instances, respiratory tract disorders are diagnosed from the findings on physical examination and the clinical manifestations. Sometimes, however, specific diagnostic tests are needed.

Blood Gas Analysis

Arterial blood gas analysis plays an important role in the investigation of pulmonary function. Arterial blood gas values most frequently determined include Pao_2, $Paco_2$, pH, and HCO_3^-. Arterial blood is more reliable than capillary or venous blood for these tests, especially in children with poor peripheral perfusion. Arterial blood gas values are used primarily to determine acid-base balance, not oxygen saturation (see Chapter 37).

Pulmonary Function Tests

Probably the most useful measures of ventilatory function are the *vital capacity* and the *expiratory flow rate*, both measured by spirometry. These tests can be performed in most children by age 6 years. Accurate measurements are difficult

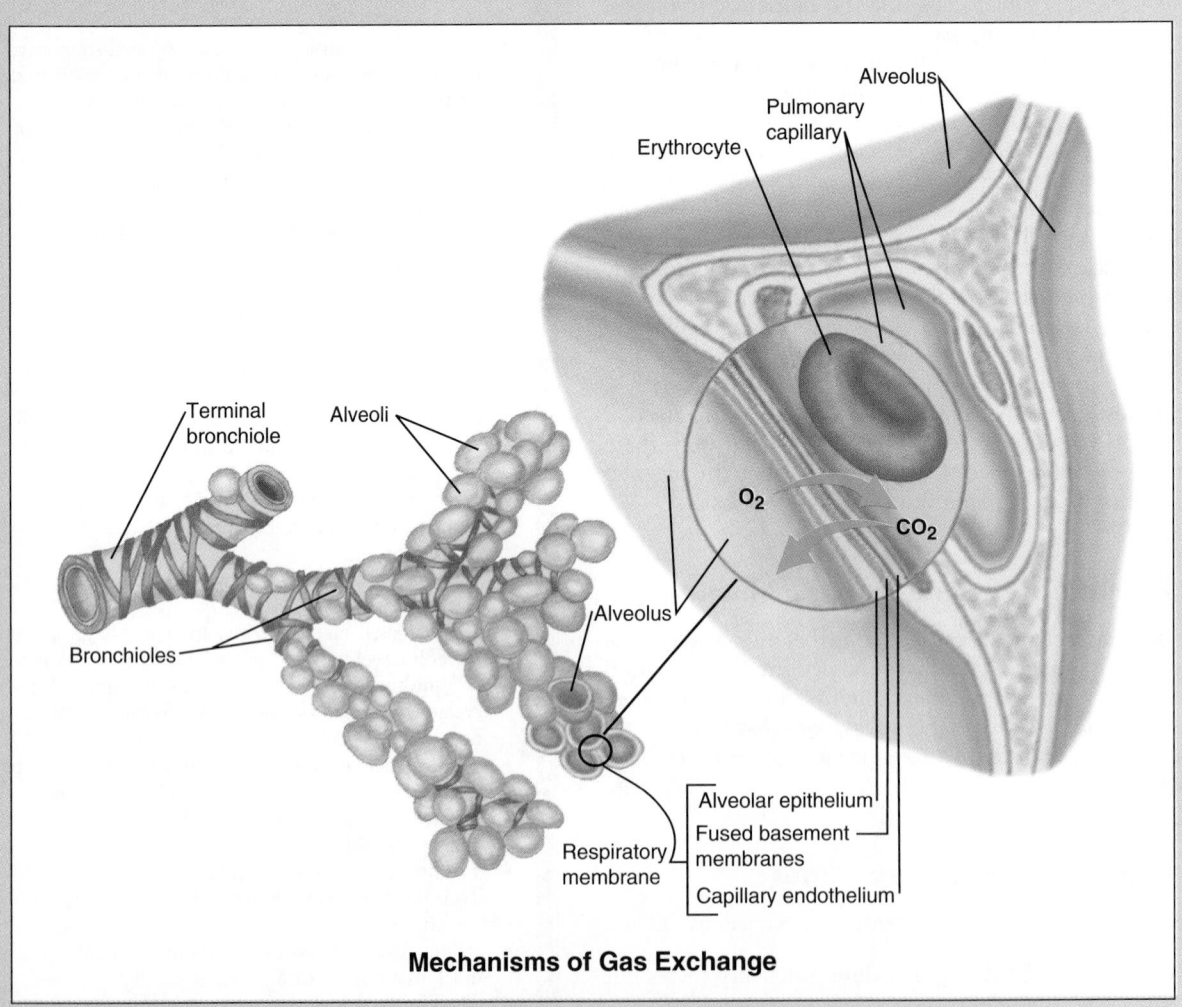

Mechanisms of Gas Exchange

Common Laboratory and Diagnostic Tests for Respiratory Disorders

Test	Description	Normal Findings	Indications	Nursing Considerations
Chest radiography, posteroanterior and lateral views	Shows airways, lungs, heart, great vessels.	Normal appearance of internal structures of the chest.	To detect respiratory disease of the lungs.	Assist in holding the child.
Computed tomography (CT)	Shows lesions in the chest wall, pleural space, mediastinum, and lung parenchyma.	Normal cross-section of lung tissue.	To image tumors or masses; to evaluate response to therapy aimed at defined lesions.	Assist with sedation and immobilization of the child. Withhold feedings 3 to 4 hours before the test because of frequent use of contrast medium.
Bronchoscopy	Provides viewing of tracheobronchial tree through a scope.	Normal appearance of tracheobronchial tree or successful removal of foreign body or mucous plugs.	To view a lesion and obtain biopsy material for culture; to remove a foreign body or mucous plugs.	Rigid bronchoscopy is usually performed under general anesthesia. Fiberoptic flexible bronchoscopy can be performed while the child is awake or sedated. Observe the child closely for signs of airway obstruction. Mist may be given to decrease swelling and edema.
Laryngoscopy	Provides direct viewing of larynx with a scope.	Normal appearance of larynx.	To identify cause of stridor and local abnormalities.	Mirror (indirect) laryngoscopy can be performed on children age 4 to 5 years or older. In infants and younger children, direct laryngoscopy or transnasal laryngoscopy with flexible bronchoscope will give much better results. General anesthesia is usually required; topical anesthesia and mild sedation may be provided for a fiberoptic examination. Fluids and foods are withheld until the effects of local anesthetic have worn off and gag reflex has returned.
Cultures	Throat, blood, nasopharyngeal, sputum.	No culture growth or normal flora only.	To isolate and identify pathogens.	See Chapter 37 for procedures.
Radioallergosorbent test (RAST) for IgE	Measures quantity of IgE antibodies in serum after exposure to specific antigens.	If the child is not allergic to the antigen, IgE antibody is not detected. A test result is positive in relation to a specific antigen if the value is above 400% of control.	To identify specific allergens; systemic reactions to insect venom, drugs, and chemicals; to monitor response to desensitization procedures. Test is also performed at the onset of asthma, hay fever, or dermatitis.	Prepare child for a peripheral blood sample to be drawn. Determine whether the child has undergone any radioisotope tests within the past week, as such tests may alter the results.

Table continued on following page

Common Laboratory and Diagnostic Tests for Respiratory Disorders Continued

Test	Description	Normal Findings	Indications	Nursing Considerations
Pilocarpine ionto-phoresis (sweat test)	Measures sweat electrolyte concentration for diagnosis of cystic fibrosis (CF). Sweating is stimulated on the child's forearm with a small electrical current and pilo-carpine; a sweat sample is then collected on preweighed, dry, sterile gauze or filter paper and the amount of sweat sodium and chloride are measured.	*Normal:* ≤40 mEQ/L *Suggestive of CF:* 40 mEq/L *Positive for CF:* ≥60 mEq/L	Used to diagnose cystic fibrosis.	No physical preparation is needed. Offer the parents and child support as they face the implications of a positive diagnosis. Inform the child and parents that the test is painless and that it is usually performed twice to ensure accurate results. Because an adequate amount of sweat is difficult to obtain from infants, the sweat test is usually unreliable in infants less than 4 weeks old.
Mantoux test	Skin test for tuberculosis. Purified protein derivative (PPD), 5 TB units (0.1 ml), is injected intradermally into the volar surface of the forearm with a short, 26- to 27-gauge needle, beveled side up. A wheal 6 to 10 mm in diameter should appear during the injection. The site is checked in 48 to 72 hours by a health care professional. Results are recorded in milli-meters (not simply as positive or negative). The reading is based on induration (hard-ness), not redness.	*Positive result:* An area of induration ≥15 mm (in children of all ages); an area of induration ≥10 mm in children less than 4 years old or at high risk for exposure; an area of induration ≥5 mm in the highest risk group. *Negative result:* The Mantoux test cannot rule out the presence of TB, particularly in young infants.	To screen and test individuals suspected of having TB or of having been exposed to TB.	Test is fairly difficult to administer. After PPD is injected, withdrawal of the needle should be delayed for 2 to 3 seconds to minimize leakage of PPD at the puncture site. In most children, skin testing will elicit a positive reaction 3 to 6 weeks after initial in-fection. Steroids and immunosuppressants given within 4 to 6 weeks can cause false negative skin test results. Positive tuberculin reactivity usually continues for the person's lifetime, even with treatment.

to obtain in younger children and infants because they are unable to follow commands. Pulmonary function tests assess the degree of pulmonary disease, response to therapy, and the presence of restrictive or obstructive disease. They are also done to test the child's response to bronchodilators should pulmonary function be affected.

The child must be given instruction and practice in blowing, pushing, and holding respirations. The child should become familiar with the mouthpiece and the nose clip to feel comfortable with their use.

Pulse Oximetry

Pulse oximetry is a simple, noninvasive, intermittent or con-tinuous method for measuring oxygen saturation for the pur-

pose of determining the need for or response to oxygen ther-apy (see Chapter 37). The goal of treatment for most respiratory conditions is an oxygen saturation greater than 95%. For children with chronic respiratory disease, how-ever, a realistic goal may be slightly lower.

Transcutaneous Monitoring

Transcutaneous monitoring continuously checks oxygen and carbon dioxide concentrations in the body through an elec-trode placed on the child's skin. Electrode sites must be changed every 3 to 4 hours to prevent burning the skin, and the machine must be recalibrated each time electrodes are changed. The readings may not be accurate if tissue per-fusion is poor.

Respiratory alterations are the most common causes of illness in the infant and child. Upper respiratory disorders affect the ear, nose, pharynx, and larynx; lower respiratory disorders include those that involve the trachea, bronchi, and lungs.

Infants and children less than 3 years old are at greater risk for developing respiratory infections than older children and adults because of their immature immune systems, smaller upper and lower airways, and underdeveloped supporting cartilage. Although most respiratory infections are self-limiting, infants and young children can quickly experience respiratory distress as mucus and edema obstruct their small airways.

Parents should be taught preventive measures, including adequate rest, good nutrition, and good hygiene, with an emphasis on hand washing. Even with the most careful hygiene and preventive practices, however, most children will experience some type of respiratory infection each year. School nurses often see children with respiratory problems in the school health office and may be the primary health caregivers for these children.

Most children can be cared for at home by their parents and do not need hospitalization. Those children who are hospitalized are being discharged from the hospital earlier in their recovery than in the past. The current health care environment underlies the need for nurses to teach parents good home care techniques, including careful observation and recognition of signs that indicate the need to contact health care providers. Parents, especially first-time parents, often are frightened by the sudden onset of respiratory symptoms, which may indicate a severe problem. Teaching them the signs and symptoms of serious illness will help them develop appropriate decision-making skills.

Children with chronic conditions have many special needs, and the child with a chronic respiratory disease is no different. Medications and treatments become a way of life for many of these children. Their activity level is often altered, and some may have a shortened life span.

The nurse plays an important role in the care of the child with a chronic respiratory disease. Beyond giving acute care to the hospitalized child, the nurse must coordinate and facilitate the child's long-term care. Because of advances being made in the treatment of chronic pediatric respiratory conditions, the treatment and care of children affected by these disorders are constantly changing and improving, requiring the nurse to stay current in these areas.

Allergic Rhinitis

Allergic rhinitis is an inflammatory disorder of the nasal mucosa. It is usually seasonal, recurrent, and triggered by specific allergens (see Chapter 41). It is sometimes referred to as *seasonal allergic rhinitis*, *seasonal pollinosis*, or *hay fever*.

Some children have symptoms year round (*perennial allergic rhinitis*).

Etiology and Incidence

Common causative agents of allergic rhinitis include dust mites, feathers, animal dander, mold spores, and pollens of trees, grasses, and weeds. There is usually a family history similar to that seen in individuals with atopic dermatitis and asthma. Unlike atopic dermatitis, however, allergic rhinitis does not predispose to the development of asthma.

The onset of allergic rhinitis usually occurs during childhood, but rarely before age 2 years. It is estimated that 5% to 10% of children have this type of allergic response (Maguire & Umetsu, 1999).

Manifestations

The classic symptoms of allergic rhinitis are watery rhinorrhea, associated with itching of nose, eyes, ears, and palate; and paroxysmal sneezing. Additional signs and symptoms include the allergic salute—an upward rubbing of the nose with the palm of the hand, which can leave a crease below the bridge (Fig. 45–1); allergic shiners—dark circles under the eyes from congestion and edema; dry lips from mouth

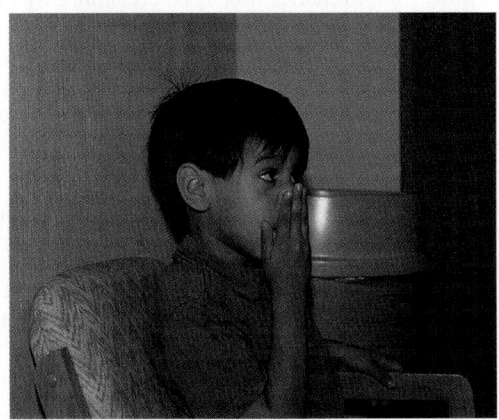

FIGURE 45–1
. . . .
Children with allergic rhinitis often have dark circles under their eyes, called allergic shiners, and may be seen rubbing their noses upward with the palm—the allergic salute. (Courtesy of Parkland Health and Hospital System Community Oriented Primary Care Clinic, Dallas, Texas.)

breathing; pale, boggy nasal mucous membranes; and nasal obstruction. Children with allergic rhinitis experience symptoms as long as they are exposed to the allergen.

It is important to distinguish allergic rhinitis from viral *nasopharyngitis* (the common cold), which is usually caused by a rhinovirus and is spread by droplet or by contact with contaminated items. Usually children with nasopharyngitis experience the associated symptoms of sore throat, fever, cough, and fatigue. The condition is self-limiting and usually resolves within 2 weeks. The quality of the nasal discharge in children with nasopharyngitis often changes from clear to cloudy or yellow. Management is supportive. Because young infants are obligatory nose breathers, the infant's blocked nasal passages can be relieved with instillation of normal saline drops followed by gentle bulb suction.

Diagnostic Evaluation

A thorough personal and family history usually elicits a description that suggests an allergic rather than infectious pattern. The nasal smear may demonstrate eosinophils. Allergy skin testing is done if signs and symptoms continue after treatment with medication. The radioallergosorbent test (RAST) is used only when skin testing is difficult because of generalized dermatitis, the child is very young, or the child is too ill for skin testing. A complete blood count might reveal elevated eosinophils, a finding associated with allergic manifestations.

Therapeutic Management

The treatment of choice is to eliminate the allergen from the child's environment. When this is impossible, as in the case of pollen in the air, medication can control symptoms. Finally, immunotherapy (allergy shots) may be considered for children whose condition is not responsive to either environmental modification or medication. Immunotherapy involves injecting the child with progressively larger doses of the allergen in an effort to reduce the magnitude of the body's allergic response. Injections are given once or twice a week until a maintenance dose is reached; monthly maintenance injections can continue for several years.

Antihistamines are given to relieve symptoms. Antihistamines are most effective when given before or very early in an allergic episode. Because they can cause drowsiness, they should be given at night. Some of the newer antihistamines (e.g., loratidine, cetirizine, fexofenadine) are long-acting and require only one or two doses daily. A decongestant can be given in conjunction with an antihistamine if nasal congestion is a problem. Short-term topical intranasal corticosteroids (e.g., beclomethasone) are quite effective in children whose condition does not respond to antihistamines and decongestants. It usually takes several days of treatment before the effects of topical corticosteroids are felt by the child. Children with severe symptoms that do not respond to treatment may be given systemic corticosteroids; relief is usually attained within 24 hours.

Nursing Considerations

Nursing care focuses on early identification of clinical signs and symptoms of allergic rhinitis and support of the thera-

---

PARENTS WANT TO KNOW

How to Implement Environmental Modification

To reduce your child's exposure to allergens, take the following measures:

Pollen and Dust

- Wash your child's sheets and blankets in hot water.
- Avoid using wool and down blankets.
- Encase pillows and mattresses in dust-proof covers.
- Replace carpet with wood, tile, slate, or vinyl.
- Replace drapes and blinds with curtains and shades.
- Replace upholstered furniture with wood or plastic.
- Keep closet doors shut.
- Cover hot air vents with filters.
- Install air cleaners.
- Use multilayer vacuum bags.
- Clean with a towel treated to attract dust.
- Run air conditioners.
- Keep household humidity at 40% to 50%.

Mold

- Clean with a mold inhibitor.
- Dry everyone's shoes thoroughly.
- Use a moisture remover in closets.
- Encourage your child to stay out of the basement.
- Replace foam rubber mattresses with springs.
- Run an air conditioner.
- Keep the humidity below 35%.
- Run a dehumidifier.
- Ventilate the house.
- Store firewood outside.
- Limit the number of indoor plants.

Dander

- Keep pets outside if possible.
- Ventilate the house.
- Install air cleaners.
- Encase mattresses and pillows in dust-proof covers.

---

peutic management of the condition. The nurse assesses and records the applicable history and helps the family identify allergens to which the child is sensitive.

Once the allergens are known, the nurse counsels parents regarding administration of medications, environmental control, and immunotherapy, as appropriate. Drowsiness, the most common side effect of antihistamines, can usually be overcome if the child takes a combination antihistamine and decongestant or takes the medication at night. Some children experience dry mucous membranes or excitability. Warm water or saline irrigations of the nasal passages can be used to moisten mucous membranes, soften crusted secretions, and wash out irritants. Saline can be mixed by adding ¼ teaspoon of salt to a cup of warm water. Saline nose drops are also available without prescription.

When specific allergens have been identified, they should be eliminated or controlled. During the pollen season the child should stay indoors as much as possible and the windows should be kept closed if the house is air conditioned. After being outdoors the child should shower and wash the hair to remove pollens from the body. Animals that have been outside may also be a source of contamination.

Receiving immunotherapy can be a traumatic experience for the child. It is often difficult for children to understand how an injection will help them. Allergy injections must be given in a physician's office because some children can experience an anaphylactic reaction to the allergy serum. Supervise the child closely for 20 to 30 minutes after the injection in case anaphylaxis develops. Keep emergency epinephrine ready.

Sinusitis

Sinusitis, although not itself a serious disorder, can lead to life-threatening complications. Inflammation and infection of the sinuses can be acute or chronic.

Etiology and Incidence

Acute sinusitis often follows an upper respiratory tract viral infection. Children with chronic sinusitis often have allergic rhinitis or acute otitis media with effusion. Hypertrophied adenoids, immune deficiencies, and foreign body

PATHOPHYSIOLOGY
· · · · · · · · · · ·
of Sinusitis

Acute sinusitis occurs when the sinus cavity is invaded by bacteria, causing mucosal inflammation and edema that block narrow sinus channels. The volume of secretions increases and the affected sinuses fill with purulent material. Inflammation and infection interfere with the protective cleansing action of the cilia covering the sinus mucous membranes. Impaired mucociliary transport leads to stagnation of secretions within the sinuses; the stagnant secretions provide a medium for bacterial growth.

Chronic sinusitis is usually a complication of acute sinusitis. Prolonged or repeated infections result in irreversible changes in the mucosal lining of the sinus. Nasal polyps, a deviated septum, and enlarged adenoids inhibit sinus drainage, which can lead to infections. The frontal and sphenoid sinuses are most often involved in children.

Infection from sinusitis can spread to the middle ear, causing otitis media. Serious complications occur when infection spreads either directly through the bone or along the venous channels of the skull into adjacent structures, such as the orbit or the central nervous system.

obstruction in the nose also predispose to sinusitis. Children with cystic fibrosis have a high incidence of sinusitis because of highly viscous mucous secretions and nasal polyps. The most common causative organisms are *Streptococcus pneumoniae*, *Hemophilus influenzae*, and *Moraxella catarrhalis*.

Sinus infections can occur in infancy as well as in childhood but are most common during the school-age years.

Manifestations

Sinusitis is characterized by signs and symptoms of a cold that do not improve after 14 days, low-grade fever, nasal congestion with purulent nasal discharge, halitosis, cough (which usually increases when the child is lying down), and headache, tenderness, and a feeling of fullness over the affected sinuses (irritability in younger children). Occasionally children experience facial edema. Children with chronic sinusitis experience many of the same symptoms except the cough is chronic and the headache is recurrent. The child's sense of taste or smell may be impaired, and the child may be fatigued.

Diagnostic Evaluation

Sinus radiographs show mucosal thickening, opacification, and air-fluid levels in children more than 1 year old. Sinus radiographs are of no value in younger children because of their small sinuses. Computed tomography (CT) provides detailed anatomic information. Because of the thick bone of the maxilla in the anterior face and the small size of the sinus, transillumination of the sinuses is not useful.

Therapeutic Management

Antibiotics are the mainstay of treatment; amoxicillin or amoxicillin-potassium clavulanate (Augmentin) are used most frequently. In addition to antibiotics, treatment includes analgesics, hydration, the application of moist heat, and decongestants. The use of antihistamines in the treatment of sinusitis is controversial. Antihistamines may be used to treat allergy symptoms associated with chronic sinusitis, but they tend to impair sinus drainage by thickening secretions. Steroid nasal sprays may be used to reduce inflammation while avoiding the rebound effect of decongestant nose drops.

Obstructive deformities such as enlarged adenoids or polyps are surgically corrected. If orbital cellulitis develops, the child should be hospitalized immediately and parenteral antibiotic therapy begun.

Nursing Considerations

The nurse should assess the location of pain or fullness. Pain can occur in the forehead, over the cheekbones or upper teeth, or may radiate to the top of the head. The nurse should inspect and palpate the face for edema, document any fever, and inspect the nose and throat for purulent discharge. The nasal mucous membranes are inspected for erythema and edema.

Nursing care focuses on teaching the parents antibiotic administration, comfort measures, how to monitor for response to treatment, and identifying complications. Emphasize the importance of the child's taking the antibiotics as prescribed. Sinus drainage is facilitated by increasing the child's intake of clear fluids and by using a bedside humidifier.

Warm moist compresses applied two to three times daily help decrease swelling and pain. Acetaminophen is given for fever and discomfort. Breathing warm mist in a hot shower or through hot, moist towels can help liquefy and mobilize nasal mucus, as can saline nose drops. The nurse should teach the parent to administer nose drops after the nasal passages have been gently cleaned. The amount, color, and consistency of nasal drainage should be noted and evaluated to determine whether the child is responding to treatment.

The child's response to treatment and the development of complications should be evaluated carefully. Advise parents to contact the physician promptly if symptoms become worse, if the child experiences any periorbital edema, or if the child does not seem to be feeling better after 3 or 4 days.

Otitis Media

Otitis media is one of the most common illnesses of infancy and childhood. The term otitis media refers to effusion and infection or blockage of the middle ear. Acute otitis media is effusion in the middle ear that occurs suddenly and is associated with other signs of illness. Otitis media with effusion refers to the presence of fluid behind the tympanic membrane without signs of infection. Otitis media with effusion often follows an episode of acute otitis media, but usually resolves after several weeks.

Etiology

The bacterial pathogens that usually cause acute otitis media are *Streptococcus pneumoniae, Hemophilus influenzae,* and *Moraxella catarrhalis.* Although viruses do not cause otitis media, they are thought to predispose the child to ear infection by altering host defenses and contributing to eustachian tube dysfunction. Allergies are also thought to precipitate otitis media.

Attendance at day care centers predisposes children to otitis media. Infants less than 1 year old who attend day care have a threefold risk of acquiring acute otitis media (Zeisel, Roberts, Neebe, et al., 1999). The use of a pacifier after age 6 months has also been identified as a risk factor (Niemelè, Uhari, & Möttönen, 1995), as has exposure to environmental smoke.

Bottle-feeding contributes to ear infection because of the position of the infant during feeding. Reflux of formula into the eustachian tube from the nasopharynx occurs when the infant swallows while supine. Breast-feeding offers some protection from ear infection by providing maternal antibodies and by decreasing the incidence of allergy; as well, the more upright position of the infant while nursing is protective against ear infection.

Incidence

The incidence of otitis media peaks between ages 6 months and 6 years, with most episodes occurring in children less than 3 years old. Most initial episodes occur at about age 6 months, when there is a decline in maternal antibody levels. Early onset of acute otitis media (during infancy) increases the risk for recurrent episodes (Montville & White, 1998).

By the end of the third year of life, 50% to 70% of all children have had at least one episode of acute otitis media. Most children under age 5 have two to three episodes of otitis media each year. Boys have a slightly higher incidence of otitis media than girls. Native American and Eskimo children are at increased risk for otitis media, perhaps because of their craniofacial structure (Montville & White, 1998). The incidence of otitis media is highest in winter and spring and lowest in the summer months.

Manifestations

Acute otitis media is characterized by

- Otalgia (earache); infants may pull their ears or roll their heads
- A bulging, opaque tympanic membrane that usually looks red, with decreased mobility; diffuse light reflex; and obscured landmarks (Fig. 45–2)
- Drainage, usually yellowish green, purulent, and foul-smelling (indicates perforation of the tympanic membrane)

These signs and symptoms might also be accompanied by irritability, sleep disturbances, persistent crying in infants, fever, vomiting, anorexia, or diarrhea (especially in infants).

Otitis media with effusion differs from acute otitis media in that there are no signs of acute infection. The tympanic membrane appears retracted, dull gray or yellow, and an air-fluid level or air bubbles may be visible through the tympanic membrane. The mobility of the tympanic membrane is decreased and landmarks are distorted. Associated signs and symptoms can be subtle and include

- Tinnitus, popping sounds
- Hearing loss (usually conductive) below 35 decibels. Delays in speech development may result from prolonged hearing loss. In the older child, hearing loss may manifest as behavior problems, poor school performance, disturbed sleep, irritability, and decreased responsiveness
- Mild balance disturbances that may result in delays in motor skills
- A flattened tracing and negative pressure on the tympanogram (a graphic representation of tympanic mobility and middle-ear pressure)

Diagnostic Evaluation

The diagnosis of otitis media is based on the history of signs and symptoms and pneumatic otoscopy. In pneumatic otoscopy, a small puff of air is blown into the ear canal through the otoscope; the examiner can discern the appearance and mobility of the tympanic membrane. In addition to pneumatic otoscopy, tympanometry can be used to confirm what was seen with the eye.

PATHOPHYSIOLOGY
• • • • • • • • • • •
of Otitis Media

The immature anatomy of the child's middle ear and eustachian tube predisposes infants and toddlers to otitis media. When the eustachian tube is obstructed, as frequently occurs with enlarged adenoids or mucosal edema from an upper respiratory tract infection, effective drainage and ventilation of the middle ear cannot occur. Air that is normally present in the middle ear is absorbed by the blood, causing a vacuum or negative pressure in the middle ear. Fluid (effusion) accumulates within the middle-ear space, creating a medium for bacterial growth. After an upper respiratory tract infection, pathogens travel from the nasopharynx to the eustachian tube. In the presence of effusion, negative pressure in the middle ear draws mucus through the eustachian tube whenever the child cries, yawns, or sucks forcefully on a nipple. Purulent fluid accumulates in the middle-ear space, causing the pressure and pain of acute otitis media.

If the eustachian tube remains nonfunctional for a prolonged period, the fluid within the middle ear becomes thick and dark (glue ear). Mild temporary conductive hearing loss (see Chapter 55) often occurs in otitis media with effusion because of the decreased mobility of the ossicles and the tympanic membrane. Permanent conductive hearing loss can result from repeated episodes of otitis media and may interfere with the development of language and cognitive skills. Chronic otitis media with effusion is the most common cause of hearing loss in children.

Complications of otitis media include conductive hearing loss and sensorineural hearing loss. The infection of acute otitis media can spread to surrounding tissues, causing mastoiditis or intracranial complications such as meningitis or brain abscess. Inflammation and pressure from otitis media may result in *tympanosclerosis* (scarring of the tympanic membrane), perforation of the tympanic membrane, and *cholesteatoma* (pus and debris in the middle ear).

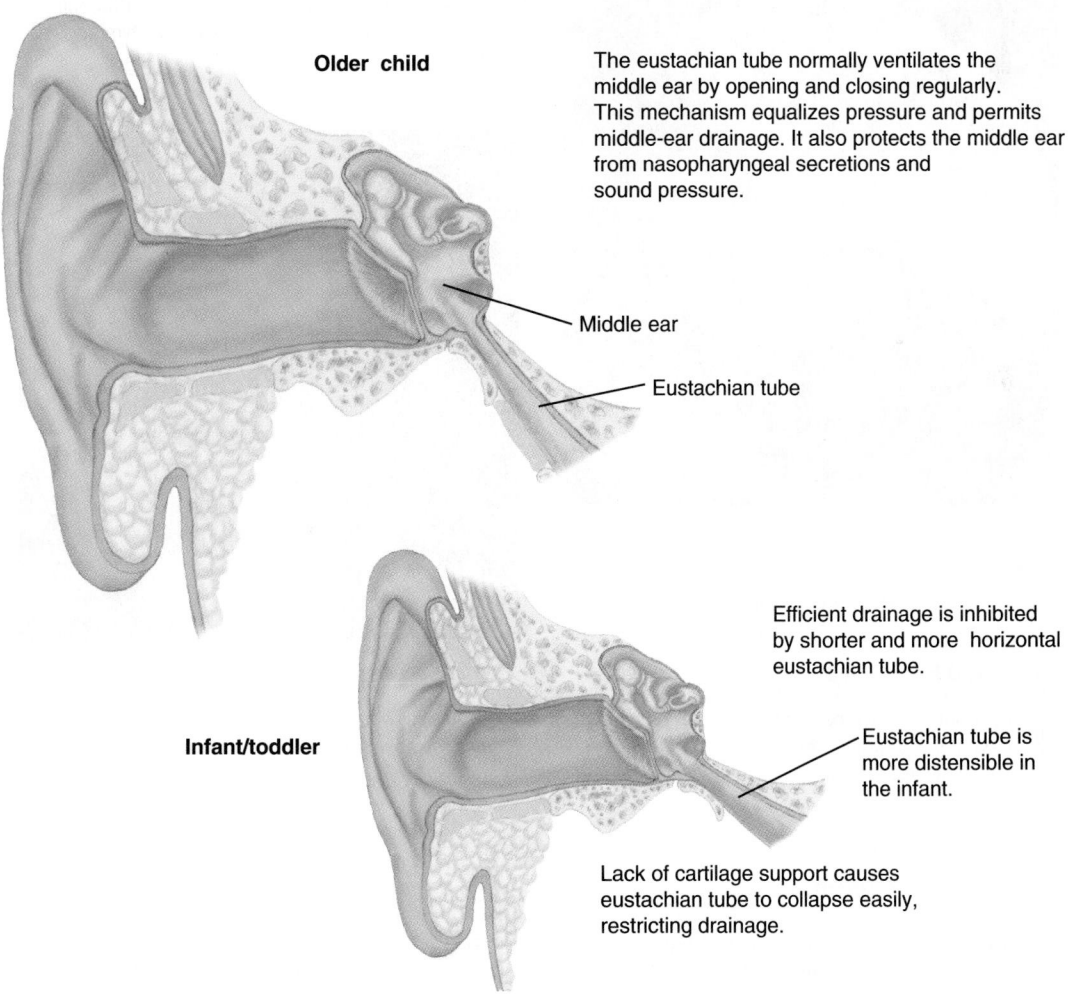

Older child

The eustachian tube normally ventilates the middle ear by opening and closing regularly. This mechanism equalizes pressure and permits middle-ear drainage. It also protects the middle ear from nasopharyngeal secretions and sound pressure.

Middle ear

Eustachian tube

Infant/toddler

Efficient drainage is inhibited by shorter and more horizontal eustachian tube.

Eustachian tube is more distensible in the infant.

Lack of cartilage support causes eustachian tube to collapse easily, restricting drainage.

◀ Normal right tympanic membrane and middle ear

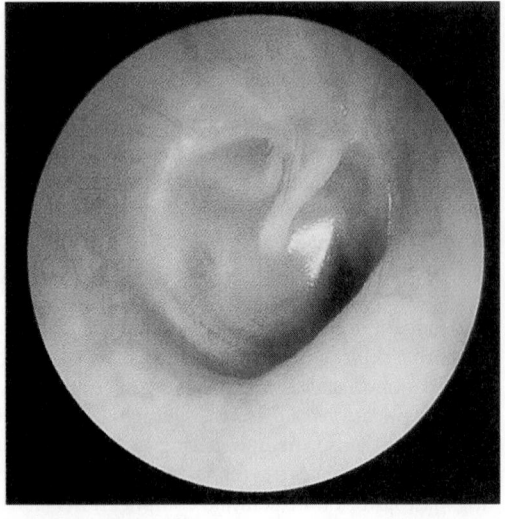

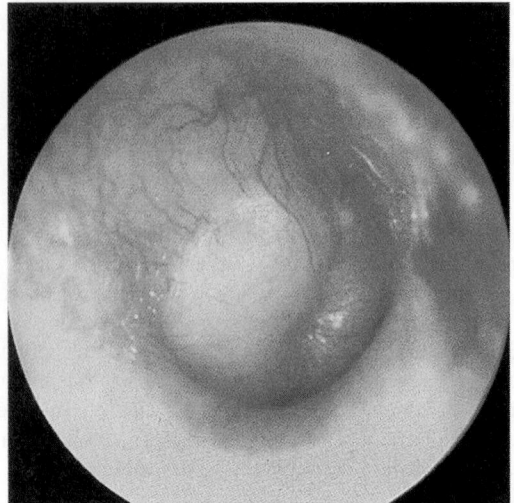

Acute otitis media: Bulging right tympanic membrane ▶

◀ Otitis media with effusion: Air-fluid level and bubbles visible through right retracted, translucent tympanic membrane

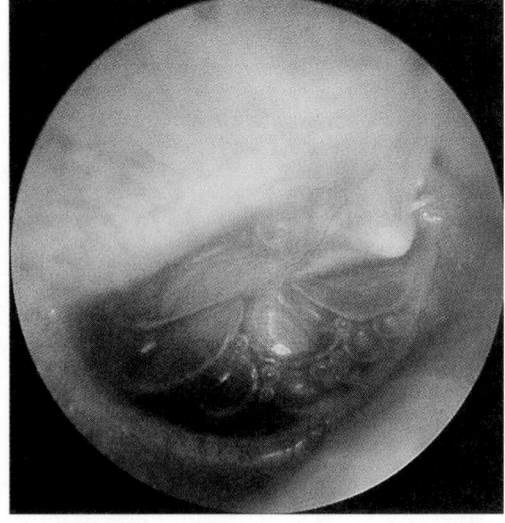

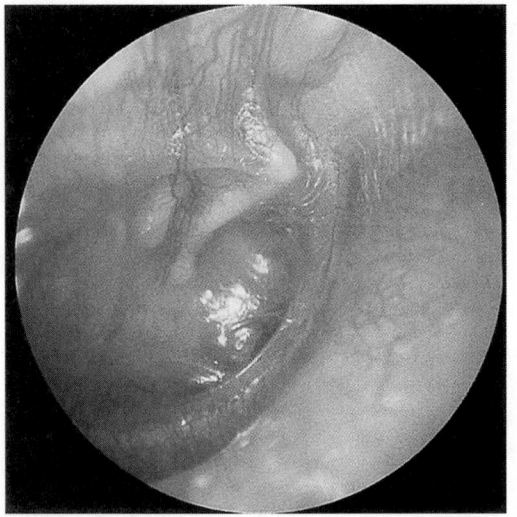

Otitis media with effusion: Severely retracted, opaque ▶
right tympanic membrane

FIGURE 45–2
. . . .
Appearance of tympanic membrane in otitis media as compared with normal tympanic membrane. (From Bluestone, C. D., & Klein, J. O. [1995]. *Otitis media in infants and children* [2nd ed.]. Philadelphia: Saunders, Color Plate Figs. 1 through 4.)

Therapeutic Management

Once diagnosed, acute otitis media is treated with a 5- to 7-day course of oral antibiotics (longer in children less than 2 years old). Amoxicillin is the initial drug of choice. Amoxicillin-clavulanate (Augmentin), effective against beta-lactamase-producing organisms resistant to amoxicillin alone, can be given to children whose infection does not begin to clear after 72 hours of treatment or if the infection persists. Alternative antibiotics such as erythromycin-sulfisoxazole (Pediazole), trimethoprim-sulfamethoxazole (e.g., Bactrim, Septra), cefaclor (Ceclor), or cefixime (Suprax) may be prescribed for penicillin-resistant organisms or in cases of penicillin allergy.

The child who has frequent, recurrent episodes of acute otitis media (three or more distinct episodes in 6 months or four or more episodes in 1 year) can be placed on prophylactic antibiotic treatment with a sulfonamide to be taken in one daily dose at bedtime (Dowell, Marcy, Phillips, et al., 1998). Prophylactic antibiotics may be given for no more than 6 months. These children should be examined monthly to monitor for middle-ear effusion. Hearing should be assessed with audiometry.

With the emergence of antimicrobial-resistant organisms, recent recommendations discourage antimicrobial treatment for children with otitis media with effusion (Dowell et al., 1998). The condition generally resolves spontaneously in approximately 3 months.

The usefulness of decongestants or antihistamines in the prevention and treatment of otitis media is controversial. Although these medications are widely prescribed, most research does not support their use except to control nasal drainage or congestion. Acetaminophen is given to help relieve pain and fever of acute otitis media.

In children with persistent ear infection despite antibiotic therapy or with otitis media with effusion that persists for more than 3 months and is associated with hearing loss, *myringotomy* with insertion of *tympanostomy tubes* (pressure equalizing, PE tubes) may be performed. During this operation, mucoid material is removed from the middle ear and a tympanostomy tube is inserted through the tympanic membrane. A tympanostomy tube is a small polyethylene tube that is inserted into the middle ear to equalize the pressure on both sides of the tympanic membrane and to keep the ear aerated. Negative pressure in the middle ear is relieved, allowing the middle-ear mucosa to return to normal and growth of the eustachian tube to occur. The tube usually falls out spontaneously in 6 to 12 months. This period may provide enough time for the effusion process to resolve, but some children need repeated insertions of tympanostomy tubes because of persistent eustachian tube dysfunction. Tympanostomy tubes are inserted under general anesthesia, usually in an outpatient surgery setting.

NURSING CARE
The Child with Otitis Media

Assessment

Ask the parent whether the child has had a recent upper respiratory tract infection or previous ear infections. Assess the child for fever and pain. Because signs of ear infection may be subtle in infants, the nurse should assess not only for obvious signs of ear pain, such as head rolling and pulling at the ear, but also for nonspecific findings, such as irritability, diarrhea, or decreased appetite. Older children may complain of pain or a feeling of fullness in the affected ear. The nurse examines the ear with a pneumatic otoscope, noting the color, mobility, and translucency of the tympanic membrane as well as the appearance of the external canal. The tympanic membrane should be inspected carefully for signs of perforation. The nurse cultures any drainage from the ear and notes the color, consistency, and odor. Hearing and language development should be assessed.

Nursing Diagnosis and Planning

The following nursing diagnoses and expected outcomes may be appropriate for the family and infant or child with otitis media:

- Pain related to inflammation and pressure in the middle ear.
  Expected Outcomes: The child will be free of pain, as evidenced by sleeping through the night, not pulling at the ears, and crying less. The child's tympanic membranes will appear shiny, pearl-gray, with normal landmarks, a visible light reflex, and normal mobility on tympanography.
- Knowledge Deficit related to incomplete understanding of the disease process and treatment regimen.
  Expected Outcomes: The parents will demonstrate methods of feeding the infant that decrease the risk of otitis media, how to keep child's ears dry if tympanostomy tubes are in place, and ways to follow the treatment regimen.
- Risk for Altered Body Temperature related to inflammation.
  Expected Outcome: The child will display a normal body temperature.
- Risk for Fluid Volume Deficit related to elevated temperature and decreased intake.
  Expected Outcome: The child will have moist mucous membranes, good skin turgor, and appropriate intake and output for age.

Interventions

Teach the parents the importance of giving antibiotics on time and for the prescribed number of days. Because the child usually feels much better after a few days of medication, parents may believe that the antibiotics are no longer necessary, and stop giving them. Increase compliance by giving written as well as oral instructions for administering medications. Providing a medication record form on which to record doses taken and a calibrated measuring device for liquid medications is also helpful.

> The nurse can enhance compliance through specific teaching about administration of antibiotics. For example, the nurse might say, "After a few days, your child may seem to be well and show no signs of the ear infection. If you stop giving the antibiotic at that time some of the germs that caused the otitis media might still be alive, and your child can experience a relapse."

The nurse also advises the parents to discard any unused antibiotic rather than save it, and not to give the child an antibiotic without consulting the physician first.

Acetaminophen can be given to relieve discomfort. The child's fluid intake should be increased if fever is present. Advise the parents to notify the physician if the child's condition has not improved after 48 hours of antibiotic treatment or if there is drainage from the affected ear. If a follow-up visit is recommended, emphasize the importance of keeping the appointment.

If the child is undergoing myringotomy with insertion of tympanostomy tubes, the nurse should prepare the child and parents as for any outpatient surgical procedure. Explain the procedure in clear terms and answer questions simply and honestly.

Postoperatively, the child is monitored for ear drainage.

A small amount of reddish drainage is normal for the first few days after surgery, but the parents should report any heavier bleeding or bleeding that occurs after 3 days. The parents should also be instructed to report any fever or increased pain. The child should avoid blowing the nose for 7 to 10 days.

Most physicians prefer that the child's ears be kept dry if tubes are in place, but some feel that a small amount of water in the ears is not harmful. Bath and lake water are potential sources of bacterial contamination, however, and chlorinated swimming pool water can be irritating to tympanic membranes with tubes. The usual recommendation is to place ear plugs or cotton balls covered with petroleum jelly in the ears during baths and shampoos. Swimming is allowed only with ear plugs and the physician's approval. Diving and swimming deep under water are prohibited. The size and appearance of the tympanostomy tubes should be described to the parents, and they should be reassured that if the tubes fall out it is not an emergency but that the physician should be notified.

Otitis media is usually a chronic problem, with frequent recurrences of infection and effusion. The nurse should teach the parents the early signs of ear infection and the importance of seeking care if these signs should occur. Because hearing impairment from middle-ear effusion can be very difficult for parents to detect, the child with chronic otitis media should undergo periodic hearing evaluations.

The nurse should teach parents methods to decrease the risk of recurrent otitis media, such as breast-feeding during infancy, discontinuing bottle-feeding as soon as possible, feeding the infant in an upright position, and refraining from giving a bottle to the infant in bed. Parents should be told not to smoke in the child's presence because passive smoking increases the incidence of otitis media.

Evaluation

- Is the child sleeping an appropriate amount of time for age?
- Did the parents complete the treatment regimen by giving the entire dose of the prescribed antibiotic and are they able to demonstrate appropriate feeding methods?
- Were follow-up appointments to determine the resolution of the otitis media kept?
- Is the child afebrile?
- Does the child appear well hydrated with moist mucous membranes and good skin turgor?

Pharyngitis and Tonsillitis

Pharyngitis, inflammation of the pharynx and surrounding lymphoid tissue, can be viral or bacterial in origin. Although pharyngitis is self-limiting and is a relatively minor disorder, streptococcal infections can have serious complications, among them rheumatic fever and acute glomerular nephritis.

Tonsillitis is the term commonly used to describe inflammation and infection of the two palatine tonsils. *Adenoiditis* refers to infection and inflammation of the pharyngeal tonsils, or adenoids, which are located above the palatine tonsils on the posterior wall of the nasopharynx. The purpose of these lymphoid tissues is to filter and protect the respiratory and digestive tracts from invasion by pathogens, but often the tonsils become a site for infection.

Etiology

Viral pharyngitis may be caused by adenoviruses, parainfluenza virus, influenza virus, coxsackieviruses, and respiratory syncytial virus. Group A beta-hemolytic streptococcus accounts for approximately 15% of pharyngitis cases. Streptococcal pharyngitis is rare before age 3 years. Streptococcal infection is spread by close droplet transmission. Tonsillitis, like pharyngitis, may be bacterial or viral in origin. The most common bacterial agent is group A beta-hemolytic streptococci.

Incidence

The incidence of pharyngitis and tonsillitis peaks between ages 4 and 7 years, when most children begin preschool and elementary school and have increased exposure to microorganisms. Group A beta-hemolytic streptococcal infection occurs most frequently in the winter and is spread more readily in crowded living situations. The incidence of tonsillitis decreases during middle childhood as the lymphoid tissue undergoes normal shrinkage.

Pathophysiology

Pharyngitis often accompanies the common cold. Tonsillitis is usually present with pharyngitis. Infection and inflammation of the tonsils cause them to enlarge. The palatine tonsils may meet in the midline (i.e., kissing tonsils) and cause difficulty swallowing and breathing. If adenoids enlarge they can obstruct the eustachian tubes, resulting in otitis media and hearing impairment. Hypertrophy of the adenoids can also block the passageway between the nose and the throat, causing mouth breathing or obstructive sleep apnea.

Manifestations

Signs and symptoms differ between viral and bacterial pharyngitis (Table 45–1). *The only reliable means of determining whether a case of pharyngitis is viral or bacterial in origin is with a throat culture.* Not all children with pharyngitis complain of a sore throat, particularly if they are of preschool age. Instead the child may complain of a stomachache or simply refuse to eat. The child with tonsillitis demonstrates the following:

- Sore throat, which may be persistent or recurrent
- Tonsils enlarged and bright red; may be covered with white exudate or cryptic plugs
- Difficulty swallowing
- Mouth breathing and an unpleasant mouth odor
- Enlarged adenoids, which may cause a nasal quality of speech, mouth breathing, hearing difficulty, otitis media, snoring, or obstructive sleep apnea

Older children and adolescents may experience a *peritonsillar abscess* associated with pharyngitis or tonsillitis. Peritonsillar abscess usually is unilateral, with the enlarged tonsil displacing the uvula to the opposite side. The child

TABLE 45–1
. . . .

Comparison of Viral and Bacterial Pharyngitis

Viral Pharyngitis	Bacterial Pharyngitis
Gradual onset	Abrupt onset (may be gradual in children < age 2 years)
Sore throat (reaches a peak on the second or third day)	Sore throat (usually severe)
Erythema and inflammation of the pharynx and tonsils (may be slight), vesicles or ulcers on tonsils	Erythema and inflammation of the pharynx and tonsils
Fever (usually low grade, but may be high)	Fever (usually high, 39.4° to 40°C [103° to 104°F], but may be moderate); begins early in illness and usually lasts 1 to 4 days
Hoarseness, cough, rhinitis, conjunctivitis, malaise, anorexia (early)	Abdominal pain, vomiting, headache
Cervical lymph nodes may be enlarged and tender	Cervical lymph nodes may be enlarged and tender
Usually lasts 3 to 4 days	Usually lasts 3 to 5 days

might refuse to talk or swallow due to severe pain that often radiates to the ear. There is a risk for airway obstruction and dehydration.

Diagnostic Evaluation

Rapid streptococcal antigen tests can accurately screen for group A streptococcal infection, but if the child's symptoms suggest a streptococcal infection, culture of a throat specimen obtained by swab should be done simultaneously. Because rapid strep tests have an approximately 20% incidence of false negative results, a throat culture should be done in symptomatic children with a negative rapid strep test. And because approximately 10% of children carry group A streptococci in their throats, a positive throat culture is not proof of active infection.

Therapeutic Management

During the acute phase of pharyngitis or tonsillitis, treatment is symptomatic, focusing on pain relief and rest. Acetaminophen or ibuprofen is used for pain; older children may find gargling with warm saline solution comforting. Cool, bland liquids are tolerated best because of the discomfort caused by swallowing solids or irritating liquids.

Antibiotics should be restricted to those children who test positive on antigen detection tests or cultures. Streptococcal pharyngitis is best treated orally with penicillin or penicillin V given two to three times daily for 10 days. Erythromycin may be used in children who are allergic to penicillin. A single intramuscular dose of procaine penicillin and benzathine penicillin G might be considered in children for whom compliance is expected to be a problem. Children placed on penicillin therapy are noninfectious to others 24 hours after therapy is initiated.

Surgical removal of the tonsils, or tonsillectomy, is controversial. Although some physicians think that a tonsillectomy is warranted in cases of recurrent tonsillitis, the prevailing attitude is more conservative, and the procedure is generally reserved for cases of upper airway obstruction, peritonsillar abscess, obstructive sleep apnea, or other serious problems. Tonsillectomy is generally not performed in children less than 3 years old because of the tendency for remaining tonsillar tissues to hypertrophy. Contraindica-

tions to tonsillectomy include active infection and cleft palate (see Chapter 43). Surgical removal of the tonsils while they are infected can result in spread of the infecting organism and sepsis. In children with cleft palate, the tonsils help prevent air escape during speech. Adenoidectomy alone may be performed in cases of recurrent otitis media secondary to eustachian tube obstruction or for persistent nasal or airway obstruction.

Many parents believe that a tonsillectomy will solve their child's problems of frequent sore throats, mouth breathing, and poor weight gain. There is no evidence that a tonsillectomy reduces the incidence of recurrent pharyngitis. The nurse should be prepared to discuss the current treatment philosophy with parents and address their concerns. If tonsillectomy is chosen as the method of treatment, the procedure is often done in a day surgery setting.

Nursing Considerations

Assessment of the child with pharyngitis or tonsillitis includes inspecting the pharynx for erythema, exudate, or petechiae. The skin should be inspected for rash and color changes. Some children with streptococcal pharyngitis have a pink, sandpaper-like rash on the trunk (see Chapter 49). The child is questioned about the onset and location of throat, ear, or abdominal pain. The parent of a preverbal child may report that the child refuses to eat or begins to cry during feedings. The nurse also assesses the child's temperature and respiratory status and asks the older child or parent about the onset of symptoms and any known contact with streptococcal infection in the school or family. Also ask whether the child has been taking any antibiotics at home, because they will interfere with the results of the throat culture.

Comfort measures to relieve throat discomfort include administering acetaminophen, warm salt water gargles (¼ teaspoon of salt per 8-ounce glass of water), and warm or cool compresses applied to the throat. The child should not be forced to eat. Offer cool, bland liquids to prevent dehydration. Soft foods such as gelatin, soup, mashed potatoes, puddings, Cream of Wheat, and flavored ice pops appeal to children the best. Bed rest is advisable while the child has a fever. The nurse should advise the parent to call the health care provider if the child has difficulty breathing or increased difficulty swallowing, or if the fever has lasted more than 3 days. If any family members develop a fever, sore throat, or headache, they should have a throat culture. Instruct the parents that leftover antibiotics from siblings or friends should never be used.

Moist mucous membranes and adequate urine output are signs of proper fluid balance. At the end of treatment the child should be free of signs of infection and show no signs of complications of the disease.

NURSING CARE
The Child Undergoing a Tonsillectomy

Preoperative Assessment

A complete history is taken with special attention given to allergy symptoms, difficulty swallowing, or airway obstruction. The child is assessed for signs of active infection (fever, elevated white blood cell [WBC] count) and redness and exudate of the throat. The child should be questioned about the presence of pain in the throat or ears. Because the tonsillar area is so vascular, any bleeding history must be recorded and communicated to the primary physician.

Laboratory results (prothrombin time, partial thromboplastin time, platelet count, hemoglobin, hematocrit, urinalysis) are reviewed and the child should be observed for loose teeth to decrease the risk of aspiration during surgery.

Preoperative Nursing Diagnosis and Planning

The following nursing diagnoses and expected outcomes may be appropriate for the child undergoing a tonsillectomy and the child's family:

■ Anxiety related to surgery.
Expected Outcome: The child and parents will exhibit a decreased level of anxiety, as evidenced by relaxed body posture and involvement in play activities.
■ Knowledge Deficit related to surgery and procedures.
Expected Outcome: The child and parents will verbalize understanding of preoperative teaching.

Preoperative Interventions

The nurse reassures the child that talking will not be a problem after surgery. Emphasize to the child that it is important to drink liquids after surgery, even though the child's throat will be sore (see also Chapter 37). Teach the child's family about postoperative pain assessment and appropriate anal-

gesia administration, because many parents undermedicate their children. Undermedication can interfere with optimal postoperative recovery (Sutters & Miaskowski, 1997). The child's ability to relax preoperatively and the family's appropriate description of the operative and recovery course comprise evaluation criteria.

Postoperative Assessment

Immediately after surgery the child should be assessed for bleeding and ability to swallow secretions. If bleeding occurs, the child is returned to surgery for recauterization. The rate and quality of respirations and breath sounds should be assessed. Vital signs, including blood pressure, should be monitored frequently (a common protocol is every 15 minutes for the first hour, hourly for 4 hours, and then every 2 to 4 hours for the next 24 hours). Suction equipment should be available, but do not suction unless there is airway obstruction. The child is assessed for bleeding (frequent swallowing, restlessness, a fast, thready pulse, or the vomiting of bright red blood). Carefully using a tongue blade and a good light source, inspect the pharynx for clots or bleeding.

Postoperative Nursing Diagnosis and Planning

The following nursing diagnoses and expected outcomes may be appropriate for the child who has undergone a tonsillectomy and the child's family:

■ Risk for Injury (hemorrhage) related to surgery.
Expected Outcome: The child will experience minimal postoperative bleeding, nausea, or vomiting.
■ Ineffective Airway Clearance related to throat discomfort.
Expected Outcome: The child will maintain a clear airway without jeopardizing the operative site.
■ Pain related to surgical removal of tonsils.
Expected Outcome: The child will describe relief from pain and be able to rest.
■ Risk for Fluid Volume Deficit related to difficulty swallowing and NPO status before surgery.
Expected Outcome: The child will have adequate fluid intake for age and will experience minimal fluid loss.

■ Knowledge Deficit related to home care.
Expected Outcome: The parents will verbalize an understanding of the care of their child at home.

Postoperative Interventions

The child should be placed in a prone or side-lying position to facilitate drainage. Although not all clinicians are in agreement, straws and forks may be withheld to prevent trauma to the surgical site. When visually assessing the site, use a flashlight for illumination and avoid using a tongue depressor if at all possible. If a tongue depressor is necessary, keep it as forward in the mouth as possible. If bleeding occurs, the child is turned to the side and the physician notified.

PARENTS WANT TO KNOW

Caring for a Child After a Tonsillectomy

- Encourage your child to participate only in quiet activities for a week after surgery.
- Encourage abundant liquid intake. Avoid citrus juices, which irritate the throat, for 10 days.
- Avoid red liquids, which will give the appearance of blood if your child vomits.
- Add full liquids (cream soups, gelatin, puddings, soups) on the second day and soft foods (mashed potatoes, soft cereals, eggs) as your child tolerates them. Avoid rough or scratchy foods (bacon, chips, popcorn), citrus foods, or spicy foods for 3 weeks.
- Encourage your child to chew and swallow, because this exercises pharyngeal muscles and promotes healing.
- Do not give your child any straws, forks, or sharp pointed toys that could be put in the mouth.
- Use acetaminophen for pain relief; your child may have a prescription for acetaminophen with codeine for sore throat. Do not use aspirin or any medicine containing aspirin because it might affect the clotting time of the blood.
- Pain should not persist past the first week. Notify your doctor if pain persists.
- Discourage your child from coughing, clearing the throat, or gargling.
- Bad mouth odor is normal and may be relieved by drinking more liquids.
- Earache and slight fever are common.
- Call your physician for any bleeding, persistent earache, or fever over 101°F (38.5°C).
- Bleeding caused by tissue sloughing during the healing process can occur 7 to 10 days after surgery. Such bleeding requires immediate medical attention.
- To protect your child from catching a cold, keep the child away from crowds for 2 weeks.
- Your child may return to school when directed by the physician, usually in about 10 days.
- Bring your child for a follow-up appointment in 1 to 2 weeks.

Vomiting of old blood (coffee grounds emesis) is common. Antiemetics are given as ordered to decrease throat pain caused by retching. If vomiting occurs, keep the child NPO for 30 minutes, and then resume clear liquids.

Nonaspirin analgesics (e.g., acetaminophen) are given as ordered. Adequate analgesia increases fluid intake. Some centers give the analgesic every 4 hours for the first 24 hours because throat discomfort is expected. An ice collar can be applied for comfort.

Provide clear, cool liquids when the child is fully awake. Citrus drinks, carbonated drinks, and extremely hot or cold liquids should be avoided because they may irritate the throat. Milk and milk products (puddings, ice cream) are avoided initially because milk products can coat the throat, causing a need to clear the throat and thus increasing the risk of bleeding. Adequate fluid intake promotes healing and maintains hydration. The nurse teaches the parents the principles of home management and ensures that the child is retaining fluids before discharging the child from the surgical unit.

Postoperative Evaluation

- Does the child have minimal bleeding, nausea, and vomiting, and are vital signs within normal limits?
- Is the child's intake and urine output normal for age?
- Are the child's complaints of pain and irritability minimal?
- Can the parents explain home care measures?

■ *Laryngomalacia (Congenital Laryngeal Stridor)*

Flaccidity of the epiglottis and supraglottic aperture and weakness of the airway walls contribute to laryngomalacia, the most common cause of inspiratory stridor in the neonatal period. Laryngomalacia may be due to immature neuromuscular development in the airway.

Manifestations

Noisy, crowing, inspiratory respiratory sounds (stridor) are present, with or without retractions. The infant does not usually become cyanotic despite the stridor. Stridor is usually present at birth, but may begin as late as age 2 months. Symptoms increase when the infant is supine or when the infant is crying. The diagnosis is based on a good history and findings on direct laryngoscopy.

Therapeutic Management

Symptoms usually resolve without treatment by age 18 to 24 months. In rare instances, endotracheal intubation or tracheostomy may be required.

Nursing Considerations

The nurse observes the neonate for stridor, retractions, and dyspnea, noting any signs of acute respiratory distress. Because some infants have feeding problems, the infant should be observed for feeding difficulties. The infant's respiratory status is assessed and findings recorded every 2 hours and as needed. Obstruction increases during crying when the child has a respiratory infection, and stridor increases when the child is supine with the neck flexed. Positioning with the neck hyperextended improves the child's breathing. A respiratory tract infection might place undue stress on the infant's system.

As part of discharge teaching, parents are taught the signs of respiratory distress so that they can monitor for changes that might indicate respiratory tract infection. If the bottle-fed infant has feeding difficulties, the parents can try using a smaller nipple. Smaller, more frequent feedings are sometimes better tolerated by infants with respiratory difficulties. Reassure the parents that the condition usually resolves by the time the child is 2 years old. The ability of parents to comfortably care for their child indicates the effectiveness of the discharge teaching.

Croup

Croup refers to a group of conditions characterized by inspiratory stridor, a harsh (brassy or croupy) cough, hoarseness, and varying degrees of respiratory distress (Table 45–2). The major types of croup are acute spasmodic croup, laryngotracheobronchitis, bacterial tracheitis, and epiglottitis. Although epiglottitis is a type of croup, it is discussed separately because it is a bacterial infection with unique symptoms and treatment.

Etiology and Incidence

Parainfluenza viruses cause most cases of viral croup. The cause of acute spasmodic croup is unknown.

Laryngotracheobronchitis, the most common form of croup, usually affects infants and toddlers. Laryngotracheobronchitis is a common cause of airway obstruction in children ages 6 months to 6 years. The incidence of croup is higher in boys than in girls, and the disease occurs more often during the winter than in other seasons.

Acute spasmodic croup occurs most often in children ages 1 to 3 years. Spasmodic croup occurs more often in anxious and excitable children. There seems to be hereditary predisposition to spasmodic croup.

Bacterial tracheitis is less common than laryngotracheobronchitis and acute spasmodic croup. It progresses from an upper respiratory tract infection and may be confused with laryngotracheobronchitis because of similar manifestations. Treatment for laryngotracheobronchitis is not effective if the child has bacterial tracheitis.

The following discussion focuses on acute spasmodic croup and laryngotracheobronchitis, the most common type of croup leading to hospitalization.

Manifestations

Croup often begins at night and may be preceded by several days of symptoms of upper respiratory tract infection. The child with laryngotracheobronchitis may have a fever along with other signs and symptoms; occasionally the fever is as high as 40°C (104°F). Children with spasmodic croup do not have a fever. Other manifestations include

- The sudden onset of a harsh, metallic cough, sore throat, inspiratory stridor, and hoarseness
- The use of accessory muscles (substernal, intercostal, suprasternal retractions) to breathe
- Frightened appearance

TABLE 45–2

Comparison of Types of Croup

	Acute Spasmodic Laryngitis (Spasmodic Croup)	Acute Laryngotracheo-bronchitis (LTB)	Acute Epiglottitis	Acute Bacterial Tracheitis
Age usually affected	1 to 3 years	3 months to 3 years	3 to 8 years	1 month to 6 years
Location of swelling and inflammation	Subglottic (below the vocal cords)	Vocal cords, subglottic, and tissue below vocal cords, including bronchi	Supraglottic (above the vocal cords)	Mucosa of the upper trachea
Cause	Viral, emotional, or genetic predisposition	Usually viral, but may be bacterial	Bacterial (usually *H. influenzae*, type b)	*Staphylococcus* (most common)
Assessment	Sudden onset, usually at night Child awakens with harsh cough, inspiratory stridor, dyspnea, and hoarseness	Gradual onset, usually at night Child awakens with harsh cough and inspiratory stridor	Sudden onset, which may rapidly progress to complete airway obstruction and death Sore throat, dyspnea	Progresses from upper respiratory infection (1 to 2 days) High fever Stridor Croupy cough Purulent secretions
Treatment	Humidity Increased fluids May treat at home	Humidity Racemic epinephrine IV fluids during respiratory distress Hospitalization may be necessary	IV antibiotics Artificial airway IV fluids Emergency hospitalization	Humidified oxygen Antipyretics IV antibiotics May require intubation

- Agitation
- Cyanosis

Symptoms are usually worse at night and better in the day; they may recur for several nights.

Diagnostic Evaluation

The diagnosis is made mainly from observation of clinical symptoms. Differentiation between viral croup and bacterial epiglottitis is very important, as treatment differs. However, the use of the *H. influenzae* b (Hib) vaccine has reduced the incidence of epiglottitis. A croup score is often used to describe the severity of respiratory distress. Arterial blood

gas values or pulse oximetry readings may be monitored to detect decreased Pao₂ levels.

Therapeutic Management

The goal of treatment is to maintain a patent airway. Children with acute spasmodic croup can usually be cared for at home. Treatment for acute spasmodic croup includes a calm approach and increased oral fluid intake if the child is not in respiratory distress. The benefits of providing mist, either from steam produced by hot running water in a closed bathroom or cool mist from a bedside humidifier, appear to provide more of a psychological effect than a physiological

PATHOPHYSIOLOGY
of Croup

Croup is a viral infection of the upper airway. Although the entire upper, or nonreactive, airway is involved to some extent in all forms of croup, each type is named according to the anatomic area most severely involved. For example, laryngotracheobronchitis affects the larynx, trachea, and bronchi. In acute spasmodic croup, the larynx is the area of most severe inflammation.

In all forms of croup, mucosal inflammation and edema cause narrowing of the airway. This narrowing is more dangerous in infants and young children than in adults because of their small airway diameter and flexible larynx, which is more susceptible to spasm.

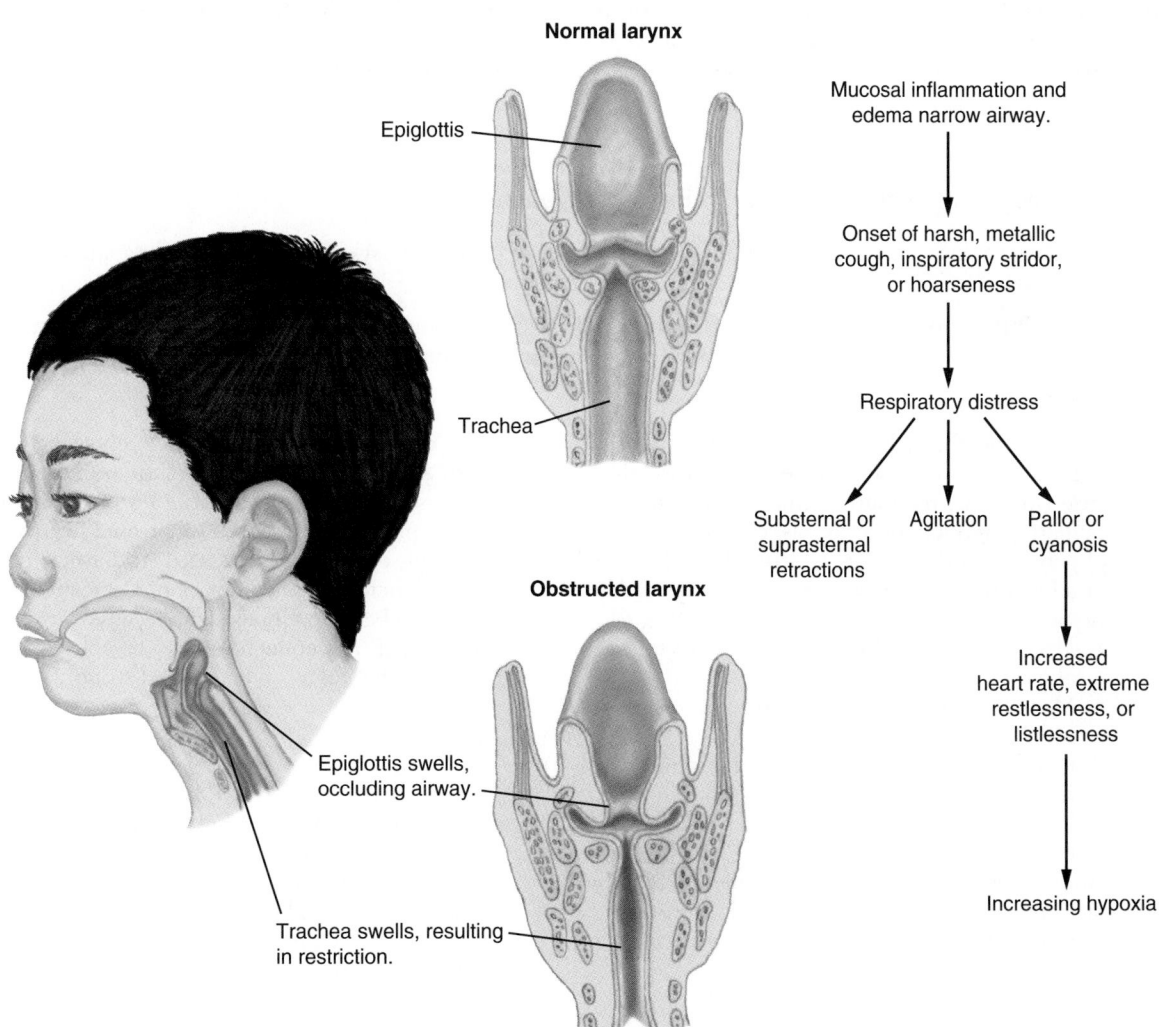

one (Grad, 1998). If mist is used, cool mist humidifiers are recommended over steam vaporizers, which pose a danger of scald burns. Taking the child out into the cool, humid night air may relieve mucosal swelling.

Crying aggravates the airway obstruction. Children who develop stridor at rest, cyanosis, severe agitation or fatigue, or moderate to severe retractions or who are unable to take oral fluids should be seen in the emergency department.

Children with laryngotracheobronchitis, usually a more severe type of croup, are more often hospitalized than those with acute spasmodic croup. Racemic epinephrine nebulized with oxygen may be given to decrease the laryngeal edema and bronchospasm. The child must be observed closely for changes in respiratory status and should not be treated with epinephrine on an outpatient basis because the effects of epinephrine are temporary. Children who receive epinephrine should be observed in the emergency department at least 3 hours after treatment and should not be discharged if stridor or retractions are present.

Corticosteroid therapy may be used in children with croup to reduce inflammatory edema and prevent destruction of ciliated epithelium. Antibiotics are not indicated unless a bacterial infection is present. Acetaminophen is given to reduce fever.

The benefits of mist-tent or hood therapy remain controversial, particularly if placing the child in a tent increases agitation. Cool mist in the room may be more effective. Intravenous (IV) fluids are given until respiratory distress subsides and the child can take adequate fluids by mouth. Sedatives are contraindicated because they depress respirations and could mask restlessness, an early sign of hypoxia.

If signs of moderate or severe hypoxia develop, the child is intubated immediately and is transferred to an intensive care unit. Usually the tube remains in place from 3 to 5 days and is removed when the child can breathe around the tube.

NURSING CARE
The Child with Croup

Assessment

A nursing history typically reveals a recent upper respiratory tract infection. Assess the child for inspiratory stridor, barking cough, hoarseness, and increased heart rate and respiratory rate. Record any signs of respiratory distress, such as the use of accessory muscles; substernal, intercostal, and suprasternal retractions; nasal flaring; restlessness and irritability; and pallor or cyanosis. Cyanosis, an increased heart rate and respiratory rate, extreme restlessness, or evidence of fatigue or listlessness may be signs of hypoxia and should be reported to the physician immediately. The lungs should be auscultated for adventitious breath sounds or areas of decreased breath sounds. Temperature and hydration status should also be assessed.

Nursing Diagnosis, Planning, Intervention, and Evaluation

Nursing Diagnosis
- Ineffective Airway Clearance related to mucosal swelling and obstruction of the upper respiratory tract.

Expected Outcome
- The child will breathe without difficulty and will have a heart and respiratory rate within normal limits for age.

Intervention

1. Monitor the child's breathing continuously for signs and symptoms of increased respiratory distress (increased respiratory rate, stridor at rest, nasal flaring, retractions, cyanosis, changes in level of consciousness or increased irritability, decreased or adventitious breath sounds, tachypnea). Additionally:
   a. *Never* leave a child with respiratory distress alone.
   b. Measure vital signs hourly and as necessary.
   c. Monitor pulse oximetry readings.
   d. Notify the physician of increased respiratory distress.
   e. If epiglottitis is suspected, call a physician and do not inspect the throat.
2. Administer humidified oxgyen at the ordered flow rate; administer mist only if ordered. Monitor pulse oximetry readings or transcutaneous oxygen concentration frequently.

Rationale

1. The child must be monitored closely to detect early signs of worsening obstruction. Extreme restlessness, listlessness, cyanosis, or a rapid, increasing respiratory rate with an increased heart rate are signs of hypoxia. Increased stridor may be a sign of increasing inflammation. Decreased stridor may also be an ominous sign, because with severe obstruction not enough air may be able to pass through the larynx to cause loud stridor.

Visual inspection may result in laryngospasm and airway obstruction.
2. Oxygen may be ordered to alleviate hypoxia and restlessness. The child's condition must be monitored closely because oxygen use can mask early signs of hypoxia and increasing obstruction.

3. Have emergency intubation equipment (e.g., intubation tray, oxygen, suction, manual resuscitation bag, valve, mask) closely available.
4. Administer aerosolized racemic epinephrine as ordered. Observe the child for response to medication. Monitor for tachycardia.

5. Keep the child as quiet as possible. Encourage parents to stay nearby or even to climb inside the mist tent (if used) with the child if the child is frightened and refuses to stay inside the tent. If the use of a tent or hood is causing distress, treatment may be more effective if the child is held by a parent and cool mist is directed toward the child's face. Maintain a calm, quiet environment. Provide a security object for the child. Observe the child closely but disturb as little as possible.
6. Support the child in an upright position with the head of the bed elevated or with the child held by the parent.

3. The child's condition can change rapidly, and respiratory arrest from airway obstruction can occur.
4. Racemic epinephrine decreases layngeal edema. Tachycardia is a side effect of adrenergic medications. The effect of racemic epinephrine lasts less than 2 hours. Children should be observed for rebound obstruction, which may occur within a few hours after administration of racemic epinephrine.
5. Crying aggravates laryngospasm and increases hypoxia. A parent's presence is an effective supportive measure for frightened, agitated infants and children. Anxiety and crying increase the airway obstruction of croup.

6. An upright position facilitates respiration by decreasing pressure from abdominal contents on the diaphragm.

Evaluation
- Are the child's respiratory rate and heart rate within normal limits for age and is the oxygen saturation greater than 95%?
- Does the child have pink mucous membranes and nail beds, and clear breath sounds with effective air movement?

Nursing Diagnosis
■ Risk for Fluid Volume Deficit related to inadequate oral intake and tachypnea.

Expected Outcome
- The child will have adequate fluid intake for age and weight.

Intervention

1. Monitor the child's hydration status with intake and output measurements and urine specific gravity. Check mucous membranes, skin turgor, and presence of tears. Weigh the child daily on the same scale and at same time of day.
2. Offer clear liquids as tolerated when the child no longer exhibits signs of respiratory distress.

3. Give liquids at room temperature.
4. Observe the child's ability to swallow, noting any respiratory distress.
5. Administer IV fluids at ordered rate. Use IV tubing with graduated fluid control chamber to guard against accidental infusion of large volumes of fluid.

6. Administer acetaminophen for fever as ordered. Monitor temperature every 4 hours.

Rationale

1. An increased respiratory rate causes insensible water loss. Difficulty swallowing leads to decreased intake.

2. Fluids are encouraged to decrease edema and the viscosity of secretions. Fluids may be given orally if stridor is mild and the child is not tachypneic. Increased oral fluids and a regular diet are offered as soon as the child's condition improves.
3. Cold liquids may increase respiratory distress.
4. Tachypnea and laryngospasm often cause dysphagia.
5. IV fluids may be ordered during the acute phase of croup to prevent dehydration. Oral fluids are contraindicated in the setting of severe respiratory distress because of the risk of aspiration and the increased stress put on the systems of the body.
6. Fever increases insensible water loss by increasing metabolic rate.

Evaluation
- Is the child taking adequate amounts of fluid?
- Does the child have urine output appropriate for age?
- Does the child have urine specific gravity of 1.002 to 1.030?
- Does the child exhibit moist mucous membranes and good skin turgor?

Nursing Diagnosis

Expected Outcomes

■ Fear related to dyspnea and hospitalization.

• The child will be less anxious, as evidenced by resting quietly, crying less, and cooperating with nursing care as appropriate for age.
• The parents will demonstrate decreased anxiety, as evidenced by their ability to assist the child to deal with stressors of hospitalization and illness.

Intervention	Rationale
1. Maintain a calm, restful environment. Organize nursing care so as to disturb the child as little as possible. Postpone unnecessary procedures until the child is in less distress. Allow periods of uninterrupted rest.	1. Anxiety and crying increase oxygen consumption and respiratory distress.
2. Encourage parents to touch and cuddle the child. Toddlers and infants like to be held when they are ill. If the child has a mist tent, parents should be told it is acceptable to sit inside the mist tent with their child. Children who are not in tents can be held in their parents' arms while mist is directed toward their faces.	2. A parent's presence is important in reducing anxiety in infants and young children.
3. Encourage parents' participation in care. Explain ways that they can make their child more comfortable and tell them that their presence is important.	3. Parents' feelings of helplessness and anxiety are decreased when they are allowed to comfort and care for their child. Participation in the child's care also helps prepare the parents for discharge and home care.
4. Provide parents with breaks as needed and assure them that their child will be cared for in their absence.	4. Caring for a child in the hospital is exhausting to parents. Fatigue magnifies feelings of anxiety and helplessness.
5. Allow the child to keep a favorite toy or blanket.	5. Familiar objects provide a sense of security for small children in the strange hospital environment.
6. Explain all treatments, equipment, and procedures to the child and parents.	6. Anxiety and fear related to lack of knowledge can be minimized by providing clear and timely explanations.
7. Allow the child and parents to ask questions and to discuss fears and concerns.	7. Cooperation is increased with understanding of the purpose of treatments. Parents are often very anxious because of the sudden onset and frightening nature of croup symptoms. Parents sometimes feel guilty for not having brought the child in for treatment sooner.
8. Use developmentally appropriate communication techniques (e.g., play, puppets).	8. A calm, empathic, caring approach is helpful in providing emotional support to the child and parents.

Evaluation

• Does the child exhibit decreased signs of agitation or being upset (less crying)?
• Does the child allow the nursing staff to provide comfort and support?
• Does the child demonstrate adequate rest and sleep patterns by not waking up during the night and showing no signs of fatigue or irritability?
• Can the child engage in age-appropriate play?
• Is the parent able to comfort the child?

Nursing Diagnosis

Expected Outcome

■ Knowledge Deficit related to course of croup and home care.

• The parents will have accurate knowledge of croup symptoms, state they are comfortable in home management of croup, and will seek assistance appropriately if symptoms become severe.

Intervention	Rationale
1. Determine the parents' level of understanding of croup and previous experiences in coping with the illness. Teach parents that once a child has had an attack, croup tends to recur. Teach parents that maintaining a stable environmental temperature and humidity and keeping the child well hydrated may help decrease the severity of attacks. Teach that croup is a viral infection, and avoiding large groups of people and practicing good health habits to prevent infection may decrease the risk of recurrence of croup.	1. Teaching about how to recognize and manage the condition increases parental control.

2. Teach parents the signs and symptoms of respiratory distress. Parents should be taught how to count respirations and how to assess for retractions and cyanosis.
  a. The child should be closely observed at all times for a worsening condition, which can occur rapidly.
  b. Parents should call the doctor if any of the following occurs in the child:
    • Increased difficulty breathing or seems to be getting worse
    • Retractions (tugging in of the skin between, above, or below the ribs with inspiration)
    • Lips turn bluish or dusky
    • Breathing cool or warm mist does not improve symptoms in 20 minutes
    • Inability to drink much over the past 24 hours
    • Drooling or difficulty swallowing
    • Fever (over 39.4° [103°F])
    • Seems exhausted, listless, or very agitated.
	2. Knowing when to seek attention prevents more serious consequences of airway obstruction.

3. Explain the possible advantage of a humidified environment in treating croup symptoms. Ways to provide humidity include the following:
  a. Hold and cuddle the child in a steamy bathroom for at least 10 minutes or until symptoms are relieved; run all the hot water faucets full force with the door closed.
  b. Place a cool mist humidifier beside the child's bed.
  c. Take the child outside into the cool, moist night air; opening the freezer door can also be effective.
	3. High humidity might help thin secretions and decrease swelling.

4. Explain the importance of adequate hydration and nutrition. If able, the child needs to drink two to four glasses (500 to 1,000 ml) of fluids daily. Sips of warm fluids during a croup attack help relax the vocal cords and thin mucus.	4. Adequate hydration is important for thinning secretions. Adequate caloric intake helps replace calories expended fighting the infection.
5. Give acetaminophen for fever. Do *not* give cough syrup or cold medicines.	5. Acetaminophen is effective in reducing fever and will help the child feel more comfortable. Cough syrups and cold medicines can dry and thicken secretions.
6. If the episode resolves, the parents should put the child back to bed and check on the child periodically throughout the night. Instruct the parents to call the physician immediately if the child seems worse or does not improve in 48 hours.	6. Close observation is essential to detect worsening of croup symptoms. Worsening of symptoms will not necessarily awaken the child.

Evaluation

• Can the parents explain the appropriate treatment of croup and when medical help is needed?

PATHOPHYSIOLOGY
. . . .
of Epiglottitis

Epiglottitis is a bacterial form of croup. The epiglottis and surrounding structures become inflamed as bacterial infection invades the soft tissue. The epiglottis becomes edematous and cherry red, and may become so swollen that it completely covers the glottis and obstructs the airway. Secretions pool in the hypopharynx and larynx. As the disease rapidly progresses, swelling becomes so severe that the child is unable to swallow and begins to drool. The child's voice is muffled and the throat is very sore. Inspiratory stridor, cough, and irritability are present. Complete airway obstruction can occur rapidly, resulting in hypoxia, acidosis, and death.

The onset of epiglottitis is usually sudden. The child may have had symptoms of a mild upper respiratory tract infection for a few days before symptoms began. Children with epiglottitis can progress from wellness to complete airway obstruction within 2 to 6 hours.

Clinical manifestations

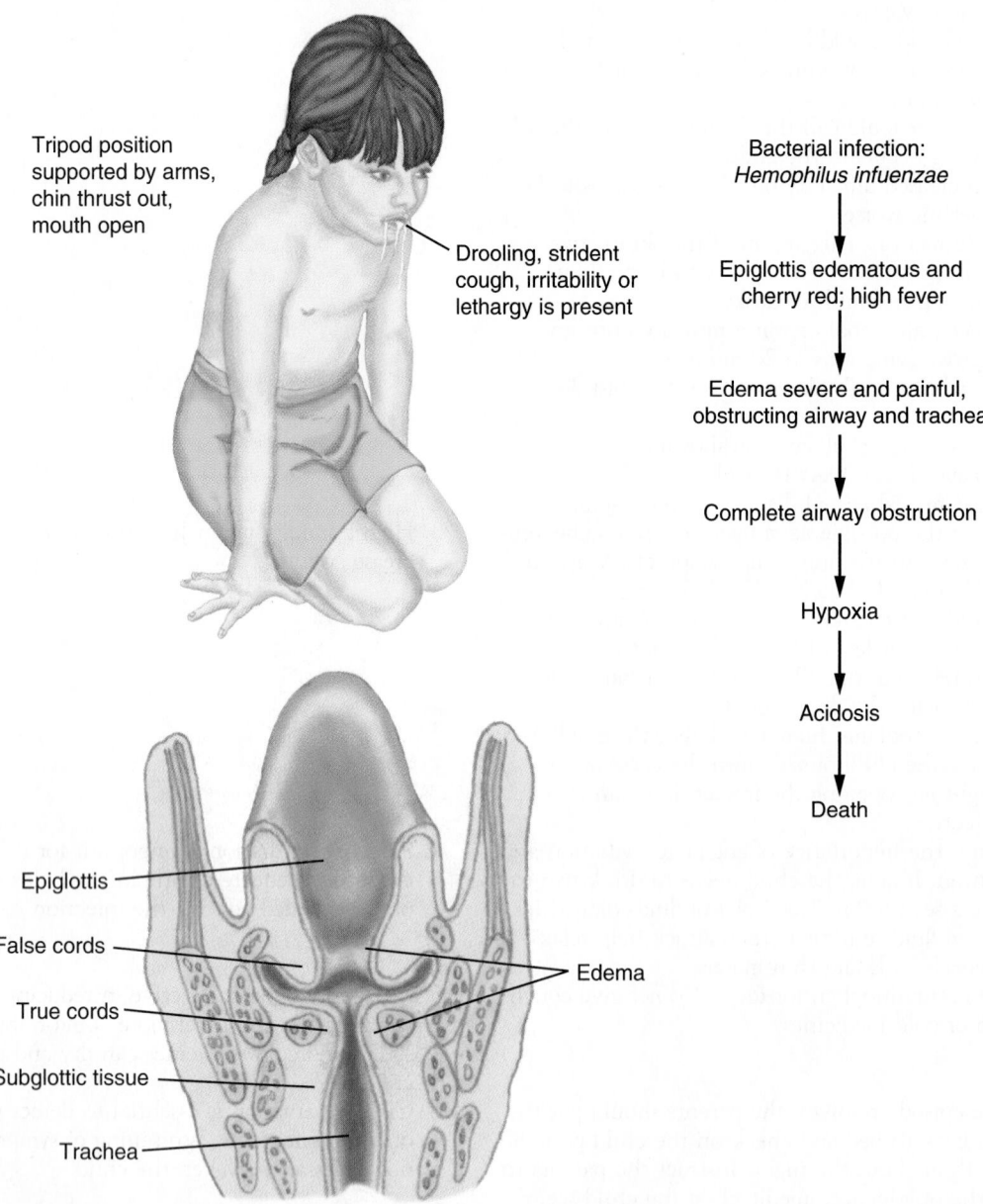

Tripod position supported by arms, chin thrust out, mouth open

Drooling, strident cough, irritability or lethargy is present

Bacterial infection: *Hemophilus infuenzae*

Epiglottis edematous and cherry red; high fever

Edema severe and painful, obstructing airway and trachea

Complete airway obstruction

Hypoxia

Acidosis

Death

Epiglottis

False cords

True cords

Subglottic tissue

Trachea

Edema

Epiglottitis

Epiglottitis (Supraglottitis)

Epiglottitis, the acute inflammation and swelling of the epiglottis and surrounding tissue, is a life-threatening, rapidly progressive condition that may cause complete airway obstruction within a few hours of onset.

Etiology and Incidence

Epiglottitis is almost always caused by *Hemophilus influenzae*. Other organisms, such as *Staphylococcus aureus*, *Hemophilus parainfluenzae*, *Streptococcus pneumoniae*, and beta-hemolytic streptococci, cause the infection less frequently. Viral epiglottitis is rare.

Epiglottitis occurs most often in children ages 3 to 7 years. The incidence is about equal in males and females. The incidence has decreased markedly with use of the Hib vaccine.

Manifestations

Unlike croup, epiglottitis has an abrupt onset with rapid progression of symptoms. Often parents report that the child was put to bed well and awakened with a severe sore throat and difficulty swallowing. The child demonstrates a high fever (39° to 40°C [102.2° to 104°F]) and appears toxic and very ill. The accompanying sore throat can progress to acute respiratory distress in a few hours. The child appears anxious and frightened and may be irritable or lethargic. One of the classic signs of epiglottitis is that the child insists on sitting upright, often in a tripod position (leaning forward supported on the arms), with the chin thrust out and the mouth open. Respiratory symptoms include nasal flaring; suprasternal, substernal, and intercostal retractions; pale skin color to cyanosis (depending on the degree of airway obstruction); and tachycardia. The epiglottis appears edematous and cherry red.

Diagnostic Evaluation

The most reliable diagnostic sign of epiglottitis is an edematous, cherry red epiglottis. However, examination and visual observation of the epiglottis are contraindicated until emergency intubation equipment and qualified personnel are available to support the child in case of sudden airway obstruction.

CRITICAL TO REMEMBER

. . . .

Cardinal Signs and Symptoms of Epiglottitis

- Drooling
- Dysphagia (difficulty swallowing)
- Dysphonia (difficulty talking)
- Distressed inspiratory efforts

Do not examine or obtain material for culture from a child's throat if epiglottitis is suspected because any stimulation with a tongue depressor or culture swab could trigger complete airway obstruction.

Do not leave a child with epiglottitis unattended.

---

struction. The child's WBC count is usually elevated (20,000 to 30,000/mm³).

Therapeutic Management

Treatment for epiglottitis should achieve a patent airway as quickly as possible. The child with epiglottitis has an edematous epiglottis, which can completely obstruct the airway at any time. Radiographs are best obtained at the bedside, where the child can be constantly monitored and emergency equipment is readily available. The danger of airway obstruction is so great that usually all invasive procedures such as venipuncture are postponed until the child is intubated. Once the airway is secured the child is transferred to the intensive care unit. Oxygenation status is closely monitored with arterial blood gas values or pulse oximetry, and humidified oxygen is administered. Mechanical ventilation is sometimes used.

Antibiotics are administered IV until the child is extubated. The usual course of treatment is 7 to 10 days. Throat and blood specimens are obtained for culture after the child is intubated. Antipyretics are given for fever.

Usually the child improves dramatically after 48 hours of antibiotic therapy and can be extubated at this time. Discharge occurs in about 3 to 7 days, and the child is sent home on a regimen of oral antibiotics.

Nursing Considerations

The nurse should continuously assess for signs of respiratory distress (stridor, nasal flaring, tachypnea, tachycardia, retractions, drooling, changes in level of consciousness, cyanosis). A sudden decrease in respiratory effort may be a sign of exhaustion and impending respiratory arrest. Arterial blood gas values and pulse oximetry findings are monitored. On pulse oximetry the oxygen saturation should remain above 95%, with the Pao₂ between 80 and 100 mm Hg.

Maintenance of a patent airway is essential. The nurse should also keep the child as calm and quiet as possible. If temperature is taken, it should be by the axillary or tympanic route rather than the oral route. The child should be supported in a position of comfort, usually sitting straight up (orthopneic); never force the child to lie down. Children who are anxious and in respiratory distress are often less fearful on their parents' laps. Parents should be encouraged to hug and comfort their child. The parents' anxiety level must be assessed and controlled because their anxiety is easily transferred to the child.

Humidified oxygen is delivered in high concentrations. Oxygen therapy is usually less upsetting if the parent holds the oxygen tubing in front of the child's face. All procedures should be explained to the parent and child clearly, calmly, and according to the child's level of understanding.

Emergency intubation equipment (oxygen, laryngoscope, endotracheal tube, suction equipment) should be immediately available in case of complete airway obstruction. Worsening of the child's condition should be reported to the physician immediately.

Antipyretics are given rectally for fever. Because of the risk of aspiration, the child is kept NPO and fluids are given IV. The nurse must closely monitor the ordered IV rate as well as the urine specific gravity and other indicators of hydration. IV antibiotics are administered as ordered.

If the child has an artificial airway, either with an endotracheal tube or a tracheostomy, the nurse must observe the child closely for respiratory distress and suction the airway as needed. The endotracheal tube must be securely taped to decrease movement of the tube and to minimize the chance of accidental extubation. Once intubated, the child needs to be restrained to prevent accidental extubation. It may be impossible to reintubate the child because of the severe swelling of the epiglottis. The endotracheal tube is usually kept in place for approximately 24 to 40 hours. After extubation, the child must be watched carefully and is usually placed in a mist tent for 24 hours before being transferred to a pediatric unit. Normal respiratory rate and rhythm and normal color serve as evaluation criteria.

Because epiglottitis progresses rapidly and acute respiratory distress is frightening, both parents and child have high anxiety levels. The nurse should care for the child calmly and efficiently and offer the family much-needed support during hospitalization. On discharge, the parents need to be taught how to administer the child's oral antibiotics. They should be reassured that epiglottitis rarely recurs. The child should be free of respiratory difficulty, resting well, and without other distress. The nurse should encourage parents of young children to have their children immunized against *Hemophilus influenzae* to decrease the risk of contracting epiglottitis.

Bronchitis

Bronchitis is a disease that rarely exists by itself but occurs together with other conditions of the upper and lower respiratory tracts. It can be confused with asthma. A cough is the major sign; it usually resolves without therapy in approximately 2 weeks.

Etiology and Incidence

Acute bronchitis is usually viral in origin. Rhinoviruses are the most common causative organisms. Other viruses thought to cause bronchitis include respiratory syncytial virus, influenza virus, parainfluenza virus, and adenovirus. Most bacterial infections occur secondary to a primary viral infection or some other airway problem. They may also occur secondary to foreign body aspiration. Air pollution has also been implicated in the disease.

The disorder is more common in young children and boys. It can occur anytime but is more common during the winter months than in other seasons.

PATHOPHYSIOLOGY
of Bronchitis

Inflammation of the trachea and major bronchi is present in bronchitis. Mucous production is increased and the mucosa is congested. Due to nonspecific leukocytic migration, purulent secretions can occur even in the absence of a bacterial infection.

Acute bronchitis is a self-limiting disease. Chronic bronchitis in children may indicate an underlying chronic respiratory dysfunction.

Manifestations and Diagnostic Evaluation

Bronchitis is characterized by the gradual onset of rhinitis and a cough that is initially nonproductive but may change to a loose cough with increased mucus production. Auscultation may reveal coarse and fine, moist crackles and high-pitched rhonchi (resembling the wheezing of asthma). Associated symptoms include malaise, low-grade fever, and increased mucus, which may be purulent.

Chest radiographs are usually normal. The diagnosis is based on the clinical picture.

Therapeutic Management

Treatment is mainly palliative and includes rest, humidification, and increased fluid intake. Exposure to cigarette smoke should be avoided. Cough suppressants are not recommended unless the child is unable to rest because of coughing. Antihistamines should be avoided because of their drying effect on secretions. Antibiotics should be given only if a bacterial infection is confirmed by culture or if the clinical picture supports the diagnosis.

Nursing Considerations

The nurse should assess temperature, appearance of secretions, and respiratory effort every 2 to 4 hours. The child's intake should be monitored, and the nurse should observe for signs of sleep deprivation related to the persistent cough.

Fluids should be encouraged by frequently offering small amounts of the child's favorite liquids, and room humidification should be provided. The child should be monitored for signs of dehydration; monitoring includes taking daily weights. Acetaminophen is administered for an elevated temperature (usually over 38.3°C [101°F]). Quiet activities should be provided for diversion.

Bronchiolitis

Bronchiolitis, or inflammation of the bronchioles, is a significant cause of hospitalization in infants less than 1 year old. Respiratory syncytial virus (RSV) is the causative agent in more than 50% of cases.

Etiology and Incidence

Infants usually acquire the disease from an older child or adult, particularly a family member or day care contact, who has a minor respiratory illness. RSV infection is easily communicable and is acquired mainly through contact with contaminated surfaces. Nosocomial outbreaks in pediatric hospitals are common. RSV can live on skin or paper for up to 1 hour, and on cribs and other nonporous surfaces for up to 6 hours. Although it is not airborne, it is highly communicable. It is usually transferred by inadequately washed hands. Meticulous hand washing decreases the spread of organisms.

In addition to RSV, other causative organisms include *Mycoplasma*, parainfluenza virus, and some adenoviruses. RSV infection occurs in annual epidemics during the winter and early spring. The incidence peaks at age 6 months. By age 2 years, nearly 100% of children will have had RSV

PATHOPHYSIOLOGY
. . . .
of Bronchiolitis

In bronchiolitis, edema and the accumulation of mucus and cellular debris cause obstruction of the bronchioles. Infants' bronchioles are very small and can become obstructed quickly. Airway resistance is increased during the inspiratory and expiratory phases of respiration due to the small air passages. Hyperinflation of the lungs results from air trapping because the bronchioles constrict during expiration. Atelectasis can occur if obstruction becomes complete and trapped air is ab-

sorbed. Normal gas exchange is impaired, and the infant becomes hypoxic. Some infants develop mild respiratory alkalosis; more frequently metabolic acidosis is observed.

The child with bronchiolitis is most acutely ill during the first 48 to 72 hours after the onset of the disease. Improvement usually occurs in a few days. Mortality is less than 1%. Some infants' lung function studies remain abnormal for months.

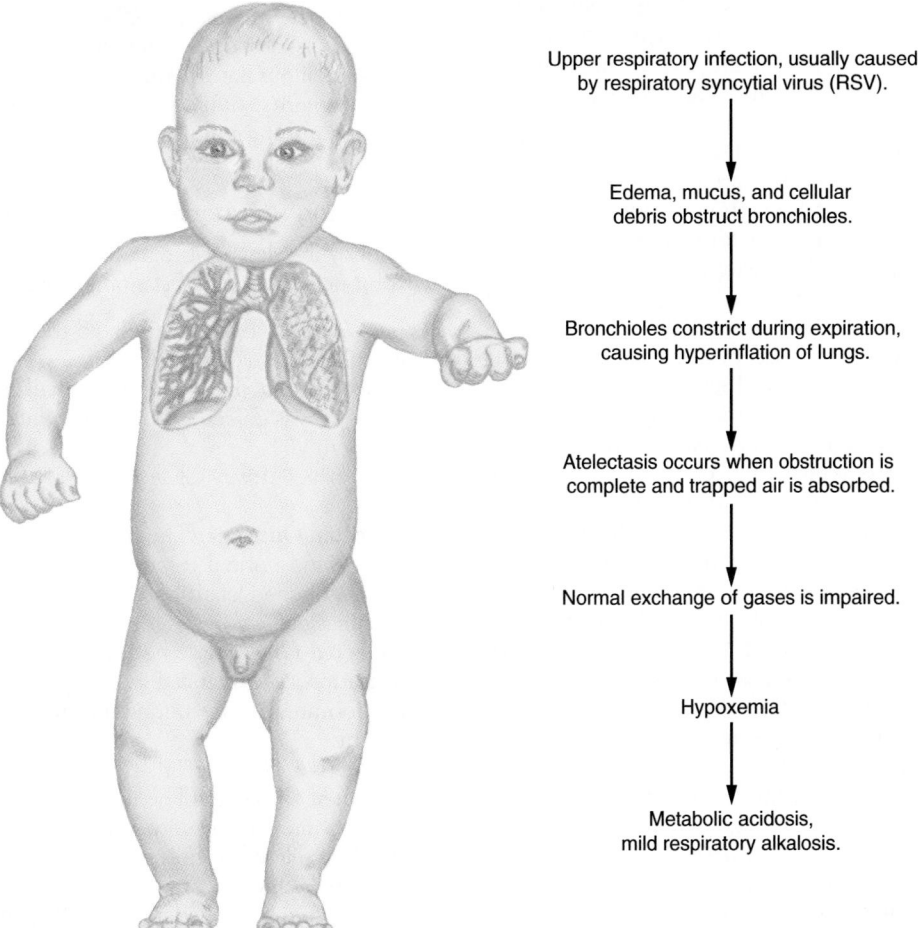

Upper respiratory infection, usually caused by respiratory syncytial virus (RSV).

↓

Edema, mucus, and cellular debris obstruct bronchioles.

↓

Bronchioles constrict during expiration, causing hyperinflation of lungs.

↓

Atelectasis occurs when obstruction is complete and trapped air is absorbed.

↓

Normal exchange of gases is impaired.

↓

Hypoxemia

↓

Metabolic acidosis, mild respiratory alkalosis.

(Wohl, 1998). Immunity does not occur, but the incidence and severity decrease with age.

Manifestations

A mild upper respiratory tract infection usually precedes the development of bronchiolitis. Serous nasal drainage, sneezing, low-grade fever, and anorexia are present for several days, followed by the onset of acute respiratory distress, manifested by the following signs and symptoms:

- Tachypnea—respiratory rates of 60 to 80 breaths/min
- Wheezing, crackles, or rhonchi
- Intercostal and subcostal retractions with or without nasal flaring
- Cyanosis

Feeding may be difficult because of increased respirations, which interfere with sucking and swallowing. The body temperature varies from hypothermic to as high as 41°C (105.8°F).

Diagnostic Evaluation

The clinical presentation and the age of the child suggest the diagnosis. Rapid virus identification can be performed on respiratory secretions obtained by nasal or nasopharyngeal washing (see Chapter 37). The diagnostic test is the enzyme-linked immunosorbent assay, or ELISA.

Chest radiographs show hyperinflation of the lungs and an increased anteroposterior chest diameter on lateral views. There are scattered areas of consolidation in some infants, a finding attributable to atelectasis secondary to obstruction or inflammation of the alveoli. In some infants the chest radiographs appear normal.

Therapeutic Management

Infants with mild bronchiolitis can be treated at home with fluids, humidification, and rest. Infants with respiratory distress are hospitalized. Treatment is supportive. Cool, humidified oxygen is delivered to relieve dyspnea, hypoxemia, and insensible water loss from tachypnea.

Parenteral administration of fluids may be necessary for acutely ill infants who are dehydrated from tachypnea or poor intake. The infant should be positioned with the head and chest at a 30- to 40-degree angle and the neck slightly extended to maintain an open airway and decrease pressure on the diaphragm.

Antibiotics are not given unless there is a secondary bacterial infection. Some health care providers use inhaled albuterol, but this has not been shown either to increase oxygenation or to hasten recovery for infants with bronchiolitis (Dobson, Stephens-Groff, McMahon, et al., 1998).

Ribavirin (Virazole) is an antiviral respiratory drug that appears to interfere with RNA and DNA synthesis, inhibiting viral replication. It is used primarily in hospitalized children with severe RSV and in high-risk children (those with congenital heart disease, chronic respiratory disease, prematurity, or immunodeficiency). Administration is via hood, face mask, or oxygen tent over 18 to 20 hours per day for a minimum of 3 days and a maximum of 7 days. The drug is most effective if administered within the first 3 days of the beginning of the disease. It is very expensive and has proved to be teratogenic in some animal studies, so pregnant health care workers or visitors should not be in the room where ribavarin is being delivered. Some caregivers experience headaches, burning nasal passages and eyes, and crystallized soft contact lenses. The efficacy of ribavirin has been questioned; more research is needed (American Academy of Pediatrics [AAP], 1996).

RSV prevention is of the utmost importance to reduce hospitalizations for young, at risk, infants and children. Intravenous RSV immune globulin (RSV-IG, RespiGam) or intramuscular RSV monoclonal antibody administered monthly throughout the RSV season has significantly reduced the hospitalization risk for premature infants (<35 weeks' gestation) less than 6 months old and children under 24 months old with chronic lung disease. Prophylaxis is done on an outpatient basis. The MMR and varicella vaccines must be postponed for 9 to 10 months following the last dose of RSV-IG.

▌ NURSING CARE
. . . .
The Child with Bronchiolitis

Assessment

The nurse should assess the infant for signs and symptoms of respiratory distress (tachypnea, dyspnea, retractions, cyanosis, nasal flaring) every 2 hours during the acute phase and as needed if changes occur. Auscultate the lungs for breath sounds. Apnea and cardiorespiratory monitoring are

indicated for the infant with acute disease. Make sure that the alarms on the cardiorespiratory monitor are set, and document any periods of apnea.

Assess the infant for signs of dehydration (dry mucous membranes, decreased urine output, sunken fontanel, weight loss) and monitor body temperature. The temperature in oxygen tents should be monitored as well as the moisture in the tent, in the tubing, and on the bedding or infant. The infant should be placed in a room near the nurses' station for easy observation.

Assess the family's understanding of the disease and family members' level of anxiety. Observe the infant for signs of anxiety, restlessness, or irritability.

Isolate the infant with RSV infection in a single room or place the infant in a room with other RSV-infected infants. Meticulous hand washing is imperative. Nurses caring for these infants should not care for other high-risk children. Maintaining contact precautions (i.e., wearing a gown and gloves) reduces nosocomial transmission of RSV.

Nursing Diagnosis and Planning

The following diagnoses may be appropriate for the infant with bronchiolitis and the infant's family:

■ Impaired Gas Exchange related to edema and increased mucus.
  Expected Outcome: The infant will have increased gas exchange, as evidenced by oxygen saturation above 95% on room air.
■ Ineffective Airway Clearance related to increased secretions.
  Expected Outcome: The infant will exhibit clear breath sounds and normal respiratory rate, depth, and rhythm.
■ Fluid Volume Deficit related to decreased intake and insensible loss.
  Expected Outcome: The infant will maintain adequate hydration, as evidenced by moist mucous membranes, a flat fontanel, urine output normal for age, and stable weight.
■ Ineffective Thermoregulation related to illness.
  Expected Outcome: The infant will demonstrate a body temperature within normal limits.
■ Anxiety related to hospitalization, dyspnea.
  Expected Outcomes: The infant will demonstrate decreased anxiety as evidenced by adequate sleep and stable vital signs. The parents will verbalize understanding of the infant's condition and be able to participate appropriately in the infant's care.

Interventions

Many hospitals are now using clinical pathways for children with respiratory disease. Figure 45–3 shows a clinical pathway for an infant with bronchiolitis. Even when using a clinical pathway, the nurse needs to focus on appropriate nursing interventions.

Facilitating Gas Exchange

The nurse monitors and documents the infant's vital signs and respiratory status every 2 hours and as needed. Particularly note the rate, quality, and depth of respirations along with any adventitious breath sounds and the presence of retractions. Close monitoring with a cardiorespiratory mon-

BRONCHIOLITIS & BRONCHIOLITIS (+) RSV
(Uncomplicated-without multi-system problems)
ICD-9 Codes 466.11 and 466.19

Expected LOS-3 Days
D#.#=Key interventions for this study.

Examples of appropriate Co-morbidities
Acute Pharyngitis
Acute Sinusitis NOS
Cellulitis
Other Specific Viral Infections
Otitis Media NOS

Examples of Co-morbidities that are not appropriate:

Asthma	Esophageal Reflux
Bronchopulmonary Dysplasia	HIV
Cardiac Conditions that extend the LOS	Pneumonia
Cerebral Palsy	Respiratory Failure
Cystic Fibrosis	Sickle Cell Anemia

Refer to Tracking Sheet for Recording

Clinical Pathway	Admission Day	Day 2	Day 3
Aspect of Care	Date ___ Unit___ ED	Date ___ Unit___	Date ___ Unit___
DAILY OUTCOME		↓ nebs if tolerated ↓ O2 if tolerated	*Discharge*

TESTS	CBC <2 mo.
	CXR
	CBG if resp distress or
	↑O2 requirements
	Possible:
	  Pertussis preps
	  Chlamydia preps
	  Viral culture
	  Blood Culture if fever (<2 mos)
		CBG if distress (↓oxygenation)
		Serum electrolytes if indicated	

CONSULTS	Case Manager:
	  Discharge needs and
	  possible home nebulizer
	Specialist:
	  Pulmonary or Infectious
	  Disease consult if hi-risk*
			Specialist if not improved

FLUID/LYTES MANAGEMENT	Possible IV fluids I/O	Hep lock if tolerating p.o.	
TREATMENTS/ PROCEDURES	*D1.0 Albuterol Nebs* Spot checks or Continuous oximeter if requiring 02 02 to keep Sat >92% Possible epi nebs CA monitor<2 mos or premature or severe respiratory distress Possible CPT	*D2.0 Albuterol or Epi Nebs* Wean 02 if tolerated Spot Check Oximetry w/vs	Albuterol or epi nebs *D3.0 Wean 02*
MEDICATIONS	*D1.2 Possible steroids* *(if hx recurrent wheezing)*	Review all IV meds and antibiotics	

CLINICAL SUPPORT	Diet p.o. if RR<60
	Contact Isolation during
	  season, even if viral studies
	  are (-) or not ordered, gown and
	  gloves when touching patient.
	R.T. to wear mask
	Education:
	  Exposure (smoke)
	  Follow-up
	  Neb treatments
		D2.1 Diet p.o. if RR <60	

Original 10/10/95   Rev. Date 11/9/95 5/1/97 8/18/97

*AAP guideline-CHD, parenchymal lung disease, infants less than 6 weeks old, prematurity, immunodeficiency, severely ill (impaired gas exchange)

Disclaimer: This clinical pathway document is provided as a general guideline for use by physicians and staff in planning the care and treatment of patients and their families. It is not intended to be and does not establish a standard of care. Each patient's care is individualized according to their specific needs.

Cook Children's Medical Center
M:\WPFILES\PATHWAYS\AUGBRONC.WPD

Privileged and Confidential Committee Document
TEX.REV.CIV.STAT.ANN. art. 4995b x 5.0

This pathway is not a permanent part of the patient's medical record.

FIGURE 45–3
. . . .
Clinical pathway for an infant with bronchiolitis. (Courtesy of Cook Children's Medical Center, Fort Worth, Texas.)

itor or continuous pulse oximeter will ensure early identification of impending respiratory distress.

Administer humidified oxygen (at 35% to 40% concentration) in the manner most comfortable for the infant (by tent, hood, mask, or nasal prongs) to decrease hypoxia and bronchial edema. Positioning the infant's head at a 30- to 40-degree upright angle with the neck slightly extended will maintain an open airway and ease respirations by decreasing pressure on the diaphragm. If the infant is in an oxygen tent, change the bedding and infant's clothes regularly to keep the infant dry. Toys that might cause static electricity are kept outside the tent; provide the infant with appropriate safe toys.

Scheduling periods of uninterrupted rest between care episodes decreases oxygen demand. Chest physiotherapy should be performed (it may require coordination with the respiratory therapy department) before, or at least 1 hour after, meals. The use of chest physiotherapy in infants is controversial because it might increase their stress and oxygen demand. Administer ribavarin if ordered.

Maintaining Fluid Balance

Most infants with bronchiolitis can take fluids orally; IV fluids are administered if respiratory distress is severe enough to risk aspiration. If the infant's nasal passages are blocked with mucus, instill saline nose drops (1 to 2 drops in each nostril, followed by gentle suctioning with a bulb syringe) prior to feeding. Offer the infant frequent, varied clear liquids (juices, Pedialyte, Ricelyte). Older infants may enjoy frozen electrolyte pops. The infant's hydration status (skin turgor, fontanel, mucous membranes) and electrolyte values are monitored and daily weights and intake and output are documented.

Reducing Fever

The nurse monitors the infant's temperature every 2 to 4 hours and as needed. Control environmental temperature by maintaining the room temperature between 72° and 75°F and dress the infant in light clothing. Fluid intake is encouraged and liquid acetaminophen or ibuprofen administered as ordered to reduce fever.

Decreasing Anxiety

Encourage the parent to stay with the infant when possible and to participate as much as possible in the infant's care. Hospital routines and all procedures and treatments should be explained to reduce fear of the unknown. Because adult anxiety can be transferred to the infant, maintain a calm environment and encourage parents to do the same. If the infant becomes anxious about being in an oxygen tent, the parent can hold the infant and direct the humidified oxygen toward the infant's face. If the infant remains in a tent, encourage the parent to play with the infant; the parent can get in the tent to maintain tactile contact with the infant. Parents need to be allowed to express concerns.

Evaluation

- Does the infant demonstrate adequate oxygenation (oxygen saturation greater than 95%), clear breath sounds, and stable respiratory status?
- Does the infant have moist mucous membranes, good

skin turgor, stable weight, a flat fontanel, and urine output of at least 1 to 2 ml/kg/hr?
- Is the infant's body temperature within normal limits?
- Does the infant demonstrate less crying or irritability and increased rest?
- Do the parents verbalize understanding of the disease, have a relaxed appearance, and demonstrate comforting behaviors toward the infant?

Pneumonia

Pneumonia is an inflammation of the lung parenchyma. It can occur as a primary or a secondary disease. Pneumonias can be classified by anatomic distribution or by the agents that cause them. Environment, immune system status, and the child's age are factors in the pathogenesis of the disease.

The two most common types of infectious pneumonia are viral and bacterial (Table 45-3). It is very difficult to differentiate clinically between viral and bacterial pneumonia. Viruses are the most common causative agents, but children with bacterial pneumonia tend to be more ill than those with viral disease. Children with chronic and acute conditions such as acquired immunodeficiency syndrome (AIDS), cystic fibrosis, congenital defects, and foreign body aspiration are at increased risk for developing pneumonia. Opportunistic infections (*Pneumocystis carinii* pneumonia) may be associated with AIDS (see Chapter 41). Secondary pneumonia can result from aspiration of hydrocarbons contained in household products or lipids (e.g., mineral oil given to treat severe constipation).

NURSING CARE
The Child with Pneumonia

Assessment

Every 2 hours, assess the child's breath sounds, respiratory rate and rhythm, color, vital signs, and degree of restlessness. Immediately report any signs of respiratory distress, including dyspnea, tachypnea, cyanosis, use of accessory muscles of breathing, diminished breath sounds, and crackles. Also note any fever, tachycardia, malaise, anorexia, discomfort, and changes in condition.

Nursing Diagnosis and Planning

The following nursing diagnoses and expected outcomes may be appropriate for the family and child with pneumonia:

- Ineffective Airway Clearance related to bronchial obstruction.
  Expected Outcome: The child will have clear airways, as evidenced by the absence of abnormal breath sounds and dyspnea.
- Ineffective Breathing Pattern related to increased mucus production.
  Expected Outcome: The child will demonstrate effective breathing, as evidenced by respiratory rate and rhythm within normal limits for age and absence of retractions.
- Impaired Gas Exchange related to increased mucus and accumulation of exudate.

TABLE 45-3
• • • • • • • • • • • •

Types of Pneumonias

Type	Etiology/Incidence	Pathophysiology	Manifestations	Therapeutic Management
Viral	Most often caused by adenoviruses, influenza viruses, cytomegalovirus (mainly in neonates), and respiratory syncytial virus (RSV). Viruses cause 80% to 85% of all pneumonias. Most common in children younger than 3 years.	Cell destruction with sloughing of cellular debris into lumen of terminal airways and alveoli causes patchy infiltrate that affects multiple lobes.	Low to high fever, cough, crackles, wheezing (more common with RSV), headache, malaise, myalgia, abdominal pain. Infiltrates seen on chest radiography. WBC <20,000/mm³. Usually lasts 5 to 7 days.	Supportive. No antibiotics are prescribed. Severely ill infants and children may be hospitalized for oxygen and fluid therapy.
Bacterial and bacterial-like	Caused primarily by *S. pneumoniae* and *S. aureas* in infants and children younger than 5 years. Pneumococcal infection is major type in children older than 5 years. Also may be caused by *H. influenzae* and group A streptococci. Other bacteria-like organisms include *Mycoplasma pneumoniae, Chlamydia pneumoniae,* and *Chlamydia trachomatis* (seen mainly in infants).	Alveoli fill with fluid and cells in a small segment or the entire lung. Bacteria enter the bloodstream via the pulmonary lymphatics. Vital capacity and lung compliance decrease as consolidation increases.	Preceded by upper respiratory infection. Abrupt onset of fever, chills, cough, decreased breath sounds, signs of respiratory distress (retractions, nasal flaring, tachypnea), restlessness and apprehension. Symptoms may be vague in infants; older children can experience gastrointestinal symptoms, chest pain, and abnormal breath sounds. Onset of the bacterial-like pneumonias may be more insidious. Radiography reveals consolidation; WBC is elevated.	IV or oral antibiotic therapy, usually with penicillins, erythromycin (for penicillin allergic children), or cephalosporins. Hospitalization for severely ill infants and children with oxygen and fluid therapy. Chest tube drainage of fluid or purulence from the pleural cavity may be necessary (particularly for children with staphylococcal pneumonia).

Expected Outcome: The child will maintain adequate gas exchange, as evidenced by decreased restlessness, appropriate oxygen saturation, and improved mucous membrane and nail bed color.

■ Fluid Volume Deficit related to fever, decreased intake, and tachypnea.

Expected Outcomes: The child will maintain fluid balance, as evidenced by moist mucous membranes, good skin turgor, urine output appropriate for age, and maintenance of age-appropriate weight.

■ Knowledge Deficit related to the disease process and home care.

Expected Outcome: The parents will verbalize an understanding of the disease process and care of the child.

■ Parental Anxiety related to infant's dyspnea and hospitalization.

Expected Outcomes: The parents will show a decrease in anxiety, as evidenced by decreased irritability and increased periods of rest. The parents will verbalize and demonstrate comfort and ease when caring for the child.

■ Pain related to coughing and difficulty breathing secondary to disease process.

Expected Outcome: The child will have decreased pain, as evidenced by less irritability, verbalization of increased comfort (if age appropriate), and a relaxed body posture.

Interventions

The severity of the illness and the cause of the disease direct the nursing care of the child with pneumonia. Some children will be cared for at home, whereas others will be hospitalized on a general pediatric unit or special care area.

For the hospitalized child, chest physiotherapy should be scheduled before meals and bedtime. Elevating the head of the bed and changing the child's position every 2 hours assist respiratory effort and promote pulmonary drainage. Older children may assume a position of comfort, but still must change their position every 2 hours. The use of infant seats should be avoided because pressure may be placed on the diaphragm, thus actually decreasing lung expansion.

The older child should be assisted with coughing and deep breathing, and splinting as necessary to ease discomfort. Oxygen should be humidified and monitored. Pulse oximetry aids in monitoring oxygen saturation and the adequacy of air exchange. A cardiorespiratory monitor is used when available.

Oral or IV fluids are given as ordered. IV fluids may be indicated when oral intake increases the stress put on an already compromised body. The nurse monitors intake and output, observes for signs of dehydration (oliguria, poor skin turgor, dry mucous membranes, sunken fontanels, weight loss). Weight should be measured daily. The specific gravity of urine is also checked.

Because conserving energy aids oxygenation, nursing care is planned to provide for periods of rest. Quiet diversional activities such as reading, puzzles, videos, and board games are suggested. The nurse maintains a quiet and cool environment and limits visitors to allow the child maximum rest. Visits by anyone with an infection should be restricted.

Administer antipyretics (acetaminophen), antibiotics, and analgesics as ordered. Normal breathing may cause discomfort. If an analgesic is not ordered, the physician should be notified of any discomfort the child experiences. Splinting of the affected side by lying on that side may decrease discomfort. Diversional activities and manipulation of the environment are often effective for pain relief.

The family and child (if of appropriate age) need to receive information about the disease and its treatment. The nurse explains all procedures and treatments and encourages the parents to stay with their child and participate in the child's care. The nurse conveys empathy for the family's feelings and concerns. The nurse also teaches the family about home management of the infant or child.

Evaluation

- Are the child's vital signs and respiratory status within normal limits?
- Is the child's oxygen saturation greater than 95%?
- Can the child comfortably participate in quiet activities and rest quietly when appropriate?
- Does the child appear hydrated, with moist mucous membranes, good skin turgor, and adequate urinary output?
- Do the parents appear relaxed, and are they able to fully participate in the child's care?
- Can the parents describe home care techniques?

PARENTS WANT TO KNOW

Home Management of the Child with Pneumonia

- Provide rest.
- Increase your child's fluid intake. Offer favorite fluids more frequently than usual, and be sure your child is urinating appropriate amounts. Warm liquids (lemonade, apple juice, Pedialyte, Ricelyte) help loosen secretions. Call your health care provider if the child's mucous membranes appear dry or if urination decreases.
- Administer acetaminophen for fever and discomfort.
- Use a cool mist humidifier.
- Administer antibiotics as ordered and give the correct dose and the entire prescribed amount.
- Avoid exposing your child to cigarette smoke.

Foreign Body Aspiration

Foreign body aspiration is seen most frequently in children ages 6 months to 5 years. Children who have objects in their mouths while they are playing, running, or laughing are at risk.

Etiology and Incidence

Children's curiosity, oral needs, and occasionally lack of supervision contribute to the occurrence of foreign body aspiration. Infants and children love to explore and investigate objects. Exploration often includes putting objects into their mouths. Children also have the uncanny ability to remove small parts from toys and to find other objects that parents thought were out of their reach (e.g., pins, screws, nuts, coins, earrings). Adults may give infants and small children foods they are not developmentally prepared to ingest (hard candy, popcorn, uncooked carrots, hot dogs, peanuts). Balloons account for a significant number of deaths from aspiration per year (Centers for Disease Control and Prevention [CDC], 1997d). Childhood aspiration can occur at any age, but most incidents occur in boys younger than 5, with a peak incidence at ages 1 to 3 years.

Pathophysiology

Most foreign bodies become lodged in the bronchi. The right main bronchus is a more common site than the left main bronchus because of its anatomic development. Objects lodged in the larynx cause edema and inflammation. Bronchial obstruction manifests as obstructive emphysema or atelectasis. Failure to remove obstructing foreign objects is almost always fatal. Most can be removed mechanically without complications; a delay in treatment can lead to aspiration pneumonia and airway trauma.

Manifestations

Immediate signs and symptoms include

- Sudden, violent coughing
- Gagging
- Wheezing
- Vomiting
- Brief episode of apnea
- Cyanosis

After aspirating a foreign object, the child may remain asymptomatic for hours or weeks. If the object is not found and removed, signs and symptoms related to edema and increased irritation and obstruction may develop. Signs and symptoms of laryngeal and tracheal obstruction include hoarseness, croupy cough, stridor, and possibly dyspnea with cyanosis. Coughing, wheezing, unilaterally decreased breath sounds, pneumonitis, and possibly respiratory arrest can indicate bronchial inflammation and obstruction.

Diagnostic Evaluation

The diagnosis is based on the history and the clinical manifestations. Fluoroscopy and chest radiography are used to reveal the presence of a foreign object in the respiratory tract.

Radiographs will reveal an opaque foreign body, and laryngoscopy or bronchoscopy confirms the diagnosis and provides an avenue for removing the object.

Therapeutic Management

Foreign bodies are removed from the respiratory tract by direct laryngoscopy or bronchoscopy. After the procedure the child should remain hospitalized for observation for laryngeal edema and respiratory distress. Cool mist is provided, and antibiotic therapy is ordered if appropriate.

Nursing Considerations

The degree of obstruction should be assessed to determine the appropriate action to take. If the child is aphonic (not speaking) and not breathing, the nurse should follow the guidelines for managing an obstructed airway (see Chapter 34). Children with a partially obstructed airway are observed for signs of increasing obstruction.

After the object has been removed, the child is observed for signs of obstruction caused by laryngeal edema and soft tissue swelling (restlessness, dyspnea). The child should be placed on a cardiorespiratory monitor.

Liquids are withheld until the child's gag reflex returns after anesthesia. Oral fluids should be started slowly and increased as the child tolerates the intake. Intake and output should be recorded. If the child refuses to drink because of a sore throat or is unable to take fluids orally, the physician should be notified so that IV fluids may be started. The parents' knowledge of respiratory distress is also evaluated before discharge.

Parental anxiety and guilt are common after an episode of aspiration. In addition to supporting the parents, the nurse assesses their knowledge of safety. Prevention is the key to reducing the incidence of aspiration. Safety is discussed at every well-child visit (see Chapters 5 through 8).

Apnea

Manifestations

Apnea is the cessation of breathing for a period of 20 seconds or longer, or for a shorter period but accompanied by bradycardia or cyanosis. True apnea differs from periodic breathing, which might be seen in premature infants. In periodic breathing, there is a shift from regular rhythmic breathing to brief episodes of apnea. This type of breathing pattern consists of three or more respiratory pauses of longer than 3 seconds, with less than 20 seconds of respiration between pauses. Rarely, periodic breathing is associated with changes in heart rate or color. Periodic breathing is very common in premature infants and decreases as the infant's gestational age increases. The cause is unknown; periodic breathing may be a normal event.

Apparent life-threatening events are sudden episodes characterized by apnea, a color change, a change in muscle tone, choking, or gagging in an infant who otherwise appears healthy. In the past, this type of occurrence was referred to as "near miss sudden infant death syndrome." This appellation was misleading. Apparent life-threatening

Indications for Home Apnea Monitoring

- The infant is a survivor of an apparent life-threatening event.
- The infant is a newborn sibling of two or more infants who have died of sudden infant death syndrome.
- The infant is premature and has symptoms of idiopathic apnea of prematurity but is otherwise ready for hospital discharge.
- The infant has a tracheostomy.
- The infant has sleep apnea syndrome caused by a neurologic disorder, periodic breathing, upper airway abnormality, or idiopathic syndrome.

Adapted from Hanly, P. (1992). Mechanisms and management of central sleeping apnea. *Lung, 170,* 1017. Reprinted by permission of Springer-Verlag.

events most often occur in infants of 37 weeks' gestational age or older while they are sleeping, feeding, or awake. Infants who have experienced such an event are usually hospitalized for observation and testing and are at increased risk for mortality (Brooks, 1998).

Two categories of true apnea events include apnea of prematurity and infant apnea (Table 45–4).

Diagnostic Evaluation

Tests are selected for the clinical indications and to rule out any underlying condition. Cardiorespiratory and neurophysiologic studies should be done. These studies include chest radiography, blood chemistry studies, electrocardiography (ECG), and electroencephalography. Pneumocardiography specifically tests for apnea by recording the heart rate and chest wall movements; however, the reliability of the test in predicting apnea has not been well established.

NURSING CARE
The Infant with Apnea

Assessment

The infant's heart rate and respirations are monitored continuously. The nurse should ascertain that the alarms on the cardiorespiratory monitor are set. Resuscitative equipment should be available.

If an apneic episode is observed, the nurse should record the time and duration of the episode, the skin color change, bradycardia, and oxygen saturation. The nurse should also describe what the infant was doing before the episode and any actions the nurse took to stimulate breathing.

Nursing Diagnosis and Planning

The following nursing diagnoses and expected outcomes may be appropriate for the family and infant with apnea:

- Ineffective Breathing Pattern related to apnea secondary to prematurity of respiratory control mechanisms (premature infant).

TABLE 45-4

. . . .

Apnea of Prematurity Compared with Infant Apnea

Etiology/Incidence	Pathophysiology	Therapeutic Management
Apnea of Prematurity		
The most common type of apnea, it occurs in neonates of 24 to 32 weeks' gestational age, with onset usually within the first week of life. It usually resolves by 38 weeks. Although the neonate's age may be related to a higher incidence of SIDS, apnea of prematurity is not considered to predict risk (Hodgman, 1998).	It varies among neonates, but may be due to upper airway obstruction, immaturity of central control mechanisms, compliant chest wall, or abnormal response during rapid eye movement (REM) sleep. Apnea often occurs during feeding because of immaturity of breathing, sucking, and swallowing coordination.	Gentle cutaneous stimulation is used to stimulate breathing in neonates with mild apnea (<10 episodes per day with little desaturation). For persistent apnea use oxygen administration, cardiorespiratory monitor; consider continuous positive airway pressure (CPAP) for neonates with severe apnea. Drug therapy may include caffeine, oral theophylline, or IV aminophylline to increase central respiratory drive and improve CO_2 sensitivity.
Infant Apnea		
Most infant apnea has no known cause. Underlying conditions such as gastroesophageal reflux, seizures, or hypoglycemia should be ruled out.	Three types: *Central*—absence of respiratory effort and air movement. *Obstructive*—apparent respiratory efforts without air movement or sound. *Mixed*—absence of respiratory effort and nasal air movement followed by resumption of respiratory effort without air movement. Short episodes of apnea are usually central apnea; apnea episodes that last 15 seconds or more are usually mixed.	If no underlying disorder is identified, home monitoring with a respiratory stimulant (caffeine, theophylline).

- Ineffective Breathing Pattern related to apnea of known or unknown etiology (term infant).
  Expected Outcome: The infant will have regular breathing patterns, as evidenced by respiratory rate and rhythm within normal limits for age.
- Parental Anxiety related to fear of infant's death.
  Expected Outcome: The parents will verbalize feelings concerning the infant's periods of apnea.
- Parental Knowledge Deficit related to unfamiliarity with apnea monitoring equipment and cardiopulmonary resuscitation (CPR).
  Expected Outcome: The parents will learn how to perform infant CPR and how to operate the apnea monitor.

Interventions

The nurse sets the heart rate parameters of the cardiorespiratory monitor according to the infant's age, and the respiratory pause at greater than 15 seconds. Resuscitative equipment should be available, and the nurse should be proficient in using it.

The apneic infant can be stimulated by gently tapping the foot or trunk or turning the infant over. The infant should not be shaken vigorously. If breathing does not resume, institute bag-and-mask ventilation.

Maintain a neutral thermal environment while the infant is hospitalized, and avoid suctioning if possible.

Several studies have shown that feeding affects ventilation. Therefore, infants should be monitored closely when being fed.

If home apnea monitoring is ordered, the family should be instructed in the use of the monitor and in CPR (Fig. 45-4). Emphasize to the parents that when the monitor alarm is triggered, they should immediately assess the infant rather than focus on the machine.

Evaluation

- Does the infant demonstrate normal respiratory rate and rhythm?
- Have the parents verbalized their fears associated with the infant's apnea?
- Have the parents demonstrated the ability to operate monitoring equipment and to perform CPR?

Sudden Infant Death Syndrome

Sudden infant death syndrome (SIDS) is defined as the sudden and unexplained death of an infant less than 1 year old. The explanation is not found despite a thorough investigation that includes a complete autopsy, examination of the death scene, and review of the clinical history. It is sometimes referred to as crib death by the public. SIDS usually occurs during sleep.

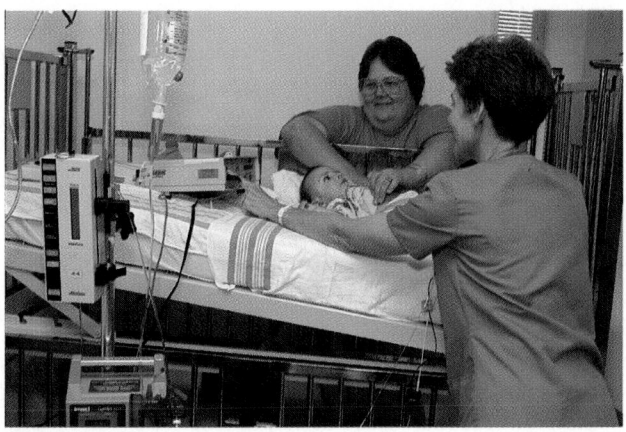

FIGURE 45–4
• • • • • • • • •
Teaching the family about using an apnea monitor and how to respond to alarms is an important element in caring for the child with infant apnea. The nurse must assess the parents' ability to tolerate the stressors of living with a child who is prone to apnea and support them as they deal with these stressors.

Etiology and Incidence

Although numerous theories have been proposed, the cause of SIDS is unknown. Proposed contributing factors include prematurity, brain stem defects, severe infant botulism, infections, reactions to immunizations, and hypersensitivity to cow's milk. Some studies have suggested a connection with lower socioeconomic status, cultural influences, lack of prenatal care, smoking, a sibling with SIDS, and season (winter).

Numerous reports from countries outside the United States have found a significant association between a prone sleeping position and the incidence of SIDS. Based on this information, the American Academy of Pediatrics (AAP) has recommended that healthy infants be placed on their sides or backs to sleep, rather than prone (AAP, 1992). Increased use of the supine and side-lying sleep positions since 1992 may correlate with a decrease in the incidence of SIDS during the same period.

Risk factors are also associated with the use of soft bed-

PATHOPHYSIOLOGY
• • • • • • • • • • • •
of Sudden Infant Death Syndrome

Autopsy findings in infants who have died of SIDS have varied widely. Nonspecific findings such as mild pulmonary edema, vascular congestion, or pulmonary inflammation are common. Other consistent findings include retarded postnatal growth, increased pulmonary arterial smooth muscle, retention of brown fat, brain stem gliosis, and intrathoracic petechiae. Partial upper airway obstruction in association with rebreathing may be an explanation for many SIDS deaths (Brooks, 1998). No single cause has been identified.

ding. Infants may suffocate by rebreathing CO_2-laden expired air when sleeping face down on soft bedding (Brooks, 1998; Gilbert-Barnes & Barnes, 1995; Kemp, Nelson, & Thach, 1994).

SIDS occurs most frequently between the second and fourth months of life, with 95% of cases occurring before age 6 months. It is more common in boys, low-birth-weight infants, and in infants from lower socioeconomic groups. It occurs more often during the winter months. Native Americans have the highest incidence, followed by African-Americans.

Manifestations

The principal manifestation of SIDS is silent death. The child may be found in any position and may be clutching bedding.

Diagnostic Evaluation

Diagnosis is confirmed through autopsy. A medical history of the infant and family should be taken. The infant is examined for signs of illness or trauma. The death scene is also investigated.

NURSING CARE
• • • • • • • • • • •
The Family of the Infant with Sudden Infant Death Syndrome

Assessment

When an infant is brought into the emergency department with suspected SIDS, there is often confusion for the family. If resuscitation was begun at home, they may assume that it was effective and that their infant is alive. Assessment of the family's understanding of the situation is necessary to plan for teaching and support. The nurse should assess the family's emotional status and coping strategies.

The nurse interviews the family in a calm, slow, and nonthreatening manner. Questions should not imply negligence or any involvement in the death. Parents need to be given time to think before they answer questions. Because the parents will be overwhelmed, questions may need to be repeated for clarity.

Nursing Diagnosis and Planning

The following nursing diagnoses and expected outcomes may be appropriate to the family of the infant victim of SIDS:

- Altered Family Processes related to death of a child.
  Expected Outcome: The parents and family will verbalize feelings related to the death of the infant.
- Ineffective Family Coping: Compromised related to death of a child.
  Expected Outcome: The parents and family will identify strengths and accept support of other family members, friends, professionals, and support groups.
- Knowledge Deficit related to cause of death.
  Expected Outcome: The parents will verbalize an understanding of the cause of their child's death.

Interventions

The nurse working with a family who has had a child die of SIDS should provide calm support. The parents are confused about the death and are trying to cope with many emotions. Most parents will experience a combination of guilt, anger, and emotional pain.

A quiet room with dim lighting and a rocking chair should be provided for the family, and someone should remain with them. Assist the family to call family, friends, or clergy. The nurse should accompany the physician when the parents are told their infant is dead. At this time the parents should also be told that the apparent cause of death is SIDS and that nothing could have been done to prevent the death. This information will help minimize feelings of guilt.

Parents should be given the opportunity to say goodbye to their child. Because the parents may not think to ask to see their infant, the nurse should provide this opportunity.

> The nurse might say, "Would you like to have some time alone with your baby? We will bring him to you and you can take as long as you would like to hold him."

The infant should be cleaned and wrapped in a blanket and brought to the parents. Parents who are not given the opportunity to hold their child and say goodbye often regret it later, but parents who do not want time alone with their baby should be respected. The nurse should accept the parents' decision in this matter. Each parent will have his or her own way of coping.

The need for an autopsy should be explained. The autopsy will verify the cause of death and confirm for the parents that they did not cause the death.

Before the parents leave the hospital, arrangements for follow-up care should be made. Many hospitals have a team consisting of a social worker, chaplain, and nurse that is called when a suspected SIDS death occurs.

Refer the family to a local SIDS program for information, support, and counseling. Nurses who are involved in home visiting can encourage the family to communicate their feelings. Siblings should not be overlooked; parents may be so overwhelmed with their own grief that they forget their other children. Another reaction might be to overprotect their other children. The nurse should guide the family in identifying the members' various responses and in treating them at the appropriate developmental level. Children in the family who perhaps resented the new baby may have tremendous guilt feelings. The loss of a sibling may be especially traumatic to a toddler, who does not understand the changes that are taking place in the family. Routines and rituals that are important to the toddler may be disrupted.

Evaluation

- Has the family joined a support group?
- Is the family able to verbalize feelings associated with the death of the child?
- Is the family using effective coping skills to work toward an understanding of the child's death?
- Has the extended family mobilized to support the family?

Asthma

Asthma, or reactive airway disease, is a leading cause of acute and chronic illness in children and the most frequent admitting diagnosis in children's hospitals. Asthma affects nearly 5 million children in the United States. Despite advances in medical treatment, the incidence and death rate from asthma have increased markedly in recent years.

Etiology

It is unclear why some children's airways are more reactive than others'. It is known, however, that heredity plays a role, because asthma tends to appear in families. Other risk factors include male sex, African-American or Latino ethnic background, crowded living conditions, poverty, prematurity, and exposure to environmental smoke (Kemper, 1997).

An asthma episode may be triggered by a variety of stimuli, among them cold air, smoke, fumes, viral infection, stress, exercise, odors, drugs (particularly aspirin and nonsteroidal anti-inflammatory drugs [NSAIDs]), or allergens. Foods are occasionally the trigger in infants, but less commonly in older children.

The immature anatomy of infants and small children predisposes them to increased distress from asthma. Children's smaller, narrower airways and decreased elastic lung recoil make them more prone to airway obstruction. The child's flexible rib cage and underdeveloped chest muscles and diaphragm lead to exhaustion when respiratory effort increases. Although asthma is not actually outgrown, the severity of asthma attacks often decreases as the child gets older because of increased airway size, improved diaphragmatic support, and better clearing of mucus. Asthma is considered a lifelong condition and may become increasingly severe after a period of remission.

Incidence

Since the early 1980s, the incidence of asthma has risen in the United States and other parts of the world. Asthma affects an estimated 14 to 15 million Americans, nearly double the 6.8 million reported in 1980, and the death rate from childhood asthma has increased by 78% (CDC, 1997b). Asthma is more common among boys than girls until puberty, when the sex difference in incidence equalizes. Although the incidence of asthma is approximately equal for whites and African-Americans, the death rate among African-Americans is almost three times higher (Yoos & McMullen, 1999).

Manifestations

The manifestations of asthma may vary. A child experiencing an asthma episode may have only a dry cough. Others, however, may exhibit one or more of the following manifestations, which may have a sudden or an insidious onset:

- Wheezing
- Dyspnea with prolonged expiration and use of accessory muscles of respiration; may also display retractions, nasal flaring, or stridor

PATHOPHYSIOLOGY

of Asthma

Asthma is a reversible obstructive airway disease characterized by:

- *Increased airway responsiveness* to a variety of stimuli
- *Bronchospasm* resulting from constriction of bronchial smooth muscle
- *Inflammation* and *edema* of the mucous membranes that line the small airways, and the subsequent accumulation of thick secretions in the airways

IMMEDIATE REACTION (EARLY PHASE RESPONSE)

Allergens or other trigger substances activate IgE receptors on sensitized airway mast cells, causing mast cell degranulation and release of chemical mediators (histamine, leukotrienes, and prostaglandins). These mediators cause bronchoconstriction shortly after exposure to the trigger; the bronchoconstriction resolves within 1 to 2 hours.

DELAYED REACTION (LATE PHASE RESPONSE)

Chemical mediators attract immune system cells (eosinophils, neutrophils, and basophils) to the respiratory tract. Infiltration by these cells and their release of additional inflammatory substances damages the epithelial and smooth muscle cells, causing airway edema, mucous plugging of small airways, and additional inflammation. Bronchoconstriction recurs and can persist for several hours. The airway hyperresponsiveness resulting from this inflammatory process can last several weeks or months.

Late asthmatic responses can occur without a previous early (immediate) response. When asthma is precipitated by nonallergic stimuli (exercise, cold air), bronchospasm usually lasts less than 1 hour and is not followed by a late response.

During an asthma episode, the mucous membranes lining the bronchioles become edematous and secrete large amounts of thick mucus. As a result, the airways narrow, leading to increased airway resistance and respiratory distress. Because small airways are normally wider on inspiration than expiration, the child is able to inhale but has difficulty exhaling through the narrowed bronchioles. Wheezing can be heard as air is forced through the narrow passages during expiration. Air becomes trapped, causing hyperinflation of the alveoli.

Airway obstruction is more severe in some parts of the lungs than in others, and air flows more easily into areas with the least resistance. The blood that flows to the less ventilated portions of the lungs is inadequately saturated with oxygen. Thus, a mismatch between ventilation and perfusion in poorly ventilated areas of the lung occurs, resulting in incompletely saturated blood entering the systemic circulation and decreased Po_2 levels (hypoxia).

As the child struggles to get enough air, respiratory rate increases (tachypnea). Tachypnea lowers carbon dioxide levels in the blood (hypocapnia). As the child tires from the increased work of breathing, hypoventilation occurs, and carbon dioxide levels increase. Increased levels of carbon dioxide in the blood (hypercapnia) during an asthma episode may be a sign of severe airway obstruction and impending respiratory failure.

- Nonproductive cough (with or without wheezing) that later becomes productive
- Tachypnea, orthopnea
- Restlessness, apprehension, diaphoresis
- Abdominal pain secondary to the strain placed on the abdominal muscles during labored breathing
- A hunched over sitting position with arms braced (tripod position)
- Fatigue and difficulty performing simple tasks, such as eating, walking, or even talking, because of shortness of breath
- A feeling of chest tightness followed by a dry cough, wheezing, and dyspnea
- Worsening of symptoms after individual goes to bed at night because of increased narrowing of the airways at night and pooling of secretions

At the beginning of the asthma episode, wheezing may be heard only with a stethoscope. As the severity of the episode increases, wheezing may be audible to the unaided ear. Children in severe respiratory distress may not demonstrate wheezing because of decreased air movement; decreased wheezing in a child who is not improving clinically may signal inability to move air. This is referred to as a silent chest and is an ominous sign during an asthma episode. With treatment, increased wheezing may actually signal that the child's condition is improving.

Diagnostic Evaluation

Wheezing is the classic symptom of asthma, but other symptoms may be present, including shortness of breath, cough, or dyspnea on exertion. Chest radiographs are usually normal except in cases of severe asthma, in which hyperinflation of the airways can be seen. Pulmonary function tests reveal a decreased forced expiratory volume in 1 second (FEV_1), increased residual volume from air trapping, and decreased vital capacity (the maximum amount of air exhaled after a maximum inhalation). Other pulmonary function test results might be altered as well. The peak expiratory flow rate (PEFR) is used to monitor children with chronic asthma. Because asthma can be triggered by gastroesophageal reflux, some children will be evaluated for its presence (see Chapter 43).

Rhinitis, sinusitis, and nasal polyps are often present in children with asthma. Eosinophilia is present in both the blood and the sputum. Skin tests are often performed to

---

CRITICAL TO REMEMBER

Emergency Asthma Management

The following symptoms indicate the need for emergency treatment of asthma:

- Worsening wheeze, cough, or shortness of breath
- A peak flow rate that decreases or does not change (even after use of an inhaled beta$_2$-agonist), or that is less than 30% to 50% of the child's predicted baseline level or personal best
- Difficulty breathing (the child's chest and neck are pulled in with each breath, or the child hunches over or struggles to breathe)
- Trouble with walking or talking
- Discontinuation of play without the ability to resume activity
- Listlessness and weak cry in an infant; refusal to suck bottle or breast
- Gray or blue lips or fingernails (in which case the child needs emergency treatment *immediately!*)

Adapted with permission from Rachelefsky, G. S. (1995). Asthma update: New approaches and partnerships. *Journal of Pediatric Health Care, 9,* 12–21.

---

identify specific allergens. The radioallergosorbent test (RAST) may be used to identify specific antigens. Arterial blood gas measurements may be ordered in patients having a severe asthma episode because of initial respiratory alkalosis and subsequent metabolic acidosis. Pulse oximetry values provide information about oxygenation.

Therapeutic Management

ACUTE ASTHMA EPISODE

A child who is experiencing an episode of wheezing along with other symptoms of asthma is usually seen at a physician's office or emergency room. First, a bronchodilator, usually a short-acting beta$_2$-adrenergic agonist like albuterol, is administered by a powered nebulizer as often as every 20 minutes for 1 hour. Close monitoring of the child's respiratory status after each course of medication assesses resolution of the episode.

If the child improves, the child can return home with an albuterol prescription and instructions for assessing respiratory status, or with instructions for administering albuterol more frequently along with routine asthma medications. If symptoms do not improve or if the asthmatic child's PEFR is less than 70% of baseline, the child should receive a dose of an oral corticosteroid (liquid preparations are available for infants). If symptoms continue to worsen, administration of the bronchodilator every 20 minutes for an additional hour is warranted. Indicators for hospital admission include

- PEFR less than 40% of baseline
- Inspiratory and expiratory wheezing

- Tachycardia and tachypnea
- Dyspnea, retractions
- Oxygen saturation 91% or lower after aggressive treatment (Kercsmar, 1998)

Once the child is hospitalized humidified oxygen is administered at 30%, either by nasal prongs or by face mask, to keep the oxygen saturation at 95% or greater. An IV line delivers fluids and provides venous access for parenteral medications (e.g., methylprednisolone). Chest radiography, arterial blood gas determinations, or pulse oximetry may be performed to further evaluate the child's oxygenation status. The child receives a bronchodilator (albuterol) by nebulizer every 1 to 2 hours initially, with the interval between doses increased as the child's condition improves. Ipratroprium bromide (Atrovent), an anticholinergic agent, has been found to be an effective bronchodilator when administered along with albuterol in children with severe exacerbations.

Increasingly severe asthma that is unresponsive to vigorous treatment measures is termed *status asthmaticus*. Status asthmaticus is a medical emergency that can cause respiratory failure and death. Hospitalization, usually in an intensive care unit, is indicated. The child is placed on a continuous cardiac-respiratory monitor and continuous pulse oximeter. Blood gas and serum electrolyte values are monitored. In addition to the previously discussed measures, the child may receive continuous nebulized albuterol, and ipratroprium bromide every 6 hours. If the child's condition does not respond to these medications, subcutaneous epinephrine (1:1,000) or subcutaneous or IV terbutaline may be administered. Some children will improve with administration of IV aminophylline.

Endotracheal intubation with mechanical ventilation may be necessary. Acidosis is corrected with IV administration of sodium bicarbonate. Antibiotics may also be administered to treat concurrent infection (such as pneumonia).

ONGOING ASTHMA

A partnership between the health care provider, parent, and child is necessary for asthma to be managed effectively. Long-term asthma treatment should minimize symptoms, prevent acute asthma episodes, avoid the side effects of therapy, and help the child maintain a normal lifestyle. Children with asthma and their parents need to be taught methods of managing asthma, including environmental control and monitoring symptoms and medication.

Environmental Control

Irritants and Allergens. Children with asthma and their parents can decrease the frequency and severity of asthma episodes by recognizing and controlling the triggers that precipitate symptoms. Common environmental irritants include cigarette smoke, smoke from wood-burning stoves and fireplaces, fumes, deodorants, overhumidified air, and perfume. Allergenic triggers, such as animal dander, seasonal pollens, and molds, often cause problems. House dust can be both an irritant and an allergen.

The extent of environmental control needed depends on the severity of the asthma. If the asthma is mild, prohibiting smoking in the house and controlling dust with frequent housecleaning may be adequate. If the child continues to have problems after these interventions, additional steps should be taken to minimize environmental triggers.

Immunotherapy (allergy shots) can be helpful in decreasing asthma symptoms caused by specific allergens the child cannot avoid. Immunotherapy is used in conjunction with, not in place of, other asthma therapies.

Exercise. Exercise is a trigger of asthma in most asthmatic children. Exercise-induced asthma may be triggered by rapid breathing of large volumes of cool, dry air (e.g., with mouth breathing during exercise). The symptoms of exercise-induced asthma usually begin after 5 to 10 minutes of exercise and often last from 30 minutes to 1 hour.

Measures to prevent exercise-induced asthma include

- Warming the air by breathing through the nose or covering the mouth and nose with a scarf when exercising in cold weather
- Using an inhaled beta$_2$-agonist or cromolyn before exercise
- Practicing techniques to decrease hyperventilation (e.g., progressive muscle relaxation, diaphragmatic breathing)

Because athletics and active play are important parts of a child's life, children with asthma should not be restricted from physical activity. Exercise not only increases physical fitness, it also enhances self-esteem and offers valuable opportunities for socialization. Swimming is frequently recommended as an ideal sport for children with asthma because the air is humidified and exhaling underwater prolongs exhalation and increases end-expiratory pressure. Other sports that do not require sustained exertion, such as gymnastics, baseball, and weight lifting, are also well tolerated, and if asthma is well controlled, the child can usually participate in any type of sport.

Infection. Viral respiratory infections are the most frequent triggers of pediatric asthma. It is advisable for children with frequent or severe asthma to avoid exposure to individuals with a viral respiratory infection. Children with asthma also benefit from influenza vaccine.

Emotions. Asthma is not caused by psychosocial problems. Emotional upset, however, can exacerbate asthma symptoms. Laughing, crying, or shouting can act as mechanical triggers of bronchoconstriction. Also, a child with asthma may become angry or frustrated and refuse to take medication or adhere to a treatment regimen. Moreover, anxiety during an episode may cause the child to hyperventilate, aggravating asthma symptoms.

Monitoring Symptoms. Asthma symptoms can best be treated if they are detected early. Children and their parents should be taught the subtle early symptoms of an asthma episode (itchy chest or chin, cough, irritability or tired feeling, increased breathing rate, dry mouth, unusually dark circles under the eyes).

A useful device for monitoring breathing capacity is the peak flowmeter, which measures the flow of air in a forced exhalation in liters per minute. Peak flow monitoring can help identify the start of an asthma episode, often before the child is aware of symptoms. It can also help determine the need for treatment modification. Home monitoring of PEFR may be performed several times a day. The results can be compared with the child's normal predicted level and with results obtained over the preceding several days, providing an objective assessment of respiratory status.

Recent studies suggest that parents and children sometimes have difficulty recognizing asthma trouble signs, and even if signs are recognized they do not make appropriate

---

. . . .
Monitoring Breathing Capacity Using a Peak Flowmeter

The peak flowmeter is a device used to monitor breathing capacity in the child with asthma. It measures the flow of air in a forced exhalation in liters per minute. Peak flow monitoring can help identify the start of an asthma episode, often before symptoms are evident. To help children monitor their asthma, a zone system can be explained as a traffic light, making it easier for them to identify and understand differences in peak flow values.

Peak Flow Zones

Personal best: _____

Green: All clear—no asthma symptoms are present (80–100% of personal best)

Yellow: Caution—acute episode may be present (50%–80% of personal best). A temporary increase in medication may be indicated. Asthma may not be under control. Medication may need to be increased.

Red: Medical alert (below 50% of personal best). An immediate bronchodilator should be taken. Practitioner should be notified if measurements do not return immediately to and stay in yellow or green zones.

HOW TO USE A PEAK FLOWMETER

1. Remove gum or food from the mouth and stand up.
2. Move the pointer on the meter to zero.
3. Hold the meter horizontally, being sure to keep your fingers away from vent holes and the marker.
4. Relax and take a few moderately slow, deep breaths. Slowly take the deepest breath possible with your mouth wide open.
5. Hold your breath while placing the mouthpiece on your tongue. Seal your lips tightly around the mouthpiece.
6. Blow out as hard and fast as possible. Give a short, sharp blast, not a slow blow. (The meter records the fastest huff, not the longest). Note the number by the marker on the numbered scale.
7. Repeat three times. Wait at least 10 seconds between attempts. (Be sure to move the pointer to zero after each try.)
8. Record the highest of the three readings.
9. Ideally, peak flow values are obtained a minimum of once a day, preferably in the morning. Peak flow measurements should be done before and after administration of an inhaled bronchodilator. The number of measurements should be increased during a flare-up.

Adapted from National Heart, Lung and Blood Institute (1991, June). *Executive summary: Guidelines for the diagnosis and management of asthma.* Washington, DC: US Department of Health and Human Services.

• • • • • • • • • •
Classification of Asthma

Mild

- Symptoms occur no more than once a week or only with exercise
- Brief episodes
- Infrequent use of bronchodilator
- Few missed school days
- Rare activity limitation
- Symptoms rarely disturb sleep (less than weekly)

Moderate

- Symptoms occur and bronchodilator used more than twice a week
- More than 9 school days missed per year
- Frequent activity limitation (most days)
- Sleep disturbed by symptoms more than twice a week

Severe

- Daily symptoms
- Daily (or almost daily) use of bronchodilator for more than 6 months per year

Adapted from Kercsmar, C. (1998). Asthma. In V. Chernick, T. Boat, & E. Kendig (Eds.), *Kendig's disorders of the respiratory tract in children* (6th ed., p. 699). Philadelphia: Saunders.

treatment accommodations (Leickly, Wade, Crane, et al., 1998; Yoos & McMullen, 1999). This observation underscores the need for thorough teaching guidelines for home asthma management, including the following:

- A written asthma plan that includes details of home management and lists indications for seeking physician or emergency room care
- Daily use of a peak flowmeter (in children more than 5 years old) to monitor pulmonary status and response to treatment
- Home initiation of inhaled beta$_2$-adrenergic agonists, and oral steroids when beta$_2$-adrenergic agonists are ineffective for resolving symptoms
- Prompt communication with the health care provider for deteriorating respiratory status or reduced response to medication (Warman, Silver, McCourt, et al., 1999)

Medications. Generally, asthma is treated with a combination of medications from two categories: bronchodilators and anti-inflammatory agents. The medication regimen is based on the classification of the child's asthma and can be changed at home according to symptoms and peak flowmeter readings. It is important to differentiate rescue medications (those used for immediate relief of an exacerbation) and routine medications.

Rescue Medications. Some medications used to relieve an asthma episode are described below.

- *Short-acting bronchodilators*—Beta$_2$-adrenergic agonists, such as albuterol (Ventolin, Proventil), metaproterenol (Alupent), and terbutaline (Brethine), cause relaxation of bronchial smooth muscle and inhibit the release of mediators from mast cells. They are delivered by metered dose inhalers or by nebulizer three or four times daily if the child is symptomatic or before exercise.
- *Anticholinergic*—Ipratropium bromide is used in combination with beta$_2$-adrenergic agonists.
- *Mast cell inhibitors*—Cromolyn sodium (Intal), an inhaled NSAID, prevents asthma symptoms by blocking the release of mast cell mediators. It can be given 30

minutes before exposure to triggers. A newer anti-inflammatory asthma medication, nedrocromil sodium (Tilade), is available for use in children age 12 years or older.
- *Systemic corticosteroids*—Prednisone or prednisolone decreases airway inflammation. They are preferably given in short bursts.

Routine Medications. The medications used for long-term, routine control of asthma are the same as those used for relief but are administered in different dosages, depending on the classification of the child's asthma. Several additional medications have become available or are being tested for asthma control.

- *Long-acting bronchodilators*—Sustained-release albuterol, salmeterol (Serevent).
- *Inhaled corticosteroids*—Beclomethasone, triamcinolone, and flunisolide deliver topical anti-inflammatory action directly to the airway.
- *Leukotriene blockers*—Zafirlukast and Zileuton diminish the mediator action of leukotrienes. They are used only in children older than 12 years.

Children with mild asthma use bronchodilators as needed for symptom relief. Children and families need to be cautioned not to overuse these medications and to notify the health care provider if the medications are needed more than twice a week or more frequently than every 3 to 4 hours during a 12 hour period.

Children with mild to moderate persistent asthma take daily anti-inflammatory medications, usually mast cell inhibitors. It can take up to 4 weeks of daily dosing to realize a therapeutic effect. In addition, beta$_2$-adrenergic agonists are used to relieve symptoms. Long-acting bronchodilators or inhaled corticosteroids are also considered. Theophylline may be given to children who do not respond to mast cell inhibitors. PEFR monitoring helps the child with mild to moderate asthma monitor symptoms and pulmonary function. The family is given a written management plan.

Children with persistent severe asthma take daily mast

. . . .
Tips on Using a Nebulizer

1. Use clean hands and a clean area.
2. Take slow, deep breaths through pursed lips to maximize deposition of aerosolized medication in the lungs.
3. Use all the medication in the nebulizer during one treatment. Do not store medication in the nebulizer for later use.
4. The length of the treatment is usually 10 to 15 minutes if the equipment is working properly and the correct amount of medication and diluent are used. If the length of treatments is prolonged, check the nebulizer or the compressor for defects.
5. Rinse the nebulizer in clean water after each treatment. Allow it to air-dry after loosely covering it with a clean paper towel. Once daily, wash the nebulizer in warm, soapy water, then rinse and soak it for 30 minutes in a disinfecting solution or a solution containing one part white vinegar and four parts water. Never store the nebulizer in a closed plastic bag until it is completely dry. Storing wet equipment promotes the growth of mold and bacteria.

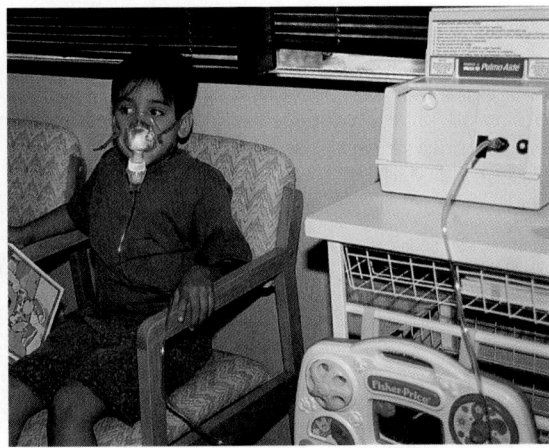

Adapted from Brim, S. (1989, January–February). A quick guide for home use of inhalant medications. *Pediatric Nursing*, 15(1), 87–94, by permission of Janetti Publications, Inc. Photo courtesy of Parkland Health and Hospital System Community-Oriented Primary Care Clinic, Dallas, Texas.

cell inhibitors, inhaled corticosteroids, and long-acting bronchodilators or leukotriene blockers. Ipratropium bromide and oral corticosteroids are considered for management.

Medication Delivery. Inhaled medications are delivered either by nebulizer or by metered dose inhaler (MDI). Both can be used for older and younger children. A spacer attached to an MDI prolongs the medication transit, effectively delivers the medication to the airway instead of the mouth, and makes it easier for younger children to use an MDI. If using a spacer, the child attaches the spacer to the outlet of the MDI, closes the lips around the spacer mouthpiece, activates the cannister, then inhales.

. . . .
How to Use a Metered Dose Inhaler

1. Stand up. Shake the inhaler well. Remove the cap.
2. Hold the inhaler upright. Hold the mouthpiece 1 to 2 inches from the lips and open your mouth wide.
3. Tilt your head back slightly and breathe out fully.
4. Place your lips tightly around the mouthpiece, press down on the inhaler, and start to breathe in slowly.
5. Breathe in slowly (3 to 5 seconds), as this allows deeper penetration of the medication.
6. Hold your breath for as long as possible, up to 10 seconds.
7. Remove the inhaler and breathe out slowly through the nose.
8. Wait at least 2 minutes and shake the inhaler again before repeating the dose.
9. Visible mist escaping from the open mouth indicates improper technique. Do not count that try. Relax and repeat.
10. Rinse your mouth with water if desired.

NURSING CARE
. . . .
The Child Hospitalized with Asthma

Assessment

The nurse begins assessment with a thorough history that includes any family history of asthma or allergy as well as past episodes of asthma, allergy, or other respiratory problems. The nurse asks the parents what treatment has been effective in previous asthma episodes. A new case of asthma may begin as a cough without wheezing. The child may have had recurrent bouts of pneumonia or sinusitis.

Assessment during an acute asthma episode should include vital signs and a careful evaluation of respiratory and oxygenation status. The nurse should note respiratory rate and effort, the presence or absence of retractions, the use of accessory muscles, nasal flaring, and pulse oximetry values. Level of consciousness is an important indicator of oxygenation and should be assessed carefully. The chest should be carefully auscultated for breath sounds, with the nurse noting any adventitious sounds or areas of diminished breath sounds. The child should be assessed for neurologic signs of impending respiratory failure (changes in consciousness, increased fatigue, somnolence). As infants and children become more hypoxic, they may not recognize or interact appropriately with their parents. Failure to resist or to cry during painful procedures is an ominous sign (Bechler-Karsch, 1994).

Because tachypnea and decreased intake of oral fluids may cause dehydration, hydration status should also be assessed (urine output, status of mucous membranes, presence of tears, skin turgor, weight).

A record of the child's routines and habits should be included in the psychosocial history. Previous hospitalizations should be documented, as a past experience may affect the child's perception of the current illness. An assessment of the family's knowledge of the disease, degree of compliance, and growth and development provides the basis for future teaching.

Nursing Diagnosis, Planning, Intervention, and Evaluation

Nursing Diagnosis
- Risk for Suffocation related to bronchospasm and mucosal edema.
- Ineffective Airway Clearance related to bronchospasm and mucosal edema.
- Impaired Gas Exchange related to air trapping in the bronchioles.

Expected Outcomes
- The child will have improved gas exchange, as evidenced by clear breath sounds, a pulse oximetry value of greater than 95% on room air, no use of accessory muscles, pink mucous membranes and nail beds, and a capillary refill time of less than 2 seconds.
- The child will be able to clear the airway, as evidenced by a respiratory rate and rhythm appropriate for the child's age, the ability to expectorate mucus, and normal vital signs for age.

Intervention

1. Monitor respiratory rate and effort, color, heart rate, and blood pressure every 15 to 30 minutes, with the interval lengthened as the child improves. Auscultate the chest for breath sounds. Monitor arterial blood gas values, pulse oximetry values, and pulmonary function test results. Notify the physician of any significant change (increased respiratory rate and effort, changes in wheezing, retractions, nasal flaring, severe cough, decreased alertness, cyanosis, increased dyspnea, or apprehension).

2. Administer humidified oxygen at the ordered flow rate. If the child has chronic carbon dioxide retention, do not exceed 2 L/min.

3. Help the child assume an upright position or position of comfort. The older child may be most comfortable leaning forward on a pillow or over-bed table.

4. Administer medications as ordered and monitor for effectiveness. Assess whether medications are effectively relieving the child's symptoms. Monitor the child for side effects.

5. Keep the child NPO during periods of respiratory distress, as ordered by the physician.

6. Maintain an IV line.

7. Ensure that respiratory treatments are given as ordered. Assess the child's breath sounds before and after treatments. Encourage the child to cough and deep breathe, especially after treatments. Suction as needed.

8. Ensure that emergency equipment is available (e.g., appropriate-size ventilation bag, endotracheal tubes, laryngoscope, emergency medication).

9. Keep the child as calm as possible. Offer support during periods of respiratory distress.

Rationale

1. Subtle changes in the child's condition may serve as an early warning of increased airway obstruction.

2. Supplemental oxygen decreases hypoxia secondary to airway edema, mucus, and bronchospasm. Administration of oxygen to a child with chronic carbon dioxide retention may lead to respiratory depression by decreasing the stimulus to breathe.

3. An upright position aids in expansion of the lungs and decreases pressure on the diaphragm.

4. Short-acting bronchodilators provide relief fairly quickly. IV methylprednisolone begins to reduce airway inflammation.

5. Oral intake is contraindicated for the child in respiratory distress because of the risk of aspiration.

6. IV access is necessary for administering medications and fluids.

7. Breathing treatments help to loosen or eliminate secretions and re-expand lung tissue. Mucus plugs can cause atelectasis and alveolar collapse.

8. The child's condition can deteriorate rapidly. Immediate resuscitation may be necessary in the event of severe respiratory distress.

9. Anxiety increases bronchospasms.

Evaluation
- Does the child maintain a patent airway?
- Is the respiratory rate within normal limits for age and is the oxygen saturation greater than 95%?
- Does the child expend minimal respiratory effort?
- Does the child have clear breath sounds with free movement of air?

Nursing Diagnosis

■ Fatigue related to hypoxia and an increased work of breathing.

Expected Outcome

• The child will exhibit decreased fatigue, as evidenced by less irritability and restlessness, uninterrupted sleep periods, and ability to perform usual activities.

Intervention	Rationale
1. Observe the child for signs and symptoms of hypoxia, including restlessness, fatigue, irritability, increased heart rate, and increased respiratory rate.	1. Irritability and agitation may be early signs of hypoxia. Prompt treatment of hypoxia decreases fatigue.
2. Organize nursing care to provide periods of uninterrupted rest and sleep.	2. Periods of quiet decrease stress and promote rest.
3. Encourage the parents' presence, particularly if the child is young.	3. The parents' presence decreases fear and anxiety.
4. Provide for the child's physical comfort. Encourage quiet, age-appropriate play activities as the child's condition improves.	4. Physical and emotional comfort confer a sense of well-being and promote rest.
5. Implement measures to relieve respiratory distress. Monitor the frequency of nebulized medications.	5. Restlessness, agitation, and inability to sleep are side effects of some asthma medications.

Evaluation

• Is the child able to play or perform usual activities without undue fatigue?

Nursing Diagnosis

■ Risk for Fluid Volume Deficit related to increased respiratory rate, diaphoresis, and decreased oral intake.

Expected Outcome

• The child will drink adequate fluid for age and weight and will not become dehydrated.

Intervention	Rationale
1. Monitor intake and output, status of mucous membranes, body weight, tearing, and urine specific gravity. Maintain urine specific gravity at 1.003 to 1.020. Monitor electrolyte levels. Observe the child's sputum for color, tenacity, and amount.	1. Rapid respiratory rate, diaphoresis, and increased pulmonary secretions may cause dehydration and increased viscosity of excretions.
2. Maintain IV infusion at the ordered flow rate. Avoid excessive amounts of fluid.	2. Adequate hydration enhances liquefaction of secretions, and thinner secretions are more easily expectorated. Excessive fluids may lead to pulmonary edema.
3. Encourage oral fluids when the respiratory distress has decreased, with the amount consumed being determined by the child's calculated needs. Offer favorite fluids. Provide liquids at the bedside.	3. Oral fluids are contraindicated during acute respiratory distress to minimize the risk of aspiration. Children are most likely to drink fluids if they are offered fluids they like.
4. Offer liquids at room temperature. Avoid milk and milk products.	4. Cold liquids may aggravate bronchospasm. Milk sometimes causes increased coughing and production of mucus.
5. Provide a humidified atmosphere.	5. Humidification helps to liquefy secretions and hydration.

Evaluation

• Does the child ingest adequate fluid for age and weight?
• Does the child maintain a urine specific gravity of 1.003 to 1.020?
• Does the child maintain pre-illness weight?
• Are moist mucous membranes and good skin turgor present?
• Does the child have adequate urinary output?

Nursing Diagnosis

■ Anxiety related to hospitalization and respiratory distress.

Expected Outcomes

• The child will exhibit reduced anxiety, as evidenced by a relaxed body position and a decrease in negative behaviors
• The parents will demonstrate reduced anxiety by verbalizing an accurate knowledge of asthma and participating in the child's care in a calm manner.

Intervention	Rationale
1. Teach the child techniques to control panic and anxiety and to slow the breathing rate (e.g., visually imagining staying calm, breathing exercises, pursed-lip breathing, belly breathing).	1. Concentration on such activities during an asthma episode calms the child and decreases the fear of suffocation.

2. Maintain a calm, quiet environment and a reassuring manner. Stay with the child. Provide care efficiently and calmly.
3. Reassure the child that there is someone nearby to assist if breathing difficulties develop. To allay any fears about going to sleep, tell the child that someone will be watching at night. Make the call light available for older children.
4. Use play therapy.

5. Encourage the parents to stay with the child. Praise the parents for rooming-in and supporting the child.
6. Keep parents informed of treatments, routines, and the child's condition.

7. Encourage expression of feelings by child and parents.
8. Avoid the use of sedatives.
9. Explain all procedures in an age-appropriate manner.

10. Facilitate trust by being truthful and acknowledging the discomfort of procedures.

2. The ability to remain calm decreases the child's oxygen demand and work of breathing.

3. Calm reassurance by the nurse can decrease the child's fear of suffocation and facilitate rest.

4. Therapeutic play allows the child to work through fears in a nonthreatening manner.
5. The presence of a familiar person can decrease fear and anxiety.
6. Reassuring the parents can help calm the child, as parental anxiety is quickly transferred to the child. Frequent and accurate updating of the child's condition reassures parents and decreases fear of the unknown.
7. Expressing feelings can help relieve stress and guilt.
8. Sedatives may depress respirations.
9. Procedures and an unfamiliar hospital setting may produce anxiety. Explanations decrease fear of the unknown.
10. Honesty fosters trust.

Evaluation
- Does the child cooperate with and participate in treatment and appear relaxed?
- Does the child obtain adequate rest and sleep?
- Do the parents verbalize decreased anxiety about the hospitalization and the child's condition?

Nursing Diagnosis
- Altered Family Processes related to the possibility of a chronic illness.

Expected Outcome
- The family will cope with the child's illness and comply with management in a way that promotes the child's normal growth and development.

Intervention

1. Provide opportunities for the family to express feelings. Recognize and accept negative feelings about the child and the illness.
2. Explore previous coping mechanisms used in times of stress.

3. Explain all procedures and treatments.

4. Keep parents informed of the child's condition.
5. Arrange for the family to meet with others affected by asthma. Identify available community resources (see Appendix L).

Rationale

1. This nonjudgmental approach helps the family work through fear, guilt, anxiety, and economic problems.
2. Identification and review of previously successful coping skills can assist the family in dealing with the present crisis.
3. A thorough explanation decreases fear of the unknown and anxiety.
4. Knowledge gives parents a sense of control.
5. Meeting others with asthma can assist with problem solving and provide support.

Evaluation
- Is the family able to provide necessary care?
- Can the family describe how to access helpful resources?

Nursing Diagnosis
- Knowledge Deficit about the disease process and home management.

Expected Outcomes
- The child will return to normal activities (exercise, play, school attendance).
- The family will describe home management principles.

Intervention

1. Determine the child's and parents' understanding of asthma. Explain unfamiliar procedures and equipment at the child's level of understanding. Teach the family about the disease, its triggers, and prescribed medications and treatments.

Rationale

1. Understanding increases compliance with treatment.

2. Help the family identify precipitating factors (e.g., exercise, infections, allergens, weather changes).
3. Explain the role of emotions and stress in the development of asthma symptoms.
4. Teach the child and family about the importance of taking medications as prescribed. Assess ability to afford medications. Provide written information and instructions about medications (names, side effects, dosages, and times of administration). Teach the family to recognize signs and symptoms that warrant notification of the physician. Reinforce the need to keep follow-up appointments.
5. Assist in developing an exercise program for the child. Medication may be needed prior to exercise. Teach the importance of a healthy lifestyle (regular exercise, adequate fluids and nutrition, rest, and prevention of infection).
6. Refer the family to a support group.

7. Teach self-management of asthma. Teach the necessary skills for home care. Encourage the child to take charge of asthma. The child should know what triggers to avoid, early warning signs of an episiode, the correct use of treatment aids (MDI, peak flowmeter), as well as proper administration of medications and techniques for stress reduction and relaxation. Encourage the child and family to participate in programs designed to develop effective self-management and decision-making skills (see Appendix L).

8. Teach the importance of follow-up care and routine health maintenance, such as keeping immunizations up to date.

2. An awareness of triggers may decrease future asthma episodes.
3. Stress and emotional upset can trigger bronchospasm.
4. Knowledge of medications increases compliance with the therapeutic regimen; compliance helps maintain serum drug levels within a therapeutic range.

5. Exercise promotes pulmonary and cardiovascular health and assists the child in leading a normal life.

6. Meeting with other children and families affected by asthma provides an avenue for expressing feelings and sharing information.
7. Knowledge of asthma decreases anxiety during acute episodes. The frequency and severity of episodes will be minimized if the child knows the appropriate actions for controlling symptoms. Learning about the condition can help decrease anxiety during episodes and increase the child's ability to take appropriate action to control symptoms. The frequency and severity of asthma episodes will be minimized if the child knows what triggers to avoid, the early warning signs of an episode, and the correct treatment of symptoms.
8. Preventing infection and practicing healthy living habits help decrease asthma triggers.

Evaluation

- Do the child and family verbalize an accurate knowledge of asthma and its treatment?
- Do the child and family keep follow-up appointments?
- Does the child resume normal daily activities?

Bronchopulmonary Dysplasia

Bronchopulmonary dysplasia (BPD) is a chronic obstructive pulmonary disease that occurs as a result of acute lung injury in some infants who have received supplemental oxygen and mechanical ventilation.

Etiology

Lung immaturity seems to be a key factor in the development of BPD, but many other factors affect its development as well. Genetic predisposition, a family history of atopic disorders, oxygen exposure (which injures immature lungs), positive pressure ventilation (which stretches lung tissue), neonatal respiratory infection, and inadequate nutrition in the very immature neonate are all risk factors for BPD (Hazinski, 1998). Infants with BPD often also have patent ductus arteriosus (see Chapter 46). Because lung development varies among infants, gestational age alone does not always predict the development of BPD.

PATHOPHYSIOLOGY

of Bronchopulmonary Dysplasia

The pressures of mechanical ventilation damage bronchial epithelium. Macrophages and polymorphonuclear inflammatory cells invade the airways, causing airway edema. Alveolar walls become thickened and fibrotic changes occur in the airways and alveoli. The continued use of oxygen affects the growth and development of lung structures, significantly reducing the number of developing alveoli.

Cystic and atelectatic areas develop in the lungs, predisposing the infant to pulmonary hypertension. There also may be loss of ciliated cells, which decreases the lungs' ability to remove mucous and leads to mucous plugs, atelectasis, and pneumonia.

Incidence

BPD is a significant cause of morbidity and mortality among very low birth weight infants (less than 1,000 g) and infants who have survived respiratory distress syndrome. It is the most frequently seen chronic lung condition in infants. The current high survival rates of low-birth-weight, preterm infants have resulted in the disorder being seen more often.

Manifestations

Manifestations of BPD include tachycardia and tachypnea related to decreased oxygenation; an increased work of breathing, retractions, and prolonged exhalation with the increased use of abdominal and accessory muscles; pallor associated with chronic hypoxia; and cyanosis and activity intolerance (feeding and handling). Affected infants also exhibit weight loss or poor weight gain related to the increased metabolic workload, hypoxia, and poor feeding; restlessness and irritability related to hypoxia; wheezing (intermittent or chronic) associated with a hyperresponsive airway; and puckering or pursing of the mouth with flaring of the nares (early signs of impending respiratory distress).

Diagnostic Evaluation

The diagnosis is based on clinical manifestations and radiographic abnormalities. Infants with respiratory symptoms that persist beyond 28 days of life, who need supplemental oxygen by 1 to 2 weeks of age and are still oxygen dependent after 28 days, or who need mechanical ventilation during the first week of life are suspected of having BPD. Chest radiographs may show infiltrates.

Therapeutic Management

Treatment goals for the infant with BPD strive to maintain adequate oxygenation to promote growth and development, prevent further lung disease, and promote healing of the damaged lungs. Treatment consists of oxygen therapy, drug therapy, and nutritional support.

Positive pressure ventilation should be discontinued as soon as possible. If mechanical ventilation is necessary to maintain life, then the lowest possible inflation pressures should be used, together with expiratory times that allow the lung to empty completely. Weaning from the ventilator may be a slow, tedious process, sometimes requiring many months to complete and often interrupted by infections and other problems (Barnhart & Czervinske, 1995).

OXYGEN THERAPY

Approximately 10% of infants with BPD will need supplemental oxygen for more than 1 year (Hazinski, 1998). Oxygen can be administered through a hood, tent, face mask, or nasal cannula. Oxygen saturation rates should be monitored closely and should be maintained between 92% and 95%. Some infants are discharged from the hospital while still oxygen dependent.

MEDICATIONS

Diuretics and fluid restriction are initiated to treat pulmonary interstitial edema. Furosemide is the most common diuretic used. Because infants with BPD often experience fluid overload and edema, fluid and electrolyte status should be monitored closely. Supplemental calcium, potassium, and chloride may be indicated for the infant receiving diuretics.

Inhaled bronchodilators, especially albuterol, when given in the early stages of BPD can lessen airway resistance and decrease the possibility of lung damage. The corticosteroid dexamethasone is often administered during weaning from mechanical ventilation. Careful monitoring during this process is needed, as dexamethasone increases lung compliance, putting the infant at risk for pulmonary barotrauma.

Infants with BPD experience frequent infections related to increased susceptibility and exposure to invasive treatments and procedures. After the initial stages of BPD, the risk of infection is probably the greatest risk to survival for these infants (Barnhart & Czervinske, 1995). Antibiotics are often needed. Ribavirin may be given to infants with respiratory syncytial virus.

NUTRITION

The infant needs increased nutritional intake for lung growth and repair beyond that required for normal infant growth. Other factors such as frequent respiratory exacerbations and feeding problems also increase caloric needs. A calorie intake of 110 to 150 kcal/kg/day to produce a weight gain of 15 to 30 g/day (Hazinski, 1998) is an appropriate goal. High-calorie formulas (24 or 27 cal/oz) assist with meeting this requirement, especially in infants in whom fluids are restricted. Medium chain triglyceride (MCT) oil or glucose polymers, if added to the formula, increase the calories per ounce.

PROGNOSIS

Most infants with BPD do improve. The mortality ranges from 10% to 25%; death usually is a result of pulmonary complications. Most infants with BPD will require ongoing therapy at home, and some will develop chronic airway hyperreactivity, which may progress to bronchial asthma. Many infants with BPD are rehospitalized during the first year of life because of acute respiratory tract infections. Infants may show a developmental delay for the first 24 to 36 months of life.

Nursing Considerations

Because of their low birth weight and possible respiratory distress syndrome, most neonates with BPD are initially cared for in a special care nursery. Nursing intervention prior to discharge includes meticulous planning for home care, coordinating referrals, and teaching home management.

Home care of the infant with BPD decreases the risk of hospital-acquired infection and reduces health care costs. Care at home also improves social development by encouraging interaction between the child and family.

Preparation for discharge and home care requires a great deal of education and reassurance. Educating the family with a chronically ill or technology-dependent child must begin early with basic care—feeding, bathing, holding, and playing. This care progresses to medical, nursing, and respiratory procedures. The infant may continue to receive supplemental oxygen at home or may have a tracheostomy. Some infants are discharged while they are still ventilator dependent. Families must be taught the necessary precautions for safe use of oxygen in the home. Before hospital discharge, the nurse contacts emergency services, utility companies, and the telephone company to notify them that a technology-dependent child will be living in their area (Fig. 45–5). Required actions

PARENTS WANT TO KNOW

About Safe Use of Oxygen at Home

SAFETY GUIDELINES

Secure the oxygen tank in an upright position.

Keep oxygen tanks at least 5 feet from heat sources and electrical devices (e.g., space heaters, heating vents, fireplaces, radios, vaporizers).

Ensure that no one smokes in the room or in the area of the oxygen tank.

Avoid using alcohol-based substances or oil to relieve dryness around your child's mouth (e.g., petroleum jelly, vitamin A & D ointment, baby oil).

Keep a fire extinguisher readily available.

Turn off both the volume regulator and the flow regulator when oxygen is not in use.

RATIONALE

Oxygen tanks are highly explosive. If a horizontally positioned tank explodes, the rapid release of oxygen can catapult it through both animate (human bodies) and inanimate objects (walls).

Smoking increases the risk of fire, which could cause the tank to explode; escaped oxygen would feed the fire.

Both alcohol and oil are flammable and increase the risk of fire.

A fire extinguisher may be needed to put out a fire immediately.

If the volume regulator is on when the oxygen is turned on, the child might receive a rapid, forceful flow of oxygen in the face that could be frightening and uncomfortable. Oxygen leakage, which might not be detected because oxygen is odorless, can cause a fire.

for contacting these services in case of emergency should be reviewed with the family.

Evaluating the family's response to the infant's illness and their coping strategies is critical for optimal home management of the infant with a chronic condition. The nurse should help the family identify physical as well as psychological strengths and weaknesses. Because the care of an infant with BPD can be extraordinarily expensive, the nurse should consider referring the family to social services for access to potential financial assistance.

ELECTRIC COMPANY
REQUEST FOR SPECIAL CONSIDERATION

Date: _____

Name: _____
Address: _____
_____

Phone: _____
Account Number: _____

Attention: Customer Service

Our infant/child, _____, is under the
care of Dr. _____ at _____
for _____. This condition(s) requires the use of a
cardiorespiratory monitor and/or other life support equipment, specifically:

_____

The necessary equipment selected for home care is equipped with a battery back-up system that will power the equipment in the event of a power failure for a **limited period of time.** If a power failure occurs, it is imperative to restore service to this home as soon as possible. Please place this home on a priority list for restoration of electric service. If you have advance warning of a temporary interruption in electric service, please notify the parents so alternative arrangements can be made. If you have questions regarding the specifications of the equipment provided, please contact our equipment provider, Pediatric Home Care Associates.

Thank you for your cooperation.

Sincerely yours,

OUR EQUIPMENT PROVIDER IS:

FIGURE 45–5

Example of a letter that can be used to notify the local public service company that a technology-dependent child is living in the service area. (Courtesy of Pediatric Home Care Associates, Garfield, NJ. From Barnhart, S. L., & Czervinske, M. P. [1995]. *Perinatal and pediatric respiratory care* [p. 662]. Philadelphia: Saunders.)

Cystic Fibrosis

Cystic fibrosis (CF), the most common lethal genetic disease in whites, is a chronic multisystem disorder affecting the exocrine glands. The mucus produced by the exocrine glands (particularly those of the bronchioles, small intestine, and the pancreatic and bile ducts) is abnormally thick, causing obstruction of the small passageways of these organs. Although CF is incurable, the life expectancy of affected children has increased dramatically. The median survival age is 30 years, making CF a disease not only of children but also of young adults. The discovery of the CF gene has brought hope for improved treatment and the possibility of eventually developing a cure for the disease.

Etiology

CF is transmitted as an autosomal recessive trait, which means that both parents must carry the gene for the child to be affected. If both parents carry the CF gene, each pregnancy has a 25% chance of producing an affected child. The CF gene has been localized to the long arm of chromosome 7.

Incidence

The incidence of CF in white children is approximately 1 in 4,000 live births (Baroni, Anderson, & Mischler, 1997). The prevalence in African-Americans is considerably lower, and CF rarely affects Latinos or Asians. It is estimated that one in 20 white Americans carry the gene for CF. Approximately two thirds of children with CF are diagnosed by the time they are 1 year old, but in many instances (ap-

proximately 10%) CF is not diagnosed until adolescence or early adulthood (Wagner & Sherman, 1997).

Manifestations

Signs and symptoms of CF, the extent of specific organ system involvement, and age at which symptoms begin vary widely among affected children. Symptoms gradually worsen as the disease progresses, and the outcome is eventually fatal.

RESPIRATORY SYSTEM

Signs and symptoms of respiratory involvement include wheezing and a dry, nonproductive cough (earliest pulmonary manifestations), repeated bouts of pneumonia and bronchitis, and purulent and copious sputum accompanying chronic bacterial infections. The cough at this stage is wet and paroxysmal and may be followed by vomiting. Crackles, wheezes, and diminished breath sounds; accessory muscle use, retractions, hypoxia, and cyanosis; and increased cough, dyspnea, tachypnea, and cyanosis occur as the disease progresses. Emphysema and atelectasis may develop as the airways become increasingly obstructed with secretions; cor pulmonale and congestive heart failure secondary to fibrotic lung changes can be seen in later stages of the disease. Spontaneous pneumothorax or hemoptysis are seen in later stages as well. Nasal polyps, sinusitis, digital clubbing (Fig. 45–6), and a barrel chest (increased anteroposterior chest diameter) are also noted.

DIGESTIVE SYSTEM

Digestive system involvement is marked by steatorrhea (frothy, foul-smelling stools two to three times bulkier than

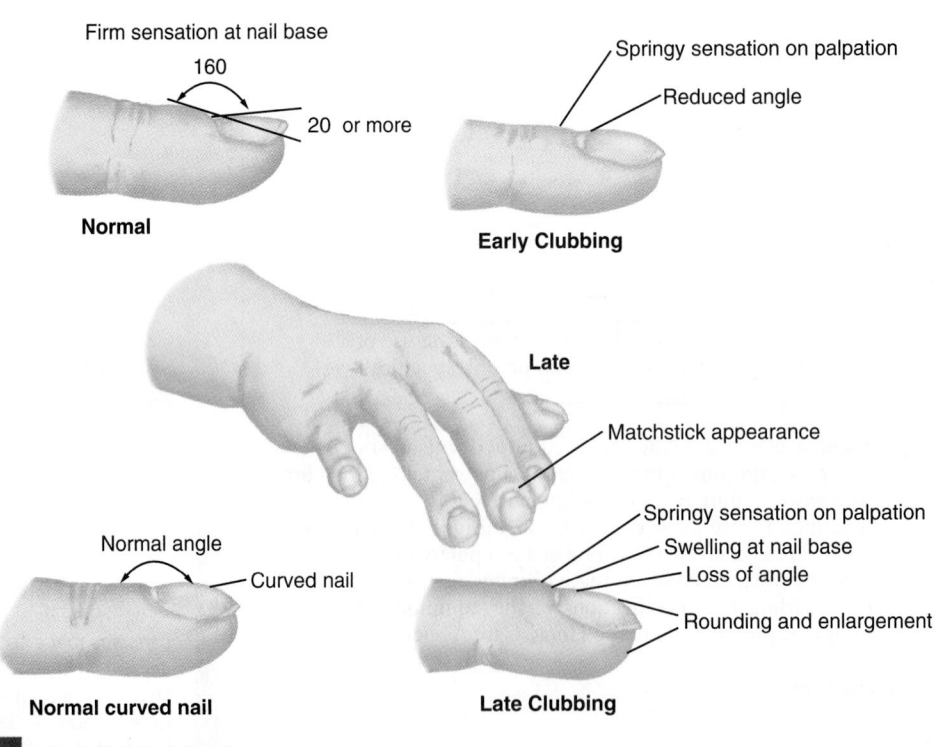

Firm sensation at nail base
160
20 or more
Normal

Springy sensation on palpation
Reduced angle
Early Clubbing

Late

Matchstick appearance

Normal angle
Curved nail
Normal curved nail

Springy sensation on palpation
Swelling at nail base
Loss of angle
Rounding and enlargement
Late Clubbing

FIGURE 45–6

Digital clubbing may be an indication of hypoxia, which often occurs in cystic fibrosis and other respiratory disorders.

of Cystic Fibrosis

Cystic fibrosis (CF) affects the exocrine glands throughout the body and causes respiratory, digestive, integumentary, and reproductive dysfunction and damage.

RESPIRATORY SYSTEM

Abnormally thick, sticky secretions cause obstruction of both the small and large airways. Stasis of secretions from bronchial obstruction provides a medium for bacterial growth. Chronic infection causes the release of toxic chemicals that damage lung tissues and alter host defenses within the airways, thus exacerbating the infection and inflammation. Inflammation may also cause bronchospasm, worsening airway blockage. Because airways dilate on inspiration and constrict on exhalation, air trapping occurs in the peripheral airways narrowed by mucous secretions. Hyperinflation is one of the first findings on chest radiographs of a child with CF. Chronic infection leads to atelectasis and eventual fibrosis and destruction of pulmonary tissue.

As the disease progresses, the lungs of almost all patients with CF eventually become colonized with *Pseudomonas aeruginosa,* an organism that can never be completely eradicated from the respiratory tract but can be controlled with vigorous antibiotic therapy. With chronic respiratory tract infection, impaired oxygen and carbon dioxide exchange causes varying degrees of hypoxia, hypercapnia, and acidosis. Fibrotic lung changes occur as the disease worsens and hypoxia increases. Alveolar hypoxia leads to pulmonary vasoconstriction, increasing pulmonary vascular resistance. Increased pulmonary vascular resistance causes the right side of the heart to work harder to pump blood into the lungs. Enlargement of the right ventricle in response to increased pulmonary resistance (cor pulmonale) results. Congestive heart failure may develop. Pulmonary complications include sinusitis, spontaneous pneumothorax, and hemoptysis. Death in patients with CF is almost always the result of respiratory failure.

DIGESTIVE SYSTEM

Eighty-five percent of patients with CF have pancreatic involvement. The pancreatic ducts, blocked by thick mucus, are unable to secrete trypsin, amylase, and lipase into the small intestine. Without these digestive enzymes, proteins, carbohydrates, and fats are poorly absorbed. Bowel obstruction from thickened intestinal mucus and pancreatic insufficiency may be present at birth (meconium ileus). The islets of Langerhans in the pancreas are normal in patients with CF, but they may decrease in number as the disease progresses and the pancreas undergoes fibrotic changes. Older children with CF sometimes develop type 1 diabetes. Abnormalities of the gallbladder are common.

INTEGUMENTARY SYSTEM

The sweat glands of children with CF secrete normal amounts of sweat. The levels of sodium and chloride in the sweat, however, are two to five times the normal range.

REPRODUCTIVE SYSTEM

Ninety-eight percent of males with CF are sterile because of obstruction of the deferent ducts and seminal vesicles. Female patients have reduced fertility because of abnormally thick cervical mucus, which impedes sperm penetration of the cervical canal.

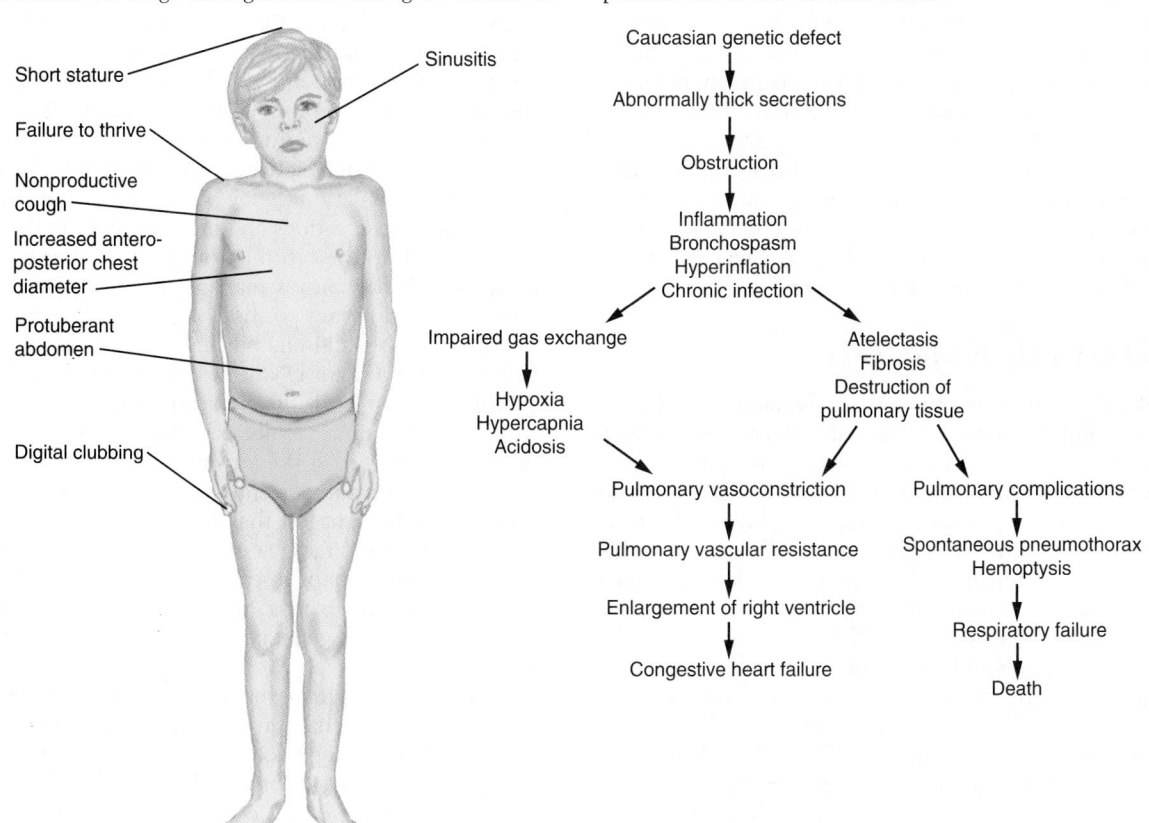

normal) and flatus. Malnutrition and growth failure are evident despite normal caloric intake; deficiencies in fat-soluble vitamins A, D, E, and K are caused by an inability to absorb fats. Vitamin A deficiency may lead to xerophthalmia and vitamin K deficiency may result in bleeding, especially in infants. Children with CF are usually thin and underweight, but with adequate treatment, most attain normal height. Fifty percent of children diagnosed with CF are assigned to less than the 10th percentile for height or weight (FitzSimmons, 1993). A protruberant abdomen, barrel chest, wasted buttocks, and thin extremities are common.

Meconium ileus in the neonate is the earliest manifestation of CF. Intestinal obstruction later in life, called meconium ileus equivalent, may occur and is the result of impacted feces at the ileocecal junction. Rectal prolapse and intussusception may also occur. Biliary cirrhosis, portal hypertension, and esophageal varices, secondary to obstruction of the bile ducts, are seen in 2% to 4% of patients. There is an increased incidence of type 1 diabetes in older individuals with CF.

EXOCRINE GLANDS

Abnormally high concentrations of sodium and chloride in sweat are an early sign of CF (mothers often report that their infants taste salty when kissed). The risk for electrolyte imbalance during hot weather is high; infants are especially prone to developing hyponatremia and hypochloremia. Many children complain of dry mouth and have an increased susceptibility to infection.

REPRODUCTIVE SYSTEM

Reproductive system involvement is marked by an average of 2 years' delay in the development of secondary sex characteristics. Young adults with CF may have difficulty becoming pregnant because of the thick cervical mucus, which acts as a barrier to sperm. This impairment of fertility should not be relied upon as a birth control method. An increased incidence of fetal loss and preterm birth and an increased neonatal mortality are also seen, although a woman with mild CF can carry a pregnancy to term with conscientious prenatal care. Sterility secondary to lack of sperm is noted in approximately 95% of male patients with CF; otherwise sexual function is normal.

Diagnostic Evaluation

CF has been called the great imitator because signs of failure to thrive and chronic respiratory infection are signs of many other childhood conditions. In some infants CF is evident at birth because of symptoms of severe bowel obstruction (meconium ileus) caused by intestinal plugging by thick, tenacious secretions. More commonly, CF is diagnosed during infancy or toddlerhood in children with poor growth; bulky, greasy stools; and frequent colds or bouts of pneumonia (Barnhart & Czervinske, 1995; Fulginiti & Lewy, 1993). The early diagnosis and treatment of CF makes a difference in the quality and length of life for these children.

The diagnosis of CF requires a positive sweat test as well as either a family history of CF or clinical signs consistent with CF. The sweat test, *pilocarpine iontophoresis*, measures the amount of sodium and chloride in sweat and is simple, painless, and reliable. It is usually performed twice to ensure accuracy. A chloride level greater than 60 mEq/L is considered to be diagnostic for CF; a level of 40 mEq/L is suggestive of CF and requires repeating the test. A sample of at least 50 mg of sweat is required for accurate results. Because this amount is difficult to obtain from small infants, the sweat test is usually not reliable in infants less than 4 weeks old.

In addition to the sweat test, the following studies are also performed: 72-hour fecal fat determination, liver function tests (ALT, AST), fasting blood glucose test, chest radiography, sputum culture (for identification of infective organisms), and pulmonary function tests.

DNA analysis of chorionic villi samples or amniotic fluid testing can establish a diagnosis prenatally. DNA analysis can also determine whether siblings of the affected child are carriers.

In newborns, screening for CF and phenylketonuria can be done simultaneously using the immunoreactive trypsinogen assay (IRT). Because the test has a high number of false positive results (Baroni et al., 1997), it has not been used widely in the United States for routine newborn screening.

Therapeutic Management

Therapy is individualized for each child and is aimed at preventing and treating pulmonary infections, maintaining optimal nutritional status, and promoting psychological adjustment. Children with CF are cared for at home most of the time. They are hospitalized during acute pulmonary infections, periodically for IV antibiotic treatment and vigorous chest physical therapy (CPT), and for end-stage disease.

RESPIRATORY PROBLEMS

Because chronic respiratory infection is a major cause of lung damage in patients with CF, treatment strives to relieve airway obstruction by mobilizing secretions, decrease the number of bacteria by removing secretions, and treat infections by administering antibiotics.

Segmental percussion and postural drainage (see Chapter 37) with inhalation therapy are performed several times a day to loosen secretions and move them from the peripheral airways into the central airways where they can be expectorated. Newer airway management techniques, such as forced exhalation and positive expiratory pressure devices, have been successful in mobilizing mucus. Mucolytic agents (inhaled recombinant DNase or Pulmozyme), inhaled bronchodilators, and anti-inflammatory agents are often used with postural drainage to decrease the viscosity of secretions or increase the size of the airways.

Exercise is an important part of pulmonary treatment. Some researchers suggest that aerobic exercise, such as jogging or swimming, may be as effective as traditional CPT in relieving pulmonary obstruction (Schidlow, 1999). Children with CF who exercise regularly have fewer pulmonary exacerbations and generally feel better than those who do not.

Antibiotics have played a major role in increasing the life expectancy of children with CF. Some physicians prescribe antibiotics prophylactically, whereas others use them only during periods of active infection. IV antibiotics are the usual treatment of choice during acute pulmonary exacerbations. Children with CF frequently need higher than usual doses of antibiotics because of their rapid metabolism of these drugs. IV antibiotics are usually administered during hospitalization, but home IV therapy is becoming more widely accepted, offering substantial savings and minimizing disruption of daily activities. Oral or aerosolized antibiotics may be used instead of IV therapy.

Steroids are sometimes prescribed when pulmonary symptoms are unresponsive to antibiotics and increased CPT. Steroids are used with caution, however, because of concern that they may worsen *Pseudomonas aeruginosa* infections. Oxygen therapy also is used with caution, as many children with CF have chronic carbon dioxide retention and are at risk for oxygen-induced carbon dioxide narcosis.

DIGESTIVE PROBLEMS

Early in the course of CF, the child may exhibit a huge appetite but not gain weight. Chronic pulmonary infections, an increased work of breathing, and malabsorption place an increased caloric and protein demand on the child with CF. The child's calorie requirements are approximately 150% of the normal recommended daily allowance (RDA). Children with CF are managed with a high-calorie, high-protein diet, pancreatic enzyme replacement therapy, fat-soluble vitamin supplements, and, if nutritional problems are severe, nighttime gastrostomy feedings or total parenteral nutrition. Fats are not restricted unless steatorrhea cannot be controlled by increased pancreatic enzymes.

Infants are usually given a predigested formula (Pregestimil or Nutramigen), which is more easily absorbed than regular formula. Formulas may also be concentrated to provide increased calories. For the older child, caloric intake may be increased with food supplements or enteral tube feedings.

Enteric-coated microencapsulated pancreatic enzyme preparations (Cotazym-S, Pancreatin, Pancrease) are administered with every meal and snack. Enzyme dosage is adjusted according to stool formation: less enzyme with constipation, more enzyme with loose, fatty stools. Bowel obstruction has been reported as being associated with high-dose enzyme replacement (lipase, 6,000 U/kg/meal) (Kuhn & Horn, 1994). Therefore, the enzyme dosage should be individualized for each child and kept as low as possible while still maintaining the child's nutritional status. Extra salt is added to the diet in extremely hot weather or when the child exercises vigorously.

NURSING CARE
· · · · · · · · · ·
The Child with Cystic Fibrosis

Assessment

The child with CF should be assessed for signs and symptoms in each of the systems usually affected by the disease, as well as for psychosocial adaptation to this chronic condition.

Respiratory Assessment

The child may have had frequent episodes of pneumonia or bronchitis. Auscultate the chest to detect any crackles, wheezes, areas of diminished breath sounds, or a prolonged expiratory phase of respiration. Note signs of long-standing respiratory difficulty, such as barrel chest or digital clubbing. The respiratory status is assessed by noting the rate, depth, and ease of respirations, from the color of the nail beds and mucous membranes, and by pulse oximetry. The characteristics of the child's cough and the color, amount, and quality of sputum should be documented, along with any fever. Exercise tolerance and the child's ability to sleep lying down at night should also be assessed.

Digestive Assessment

The nurse weighs and measures the child, plotting the results on a standardized growth chart. Signs of malabsorption, such as steatorrhea, frequent infections, fatigue, and a protuberant abdomen with thin extremities, should be noted. A diet history is useful in assessing the child's caloric intake. The use of vitamins and dietary supplements should be recorded. Determining the number and consistency of stools assesses the adequacy of intestinal enzyme replacement. Because ulcers and intestinal obstruction often accompany CF, complaints of abdominal pain, blood in the stools, and constipation should be noted. Use of antacids, H_2-receptor blockers, or antireflux medications should also be assessed.

Reproductive Assessment

Girls should be assessed for vaginal itching or drainage, which may indicate a vaginal infection. Contraception should be discussed with adolescents.

Nursing Diagnosis and Planning

The following nursing diagnoses often apply to children with CF:

- Ineffective Airway Clearance related to increased pulmonary secretions.
  Expected Outcome: The child will be able to remove secretions from the airway.
- Impaired Gas Exchange related to air trapping within the alveoli secondary to obstruction of the airways by thick mucus.
  Expected Outcome: The child will maintain an oxygen saturation level of greater than 95%.
- Risk for Infection related to tenacious secretions and altered body defenses.
  Expected Outcome: The child will remain free of infection.
- Altered Nutrition: Less Than Body Requirements, related to poor intestinal absorption of nutrients.
  Expected Outcome: The child's nutritional status will improve and the child will exhibit normal growth; the child's stools will be of normal consistency, frequency, and color.
- Activity Intolerance related to pulmonary congestion and poor absorption of nutrients.
  Expected Outcome: The child will rest comfortably and engage in age-appropriate activities.
- Self-Esteem Disturbance related to physical changes from chronic illness.
  Expected Outcome: The child will demonstrate a positive self-concept and feelings of independence as demonstrated by participating in self-care.

■ Ineffective Individual/Family Coping: Compromised, related to chronic illness.
Expected Outcome: The child and family will comply with the treatment regimen, verbalize feelings about the impact of the illness on their lives, and use available support systems and community resources.

■ Anticipatory Grieving related to a potentially fatal diagnosis.
Expected Outcome: The child and family will make realistic plans for the future and be able to discuss feelings about the anticipated death.

Interventions

Facilitating Airway Clearance and Gas Exchange

Perform CPT every 4 hours, just before bedtime, and as needed; perform treatments at least 1 hour before or 2 hours after meals to reduce gastrointestinal upset. The child's respiratory status should be determined before and after CPT. Note the child's tolerance of the procedure. Teach "huffing" (forced expiration) to mobilize secretions. The child should take a deep breath, then exhale rapidly while whispering the word huff. Administer ordered bronchodilators or mucolytics in conjunction with CPT or as ordered.

To facilitate gas exchange, administer humidified, low-flow (2 L/min or less) oxygen as ordered. The recommended amount of oxygen should not be exceeded because too much oxygen administered to children who are chronically hypoxic can depress respirations. Elevate the head of the bed or support the child in an upright position if the child is dyspneic. Be sure to stay with the child during coughing episodes.

Preventing Infection

Children with CF are prone to respiratory infection, especially airway colonization with *P. aeruginosa,* and oral or inhaled antibiotic therapy may be routine. IV antibiotics may be required during acute exacerbations. Pay meticulous attention to hygiene measures, especially hand washing, and teach the child and family to do the same. Monitor the child for signs of respiratory infection (fever, chills, increased respirations, dyspnea, cough, purulent secretions, increased WBC count). Advise the family to avoid exposing the child to others who are ill. Children with CF should receive all routine childhood immunizations at ages recommended by the American Academy of Pediatrics (Appendix F). An annual influenza vaccine is also appropriate, based on recommendations by the Centers for Disease Control and Prevention.

Providing Optimal Nutrition for Growth

Provide a well-balanced diet that is high in calories, protein, and carbohydrates and that includes the child's favorite foods. Oral or enteral high-calorie supplements can increase the child's calorie intake.

The child needs to take pancreatic enzymes as ordered within 30 minutes of eating all meals and snacks. The child should not mix the enzymes with hot or starchy foods because enzymes are inactivated by heat. Older children may take enteric-coated pancreatic enzyme capsules or enzyme beads. For children who cannot swallow capsules, mix the enzyme with a small amount of a nonprotein food. Because prolonged contact with enzyme powder may cause excoriation of oral mucosa, wipe off any powder that remains on the child's lips. Advise the family to note the color, consistency, and frequency of the child's stools because enzyme replacement is correlated with the child's bowel elimination pattern (e.g., one to two stools daily in older children; more often in infancy is an acceptable pattern). The enzyme dosage should be increased when high-fat foods are eaten. Administer multivitamins, water-miscible, fat-soluble vitamins, and iron supplements as ordered. Monitor the child's appetite and food intake. Extra salt and fluid are required when the weather is hot.

Promoting Increased Exercise Tolerance

For the child in acute exacerbation, provide rest periods between treatments and organize nursing care to ensure periods of uninterrupted rest. The child's activity level is increased as tolerated, and arrange age-appropriate activities geared to the child's energy level. When the child is feeling well, encourage active play and activities, such as swimming and gymnastics.

Meeting the Child's and Family's Emotional Needs

Encourage the child to express feelings about the chronic illness and its effect on feelings of self-worth. This is especially important for adolescents who keep secrets about their illness as a way to cope with feelings about being different (Christian & D'Auria, 1997). Helping the child identify personal strengths and areas of accomplishment will increase the child's self-esteem. Teach parents the importance of fostering independence in their child. As the child grows, encourage discussion about areas of concern, such as dating, sexuality, and peer acceptance. Assist families with the child's transition from pediatric to adult health care providers.

Introducing the family to other families affected by CF can increase problem-solving strategies and facilitate support. Provide information about available community resources, such as the Cystic Fibrosis Foundation and the American Lung Association. The family also should be encouraged to communicate with personnel at the child's school to ensure coordination of care between home and school.

Although tremendous progress has been made in treating CF, it remains a chronic disease with no cure. Provide the family with honest information about the disease and its prognosis. Refer the family for counseling and listen if they wish to discuss feelings about the disease, the future, and death.

Home Care

Preparation for home care involves teaching family members how to carry out CPT, how to provide breathing treatments, and how to give medications at home. Written instructions should describe the specifics of all aspects of the child's care. Families may need assistance in obtaining home care equipment.

Evaluation

• Does the child exhibit improved breath sounds, oxygen saturation greater than 95% on room air, and stable respiratory status?

- Are the child's body temperature and white blood cell count within normal limits? Has the sputum amount decreased?
- Is the child growing in height and weight along the normal growth curve?
- Are the child's stools of normal consistency, frequency, and color?
- Is the child able to engage in appropriate physical activity?
- Does the child appear to be developing age-appropriate cognitive, emotional, and social skills and appropriate level of self-care?
- Does the child demonstrate an attitude of acceptance of self and of the illness?
- Does the family demonstrate appropriate coping strategies, compliance with the child's treatment plan, and the ability to access needed resources?
- Can the parents demonstrate CPT, inhalation therapy, and other treatments to be performed at home?
- Are the child and family able to appropriately express feelings of anger, sadness, and fear without guilt?

Tuberculosis

Tuberculosis (TB) is a reportable contagious disease with a high morbidity and mortality throughout the world. Its incidence was declining until 1985, when it again began to rise. The World Health Organization has declared TB a global crisis (Ott et al., 1995).

Etiology

Mycobacterium tuberculosis, an acid-fast bacillus, causes TB. Contamination occurs chiefly through inhalation of droplets from a person with active TB. Droplets produced by coughing and sneezing remain suspended in the air. When they are inhaled, they can reach the bronchioles and alveoli.

The risk for infection by the organism is thought to depend on several physiologic and socioeconomic factors. Most children are infected by a family member, babysitter, or other person with whom they have frequent contact.

Incidence

Almost 1.3 million cases and 450,000 deaths from tuberculosis occur among children each year. More than two thirds of the reported cases in the United States now occur in urban, low-income areas and in nonwhite racial and ethnic groups (AAP Committee on Infectious Diseases, 1997). In the pediatric population, TB occurs most commonly in infants and adolescents and in children with immunosuppressive conditions. Of particular concern is the increase in multi-drug-resistant (MDR) TB, which develops primarily in persons who do not take medications as prescribed (Ott et al., 1995).

Manifestations

Children ages 3 to 15 years are usually asymptomatic, have normal chest radiographs, and can be identified only through a positive skin test. Some children experience malaise, fever, night sweats, a slight cough, weight loss, anorexia, lymphadenopathy, or more specific symptoms related to the site of extrapulmonary infection (e.g., kidneys, brain, bone).

PATHOPHYSIOLOGY
of Tuberculosis

The bacillus multiplies in lung tissue, alveoli, and regional lymph nodes. After an incubation period of 2 to 12 weeks, hypersensitivity develops; at that time the infected child will test positive on skin tests. Most infected children are asymptomatic at the time of the initial positive skin test result.

The *disease* of TB is differentiated from TB *infection* by the presence of clinical manifestations. The risk of developing TB disease is highest in the first 2 years after infection, but many infected children never progress to clinical disease.

The immunologic response of most people is usually strong enough to keep the bacteria from multiplying and spreading. If the host response is adequate, the organism is walled off and the tubercle becomes a healed calcified mass. TB bacilli can remain dormant and cause active disease at a later time if the child's resistance is lowered. If the lesion does not heal and is not walled off, it may continue to enlarge and spread into nearby tissues, or it may enter the blood and spread to other sites (middle ear, brain, kidney, bones, joints, and skin).

TB disease destroys host tissue. When tubercle bacilli multiply, they may damage tissue so badly that the center of the infected area turns to liquid pus. When this liquid escapes through an airway, it is coughed up as sputum, leaving a tiny hole (cavitation) in the lung. This bacteria-laden sputum is infectious. Only rarely do children develop active pulmonary TB with cavitation, and only in such instances is the child infectious to others (Ott, Horn, & McLaughlin, 1995). Because children with primary pulmonary TB have small lesions and minimal cough they are not contagious (AAP Committee on Infectious Diseases, 1997). The duration of infectivity of treated adults and adolescents depends on the drug susceptibility of the infecting organism and cough frequency. Although infectivity usually lasts only a few weeks after treatment is begun, it may last longer if the person fails to take the prescribed medication or is infected with a resistant strain.

Diagnostic Evaluation

Skin testing is the initial method of screening and testing for TB. In most children skin testing will produce a positive reaction 2 to 12 weeks after the initial infection and, once positive, tuberculin reactivity usually continues throughout life, even with treatment.

Skin testing with 5 tuberculin unit (TU) purified protein derivative (PPD) (Mantoux test) is the preferred method of screening. The PPD is administered by intradermal injection on the forearm. The skin reaction is read by an experienced professional 48 to 72 hours after placement. A 15-mm induration in any child older than age 4 years is considered a positive sign of TB. Induration of more than 5 mm suggests TB in certain populations of children. A neg-

· · · · · · · · · ·
Risk Factors for the Development of Tuberculosis

- Contact with adults with infectious TB
- Chronic illness, immunosuppression, HIV infection
- Malnutrition
- Age (infancy and adolescence)
- Nonwhite racial and ethnic groups; immigration from areas with a high incidence of TB
- Urban, low-income living conditions
- Incarcerated adolescents
- Children in close contact with any of the following groups of adults: HIV-infected persons, users of IV or other street drugs, poor or medically indigent city dwellers, residents of nursing homes, migrant farm workers

ative tuberculin skin test does not rule out TB, particularly in infants.

Children with positive skin test results undergo follow-up examinations, which include periodic chest radiography and sputum cultures and smears. Because children often swallow sputum rather than expectorate it, gastric washings to obtain swallowed sputum are sometimes done. A thorough history should be obtained, and all contacts of the affected child should be tested for the disease.

· · · · · · · · · ·
Definition of a Positive Mantoux Skin Test in Children

AREA OF INDURATION ≥5 MM

- Children in close contact with persons who have known or suspected infectious cases of tuberculosis (TB)
- Children suspected of having TB disease (based on positive chest x-ray findings or clinical manifestations of TB)
- Children with immunosuppressive conditions or HIV infection

AREA OF INDURATION ≥10 MM

- Children younger than 4 years
- Children with chronic illness (malignant disease, diabetes mellitus, chronic renal failure, malnutrition)
- Children known to have environmental exposure (those born [or with parents born] in regions of the world where TB is highly prevalent; those in close contact with adults who are HIV-infected, homeless, IV drug users, migrant farm workers, nursing home residents, or incarcerated/institutionalized persons)

INDURATION ≥15 MM

- Children 4 years old or older without any risk factors

Modified from American Academy of Pediatrics Committee on Infectious Diseases. (1997). *Report of the Committee on Infectious Diseases (1997 red book)* (24th ed., p. 545.) Elk Grove Village, IL: Author. Used with permission of the American Academy of Pediatrics.

Therapeutic Management and Nursing Considerations

TUBERCULOSIS DISEASE

A 6-month course of antituberculous medications (isoniazid [INH], rifampin, and pyrazinamide for the first 2 months, INH and rifampin for the next 4), optimal nutrition, and preventing of exposure to infection, which could further compromise the child's already challenged immune system, are the mainstays of treatment. Most children are treated at home. The nurse needs to emphasize to the family the importance of following the prescribed medication regimen meticulously and for the appropriate length of time, because inappropriate medication dosing contributes to the growth of drug-resistant organisms.

Children with TB may be hospitalized, depending on the severity of the disease, the age of the child, the need for more extensive testing, or the child's family and social environment. Unless the child is acutely ill, bed rest is not required. Isolation is not usually required because children with TB are rarely contagious.

TUBERCULOSIS INFECTION

After a chest radiograph is obtained, asymptomatic children with positive tuberculin tests and no previous history of TB receive INH for at least 6 to 9 months. For children with HIV infection, a minimum of 12 months of treatment is recommended. Children with drug-resistant TB need an individualized treatment regimen. Household contacts (especially children less than 4 years old), immunosuppressed contacts, and contacts who were exposed during the previous 3 months should undergo skin testing and chest radiography. Even if the skin test is negative, asymptomatic contacts should receive INH for at least 12 weeks after contact has been broken until the negative skin test can be confirmed (AAP Committee on Infectious Diseases, 1997). Reporting cases of TB is required by law in all states in the United States. Nurses should assist in searching for the source case and others infected by the source case.

Bacillus Calmette-Guérin (BCG) vaccine is the only anti-TB vaccine available. Unfortunately, the BCG vaccine varies in the immunity it provides and has resulted in serious reactions. In the United States, it is used mainly for children with negative chest x-rays and skin test results who have had repeated exposures to TB, and for asymptomatic HIV-infected children, who are at increased risk for developing TB.

PREVENTION AND SCREENING

Case finding is the most important factor in preventing transmission of TB in children (Gaffney & Carneiro, 1994). Because most children are infected by a family member, the best way to stop transmission of the disease is to identify those who are infected and to provide TB therapy (Ott et al., 1995).

Early detection of the disease is accomplished by screening. Children at high risk for TB should be tested annually with the Mantoux test. Annual skin testing of children in low-prevalence areas who have no risk factors is not indicated.

KEY CONCEPTS

- Infants and children less than 3 years old are at increased risk for developing respiratory tract infections because of their immature immune system, smaller airways, and underdeveloped supporting cartilage.
- At birth the neonate must inflate the lungs, establish continuous breathing, and transfer the gases needed to meet metabolic needs.
- The severity of allergic rhinitis can be decreased through the early identification and treatment of manifestations.
- Respiratory obstruction increases during crying, and stridor increases when the child is supine with the neck flexed.
- The only reliable way to determine whether pharyngitis is viral or bacterial in origin is with a throat culture.
- Manifestations of bleeding after a tonsillectomy include frequent swallowing, restlessness, a fast, thready pulse, and the vomiting of bright red blood.
- The mucosal edema associated with croup can sometimes be decreased by steam from hot running water in a closed bathroom or a cool humidifier, or by taking the child out into the cool, humid night air.
- Children with croup who develop stridor at rest, cyanosis, severe agitation or fatigue, or moderate to severe retractions or who are unable to take oral fluids should be seen in the emergency department.
- The four *D*s of epiglottitis are *d*rooling, *d*ysphagia, *d*ysphoria, and *d*istressed inspiratory efforts.
- Visual examination of the epiglottis is contraindicated if epiglottitis is suspected because the examination tools can provoke laryngospasm and airway obstruction.
- Because respiratory syncytial virus infection is highly communicable, during RSV season infected children should be placed in contact isolation. Good hand washing should be emphasized and gowns worn when there is a chance clothing might be soiled.
- Oxygen needs can be decreased in the child in respiratory distress by scheduling nursing care to allow the child periods of rest.
- If a child is aphonic and not breathing, the guidelines for management of an obstructed airway should be followed.
- During an apneic episode the time and duration of the episode, color change, bradycardia, oxygen saturation, what the infant was doing before the apneic period, and any actions that stimulated breathing should be recorded.
- Healthy infants should be placed on their sides or backs for sleeping to reduce the risk of SIDS.
- When interviewing parents of an infant suspected of dying of SIDS, the nurse should avoid any implication of guilt on the part of the parents.
- Asthma is the most common chronic disease of childhood. Asthma is characterized by bronchospasm, edema of the bronchiolar mucous membranes, and increased secretion of mucus in the airways.
- Asthmatic symptoms signaling spasm of the smooth muscle of the bronchi and bronchioles may be triggered by a variety of stimuli, including allergens, cold air, weather changes, infection, exercise, fatigue, and emotional distress.
- Status asthmaticus, or continued severe respiratory distress despite medical treatment, places the child in imminent danger of respiratory arrest and requires immediate hospitalization.
- Nursing care of the child with a severe asthma episode includes administration of inhaled or IV bronchodilators or corticosteroids, as ordered; providing oxygen therapy; providing IV fluids; and assisting with intubation and mechanical ventilation.
- Nursing care of the child with chronic asthma includes administration of prescribed medications and treatments and education of the child and family about medications, how to avoid triggers of asthma symptoms, how to recognize early warning signs of an asthma episode, and measures that can be taken to prevent severe asthma episodes.
- Bronchopulmonary dysplasia (BPD) is a chronic obstructive pulmonary disease characterized by thickening of the alveolar walls and bronchiolar epithelium. BPD occurs primarily in premature and low-birth-weight infants who have been mechanically ventilated with high concentrations of oxygen for prolonged periods of time.
- Nursing care of the infant with BPD includes supportive interventions to maintain adequate oxygenation and the provision of appropriate stimulation to promote normal growth and development.
- Cystic fibrosis (CF) is an inherited (autosomal recessive), multisystem disorder characterized by widespread dysfunction of the exocrine glands. Abnormal secretion of thick, tenacious mucus causes obstruction and dysfunction of the pancreas, lungs, salivary glands, sweat glands, and reproductive organs.
- Nursing care of the child with CF includes maintaining a patent airway by administering bronchodilators and performing or supervising respiratory treatments, administering antibiotics and pancreatic enzymes, and teaching the child and family about CF and its treatment.
- Nursing care of the child with tuberculosis (TB) includes administering and evaluating TB skin tests and administering anti-TB medications as ordered. The nurse also instructs the child and family about the importance of adequate rest, a nutritionally adequate diet, and compliance with the medication regimen, as well as ways to prevent the transmission of TB infection.

ANSWERS TO CRITICAL THINKING EXERCISE 45-1

1. Children often leave the hospital with pain medication (usually liquid acetaminophen with codeine) ordered PRN. Ordering the medication this way relies on the parent or caregiver to assess the child's pain before administering the analgesic. Further research is needed to determine how well parents understand and accurately assess their child's pain during the initial postoperative period. In addition, undermedication can be related to the following:
   - Inadequate doses ordered
   - Parental fear of overmedication

   - Parents' fear that the child will become addicted to the medication
   - Inadequate instructions for medicating
   - Expectations regarding the amount of pain associated with the procedure
   - Difficulty getting the child to swallow the medication (Sutters & Miaskowski, 1997)

2. Inadequate pain relief can adversely affect the child's behavior and ability to rest. In the child who has had a tonsillectomy, more serious effects are related to the re-

fusal of fluids. Because children who have had tonsils removed can experience moderate to severe postoperative pain, medication should be administered regularly around-the-clock and not PRN for most effective postoperative progress. Nurses should emphasize this to parents prior to discharge. If the facility allows, a postoperative phone call to the child's home to inquire about the child and remind the parent about continuous pain relief may be helpful.

REFERENCES AND READINGS

Adams, E., Chavez, G., Steen, D., et al. (1998). Changes in the epidemiologic profile of sudden infant death syndrome as rates decline among California infants: 1990-1995. *Pediatrics, 102*(6), 1445-1451.

Agudo, A., Bardagi, S., Romer, P., & Gonzalez, C. (1994). Exercise-induced airways narrowing and exposure to environmental tobacco smoke in school children. *American Journal of Epidemiology, 140*, 409-417.

Aitkin, M. (1992). Recombinant DNAse inhalation in normal and cystic fibrosis subjects: A phase study. *Journal of the American Medical Association, 267*(14), 1947-1981.

Akers, P., & Kuhn, R. (1997). Pediatric asthma update: Current therapy and new agents. *Pediatric Nursing, 23*(3), 310-313.

American Academy of Pediatrics. (1992). *AAP Task Force on Infant Positioning and SIDS.* Elk Grove Village, IL: Author.

American Academy of Pediatrics. (1994). AAP reaffirms non-prone sleeping position endorsement. *AAP News, 10*, 2.

American Academy of Pediatrics. (1996). SIDS decline linked to parents' actions. *AAP News, 12*, 1.

American Academy of Pediatrics. (1997). Does bed sharing affect the risk of SIDS? *Pediatrics, 100*(2), 272.

American Academy of Pediatrics. (1998). Prevention of respiratory syncytial virus infections: Indications for the use of Palivizumab and update on the use of RSV-IGIV. *Pediatrics, 102*(5), 1211-1216.

American Academy of Pediatrics Committee on Infectious Diseases. (1993). Use of ribavirin in the treatment of RSV. *Pediatrics, 92*(3): 501-504.

American Academy of Pediatrics Committee on Infectious Diseases. (1994). Screening for tuberculosis in infants and children. *Pediatrics, 93*(1), 131-134.

American Academy of Pediatrics Committee on Infectious Diseases. (1997). *Report of the Committee on Infectious Diseases (1997 red book)* (24th ed.). Elk Grove Village, IL: American Academy of Pediatrics.

American Thoracic Society Medical Section of the American Lung Association and Centers for Disease Control and Prevention. (1994). Treatment of tuberculosis and tuberculosis infection in adults and children. *Journal of Respiratory and Critical Care Medicine, 149*(5), 1359-1374.

Autio, L., & Rosenwo, D. (1999). Effectively managing asthma in young and middle adulthood. *The Nurse Practitioner, 24*(1), 100.

Bandla, H., Davis, S., & Hopkins, N. (1999). Lipoid pneumonia: A silent complication of mineral oil aspiration. *Pediatrics, 103*(2), e19.

Barnes, L. P. (1993). Tuberculosis: Implications for patient teaching. *MCN: American Journal of Maternal/Child Nursing, 18*, 224.

Barnhart, S. L., & Czervinske, M. P. (1995). *Perinatal and pediatric respiratory care.* Philadelphia: Saunders.

Baroni, M., Anderson, Y., & Mischler, E. (1997). Cystic fibrosis newborn screening: Impact of early screening results on parenting stress. *Pediatric Nursing, 23*(2), 143-150.

Bechler-Karsch, A. B. (1994). Assessment and management of status asthmaticus. *Pediatric Nursing, 20*(3), 217-223.

Behrman, R. E., Kliegman, R. M., & Arvin, A. M. (Eds.). (1996). *Nelson textbook of pediatrics* (15th ed.). Philadelphia: Saunders.

Brenton, S. (1997). RSV specimen collection methods: Nasal vs. nasopharyngeal. *Pediatric Nursing, 23*(6), 621-622.

Brim, S. (1989, January-February). A quick guide for home use of inhalant medications. *Pediatric Nursing, 15*(1), 87-94.

Brooks, J. (1998). SIDS and ALTE. In V. Chernick, T. Boat, & E. Kendig (Eds.), *Kendig's disorders of the respiratory tract in children* (pp. 1166-1172). Philadelphia: Saunders.

Bye, M. R., Ewig, J. M., & Quittell, B. E. (1994). Cystic fibrosis. *Lung, 172*, 251-270.

Capen, C., & Sherman, J. (1998). Fatal asthma in children: A nurse managed model for prevention. *Journal of Pediatric Nursing, 13*(6), 356-366.

Capen, C. L., Dedlow, E. R., Robillard, R. H., Fuller, B. M., & Fuller, C. P. (1994). The team approach to pediatric asthma education. *Pediatric Nursing, 20*(3), 231-237.

Carlson, J. (1993). The psychologic effects of sudden infant death syndrome on parents. *Journal of Pediatric Health Care, 7*, 77-81.

Carlson, L., & Fall, P. (1998). Otitis media: An update. *Journal of Pediatric Health Care, 12*(6), 313-319.

Carter, E., Maurice, C., Chesrown, S., Shieh, G., Reilly, K., & Hendeles, L. (1993). Efficacy of intravenously administered theophylline in children hospitalized with severe asthma. *Journal of Pediatrics, 122*, 470-476.

Centers for Disease Control and Prevention. (1997a). Case definitions for infectious conditions under public health surveillance. *Morbidity and Mortality Weekly Report, 46*(RR-10), 1-55.

Centers for Disease Control and Prevention. (1997b, Aug. 8). Facts about asthma. Atlanta, GA: Author.

Centers for Disease Control and Prevention. (1997c). Screening for tuberculosis and tuberculosis infection in high-risk populations: Recommendations of the Advisory Council for the Elimination of Tuberculosis. *Morbidity and Mortality Weekly Report, 46*(RR-11), 18-34.

Centers for Disease Control and Prevention. (1997d). Toy-related injuries. *Morbidity and Mortality Weekly Report, 46*(50), 1185-1189.

Chernick, V., Boat, T., & Kendig, E. (Eds.). (1998). *Kendig's disorders of the respiratory tract in children* (6th ed.). Philadelphia: Saunders.

Chessare, J., Hunt, C., & Bourguignon, C. (1995). A community-based survey of infant sleep position. *Pediatrics, 96*(5), 893-896.

Chiocca, E. (1994). RSV and the high risk infant. *Pediatric Nursing, 20*(6), 565-568.

Christian, B., & D'Auria, J. (1997). The child's eye: Memories of growing up with cystic fibrosis. *Journal of Pediatric Nursing, 12*(1), 3-12.

Cohen, B., & Brady, M. (1992). Practices surrounding ribavirin administration. *Pediatric Nursing, 18*(3), 253–257.

Conte, V. H. (1992). Bronchopulmonary dysplasia. In P. L. Jackson & J. A. Vessey (Eds.), *Primary care of the child with a chronic condition.* St. Louis: Mosby.

Cunha, B. (1998a). Acute sinusitis. *Emergency Medicine, 29,* 134.

Cunha, B. (1998b). Peritonsillar abscess. *Emergency Medicine, 29,* 170–171.

Davis, B., Moon, R., Sachs, H., & Ottolini, M. (1998). Effects of sleep position on infant motor development. *Pediatrics, 102*(5), 1135–1140.

Davis, P., Drumm, M., & Konstan, M. (1996). Cystic fibrosis. *American Journal of Respiratory and Critical Care Medicine, 154*(5), 1229–1256.

Dobson, J., Stephens-Groff, S., McMahon, S., et al. (1998). The use of albuterol in hospitalized infants with bronchiolitis. *Pediatrics, 101*(3), 361–368.

Dowell, S., Marcy, S., Phillips, W., et al. (1998). Otitis media: Principles of judicious use of antimicrobial agents. *Pediatrics, 101*(Suppl. 1), 165–171.

Eddy, M., Carter, B., Kronenberger, W., et al. (1998). Parent relationships and compliance in cystic fibrosis. *Journal of Pediatric Health Care, 12*(4), 196–202.

Feder, H., Gerber, M., Randolph, M., et al. (1999). Once-daily therapy for streptococcal pharyngitis with amoxicillin. *Pediatrics, 103*(1), 47–51.

FitzSimmons, S. C. (1993). The changing epidemiology of cystic fibrosis. *Journal of Pediatrics, 122*(1), 1–9.

Froese-Fretz, A. (1998). Children with asthma. *Journal of the Society of Pediatric Nurses, 3*(1), 45–46.

Fulginiti, V., & Lewy, J. (1993). Pediatrics: Update on cystic fibrosis. *Journal of the American Medical Association, 210*(2), 246–248.

Gaffney, K., & Carneiro, D. (1994). Think TB: New focus for family assessment. *Pediatric Nursing, 20,* 36–38.

Gibson, E., Cullen, J., Spinner, S., Rankin, K., & Spitzer, A. (1995). Infant sleep position following new AAP guidelines. *Pediatrics, 96*(1), 69–72.

Gilbert-Barnes, E., & Barnes, L. (1995). Sudden infant death: A reappraisal. *Contemporary Pediatrics, 12*(4), 88–107.

Grad, R. (1998). Acute infections producing upper airway obstruction. In V. Chernick, T. Boat, & E. Kendig (Eds.), *Kendig's disorders of the respiratory tract in children* (pp. 447–460). Philadelphia: Saunders.

Gray, P. H., & Rogers, Y. (1994). Are infants with bronchopulmonary dysplasia at risk for sudden infant death syndrome? *Pediatrics, 93*(5), 774–777.

Hall, C. B. (1993). Respiratory syncytial virus: What we know now. *Contemporary Pediatrics, 11,* 92–110.

Hanly, P. (1992). Mechanisms and management of central sleeping apnea. *Lung, 170,* 1017.

Haviland, M. (1997). Making sense of the β-agonist debate: A guide for nurse practitioners. *Journal of Pediatric Health Care, 11*(5), 215–221.

Hazinski, T. (1998). Bronchopulmonary dysplasia. In V. Chernick, T. Boat, & E.

Kendig (Eds.), *Kendig's disorders of the respiratory tract in children* (pp. 364–388). Philadelphia: Saunders.

Hegland, A. (1997). Two high-risk infant groups targeted for RSV-IGIV therapy. *AAP News, 13*(2), 1.

Hiatt, P., Grace, S., Kozinetz, C., et al. (1999). Effectiveness of RSV-IVIG in premature infants: Success in the home. *Pediatrics, 103*(3), 619–626.

Hodgman, J. (1998). Apnea of prematurity and risk for SIDS. *Pediatrics, 102*(4), 969–971.

Jackson, M. (1993). Tuberculosis in infants, children, and adolescents: New dilemmas with an old disease. *Pediatric Nursing, 19*(5), 437–442.

Kelly, K. (1998). Integration of holistic nursing care in the treatment of asthma: A case study. *Journal of Emergency Nursing, 24,* 489–491.

Kemp, J., Nelson, V., & Thach, B. (1994). Physical properties of bedding that may increase risk of sudden infant death syndrome in prone sleeping infants. *Pediatric Resident, 36,* 7–11.

Kemper, K. (1997). A practical approach to chronic asthma management. *Contemporary Pediatrics, 14*(8), 86–106.

Kercsmar, C. (1998). Asthma. In V. Chernick, T. Boat, & E. Kendig (Eds.), *Kendig's disorders of the respiratory tract in children* (pp. 688–730). Philadelphia: Saunders.

Kuhn, R. J., & Horn, L. (1994). Pancreatic enzyme therapy in patients with cystic fibrosis: The high dose lipase issue. *Pediatric Nursing, 20*(8), 623–624.

Ladebauche, P. (1997). Managing asthma: A growth and development approach. *Pediatric Nursing, 23*(1), 37–43.

Lara, M., Duan, N., Sherbourne, C., et al. (1998). Differences between child and parent reports of symptoms among Latino children with asthma. *Pediatrics, 102*(6), e63.

Leickly, F., Wade, S., Crain, E., et al. (1998). Self-reported adherence, management behavior, and barriers to care after an emergency department visit by inner city children with asthma. *Pediatrics, 101*(5), e8.

Light, M. J. (1994). rhDNase and cystic fibrosis: The penultimate step. *RT: Journal of Respiratory Care Practitioners, 7,* 45–48.

Loutzenhiser, J. K., & Clark, R. (1993). Physical activity and exercise in children with cystic fibrosis. *Journal of Pediatric Nursing, 8*(2), 112–119.

Lurie, N., Straub, M., Goodman, N., & Bauer, E. (1998). Incorporating asthma education into a traditional school curriculum. *American Journal of Public Health, 88*(5), 822–823.

Maguire, P., & Umetsu, D. (1999). Allergic rhinitis. In F. Burg, E. Wald, J. Ingelfinger, & R. Polin (Eds.), *Gellis & Kagan's current pediatric therapy* (16th ed., pp. 1047–1051). Philadelphia: Saunders.

McCoy, K. (1993). Pediatric parenchymal diseases. In P. Koff, D. Eitzman, & J. Neu (Eds.), *Neonatal and pediatric respiratory care* (pp. 97–98). Philadelphia: Saunders.

McMillan Jackson, M., & McLeod, R. (1998). Tuberculosis in infants, children, and adolescents: An update with case studies. *Pediatric Nursing, 23*(5), 411–419.

Meng, A., Tiernan, K., Bernier, M., & Brooks, E. (1998). Lessons from an evalua-

tion of an asthma day camp. *MCN: American Journal of Maternal/Child Nursing, 23*(6), 300–305.

Miller, V., Rice, J., DeVoe, M., & Fos, M. (1998). An analysis of program and family costs of case managed care for technology-dependent infants with bronchopulmonary dysplasia. *Journal of Pediatric Nursing, 13*(4), 244–250.

Mischler, E., Wilford, B., Fost, N., et al. (1998). Cystic fibrosis newborn screening: Impact on reproductive behavior and implications for genetic counseling. *Pediatrics, 102*(1), 44–52.

Mitchell, S. (1996). Infants with bronchopulmonary dysplasia: A developmental perspective. *Journal of Pediatric Nursing, 11*(3), 145–151.

Montville, N., & White, M. (1998). Diagnosis and pharmacological management of acute otitis media. *Pediatric Nursing, 23*(5), 423–429.

National Heart, Lung and Blood Institute. (1991, June). *Executive summary: Guidelines for the diagnosis and management of asthma.* Washington, DC: US Department of Health and Human Services.

National Jewish Center for Immunology and Respiratory Medicine. (1995). Patient education material. Denver, CO: Author.

Newacheck, P., & Halforn, N. (1998). Prevalence and impact of disabling chronic conditions in childhood. *American Journal of Public Health, 88*(4), 610–615.

Niemelè, M., Uhari, M., & Möttönen, M. (1995). A pacifier increases the risk of recurrent acute otitis media in children in day care centers. *Pediatrics, 96*(5), 884–888.

O'Brien, K., Dowell, S., Schwartz, B., et al. (1998a). Acute sinusitis: Principles of judicious use of antimicrobial agents. *Pediatrics, 101*(Suppl. 1), 174–177.

O'Brien, K., Dowell, S., Schwartz, B., et al. (1998b). Cough illness/bronchitis: Principles of judicious use of antimicrobial agents. *Pediatrics, 101*(Suppl. 1), 178–181.

Oertel, M. (1996). Respigam: An RSV immune globulin. *Pediatric Nursing, 22*(6), 525–528.

O'Sullivan, B. (1994). Respiratory injury after hydrocarbon poisoning. In D. Schidlow & D. Smith (Eds.), *A practical guide to pediatric respiratory diseases.* Philadelphia: Hanley & Belfus.

Ott, M. J., Horn, M., & McLaughlin, D. (1995). Pediatric TB in the 1990s. *MCN: American Journal of Maternal/Child Nursing 20*(1), 16–20.

Owen, A. (1998). Respiratory assessment revisited. *Nursing, 28*(4), 48–49.

Owen, C. (1999). New directions in asthma management. *American Journal of Nursing, 99*(3), 26–33.

Paradise, J. (1995). Managing otitis media: A time for change. *Pediatrics, 96*(4), 712–715.

Pass, R. (1998). Respiratory virus infection and otitis media. *Pediatrics, 102*(2), 400–401.

Rachelefsky, G. S. (1995). Asthma update: New approaches and partnerships. *Journal of Pediatric Health Care, 9,* 12–21.

Rhodes, A. M. (1993). TB: Public health statutes. *MCN: American Journal of Maternal/Child Nursing, 18,* 225.

Russell, M., Reinbold, J., & Maltby, H. (1996). Transferring to adult health care: Experiences of adolescents with cystic fibrosis. *Journal of Pediatric Nursing, 11*(4), 262–268.

Ryan-Wenger, N. M., & Walsh, M. (1994). Children's perspective on coping with asthma. *Pediatric Nursing, 20*(3), 224–228.

Schidlow, D. (1999). Cystic fibrosis. In F. Burg, J. Ingelfinger, E. Wald, & R. Polin (Eds.), *Gellis and Kagan's current pediatric therapy* (16th ed., pp. 541–546). Philadelphia: Saunders.

Schmidt, B. (1999). *Instructions for pediatric patients.* Philadelphia: Saunders.

Schwartz, B., Marcy, M., Phillips, W., et al. (1998). Pharyngitis: Principles of judicious use of antimicrobial agents. *Pediatrics, 101*(Suppl. 1), 171–174.

Spiers, P., & Guntheroth, W. (1994). Recommendations to avoid the prone sleeping position and recent statistics for sudden infant death syndrome in the United States. *Archives of Pediatric Adolescent Medicine, 149*, 141–146.

Spitzer, A. (1996). SIDS and recurring apnea. In F. Burg, J. Ingelfinger, E. Wald, & R. Polin (Eds.), *Gellis and Kagan's current pediatric therapy* (15th ed., pp. 161–162). Philadelphia: Saunders.

Sutters, K., & Miaskowski, C. (1997). Inadequate pain management and associated morbidity in children at home after tonsillectomy. *Journal of Pediatric Nursing, 12*(3), 178–185.

Wagner, M., & Jacobs, J. (1997). Improving asthma management with peak flow meters. *Contemporary Pediatrics, 14*(8), 111–119.

Wagner, M., & Sherman, J. (1997). Cystic fibrosis and the general pediatrician. *Contemporary Pediatrics, 14*(2), 89–109.

Warman, K., Silver, E., McCourt, M., & Stein, R. (1999). How does home management of asthma exacerbations by parents of inner-city children differ from NHLBI guideline recommendations? *Pediatrics, 103*(2), 422–427.

Williams, M. (1996). An educational approach to successful management of childhood asthma as a chronic illness. *Journal of Pediatric Nursing, 11*(5), 335–336.

Williams, S., Mitchell, E., & Scragg, R. (1997). Why is sudden infant death more common at weekends? The New Zealand National Cot Death Study Group. *Archives of Disease in Childhood, 77*, 415–419.

Willinger, M., Hoffman, H., & Hartford, R. (1994). Infant sleep position: Risk for sudden infant death syndrome. *Pediatrics, 93*(5), 814–819.

Wohl, M. (1998). Bronchiolitis. In V. Chernick, T. Boat, & E. Kendig (Eds.), *Kendig's disorders of the respiratory tract in children* (pp. 473–483). Philadelphia: Saunders.

Yoos, H. L., McMullen, A., Bezek, S., et al. (1997). An asthma management program for urban minority children. *Journal of Pediatric Health Care, 11*(2), 66–74.

Yoos, H. L., & McMullen, A. (1999). Symptom perception and evaluation in childhood asthma. *Nursing Research, 48*(1), 2–7.

Zeisel, S., Roberts, J., Neebe, E., et al. (1999). A longitudinal study of otitis media with effusion among 2- to 5-year old African-American children in child care. *Pediatrics, 103*(1), 15–19.

46

• • • • • • • • • • • •

The Child with a Cardiovascular Alteration

- Describe the circulatory changes that occur during and after the birth process.
- Describe the anatomy and physiology of the normally functioning heart.
- Differentiate symptoms of right- and left-sided heart failure.
- Identify nursing interventions that decrease the workload of the myocardium in children with heart failure.
- Identify the nurse's role in discharge planning for the child with congestive heart failure.
- Discuss the physiology of congenital cardiac lesions.
- Discuss the unique presentation behaviors of infants and children with a congenital heart defect.
- Implement the nursing diagnoses specific to caring for infants or children with a congenital heart defect.
- Discuss nursing interventions as they relate to specific nursing diagnoses commonly implemented when caring for a child with a congenital heart defect.
- Describe nursing care for the child with rheumatic fever.
- Identify priority nursing interventions when caring for a child with Kawasaki disease.
- Identify nursing interventions that support the management of primary and secondary hypertension.
- Utilize appropriate screening tools and identify diagnostic aids in determining the etiology of hypertension.

DEFINITIONS

afterload The amount of resistance against which the heart pumps.

angioplasty Procedure that dilates vessels.

arrhythmia Abnormal rhythm of the heart; may be used interchangeably with dysrhythmia.

artery Vessel that carries blood away from the heart.

atresia Absence of a normal opening or vessel.

bradycardia Heart rate that is slow for age.

cardiac output The factor of the amount of blood pumped from the heart (stroke volume) and the heart rate.

cardiomegaly An enlarged heart.

central venous pressure Pressure measured in the right atrium; helpful in determining the amount of circulating blood volume.

chronotropic Affecting the time or rate.

compensation Maintenance of an adequate blood flow without distressing symptoms, accomplished by cardiac and circulatory adjustments such as tachycardia, cardiac hypertrophy, and increased blood volume from sodium and water retention.

decompensation Inability of the heart to maintain adequate circulation, marked by dyspnea, venous engorgement, cyanosis, and edema.

dilation To make larger using artificial means (such as a balloon catheter).

dysrhythmia Disturbance of rhythm.

gradient Difference.

hypertrophy Enlargement or thickening of the wall of an organ (such as the heart).

inotropic Affecting the force of muscular contractions.

ischemia Deficiency of blood supply to an organ.

murmur A sound in the cardiac cycle caused by turbulent blood flow.

myocardial contractility Ability of myocardial cells and tissues to shorten in response to an appropriate stimulus; force of contraction of the myocardium.

oxygen saturation A measure of the degree to which oxygen is bound to hemoglobin.

palpitations Sensation of rapid or irregular heartbeat.

preload Amount of stretch of the myocardial fibers before contraction; most easily measured by determining central venous pressure.

pulmonary edema Collection of excessive fluid in the alveoli of the lungs.

pulmonary hypertension Increased pressure in the pulmonary arteries and arterioles.

pulmonary vascular resistance Amount of resistance in the pulmonary vascular bed against which the right heart must pump.

pulmonary venous congestion Increased pulmonary pressure leading to the accumulation of excessive fluid and blood in the pulmonary veins.

regurgitation Abnormal backward flow of blood through a heart valve.

shunt Abnormal blood flow from one side of the heart to the other.

stenosis Narrowing or constriction of an opening (such as a heart valve).

systemic vascular resistance Amount of resistance in the systemic vascular bed against which the left heart must pump.

systemic venous congestion Increased systemic venous pressure leading to the accumulation of excessive fluid in the systemic veins.

tissue perfusion Amount of blood flow distributed to an area.

valve An opening, covered by membranous flaps, between two chambers of the heart or between a chamber of the heart and a blood vessel; when closed, no blood normally passes through the opening.

valvuloplasty Mechanical procedure to open a valve.

Review of the Heart and Circulation

Normal Cardiac Anatomy and Physiology

The heart is a muscular pump divided into four chambers. The two upper chambers are the atria and the two lower chambers are the ventricles. Valves, veins, and arteries connect the chambers; they provide for the oxygenation of blood in the lungs and subsequent distribution of the blood to the body tissues.

Electricity is required for the heart's pumping mechanism to work. This electricity is initiated by a group of cells called the sinus node. The electrical impulse initiated sends a message to the relay station, the atrioventricular node, which then carries the impulse to the ventricles through the His bundle, the bundle-branch system, and finally the Purkinje fibers.

Each cardiac cycle consists of this electrical activity, which produces depolarization and subsequent repolarization of the cardiac muscle—more simply, a heartbeat. During each cycle, unoxygenated blood returns to the heart via the superior and inferior venae cavae. It enters the right atrium, travels through the tricuspid valve, and into the

right ventricle. The blood is then pumped through the pulmonary valve into the pulmonary artery, then travels through the pulmonary system (the lungs) for the removal of carbon dioxide and the addition of oxygen. The blood leaves the lungs via the pulmonary veins and travels through the left atrium by way of the mitral valve, and into the left ventricle. The left ventricle pushes the blood into the aorta, which then delivers blood to the rest of the body. The pressures in the left side of the heart are four to five times higher than those in the right side. A malformation or anomaly in any of the heart's structures may affect blood flow and subsequent hemodynamic stability.

Fetal Circulation

Fetal circulation differs from neonatal circulation in three areas: the process of gas exchange, the pressures within the systemic and pulmonary circulations, and the existence of anatomic structures that assist in the delivery of oxygen-rich blood to vital organ systems.

In the fetus, oxygenation (gas exchange) takes place at the placenta. Oxygen and nutrients are carried by the umbilical vein through the liver to the inferior vena cava.

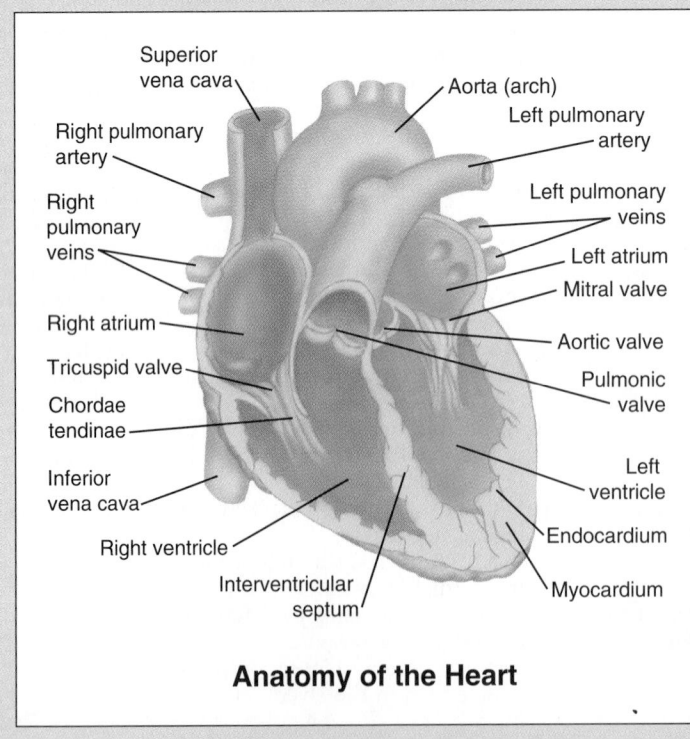

Anatomy of the Heart

A small amount of blood travels into the hepatic circulation via a fetal structure, the ductus venosus, to provide oxygen and nutrients to the hepatic tissue. Liver function is minimal in the fetus, so very little blood supply is required.

The inferior vena cava empties blood into the right atrium. The trajectory (direction) of the blood flow, as well as the pressure in the right atrium, propels this blood through a second fetal structure, the foramen ovale, into the left atrium. This richly oxygenated blood travels through the left ventricle into the aorta, feeding the coronary arteries and the brain, the two most oxygen-needy organ systems.

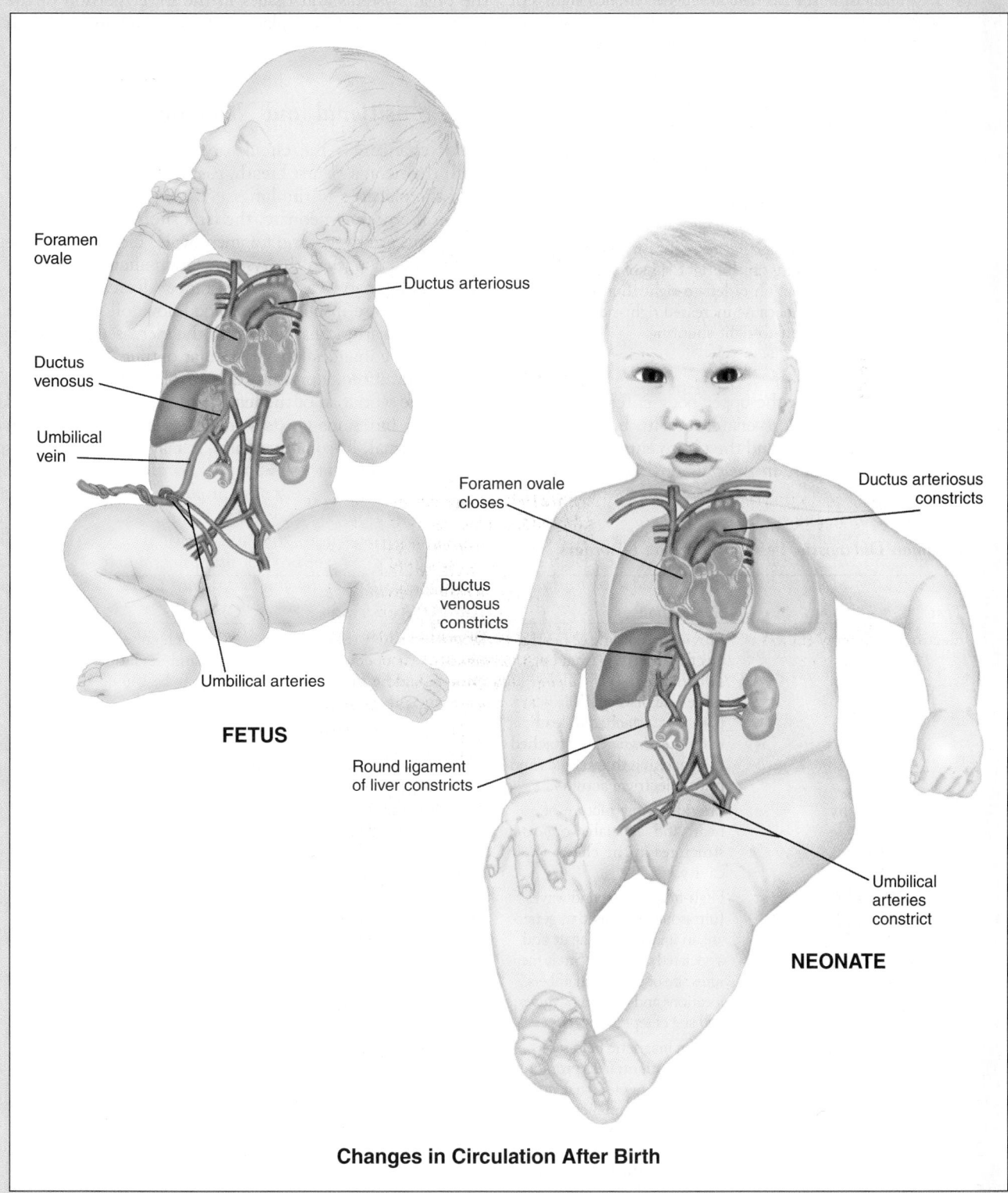

FETUS

NEONATE

Changes in Circulation After Birth

Heart disease in children is either congenital heart disease or acquired heart disease. Congenital heart disease denotes one or more structural abnormalities that develop before birth, although the clinical symptoms may not be present in the newborn period. Acquired heart disease develops over time and may be seen both in children with normal hearts and in those with congenital heart disease.

The nurse's role is very important in the astute and vigilant monitoring of a child with potential cardiovascular alterations. The degree of change in acuity and the speed of decompensation are much greater in infants and children than in any other age group. Thus, the skill required of the pediatric nurse in assessing, monitoring, and delivering prompt treatment is an unparalleled nursing challenge.

Cardiovascular Assessment

Serious cardiac lesions become symptomatic early in infancy. Remarkable technological advances in the understanding of the cardiovascular system's function and needs have led to refinements in the tools and techniques for detecting and diagnosing congenital heart defects. Invasive procedures are required only in the most extreme cases (see p. 1252 for common diagnostic tests). Nevertheless, no tool or technique replaces taking a good history of both the child and the parents and performing a thorough physical examination (Table 46–1).

The cardiac assessment should take place in a non-threatening environment with a parent present, if possible. Parents know their children best, and they can offer subtle clinical information that may not be evident on examination. The nurse needs to establish an atmosphere of trust: cardiac assessment is best and most easily performed on a cooperative infant or child.

The room should be warm, because peripheral perfusion is affected by ambient temperature (Engel, 1997). A well-lighted room is also necessary. Natural light from windows will allow the nurse to accurately assess skin color.

The assessment should begin with the least threatening interventions—the history and inspection. During the parent interview, the child has the opportunity to observe the interaction between nurse and parent and has time to become comfortable with the nurse's presence. The child should be allowed to participate in the assessment and encouraged to touch and inspect each piece of equipment to be used during the examination.

Assessment progresses from inspection to auscultation to palpation; each step requires more touching. The nurse must remember to warm the stethoscope used for auscultation, as well as the hands prior to touching the child's skin. This is particularly important when assessing a resting infant, who may become startled by the cold touch of the hands and stethoscope.

TABLE 46–1
. . . .

Cardiac Assessment

Parameter	Assessment Guidelines	Findings/Comments
Health history	Inquire about a family history of congenital heart disease.	There is an increased incidence of congenital heart disease within families.
	Ask about maternal illnesses, infections, medications taken during pregnancy.	Chronic maternal illness, perinatal infections, and certain medications have been linked to congenital heart disease.
	Discuss feeding difficulties (in infants), frequency of respiratory infections, poor weight gain, fatigue, exercise intolerance.	Poor weight gain and failure to thrive are often associated with cardiac disease.
Inspection	**Color:** Assess skin color in natural light, if possible. Pay special attention to hands and feet, face, mucous membranes, and nail beds.	Cyanosis, pallor, mottling, or ruddiness may indicate cardiac disease. Clubbing of nail beds indicates chronic hypoxia.
	Activity level: Assess child while either sitting or lying down.	Lethargy or restlessness may indicate poor cardiac function.
	Observe level of activity and position of comfort.	Squatting indicates hypoxia.

1254

TABLE 46-1
• • • • • • • • • • •

Cardiac Assessment Continued

Parameter	Assessment Guidelines	Findings/Comments
Inspection (*cont.*)	**Chest:** Assess precordial activity and chest movement.	Point of maximal impulse (apical pulse) may be seen in thin children. It is found at the 4th intercostal space in young children and the 5th intercostal space in children older than 7 years (Engel, 1997). An active precordium may indicate cardiac disease.
	Respiratory pattern: Observe work of breathing at rest. Look for signs of respiratory difficulty (grunting, retractions, nasal flaring, crackles).	Increased work of breathing and respiratory difficulty may indicate congestive heart failure.
Auscultation	**Heart sounds:** Auscultate using both bell of stethoscope (for low-pitched sounds) and diaphragm (for high-pitched sounds).	Heart tones should be synchronous with radial pulse. Rhythm normally is regular. Ask the older child to briefly hold breath to allow the nurse to hear more clearly.
	Identify 1st and 2nd heart sounds.	S_1 is heard best at apex of heart. S_2 is heard best at base (right and left of sternum at 2nd intercostal space).
	Identify additional heart sounds (S_3 and S_4). These are best assessed with child lying on the left side.	S_3, a ventricular flow sound, is a normal finding (Engel, 1997). S_4, a gallop, indicates cardiac failure.
	Identify presence of murmurs, clicks, precordial friction rubs.	Murmurs are caused by turbulent blood flow. Murmurs are described according to location, timing within cardiac cycle, intensity, and pitch.
Palpation	**Temperature:** Compare temperature of trunk with extremities.	Cooler extremities often indicate poor perfusion due to decreased cardiac output. If room is cold, cool extremities may indicate vasoconstriction to conserve heat.
	Pulses: Compare central and distal pulses. Assess pulses in all four extremities.	Peripheral pulses may be diminished if cardiac output is impaired. Weak or absent pulses in the lower extremities may indicate coarctation of the aorta.
	Blood pressure: Assess in all four extremities during initial assessment.	Discrepancies between upper and lower extremity blood pressure may indicate cardiac disease.
	Capillary refill: Assess capillary filling in extremities; use fingertips to compress skin.	Normal is less than 2 seconds.
	Chest: With fingertips, locate the point of maximal impulse (PMI). Assess for presence of vibratory thrills or friction rubs.	Lower PMI may indicate cardiac enlargement (Engel, 1997). Thrills, described as a palpable murmur, feel like the belly of a purring cat. Friction rubs, caused by the presence of fluid in the cardiac or pleural space, produce a grating sensation.
	Abdomen: Locate the liver border. It should be at or slightly below the right costal margin in infants and young children.	Normally the border should be firm and smooth. Liver may be boggy with a poorly defined edge when congestive heart failure is present.
Percussion	Percussion of the chest may help define heart borders but is usually deferred.	PMI is a better indication of heart size (Engel, 1997). A thorough cardiac workup will include chest radiography and ECG.

Cyanosis

Significant congenital heart disease manifests with cyanosis (hypoxemia) or congestive heart failure. Cyanosis, a bluish discoloration of the skin, nail beds, and mucous membranes, appears when tissues are deprived of adequate amounts of oxygen. Cyanosis becomes visible when approximately 5 g Hgb/100 ml blood circulates unbound to oxygen (O'Brien & Smith, 1994) and the measured oxygen saturation drops below 85% (Nadas, 1992). The degree of cyanosis varies; some children will appear pale and mildly cyanosed, while others will be quite dusky.

Cardiac lesions produce cyanosis when blood from the venous system enters the arterial system without passing through the lungs. This event occurs when (1) blood flow to the lungs is restricted, (2) blood return from the lungs is restricted, or (3) mixing of arterial and venous blood occurs within the chambers of the heart.

The clinical consequence of cyanosis include polycythemia, anemia, clotting abnormalities, hypercyanotic episodes, central nervous system injury, dehydration, and developmental delay. Polycythemia is a compensatory response of the body to chronic hypoxia. The body attempts to improve tissue oxygenation by increasing the oxygen-carrying capacity of the blood—in other words, by producing additional red blood cells.

Accelerated red blood cell production increases the viscosity of the blood and crowds the vascular space so there is less room for plasma and clotting factors. Children who are polycythemic are at greater risk for bruising and prolonged bleeding. They are also more likely to become dehydrated when they experience vomiting or diarrhea.

Increased blood viscosity makes the peripheral circulation sluggish and places the child at risk for central nervous system injury from a brain abscess or cerebrovascular accident. Depletion of iron stores may also result, and anemia may develop if iron is not available to participate in hemoglobin formation.

Hypercyanotic Episode

By far the most clinically significant and dramatic event seen in children with cyanotic heart disease is the hypercyanotic episode. These events are often called "tet spells" because they frequently occur in children with unrepaired tetralogy of Fallot. The exact cause is unknown, but it is thought that the child experiences acute spasms of the right ventricular outflow tract (infundibulum) that dramatically decrease pulmonary blood flow and increase right-to-left shunting (O'Brien & Baker, 1999).

Hypercyanotic episodes are seen most frequently in the first year of life and seem to occur mainly in the morning. Often the episode is preceded by crying, feeding, or defecation (Spilman & Furdon, 1998). Episodes are characterized by a worsening of cyanosis and an increase in respiratory rate. The infant becomes agitated and may eventually lose consciousness. Frequent or prolonged episodes may lead to diminished cerebral oxygenation and brain damage.

Treatment of the episode includes calming the infant, placing the infant in the knee-chest position, and administering oxygen. Giving morphine sulfate may relieve infundibular spasm. Ultimately, though, hypercyanotic episodes

indicate the need to surgically repair or palliate the defect (Zuberbuhler, 1995).

■ NURSING CARE
The Child with Cyanosis

Assessment

Assessment of cyanosis starts with an evaluation of the child's general appearance. Cyanotic children often are smaller than their peers and may demonstrate clubbing, thickening and flattening of the fingertips and toes (see Fig. 45–6) due to polycythemia. Visible cyanosis is most easily seen in natural light and is evaluated by observing the skin of the hands, feet, and face as well as the mucous membranes of the mouth and conjunctiva.

The child often becomes dyspneic during feeding, crying, and other exertional activities and may have difficulty keeping up with peers. Cyanotic children experience frequent respiratory infections, miss more school days, and may, as a result, academically lag behind their classmates. They are also at greater risk for developing bacterial endocarditis and need ongoing antibiotic prophylaxis.

Nursing Diagnosis and Planning

Nursing diagnoses typical for the child with cyanosis and the child's family include the following:

■ Family Knowledge Deficit related to the impact of a life-threatening illness.
  Expected Outcome: The parents will verbalize adequate knowledge of the disease process, treatment, and interventions and will demonstrate the ability to perform home care treatments, including medication administration.
■ Altered Family Process related to impact of a life-threatening disease.
  Expected Outcome: The parents will express positive feelings for their child and for each other and will demonstrate the ability to meet the needs of the child, each other, and other family members.
■ Altered Growth and Development related to repeated episodes of decreased oxygenation or of inadequate oxygen to meet body needs.
  Expected Outcome: The child will perform motor, social, and expressive skills typical of age group within the scope of the child's present capabilities; the parents will verbalize an understanding of developmental delay or deviation and plans for intervention.
■ Altered Tissue Perfusion related to hypercyanotic episodes.
  Expected Outcome: The child will remain free of decreased tissue perfusion, as evidenced by the absence of profound cyanosis, a normal activity level and affect for child, and a normal respiratory status and oxygenation for child.
■ Risk for Infection related to the presence of infection-promoting conditions.
  Expected Outcome: The child will remain free of endocardial infection; the parents will verbalize an understanding of antibiotic prophylaxis.

Interventions

Cyanotic heart disease is usually diagnosed very early in life. The initial nursing interventions are directed toward stabilizing the child's hemodynamic status and preparing the child for surgical intervention. Pulmonary blood flow in cyanotic heart disease may depend on the persistence of the ductus arteriosus. Prostaglandin E_1 (PGE_1), a vasodilator, is often administered intravenously (IV) to maintain ductal patency. The nurse is responsible for monitoring PGE_1 infusion flow and evaluating peripheral perfusion and respiratory status. The nurse assesses IV line patency and inspects IV tubing for the presence of air. The use of an air filter is recommended (O'Brien & Smith, 1994).

Parental teaching and support at the time of diagnosis are paramount. Parents receive complicated information and are often asked to make important decisions that may affect their child's current therapy and, perhaps, future interventions. Parents need simple yet thorough explanations to help them make informed choices. The nurse may need to repeat the information several times. Help parents identify sources of emotional support and encourage communication within the family.

Parents of children with cardiovascular disease may be anxious and overprotective of their children. Knowing this, the nurse has a responsibility to educate parents about their child's disease and to stress the importance of the child interacting with the environment as normally as possible. For effective planning and provision of care, the disease must be placed in the context of the family's life.

In the cyanotic child, careful monitoring of fluid status is necessary to prevent hemoconcentration. Intake and output are closely monitored and daily weights are recorded during hospitalization. Teach parents to recognize illnesses that place their child at risk for dehydration and to seek medical attention when their child experiences fluid losses.

Parents are concerned about worsening cyanosis and fear hypercyanotic episodes. Teach parents to recognize events that may trigger an episode and to respond calmly and place the infant in a knee-chest position. Remind parents that there is no need to strictly limit their child's physical activity since most cyanotic children will do so themselves (Holt, 1998).

Prevention of bacterial endocarditis is accomplished through antibiotic prophylaxis. Parents may be given copies of the American Heart Association's guidelines for bacterial endocarditis prophylaxis.

Cyanotic children are prone to frequent respiratory infections. Respiratory infections may increase cardiac workload and compromise cardiac effectiveness. Careful hand washing is necessary to reduce the risk of infection. Teach parents to avoid crowded areas and contact between their child and other people with respiratory infections.

Evaluation

- Has the cyanosis lessened or remained unchanged with medical or surgical treatment?
- Is the child showing a steady increase in physical growth and attaining age-appropriate developmental goals?
- Have the parents demonstrated an understanding of the child's cardiac defect?

- Are the parents able to monitor their child's condition, provide home treatments, administer medications, and support the child's fluid and nutritional needs?
- Is the child free of signs and symptoms of infection?
- Is the family expressing feelings and supporting each other and the child?

Congestive Heart Failure

Congestive heart failure (CHF) is a clinical syndrome that reflects the heart's inability to pump sufficiently to meet the metabolic demands of the body. The heart becomes overloaded and is unable to deliver adequate cardiac output. In infants and children, inadequate cardiac output is most commonly caused by congenital heart defects that produce an excessive volume or pressure load on the myocardium (Kohr & O'Brien, 1995).

In infants and children, CHF occurs most often in association with a diagnosis of congenital heart disease. A variety of acquired conditions, however, may also cause CHF. The most common of these conditions are rheumatic heart disease, endocarditis and myocarditis, cardiomyopathies, and severe dysrhythmias.

Manifestations

The clinical manifestations of right-sided heart failure develop over time and include periorbital and facial edema, hepatomegaly, splenomegaly, ascites, wheezing, and neck vein distension (in children). Manifestations of left-sided heart failure include tachypnea, dyspnea, crackles, intercostal muscular and sternal retractions, and wheezing. Manifestations of right- and left-sided heart failure include tachycardia, cardiomegaly, a gallop heart rhythm, decreased peripheral perfusion, excessive diaphoresis, a sudden, large weight gain, decreased urine output, and cyanosis or pallor.

The earliest clinical manifestations of CHF are often subtle. The infant may have difficulty feeding, owing to decreased cardiac output and an increased work of breathing. Feedings take longer, use more energy, and result in fewer calories consumed. Feedings provide little satisfaction. The

PATHOPHYSIOLOGY

of Congestive Heart Failure

In children with CHF, a combination of both left-sided and right-sided heart failure is usually present. In left-sided failure, the left ventricle is unable to effectively pump blood to the systemic circulation. The blood then backs up into the left atrium and pulmonary veins, causing increased left atrial and pulmonary venous pressure. The lungs become congested with blood, which leads to *pulmonary edema*.

In right-sided failure, the right ventricle is unable to pump blood adequately to the pulmonary arteries and the pulmonary vasculature. This causes less blood to be oxygenated and increases the right atrial and systemic venous pressures. The end result is that when the heart is overloaded, it is unable to deliver adequate cardiac output.

baby tires easily, is frequently fussy, and has difficulty sleeping. Over time, the infant fails to gain weight.

Decreased cardiac output places a greater demand on the heart to provide adequate amounts of oxygen to the tissue. Tachycardia results as a compensatory mechanism. Tachycardia, however, increases myocardial oxygen consumption, shortens the heart's resting phase, and decreases coronary blood flow (Bernstein, 1996; O'Brien & Baker, 1999).

The infant also responds to decreased cardiac output by increasing peripheral vascular resistance and limiting blood flow to certain organ systems. Mesenteric and renal blood flows are diminished. The kidneys respond by activating the renin-angiotensin-aldosterone mechanism, which ultimately results in sodium and water reabsorption. This leads to fluid retention, and edema develops.

Pulmonary congestion increases the work of breathing and results in respiratory distress. Nasal flaring, grunting, and retractions are frequently seen. The infant or child has difficulty eating, sleeping, and carrying on activities of daily living. The child may develop a dry, hacking cough, and crackles may be heard on auscultation.

Diagnostic Evaluation

The diagnosis of CHF is established on the basis of clinical manifestations, chest radiographic appearance, electrocardiography (ECG), and echocardiography. Laboratory studies that may be indicated to determine the presence of heart failure in children include determinations of arterial blood gas values, serum electrolyte levels, complete blood cell count, sedimentation rate, serum glucose and calcium levels, and urinalysis.

Therapeutic Management

The management of CHF is directed toward decreasing cardiac workload and improving cardiac output. Pharmaco-

---

PARENTS WANT TO KNOW

About Administering Digoxin

Medication:	Digoxin (Lanoxin)
Your child's dosage:	_____
What it does:	• Digoxin (Lanoxin) helps the heart pump blood more forcefully. Also, it will help the heart beat slower if it is beating too fast.
What you need to know:	• Digoxin (Lanoxin) should be taken about the same time each day. If you need to administer digoxin two times a day, doses should be given about 12 hours apart.
	• If the dose is spit back or vomited immediately, you may repeat the dose. If vomiting occurs more than 15 minutes after the digoxin was given, do not repeat it; just give the next dose at the regular time.
	• Draw up the dose in the syringe as you have been taught. Do not use the dropper provided with the medicine.
Things to watch for:	• Frequent vomiting can be a sign that children have too much digoxin in their system. If your child begins to vomit frequently or refuses to eat all day, do not give the digoxin and call your heart doctor.
What to do if you miss a dose:	• If it has been more than 4 hours since the scheduled time, wait until the next dose. If it has been less than 4 hours, give the medicine.
	• If more than two doses are missed, call the heart doctor to see if any changes need to be made.

• Refill your prescription 1 week before it runs out. Ask for a new prescription at your physician visits.
• Keep this and all medicines out of reach of children.

Adapted and used with permission from Cook Children's Medical Center, Department of Cardiology, Fort Worth, Texas. Developed by V. Zeigler, RN, MSN, V. Carter, RN, and S. Williams, RN, MSN.

Feeding the Infant or Child with Congestive Heart Failure

Feed the infant or child in a relaxed environment. The infant with CHF tends to tire easily during feedings. Frequent, small feedings may be less tiring. If the child is unable to consume an appropriate amount during a 30-minute feeding period every 3 hours, nasogastric feeding should be considered.

Molly, a 2-month-old infant, is seen in the pediatrician's office. She has gained 1 lb since birth and has a murmur. She is admitted to the pediatric unit with a diagnosis of congestive heart failure. You will obtain a health history and perform an admission assessment.

1. What specific questions should Molly's parents be asked about her feeding patterns and behavior?
2. What physical assessment findings would you expect in an infant with congestive heart failure?
3. List nursing interventions that would address Molly's nutritional and comfort needs.

logic agents used include positive inotropes, diuretics, and afterload-reducing drugs.

Initial drug therapy usually begins with digoxin. Digoxin is a cardiac glycoside that increases cardiac output and improves cardiac effectiveness by several mechanisms. It has a positive inotropic effect that strengthens the force of ventricular contractions. It has a negative chronotropic effect that slows the heart rate and conduction of cardiac impulses through the atrioventricular (AV) node, allowing the ventricles more time to fill with blood. It also improves blood flow to the kidneys and supports and enhances diuresis.

Digoxin may be administered IV or orally. The effectiveness of digoxin depends on achieving and maintaining a therapeutic serum drug level. A loading or digitalizing dose is administered in divided doses over 24 hours and maintenance doses are given daily, usually in two divided doses.

Diuretics are administered to eliminate excess water and sodium and to reduce cardiac workload. These drugs may also eliminate potassium, placing the child at risk for hypokalemia. Potassium supplements are often given in tandem with diuretics to replace these losses.

Vasodilators such as captopril or enalapril may be used to relax vascular smooth muscles and reduce afterload (Talner, 1995). This class of vasodilators is called angiotensin-converting enzyme (ACE) inhibitors because they block the conversion of angiotensin I to angiotensin II and reduce vasoconstriction.

NURSING CARE

The Child with Congestive Heart Failure

Assessment

Assessment of the child with CHF includes close monitoring of vital signs and a thorough cardiovascular examination. Recognizing the early signs of CHF will expedite early treatment and prevent decompensation to a more severe state. The early symptoms of tachypnea, poor feeding, and diaphoresis during feeding should be noted and the physician alerted as soon as possible.

Nursing Diagnosis, Planning, Intervention, and Evaluation

Nursing Diagnosis	■ Altered Tissue Perfusion related to increased cardiac workload.
Expected Outcome	• The child will have adequate tissue perfusion, as evidenced by pink mucous membranes and nail beds, a capillary refill time of less than 2 seconds, easily palpable peripheral pulses, and an activity level within the normal limits of the defect.

Intervention	Rationale
1. Assess peripheral perfusion by palpating peripheral pulses, noting any color changes and capillary refill time.	1. Poor peripheral perfusion is usually evident from decreased or absent pulses or blood pressure in the extremities. Color and temperature changes (e.g., cyanosis, coolness, mottling) may be present in all extremities. Prolonged capillary refill time is an additional sign of poor perfusion.
2. Maintain a neutral thermal environment; use a warmer bed or isolette for the newborn; treat fever promptly.	2. Episodes of hypothermia or hyperthermia increase oxygen demands and increase the cardiac workload.
3. Time nursing interventions to disturb the infant or child as little as possible. Anticipate and respond to stressful events quickly.	3. Rest periods reduce cardiac workload and maximize oxygen delivery; stress places a higher oxygen demand on the heart. Organizing nursing activities decreases the child's stress and fatigue.

4. Administer digoxin (Lanoxin) as prescribed. Ascertain that the dosage is within safe limits. Count the apical rate for 1 full minute. Check the dosage with a second nurse. Observe for signs of toxicity.

4. Digoxin is effective within a narrow therapeutic range (1.0 to 2.0 ng/ml [Artman, 1995]). Safety in dosing is achieved by double-checking the dose and counting the heart rate. Withhold the dose and notify physician if the heart rate is less than 90 to 100 BPM in infants or less than 70 to 85 BPM in children (O'Brien & Baker, 1999). Digoxin toxicity usually manifests with vomiting.

Evaluation
- Are mucous membranes and nail beds pink?
- Is the capillary refill time less than 2 seconds?
- Are peripheral pulses easily palpated, and is the child alert and active?

Nursing Diagnosis
■ Fluid Volume Excess related to left and right ventricular overload and ineffective pumping.

Expected Outcome
- The infant or child exhibits evidence of fluid loss (e.g., frequent urination, weight loss, inadequate balance between intake and output).

Intervention

1. Administer diuretics as prescribed, ensuring correct dosage, route, and effectiveness.

2. Maintain accurate intake and output records.

3. Maintain fluid restriction, if ordered.

4. Using the same scales, weigh the child daily at approximately the same time. Notify the physician of excessive weight gain (more than 50 g/day in infants; more than 200 g/day in children).
5. To prevent skin breakdown associated with edema, provide skin care and change position frequently.
6. Assess for increased or decreased edema.

7. Monitor serum electrolyte levels, especially potassium.

Rationale

1. Diuretics help the body get rid of excess fluid. Their effectiveness is evaluated from the urine output, either by measuring the amount of urine or by weighing diapers.
2. The fluid intake and output should be about the same. If intake grossly exceeds output, the diuretics may not be effective, the child may need fluid restriction, or both.
3. Fluid restriction will decrease pulmonary and liver edema.
4. Excess fluid volume is not always overtly visible. Weight changes may indicate fluid retention. Weighing the infant or child on the same scales at the same time each day ensures consistency.
5. Edematous areas are extremely prone to skin breakdown due to stretching and opacity. Frequent position changes will prevent undesirable pooling of fluid in certain areas.
6. Changes in the amount of edema can indicate the effectiveness or ineffectiveness of therapies, interventions, and nursing care.
7. Diuretics may stimulate potassium loss.

Evaluation
- Is the child urinating frequently?
- Has the child lost weight?
- Are intake and output balanced?

Nursing Diagnosis
■ Ineffective Breathing Pattern related to pulmonary congestion.

Expected Outcome
- The child will demonstrate a respiratory rate within normal limits for age, will breathe easily, and will have satisfactory rest periods. Color will remain pink.

Intervention

1. Assess respiratory rate and rhythm, the presence or absence of nasal flaring, the use of accessory muscles, and the presence or absence of crackles or rhonchi.
2. Position the infant or child with the head of the bed elevated 30 to 45 degrees. Avoid clothing that constricts the chest.
3. Administer oxygen as often as ordered.

4. Plan nursing interventions to allow maximum rest for the child. Do not perform multiple interventions at any one time.

Rationale

1. Infants and children with CHF experience changes in their breathing pattern due to increased fluid retention in the lungs, liver, and other areas of the body when the child is at rest.
2. An elevated position lowers the diaphragm and maximizes chest expansion.

3. Supplemental oxygen administration improves oxygen saturation and delivery to tissues.
4. Organizing nursing activities decreases the child's stress and fatigue.

Evaluation	• Is the child's respiratory rate within normal limits for age? • Are the child's mucous membranes and nail beds pink? • Is the child breathing easily?
Nursing Diagnosis	■ Altered Nutrition: Less Than Body Requirements related to increased energy expenditure.
Expected Outcome	• The infant or child will demonstrate appropriate weight gain and no significant loss of weight over a short period.

Intervention

1. Weigh the infant or child daily or before and after each feeding for breast-fed infants. Use the same scale.
2. Feed smaller volumes of concentrated formula (24 to 28 cal/oz) every 3 hours; ensure adequate free water and protein composition of 8% to 10%.

3. Use soft, large-hole nipples for feedings.

4. Implement gavage feedings if the infant tires before the recommended amount of feedings is consumed.
5. Time feedings to allow for adequate rest. Every 3 hours is optimal.

Rationale

1. Using the same scale ensures consistency.

2. Increased caloric content of formula increases caloric consumption and enhances weight gain. Commercially prepared formulas will provide adequate protein composition of 8% to 10% (Gaedeke-Norris & Hall, 1994).
3. Infants with CHF tire easily. A soft nipple with a large hole facilitates easy sucking and decreases energy expenditure during feeding.
4. Gavage feedings decrease energy expenditure and allow calories consumed to be used for growth.
5. Frequent disturbances increase oxygen consumption. Too frequent feedings disturb rest, whereas less frequent feedings require increased intake, which tires the infant.

Evaluation	• Has the infant or child maintained a steady weight gain?
Nursing Diagnosis	■ Knowledge Deficit related to disease process, treatment, interventions, and home care.
Expected Outcome	• Parents will verbalize understanding of cardiac defect and current and future interventions and will demonstrate an ability to perform treatments, including medication administration.

Intervention

1. Assess parents' readiness to learn and need to know.

2. Provide brief, factual explanations of the child's defect or any treatments and interventions. Do so frequently.
3. Allow the parents and child to verbalize feelings and concerns related to hospitalization.

4. Teach the parents to administer all necessary cardiac medications and explain their associated actions and potential adverse effects. Provide demonstrations and obtain return demonstrations by parents. Explain the use of oral syringes for accurate measurement of drugs.
5. Provide parents with written information when available.

6. Assess parents' understanding of instructions through return demonstrations and repeated information.

Rationale

1. A baseline assessment of prior knowledge should be considered before developing any teaching plan. If parent is not ready, learning will not occur.
2. Parents are most likely to retain simple, repetitive explanations.

3. Hospitalization is a frightening experience. By allowing verbalization of feelings and concerns related to the experience, nurses can assist in allaying fears and addressing concerns.
4. Family members should be taught how to administer all cardiac medications before discharge. This allows for questions and answers and evaluation of their home care techniques.

5. Written information provides an adjunct to individual teaching and a reference for the caregiver at home. Written information can be referred to during less stressful times, when it may be more likely to be retained.
6. Return demonstrations and repeated information validate that learning has occurred and that the parents are competent to provide care.

Evaluation	• Have the parents verbalized adequate and correct knowledge of the diagnosis and interventions? • Have the parents demonstrated confidence and competence in caregiving activities, including medicine administration?

Congenital Heart Disease

The most common cardiac problems in children result from congenital heart disease—structural or functional defects within the heart that are present at birth. The precise etiology of congenital heart disease is not known. Investigations into environmental and genetic causes are in progress. The genetic component of congenital heart disease has been investigated more thoroughly than the environmental aspect. A family history of congenital heart disease increases the risk of giving birth to a child with congenital heart disease. Siblings of a child with congenital heart disease have a 2% to 6% incidence (Bernstein, 1996) and the incidence may be even higher if one of the parents has a cardiac lesion (Brook, 1998). Teratogenic factors include exposures to certain drugs, as well as chronic maternal illnesses such as diabetes mellitus.

Classification of Congenital Heart Disease

Congenital heart disease is frequently divided into two major categories, acyanotic lesions and cyanotic lesions. Not all cardiac defects fall easily into one of these categories and not every child with a specific lesion will manifest the typical clinical picture of that defect. Complex lesions combine elements of several defects and frequently require a creative management plan.

Acyanotic Lesions

Acyanotic lesions are cardiac defects that generally do not produce cyanosis. The clinical signs are not always apparent at birth; they may manifest at any time during infancy or early childhood. Acyanotic lesions are further subdivided into left-to-right shunting lesions and obstructive or stenotic lesions.

LEFT-TO-RIGHT SHUNTING LESIONS

Intracardiac shunting occurs when the blood flow is forced by a higher pressure to go through an opening that is not normally present. In the case of left-to-right shunts, blood is shunted to the right side of the heart because the left side is normally functioning under a higher pressure than the right side. This shunting allows oxygenated and unoxygenated blood to mix. This results in increased pulmonary blood flow because the abnormal communication or opening sends more blood to the right side of the heart (through the opening) than normal.

The physiologic effects of left-to-right shunting include excessive pulmonary blood flow, increased cardiac workload, and right ventricular strain, dilation, and hypertrophy. The clinical consequences may include CHF, pulmonary hypertension, and infective endocarditis.

The four common lesions that result in left-to-right shunts are atrial septal defects (ASDs), ventricular septal defects (VSDs), patent ductus arteriosus (PDA), and atrioventricular canal defects (AVCs).

Patent Ductus Arteriosus

Incidence and Pathophysiology. Patent ductus arteriosus (Fig. 46–1) accounts for approximately 10% of all congenital heart disease. In the preterm infant, however,

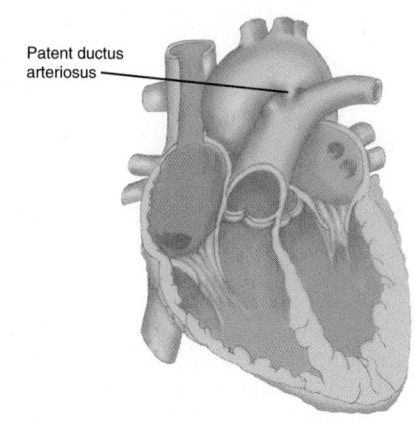

Patent ductus arteriosus

FIGURE 46–1

Patent ductus arteriosus.

the incidence is much higher. This lesion is marked by failure of the fetal ductus arteriosus to close completely after birth. Normally, the ductus arteriosus constricts within hours of birth (functional closure) and degenerates to a ligament (anatomic closure) within the first few weeks of life.

Altered Hemodynamics. Blood from the aorta flows into the pulmonary arteries to be reoxygenated in the lungs and returned to the left atrium and left ventricle. The effects of this altered circulation include increased workload on the left side of heart and increased pulmonary vascular congestion.

Manifestations. Term infants are often clinically asymptomatic, but a machinery-like murmur may be heard throughout both systole and diastole. This murmur may be accompanied by a suprasternal thrill. Continuous "runoff" of the aortic blood flow to the pulmonary arteries produces a widened pulse pressure and bounding pulses. The heart will be enlarged on chest radiographs and the infant may experience frequent respiratory tract infections, growth retardation, and fatigue.

Preterm infants frequently present with CHF and respiratory distress. They may have increased oxygen requirements and may need ventilatory support.

Therapeutic Management. The symptomatic newborn is treated with digoxin and diuretics to control CHF. The infant should be given ample rest periods to conserve energy and reduce oxygen requirements and placed in a position of comfort. The mortality is very low, less than 1%.

Medical Management. Ductal closure may be achieved by the use of indomethacin (Indocin), a prostaglandin inhibitor that promotes ductal constriction.

Surgical Management. Surgical closure is performed through a left thoracotomy. The ductus is divided and ligated. Surgery is usually performed within the first year of life to decrease the risk of bacterial endocarditis.

Atrial Septal Defect

Incidence and Pathophysiology. Atrial septal defect (Fig. 46–2) accounts for approximately 10% of all congenital heart disease. It is more frequently seen in females than in males. This lesion consists of an abnormal opening between the atria. There are three types: (1) ostium secundum (ASD2°), which is located in the middle of the atrial septum (fossa ovalis) and the most common type seen; (2) ostium primum (ASD1°), which is located low in the atrial septum, results from a defect in endocardial tissue formation, and is often associated with a VSD and AV valve malformation; and (3) sinus venosus, which is located high in the septum close to the SVC and frequently is associated with an anomalous right-sided pulmonary vein.

Altered Hemodynamics.   Pressure in the left atrium exceeds that in the right atrium, causing blood to flow left to right through the defect. Pulmonary blood flow is increased.

Manifestations.   Many children are asymptomatic but, over time, may experience fatigue and dyspnea on exertion. A characteristic systolic murmur is heard that is produced by increased blood flow across the pulmonary valve. A large defect may produce CHF, and pulmonary vascular disease may develop later in life if the lesion is unrepaired. Atrial dysrhythmias have been reported, usually as the result of atrial enlargement. The perioperative mortality is generally less than 1%.

Therapeutic Management.   The asymptomatic child is followed by the cardiologist. Bacterial endocarditis prophylaxis will be provided when indicated.

Medical Management.   Nonsurgical closure may be attempted by cardiac catheterization using a prosthetic umbrella patch.

Surgical Management.   Surgical closure using either sutures or a prosthetic patch is performed on an elective basis early in childhood. This is an open heart procedure in which cardiopulmonary bypass is used.

Ventricular Septal Defect

Incidence and Pathophysiology.   Ventricular septal defects (Fig. 46–3) account for approximately 25% of all congenital heart disease. It is the most commonly seen cardiac lesion and is often accompanied by other cardiac defects. The lesion consists of an abnormal opening between the right and left ventricles, which may vary in size from a minuscule hole to complete absence of the septum, resulting in a common ventricle.

Altered Hemodynamics.   High pressure in the left ventricle forces blood through the defect into the right ventricle, resulting in increased pulmonary blood flow and higher than normal pulmonary artery pressures.

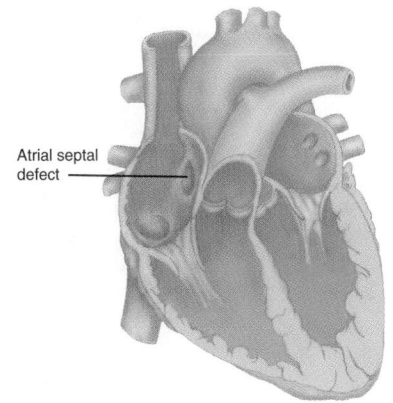

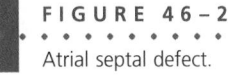

FIGURE 46–2
Atrial septal defect.

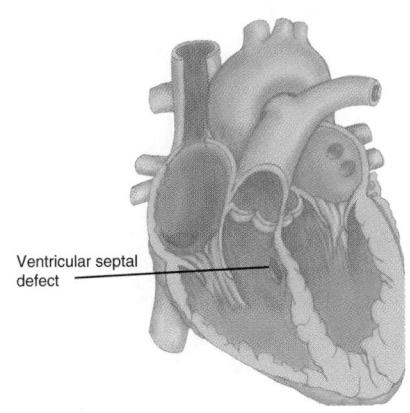

FIGURE 46–3
Ventricular septal defect.

Manifestations.   Signs and symptoms vary with the size of the defect and the presence of associated cardiac lesions. Clinical symptoms are usually not seen at birth because of continued high pulmonary vascular resistance in the newborn. Infants with moderate to large defects will become symptomatic within the first few weeks of life. Children with small defects will remain asymptomatic.

A characteristic loud, harsh, systolic murmur is heard on auscultation. The murmur is often associated with a palpable thrill. In children with large defects, a gallop rhythm may be present.

Infants with moderate to large defects may develop CHF that is accompanied by poor feeding and failure to thrive. Pulmonary stenosis or valvular insufficiency may also be present. There is a significant risk of progressive pulmonary vascular disease in patients with large defects.

Therapeutic Management.   From 20% to 60% of all VSDs close spontaneously. Children with small lesions will be followed by the cardiologist and receive antibiotic prophylaxis when indicated. Mortality varies with the size of the defect and the presence of other cardiac lesions. Isolated lesions are associated with a mortality of less than 5%. Postoperative complications include residual VSD and rhythm disturbances.

Medical Management.   Infants who develop CHF are managed with digoxin and diuretics. Nutritional status is a concern, and supplements are often added to the infant's formula to increase caloric intake.

Surgical Management.   Young infants with severe intractable CHF and failure to grow may be candidates for pulmonary artery banding. In this palliative procedure a band is placed around the main pulmonary artery, decreasing pulmonary blood flow, reducing the severity of CHF, and decreasing the risk of pulmonary vascular disease. The trend today, however, is to perform corrective surgery earlier in life, and consequently pulmonary artery banding is performed less frequently than in the past.

Total correction is accomplished by placing a purse-string suture around small defects and placing a prosthetic patch over moderate and large defects. Both procedures require cardiopulmonary bypass. The surgical approach is usually through the right atrium to avoid a right ventricular incision and maintain contractility of the ventricle.

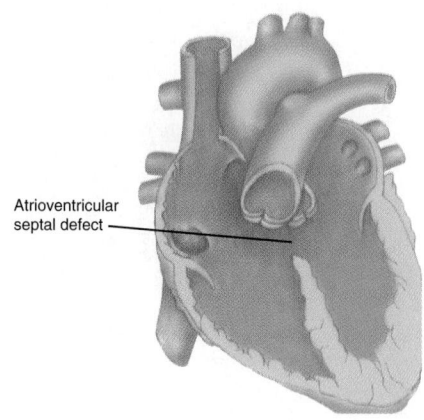

FIGURE 46–4
Atrioventricular septal defect.

Atrioventricular Septal Defect

Incidence and Pathophysiology. Atrioventricular septal defects (Fig. 46–4) account for 4% to 5% of all congenital heart disease and are often associated with Down syndrome. Inappropriate development of the endocardial cushion tissue produces abnormalities in the atrial and ventricular septa and the AV valve. The two most common classifications are partial/incomplete, marked by an ostium primum ASD and a cleft in the mitral valve, and complete, marked by a common AV valve orifice as well as ASD and VSD. The term canal has been used to describe this lesion because the defect creates a large opening in the center of the heart.

Altered Hemodynamics. The direction and magnitude of the intracardiac shunting are determined by the combination of defects and the difference between aortic and pulmonary pressures. Partial defects produce left-to-right shunting with increased pulmonary blood flow and the risk of CHF; complete defects produce CHF due to greatly increased pulmonary blood flow. Mixing of oxygenated and unoxygenated blood also occurs, so mild cyanosis may be seen.

Manifestations. The child with a partial defect may be asymptomatic. A systolic pulmonary murmur, however, may be heard. The symptoms seen in a child with a complete defect depend on the pulmonary artery pressure. If it is high, the child will experience cyanosis upon exertion; if low, CHF will be present.

Therapeutic Management
Medical Management. Congestive heart failure is treated symptomatically with digoxin and diuretics.
Surgical Management. If the child with a partial defect is asymptomatic, an elective surgical repair is planned in infancy or early childhood. The ostium primum defect is closed with a prosthetic patch and the mitral valve is repaired. The infant with a complete defect may require surgery at an early age if the left ventricle is small, CHF is intractable, or pulmonary vascular resistance is high. Total correction involves closing the atrial and ventricular septal defects and constructing two AV valves. If the mitral valve remains defective, a replacement valve may be used. Correction is performed before the child is 2 years old to prevent irreversible pulmonary vascular damage.

The surgical mortality may be as high as 10%. Postoperative complications include dysrhythmias and mitral valve regurgitation.

STENOTIC LESIONS

Stenosis is the narrowing or constriction of an opening. Stenosis can occur in a valve or a vessel. The narrowing or constriction results in obstruction of blood flow through this area.

The physiologic effects of obstructive or stenotic lesions include increased cardiac workload and ventricular strain; the clinical consequences of these lesions include CHF, decreased cardiac output, and pump failure. Stenotic lesions include pulmonary stenosis, aortic stenosis, and coarctation of the aorta.

Pulmonary Stenosis

Incidence and Pathophysiology. Obstruction of the right ventricular outflow tract and pulmonary arterial tree occur either isolated or in combination with other cardiac lesions in 25% to 30% of all congenital heart disease (Rocchini & Emmanouilides, 1995). Isolated valvular pulmonary stenosis accounts for 8% to 10% of cardiac defects (Fig. 46–5). The lesions are marked by narrowing at the entrance to the pulmonary artery, which may be valvular, subvalvular, or supravalvular.

Altered Hemodynamics. Resistance to blood flow at the right ventricular outflow tract decreases pulmonary blood flow and leads to right ventricular hypertrophy. High right ventricular pressure may cause blood to back up into the right atrium, increasing pressure and forcing the foramen ovale open to allow blood to flow from right to left atrium.

Manifestations. Many children are clinically asymptomatic. They present with a systolic ejection murmur that may be accompanied by a palpable thrill. The heart is enlarged on chest radiographs.

Children with moderate to severe pulmonic stenosis may experience exercise intolerance. Severe pulmonary stenosis manifests with right ventricular failure, CHF, and, if there is right-to-left shunting through the foramen ovale, mild to moderate cyanosis.

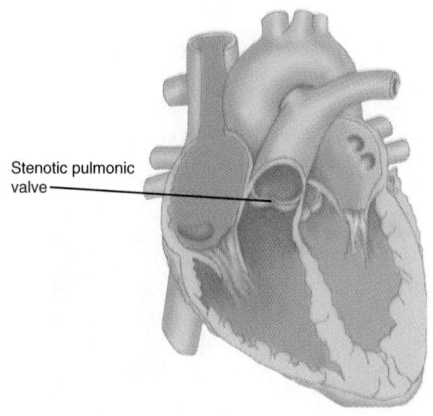

Stenotic pulmonic valve

FIGURE 46–5
Pulmonary stenosis.

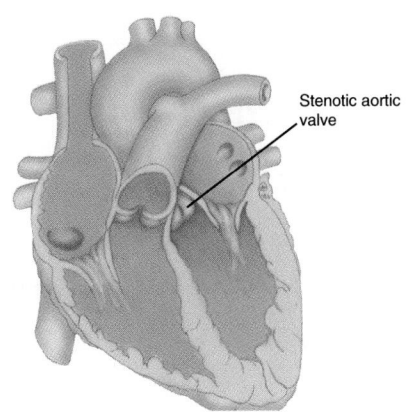

FIGURE 46–6
• • • • • • • • •
Aortic stenosis.

Therapeutic Management

Medical Management. In the clinically asymptomatic child, cardiac follow-up and appropriate antibiotic prophylaxis are the usual treatment. Over time, children with moderate pulmonic stenosis may develop a larger pressure gradient across the pulmonary valve.

Surgical Management. Pulmonary balloon valvuloplasty may be performed in the cardiac catheterization laboratory to reduce the gradient. Pulmonary balloon valvuloplasty is the treatment of choice for most children, even newborns with critical pulmonic stenosis (Rocchini & Emmanouilides, 1995; Wood, 1998). Surgical valvotomy is performed when balloon dilation is unsuccessful. The mortality is very low for both surgical repair and balloon valvuloplasty.

Aortic Stenosis

Incidence and Pathophysiology. Aortic stenosis (Fig. 46–6) accounts for 5% of all congenital heart disease. It is three times more common in males than females (Bernstein, 1996). In this lesion the aortic valve is thickened and rigid, with some fusion of the commissures (leaflets); the valve frequently is bicuspid.

Altered Hemodynamics. Stricture creates a pressure gradient across the aortic valve. Blood flow at rest is frequently unaffected due to a supranormal cardiac pump function (Friedman, 1995). With activity and increased oxygen demands, however, cardiac output and myocardial blood flow are diminished.

Manifestations. Aortic stenosis may be classified as mild, moderate, or severe, depending on the degree of stricture and the pressure gradient across the aortic valve. The diagnosis may be made with echocardiography or cardiac catheterization.

Severe aortic stenosis often manifests in early infancy and is called critical aortic stenosis. The infant exhibits profoundly decreased cardiac output with faint peripheral pulses, poor peripheral perfusion, severe CHF, and feeding difficulties. Older children with severe aortic stenosis experience significant angina, dizziness, and syncope on exertion. Sudden death has been reported (Bernstein, 1996).

Children with mild to moderate aortic stenosis are frequently clinically asymptomatic and enjoy normal growth and development. A systolic ejection murmur, sometimes accompanied by a thrill, is heard on examination. Cardiomegaly is seen on chest radiographs.

Therapeutic Management. Mild valvular aortic stenosis usually produces no clinical symptoms.

Medical Management. Children are followed by the cardiologist and treated with antibiotic prophylaxis. Aortic balloon valvuloplasty is performed to treat moderate to severe aortic stenosis. This procedure may prevent left ventricular dysfunction and reduce the risk of sudden death. Physical activity is limited in this group of children.

Surgical Management. Surgical valvotomy may be performed in infants and children with severe aortic stenosis. Many children experience aortic valvular insufficiency and restenosis following either surgical or balloon procedures and may need additional surgery. A valve replacement may prove necessary.

Coarctation of the Aorta

Incidence and Pathophysiology. Coarctation of the aorta (Fig. 46–7) accounts for 5% to 10% of congenital heart disease. Many children with coarctation of the aorta have a bicuspid aortic valve that may later become stenotic. This lesion consists of localized constriction of the aorta at or near the insertion site of the ductus arteriosus. This increases afterload and reduces cardiac output. It is caused by improper development of the aortic segment.

Altered Hemodynamics. Constriction impedes systemic blood flow, reducing cardiac output and creating pulmonary congestion through pooling of blood in the left side of the heart. Aortic pressure is high proximal to the constriction and low distal to the constriction. Collateral blood vessels develop over time to provide channels for blood flow past the constricted area.

Manifestations. The clinical symptoms seen are directly related to the severity of the constriction and the presence of associated cardiac lesions. The newborn with severe coarctation of the aorta will present with signs of poor lower body perfusion, metabolic acidosis, and CHF. If a patent ductus arteriosus persists, there may be right-to-left shunting, and differential cyanosis (significant differences in color and oxygen saturation between upper and lower body parts) may result.

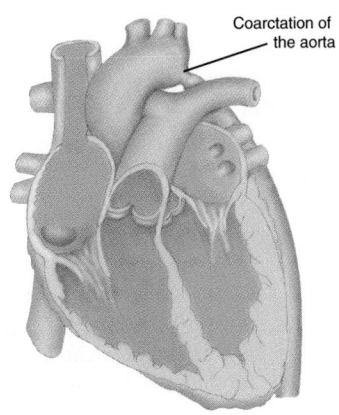

FIGURE 46–7
• • • • • • • • •
Coarctation of the aorta.

Children who are diagnosed after infancy are frequently asymptomatic. They may be referred to the cardiologist after systemic hypertension is detected on routine screening. The classic finding in these children is a disparity in pulses and blood pressures between the upper and lower extremities. Frequently, femoral pulses are weak or absent. The child may describe weakness, tingling in the lower extremities, and muscle cramps on exertion. A systolic murmur may be heard on auscultation and may be accompanied by an ejection click or thrill.

Therapeutic Management. The symptomatic newborn is treated with digoxin and diuretics to manage CHF.

Medical Management. The infant may also receive PGE_1 infusions to maintain ductal patency and improve perfusion to the lower body. Definitive treatment (balloon dilation or surgery) is indicated following stabilization (Beekman, 1995; Bernstein, 1996).

Surgical Management. Elective surgical coarctation repair at age 3 to 5 years is recommended for asymptomatic children (Beekman, 1995). The repair is performed through a left thoracotomy. Several surgical techniques are available: end-to-end anastomosis if the constricted area is short; use of a prosthetic patch to widen the constriction; or a subclavian flap in which the left subclavian artery provides the patch. Children undergoing the subclavian flap procedure will no longer have a palpable pulse in their left arm.

The mortality following surgical repair of isolated coarctation of the aorta in both infants and children is negligible, almost 0% (Beekman, 1995). The rate of restenosis, however, is significant, especially in children whose repairs were performed in infancy (Wood, 1998). These children may benefit from balloon dilation performed in the cardiac catheterization laboratory.

Cyanotic Lesions

Cyanotic lesions permit unoxygenated blood to enter the systemic circulation. Infants with cyanotic heart lesions become symptomatic within the first few days of life, when the ductus arteriosus begins to close (Spilman & Furdon, 1998). They often need emergency management with drugs or surgical intervention to survive the neonatal period.

PGE_1, a vasodilating drug, is often administered to reestablish patency of the ductus arteriosus and restore pulmonary blood flow. Continuous infusion of the drug may improve arterial oxygen saturation and tissue perfusion, allowing the infant to be stabilized in anticipation of further diagnostic and treatment interventions.

CYANOTIC LESIONS WITH DECREASED PULMONARY BLOOD FLOW

Cyanotic lesions with decreased pulmonary blood flow include tricuspid atresia, pulmonary atresia, and tetralogy of Fallot. These types of lesion arise from an error in fetal development that results in hypoplasia, malalignment, or obstruction on the right side of the heart. Pulmonary blood flow is frequently dependent on a patent ductus arteriosus. The physiologic consequences of these lesions include hypoxemia, increased cardiac workload, and ventricular strain. The overwhelming clinical consequence is hypoxemia resulting in cyanosis. The cyanosis is profound, often intensi-

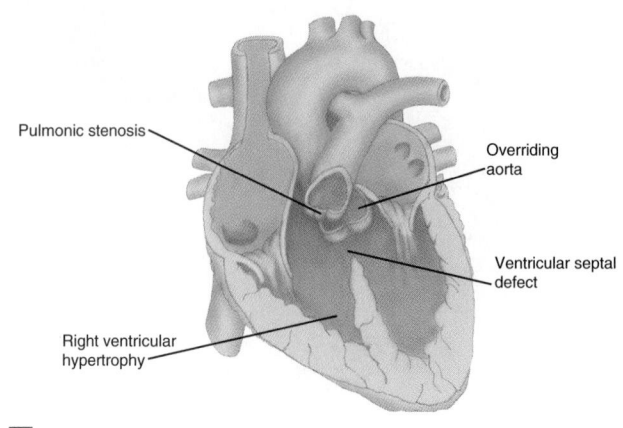

FIGURE 46–8
. . . .
Tetralogy of Fallot.

fied by crying, and not satisfactorily relieved by oxygen administration.

Tetralogy of Fallot

Incidence and Pathophysiology. Tetralogy of Fallot (Fig. 46–8) accounts for 8% to 10% of all congenital heart disease and is the most common cyanotic lesion seen in the first year of life (K. E. Paul, 1995; Spilman & Furdon, 1998). Malalignment of the ventricular septum during fetal development results in the constellation of four characteristics of this lesion: (1) nonrestricted VSDs, (2) pulmonic stenosis, (3) overriding of the aorta, and (4) hypertrophy of the right ventricle.

Altered Hemodynamics. Pulmonic stenosis impedes blood flow to the lungs, thereby increasing right ventricular pressure and workload and forcing unoxygenated blood through the VSD and directly into the aorta.

Manifestations. The degree of pulmonic stenosis governs the onset and severity of the symptoms. If pulmonic stenosis is mild, there is little or no right-to-left shunting. This is known as "pink tet."

Some infants present as cyanotic newborns. When antegrade pulmonary blood flow is severely impeded, blood flow to the lungs is dependent on a patent ductus arteriosus. As this structure closes, the newborn becomes profoundly cyanotic.

Other infants become visibly cyanotic over the first few months of life. They tire easily, especially with exertion, and may have difficulty feeding and gaining weight. In time, these infants may have hypercyanotic episodes, as well as other clinical signs of chronic hypoxemia (see p. 1256). Auscultation reveals a systolic murmur, often accompanied by a palpable thrill. The heart is boot-shaped on chest radiographs due to poor development of the pulmonary artery.

Therapeutic Management. The symptomatic newborn frequently needs continuous PGE_1 infusion to maintain ductal patency. Definitive surgical intervention is necessary in the first days of life.

Medical Management. Older infants need very close monitoring for signs and symptoms of worsening hypoxemia. Illnesses that put them at risk for dehydration must be treated promptly. Hemoglobin levels and hematocrit values are frequently evaluated. Worsening hypoxemia is often accompanied by the appearance or escalation in frequency of hypercyanotic episodes, heralding the need for surgical intervention.

Surgical Management. Choices in surgical management include palliative procedures to increase pulmonary blood flow or a definitive intracardiac repair. In recent years, primary repair during infancy has become the treatment of choice, with surgery scheduled at 3 to 12 months of age (Zuberbuhler, 1995).

Some symptomatic newborns are poor candidates for primary repair. These infants may benefit from the surgical creation of a systemic-pulmonary artery shunt to increase pulmonary blood flow. The most commonly performed is the modified Blalock-Taussig procedure. Surgical mortality in all procedures is low, less than 5% (Bernstein, 1996). The most common postoperative complications are rhythm disturbances, primarily right bundle-branch block and AV block.

Tricuspid Atresia

Incidence and Pathophysiology. Tricuspid atresia (Fig. 46–9) represents approximately 2% to 3% of all congenital heart disease. Additional cardiac anomalies are seen in 20% of patients with this lesion (Rosenthal & Dick, 1995). In this lesion, the tricuspid valve does not develop.

Altered Hemodynamics. Absence (atresia) of the tricuspid valve forces all of the blood entering the right atrium to be shunted through the foramen ovale into the left atrium, bypassing the lungs. Oxygenation takes place by retrograde flow through a persistent patent ductus arteriosus.

Manifestations. Profound cyanosis is present in the neonate and is usually visible within the first few hours of life. A systolic pulmonary murmur is often heard.

Therapeutic Management

Medical Management. Pulmonary blood flow is reestablished through continuous PGE$_1$ infusion. The infant is stabilized and readied for surgery.

Surgical Management. The newborn requires a systemic-pulmonary artery shunt to provide adequate pulmonary blood flow. This is the first procedure in a three-stage effort to palliate this defect.

A bidirectional Glenn procedure is performed at 4 to 6 months of age, once the pulmonary arteries have reached an adequate size. In this procedure the superior vena cava

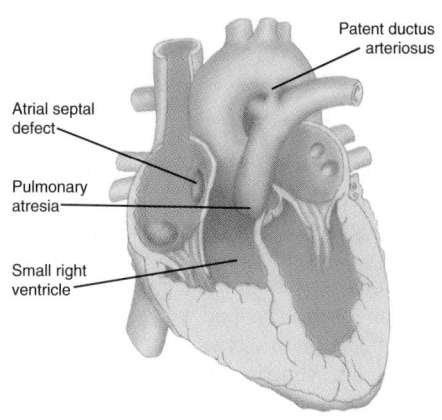
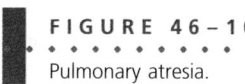

FIGURE 46–10

Pulmonary atresia.

is connected to the pulmonary arteries, thereby reducing left ventricular overload by one third (Rosenthal & Dick, 1995).

The third procedure, the modified Fontan operation, is performed between ages 18 months and 3 years. Blood is directly channeled from the inferior vena cava to the pulmonary arteries.

Surgical mortality has declined and is now reported to be 4% to 8% (Rosenthal & Dick, 1995). Postoperative complications include elevated systemic venous pressures and pericardial and pleural effusions.

Pulmonary Atresia

Incidence and Pathophysiology. Pulmonary atresia (Fig. 46–10) accounts for approximately 3% of congenital heart disease (Freedom, 1995). Failure of the pulmonary valve to develop, accompanied by hypoplastic development of the pulmonary artery and right ventricle, causes this lesion.

Altered Hemodynamics. Atresia of the pulmonary valve forces all of the blood entering the right ventricle to be propelled retrograde to the right atrium and shunted through the foramen ovale to the left atrium. Oxygenation of the blood occurs through retrograde flow via a persistent patent ductus arteriosus.

Manifestations. Profound cyanosis is seen during the early neonatal period. Survival depends on the presence of a patent ductus arteriosus. On auscultation, the second heart sound (S$_2$) is single. Occasionally, if patent ductus is present, a soft systolic murmur or continuous murmur is heard.

Therapeutic Management

Medical Management. The newborn requires continuous PGE$_1$ infusion to maintain ductal patency. The primary treatment of this lesion is surgical.

Surgical Management. Early surgical intervention involves pulmonary valvotomy and the creation of a systemic-pulmonary artery shunt (Bernstein, 1996). These interventions may encourage growth of the right ventricular chamber. If successful, future surgical repair is aimed at further dilating the pulmonary valve and enhancing the right ventricle with a patch. If the right ventricle remains very small, the surgical procedure of choice is the modified Fontan procedure.

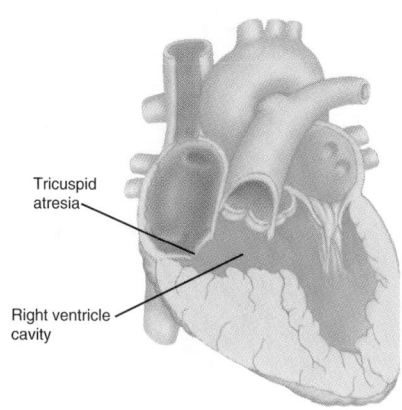

FIGURE 46–9

Tricuspid atresia.

Surgical mortality ranges from 19% after the first procedure to 36% after both procedures (Freedom, 1995). Some families may consider cardiac transplantation as a future option.

CYANOTIC LESIONS WITH INCREASED PULMONARY BLOOD FLOW

These defects result from failure of the heart to correctly divide into separate pulmonary and systemic circuits during fetal development (J. B. Smith, Baker, Moynihan, et al., 1996). Mixing of arterial and venous blood occurs. The physiologic effects of this type of defect include increased cardiac workload, ventricular strain, and decreased cardiac output. The clinical consequences include cyanosis and CHF.

The infant with this type of lesion may appear ruddy or mildly cyanotic. Often the work of breathing is increased, and respiratory distress may develop. If systemic circulation is compromised, the infant may be dusky or gray in color and present in cardiogenic shock. Lesions representative of this category include truncus arteriosus and hypoplastic left heart syndrome.

Truncus Arteriosus

Incidence and Pathophysiology. Truncus arteriosus (Fig. 46–11) accounts for 1% to 4% of all congenital heart disease (J. B. Smith et al., 1996). It is marked by incomplete division of the common great vessel. A single large vessel gives rise to the pulmonary, systemic, and coronary circulations. A VSD is present; the vessel overrides this defect and receives blood from both right and left ventricles (Bernstein, 1996). There are four classifications of truncus arteriosus, with type I being most common.

Altered Hemodynamics. A common ventricular outflow tract mixes both oxygenated and unoxygenated blood. The common great vessel sends this mixed blood to the systemic, pulmonary, and coronary circulations. Oxygen saturation depends on the volume of pulmonary blood flow: the greater this flow, the higher the saturation.

Manifestations. The infant presents, often in the neonatal period, with CHF and some degree of cyanosis. The volume of pulmonary blood flow determines the severity of symptoms. Unrestricted flow to the pulmonary artery results in pulmonary congestion and severe CHF. If pulmonic stenosis is present, pulmonary blood flow is limited, and cyanosis increases.

A harsh systolic murmur, due to the VSD, is heard, accompanied by a thrill. The opening of the single truncal valve may produce a click. The infant may also have bounding pulses and a widened pulse pressure.

Therapeutic Management

Medical Management. Medical management is aimed at reducing the effects of CHF and preventing polycythemia. CHF is treated with digoxin and diuretics; however, diuretic therapy is closely monitored to prevent hemoconcentration. Surgical repair is performed at approximately six weeks of age (Mair et al., 1995).

Surgical Management. Newborns who do not respond to early medical management may benefit from pulmonary artery banding; however, there are known risks and complications associated with this procedure (Mair et al., 1995), and total corrective surgery is preferred.

The corrective repair closes the VSD and directs the right ventricular blood through a conduit to the pulmonary artery. A valvuloplasty of the truncal valve may be performed to improve valvular competence.

The surgical mortality has been reported to be 5% to 10% in patients who do not have associated malformations (Mair et al., 1995). Lifelong antibiotic prophylaxis is necessary, and a future truncal valve replacement may be needed.

Hypoplastic Left Heart Syndrome

Incidence and Pathophysiology. Hypoplastic left heart syndrome (Fig. 46–12) accounts for 7% of all congenital heart disease (J. B. Smith et al., 1996). It is seen more frequently in males than in females. Approximately 95% of all affected infants who are untreated will die within the first months of life (Freedom & Benson, 1995).

Hypoplastic left heart syndrome results from inadequate development of the left side of the heart, resulting in only one effective ventricle. The syndrome may include aortic valve atresia, hypoplasia of the left ventricle, atresia or hypoplasia of the ascending aorta, and mitral valve stenosis or atresia. Most infants have an intact ventricular septum (Bernstein, 1996).

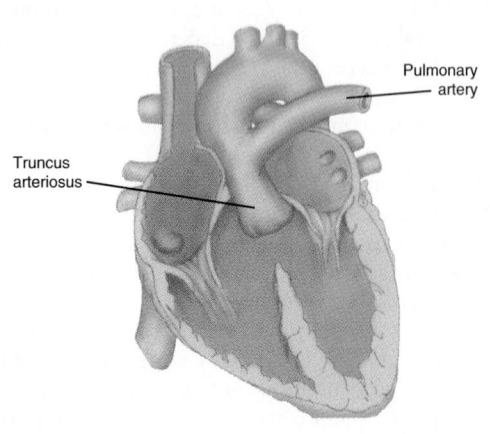

FIGURE 46–11

Truncus arteriosus.

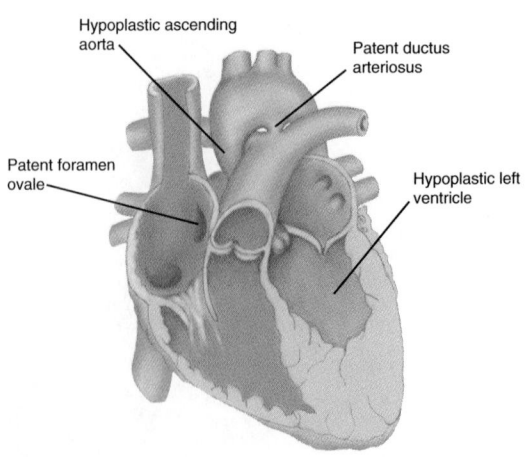

FIGURE 46–12

Hypoplastic left heart syndrome.

Altered Hemodynamics. Pulmonary venous blood return is unable to flow through the left side of the heart. It is shunted left to right through a patent foramen ovale into the right atrium. Mixed blood travels though the right ventricle to the pulmonary artery. Systemic and coronary circulations are supplied through a patent ductus arteriosus.

Manifestations. Most infants present within the first few days of life with CHF and, as the ductus arteriosus begins to close, systemic hypoperfusion and shock. The infant appears grayish blue in color, with dyspnea and hypotension.

Therapeutic Management. Because this lesion proves fatal in over 90% of all untreated infants, surgical intervention is indicated.

Medical Management. Emergency management addresses correction of the acid-base and electrolyte balances and re-establishment of ductal patency with PGE_1.

Surgical Management. Two surgical courses are available. Cardiac transplantation, as a single, definitive correction, has been successful, with an 85% operative survival rate and an 81% 5-year survival rate (Freedom & Benson, 1995). The scarcity of neonatal donor hearts, however, greatly limits the number of infants who may receive transplants.

A three-stage repair has been developed that palliates the condition. The first stage, the Norwood procedure, provides unobstructed blood flow from the right ventricle to the aorta with pulmonary blood flow supplied through a systemic-pulmonary artery surgical shunt. This procedure is performed during the neonatal period.

The second stage, a bidirectional Glenn procedure, is performed at approximately 6 months of age (see p. 1267). The palliation is completed within the first 2 years of life with a modified Fontan procedure (see p. 1267). Surgical mortality for the staged procedure varies widely among institutions. Recent reports suggest the 4-year survival following staged repair to be greater than 50% (Freedom & Benson, 1995).

MIXED LESIONS

Types of Mixed Lesions. Not all cyanotic lesions fall easily into one of these two categories. A small number of cardiac defects have variable pulmonary blood flow and require mixing of atrial and venous blood to support survival. Infants born with these cardiac lesions demonstrate severe cyanosis and pulmonary congestion. An example of this type of defect is transposition of the great arteries.

Transposition of the Great Arteries
Incidence and Pathophysiology. Transposition of the great arteries (Fig. 46–13) accounts for 5% to 7% of all congenital heart disease. It is more common in males than in females. About 45% of affected children have a coexisting VSD (M. H. Paul & Wernovsky, 1995). Improper separation and rotation of the common truncal vessel in fetal life cause this defect. The right ventricle gives rise to the aorta and the left ventricle gives rise to the pulmonary artery.

Altered Hemodynamics. In this defect, the pulmonary and systemic circulations exist in parallel. Systemic venous blood (unoxygenated) travels through the right atrium

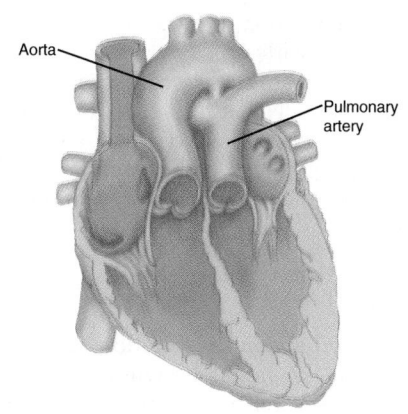

Aorta

Pulmonary artery

FIGURE 46–13
• • • • • • • • •
Transposition of the great arteries.

and right ventricle into the aorta. Pulmonary venous blood (oxygenated) recirculates through the left side of the heart and through the lungs. Survival depends on mixing of these two circulations through the fetal structures—the foramen ovale and ductus arteriosus.

Manifestations. Most newborns present with cyanosis during the few hours or days of life. They demonstrate hypoxemia with a minimal response to oxygen administration. Prompt diagnosis and treatment are paramount for survival.

Therapeutic Management

Medical Management. A continuous infusion of PGE_1 is begun to maintain ductal patency and support interatrial mixing of oxygenated and unoxygenated blood. A Rashkind balloon atrial septostomy may be performed on some infants. This procedure, performed in the cardiac catheterization laboratory, tears a hole in the atrial septum and enhances mixing of blood.

Surgical Management. The current surgical treatment of choice is the arterial switch procedure (Bernstein, 1996). This procedure anatomically corrects the defect by placing the pulmonary artery and aorta in their proper anatomic positions over the right ventricle and left ventricle, respectively. The arterial switch survival rate is 90% to 95% for uncomplicated lesions (Bernstein, 1996).

Early surgical techniques (the Mustard and Senning procedures) attempted to physiologically correct the defect by channeling atrial blood to the appropriate ventricle and restoring serial circulation (right ventricle to lungs to left atrium and ventricle to aorta). Early postoperative survival following this kind of procedure has been very good, 85% to 90% (Bernstein, 1996). Survivors may have significant difficulties with systemic venous congestion and atrial rhythm disturbances.

The Child Undergoing Cardiac Surgery

Most cardiac lesions are amenable to palliative or corrective repair, and the child with congenital heart disease is likely to undergo a surgical procedure at some point during infancy or childhood. The timing of surgery is dictated by the child's clinical condition, but the trend in recent years is to intervene at an early age.

Families anticipate surgery as a means of achieving a more normal lifestyle, but they also experience anxiety about the child's postoperative course and ultimate outcome. The nurse can help both the child and the parents cope with this stressful and traumatic event through support and education.

Preoperative Preparation

Preoperative teaching and preparation acquaint the child and family with the hospital environment and expected perioperative care as well as foster positive coping strategies. The family should receive written information that describes the course of events throughout the hospitalization. It is important to evaluate the family's understanding of the surgical procedure and its expected outcomes.

The parents and child should tour the intensive care unit (Fig. 46–14). This preparation allows them to become familiar with the physical environment as well as the noise and activity level. The visit should allow time for the family to meet members of the nursing staff and see equipment that will be used in the child's postoperative care.

Monitors, ventilators, and tubes should be described and shown to the family. Parents should be reminded that invasive monitoring lines, chest tubes, and an endotracheal tube are inserted during surgery while the child is anesthe-

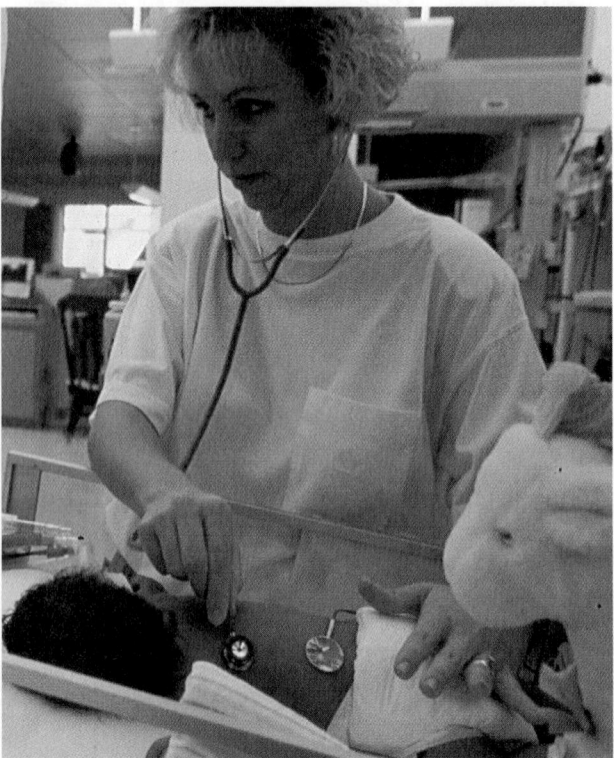

FIGURE 46–14

If a visit to the intensive care unit is age appropriate, the family and child should participate in a visit before the child undergoes cardiac surgery. The experience prepares the family for the sights and sounds of the unit.

tized, and should be reassured that these tubes and lines will be removed as soon as the child's condition permits.

The sequence of events surrounding the day of surgery—when and where to arrive and where to wait during the procedure—should be reviewed. Parents should be assured that they will receive updates about their child's condition throughout the procedure and will be permitted to visit soon after the surgery is completed.

Postoperative Management

Postoperative nursing management includes promoting hemodynamic stability and healing, providing comfort and emotional support, and preventing complications. Early postoperative care in the intensive care unit involves consistent monitoring of vital signs and cardiac output and frequent multisystem assessments.

MONITORING CARDIAC OUTPUT
The child's cardiac output is monitored through the assessment of vital signs and peripheral perfusion. Signs of low cardiac output include coolness and mottling of extremities, diminished peripheral pulses, delayed capillary refill time, hypotension, decreased urine output, and changes in level of consciousness.

The components of cardiac output are heart rate, preload, contractility, and afterload. Problems with one or more of these components may develop during the early postoperative period. Changes in heart rate or rhythm affect cardiac function, and antiarrhythmic drugs or temporary cardiac pacing may be instituted to correct transient postoperative rhythm disturbances. Blood loss and leakage of fluid into the interstitial space influence preload. Transfusions of blood products and colloids are sometimes needed to maintain adequate circulating blood volume. Acid-base and electrolyte imbalances, as well as hypoxia, adversely affect contractility. Correction of these abnormalities may improve cardiac function, but some children will need continuous infusion of inotropic medications to support cardiac output. Changes in systemic and pulmonary vascular resistance influence afterload, and the use of vasodilators, such as nitroprusside, sometimes proves necessary.

SUPPORTING RESPIRATORY FUNCTION
During cardiopulmonary bypass, the lungs are deflated, placing the child at risk for postoperative atelectasis. Also, fluid may accumulate in the pleural interstitial space at this time. Initially, the child may remain intubated, mechanical ventilation may be instituted to re-expand alveoli and promote adequate gas exchange.

Airway patency is maintained through prudent suctioning of the endotracheal tube. The nurse must pay strict attention to oxygen saturation readings during the procedure to avoid episodes of transient hypoxia. Frequently, the child receives bolus or continuous infusions of sedative medications to help maintain comfort during this time.

On extubation, the child is encouraged to deep breathe and cough. Incentive spirometry is often used to enhance lung expansion. Supplemental oxygen is administered initially, then tapered off as the child's condition permits. Pain medication is given before treatments and pulmonary exercises to allow the child to participate with minimal discomfort. The child can be encouraged to splint the chest during coughing by hugging a favorite stuffed animal.

Chest tubes are placed during surgery to evacuate drainage and air and assist with lung re-expansion. These tubes are inserted in either the mediastinal or pleural space, depending on the surgical approach, and are removed when lung re-expansion is confirmed and drainage has ceased.

Initial chest tube drainage is bloody and changes to serosanguineous then serous over time. Drainage is heaviest during the first 12 to 24 hours postoperatively, and hourly measurements of drainage and evaluation of color are performed. Increased chest tube drainage may indicate surgical bleeding or clotting abnormalities and must be strictly monitored and rapidly resolved.

Chest tubes are uncomfortable while in place; they restrict movement and cause discomfort when the child's position is changed. Chest tube removal is a painful experience, and the child should be premedicated with an opiate analgesic before the procedure is performed.

MAINTAINING FLUID AND ELECTROLYTE BALANCE

Cardiac surgery and cardiopulmonary bypass affect fluid and electrolyte status. Blood loss and fluid shifts reduce circulating blood volume. Cardiopulmonary bypass stimulates secretion of aldosterone and antidiuretic hormone (ADH), resulting in water and sodium retention and potassium loss (Holt, 1998). Stress can increase calcium deposition in bone, placing the child at risk for hypocalcemia.

Accurate recording of intake and output monitors fluid balance. Urine output is measured hourly and weight is measured daily. Fluid requirements are calculated based on the child's weight. The child with fluid volume deficit may require fluid boluses of crystalloid, colloid, or blood, while the child with fluid volume excess may require fluid restriction and diuretic therapy.

Electrolyte imbalances adversely affect cardiac contractility. Serum electrolyte values are determined at regular intervals in the early postoperative period, and IV boluses of calcium or potassium are administered to correct abnormalities. These medications are delivered through a centrally placed venous line and given according to precise guidelines.

PROMOTING COMFORT

Postoperative pain management is one of the most important nursing concerns in the care of the child undergoing cardiac surgery. The experience is frightening to both the child and parents. Parents worry that their child will be in constant, severe pain following the procedure.

Optimal pain management in the initial postoperative period is frequently accomplished through the use of a continuous IV infusion of an opiate analgesic, such as morphine sulfate or fentanyl. This infusion is often accompanied by the administration of sedatives. This combination of drugs provides pain control and allows the child to rest.

Once invasive monitoring lines and tubes have been removed, pain control can usually be achieved through the

---

PARENTS WANT TO KNOW

About Care After Heart Surgery

Activity

- Resume regular nap and sleep schedules and play activities (infants).
- Omit play outside for several weeks, allowing inside play as tolerated.
- Avoid activities where the child could fall (like riding tricycles, bicycles, swinging, or sliding) for 2 to 4 weeks after hospital discharge.
- Resume regular bedtime (children).
- Avoid large crowds of people for 1 week after discharge (including day care and church).

Diet

- Resume regular formula/milk and baby foods (infant).
- Do not give any new foods until after the first checkup (infant).
- If baby eats table foods, follow a no-added-salt diet (infant).
- Follow a no-added-salt diet until checkup (children).
- Appetite should pick up at home.

Incision

- Bathe infant/child with soap and water in the usual way. Do not use a bandage.
- No creams, lotions, or powders on incision until it is completely healed and without scabs.

School

- Child may return to school the third week after hospital discharge.
- The child should go to school for half days for the first few days.
- No physical education until 2 months after the operation.

When to Call the Doctor

- Faster, harder breathing than normal when child is at rest
- New, frequent coughing
- Turning blue or bluer than normal
- Frequent vomiting or diarrhea
- Pain worse instead of better
- Appetite worse than at time of discharge
- Any new swelling, redness, or drainage of the incision
- Temperature above 100.5°F

Checkup

- An appointment should be made for a 2-week follow-up at the time of discharge.

use of oral analgesics. Acetaminophen with or without an opiate additive is frequently the drug of choice. The incision site sometimes determines the amount of pain medication the child will need to remain comfortable. A thoracotomy incision usually divides muscle and necessitates spreading of the ribs for exposure; children who have undergone this surgical approach frequently experience more postoperative discomfort than those who have had a midsternotomy incision.

Pain assessments should be performed frequently throughout the hospitalization. Preverbal children are unable to express their discomfort and older children may not be able to accurately describe their pain. Pain assessment tools should be used to accurately assess the child's pain. The nurse also must be alert to nonverbal pain behavior, which includes restlessness and irritability, difficulty resting and sleeping, guarding, rigidity, resistance to move, an increase in heart rate and blood pressure, and disinterest in eating and other activities. Consulting the parents can help the nurse validate the assessment. Parents know their child best and are familiar with their child's response to stressful situations.

PROMOTING HEALING AND RECOVERY
A balance between rest and activity is necessary to promote healing. Children often experience fatigue during their postoperative recovery and may benefit from a planned schedule of progressive activity. Parents should be encouraged to allow their child to gradually resume his or her preoperative activity level. Regularly scheduled administration of pain medication provides comfort, allows the child to rest, and reduces fatigue and anxiety.

Nutritional intake is monitored and the child is encouraged to resume normal eating patterns. While hospitalized, some children will receive a low-salt diet; when they are discharged, parents may be asked to follow a no-added-salt regimen for a short time.

Acquired Heart Disease

Types of Acquired Heart Disease

Acquired heart disease encompasses cardiac conditions that are not present at birth. Although children with congenital heart disease may develop acquired cardiac problems, such as dysrhythmias and bacterial endocarditis, children with structurally normal hearts may be affected by these conditions as well. Some factors that play a role in triggering these problems include genetic tendencies, autoimmune responses, and infection.

Bacterial Endocarditis

Bacterial (infective) endocarditis is an inflammation resulting in infection of the valves, endothelium, and endocardium. It is caused by a bacterial or occasionally fungal agent.

ETIOLOGY
Bacterial endocarditis most commonly occurs in children with congenital heart disease. Those with prosthetic heart

---

PATHOPHYSIOLOGY
• • • • • • • • • • •
of Bacterial Endocarditis

Children with congenital heart defects experience a pressure gradient within the structures of their heart. This pressure gradient causes turbulence, which may result in damage or disruption of the endocardium or endothelium. A fibrin clot composed of fibrin and entrapped platelets may form at the site of the disruption. If bacteria are present, this clot may also entrap circulating microorganisms and cause a vegetation to form. The vegetation increases in size as the microorganisms, fibrin, and platelets proliferate within a protective sheath of fibrin. The contained and protected bacteria can quickly destroy the surrounding tissue and valve structures.

Data from Dajani, A. S., & Taubert, K. A. (1995). Infective endocarditis. In G. C. Emmanouilides, A. J. Moss, & F. H. Adams (Eds.), *Moss and Adams' heart disease in infants, children, and adolescents: Including the fetus and young adult* (5th ed., pp. 1541–1553). Baltimore: Williams & Wilkins; Estlow, M. M. (1998). Prevention of infective endocarditis in the pediatric congenital heart population. *Pediatric Nursing, 24*(3), 205–225.

---

valves, complex cyanotic heart disease, or surgically constructed systemic-pulmonary artery shunts or conduits and those with a previous history of endocarditis are at greatest risk (Dajani, Taubert, & Wilson, 1997). Valvular disease, either acquired (due to rheumatic fever) or congenital, also predisposes to the development of bacterial endocarditis (Dajani & Taubert, 1995). The bacterial organisms most commonly responsible are gram-positive organisms, including *Streptococcus viridans, Staphylococcus aureus,* and *Staphylococcus epidermidis.* Occasionally, fungi such as *Candida* may be identified on culture (Dajani & Taubert, 1995).

INCIDENCE
The incidence of bacterial endocarditis in neonates has increased over the past decade. This increase is probably attributable to the increased survival of at-risk neonates and the use of indwelling vascular catheters (Doerr & Starke, 1996). Bernstein (1996) enumerates reasons why endocarditis is still a cause of morbidity and mortality, despite the use of prophylactic antibiotics:

• The infecting agents have changed.
• Some physicians and dentists remain unaware of the threat of the disease and preventive measures available.
• The diagnosis may be difficult to make when delayed.
• Groups at increased risk have emerged, including IV drug users, survivors of cardiac surgery, and children and infants with lowered resistance who need intravascular catheters.

MANIFESTATIONS
The clinical manifestations of bacterial endocarditis include heart murmur; fever, malaise, or sweating; signs and symptoms of heart failure; anemia; increased sedimentation rate; myalgias and arthralgias; headache; and anorexia.

DIAGNOSTIC EVALUATION

The diagnosis of bacterial endocarditis is primarily established on the basis of a blood culture that yields the causative organism and on visualization of a *vegetation* (an abnormal growth of tissue) on echocardiographic studies. Other laboratory tests that may help to confirm the diagnosis are an elevated sedimentation rate and C-reactive protein level. ECG is usually not helpful in the diagnosis of bacterial endocarditis (Dajani & Taubert, 1995).

THERAPEUTIC MANAGEMENT

Prevention is the most important therapeutic management for bacterial endocarditis. Children at risk should establish and maintain a good oral hygiene routine to reduce the incidence of periodontal infections. Prior to any procedure that may increase the risk of introduction of organisms into the blood, bacterial endocarditis prophylaxis is recommended. Examples include dental procedures that may induce gingival or mucosal bleeding, as well as certain respiratory, genitourinary, and gastrointestinal procedures.

Treatment for bacterial endocarditis includes parenteral administration of antibiotics for 2 to 6 weeks, depending on the pathogen involved and the clinical circumstances. The prolonged course of antibiotics is necessary because the bacteria in the vegetations are protected from phagocytic and other host defense mechanisms, and the density of bacteria is very high (Dajani & Taubert, 1995).

Surgical interventions, such as excision of the vegetation and, in some circumstances, removal of an infected valve and other structures, may be indicated. The child should be evaluated for circulatory compromise, and surgical intervention should be addressed before the child's condition deteriorates significantly (Dajani & Taubert, 1995; O'Brien & Baker, 1999).

NURSING CARE

The Child with Bacterial Endocarditis

Assessment

Assessment of the child with bacterial endocarditis requires close monitoring of temperature elevations and vital signs. Vital signs should be monitored every 2 to 4 hours, along with a thorough cardiovascular assessment. A murmur may or may not be present. If it is present, any change in the murmur should be reported to the physician.

Nursing Diagnosis and Planning

Nursing diagnoses for the child with bacterial endocarditis include the following:

- Altered Tissue Perfusion (Peripheral) related to hemodynamic instability as a result of impaired valvular or myocardial function.
  Expected Outcome: The child will have adequate tissue perfusion, as evidenced by pink mucous membranes and nail beds, a capillary refill time of less than 2 seconds, strong peripheral pulses, vital signs within normal limits, and a level of consciousness within normal limits.
- Hyperthermia related to bacterial infection.
  Expected Outcome: The child will maintain a body temperature that is within normal limits.

Recommendations for Bacterial Endocarditis Prophylaxis

DEFECTS REQUIRING PROPHYLAXIS

- Prosthetic cardiac valves
- Previous bacterial endocarditis, even without heart disease
- Most congenital heart malformations
- Acquired valve abnormalities due to surgery, heart disease, rheumatic fever
- Hypertrophic cardiomyopathy
- Persistent VSD despite surgery
- First 6 months after congenital heart disease repair

DEFECTS NOT REQUIRING PROPHYLAXIS

- Isolated ostium secundum ASD
- Beyond first 6 months after ASD, VSD, or PDA repair
- Mitral valve prolapse *without* regurgitation
- Physiologic/functional heart murmurs
- Previous Kawasaki disease *without* valvular dysfunction
- Previous rheumatic fever *without* valvular dysfunction
- Cardiac pacemakers and implanted defibrillators

PROCEDURES REQUIRING PROPHYLAXIS

- All dental procedures likely to induce gingival or mucosal bleeding, including professional teeth cleaning (not simple adjustment of orthodontic appliances or shedding of deciduous teeth)
- Tonsillectomy and/or adenoidectomy
- Surgical procedures or biopsy involving respiratory or intestinal mucosa
- Incision and drainage of infected tissue
- Genitourinary and gastrointestinal procedures, including most diagnostic and therapeutic procedures that are invasive (sclerotherapy for esophageal varices, esophageal dilation, cystoscopy, urethral dilation, urethral catheterization or surgery if urinary tract infection is present, and prostatic surgery)

Adapted from Dajani, A. S., et al. (1997). Prevention of bacterial endocarditis: Recommendations by the American Heart Association. *JAMA 277*(22), 1794–1801. Copyright 1997, American Medical Association.

- Pain (headaches, arthralgias, myalgias) related to hyperthermia.
  Expected Outcome: The pain associated with headaches, arthralgias, and myalgias will be reduced or eliminated.
- Family Knowledge Deficit related to home care of the child with bacterial endocarditis.
  Expected Outcome: The parents will be able to administer medications and monitor the child's condition.

Interventions

The child will need vigilant monitoring of vital signs, peripheral perfusion, and hemodynamic stability. Any change in the heart murmur or in tissue perfusion should be immediately reported to the physician. The child's activity level may be diminished, necessitating assistance with activities of daily living. Opportunities for quiet activities such as reading, watching videos, drawing, and doing puzzles should be provided.

The child's temperature should be monitored every 2 to 4 hours and plotted on a graph. If the child is receiving an aminoglycoside antibiotic, serum peak and trough levels should be monitored. The nurse must administer the antibiotics at the appropriate time, with trough levels determined 15 minutes before and peak levels determined 1 hour after the dose is administered. Acetaminophen is administered as needed for fever, as ordered by the physician, once the initial blood samples have been drawn for culture. Acetaminophen may also be administered for persistent headaches, arthralgias, and myalgias. Reassure the child and parents that the aches and malaise will resolve eventually.

The child may be discharged home receiving parenteral antibiotic therapy. It is imperative that the parents have access to adequate community resources. The nurse must confirm that they have undergone formal instruction in the use of the IV mode selected (e.g., heparin lock, Port-a-Cath, Hickman catheter, or percutaneous line) and the proper administration of antibiotics. Provide reassurance and support to the family and child regarding the extensive and lengthy therapy that will be needed.

Evaluation

- Have the child's vital signs improved?
- Are the blood culture results negative?
- Have symptoms of malaise, arthralgia, myalgia, and fever subsided?
- Does the child have a capillary refill of less than 2 seconds?
- Are the parents demonstrating the ability to manage their child's condition at home?

Rheumatic Fever

Rheumatic fever is an inflammatory autoimmune condition that affects the connective tissue of the heart, joints, subcutaneous tissues, or blood vessels of the central nervous system. The most serious complication is rheumatic heart disease, which affects the cardiac valves, most commonly the mitral valves, causing scarring and permanent damage.

Etiology

Rheumatic fever characteristically manifests 2 to 6 weeks after an untreated or partially treated group A beta-

---

PATHOPHYSIOLOGY
• • • • • • • • • • • •
of Rheumatic Fever

A current and popular theory suggests that colonization of the pharynx by group A beta-hemolytic streptococci triggers an abnormal immunologic response in patients who develop rheumatic fever. Sensitized B cells produce antistreptococcal antibodies that form immune complexes. These immune complexes then cross-react with cardiac tissue, initiating a myocardial and valvular inflammatory response.

From Ayoub, E. M. (1995). Acute rheumatic fever. In G. C. Emmanouilides, A. J. Moss, & F. H. Adams (Eds.), *Moss and Adams' heart disease in infants, children, and adolescents: Including the fetus and young adult* (5th ed., pp. 1400–1416). Baltimore: Williams & Wilkins.

---

hemolytic streptococcal infection of the upper respiratory tract. The initial infection may or may not produce symptoms of pharyngitis (Ayoub, 1995). There may be predisposing genetic factors. Crowding, particularly in the bedroom and classroom, also increases the risk (Todd, 1996).

Incidence

Rheumatic fever is a disease in transition. Its incidence decreased dramatically in the late 1960s and 1970s but unexpectedly rose in the middle to late 1980s (Ayoub, 1995; Todd, 1996). Rheumatic fever is most often seen in susceptible children between the ages of 5 and 15 years, and the annual incidence in the United States is less than 1 per 10,000 (Ayoub, 1995). Rheumatic fever is seasonal in occurrence, with most new cases seen in late winter and spring. The disease is slightly more common in girls than in boys and in African-American children than in Caucasians.

Manifestations

Major manifestations of rheumatic fever include the following (Fig. 46–15):

- Polyarthritis—tender, painful joints, especially in the elbows, knees, ankles, and wrists; usually seen in the acute febrile period (first 1 to 2 weeks of illness)
- Carditis—inflammation of all parts of the heart, primarily the mitral valves; characterized by a cardiac murmur, CHF, and a pericardial friction rub
- Chorea—involuntary movements of the legs, arms, and face (including speech muscles) indicating central nervous system involvement
- Erythema marginatum—red skin lesions that start as flat or slightly raised macules, usually over the trunk, and spread peripherally
- Subcutaneous nodules—small, nontender lumps, often located over the joints

Although arthritis is the most common manifestation, carditis is by far the most serious, as it is the major cause of morbidity and mortality during both acute and chronic phases of the disease. Cardiac valvular disease is the major complication of rheumatic fever (Todd, 1996).

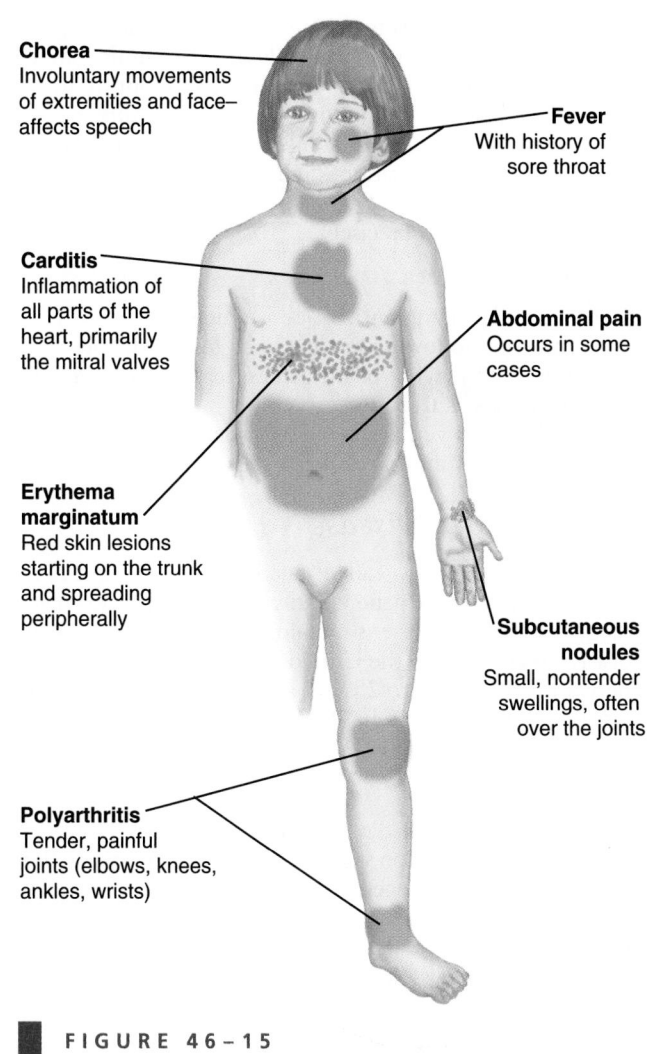

Chorea
Involuntary movements
of extremities and face–
affects speech

Fever
With history of
sore throat

Carditis
Inflammation of
all parts of the
heart, primarily
the mitral valves

Abdominal pain
Occurs in some
cases

**Erythema
marginatum**
Red skin lesions
starting on the trunk
and spreading
peripherally

**Subcutaneous
nodules**
Small, nontender
swellings, often
over the joints

Polyarthritis
Tender, painful
joints (elbows, knees,
ankles, wrists)

FIGURE 46–15

Clinical manifestations of rheumatic fever.

Diagnostic Evaluation

A diagnosis of rheumatic fever is confirmed by the presence of two major manifestations or one major and two minor manifestations from the Jones criteria, plus evidence of a recent streptococcal infection on one of the following positive diagnostic studies: antistreptolysin O titer, streptozyme, or anti-DNAse B assay. Other test results that may indicate inflammation include increases in C-reactive protein levels, antihyaluronidase levels, and the erythrocyte sedimentation rate. In patients with suspected carditis, a chest radiograph may show enlargement of the heart. An electrocardiogram will show rhythm abnormalities and evidence of myocarditis, and an echocardiogram will demonstrate the size and location of lesions.

Therapeutic Management

The management of rheumatic fever includes eradication of the streptococcal bacteria and treatment of other symptoms, such as inflammation, CHF, and chorea. Penicillin is the drug of choice. Erythromycin may be used in penicillin-

---

Diagnosis of Acute Rheumatic Fever by the Jones Criteria—1992 Update

MAJOR MANIFESTATIONS

Carditis
Polyarthritis
Chorea
Erythema marginatum
Subcutaneous nodules

MINOR MANIFESTATIONS

Fever
Arthralgia
Elevated erythrocyte sedimentation rate (ESR) or positive C-reactive protein (CRP)
Prolonged P-R interval

Plus supporting evidence of preceding streptococcal infection: history of recent scarlet fever, positive throat culture for group A streptococcus, increased antistreptolysin-O (ASO) titer, or other streptococcal antibodies.

Adapted from Todd, J. (2000). Group A streptococcus. In R. E. Behrman, R. M. Kliegman, & H. B. Jenson (Eds.), *Nelson textbook of pediatrics* (16th ed., p. 808). Philadelphia: Saunders.

---

allergic children. Prescribed anti-inflammatory agents include aspirin or corticosteroids (aspirin should not be given to a child who has chickenpox or other viral infection). The duration of therapy is tailored to meet the needs of the child. The child should receive antibiotic prophylaxis for 5 years or through adolescence, whichever is greater. Penicillin is the drug of choice.

NURSING CARE

The Child with Rheumatic Fever

Assessment

Initially, the nurse determines whether the child or any family members have had a sore throat or unexplained fever within the past 2 months. The child should be monitored for cardiac complications throughout the course of hospital-

---

CRITICAL TO REMEMBER

Streptococcal Prophylaxis for the Child with Rheumatic Fever

Streptococcal prophylaxis for 5 years or through adolescence, whichever is greater, is the most important aspect of therapeutic management because damaged valves can become further damaged with repeated infections. Intramuscular penicillin, administered monthly, is the drug of choice. Alternatives include oral penicillin taken twice daily or sulfadiazine taken orally once a day for children who are sensitive to penicillin.

ization. Temperature, pulse, respiration, and blood pressure are assessed and the child is observed for signs of carditis, including shortness of breath, edema of the face, abdomen, or ankles, and precordial pain. Examination of the joints may reveal very tender elbows, knees, ankles, and wrists, with small lumps. Assessment of pain using a self-report assessment tool provides additional information (see Chapter 39). Children with rheumatic fever may have red skin lesions spreading peripherally from the trunk. When questioned, parents may report the child has had rapid, purposeless, involuntary movements.

Nursing Diagnosis and Planning

Nursing diagnoses for the child with rheumatic fever include the following:

- Knowledge Deficits related to medications and activity restrictions.
  Expected Outcome: The child will comply with the medication regimen and activity restrictions.
- Ineffective Individual Coping related to confinement.
  Expected Outcome: The child will participate in quiet activities and maintain social contact.
- Pain related to polyarthritis.
  Expected Outcome: The child will verbalize increased comfort.
- Risk for Injury related to subsequent streptococcal infection.
  Expected Outcome: The child will inform parents at the first sign of a sore throat.

Interventions

The nurse administers antibiotics, analgesics, and antipyretics as ordered and reports to the physician any fever or pain. In addition to medications, children with rheumatic fever require bed rest during the acute febrile stage of the illness. Children should not return to school while there is clear evidence of rheumatic activity. While the child's activities are restricted, the nurse and family should talk about limiting visitors and phone calls and arranging for quiet yet enjoyable activities. Family members and friends may provide board, card, and computer games, movies, puzzles, crafts, models, and riddle books for the school-age child. Such activities will help minimize activity as well as cardiac output. The affected child may develop a daily schedule that includes rest periods interspersed with these diverse activities and some limited exercise (e.g., passive range-of-motion exercises). An art or play therapist can work with the child who is extremely anxious because of confinement. Such anxiety may place undue stress on the heart.

Nursing comfort measures include alternating application of heat and cold to affected joints, repositioning, massage, and providing distraction using guided imagery and relaxation. Seizure precautions are warranted if the child is experiencing chorea. At home, parents must practice safety measures. For example, the child who cannot control movements may need to sleep on a mattress on the floor and may need assistance going up and down stairs. The child may be embarrassed by uncontrolled movements, especially in front of peers, and will need reassurance that these symptoms are temporary.

Emphasize to parents the importance of completing the entire course of antibiotic prophylaxis. The family may be allowed to offer an older child a choice of monthly injections versus daily oral administration. If the child chooses the oral route, instruct the family about the required dose, frequency of administration, duration, effects, and side effects, as well as potential cardiac complications if the regimen is not followed precisely.

Evaluation

- Is the child taking antibiotics as ordered?
- Is the child following modified bed rest guidelines?
- Is the child playing board games, reading, and visiting with friends as tolerated?
- Has the child verbalized a decrease in pain?
- Has the child informed the parents of a sore throat?

Kawasaki Disease

Kawasaki disease, also called mucocutaneous lymph node syndrome, is a febrile generalized vasculitis of unknown etiology. Kawasaki disease is a major cause of acquired heart disease in children in the United States, affecting the coronary arteries in 20% to 25% of all children with Kawasaki disease (Rubin & Cotton, 1998).

Etiology

The cause of Kawasaki disease remains unknown. However, the clinical presentation suggests a hypersensitivity reaction to an environmental agent or a microorganism. There may be a correlation with rug shampooing, dust mites, or proximity to stagnant water (Belkengren & Sapala, 1997). Kawasaki disease also has a seasonal component; it is diagnosed most often in late winter and early spring.

Incidence

Kawasaki disease is seen most frequently in children less than 5 years old, with a peak incidence in the United States at 18 to 24 months (Rubin & Cotton, 1998). Historically, Kawasaki disease has rarely been seen in children over 8 years of age, but recent studies have identified an older population of affected children. These children are frequently diagnosed later in the course of the disease and appear to have a greater morbidity and mortality from coronary artery complications (Momenah et al., 1998). Affected boys outnumber girls 1.5 to 1, with an increased incidence in Asian children (Takahashi, 1995).

Manifestations

Kawasaki disease manifests in three phases. The acute stage lasts approximately 10 to 14 days and is characterized by a prolonged fever that persists longer than 5 days. The fever is generally 38.3° to 39.9°C (101° to 104°F) and is unresponsive to antibiotic treatment. Other clinical signs include bilateral, nonpurulent conjunctivitis; changes in the mouth (i.e., erythema, fissures, and crusting of the lips; strawberry tongue); changes in the peripheral extremities, such as induration of the hands and feet and erythema of the palms and soles; erythematous rash (Fig. 46–16); and enlarged cervical lymph nodes.

PATHOPHYSIOLOGY
· · · · · · · · · · · ·
of Kawasaki Disease

In the acute phase of Kawasaki disease, there are more helper T cells than suppressor T cells, and increased numbers of B cells spontaneously secrete IgG and IgM. Antibody-antigen complexes form and are thought to bind to the vascular epithelium, causing inflammation of the vessels and increased platelets, which result in clot formation. Vascular changes in the myocardium and coronary arteries may lead to aneurysms and myocardial infarction, resulting in death.

From Levin, M., Tizard, E. J., & Dillon, M. T. (1991). Kawasaki disease: Recent advances. *Archives of Diseases in Children, 66*(12), 1369–1372.

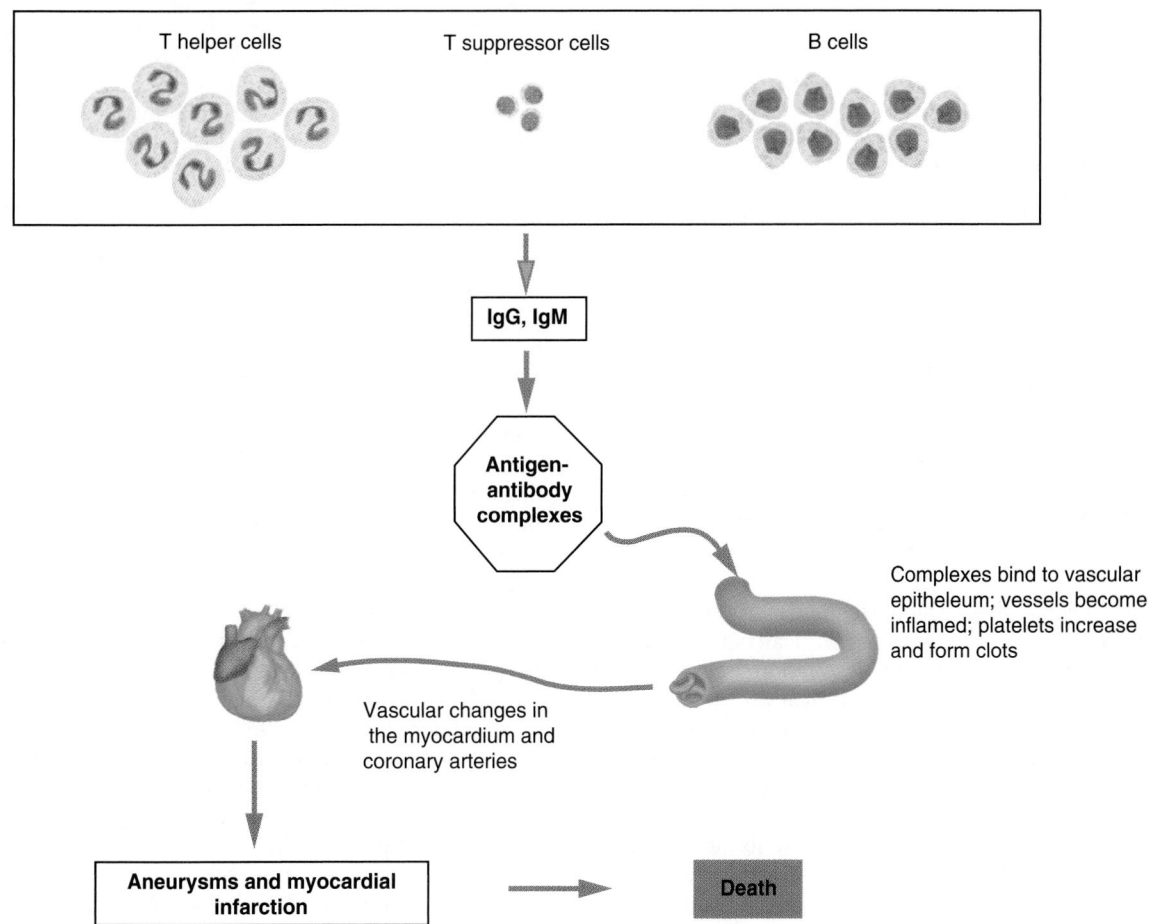

The second or subacute phase lasts approximately 10 days. The fever disappears and most symptoms resolve. The phase is characterized by extreme irritability, anorexia, lip cracking and fissuring, desquamation of the fingers and toes, arthritis and arthralgia, and cardiovascular manifestations (Rubin & Cotton, 1998; Takahashi, 1995).

Coronary aneurysm formation begins early in the second phase. A baseline echocardiogram at diagnosis with repeated studies during week 3 of the illness and again 1 month later will help identify the development of coronary artery involvement (Rubin & Cotton, 1998).

The final or convalescent stage begins on day 26 and lasts until the erythrocyte sedimentation rate returns to normal and all signs of illness have disappeared. Deep transverse grooves, called Beau's lines, may appear on the child's nails.

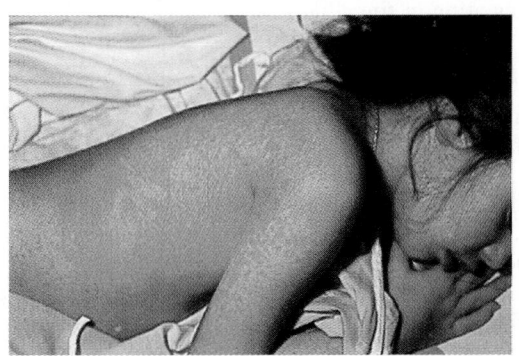

FIGURE 46-16
· · · · · · · · · ·
Erythematous rash of Kawasaki disease. (From Lookingbill, D. P., Marks, J. G., Jr. [1992]. *Principles of dermatology* [2nd ed., p. 223]. Philadelphia: Saunders.)

Diagnostic Evaluation

Fever of 5 days' duration in conjunction with four of the five primary clinical findings as described for the acute phase establishes the diagnosis of Kawasaki disease (Belkengren & Sapala, 1997; Holt, 1998; Takahashi, 1995). Laboratory data are nonspecific. The white blood cell (WBC) count is elevated during the acute phase, as is the erythrocyte sedimentation rate and C-reactive protein level. Platelet levels rise during the subacute phase. Aneurysms are detected with echocardiography.

Therapeutic Management

Therapeutic management is directed toward preventing or reducing the coronary artery damage from Kawasaki disease. At diagnosis, gamma-globulin is given IV in a dosage of 2 gm/kg over a 12-hour infusion (Rubin & Cotton, 1998). High-dose aspirin therapy is begun at the same time. Initially, the dosage is 80 to 100 mg/kg/day until fever resolves. The dosage is reduced to 3 to 5 mg/kg/day once daily and continued through weeks 6 to 8 of the illness. If coronary artery abnormalities are identified, this dosage is continued indefinitely (Belkengren & Sapala, 1997).

NURSING CARE
The Child with Kawasaki Disease

Assessment

During the acute phase, the nurse must monitor the child's cardiac status closely, looking for clinical signs and symptoms of CHF. Changes in pulse, respiration, blood pressure, and color, along with shortness of breath, chest pain, and decreased activity, may suggest cardiac complications. It is important to examine the child's eyes, mouth, and skin for signs of infection and the joints for redness, swelling, and tenderness.

The nurse should determine the parents' anxiety level. Parents are often frightened by how sick the child is and the threat of a possibly devastating outcome. Families appreciate talking about their fears, learning about the cause of the illness, the treatment plan, and the prognosis, and participating in the child's care.

Nursing Diagnosis and Planning

Nursing diagnoses for the child with Kawasaki disease and the family include the following:

■ Risk for Fluid Volume Deficit related to fever.
  Expected Outcome: The child will maintain fluid and electrolyte balance.
■ Pain related to fever, skin manifestations, and joint inflammation.
  Expected Outcome: The child will rest comfortably.
■ Fear related to changes in the child's behavior and uncertainty about the long-term prognosis.
  Expected Outcome: The parents and child will discuss their fears related to having a serious disease with a long recuperative period.

Interventions

The nurse should administer aspirin with milk or food and intravenous immune globulin (IVIG) as ordered. Often a test dose of IVIG is given before an infusion is initiated. During the test, as well as during the infusion, it is important to monitor the child's vital signs and any adverse reactions to IVIG, including facial flushing, tightness in the chest, chills, dizziness, nausea, vomiting, diaphoresis, and hypotension. Blood pressure is checked every 15 minutes for the first hour and every 30 minutes thereafter until the infusion is complete. A precipitous fall in blood pressure may occur 30 to 60 minutes after the infusion has begun and is often related to the rate of infusion. The physician will usually lower the prescribed rate of infusion if such a reaction occurs and may order diphenhydramine (Benadryl) and acetaminophen to control side effects. Epinephrine is given for anaphylactic reactions. IVIG may interfere with achieving immunity from live-virus vaccines, so some immunizations (e.g., measles-mumps-rubella) should be delayed for 5 months following IVIG therapy (Rubin & Cotton, 1998).

Nursing care focuses on comfort measures and adequate hydration. The nurse and parents must encourage fluid intake by offering frozen Popsicles or ice to numb affected mucous membranes; giving liquids that are high in calories and low in acid through a straw (avoiding citrus drinks and sodas), and applying topical anesthetics 15 to 60 minutes before offering favorite foods that are soft and bland. The nurse or family provides mouth care following any intake other than water, and applies salve to soothe cracked, dry lips.

Sponge baths with tepid water often decrease fever and relieve discomfort from skin manifestations. Because desquamation increases the risk of infection, it is important to keep the child's skin clean and dry and to avoid soap irritants. If itching is severe, the physician should be notified.

Toddlers and preschool children fear hospitalization and body changes, often exhibiting regressive behavior and sleeping poorly. Feeding, skin care, and position changes may cause pain. The nurse and family can work together to manage the child's pain by planning care so that everything that requires touching the child is done at once, and by arranging for rest periods in between care episodes. It may help to line the bed with soft blankets from home and to use the palms of the hands when lifting the child. Even in the hospital, it is possible to keep the environment calm by talking in gentle tones, playing soft music, restricting visitors and phone calls, and avoiding bright overhead lights. Assure the family that pain and irritability will eventually resolve, and praise their hard work in keeping the child comfortable. Discharge instructions should include provisions for a cardiac follow-up examination. Parents' fears can be decreased through an understanding of the disease and treatment.

Evaluation

• Is the child taking adequate amounts of fluid and maintaining electrolyte balance?
• Are the parents able to verbalize their fears, and discuss the course of the illness and their commitment to follow-up care?
• Is the child experiencing periods of uninterrupted rest?

About Kawasaki Disease

Review the following at the time of hospital discharge of a child diagnosed as having Kawasaki disease:

Skin

- Rinse with water only.
- Avoid soaps and lotions.
- Use salve on the lips.
- Call the physician for severe itching.

Temperature

- Record the child's temperature in the A.M. and P.M. before giving aspirin.
- Bring the temperature chart to all physician's appointments.

Arthritis

- Look for hot, reddened joints.
- Observe for pain with touch or movement.
- Elevate affected joints.
- Call the physician if the child refuses to walk.

Heart

- Offer a low-cholesterol diet.
- Give aspirin as ordered.
- Call the physician for bleeding or bruising, color changes, shortness of breath, chest pain, or decreased activity level.

Personality

- Discuss personality changes with household members.
- Provide support and reassurance.
- Encourage quiet activities and rest periods.
- Eliminate stimulation at naptime and bedtime.
- Play soft music and use dim lights.

Anorexia

- Offer liquids high in calories but low in acid.
- Avoid citrus juices and sodas.
- Give bland foods initially.
- Prepare favorite dishes.

Adapted from Lux, K. M. (1991). New hope for children with Kawasaki disease. *Journal of Pediatric Nursing, 6,* 159–165.

Hypertension

Hypertension is defined as an average systolic and/or average diastolic blood pressure that exceeds or is equal to the 95th percentile for age and sex, based on measurements obtained on at least three occasions. Normal blood pressure is defined as a systolic and/or diastolic pressure that is less than the 90th percentile for age and sex (see Appendix J).

The two primary categories of hypertension are essential (primary or idiopathic) and secondary (symptom of underlying disease).

Etiology

Essential hypertension is considered an inherited disorder. In essential hypertension, elevated blood pressure may be a response to environmental stimuli. Both adults and children with primary hypertension exhibit exaggerated blood pressure responses to physical and emotional stresses as compared with normotensive individuals (those having a normal blood pressure). Some individuals (particularly the African-American population) with essential hypertension also have a blood pressure increase in response to increased levels of sodium. There is also evidence of a basic defect in the sodium ion transport mechanism in patients with essential hypertension (Feld & Verga, 1997).

Height and weight are additional determinations of blood pressure in children. Children with elevated blood pressure are usually taller and heavier than their age-matched peers. Obesity is a common concurrent condition in children with hypertension (Sharma & Sinaiko, 1995).

The causes of secondary hypertension in children include coarctation of the aorta, endocrine disorders, bron-

of Hypertension

Systolic pressure reflects the stroke volume of the heart, the rate of blood ejected, and the elasticity of the aorta. Diastolic pressure reflects the resting pressure of the arterial system and is affected by the peripheral vascular resistance or the diameter of the arteries and the heart rate. An increase in the heart rate decreases the diastolic or ventricular filling time. Together, these measurements form the arterial blood pressure and provide information about arterial function.

Hypertension, or increased arterial blood pressure over time, may produce cardiac enlargement and subsequent cardiac failure, cerebrovascular disease, renal disease and failure, retinal disease, and accelerated atherosclerosis and coronary heart disease. These effects are predominantly seen with primary or essential hypertension.

chopulmonary dysplasia, and various renal and renovascular diseases. Coarctation of the aorta is the most common cardiovascular cause of hypertension. Renal arterial disease in the neonate is usually caused by renal artery thrombosis secondary to the use of umbilical artery catheters or polycythemia. Renal parenchymal disease is a common cause of hypertension in all age groups.

Incidence

Few documented studies in the pediatric population have determined the incidence of hypertension, but prevalence appears to be low prior to adulthood (Sharma & Sinaiko, 1995). Studies have reported that screening of well children for hypertension finds less than 2% of school-age children affected (Fixler & Laird, 1983; Sinaiko, Gomez-Marin, & Prineas, 1989). Blood pressure does not appear to differ significantly by racial group in children, a finding different from that in adults (Celebrado & Kaskel, 1997; Sharma & Sinaiko, 1995).

Manifestations

Children with primary hypertension rarely have clinical evidence of disease; the elevated blood pressure is usually detected on a routine physical examination. High elevations of blood pressure, however, can lead to the following manifestations:

- Essential or primary hypertension—dizziness, headaches, epistaxis, visual disturbances, neurologic deficits (late sign), extremity weakness, and cerebrovascular accident.
- Secondary hypertension—*Renal:* weight loss or failure to gain weight, facial or pretibial edema, pale mucous membranes, and unilateral or bilateral abdominal mass. *Cardiovascular:* absent or decreased femoral pulses, decreased blood pressure in the lower extremities compared to the upper extremities, cardiomegaly, murmur, and signs and symptoms of CHF.

Diagnostic Evaluation

Differentiating primary or essential hypertension from secondary hypertension requires a comprehensive physical examination and a complete medical history. Blood pressure measurements are done on all four extremities and repeated twice if elevated. Blood tests (CBC count, urinalysis, and blood urea nitrogen, creatine, uric acid, and electrolyte levels), echocardiography, ultrasonography of the kidneys, and arteriography may be performed to rule out any diseases that may be causing secondary hypertension.

The diagnosis of primary or essential hypertension is established primarily by excluding an underlying disease. In a hypertensive child with a family history of hypertension and a diagnosis established in the pre-adolescent or adolescent period it is more likely the child will have primary hypertension as opposed to secondary hypertension (O'Brien & Baker, 1999).

Therapeutic Management

PRIMARY HYPERTENSION

Treatment of primary, or essential, hypertension in children emphasizes control or elimination of risk factors. Lifestyle counseling and modification targets nonpharmacologic therapy that includes weight reduction, physical conditioning, dietary modifications, and stress modification. If the nonpharmacologic treatments are maximized, the need for pharmacologic therapy in children with hypertension should be less than 1% (Second Task Force on Blood Pressure Control in Children, 1987).

Weight Reduction. There is a direct relationship between obesity and hypertension in children and adolescents. The relationship between obesity and hypertension may be due in part to increased sympathetic nervous system activity. Weight reduction reduces this activity and plays a role in lowering blood pressure (Feld & Waz, 1997). Weight loss requires a program of diet, exercise, and lifestyle changes and may be difficult to accomplish. Success frequently depends on support from health care professionals, nutritionists, and, most important, family members.

Physical Conditioning. An exercise program should be initiated in conjunction with a dietary weight reduction plan. Not only does exercise facilitate weight loss, it also lowers blood pressure, an effect that is independent of weight loss. It has been found that 30 minutes of aerobic exercise three times per week may result in a consistently lower resting blood pressure. In adolescents, weight lifting may also lower blood pressure. Any weight-lifting or aerobic exercise program should be initiated under the supervision of a physician.

Dietary Modification. Moderate sodium restriction is recommended in hypertensive children and adolescents. The degree of sodium restriction necessary to decrease blood pressure effectively has not been established, but it is recommended that the dietary intake should be not greater than 5 to 6 g/day (Second Task Force on Blood Pressure Control in Children, 1987).

Studies have suggested a relationship between potassium and calcium levels and hypertension. Some researchers believe that both dietary potassium and calcium supplements may play a role in reducing blood pressure (Feld & Waz, 1997; Sharma & Sinaiko, 1995).

Evidence shows an association between alcohol and hypertension. The mechanism for this association is currently being studied, but it is believed to be related to the role of the renin-angiotensin system and neurotransmitters. Smoking also produces an aldosterone-like hypertension in young people. Therefore, avoidance of alcohol and tobacco is recommended.

Relaxation Techniques. Relaxation techniques and biofeedback have resulted in modest reductions in blood pressure in the adult population. Information on the efficacy of these techniques in children is not yet available. The Second Task Force on Blood Pressure Control in Children (1987), however, states that reducing undue environmental stress and providing support for coping with family and school difficulties may be effective strategies for blood pressure control.

Pharmacologic Treatment. Pharmacologic treatment of primary hypertension may be indicated if there is significant diastolic hypertension, evidence of target organ injury, and clinical signs or symptoms related to blood pressure elevation. The primary drugs used are alpha- and beta-adrenergic receptor blockers; diuretics; vasodilators, including calcium-channel blockers; and ACE inhibitors.

SECONDARY HYPERTENSION

Treatment of the underlying process is the focus of therapy in secondary hypertension. If the secondary disease is coarctation of the aorta or is renovascular in nature, surgery may be indicated. Therapy in patients with renal parenchymal or endocrine pathology focuses on the disease process; effective treatment will result in secondary control of blood pressure.

NURSING CARE
The Child with Hypertension

Assessment

Blood Pressure Screening

Blood pressure screening should be initiated when a child is 3 years old and should continue through adolescence. Blood pressure should be checked at least yearly. The environment should be as quiet as possible when auscultating the blood pressure, and the child's arm should be supported at the heart level. If an elevated blood pressure is found, measurement should be repeated two more times, allowing a 2- to 3-minute interval between blood pressure checks.

Physical Assessment

Assessment of a child with hypertension includes inspection of the skin to detect any evidence of edema, ascertain the color of mucous membranes, and document the presence or absence of café au lait spots or moon face. Any of these findings may indicate an underlying disease that may be the cause of the hypertension. The pulses should be palpated for symmetry and strength. A child with coarctation of the aorta may have bounding upper extremity pulses and diminished or absent femoral and pedal pulses. The heart is auscultated to determine the heart rate and to detect any heart murmur or gallop. The abdomen is auscultated for bruits. A neurologic examination is indicated in children with acute, severe hypertension to detect a possible cerebrovascular accident.

Nursing Diagnosis and Planning

Nursing diagnoses for the child with hypertension include the following:

■ Altered Tissue Perfusion (peripheral and cardiovascular) related to elevation in systolic and/or diastolic arterial blood pressure.
Expected Outcome: The child will maintain normal tissue perfusion with blood pressure at a controlled level (below the 95th percentile for age).
■ Ineffective Management of Therapeutic Regimen, Noncompliance related to restrictions on diet, motivation for physical conditioning, and a possible medication regimen.
Expected Outcome: The child will adhere to dietary, physical conditioning, and medication therapy.

Interventions

Nursing interventions focus on education and support of the family and adhering to the treatment regimen. The nurse may consult a dietician and collaboratively develop a teaching plan regarding a low-sodium and weight-reduction diet, if ordered. When counseling the family and child about dietary modifications, it is important to include the whole family in making the necessary dietary changes. Motivation and compliance will be much improved if all family members support the change in diet.

If a physical conditioning program is prescribed, physical activities the child enjoys are identified so that those activities can be incorporated into the conditioning plan. Other family members or friends are encouraged to join the child in the exercise program. Praise the child for progress in weight loss and increased endurance. Encourage the child to vent feelings about any possible problems related to home or school situations. Discuss methods for facilitating relaxation that may be helpful during periods of stress.

The child who is hospitalized with acute, severe hypertension may require medications. Once the child has been stabilized after an acute hypertensive crisis, oral antihypertensive medications will likely be prescribed. During discharge planning, reinforce the importance of compliance with the medication regimen and of periodic follow-up evaluations.

Evaluation

• Does the child maintain a blood pressure below the 95th percentile for age?
• Has the child maintained weight loss?
• Is the child adhering to a low-sodium diet?
• Is the child complying with the medication regimen?

Dysrhythmias

The identification of dysrhythmias in children is similar to that in adults. ECG findings are the same in children as in adults with a few variations. The heart rate is usually faster in both normal and abnormal rhythms and increases from birth to about 2 months of age, then gradually decreases with age. The QRS and PR intervals are usually shorter and increase with age.

Etiology

There are numerous causes of cardiac rhythm disturbances. Although many dysrhythmias are associated with underlying congenital heart disease, a number of children will have structurally normal hearts.

Dysrhythmias may be seen in the postoperative period following repair or palliation of a cardiac lesion. Tachydysrhythmias are frequently caused by injury to the conduc-

PATHOPHYSIOLOGY
• • • • • • • • • •
of Dysrhythmias

Dysrhythmias may be marked by a rapid heart rate (*tachy*) or a slow heart rate (*brady*).

Tachydysrhythmias. Primary tachydysrhythmias may originate in either the atria or the ventricles. The most common atrial tachydysrhythmia is supraventricular tachycardia (SVT). SVT is triggered by an atrial ectopic focus (a group of irritable cells somewhere in the atrium) or a reentry circuit (accessory pathway permitting abnormal conduction within the heart). Ventricular tachycardia is uncommon; it is seen in prolonged QT syndrome or pre- or postoperative children with underlying structural heart disease.

Bradydysrhythmias. Most often bradydysrhythmias are related to hypoxia resulting from respiratory failure or arrest. Primary cardiac bradydysrhythmias usually result from damage to the sinus node or the conduction pathway between the atria and the ventricles (AV block).

Data from Zeigler, V. L. (1994b). Supraventricular tachycardia in children: A challenge for pediatric nurses. *Journal of Pediatric Nursing, 9*(5), 288–298; Chameides, L., & Hazinski, M. F. (1997). *American Heart Association pediatric advanced life support* (3rd ed., pp. 7.1–7.15). Dallas: American Heart Association.

tion system during surgery, suture placement close to the conduction system, ischemia, or edema; bradydysrhythmias often result from damage to the sinus node, AV node, or bundle of His (Zeigler, 1994a). Postoperative patients are also at risk for acid-base and electrolyte imbalances, which may trigger rhythm disturbances.

Underlying acquired heart disease, such as myocarditis or cardiomyopathy, sometimes produces dysrhythmias. Noncardiac causes of rhythm disturbances include fever, temperature instability, hypoxia, metabolic disturbances, increased intracranial pressure, and drug therapy or reactions.

Incidence

Dysrhythmias in children are not uncommon, and most are not life-threatening. Approximately 1% to 5% of all newborns will demonstrate an irregular heart rate or rhythm within the first week of life; most are transient and rarely require treatment (Page & Hosking, 1997). Supraventricular tachycardia (SVT) is the most common primary symptomatic rhythm disturbance seen in infants and children (Page & Hosking, 1997; Zeigler, 1994b). It is believed that life-threatening rhythm disturbances are more often the result rather than the cause of cardiovascular emergencies (Chameides & Hazinski, 1997).

Manifestations

The American Heart Association and the American Academy of Pediatrics (Chameides & Hazinski, 1997) classify rhythm disturbances according to their effect on central pulses:

fast pulse rate:	tachydysrhythmia
slow pulse rate:	bradydysrhythmia
absent pulse:	pulseless arrest (collapse rhythm)

In all three classes, cardiac output is diminished. The clinical presentation represents low output syndrome with poor end-organ perfusion. The earliest signs and symptoms may be subtle; later they can be quite dramatic. Clinical manifestations for the infant and toddler may include poor feeding, irritability, lethargy, poor peripheral perfusion (diminished pulses, mottling, cool extremities, delayed capillary refill time), and CHF.

In older children palpitations, dizziness, syncope, and exercise intolerance are often demonstrated. In general, older children tolerate rhythm disturbances more easily and for longer periods of time. Infants become symptomatic sooner and demonstrate more dramatic and serious clinical signs.

Diagnostic Evaluation

The primary tool in diagnosing pediatric dysrhythmias is the 12-lead ECG. Twenty-four-hour Holter monitoring and transtelephonic monitoring may be useful in documenting specific episodes of cardiac rhythm disturbances.

Therapeutic Management

Pediatric rhythm disturbances should be treated as emergencies *only* if they compromise cardiac output or have the potential to degenerate into lethal (collapse) rhythms (Chameides & Hazinski, 1997). Management strategies include drug therapy, radiofrequency ablation, cardioversion, and pacemakers; the choice of treatment is guided by the origin of the dysrhythmia and the clinical consequences.

SUPRAVENTRICULAR TACHYCARDIA

Children who are asymptomatic and hemodynamically stable are treated conservatively. Vagal maneuvers may be used to terminate an episode of SVT by eliciting the diving reflex. Immersing the child's face in ice water stimulates a vagal response that may stop the tachycardia; placing an ice bag over the infant's face for 10 to 15 seconds accomplishes the same result (Zeigler, 1994b). Antiarrhythmic drug therapy may be successful in suppressing further episodes. As many as 30% of affected children "outgrow" this tachycardia as they pass beyond infancy (Zeigler, 1994b). Children who continue to have episodes of SVT may benefit from radiofrequency ablation of the ectopic focus or accessory pathway.

Infants and children who are hemodynamically unstable require emergency intervention. If vascular access is present, the drug adenosine may be given. Adenosine is an effective anti-arrhythmic due to its ability to slow conduction through the AV node and, in many cases, successfully terminate episodes of SVT rapidly and safely (Chameides &

Hazinski, 1997). Synchronized cardioversion, however, remains the treatment of choice for the child with profound cardiovascular compromise.

VENTRICULAR TACHYCARDIA

The emergency management of ventricular tachycardia in children who have a palpable pulse is synchronized cardioversion. Children without a pulse require defibrillation. Lidocaine, 1 mg/kg, may be administered before cardioversion, followed by a continuous infusion of the drug to prevent further episodes (Chameides & Hazinski, 1997). Once the tachycardia has been terminated, underlying causes should be explored.

BRADYDYSRHYTHMIAS

Most episodes of bradydysrhythmia are due to noncardiac causes. Airway management, oxygenation, ventilation, and cardiac compressions, if indicated, may successfully resolve the event. The use of epinephrine or atropine (or both) may be indicated if the rhythm has not improved once oxygenation and ventilation have been re-established.

Primary cardiac bradyarrhythmias are managed in the same manner. Temporary or permanent cardiac pacing may be necessary to maintain adequate cardiac output.

ABSENT RHYTHMS

The classification of absent or collapse rhythms includes asystole, ventricular fibrillation, and pulseless electrical activity. Asystole, the absence of electrical cardiac activity, is treated by initiating cardiopulmonary resuscitation (CPR) (see Chapter 34). Epinephrine is administered to stimulate cardiac activity. The drug may be given IV, intraosseously or through an endotracheal tube.

Ventricular fibrillation is rare in children and frequently due to underlying cardiac disease. The emergency management of episodes of ventricular fibrillation is defibrillation and CPR. Drugs administered during resuscitation efforts include epinephrine, lidocaine, and other antiarrhythmic agents.

Pulseless electrical activity indicates a hemodynamically compromised state in which cardiac electrical activity is unable to generate effective myocardial contraction and cardiac output. The underlying cause is usually noncardiac and must be identified and corrected for the child to survive the episode. Causes include severe hypoxia or acidosis, hypovolemia, tension pneumothorax, and cardiac tamponade. Emergency management includes CPR, administration of epinephrine, and discovery of the underlying cause (Chameides & Hazinski, 1997).

NURSING CARE
. . . .
The Child with Dysrhythmias

Assessment

Children with dysrhythmias require a thorough cardiovascular assessment because they are prone to developing car-

diogenic shock. In a stable or compensated child with dysrhythmias, it is important to obtain a comprehensive and accurate history of activity tolerance. Older children may have unexplained episodes of dizziness, palpitations, or syncope.

Nursing Diagnosis and Planning

Nursing diagnoses for the child with dysrhythmias include the following:

- Altered Tissue Perfusion related to decreased ventricular filling or decreased rate of heart contractions, leading to inadequate cardiac output.
  Expected Outcome: The child will have pink mucous membranes and nail beds, brisk capillary refill, and good-quality pulses.
- Risk for Injury related to episodes of syncope.
  Expected Outcome: The child will remain free of episodes of syncope and injury.
- Knowledge Deficit related to care of a child with a potentially fatal condition.
  Expected Outcome: The family will demonstrate an understanding of medication administration, an ability to identify signs and symptoms indicative of dysrhythmias, and be able to perform CPR.

Interventions

Nursing interventions involve immediate care of the child who is experiencing the dysrhythmias, as well as education of the child and family. The child and family will need information regarding monitoring for future signs and symptoms of dysrhythmias, administering medications as ordered, and appropriate emergency measures to initiate, including CPR, once the child has been discharged from the hospital.

Education of the child and family is imperative for those children with life-threatening dysrhythmias. Teach the child to identify the signs and symptoms of dysrhythmia, including palpitations, dizziness, and fatigue. These signs and symptoms should be reported to the parent or teacher as soon as possible and medical attention should be sought. Children who take antiarrhythmics at home need to adhere to the prescribed medication schedule closely and must be careful not to skip any doses. Parents and teachers also need to be aware of signs and symptoms that may indicate early appearance of dysrhythmias. All caretakers should complete a formal course in CPR.

Evaluation

- Have the child, parents, and other caregivers received instructions about and demonstrated an understanding of medications, activity limitations, and the possibility of a life-threatening episode?
- Are the child's pulses of good quality and mucous membranes pink?
- Has the child remained free of injury related to falling secondary to syncope?

KEY CONCEPTS

■ With the neonate's first breath, gas exchange is transferred from the placenta to the lungs. The fetal shunts (ductus venosus, ductus arteriosus, foramen ovale) close and resistance to flow in the pulmonary system decreases as systemic resistance increases. Pulmonary vascular resistance decreases and a marked increase in pulmonary blood flow follows.

■ Stenosis can occur in a valve or a vessel and result in obstruction of blood flow through the area.

■ In left-to-right shunts, blood is shunted to the right side of the heart because the pressure is higher on the left side. Oxygenated and unoxygenated blood mixes.

■ Poor weight gain with failure to thrive is a common sign of congenital heart disease.

■ Hypercyanotic episodes, or "tet spells," are characterized by increased respiratory rate, depth of respiration, and hypoxemia.

■ Assessment of the family of a child with a congenital cardiac defect should begin at diagnosis and continue throughout the care of the child.

■ Common nursing diagnoses associated with infants with congenital heart defects and their parents include activity intolerance, knowledge deficit, anxiety, altered family processes, risk for infection, pain, and risk for altered health maintenance.

■ Signs of right-sided heart failure include ascites, liver and spleen enlargement, edema, and neck vein distension. Signs of left-sided heart failure include dyspnea, rales, tachypnea, intercostal muscular and sternal retractions, and wheezing. Signs of both left- and right-sided heart failure are tachycardia, cardiomegaly, gallop rhythm, decreased peripheral perfusion, excessive diaphoresis, and weight gain.

■ Measures to decrease the workload on the heart include limiting the time the child is allowed to bottle-feed or nurse, elevating the head of the bed, allowing for uninterrupted rest periods, and providing oxygen during stressful periods.

■ It is imperative to educate parents regarding medications, monitoring for signs and symptoms of congestive heart failure, and decreasing stress in the environment as the family is prepared for home discharge with infants or children with congestive heart failure.

■ Prophylaxis with penicillin for 5 years or through adolescence, whichever period is longer, is the most important aspect of therapeutic management for rheumatic fever. Intramuscular injection is the route of choice. Oral medication is an alternative, if given precisely and faithfully.

■ In Kawasaki disease, coronary aneurysms may occur about 11 days after the onset of fever. Nursing management includes administering intravenous immune globulin and aspirin to reduce the formation of the aneurysms and fever.

■ The initial management of children with primary hypertension includes diet modification, reduction of weight (when needed), physical conditioning, and relaxation techniques.

■ An appropriate-sized blood pressure cuff, two repeat blood pressure readings on all four extremities, and a careful medical history are important in assessment for a diagnosis of hypertension.

■ The heart rate in a child is usually faster in both normal and abnormal rhythms and increases from birth to 2 months of age, then gradually decreases with age.

ANSWERS TO CRITICAL THINKING EXERCISE 46-1

1. Appropriate questions to ask concerning infant feeding patterns include these:
   • How often does she eat?
   • How much does she eat at each feeding?
   • Does she tire easily?
   • Does she require frequent rest periods?
   • Do you notice beads of perspiration on her forehead during feedings?
   • Do you notice any change in her color or respiratory pattern during feedings?
   • Does she raise her eyebrows or wrinkle her forehead during feedings?

2. Some frequently seen physical assessment findings associated with congestive heart failure include tachycardia; tachypnea; increased work of breathing—nasal flaring, grunting, use of accessory muscles; pulmonary congestion, crackles; dry cough; hepatomegaly; distended neck veins; and periorbital, facial, or generalized edema.

3. Nutritional nursing care would include:
   • Enlarging the nipple hole to reduce the energy needed to suck.
   • Feeding every 3 hours, allowing rest periods between feedings.
   • Increasing the caloric content of the formula.
   You may need to provide supplemental feedings at night through a nasogastric tube.

   Comfort measures include allowing rest periods between feedings. Do not overtire infants with multiple interventions at any one time. Place infants and children in a position of comfort, usually with the head of the bed elevated to decrease the work of breathing.

REFERENCES AND READINGS

American Academy of Pediatrics. (1987). Report of the Second Task Force on Blood Pressure Control in Children. *Pediatrics, 79*(1), 1–25.

Artman, M. (1995). Pharmacologic therapy. In G. C. Emmanouilides, A. J. Moss, & F. H. Adams (Eds.), *Moss and Adams' heart disease in infants, children, and adolescents: Including the fetus and young adult* (5th ed., pp. 375–378). Baltimore: Williams & Wilkins.

Ayoub, E. M. (1995). Acute rheumatic fever. In G. C. Emmanouilides, A. J. Moss, & F. H. Adams (Eds.), *Moss and Adams' heart disease in infants, children, and adolescents: Including the fetus and young adult* (5th ed., pp. 1400–1416). Baltimore: Williams & Wilkins.

Baker, A. (1994). Acquired heart disease in infants and children. *Critical Care Nursing Clinics of North America, 6*(1), 175–186.

Beekman, R. H. (1995). Coarctation of the aorta. In G. C. Emmanouilides, A. J. Moss, & F. H. Adams (Eds.), *Moss and Adams' heart disease in infants, children, and adolescents: Including the fetus and young adult* (5th ed., pp. 1111–1133). Baltimore: Williams & Wilkins.

Belkengren, R., & Sapala, S. (1997). Pediatric management problems. *Pediatric Nursing, 23*(4), 4094–4095.

Bernstein, D. (1996). The cardiovascular system. In R. E. Behrman, R. M. Kliegman, & A. M. Arvin (Eds.), *Nelson's textbook of pediatrics* (15th ed., pp. 1262–1374). Philadelphia: Saunders.

Brook, M. (1998). The cardiovascular system. In R. E. Behrman & R. M. Kliegman (Eds.), *Nelson's essentials of pediatrics* (3rd ed., pp. 497–544). Philadelphia: Saunders.

Celebrado, N. C., & Kaskel, F. (1997). Measurement of blood pressure. In L. G. Feld (Ed.), *Hypertension in childhood* (pp. 9–37). Boston: Butterworth-Heinemann.

Chameides, L., & Hazinski, M. F. (1997). *American Heart Association pediatric advanced life support* (3rd ed., pp. 7.1–7.15). Dallas: American Heart Association.

Dajani, A. S., & Taubert, K. A. (1995). Infective endocarditis. In G. C. Emmanouilides, A. J. Moss, & F. H. Adams (Eds.), *Moss and Adams' heart disease in infants, children, and adolescents: Including the fetus and young adult* (5th ed., pp. 1541–1553). Baltimore: Williams & Wilkins.

Dajani, A. S., Taubert, K. A., & Wilson, W. (1997). Prevention of bacterial endocarditis: Recommendations by the American Heart Association. *JAMA, 227*(22), 1794–1801.

DeJong, M. J. (1998). Infectious endocarditis. *American Journal of Nursing, 98*(5), 34–35.

Doerr, C., & Starke, J. (1996). Infective endocarditis. In J. Ingelfinger, E. Wald, & R. Polon (Eds.), *Gillis and Kagan's current pediatric therapy* (16th ed.). Philadelphia: Saunders.

Engel, J. (1997). Pocket guide to pediatric assessment (3rd ed., pp. 3–17, 167–180). St. Louis: Mosby.

Estlow, M. M. (1998). Prevention of infective endocarditis in the pediatric congenital heart population. *Pediatric Nursing, 24*(3), 205–225.

Feld, L. G., & Verga, P. A. (1997). Causes of hypertension in children. In L. G. Feld (Ed.), *Hypertension in childhood* (pp. 39–65). Boston: Butterworth-Heinemann.

Feld, L. G., & Waz, W. R. (1997). Nonpharmacologic therapy of hypertension. In L. G. Feld (Ed.), *Hypertension in childhood* (pp. 111–131). Boston: Butterworth-Heinemann.

Feldt, R. H., Porter, C. J., Edwards, W. D., et al. (1995). Atrioventricular septal defects. In G. C. Emmanouilides, A. J. Moss, & F. H. Adams (Eds.), *Moss and Adams' heart disease in infants, children, and adolescents: Including the fetus and young adult* (5th ed., pp. 704–724). Baltimore: Williams & Wilkins.

Fixler, D. E., & Laird, W. P. (1983). Validity of mass blood pressure screening in children. *Pediatrics, 72,* 459–463.

Freedom, R. (1995). Pulmonary atresia with intact ventricular septum. In G. C. Emmanouilides, A. J. Moss, & F. H. Adams (Eds.), *Moss and Adams' heart disease in infants, children, and adolescents: Including the fetus and young adult* (5th ed.). Baltimore: Williams & Wilkins.

Freedom, R. M., & Benson, L. N. (1995). Hypoplastic left heart syndrome. In G. C. Emmanouilides, A. J. Moss, & F. H. Adams (Eds.), *Moss and Adams' heart disease in infants, children, and adolescents: Including the fetus and young adult* (5th ed., pp. 1133–1153). Baltimore: Williams & Wilkins.

Friedman, W. F. (1995). Aortic stenosis. In G. C. Emmanouilides, A. J. Moss, & F. H. Adams (Eds.), *Moss and Adams' heart disease in infants, children, and adolescents: Including the fetus and young adult* (5th ed., pp. 1087–1111). Baltimore: Williams & Wilkins.

Gaedeke-Norris, M. K., & Hill, C. S. (1994). Nutritional issues in infants and children with congenital heart disease. *Critical Care Nursing Clinics of North America, 6*(1), 153–163.

Graham, T. P., & Gutgesell, H. P. (1995). Ventricular septal defects. In G. C. Emmanouilides, A. J. Moss, & F. H. Adams (Eds.), *Moss and Adams' heart disease in infants, children, and adolescents: Including the fetus and young adult* (5th ed.). Baltimore: Williams & Wilkins.

Hinocki, K. W. (1998). Congenital heart disease: Effects on the family. *Neonatal Network, 7,* 1–10.

Holt, C. F. (1998). Alterations in cardiovascular status. In V. R. Bowden, S. B. Dickey, & C. S. Greenberg (Eds.), *Children and their families: The continuum of care* (pp. 782–862). Philadelphia: Saunders.

Kirsten, D. (1996). Patent ductus arteriosus in the preterm infant. *Neonatal Network, 15*(2), 19–26.

Kohr, L., & O'Brien, P. (1995). Current management of congestive heart failure in infants and children. *Nursing Clinics of North America, 30*(2), 261–290.

Levin, M., Tizard, E. J., & Dillon, M. T. (1991). Kawasaki disease: Recent advances. *Archives of Diseases in Children, 66*(12), 1369–1372.

Lux, K. M. New hope for children with Kawasaki disease. *Journal of Pediatric Nursing, 6,* 159–165.

Mair, D. D., Edwards, W. D., Julsnid, P. R., et al. (1995). Truncus arteriosus. In G. C. Emmanouilides, A. J. Moss, & F. H. Adams (Eds.), *Moss and Adams' heart disease in infants, children, and adolescents: Including the fetus and young adult* (5th ed., pp. 1036–1041). Baltimore: Williams & Wilkins.

Momenah, T., Sanatania, S., Potts, J., et al. (1998). Kawasaki disease in the older child. *Pediatrics, 102*(1), 7–13.

Moody, L. Y. (1997). Pediatric cardiovascular assessment and referral in the primary care setting. *The Nurse Practitioner, 22*(1), 120–134.

Nadas, A. S. (1992). Hypoxemia. In Fyler, D. C. (Ed.), *Nadas' pediatric cardiology* (pp. 73–76). Philadelphia: Hanley-Belfus.

O'Brien, P., & Baker, A. L. (1999). The child with cardiovascular dysfunction. In D. L. Wong et al. (Eds.), *Whaley and Wong's nursing care of infants and children* (6th ed., pp. 1583–1649). St. Louis: Mosby.

O'Brien, P., & Smith, P. A. (1994). Chronic hypoxemia in children with cyanotic heart disease. *Critical Care Nursing Clinics of North America, 6*(1), 215–226.

Page, J., & Hosking, M. (1997). An approach to the neonate with sudden dysrhythmia: Diagnosis, mechanisms, and management. *Neonatal Network, 16*(6), 7–17.

Paul, K. E. (1995). Recognition, stabilization, and early management of infants with critical congenital heart disease in the first days of life. *Neonatal Network, 14*(5), 13–19.

Paul, M. H., & Wernovsky, G. (1995). Transposition of the great arteries. In G. C. Emmanouilides, A. J. Moss, & F. H. Adams (Eds.), *Moss and Adams' heart disease in infants, children, and adolescents: Including the fetus and young adult* (5th ed., pp. 1154–1245). Baltimore: Williams & Wilkins.

Pelech, A. N. (1998). The cardiac murmur: When to refer? *Pediatric Clinics of North America, 45*(1), 107–122.

Porter, C. J., Feldt, R. H., & Edwards, W. D., et al. (1995). Atrial septal defects. In G. C. Emmanouilides, A. J. Moss, & F. H. Adams (Eds.), *Moss and Adams' heart disease in infants, children, and adolescents: Including the fetus and young adult* (5th ed., pp. 687–703). Baltimore: Williams & Wilkins.

Rocchini, A. P., & Emmanouilides, G. C. (1995). Pulmonary stenosis. In G. C. Emmanouilides, A. J. Moss, & F. H. Adams (Eds.), *Moss and Adams' heart disease in infants, children, and adolescents: Including the fetus and young adult* (5th ed., pp. 930–962). Baltimore: Williams & Wilkins.

Rosenthal, A., & Dick, M. (1995). Tricuspid atresia. In G. C. Emmanouilides, A. J. Moss, & F. H. Adams (Eds.), *Moss and Adams' heart disease in infants, children, and adolescents: Including the fetus and young adult* (5th ed., pp. 902–918). Baltimore: Williams & Wilkins.

Rubin, B., & Cotton, D. M. (1998). Kawasaki disease: A dangerous acute childhood illness. *The Nurse Practitioner, 23*(2), 34–48.

Second Task Force on Blood Pressure Control in Children. (1987). Report of the Second Task Force on Blood Pressure Control in Children: National Heart, Lung, and Blood Institute—1987. *Pediatrics, 79*(1), 1–25.

Sharma, A., & Sinaiko, A. R. (1995). Systemic hypertension. In G. C. Emmanouilides, A. J. Moss, & F. H. Adams (Eds.), *Moss and Adams' heart disease in infants, children, and adolescents: Including the fetus and young adult* (5th ed., pp. 1641–1659). Baltimore: Williams & Wilkins.

Sinaiko, A. R., Gomez-Marin, O., & Prineas, R. J. (1989). Prevalence of "significant" hypertension in junior high school-aged children. *Journal of Pediatrics, 114,* 664–669.

Smith, J. B., Baker, A. L., Moynihan, P. J., Lincoln, P., & Kane, P. L. (1996). Cardiovascular critical care problems. In M. A. Q. Curley, J. B. Smith, & P. A. Maloney-Harmon (Eds.), *Critical care nursing of infants and children* (pp. 557–618). Philadelphia: Saunders.

Smith, K. M. (1997). The innocent heart murmur in children. *Journal of Pediatric Health Care, 11*(5), 207–214.

Spilman, L. J., & Furdon, S. A. (1998). Recognition, understanding, and current management of cardiac lesions with decreased pulmonary bloodflow. *Neonatal Network, 17*(4), 7–18.

Stollerman, G. H. (1997). Rheumatic fever. *Lancet, 349,* 935–942.

Takahashi, M. (1995). Kawasaki syndrome. In G. C. Emmanouilides, A. J. Moss, & F. H. Adams (Eds.), *Moss and Adams' heart disease in infants, children, and adolescents: Including the fetus and young adult* (5th ed., pp. 1390–1399). Baltimore: Williams & Wilkins.

Talner, N. S. (1995). Heart failure. In G. C. Emmanouilides, A. J. Moss, & F. H. Adams (Eds.), *Moss and Adams' heart disease in infants, children, and adolescents: Including the fetus and young adult* (5th ed., pp. 1746–1775). Baltimore: Williams & Wilkins.

Teitel, D. F., & Cassidy, J. W. (1995). Fetal and post-natal circulations: Systemic circulation. In G. C. Emmanouilides, A. J. Moss, & F. H. Adams (Eds.), *Moss and Adams' heart disease in infants, children, and adolescents: Including the fetus and young adult* (5th ed., pp. 47–59). Baltimore: Williams & Wilkins.

Todd, J. (2000). Group A streptococcus. In R. E. Behrman, R. M. Kleigman, & H. B. Jenson (Eds.), *Nelson textbook of pediatrics* (16th ed., p. 808). Philadelphia: Saunders.

Wood, M. K. (1998). Acyanotic cardiac lesions with normal pulmonary blood flow. *Neonatal Network, 17*(3), 5–11.

Zeigler, V. L. (1994a). Postoperative rhythm disturbances. *Critical Care Nursing Clinics of North America, 6*(1), 227–235.

Zeigler, V. L. (1994b). Supraventricular tachycardia in children: A challenge for pediatric nurses. *Journal of Pediatric Nursing, 9*(5), 288–298.

Zuberbuhler, J. R. (1995). Tetralogy of Fallot. In G. C. Emmanouilides, A. J. Moss, & F. H. Adams (Eds.), *Moss and Adams' heart disease in infants, children, and adolescents: Including the fetus and young adult* (5th ed., pp. 998–1018). Baltimore: Williams & Wilkins.

47

The Child with a Hematologic Alteration

After studying this chapter, you should be able to:

- Describe the anatomy and physiology of the hematopoietic system.
- Discuss the pediatric differences related to blood.
- Discuss the role of the nurse in the prevention of iron deficiency anemia.
- Describe common factors in the care of a child with anemia.
- Discuss the pathology and therapeutic management of common hematologic alterations.
- List possible nursing diagnoses for children with hematologic alterations.
- Describe possible nursing care for children with hematologic alterations.

DEFINITIONS

autoimmune disorder A disorder in which the body launches an immunologic response against itself.

chelation Binding of a metallic ion with a structure so that the ion is inactivated.

erythropoiesis Production of erythrocytes.

extramedullary Outside the bone marrow.

granulocytes Polymorphonuclear leukocytes (neutrophils, eosinophils, or basophils).

hematopoiesis Production of blood cells; normally occurs in the bone marrow, but may occur in extramedullary sites.

hemolysis Breakdown of red blood cells.

hemosiderosis Focal or general increase in tissue iron stores without associated tissue damage.

pancytopenia A reduction in all types of blood cells.

reticulocyte Immature red blood cell; normal value for children is 1%.

reticuloendothelial system The collection of cells, throughout the body, that are capable of phagocytosis.

Nursing Diagnosis, Planning, Intervention, and Evaluation

Nursing Diagnosis	■ Altered Tissue Perfusion related to anemia.
Expected Outcome	• The child will have adequate or optimal tissue perfusion, as evidenced by a normal level of consciousness, vital signs within normal range for age, oxygen saturation of 95% or greater, and a urine output of at least 1 to 2 ml/kg/hr.

Intervention	Rationale
1. Examine the child for signs of decreased tissue perfusion by assessing level of consciousness, activity level, vital signs, respiratory effort, capillary refill time, mucous membrane color, urine output, and oxygenation saturation. Document findings and report any abnormalities to the physician.	1. Visible deterioration in tissue perfusion is an early warning sign that vital organs are not receiving enough oxygen.
2. Administer RBCs as ordered.	2. RBCs are used *only* in children with severe anemia, and after a reliable response to iron therapy has not been demonstrated. When administered, RBC transfusions deliver needed cells without the risk of volume overload associated with whole blood transfusion.

Evaluation	• Did the child experience deterioration in level of consciousness, cardiac output, urine output, or activity level? • Has the child maintained an oxygen saturation level of 95% or greater? • Can parents describe an iron-rich diet appropriate for the child's age?
Nursing Diagnosis	■ Altered Nutrition: Less Than Body Requirements related to parents' poor knowledge of age-appropriate nutritional needs.
Expected Outcome	• The child's iron, hemoglobin, and hematocrit levels will be normal within 6 weeks after initiation of therapy.

Intervention	Rationale
1. Assess the child's past and current nutritional history. Instruct the caregiver to continue to give infant iron-fortified formula or breast feed and give supplementary iron-fortified foods until age 12 months. In a child older than age 12 months, milk intake should be decreased to 24 oz/day or less.	1. Therapy is based on the child's history. Cow's milk is poorly digested and is not rich in iron. The American Academy of Pediatrics (AAP) recommends continuing breast milk or iron-fortified formula until age 12 months. Decreasing milk intake will encourage the consumption of other iron-rich foods.
2. Begin the child on iron-fortified formula and, if old enough, iron-rich foods. Depending on the child's age, suggest intake of liver, dried beans, Cream of Wheat, iron-fortified cereal, apricots, prunes, egg yolks, and leafy dark green vegetables.	2. Iron-fortified formula and food will establish healthier eating habits.
3. Administer vitamin C as ordered, and encourage intake of foods rich in vitamin C.	3. Vitamin C increases the absorption of iron by the body.
4. Administer oral iron supplements as ordered by the physician. Iron is usually given in three divided doses between meals. Encourage administration on an empty stomach, with fruit juice, and avoid administration with milk, formula, and cereals.	4. The immediate need is to increase iron intake beyond that absorbed from formula or food. An acid stomach environment facilitates absorption.
5. Administer iron through a straw or medicine dropper placed at the back of the mouth. Brush or wipe teeth after administration.	5. Iron temporarily stains teeth.
6. Instruct parents to keep iron supplements out of reach of children.	6. Iron poisoning is possible with overdose. This can be serious, possibly even fatal.
7. Monitor the child's laboratory values, including reticulocyte count and hemoglobin level.	7. Reticulocyte count should peak in 5 to 7 days. It serves as an objective test for determining the parents' degree of compliance with therapy. The hemoglobin level should increase in 4 to 30 days (Behrman et al., 1996).

8. Instruct parents to expect dark, black stools, and inquire about their presence.

9. Obtain a social services consult for enrollment in a federal or state social services program, if warranted.

8. The absence of tarry stools may indicate lack of compliance with therapy.

9. Poor nutritional habits may be attributable to a lack of resources.

Evaluation

- Has the child experienced a recurrence of iron deficiency anemia?
- Does the child have normal iron, hemoglobin, and hematocrit levels, and do the child and family demonstrate a change in eating habits?

Nursing Diagnosis

■ Knowledge Deficit concerning age-appropriate nutritional intake.

Expected Outcome

- The parents will effectively administer iron and will demonstrate or confirm an appropriate change in the child's diet.

Intervention	Rationale
1. Explain the need for iron in the manufacture of RBCs, the effect of iron therapy on laboratory test results, the potential outcome with no intervention, the lack of iron in cow's milk, and iron's effect on the body.	1. Providing explanations of the rationale for therapy can often help improve compliance with therapy.
2. Obtain a nutritional consult.	2. The dietician will reinforce the principles of good dietary habits. Preventing iron deficiency anemia is the goal of nursing care.
3. Teach parents the appropriate method for administering iron. (See Parents Want to Know About Home Care of a Child with Iron Deficiency Anemia.)	3. Do not assume the parents are able to administer iron effectively. Evaluate their technique of medication administration and offer suggestions as necessary.

Evaluation

- Can the parents demonstrate compliance with the prescribed therapy and verbalize appropriate questions?

■ Sickle Cell Disease

Sickle cell disease (SCD) is the generic term that refers to a group of genetic disorders characterized by the production of sickle hemoglobin (HbS), chronic hemolytic anemia, and ischemic tissue injury. The more common forms of sickle cell disease include homozygous HbSS disease (sickle cell anemia), HbC disease (sickle C disease), and the sickle beta-thalassemia syndromes. SCD is an inherited, lifelong disease that primarily affects African-Americans but can also occur in individuals of Mediterranean, Indian, and Middle Eastern descent. Morbidity and mortality from the severe forms of the disease have decreased as a result of newborn screening for the disease, routine prophylactic penicillin administration, and pneumococcal and *Hemophilus influenzae* vaccines.

Etiology

SCD is a group of hemoglobinopathies in which normal hemogloblin is partially or totally replaced by an abnormal hemoglobin, hemoglobin S (HbS). They are inherited, autosomal recessive diseases (see Chapter 9). If one parent has the HbS trait and the other parent is normal, each pregnancy has a 50% risk of having the child inherit the trait. If each parent carries the trait, there is a 25% chance that the child will be normal, a 50% chance that the child will carry the trait, and a 25% chance that the child will have the disease. The carrier state of SCD—sickle

cell trait—may produce clinical symptoms in times of extreme stress, as the carrier state may reflect a high portion of HbS.

Incidence

There appears to be a geographic variable in the incidence of SCD. Among African-Americans the incidence of sickle cell trait is 7% to 13%, whereas the incidence among East Africans is as high as 45% (Kline & Mooney, 1998). It has been proposed that the sickle trait may be a protective mechanism against the lethal forms of malaria in the malaria-endemic zones of the Mediterranean and Africa.

Manifestations

All of the clinical manifestations of SCD are a result of the obstructions caused by the sickled RBCs and the increased destruction of sickled and normal RBCs caught in microcirculation obstructions. Large amounts of fetal hemoglobin (HbF) present in the first few months of life obscure the presence of HbS, so that symptoms of the disease usually do not appear until age 4 to 6 months.

The disease affects most organ systems. Delayed puberty and growth are common. The child usually has small stature throughout adolescence but attains normal growth in the early 20s.

The general manifestations of SCD (chronic hemolytic

the life span of their sickled RBCs is shortened. Prenatal diagnosis is an option and is done using chorionic villus sampling at 8 to 10 weeks' gestation or amniocentesis at 15 weeks' gestation.

Therapeutic Management

In SCD, the spleen often does not function properly or has been surgically removed owing to complications. Functional or actual asplenia places children and adults with SCD in an immunocompromised state. Bacterial septicemia is associated with a 15% mortality in children with SCD under the age of 3 years (Cooperative Study of Sickle Cell Disease, 1995; Wang et al., 1996). The bacteria *Streptococcus pneumoniae* and *Hemophilus influenzae* are normally destroyed by the reticuloendothelial system of the spleen, but because children with SCD do not have a properly functioning spleen, they are considered to be more susceptible to infection with these bacteria.

The natural history of splenic dysfunction in children with HbSS places them at higher risk for fulminant septicemia and death during the first 3 years of life than children with HbC. Prophylactic daily penicillin therapy is recommended in all children with suspected or actual diagnosis by age 2 months and is continued until at least age 5 years (AAP Committee on Infectious Diseases, 1997a). Although views regarding the use of penicillin differ, some experts will continue penicillin prophylaxis throughout childhood in high-risk patients with asplenia. The pneumococcal vaccine is recommended at age 2 years, with revaccination after 3 to 5 years for children age 10 years or younger and for older children who were immunized at least 5 years earlier (AAP Committee on Infectious Diseases, 1997a). *H. influenzae* vaccine is recommended at 2 months of age, as in healthy children, and to all previously unimmunized children with asplenia (AAP Committee on Infectious Diseases, 1997a). The hepatitis B series should be given because of the number of transfusions these children receive. Moreover, they should receive the influenza vaccine annually (AAP Committee on Infectious Diseases, 1997b).

The treatment of SCD focuses on prompt diagnosis, education about the disease, prevention of exacerbations, and supportive care during crises (hydration, oxygenation, analgesia, and RBC transfusion). Additional therapies currently under investigation include erythrocytapheresis (removal of sickled erythrocytes via an exchange transfusion technique), phenotyping RBCs for transfusion ("tissue typing" blood products that can potentially reduce alloimmunization), and hydroxyurea administration (augments HbF, which interferes with the RBC sickling process).

Research toward a cure continues; especially promising may be gene therapy. Another promising area of research is hematopoietic stem cell transplantation (HSCT) (marrow transplantation). HSCT has been successful with strict candidate selection criteria. There are logistical and ethical issues related to this curative strategy. Table 47–1 presents the therapeutic management of SCD.

▌ NURSING CARE
• • • • • • • • • •
The Child with Sickle Cell Disease

Assessment

On initial diagnosis, the subjective data usually include parental concern that the child is in pain. The parents may have noticed swelling of the joints or the child's refusal to move an extremity, or the child's crying out when a joint is moved or touched. Fever and irritability may accompany the pain. Parents of a child already diagnosed with SCD who have been educated about the signs of complications will give a much more detailed history of the present illness. A nurse familiar with the child can become adept at assessing the severity of that child's condition. The presence of SCD does not eliminate other serious causes of pain.

Despite teenagers' ability to verbalize symptoms, assessment of adolescents who are experiencing pain is a unique challenge. During the developmental time in their life when they most want to fit in with their peer group, teenagers with SCD are different. After the initial pain of an episode has subsided, teens may seek attention from health care providers in an attempt to avoid their peer group, verbalizing continued symptoms that would make them unable to return to their normal activities. Objective data will vary according to the type of painful episodes. Meperidine (Demerol) is no longer recommended for long-term pain management because of its side effects. Morphine is the current drug of choice.

Parents should be taught to assess the size of the child's spleen for close monitoring of the child's condition.

Nursing Diagnosis, Planning, Intervention, and Evaluation

Nursing Diagnosis	■ Altered Tissue Perfusion related to vaso-occlusion and anemia.
Expected Outcomes	• The child's oxygen saturation level will be maintained at 95% or greater.
	• The child will exhibit no long-term complications from a lack of oxygen.

Intervention	Rationale
1. Assess the child's vital signs and respiratory status every 4 hours and as needed.	1. Respirations are assessed frequently to detect changes in respiratory status quickly. Signs of respiratory decompensation include increasing respiratory rate, increased work of breathing, decreased oxygenation saturation, poor color, and altered level of consciousness. Change in level of consciousness often indicates poor perfusion or oxygenation of the brain.
2. Use pulse oximetry.	2. Oxygen saturation levels are monitored with pulse oximetry.
3. Administer oxygen as ordered to keep saturation levels at 95% or greater.	3. Delivering oxygen helps ease the child's work of breathing and facilitates tissue oxygenation. Oxygen does not reverse the sickling process but may prevent more sickling.
4. Elevate the head of the bed to a comfortable level and encourage deep breathing.	4. Raising the head of the bed facilitates chest expansion by decreasing pressure on the diaphragm. Children with chest syndrome have shallow respirations and exhibit guarding (see Table 47–1).
5. Assess level of comfort frequently and administer analgesia.	5. Painful crises can affect level of comfort. In particular, chest crises may impede full diaphragmatic excursion and encourage shallow, ineffective respirations.
6. Administer RBCs as ordered.	6. Transfusions of normal RBCs will increase the oxygen-carrying capacity of the blood and decrease the relative amount of sickled cells.

Evaluation	• Is the child able to resume usual activities?
	• Can the child maintain an oxygen saturation level of 95% or greater?

Nursing Diagnosis	■ Pain related to vaso-occlusion.
Expected Outcome	• The child will have decreased pain, as evidenced by a lowered score on the selected pain assessment tool.

Intervention	Rationale
1. Assess pain every 1 to 2 hours and more frequently if needed, using a pain assessment tool appropriate for the child's age.	1. Pain can be very severe in vaso-occlusive crisis and is relieved for only short periods of time. An assessment tool is helpful in determining the child's level of discomfort.
2. Administer analgesics as ordered.	2. Analgesics may be administered intermittently, via a patient- or parent-controlled analgesic pump, or by continuous infusion.
3. Increase oral fluids, if able to tolerate, and administer fluids intravenously at a rate that is 1½ to 2 times the maintenance rate.	3. Increased fluid volume helps reduce the viscosity of the blood, thus alleviating sites of vascular occlusion and preventing further sickling secondary to dehydration.
4. Administer RBCs as ordered.	4. This measure increases oxygen-carrying capacity to prevent further sickling and microvascular ischemia.
5. Incorporate the use of age-appropriate nonpharmacologic pain relief measures.	5. Comfort measures often help distract the patient from discomfort (see Chapter 39).

Evaluation	• Does the child verbalize or demonstrate decreased pain?
	• Does review of the child's pain assessment tool show a decrease in discomfort?

NURSING CARE
The Child with von Willebrand Disease

Assessment

A careful history detailing episodes of bruising and bleeding is essential. Possible causes of any previous episodes of bleeding, if any can be identified, should also be discussed. Ask how many times the child has experienced a nosebleed, how long the child bleeds from "normal" trauma, and whether there is a history of prolonged bleeding associated with surgery or trauma associated with prolonged bleeding.

Physical examination usually reveals a normal child except for evidence of bruising greater than expected for the degree of trauma experienced. If the child is being seen after a major bleeding episode, signs of hemorrhage or a decreased hemoglobin level (or both) will be seen.

Nursing Diagnosis and Planning

The following nursing diagnoses and expected outcomes may be appropriate following assessment of the child with von Willebrand disease:

- Risk for Injury related to hemorrhage due to platelet adhesion dysfunction.
  Expected Outcome: The child will experience no life-threatening episodes of hemorrhage.
- Knowledge Deficit related to the disorder.
  Expected Outcome: The child and family will verbalize an understanding of the disorder and its chronic nature.

Intervention

Education of the family is aimed at producing an understanding of the precautions to take with the child, as well as knowledge of when prophylactic therapy should be given prior to elective procedures. The child should wear a Medic Alert tag at all times. The family should be referred to the Hemophilia Foundation for support services (see Appendix L). Avoidance of prescription and over-the-counter medications that affect platelet function, such as aspirin, is also recommended.

The degree of activity limitation will depend on the severity of the disorder. Limitations may include avoidance of contact sports, especially football.

Evaluation

- Are episodes of bleeding minimal and controlled?
- Does the family communicate an understanding of the importance of avoiding medications that affect platelet function and avoiding activities that increase the risk of bleeding?

Immune Thrombocytopenic Purpura

Immune thrombocytopenic purpura (ITP) is a hematologic disorder resulting in a reduction in and destruction of platelets. This disorder may be seen by nurses in both inpatient and outpatient settings, depending on the severity of the illness. With greater recognition of the immunologic component of this disease, the name of the disease has been changed from *idiopathic* to *immune* thrombocytopenic purpura.

Pathophysiology

ITP is an autoimmune disorder resulting in both destruction of circulating platelets and decreased production of platelets by the bone marrow. ITP may be acute and self-limiting, or it may be chronic, requiring therapy.

Etiology and Incidence

The cause of ITP is unknown, but it typically occurs after a febrile, viral illness. The peak age of onset for ITP is 2 to 5 years, and it occurs with equal frequency in male and female patients (Imbach, Kühne, & Holländer, 1997).

Manifestations

Clinical manifestations of ITP include excessive bruising and petechiae, especially involving the mucous membranes and sclera (Fig. 47–2).

Diagnostic Evaluation

The initial diagnostic evaluation should include a thorough history and a CBC, including evaluation of a peripheral blood smear. The history should include information about any medications the child has taken that could cause thrombocytopenia, and any instances of illness, especially febrile illness, in the past month. In an affected child, the initial CBC will reveal a low platelet count, often below 50,000/mm³, but the results will otherwise be normal. The physical examination findings will be normal, aside from the signs of bleeding.

If any data in the history or CBC are suggestive of a diagnosis other than ITP, the physician may obtain a bone marrow aspirate to rule out an oncologic disorder and to determine whether megakaryocytes, the precursors of platelets, are present. Routine bone marrow examination is not warranted in a child with findings consistent with acute ITP.

Physical examination of the affected child reveals

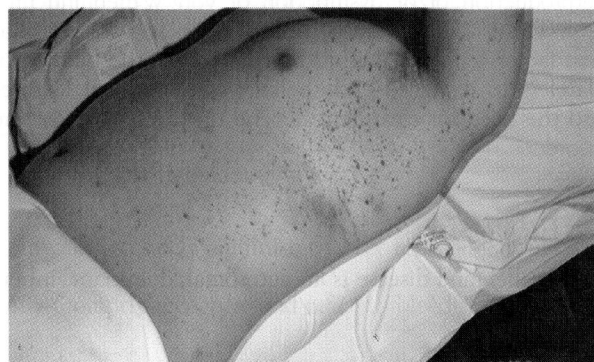

FIGURE 47-2

Multiple petechiae are characteristic of immune thrombocytopenic purpura. This disorder results in the destruction of circulating platelets and decreased bone marrow production of new platelets. (Courtesy of Cook Children's Medical Center, Fort Worth, Texas.)

bruising and petechiae, the severity of which depends on how low the platelet count is and the child's tolerance of the low platelet count. The spleen and liver are generally normal in size. The greatest risk of a low platelet count is intracranial hemorrhage, so a neurologic assessment is important.

Therapeutic Management

The goal of treatment is to prevent rare, life-threatening bleeding events such as intracranial bleeding. Additional goals include restoration of the platelet count to above 20,000/mm^3 in children with mucocutaneous bleeding and a reduction in the duration of thrombocytopenia. Treatment is based on the child's presenting condition.

Most cases are self-limiting, with a normal platelet count returning within 6 months with no therapy (George et al., 1996; Warrier et al., 1997). However, some physicians prefer to initiate treatment at the time of diagnosis.

Depending on whether the child is an inpatient or outpatient, intravenous or oral steroids may be administered over a 2- to 4-week period. For unknown reasons, the steroids block the autoimmune destruction of platelets. The other drug that may be used to treat ITP is intravenous immune globulin (IVIG), administered once daily for 3 days. Often, the platelet count is dramatically increased after one dose of IVIG.

ITP is considered to be acute if recovery of a normal platelet count is seen within 6 months. The condition becomes chronic if it lasts longer than 6 months. Children with chronic ITP may initially respond to steroids with an increase in platelet count, but it will not reach normal levels. These children may go for long periods without experiencing problems with excessive bleeding or a low platelet count; the count will then begin to decline again, at which time steroid therapy should be resumed.

When steroids and IVIG do not control the thrombocytopenia in a child with chronic ITP, a splenectomy may

be indicated. Splenectomy will cure most children with chronic ITP because the spleen synthesizes the antiplatelet antibody that results in the destruction of circulating platelets. The risk associated with removal of the spleen is sepsis from those organisms that the spleen's reticuloendothelial system fights. Without the spleen, the body's ability to fight *Streptococcus pneumoniae*, *Hemophilus influenzae*, and *Neisseria meningitidis* is limited. This limitation is greater in children under age 5 years, so ITP is managed without splenectomy, if possible, until age 5 years. Platelet transfusions are given only in children when active, uncontrolled bleeding occurs.

NURSING CARE

The Child with Immune Thrombocytopenic Purpura

Assessment

Parents usually bring their child to the physician because they have noticed excessive bruising or a "red rash" in the child's mouth or on the child's body. Although this "rash" may look remarkable to a nurse, it often evolves so gradually that it escapes the immediate notice of a parent who sees the child every day. As a result, health care may not be sought until very significant bruising and petechiae, even hematomas, are present.

Affected children usually demonstrate normal activity levels for their age, as they do not "feel bad." Assessment should include observation for signs of any further bruising or bleeding, including epistaxis, hematuria, or blood in the stools, as well as for signs of a decreasing level of consciousness, which could indicate intracranial hemorrhage.

Nursing Diagnosis and Planning

The following nursing diagnoses and expected outcomes may be appropriate following assessment of the child with ITP:

- Risk for Injury related to hemorrhage due to low platelet count.
  Expected Outcome: The child will exhibit no signs of active bleeding or intracranial hemorrhage.
- Risk for Infection related to chronic use of steroids, or to splenectomy.
  Expected Outcome: The child will respond rapidly to treatment for infections.
- Knowledge Deficit related to the disorder and its therapeutic management.
  Expected Outcome: The child and family will verbalize an understanding of ITP and the treatment plan.

Interventions

The family is referred to a nursing care center to carry out medical treatments, and the family is educated about ITP and home care.

Often, an intravenous access line is established for the purpose of administering intravenous steroids or IVIG. It can be quite challenging to establish intravenous access in children with ITP because merely puncturing the skin may result in a hematoma, which may be confused with "blow-

---

PARENTS WANT TO KNOW

About Home Care of the Child with Immune Thrombocytopenic Purpura

- Eliminate participation in high-risk activities such as contact sports, bicycle riding, roller skating, and diving if the child's platelet count is low.
- Avoid medications that can affect platelet function.
- Use an extra-soft toothbrush if the platelet count is less than 20,000/mm^3.
- Establish an age-appropriate, safe home environment.
- Pad table corners.
- Pad crib rails.
- Offer extra joint padding on clothes.
- For additional resources and information, contact national organizations (for example, the ITP Society of the Children's Blood Foundation; see Appendix L).

ing" the vein. Careful flushing of the intravenous catheter with normal saline will confirm proper placement of the catheter.

Restricting the activity of toddlers and young children can be a challenge. Extra-soft-bristle toothbrushes or toothettes should be used on all children whose platelet count is less than $20,000/mm^3$. Until the platelet count returns to normal, activities such as bicycle riding, contact sports, and roller skating should be curtailed.

Education includes teaching the family about the disease process of ITP; the side effects of steroids and IVIG, if used; the need to restrict the child's activity; and the importance of proper follow-up evaluations. Parents should be instructed regarding the signs and symptoms of infection, as steroids may mask an infection. (See also Parents Want to Know about Home Care of the Child with Immune Thrombocytopenic Purpura.)

If the child has had a splenectomy, pneumococcus vaccine or daily penicillin (or both) should be administered. Any signs and symptoms of infection should be reported immediately to the physician so that proper therapy can be initiated before the infection becomes life-threatening.

Evaluation

- Have areas of ecchymosis and petechiae decreased?
- Does the family verbalize and implement a plan of care that decreases the risk of the child incurring an injury that is likely to cause hemorrhage?
- Does the family respond quickly to early signs of infection by notifying the primary health care provider?

Disseminated Intravascular Coagulation

Disseminated intravascular coagulation (DIC) is an acquired hemorrhagic syndrome characterized by uncontrolled formation and deposition of fibrin thrombi, and by the resulting consumption of clotting factors leading to uncontrolled bleeding. In children, DIC occurs without the overwhelming mortality that occurs in adults. The key to recovery is identification and treatment of the underlying cause of the DIC.

Etiology

DIC is triggered by any factor that causes endothelial damage, liberation of tissue thromboplastin, circulating endo-toxins, or immune complexes. In children the most common causes are trauma, hypoxia, necrotizing enterocolitis, shock, liver disease, overwhelming viral or bacterial infections, and acute promyelocytic leukemia.

Manifestations

Manifestations of DIC involve an insidious onset, corresponding to platelet count and fibrinogen levels. Early indicators include excessive bruising and petechiae, oozing from puncture sites, oozing from sites of mild tissue trauma (e.g., site of insertion of a nasogastric tube), and mild gastrointestinal bleeding. As the disease progresses, manifestations of

PATHOPHYSIOLOGY

of Disseminated Intravascular Coagulation

Disseminated intravascular coagulation (DIC) is a consumptive disorder caused by abnormal activation of the clotting mechanism, which causes rapid depletion of platelets, prothrombin, and fibrinogen. It is a pathologic syndrome resulting from the formation of thrombin, subsequent activation and consumption of certain coagulant proteins, and the production of fibrin thrombi. DIC manifests with diffuse microvascular coagulation secondary to depletion of clotting factors, resulting in impaired hemostasis.

The pathophysiology of DIC is complicated and often not easily understood, as both excessive bleeding and excessive clotting are occurring at the same time. The syndrome of DIC leads to deposition of platelet and fibrin plugs in the vasculature and the simultaneous depletion of platelets and clotting factor proteins.

The process of blood coagulation follows either an intrinsic or an extrinsic pathway (Nathan & Oski, 1999). Both pathways ultimately lead to the common pathway of prothrombin forming thrombin, which, in the presence of fibrinogen, forms fibrin. Alternately, fibrinolysis (clot destruction) requires the presence of thrombin. During this process, the enzyme plasmin lyses fibrin into fragments called fibrin degradation products (FDPs), which interfere with the ability of platelets to adhere to one another. In DIC, initiation of the clotting process is stimulated by endothelial damage or some form of tissue injury. Platelets and clotting factors are subsequently depleted. As clotting is stimulated, the body perceives the need to produce substances to dissolve those clots, and there is an increase in the end result of clot lysis, FDPs. The overstimulation of both of these normal processes has three major effects on the body:

- Increased, uncontrolled bleeding resulting from the depletion of platelets and clotting factors and overstimulation of the fibrinolytic process.
- Anemia caused by the excessive bleeding and the mechanical fragmentation of RBCs.
- Organ damage secondary to the formation of emboli.

• • • • • • • • • • •
Confirmatory Laboratory Findings in Disseminated Intravascular Coagulation

- Decreased RBC count
- Low platelet count noted on CBC count
- RBC fragments on the smear
- Prolonged prothrombin time
- Decreased fibrinogen level
- Elevated levels of fibrin degradation products (e.g., D-dimer)

DIC include purpural rash, worsening of bleeding, hemoptysis, hypoxemia, oliguria progressing to renal failure, progressive organ failure, and intracranial hemorrhage.

Diagnostic Evaluation

The diagnosis of DIC is confirmed by laboratory testing.

Therapeutic Management

To control DIC, the clinician must identify and then treat the underlying cause of the condition. Treatment then becomes symptomatic and directed at replenishing consumed coagulation factors. Depleted coagulation factors are replaced (e.g., cryoprecipitate, fresh frozen plasma [FFP]) to normalize the PT by replacing fibrinogen and other clotting factors. RBCs and platelet transfusions can aid in replacing cells lost in hemorrhage. Exchange transfusions may be used in neonates to minimize the excessive fluid volume required by replacing platelets, clotting factors, and RBCs. Vitamin K may also be administered to normalize the PT. The most familiar drug used to dissolve clots is heparin. However, heparin has a controversial role in the treatment of childhood DIC except in that associated with acute promyelocytic leukemia.

NURSING CARE
• • • • • • • • • • •
The Child with Disseminated Intravascular Coagulation

Assessment

DIC typically develops in a child who is already hospitalized. The subjective and objective data assessed will depend entirely on the initial illness. The nurse must be cognizant of the patient who is at risk for DIC. Evidence of bleeding at any site of integumentary interruption and at every orifice should be assessed. The nurse should also note any changes in the pattern of vital signs. Adequate tissue perfusion should be confirmed, as normal function of an organ is the end result of sufficient oxygenation of that organ. Children with full clinical manifestations of DIC are typically cared for in an intensive care setting owing to the complex multisystem sequelae and management of DIC.

Nursing Diagnosis and Planning

The following nursing diagnoses and expected outcomes may be appropriate following assessment of the child with DIC:

- Risk for Injury related to hemorrhage due to depletion of clotting factors and platelets and increased circulating fibrin degradation products (FDP).
  Expected Outcome: The child will receive prompt appropriate treatment for bleeding.
- Risk for Injury related to organ damage due to emboli formation obstructing adequate blood flow.
  Expected Outcome: The child will maintain adequate cardiac output and tissue perfusion.
- Anxiety related to illness.
  Expected Outcome: The family will demonstrate positive coping mechanisms.

Interventions

Any areas of active bleeding should be located promptly and pressure applied, if possible. Continue to monitor the child for overt and covert signs of bleeding. Care should be taken to avoid any unnecessary tissue trauma or injury. Intravenous lines and indwelling tubes should be secured and protected to eliminate the additional trauma caused by reinsertion. Frequent monitoring of vital signs is necessary to identify changing patterns and ensure adequate cardiac output and end-organ perfusion. Laboratory results are also monitored carefully, with particular attention to the trending of values. Medical orders are followed with regard to the administration of medicines, blood products, and treatments, including monitoring of patient tolerance and outcomes. Because hypoxemia and acidosis may actually cause DIC, adequate ventilation must be ensured to prevent or reduce compromised respiratory function.

The morbidity and mortality of children with DIC depend on the underlying causative condition. With prompt recognition of both the underlying cause and diagnosis of DIC, and with proper management of both, these children can have favorable outcomes.

Evaluation

- Were early signs of DIC identified, and was the child transferred to an intensive care unit for specialized care?
- Are the child's organs functioning?
- Are the child's vital signs within normal limits for age?
- Has the family asked questions about DIC, mobilized support systems, and discussed their fears related to the child's condition?

Aplastic Anemia

Aplastic anemia is a condition in which the bone marrow ceases production of the cells it normally manufactures. The result is peripheral *pancytopenia*.

Etiology and Incidence

Aplastic anemia can be congenital, acquired, or idiopathic. Several rare, inheritable disorders are characterized by aplastic anemia. The most common of these is Fanconi's anemia. Aplastic anemia can also be acquired; a number of agents and conditions have been implicated. These most often include drugs or chemicals and less often radiation exposure, viruses, and immune diseases. Most cases of aplastic anemia in children are idiopathic. If the disease is acquired, the causative agent damages the bone marrow, preventing

PATHOPHYSIOLOGY
. . . .
of Aplastic Anemia

Aplastic anemia is characterized by cessation of hematopoiesis by the bone marrow of granulocytes, erythrocytes, and megakaryocytes. The disease may be classified as mild, moderate, or severe, depending on how low the values are for absolute neutrophil count, platelet count, and absolute reticulocyte count. The diagnosis of severe aplastic anemia requires two of the following anomalies: granulocyte count less than 500/µl, platelet count less than 20,000/µl, and reticulocyte count below 1% (after correction for hematocrit). In addition, the bone marrow biopsy must contain less than 25% of the normal cellularity (Alter & Young, 1998).

the development of granulocytes, RBCs, and platelets. Aside from antineoplastic agents, the drug used in pediatric care that most commonly causes aplastic anemia is chloramphenicol. Acquired aplastic anemia has a poorer prognosis with a more rapid progression than the primary types.

Annually, in the United States and Europe, the incidence of aplastic anemia is two cases per million per year. Leukemia, by comparison, has an incidence of 50 cases per million per year (Nathan & Oski, 1998).

Manifestations

The clinical manifestations of aplastic anemia include petechiae, bruising, pallor, epistaxis, fatigue, tachycardia, and infection.

Diagnostic Evaluation

Although the diagnosis of aplastic anemia may be suspected from the child's history and the results of a CBC, bone marrow aspiration and biopsy must be performed to confirm the diagnosis. Biopsy results should reveal the presence or absence of precursors of the mature cells found in a peripheral blood sample. In aplastic anemia, these precursors are notably absent from the marrow sample. This type of marrow is described as hypocellular and often contains a predominance of lymphocytes.

Therapeutic Management

If the aplastic anemia is determined by history to be acquired, exposure to the causative agent is discontinued immediately. Treatment then is based on symptoms. Platelet and RBC transfusions may be ordered. Granulocyte transfusions are not used due to their short life span in the circulation. If symptoms of infection are present, antibiotics are administered after appropriate cultures are obtained.

Drugs used to treat aplastic anemia include steroids, cyclosporin, and antithymocyte globulin (ATG)/antilymphocyte globulin (ALG) and colony-stimulating factors. Although these drugs are usually the first course of therapy, allogeneic marrow transplantation remains the treatment of choice for patients with severe aplastic anemia for whom a suitable donor has been identified (Vlachos & Lipton,

1996). See Chapter 48 for a discussion of marrow transplantation.

NURSING CARE
. . . .
The Child with Aplastic Anemia

Assessment

The subjective assessment usually elicits parents' observations of bruising immediately after an event that would not normally result in a bruise. An observant parent may have noticed petechiae in the child's mouth while assisting the child in brushing the teeth. Information should be elicited about drugs recently taken or recent exposures to environmental substances outside the child's usual realm in an effort to determine possible drug- or chemical-related causes for the pancytopenia.

Petechiae, bruising, pallor, lethargy, and tachycardia are the usual abnormal findings and are directly related to the degree of pancytopenia. Otherwise, the results of the physical assessment are usually normal.

Nursing Diagnosis and Planning

The following nursing diagnoses and expected outcomes may be appropriate for the child with aplastic anemia:

- Risk for Infection related to granulocytopenia.
  Expected Outcome: The child will remain free of infection.
- Risk for Injury related to bleeding due to thrombocytopenia.
  Expected Outcome: The child will not experience episodes of major bleeding.
- Altered Tissue Perfusion related to anemia.
  Expected Outcome: The child's demand for oxygen will be balanced with the body's supply.
- Knowledge Deficit related to the disease process.
  Expected Outcome: The child and family will verbalize an understanding of the disease process and its potential complications.

Interventions

Nursing care initially focuses on providing supportive care and preventing any serious physiologic sequelae of pancytopenia. Because of the increased risk of bacterial infection, affected children should be assigned to private rooms and instructed in meticulous hand washing. Precautionary measures should be taken as for any individual with a low platelet count, including no injections, no rectal temperatures, use of an extra-soft-bristle toothbrush or toothette, abstinence from any contact sports or activity, and periodic assessment for increased bleeding.

Physicians' orders should be followed with regard to blood transfusions, acquisition of blood cultures, and administration of antibiotics. Usually, the platelet count will be maintained at a level greater than 20,000/mm³ to prevent intracranial hemorrhage or signs of active bleeding. The hemoglobin level is typically maintained above 7 g/dl. If any symptoms of infection are present, blood should be drawn for culture. The need for other cultures will depend on the child's symptoms.

Antibiotics should be administered immediately to a

febrile child with neutropenia, owing to the risk of rapid, overwhelming sepsis. Children who are hospitalized, febrile, and neutropenic should be assessed frequently for signs of septic shock. Assessment includes the quality of peripheral pulses compared to central pulses, extremity temperature, capillary refill time, level of consciousness, and vital signs.

Education of the family and child should include information about the disease process and the complications that should be reported promptly to the health care provider. Often, referral is made to a marrow transplant center. If so, intense pretransplant education is indicated. The Aplastic Anemia Foundation of America is a good source of informa-

tion for children, parents, and health care providers (see Appendix L). Follow-up studies should include frequent CBC and physical examinations.

Evaluation

- Has the family received instruction regarding the disease and home care and verbalized an understanding of the information?
- Has the child remained free from infection?
- Has the child experienced any major bleeding?
- Is the child able to participate in age-appropriate activities?

KEY CONCEPTS

- For RBCs to carry oxygen, there must be an adequate amount of hemoglobin, the level of which depends on sufficient circulating iron.
- Anemia results from blood loss, decreased production of RBCs or hemoglobin, or increased destruction of RBCs.
- Caring for children with blood disorders requires an understanding of the anatomy and physiology of blood and blood-forming tissues, genetics, and the care of children with a chronic disease.
- The number of RBCs varies according to age, gender, and the altitude at which a person lives.
- Iron deficiency anemia can largely be prevented by teaching parents the importance of providing iron-fortified formula or breast milk with iron supplementary foods, such as iron-fortified cereal, to children until age 12 months.

- Morphine is the drug of choice for children with pain secondary to a "painful episode" associated with sickle cell disease.
- Complications associated with sickle cell anemia can be reduced through early screening, parent/child education, routine immunizations, pneumococcal and influenza immunizations, penicillin prophylaxis, and early diagnosis and management of complications.
- Children with decreased platelet counts and factor disorders should not receive aspirin or have their temperature taken rectally. Invasive procedures should be done only when necessary and then only with extreme caution to avoid hemorrhage.
- Factor prophylaxis is warranted in infants and young children with hemophilia who are at risk for developing joint problems secondary to bleeding.

- Bleeding associated with hemophilia is treated with rest, ice, elevation, compression, and factor replacement, as necessary.
- Education of the family about home care for the child with hemophilia should include information on the management of bleeding episodes, environmental safety, administration of medications, health promotion, and normal growth and development.
- Educating the family of a child with ITP about the need to restrict activity and to provide protection is a major nursing challenge.
- Treatment of DIC is directed toward treating the cause of the condition.
- Nursing care of the child with aplastic anemia focuses on the prevention of infection secondary to pancytopenia.

ANSWERS TO CRITICAL THINKING EXERCISE 47-1

1. Mrs. Anders is probably most concerned about Jacob's cough and fever. For that reason, the nurse will want to address the acute illness and then approach Mrs. Anders about concerns related to the anemia. Nurses must be sensitive to what parents perceive as priorities and should address those needs, so that the parents will be able to give their attention to other concerns. In this case, even if Jacob has a minor common cold, the nurse can provide Mrs. Anders with information that will make Jacob more comfortable and then approach the treatment of anemia.

2. Although the priority is to take action related to the acute disease, it is also a time to assess the child and to provide preventive care. Some families see health care providers only when they are ill. Knowing the severity of the acute illness, the nurse can determine what can be achieved during the visit and what warrants a follow-up.

3. It is an opportunity to start or update a child's health records through assessment of the child and communicating with the parent and the child, if age appropriate. Such a visit also provides an

opportunity to administer immunizations, if the child is not too ill, and to provide anticipatory guidance related to nutrition, safety, growth and development, and preventive care. For Jacob, the nurse will want to do a thorough nutrition assessment to determine if diet is the causative factor in the anemia. To increase the chance of compliance, a system of tracking children with diseases that need long-term treatment should also be in place.

REFERENCES AND READINGS

Adams, D. M., Schultz, W. H., Ware, R. E., & Kinney, T. R. (1996). Erythrocytapheresis can reduce iron overload and prevent the need for chelation therapy in chronically transfused pediatric patients. *Journal of Pediatric Hematology/Oncology,* 18(1), 46–50.

Alter, B. P., & Young, N. S. (1998). The bone marrow failure syndrome. In D. G. Nathan & S. H. Orkin (Eds.), *Nathan and Oski's hematology of infancy and childhood* (5th ed., pp. 237–335). Philadelphia: Saunders.

American Academy of Pediatrics Committee on Infectious Diseases. (1997a). Active and passive immunization. In G. Peter (ed.), *Report of the committee on infectious diseases: 1997 Red book* (24th ed., pp. 1–68). Elk Grove Village, IL: American Academy of Pediatrics.

American Academy of Pediatrics Committee on Infectious Diseases. (1997b). Section III: Summaries of infectious diseases. In G. Peter (ed.), *Report of the committee on infectious diseases: 1997 Red book* (24th ed., pp. 129–592), Elk Grove Village, IL: American Academy of Pediatrics.

American Academy of Pediatrics Committee on Nutrition. (1998). *Pediatrics nutrition handbook* (4th ed). Elk Grove Village, IL: American Academy of Pediatrics.

Behrman, R. E., Kliegman, R. M., & Arvin, A. (Eds.). (1996). *Nelson textbook of pediatrics* (15th ed.). Philadelphia: Saunders.

Burke, S. M. (1996). Hydroxyurea in sickle cell anemia. *American Journal of Maternal-Child Nursing,* 21(4), 210.

Cahill, M. (1996). Hematologic problems in pediatric patients. *Seminars in Oncology Nursing,* 12(1), 38–50.

Cahill-Alsip, C., & McDermott, B. (1996). Hematologic critical care problems. In M. A. Curley, J. B. Smith, & P. Moloney-Harmon (Eds.), *Critical care nursing of infants and children* (pp. 793–818). Philadelphia: Saunders.

Camitta, B. M., Thomas, E. D., Nathan, D. G., Santos, G., Gordon-Smith, E. D., Gale, R. P., Rappeport, J. M., & Storb, R. (1976). Severe aplastic anemia: A prospective study of the effect of early marrow transplantation on acute mortality. *Blood,* 48(1), 63–70.

Conner-Warren, R. L. (1996). Pain intensity and home pain management of children with sickle cell disease. *Issues in Comprehensive Pediatric Nursing,* 19, 183–195.

Cooperative Study of Sickle Cell Disease [Gill, F. M., Sleeper, L. A., Weiner, S. J., Brown, A. K., Bellevue, R., Grover, R., Pegelow, C. H., & Vichinsky, E.]. (1995). Clinical events in the first decade in a cohort of infants and children with sickle cell disease. *Blood,* 86, 776–783.

Curley, M. A., Smith, J. B., & Moloney-Harmon, P. (Eds.). (1996). *Critical care nursing of infants and children.* Philadelphia: Saunders.

Day, S. W., Brunson, G. E., & Wang, W. C. (1997). Successful newborn sickle cell trait counseling program using health department nurses. *Pediatric Nursing,* 23(6), 557–561.

Diav-Citrin, O., & Koren, G. (1997). Oral iron chelation with deferiprone. *Pediatric Clinics of North America,* 44(1), 235–247.

DiMichele, D. (1996). Hemophilia 1996: New approach to an old disease. *Pediatric Clinics of North America,* 43(3), 709–732.

George, J. M., Woolf, S. H., Raskob, G. E., Wasser, J. S., Aledort, L. M., Ballen, P. J., Blanchette, V. S., Bussel, J. B., Cines, D. B., Kelton, J. G., Lichtin, A. E., McMillan, R., Okerbloom, J. A., Regan, D. H., & Warrier, I. (1996). Idiopathic thrombocytopenic purpura: A practice guide-line developed by explicit methods for The American Society of Hematology. *Blood,* 88, 3–40.

Golden, C., Styles, L., & Vichinsky, E. (1998). Acute chest syndrome and sickle cell disease. *Current Opinion in Hematology,* 5(2), 89–92.

Guyton, A. C., & Hall, J. E. (1996). *Textbook of medical physiology* (9th ed). Philadelphia: Saunders.

Hilliard, L. M., Lounsbury, A. E., & Howard, T. H. (1998). Erythrocytapheresis limits iron accumulation in chronically transfused sickle cell patients. *American Journal of Hematology,* 59(1), 28–35.

Honig, G. H. (1996). Hemoglobin disorders. In R. E. Behrman, R. M. Kliegman, & A. Arvin (Eds.), *Nelson textbook of pediatrics* (15th ed., pp. 1401–1404). Philadelphia: Saunders.

Hoppe, C., Styles, L., & Vichinsky, E. (1998). The natural history of sickle cell disease. *Current Opinion in Pediatrics,* 10(1), 49–52.

Imbach, P. A., Kühne, T., & Holländer, G. (1997). Immunologic aspects in the pathogenesis and treatment of immune thrombocytopenic purpura in children. *Current Opinion in Pediatrics,* 9, 35–45.

Johnson, F. L. (1996). What is the most effective treatment of children with severe aplastic anemia who lack a matched sibling donor? *Bone Marrow Transplantation,* 18, S30–S44.

Johnston, H. S. (1999). Beta-thalassemia. In F. D. Burg, E. R. Wald, J. R. Ingelfinger, & R. A. Polin (Eds.), *Gellis & Kagen's current pediatric therapy* (pp. 693–694). Philadelphia: Saunders.

Kline, N. E., & Mooney, K. H. (1998). Alteration of hematologic function in children. In K. L. McCance & S. E. Huether (Eds.), *Pathophysiology: The biologic basis for disease in adults and children* (3rd ed., pp. 935–945). St. Louis: Mosby.

Lane, P. A. (1996). Sickle cell disease. *Pediatric Clinics of North America,* 43(3), 639–665.

Lee, G. R., Foerster, J., Lukens, J. N., Paraskevas, F., Greer, J., & Rodgers, G. M. (Eds.). (1999). *Wintrobe's clinical hematology* (10th ed.). Baltimore: Williams & Wilkins.

Medeiros, D., & Buchanan, G. (1996). Current controversies in the management of idiopathic thrombocytic purpura during childhood. *Pediatric Clinics of North America,* 43(3), 757–772.

Nathan, D. G., & Oski, S. H. (1998). Nathan & Oski's *hematology of infancy and childhood* (5th ed.) Philadelphia: Saunders.

Ohene-Frempong, K., & Smith-Whitley, K. (1997). Use of hydroxyurea in children with sickle cell disease: What comes next? *Seminars in Hematology,* 34(3), 30–41.

Parker, R. I. (1997). Etiology and treatment of acquired coagulopathies in the critically ill adult and child. *Critical Care Clinics,* 13(3), 591–609.

Rogers, M. C. (Ed.). (1992). *Textbook of pediatric intensive care* (3rd ed.). Baltimore: Williams & Wilkins.

Rohaly-Davis, J., & Johnston, K. (1996). Hematologic emergencies in the intensive care unit. *Critical Care Nursing Quarterly,* 18(4), 35–43.

Souid, A. K., & Sadowitz, D. (1995). Acute childhood immune thrombocytopenic purpura. *Clinical Pediatrics,* 34, 487–494.

Storb, R. (1997). Hematopoietic stem cell transplantation in nonmalignant disease. *Journal of Rheumatology,* Suppl. 48, 30–35.

Styles, L. A., & Vichinsky, E. P. (1997). New therapies and approaches to transfusion in sickle cell disease in children. *Current Opinion in Pediatrics,* 9(1), 41–45.

Tarantino, M. D., Madden, R. M., Fennewald, D. L., Patel, C. C., & Bertolone, S. J. (1999). Treatment of childhood acute immune thrombocytopenic purpura with anti-D immune globulin or pooled immune globulin. *The Journal of Pediatrics,* 134(1), 21–26.

U.S. Department of Health and Human Services, Agency for Health Care Policy and Research. (1993). *Sickle cell disease: Screening, diagnosis, management, and counseling in newborns and infants.* Rockville, MD: Author.

Vermylen, C., & Cornu, G. (1997). Hematopoietic stem cell transplantation for sickle cell anemia. *Current Opinion in Hematology,* 4(6), 377–380.

Vichinsky, E. P. (1997). Hydroxyurea in children: Present and future. *Seminars in Hematology,* 34(3), 22–29.

Vlachos, A., & Lipton, J. M. (1996). Bone marrow failure in children. *Current Opinion in Pediatrics,* 8(1), 33–41.

Wang, W. C., Wong, W. Y., Rogers, Z. R., Wilimas, J. A., Buchanan, G. R., & Powars, D. R. (1996). Antibiotic-resistant pneumococcal infection in children with sickle cell disease in the United States. *Journal of Pediatric Hematology/Oncology,* 18(2), 140–144.

Warrier, I., Bussel, J. B., Valadex, L., Barbosa, J., Beardsley, D. S., & the Low-Dose IVIG Study Group. (1997). Safety and efficacy of low-dose intravenous immune globulin (IVIG) treatment for infants and children with immune thrombocytopenic purpura. *Journal of Pediatric Hematology/Oncology,* 19(3), 197–201.

Weatherall, D. J. (1997). The thalassaemias. *British Medical Journal,* 314, 1675–1678.

Werner, E. J. (1996). Von Willebrand disease in children and adolescents. *Pediatric Clinics of North America,* 43(3), 683–706.

48

The Child with Cancer

DEFINITIONS

blast cell   Immature white blood cell, such as a lymphoblast, myeloblast, or monoblast.

cellular immunity   Immunologic response to an antigen that results in increased production of T lymphocytes by the thymus.

clean margins   Evidence of normal, disease-free tissue in the outermost layer of cells of a surgical sample.

hepatosplenomegaly   Enlargement of the liver and spleen, detected by palpation of the abdomen.

humoral immunity   Immunologic response to an antigen that results in production of B lymphocytes.

immunosuppression   A weakening or cessation of the body's normal immune response.

intrathecal   Within the spinal column.

lymphadenopathy   Swelling of the lymph nodes, detected by palpation.

neutropenia   A decrease in the number of circulating neutrophils that results in a decreased ability of the body to fight infection.

protocol   A systematic plan of care, including drug therapy and follow-up care, that is based on research in cancer therapy.

thrombocyte   Platelet; necessary for blood clotting.

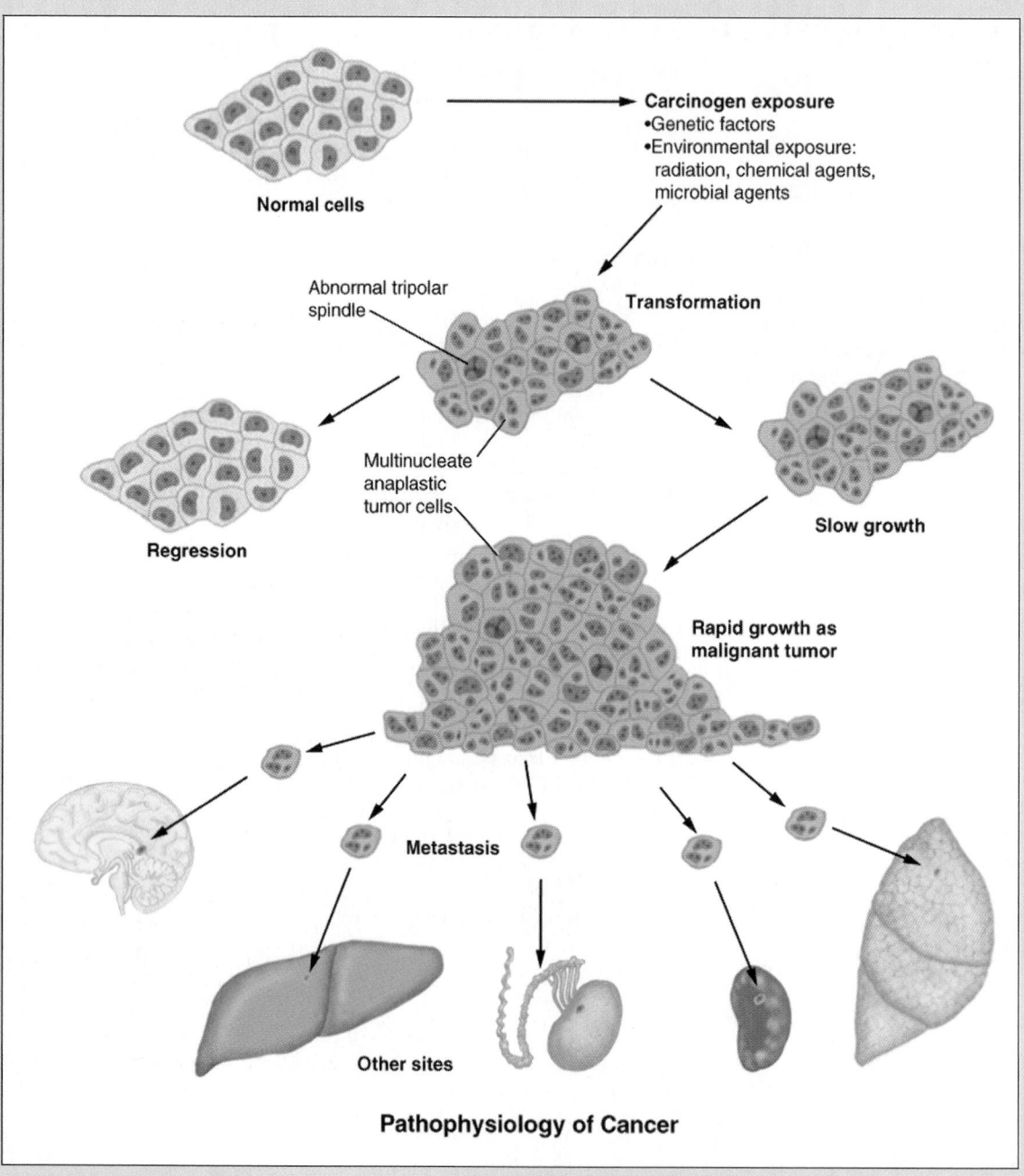

Pathophysiology of Cancer

Review of Cancer

A neoplasm is any tumor that arises from new, abnormal growth. A tumor may be benign or malignant. Cancer is always malignant. The distinguishing feature of cancer is its ability to invade surrounding tissue and metastasize. Cancerous cells grow progressively; they have lost the ability to perform their intended functions because of changes in the cell's DNA resulting in "wrong" information being transmitted. As the cancerous cells proliferate, they crowd out normal cells and compress vascular structures and vital organs, which results in symptoms.

The cause of most childhood cancers is unknown. It is currently believed the underlying cause of cancer is genetic. Alterations in normal DNA occur that predispose the indi-

vidual to the development of cancer. A small percentage of cancers are associated with an inherited predisposition related to chromosomal abnormalities (Quesnel & Malkin, 1997). A second, more controversial hypothesis holds that cancer develops as a result of failure of the immune system to distinguish between normal and abnormal cells. In addition to heredity, known carcinogens such as radiation, physical irritation, and chemical irritants contribute to the development of cancer. Certain environmental exposures known to cause cancer in adults have little correlation with the development of cancer in children.

Cancer cells spread in one of two ways: (1) by *invasion*, in which the cells grow in an unrestricted, disorderly fashion at the site of origin, and (2) by *metastasis*, in which the cells grow in sites other than the site of the primary cancer.

• • • • • • • • • • •

Diagnostic Tests and Procedures for Cancer

Test	Description	Purpose	Nursing Considerations
Bone marrow aspiration	Bone marrow is aspirated from the anterior or posterior iliac crests (the tibia is sometimes used in infants).	Pathologic examination of the aspirated material shows the presence, absence, and ratio of cells that are specific to and diagnostic of certain diseases. Some of the conditions that can be diagnosed include leukemia, specific vitamin deficiencies, neoplastic diseases in which the marrow is invaded by tumor cells, and agranulocytosis.	Describe the procedure to the child and parents. Allow parents to stay with the child if they wish. Depending on the protocol of the facility, the child may receive a wide range of sedative or anesthetic agents. Some centers use local anesthesia with no systemic sedation; others use a combination of a sedative and an analgesic. The child should be told that some discomfort will be felt when the needle is inserted and the marrow aspirated, but that the discomfort will last only a few seconds. Apply a dressing to the area. If the child's platelet count is below 50,000/mm^3, use a pressure dressing.
Positron emission tomography (PET)	This study combines conventional nuclear medicine techniques with tomography and adds double-photon imaging, which images metabolic activity.	PET is used mainly to evaluate brain and cardiac function. Brain metabolism indicates tissue viability, and PET can help identify the degree of malignancy present.	Be sure the patient is not pregnant. Younger children may need sedation. Older children should be told about the scan and allowed to see the equipment.
Single-photon emission computed tomography (SPECT)	This study combines the techniques of conventional nuclear medicine imaging with that of CT using gamma-emitting radioactive isotopes.	SPECT displays a normal organ in axial, parasagittal, and coronal sections.	Same as for PET

Note: See Chapter 52 (CT, lumbar puncture, MRI) and Appendix E (CBC, serum chemistry, urinalysis) for other common tests used in the care of the child with cancer.

Cardinal Signs and Symptoms of Cancer in Children

OVERT SIGNS

- A mass
- Purpura
- Pallor
- Weight loss
- Squint or change in the eye
- Vomiting in early morning
- Recurrent or persistent fever

SIGNS AND SYMPTOMS THAT MAY BE COVERT

- Bone pain
- Headache
- Persistent lymphadenopathy
- Change in balance, gait, or personality
- Fatigue, malaise

Tumor staging is based on the results of diagnostic studies and in some cases surgical examination. Staging describes the extent of disease locally, regionally, and systemically and guides the therapy for most solid tumors. Each tumor has its own specific system of staging, which assists in determining treatment and prognosis.

Cancer is uncommon in children; nevertheless, it is the leading cause of death due to disease in childhood. Cancer in children is often difficult to diagnose, and health care providers must be aware of the clinical manifestations that should raise the suspicion of cancer. The signs and symptoms depend on the child's age, the type of tumor, and the extent of the disease. Testing, diagnosis, and initiation of treatment may occur within a very short period, which can be devastating to the child and family. The nurse becomes the informational lifeline for the child and family as they go through the treatment process.

▮ Childhood Cancer and Its Treatment

Children with cancer are treated in a multidisciplinary setting. The pediatric oncology nurse plays a prominent role in the care of the child with cancer and the child's family. Nurses support and educate children and their families as they move through a process that is stressful and of long duration. Pediatric oncology nurses are challenged to maintain a high level of technical competence and to provide psychological support for the child and family. Working with children with cancer can be an emotional experience, and the nurse must have a support system and be aware of personal limitations.

Incidence

Cancer is the second leading cause of death during childhood, following accidents. Fourteen childhood cancers per 100,000 children under age 15 years and 20 cancers per 100,000 children ages 15 to 19 years are diagnosed each year (Landis, Murray, Bolden, et al., 1998). The goal of treatment is to cure the child with a minimum of long-term side effects. Treatment challenges include maintaining normal growth and development of the child, which can be affected by cancer treatments.

The cardinal signs of cancer in children are different from those in adults (see p. 1316). Most cancers in adults are carcinomas, and more screening tools are available for early detection. In children, however, most cancer signs and symptoms resemble those of common childhood illnesses, and children often are not brought for medical care until obvious signs and symptoms are present. Primary care providers are understandably reluctant to think about cancer as the cause of the child's illness.

A great deal of research has been done over the past 30 years to improve the outcome for children with cancer. Current survival rates are attributed to cooperative, systematic research through the Pediatric Oncology Group, the Children's Cancer Group, and the International Society for Pediatric Oncology. Each group meets twice a year to develop new protocols and monitor the results of current protocols; subgroups meet as needed throughout the year. Research shows that children have better outcomes if they are treated according to a scientific protocol that directs when in the treatment course drugs are to be given, how frequently, and in what dosages, as well as which diagnostic and follow-up studies are to be done and how often.

Because of the efforts of cooperative pediatric clinical trials, approximately 72% of children diagnosed with cancer will survive 5 years or longer after the diagnosis is made (Landis et al., 1998). This figure represents a 40% increase in long-term survival from the 1960s (Wingard, 1997). It is estimated that by the year 2000, there will be over 100,000 adult survivors of childhood cancer. This knowledge has renewed emphasis on identifying the long-term sequelae of cancer treatment in children and intervening in a timely fashion.

Even after apparently successful treatment of cancer in children, cancer may recur shortly after therapy is completed to years later. A second tumor may represent recurrence of the original disease or a new (or second) malignancy. For example, some children with acute lymphocytic leukemia (ALL) relapse with acute myelocytic leukemia (AML). Some children with ALL who were treated with prophylactic irradiation of the central nervous system (CNS) relapse with brain tumors. Thus, once therapy is complete, emphasis shifts to monitoring for the late effects of treatment and the early recurrence of disease.

Therapeutic Management

Chemotherapy, surgery, and radiation therapy are the primary treatment modalities for children with cancer. Bone marrow transplantation, stem cell transplantation, and biologic response modifiers are reserved for a specific subpopulation of children with cancer.

CHEMOTHERAPY

Chemotherapy is the use of drugs (antineoplastic agents) to kill cancer cells. Different drugs have different side effect profiles and modes of action. Combinations of drugs known individually to be active against the specific disease are used. Additionally, tumors have the ability to develop resistance to chemotherapy agents, so a variety of drugs are frequently used. Chemotherapy may be given orally, intravenously, intramuscularly, subcutaneously, or intrathecally (via the spinal column). Rarely, it may be given directly into a body cavity (i.e., intra-arterially, intraperitoneally, or intrathecal) for direct action. Depending on the protocol, a child may be hospitalized for chemotherapy, receive it on an outpatient basis, or be treated at home.

The drugs used in chemotherapy treatment do not differentiate between normal cells and cancer cells. The cytotoxic effects of the drugs affect rapidly dividing healthy cells as well as cancer cells. Rapidly dividing cells include cells that make up the hair follicles, bone marrow, and mucosa. Each child is an individual and may be more or less sensitive to the side effects of the drugs; dosages of a particular drug may need to be altered in individual cases because of toxic side effects.

The side effects of chemotherapy represent challenges to caregivers and are due to the effect of chemotherapy on

• • • • • • • • • • •

Common Side Effects of Chemotherapy and Radiation Therapy

Chemotherapeutic drugs and radiation therapy affect normal as well as abnormal cells, primarily cells that divide rapidly, such as cells of the GI tract, hair follicles, and bone marrow. As a result, children undergoing these therapies frequently experience the following:

CHEMOTHERAPY SIDE EFFECTS

- Bone marrow suppression
- Alopecia
- Malaise/fatigue
- Nausea
- Vomiting
- Anorexia
- Stomatitis

RADIATION SIDE EFFECTS

- Skin reactions
- Fatigue
- Bone marrow suppression
- Nausea
- Vomiting
- Anorexia
- Mucositis

SIDE EFFECTS OF RADIATION TO THE BRAIN

Acute (During and Shortly After Irradiation)

- Brain edema
- Transient increase in neurologic symptoms
- The general radiation side effects listed in this table

Subacute (1 to 6 Months After Irradiation)

- Somnolence syndrome—pronounced drowsiness, nausea, and malaise (typically 4 to 8 weeks after completing radiation therapy)
- Fever
- Irritability
- Ataxia
- Anorexia
- Dysphasia
- Dizziness

Late Effects (over 6 Months)

- Morphologic changes—cerebral atrophy, white matter degeneration, necrosis calcification
- Functional changes—encephalopathy, neuropsychological deterioration, focal neurologic deficits
- Alopecia within the radiation field

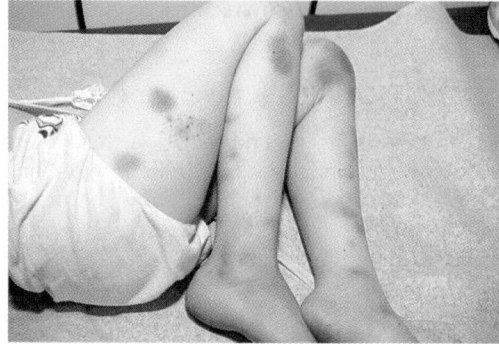

Suppression of the bone marrow in chemotherapy or radiation therapy reduces the cells produced by this organ. Low platelet levels lead to spontaneous bruising, as shown here. Nosebleeds and bleeding of the gums are other consequences. The nurse must make a special effort to observe for bruising in dark-skinned children because it will be more difficult to see.

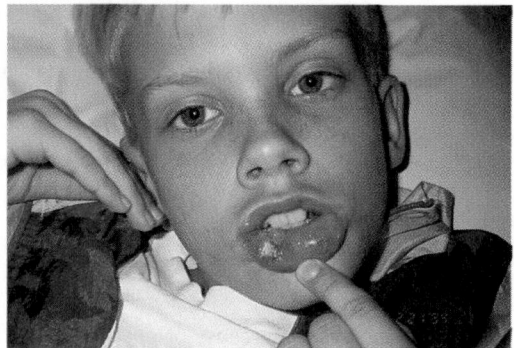

Mucositis (inflammation of the mucous membranes) and mouth ulcers are common side effects of chemotherapeutic drugs. Any mucous membrane can be affected.

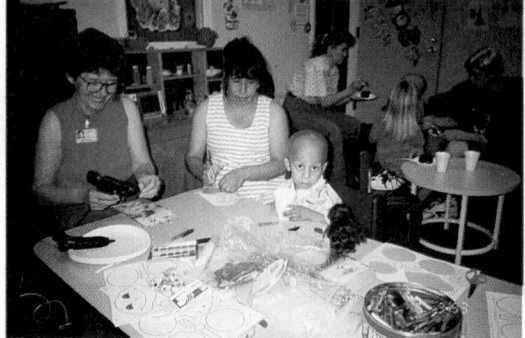

Hair loss is a distressing side effect of cancer treatment. School-age children and adolescents are most likely to feel this distress. Activities such as crafts or play groups help children feel more normal and provide interaction with others.

Photos courtesy of Cook Children's Medical Center, Fort Worth, Texas.

the more rapidly dividing cells of the hematopoietic system, the gastrointestinal (GI) tract, and integumentary system.

Bone marrow cells are one of the rapidly proliferating tissues adversely affected by many chemotherapy agents. Bone marrow production may become suppressed, resulting in neutropenia, anemia, or thrombocytopenia. The nadir—the time of the greatest bone marrow suppression—generally occurs 7 to 10 days after chemotherapy administration, depending on the specific agent used. The greatest concern during the period of bone marrow suppression is infection.

Neutropenia places the child with cancer at risk for the development of opportunistic infections. Opportunistic infections are those caused by nonpathogenic bacteria and fungi that, because of the child's compromised immunity, are able to invade and cause infection. Bacteria, generally present on the skin and within the gut, may invade the bloodstream via a break in the skin and lead to a life-threatening infection. In the absence of white blood cells (WBCs), the usual inflammatory response (erythema, edema, and swelling) indicative of an infection is not present. Fever is frequently the only indication of infection. Health care providers and families must remain acutely aware of elevated body temperature and breaks in the skin during periods of neutropenia.

The treatment of nausea and vomiting was revolutionized in 1992 with the release of the class of antiemetic drugs called 5-HT3 serotonin antagonists. These drugs include ondansetron (Zofran), granisetron (Kytril), and dolasetron (Anzemet). They have been more effective in combating chemotherapy-induced nausea and vomiting than earlier antiemetics.

Anorexia is associated not only with nausea, but also with a change in taste experienced by some people in response to certain chemotherapeutic agents. Some children use anorexia as a way to exert what little control they have left after the diagnosis. At the time of diagnosis, parents must be taught strategies that may avert aggressive nutritional supplementation. Strategies such as offering small, frequent meals high in calories and protein will help keep the child's weight from falling.

Treatment-related fatigue, common in adult cancer patients, is poorly reported in children and adolescents. Normal activities are important to keep spirits and energy levels high. Allow friends to visit the child as tolerated. Encourage video games, movies, and playroom or teen lounge activities with others of the same age. Allow the hospital routine to be as close to the child's home routine as possible.

Hair loss has a tremendous psychological effect, especially on school-age children and adolescents. Some chemotherapeutic agents do not produce hair loss, but most do. Other side effects are specific to the agent being used and the dose.

Nurses administering chemotherapeutic agents should be trained by the institution in which they work. Currently, there is no nationally recognized chemotherapy administration certification program. Nursing responsibilities and precautions related to chemotherapy administration are detailed in the box.

SURGERY

Surgery is frequently part of cancer therapy for children. The surgery may be limited to a biopsy. The purpose of a biopsy is to obtain a small piece of the tumor for microscopic examination. Examination of the tissue by a pathologist confirms the tumor type and influences therapy decisions. Surgery may also be used to *debulk* or *resect* a solid tumor mass. In some diseases the tumor cannot be resected at the beginning of therapy. After the child has received some chemotherapy the mass may decrease in size, and a less extensive surgical procedure may be performed (see Chapter 37 for a discussion of preoperative care).

RADIATION THERAPY

Radiation therapy may be given palliatively in low doses to prevent further growth of a tumor or curatively to eradicate disease. Total body irradiation is sometimes given before bone marrow transplantation in an attempt to eradicate microscopic disease and promote bone marrow suppression. Radiation therapy may be given in hyperfractionated doses, in which the daily dose is split into smaller doses given more frequently in an attempt to minimize side effects.

The side effects of radiation therapy depend on the dose and treatment site and, as with chemotherapy, are a result of radiation's effect on healthy, rapidly dividing cells. These side effects usually appear 7 to 10 days after the initiation of therapy and dissipate within days or a few weeks of cessation of radiation therapy. The decision regarding radiation dose, frequency, and location depend on the purpose of the radiation therapy and the disease process being treated.

Preparing the child and family for radiation entails educating them about the process and the side effects. Some institutions provide a pre-radiation therapy tour so that children may experience the room and surroundings before therapy. During the tour, children should be shown the win-

• • • • • • • • • •
Nursing Responsibilities and Precautions for Chemotherapy

- Know OSHA guidelines for administration of antineoplastic agents.
- Measure child's height and weight accurately.
- Confirm body surface area (BSA, in m^2) calculation used to calculate dosages.
- Always double-check the ordered dosage against the BSA.
- Always double-check the ordered dosage against protocol recommendations.
- Always double-check the medication against the *original* physician's order.
- A complete blood count should be obtained within 48 hours preceding administration of chemotherapy.
- The white blood cell and platelet counts need to be at a predetermined level before chemotherapy is given.
- Know the potential side effects of the drugs being administered and appropriate actions to ameliorate those effects.
- Ensure the patency of IV tubing before giving drugs by checking for blood return.
- If using an implantable infusion device, ensure needle placement is secure and blood returns.
- Vesicants (agents that produce blisters) should be given through a fresh IV site.
- Have emergency drugs available.

dow or monitor through which they will be observed while undergoing radiation treatment alone in the room. Some children need to be sedated for radiation treatments; others can be coached to lie still with the help of child life specialists and parents. The child must lie still for prolonged periods because the radiation oncologist must control the depth and peripheral margins of the radiation site very carefully.

Erythema within the area being treated with radiation is the most common side effect. The parents' first reaction to the erythematous skin that is evident after radiation therapy may be to apply lotion. Some lotions will worsen the skin's reaction to radiation. Remind parents to use only approved lotions or creams on the skin. Loose clothing may be more comfortable. Sun protection is essential while the child is undergoing radiation treatments. Fatigue associated with therapy may necessitate more frequent rest periods than parents are used to their child taking. Anorexia, nausea, and vomiting commonly occur; parents need to be creative in meal planning to prevent dehydration and weight loss. Radiation therapy will also cause bone marrow suppression, to a degree that depends on the dose and treatment site. The results of laboratory tests should be closely monitored during a course of radiation therapy for evidence of neutropenia, anemia, and thrombocytopenia.

BONE MARROW AND STEM CELL TRANSPLANTATION

In recent years, bone marrow or stem cell transplantation has become accepted therapy for the treatment of several hematologic and oncologic disorders. Transplantation allows physicians to give extremely high doses of chemotherapy (with or without irradiation) without regard for bone marrow recovery.

Bone marrow transplantation (BMT) uses bone marrow to reconstitute immunologic function after high-dose chemotherapy. Stem cell transplantation uses a unique immature cell present in the peripheral circulation to restore immunologic function in a similar manner. Stem cells are precursor cells that are able to differentiate into any type of hematologic cell.

The healthy bone marrow or stem cells are infused into the bloodstream and migrate to the marrow space to replenish the patient's immunologic function. The source of marrow or stem cells depends on the disease process being treated.

Collection of bone marrow is considered a surgical procedure. The donor undergoes general anesthesia for aspiration of the bone marrow, which is then processed in the laboratory and frozen until it is infused into the recipient.

Stem cell collection is frequently accomplished in the outpatient setting. Patients are monitored for blood cell count recovery and the presence of immature cells after priming chemotherapy. The donor's tissue may be stimulated to produce these immature stem cells with granulocyte colony-stimulating factor (G-CSF), a biologic response modifier described in the next section. A pheresis machine is used to remove the immature stem cells by centrifugation of the blood. The unused portion of the blood is returned to the donor. Collection is complete when the appropriate

number of immature cells has been collected. This process may take 1 to several days or collection periods.

There are three types of transplant—syngeneic, autologous, and allogeneic. The type used depends on the child and on the disease's effect on the bone marrow. Rarely, a child will have an identical twin and can receive a syngeneic transplant. In autologous transplantation, patients are their own donors. The child's own unaffected bone marrow or stem cells are collected prior to the high-dose chemotherapy. In allogeneic BMT, a donor with a tissue type matching the child's tissue type is found. Only 35% of the population have a non-twin sibling with matching tissue type (O'Connell & Schmit-Pokorny, 1997), so a national or international search through the National Marrow Donor Program may be conducted to look for an unrelated matched donor.

The major problem associated with allogeneic transplantation is graft-versus-host disease (GVHD). GVHD is caused when the infused immunocompetent bone marrow cells recognize the recipient's tissue as foreign. GVHD may affect numerous organ systems. Individuals may exhibit a wide variety of signs associated with GVHD, such as mild to severely elevated liver enzyme levels, mild to copious diarrhea, and maculopapular skin reactions ranging from rashes to full skin desquamation. Antirejection drugs are given to help prevent GVHD from occurring.

In preparation for a transplant, the patient begins a regimen of chemotherapy and radiation therapy (called *conditioning*) to try to eradicate any disease from the body. WBC, red blood cell (RBC), and platelet counts begin to drop as the chemotherapy and radiation therapy exert their effects on the bone marrow. When the conditioning phase is over, the patient receives the thawed marrow or stem cells by intravenous (IV) infusion. The production of WBCs, RBCs, and platelets from the transplantation of normal cells is evidence that the marrow has *engrafted*, or been accepted by the body.

Once the marrow is infused, nursing care focuses on preventing profoundly immunosuppressed children from developing life-threatening infections until the marrow has engrafted and the children are producing their own WBCs with which to fight infection. The waiting game begins for parents and child until the daily complete blood count (CBC) begins to show signs of marrow engraftment.

Common complications in the days and weeks after BMT include mucositis, diarrhea, fevers, and nosebleeds. Children receive parenteral nutritional support because most will not be able to take food and fluids due to severe mucositis and GI discomfort and diarrhea.

In many centers, the initial post-transplantation management includes strict isolation. High-efficiency particulate air (HEPA) filters are used to clean the air in the child's room to eliminate many viruses, molds, and fungi that a person with a normal immune system would be able to handle. Regimented oral and skin care are required. Strict intake and output measurements are made. Vital signs are monitored frequently. Blood products are administered several times a week while waiting for the child's marrow to become active. Many different medications are given to prevent infections, GVHD, peptic ulcers, and other complications of treatment.

Children are not discharged home until their WBC count is sufficient to fight infections, and even then they must be considered immunosuppressed for months. Home care may include nutritional support, platelet transfusions, IV immune globulin (IVIG), and antiviral medications. The child must wear a mask when venturing out in public. Different institutions have different standards for discharge home. Home care varies as well. Follow-up visits are initially biweekly and continue for months.

Transplantation is currently standard therapy for children in first remission with Philadelphia chromosome-positive ALL (a genetically determined ALL with a 90% relapse rate), AML, and stage IV neuroblastoma, as well as for children with chronic aplastic anemia and severe combined immunodeficiency syndrome. Transplantation is also used for children with solid tumors, Hodgkin's disease, and non-Hodgkin's lymphoma resistant to conventional chemotherapy and radiation therapy, as evidenced by relapse while the child is receiving therapy.

BIOLOGIC RESPONSE MODIFIERS

The most recent addition to cancer therapy are the biologic response modifiers. Biologic response modifiers are naturally occurring substances found in small quantities in the body that influence immune system functions (e.g., colony-stimulating factors [CSFs]).

Used to enhance cell recovery, different CSFs work on different types of blood cells to reduce the time and severity of bone marrow suppression. They may reduce the length of time a child must be hospitalized for fever and neutropenia by causing the production of neutrophils. CSFs are used in conjunction with high doses of chemotherapy, known to cause neutropenia. CSFs may reduce bone marrow recovery time, enabling the chemotherapeutic regimen to continue as scheduled for maximum effectiveness. Other CSFs may promote the recovery of platelets or RBCs, which can reduce the need for blood products.

Over the past few years, a number of immune modulating agents have been examined in the laboratory, with very few translating into clinically beneficial treatment modalities. Interleukin, a protein that mobilizes the immune response, monoclonal antibodies, interferon, and activated T-cell antigens are all in ongoing clinical trials to evaluate their role in the treatment of cancer (Lum, 1999).

▋ Leukemia

Leukemia is the disease that most often comes to mind when one discusses childhood cancer. Leukemia is a proliferation of immature WBCs and is the most common form of cancer in children under age 15 years. Considerable progress in its treatment has been achieved through years of research.

Etiology

Leukemia most likely arises from a fundamental alteration in the genetic makeup of the stem cell. All cells produced from the altered stem cell have the defect. These cells tend to replicate quickly, forming immature or blast cells in the bone marrow that are then released into the peripheral circulation, crowding other cells produced. The blast cells do not respond properly to the body's feedback mechanism and continue to replicate in great numbers. When karyotyped, the leukemic cells in over 90% of children with the disease reveal chromosomal abnormalities (Friebert & Shurin, 1998a).

Children with Down syndrome have a risk of developing leukemia up to 15 times greater than other children (Margolin & Poplack, 1997). The twin of a child who has had ALL also has a slightly higher likelihood of developing the disease than other children. For monozygous twins, the unaffected twin has a 25% risk of developing the disease in the first year after the affected twin is diagnosed. At age 7 years, the unaffected twin's risk drops to that of the general population (Friebert & Shurin, 1998a).

Incidence

Approximately 3,000 new cases of childhood leukemia are diagnosed each year (Friebert & Shurin, 1998a; Margolin & Poplack, 1997). ALL accounts for 80% of all cases of leukemia, AML for 15% to 20%, and chronic myelocytic leukemia is rare (Friebert & Shurin, 1998a). The peak incidence occurs between ages 2 and 5 years for ALL. Leukemia is more common in boys than girls.

Manifestations

Clinical manifestations of leukemia include fever, pallor, excessive bruising, bone or joint pain (usually leg pain), lymphadenopathy, malaise, hepatosplenomegaly, abnormal WBC counts (either lower or higher than normal for age), and mild to profound anemia and thrombocytopenia. The severity of the clinical manifestations varies with the cell type of leukemia and the length of time before diagnosis.

Diagnostic Evaluation

The diagnosis can be strongly suspected from a history of the clinical manifestations and an initial CBC. The confirmatory test for leukemia is microscopic examination of bone marrow obtained by bone marrow aspiration and biopsy (see Chapter 37). A bone marrow aspirate alone usually provides sufficient material to establish the diagnosis of ALL. A lumbar puncture is also done to look for blast cells in the spinal fluid that are indicative of CNS disease. Serum electrolyte levels are determined to ensure metabolic stability before chemotherapy is initiated. An elevated uric acid level, indicating rapid cell turnover, may be expected if the WBC count is very high.

Therapeutic Management

Combination chemotherapy is the preferred treatment for leukemia. The period of treatment varies according to the cell type but usually lasts 2 to 3 years and is divided into phases: induction, consolidation, and maintenance. The aim of the first month of chemotherapy treatment, or induc-

PATHOPHYSIOLOGY
of Leukemia

In leukemia, normal bone marrow is replaced by malignant *blast cells*. As the blast cells take over the bone marrow, eventually RBC and platelet production is affected and the child becomes anemic and thrombocytopenic. The reticuloendothelial system is affected, disturbing the body's defense system and rendering these children unable to fight infections normally. The symptoms of the disease reflect bone marrow failure and organ infiltration.

In addition to being present in the blood and bone marrow, leukemia cells infiltrate extramedullary sites, most commonly the CNS and the testicles. Although it is not common to see extramedullary leukemia at time of diagnosis, these are common sites of relapse.

Leukemias are classified by the type of WBC affected. Broadly, acute leukemias are classified as acute lymphocytic leukemia (ALL) and acute nonlymphocytic leukemia (ANLL). ALL originates from B lymphocytes (B-cell ALL), T lymphocytes (T-cell ALL), or is classified as common ALL, which has a B-cell lineage. ANLL is also known as acute myelocytic leukemia (AML) and can be further classified as acute promyelocytic leukemia (APL), acute myelomonocytic leukemia (AMMoL), and acute monocytic leukemia (AMoL). ANLL tends to be less responsive to therapy, more aggressive and difficult to treat, and more likely to result in relapse than ALL.

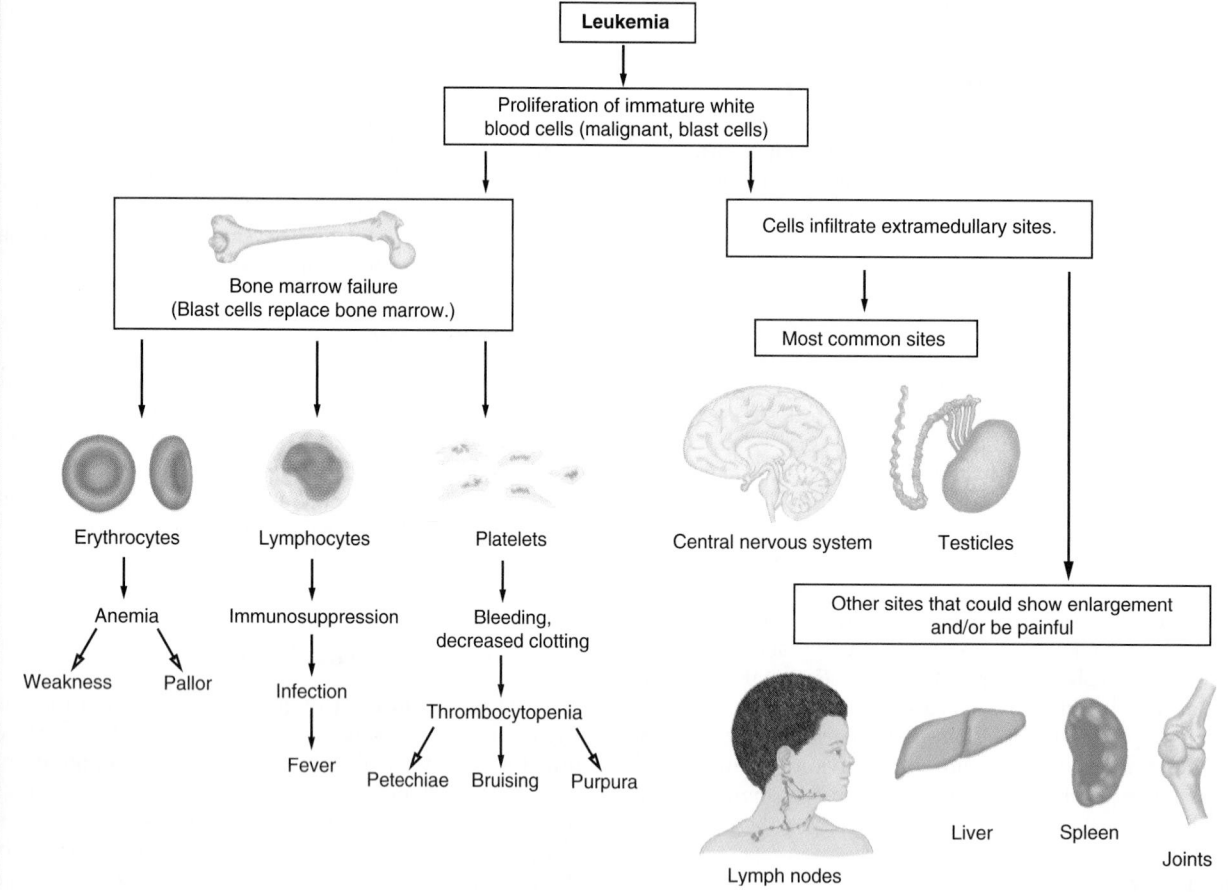

tion, is to induce remission. Remission is the reduction of immature blast cells in the bone marrow to less than 5%. About 95% of children achieve remission within 1 month (Friebert & Shurin, 1998b). The goal of therapy following remission is to maintain remission and to prevent disease in sanctuary sites. Sanctuary sites include the testes and CNS. They are referred to as "sanctuary" because systemic therapy is poorly delivered to these areas. Before induction, the child is treated for presenting signs, which may include sepsis, anemia, hemorrhage, and metabolic abnormalities.

REMISSION INDUCTION
During induction, the hospitalized child receives the first doses of chemotherapy while the response to the drugs is assessed. Remission can be verified within the first 28 days after the initiation of chemotherapy by sequential bone marrow aspirates and lumbar punctures. If a significant number of blast cells is still present, a new and stronger drug regimen is given. The presence of more than 5% blasts in the marrow at day 28 is an ominous sign, indicative of a poorer prognosis.

The particular drugs used, their dose, route, and scheduling depend on the *protocol* that will be used for that specific type of leukemia. Children are placed into prognostic categories with specifically tailored therapies. Before the child receives chemotherapy, allopurinol and IV fluids with sodium bicarbonate are given to decrease the serum uric acid level and alkalinize the urine. This is especially important when the WBC count is very high. As WBCs break down in reaction to chemotherapy, they release uric acid into the serum, which can compromise kidney function. Steroids are used in induction therapy for ALL, as are vincristine, daunorubicin, and asparaginase. Induction therapy for AML includes cytarabine (ara-C) and an anthracycline such as daunorubicin or doxorubicin. Intrathecal chemotherapy is given prophylactically to prevent relapse in the CNS.

CONSOLIDATION

Consolidation chemotherapy begins after remission is obtained and entails administering cyclic doses of drugs. Treatment may be given on an inpatient or an outpatient basis, depending on the protocol. Interim maintenance and delayed intensification therapy are provided on an outpatient basis; the intensity of the therapy depends on the cell type. The average length of consolidation chemotherapy is four weeks.

MAINTENANCE

Maintenance therapy begins after the completion of remission induction and consolidation therapy. Combined drug regimens are used. CBC counts are determined and lumbar punctures are performed periodically when chemotherapy is given intrathecally. Various studies have shown improved event-free survival rates when intensive therapy consisting of "reinduction" and "reconsolidation" therapy was added early in the maintenance phase. This is called *delayed intensification* therapy and occurs after an interim maintenance phase. Treatment is given on an outpatient basis. Children are usually healthy and able to lead normal lives by the time they reach this phase of treatment. Generally, after the initial induction and consolidation phases, girls are treated for 2 years and boys for 3 years. Boys are treated a year longer because they are at higher risk for relapse. Children who experience relapse while on maintenance therapy have a poor prognosis. If relapse occurs, an attempt is made to reinduce a remission, usually with different chemotherapeutic agents.

RELAPSE

The gonads and the CNS are the most common sites of extramedullary relapse. Therapy includes a more aggressive regimen. The more relapses the child has, the less likely it is that a cure will be attained.

NURSING CARE
The Child with Leukemia

Assessment

Subjective data almost always reveal an insidious onset of symptoms. The parents may state they realized their child was less active than normal. A persistent or recurrent fever of unknown cause is often in the history. The parents may have suddenly noticed their child had more bruises than usual. Sometimes the child has complained intermittently of a stomachache that the parents attributed to school avoidance. Leg pain may have been attributed to growing pains or laziness. Parents commonly express guilt because they did not recognize anything was wrong with their child sooner or, if they did notice, the manifestations were so vague they delayed seeking treatment. Psychosocial assessment of the family is carried out throughout the care of the child.

The nurse should observe both the child's and the parents' reactions to the disease. The emotional maturity of the child and the family will affect how each person copes with the illness and treatment. The child's chronological age and stage of development as well as previous experience with the health care system are critical factors in the assessment.

Parents who are unable to cope with the disease and who display a high level of anxiety will transfer this anxiety to their child. Children who have had previous negative experiences associated with hospitals, nurses, and doctors may exhibit increased anxiety. Families who have had a relative who had cancer and perhaps died will exhibit increased anxiety and need for support, even if the relative was an older person. The nurse's role is to identify and respond to these needs.

Children often present with fever. Fatigue, pallor, bruising on the extremities, petechiae in the mouth and sclera, and hepatosplenomegaly are common signs and symptoms. Children with very high WBC counts or AML may present with more pronounced manifestations. The mental and neurologic status of the child is assessed because of the risk of infiltration into the CNS.

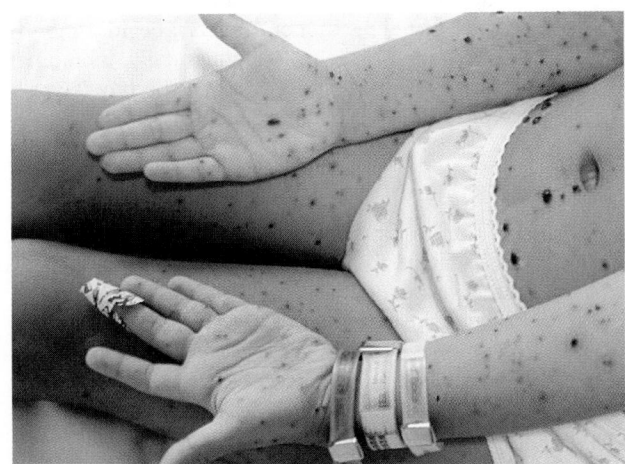

FIGURE 48–1

Varicella (chickenpox) can be deadly in the immunocompromised child. Thrombocytopenia (low platelet count) associated with chemotherapy can cause the varicella lesions to be hemorrhagic, like those shown here. Secondary infections of the lesions are also common because of low WBC counts. (Courtesy of Cook Children's Medical Center, Hematology-Oncology Clinic, Fort Worth, Texas.)

Nursing Diagnosis, Planning, Intervention, and Evaluation

Nursing Diagnosis   ■ Risk for Infection related to the immunosuppressed state.

Expected Outcomes
- The child will be free of signs of infection, as evidenced by an afebrile state, no redness of the integument, no redness or swelling at the site of insertion of a central venous catheter, and negative culture results.
- Parents and child will recognize and verbalize early signs of infection.

Intervention	Rationale
1. Monitor vital signs every 4 hours and as necessary if the child is hospitalized. Instruct parents to measure the child's temperature as needed at home (by the oral, axillary, or tympanic routes only).	1. In the absence of WBCs, an elevated temperature may be the only evident sign of infection. The risk of injury to the fragile mucous membranes is so great that only oral, tympanic, or axillary routes should be used to measure temperatures. Rectal abscesses can easily occur to friable rectal tissue. Temperatures should not be measured rectally.
2. Practice proper hand washing, and teach this to the family.	2. Proper hand washing is the best way to prevent the spread of infection.
3. Inspect the child's skin daily for breaks and redness.	3. Some neutropenic patients will not produce erythema or purulent drainage. Because pus is made of WBCs, drainage cannot be used as a sign of infection. Skin provides a barrier against infection.
4. Inspect the child's mouth daily for oral ulcers and inspect the perineum for fissures. Teach older children to do self-examination. No suppositories should be given.	4. The mucous membranes are fragile and easily affected by chemotherapy and irradiation. Mouth ulcers and rectal abscesses are common side effects of chemotherapy and radiation therapy and potential sites for bacteria entry because of the impaired mucosa.
5. Encourage regular bowel habits.	5. Decreased activity, altered nutrition, and certain medications may predispose to constipation. The passage of hard stool may traumatize delicate rectal mucous membranes and create a potential site for entry of bacteria.
6. Teach the parents and child meticulous oral hygiene at diagnosis. a. Use a soft-bristled toothbrush or toothettes. b. Perform oral hygiene four times a day. c. If the platelet count is low, use a cotton-tipped applicator instead of a toothbrush.	6. Preventing dental caries and ulcerations on fragile oral mucosa will help prevent infections.
7. At the first signs of mouth ulcers, begin a mouth care regimen three to four times daily, including an antifungal drug as ordered by the physician. Avoid alcohol-containing mouthwashes.	7. Fungal infections originating from the mouth or GI tract can quickly become disseminated in immunosuppressed children. Over-the-counter mouthwashes may have a high alcohol content and may be drying to oral mucosa, thus increasing the risk of breaking down the protective barrier of the skin.
8. For the hospitalized neutropenic child, allow flowers or plants to be kept in the room only if institutional protocol allows. Do not use humidifiers.	8. Standing water and damp soil harbor *Aspergillus* and *Pseudomonas,* to which these children are very susceptible.
9. Change any dressings and IV lines using sterile techniques.	9. Because the child with neutropenia is not able to fight infection normally, extra precautions must be taken.
10. The child should not receive live-virus vaccines. Siblings should receive inactivated polio vaccine but may receive live measles-mumps-rubella (MMR) vaccine.	10. Live virus is shed in the stool after administration of the polio vaccine. The live MMR vaccine could produce infection in the severely immunocompromised child, but no virus shedding occurs to create a threat if given to the sibling.
11. Keep any child with chickenpox or any child who has been exposed to the virus away from the child with cancer. Inform the teacher of the importance of notifying parents immediately if a case of chickenpox occurs in another child at school. Encourage vaccination of siblings who have not had varicella, to create herd immunity.	11. Immunocompromised patients are unable to fight varicella adequately. Chickenpox can be deadly to the immunocompromised child (Fig. 48–1). If a child who has not had chickenpox is exposed to someone with varicella, the child should receive varicella-zoster immune globulin within 96 hours of exposure.

12. Obtain specimens for culture as ordered, and monitor the results.

13. Administer acetaminophen for fever.

14. Administer antibiotics as ordered after culture results are available.

12. Physicians will order blood, urine, stool, and wound cultures, as signs appear when the neutropenic child has fever.

13. Aspirin and ibuprofen given to a child who is thrombocytopenic can cause platelet dysfunction.

14. Cultures identify the specific organism so that the most effective antibiotic can be given. Appropriate antibiotic treatment should begin promptly.

Evaluation

- Has the child remained free of signs of infection?
- Have the child and parents promptly recognized and responded to warning signs of infection?

Nursing Diagnosis

■ Risk for Injury related to abnormal blood profile.

Expected Outcomes

- The child will have no excessive, uncontrolled bleeding.
- Parents and child will understand risk for hemorrhage as evidenced by their ability to respond appropriately to bleeding.

Intervention

1. Apply gentle, firm pressure to any puncture sites. Apply a pressure dressing to sites of bone marrow aspiration.
2. If the child is severely thrombocytopenic (platelet count less than 20,000/mm³), take the following steps:
   a. Limit any activity that could result in head injury; encourage the child to participate in quiet activities (e.g., reading books, watching videos, coloring). No contact sports.
   b. Provide a soft-bristled toothbrush only or toothettes.
   c. Give stool softeners to prevent straining with constipation.
   d. Do not use suppositories.
   e. Check urine and stools for blood.
3. Teach the child how to control nosebleeds and to blow the nose gently.

Rationale

1. Additional pressure may be needed to stop bleeding if the platelet count is low.

2. A decreased platelet count increases the risk for bleeding. There is a potential risk for intracranial hemorrhage.

3. One of the most common sites of bleeding is the nose. Blood loss can be reduced through avoidance of nosebleeds.

Evaluation

- Has the child experienced excessive bleeding?
- Have the parents demonstrated what to do for a nosebleed?
- Can the child or parents promptly recognize and respond to bleeding?

Nursing Diagnosis

■ Altered Nutrition: Less than Body Requirements related to nausea and vomiting or mucositis.

Expected Outcomes

- The child will have a growth rate appropriate for age.
- The child will experience no more than 5% weight loss.

Intervention

1. Administer antiemetics prophylactically and as needed, as ordered.
2. When the child is nauseated, offer cool, clear liquids. Be creative with the liquids offered to make them more interesting and inviting.
3. Offer small, frequent meals of high protein and high calorie content. Fortify foods with nutritional supplements. Allow the family to bring favorite foods to the hospital.
4. Do not offer favorite foods when the child is nauseated.
5. Administer ordered mouth analgesics before oral intake.

Rationale

1. Antiemetics will decrease or prevent vomiting.

2. Cool liquids are soothing and better tolerated than hot ones and they avoid the risk of burning fragile mucosa.

3. Small, frequent meals are better tolerated than large ones. Protein promotes tissue healing. High calories are needed for growth. Children are more likely to eat their favorite foods.

4. Foods eaten within hours of nausea will be associated with being sick.

5. If mouth sores are present, analgesics will increase comfort and provide interest in eating.

6. Monitor daily weight. Keep strict intake and output records. Weigh the infant's diapers.

6. Strict measurements ensures adequate intake and provides an objective assessment to alert the nurse that further interventions may be needed.

7. Involve the child in food selection.

7. Food selection allows the child control over as much as possible and may increase interest and participation in eating.

8. Include a dietician in the nutritional assessment and evaluation.

8. A dietician provides specialized input into developing and evaluating nutritional status.

Evaluation

- Did the child experience no more than 5% weight loss?
- Has growth progressed appropriately for age?

Nursing Diagnosis

- ■ Knowledge Deficit related to the disease process and treatment plan.

Expected Outcome

- The child and parents will verbalize an understanding of the diagnosis and demonstrate compliance with treatment.

Intervention

1. Assess the child's and parents' readiness for learning. Create an environment of learning.

2. On initial diagnosis and during subsequent follow-up visits, spend time with the family, repeating and explaining the diagnosis, its sequelae, and its treatment. Offer written literature, or offer to tape educational sessions (see p. 1329).

3. Keep explanations at the family's level of understanding.

4. Offer encouragement for parents' recognition of danger signs and parents' appropriate use of medical care.

Rationale

1. On initial diagnosis, family members may need time to adjust before they are ready for education. Offer written supporting information.

2. Education is ongoing and will need reinforcing with stressed parents. Explaining the treatment rationale and sequelae helps ensure compliance with therapy. Written or taped information can be reviewed later for better absorption.

3. Vary explanations to meet the family's educational level.

4. Praise reinforces behavior. Parents want to know they are doing the right thing for their child.

Evaluation

- Have the parents and child demonstrated an understanding of the treatment protocols by complying with therapy and seeking appropriate medical care for danger signs?

Nursing Diagnosis

- ■ Body Image Disturbance related to hair loss.

Expected Outcomes

- The child will adapt to alopecia, as evidenced by a return to socialization.
- The child will discuss concerns related to hair loss.

Intervention

1. Instruct the child and parents on the progression of hair loss and potential changes in color and texture when the hair regrows. Suggest obtaining a wig before hair is lost or a clipping of hair with a recent photograph.

2. Encourage verbalization of feelings about hair loss. Enlist the help of a child life specialist to engage the child in play therapy.

3. Discuss ways to minimize the reaction to alopecia by promoting creative solutions, such as hats, wigs, or scarfs.

4. Make visits to the child's classroom.

5. Encourage a return to school as soon as possible.

Rationale

1. Reassure that hair loss is temporary for most cancers, but some cranial irradiation can result in patches of permanent hair loss. Matching a wig to original hair color, texture, and style is easier before hair is lost.

2. Allowing the child to verbalize concerns about returning to a social environment or school is an assessment tool for the nurse. Play therapy is a safe way for the child to express feelings and fears.

3. Allowing children to create their own headpieces may minimize the negative impact of hair loss.

4. Preparation of classmates for the child's school reentry will lessen classmates' negative reactions, fears, anxiety, and lack of understanding. It will also increase the support they can give the ill child.

5. The sooner the child returns to school, the less likely the child will begin a pattern of absenteeism. If the child returns to school before major body changes take place, the changes may not be so noticeable to the other children, thus decreasing undesirable reactions.

Evaluation

- Is the child involved in prediagnosis social life?
- Has the child discussed hair loss and feelings connected with body image?

Nursing Diagnosis

■ Ineffective Individual/Family Coping related to chronic illness.

Expected Outcomes

- The child will comply with the treatment plan.
- The parents will verbalize concerns about the impact of the illness on their family.
- The child and parents will use available support systems and community resources.

Intervention	Rationale
1. Teach the family the necessity of adhering to the protocol. Teach the warning signs of problems to watch for and how to access after-hours emergency care.	1. Conscientious application of the treatment plan increases the chance of a positive outcome.
2. Listen and encourage the child and family to verbalize their feelings and express their concerns. Answer questions honestly and openly.	2. Identifying concerns and clarifying misconceptions will help families cope with the stress of chronic illness.
3. Introduce the family to other families of children with cancer.	3. Families of other children with cancer can offer suggestions and support.
4. Consult social services and a chaplain or appropriate religious figure.	4. The financial and emotional burden of caring for a child with cancer can be overwhelming.
5. Offer a list of local support groups appropriate to the child's age and the family's individual needs.	5. Support groups of individuals in similar situations can provide much comfort and support to the child and the family.

Evaluation

- Has the family complied with the treatment plan?
- Do the family and child verbalize appropriate concerns and questions?
- Does the family utilize appropriate resources?

Nursing Diagnosis

■ Pain related to the disease process and procedures.

Expected Outcome

- The child will experience decreased discomfort, as evidenced by periods of uninterrupted rest, verbalization of increased comfort, and participation in play activities.

Intervention	Rationale
1. Explain procedures to the child before performing them.	1. Honest explanations build rapport and reduce fear.
2. Assess for symptoms of pain, such as inactivity for age, increased heart rate or blood pressure, grimacing, verbalization of discomfort, irritability, and crying. Use a pain assessment tool when appropriate for age.	2. Younger children will not be able to verbalize pain. Stoic children may not express discomfort. Nurses must watch for physiologic signs of pain.
3. Administer comfort measures as needed, such as positioning, adjusting room temperature, and offering distractions appropriate for age.	3. Comfort measures can decrease the perception of pain and even decrease the amount of analgesic needed.
4. Administer analgesics promptly as ordered. Use topical anesthetics for procedural pain.	4. Analgesics reduce the pain of procedures and of the disease. Delays in pain administration can increase anxiety and, thus, increase pain.
5. Explain the pain control regimen to the parents and child, as age appropriate.	5. Parents know their child and can assist the nurse in assessing pain and reporting it promptly.
6. Notify the physician if pain relief is not obtained with the ordered dose of analgesic.	6. Pain tolerance varies greatly among children. Dosage increases may be needed, especially in the child with chronic pain or a dying child.
7. Elicit a child life specialist's help before and during procedures.	7. Child life specialists are trained to use distraction techniques with children and represent a "safe" person for the child to be with during repeated painful procedures.
8. Administer antianxiety drugs as ordered (see Chapter 39 for more information related to pain management in children).	8. Especially in the adolescent patient, anticipation of a painful procedure may worsen the pain. Giving an antianxiety drug may help calm the child so the procedure is better tolerated.

Evaluation
- Does the child express decreased levels of discomfort?
- Is the child joining other children in play?

Nursing Diagnosis
■ Impaired Skin Integrity related to radiotherapy, chemotherapy, and immobility.

Expected Outcome
- The child's skin will remain intact.

Intervention	Rationale
1. Assess the child's skin each shift.	1. Skin erythema is common with radiation therapy but should not progress to skin breakdown.
2. Use only approved lotions and creams on the skin, and instruct parents in the same.	2. Some commercial lotions can increase skin irritation and redness.
3. Avoid excessive scrubbing of skin, hot water, and abrasive soaps.	3. Friction may increase skin breakdown. Hot water is uncomfortable to irritated tissue.
4. Offer loose clothing of soft materials.	4. Tight clothing or abrasive fabrics may further irritate the skin.
5. Notify the physician if skin breakdown occurs.	5. Additional orders for therapeutic creams may be needed.
6. If the child is immobile, gently turn and vary the position at least every 2 hours.	6. Immobility may increase pressure on skin and promote breakdown.

Evaluation
- Has the child's skin remained intact?

Nursing Diagnosis
■ Altered Mucous Membrane related to chemotherapy and radiation therapy.

Expected Outcome
- The child will show no signs of oral mucositis or rectal ulceration.

Intervention	Rationale
1. Assess the child's mouth and anus each shift for ulcers, erythema, or breakdown. Teach the parent or child, if age appropriate, the same. Report ulcerations to the physician.	1. A breakdown in mucous membranes usually begins with erythema and progresses to ulcerations. Home care should include this assessment for the duration of therapy. Additional medications, mouth rinses, or ointments will be ordered if ulcerations occur.
2. Do not take a rectal temperature in a child undergoing chemotherapy or radiation therapy. Do not take oral temperatures if mouth ulcers are present. Teach parents how to take accurate axillary or tympanic temperatures.	2. The introduction of a thermometer into the rectum or mouth of a child with fragile mucous membranes, no matter how carefully done, can tear tissue.
3. Begin meticulous mouth care, avoiding alcohol-based mouthwashes, several times a day with a soft-bristled toothbrush or toothettes.	3. Frequent mouth care will help remove bacteria from the oral mucosa, decreasing the risk of infection of irritated tissue.
4. If the rectum becomes irritated, begin sitz baths several times a day and after bowel movements.	4. Lukewarm sitz baths keep the perineum clean and soothe irritated tissue.
5. In diaper-wearing children, use only diaper wipes that do not contain alcohol or perfumes. If the perineum is very irritated, use only warm water wipes of the area.	5. Alcohol and perfumes will further irritate the skin and can cause great discomfort. Very few commercial diaper wipes are safe for these children.
6. Offer bland, nonirritating foods and cool liquids.	6. Citrus products may be very painful to an ulcerated mouth, as may spicy foods. Cool liquids are soothing. Ice pops and slushes are usually well tolerated.

Evaluation
- Has the child exhibited signs of mucosal breakdown?

■ Wilms' Tumor (Nephroblastoma)

Wilms' tumor, or nephroblastoma, is the most common renal tumor in children. Much research has been done on this disease, and the subsequent changes in therapy have resulted in favorable outcomes.

Pathophysiology

Wilms' tumor arises from the renal parenchyma of the kidney and grows very rapidly. It may occur unilaterally or bi- laterally. At the initial diagnosis the disease is usually local, but occasionally there are metastases to other organs. The lungs are the most common site of metastasis. As with other tumors, a staging system to direct treatment exists.

Etiology

The cause of Wilms' tumor is unknown. Most Wilms' tumors occur in children with no unusual physical features and no family history of the disease. These are considered

Caring for the Child with Cancer

- Reinforce teaching concerning diagnosis, treatment, and side effects of chemotherapy.
- Encourage parents to participate actively in the child's care.
- Provide written and verbal instructions concerning home care and provide ample opportunity for parents to give return demonstrations of
  - Central venous access dressing changes
  - Oral medication administration
  - Assessment of oral mucous membranes
  - Temperature measurement by axillary, oral, and tympanic routes.
- Teach the signs and symptoms of infection and bleeding that require immediate treatment and how to access after-hours emergency treatment.
- Provide phone numbers needed for questions concerning the diagnosis, treatment, and the side effects of chemotherapy.
- Make appropriate referrals to social services, a chaplain or other religious figure, and a home health nursing agency.
- Encourage parents to use community resources.
- Stress the importance of preventing infection and bleeding and the need for follow-up visits. Note that many visits will involve drawing blood to monitor WBC and platelet counts.

sporadic cases. In some cases, however, a genetic predisposition exists. Approximately 1% to 2.5% of children who develop this disease have a familial predisposition. It is known to be associated with other congenital anomalies, such as Beckwith-Wiedemann syndrome, genitourinary anomalies, hemihypertrophy, microcephaly, mental retardation, and sporadic aniridia (Petruzzi & Green, 1997). There are two prognostic groups: approximately 85% of the cases have a favorable histology, and a much smaller group has an unfavorable histology (Petruzzi & Green, 1997).

Incidence

The annual incidence is 8.1 cases per 1 million white children. The incidence is higher in African-Americans and lower in East Asians, with approximately 400 new cases diagnosed annually (Green, Coppes, Breslow, et al., 1997). The mean age at diagnosis for unilateral Wilms' tumor is 46.9 months for girls and 41.5 months for boys. In general, children diagnosed with bilateral Wilms' tumor are younger than those diagnosed with unilateral disease (Green, D'Angio, Beckwith, et al., 1996).

Manifestations

The clinical manifestations of Wilms' tumor include a mobile abdominal mass, microscopic or gross hematuria, hypertension, abdominal pain, fatigue, anemia, and fever. The lungs are the primary site for distant metastasis.

Diagnostic Evaluation

The diagnosis can be suspected from a good history. Abdominal ultrasonography (US) is the initial study done to detect a solid intrarenal mass. Abdominal computed tomography (CT) or magnetic resonance imaging (MRI), chest radiography, and chest CT are done to confirm the diagnosis. The CBC count, electrolytes, blood urea nitrogen, and creatinine levels are determined and urinalysis is performed. A definitive diagnosis is made at the time of surgery on the basis of pathologic findings.

Therapeutic Management

After a thorough diagnostic workup, a nephrectomy of the involved kidney and lymph node sampling are done. In the few cases in which complete surgical resection cannot be done at the time of diagnosis, biopsies only are performed, followed by preoperative chemotherapy. The goal in these children is to reduce the tumor size before definitive surgery is performed. Radiation therapy is added to the treatment of tumors that respond poorly to chemotherapy. The surgeon preserves as much of the renal parenchyma as possible and takes care there is no spillage of the tumor in the surgical process, which would necessitate more aggressive treatment (Green et al., 1997). After pathologic study of the surgical specimen, the tumor stage directs the therapeutic management of the child. Chemotherapy alone or in combination with radiation therapy is used to treat these children.

Survival rates for Wilms' tumor are much better than for many other forms of cancer. Histologic features remain the most important determinant of prognosis. Long-term survival rates for children with tumors with a favorable histology approach, and in some cases exceed, 90% (Green et al., 1997).

The Child with Wilms' Tumor

Assessment

Parents often report that when bathing their child they noticed the child's stomach seemed swollen. Some parents will state the diaper no longer fit easily around the child's abdomen. More often than not, the child's activity level and appetite have not changed. Except for a palpable abdominal mass that usually does not cross the midline, the physical examination of the child is normal.

Assessing the Child with a Wilms' Tumor

The tumor mass should not be palpated during the assessment due to the risk of rupturing the protective capsule. Excessive manipulation can cause seeding of the tumor and spread of cancerous cells.

Nursing Diagnosis and Planning

The following nursing diagnoses and expected outcomes apply to the child with Wilms' tumor and the child's family:

- Anxiety related to surgery with nephrectomy.
  Expected Outcome: The child and parents will express decreased anxiety about the outcome of surgery.
- Risk for Infection related to surgical interventions.
  Expected Outcome: The child will exhibit no signs and symptoms of infection.
- Knowledge Deficit related to the disease process and treatment plan.
  Expected Outcome: The child and parents will verbalize an understanding of the disease process and treatment plan.

Interventions

Because the child usually feels well, nursing care initially focuses on preoperative teaching of the parents and child. A sign should be placed on the bed warning against palpating the abdomen. A nephrectomy is a serious surgical procedure, and family members will have anxiety about the child losing a kidney. Nurses must offer support and reassurance.

Monitor the child for GI activity, bowel sounds, stool production, abdominal distension, signs and symptoms of infection, hemorrhage, and changes in blood pressure. Careful assessment of output by the remaining kidney is important. Strict intake and output measurements are made and totaled at least every 4 hours. These children will probably return from surgery with a nasogastric (NG) tube in place and with an order for replacement IV fluid for the NG drainage. Typically, NG tube output is totaled every 4 hours; that total is divided by 4, and either the resulting number is added to the current IV fluid rate or another IV solution is hung so that the amount lost by NG drainage is replaced over the next 4 hours. The process is repeated until the NG drainage has slowed enough that it does not affect overall fluid and electrolyte balance. The replacement fluid usually contains potassium because gastric contents are potassium rich. Serum electrolyte levels are checked every 8 to 12 hours during this process (see Chapter 37 for additional information on general postoperative care).

Once the tumor has been staged, the child is assigned to the appropriate therapeutic protocol. Teaching should center on the sequencing of tests and drugs on that protocol. Support for family members and assessment of their coping skills continues throughout therapy. Therapy for Wilms' tumor is usually accomplished on an outpatient basis (see p. 1324 for related nursing care).

Evaluation

- Are the parents and child using coping skills and mobilizing support systems?
- Is the family asking questions and sharing concerns and fears?
- Has the child remained free of infection and other complications of surgery?

Hodgkin's Disease

Hodgkin's disease is a neoplasm of lymphatic tissue. It is less common in children than non-Hodgkin's lymphoma. The presence of giant multinucleated cells (Reed-Sternberg cells) is the hallmark of Hodgkin's disease.

Etiology

The cause is unknown; however, the possibility of an infectious agent is being investigated (Hudson & Donaldson, 1997a). Herpesvirus 6, cytomegalovirus, and Epstein-Barr virus have been associated with Hodgkin's disease, but the exact relationship is unknown.

Incidence

In the United States, Hodgkin's disease is the fifth most common malignant tumor in both African-American and Caucasian children less than 15 years old. The overall incidence across the age range shows a slight male predominance, most marked in children less than 10 years old (Hudson & Donaldson, 1997b). Hodgkin's disease is extremely uncommon in children less than 5 years old. The diagnosis is usually made in the teenage to adult years.

Manifestations

Painless, firm movable adenopathy in the cervical and supraclavicular regions is the most common presentation. Mediastinal involvement, with or without airway obstruction, occurs in two thirds of children. Constitutional symptoms include fever, drenching night sweats, and weight loss (20% to 30% of children). Other manifestations include hepatosplenomegaly and fatigue.

Diagnostic Evaluation

Biopsy of an involved lymph node and histologic classification of the tissue confirm the diagnosis. The CBC, sedimentation rate, and serum ferritin and transferrin levels are determined, and renal and liver function tests are performed. A gallium scan is done to look for extent of disease. Gallium is a staging study as well as an excellent disease response marker when the tumor takes up gallium at diagnosis. Chest radiography and CT of the chest, abdomen, and pelvis are done to determine the extent of disease. Bilateral bone marrow aspirations and biopsies are done if constitutional symptoms are present.

A surgical staging laparotomy used to be performed commonly. It is an invasive surgical procedure that involves splenectomy, liver biopsy, and sampling of the retroperitoneal and pelvic nodes, and that defines the extent of disease more precisely than radiographic studies alone. Now that most pediatric patients receive systemic chemotherapy as part of their treatment, precise staging is less important. Because of the potential complications, a staging laparotomy is avoided unless the findings would significantly alter therapy (Hudson & Donaldson, 1997a).

Some manifestations are of prognostic significance, and staging takes them into account. Children with unexplained weight loss of more than 10% body weight in the preceding 6 months, unexplained fevers above 38.0°C (100.4°F), and night sweats are considered to have B disease, as opposed to A (asymptomatic) disease. The presence of B symptoms is thought to negatively impact prognosis (Hudson & Donaldson, 1997b). There are four stages, with stage I having the most favorable prognosis and stage IV the least favorable.

PATHOPHYSIOLOGY
of Hodgkin's Disease

Hodgkin's disease originates in a single lymph node or a group of lymph nodes in the same anatomic region. Hodgkin's disease is characterized by giant multinucleated cells called Reed-Sternberg cells that are thought to represent activated B and T lymphocytes (see Chapter 41 Clinical Reference pages). *Humoral immunity* remains normal in these patients, but they exhibit altered *cellular immunity*. Hodgkin's disease spreads predictably from lymph nodes to nonnodal sites such as the spleen, liver, bone, bone marrow, lungs, and mediastinum.

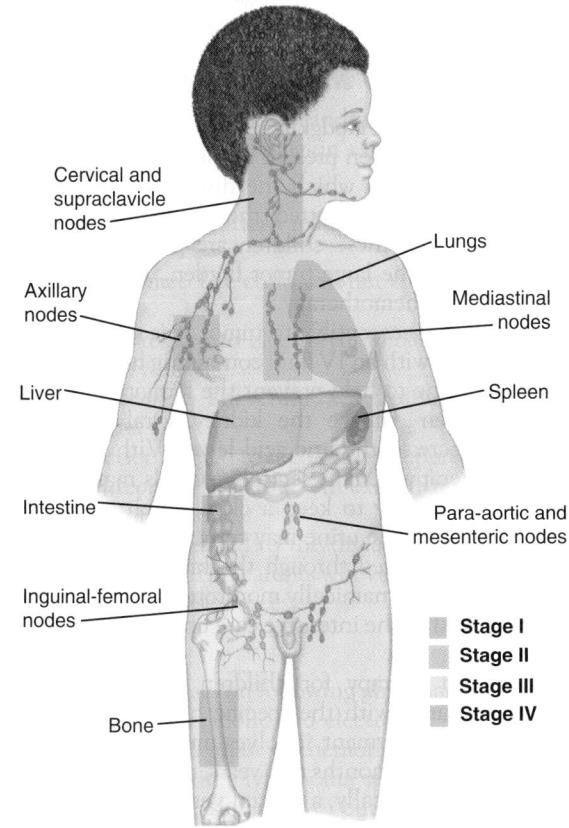

Cervical and supraclavicle nodes

Lungs

Axillary nodes

Mediastinal nodes

Liver

Spleen

Intestine

Para-aortic and mesenteric nodes

Inguinal-femoral nodes

Stage I
Stage II
Stage III
Stage IV

Bone

Therapeutic Management

Therapy depends on the child's age at diagnosis, disease stage, and histologic type. If the mediastinal disease is expansive, it may compromise respiration. Radiation therapy may be used to shrink the tissue before the child undergoes general anesthesia.

Most children are treated with chemotherapy alone or chemotherapy and radiation therapy. If the disease is detected in a single site, radiation therapy may be used as a single treatment in fully grown patients. Long-term survival rates in excess of 90% can be expected with stage I and II disease. For stages III and IV disease, the long-term survival rates are 80% and 70%, respectively (Hudson & Donaldson, 1997a).

NURSING CARE
The Child with Hodgkin's Disease

Assessment

When asked about activity level, children with Hodgkin's disease may report not noticing any change until it was brought to their attention, because the onset is insidious. Typically, the child noticed lumps around the neck while bathing. Initial assessment of these children includes a thorough lymph node examination. Depending on the severity of the mediastinal disease, the respiratory system should be assessed for a change in status with the child both sitting and lying down. Preoperative teaching is done to prepare the child for the biopsy. Assessment for future educational preparation is done.

Nursing Diagnosis and Planning

The following nursing diagnoses and expected outcomes apply to the child with Hodgkin's disease and the child's family:

■ Risk for Infection related to immunosuppressed state and, if performed, surgery and splenectomy.
Expected Outcome: The child will experience no signs or symptoms of infection.
■ Ineffective Breathing Pattern related to mediastinal disease (if present).
Expected Outcome: The child will experience no severe respiratory distress.
■ Knowledge Deficit related to the disease process.
Expected Outcome: The parents will verbalize an understanding of the disease process and their fears.

Interventions

Initially, the nurse will need to prepare the child for the diagnostic procedures and a surgical biopsy. A central venous catheter may be inserted at the time of diagnosis. In older children a peripheral IV line may be placed at the time of each chemotherapy treatment so they do not need a central venous catheter.

At least two thirds of children present with some degree of mediastinal involvement (Hudson & Donaldson, 1997a). Management of the airway is a concern if the child has any mediastinal disease.

A staging laparotomy with splenectomy is generally avoided. If it is required, however, these children need special care. The spleen removes organisms such as *Streptococcus pneumoniae* and *Hemophilus influenzae*. Without the spleen, these organisms can produce fulminating infections. Ideally, children who undergo splenectomy receive a pneumoccocal and *Hemophilus influenzae* type B immunization before the procedure. Postoperative care includes assessing for bleeding at dressing sites and administering prophylactic antibiotics.

Induction chemotherapy is begun as soon as the child is stable and staging of disease has been completed. If there is airway compromise, radiation therapy will be given locally to provide immediate relief.

Education includes an explanation of the therapeutic protocol. Questions should be answered honestly. Realistic expectations of response to therapy will help parents deal

PATHOPHYSIOLOGY
. . . .
of Brain Tumors

The histology of brain tumors ranges from benign to highly malignant. The impact of these tumors on the brain may have little to do with their relative malignancy and everything to do with the size of the tumor and the area of the brain affected.

Most brain tumors arise in the posterior fossa.

About 50% of tumors are astrocytomas, 25% are medulloblastomas, 11% are brain stem gliomas, and 9% are ependymomas (Heideman et al., 1997). Prognostic percentages vary with the type of tumor, the amount resected, metastatic spread, age and physical status of the child, and the individual response to therapy.

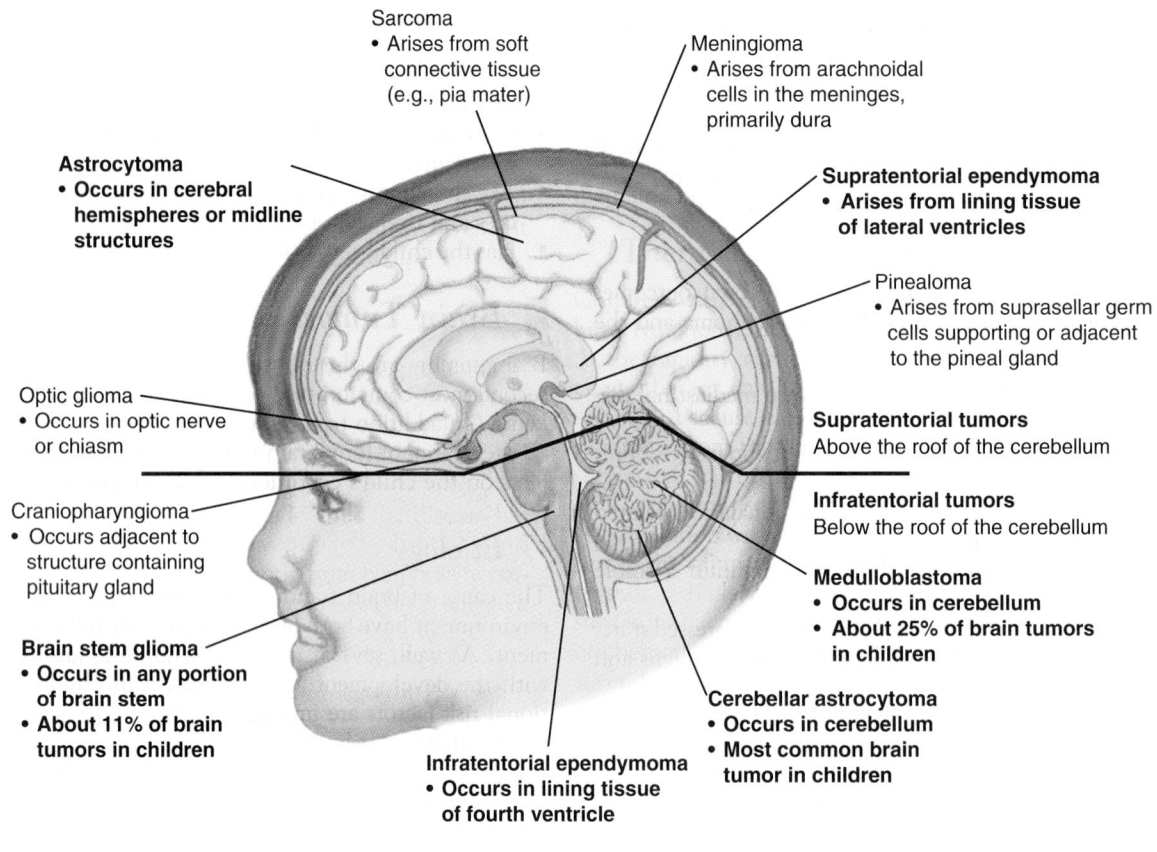

Sarcoma
• Arises from soft connective tissue (e.g., pia mater)

Meningioma
• Arises from arachnoidal cells in the meninges, primarily dura

Astrocytoma
• Occurs in cerebral hemispheres or midline structures

Supratentorial ependymoma
• Arises from lining tissue of lateral ventricles

Pinealoma
• Arises from suprasellar germ cells supporting or adjacent to the pineal gland

Optic glioma
• Occurs in optic nerve or chiasm

Supratentorial tumors
Above the roof of the cerebellum

Infratentorial tumors
Below the roof of the cerebellum

Craniopharyngioma
• Occurs adjacent to structure containing pituitary gland

Medulloblastoma
• Occurs in cerebellum
• About 25% of brain tumors in children

Brain stem glioma
• Occurs in any portion of brain stem
• About 11% of brain tumors in children

Cerebellar astrocytoma
• Occurs in cerebellum
• Most common brain tumor in children

Infratentorial ependymoma
• Occurs in lining tissue of fourth ventricle

Location of brain tumors in children. Boldface labels indicate the most frequently occurring tumors in children.

• cranial enlargement and a bulging fontanel in infants
• nuchal rigidity
• subtle behavioral changes (including irritability)
• altered school performance

Diagnostic Evaluation

Once a tumor is suspected, MRI, CT, single-photon emission computed tomography (SPECT), or positron emission tomography (PET) may be done. MRI is currently the imaging modality most commonly used to evaluate brain tumors. During MRI, the child must lie motionless inside a dark tunnel for approximately 1 hour. This is especially difficult for young children. Infants, toddlers, and sometimes older children need sedation. Spinal MRI is done to look for metastatic disease in the spine. Cerebrospinal fluid (CSF) is examined for the presence of tumor cells.

Usually the diagnosis is suspected from the child's signs and symptoms and the location of the tumor. Pathologic examination confirms the tissue type and tumor diagnosis.

Therapeutic Management

Initial intervention for a child with a brain tumor is debulking, or the surgical removal of as much of the tumor as is possible while minimally disturbing the surrounding brain tissue so that the child's neurologic functioning is preserved to the highest degree possible. Complete removal of the tumor is associated with the best prognosis. In the case of a brain stem tumor, the risk to neurologic function outweighs the benefit of debulking, so surgery may not be done. Depending on the location of the tumor and the extent of surgical resection, a ventriculoperitoneal shunt may be inserted to relieve the hydrocephalus, thus relieving some of the symptoms. Children with supratentorial tumors are at risk for seizures from the tumor itself or from scar tissue formation after surgery. These children are prescribed anticonvulsants with monitoring of therapeutic levels.

Therapy depends on the type of tumor, its location, and the amount of residual tumor after surgery. Therapy frequently consists of surgery, radiation therapy, and chemotherapy. Imaging is performed at intervals to help determine the response to therapy.

NURSING CARE

The Child with a Brain Tumor

Assessment

Because most pediatric brain tumors arise in the posterior fossa, symptoms are related to increased intracranial pressure (ICP) and hydrocephalus as well as to impaired balance or brain stem function.

Parents may express guilt for not paying attention to their child's complaints of headaches. These children are initially seen with neurologic symptoms. A thorough neurologic assessment should be performed (see Chapter 33). Before the child is allowed to get out of bed without help, the child's safety should be assessed. Children who have had insidious loss of visual function may have learned to compensate well; excellent nursing assessment skills will be needed to determine that loss. Seizure precautions should be considered for any child with a brain tumor, both preoperatively and postoperatively.

Depending on the length of time the child has been feeling ill, weight loss and poor nutrition may be present. Assess nutritional status, growth, and development throughout treatment.

Nursing Diagnosis and Planning

The following nursing diagnoses and expected outcomes may be appropriate for the child with a brain tumor and the child's family:

- Pain related to increased ICP.
  Expected Outcome: The child will verbalize a decrease in the severity of headaches.
- Risk for Infection related to surgery.
  Expected Outcome: The child will exhibit no signs of infection.
- Anxiety (child and parent) related to the surgery and diagnosis.
  Expected Outcome: The child and parents will exhibit decreased anxiety about the outcomes of surgery and therapy.
- Knowledge Deficit related to the disease process.
  Expected Outcome: The parents will verbalize an understanding of the disease process.
- Body Image Disturbances related to a shaved head and hair loss.
  Expected Outcome: The child will demonstrate appropriate coping techniques for hair loss and a return to socializing.

Interventions

When a child is suspected of having a brain tumor, the fear and anxiety are tremendous because of the potential neurologic impact of surgery and the fear of treatment failure and death.

Preoperative Care

Preoperative teaching at the child's developmental level prepares the child and family for the potential outcomes of surgery. The child should be educated about anesthesia and should be prepared to spend some time in the intensive care unit after surgery. (See Chapter 37 for a discussion of preoperative care.)

The child's head will be shaved before surgery. Although every effort is made to shave only as much hair as is necessary, shaving may still be traumatic for the child. The nurse should be aware of this and assist the child in verbalizing fears. Some children enjoy wearing a favorite cap or hat or making an outing of going to buy a hat. Prepare the child to wake up with a large dressing covering the head.

Postoperative Care

Postoperatively the child is at risk for increased ICP related to cerebral edema, hydrocephalus, or hemorrhage. Check and record vital signs, mental status, and neurologic status frequently. Pay special attention to the child's temperature, which may be elevated because of hypothalamic or brain stem involvement following surgery (the brain stem is not surgically manipulated but may become edematous following resection of adjacent tissues). A cooling blanket should either be in place on the bed or readily available in case the child becomes hyperthermic.

Assess the child for signs of bleeding. Internal bleeding manifests through changes in parameters associated with increasing ICP (i.e., mental status and neurologic status changes or, much later, abnormal pupil size, blood pressure, and respiratory pattern). Note any external bleeding on the dressing. Assess the back of the dressing for posterior pooling of blood. It is helpful to know the amount of expected drainage, especially if a drain has been placed in the wound. Circle areas of drainage to monitor the amount of drainage, and reinforce the dressing. Colorless drainage indicates CSF and should be reported immediately.

Postoperative positioning is prescribed by the surgeon. The location and size of the tumor are factors in determining the child's position. The head of the bed may be elevated to promote drainage of CSF, or the child may be required to lie flat. When turning the child, take care not to place tension on the suture line if it is in an area that movement will affect. Never place the child in the Trendelenburg position because it increases ICP and the risk of bleeding. In the event of shock, notify the surgeon immediately, before changing the child's position.

Many children return from the surgical suite with external ventricular shunts in place. The external drains must be maintained at appropriate levels and CSF measured accurately. Grossly bloody fluid may indicate a ventricular hemorrhage and should be reported immediately (Shiminski-Maher & Shields, 1995). From 30% to 40% of children with brain tumors will develop hydrocephalus, requiring placement of a permanent shunt catheter (Ryan &

Functional Deficits Following Surgery for a Brain Tumor

After surgery, the child should be assessed for the following functional deficits:

- Ataxia, including head control and truncal stability
- Bilateral extremity strength and purposeful movement
- Speech
- Ability to swallow
- Vision and hearing
- Presurgical development task mastery
- Receptive and expressive language

If the deficits are significant, the child may need rehabilitative therapy to regain function.

Shiminski-Maher, 1995). (Chapter 52 addresses care of the child with a shunt.)

The child may have a severe headache due to cerebral edema. A quiet environment without bright lighting should be provided, together with comfortable positioning within the limits of the child's condition. Analgesia should be provided according to the surgeon's protocol. The analgesic agent will vary from morphine to Tylenol (acetaminophen). (See Chapter 39 for a discussion of pain management.)

After the child's condition has been stabilized, assess the child for functional deficits resulting from surgery. These deficits are somewhat predictable if the involved area of the brain and the function of that area are known. If the deficits are significant, rehabilitative therapy may be necessary to help the child regain function.

Depending on the type and extent of the tumor and the child's age, radiation therapy, chemotherapy, or both may be provided after recovery from surgery. Some brain tumors that can be completely resected are not further treated, but the child is carefully monitored with serial MRIs. Often, however, further treatment is necessary. Radiation therapy is avoided in children less than 3 to 5 years old because of the toxic effects on developing brain tissue (Shiminski-Maher & Shields, 1995). The side effects of radiation therapy to the brain merit special attention (see p. 1318). It is important for families to be aware of its potential side effects and to understand that acute side effects will resolve.

Over the past decade, chemotherapy has emerged as treatment for pediatric brain tumors, either in conjunction with radiation therapy or alone. Its use has increased survival rates as much as twofold (Shiminski-Maher & Shields, 1995). Chemotherapy may be delivered on an inpatient or outpatient basis, depending on the intensity (see p. 1324 for related nursing care).

Evaluation

- Are there both verbal and nonverbal indications of a positive comfort level?
- Is the family able to discuss the treatment plan and concerns related to the disease and treatment plan?
- Has the child remained free of infection?
- Is the child relating with peers in the same manner as before the diagnosis and hospitalization?

- Have the child and family expressed decreased levels of stress and the ability to rely on coping strategies?

Neuroblastoma

Neuroblastoma is a solid tumor found only in infants and children. Children less than 12 months old and those with a lower stage of disease have a more favorable prognosis.

Pathophysiology

The embryonal tumor arises from neural crest cells, which normally develop into the sympathetic nervous system and the adrenal medulla. Typically the tumor infringes on adjacent normal tissue and organs. Greater understanding of the cytogenetic makeup of this tumor has given researchers insight into prognostic indicators, which help with treatment planning.

Etiology

The cause of neuroblastoma is unknown. Its prevalence is similar in various countries around the world, suggesting that environmental factors do not cause the disease. There is evidence that a familial form of neuroblastoma may occur; children in families with one or more affected members may be at increased risk for the development of neuroblastoma.

Incidence

Neuroblastoma occurs at a rate of 8.7 per 1 million children, or 500 to 600 new cases diagnosed each year in the United States (Castleberry, 1997). It is more common in boys than in girls, and more common in white children than in African-American children. The peak age of presentation is 22 months, with 97% of children diagnosed before age 10 years. About 80% of patients present with metastases (Kusumakumary, Ajithkumar, Ratheesan, et al., 1998) to the bone, bone marrow, liver, or lung.

Manifestations

The manifestations of neuroblastoma depend on the extent of disease and the location of the tumor. In 65% of cases a primary abdominal mass and a protuberant firm abdomen are present (Kusumakumary et al., 1998). Other manifestations include impaired range of motion and mobility, pain and limping, and a large abdominal mass, which can disrupt bowel and bladder function. Chest tumors may produce cough and decreased chest expansion, with respiratory compromise. Compression of the superior vena cava results in facial and periorbital edema. Spinal cord compression may cause inability to walk and impaired bowel and bladder function. Drooping eyelids or small pupils may be evident, as are "dancing" eye movements, myoclonic jerks and bruising.

Diagnostic Evaluation

The diagnostic workup includes chest radiography, CT of the chest, abdomen, and pelvis, and skeletal scintigraphy to determine the extent of disease. Bone marrow aspiration and biopsy, usually of both posterior iliac crests, are done to evaluate marrow involvement.

Tumor samples will be sent to special reference laboratories to look at the genetic makeup of the tumor. Genetic information helps determine the prognosis and treatment plan.

Therapeutic Management

The treatment of neuroblastoma depends on the presence and extent of metastasis. The International Staging System for Neuroblastoma is used to compare patients. Staging criteria include the extent and location of metastases, lymph node involvement, and whether the tumor is unilateral or crosses the midline. Early-stage disease without metastasis may require only surgical excision of the tumor and follow-up evaluations. Children with later-stage, poor-prognosis disease may undergo surgery to obtain tissue samples or for tumor debulking for pain control, not for resection of the tumor or tumors.

Age at diagnosis is also an important prognostic indicator. Children diagnosed before they are 1 year old have a better prognosis than children diagnosed at a later age. Neuroblastomas that occur in infants less than 1 year old have a high rate of spontaneous regression and may be watched carefully or treated with low-dose chemotherapy (Castleberry, 1997).

After staging, treatment plans may include radiotherapy to tumor sites and systemic chemotherapy for several months. Another attempt may be made to resect the tumor after combination chemotherapy has been administered to reduce the tumor size. Autologous BMT has been found to be effective in children with advanced-stage disease (Stram, Matthay, O'Leary, et al., 1996).

Children with stage I or II disease and who are without poor prognostic factors have a cure rate of 80% to 90%. Children with disseminated disease and who are over 1 year old have a survival rate of 10% to 30% (Brodeur, Maris, Yamashiro, et al., 1997).

NURSING CARE
The Child with Neuroblastoma

Assessment

Parents may state their child has wanted to be held more often than usual. Activity level and appetite are usually decreased. Children with neuroblastoma typically appear pale, very irritable, and uncomfortable. Because of large abdominal tumors, many present with protuberant abdomens in which hard masses crossing the midline can be palpated. Range of motion and mobility are often impaired, so much so that the child cannot bear weight. If the tumor is compressing a nerve, neurologic changes may be noted. If the tumor is causing compression within the abdomen, vascular drainage may be compromised.

Nursing Diagnosis and Planning

The following nursing diagnoses and expected outcomes may be appropriate for the child with a neuroblastoma and the child's family:

- Pain related to tumor pressure.
  Expected Outcome: The infant will exhibit decreased crying and a relaxed body position.
- Anxiety (parents) related to a diagnosis of cancer, surgery, and treatment plan.
  Expected Outcome: The parents will express decreased anxiety about the outcomes of therapy.
- Knowledge Deficit related to the disease process.
  Expected Outcome: The parents will verbalize an understanding of the disease process.

Interventions

Nursing care focuses initially on support of family members as they react and adjust to the diagnosis of cancer. The nurse facilitates the educational process to allay fears of the unknown. The initial care of the child includes pain management, both preoperatively and postoperatively. Expect the child with an abdominal tumor to return from surgery with an NG tube in place. Assess the wound carefully for bleeding and signs of infection. (Postoperative care of the child is discussed in Chapter 37.)

Typically, later-stage disease will be treated immediately postoperatively with chemotherapy. With responsive tumors, improvements in the child's disposition will result very quickly (see p. 1324 for additional nursing care).

Evaluation

- Has the infant exhibited decreased crying and irritability?
- Does the infant rest quietly and comfortably in the parent's arms and have uninterrupted periods of rest?
- Are the parents asking questions related to the child's disease and treatment and seeking the support of family and friends?
- Are the parents verbalizing their fears and indicating the existence of coping skills?

Osteosarcoma

Osteosarcoma, or osteogenic sarcoma, is the most common bone malignancy in children, and a very aggressive tumor. The symptoms of this disease in its earliest stage are almost always attributed to extremity injury or normal growing pains. Typically, trauma brings the tumor to the attention of medical personnel.

Pathophysiology

Osteosarcoma originates from bone-producing cells, which invade the medullary canal of the bone and form a solid tumor. Lesions of the distal femur and around the knee account for 42% of all osteosarcoma (Meyer & Gorlick, 1997).

Etiology

The cause of osteosarcoma is unknown, although associations have been made between radiation therapy for other diseases and osteosarcoma. Familial tendencies have been seen, suggesting that genetic factors are involved (Pratt, Meyer, Luo, et al., 1997).

Incidence

The incidence of osteosarcoma peaks in the teenage years, and the rapid bone growth of the adolescent growth spurt is associated with the development of this tumor. Osteosarcoma occurs in girls at an earlier age than in boys, which corresponds to the earlier maturation of girls. Before adolescence osteosarcoma is rare but occurs with equal frequency in boys and girls (Meyer & Gorlick, 1997). In about 20% of children the disease has metastasized at the time of diagnosis, usually to the lungs (Meyer & Gorlick, 1997).

Manifestations

Manifestations of osteosarcoma include progressive, insidious, or intermittent pain at the tumor site; a palpable mass; limping, if a weight-bearing limb is affected; progressive, limited range of motion; and eventually pathologic fractures at the tumor site.

Diagnostic Evaluation

Initially, radiographs of the primary site and chest are taken, then CT or MRI and skeletal scintigraphy are performed. The CT scan includes the chest to search for pulmonary metastases, which helps with staging the disease. A biopsy of the tumor must be performed with great care so that there is no local contamination of tissue by tumor. Laboratory tests include a CBC, chemistries, and serum alkaline phosphatase (ALP) and lactate dehydrogenase (LDH) determinations. Higher levels of the enzymes ALP and LDH correlate with a higher probability of treatment failure.

Therapeutic Management

The goals of therapy are to remove the tumor and to prevent the spread of disease. Osteogenic sarcoma is treated with a combination of surgery and chemotherapy. Chemotherapy is administered before and after surgery. Radiation therapy is used only for palliative pain control in advanced-stage disease because osteosarcoma is generally unresponsive to irradiation.

Amputation was once the standard surgical intervention and is still necessary in some cases. Occasionally favorable tumor location allows specially trained orthopedic surgeons to perform a complex limb-salvage operation. The affected tissue is removed with the certainty of clean margins, while limb function is preserved. The diseased bone is removed, and either bone grafts or surgically placed orthopedic devices are implanted.

Early research on this disease found that 90% of patients developed recurrent disease after surgery alone. This finding alerted physicians to the presence of microscopic disease. Therefore, after surgery, chemotherapy is continued even if the surgical procedure appears to have been successful. Chemotherapy is aimed at preventing the spread of disease by killing any microscopic tumor cells present anywhere in the body.

The extent of disease at diagnosis, elevated LDH and ALP levels, and tumor necrosis found on surgical resection are the three most significant prognostic indicators. The cure rate is about 75% for children without overt metastases at diagnosis (Meyer & Gorlick, 1997). The 20% of children

with metastatic disease at diagnosis have a substantially poorer outcome.

NURSING CARE
The Child with Osteosarcoma

Assessment

Subjective data to be gathered include a history of any injury to the affected limb and a history of discomfort. By the time children with osteosarcomas come to medical attention, they may be in considerable pain from the tumor. Warmth, erythema, and tenderness at the site of tumor are not uncommon. If the swelling is great, the skin may appear shiny and taut, with dilated blood vessels. Lung involvement is usually asymptomatic.

To prepare the child for outcomes of surgery, an assessment of physical activity and sports involvement is essential, as is the psychosocial history. As for any child with cancer, body image changes, especially if the affected limb must be amputated, are of paramount importance. Preoperatively, the nurse should not only assess children's values and fears, but should also begin the process of preparing children for what they will look like after surgery.

Nursing Diagnosis and Planning

The following nursing diagnoses and expected outcomes may be appropriate for the child with an osteosarcoma and the child's family:

- Pain related to disease process and procedures.
  Expected Outcome: The child will verbalize adequate pain control using a pain assessment tool.
- Fear and Anxiety related to loss or impairment of a limb and a diagnosis of cancer.
  Expected Outcome: The child and parents will express decreased fears and anxiety related to the surgery and diagnosis.
- Risk for Infection related to chemotherapy or surgery.
  Expected Outcome: The child will exhibit no signs and symptoms of infection.
- Body Image Disturbance related to loss or impairment of a limb.
  Expected Outcome: The child will return to appropriate social situations.
- Impaired Physical Mobility related to loss or impairment of limb function.
  Expected Outcome: The child will adapt to physical impairment with assistance, with a return of mobility.
- Knowledge Deficit related to the disease process.
  Expected Outcome: The child and parents will verbalize an understanding of the disease process.

Interventions

Initial care is focused on making the child comfortable. Preoperative teaching is extensive and procedure specific. If limb salvage is the procedure of choice, the surgeon and nurse will spend considerable time with the family explaining what is to be done. The nurse reinforces the preoperative and postoperative teaching.

In addition to the usual postoperative care, pain, infection, and potential hemorrhage are nursing concerns. The potential for postoperative pneumonia may be greater in the child with pulmonary metastases than in the child without such metastases.

If amputation occurs, phantom limb pain is a temporary condition some children may experience. This sensation of burning, aching, or cramping in the missing limb is most distressing to the child. The child needs to be reassured that the condition is normal. Numerous pharmacologic agents are available to help with postoperative neurogenic pain.

The child who undergoes amputation will be fitted with a permanent prosthesis once the surgical site has thoroughly healed. To begin to mold the stump for that, a temporary prosthesis may be used. A temporary prosthesis enables the child to maintain use and strength of surrounding muscles in preparation for the permanent device. A prosthesis will address the issue of body image disturbance and enable the child to become independent in activities of daily living faster. Prepare the child for extensive work with physical therapists to achieve mobility with the prosthesis. Teenagers especially may become discouraged if they expect the prosthesis to enable them to move normally. Prepare them for a limp or for awkward movements with the prosthesis.

Assist the child to verbalize feelings about changes in body image and function. Involve the child in age-appropriate decision making concerning care. Encourage interaction with other children of the same age who have the same disease (support groups). Provide opportunities for the family to participate in the care of the child and to provide support and encouragement.

Follow-up outpatient visits need to include a careful assessment of psychosocial adjustment. Questions should include the topics of social interactions, school attendance and performance, and behavioral changes (see p. 1324 for related nursing care).

Evaluation

- Is the child experiencing discomfort related to the surgical procedures?
- Are the family and child discussing fears related to the disease and treatment?
- Is the child relating with peers?
- Has the child adapted to the physical impairment, with a return to mobility?
- Is the child free of infection?
- Are the child and family asking questions related to the disease process?
- Does the family and child verbalize an understanding of the treatment of the tumor?

Ewing's Sarcoma

Ewing's sarcoma is the second most common bone tumor seen in children. The diagnosis is often challenging to make because this disease mimics infection and may be difficult to differentiate from other malignancies. Ewing's sarcoma may also manifest as a soft tissue mass.

Pathophysiology

The diagnosis of Ewing's sarcoma is made after all other small round cell tumors have been excluded. Ewing's sarcoma has no defining characteristics. Like osteosarcoma, this tumor invades the bone and is found most often in the midshaft of long bones, especially the femur, vertebrae, ribs, and pelvic bones (Grier, 1997). Gross metastasis is uncommon at diagnosis but does occur, most often to the lungs, bones, or bone marrow. As with osteosarcoma, microscopic disease is thought to be present early in the disease process.

Etiology

The cause is unknown. No genetic predispositions have been shown.

Incidence

The incidence of Ewing's sarcoma is 1.7 per 1 million white children per year. The disease is very uncommon in African-American and Chinese children (Grier, 1997). Ewing's sarcoma is rare in children less than 5 years old and adults more than 30 years old. The incidence peaks between ages 10 and 20.

Manifestations

Manifestations of Ewing's sarcoma include pain, soft tissue swelling around the affected bone, and fever. If metastatic disease occurs, anorexia, fever, malaise, fatigue, and weight loss are seen. If vertebral tumor is present, neurologic symptoms will be seen. If a rib tumor is present, respiratory symptoms may be seen.

Diagnostic Evaluation

The diagnostic workup is the same as for osteosarcoma, and biopsy is necessary to differentiate Ewing's sarcoma from other neoplastic processes.

Therapeutic Management

Treatment begins with chemotherapy to decrease the tumor bulk, followed by surgical resection of the primary tumor. Clinicians debate whether to manage the primary tumor site with surgery or radiotherapy because this tumor is so sensitive to radiation. Consideration is given to the expendability of the bone involved when surgery is a treatment option, versus the potential late effects of radiation. Ribs and the proximal fibula are considered expendable and may be removed to excise the tumor without affecting function. Cure rates exceed 70% in children with small extremity tumors and no metastases (Meyer & Marina, 1996). With gross metastasis, the cure rate is dramatically decreased.

NURSING CARE
The Child with Ewing's Sarcoma

Nursing care is similar to that for children with osteosarcomas, with the addition of care for the child receiving radiotherapy (see pp. 1318 and 1324 for related nursing care).

Rhabdomyosarcoma

Rhabdomyosarcoma is a malignancy of muscle, or striated tissue, that most often occurs periorbitally, in the head and neck in younger children, or in the trunk and extremities in older children. Long-term survival rates vary with the age of the patient, the histologic type, and the location of the tumor.

Pathophysiology

Four histologic subtypes of rhabdomyosarcoma exist. The embryonic type accounts for 50% to 60% of the tumors and has the best prognosis. About 20% of cases are of the alveolar type, which is most often found in the perineal area, trunk, and extremities and has the worst prognosis. The pleomorphic type is very rare in children. Some 10% to 20% of tumors are considered undifferentiated (Wexler & Helman, 1997).

The prognosis depends on several factors other than histologic type. If the tumor is in a location where manifestations appear early, rather than deeply buried in a body cavity, the prognosis is better because the tumor is usually found before it has metastasized. Abnormalities in the DNA content of the tumor cells have prognostic significance. Staging of the tumor is based on whether the tumor was resected completely, resected with residual microscopic disease, incompletely resected, or had metastasized to distant sites (McHugh & Boothroyd, 1999). Local failure is more common if the tumor cannot be completely resected.

Etiology

Although the exact etiology is unknown, rhabdomyosarcoma has been associated with familial cancer syndromes. There is a higher incidence of maternal breast cancer in mothers of children with rhabdomyosarcoma.

Incidence

Rhabdomyosarcoma is the most common soft tissue malignancy in children and accounts for 5% to 10% of all malignant solid tumors in children (Pappo, Shapiro & Crist, 1997). The annual incidence in the United States is estimated at 4.3 cases per 1 million white children and 3.3 cases per 1 million African-American children. Two age groups predominate, 2 to 6 years and 15 to 19 years (Pappo et al., 1997).

Manifestations

The manifestations of rhabdomyosarcoma depend on the tumor location. Soft to hard, nontender, relatively immobile masses may be mistaken for a traumatic hematoma. If the lesion is periorbital, visual changes are present; the child may have ptosis, exophthalmos, or proptosis (bulging). Cranial nerve involvement may occur. If the lesion affects an extremity, range of motion will be limited. In the case of pelvic tumors, the function of organs around the tumor is disrupted.

Diagnostic Evaluation

The diagnosis is made after biopsy or attempted surgical resection of the tumor, and a decision about treatment is made, depending on the location of the tumor. CT, skeletal scintigraphy and bone marrow aspiration and biopsy are performed to determine the extent of metastasis. Laboratory studies include a CBC, urinalysis, and renal and liver function tests.

Therapeutic Management

Rhabdomyosarcoma is treated with chemotherapy, surgery, and radiation therapy. Chemotherapy is used to decrease the tumor bulk and reduce the extent and morbidity of surgery. After surgical removal of the tumor, additional chemotherapy is provided. Like Ewing's sarcoma, microscopic rhabdomyosarcoma is often present at the time of diagnosis. Discontinuation of chemotherapy after removal of the tumor generally results in recurrent disease. Tumor cells not removed by surgery are referred to as *residual disease*. Radiation therapy is used for children who have residual disease or whose tumor was not resectable. About 80% of children with metastatic disease at the time of diagnosis relapse (Pappo et al., 1997).

■ NURSING CARE
The Child with Rhabdomyosarcoma

Assessment

Parents may relate that their first indication that something was wrong was a decreased activity level in a young child unable to verbalize pain. If the tumor is more superficially located, parents may have discovered a lump or swelling.

The physical examination findings will depend on the location of the tumor, but typically a soft to hard, nontender mass will be palpated. The surrounding lymph nodes should be palpated for enlargement, which may indicate tumor involvement. The CBC is usually normal unless the tumor has extended into bone marrow, causing a decrease in hemoglobin values.

Nursing Diagnosis and Planning

The following nursing diagnoses and expected outcomes apply to the child with rhabdomyosarcoma and the child's family:

- Anxiety (family/child) related to the surgical procedure and outcome.
  Expected Outcome: The child and parents will express decreased anxiety about the surgical procedure and outcomes.
- Risk for Infection related to chemotherapy or surgery.
  Expected Outcome: The child will exhibit no signs or symptoms of infection.
- Knowledge Deficit related to the disease process and treatment plan.
  Expected Outcome: The child and parents will verbalize an understanding of the disease process and treatment.

Interventions

Nursing care initially focuses on support of family members as they react and adjust to the diagnosis of cancer. Second, the nurse facilitates the educational process to allay fears of the unknown.

Postoperative care of the biopsy or surgical site involves careful observation for signs of infection, hemorrhage, and edema. If surgery entailed excision of an abdominal or pelvic tumor, the child will return from the surgical suite with an NG tube and possibly drains in place. Typically, a central venous catheter is placed at the time of surgery to facilitate chemotherapy administration (see p. 1318 for care of the child receiving chemotherapy or radiation therapy).

Follow-up care involves periodic CT or MRI studies to assess tumor response to therapy and to monitor any development of disease progression. Most relapses occur within 2 years of diagnosis and during therapy, although relapses have been reported as late as 6 years after diagnosis (Pappo et al., 1997) (see p. 1324 for related nursing care).

Evaluation

- Is anxiety decreased in the family and the child?
- Is the family supported by extended family members and friends, and are they asking questions related to the child's disease and care?
- Has the child remained free of infection?
- Does the child display a relaxed, comfortable body posture while relating with peers and family members?
- Can the child and family verbalize an understanding of the disease process and treatment?

Retinoblastoma

Retinoblastoma is a rare, malignant tumor of the eye found only in children. Observant parents may bring this disease to the attention of the physician when they look at a photograph and see a white reflection in one of the child's eyes instead of the normal red color when the camera flash is reflected off the retina.

Pathophysiology

The tumor develops on the retina, growing inward toward the vitreous humor or out toward the subretinal space. Retinoblastoma can develop at a single site, but more commonly there are multiple independent tumors. The process of cells breaking off from the main mass and forming additional independent tumors is called *seeding*. Bilateral disease is present in less than 30% of cases. Extension of the tumor down the optic nerve into the CNS occurs rarely. In the United States, most cases of retinoblastoma are diagnosed before the tumor has metastasized beyond the intraocular space (Donaldson, Egbert, Newsham, et al., 1997).

As for other cancers, a staging system has been developed to standardize descriptions of extent of disease and direct treatment regimens.

Etiology

Retinoblastoma results from a genetic mutation. The majority of these genetic mutations are sporadic, occurring within a single retinal cell that then multiplies to form the tumor. Familial retinoblastoma occurs in individuals who have a germline mutation. The mutation that causes familial disease has been isolated to chromosome 13. Advances in genetic studies of this disease have led to genetic research on other forms of childhood cancer.

Incidence

The incidence is 1 in 20,000 live births, with an equal distribution between sexes and across races. Approximately 80% of cases are diagnosed before age 3 to 4 years (Donaldson et al., 1997).

Manifestations

Manifestations of retinoblastoma include leukokoria, or cat's-eye reflex; vision loss; pain, redness, and inflammation of the eye; strabismus; and squinting.

Diagnostic Evaluation

The diagnosis is usually made by detecting leukokoria on routine examination. In children with a family history of retinoblastoma, the diagnosis usually follows routine funduscopic examination under general anesthesia. CT of the orbits and head to search for extraocular spread of tumor should be performed in a child with suspected retinoblastoma. Skeletal scintigraphy, bone marrow aspiration and biopsy, and lumbar puncture generally are not necessary unless there is clinical evidence of metastasis (Scott, O'Brien, Murray, et al., 1997).

Therapeutic Management

The goal of current treatment of retinoblastoma is not only to save the child's life, but also to preserve the globe and useful vision (Zhao et al., 1998). Enucleation, or removal of the eye, was standard therapy but is becoming less frequent as nonsurgical therapies improve. Enucleation may be indicated if the child has no chance for useful vision even if the tumor is destroyed. Another indication is failure of nonsurgical treatment. A disadvantage of enucleation in children under 3 years of age is that the orbit ceases to grow normally after the eye is removed and will look increasingly sunken as the child's face continues to grow.

External beam radiation therapy is now the reference standard in the treatment of many retinoblastomas (Donaldson et al., 1997). The disadvantages of radiation therapy are cosmetic deformities resulting from abnormal growth of the areas of skull exposed to radiation and a higher risk of secondary malignancies in children with familial retinoblastoma.

The role of chemotherapy in treating intraocular disease has been disappointing because intraocular penetration of systemic drugs is poor and the tumors often develop multidrug resistance. Preliminary results using chemotherapy in combination with cyclosporin therapy, laser therapy, and cryosurgery show promise of curing many children, without requiring external beam radiation therapy or enucleation (Gallie, Budning, DeBoer, et al., 1996; Pratt, 1998). Chemotherapy is used to treat metastatic disease, although not usually with long-term cure. The long-term survival rate among children with retinoblastoma is excellent. The 5-year survival rate for children with disease that does not extend to extraocular sites exceeds 85% (Donaldson et al., 1997).

NURSING CARE
· · · · · · · · · ·
The Child with Retinoblastoma

Assessment

Except for leukokoria (a whitish reflex in pupillary area), the findings on physical examination are usually normal.

Nursing Diagnoses and Planning

The following nursing diagnoses and expected outcomes apply to the child with retinoblastoma and the child's family:

- Anxiety (child and family) related to cancer and enucleation or fear of blindness.
  Expected Outcome: The child and family will express decreased anxiety about outcomes of therapy.
- Sensory/Perceptual Alterations (Visual) related to visual changes caused by the tumor or enucleation.
  Expected Outcome: The child will develop compensatory mechanisms for vision.
- Knowledge Deficit related to the disease process and treatment.
  Expected Outcome: The child and parents will verbalize an understanding of the disease process and the treatment plan.

Interventions

Nursing care initially focuses on support of family members as they react and adjust to the diagnosis of cancer. Second, the nurse facilitates the educational process to allay fears based on unknowns.

Postoperative care of the enucleated orbit entails careful observations for signs of infection, hemorrhage, and edema. The child will wear a patch over the socket for about 1 week postoperatively. To preserve the shape of the orbit for prosthesis, which will be fitted 5 to 6 weeks after surgery, a conformer is placed in the orbit. Nursing interventions include teaching the parents (and child, if old enough) how to remove, clean, and reinsert first the conformer, then the prosthesis.

Whatever the extent of involvement by tumor or the treatment modality used, careful follow-up monitoring by retinal examination under anesthesia and CT is indicated. Genetic counseling is recommended. If the retinoblastoma is found to be genetically inherited, siblings should be periodically examined, as should any offspring subsequently produced when the affected child reaches adulthood.

Children with familial retinoblastoma have a high incidence of developing second malignancies later in life because of the genetic origin of the disease. Although no specific screening is recommended, symptoms should be carefully evaluated with a high index of suspicion (see p. 1324 for nursing care).

Evaluation

- Are the child and family verbalizing their understanding of the disease and the treatment plan?
- Is the child able to relate to peers and family?
- Are the child and family verbalizing fears and a decrease in anxiety?
- Is the child able to compensate for loss of vision and continue daily activities?

KEY CONCEPTS

- The signs and symptoms of childhood cancer vary according to the child's age, the type of tumor, and the extent of the disease.
- Childhood cancer is difficult to diagnose because most symptoms can be attributed to common childhood illnesses.
- Children typically have longer treatment plans than adults with cancer because of their increased metabolic rate, resulting in an increased rate of cell turnover.
- Fatigue is a common side effect of radiation therapy, and the child may need longer or more frequent periods of rest.
- There are three types of bone marrow transplantation: syngeneic (from an identical twin), autologous (from child's own marrow), and allogeneic (from another donor).
- Nursing care of children with bone marrow transplants focuses on preventing infection until the marrow engrafts and the children produce their own white blood cells with which to fight infection.
- Biologic response modifiers are naturally occurring substances found in the body that influence the immune system.
- Chemotherapy is the preferred treatment for leukemia and is divided into phases: remission induction, consolidation, delayed intensification, and maintenance.
- Common nursing diagnoses associated with the child with cancer include Risk for Infection; Altered Nutrition; Less than Body Requirements; Knowledge Deficit; Ineffective Family/Individual Coping; Pain; Impaired Skin Integrity; Body Image Disturbance; and Altered Oral Mucous Membrane.
- The mouth and anus are at increased risk for breakdown in the child receiving chemotherapy or radiation therapy. Temperatures should not be measured rectally, and meticulous mouth and anal care should be given.
- The abdomen of a child with a Wilms' tumor should not be palpated because excessive manipulation can cause seeding of the tumor if the protective capsule is ruptured.
- Postoperatively, the child with a brain tumor is at risk for increased intracranial pressure related to edema, hydrocephalus, or hemorrhage. Vital signs and mental and neurologic status are checked frequently.
- A cooling blanket should be available postoperatively for the child who has undergone brain surgery because of the risk of hyperthermia resulting from hypothalamic or brain stem involvement.
- A quiet environment should be provided for the child who has undergone brain surgery. The position of the child is usually determined by the physician and depends on the location and size of the tumor.

REFERENCES AND READINGS

Ablin, A. R. (Ed.). (1997). *Supportive care of children with cancer* (2nd ed.). Baltimore, MD: Johns Hopkins University Press.

Abramovitz, L. Z., & Senner, A. M. (1995). Pediatric bone marrow transplantation update. *Oncology Nursing Forum 22*(1), 107–115.

Altman, A. J. (1997). Chronic leukemias of childhood. In P. A. Pizzo & D. G. Poplack (Eds.), *Principles and practice of pediatric oncology* (pp. 483–504). Philadelphia: Lippincott–Raven.

Brodeur, G., Maris, J., Yamashiro, D., Hogarty, M., & White, P. (1997). Biology and genetics of human neuroblastomas. *Journal of Pediatric Hematology/Oncology, 19*(2), 93–101.

Castleberry, R. (1997). Biology and treatment of neuroblastoma. *Pediatric Clinics of North America, 44*(4), 919–937.

Donaldson, S. S., Egbert, P. R., Newsham, I., & Cavenee, W. K. (1997). Retinoblastoma. In P. A. Pizzo & D. G. Poplack (Eds.), *Principles and practice of pediatric oncology* (pp. 699–716). Philadelphia: Lippincott–Raven.

Foley, G. V., Fochtman, D., & Mooney, K. H. (Eds.). (1993). *Nursing care of the child with cancer* (2nd ed.). Philadelphia: Saunders.

Friebert, S. E., & Shurin, S. B. (1998a). Acute lymphocytic leukemia: Diagnosing acute lymphocytic leukemia in children. *Patient Care, 32*(10), 100.

Friebert, S. E., & Shurin, S. B. (1998b). Acute lymphocytic leukemia: Treatment and ongoing care. *Patient Care, 32*(11), 183.

Gallie, B. L., Budning, A., DeBoer, G., Thiessen, J. J., Koren, G., Verjee, Z., Ling, V., & Chan, H. S. L. (1996). Chemotherapy with focal therapy can cure intraocular retinoblastoma without radiotherapy. *Archives of Ophthalmology, 114*, 1321–1328.

Grier, H. (1997). The Ewing family of tumors: Ewing's sarcoma and primitive neuroectodermal tumors. *Pediatric Clinics of North America, 44*(4), 991–1004.

Golub, T. R., Weinstein, H. J., & Grier, H. E. (1997). Acute myelogenous leukemia. In P. A. Pizzo & D. G. Poplack (Eds.), *Principles and practice of pediatric oncology* (pp. 463–482). Philadelphia: Lippincott–Raven.

Green, D. M., Coppes, P. E., Breslow, N. E., Grundy, P. E., Ritchey, M. L., Beckwith, J. B., Thomas, P. R. M., & D'Angio, G. J. (1997). Wilms tumor. In P. A. Pizzo & D. G. Poplack (Eds.), *Principles and practice of pediatric oncology* (pp. 733–760). Philadelphia: Lippincott–Raven.

Green, D. M., D'Angio, G. J., Beckwith, J. B., Breslow, N. E., Grundy, P. E., Ritchey, M. L., & Thomas, P. R. M. (1996). Wilms tumor. CA: *A Cancer Journal for Clinicians, 46*(1), 46–63.

Heideman, R. L., Packer, R. J., Albright, L. A., Freeman, C. R., & Rorke, L. B.

(1997). Tumors of the central nervous system. In P. A. Pizzo & D. G. Poplack (Eds.), *Principles and practice of pediatric oncology* (pp. 633–698). Philadelphia: Lippincott–Raven.

Hudson, M. M., & Donaldson, S. S (1997a). Hodgkin's disease. *Pediatric Clinics of North America, 44*(4), 891–906.

Hudson, M. M., & Donaldson, S. S. (1997b). Hodgkin's Disease. In P. A. Pizzo & D. G. Poplack (Eds.), *Principles and practice of pediatric oncology* (pp. 523–544). Philadelphia: Lippincott–Raven.

Kusumakumary, P., Ajithkumar, T., Ratheesan, K., Chellam, V., & Nair, M. (1998). Pattern and outcome of neuroblastoma: A 10 year study. *Indian Pediatrics, 35*(3), 223–229.

Landis, S., Murray, T. Bolden, S., & Wingo, P. (1998). Cancer statistics, 1998. CA: *A Cancer Journal for Clinicians, 48*(1), 6–29.

Lum, L. (1999). T cell-based immunotherapy for cancer: A virtual reality? CA: *A Cancer Journal for Clinicians, 49*(2), 74–100.

Margolin, J. F., & Poplack, D. G. (1997). Acute Lymphoblastic Leukemia. In P. A. Pizzo & D. G. Poplack (Eds.), *Principles and practice of pediatric oncology* (pp. 409–462). Philadelphia: Lippincott–Raven.

McHugh, K., & Boothroyd, A. (1999). The role of radiology in childhood rhabdomyosarcoma. *Clinical Radiology, 54*(1), 2–10.

Meyer, P., & Gorlick, R. (1997). Osteosarcoma. *Pediatric Clinics of North America, 44*(4), 973–989.

Meyer, W., & Marina, N. (1996). Ewing's sarcoma/peripheral neuroepithelioma. In R. E. Behrman, R. M. Kliegman, & A. M. Arvin (Eds.), *Nelson textbook of pediatrics* (15th ed., pp. 1468–1470). Philadelphia: Saunders.

O'Connell, S., & Schmit-Pokorny, K. (1997). Blood and marrow stem cell transplantations: Indications, procedure, process. In M. Bakitas Whedon & D. Wujcik (Eds.), *Blood and marrow stem cell transplantation: Principles, practice and nursing insight* (2nd ed., pp. 66–99). Boston: Jones & Bartlett.

Pappo, A., Shapiro, D., & Crist, W. (1997). Rhabdomyosarcoma: Biology and treatment. *Pediatric Clinics of North America, 44*(4), 953–972.

Petruzzi, M. J., & Green, D. M. (1997). Wilms' tumor. *Pediatric Clinics of North America, 44*(4), 939–952.

Pratt, C. B. (1997). Familial osteosarcoma or osteosarcoma as part of a spectrum of familial tumors? *Proceedings of the annual meeting of the American Society of Clinical Oncologists, 16*(A), 1929.

Pratt, C. B. (1998). Use of chemotherapy for retinoblastoma. *Medical and Pediatric Oncology, 31*, 531–533.

Pratt, C. B., Meyer, W. H., Luo, X., & Cain, A. M. (1997). Second malignant neoplasms in survivors of osteosarcoma. *Cancer, 80*(5), 960–965.

Quesnel, S., & Malkin, D. (1997). Genetic predisposition to cancer and familial cancer syndromes. *Pediatric Clinics of North America, 44*(4), 791–808.

Ryan, J. A., & Shiminski-Maher, T. (1995). Hydrocephalus and shunts in children with brain tumors. *Journal of Pediatric Oncology Nursing, 12*(4), 223–229.

Sandlund, J. T., Downing, J. R., & Crist, W. M. (1996). Non-Hodgkin's lymphoma in childhood. *New England Journal of Medicine, 334*(19), 1238–1248.

Sawada, T. (1997), Measurement of urinary vanillylmandelic acid (VMA) and homovanillic acid (HVA) for diagnosis of neural crest tumors. *Pediatric Hematology and Oncology, 14*(4), 291–293.

Scott, I. U., O'Brien, J. M., & Murray, T. G. (1997). Retinoblastoma: A review emphasizing genetics and management strategies. *Seminars in Ophthalmology, 12*(2), 59–71.

Shad, A., & Magrath, I. (1997). Non-Hodgkin's lymphoma. *Pediatric Clinics of North America, 44*(4), 863–90.

Shad, A., & Magrath, I. T. (1997). Malignant non-Hodgkin's lymphomas in children. In P. A. Pizzo & D. G. Poplack (Eds.), *Principles and practice of pediatric oncology* (pp. 545-588). Philadelphia: Lippincott–Raven.

Shiminski-Maher, T., & Shields, M. (1995). Pediatric brain tumors: Diagnosis and management. *Journal of Pediatric Oncology Nursing, 12*(4), 188–198.

Stewart, E., & Cohen, D. (1998). Central nervous system tumors in children. *Seminars in Oncology Nursing, 14*(1), 34–42.

Stram, D., Matthay, K., O'Leary, M., Reynolds, C., Haase, G., Atkinson, J., Brodeur, G., & Seegar, R. (1996). Consolidation chemoradiotherapy and autologous bone marrow transplantation versus continued chemotherapy for metastatic neuroblastoma: A report of two concurrent children's cancer group studies. *Journal of Clinical Oncology, 14*, 2417–2426.

Vernon-Levett, P., & Geller, M. (1997). Posterior fossa tumors in children: A case study. *AACN Clinical Issues, 8*(2), 214–226.

Wexler, L., & Helman, L. (1997). Rhabdomyosarcoma and the undifferentiated sarcomas. In P. A. Pizzo & D. G. Poplack (Eds.), *Principles and practice of pediatric oncology* (pp. 799–829). Philadelphia: Lippincott–Raven.

Wingard, J. (1997). Bone marrow to blood stem cell: Past, present, future. In M. Bakitas Whedon & D. Wujcik (Eds.), *Blood and marrow stem cell transplantation: Principles, practice and nursing insight* (2nd ed., pp. 3–24). Boston: Jones & Bartlett.

Zhao, D., Shields, C. L., Shields, J. A., & Gunduz, K. (1998). New developments in the management of retinoblastoma. *Journal of Ophthalmic Nursing and Technology, 17*(1), 13–18.

49

The Child with an Integumentary Alteration

LEARNING OBJECTIVES

After studying this chapter, you should be able to:

- Describe the anatomy and physiology of normal skin.
- Describe any differences between the newborn, child, and adult's skin.
- Identify common skin disorders of infants and children.
- Discuss the manifestations of and treatment for such skin disorders as bacterial, fungal, and viral infections; infestations; inflammatory disorders; acne vulgaris; and insect bites and stings.
- Discuss common causes of burns in children and the prevention of burn injuries.
- Describe the implications of burn injuries in children.
- Discuss the classifications of depth, extent, and severity of a burn injury.
- Describe the therapeutic management and nursing care of children with minor burns.
- Apply the nursing process to the care of infants and children with skin disorders.

DEFINITIONS

alopecia Hair loss.

apocrine sweat glands Secretory glands located in the axillae and genital regions that become active at puberty and respond to emotional and sexual stimulation.

debridement Removal of foreign material and devitalized or contaminated tissue from a traumatic or infected lesion to expose healthy tissue.

desquamation Sloughing of the skin in scales or sheets; can lead to loss of the deeper skin layers.

ecchymosis Discoloration of the skin or mucous membranes caused by leakage of blood into the subcutaneous tissue.

eccrine sweat glands Secretory glands distributed over the body that secrete sweat.

erythema Redness of the skin.

eschar Sloughing produced by a thermal burn or corrosive application.

excoriation Scratch or abrasion of the skin.

hydrotherapy Therapy entailing water soaks to clean wounds, which removes old dressings, and softens dead tissue for easier removal.

intertrigo Maceration of two closely apposed skin surfaces.

keratosis Overgrowth and thickening of the cornified epithelium.

lichenification Thickening and hardening of the skin with accentuation of skin markings; often the result of chronic scratching.

petechiae Tiny, flat, purplish red spots on the skin surface resulting from minute hemorrhages within the dermis.

pruritus Itching.

urticaria (hives) Vascular reaction of the skin characterized by pruritic wheals, often caused by allergy or emotional stress.

Review of the Integumentary System

A knowledge of integumentary structure and function is necessary for the nurse to understand the changes that occur with disease. There are a number of important differences between the skin of infants and young children and that of adults.

The skin is the body's largest organ. It has five major functions: (1) to protect the deeper tissues from injury, drying, and invasion by foreign matter, (2) to regulate temperature, (3) to aid in excretion of water, (4) to aid in production of vitamin D, and (5) to initiate the sensations of touch, pain, heat, and cold.

The skin is composed of two layers: the outer *epidermis* and the inner supportive *dermis*. Beneath these layers is the *subcutaneous layer*, which is composed largely of adipose tissue.

The *epidermis* is nonvascular stratified epithelium. It is divided into two major layers. The outermost layer, the *stratum corneum*, is a tough, horny collection of dead keratinized cells that have migrated up from the underlying layers. *Keratin*, a fibrous protein, is also the principal component of the nails and hair. Skin cells are constantly being shed and replaced with new cells from from the layers below.

The *stratum basale*, or basal cell layer, anchors the epidermis to the dermis. This innermost layer contains melanocytes, the source of melanin, the pigment that gives skin its color. The epidermis is completely replaced every 4 weeks.

The *dermis*, composed of tough connective tissue, contains lymphatics and nerves. The highly vascular dermis nourishes the epidermis.

Appendages from the epidermis—sebaceous glands, sweat glands, and hair follicles—are embedded in the der-

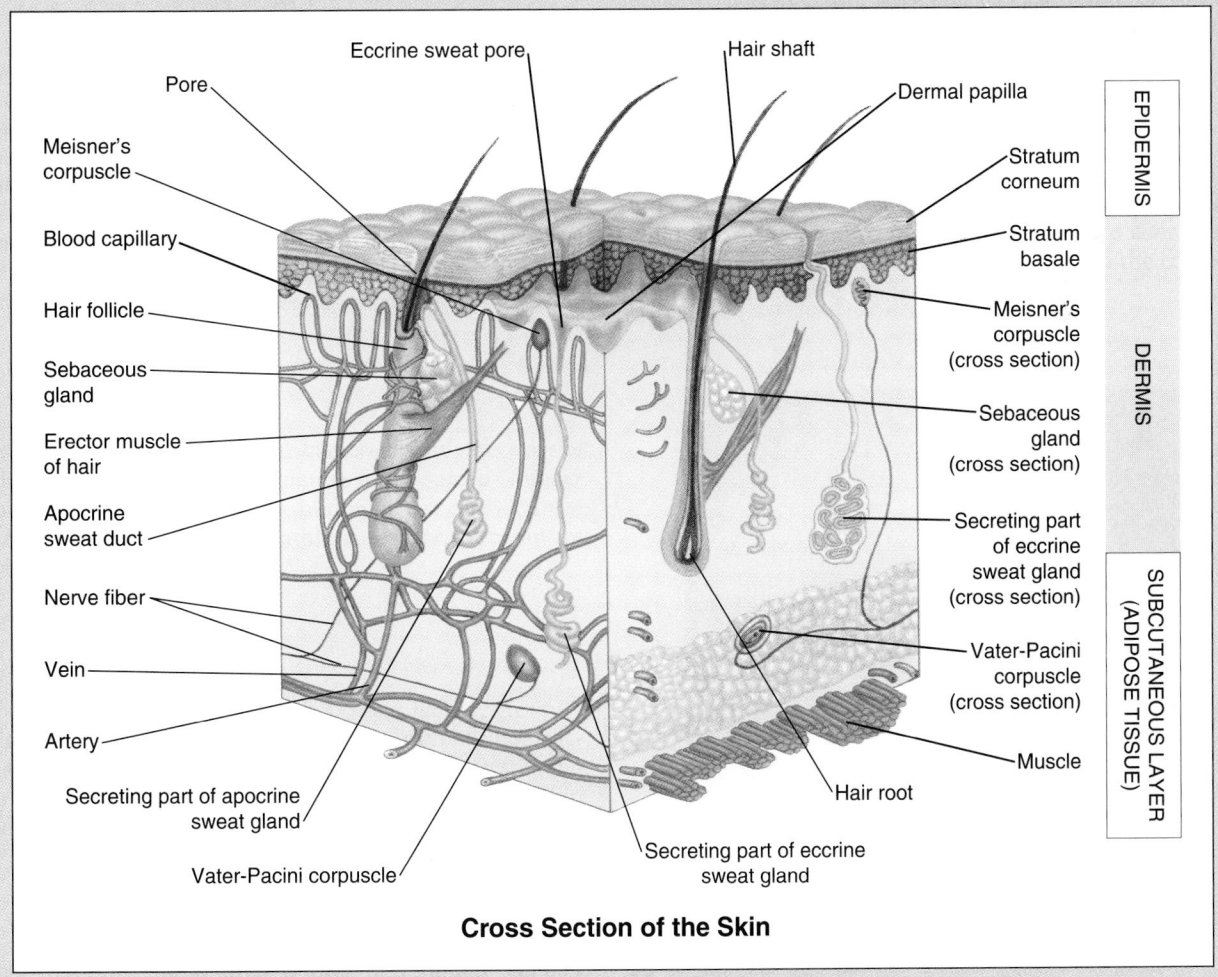

Cross Section of the Skin

PATHOPHYSIOLOGY
• • • • • • • • • • • •
of Tinea Infection

Tinea infection occurs when the fungus causing tinea invades the hair, the stratum corneum of the skin, or the nails.

In *tinea capitis*, the fungus invades the hair shafts, causing the hairs to become brittle and to break off at the level of the scalp, leaving an area of stubby, black-dotted alopecia. An immune reaction to the fungus may develop in the form of a *kerion*, a boggy, red, tender scalp mass that may contain *Staphylococcus aureus* and is often accompanied by fever and lymphadenopathy. Children with allergies seem to be more susceptible to tinea capitis.

Tinea corporis (ringworm) is a fungal infection of the face, trunk, or extremities. It can be transmitted by humans or by dogs and cats. Most lesions of tinea corporis clear without treatment in several months, but some may become chronic.

Tinea cruris (jock itch) is characterized by an intense inflammatory reaction with severe pruritus.

Tinea pedis (athlete's foot) may become chronic, particularly in adolescents who wear nonventilated athletic shoes. Tinea lesions may become secondarily infected with bacteria or *Candida*.

Manifestations

Common manifestations of tinea capitis include erythema and scaling of the scalp, as well as one or more round patches of alopecia that slowly increase in size. Small papules at the base of hair follicles become crusting pustules and red scales. Thick, broken hairs close to the scalp surface result in patches of "black dot" alopecia. Mild pruritus and a kerion from an allergic reaction to the fungus may be present. Surrounding lymph nodes may be enlarged.

Tinea corporis may be marked by ring-like plaques with pale centers and scaly, red margins, especially on the trunk, face, and extremities; lesions, usually $\frac{1}{2}$ to 1 inch in diameter; and pruritus.

Manifestations of tinea cruris may include pink papules and scales on the inner thighs, groin, scrotum, and buttocks (but not the penis). Pruritus is also present.

Tinea pedis may produce fine vesiculopustular or scaly lesions on the soles of the feet, between the toes, and under the nails. Peeling, fissures, and maceration appear in severe cases, and pruritus and burning are present.

Diagnostic Evaluation

Most tinea infections can be diagnosed from the clinical appearance of the lesions. Fungal cultures or microscopic examination of skin scrapings prepared with potassium hydroxide (KOH) confirm the diagnosis. In the past, tinea infections were diagnosed when the lesions fluoresced under an ultraviolet Wood's light. However, the most common organism causing tinea today, *Trichophyton tonsurans*, does not fluoresce. *Microsporum* lesions fluoresce as a bright blue-green.

Therapeutic Management

TINEA CAPITIS

For treatment to be effective, medication must penetrate the hair follicles. Topical therapy alone is not effective for tinea capitis. Oral griseofulvin, 10 to 20 mg/kg/day for 6 to 8 weeks, is the treatment of choice. Because griseofulvin is insoluble in water, its absorption is increased if it is taken with a high-fat meal or with milk. Ketoconazole (Nizoral) may be prescribed for children who cannot tolerate griseofulvin or who fail to respond to it. Ketoconazole is used with caution in children because of the risk of hepatotoxicity when prescribed for long-term therapy. Selenium sulfide shampoo (Selsun Blue, Exsel) should be used twice a week for 2 weeks to eliminate spores.

TINEA CORPORIS

Local treatment is usually effective for tinea corporis. Antifungal preparations such as clotrimazole (Lotrimin) or miconazole (Micatin) can be used three times daily until the lesions have been gone for 1 week. Infected pets should be treated as well. Micatin cream should be applied to visible ringworm patches on the pet's skin. If no patches are seen but ringworm recurs in the child, Micatin powder should be applied to the pet's entire fur twice weekly for 3 weeks. The child should avoid close contact with the infected pet. Natural immunity develops in animals after 4 months (Schmitt, 1999). Extensive cases of tinea corporis might require systemic antifungal treatment with griseofulvin or other systemic antifungal agent.

TINEA CRURIS

Management for tinea cruris is similar to that for tinea corporis. Topical antifungal preparations should be applied twice daily to the lesions and at least 1 inch beyond the borders. Care should be taken to apply the medication to all creases, and the adolescent should be advised to wear loose clothing.

TINEA PEDIS

A prescribed topical antifungal agent such as clotrimazole (Lotrimin), miconazole (Monistat), or oxiconazole (Oxistat) is applied twice daily until the lesions have been cleared for 1 week. If the lesions do not respond to topical therapy, oral griseofulvin may be given, 5 to 10 mg/kg/day for a month or longer, to promote healing. Newer systemic antifungals, such as itraconazole (Sporanox), have demonstrated improved success over a shorter time period than griseofulvin (Gallas & Levy, 1998), but administration of this medication requires baseline and follow-up liver function tests. If the affected area is inflamed and oozing, soaking the feet in Burow's solution can promote healing.

NURSING CARE
• • • • • • • • • • •
The Child with a Tinea Infection

Assessment

Obtain a history that includes a description of the skin lesions and possible contacts. Animals the child has played with should be carefully inspected for ringworm. The child's siblings and playmates should also be examined, as children often share hairbrushes, hats, and barrettes, increasing the spread of infection.

Nursing Diagnosis and Planning

- Impaired Skin Integrity related to inflammation and scratching of lesions.
  Expected Outcomes: The child will exhibit intact skin over impaired areas. The skin lesions will exhibit progressive healing.
- Altered Comfort related to pruritic lesions.
  Expected Outcome: The child will remain calm and exhibit no evidence of discomfort or pruritus.
- Knowledge Deficit of the cause, treatment, and spread of the infection related to lack of information.
  Expected Outcomes: The child and family will verbalize accurate information about the child's skin condition. The child and family will demonstrate behaviors that prevent spread of the fungus. Treatments will be performed correctly.

Interventions

Adequate teaching is essential for successful treatment of tinea infection. In addition to teaching therapeutic management techniques specific for the child's particular type of tinea, emphasize to the parent that any prescribed oral medication regimen must be followed meticulously. Tinea infections are sometimes difficult to eradicate; discontinuing medication too soon risks reoccurrence. Treatment sometimes continues for as long as 6 to 8 weeks. It is also important to advise the parent and the older child that the child taking griseofulvin must avoid sun exposure because griseofulvin makes the skin more susceptible to a photosensitivity reaction. If the child is taking itraconazole, the parent must ensure the child undergoes the recommended liver function studies.

Fungus thrives in a warm, moist environment, so it is important to keep infected areas as dry as possible. Teaching proper hygiene is essential for preventing and treating fungal infections. Teach children to avoid sharing personal items such as combs, hats, and hair ornaments. Children with tinea infections should sleep alone and should not share towels and washcloths with others. Feet should be

washed daily and kept dry. Advise children to allow their nonventilated athletic shoes to dry thoroughly between wearings. Heavy cotton socks absorb sweat and keep the feet dry. If tinea pedis is present, the child should change socks at least twice a day and go barefoot, or wear sandals as much as possible. Talcum powder or antifungal powder applied twice daily might help keep feet dry.

Tinea cruris heals much faster if the groin area is kept dry. Loose-fitting cotton underwear should be worn, and athletic supporters and underwear should be washed frequently. The rash should be washed each day with plain water and carefully dried. Soap should be avoided. Scratching delays healing, so instruct the child to avoid scratching the area. Reassure the young man and his parents that tinea cruris is not associated with sexually transmissible disease.

Instruct parents to call the physician if the infection has not cleared up in 4 weeks or if it continues to spread after a week of treatment. Reassure parents that fungal infection is not an indication of poor hygiene or neglect.

Evaluation

- Does the child have clean, intact skin?
- Is the child comfortable and without pruritus?
- Do the child and parents perform treatments correctly and verbalize ways to prevent the spread of infection?

■ *Herpes Simplex Virus Type 1 Infection*

Herpes simplex virus type 1 (HSV-1) is responsible for a common, contagious, and often recurrent infection of the skin and mucous membranes. This infection can be asymptomatic or symptomatic and extremely painful. A wide spectrum of disease is caused by HSV-1: the common fever blister or cold sore (herpes labialis), corneal lesions, genital lesions (rare in children), and central nervous system infection.

Etiology

HSV-1 is transmitted by infected body fluids and secretions coming in contact with breaks in the skin or mucous mem-

---

THE CHILD AND PARENTS WANT TO KNOW

Home Care for a Child or Adolescent with a Tinea Infection

When providing information to the parent or older child with tinea, emphasize the following:

- Keep the infected areas as dry as possible.
- Do not share personal items such as towels, washcloths, combs, hats, or hair ornaments.
- **Athlete's foot:** Wash the feet daily and keep them dry. Nonventilated athletic shoes should dry thoroughly between wearings. Wear heavy cotton socks, and change socks at least twice a day. Talcum powder or antifungal powder applied twice daily might help keep feet dry.

- **Jock itch:** Keep the groin area dry. Wear loose-fitting cotton underwear. Wash athletic supporters and underwear frequently. Wash the rash each day with plain water and dry carefully. Do not use soap on the affected area. Avoid scratching.
- Continue to take oral medication as directed, even if the condition has improved. Discontinuing medication too soon can allow the infection to reappear.
- Call your physician if the infection has not cleared up in 4 weeks or if it continues to spread after a week of treatment.

branes. Delivery through an infected birth canal can cause infection in newborns. HSV-1 can be transmitted by nurses who fail to practice careful hand washing. Children with burns, eczema, or diaper rash or those who are immunosuppressed are particularly susceptible to HSV-1 infection.

Incidence

HSV-1 is widespread. An initial HSV-1 infection commonly occurs by the time a child reaches age 5 (Gallas & Levy, 1998). HSV infections in children are usually caused by HSV-1. Infection with HSV-2, which primarily affects the anal-genital area, is rare before age 14. Child sexual abuse should be considered in any child with a genital herpes infection. Herpes infections are more common in lower socioeconomic groups.

Manifestations

HERPES LABIALIS ("COLD SORE," "FEVER BLISTER")

Prodromal symptoms of herpes labialis are burning, itching, or tingling; these symptoms occur up to several days before

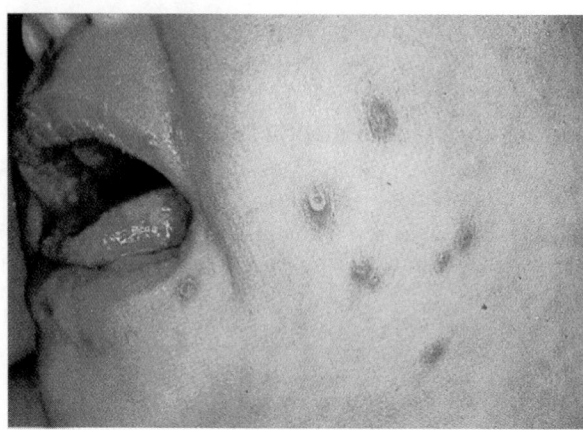

FIGURE 49–5

Herpes simplex infection in an infant. (From Feigin, R. D., & Cherry, J. D. [Eds.]. [1992]. *Textbook of pediatric infectious diseases* [3rd ed., p. 773]. Philadelphia: Saunders.)

lesions appear. Symptoms appear 2 days–2 weeks after exposure. Lesions appear in clusters of fluid-filled vesicles that ulcerate, dry, and crust within 7 to 14 days (Fig. 49–5). Usually one or two lesions are present on the lips, tongue, gingiva, or buccal mucosa. Pruritus and pain are present. Approximately 85% of active HSV-1 infections are asymptomatic.

HERPETIC GINGIVOSTOMATITIS

Herpes gingivostomatitis is a severe oral infection that affects children under age 5. Vesicles and ulcerations, an edematous throat, and enlarged, painful cervical lymph nodes are seen. Associated signs and symptoms include chills, fever, malaise, bad breath, and drooling.

HERPETIC OCULAR INFECTION

Herpetic ocular infection causes irritation and inflammation of the conjunctiva or cornea with associated tearing and photophobia. Vesicles appear on the eyelid and mucous membranes of the eye.

HERPETIC WHITLOW

Symptoms of herpetic whitlow appear 3 to 7 days after exposure and include vesicles, swelling, pruritus, and severe pain of the affected fingers. Discomfort may continue for weeks after the vesicles have healed.

Diagnostic Evaluation

Clinical manifestations and the child's history can suggest the diagnosis. A Tzanck smear can confirm a herpes infection, but a positive smear cannot differentiate between varicella-zoster virus and HSV-1, and a negative smear does not rule out HSV infection. Tissue culture is a more reliable method of diagnosis.

Therapeutic Management

Treatment is symptomatic. The child with oral HSV-1 infection is usually cared for at home if able to take adequate fluids. If the child becomes dehydrated, IV fluids are needed.

Topical or oral acyclovir (Zovirax), if given early

PATHOPHYSIOLOGY

of Herpes Simplex Type 1 Infection

There are four types of human herpesviruses: herpes simplex virus (HSV types 1 and 2), cytomegalovirus (CMV), Epstein-Barr virus (EBV, which causes infectious mononucleosis), and varicella-zoster virus. HSV-1 causes the "oral" type of herpes and usually affects areas above the waist, producing "cold sores," "fever blisters," and corneal lesions. HSV-2 affects areas below the waist (anal-genital area). However, either type can affect any region of the body. After an initial HSV-1 infection the virus remains dormant but alive within nerve cells innervating that portion of the skin originally infected. Fever, stress, trauma, sun exposure, menstruation, or immunosuppression can reactivate the virus. When reactivated, the virus migrates to the skin area innervated by the ganglia that harbor it, near the site of the initial infection. The recurrent infection can be symptomatic or asymptomatic, but it is just as contagious as the initial infection. Recurrent infections tend to be less severe than the initial infection.

The immune status of the host determines the severity of HSV infection. HSV-1 infection in the newborn or immunocompromised child can be fatal. HSV-1 is the most common cause of viral encephalitis in children.

Herpetic whitlow, a painful HSV-1 infection of the fingers, can be transmitted to a nurse during oral or tracheal care of a child with herpes infection. Thumb-sucking children with oral HSV-1 infection can also develop this condition. Health care personnel with herpetic whitlow should not have patient contact until the infection has healed because the infection is highly contagious.

enough in the course of the infection, can reduce the time to recovery. Although there is no cure for HSV-1 infection, acyclovir (Zovirax) given IV may be used in immunocompromised children, neonates, and children with encephalitis or ocular HSV to decrease the severity of the infection.

Antibiotic ointment may be used to treat secondary bacterial infection of lesions. Corticosteroids are contraindicated because they can worsen HSV-1 infection. Oral or rectal acetaminophen with or without codeine may be prescribed, and topical anesthetics may be dabbed on lesions to help relieve pain. A prescribed anesthetic mouth rinse of equal parts of diphenhydramine (Benadryl) elixir, Kaopectate, and 2% viscous lidocaine may decrease pain and help the child eat.

▌ NURSING CARE
The Child with a Herpes Simplex Type 1 Infection

Assessment

Obtain a history and ask the parent or child about previous HSV infections or contact with an infected person. Examine the skin carefully for lesions. Inspect the eyes for corneal ulcerations and edema, and assess the child's vision for blurring and photophobia. Referral to an ophthalmologist is necessary for suspected ocular HSV-1 infection. For the child with herpes gingivostomatitis, pay particular attention to assessing hydration status.

Nursing Diagnosis and Planning

- Impaired Skin Integrity related to inadequate secondary defenses.
  Expected Outcomes: The child will demonstrate healing of lesions. The child will have no other signs of infection.
- Pain related inflammation and infection.
  Expected Outcome: The child will have minimal pain, as evidenced by adequate fluid intake, decreased verbalization of pain, and decreased restlessness and irritability.
- Risk for Infection related to changes in skin integrity.
  Expected Outcome: The child will have no signs of secondary bacterial infection, as evidenced by healing lesions and normal body temperature.
- Risk for Fluid Volume Deficit related to painful oral lesions.
  Expected Outcomes: The child will maintain urine output of at least 1 to 2 ml/kg/hr and exhibit moist mucous membranes and good skin turgor.

Interventions

Children with oral HSV-1 infection may be extremely uncomfortable. Swallowing can cause severe pain, and dehydration is a real danger. Advise parents to contact the physician if the child develops signs of dehydration. Fluid intake is very important, and the child must be encouraged to drink. Frozen ice pops, noncitrus juices, milk, and flattened soft drinks are best. Frequent small feedings of bland, soft foods can be offered. Parents may need to be reassured that a few days without solid food will not harm the child as long as fluid intake is adequate.

To prevent secondary infection, the child's mouth should be rinsed often with normal saline or one-quarter-strength hydrogen peroxide, especially after eating. Oral or rectal acetaminophen with codeine can be given as ordered for pain and fever. Topical anesthetics, such as viscous lidocaine, must be used with caution. Overuse of topical anesthetics in small children might depress the gag reflex and increase the risk of aspiration.

Hospitalized children infected with HSV-1 should be placed on contact precautions. The child is considered contagious until the scabs from visible lesions have fallen off. Because scabs do not form on mucous membranes, these lesions are considered contagious until they are completely healed. It is important to remember that active HSV infections may be asymptomatic.

All personnel who have contact with the child should follow standard precautions and be particularly careful when touching the child near the lesions, during oral care or suctioning, and when handling bed linens or objects that might be contaminated with saliva or secretions from the lesions. Careful hand washing is essential.

Parents should take similar precautions when caring for the child at home to prevent spread of infection. Advise the parents to wash bottles, nipples, toys, eating utensils, and towels in hot, soapy water or in a dishwasher, if available. Family members should not share any of these items with the infected child.

Because the infection can be spread to other parts of the body, the child should not put his or her fingers near the mouth or infected area. Elbow restraints may be necessary for children too young to understand this. The child with HSV-1 infection is usually miserable and needs generous cuddling and comforting despite the infectious condition.

Evaluation

- Are lesions healed, with no sign of infection spread?
- Does the child demonstrate increased comfort?
- Is the child properly hydrated?
- Can the parent or caregiver describe infection control measures?

▌ Lice Infestation

Pediculosis, infestation of lice on the scalp or body, is a major and most exasperating problem in schools today. Although pediculosis is not a serious health problem, it causes much embarrassment and often elicits an emotional reaction among parents and school personnel.

Etiology

Lice live only on humans and are transmitted by direct contact with infected persons and indirect contact with the infected person's belongings (e.g., brushes, hats). Lice cannot jump like fleas. Clean hair is no deterrent to head lice. It has been said that the healthiest lice live on the healthiest heads.

Incidence

Approximately 5 million cases of infested schoolchildren are reported each year in the United States, although this probably represents only a small proportion of the actual cases (O'Brien, 1998). Approximately 20% of schoolchildren in an individual school will be affected during an

PATHOPHYSIOLOGY

of Pediculosis

Pediculosis may involve the scalp (pediculosis capitis), the body (pediculosis corporis), and the pubic area and eyelashes (pediculosis pubis). A specific type of louse, each of which has a similar life cycle, causes each of these infestations. All lice pierce the skin and suck blood. Severe itching caused by bites can predispose the child to secondary infection.

Head and pubic lice spend their life cycles on the skin of the human host; body lice live in clothing, coming to the skin only to feed. The female head louse lays eggs (nits) at the base of the hair shaft. The egg is covered with a gelatinous material, which hardens to semi-opaque, tiny pearly, whitish masses that are stuck tight to the hair shaft (see Fig. 49–6). Eggs incubate for about 1 week, and lice reach sexual maturity in about 2 weeks.

Pediculosis pubis is spread through sexual contact. Half of all patients with pediculosis pubis have another sexually transmitted disease, usually gonorrhea.

Lice may spread as long as the lice and nits remain alive on the infested person or belongings. Lice can live only 48 hours off the human host. Nits shed into the environment are capable of hatching for 10 days.

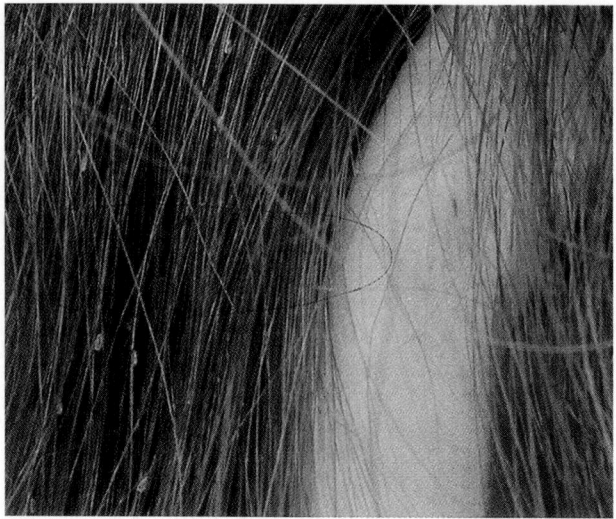

FIGURE 49–6

Head lice (pediculosis capitis). Note the nits attached to the hair shafts. (From Calen, J. P., Greer, K. E., Hood, A. F., Paller, A. S., & Swinyer, L. J. [1993]. *Color atlas of dermatology* [p. 373]. Philadelphia: Saunders.)

epidemic (Brainerd, 1998). Pediculosis rarely occurs in African Americans. Girls are affected twice as often as boys. All socioeconomic groups are affected. The peak incidence is in preschool and young school-age children. Pubic lice are usually seen in adolescents or young adults and are generally transmitted by sexual contact.

Manifestations

PEDICULOSIS CAPITIS (HEAD LICE)

Nits are visible and are attached firmly to the hair shafts near the scalp. They are tiny silvery or grayish white specks resembling dandruff but are more difficult to remove. They are commonly found behind the ears and at the nape of the neck. In active infestation, nits are found approximately one-quarter to one-half inch away from the scalp surface (Fig. 49–6). Adult lice are difficult to see and appear as small gray specks 1 to 2 mm long that crawl very fast to avoid light. Scattered lesions on the scalp or back of the neck, or both, cause intense pruritus. These lesions are often associated with posterior cervical lymph adenopathy. Secondary scalp infection may develop from scratching.

PEDICULOSIS CORPORIS (BODY LICE)

Papular, rose-colored dermatitis, causing intense pruritus, appears on the skin in areas under tight clothing. Nits attach firmly to seams of the child's clothing or bedding.

PEDICULOSIS PUBIS (PUBIC LICE OR CRAB LICE)

Pediculosis pubis are lice that can be found in pubic hair, facial hair, axillae, and on the body surface. The presence of pubic lice in the eyebrows or eyelashes of a prepubescent child suggests sexual abuse (Urbach, 1999). Pubic lice also cause intense pruritus. *Maculae cerulae* (blue spots) may be seen on the thighs and trunk in cases of heavy infestation. Dark brown spots on underwear and sheets are insect waste materials.

Diagnostic Evaluation

The diagnosis of head lice is made by identification of nits or lice on the scalp. The examiner parts the hair with two tongue depressors and moves from side to side and front to back, paying particular attention to the crown, behind the ears, and the nape of the neck. The exposed scalp should be carefully examined under bright light or in a sunny area. A magnifying glass can assist in identification. Unlike dandruff, nits are not easily removed from hair shafts. Pubic lice are diagnosed from a history of symptoms and visual inspection.

Therapeutic Management

Management of the child with pediculosis involves a three-tiered approach: (1) killing the active lice, (2) removing nits, and (3) preventing spread or recurrence by managing the environment.

KILLING ACTIVE LICE

Approaches to treating pediculosis have changed recently as a result of the development of pediculocide-resistant strains of lice and because prescription lindane (Kwell) can be neurotoxic if absorbed through the skin. Over-the-counter products containing pyrethrins (RID, Triple X, R&C, Pronto) are safe and effective. Because they lack residual activity (that is, they do not stay in the hair after treatment), treatment with these products must be repeated 1 to 2 weeks after the initial treatment.

An over-the-counter pediculocide, permethrin 1% (Nix), kills head lice and pubic lice and eggs with one application and has residual activity for 10 days. Nix is applied to the hair after shampooing, and as a lotion to pubic hair, and left for 10 minutes before it is rinsed out. The hair should not be shampooed for 24 hours after the treatment. Treatment is required for sexual contacts of a person with pubic lice, along with testing for other sexually transmitted diseases.

Body lice are treated with a prescription drug or an over-the-counter medication (RID, Pyrinate200, Triple X), following the manufacturer's instructions. Clothing and bedding should be dusted with lindane or other recommended powder, then washed in hot water and dried for 20 minutes at a hot dryer setting.

For resistant head lice, some cases respond to a treatment of 5% permethrin (Elimite) left on under a shower cap overnight (Kronemyer, 1997). Systemic or topical ivermectin, an antiparasite medication, has the side effect of effectively killing lice, but it has not been approved for children who weigh less than 15 kg (Estrada, 1998). This medication kills active lice but not eggs. Some practitioners have had success with systemic trimethoprim-sulfamethoxazole (Bactrim) (Kronemyer, 1997). Finally, various electric combs are able to detect and kill active lice (O'Brien, 1998).

REMOVING NITS
Unless the eggs are examined under a microscope, it is nearly impossible to tell whether treated nits have been killed. To ensure that living eggs will not hatch, all nits should be removed from the child's hair. Using a very fine-toothed metal comb releases the egg from the hair shaft.

ADDRESSING THE ENVIRONMENT
Environmental objects, clothing, and bedding should be treated or washed. It is most important to examine and treat family members and others who might be in close contact with the infested child. Meticulous vacuuming of carpets in classrooms with affected children will help prevent continuation of an epidemic.

NURSING CARE
The Child with Pediculosis

Assessment
Examine children for lice in an unobtrusive and private manner. In a school setting, classmates should be brought to the school nurse's office and admitted one at a time, rather than being seen together in a general check in a classroom setting. Use disposable tongue depressors or Popsicle sticks to part the hair, and discard these implements between children. Check all family members for the presence of nits or lice.

Assess adolescents with pubic lice for signs of other sexually transmitted diseases and ask about sexual contacts, because they will need treatment as well.

Nursing Diagnosis and Planning
- Pain related to inflammatory response and pruritus.
  Expected Outcome: The child will rest comfortably and be free of scratching.
- Risk for Infection related to scratching of scalp.
  Expected Outcome: The child will have no signs of secondary bacterial infection, as evidenced by intact skin and normal-sized cervical lymph nodes.

- Knowledge Deficit about treatment of lice infestation and the prevention of recurrence related to anxiety or incomplete information.
  Expected Outcomes: The child and/or family will carry out the prescribed treatment. The parent will demonstrate measures taken to prevent re-infestation.

Interventions
Advise parents to carefully follow printed directions that come with an over-the-counter pediculocide product, or to follow the physician's recommendation for using prescription products. Depending on the product used, retreatment might be necessary after 7 to 10 days. Caution parents against applying the medication more frequently than the directions recommend.

> Reassure parents that lice infestation does not reflect poor hygiene or low socioeconomic status. Advise them that it is necessary to notify the school nurse if the child is infested.

Teach parents to remove nits by back-combing with a fine-toothed comb. An hour before combing, nits can be loosened with a mixture of half vinegar and half water. It is easier to comb the child's hair for nit removal when the hair is damp, rather than wet or dry. Over-the-counter products such as Step 2 and Clear dissolve chitin, the substance that attaches nits to hair shafts. The goal is to remove all nits, leaving none with the potential to hatch. Many schools have a "no nit" policy, which requires that a child be free of all nits prior to reentry. Lice and nits can be removed from eyelashes by applying petrolatum to the eyelashes twice a day for 8 days.

Advise parents to wash clothing (especially hats and jackets), bedding, and linens in hot water and dry at a hot dryer setting. Dress-up clothes used at home or school and bicycle helmets should be treated as well. Items that cannot be washed should be dry-cleaned or sealed in plastic bags and kept in a warm place for 2 to 3 weeks.

Antilice sprays used for furniture and other environmental objects should *never* be used on a child. Thorough home cleaning is necessary to remove any remaining lice or nits. Parents should vacuum floors, play areas, and furniture to remove any hairs that might carry live nits. Combs and brushes should be boiled or soaked in antilice shampoo or hot water (above 140°F) for at least 10 minutes. Routinely teach children not to share hats, combs, or hair ornaments with other children. At school, individually assigned lockers or separate hooks for coats can help inhibit spread of lice.

The child should be rechecked in 7 to 10 days for infestation. Advise parents to call the physician if itching interferes with the child's sleep, if the condition does not clear up after 1 week, or if scalp lesions look infected. The National Pediculosis Association provides information about this disorder (see Appendix L).

Evaluation
- Is the child free of infestation?
- Do parents carry out the prescribed treatments?
- Can parents describe measures to prevent the spread of lice to others?

CRITICAL THINKING EXERCISE 49-1

The pediatric clinic receives a phone call from an obviously upset mother about her 4-year-old daughter, who is in preschool. This is the third time in a month that the parent has been called at work to take her child out of school because the child was found to have lice. The mother states that she has properly treated her daughter and other family members, and she insists the child is catching the condition from someone at school. The school maintains that no other child has this problem.

1. What should be the nurse's approach to this mother?
2. What kind of information will the nurse need to obtain to help this mother with her problem?

Mite Infestation (Scabies)

Scabies, or "itch mite," is a contagious condition that has been recognized for many centuries. It results from infestation with *Sarcoptes scabiei*.

Etiology

Scabies is transmitted by close personal contact with infected persons. Persons who share a bed or live in crowded conditions are likely to transmit scabies to each other. The scabies mite cannot survive for more than 3 days away from the human skin. For that reason, transmission of scabies by bedding or clothing is infrequent.

Incidence

Scabies is widespread throughout the United States and is prevalent in many schools. All socioeconomic groups are affected.

Pathophysiology

The female mite burrows into the epidermis, lays her eggs, and dies in the burrow after 4 to 5 weeks. The eggs hatch in 3 to 5 days, and larvae migrate to the skin surface to mature and complete the life cycle. The mites, eggs, and their excrement cause intense pruritus. One of the major complications of scabies is impetigo secondary to scratching.

Manifestations

Intense pruritus occurs, especially at night. Infants may be cranky, sleep fitfully, and rub their hands and feet together. Burrows (fine, grayish, thread-like lines) can be difficult to see because they are usually obscured by secondary changes of excoriation and inflammation. Papules, vesicles, and nodules are common (Fig. 49–7), and located mainly on the wrists, in the finger webs, on the elbows, in the umbilicus, in the axillae, in the groin, and on the buttocks. In infants the head, palms, and soles may be affected. Lesions often become secondarily infected from scratching. Scabies can be found on more than one family member.

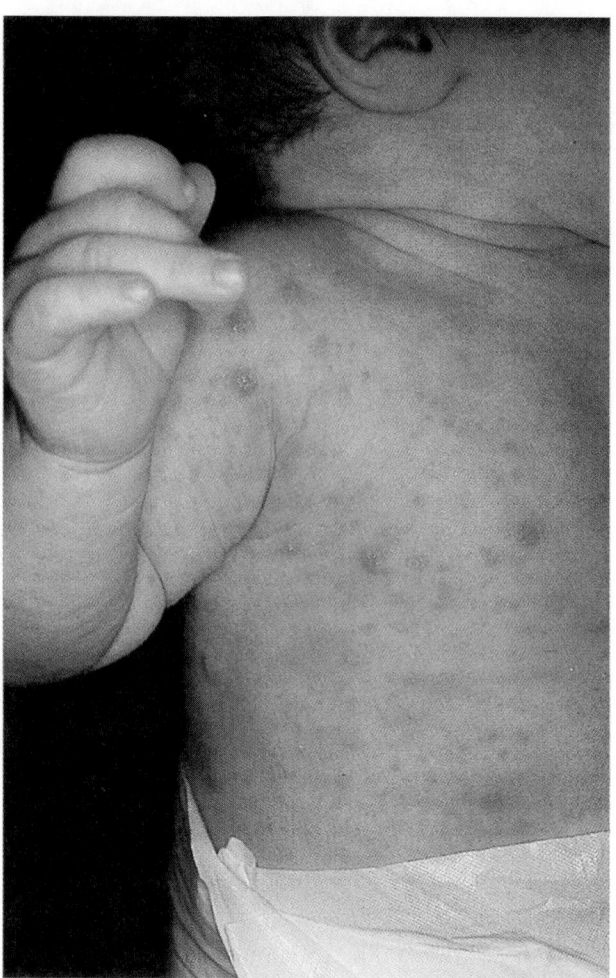

FIGURE 49-7

Scabies lesions on an infant. (From Calen, J. P., Greer, K. E., Hood, A. F., Paller, A. S., & Swinyer, L. J. [1993]. *Color atlas of dermatology* [p. 301]. Philadelphia: Saunders.)

Diagnostic Evaluation

A history of intense pruritus, especially at night, is suggestive. The diagnosis is made by microscopic examination of scrapings of the lesions.

Therapeutic Management

Scabies can be treated with topical application of either permethrin 5% (Elimite) or lindane cream (Kwell, Scabene). Because of the risk of neurotoxicity, lindane should not be used in children under age 2 or in pregnant women. The medication is applied to the body and head, avoiding the eyes and mouth. The medication must remain on the child for 8 to 14 hours to be effective, so applying it at bedtime is most effective. It is washed off in the morning. Retreatment in a week is usually recommended. Pruritus may last for several days to weeks after treatment and can be relieved with corticosteroid cream (e.g., hydrocortisone cream) and oral antihistamines.

Family members, even if asymptomatic, and day care contacts (except for pregnant women) should also be treated. The child's bedding and clothing should be washed in hot water in a fashion similar to the environmental treatment for pediculosis.

NURSING CARE
The Child with Scabies

Assessment
Inspect the child's hands, elbows, umbilicus, groin, and buttocks for burrows. Burrows may be difficult to see, however, and complaints of persistent itching may be the only symptom. Evaluate an adolescent with scabies for sexually transmitted disease.

Nursing Diagnosis and Planning
- Risk for Impaired Skin Integrity related to pruritus.
  Expected Outcome: The child will demonstrate no increased redness, irritation, or abrasions.
- Risk for Infection related to scratching of lesions.
  Expected Outcome: The child will have no signs of secondary bacterial infection, as evidenced by normal body temperature and intact skin.

Interventions
Instruct parents to use the scabicide according to manufacturer's instructions. The lotion is applied all over the child's body, including the soles of the feet, the scalp behind the ears, in intertriginous areas, and under the toenails and fingernails. The lotion should be kept on for the recommended time (4 to 8 hours for lindane and 8 to 14 hours for Elimite), and then the child should be bathed. Infants should be clothed during treatment so they will not lick their skin. To minimize absorption and the risk of toxic effects from lindane, the lotion should not be applied for at least ½ hour after bathing and should be applied only to cool, dry skin.

Advise the parent that persistent itching following treatment is not a sign of reinfestation or an indication for repeated application. Overuse of lindane can lead to neurotoxicity.

Scabies is usually cured with one treatment. Severe infestations may require a repeat application in 1 week. Clothing and bed linen should be dry-cleaned or washed in hot water and dried at a hot dryer setting.

Evaluation
- Is the child's skin intact and free of infestation?
- Is the child free from signs of secondary infection?

Atopic Dermatitis

Atopic dermatitis, or eczema, is a common chronic, allergic, inflammatory disease of the skin characterized by severe pruritus and various other manifestations. Atopic dermatitis can have distressing psychosocial effects on the child and family.

Etiology
The cause of atopic dermatitis is unknown, but the disease is thought to be genetically determined. Contributing factors include an inherited tendency for dry, sensitive skin, allergy, and emotional stress. Most children with atopic dermatitis have a family history of asthma, hay fever, or atopic dermatitis, and 50% to 80% of children with atopic dermatitis develop asthma or allergic rhinitis (Eigenmann et al., 1998). Although the role of allergy in etiology of atopic dermatitis is controversial, IgE-mediated food allergy has been shown to be an exacerbating factor in some children.

Incidence
Atopic dermatitis is a common condition that affects 5% to 10% of young children (Adinoff & Clark, 1996). The condition usually begins in infancy and clears by age 2 or 3 years. Some children continue to have signs into childhood, with a rash pattern that differs from the rash seen during infancy. Atopic dermatitis affects all races. It is most common in urban areas. Symptoms tend to be worse during winter months.

Manifestations
During infancy, erythematous areas of oozing and crusting appear first on the cheeks, then on the forehead, scalp, and extensor surfaces of the arms and legs (Fig. 49–8). Papulovesicular rash and scaly, red plaques become excoriated and lichenified. The affected scalp area resembles seborrheic dermatitis, but unlike seborrheic dermatitis, atopic dermatitis is intensely pruritic. Infants begin manifesting symptoms at approximately age 1 to 4 months.

If the condition persists into childhood or adolescence, the skin appears scaly. The flexor surfaces of the wrists, ankles, knees, and elbows are affected, as are the neck creases, eyelids, and the dorsal surfaces of the hands and feet. There may be acute weeping areas, with or without secondary infection. Chronic lichenification results from persistent scratching.

Children and adolescents with atopic dermatitis more readily experience intense itching, especially in response to sweating or contact with irritating fabrics such as wool. Emotional upset increases sweating and precipitates itching and scratching. Dry skin is a hallmark of this condition.

PATHOPHYSIOLOGY
of Atopic Dermatitis

Atopic dermatitis is an allergic skin condition. The skin of affected children releases twice as much histamine as that of normal children. The high levels of histamine trigger an inflammatory response, resulting in erythema, edema, and intense pruritus. Scratching increases itching, leading to an "itch-scratch-itch" cycle. Continual scratching and rubbing excoriates and damages the skin. Oozing, weeping, crusting, and cracking lesions develop. The skin of children with atopic dermatitis carries a higher than normal colonization of *Staphylococcus aureus*, and secondary infection is common. Impetigo and viral infections (herpes, molluscum contagiosum) occur frequently in these children.

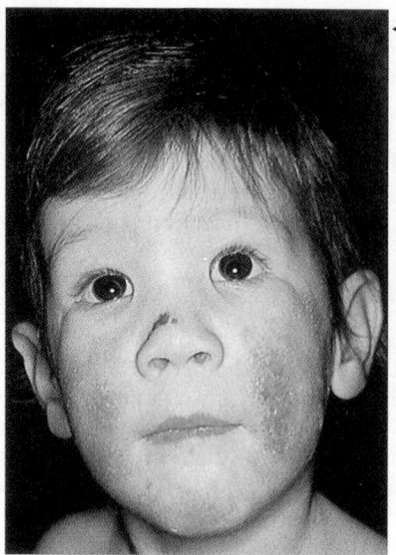

◀ Lesions on cheeks often spread to the forehead, scalp, and extensor surfaces of arms and legs.

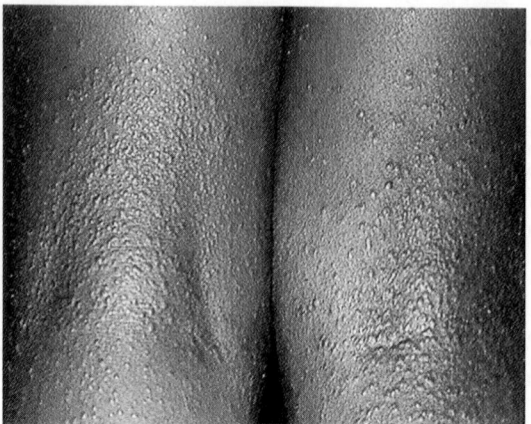

Flexor surfaces of wrists, ankles, knees, and elbows may be affected in the childhood form of the disease.

FIGURE 49–8

Atopic dermatitis, an allergic skin condition, affects 10% to 15% of children. It usually begins in infancy and clears by age 2 to 3 years, but can continue into childhood. (From Hurwitz, S. [1993]. *Clinical pediatric dermatology: A textbook of skin disorders of childhood and adolescence* [2nd ed., pp. 49, 51]. Philadelphia: Saunders.)

Diagnostic Evaluation

The diagnosis is based on the clinical features of intense pruritus, the appearance of the lesions, the pattern of remissions and exacerbations, and a family history of allergy. IgE levels and eosinophils are often elevated. Skin testing for food allergies—usually milk, eggs, wheat, soy, peanuts, and fish—can help identify potential food triggers.

Therapeutic Management

The main goals of treatment are to control itching and scratching, moisturize the skin, prevent secondary infection, and remove irritants and allergens. Control of pruritus includes avoiding trigger factors such as overheating, soaps, wool clothing, and other skin irritants. Oral antihistamines such as hydroxyzine (Atarax), diphenhydramine (Benadryl), and loratidine (Claritin) can be used to help break the "itch-scratch-itch" cycle. Because in most children with atopic dermatitis the itching is more severe at night, antihistamines should be given before bedtime. Secondary infection is treated with antibiotic therapy.

Proper skin hydration is essential. Bathing and the use of wet compresses and occlusive creams and ointments are the mainstays of treatment. In humid climates, bathing should be as infrequent as possible, and only lukewarm water and mild, nonperfumed soap (e.g., Purpose, Dove, Basis) should be used. Emollients such as Eucerin cream or petroleum jelly applied several times a day help the skin retain moisture. The child who lives in a dry climate should bathe frequently (several times a day), using a hydrophilic agent such as Cetaphil instead of soap, and should moisturize with a moisturizing ointment or cream immediately after bathing. Applying the moisturizer while the skin is still damp hydrates the skin. The child should avoid using lotions that contain alcohol, because these can contribute to skin dryness.

Anti-inflammatory corticosteroid creams (Aristocort, Kenalog) are prescribed for inflamed or lichenified areas. These creams are more effective when applied after bathing. The lowest potency that controls signs should be used.

Identifying and eliminating allergens can be helpful. Allergy-proofing the home might be recommended (see Chapter 45). Because allergy to certain foods is an exacerbating factor in some children, those foods should be eliminated from the diets of sensitive infants. Breast-feeding for the first year is recommended for infants at risk for allergy. Solid foods should not be introduced until the infant is at least 6 months old.

NURSING CARE
The Child with Atopic Dermatitis

Assessment

Obtain a thorough history that includes information about allergies in the family. Question parents about any environmental or dietary factors that seem to worsen the child's condition. Determine what treatments have been tried, and their effectiveness. Examine skin lesions for type, distribution, and evidence of any secondary infection. Assess the child's comfort level and the family's feelings and coping methods.

Nursing Diagnosis and Planning

- Impaired Skin Integrity related to environmental and immunologic factors.
  Expected Outcome: The child's skin will exhibit decreased evidence of excoriation.
- Pain related to dry skin, secondary infection, and external irritations.
  Expected Outcomes: The child will exhibit reduced skin dryness and irritation. The child will experience minimal pain and pruritus, as evidenced by decreased irritability, absence of scratching, and uninterrupted periods of sleep.
- Risk for Infection related to skin excoriation.
  Expected Outcome: The child will have no signs of secondary bacterial infection, as evidenced by a normal body temperature and absence of purulent drainage.
- Knowledge Deficit about controlling itching, preventing secondary infection, and identifying aggravating factors related to anxiety or incomplete understanding of information.
  Expected Outcomes: The child and family will identify and eliminate allergens and aggravating factors. The family will carry out prescribed treatments correctly. Family members will express any anxiety related to the child's condition.
- Altered Family Processes related to child's pruritus and involved treatment.
  Expected Outcome: The child and family will discuss their feelings and concerns.

Interventions

Care of the child with atopic dermatitis is demanding, and the entire family routine may revolve around the affected child. Parents need support and reassurance as they care for an uncomfortable, often irritable child (see Chapter 36).

Keeping the child's skin hydrated will help relieve itching. Instruct parents to apply moisturizing creams such as Eucerin, Nivea, or Vaseline Dermatology Formula several times a day and immediately after the child is bathed. Reassure parents that moisturizing creams contain no harmful drugs and should be applied whenever the child's skin looks dry. Soaks and cool, wet compresses are soothing and can be applied to remove crusts, reduce inflammation, and dry weeping areas. Provide parents with explicit instructions on the use of soaks and topical medications. Strips of old cotton sheets moistened in lukewarm or cool tap water work well for wet dressings. Wet compresses should not be used for more than 3 days.

Rough clothing can aggravate eczema, particularly wool or other fabrics that cause sweating. Soft cotton or cotton-polyester blends are tolerated best. Undergarments with irritating seams can be turned inside out so that the soft seam is against the skin. Heat and sweating increase pruritus, so instruct parents to be careful not to "bundle up" the child in heavy blankets or clothing. Because detergents and fabric softeners can also aggravate atopic dermatitis, clothes should be washed in mild detergent and rinsed twice.

Advise the parents to keep the child's fingernails clean and short. Cotton gloves or mittens might be needed to prevent excoriation from scratching but should be used with caution, preferably only at night, because overuse could interfere with fine motor development. Lightweight long-sleeved tops and one-piece outfits discourage scratching.

The child's skin must be kept clean to minimize secondary infection. Avoid using soap. Bath oil or emulsifying ointment can be used as a soap substitute but must be used with caution because these cause both the child and the tub to become slippery. Tepid bathwater helps prevent the child from becoming overheated and itchy. Instruct parents to contact the physician at the earliest signs of skin infection (weeping skin, pustules) and to administer topical and oral antibiotics as prescribed.

Swimming can be beneficial for some children if a moisturizer is applied before swimming and immediately upon exiting the pool. Prolonged immersion in water (more than 20 minutes) can have a drying rather than a hydrating effect. A humidifier in the child's room during winter months may decrease skin dryness. The child should avoid sun exposure.

Children and families of children with atopic dermatitis exhibit frustration when the condition does not resolve quickly. The parent or child might be concerned about the child's appearance as well as the child's discomfort.

> Help parents take control of the child's condition by empowering them with knowledge about therapeutic management. Allowing parents to verbalize frustrations and helping them learn management techniques that do not disrupt family routine are important interventions.

It might be necessary to teach an older child stress-reduction techniques to be used in times of emotional upset. A resource for families of a child with atopic dermatitis is the Eczema Association for Science and Education.

Evaluation

- Is the child's skin intact, with decreased pruritis and pain?
- Do parents carry out prescribed treatments correctly?
- Are parents able to demonstrate appropriate coping techniques?
- Can the child demonstrate stress-relief measures to decrease itching?

■ *Seborrheic Dermatitis*

Seborrheic dermatitis, or "cradle cap," is a chronic inflammatory skin condition seen frequently in infants. It often begins in the first 2 to 3 weeks of life and usually disappears by age 12 months. Seborrhea in older children might appear on the face, behind the ears, around the umbilicus, or in any other area with a large number of sebaceous glands. Although its cause is unknown, it appears to be related to sebaceous gland dysfunction.

Seborrheic dermatitis is characterized by nonpruritic, oily yellow scales that block sweat and sebaceous glands, causing retained secretions and inflammation in affected areas (Fig. 49–9). Confluent erythema might be present in the diaper and intertriginous areas and around the umbilicus (Fig. 49–10). Often, there is overgrowth of normal skin bacteria and yeast, which increases inflammation and leads to secondary infection.

The nurse inspects the infant's scalp or other affected areas for lesions and inflammation and questions parents about frequency and technique of washing the infant's scalp. Instruct the parents to remove the scales daily by shampooing with a mild baby shampoo or an over-the-counter antiseborrheic shampoo containing sulfur and sali-

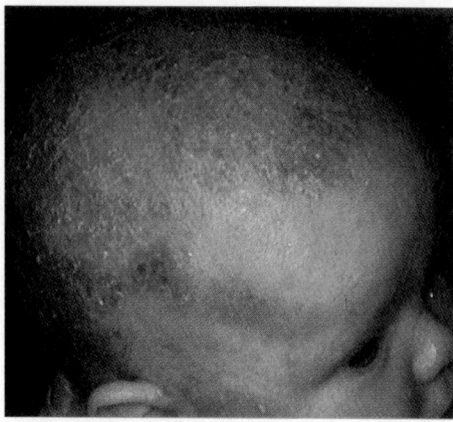

cylic acid (Fostex Medicated Cleansing, P&S, Sebulex), selenium, or tar (Neutrogena T/Gel, Polytar). Massaging the scalp with warm mineral oil before shampooing helps loosen scales. Using a fine-toothed comb or a clean, soft-bristle toothbrush during the shampoo also helps loosen scales. Eyelid dermatitis (blepharitis) is treated with warm tap water compresses and cleansing with "no tears" baby shampoo. Care must be taken to keep topical medications out of the infant's eyes.

Teach the parents the importance of good hygiene of the infant's scalp and skin to prevent recurrence. Reassure them that the fontanel is not fragile and will not be damaged by gentle pressure and washing. Advise the parents to contact the physician if the sites become infected. Skin lesions that do not clear with frequent washing can be treated with hydrocortisone cream applied twice daily.

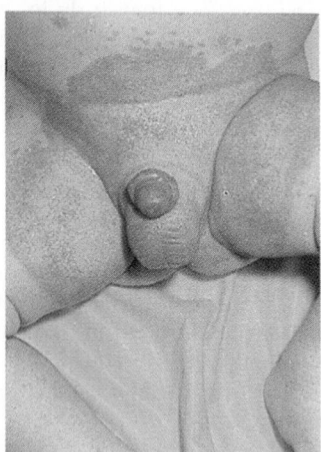

Seborrheic dermatitis of the diaper area is often secondarily infected with *Candida albicans* and requires appropriate treatment. Lotions and creams tend to aggravate the condition and should not be used.

Contact Dermatitis

Contact dermatitis is a skin inflammation that results from a body part's direct contact with an irritant.

Etiology

Contact dermatitis can be caused by hundreds of substances. Among the most common causes of contact dermatitis are rubber products, clothing dyes, nickel (in jewelry, bra strap hooks, jean fasteners), and plant oils. Scented or strongly alkaline soaps, skin lotions, cosmetics, and wool clothing also are irritating to many children.

Diaper dermatitis (diaper rash) is a contact dermatitis from irritants such as moisture, friction, and chemical substances in the diaper area. Urine ammonia, formed from the breakdown of urea by fecal bacteria, is extremely irritating to sensitive infant skin. Ammonia by itself does not cause skin breakdown. Only skin damaged by infrequent diaper changes and constant urine and feces contact is prone to damage from ammonia in urine. Inadequate fluid intake, heat, and detergents in diapers aggravate the condition.

Incidence

Irritant contact dermatitis is more common in children than allergic contact dermatitis. Diaper rash occurs in about 10% of infants and is most common between ages 7 and 9 months. Some infants seem predisposed to diaper dermatitis.

PATHOPHYSIOLOGY
. . . .
of Contact Dermatitis

Contact dermatitis is an inflammatory reaction of the skin caused by either direct exposure to an irritant (*irritant contact dermatitis*) or as a result of a delayed hypersensitivity response to an allergen (*allergic contact dermatitis*).

Irritant contact dermatitis can occur in any person who has repeated or prolonged contact with a primary irritant. Examples of primary irritants include citrus juices, detergents, bubble bath formulations, and urine. Diaper dermatitis is an example of irritant dermatitis that results from prolonged exposure to urine. Teething infants can develop dermatitis on the face and neck folds from drooling.

Allergic contact dermatitis, a delayed hypersensitivity reaction, occurs in susceptible individuals who are sensitized to a substance by a previous exposure to the contact allergen. *Rhus dermatitis* (caused by poison ivy, oak, and sumac), the most common type of allergic contact dermatitis in children, is caused by oleoresins contained in all parts of the plant. Lesions appear several hours to several days after contact.

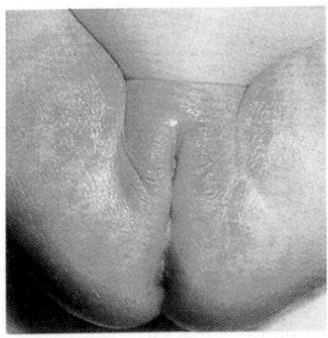

FIGURE 49-11

Contact diaper dermatitis. (From Moschella, S. L., & Hurley, H. J. [1992]. *Dermatology* [3rd ed., p. 239]. Philadelphia: Saunders.)

Manifestations

Manifestations of irritant contact dermatitis include dry, inflamed, and pruritic skin. The distribution of lesions correlates with the skin surface in contact with the offending agent (e.g., watchband, clothing). Diaper dermatitis begins with erythema in the perianal region and possibly excoriating and progressing to macules and papules, which form erosions and crusts (Fig. 49-11). Manifestations of allergic contact dermatitis include blistering, weeping lesions over an area of inflamed skin, intense pruritus, and crusted, scaly lesions that heal in 10 to 14 days without treatment. Rhus dermatitis may cause severe systemic reactions.

Diagnostic Evaluation

The characteristic appearance of the lesions and a history of exposure to an irritating substance establish the diagnosis. Skin testing might be performed in children with persistent or recurrent dermatitis.

Therapeutic Management

Discontinuing exposure to the offending agent treats contact dermatitis. The skin should be washed thoroughly if any irritant remains on the skin. Cool compresses of tap water or Burow's solution can soothe weeping, crusting lesions. Steroid cream (e.g., triamcinolone 0.1% or fluocinolone 0.025%) may be applied several times daily after application of compresses. Severe contact dermatitis might require treatment with oral steroids, which should be tapered gradually. Desensitization therapy is usually not effective in managing contact dermatitis.

NURSING CARE
The Child with Contact Dermatitis

Assessment

Investigate new or continuing exposure to any potentially irritating substances. Assessment of skin lesions includes noting their distribution and configuration, and looking for evidence of pruritus.

For a child with diaper dermatitis, carefully inspect the diaper area, noting the type and extent of lesions. It is important to evaluate the infant's hygiene as well as the parents' knowledge of care related to the infant's skin integrity. Question parents about the type of diapers used, laundering practices, and frequency and method of cleaning the diaper area. Any recent changes in the infant's care such as new foods, soaps, detergents, or lotions should be investigated.

Nursing Diagnosis and Planning

- Pain related to skin inflammation.
  Expected Outcomes: The child will have reduced skin irritation as evidenced by decreased excoriation and increased healing. The child will exhibit minimal pain and pruritus, as evidenced by decreased irritability, absence of scratching, and uninterrupted periods of sleep.
- Risk for Infection related to scratching of pruritic lesions.
  Expected Outcome: The child will have no signs of secondary bacterial infection, as evidenced by clear intact skin.
- Knowledge Deficit of management and prevention of future skin inflammation related to incomplete understanding of therapeutic principles.
  Expected Outcome: The child and family will identify and avoid irritating substances and carry out prescribed treatments correctly.

Interventions

Nursing care of the child with contact dermatitis is directed toward relieving itching, preventing infection, and identifying and removing offending substances. Cool compresses, antipruritic lotions (Calamine), and tepid Aveeno baths provide some relief from itching. Prescribed topical steroid creams should be applied in a thin layer after moisturizing with wet compresses to relieve inflammation. Antihistamines such as diphenhydramine (Benadryl) or hydroxyzine (Atarax) also help the child rest. Because overheating increases itching, advise the parents to occupy the child with quiet activities and to keep the room temperature at a comfortable level.

Reassure the parents and child that the lesions are not contagious and cannot be spread to others or to other parts of the body by scratching. Oils from rhus plants (poison ivy, oak, and sumac) that adhere to the skin, under the fingernails, and on clothing can cause new lesions if they are not removed with soap and water. Lesions can become secondarily infected, so the skin should be kept clean and every effort should be made to prevent scratching. Instruct the parents to contact the physician if the child develops a fever or if the lesions become purulent.

Contact dermatitis is prevented by avoiding offending substances. Children should be taught to recognize plants of the rhus group. If the child is exposed to these plants, rinse the skin with cool water immediately (within 15 minutes) and wash clothing in hot, soapy water. Oleoresins in the plants can be spread not only by direct contact with the plant, but also in the smoke of burning leaves or by touching pets that have contacted the plants.

Avoiding known irritants such as cosmetics, jewelry, and canvas athletic shoes can prevent other types of contact dermatitis. Nickel-sensitive children can usually tolerate 14-karat gold or sterling silver jewelry. Pierced earrings should have hypoallergenic or surgical stainless steel posts.

Diaper dermatitis is much easier to prevent than to treat. Successful treatment and prevention of diaper rash, regardless of the cause, depend on cleaning the diaper area thoroughly and keeping the skin dry. Prompt, gentle cleaning after each voiding or defecation with water and mild soap (Dove, Neutrogena Baby Soap) rids the skin of ammonia and other irritants and decreases the chance of skin breakdown and infection. Careful attention should be given to skin folds and creases. The parent should pat the skin dry with a soft cloth towel after washing. Air drying the skin and frequently exposing the skin to air and light promotes healing of diaper rash. During bouts of diaper rash, the diaper may be left off during nap times.

A bland, protective ointment (A and D, Desitin, zinc oxide) can be applied to clean, dry, intact skin to help prevent diaper rash. Ointments should not be applied to inflamed areas, because they retain moisture. Steroid creams may be indicated for severe dermatitis but should be used for only 7 to 10 days, as prescribed.

Frequent diaper changes decrease irritation from urine and feces. Encourage the parents to check the newborn's diaper every hour and the older infant's diaper every 2 hours. Using disposable diapers does not eliminate the need for frequent diaper changes. Although the "wicking" action of disposable diapers pulls moisture away from the skin toward the liner, ammonia and other by-products are left behind on the infant's skin, causing irritation. Rubber or plastic pants increase skin breakdown by holding in moisture and should be used infrequently.

If cloth diapers are laundered at home, the parents should wash them in hot water, using a mild soap and double rinsing. Soaking diapers before washing in a quaternary ammonium compound (Diaperene) decreases ammonia in the diapers. Using one-quarter cup of vinegar in the rinse is also helpful.

Advise parents to contact the physician if the rash does not improve in 3 days with treatment, if the rash becomes solid and bright red, if the rash becomes raw or bleeds, if blisters or boils develop, or if the infant develops a fever (over 37.8°C, or 100°F).

Evaluation

- Is the child's skin intact, with healed lesions and no evidence of infection or pain?
- Do the parents demonstrate understanding of proper skin and diaper area care?

▎ Acne Vulgaris

Acne is an inflammatory disease of the skin that involves the sebaceous glands and hair follicles. Although acne is generally perceived as a minor disorder, it can cause significant anxiety and emotional pain for the affected adolescent. The disfiguring lesions of acne, although temporary, can lead to physical and emotional scarring.

Etiology

Although the exact cause is unknown, many variables seem to play a role in the development of acne lesions, including heredity, hormonal influences, and emotional stress. Foods do not appear to cause or increase the severity of acne. Acne is unrelated to the general cleanliness of the skin.

PATHOPHYSIOLOGY
of Acne Vulgaris

Acne begins when sebaceous glands, stimulated by androgens at the onset of puberty, enlarge and secrete increased amounts of sebum. The sebaceous glands become plugged and dilated with sebum. When the enlarged gland is open to the skin surface, an open comedone, or blackhead, is formed. The characteristic black color is not a result of poor hygiene but is produced as fatty acids are oxidized on the skin. If the gland does not have an opening, a closed comedone, or whitehead, is formed. Closed comedones are small, nonerythematous papules just beneath the skin surface. Because a closed comedone has only a microscopic opening on the skin surface, pressure from excess sebum and keratin causes the comedone walls to rupture. Fatty acids produced by bacterial action on sebum are released into the surrounding tissues, causing inflammation. If the rupture occurs close to the surface, a pustule is formed. Ruptures deep in the dermis result in cysts and abscesses, which can lead to significant scarring.

Bacteria, particularly *Propionibacterium acnes*, play a role in the development of acne lesions by increasing inflammation and disrupting the integrity of the follicle walls.

Incidence

Acne affects approximately 85% of adolescents. Although acne may begin at any age, it usually develops during puberty and lasts into early adulthood. Acne is more common in males than in females. It tends to improve in summer and flare up in winter.

Manifestations and Diagnostic Evaluation

Acne consists of closed whiteheads, blackheads, papules, pustules, and nodules (Fig. 49–12). Not all adolescents experience all types of acne, and treatment is based on the type experienced. The areas most often affected are the face, neck, back, shoulders, and upper chest. The diagnosis is based on examination of the lesions and the child's history.

Therapeutic Management

The goal of treatment is to prevent scarring and to promote a positive self-image in the adolescent. Treatment must be individualized according to the severity of the condition, the types of lesion present, and the adolescent's sex. Improvement usually begins in 4 to 6 weeks, so the adolescent needs support to keep from feeling discouraged after treatment begins. Three to five months are needed for optimal results.

Topical therapy with a variety of agents is the primary treatment for acne. Commonly used agents include benzoyl peroxide, which reduces fatty acid production and is bactericidal for *Propionibacterium acnes*, and tretinoin (RetinA), a vitamin A derivative. Tretinoin reduces comedone formation and eliminates the lesions already present. Benzoyl

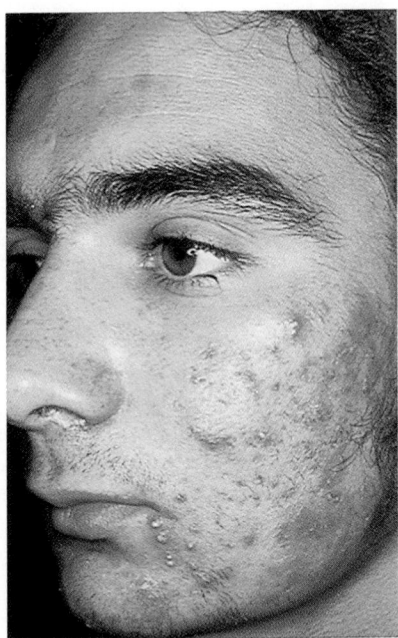

FIGURE 49–12

An adolescent with acne vulgaris. (From Hurwitz, S. [1993]. *Clinical pediatric dermatology: A textbook of skin disorders of childhood and adolescence* [2nd ed., p. 137]. Philadelphia: Saunders.)

peroxide comes in a gel, cream, lotion, or soap in various strengths. Lower-potency formulas are available over-the-counter. Tretinoin is available in cream, gel, or liquid form by prescription. Sunscreen should be used with tretinoin to reduce photosensitivity. When applied together to the skin, benzoyl peroxide and tretinoin have a potentially offsetting effect and can reduce the overall effectiveness of each individual agent. For this reason, the physician may order that the two medications be applied on alternate days or that benzoyl peroxide be applied in the morning and tretinoin at bedtime.

Topical antibiotics, particularly tetracycline and erythromycin, decrease the number of *P. acnes* organisms in hair follicles and are often used for inflammatory acne. Because strains of *P. acnes* are becoming resistant to topical antibiotics, other topical agents are tried first (Landow, 1997). Topical antibiotics are preferred over systemic antibiotics.

Oral antibiotics (tetracycline, minocycline, erythromycin, clindamycin) might be prescribed for adolescents with severe inflammatory acne or those who are unresponsive to topical treatment. Exposure to sunlight should be avoided if tetracycline is used. Oral isotretinoin (Accutane) has dramatically improved the condition of adolescents with severe, nodular/cystic acne. This drug suppresses sebum production and sebaceous gland activity. Because of the severity of side effects, isotretinoin is not indicated for all adolescents. Side effects include cataracts, cheilitis, dry skin, pruritus, conjunctivitis, nosebleeds, and depression. Young women who anticipate becoming pregnant should not take isotretinoin because of its teratogenic effects. Sexually active female adolescents should use an effective form of contraception from the month before treatment until 1 month after discontinuing treatment. A negative pregnancy test must be obtained before initiating therapy. Informed consent is recommended for treatment with isotretinoin.

Estrogen may be prescribed for young women who are unresponsive to antibiotic therapy or who cannot take isotretinoin. The dermatologist may mechanically express comedones. The adolescent should be cautioned not to pick or squeeze lesions. Although scars cannot be completely removed, techniques such as dermabrasion, plastic repair, and collagen implants may improve appearance.

NURSING CARE
The Adolescent with Acne Vulgaris

Assessment

Obtain a history that includes such information as how long acne lesions have been present and the effect of menses, clothing, and stress on the severity and frequency of the lesions. Investigate any acne treatments that have been tried and their effectiveness. It is important to establish how often the adolescent washes the skin and hair and the type of cleansing agents used. Inquire about whether the adolescent uses cosmetics on a regular basis, and what type of cosmetics are used. Try to assess the adolescent's understanding of the development and treatment of acne.

Examine the adolescent's face, chest, back, and neck for lesions. The depth of tissue involvement and the presence of pustules, papules, cysts, and scars should be noted. The adolescent's feelings about appearance and self-image should be explored.

Nursing Diagnosis and Planning

- Impaired Skin Integrity related to increased sebaceous gland secretions, hormonal changes, and the action of bacteria on the contents of clogged follicles.
  Expected Outcome: Affected areas will exhibit signs of healing.
- Risk for Infection related to inflammation of skin lesions.
  Expected Outcome: The adolescent will have no signs of secondary bacterial infection, as evidenced by clear, intact skin.
- Body Image Disturbance related to appearance of skin lesions.
  Expected Outcome: The adolescent will verbalize feelings and concerns.
- Knowledge Deficit about skin care and treatment regimen related to being too embarrassed to ask questions.
  Expected Outcome: The adolescent will carry out the prescribed treatment regimen to control excessive sebaceous gland activity.

Interventions

Because acne is a long-term condition, the affected adolescent needs support and encouragement if the treatment regimen is to be effective. Improvement may take as long as 12 weeks, and exacerbations are common. Although there is no cure for acne, much can be done to control inflammation and reduce scarring.

Explain the cause of acne and the rationale for treatment at the outset, so the adolescent can help plan the treatment regimen. Providing written instructions and involving the adolescent in care can help improve compliance. The treatment must be individualized, but all treatment regimens include measures to reduce oil on the skin. Gently cleaning the face twice a day with mild antibacterial soap and shampooing the hair daily are important facets of care. Warn the adolescent to avoid vigorous scrubbing and picking or squeezing of lesions, which can rupture pilosebaceous ducts and cause secondary infection. Teach the adolescent how to apply topical medications and caution against overusing these products to speed results. Because oily cosmetics and creams add to the plugging of follicles, only water-based cosmetics should be used.

A healthy lifestyle, including adequate rest, exercise, and a balanced diet, promotes healing of lesions. Explore the adolescent's feelings about appearance and coping mechanisms. Reinforce positive self-image and self-esteem. Concerns and fears should be openly discussed, and myths about acne dispelled. Provide parents with needed information about acne to clear up misconceptions and to prevent needless nagging of the adolescent.

Evaluation

- Do the acne lesions exhibit signs of healing without signs of infection?
- Does the adolescent carry out the treatment regimen to control acne and prevent scarring?
- Is the adolescent able to express feelings and concerns about possible change in body image?
- Does the adolescent appear confident and assured as the process of healing is occurring?

Miscellaneous Skin Disorders

There are a number of less common skin disorders of varied causes and manifestations. These disorders, along with their manifestations, management, and special considerations, are listed in Table 49–1.

TABLE 49–1

Miscellaneous Skin Disorders

Disorder/Etiology	Manifestations	Management	Comments
Stevens-Johnson Syndrome, Erythema Multiforme			
Acute, sometimes recurrent autoimmune disease. May be triggered by infections or medications such as sulfonamides or anticonvulsants. New lesions continue to erupt for 2–3 weeks, followed by healing during the next 6 weeks.	Following a prodromal respiratory illness, bullae appear on the lips, mouth, eyes, and genitals. Fever, chills, malaise, neutropenia, anemia, weakness. Purulent conjunctivitis is common. Skin lesions rupture and may lead to significant fluid loss.	Withdraw the triggering medication. Treatment of skin lesions similar to treatment of extensive burns: aseptic technique, IV fluids, air/fluid bedding, nutritional support, and pain management. Give antibiotics for secondary infections. Obtain ophthalmology consultation for eye lesions.	Reassure child that the skin lesions will disappear. Inform parents about the possibility of recurrence and encourage them to avoid any implicated medications.
Psoriasis			
Chronic, inflammatory rash caused by rapid proliferation of keratinocytes. Hereditary predisposition; onset in first two decades of life. Remissions and exacerbations; lasts throughout life. Exacerbations associated with stress. Arthritis is sometimes a complication.	Pruritus; erythematous, elevated plaques and silvery scales on the scalp, face, knees, elbows, and gluteal folds. Scales are attached at the center rather than edges and may bleed when removed.	Topical corticosteroids and tar preparations; keratolytic agents. Exposure to ultraviolet light and sunlight. Skin care to prevent secondary infection. Keratolytic agents enhance penetration of topical steroids. Sunlight may cause phototoxic reactions with tar preparations. To prevent tar folliculitis, tar should be applied down an extremity rather than up.	There is no cure for psoriasis. A resource for families of children with psoriasis is in Appendix L.
Pityriasis Rosea			
Acute, inflammatory, self-limited skin disorder. Etiology unknown; may be viral.	Sudden eruption of salmon-pink, irregular patches on trunk and proximal portions of extremities. Symmetric distribution of lesions, "Christmas tree" appearance on back. "Herald patch" precedes rash by 7–10 days.	No treatment required for asymptomatic children. Pruritus can be treated with antipruritic lotions, ultraviolet light, or sunlight.	Child generally feels well. Rash may last 6–12 weeks.

TABLE 49-1

. . . .

Miscellaneous Skin Disorders Continued

Disorder/Etiology	Manifestations	Management	Comments
Warts			
Skin infection caused by human papillomavirus (HPV). Incubation period is 1–6 months. Can persist from a few months to 5 or more years.	Painless, hyperkeratotic papule. Begins as a round, flesh-colored papule; later becomes brown or tan with a rough surface. Most common sites: dorsum of hands, fingers, feet, face, and genitalia.	Various methods of treatment: daily application of lactic acid and salicylic acid (e.g., Compound W); freezing with liquid nitrogen; topical application of cantharidine for plantar or periungual warts.	Most warts disappear without treatment in 2–3 years. With treatment they usually resolve in 2–3 months. Picking at warts may cause them to spread to other areas of the body. Warts are not highly contagious to other people. Immunocompromised children are more susceptible to warts.
Molluscum Contagiosum			
Viral infection of the skin and mucous membranes. Transmitted by skin-to-skin and fomite-to-skin contact. May be transmitted by sexual contact.	Begin as pinpoint papules which increase in size to 2–3 mm or larger. Firm, solid, pink papules changing into soft, waxy, umbilicated papules. Curd-like core of the lesion can be expressed. Most common sites: face, trunk, extremities, oral mucous membranes, conjunctiva, and genitalia.	Lesions may be treated with cantharidin or liquid nitrogen. Treatment can be repeated once or twice a month, depending on the rate of appearance of new lesions. Condition usually responds well to treatment.	Lesions may be spread to other parts of the body and may be transmitted to others. Lesions disappear spontaneously over time. Children with eczema or impaired immunity are at risk for generalized spread of lesions.
Frostbite			
Freezing of tissue resulting from exposure to extreme cold. Exposed areas (fingers, toes, nose, cheeks, ears) are most often affected. Cold causes arteriolar vasoconstriction, resulting in tissue anoxia and destruction.	*Early signs:* Blanching of skin; stinging sensation followed by numbness and white, mottled appearance. Area feels cold, hard; may be without sensation. *First-degree:* Redness and discomfort with return to normal in a few hours. *Second-degree:* Redness; blisters and bullae 24–48 hours after rewarming. Pain during rewarming. *Third-degree:* Cyanosis and mottling, followed by redness and swelling. Necrosis of epidermis, dermis, and subcutaneous tissue. Sensation is absent. Pain during rewarming. *Fourth-degree:* Complete necrosis with gangrene, possible loss of body part.	Immediately cover affected areas with warm hands and warm clothing. Massaging areas causes further damage and should be avoided. Rapidly rewarm areas by immersion in a warm water bath (90–106°F) until all frozen tissues are thawed and the skin appears flushed. Pain during thawing can be severe and should be treated with analgesics and sedatives. Severely damaged areas are treated as burns.	Children in cold climates should be taught to prevent frostbite by wearing adequate warm, layered clothing, hat, gloves, and two pairs of socks (one cotton, one wool). Children should be taught to warm themselves when hands or feet begin to sting. Young children should not be allowed to play outside in extremely cold temperatures.
Foreign Bodies			
Skin injury due to penetration of splinters, gravel, cactus spines, bee stingers, glass, or other foreign objects.	Pain, erythema, possible secondary infection. Foreign body may or may not be visible.	Area surrounding foreign body should be washed with soap and water before removal. Superficial splinters can be removed with a needle and tweezers disinfected with alcohol or flame.	Deeply embedded foreign bodies, fishhooks, and other difficult to remove objects may require medical attention. Tetanus prophylaxis may be indicated.

Insect Bites or Stings

Insects are found almost everywhere, and children often come in contact with them during play. The bites of most insects are not serious, usually causing only itching and mild pain. Severe systemic reactions can occur in sensitized children, however. Approximately 2 million people in the United States are severely allergic to venomous stinging insects. The prevalence may be as high as 1% of all children (Golden, 1996). Approximately 50 people die each year from allergic reactions to insect stings (Golden, 1996). Children who are allergic to insect stings should wear identification describing the allergy and outlining appropriate treatment. An emergency kit containing an antihistamine, epinephrine, and a syringe should be kept immediately available for such children. Parents should check the expiration date on the kit and replace it if it is outdated. (See Chapter 41 for a discussion of allergic reactions.)

Arachnids (scorpions, spiders, ticks, and mites) are found in areas where children play. Most arachnids are not dangerous or aggressive. In the United States only one type of scorpion and two types of spiders (black widow and brown recluse) cause life-threatening reactions.

Topical insect repellents are usually safe and effective in preventing insect bites. Repellents containing high concentrations of diethyltoluamide (DEET) should not be used on small children because of the risk of toxic encephalopathy. Such repellents should not be applied near the face, and children should be cautioned not to put their fingers in their mouths when wearing DEET.

The bites and stings of common insects and arachnids are discussed in Table 49–2. The table includes information on manifestations, treatment, and prevention.

TABLE 49–2

Skin Lesions Caused by Insects and Arachnids

Agent/Characteristics	Manifestations	Treatment and Prevention
Insects		
Mosquitoes, Fleas, Flies, Gnats		
Foreign protein in insect's saliva is injected as insect pierces skin to suck blood.	Itching, erythema, small wheal. Allergic reaction may occur.	Apply antipruritic lotions and cool compresses to relieve itching. Give antihistamines if needed for sleep. **Prevention:** Wear insect repellent when contact is anticipated. Treat potential breeding places (standing water for mosquitoes; pets, furniture, yard for fleas).
Hymenoptera (Bees, Wasps, Hornets, Yellow Jackets, Fire Ants)		
Venom is injected through a stinger.	Histamine and foreign proteins in venom cause local reaction of pain, swelling, redness, and itching. Systemic allergic reactions may be manifested by nausea, generalized edema, respiratory distress, and shock.	Carefully remove stinger by scraping it out horizontally. Avoid squeezing stinger, as more venom will be released. Wash with soap and water. Paste made of powdered meat tenderizer and water is soothing. Apply ice and analgesics for discomfort, antihistamines for itching. For a systemic allergic reaction, give epinephrine and corticosteroids immediately; transport to emergency facility. Children allergic to hymenoptera should wear medical identification. **Prevention:** Treat known hives or nests. Avoid wearing colorful clothing and perfumes when outside.
Arachnids		
Brown Recluse ("Fiddle Back") Spider		
Yellowish to reddish brown with a violin-shaped mark on its back. Venom injected by fangs. Bites only when threatened. Lives in dark, protected areas (woodpiles, basements, closets, trash heaps).	Mild stinging at time of bite. Within 2–8 hours, area around bite becomes painful and erythema develops, followed by a blister. Venom is necrotoxic. Edema, redness, and purpura may involve entire limb.	Immobilize and elevate affected extremity. Cool compresses, analgesics, tetanus prophylaxis. Observe for secondary infection. Skin graft may be necessary for large ulcers.

TABLE 49–2

Skin Lesions Caused by Insects and Arachnids Continued

Agent/Characteristics	Manifestations	Treatment and Prevention
	Central portion of lesion develops an indurated wheal that progresses to deep, sloughing ulcer in 7–14 days. Ulcer often does not heal for several months. Usually results in a scar.	No antivenin available. **Prevention:** Avoid areas inhabited by spiders.
Black Widow Spider Shiny black with a red hourglass-shaped mark on abdomen. Female's venom is very poisonous to humans. Males do not bite. Female builds irregular web in dark, sheltered spots and aggressively defends eggs.	Bite may be painless initially. Within 1 hour pain develops at site. Severe muscle pains and numbness spread from bite, and puncture site becomes red, swollen, and pruritic. Neurotoxic venom enters the bloodstream within an hour, causing dizziness, headache, nausea, vomiting, cramps, tremors, and rapid, shallow respirations. Shock and renal failure may develop in young children.	Hospitalization for children. Antivenin if no allergy to horse serum. Supportive care, including IV calcium gluconate, morphine, and muscle relaxants. Tetanus prophylaxis. **Prevention:** Avoid areas infested by spiders (woodpiles, outhouses).
Ticks Brown or gray. Live in fields, pastures, woods. Feed on blood of humans, dogs, livestock, or deer. Larvae feed on rodents. Tick buries head and mouthparts in the skin to suck blood.	Bites may cause local reactions or, rarely, systemic reactions (tick fever or tick paralysis). Ticks can transmit Lyme disease, Rocky Mountain spotted fever, Q fever, and tularemia.	**Methods to remove ticks:** Remove with tweezers as close to the skin as possible, taking care to remove head. If mouthparts remain, remove with sterile needle. Wash site with soap and water. There is some evidence that prompt removal of ticks decreases chance of transmission of disease. **Prevention:** Wear long sleeves and pants and use insect repellent when walking in tick-infested areas. Inspect clothing and hair for ticks after walking through fields or woods.
Scorpion Most scorpions are not dangerous. They rarely attack humans unless accidentally disturbed or stepped on. If disturbed, they inflict a painful sting. One type, *C. sculpturatus*, is extremely poisonous and its sting can be fatal. It is found in Arizona. Scorpions are found mainly in the southwestern U.S. Scorpions hide by day in basements, garages, closets, and crevices. Some varieties burrow and hide in gravel or children's sandboxes.	Sting is extremely painful. Local reaction of swelling at puncture site. Some species cause systemic reactions: tachycardia, hypertension, arrhythmias, irritability, seizures, pulmonary edema, coma. Fatal reactions most often occur in children under age 3 years.	Ice packs and tourniquet applied proximal to the site slow the spread of venom. Wound should not be excised. Topical steroids and antihistamines are used to relieve symptoms. For severe reactions, provide supportive care for pain, shock, and seizures. Narcotic analgesics act synergistically with scorpion venom and are contraindicated. Antivenin is given for systemic reactions (available from the Antivenom Production Laboratory, Arizona State University). **Prevention:** Wear shoes to prevent stepping on scorpions. Inspect shoes and clothing before dressing. Apply creosote to garages, basements.
Chiggers (Harvest Mites) Live in tall grass and underbrush. Chiggers burrow into hair follicles and skin pores to feed.	Tend to concentrate in warm areas where clothing is snug (underwear elastic). Cause erythematous papules and intense itching.	Antipruritic agents. Prevention of secondary infection. **Prevention:** Insect repellent on clothing, ankles, and legs.

Burn Injuries

Burn injury may involve a small, painful area that hurts until healing occurs or it may involve most of a child's body, with resulting severe trauma or death. Infants and toddlers are at greatest risk for sustaining burns because they are totally dependent on others for safety.

Pediatric Differences in the Effects of Burn Injury

- Very young children who have been severely burned have a higher mortality rate than older children and adults with comparable burns.
- Because a child's skin is thinner than an adult's, lower burn temperatures and shorter exposure to heat or chemicals can cause a more severe burn.
- A larger body surface area as compared with adults places severely burned children at increased risk for fluid and heat loss. Children are also at increased risk for dehydration and metabolic acidosis secondary to diarrhea, evaporative water loss, and increased fluid requirements.
- The higher proportion of body fluid to mass in children increases the risk of cardiovascular problems because of their less effective cardiovascular response to changing intravascular volume.
- Burns involving more than 10% TBSA require a form of fluid resuscitation (Reeves et al., 1994).
- Infants and children are at increased risk for protein and calorie deficiency because they have smaller muscle mass and lower body fat than adults. If they are not eating and their metabolism is increased, their protein and calorie needs will not be met.
- Hypertrophic scarring is more severe and scar maturation is prolonged (Reeves et al., 1994).
- An immature immune system means an increased risk of infection for infants and young children.
- A delay in growth may follow extensive burns.
- In children, Curling (gastroduodenal) ulcer occurs in the third or fourth week post burn, which is later than in adults.

Recovery from a major burn injury requires many months, and the child's appearance might be altered for life. Caring for a burned child entails a multidisciplinary approach with a focus on the child and the family. Nursing care entails treating the physical injury and its psychological effects on the child and family members. The challenges of burn nursing begin with acute burn care but continue through the rehabilitation phase until the child is restored to optimal function.

Etiology

Burn injuries in children can be accidental or nonaccidental. In children younger than age 5, accidental burns are likely to occur as a result of environmental situations that are not controlled by caretakers. The young child's curiosity and increasing mobility contribute to the risk (Table 49–3). A child can start a fire by playing with matches or flammable materials near open fires, or a child might be the victim of a house fire while sleeping or might be accidentally scalded or electrocuted. (See Chapter 4 for a discussion of safety.) Either neglectful supervision or purposeful abuse can cause nonaccidental burns.

The extent of the injury determines whether the problem is local or systemic. Other factors such as the location of the burned area, whether it is an electrical injury, a concurrent inhalation injury, or trauma, and whether there is a preexisting medical disease contribute to morbidity and mortality. Morbidity and mortality are higher in children who have been burned than in adults.

Incidence

Fire and burn injuries are the third leading cause of accidental deaths in children ages 1 to 14 years in the United States (Centers for Disease Control and Prevention, 1997). In children younger than age 4, 66% of burns result from scalds and 14% from flame injury (Dickerson, Gordon, & Walter, 1998). The rest of the burn injuries are due to electrical and chemical causes. Approximately 16% of burn injuries are related to child abuse (Herrin & Antoon, 1996).

TABLE 49–3

Age-Related Risks for Burn Injury

Age	Injury Type	Risk Factors
<5 years	Flame	Playing with matches and cigarette lighters Playing with fires in fireplaces, barbecue pits, trash fires
	Scald	Kitchen injury from tipping scalding liquids Bathtub scalds associated with lack of supervision or child abuse *Most who are pediatric burn patients are infants and toddlers less than 3 years old burned by scalding liquids*
5 to 10 years	Flame	Male children at increased risk Often associated with fire play and risk-taking behaviors
	Scald	Female children at increased risk Likely to occur at home in kitchen or bathroom
Adolescent	Flame	Injury associated with male peer-group activities involving gasoline or other flammable products Gasoline sniffing possibly involved Rarely occurs in female adolescents except in house fires or automobile accidents
	Electrical	Occurs most often in male adolescents involved in dare-type behaviors, such as climbing utility poles or antennas In rural areas, may be associated with moving irrigation pipes that touch an electrical source

Most children with severe burns are treated in burn centers. The American Burn Association has outlined criteria for referral to a burn center.

Pathophysiology

Burn injuries are described using three parameters: depth of tissue damage, extent of injury, and severity. The combination of these factors determines referral and therapeutic management decisions.

DEPTH OF BURN INJURY

Depth of burn injury describes local tissue damage and is largely a factor of the duration of exposure and the temperature or destructive potential of the agent causing the damage. Depth of injury is classified as superficial (first degree), partial thickness (second degree), or full thickness (third degree) (Table 49–4).

Partial-thickness thermal, chemical, or electrical injury to the skin interferes with the skin's ability to carry out its normal physiologic functions of protection from infection or injury and preservation of fluid balance and temperature regulation. In addition, deep tissue injury damages sensory nerve endings and local circulatory patterns, and adversely affects the skin's ability to regenerate or synthesize vitamin D.

EXTENT OF BURN INJURY

The extent of injury refers to the percent of total body surface area (TBSA) burned. The standard "rule of nines" used in adults gives an inaccurate estimate for children because of the differences in body proportion between children and adults. When using the rule of nines in children, 9% is taken from the legs and added to the head for a child up to 1 year of age. Each subsequent year, 1% is returned to the legs until, at approximately age 9, the child's head is in proportion to an adult's (Miller, Richard, & Staley, 1994). Many burn facilities use the Lund and Browder chart, which is a body surface chart corrected for age (Fig. 49–13). Another, more recently developed formula is to estimate the burn percentage by calculating the complete palmar surface of the child's hand. The area of the palmar surface equals 1% of the total body surface area (Kumar, 1999; Nagel & Schunk, 1997).

SEVERITY OF BURN INJURY

Severity of burn injury is determined by the degree to which the skin's physiologic functions are disrupted beyond the body's normal ability to respond with compensatory mechanisms. Burn injuries are classified as minor, moderate uncomplicated, and major. The severity of burn injury is related to a combination of factors, including age, medical history, extent and depth of burn, special care of the body area involved (e.g., face or hands), and the presence of concomitant trauma, such as fractures or head injury, sustained at the time of the burn. Burn severity relates to the child's eventual morbidity or mortality status.

Manifestations

Table 49–5 lists the clinical manifestations associated with burns of different severity.

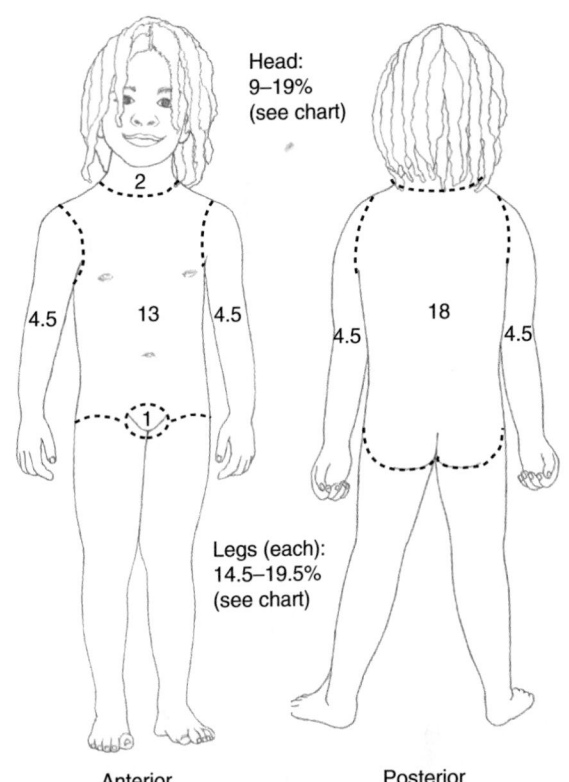

Head:
9–19%
(see chart)

Legs (each):
14.5–19.5%
(see chart)

Anterior   Posterior

Child Burn Size Estimation Table
(percent total body surface area)

Burn area	Age (years)				
	1	**1–4**	**5–9**	**10–14**	**15**
Head	19	17	13	11	9
Neck	2	2	2	2	2
Anterior trunk	13	13	13	13	13
Posterior trunk	18	18	18	18	18
Genitalia	1	1	1	1	1
Upper extremity (each)	9	9	9	9	9
Lower extremity (each)	14.5	15.5	17.5	18.5	19.5

FIGURE 49–13

Calculating total body surface area (TBSA) burned in children. The standard "rule of nines" and standard body surface charts must be adapted because of the difference in body proportions between adults and children. (Child Burn Size Estimation Table reprinted from Lund, C. C., & Browder, N. C. [1944]. Estimation of burn size. *Surgery, Gynecology, and Obstetrics, 79,* 352–358. By permission of *Surgery, Gynecology, and Obstetrics,* now known as the *Journal of the American College of Surgeons.*)

Therapeutic Management

SUPERFICIAL BURN INJURIES

The most common cause of a superficial (epidermal layer only) burn is sunburn. Although uncomfortable, sunburn rarely requires intensive burn treatment. Cool compresses and application of soothing topical lotions (especially those containing aloe) or mild topical corticosteroids (Prose & Antaya, 1998), provide symptomatic treatment. If the discomfort is disturbing the child's sleep, acetaminophen or ibuprofen can provide relief.

Preventing sunburn is especially important in children

TABLE 49-4
Depth of Burn Injury

	Superficial (First Degree)	Partial-Thickness (Second Degree) Superficial	Partial-Thickness (Second Degree) Deep	Full-Thickness (Third Degree)
Morphology	Destruction of epidermis; physiologic functions remain intact	Destruction of epidermis and some dermis	Destruction of epidermis and dermis	Destruction of epidermis, dermis, and underlying tissue; may include fascia, muscle, tendon, and bone
Blister formation	After 24 hours (e.g., from sunburn)	Within minutes; thin-walled, fluid-filled	May or may not appear as fluid-filled blisters; often, they are flat, dehydrated, and tissue paper–like. Body fluids lost through burn tissue must be replaced	Rare; may appear as a tissue paper–like layer that is flat and dehydrated
Appearance	Peels after 24–48 hours	Red to pale ivory, moist surface	Mottled, waxy white, dry surface	White, cherry red, or black
Healing time	3–7 days	7–21 days if no infection develops	30 days to several months if no infection; if infected, this type of burn may convert to full thickness	Will not heal; skin grafting required. Very small areas may heal from edges after a period of weeks
Patient reaction	Moderate discomfort, pain; chills; nausea; vomiting	May cause considerable pain	Severe pain upon exposure to air or water because nerve endings are intact	No pain in area of full-thickness burn because nerve endings are destroyed; surrounding areas of lesser depth are painful
Scarring	None	Minimal; influenced by genetic predisposition	Greatest because the slow healing of these burns increases scar tissue. Scar formation is influenced by genetic predisposition	Autograft scarring is minimized by early excision and grafting. Scar formation is influenced by genetic predisposition

TABLE 49–5

Classification of Severity of Burn Injury in Children

Type of Injury	Clinical Manifestations
Minor	
Partial-thickness burn of <10% total body surface area (TBSA)	Localized pain and blister formation in the area of injury; white or black full-thickness injury
Full-thickness burn of <2% TBSA that does not involve special care areas (eyes, ears, face, hands, feet, perineum, joints)	No systemic effects
Excludes electrical injury, inhalation injury, concurrent trauma, all poor-risk children (e.g., those of extremely young age or with intercurrent disease)	Little or no scarring, except in areas of full-thickness injury
Moderate, Uncomplicated	
Partial-thickness burns of 10%–20% TBSA	Open wound that is a potential source of infection and a site for loss of fluids and electrolytes
Full-thickness burns of <10% TBSA that do not involve special care areas	Pain that may interfere with routines of daily living
Excludes electrical injury, inhalation injury, concurrent trauma, all poor-risk children (e.g., those of extremely young age or with intercurrent disease)	Wound healing rate influenced by nutritional status
	Possible scarring in areas of partial and full-thickness injuries
Major	
Partial-thickness burns of >20% TBSA	Life-threatening injuries with risk for severe complications and death
All full-thickness burns of ≥10% TBSA	Volatile hospital course characterized by periods of relative physiologic stability followed, within hours, by life-threatening emergencies such as shock
All burns involving eyes, ears, face, hands, feet, perineum, or joints	Repeated operative procedures for skin grafting that are accompanied by major blood loss requiring multiple transfusions
All inhalation injury, electrical injury, concurrent trauma, all poor-risk patients	Potential risk for infection, either of the burn wound or related to pulmonary complications or systemic sepsis, until wound closure is achieved over 80% of the TBSA
	Much higher mortality associated with burn injury accompanied by inhalation injury than with burn injury alone

because frequent sunburn causes long-term damage to the skin. Children who are susceptible to sunburn are also susceptible to the later development of melanoma (Prose & Antaya, 1998). Children should avoid sun exposure, especially between the hours of 10 A.M. and 3 P.M. during the summer. If exposure is likely during that time, parents should apply an appropriate ultraviolet A- and ultraviolet B-protective sunscreen with a sun protection factor greater than 15. Waterproof sunscreens are available for children who like to run in and out of the water, but frequent applications of sunscreen are still desirable. Sunscreen is contraindicated for infants under age 6 months. Parents should keep infants in the shade, away from reflecting sun rays.

MINOR PARTIAL-THICKNESS BURN INJURIES

In general, children with a minor burn injury are treated as outpatients in a physician's office, clinic, or hospital physi-

cal therapy department unless the extent of injury warrants hospital admission. Therapy is aimed at promoting wound healing, preventing infection, and providing pain relief. Burn wound care requires aseptic technique. Because anaerobic and aerobic bacteria can grow at the interface between burned and healthy tissue, tetanus toxoid is given to children whose immunizations are not up-to-date.

Wound Cleaning. Burn wounds receive care at least daily until closure is achieved. After old dressings are removed, the burned skin is cleaned with sterile saline or mild soap and water. If the child is hospitalized, hydrotherapy (Fig. 49–14) can be used to remove old dressings and clean the wound and the child. During this cleaning process, the child can perform active range-of-motion exercises. Hydrotherapy can be done in a tank, tub, or shower. Some facilities use disposable plastic liners to prevent contamination between uses. Hydrotherapy should last no longer than 20 minutes to prevent electrolyte loss (through skin into water, secondary

Burn Center Referral Criteria

The American Burn Association has identified the following injuries as those requiring referral to a burn center. Patients with these burns should be treated in a specialized burn facility after initial assessment and stabilization in an emergency department.

- Second- and third-degree burns of more than 10% BSA in patients under 10 or over 50 years old.
- Second- and third-degree burns of more than 20% BSA in all other age groups.
- Second- and third-degree burns with serious threat of functional or cosmetic impairment that involve the face, hands, feet, genitalia, perineum, and major joints.
- Third-degree burns of more than 5% BSA in any age group.
- Electrical burns, including lightning injury.
- Chemical burns with serious threat of functional or cosmetic impairment.
- Inhalation injury with burn injury.
- Circumferential burns of an extremity and/or the chest.
- Burned children should be transferred to a hospital with qualified personnel and equipment.
- Any burn patient with coexisting trauma, such as fractures, in which the burn injury poses the greatest risk of morbidity or mortality. However, if the trauma poses the greater immediate risk, the patient may initially be treated in a trauma center until stable, before being transferred to a burn center. Burn care may be provided simultaneously, or transfer may be accomplished after the burn patient has recovered from the immediate effects of the associated mechanical trauma. Should the burn injury present the dominant threat to mortality and the greatest risk of morbidity, then transfer to the burn center is appropriate. Physician judgment will be necessary in such situations and should be in concert with the regional medical control plan.

Preexisting medical conditions frequently complicate burn management and prolong recovery.

Patients at the extremes of age are subject to variable physiologic response to thermal injury. Infants and elderly patients are less tolerant of thermal, electrical, or chemical injuries. The burn team approach utilizing physicians, nurses, psychologists, dietitians, and physical and occupational therapists has a significant influence on the outcome of major burn and electrical injuries.

STABILIZATION IN PREPARATION FOR TRANSFER

Once the decision has been made to transfer a burn patient, it is essential that the patient be properly stabilized prior to the transfer process.

Nebraska Burn Institute. (1994). ABLS (Advanced Burn Life Support) Course. Lincoln, NE: Author.

to osmosis). The room temperature is kept warm, and the child is covered and dried immediately after the procedure.

Debridement. *Debridement* is the removal of dead material within a wound to promote healing. In a burn injury, there is necrosis of skin and subcutaneous tissue. The burned tissue is called *eschar*. Eschar releases chemical mediators that stimulate leukocytes to digest debris, but this also damages capillaries and skin elements. Necrotic tissue within a wound prolongs inflammation and slows healing and epidermal coverage (Saffle & Schnebly, 1994).

Initial debridement might be performed in the office, emergency department, or hydrotherapy treatment room. The burned area is debrided of loose debris and necrotic tissue. Blisters usually are left intact and debrided only after

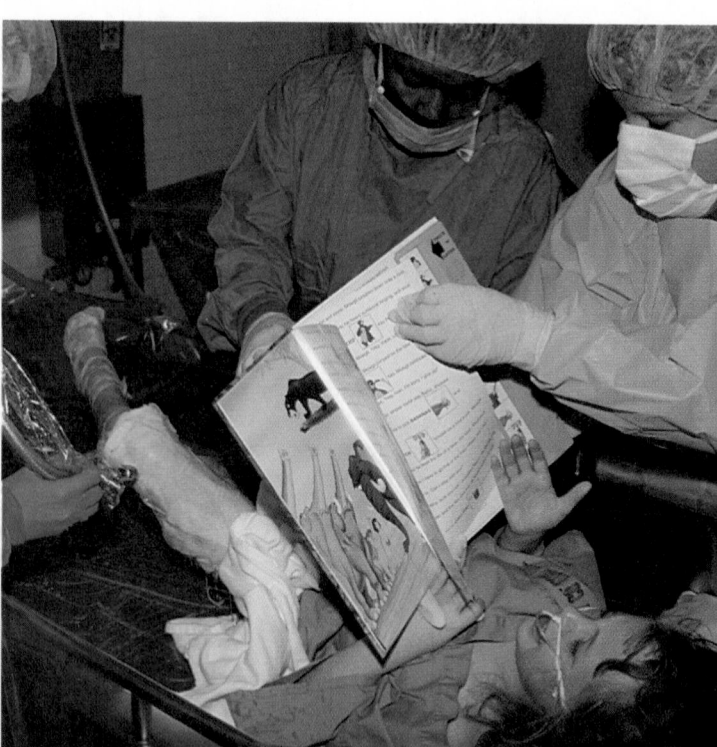

FIGURE 49–14

Burn dressings can be changed in the hydrotherapy room. The room is kept warm because children who have been burned have poor body temperature control. The child life therapist reads a book to the child to distract her from the discomfort associated with the procedure. (Courtesy of Parkland Health and Hospital System, Dallas, Texas.)

TABLE 49-6

Topical Antimicrobial Agents Commonly Used for Burns

Agent	Advantages	Side Effects/Disadvantages	Nursing Considerations
Silver nitrate solution	Effective against most gram-positive and some gram-negative organisms	Hyponatremia, hypokalemia, hypochloremia Decreased penetration of eschar Not effective against established infection Requires large, bulky dressings which limit mobility	0.5% solution in distilled water applied to wet dressing every 2 hours Dressing changes twice daily
Mafenide acetate cream (Sulfamylon)	Effective against a wide range of gram-positive and gram-negative organisms Rapidly diffuses through eschar (improved effectiveness in established infections) Permits open treatment of wound, thus increasing mobility	Painful on application May cause hypersensitivity reaction in 5%–7% of patients Associated with acid-base derangements	Applied to cleansed wound 1 to 2 times per day Treated area left open because wrapping causes maceration
Silver sulfadiazine cream (Silvadene)	Effective against a wide range of gram-positive and gram-negative organisms Soothing on application Softens eschar and increases joint mobility Absorbed slowly, reducing the possibility of nephrotoxicity	May cause hypersensitivity reaction in 5%–7% of patients Associated with initial decrease in leukocyte count	Applied to cleansed wound 1 to 3 times per day Wound may be left open or covered with light dressing

Adapted from Marvin, J. A. (1991). Burn injuries and skin trauma. In M. L. Patrick, S. L. Woods, R. F. Craven, J. S. Rokosky, & P. M. Bruno (Eds.), *Medical-surgical nursing: Pathophysiological concepts* (2nd ed., p. 1854). Philadelphia: Lippincott.

they open (Brady & Dunn, 1996; Kumar, 1999). Old creams and ointments must be removed as part of the debridement, and loose tissue is trimmed around the burned area.

Application of Antimicrobial Agents and Dressings. Topical antibacterial agents (Table 49–6) are placed on burn wounds to penetrate the eschar and to control bacterial growth in and around the burn wound. Silver sulfadiazine (Silvadene) is the most commonly used topical agent, but it is not typically used on the face or on electrical burns. Facial burns are covered with a light layer of antimicrobial ointment. Mafenide (Sulfamylon) is the topical agent of choice for burns to the ear or electrical burns because of its deep penetration into the eschar. Sulfamylon should not be applied to the face.

Following application of the topical antibacterial, a dressing usually is applied. Depending on the burn care protocol, dressings are changed one to three times daily. Because exposed nerve endings can cause significant pain, wound assessment and care should be done as quickly as possible. Narcotic or nonnarcotic pain medications are administered 20 to 30 minutes prior to dressing changes to ensure maximum pain control at the time of the procedure. The Child Life Specialist can assist with teaching the child how to use nonpharmacologic pain relief techniques.

Besides pain control, measures to maintain the child's core body temperature, minimize shivering, and conserve energy also must be implemented as part of wound care activities. To the degree possible, the child's capacity for self-

care should be optimized. Allowing the child to remove dressings provides a measure of control.

Aseptic technique is used during dressing changes. After dressings are applied to burn wounds, isolation is not necessary, and the child does not need to be restricted to a room or to an area of the hospital.

Depending on the depth and extent of the burn, the physician might choose to cover the area with a biologic or synthetic dressing to reduce the chance of infection, provide pain relief, reduce evaporative fluid and heat loss, and promote healing. Such dressings are best used for partial-thickness burns. Commonly used biologic dressings include human skin, pig skin, and fresh human amniotic membrane (from the placenta). Synthetic dressings include plastic films, hydrocolloids, hydrogels, and collagen-impregnated dressings. The major risk associated with these dressings is infection; thus, the wound must be clean and dry prior to dressing application.

NURSING CARE

The Child with a Minor Partial-Thickness Burn

Assessment

In the first few seconds after the arrival of a child who has been burned, a determination is made as to the severity of the burn. If the burn is of minor or moderate uncomplicated severity, care focuses on pain management and wound care. Take vital signs, paying special attention to the child's body temperature. Without skin the burned child, especially if very young, rapidly loses heat to the atmosphere and is at risk for hypothermia. The child should be awake, alert, and oriented unless some condition other than an uncomplicated burn injury exists.

Assessment for pain intensity takes place on a scheduled basis, and interventions to control pain are implemented as needed. Assess the wound with each dressing change, and document any signs of decreased circulation or infection. Assessment also includes range-of-motion abilities and the frequency and effectiveness of any physical therapy treatments. It is important to assess the child's ability to assume independent activities, particularly when the burn affects the child's extremities. Young children tend to protect injuries, so the child might need encouragement to move appropriately.

Nursing Diagnosis, Planning, Intervention, and Evaluation

Nursing Diagnosis
- Impaired Skin Integrity related to the burn.

Expected Outcome
- The burn will heal without infection, as evidenced by restoration of the epithelial layer.

Intervention

1. Clean and debride the wound daily and apply antimicrobial ointments and dressings as ordered. Observe and assess the site and record findings.
2. Maintain aseptic technique for wound care by wearing protective gear and practicing meticulous hand-washing techniques.
3. Promote adequate fluid and nutritional intake. Offer high-calorie, high-protein meals and snacks. Provide foods that the child likes. Arrange the timing of meals so that they do not immediately precede or follow painful or distressing events.
4. Perform active and passive range-of-motion exercises of the affected parts of the child's body.
5. Make sure that the child's tetanus toxoid immunizations are current.

6. Monitor the child for signs and symptoms of infection: changes in sensorium, hypothermia, fever, or a change in wound appearance (drainage or odor). Obtain specimens for culture if ordered.
7. Administer vitamins and minerals (A, B, C, iron, and zinc) as ordered.
8. Instruct the child and parents to keep the healed burn wound out of the sun for at least a year.

Rationale

1. Infection can be prevented by removing bacterial contamination, exudate, and previously applied medication.
2. Cross-contamination of burn wounds from other patients or staff increases the risk of sepsis.

3. Healing occurs only in the presence of a positive nitrogen balance. The child's protein and calorie needs are elevated because of increased metabolism and catabolism.

4. Use of the burned area promotes edema reabsorption and prevents contracture deformity.
5. Anaerobic bacteria can cause infection at the interface between the burn wound and healthy tissue.
6. Early detection of infection will ensure prompt treatment.

7. Vitamin and mineral supplements facilitate wound healing and epithelialization.
8. Burned skin is more sensitive to sunlight, which increases the risk of sunburn.

Evaluation
- Does the burn wound shows signs of progressive healing?
- Is the tissue pink and free from exudate?
- Have blistered areas resolved?
- Is the child free of fever and other signs of infection?

Nursing Diagnosis
- Pain related to thermal injury and related procedures.

Expected Outcome
- The child will remain free from pain, except during procedures and physical therapy, as evidenced by age-appropriate behaviors, adequate nutritional intake, and appropriate sleep patterns and will begin to assume age-appropriate activities.

Intervention

1. Determine the child's pain level using an age-appropriate assessment tool (see Chapter 39).

2. Administer pain relief measures and medication on a scheduled basis, rather than on demand. Premedicate the child at least 20 to 30 minutes before painful procedures.

Rationale

1. The child's developmental stage affects response to pain and the child's response to various pain assessment tools is related to developmental level.
2. The fact that burns hurt is irrefutable, so there is no need to wait until pain is behaviorally indicated before administering medication.

3. Minimize the time spent on wound manipulation and exposure.

4. Use nonpharmacologic pain reduction measures (see Chapter 39).

5. Perform passive and active range-of-motion exercises. Be careful that dressings are applied so as to preserve function of body parts.

3. Exposure of the burned area to air or water causes pain because the nerve endings are exposed. Dressing changes should be done as quickly as possible to minimize pain.

4. Distraction, relaxation techniques, therapeutic touch, and other measures may help alleviate pain.

5. Exercise, although painful in the acute stage, reduces the likelihood of contracture formation and increases functional ability.

Evaluation

- Except during times of direct wound care and physical therapy, is the child pain free, as evidenced by normal sleep, play, and eating patterns?
- Is the child able to cooperate with dressing changes and range-of-motion exercises?

Nursing Diagnosis

■ Risk for Fluid Volume Deficit related to loss of skin integrity in the area of the burn and resulting fluids shifts.

Expected Outcome

- The child will maintain normal fluid and electrolyte balance, as evidenced by intake and output measurements and serum electrolyte values within normal ranges.

Intervention	Rationale
1. Administer fluids orally or IV as ordered.	1. Fluids help maintain capillary circulation to the viable skin appendages and general circulation to the vital organs. Fluid replacement continues until wound coverage is achieved.
2. Instruct the parents to monitor the child's intake and output frequently.	2. Close monitoring is necessary to determine whether fluid resuscitation is necessary or adequate. Fluid intake sufficient to produce 1 to 2 ml/kg/hr of urine ensures adequate tissue perfusion.
3. Weigh the hospitalized child daily.	3. Weight is an accurate measurement of hydration status. Increasing weight indicates fluid overload.
4. Monitor laboratory values for elevated electrolyte or hemoglobin levels.	4. Early identification of abnormal laboratory values permits early treatment of fluid volume imbalances.

Evaluation

- Is the child voiding at least 1 to 2 ml/kg/hr?
- Are serum electrolyte values within normal ranges?
- Does the child appear well hydrated?
- Does the child take fluids well?

Nursing Diagnosis

■ Risk for Infection related to scratching.

Expected Outcome

- The child will not complain of itching and will express understanding of the danger of scratching healing tissue.

Intervention	Rationale
1. Administer antihistamines as ordered.	1. Itching persists for several months after burns heal, as new nerve endings and dermal elements reestablish themselves. Antihistamines such as diphenhydramine hydrochloride (Benadryl) reduce itching.
2. Apply soothing lotions such as Nivea or Eucerin to healing skin.	2. These lotions reduce dryness, which is a factor contributing to itching.
3. Keep the child's hands clean at all times and the fingernails cut short. Encourage the child not to scratch or rub healing skin.	3. These actions reduce the risk of impairing skin integrity.

Evaluation

- Is the child's skin intact and healing as expected?
- Is itching reduced?

Nursing Diagnosis
■ Body Image Disturbance related to altered appearance of the healing burn.

Expected Outcomes
• The child will reenter previous social settings and express a feeling of comfort in these areas.
• The family will provide emotional support for the child.
• The child will discuss feelings about others' reactions to the change in appearance.

Intervention	Rationale
1. Encourage the child to verbalize feelings about appearance and about returning to school.	1. Identifying the child's concerns and anxieties is the first step in developing effective coping strategies.
2. Provide honest answers to the child's questions regarding appearance.	2. Honesty builds trust and helps the child develop realistic expectations.
3. Encourage the family's involvement in the child's care.	3. Family involvement provides support for the child and decreases the child's feelings of separation from significant others.
4. Encourage the child to provide age-appropriate self-care.	4. Participating in self-care helps increase self-esteem.
5. Identify support systems and coping mechanisms used in previous times of stress or crisis.	5. Strategies that were previously effective can be mobilized to aid the child and family through a stressful period.
6. Engage the assistance of a child life specialist to work with the child to identify feelings.	6. Children can often best express feelings through play and art.
7. Discuss ways in which the child can "cover up" any disfigurement through clothing and makeup.	7. Cosmetics can decrease or minimize the disfigurement.
8. Visit the child's school prior to the child's return.	8. Visiting the school will prepare the child's classmates for the changes in the child's appearance and engage them in making the reentry a positive experience through acceptance.

Evaluation
• Does the child express a desire to reengage social contacts?
• Is the child able to express fears related to the reactions of others?
• Does the family support the child emotionally and encourage the child to express feelings?

PARENTS AND CHILDREN WANT TO KNOW

Measures to Prevent and Initially Manage a Burn

Prevention

1. Have periodic fire drills to teach your children how to evacuate the house in the event of a fire.
2. Place child identification stickers, which can be obtained from most fire departments, on the outside of the bedroom door and in one window of each child's bedroom.
3. Identify two or more exits from each room and a location to meet outside the house. Emphasize to your children that they should not return to the house under any circumstances, even if another family member or pet remains in the house.
4. Be sure your child understands "stop, drop, and roll" as a measure to stop the burning process.
5. Be sure to keep all matches and lighters out of reach. Check electrical cords regularly. Use outlet covers if children under age 5 are in the house.
6. Check smoke detectors regularly and keep them clean. Replace the batteries regularly if they are battery operated.
7. To reduce the number of scald burns, turn the hot water heater thermostat down to 120°F.
8. Turn pot handles in and use back burners on the stove whenever possible.
9. Do not seat a child on your lap while you are drinking a hot liquid.
10. Keep your children away from outdoor grills and indoor wood- or coal-burning stoves. Keep older infants from crawling near floor heating grates.

Initial Emergency Burn Management

1. Apply cool compresses or submerge minor burns in cool water, not ice.
2. To prevent scalding, remove clothing soaked with hot water as quickly as possible.
3. Contact the physician for any child with a burn that has blistered.
4. Cover a child who has a major burn with a clean sheet while waiting for emergency personnel.
5. Do not try to remove clothing that is adhering to burned skin.

Home Care for a Child with Burns

Often it is the parents' responsibility to care for the burn wound at home, supported by daily visits to the office or clinic for debridement and wound assessment.

Parents will need to know the following to adequately care for the child:

- Type of cleaning method used to remove old antimicrobial ointment.
- Where to obtain the topical ointment and dressing supplies.
- How often to visit the office or clinic (the nurse provides the phone number and a list of scheduled appointments).

Teach the parents the following:

- Use principles of aseptic technique. Use sterile gloves and applicators, and know where to obtain these supplies. Know how to put on the gloves; give a return demonstration.
- Give the child medication for pain (if needed) 20 to 30 minutes before doing the dressing change. Enlist other family members to provide distraction or to help hold the child.
- Wash the area with mild soap and tepid water or sterile saline. The old dressing can be soaked in tepid water to loosen it and decrease the discomfort of its removal.
- Apply the prescribed ointment and a light gauze dressing. Cover the area with a tubular net bandage if possible, rather than wrapping with flexible gauze.
- To recognize signs and symptoms of infection, provide adequate fluids, and be sure the child's nutritional needs are met.
- Encourage the child in activities appropriate for age and development.
- Keep follow-up appointments.

Major Burn Injuries and Associated Conditions

For a child with a major burn injury, initial assessment and care focus on the ABCs—establishing and maintaining the child's airway, breathing, and circulation. After an airway and IV access have been established, a catheter is inserted into the bladder to begin hourly urine output measurements, and a nasogastric tube is inserted into the stomach to prevent aspiration.

Burn shock is a hypovolemic condition that develops after burn injury affecting more than 15% to 20% of TBSA in children. Mechanisms of burn shock are not well understood, but the sequence of major burn injury followed by massive capillary leakage of circulating fluid into the surrounding tissues is well recognized.

Within minutes of a major burn injury, all of the capillaries in the circulatory system, not just those in the area of the burn, lose their capillary seal, resulting in leakage of intravascular body fluid into the interstitial spaces. Erythrocytes and leukocytes remain in the circulation and produce an elevated hematocrit and leukocyte count. The process of burn shock continues for approximately 24 to 48 hours, at which time the capillary seal is restored.

Treatment for burn shock is aimed at supporting the patient through the period of hypovolemic shock until capillary integrity is restored. To maintain adequate circulating volume, IV fluids are administered at a rate greater than the rate of fluid loss. Many formulas can be used to calculate the rate of fluid administration. The most common is the Parkland formula for fluid resuscitation. Ringer's lactate is the IV fluid of choice because it most closely approximates the composition of the extracellular fluid being lost.

Because urine output reflects end-organ tissue perfusion, IV fluids are administered at a rate sufficient to maintain the child's urine output at 1 to 2 ml/kg of body weight/hr. Inadequate urine output during burn shock is usually due to insufficient administration of resuscitative fluids. Renal failure is not an expected component of burn shock if an

Parkland Formula for Fluid Resuscitation for Burn Shock

4 ml Ringer's lactate solution
× kg body weight
× % total body surface area (TBSA) burn

One half of total is administered in the first 8 hours post burn
One fourth of total is administered in the second 8 hours post burn
One fourth of total is administered in the third 8 hours post burn

During the first 24 hours post burn, Ringer's lactate solution is administered IV using the formula as a guideline. In addition, provide daily maintenance volume necessary to ensure adequate urinary output. The criterion for successful burn shock fluid resuscitation is based on an hourly urine output of 1 ml/kg/hr in children. Time is calculated from the time of injury, not from the time of admission.

Example: A 10-kg child with a 50% TBSA burn

4 ml × 10 kg × 50% TBSA burn = 2,000 ml
or 2 liters of Ringer's lactate in 24 hours

Administer: 1,000 ml in first 8 hours at 125 ml/hr
500 ml in second 8 hours at 62 ml/hr
500 ml in third 8 hours at 62 ml/hr

In the event that fluid resuscitation is delayed, one half of the amount is still administered in the remaining time. For example, if fluids are not started until 2 hours after the injury, one half of the fluids are administered in the next 6 hours.

From Baxter, C. R. (1974). Fluid volume and electrolyte changes of the early postburn period. *Clinics in Plastic Surgery, 1,* 693–709.

TABLE 49-7
• • • • • • • • • • • • •

Body System Alterations Following Moderate to Severe Burns

System/Alteration	Cause	Management
Respiratory		
Upper airway tissue injury with respiratory distress and possible obstruction	Edema from inhalation of superheated air	Establish adequate airway, provide moist mist with oxygen as needed
Lower airway tissue injury	Inhalation of smoke	Give oxygen as needed, place child in a head-elevated position, intubate with ventilatory support if necessary
Carbon monoxide inhalation and hypoxia	End products of combustion	Give 100% oxygen by mask; intubate and provide ventilatory support if necessary
Limited chest expansion	Circumferential burns	Escharotomy
Cardiovascular		
Fluid volume deficit with decreased cardiac output; tachycardia	Fluid shifts from vascular to interstitial compartment; massive leaking of fluid through the burn wound	Provide fluid and electrolyte replacement with or without colloids; goal is to achieve urinary output of 1–2 ml/kg/hr and good capillary refill
Initial vasodilation, then vasoconstriction	Compensatory mechanism to preserve fluid volume and prevent shock	
Edema, compartment syndrome	Increased fluid in interstitial spaces	
Elevated hemoglobin and hematocrit	Hemoconcentration caused by fluid loss	
Increase followed by decrease in serum potassium	Release of destroyed tissue cells into extracellular space	
Decreased serum sodium	Trapped in edema fluids	
Gastrointestinal		
Gastric dilation and paralytic ileus	Decreased perfusion to GI tract as a result of hypovolemia	Restore fluid and electrolyte balance
Thirst	Hypovolemia	
Renal		
Oliguria, elevated blood urea nitrogen and creatinine values	Reduced circulation to kidneys	Adequate fluid resuscitation
Risk for acute tubular necrosis	Obstruction of renal tubules	
Metabolic		
Increased metabolic rate with elevated body temperature and massive evaporative heat loss	Insult of open wound	Provide caloric requirements 2 to 3 × basal requirements; provide high-protein diet or protein supplements; tube feed or use parenteral nutrition as necessary; provide vitamin C and vitamin A supplements
Catecholamine release	Burn stress; increased temperature and metabolic rate	
Hyperglycemia	Mobilization of glucagon and decreased insulin production	
Hematologic		
Decreased hematocrit follows initial hematocrit increase (from hemoconcentration)	Increased red blood cell (RBC) hemolysis, decreased RBC production, blood loss from wound care	Packed red blood cell transfusion for low hematocrit
Coagulation disorders	Decreased platelet count and serum clotting factors	
Increased immature neutrophils to digest products of injury	Depletion of mature neutrophils	
High risk for infection, wound sepsis, and septic shock (disorientation, fever, diminished bowel sounds are first signs, temperature falls below normal as body resistance to infection decreases)	Open wound; altered protective mechanisms; decreased circulation to the skin	Burn excision and debridement followed by application of topical antimicrobial agents; may need biologic or synthetic skin coverings, graft
Pain		
	Tissue injury exposing nerve endings; edema; burn treatments	Meticulous pain management both round-the-clock and prior to treatments

adequate volume of IV fluids is being administered for burn shock resuscitation. It should be recognized that the Parkland formula and other burn shock fluid resuscitation formulas are guidelines; individual children may need more than 4 ml/kg/% TBSA burn during the first 24 hours after the burn.

Table 49–7 lists additional physiologic effects caused by moderate to major burns. Once a child with a moderate or major burn has been stabilized, the child usually is transferred to a burn center for specialized care.

Electrical Injury and Associated Conditions

Electrical injury is a major injury that often results in instant death, as the electrical current disrupts the electrical rhythm of the heart. The child who does not die instantly is at risk for four major complications during the acute phase:

- Cardiac arrest or arrhythmia
- Tissue damage
- Myoglobinuria (globulin from muscle serum)
- Metabolic acidosis

CARDIAC ARREST OR ARRHYTHMIA

The immediate risk is cardiac arrest or arrhythmia secondary to damage to the heart's electrical conduction system. If cardiac arrest occurs, standard cardiac life support measures are initiated (see Chapter 34).

TISSUE DAMAGE

The electrical current follows the path of least resistance through the body. Entering through the skin, electricity causes heat damage to the skin layers, bone, nerves, tendons, and blood vessels. The heat of the electrical current coagulates blood vessels and leaves the affected area without blood supply. Gangrene develops in necrotic tissue unless it is removed. Amputation is necessary in more than 90% of children sustaining electrical injuries. The location of the damage depends on the child's position and exposure. Electricity may enter one hand and exit from the other, for example, or it may travel through the body and exit from one or both legs. The greatest damage occurs at the entrance and exit sites.

MYOGLOBINURIA

Myoglobinuria develops from release into the blood of products found in normal muscle; the release can be occasioned by electrical injury. Myoglobin is a large molecule that can mechanically obstruct the renal tubules and lead to acute tubular necrosis unless large amounts of IV fluid are administered to flush the myoglobin out of the kidney. Osmotic diuretics may be administered to promote increased urine volume. IV fluid is administered at a rate that maintains urine output at 2 ml/kg/hr until the myoglobinuria resolves.

METABOLIC ACIDOSIS

Metabolic acidosis follows electrical injury because of the associated cellular destruction and hypovolemic shock. Ringer's lactate, the fluid used for fluid resuscitation, contains sufficient bicarbonate to manage the acidosis that accompanies burn shock, but not enough to correct that associated with shock following electrical injury (i.e., pathophysiologic hypovolemic shock, not a "shock" from the electrical current).

OTHER COMPLICATIONS

The four complications just described usually resolve within 24 hours after injury. Other complications that follow electrical injury include loss of short-term memory and altered emotional states. The child can usually remember events up to the time of injury, including the names of family members, and his or her address, telephone number, and personal information, but is unable to recall more recent events. This loss of memory can be distressing to the child and frustrating to the family. For example, the child may be unable to remember visits by the family and so may feel abandoned by them. It is difficult for the child to follow instructions because of the inability to retain instructions, and this may lead to difficulty in planning care. Altered emotional states may include an absence of affect and blank stares, or the opposite type of emotional response—manic behavior, hyperactivity, swearing, physical violence, and feelings of paranoia. Emotional responses usually become normal after about a week but may persist longer in some children. The electrical injury need not be to the head for these altered states to occur.

The long-term sequelae of electrical injury include gait pattern instability and ocular cataracts. In addition to adaptation to any amputations, neurologic deficits may lead to gait pattern instability and alterations in depth perception and other spatial orientation. Ocular cataracts may occur in one or both eyes at varying times from 3 months to 18 months of injury. In the very young child, changes in visual acuity may not be noticed; therefore, regular eye examinations should be scheduled every 3 months for the first year.

■ KEY CONCEPTS
. . . .

- The functions of the skin include protection, thermoregulation, excretion, production of vitamin D, and sensation.
- The skin comprises two layers, the outer epidermis and the inner supportive dermis. The dermis contains blood vessels, nerves, and sweat glands. Beneath these layers is subcutaneous tissue, which attaches the dermis to the underlying structures.
- Developmental differences cause the skin of infants and children to be more susceptible to external irritants and infection than adults' skin.
- Impetigo, the most common skin infection of childhood, is highly contagious. Nursing care includes administration of topical or oral antibiotics and education regarding good hand washing and careful hygiene to prevent spread of infection.
- Because the fungus that causes tinea thrives where it is moist and warm, infected areas should be

kept as dry as possible. Proper hygiene should be taught and maintained to minimize the spread of infection.

■ Herpes simplex virus is transmitted by infected body fluids coming in contact with breaks in the skin or mucous membranes. Careful hand washing and attention to hygiene decrease the risk of spreading infection.

■ Preventing reinfestation is a primary goal in the treatment of pediculosis.

■ Nursing care for the child with eczema includes frequent skin moisturizing and cautioning against the use of clothing, fabrics, or soaps that might irritate the skin. Identifying and eliminating allergens may be helpful.

■ Diaper dermatitis is much easier to prevent than to treat. Successful treatment and prevention of diaper rash entail thorough cleansing of the diaper area and keeping the skin dry.

■ Nursing care of the adolescent with acne includes teaching about regular, gentle cleansing of the skin, applying topical medications, and encouraging a healthy lifestyle with adequate rest, exercise, and a balanced diet. The nurse must be sensitive to the effect of acne on the adolescent's self-image.

■ Insect bites and stings can cause severe systemic reactions in a sensitized child.

■ Young children are at increased risk for burn injuries because they are curious, mobile, and totally dependent on their caretakers for safety.

■ The extent of a burn injury (depth and severity) determines whether the child will experience a local or a systemic reaction.

■ The depth of a burn injury is classified as superficial (first degree), partial thickness (second degree), or full thickness (third degree).

■ In comparison with adults, children who sustain burn injuries are at increased risk for fluid and heat loss, hypertrophic scarring, cardiovascular problems, infection, and protein and calorie deficiency.

■ In calculating the total body surface area burned, a body surface chart that is corrected for age should be used.

■ A minor burn wound should be cleaned with mild soap and water, debrided of loose debris and tissue, and covered with an antimicrobial ointment and a sterile dressing.

■ After stabilization, a child with a major burn is cared for in a burn treatment center because of multiple body system complications.

ANSWER TO CRITICAL THINKING EXERCISE 49–1

1. The nurse should first ask the mother what symptoms, if any, the child is experiencing. If the child is symptomatic with pruritus and visible nits or lice, treatment failure is a possibility. The nurse needs to ask what pediculocide was used, whether nits were fully combed out, whether family members were treated, and what environmental measures were taken to prevent reinfestation in the home. If the parent has followed the instructions meticulously, the nurse needs to explore other areas. Because of the child's age, the nurse needs to question whether the mother has treated her daughter's dress-up clothes and hair ornaments as well as the usual bedding, clothing, combs, brushes, and furniture. If it appears the management has been thorough, the child may have developed pediculocide-resistant lice and will need a slightly different approach.

2. If the child is not symptomatic, the school official may be seeing dead nits in the child's hair. The nurse needs to ask the mother about the treatment used and whether all the nits were removed. Removing nits is especially difficult in preschool children because it is time-consuming, and these young children find sitting still that long difficult. Also, many preschool girls have long hair, which can prolong the process. The nurse should advise the mother to remove all the nits and check her child regularly to be sure they are all gone. The nurse can give the mother suggestions about the most effective method of nit removal and encourage the mother to be persistent. Positive reassurance and encouragement are most important.

REFERENCES AND READINGS

Abdullah, A., Blakeny, P., Hunt, R., Broemeling, L., Phillips, L., Herndon, D., & Robson, M. (1994). Visible scars and self-esteem in pediatric patients with burns. *Journal of Burn Care and Rehabilitation, 15*(2),164–168.

Adinoff, A., & Clark, R. (1996). Atopic dermatitis. In C. W. Bierman, D. Pearlman, G. Shapiro, & W. Busse (Eds.), *Allergy, asthma, and immunology from infancy to adulthood* (pp. 613–632). Philadelphia: Saunders.

Barber, N. (1996). Dermatological diseases. In C. Burns, N. Barber, M. Brady, & A. Dunn (Eds.), *Pediatric primary care: A hand-book for nurse practitioners* (pp. 737–769). Philadelphia: Saunders.

Brady, M. (1996). Atopic disorders and rheumatic diseases. In C. Burns, N. Barber, M. Brady, & A. Dunn (Eds.), *Pediatric primary care: A handbook for nurse practitioners* (pp. 491–512). Philadelphia: Saunders.

Brady, M., & Dunn, A. (1996). Common injuries and poisonings. In C. Burns, N. Barber, M. Brady, & A. Dunn (Eds.), *Pediatric primary care: A handbook for nurse practitioners* (pp. 831–854). Philadelphia: Saunders.

Brainerd, E. (1998). From eradication to resistance: Five continuing concerns about pediculosis. *Journal of School Health, 68*(4), 146–150.

Carrougher, G. J. (1993). Inhalation injury. *AACN Clinical Issues in Critical Care Nursing, 4,* 367–377.

Centers for Disease Control and Prevention (1997). Recommended framework for presenting injury mortality data. *Morbidity and Mortality Weekly Report, 46*(RR-14), 11.

Childs, N. (1998). Spider bites: What to look for this summer. *Pediatric News, 32*(5), 29.

Clark, K., et al. (1997). Burn abuse. *Pediatric Emergency Care, 13*(4), 259–261.

Cohen, B. (1997). Warts and children: Can they be separated? *Contemporary Pediatrics*, 14(2), 128–149.

Cooley, S., Atkinson, P., Parks, D., & Hebert, A. (1998). Management of acne vulgaris. *Journal of Pediatric Health Care*, 12(1), 38–40.

Dickerson, P., Gordon, M., & Walter, P. (1998). Burns. In M. Slota (Ed.), *Core curriculum for pediatric critical care nursing* (pp. 652–675). Philadelphia: Saunders.

Drolet, B., & Esterly, N. (1999). Atopic dermatitis. In F. Burg, E. Wald, J. Ingelfinger, & R. Polin (Eds.), *Gellis & Kagan's current pediatric therapy* (16th ed., pp. 954–955). Philadelphia: Saunders.

Eigenmann, P., Sicherer, S., Borkowski, T., Cohen, B., & Sampson, H. (1998). Prevalence of IgE-mediated food allergy among children with atopic dermatitis. *Pediatrics*, 101(3), e8.

Engelhardt, V., & Clark, S. (1994). Early enteral feeding of a severely burned pediatric patient. *Journal of Burn Care and Rehabilitation*, 15(3), 293–297.

Estrada, B. (1998). Head lice: What about Ivermectin? *Infections in Medicine*, 15(12), 823.

Faldmo, L., & Kravitz, M. (1993). Management of acute burns and burn shock resuscitation. *AACN Clinical Issues in Critical Care Nursing*, 4, 351–366.

Fallat, M. E., & Rengers, S. J. (1993). The effect of education and safety devices on scald burn prevention. *The Journal of Trauma*, 34(4), 560–563.

Gallas, S., & Levy, M. (1998). Viral and fungal skin infections. In R. Feigin & J. Cherry (Eds.), *Textbook of pediatric infectious diseases* (4th ed., Vol. 1, pp. 753–785). Philadelphia: Saunders.

Golden, D. (1996). Allergic reactions to insect stings. In C. W. Bierman, D. Pearlman, G. Shapiro, & W. Busse (Eds.), *Allergy, asthma, and immunology from infancy to adulthood* (pp. 348–354). Philadelphia: Saunders.

Helvig, E. (1993). Pediatric burn injuries. *AACN Clinical Issues in Critical Care Nursing*, 4, 433–442.

Herndon, D., Rutan, R., & Rutan, T. (1993). Management of the pediatric patient with burns. *Journal of Burn Care and Rehabilitation*, 14(1), 38.

Herrin, J. T., & Antoon, A. Y. (1996). Burn injuries. In R. Behrman, R. Kliegman, & A. Arvin (Eds.), *Nelson textbook of pediatrics* (15th ed., pp. 270–277). Philadelphia: Saunders.

Hurwitz, S. (1993). *Clinical pediatric dermatology* (p. 68). Philadelphia: Saunders.

Kravitz, M. (1993). Immune consequences of burn injury. *AACN Clinical Issues in Critical Care Nursing*, 4, 399–413.

Kravitz, M. (Ed.). (1993). Burn care. *AACN Clinical Issues in Critical Care Nursing*, 4, 349–442.

Kronemeyer, B. (1997). Lice more resistant than ever before. *Infectious Diseases in Children*, 10(7), 26.

Kumar, V. (1999). Burns in childhood. In F. Burg, E. Wald, J. Ingelfinger, & R. Polin (Eds.), *Gellis and Kagan's current pediatric therapy* (16th ed., pp. 1171–1172). Philadelphia: Saunders.

Landow, K. (1997). Dispelling myths about acne. *Postgraduate Medicine*, 102(2), 94–111.

Lewis, A. M. (1999). Managing common pediatric emergencies. *Nursing 99*, 29(1). On line: www.springnet.com/content/nursing/9901.

Mayes, T., Gottschlich, M., Khoury, J., & Warden, G. (1996). Evaluation of predicted and measured energy requirements in burned children. *Journal of the American Dietetic Association*, 96(1), 24–29.

McCain, D., & Sutherland, S. (1998). Nursing essentials: Skin grafts for patients with burns. *American Journal of Nursing*, 98(7), 34–38.

Melish, M., & Bertuch, A. (1998). Bacterial skin infections. In R. Feigin & J. Cherry (Eds.), *Textbook of pediatric infectious disease* (4th ed., Vol. 1, pp. 741–752). Philadelphia: Saunders.

Meyer, W., Blakeney, P., Moore, P., Murphy, L., Robson, M., & Herndon, D. (1994). Parental well-being and behavioral adjustment of pediatric survivors of burns. *Journal of Burn Care and Rehabilitation*, 15(1), 62–68.

Miller, S., Richard, R., & Staley, M. (1994). Triage and resuscitation of the burn patient. In R. Richard & M. Staley (Eds.), *Burn care and rehabilitation: Principles and practice* (pp. 105–118). Philadelphia: Davis.

Molter, N. (1993). When is burn injury healed? Psychosocial implications of care. *AACN Clinical Issues in Critical Care Nursing*, 4, 424–432.

Moskowitz, H., & Meissner, C. (1997). Tickborne diseases: Warm weather worry. *Contemporary Pediatrics*, 14(8), 33–49.

Nagel, T., & Schunk, J. (1997). Using the hand to estimate the surface area of a burn in children. *Pediatric Emergency Care*, 13(4), 254–255.

O'Brien, E. (1998). Detection and removal of head lice with an electronic comb: Zapping the louse! *Journal of Pediatric Nursing*, 13(4), 265–266.

Ou, L., Lee, S., Chen, Y., Yang, R., & Tang, Y. (1998). Use of Biobrane in pediatric scald burns: Experience in 106 children. *Burns*, 24(1), 49–53.

Peters, S. (1997). Treating dermatitis in children: The role of topical corticosteroids. *Advances for Nurse Practitioners*, 5(2), 50–51.

Peterson, K. (1998). Erythema multiforme, Stevens-Johnson syndrome, and toxic epidermal necrolysis. *Pediatric Pharmacotherapy* [On-line], 4(11). Available: www.medscape.com/UVA/PedPharm/1998/v04.n11/pp0411.01.pete/pp0411.01.pete-01.html.

Prose, N., & Antaya, R. (1998). Damaging effects of solar radiation. In L. Finberg (Ed.), *Saunders manual of pediatric practice*. Philadelphia: Saunders.

Reeves, S., Warden, G., & Staley, M. (1994). Management of the pediatric burn patient. In R. Richard & M. Staley (Eds.), *Burn care and rehabilitation: Principles and practice* (pp. 499–530). Philadelphia: Davis.

Reynolds, E. M., Ryan, D. P., & Doody, D. P. (1993). Mortality and respiratory failure in a pediatric burn population. *Journal of Pediatric Surgery*, 28(10), 1326–1331.

Rieg, L. S. (1993). Metabolic alterations and nutritional management. *AACN Clinical Issues in Critical Care Nursing*, 4, 388–398.

Sadow, K., & Chamberlain, J. (1998). Blood cultures in the evaluation of children with cellulitis. *Pediatrics*, 101(3), e4.

Saffle, J., & Schnebly, W. A. (1994). Burn wound care. In R. Richard & M. Staley (Eds.), *Burn care and rehabilitation: Principles and practice*. Philadelphia: Davis.

Schmitt, B. D. (1999). *Instructions for pediatric patients*. Philadelphia: Saunders.

Scholer, S., Hickson, G., Mitchel, E., & Ray, W. (1998). Predictors of mortality from fires in young children. *Pediatrics*, 101(5), E12.

Stephenson, M. (1997). When treating lice, don't forget to remove nits. *Infectious Diseases in Children*, 10(7), 32–33.

Uitvlugt, N., & Ledbetter, D. (1995). Treatment of pediatric burns. In R. Arensman (Ed.), *Pediatric trauma* (pp. 173–199). New York: Raven Press.

Urbach, A. (1999). Pediculosis. In F. Burg, E. Wald, J. Ingelfinger, & R. Polin (Eds.), *Gellis & Kagan's current pediatric therapy* (16th ed., pp. 976–977). Philadelphia: Saunders.

Vernon, P. (1997). The heartbreak of psoriasis: No laughing matter. *Journal of Pediatric Health Care*, 11(1), 32–33.

Weber, J. M., & Tompkins, D. M. (1993). Improving survival: Infection control and burns. *AACN Clinical Issues in Critical Care Nursing*, 4, 414–423.

50

The Child with a Musculoskeletal Alteration

LEARNING OBJECTIVES

After studying this chapter, you should be able to:

- Demonstrate an understanding of the anatomy and physiology of an infant or young child's musculoskeletal system.
- Describe the pathology, etiology, manifestations, diagnostic evaluation, and therapeutic management of common pediatric musculoskeletal alterations.
- Select relevant criteria to determine the etiology and diagnosis of common pediatric musculoskeletal alterations.
- State appropriate nursing diagnoses for the child with alterations in musculoskeletal function.
- Identify characteristic behaviors that indicate alterations in musculoskeletal functioning.
- Summarize the treatment modalities used to manage the child with musculoskeletal alterations.
- Design, implement, and evaluate appropriate nursing interventions for the child with altered musculoskeletal functioning.

DEFINITIONS

abduction Movement away from the midline.

acetabulum The hip socket in the pelvis.

adduction Movement toward the midline.

ankylosis Condition in which a joint is stiff or difficult to move.

anomaly Abnormality.

autologous blood transfusion Transfusion of one's own, previously harvested blood.

avascular necrosis Tissue damage secondary to inadequate blood supply.

crepitus A grating sensation at a fracture site that occurs when the ends of a broken bone move.

dislocation Displacement of a bone from its normal articulation within a joint.

dysplasia Abnormal development.

external fixation Placement of pins, screws, or bars through bone and soft tissue to immobilize or correct a deformity.

internal instrumentation Placement of instruments inside the body to immobilize parts.

inversion A turning toward the midline.

orthoses Braces, external supports, or artificial limbs made by a specialist to meet individual needs.

ossification Formation of bone from osseous tissue or cartilage.

osteoblastic Activity by osteoblasts that promotes bone formation.

osteochondrosis Disorders of the epiphyses in which there is an interruption of the blood supply.

osteoclastic Activity by osteoclasts that absorbs and removes old bony tissue.

osteotomy Surgical cutting of bone.

paresthesia Sensation of numbness and tingling.

Pavlik harness A device that holds an infant's hips in flexion and external rotation.

plantar flexion Bending toward the sole of the foot.

polydactyly Extra fingers or toes.

pseudarthrosis Failure of the bones to fuse.

reduction Repositioning of bone fragments into normal alignment. Application of a device or mechanism that will maintain alignment of bone until healing occurs.

spica cast Cast used to immobilize the hips; extends from above the waist to the knees or ankles.

subluxation Partial dislocation of a joint.

superior mesenteric artery syndrome A condition resembling intestinal obstruction caused by reduced blood supply to a segment of the mesentery.

syndactyly Fusion or webbing of two or more fingers or toes.

valgum Abnormal position of a limb that involves bending away from the midline of the body. Genu valgum results in knock-knees.

varum Abnormal position of the limb that involves bending toward the midline of the body. Genu varum results in bowlegs.

Review of the Musculoskeletal System

Bones, joints, muscles, and cartilaginous tissues make up the musculoskeletal system. To understand alterations in musculoskeletal function it is first necessary to understand normal musculoskeletal structure and function, as well as patterns of growth and development.

Skeletal System

The bony skeleton provides a surface for the attachment of muscles, tendons, and ligaments. The pulling action on individual bones makes it possible for us to move. The human skeletal system consists of 206 bones, which are classified as long bones (e.g., humerus, radius), short bones (e.g., carpals, tarsals), flat bones (e.g., ribs), irreg-

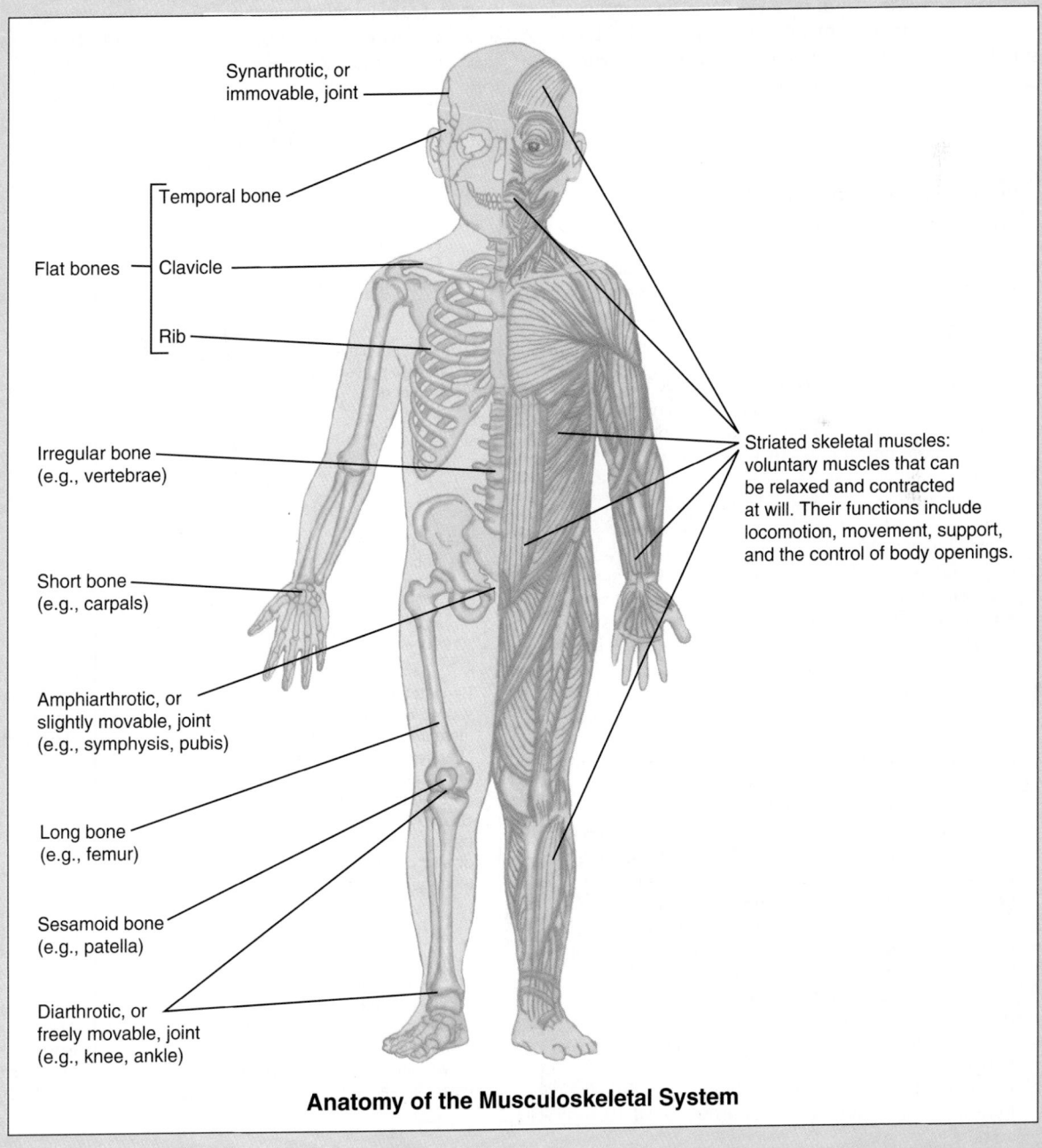

Anatomy of the Musculoskeletal System

ular bones (e.g., vertebrae), and sesamoid bones (e.g., kneecap).

Each long bone consists of a diaphysis (shaft) with an epiphysis (secondary ossification center) at each end. The muscles attach here and are responsible for joint stability. The metaphysis, or wide portion of the bone, is responsible for growth. The metaphysis consists of cartilage and actively produces bone. Periosteum, a vascular connective tissue, covers the bone. The medullary cavity is located in the center of the diaphysis.

Articular System

The joints, which are composed of connective tissue and cartilage, connect bones to one another and enable great freedom of movement. Joints are classified by their degree of movement: synarthrotic, or immovable (e.g., the skull), amphiarthrotic, or slightly movable (e.g., the symphysis), and diarthrotic, or freely movable (e.g., the knee). Muscles help stabilize joints and maintain contact between articular surfaces. The shape of the two ends of each muscle and of

the joint determine the extent of movement or articulation. Ligaments bind one bone firmly to another, and the joints are further stabilized by the overlying tendons and muscles.

Muscular System

Muscle, which is composed of elongated fibers, produces movement by contraction. The three types of muscle are smooth muscle, found primarily in the internal organs; striated muscle or skeletal muscle, so called because of its striped appearance under the microscope; and cardiac, or heart, muscle.

Cartilage

Cartilage is dense connective tissue that develops at the epiphysis and is capable of withstanding considerable tension. The skeleton of an embryo is mostly cartilage. In time it will largely convert to bone by ossification. Bone is necessary for longitudinal growth. Growth in the length of the long bones continues at the epiphysis until adult height is reached. The epiphyseal plate absorbs shock, protecting the joint surfaces from serious fractures.

Pediatric Differences in the Musculoskeletal System

- Muscle tissue is almost completely developed at birth. Growth occurs because of an increase in size rather than number of the muscle fibers.
- In the fetus, bony tissue begins to develop as closely packed connective tissue. Connective tissue is replaced by cartilage, and cartilage is replaced by mineral salts, which give rise to solid bone. The infant's bones are only 65% ossified at 8 months of age and are neither as firm nor as brittle as those of the older child.
- New bony tissue is produced during periods of growth. The rate of growth varies at different ages. Skeletal growth is stimulated by pituitary growth hormone. Growth of the long bones occurs at the epiphyses, which are located at the ends of the bones and separated from the main portion of the bone by cartilage during the period of growth. Injury to the epiphyses can cause growth disturbances.
- Growing bones produce callus and heal quickly, making internal fixation of fractures unnecessary in most children. Fractures in children less than 1 year old are unusual because a large amount of force is necessary; abuse or underlying pathophysiology is often the cause of fractures in infants.
- The skull is not rigid during infancy, and the sutures of the cranium do not fuse completely until approximately 16 to 18 months of age. Increased intracranial pressure can separate the sutures, causing the infant's head to enlarge.
- Postural changes during infancy and childhood result from the development of neurologic control, bone and muscle growth, and the laying down of adipose tissue. Postural changes are a good indication of the level of development of the musculoskeletal and neurologic systems.
- Because soft tissues are resilient in children, dislocations and sprains are less common than in adults.

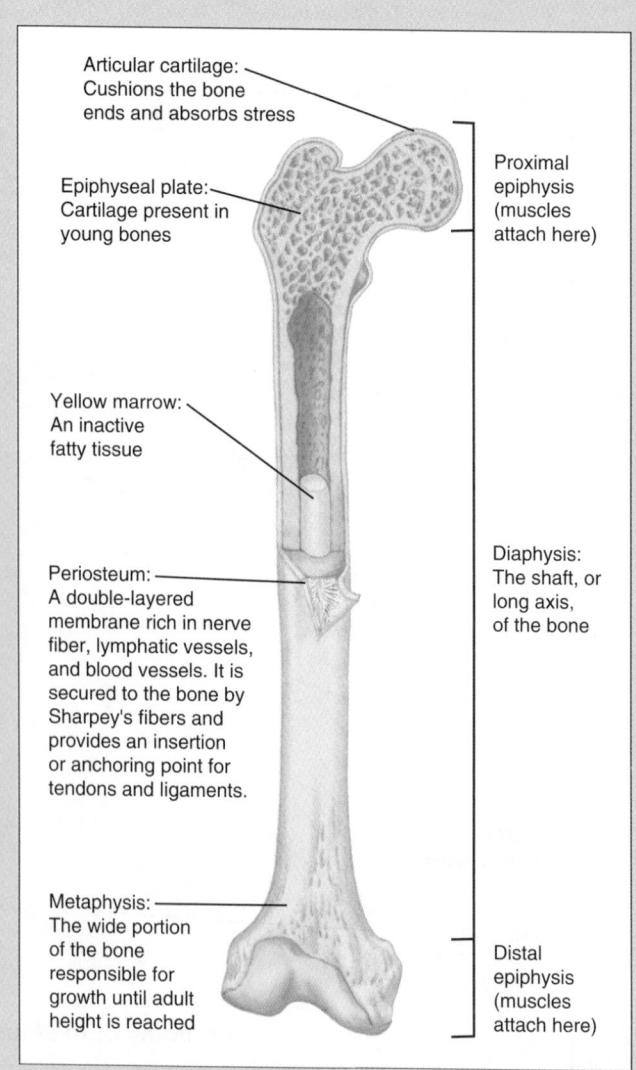

Articular cartilage: Cushions the bone ends and absorbs stress

Epiphyseal plate: Cartilage present in young bones

Yellow marrow: An inactive fatty tissue

Periosteum: A double-layered membrane rich in nerve fiber, lymphatic vessels, and blood vessels. It is secured to the bone by Sharpey's fibers and provides an insertion or anchoring point for tendons and ligaments.

Metaphysis: The wide portion of the bone responsible for growth until adult height is reached

Proximal epiphysis (muscles attach here)

Diaphysis: The shaft, or long axis, of the bone

Distal epiphysis (muscles attach here)

• • • • • • • • • •

Common Diagnostic and Laboratory Tests and Procedures for Musculoskeletal Disorders in Children

Test	Purpose/Description	Nursing Implications

Radiography (x-ray)	For detection of abnormalities or to determine bone age. X-rays (gamma radiation) pass through the body, reach the film on the other side of the body, and turn the film black. Areas filled with air appear dark on the film. Different densities of tissue absorb various amounts of radiation. The four densities of x-ray are:
	  air: blackish
	  fat: dark gray
	  water: lighter gray
	  bone: whitish
		Food and fluids are not usually restricted. Clothing and jewelry should be removed; a paper or cloth gown is worn. Young children may require immobilization. Adequate preparation is essential to ensure cooperation.

Arthrography	To evaluate suspected joint damage such as tears of cartilage. Dye is injected into the joint, usually the knee, sometimes the shoulder or other joint.	Performed under local anesthesia. Check for allergies to iodine. May have mild to moderate discomfort after the procedure. Joint should rest for about 12 hours; compression dressing may be applied after procedure to reduce swelling.
Radionuclide scintigraphy (bone scan)	To detect tumors, infection, inflammation. Radioactive material given IV. In 2 to 4 hours the entire body is scanned, front, and back.	Young children need sedation. Encourage fluids 2 to 4 hours before the test to ensure the child is well hydrated and to quickly eliminate radioactive material not absorbed by the bones. Child must void before the scan so that the pelvic bones can be seen.
Computed tomography (CT)	To visualize anatomic details. Narrow-beam x-rays are used to scan an area in successive layers. A computer processes readings and converts them to a picture shown on a screen, which is stored on disks. A three-dimensional cross section of body parts is shown.	Although the procedure is painless, it may be frightening. Child must remain still during procedure, so young children need sedation. Contrast medium may or may not be used. Tell the child the machine looks and sounds like a clothes dryer or washing machine.
Magnetic resonance imaging (MRI)	Clearly defines organ structures; shows changes in tissue such as edema, blood flow patterns, or infarcts. Demonstrates marrow, bone and soft tissue tumors, structure of muscles, ligaments, and bones. Huge magnet and radio waves create an energy field that can be translated into a visual image. Child is placed on a moving stretcher, which is pushed into the large cylinder that contains the magnet. A variety of noises will be heard during the procedure.	Food and fluids are not restricted. Study is not done in patients with metal implants, pacemakers, or prostheses. Procedure may take an hour or more, so young children need sedation. Child should void before procedure. Adequate preparation, relaxation techniques, and parental presence decrease fear and feelings of claustrophobia.
Arthroscopy	To image the inside of a joint for diagnosis of injury or minor surgical repairs. Normally, arthrography is performed before arthroscopy. Fiberoptic endoscope is inserted to examine interior of joint.	Requires local or general anesthesia. Child must be NPO for 8 hours before the test if general anesthesia is used; NPO recommendations for local anesthesia vary with the practitioner. Prepare child for postoperative dressings, altered mobility, pain. Assess for infection. Prophylactic antibiotics may be ordered. Use ice bags postoperatively to reduce swelling.
Joint aspiration	Fluid is withdrawn for analysis, usually for detection of infection or to relieve pain.	Requires local anesthesia. Prepare patient for some discomfort during and after procedure.

Common Diagnostic and Laboratory Tests and Procedures for Musculoskeletal Disorders in Children
Continued

Test	Purpose/Description	Nursing Implications
Ultrasound	To demonstrate body tissue structure or for wave-form analysis of Doppler studies. Doppler probe is held over the skin surface or in a body cavity to produce an ultrasound beam in the tissues. Echoes reflected from the tissues are transformed by computer into a visual image or audible sounds (Doppler).	Noninvasive; food and fluid are not restricted, except in small infants, who may be NPO for 2 to 3 hours before the procedure so they can eat during the test.
Alkaline phosphatase (ALP) assay	ALP is an enzyme found mainly in liver, bone, placenta, and kidney; levels may be elevated in bone disease, fractures, trauma, or liver disease, and may also be elevated during periods of rapid growth. Determinations may be ordered to differentiate between bone and liver problems.	Nonfasting
Creatine kinase (CK) assay	CK is an enzyme found in heart and skeletal muscle, and the CK assay is a specific test for cardiac and muscle damage. Levels are elevated in trauma, myocardial infarction, muscular dystrophy. Determinations may be ordered to differentiate between cardiac (MB) and skeletal (MM) CK.	Nonfasting
Rheumatoid factor (RA) assay	RA is a macroglobulin antibody that may be responsible for the destructive changes associated with RA. A positive assay for RA factor supports the possible diagnosis of JA.	Nonfasting
C-reactive protein (CRP) assay	CRP appears in blood due to an inflammatory process. It is not seen in healthy people. The assay is nonspecific, merely indicating the presence of inflammation.	Nonfasting
Erythrocyte sedimenation rate (ESR)	ESR is the rate at which erythrocytes settle out of unclotted blood. Inflammation and necrotic problems cause an elevation in ESR levels.	Nonfasting

usculoskeletal problems affect muscles, bones, joints, and tendons, all of which are necessary for movement and therefore are critical to a child's development. Many musculoskeletal problems occur because of vigorous motor activities that are part of a child's daily life, but the rapid growth of the skeletal system plays a significant role as well. Most musculoskeletal problems are short term, but a number of chronic musculoskeletal conditions require long-term treatment and nursing assistance.

Casts and Traction

Casts or traction are applied to immobilize a bone or joint, thereby achieving a more functional position or to rest the area during bone healing. Because many musculoskeletal problems require the application of traction or a cast, the nurse needs to understand general principles of care.

Casts

A cast provides support and maintains anatomic position for bone healing or correction of a deformity. Casts may also be used to ensure compliance with treatment protocols. Materials most frequently used for casting are plaster of paris or synthetic materials, such as fiberglass. Plaster of paris is a heavier material that molds easily to the extremity and is less expensive than synthetic materials. It also takes 24 hours or more to dry. Plaster of paris is not water resistant; when wet, a cast made of plaster of paris will begin to disintegrate.

Synthetic casts are more expensive, but they dry quickly and are lighter and water resistant (Fig. 50–1). They also come in varied colors and patterns that appeal to young children. Should a synthetic cast become wet, inadequate air flow under the cast prevents thorough drying of the skin, and damp skin is more susceptible to skin breakdown. Also, synthetic casts do not mold well to the body and are not recommended for young children or those with serious fractures.

Most casts are applied on an outpatient basis. The size of the cast is determined by the type of fracture and the amount of weight bearing the extremity can tolerate. Short or long leg or arm casts are generally used for fractures of the upper and lower limbs. Fractures of the hip and knee may require a body or spica cast.

Equipment needed for cast application includes

- Tubular gauze (stockinette)
- Casting material (rolls or strips)
- Water

The tubular gauze is placed over the extremity to be casted and the limb is held in the appropriate position. After soaking the casting material in water, the physician applies the strips over the gauze, bringing the end of the gauze over the end of the casting material to provide a smooth edge. A chemical reaction between the casting material and the water will cause a feeling of warmth as the cast is applied.

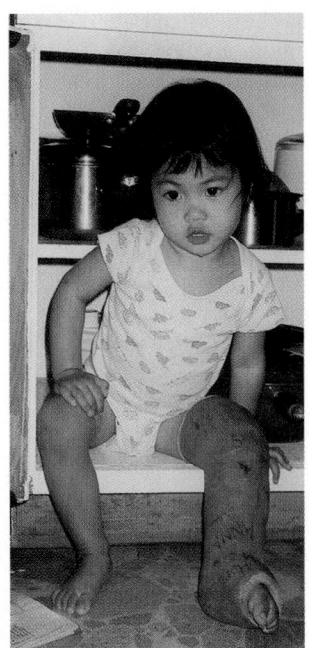

FIGURE 50–1
. . . .
Child in a synthetic cast.

Traction

Effective immobilization may also be achieved through the use of traction. Traction is a pull or force exerted on one part of the body; in treatment, traction may be applied to the spine, pelvis, or long bones of the upper and lower extremities. The angle formed by the placement of the pulley on the bed frame and the angle of the involved joint determine the direction of the pull or force.

Once the direction of the pull or force has been determined, it is important to direct the traction along the long axis of the bone. Traction can be applied to the skin or the bone. Some traction, such as halo femoral traction used for spinal problems, exerts a force without the use of weights.

An opposing pull or force (countertraction) must be provided at the same time if the traction is to be effective. Countertraction results in a two-way pull that maintains alignment of the affected extremity. The child's weight is usually sufficient to provide the countertraction. If body weight is not sufficient, additional weights may be used. Depending on the age of the child, restraining devices may be needed to maintain countertraction.

The part of the bed that holds the traction apparatus is tilted or elevated, thereby assisting with countertraction. For example, if the leg were being placed in traction, the foot of the bed would be elevated. Otherwise the child would slide in the direction of the traction, disrupting the alignment of the extremity and reducing the effectiveness of treatment. Also, the mattress should be firm and a bed board or footplate may be necessary to prevent flexion.

The disadvantages of traction include the need for hospitalization and prolonged immobility. Currently, the use of traction for some musculoskeletal conditions is being replaced by early casting and percutaneous pinning.

Traction may be described as either continuous or intermittent. Continuous traction exerts a constant pull and is used for fractures and dislocations. Intermittent traction provides a periodic pull or force and is used for contractures, low back pain, or muscle spasm. *The nurse should always assume that traction is continuous unless the physician states otherwise.* The removal of traction that was intended to be continuous could prove harmful to the child and result in poor healing. The nursing care plan should always reflect the frequency and amount of time intermittent traction may be removed. When removing the traction apparatus, the nurse must use the hands to maintain manual traction and pull on the body part.

Traction may also be described as running or balanced. Running, or straight, traction exerts a pull on the affected part without balanced support from a sling or splint. The child's weight provides the countertraction. Balanced, or suspension, traction also exerts a pull on the affected part but the extremity is supported by a sling or splint. Countertraction is provided through the use of weights and pulleys attached to the sling or splint. When balanced traction is applied, the pull remains constant, even when the child moves. The countertraction offsets any movement and results in fewer problems with immobility. Both balanced and running traction may be applied to either the skin or bone.

Types of Skin Traction

BUCK EXTENSION

Purpose: Used to treat some fractures, hip disorders, contractures, and muscle spasms.
Description: Continuous or intermittent boot or circular wrap is applied to the skin. Traction is applied to boot or wrap. Rolled towels are placed on the external surface of the knee to prevent external rotation of the affected leg. Countertraction is provided by elevating the foot of the bed.

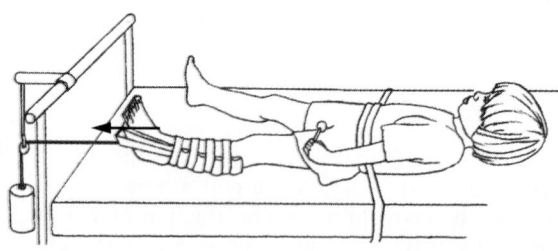

BRYANT TRACTION

Purpose: Used to treat congenital hip dysplasia and fractured femurs in children younger than 2 to 3 years; it is not being used as frequently because of the increased risk of circulatory compromise.
Description: Intermittent traction. Child is supine with legs flexed slightly less than 90 degrees, thus relaxing the hamstrings. Spreader bar or footplate is used to keep traction straps away from the ankles. The sacrum should be off the mattress.

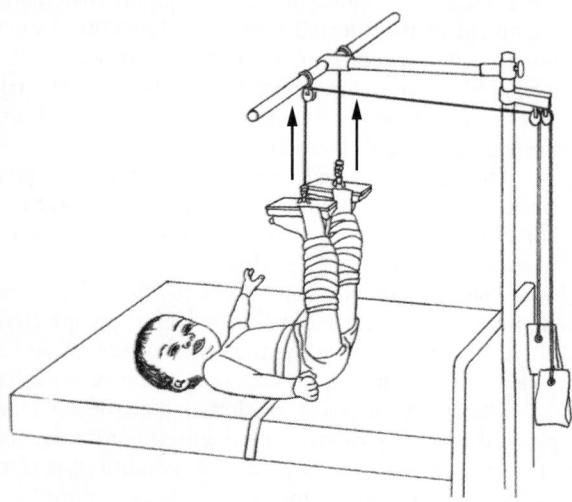

RUSSELL TRACTION

Purpose: Used to stabilize fractured femurs until callus forms.
Description: Continuous traction. Knee slightly flexed and supported with sling. Trapeze overhead may be used by child for repositioning and upper extremity muscle integrity.

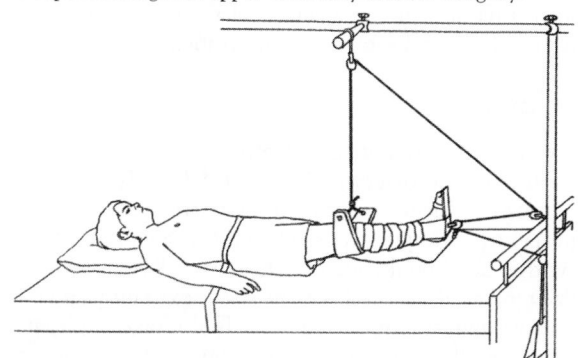

CERVICAL TRACTION

Purpose: Used to treat muscle or nerve irritation of shoulders and upper arms.
Description: May be continuous or intermittent. Maintains the head in extension via a halter: front straps fit under the chin, rear straps rest at base of skull. Spreader bar equalizes force of pull. Elevating the head of the bed 20 to 30 degrees helps correct alignment.

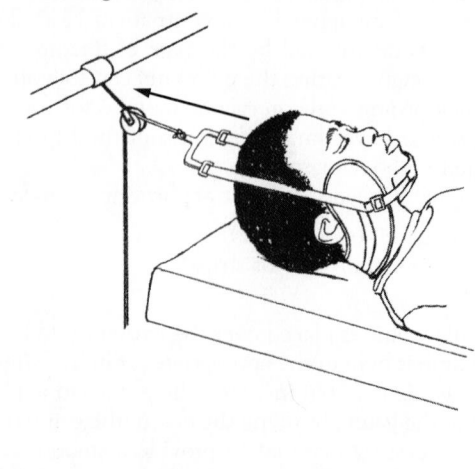

SKIN TRACTION

Skin traction exerts force directly on the body surface. It is noninvasive, well tolerated, and does not require anesthesia. Skin traction is most effective with children who weigh less than 30 pounds or are younger than age 2 to 3 years. It can be applied to the pelvis, spine, or extremities (usually the long bones). Skin traction is preferred for conditions in which invasive procedures are contraindicated, such as hemarthrosis due to hemophilia. Foam rubber straps, adhesive moleskin, or cloth belts are applied to the skin and then attached to the weights and pulleys. Sometimes an elastic bandage is wrapped around the skin to hold the traction apparatus in place. If skin traction to the lower leg is needed, a foam rubber boot may be used; the fit should be secure.

The effectiveness of skin traction is determined by the amount of pull that can be placed on the extremity. For this reason, skin traction is not appropriate if the child has a skin infection, an open wound, or extensive tissue damage. Skin breakdown may also develop. Spraying the skin with tincture of benzoin before the traction is applied may protect against skin irritation.

If the traction has not been set up correctly, neurovascular impairment may occur. Hyperextension of the knee and elastic bandages that have been wrapped too tightly are the most common causes of this problem. A thorough assessment of the traction apparatus as well as the extremity should be conducted at least once a shift as a preventive measure.

SKELETAL TRACTION

Skeletal traction (Fig. 50–2) exerts greater force than skin traction and can be physiologically tolerated for longer periods of time. Traction is maintained via a metal device that is inserted into the bone. This is accomplished by introducing a Kirschner wire or Steinmann pin into the bone or Crutchfield tongs into the skull.

The insertion site of these stainless steel wires, pins, or tongs is determined by the fracture site. Common sites for skeletal traction include the skull, the proximal end of the ulna, and the distal end of the femur, as well as the tibia

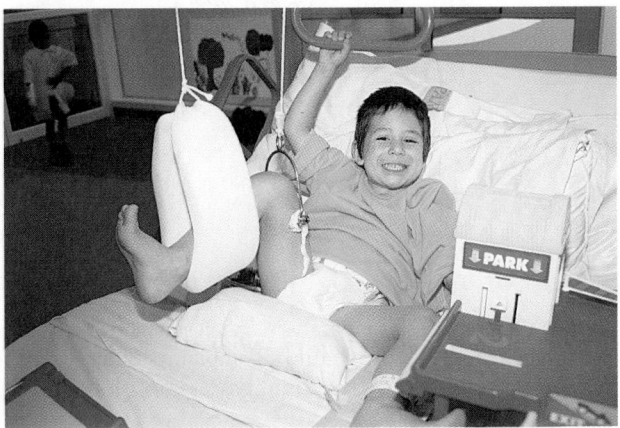

FIGURE 50–2

Skeletal traction is used to reduce and immobilize fractures and allows greater pull than would be possible with skin traction. Osteomyelitis may be a serious complication because skeletal traction is invasive. (Courtesy of Parkland Health and Hospital System, Dallas, Texas.)

> ### CRITICAL TO REMEMBER
>
> ### The Child in a Cast or Traction
>
> Tissue ischemia and nerve damage are serious complications that may accompany immobilization in a cast or traction. Skin color and temperature, movement and sensation of the extremity, quality of pulses, and capillary refill time of the extremity are related to neurovascular status and should be assessed carefully; problems must be handled quickly to prevent permanent disabilities.
>
> The five P's of vascular impairment can be used as a guide when assessing neurovascular problems:
>
> Pain
> Pallor
> Pulselessness
> Paresthesia
> Paralysis
>
> Pain or a burning sensation unrelieved by analgesia or nursing interventions may be an indication of tissue ischemia. Prompt intervention is crucial if neurovascular impairment is to be prevented. This type of complaint must be referred to the physician.

and heel. *Internal fixation*, or the direct application of hardware to the bone, is common in skeletal traction. It helps maintain correct alignment of the bony fragments and assists in proper healing. General anesthesia is required for internal fixation.

The most serious complication associated with skeletal traction is *osteomyelitis*, an infection involving the bone. Organisms gain access to the bone systemically or through the opening created by the metal pins or wires used for traction. Osteomyelitis may also occur with any open fracture. Clinical manifestations include complaints of localized pain, swelling, warmth, tenderness, or unusual odor. An elevated temperature may accompany the symptoms. To decrease the risk of infection at the pin sites, some facilities have an institutional protocol for frequent pin site care (once a day or more). This procedure involves cleaning the skin around pin sites (usually with half strength hydrogen peroxide), followed by application of an antibiotic ointment and a gauze pad.

Skeletal traction is always continuous. If the force of the traction were altered, the muscles would contract and fracture alignment would be disrupted. The tissues around the fracture could also be injured.

NURSING CARE

The Child in a Cast or Traction

Assessment

Prior to application of a cast or traction, assess the child's and parent's knowledge about the procedure. Also assess the child's skin and note the presence of any bruises or abrasions that might be covered by the cast.

• • • • • • • • • •
Types of Skeletal Traction

CRUTCHFIELD TONGS

Purpose: To stabilize fractures or displaced vertebrae in cervical and thoracic areas.

Description: Tongs are inserted on either side of the head through drill holes. The center of the curved metal bar must extend along the same planes as the spinal cord. Traction pull is always along the axis of the spine. The child must maintain straight body alignment.

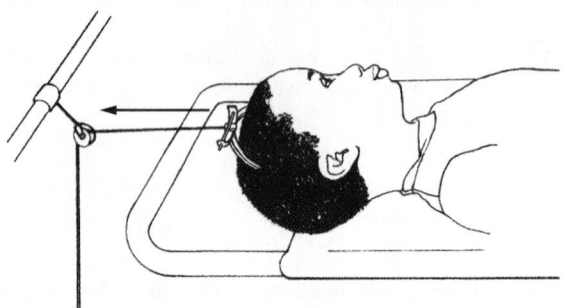

BALANCED SUSPENSION

Purpose: Suspends and immobilizes a leg without applying traction to the body.

Description: May be applied to a hip, tibia, fibula, or femur. The leg is supported by a Pearson attachment and a Thomas splint. A Thomas splint is a padded ring that fits around the upper leg; a Pearson attachment meets the Thomas splint at the knee and supports the lower leg. A canvas sling may be used to further support the lower leg.

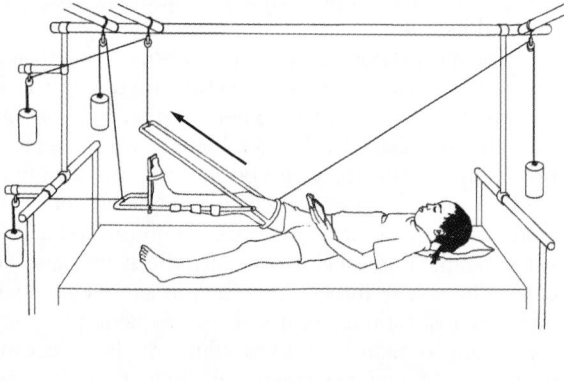

90/90 FEMORAL TRACTION

Purpose: Most commonly used traction for complicated fractures of the femur; most effective in children more than 6 years old. Within 2 to 3 weeks, callus formation is sufficient to allow application of a spica cast.

Description: A pin or wire is inserted through the distal femur; the lower leg may be casted.

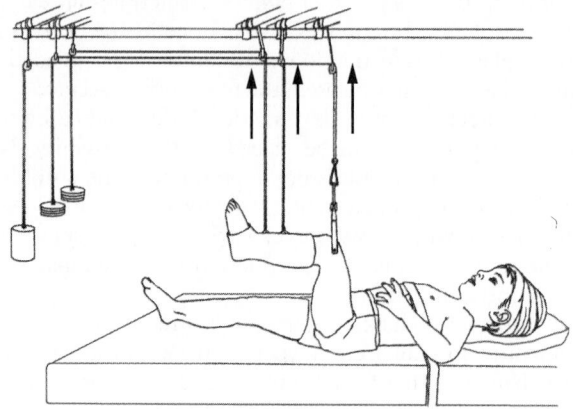

DUNLOP TRACTION

Purpose: Used to treat supracondylar fractures of the humerus.

Description: A pin is inserted through the distal humeral fragments. The elbow is flexed at a 90-degree angle with the forearm in neutral position.

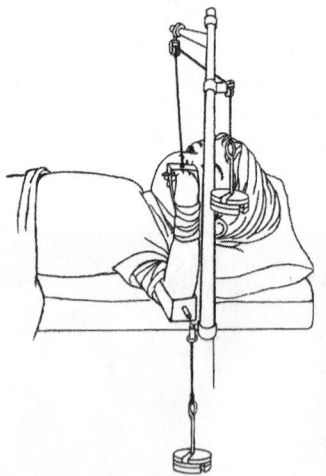

After the cast or traction is applied, perform a neurovascular assessment at least every 1 to 2 hours during the first 48 hours. Assess the strength of the pulse distal to the cast or traction site and compare it with the pulse in the uninvolved extremity. A sluggish capillary refill time usually indicates neurovascular impairment.

Signs of circulatory impairment include coldness, pallor, blueness of the extremity, swelling, loss of motion, and numbness and tingling of the extremity. Paresthesia, or numbness and tingling, can be assessed by touching the fingers or toes and noting any decrease or loss in feeling. Paresthesia is of serious concern because paralysis can result if the problem is not corrected. Report a child's complaints of a pins-and-needles sensation or of the extremity "feeling asleep."

> Because young children are not always able to describe a feeling or sensation, avoid questions such as "Do you feel this?" Asking a child to wiggle the fingers or toes is an appropriate way to determine motor impairment.

Motor function and sensation distal to the cast or traction should be assessed frequently.

Nursing Diagnosis, Planning, Intervention, and Evaluation

| Nursing Diagnosis | ■ Risk for Injury related to neurovascular impairment or infection from cast or traction. |

Expected Outcomes
• The child's neurovascular integrity will be maintained or supported.
• The child will be free of complications from infection.

Intervention	Rationale
1. Monitor neurovascular status by determining color, temperature, sensation, motion, capillary refill time (normal is less than 2 seconds), and pulsation every 1 to 2 hours and as necessary; insert one finger between the cast and skin to check for cast tightness. Compare the quality of the pulse distal to the affected site with the pulse in the uninvolved extremity.	1. Casts or traction devices may compress or restrict nerves or arteries, impeding healing and causing serious ischemic and circulatory problems. Swelling generally peaks 1 to 2 days after application of a cast.
2. Maintain correct body alignment. For a child in traction, draw a line on the sheet and ask the parents to keep the child above that line.	2. Proper alignment prevents pressure on the affected extremity and promotes healing.
3. Monitor the type and duration of pain. Ask parents how the child normally reacts to pain. Be alert to preverbal children and their expressions of pain; irritability, inability to move or wiggle their toes, or color changes in a distal extremity are typical signs.	3. A complaint of burning pain or pain unrelieved by analgesic medication is an indicator of ischemia and nerve injury. Prompt intervention is crucial to prevent neurovascular impairment.
4. Maintain cast integrity by supporting the drying cast with pillows. Reposition every 2 to 4 hours; turn the cast with the palms of the hands. A dry cast should sound hollow when tapped and should be cool to the touch. Keep plaster casts dry. Monitor for fever, cast hot spots, or unusual odor from the cast.	4. An intact cast provides support and controls the position of the involved extremity. Supporting the cast with pillows helps maintain correct position. Repositioning enhances drying. Using the palms prevents denting the cast. Any area of warmth (hot spot) or odor from inside the cast can indicate infection, and the physician should be notified.
5. Elevate the casted extremity above heart level; apply ice to cast as needed. If swelling persists after elevation, notify physician.	5. Elevating the extremity will reduce venous pooling; ice will reduce swelling and edema.
6. Circle any drainage on the cast and report any increase to the physician.	6. Drainage on a cast could indicate complications secondary to an open reduction.
7. Maintain traction integrity by ensuring all weights and pulleys are hanging free and do not touch the floor or bed. Elevate the head or foot of the bed as indicated to maintain countertraction. Do not release the traction without a physician's order. Restrain child to maintain proper alignment (restraints should be used only if absolutely necessary for safety). Document that the correct amount of weight is in use by checking with the physician's order.	7. Effective traction prevents movement of the affected limb and maintains skeletal alignment during healing. The correct amount of weight is necessary to maintain bone position.

Evaluation
• Does the child have appropriate skin color as compared to the unaffected extremity?
• Is there equal warmth and sensation in both extremities?
• Is the child free of pain?
• Are there equal and strong pulses in both extremities (if appropriate)?
• Is the capillary refill time less than 2 seconds?

| Nursing Diagnosis | ■ Risk for Impaired Skin Integrity related to immobilization. |
| Expected Outcome | • The child's skin will remain intact, particularly over bony prominences. |

Intervention	Rationale
1. Examine the skin condition, especially over bony prominences, at least once a shift.	1. Regular skin examination can identify problem areas early and prevent the development of decubitus ulcers.

2. Reposition the child every 2 hours and as needed. Encourage use of a trapeze to facilitate independent movement.
3. Examine the skin around traction pin sites at least once a shift; perform pin care according to hospital protocol.
4. Wash and dry the child at least twice a day; massage the skin with circular movements; remove excess lotion with a towel. Do not use powder or talc because it tends to collect moisture and irritate the skin.
5. Place an egg-crate or sheepskin mattress under the back and lower legs; use water-filled gloves under the heels to prevent skin breakdown.
6. Petal the edges of the cast with adhesive tape or moleskin. Use adhesive moleskin or other adhesive tape 1 to 2 inches wide and cut into strips approximately 3 to 4 inches long. Round one edge. Beginning with the straight end of the strip, place it on the inside of the cast edge; the rounded or petaled end is brought up and over the cast edge so it is on the outside of the cast. Overlap each strip on the previous one.
7. Protect the skin under the cast from moisture. Avoid getting the cast wet (no swimming, baths, or showers); cover the cast with plastic and waterproof tape if it is likely the child may get the cast wet (e.g., playing or due to bladder incontinence).
8. Monitor the types of toys the child uses. Do not allow a young child to play with small toys that could be hidden inside a cast or underneath the child. Supervise feeding because food may be hidden in the cast as well.

2. Frequent turning reduces pressure on sensitive skin.
3. Tenting, or adherence of the skin to pins, results in skin breakdown and openings for organism entry. Pin care can prevent tenting.
4. Skin that is clean and dry is less likely to develop decubiti. Frequent massage increases circulation to the skin and reduces the likelihood of skin breakdown.
5. These actions relieve pressure over bony prominences.
6. Infants' and children's skin is fragile and prone to injury from rough or jagged cast edges.
7. Damp or moist skin inside a cast is an excellent environment for bacterial growth. Persistent dampness alters skin integrity and can disintegrate a plaster cast.
8. Objects or food hidden inside a cast place pressure on the skin and can lead to irritation and skin breakdown.

Evaluation
• Is the child's skin smooth amd without evidence of redness, irritation, or tissue breakdown?

Nursing Diagnosis
■ Impaired Physical Mobility related to cast or traction care.

Expected Outcome
• The child will experience minimal physiologic problems as a result of immobilization.

Intervention
1. Test muscle strength and joint mobility every shift and as needed.
2. Encourage active range-of-motion and stretching exercises of unaffected extremities as appropriate. Consult the physician regarding the need for occupational therapy and the use of splints or footboards.
3. Apply elastic stockings or TEDS.
4. Plan age-appropriate play activities that require the use of unaffected extremities. When the cast is fully dry, give the child and friends colored markers to decorate the cast.
5. Offer frequent small feedings of foods high in protein and calcium (milk, cheese, yogurt, green vegetables, puddings).
6. Maintain hydration levels that are age appropriate. Offer juices (cranberry, apple) and acid ash foods (cereal, meats) that will acidify the urine.

Rationale
1. Baseline data are essential if an appropriate plan of care is to be developed for the child.
2. Inactive muscles lose tone and strength at a rate of 3% to 5% a day, which may lead to loss of muscle mass and tissue breakdown. Joints become fibrotic from disuse, which leads to muscle shortening and joint contractures; exercise facilitates the movement of calcium into the bone.
3. Elastic stockings promote venous return and decrease circulatory stasis.
4. Exercise will strengthen and enhance muscle and joint integrity while assisting with normal developmental needs.
5. A diet high in calcium and protein will reduce problems associated with a negative nitrogen balance and increased bone catabolism.
6. Encouraging fluids reduces problems associated with hypercalcemia, renal calculi, and stasis of respiratory secretions. Acid urine inhibits growth of microorganisms.

7. Observe for urine output of 1 to 2 ml/kg/hr. Check urine for protein, blood, and specific gravity as ordered.
8. Monitor bowel sounds and elimination pattern. Provide increased roughage in the diet and offer favorite foods. Determine the child's usual bowel patterns; determine the character of the stool (amount, color, consistency, time). Position the child as upright as possible during defecation. Administer stool softeners and mild laxatives as needed; use familiar words for defecation.
9. Monitor respiratory status at least once a shift. Encourage coughing and deep breathing through the use of such games as blowing bubbles, pinwheels, or magic tricks. Older children may use the triflow or incentive spirometer as needed.

7. Adequate renal output reduces the incidence of urinary tract infections secondary to urinary stasis and assists in reducing renal calculi.
8. Immobility decreases peristalsis and increases problems with constipation. Increasing dietary fiber keeps the stool soft. Assisting the child to defecate in as normal a position as possible and using appropriate terminology to assess the need for defecation is important for children.
9. Immobility places the child at risk for stasis of secretions, which may lead to pneumonia or atelectasis.

Evaluation
- Does the child display normal muscle and joint function in the unaffected extremities?
- Are cardiac or respiratory complications absent?
- Does the child display age-appropriate nutritional, bowel, and bladder habits?

Nursing Diagnosis
■ Altered Growth and Development related to anxiety, diversional activity deficit, immobility, and hospitalization.

Expected Outcomes
- The family will verbalize feelings and concerns regarding the child's hospitalization and immobility.
- The child will exhibit developmentally appropriate behaviors.
- The parents will support and maintain appropriate developmental behavior for their child.

Intervention

1. Determine and acknowledge the extent of the child's and parent's anxiety and, when possible, model appropriate behaviors or teach activities that reduce anxiety.
2. Maintain a calm, consistent environment. Organize nursing care to allow periods of developmentally appropriate activities. When possible, assign the same nursing personnel.
3. Recognize the child's need to regress in response to the injury or hospitalization. Accept the behavior and assist the child to regain prior developmental stages when ready.

4. Encourage parents to stay with the child. If the parents cannot stay, encourage them to leave an article of clothing or other personal item with the child. Audio tapes of parents reading favorite stories are also helpful.
5. Explain all routines and procedures to the child and parents. Continue to offer explanations until the child and parents express understanding.

6. Involve the parents in the care of the child when appropriate. Begin teaching the family about home care on the first day of hospitalization.

Rationale

1. Such data provide information about family strengths and nursing care needs. Modeling behaviors provide a visual teaching tool.

2. Anxiety can be transferred to the child from a parent or staff person. A consistent caregiver will provide a sense of security to the child.

3. Schedules, routines, and rituals offer a sense of security to the young child. Hospitalization and injuries interrupt these routines and create stressful situations that impact on the child's ability to perform self-care activities such as toileting, sleeping, discipline, and feeding. Regression in response to stress is normal in young children.
4. The presence of a parent or significant family member can reduce the fear of separation and foster a sense of security. If the parent cannot be present, reminders are helpful.

5. The unknown is a powerful influence on the child and increases anxiety; the presence of anxiety decreases the child's and parents' ability to process and analyze information.
6. Encouraging the parents to participate in the child's care increases their sense of control and provides the child with a sense of security.

7. Provide age-appropriate play or diversional activities. When possible, involve the parents in the child's play. Encourage expressive activities such as throwing balls through a hoop or bean bags into a basket, pounding boards to reduce stress and anxiety, or using modeling clay or play dough or painting to release frustration. If available, allow the child to play with remote control toys to give the child a feeling of mobility. Use therapeutic play: activities such as applying a cast to a doll, puppet play, storytelling utilizing pictures the child has drawn, or role-playing.

8. When possible use age-appropriate dishes and cups for the young child. Let the child wear his or her own clothing; slit the sides of the jeans and shorts and sew Velcro closures on the legs. Allow the young child a transitional object in bed; use a night-light and when possible follow nighttime rituals. Encourage therapeutic play with the preschool child; if possible, place two preschoolers in the same room. Recognize the preschooler's use of magical thinking and encourage expressive play when dealing with the stress of immobility.

9. Provide the school-age child and adolescent with opportunities for keeping up with schoolwork. Ask teachers or peers to tape record classes. Encourage the child to maintain activities related to organizations like Boy Scouts or Girl Scouts, if possible. Monitor time spent watching television or playing video games. Encourage involvement in hobbies and when possible select a roommate close in age.

10. Provide a change in the child's environment frequently. Move the infant's bed to take advantage of a different view or transport the infant outside the room in a stroller or wagon. Wheel an older child who is in traction to the playroom in the bed. Encourage motor activities of unaffected extremities.

7. Therapeutic play provides a safe and effective mechanism for reducing the stress of hospitalization and immobility. Therapeutic play puts the child in charge, provides a sense of control, and presents the child with opportunities to make choices. Play helps the child work through fears and anxieties.

8. The use of familiar objects and maintaining routines provides the child with a sense of security and belonging; allowing contact with friends and family members reassures the child and provides opportunities to enhance and support appropriate developmental behaviors.

9. Maintaining routines and helping the older child and adolescent maintain school activities provides opportunities for independence and productivity. Tutoring as well as Big Sister/Big Brother programs in the school can be very beneficial to the immobilized child. Appropriately relating to the school-age child or adolescent reinforces developmentally appropriate behavior as well as validating the child's importance.

10. The immobilized child suffers from a lack of environmental stimuli and restricted movement. Regardless of age, the restrained child is constantly struggling between dependence and independence and needs opportunities to exert autonomy.

Evaluation

- Does the child appear to be developing normally, as evidenced by decreased crying or acting-out behaviors, increased cooperation with self-care activities, and normal sleep habits?
- Do the child and parents verbalize increased trust toward health care providers?
- Does the child verbally or through play disclose feelings or concerns regarding the injury or hospitalization?
- Do the parents accept the child's regressive behaviors and become more involved in the child's care?

Nursing Diagnosis

■ Knowledge Deficit about the child's home management related to incomplete understanding of cast care.

Expected Outcome

- The parents will verbalize accurate knowledge of treatment, increased confidence with home care of the child, and an awareness of problems that may occur and the appropriate actions to take.

Intervention

1. Determine parents' level of understanding regarding cast care and their past experiences in caring for a child in a cast.

2. Provide verbal and written discharge instructions. Instruct parents to protect the cast from damage by keeping food and small objects away from the cast, never to allow the child to scratch under the cast, and keep the cast from getting wet.

Rationale

1. Developing a teaching plan for the parents cannot begin until the parents' knowledge level is determined and the nurse can identify areas to emphasize or clarify.

2. Providing parents with information will increase their self-confidence and assist them in caring for their child in a safe and appropriate manner. Written instructions remind parents of what has been taught. Parental anxiety may interfere with the ability to remember.

3. Discuss self-care activities with the parents and child (if age appropriate) as well as modifications in home and school routines. Refer to appropriate resources for crutch walking as well as appropriateness of isotonic and isometric exercises. Refer to an occupational therapist, if needed, to assist with adaptive devices for the performance of activities of daily living and to increase the child's independence.

4. Review the neurovascular assessment and identify appropriate resources for the parents to contact if problems occur. Identify potential problems related to skin breakdown and infection. Follow up all teaching with return demonstrations if appropriate.

5. Assist parents in understanding the impact of immobility on the child's growth and development.

3. Anticipatory guidance reduces parental anxiety and facilitates the transition from hospital to home.

4. Parents need to be instructed about potential complications and available resources.

5. It is important that parents realize that despite the cast, there are many ways they can enhance their child's development.

Evaluation

- Can the parents manage the transition from hospital to home smoothly and without problems, as evidenced by safe and effective home care?
- Are the parents able to describe age-appropriate developmental behaviors in the child?
- Can the parents and child express the importance of follow-up care and the impact of immobility on the child's growth and development?

PARENTS AND CHILD WANT TO KNOW
Home Care for the Child in a Cast

Check the edges of the cast.

- If they appear rough or are irritating the skin, "petal" the cast by overlapping moleskin or adhesive tape (1 to 2 inches in width; 3 to 4 inches in length with one rounded edge) around the cast edges.

To assist with drying the cast,

- Place your child on a firm mattress.
- Support the cast and adjacent joints with pillows.
- For a plaster cast, reposition every 2 to 4 hours to ensure thorough drying.
- Lift the cast using the palms of your hands.
- You may direct a fan toward the cast to facilitate drying.
- Once dry, the cast should sound hollow and be cool to the touch.

Swelling generally peaks within 24 to 48 hours. To prevent problems,

- Apply ice to the casted area (be sure to keep melting ice from touching the cast or leaking underneath).
- Elevate the extremity with pillows.
- Apply pressure to the child's nail bed and count how long it takes for the color to return (it should take no longer than 2 seconds). Repeat every 2 to 3 hours for the first 24 to 48 hours.
- The casted extremity should be the same color and temperature as the other extremity.
- Check each finger or toe for sensation and movement several times a day for 2 days.

Protect the cast.

- If given permission to bathe or shower, be sure to cover the cast with plastic to keep the cast dry.
- Do not put anything inside the cast. Keep small toys and sharp objects away from the cast.

Contact the physician if

- The cast feels warm, hot, or has an unusual smell or odor.
- Any drainage or blood suddenly appears on the cast.
- You feel (or the child complains of) pain, burning, numbness, or tingling, or if the extremity changes color or temperature.

When it is time for the cast to be removed,

- Explain the cast removal to your child. The cast cutter works by vibrations that create heat and a tickling feeling on the skin. It sometimes sounds loud, so you need to provide reassurance if your child is afraid of loud noises.
- Allow time for the child to adjust to the cast cutter. Ask the technician or doctor if your child can examine the cast cutter and see how it works ahead of time. Sometimes children are allowed to remove a doll's cast with supervision.
- Once the cast is removed, the skin will be dry and flaky. Wash the area with warm water and soap.
- The extremity will be stiff for a while and will look smaller because the muscles haven't been used. It may need to be supported with a sling. Normal movement will correct the stiffness.

Limb Defects

Limb defects are common in children and are a concern for parents. Most alterations of arms and legs are mild variations of normal posturing, but some are severe anomalies or abnormalities.

Etiology and Incidence

Limb defects result from birth anomalies and sometimes from trauma. These defects take many forms, including webbing (*syndactyly*) or extra digits (fingers or toes; *polydactyly*), congenital absence of all or part of an extremity, *genu valgum* (knock-knees) and *genu varum* (bowlegs), and clubfoot. Bowlegs are common in sturdily built infants and toddlers (Fig. 50–3). This condition is also associated with tibial torsion, a normal variation in toddlers. Knock-knees are often seen in the preschool-age group. The structure and function of congenitally malformed limbs can be improved with therapy, but the affected limbs seldom become normal.

Trauma to or infection of an extremity may result in a variety of difficulties. Leg length discrepancy can be a result of trauma, infection, or radiation therapy, because the unaffected limb continues to grow.

Pathophysiology

Mild limb defects most frequently occur secondary to extrinsic pressure, such as in utero positioning, or to the sitting

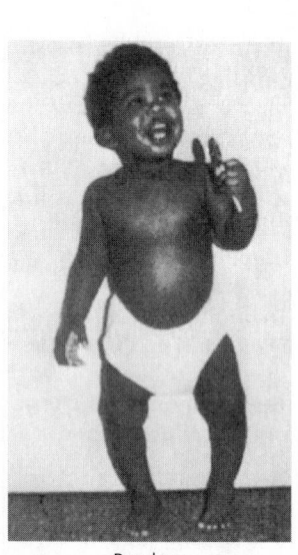
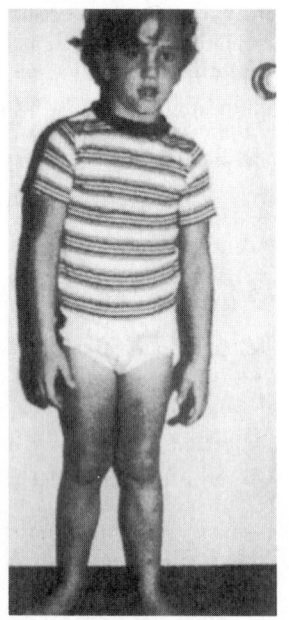

Bowlegs   Knock-Knees

FIGURE 50–3

In the child with genu varum, or bowlegs, there is a persistent space between the knees when the ankles are together. Genu varum is a normal finding for 1 year after the child begins walking. In the child with genu valgum, or knock-knees, there is a space between the ankles when the knees are together. Genu varum occurs as a normal variation in children 2 to 3½ years old. To remember the terminology, link the *r*s and *g*s: genu varum—knees apart; genu valgum—knees together. (From McDade, W. [1977, November]. Bowlegs and knock knees. *Pediatric Clinics of North America*, 24(4), 831.)

and sleeping postures of young children. Heredity may also play a part in mild limb defects. These disorders are usually cosmetic, although occasionally function is altered as well. They tend to correct as the child grows.

Diagnostic Evaluation

Severe congenital defects are readily apparent at birth. Mild defects and deformities that develop over time are usually identified by parents or school nurses and are evaluated by specialized clinicians. Radiographs may be necessary to fully evaluate limb defects and assist with developing a treatment plan.

Therapeutic Management

Mild limb deformities often resolve without treatment. Exercises, splints, special shoes, or casts may be prescribed. Surgical intervention may be required for severe deformities to release tendons, reposition bones, reconstruct parts, retard growth of an extremity, or augment growth of a limb. In some situations, long-term immobility of an extremity is necessary using casts or external fixation. Orthoses or physical therapy may be prescribed for specific needs.

Nursing Considerations

Nursing care varies with the defect and its treatment. Parents may need reassurance about the outcome of their child's therapy. The nurse should reinforce the principles of therapy, teach parents to carry out treatments at home, and encourage parents to persist with the treatment regimen even if the child does not like it. For example, exercises, special appliances, or braces may require daily use. Children in casts will require specialized home care. Parents may be referred to an orthotist for construction of a device to assist with the child's function or mobility. Periodic follow-up is often necessary to reinforce correct use of appliances and care of the skin.

Clubfoot

Clubfoot is a congenital malformation of the lower extremity that affects the lower leg, ankle, and foot.

Etiology and Incidence

Clubfoot shows a genetic predisposition and a multifactorial etiology. Children with certain neuromuscular disorders, such as myelomeningocele, are especially at risk. Clubfoot occurs in 1 in 1,000 births. Males are more commonly affected than females, in a 2:1 ratio.

Manifestations and Diagnostic Evaluation

The clinical manifestations of clubfoot include a plantar-flexed foot, with an inverted heel and adducted forefoot (Fig. 50–4), unilateral or bilateral defect, and a rigid limb that cannot be manipulated into a neutral position. Clubfoot is distinguished from *metatarsus adductus*, a nonrigid medial deviation of the midfoot. Clubfoot is readily apparent on clinical examination at birth.

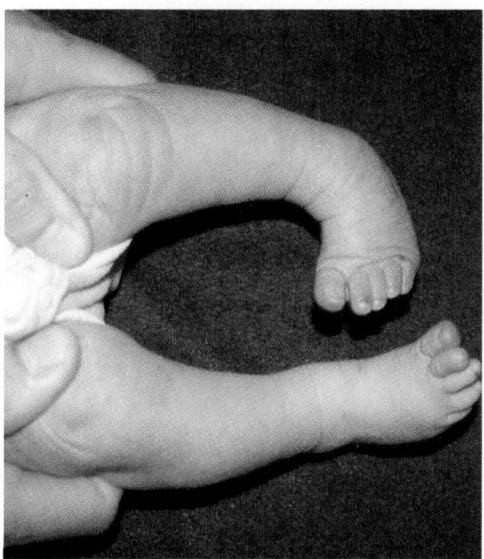

FIGURE 50–4

An infant with left clubfoot. Note the positional difference between the two feet.

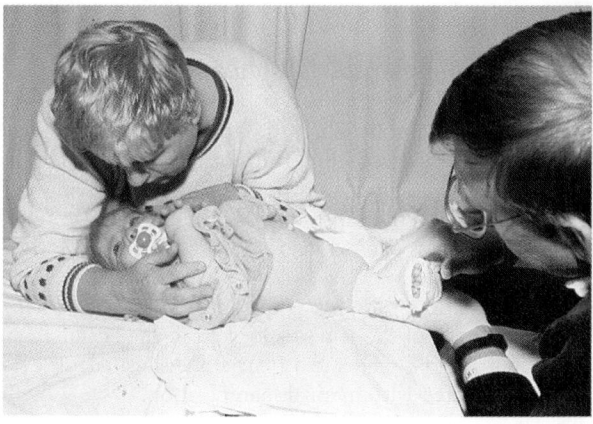

FIGURE 50–5

In the infant with clubfoot, serial manipulation and casting are started as soon after birth as possible to take advantage of the natural pliability of the neonate's bones. Long-term casting with frequent cast changes places great responsibility on the parents. (Courtesy of Cook Children's Medical Center, Fort Worth, Texas.)

Therapeutic Management

Treatment for clubfoot is started as soon after birth as possible. Serial manipulation and casting are performed at least weekly. If sufficient correction is not achieved in 3 to 6 months, surgery is usually indicated. Some malformations respond readily to treatment; other, more severe forms respond less well to even vigorous and prolonged therapy. Although early treatment may result in a foot that appears normal, recurrence is common. For this reason, long-term follow-up, until the child reaches skeletal maturity, is essential because further treatment may be indicated. Even with aggressive treatment, the foot is seldom completely normal. Lifelong atrophy of the calf is common, and the foot is usually a half size smaller than the other (Hoffinger, 1996).

Treatment for infants with metatarsus adductus, however, usually involves passive stretching exercises. Parents are instructed to perform these exercises several times a day in conjunction with some aspect of the infant's care routine, such as at each feeding or when diapers are changed. Occasionally a brace, cast, or straight-last shoes may be needed. Many children outgrow this deformity with little treatment.

Nursing Considerations

Nursing interventions are related to the stage of treatment. Initially, parents need help understanding clubfoot and the possibile treatments and outcomes. They also may need help acknowledging their disappointment in having a less than perfect baby. The nurse can encourage parents to discuss and recognize each other's unique strategies for coping. Long-term casting with frequent cast changes places great responsibility on the parents (Fig. 50–5). The nurse should assess their ability to adequately monitor the child for complications and pursue long-term follow-up.

If surgery is needed, the nurse oversees pain management in the immediate postoperative period. Initially, an intrave-

nous analgesic is used, with progression to an oral analgesic such as codeine and then to non-aspirin-containing, non-narcotic analgesics. Elevate the child's feet postoperatively, and apply ice bags to reduce swelling and pain. Assess the neurovascular status of the toes at least every 1 to 2 hours in the immediate postoperative period. Parents will need help positioning the infant for comfortable feeding.

The nurse also teaches parents how to keep the cast clean and dry at home. Parents should be taught how to bathe and diaper the infant without soiling or wetting the cast. When cast changes are done on an outpatient basis, parents need to learn how to assess the child's neurovascular status and when to seek help.

The nurse may refer the family to the local visiting nurse agency. Because clubfoot can recur, all children with this condition require interval follow-up until they reach skeletal maturity.

Developmental Dysplasia of the Hip

Developmental dysplasia of the hip has traditionally been known as congenital dislocation of the hip. Developmental dysplasia of the hip is a condition in which the head of the femur (ball) is improperly seated in the acetabulum (hip socket) of the pelvis. Hip dysplasia varies in severity from very mild to severe dislocation. Developmental dysplasia of the hip can be present at birth (congenital), but in some children it develops after birth; hence the term developmental.

Etiology

Developmental dysplasia of the hip appears to be multifactorial in origin. Genetic factors and pre- and postnatal positioning seem to be related. Laxity of the ligaments holding the femur head within the acetabulum may be the major underlying predisposing factor (Novacheck, 1996).

PATHOPHYSIOLOGY

. . . .

of Developmental Dysplasia of the Hip

In the normal infant hip, the head of the femur is well seated in the acetabulum (hip socket) and is stable. Developmental dysplasia of the hip occurs in varying degrees, ranging from instability of the hip joint to frank dislocation, as defined below.

- Instability of the hip is the appropriate term when the head of the femur is located in the acetabulum but may be subluxated (partially dislocated) or even dislocated with manual manipulation.

- Subluxation of the hip occurs when the head of the femur is positioned under the edge of the acetabulum. It is not well seated in the acetabulum, yet neither is it completely dislocated.
- Dislocation of the hip occurs when the head of the femur lies outside of the acetabulum. It can occur as a late stage of developmental dysplasia of the hip, or it can occur in children with certain neuromuscular disorders.

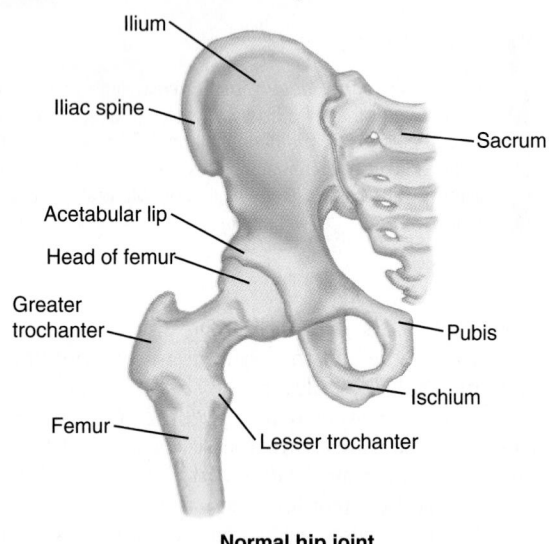

Normal hip joint

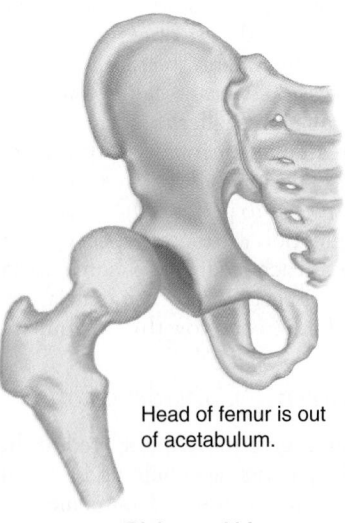

Ligaments of normal hip joint

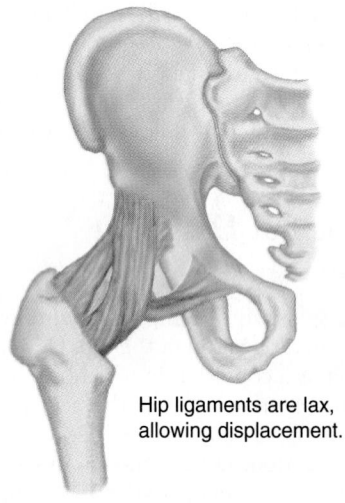

Hip ligaments are lax, allowing displacement.

Unstable hip

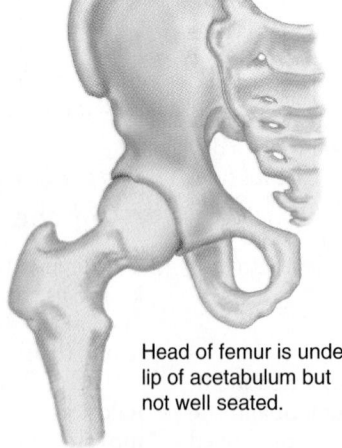

Head of femur is under lip of acetabulum but not well seated.

Subluxated hip

Head of femur is out of acetabulum.

Dislocated hip

Incidence

The incidence of developmental dysplasia of the hip varies greatly among people of different races. It is less common in African-American and Asian infants and more common in Native Americans. It is most common in whites, in females, and in first-born infants. It is marked by a familial tendency. The condition is associated with breech deliveries. The overall incidence is difficult to determine because it varies with age and the severity of the problem (Harcke, 1999).

Manifestations

The manifestations of developmental dysplasia of the hip vary according to age. In neonates, laxity of the ligaments around the hip allows the femoral head to be displaced from the acetabulum upon manipulation. Infants beyond the newborn period exhibit asymmetry of the gluteal skin folds when the infant is lying and the legs are extended against the examining table (or when the infant is held upright with the legs dangling). There is a limited range of motion in the affected hip, as well as asymmetric abduction when the child is placed supine with the knees and hips flexed. The femur on the affected side appears to be short. The walking child displays minimal to pronounced variations in gait, with lurching toward the affected side.

Diagnostic Evaluation

Because of the complexities of diagnosis, screening for developmental dysplasia of the hip should be done at birth and during each routine infant well-child visit by a well-trained nurse or physician.

The diagnosis of developmental dysplasia of the hip in the neonate can be very difficult to make because the signs and symptoms may be very subtle. In affected newborns, the hip joints appear lax rather than completely dislocated. The Ortolani and Barlow maneuvers (see Chapter 22) can be done to assess subluxation or laxity, but the results are not diagnostically valid after the infant is 1 month old (Harcke, 1999). Radiography is not useful in the neonate because bony ossification is not complete. Ultrasonography is now used to assist with the diagnosis of developmental dysplasia of the hip (Rosendahl, Aslaksen, Lie, et al., 1995). Computed tomography (CT) and magnetic resonance imaging (MRI) may also be helpful, but use of these studies is limited.

In the older infant, the physical signs of developmental dysplasia of the hip are different. The symptoms change from lax ligaments to contractures and stiffness in the affected hip joint(s). Limited abduction on the affected side(s) is a major diagnostic sign. Any abnormalities in an older child's gait need to be carefully evaluated as possible signs of the condition. Radiography is more useful in establishing the diagnosis in older infants and children than in very young infants.

Bilateral dysplasia is always more difficult to identify than unilateral dysplasia because there is no normal hip that can be used for comparison. Interestingly, many unstable hips resolve spontaneously. If untreated, only about 20% will settle into a dislocated position.

Therapeutic Management

Early diagnosis and treatment of developmental dysplasia of the hip are important to maximize the likelihood of a successful outcome. Treatment depends on the age of the child at the time of diagnosis and on the severity of the dysplasia. Because the musculoskeletal development of the neonate is immature, early diagnosis and successful treatment of developmental dysplasia of the hip can result in a normal or near normal hip.

In the neonatal period, treatment involves splinting the hips with a Pavlik harness to maintain flexion and abduction and external rotation. The Pavlik harness consists

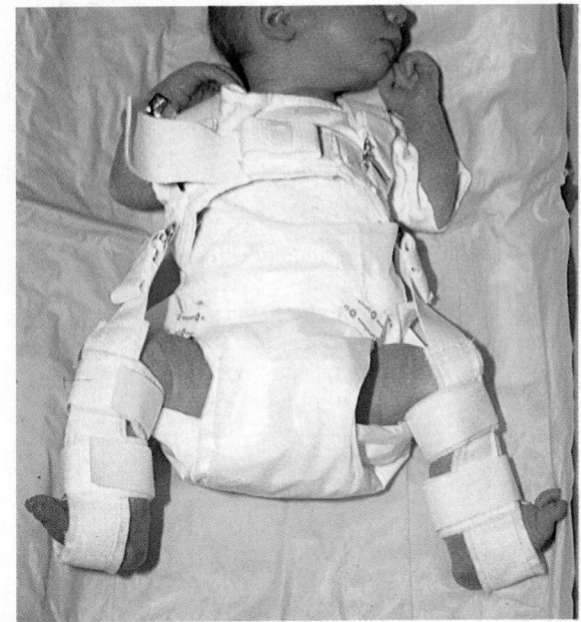

FIGURE 50–6

An infant in a Pavlik harness to treat developmental dysplasia of the hip.

of chest and shoulder straps and foot stirrups (Fig. 50–6). Initially the harness is worn continuously. Positioning in the harness promotes development of a functional hip socket and a well-formed femoral head. This splinting may be the only treatment necessary to allow the hip to mold and grow normally. Hips that remain unstable become progressively deformed as the skeleton matures, resulting in functional disability. Parents must be taught the proper use of the harness, because improper positioning of the infant's hip can cause interruption of the blood supply to the head of the femur, resulting in avascular necrosis (tissue damage secondary to an inadequate blood supply). In addition, skin care, techniques for holding and feeding, and the importance of vigilant follow-up must be emphasized.

Treatment is more complicated when the condition is diagnosed after the newborn period. Traction or surgery to release muscles and tendons is usually necessary to allow adequate control of the hip joint. The procedure is followed by positioning and immobilization in a spica cast. For profoundly affected children, traction is often followed by osteotomy (surgical cutting of the bone) and repositioning of the femur. After surgery, long-term immobilization in a spica cast is necessary until healing is achieved. Radiographs show the progress achieved with treatment. Follow-up monitoring is essential, as the treatment may have to be modified.

■ NURSING CARE

The Child with Developmental Dysplasia of the Hip

Assessment

All infants should be assessed for developmental dysplasia of the hip during routine neonatal and well-child visits to ensure prompt diagnosis and treatment. Assessment proce-

CARING FOR NICOLE, A CHILD IN A SPICA CAST

◆ ◆ ◆ ◆ ◆

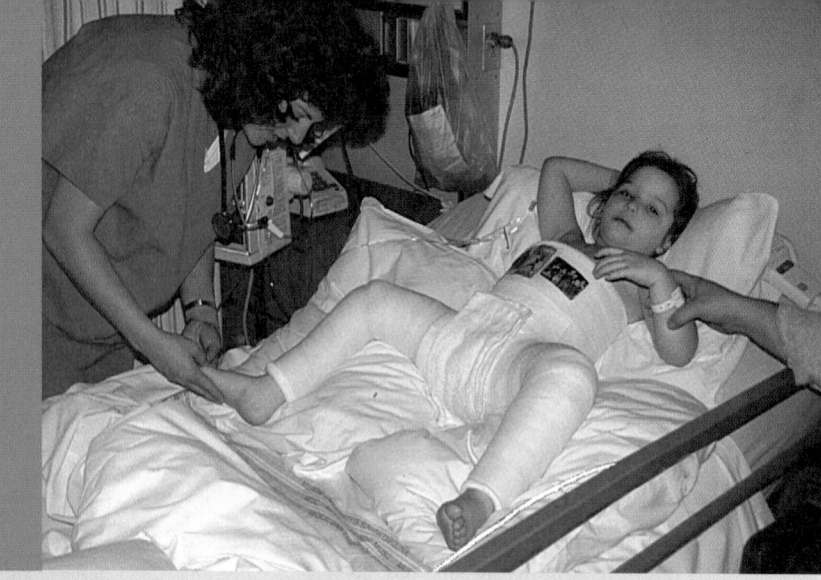

Four-year-old Nicole is immobilized in a spica cast after hip surgery. She receives IV morphine for pain. The therapies imposed by surgery and casting can lead to complications of respiration, elimination, skin breakdown, nutrition, and boredom. These potential complications, along with Nicole's growth and developmental needs, present challenges to her parents and the nurses caring for her.

Nicole is positioned to her level of comfort with pillows at her back. A folded pillow under each leg keeps her heels from pressing against the mattress, thereby preventing pressure points. If Nicole were a few years younger, she would not be able to tell her caregivers where to place pillows for comfort or if her heels or toes were hurting or bent. Particular attention to potential pressure points is necessary with preverbal children.

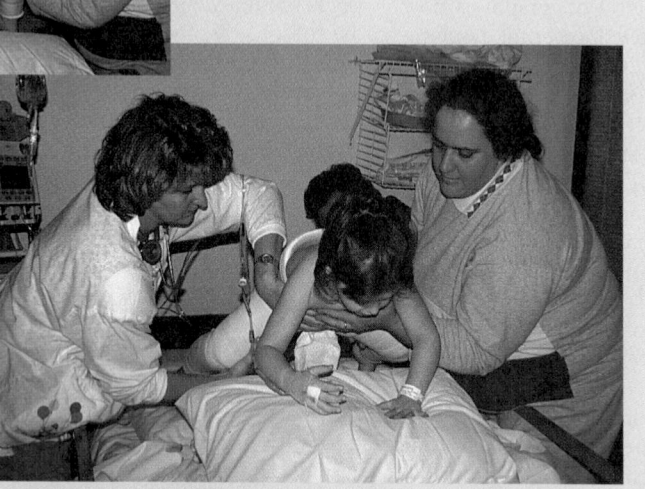

Three people are needed to turn Nicole: two to lift and turn her and a third to reposition pillows. Nicole is repositioned every 2 hours to prevent respiratory stasis. The crossbar between the legs of a spica cast (not present on this cast) should not be used as a handle when lifting the child. Once the child is feeling better and develops trust that she will not be dropped, repositioning is less frightening for her.

When prone, Nicole has a pillow under her chest to keep her face off the mattress and to allow her head mobility. A pillow under each leg keeps her feet and toes free. The prone position provides independence and increases Nicole's perception of control.

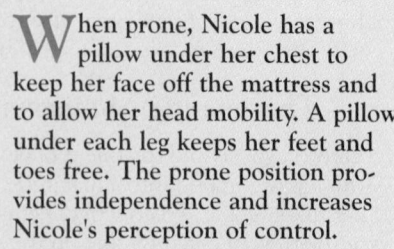

To prevent aspiration, Nicole eats in a prone position. Because independence and autonomy are important to children, every opportunity to enhance the child's independence should be encouraged. Food should be served in bite-sized pieces; finger foods may be preferred. Straws are used for liquids. The child should not be left unattended while eating.

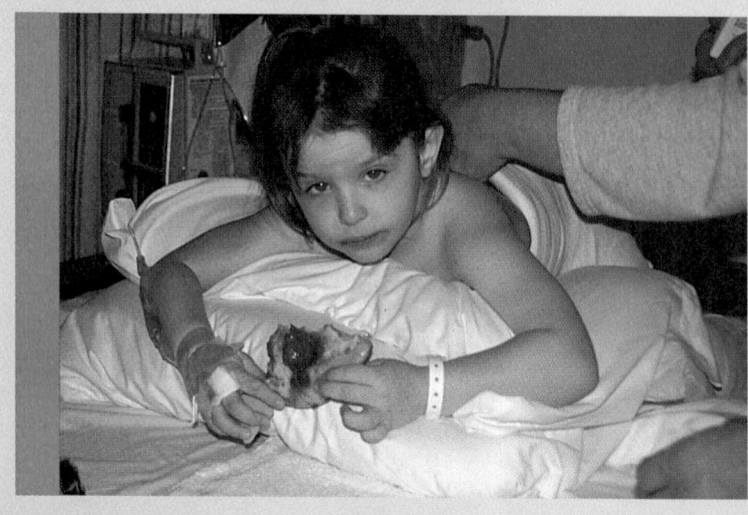

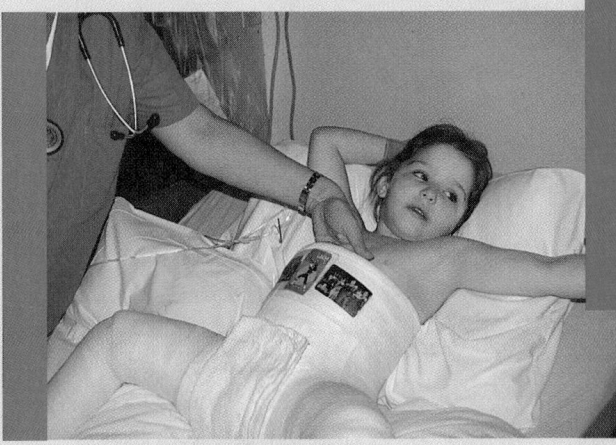

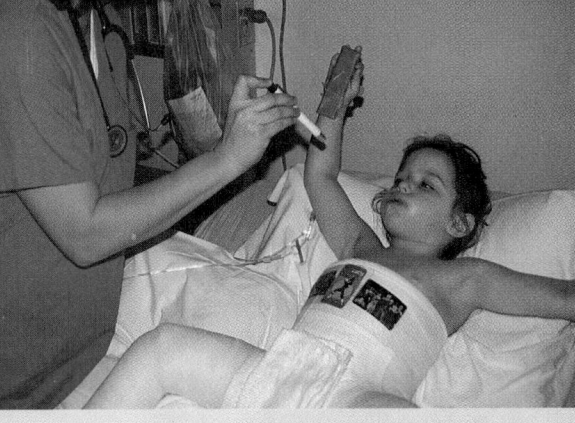

Nicole's nurse assesses her respiratory status. The cast must allow adequate room for respiratory excursion. Note that the nurse is able to fit several fingers under the edge of the cast around Nicole's chest. Respiratory assessment is performed at least every 8 hours. Deep breathing should be accomplished every 2 to 4 hours in the immediate postoperative period. Here the nurse asks Nicole to "blow out the light." Pinwheels, soap bubbles, and other tricks may be used to encourage deep breathing. In young children, crying provides the exercise of deep breathing.

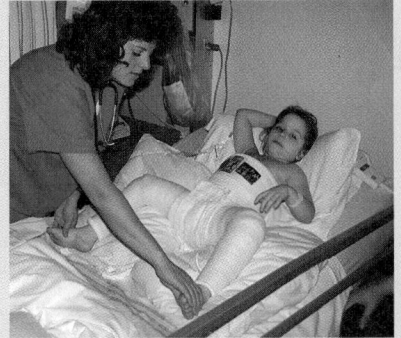

The nurse performs neurologic checks to ensure the adequacy of circulation and sensation in Nicole's feet. The nurse assesses bilaterally for color, temperature, sensation, swelling, and pulses.

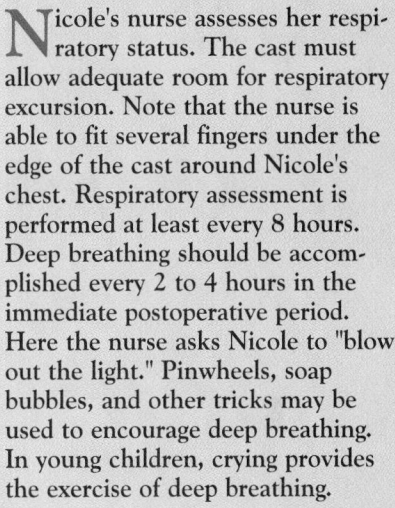

After Nicole is discharged from the hospital, her safety on the trip home is ensured by a special car-seat restraint available for children in spica casts. Whenever she travels in the car, Nicole is secured safely with this restraint.

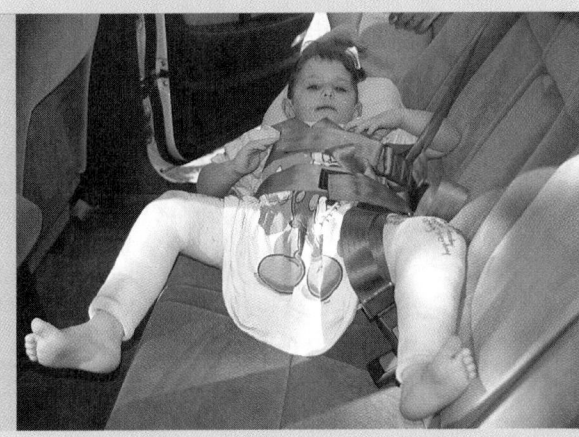

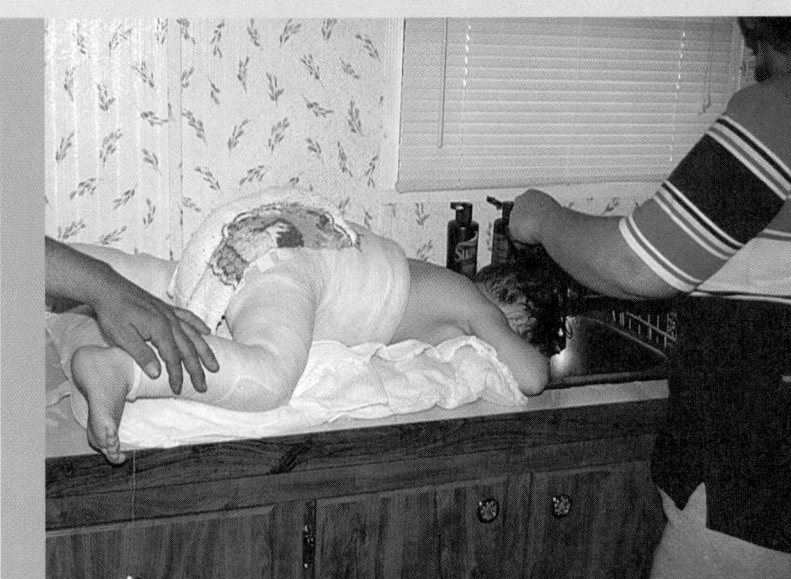

Before Nicole's discharge, her parents were instructed in body mechanics to prevent injury when lifting and turning Nicole in her heavy cast. At home, Nicole's mother washes her hair at the kitchen sink. Towels are used for comfort and to prevent water from running under the cast. Nicole is never left unattended on the kitchen counter or in other high places. To prevent burning Nicole, her mother is careful to check the water temperature.

CONTINUED

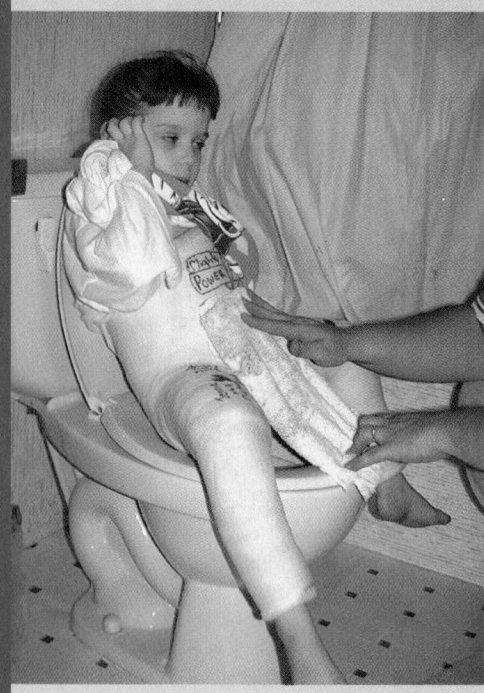

Nicole's mother has devised a system for toileting at home. Keeping Nicole in an upright position prevents soiling of the cast. Attention to bowel function is important, as constipation is a potential problem. Increased dietary fiber and fluid intake, including prune juice, is usually adequate to promote regularity.

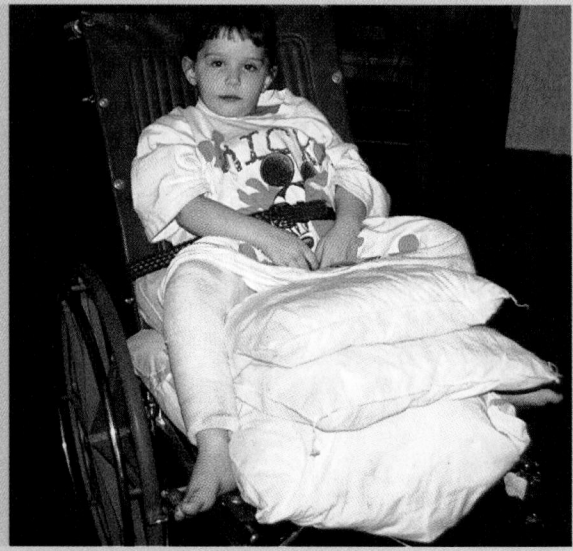

With pillows for positioning and comfort, Nicole uses a wheelchair for mobility. A younger child in a spica cast may be placed in a wagon padded with pillows. Children in wheelchairs and wagons should be strapped in to prevent falls. A child in a spica cast may also be placed on a blanket on the floor in an area of activity. This effort decreases the child's sense of isolation by increasing interactions with family members and friends.

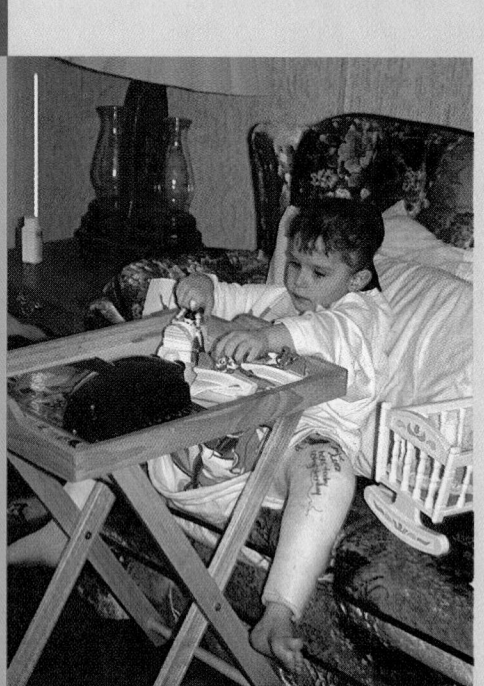

Nicole is usually dressed in large T-shirts, which are soft, absorbent, and easy to put on and take off. Although Nicole is continent, a disposable diaper is taped under her perineal area in place of underpants. Clothing may be adapted with Velcro closures. Socks are used when needed to keep Nicole's feet warm.

Age-appropriate activities help the immobilized child pass the time and can challenge and enhance development. Dolls, books, and coloring interest Nicole. At home, Nicole prefers to sit on the edge of the couch. She is never left alone and is old enough to request assistance if she feels herself sliding.

Photographs courtesy of Judy Gross and Children's Hospital, Orthopediatric Unit, Medical University of South Carolina, Charleston, South Carolina.

dures are complex and vary with the age of the child. Once the diagnosis is established, nursing assessment is directed to the parents' knowledge level, their anxiety and coping abilities, and ensuring that the treatment regimen is followed.

> Because the needs of children with musculoskeletal disorders are often long term, parents usually have a good understanding of their child's progress. Questions such as "What concerns do you have about your child's progress today?" or "How are you doing at home?" acknowledge that the parents' feelings and ideas are valued and important. Information generated by such questions can become the focus for assessment and further intervention.

Monitor the skin integrity of an infant in a Pavlik harness or cast. When surgery becomes necessary, nursing priorities shift to an assessment of lower extremity circulation and pain.

Nursing Diagnosis and Planning

The following nursing diagnoses and expected outcomes may be appropriate for the family and the child with developmental dysplasia of the hip:

- Knowledge Deficit about the diagnosis of developmental dysplasia of the hip and its treatment related to incomplete understanding of the child's condition.
  Expected Outcomes: The parents will demonstrate the therapeutic and safe use of a Pavlik harness. The parents will verbalize how to care for their child in a spica cast, and on follow-up visits the cast will be reasonably clean and dry and the child's skin will be clear and intact, without abrasions or sores. The parents will demonstrate proper technique for diapering and dressing the child in a spica cast.
- Anxiety (Parental) related to having a less than perfect child and the need to provide complex care for an extended period of time.
  Expected Outcomes: The parents will describe developmental dysplasia of the hip and its treatment in lay terms to other family members; carry out treatment regimens, demonstrating increased self-confidence in the care of their child; treat the child as normally as possible; and interact with health care providers and others in a calm and friendly manner.
- Risk for Impaired Skin Integrity related to skin chafing by the Pavlik harness or cast.
  Expected Outcome: The child's skin will remain clear and free from lesions.
- Altered Tissue Perfusion (Lower Extremities) related to impaired circulation secondary to surgery or casting.
  Expected Outcome: The circulation to the child's feet and toes will remain adequate.
- Risk for Injury related to difficult positioning of a child in infant-carrying devices (infant seats, strollers, car seats).
  Expected Outcome: The child will be safe from falls and will be adequately restrained when traveling in an automobile.
- Knowledge Deficit about home care related to depth of presented information.

Expected Outcome: The family will successfully manage treatment at home.

Interventions

Teaching About the Pavlik Harness

Demonstrate and teach the parents the proper care and application of the Pavlik harness, including how to position and fasten the chest halter. Place the child's leg and foot into the stirrup and straps, and connect the straps to the halter. Because the requirements for harness use may change during therapy, teaching, demonstration, and return demonstration are essential at every visit. Harness straps should be secure enough to keep the child's hips flexed, without being tight. The harness should be worn 23 hours a day and should be removed only according to physician recommendation. The hips and buttocks should be carefully supported if the infant is out of the harness. Encourage the parents to hold and cuddle the infant as much as possible. An infant in a Pavlik harness can be fed in the usual positions, with the parent carefully supporting the lower extremities during the feeding.

Teach parents to protect the child's skin and legs under the harness. A long T-shirt ("onesie") under the halter reduces harness rubbing. The use of long socks and Webril around the shoulder straps is helpful. The diaper should go on under the harness as well. Teach the parents to inspect the child's skin frequently for reddened or irritated areas and to reposition the child frequently.

Teaching About Spica Cast Care

Caring for a child in a spica cast is similar to caring for a child in any other type of cast (discussed previously), with some additional adaptations. Because the cast covers the entire lower half of the child's body, with the exception of the perineal opening, managing the child's elimination is a challenge. Excess urine can trickle under the cast, irritating and macerating the skin, resisting drying, and becoming malodorous. Advise the family to tuck a disposable diaper underneath the cast edges at the circular perineal opening; alternatively, sheet plastic is tucked under the cast opening and brought over the cast edge to the outside. Tuck sanitary napkins under the plastic and cover with a disposable diaper. Elevating the head of the bed helps urine and feces drain downward and away from the cast.

Monitor the child's neurovascular status frequently and teach the family the signs of neurovascular compromise. Fever, wound drainage, and discomfort may be signs of infection and should be reported promptly. Teach the family ways to provide environmental and developmental stimulation (e.g., by moving the child to different areas during the day, placing the child's bed near a window, placing appropriate toys within reach, providing age-appropriate activities). Explain the importance of feeding the child a diet high in fluids, calories, calcium, protein, and fiber. Instruct the parents about ways to dress their child to accommodate climate, style, and other needs (e.g., by fitting socks over the toes of the cast, using Velcro closures on pants and shorts, using clothing made of stretch fabrics). Give the parents the name and telephone number of an easily accessible health care provider in case questions arise at home.

Alleviating Anxiety

Communicate information to parents in a clear, kind, and straightforward manner because complex or ambiguous messages raise anxiety. Adjust teaching to accommodate parents' need for information and support. Reduce waiting time during follow-up visits and express interest in the child and parents. Providing reliable, respectful, and empathic care builds trust and reduces stress.

Preventing Injury

Assume a proactive role and advise parents of the potential for injury and the importance of taking safety precautions. Most infant-carrying devices are not suitable or safe for infants in spica casts. Assist parents in identifying strategies for transporting their infant in a safe and comfortable manner, including the use of a car seat that can accommodate the wide leg spread caused by the spica cast. During waking hours, suggest placing the child on an open area of the floor that has been covered with a blanket, as an alternative to an infant seat. Remind parents that the child must not be left unattended; infants and young children often develop a surprising ability to move, despite the restrictions imposed by a cast.

Evaluation

- Do the parents demonstrate the use of the Pavlik harness or spica cast in a safe and therapeutic manner?
- Can the parents describe developmental dysplasia of the hip and its treatment in lay terms to other family members, carry out the prescribed therapy to the greatest extent possible, and treat the child as a normal developing child?
- Do the parents seek recommended health care and keep follow-up appointments?
- Is the child's skin clear and free of lesions or breakdown?
- Are the child's toes warm and pink with capillary refill less than 2 seconds; can the child move the toes freely?
- Do the parents and child appear calm and able to participate in care?
- Does the child remain injury free?

▌ Legg-Calvé-Perthes Disease

Legg-Calvé-Perthes disorder, also known as osteochondritis deformans juvenilis or coxa plana, is a self-limiting disorder in which there is avascular necrosis of the femoral head. The child suffers from a painful limp that is exacerbated by activities such as walking or running.

Etiology

Although the cause of Legg-Calvé-Perthes disease is unknown, it is widely accepted to be a disorder of growth. Children with Legg-Calvé-Perthes disease are usually of shorter than average height; many of these children were low-birth-weight infants as well (less than 2.5 kg or 5.5 lb). Some studies have found a correlation between elevated free thyroxine levels and the degree of femoral head involvement (Koop & Quanbeck, 1996).

PATHOPHYSIOLOGY
• • • • • • • • • • •
of Legg-Calvé-Perthes Disease

A disturbance in the blood supply to the femoral epiphysis results in avascular necrosis of the femoral head. The most serious problem associated with Legg-Calvé-Perthes disease is the risk of permanent deformity. If the femoral head protrudes outside the acetabulum and the healing process within the femoral head is incomplete, over time the femoral head will flatten and take on a misshapen appearance. This could lead to later problems with arthritis.

The disorder is considered to be self-limiting and is classified by the extent of femoral head involvement and by disease stage. The disorder usually progresses through four stages, each generally lasting 1 to 2 years.

During stage 1, synovitis, the epiphysis begins to show the results of ischemia. The synovitis produces stiffness and pain. Necrosis begins; radiographs show a reduction in size and increased density of the femoral head. Once necrosis occurs, the bone weakens and dies, causing collapse of the femoral head. Stage 2 is the fragmentation stage in which avascular bone is reabsorbed. Healing occurs as new bone is formed. During the re-ossification stage, stage 3, the femoral head and neck begin to re-form. Stage 4, or the stage of reconstitution, results in final healing.

Incidence

The incidence of Legg-Calvé-Perthes disease is approximately 1 in 12,000. It is more likely to occur in boys than in girls (Koop & Quanbeck, 1996), and in boys it occurs most frequently between ages 4 and 8 years, with an average age at onset of approximately 6 years. Unilateral hip involvement is more common than bilateral involvement. This disease is rare in African-Americans and Asians.

Manifestations

Manifestations of Legg-Calvé-Perthes disease include complaints of hip or knee soreness or stiffness; the pain may be intermittent. A painful limp, quadriceps muscle atrophy, and pain of insidious onset may also be present.

Diagnostic Evaluation

The diagnosis is made by radiographic examination. A bone scan or MRI study may reveal necrosis and irregularity of the femoral head. However, in the vast majority of cases plain radiographs of the femoral head will disclose the problem.

Therapeutic Management

Treatment strives to maintain the spherical shape of the femoral head as it regenerates and to reduce the risk of permanent stiffness and degenerative arthritis. The femoral head is maintained in the acetabulum and protected from the stress of weight bearing during the healing process. In addition, synovitis should be reduced to improve range of motion. Some physicians, however, do not believe that weight bearing is harmful as long as the femur remains in the acetabulum. There is some lack of consensus as to whether treatment alters the course of the disorder (Koop & Quanbeck, 1996).

Because Legg-Calvé-Perthes disease is first identified from the child's complaints of a painful, stiff hip joint, the physician may recommend non-weight-bearing, range-of-motion exercises and bed rest. If improvement is not seen within a week to 10 days and the child is still unable to abduct the hip, alternative methods of treatment are considered.

For children with severe necrosis, the femoral head is abducted and internally rotated in relation to the acetabulum through some type of containment device that uses the acetabulum to maintain the spherical shape of the femoral head. Containment prevents the acetabulum from rubbing against the weakened portion of the femoral head and creating a flat shape. Methods of containment usually include bracing or surgical intervention.

The position of the femoral head is maintained in the acetabulum by abducting the leg. The child is fitted with an abduction brace that prevents weight bearing on the affected side while allowing the hip to move freely. Also, non-weight-bearing exercises are needed to maintain muscle integrity while the child wears the brace during a period of up to 1 to 3 years.

Surgical procedures include an osteotomy, which places the femur more securely into the acetabulum, or an innominate osteotomy, which rotates the acetabulum to completely cover the femoral head. Many physicians recommend surgical intervention because it reduces treatment time and eliminates problems with compliance.

NURSING CARE
The Child with Legg-Calvé-Perthes Disease

Assessment

Assessment of a child with Legg-Calvé-Perthes disease reveals loss of internal hip rotation and limited abduction. The nurse should determine how long the child has been limping as well as the pattern, timing, and severity of the pain. The pain may be referred to the thigh or knee. The child will describe the pain as increasing with activity and decreasing with rest. Physical examination of the extremity may reveal muscle wasting of the thigh and buttock, a reflection of disuse. Shortening of the extremity on the affected side indicates collapse of the femoral head.

Nursing Diagnosis and Planning

The following nursing diagnoses and expected outcomes may be appropriate following assessment of the child with Legg-Calvé-Perthes disease:

- Risk for Injury related to necrosis and collapse of the femoral head.
  Expected Outcome: The child will remain free of injury.
- Impaired Physical Mobility related to the disease process and activity restrictions.
  Expected Outcome: The child will tolerate activity restrictions and comply with treatment regimen.

- Risk for Impaired Skin Integrity related to the brace.
  Expected Outcome: The child will maintain skin integrity.
- Body Image Disturbance related to the corrective brace.
  Expected Outcome: The child will have an increased sense of self-esteem and self-worth; the child will exhibit age-appropriate behaviors.
- Knowledge Deficit about the condition and home management related to insufficient prior information.
  Expected Outcomes: The parents will provide safe home care, demonstrate the correct use of the brace or crutches, perform neurovascular assessments, and provide age-appropriate activities for their child.

Interventions

Facilitating Appropriate Activity

Activity restrictions are one of the most problematic areas in the care of a child with Legg-Calvé-Perthes disease. The child may become frustrated and angry when unable to meet the physical and social demands of peers. Initially the child may appear to adjust to the lifestyle restrictions, but the nurse must be alert to subtle indicators of rebelliousness and uncooperative behavior. Other children will adapt quickly to the appliance they wear and demonstrate incredible activity levels. Never construe a child's refusal to comply with treatment regimens as maladaptive behavior. The demand to keep up with their peers is sometimes so great that children are simply unable to make cognitively appropriate choices regarding their health.

Returning to school with a brace poses unique problems as well. The school nurse and the child's teacher should be involved in the discharge planning because it is important that the child participate in as many school-related activities as possible. Acknowledging the child's mobility limitations and working with school officials to identify appropriate alternatives will ensure a successful school reentry. Emphasizing hobbies and other creative activities provides ways for the child to excel and feel a sense of accomplishment.

Teaching Home Management

Because the child will receive the greater part of care as an outpatient, nursing care should focus on home care and management of the appliance selected for therapy. Parents will need information concerning the purpose, application, and care of the appliance. The family must clearly understand the issue of compliance and the role it will play in the healing process. Parents will need to learn how to perform neurovascular assessments. Also, safety issues regarding the child's mobility when wearing the brace should be identified. The physical therapist and occupational therapist are important resources for the parents.

The purpose of any brace used to treat Legg-Calvé-Perthes disease is to distribute the child's weight to the ischial tuberosities. By design, the appliance places additional stress on the child's skin. Advise the parent to assess the child's skin condition frequently and identify any friction areas. Teach parents to check bony prominences; any reddened area on the skin that persists longer than 20 to 30 minutes demands immediate attention.

Mild soaps (Dove, Cetaphil) should be used during bathing; do not use moisturizers on pressure areas. Instead, rubbing alcohol (70%) is recommended to toughen the skin. If lotion or moisturizers are used on the skin, it is important to wipe the excess off to prevent skin breakdown. Bony prominences should not be massaged. Place protective foam or transparent dressings over susceptible areas. If appropriate, protective clothing may be worn under the brace, but keep the clothing as free from wrinkles as possible.

Evaluation

- Has the hip healed without complications or additional injury?
- Does the child exhibit normal joint and muscular integrity?
- Does the child participate in age-appropriate peer and school-related activities, within activity limitations?
- Is the child's skin intact, smooth, clear, and free from pressure areas?
- Do the parents verbalize an understanding of the child's treatment regimen?
- Are the parents able to provide developmentally appropriate activities for their child?

Slipped Capital Femoral Epiphysis

Slipped capital femoral epiphysis is a condition that affects the upper (capital) femoral growth plate. It is a hip disorder related to growth, particularly during adolescence.

Etiology and Incidence

The cause of slipped capital femoral epiphysis is unknown. Slippage appears to be related to increased stress on the proximal femur at a time when the epiphyseal plate is thinning in preparation for eventual closure. The weakness of the growth plate may be related to adolescent hormonal imbalance and is seen most frequently in adolescents who are tall and heavy for their age but have not yet developed secondary sex characteristics.

The annual incidence of slipped capital femoral epiphysis is up to 10.8 per 100,000 (Benchot, 1996). The average age at onset is 11½ years for girls and 13 years for boys, but boys are affected twice as often as girls. There may be an increased incidence in families. The majority of affected adolescents exceed the 95th percentile for weight and the 90th percentile for height. Although initially the condition is unilateral, it can become bilateral.

Pathophysiology

The epiphyseal plate begins to thin in response to hormonal influences during adolescence. Eventually the plate closes completely, when the adolescent has reached skeletal maturity. Increased body weight and height place more stress on the epiphyses, causing a relative displacement (slip) of the femoral neck from the femoral head; the movement appears to be in a posterior and inferior direction. In most instances the slippage occurs gradually.

CRITICAL THINKING EXERCISE 50–1

Children often come to the ambulatory care setting complaining of hip or knee pain and walking with a limp.

Compare and contrast the three common hip disorders in children.

Manifestations and Diagnostic Evaluation

The classic manifestations of slipped capital femoral epiphysis include a limp, gait disturbance, and pain. The pain usually is in the groin, thigh, or knee; it is intermittent and worse with activity. The leg often is externally rotated. Because the adolescent often presents with knee pain, hip involvement may be overlooked. Presenting symptoms along with characteristic growth signs suggest the diagnosis, so hip disease should be ruled out in adolescents who present with knee pain. Radiographs confirm the diagnosis. Radiographs are obtained with the legs in a frog-leg position.

Therapeutic Management and Nursing Considerations

Treatment is usually surgical: a screw inserted across the growth plate secures the femoral head and prevents further slippage. More severe slips may require reconstruction of the femoral head, followed by pinning.

As soon as the diagnosis is made, the adolescent is admitted to the hospital and placed on bed rest to prevent exacerbation of the slip. Often Buck extension is used preoperatively to relieve muscle spasms and keep the hip in alignment. Postoperatively, the adolescent uses crutches with partial weight bearing for 2 to 6 weeks. The screw or pin usually is removed after several years.

The nurse should assess adolescents for slipped capital femoral epiphysis any time an adolescent complains of knee or thigh pain. Interventions are similar to those for any child in traction or undergoing surgery. Postoperatively, the adolescent needs to be taught isometric exercises and crutch walking. Weight control may be an issue; the adolescent needs to learn to develop good nutritional habits and avoid high-calorie foods. Referral to a dietician may be helpful. Provide the adolescent and parent with written instructions prior to discharge.

Fractures

Although fractures are not always serious, they are important because they may lead to life-threatening complications. A fracture is a break or disruption in a bone's continuity. Generally, fractures occur when excessive or traumatic force exceeds the strength of the bone.

Etiology

Fractures in children usually result from increased mobility and inadequate or immature motor and cognitive skills. They may result from trauma (falls, motor vehicle accidents, sports injuries, child abuse) or bone diseases that result in abnormally fragile bones (e.g., osteogenesis imperfecta).

An understanding of growth and development is helpful when assessing trauma in specific age groups. For example, fractures in infancy are generally rare because of the cartilaginous quality of the skeleton. Fractures in infants are usually the result of trauma during birth or nonaccidental trauma. Therefore, fractures in infants warrant further investigation to rule out the possibility of child abuse.

Accidental injury is the leading cause of death in children of all ages (see Chapter 34). Trauma, probably the most ominous threat to children today, frequently causes fractures.

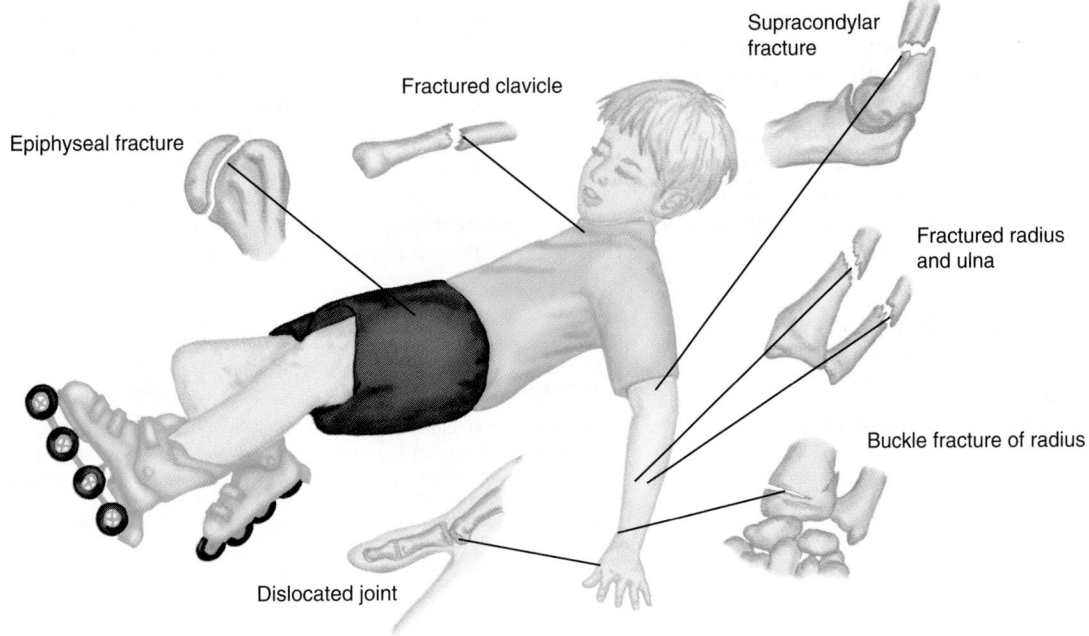

FIGURE 50–7

Upper extremity fractures in children often occur when the child attempts to break a fall with an outstretched arm.

In fact, musculoskeletal trauma accounts for half of injury-related emergency room visits (England & Sundberg, 1996).

The other major cause of children's fractures is falls. Because children attempt to protect themselves, the outstretched arm receives the full force of the fall (Fig. 50–7). This type of fall can affect every part of that outstretched arm (wrist, elbow, shoulder).

A fractured clavicle may occur at any age. Lack of movement or a pseudoparalysis of the upper arm may be the only sign in an infant who has sustained a fractured clavicle during birth. An older child will complain of pain and will experience a swelling on the clavicle at the point of the fracture. A supracondylar humeral fracture is a serious injury because it may lead to circulatory impairment, cellular necrosis, and ischemic contracture (Volkmann's contracture).

Regardless of the cause of the fracture, it is important to remember that a child with an uncomplicated fracture should not present with signs of shock. If shock is evident, more than likely there is a more serious problem, and a thorough assessment is required.

Incidence

Because the daily actions of children include numerous gross motor activities that place them at risk for injuries, fractures are common during childhood and adolescence.

PATHOPHYSIOLOGY

of Fractures

When a fracture occurs, the break in the continuity of the bone results in bone fragmentation and injury to the surrounding tissues. Torn blood vessels cause bleeding from the bone and tissues around the bone fragments. As blood clots at the site, fibrin strands provide a network for healing. Osteoblasts begin forming in immense numbers almost immediately after the injury. This increased osteoblastic activity results in the formation of new bone matrix between the bone fragments. Calcium salts are deposited in the new bone matrix, forming a *callus*. The callus is responsible for stability and support of the fracture while healing occurs. Gradually the callus is formed into new bone. Remodeling, or correction of an injury at the fracture site through the buildup of callus, occurs more rapidly in growing children.

Fractures are referred to as simple or compound. A fracture that is *simple* (closed) is characterized as intact with no breaks in the skin. If wounds accompany a simple fracture, they are usually superficial or unrelated to the fracture. The nurse should never assume, however, that a simple fracture does not warrant close assessment. It is quite possible that other problems associated with the injury exist. For example, if hemorrhage occurs, it would be internal.

A systemic risk associated with fractures, especially multiple fractures or femur fractures, is emboli. Emboli can form from postinjury bleeding with clotting or from fat droplets, shed from the fractured bone marrow (fat embolism), that enter the circulatory system and travel to the lungs or brain.

(continued)

Fractures in which the skin, subcutaneous tissue, or muscle has been broken are called *compound* (open) fractures. Infection is a risk with this type of fracture because organisms can enter the fracture site through the wound. Children with compound fractures are at risk for blood loss secondary to external hemorrhage.

Epiphyseal injuries occur when a break or fracture occurs between the shaft of the bone and epiphyseal plate. In a growing bone, the region of least resistance to stress is the area between the metaphysis and the cartilaginous epiphyseal plate. The amount of growth arrest associated with an epiphyseal injury is determined by the extent of the damage to the epiphyseal plate. If the germinal cells remain with the epiphysis and appear uninjured, healing is rapid and growth is seldom affected. If the germinal layer is destroyed, however, growth disturbances will occur. The Salter-Harris classification system classifies epiphyseal growth plate injuries and their associated risk of growth disturbance.

Pediatric fractures are seldom complete breaks. Rather, children's bones tend to bend or buckle because of increased flexibility. This flexibility is due to a thicker periosteum and increased amounts of immature bone.

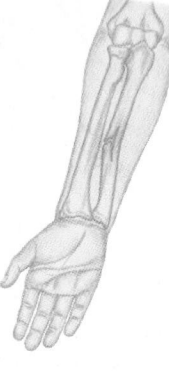

Greenstick

Break occurs through the periosteum on one side of the bone while only bowing or buckling on the other side. Seen most frequently in forearm.

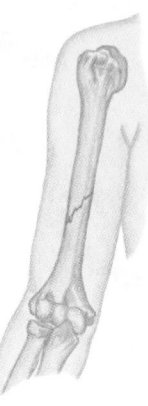

Spiral

Twisted or circular break that affects the length rather than the width. Seen frequently in child abuse.

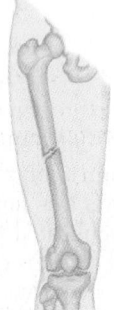

Oblique

Diagonal or slanting break that occurs between the horizontal and perpendicular planes of the bone.

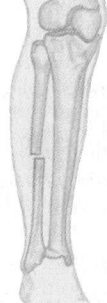

Transverse

Break or fracture line occurs at right angles to the long axis of the bone.

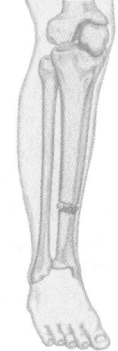

Comminuted

Bone is splintered into pieces. This is a rare occurrence in children.

Physeal growth plate injuries: Salter-Harris classification. Epiphyseal fractures are common in children.

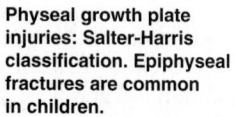
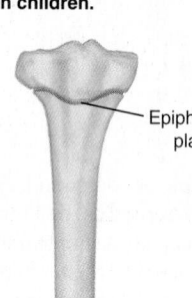

Epiphyseal plate

Epiphyseal plate

Type I

Epiphysis is completely separated from the metaphysis without fracture.

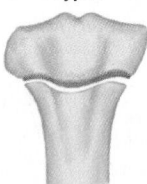

Type II

Transverse fracture extends through the separated epiphyseal plate, producing triangular break.

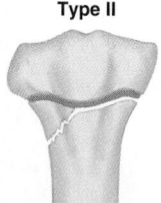

Type III

Fracture extends through part of the epiphyseal plate into the joint.

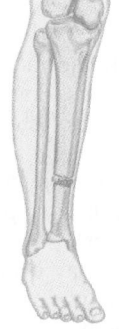

Type IV

Fracture extends through the epiphyseal plate and through the metaphysis.

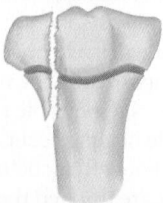

Type V

Epiphyseal plate is crushed, causing cell death in growth plate.

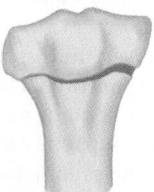
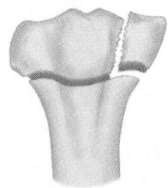

Children between ages 5 and 9 are most likely to experience fractures, particularly of the hip and femur, related to motor vehicle accidents (see Chapter 34). The most common sites of fractures in children are the ulna, clavicle, tibia, and femur. Epiphyseal fractures are also common in children. A severe epiphyseal fracture can interfere with bone growth.

Manifestations

The signs and symptoms of a fracture vary with the location, type, and cause of the injury. General manifestations include pain or tenderness at the site, immobility or decreased range of motion, deformity of the extremity, and edema. Other signs and symptoms include crepitus, ecchymosis, erythema, muscle spasm, and inability to bear weight.

Diagnostic Evaluation

Local signs and symptoms of a fracture are not always present, which may make assessment of a fracture difficult. Radiography of the skeleton is the most effective tool for determining the type and location of a fracture. Often a radiograph of the unaffected extremity is obtained for comparison purposes, especially when the physician is trying to determine whether a line on the radiograph represents a fracture or merely an epiphyseal line. Because the periosteum of children's bones is thicker and stronger than in adults, it is less likely to displace at the fracture site. Consequently, the fracture may not be visible on radiographs until healing begins. Radiographs are also obtained after fracture reduction and during the healing process to assess progress.

Therapeutic Management

The key to healing is correct fracture reduction and retention. *Reduction* is the repositioning of the bone fragments into normal alignment. *Retention* entails the application of a device or mechanism that maintains alignment until healing occurs.

REDUCTION METHODS

Fractures are treated by either closed or open reduction. Closed reduction is accomplished by manual alignment of the fragments followed by immobilization. Simple or closed fractures are treated by closed reduction. Hospitalization is seldom necessary for closed reduction, and most of these fractures heal without complications.

Open reduction entails the surgical insertion of internal fixation devices such as rods, wires, or pins that help maintain alignment while healing occurs. External fixation devices (e.g., Ilizarov external fixator) may also be used to lengthen bones and correct angular deformities that involve bone and soft tissue. External fixators allow for periodic changes in alignment and length of the bone. In fact, external fixation devices are becoming so common in the treatment of fractures that traction is infrequently used. Because the screws of the external fixator pass through the skin to anchor in the bone, meticulous assessment of entry sites is necessary. Pin care may be recommended to prevent infection. General anesthesia is necessary for removal of external fixation devices.

When open reduction is employed, hospitalization is required and the child is monitored for postoperative complications. Complications after open reduction include delayed healing and nonunion. Infections may also interfere with recovery. Close assessment by the health care team as well as strict adherence to sterile technique during dressing changes can decrease the risk of postoperative problems and promote healing.

RETENTION

Once correct alignment of the fracture is achieved, it is imperative to protect the fracture site as well as maintain position of the fragments. This is accomplished through the application of a cast or, in certain situations, traction, which effectively immobilizes the area while healing occurs.

Nursing Considerations

INITIAL TRAUMA ASSESSMENT

Nursing assessment of the child with a traumatic fracture should begin with a thorough assessment of the child's airway, breathing, and circulation (see Chapter 34). Once this is done, obtain a history of the circumstances surrounding the fracture. Determining the cause of any fracture is important because nonaccidental trauma may be involved. Both a complete history of how the fracture occurred and physical findings are important if child abuse is suspected.

Examine the fracture site for bruising, skin lacerations, and swelling. Generally the child will favor the extremity, even to the point of cradling or supporting it. Often the child will complain of numbness and tingling distal to the fracture site. Movement may be limited. The area of the fracture is important to determine because growth plate injuries are not always evident on radiographs.

ASSESSING FOR COMPARTMENT SYNDROME

Serious complications such as nerve compression, circulatory impairment, or compartment syndrome can result from swelling caused by trauma or an immobilizing device. The muscles and nerves of the upper and lower extremities are enclosed in compartments that are surrounded by tough, inelastic fascia. *Compartment syndrome* occurs when swelling causes pressure within this closed space to rise. The increased pressure compromises circulation to the muscles and nerves within the compartment and can result in paralysis and necrosis of tissues. Signs of compartment syndrome include severe pain, often unrelieved by analgesics, and signs of neurovascular impairment. Compartment syndrome is not uncommon in forearm fractures; therefore, assess the quality of the radial pulse and the child's ability to extend the fingers. If extending the fingers produces pain, notify the physician. When assessing a complaint of pain, make a distinction between pain related to the fracture and burning sensations distal to the fracture. Pain associated with compartment syndrome usually is described as more intense than would be expected from the severity of the injury and it does not remit with analgesics. Because children who sustain fractures are treated with casts or traction, nursing diagnoses, planning, intervention, and evaluation are the same as for any child in a cast or traction.

Soft-Tissue Injuries: Sprains, Strains, and Contusions

Soft-tissue injuries are common among children. They are usually due to accidents during play or athletic activities.

Etiology

Sprains occur as a result of trauma to a joint in which ligaments are stretched or partially or completely torn. *Strains*, also known as pulls, tears, or ruptures, result from an excessive stretch of muscle. *Contusions* occur when soft tissue, muscle, or subcutaneous tissues are damaged. Sprains and contusions frequently accompany each other. *Dislocations* occur when a joint is disrupted in such a way that articulating surfaces are no longer in contact.

Incidence

Sprains are not frequently seen in young children because of their poorly developed epiphyseal plate. A twisting or turning injury will more likely result in a fracture than a sprain because the epiphyseal plate is weaker. Sprains and strains are more commonly seen in adolescents and are frequently the result of athletic injuries. In general, sprains and contusions are more likely to occur with more physical or violent sports activities.

Manifestations and Diagnostic Evaluation

Manifestations of soft tissue injuries include pain, swelling, localized tenderness, limited range of motion, poor weight bearing, and a pop or snapping sound (sprain). The diagnosis is based on the clinical picture. An x-ray, however, may be ordered to rule out a fracture.

Therapeutic Management

Control of swelling and the prevention of further injury are tantamount with sprains and contusions. Swelling can inhibit healing by keeping the ligament ends apart and increasing fibrous scarring. The earlier that treatment is initiated, the less severe the swelling and immobility become.

CRITICAL TO REMEMBER
· · · · · · · · · · ·
The Child with a Soft-Tissue Injury

The first 6 to 12 hours after soft-tissue injury are the most important in controlling swelling and reducing muscle damage. Treatment of soft-tissue injuries is summarized in the acronyms RICE or ICES:

R = Rest
I = Ice
C = Compression
E = Elevation

I = Ice
C = Compression
E = Elevation
S = Support

The injured area should be wrapped immediately with a thin layer of elastic bandage or elastic wrap to support the joint and control the swelling. To reduce the swelling, ice is applied to the injured area, with additional wrap being used to secure the ice. Ice should be applied for no longer than 20 minutes every 1 to 4 hours, even though the effects of the ice can last as long as 5 to 6 hours. Ice is used for several days. Nonsteroidal anti-inflammatory drugs (NSAIDs) alleviate pain and reduce inflammation.

For more severe soft tissue injury, the child should avoid weight bearing for 3 days; crutches may be necessary to be sure the child does not bear weight. An air cast may be used over the elastic wrap; the child will use the air cast for several weeks while the joint is healing. When the swelling and pain have diminished, the child can begin stretching and isometric exercises to improve joint stability.

Immobilization of the injured joint and cold application are generally very effective in the treatment of incomplete ligament tears. A complete rupture could require surgery to prevent excessive scar formation and long-term joint mobility problems. Application of a cast or splint for 4 to 5 weeks may also be necessary, especially for knee injuries.

Nursing Considerations

One of the major functions of the nurse when assessing a sprain is to determine the severity of the injury. Assess the child for neurovascular impairment as well as for diminished range of motion. The initial examination may reveal localized tenderness over the injured joint as well as limited joint mobility.

Analgesics such as ibuprofen or acetaminophen are appropriate for pain management. Distraction as well as age-appropriate play activities can be very effective in managing a child's pain.

The nurse needs to keep the extremity elevated above the heart. This position enhances venous return and aids in reducing the swelling. Pillows placed beneath the extremity will provide support as well as comfort. When applying the elastic wrap, assess neurovascular status because it is possible to apply the wrap too tightly.

Stretching and strengthening exercises are helpful in maintaining joint and muscle integrity. These exercises are done passively at first. As healing progresses, teach the child active stretching and strengthening exercises. Asking parents for a return demonstration helps evaluate the effectiveness of teaching. Physical therapy referrals may be helpful as well.

The amount of time needed for healing is determined by the severity of the injury. Weight bearing is increased gradually as the pain subsides. More severe injuries may require partial weight-bearing exercises, with full weight bearing introduced once the swelling has resolved. Sports activities may be restricted for 3 to 8 weeks.

Review the principles of rest, support, and the application of ice with the parents and child. If wraps, splints, or air casts are used, teach the parents and child how to assess neurovascular status. If crutches are required, review the principles of crutch walking with both the parents and the child. Make sure all family members understand activity and sports restrictions. Discuss follow-up appointments and the importance of adhering to activity restrictions until the injury has healed and the child has been cleared for sports.

Osgood-Schlatter Disease

The classic picture of Osgood-Schlatter disease is bilateral knee pain that is exacerbated by running, jumping, or climbing stairs in a very active adolescent boy who is involved in sports activities. The child will point to the tibial tubercle as the site of pain.

Etiology, Incidence, and Pathophysiology

The etiology of Osgood-Schlatter disease is believed to be related to repetitive stress from sports-related activities, combined with overuse of immature muscles and tendons over an extended period of time and an imbalance in the strength of the quadriceps muscle during adolescent growth. Osgood-Schlatter disease occurs in boys and girls between ages 8 and 16 years, although it is more common in boys. Usually both knees are involved.

During the adolescent growth spurt, overuse trauma causes inflammation in the tibial tubercle at the tendon insertion site. This causes tendinitis of the distal infrapatellar tendon. Without treatment, the tubercle enlarges and can cause later functional and cosmetic problems.

Manifestations and Diagnostic Evaluation

Osgood-Schlatter disease is characterized by the insidious onset of knee pain and tenderness, followed by swelling of the tibial tubercle and difficulty with weight bearing. The diagnosis is based on the clinical picture and x-ray examination.

Therapeutic Management

Treatment is conservative because the disorder is usually self-limiting. Avoiding activities such as kneeling, bicycling, and running provides adequate pain control. In some cases the physician may suggest wrapping the affected knee with elastic bandages. This limits knee flexion, reduces swelling, and provides time for healing. Physical therapy for quadriceps stretching and strengthening might be required.

In severe cases, ice, heat, and NSAIDs are helpful. A knee immobilizer or casting with the knee in full extension may be necessary to decrease pain. Activity may be restricted for 6 weeks or more. Improvement generally is seen within 6 to 8 weeks, and the problem disappears once growth stops.

NURSING CARE
. . . .
The Child with Osgood-Schlatter Disease

Assessment

Since Osgood-Schlatter disease develops in response to repetitive stress from sports-related activities, the nurse should obtain a thorough history of the child's activities.

Examine the knee for pain, tenderness, and swelling over the proximal tibia.

Pain that is aggravated by activities that require kneeling, running, or climbing stairs is an important feature of this disease. Inability to shift from a squatting position to a standing position without experiencing pain is highly significant. When asked to identify the area that hurts, the child will point to the tibial tubercle.

Nursing Diagnosis and Planning

The following nursing diagnoses and expected outcomes may be appropriate following assessment of the child with Osgood-Schlatter disease:

- Noncompliance related to age and activity restrictions. **Expected Outcome:** The child will comply with activity restrictions.
- Self-Esteem Disturbance related to decreased physical mobility and reduced involvement in age-appropriate activities. **Expected Outcome:** The child will maintain peer activities and involvement in school activities.
- Knowledge Deficit (parental) about home care and therapeutic regimen, related to unfamiliarity with the condition and its management. **Expected Outcome:** The parents will verbalize an understanding of the child's treatment plan and identify concerns or issues regarding home care.

Interventions

Nurses working with school-age children and adolescents should have a clear understanding of Osgood-Schlatter disease so that a simple complaint of knee pain is not overlooked or incorrectly diagnosed, resulting in more serious problems later.

The restrictions placed on the child's activity may interfere with the healthy development of peer relationships and self-esteem. Missing school or sports-related activities, limited interactions with peers, or even the need for special arrangements to participate in a peer-related activity contribute to the child's sense of isolation and alienation. Continued contact with peers is important to help the child achieve age-appropriate developmental tasks.

Parents need to be encouraged to express their fears and concerns. Since prevention of sports-related injuries should be the primary concern among all those involved in youth athletic participation, injury prevention education should be provided by the school nurse to all children involved in athletics (Ostrum, 1993).

Reassure parents that the child will outgrow this problem. Although Osgood-Schlatter disease is self-limiting, activity restrictions must be clearly understood by the parents. Before the child resumes athletics, the parents and child should discuss the advisability of such activities with their physician. Hamstring stretching exercises may be helpful, but frequently physical therapy is required. This can prove to be expensive.

Evaluation

- Does the child have full range of motion after treatment and healing?
- Is the child free of pain?

- Do the parents verbalize an understanding of the child's treatment regimen?
- Do the parents provide developmentally appropriate activities for their child, within activity limitations and does the child comply with activity restrictions?

Osteogenesis Imperfecta

Etiology

Osteogenesis imperfecta, also known as brittle bone disease, is an inherited disorder characterized by connective tissue and bone defects. Depending on the type of inheritance pattern, the child's symptoms will be more or less severe.

Manifestations

In the most common type of osteogenesis imperfecta (type 1, or autosomal dominant), the child experiences osteoporosis, excessive bone fragility, blue sclerae, discolored teeth, and deafness by age 20 to 30 years as a result of problems with bony ear structures. The child's skin may appear transparent. Eventual adult height is shorter than average. By far the most common sign is frequent fractures. Sometimes the excessive number of old fractures can raise suspicion of child abuse in health care personnel unfamiliar with the disease.

Diagnostic Evaluation

Clinical evaluation is very helpful in diagnosing osteogenesis imperfecta, with x-rays identifying current or healed fractures. Genetic testing may be ordered to rule out hereditary problems as well as to advise the parents on the risk of the disease for other children.

Therapeutic Management

Treatment strives to maintain the integrity of the musculoskeletal system and prevent fractures. Various approaches, including traction, casting, fixation, and other orthopedic stabilizing methods, are used.

Nursing Considerations

The child with osteogenesis imperfecta has a history of multiple fractures and delayed growth. The extremities may have an angular deformity secondary to old fractures. Upon examination, the nurse may note deformities of the leg and kyphoscoliosis. The child will appear short because of com-

PATHOPHYSIOLOGY
. . . .
of Osteogenesis Imperfecta

In osteogenesis imperfecta, there is a biochemical defect in the synthesis of collagen. Because collagen is an essential component of connective tissue, the abnormal collagen results in the incomplete development of bones, teeth, ligaments, and sclerae. Bones are brittle and extremely fragile, and fracture easily.

pression fractures of the spine, and joint mobility will be unusual due to relaxed ligaments. The child's teeth may appear discolored due to abnormal enamel. Too often, because of the child's appearance, people assume that the child is cognitively impaired. Children with osteogenesis imperfecta have normal or above normal intelligence.

No effective treatment has been developed for osteogenesis imperfecta; therefore providing care for a child with this disease requires attention to detail and the use of anticipatory guidance.

Identifying mobility issues that affect the child's functioning is important. Highest priority is given to preventing fractures and maintaining muscle and joint integrity. Gentle turning, passive range-of-motion exercises, daily skin care, and thorough assessment of high-stress areas of the body are necessary to protect the child from fractures and related complications.

Excessive weight gain can place undue stress on the musculoskeletal system. Maintaining optimal physiologic functioning is critical if the complications of osteogenesis imperfecta are to be avoided. Instruct parents about nutritional guidelines that support healthy growth and development, including emphasizing high-calcium foods. If necessary, calcium, magnesium, and vitamin supplements may be added to the diet.

Because each child is different, responses to the disease will vary. Coping with a chronic illness (see Chapter 36) that involves repeated hospitalizations and restricted mobility places incredible stress on the child and family. Learning how to accept the illness and how to adapt to the demands of the disease while meeting the needs of the family stresses the parents' ability to cope. The nurse needs to become aware of family dynamics, determine how the illness is affecting the family system, and assess the effectiveness of current coping strategies. Once this is done, appropriate interventions should be developed to address problematic areas.

Parents will need assistance with dressing and bathing the child. Clothing may have to be altered to allow for ease in dressing and undressing. If the child is to be discharged with a cast, the nurse should review the principles of cast care and assessment of neurovascular status. Because of the risk of accidental fractures, the nurse should review the principles of safety during play and normal activities. A home referral may be appropriate to assist the family in the transition from hospital to home.

Osteomyelitis

Osteomyelitis is a bacterial infection of the bone that involves the cortex or marrow cavity. It is classified as acute or chronic. Osteomyelitis is considered chronic if the infection persists longer than a month or does not respond to the initial antibiotic protocol. Regardless of advances in antibiotic treatment, osteomyelitis is a serious problem that can be very difficult to diagnose and, if inadequately treated, results in high morbidity.

Etiology

Bacteria infiltrate the bone through endogenous routes (e.g., skin or respiratory infections, abscessed teeth, acute otitis media) or exogenous routes (e.g., injury or surgical procedures). The infection is usually the result of vascular

PATHOPHYSIOLOGY
of Osteomyelitis

Osteomyelitis occurs most frequently in the metaphyseal region of the long bones, especially the femur or tibia. Bacteria enter the metaphysis via the osseous circulation, and the inflammatory process begins. Pus forms and spreads toward the medullary canal as well as the cortex of the bone. Because the periosteum of a child's bone is thick and easily displaced, pus quickly spreads along the shaft of the bone. Involucrum, or new bone, will develop in an attempt to isolate the infection. As a result, the cortex of the bone becomes devascularized and the area of necrotic bone detaches to form a separate area called a sequestrum (Herndon, 1993).

Large sections of sequestrum may eventually become honeycombed with cavities or sinuses that contain infective material. These cavities are so effectively walled off that antibiotic therapy may not be successful. Thus it is possible for osteomyelitis to recur in a chronic form.

spread of the bacteria. Osteomyelitis also may occur as a result of direct entry (open fracture) or injury to surrounding soft tissues (cellulitis). External fixation devices and skeletal traction can also lead to osteomyelitis. Although strict adherence to aseptic techniques and frequent assessments of pin sites have greatly controlled this problem, the development of osteomyelitis can be a serious deterrent to successful healing.

The most common causative organism in all ages is *Staphylococcus aureus. Streptococcus pneumoniae, Hemophilus influenzae* (in infants), and *Escherichia coli* and group B streptococci (in neonates) also are responsible for osteomyelitis. The most common causative organism for osteomyelitis in children with sickle cell anemia is *Salmonella.*

Incidence

Osteomyelitis may occur at any age, but yearly it affects 1 in 5,000 children under the age of 13 years (Sonnen & Henry, 1996). Boys are affected at least two times as often as girls. Although osteomyelitis is more likely to occur during growth spurts, the age groups typically affected are preschoolers and adolescents.

Manifestations

The manifestations of osteomyelitis in infants can be vague and nonspecific, such as fever, irritability, and feeding difficulties. Some infants demonstrate signs of sepsis. In the older child the major signs and symptoms include pain, warmth, and tenderness localized over the site of infection; favoring the affected extremity; erythema; limited range of motion; and systemic manifestations such as fever and lethargy.

Diagnostic Evaluation

Osteomyelitis is diagnosed from a positive blood culture, bone purulence, localized edema or erythema, or a positive

imaging study (Sonnen & Henry, 1996). The erythrocyte sedimentation rate (ESR), which indicates an inflammatory process, is usually elevated. An elevated white blood cell count may or may not be present. Bone changes may not be apparent on x-ray until 7 to 14 days after the onset of symptoms (Herndon, 1993). Bone scans are helpful in localizing the area of increased vascularity.

Therapeutic Management

Once a culture has been done and the organism's sensitivity to antibiotics determined, antibiotic treatment is initiated. Controversy exists regarding the length of time required for antibiotic therapy, the need for intravenous versus oral antibiotics, and the role of bactericidal antibiotics and therapeutic blood levels. Nevertheless, it is generally recommended that therapy for osteomyelitis requires 4 to 6 weeks of high-dose parenteral therapy, preferably through a peripherally inserted central catheter (PICC).

Because the antibiotics are administered over an extended period of time and high-dose therapy may be necessary to obtain the desired outcome, assessing the child's response to the antibiotics is an integral part of the treatment protocol. Peak and trough serum antibiotic levels are monitored closely. Renal and hepatic function should be monitored, and blood cell counts done frequently to determine bone marrow activity. Children receiving aminoglycosides should be assessed periodically for side effects such as ototoxicity and nephrotoxicity.

To limit the spread of infection and to promote healing, the child is placed on complete bed rest. The extremity may be immobilized with a splint or bivalved cast. Surgical intervention may be necessary if an abscess is present or if the infection fails to respond to antibiotics. Invasive procedures include draining the abscess, debriding necrotic tissue, and performing a sequestrectomy (removal of the sequestrum). Osteomyelitis of the proximal femur generally requires some type of surgical decompression because septic arthritis of the hip may accompany this infection. Aseptic technique is critical after any type of orthopedic surgery because a secondary infection could inhibit the healing process.

NURSING CARE
The Child with Osteomyelitis

Assessment

Although it may be difficult for parents to recall every injury their child has suffered, a thorough history of recent falls or traumas is helpful in determining the source of the infection. The nurse should carefully examine the affected area and note any pain, tenderness, erythema, or swelling. Usually the child will appear to protect the extremity, even tensing adjacent muscles and demonstrating reluctance to straighten or move the extremity.

Nursing Diagnosis and Planning

The following nursing diagnoses and expected outcomes may be appropriate following assessment of the child with osteomyelitis:

■ Risk for Injury related to neurovascular impairment and complications related to antibiotic therapy.

Expected Outcome: The child will remain free from injury, as evidenced by neurovascular functioning and the absence of iatrogenic problems.

- Pain related to the infectious process.
  Expected Outcome: The child will experience a decrease in pain.
- Impaired Physical Mobility related to the infectious process and activity restrictions.
  Expected Outcome: The child will accept the activity restrictions, as evidenced by increased compliance with treatment plan.
- Altered Growth and Development related to hospitalization and immobility.
  Expected Outcome: The child will exhibit age-appropriate growth and developmental behavior, increased self-care behavior, and normal sleep patterns.
- Knowledge Deficit about home management of long-term antibiotic therapy related to unfamiliarity with the procedure.
  Expected Outcomes: The parents will demonstrate the correct administration of antibiotics, verbalize reportable adverse effects, and identify any other concerns or issues regarding home care.

Interventions

Chart the child's neurovascular and pain status at least once a shift. Because any movement of the involved extremity will be accompanied by discomfort, the extremity should be immobilized and supported with pillows. When moving or turning is necessary, ask the child what is the most comfortable way to achieve position changes. If the child is preverbal or not able to explain, the nurse should consult the parents. During the acute phase, the pain may be quite severe and the child should be premedicated with an analgesic before any repositioning.

Administering Intravenous Antibiotics

Because it is important to maintain a long-term intravenous site for antibiotic administration, the nurse carefully and frequently monitors the site for signs of complications (see Chapter 37) and flushes the line according to facility protocol.

The nurse should have a thorough knowledge of the antibiotic being given. This includes calculating dosage based on body weight or surface area, reviewing side and adverse effects, and determining if therapeutic blood levels are required. If the level of drug in the patient's blood exceeds the therapeutic range, the antibiotic should be withheld and the physician notified. Notify the physician also if the level is below the therapeutic level.

Because the child will probably be receiving multiple antibiotics, compatibility is important. Allergies and any problems the parents may have encountered during previous antibiotic administration should be noted. Periodically the nurse should review current laboratory data to ensure adequate liver and kidney function. A complete blood cell count and ESR should be measured on a regular basis to evaluate the child's response to treatment.

Providing Wound Care

Standard precautions should be maintained at all times. Sterile technique and appropriate removal of soiled materials should be strictly enforced. Children with surgical wounds or drains need close monitoring. Drainage should be measured as accurately as possible and recorded at the end of the shift. The color and consistency of the drainage and any unusual odor should be noted in the nurses' notes. A description of the wound should also be included.

Maintaining Activity Limitations

Bed rest or non-weight-bearing is very important to prevent spread of the infection. Returning the child to full weight-bearing and self-care activities is determined by the child's response to treatment and by the physician's assessment of the healing process.

Immobility can diminish the child's appetite. Meeting the child's nutritional needs is essential to facilitate growth and development and to assist with the healing process. The child should receive a diet high in calories and protein. Frequent small meals and food that has been brought from home are helpful in stimulating the child's appetite.

Teaching Home Management

If the child is to receive intravenous antibiotic therapy at home, teach the parents how to set up the medication and how to ensure the infusion is being administered safely. Plan the teaching to fit the parents' schedule, and pay particular attention to signs of frustration or anxiety. Repetitive questions, poor eye contact, and nervous gestures are indicators that anxiety may be interfering with the parents' ability to retain information. Allow parents to express feelings of concern and give them positive feedback as they learn procedures. A return demonstration is the most effective way to evaluate teaching effectiveness. Make a home care referral to assist the family with the intravenous infusions.

Occasionally, children who have had a favorable clinical response to intravenous antibiotics will be discharged with a course of oral antibiotics. It is imperative to discuss adherence to the medication regimen with the parents. Emphasize the importance of follow-up care. A referral to a home care agency would be appropriate.

Promoting Optimal Development

Developmental issues need to be addressed by the nurse. If the child is to remain at home with restricted activity, the family must clearly understand how the restrictions aid the healing process. Discuss age-appropriate activities that will maintain current developmental levels. If the child is exhibiting any residual fears or concerns related to hospitalization, therapeutic play activities may be needed. School-age children need to continue with their schoolwork and maintain contact with their friends. Advise and arrange for tutoring as soon as possible. Resources available to homebound children should be explored with the parents.

Evaluation

- Is the neurovascular function of the extremity intact after treatment and healing?
- Can the child exhibit full range of motion and weight bearing without pain?
- Does the child participate in self-care?
- Do the parents verbalize an understanding of home care?
- Do the parents provide developmentally appropriate activities for their child?

Juvenile Arthritis

Juvenile arthritis, formerly known as juvenile rheumatoid arthritis, is an autoimmune inflammatory disease with no known cause. The term juvenile rheumatoid arthritis is misleading because it implies a positive rheumatoid factor (RF+), which is not always present in children with the disease. Because arthritis in children can appear in a number of different forms, each with a different treatment protocol and prognosis, the more accurate term is juvenile arthritis.

Regardless of which term is used, there is overwhelming consensus that this is a multisystemic disorder that affects the body's connective tissue. It is characterized by joint swelling with limited range of motion, accompanied by pain, tenderness, and inflammation of one or more joints. For diagnostic purposes, the symptoms must be present for 6 weeks or more.

Juvenile arthritis, one of the more common chronic diseases in children, is the leading cause of blindness and disability in children. Juvenile arthritis is not a childhood version of rheumatoid arthritis. Rather, the onset and course of the disease are very clearly defined. The prognosis is considered good, but success is influenced by how well the child's growth and developmental needs are integrated into the treatment plan.

Etiology

Despite extensive research, the cause of juvenile arthritis remains unknown. Infection, trauma, and emotional stress, frequently cited as factors that may trigger the autoimmune response, occur with such frequency in all children that a relationship is difficult to demonstrate. Genetic factors called human leukocyte antigens (HLAs) are believed to play a role in the development of juvenile arthritis (Hollister, 1995).

PATHOPHYSIOLOGY
. . . .
of Juvenile Arthritis

The synovial joints are the primary structures involved in this rheumatic process. Normally, synovial joints are movable and contain synovium, a highly vascular tissue that produces a clear viscous synovial fluid that nourishes and lubricates articular cartilage. In juvenile arthritis, immune complexes in blood and synovial tissue initiate the inflammatory response, producing inflammatory cytokines. Phagocytosis and accumulation of immune complexes cause chronic inflammation and joint destruction.

As the synovium becomes inflamed, excessive fluid is produced. Unlike normal synovial fluid, this fluid is thin and watery. The synovium swells, and thickened villi and nodules protrude into the joint cavity. Pannus formation occurs over the articular cartilage.

Periarticular structures outside the joint may also become involved. With further deterioration, the articular cartilage and contiguous bone become eroded and destroyed.

Incidence

Juvenile arthritis affects approximately 1 in 1,000 to 1 in 1,500 children in the United States (O'Neil, 1998). It occurs before age 16, although most cases have their onset between the toddler and the adolescent years. Juvenile arthritis seldom occurs before age 6 months and is more than twice as likely to occur in girls than boys.

Manifestations

Intermittent joint pain that lasts longer than 6 weeks in more than one joint suggests juvenile arthritis. The joints may appear painful, stiff, swollen, warm to the touch (no redness), and with limited range of motion. Stiffness is worse in the morning or after a prolonged period of rest (gel phenomenon). Table 50–1 lists associated signs and symptoms of the juvenile arthritis subtypes. *Uveitis*, or inflammation of the eye structures in the uveal tract, can cause blindness.

Diagnostic Evaluation

The early diagnosis of juvenile arthritis relies on recognizing the several modes of onset and incidence patterns. The character, frequency, and severity of the systemic and articular manifestations are also critical to the diagnosis. Rheumatoid factor (RF), antinuclear antibodies (ANA), an elevated ESR, and C-reactive protein (CRP) may or may not be present, according to the type of juvenile arthritis. Certain types of juvenile arthritis are specific HLA antigen positive. Uveitis is diagnosed by slit lamp examination.

Therapeutic Management

Therapeutic management is supportive and directed toward preserving joint function, controlling the inflammatory process, minimizing deformity, and reducing the impact of the disease on the child's development. Drug therapy, physical and occupational therapy, family education regarding home care, and developmental interventions are the treatments of choice. It is important to remember that none of these treatment modalities is curative. When they are used appropriately, however, synovitis can be reduced, mobility increased, and the child's growth and developmental needs addressed appropriately.

DRUG THERAPY

The major groups of drugs used to suppress the inflammatory process and control pain are the NSAIDs, such as ibuprofen, naproxen sodium (Naprosyn), tolmetin sodium (Tolectin), and aspirin. For children who do not respond well to NSAIDs and who have severe disease, the slower-acting antirheumatic drugs (SAARDs), such as hydroxychloroquine, gold salts, or penicillamine, can be given alone or in conjunction with the NSAIDs. Corticosteroid (e.g., prednisone) use is limited in the treatment of juvenile arthritis. Despite anti-inflammatory properties, their use neither cures juvenile arthritis nor prevents long-term joint damage. Moreover, the chronic side effects that frequently occur can be problematic for children (see Chapter 41). Indications for use are limited to life-threatening complications

T A B L E 5 0 – 1

Major Types of Juvenile Arthritis

Type	Incidence	Sex Affected	Age	Joints Affected	Other Manifestations	Labortory Values	Prognosis
Systemic	10%–20%	Males and females equally affected	Any	Few to multiple	High fever (especially in the evening), chills, rash on trunk and extremities, enlarged liver and lymph nodes, pericarditis/pleuritis, leukocytis, abdominal pain, anemia, arthralgias before arthritis begins	↑ WBC, ↓ Hct, ↑ ESR, ↑ CRP, RF negative, ANA negative	Approximately 20% develop chronic joint disease
Polyarticular, rheumatoid factor positive	5%; may be familial	90% girls	>8 years old	Any or multiple large and small joints, upper and lower extremities, symmetric pattern	Rapid, severe course; rheumatoid nodules (palpable near elbows); low fever; slight anemia	↑ ESR, RF positive	Early joint erosion, with many having permanent disability
Polyarticular, rheumatoid factor negative	20%–30%	70%–75% girls	Early childhood; school age	Multiple large and small joints	Arthritis persists, loss of bone mass, small percentage with iridocyclitis, growth disturbances, low fever, malaise, anorexia, anemia	↑ ESR, RF negative	Small percentage have joint damage
Pauciarticular oligo-arthritis	40%–55%; may be familial	Girls: 20%–35% will develop a polyarticular course after approximately 3 years	Early childhood	Knees, ankles, elbows, (fewer than four joints), asymmetrical pattern	Chronic uveitis with occasional loss of vision, malaise, low fever, slight anemia; slightly enlarged liver, spleen, and lymph nodes during active disease	HLA-DR5 antigen positive ANA positive	Those with polyarticular course have more severe functional problems
		Boys: Many develop spondyloarthropathies	Late childhood	Large joints of lower extremities, hips, spine	Small percentage have acute uveitis	HLA-B27 antigen positive	

Abbreviations: WBC, white blood cell count; Hct, hematocrit; ESR, erythrocyte sedimentation rate; CRP, C-reactive protein; RF, rheumatoid factor; ANA, antinuclear antibody.

Adapted from Schulte, B., Price D., & James, S. (1997). *Thompson's pediatric nursing: An introductory text* (p. 344). Philadelphia: Saunders.

of juvenile arthritis such as pericarditis, profound anemia, and vasculitis.

Immunosuppressive and cytotoxic agents have been effective in the treatment of certain children with juvenile arthritis. Immunosuppressive agents (e.g., cyclophosphamides, methotrexate, chlorambucil) are reserved for children with crippling juvenile arthritis and in whom the disease is unresponsive to conventional treatment.

PHYSICAL AND OCCUPATIONAL THERAPIES

By controlling the synovitis of juvenile arthritis, drug therapy plays a role in preventing additional musculoskeletal problems. Preserving muscle integrity and joint mobility is equally important. Juvenile arthritis places the child at risk for impaired mobility, contractures, and altered growth and development.

Rehabilitation is designed to prevent such problems from occurring. A program of rest, proper positioning, and exercises (strengthening, active and passive range-of-motion, and resistive exercises) has been developed by occupational and physical therapists. To ensure compliance when developing an exercise program, the therapist considers the child's interests as well as school and extracurricular activities.

To maximize the effectiveness of the exercise program, the strengths and limitations of the child's joints must be thoroughly evaluated. With this information, an individualized exercise program can be developed. Swimming is an excellent exercise for the child. The warmth of the water coupled with the mild resistance it provides makes swimming the perfect medium for strengthening and range-of-motion exercises while protecting the joint.

Children are naturally active, and children with juvenile arthritis are no different. Activity helps maintain normal muscle and joint integrity. During remissions of the disease, the youthful activity level assists with maintaining muscle strength. During painful exacerbations of the disease, however, the child's natural reaction is to rest the painful joint. Inactivity could lead to muscle wasting and flexion deformity. Hot or cold packs, splinting, and positioning the affected joint in a neutral position help reduce the pain during painful episodes. Although resting the extremity is appropriate, it is important to begin simple isometric or tensing exercises as soon as the child is able. These exercises are appropriate during exacerbations of the disease because they do not involve joint movement.

Besides physical and occupational therapy, several other treatment modalities have proved effective. Ultrasound, cold, and electrical stimulation assist in controlling the child's pain and increasing joint mobility. Heat also helps reduce joint stiffness and muscle spasm because the fibrous tissue found in joints and tendons yields better to stretching when it is heated. Examples of heat therapies are hot baths, whirlpools, hydrocollator packs, and paraffin baths.

SURGICAL TREATMENT

Surgical intervention is considered when the child or adolescent is having problems with joint contractures and unequal growth of extremities. This type of treatment can range from diagnostic procedures such as arthroscopic examination or open biopsy to soft tissue release (*tenotomy*) for contractures. Surgery to correct leg length discrepancies as well as arthroplasty and joint replacement may also be necessary.

NURSING CARE
. . . .
The Child with Juvenile Arthritis

Assessment

Most children with juvenile arthritis are managed successfully at home, and hospital admission is not needed. The nursing assessment focuses on the status of the affected joints, the physical restrictions placed on the child, the level and intensity of the pain, and the child's and family's response to the disease process.

Examine affected joints for warmth, tenderness, pain, and limited range of motion. Because children are not always able to clearly identify the problem, be alert for irritability, guarding of the painful joints, or refusal to bear weight. The child may limp or favor the extremity.

Pain is a major component of this disease. Attempt to determine the intensity and severity of the pain. It is important to remember that the nonverbal child cannot report pain. The parent may describe the child as very fussy and irritable in the morning. The young child may be reluctant to walk and want to be carried. Help the family determine what activities increase the pain as well as what the child does when the pain starts. Explore with the child methods that may relieve the pain, and whether they are effective.

Assess joint stiffness as well as the duration of the stiffness and the child's description of how difficult it is to move around after periods of inactivity.

Assess the child for any indication of systemic involvement, such as a history of temperature elevations, especially in the late afternoon or evening, and determine whether a rash occurs with the fever. Anorexia, weight loss, and failure to grow may be the first indicators that something is wrong. The parent may report that the child is not sleeping at night or may simply describe the child as irritable and fussy. Lethargy and malaise may also occur.

During the physical examination, assess for lymphadenopathy, hepatosplenomegaly, and visual problems. Uveitis will be apparent only on slit lamp examination. An accurate height and weight should be obtained and, if possible, past growth parameters should be plotted on a growth chart to determine alterations in growth. Cardiac and respiratory system assessments provide baseline information that will allow early detection of pericarditis and pleuritis.

Nursing Diagnosis and Planning

The following nursing diagnoses and expected outcomes may be appropriate to the child and family:

■ Risk for Injury related to joint inflammation and medications.
   Expected Outcome: The child will remain free from injury; the effects of inflammation will be reduced.
■ Pain related to the inflammatory process and painful joint and muscle weakness.
   Expected Outcome: The child's pain will decrease.

- Impaired Physical Mobility related to inflammation of the joint and associated muscle weakness.
  Expected Outcome: The child will accept activity restrictions and comply with the exercise program.
- Altered Growth and Development related to activity intolerance.
  Expected Outcomes: The child will exhibit age-appropriate behaviors. The parents will support and maintain appropriate developmental activities for their child.
- Body Image Disturbance related to activity intolerance.
  Expected Outcome: The child will maintain relationships with peers and participate in age-appropriate activities when able.
- Knowledge Deficit about the care and treatment of juvenile arthritis related to unfamiliarity with the condition.
  Expected Outcome: The parents will demonstrate safe home care, adherence to treatment regimen, and understanding of the exercise program.

Interventions

Preventing Injury

Assist the family to identify when the child's condition has exacerbated. Teach positioning of inflamed joints, appropriate application of heat or cold, and how to support and protect the affected joints. Emphasize that isometric exercises and passive range-of-motion exercises will prevent contractures and deformities.

Because some of the medications used to treat juvenile arthritis cause immunosuppression, teach parents to recognize the signs of immunosuppression and notify the physician as appropriate. Some childhood immunizations may need to be postponed. Because the combination of aspirin and viral infection can predispose the child to Reye's syndrome (see Chapter 52), aspirin should be discontinued if the child is experiencing a viral illness. As long as the child is not immunosuppressed, administer varicella and influenza vaccines to prevent these viral infections.

Emphasize regular visits to the ophthalmologist to prevent complications from uveitis. In general, children with juvenile arthritis should undergo slit lamp examinations every 6 months; children with pauciarticular juvenile arthritis should be seen more frequently (O'Neil, 1998).

Managing Pain

Teach parents to identify both verbal and nonverbal pain indicators. Nonverbal cues are more difficult to recognize but may include restlessness, withdrawal, decreased attention span, increased crying, and decreased sleep. Maintaining a therapeutic blood level of pain medication is the most effective way to ensure maximum comfort.

Nonpharmacologic pain relief measures such as diversion, splinting, heat or cold application, imagery, and meditation can be useful for some children. Remember to encourage parents to continue with isometric exercises.

Promoting Mobility

Assist the parents to learn the exercise program. Be sure that the program is developmentally appropriate and fun for the child. Teach the parents how to assess joint mobility and to maintain correct body alignment. The child might need elastic stockings if prolonged inactivity is expected. Encourage a diet high in fiber, protein, and calcium and an adequate fluid intake. Discuss with the parent and child age-appropriate play activities that involve the unaffected extremities; aerobic activities will prevent stasis of respiratory secretions.

Facilitating Emotional and Social Development

Acknowledge the child's and family's anxiety and allow family members to express concerns. Encourage such expressive therapeutic activities as pounding boards, bean bag throws, clay, painting, story composing, and doll play. Therapeutic play provides a safe and effective mechanism for reducing the stress of immobility. The nurse should recognize that age, sex, and self-concept play a role in a child's adjustment to chronic illness. Use anticipatory guidance to assist the child in developing coping mechanisms that will foster the development of optimism and a sense of personal competence.

Communicate with the school nurse about scheduling necessary rest periods for the child during the school day. The child might enjoy a short period of quiet activity in the school health office if allowed to bring a friend. Because stiffness is more prominent in the morning, the child may need additional time to get ready for school. School nurses can help the child's daily transition to school by communicating with teachers about the child's needs.

Assisting the child to identify strengths and areas of accomplishments increases self-esteem. Identify creative hobbies or activities that will enhance the child's sense of self-worth.

Family Education

As part of the multidisciplinary approach, the nurse must take an active part in helping the parents and child learn how to cope with and adapt to the limitations of the disease. Because the greater part of the child's care will take place in the home, the success of the therapeutic plan will be determined by the parents. Planning begins as soon as possible in the course of the illness. The parents should be involved in as many nursing activities as possible. This will reduce their anxiety and increase their sense of control over a very frightening situation. Provide verbal and written instructions and use return demonstrations to ensure parental understanding of procedures. Coordinate referrals and physical therapy with the child's and parents' routines and schedules.

Evaluation

- Is the child free from joint inflammation and residual deformity, and does the child demonstrate age-appropriate range of motion and muscle strength?
- Does the child experience pain control, as evidenced by increased sleep, decreased restlessness and irritability, and increased participation in age-appropriate activities?
- During an exacerbation, is the child able to accept activity restrictions and increase compliance with the exercise program?
- Is the child free from respiratory problems or other problems associated with immobility?

- Is the child able to perform self-care activities appropriate for age?
- Do the parents demonstrate the ability to facilitate the child's growth and development within the limitations posed by the child's disease?
- Do the child and parents verbalize an increased trust of health care providers?
- Does the child demonstrate age-appropriate behaviors, increased social interactions with friends, and appropriate adaptation to school?
- Are the parents able to articulate and demonstrate solutions to care problems encountered in the home?

Muscular Dystrophies

Muscular dystrophies are a group of progressively degenerative, inherited diseases that affect the muscle cells of specific muscle groups, causing weakness and atrophy. They vary in pattern of inheritance and age at onset, but most are identified in early childhood and are characterized by progressive muscle weakness (Table 50–2). Duchenne muscular dystrophy is the most common of several forms of muscular dystrophy.

Etiology

Muscular dystrophies are inherited in various genetic patterns. Duchenne muscular dystrophy is a sex-linked recessive disorder and therefore it affects only males. Females are carriers and pass the defect on to their male children.

Incidence

Duchenne muscular dystrophy occurs in 1 in 3,000 male children. Spontaneous mutations are responsible for 30% or more of those affected; therefore, many of these children have no family history of the disorder. Other forms of muscular dystrophy are less common, with varying patterns of inheritance.

Pathophysiology

Over time, muscle fibers degenerate and are replaced by fat and connective tissue. Progressive weakness and wasting of symmetric groups of skeletal muscles result in increasing disability and deformity.

Manifestations

Progressive, symmetric muscle wasting and weakness without loss of sensation first appear after walking is achieved (usually 3 to 7 years). The child must use the Gower maneuver to rise from the floor (child puts hands on knees and moves the hands up legs until standing erect). The child has a waddling, wide-based gait. The muscles of the pelvis and shoulders are most often affected in Duchenne muscular dystrophy. The calf muscles are characteristically weak but hypertrophied. Increasing disability and deformities include hip and knee contractures, foot deformities, scoliosis, and lordosis; walking ability (Duchenne) is lost by age 9 to 12 years. Associated signs and symptoms include moderate obesity, decreased IQ, and shortened life span. Cardiopulmonary complications are the most common cause of death.

Diagnostic Evaluation

Children with a positive family history are especially at risk for muscular dystrophy and should be monitored for clinical symptoms, which generally do not appear until the preschool years. Serum creatine kinase (CK) levels are elevated in the early stages of the disease and then decrease as muscle bulk decreases. Electromyography and muscle biopsy may also assist with the diagnosis. The gene locus for Duchenne muscular dystrophy has been identified, which makes it easier to determine whether a woman is a carrier.

Therapeutic Management

The therapeutic management of the child with a muscular dystrophy is aimed at maintaining ambulation and independence for as long as possible as muscle weakness progresses. Contractures further reduce mobility and independence. Surgery, bracing, and physical therapy contribute to keeping the child as mobile as possible. Later, therapy is directed toward maximizing sitting capabilities, respiratory function, and self-care. Preventing obesity in order to facilitate mobility and care is a priority. Prompt attention to infection, especially of the respiratory tract, is essential.

Nursing Considerations

Where there is a family history of muscular dystrophy, infants and young children need to be monitored carefully for its occurrence. When a diagnosis is made, nursing interventions can become a major source of support for these children and their families. The family's ability to cope with chronic illness and the poor prognosis of muscular dystrophy needs to be assessed. Over time, the child's mobility and self-care abilities should be monitored to ensure independence for as long as possible. The potential for weight gain and respiratory tract infection and the adequacy of support systems must be regularly assessed.

Nursing interventions for the child with muscular dystrophy include coordinating a variety of health care services. Anticipating the child's future needs requires a sensitive yet knowledgeable approach. Maintenance of activity and self-care functions is important to the child and the family, and independence must be fostered, within the limits of safety. Activities such as swimming, which promote range of motion and mobility for as long as possible, are helpful. As the disease progresses and movement is increasingly restricted, the nurse can suggest activities that take less energy but keep the child involved with peers.

Because children in the late stages of muscular dystrophy have difficulty moving, the nurse and family should assist with position changes every 2 hours to prevent injury to the skin and other tissues from prolonged pressure. Adequate fluid intake must be encouraged to prevent urine stasis. A bowel regimen, including stool softeners or laxatives, may be necessary.

The home environment, including bathing and toileting facilities, may need to be modified to allow wheelchair mobility. Creative approaches to clothing can simplify dressing while meeting the needs of a child trying to fit in with peers.

Specific suggestions about dietary modifications to control weight may be necessary. The nurse can educate fami-

TABLE 50-2

Muscular Dystrophies of Childhood

Type	Onset/Progression	Inheritance/Incidence	Clinical Manifestations
Duchenne	Onset: 1–4 years. Rapidly progressive; loss of walking by 9 to 10 years; death in late teens from respiratory failure, heart failure, pneumonia.	X-linked recessive Most common hereditary neuromuscular disease. Affects all races. Incidence: 1 in 3,000 male infants	Progressive generalized weakness and muscle wasting affecting limb and trunk muscles first; calves often enlarged; waddling gait; lordosis; cardiomyopathy; Gower maneuver; mental retardation common.
Myotonic (Steinert disease)	Onset: In severe neonatal form: weakness at birth, may have paralysis of diaphragm. If child survives early weeks of life, steady improvement in motor function over the first decade, usually developing ability to walk. Often survive to late adulthood.	Autosomal dominant Incidence: 1 in 30,000	In the severe neonatal form, hypotonia and weakness are evident at birth. Others may appear normal at birth. Mild weakness in first few years, with progressive wasting of distal muscles. Myotonia worsened by cold, fatigue, stress. Mental retardation in about half of cases.
Becker	Onset: 5–10 years. Slowly progressive; maintain walking past early teens; life span into third decade.	X-linked recessive Incidence: 1 in 20,000 births	Almost identical to Duchenne but less severe; child is mobile until late teens; normal intelligence.
Congenital	Onset: Birth. Typically slow but variable; many do not attain walking. Shortened life span.	Autosomal recessive Incidence: Rare	Generalized muscle weakness with possible joint deformities; hypotonia. Mental retardation and seizures common in types with CNS disease.
Facioscapulohumeral (FSH, or Landouzy-Dejerine disease)	Onset: First decade. Slowly progressive loss of walking in later life; variable life expectancy; disease may span many decades.	Autosomal dominant or recessive Incidence: 3–10 per million births	Earliest and most severe weakness occurs in facial and shoulder girdle muscles. May be unable to close eyes completely during sleep. Progressive disability, leading to inability to walk. May be mild, causing minimal disability.
Emery-Dreifus (scapuloperoneal or scapulohumeral)	Onset: Middle childhood to early teens. Progression is very slow; many survive to late adulthood.	X-linked recessive Incidence: Rare	Contractures of elbows and ankles develop early; shoulder muscles become wasted. Slowly progressive, with eventual cardiac abnormality.

lies about how to make dietary changes without making food a source of controversy. To reduce the chance of life-threatening respiratory infections, the child needs to be protected from children with respiratory and contagious diseases. As disability progresses, pulmonary hygiene and respiratory exercises are needed to maintain respiratory function.

Regular monitoring by a multispecialty team helps meet the varying needs of the child and family as the child's condition changes. Therapy is individualized to address the specific needs of the child. Genetic screening and counseling are recommended for parents and siblings of children with muscular dystrophy.

Parents must be taught how to perform basic nursing tasks and referred to agencies that can assist with home care and equipment such as a motorized wheelchair. Extended family and support groups such as the Muscular Dystrophy Association of America (see Appendix L) can provide needed emotional support and specific assistance as parental energies are exhausted. In addition, the needs of the grieving family should be addressed.

Scoliosis

Although scoliosis is defined as lateral curvature of the spine, it is in fact a three-dimensional deformity involving rotation of the vertebral bodies. The forces of a curved spine on the structure of the body cause the rib cage to become misshapen. The body develops a compensatory curve to maintain posture and balance. Scoliotic curves are measured in degrees: a curve of less than 20 degrees is a slight curve, a curve of more than 40 degrees usually requires surgery, and a curve of more than 80 degrees compromises respiratory function and is considered severe.

Incidence

The incidence of scoliosis varies with the cause. Idiopathic scoliosis is a common disorder, affecting approximately 10% of the population. Most cases of idiopathic scoliosis are of no clinical significance and go undetected. Idiopathic scoliosis is most common in females and in families in which another member is affected. The incidence of congenital scoliosis is variable. It is believed to be caused by a variety of factors and is also associated with certain other congenital anomalies. Scoliosis is relatively common in children with neuromuscular disorders.

Manifestations

The clinical manifestations of scoliosis include a visible curve of the spine (Fig. 50–8), a rib hump when the child is bending forward, an asymmetric rib cage, and uneven shoulder or pelvic heights and prominence of the scapula or hip. There is a difference in the space between the arms and the trunk when the child is standing, as well as an apparent leg-length discrepancy. In severe cases the child experiences reduced vital capacity (see Chapter 33 for a discussion of screening for scoliosis).

Diagnostic Evaluation

Scoliosis may be detected at any time during childhood or adolescence. It is often first discovered during routine screening for scoliosis either at school or a physician's office. Clinical manifestations should lead to more thorough as-

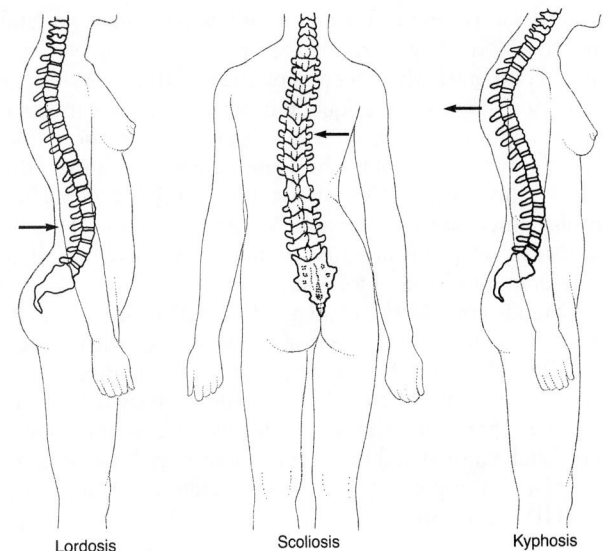

Lordosis   Scoliosis   Kyphosis

FIGURE 50–8

Most spinal abnormalities in children are abnormal curvatures. In *scoliosis,* the spine curves laterally and the vertebrae rotate, pulling the ribs along. *Kyphosis* is a front-to-back rounding, usually of the thoracic spine; it is often accompanied by scoliosis. *Lordosis* is an exaggerated concave curvature of the spine, usually in the lumbar area. (From Ignatavicius, D. D., Workman, M. L., & Mishler, M. A. [1995]. *Medical surgical nursing: A nursing process approach* [2nd ed., p. 1399]. Philadelphia: Saunders.)

sessment of the spine. Radiographic examination of the thorax will confirm the diagnosis and add information to be considered in planning treatment. In addition, children with disorders commonly associated with scoliosis should be monitored for the development of spinal deformity.

Therapeutic Management

The treatment of scoliosis is complex. Depending on the extent of the curve, the child's age and projected growth, and presence of associated complications, treatment options include regular and periodic observation with radiographic evaluation, bracing, or spinal fusion surgery. Although mild curvatures may never progress to the point that treatment is warranted, the curvature can become increasingly pronounced, which is why children must be examined regularly over the long term.

BRACING

In the past, bracing was used extensively in the treatment of scoliosis, and it may still be used today to stabilize some mild curves. Studies on the effects of bracing have not conclusively established that bracing is more effective in altering the natural course of scoliosis than monitoring without bracing (Noonan, Weinstein, Jacobson, et al., 1996). If used, the brace must be worn 18 to 23 hours a day. The child's skin needs to be meticulously monitored for signs of breakdown.

SURGERY

Spinal fusion is used to treat severe scoliosis. Because fusion results in cessation of growth of the fused vertebrae, it is

---

PATHOPHYSIOLOGY

of Scoliosis

Most cases of scoliosis can be classified into three major categories, which offer some insight into the causes of the disorder. *Idiopathic scoliosis* is the predominant form of scoliosis. Although there is no recognizable cause for idiopathic scoliosis, the disease appears to have a genetic component. Most idiopathic scoliosis occurs in adolescent girls and tends to progress more rapidly during growth spurts, such as the period immediately preceding menarche. Idiopathic scoliosis can also occur in other age groups. *Congenital scoliosis* is another major category of scoliosis. It is the result of vertebral abnormalities, such as hemivertebra or vertebral bars, and is associated with other congenital anomalies. A third category of scoliosis is *paralytic scoliosis*. This type of scoliosis is relatively common in individuals with certain neuromuscular diseases, such as cerebral palsy, muscular dystrophy, paraplegia, or quadriplegia. Scoliosis may also develop in children with certain other disorders, such as osteogenesis imperfecta, juvenile arthritis, and spinal cord tumors, and it may also occur secondary to radiation therapy.

delayed for as long as possible to allow maximum skeletal growth. Many new surgical techniques have shown improved outcomes while decreasing the length of hospitalization. Most surgical techniques rely on some form of internal instrumentation—rods or wires—that corrects the deformity (curve) and holds the spine immobile during the long healing period. Operations are usually accomplished through incisions in the back (for posterior fusion); some surgeons prefer the anterior thoracic approach. An iliac bone graft can be used for the fusion.

Significant blood loss may occur during spinal fusion procedures, and replacement of blood is frequently necessary. Because spinal fusion for scoliosis is a planned procedure, children are often able to donate their own blood in the weeks preceding the surgery for use at the time of surgery. Such autologous blood transfusions have become commonplace in response to the human immunodeficiency virus (HIV) epidemic.

PROGNOSIS

With close monitoring and follow-up, the treatment outcomes for idiopathic scoliosis are excellent. The older the child is at the time of treatment, the more successful the ultimate result is likely to be. The prognosis for congenital scoliosis is variable and depends on the underlying defect. The treatment of scoliosis in children with neuromuscular disorders is a challenge, and outcomes are variable. These children must be monitored for an indefinite period for the possibility of curve progression.

COMPLICATIONS

A variety of complications can occur during treatment for scoliosis. Braces can cause skin irritation and even pressure sores. Neurologic damage can result from mechanical injury during surgery or from stretching of the spinal column during correction. Although electronic monitoring (somatosensory evoked potentials) during surgery helps reduce the possibility of spinal cord damage intraoperatively, postoperative sensation and motor function are the only definitive indicators of neurologic function.

Another complication in the surgical treatment of scoliosis is superior mesenteric artery syndrome. This disorder is caused by mechanical changes in the position of the patient's abdominal contents, resulting from lengthening of the body. It results in a syndrome of emesis and abdominal distension similar to that which occurs with intestinal obstruction or paralytic ileus; therefore, postoperative vomiting warrants attention. Fluid or electrolyte imbalances can also occur in the postoperative period, as can atelectasis and sluggish bowel function. Superficial or deep wound infection also is possible. The major long-term complication of spinal fusion is pseudarthrosis, or failure of one or more segments of the spine to fuse.

NURSING CARE
· · · · · · · · · · · ·
The Child with Scoliosis

Assessment

Nurses are involved in the routine screening of children and adolescents for scoliosis in acute care settings, outpatient

settings, and schools. School nurses screen children for scoliosis, usually beginning in the fourth grade. For children who have been diagnosed but are not undergoing treatment, periodic evaluation is necessary to monitor possible progression of the curve. For those undergoing treatment, assessment focuses on determining the child's and parents' level of knowledge about scoliosis. It also involves assessing for body image concerns, anxiety about the various treatment modalities, compliance with prescribed treatments, including bracing, and an understanding of the many issues surrounding spinal fusions.

Children undergoing nonsurgical treatment and their families must understand and correctly apply treatment measures and be committed to compliance. For example, children who wear a brace need to be monitored closely to ensure that treatment goals are being met. The drawbacks of braces include discomfort in warm weather and skin irritation. Adolescent girls may find braces cosmetically offensive, and cooperation is often a problem. Clothing modifications are necessary if compliance is to be expected.

Children undergoing spinal fusion have special needs in the perioperative period. Preoperatively, explanations about the procedures and the care anticipated are aimed at reducing the anxiety and fear surrounding surgery. The nurse also may coordinate autologous blood donation.

> For example, "Many girls facing surgery are nervous about what it will be like to have this operation. Perhaps you would like to know more about what it will be like."

In the immediate postoperative period, children are monitored closely to determine the cardiovascular and neurologic status of the lower extremities, as well as to assess pain, fluid status, bleeding, and return of bowel function. Assess all extremities for color, circulation, capillary refill, warmth, sensation, and motion. Perform neurovascular checks every 2 hours for the first 24 hours and then every 4 hours for the next 48 hours. Check and record the quality of pedal pulses every hour for 48 hours. Short-interval monitoring is especially important if the anterior thoracic approach has been used and the child has a chest tube. Pulmonary hygiene measures, including turning, coughing, and deep breathing, various incentive spirometry measures, and log rolling the child from side to side every 2 hours, are also an essential nursing task in the immediate postoperative period. Most children are cared for in the intensive care unit for several days postoperatively.

As the child stabilizes postoperatively, mobility increases quickly, and the diet can be progressed with monitoring of gastrointestinal status. Children must understand the function and use of orthoplast jackets that may be used postoperatively. A cotton T-shirt between the plastic and the skin reduces discomfort and irritation. The nurse may suggest ways clothing can be adapted to accommodate the jacket while being attractive and acceptable.

It is not unusual for children to be discharged from the hospital by the fifth postoperative day. Because the treatment of scoliosis is a long-term process and can affect a child for most of the growing years, close monitoring is important to ensure positive outcomes.

Nursing Diagnosis, Planning, Intervention, and Evaluation

Nursing Diagnosis	■ Knowledge Deficit related to lack of information about the natural history of scoliosis and the treatment modalities available.
Expected Outcome	• The child and family will express an understanding of what has been taught about scoliosis, including the reasons for therapy, demonstrate the skills taught (such as performance of prescribed exercise), ask appropriate questions that indicate a knowledge of scoliosis and treatment (e.g., "Will I be able to play basketball?"), and follow through with needed therapy.

Intervention	Rationale
1. Determine the child's and family's knowledge of scoliosis and treatment modalities.	1. Teaching needs to begin at the client's level of understanding.
2. Teach the child and family about scoliosis, its signs and symptoms, progression, and treatment.	2. Knowledge and understanding increase motivation and compliance with treatment while reducing anxiety.
3. Identify the child's and family's areas of concern (e.g., activity restriction, operative concerns, outcomes of therapy).	3. Teaching will be most effective if it is directed at the individual's needs.
4. Select instructional methods that are appropriate for the child's developmental level (e.g., puppets, audiovisuals).	4. Learning styles vary with individual interest and abilities.
5. Communicate clearly and honestly.	5. A clear and honest approach establishes trust between the staff and family and promotes confidence in the effectiveness of treatment.
6. Explain the reason for the various interventions (such as turning in the postoperative period).	6. Children are more cooperative in the postoperative period if they know the reason for interventions.
7. Have the child (or parents) demonstrate specific skills (such as recumbent log rolling).	7. Demonstration allows the nurse to evaluate learning and children to gain confidence in their ability to perform the maneuver.
8. Encourage the child to ask questions and discuss concerns. Correct any inaccurate information. Allow the child to handle equipment.	8. Children use their senses to learn. Receiving answers to questions reduces anxiety and clarifies information.
9. Include the parents in teaching.	9. Parents will develop confidence in the care of their child and show reduced levels of anxiety. If parents are less anxious, the child will be as well.

Evaluation	• Are the child and family able to express an understanding of scoliosis and its treatment, ask appropriate questions, demonstrate the skills taught, and follow through with required therapy?
Nursing Diagnosis	■ Body Image Disturbance related to a postural deformity, to bracing, or to a surgical scar on the back.
Expected Outcomes	• The child will talk about feelings about the effect of the scoliosis on body perception and the brace or surgical scar on self-image. • The child will demonstrate confidence in abilities (academic, extracurricular activities, or other qualities).

Intervention	Rationale
1. Encourage the child or teen to talk about the diagnosis, treatment, and feelings about the experience.	1. This allows assessment of the child's perceptions and provides opportunities to clarify misconceptions and to vent feelings.
2. Encourage conversation that focuses on the child's body perception.	2. This allows the nurse to provide emotional support and may ease anxiety.
3. Encourage the child to discuss experiences with friends.	3. Friends are likely to be very supportive and helpful if they know something about the disorder and the child's experiences.
4. Provide information about the disorder and the treatment. Encourage the child to consider an activity that can be mastered and create a sense of accomplishment (e.g., science club).	4. Activities help the child gain a sense of control over the experience.
5. During hospitalization, provide privacy to the greatest extent possible.	5. Children and teens are very modest.

Evaluation
• Does the child demonstrate acceptance of body changes and express confidence in abilities?

Nursing Diagnosis
■ Anxiety related to impending surgery.

Expected Outcome
• The child will discuss anxiety and identify effective coping mechanisms to address it.

Intervention

1. Determine whether the child is anxious about surgery.
2. Initiate a conversation with the child about how anxiety makes one feel and how anxiety is a normal response to anticipated surgery.
3. Assist the child with identifying and using positive and effective means for resolving anxiety (e.g., talking with a friend, exercising or engaging in other activities, practicing relaxation techniques).
4. Identify and provide an alternative to negative behaviors associated with anxiety (e.g., verbal outbursts, physical aggression, withdrawal).

Rationale

1. The child may not be anxious or may be hiding anxiety.
2. The child may need permission to discuss anxiety and assistance verbalizing feelings. Children need to be assured that they are normal.
3. In role-modeling for the child and discussing various possibilities for coping, the nurse allows the child to find a comfortable means for expressing feelings.
4. The child needs to understand that there are acceptable and unacceptable ways to express one's feelings.

Try telling the child "It's OK and normal to be anxious about surgery. This is hard for your parents, too. Let's talk about ways you might let your parents know how you are feeling."

---

5. Reassure the child about specific fears ("Can my mom be with me?" "Will I get a shot?").
6. Determine the child's need for specific information, and teach accordingly.

5. Reassurance and conversation may help resolve some fears.
6. Fears about the unknown may be reduced by increasing knowledge.

Evaluation
• Is the child able to identify the source of anxiety and demonstrate ways of coping effectively with the anxiety?

Nursing Diagnosis
■ Pain related to the operative procedure.

Expected Outcome
• The child will indicate decreasing amounts of pain as measured on a pain scale, appear calm and relaxed, and turn, cough, and deep breathe effectively with assistance.

Intervention

1. Monitor the child's pain level frequently in the postoperative period (statements of pain, anxiety, an inability to cough, hyperalertness, reluctance or refusal to move, or sweating may indicate pain).
2. Provide prescribed analgesics in a timely manner (children usually receive morphine by a patient-controlled technique for several days).

3. Assist family members in understanding the child's experience and interventions.

4. Explore alternative means for relieving pain (using anxiety-reducing techniques, dimming the room lights, reducing stimuli, playing music, therapeutic touching).
5. Determine the child's response to pain relief measures and communicate with the physician about possible adjustments, if needed (see Chapter 39).

Rationale

1. Children and adolescents may be unable or unwilling to verbalize their pain.

2. The appropriate and timely use of analgesics provides optimal control of pain. Pulses of additional medication may be required if PCA is not properly effective.
3. When parents understand and can participate in the child's care, they can provide support to the child and encourage nonpharmaceutical pain relief measures.
4. Alternative therapy may be very effective.

5. Adjustments may be necessary to achieve optimal pain relief.

| Evaluation | • Can the child use a pain scale to demonstrate decreasing pain?
• Does the child appear calm and relaxed?
• Is the child able to turn, cough, and deep breathe effectively with assistance? |

| Nursing Diagnosis | ■ Knowledge Deficit about home care related to unfamiliarity with spinal fusion. |

| Expected Outcome | • The family and child will successfully manage treatment at home. |

Intervention	Rationale
1. Teach the family and child the correct technique for wound care. Discuss the importance of a well-balanced diet.	1. Proper wound care and good nutrition promote healing and decrease the chance of infection.
2. Discuss activity restrictions (usually, these children cannot ride a bike, use in-line skates, ski, or lift more than 10 lb). Show the child how to perform activities without twisting or bending at the waist.	2. Home care instructions for activity are important to reduce the possibility of complications. Activity restrictions are usually maintained for 6 to 9 months, depending on the type of surgery and the physician.
3. Instruct the family and child to be alert for unfavorable signs, such as skin breakdown, pain, or difficulty breathing, and inform them about problems that can be anticipated and what to do if they occur.	3. Home care instructions reduce the possibility of complications.
4. Provide the name and phone number of an easily accessible health care provider in case questions arise at home. Inform the family about community resources available.	4. Access to a health care provider and community resources decreases anxiety and improves compliance with treatment.
5. Schedule a follow-up appointment prior to discharge. Emphasize the importance of keeping appointments.	5. Periodic evaluation is important to recovery.

| Evaluation | • Can the family demonstrate the procedures necessary to care for the child at home?
• Is the family aware of sources of help, if needed?
• Does the family keep follow-up appointments? |

Kyphosis

Kyphosis is defined as a front-to-back rounding of the thoracic spine. Mild kyphosis occurs normally and in varying amounts. It may be a postural deviation related to self-consciousness that is manifested by round shoulders. Although kyphosis usually occurs in the thoracic area, it can occur in other areas of the spine, and it becomes especially problematic when it progresses uncontrollably and results in neurologic damage or reduced respiratory function. Kyphosis is often accompanied by scoliosis, although the reverse is not necessarily true.

Etiology and Incidence

Kyphosis can occur as a postural defect (idiopathic), as a result of structural abnormalities of the vertebral bodies of the spine, or secondary to certain neuromuscular disorders, such as myelomeningocele, or to other factors, such as tumors, surgery, or radiation therapy.

Postural kyphosis is found in about 4% of otherwise healthy adolescents. The incidence of kyphosis that occurs secondary to other conditions and disorders and that is severe enough to treat is variable.

Manifestations

The clinical manifestations of kyphosis include a visually appreciable humpback or convex deformity that predominantly affects the thoracic area, but may involve a lower portion of the spine (Fig. 50–8).

Diagnostic Evaluation

The diagnosis of kyphosis is relatively easy to establish from visual examination of the spine. It is often associated with other conditions, necessitating a comprehensive analysis of its cause.

Therapeutic Management and Nursing Considerations

Exercises may be recommended for mild postural curves. The treatment for severe kyphosis is similar to the treatment for scoliosis. Because the two conditions are often found in the same child, treatment is directed toward both conditions. In children who have not yet reached skeletal maturity and whose curves are flexible, casting or bracing may be attempted first. For complex progressive curves, spinal fusion frequently becomes necessary.

Nursing care of the child with kyphosis, including home care, is based on the same principles as outlined for scoliosis management.

Lordosis

Lordosis is an exaggerated concave curvature of the spine, usually in the lumbar area, where a mild concave curve is normal. Occasionally it occurs in other areas of the spine, in which case it is not considered normal, as it can compress vital organs, such as the heart and lungs, and may require immediate intervention.

Etiology and Incidence

Lumbar lordosis by itself is usually not severe enough to cause concern. It may, however, occur secondary to other defects, such as hip flexion contracture, muscular dystrophy, obesity, or developmental dysplasia of the hip. Lordosis is a frequent complication of myelomeningocele and several other neuromuscular disorders (see Chapter 52).

The incidence of lordosis is variable and depends on the presence of associated conditions.

Manifestations and Diagnostic Evaluation

The clinical manifestations of lordosis include an exaggerated concave curve in the lumbar area, pain in the lower back, and an accompanying defect, such as developmental dysplasia of the hip, hip flexion contracture, or obesity.

A diagnosis of lordosis is confirmed by physical examination and radiographic studies.

Therapeutic Management and Nursing Considerations

Treatment for lordosis depends on its cause, but treatment modalities are grounded on the principles outlined for scoliosis management.

The nursing care for children with lordosis, including home care, is similar to that outlined for children with scoliosis. In addition, accompanying disorders must be monitored and treated concurrently.

KEY CONCEPTS

- Musculoskeletal problems are frequently caused by trauma. Therefore, nursing assessment should always begin with the child's airway, breathing, and circulation.
- The cause of the musculoskeletal injury must be determined because nonaccidental trauma or child abuse may be involved.
- The neurovascular assessment of a child in traction or a cast includes assessment of skin color, capillary refill time, temperature, and sensation in the extremity. The quality of the pulse distal to the site should also be evaluated and compared with that of the uninvolved extremity.
- When evaluating neurovascular status, remember to assess for the five P's of ischemia—pain, pallor, pulselessness, paresthesia, and paralysis.
- Commonly seen musculoskeletal developmental disorders include clubfoot, developmental dysplasia of the hip, Legg-Calvé-Perthes disease, and slipped capital femoral epiphysis. Each often requires splinting, traction, bracing, casting, or a combination of these.
- Treatment for Legg-Calvé-Perthes disease maintains the femoral

head in the acetabulum and protects the hip from the stress of weight bearing during the healing process.
- Nursing outcomes for the child with Legg-Calvé-Perthes disease include compliance with activity restrictions, facilitating home care and management of the appliance selected for treatment, and promoting age-appropriate cognitive and emotional development.
- In an open fracture (marked by a wound or break in the skin) the possibility of infection is increased.
- Immobilization of fractures involves repositioning the bone fragments (reduction) and applying a cast or traction to maintain alignment (retention) until healing occurs.
- Osteogenesis imperfecta places the child at risk for pathologic fractures, bony deformities due to bending and bowing of softened bones, and kyphoscoliosis.
- Nursing outcomes for the child with osteogenesis imperfecta include keeping the child free from injury, the development of healthy coping behaviors, and maintenance of developmental integrity.

- Treatment for Osgood-Schlatter disease is conservative and involves limiting activities that require bending or kneeling. These restrictions may interfere with the achievement of developmental milestones and may result in isolation and alienation.
- Nursing care of the child with Osgood-Schlatter disease involves promoting compliance, reassuring the child that the problem is self-limiting, and assisting the child to achieve age-appropriate developmental tasks.
- Nursing care of the child with osteomyelitis includes assessment and documentation of the child's status, support and immobilization of the extremity, administration of antibiotics without iatrogenic injury, and careful monitoring of the infusion equipment and intravenous site.
- Therapeutic management of juvenile arthritis is supportive and directed toward preserving joint function, controlling the inflammatory process, minimizing deformity, and reducing the impact of the disease on the child's development.

■ Nursing outcomes for a child with juvenile arthritis include keeping the child free from injury, pain control, enhancing physical mobility, and promoting age-appropriate developmental behaviors.

■ Nursing outcomes for a child with muscular dystrophy include maintaining physical activity, promoting respiratory function, weight management, and reducing the impact of the disease on the child's development.

■ Scoliosis, kyphosis, and lordosis are spinal abnormalities that require long-term assessment and management. Each has the potential for altering a child's body image, so nursing interventions must address emotional as well as physical consequences of these disorders.

ANSWERS TO CRITICAL THINKING EXERCISE 50–1

The following summary compares the three common hip disorders.

	Developmental Dysplasia of the Hip	Legg-Calvé-Perthes Disease	Slipped Capital Femoral Epiphysis
Age at onset	Infancy, early childhood	Preschool, young school age	Adolescence
Manifestations	Hip instability, as evidenced by Barlow or Ortolani signs; limp or waddling gait in the older child; limited abduction on affected side	Presence of synovitis and necrosis on x-rays; limp; intermittent knee or hip soreness; child small for age; limited internal rotation and abduction on affected side	Radiographic demonstration of slippage; limp; intermittent knee or thigh pain that worsens with exercise; child large for age; external rotation of the affected leg

Joint synovitis, or septic hip, is a condition that can span age groups. Hip pain and joint limitation are prominent manifestations. Pain is of more acute onset and may be accompanied by fever and laboratory signs of inflammation.

REFERENCES AND READINGS

Abramson, S. J. (1992). Real ultrasonographic evaluation of the infant hip. *Orthopaedic Nursing, 11*(1), 723.

Allington, N. J., & Bowen, J. R. (1996). Adolescent idiopathic scoliosis: Treatment with the Wilmington brace. A comparison of fulltime and part-time use. *Journal of Bone and Joint Surgery, 78A*(7), 1056–1062.

Allshouse, M., Rouse, T., & Eichelberger, M. (1993). Childhood injury: A current perspective. *Pediatric Emergency Care, 9*(3), 159–164.

American Academy of Pediatrics. (1998). In-line skating injuries in children and adolescents. *Pediatrics, 101*(4), 720–722.

Anderson, B. (1999). *Office orthopedics for primary care diagnosis and treatment* (2nd ed.). Philadelphia: Saunders.

Andrews, J. (1997). Making the most of the sports physical. *Contemporary Pediatrics, 14*(3), 182–205.

Barlow, T. G. (1962). Early diagnosis and treatment of congenital dislocation of the hip. *Journal of Bone and Joint Surgery, 44B*(2), 292–301.

Benchot, R. (1996). The adolescent with slipped capital femoral epiphysis. *Journal of Pediatric Nursing, 11*(3), 175–182.

Boachie-Adjei, O., & Lonner, B. (1996). Spinal deformity. *Pediatric Clinics of North America, 43*(4), 883–898.

Brosnan, H. (1991). Nursing management of the adolescent with idiopathic scoliosis. *Nursing Clinics of North America, 26*(1), 17–31.

Bruce, R. (1996). Torsional and angular deformities. *Pediatric Clinics of North America, 43*(4), 867–881.

Bubulka, G. M., & Cipolla, F. (1991). Preparing for pediatric emergencies. *Journal of Emergency Nursing, 17*(4), 236–240.

Cady, R. (1997, March). Subtle symptoms help unmask serious hip disorder. *AAP News*, 18–19.

Campbell, L. S., & Campbell, J. D. (1991). Musculoskeletal trauma in children. *Critical Care Nursing Clinics of North America, 3*(3), 445–456.

Carlino, H. (1991). The child with an Ilizarov external fixator. *Pediatric Nursing, 17*(4), 355–358.

Cotton, L. A. (1991). Unit rod segmental spinal instrumentation for the treatment of neuromuscular scoliosis. *Orthopaedic Nursing, 10*(5), 17–23.

Davids, J. (1996). Pediatric knee: Clinical assessment and common disorders. *Pediatric Clinics of North America, 43*(5), 1067–1089.

DiFiori, J. (1999). Overuse injuries in children and adolescents. *Physician and Sports Medicine, 27*(1), 75–89.

England, S., & Sundberg, S. (1996). Management of common pediatric fractures. *Pediatric Clinics of North America, 43*(5), 991–1012.

Fife, R. Z. (1993). Methotrexate use in juvenile rheumatoid arthritis. *Orthopaedic Nursing, 12*, 32–36.

Fink, C., Fernandez-Vina, M., & Stastny, P. (1995). Clinical evidence that juvenile arthritis is not a single disease. *Pediatric Clinics of North America, 42*(5), 1155–1167.

Gagliardi, B. A. (1991). The impact of Duchenne muscular dystrophy on families. *Orthopaedic Nursing, 10*(5), 41–48.

Giannini, E., & Cawkell, G. (1995). Drug treatment in children with juvenile rheumatoid arthritis: Past, present, and future. *Pediatric Clinics of North America, 42*(5), 1099–1125.

Green, M., Haggerty, R., & Weitzman, M. (1999). *Ambulatory pediatrics* (5th ed.). Philadelphia: Saunders.

Hall, D. E. (1992). Sports injuries. In R. A. Hoekelman, S. B. Friedman, N. M. Nelson, & H. M. Seidel (Eds.), *Pediatric primary care*. St. Louis: Mosby.

Harcke, H. (1999). Developmental dysplasia of the hip: A spectrum of abnormality. *Pediatrics, 103*(1), 152–153.

Hart, K. (1994). Using the Ilizarov external fixator in bone transport. *Orthopaedic Nursing, 13*(1), 35–40.

Hartley, B., & Fuller, C. (1997). Juvenile arthritis: A nursing perspective. *Journal of Pediatric Nursing, 12*(2), 100–109.

Herndon, W. (1993). Acute osteomyelitis and septic arthritis. In J. Surpure (Ed.), *Synopsis of pediatric emergency care*. Boston: Andover Medical.

Hoffinger, S. (1996). Evaluation and management of pediatric foot deformities. *Pediatric Clinics of North America, 43*(5), 1091–1111.

Hollister, J. R. (1995). Rheumatic diseases. In W. W. Hay, J. R. Groothuis, A. R. Hayward, & M. J. Levin (Eds.), *Current pediatric diagnosis and treatment* (12th ed.). East Norwalk, CT: Appleton & Lange.

Hsu, L. C., & Upadhyay, S. S. (1994). Effect of spinal fusion on growth of the spine and lower limbs in girls with adolescent idiopathic scoliosis. *Journal of Pediatric Orthopaedics, 14*(5), 564–568.

Hughes, R. B., & D'Ambrosia, K. (1993). Nursing management of a child with juvenile rheumatoid arthritis. *Orthopaedic Nursing, 12,* 17–22.

Jones-Walton, P. (1991). Clinical standards in skeletal pin site care. *Orthopaedic Nursing, 10*(2), 12–17.

Koop, S., & Quanbeck, D. (1996). Three common causes of childhood hip pain. *Pediatric Clinics of North America, 43*(5), 1053–1065.

Kyzer, S. P. (1991). Congenital idiopathic clubfoot. *Orthopaedic Nursing, 10*(4), 11–18.

Ledwith, C. A., & Fleisher, G. R. (1992). Slipped capital femoral epiphysis without hip pain leads to missed diagnosis. *Pediatrics, 89*(4), 660–662.

Levy, J., & Ward, W. T. (1993). Pediatric femur fractures: An overview of treatment. *Orthopaedics, 16,* 183–190.

MacEwen, D., Kasser, J., & Heinrich, S. (1993). *Pediatric fractures: A practical approach to assessment and treatment.* Baltimore: Williams & Wilkins.

Macias, C., Bothner, J., Wiebe, R. (1998). A comparison of supination/flexion to hyperpronation in the reduction of radial head subluxations. *Pediatrics, 102*(1), e10.

Mansfield, M. J., & Emans, S. J. (1993). Growth in female gymnasts: Should training decrease during puberty? *Journal of Pediatrics, 122*(2), 237–240.

Martinez, A. G., Weinstein, S. L., & Dietz, F. R. (1992). The weight-bearing abduction brace for the treatment of Legg-Perthes disease. *Journal of Bone and Joint Surgery, 74A,* 12–21.

Mason, K. J. (1991). Congenital orthopedic anomalies and their impact on the family. *Nursing Clinics of North America, 26*(1), 1–16.

Meehan, P. L., Angel, D., & Nelson, J. M. (1992). The Scottish-Rite abduction orthosis for the treatment of Legg-Perthes disease. *Journal of Bone and Joint Surgery, 74A,* 2–11.

Nance, D. K., & Mardjetko, S. M. (1994). Technical aspects and nursing considerations of limb lengthening. *Orthopaedic Nursing, 13*(1), 21–33.

National Youth Sports Foundation for the Prevention of Athletic Injuries, Inc. (1993). *Fact sheet—Youth sports injuries.* Needham, MA: Author.

Noonan, K. J., Weinstein, S. L., Jacobson, W. C., & Dolan, L. A. (1996). Use of the Milwaukee brace for progressive idiopathic scoliosis. *Journal of Bone and Joint Surgery, 78A*(4), 557–567.

Novacheck, T. (1996). Developmental dysplasia of the hip. *Pediatric Clinics of North America, 43*(4), 829–847.

Nypaver, M., & Treloar, D. (1994). Neutral cervical spine positioning in children. *Annals of Emergency Medicine, 23*(2), 208–211.

O'Neil, K. (1998). Juvenile arthritis. In L. Finberg (Ed.), *Saunders manual of pediatric practice.* Philadelphia: Saunders.

Ostrum, G. (1993). Sports-related injuries in youth: Prevention is the key and nurses can help. *Pediatric Nursing, 19*(4), 333–342.

Page, G. G. (1991). Chronic pain and the child with juvenile rheumatoid arthritis. *Journal of Pediatric Health Care, 5*(1), 18–23.

Puno, R. M., Mehta, S., & Byrd, J. A. (1994). Surgical treatment of idiopathic thoracolumbar and lumbar scoliosis in adolescent patients. *Orthopaedic Clinics of North America, 25*(2), 275–286.

Randolph, C. (1998). Considerations for the orthopedic nurse in diagnosis and treatment of adolescent sports injuries. *Nursing Clinics of North America, 33*(4), 615–628.

Rang, M. (1993). Perthes disease. In D. Wenger & M. Rang (Eds.), *The art and practice of children's orthopaedics.* New York: Raven Press.

Reed, L. J., & Keegan, M. J. (1993). Fat embolism syndrome: A complication of trauma. *Critical Care Nursing, 13*(3), 33–37.

Rosendahl, K., Aslaksen, A., Lie, R. T., & Markestad, T. (1995). Reliability of ultrasound in the early diagnosis of developmental dysplasia of the hip. *Pediatric Radiology, 25*(3), 219–224.

Saperstein, A., & Nicholas, S. (1996). Pediatric and adolescent sports medicine. *Pediatric Clinics of North America, 43*(5), 1013–1033.

Schafermeyer, R. (1993). Pediatric trauma. *Emergency Medicine Clinics of North America, 11*(1), 187–205.

Schultz, D. (1995). The role of the neuroscience nurse in lumbar fusion. *Journal of Neuroscience Nursing, 27*(2), 90–95.

Shoppee, K. (1992). Developmental dysplasia of the hip. *Orthopaedic Nursing, 11*(5), 30–36.

Sipos, D. A. (1993). M. P. implants for rheumatoid arthritis of the hand. *Orthopaedic Nursing, 12*(5), 7–14.

Sonnen, G., & Henry, N. (1996). Pediatric bone and joint infections: Diagnosis and antimicrobial management. *Pediatric Clinics of North America, 43*(4), 933–947.

Sonzogni, J. J., & Gross, M. (1993). Hip and pelvic injuries in the young: Fractures and special disorders, part 2. *Emergency Medicine, 25*(8), 18–20.

Speers, A. T., & Speers, M. (1992). Care of the infant in a Pavlik harness. *Pediatric Nursing, 18*(3), 229–232.

Staheli, L. (1992). *Fundamentals of pediatric orthopedics.* New York: Raven Press.

Stout, J. D., Bandy, P., Feller, N., Stroup, K. B., & Bull, M. J. (1992). Transporting resources for pediatric orthopaedic clients. *Orthopaedic Nursing, 11*(1), 34–40.

Theiss, S. M., Lonstein, J. E., & Winter, R. B. (1996). Wound infections in reconstructive spine surgery. *Orthopaedic Clinics of North America, 27*(1), 105–110.

Unkila-Kallio, L. (1994). Serum C-reactive protein, erythrocyte sedimentation rate, and white blood cell count in acute hematogenous osteomyelitis of children. *Pediatrics, 93*(1), 59–62.

Weiner, D. (1993). *Pediatric orthopedics.* New York: Churchill Livingstone.

White, P. H., & Ansell, B. M. (1992). Methotrexate for juvenile rheumatoid arthritis. *New England Journal of Medicine, 326*(16), 1077–1078.

Winter, R. B. (1994). The pendulum has swung too far: Bracing for adolescent idiopathic scoliosis in the 1990s. *Orthopaedic Clinics of North America, 25*(2), 195–204.

51

◆ ◆ ◆ ◆ ◆ ◆ ◆ ◆ ◆ ◆

The Child with an Endocrine Alteration

LEARNING OBJECTIVES

After studying this chapter, you should be able to:

- List the six major hormones of the endocrine system.
- Describe the negative feedback system.
- Discuss nursing strategies to improve compliance with medications.
- Describe the signs and symptoms of hypothyroidism versus hyperthyroidism.
- Compare and contrast the relationship between diabetes insipidus and syndrome of inappropriate antidiuretic hormone as they relate to water metabolism.
- Describe the psychosocial issues concerning children with precocious puberty.
- Identify the role of insulin in the metabolism of carbohydrates, fats, and proteins in both the fasting and postprandial state.
- Compare and contrast type 1 diabetes mellitus (insulin-dependent diabetes mellitus) and type 2 diabetes mellitus (non–insulin-dependent diabetes mellitus).
- Identify management goals for the child with type 1 diabetes mellitus.
- List the nursing diagnoses associated with type 1 diabetes mellitus.
- Identify the child/family teaching needs associated with home management of type 1 diabetes mellitus.
- Identify the role and nursing implications of insulin therapy, diet therapy, exercise, self-monitoring of blood glucose, and urine ketone monitoring in the management of diabetes.
- Describe the signs, symptoms, causes, and treatment of hypoglycemia and hyperglycemia.
- Identify the pathophysiology of diabetic ketoacidosis, treatment, and nursing care of the child in diabetic ketoacidosis.

DEFINITIONS

beta cells   Specialized cells in the pancreas that manufacture and secrete insulin; thought to be the target of the autoimmune destructive process of type 1 diabetes mellitus.

diabetic ketoacidosis (DKA)   Metabolic consequence of severe insulin deficit; marked by hyperglycemia, acidosis, and ketosis.

euthyroid   Having normal thyroid function.

gland   An organ or structure that secretes a substance or hormones to be used in some other part of the body.

glucagon   A hormone produced by the alpha cells of the pancreas; counteracts the action of insulin by converting liver stores of glycogen to blood glucose, resulting in an elevation of the blood glucose level.

glucose   The substrate of choice for cellular energy; the breakdown product of carbohydrate.

glycosuria   Glucose in urine; occurs when the blood glucose level exceeds the renal threshold and glucose "spills" into the urine.

glycosylated hemoglobin   A laboratory test used to evaluate glycemic control by measuring glycosylation (or sugar coating) on the hemoglobin portion of the red blood cell; offers a 3-month average of blood glucose control.

honeymoon phase   An early stage of diabetes characterized by relatively small exogenous insulin requirements to maintain normal blood glucose.

hormone   A chemical substance produced by one gland or tissue and carried by the blood to other tissues or organs, where it causes a specific effect.

hyperglycemia   Blood glucose levels above 120 mg/dl (fasting) or 200 mg/dl (random).

hypoglycemia   Blood glucose levels below 70 mg/dl.

hypothalamus   Portion of the brain that secretes releasing factors to the pituitary gland for the maintenance of endocrine/metabolic activities.

idiopathic   For unknown reasons.

ketone/ketoacid   An acid manufactured by the liver in response to starvation (in diabetic child, a result of insulin deficit); produced from fat stores, can be used for energy when glucose is unavailable.

Kussmaul respiration   Deep, rapid respiration seen with DKA, in which CO_2 is expelled in a respiratory compensation for acidosis; also described as *air hunger*.

pituitary   An endocrine gland attached to the base of the brain that secretes numerous hormones; often referred to as *the master gland*.

Review of the Endocrine System

Various tissues that produce and secrete chemicals called *hormones* comprise the endocrine system. The hormones stimulate and regulate the actions of other tissues, the target tissues.

The endocrine system and the autonomic nervous system function in tandem to regulate growth, metabolism, and reproduction. The hypothalamic–pituitary axis controls their activities. The autonomic nervous system reacts to a stimulus, transmitting its message to the hypothalamus. In turn, the hypothalamus manufactures and secretes the appropriate hormonal factors. These are transmitted to the anterior pituitary gland, which then stimulates or inhibits the release of the involved hormones.

The principle of feedback control is involved in hormone production and secretion. In negative feedback, increasing levels of a specific hormone begin to inhibit the system responsible for releasing that hormone. As the hormonal secretion rises, there is a corresponding decrease in secretion production of its stimulating hormone. Conversely, when there is too little circulating hormone, the target gland is stimulated to secrete additional hormone.

The pituitary gland is composed of an anterior lobe and a posterior lobe. The anterior pituitary lobe secretes six hormones: adrenocorticotropic hormone (ACTH), thyroid-

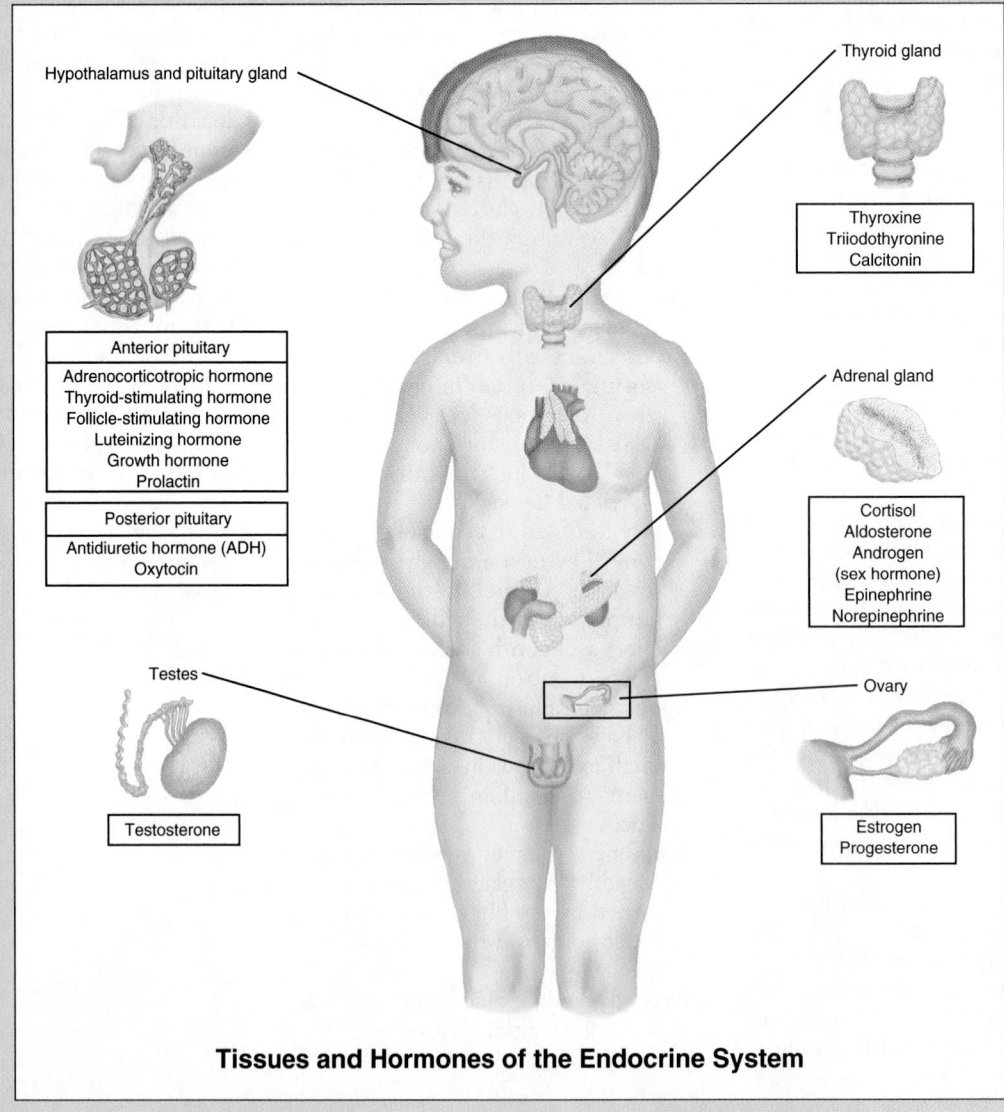

Hypothalamus and pituitary gland

Thyroid gland

Thyroxine
Triiodothyronine
Calcitonin

Anterior pituitary

Adrenocorticotropic hormone
Thyroid-stimulating hormone
Follicle-stimulating hormone
Luteinizing hormone
Growth hormone
Prolactin

Posterior pituitary

Antidiuretic hormone (ADH)
Oxytocin

Adrenal gland

Cortisol
Aldosterone
Androgen
(sex hormone)
Epinephrine
Norepinephrine

Testes

Testosterone

Ovary

Estrogen
Progesterone

Tissues and Hormones of the Endocrine System

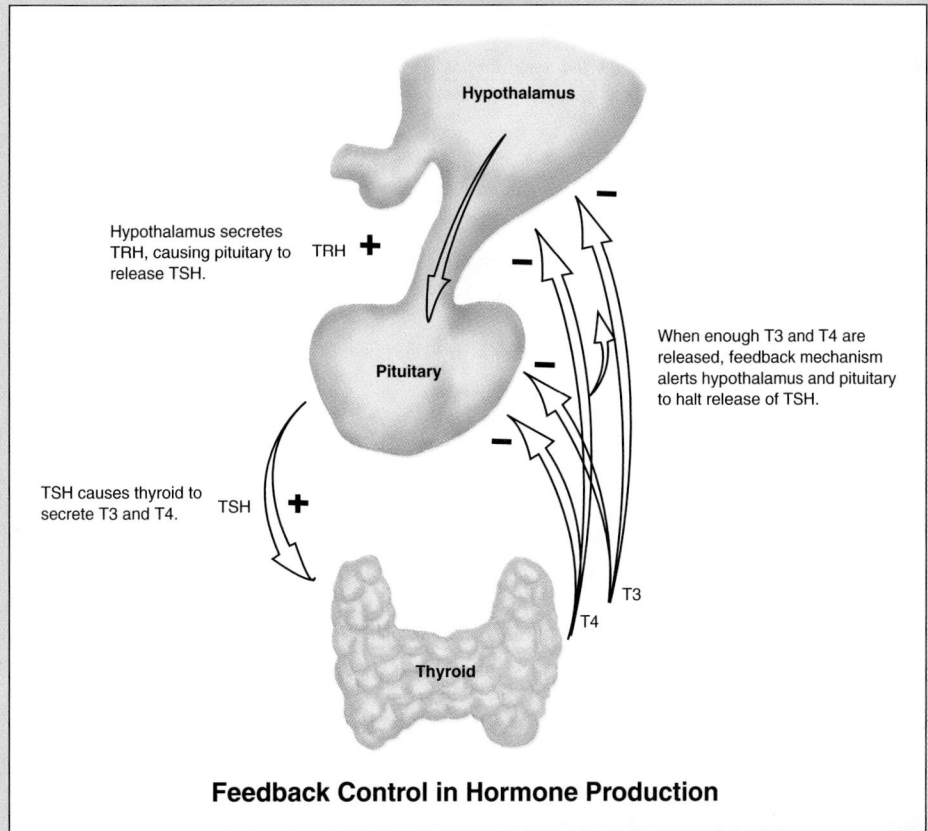

Feedback Control in Hormone Production

Hypothalamus

Hypothalamus secretes TRH, causing pituitary to release TSH.

TRH **+**

Pituitary

TSH causes thyroid to secrete T3 and T4.

TSH **+**

When enough T3 and T4 are released, feedback mechanism alerts hypothalamus and pituitary to halt release of TSH.

T3
T4

Thyroid

stimulating hormone (TSH), follicle-stimulating hormone (FSH), luteinizing hormone (LH), growth hormone (GH), and prolactin. Four of these hormones—ACTH, TSH, LH, and FSH—in turn stimulate their target glands to secrete the appropriate specific hormones. The posterior pituitary lobe stores antidiuretic hormone (ADH) and oxytocin, which are synthesized by the hypothalamus.

Disruption in the neurologic or chemical control of hormone secretion causes an endocrine disorder. Possible underlying causes include malfunction of the nervous system, the hypothalamus, the pituitary gland, or the target gland. Congenital, infectious, neoplastic, autoimmune, or idiopathic factors may play a role.

▌ *Diagnostic Tests and Procedures*

Diagnosing endocrine dysfunction usually involves laboratory testing. Serum hormone levels are measured to deter-

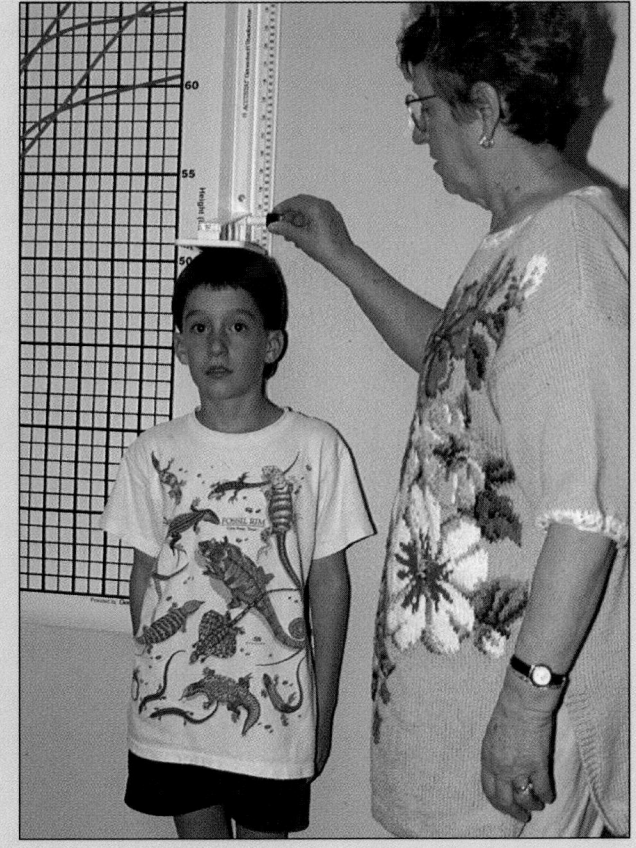

Pediatric Differences in the Endocrine System

- The endocrine system is less developed at birth than any other body system.
- Hormonal control of many body functions is lacking until 12 to 18 months of age. As a result, infants might manifest imbalances in concentration of fluids, electrolytes, amino acids, glucose, and trace substances.

Common Laboratory and Diagnostic Tests for Endocrine System Dysfunction

Test	Description	Normal Findings	Indications	Preparation and Nursing Considerations
Blood				
Growth hormone test	An agent such as insulin, arginine, or clonidine is given to stimulate release or production of GH	One or more peak GH levels greater than 7 ng/ml	Evaluate GH production, identify GH deficiency	Time specific; specimens must be drawn accurately NPO after midnight before test Notify physician if severe or prolonged hypoglycemia develops when insulin is given as stimulating agent
Cosyntropin test (Cortrosyn)	IV cosyntropin (ACTH) is given after baseline cortisol is measured to test ability of adrenal gland to respond to ACTH	A rise of cortisol level equal to double baseline; maximum cortisol level <18 μg/dl indicates insufficiency	Evaluate adrenal production of cortisol (may be associated with GH deficiency or hypopituitarism) Identify adrenal insufficiency	NPO after midnight Blood samples must be drawn before and after cosyntropin is given
Diagnostic				
Water deprivation study	Child is deprived of water and other fluids for 7 hr	Decreased urine output Increased urine specific gravity Normal serum sodium	Confirm diagnosis of diabetes insipidus	Strictly monitor serum sodium and urine osmolality Stop test if significant weight loss, or change in vital signs or neurologic status develop Weigh child before, during, and after test
Radiologic				
Bone age radiograph	Radiographic study of wrist to determine bone maturation.	Bone age consistent with chronologic age	Delayed bone age may indicate GH deficiency or hypothyroidism; advanced bone age may be associated with precocious puberty	None
Computed tomography/magnetic resonance imaging of brain	Noninvasive imaging techniques to identify structures/abnormalities of the brain	Normal structures	Determine presence of tumors or cysts, or structural abnormalities that may be affecting either hypothalamus or pituitary gland	May require sedation
Pelvic ultrasound study	Noninvasive sound waves identify anatomy of pelvic structures/abnormalities	Normal structures	Identify tumors/cysts within ovaries or adrenal glands in disorders associated with puberty	May require full bladder

ACTH, adrenocorticotropic hormone; GH, growth hormone; NPO, nothing by mouth.

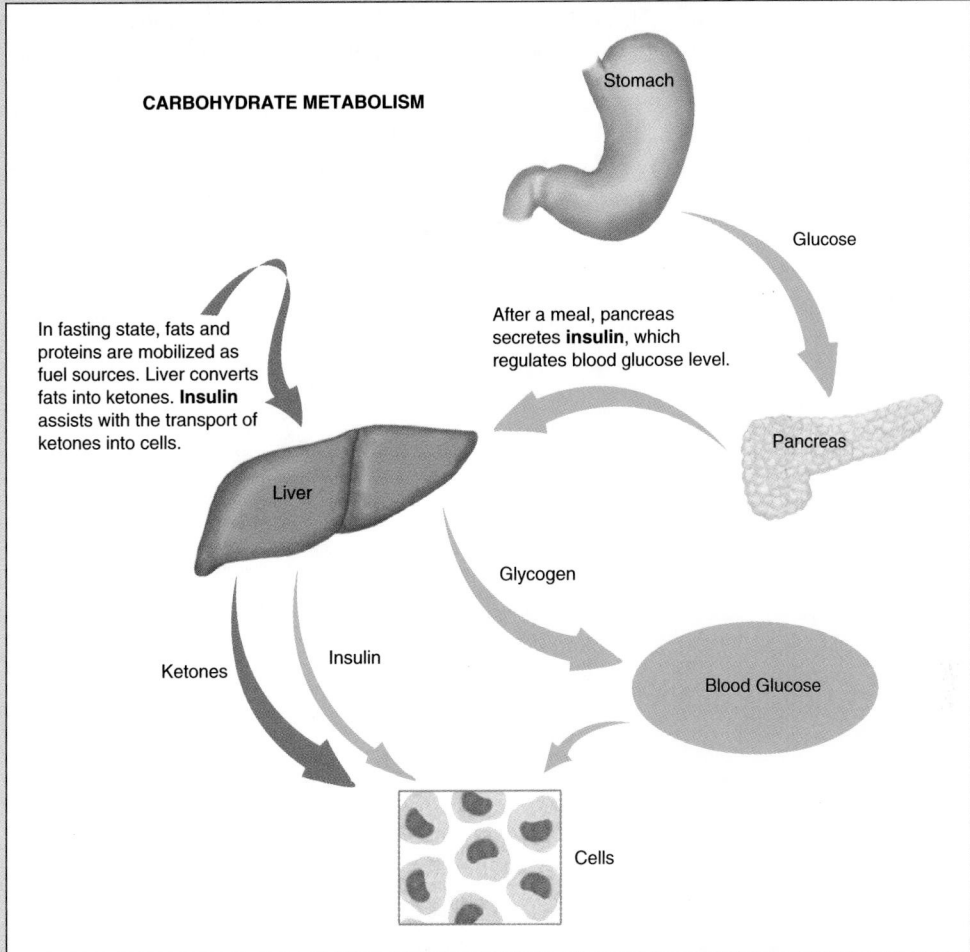

CARBOHYDRATE METABOLISM

Stomach

Glucose

After a meal, pancreas secretes **insulin**, which regulates blood glucose level.

Pancreas

In fasting state, fats and proteins are mobilized as fuel sources. Liver converts fats into ketones. **Insulin** assists with the transport of ketones into cells.

Liver

Glycogen

Ketones   Insulin

Blood Glucose

Cells

mine if the amounts are adequate, deficient, or excessive. Laboratory screening is useful for diagnosis of disease, as well as for monitoring children on hormone therapy.

Normal hormone levels are related to the child's age and stage of puberty. Because hormones are secreted at various times during the day or on a circadian rhythm, random blood samples may be difficult to interpret. Stimulation testing frequently demonstrates more accurate and definitive test results. With stimulation testing, a releasing factor or other agent is given to trigger the release or inhibition of a specific hormone. Serial blood sampling identifies the peak or trough level of the hormone, aiding in more accurate interpretation.

Other diagnostic tests include radiography and imaging techniques. Bone age radiographs can determine bone maturation and growth potential. Computed tomography scans and magnetic resonance imaging are used to determine the presence of tumors or cysts affecting the hypothalamus, pituitary, or target glands.

Accurate measurement of height and weight is essential when assessing the child for endocrine function. Evaluation of sexual development according to Tanner stages is also a part of the diagnostic workup (see Table 8–2). Developmental milestones and school performance should also be monitored because delays might be associated with endocrine disorders.

Physiology of Carbohydrate Metabolism

Glucose is the primary source of energy for body cells. Glucose can be stored in the fat tissues and, as glycogen, in

Actions of Insulin

Anabolic Actions of Insulin	Catabolic Consequences of Insulin Deficit
Promotes glucose as a fuel source	Promotes fats and proteins as fuel sources
Promotes storage of glucose as glycogen	Allows glycogen stores to be broken down
Prevents breakdown of fat stores	Allows fat stores to be depleted
Increases protein synthesis	Allows protein breakdown into amino acids

muscle or liver cells. Because only small amounts of glucose can be stored, the body must maintain a minimum blood glucose level.

Insulin, a hormone, is secreted by the beta cells of the pancreas. Its main function is to regulate the blood glucose level by controlling the rate of glucose uptake by cells. Little or no insulin is secreted by the beta cells when a person is in the fasting state; greater quantities are secreted after the person has eaten a meal. In the fasting state, with relatively small quantities of available insulin, the body mobilizes fats and proteins to be used as fuel sources. The liver then converts the fats into ketoacids, or ketones. With the assistance of insulin, the ketones are transported into the cells and are used as an alternative source of fuel for bodily functions. This process ensures an energy source during periods of fasting.

Some endocrine disorders, such as precocious puberty and growth hormone deficiency, are most often seen in an outpatient setting. Others, such as diabetes mellitus, are managed in both inpatient and outpatient settings. Because several disorders require long-term management, the nurse's priority is teaching and advocacy. Addressing psychological needs must be a priority for a child with a disorder that affects appearance.

■ Congenital Hypothyroidism

Congenital hypothyroidism is a condition in which the thyroid gland does not produce sufficient thyroid hormone to meet the body's metabolic needs. The condition is present from birth and, if not treated, can lead to mental retardation.

Etiology

Congenital hypothyroidism is caused by an absent (aplastic) or underdeveloped (lingual) thyroid gland. For unknown reasons, the fetal thyroid gland fails to develop or does not fully develop. Other causes may be hypothalamic or hypopituitary disorders in which there is insufficient thyroid-stimulating hormone (TSH) to stimulate the thyroid gland. Maternal intake of medications during pregnancy or exposure to radiation can cause transient or permanent hypothyroidism in the infant.

Incidence

Congenital hypothyroidism occurs in 1:4,000 births, as detected by newborn screening. Because untreated hypothyroidism causes mental retardation, most states have mandatory newborn screening programs to diagnose hypothyroidism before symptoms occur. Early detection and treatment favors increased intellectual function. Although most occurrences are spontaneous, approximately 10% have a genetic cause (Fort, 1996).

Manifestations

The infant with congenital hypothyroidism may display the following signs (Fig. 51–1): skin mottling, a large fontanel, large tongue, hypotonia/slow reflexes, and a distended abdomen. Other signs and symptoms include prolonged jaundice, lethargy, constipation, feeding problems, coldness to touch, umbilical hernia, hoarse cry, and excessive sleeping. The infant with congenital hypothyroidism may have none of these signs or symptoms; screening is essential for recognizing these infants.

Diagnostic Evaluation

Congenital hypothyroidism is usually diagnosed by newborn screening. Ideally, testing should be done at 3 to 6 days of

PATHOPHYSIOLOGY

of Congenital Hypothyroidism

The thyroid gland is a butterfly-shaped gland located in front of the neck. Thyroid-stimulating hormone (TSH), secreted by the pituitary, induces the thyroid to produce thyroxine (T_4) and triiodothyronine (T_3). The thyroid traps iodine and produces T_4, which is essential for normal growth and development, especially brain development, in the first 2 years of life. Immediately after delivery, there is a dramatic increase in TSH, most likely related to the stress of the birth process. Within the first week of life, the TSH level gradually falls.

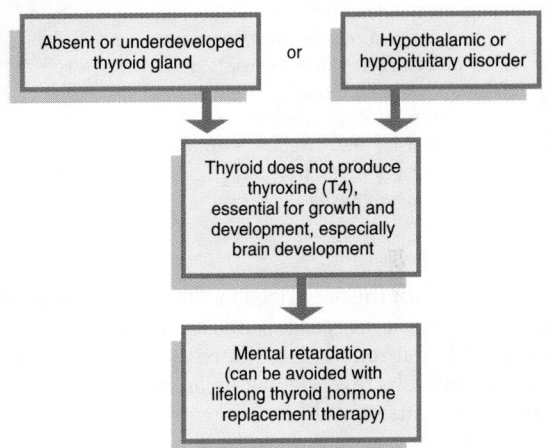

Underdevelopment of the thyroid gland or a hypothalamic or hypopituitary disorder causes inadequate production of T_4, which is essential for brain development. If not treated, this can cause mental retardation in the developing child. An infant with congenital hypothyroidism has an elevated TSH and a low T_4.

age. Tests done 24 to 48 hours after delivery may be falsely interpreted because of the rise in TSH immediately after birth.

Thyroid scans can identify any functioning thyroid tissue. Treatment should *never* be delayed while waiting for scan results.

Therapeutic Management

Treatment of congenital hypothyroidism consists of lifelong thyroid hormone replacement, usually in the form of levothyroxine. It is given as a single daily oral dose that varies with age. The dosage is titrated to suppress TSH and maintain thyroxine (T_4) in the upper half of the normal range (Fort, 1996).

■ NURSING CARE

The Infant with Congenital Hypothyroidism

Assessment

Nursing care of the infant with congenital hypothyroidism involves assessing growth and development and ensuring

FIGURE 51–1

This infant with congenital hypothyroidism fed poorly and was constipated. She was very lethargic and had no social smile and no head control. In the pretreatment photograph, notice her puffy face, large tongue, dull expression, and hirsute forehead. The post-treatment photograph shows decreased facial puffiness, decreased hirsutism of the forehead, and an alert appearance. Newborn screening for hypothyroidism is important because treatment should begin in the first weeks of life to prevent mental retardation and other problems. Treatment consists of lifelong thyroid hormone replacement. (From Behrman, R. E., Kliegman, R. M., & Arvin, A. M. [1996]. *Nelson textbook of pediatrics* [15th ed., p. 1592]. Philadelphia: Saunders.)

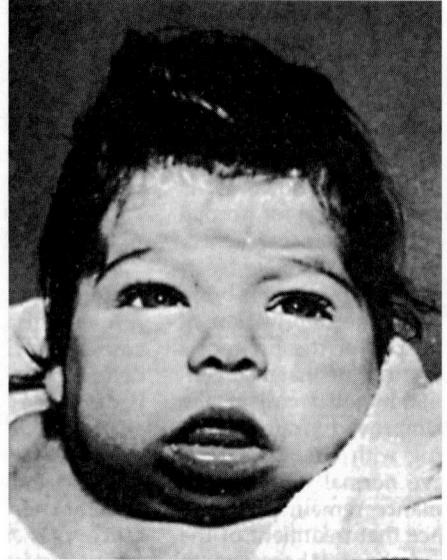

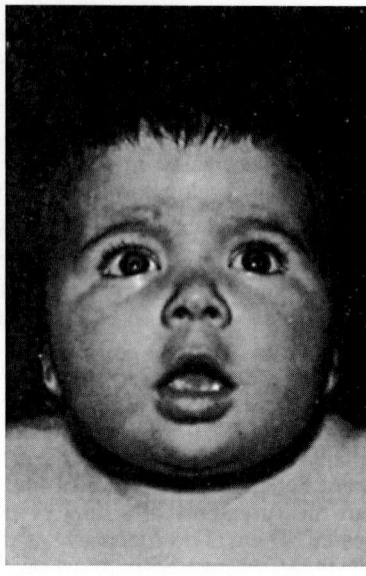

◀ Untreated congenital hypothyroidism in a 6-month-old infant

Four months after treatment ▶

compliance with the prescribed medication regimen. Nurses play a major role in recognizing the infant with hypothyroidism. Mental retardation caused by untreated hypothyroidism cannot be reversed, but it can be prevented through early identification and proper treatment. In general, infants with hypothyroidism are evaluated every month for the first year of life, and then every 3 to 6 months thereafter. The nurse should obtain accurate measurements of height, weight, and head circumference at each visit. Frequent developmental assessment is also essential.

Nursing Diagnosis and Planning

The following nursing diagnoses and expected outcomes may be appropriate for the infant with congenital hypothyroidism.

■ Knowledge Deficit related to the congenital disorder.
Expected Outcomes: The parents will demonstrate the ability to monitor their infant for signs and symptoms of hypothyroidism and hyperthyroidism; verbalize an understanding of normal growth and development mile-

---

CRITICAL TO REMEMBER

The Child with Congenital Hypothyroidism

• Untreated hypothyroidism leads to mental retardation.
• Thyroxine (T_4) and thyroid-stimulating hormone (TSH) levels vary with age, but any infant with a low T_4 and a TSH value exceeding 40 μU/ml is considered to have primary hypothyroidism until proven otherwise (American Academy of Pediatrics, 1993).

---

stones; give thyroid medication properly; and verbalize understanding of the child's lifelong needs and routines.
■ Altered Growth and Development related to disease process.
Expected Outcome: The infant will demonstrate growth and developmental milestones appropriate for age.
■ Ineffective Thermoregulation related to decreased basal metabolic rate.
Expected Outcome: The infant will maintain normal body temperature.

Interventions

Instruct family members on the importance of medication compliance. Emphasize that the medication is necessary for the child's growth, especially for the rapidly developing brain.

Teach the family how and when to administer the medication. Levothyroxine is given orally as a single daily dose. The medication can be dissolved in a small amount of water and given by syringe, or placed into the nipple of a baby bottle along with a small amount of formula. Warn the caregiver not to dissolve the medication in a large amount of formula because, if the formula is unfinished, the infant will not receive the full dosage. When the infant is older, the medication can be given in a spoonful of cereal or baby food. If the infant or child vomits within 1 hour of taking medication, the dose should be readministered. Frequently missed doses can lead to developmental delays and poor growth.

Also, teach the parents the signs and symptoms of both hypothyroidism and hyperthyroidism and when to notify the physician if symptoms occur. Hyperthyroidism can develop in infants receiving too much medication. Parents need to be taught to count their child's pulse and to notify their health care provider if the rate is greater than the recommended parameter.

Because hypothyroidism is a lifelong condition, school-age children and teenagers should be made aware of the importance of taking their medication and of keeping regular follow-up visits with the physician.

Evaluation

- Has the infant exhibited any signs or symptoms of hypothyroidism or hyperthyroidism?
- Is the child developing appropriately for age according to growth charts and Denver Developmental Screening Test (DDST) scores?
- Does the child have normal results on thyroid function tests?
- Is the child's body temperature within normal limits?
- Have the parents verbalized an understanding of their child's lifelong needs and routines?

Acquired Hypothyroidism

Hypothyroidism is a condition in which the thyroid gland produces an inadequate amount of thyroid hormone to meet the body's metabolic needs.

Etiology

Hashimoto's thyroiditis, a common cause of acquired hypothyroidism, is usually associated with a goiter. Other primary causes of hypothyroidism include surgical thyroidectomy, radioactive iodine therapy for hyperthyroidism, radiation therapy for malignancies, and excessive iodine ingestion. Less frequently, decreased TSH secretion by the pituitary gland or decreased thyrotropin-releasing hormone secretion by the hypothalamus causes hypothyroidism.

Thyroiditis is the most common cause of acquired hypothyroidism in children and adolescents. It often occurs in families with a history of thyroid disease. Other family members may have positive thyroid antibodies. Thyroiditis is more common in girls.

Pathophysiology

In contrast to congenital hypothyroidism, adverse effects from hypothyroidism acquired after 2 to 3 years of age are often reversible. Goiter, an enlarged thyroid gland one to two times normal size, occurs in response to TSH secretions.

Manifestations

Manifestations of hypothyroidism include goiter (one lobe usually larger than the other); dry, thick skin and coarse hair; tiredness/fatigue; cold intolerance; constipation; weight gain; decreased linear growth; edema of face, eyes, and hands; and irregular or delayed menses.

Diagnostic Evaluation

Hypothyroidism is diagnosed by elevated TSH and low T_4. Elevated TSH is the most sensitive indicator of primary hypothyroidism.

Thyroiditis is diagnosed by the presence of circulating thyroid antibodies and is usually associated with a firm goiter. Initially, TSH is elevated with normal T_4, although, over time, T_4 decreases. With secondary or tertiary hypo-

thyroidism, TSH is not elevated; therefore, thyrotropin-releasing hormone stimulation testing is usually required for diagnosis.

Therapeutic Management

Management of hypothyroidism involves thyroid hormone replacement, usually with levothyroxine. Dosage varies according to the child's age and weight, and is given as a single daily dose. The dose is titrated to maintain T_4 in the upper half of the normal range and to suppress TSH.

■ NURSING CARE
The Child with Acquired Hypothyroidism

Assessment

Care of the child with acquired hypothyroidism includes assessing response to treatment and compliance with the medication regimen. With proper treatment, the goiter should decrease in size. Signs and symptoms of hypothyroidism should also resolve with adequate thyroid hormone replacement. Monitoring height, weight, and performance on the DDST at each visit assesses the child's growth and development. The nurse should monitor school performance as well.

Nursing Diagnosis and Planning

The following nursing diagnoses and expected outcomes may be appropriate for a child with acquired hypothyroidism:

- Constipation related to decreased basal metabolic rate secondary to hypothyroidism.
  Expected Outcome: The child will maintain normal bowel movements.
- Activity Intolerance related to fatigue.
  Expected Outcome: The child will be able to exercise at the same level as peers.
- Altered Nutrition: More Than Body Requirements related to weight gain/obesity.
  Expected Outcome: The child will grow and gain weight at an age-appropriate rate.
- Ineffective Thermoregulation related to decreased basal metabolic rate secondary to hypothyroidism.
  Expected Outcome: The child will maintain normal body temperature.

Interventions

Parents and school-age and older children should be instructed on the correct dose and timing of thyroid medication. Thyroid hormone levels are usually checked every 3 to 6 months. Laboratory values within the normal range indicate good response to therapy. Instruct parents on the signs and symptoms of hypothyroidism and hyperthyroidism and to notify the physician if symptoms occur.

Evaluation

- Does the child have normal results on thyroid function tests?
- Has the child maintained normal bowel movements?
- Can the child tolerate exercise at the same level as peers?

- Has the child maintained age-appropriate height and weight?
- Has the child maintained normal body temperature?

Hyperthyroidism (Graves' Disease)

Graves' disease is an autoimmune condition in which excessive thyroid hormones are produced by an enlarged thyroid gland. It is the most common cause of hyperthyroidism in children.

Incidence

Graves' disease accounts for 5% to 10% of thyroid disorders in children (Dallas, 1996). The female-to-male ratio is approximately 4:1. There may also be a familial tendency toward Graves' disease. Children with autoimmune disease are at risk for other autoimmune disorders.

Pathophysiology

Circulating autoantibodies known as thyroid-stimulating immunoglobulins stimulate the thyroid gland to make tri-iodothyronine (T_3) and T_4. These antibodies attach themselves to the TSH receptor sites on the thyroid gland, resulting in excessive thyroid hormone production. The cause of antibody production is unknown.

Manifestations

The following manifestations are common in Graves' disease: goiter, increased appetite with weight loss, nervousness, diarrhea, increased perspiration/heat intolerance, increased heart rate, palpitations, tremors, exophthalmos, poor attention span, and behavior/school problems.

Diagnostic Evaluation

Elevated serum T_4 levels and suppressed TSH levels, associated with symptoms of hyperthyroidism, suggest Graves' disease. Autoantibodies usually are positive. Thyroid uptake of radioactive iodine is increased.

Therapeutic Management

The three approaches to the management of Graves' disease include antithyroid drug therapy, radioactive iodine, and surgery. Antithyroid drug therapy with propylthiouracil or methimazole is the treatment of choice for childhood hyperthyroidism. These drugs act by blocking thyroid hormone production by the thyroid gland. The medications usually are given three times a day and lower thyroid hormone levels in several weeks. Minor adverse effects include arthralgia, skin rash, pruritus, and gastric intolerance. Major adverse effects may include neutropenia, hepatotoxicity, and hypothyroidism.

A second approach to management is oral radioiodine treatment. Radioactive iodine (I-131) is given as an oral solution. With this therapy, the radioactive iodine is absorbed and concentrated by the thyroid gland, destroying the thyroid tissue in approximately 6 to 18 weeks. Hyperthyroid symptoms may intensify briefly after treatment. Hy-

pothyroidism can result once the thyroid gland is radiated, necessitating thyroid replacement therapy.

Subtotal or partial thyroidectomy, the surgical removal of thyroid gland tissue, is the third form of management. Lugol's solution (potassium iodide), given 10 to 14 days before surgery, decreases the gland's vascularity. Surgery carries the risk of injury to the parathyroid glands, resulting in hypocalcemia. Calcium levels are monitored after surgery.

Recurrence of hyperthyroidism is uncommon but possible. There is also a 60% to 80% chance for development of hypothyroidism, which can be treated with thyroid replacement therapy.

Follow-up evaluations correlate with response to therapy. As thyroid functions normalize, follow-up endocrine evaluations are recommended once or twice per year.

NURSING CARE

The Child with Hyperthyroidism

Assessment

The treatment goal consists of normalizing thyroid hormone levels, alleviating symptoms of hyperthyroidism, and decreasing the goiter. The nurse should assess for compliance with medication therapy. Determine that the family understands that medical therapy might take several weeks to decrease thyroid hormone action. Propranolol, a beta-adrenergic blocker, may be prescribed to decrease adrenergic symptoms (tachycardia, heat intolerance, tremor) until the antithyroid medication is effective. Monitor the child for signs of adrenergic symptoms.

A child being treated with propylthiouracil has an increased risk of neutropenia and hepatotoxicity; regular blood counts and liver function studies are done to assess these risks. Assess the child for fever, joint pain, edema, rash, or excessive bruising. A child who acquires a fever or sore throat while receiving propylthiouracil should be evaluated by a physician and a complete blood count should be obtained.

Nursing Diagnosis and Planning

The following nursing diagnoses and expected outcomes may be appropriate for a child with hyperthyroidism:

- Ineffective Management of Therapeutic Regimen (Individual) related to noncompliance with medication.
  Expected Outcome: The child will comply with the medication regimen.

Hypothyroidism Versus Hyperthyroidism

Hypothyroidism	Hyperthyroidism
• Tiredness/fatigue	• Nervousness/anxiety
• Constipation	• Diarrhea
• Cold intolerance	• Heat intolerance
• Weight gain	• Weight loss
• Dry, thick skin	• Smooth, velvety skin
• Edema of face, eyes, hands	
• Decreased growth	

- Altered Nutrition: Less Than Body Requirements related to increased metabolic rate.
  Expected Outcome: The child will maintain weight appropriate for age and height.
- Diarrhea related to increased basal metabolic rate secondary to hyperthyroidism.
  Expected Outcomes: The child will be euthyroid, as evidenced by normal results on thyroid function tests; the child will have normal bowel movements.
- Risk for Activity Intolerance related to loss of muscle mass from increased basal metabolic rate secondary to hyperthyroidism.
  Expected Outcome: The child will be able to exercise at the same level as peers.
- Sleep Pattern Disturbance related to increased metabolic rate secondary to hyperthyroidism.
  Expected Outcome: The child will sleep through the night without waking.
- Risk for Altered Body Temperature related to increased basal metabolic rate secondary to hyperthyroidism.
  Expected Outcome: The child will maintain normal body temperature.

Interventions

The antithyroid drugs propylthiouracil and methimazole are usually given two or three times per day. This regimen may be difficult for some children to follow. Advise the use of pill dispensers and a watch with an alarm to remind the child to take the medication at specific times. The endocrinologist should evaluate the child and monitor thyroid function every 2 to 3 months while the child is undergoing treatment. Normal thyroid function tests and alleviation of symptoms indicate good response to therapy.

Once the child is euthyroid and asymptomatic, evaluation should occur once or twice a year. Medical therapy may be tapered after 3 years to evaluate for remission. Contact sports should be limited while the child is being treated to decrease the possibility of damage to the liver.

Evaluation

- Does the child have normal results on thyroid function tests?
- Is the child free of symptoms of hyperthyroidism?
- Is the child growing at an age-appropriate rate?
- Does the child demonstrate normal bowel movements?
- Is the child able to exercise at an age-appropriate level?
- Does the child sleep throughout the night?
- Has the child maintained a normal body temperature?

Diabetes Insipidus

Diabetes insipidus is an inability to concentrate urine because of a deficiency of vasopressin, also known as antidiuretic hormone (ADH).

Etiology

Diabetes insipidus commonly results from head trauma, tumors, or infection in the area of the hypothalamus. The most common type of tumor involving the hypothalamus that causes diabetes insipidus is craniopharyngioma.

Cranial radiation for treatment of tumors also may lead to ADH deficiency. Other causes include infections of the central nervous system such as meningitis or encephalitis, and congenital malformations, such as septic optic dysplasia or hypopituitarism.

Incidence

Head trauma and surgical resection of suprasellar tumors account for most cases of diabetes insipidus. Permanent diabetes insipidus develops in approximately 50% of children who have sustained trauma to the sella turcica. Transient or permanent diabetes insipidus is related to the percentage of damage to the vasopressin neurons (Muglia & Majzoub, 1996).

Manifestations

Increased urination (polyuria) and excessive thirst (polydipsia) are the classic manifestations of diabetes insipidus. Other signs and symptoms include nocturia and dehydration.

Diagnostic Evaluation

Diagnostic criteria include polyuria with associated hypernatremia (>150 mEq/L) and low urine specific gravity (<1.005) in the absence of hyperglycemia. Urine should be checked for glucose to rule out hyperglycemia as a cause of increased urine output.

A water deprivation test may also be necessary to confirm the diagnosis. In this 7-hour procedure, the child is deprived of water. A normal response is decreased urine output with a high urine specific gravity and no change in serum sodium. In diabetes insipidus, when fluid is restricted, the child continues to have large amounts of dilute urine, evidenced by low urine specific gravity. The serum sodium level also increases. To ensure the child's safety, this test is done in a hospital setting with frequent monitoring of serum sodium, hematocrit, and osmolality. Urine osmolality and output are also measured. The child is weighed at the beginning, middle, and conclusion of the water deprivation test. *Water deprivation should be stopped if the child loses 3% to 5% of baseline body weight, becomes dehydrated, or demonstrates a significant change in vital signs or neurologic status.*

Therapeutic Management

Treatment involves maintaining fluid balance and administering synthetic vasopressin (DDAVP). The dose of DDAVP ranges from 5 to 20 μg/kg/day in two doses. It is administered either intranasally, through a soft, flexible tube or metered spray, or by subcutaneous injection. The concentration of intranasal DDAVP is 100 μg/ml; the concentration of subcutaneous DDAVP is 4 μg/ml.

Dosage is individualized based on the child's age, size, urine output, and urine specific gravity. The subcutaneous dose is 10% of the intranasal dose. The duration of action varies from 12 to 24 hours. Doses are timed so that before the next dose, the child is allowed to have mildly increased urination. This helps prevent overtreatment and water retention. Parents are often taught to measure urine specific gravity at home to monitor effectiveness of treatment.

PATHOPHYSIOLOGY
. . . .
of Diabetes Insipidus

Antidiuretic hormone (ADH) is produced in the hypothalamus, transported through the pituitary stalk, and stored in the posterior pituitary. It is carried through the blood to the kidneys, where it acts on the distal tubules and collecting ducts to increase reabsorption of free water, thereby concentrating urine and decreasing urinary output.

Antidiuretic hormone is under the control of osmoreceptors in the anterior pituitary. These osmoreceptors operate on a negative feedback system based on serum osmolality, particularly sodium concentration. When the osmolality is low, production of ADH decreases, causing increased urine output and normalizing osmolality; conversely, when osmolality is increased, ADH production increases, causing water retention and decreasing urine output. In diabetes insipidus, a deficiency of ADH makes the body unable to conserve water, which results in large volumes of dilute urine. Loss of free water leads to an increase in serum sodium concentration. If the child has an intact thirst center, increasing oral intake might compensate for the large fluid loss. If the thirst drive is not intact or the child is unable to drink enough, the child may become dehydrated and have a high serum sodium level.

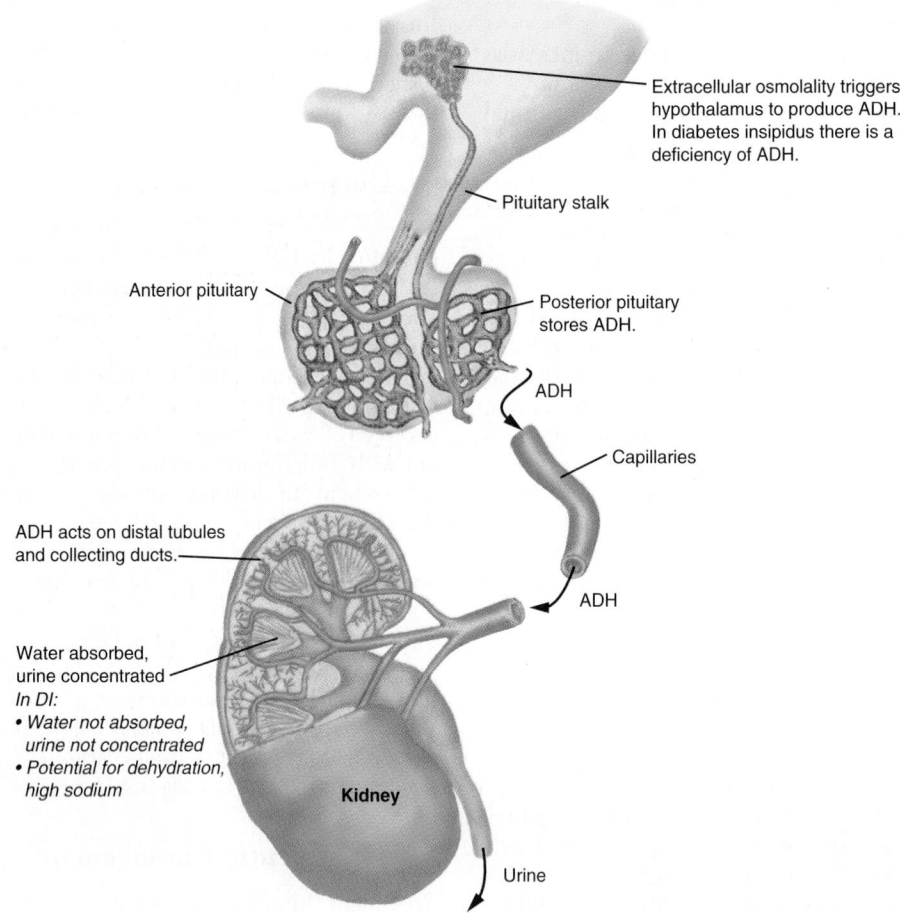

Extracellular osmolality triggers hypothalamus to produce ADH. In diabetes insipidus there is a deficiency of ADH.

Pituitary stalk

Anterior pituitary

Posterior pituitary stores ADH.

ADH

Capillaries

ADH

ADH acts on distal tubules and collecting ducts.

Water absorbed, urine concentrated
In DI:
• Water not absorbed, urine not concentrated
• Potential for dehydration, high sodium

Kidney

Urine

A child with an intact thirst center is able to self-regulate fluid needs and intake. If the child is not able to recognize thirst because of head trauma/surgery, the physician may prescribe a 24-hour fluid requirement.

Nursing Considerations

Nursing care involves assessing the parents' and child's understanding of diabetes insipidus. Educate the family about the basic pathophysiology of water metabolism and the cause of diabetes insipidus. Include a description of symptoms. Instruct the parent about symptoms indicating the need for DDAVP (increased thirst, polyuria, and dehydration), as well as symptoms of excessive DDAVP (decreased urine output, headaches, and water retention).

Teach the family the proper administration of DDAVP and observe a return demonstration of medication administration. If appropriate, instruct the family in using a refractometer to measure urine specific gravity. The child should wear a Medic Alert bracelet noting the diagnosis of diabetes insipidus. The child's teachers need to be aware of the diagnosis and must allow the child free access to water and toilet facilities. Advise the family to watch the child closely for signs of dehydration.

Syndrome of Inappropriate Antidiuretic Hormone

Syndrome of inappropriate ADH (SIADH) results from the excessive production or release of ADH, or vasopressin.

Etiology

Childhood SIADH usually is caused by disorders affecting the central nervous system, including infections (e.g., meningitis), head trauma, and brain tumors. SIADH is rare in children and is usually related to an underlying cause. Surgery for brain tumors may cause the child to experience transient SIADH. Often a triple response occurs after surgery: initially, the child has diabetes insipidus, then experiences temporary SIADH, and then returns to diabetes insipidus (Muglia & Majzoub, 1996). SIADH is usually transient and resolves when the underlying condition is corrected.

Manifestations

Certain manifestations occur with SIADH. These include decreased urine output, increased urine specific gravity, fluid retention, weight gain, hyponatremia, and increased urine osmolality.

Diagnostic Evaluation

Syndrome of inappropriate ADH should be suspected in children with central nervous system involvement, such as infections or head trauma, who have decreased urine output despite adequate intake. Laboratory diagnosis includes evidence of hyponatremia, hypochloremia, and low serum osmolality. Urine osmolality is usually greater than serum osmolality. Urine specific gravity is greater than 1.030. Adrenal, thyroid, and renal function studies can rule out other causes of hyponatremia.

Therapeutic Management

Initial treatment is correction of the underlying cause. The physician orders fluid limitations to correct hyponatremia.

PATHOPHYSIOLOGY

of Syndrome of Inappropriate Antidiuretic Hormone

Excessive antidiuretic hormone results in the kidney reabsorbing too much free water. This causes decreased output of concentrated urine, evidenced by a high urine specific gravity (>1.030). The excess water also causes an expanded fluid volume and a low serum sodium level. Once the sodium level falls below 125 mEq/L, the child can become symptomatic and experience anorexia, nausea, weakness, weight gain, confusion, and irritability.

Signs of Hyponatremia

Mild (Early)	Moderate	Severe
Anorexia	Confusion	Seizures
Headache	Irritability	Coma
Nausea	Lethargy	
Vomiting	Altered level of consciousness	

A child with severe hyponatremia may need intravenous infusion of sodium chloride. Drug therapy usually is not indicated for transient SIADH. Medications such as lithium and demeclocycline block the action of ADH at the renal collecting tubules and have been used in the management of chronic SIADH.

Nursing Considerations

The nurse should assess the child with SIADH for signs and symptoms of fluid overload, including edema, weight gain, urine specific gravity greater than 1.030, and dilutional hyponatremia. If the child is hyponatremic, monitor neurologic status by assessing level of consciousness and observing for headache, irritability, or seizures.

The child with fluid overload is at risk for injury related to seizures caused by hyponatremia. Interventions are directed toward maintaining fluid balance and preventing injury.

Assess the child's hydration and neurologic status every 2 to 4 hours. Carefully maintain strict fluid restrictions and document intake and output. Weigh the child daily to monitor fluid retention.

The child may have difficulty complying with the fluid restrictions. Explain to the child and parents the need for limited fluids and that the restriction is temporary. The nurse may give the child hard sugarless candies or apply wet washcloths to help keep mucous membranes moist.

Diet should include foods with high sodium content because extra sodium can help correct hyponatremia. Keep

---

Diabetes Insipidus Versus Syndrome of Inappropriate Antidiuretic Hormone (SIADH)

Diabetes Insipidus (High and Dry)	SIADH (Low and Wet)
• Increased urination	• Decreased urination
• Increased thirst	• Hypertension
• Nocturia	• Weight gain
• Dehydration	• Fluid retention
• Hypernatremia	• Hyponatremia
• Urine specific gravity <1.005	• Urine specific gravity >1.030
• Elevated serum osmolality (>300 mOsm/kg)	• Decreased serum osmolality (<280 mOsm/kg)
• Decreased urine osmolality	• Increased urine osmolality

in mind, however, that salty foods such as chips might make the child thirsty.

Closely monitor serum electrolyte levels as ordered by the physician. Alert the physician immediately to any change in neurologic status. Because severe hyponatremia can cause seizures, initiate seizure precautions if the serum sodium level drops below 125 mEq/L.

Evaluation of the child with SIADH should address a balanced intake and output, stable weight, and normal se-

rum sodium levels. Urine specific gravity should be maintained between 1.010 and 1.020.

Precocious Puberty

Precocious puberty refers to early onset of puberty, occurring before 8 years of age in girls and before 9 years of age in boys. It is defined as the premature appearance of secondary sexual characteristics, accelerated growth rate, and ad-

PATHOPHYSIOLOGY
of Precocious Puberty

Puberty occurs when the hypothalamus releases gonadotropin-releasing hormone (GnRH). This stimulates the pituitary gland to release luteinizing hormone (LH) and follicle-stimulating hormone (FSH). In girls, FSH stimulates formation of ovarian follicles to produce estrogen. Estrogen is necessary for the development of secondary sexual characteristics, such as breast development and maturation of the vagina and labia. LH is involved in the process of ovulation. In boys, FSH triggers the testes to support the development of sperm. LH stimulates the production of testosterone, which is necessary for the development of sexual characteristics and sperm production. Puberty development is classified according to Tanner stages I through V

(see Table 8–2). The adrenal glands produce the hormone dehydroepiandrosterone (DHEA), which causes pubic and axillary hair growth. During puberty, there is also an increase in growth rate, or a "growth spurt," in which a child grows an average of 4 to 6 inches per year.

In precocious puberty, the sex hormones that accelerate growth also cause the bone plates to close early. Bone usually fuses at 14 years of age for girls and 17 years for boys. With true precocious puberty, children have hormonal changes that mimic the onset of normal puberty. These hormonal changes may be central, arising from the hypothalamus, or peripheral, arising from the ovaries, testes, or adrenal glands.

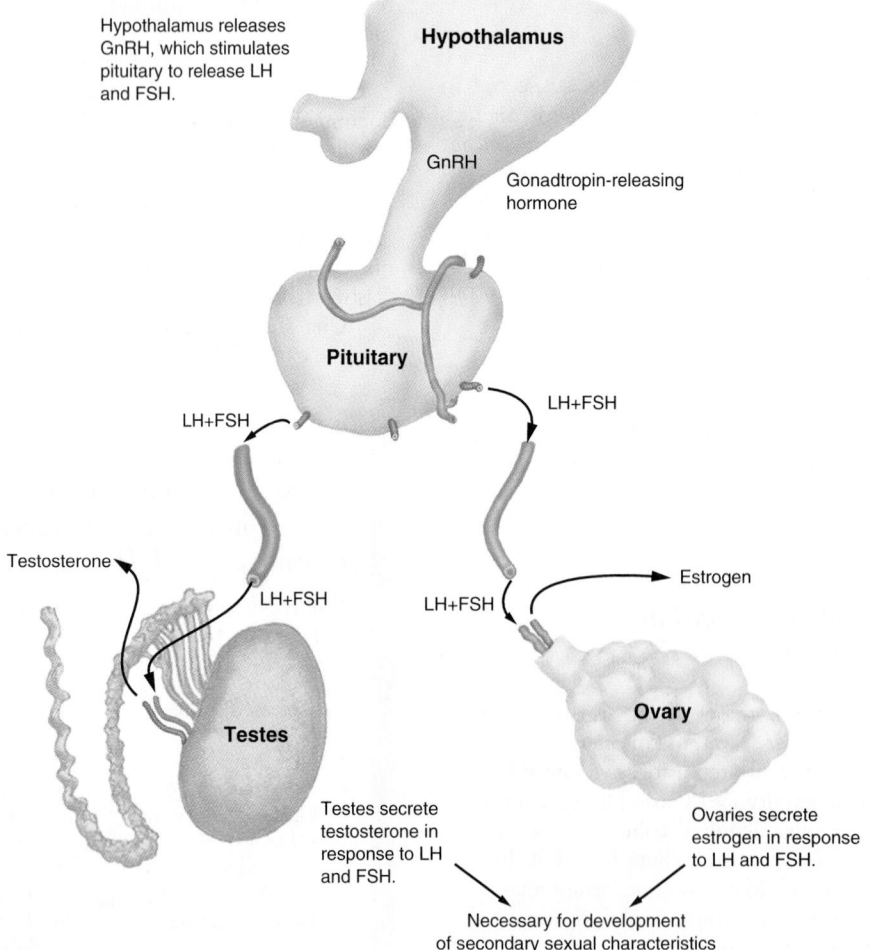

Hypothalamus releases GnRH, which stimulates pituitary to release LH and FSH.

Hypothalamus

GnRH — Gonadtropin-releasing hormone

Pituitary

LH+FSH   LH+FSH

Testosterone

LH+FSH   LH+FSH   Estrogen

Testes   **Ovary**

Testes secrete testosterone in response to LH and FSH.

Ovaries secrete estrogen in response to LH and FSH.

Necessary for development of secondary sexual characteristics

vanced bone maturation. The major consequence of precocious puberty is rapid bone growth, which causes early growth plate fusion and ultimately short stature in adulthood.

Etiology

Central, or true precocious puberty can be idiopathic or caused by central nervous system tumors (most commonly hamartomas), head trauma, or cranial radiation. Peripheral causes include abnormalities or tumors of the adrenal glands, ovaries, or testes. Congenital adrenal hyperplasia, a genetic disorder of the adrenal pathway, is the most common cause of peripheral precocious puberty. McCune-Albright syndrome may cause early puberty in girls; the genetic disorder familial testotoxicosis causes early puberty in boys.

Incidence

Precocious puberty occurs more frequently in girls; approximately 70% of cases are idiopathic, although boys have a higher incidence of central nervous system lesions. Both boys and girls can have hypothalamic hamartomas.

Manifestations

Manifestations of precocious puberty reflect sex differences:

Girls	Boys
• Breast development	• Testicular enlargement
• Pubic hair	• Penile enlargement
• Axillary hair	• Pubic hair
• Enlargement of vagina, uterus, and ovaries	• Axillary/chest hair
• Acne	• Facial hair
• Adult body odor	• Acne
• Growth spurt	• Adult body odor
• Moodiness	• Deepening of voice
• Onset of menstrual periods	

Diagnostic Evaluation

Diagnosis of precocious puberty begins with a thorough history, including onset of sexual characteristics, and a physical examination. Blood tests are then necessary to evaluate for elevated levels of luteinizing hormone (LH), follicle-stimulating hormone (FSH), testosterone, and estrogen. Unfortunately, because these hormones are released in small bursts during the day, random samples may not be adequate.

The gonadotropin-releasing hormone (GnRH) stimulation test is a more accurate and definitive test in determining the role of the pituitary gland during early puberty. Synthetic GnRH is administered intravenously to stimulate the release of LH and FSH from the pituitary gland. Serial samples of LH and FSH are then obtained over a 2-hour period. Before the onset of puberty, the FSH peak is higher than the LH peak. With the onset of puberty, the LH peak is higher than the FSH peak.

Radiographic studies also support diagnosis of precocious puberty. Radiographs of the wrist determine bone age and maturation and can assist in predicting final adult height. Skull radiographs screen for central nervous system lesions, although computed tomography scans and magnetic resonance imaging are more accurate in visualizing tumors. Abdominal and pelvic ultrasound are beneficial in diagnosing adrenal and ovarian tumors or cysts. Pelvic ultrasound also provides evidence of pubertal changes in the uterus and ovaries. Finally, isolated pubic hair development and elevated androgen hormone levels suggest an adrenal origin for premature sexual hair growth.

Therapeutic Management

Treatment aims to stop or reverse the development of secondary sexual characteristics and to maximize adult height. Current therapy for central (or pituitary-initiated) precocious puberty involves administration of a GnRH agonist, or blocker. GnRH blockers inhibit the binding of GnRH to the pituitary gland, causing decreased production of the pubertal hormones and slowing or reversing sexual development.

Several commercially available GnRH agonists can be administered either intranasally or by a monthly intramuscular injection. Once therapy is initiated, GnRH secretion is suppressed within 2 to 4 weeks. The accelerated growth rate and bone maturation slow, and some secondary sexual characteristics regress within the first year of treatment. Noncompliance with medication therapy can promote pubertal changes rather than suppress puberty.

There is no evidence suggesting that GnRH agonist therapy interferes with the child's reproduction in the future. Once therapy is discontinued pubertal progression resumes. For children with peripheral precocious puberty, treatment is aimed at correcting the underlying cause.

NURSING CARE
The Child with Precocious Puberty

Assessment

Nursing care of the child with precocious puberty addresses the physical and behavioral changes associated with puberty. A nurse working with these children may notice that they feel more comfortable around older children rather than peers of their own age. They often experience teasing about their bodies and may limit social activities such as swimming. Boys often exhibit aggressive behavior. Children who go through early puberty appear older than their chronologic age and are often treated accordingly by adults. Because of their mature appearance, children with precocious puberty are at greater risk for sexual abuse.

> If a child appears embarrassed or uncomfortable when being interviewed about sexual development, the nurse should explain to the child: "Everyone goes through body changes when growing up; it's just that these changes are happening to you sooner than most children. Can you tell me in your own words how you feel about your body?"

Nursing Diagnosis and Planning

The following nursing diagnoses and expected outcomes may be appropriate for the child with precocious puberty:

■ Knowledge Deficit about medication administration related to inadequate understanding of intramuscular or intranasal GnRH agonist.
  Expected Outcome: The caregiver will give an appropriate return demonstration of medication administration technique.
■ Altered Sexuality Patterns related to early puberty.
  Expected Outcome: The child will discuss feelings related to sexual development.
■ Body Image Disturbance related to early sexual development.
  Expected Outcome: The child will verbalize acceptance of body appearance.
■ Impaired Social Interaction related to appearing older than chronologic age.
  Expected Outcome: The child will exhibit age-appropriate behaviors and social interactions.

Interventions

Many parents may not be comfortable with their child's early development. The nurse assists with explaining the stages of puberty and each stage's associated behavioral changes. The nurse teaches parents that the child is experiencing normal changes at an unusual time.

Explanations given to the child should be geared to chronologic age. The nurse can direct the parent to books that explain sexual maturation in terms the child can understand. Psychological counseling might be necessary to help the family deal with the sensitive issues of sexuality.

The nurse also teaches the family about the prescribed medication regimen. In some instances, the parent is taught how to administer monthly injections. These might be stressful for the young child. The nurse demonstrates appropriate injection technique and teaches the child coping strategies to be used when the injection is given.

Evaluation

• Can the parents demonstrate proper medication administration?
• Has the child verbalized an understanding of body changes?
• Have the child and parents verbalized their concerns about their child's early sexual development?
• Is the child free of sexually precocious behavior?

▌ Growth Hormone Deficiency

Growth hormone (GH) deficiency results from inadequate production or secretion of GH, causing poor growth and short stature.

Etiology

Growth hormone deficiency may be isolated or may be associated with an underlying cause. Such causes include hypopituitarism, brain tumors (most commonly craniopharyngioma), and cranial irradiation. Other disorders associated with short stature that may respond to GH therapy include Turner's syndrome and chronic illnesses, such as renal disease.

PATHOPHYSIOLOGY
· · · · · · · · · · ·
of Growth Hormone (GH) Deficiency

Hormones such as GH, thyroxine, cortisol, and sex hormones influence growth. The hypothalamus secretes GH-releasing factor, which stimulates the pituitary gland to release GH. This hormone is secreted in pulses throughout the day, with increased secretion during the night. In the presence of hypoglycemia, GH is secreted to counteract insulin and raise the blood glucose level. Many children with GH deficiency may present with hypoglycemia.

Most children with short stature have constitutional growth delay. Children with short stature or poor growth rates may also be deficient in other hormones. Normal thyroid function is essential for growth; therefore, hypothyroidism may also present with short stature. Sex hormones are required for the growth spurt and sexual maturation that occurs with puberty. Children lacking more than one hormone produced by the pituitary gland are referred to as having hypopituitarism. Rate of growth and final adult height depend on factors such as family heights and nutrition. Any child growing less than 5 cm per year should be referred to an endocrinologist for further evaluation.

Incidence

The incidence of GH deficiency is approximately 1 in 10,000 to 20,000 children. In the United States, approximately 30,000 children are being treated with GH replacement.

Manifestations

These manifestations are typical of GH deficiency: height less than fifth percentile for age and sex, immature/cherubic facies, high-pitched voice, delayed puberty, hypoglycemia, and micropenis (associated with hypopituitarism).

Diagnostic Evaluation

Diagnosis of GH deficiency begins with careful measurements of growth over an extended period (usually 6 to 12 months). Height should be measured on a consistent scale, preferably with a calibrated stadiometer.

Initial screening involves thyroid function tests, complete blood count, somatomedin-C (an indirect measurement of GH level), and a bone age radiograph. Normal thyroid function is essential for adequate growth; thyroid studies are essential when evaluating for short stature. Complete blood count and other specific blood screening for any systemic/chronic illness should be done.

Because GH is normally secreted in pulses throughout the day and night, stimulation testing is necessary to confirm the diagnosis of GH deficiency. Agents used in provocative testing to stimulate GH production include insulin, arginine, clonidine, glucagon, and L-dopa. Once the stimulating agent is given, serial GH levels are drawn. Although criteria vary between agencies, a GH level below 7 ng/ml usually indicates GH deficiency. Two positive tests are required for diagnosis.

Therapeutic Management

A child with GH deficiency requires replacement therapy. Synthetic GH comes in a powdered form that must be diluted for administration. It is given as a subcutaneous injection six or seven times per week, usually in the evening. Dosage ranges from 0.18 to 0.3 mg/kg/wk, depending on the child's age and response to therapy. Once diluted, GH must be stored at 36° to 46°F. Treatment is usually considered effective if the child exhibits a height increase of 2 cm/yr over the pretreatment growth rate. The earlier treatment is initiated, the greater the child's height potential. Treatment is continued until the child's growth plates close or the child reaches his or her predicted final height. GH should not be administered to short-statured children who do not demonstrate GH deficiency. Administering GH to these children causes an initial height spurt but does not appreciably affect the child's adult height (Allen, 1999).

NURSING CARE
The Child with Growth Hormone Deficiency

Assessment

Nursing care of the child with GH deficiency includes assessment of family attitudes and perceptions. Parental attitudes regarding the child's size can influence the child's self-esteem. Assess the child's attitude about height. Are height and growth issues voiced more by the parent or by the child? If parents place excessive emphasis on height, the child may be more self-conscious or demonstrate low self-esteem. Height issues might affect a child's psychosocial adjustment, as demonstrated by poor school performance and lack of involvement in extracurricular activities. Often, short children appear younger and are often treated as such by adults, or may be teased by their peers.

> When assessing a child with short stature, the nurse should ask the child if height causes any problems at school. For example, the nurse might ask, "Have you ever been teased or been in any fights at school because of your height?"

Once the child is on therapy, the nurse should assess compliance with the medication regimen, injection tech-

nique, and medication preparation and storage. These should be reviewed periodically and with each dosage change. As children with this problem mature, they might elect to learn to self-administer injections.

Nursing Diagnosis and Planning

The following nursing diagnoses and expected outcomes may be appropriate for the child with GH deficiency:

■ Altered Growth and Development related to GH deficiency.
Expected Outcome: The child will exhibit increased growth rate.
■ Body Image Disturbance related to short stature.
Expected Outcome: The child will demonstrate acceptance of body image.
■ Self-Esteem Disturbance related to short stature.
Expected Outcome: The child will demonstrate appropriate feelings of self-esteem.
■ Ineffective Management of Therapeutic Regimen: Families, related to noncompliance with daily injection.
Expected Outcome: The child/parents will comply with the injection schedule.

Interventions

The nurse reassures the child and parents that compliance with the injections will improve growth rate. It is also helpful to remind children that the injections are temporary and are helping them to grow. Keeping a growth chart at home and needing larger clothing sizes are physical signs the child can use to monitor growth. These indicators also assist with compliance.

The nurse has an important role in educating children and families about the proper dilution and administration of the GH. Demonstrate injection technique to the caregiver and request a return demonstration.

Effectiveness of therapy is evaluated by growth rate. Children are evaluated approximately every 3 months by the endocrinologist. Accurate measurements of height are essential to evaluate efficacy. Using a growth chart helps to identify growth velocity. Therapy is continued until the child reaches predicted adult height or there is radiographic evidence of growth plate fusion.

Evaluation

- Has the child exhibited increased growth rate?
- Does the child verbalize feelings regarding body image/self-esteem?
- Is the child/family compliant with injection schedule?

CRITICAL TO REMEMBER
Growth Hormone (GH) Deficiency

Criteria for suspecting GH deficiency:

- Consistently poor growth (<5 cm/yr)
- Growth more than two standard deviations from the mean for height
- Downward deviation from the previous growth curve

CRITICAL THINKING EXERCISE 51–1

Periodically, the media have drawn attention to the use of growth hormone. Parents of young teenage boys often are concerned about their child's present and eventual height. Boys who are significantly shorter than their peers during early adolescence can experience altered self-esteem.

How should a nurse respond if a parent asks whether giving growth hormone to their short son will increase his eventual height?

Congenital Adrenal Hyperplasia

Congenital adrenal hyperplasia (CAH) is a family of diseases in which the adrenal gland is not able to manufacture glucocorticoid, but instead produces excess androgen. It is caused by a defect in the enzymatic pathway of steroid production. Instead of producing glucocorticoid, excessive amounts of androgens are produced in response to increasing pituitary adrenocorticotropic hormone (ACTH) stimulation. Mineralocorticoid production may be normal or low. Infants with "salt-wasting" CAH may experience a hypovolemic crisis precipitated by low sodium levels. Several enzymatic defects have been identified, the most common being 21-hydroxylase deficiency. CAH is an autosomal recessive disease.

Manifestations

Congenital adrenal hyperplasia is marked by ambiguous genitalia of the newborn female infant; postnatal virilization in both sexes; salt-wasting crisis (first few weeks of life) with low serum sodium, high serum potassium, and vascular collapse; advanced bone age with ultimate adult short stature; menstrual irregularities; and delayed menses.

Diagnostic Evaluation

The findings of ambiguous genitalia in the newborn infant should raise the possibility of CAH. The diagnosis is confirmed by elevated values of 17-hydroxyprogesterone, a glucocorticoid precursor. Many states include CAH in the newborn screen. Determining newborn serum sodium levels in the infant with diagnosed or suspected CAH is important in identifying and treating a potential salt-wasting crisis. Serum renin levels evaluate mineralocorticoid deficit.

Therapeutic Management

Treatment for CAH involves lifelong glucocorticoid therapy. Oral glucocorticoid (hydrocortisone acetate, cortisone acetate) dosage is prescribed based on body size, and is given three times per day. A suspension is available for infants, tablets for older children. For children requiring mineralocorticoid replacement, fludrocortisone acetate is prescribed, taken once daily. Therapy is evaluated with serum 17-hydroxyprogesterone levels, and renin levels if mineralocorticoid replacement therapy is required. Special sick day instructions should be provided to the family. The glucocorticoid dosage is usually doubled or tripled when the child is ill or undergoing a surgical procedure. Bone age radiographs are performed yearly to assess bone maturity; poor compliance or undertreatment result in advanced bone age.

Nursing Considerations

All newborn girls should be assessed for ambiguous genitalia: fused labia, enlarged clitoris, or migration of urethral opening. Infant boys with unexplained dehydration and elevated serum sodium should be considered to have adrenal insufficiency, requiring careful assessment of fluid and electrolyte status.

Infant girls with ambiguous genitalia might require reconstructive surgery. Depending on degree of virilization, surgical correction may be recommended in infancy or in early puberty. If appropriate, reassure parents that the infant has appropriate internal structures, and that external structures can be corrected surgically. Allow them to express any concerns and encourage parent–infant attachment.

Assess older children receiving glucocorticoid replacement therapy for growth and signs of early puberty. Noncompliance can cause early virilization, increased growth velocity, ultimate short adult height, and menstrual irregularities in girls. Blood pressure monitoring is important for children receiving mineralocorticoid replacement therapy.

Instruct parents about replacement hormone administration and the timing of medication. A suspension is available for infants, tablets for older children. Develop a plan for sick day dosage of medication. The infant with salt-wasting CAH may require salt supplements; the family needs instruction on preparation of the supplement.

Follow-up evaluations with the endocrinologist are scheduled every 2 to 3 months in infancy and every 6 months in the older child. Parents of the child with CAH should be referred to a genetics counselor if planning more pregnancies because future children are at risk for CAH. In-utero treatment is available.

Encourage the adolescent to assume increasing responsibility for medication administration. Emphasize the importance of compliance. Surgical genital reconstruction and vaginal dilatation may be required in the adolescent years. Careful explanations of procedures reassure affected adolescents that they are "normal."

Type 1 Diabetes Mellitus

Type 1 (formerly termed *insulin-dependent*) diabetes mellitus results when the pancreas is unable to produce and secrete insulin. This form of diabetes, the most common childhood endocrine disorder, presents challenges in the areas of teaching, management, and compliance. Because of recent changes in the health care delivery system, meeting the needs associated with management of type 1 diabetes mellitus has become more complicated. Unless the newly diagnosed child is in diabetic ketoacidosis (DKA), the child may not be hospitalized. The nurse must develop a plan of care that involves family education, in either an inpatient or outpatient setting. Including the family in the child's care and support must be part of planning and implementation of nursing care. Because type 1 diabetes mellitus is a chronic disease, see Chapter 36 for a discussion of that aspect of care.

Etiology

Type 1 diabetes mellitus is an autoimmune process that results in the destruction of the insulin-secreting cells of the pancreas. A genetic predisposition plus an environmental or viral trigger are thought to initiate the autoimmune destructive process. Current research focuses on identifying specific genes that may affect a person's susceptibility to type 1 diabetes mellitus, as well as exploring methods of interrupting or preventing the autoimmune response in susceptible people (first-degree relatives of a diabetic person). No prevention or cure is available.

PATHOPHYSIOLOGY
of Type 1 Diabetes Mellitus

In the absence of insulin, the metabolism of fats, proteins, and carbohydrates is impaired. Glucose is unable to move into the intracellular space, resulting in hyperglycemia. As blood glucose levels exceed the renal threshold, glucose is "spilled" into the urine through osmotic diuresis, resulting in polyuria. Excessive thirst follows in response to fluid loss. Fatigue, hunger, and weight loss also accompany the onset of type 1 diabetes mellitus because cellular starvation continues in the absence of insulin.

Ketones (ketoacids), manufactured by the liver from adipose tissue, are produced in response to cellular starvation. In the absence of insulin, ketones are also unavailable to the cell for nourishment. Increasing blood levels of ketones (ketonemia) result in ketoacidosis.

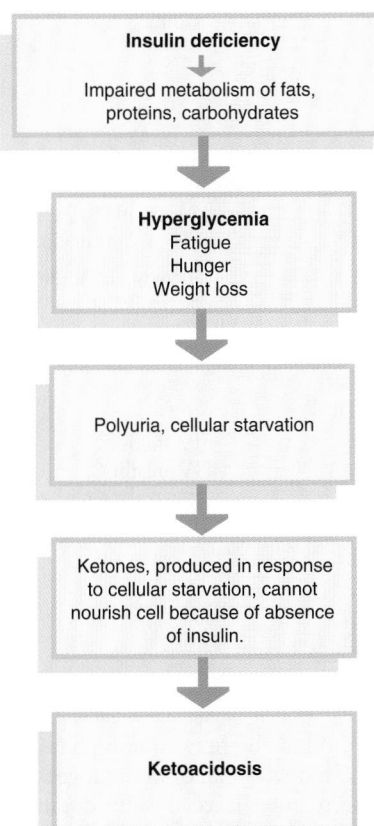

Incidence

The incidence of type 1 diabetes mellitus in the United States is 1.7 in 1,000 people, with approximately 13,000 new cases diagnosed every year (American Diabetes Association, 1999). This incidence decreases to 5 per 100,000 for the population older than 20 years of age. The risk of diabetes increases to 1 in 20 if the person has a first-degree relative (parent or sibling) with type 1 diabetes mellitus, and increases to 1 in 3 if an identical twin has the disease. The average age of onset is during the school age period. Type 2 (or non–insulin-dependent diabetes mellitus), which is not an autoimmune condition, is more prevalent in people older than 40 years of age, but is being seen more frequently in adolescents.

Manifestations

The classic initial symptoms of hyperglycemia, known as the "three P's," include polyuria (or enuresis in a toilet-trained child), polydipsia, and polyphagia. The child experiences weight loss (despite increased food intake), fatigue, and blurred vision.

If the condition progresses without intervention, the child can exhibit the following signs of ketoacidosis: nausea/vomiting, abdominal pain, acetone (fruity) odor to breath, dehydration, increasing lethargy, Kussmaul respirations, and coma.

Children who receive insulin for treatment of type 1 diabetes mellitus can experience hypoglycemia. Table 51–1 compares hypoglycemia, hyperglycemia, and ketoacidosis.

Diagnostic Evaluation

Diagnosis of type 1 diabetes mellitus is based on a clinical picture of hyperglycemia (and acidosis, if present) combined with the laboratory data of a fasting serum glucose exceeding 120 mg/dl and a random serum glucose exceeding 160 mg/dl. Ketonuria, although not diagnostic, is a frequent finding, as is glycosuria. Glucose tolerance testing is rarely used in diagnosing type 1 diabetes mellitus. The glycosylated hemoglobin value is elevated in response to prolonged elevations of blood glucose.

Therapeutic Management

The goals of diabetes management include

- Facilitating appropriate growth (height and weight)
- Maintaining an age-appropriate lifestyle
- Achieving near-normal glycosylated hemoglobin
- Preventing acute complications (hypoglycemia, hyperglycemia)

INSULIN THERAPY
The child with type 1 diabetes mellitus loses the ability to make insulin through an autoimmune destruction of the insulin-producing cells, the beta cells. Symptoms of hyperglycemia become evident when most of the beta cells are destroyed. After initiation of insulin therapy, the child may experience a "honeymoon" phase, characterized by hypoglycemia and a decreasing need for insulin. This may last from a few weeks to a year or longer. It is important to prepare the child and family for the possibility of a honeymoon phase both to avoid the misconception that the diabetes is "going away" and to provide instruction on recognition and treatment of hypoglycemia.

The goal of insulin therapy is to replace the insulin the child is no longer able to make. Synthetic human insulin, made by recombinant DNA technology, is free of animal impurities and is recommended for children. Oral hypogly-

TABLE 51–1

Comparison of Hypoglycemia, Hyperglycemia, and Ketoacidosis

Descriptor	Hypoglycemia	Hyperglycemia	Ketoacidosis
Onset	Rapid	Slow	Slow

Signs and symptoms	*Adrenergic signs:*
	Trembling
	Sweating
	Tachycardia
	Pallor
	Clammy skin
	Hunger
		Increased urination
		Increased thirst
		Fatigue
		Weight loss (gradual, over
		   several weeks)
		Blurred vision
			Hyperglycemia signs plus:
			Abdominal pain
			Chest pain
			Kussmaul respirations
			Nausea and vomiting
			Acetone (fruity) breath odor
			Signs and symptoms of dehydration:
			Dry lips and mucous
			   membranes
			Sunken eyes
			Sudden weight loss
			Decreased urination

Sensorium	*Neuroglycopenic symptoms:*
	Personality change
	Irritability
	Drunken behavior
	Decreasing level of
	   consciousness, to loss
	   of consciousness
	Seizure activity
		Normal sensorium	Increasing lethargy
			Decreasing level of
			   consciousness
			Coma

Laboratory data	Blood glucose <70 mg/dl Urine ketones negative or trace	Serum glucose >160 mg/dl	Serum glucose >300 mg/dl Urinary ketones positive Serum pH <7.25 Serum ketones positive

Causes	Too much insulin
	Excessive activity without
	   eating extra carbohydrate
	Missed or delayed meal
		Excessive intake of
		   carbohydrate
		Little or no exercise
		Inadequate amount of insulin
		Increased stress, either
		   emotional or physical
			Inadequate amount of insulin
			Excessive stress

Treatment	15 g oral carbohydrate
	*For loss of consciousness or
	   seizure activity:*
	Glucagon subcutaneously or
	   intramuscularly
	IV glucose
		Insulin
		Exercise
			IV fluids
			IV insulin
			Electrolyte replacement

Abbreviation: IV, intravenous.

cemic agents, although useful in the treatment of type 2 diabetes, are not effective in the treatment of type 1 diabetes.

The choice of insulin types and schedule of injections is based on the child's needs (Table 51–2). Daily self-monitoring of blood glucose aids in defining insulin require-

ments. The child in the honeymoon phase needs less insulin than the child who makes no endogenous insulin. The pubertal child requires larger insulin dosages.

Schedule. The Diabetes Control and Complications Trial Research Group (DCCT Research Group, 1993) concluded that long-term diabetic complications can be minimized by intensive treatment. This treatment, defined as three or more injections of insulin per day (or the use of a continuous insulin infusion pump), mimics physiologic delivery of insulin. Three injections per day have become the most frequently used insulin therapy for the child: intermediate-acting combined with rapid-acting insulin injected before breakfast, rapid-acting insulin injected before the evening meal, and intermediate-acting insulin injected before bed. The peak actions of these insulins are timed to correspond to the child's usual mealtimes and snack time to minimize the possibility of hypoglycemia (Fig. 51–2).

TABLE 51–2

Insulin Action by Type (Humulin)

Type	Onset	Peak	Duration
Lispro	15–30 min	60–90 min	2–3 hr
Regular	30 min	2–4 hr	4–6 hr
NPH or Lente	2–4 hr	6–8 hr	12–24 hr
Ultralente	>2 hr	Variable	24–36 hr

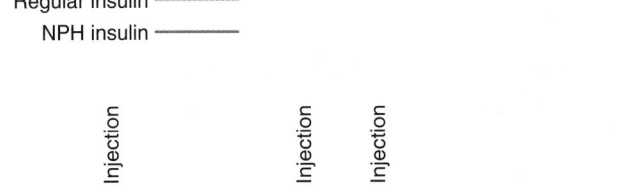

Regular insulin ········
NPH insulin ————

FIGURE 51–2
• • • • • • • • • •
For children with type 1 diabetes mellitus, three injections of insulin per day is the usual therapeutic regimen. Peak action of these injections is timed to correspond with the child's usual meal and snack time to minimize the chance of hypoglycemia.

Administration. Because insulin is a protein, and would be digested if taken orally, it is given parenterally. Insulin is administered by subcutaneous injection into the adipose tissue over large muscle masses: the back of the arms, the top and outer portion of the thighs, the abdomen, and the hip (Fig. 51–3). To avoid injecting into the muscle

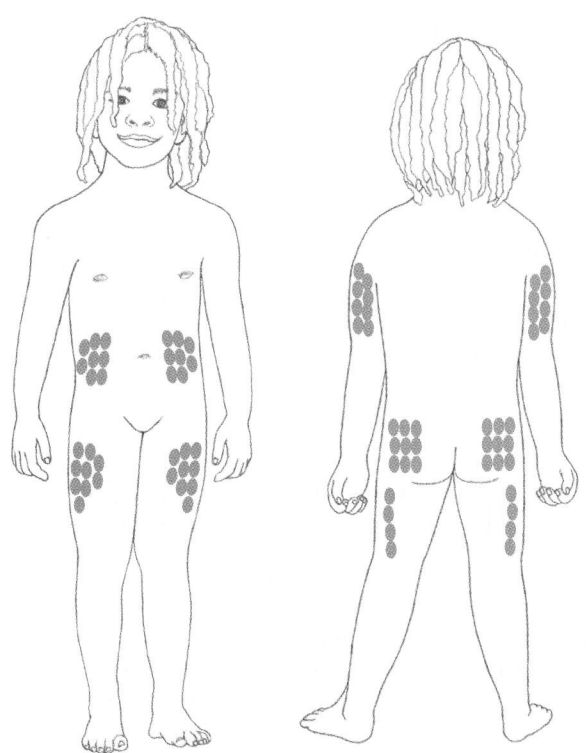

Insulin Absorption by Sites

Most rapid ————————➡————————— Least rapid

Abdomen ➡ Arms ➡ Hips ➡ Thighs

FIGURE 51–3
• • • • • • • • • •
Rotation of insulin injection sites. (Adapted from Albisser, A. M., & Sperlich, M. [1993]. Adjusting insulins. *Diabetes Educator, 18*(3), 211–227.)

or vascular space, use a 45-degree angle of injection with the 1/2-inch needle, or a 90-degree angle with the 5/16-inch needle. Rotation of injection sites helps prevent adipose hypertrophy (fatty lumps), which absorb insulin poorly. Various injection sites absorb insulin at slightly different rates. Absorption is also affected by the amount of exercise the underlying muscle engages in and by body temperature. To help decrease day-to-day variations in absorption, the child should use one location within a major site for the morning injection, then rotate to another location within the site for the evening injection and a third location for the bedtime injection.

Insulin can be administered by an insulin syringe, air injector, or insulin pump. Disposable syringes are to be used one time and safely discarded (with the syringe placed in a puncture-resistant, opaque container before placing in the trash).

The air injector uses compressed air to deposit the insulin within the fatty tissue, without the use of a needle. The child or family must learn to use the device correctly: to load insulin, adjust pressure settings to avoid intramuscular delivery, and clean properly.

The insulin pump is a device that provides a continuous infusion of rapid-acting insulin. The device comprises a computer, a reservoir of rapid-acting insulin, and thin tubing through which the insulin is delivered by a small needle inserted into the abdomen. A continuous basal rate of insulin infusion is maintained, and bolus dosages are infused as determined by blood glucose testing. The pump most closely mimics physiologic delivery of insulin and provides a more flexible lifestyle. This option may appeal to adolescents, but the candidate for insulin pump therapy must be willing meticulously to measure blood glucose throughout the day (and often night) to avoid hypoglycemia and to respond to hyperglycemia. Dietary recommendations are different for children or adolescents using an insulin pump and are based on carbohydrate counting (American Diabetes Association, 1999).

NUTRITION THERAPY

The goal of nutrition therapy is to promote normal growth, encourage good nutrition, prevent complications, and maintain near-normal blood glucose levels. Because the insulin dosage is balanced with food intake, the diet plan should stress a consistent intake, particularly of carbohydrate food products. The diet therapy chosen should be easy to understand and should help the child and family learn to make healthy food choices. The meal plan is based on the child's diet history. As the child grows, the meal plan is tailored to meet changing dietary needs.

EXERCISE

Exercise is an important aspect of diabetes management. Exercise enhances the action of insulin in lowering blood glucose levels. The child with diabetes should be encouraged to participate in age-appropriate sports. Early enjoyment of a sport or activity can promote a lifelong active lifestyle. Because exercise lowers glucose levels, the child must be taught how to prevent hypoglycemia. The child should try to schedule activities to avoid exercising when an insulin dose is peaking. Maintaining proper hydration while exercising is very important.

Teach the family to add extra snacks of 15 to 30 g carbohydrate for each 45 to 60 minutes of exercise. Coaches and teammates should be taught how to recognize and treat hypoglycemia. Delayed or nocturnal hypoglycemia can occur after strenuous activity. Additional carbohydrate might be required after exercise to maintain blood glucose levels. The child should always wear medical alert identification.

BLOOD GLUCOSE MONITORING

Self-monitoring of blood glucose provides an objective tool to assist with diabetes control. Monitoring is recommended before meals and before the bedtime snack. More frequent monitoring may be useful during prolonged exercise, during an illness, or if nighttime hypoglycemia is suspected.

Blood glucose goals must be tailored to the abilities of the family and the age of the child. Goals for the infant or toddler are usually liberalized to aid in preventing severe hypoglycemia. Preprandial blood glucose goals include

- Nondiabetic: 70 to 110 mg/dl
- Children with type 1 diabetes mellitus: 80 to 150 mg/dl
- Infants/toddlers: 100 to 200 mg/dl

The identified goals are a target range; not all glucose levels fall in this range, even in the child with excellent diabetes control.

Glucose test results should be recorded in a glucose diary or record book. Patterns or trends in blood glucose levels outside of the target range indicate a need to adjust the insulin dose. Three or four days of a consistent pattern of glucose values (e.g., 200 mg/dl before the evening meal for 3 consecutive days) indicates a need to increase the appropriate insulin. The health care team may provide the family with guidelines for increasing insulin dose based on blood glucose patterns.

Blood glucose meters are accurate only if used according to manufacturers' recommendations. Regardless of the brand selected, quality control procedures must be performed as recommended. Test supplies must be stored according to manufacturers' specifications and discarded when outdated. (Figure 37–11 shows the finger stick method for obtaining a small blood sample.)

DEVELOPMENTAL ISSUES

Infant and Toddler. The infant or toddler with type 1 diabetes poses special challenges for diabetes management. The burden of management falls on the parents or other caregivers. Achieving consistency in dietary intake with the infant can be quite difficult. Inconsistent intake, particularly of carbohydrates, contributes to blood glucose variability. Food control issues can easily become a battleground between the child and the parent. A diet strategy that stresses carbohydrate consistency rather than specific food groups offers more flexibility than a structured meal plan.

Allow the toddler to participate in making food choices (from perhaps two or three options) to offer the child a sense of control. The signs and symptoms of hypoglycemia are difficult to recognize in the infant or might be mistaken for the toddler's temper tantrum. The glucose goals for this age group are liberalized to avoid episodes of severe hypoglycemia.

Establishing rituals and routines helps the toddler feel

CRITICAL TO REMEMBER

Managing the Child with Type 1 Diabetes Mellitus

Insulin

- Store insulin in a cool, dry place. Do not freeze or expose to excessive heat or agitation.
- Check the expiration date on the vial before using.
- Once opened, date the vial and discard as recommended.
- When mixing two different types of insulin, inject the appropriate amount of air into both vials, then withdraw the short-acting (clear) insulin first.

Nutrition

- Meals and snacks are balanced with insulin action.
- Both the timing of the meal or snack and the amount of food are important in avoiding hyperglycemia or hypoglycemia.
- Adherence to a daily schedule that maintains a *consistent* food intake combined with consistent insulin injections aids in achieving metabolic control.

Exercise

- Avoid exercising during insulin peak.
- Add extra 15- to 30-g carbohydrate snacks for each 45 to 60 minutes of exercise.

Blood Glucose Monitoring

- Record blood glucose results in a diary.
- A 3- to 4-day alteration in glucose levels requires an adjustment of insulin dose.

---

more in control. Encourage the parent to have a specific place to perform the blood test and a special place to keep supplies. Toddlers feel more in control if they are able to predict and participate in diabetes activities (Table 51–3).

Preschooler. The preschool years are characterized by increasing motor maturity, a widening social circle, and magical thinking. The preschooler can understand simple explanations regarding diabetes. Such explanations help to allay fears that the diabetes was caused by the child's being "bad." Play therapy using dolls and diabetes equipment helps the preschooler express concerns regarding injections and finger sticks.

The preschooler has a more predictable appetite than the toddler and is frequently willing to try new foods. Nonetheless, supervision is necessary to ensure that meals and snacks are eaten, especially if the child is in a day care setting with many distractions.

The preschooler may be able to identify the feelings associated with hypoglycemia. Use the child's description as a code word for the onset of hypoglycemia symptoms. Preschoolers' preference for high-energy activities puts

TABLE 51–3

Examples of Delegation of Diabetes Tasks (with Supervision)

Developmental Characteristics	Diabetes Task	Diet Task
Toddler/Preschooler		
Likes rituals Finicky eater Not yet able to understand need for insulin	Chooses and cleans finger for puncture Helps by holding still for injection Identifies a word or phrase to describe a feeling of hypoglycemia	Helps by choosing foods
School-Age Child		
Thinking is present oriented Spending large amounts of time away from parents Begins to develop self-concept	Performs finger puncture and blood glucose test Chooses injection site according to rotation schedule Pushes plunger on insulin syringe after the needle is inserted by parent or gives own injection Performs ketone test	Recognizes need to eat on time to avoid hypoglycemia Knows treatment for hypoglycemia
Early Adolescent		
Looks to peer group for identity Needs to conform to peer group norms Increased risk-taking behaviors	Records blood glucose values in diary Draws up insulin with supervision Performs insulin injection	Knows meal plan Can choose correct foods for snack Adds extra snack for increased activity
Middle/Late Adolescent		
Future oriented Wants to take charge of life Able to recognize consequences of behaviors and choices Emotional separation from parents	Draws up and injects insulin Looks for patterns in blood glucose values Recognizes when to test for ketones Initiates treatment for ketones (fluids)	Can plan meals and snacks based on meal plan Can choose appropriate foods at a party

them at risk for hypoglycemia. The caregiver should be prepared with readily available carbohydrate foods as well as emergency medications.

School-Age Child. The school-age child and family face the challenge of incorporating diabetes care within a busy school day. To avoid singling the child out, the diabetes care should be as unobtrusive as possible while still maintaining a safe environment for the child. The family should communicate with school personnel about the child's diabetes. A school nurse or health aide should be identified to supervise prelunch blood glucose monitoring, to assist with insulin injections, and to educate other school personnel in recognizing and treating hypoglycemia. Schools vary on the availability of nursing services. Parents may have to work with school personnel to identify appropriate staff to supervise their child's diabetes care.

Planning ahead for field trips, school parties, and athletic events allows the child with diabetes to participate safely in age-appropriate activities. For example, the child who has soccer practice three afternoons per week needs to plan how to prevent hypoglycemia during practice.

Adolescent. The developmental milestones of the adolescent are often in conflict with the recommendations for achieving diabetes control. The young adolescent is concerned with body image and peer group acceptance, and is moving away from the family for support and identity. Clothing, diet, lifestyle, and speech are areas in which the early adolescent strives to conform to peers.

The mid-adolescent is open to risk-taking behaviors and is more openly challenging of parental authority. By late adolescence, the person becomes more future oriented, with behaviors based more on abstract morals and less on peer group demands.

These normally recognized milestones become dilemmas when diabetes control is affected. Missed injections, omitted blood tests, irregular meals, and dietary splurges are frequent complaints of parents of diabetic adolescents.

The parents and their adolescent must accept that diabetes responsibility increasingly shifts to the adolescent. Encourage parents to work as partners with the adolescent to achieve diabetes control. Identify what is important to the adolescent, and use that information as a tool to motivate compliance. The adolescent is not motivated by predictions of complications in the distant future. Rather, motivation should focus on issues important to the adolescent: personal appearance, athletic ability, strength/muscle mass, endurance, or ideal weight.

DELEGATING DIABETES RESPONSIBILITIES

Children with diabetes are functionally able to perform diabetes skills far sooner than they can cognitively understand the implications of the activity or consequences of omitting the activity. Transfer of responsibility should be on a step-by-step basis, according to the child's cognitive understanding and functional abilities. Diabetes responsibilities shift from full parent responsibility to a partnership between parent and child, then to the acceptance of responsibility by the young adult. Delegating diabetes responsibility at an inappropriate age results in poor diabetes control and frequent bouts of DKA. The importance of ongoing parental support and supervision cannot be overemphasized.

NURSING CARE

The Child with Type 1 Diabetes Mellitus

Assessment

Nursing assessment of the child diagnosed with type 1 diabetes mellitus begins with a careful history. Identify signs and symptoms of hyperglycemia—the three P's. Daytime polydipsia and polyuria may not worry a parent, but enuresis or accidents in the previously toilet-trained child and nighttime requests for water spark concern. New-onset diabetes is frequently overlooked in light of specific symptoms. A urinary tract infection might be suspected based on urinary frequency. An infective process frequently accompanies the onset of diabetes, but is not the cause of the diabetes. The stress associated with an infection can compromise the function of the remaining insulin-secreting cells. A history of weight loss or fatigue is also a common parental observa-

tion. Nausea and vomiting are present in the child who is acidotic. Ask about other medications used. Glucocorticoids and some chemotherapeutic agents can cause hyperglycemia.

Physical assessment should include signs and symptoms of dehydration: dry mucous membranes, flushed skin, acute weight change, absence of tearing, or poor skin turgor. Identify the time of most recent voiding. Oliguria is a significant finding in the assessment of dehydration.

Assess for signs and symptoms of acidosis: abdominal pain, nausea and vomiting (which also contribute to dehydration), Kussmaul respirations coupled with a fruity breath odor, or decreasing level of consciousness (LOC). Ongoing assessment of the child in acidosis should include vital signs, LOC, and intake and output. Vital signs and LOC should be monitored frequently until stable.

Assess the family's knowledge of diabetes. For the newly diagnosed child, prepare the family to participate in a diabetes education program to learn home care skills. Encourage parents to arrange for time away from work and school to participate. Assess the family's ability to cope with the diagnosis of a chronic disease. Identify usual methods of coping with stress and usual support systems. Explore the availability of financial resources to meet the child's health care needs.

FAMILIES WANT TO KNOW

About Home Management of Type 1 Diabetes Mellitus

The child and family are understandably overwhelmed with questions and fears about the diagnosis. Encourage all family members to participate. Choose a comfortable location subject to few interruptions. Provide appropriate literature and materials for family members. Videotapes, booklets, and pamphlets should be developmentally appropriate. Educational materials for the parent should also match the parent's literacy skills.

The family needs to know the following. The accompanying checklist of outcomes evaluates level of understanding.

- General information about type 1 diabetes mellitus
- How to administer and store insulin
- How to monitor blood glucose levels, using the equipment properly
- Signs and management of hypoglycemic episodes
- Signs and management of hyperglycemia
- Strategies for when the child is ill
- Nutrition and exercise principles
- Potential long-term complications
- Available resources for emotional and physical support

All family members should be given the opportunity to practice skills taught. Practicing procedures on themselves or each other helps allay family fears and allows the child to supervise as a family member performs the procedure. Help develop problem-solving skills by using various scenarios that encourage decision making. Because education is an ongoing process, the family needs a contact person to whom they can turn for advice and support.

Outcomes

General Information
The child and family will be able to

1. Describe the action of insulin in the body.
2. Describe the characteristics of type 1 versus type 2 diabetes.
3. Identify three factors that can be used to control blood glucose levels.

Medication Therapy
The child and family will be able to

1. Name the child's insulin and identify the onset, peak, and duration of action.
2. State the storage recommendations for insulin.
3. State the recommended expiration date of the insulin.
4. Demonstrate accurate syringe preparation for a single type of insulin.
5. Demonstrate syringe preparation using two types of insulin.
6. Demonstrate subcutaneous insulin injection technique.
7. Identify insulin injection sites and describe a pattern of rotation.
8. Identify a plan for safe syringe disposal.
9. Identify recommended insulin dosages and injection times.

Home Glucose Monitoring
The child and family will be able to

1. Identify nondiabetic blood glucose levels and target goals for good glucose control.
2. Demonstrate the use, calibration, control testing, and cleaning of the blood glucose monitor.
3. Identify a plan for recording blood glucose values.

Hypoglycemia
The child and family will be able to

1. Identify the signs and symptoms of a hypoglycemic reaction.
2. Describe appropriate treatment for both a mild and severe hypoglycemic reaction.
3. Identify three potential causes of a hypoglycemic reaction.
4. Identify the importance of medical emergency identification.
5. Describe typical blood glucose trends during the honeymoon phase.

Hyperglycemia/Sick Day
The child and family will be able to

1. Identify the signs and symptoms of hyperglycemia.
2. Identify strategies to control hyperglycemia.
3. Describe the possible effects of stress or illness on diabetes control.
4. Demonstrate the procedure for urinary ketone testing.

5. State when to test for urinary ketones.
6. State basic treatment for urinary ketones.
7. Describe the signs and symptoms requiring physician/health care team contact.

Exercise
The child and family will be able to

1. State the effect of exercise on blood glucose levels.
2. State the benefits of and precautions for exercise.
3. Identify the relationship of diet, exercise, and insulin on blood glucose control.
4. Generate a home schedule that identifies mealtimes, blood test times, and insulin injection times.

Complications
The child and family will be able to

1. Identify the role of glucose control in the prevention or delay of diabetes-related complications.
2. Identify appropriate health care follow-up for the child with diabetes.

Psychological Adjustment/Family Involvement
The child and family will be able to create a plan for the entire family to participate in diabetes care and management.

Community Resources
The child and family will be able to identify available community resources for ongoing diabetes education and support.

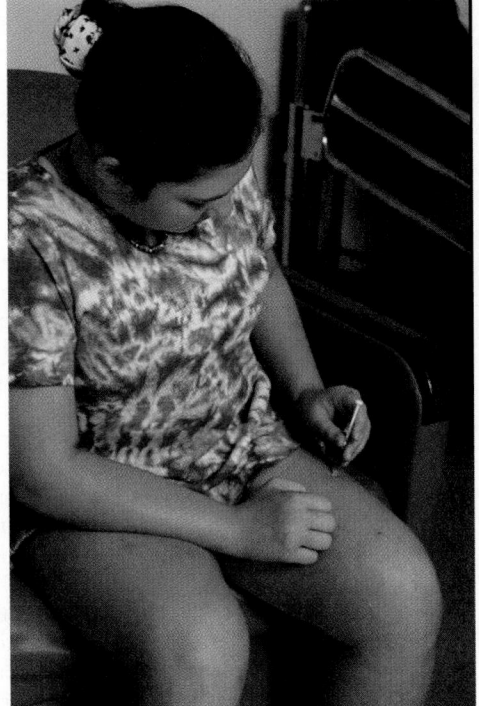

When other parts of the treatment regimen have become ▶ familiar, the injections can be taught. Initially, self-injecting insulin will be scary for the school-age child. It is usually advisable to start with the parent inserting the needle and the child pushing the plunger. The child can then progress to performing self-injection.

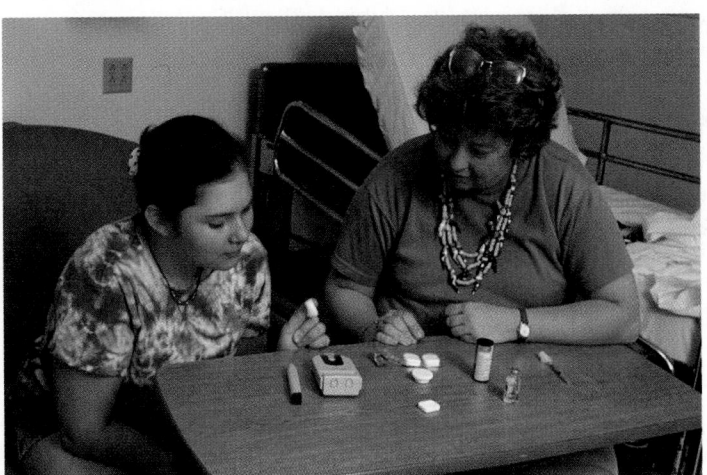

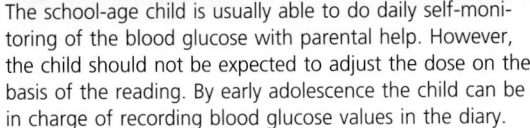

The school-age child is usually able to do daily self-monitoring of the blood glucose with parental help. However, the child should not be expected to adjust the dose on the basis of the reading. By early adolescence the child can be in charge of recording blood glucose values in the diary.

Nursing Diagnosis, Planning, Intervention, and Evaluation

Nursing Diagnosis

■ Knowledge Deficit related to unfamiliarity with home care needs of the child with type 1 diabetes mellitus.

Expected Outcome

• The child and family will be able successfully to manage diabetes, as evidenced by demonstration of skills and verbalization of concepts necessary for home care.

Intervention

1. Identify barriers to learning that might hinder the family's ability to learn home care information. Barriers could include issues such as language fluency, literacy, employment pressures, and child care. These issues should be addressed before initiating education.
2. Identify learning objectives with the family.

3. Present information at a developmentally appropriate level for the child.

Rationale

1. Identifying and addressing these issues optimizes the learning ability of the family. For example, provide appropriate written materials for the person with low literacy skills.

2. A written list of specific objectives helps the family prioritize education, as well as provides a sense of accomplishment as learning objectives are met.
3. The child must cognitively understand diabetes. More advanced information can be presented as the child matures.

Evaluation

• Can the child and family successfully manage home care, as evidenced by demonstrations of skill mastery and verbalization of home care concepts?

Nursing Diagnosis

■ Altered Family Processes related to the chronic health care needs of a child with type 1 diabetes mellitus.

Expected Outcome

• The family will recognize/identify stresses and construct strategies for dealing with the stress of a chronic disease.

Intervention

1. Assist family to identify age-appropriate diabetes skills for the child and the responsibilities of the parent.

2. Assist the child and family to identify behaviors that the child recognizes as supportive. Supportive family behaviors might include the following: all family members follow the child's meal plan, avoid having sweets in the home, offer to record blood glucose levels in the diary for the child, or recognize and praise the child's attempts at adherence.
3. Identify community support systems available for the family. For the child with diabetes, summer diabetes camp and age-specific support groups are invaluable for motivation and building self-esteem. A parent support group or participation in fundraising activities in a local diabetes community group can provide support for other family members.
4. Identify a "vacation" plan in which the major caregiver can take a break from diabetes responsibilities. The ongoing, day-to-day responsibility of diabetes management can be shared between parents, siblings, and others. Although total responsibility might not be delegated, perhaps the child (or parent) can take a break from one aspect of responsibility as another family member takes on the responsibility.

Rationale

1. Delegation of responsibilities should occur as the child is both able to perform the skill and to understand the implications of the skill. Parental support and supervision is essential for all children for successful home management of diabetes.
2. Discussions of family support help involve all family members in the child's care, as well as give the child the opportunity to identify supportive behaviors. Adaptation is enhanced by focusing on the strengths of the child and family.

3. Community resources offer a variety of opportunities for support, as well as an alternative to relying solely on family coping skills (see Appendix L).

4. Taking responsibility for diabetes control is very stressful and demanding. Sharing responsibilities among family members helps prevent burnout, discouragement, and frustration.

Evaluation
- Can the child and family verbalize a plan for sharing diabetes responsibility?

Nursing Diagnosis
- Altered Nutrition: Less Than Body Requirements related to insulin deficit.

Expected Outcome
- The family will demonstrate ability to use insulin therapy, diet therapy, and glucose self-monitoring to maximize nutritional status.

Intervention	Rationale
1. Teach family the action of food (carbohydrates, fats, and proteins) on blood glucose level: carbohydrates raise blood glucose levels, fats and proteins have minimal effects on glucose levels.	1. Understanding the relationship of food to blood glucose levels will help the family recognize the rationale for adhering to the diabetic diet.
2. Based on the child's usual schedule, generate a daily schedule that includes times for blood glucose test, medication, meals, and snacks.	2. Consistency in timing of meals and snacks in relation to insulin injections is essential. Encouraging child and family input into this aspect of planning will impart a sense of control, as well as promote compliance.
3. Ask the child to identify favorite foods and demonstrate how to incorporate these into the meal plan.	3. Most foods can be incorporated into the meal plan, even if only in small amounts. Allowing small amounts of favorite "treats" can encourage compliance.
4. Observe whether the child's hunger is satisfied on the prescribed diet. Instruct the child/parent to notify the nutritionist if the meal plan forces the child to overeat, or if the child is persistently hungry. Utilize appropriate growth chart to track the child's height and weight with respect to age.	4. The meal plan is tailored to the child and the child's activity level. Nutritional needs vary with age, as well as with variations in activity level. For example, a morning gym class may require that the child add a mid-morning snack.
5. Discuss the relationship between insulin, food (carbohydrate), and exercise. Identify ideal blood glucose goals for the child. Present an example situation in which the blood glucose is out of the ideal range, and encourage the family to identify possible options using diet, insulin, and/or exercise to more closely attain the blood glucose goal.	5. Diet, exercise, and insulin therapy are the tools of diabetes management. This exercise will develop problem-solving skills within the family and provide a sense of competency.
6. Instruct the family to plan 3 or 4 days of menus based on the meal plan. Both the type of food as well as amount of food should be included.	6. This exercise will help the family operationalize the diet instructions.

Evaluation
- Is the child's height and weight appropriate for age compared with growth chart percentiles?
- Is the child free of episodes of severe hypoglycemia or hyperglycemia?

Nursing Diagnosis
- Risk for Injury related to hypoglycemia or hyperglycemia.

Expected Outcome
- Family members will demonstrate knowledge of the signs, symptoms, and treatment of hypoglycemia and hyperglycemia and will initiate appropriate treatment.

Intervention	Rationale
For hypoglycemia—blood glucose below 70 mg/dl	
1. Teach the child and family to recognize the signs and symptoms of hypoglycemia (see Table 51–1). School personnel should also be involved in teaching. The school nurse, if available, can play a key role in the care of a child with diabetes.	1. Signs and symptoms of hypoglycemia should prompt the child or parent to test the blood glucose level. Some children do not display adrenergic signs of hypoglycemia. Neuroglycopenic signs (altered sensorium) may be the only clues to hypoglycemia in these children. These signs are very hard for the child to recognize, but can be observed by a parent or teacher. Blood glucose goals for this child may need to be modified to prevent hypoglycemia unawareness.

2. Treat hypoglycemia promptly with 15 g of easily digested carbohydrate. If symptoms are not relieved (or blood glucose level is not above 80 mg/dl) in 15 minutes, repeat the treatment. If the hypoglycemia occurs during the night, treat with 30 g carbohydrate: 15 g simple carbohydrate and 15 g complex carbohydrate with protein. Examples of 15 g of carbohydrate include 4 ounces of real fruit juice, 6 ounces of regular cola, 6 Life Savers, or a commercial glucose product.

3. Help the child and family identify strategies to prevent hypoglycemia based on common causes of hypoglycemia: missed or delayed meal, excess insulin, extra exercise without increasing carbohydrate intake. Encourage the family to teach the signs and symptoms of hypoglycemia and necessary treatment to school personnel and day care workers. Help the child prepare to explain hypoglycemia to friends. Compile a diabetes box for school and day care. The box should contain carbohydrates for treating hypoglycemia as well as written information. Instruct the child to wear medical alert identification at all times.

4. Teach the parents how to treat severe hypoglycemia. For the unconscious child or the child having a seizure, a small amount of glucose gel (cake frosting or honey will also work) can be rubbed on the inner cheek and gums. Avoid placing a large amount of gel in the mouth, because the child could choke. Glucagon (available by prescription as Glucagon Emergency Kit from Eli Lilly Co.) can be injected subcutaneously or intramuscularly. Inject 1 mg for the child weighing over 50 lb or 20 to 30 μg/kg for the child weighing under 50 lb. The onset of action is 10–15 minutes. Position the unconscious child on the side. Once conscious, the child needs a large snack to replace lost glycogen stores.

For hyperglycemia—blood glucose levels higher than target range

1. Teach the family to recognize potential causes of hyperglycemia: inadequate insulin, increased dietary intake, decreased exercise, and stress response (either emotional or physical stress such as illness).

2. Instruct family on sick day diabetes management, including when and how to test for urinary ketones. Identify a home treatment plan for ketones, and identify precautions for vomiting.

3. Identify strategies to prevent or treat hyperglycemia.

2. Prompt treatment reduces the possibility of a severe reaction. Candy bars, donuts, and cookies are poor treatment choices because of their high fat content, which can delay carbohydrate digestion. The child could also interpret these treats as a reward for hypoglycemia.

3. Many episodes of hypoglycemia can be avoided by careful planning and anticipating potential situations that could result in hypoglycemia. Instruction on the signs, symptoms, and treatment of hypoglycemia is essential information to be shared with people caring for the child. Hypoglycemia is a potential emergency that requires prompt recognition and treatment.

4. The unconscious child or the child having a seizure requires prompt treatment. Glucagon is a pancreatic hormone that opposes the action of insulin and promotes the conversion of liver glycogen to blood glucose. The child is positioned on the side to prevent aspiration. Both severe hypoglycemia and glucagon administration can result in nausea with vomiting.

1. Anticipating situations that might result in hyperglycemia can help the family plan for such events. The signs and symptoms of hypoglycemia and hyperglycemia can be difficult to distinguish from one another. Test blood glucose before treating to verify glucose level. *If testing is impossible, treat for hypoglycemia.*

2. Testing for ketones when ill or when blood glucose is 250 mg/dl or higher aids in detecting insulin deficit. Ketones are treated with (calorie-free) fluids, and additional rapid-acting insulin as ordered by the physician. Nausea with vomiting leads to dehydration and cannot be treated with oral fluids. The physician must be notified if the child is vomiting.

3. Consistency in diet, exercise, and insulin injection times aids in preventing hyperglycemia. Persistent hyperglycemia may indicate a need for an insulin dosage adjustment. The growing child needs periodic increases in baseline insulin dosages.

Evaluation

- Are the child and family able correctly to recognize and promptly treat hypoglycemia and hyperglycemia?

*Sick Day Rules for the Child
with Type 1 Diabetes Mellitus*

1. Always give the insulin injection, even if the child does not have an appetite. If you believe that the child will become hypoglycemic with the usual dose, contact the physician or nurse educator for specific instructions. If ordered, use sliding-scale rapid-acting insulin for hyperglycemia, every 3 to 4 hours.
2. Test blood glucose level at least every 4 hours, and more often for persistent hypoglycemia or hyperglycemia.
3. Test for urinary ketones with each voiding. Notify the physician or nurse educator if moderate or large amounts of urinary ketones are present. Additional regular insulin may be ordered.
4. Encourage calorie-free liquids. If ketones are present, liquids are essential to aid in clearing.
5. Follow the child's usual meal plan. If the child has a poor appetite, a sick day diet consisting of simple carbohydrates can be substituted. Try to replace the usual grams of carbohydrate with simple carbohydrate foods.
6. Encourage rest—especially if urinary ketones are present. Exercising while ketones are present results in increased ketone formation.
7. Notify the physician or nurse educator for:
   • Nausea and vomiting
   • Fruity odor to the breath
   • Deep, rapid respirations
   • Decreasing level of consciousness
   • Moderate or high urinary ketones
   • Persistent hyperglycemia

Diabetic Ketoacidosis

Diabetic ketoacidosis is the metabolic consequence of a severe insulin deficit.

Etiology

Diabetic ketoacidosis results from an absolute or relative insulin deficit. In the younger diabetic child, the most common cause is insulin resistance, such as a stress response initiated by an infection. In the adolescent, the most common cause is missed insulin injection(s).

Manifestations

Table 51–1 lists signs and symptoms of DKA, which include abdominal and chest pain, nausea/vomiting, fruity breath, decreased LOC, Kussmaul respirations, and symptoms of dehydration.

Diagnostic Evaluation

Diabetic ketoacidosis is confirmed by the following test results:

• Blood glucose: elevated
• Arterial or venous pH: low
• Urinary ketones: large
• Serum ketones (beta-hydroxybutyric acid): elevated
• Serum potassium: elevated, normal, or low
• Serum phosphorus: low
• White blood cell count: elevated, especially with infection
• Serum CO_2: low

NURSING CARE

The Child in Diabetic Ketoacidosis

Assessment

Assessment of the child in DKA includes assessing the child's level of consciousness, hydration status, respiratory status, and weight. If the child has a known history of type 1 diabetes mellitus, obtain the following data:

• Most recent blood glucose values
• History of urinary ketones, and the steps taken to manage ketones at home
• Usual insulin dosages, and the time and amount of the most recent injection
• Time of last meal and amount of food eaten
• Identification of the family member usually given the responsibility for injections and blood tests
• The family's understanding of the daily management of diabetes
• Usual sick day management plan

Nursing Diagnosis, Planning, Intervention, and Evaluation

Nursing Diagnosis	■ Fluid Volume Deficit related to abnormal fluid losses through diuresis and emesis.
Expected Outcome	• The child will be safely rehydrated as evidenced by normal weight, skin turgor, urine output, and moist mucous membranes.

Intervention

1. Determine the child's hydration status, evaluating weight, skin turgor, mucous membranes, and urine output.
2. Encourage calorie-free fluids if the child is not nauseated. Initiate intravenous (IV) fluids as ordered. Normal saline is the initial fluid used, followed by half-normal saline.

Rationale

1. Identifies baseline hydration status. A comparison of the child's usual weight with the admission weight provides an estimation of percent of total body fluid loss.
2. Rehydration is the initial step in resolving DKA. If acidosis has resulted in nausea and vomiting, IV fluids are required. Fluid losses occur primarily from the osmotic diuresis occurring with hyperglycemia. Emesis can also contribute to fluid loss. Normal saline is the initial IV rehydration fluid. Although normally a hypertonic solution compared with blood, it is isotonic in states of dehydration.

3. Maintain strict intake and output monitoring.

4. Observe for edema or pulmonary congestion during rehydration.

5. Weigh on arrival and frequently during rehydration (every 8 hours may be appropriate).

3. Accurate intake and output records are essential in calculating rehydration status.

4. These signs indicate overhydration.

5. A comparison of the admission weight with the child's usual weight provides an indication of hydration status. Follow-up weights provide ongoing assessment.

Evaluation

- Is the child safely rehydrated as evidenced by normal weight, urine output, skin turgor, and moist mucous membranes?

Nursing Diagnosis

■ Risk for Injury related to altered acid–base balance from lack of insulin, leading to ketone production and acidosis.

Expected Outcome

- The child will experience a resolution of ketosis and acidosis, as evidenced by laboratory results and clinical assessment.

Intervention

Rationale

1. Test all urine samples for the presence of ketones. Monitor the child's breath for acetone. Observe respirations to identify Kussmaul respirations.

1. The presence of urinary ketones indicates possible acidosis. Serum ketone analysis, or beta-hydroxybutyric acid, is a direct measurement of ketone activity. The liver produces three ketoacids: beta-hydroxybutyric acid, acetoacetate, and acetone. Acetone, the weakest of the acids, is expelled by the lungs and can be assessed as a fruity smell to the child's breath. High acid levels trigger a rapid and deep respiration (Kussmaul respirations) in an effort to remove excessive acetone.

2. Encourage calorie-free fluids, if the child is able to drink. If ordered, begin IV fluids.

2. Fluids are essential in flushing ketones as well as in maintaining hydration. In severe dehydration, the osmotic pull of the blood glucose helps to hold fluid in the bloodstream, thus preventing circulatory shock. Insulin is not given until rehydration has begun to diminish the risk of circulatory shock.

3. Initiate IV insulin therapy as ordered. Prime the IV tubing according to institution protocol.

3. Insulin therapy is initiated after rehydration has begun. A continuous IV infusion of regular insulin is titrated to keep blood glucose in a safe range while avoiding hypoglycemia. Insulin therapy inhibits the production of ketones. Subcutaneous insulin is not an appropriate therapy for the dehydrated child. With dehydration, peripheral vessels constrict, resulting in poor absorption and distribution of the insulin. Insulin adheres to the plastic of the IV bag and tubing, and it is not known whether this affects therapy. Some clinicians recommend priming the IV tubing with the insulin solution and flushing with a fresh solution before delivery. This technique saturates the binding sites of the plastic and provides nonfluctuating insulin delivery.

4. Monitor blood glucose frequently.

4. IV insulin acts rapidly. A continuous infusion of insulin could quickly result in hypoglycemia.

5. Provide glucose-containing IV fluids as ordered.

5. Insulin is needed to inhibit ketone formation. Even though blood glucose values may be in an acceptable range, the insulin infusion must continue until the serum ketones are cleared. To prevent hypoglycemia, glucose is added to the saline hydration solutions.

Evaluation

- Within 24 hours of admission, does the child display any evidence of ketosis (ketonuria, fruity breath, elevated blood glucose)?

| Nursing Diagnosis | ■ Risk for Injury related to electrolyte imbalance from emesis and acidosis. |
| Expected Outcome | • The child will not experience adverse consequences of electrolyte abnormalities, as evidenced by normal serum sodium and potassium values. |

Intervention

Rationale

1. Monitor potassium levels closely, looking for signs and symptoms of hyperkalemia, including bradycardia, muscle weakness, hyperreflexia, and respiratory arrest. Also monitor for signs and symptoms of hypokalemia, including muscle weakness, fatigue, hypotension, and hyporeflexia.

1. During acidosis, potassium moves out of the cell and into the intravascular spaces. Intravascular potassium is lost through diuresis. Initially, serum potassium levels may appear in an acceptable range, but this does not reflect the lost intracellular potassium. As rehydration and correction of acidosis begins, potassium moves back into the cells, resulting in lower serum levels. Serum potassium levels are obtained frequently (every 1–2 hours initially) during treatment of DKA to adequately assess potassium needs. See Chapter 42 for further discussion.

2. Use cardiac monitor to determine abnormal electrocardiogram resulting from altered potassium levels. Hypokalemia produces prolonged ST segment; notched, flat, or inverted T waves; and dysrhythmias. Hyperkalemia produces flattened P wave or peaked T wave and ventricular fibrillation.

2. Hypokalemia or hyperkalemia can cause a medical emergency, requiring rapid response.

3. After verifying urine output, initiate potassium therapy as ordered. If the child is anuric, notify the physician and do not give potassium.

3. Renal failure can result from severe dehydration. If the child is anuric, potassium is retained, causing abnormal serum levels. Replacement therapy must be done cautiously.

| Evaluation | • Does the child maintain a stable fluid and electrolyte balance, with serum sodium and potassium levels within normal limits? |

| Nursing Diagnosis | ■ Risk for Injury related to cerebral edema from resolving DKA. |
| Expected Outcome | • The child will not experience adverse consequences of cerebral edema, as evidenced by appropriate level of consciousness. |

Intervention

Rationale

1. Observe child frequently for signs of cerebral edema: complaints of headache, decreasing level of consciousness, or unequal, fixed, or dilated pupils. Notify physician of any changes from the baseline assessment.

1. Cerebral edema is a complication of resolving DKA that can result in brain damage or death. The causes are unclear, but may be related to overhydration; rapid fluid shifts, particularly into the cerebral intracellular space; and electrolyte imbalance. Frequent neurologic checks aid in prompt recognition and prevention of neurologic deficits.

2. Monitor blood glucose values frequently (hourly) when IV insulin is being infused.

2. Blood glucose values should not drop more than 50–100 mg/dl/hr to prevent rapid osmotic shifts. As the serum glucose approaches the mid-200s, glucose will be added to the IV fluids. Blood glucose levels are maintained in the mid-200s for the duration of the IV insulin therapy.

| Evaluation | • Does the child demonstrate appropriate neurologic status and absence of signs of cerebral edema? |

| Nursing Diagnosis | ■ Knowledge Deficit related to home management during sick days. |
| Expected Outcome | • The family will promptly recognize and respond to situations requiring sick day management. |

Intervention

Rationale

1. Teach the family how and when to test for urinary ketones
   • When blood glucose level exceeds 250 mg/dl.
   • When the child is ill.

1. Ketones are formed in response to an insulin deficit. Either high glucose values or illness could be associated with insulin deficit.

2. Instruct family about sick day management.

3. Identify situations requiring the family to contact the diabetes health care team, including nausea with vomiting, high levels of urinary ketones, procedures requiring NPO status, and signs of acidosis.
4. Provide the child and family with phone numbers of appropriate health care professionals for questions on sick day management.
5. Frequent bouts of DKA require evaluation of home care knowledge, compliance with recommended regimen, home supervision, and coping skills.

2. Stress, either from an infection or the environment, can cause hyperglycemia and uncontrolled diabetes. Early recognition and treatment of ketones can prevent acute complications.
3. Early intervention is essential in preventing acidosis and its sequelae. The family can initiate outpatient management of ketones with direction from the diabetes team.

4. The child and family should know whom to call and how to reach the appropriate health care professional for guidance during sick days.
5. Frequent episodes of DKA may reflect poor compliance, poor understanding of home care needs, inappropriate or absent parental supervision, or depression. A team approach (including nurse educator, nutritionist, social worker, psychologist, physician) can address many of these issues.

Evaluation

• Can the child and family promptly recognize and respond appropriately to situations requiring sick day management?
• Is the child able to prevent DKA?

Long-Term Health Care Needs for the Child with Type 1 Diabetes Mellitus

Serious complications are associated with long-term diabetes: retinopathy, nephropathy, neuropathy, and cardiovascular disease. Studies have demonstrated that strict metabolic control of diabetes may decrease the onset or severity of complications by 35% to 70% (DCCT Research Group, 1993). A team approach to diabetes management can best provide the tools to achieve metabolic control. The team includes the physician specialist, nurse educator, dietician,

and behavioral specialist. Regular checkups and telephone contact with the diabetes team are essential to address the needs of the growing child.

Routine health care for the child with diabetes should also include yearly dental and ophthalmologic evaluations, as well as prophylactic interventions such as influenza vaccinations. Other referral sources should be used as specific needs are identified.

Diabetes research is aimed at preventing diabetes and finding a cure after diagnosis. Multiple immune intervention strategies are being identified and tested, and islet cell transplantation research holds promise for a cure.

KEY CONCEPTS
. . . .

■ The six major hormones of the endocrine system are adrenocorticotropic hormone (ACTH), thyroid-stimulating hormone (TSH), follicle-stimulating hormone (FSH), luteinizing hormone (LH), growth hormone (GH), and prolactin.
■ The pituitary gland stimulates target organs to produce specific hormones. When sufficient hormone is produced, the gland signals the pituitary to stop stimulation. This mechanism is referred to as negative feedback.
■ To improve compliance with daily medications, the nurse may suggest using pill dispensers or a watch with an alarm as a reminder to take medication at specific times.

■ Signs and symptoms of hypothyroidism include fatigue, constipation, cold intolerance, weight gain, dry thick skin, edema, and poor growth. Signs and symptoms of hyperthyroidism include nervousness, diarrhea, heat intolerance, weight loss, smooth, velvety skin, exophthalmos, and increased appetite.
■ Diabetes insipidus is an inability to concentrate urine due to a deficiency of antidiuretic hormone. Diabetes insipidus is characterized by polyuria, dehydration, increased serum sodium, and a low urine specific gravity. In comparison, syndrome of inappropriate antidiuretic hormone (SIADH) results from excessive production of

antidiuretic hormone. This is evidenced by decreased urine output, increased urine specific gravity, and decreased serum sodium.
■ Psychosocial issues concerning children with precocious puberty include self-consciousness about their bodies, being treated as older than their chronologic age, and aggressive behavior by boys.
■ Congenital adrenal hyperplasia (CAH) should be considered in any neonate with unusual-appearing genitalia.
■ In the absence of insulin, the metabolism of fats, proteins, and carbohydrates is impaired, and glucose is unable to move into the intracellular space, resulting in hyperglycemia.

■ Both type 1 and type 2 diabetes mellitus involve abnormal carbohydrate metabolism, but risk related to age of onset, body size, gender, and ethnic background, and treatment are different for the two types of diabetes.

■ The goals of diabetes management are to maintain appropriate height and weight, maintain age-appropriate lifestyle, maintain near-normal glycosylated hemoglobin, and prevent acute complications of hypoglycemia and hyperglycemia.

■ Common nursing diagnoses associated with type 1 diabetes mellitus

include Knowledge Deficit, Altered Family Processes, Altered Nutrition, and Risk for Injury related to hypoglycemia and hyperglycemia.

■ Teaching needs associated with home management of type 1 diabetes mellitus are related to the disease process, medication, home glucose monitoring, hypoglycemia, hyperglycemia, exercise, complications, and support services.

■ There are adrenergic and neuroglycopenic clinical manifestations of hypoglycemia. Hypoglycemia should be treated with 15 g of easily digested carbohydrate.

■ Hyperglycemia is caused by an inadequate amount of insulin, increased dietary intake, decreased amount of exercise, and a response to emotional or physical stress. Persistent hyperglycemia may indicate a need for an insulin dosage adjustment.

■ Nursing diagnoses related to care of the child in diabetic ketoacidosis (DKA) include Fluid Volume Deficit, Risk for Injury related to altered acid–base balance, Risk for Injury related to electrolyte imbalance, Risk for Injury related to cerebral edema, and Knowledge Deficit.

ANSWER TO CRITICAL THINKING EXERCISE 51–1

Signs of growth hormone (GH) deficiency, or another underlying disorder affecting growth, are related to the rate of the child's growth, not to the height measurement itself. If, over a period of 6 to 12 months of careful growth measurement, the child demonstrates a marked downward deviation of a previous growth rate along with other signs of GH deficiency,

then the child would need to be referred for diagnostic evaluation.

Children grow and mature at varying rates, depending on genetic and environmental factors. Many boys do not begin their growth spurts until the late teen years but still attain an adequate adult height. Some children have a familial tendency toward short stature, not related to any underlying

disorder. One way of estimating a child's eventual adult height (within 2 to 3 inches) is to add the mother's and father's height (in inches) and divide by 2. To this, add 2.5 inches (boys) or subtract 2.5 inches (girls). Emphasize to a worried parent that administration of GH will not help a child who does not have a true GH deficiency.

REFERENCES AND READINGS

Albisser, A. M., & Sperlich, M. (1993). Adjusting insulins. *Diabetes Educator, 18*(3), 211–227.

Allen, D. B., Blizzard, R. M., & Rosenfeld, R. G. (1995). The use—and misuse—of growth hormone. *Contemporary Pediatrics, 12*(9), 45–46, 49–50, 53–54 passim.

Allen, D. B. (1999). Short stature. In F. Burg, E. Wald, J. Ingelfinger, & R. Polin (Eds.), *Gellis & Kagan's current pediatric therapy* (16th ed., pp. 733–734). Philadelphia: Saunders.

American Academy of Pediatrics, American Thyroid Association. (1993). Newborn screening for congenital hypothyroidism: recommended guidelines. *Pediatrics, 91*, 1203–1209.

American Diabetes Association. (1999). Clinical Practice Recommendations 1999. *Diabetes Care, 22*(Suppl. 1). Available on-line: http://www.diabetes.org/diabetescare/supplement199/

Angelucci, P. A. (1995). Caring for patients with hypothyroidism. *Nursing, 25*(5), 60–61.

Anonymous. (1998). Critical care: A quick check of the endocrine system. *Nursing, 28*(7), 12–13, 32.

Armentrout, D. (1995). Neonatal diabetes mellitus. *Journal of Pediatric Health Care, 9*, 75–78.

Aronson, R., Ehrlich, R., Bailey, J., & Rovet, J. (1990). Growth in children with congenital hypothyroidism detected by neonatal screening. *The Journal of Pediatrics, 116*(1), 33–37.

Bianco, C. M. (1996). Clinical snapshot: Diabetes insipidus. *American Journal of Nursing, 96*(8), 30–31.

Bode, H. H., Crawford, J. D., & Danon, M. (1996). Disorders of antidiuretic hormone homeostasis. In F. Lifshitz (Ed.), *Pediatric endocrinology* (3rd ed.). New York: Marcel Dekker.

Boland, E., Ahern, J., & Grey, M. (1998). A primer on the use of insulin pumps in adolescents. *Diabetes Educator, 24*(1), 78–86.

Bradshaw, K. D. (1997). Diagnosing and treating precocious puberty. *Hospital Medicine, 33*(9), 40–44, 47–49, 71–72.

Coates, V., & Boore, J. (1998). The influence of psychological factors on the self-management of insulin-dependent diabetes mellitus. *Journal of Advances in Nursing, 27*(3), 528–537.

Conners, M. H. (1997). Growth in the diabetic child. *Pediatric Clinics of North America, 44*(2), 301–306.

Dallas, J. S., & Foley, T. P. (1996). Hyperthyroidism. In F. Lifshitz (Ed.), *Pediatric endocrinology* (3rd ed.). New York: Marcel Dekker.

Faulkner, M. (1996). Family responses to children with diabetes and their influence on self-care. *Journal of Pediatric Nursing, 11*(2), 82–92.

Fort, P., & Brown, R. S. (1996). Thyroid disorders in infancy. In F. Lifshitz (Ed.), *Pediatric endocrinology* (3rd ed.). New York: Marcel Dekker.

Greg, M., et al. (1999). Coping skills training for youths with diabetes on intensive therapy. *Applied Nursing Research, 12*(1), 3–12.

Grey, M., Cameron, M., Lipman, T., & Thurber, F. (1994). Initial adaptation in children with newly diagnosed diabetes and healthy children. *Pediatric Nursing, 20*(1), 17–21.

Grunt, J., & Schwartz, D. (1992). Growth, short stature, and the use of growth hormone: Considerations for the practicing pediatrician. *Current Problems in Pediatrics, 22*(9), 390–409.

Harrell, G. B., & Murray, P. D. (1998). Diagnosis and management of congenital hypothyroidism. *Journal of Perinatal and Neonatal Nursing, 11*(4), 75–85.

Hatton, D. L., Canam, C., Thorne, S., & Hughes, A. M. (1995). Parents' perception of caring for an infant or toddler with diabetes. *Journal of Advanced Nursing, 22*(3), 569–577.

Henry, J. (1992). Routine growth monitoring and assessment of growth disorders. *Journal of Pediatric Health Care, 6*(5), 291–301.

Review of the Central Nervous System

Embryologic Development

The nervous system is one of the first systems to form in utero. By the fourth week of gestation the neural tube has closed at the anterior end to form the brain and at the posterior end to form the spinal cord.

During the second month of gestation the brain becomes the prominent body structure. It grows rapidly and continues to grow until around the fifth year of life. There appear to be two periods of rapid brain cell growth during gestation. Between the 15th and 20th weeks of gestation the number of neurons increases significantly. At 30 weeks

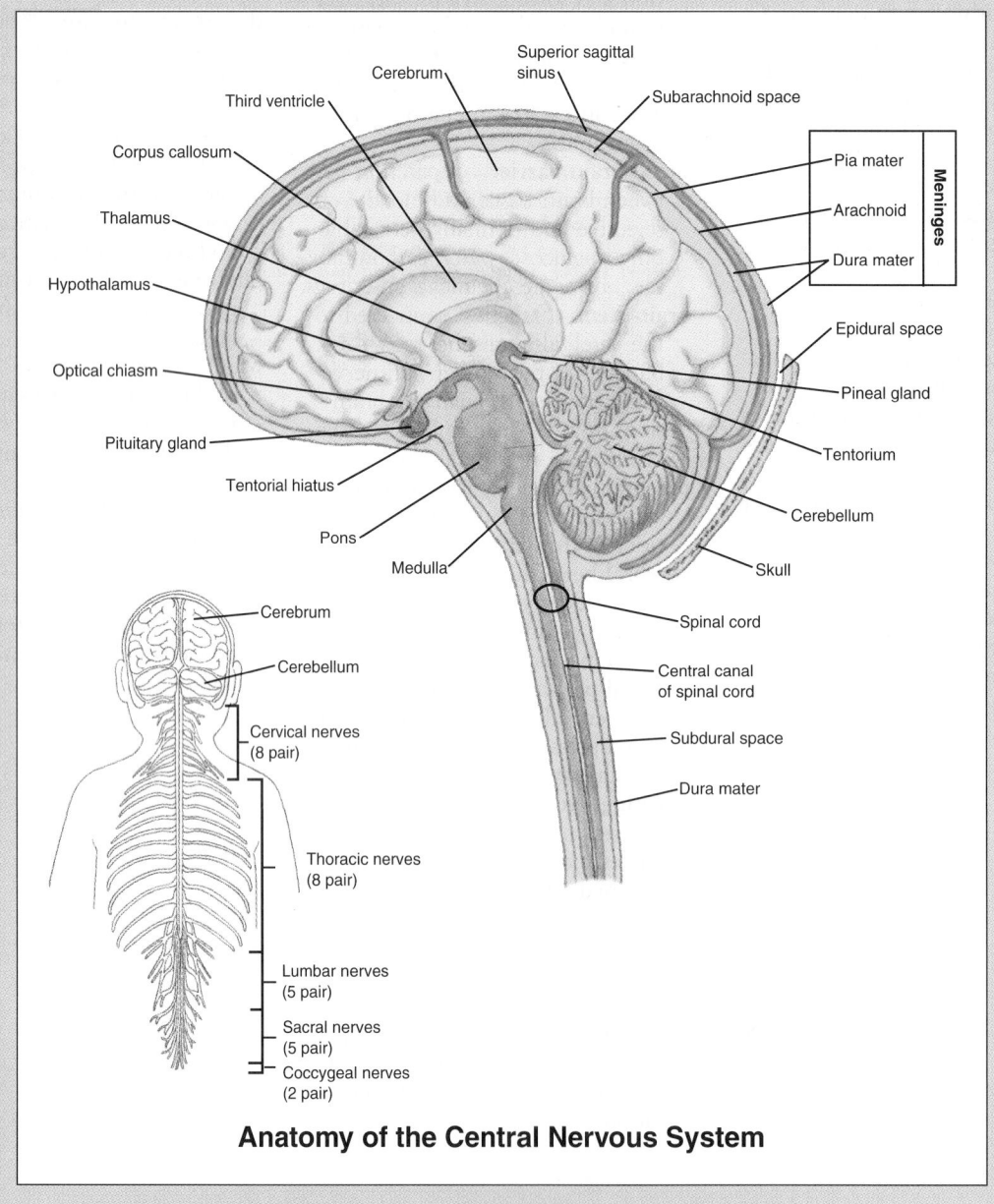

Anatomy of the Central Nervous System

Pediatric Differences in the Central Nervous System

- The brain constitutes 12% of a newborn's body weight, in contrast to only 2% of an adult's body weight.
- The brain of a term infant is two-thirds the weight of an adult's brain. By age 1, it weighs 80% as much as an adult's brain, and by age 6, approximately 90% as much as an adult's brain.
- An infant has about 50 ml of cerebrospinal fluid, compared with 150 ml in an adult.
- The peripheral nerves are not completely myelinated by birth. As myelinization progresses, so does the child's coordination and fine muscle movements.
- The head circumference in a term infant is 34 to 35 cm. By age 6 months the head circumference is 44 cm, and by age 12 months it is 47 cm.
- Papilledema rarely occurs in infancy because of the open fontanels and sutures, which can expand with increased intracranial pressure.
- The primitive reflexes of Moro, grasp, and rooting, present at birth, disappear at various times during the first 5 months. These primitive reflexes may reappear with neurologic disease.

the number of neurons increases again, continuing through 1 year of age. Appropriate prenatal care during periods of rapid neuronal increase can prevent developmental neurologic deficits.

The Myelin Sheath

Myelin, the fatty substance that surrounds the nerves of both the central and the peripheral nervous systems, begins to form at about the 16th week of gestation. Myelin insulates the nerves and helps to conduct electrical impulses. Coordination of fine and gross motor skills progresses with the deposition of the myelin sheath. Nerve fibers can conduct impulses in the absence of myelin; however, the impulses travel more slowly. Gross motor skills develop before fine motor skills, as coordination and control advance throughout childhood. The myelin sheath can be destroyed by disease, drugs, and the aging process itself.

The Neural System

The neural system develops multiple connections between the areas of the brain that control specific functions, including vision, hearing, motor function, sensation, coordination, and speech. Each function is under the control of a specific area of the brain. The right half, or hemisphere, of the brain controls the left side of the body and is concerned with the social aspects of perception, intuition, and experience; the left hemisphere controls the right side of the body and is largely concerned with language acquisition and use and logical, verbal reasoning.

The neonate's neurologic system functions at a subcortical level. Spinal cord reflexes such as sucking and cardiorespiratory functions are present; cortical functions, including memory and coordination, are only partially developed.

The Axial Skeleton

The axial skeleton protects the underlying structures of the central nervous system (CNS). For convenience of study, the bones of the skull and the vertebral column are divided into regions that form the wall of the cranial cavity and the spinal column. The frontal, occipital, temporal, and parietal bones form the cranial vault. The floor of the cranial vault is composed of three compartments or fossae—the anterior, middle, and posterior fossae. The anterior fossa houses the frontal lobes of the brain, the middle fossa contains the upper brain stem and the pituitary gland, and the posterior fossa contains the lower brain stem. Blood vessels and cranial nerves enter and leave the skull through the foramina.

At birth the skull plates are not fused but are separated by nonossified spaces called fontanels. The posterior fontanel usually fuses by age 2 months and the anterior fontanel by 16 to 18 months. The fontanels allow the cranium to expand in response to rapid brain growth. Before fusion of the fontanels and sutures, an increase in intracranial pressure (ICP) will produce an increase in head circumference.

Because brain growth is rapid during infancy, it is difficult to predict the long-term sequelae of neurologic insults that occur to infants. Brain growth can be assessed through head circumference measurements. These measurements are an important part of the routine physical examination of children and should be plotted on a growth chart, for insufficient or excessive head and brain growth could indicate a potential neurologic problem. Premature closing of the fontanels or sutures can cause massive neurologic damage, and continued evaluation by the physician will be needed.

The Meninges

Three membranes surround the brain and spinal column. The outer layer is the dura mater, a fibrous connective tissue structure containing many blood vessels and fibroblast-like cells that secrete collagen to produce a tough, protective membrane (Martin, 1996). The dura mater consists of two layers having outer and inner meningeal components. Between the periosteum of the bone and the dura mater lies the epidural space. Sheets of dura also extend downward and inward to form partitions within the cranium. The falx cerebri separates the cerebral hemispheres, and the falx cerebelli separates the cerebellar hemispheres.

The tentorium is a tent-like structure that separates the cerebellum from the occipital lobe of the cerebrum. The large gap through which the brain stem passes is the tentorial hiatus.

The middle layer is the arachnoid, a delicate, avascular, web-like, serous membrane loosely covering the brain. Between the arachnoid and the dura lies the subdural space, which contains a small amount of fluid, just sufficient to prevent adhesion of the two membranes.

. . . .

Cerebrospinal Fluid Analysis in Children: Normal Findings

	Neonate		Child over
Parameter Evaluated	Preterm	Full term	6 months
White blood cells (per mm³)	≤25	≤7	≤5
Protein (mg/dl)	<150	<170	<40
Glucose (mg/dl)	>30	>60	>40
Red blood cells (per mm³)	>1,000	<800	<5
Pressure (mm Hg)	50–80	50–80	100–280

The innermost layer is the pia mater. It is a delicate, transparent membrane that adheres closely to the outer surface of the brain. The pia mater is a vascular membrane, consisting of arteries and veins.

Between the pia mater and the arachnoid is the subarachnoid space, which is filled with cerebrospinal fluid (CSF). The CSF acts as a cushion to reduce the force of trauma on the brain.

The Brain

The three sections of the brain are the cerebrum, the cerebellum, and the brain stem. The cerebrum is the largest component, filling the upper portion of the skull. It is divided into two hemispheres, right and left, which are separated by a longitudinal fissure. The two hemispheres are joined by a thin sheet of membrane called the corpus callosum. The cerebral hemispheres are further divided into lobes in relation to the cranial bones: frontal, parietal, temporal, and occipital. The cerebrum also includes part of the thalamus, hypothalamus, basal ganglia, and the olfactory and optic nerves.

The cerebellum is composed of white and gray matter. It is attached to the brain stem by paired bundles of fibers. The brain stem consists of the midbrain, the pons, the medulla, the thalamus, and the third ventricle.

The Cranial Nerves

Twelve pairs of cranial nerves arise from the brain and brain stem, each with a specific function. Testing these nerves can indicate the location and degree of CNS injury (see Chapter 33).

The Spinal Cord

The spinal cord is described as segmented into the cervical, thoracic, lumbar, and sacral regions. The spinal nerves are named for their corresponding vertebral segments.

The spinal cord transmits signals to and from the brain and responds to local sensory information through automatic motor responses called reflexes. The simplest type of spinal cord response is the reflex arc. Sensation is transmitted to the spinal cord from a sensory nerve fiber. It synapses with a motor neuron in the same cord segment, causing a muscle or tendon contraction in the corresponding motor nerve. Deep tendon reflexes are examples of the reflex arc.

Sensory innervation occurs as sensory nerves carrying body sensations enter the spinal cord on the dorsal surface. Most sensory fibers for pain and temperature ascend to the brain by way of lateral spinal tracts. Sensory fibers for touch and pressure ascend through anterior tracts. Almost all sensory fibers pass through the thalamus, where the perceptions

. . . .

Cerebrospinal Fluid Analysis: Findings in Pathologic Conditions

Condition	Appearance	Pressure	Cells	Protein	Glucose/Other
Traumatic tap	Bloody; supernatant fluid clear	Normal	Any red blood cells	4 mg/dl rise per 5,000 red cells	NA
Acute bacterial meningitis	Cloudy to milky or xanthochromatic	Usually elevated	Polymorphonuclear cells from 100–60,000/mm³	100–500 mg/dl	Decreased compared to blood
Viral meningitis	Clear	Normal or increased	0 to a few hundred/mm³, mostly leukocytes	50–200 mg/dl	Normal
Encephalitis	Clear and colorless	Normal or slightly elevated	Normal or increased	50–200 mg/dl	<40 mg/dl
Subdural hematoma	Yellow to clear and colorless	Increased	Normal	Normal or increased	Normal
Diabetic coma	Clear and colorless	Decreased	Normal	Normal or slightly increased	May be 200–300 mg/dl

Common Diagnostic Tests and Procedures for Neurologic Disorders in Children

Test	Description	Purpose	Nursing Considerations
Computed tomography (CT Scan)	Produces computer image of horizontal and vertical cross-sections of brain at any axis.	Identifies abnormal tissue and structures, as in brain tumor, bleeding, or hydrocephalus.	An IV line may need to be inserted if contrast medium is used. Notify the radiologist if the child is allergic to iodine. The child may be sedated if necessary.
Angiography	After IV contrast dye is injected a clear image of the vessels is obtained, as the computer eliminates all tissue that has not been infused by the contrast dye.	Shows vascular abnormalities.	May be NPO. Notify the radiologist if the child is allergic to iodine. Obtain signed permission form. There are restrictions on activity after the test.
Echoencephalography	Echoes from ultrasonic waves are recorded as they reflect off various surfaces of the skull.	Identifies abnormal structure, position, and function.	Painless procedure. No preparation.
Electroencephalography (EEG)	Electrodes placed on the scalp conduct and amplify electrical activity; electrical potential of the brain is measured and recorded.	Identifies abnormal electrical brain discharges, as in seizures.	Child may have regular diet or fluids, but no caffeine or stimulants. Hair should be clean. Tell the child the procedure is painless.
Lumbar puncture (LP)	CSF pressure is measured and a specimen obtained as a needle is inserted into the subarachnoid space between L3 and L4.	Measures pressure, and analysis of CSF identifies infections. Procedure may be used to administer medications.	Obtain signed consent. Instruct the child to lie on the side with the knees up to chest. After the procedure, the child lies flat.
Magnetic resonance imaging (MRI)	Produces computer images of the brain by means of radiofrequency emissions from certain elements.	Demonstrates morphological features of tissue and structures with degree of detail not achievable by other methods.	The procedure is painless, but the child may be sedated if necessary. Inform child that loud clicking noises will be heard. The child's head will be restrained.
Nuclear brain scan (Single photon emission computed tomography, SPECT)	A radioactive substance injected IV (the amount of the substance measured and recorded). Abnormal uptake indicates abnormal tissue or structure.	Identifies focal brain lesions and demonstrates CSF pathways.	The child needs to remain still during the test. An IV line is needed.

of touch, pressure, and temperature are interpreted. Perceptions of texture, size, and weight are interpreted in the cortex.

Motor nerves are stimulated to respond after the brain receives a signal from a sensory nerve. The motor nerves cross over to the contralateral (opposite) side of the spinal cord from which they originate, then exit on the ventral surface of the spinal cord. The side of the body contralateral to the injured side of the brain will be the side affected by injury.

Functional differences exist between the upper and lower motor neurons, so that the outcome of a spinal cord injury is affected by the site of the injury. An injury between the brain and the dendrites (the nerve fibers that carry impulses toward the cell body) will render the brain incapable of signaling the muscle cells to cease responding reflexively, and the muscle will become contracted, or spastic. If the injury is to a section of the nerve between the muscle and axons (the nerve fibers that carry impulses away from the

cell body), the muscles will become incapable of responding reflexively, causing them to become flaccid.

Cerebrospinal Fluid

CSF is a clear liquid produced in the choroid plexus of the ventricles. The CSF aids in protecting the brain, spinal cord, and meninges by acting as a watery cushion surrounding them, to absorb the shocks to which they are exposed. It is reabsorbed through the arachnoid villi into the venous sinuses.

Cerebral Blood Flow

The internal carotid arteries supply blood to all parts of the brain. Approximately 17% of cardiac output and 20% of body oxygen are transported to the brain. The brain requires approximately ten times the oxygen used by the rest of the body.

Cerebral blood flow (CBF) is controlled by *cerebral perfusion pressure* (CPP), which is the difference between the mean arterial blood pressure and ICP.

Autoregulation, or self-regulation, is a unique physiologic ability. It allows cerebral arteries to change diameter in response to changes in the CPP. The cerebral vessels can maintain a steady blood flow to the brain during alterations in blood pressure and perfusion; however, autoregulation fails when the limits of cerebrovascular dilation are reached.

Autoregulation may be impaired as a result of trauma or ischemia. It is influenced significantly by changes in Pao_2 and $Paco_2$. An increase in $Paco_2$ (above 40 mm Hg) produces cerebral vasodilation and an increase in cerebral blood flow. A decrease in $Paco_2$ (25 to 30 mm Hg) causes cerebral vasoconstriction and thus reduces blood flow to the brain. Alterations in Pao_2 between 80 and 100 mm Hg have little effect on cerebral blood flow, though hypoxia will dramatically increase cerebral blood flow.

The Child with a Nervous System Disorder

Assessment

The child with a neurologic injury or illness needs a complete neurologic assessment (see Chapter 33 for assessment of the cranial nerves). Test the child's level of consciousness, cerebral function, cerebellar function, and orientation. Note the child's mood and behavior. Knowledge of normal developmental milestones, as measured by the Denver Developmental Screening Test II (DDST-II) is essential (see Chapter 4 and Appendix I). The child's level of consciousness may be assessed using the Glasgow Coma Scale (GCS) modified for children. The child's interaction with the family and the environment will also yield information about level of consciousness. Note lethargy, drowsiness, hyperactivity, tremors, or jitteriness.

Assess balance, coordination, and motor skills by observing the child's behaviors, particularly while the child is dressing or playing. Coordination can be assessed by the finger-to-nose test, by observing the child throw a ball or handle a pencil, or using rapidly alternating movements. Observe the child's walking gait for hemiplegia, scissor gait, or an abnormally wide-spaced gait. Observe and record the child's muscle development, strength, and tone. Test deep tendon reflexes and range of motion of all joints. Check the sensory function of the face, trunk, arms, and legs. Test both sides of the child for vibration, superficial tactile sensation, superficial pain, and temperature.

Care of the child with neurologic problems requires knowledge of neuroanatomy, neurophysiology, and normal growth and development. The nurse plays an important role in the early recognition of pediatric neurologic problems, some of which have the potential for devastating long-term outcomes. The nurse assesses the child's condition by comparing the child's normal behavior with current behavior. The family is an invaluable source of information about the child's normal behavior and how current behavior deviates from that norm. The child and the family need support and understanding because the child's illness represents a crisis in their lives. The family's ability to respond and influence the child's coping mechanisms will directly influence the recovery and adaptation process.

Many conditions of the nervous system share common assessment data, diagnoses, and interventions. Principles of nursing care for the child with a nervous system disorder can be applied to a variety of situations.

Nursing Diagnosis, Planning, Intervention, and Evaluation

Nursing Diagnosis	■ Altered Cerebral Tissue Perfusion related to alteration of arterial or venous blood flow, cerebral infarction, hemorrhage, hematoma, increased intracranial pressure (ICP), cerebral edema, seizures, hypoventilation, or increased cerebral metabolism.
Expected Outcomes	• The child will have improved cerebral perfusion, no cranial nerve deficits, improved or normal level of consciousness, vital signs in baseline normal, and GCS score within normal limits. • The child will demonstrate appropriate behavior or thought patterns for age.

Intervention	Rationale
1. Determine a baseline age and developmental level of child.	1. Baseline age and developmental level will help the nurse gauge changes in neurologic status.
2. Perform a baseline neurologic and level of consciousness assessment and measure vital signs on admission.	2. Changes in neurologic signs can indicate deterioration or improvement in status. Changes are compared to baseline.
3. Monitor factors that may further increase cerebral edema and ICP (hypoxia, fever, seizures, hypotension, hypercapnia).	3. Monitoring these factors allows for correction of conditions that increase ICP and keeps cerebral metabolic needs to a minimum.
4. Maintain head of bed at a 30- to 45-degree angle.	4. Venous outflow drainage of the brain is facilitated by gravity.
5. Avoid the prone position, neck flexion, or hip flexion.	5. All of these positions tend to increase ICP. Lying flat in bed increases ICP. Neck flexion kinks the jugular vein where venous drainage occurs. Hip flexion can increase intra-abdominal or intrathoracic pressure, thus increasing ICP.
6. Organize nursing care around periods of low ICP.	6. Nursing care such as suctioning, bathing, and repositioning increases ICP.

7. Monitor pupil size and reactivity every hour, as needed, or as ordered.
8. Measure head circumference daily or as needed and record on growth chart, if age appropriate.
9. Palpate the anterior fontanel every shift, if age appropriate.
10. Palpate the cranial suture lines every shift, if age appropriate.
11. Observe the infant for irritability, lethargy, feeding intolerance, and decreasing GSC score.
12. Place emergency equipment (oxygen, suction, bag-valve-mask) near the child's room or at the bedside.
13. Monitor intake and output hourly.

14. Check urine specific gravity every 4 to 6 hours or as needed. Notify the physician if the urine specific gravity is above 1.030 or below 1.010, or if output is below 1 ml/kg/hr or above 2 ml/kg/hr.

7. An increase in pupil size and reactivity might indicate an increase in ICP.
8. If fontanels are open, cranial expansion takes place when the CSF is under pressure.
9. An increase in fontanel size and tenseness may indicate an increase in CSF accumulation.
10. The cranial sutures may separate with an increase in CSF volume or pressure.
11. All are signs of increasing ICP and deteriorating neurologic status.
12. Increased ICP can cause apnea and may lead to cardiopulmonary arrest.
13. Imbalance in fluid volume associated with increased ICP can be corrected earlier.
14. Urine specific gravity normally is 1.010 to 1.030, and normal urine output is 1 to 2 ml/kg/hr. With increasing ICP, diabetes insipidus or syndrome of inappropriate antidiuretic hormone (SIADH) may occur (Behrman, Kliegman, & Arvin, 1996).

Evaluation

- Does the child demonstrate a normal respiratory rate and pattern and vital signs?
- Does the child demonstrate an improved level of consciousness?
- Does the child have normal urine output and normal urine specific gravity?
- Does the child show intact cranial nerve function, an optimum level on the GCS, and behavior and thought patterns appropriate for age?

Nursing Diagnosis

■ Altered Nutrition: Less than Body Requirements related to restricted intake, neurologic impairment, swallowing or chewing difficulty, risk for aspiration, nausea, or vomiting.

Expected Outcome

- The child will maintain stable or normal weight for age and height; exhibit normal serum proteins, moist mucous membranes, and adequate urine output; and be free of nausea and vomiting.

Intervention

1. Weigh the child daily on the same scale, at the same time of day, and in the same clothes. Record on a growth chart.

2. Monitor skin turgor, mucous membranes, eye orbits, urine output, urine specific gravity, and serum and urine electrolyte values.
3. Position the child or infant upright after feedings. If the child is old enough and the ICP is not elevated, the head should be slightly flexed and facing forward. Arms should be positioned forward with feet placed on a firm surface.
4. Provide a flexible feeding schedule with small feedings of favorite foods.
5. Minimize handling around feeding times.

6. If swallowing is impaired, assist the child with chewing by holding the child's chin and jaw.

7. Determine the child's level of consciousness before giving liquids.
8. Consult a dietician.

Rationale

1. Changes in weight indicate alterations in fluid balance and nutritional status. Being consistent with timing and type of clothing enhances accurate comparison. The nurse should weigh only if the procedure does not increase ICP.
2. These are indicators of fluid and electrolyte status.

3. Proper positioning will decrease the risk of aspiration, enhance comfort, prevent contractures, and provide for safety while feeding.

4. These techniques facilitate digestion and the ability to maintain adequate caloric intake.
5. Minimal handling during feeding decreases the likelihood of vomiting and aspiration.
6. Swallowing may be facilitated by this method, because it keeps the child's head stabilized in an appropriate anatomic position.
7. A decreased level of consciousness may cause aspiration with swallowing.
8. The dietician will advise how best to meet metabolic demands and plan the most efficient way to get calories.

9. Verify placement of any oral or nasogastric tube before tube feedings are initiated.
10. Obtain order to medicate for nausea and vomiting if necessary.

9. Incorrect placement of a nasogastric tube will result in placing feedings into the lungs.
10. The child will be more likely to tolerate feedings when nausea is controlled.

Evaluation

- Does the child show normal growth for age, with no weight loss?
- Is the child free from nausea and vomiting?
- Does the child have age-appropriate caloric intake daily?
- Does the child have proper hydration with moist mucous membranes?

Nursing Diagnosis

■ Risk for Impaired Skin Integrity related to neuromuscular impairment, decreased level of consciousness, inadequate physical activity, immobility, or improper fluid or nutritional intake.

Expected Outcomes

- The child will demonstrate a progressive increase in or adequate physical activity, optimal range of motion, and no skin breakdown.
- The parents will participate in their child's care.

Intervention

1. Use an egg crate mattress or special flotation mattress to protect bony prominences. Reposition every 2 hours and as needed. Check for redness and pressure areas.
2. Observe skin condition every 2 hours with the repositioning of the child or infant.
3. Avoid putting temperature probes, cardiac monitor leads, or excessive tape over a shunt site.
4. Encourage parents or caregivers to participate in passive range-of-motion exercises for the child, if appropriate.

5. If braces or splints are used, assess the skin before and after the splints or assistive devices are put on and taken off.
6. Implement a daily skin care regimen. Teach parents or family to check skin frequently.

Rationale

1. The child with a depressed level of consciousness may not be active, and immobility can cause skin breakdown.

2. Prolonged pressure on the skin will quickly lead to its breakdown.
3. Irritation from adhesives will contribute to skin breakdown and possible infection.
4. Participating in the child's care enhances the parents' control and the child's sense of well-being. Passive range-of-motion exercises provide emotional and physical support for the child and increase the child's activity.
5. Correct application of braces will minimize pressure points and reduce skin breakdown.

6. Bathing, moisturizing, and inspecting the skin will preserve skin integrity.

Evaluation

- Does the child have intact, clean, dry skin without pressure areas or sores?
- Is the child able to participate in his or her own care as tolerated?
- Do the parents or caregivers participate in the child's skin care regimen?
- Are the parents or caregivers able to assist in passive range-of-motion activities for the child?

Nursing Diagnosis

■ Parental Anxiety related to change in the child's health status, threat to self-concept, behavior changes, possible injury, social isolation, seizures, neurologic impairment, or lack of privacy.

Expected Outcome

- The parents will demonstrate management of anxiety, maintain social and personal relationships, verbalize relaxation, verbalize feelings about the child's neurologic impairment, and demonstrate coping skills.

Intervention

1. Keep the parents informed of the child's progress, prognosis, and plan of care. Encourage parents to talk about concerns and ask questions. Allow parents to make decisions where possible.
2. Encourage parents to participate actively in activities of daily living (oral hygiene, bathing, feeding, etc.).
3. Orient the parents to hospital routine and refer to clergy, social worker, and other team members.

Rationale

1. Control over any event of the child's care helps the parents feel they are part of the caregiving team and will lessen their anxiety.

2. Touching the child and active participation in the child's care lower parental anxiety.

3. A familiar environment is less threatening and will enable the family to better deal with the child's condition and prognosis.

4. Encourage rooming-in when possible.

4. Rooming-in will involve the parents more in the child's care, make them part of the health care team, and decrease the child's anxiety.

5. Assist with anxiety reduction techniques such as relaxation techniques, music, and guided imagery.

5. Such techniques facilitate coping and stress reduction.

Evaluation

- Do the parents participate in caregiving for their child when possible?
- Do the parents meet with the health care team periodically?
- Are the parents able to discuss concerns and fears?
- Do the parents plan with the team for the child's future and participate in decision making?
- Are the parents able to state reduced feelings of loneliness?
- Do the parents demonstrate coping and problem-solving skills?

Nursing Diagnosis

■ Knowledge Deficit related to unfamiliarity with infectious process, disease process, medication regimen, dietary or fluid needs, measures for prevention, or chronic illness of a child or infant.

Expected Outcomes

- The child and parents will state age-appropriate, realistic factors about the child's condition, will list factors to decrease neurologic deficits and measures to prevent further occurrences of illness, and will demonstrate medication administration and nutritional adaptations.
- The family will demonstrate that the grieving process has begun.

Intervention

1. Allow time for teaching. If the child is to undergo an operation, do preoperative teaching for the parents as well.

2. Determine the parents' understanding of the child's disability, including the child's need for physical, speech, or occupational therapy.

3. Put parents in touch with community support groups.
4. Supply the parents with phone numbers to call for needed information once they are home.

5. Teach the parents important signs and symptoms of the child's condition, side effects of medications, and when to call the physician or nurse. Provide written instructions.

6. Review the signs and symptoms of wound infection.
7. Review with the parents the signs and symptoms of urinary tract retention or infection.

Rationale

1. Teaching answers questions and reinforces information given to the parents by the physician. It includes the parents in the learning experience.

2. Parents need to understand the intellectual and physical abilities and disabilities of their child to give informed consent or reinforce the need for therapies.

3. Support can be gained by seeing or hearing how others coped with similar situations.
4. Health care workers can help parents feel in touch and educate them at the same time by discussing the child's condition on the telephone.

5. The parents need to state important signs and symptoms that indicate a change in the child's condition and be aware of when to seek medical attention. Anxiety reduces learning and attention span. A written copy of signs and symptoms provides an ongoing resource that can be referred to later.

6. Until the surgical incision is healed, the risk of infection is present.
7. Due to retention and reflux the child might be at risk for urinary tract infections.

Evaluation

- Can the parents discuss the child's care appropriately?
- Are the parents able to list situations in which the child should be seen by the physician or nurse?
- Do the parents know how to contact community support?
- Can the parents demonstrate required adaptation?
- Does the family appropriately express feelings of grief and demonstrate progress toward acceptance?

of Increased Intracranial Pressure

The major pathophysiologic changes associated with increased intracranial pressure (ICP) result from alterations in the brain, cerebrospinal fluid (CSF) dynamics, and cerebral bloodflow. To maintain cerebral pressure and volume within normal range, changes in one or more of the contents of the cranium must be compensated for by changes in the others; this is referred to as the Monroe-Kellie doctrine.

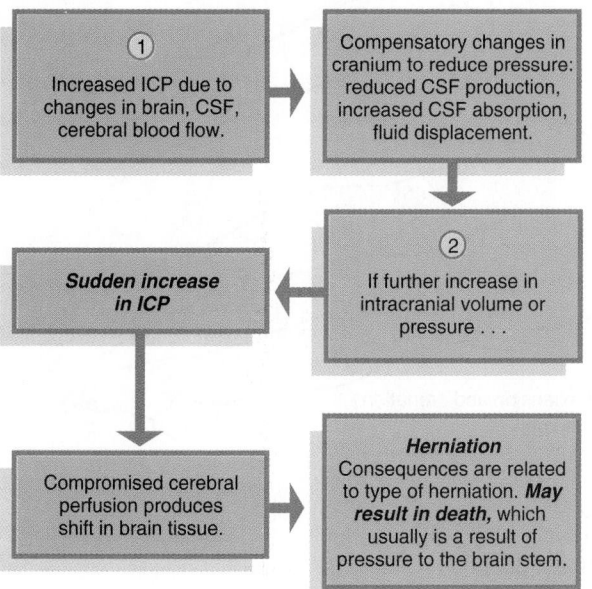

Compensatory mechanisms include a reduction in CSF production, an increase in CSF absorption, and a reduction in cerebral mass as a result of fluid displacement. Once the limits of compensation are reached, any further increase in volume or pressure will cause a sudden

increase in ICP and an associated decline in the child's clinical status. Ultimately, increased ICP will compromise cerebral perfusion and produce shifting of brain tissue, causing herniation. The consequences of herniation depend on its severity and location.

There are four types of herniation. *Transtentorial herniation* occurs when part of the brain herniates downward and around the tentorium cerebelli. It may be unilateral or bilateral and may involve anterior or posterior portions of the brain. If a large amount of tissue is involved, it may cause death because vital brain structures are compressed and become unable to perform their functions.

Temporal lobe herniation, or uncal herniation, refers to a shifting of the temporal lobe laterally across the tentorial notch. This produces compression of the third cranial nerve and ipsilateral pupil dilation. If pressure continues to rise, flaccid paralysis, pupil dilation, pupil fixation, and death will result.

Tonsillar herniation occurs when the cerebellar tonsils herniate through the foramen magnum. The child will develop nuchal rigidity, shoulder or arm numbness, and changes in heart and respiratory rates and patterns. *Arnold-Chiari malformation*, a condition sometimes associated with hydrocephalus, includes herniation of the cerebellar tonsils.

Brain stem herniation through the foramen magnum results in death as a result of compression of vital cardiorespiratory centers.

Infants are somewhat able to compensate for increasing ICP because their cranial sutures remain open. *Craniosynostosis* is premature closure of the cranial sutures. This abnormal skull development causes an abnormally shaped skull. In some cases, craniectomy is needed to manage the increased ICP.

Increased Intracranial Pressure

Intracranial pressure reflects the pressure exerted by the blood, brain, cerebrospinal fluid (CSF), and any other space-occupying fluid or mass. Increased ICP results from a disturbance in autoregulation and is defined as pressure sustained at 20 mm Hg or higher.

Etiology

Alterations in the brain can result from a space-occupying lesion such as a brain tumor or hematoma. The brain can swell as a result of head trauma, infection, or a hypoxic episode. Overproduction of fluid, malabsorption of fluid, or a communication problem within the system can disrupt CSF dynamics.

Manifestations

Signs and symptoms of increased ICP differ according to the child's developmental level. Late signs of increased ICP

Developmental Manifestations of Increased ICP

Infant

- Poor feeding or vomiting
- Irritability or restlessness
- Lethargy
- Bulging fontanel
- High-pitched cry
- Increased head circumference
- Separation of cranial sutures
- Distended scalp veins
- Eyes deviated downward ("setting sun" sign)
- Increased or decreased response to pain

Child

- Headache
- Diplopia
- Mood swings
- Slurred speech
- Papilledema (after 48 hours)
- Altered level of consciousness
- Nausea and vomiting, especially in the morning

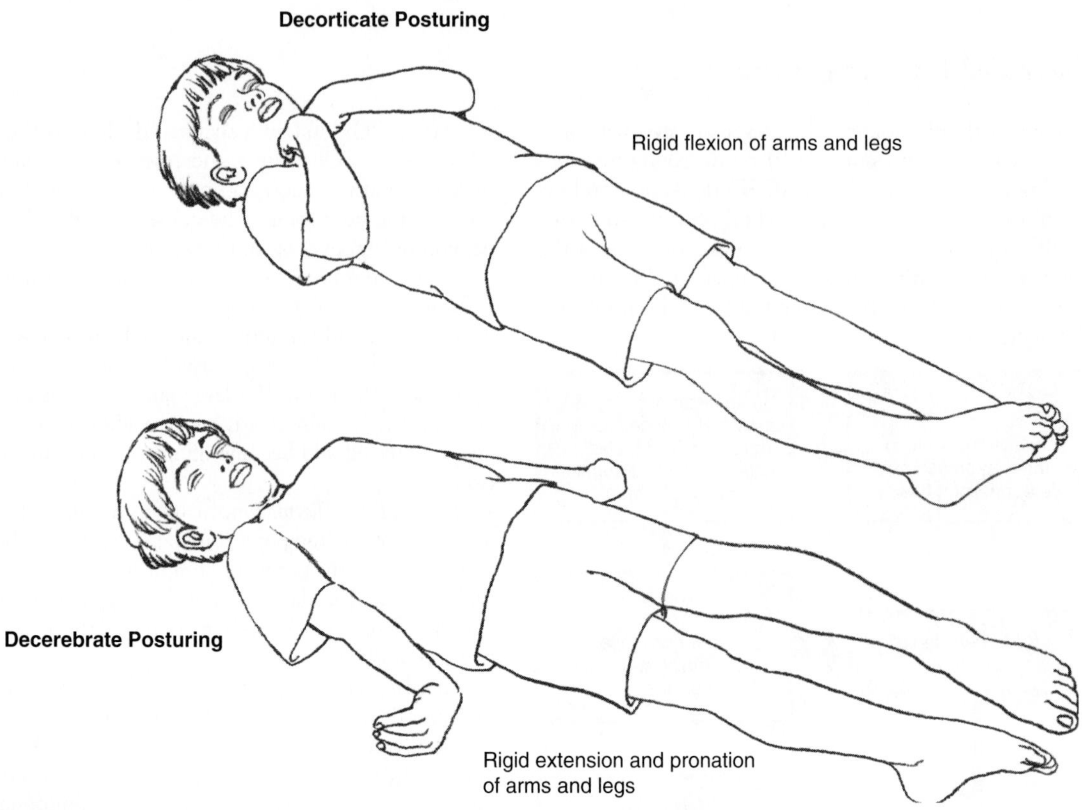

Decorticate Posturing

Rigid flexion of arms and legs

Decerebrate Posturing

Rigid extension and pronation of arms and legs

FIGURE 52–1
· · · · · · · · · ·
Decorticate and decerebrate posturing.

include tachycardia that leads to bradycardia, apnea, systolic hypertension, widening pulse pressure, and decorticate or decerebrate posturing (Fig. 52–1).

Diagnostic Evaluation and Therapeutic Management

Diagnostic tests for increased ICP include computed tomography (CT), magnetic resonance imaging (MRI), lumbar puncture, electrolyte and arterial blood gas determinations, a complete blood count (CBC), electroencephalography (EEG), and radiography. Normal blood gas levels are a Pao_2 above 80 mm Hg and a $Paco_2$ below 45 mm Hg in a child with normal ICP. Passive hyperventilation is an initial treatment for the child with increased ICP because it lowers the $Paco_2$, causing cerebral vasoconstriction and decreased fluid. The goal of hyperventilation is to achieve a $Paco_2$ between 30 and 35 mm Hg (Geraci & Geraci, 1996).

The management of increased ICP is directed toward treating the underlying cause of increased ICP, reducing the volume of the CSF, preserving cerebral metabolic function, and avoiding situations that increase ICP.

The head of the child's bed should be elevated 30°. In addition to being treated with hyperventilation, the child may be given an osmotic diuretic (e.g., mannitol), hypothermia, or dexamethasone.

NURSING CARE
· · · · · · · · · · ·
The Child with Increased Intracranial Pressure

Assessment

Assessment of the child with increased ICP requires astute clinical observation. Common signs and symptoms may not occur until the ICP is significantly elevated and the child's condition is deteriorating rapidly.

· · · · · · · · · ·
Instruments for Monitoring Increased ICP

- **Subarachnoid bolt:** The end of the bolt is placed in the subarachnoid space. The top of the bolt is attached to a transducer to conduct a waveform to the monitor. The neurosurgeon adjusts the transducer to produce a waveform on the monitor.
- **Intraventricular catheter:** The catheter is placed in the lateral ventricle or subarachnoid space. The catheter provides a method for measuring pressure as well as a conduit to drain off extra fluid into the drainage bag. The manometer and drainage bag are part of a sterile closed system.

Nursing care depends on the progression of central nervous system (CNS) involvement. The assessment parameters are those common to all children with an underlying neurologic problem. The nurse should focus special attention on level of consciousness, behavior, pupil status, cranial nerve function, motor function, reflexes, and vital signs.

Level of Consciousness

The nurse should assess and document a baseline level of consciousness. Information about the child's normal behavior should be obtained from the parents or primary caregivers. Serial observations are made to assess changes in the child's condition.

The Glasgow Coma Scale is a standardized scale, which in a modified form is frequently used to assess level of consciousness in infants and children. It consists of a three-part assessment: eye opening, verbal response, and motor response (Table 52–1). Each level of response is assigned a number value. When the assessment of each response is complete, the scores are totaled, providing an objective measure of the child's level of consciousness. The total numeric scores range from 15, indicating no change in level of consciousness, to 3, indicating a deep coma and poor prognosis.

CRITICAL TO REMEMBER

Standard Terms for Level of Consciousness

Level of consciousness should be described by the nurse using standard terminology:

Full consciousness: Awake, alert, oriented, interacts with environment.
Confused: Lacks ability to think clearly and rapidly.
Disoriented: Lacks ability to recognize place or person.
Lethargic: Awakens easily but exhibits limited responsiveness.
Obtunded: Sleeps unless aroused, and once aroused has limited interaction with the environment.
Stupor: Requires considerable stimulation to arouse.
Coma: Vigorous stimulation produces no motor or verbal response.

Behavior

Changes in the child's normal behavior pattern may be an important early sign of increased ICP. Parents often are the first to notice a change in the child's behavior; therefore, a parent's comment that "he isn't acting like himself" should be taken seriously. The child who no longer recognizes parents, cannot follow commands, or has minimal response to pain is deteriorating. Decreased responsiveness to painful stimuli is a significant sign of alteration in level of consciousness.

Pupil Evaluation

Pupil evaluation is done to detect increasing ICP. As ICP rises, compression of the third cranial nerve occurs, resulting in pupil dilation with sluggish or absent constriction in response to light. When evaluating pupils, be aware that some medications can affect pupillary reactions. Atropine will cause the pupils not to react to light.

Motor Function

The child with increased ICP will exhibit changes in motor function. Purposeful movement will decrease, and abnormal posturing may be observed. *Decorticate posturing* refers to flexion of the upper extremities (elbows, wrists) and extension of the lower extremities. Plantar flexion of the feet may also be observed. This type of posturing implies an injury to the cerebral hemispheres. *Decerebrate posturing* involves extension of the upper extremities with internal rotation of the upper arm and wrist. The lower extremities will extend, with some internal rotation noted at the knees and feet. This type of posturing is indicative of damage to more areas of the brain, such as the diencephalon, midbrain, or pons. The progression from decorticate to decerebrate posturing usually indicates deteriorating neurologic function and warrants physician notification. Flaccid paralysis indicates further deterioration in the child's condition.

TABLE 52–1

Glasgow Coma Scale Modified for Children

Child	Infant
Eyes	
4 Opens eyes spontaneously	Opens eyes spontaneously
3 Opens eyes to speech	Opens eyes to speech
2 Opens eyes to pain	Opens eyes to pain
1 No response	**No response**
_____ = Score (Eyes)	
Motor	
6 Obeys commands	Spontaneous movements
5 Localizes	Withdraws to touch
4 Withdraws	Withdraws to pain
3 Flexion	Flexion (decorticate)
2 Extension	Extension (decerebrate)
1 No response	**No response**
_____ = Score (Motor)	
Verbal	
5 Oriented	Coos and babbles
4 Confused	Irritable cry
3 Inappropriate words	Cries to pain
2 Incomprehensible words	Moans to pain
1 No response	**No response**
_____ = Score (Verbal)	
_____ = Total Score (Eyes, Motor, Verbal) Scores will range from 3 to 15.	

Reprinted from James, H. E., Anas, N. G., & Perkin, R. M. (1985). *Brain insults in infants and children.* Orlando, FL: Grune & Stratton.

Vital Signs

Vital signs should be measured regularly, every 15 minutes to 2 hours, depending on the status of the child. Particular attention should be given to careful measurement of blood pressure, pulse, and respiratory rate. Significant changes in vital signs should be reported immediately. Temperature elevation may occur in children with increased ICP. Initiating measures to decrease elevated temperatures (>40°C; >103.9°F) should be a priority in care.

Cushing's response is usually apparent just before or at the time of brain stem herniation. *Cushing's response* consists of an increased systolic blood pressure with widening pulse pressure, bradycardia, and a change in respiratory rate and pattern. This usually indicates an alteration in brain stem perfusion, with the body attempting to improve cerebral blood flow by increasing blood pressure.

In children Cushing's response is a late sign of increased ICP.

As ICP rises, the child's baseline respiratory pattern may change, exhibiting Cheyne-Stokes respiration, central neurogenic hyperventilation, or apneustic breathing. *Cheyne-Stokes respiration* refers to a pattern of breathing characterized by increasing rate and depth, then decreasing rate and depth with a pause of variable length. The cycle will be repeated again and again. *Central neurogenic hyperventilation* is identified by a rapid rate despite normal arterial blood gas values. This type of breathing pattern usually indicates midbrain or pontine involvement. *Apneustic breathing* occurs when the child demonstrates prolonged inspiration and expiration. As Cushing's response occurs, the child will develop apnea. The cerebral perfusion pressure is the mean arterial blood pressure minus ICP (Hickey, 1992).

Nursing Diagnosis, Planning, Intervention, and Evaluation

Nursing Diagnosis ■ Risk for Infection related to invasive lines and procedures.

Expected Outcome • The child will remain afebrile and have a normal white blood cell (WBC) count, no evidence of meningitis or pneumonia, no CSF drainage or purulent drainage, and no urinary tract infection.

Intervention	Rationale
1. Maintain strict asepsis when manipulating ventriculostomy drainage system.	1. Asepsis helps prevent an infection of the catheter site and CSF (see Chapter 51).
2. Monitor invasive sites for redness or drainage.	2. These are signs of infection.
3. Monitor temperature, WBC count, appearance on chest radiographs, and urinalysis results for signs of infection.	3. Steroids given to decrease ICP may mask infection and decrease immunity to infectious organisms.
4. Use aseptic techniques with a Foley catheter.	4. Children on bed rest or who are immobilized are prone to urinary tract infection.

Evaluation
• Is the child's temperature within normal limits?
• Is the child free from signs of infection?

Nursing Diagnosis ■ Fluid Volume Deficit related to restricted intake, inability to swallow, and change in mental status.

Expected Outcome • The child will have moist mucous membranes, serum osmolality and electrolyte values within normal limits for age, and intake and output normal for age.

Intervention	Rationale
1. Monitor intake and output and urine specific gravity. Notify physician of a urine output less than 1 ml/kg/hr or greater than 2 ml/kg/hr.	1. SIADH or diabetes insipidus can occur with stress, surgery, brain dysfunction, or some medications.
2. Administer fluids within fluid restrictions.	2. Fluid restriction aids in decreasing extracellular fluid volume, which in turn decreases ICP.
3. Administer medications as ordered.	3. Osmotic and loop diuretics (mannitol, furosemide) will decrease cerebral edema by increasing fluid excretion.
4. Monitor serum sodium, electrolytes, and serum osmolality.	4. These levels indicate fluid status and help identify measures to take to keep electrolytes in balance. Hyponatremia will cause cerebral edema.

Evaluation
• Does the child demonstrate appropriate fluid balance and normal electrolyte levels?
• Is urinary output at 1 to 2 ml/kg/hr?

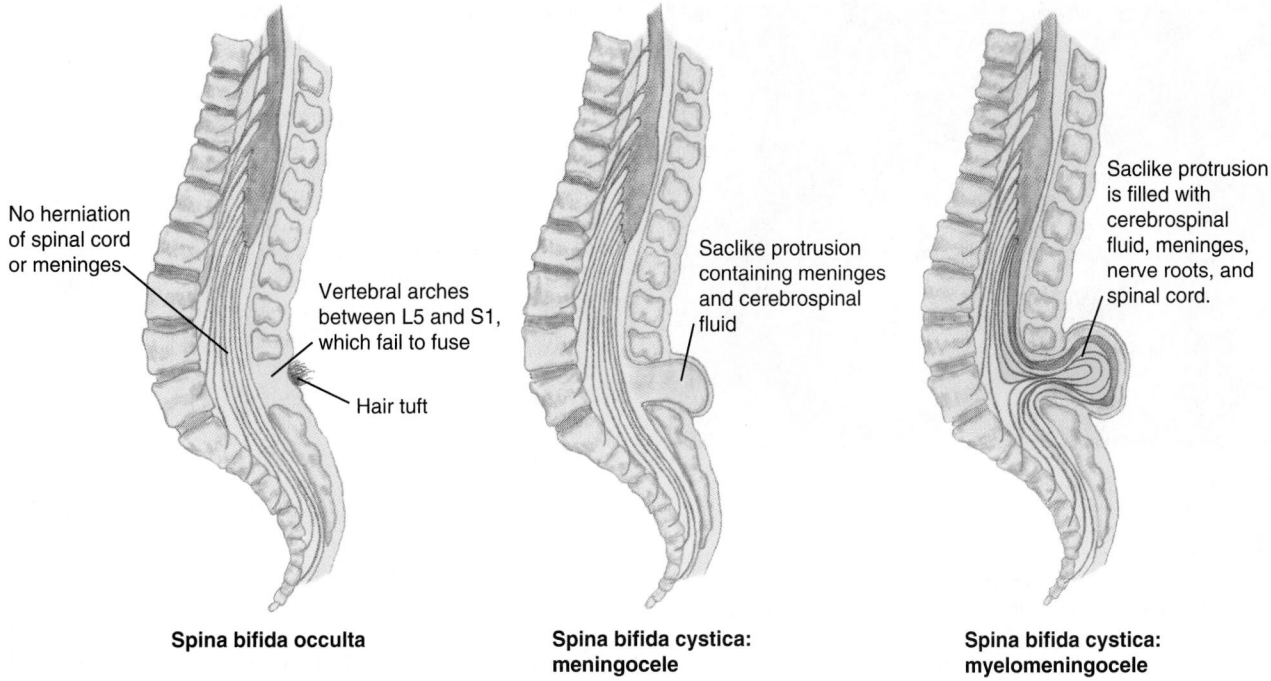

Spina bifida occulta

No herniation of spinal cord or meninges

Vertebral arches between L5 and S1, which fail to fuse

Hair tuft

Spina bifida cystica: meningocele

Saclike protrusion containing meninges and cerebrospinal fluid

Spina bifida cystica: myelomeningocele

Saclike protrusion is filled with cerebrospinal fluid, meninges, nerve roots, and spinal cord.

FIGURE 52-2

Three forms of spina bifida.

Spina Bifida

Spina bifida is a congenital neural tube defect in which there is incomplete closure of the vertebrae and neural tube during fetal development. Spina bifida is classified as spina bifida occulta and spina bifida cystica (Fig. 52–2). Spina bifida occulta usually occurs between the L5 and S1 vertebrae, with failure of the vertebrae to completely fuse. The child may have no sensory or motor defects. The only clinical manifestation that may appear is a dimple, a small tuft of hair, a hemangioma, or a lipoma in the lower lumbar or sacral area. These defects may be detected accidentally on routine radiographs.

Spina bifida cystica results in incomplete closure of the vertebrae and neural tube, evidenced by a sac-like protrusion in the lumbar or sacral area with varying degrees of nervous tissue involvement. Spina bifida cystica is further described as meningocele, myelomeningocele, lipomeningocele, and lipomeningomyelocele. Meningocele is a sac-like protrusion filled with spinal fluid and meninges. The most severe form of meningocele is myelomeningocele, in which the sac is filled with spinal fluid, meninges, nerve roots, and spinal cord.

Etiology and Incidence

The cause of spina bifida is unknown in most cases. Evidence suggests that there may be a genetic predisposition. Maternal folic acid deficiency has been strongly linked to neural tube defects. Daily consumption of folic acid by all women of childbearing age is recommended (see Chapter 15). Evidence of a viral origin has prompted research, but no cause or preventive measures have been identified.

The incidence is 1 to 5 per 1,000 live births. There is variability in geographic locations within the United States and worldwide (Hobdell, 1996).

Manifestations

In addition to the appearance of the lesion, manifestations relate to the degree of deficit, which is determined by the level of the lesion (Fig. 52–3).

T12:	Flaccid lower extremities, decreased sensation and lack of bowel control, incontinence and dribbling of urine
L1–L3:	Hip flexion, flail feet
L2–L4:	Hip adduction
L3–S2:	Hip adduction, hip extension, knee flexion
S3 and below:	No motor impairment
Sacral roots:	Plantar flexion

PATHOPHYSIOLOGY

of Spina Bifida

During the fourth week of gestation (days 24 to 28) ventral induction of the neural tube fails to occur. The degree of impairment corresponds to the level of the defect on the spinal cord and the size of the defect. Ninety percent of spinal cord lesions are at or below the L2 vertebra. The lesion results in paralysis, partial paralysis, or varying sensory defects. Club feet, scoliosis, contracture, and dislocation of the hips may also be associated with the defect. Associated malformations include hydrocephalus and Arnold-Chiari malformation.

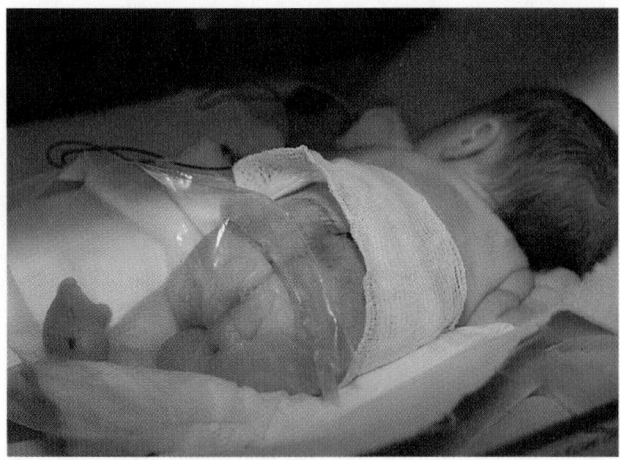

FIGURE 52-3

This infant has a repaired myelomeningocele. Note the left clubfoot. This deformity often accompanies the defect because normal intrauterine movement does not occur in the fetus with spina bifida, interfering with the development of the extremities. The legs are flaccid, and normal neonatal flexion is absent. The infant is also incontinent, dribbling stool and urine constantly. Hydrocephalus also commonly accompanies these neural tube defects. (Courtesy of Parkland Health & Hospital System, Dallas, Texas.)

Children with spina bifida are at high risk for developing latex allergies because of frequent exposure to latex during catheterizations and multiple operations. Latex allergy is estimated to occur in 18% to 60% of children with spina bifida. Allergic reactions can range from mild signs and symptoms to anaphylactic shock. Children should be tested for latex allergy, and precautions should be taken from birth to decrease exposures. The nurse should check equipment for latex and choose nonlatex alternatives.

Diagnostic Evaluation

Diagnostic tests include determining alpha-fetoprotein levels in blood at 16 to 18 weeks of gestation. If the alpha-fetoprotein screen is abnormal, amniocentesis and fetal ultrasound are performed (see Chapter 16). After delivery, a CT scan or myelography may be done.

Therapeutic Management

Immediate surgical closure is the most common choice of treatment. The rationale for immediate surgical closure is to decrease the risk of infection, morbidity, and mortality. Other benefits are improved prognosis without further cord deterioration, and earlier and easier physical handling and bonding. In addition, new microsurgical techniques while the fetus is still in the womb are showing great promise.

NURSING CARE
The Child with Spina Bifida

The sac-like protrusion of the meningocele should be assessed and the lesion measured. The nurse should measure the infant's head circumference and palpate the anterior fontanel for fullness. The infant should be in a prone position to avoid stress or pressure on the sac. A roll is placed under the infant's ankles to maintain foot alignment, and a roll is placed between the knees with the hips slightly flexed to maintain hip alignment and decrease tension on the sac.

Assessment

Continuous baseline and neurologic assessment of the infant is necessary. Assess the infant's overall tone, taking special note of spontaneous movement of the extremities. The motor examination is done with the infant at rest, using painful stimuli from the torso downward. Observe for voluntary movement below the level of the lesion.

The infant is at risk for infection before the sac is closed. Therefore, the infant's temperature must be monitored every 1 to 2 hours. Note signs of infection along with irritability, lethargy, or nuchal rigidity. A sterile saline dressing is placed over the sac to maintain the moisture of the sac and its contents. A risk of infection remains, however, and the dressing needs to be changed on a regular schedule or whenever soiled. Record the appearance of the sac and contents with each dressing change.

Nursing Diagnosis, Planning, Intervention, and Evaluation

Nursing Diagnosis	■ Risk for Impaired Skin Integrity related to presence of sac.
Expected Outcome	• The child will have no pre- or postoperative infection and will not develop pressure sores.

Intervention	Rationale
1. Use a special mattress or pad for infant's bed.	1. Special bedding can help alleviate pressure points caused by the required prone position.
2. Assess the infant's skin and reposition frequently. Change the diaper and clean the area when soiled.	2. Keeping the infant's diaper open will enable frequent cleaning of the perineal area because oozing of stool and dribbling of urine may occur.
3. Use stoma adhesive on each side of the lesion; consult the stoma therapist if needed.	3. Frequent dressing changes can irritate the skin, and the potential for irritation will be less if the tape is stuck to the stoma adhesive. The stoma therapist may make special recommendations for neonatal skin needs.

Evaluation
- Does the infant exhibit any signs of skin breakdown?
- Are the perineal area, incision site, and buttocks clean and dry?

Nursing Diagnosis
■ Risk for Infection related to the open sac and the operative procedure.

Expected Outcomes
- The child will have no drainage from the sac and no areas of redness preoperatively.
- The child will remain afebrile, and will maintain a WBC count within normal limits.

Intervention	Rationale
1. Monitor vital signs. Observe the sac for redness and clear or purulent drainage.	1. These are signs of infection that need to be documented and reported to the physician.
2. Begin feedings postoperatively when bowel sounds are present.	2. Adequate nutrition is needed for healing; feeding cannot begin until peristalsis is established.
3. Maintain sterile dressings over the sac or incision site.	3. Sterile dressings will facilitate healing and decrease the risk of infection.
4. Frequently reposition the infant.	4. Repositioning the infant will decrease the chance of pressure sores or stress on the incision.

Evaluation
- Does the infant's sac remain intact preoperatively?
- Is the infant infection free (afebrile, calm, able to eat)?
- Does the incision site appear intact and without redness or drainage?

Nursing Diagnosis
■ Impaired Physical Mobility related to neuromuscular impairment.

Expected Outcomes
- The child will learn to use appropriate mobilization devices and will maximize abilities to be mobile.
- The child will achieve appropriate developmental milestones.

Intervention	Rationale
1. Determine and record physical impairments and abilities. Note the activities in which the child can participate and encourage as much activity as is tolerated.	1. This documentation notes advances or regression in activities or the child's abilities. Encouraging activity maintains muscle tone.
2. Maintain splints, braces, and casts. Use wheelchairs, walkers, and other assistive devices as needed.	2. These aids may be used for proper alignment and to decrease contractures. Other devices may increase independence and mobility.
3. Ensure that the child attends therapy classes and participates fully. Encourage self-care.	3. Therapy and self-care help prevent contractures, encourages independence, and increases self-esteem.
4. Refer the family to the Spina Bifida Association (see Appendix L).	4. Support groups can help families cope with the stresses of a chronic condition.

Evaluation
- Does the child enjoy mobility as desired, and as allowed by impairments?
- Do the parents handle the child and encourage occupational and physical therapy?
- Do the parents encourage the child's maximum development?

Nursing Diagnosis
■ Altered Urinary Elimination related to the neuromuscular impairment.

Expected Outcome
- The child will be free of urinary infections; urine will be clear and odor free.

Intervention	Rationale
1. Observe urinary stream.	1. Urinary dribbling indicates interrupted innervation to the bladder.
2. Maintain moist mucous membranes. Offer adequate fluids.	2. Good hydration will help prevent urinary tract infections.
3. Teach and maintain regular toilet habits. Use intermittent clean catheterization to keep bladder empty if necessary.	3. Regular toilet habits facilitate complete and regular emptying of the bladder and help prevent urine retention and urinary tract infections.
4. Check urinary frequency, input and output, and specific gravity.	4. These values may be initial indicators of urinary pattern alteration.

Evaluation
- Has the child established regular voiding patterns?
- Is the urinalysis normal?

Nursing Diagnosis
■ Constipation related to sensory deficit and neurologic impairment.

Expected Outcome
• The child will have regular bowel movements.

Intervention	Rationale
1. Observe and record the infant or child's anal opening and pattern of bowel movements.	1. Absence of rectal sphincter tone indicates abnormal bowel function; noting the pattern will alert caregivers to implement a bowel program.
2. Monitor for abdominal distension, vomiting, and poor feeding.	2. These signs may indicate constipation.
3. Develop a bowel program: give a suppository before breakfast and have the child sit on toilet after breakfast. May need to stimulate the anal sphincter.	3. A bowel program will ensure elimination needs are met.
4. Consult a dietician to be sure the diet provides adequate fluid and fiber.	4. Fluid and fiber facilitate softer stools and easier passage.

Evaluation
• Is the child free of constipation or impaction, as evidenced by regular bowel movements?

PATHOPHYSIOLOGY
• • • • • • • • • • •
of Hydrocephalus

Cerebrospinal fluid (CSF) is produced primarily by the choroid plexus, which lines the lateral ventricles. CSF circulates through the ventricular system and flows into the subarachnoid space around the brain and the spinal cord. It is then reabsorbed within the subarachnoid spaces.

Hydrocephalus results when there is either (1) impaired absorption of CSF within the subarachnoid space (communicating hydrocephalus) or (2) obstruction of CSF flow within the ventricles that prevents CSF from circulating around the spinal cord and the subarachnoid space (noncommunicating hydrocephalus). Hydrocephalus may rarely be caused by overproduction of CSF by a tumor of the choroid plexus.

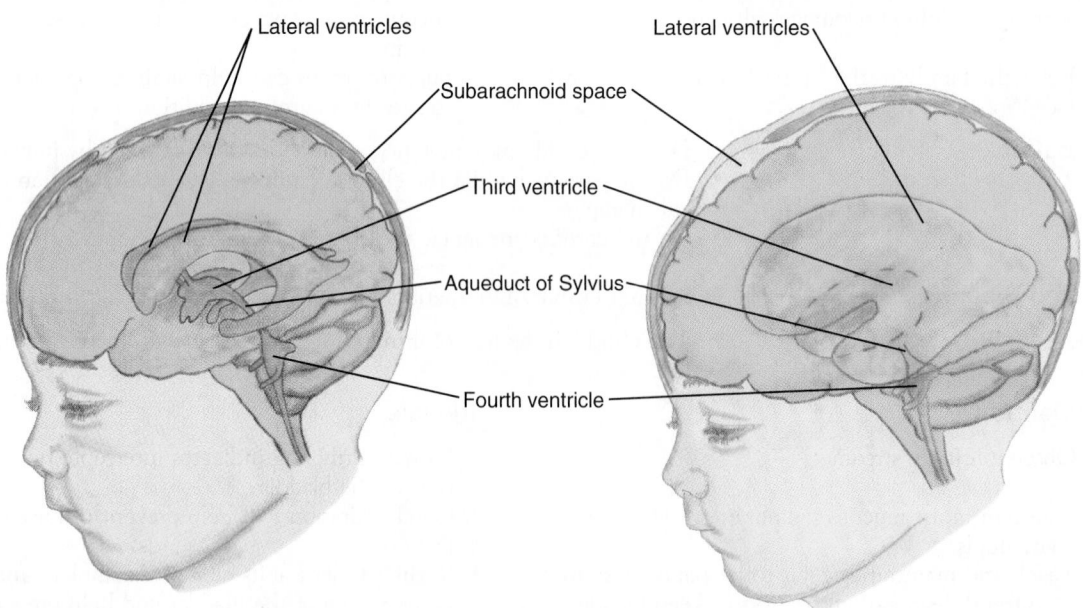

Lateral ventricles
Subarachnoid space
Lateral ventricles
Third ventricle
Aqueduct of Sylvius
Fourth ventricle

Normal ventricles/normal CSF circulation

Impaired flow of CSF, enlarged lateral and third ventricles, stenosis of aqueduct

Hydrocephalus

Hydrocephalus develops as a result of an imbalance between the production and absorption of CSF. As excess CSF accumulates in the ventricular system, the ventricles become dilated, and the brain is compressed against the skull. This results in enlargement of the skull if the sutures are open, or signs and symptoms of increased ICP if the sutures are fused.

Etiology

Hydrocephalus may be congenital, acquired, or of unknown etiology. In infancy, hydrocephalus is most often congenital or related to prematurity. Congenital hydrocephalus results from developmental defects such as Arnold-Chiari malformations, congenital arachnoid cysts, congenital tumors, or aqueductal stenosis. In premature infants neonatal meningitis or subarachnoid hemorrhage may result in hydrocephalus. Hydrocephalus is often associated with myelomeningocele. Intrauterine infection and perinatal hemorrhage cause hydrocephalus in some infants. In older children hydrocephalus is usually acquired as a complication of meningitis, tumor, or hemorrhage.

Incidence

The incidence of hydrocephalus in infancy is 5.8 per 10,000 births. The incidence of hydrocephalus with spina bifida is considered to be 3 to 4 per 1,000 births. Obstructive, or noncommunicating, hydrocephalus accounts for 99% of all cases of hydrocephalus in children.

Manifestations and Diagnostic Evaluation

Because of anatomical differences between infants and children, manifestations of hydrocephalus differ according to developmental stage (Table 52–2).

Diagnostic tests for hydrocephalus include serial measurements of head circumference, CT, MRI, and lumbar puncture.

Therapeutic Management

Therapy strives to prevent further CSF accumulation and reduce disability and death. The objective is to bypass the blockage and drain the fluid from the ventricles to an area where it may be reabsorbed. A *ventriculoperitoneal shunt*, or tube leading from the ventricles out of the skull and passing under the skin to the peritoneal cavity, accomplishes this (Fig. 52–4). An alternative shunt, the *ventriculoatrial shunt*, which is used in older children, drains the fluid from the ventricles to the right atrium of the heart.

TABLE 52–2
• • • • • • • • • • •

Early and Late Manifestations of Hydrocephalus

Early	Late
Infant	
Rapid growth—increase in head circumference above the normal growth curve	"Setting sun" sign: sclera visible above the iris
Full, bulging anterior fontanel	Frontal bone enlargement or bossing
Irritability	Vomiting; difficulty swallowing or feeding
Poor feeding	Increased blood pressure, decreased heart rate
Distended, prominent scalp veins	Altered respiratory pattern
Widely separated cranial sutures	Shrill, high-pitched cry
	Sluggish or unequal pupillary response to light
Child	
Strabismus	Seizures
Frontal headache that occurs in the morning and is relieved by emesis or by sitting upright	Increased blood pressure
	Decreased heart rate
Nausea and vomiting that may be projectile	Alteration in respiratory pattern
Diplopia	Blindness from herniation of the optic disc
Restlessness	Decerebrate rigidity
Behavior or personality changes	
Ataxia	
Papilledema	
Irritability	
Sluggish and unequal pupillary response to light	
Confusion	
Changes in schoolwork	
Lethargy	

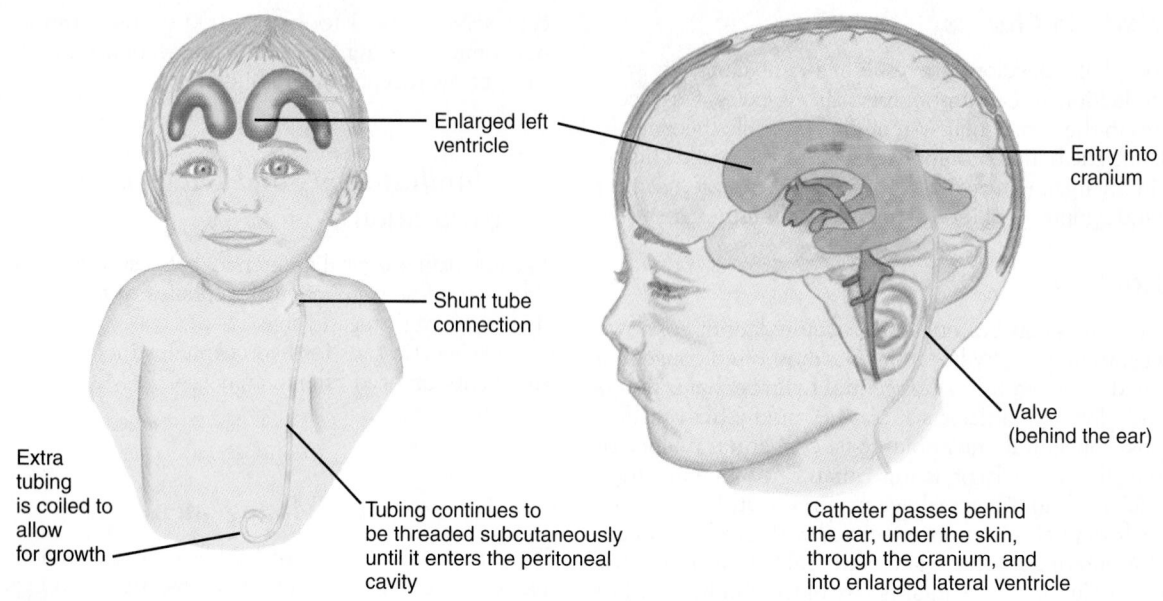

Enlarged left
ventricle

Entry into
cranium

Shunt tube
connection

Extra
tubing
is coiled to
allow
for growth

Tubing continues to
be threaded subcutaneously
until it enters the peritoneal
cavity

Valve
(behind the ear)

Catheter passes behind
the ear, under the skin,
through the cranium, and
into enlarged lateral ventricle

FIGURE 52–4

A ventriculoperitoneal shunt is implanted in the child with hydrocephalus to prevent excess
accumulation of CSF in the ventricles. The tubing diverts the CSF from the ventricles into the
peritoneal cavity, where it is reabsorbed. Nursing care of the child with a ventricular shunt
includes monitoring for infection and pain, administering antibiotics and pain medications as
ordered, and teaching the family how to change dressings and how to recognize shunt problems.

NURSING CARE

The Child with Hydrocephalus

The care of the child with hydrocephalus includes giving
medications to decrease CSF production. Because most cases
of hydrocephalus require shunting to drain the excess CSF,
however, most of the nursing care will be postoperative.

Assessment

When an infant is born with hydrocephalus, signs may be
apparent at birth or signs of an obstruction may appear over
the next few months. The first symptom may be an abnormal
head circumference. The head circumference should be measured daily or more frequently, depending on the child's condition, and should be recorded and plotted on a graph. To
facilitate accuracy when different personnel take the measurement, make a pen mark on the scalp where the tape measure is placed. The tape measure is usually placed just above

the top of the ears and around the head, around the mid-
forehead and the most prominent portion of the occiput.

Palpate the infant's anterior fontanel for size, bulging,
tenseness, and cranial suture separation. The fontanel is assessed with the baby sitting upright and quiet. It may bulge
or pulsate if the infant is crying.

Observe the infant's behavior when the fontanel is full
or tense. Ask the parent if the baby is irritable, lethargic,
or if any change in feeding behavior has been noticed. Ask
if the infant has had any seizures. Vital signs are assessed
to identify any changes from the infant's baseline measurements.

If the child is older, any change in level of consciousness, personality, interaction with the environment, or
sleep patterns or delays in developmental milestones need
to be explored with the parents. Note complaints of headache that may be relieved when the child sits upright, and
vomiting of unexplained origin. If the child has a history
of vomiting, hydration status also should be assessed.

Nursing Diagnosis, Planning, Intervention, and Evaluation

Nursing Diagnosis	■ Risk for Infection related to shunt surgical placement.
Expected Outcomes	• The child will maintain a normal temperature, have a clean, dry suture line, tolerate feedings well, and exhibit no signs of increased ICP. • The parents will demonstrate infection control measures.

Intervention	Rationale
1. Monitor temperature every 1 to 2 hours and as needed. Observe for decreased level of conscious- ness and vomiting. Also monitor for swelling or redness along the shunt tract.	1. These are the first signs of an infection.

2. Observe head, abdominal, and chest dressings for drainage. Test drainage for glucose with a Dextrostix, or check for a halo sign on gauze.
3. Position the child off the shunt site so that no weight is placed on the valve for the first 2 days.
4. Administer intravenous (IV) antibiotics as ordered and monitor serum levels to prevent subtherapeutic or toxic levels.
5. Teach the parents the dressing change technique, and show them how to recognize shunt infection.

2. Drainage could be CSF, indicating a route for infection to reach the brain. CSF contains glucose and makes a halo on gauze.
3. Careful placement prevents skin breakdown and reduces the risk of infection.
4. *Staphylococcus epidermidis* infection is the major complication of shunts.
5. Parents need to know how to care for their child at home and when to seek medical attention.

Evaluation

- Is the child infection free, as evidenced by a normal body temperature?
- Does the child have a clean, dry suture site?
- Can the parent demonstrate dressing changes using aseptic technique and state the signs of infection?

Nursing Diagnosis

■ Pain related to operative procedure.

Expected Outcome

- The child will exhibit pain relief, as evidenced by stable vital signs, sleeping restfully, playing whenever possible, and verbalizing pain relief.

Intervention

1. Determine child's pain level, activity, and irritability, and give pain medications as needed. Administer analgesics (e.g., codeine) as ordered if needed.
2. Hold, cuddle, and distract the child. Teach therapeutic play to family members and caregivers.

Rationale

1. Pain relief will help decrease crying, ICP, and metabolic demands. Codeine does not interfere with the child's level of consciousness.
2. Nonpharmacologic methods of pain management also decrease ICP.

Evaluation

- Does the child smile and react with the caregivers?
- Are the child's vital signs normal for age?
- Does the older child express pain relief or choose a lower value on a pain assessment scale?

Nursing Diagnosis

■ Parental Knowledge Deficit related to unfamiliarity with home care and signs and symptoms of shunt malfunction or complications.

Expected Outcome

- The parents will demonstrate assessment of the child's level of consciousness and discuss the shunt's purpose and function.

Intervention

1. Assess the parents' knowledge of changes in the child's level of consciousness. Begin teaching at their level of understanding.
2. Teach the parents to observe the child for abdominal distension or discomfort (Williams, Hays, & McCool, 1996).
3. Teach the parents to observe for poor feeding, nausea or vomiting, elevated temperature, and skin redness or tenderness and report these to the physician.
4. Teach parents safety measures for use in home care, playing, and in the car (padded seats).
5. Emphasize the importance of neurosurgical follow-up care.

Rationale

1. Parents need to understand that shunt malfunction will cause increased ICP.
2. Shunt placement may cause a paralytic ileus or peritonitis.
3. These are all signs of an infection.

4. It is important to provide anticipatory guidance for the growing child.
5. The shunt may need revision as the child grows.

Evaluation

- Can the parents discuss care of child with a shunt?
- Are the parents able to describe signs of shunt malfunction?

Cerebral Palsy

Cerebral palsy, also known as static encephalopathy, is a chronic, nonprogressive disorder of posture and movement. It is characterized by difficulty in controlling the muscles due to an abnormality in the extrapyramidal or pyramidal motor system (motor cortex, basal ganglia, cerebellum).

Etiology and Incidence

The damage to the motor system can occur prenatally, perinatally, or postnatally. Approximately two per 1,000 live births in the United States result in a child with cerebral palsy.

Manifestations

The manifestations of cerebral palsy may vary, and one or more of the following may be observed in any one child: persistence of primitive reflexes, delayed gross motor development, and lack of progression through the developmental milestones. Abnormal posturing with inability to maintain normal posture and balance and spasticity or uncontrollable movements in the extremities may be present. Also documented are disturbances of gait (particularly ataxia and toe walking), seizures, attention deficit disorder, sensory impairment, failure of automatic reactions (equilibrium), and speech and swallowing impairments.

Diagnostic Evaluation and Therapeutic Management

Diagnostic tests include EEG, CT or MRI, electrolyte levels, metabolic workup, and a thorough neurologic examination. Persistent primitive reflexes are seen, as are abnormal muscle tone and posture and abnormal motor development.

. . . .
Factors Associated with Cerebral Palsy

Prenatal

Maternal diabetes
Rh or ABO incompatibility
Rubella in the first trimester
Genetic
Intrauterine ischemic event
Toxoplasmosis
Cytomegalovirus
Congenital brain abnormality

Perinatal

Asphyxia
Low birth weight
Prematurity
Precipitous delivery
Pregnancy-induced hypertension
Birth trauma
Anoxia
Prolonged labor
Perinatal metabolic condition (diabetes)
Intracranial hemorrhage

Postnatal

Infections
Trauma
Stroke
Poisoning

The goal of managing the child with cerebral palsy is early recognition and intervention to maximize the child's abilities. Cerebral palsy often is not diagnosed before age 2 years. Through repetition, new brain pathways develop through alternative receptor sites to achieve proper motor

PATHOPHYSIOLOGY
. . . .
of Cerebral Palsy

A number of neuromuscular disabilities are associated with cerebral palsy. The alteration in voluntary muscular control is related to a cerebral insult. The area of the brain that has been injured determines the type of neuromuscular disability.

There are five classifications of cerebral palsy: dyskinetic, spastic, ataxic, rigid, and mixed. *Dyskinetic (athetoid) palsy* refers to an injury in the basal ganglia. Slow, writhing, uncontrolled, involuntary movements involving all extremities characterize this type.

Spastic cerebral palsy is the most common type. The affected area of the brain is the cortex. Spastic cerebral palsy is characterized by increased deep tendon reflexes, hypertonia, flexion, and sometimes contractures. The child's muscles are very tense, and any stimulus may cause a sudden jerking movement. The child has to make a conscious effort to relax. Scissor gait, hip flexion with adduction and internal rotation, or toe walking due to tight heel cords may be present.

In *ataxic cerebral palsy*, the affected area of the brain

is the cerebellum. This type of cerebral palsy is characterized by a loss of coordination, equilibrium, and kinesthetic sense. Overall, the child appears clumsy.

Rigid/tremor/atonic cerebral palsy is relatively rare in children. The child pictured has rigidity of both flexor and extensor muscles. In a child with tremors, the tremors are apparent both at rest and during movement. The prognosis for a child with this type of cerebral palsy is poor because of associated deformities and lack of active movement.

Approximately half of children with cerebral palsy have some degree of mental retardation and other disabilities. Other than epilepsy and mental retardation, problems with learning, poor attention span, hyperactivity, hearing or visual loss, and emotional problems may be seen. Gastroesophageal reflux may be a problem (see Chapter 43). There is a high expenditure of calories with the intense movements, and difficulty feeding leads to a calorie deficit.

function. The child may be intellectually intact, but this may be overlooked because of the child's physical limitations.

A multidisciplinary health care team approach is necessary to meet the many needs of the child with cerebral palsy. The team includes the child and family, a pediatrician, neurologist, orthopedic surgeon, nurse, speech and hearing therapist, social worker, occupational physical therapist, and educators.

NURSING CARE
The Child with Cerebral Palsy

Nursing care of the child with cerebral palsy entails a multidisciplinary approach. Family teaching includes techniques for feeding, carrying, dressing, bathing, and playing with the child and the use of adaptive equipment.

Assessment

The most important component of assessment is identifying the condition. The infant identified to be at risk is then monitored for irritability, feeding difficulties, delayed development, poor motor development, abnormal posturing, persistence of infant reflexes, ataxic gait, and poor muscle tone. Assessing the child's response to therapy is important. Monitoring and documenting progress or lack of progress is just as important as identifying problems.

The nurse needs to be aware of normal growth and development, with special attention to developmental milestones. Delay in reaching these milestones is one of the key indicators of cerebral palsy (Burns et al., 1996).

Nursing Diagnosis, Planning, Intervention, and Evaluation

Nursing Diagnosis
- Impaired Physical Mobility related to spasticity and muscle weakness.

Expected Outcome
- The child will maximize ability for movement, be free of contractures or injuries, and be free of complications from immobility.

Intervention

1. Reinforce physical therapy exercises to strengthen and help coordination of muscles.
2. Encourage parents to be active in the child's daily physical and occupational therapy.
3. Observe and record the child's response to physical therapy.
4. Determine the need for special equipment for reading, writing, eating, and mobility.

Rationale

1. Early intervention and consistent therapy will facilitate proper posture and circumvent the development of contractures.
2. Active involvement in the child's care empowers the parents.
3. Changes in therapy may be made in a timely fashion for a higher degree of success.
4. The use of special equipment will improve the chance for successful self-care.

Evaluation
- Does the child demonstrate improved mobility and self-care?
- Can the parents demonstrate physical therapy techniques used for their child?

Nursing Diagnosis
- Altered Growth and Development related to neuromuscular impairment.

Expected Outcome
- The child and family will explore ways to learn and will participate with other children in some activities.

Intervention

1. Monitor the child's developmental level and intelligence.
2. Encourage early intervention and participation in school programs.
3. Communicate and interact with the child at the child's functional level, not chronological age.

Rationale

1. The child with cerebral palsy should be given opportunities to learn and should be exposed to new experiences in order to maximize developmental progress.
2. Interventions by multidisciplinary groups will maximize the child's potential for learning.
3. A child with normal intelligence can understand age-appropriate communication and speech, but a child with decreased intelligence might have a different cognitive understanding than age would indicate.

Evaluation
- Does the child attend public school and play with peers whenever possible?
- Does the child receive physical, speech, and occupational therapy at school?
- Do the parents maximize the child's potential?

Nursing Diagnosis	■ Risk for Injury related to spasticity, uncontrolled muscle movements, or seizures.
Expected Outcome	• The child will have a safe environment and not be injured.

Intervention	Rationale
1. Provide a safe environment; remove sharp objects.	1. Providing a safe environment will reduce the risk of injury.
2. Have the child wear a protective helmet if the child falls frequently.	2. A helmet protects against head injury.
3. Implement bedside seizure precautions. (Do not pad the rails with pillows.)	3. Keeping suction, oxygen, and airway equipment at the bedside and padding the side rails help prevent injury, and allow for resuscitation of the child if necessary. Pillows should not be used as pads because they may cause suffocation.
4. Provide safe toys that are appropriate for age and developmental level.	4. No sharp, very small, or easily shattered toys should be allowed for the child who may fall due to erratic movements.
5. Position the child upright after meals.	5. An upright position prevents aspiration secondary to gastroesophageal reflux.

Evaluation	• Does the child remain free from injury? • Do the parents demonstrate safety measures for the child?

Nursing Diagnosis	■ Impaired Verbal Communication related to neuromuscular impairment and difficulty with articulation.
Expected Outcome	• The child will appropriately express needs and will develop methods for communicating with others.

Intervention	Rationale
1. Use flash cards and talking boards to facilitate communication.	1. Teaching aides help reinforce language and speech development and increase self-esteem.
2. Refer the child to a speech therapist.	2. Early intervention will maximize speech capabilities.
3. Encourage and reinforce speech therapy techniques, nonverbal methods of communication, proper feeding techniques, and jaw control.	3. These techniques facilitate communication and decrease the child's frustration at not being understood. They also facilitate the goals of speech therapy.
4. Encourage parents to convey in detail the child's communication techniques any time the child is in a new situation.	4. Sharing the child's communication techniques helps the child adjust to new situations.

Evaluation	• Does the child participate in groups using appropriate communication? • Does the child use various methods to communicate? • Do the parents allow time for the child to respond to questions and conversations? • Have the parents learned the same communication method that the child uses?

■ Head Injury

Head injury refers to the pathologic result of any mechanical force to the scalp, skull, meninges, or brain.

Types of Head Injuries

Types of head injury include the following:

• *Closed head injury:* Nonpenetrating injury to the head in which there is no break in the integrity of the barrier between the outside environment and the intracranial cavity.
• *Open head injury:* Penetrating injury to the head in which there is a break in the integrity of the barrier (skull, meninges) between the outside environment and the intracranial cavity. Infection will be a major concern.
• *Coup injury:* Cerebral injury sustained directly below the site of impact.
• *Contracoup:* Cerebral injury sustained in the region or pole opposite the site of impact. The injury is caused by the rapid movements of the semisolid brain within the cranial vault.
• *Missile injury:* Penetrating injury of the skull or brain, most often caused by a bullet.
• *Impalement injury:* Penetrating injury caused by a pierce to the scalp, skull, or brain with something sharp.

SKULL FRACTURES

Skull fractures include the following types:

- *Linear:* Straight-line fracture; dura is not involved.
- *Depressed:* Bone is pressing downward, indented.
- *Basilar:* Fracture of the base of the skull. Symptoms are Battle's sign, raccoon eyes, rhinorrhea, otorrhea, and hemotympanum (blood behind the eardrum).
- *Comminuted:* Fragmentation of the bone into many pieces or a multiple fracture line.

CONTUSION

Contusions are petechial hemorrhages along the superficial aspects of the brain. They may occur at the site of impact or in association with a lesion remote from the site of direct impact.

CONCUSSION

A concussion is a transient and reversible neuronal dysfunction, with instantaneous loss of awareness and responsiveness.

INTRACRANIAL HEMORRHAGE

Intracranial hemorrhages include two types:

- *Epidural:* Blood accumulates between dura and skull. Arterial damage is the usual type of injury; therefore the hemorrhage is fast.
- *Subdural:* Blood accumulates between the dura and the cerebrum. A subdural hemorrhage can be acute or chronic (Fig. 52–5).

Incidence

Multiple trauma is the leading cause of death in children beyond infancy. Approximately 200,000 children are hospitalized yearly in the United States for evaluation and treatment of a head injury. Common causes of head injuries include car accidents, bicycle collisions, falls, sports injuries, beatings, and gunshot wounds.

Classification of Severity of Head Injuries

MILD HEAD INJURY (GLASGOW COMA SCALE SCORE OF 13–15)

- Possible headache and cognitive deficits (especially affecting memory)
- Possible stress intolerance

MODERATE HEAD INJURY (GLASGOW COMA SCALE SCORE OF 9–12)

- Headache, memory deficits, cognitive deficits, difficulty with activities of daily living; occasionally results in death

SEVERE HEAD INJURY (GLASGOW COMA SCALE SCORE OF 3–8)

- Posttrauma syndromes and cognitive, emotional, motor, and sensory deficits due to irreversible brain injury
- Long-term care or support in the community usually needed

Manifestations

Head injuries are classified as minor, moderate, or severe as correlated with the Glasgow Coma Scale. Minor head injuries exhibit the following manifestations: possible change in level of consciousness, transient period of confusion, irritability, vomiting, somnolence, and headache. Moderate to severe head injuries are marked by altered mental states, changes in vital signs, signs of increased ICP, retinal hemorrhage, hemiparesis, and papilledema.

Diagnostic Evaluation

A complete history of the event helps to determine the mechanism of injury and whether the child lost consciousness. Radiographs are obtained to ascertain there is no cer-

---

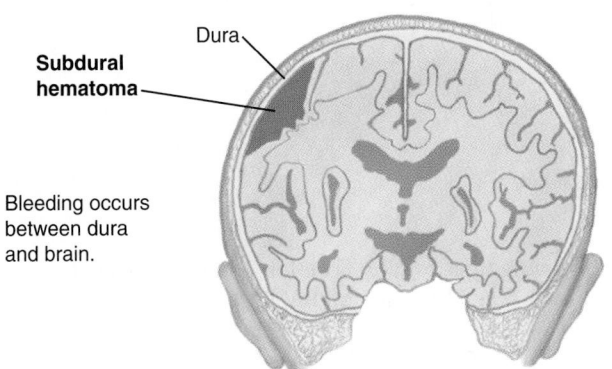

Subdural hematoma — Dura

Bleeding occurs between dura and brain.

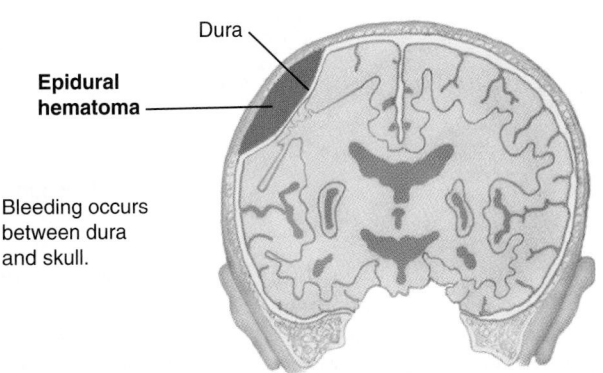

Epidural hematoma — Dura

Bleeding occurs between dura and skull.

FIGURE 52–5

Subdural and epidural hematomas are the two most common cranial hematomas; one or the other occurs in 6% to 7% of head-injured children. A *subdural hematoma* is often caused when the head strikes an immovable object. However, in an infant a subdural hematoma may result from aggressive shaking (a form of child abuse); retinal hemorrhage is also a classic sign of shaking injury in infants. With *epidural hematoma,* a rapid decline in neurologic function may occur 4 to 8 hours after a brief period of lucidity. If untreated, the increased ICP can cause death in a short period of time.

PATHOPHYSIOLOGY
of Head Injury

The cranium is a rigid structure that contains blood, brain tissue, and cerebrospinal fluid (CSF). The pressure exerted by these components on the cranium is between 4 and 15 mm Hg. According to the Monroe-Kellie doctrine, an increase in one of these components must be accompanied by a decrease in one of the others to maintain ICP within normal range. Cerebral function is dependent on adequate delivery of nutrients such as oxygen, glucose, and other substrates; an abnormal increase in ICP will interfere with the balance and delivery of these nutrients.

Head injuries are either primary or secondary. Primary head injuries are damage sustained at the time of injury; secondary head injuries refer to the consequences of the primary injury, particularly increased ICP. The severity of the injury depends on the amount of stress to the cranium and brain. Head injuries include concussions, contusions, lacerations, fractures, and hematomas.

Motor vehicle collisions, falls, sports injuries, child abuse, and neglect cause most head injuries in children. *Acceleration-deceleration* is the term used to describe the mechanism of injury. The shearing force of the initial impact moves the brain forward, followed by a countering, backward movement of the brain in the skull. The shearing force produces bruising, tearing, and bleeding. Shaken baby syndrome, a type of child abuse, may result in epidural hematomas and retinal hemorrhages (see Chapter 53).

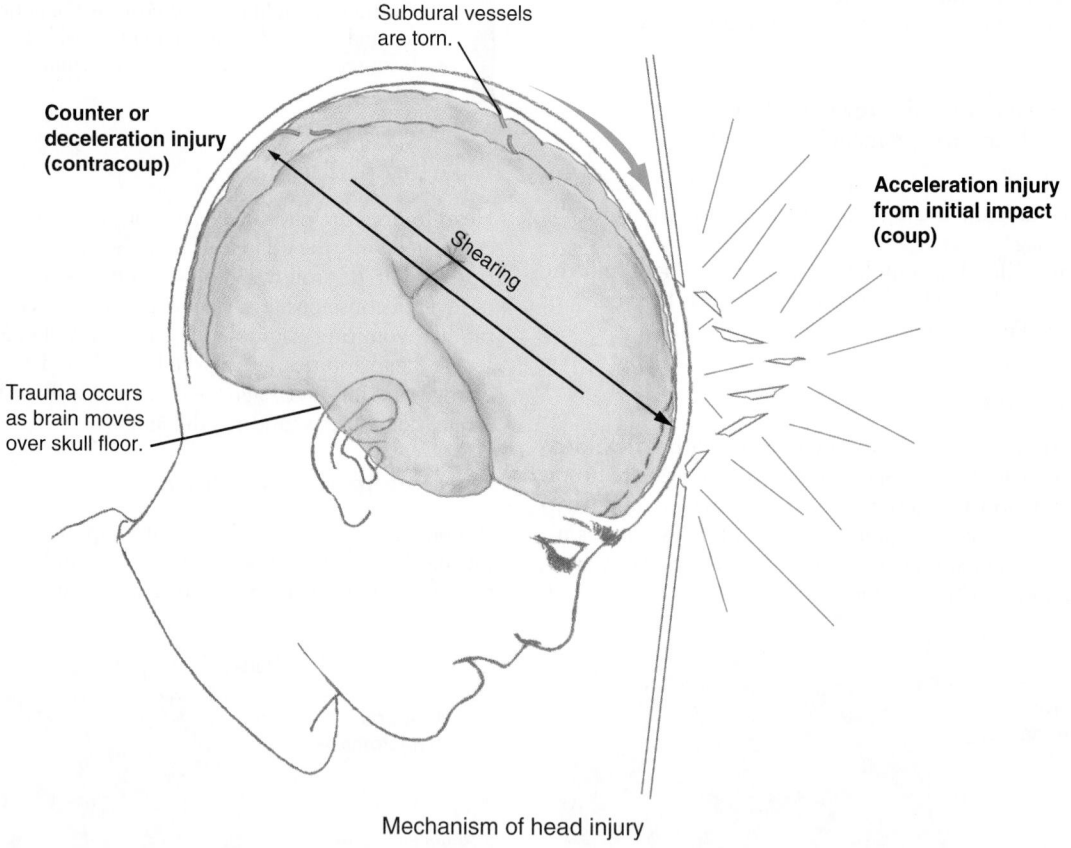

Subdural vessels are torn.

Counter or deceleration injury (contracoup)

Acceleration injury from initial impact (coup)

Shearing

Trauma occurs as brain moves over skull floor.

Mechanism of head injury

vical spinal cord injury; radiographs are followed by a complete neurologic examination. Any indication of increased ICP is quickly reported to the physician. CT or MRI is the most precise study with which to diagnose the specific kind of head injury sustained.

Therapeutic Management

Initial management of the child with a head injury includes assessing ventilatory function, neurologic status, and any other injuries present (see Chapter 34). Interventions to maintain vital functions are provided until all injuries are determined. Increased ICP or seizures may develop in a child with a head injury. The long-term outcome of a head injury is related to the child's GSC score.

NURSING CARE
The Child with a Head Injury

Assessment

Initial assessment of the child with a head injury includes the ABCs—evaluation of airway, breathing, and circulation (see Chapter 34). The child's neck is immobilized as special attention is given to the cervical spine. Obtain and record baseline

PARENTS WANT TO KNOW

Guidelines for the Child with a Head Injury

Apply ice to the child's head to prevent swelling. Clean any scrapes or cuts with soap and water. Encourage the child to rest, and limit foods if the child is vomiting. You will need to watch the child carefully for 2 days. For 2 nights waken the child once at your bedtime and once 4 hours later. Check that the child becomes alert and can answer questions appropriately.

Call the doctor immediately after the injury if the child

- has bleeding that does not stop after pressure has been applied for 10 minutes
- needs sutures
- is less than a year old
- had a seizure after the head injury
- was unconscious or confused
- has a severe headache or vomiting

- has slurred speech or blurred vision
- has blood or watery fluid coming from the ear or nose
- has unequal pupils or crossed eyes
- has difficulty walking or crawling, or weakness in the arms
- has other symptoms that concern you

Postconcussion Syndrome
Some children who have had a head injury can experience an after effect called postconcussion syndrome. If your child has this condition, your child may be upset easily and may be irritable if tired or stressed. Memory problems are common, as are learning difficulties, double vision, dizziness, headaches, fatigue, and light sensitivity. These symptoms may last many months.

Data from Schmitt, B. D. (1999). *Instructions for pediatric patients* (2nd ed., p. 138). Philadelphia: Saunders.

---

vital signs, and obtain further signs as indicated by the child's clinical condition. A complete history and comprehensive neurologic examination should be completed. Assess the child's level of consciousness (with the Glasgow Coma Scale), pupil size, and pupil reactivity to light.

Test cranial nerve function to identify deficits resulting from the injury and to monitor for increased ICP. The clinical signs and symptoms of increased ICP, with or without actual measurement of the ICP, will determine both the clinical status of the child and the medical and nursing interventions. Nasotracheal suctioning is contraindicated in a child with a basilar skull fracture. Because of the nature of the injury the suction catheter could be introduced into the brain.

The child with a head injury can experience a post-injury alteration in antidiuretic hormone (ADH). Possibly as a result of injury to the hypothalamus or posterior pituitary, the child can exhibit signs of excess ADH (syndrome of inappropriate diuretic hormone, SIADH), or deficit of ADH (diabetes insipidus) (see Chapter 51). Any child with a head injury needs to be addressed for fluid and electrolyte alteration. Nursing care of the child with a head injury is similar to nursing care of any child with increased ICP.

Nursing Diagnosis, Planning, Intervention, and Evaluation

Nursing Diagnosis

■ Risk for Fluid Volume Deficit related to diabetes insipidus.

Expected Outcomes

- The child will have a urine output of 1 to 2 ml/kg/hr and will maintain serum sodium levels between 135 and 145 mEq/L.
- The parents will describe the signs of diabetes insipidus.

Intervention	Rationale
1. Carefully monitor IV fluid intake.	1. The child with head injury is at risk for diabetes insipidus.
2. Accurately determine and record intake and output. An indwelling urinary catheter may be needed, or diapers can be weighed before and after use.	2. Monitoring intake and output documents fluid loss.
3. Monitor for other fluid losses, diarrhea, or vomiting. Notify the physician and replace fluids as prescribed.	3. Monitoring other fluid losses prevents dehydration and hypovolemic shock.
4. Teach parents about the signs of diabetes insipidus.	4. Early recognition of signs and symptoms improves outcomes.

Evaluation

- Does the child sustain minimal weight loss (less than 3% of total preinjury body weight)?
- Are the child's mucous membranes moist?
- Is the child voiding adequately, and is the skin turgor normal?
- Can the parents describe observations that might indicate diabetes insipidus?

Nursing Diagnosis
Expected Outcomes

- Fluid Volume Excess related to SIADH.

- The child will have a urine specific gravity of between 1.002 and 1.030, a serum sodium value of 135 to 145 mEq/L, and a serum osmolality of between 275 and 295 mOsm/kg.
- The parents will describe the signs of SIADH.

Intervention	Rationale
1. Restrict fluid intake as prescribed.	1. Restriction of fluid intake prevents fluid overload and complications of hyponatremia such as cerebral edema and increased ICP.
2. Monitor electrolytes and serum osmolality. Monitor intake and output, daily weights, urine specific gravity.	2. Monitoring fluids and electrolytes allows for early recognition and correction of fluid overload.
3. Keep an IV line patent. Change IV fluids as prescribed.	3. A patent IV line allows the nurse to manipulate IV fluids to maintain homeostasis.
4. Teach parents about signs and symptoms of SIADH.	4. Parents may assist the health care team by monitoring for signs and symptoms of SIADH once the child is discharged from the hospital or rehabilitation hospital.

Evaluation

- Does the child maintain normal electrolytes and urine specific gravity, and appear appropriately hydrated?
- Can the parents discuss observations to be made at home to monitor for SIADH?

Spinal Cord Injury

Spinal cord injury can result from any trauma or injury to the spinal cord or to its vascular supply or venous drainage.

Etiology

Spinal cord injuries in children are usually caused by motor vehicle accidents, falls, diving accidents, sports injuries, gunshot or knife wounds, or attempted suicide. In the infant, a common cause of spinal cord injury is intentional aggressive shaking by an older person.

Incidence

Although spinal cord injuries are less common in children than in adults, 75% of spinal cord injuries in children occur

PATHOPHYSIOLOGY
of Spinal Cord Injury

Spinal cord injuries occur in children when vertebral bodies are fractured or subluxation of the vertebra occurs. Subluxation results in malalignment of contiguous vertebrae, so that the spinal cord is compressed. The cord may be crushed, stretched beyond tolerance, or completely divided. All neurons carrying sensations from those parts of the body below the lesion are unable to pass their message on to the brain. A severe cord injury will cause complete paralysis and complete loss of sensation below the severed level.

Flaccid paralysis of the affected limbs immediately follows a spinal cord injury. Paralysis is due to spinal shock, which can last 3 weeks or more. The flaccidity changes to spasticity when the spinal shock resolves.

in the cervical spine, between the occiput and C3. Young children are more susceptible to upper spinal cord injury because of the larger head size in relation to body size. As the child grows older the site of the spinal cord injury moves distally.

Manifestations

Manifestations of spinal cord injury include loss of some or all movement or sensation below the level of injury, respiratory depression or apnea, hypotension and bradycardia, hypothermia, and neck pain.

Diagnostic Evaluation

After the nurse takes the history of the injury and performs a complete neurologic examination, the extent of the spinal cord injury will be determined with radiography, or MRI. The extent of motor or sensory deficit may resolve somewhat as spinal shock resolves.

Therapeutic Management

Treatment includes steroid therapy, which may be administered within 8 hours of the injury as a bolus of 30 mg/kg followed by a continuous infusion of 5.4 mg/kg/hr for 23 hours. Other treatments include halo traction (Fig. 52–6) or Gardner-Wells tongs for unstable injuries, subluxation, or until surgical stabilization can be performed.

NURSING CARE
The Child with a Spinal Cord Injury

Assessment

The spine must be immobilized before any attempt is made to move the child. The airway is assessed immediately, and

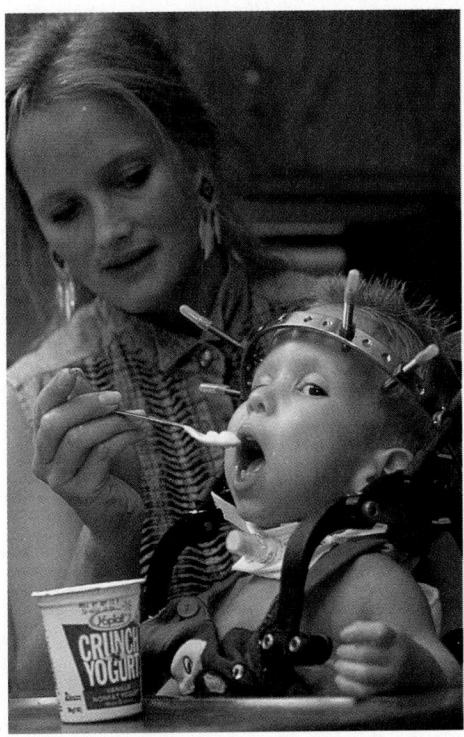

FIGURE 52–6
. . . .
Children who have injuries or birth defects that involve the upper spine may be placed in halo traction to stabilize the spine and prevent added nerve damage. Spinal cord injury is a catastrophic event for the child and family, who will need intense nursing support and education as well as referral to support groups. (Courtesy of Cook Children's Medical Center, Fort Worth, Texas.)

if intubation is necessary it is done without hyperextending the neck. Next, assess circulation, keeping in mind that hypotension may be a result of either hypovolemia or neurologic shock. Bradycardia and hypothermia may ensue. Attempt to maintain the body temperature and keep the child well oxygenated.

The neurologic assessment includes evaluating mobility, sensation, and reflexes. The injury may be complete or incomplete. In a complete spinal cord injury the cord is completely severed and there is no spinal innervation below the injury. With an incomplete spinal cord injury the cord has some function remaining. The neurologic assessment is ongoing and carefully documented so that changes can be dealt with in a timely fashion. The child is then assessed for trauma to other systems.

Nursing Diagnoses and Planning

The following nursing diagnoses and expected outcomes may be appropriate following assessment of the child with spinal cord injury:

■ Ineffective Breathing Pattern related to weakness or paralysis of respiratory muscles following spinal cord injury. *Expected Outcome:* The child will have arterial blood gas values within normal limits, stable vital signs, and motor and sensory function.

■ Risk for Impaired Skin Integrity related to immobility.

Expected Outcome: The child will have no evidence of skin breakdown.

■ Anxiety related to having an acute illness or having a child with an acute illness.

Expected Outcome: The child and parents will verbalize what the spinal cord injury means to them.

■ Altered Family Processes related to having a child with an acute and chronic injury.

Expected Outcome: The parents will participate in the child's care.

Interventions

The goal of nursing care is to minimize the potential for further injury, prevent the sequelae of immobility, and promote maximal spinal cord recovery. The spinal cord is immobilized with the use of tongs or halo traction. The child will remain in traction for several weeks. The nurse is responsible for maintaining proper alignment by monitoring the status of the traction every 1 to 2 hours. Towels and rolls can be useful to help position the child. The nurse should perform a motor and sensory assessment after each change of position (see Chapter 50).

If the child's situation becomes unstable, surgical stabilization may become necessary. Progressive neurologic deterioration is the major indicator for surgery.

The immobilized and neurologically impaired child is at risk for respiratory complications as a result of muscle weakness and immobility. Respiratory status and pulse oximetry are assessed and recorded every 1 to 2 hours. Supplemental oxygen may be indicated. Nebulizer, incentive spirometry, and intermittent positive-pressure breathing (IPPB) may be ordered. Some children may need a tracheostomy and mechanical ventilation if the respiratory muscles are involved or if weaning from the ventilator is slow and difficult to accomplish.

The nurse assesses perfusion by monitoring vital signs, color, skin temperature, and input/output. Because of bladder muscle weakness or paralysis, an indwelling urinary catheter facilitates bladder emptying and accurate measurement of intake and output, which is monitored hourly. If alterations in perfusion occur, the child will receive crystalloids by bolus infusion. Vasopressors such as dopamine and dobutamine may also be used.

The spinal cord–injured child may have a problem with body temperature control, and so should be warmed or cooled as appropriate. If the child has an elevated temperature, samples of wound material and blood are obtained for culture. Sputum cultures may be necessary. Antipyretic and broad-spectrum antibiotic therapy is initiated after the specimens are sent to the laboratory.

The child may have a nasogastric tube in place. The nurse will maintain tube patency and monitor and record drainage. The pH of the gastric fluid may be tested and the child treated with antacids, sucralfate (carafate), or histamine blockers. The child is at risk for stress ulcers and gastrointestinal hemorrhage. A bowel regimen will be initiated and maintained to prevent impaction. Bowel training includes ingestion of a high-fiber diet (when the child is able to eat), the use of stool softeners, and increased water intake. While the indwelling catheter is in place, care is taken to prevent infection. Intermittent catheterization may eventually be initiated if necessary.

Inspect the child's skin frequently and administer skin care each time the child is repositioned. Pressure on the bony prominences is minimized with the use of special mattresses and padding.

Adequate nutrition is essential to the healing process. Caloric intake is monitored, and the child may receive nutrition by oral intake, tube feeding, or total parenteral nutrition. A good indicator of a favorable response to the nutrition is timely healing of wounds.

Spinal cord injury is a catastrophic event. The life of the child and family has been suddenly and permanently altered. They will need intense assistance and support. These goals can be achieved through therapeutic play, promotion of independent functioning, referral to a multidisciplinary rehabilitation team, referral to support groups, and thorough discharge planning and home care teaching.

Evaluation

- Has the child's neurologic function improved?
- Are bodily functions (respiration, elimination, muscle strength) maintained as normally as possible?
- Do the child and parents verbalize feelings and emotions about the injury and the prognosis?
- Is the child's skin intact?
- Do the parents demonstrate ability to provide physical and emotional support for the child?

Seizure Disorders

A seizure consists of brief paroxysmal behavior that is due to excessive abnormal discharge of neurons. Epilepsy is marked by recurrent seizure activity that does not occur in association with an acute illness. There are two types of seizures, partial (focal) or generalized. Partial seizures occur in one part of the brain and may or may not alter consciousness. Generalized seizures occur over the entire brain and do alter consciousness.

Etiology

Seizures are symptomatic of altered neuronal activity in the CNS. Seizures can occur for many reasons, and are categorized as primary or secondary. Primary seizures occur in the absence of any underlying brain structural abnormality. Primary seizures are linked to genetic predisposition and include febrile seizures, absence seizures, and benign seizures of the newborn. Secondary, or symptomatic, seizures are usually provoked by some temporary or permanent structural or metabolic abnormality. Cerebral lesions, malformations, metabolic disorders, acquired causes (e.g., anoxia, trauma, stroke), infections, degenerative disorders, and toxic disturbances are linked to secondary seizures. Approximately 50% of childhood seizures are idiopathic, meaning they have no known cause.

Incidence

An estimated six in 1,000 children will have seizures before age 18 years. An estimated 3% to 4% of children age 6 months to 3 years will have a febrile seizure. Sixty percent of children with epilepsy experience the onset of seizures before their 18th birthday. Neonatal seizures occur in approximately 20% of preterm infants.

Pathophysiology

During a seizure there is excessive, self-limiting neuronal discharge. The result of this discharge is activation of associated motor or sensory organs. The extent of the seizure depends on the location and extent of the abnormal neuronal discharges. The brain consists of millions of nerve cells; electrical impulses are sent through many of these cells by means of neurotransmitters. When numerous nerve cells fire abnormally at the same time, a seizure may result.

Manifestations

There are many types of seizures. The International Classification of Seizures is used to divide seizures into two groups: generalized and partial. In addition, some other types of seizures are seen in children.

Febrile seizures are generally seen in young children. Only about one third of these children ever have another seizure, and about 3% of this group of children develop epilepsy. The height and rapidity of temperature elevation seem to be factors in precipitating febrile seizures. The temperature is usually elevated above 38.8°C (101.8°F). The seizure activity occurs during the temperature rise rather than after prolonged elevation. Simple febrile seizures are familial and probably transmitted by autosomal dominant inheritance (Fenichel, 1997). Ninety percent of febrile seizures occur as a result of fever caused by otitis media, pharyngitis, and adenitis. The family of a child who experiences a febrile seizure should be given information about these seizures and instructed what to do if another seizure occurs.

Neonatal seizures are usually caused by an underlying pathological process. The most frequent cause of neonatal seizures is perinatal asphyxia leading to hypoxic-ischemic encephalopathy, which accounts for as many as 65% of neonatal seizures. Another 15% of cases can be attributed to intracranial hemorrhage. Other causes include metabolic disturbances, meningitis, cerebral infarcts, drug withdrawal, hyperthermia, hypoglycemia, sodium and potassium imbalances, congenital anomalies of the CNS, and inherited syndromes.

The mechanism of neonatal seizures is not clearly understood. Possible explanations include an excess of excitatory neurotransmitter compared with inhibitory neurotransmitter, altered permeability of the neuronal membrane inhibiting sodium movement, and an imbalance between depolarization and repolarization of the neurons. Because of the overall anatomic and physiologic immaturity of the nervous system in the neonate, well-organized generalized seizures are rare.

Because of the lack of myelinization of fiber tracts, neonates do not experience the same type of tonic-clonic seizure an older child experiences. Seizures in neonates may produce subtle signs, such as sustained eye opening, tonic horizontal deviation of the eyes, blinking or eyelid fluttering, sucking, smacking, drooling, tongue thrusting, pedaling movements of the legs, swimming movements of the arms, and apnea. These manifestations are more common

International Classification of Seizures

GENERALIZED SEIZURES

Onset starts at any age. Clinical features indicate involvement of both cerebral hemispheres. Consciousness is impaired.

TONIC-CLONIC SEIZURES

Formerly called grand mal seizures, tonic-clonic seizures cause an abrupt arrest of activity and impairment of consciousness.

The *tonic phase* consists of a sustained, generalized stiffening of muscles, including the diaphragm, lasting a few seconds.

The *clonic phase* is symmetrical and rhythmic, consisting of alternating contraction and relaxation of major muscle groups. This phase usually ends spontaneously in less than 5 minutes. Respirations are irregular and may be stridorous. Sphincter incontinence may or may not be present.

The tonic-clonic seizure is followed by a variable period of confusion, lethargy, and sleep.

ATONIC SEIZURES

Atonic seizures cause an abrupt loss of postural tone, impairment of consciousness, confusion, lethargy, and sleep.

MYOCLONIC SEIZURES

Myoclonic seizures are brief, random contractions of a muscle group. They can occur on both sides of the body, and may occur singly or in clusters. Impairment of consciousness might occur during myoclonic seizures. Onset can occur as early as age 2 months, but myoclonic seizures are more frequently seen in school-age children or adolescents than in very young children. Myoclonic seizures that occur during infancy are called infantile spasms; those that occur during adolescence are denoted juvenile myoclonic epilepsy.

ABSENCE SEIZURES

Formerly called petit mal seizures, absence seizures are very brief episodes of altered consciousness. There is no muscle activity except for eyelid fluttering, twitching, or head bobbing. The child has a blank facial expression. Absence seizures last only 5 to 10 seconds, but they may occur one after another several times a day. The onset of absence seizures usually does not occur before age 5. Children usually outgrow absence seizures during adolescence.

PARTIAL SEIZURES

Onset starts at any age. The clinical features suggest that only a limited functional area in one hemisphere of the brain is involved, and therefore symptoms are seen on only one side of the body. Partial seizures begin focally but may become generalized when the electrical impulses are passed across the corpus callosum to the other hemisphere. Partial seizures are further divided into those with or without change in level of consciousness.

Simple Partial Seizures. Simple partial seizures consist of motor, autonomic, or sensory symptoms. There is no change in level of consciousness with simple partial seizures. Symptoms may include an odd taste in the mouth or odd smell, abdominal discomfort, unexplained feelings of fear or dread, or motor movements. This type of seizure may last 20 seconds to several minutes.

Complex Partial Seizures. Complex partial seizures may begin with or without an aura. The aura is a simple partial seizure. Symptoms include impaired consciousness, transient staring, altered mental status, and feelings of unreality, detachment, and disrupted memory. There may be distortions of perception or hallucinations, teeth grinding, lip smacking, chewing, swallowing, scratching, or pulling at shirt buttons. Tonic-clonic movements of one side of the body may also be seen. The average duration of a complex partial seizure is 1 to 5 minutes. A complex partial seizure is followed by a variable period of confusion, lethargy, and sleep.

Adapted from Behrman, R. E., Kliegman, R. M., & Arvin, A. M. (1996). *Nelson textbook of pediatrics* (15th ed.). Philadelphia: Saunders.

in preterm infants and infants with hypoxic ischemic encephalopathy. Neonatal seizures also can be focal, tonic, or myoclonic, with jerking movements of the extremities.

Diagnostic Evaluation

The child's health history and family history are important parts of the initial workup. A thorough description of the child's behavior before, during, and after the seizure activity is important to delineate the type of seizure. Video recording and EEG monitoring will help identify the seizure. Serum electrolyte determinations, CBC, blood glucose determination, lumbar puncture, and other laboratory tests can help uncover metabolic causes. CT and MRI will indicate trauma, tumor, or congenital malformation. In neonates, several other laboratory tests may be included, such as TORCHS (see Chapter 30) titers, to exclude congenital viral infections, as well as amino acid and organic acid studies to exclude inborn errors of metabolism.

Therapeutic Management

The basic tenet of treatment for seizures is to treat the whole child. The goals are to identify and correct the cause of the seizure, eliminate the seizure with a minimum of side effects and using the least amount of medication, and normalize the child's and family's life.

Common Seizure Medications

Partial Seizures	Generalized Seizures
Carbamazepine	Valproic acid
Valproic acid	Clonazepam
Felbamate	Phenytoin
Phenytoin	Ethosuximide
Topiramate	
Gabapentin	
Lamotrigine	

CRITICAL TO REMEMBER

Observations and Nursing Care During a Seizure

- As the seizure begins, look at your watch, or a clock. It is important to be able to describe how long seizure activity lasts.
- Protect the child from injury by loosening clothing at the neck and turning the child gently onto the side. Do not restrain the child or insert any object into the child's mouth.
- Carefully observe where the seizure begins, its progression, and how it ends.
- Be able to describe any preceding or accompanying sensory or motor manifestations.
- When the seizure is over, allow the child to rest, if the child desires. Record the child's behavior before, during, and after the seizure and the approximate duration of the seizure.
- In neonates, if the movement can be initiated by a stimulus, such as touch, it is probably a tremor. If it cannot be stopped or controlled with gentle restraint or passive flexion, it is probably a seizure.

NURSING CARE

The Child with Seizures

Assessment

A detailed history that includes the prenatal, perinatal, and neonatal periods is important in determining factors precipitating seizure activity. Pathologic precipitating factors include hypoxia, cerebral trauma, high fever, lead poisoning, metabolic disorders, brain tumors, birth trauma, and CNS infections. Nonpathologic factors include overhydration, oversedation, drug abuse, sleep deprivation, antihistamine drug use, alcohol intoxication, and family history.

Seizures often are not witnessed by the health care professional. The parents should be asked about the child's age at onset of the seizure activity, time of onset, precipitating events, and the child's behavior before and after the seizure. A detailed description of the seizure itself is essential, including the child's behaviors during the seizure, how the seizure progresses, how long it lasts, and the child's behavior after the seizures.

The child is given a comprehensive physical examina-

PARENTS WANT TO KNOW

Guidelines for the Child or Adolescent Taking Seizure Medication

- Oral care is very important for children taking Dilantin, because Dilantin can cause gum problems. Your child should brush and floss after every meal, using a soft brush. Take your child to the dentist every 3 to 6 months for a checkup and teeth cleaning.
- Once your child has started taking the medication your child will need to have blood levels monitored to determine that the medication has reached and maintained a therapeutic level and to monitor for a toxic level. Additionally, your child may need other blood tests to be sure the medication is not harming the liver or blood cells. Take your child for blood level tests periodically as your doctor recommends, if a seizure occurs, or if side effects are noticed.
- If your child is taking valproic acid, be alert for any signs of unusual bleeding or bruising. Valproic acid can affect the platelets (cells that help the blood clot) and cause the platelet counts to drop.
- Be sure your child does not suddenly stop taking antiepileptic medications without discussing it with a doctor or nurse. Suddenly stopping medications can cause the child to have a seizure or status epilepticus.
- Some states require a driver to be seizure free for 6 months to 1 year to obtain a driver's license. If your child is of driving age, discuss this with your health care provider.
- Birth control pills might be less effective while taking anti-epileptic medications. If sexually active, your adolescent should consult a nurse or physician for additional forms of birth control.
- Alcohol, marijuana, and street drugs will lower the seizure threshold. It is best to avoid or limit these drugs.

tion with special emphasis on the neurologic system. Parameters include assessment of behavior, motor skills, and developmental level. The child and family's emotional response to the seizure disorder is assessed at this time.

The nursing care of the child with seizures is both acute and long term. Acute management includes identification of the type of seizure and factors that precipitated the event. Long-term management focuses on medication administration and education.

Nursing Diagnosis, Planning, Intervention, and Evaluation

Nursing Diagnosis	■ Risk for Injury related to seizure activity.
Expected Outcomes	• The child will remain uninjured after a seizure. • The parents will discuss seizure prevention and will demonstrate first aid for seizures.

Intervention	Rationale
1. Pad side rails with blankets and keep bed in low position. Place child on a soft surface if not in bed. Remove sharp objects and keep furniture out of the way.	1. These actions modify the environment to make it safer for the child during the seizure.

2. Do not put anything into the child's mouth during a seizure.
3. Place the child on the side in a lateral position. Do not restrain the child. Loosen clothing around the child's neck.

4. Record the time of seizures, precipitating factors, types of behavior observed during the seizure, bladder or bowel incontinence, and frequency of seizures.
5. Stay with the child.

6. If the seizure lasts longer than 5 minutes, notify a physician.

2. Forcing something into the child's mouth may cause injury to the child's mouth, gums, or teeth.
3. Positioning the child on the side will prevent aspiration, as the saliva drains out the corner of the child's mouth. Restraints could cause injury to the child. The nurse or family may gently guide or protect the child's movements and may suction the child's mouth after the seizure is over.
4. These observations help pinpoint the focus of the seizure and will help the physician treat the seizure correctly.
5. Staying with the child reduces the risk of injury and allows for observation and documentation of the seizure.
6. Medication may need to be administered to stop prolonged seizures. Remember that the main side effect of diazepam (Valium) and lorazepam (Ativan) is respiratory depression.

Evaluation
- Does the child remain injury free?
- Are seizures monitored and documented?
- Can the parents demonstrate first aid for seizures?

Nursing Diagnosis
- Knowledge Deficit related to having a seizure disorder.

Expected Outcome
- The child and parents will discuss seizures and physical, emotional, and educational needs.

Intervention

1. Determine the child's and parent's educational needs.
2. Provide an individual teaching plan for the child and parents for handling seizures.
3. Explore actual and potential problems that may arise and interfere with treatment.

4. Measure outcomes of education to ensure that learning has taken place and is facilitating acceptance.
5. Refer to an epilepsy support group. (See Appendix L for a list of resource organizations.)
6. Educate the child and parents about the medication regimen. Emphasize the importance of complying with medical treatment.
7. Identify the side effects of the medication and when medical attention should be sought.

8. Point out the hazards of noncompliance with medications. Encourage the parents and child not to discontinue medications even if the child is seizure free.
9. Emphasize to the child and parents the importance of regular medical evaluation and follow-up, including measurement of blood levels of the medication and evaluating for toxicity or side effects.
10. Inform the parent about the need for an identification band for the child.

11. Encourage the family to find alternative activities besides contact sports for the child. The child should avoid swimming or climbing alone. Identify the child's strengths, not what the child cannot do.

Rationale

1. Determining educational needs provides baseline information in order to develop a teaching plan.
2. An individualized teaching plan ensures that what is needed by the child and parents will be taught.
3. Exploring possible problems facilitates adjustment and normalizes life; it also provides anticipatory guidance.
4. Evaluation of teaching is an ongoing process to ensure continued learning.
5. Social support is helpful for some families and may promote adjustment to lifestyle changes.
6. The goal of pharmacologic management is to raise the seizure threshold, thus preventing seizures.

7. Knowledge of what is expected and normal will facilitate proper use and compliance with medication.
8. Noncompliance will affect the serum levels of anticonvulsants and may cause a seizure to occur.

9. Regular medical follow-up facilitates maintenance of appropriate therapeutic blood levels of anticonvulsants and identification of side effects of medication.
10. Identification bands alert others to the child's condition in an emergency. If the child has a seizure in a public place, the identification band will inform passers-by of what to do for the child.
11. Appropriate activities will reduce the risk of injury while promoting a positive self-image.

12. Encourage verbalization of fears and concerns about having seizures.
13. Teach the child and parent to educate other family members, friends, and teachers about seizures.

12. This therapeutic communication may identify issues that need to be addressed.
13. Accurate information reduces the stigma associated with epilepsy.

Evaluation

- Does the child discuss having seizures, fears and concerns about seizures, and life with them?
- Does the child participate in the medical regimen by discussing medication side effects and dosage?
- Does the child demonstrate a positive self-image?
- Is the family able to demonstrate safety principles for the child with seizures?
- Does the family administer anticonvulsants safely and appropriately, and know when to call the physician?

Status Epilepticus

Status epilepticus is a pediatric emergency. It is marked by prolonged seizure activity, in the form of either a single seizure lasting 10 minutes or more or recurrent seizures lasting more than 30 minutes with no return to a normal level of consciousness between seizures. The most common form of status epilepticus is generalized status, which has the highest potential for complications and possible death.

Etiology

The causes of status epilepticus are many. Acute CNS injury from head trauma, meningitis, or electrolyte imbalance frequently precipitates status epilepticus. The condition can also be caused by toxins and specific medications. Other causes are chronic CNS injury and sudden withdrawal from anticonvulsants.

Incidence

Status epilepticus occurs in 5% to 10% of children with epilepsy. The most common cause in children under age 3 years is febrile status epilepticus.

Pathophysiology

Status epilepticus is caused by the random discharge of large numbers of neurons firing abnormally. The discharges cause abnormal repetitive motor activity. In the CNS the metabolic rate increases, glucose stores are depleted, and oxygen consumption increases. If cerebral metabolic demands are not met, these changes cause neuronal injury. Prolonged seizures cause lactic acidosis, an altered blood-brain barrier, and increased ICP.

Manifestations

See the International Classification of Seizures on p. 1495.

Diagnostic Evaluation

Diagnostic laboratory tests should include blood glucose, arterial blood gases, electrolytes, anticonvulsant drug levels, a toxicology screen, and possibly lumbar puncture. Results may be similar to those of the child with increased ICP.

Therapeutic Management

Generalized tonic-clonic status epilepticus is a medical emergency. Treatment consists in maintaining optimal respiratory and hemodynamic function and identifying and treating the causes of the seizure activity. Diazepam (Valium) or lorazepam (Ativan) are given IV. If IV access cannot be obtained, medication can be given orally or rectally. Clorazepate dipotassium (Tranxene) can be given orally for cluster seizures. Fosphenytoin (Cerebyx) or phenobarbitol may be given IV as a second round of drugs if Valium or Ativan does not stop the seizures. The intramuscular route is not used as it is unpredictable.

NURSING CARE
The Child with Status Epilepticus

Assessment

On arrival at the hospital, the child will exhibit seizure activity and have unstable vital signs. Along with general seizure precautions, this child requires rapid assessment and vigorous supportive therapy. Supportive measures include assessing and maintaining a patent airway, and administration of oxygen. IV hydration and drug therapy are initiated to arrest the seizure activity.

Nursing Diagnoses and Planning

The following nursing diagnoses and expected outcomes may apply to the child with status epilepticus:

- Impaired Gas Exchange related to decreased respirations associated with seizures.
  Expected Outcome: The child's pulse oxygen saturation will remain above 95%.

CRITICAL TO REMEMBER

Drug Therapy for Generalized Tonic-Clonic Status Epilepticus

Generalized tonic-clonic status epilepticus is a medical emergency. Diazepam (Valium) or lorazepam (Ativan) are given intravenously. Intravenous diazepam must be given directly into the vein (not the tubing, because it interacts with plastic), at a rate no greater than 1 mg/min. It should not be mixed with other drugs or solutions, and it can be diluted only with normal saline. Resuscitation equipment should be at the bedside and the child's respirations closely monitored during IV administration.

- Ineffective Breathing Pattern related to loss of muscle control associated with seizures.

  Expected Outcome: The child's pulse oxygen saturation will remain at 95%.

- Ineffective Airway Clearance related to possible aspiration during seizure.

  Expected Outcome: The child will have clear breath sounds.

- Altered Cerebral Tissue Perfusion related to lactic acidosis with prolonged seizure activity.

  Expected Outcome: The child's level of consciousness will return to normal.

Interventions and Evaluation

Nursing interventions and evaluation are similar to those described for the child with epilepsy.

Meningitis

Meningitis is the most common infectious process of the CNS. It may occur as a primary disease or as a result of complications of neurosurgery, trauma, systemic infection, or sinus or ear infections. A wide variety of bacteria and viruses can be responsible for the primary infection. Earlier diagnosis and improved antibiotic therapy have reduced the mortality and incidence of complications from bacterial meningitis.

Etiology

The primary organisms responsible for causing bacterial meningitis vary according to age. Among children ages 2 months to 12 years, three pathogens seem to be the most prevalent. *Hemophilus influenzae* type B, *Neisseria meningitidis*, and *Streptococcus pneumoniae* cause 95% of cases of purulent meningitis in this age group. Tuberculous meningitis also is becoming more common in this age group. These types of meningitis usually result from extension of a localized infection, such as otitis media, sinusitis, pharyngitis, or pneumonia, into the CSF. The organisms primarily responsible for neonatal meningitis are group B streptococci and *Escherichia coli*.

Organisms also may be introduced directly after an injury in which the skin is broken and communication between skin, sinuses, and CSF occurs. Entry may occur in association with a lumbar puncture, skull fracture, or surgery.

Meningococcal meningitis caused by *Neisseria* usually occurs in older children and adolescents. Because it is transmitted primarily by droplet infection, the risk increases as the number of contacts increases.

Viral meningitis is associated with such viruses as mumps, paramyxoviruses, herpesviruses, and enteroviruses. In rare cases, protozoa or fungi are the infecting organisms. These types of meningitis are seen most frequently in children with AIDS.

Incidence

Meningitis most commonly affects children between ages 1 month and 5 years, but it can occur at any age. Boys are affected more frequently than girls, and risk factors increase where individuals are in close contact with one another (as in day care centers, college dormitories, or in large families in

PATHOPHYSIOLOGY
. . . .
of Meningitis

Meningitis is an inflammation of the meninges of the brain that results from a pathogen entering the CNS and causing a toxic response. As the process continues, increased intracranial pressure (ICP) develops, along with subdural empyema. If the infection spreads to the ventricles, edema and tissue scarring around the ventricle causes obstruction of the CSF and subsequent hydrocephalus.

This process can happen very rapidly because CSF is an excellent growth medium for bacteria, containing nutrient substances such as protein and glucose. Leukocytes are unable to function as a defense mechanism in the fluid environment of the CSF. Leukocytes require a tissue surface to destroy bacteria, so there is little defense to stop the growth of bacteria, and they can multiply quickly.

As the infection spreads farther into brain tissue, changes occur in the permeability of capillaries and blood vessels in the dura mater. These changes lead to increased passage of albumin and water into the subdural space, with a subsequent accumulation of protein and fluid. This results in a further increase in ICP.

The most common neurologic sequelae of meningitis are hearing loss, mental retardation, seizures, visual impairment, and behavioral problems (Behrman et al., 1996). Other complications include cranial nerve dysfunction, brain abscess, and the syndrome of inappropriate secretion of antidiuretic hormone (SIADH).

small dwellings). There is a higher incidence among African-American children than Caucasian children. The incidence of *H. influenzae* type B infection related to meningitis has declined rapidly with the immunization of infants.

Manifestations

Signs and symptoms of meningitis vary according to the age of the child and the duration of the preceding illness. There is no single hallmark sign or symptom.

The clinical signs of meningitis in the neonate include poor feeding, poor sucking, vomiting, diarrhea, poor muscle tone, poor cry, hypothermia or hyperthermia, apnea, seizures, sepsis, disseminated intravascular coagulation, a full, tense, and bulging fontanel, and lethargy.

Clinical signs of meningitis in the infant and child include fever, poor feeding, vomiting, irritability, seizures, a high-pitched cry, a bulging anterior fontanel, and lethargy. In the neonate, infant, and young child the symptoms of meningitis are frequently vague and nonspecific.

Early clinical signs of meningitis in children and adolescents include severe headache, photophobia, nuchal rigidity, fever, altered level of consciousness (lethargy, irritability), poor feeding, vomiting, diarrhea, agitation, and drowsiness. Muscle or joint pain and purpura may be noted. Kernig's sign (pain with extension of leg and knee; Fig. 52–7) and Brudzinski's sign (flexion of head causing flexion of hips and knees; Fig. 52–7) are often exhibited. Addition-

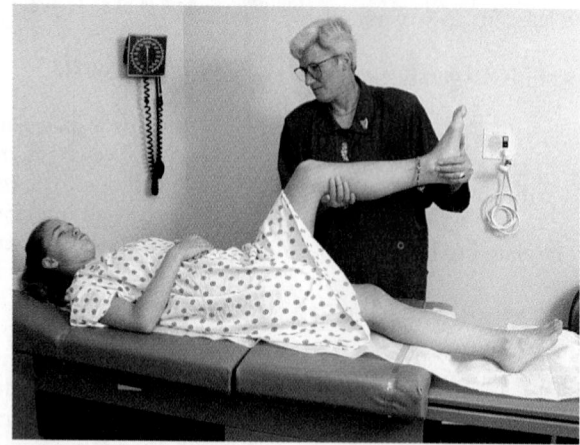

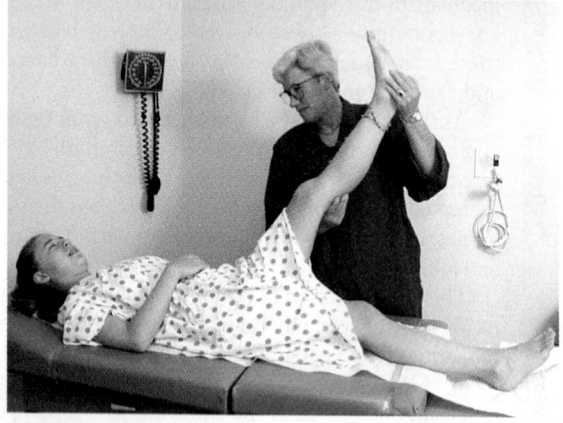

Kernig's Sign

The child can easily extend the leg when in the supine position. However, when the thigh is flexed toward the abdomen, pain prevents complete extension of the leg.

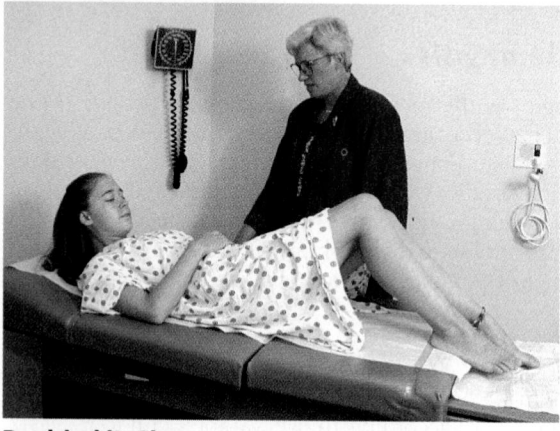

Brudzinski's Sign

In the supine position, the child bends her head toward her chest. (In a younger child, the nurse can bend the child's head.) This action usually produces involuntary hip and knee flexion in the child with meningitis.

FIGURE 52–7
• • • • • • • • • •
As part of the assessment for meningitis, the nurse can attempt to elicit Kernig's sign and Brudzinski's sign. Both are early signs of meningitis in children and adolescents. (Courtesy of Parkland Health & Hospital System, Dallas, Texas.)

ally, petechial or purpuric rash (meningococcal infection) may be observed.

Late clinical signs of meningitis in children and adolescents include changes in level of consciousness and seizures.

Diagnostic Evaluation

The diagnosis is made by testing CSF obtained by lumbar puncture. Findings usually include increased CSF pressure, cloudy CSF (in the case of bacterial meningitis), high protein concentration, and low glucose level. Blood cultures may be done, and nose and throat cultures are occasionally helpful if the CSF is negative.

Therapeutic Management

Acute bacterial meningitis is a medical emergency requiring early recognition and prompt, aggressive management. Isolation is begun and maintained for at least 24 hours after antibi-

otics are given. Prompt initiation and uninterrupted IV administration of appropriate antibiotics is essential in cases of suspected bacterial meningitis. Treatment is started before the causative organism is identified because cultures may take up to 3 days to yield results. It is vital to start antibiotics early because delay could be fatal. Antibiotic therapy is based on the age of the child, the pathogen most frequently encountered in that age group, and the initial appearance of the CSF. If IV access is difficult to achieve, the first dose of antibiotics should be administered intramuscularly.

Treatment for neonatal bacterial meningitis consists of ampicillin and an aminoglycoside or a third-generation cephalosporin. For older children and adolescents, the treatment of choice is ampicillin and penicillin G. The initial antibiotic must be a broad-spectrum drug to cover most of the suspected pathogens. When the culture and sensitivity test results are available, treatment regimens may have to be changed. The treatment for viral meningitis is symptomatic and supportive, usually with complete recovery.

NURSING CARE

The Child with Meningitis

Assessment

The information from the history and physical examination will provide baseline data, along with a complete neurologic assessment that includes evaluating for the presence or absence of headaches, photophobia, hearing loss, seizure activity, changes in level of consciousness, changes in pupil reactions and size, nuchal rigidity, and muscle flaccidity. Personality changes and irritability may be noted. It is also important to note any food and fluid intake, nausea, vomiting, or loss of appetite. The nurse should review the history for recent immunizations or recent illnesses, such as upper respiratory tract infections, otitis media, surgery, skull fracture, or previous lumbar puncture.

Early recognition and treatment of complications can substantially reduce the morbidity and mortality. Thorough knowledge of the disease process is important, and assessments must be complete, frequent, and alert to any changes in the child's condition. Assessment of peak and trough antibiotic levels are important to prevent ototoxicity from aminoglycosides.

Nursing Diagnosis and Planning

Nursing diagnoses that apply to the child with meningitis include those common to other neurologic disorders. Care related to these nursing diagnoses is detailed on pp. 1471 to 1474. The nursing diagnosis specific to the child with meningitis is

■ Knowledge Deficit related to seriousness of meningitis, possible residual neurologic deficits, home management, and prophylaxis.
  Expected Outcome: The parents will discuss the disease process and possible sequelae, treatment, home management, and possible implications for spread of the disease.

Interventions

Discuss the disease process and prognosis with the parents after assessing their existing knowledge. It is important to

---

CRITICAL TO REMEMBER

Guidelines for the Child with Meningitis

- The close contacts of the child with *Hemophilus influenzae* infection need prophylactic treatment with rifampin.
- Anyone who spent at least 4 hours with the child in the 5 to 7 days preceding a child's hospitalization with *H. influenzae* needs prophylactic treatment if not already immunized.
- All close contacts of children with *Neisseria meningitidis* need prophylactic treatment, regardless of age or immunization status.
- Rifampin colors the urine and sweat red-orange, and will stain contact lenses.

CRITICAL THINKING EXERCISE 52–1

Pediatric nurses in the community often are in a position to answer questions about childhood illnesses. Recently, parents of high school children received a notice from the school nurse that a male student had been diagnosed with meningococcal meningitis. The nurse recommended that parents should be watchful but not overly concerned. Her letter advised parents to watch their children for 2 weeks and call the physician at any sign of illness.

1. Is this course of action prudent?
2. If so, why? If not, why not?

---

teach the family about the possible complications and sequelae of meningitis. Discuss the importance of follow-up care.

It is necessary to provide prophylaxis for the ill child's close contacts. Ask the parents to identify others exposed to meningitis, and refer them for treatment. Close contacts should not wait for signs of meningitis to develop but should seek prompt medical attention because they may be incubating the infection.

Instruct the parents about prescribed medications and treatments. Document instructions and request a return demonstration by parents or caregiver. The parents will be anxious and grieving about the child's illness and outcome; learning will be difficult. To be sure the parents have learned, watch them perform the necessary procedures.

Complications of meningitis may include hydrocephalus, vision and hearing loss, delayed growth and development, seizures, subdural effusions, and cranial nerve palsy.

Evaluation

- Can the parents demonstrate the ability to administer the child's treatments and medication?
- Do the parents discuss the disease and treatments?
- Have the parents referred close contacts for treatment?

Neurologic Conditions Requiring Critical Care

A number of neurologic conditions, including encephalitis, Reye's syndrome, Guillain-Barré syndrome, botulism, and tetanus, require critical nursing care. Children with these conditions are frequently admitted to hospital critical care units where the care is specialized (Table 52–3).

Headaches

Headaches are a common complaint in children of all ages. Seventy-five percent of all children will suffer a significant headache before age 15 (Winner, 1997).

Etiology

The three primary sources of recurrent headache are vascular, tension related, and increased ICP (Table 52–4).

TABLE 52 – 3

Neurologic Conditions Requiring Critical Care

Condition	Pathophysiology, Etiology, and Incidence	Manifestations	Therapeutic Management	Nursing Considerations
Encephalitis	Inflammation caused by infection or toxin and resulting in cerebral edema and neurologic dysfunction. Numerous agents are causative. Peak incidence is in middle to late childhood.	Headache, irritability, lethargy, altered level of consciousness, nuchal rigidity, seizures, fever, malaise, dizziness, nausea and vomiting, ataxia, sensory disturbances.	Diagnosed by lumbar puncture and cerebrospinal fluid (CSF) culture, electroencephalographic (EEG) alterations are not unusual. Care includes hospitalization and monitoring for increased intracranial pressure (ICP). Medication: cephalosporin or acyclovir (depending on causative agent), anticonvulsants.	Care is similar to that for any child with increased ICP. Care also includes fever management with antipyretics and tepid baths; pharmacologic and nonpharmacologic headache relief measures; maintenance of fluid and electrolyte balance; providing support to anxious family members; assisting the family to manage any long-term neurologic deficits; and facilitating grieving for the family of a child with a poor prognosis.
Reye syndrome	Exposure to viral agent or toxin in at-risk children leads to liver cell damage with rising serum ammonia levels. The toxic serum ammonia levels result in cerebral dysfunction (encephalopathy and cerebral edema), fluid and electrolyte and acid-base imbalances, and coagulopathies. The average age at onset is 6 to 7 years. Reye syndrome might be related to administration of aspirin to children with viral disease.	Antecedent viral infection; malaise, nausea, vomiting, progressive neurologic deterioration. Laboratory tests: elevated serum ammonia levels, liver dysfunction on biopsy, hypoglycemia, altered coagulation times, increased ICP with respiratory dysfunction. Reye syndrome is clinically staged from I (lethargy) to V (coma with flaccidity/decerebrate posturing), according to degree of altered consciousness.	Care includes hospitalization for monitoring of neurologic status, increasing ICP, hydration and acid-base balance, and cardiorespiratory status.	Care is similar to that for any child with increasing ICP, with the potential addition of mechanical respiratory support. Accurate, continuous monitoring of neurologic and cardiorespiratory status is essential because the child's condition can deteriorate suddenly. Fluid replacement is achieved with IV hypertonic solutions if ICP is not increased. Protect the child from coagulopathy-related injury. Provide support and anxiety relief measures for family members. Discourage the use of aspirin-containing products.

Guillain-Barré syndrome (post-infectious polyneuritis)	Rare (1 per 100,000 people per year), progressive motor weakness associated with antecedent infection or immunization producing demyelization of motor and sometimes sensory nerves; affects all ages.	Numbness, tingling, and weakness of the lower extremities; ascending loss of deep tendon reflexes with flaccid paralysis; autonomic instability with blood pressure fluctuations, hypotension, and dysrhythmias; bowel and bladder incontinence; cranial nerve dysfunction; neuromuscular impairment; respiratory failure. Recovery can take months to years; neuromuscular impairment improves in descending order as healing occurs.	Care is primarily supportive, with attention to neurologic, respiratory, and cardiovascular systems and timely recognition of deteriorating status. Plasmaphoresis may be beneficial. Most deaths are attributed to respiratory failure.	Establish the antecedent factor. Perform frequent neurologic, cardiovascular, and respiratory assessments and pulse oximetry with daily pulmonary function testing. Keep appropriate emergency and ventilatory support equipment at the child's bedside. Frequent chest physiotherapy and other techniques help prevent the consequences of immobility. Ensure the child is receiving adequate nutrition (NG tube or gastrostomy feedings might be necessary). Anticoagulants may be given if risk of pulmonary embolism is high. Provide anxiety relief for the child and parents, and facilitate the child's development.
Botulism	Food poisoning caused by Clostridium botulinum toxin. The source is honey (in infants) or improperly sterilized canned foods.	CNS symptoms 12 to 36 hours after ingestion: weakness, headache, double vision, vomiting, difficulty talking, respiratory paralysis, decreased deep tendon reflexes, impaired gag reflex.	Care is supportive and includes respiratory support and administering antitoxoid. Recovery after treatment takes an average of 1 month.	Advise parents not to give infants honey or syrup in their milk or water. Educate the public about proper food preparation techniques.
Tetanus (lockjaw)	Caused by endotoxin produced by the anaerobic, spore-forming, gram-positive bacillus Clostridium tetani. Entry sites include puncture wounds, burns, lacerations, and compound fractures. The incubation period is 3 days to 3 weeks.	Painful muscular rigidity of masseter and neck muscles, facial spasms, dysphagia, laryngospasm, severe pain, respiratory arrest.	Care includes ventilatory and respiratory support. Medication: diazepam (Valium) or lorazepam (Ativan) for seizures; tetanus immune globulin.	Assess the child's ventilatory and neurologic status and provide respiratory support as needed. Provide fluids and electrolytes; seizure precautions; quiet environment. Educate the child and family about immunizations.

TABLE 52–4

Etiology of Recurrent Headache

Vascular headache
  Migraine
  Arteriovenous malformations
Tension-type headache
  Stress
Headache due to increased intracranial pressure
  Space-occupying lesion
  Idiopathic intracranial hypertension (pseudotumor
    cerebri)
Other causes
  Systemic diseases
  Sinusitis
  Ocular diseases
  Temporomandibular joint disease

Data from Singh, B. V., & Roach, E. S. (1998). Diagnosis and management of headaches in children. *Pediatrics in Review*, *19*(4), 132–135.

Incidence

Migraine (vascular) headaches occur in close to 5% of children. Tension-type headaches are seen in about 15% of children, and 30% suffer from nonmigrainous headaches (Singh & Roach, 1998). Migraine in preadolescents is equally prevalent in males and females, but in adolescents the prevalence greatly increases for females. A family history of headache is noted in a majority of these cases.

Manifestations

Headaches related to increased ICP have been addressed in the earlier discussion about increased ICP.

MIGRAINE

Symptoms range from mild, in which case the child may continue with daily activities, to episodes that force the child to go to a quiet, dark room. In some cases an aura may occur before the headache begins. The aura may include seeing flashing lights; smelling specific odors; blurry, double, or lost vision; and tingling in the arms or legs. Once the headache begins the most common symptoms include throbbing pain, typically on one side of the head, nausea and vomiting, irritability, abdominal pain, photophobia, and phonophobia. The pain can last from minutes to several hours.

TENSION-TYPE HEADACHES

The pain associated with tension-type headaches is usually more generalized than that of a migraine. The child may describe the pain as a band-like tightness or pressure, tight neck muscles, or soreness of the scalp. Nausea is rare, but fatigue and dizziness are common. These headaches may last for days or weeks but usually do not interfere with the child's regular activities.

Diagnostic Evaluation

Evaluation of the child's blood pressure and measurement of the child's head size (for evidence of chronically in-creased ICP) should be done. A detailed neurologic exam should be performed, with special attention given to auscultation for a bruit in the head (suggesting an arteriovenous malformation), assessing mental status, and examining both optic discs for papilledema. CT or MRI may be performed in children with chronic headaches or those with abnormalities found on the neurologic examination.

NURSING CARE

The Child with Headaches

Assessment

A detailed history of the child's headache and preheadache events is important to determine precipitating factors. A social history of the child and family may identify triggering stressors (e.g., divorce, move to a new school, loss of a family member, friend, or pet). The child should receive a comprehensive physical examination with emphasis on the neurologic system.

Nursing Diagnosis and Planning

Nursing diagnoses that may apply to a child with a headache include those common to other neurologic disorders:

- Knowledge Deficit related to management of a child with a headache and medication regimen.
  Expected Outcome: The child and parents will discuss headaches and educational needs.
- Risk of Injury related to headache symptoms (change in vision, dizziness).
  Expected Outcome: The child will remain free of injury after headache. Parents will verbalize a safety plan for the child during headache and a medication regimen.
- Pain related to underlying contributing factors.
  Expected Outcome: The child will identify triggering factors and demonstrate appropriate nonpharmacologic approaches.

Interventions

Certain factors may trigger the onset of a headache. Triggers may include stress, food, menstruation, visual stimuli, fatigue, and certain medications. The child and family need to be educated about lifestyle changes that will lower stress, and about avoiding other triggers. Keeping a diary of the child's headaches and preheadache events will aid in identifying the triggers specific for the child.

For mild or infrequent migraines and tension headache, common analgesics such as acetaminophen or ibuprofen may be effective. For a more severe migraine, treatment may include naproxen, metoclopramide or combination drugs containing sympathomimetic drugs, sedatives, and analgesics. If children have two or more severe migraine headaches per month, they may need daily prophylactic medication. Commonly used prophylactic medications include amitriptyline and propranolol. Psychological evaluation followed by relaxation therapy, counseling, and biofeedback therapy may be helpful for some children.

The nursing care for a child with headaches is acute and long term. Acute management includes placing the child in a dark, quiet environment and medication administration. Long-term management focuses on education about and elimination of trigger factors, and medication administration.

Evaluation

- Do the child and parents demonstrate an understanding of the management of headache and the medication regimen?

- Do the child and parents understand the need for following a safety plan to prevent injury during headache and medication?
- Are the child and parents learning to eliminate headache trigger factors?
- Can the child demonstrate and benefit from relaxation therapy and biofeedback?

KEY CONCEPTS

- The CNS is composed of the brain and spinal cord, which are protected by bony coverings, the skull and vertebral column. The skull has several bones that are not fused at birth and do not fuse until 12 to 18 months of life. The brain and spinal cord are also covered by the meninges, a fibrous connective tissue structure that contains many blood vessels.
- Cerebrospinal fluid surrounds the brain and spinal cord. The brain consists of the cerebrum, cerebellum, and brain stem.
- The peripheral nervous system consists of 12 pairs of cranial nerves and 31 pairs of spinal nerves. The autonomic nervous system consists of the sympathetic and parasympathetic systems, which are in control of the body's automatic functions.
- The physiologic process of autoregulation helps the body regulate blood flow. When autoregulation fails to change vascular diameter in response to changes in cerebral perfusion pressure, cerebrovascular dilation is impaired and cerebral blood flow decreases.
- Hypercapnia or hypoxia lead to cerebral dilation and increased ICP. Hypocapnia leads to cerebral arterial constriction and decreased ICP.
- An infant's brain is two-thirds the size of an adult's brain. The brain grows to 80% of adult size by age 1 year.
- Head circumference can change in the infant and young child, but the head of the adolescent and adult is unyielding. This change has implications for head circumference measurement for growth and development in the infant and young child.

- The spinal cord, cranial nerves, and peripheral nerves get longer during childhood; the spinal cord terminates at L3 in the newborn and L1 to L2 in the adult.
- Myelinization of nerves begins in the third month of gestation and is completed in adolescence, as demonstrated by progressive development and coordination.
- Neurologic changes may be more subtle in the infant or child than in the adult and may be indicated by irritability or poor feeding behaviors.
- The neurologic examination assesses level of consciousness, pupil size and reaction to light, cranial nerve function, motor and sensory functions, respiratory status and function, vital signs, and head circumference.
- Different seizure types are treated with specific anticonvulsants to achieve optimal seizure control. Anticonvulsants have many side effects, which may include blood dyscrasias, liver damage, weight gain, abdominal upset, gum hypertrophy, and cosmetic changes. The CBC and liver enzyme levels should be determined routinely.
- When anticonvulsants are given IV, the most common side effect is respiratory depression. Mannitol and furosemide (Lasix) are diuretics that are used to help decrease ICP. Their effect is monitored with serum electrolyte levels and serum osmolality.
- Measures to prevent cerebral edema range from preventing trauma by encouraging the use of seat belts and helmets and teaching bicycle safety to discouraging risk taking and driving under the influence of alcohol or drugs.

- Cerebral edema is decreased by hyperoxygenating and hyperventilating the child, administering diuretics, elevating the head of the bed 30 to 45 degrees, keeping the child in good alignment so that venous drainage is not impaired, and reducing agitation and noxious stimuli.
- Abnormal posturing is an ominous neurologic sign. Flexion (decorticate) posturing refers to flexion of the upper extremities, arms, hands, and wrists. The child's legs are extended. Flexion indicates cortical damage. Extension (decerebrate) posturing refers to extended arms that are inwardly rotated and extended legs. Extension indicates damage to a greater area of the brain, theoretically extending to the brain stem.
- Impaired absorption of CSF in the arachnoid villi secondary to meningitis or subarachnoid hemorrhage is referred to as communicating hydrocephalus. Blockage of the flow of CSF through the ventricular system, most commonly related to tumor or developmental defect, is referred to as noncommunicating hydrocephalus. Changes in the brain include enlarged ventricles and ICP. If the cranial sutures are not ossified the head circumference will be abnormally large.
- Teaching for the child with a neurologic deficit and family is begun after the child's and family's needs have been assessed. The family's grieving may be verbalized; emotions and fears should be expressed and validated. The nurse reinforces information that has been supplied by other members of the health care team.

■ The nurse encourages parents in their caregiving efforts, when appropriate; assists the family in setting realistic goals for the child; and identifies support systems and refers to community agencies.

■ The nurse has family members demonstrate skills necessary for home care and encourages therapeutic play, which can promote peer contact, when possible

and appropriate. The nurse provides incentives for accomplishments and points out the child's positive qualities and coping mechanisms.

ANSWERS TO CRITICAL THINKING EXERCISE 52–1

1. The course of action is a prudent one. It is often difficult to alert large numbers of people while at the same time not creating panic. Although meningococcal meningitis can be serious in children, it is not so highly communicable that prophylaxis for the entire school would be required. For high school students, it is generally not necessary to provide prophylaxis, even to classmates. The illness is transmitted through close or intimate contact and through contact with the ill person's oral secretions. Family members and other close personal contacts should receive rifampin or ceftriaxone prophylaxis.

2. If the student were a nursery school student or in a day care setting, the risk of coming in contact with oral secretions would be higher. Kissing or sharing eating utensils can transmit the illness, so prophylaxis should be considered for the teen's girlfriend. Also, if the ill teen is a member of a sports team, prophylaxis should be considered for the other members of the team because they share water bottles during practice and games. The parents of the other students should know the signs of meningitis and be given criteria for when to call their physician. Immunization against meningococcal meningitis is available. It should be considered for college-bound students, although universal vaccination for college students is not recommended at this time.

REFERENCES AND READINGS

Austin, J. K. (1996). A model of family adaptation to new onset childhood epilepsy. *Journal of Neuroscience Nursing, 28*(2), 82–92.

Bachman, D. L. (1992). The diagnosis and management of common neurologic sequelae of closed head injury. *Journal of Head Trauma Rehabilitation, 7*(2), 50–59.

Barker, E. (1994). *Neuroscience nursing.* St. Louis: Mosby.

Baron, M. C. (1991). Advances in the care of children with brain tumors. *Journal of Neuroscience Nursing, 23,* 39.

Behrman, R. E., Kliegman, R. M., & Arvin, A. M. (1996). *Nelson textbook of pediatrics* (15th ed.). Philadelphia: Saunders.

Bernes, S. M., & Kaplan, A. M. (1994). Evolution of neonatal seizures. *Pediatric Clinics of North America, 41*(5), 1069–1104.

Burns, C. E., Barber, N., Brady, M. A., & Dunn, A. M. (1996). *Pediatric primary care: A handbook for nurse practitioners.* Philadelphia: Saunders.

Bysshi, J. (1993). Bacterial meningitis: Why vigilance must continue. *Professional Care of Mother & Child, 3,* 222.

Carno, M. (1994). Meningococcemia: Recognizing and reducing complications in pediatric patients. *AACN Clinical Issues in Critical Care Nursing, 5,* 276.

Celand, R. T. (1998). Diagnosing pediatric epilepsy: An update for the primary care clinician. *The Nurse Practitioner, 23*(3), 69.

Colantonio, A., Dawson, D., & McLellan, B. (1998). Head injury in young adults: Long term outcome. *Archives of Physical Medicine and Rehabilitation, 79*(5), 550–558.

DeRogetes, H. (1993). A different reflection . . . growing up with cerebral palsy. *Nursing Outlook, 41,* 235.

Divertie, V. C. (1996). Recurrent headaches in children. *MCN: American Journal of Maternal/Child Nursing, 21*(5), 235–240.

Dormans, J. P. (1993). Orthopedic management of children with cerebral palsy. *Pediatric Clinics of North America, 40,* 645.

Failla, S., & Todaro, A. W. (1992). Planning for a child with hydrocephalus: A guide for school nurse. *Journal of School Health, 62*(3), 107–108.

Faller, N. A., & Smith, K. (1992). Bowel and bladder management in a child. *Journal of ET Nursing, 19*(1), 36.

Fecht-Gramley, M. E. (1995). Emergency pediatric head trauma. *American Journal of Nursing, 95,* 54.

Fenichel, G. M. (1997). *Clinical pediatric neurology: A signs and symptoms approach.* Philadelphia: Saunders.

Geraci, E., & Geraci, R. (1996). A look at recent hyperventilation studies: Outcomes and recommendations for early use in the head-injured patient. *Journal of Neuroscience Nursing, 28*(4), 222–233.

Graves, C., Hayes, V. E. (1996). Do nurses and parents of children with chronic conditions agree on parental needs? *Journal of Pediatric Nursing, 11,* 288–299.

Greif, L., & Miller, C. L. (1991). Shunt lengthening: A descriptive review. *Journal of Neuroscience Nursing, 23*(2), 120–124.

Harper, J. (1988). Use of steroids in cerebral edema: Therapeutic implications. *Heart and Lung, 17,* 70.

Hazinski, M. F. (1991). *Nursing care of the critically ill child.* St. Louis: Mosby–Year Book.

Heaton, G. M., & Daddarco, J. B. (1992). Principles of intracranial pressure monitoring. *NAACOGS Clinical Issues in Perinatal and Women's Health Nursing, 3*(3), 498–504.

Herf, C., Nichols, J., Fruh, S., Holloway, B., & Anderson, C. (1998). Meningococcal disease: Recognition, treatment, and prevention. *The Nurse Practitioner, 23*(8), 30.

Hickey, J. V. (1992). *The clinical practice of neurological and neurosurgical nursing* (3rd ed.). Philadelphia: Lippincott.

Hilton, G. (1998). Pharmacologic management of seizures disorders. *Clinical Excellence for Nurse Practitioners, 2*(3), 133–139.

Hobdell, E. F. (1996). Perceptual accuracy and gender-related differences in parents of children with myelomeningocele. *Journal of Neuroscience, 27*(4), 240–244.

Kirk, E. A., et al. (1992). Effects of a nursing education intervention on parents' knowledge of hydrocephalus and shunts. *Journal of Neuroscience Nursing, 24*(2), 99–103.

Kurtz, M. J. (1993). Case study of an adolescent spinal cord injury patient. *Rehabilitation Nursing, 18,* 237.

Lascelles, M. A., Cunningham, S., McGrath, P., & Sullivan, M. (1989). Helping adolescents manage migraine headaches. *American Journal of Nursing, 89*(9), 1215–1216.

Lee, S. (1989). Intracranial pressure changes during positioning of patients with severe head trauma. *Heart and Lung, 18,* 411.

Leger, R. R., & Meeropol, E. (1992). Children at risk: Latex allergy and spina bifida. *Journal of Pediatric Nursing, 7,* 371–376.

Maria, B. L. (1999). *Current management in child neurology.* London: Decker.

Martin, J. H. (1996). *Neuroanatomy: Text and atlas* (2nd ed.). Stamford, CT: Appleton & Lange.

Merenstein, G. B., & Gardner, S. L. (1993). *Handbook of neonatal intensive care* (3rd ed.). St Louis: Mosby–Year Book.

Moore, P. C. (1988). When you have to think small for a neurologic exam. *RN, 6,* 38.

Morrison, C. (1987). Brain herniation syndromes. *Critical Care Nurse, 5,* 34.

Morrow, J. D. (1995). Treatment of the infant with myelomeningocele. *Journal of Pediatric Nursing, 10,* 99.

Paratz, J., et al. (1993). Intracranial dynamics in preterm infants and neonates. *Australian Journal of Physiotherapy, 39,* 171.

Peterson, P. M., Raven, K., Brown, J., & Cole, J. (1994). Spina bifida: The transition into adulthood begins in infancy. *Rehabilitation Nursing, 19*(4), 229–238.

Pieper, P. (1994). Pediatric trauma: An overview. *Nursing Clinics of North America, 29,* 563.

Quagliarello, V. J., & Scheld, W. M. (1997). Treatment of bacterial meningitis. *New England Journal of Medicine, 336*(10), 708–716.

Reimer, M. (1989). Head injured patients: How to detect early signs of trouble. *Nursing 89, 19,* 34.

Rekate, H. L. (1997). Recent advances in the understanding and treatment of hydrocephalus. *Seminars in Pediatric Neurology, 4*(3), 167–178.

Rising, C. J. (1993). The relationship of certain nursing activities to intracranial pressure. *Journal of Neuroscience Nursing, 25,* 302.

Roddy, S. P., Cohn, S., Moller, B., Duncan, S., Gosche, J., & Seashore, J. (1998). Minimal head trauma in children revisited: Is routine hospitalization required? *Pediatrics, 101*(4), 575–577.

Rolak, L. A. (1993). *Neurology secrets.* St. Louis: Mosby.

Samuelson, J. J., et al. (1992). Stress and coping in families of children with myelomeningocele. *Archives of Pediatric Nursing, 6*(5), 287–295.

Scheinblum, S. T., & Hammond, M. (1990). The treatment of children with shunt infections: Extraventricular drainage system care. *Pediatric Nursing, 16*(2), 139–145.

Schmitt, B. D. (1999). *Instructions for pediatric patients* (2nd ed.). Philadelphia: Saunders.

Sheth, D. P. (1997). Hypocalcemic seizures in neonates. *American Journal of Emergency Medicine, 15*(7), 638–641.

Shiminski-Maher, E., et al. (1994). Current trends in the diagnosis and management of hydrocephalus in children. *Journal of Pediatric Nursing, 9,* 74.

Shpritz, D. W. (1994). Practical points in understanding ICP. *Journal of Post Anesthesia Nursing, 9,* 357.

Silverstein, S. D. (1990). Twenty questions about headaches in children and adolescents. *Headache, 30,* 716–724.

Singh, B. V., & Roach, E. S. (1998). Diagnosis and management of headaches in children. *Pediatrics in Review, 19*(4), 132–135.

Stewart-Amedei, C. (1988). What to do until the neurosurgeon arrives. *Journal of Emergency Nursing, 14,* 296.

Swoboda, K., & Drislane, F. (1994). Seizure disorders: Syndromes, diagnosis and management. *Contemporary Therapy, 20,* 67.

Terry, D., & Nisbet, K. (1991). Nursing care of the child with external ventricular drainage. *Journal of Neuroscience Nursing, 23*(6), 347–355.

Volpe, J. J. (1995). *Neurology of the newborn* (3rd ed.). Philadelphia: Saunders.

Vos, H. (1993). Making headway with intracranial hypertension. *American Journal of Nursing, 2,* 28.

Walsh, E., & Ioli, J. (1994). Childhood near drowning: Nursing care and primary prevention. *Pediatric Nursing, 20*(3), 265.

Werdman, M. J. (1994). Pediatric drowning. *Emergency, 26,* 28.

Whiting, S. (1994). A child's first seizure: Should you treat it? *Medical Clinics of North America, 17,* 55.

Wildrick, D., Parker-Fisher, S., & Morales, A. (1996). Quality of life in children with well-controlled epilepsy. *Journal of Neuroscience Nursing, 28*(3), 192–198.

Williams, D. G., Hayes, J., & McCool, S. (1996). Shunt infections in children: Presentation and management. *Journal of Neuroscience Nursing, 28*(3), 155–162.

Wilson, W. (1993). Meningitis in childhood. *Pediatric Nursing, 6,* 23–28.

Winner, P. K. (1997). Headaches in children: When is a complete diagnostic workup indicated? *Postgraduate Medicine, 101*(5), 81–85.

Wolman, C., et al. (1994). Factors influencing self-esteem and self-consciousness in the adolescent with spina bifida. *Journal of Adolescent Health, 15,* 543.

Zickler, C. F., & Dodge, N. N. (1994). Office management of the young child with cerebral palsy and difficulty growing. *Journal of Pediatric Health Care, 8,* 111.

Ziemba, S. K. (1995). Clinical snapshot: Seizures. *American Journal of Nursing, 95,* 32.

Zimmerman, S., & Gildea, J. (1985). *Critical care pediatrics.* Philadelphia: Saunders.

53

The Child with a Psychosocial Disorder

LEARNING OBJECTIVES

After studying this chapter, you should be able to:

- Identify common characteristics of anxiety and depression.
- Identify the factors and behaviors of separation anxiety.
- Identify the factors and behaviors that correlate with childhood depression, suicide, or suicide attempts.
- Develop a nursing care plan for a child at risk for suicide or for support of the family of a child who has committed suicide.
- Discuss the symptoms, causes, risk factors for, and psychological dynamics associated with eating disorders.
- Develop a nursing care plan for a child with an eating disorder.
- Identify the primary symptoms and manifestations of attention-deficit hyperactivity disorder (ADHD).
- Develop a nursing care plan for children and families with ADHD.
- Identify signs and symptoms of various types of substance abuse.
- Describe family characteristics and social factors that contribute to physical, emotional, and sexual abuse of children.
- Identify the nurse's responsibilities for the safety and welfare of children relative to emotional, physical, and sexual abuse.
- Develop a nursing care plan for a child who has been abused.
- Develop a nursing care plan for a child who has failed to thrive.

DEFINITIONS

abuse Nonaccidental physical injury or a nonaccidental act of omission by a parent or person responsible for the care of a child; may include physical injury, sexual molestation, neglect, or emotional injury.

comorbidity The simultaneous co-occurrence of two different but interactive conditions in a single individual.

double message A verbal message that contradicts the underlying tone or meaning of the message.

substance abuse Excessive or inappropriate use of medication to modify mood or behavior or in a manner that results in social, occupational, psychological, or physical problems, or in a situation that creates a physical hazard.

substance addiction Physical or psychological dependence on a substance, with continued use even when it is known to impair cognitive or social functioning.

substance dependence A physical or psychological craving for a chemical substance, the cessation of which causes withdrawal symptoms.

suicide Voluntary and intentional cessation of one's life.

suicide attempt Any actions taken by an individual toward self that will result in death if not interrupted.

suicide gesture A suicide attempt that is undertaken primarily to get attention rather than to actually take one's life; nonetheless, it is still considered a serious behavior.

suicide threat A statement or behavior that usually occurs prior to overt suicidal activity.

violence The use of extreme force or a destructive action that results in injury, discordance, or outrage, or engaging in sudden intense activity to the point of loss of control.

Overview of Childhood Psychopathology

Neurobiologic, family, and sociocultural factors can contribute to the development of psychosocial disorders in children. Neurobiologic factors are briefly reviewed here; family, social, and cultural factors are discussed in the text in conjunction with the various disorders presented.

Neurobiologic Factors

For disorders with a psychological basis, the primary organ involved is the brain, together with chemicals produced and used by the brain to initiate specific actions. These actions include memory, learning, attention and concentration, mood, and cognition. Because the brain develops throughout childhood, significant changes in the anatomy and physiology of the brain also occur. The most significant changes affecting psychosocial development include myelinization, growth of new tissue, and extension of the neural system throughout the brain. (See p. 1466 for a review of brain anatomy and physiology.)

The brain increases in tissue mass and size throughout childhood and adolescence. The increase in the size of the brain results in an increased potential for memory and complex cognitive reasoning, as well as the capacity to learn new skills and acquire new information. Cognitive development proceeds from the simple to the complex, and from the concrete to the abstract.

The effect of brain damage depends on several factors. One of the most significant factors is the maturational stage of the brain at the time the damage occurs. Early damage spares more language functions but may cause changes in all subsequent areas of development related to the specific area of brain that is injured. Another factor is the length of time the brain tissue is impaired (as a result of swelling, hemorrhage, or tissue destruction). Finally, the specific area of the brain that is damaged may determine the specific areas of deficit. One factor that is not directly related to actual tissue damage but is clearly related to effects on behavior is the individual's perception of an experience, which is encoded in the brain's memory system and used as a basis for later behaviors.

Manifestations of Psychopathology

Psychosocial disorders are responses to stress and may be manifested as disturbances in feeling (e.g., depression, anxiety), in body functions (e.g., encopresis, enuresis), in behavior (e.g., conduct disturbance, school avoidance, or

Psychosocial Disorders Typically Manifested in Childhood

- Mental retardation (see Chapter 54)
- Pervasive developmental disorders, autistic disorder
- Learning disorders: reading, arithmetic, and other skills
- Disruptive behavior disorders: attention-deficit hyperactivity disorder, conduct disorder, oppositional defiant disorder
- Anxiety disorders: separation anxiety disorder, post-traumatic stress disorder, phobias, obsessive-compulsive disorder
- Mood disorders: depression, bipolar disorder
- Eating disorders: anorexia nervosa, bulimia nervosa, pica, obesity, rumination disorder of infancy
- Tic disorders: Tourette disorder, chronic motor or vocal tics, transient tics
- Elimination disorders: functional encopresis, functional enuresis (see Chapters 43 and 44)
- Communication disorders: receptive or expressive language disorders, cluttering, stuttering, elective mutism

Data from American Psychiatric Association. (1994). *Diagnostic and statistical manual of mental disorders* (4th ed.). Washington, DC: Author; Johnson, B. S. (1995). *Psychiatric-mental health nursing*. Philadelphia: Lippincott.

passive-aggressive behaviors), or in performance (learning problems). The manner in which an individual responds to stress depends on multiple factors.

INDIVIDUAL RESPONSES TO STRESS
Factors that influence responses to stress include

- Temperament
- Developmental level
- The nature and duration of the stress
- Past experiences
- Coping and adaptive abilities of the family

Diagnostic Evaluation

Diagnosing psychosocial disturbance in a child is difficult, for several reasons. First, young children normally exhibit a wide range of emotional and social behaviors. Even through adolescence, the individual is maturing and developing in terms of coping skills, attitudinal responses, and perspective. During childhood, there is marked inconsistency and unpredictability in behavioral responses to various situations. Also, during examinations, both the child and the adolescent are markedly affected by their relationship and level

Mental Status Examination of Children

- Appearance: dress, gestures, posture, tics, or other repetitive movements; physical presentation, such as age, stature, race, age-appropriate behaviors
- Ability to attend to task
- Mood or affect: predominant feelings, mood fluctuations, mood congruence with verbalizations
- Manner of relating to the examiner: exploration of their understanding of the purpose of the interview, approach or avoidance behaviors, use of play materials available, verbalizations
- Intellectual skills: problem-solving abilities, conceptualization of causality, body image, memory, judgment, general fund of knowledge, insight (findings are compared with developmental norms)
- Capacity for imaginative thinking and play
- Sensorimotor development: fine and gross motor skills, symmetry and coordination of movement, hand and eye dominance, right-left discrimination
- Perceptions and thought content: presence or absence of suicidal-homicidal ideation, intent, plan; delusions or illusions; hallucinations
- Speech: fluency, tone, volume, age appropriateness

Common Laboratory and Diagnostic Tests for Psychosocial Disorders in Children and Adolescents

- **Urine tests:** Used to assess for specific drugs excreted by the kidneys.
- **Blood and serum tests:** Used to assess the long-term effects of malnutrition, evidence of specific drugs or ingested chemicals, and the potency of selected pharmacotherapeutic agents prescribed for symptom reduction.
- **Radiographs of the skull and long bones:** Frequently used to identify current and previous fractures, which are common signs of physical abuse.
- **Genital and anal examinations:** Performed by a physician and used, together with slides of secretions, to help determine whether sexual abuse has occurred.
- **Measurement of subcutaneous tissue:** May be ordered if physical neglect associated with malnutrition is suspected.

of comfort with the examiner and by the setting. Finally, children and adolescents are affected and shaped by their relationships with parents and other social figures. For a thorough assessment of psychosocial disorders, a structured mental status examination of the child must be completed. Various laboratory and diagnostic tests may also be appropriate. The results of these tests will help determine whether pharmacologic intervention may be effective.

Pediatric nursing includes a number of disorders and conditions that are best viewed as psychosocial disorders, as they primarily involve the way in which the child or adolescent relates to others and copes with stress. Most psychosocial disorders have a familial or biologic predisposition that may be triggered if the environment is demanding or unsupportive. Physical stressors such as birth defects, physical injuries, and chronic illness may produce psychosocial disorders. Emotional stressors such as inconsistent or contradictory child-rearing practices, marital conflict, or neglect may also contribute to psychiatric disorder development. Some psychosocial disorders, such as fragile X syndrome, are inheritable disorders. Other disorders are primarily related to an inaccurate or inappropriate relationship between the child and significant others in the social environment. Research consistently shows that psychosocial disorders are caused by a combination of predisposing or inherent factors and environmental or interactional factors.

Anxiety and Depression

Mood or affective disturbances in children and adolescents are generally of two types: anxiety or depression. It is difficult to differentiate between anxiety and depressive disorders in children, for several reasons. In children and adolescents, the behavioral presentation of both disorders may be similar. For example, the child who is anxious may be withdrawn, tearful, unwilling to engage in play, or prone to acting aggressively toward others. These same symptoms typically occur in children who are depressed. Moreover, it is often difficult to differentiate between normal mood changes secondary to normal developmental maturation and adaptation and abnormal, persistent mood disturbances. Generally, however, mood disturbance is more intense and persistent and interferes with social relations and daily functioning. Finally, the child or adolescent may have both anxiety and depression.

Anxiety Disorders

Anxiety is one of the most common categories of psychopathology in childhood. Anxiety is expected and normal in children at specific times in development. For example, infants and children up to preschool age often show intense distress at times of separation from their parents or family members. It is not uncommon for young children to have short-lived fears related to darkness, storms, animals, and imaginary situations. Whereas school-age children typically express anxiety or fear of bodily harm or potentially real worries (thunder and lightning), adolescents may exhibit anxiety regarding social situations and acceptance. When worry and distress become overwhelming and begin to interfere with daily functioning, anxiety becomes pathologic and warrants serious intervention.

SEPARATION ANXIETY AND SCHOOL REFUSAL

The essential feature of separation anxiety is disabling anxiety about being apart from one's parents or away from home (American Academy of Child and Adolescent Psychiatry [AACAP], 1997). It may develop spontaneously or under stress (e.g., in temporal relation to a move or a death in the family) and may last for several years, waxing and waning. These children frequently fear that if they are apart from their parents, harm will come to the parent or themselves. Separation anxiety occurs in approximately 4% of children and young adults (American Psychiatric Association [APA], 1994).

Persistent reluctance or refusal to go to school or elsewhere may be the primary reason why families seek intervention. Unlike truants, who are relatively fearless and avoid school to pursue other interests, children with separation anxiety stay home or attempt to remain with their parents. The child may complain of physical symptoms, cry, plead, or even exhibit panic symptoms shortly before time for school approaches, but the symptoms subside after the child is allowed to stay home, only to reappear the next morning. Sometimes the child may simply refuse to leave the home.

School refusal may also be related to a *social phobia*, whereby individuals avoid social or performance situations to such a degree that their daily routine is affected (e.g., by refusing to participate in physical education exercises or by failing to raise their hands to ask a question in class). School refusal is also discussed in Chapter 7.

OTHER ANXIETY DISORDERS

In addition to separation anxiety, anxiety disorders present as other specific disorders. Anxiety may be so intense that the child experiences a sense of panic, in which case the disorder may be termed *panic disorder*. One type of panic disorder that follows a specific and terrifying event is *posttraumatic stress disorder*. Symptoms of this disorder include intense fear, helplessness, or horror, along with physiologic symptoms of increased arousal. The individual demonstrates persistent avoidance of stimuli associated with the traumatic event. This disorder is frequently seen in children who have been sexually or physically abused. Obsessive-compulsive disorder may manifest in children as in adults as intrusive, unwanted thoughts that create mounting tension that is relieved only by repetitive, compulsive actions. These acts are designed to relieve the anxiety the child usually realizes is irrational.

Depressive Disorders

Depressive disorders are also varied and are specified according to the intensity or duration of depressive symptoms or the particular behaviors displayed by the individual. Children or adolescents who exhibit a depressed or irritable mood for at least 1 year meet the criteria for *dysthymic disorder*. If the child experiences chronic, fluctuating mood disturbances for 1 year, *cyclothymic disorder* or *bipolar mood disorder* may be diagnosed. If the clinical presentation includes a 2-week (or longer) episode of depressed or irritable mood in addition to disturbances in appetite, sleep, psychomotor activity, energy, or self-esteem, the child meets the criteria for *major depressive disorder*. A psychiatric nursing text should be consulted for more detailed information about these specific disorders.

Psychophysiology

Research supports the view that both anxiety and depression have a biologic basis. Among the biochemical agents that appear to modulate mood are monoamines, including catecholamines and indolamines, and neurotransmitters, such as norepinephrine, serotonin, and acetylcholine. The limbic region in the brain is considered to be the seat of emotions, and chemical or physical alterations in this region have been found to affect mood as well as some other characteristics, such as energy, self-valuation, and sleep patterns.

Etiology

Affective disorders have been shown to have a genetic basis. Having a first-degree relative with an anxiety or depressive disorder may predict an increased risk of the disorder in offspring. A family history of suicide or depression (particularly parental) is a significant risk factor (Lombroso, Pauls, & Leckman, 1994; U.S. Public Health Service [USPHS], 1997).

Psychosocial theories emphasize the importance of the interaction within the family system, behavioral patterns of the individual, and interpersonal factors in the development of depression. There is evidence that children and adolescents with a history of verbal, physical, or sexual abuse, frequent separation from or loss of loved ones, incarceration, pregnancy, lower socioeconomic status, homosexuality, chronic illness, behavioral disorders, and dysfunctional families are more likely than peers with healthy family patterns to develop anxiety or depressive disorders (Brage, Campbell-Grossman, & Dunkel, 1995; Donnelly, 1998; USPHS, 1997).

Incidence

Current epidemiologic information about anxiety disorders indicates that 7% to 15% of individuals younger than 18 are affected (Costello & Angold, 1995).

The incidence of major depression and dysthymic disorder is estimated at 1% in preschoolers, 2% in school-age children, and 4% to 15% in adolescents (AACAP, 1998; Bowers, 1998; Brage et al., 1995). Bipolar disorder occurs in approximately 1% of adolescents, but retrospective studies suggest a higher incidence (Lewinsohn, Klein, & Seeley, 1995). Bipolar disorder develops in 20% to 40% of children and adolescents with depressive disorders (AACAP, 1998).

Manifestations

The clinical manifestations of anxiety or depressive disorders include sad or irritable mood, diminished interest in daily activities, significant weight loss or gain, insomnia or hypersomnia, psychomotor agitation or retardation, and fatigue or loss of energy. Feelings of worthlessness, hopelessness, or excessive guilt, as well as diminished ability to think or concentrate, are exhibited. Somatic complaints, such as recurrent abdominal pain or headaches, with no physical cause are common. Recurrent thoughts of death or suicide are sometimes reported.

Therapeutic Management

Antidepressants, particularly selective serotonin re-uptake inhibitors (SSRIs), are frequently prescribed for anxiety and depressive disorders. The most effective treatment, however, combines medication and the child's and family's exploration of situations and environmental factors that are related to the child's symptoms. Individual and family therapy are essential for children with suicidal ideation or persistent mood disturbances. It is common for both anxiety disorder and mood disorders to recur. Social skills training or group therapy may be most helpful for social anxiety. School phobia is treated by insisting that the child attend school, offering interventions during school time to reduce anxiety symptoms, and refusing to pick up the child from school, even if the child insists. This form of intervention is a type of desensitization therapy. Other strategies for decreasing anxiety or depressive symptoms include relaxation therapy, distraction strategies, self-talk, or cognitive strategies, as well as support from adults or friends who are safe and reassuring.

NURSING CARE

The Child with Anxiety or Depression

Assessment

A thorough history should be obtained from the child and the family. Initially it may be necessary to interview the child in front of the parents, but once the child becomes more comfortable with the nurse, time alone with the child should be offered. The interview should cover both the child's mood and events related to those moods, physiologic symptoms, patterns of daily activities, identification of stressors, and information about the duration, frequency, and intensity of symptoms. Suicidal ideation or plans should be assessed by asking both direct and indirect questions.

Questions about the family environment should seek to identify those with whom the child relates most easily as well as family interaction patterns. It is important to explore any family history of mood disturbance, as well as other emotional problems or substance abuse problems.

Several self-reporting instruments and interview schedules are available for the specific assessment of anxiety and depression. They are used to assess and quantify progress or regression of treatment.

Nursing Diagnosis and Planning

The following nursing diagnoses apply to the child with anxiety or depression:

- Ineffective Individual Coping related to loss of energy, sleep disturbance, biochemical imbalance, or loss of control.
  Expected Outcome: The child will display adaptive ability to attend to activities of daily living.
- Self-Esteem Disturbance related to cognitive distortions,

inability to manage daily events, and a sense of hope-lessness or guilt.

Expected Outcome: The child will relate an increase in self-confidence and an increase in positive feelings about self.

- Risk for Violence: Self-Directed, related to suicidal ide-ation, guilt, or hopelessness.

Expected Outcome: The child will report a decrease in the frequency or severity of depressed or anxious moods.

- Sleep Pattern Disturbance related to anxiety, depression, and inactivity.

Expected Outcome: The child will express feelings of being well rested and show no signs of sleep deprivation (e.g., irritability, lethargy, restlessness).

Interventions

The nurse is part of a team that offers support for the entire family while exploring the factors that contribute to the emotional distress in the child. The nurse should identify specific changes in the environment and interaction pat-terns that could support a sense of control and positive re-gard for the child. Privacy and space for the child or family members to discuss their feelings as treatment progresses should be made available on a regular basis.

If the child needs hospitalization, admission will gener-ally be to a psychiatric unit where specialized nursing is available. Mood disturbances often are identified on pediat-ric units, in outpatient clinics, or in school systems. Educat-ing parents and teachers about depression and anxiety in childhood is an important service for nurses to provide to the community.

Evaluation

- Does the child report feeling happier, less sad, or less upset?
- Does the child exhibit normal patterns of eating and sleeping?
- Does the child exhibit an energy level that allows for interactions, play, and work?
- Does the child seem interested in people and events?
- Does the child communicate positive statements about self?

Suicide

Suicide is the third leading cause of death among adoles-cents between 15 and 19 years old and the sixth among children 5 to 14 years old (USPHS, 1997). Parents often underestimate the severity of warning signs, particularly de-pression, substance abuse, or other psychological disorders, until a child actually attempts suicide or succeeds. Risk fac-tors for suicide are depression, a family history of psychiatric disorders (especially depression and suicide), and previous attempts. Other significant risk factors are chronic medical illness, family violence, substance abuse, poor impulse con-trol, poor school performance, homosexuality, and access to firearms in the household (AACAP, 1998; Woods, Lin, Middleman, et al., 1997).

Psychopathology

Most adolescent suicide attempts are impulsive; however, any verbalization or gesture of suicide should be taken very

> ### CRITICAL TO REMEMBER
> #### Threats of Suicide
>
> A suicide gesture or threat should *never* be ignored. The child should be encouraged to discuss the thought specifically in order to determine if there is a plan and the lethality of the plan. Help should be obtained from qualified health professionals.

seriously. It is estimated that two thirds of adolescents who attempt suicide have high intent and a strong wish to die. The motive may be a desire to influence others, gain atten-tion, communicate love or anger, or escape a difficult or painful situation (Kienhorst, deWilde, Dielestra, et al., 1995).

The development of a concept of mortality and death follows the general laws of the development of cognitive and affective abilities, from the concrete to the abstract. Up to age 6, it is unlikely that a child has any realistic concept of death or looks for it in an active way. There are children as young as 3 years of age, however, who have tried to com-mit suicide and apparently understood what they were do-ing. Between ages 6 and 8, children abandon an egocentric view and discover that death is one of many events out of an individual's control. From age 9 on, the child begins to view death as inevitable and universal.

Etiology

Underlying depression and poor self-concept appear to be the most significant factors contributing to suicide, regard-less of age or sex. Long-standing family dysfunction is gener-ally present, with emotional detachment and isolation be-tween family members. The suicide victim is typically a vulnerable individual who, under stress, seeks and finds a way to die. The individual is for some reason unable to elicit adequate adult support to stop the suicide process.

Incidence

Estimates of the prevalence of suicidal *ideation* are 19% in males and 23% in females. The prevalence of *suicide attempts* is 5% in males and 13% in females. For completed suicides, the male-female ratio is 5:1 (Centers for Disease Control and Prevention, 1995). The higher incidence of completed suicides in males may be related to the more violent meth-ods of suicide used by boys. It is common for suicides to occur in a cluster within a community.

Of significant importance, gay and lesbian youths are two to three times more likely to attempt suicide than their heterosexual peers. Suicide is the leading cause of death in this group, which accounts for 30% of teen suicides (Garofalo, Wolf, Kessel, et al., 1998).

Manifestations and Risk Factors

The risk of suicide should be considered if the following are present:

- Suicidal clues, such as cryptic verbal messages, giving away of personal items, and changes in expected patterns of behaviors (e.g., sudden calmness in a normally anxious teenager)
- Specific statements about suicide or self-harm
- Preoccupation with death, often manifested by an interest in death themes in literature and art
- Frequent risk-taking or self-abusive behaviors
- Use of alcohol or drugs to cope
- Overwhelming sense of guilt or shame
- Obsessional self-doubt
- Open signs of mental illness manifested as delusions or hallucinations
- Significant change or a major life event that is internally disruptive
- History of physical or sexual abuse
- Homosexuality, especially if the teen discovers same-sex orientation early in adolescence, experiences violence due to homosexual identity, or is rejected by family members as a result of sexual orientation (Hammelman, 1993).

Therapeutic Management

Suicide prevention is viewed as the most significant mental health contribution and is promoted at local, state, and federal levels. Prevention is offered through multimedia educational presentations in schools, through support groups at local mental health centers, through community emphasis on stress reduction, through social affiliations, and through networking with support systems.

Screening for depression, both at school and in the health care system, is one of the most significant prevention strategies. Most individuals who commit suicide have offered at least veiled information about their suicidal ideation or feelings of despair to classmates, teachers, or health care providers.

Following a child's suicide, counseling services must be provided to family members and immediate friends of the child. It is important that these services be offered quickly, preferably within the first 24 hours after the suicide, and that counselors remain available for a year following the event. Grieving and emotional adjustment often take several months and may peak around the anniversary of the suicide event.

Children or adolescents with persistent suicidal ideation should undergo a thorough psychiatric evaluation by a mental health professional. The child may need pharmacotherapeutic agents, such as antidepressants or antipsychotic medications. The use of medications in children and adolescents at risk for suicide requires close monitoring and allocation in small doses, because they could be used in a suicide attempt or act.

NURSING CARE

The Child or Adolescent at Risk for Suicide

Assessment

The risk of suicide is best assessed using a systematic approach to behaviors, attitudes, and risk factors. Several in-

Questions to Assess Suicide Potential

1. Have you ever thought of trying to hurt yourself? How might you do this?
2. Have you ever thought of killing yourself? How might you do this?
3. Have you known anyone who has committed suicide? When did this occur? What was it like for you?
4. Do you have access to firearms? Knives?
5. Do you ever do things to deliberately place yourself in danger, such as driving when you are drunk or playing Russian roulette with a gun?
6. Have you ever told anyone about wanting to kill yourself?
7. Have you ever been hospitalized for suicidal behavior?
8. How do you feel right now?

struments have been developed to assess lethality and potentiality, which lessens the likelihood of overlooking contributing factors. The instruments are similar and explore risk factors, stressors, lethality of method, coping mechanisms, and support systems. Subtle symptoms of depression or anxiety, such as decreased energy or persistent restlessness, should also be considered. It is important to explore thought content and organization, awareness and expression of feelings, perceived level and types of stress, perceived availability of support resources, prior suicidal behaviors, and medical status.

Nursing Diagnosis and Planning

The following nursing diagnoses apply to the child or adolescent at risk for suicide:

- Risk for Self-Directed Violence related to a desire to cease emotional pain, to solicit the attention of others, or to avoid responsibility.
  Expected Outcome: The child or adolescent will use effective communication techniques to express needs and feelings and verbalize that there are solutions to problems.
- Self-Esteem Disturbance related to a sense of failure and hopelessness about the ability to change self or circumstances.
  Expected Outcome: The child or adolescent will elicit the necessary support from others to meet the needs of attention, belonging, and worth.
- Anxiety related to current or anticipated events.
  Expected Outcome: The child or adolescent will recognize own anxiety and will use effective coping mechanisms.
- Altered Family Processes related to relational disturbance or possible abuse or neglect.
  Expected Outcome: The child or adolescent and family will mobilize support systems in an effective manner to reduce the likelihood of another suicide decision.
- Ineffective Individual Coping related to a sense of despair or limited availability of support.
  Expected Outcome: The child or adolescent and family will develop a suicide prevention plan.

Interventions

The approach to therapy should be empathic and nonjudgmental to decrease the child's or adolescent's sense of isolation and rejection. The nurse should adopt a voice and demeanor that are clear, direct, and supportive. Being emotionally and physically available, offering opportunities to discuss feelings and the suicidal event, and removing potentially harmful objects will help protect the youth from self-injury.

The nurse should suggest different coping strategies, such as choosing alternative activities when impulses arise and remaining near other people. The nurse can help the child identify specific feelings and effective ways to manage those feelings. It is important for the nurse to assess how closely a child needs to be monitored throughout the day, realizing that the potential for self-harm fluctuates.

To allow a balance between the need to explore personal issues and the need for social support, anticipatory guidance related to grieving for families of suicidal or potentially suicidal individuals is best provided on both an individual and a group basis. Grieving will occur even if the suicide attempt was unsuccessful. Individual and family therapy will also provide an opportunity to explore contributory factors that can be altered to reduce the suicide potential. Working with the parents, together with other therapeutic team members, will help the parents regain their ability to assist their child and manage the home environment. It is important to increase the adult-child interactions, thereby decreasing the risk of another suicide attempt.

Evaluation

- Is the child or adolescent able to identify times when suicidal potential is greatest and to seek help during these times?
- Does the child or adolescent participate in activities that reduce feelings of despair and hopelessness?
- Does the child or adolescent display evidence of positive self-esteem?
- Is the family able to identify warning signs of suicidal risk?
- Does the family support one another?
- Has the child or adolescent developed coping mechanisms?

Eating Disorders: Anorexia Nervosa and Bulimia Nervosa

Eating disorder is a general term that encompasses anorexia nervosa, bulimia nervosa, pica, obesity, and rumination disorders. Anorexia nervosa and bulimia nervosa are the two most common eating disorders in children (obesity is discussed in Chapter 7). Anorexia and bulimia have overlapping features and similar causes, which supports viewing these disorders as a continuum.

Anorexia nervosa is characterized by a deliberate refusal to maintain adequate body weight, a distorted body image, and amenorrhea (in females). The term anorexia is a misnomer, as the individual rarely experiences loss of appetite. *Bulimia nervosa* is characterized by recurrent episodes of binge eating; a sense of lack of control over eating binges;

self-induced vomiting or excessive use of laxatives, diuretics, or emetics to prevent weight gain; and a persistent overconcern with body image. Children and adolescents with eating disorders typically report shame and guilt about many life experiences, but especially eating.

Individuals with severe eating disorders have a mortality rate up to 20% from complications of the disorder or from suicide (Comerci, 1999). Treatment resistance is very high in individuals with anorexia and bulimia, because all of their psychological and sociologic experiences are framed by their body image and self-esteem and because of secondary gains such as attention, admiration, envy, and control over others through eating patterns. Unfortunately, in addition to the eating disorder, about 50% of these children and adolescents also meet criteria for other serious psychiatric disorders, such as major depression or a personality disorder.

Ritualistic behaviors are common in these children and adolescents, particularly around issues of food. For example, the child or adolescent may eat only at a particular time of day, eat foods only in a certain order, or insist on washing all foods before eating them. The rituals are often an attempt to control the portions, fat content, or nutrients ingested. The rituals also serve to enhance the individual's sense of control over food or dietary intake.

The child or adolescent will go to extreme measures to prevent others from becoming aware of the weight loss or lack of food intake. They may ingest large amounts of water or insert heavy objects in the vaginal cavity prior to weighing in order to give the impression of weight gain. The child or adolescent may eat in front of people and then go to the bathroom to purge themselves after the meal.

Etiology

Disordered eating emerges from multiple risk factors. One of the most salient factors appears to be enmeshed family relationships in which the child is considered to be an extension of the parent or is viewed as a means of meeting the parents' needs rather than being allowed to develop as an autonomous individual. The disorder is more common among sisters and mothers of those with the disorder than in the general population, suggesting some familial predisposition.

The development and severity of the individual's risk for eating disorders appear to be related to the child's re-

---

PATHOPHYSIOLOGY
• • • • • • • •
of Eating Disorders

Frequently, impaired carbohydrate metabolism in the hypothalamic-pituitary axis is noted in individuals with an eating disorder. The conversion of thyroxine (T_4) to triiodothyronine (T_3) is inadequate. Phosphate concentrations are inadequate, especially in patients with severe anorexia complicated by bulimic episodes. Individuals with eating disorders commonly experience hypokalemia, hypochloremia, hyponatremia, alkalosis, dental enamel erosion, parotid and salivary gland enlargement, decreased transferrin levels, and malabsorption complications.

sponse to biologic maturity and to the psychological and social demands of sexual development. Other significant risk factors are earlier pubertal maturation and higher body fat, depressive tendencies, concurrent psychological disturbance, alterations in brain neurotransmitters, subsequent eating problems, cultural expectations to be thin, and the individual's pervasive sense of ineffectiveness (Graber, Brooks-Gum, Parkoff, et al., 1994; Jarry & Vaccarino, 1996).

Individuals with eating disorders usually have a family history of affective disorders. The family dynamics for male anorexics are reported to include poor father-son relationships, with the father typifying the strong, cultural image, and a mother who is overinvolved, overprotective, and overdependent on the mother-son relationship.

Incidence

Bulimia nervosa appears to be more prevalent than anorexia nervosa, with as many as 2% to 8% of the female adolescent population reporting symptoms. For girls between the ages of 12 and 18 years, the reported incidence of eating disorders of some type is approximately 1 in 1,000. Eating disorders are rarer in boys; only 1 in 10 individuals with an eating disorder is male.

Manifestations

ANOREXIA NERVOSA

The hallmark of anorexia nervosa is the refusal to maintain a body weight that exceeds the minimal weight recommended for height (15% below expected weight). Intense preoccupation with and unrelenting fear of obesity and a disturbed body image (weight, size, or shape) that is obviously contrary to reality (Fig. 53–1) are also observed. Other clinical manifestations in females include at least three missed menstrual periods (primary or secondary amenorrhea), a misperception of internal and external stimuli, particularly food-related cues, such as hunger; overwhelming feelings of ineffectiveness and inadequacy; lanugo, dry or flaky skin, and dull, brittle hair; and fatigue and muscle wasting.

Boys with eating disorders demonstrate many behavior patterns similar to girls', including weight loss through excessive dieting, compulsive activities, and purging to get strong or to develop an athletic build (rather than to be thin, as reported by females).

BULIMIA NERVOSA

The clinical manifestations associated with bulimia nervosa include recurrent episodes of binge eating; a sense of lack

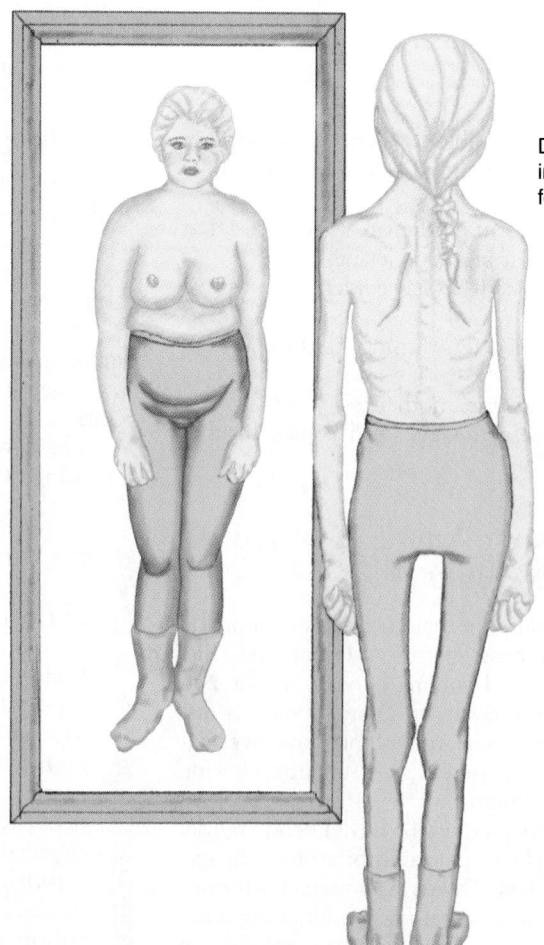

Distorted body image results in extreme need to control food intake.

Amenorrhea
Lanugo
Fatigue
Constipation
Dry, flaky skin
Severe caries
Dull, brittle hair
Muscle wasting

FIGURE 53–1

In anorexia nervosa, the adolescent refuses to maintain adequate body weight, partly because of a distorted body image: she perceives herself as overweight when in fact she is below minimum weight.

of control over eating behaviors during binges; and strategies that prevent weight gain (self-induced vomiting; use of laxatives, diuretics, or emetics; fasting; vigorous and excessive exercise). A minimum of two binge eating episodes per week for at least 3 months and persistent overconcern with body shape and weight are also common factors. These individuals are also at increased risk for tooth erosion secondary to the effects of acidic content on the teeth from the subsequent vomiting.

Diagnostic Evaluation

An electrocardiogram and chest radiograph are typically obtained if symptoms of bradycardia, hypotension, or hypothermia are noted. Complete liver and renal function tests, thyroid function tests, and serum electrolyte studies are usually included in the medical workup.

Therapeutic Management

The treatment of eating disorders initially focuses on the secondary effects of self-induced vomiting, excessive use of diuretics and laxatives, and insufficient nutrients to sustain the function of body systems. Electrolyte levels and body chemistry values should be stabilized to prevent sustained damage to body systems, especially the cardiac, respiratory, and gastrointestinal systems. Adequate caloric intake is the next major goal of treatment and often requires strict patient monitoring to prevent sabotage of medical treatment. Ongoing intensive and highly individualized therapy helps the adolescent cope with complex issues. Finally, alteration of misperceptions about body image and a reorientation to issues of control and self-management are necessary. Follow-up therapy for the individual and family is indicated for a period of several months to 3 years.

NURSING CARE

The Child or Adolescent with an Eating Disorder

Assessment

Children and adolescents with eating disorders typically have varying degrees of mistrust, ambivalence, and denial. It is generally better if the assessment is conducted in a structured and concrete manner (rather than as an open-ended exploration), with an emphasis placed on alliance building and periodic review of the assessment process for the child or adolescent. Determining motivations for changing behaviors is crucial, and motives should be assessed for each specific behavior (i.e., weight gain, induced vomiting, altered self-perception of body). A mental status examination should also be included, as the side effects of restrictive dieting can impair cognitive functioning and perpetuate affective disturbances. Any history of self-injury should be noted. The nurse should assist the child or adolescent in gaining an understanding of impulse control problems and ritualistic and compulsive behaviors.

The medical history and physical assessment should be comprehensive, focusing on any medically based illness that mimics an eating disorder or exists concomitantly. Psycho-

logical assessment of body image and identification of problems, substance abuse, and social support systems utilized by the adolescent are important components of the assessment. A family history of eating disorders or other psychiatric illnesses should be noted. Family dynamics, including level or quality of interaction, support, discipline, and differentiation of members, should be explored in depth. Previous treatment attempts and coping strategies should also be identified.

Nursing Diagnosis and Planning

The following nursing diagnoses apply to the child or adolescent with an eating disorder:

- Altered Nutrition: Less Than Body Requirements, related to inadequate intake, malabsorption from extended periods of starvation, or distorted body image.
  Expected Outcome: The child or adolescent will gain sufficient weight or maintain an adequate weight to sustain systemic homeostasis and physiologic health.
- Anxiety, Fear, or Powerlessness related to weight gain, sense of self-inadequacy, and lack of control over body and self.
  Expected Outcome: The child or adolescent will demonstrate the ability to seek help with anxiety management and will demonstrate improved coping strategies, including open expression of feelings.
- Risk of Activity Intolerance or Sleep Pattern Disturbance related to fatigue, depression, and an excessive drive to exercise and expend energy.
  Expected Outcome: The child or adolescent will establish improved sleeping and activity patterns with a corresponding improvement in affect, energy, and sense of well-being.
- Fluid Volume Deficit related to excessive use of diuretics or laxatives and/or inadequate fiber and fluid intake.
  Expected Outcome: The child or adolescent will have electrolyte levels that are within normal limits, normal skin turgor, and moist mucous membranes.

Interventions

Children and adolescents with severe eating disorders may need to be hospitalized to achieve physiologic stability. These children are then generally transferred to a day treatment program. Care focuses on restructuring cognitive perceptions, reducing opportunities to engage in ritualistic and self-injurious behaviors, and re-establishing physiologic homeostasis. The programs typically include interventions that enlist the adolescent's cooperation in a refeeding program. Nutritional consultation is provided to facilitate gradual weight gain. Intake and output, weight gain, vital signs, laboratory values, electrolyte status, and cardiac status are carefully monitored.

Support in exploring refeeding sensations of fullness, bloating, and delayed gastric emptying and help tolerating these feelings and body sensations is important. The nurse and adolescent jointly participate in monitoring affect, mood, and potential for suicide. They also agree to a contract specifying necessary interventions to ensure safety, as well as to monitor daily food intake and feelings. These interventions may take the form of interacting with the staff at regular intervals or agreeing to approach the staff if suicidal ideation is present. The nurse will need to validate the adolescent's feelings of ambivalence, fear, and powerlessness. If hyperalimentation or nasogastric tube feedings are needed for adequate nutritional intake, the nurse should support the adolescent and monitor feedings. Finally, the nurse should provide educational information about the short- and long-term effects of starvation.

The nurse is likely to participate in providing or supporting psychological treatments, such as individual, group, and family therapy sessions. Especially in the early phase of treatment, the adolescent may be very resistant to efforts to increase nutritional intake and may resort to denial, trickery, or manipulation to prevent a weight increase or thwart adherence to dietary regimens. It may be necessary to observe the adolescent following meals to prevent episodes of purging.

The family should be informed and involved in treatment goals and progress. Participation in family therapy is generally a required part of the treatment plan, as the cause may be directly related to family interactional patterns. The nurse should support the family in voicing concerns while encouraging them to view the adolescent as having an independent identity and sense of control.

Evaluation

- Does the child or adolescent demonstrate an increase in food consumption adequate to sustain growth and developmental needs?
- Has the child or adolescent reduced bingeing or purging activities?
- Can the child or adolescent demonstrate a positive alteration in self-perceptions and body image, as evidenced by verbalizing an increased sense of self-control and decreased anxiety about the present and the future?
- Does the child or adolescent demonstrate a decrease in ambivalence and mistrust about self and significant others?
- Does the child show increased energy and display appropriate affect?
- Are electrolyte levels within normal limits and mucous membranes moist?

Attention-Deficit Hyperactivity Disorder

Attention-deficit hyperactivity disorder (ADHD) is the most common chronic behavioral disorder of children and accounts for 50% of the children seen in child psychiatric clinics (Cantwell, 1996). ADHD is associated with significant problems in three specific areas: (1) attention and concentration, (2) impulse control, and (3) overactivity. Over the years it has variously been called postencephalitic behavior disorder, restlessness syndrome, hyperkinetic impulse disorder, minimal brain dysfunction, and hyperactive child syndrome. There is increasing evidence that developmental failure in brain circuitry underlies the impulsivity and hyperactivity, or poor response regulation and inhibition (Barkley, 1997).

Referrals for ADHD may be made by parents or teachers. Of concern are not only the primary symptoms, which often result in frequent injuries, poor scholastic performance, and low performance motivation, but also the associated symptoms, which may include anxiety or depression, aggressiveness toward peers, and antisocial or oppositional defiance toward authority figures.

A single individual affected with ADHD may exhibit wide variations in response to the environment. For example, a child with ADHD is likely to perform poorly on a highly complex task. If the structure is rigid or if behavior is severely restricted, the child with ADHD becomes increasingly frustrated and distinguishable from unaffected children. If instructions are repeated frequently or if the task is novel or unfamiliar, the child's performance tends to improve. Immediate reinforcement is very important because these children require much higher rates of reinforcement than their same-age peers. Fatigue may also affect the degree to which ADHD symptoms are exhibited.

Etiology

ADHD occurs more commonly in first-degree biologic relatives of people with the disorder than in the general population, which suggests a genetic predisposition for the disorder. Other central nervous system abnormalities, such as the presence of neurotoxins and epilepsy, or other neurologic disorders are thought to be predisposing factors, although less than 5% of children with ADHD have definitive neurologic findings. Chaotic or abusive environments may predispose to the appearance of ADHD.

Incidence

Estimates of the incidence of ADHD range from 1% to 20%, but the general consensus is that 3% to 5% of children are accurately diagnosed with ADHD. Symptoms generally occur early in childhood, with the mean age at onset 3 or 4 years (Kendall, 1997). Sex ratios also vary, but a 6:1 boy-girl ratio is most often cited for clinic-referred samples. In epidemiologic studies the male-female ratio is approximately 3:1 among nonreferred children displaying these symptoms. Aggressive and antisocial behaviors are thought to explain the higher rate of referrals of boys.

Manifestations

The child with ADHD typically exhibits the following manifestations (APA, 1994):

- Fidgeting with hands or feet; squirming in seat
- Easily distracted by internal or external stimuli

PATHOPHYSIOLOGY

of Attention-Deficit Hyperactivity Disorder

Inconclusive but consistent evidence indicates that the basis of ADHD is a sluggish or underreactive neurologic, electrophysiologic response to stimulation. Prefrontal and limbic system connections in the brain are viewed as the likely locations for neurologic functional abnormalities. The most likely neurochemical transmitter associated with ADHD appears to be dopamine, brain levels of which are decreased.

- Difficulty awaiting turns in games or group situations
- Blurting out answers to questions before the questions have been completed
- Difficulty following through on instructions from others, even when instructions are clearly understood
- Difficulty sustaining attention in tasks or play activities
- Shifting from one uncompleted activity to another
- Difficulty playing quietly
- Talking excessively
- Interrupting or intruding on others
- Seeming not to listen to what is being said
- Losing things necessary for tasks or activities at school or at home (pencils, books, clothes, assignments)
- Engaging in physically dangerous activities without considering the possible consequences, but not for the express purpose of thrill seeking

Diagnostic Evaluation

Although high-resolution magnetic resonance imaging (MRI) and blood and urine studies of metabolites of brain neurotransmitters have been performed in individuals with ADHD, none of these tests has provided consistent information. The diagnosis of ADHD is currently established on the basis of reports by the client, parent, and teacher. The behaviors and symptoms of ADHD must be present in two out of three areas—home, school, or social situations—to support the diagnosis. These reports are coupled with psychological assessments conducted while the child is completing tasks requiring vigilance, attention, and concentration, as well as those involving delayed gratification. Clinical interviews may be coupled with clinical trials of psychopharmacologic agents, such as methylphenidate (Ritalin) or dextroamphetamine (Dexedrine), to determine the child's behavioral response.

Therapeutic Management

The goal of therapeutic management is to reduce the frequency and intensity of unsocialized behaviors. This requires achieving a balance between the child's temperament and environmental demands, expectancies, and supports. Therefore, treatment interventions must be targeted at enhancing the child's capabilities and self-esteem. Expectations that may be appropriate for a child without ADHD— "he should be able to sit still in school for 40 minutes," or "she should be able to handle 1 hour of homework"—may need to be modified for the child with ADHD. In every case, the nurse should work with the parents to modify the environment and develop strategies that foster competencies in the child. Most clinicians combine psychopharmacotherapy with behavior-oriented family therapy to achieve alterations in the child's internal functioning and external environment. Stimulant medications commonly used as part of the treatment plan include Ritalin, Dexedrine, and Adderal. Psychostimulants are most effective when used in conjunction with behavior and psychosocial therapy.

Some parents and professionals prefer more conservative approaches, such as dietary changes; however, researchers have concluded that food additives and sugars do not have significant clinical influences on most children with ADHD (Cantwell, 1996). Medication is typically adminis-

tered during the school day, but it has become increasingly recognized that attention, concentration, and alertness are needed for any learning task, such as learning to play baseball or learning to drive a car. The side effects and potency of the medications used to treat ADHD often make parents and physicians hesitant to administer medications other than during critical learning periods.

NURSING CARE
The Child with Attention-Deficit Hyperactivity Disorder

Assessment

The nurse should document the typical behavior of the child playing alone and with other children, during mealtimes, and while the parent is on the telephone or occupied with chores. The length of time it takes the child to bathe or dress and how often the child becomes distracted during these tasks are also explored. These behaviors are then compared to those exhibited when the child is engaged in highly stimulating activities and activities with frequent feedback, such as video and computer games. The child's behavior is also compared during novel versus routine activities.

The child's developmental and family history is explored in detail, with the nurse noting the age at which the child began to exhibit independent behaviors such as walking, getting out of bed alone, and exploring the environment. It is not uncommon for children with ADHD to explore the environment at an early age, with only limited need to return to the caregiver for support or approval. Family members diagnosed with ADHD or who exhibit similar behaviors are noted. Parents should be given self-report inventories, such as the Child Behavior Checklist, Conners Teacher Rating Scale—Revised, or the School Situations Questionnaire, to complete and return to the appropriate professional.

Observation within the home or school setting is likely to generate the most valid information, as the clinic environment may be unfamiliar and, by the nature of the disorder, may inhibit the child's natural tendency to explore, become distracted, or display limited motivation in task completion.

Nursing Diagnosis and Planning

The following diagnoses apply to the child with ADHD and the child's family:

- Impaired Social Interaction related to impulsivity, poor self-management skills, and aggressive behaviors. *Expected Outcome:* The child will improve impulse control and ability to sustain attention on tasks.
- Risk for Injury related to impulsivity, limited judgment skills, or excessive need for mobility and stimulation. *Expected Outcome:* The child will remain safe from injury as a result of adequate supervision and the provision of safe ways to meet the child's need for increased activity and movement.
- Ineffective Family Coping: Compromised or Disabling, related to the need for consistent and close supervision of the child, hyperactivity of the child, or social stigma of having a child with impulsive or aggressive behaviors.

Expected Outcome: The family will discuss the child's needs and a plan to provide the needed support.

■ Knowledge Deficit related to perceptions that the child is willfully defiant or disobedient in following directions or in limit testing.

Expected Outcome: The family will discuss the child's disease and display an understanding of the disease process and treatment.

Interventions

The primary nursing intervention for the child with ADHD is to teach the family about the disorder. Emphasis is placed on reducing the parents' blame and guilt about the child's problems and altering their perceptions that the child intentionally misbehaves or lacks motivation to learn or achieve. Teaching demonstrates ways to provide frequent positive reinforcement. Also, instruction about medications is important for both parents and child, as well as the adaptations in environment that are needed to allow the child to practice new skills.

The nurse may facilitate communication between the family and the school about ways to accommodate the child's shortened attention span and increased need for mobility and frequent breaks. Often cognitive-behavioral therapy, provided by a specially trained professional, is helpful in identifying specific exercises that can reduce bothersome traits. Support groups for parents can help families cope with the child with ADHD and modify their interactions with and expectations of the child.

Ordinarily, positive effects of medication are seen within 1 to 2 weeks when medication is taken as prescribed. It is common for the family to observe a rapid change in the child's behavior and experience relief as manifestations subside. Ongoing support is required because this disorder is lifelong and progress in self-control and behavioral patterns is usually slow. Parents may need to be actively involved in dispensing medication, even through adolescence, because children fluctuate in their willingness to comply with therapy. Affected children also may have difficulty remembering to take the medication because of the attentional deficits characteristic of the disorder.

Evaluation

- Does the child comply with the cognitive strategies designed to increase self-control, as evidenced by a decrease in impulsivity?
- Does the child comply with the pharmacologic regimen, which is aimed at increasing the child's ability to attend and concentrate at school or in attention-demanding situations?
- Does the child complete school assignments in less time than formerly, with less distractibility?
- Does the child demonstrate increased skill in peer relations, as evidenced by fewer conflicts and more frequent positive statements to and about peers?
- Does the family demonstrate acceptance of the child and the special needs of the child?
- Does the family demonstrate an increased acceptance of the child's condition as a medical problem, rather than a social or behavioral problem?
- Does the family provide a safe and supportive environment within the home, as evidenced by adequate super-

- - - - - - - - - -
Phases of Substance Abuse
PHASE 1: EXPERIMENTATION

The drug is taken to see what it does, or to appease peers.

PHASE 2: EARLY DRUG USE

A specific drug or various drugs are used with some regularity for their pleasurable effects or to reduce anxiety. Social use of drugs typically falls into this category.

PHASE 3: TRUE DRUG ADDICTION

Drugs are used regularly, and physical dependence begins if it is characteristic of the drug. Social functioning revolves around a drug focus.

PHASE 4: SEVERE DRUG ADDICTION

The physical condition of the addict deteriorates. All activities are related to obtaining or using the drug, with isolation from nondrug culture.

vision and opportunities for meeting the child's mobility needs in a safe manner?
- Does the family comply with the medication regimen?

Substance Abuse

Chemical agents that are typically abused by children and adolescents include alcohol, hallucinogens, sedatives, analgesics, anxiolytics, steroids, and stimulants. The substance abused depends on its availability and cost, as well as on social influences and parental behaviors or tolerance of drug use. Most professionals differentiate between *substance abuse* and *substance addiction.* However, the basic treatment concerns are similar. Substance abuse is generally considered to increase over time.

Etiology

Productive analysis of substance abuse considers risk factors, which include social, personal, and familial factors. Substance abuse and substance dependence tend to cluster in families, with clinical evidence of genetic influences. For alcohol as for most other drugs, there also is some evidence that substance abuse often represents the individual's attempt to cope with anxiety generated by impaired social

PATHOPHYSIOLOGY
- - - - - - - - -
of Substance Abuse

The primary effect of substance abuse is on the brain and residually on the rest of the body. The actual action depends on the type of substance used, as substances act in accordance with their specific chemical composition. For example, alcohol affects the entire brain by decreasing its responsiveness.

TABLE 53-1

Commonly Abused Drugs and Their Effects

Drug	Expected Behaviors/Effects	Special Considerations
Tobacco	Chronic cough, wheezing, increased phlegm production, atherosclerosis	Considered a gateway drug; initial use usually begins in elementary school
Alcohol	Amount-related effects include euphoria followed by depression or hostility, decreased inhibitions, impaired judgment, incoordination, and slurred speech	Considered a gateway drug; easily accessible
Marijuana	Relaxation, mild euphoria, loss of inhibition, decreased motivation, red eyes, dry mouth	Considered a gateway drug
Opiates	Euphoria, elation, pain relief, detachment and apathy, drowsiness, constricted pupils, constipation, slurred speech, impaired judgment	Long-term apathy about self, often leading to physical malnutrition and dehydration; criminal behaviors associated with obtaining drugs likely to occur; infections at injection sites common
Barbiturates	Similar to those associated with alcohol	Often used in conjunction with stimulants; may have a paradoxical effect of hyperactivity in children
Amphetamines	Euphoria, hyperactivity, agitation, irritability, insomnia, weight loss, tachycardia, hypertension	May have a paradoxical effect of depression in children
Cocaine	Euphoria, elation, agitation, hyperactivity, irritability, pressured speech, grandiosity, tachycardia, hypertension diaphoresis, anorexia, weight loss, insomnia	Psychotic behavior possible if the dose is large; can be fatal if combined with other drugs
Hallucinogens	Distorted perceptions, heightened awareness, hallucinations, illusions, depersonalization, dilated pupils, hypertension, increased salivation	Psychotic behaviors, panic flashbacks long after drug use ceases, self-destructive behaviors
Phencyclidine hydrochloride (PCP)	Euphoria, distorted perceptions, agitation, violence, antisocial behaviors, hypertension, increased salivation, increased pain response	Panic, irrational behaviors, psychosis

skills, low self-esteem, poor interpersonal relationships, or lack of adaptive behaviors. Some psychosocial disorders, such as ADHD, depression, and conduct disorder, are associated with an increased risk of substance abuse.

Incidence

Great variation exists in the types of substances abused across sex and age (Table 53–1). Typically, boys consume alcohol more than girls do. Female junior high school students are increasing their use of tobacco, whereas tobacco use by their male counterparts has remained consistent.

Based on findings from the 1998 national survey of nearly 50,000 students, the National Institute on Drug Abuse concluded that illicit drug use appears to be decreasing after 6 years of steady increase. Declines in use of marijuana, amphetamines (speed, crystal meth), hallucinogens (LSD, MDMA or ecstasy), and inhalants were significant. Use of heroin, cocaine, tranquilizers, alcohol, and tobacco remains the same (Johnston & Buchanan, 1998).

Illicit drug use, including alcohol and tobacco, remains high despite reports of declining use among adolescents.

Daily cigarette smoking among 12th graders was over 22% in 1998, with Caucasians accounting for the highest percentage (41.7%) and African-Americans the lowest (14.9%). It is estimated the 90% of adolescents have tried alcohol by the time they reach adulthood. Experimentation with marijuana, the most widely used illicit drug, is reported in nearly a quarter of 8th graders and approximately half of 12th graders (AACAP, 1998; Johnston & Buchanan, 1998). Research consistently supports the hypothesis that

CRITICAL TO REMEMBER

Risks for Substance Abuse

Family systems that are closed to outsiders, that have a history of psychiatric disturbance, including substance abuse, or that have poor communication skills are at risk for creating an environment in which substance abuse in youth is perpetrated.

drug use progresses from beer or wine to cigarettes or hard liquor and then marijuana, followed by other illicit drugs (Chatlos, 1996). These substances are sometimes referred to as gateway substances.

Public awareness and emphasis on treatment and prevention seem to be working, even though they had very limited impact on teenagers in the 1990s. An awareness of the possibility of substance abuse is the responsibility of the parent, teacher, and health professional. Knowing the clinical behavioral manifestations of substance abuse is essential, and much information is readily available to adults interested in prevention and early identification.

Manifestations

The clinical manifestations of substance abuse are marked by increased antisocial behavior as the desire for social conformity and acceptance decreases and the need for the substance increases. Behaviors that may indicate substance abuse problems include irregular school attendance, low grades or poor school performance, aggressive or rebellious behavior, excessive dependence on peer influence, and deterioration of relationships with family members or former friends. Rapid or extreme changes in behavior or mood and loss of interest in hobbies, sports, or other favorite activities are often observed. Lack of parental support and supervision, as well as changes in eating or sleeping patterns that increase as manipulative behaviors increase, especially those that are related to the need to acquire desired substances, may also be involved.

Therapeutic Management

Treatment in a center specifically designed for substance abuse is recommended and includes individual, group, and family therapy. Participation in Alcoholics Anonymous or Narcotics Anonymous is advocated. These organizations also offer support groups geared toward helping family members with programs that promote alterations in the family system that may decrease the likelihood of relapse.

NURSING CARE
The Child or Adolescent with a Substance Abuse Problem

Assessment

Physical assessment should include evaluation of the adolescent's respiration rate, heart rate, blood pressure, activity

---

CRITICAL TO REMEMBER

Relapse Among Substance Abusers

Substance abusers' rates of refusal to adhere to therapeutic recommendations, together with resulting relapses, are quite high. More than 50% of those completing a course of treatment continue to abuse substances throughout their lifetimes.

---

level (hyperactive or hypoactive), mood, affect, judgment, speech, sensory responses, and memory. A thorough history of current and past drug use should be obtained. A family and social history, a medical history, and a legal history (e.g., past and current charges related to substance abuse) should be obtained.

Nursing Diagnosis and Planning

The following diagnoses apply to the child or adolescent with a substance abuse problem:

■ Altered Thought Processes related to the specific effects of the particular substance involved.
  Expected Outcome: The child or adolescent will maintain orientation to time, place, and person.
■ Sensory/Perceptual Alterations related to the specific effects of the particular substance involved.
  Expected Outcome: The child or adolescent will not experience falls or other injuries related to sensory or perceptual changes.
■ Anxiety related to a decrease in sense of control over self or the environment.
  Expected Outcome: The child or adolescent will express increased feelings of self-worth and the ability to change behavior.
■ Ineffective Individual Coping related to limited development of effective social interactions and problem-solving skills.
  Expected Outcome: The child or adolescent will identify current stressors leading to substance use or abuse.
■ Impaired Social Interaction related to anxiety or limited social skills.
  Expected Outcome: The child or adolescent will identify alternative activities, people, and social situations that promote nonuse of abuse substance.
■ Self-Esteem Disturbance related to limited social skills, ineffective coping skills, or a poor sense of self-management.
  Expected Outcome: The child or adolescent will replace substance abuse with more appropriate social skills and develop meaningful relationships with nonabusing peers and family members.

Interventions

The nurse's responsibilities in caring for children or adolescents with substance abuse problems depend on the severity of the abuse and the treatment goals. If the nurse is the first to encounter the abuse, notification of the family and referrals for treatment should be initiated. If the youth has been identified as a substance abuser and referred to a treatment facility, the nurse's primary responsibility will be to stabilize the adolescent's physiologic status and support recommendations for treatment. Explaining the expectations and the types of service offered is important, because most treatment programs increase adolescent and family responsibilities over time.

Initially, maintaining safety and an optimal level of physical comfort is necessary, especially if detoxification is required. This includes close observation, removal of any potentially dangerous items, and monitoring vital signs. Being readily available to discuss thoughts, concerns, and perceptions is important to create an emotional sense of safety.

Additional interventions include educating the child or adolescent and family members about necessary laboratory tests and providing ongoing information about the nature of substance abuse.

Another significant nursing intervention is to assist the child or adolescent and family in developing social support systems and refer them to appropriate resources that can offer additional support as they make long-term changes in their social and emotional patterns of relating. It is also essential to help the youth assume responsibility for the substance abuse problem, rather than passing the blame on to others. Providing emotional support for the youth and family as they develop insight into their behaviors and the need for changes is important because these changes are often difficult to affect.

The relapse rate among youthful substance abusers is extremely high, and success in a short-term treatment program is not necessarily an indicator of long-term control. The incidence of relapse is generally reduced if the child and family maintain active, long-term involvement in support groups such as Alcoholics Anonymous, Ala-Teen, Ala-Tot, and Narcotics Anonymous. Tough Love support groups for parents may also be beneficial in providing counsel and support.

Evaluation

- Has the child or adolescent remained substance free?
- Does the child or adolescent demonstrate an increased sense of self-confidence?
- Has the child or adolescent assumed responsibility for changing behaviors related to the substance abuse?
- Does the child or adolescent show improvement in peer and family relationships?
- Is the child or adolescent participating in daily activities?
- Is the child or adolescent able to identify stressors and use appropriate coping mechanisms?
- Has the child or adolescent remained injury free secondary to sensory or perceptual changes?

Child Abuse

Child abuse includes emotional abuse, physical abuse, and neglect, as well as sexual exploitation or molestation by caretakers or other individuals.

Physical Abuse and Neglect and Emotional Abuse

ETIOLOGY

Family dysfunction underlies most forms of child abuse. The family profile varies with the type of abuse, although it is

---

CRITICAL TO REMEMBER

Denial of Abuse

It is common for the abuser, the noninvolved parent, and the child to deny the abuse. Each may deny the event, awareness of the event, impact of the event, or any responsibility for the event.

Characteristics of the Abusive Family

- Isolation from community and social groups
- Intense competition for emotional resources within the family, such as affection, attention, and nurturance
- Low levels of differentiation among family members
- Low trust for outsiders and family members
- Unpredictable and unstable family environment
- Conflict resolution generally achieved through aggression or power struggle between family members
- Present focus and crisis-oriented actions for immediate gratification
- Communication often characterized by mixed or double messages, threats, or a focus on nonverbal communication rather than direct verbalization
- Family roles that are typically fixed and traditional, with rigid rules
- Frequent domination by a single family member who maintains control through manipulation, intimidation, deceit, and aggression

---

not uncommon for multiple types of abuse to exist in a single family. Generally, the dysfunctional family dynamics are multigenerational and involve both parents.

Socioeconomic factors also appear to influence the incidence and etiology of child abuse, with increased child abuse observed during periods of economic hardship or external stress. The typical perpetrator is a direct relative of the child, usually the parent (77%) or primary caretaker, is under age 40 (80%), and is female (66%) (National Committee to Prevent Child Abuse [NCPCA], 1997). Often this individual has limited coping skills and was abused as a child or teenager. The typical profile of an abused child is more difficult to determine. Some research indicates that the typical abused child is less than 5 years old, often has mild physical abnormalities, is developmentally or physically delayed, has a difficult temperament, or reminds the abuser of someone else. A parent is 100 times more likely to kill a stepchild than a biologic child.

INCIDENCE

In the past 10 years, child abuse reports to Child Protective Services (CPS) have increased 45%. This increase has been attributed to the public's, teacher's, and clinician's increased awareness and willingness to report, rather than to an actual increase in prevalence (NCPCA, 1997).

In 1996, almost 1 million children were identified as victims of substantiated abuse or neglect. Of those identified, 52% suffered from neglect; 24% were physically abused; 12% were victims of sexual abuse; and 3% were abused emotionally. The national rate of victimization is 15 per 1,000 children (NCPCA, 1997).

Approximately 1,000 children died from maltreatment in 1996. Seventy-seven percent were less than 5 years old, and 45% were less than 1 when they died (Daro & Wang, 1997).

MANIFESTATIONS

Physical Indications of Abuse.   Physical indicators of abuse include unexplained bruises or welts that appear in various stages of healing, often in clustered patterns that

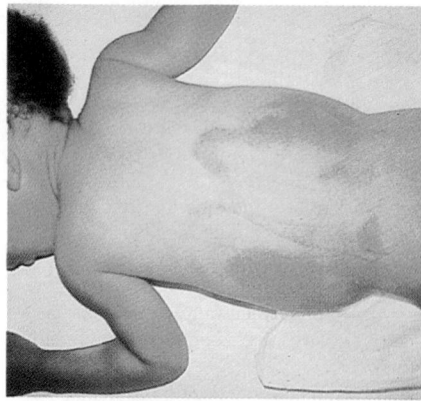

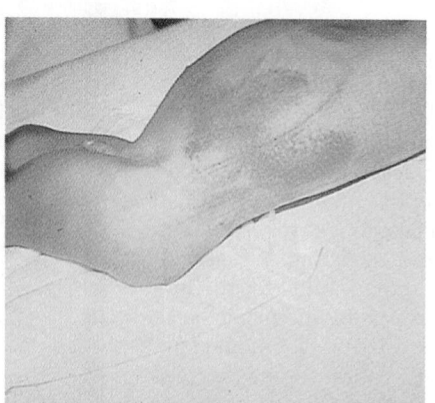

Nonaccidental distribution of bruises—All four surfaces of the mid-body are involved, but there are no bruises on arms and legs.

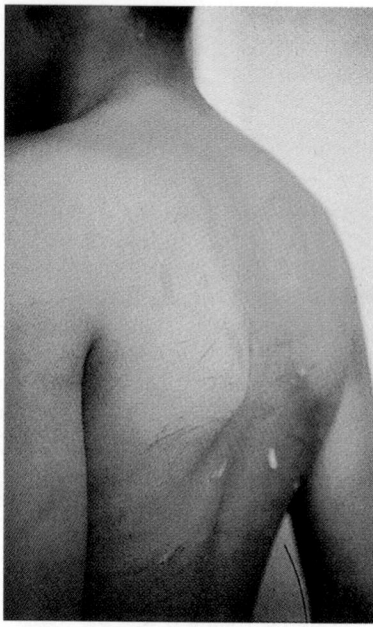

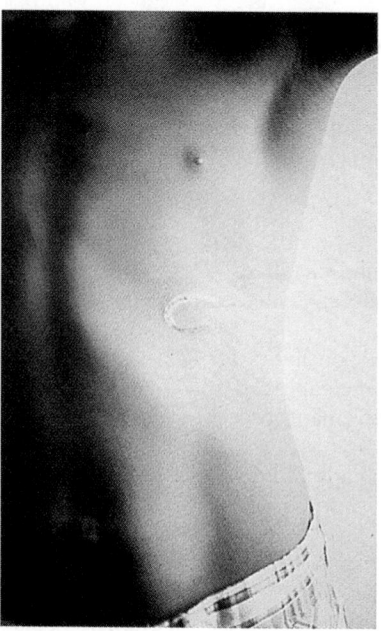

Pattern of injury—Linear scars of various ages indicate repeated abuse using a switch or whip. The loop pattern on the boy's anterior torso is consistent with a looped electrical cord used as a whip.

Scald burn of shoulder and neck—The typical distribution of a scald burn in a toddler. This type of injury occurs when a toddler pulls a cup of coffee or pan of water off a stove.

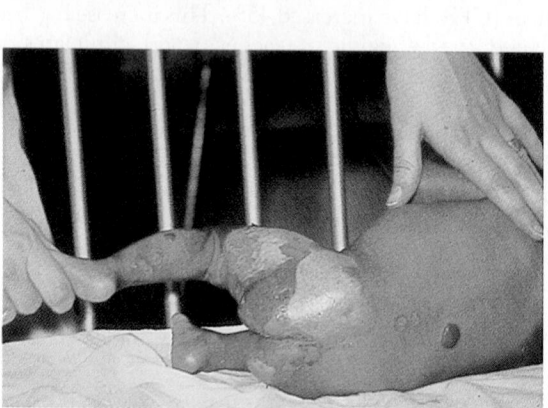

Nonaccidental immersion scald—Involvement of virtually the entire posterior surface of the legs indicates that the legs were held under scalding water; even an infant this young would flex the knees to avoid the hot water.

FIGURE 53–2
· · · · · · · · · · ·
Physical signs of child abuse. The nurse should be alert for the typical behavioral indicators of abuse. (Courtesy of Barbara Tenney, M.D. From Henry, M. C., & Stapleton, E. R. [1992]. *EMT: Prehospital care* [p. 675]. Philadelphia: Saunders.)

reflect the shapes of the articles used to inflict injury, and unexplained burns, especially on the soles, palms, back, or buttocks; immersion burns may be seen (sock-like, glove-like, or doughnut shaped) on buttocks or genitals (Fig. 53–2). Other signs may include infected burns, which indicate a delay in seeking treatment, and bald patches on the scalp. Unexplained fractures of the skull, nose, or facial structures or multiple or spiral fractures or dislocations, as well as numerous fractures in various stages of healing, are also significant.

Behavioral Indicators of Abuse. Behavioral indicators of abuse include a child's wariness in response to adult contact, apprehension when others cry or lack of crying when approached by a stranger or examiner, and fear of parents or of going home. Extreme aggressiveness or withdrawal, vacant or frozen stares, monosyllabic responses to questions, and lying very still when surveying surroundings may be observed. A capacity to engage only in superficial relationships, manipulative behaviors to get attention, inappropriate or precocious maturity, and indiscriminate seeking of attention may also be reactions to abusive situations.

Physical Indicators of Neglect. Children suffering from neglect will probably show inadequate weight gain for age, poor growth pattern, and failure to thrive. They may exhibit constant hunger, poor hygiene, wasting of subcutaneous tissue, and bald patches on the scalp, and they may be dressed in clothes that are not seasonally suitable (e.g., no coat or shoes in winter). Reports of lack of supervision for long periods of time, permission to engage in unsafe activities, or abandonment may also accompany a neglected child.

Behavioral Indicators of Neglect. A child who begs or steals food, has inconsistent school attendance or comes very early and stays very late at school, or is constantly fatigued or listless in class may be exhibiting the effects of neglect. Other behavioral indicators of neglect include assuming adult responsibilities or roles, alcohol or substance abuse, and delinquency.

Physical Indicators of Emotional Abuse. Children who have been emotionally abused may exhibit speech disorders, lags in physical development, failure to thrive, or hyperactive and disruptive behaviors.

Behavioral Indicators of Emotional Abuse. Behavioral indicators of emotional abuse may include habit disorders (sucking, biting, rocking), conduct or learning disorders, overly adaptive or compliant behaviors (withdrawal, aggression). Neurotic traits including sleep disorders, inhibition of play, and unusual fearfulness, as well as psychoneurotic reactions such as hysteria, obsession, compulsions, phobias, and hypochondriasis, are also observed. Suicide attempts may also be indicative of emotional abuse.

Shaken Baby Syndrome

Shaken baby syndrome is a widely recognized form of child abuse that is caused by vigorous shaking of the infant held by the extremities or shoulders. This type of physical abuse leads to whiplash-induced intracranial and intraocular bleeding. There is generally no external sign of head trauma, which makes this syndrome difficult to detect. The most common trigger of severe shaking is crying, especially if the child is colicky. Shaken baby syndrome should be considered in infants who present with failure to thrive, seizures, apnea, respiratory irregularities, coma, or vomiting associated with drowsiness or lethargy (Chiocca, 1995; Kelley & Beauchesne, 1998).

Munchausen Syndrome by Proxy

Munchausen syndrome by proxy is the most difficult form of child abuse to diagnose. It is often inflicted by the mother or primary caretaker. The caretaker falsifies illness in the child through simulation or production of illness and then takes the child for medical care, claiming no knowledge of how the child became ill. The most common reasons these caretakers give for seeking medical treatment are bleeding, seizures, central nervous system depression, apnea, diarrhea, vomiting, fever, and rash. Long-term mortality in these cases is as high as 15%. Under the supervision of other adults, the child exhibits no symptoms and may appear normal and healthy. The parent's behavior reflects a serious disturbance that requires specialized psychiatric treatment and removal of the child from the parents' care. A multidisciplinary team is the best approach to diagnosing this disorder (Krugman, Wilson, & Krugman, 1998).

Sexual Abuse

INCIDENCE

Victims of sexual abuse are usually between 6 and 9 years old at the onset of the abuse. The accepted ratio of three females to every male, however, may represent less than the actual incidence for boys.

Children often cope with sexual victimization through an accommodation syndrome, in which the coping mecha-

---

> ### CRITICAL THINKING EXERCISE 53–1
>
> Matthew, age 2, is brought to the emergency department by his mother, Mrs. Jackson, and her boyfriend. Mrs. Jackson tells the nurse that Matthew has been crying and holding his arm since she picked him up at the baby-sitter's earlier in the evening. Upon further questioning, Mrs. Jackson states that "Matthew is all boy. You have to watch him every minute or he is into something. He is constantly climbing and falling."
>
> Upon examination the nurse notes several bruises on Matthew's right leg and right arm. He also has a small abrasion on his nose. Mrs. Jackson is holding Matthew and seems concerned, as does her boyfriend. Matthew quiets when his mother holds him and drifts off to sleep. Mrs. Jackson's boyfriend leaves the room and returns with a snack for both Matthew and Mrs. Jackson. He offers to hold Matthew.
>
> 1. What are some of the possible reasons Matthew is crying and holding his arm? Support your assumptions with rationales.
> 2. If the nurse suspects child abuse, what added assessments should be performed?
> 3. What legal responsibility does the nurse have in cases of suspected child abuse?

nisms become the child's normal behaviors in response to an abnormal event. There is nothing the child can do to prevent the abuse. The initial strategy involves secrecy because the child realizes the situation lacks social acceptance. This awareness dominates the child's sense of self, and the child experiences a great deal of guilt. The guilt may be intensified by the child's ambivalence about pleasure that may be experienced during the event. The secrecy is typically reinforced by threats that the child, the perpetrator, or another loved one will "get into trouble."

The second behavioral response arises from the child's sense of helplessness. The child feels responsible for holding the family system together and feels isolated from peers because of shame and guilt, so the child plays possum, pretending to be asleep or unaffected by the sexual abuse. This is the child's attempt to manage the intrusion experienced.

In order to cope with an enduring sense of entrapment, the child takes responsibility for the abuse. This strategy involves minimizing the pain, because as long as the child is accessible, the molestation continues. Almost universally, sexually abused children believe that the reason the abuse continues is because they are bad, rather than placing the responsibility on the perpetrator.

Sexually abused children often dissociate during the abuse to avoid feelings or physical pain. Frequently the child will make veiled attempts at disclosure or will delay disclosure in order to keep the abuse secret and avoid the risk of alienating significant others. The child fears that the consequences of revealing the abuse will be worse than keeping the secret. In fact, most sexually abused children keep the abuse secret throughout their lives, unless there is some intervention from outside the abusive system. Finally, the sexually abused child typically retracts the revelation of abuse once it has been made, out of fear of ridicule, retaliation, attending court, or losing contact with a loved one.

MANIFESTATIONS

Physical Indicators of Sexual Abuse. The sexually abused child may exhibit difficulty walking or sitting; torn, stained, or bloody underclothing; pain, swelling, or itching of genitals; and pain on urination. Additional physical signs include bruises, bleeding, or lacerations involving the external genitalia, vagina, or anal area, and vaginal or penile discharge. Sexually transmitted disease, poor sphincter tone, and excessive masturbation may also be present.

◀ Note the communication techniques designed to reassure the child and give the child some power. The little girl is not immediately positioned for a genital examination. The physician first sits to talk with the child at her eye level and makes eye contact with her.

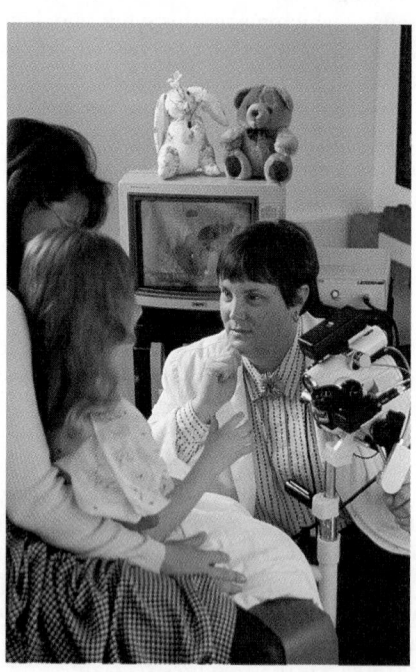

Drawings may help to identify the abused ▶ child and assist in therapy. Art can also help the child express what cannot be expressed in words.

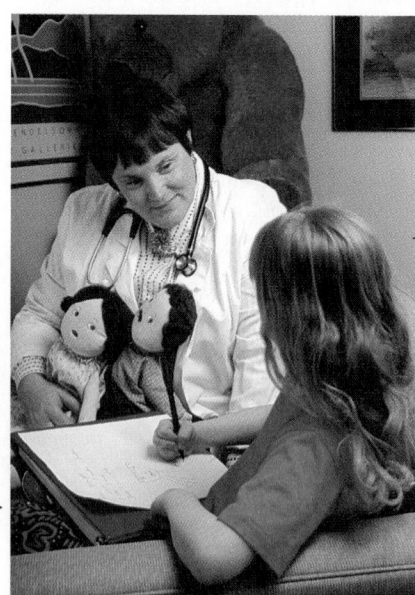

FIGURE 53–3

Disclosure of abuse may be slow because the child often has difficulty trusting any adult. Identification of sexual abuse requires particular sensitivity, as physical examination of the child's genitals to detect signs of injury or sexually transmitted disease can be frightening for the child, who associates handling of the genitals with pain or shame. Anatomically correct dolls are often used in the assessment of abuse within a family. These dolls help children express what they cannot express in words; young children in particular have a limited vocabulary to use when describing the events that have occurred. (Courtesy of Cook Children's Medical Center, Fort Worth, Texas.)

Behavioral Indicators of Sexual Abuse. The sexually abused child may demonstrate an unwillingness to change clothes or participate in gym activities; withdrawal, fantasy, or infantile behavior; or bizarre, sophisticated, or unusual sexual behavior or knowledge. Promiscuity, poor peer relations, delinquency or running away, depression or suicidal ideation, gestures, or attempts are often observed. These behaviors may coincide with aggression, a change in school performance, or sleep disturbances or nightmares. Additionally, eating disturbances (obesity, anorexia, bulimia), self-destructive behaviors (substance abuse, self-mutilation), and sexual acting out toward a younger child are sometimes present.

NURSING CARE
The Abused Child

Assessment

The nurse should conduct a thorough evaluation for skin integrity, including examination of the scalp, bottoms of the hands and feet, front and back of the trunk, and genitals. A baseline measurement of height and weight should be obtained, along with documentation of the birth weight for infants. An assessment of the child's anxiety level, ability to relate to the examiner, and emotional tone is also crucial. In addition, an assessment of the family support system, including patterns of interaction, belief systems, and social support systems, should be conducted.

During the physical assessment, information about bruises, injuries, and sexual abuse should be requested in a nonemotional, matter-of-fact manner with particular attention to the child's need for privacy and dignity. Comments made by the child should be written down verbatim, since disclosure of abuse is often subtle, and this information may be used in legal proceedings at a later time. Assessment should include an account of written or verbal contact with teachers, relatives (including both parents, siblings, and grandparents), and others who have been involved with the child over an extended period of time.

Trust may be enhanced by answering questions directly and specifically, assuming a nonjudgmental and supportive stance throughout all interactions, and acting as an advocate for the holistic care of the child as well as of the family. Recognition of the child's low self-esteem, feelings of inadequacy, and fear will enable the nurse to relate in a manner that is supportive. The child will need encouragement to make self-care decisions and to discuss thoughts and feelings, which may have been repressed in order to survive the trauma (Fig. 53–3). The child may also feel affection for the perpetrator and believe that the abuse is a necessary part of the relationship.

When sexual abuse is suspected, the child and parent should be interviewed in the same manner as described for physical abuse. The nurse should observe for clinical manifestations of sexual abuse in a manner that provides dignity and respect for both the child and the parent. Assessment tools are available that identify behaviors typical of the child who has been sexually abused.

Nursing Diagnosis, Planning, Intervention, and Evaluation

Nursing Diagnosis	■ Altered Parenting related to immaturity, lack of knowledge, apathy on the part of parental caregivers, or limited or negative past parenting experience.
Expected Outcome	• The family will express an understanding of positive parenting models and will respond to the child's needs in a timely and appropriate manner.

Intervention	Rationale
1. Assess the parents' strengths and weaknesses, normal coping mechanisms, and the presence or absence of support systems. Special attention should be paid to the following: a. Expectations with regard to the child b. Comforting behaviors c. Response to the child d. General knowledge about the child	1. To provide optimal care for the child, involvement of the family is crucial. By understanding the needs of the family, the nurse can develop a plan of care, including referral to appropriate supportive agencies.
2. Discuss with the parents the parenting they received as children.	2. Parenting is a learned behavior.
3. Observe the parents' interactions with the child.	3. Although parents may verbalize a positive relationship with their child, observation of actual interactions provides a more realistic view of the parent-child relationship.
4. Provide an accepting environment.	4. Communication is encouraged by demonstrating acceptance.
5. Provide information regarding normal growth and development for parents.	5. Parents who are abusers often have unrealistic expectations of their children, in part because of their lack of knowledge regarding growth and development.

6. Include role modeling as a method of teaching parenting.

7. Devote part of the time spent with the child and family to focusing on the child's positive attributes (e.g., "You are such a pretty little girl," or "Look at that wonderful smile").
8. Encourage the parents to participate in the care of the child. Reinforce positive behaviors.

6. By observing the way the nurse touches and talks to the child in an affirming manner, the parents can observe firsthand the child's response to positive parenting-type skills.
7. Parents' negative perceptions of the child, which may be based on their own life experiences, can be altered by viewing the child through another's eyes.
8. Strategies that encourage and reinforce positive parental participation in child care build self-esteem and confidence in parenting skills.

Evaluation

- Do the parents interact appropriately with the child through verbal, physical, and visual contact?
- Have the parents verbalized an understanding of normal growth and development?
- Do the parents verbalize positive statements regarding the child?
- Do the parents bring the child in for follow-up visits?

Nursing Diagnosis

- ■ Fear and/or Powerlessness related to the possible outcomes of disclosure, sense of shame and possible loss of family.

Expected Outcome

- The child will verbalize the source of fear and will express feelings related to shame and fear of loss of family.

Intervention

1. Reassure the child in regard to personal safety.
2. Identify specific strategies the child can use to maintain a sense of stability (i.e., stay with a trusted adult, refuse to answer intrusive questions, limit exposure to adults who are not trusted).
3. Acknowledge the child's fear.

4. Spend time with the child. Use both verbal and nonverbal forms of communication.
5. Offer choices, when available, regarding activities of daily living, recreation time, and time with other children and adults.

Rationale

1. Verbal reassurance can provide a sense of security.
2. By providing some viable options, the nurse can help the child begin to gain a sense of control over the experience.

3. Acknowledgment helps the child identify feelings and opens up new areas of communication.
4. Actions of support provide comfort and encourage verbalization of feelings.
5. Being offered choices gives the child a sense of control and diminishes feelings of powerlessness.

Evaluation

- Does the child participate in play activities?
- Has the child verbalized specific fears related to abuse and disclosure?
- Has the child verbalized fears related to being removed from the family?

Nursing Diagnosis

- ■ Knowledge Deficit related to the developmental abilities of the child, external support resources, or ways to manage internal and external stressors.

Expected Outcome

- The family will verbalize an understanding of the child's developmental and emotional needs in a framework that is oriented to the child's welfare and will identify support systems.

Intervention

1. Assess the parents' knowledge of child growth and development.
2. Serve as a role model for positive parenting skills.

3. Assist the family in identifying stressors and the support systems and resources that may help decrease the parents' stress level.
4. Refer the family to pertinent support groups, such as Parents Anonymous.
5. Involve the parents in the care of the child.

Rationale

1. A baseline assessment must be done in order to develop a plan of care.
2. Learning can be enhanced through observing the application of parenting skills, which is more effective than listening to a lecture.
3. If the parents' level of stress is decreased, the risk of abuse is decreased.

4. Lack of support and isolation are common among abusive families. A support group may decrease isolation.
5. Participation in care will provide opportunities for positive reinforcement, teaching, and increased emotional attachment to the child.

6. Provide education in the areas of
   a. Growth and development
   b. Nutrition
   c. Care related to activities of daily living
   d. Routine well-child care
   e. Manifestations of illness
   f. Need for care and loving
7. Provide a consistent caregiver from among the nursing staff.

6. Education in parenting skills may decrease unrealistic expectations, increase awareness of the needs of children, and increase the chances of positive parenting. Parents may not have had positive parenting role models as children.

7. Consistency of care increases the child's feelings of trust and security and provides increased opportunities for the child to verbalize feelings.

Evaluation

- Do the parents verbalize an understanding of child growth and development?
- Have the parents joined a support group?

Nursing Diagnosis

■ Risk for Injury related to a family with a history of physical abuse, physical neglect, emotional abuse, or sexual abuse.

Expected Outcomes

- The child will remain free from physical or psychological injury and neglect.
- The family will seek psychological support to overcome the problem of abuse.

Intervention

1. Assess the child's physical and mental status.

2. Observe the interactions between child and family.
3. Obtain a thorough history.

4. Use a nonthreatening, nonjudgmental manner when interacting with the child's parents.

5. Report all cases in which abuse is suspected.

6. Assist in removing children from an unsafe environment.

7. Document the following:
   a. Results of the child's physical assessment
   b. Observations of interactions between the child and family and between the child and other adults, as well as the child's reaction to hospitalization or the health care setting
   c. Direct comments made by the child and the family that pertain to the child or the child's injury
   d. Child's developmental level
8. If the child is removed from the home, provide the child and family with support and opportunities to verbalize feelings. Play therapy may be used effectively with children.

Rationale

1. All children should undergo a thorough physical assessment on presentation to the health care setting and should be assessed for bruises, burns, scars, and other signs of abuse. Children may enter the health care system for reasons other than injury.
2. Subtle signs of abuse may be detected in the way the child interacts with the abuser and other adults.
3. Frequent presentation of the child for injuries or signs of healed injuries may indicate a pattern of abuse.
4. By building a trusting relationship with the parents, the nurse can help the child. If the parents become suspicious or alienated, they may deny the child access to health care. They will become defensive, and will not be open to teaching.
5. All 50 states require health care professionals to report all cases of suspected abuse.
6. Suspected abuse should be evaluated immediately so that the child can be removed to an environment that is safe, thereby preventing further injury.
7. Objective documentation is essential in all cases of suspected abuse.

8. Children who are removed from the custody of their parents will grieve their loss. Parents will need support in dealing with guilt and loss.

Evaluation

- Does the child remain free of inflicted injury?
- Has the child been placed in a safe environment?
- Has the child verbalized feelings regarding placement outside the home?
- Has the family sought psychological counseling?

Failure to Thrive

Most clinicians agree that failure to thrive is not an actual diagnosis but rather a term that describes a cluster of concurrent symptoms. In practice, if a child's weight falls below the fifth percentile or drops more than two major percentile groups, or if the average daily growth gain in grams is less than normal values, the child is considered to be at risk for failure to thrive, and a more thorough evaluation is warranted.

PATHOPHYSIOLOGY
. . . .
of Failure to Thrive

Three types of failure to thrive are typically described: organic, nonorganic, and mixed failure to thrive.

Organic failure to thrive is marked by failure to gain weight secondary to physical factors. These physical factors may be a specific physiologic impairment, such as a congenital heart defect, gastrointestional disorder, or endocrine disorder. Alternatively, the physical factor may be a chronic infection, a central nervous system abnormality, a chromosomal disorder, or a metabolic disorder.

Nonorganic failure to thrive is a diagnosis applied in the absence of a history contributing to, or physical or laboratory findings suggestive of, an organic disease capable of causing failure to gain weight. Generally, environmental factors influence a child's intake or use of calories. This form of the disorder is commonly believed to result from a complex interactive pattern between the infant and the primary caregivers.

Mixed failure to thrive is caused by a combination of organic and inorganic factors. The initial problem may be physical, such as respiratory distress, which limits effective suckling. This difficulty in turn interferes with the caregiver's sense of adequacy and ability to provide nurturing care to the infant. The infant becomes more irritable and difficult to manage, further increasing the caregiver's sense of inadequacy.

Persistent failure to gain weight is considered to originate with malnutrition. The long-term effects of undernutrition, regardless of the cause, may include secondary immune system dysfunction, deficiencies in micronutrients, and developmental delays in all major areas. Associated immune system dysfunctions include reductions in complement, secretory immunoglobulin A (IgA), and T-cell function. Affected children may have repeated gastrointestinal or respiratory infections, with each episode raising the child's caloric needs and lowering intake, resulting in even greater vulnerability. Micronutrient deficiencies often complicate undernutrition by causing anemia and rickets. Iron and calcium deficiencies tend to increase lead absorption, which can lead to constipation, abdominal pain, or anorexia. Zinc deficiency impairs growth directly and can also interfere with tastebud function. Chronic undernutrition in the first 2 years of life can result in limited brain size, a reduction in neuronal number, and decreased synaptic complexity. Acquired microcephaly may persist even when somatic growth recovers.

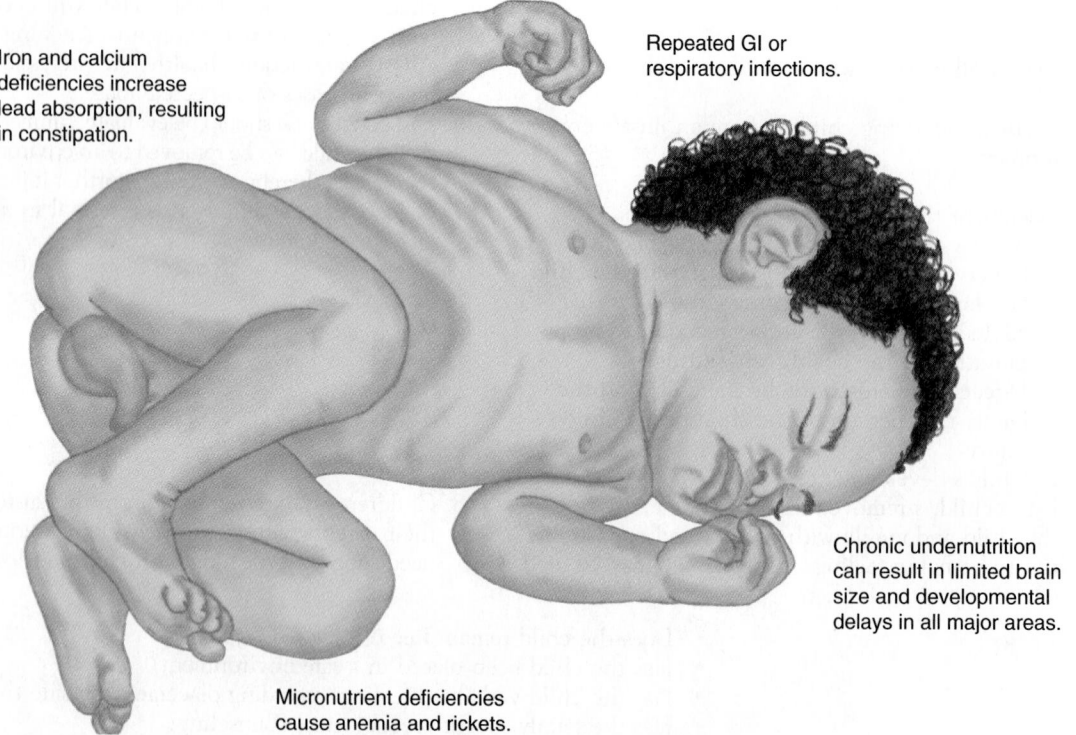

Iron and calcium deficiencies increase lead absorption, resulting in constipation.

Repeated GI or respiratory infections.

Chronic undernutrition can result in limited brain size and developmental delays in all major areas.

Micronutrient deficiencies cause anemia and rickets.

Etiology

Nonorganic failure to thrive is thought to be caused by multiple factors, including poverty, maternal depression, poor social support systems, poor bonding or maladaptive interactions between the child and mother, and irritable, resistant to touch infants (MacPhee & Schneider, 1996; Steward & Garvin, 1997). Although mothers of children with nonorganic failure to thrive often report abuse and neglect in their own childhoods, increased life stress, and negative partner relationships, these factors have not been distinct enough to explain nonorganic failure to thrive (Steward & Garvin, 1997). A maladaptive parent-infant relationship, in which the parent displays impaired skills in reading or responding to the infant's cues, is the most commonly observed risk factor for nonorganic failure to thrive. The infant has difficulty eliciting attention and appropriate care, often becoming irritable or stiff, or exhibits feeding difficulties. These symptoms are difficult for new parents to manage, resulting in parental anxiety and difficulty in bonding emotionally with the infant.

Incidence

From 1% to 5% of hospitalized infants are listed as being admitted for failure to thrive; however, these estimates of occurrence may be low. Children hospitalized with a diagnosis of failure to thrive, 2 years old and younger, demonstrated some degree of malnutrition (34.9%). (Hendricks, Duggan, Gallagher, et al., 1995). Although failure to thrive occurs in children of all social classes, a disproportionate number of these children are from low-income families.

Manifestations and Risk Factors

PHYSICAL INDICATORS

Physical indicators of failure to thrive include weight below the fifth percentile, a sudden or rapid deceleration in the growth curve, delay in reaching developmental milestones, and decreased muscle mass. Muscular hypotonia, abdominal distension, generalized weakness, and cachexia (general ill health and malnutrition) are additional signs.

BEHAVIORAL INDICATORS

Behavioral indicators of failure to thrive include avoidance of eye contact, avoidance of physical touch, intense watchfulness, and sleep disturbances. Lack of age-appropriate stranger anxiety, inappropriate lack of preference for own parents, and disturbed affect, such as apathy, extreme irritability, and extreme compliance, may also be observed. Repetitive self-stimulating behaviors, such as rocking, head banging, intense sucking, intense chewing on fingers or hands, and head rolling are also seen.

Diagnostic Evaluation

The differential diagnosis is generally made by a multidisciplinary team whose initial task is to search for an organic cause of the growth failure. If no cause is identified, the approach is to diagnose by response. Nutrition and nurturing are provided in a consistent manner, and if the infant gains the expected weight, nonorganic failure to thrive is considered to be the appropriate diagnosis.

Therapeutic Management

Treatment provides nutritional therapy to increase the child's caloric intake. The goal is for the child to grow at two to three times the average rate for age. Daily multivitamin supplements with minerals are often prescribed to ensure that specific nutritional deficiencies do not occur in the course of rapid growth. Caloric enrichment of food is essential, and formula may be concentrated in titrated amounts up to 24 calories per ounce. Greater concentrations can lead to diarrhea and dehydration.

NURSING CARE
. . . .

The Child with Failure to Thrive

Assessment

The initial assessment should include a complete history of the presenting problem, with an emphasis on age at onset, recent changes in the child's routines (i.e., travel out of the country), and attendance at large day care centers or shelter-type living environments. The nurse should also obtain information about any chronic nasal obstruction, episodes of bronchitis or wheezing, or other respiratory difficulties. Information about stool frequency, consistency, and any discomfort associated with excretion should be documented. A thorough dietary history should include all drinks, meals, and snacks consumed by the child, as well as where, when, how, and by whom the child is typically fed. The nurse should explore possible reasons for low intake, such as recurrent infections or medical complications of earlier episodes of malnutrition. Common dietary patterns may be overlooked if the dietary history is not carefully investigated.

The physical examination should focus especially on the skin, hair, nails, and mucous membranes of the child to identify signs of malnutrition. Also, the nurse should look for lesions that could interfere with eating, such

. . . .

Common Reasons for Inadequate Nutritional Intake in Infants and Children

- Overdilution of formula
- Large quantities of cereal or baby food in bottles
- Excessive intake of fluids other than formula or milk
- Selection of foods with inappropriate texture for infant's stage of development
- Infrequent feedings, especially in children who are temperamentally quiet or undemanding
- No set feeding times
- No high chair
- Frequent small sips from a bottle (grazing)
- Distractions during feedings (television or social interactions)
- Struggles over feeding between caregiver and child

About Effective Feeding Practices

Almost all children at one time or another do not eat as well as parents would like. If you are concerned about your child's eating, these guidelines may help:

- Children do well with schedules. Try to maintain consistent mealtimes and snack times each day.
- Children need to eat often, not constantly. Offer something every 2 to 3 hours, allowing three meals and two to three snacks per day.
- Make sure your child can easily reach the food served. Use a high chair, phone books, or small table.
- Allow children to feed themselves. Try very small amounts at first. Offer seconds later. Expect messiness, and prepare in advance for easy cleanup (use bibs, newspapers under the high chair, or whatever works for you). If you are worried that little food actually gets into the child's mouth, use two spoons: one for the baby to control, and one for you to use for feeding.
- Don't force-feed, bribe, or cajole! These approaches will backfire.
- Don't worry if your child wants to eat the same food every day; many children are like that. Variety is not important to a toddler's nutrition. What matters is the total caloric and protein intake.
- At mealtimes, offer solids first. Liquids are filling and provide fewer calories.
- Limit the amount of juice, water, and carbonated drinks consumed. Offer milk or formula instead.
- Offer foods that are easy for your child to handle. Finger foods, such as Cheerios, french fries, slices of banana, and peas, are ideal. Make sure pieces are small to avoid the child's choking.
- For more calories per bite, add margarine, mayonnaise, gravies, and grated cheese to foods. For snacks, use peanut butter, cheese, pudding, bananas, or dried fruit.
- Limit the consumption of junk foods such as soda, chips, and candy. They take up valuable space in the stomach without providing nutrients.
- Eat with your child or allow your child to eat with others, so that meals and snacks can be fun.

Adapted with permission from Frank, D. A., Silva, M., & Needlman, R. (1993, February). Failure to thrive: Mystery, myth, and method. *Contemporary Pediatrics, 10*, 121.

as dental caries, tongue enlargement, mandibular hypoplasia, unrecognized submucosal cleft palate, or tonsillar hypertrophy.

The nurse should complete a thorough psychosocial history that focuses on income, family (dis)organization, social isolation, stress factors, support systems, and family psychopathology, such as maternal depression, family violence, or alcoholism. It is important to ask about the availability of food, especially around the time of arrival of a paycheck or other forms of income. Finally, the psychosocial history should include questions about facilities for storing and preparing food.

Assessment of infant-parent interactions should focus on the ways in which the child is held and fed, how eye contact is initiated and maintained, and the facial expressions of both the child and the caregiver during interactions. Observations of various kinds of interactions are important, too, and should include play, talk, and touch by both the child and caregiver, as well as the other's reaction to these attempts to engage in interaction. The nurse should note the responses of the caregiver to the child's cues, such as when the child cries, reaches out, or looks toward the caregiver. A feeling of synchrony or harmony should be sensed in the interaction.

Nursing Diagnosis, Planning, Intervention, and Evaluation

Nursing Diagnosis

- Altered Nutrition: Less Than Body Requirements, related to insufficient intake of calories, incomplete absorption of nutrients, impaired interactions with caregivers, or inadequate care by caregivers.

Expected Outcomes

- The child will experience normal growth and development for age and sex.
- The child's caloric intake will increase.

Intervention

1. Monitor the child's nutritional status.
   a. Document physical alterations, especially changes in physical status during or after feedings.
   b. Document the child's feeding patterns.
   c. Document the nature of parent-child interactions, especially before, during, and after feedings.

Rationale

1. Fatigue, colic, or respiratory distress may indicate an underlying cause of the disorder. Subtle deficits may have a significant bearing on nutritional intake. Psychological components revealed in the context of interactions may be the most significant indicators of the cause for undernutrition.

2. Encourage the caregiver to discuss both positive and negative feelings about care, procedures, and interactions with the child.

3. Increase the child's caloric intake by feeding the child on demand or increasing intake as tolerated, offering high-protein snacks between meals, offering small portions of a wide variety of food at mealtimes, teaching the child healthy mealtime behaviors (decrease distractions, make mealtime pleasurable), planning naps or rest periods, and intervening in the event of fretfulness or crying.

4. Monitor the child's intake and output.

5. Weight should be measured daily at the same time, using the same scales, and with the child dressed in the same amount of clothing each time.

6. Provide a consistent caregiver from the nursing staff.

2. The caregiver may be unaware of some of the underlying feelings that may be affecting the infant-caregiver relationship.

3. The child's intake must be greater than the infant's caloric expenditure.

4. Fluid loss may affect daily weight patterns.

5. This approach reduces the effect of various factors that influence weight measurements.

6. This strategy increases trust and provides the child with an adult who anticipates needs, thus decreasing the child's level of frustration.

Evaluation

- Is the child attaining developmental milestones?
- Does the child eat the food offered?
- Do the parents participate in feeding the child?
- Does the child's physical growth show an increase?

Nursing Diagnosis

■ Knowledge Deficit related to lack of experience and of positive parenting training.

Expected Outcomes

- The caregiver will hold and maintain eye contact with the child.
- The parent will participate in feeding the child.
- The parents will express realistic expectations of the child based upon the child's developmental needs.

Intervention

1. Provide instruction in child care, being sure to model appropriate adult-child interactions. Include techniques for holding, touching, and feeding the child.

2. Exhibit a positive attitude toward the parents.

3. Provide information regarding normal growth and development.

4. Provide for rooming-in with the child.

5. Teach the parents ways to increase the child's caloric intake and to minimize the control issues associated with mealtimes.

Rationale

1. Instruction, coupled with modeling and practice, will facilitate integration of information.

2. Acceptance increases trust and fosters openness to learning.

3. Parents may lack an understanding of normal growth and development and may have unrealistic expectations of the child.

4. This arrangement allows the nurse to observe parent-child interactions and provide further teaching if necessary.

5. Lack of previous experience and knowledge may result in ineffective parenting skills.

Evaluation

- Have the parents been observed interacting appropriately with the child during meals?
- Do the parents verbalize an openness to learning new techniques of feeding?
- Are the parents holding and touching the child?
- Have the parents asked questions related to parenting?

KEY CONCEPTS

■ In children and adolescents, the behavioral manifestations of anxiety and depression may be similar. Individuals with both diagnoses may be withdrawn, tearful, unwilling to engage in play, and aggressive toward others.

■ It is difficult to differentiate between normal mood changes secondary to developmental maturation and abnormal, persistent mood disturbances.

■ Separation anxiety and school avoidance need to be addressed if the problem becomes persistent or debilitating. Such anxiety is characterized by excessive fear, even panic, of being away from the parent or home.

■ A suicide gesture or statement should never be ignored.

■ Protecting a child or adolescent from inflicting harm to self involves being emotionally and physically available, offering opportunities to discuss feelings and the suicidal event, and removing potentially harmful objects.

■ Support for grieving families of suicidal or potentially suicidal individuals is best provided on both an individual and a group basis to allow exploration of personal issues and social support.

■ Anorexia nervosa is characterized by a deliberate refusal to maintain adequate body weight, a distorted body image, and amenorrhea (in female patients).

■ One common factor among children with an eating disorder is a family system in which the individual is considered to be an ex-

tension of the parent, or serves as a means of meeting the parents' needs, rather than being allowed to develop as an autonomous individual. The mother tends to be overprotective, lacking in empathy, and overly invested in the daily activities of the child. The father is often emotionally distant from the mother and the child.

■ The focus of care for an adolescent with an eating disorder involves restructuring cognitive perceptions, reducing opportunities for engaging in ritualistic and self-injurious behaviors, and reestablishing physiologic homeostasis.

■ During the early treatment phase of eating disorders, it may be necessary to observe the adolescent following meals to prevent episodes of purging.

■ Attention-deficit hyperactivity disorder (ADHD) is a developmental disorder characterized by developmentally inappropriate degrees of inattention, overactivity, and impulsivity.

■ Support groups are important in assisting families to cope with and modify expectations and interactions involving the child with ADHD.

■ Educating the family about ADHD is a crucial component of caring for the child with this disorder.

■ Low grades, irregular school attendance, aggressive or rebellious behavior, deteriorating relationships with family members or former friends, rapid or extreme changes in behaviors or mood, and loss of

interest in hobbies, sports, or other activities are some common signs of substance abuse.

■ An individual with a substance abuse problem, together with the family, should receive help in developing social support systems, with referral to appropriate resources that can offer additional support as they attempt to make long-term changes in their social and emotional patterns of relating.

■ Child abuse tends to increase during times of economic hardship or external stress. Abusive families are often isolated, lack a support system, exhibit low levels of trust, resolve conflict through aggression, assume fixed and traditional roles within the family, and establish rigid rules.

■ All suspected child abuse must be reported to the appropriate authorities.

■ Abusive parents often have unrealistic expectations of their children, which may relate to lack of knowledge of normal growth and development.

■ Role-modeling positive parenting skills is an effective intervention in the care of the child who has been abused.

■ The assessment of infant-parent interactions in cases of nonorganic failure to thrive should include observation of the ways in which the child is held and fed, how eye contact is initiated and maintained, and the facial expressions of both the child and the caregiver during interactions.

ANSWERS TO CRITICAL THINKING EXERCISE 53–1

1. Matthew may have fallen while at the baby-sitter's or even at home and either sprained or fractured his arm. Two-year-olds are curious and also like to climb. Children get frequent scrapes and bruises at this age. Because of the injured arm, bruises, and abrasion, physical abuse is also a possibility.

2. Matthew should be assessed for other bruises in various stages of healing or clustered in patterns re-

flecting the shape of a hand or an article that may have caused the bruise. The nurse must determine if the injury matches the description of the cause.

   The nurse should also check for records of other emergency department visits for injuries or signs of old fractures on Matthew's radiographs. In addition, she should gather information about the baby-sitter: has any other injury oc-

curred while Matthew was in the sitter's care? What explanation did the sitter give for Matthew's behavior when his mother picked him up?

   During the interview, the nurse should observe both Mrs. Anderson and her boyfriend to assess their relationship with Matthew. Do they comfort him? Do they respond to his needs? Do they seem overly concerned about the injury?

Matthew's behavior is not typical of an abused child. He seeks comfort from his parent and does not appear apathetic. If at the end of the interview, history, assessment, and diagnostic testing it is determined that an adult did not inflict the injury, the nurse should use the opportunity to explore ways that the injury could have been prevented. The roles of mother, sitter, and boyfriend should be incorporated into the discussion.
3. If the nurse suspects child abuse, it must be reported to child protective services.

REFERENCES AND READINGS

American Academy of Child and Adolescent Psychiatry. (1997). Practice parameters for the assessment and treatment of children and adolescents with anxiety disorders. *Journal of the American Academy of Child and Adolescent Psychiatry, 36*(Suppl. 1-10).

American Academy of Child and Adolescent Psychiatry. (1998). Practice parameters for the assessment and treatment of children and adolescents with depressive disorders. *Journal of the American Academy of Child and Adolescent Psychiatry, 37*(Suppl. 10).

American Psychiatric Association. (1994). *Diagnostic and statistical manual of mental disorders* (4th ed.). Washington, DC: Author.

Barkley, R. A. (1997). *Attention-deficit hyperactivity disorder* (3rd ed.). New York: Guilford Press.

Bowers, R. (1998). Child and adolescent affective disorders and their treatment. In W. M. Klyklo, J. Kay, & D. Rube (Eds.), *Clinical child psychiatry* (pp. 171–204). Philadelphia: Saunders.

Brage, D., Campbell-Grossman, C., & Dunkel, J. (1995). Psychological correlates of adolescent depression. *Journal of Child and Adolescent Psychiatric Nursing, 4*, 23–30.

Cantwell, D. P. (1996). Attention deficit disorder: A review of the past 10 years. *Journal of the American Academy of Child and Adolescent Psychiatry, 35*, 978–987.

Centers for Disease Control and Prevention. (1995). Youth risk behavior surveillance—United States. *Morbidity and Mortality Weekly Report, 44*(55-1), 1–56.

Chatlos, J. C. (1996). Recent trends and a developmental approach to substance abuse in adolescents. *Child and Adolescent Psychiatric Clinics of North America, 5*(1), 1–27.

Chiocca, E. (1995). Shaken baby syndrome: A nursing perspective. *Pediatric Nursing, 21*(1), 33–37.

Cicchetti, O., & Toth, S. (1995). A developmental psychopathology perspective on child abuse and neglect. *Journal of the American Academy of Child and Adolescent Psychiatry, 34*(5), 541–562.

Comerci, G. (1999). Disordered eating behavioral: Anorexia nervosa, bulimia nervosa, cyclic vomiting syndrome, and rumination disorder. In M. D. Levine, W. B. Carey, & A. C. Crocker (Eds.), *Developmental-behavioral pediatrics* (3rd ed., pp. 380–391). Philadelphia: Saunders.

Costello, E. J., & Angold, A. (1995). Epidemiology. In J. S. March (Ed.), *Anxiety disorders in children and adolescents* (pp. 109–129). Philadelphia: Saunders.

Daro, D., & Wang, C. T. (1997). *Current trends in child abuse reporting and fatalities: The results of the 1996 annual fifty-state survey.* Chicago: National Committee to Prevent Child Abuse.

Dashiff, C. (1995). Understanding separation anxiety. *Journal of Child and Adolescent Psychiatric Nursing, 8*(2), 27–38.

Devlin, B. K., & Reynolds, E. (1994, March). Child abuse. *American Journal of Nursing, 3*, 26–32.

Donnelly, C. (1998). Anxiety disorders in childhood and adolescence. In W. M. Klyklo, J. Kay, & D. Rube (Eds.), *Clinical child psychiatry* (pp. 205–229). Philadelphia: Saunders.

Finkelhor, D. (1979). *Sexually victimized children.* New York: Free Press.

Finkelhor, D., & Berliner, L. (1995). Research on the treatment of sexually abused children: A review and recommendations. *Journal of the American Academy of Child and Adolescent Psychiatry, 34*(11), 1408–1422.

Garofalo, R., Wolf, R. C., Kessel, S., Palfrey, J., & DuRant, P. H. (1998). The association between health risk behaviors and sexual orientation among a school-based sample of adolescents. *Pediatrics, 101*, 895–902.

Graber, J. A., Brooks-Gum, J., Parkoff, R., & Warren, M. P. (1994). Prediction of eating problems: An 8 year study of adolescent girls. *Developmental Psychology, 30*, 823–834.

Hammelman, T. L. (1993). Gay and lesbian youth: Contributing factors to serious attempts or considerations of suicide. *Journal of Gay and Lesbian Psychotherapy, 2*, 77–89.

Hendricks, K. M., Duggan, C., Gallagher, L., et al. (1995). Malnutrition in hospitalized pediatric patients. *Archives of Pediatric and Adolescent Medicine, 149*, 1118.

Jarry, J. L., & Vaccarino, F. J. (1996). Eating disorder and obsessive-compulsive disorder: Neurochemical and phenomenological commonities. *Journal of Psychiatric Neuroscience, 21*, 36.

Johnson, B. (1995). *Psychiatric-mental health nursing.* Philadelphia: Lippincott.

Johnston, L. D., & Buchanan, J. G. (1998, Dec. 18). National survey results on drug use. Monitoring the Future, 1975–1998 [Press release]. Ann Arbor, MI: University of Michigan Institute for Social Research.

Kelley, B., & Beauchesne, M. (1998). Children and violence. *Journal of the Society of Pediatric Nurses, 3*(3), 127–129.

Kelly, S. J. (1998). Stress and coping behaviors of substance-abusing mothers. *Journal of the Society of Pediatric Nurses, 3*(3), 103–110.

Kendall, W. (1997). The use of qualitative methods in the study of wellness in children with attention deficit hyperactivity disorder. *Journal of Child and Adolescent Psychiatric Nursing, 10*(4), 27–38.

Kienhorst, I., deWilde, E. J., Dielestra, F. W., et al. (1995). Adolescents' image of their suicide attempt. *Journal of the American Academy of Child and Adolescent Psychiatry, 34*(5), 623–628.

Krugman, S. D., Wilson, L. S., & Krugman, R. D. (1998). Facing facts: Child abuse and pediatric practice. *Contemporary Pediatrics, 15*(8), 131–144.

Lewisohn, P. M., Klein, D. L., & Seeley, J. R. (1995). Bipolar disorders in a community sample of older adolescents: Prevalence, phenomenology, comorbidity, and care. *Journal of the American Academy of Child and Adolescent Psychiatry, 34*, 454–463.

Lombroso, P. J., Pauls, D. L., & Leckman, J. F. (1994). Genetic mechanisms in childhood psychiatric disorders. *Journal of the American Academy of Child and Adolescent Psychiatry, 33*(7), 921–938.

MacPhee, M., & Schneider, J. (1996). A clinical tool for nonorganic failure to thrive feeding interactions. *Journal of Pediatric Nursing, 11*(1), 29–38.

Mascari, M. E. (1998). Walking a thin line: Managing care for adolescents with anorexia and bulimia. *MCN: American Journal of Maternal/Child Nursing, 23*(3), 130–140.

Messer, S. C., & Beidel, D. C. (1994). Psychosocial correlates of childhood anxiety disorders. *Journal of the American Academy of Child and Adolescent Psychiatry, 33*(7), 975–983.

National Committee to Prevent Child Abuse. (1997). *Child abuse and neglect statistics from the National Committee to Prevent Child Abuse.* Chicago: Author.

National Research Council, Food and Nutrition Board. (1989). *Recommended daily allowances.* Washington, DC: National Academy of Sciences.

Steward, D. K., & Garvin, B. J. (1997). Nonorganic failure to thrive: A theoretical approach. *Journal of Pediatric Nursing, 12*(6), 342–347.

U.S. Public Health Service. (1997). Depression: Putting prevention into practice. *Journal of the American Academy of Nurse Practitioners, 9*(9), 431–435.

Woods, E. R., Lin, Y. G., Middleman, A., Beckford, P., Chase, L., & DuRant, R. H. (1997). The associations of suicide attempts in adolescence. *Pediatrics, 99*(6), 791–796.

54

The Child with a Cognitive Deficit

LEARNING OBJECTIVES

After studying this chapter, you should be able to:

- Identify the various causes of mental retardation.
- Identify specific tools used in assessing the presence and degree of mental retardation.
- Identify educational and support resources for families with a child who is mentally retarded or developmentally delayed.
- Develop appropriate nursing strategies for supporting the family and child with mental retardation or developmental delay.
- Develop nursing strategies for families caring for a child with Down syndrome.
- Identify behavioral characteristics and appropriate nursing actions when working with a child with fragile X syndrome.
- Identify the basic diagnostic criteria for autism.
- Explain the ways autism differs from other types of pervasive developmental disorders.
- Identify the major considerations in working with the family of an autistic child.
- Develop home care interventions appropriate to the family's abilities and the developmental needs of a child with a cognitive deficit.

DEFINITIONS

comorbidity   The occurrence of two or more different disorders in the same individual. Children with cognitive impairments often have co-existing psychiatric disorders.

echolalia   Stereotyped repetition of another person's words or phrases.

functional age   The age equivalent at which the child is actually able to perform specific self-care or relational tasks. For example, the child may be 6 years old chronologically but only able to perform skills representative of children 4 years old. The child's functional age would then be 4 years.

intelligence   The innate capacity of the individual; what individuals can do relative to learning, thinking, and problem solving; results obtained on intelligence tests that measure specific skills, such as verbal, nonverbal, or mechanical abilities.

mutation   Variation in a gene that affects its function.

pervasive developmental disorders (PDDs)   Infant and childhood disorders characterized by severe and pervasive impairment in several areas of development in a manner distinctly deviant from the individual's developmental level or mental age (American Psychiatric Association, 1994).

premutation   A small, but abnormal, increase in the number of base pairs on a chromosome.

Common Diagnostic Tests for Cognitive Disorders

Test	Description	Normal Findings	Indications	Nursing Implications
Vision Test	Assessment of vision, ocular pressure, and structural defects	Normal vision, normal structures	Children with Down syndrome; 40%–45% have refractive errors, cataracts, or other visual problems	Explain pupil dilation. Provide protective eyewear following the examinations.
Hearing Test	Assessment of perception of sound frequency and volume	Normal hearing range	Children with Down syndrome; 70%–80% have hearing defects	Explain the test in simple terms.
			Children with autism and pervasive developmental disorder (PDD); often appear to have defective hearing, despite normal hearing function, so hearing tests should be conducted	The test may require that the child wear a headphone, which may be difficult to tolerate.
Thyroid Studies	Blood serum tests to determine thyroid levels	Ages 1–3 years: 6.8–13.5 µg/dl Ages 3–10 years: 5.5–12.8 µg/dl Puberty–adulthood: 4.2–13.0 µg/dl	Children with Down syndrome; slowed growth rates are common	These studies should not be performed within 7 days of a radionuclide scan.
Adaptive Behavior Scales*	Assessment of language, motor, social, and self-care skills	Age-expected skills within 1 standard deviation (SD) from the mean	Children with suspected developmental delays	Explain the test and how results will be interpreted.
IQ Tests†	Assessment of cognitive abilities	Age-normal skills within 1½ SD from the mean	Children with suspected developmental delays	Explain the test and how results will be interpreted.
Bone Roentgenography	Assessment of bone plates and joint spaces	Age-expected bone age	Children with Down syndrome; decreased growth rate is common	The child must be motionless during the study.
Brain Sonography	Ultrasonogram of cranium	Normal position of brain's midline structures and normal blood flow velocity, no hemorrhages	Microcephaly or macrocephaly, misshapen cranium, family history of hydrocephaly	The child must be supine. Any jewelry or metal objects should be removed from the child's head. The child may need sedation or may need to be restrained, as this procedure takes 1 hour to complete. Explain to the child that the test is not painful. Keep the child warm during the procedure.

Table continued on following page

Common Diagnostic Tests for Cognitive Disorders *Continued*

Test	Description	Normal Findings	Indications	Nursing Implications
Genetic Analysis	Cytogenic bonding, culture media analysis	Normal findings for gene product analysis	Suspected genetic or neoplastic disorders	Allow the child an opportunity to ask questions and express concerns about the possible results and implications of the testing.
Computed Tomography (CT)	Special noninvasive radiographic technique that images brain tissue in very thin sections	No blood clots, tumors, or infections	Impaired development, such as microcephaly; family history of central nervous system malformations; possible tumors or subdural hematomas	The child may need to be sedated or restrained and will need to assume supine position. CT scans require the use of contrast medium and so require informed consent.
Magnetic Resonance Imaging (MRI)	Noninvasive method used to create images corresponding to density of tissue	Normal anatomy and physiology of the brain and spinal column	Same as for CT	The test requires informed consent. Remove metal or magnetic objects from the child before the study. Sedation of the child is usually required.
Positron Emission Tomography (PET)	Noninvasive means of comparing cerebral brain flow and metabolic changes. Used to localize seizure foci, visualize brain hemodynamics, and study brain pharmacology using radioisotopes	Normal metabolism of glucose in brain, normal blood flow and electrical activity	Seizures, hydrocephaly, evidence of cerebral dysfunction	The test requires informed consent. The child will need to be sedated. Liquids may be limited before the procedure. If not in diapers, the child will need to void before the procedure. Parents may be able to remain with the child during the procedure.

* Adaptive behavior scales include the American Association on Mental Retardation (AAMR) test, the Minnesota Child Development Inventory Profile (MCDI), the Denver Developmental Screening Test (DDST-II), the Wechsler Preschool and Primary Scale of Intelligence (WPPSI), the Wechsler Intelligence Scale for Children (WISC-III), and the Wechsler Adult Intelligence Scale—Revised (WAIS-R).

† IQ tests include the Bayley Scales (birth to 3 years), the Stanford-Binet Scale (2 years and older), the WPPSI (3 to 6 years), the WISC-III (6 to 16 years), and the WAIS-R (16 years and older).

Children with cognitive deficits have significant impairments in measured intelligence and adaptive behavior. Cognitive impairments can be a result of malformations of the brain and central nervous system, injury, infections, anoxia, or poisoning, or the cause may be unknown. Specific disabilities are differentiated on the basis of an assessment of language, cognition, academic ability, self-help skills, social behaviors, and motor performance.

A cognitive impairment may be classified as a general delay, as in mental retardation, or as a part of a larger constellation of failures in skill acquisition, as in pervasive developmental disorders (PDDs). There is considerable overlap within several cognitive-related disorders. For example, children with autism, a specific disorder classified as a PDD, are often moderately or severely mentally retarded.

The family of a child with a cognitive deficit must cope with frequent and exceptionally high demands. The family is confronted with serious medical and environmental issues that rarely seem to be solved, only managed. Independence and self-management should be emphasized throughout childhood and adolescence so that, as the individual reaches adulthood, the possibility of independent living and gainful employment can be maximized.

The nurse is an integral part of the multidisciplinary team that manages the care of a child with a cognitive deficit. The nurse is involved in early assessment of the child, support of the family, assistance with self-care training and behavioral training, referral to support services, and providing the necessary nursing care for other disabilities the child may have. School and community nurses need a broad range of knowledge to support children who have multiple cognitive and physical deficits.

▋ Mental Retardation

The term "mental retardation" is often misunderstood and considered derogatory because some believe the definition is based only on "below normal intelligence (IQ) and that retarded persons are unable to learn or care for themselves" (American Academy of Child and Adolescent Psychiatry [AACAP], 1995). Mental retardation is not diagnosed, however, unless the person has "significantly sub-average general intellectual functioning existing concurrently with deficits in adaptive functioning and manifested before age eighteen" (American Psychiatric Association [APA], 1994). Other terms used to describe individuals with mental retardation are "mentally handicapped," "developmentally delayed," and "mentally deficient." The term applied usually reflects more the discipline of the professional assigning the diagnostic label rather than manifestations (Elder, 1994).

When standardized tests of intelligence are used, subaverage general intellectual functioning refers to an IQ score of 70 or below. Adaptive functioning refers to effective coping with common life demands, as well as the ability to maintain acceptable community standards of personal independence expected of individuals of the same age group, sociocultural background, and community setting. For a diagnosis of mental retardation to be assigned, deficits must occur in two of the following ten adaptive skill areas: "communication, self-care, home living, social/interpersonal skills, use of community resources, self-direction, functional academic skills, work, leisure, health, and safety" (APA, 1994).

The American Association on Mental Retardation (AAMR), the leading professional organization in the area of mental retardation, has proposed that this definition be modified to include individuals with an intellectual functioning score of 70 to 75. The AAMR has also suggested reducing the number of levels to two, mild and severe, rather than the current four (mild, moderate, severe, and profound) (Luckasson, 1992). The AAMR's definition focuses more on adaptive behaviors than on intellectual functioning; therefore, intelligence scores may become irrelevant if adaptive skills are not affected (Fredricks & Williams, 1998).

Developmental Disabilities and Child Abuse

There appears to be a significant relationship between developmental disabilities and child abuse. Among children with developmental disabilities, 11.5% are abused, compared with 1.5% of nondisabled children (Verdugo, Bermejo, & Fuertes, 1995). Possible reasons for this strong relationship are the intense stress experienced by families of disabled children, parental isolation, and unrealistic expectations for the child's performance due to a lack of knowledge about normal growth and development.

Evidence also suggests that abuse can result in developmental disabilities or handicapping conditions. Despite available funding and support groups, families of children with developmental delays often feel isolated from supportive services and report that professionals have limited understanding of their children's needs. These factors further perpetuate the sense of helplessness and lack of control in these family systems.

Defining Cognitive Impairment

Cognitive impairment is a general term that denotes limitations in intellectual and functional abilities. Intelligence is a difficult concept, defined in a number of ways. The nurse needs to determine the meaning of the word as it is used by the professional and by the parent. Often, the child's IQ has little meaning for the parent, so the nurse must explain its meaning and purpose. Mental age or functional age are terms often used to compare a child's mental ability with the expected abilities of other children of the same chronological age. This score also gives some information about the level of cognitive understanding. For example, if an individual has a mental age of 5 years, the nurse's explanations

Safety for the Child with a Cognitive Impairment

Safety is a persistent concern of parents, teachers, and health professionals caring for cognitively impaired children. The child's maturation in anticipating danger, in problem solving, and in judgment are generally impaired across the life span. Children with motor disabilities are often unable to perform skills in ways that foster safety.

peers. Among preschool-age children, however, injuries are less common in those with cognitive impairment, as the parents of these children are very protective and the children have less exposure to risk.

There appear to be no sex differences in the risk for injury among this population (Sherrard, Tonge, & Einfeld, 1997). Table 54–1 presents some safety issues to be taught in the home and in the community. Although the learning needs of cognitively impaired children are similar to those of children without disabilities, children with cognitive impairments may need prolonged teaching, more demonstration during teaching, frequent verbal and visual reminders, and more practice.

need to be simple and specific. If the individual has a mental age of 12 years, however, the nurse's explanations can provide more description and detail and can require some degree of inductive reasoning.

Functional age does not include the individual's life experience or functioning in adaptive skills. For example, an adult with a functional age of 12 does not "have the mind of a 12-year-old" because that individual may have been affected by environmental experiences such as job training and group living situations.

Safety Challenges

Cognitively impaired children are, by definition, less capable of managing environmental challenges than their unimpaired peers. Because of impaired functioning, injuries are generally more common in these children than in same-age

Legal and Educational Considerations

Mental retardation has been a greater consideration in legal, administrative, and educational spheres than in medical diagnosis and treatment. Indeed, under many insurance plans, the single diagnosis of mental retardation does not qualify as a medical condition, and funds are not available for treatment.

The medical criteria, and the terminology used, are often somewhat different from the educational criteria used to identify mentally retarded students. In addition, the educational system uses slightly different criteria for placement in the classroom, which is usually based on intellectual testing. The IQ score is an important measure in education, as it either limits or makes accessible various resources to the child. Public laws (PL 94-142 and PL 99-457) define and limit the placement of students in the school system, emphasizing the least restrictive environment for learning and

TABLE 54–1

Safety Concerns for Developmentally Delayed or Impaired Children

Site of Concern	Possible Injury	Education/Training Issues
Home		
Kitchen	Burns Poisoning	*Preschool age:* Preventive education (i.e., instruct not to touch hot stove, not to ingest toxic substances) *Elementary school age:* Safe use of equipment, basic safety *High school age:* Cooking safety, emergency precautions
Bathroom	Falls Burns Cuts	*Elementary school age:* Tub safety, precautions on wet floors *High school age:* Safe use of hair care equipment, shaving utensils, and similar objects
General		*Preschool and elementary school age:* Avoidance of electrical outlets, safe passage around objects
Outdoors		
Yard or playground	Animal bites Poisoning Abduction	*Preschool age:* Staying within boundaries, appropriate response to strange animals and people, safe use of equipment, avoidance of ingestion of berries *Elementary school age:* Stranger safety, bicycle safety, traffic safety, water safety
Vehicles	Cuts Falls Serious injury	*Preschool and elementary school age:* Seat belt use, keeping hands in car *High school age:* Traffic safety

the greatest inclusion with nonimpaired children possible. Educational services for children with mental or physical disabilities are ensured from birth through age 21. When working with these children and families, the nurse may need to serve as a resource for helping families locate advocacy services for their children.

Comorbidity with Psychiatric Conditions

Psychiatric comorbidity is common in people with mental retardation. Prevalence estimates for mental disorders and mental retardation are up to 70% (King & State, 1998). Brain malfunctions that cause cognitive deficits frequently affect those areas of the brain that monitor emotional states. The most frequent accompanying diagnoses include disruptive behavioral disorders, depression, and atypical psychosis (Feinstein & Reiss, 1996).

Etiology

Mental retardation may be the result of congenital or early environmental factors, but it may also be secondary to head injury, asphyxia, intracranial hemorrhage, infections, poisoning, or the presence or treatment of a brain tumor. Mental retardation has more than 350 known causes, but its specific cause is unknown in nearly half of all cases (Luckasonn, 1992).

As medical technology advances, a medical basis for cognitive and adaptive impairments is found in an increasing proportion of mentally retarded children. Often the cause is a subtle but nonetheless significant biologic factor, such as minor chromosomal abnormalities, rare genetic syndromes, subclinical lead intoxication, nutritional deficiencies, or exposure to numerous prenatal risks or trauma. Evidence suggests that early neurodevelopmental functioning and later neurologic integrity and intellectual ability are strongly associated. Low socioeconomic status and related factors have also been consistently reported as influencing cognitive function.

Incidence

Mental retardation occurs in 1% to 3% of the general population. Mental retardation is 10 times more common than cerebral palsy, 25 times more common than blindness, and 28 times more common than neural tube defects (Batshaw, 1997). Among those diagnosed with mental retardation, 85% display only mild cognitive impairment, 10% are classified as moderately mentally retarded, 3% to 4% are severely mentally retarded, and 1% to 2% are profoundly mentally retarded. This distribution has clinical significance in that most families are able to care for mildly to moderately impaired children and adolescents at home.

Because a diagnosis of mental retardation is based concurrently on adaptive behavior, not just IQ, the epidemiology varies throughout the life cycle. An increased incidence of retardation is reported in the early school years, then the incidence declines in late adolescence as the children leave the formal education setting and are assimilated into the adult world. Most impaired individuals are able to

---

. . . .
Causes of Mental Retardation

HEREDITARY ORIGIN (5%)

Inborn errors of metabolism: Galactosemia, Tay-Sachs disease, phenylketonuria
Hereditary syndromes: Muscular dystrophy, tuberous sclerosis, neurofibromatosis
Chromosomal aberrations: Down syndrome, fragile X syndrome
Familial retardation of probable polygenic origin

EARLY EMBRYONIC ALTERATIONS (30%–35%)

Sporadic chromosomal changes: Down syndrome
Multiple congenital anomalies: Congenital hypothyroidism
Prenatal influence syndrome: Intrauterine infections, drugs, HIV, unknown forces
Intrauterine infections: Congenital rubella, toxoplasmosis, herpes

EARLY INTRAUTERINE OR NEONATAL ALTERATIONS (10%–15%)

Fetal malnutrition: Placental insufficiency, pregnancy-induced hypertension, drug addiction, maternal uterine cancer, multiple pregnancy
Neonatal conditions: Prematurity, neonatal asphyxia, hyperbilirubinemia, hypoglycemia, central nervous system hemorrhage, ABO incompatibilities

ACQUIRED CHILDHOOD CONDITIONS OR DISEASES (3%–5%)

Complications of infections: Meningitis, encephalitis, pertussis, varicella
Lead poisoning
Cranial trauma
Cerebral tumors
Cardiac arrest
Asphyxiation

ENVIRONMENTAL PROBLEMS AND BEHAVIORAL SYNDROMES (20%)

Psychosocial deprivation
Parental neurosis, psychosis, character disorder
Childhood psychosis, autism, other pervasive developmental disorders

UNKNOWN CAUSES (30%–35%)

Data from King, B. H., State, M. W., Shah, B., Davanzo, P. O., & Dykens, E. (1997). Mental retardation: A review of the past 10 years. Part I. *Journal of the American Academy of Child and Adolescent Psychiatry, 36*(12), 1656–1663; American Psychiatric Association. (1994). *Diagnostic and statistical manual of mental disorders* (4th ed.). Washington, DC: Author.

marry (often to individuals with normal intellectual functioning), maintain employment, and have satisfying relationships.

Manifestations

The cardinal sign of mental retardation is delayed achievement of developmental milestones. Specific congenital malformations often result in specific clinical manifestations. In addition, the severity of the mental retardation affects the types and frequency of problem behaviors.

In addition to general clinical manifestations based on the degree of impairment, many syndromes are characterized by particular features, which are helpful in determining the cause of the cognitive impairment. The two most common genetic disorders in which mental retardation is a central feature are Down syndrome and fragile X syndrome (see pp. 1546 and 1550).

Many disabilities associated with mental retardation can further limit a child's adaptive skills. These deficits include cerebral palsy, visual deficits, seizure disorders, communication deficits, feeding problems, PDDs, failure to thrive, or attention deficit/hyperactivity disorder. Speech and language development are often profoundly affected. Seizure disorders frequently develop as the child matures.

Although mentally retarded children can be generally healthy, the presence of associated deficits may place these children at increased risk for illness (Fig. 54–1). For example, if a mentally retarded child also has cerebral palsy, the risk for gastroesophageal reflux and aspiration pneumonia is high. Motor or swallowing problems may result in inadequate oral intake or insufficient weight gain.

Diagnostic Evaluation

Diagnostic evaluations may be performed in utero, during the neonatal period, or after the child fails to achieve expected developmental milestones. Tests may be general or specific for the neurologic or cognitive area in question. Several neuropsychological tests assess the individual's current level of functioning and help the clinician anticipate persistent cognitive deficits. These tests—which may

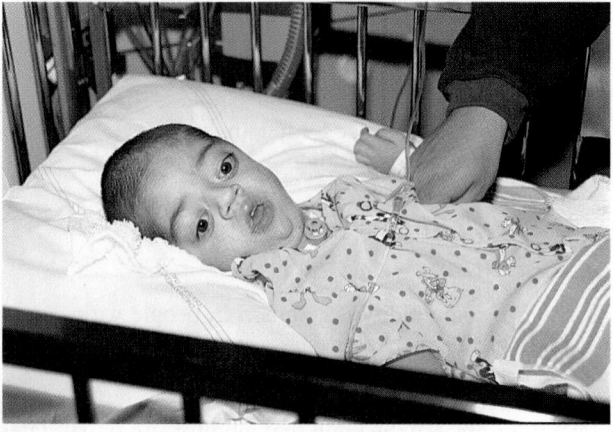

FIGURE 54–1

Children with cognitive deficits may have other dysfunctions as well. The family of a cognitively impaired child often experiences ongoing grieving because the child does not meet their expectations. This child has Marshall-Smith syndrome, which does not appear to be hereditary. His bones ossified unusually early, necessitating a craniotomy to allow greater brain development. He has a tracheostomy because of respiratory difficulties associated with an abnormally developed larynx. A gastrostomy button facilitates his nutrition. (Courtesy of Children's Medical Center, Dallas, Texas.)

involve pencil-and-paper tasks, motor tasks, sensory tasks, or some degree of cognitive processing—help to determine both the severity and type of cognitive impairment. Learning disabilities are often identified using some of these same instruments, and many are available through the school system. Nurses can also learn to administer developmental screening tools, such as the Denver Developmental Screening Test II (DDST-II) (see Chapter 4 and Appendix I).

Often, the diagnosis of mental retardation is not made until the child enters school and experiences significant academic failure, prompting formal psychological testing. Routine assessment of development during pediatric visits, however, is the best method of early detection.

Therapeutic Management

Medical strategies are directed toward preventing and treating infections, correcting structural deformities, and treating associated behaviors, such as aggressiveness. Corrective measures might include congenital heart surgery for malformations, inserting tympanostomy tubes, or placing splints for joints that are hypotonic and hyperextended. Frequently, antibiotics are given prophylactically to reduce the likelihood of infections. The treatment of behavioral difficulties and psychosocial disturbances may involve administration of medications.

Therapeutic management largely depends on community and educational resources. Obtaining services for these children, however, requires multidisciplinary efforts and strong advocacy on the part of both parents and professionals.

> **· · · · · · · · · · ·**
> ## Problems Related to Mental Retardation
> ### MILD MENTAL RETARDATION
> - Self-esteem issues related to presence or absence of physical features, largely determined by the cause of the cognitive disability
> - Social isolation and loneliness
> - Depression
>
> ### SEVERE MENTAL RETARDATION
> - Self-injury
> - Fecal smearing
> - Tearing of personal clothes and objects
> - Severe temper tantrums
> - Disrobing

Expected Skills According to IQ Scores

NORMAL (IQ: 85–115)

- Normal-age skills across all domains

BORDERLINE (IQ: 68–84)

- Early milestones achieved
- Likely to be noticed when school performance is monitored
- Vocational skills adequate for competitive employment

MILD MENTAL RETARDATION (IQ: 52–67)

- Slight delay in achieving developmental milestones
- No alteration in sequence of skill acquisition
- Likely to require special education services with an emphasis on vocational and self-maintenance skills
- Able to form and maintain adult relationships

MODERATE MENTAL RETARDATION (IQ: 36–51)

- Noticeable delay in motor and speech development

- Early and persistent training in self-care required
- Supervision required for complex activities or problem solving

SEVERE MENTAL RETARDATION (IQ: 20–35)

- Marked delay in all motor skills
- Limited expressive speech, even though some receptive language skills may be present
- Constant supervision required

PROFOUND MENTAL RETARDATION (IQ: 0–19)

- May be able to walk
- May have primitive speech
- Constant supervision required

Adapted from Batshaw, M. (1997). *Children with disabilities*. Baltimore: Paul H. Brooks.

NURSING CARE

The Child Who Is Mentally Retarded

Assessment

The Child

When assessing cognitive skills and level of adaptive functioning, the nurse needs to become familiar with age-expected abilities that can be used as a standard for comparison (see Chapters 5 through 8). Life experiences also affect a child's abilities. Children who have had limited exposure to social rules and limited opportunities for thinking about their experiences will talk and act differently from children who have had more practice in these areas. Alternating between questions and demonstrations may be helpful in maintaining the child's interest in the assessment.

Look directly at the child and speak in a direct and simple yet noncondescending manner. Ask the child for as much of the necessary information as possible rather than relying solely on the parents to provide the information. As the child speaks, attend to the child's level of communication, skill in using words to communicate, and ability to follow one-step commands or more complicated requests.

The Family

Assessing the family's level of functioning is crucial. Specific concerns include coping skills available and typically used and the family's awareness of and involvement in addressing the needs of the child. The child may come from a home where the parents have below-average intellectual functioning; or the parents may be young and lack understanding of development, making them less aware of their child's abilities and functional deficits. Social and financial resources need to be explored in a manner that is informa-

tive but does not invade privacy. A matter-of-fact approach is helpful in assessing how the family meets the basic needs of each member and manages the exceptional needs of the cognitively impaired child. This part of the assessment may be lengthy, as it may be necessary to assist the family in seeking long-term assistance for meeting the child's medical, psychological, and social needs.

The family's interactional patterns should be assessed on an ongoing basis. The family's level of coping with the diagnosis or current situation should also be assessed. Families with mentally retarded children experience grief much as do families of children with other chronic illnesses (see Chapter 36). This grief cycle begins with disbelief and denial, then progresses to anger. A search for answers generally follows. When no specific cause of the disorder can be identified, this process is particularly difficult. The family then becomes preoccupied with the child's disabilities and symptoms. Finally, the family begins to identify the child's strengths and resources and moves toward a sense of integration and homeostasis. This process is repeated with each new developmental stage or situational setback, such as surgery or illness. The goal is for the family system to adjust to accommodate the child, and for the child to receive safe, nurturing care and the opportunity to develop skills to the greatest degree possible.

An interdisciplinary approach is critical for the effective management of children with cognitive impairments. The team generally includes physicians, nurses, psychologists, speech and language pathologists, educational and recreational professionals, and possibly physical therapists and occupational therapists. In addition to nursing care, the family may be referred for genetic counseling and supportive psychotherapy. The assessment should identify the need for other team members or auxiliary services. Long-term services may include respite care, in-home services, parent training, and support groups.

Nursing Diagnosis, Planning, Intervention, and Evaluation

Nursing Diagnosis
■ Risk for Injury related to level of self-care skills and inability to anticipate danger.

Expected Outcome
• The child will avoid self-injury or accidental injury.

Intervention

1. Provide anticipatory guidance relative to the child's developmental abilities to perform or understand.

2. Keep safety rails up on hospital beds and on the bed at home if the child is predisposed to falling or roaming at night. Provide child-sized furniture and select age- and skill-related play equipment.

3. Give simple explanations about unsafe areas in the environment. Use the child's cognitive level as a key to what the child can understand or the degree of unsupervised freedom that can safely be allowed.

Rationale

1. Parents may not be able to anticipate the child's cognitive or functional level accurately, particularly if the parents are inexperienced or have limited cognitive skills themselves.

2. These strategies help to prevent accidental falls, as these children are accident prone and have limited ability to assess the environment for safety.

3. Young or cognitively delayed individuals can understand concrete explanations.

Evaluation
• Has the child remained safe and not sustained any injury?

Nursing Diagnosis
■ Knowledge Deficit (family members) related to the cause and likely outcomes of the child's cognitive disabilities, available support systems, or information about sexuality, vocational options, leisure skills, and so on.

Expected Outcome
• The family will access and use personal and community resources to increase the child's ability to develop personal skills for appropriate social, leisure, and vocational abilities.

Intervention

1. Provide information that is simple, concrete, and solution focused.
2. Explain medical terms without assuming that the family knows the terminology. Give explanations to both the child and the parents. Use demonstrations and therapeutic play.
3. Select skills that enhance self-care and socially appropriate behaviors. As the child reaches puberty, provide simple information about sexuality and physical changes. Support training in leisure skills.
4. Identify for the parents local and national resources for the home care, education, and training of mentally retarded individuals.

5. Provide parents with anticipatory guidance about developmental milestones and anticipated skills, including safety, sexuality, skills that can be expected, and behavioral changes throughout the developmental process.

Rationale

1. Hospitalization is stressful and may impair the family's adaptive coping skills.
2. The child may have a limited capacity to understand words but may be able to understand a demonstration.

3. Education that is practical and functional for the child's mental and chronological age fosters self-esteem, compliance, and cooperation.

4. Additional services will be needed as the child grows or needs more specialized training. Families may have to find out-of-home placement if the child's disability is severe or destructive to the family.
5. Parents may have unrealistic expectations or expect too little from the child.

Evaluation
• Has the family used the resources available in the community to maximize the child's abilities?

Nursing Diagnosis
■ Impaired Social Interaction related to an inability to initiate and maintain social relationships.

Expected Outcome
• The child will have relationships with family and peers and will have solitary leisure skills.

Intervention

1. Encourage the parents to support the child in participating in group activities that promote peer interactions (Special Olympics, special camps, etc.) (Fig. 54–2). The family will arrange social activities with other children (e.g., visiting the park with friends, inviting friends to the home to play).

Rationale

1. To accommodate to social expectations and demands, children who are mentally retarded need to be exposed to nonimpaired children as well as to children with similar handicaps.

2. Encourage the parents to participate in interactive activities, such as reading books and playing, on a regular basis.

2. Families are likely to limit interactions, as the child offers reduced reinforcements in social situations.

Evaluation

• Has the child demonstrated a sense of pleasure in social interactions with family members and with other individuals within his or her social sphere?

Nursing Diagnosis

■ Ineffective Family Coping: Compromised or Disabling, related to excessive emotional and financial strain on family members caring for a cognitively impaired individual, lack of acceptance by society, or an extended grieving process associated with a chronic disability.

Expected Outcome

• The family will express self-satisfaction in their family management and will have social acceptance within the community.

Intervention

1. Provide anticipatory and ongoing support for the grieving process. Parents should be told the diagnosis and needed information as quickly as possible. This information should be given when both parents or supportive family members are available. Information may need to be explained in different ways (orally, in writing, with videos) to help parents grasp the meaning of the diagnosis.
2. Assist in identifying appropriate resources for social interactions and social training (early intervention programs, special education programs, recreational programs for mentally retarded children, and so forth).
3. Identify and refer the family to appropriate community resources for both emotional support and family/child education. The nurse may need to act as an advocate and referral center (about support groups, education consultants, home health agencies).
4. Assist family members in identifying realistic short- and long-term goals for the child and themselves. Encourage the family to express feelings and concerns; provide hope when appropriate.
5. Educate the parents in monitoring the child for alterations in health status. Help the family recognize nonverbal signs of discomfort.
6. Assist family members in exploring their choices for home care, a group home, or a residential facility.

Rationale

1. Families typically experience a cycle of grieving that is repeated when milestones are not reached or when the child experiences an illness or a change in behavior.

2. Mildly and moderately retarded individuals often experience loneliness and depression as a result of insufficient stimulation and social contact. Such programs can assist the child in reaching maximum potential.
3. The grieving process and the need to accommodate to the child's skill level are ongoing; families often feel isolated and helpless in locating necessary resources.

4. Stress, grieving, and limited knowledge may impair the family's ability to set reasonable goals itself.

5. The child may be unable to verbalize pain typically associated with ear infections, colds, or major illnesses.
6. Families may hesitate to discuss care options out of fear of being perceived as uncaring or unable to provide home care.

Evaluation

• Do the child and family have the ability to manage the anxiety and grieving experience as they understand the diagnosis and the severity of the disorder?
• Does the family accommodate the child in the family system in a manner that facilitates growth and maturity to the greatest degree possible?
• Does the family seek medical attention when needed and use several resources to meet the child's social, emotional, educational, and medical needs?
• Is the family able to meet financial responsibilities?
• Does the family participate in social activities outside the family?

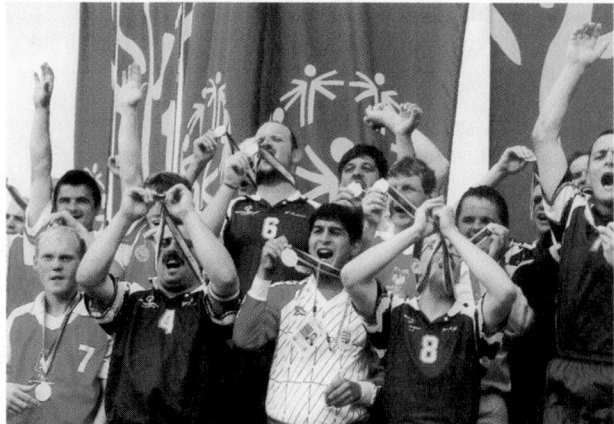

FIGURE 54-2
• • • • • • • • • •
Special Olympics International is the largest recreational program in the world for people with mental retardation. With more than one million athletes in 125 countries, Special Olympics offers opportunities for social interaction with peers and assists mentally retarded children in reaching their maximum potential. (Courtesy of Special Olympics, Inc.)

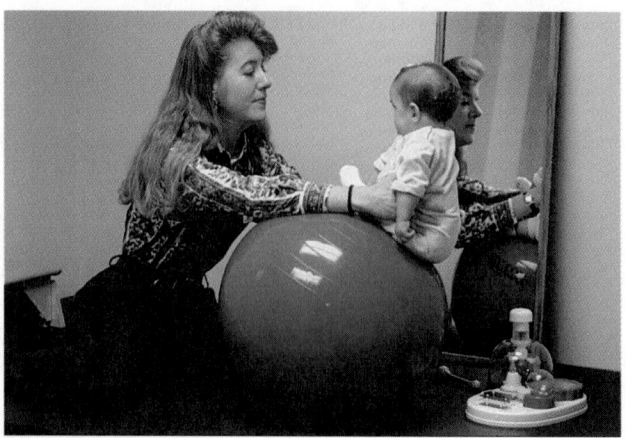

FIGURE 54-3
• • • • • • • • • •
Children with delayed motor or cognitive function, whether temporary or pervasive, benefit from early and vigorous therapy to help them reach their maximum development. (Courtesy of Cook Children's Medical Center, Fort Worth, Texas.)

Down Syndrome

The most common genetic disorder causing moderate to severe mental retardation is Down syndrome (trisomy 21). The assessment and nursing interventions for mentally retarded individuals are applicable to these individuals. Additional considerations, however, apply to those identified as having Down syndrome.

Depending on the severity of the symptoms, the most common experience is for parents to rear the child at home until early adulthood, after which group home placement is an option. Supported employment is encouraged, and parents are typically advised to initiate vocational training in elementary school. The partnership of parents and professionals is vital in managing the symptoms and in providing the comprehensive services that are needed.

Services required throughout the life span include education and vocational training, transitional services, respite care, social services, financial supplements, psychotherapy, and preventive or corrective medical care. This array of needed services may be overwhelming to the family, and the potential for frustration on the part of both the parents and the professional team is high. Communication and coordination of services are considered primary tasks for each team member (Fig. 54-3).

Etiology

Although the specific cause is unknown, late maternal age has been consistently identified as one of the most significant factors associated with Down syndrome. The risk of a 35-year-old woman bearing a child with trisomy 21 is 1 in 250. By age 48, the risk increases to 1 in 11. As a result of early screening for women who are at high risk for having a child with Down syndrome, most of these children are now born to women less than 35 years old. Women having

children after age 35 account for 20% to 25% of Down syndrome cases but for only 7% of overall births each year (Cohen, 1999).

Several chromosomal alterations that result in Down syndrome have been identified. In 97% of Down syndrome cases, nondisjunction, a failure of the chromosomes to separate normally during meiosis, occurs. The remaining 3% result from chromosome 21 translocating to chromosome 14 or 22. Translocation is caused by an inherited factor. Translocator carrier parents are at increased risk of producing

PATHOPHYSIOLOGY
• • • • • • • • • • •
of Down Syndrome

Trisomy 21, or Down syndrome, occurs when three representatives of chromosome 21 are present instead of the usual two. There is some evidence that a particular region of chromosome 21 is responsible for the facial features, heart defects, mental retardation, and dermatologic changes. Many of the malformations in this disorder result from incomplete rather than abnormal embryogenesis. Examples include malformations of the atrioventricular canal, tracheoesophageal fistula, and imperforate anus. Alterations in neurotransmitters, particularly in the cholinergic system, are responsible for the premature aging and Alzheimer's-type dementia that are common in individuals with Down syndrome.

A number of medical problems in the newborn period can seriously compromise health and survival. If the child survives these complications, a number of less serious difficulties are generally encountered in childhood.

Medical Conditions Associated with Down Syndrome

CONDITIONS FREQUENTLY IDENTIFIED DURING THE NEONATAL PERIOD

Cardiac conditions
- Endocardial cushion defect
- Tetralogy of Fallot
- Atrial septal defects
- Patent ductus arteriosus
- Ventricular septal defects

Gastrointestinal conditions
- Tracheoesophageal fistula
- Pyloric stenosis
- Imperforate anus
- Duodenal atresia
- Aganglionic megacolon (Hirschsprung's disease)

Congenital cataracts
Hypothyroidism
Dysplastic hips
Leukemia-like conditions

CONDITIONS FREQUENTLY IDENTIFIED DURING CHILDHOOD

Endocrine disorders
- Decreased growth
- Obesity secondary to overeating, underexercise, or undetected hypothyroidism
- Thyroid dysfunction
- Infertility (male)

Alopecia
Thin hair
Sensitive skin and propensity for rashes
Ophthalmic problems, such as myopia, strabismus, nystagmus, cataracts, blepharitis, and keratoconus
Chronic serous otitis media
Hematologic abnormalities
- Subtle immune deficiencies
- Acute nonlymphoblastic leukemia
- Acute lymphoblastic leukemia

Craniofacial defects
- Malocclusions
- Delayed tooth eruption
- Periodontal disease and gingivitis
- Bruxism
- Sinusitis and rhinitis
- Sleep apnea secondary to cranial malformations

Musculoskeletal abnormalities
- Hypotonia
- Joint laxity and dislocations
- Atlantoaxial subluxation or dislocation

Sensory deficits
Seizure disorders
Psychiatric disorders, particularly adjustment reaction disorders, anxiety disorders, depression, behavior disorders, dementia
Pervasive developmental disorders

---

multiple offspring with Down syndrome (McCance & Huether, 1994).

Incidence

In the United States, more than 300,000 individuals have Down syndrome, with up to 10,000 new cases occurring each year. This syndrome accounts for one third of all cases of moderate to severe mental retardation. The prevalence of Down syndrome is 1.2 in 1,000 live births (State, King, & Dykens, 1997). Affected boys outnumber girls 1.3:1.0. As a result of increased prenatal diagnosis, approximately 40% of fetuses with Down syndrome in women age 35 or older are now aborted voluntarily. This trend has resulted in a recent decrease in the birth rate of children with Down syndrome.

Manifestations

Certain facial features are common in children with Down syndrome:

- Brachycephaly (disproportionate shortness of the head)
- Flat profile
- Upward slanted palpebral fissures
- Inner epicanthal folds
- Wide, flat nasal bridge
- Speckled irises
- Narrow, high-arched palate
- Protruding tongue
- Small, short ears, which may be low-set
- Delayed teeth eruption and frequently poor alignment

Body features associated with Down syndrome include

- Short stature
- Short, broad hands
- Simian line (single transverse palmar crease)
- Clinodactyly (in-curved little finger)
- Broad, stubby feet with plantar crease
- Wide gap between 1st and 2nd toes
- Short, broad neck
- Likelihood of diastasis recti abdominis and umbilical hernia
- Small penis in males, bulbous vulva in females
- Dry skin with tendency to crack and fissure
- Hyperextensibility of joints and hypotonicity of muscles
- 15% have atlantoaxial instability (i.e., at the first and second cervical vertebrae)

Down syndrome is associated with intellectual, language, and social dysfunctions, including

- Mild to severe mental retardation, with intellectual abilities that continue to decline with age
- Onset of Alzheimer's-type dementia with increasing age
- Language development characterized by particular difficulty with grammar but general strength in pragmatic language (social usage) (pragmatic language includes

such skills as maintaining the conversation on a specific topic and taking turns during conversation)
- Social skills that surpass expected skills based on intellectual capacity
- Social skills and adaptive self-care skills that decline with age
- A limited ability to use the environmental cues available (i.e., infrequent scanning and use of only a few referential cues, such as eye contact with the primary caregiver, which often results in an inability to extract the information needed to draw conclusions)
- Blunted affect
- Fewer disruptive behaviors than with other chromosomal disorders (Cohen, 1999; State, King, & Dykens, 1997).

Diagnostic Evaluation

Down syndrome is usually evident at birth because of the characteristic prominent features, although if the diagnosis is questionable, chromosomal analysis is conducted. Other diagnostic tests are conducted on the basis of the associated features, such as nasopharyngeal abnormalities or cardiac defects.

To rule out associated disorders and to detect frequently encountered difficulties, clinicians recommend that the child be monitored frequently throughout the first 12 months of life, with an emphasis on gastrointestinal and cardiac symptoms. The diagnosis often requires a full cardiac workup initially and an electrocardiogram at the end of the first year. In the second to fourth years of life, the medical emphasis is on sleep and behavioral difficulties, along with annual thyroid screening and ophthalmologic assessment. Generally, the child is referred for dental assessments at 24 months and should be re-evaluated medically and behaviorally at least annually throughout childhood.

Therapeutic Management

The management of Down syndrome is manifestation specific, as there is no cure for the disorder. Surgery to correct cardiac abnormalities, gastrointestinal malformations, and craniofacial deviations has been used to prolong life, alleviate discomfort, and decrease the likelihood of further medical complications. Neck radiography should be performed prior to participating in any sports because of the risk of children with Down syndrome having atlantoaxial instability.

NURSING CARE
The Child with Down Syndrome

Assessment

Neonatal assessment is crucial in diagnosing Down syndrome on the basis of physiologic characteristics (see Chapter 22). Assessment for Down syndrome is based on family history, especially the mother's age. If Down syndrome is suspected or already confirmed on the basis of earlier genetic testing, serum alpha-fetoprotein levels, or amniotic fluid samples, an assessment is conducted to determine the severity of the manifestations and the family's ability to cope with and accommodate the needs of the infant. Assessment for mental retardation is also appropriate for the child with Down syndrome.

A thorough physical examination should be conducted including hearing and vision examinations. Children with Down syndrome are at increased risk for hearing deficits and refractive errors or cataracts.

If a child with Down syndrome is hospitalized for surgical repair, infections, or injury, assess the child's typical coping patterns, to support strategies already in place. Children with Down syndrome prefer routine and consistency, so an assessment of their daily routine is important; include times and habits related to mealtimes, bathing, and order of dressing.

Assessing the child's understanding of language and ability to communicate is important in order to provide information that the child can understand. Knowing the child's words for specific body functions, such as voiding, defecating, or sleeping, will allow for greater comfort for the hospitalized child. It is important to assess the child's learning abilities before initiating any education or procedure-related play.

The child's motor skills are assessed to determine what procedures will be necessary to ensure the child's safety. Children with Down syndrome often are awkward and somewhat uncoordinated, which increases the likelihood of their falling. Self-stimulating behaviors (e.g., picking at the arm) need to be identified, as they are often used as coping strategies but may also be self-injurious. Sensory deficits, such as vision or hearing difficulties, should be identified as part of the routine assessment. Such deficits can be detected through close observation as the child reaches for objects, by listening to conversation, or by speaking the child's name. The child with Down syndrome, however, may respond to sensory stimuli less noticeably than unimpaired children or with dulled affect, even if hearing or vision deficits are not present.

> Health care professionals may forget the importance of discussing normal aspects of the child with parents. For example, the nurse may state, "Billy has the most beautiful eyes. They seem to light up when he sees someone he knows."

An assessment of the environment will help determine whether it is conducive to safety and provides sufficient stimulation. Affected children frequently do not seek out stimulation and may need encouragement through colors, sound, and motion. An assessment of social behaviors is also important and should include play, social judgment skills, and social interest in the environment. The child may demonstrate inappropriate behaviors like those associated with severe mental retardation. Moreover, the child's natural curiosity may be diminished as a result of fear or frustration.

Nursing Diagnosis, Planning, Intervention, and Evaluation

Nursing Diagnosis	■ Altered Parenting related to the child's delayed development, physical appearance, and medical complications.
Expected Outcome	• The family will develop satisfying and supportive relationships that meet the physical and emotional needs of each family member.

Intervention	Rationale
1. Offer assistance and support to parents by giving clear explanations.	1. Understanding increases compliance and competence.
2. State clearly what you observe about the child's behaviors and skills.	2. Parents may not understand their child's limitations or may be in denial. Identifying behaviors and skill level may increase understanding.
3. Assist in identifying positive features and behaviors in the child.	3. Parents are often fearful of how others will respond to their child and may need encouragement to identify the child's positive characteristics.

Evaluation	• Are parent-child interactions positive and mutually satisfying? • Do the parents demonstrate acceptance of the child's disabilities, with a tolerance for delayed skill development? • Do the parents show an interest and willingness to help the child learn new skills through demonstration, repetition, and much positive feedback?

Nursing Diagnosis	■ Self-Care Deficit related to cognitive immaturity.
Expected Outcome	• The child will meet his or her own needs related to toileting, feeding, bathing, and dressing.

Intervention	Rationale
1. Keep the environment as routine as possible. Obtain information about the child's home routines and record it in the care plan so that the information can be accessed easily.	1. A change in routine often results in excessive frustration and decreased coping abilities.
2. The plan of care is based on the child's cognitive and motor abilities rather than on chronological age. Observe the child for signs of readiness to learn a new task (reaching for a cup, attempting to dress self, and so forth).	2. The child's skills may be age-appropriate in some areas but markedly delayed in others. Self-care should be encouraged.
3. Adaptive tools for dressing, bathing, and eating may be necessary.	3. The child's level of coordination, muscle strength, and dexterity may not allow the child to zip, button, or feed self in the usual way.

Evaluation	• Does the child demonstrate continued development and use of self-care skills already present? • Does the child have a sense of mastery and competency with the learning of new skills?

Nursing Diagnosis	■ Altered Growth and Development related to poor sucking abilities or mouth deformities, flaccid facial muscles, or other abnormalities.
Expected Outcome	• The child will maintain a steady growth velocity pattern throughout childhood.

Intervention	Rationale
1. Explore options for fluid and calorie intake; use special bottles or adaptive utensils as needed as the child develops.	1. Breast-feeding may not be possible if the child's muscle tone or sucking reflex is immature. Because of facial, mouth, or trunk abnormalities, the child may not have the strength or ability to use ordinary eating or drinking tools.
2. Refer the parents for nutritional consultation as necessary. Provide resources for behavioral training to encourage intake of new foods or the acquisition of new skills.	2. The child with Down syndrome likes to maintain routines and is often resistant to food or environmental changes.

Evaluation	• Does the child exhibit a normal growth pattern appropriate for age and abilities?

Fragile X Syndrome

Fragile X syndrome is the most common inherited cause of mental retardation. It accounts for 10% to 12% of all mental retardation in males. The disorder usually does not manifest as mental retardation in females, but a female carrier normally passes the fragile X chromosome to the offspring. This syndrome has a unique profile of behavioral and cognitive patterns.

Etiology

The gene that causes fragile X syndrome is located on the X chromosome. Typically, a female child receiving the X chromosome having a fragile site will become a carrier and will be mildly affected, if at all. The female may continue to pass on the abnormal X chromosome. A male, however, will usually exhibit the full effects if he receives the abnormal gene (State, King, & Dykens, 1997). Transmission occurs through carrier mothers and not through an unaffected "carrier" father.

Incidence

Fragile X syndrome affects approximately 1 in every 1,000 male children and 1 in every 3,000 female children (King & State, 1998; Laxova, 1994). As many as 1 in 259 females carry the fragile X gene, either as a premutation or as a full mutation (Hagerman, 1999). In general, only males exhibit the full effects of the X-linked recessive disorder because their single X chromosome has the abnormal gene. Approximately 50% to 70% of females with the full genetic mutation manifest cognitive defects, usually with borderline to mild mental retardation.

Manifestations

Physical features associated with fragile X syndrome include

- Facial dysmorphism, with large or prominent ears and a long, narrow face; a head circumference that may be disproportionate to height and weight; lowered epicanthic folds; and prominent nasal alae (cartilaginous flap on outer side of each nostril)
- Postpubertal macro-orchidism
- Flat feet
- Lax ankles
- Hyperextensible fingers
- Extremely soft and smooth skin
- Mitral valve prolapse (common)

PATHOPHYSIOLOGY
of Fragile X Syndrome

Fragile X syndrome is caused by an underlying single gene defect. There is an abnormality in the *FMR1* (fragile X mental retardation) gene in all affected individuals. There are excessive repetitions of the CGG sequences in affected individuals.

Intellectual, language, and social dysfunctions associated with fragile X syndrome include the following characteristics:

- Autistic-like behaviors, such as gaze avoidance, hand flapping, echolalia, and abnormal speech patterns
- Hyperkinetic behaviors, including restlessness, agitation, and attention deficits
- Hand biting
- Sensory motor integration deficits, such as poor coordination, motor planning deficits, and tactile defensiveness
- *In boys:* Cognitive deficits in the moderate to severe range, strengths in visual memory but weakness in auditory processing abilities and abstract reasoning, improved performance with simultaneous rather than sequential processing, language delays, perseveration, tangential speech, and other communicative disorders
- *In girls:* Generally only mild cognitive deficits but with many variations
- High degree of disruptive behaviors, including temper tantrums, self-injurious behaviors, extreme agitation
- Progressive dementia (American Academy of Pediatrics [AAP], 1996; Baumgardner et al., 1995; King & State, 1998)

Diagnostic Evaluation

DNA testing is the definitive method of diagnosing fragile X syndrome. Identification of the *FMR1* gene mutation allows diagnosis in both carriers and those affected (Hagerman, Kimbro, & Taylor, 1998). Individuals with mental retardation of unknown cause or learning disabilities, together with manifestations of fragile X syndrome, should be considered for fragile X testing.

Therapeutic Management

Treatment is provided through various types of therapy. Special education, vocational programs, and behavioral management classes are important to assess overall development. Speech and language evaluation and therapy are generally prescribed during the first year of life and are made available on an ongoing basis. Sensorimotor integration therapy may be offered to enhance motor planning, joint stability, coordination, and integration of visual, auditory, and tactile information. Sensorimotor therapy is considered to be the intervention of choice for learning disabilities.

Nursing Considerations

The nursing care of individuals with fragile X syndrome is similar to care for mentally retarded children, but with specific attention to the behavioral and cognitive difficulties presented by the individual child. The plan should include a multidisciplinary team approach to assessment. Anticipatory guidance should be provided, with a review of the support groups and services available. Special education services will be necessary to address the child's specific cognitive and academic difficulties, as well as to foster continued skill development and to reduce the stress created in the typical educational setting. Remediation services should include behavioral interventions specific to the child's needs, speech and language assistance, and possibly occupational and physical therapy to address visual-motor and motor skill deficits. Family members of individuals with fragile X syndrome should receive genetic counseling and testing.

Assessment for other related abnormalities, such as cleft palate, foot deformities, hip dislocations, and other conditions involving joint hyperextensibility, hernias, and hypertonia, should also be performed. Seizures occur in 17% to 50% of these children, so medications and educating the family about seizure disorders may be warranted.

Autism

Autism is the most severe condition classified as a *pervasive developmental disorder* (PDD) by the American Psychiatric Association (1994). PDDs are disorders characterized by "severe and pervasive impairment in several areas of development: reciprocal social interaction skills, communication skills, or the presence of stereotyped behavior, interests, and activities" (APA, 1994). Typically, these conditions are evident in the first 12 months of life, but they may be overlooked if gross motor skills are progressing normally. Frequently they occur concurrently with a diverse group of other medical conditions. Other conditions included in this category are Rett syndrome and childhood thought disorders, formerly known as childhood schizophrenia, symbiotic psychosis, and childhood psychosis. Autism is the most severe of these disorders, but it is not the most frequently encountered disorder among PDDs.

There is no evidence that autism can be cured, so treatment is generally lifelong and is characterized by varying degrees of success. Children with IQs of less than 50 generally remain cognitively stable. In those with IQs above 50, the outcome varies, depending on education and early treatment. Research indicates that language functions rather than social behaviors can be used most successfully to predict short-term outcomes. The early onset of social symptoms does not necessarily indicate greater severity of symptoms, lower intelligence, or insecure attachments.

Etiology

The cause of autism is unknown, but it is believed that the disorder can be caused by a wide range of prenatal, perinatal, and postnatal conditions, including maternal rubella, untreated phenylketonuria, tuberous sclerosis, anoxia during birth, encephalitis, and fragile X syndrome (Barton & Volkmar, 1998). It was once believed that family child-rearing practices and parental personality characteristics influenced the development of autism, but no controlled studies confirm this view. Because siblings are more likely to develop the disorder than children in the general population, genetic factors are believed to play a role.

Incidence

Autism affects 10 to 15 children in every 10,000 and is three to four times more common in boys than in girls. No differ-ences in incidence have been correlated with race, socioeconomic level, or culture.

Manifestations

Autism is a severely incapacitating, lifelong developmental disability that is characterized by a qualitative impairment in four developmental areas:

- Disturbance in the rate and appearance of physical, social, and language skills
- Abnormal responses of the body sensations
- Thinking capacity, but with absent or delayed speech and language
- Abnormal ways of relating to people, objects, and events

A child may have a vast vocabulary yet have no comprehension of the meaning of the words. Another child may be able to solve intricate mathematical problems but not be able to make change from a dollar. Children may seem oblivious to the sound of their own names but may come running into the room at the sound of a truck. Generally, they show a fixed, unchanging response to a particular stimulus. Self-stimulation is common and generally involves repetition of a particularly pleasing sensory stimulus, such as twirling a toy or rubbing the top of the head. The autistic child typically repeats an act, such as fingering an object or continuously spinning around, rather than responding to a new stimulus.

Apparently, interest is limited by nature, rather than by choice, to an extremely narrow range. The child with autism generally overreacts to any change within the environment. Often, autistic children do not have a typical sense of personal space and so may touch others on the face or stand face to face, with noses touching, even when encountering a total stranger.

Autism is usually apparent to parents before age 3, although a period of apparently normal development may be followed by rapid deterioration. There is a wide range in the degree of impairment produced. Autism shares some similarities with the characteristic presentation of what has been called childhood schizophrenia and mental retardation, but with definitive differences. These differences are outlined in Table 54–2. Seventy-five percent of autistic individuals are mentally retarded. A few individuals with autism also have an extremely developed skill in a particular area, such as music or mathematics. These individuals are sometimes known as idiot savants because they have both a severe cognitive deficit and an extraordinary cognitive skill or expertise.

Social behaviors associated with autism include

- Marked lack of awareness of the existence or feelings of others (e.g., individual ignores emotions of others)
- Lack of or abnormal amount of comfort seeking at times of distress (e.g., individual does not show pain when hurt)
- Lack of or abnormal imitation of others' actions
- Lack of or abnormal social play (generally plays alone or involves others only as mere objects)
- Gross impairment in social peer relationships (appears not to want or need friends)

TABLE 54-2

Differential Diagnosis of Autism, Mental Retardation, and Schizophrenia

Autism	Mental Retardation
Peaked skill profile	Flat skill profile
Lack of imitative skills	Imitation skills and gesturing
Nonsocial behaviors with little initiation	Social behavior, initiation of social contact
Abnormal communication and language	Limited language ability but sufficient for communication
Development seizures possible during adolescence	Usually no seizures, Alzheimer's-type dementia in adulthood

Autism	Schizophrenia
Onset before age 30 months	Onset during pubescence or adolescence
No remissions	Remissions and relapses
Hallucinations/delusions rare	Hallucinations/delusions common
Absence of thought disorder	Thought disorder
No family history of schizophrenia	Family history of schizophrenia
Self-stimulating behaviors	Odd behavior but no self-stimulating behaviors
Medications of limited use	Medications often helpful in reducing symptoms

The child with autism typically exhibits the following language characteristics:

- Lack of or impaired verbal communication and abnormalities in the production of speech (inappropriate volume, pitch, rate, rhythm, or intonation, such as a monotone voice or echolalia)
- Markedly abnormal nonverbal communication (i.e., the child uses no gestures or behavioral cues)
- Absence of imaginative play (no imitative or dramatic role playing)
- Impaired interactive speech and communication (the child does not allow for the normal give-and-take of conversation and tends to become preoccupied with a given subject or word out of context with the conversation)

The child with autism also exhibits a restricted behavioral repertoire, including

- Stereotyped body movements (e.g., spinning around, head banging, "flapping," rocking)
- Persistent preoccupation with characteristics of objects (smell, taste, texture) or an abnormal attachment to objects (e.g., piece of string, picture of a whale)
- Marked distress over a minor change in the environment (e.g., exhibiting tantrums when a light is turned on, refusing to look at a teacher who is wearing a new dress)
- Unreasonable insistence on routine (e.g., following a schedule exactly to the minute or second, refusal to attend an assembly during a scheduled mathematics class)
- Self-injurious behaviors (e.g., biting, picking at skin, scratching eyes)
- Marked restriction in range of interests (e.g., may repeat-

edly align objects and cannot be diverted from doing so) (APA, 1994; Dawson et al., 1998)

Diagnostic Evaluation

A diagnosis of autism is usually established on the basis of manifestations. Often, the family is interviewed initially, followed by observation of the child alone, with the parent, and interacting with the examiner or others in the environment. Interviews are coupled with observations and clinician's rating scales. The onset of characteristic delays or of abnormal functioning must occur before age 3.

Therapeutic Management

Early identification of autism is essential. Treatment generally entails placement in an environment that facilitates interaction and promotes replacement of stereotypical behaviors with more normal behaviors. Behavioral methods are typically used. Autistic people have a normal life span; consequently, they require significant financial resources for treatment and supervision.

Because of the severity of the social impairment and the ineffectiveness of normal environmental interventions, affected children are usually referred to special programs designed to offer stimulation, modify stereotypical behaviors, or establish routines for teaching as soon as the disorder has been identified. Programs usually focus on safety precautions for self-injurious behaviors, such as head banging, and the promotion of communication. Facilitative communication through the use of picture boards or keyboards is controversial but has been used in many educational settings to help these children interact with their environment.

NURSING CARE
The Child with Autism

Assessment

Since there are no classic physical features that highlight autism, the nurse must assess the child with possible autism as if no physical or cognitive deficits are present. This is done prior to establishing a diagnosis. The primary characteristic of autism is lack of social interaction and awareness. For this reason, if the child is very young, the nurse who interacts only with the child's parents is unlikely to be aware of the child's degree of social disengagement. If the child has already been diagnosed as having autism and the purpose of assessment is to determine the severity of the disorder—or the assessment occurs before a procedure or hospitalization—it is performed in the same manner as with any normal child. The nurse, however, will quickly become aware of the child's social detachment or lack of language as the assessment continues.

A systematic exploration of the child's skills and comparison with developmental norms is essential. For the staff nurse, this process may include evaluating the child's ability to feed self, dress, and toilet. The assessment should include the child's interactive patterns and verbalization skills. The child's motor skills will be important to note also, as these have major implications for safety and self-care. For initial, generalized screening, the DDSI-II may be helpful (see Chapter 4). A family history of autism or other mental disorders, family coping skills, and available social support systems should also be assessed.

Nursing Diagnosis and Planning

The following nursing diagnoses may be appropriate following assessment of the child with autism.

- Risk for Injury related to an inability to anticipate danger, a tendency for self-mutilation, and sensory perceptual deficits.
  Expected Outcome: The child will maintain integrity of skin and avoid self-injury or accidental injury.
- Impaired Social Interaction related to an inability to initiate and maintain social relationships and to limited verbal skills.
  Expected Outcome: The child will develop understandable and socially acceptable ways to communicate needs and wants.
- Altered Thought Processes related to an inability to perceive self or others accurately and to cognitive and perceptual dysfunction.
  Expected Outcomes: The child will show interest in surroundings, be able to acknowledge others in the environment, demonstrate orientation to person, place, and time, and perform activities of daily living appropriate to this orientation

Interventions

When working with autistic children, the nurse needs to work closely with the family to determine the child's routines, habits, and preferences. The nurse should write down

---

CRITICAL TO REMEMBER
Maintaining Routine for the Child with Autism

Children with autism often are unable to tolerate even the slightest change in routine and may become withdrawn, self-abusive, or violent if their routines are altered.

---

any specific cues that will help the child remain oriented to the environment and will facilitate tolerance to change. For example, the nursing staff should be limited to as few individuals as possible. The child may need to perform toileting and self-care activities in a particular order. The child may need an environmental cue, such as stroking a favorite blanket, before being able to move from one activity to the next. The nurse can generally evaluate the child's tolerance of the situation by monitoring signs of anxiety or emotional comfort, as evidenced by such behaviors as attending or observing the nurse in the room or demonstrating a willingness to participate in self-care.

The nurse must work closely with the family to determine the specific ways in which the child communicates. The child may use sign language or pictures to specify needs if no verbal skills are developed. Children with autism are often reluctant to initiate or sustain direct eye contact, so the nurse may interpret this behavior as meaning that the child is not listening or is unaware of what is being said. In addition, the child may answer questions after several minutes' delay. The nurse should identify these behaviors, allow extra time, and be alert to differences in communication styles. Children with autism generally understand much more language than they are able to use expressively themselves.

The child who demonstrates a tendency for head banging may need a helmet or side rolls. Wrist restraints may be necessary if the child is unable to remain in the bed at night. The nurse should help the parents understand and explain to their child any safety precautions that are unfamiliar to the child. The presence of a parent or older sibling is almost always necessary when an autistic child is hospitalized. Evaluating the child for safety is an ongoing nursing function. Reducing the adjustment demands for the child may be necessary if the nurse recognizes behaviors indicating stress or anxiety.

Evaluation

- Has the child remained free of injury?
- Has the child developed a way to communicate needs?
- Does the child demonstrate an interest in surroundings?
- Does the child acknowledge the presence of others in the environment?
- Has the child developed the ability to perform activities of daily living?
- Has the child accommodated to the hospital setting by adjusting to the change in environment and schedule?

KEY CONCEPTS

■ Children with a cognitive deficit experience limitations in social interactions, use of language for self-expression, and self-care abilities. If these limitations are severe, the child will need the care of mature, caring adults throughout his or her life.

■ Children with cognitive deficits have many normal needs, including the need for positive attention and opportunities for self-discovery and growth. The nurse needs to work closely with the family to identify the child's specific patterns of interacting with the environment. This is done by asking relevant, clear questions about how the child communicates and perceives experiences.

■ Another nursing consideration is that families with a cognitively impaired child experience repeated stress and grief as the child continues to fail to reach developmental expectations.

■ The nurse can be most helpful by offering family members an opportunity to discuss feelings and by identifying resources to help meet the child's needs. The nurse may act as an advocate for the parents in the school system and the community.

■ Mental retardation may be the result of congenital or early environmental factors, or it may occur secondary to head injury, asphyxia, intracranial hemorrhage, infections, poisoning, or the presence or treatment of a brain tumor.

■ Several neuropsychological tests are available to assess levels of mental retardation. The best method of early detection is by assessing development during routine pediatric preventive care visits.

■ Parents of children with cognitive deficits should be provided with anticipatory guidance relative to their child's developmental abilities.

■ Changes in routine can cause frustration for the child with Down syndrome.

■ The family of a child with Down syndrome may need assistance in identifying and obtaining adaptive tools for dressing, bathing, and eating.

■ The family of a child with Down syndrome should be encouraged and assisted in helping the child learn new skills through demonstration, repetition, and positive feedback.

■ Children with fragile X syndrome exhibit autistic-like behaviors, such as gaze avoidance, hand flapping, echolalia, and abnormal speech patterns. In addition, affected children have poor coordination, hyperkinetic behaviors, and cognitive deficits that are moderate to severe.

■ Autism is characterized by an impairment in the rate and appearance of physical, social, and language skills; abnormal responses of the body sensations; thinking capacity, but with absent or delayed speech and language; and abnormal ways of relating to people, objects, and events.

■ Autism shares similarities with childhood schizophrenia and mental retardation, but there are definitive differences.

■ When working with children with autism, the nurse needs to work with the family to determine the child's routines, habits, and preferences.

REFERENCES AND READINGS

American Academy of Child and Adolescent Psychiatry. (1995). *Facts for families #23: Children who are mentally retarded.* Washington, DC: Author.

American Academy of Pediatrics. (1996). Health supervision for children with fragile X syndrome. *Pediatrics, 98*(2), 297–300.

American Psychiatric Association. (1994). *Diagnostic and statistical manual of mental disorders* (4th ed.). Washington, DC: Author.

Barton, M., & Volkmar, K. (1998). How common are known medical conditions associated with autism? *Journal of Autism and Developmental Disorders, 28*(4), 273–278.

Batshaw, M. (1997). *Children with disabilities.* Baltimore: Paul H. Brooks.

Bauer, S. (1995). Autism and the pervasive developmental disorders: Part 1. *Pediatrics in Review, 16*(4), 130–136.

Bauer, S. (1995). Autism and the pervasive developmental disorders: Part 2. *Pediatrics in Review, 16*(5), 168–176.

Baumgardner, T. L., Reiss, A. L., Freund, L. S., & Abrams, M. T. (1995). Specification of the neurobehavioral phenotype in males with fragile X syndrome. *Pediatrics, 95,* 744–752.

Cohen, W. I. (1999). Down syndrome: Care of the child and family. In M. D. Levine, W. B. Carey, & A. C. Crocker (Eds.), *Developmental-behavioral pediatrics* (3rd ed., pp. 240–248). Philadelphia: Saunders.

Dawson, G., Meltzoff, A. N., Osterling, J., & Rinaldi, J. (1998). Neuropsychological correlates of early symptoms of autism. *Child Development, 69*(5), 1276–1285.

Dykens, E. M., Rosner, B. A., & Butterbaugh, G. (1998). Exercise and sports in children and adolescents with developmental disabilities. *Child and Adolescent Psychiatric Clinics of North America, 7*(4), 757–771.

Elder, J. H. (1994). Beliefs held by parents of autistic children. *Journal of Child and Adolescent Psychiatric Nursing, 7,* 9–16.

Feinstein, C., & Reiss, A. L. (1996). Psychiatric disorder in mentally retarded children and adolescents. *Child and Adolescent Psychiatric Clinics of North America, 5*(4), 827–852.

Fink, L. (1995). Mental retardation. In B. S. Johnson (Ed.), *Child, adolescent and family psychiatric nursing.* Philadelphia: Lippincott.

Fredricks, D. W., & Williams, W. L. (1998). New definitions of mental retardation for the American Association of Mental Retardation. *Image: Journal of Nursing Scholarship, 30,* 53–56.

Hagerman, R. J. (1999). Chromosomal disorders. In M. D. Levine, W. B. Carey, & A. C. Crocker (Eds.), *Developmental-behavioral pediatrics* (3rd ed., pp. 230–239). Philadelphia: Saunders.

Hagerman, R. J., Kimbro, L. T., & Taylor, A. K. (1998). Fragile X syndrome: A common cause of mental retardation and premature menopause. *Contemporary Ob/Gyn, 43*(1), 53–54.

King, B. H., & State, M. W. (1998). Mental retardation. In W. M. Klykylo, J. Kay, & D. Rube (Eds.), *Clinical child psychiatry* (pp. 356–378). Philadelphia: Saunders.

Laxova, R. (1994). Fragile X syndrome. *Advances in Pediatrics, 41,* 305–341.

Luckasson, R. (Ed.). (1992). *Mental retardation: Definition, classification and systems of support* (9th ed.). Washington, DC: American Association on Mental Retardation.

McCance, K. L., & Huether, S. E. (1994). *Pathophysiology: The biologic basis for disease in adults and children.* St. Louis: Mosby.

Sherrard, J., Tonge, B. J., & Einfeld, S. L. (1997). Behaviours in young people with intellectual disability: Preliminary findings and implications for injury. *Journal of Intellectual and Developmental Disability, 22*(1), 39–48.

State, M. W., King, B. H., & Dykens, E. (1997). Mental retardation: A review of the past 10 years. Part II. *Journal of the American Academy of Child and Adolescent Psychiatry, 36*(12), 1664–1671.

Verdugo, M. A., Bermejo, B. G., & Fuertes, J. (1995). The maltreatment of intellectually handicapped children and adolescents. *Child Abuse and Neglect, 19*(2), 205–215.

## 55

The Child with a Sensory Alteration

LEARNING OBJECTIVES

After studying this chapter, you should be able to:

- Describe the structure and function of the eye and ear.
- Describe the specific information required in a health history for a child with potential sensory deficits.
- Define the nurse's role in assessing for sensory deficits.
- Describe specific nursing care for children with health problems affecting the eye and ear.
- Describe how alterations in the sensory organs affect the child's ability to communicate.
- Identify potential growth and development interruptions that may occur with problems affecting the sensory organs.

DEFINITIONS

amblyopia Reduced visual acuity not correctable by refractive means and not attributable to structural or pathologic ocular anomalies.

astigmatism Abnormal curvature of the cornea or the lens.

cataract A loss of transparency of the crystalline lens or its capsule.

central hearing loss Result of damage to the conduction system between the brainstem and cerebral cortex.

concomitant strabismus Not of paralytic origin, remains constant for all directions of gaze.

conductive hearing loss Reversible loss caused by damage, inflammation, or obstruction to outer or middle ear. Sound is prevented from progressing across middle ear.

congenital (infantile) glaucoma Increased intraocular fluid pressure that occurs during first 3 years of life because of a defect in the drainage network of the eye.

diplopia Double vision.

hyphema A hemorrhage or sanguineous exudate in the anterior chamber of the eye.

mixed hearing loss Combination of conductive and sensorineural loss.

nonconcomitant strabismus Angle of deviation varying with direction of gaze due to paralysis or paresis of one or more extraocular muscles.

nystagmus Involuntary eye movements that make the eyes appear to be darting back and forth.

ophthalmia neonatorum Conjunctivitis noted in the first few weeks of life, usually gonococcal or chlamydial.

secondary glaucoma Increased intraocular fluid pressure that occurs after 3 years of age and may be the result of disease or surgery.

sensorineural hearing loss Result of damage or malformation of the middle ear or auditory nerve. Hearing loss is usually permanent.

strabismus "Squint" or "lazy eye"; a condition in which the eyes are not straight because of lack of coordination of the extraocular muscles; most often due to muscle imbalance or paralysis of the extraocular muscles but may also result from conditions such as a brain tumor, myasthenia gravis, or infection.

subconjunctival hemorrhages Bleeding situated beneath the conjunctiva. In children, most frequent cause is trauma or after severe coughing or sneezing episodes (Valsalva maneuvers). Also caused by infection with *Streptococcus pneumoniae* and *Hemophilus influenzae*.

visual accommodation Ability to focus on distant and near objects.

Review of the Eye

Structure and Function

The eye is attached to the skull by six accessory muscles. These are used to move the eye to achieve vision. Ciliary muscles function to alter the shape of the eye to provide focus and accommodation at various distances. Cranial nerves II, III, IV, V, and VI all affect the eye.

The orb, or eye, is made up of several parts. The cornea is the clear area located in the front of the eye, where light enters the eye. The cornea and sclera (white outer covering) make up the eye's outer layer. The middle layer is composed of the choroid (vascular lining), the lens (a clear structure that changes shape to allow accommodation of light on the retina), and the iris (the colored muscular ring located behind the cornea that expands or contracts to control the amount of light entering the eye). The inner layer of the eye is known as the retina. This area contains the rods and cones. These receive light impulses and transmit them through the optic nerve (cranial nerve II) to the brain. The macula contains the greatest concentration of nerve endings. The cornea and lens focus light onto the macula. The optic disk is the area where the optic nerve enters the eye.

Neonatal Development

The eyes begin to develop at approximately 22 days' gestation. The critical period for development is considered to be 22 to 50 days. Congenital abnormalities appear to be caused by either genetic or environmental factors or by a combination of the two. The eye is especially sensitive to teratogens, in particular to infections such as cytomegalovirus and rubella.

Review of the Ear

Structure and Function

The ear is divided into three parts: the outer, middle, and inner ear. The outer ear includes the auricle and external ear canal. It is separated from the middle ear by the tympanic membrane (eardrum). The tympanic membrane vibrates to conduct sound waves to the middle ear. The middle ear contains the bones of hearing—the malleus (hammer), incus (anvil), and stapes (stirrup). These bones conduct sound waves from the tympanic membrane to the inner ear. The inner ear contains the nerve endings that conduct sound impulses to the brain. These are located in a snail-shaped chamber (the cochlea) that is filled with fluid. The inner ear also controls balance. The eustachian tube connects the middle ear with the nasopharynx. It functions to allow fluids to drain into the nasopharynx and to assist in equalizing pressure between the outer and middle ear.

Neonatal Development

The ear begins to develop during the third week of gestation. The critical period for the development of the ear is

Pediatric Differences in the Sensory Organs

Development of the eye is not complete at birth, but the newborn is able to fixate, follow an object to midline, and react to a change in intensity of light.

By 3 months of age, the infant can follow moving objects. By 4 months of age, the infant can recognize familiar objects.

Binocularity, the ability to fixate on one visual field with both eyes, is not present at birth but is established by 6 months of age. Frequent eye crossing after 6 months of age is abnormal and indicates strabismus.

Visual acuity changes with age:

4 months	20/50 to 20/80
1 year	20/40 to 20/70
4 years	20/30 to 20/40
5 years	20/20 to 20/30

Lacrimal glands are not fully developed at birth. Tears are not often present with crying until after 1 to 3 months. Temporary obstruction of lacrimal ducts may cause overflow of tears.

The size of the orbits doubles by the time the child is 1 year of age and doubles again by 6 years. Eye growth is completed at 10 to 12 years of age.

Development of the ear begins during the third week of gestation and is complete by the third month of embryonic life. Infection or other insult to the fetus during this time can cause irreparable damage to the ear. Ear development occurs at the same time as kidney development, so malformation in one system may indicate problems in the other. An infant as young as 3 days of age is able to distinguish between familiar and unfamiliar sounds and can recognize the mother's voice. The infant can distinguish between frequently heard words and other words (nonsense language) by 1 year. Basic auditory skills are in place by 3 years of age. Hearing can be evaluated by audiometry testing by this age.

Infants can imitate sounds heard by 3 to 5 months of age. Verbal dialogue similar to an adult's is noted by approximately 6 months of age.

Infants and young children have shorter, more horizontal, and more flaccid eustachian tubes, predisposing them to otitis media.

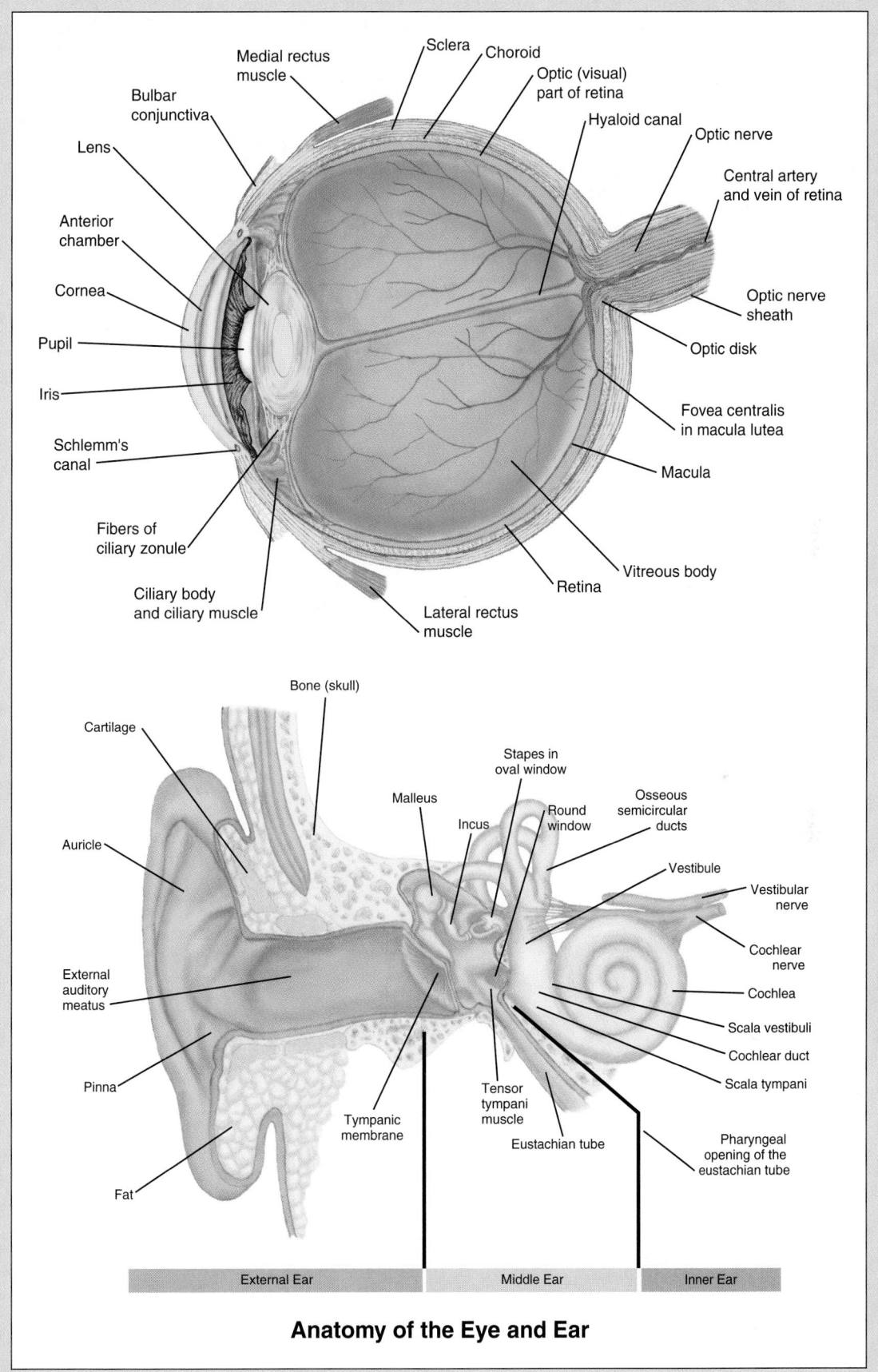

Anatomy of the Eye and Ear

between 4 and 6 weeks' gestation. Like the eye, the ear is very sensitive to teratogens. It is innervated by the acoustic nerve (cranial nerve VIII). Congenital deafness appears to be largely due to genetic factors.

▮ Speech Development

Because the fetus is capable of hearing during the second trimester of pregnancy and is able to hear voices and the mother's heart beat, the infant is born with the ability to be sensitive to variations of speech. Adequate hearing is essential for the development of speech. The infant begins to coo and vocalize quite early (birth to 4 months). Babbling begins at approximately 4 to 6 months. Babbling is followed by receptive language development (understanding words) and expressive language development (saying words; see Chapters 5, 6, 7, and 8 for specifics of speech development). Any hearing impairment can interfere with speech development, as can any alteration affecting the oral cavity.

Because a child learns so much through the senses, deficits in hearing and vision can have profound effects on development. Appropriate screening and early interventions are crucial. Early identification of vision and hearing deficits allows for early intervention, either correction or the provision of adaptive measures, so that the child's "normal" growth and development may be preserved. Because a child cannot report sensory deficits, nurses must assess carefully for alterations in vision or hearing.

The health history of a child with a potential sensory deficit is essentially the same for any child (see Chapter 33) but should also include some additional pieces of information:

- Thorough prenatal history
- Growth and developmental history
- Past history of any infections (including treatment, because many medications can cause sensory deficits)
- Previous trauma to the eye or ear
- Changes noted in behavior (such as rubbing the eyes, turning up the volume on the television, decreased attention span)
- Changes in appearance (red, inflamed eyes, drainage from the eye or ear)
- Physical complaints (complaints of ear or eye pain, headache, nausea and vomiting)

After carefully reviewing the health history, the nurse performs a thorough physical examination using age-appropriate measures of vision and hearing acuity (see Chapter 33).

Disorders of the Eye

The nurse has a very important role in the prevention and early detection of eye problems. All children should have vision screening done according to the following schedule (Bacal, Rousta, & Hertle, 1999):

- At birth—external and internal appearance, red reflex, fixation
- Age 3 to 6 months—fixation and ability to follow, alignment (corneal light reflex, photoscreening)
- Age 3½ years—visual acuity, using developmentally appropriate charts (Allen chart, picture chart, tumbling E)
- Visual acuity at the kindergarten examination (age 5 years) and then periodically throughout the school years

Careful attention to behavioral and appearance changes as well as physical complaints assists in the early detection and treatment of eye disorders. Children who have any symptoms should be referred for further evaluation.

. . . .

Signs and Symptoms of Potential Eye Problems

BEHAVIORAL

- Rubbing eyes excessively
- Shutting or covering one eye when reading or concentrating
- Tilting head or thrusting head forward to see
- Difficulty in reading or doing close-up tasks
- Increased incidence of blinking, especially when doing close-up tasks
- Inability to see distant objects clearly
- Squinting or frowning to see

APPEARANCE

- Crossed eyes
- Redness or swelling
- Drainage
- Excessive tearing
- Recurring infections

PHYSICAL COMPLAINTS

- Inability to see
- Headaches, dizziness, nausea/vomiting with close-up tasks
- Double vision
- Blurred vision

Adapted from Gerali, P. S. (1991). Childsight: Helping children grow up with good vision. *Journal of Ophthalmic Nursing and Technology, 10,* 222–223.

Nursing Considerations for the Child with a Refractive Error

Refractive errors cause vision disturbances from alterations in the path of light rays through the eye. They usually result from an abnormally shaped orb; the orb may be flattened or elongated (Table 55–1). Refractive errors are often discovered when a child squints or frowns, or moves objects so that they are more easily seen. A teacher or complaints from the child may also alert parents. *Legal blindness* is defined as a correction of 20/200 or less in the better eye or a visual field of 20 degrees or less.

Nurses should assess children's vision at every well-child visit. Visual acuity can be reliably tested in a cooperative child as young as 3 years of age. When testing visual acuity, the nurse needs to remember that a vision discrepancy of two lines or more on the vision chart, even if one eye tests normal, is cause for referral. A child with this discrepancy could have *anisometropia*, or large refractive discrepancy between eyes. If not corrected, this condition can lead to amblyopia.

Corrective lenses are used to improve the child's vision. Glasses should be impact resistant and have "spring-loaded" frames that are less likely to be bent or warped. Because the bridge of the nose is flat, cable temples (ear pieces that wrap around the ear) are recommended in children younger than 4 years of age (Catalano & Nelson, 1994). Straps can also

TABLE 55–1

Types of Refractive Disorders

Refractive Error	Description	Clinical Manifestations	Treatment
Myopia	Near-sightedness Ability to see close objects more clearly than those at a distance Caused by the image focusing in front of the retina	Difficulty seeing the blackboard or TV clearly Decreased interest in activities requiring distance vision Squinting, head tilting, holding books close to eyes Decreased attention span, poor school performance	Treated with biconcave lenses New lenses may be required every year or two as the child grows
Hyperopia	Far-sightedness Ability to see distant objects more clearly than those close up Caused by the image focusing beyond the retina	Most children are normally hyperopic until approximately 7 years of age but are able to accommodate to see clearly Strabismus or amblyopia may develop from prolonged hyperopia	Most young children with hyperopia need no correction If correction is required, convex lenses are used
Astigmatism	Unequal curvature of the cornea or the lens, causing light rays to bend in different directions May coexist with myopia or hyperopia	Mild astigmatism may be asymptomatic Manifestations may be similar to myopia	Treated with special lenses to compensate for the unequal curvature of the cornea

be used to help hold the glasses in place. Special prescription sports goggles are available for athletes. Both gas-permeable and soft contact lenses provide an alternative for children old enough and responsible enough to care for contacts independently.

The nurse needs to teach parents and children about appropriate care of corrective lenses, and should educate parents and children about recognizing and intervening with vision problems early.

Nursing Considerations for the Child with Color Blindness

Color "blindness," or color deficiency, occurs in 8% of the population and affects primarily boys. It affects the ability to distinguish between colors within certain groups such as red, blue, and green.

Testing should be done if the clinician suspects a problem (i.e., a suspected optic nerve or retinal dysfunction) or the family has a history of color blindness. Testing is routine in preschool boys (Catalano & Nelson, 1994). The most common detection test is the pseudoisochromatic (color confusion) test, in which color plates include patterns that are hidden to a person with a color deficit. Pseudoisochromatic plates are also available for children who cannot yet read. If a problem is detected, more sophisticated testing may be necessary to determine the exact type of color blindness. Although color blindness has no cure, certain types of tints used in contact lenses and glasses can help the child discriminate color differences.

Because color blindness cannot be cured, nursing care

CHILDREN AND PARENTS WANT TO KNOW

How to Care for Corrective Lenses

- To prevent warping of the frame, always remove your eyeglasses with both hands.
- To prevent scratches, never lay eyeglasses face down.
- Use only the recommended method for cleaning eyeglass lenses; paper towels and other dry cloths can scratch your lenses.
- If a harness is used to hold your infant's glasses in place, take care to avoid getting the elastic bands too tight.
- Never replace missing screws with paper clips or wires because these may come loose and cause eye trauma. Eyeglass repair kits are available at your local pharmacy.

- Eyeglasses are too small for your child when the bend of the side piece is in front of the ear.
- Always follow the doctor's instructions for cleaning and disinfecting contact lenses. Use the solution recommended for your type of lenses.
- Always wash your hands before inserting or removing contact lenses to prevent infection.

Adapted from Catalano, R. A., & Nelson, L. B. (1990). *Pediatric ophthalmology: A test atlas.* East Norwalk, CT: Appleton and Lange.

Vision Screening

- Thoroughly explain the procedure to the child before beginning. If using a picture chart, show the child the pictures and ask the child to identify them. Children might have different names for the same picture.
- Take the child to a quiet, nondistracting area that has been marked for the appropriate distance from the chart.
- Have the child cover one eye. Use a colorful, opaque cover that completely blocks the child's vision. The parent can help hold the cover in place.
- Point to a picture (letter, number) on a line that the child can probably see readily and move to smaller lines. Vary the direction (left to right, right to left) to reduce the likelihood that the child is memorizing the symbols.

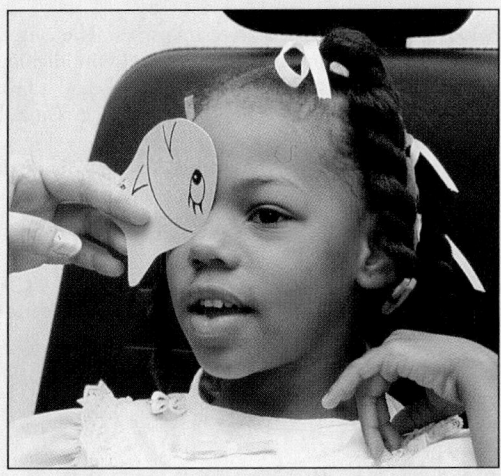

- Give positive feedback. Perform the test as quickly as possible because small children lose interest quickly.
- Test both eyes. Refer if there is a discrepancy of two lines, or if the child tests in the abnormal range on two successive screenings.

focuses on adaptive and supportive measures. Encourage parents to have children tested if they have a family history of color blindness or if the nurse suspects the child is having trouble distinguishing colors.

Parent/child education is very important for the child with color blindness. Teaching should focus on alternative ways to discriminate the deficient colors. For the older child who can dress without assistance, clothes can be labeled or organized consistently in the closet and bureau so that items can be coordinated easily.

Safety is a major concern for the color-blind child. For example, the child who cannot distinguish red and green must learn another way to distinguish traffic signals and other warning lights. Finally, anticipatory guidance is some-

times related to appropriate career choices. For example, color blindness may prohibit an adult from becoming a pilot, police officer, or fire fighter.

Nursing Considerations for the Child with a Blocked Lacrimal Duct

A blocked lacrimal (tear) duct is characterized by excessive tearing (epiphora) and crusting, or "mattering," of the eyelids on awakening. Parents may also notice a small mass just below the inner aspect of the eye. Treatment usually consists of massaging the duct. If the duct remains blocked despite massaging or remains blocked after 1 year of age, surgical opening of the duct is indicated.

The nurse should carefully assess the mucoid drainage. In a noninfected duct, the drainage is usually white or clear. If the duct has become infected, however, the drainage may be green or yellow. If the drainage appears infected, antibiotic eye drops or ointment are indicated.

The nurse teaches the parent about the proper technique for lacrimal massage. This process involves washing hands thoroughly and placing the index finger over the lacrimal duct (at the inner aspect of the eye by the bridge of the nose) and "milking," or gently massaging the duct, in an upward motion. Emphasize that massaging down the nasal bone has very little effect on the duct because the lacrimal system is intraosseous and unaffected by massage. Other teaching includes monitoring for signs and symptoms of infection.

Nursing Considerations for the Child with Strabismus

Strabismus (squint, lazy eye) is a condition in which the eyes are not aligned because of lack of coordination of the extraocular muscles. It is present in 2% to 5% of newborns (Huddleston, 1994). Strabismus is most often due to muscle imbalance or paralysis of the extraocular muscles but may also result from conditions such as a brain tumor, myasthenia gravis, or infection. Approximately 50% of children with strabismus have a family history of the condition. The type of deviation noted defines strabismus. When assessing infants for strabismus, the nurse needs to remember that strabismus is normal in the young infant but should not be present after approximately 4 months of age.

When both eyes are unable to focus simultaneously, the brain suppresses the image from the deviating eye to avoid double vision (diplopia). Amblyopia, or decreased vision in the deviated eye, can develop if strabismus is not treated early. If untreated amblyopia occurs in a child younger than age 4 years of age (the critical period for development of the visual cortex), permanent loss of vision in the deviated eye can result. Because the child loses binocular vision, depth perception may also be impaired. Early detection and treatment of strabismus are essential to prevent loss of vision.

The Hirschberg test, cover–uncover test, and the alternate-cover tests (see Chapter 33) are used in the diagnosis of strabismus (Castiglia, 1994; Bacal & Hertle, 1998). The nurse may suspect strabismus when the child complains of frequent headaches, squints, or tilts the head to see. Chil-

Types of Strabismus

Nonparalytic (nonconcomitant) strabismus: Most common type of strabismus in children. Constant deviation in all fields of gaze, not associated with eye muscle paralysis. All extraocular muscles function but are not coordinated. Child has difficulty seeing at close range and often squints. Accommodative nonparalytic strabismus may develop between 2 and 4 years of age as a result of a large refractive error.

Paralytic (concomitant) strabismus: Caused by a weakness or paralysis of one or more of the extraocular muscles. The eye appears crossed when turned in the direction of the affected muscle. May cause headache, uncoordination. Diplopia may cause child to close one eye or tilt head.

Esotropia (convergent): The eye turns inward, most common type of strabismus in infants. May occur with hyperopia as the eyes compensate for the refractive error by overconvergence.

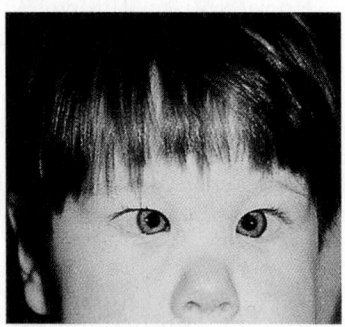

Infant with early-onset esotropia. The deviation may not be apparent until age 3 or 4 months.

Exotropia (divergent): The eyes turn away from the midline, occurs most often when the child attempts to focus on a distant object. May be present at birth.

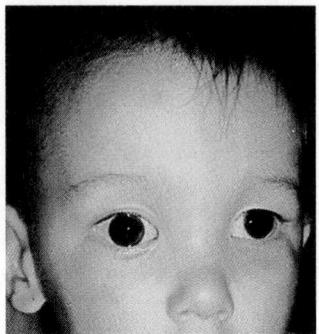

Child with left exotropia. Most exodeviations in childhood are intermittent.

Pseudostrabismus: Not a true strabismus. The eyes appear to deviate inward but are actually in alignment. Facial features, such as epicanthal folds and a broad, flat nasal bridge, can give the appearance of misalignment.

Phoria: A tendency for the eye to deviate. More evident during times of stress, fatigue, or illness.

Tropia: A continuous misalignment of the eye.

Photographs from Albert, D. M., & Jakobiec, F. A. (Eds.). (1994). *Principles and practice of ophthalmology* (pp. 2731, 2733). Philadelphia: Saunders.

---

dren with family members with strabismus should be regularly assessed for development of the condition.

Treatment of strabismus may include special glasses, vision therapy, patching, surgery, or pharmacologic therapy. If the deviation is caused by hyperopia, corrective lenses are indicated to correct vision. Eyeglasses with specially ground prism power may also be indicated. These glasses correct vision in the affected eye so that the brain receives the same image from both eyes.

Patching may also be used to strengthen the weak eye. In this treatment, the "good" eye is patched, so that the child uses the weaker eye. Patching is most successful when done during the preschool years (American Academy of Ophthalmology, 1994). The schedule for patching is individualized; a common regimen is an initial patching for a period equal to 1 week for every year of the child's age (Jockin, 1999). The child usually must wear the patch for nearly 24 hours a day (Bacal & Hertle, 1998). The patching regimen is prescribed by the ophthalmologist.

Compliance with the patching regimen is essential. Teaching should explain the reasons for patching or corrective lenses, the expected results of wearing the patch or lens, correctly placing the patch, the number of hours per day the patch or lens is to be worn, and the expected length of treatment. The child needs to understand that wearing the

PARENTS WANT TO KNOW

Information About Eye Patching

- Your child will need to wear the eye patch for the exact time your doctor has prescribed. Not complying with the full wearing time could interfere with the treatment.
- Prescribed patching will not harm your child's stronger eye but will force the muscles of the weaker eye to be used.
- Apply the patch directly to your child's face, being sure to cover the whole eye. Do not leave any openings through which the child can peek.
- If your child wears eyeglasses as well, put the glasses on over the patch.
- It can be frustrating for the child to have to wear the patch. Try to be patient, understanding, and supportive. It is essential that patching be nonnegotiable. Find decorative patches or put your own decoration on the patch. Praise your child frequently for complying with the treatment.

patch or lens is not negotiable. The nurse often must teach parents strategies for dealing with resistant behaviors.

Surgery may be indicated to realign the weakened muscles. It is most often indicated when amblyopia is present (Castiglia, 1994) and should be performed before the child is 2 years of age. The stronger eye may be patched before surgery to treat any existing amblyopia, but surgery can be done before the amblyopia treatment begins (Bacal & Hertle, 1998). Surgery may be required only on the weakened eye or on both eyes. More than one surgery may be necessary. During the surgery, small incisions are made, and the weakened muscles are tightened.

If the child is to have a surgical correction, the nurse should prepare the child and parents before surgery for what to expect after surgery and should provide information about dressing changes, eye drops, corrective lenses, and any other postoperative treatments that may be required. Interventions are similar to those for any child having eye surgery.

Finally, botulinum toxin (Botox) was approved in 1989 by the U.S. Food and Drug Administration as an alternative to surgery. The toxin is injected into the eye muscle and produces temporary paralysis. This condition allows the muscles opposite the paralyzed muscle to straighten the eye. With successful treatment, once the medication wears off (in approximately 2 months), the correction remains. The most common side effect is a drooping eyelid (ptosis), which resolves spontaneously (Castiglia, 1994).

Nursing Considerations for the Child with Glaucoma

Glaucoma is a condition in which the intraocular fluid pressure of the eye is increased. This pressure increase, if left untreated, leads to atrophy of the optic disk and, ultimately, blindness.

There are two types of glaucoma in children. Congenital, or infantile, glaucoma occurs during the first 3 years of life and is due to a defect in the drainage network of the eye. Greater than 50% of all infantile glaucoma is of this type (Catalano & Nelson, 1994). Secondary glaucoma refers to disease that occurs after 3 years of age and may be the result of inherited disease or may occur after disease (e.g., congenital rubella), trauma, or cataract removal (Wagner, 1994).

Clinical signs of glaucoma include excessive tearing, light sensitivity, blepharospasm (muscle spasm causing involuntary closing of the eyelid), and enlargement of the globe and cornea (Wagner, 1997). Parents often note excessive tearing or corneal haziness due to edema and bring the child in for clinical evaluation. The child may also be brought to the practitioner for what appears to be conjunctivitis, or "pinkeye."

Physical examination includes an assessment of visual acuity, measurement of intraocular pressure (tonometry), assessment of corneal diameter and clarity, and an examination of the retina to assess for optic nerve cupping. Any infant with a visible iris diameter greater than 10.5 mm should be evaluated. If retinal edema is present, the light reflex is diffuse. Because young children may not be able to cooperate during an examination, they are often sedated.

Intraocular pressure should be measured only under light sedation, however, because deeper sedation may alter readings (either high or low, depending on the agent used).

The preferred treatment for childhood glaucoma is surgery. Medications to clear the cornea may be used before surgery to allow better visibility. Surgery should be done as soon as possible after diagnosis to prevent loss (or further loss) of vision. The goal of surgery is to increase the outflow of the aqueous humor from the anterior chamber. Medications such as cholinergic agents, beta-adrenergic blocking agents, or adrenergic agents may be indicated after surgery to maintain a low intraocular pressure.

Prognosis varies from child to child. The earlier the onset of glaucoma, the poorer the prognosis (Wagner, 1994). Over half of children who have glaucoma at birth and 20% of those with later onset will be legally blind in the affected eye(s) (Wagner, 1994). Approximately one third of children who undergo successful surgery will have vision better than 20/50 (Wagner, 1994). Decreased vision may result from damage to the optic nerve, opacity of the cornea or lens, or amblyopia resulting from refractive errors.

Nursing interventions are similar to those for any child having eye surgery. Postoperative nursing care includes monitoring for signs and symptoms of increased intraocular pressure (pain, nausea and vomiting, increased inflammation) and administering any ordered medications such as miotic eye drops (used to constrict the pupils) and antibiotic ointments or eye drops. If the child's eyes are patched, the nurse pays special attention to the resulting sensory deficits.

Patient/parent education is essential to maintain the appropriate intraocular pressure and prevent complications (including blindness). Education includes the use of any prescribed medications, patching, and any other measures designed to correct refractive errors. The importance of returning for follow-up care should be emphasized. The child and caregivers should also be taught signs and symptoms of increasing intraocular pressure. Any signs of increasing intraocular pressure or infection should be reported immediately to the ophthalmologist.

Nursing Considerations for the Child with a Cataract

A cataract is an opacity, or loss of transparency, of the lens. Causes include an inherited tendency (usually an autosomal dominant trait), infection (e.g., rubella), trauma, or a metabolic imbalance. Cloudiness of the lens may be noted during examination in the newborn nursery (indicated by a white instead of red reflex) or by parents. Ophthalmoscopy may reveal a dark spot in the lens. Parents may note that the infant exhibits visual inattentiveness and come in for an evaluation. Other clinical signs include nystagmus and strabismus.

The cataract alters vision because it does not allow a sharp, clear image to be formed on the retina. Early intervention (before 3 months of age) for the infant born with cataracts is crucial to allow vision to develop normally (Wagner, 1997).

Treatment for cataracts is the surgical removal of the opaque lens. The resultant hyperopia is then dealt with using a contact lens or an intraocular lens implant. Glasses may also be used to correct the resultant vision problem.

Amblyopia may also be present. In this case, the normal eye may be patched after surgery to develop the weakened eye.

Postoperative interventions are directed toward avoiding increased intraocular pressure. Measures include preventing coughing, straining, vomiting, and touching the operative site. A patch and "hard shield" are usually in place after surgery to prevent injury to the operative site. To prevent edema and pressure on the site, the nurse should elevate the head of the bed slightly and avoid placing the child with the affected eye in a dependent position (Symanski, Newman, & Bachynski, 1994). Monitor the child for signs and symptoms of infection (fever, drainage, redness). Medications, including antibiotics, mydriatics, and steroids, may be used after surgery.

Postoperative teaching includes how to insert, remove, and care for the child's contact lens. Parents need to be taught the signs and symptoms of infection and increasing intraocular pressure. To provide visual stimulation to the affected eye and prevent further loss of vision, the importance of complying with the patching regimen should also be emphasized. Finally, the nurse teaches the importance of returning for follow-up visits to ensure that the lens fits correctly, the vision correction is appropriate, and there are no signs and symptoms of complications.

Nursing Considerations for the Child with an Eye Infection

CONJUNCTIVITIS

Conjunctivitis ("pinkeye") is an inflammation of the conjunctiva (the clear, membranous lining of the lid and sclera). Signs and symptoms of conjunctivitis may include itching, burning, light sensitivity (photophobia), "scratchy" eyelids, redness, edema, and discharge. It is usually caused by either allergy or infection. Accurate diagnosis before treatment is important because inappropriate treatment can lead to complications.

Conjunctivitis noted in the first few weeks of life is called *ophthalmia neonatorum*. In infants, conjunctivitis occurring in the first 24 hours of life is usually due to chemical irritation from infection prophylaxis administered soon after birth (see Chapter 23). Either infection or a blocked lacrimal duct can cause conjunctivitis that occurs after the first 24 hours. Infants acquire infection during birth (from passing through the birth canal) or after birth. *Chlamydia* is responsible for most eye infections noted in infants (Wagner, 1997). Medical treatment should be directed at the cause of the infection. Antibiotic or antiviral eye drops or ointments are most often used to treat infectious conjunctivitis. If *Chlamydia* is the cause, however, systemic antibiotics are also used to prevent pneumonia.

Conjunctivitis in older children may have a variety of etiologies. Among them are allergy, infection, and trauma. Organisms most frequently implicated in bacterial conjunctivitis include *Hemophilus influenzae* and *Streptococcus pneumoniae*. As with the infant, treatment depends on the cause. The nurse obtains a detailed history to help determine the cause. Infection should be suspected if the child has recently been exposed to another person with conjunctivitis or has an upper respiratory infection (Catalano & Nelson, 1994). Itching often identifies the cause as an allergic response. Chlamydial conjunctivitis is rare in older children. It may be suspected, however, in a sexually active adolescent with chronic infection that is unresponsive to other treatment (King, 1993). A diagnosis of chlamydial conjunctivitis in a child who is not sexually active should signal the health care provider to assess the child for possible sexual abuse (Catalano & Nelson, 1994).

Medical management depends on the cause of the conjunctivitis. If the cause is infection, antibiotic or antiviral eye drops or ointment may be prescribed. If allergies are suspected, antihistamines, either oral or in the form of eye drops, may be indicated. In severe cases of allergic conjunctivitis, steroid eye drops and cromolyn sodium eye drops may be helpful. The steroid eye drops are tapered over approximately 7 days. Because steroids can worsen the severity of many infections, they are used with caution and only for a short time. Long-term use of steroids has been associated with an increased risk of cataract and glaucoma (Catalano & Nelson, 1994).

Teach parents to keep the child's eye clean and to administer any prescribed medications (see Chapter 38). Because bacterial and viral conjunctivitis is extremely contagious, the nurse teaches infection control measures. These include good hand washing and not sharing towels and washcloths. Bottles of eye medication should never be shared with another person. The tip of the dropper or ointment tube should not touch the child's eye or eyelid during administration. The child should also be kept home from school or day care until 24 hours after antibiotics are started.

Preventing injury from rubbing the eye is also important. Mittens may be used for infants. These may be fashioned from booty-type socks or may be commercially made mittens. Distraction and constant reminding are recommended for toddlers and older children. If the child wears contact lenses, advise discontinuing them until the infection has completely cleared. Securing new contact lenses eliminates the chance of reinfection from contaminated contact lenses and also lessens the risk of a corneal ulceration. Eye makeup should also be discarded and replaced, because the chance of reinfecting eyes from contaminated makeup is high. Mascara should be replaced routinely at least every 3 months.

If the conjunctivitis is allergic in origin, cool compresses and dark glasses may also help to lessen the irritation and photophobia. If cromolyn sodium eye drops are prescribed, parents should be taught to begin using them *before* the allergy season because they have little effect on an active inflammatory process (King, 1993). Ophthalmic nonsteroidal anti-inflammatory preparations may also be helpful.

PERIORBITAL CELLULITIS

Orbital cellulitis is caused by an infection of the soft tissues of the orbit. It may occur as a result of trauma or an infection of the ethmoid sinus. Clinical signs and symptoms include severe eyelid edema, erythema, and an anteriorly displaced eye. The child is febrile and has an elevated white blood cell count.

Treatment includes intravenous antibiotics after appropriate cultures have been taken. If the area is painful, analgesics might also be prescribed. Children with periorbital cellulitis need to be admitted to the hospital for observation and treatment because of the potential for rapid progression (Steinkuller, Edmond, & Chen, 1998). Left untreated, the infection causing the periorbital cellulitis can spread to the optic nerve directly to the brain, causing meningitis.

Nursing care involves administering prescribed medications and monitoring the child receiving intravenous therapy. The child should also be carefully monitored for signs and symptoms that the infection is spreading. This includes a thorough neurologic assessment. Finally, the nurse assesses the child's pain status frequently. Hot packs four times a day and prescribed analgesics as ordered can relieve pain.

CORNEAL ULCER

Corneal ulcers are usually caused by ocular infection. Signs and symptoms include pain, tearing, purulent discharge, and blurred vision. Risk factors for corneal ulceration include trauma, extended wearing of soft contact lenses, surgical procedures, and viral infection in the eye. Immunosuppression and prolonged use of topical antibiotics in the eye also increase the risk of corneal ulceration (Catalano & Nelson, 1994).

Treatment includes aggressive topical antibiotic therapy. Cultures are common and treatment is started with a potent new generation of fluoroquinolones: ciprofloxacin, oflaxacin, and norfloxacin.

The nurse teaches the parent about administration of any prescribed medications and the cause and prevention of future ulcerations. The parent needs to discourage the child from rubbing the eyes (which can worsen the injury). The child who wears contact lenses should avoid wearing them until the ulceration and infection are completely healed. Any lenses worn during the episode should be discarded.

Nursing Considerations for the Child with Eye Trauma

CORNEAL ABRASION

Corneal abrasions usually result from a scraping or tearing of the cornea by foreign bodies, contact lenses, paper, and fingernails. The child may present with light sensitivity, pain, excessive tearing, and decreased vision. The abrasion is diagnosed by instilling a fluorescein dye in the eye and examining the eye under a blue filtered light (Wood's lamp) to highlight the injury. If foreign bodies remain in the eye, they should be removed.

If the abrasion is a small one, treatment may consist only of the instillation of antibiotic ointment four times a day for 1 to 2 days with a follow-up evaluation to check healing. Larger abrasions require patching for 24 hours. Referral to an ophthalmologist should be considered with any large abrasion or with the suspicion of a penetrating injury. Many authorities now recommend no patching unless the wound is very large. If patched, the eye should be examined in 24 hours. Failure to treat an abrasion may result in loss of visual acuity or permanent scarring and opacity of the cornea.

Parent education is very important in caring for the child with a corneal abrasion. Because an abrasion increases the risk of infection, parents should be taught the importance of administering antibiotics as prescribed. The child should not rub the eye because rubbing can worsen an abrasion. If the eye is patched, advise the parents not to remove the patch for 24 hours, even to instill ointment. Keeping the patch in place prevents further damage to the eye from blinking. The nurse also reinforces injury prevention, especially wearing safety goggles during sports and other activities, such as wood working.

SUBCONJUNCTIVAL HEMORRHAGE

Subconjunctival hemorrhages present as red areas beneath the conjunctiva. They are often the result of Valsalva maneuvers such as coughing, vomiting, or straining. Subconjunctival hemorrhages resolve on their own within 2 to 3 weeks and require no treatment. Although they often appear worse than they are, they may be associated with other ocular or physical problems and should be evaluated.

Because these hemorrhages resolve on their own, care is aimed at reassurance. Parents should be told that the hemorrhage will appear to grow larger in the first few days because of the effects of gravity (Catalano & Nelson, 1994).

HYPHEMA

A hyphema is a hemorrhage resulting from a blow to the eye. Symptoms include a recent history of injury, pain, light sensitivity, decreased vision, the presence of floaters, and excessive tearing. The child is usually sleepy. If there is no known history of injury, the child should be assessed for a bleeding disorder, anticoagulant therapy, renal or hepatic disease, retinoblastoma, or child abuse. An examination of the eye reveals blood in the anterior chamber (between the cornea and iris) of the eye. Traumatic hyphema usually fills less than one third of the anterior chamber.

Recommendations for management vary. Treatment usually includes hospitalization, bed rest, sedation, and patching of both eyes. Because of the risk of a rebleed between the third and fifth days, bed rest and patching are often recommended (Hertle, 1999) for at least that length of time. Medications such as steroid eye drops, antifibrinolytic eye drops (tranexamic acid is best for pediatric use), antiglaucoma medications, and cycloplegic eye drops (atropine) may also be used.

Careful assessment is required for the child with a hyphema. Assess the eye frequently for a secondary hemorrhage, or rebleed. This condition is characterized by an increase in size of the hyphema, with bright red "new" blood noted over the existing clot. The child should also be monitored for signs and symptoms of increasing intraocular pressure (pain, nausea and vomiting, increased inflammation). The child should be monitored closely for side effects of medications, which include nausea and vomiting, orthostatic hypotension, tinnitus, and hematuria (Catalano & Nelson, 1994).

The child is usually restricted to bed rest with bathroom privileges. Elevating the head of the bed 30 to 40 degrees helps settle the hyphema in the inferior anterior chamber angle. Television viewing may or may not be allowed, and reading and other near activities are usually forbidden.

Therefore, boredom is a problem for most children. Offer diversional activities that do not involve reading or straining the eyes, such as music and books on tape. If both eyes are patched, the nurse orients the child to the environment and provides for safety.

Discharge teaching includes use of prescribed home medications, patching regimen (the eye is usually patched at night for 2 weeks after discharge), and prevention of further injury. The child's eye should be protected with a shield if an eye patch is worn at night. The child can usually return to all normal activities 1 month after the injury, but eye protection should be worn during high risk activities for the rest of the child's life (Catalano & Nelson, 1994). The nurse should also emphasize the importance of follow-up because the child is at risk for complications such as glaucoma and cataracts.

CHEMICAL BURNS

Chemical burns constitute an ocular emergency. Burns may occur from any of a number of common household items such as bleach, ammonia, drain opener, and oven cleaner.

Initial care of the child with a chemical burn to the eyes is focused on immediate irrigation with water or saline to prevent further injury. If the chemical is alkaline, the irrigation may continue for several hours because the damaging action of alkaloids may be prolonged. If the burn is mild, irrigation should continue for at least 30 minutes, using at least 2 L of irrigant, and for 2 to 4 hours or with at least 10 L of irrigant if the burn is severe (Catalano, 1993). The cornea may appear cloudy after an alkali burn. Irrigation of a frightened, hurting child's eyes can be very difficult. Helping the child lean over a water fountain that is spraying upward makes the task easier.

Further treatment may include referral to an ophthalmologist for topical steroids, medications to dilate the pupils and decrease the risk of adhesions, antibiotic ointment, and patching. Oral antibiotics and analgesics may also be indicated. Nursing care focuses on prescribed medical treatments, comfort measures, and injury prevention (particularly if both of the child's eyes are patched).

Discharge teaching focuses not only on the prescribed medical treatments but on the importance of compliance with long-term follow-up and injury prevention. Follow-up care includes monitoring visual acuity and monitoring for side effects, such as increased intraocular pressure and cataracts.

◼ Eye Surgery

Several eye disorders seen in infancy and childhood require surgical correction. Any surgical procedure is stressful for the child and family. Eye surgery is particularly stressful because the child's visual fields or acuity may be greatly reduced or absent for a period. If both eyes are affected, the child's ability to maneuver and perform activities of daily living independently is also affected.

The nurse should pay special attention to education. If the child is going home with patches, drops, or any other procedure that must be performed, the family needs to know how to perform this care and should also know the safety precautions involved.

NURSING CARE

The Child Having Eye Surgery

Assessment

Assessment of the child and family begins with determining their understanding of the planned surgical procedure and why this is necessary. This includes assessing their knowledge of the care that will be necessary after discharge, as well as any changes to expect. These might include home schooling if both eyes are affected. Understanding of safety principles should also be addressed at admission and should be reinforced during the child's hospitalization. Finally, the nurse assesses understanding of any special adaptations for procedures and begins teaching at the time of admission.

Nursing Diagnosis, Planning, Intervention, and Evaluation

Nursing Diagnosis

■ Sensory/Perceptual Alterations: visual impairment related to eye patching or surgical procedure.

Expected Outcomes

• The child and family will describe any anticipated visual changes.
• The child and parents will become familiar with the surroundings and will be prepared for unfamiliar sights and sounds.
• The child will remain alert and oriented to time and self.

Intervention	Rationale
1. Prepare the child and family before surgery for any changes expected in vision, including blurred vision or patched eyes.	1. Preoperative preparation allows the child and family to know what to expect, thus lessening anxiety.
2. Before surgery, orient the child and family to the surroundings, including the recovery room and hospital room.	2. Preoperative orientation to surroundings allows the child a feeling of familiarity during the postoperative period.
3. Provide reality orientation (time, day) for the child during the postoperative period, especially if vision is impaired or eyes are patched.	3. Providing a sense of time passage, and orienting to day and night prevents the child from becoming disoriented and confused.
4. Provide emotional support and allow expression of feelings of anger and frustration, often through play therapy and therapeutic communication.	4. Allowing the child and family to express their fears and frustrations in a "healthy" manner provides an appropriate outlet and encourages the use of other senses.

Evaluation

• Do the child and family express understanding of vision changes?
• Are the child and parents oriented to surroundings?
• Does the child remain alert and oriented to time and self?

Nursing Diagnosis

■ Risk for Injury related to increased intraocular pressure resulting from bleeding, edema, hematoma, postoperative vomiting.

Expected Outcomes

• The child will not experience a physical injury and will wear eye patches or shields as ordered.
• The child will not experience nausea or vomiting.

Intervention	Rationale
1. Fully orient the child to surroundings and ensure that unsafe objects are removed from the environment.	1. Orienting the child to the environment and ensuring that the environment is safe prevents falls and other injuries when the child is out of bed.
2. Ensure that the child wears eye patches or shields as ordered.	2. Eye patches and shields are often prescribed to prevent any further injury to the eye.
3. Encourage the parents to remain with the child and prevent the child from rubbing the eyes. Restraints are used as a last resort to prevent injury.	3. Rubbing the eyes can damage the surgical site. If restraints are needed, elbow restraints provide protection without total restriction.
4. Monitor for signs and symptoms of increased intraocular pressure. Give ordered antiemetics if the child is nauseous. Administer intravenous fluids until the child is stable.	4. Increasing intraocular pressure can damage the eye and seriously impair vision. Vomiting can increase intraocular pressure.

Evaluation

• Does the child remain free of physical injury?
• Does the child wear eye patches or shields as ordered?
• Is the child free from nausea or vomiting?

Nursing Diagnosis	■ Risk for Infection related to surgical incision.
Expected Outcome	• The child will not experience complications related to infection.

Intervention	Rationale
1. Monitor the child for signs and symptoms of infection, including redness, drainage, fever, and excessive tearing or edema.	1. These are physical signs that a postoperative infection is developing in the eye.
2. Administer antibiotic therapy as ordered.	2. Antibiotics may be used as prophylaxis against infection.

Evaluation	• Have any signs and symptoms of infection been reported and treated immediately?
	• Is the child free from fever, redness, or eye drainage?

Nursing Diagnosis	■ Pain related to surgical procedure.
Expected Outcome	• The child will experience minimal discomfort during the postoperative period, as evidenced by acceptable pain scale rating, normal vital signs, and participation in quiet activities.

Intervention	Rationale
1. Monitor the child frequently (every 2–4 hours while awake) for pain using an age-appropriate pain scale. Monitor physiologic signs of pain in the young child (increased pulse, restlessness, inability to sleep, inability to play).	1. Pain can increase anxiety and restlessness that could lead to increased intraocular pressure. The young child who would ordinarily use a visual scale to rate pain is unable to do so if eyes are patched.
2. Administer pain medications as ordered.	2. Pain control decreases the child's need to rub or touch the eyes, which can cause trauma to the surgical site.
3. Provide nonpharmacologic pain relief measures such as ice pack and moist heat as indicated. Use distraction techniques frequently (music, stories).	3. Nonpharmacologic pain relief measures can replace or augment pharmacologic measures. Verbal distraction techniques can decrease pain and take the child's mind away from the bandages.

Evaluation	• Does the child express relief of pain using an age-appropriate pain scale?
	• Are the child's vital signs within normal limits, and can the child participate appropriately in quiet activities?

■ *Hearing Loss in Children*

Etiology

Damage to, or impairment of, any part of the ear can cause hearing loss. Four types of hearing loss have been identified: conductive, sensorineural, mixed, and central. Each has a different treatment regimen and response to intervention.

Incidence

In areas that mandate newborn hearing screening, the incidence of newborns diagnosed with hearing loss is 1 to 4 newborns per 1,000. A recent study suggests that as many as 14.9% of children 6 to 19 years of age experience slight hearing loss, particularly at the upper and lower frequencies (Nisak et al., 1998).

Diagnostic Evaluation

Evidence suggests that infants with hearing loss who have been identified and treated before 6 months of age have a better prognosis than those for whom treatment has been delayed. Using risk criteria for screening infants for hearing loss helps identify only approximately 50% of infants af-

. . . .
Types and Etiology of Hearing Loss

Conductive: Outer or middle ear affected by damage, inflammation, or obstruction. Sound conduction is prevented from progressing from the outer ear to the inner ear. May be the result of excessive cerumen (wax), foreign bodies, perforated tympanic membrane, or otitis media (with or without effusion). Hearing loss is often temporary and reversible.

Sensorineural: Result of damage or malformation of structures of the inner ear and/or auditory nerve. May be result of infection (meningitis or intrauterine), heredity, exposure to loud noise, ototoxic medications, or prematurity. Meningitis causes 6% to 13% of acquired hearing loss in children (Roizen, 1999). Hearing loss is usually permanent.

Mixed: Combination of conductive and sensorineural loss. Conductive loss is often reversible, whereas sensorineural loss is not.

Central: Result of damage to the conduction system between the auditory nervous system and cerebral cortex. May be result of trauma, neurovascular changes, or brain tumors. May cause difficulty in differentiation of sounds, auditory memory.

PATHOPHYSIOLOGY
of Hearing Loss

Adequate hearing depends on intact auditory structures and quality of sound. Sound is described in terms that combine volume (expressed in decibels [dB]) and pitch, or frequencies (expressed in hertz [Hz]). Normal speech ranges in volume between 10 and 60 dB. Normal hearing ranges from −10 to +15 dB at a variety of frequencies. Most people can hear frequencies between 10 and 20,000 Hz but are particularly sensitive to sounds between 1,000 and 2,000 Hz (Nash et al., 1997). Hearing loss is categorized as follows:

Slight	Failure to hear at 16 to 25 dB
Mild	Failure to hear at 26 to 40 dB
Moderate	Failure to hear at 41 to 55 dB
Moderately Severe	Failure to hear at 56 to 70 dB
Severe	Failure to hear at 71 to 90 dB
Profound	Failure to hear at >90 dB

A child with moderate hearing loss has difficulty hearing speech beyond a distance of 3 to 5 feet (Nash et al., 1997). This deficit obviously poses problems for unidentified school children, who miss most of what a teacher says in a classroom.

fected. The Joint Committee on Infant Hearing has recommended that all infants with hearing loss be identified before 3 months of age and receive intervention before 6 months of age (Folsom & Diefendorf, 1999). Several states in the United States have passed legislation making newborn hearing screening mandatory; many others are considering doing the same.

Hearing screening for infants is challenging because of their inability to give accurate behavioral cues indicating intact hearing. Assessing hearing in the newborn or young infant often relies on eliciting a startle reflex with a loud noise. It is difficult, however, to be certain that the response is actually due to the sound itself. Two hearing screening tests can accurately identify infants with hearing deficits: the auditory brainstem response and the evoked otoacoustic emissions test. Newer equipment has made it possible for these tests to be completed quickly and accurately in the hospital nursery (Schuman, 1998). Both tests have a pass/refer option. If the infant fails after two tries (2 weeks apart), referral to an audiologist for more accurate testing is required. More sophisticated testing, such as visual reinforcement audiometry or conditioned-play audiometry, are done by audiologists.

Hearing testing in the older child (3 years and older) is done by audiometry. The child is presented tones of varying frequencies at a standard volume. A quick screening test done in a physician's office with a hand-held audiometer tests frequencies of 500, 1,000, 2,000, and 4,000 Hz at 25 dB. If the child fails the screening, particularly at lower frequencies, a tympanogram might indicate middle ear effusion (see Chapter 45). The problem with office audiometric screening is that it can miss hearing loss at higher frequencies, which is usually sensorineural. When doing audiometry screening of children, therefore, the nurse should per-

---

Risk Factors Indicating the Need for Hearing Screening

NEONATES (BIRTH TO 28 DAYS)

- Family history of inherited sensorineural hearing loss
- Intrauterine infections such as rubella, cytomegalovirus, and toxoplasmosis
- Craniofacial abnormalities
- Birth weight <1.5 kg (3.3 lb)
- Hyperbilirubinemia requiring exchange transfusion
- Ototoxic medications given in multiple courses or with loop diuretics
- Bacterial meningitis
- Apgar scores of 0 to 4 at 1 minute or 0 to 6 at 5 minutes
- Mechanical ventilation for 5 or more days
- Any findings associated with a syndrome that includes hearing loss

INFANTS DEVELOPING CERTAIN CONDITIONS ASSOCIATED WITH HEARING LOSS (29 DAYS TO 2 YEARS)

- Hearing, speech, language, or developmental delay
- Infections associated with sensorineural hearing loss
- Head trauma resulting in loss of consciousness or skull fracture
- Any findings associated with a syndrome that includes hearing loss

- Ototoxic medications given in multiple courses or with loop diuretics
- Recurrent otitis media with effusion lasting at least 3 months

INFANTS (29 DAYS TO 3 YEARS) NEEDING PERIODIC HEARING SCREENING

Sensorineural

- Family history of inherited sensorineural hearing loss
- Intrauterine infections such as rubella, cytomegalovirus, and toxoplasmosis
- Neurofibromatosis type II or other neurodegenerative disorder

Conductive

- Recurrent otitis media with effusion lasting at least 3 months
- Anything that affects eustachian tube function
- Neurodegenerative disorders

Adapted from Joint Committee on Infant Hearing. (1994). 1994 Position statement. *ASHA, 36*(12), 38–41.

• • • • • • • • • •
Hearing Tests Used for Infants

AUDITORY BRAINSTEM RESPONSE

• Electrodes, which record brain wave activity, are placed on the infant's head.
• Foam-padded earphones are placed over the ears.
• The earphones sound a click at a 35-dB volume. The resulting brain wave measurement is compared with the brain wave measurement from a normal infant.
• More accurate testing can be done with more electrodes and clicks of varying intensities. The auditory brainstem response does not test hearing directly, but tests the function of the auditory system and hearing sensitivity in the middle to high frequency ranges (Folsom & Diefendorf, 1999)
• The test takes from 10 minutes to 1 hour to administer, depending on the underlying testing objective.

EVOKED OTOACOUSTIC EMISSIONS

• This test assesses the integrity of the inner ear structures by recording sounds (otoacoustic emissions) that are generated by the inner ear. It cannot assess the degree of hearing loss, but can assess whether hearing is present.
• An ear probe, which contains a sound transmitter and microphone, is attached to a computer and placed in the ear.
• Click sounds evoke the emissions, which are displayed on the computer screen.
• Emissions are present in infants who can hear at 20 dB, but not present in infants who hear only at 35 to 45 dB (mild to moderate hearing loss)(Folsom & Diefendorf, 1999).
• The test takes approximately 5 minutes to administer.

form the test in a quiet environment and determine ahead of time what signal the child will use to indicate hearing the tone.

Therapeutic Management

The goals of identification and management of infants and children with hearing loss are directed toward maximizing language development and preventing later problems with school performance and social interaction. Treatment of hearing loss depends on the type of loss. Conductive hearing

CRITICAL THINKING EXERCISE 55–1
• • • • • • • • •

At the recommendation of the Joint Committee on Infant Hearing, five states in the United States and many areas of Canada have implemented mandatory newborn infant hearing screening programs. As part of these programs, newborns are screened before hospital discharge. Consider the advantages and disadvantages of this issue. Should nurses advocate that their states implement similar programs?

loss is managed by medical or surgical correction of the underlying problem (otitis, cerumen).

Sensorineural hearing loss, which is seldom reversible, requires a different approach. Hearing aids are often recommended for these children. The type of aid chosen depends on the specific needs of the child. The aid should provide the best acoustics and be cosmetically appropriate. For example, an adolescent seldom chooses a body-type hearing aid if an "ear level" aid (one inserted into the ear canal) suffices. The four types of hearing aids most commonly used for pediatric patients are the "behind the ear," the "ear level" (in the ear), eyeglass (aids attached to the temples of eyeglass frames), and body (a box with wires connected to an earmold). Infants and young children often do better with ear-level hearing aids. Infants diagnosed with hearing loss need to begin wearing hearing aids as soon as possible to help facilitate language development.

Cochlear implants offer new options for children with sensorineural hearing loss. The implant is a small electronic device surgically implanted in the cochlea. It delivers electrical stimulation to the inner ear, causing nerve impulses to travel to the brain, where they are interpreted as normal sound. Cochlear implants are considered for profoundly deaf children who are not helped by hearing aids. Because the implant can destroy any residual hearing, it is used only in one ear (Brookhouser, Beauchaine, & Osberger, 1999).

Nursing Considerations for the Child with Hearing Loss

Assess the child's hearing at each well-child visit and with any complaint specific to ears, including otitis media (see Chapter 45). Note an infant's response to bells, rattles, clapping of hands, or horns held approximately 12 inches from the ear. Older children can be asked to repeat whispered words or phrases or listen for a ticking watch. Begin audiometry testing at 3 years of age or younger in a cooperative child.

Assess language skill development. Deaf infants babble like hearing infants until approximately 5 to 6 months of age, when babbling is noted to cease in deaf children. The nurse also questions parents about the child's attention span, disruptive behavior, and other behaviors such as increasing the volume on the television. If the child appears to have hearing loss or is lagging behind in developmental milestones, refer for further evaluation by an audiologist and ear, nose, and throat physician.

When caring for a hearing-impaired child, the nurse should do the following:

• If the child has a hearing aid, encourage its use. Make sure it is in place before beginning to speak.
• Look directly in the child's face. To enhance lip reading, have the child's complete attention before beginning to speak.
• Speak clearly. Slow speech slightly. Do not speak loudly.
• Eliminate background noise.
• Use visual aids to assist communication. These include pictures, hands, and written messages for older children.
• If the child uses American Sign Language to communicate, have a diagram of commonly used words readily

available. Use an interpreter for more complex discussions.

An important nursing responsibility is to educate parents about preventable hearing loss. Mild sensorineural hearing loss can occur from exposure to loud noises such as from firecrackers, firearms, loud infant squeak toys, outdoor yard equipment, boat and snowmobile motors, and rock music. People exposed to loud sounds over long periods need to wear protective ear coverings (e.g., ear plugs, mufflers). Advise teens to decrease exposure to loud rock music and to turn music volume down, especially when listening through ear phones.

Language Disorders

Until 10 months to 1 year of age, a child is considered prelingual. The sounds the child makes have no direct meaning or connection to future language. They are, instead, practice of a learned skill. Before approximately 6 months of age, infants make few sounds other than crying. At approximately 4 to 6 months of age, however, they enter the babbling phase. These are the cooing, happy sounds that an infant makes when content. The first words appear at approximately 10 months to 1 year of age. First sentences appear at approximately 18 months of age. By 2 years of age, most children have at least a 50-word vocabulary.

Girls have more rapid language development until approximately 3 years of age, when the difference disappears. By adolescence, however, girls again show superior verbal skills. Although a relationship exists between developmental delay and verbal skills, the relationship between language development and intelligence is unclear. There seems to be no scientific evidence that a child who talks early is brighter than one who does not. Children who talk very early do appear, however, to be "bright," whereas those who talk extremely late appear to have some developmental delay.

Language disorders in the child are usually of two types. The first is the inability to comprehend (receptive disorder). The second is a disorder in which the child cannot express thoughts through speech (expressive disorder). Receptive

---

PARENTS WANT TO KNOW

How to Encourage Language Development

Talk
Talking to your child is necessary for language development. Because children usually imitate what they hear, how much you talk to your child, what you say, and how you say it affects how much and how well your child talks.

Look
Look directly at your child's face and wait until your child pays attention before you begin talking.

Control Distance
Be sure that you are close to your child when you talk (no farther than 5 feet). The younger the child, the more important it is to be close.

Loudness
Talk slightly louder than you normally do. To remove background noise, turn off the radio, TV, dishwasher.

Be a Good Speech Model
- Describe daily activities to your child as they occur.
- Expand what your child says. For example, if your child points and says "car," you say, "Oh, you want the car."
- Add new information. You might add, "That car is little."
- Build vocabulary. Make teaching new words and concepts a natural part of every day's activities. For example, use new words while shopping, taking a walk, or washing dishes.
- Repeat your child's words using adult pronunciation.

Play and Talk
Set aside some times throughout each day for play time for just you and your child. Play can be looking at books, exploring toys, singing songs, coloring, and so on. Talk to your child during these activities, keeping the conversation at your child's level.

Read
Begin reading to your child at a young age (under 12 months). Ask a librarian for books that are right for your child's age. Reading can be a calming-down activity that promotes closeness between you and your child. Reading provides another opportunity to teach and review words and ideas. Some children enjoy looking at pictures in magazines and catalogs.

Do Not Wait
Your child should have the following skills by these ages:

- 18 months: 3-word vocabulary
- 2 years: 25- to 30-word vocabulary and several 2-word sentences
- 2½ years: At least a 50-word vocabulary and 2-word sentences consistently

If your child does not have these skills, tell your doctor. A referral to an audiologist and speech pathologist may be indicated. Hearing and language testing may lead to a better understanding of your child's language development.

From Northern, J. L., & Downs, M. P. (1991). *Hearing in children* (4th ed., pp. 26–27). Baltimore: Williams & Wilkins. Adapted from *Suggestions for parents*, Noel Matkin, PhD.

disorders result from some type of central nervous system failure. This may be the result of trauma, a congenital malformation, or other failure of language development. This child cannot express symbols and abstract ideas in spoken words or in a logical manner.

Expressive disorders are most often of three types. The first is a disorder of the voice. This is an alteration in the pitch and intonation that may result from a medical condition such as a cleft palate. The second is a defect of articulation, or the way in which words are pronounced. This is the most common type of speech defect and may be related to neuromuscular disease or to structural abnormalities of the nose, throat, and mouth. It may also be idiopathic. Finally, fluency disorders interrupt the flow of normal speech. Included in this category are lisping and stuttering. If stuttering persists after 5 years of age, the child should receive appropriate referrals for speech evaluation (Fig. 55–1).

As with screens for hearing loss, the nurse should assess the child's communication patterns with each well-child visit. Any problems should be noted and referrals made to provide appropriate intervention as soon as possible. Encourage parents to take measures to encourage speech and prevent speech problems.

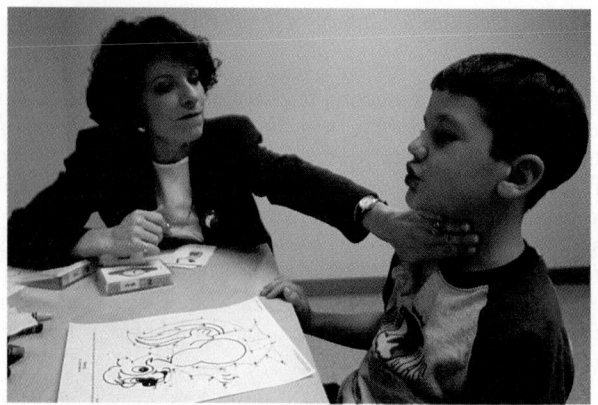

FIGURE 55–1

Expressive speech disorders include disorders of voice, articulation, and fluency. A speech therapist works with the child to help the child speak more clearly and be better understood. Early intervention is very important to correct speech disorders. The nurse should therefore assess speech patterns during each health screening visit. Referrals should be made for any problems noted. (Courtesy of Cook Children's Medical Center, Fort Worth, Texas.)

KEY CONCEPTS

■ Anything that alters a child's sensory perception can adversely affect growth and development.

■ Sense organs develop very early and are sensitive to teratogens. Any interference with development can result in later sensory alteration.

■ Special care should be taken when caring for the child with sensory alterations. Orientation to a new environment is critical in preventing stress and possible injury.

■ Most screenings for sensory alterations are noninvasive and relatively painless.

■ Parent education and support are critical in assisting the child with sensory alteration to develop as normally as possible.

■ Early intervention for the child with sensory alterations allows for more normal growth and development.

■ Health teaching should include injury prevention.

ANSWER TO CRITICAL THINKING EXERCISE 55–1

With any new program, it is important to look at the cost-benefit ratio. The benefits of this program cannot be argued. The costs can be high, but the increased initial cost could decrease later costs associated with intervention, rehabilitation, and emotional stress for the child and family.

Advantages
• With this program, the approximately 1 to 4 per 1,000 infants who are deaf at birth might be identified early enough to begin intervention.

• Deafness in the newborn is difficult to diagnose by behavior alone because responding to loud noises with a startle or blink might be related more to vibration than actual hearing.

• Delayed diagnosis compromises language development and future school performance.

• Only 50% of infants with deafness are identified under the risk referral criteria currently recommended.

• Diagnosis and intervention before the infant is 6 months old greatly improve outcomes.

Disadvantages
• Equipment to do valid testing on newborns is expensive. Not all institutions could afford to implement a program without some monetary assistance.

• Depending on the test used, additional personnel might be required.

• Follow-up by the parent cannot be mandated. Tracking those who do not follow up could require additional personnel and paper work.

REFERENCES AND READINGS

American Academy of Ophthalmology. (1994). Strabismus: Etiology, diagnosis, and treatment. *Journal of Ophthalmic Nursing and Technology, 13*(3), 121–123.

Bacal, D., & Hertle, R. (1998). Don't be lazy about looking for amblyopia. *Contemporary Pediatrics, 15*(6), 99–107.

Bacal, D., Rousta, S., & Hertle, R. (1999). Why early vision screening matters. *Contemporary Pediatrics, 16,* 155–163.

Besinger, R. (1992). Color vision testing. *Journal of Ophthalmic Nursing and Technology, 11*(4), 161–163.

Brookhouser, P., Beauchaine, K., & Osberger, M. (1999). Management of the child with sensorineural hearing loss. *Pediatric Clinics of North America, 46,* 121–141.

Castiglia, P. T. (1994). Strabismus. *Journal of Pediatric Health Care, 8,* 236–238.

Catalano, R. A. (1993). Eye injuries and prevention. *Pediatric Clinics of North America, 40,* 827–839.

Catalano, R. A., & Nelson, L. B. (1994). *Pediatric ophthalmology: A text atlas.* Norwalk, CT: Appleton & Lange.

Finitzo, T., & Crumley, W. (1999). The role of the pediatrician in hearing loss. *Pediatric Clinics of North America, 46,* 15–34.

Flax, J., & Rapin, I. (1998). Evaluating children with delayed speech and language. *Contemporary Pediatrics, 15*(10), 164–172.

Folsom, R., & Diefendorf, A. (1999). Physiologic and behavioral approaches to pediatric hearing assessment. *Pediatric Clinics of North America, 46,* 107–120.

Gerali, P. S. (1991). Childsight: Helping children grow up with good vision. *Journal of Ophthalmic Nursing and Technology, 10*(5), 222–223.

Hertle, R. (1999). Anterior segment. In F. Burg, E. Wald, J. Ingelfinger, & R. Polin (Eds.), *Gellis and Kagan's current pediatric therapy* (16th ed., pp. 1010–1012). Philadelphia: Saunders.

Huddleston, K. (1994). Strabismus repair in the pediatric patient. *AORN Journal, 60,* 754–755, 757–760.

Jockin, Y. (1999). Strabismus. In F. Burg, E. Wald, J. Ingelfinger, & R. Polin (Eds.), *Gellis and Kagan's current pediatric therapy* (16th ed., pp. 1016–1017). Philadelphia: Saunders.

Joint Committee on Infant Hearing. (1994). 1994 position statement. *ASHA, 36*(12), 38–41.

King, R. A. (1993). Common ocular signs and symptoms in childhood. *Pediatric Clinics of North America, 40,* 753–766.

Kramer, S. J., & Williams, D. R. (1993). The hearing-impaired infant and toddler: Identification, assessment, and intervention. *Infants and Young Children, 6*(1), 35–49.

Kratz, I. (1997). Using equipment in unfamiliar clinical settings: Audiology screening. *Journal of Pediatric Nursing, 12,* 307–310.

Kravitz, L., & Selekman, J. (1992). Understanding hearing loss in children. *Pediatric Nursing, 18,* 591–594.

Lavrich, J. B., & Nelson, L. B. (1993). Diagnosis and treatment of strabismus disorders. *Pediatric Clinics of North America, 40,* 737–752.

McCartney, P. (1999). Newborn hearing screening: What nurses think. *MCN: American Journal of Maternal/Child Nursing, 24,* 48.

Nash, D., Schochat, E., Rozycki, A., & Musiek, F. (1997). When loud noises hurt. *Contemporary Pediatrics, 14*(6), 97–109.

Nisak, A., Kieszak, S., Holmes, A., Esteban, E., Rubin, C., & Brody, D. (1998). Prevalence of hearing loss among children 6 to 19 years of age: The third national health and nutrition examination survey. *JAMA, 279,* 1071–1075.

Robinson, B., Bobier, W., Martin, E., & Bryant, L. (1999). Preschool vision screening program. *American Journal of Public Health, 89,* 193–197.

Roizen, N. (1999). Etiology of hearing loss in children. *Pediatric Clinics of North America, 46,* 49–64.

Schuman, A. (1998). Universal newborn hearing screening: The time is right. *Contemporary Pediatrics, 15*(7), 49–60.

Stein, L. (1999). Factors influencing the efficacy of universal newborn hearing screening. *Pediatric Clinics of North America, 46,* 95–105.

Steinkuller, P., Edmond, J., & Chen, R. (1998). Ocular infections. In R. Feigin & J. Cherry (Eds.), *Textbook of pediatric infectious diseases* (pp. 786–806). Philadelphia: Saunders.

Symanski, M. E., Newman, C. O., & Bachynski, B. N. (1994). Treating congenital cataracts. *MCN: American Journal of Maternal/Child Nursing, 19,* 335–338.

Tomaski, S., & Grundfast, K. (1999). A stepwise approach to the diagnosis and treatment of hereditary hearing loss. *Pediatric Clinics of North America, 46,* 35–48.

Trobe, J. D. (1993). *The physician's guide to eye care.* San Francisco: American Academy of Ophthalmology.

Wagner, R. S. (1994). Glaucoma in children. *Pediatric Clinics of North America, 40,* 855–867.

Wagner, R. S. (1997). Eye infections and abnormalities: Issues for the pediatrician. *Contemporary Pediatrics, 14*(6), 137–153.

Wilson, M. (1999). Cornea. In F. Burg, E. Wald, J. Ingelfinger, & R. Polin (Eds.), *Gellis and Kagan's current pediatric therapy* (16th ed., pp. 1008–1010). Philadelphia: Saunders.

Appendixes

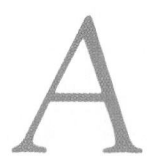

NANDA-Approved Nursing Diagnoses

This list represents the NANDA-approved nursing diagnoses for clinical use and testing.

Pattern 1: Exchanging

1.1.2.1	Altered Nutrition: More Than Body Requirements
1.1.2.2	Altered Nutrition: Less Than Body Requirements
1.1.2.3	Altered Nutrition: Risk for More Than Body Requirements
1.2.1.1	Risk for Infection
1.2.2.1	Risk for Altered Body Temperature
1.2.2.2	Hypothermia
1.2.2.3	Hyperthermia
1.2.2.4	Ineffective Thermoregulation
1.2.3.1	Dysreflexia
* 1.2.3.2	Risk for Autonomic Dysreflexia
★ 1.3.1.1	Constipation
1.3.1.1.1	Perceived Constipation
1.3.1.1.2	Colonic Constipation (deleted in 1998)
★ 1.3.1.2	Diarrhea
★ 1.3.1.3	Bowel Incontinence
* 1.3.1.4	Risk for Constipation
1.3.2	Altered Urinary Elimination
1.3.2.1.1	Stress Incontinence
★ 1.3.2.1.2	Reflex Urinary Incontinence
1.3.2.1.3	Urge Incontinence
★ 1.3.2.1.4	Functional Urinary Incontinence
1.3.2.1.5	Total Incontinence
* 1.3.2.1.6	Risk for Urinary Urge Incontinence
1.3.2.2	Urinary Retention

# 1.4.1.1	Altered Tissue Perfusion (Specify type: Renal, Cerebral, Cardiopulmonary, Gastrointestinal, Peripheral)
* 1.4.1.2	Risk for Fluid Volume Imbalance
1.4.1.2.1	Fluid Volume Excess
1.4.1.2.2.1	Fluid Volume Deficit
1.4.1.2.2.2	Risk for Fluid Volume Deficit
1.4.2.1	Decreased Cardiac Output
★ 1.5.1.1	Impaired Gas Exchange
★ 1.5.1.2	Ineffective Airway Clearance
★ 1.5.1.3	Ineffective Breathing Pattern
1.5.1.3.1	Inability to Sustain Spontaneous Ventilation
1.5.1.3.2	Dysfunctional Ventilatory Weaning Response
1.6.1	Risk for Injury
1.6.1.1	Risk for Suffocation
1.6.1.2	Risk for Poisoning
1.6.1.3	Risk for Trauma
1.6.1.4	Risk for Aspiration
1.6.1.5	Risk for Disuse Syndrome
* 1.6.1.6	Latex Allergy Response
* 1.6.1.7	Risk for Latex Allergy Response
1.6.2	Altered Protection
# 1.6.2.1	Impaired Tissue Integrity
★ 1.6.2.1.1	Altered Oral Mucous Membrane
# 1.6.2.1.2.1	Impaired Skin Integrity
# 1.6.2.1.2.2	Risk for Impaired Skin Integrity
* 1.6.2.1.3	Altered Dentition
1.7.1	Decreased Adaptive Capacity: Intracranial
1.8	Energy Field Disturbance

Pattern 2: Communicating

# 2.1.1.1	Impaired Verbal Communication

Pattern 3: Relating

3.1.1	Impaired Social Interaction
3.1.2	Social Isolation
3.1.3	Risk for Loneliness
★ 3.2.1	Altered Role Performance
★ 3.2.1.1.1	Altered Parenting
★ 3.2.1.1.2	Risk for Altered Parenting
3.2.1.1.2.1	Risk for Altered Parent/Infant/Child Attachment
3.2.1.2.1	Sexual Dysfunction
★ 3.2.2	Altered Family Processes
★ 3.2.2.1	Caregiver Role Strain
3.2.2.2	Risk for Caregiver Role Strain
3.2.2.3.1	Altered Family Processes: Alcoholism
3.2.3.1	Parental Role Conflict
3.3	Altered Sexuality Patterns

Pattern 4: Valuing

4.1.1	Spiritual Distress (Distress of the Human Spirit)
* 4.1.2	Risk for Spiritual Distress
4.2	Potential for Enhanced Spiritual Well-Being

Pattern 5: Choosing

★ 5.1.1.1	Ineffective Individual Coping
★ 5.1.1.1.1	Impaired Adjustment

5.1.1.1.2 Defensive Coping
5.1.1.1.3 Ineffective Denial
5.1.2.1.1 Ineffective Family Coping: Disabling
5.1.2.1.2 Ineffective Family Coping: Compromised
5.1.2.2 Family Coping: Potential for Growth
5.1.3.1 Potential for Enhanced Community Coping
★ 5.1.3.2 Ineffective Community Coping
5.2.1 Ineffective Management of Therapeutic Regimen: Individuals
5.2.1.1 Noncompliance (specify)
5.2.2 Ineffective Management of Therapeutic Regimen: Families
5.2.3 Ineffective Management of Therapeutic Regimen: Community
5.2.4 Ineffective Management of Therapeutic Regimen: Individual
5.3.1.1 Decisional Conflict (specify)
5.4 Health-Seeking Behaviors (specify)

Pattern 6: Moving

★ 6.1.1.1 Impaired Physical Mobility
6.1.1.1.1 Risk for Peripheral Neurovascular Dysfunction
6.1.1.1.2 Risk for Perioperative Positioning Injury
6.1.1.1.3 Impaired Walking
6.1.1.1.4 Impaired Wheelchair Mobility
* 6.1.1.1.5 Impaired Transfer Ability
6.1.1.1.6 Impaired Bed Mobility
6.1.1.2 Activity Intolerance
★ 6.1.1.2.1 Fatigue
6.1.1.3 Risk for Activity Intolerance
★ 6.2.1 Sleep Pattern Disturbance
6.2.1.1 Sleep Deprivation
6.3.1.1 Diversional Activity Deficit
6.4.1.1 Impaired Home Maintenance Management
6.4.2 Altered Health Maintenance
6.4.2.1 Delayed Surgical Recovery
6.4.2.2 Adult Failure to Thrive
★ 6.5.1 Feeding Self-Care Deficit
★ 6.5.1.1 Impaired Swallowing
6.5.1.2 Ineffective Breastfeeding
6.5.1.2.1 Interrupted Breastfeeding
6.5.1.3 Effective Breastfeeding
6.5.1.4 Ineffective Infant Feeding Pattern
★ 6.5.2 Bathing/Hygiene Self-Care Deficit
★ 6.5.3 Dressing/Grooming Self-Care Deficit
★ 6.5.4 Toileting Self-Care Deficit
6.6 Altered Growth and Development
6.6.1 Risk for Altered Development

6.6.2 Risk for Altered Growth
6.7 Relocation Stress Syndrome
6.8.1 Risk for Disorganized Infant Behavior
★ 6.8.2 Disorganized Infant Behavior
6.8.3 Potential for Enhanced Organized Infant Behavior

Pattern 7: Perceiving

7.1.1 Body Image Disturbance
7.1.2 Self-Esteem Disturbance
7.1.2.1 Chronic Low Self-Esteem
7.1.2.2 Situational Low Self-Esteem
7.1.3 Personal Identity Disturbance
7.2 Sensory/Perceptual Alterations (Specify: Visual, Auditory, Kinesthetic, Gustatory, Tactile, Olfactory)
7.2.1.1 Unilateral Neglect
7.3.1 Hopelessness
7.3.2 Powerlessness

Pattern 8: Knowing

8.1.1 Knowledge Deficit (specify)
8.2.1 Impaired Environmental Interpretation Syndrome
8.2.2 Acute Confusion
8.2.3 Chronic Confusion
8.3 Altered Thought Processes
8.3.1 Impaired Memory

Pattern 9: Feeling

9.1.1 Pain
9.1.1.1 Chronic Pain
* 9.1.2 Nausea
9.2.1.1 Dysfunctional Grieving
9.2.1.2 Anticipatory Grieving
* 9.2.1.3 Chronic Sorrow
9.2.2 Risk for Violence: Directed at Others
9.2.2.1 Risk for Self-Mutilation
9.2.2.2 Risk for Violence: Self-Directed
★ 9.2.3 Post-Trauma Syndrome
★ 9.2.3.1 Rape-Trauma Syndrome
9.2.3.1.1 Rape-Trauma Syndrome: Compound Reaction
9.2.3.1.2 Rape-Trauma Syndrome: Silent Reaction
* 9.2.4 Risk for Post-Trauma Syndrome
# 9.3.1 Anxiety
* 9.3.1.1 Death Anxiety
# 9.3.2 Fear

B

• • • • • • • • • • •

Infection Control in Maternity, Pediatric, and Women's Health Care

Pathogens such as human immunodeficiency virus (HIV) and hepatitis B virus (HBV) have resulted in significant changes in infection control. Early infection control practices were based on segregation of infected persons or on disease-specific categories of isolation such as respiratory isolation, wound and skin precautions, or blood precautions. The major shortcoming of these systems was that they were applied after the infection status of the person was known. They also involved placing warning signs on the door to the infected person's room, which compromised the person's privacy.

The increasing prevalence of HIV and HBV infections required a new approach because these pathogens could be transmitted long before signs and symptoms of infection became evident. To prevent transmission of blood-borne pathogens to caregivers, the infection control practice of *universal precautions* was established. Universal precautions stressed that all clients were to be presumed infectious for HIV and other blood-borne pathogens. Universal precautions required the use of protective equipment if contact with certain body fluids, or articles contaminated with these fluids, was likely. A major advantage of universal precautions was that they could protect the health care worker from infection with blood-borne pathogens when the client's infection status was unknown. A shortcoming of universal precautions was that the guidelines did not address sources of infection other than blood-borne. Universal precautions did, however, specify the use of general infection control practices, such as hand washing.

Because *all* body substances may contain pathogens, the more comprehensive guidelines of *body substance isolation* were adopted by many hospitals in the late 1980s. These guidelines specified the use of barriers, primarily gloves, for contact with all moist body substances, mucous membranes, and nonintact skin. The guidelines also included placing signs on doors instructing visitors and other medical personnel to check with the nurse before entering the rooms of clients who might have had infections transmitted by the airborne route. The advantages of the body substance isolation guidelines were that they protected the client's privacy better and they protected workers from more pathogens than universal precautions alone did.

New Infection Control Guidelines

The newest guidelines for infection control have two levels of protection. The first level, *standard precautions*, combines features from universal precautions and body substance isolation guidelines and applies to all clients. Standard precautions specify the use of personal protective equipment for potential contact with

> Blood
> All body fluids, secretions, and excretions except sweat
> Nonintact skin
> Mucous membranes

Hand washing before and after care is essential. Immediate, thorough hand washing should follow unexpected contact with body substances.

The second level of protection, *transmission-based precautions*, is used for the care of specific clients. Transmission-based precautions are designed to limit the spread of pathogens that may not be confined by the use of standard precautions. These pathogens can be spread by air, droplets (such as with breathing, coughing, or sneezing), or contact with dry skin or contaminated surfaces. Transmission-based precautions are used in addition to standard precautions.

Gloves are a major component of personal protective equipment, but gloves do not prevent injuries from needles or sharp instruments. Caregivers should not recap needles, purposely bend or break them by hand, remove them from disposable syringes, or otherwise manipulate used needles and other sharp instruments by hand. After use, disposable syringes and needles, scalpel blades, and other sharp items are placed in puncture-resistant containers for disposal.

Sources of Infection in Maternity, Pediatric, and Women's Health Care

Nursing care of the woman, infant, or child includes many situations in which the nurse must expect exposure to pathogens, both blood-borne and other infectious agents:

- Handling tissue specimens or specimens of body secretions
- Surgical procedures (scrub personnel near the operative site need more protective equipment than circulating personnel)
- Contact with nonintact skin, including surgical incisions
- Contact with mucous membranes, such as during vaginal or rectal examinations or assessment of the mouth
- Parenteral procedures, such as venipunctures, injections, finger sticks, and heel sticks

- Application of medication to nonintact skin or mucous membranes, such as placement of rectal or vaginal suppositories, application of topical preparations, infant eye prophylaxis, and care of the umbilical cord
- Preoperative shaving, perineal care, enemas
- Handling linens, gowns, underpads, perineal pads, and dressings; during the intrapartum and postpartum periods, these items are likely to be contaminated with amniotic fluid, blood, or both
- Handling the infant before the first bath is given
- Changing diapers and cleaning the diaper area
- Assessing breasts or contact with colostrum or breast milk
- Suture or staple removal

C

Effects of Drug Use During Pregnancy and Breast-Feeding

FDA Pregnancy Risk Categories

The U.S. Food and Drug Administration (FDA) has assigned pregnancy risk categories to many drugs on the basis of (1) their known relative safety or danger to the fetus and (2) whether safer alternative drugs exist. For many drugs, little is known about the fetal risk. The categories are as follows:

A: No evidence of risk to the fetus.
B: Animal reproduction studies have not demonstrated a risk to the fetus. No adequate and well-controlled studies have been done in pregnant women. Or animal studies show adverse effect on the fetus, but human studies with pregnant women have not demonstrated a risk to the fetus in any trimester of pregnancy.

C: Animal reproduction studies have shown an adverse effect on the fetus but no adequate, well-controlled studies have been done in humans. Potential benefits may warrant use of the drug in pregnant women despite fetal risks.
D: There is positive evidence of human fetal risk based on adverse reaction data, but potential benefits may warrant use of the drug in pregnant women despite fetal risks. Essentially, no safer alternatives to the drug are available.
X: There is positive evidence of human fetal risk based on animal or human studies and/or adverse reaction data. The risks of using the drug in pregnant women clearly outweigh potential benefits. Safer alternatives to these drugs may be available.

Drug Use During Lactation

The effects of many drugs when used during lactation have not been studied. In general, if a drug is safe for use in infants, it is probably safe for the lactating woman to take. Other drugs are known not to be excreted in breast milk or to be excreted in an inactive form or in very low concentrations. Modifying the time of maternal ingestion may reduce transfer of the drug to the infant. Other drugs are undesirable because they suppress lactation.

The American Academy of Pediatrics (AAP) has established classifications for safety of some drugs during lactation. The categories are as follows:

AAP compatible: Usually compatible with breast-feeding
AAP contraindicated: Contraindicated for use in breast-feeding mothers
AAP reason for concern: Reports of infant side effects cause concern about use in breast-feeding mothers

Check for updated medication information when giving a drug to a pregnant or lactating woman.

Drug Use During Pregnancy and Lactation

Drug	Use During Pregnancy	Use During Breast-Feeding
Analgesics		
Aspirin	Risk category D. May prolong pregnancy because of its antiprostaglandin effects. May cause bleeding disorders in mother or newborn if used during late pregnancy.	AAP reason for concern. Toxicity unlikely in normal doses, but higher doses could cause bleeding in infant.
Acetaminophen	Risk category B. Problems have not been documented, but drug does cross placenta. Use with caution.	AAP compatible. Very small amounts are secreted into breast milk.
Narcotic analgesics (butorphanol, hydrocodone, meperidine, morphine, nalbuphine, propoxyphene)	Butorphanol: risk category B first two trimesters; category D last trimester. Associated with sinusoidal monitor patterns. Risk category B: meperidine, morphine, nalbuphine Risk category C: hydrocodone, propoxyphene	Most narcotics given briefly and in therapeutic doses are compatible with breast-feeding. Infant lethargy and poor feeding may be noted with large doses. Prolonged use may result in infant drug dependence and subsequent withdrawal when the mother no longer takes the drug.

Drug Use During Pregnancy and Lactation Continued

Drug	Use During Pregnancy	Use During Breast-Feeding
Analgesics (cont.)		
	Neonatal respiratory depression is the most significant adverse effect when narcotic analgesics are used during labor. Neonatal withdrawal may occur if the woman is addicted to the narcotic.	
Nonsteroidal anti-inflammatory drugs (NSAIDs) (fenoprofen, flurbiprofen, ibuprofen, indomethacin, ketoprofen, naproxen)	Risk category B. Not recommended after 34 weeks. May prolong pregnancy or labor because of antiprostaglandin effects. Associated with premature closure of ductus arteriosus in fetus.	Ibuprofen and indomethacin are AAP compatible. All should be used cautiously owing to potential for infant bleeding. Ketoprofen and naproxen have long half-lives and may remain in the blood a long time.
Antiallergic and Antiasthmatic Drugs (See also Hormones, Corticosteroids)		
Antihistamines	Risk category B: chlorpheniramine, clemastine, cyproheptadine, loratadine, meclizine Risk category C: astemizole, brompheniramine, diphenhydramine, phenylephrine, phenylpropanolamine, terfenadine, triprolidine	All should be used with caution. Most are safe, but may cause infant drowsiness. If this adverse effect occurs, a different drug may be tried. Clemastine is rated as AAP reason for concern and is contraindicated.
Cromolyn	Risk category B	Minimal oral absorption, so it is unlikely to adversely affect infant.
Epinephrine	Risk category C	Unlikely to be absorbed in infant's gastrointestinal tract after early newborn period, or if preterm.
Metaproterenol (Alupent)	Risk category C	Unknown whether secreted in milk; use cautiously.
Anticoagulants		
Heparin	Risk category C. Does not cross placenta. Anticoagulant of choice during pregnancy	AAP compatible. Not excreted in breast milk.
Warfarin (Coumadin)	Risk category D. Associated with facial abnormalities and neurologic deficits. Traumatic intracranial hemorrhage may occur in neonate if ingested near term. If used, it is typically avoided between 6 and 12 weeks' gestation and for 2 to 3 weeks before term.	AAP compatible, but should be used with caution. Very small amounts secreted in milk. No reported bleeding abnormalities in infant, but observe for bruising or petechiae.
Anticonvulsants		
Carbamazepine (Tegretol)	Risk category C. Associated with craniofacial abnormalities, under-developed fingernails, neural tube defects, and developmental delay.	AAP compatible. Small amounts secreted in breast milk; accumulation does not seem to occur. Observe infant for sedation.
Magnesium sulfate	Risk category A (category C shortly before birth). Infants exposed to magnesium sulfate shortly before birth may exhibit respiratory depression, hypotonic muscle tone, depressed reflexes, hypocalcemia, or cardiac dysrhythmias.	AAP compatible. Moderate amounts secreted in milk, but most remains in infant's gastrointestinal tract. Milk levels return to normal about 24 hours after drug is stopped.
Phenobarbital	Risk category D. Fetal addiction with subsequent withdrawal is possible but rare at dose levels used for seizure control. Abnormalities similar to those seen in infants exposed to carbamazepine, phenytoin, and valproic acid have been reported.	AAP reason for concern. Significant amounts accumulate in infant's plasma. Psychomotor delay and sedation possible. Use cautiously.

Table continued on following page

• • • • • • • • • • •

Drug Use During Pregnancy and Lactation *Continued*

Drug	Use During Pregnancy	Use During Breast-Feeding
Anticonvulsants (*cont.*)		
Phenytoin (Dilantin)	Risk category D. The fetal hydantoin syndrome includes prenatal-onset growth deficiency, small head, mental retardation, craniofacial and other anomalies, underdeveloped nails or distal phalanges.	AAP compatible. Minimal effects if maternal dose is low. Observe for sedation and decreased sucking.
Trimethadione (Tridione)	Risk category D. Fetal risk for malformations is greater than with other anticonvulsants. Associated with developmental delay, craniofacial abnormalities, cardiovascular and other internal abnormalities.	Enters breast milk. Use cautiously.
Valproic acid (Depakene)	Risk category D. Associated with neural tube defects, craniofacial abnormalities.	AAP compatible. Secreted in small amounts. May cause drowsiness. Used for infant seizures.
Antidiabetic Agents		
Insulin	Risk category B. Insulin is only appropriate drug to control diabetes during pregnancy because it does not cross placenta.	AAP compatible. Any insulin secreted would be destroyed in infant's gastrointestinal tract.
Oral hypoglycemic agents	Contraindicated; cross placenta. Insulin controls blood glucose levels without crossing placenta. May cause prolonged neonatal hypoglycemia.	Safety not established for most. Observe for infant hypoglycemia.
Antihypertensives (See also Diuretics, because these drugs are often used to treat hypertension)		
ACE inhibitors (benazepril, captopril, enalapril, fosinopril, ramipril)	Risk category D. Suspected teratogenic effects. May reduce uteroplacental perfusion and cause fetal hypotension. Renal malformations with anuria, leading to oligohydramnios, lung hypoplasia, and cranial and facial deformities, have been reported.	Use with caution. Captopril and enalapril are AAP compatible. Small amounts are transferred to infant. Observe infant for hypotension.
Beta-adrenergic blockers (acebutolol, atenolol, betaxolol, labetalol, metoprolol, nadolol, penbutolol, pindolol, propranolol, timolol)	Risk category C, except acebutolol and pindolol, which are risk category B. Possible fetal or neonatal effects include transient bradycardia, respiratory depression, and hypoglycemia.	AAP compatible, but potentially hazardous: acebutolol, labetalol, nadolol, timolol. Observe infant for pharmacologic effects if mother is taking a beta-adrenergic blocker: hypotension, bradycardia, sedation, and fatigue may occur.
Calcium channel blockers (amlodipine, diltiazem, nicardipine, nifedipine, nimodipine, verapamil)	Risk category C. Hypotensive effects may reduce uteroplacental perfusion and may lead to fetal heart failure and atrioventricular block. Nifedipine has been used on an investigational basis to inhibit preterm labor.	Drugs excreted in breast milk. AAP compatible: diltiazem, nifedipine, and verapamil. Use with extreme caution; overdoses in young children are very dangerous. Observe for hypotension and bradycardia. Delaying nursing for 3–4 hours after the *non-sustained-release* form may reduce transfer to infant.
Centrally acting sympatholytics (clonidine, guanabenz, guanfacine, methyldopa)	Risk category C, except for guanfacine (risk category B).	Methyldopa is AAP compatible. Others should be used cautiously, as safety is not established. Observe for hypotension and sedation.
Vasodilators (hydralazine, minoxidil)	Risk category C. No adverse fetal effects associated with long-term use. Excessive hair has been reported.	Listed drugs are AAP compatible.

Drug Use During Pregnancy and Lactation Continued

Drug	Use During Pregnancy	Use During Breast-Feeding
Antimicrobials		
Aminoglycosides (gentamicin, kanamycin, neomycin, streptomycin)	Risk categories C and D. Associated with hearing loss and renal toxicity.	AAP compatible: kanamycin and streptomycin. Most drugs in this class are poorly absorbed orally.
Azithromycin (Zithromax)	Risk category B. Chemically related to erythromycin.	Only small amounts are likely to be ingested by infant.
Cephalosporins	Most are risk category B.	Secretion into milk is generally poor. Observe for diarrhea.
Chloramphenicol	Risk category C. Not recommended for use at term because it is associated with neonatal "gray baby syndrome" (rapid respiration, ashen and pale color, poor feeding, abdominal distension, vasomotor collapse, death).	AAP reason for concern. Generally contraindicated in breast-feeding mothers. May cause infant sensitivity.
Erythromycins	Risk category B. Little transfer to fetus across placenta, which limits the drugs' usefulness for treating syphilis.	AAP compatible. May cause alteration in gastrointestinal flora, allergies, interference with infant's cultures for infection.
Fluoroquinolones (includes ciprofloxacin, norfloxacin, ofloxacin)	Risk category C. Animal studies have shown joint abnormalities.	Contraindicated. Possible association with cartilage damage and colitis.
Metronidazole (Flagyl)	Risk category B. However, not recommended to treat *Trichomonas* infections during first trimester.	AAP reason for concern (primarily for oral form). Breast-feeding may be discontinued for 12–24 hours to allow mother to excrete last dose, then restarted.
Nitrofurantoin (Macrodantin)	Risk category B. Use should be avoided near term because it may cause hemolytic anemia in newborn.	AAP compatible for older infants. Should avoid if infant is younger than 1 month. Risk for hemolytic anemia if infant has an enzyme (G6PD) deficiency.
Penicillins (includes amoxicillin, ampicillin, penicillin G)	Risk category B. No reported adverse fetal effects. Penicillins combined with beta-lactamase inhibitors (Augmentin, Timentin, Unasyn) have not been adequately studied, although fetal effects are unlikely.	Penicillins are AAP compatible. Observe for infant diarrhea or development of sensitivity.
Sulfonamides	Risk category B (D near term). May result in neonatal hyperbilirubinemia.	Potentially hazardous. Sulfisoxazole is considered compatible, but all should be used with great caution. Associated with jaundice, diarrhea, rash.
Tetracyclines	Risk category D. Can interfere with tooth enamel formation and cause discolored teeth. Prenatal exposure does not affect permanent teeth.	AAP compatible for short periods. Tooth discoloration, slowed bone growth, and altered bowel flora are possible.
Antineoplastics		

Few cases have been studied because of the relative rarity with which these drugs are used in women of childbearing age. Therefore, their relative safety or danger cannot be accurately determined. Additionally, reported congenital defects may be more related to the mother's serious disease than to the drug itself.

Alkylating agents	Probable association with fetal anomalies. Risk category D	Contraindicated
Antimetabolites	Risk category D. Methotrexate is contraindicated for treatment of psoriasis or rheumatoid arthritis during pregnancy (risk category X).	Contraindicated
Tamoxifen (Nolvadex)	Risk category D	Contraindicated

Table continued on following page

Drug Use During Pregnancy and Lactation Continued

Drug	Use During Pregnancy	Use During Breast-Feeding
Antituberculosis Agents (See also Antimicrobials)		
Ethambutol	Risk category B. No evidence of increased abnormalities. Fetal effects of combinations of ethambutol with other antituberculosis drugs are unknown.	AAP compatible. Concentration in breast milk is similar to that in maternal serum, so caution is indicated.
Isoniazid	Risk category C	AAP compatible, but infant should be observed for liver toxicity and neuritis.
Pyrazinamide	Risk category C. Safety is not established; however, most authorities recommend the drug because it is rapid and highly effective	Use cautiously.
Rifampin	Risk category C	AAP compatible. No reported adverse effects
Antitussives and Expectorants		
Dextromethorphan	Risk category C at therapeutic levels	Unlikely to pass into milk enough to provide clinically significant levels in the infant.
Guaifenesin	Risk category C	Untoward effects not reported.
Antiviral Agents		
Acyclovir	Risk category C	AAP compatible. Few reported toxic effects. If topical drug is used on nipples, wash thoroughly before nursing.
Ribavirin (Virazole)	Risk category X. Administered by aerosol. Women who are pregnant or who may become pregnant should avoid exposure.	Not known whether drug is excreted in milk.
Zidovudine (formerly called AZT)	Risk category C. Given to HIV-seropositive women to reduce risk for perinatal transmission of the virus.	The Centers for Disease Control and Prevention currently recommend that HIV-positive mothers not breast-feed.
Bronchodilators		
Albuterol	Risk category C	Small amounts likely to be secreted. Observe infant for tremors and excitement.
Terbutaline (Brethine)	Risk category B. Also used in treatment of preterm labor	AAP compatible. Observe infant for tremors and nervousness.
Theophylline	Risk category C	AAP compatible. Excreted in milk. May result in infant irritability, insomnia, and fretfulness.
Cardiac Glycosides		
Digoxin	Risk category C	AAP compatible
Decongestants		
Ephedrine, epinephrine, triprolidine, phenylephrine	Risk category C	Use with caution. May cause irritability in infant.
Pseudoephedrine	Risk category C	AAP compatible. Minimal amounts secreted in milk.
Diuretics		
Furosemide (Lasix)	Risk category C	Effects unknown but probably minimal. May reduce milk production.
Thiazides	Risk categories B and C. Decreased intravascular volume may reduce uteroplacental perfusion. Metabolic disturbances and thrombocytopenia may occur in mother and fetus.	AAP approved: chlorothiazide; hydrochlorothiazide. May reduce milk production.

Drug Use During Pregnancy and Lactation *Continued*

Drug	Use During Pregnancy	Use During Breast-Feeding
Hormones		
Corticosteroids	Risk category C (prednisone category B). Prednisone is agent of choice for asthmatic woman who needs steroids. Betamethasone and dexamethasone are used to accelerate maturation of fetal lungs if preterm delivery is likely.	Prednisone is AAP approved. Potentially hazardous in high doses or with long-term use. Delay nursing 4 hours after dose to reduce transfer to infant. Do not apply topically to nipples.
Estrogens	Risk category X. Diethylstilbestrol (DES) is associated with development of vaginal cancer in female offspring during adolescence or adulthood.	AAP approved. Reduces milk volume and protein content. Try to delay drug until breast-feeding is firmly established. DES should not be used.
Oral contraceptives (estrogen-progestin combinations)	Risk category X. Doses much higher than those used in oral contraceptives are associated with masculinization of the female fetus's genitalia.	AAP approved, but best to avoid use until lactation is well established, or drugs may decrease milk quantity and quality.
Clomiphene citrate (Clomid)	Risk category X. Questionable association with neural tube defects. Drug is discontinued after pregnancy is achieved.	Has been tested as a lactation suppressant, but not prescribed for this purpose. Unlikely to be prescribed during lactation because it is given for infertility.
Psychoactive Drugs		
Benzodiazepines	Most are risk category D. The following benzodiazepines are risk category X and contraindicated during pregnancy: estazolam, quazepam, temazepam, and triazolam. Some reports of mild facial abnormalities and developmental delay, but no conclusive studies.	Potentially hazardous. Preferred drugs in this class are lorazepam or oxazepam.
Fluoxetine (Prozac)	Risk category B	Effect on nursing infants is unknown, but is cause for concern.
Lithium	Risk category D. Slightly increased risk for cardiac abnormalities.	AAP contraindicated
Meprobamate	Contraindicated. Associated with a significant increase in malformations. Equagesic contains meprobamate.	Concentrations in milk are higher than in maternal serum. May cause sedation in infant.
Phenothiazines (chlorpromazine, perphenazine, prochlorperazine, thioridazine, trifluoperazine)	Risk category C. Risk of malformations is uncertain. Continued use during pregnancy should be carefully evaluated.	AAP reason for concern; some sources say these drugs are probably safe in usual doses. Observe infant for sedation or jerking movements.
Tricyclic antidepressants	Risk categories C and D. Most likely are not teratogenic.	Use with caution. Probably safe in usual doses. Desipramine and nortriptyline are preferred. Some sources consider these drugs contraindicated for breast-feeding mothers.
Thyroid Drugs		
Antithyroids (methimazole, propylthiouracil [PTU])	Risk category D. May result in neonatal goiter or hypothyroidism, although uncommon at usual therapeutic doses. Methimazole has possible association with scalp defects.	AAP compatible. Propylthiouracil is preferred drug.
Iodine, iodides	Risk category C. Long-term exposure may produce fetal thyroid enlargement.	Use with caution. May cause rash or suppress infant's thyroid function. Large quantities of iodides are contraindicated.
Thyroid replacement hormones (levothyroxine, liothyronine, liotrix)	Risk category A. Cross placenta only to limited extent.	Small amounts secreted in milk. Observe infant for nervousness and agitation. Infant should have periodic thyroid studies.

Table continued on following page

• • • • • • • • • • •

Drug Use During Pregnancy and Lactation *Continued*

Drug	Use During Pregnancy	Use During Breast-Feeding
Vitamins and Retinoids		
Retinoids (etretinate [Tegison], isotretinoin [Accutane])	Risk category X. Related to vitamin A. Associated with severe fetal malformations (microcephaly, ear abnormalities, cardiac defects, central nervous system abnormalities). Etretinate has a long half-life and may have fetal effects up to 18 months after drug is stopped.	Not recommended.
Vitamin A	Risk category A (X at high doses). Excess intake may lead to abnormalities noted for etretinate and isotretinoin.	Breast milk usually supplies sufficient vitamin A to infant. Mother should not take more than 5,000 units per day.
Vitamin B$_6$ (pyridoxine)	Risk category A. Large doses could produce pyridoxine deficiency in infant.	AAP compatible, but a maximum of 10 mg/day should be prescribed, and only for women having deficiencies.
Vitamin D	Risk category C (D at high doses). Excess intake associated with malformations, including aortic stenosis, facial abnormalities, and mental retardation.	AAP compatible. Should be supplemented with caution. High doses could cause high infant calcium levels.
Miscellaneous Drugs		
Nicotine gum; nicotine transdermal	Nicotine gum: category X; nicotine transdermal: category D	Nicotine levels from drug may be less than those from smoking, *if* the mother does not smoke at all. Smoking plus use of nicotine-containing drugs could lead to high levels in infant. Observe infant for shock, vomiting, diarrhea, tachycardia, and restlessness.

BIBLIOGRAPHY
• • • • • • • • • •

American Academy of Pediatrics Committee on Drugs. (1994). Transfer of drugs and other chemicals into human milk. *Pediatrics, 93*(1), 137–150.

Andres, R. L. (1999). Social and illicit drug use during pregnancy. In R. K. Creasy & R. Resnik (Eds.), *Maternal-fetal medicine: Principles and practice* (4th ed., pp. 145–164). Philadelphia: Saunders.

Caldwell, J. (1996). Hyperthyroidism during pregnancy: Nursing care issues. *Journal of Obstetric, Gynecologic and Neonatal Nursing, 25*(5), 395–400.

Corbett, J. V., & Kenney, C. (1995a). Anticoagulants during pregnancy. *MCN: American Journal of Maternal/Child Nursing, 20*(1), 56.

Corbett, J. V., & Kenney, C. (1995b). Zidovudine in pregnancy. *MCN: American Journal of Maternal/Child Nursing, 20*(2), 122.

Cunningham, F. G., MacDonald, P. C., Gant, N. F., Leveno, K. J., Gilstrap, L. C., Hankins, G. D. V., et al. (1997). *Williams obstetrics* (20th ed.). Norwalk, CT: Appleton & Lange.

Goldaber, K. G. (1997). Psychotropics. *Seminars in Perinatology, 21*(2), 154–159.

Hale, T. (1996). *Medications and mothers' milk* (1998–1999 ed.). Amarillo, TX: Pharmasoft Medical Publishing.

Hodgson, B., & Kizior, R. (1998). *Nurse's drug handbook*. Philadelphia: Saunders.

Jones, K. L. (1999). Effects of therapeutic, diagnostic, and environmental agents. In R. K. Creasy & R. Resnik (Eds.), *Maternal-fetal medicine: Principles and practice* (4th ed., pp. 132–144). Philadelphia: Saunders.

Malone, F. D., & D'Alton, M. E. (1997). Drugs in pregnancy: Anticonvulsants. *Seminars in Perinatology, 21*(2), pp. 114–123.

Mastrobattista, J. M. (1997). Angiotensin converting enzyme inhibitors in pregnancy. *Seminars in Perinatology, 21*(2), 124–134.

Minkoff, H. L. (1999). Human immunodeficiency virus. In R. K. Creasy & R. Resnik (Eds.), *Maternal-fetal medicine: Principles and practice* (4th ed., pp. 725–735). Philadelphia: Saunders.

Ramin, S. M., Ramin, K. D., & Gilstrap, L. C. (1997). Anticoagulants and thrombolytics during pregnancy. *Seminars in Perinatology, 21*(2), 149–153.

Rebar, R. W. (1999). The breast and the physiology of lactation. In R. K. Creasy & R. Resnik (Eds.), *Maternal-fetal medicine: Principles and practice* (4th ed., pp. 106–121). Philadelphia: Saunders.

Simpkins, S. M., Hench, C. P., & Ghatia, G. (1996). Management of the obstetric patient with tuberculosis. *Journal of Obstetric, Gynecologic and Neonatal Nursing, 25*(4), 305–312.

D

Laboratory Values in Pregnant and Nonpregnant Women and in the Newborn

Laboratory Values in Pregnant and Nonpregnant Women

Value	Nonpregnancy	Pregnancy
Blood volume, total	60–80 ml/kg	Increases 45%
Plasma volume	40–50 ml/kg (average, 4,700 ml total)	Increases 45% by 32 weeks (4,700–5,200 ml total)
Red blood cell mass	20–30 ml/kg	Increases 20%–30% (average total increase of 250–450 ml)
Red blood cell count	3.8–5.1 million/mm^3	Increases 20%–30%, 4.5–6.5 million/mm^3
Hemoglobin	12–16 g/dl	11–12 g/dl (<11 g/dl in late pregnancy suggests anemia)
Hematocrit, packed cell volume	35%–45%	33%–46%
White blood cell count	5,000–10,000/mm^3	5,000–12,000/mm^3; rises during labor and postpartum up to 25,000/mm^3
Platelets	150,000–400,000/mm^3	Slight decrease (values <100,000/mm^3 are considered abnormal); marked increase 3–5 days after birth
Prothrombin time	11–15 sec	Slight decrease
Activated partial thromboplastin time	21–35 sec	Slight decrease
Fibrinogen	200–400 mg/dl	300–600 mg/dl
Glucose, serum Fasting	65–110 mg/dl	Averages 74 ± 2.7 mg/dl
Postprandial	2 hr: 65–139 mg/dl	Screening glucose challenge test: <140 mg/dl 1 hr: <190 mg/dl 2 hr: <165 mg/dl
Creatine, serum	0.83 mg/dl	End of first trimester: 0.73 mg/dl Late pregnancy: 0.50 mg/dl
Creatinine clearance, urine	71–121 ml/min	110–150 ml/min

Data from Creasy, R. K., & Resnik, R. (1999). *Maternal-fetal medicine: Principles and practice* (4th ed.). Philadelphia: Saunders; Cunningham, F. G., MacDonald, P. C., Gant, N. F., Leveno, K. J., Gilstrap, L. C., Hankins, G. D. V., et al. (1997). *Williams obstetrics* (20th ed.). Norwalk, CT: Appleton & Lange; Fischbach, F. (1996). *A manual of laboratory and diagnostic tests* (5th ed.). Philadelphia: Lippincott; Harvey, M. G. (1999). Physiologic changes during pregnancy. In L. K. Mandeville & N. H. Troiano (Eds.), *High-risk and critical care intrapartum nursing*. Philadelphia: Lippincott; and Tietz, N. W. (1995). *Clinical guide to laboratory tests* (3rd ed.). Philadelphia: Saunders.

Laboratory Values in the Newborn

Test, Specimen, and Unit of Measure	Age	Normal Ranges	Test, Specimen, and Unit of Measure	Age	Normal Ranges		
Red blood cell	Cord	3.9–5.5	Lymphoctyes (%)		25–33		
count, whole	1–3 days	4.0–6.6	Monocytes (%)		3–7		
blood (million/	1 wk	3.9–6.3	Eosinophils (%)		1–3		
mm^3)	1 mo	3.0–5.4	Basophils (%)		0–0.75		
Hemoglobin,	1–3 days (cap)	14.5–22.5	Platelet count,	Newborn	84–478		
whole blood	2 mo	9.0–14.0	whole blood	>1 wk	150–400		
(g/dl)			(thousand/				
Hematocrit,	1 day (cap)	48–69	mm^3)				
whole blood	2 days	48–75	Glucose, serum	Cord	45–96		
(%)	3 days	44–72	(mg/dl)	Newborn,	40–60		
	2 mo	28–42		1 day			
White blood	Birth	9.0–30.0		Newborn,	50–90		
cell count,	24 hr	9.4–34.0		>1 day			
whole blood	1 mo	5.0–19.5				**Preterm**	**Full-Term**
(thousand/							
mm^3)			Bilirubin, total	Cord		<2.0	2.0
White blood cell			serum (mg/dl)	0–1 day		<8.0	<6.0
differential				1–2 days		<12.0	<8.0
count, whole				2–5 days		<16.0	<12.0
blood				>5 days		<2.0	0.2–1.0
Myelocytes (%)		0	Bilirubin, direct			0–0.02	
Neutrophils		3–5	(conjugated)				
("bands") (%)			serum (mg/dl)				
Neutrophils		54–62					
("segs") (%)							

Adapted from Behrman, R. E. (Ed.). (1996). *Nelson textbook of pediatrics* (15th ed.). Philadelphia: Saunders.

To conserve space, the following common abbreviations are used.

ABBREVIATIONS

Ab	absorbance
AU	arbitrary unit
CKBB	brain isoenzyme of creatine kinase
CKMB	heart isoenzyme of creatine kinase
d	diem, day, days
F	female
g	gram
hr	hour, hours
Hb	hemoglobin
HbCO	carboxyhemoglobin
IU	International Unit of hormone activity
L	liter
M	male
MCV	mean corpuscular volume
mEq/L	milliequivalents per liter
min	minute, minutes
mm^3	cubic millimeter; equivalent to microliter (μl)
mm Hg	millimeters of mercury
mo	month, months
mol	mole
mOsm	milliosmole
MW	relative molecular weight
N	nitrogen
Pa	pascal
pc	postprandial
RBC	red blood cell(s); erythrocyte(s)
RT	room temperature
s	second, seconds
U	International Unit of enyzme activity
vol	volume
WBC	white blood cell(s)
wk	week, weeks
yr	year, years

SYMBOLS

$>$	greater than
$\geq$	greater than or equal to
$<$	less than
$\leq$	less than or equal to
$\pm$	plus or minus
$\cong$	approximately equal to

ABBREVIATIONS FOR SPECIMENS

S	serum
P	plasma
(H)	heparin
(LiH)	lithium heparin
(E)	EDTA
(C)	citrate
(O)	oxalate
W	whole blood
U	urine
F	feces
CSF	cerebrospinal fluid
AF	amniotic fluid
(NaC)	sodium citrate
(NH_4H)	ammonium heparinate

E

Common Pediatric Laboratory Tests and Normal Values

KEY TO COMMENTS

30°, 37°	temperature of enzymatic analysis (Celsius)
a	colorimetry
b	Ektachem, proprietary analytic system of Johnson & Johnson Clinical Diagnostics, Inc.
c	enzyme-amplified immunoassay
d	values obtained are significantly method dependent
e	nephelometry
f	cation-exchange chromatography
g	values in older males higher than those in older females
h	ion-selective electrode
i	fluorescence polarization
j	enzymatic assay

Prefixes Denoting Decimal Factors

Prefix	Symbol	Factor
mega	M	10^6
kilo	k	10^3
hecto	h	10^2
deka	da	10^1
deci	d	10^{-1}
centi	c	10^{-2}
milli	m	10^{-3}
micro	μ	10^{-6}
nano	n	10^{-9}
pico	p	10^{-12}
femto	f	10^{-15}

Adapted from Behrman, R. E., Kliegman, R. M., & Arvin, A. M. (1996). Nelson textbook of pediatrics (15th ed., pp. 2033–2058). Philadelphia: Saunders.

Common Laboratory Tests and Normal Values

Test	Specimen	Reference Range (Conventional Units)	Factor	Reference Range, International Units (SI)	Comments
Acetaminophen	S, P(H, E)	Therapeutic concentration 10–30 µg/ml; Toxic concentration >200 µg/ml	× 6.62	66–200 µmol/L; >1,300 µmol/L	i z
Activated partial thromboplastin time (APTT)	P(C)	25–35 s; Infant: <90 s		25–35 s; Infant: <90 s	
Adrenocorticotropic hormone (ACTH)	P(H)	Cord blood 130–160 pg/ml; 1–7 d postnatal 100–140 pg/ml; Adult 0800 hr 25–100 pg/ml; 1800 hr <50 pg/ml	× 1	130–160 µg/L; 100–140 µg/L; 25–100 µg/L; <50 µg/L	37° s b
Alanine aminotransferase (ALT, SGPT)	S	0–5 d 6–50 U/L; 1–19 yr 5–45 U/L	× 1	6–50 U/L; 5–45 U/L	
Albumin	P	Premature 1 d 1.8–3.0 g/dl; Full-term <6 d 2.5–3.4 g/dl; <5 yr 3.9–5.0 g/dl; 5–19 yr 4.0–5.3 g/dl	×10	18–30 g/L; 25–34 g/L; 39–50 g/L; 40–53 g/L	
	U	4–16 yr 3.35–15.3 mg/24 hr/1.73 m²			c
Ammonia nitrogen	CSF	10–30 mg/dl		100–300 mg/L	
	S, P(LiH)	Neonate 90–150 µg N/dl; 0–2 wk 79–129 µg N/dl; >1 mo 29–70 µg N/dl; Thereafter 15–45 µg N/dl; 1–90 d 59–202 µg N/dl; 3 mo–3 yr 48–195 µg N/dl	× 0.714	64–107 µmol/L; 56–92 µmol/L; 21–50 µmol/L; 11–32 µmol/L; 42–144 µmol/L; 34–139 µmol/L	j f
	U	500–1,200 mg N/24 hr	× 0.0714	36–86 mmol/d	
Amphetamine	S, P(H, E)	Therapeutic concentration 20–30 ng/ml; Toxic concentration >200 ng/ml	× 7.396	150–220 nmol/L; >1,500 nmol/L	
Antistreptolysin-O titer (ASO titer)	S	≤166 Todd units; 170–330 Todd units in school-age children			
Base excess	W(H)	Neonate (−10)–(−2) mmol/L; Infant (−7)–(−1) mmol/L; Child (−4)–(+2) mmol/L; Thereafter (−3)–(+3) mmol/L		(−10)–(−2) mmol/L; (−7)–(−1) mmol/L; (−4)–(+2) mmol/L; (−3)–(+3) mmol/L	
Bicarbonate	S, P	Arterial 21–28 mmol/L; Venous 22–29 mmol/L		21–28 mmol/L; 22–29 mmol/L	
Bilirubin	S, P				

Bilirubin — Total (S), Factor × 17.10

	Conventional Units Premature	Conventional Units Full-Term	SI Premature	SI Full-Term
Cord blood	<2.0 mg/dl	<2.0 mg/dl	<34 µmol/L	<34 µmol/L
0–1 d	<8.0 mg/dl	<6.0 mg/dl	<137 µmol/L	<103 µmol/L
1–2 d	<12.0 mg/dl	<8.0 mg/dl	<205 µmol/L	<137 µmol/L
2–5 d	<16.0 mg/dl	<12.0 mg/dl	<274 µmol/L	<205 µmol/L
>5 d	<2.0 mg/dl	0.2–1.0 mg/dl	<34 µmol/L	3.4–17.1 µmol/L

Analyte	Specimen	Condition	Conventional Units	Factor	SI Units
Conjugated	U, AF		Negative	×17.10	Negative
		28 wk	<0.075 mg/dl (or Ab450 <0.048)		<1.3 μmol/L (or Ab450 <0.048)
		40 wk	<0.025 mg/dl (or Ab450 <0.02)		<0.43 μmol/L (or Ab450 <0.02)
			0–0.2 mg/dl		0–3.4 μmol/L
Bleeding time (BBT)					
Ivy	S		Normal 2–7 min; Borderline 7–11 min		Normal 2–7 min; Borderline 7–11 min
Simplate (G–D)			2.75–8 min		2.75–8 min
Blood volume	W(H)		M 52–83 ml/kg; F 50–75 ml/kg	×0.001	M 0.052–0.083 L/kg; F 0.050–0.075 L/kg
C-reactive protein [c]	S	Cord blood	52–1,330 ng/ml	×1	52–1,330 μg/L
		2–12 yr	67–1,800 ng/ml		67–1,800 μg/L
Calcium, ionized (Ca)	S, P(H), W(H)	Cord blood	5.0–6.0 mg/dl	×0.25	1.25–1.50 mmol/L
		Neonate 3–24 hr	4.3–5.1 mg/dl		1.07–1.27 mmol/L
		24–48 hr	4.0–4.7 mg/dl		1.00–1.17 mmol/L
		Thereafter	4.8–4.92 mg/dl, or	×0.25	1.12–1.23 mmol/L
			2.24–2.46 mEq/L	×0.5	1.12–1.23 mmol/L
Calcium, total	S	Cord blood	9.0–11.5 mg/dl	×0.25	2.25–2.88 mmol/L
		Neonate 3–24 hr	9.0–10.6 mg/dl		2.3–2.65 mmol/L
		24–48 hr	7.0–12.0 mg/dl		1.75–3.0 mmol/L
		4–7 d	9.0–10.9 mg/dl		2.25–2.73 mmol/L
		Child	8.8–10.8 mg/dl		2.2–2.70 mmol/L
		Thereafter	8.4–10.2 mg/dl		2.1–2.55 mmol/L
	U	Ca in diet		×0.025	
		Ca-free	5–40 mg/24 hr		0.13–1.0 mmol/24 hr
		Low to average	50–150 mg/24 hr		1.25–3.8 mmol/24 hr
Carbon dioxide	W(H)	Neonate	27–40 mm Hg	×0.1333	3.6–5.3 kPa
		Infant	27–41 mm Hg		3.6–5.5 kPa
Partial pressure (Pco₂)		Thereafter M	35–48 mm Hg		4.7–6.4 kPa
		F	32–45 mm Hg		4.3–6.0 kPa
Total (tco₂)	S, P(H)	Cord blood	14–22 mmol/L	×1	14–22 mmol/L
		Premature	14–27 mmol/L		14–27 mmol/L
		Neonate	13–22 mmol/L		13–22 mmol/L
		Infant	20–28 mmol/L		20–28 mmol/L
		Child	20–28 mmol/L		20–28 mmol/L
		Thereafter	23–30 mmol/L		23–30 mmol/L
Carbon monoxide	W(E)	Nonsmokers	<2% HbCO	×0.01	HbCO fraction <0.02
		Smokers	<10%		<0.10
		Lethal	>50%		>0.5

Table continued on following page

Common Laboratory Tests and Normal Values *Continued*

Test	Specimen	Reference Range (Conventional Units)	Factor	Reference Range, International Units (SI)	Comments
Cerebrospinal fluid					
Pressure	CSF			70–180 mm H$_2$O	
Volume	CSF	Child 60–100 ml; Adult 100–160 ml	× 0.001	0.06–0.10 L; 0.1–0.16 L	
Chloral hydrate	S	As trichloroethanol; Therapeutic concentration 2–12 µg/ml; Toxic concentration >20 µg/ml	× 6.694	13–80 µmol/L; >134 µmol/L	j
Chloride	S, P(H)	Cord blood 96–104 mmol/L; Neonate 97–110 mmol/L; Thereafter 98–106 mmol/L	× 1	96–104 mmol/L; 97–110 mmol/L; 98–106 mmol/L	
	CSF	118–132 mmol/L	× 1	118–132 mmol/L	
	U	Infant 2–10 mmol/24 hr; Child 15–40 mmol/24 hr; Thereafter 110–250 mmol/24 hr (varies greatly with Cl intake)	× 1	2–10 mmol/24 hr; 15–40 mmol/24 hr; 110–250 mmol/24 hr	
	Sweat	Normal <40 mmol/L; Borderline 45–60 mmol/L; Cystic fibrosis >60 mmol/L	× 1	<40 mmol/L; 45–60 mmol/L; >60 mmol/L	
Cholesterol, total	S	1–3 yr 45–182 mg/dl; 4–6 yr 109–189 mg/dl	× 0.0259	1.15–4.70 mmol/L; 2.80–4.80 mmol/L	
	S		× 0.0259		
Clotting time, Lee-White, 37°C	W	Glass tubes 5–8 min (5–15 min at RT); Silicone tubes About 30 min prolonged		Glass tubes 5–8 min (5–15 min at RT); Silicone tubes About 30 min prolonged	
Creatine kinase	S	Cord blood 70–380 U/L; 5–8 hr 214–1,175 U/L; 24–33 hr 130–1,200 U/L; 72–100 hr 87–725 U/L; Adult 5–130 U/L	× 1	70–380 U/L; 214–1,175 U/L; 130–1,200 U/L; 87–725 U/L; 5–130 U/L	
Creatine kinase isoenzymes	S	CKMB: Cord blood 0.3–3.1%; 5–8 hr 1.7–7.9%; 24–33 hr 1.8–5.0%; 72–100 hr 1.4–5.4%; Adult 0–2%. CKBB: 0.3–10.5%; 3.6–13.4%; 2.3–8.6%; 5.1–13.3%; 0			30°g
Creatinine, plasma Jaffe, kinetic, or enzymatic	S, P	Cord blood 0.6–1.2 mg/dl; Neonate 0.3–1.0 mg/dl; Infant 0.2–0.4 mg/dl; Child 0.3–0.7 mg/dl; Adolescent 0.5–1.0 mg/dl; Adult M 0.6–1.2 mg/dl, F 0.5–1.1 mg/dl	× 88.4	53–106 µmol/L; 27–88 µmol/L; 18–35 µmol/L; 27–62 µmol/L; 44–88 µmol/L; M 53–106 µmol/L, F 44–97 µmol/L	

Test	Specimen	Condition	Conventional value	Factor	SI value	Notes
Jaffe, manual	S, P		0.8–1.5 mg/dl	× 88.4	70–133 µmol/L	
	AF	After 37 wk gestation	>2.0 mg/dl	× 88.4	>180 µmol/L	d b
Creatinine, urinary	U	Premature	8.1–15.0 mg/kg/24 hr	× 8.84	72–133 µmol/kg/24 hr	
		Full-term	10.4–19.7 mg/kg/24 hr		92–174 µmol/kg/24 hr	
		1.5–7 yr	10–15 mg/kg/24 hr		88–133 µmol/kg/24 hr	
		7–15 yr	5.2–41 mg/kg/24 hr		46–362 µmol/kg/24 hr	
Creatinine clearance (endogenous)	S, P, U	Neonate	40–65 ml/min/1.73 m^2			
		<40 yr				
		M	97–137 ml/min/1.73 m^2			
		F	88–128 ml/min/1.73 m^2			
		Decreases	~6.5 ml/min/decade			
Diazepam	S, P(H, E) at trough	Therapeutic concentration	100–1,000 ng/ml	× 3.512	350–3,500 nmol/L	
		Toxic concentration	>5,000 ng/ml		>17,500 nmol/L	
Digoxin	S, P(H, E) (12-hr post)	Therapeutic concentration		× 1.281		i c
		CHF	0.8–1.5 ng/ml		1.0–1.9 nmol/L	
		Arrhythmias	1.5–2.0 ng/ml		1.9–2.6 nmol/L	
		Toxic concentration				
		Child	>2.5 ng/ml		>3.2 nmol/L	
		Adult	>3.0 ng/ml		>3.8 nmol/L	
Eosinophil count	W(E, H) capillary		50–350 cells/mm^3 (µl)	× 10^6	50–350 × 10^6 cells/L	

Test	Specimen	Condition	Millions of cells/mm^3 (µl)	Factor	× 10^{12} cells/L
Erythrocyte count (RBC count)	W(E)	Cord blood	3.9–5.5	× 1	3.9–5.5
		1–3 d (capillary)	4.0–6.6		4.0–6.6
		1 wk	3.9–6.3		3.9–6.3
		2 wk	3.6–6.2		3.6–6.2
		1 mo	3.0–5.4		3.0–5.4
		2 mo	2.7–4.9		2.7–4.9
		3–6 mo	3.1–4.5		3.1–4.5
		0.5–2 yr	3.7–5.3		3.7–5.3
		2–6 yr	3.9–5.3		3.9–5.3
		6–12 yr	4.0–5.2		4.0–5.2
		12–18 yr			
		M	4.5–5.3		4.5–5.3
		F	4.1–5.1		4.1–5.1
		18–49 yr			
		M	4.5–5.9		4.5–5.9
		F	4.0–5.2		4.0–5.2

Table continued on following page

Common Laboratory Tests and Normal Values *Continued*

Test	Specimen	Reference Range (Conventional Units)		Factor	Reference Range, International Units (SI)		Comments
Erythrocyte sedimentation rate (ESR)	W(E)						
Westergren, modified		Child	0–10 mm/hr		0–10 mm/hr		
		Adult					
		M <50 yr	0–15 mm/hr		0–15 mm/hr		
		F <50 yr	0–20 mm/hr		0–20 mm/hr		
Wintrobe		Child	0–13 mm/hr		0–13 mm/hr		
		Adult					
		M	0–9 mm/hr		0–9 mm/hr		
		F	0–20 mm/hr		0–20 mm/hr		
			41–54%	× 1	41–54 AU		
Fat, fecal	F (72 hr)	Infant, breast-fed	<1 g/24 hr		<1 g/24 hr		
		0–6 yr	<2 g/24 hr		<2 g/24 hr		
		Adult					
		Normal diet	<7 g/24 hr		<7 g/24 hr		
		Fat-free diet	<4 g/24 hr		<4 g/24 hr		
		Coefficient of Fat Absorption (%)		× 0.01	*Absorbed Fraction*		
		Infant					
		Breast-fed	>93		>0.93		
		Formula-fed	>83		>0.83		
		>1 yr	≥95		≥0.95		
α-Fetoprotein (AFP)	S maternal	*Pregnancy (wk)*	*Median*	× 1		*Median*	
		15	34 ng/ml			34 μg/L	
		16	38 ng/ml			38 μg/L	
		17	44 ng/ml			44 μg/L	
		18	49 ng/ml			49 μg/L	
		19	56.5 ng/ml			56.5 μg/L	
		20	66 ng/ml			66 μg/L	
	AF		*Mean*				
		15	13.5 ± 3.42 μg/ml				
		16	11.7 ± 3.38 μg/ml				
		17	10.3 ± 3.03 μg/ml				
		18	9.5 ± 3.22 μg/ml				
		19	7.1 ± 2.86 μg/ml				
		20	5.0 ± 2.45 μg/ml				
Fibrinogen	P(NaCl)	Neonate	125–300 mg/dl	× 0.01	1.25–3.00 g/L		
		Adult	200–400 mg/dl		2.00–4.00 g/L		
Galactose	S	Neonate	0–20 mg/dl	× 0.0555	0–1.11 mmol/L		
	P	5 mo–17 yr	0.0–0.5 mg/dl		0.0–0.03 mmol/L		
	U	Neonate	≤60 mg/dl	× 0.0555	≤3.33 mmol/L		
		Thereafter	14 mg/24 hr	× 0.00555	<0.08 mmol/24 hr		j

Test	Specimen		Normal (Conventional)	Diabetic (Conventional)	Factor	Normal (SI)	Diabetic (SI)
Glucose	S	Cord blood	45–96 mg/dl		× 0.0555	2.5–5.3 mmol/L	
		Neonate 1 d	40–60 mg/dl			2.2–3.3 mmol/L	
		>1 d	50–90 mg/dl			2.8–5.0 mmol/L	
		Child	60–100 mg/dl			3.3–5.5 mmol/L	
		Adult	70–105 mg/dl			3.9–5.8 mmol/L	
		Adult	65–95 mg/dl			3.6–5.3 mmol/L	
	W(H)		40–70 mg/dl			2.2–3.9 mmol/L	
Quantitative, enzymatic	CSF						
Qualitative	U		<0.5 g/24 hr		× 5.55	<2.8 mmol/24 hr	
Glucose, 2 hr pc	U		Negative			Negative	
	S		<120 mg/dl		× 0.0555	<6.7 mmol/L	
		(For diabetes, see Glucose tolerance test, oral)					

Glucose tolerance test (GTT), oral	S		Normal	Diabetic	Factor	Normal	Diabetic
Adult dose: 75 g		Fasting	70–105 mg/dl	>115 mg/dl	× 0.0555	3.9–5.8 mmol/L	>6.4 mmol/L
Child dose: 1.75 g/kg of ideal weight up to maximum of 75 g		60 min	120–170 mg/dl	≥200 mg/dl		6.7–9.4 mmol/L	≥11 mmol/L
		90 min	100–140 mg/dl	≥200 mg/dl		5.6–7.8 mmol/L	≥11 mmol/L
		120 min	70–120 mg/dl	≥140 mg/dl		3.9–6.7 mmol/L	≥7.8 mmol/L

Growth hormone (hGH, somatotropin)	S, P(E, H)			Factor	
		Neonate 1 d	5–23 ng/ml	× 1	5–53 µg/L
		1 wk	5–27 ng/ml		5–27 µg/L
		1–12 mo	2–10 ng/ml		2–10 µg/L
	Fasting, at rest	Child	<0.7–6 ng/ml		<0.7–6 µg/L
		Adult	<0.7–6 ng/ml		<0.7–6 µg/L

Hematocrit (HCT, Hct)	W(E)		Percent Packed Red Cells (Vol. Red Cells/Vol. Whole Blood Cells × 100)	Factor	Volume Fraction (Vol. Red Cells/Vol. Whole Blood)
Calculated from MCV and RBC (electronic displacement or laser)		1 d (capillary)	48–69%	× 0.01	0.48–0.69
		2 d	48–75%		0.48–0.75
		3 d	44–72%		0.44–0.72
		2 mo	28–42%		0.28–0.42
		6–12 yr	35–45%		0.35–0.45
		12–18 yr M	37–49%		0.37–0.49
		F	36–46%		0.36–0.46
		18–49 yr M	41–53%		0.41–0.53
		F	36–46%		0.36–0.46

Table continued on following page

Common Laboratory Tests and Normal Values *Continued*

Test	Specimen	Reference Range (Conventional Units)	Factor	Reference Range, International Units (SI)	Comments
Hemoglobin (Hb)	W(E)	1–3 d (capillary)	× 0.155	2.25–3.49 mmol/L	MW Hb = 64,500
		2 mo		1.40–2.17 mmol/L	
		6–12 yr		1.78–2.40 mmol/L	
		12–18 yr			
		M		2.02–2.48 mmol/L	
		F		1.86–2.48 mmol/L	
		18–49 yr			
		M		2.09–2.27 mmol/L	
		F		1.86–2.48 mmol/L	
	P(H)	<10 mg/dl	× 0.155	<1.55 µmol/L	
		<3 mg/dl with butterfly set-up and 18G needle		<0.47 µmol/L with butterfly set-up and 18G needle	
Hemoglobin A	U	Negative		Negative	
Hemoglobin F	W(E, C, H)				
Alkali denaturation	W(E)	>95%	× 0.01	Fraction of hemoglobin >0.95	
		1 d	× 0.01	0.62–0.92 mass fraction	
		5 d		0.65–0.88 mass fraction	
		3 wk		0.55–0.85 mass fraction	
		6–9 wk		0.31–0.75 mass fraction	
		3–4 mo		<0.02–0.59 mass fraction	
		6 mo		<0.02–0.09 mass fraction	
		Adult		<0.02 mass fraction	
Immunoglobulin A (IgA)	S	62–92% HbF			e
		65–88% HbF			
		55–85% HbF			
		31–75% HbF			
		<2–59% HbF			
		<2–9% HbF			
		<2% HbF			
		Cord blood	× 10	14–36 mg/L	
		1–3 mo		13–530 mg/L	
		4–6 mo		44–840 mg/L	
		7 mo–1 yr		110–1,060 mg/L	
		2–5 yr		140–1,590 mg/L	
		6–10 yr		330–2,360 mg/L	
		Adult		700–3,120 mg/L	
Immunoglobulin D (IgD)	S	Neonate	× 10	None detected	
		Thereafter		0–80 mg/L	
Immunoglobulin E (IgE)	S	M	× 1	0–230 kIU/L	
		F		0–170 kIU/L	
Immunoglobulin G (IgG)	S	Cord blood	× 0.01	6.36–16.06 g/L	e
		1 mo		2.51–9.06 g/L	
		2–4 mo		1.76–6.01 g/L	
		5–12 mo		1.72–10.69 g/L	
		1–5 yr		3.45–12.36 g/L	
		6–10 yr		6.08–15.72 g/L	
		Adult		6.39–13.49 g/L	
Immunoglobulin M (IgM)	S	Cord blood	× 10	63–250 mg/L	e
		1–4 mo		170–1,050 mg/L	
		5–9 mo		300–1,260 mg/L	
		10 mo–1 yr		410–1,730 mg/L	
		2–8 yr		430–2,070 mg/L	
		9–10 yr		520–2,420 mg/L	
		Adult		560–3,520 mg/L	

Additional conventional unit values (IgA / IgG / IgM rows):
Immunoglobulin A: Cord blood 1.4–3.6 mg/dl; 1–3 mo 1.3–53 mg/dl; 4–6 mo 4.4–84 mg/dl; 7 mo–1 yr 11–106 mg/dl; 2–5 yr 14–159 mg/dl; 6–10 yr 33–236 mg/dl; Adult 70–312 mg/dl.
Immunoglobulin D: Neonate None detected; Thereafter 0–8 mg/dl.
Immunoglobulin E: M 0–230 IU/ml; F 0–170 IU/ml.
Immunoglobulin G: Cord blood 636–1,606 mg/dl; 1 mo 251–906 mg/dl; 2–4 mo 176–601 mg/dl; 5–12 mo 172–1,069 mg/dl; 1–5 yr 345–1,236 mg/dl; 6–10 yr 608–1,572 mg/dl; Adult 639–1,349 mg/dl.
Immunoglobulin M: Cord blood 6.3–25 mg/dl; 1–4 mo 17–105 mg/dl; 5–9 mo 33–126 mg/dl; 10 mo–1 yr 41–173 mg/dl; 2–8 yr 43–207 mg/dl; 9–10 yr 52–242 mg/dl; Adult 56–352 mg/dl.

Analyte	Specimen	Reference population	Conventional — M (mg/dl)	Conventional — F (mg/dl)	Conversion factor	SI — M (mmol/L)	SI — F (mmol/L)	Notes
Iron	S	Neonate	100–250 µg/dl		× 0.179	17.90–44.75 µmol/L		
		Infant	40–100 µg/dl			7.16–17.90 µmol/L		
		Child	50–120 µg/dl			8.95–21.48 µmol/L		
		Thereafter M	50–160 µg/dl			8.95–28.64 µmol/L		
		F	40–150 µg/dl			7.16–26.85 µmol/L		
		Intoxicated child	280–2,550 µg/dl			50.12–456.5 µmol/L		
		Fatally poisoned child	>1,800 µg/dl			>322.2 µmol/L		
Iron-binding capacity, total (TIBC)	S	Infant	100–400 µg/dl		× 0.179	17.90–71.60 µmol/L		
		Thereafter	250–400 µg/dl			44.75–71.60 µmol/L		
17-Ketogenic steroids (17-KGS)	U	0–1 yr	<1.0 mg/24 hr		× 3.467	<3.5 µmol/24 hr		Conversion based on dehydroepi-androsterone, MW 288
		1–10 yr	<5 mg/24 hr			<17 µmol/24 hr		
		11–14 yr	<12 mg/24 hr			<42 µmol/24 hr		
		Thereafter M	5–23 mg/24 hr			17–80 µmol/24 hr		
		F	3–15 mg/24 hr			10–52 µmol/24 hr		
Ketone bodies								
Qualitative	S		Negative			Negative		
Qualitative	U		Negative			Negative		
Quantitative	S		0.5–3.0 mg/dl		× 10	5–30 mg/L		
LDL-cholesterol (LDLC)	S, P(E)	Cord blood	10–50	10–50	× 0.0259	0.26–1.30	0.26–1.30	
		1–9 yr	60–140	60–150		1.55–3.63	1.55–3.89	
		10–19 yr	50–170	50–170		1.30–4.40	1.30–4.40	
		20–29 yr	60–175	60–160		1.55–4.53	1.55–4.14	
		30–39 yr	80–190	70–170		2.07–4.92	1.81–4.40	
		40–49 yr	90–205	80–190		2.33–5.31	2.07–4.92	
		Recommended (desirable) range for adults	<130 mg/dl			1.68–4.53 mmol/L		
Lead	W(H)	Child	<10 µg/dl		× 0.0483	<0.48 µmol/L		
		Adult	<40 µg/dl			<1.93 µmol/L		
		Acceptable for industrial exposure	<60 µg/dl			<2.90 µmol/L		
		Toxic	≥100 µg/dl			≥4.83 µmol/L		
	U (24-hr)		<80 µg/dl		× 0.00483	<0.39 µmol/L		
Leukocyte count (WBC)	W(E)		× 1,000 cells/mm³ (µl)			× 10⁹ cells/L		
		Birth	9.0–30.0			9.0–30.0		
		24 hr	9.4–34.0			9.4–34.0		
		1 mo	5.0–19.5			5.0–19.5		
		1–3 yr	6.0–17.5			6.0–17.5		
		4–7 yr	5.5–15.5			5.5–15.5		
		8–13 yr	4.5–13.5			4.5–13.5		
		Adult	4.5–11.0			4.5–11.0		

Table continued on following page

Common Laboratory Tests and Normal Values *Continued*

Test	Specimen	Reference Range (Conventional Units)	Factor	Reference Range, International Units (SI)	Comments
Leukocyte differential	W(E)				
Myelocytes		0	× 0.01	0	
Neutrophils—"bands"		3–5%		0.03–0.05 no. fraction	
Neutrophils—"segs"		54–62%		0.54–0.62 no. fraction	
Lymphocytes		25–33%		0.25–0.33 no. fraction	
Monocytes		3–7%		0.03–0.07 no. fraction	
Eosinophils		1–3%		0.01–0.03 no. fraction	
Basophils		0–0.75%		0–0.0075 no. fraction	
Mean corpuscular hemoglobin concentration (MCHC)	W(E)		× 0.0155		
		Birth — 31–37 pg/cell		0.48–0.57 fmol/cell	
		1–3 d (capillary) — 31–37 pg/cell		0.48–0.57 fmol/cell	
		1 wk–1 mo — 28–40 pg/cell		0.43–0.62 fmol/cell	
		2 mo — 26–34 pg/cell		0.40–0.53 fmol/cell	
		3–6 mo — 25–35 pg/cell		0.39–0.54 fmol/cell	
		0.5–2 yr — 23–31 pg/cell		0.36–0.48 fmol/cell	
		2–6 yr — 24–30 pg/cell		0.37–0.47 fmol/cell	
		6–12 yr — 25–33 pg/cell		0.39–0.51 fmol/cell	
		12–18 yr — 25–35 pg/cell		0.39–0.54 fmol/cell	
		18–49 yr — 26–34 pg/cell		0.40–0.53 fmol/cell	
Mean corpuscular hemoglobin	W(E)	*Percentage Hb/cell or g Hb/dl RBC*	× 0.155	*mmol Hb/L RBC*	
		Birth — 30–36		4.65–5.58	
		1–2 wk — 29–37		4.50–5.74	
		1–2 mo — 28–38		4.34–5.89	
		3 mo–2 yr — 29–37		4.50–5.74	
		2–18 yr — 30–36		4.65–5.58	
		>18 yr — 31–37		4.81–5.74	
		31–37		4.81–5.74	
Mean corpuscular volume (MCV)	W(E)		× 1		
		Birth — 95–121 μm³		95–121 fl	
		1–3 d (capillary) — 70–86 μm³		70–86 fl	
		0.5–2 yr — 77–95 μm³		77–95 fl	
		6–12 yr			
		12–18 yr			
		M — 78–98 μm³		78–98 fl	
		F — 78–102 μm³		78–102 fl	
		18–49 yr			
		M — 80–100 μm³		80–100 fl	
		F — 80–100 μm³		80–100 fl	
Occult blood	F	Negative (>2 ml blood/24 hr in ~ 100–200 g stool)		Negative	
	U	Negative		Negative	
Osmolality	S	Child and adult: 275–295 mOsm/kg H_2O		275–295 mOsm/kg H_2O	
	U	50–1,400 mOsm/kg H_2O, depending on fluid intake. After 12 hr of fluid restriction, normal range is >850 mOsm/kg H_2O			
	U (24-hr)	300–900 mOsm/kg H_2O			
Oxygen, partial pressure of (PO_2)	W(H), arterial		× 0.133		
		Birth — 8–24 mm Hg		1.1–3.2 kPa	
		5–10 min — 33–75 mm Hg		4.4–10.0 kPa	
		30 min — 31–85 mm Hg		4.1–11.3 kPa	
		>1 hr — 55–80 mm Hg		7.3–10.6 kPa	
		1 d — 54–95 mm Hg		7.2–12.6 kPa	
		Thereafter (decreases with age) — 83–108 mm Hg		11–14.4 kPa	

Determination	Specimen	Category	Conventional	Conversion factor	SI Units	Comments
Oxygen saturation	W(H), arterial		85–90%	× 0.01	0.85–0.90 Saturated fraction	
	W(NaCl)		95–99%		0.95–0.99 Saturated fraction	
Partial thromboplastin time (PTT)						
Nonactivated			60–85 s (Platelin)		60–85 s	
Activated			25–35 s (differs with method)		25–35 s	
Phenobarbital	S, P(H, E) at trough	Therapeutic concentration	15–40 µg/ml	× 4.306	65–170 µmol/L	i c
		Toxic concentration				
		Slowness, ataxia, nystagmus	35–80 µg/ml		150–345 µmol/L	
		Coma				
		With reflexes	65–117 µg/ml		280–504 µmol/L	
		Without reflexes	>100 µg/ml		>430 µmol/L	
Phenylalanine	S	Premature	2.0–7.5 mg/dl	× 60.54	120–450 µmol/L	
		Neonate	1.2–3.4 mg/dl		70–210 µmol/L	
		Thereafter	0.8–1.8 mg/dl		50–110 µmol/L	
	U	10 d–2 wk	1–2 mg/24 hr	× 6.054	6–12 µmol/24 hr	
		3–12 yr	4–18 mg/24 hr		24–110 µmol/24 hr	
		Thereafter	Trace–17 mg/24 hr		Trace–103 µmol/24 hr	
Plasma volume	P(H)	M	25–43 ml/kg	× 0.001	M 0.025–0.043 L/kg	
		F	28–45 ml/kg		F 0.028–0.045 L/kg	
Platelet count (thrombocyte count)	W(E)		Neonate 84–478 × 10³/mm³ (µl) (after 1 wk same as adult)	× 10⁶	84–478 × 10⁹/L	
			Adult 150–400 × 10³/mm³ (µl)		150–400 × 10⁹/L	
Potassium	S	<2 mo	3.0–7.0 mmol/L	× 1	3.0–7.0 mmol/L	h
		2–12 mo	3.5–6.0 mmol/L		3.5–6.0 mmol/L	Increased by hemolysis
		>12 mo	3.5–5.0 mmol/L		3.5–6.0 mmol/L	Serum values systematically higher than plasma values
	P(H)				3.5–4.5 mmol/L	
	U (24-hr)		2.5–125 mmol/L (varies with diet)		2.5–125 mmol/L (varies with diet)	
Protein						
Total	S	Premature	4.3–7.6 g/dl	× 10	43–76 g/L	
		Neonate	4.6–7.4 g/dl		46–74 g/L	
		1–7 yr	6.1–7.9 g/dl		61–79 g/L	
		8–12 yr	6.4–8.1 g/dl		64–81 g/L	
		13–19 yr	6.6–8.2 g/dl		66–82 g/L	
Total urinary	U (24-hr)		1–14 mg/dl	× 10	10–140 mg/L	
			50–80 mg/24 hr (at rest)		50–80 mg/24 hr (at rest)	
			<250 mg/24 hr after intense exercise		<250 mg/24 hr after intense exercise	
Total protein (column)	CSF	Lumbar	8–32 mg/dl	× 10	80–320 mg/L	

Table continued on following page

Common Laboratory Tests and Normal Values *Continued*

Test	Specimen	Reference Range (Conventional Units)	Factor	Reference Range, International Units (SI)	Comments
Prothrombin time (PT) One-stage (quick)	W(NaC)	In general, 11–15 s (varies with type of thromboplastin) Neonate: prolonged by 2–3 s		11–15 s Neonate: prolonged by 2–3 s	
Two-stage modified (Ware and Seegers)	W(NaC)	18–22 s		18–22 s	
RBC count. See Erythrocyte count					
Red cell volume	W(H)	M 20–36 ml/kg F 19–31 ml/kg	× 0.001	0.020–0.036 L/kg 0.019–0.031 L/kg	
Reticulocyte count	W(E, H, O)	Adults 0.5–1.5% of erythrocytes, or 25,000–75,000/mm³ (μl)	× 0.01 × 10⁶	0.005–0.015 number fraction 25,000–75,000 × 10⁶/L	
	W (capillary)	1 d 0.4–6.0%	× 0.01	0.004–0.060 number fraction	
		7 d <0.1–1.3%		<0.001–0.013 number fraction	
		1–4 wk <1.0–1.2%		<0.001–0.012 number fraction	
		5–6 wk <0.1–2.4%		<0.001–0.024 number fraction	
		7–8 wk 0.1–2.9%		0.001–0.029 number fraction	
		9–10 wk <0.1–2.6%		<0.001–0.026 number fraction	
		11–12 wk 0.1–1.3%		0.001–0.013 number fraction	
Salicylate	S, P(H, E) at trough	Therapeutic concentration 15–30 mg/dl Toxic concentration >30 mg/dl	× 0.0724	1.1–2.2 mmol/L >2.2 mmol/L	
Sedimentation rate. See Erythrocyte sedimentation rate					
Sickle cell tests Sodium metabisulfite Dithionite test	W(E, H, O) W(E, H, O)	Negative Negative			
Sodium	S, P(LiH, NH₄H)	Neonate 134–146 mmol/L Infant 139–146 mmol/L Child 138–145 mmol/L Thereafter 136–146 mmol/L	× 1	134–146 mmol/L 139–146 mmol/L 138–146 mmol/L 136–148 mmol/L	
	U (24-hr)	(depending on diet) 40–220 mmol		40–220 mmol	
	Sweat	Normal <40 mmol/L Indeterminate 45–60 mmol/L Cystic fibrosis >60 mmol/L	× 1	<40 mmol/L 45–60 mmol/L >60 mmol/L	
Specific gravity	U	Adult 1.002–1.030 After 12-hr fluid restriction >1.025		1.002–1.030 >1.025	
	U (24-hr)	1.015–1.025		1.025	
Theophylline	S, P(H, E)	Therapeutic concentration, bronchodilator 10–20 μg/ml	× 5.550	56–110 μmol/L	i j
		Premature apnea 5–10 μg/ml Toxic concentration >20 μg/ml		28–56 μmol/L >110 μmol/L	
Thrombin time	W(NaC)	Control time ±2 s when control is 9–13 s		Control time ±2 s when control is 9–13 s	

Test	Specimen		Conventional Units	Factor	SI Units
Thyroxine Total	S	Full-term infant		× 12.8700	
		1–3 d	8.2–19.9 µg/dl		106–256 nmol/L
		1 wk	6.0–15.9 µg/dl		77–205 nmol/L
		1–12 mo	6.1–14.9 µg/dl		79–192 nmol/L
		Prepubertal child			
		1–3 yr	6.8–13.5 µg/dl		88–174 nmol/L
		3–10 yr	5.5–12.8 µg/dl		71–165 nmol/L
		Pubertal children and adults	4.2–13.0 µg/dl		54–167 nmol/L
Free	S	Neonate		× 12.87	
		3 d	2.0–4.9 ng/dl		26–631 pmol/L
		Infant			
		1–12 mo	0.9–2.6 ng/dl		12–33 pmol/L
		Prepubertal child	0.8–2.2 ng/dl		10–28 pmol/L
		Pubertal children and adults	0.8–2.3 ng/dl		10–30 pmol/L
Thyroxine, total	W	Neonatal screen (filter paper)	6.2–2.2 µg/dl		

Tourniquet test

Conventional:
<5–10 petechiae in 2.5-cm circle on forearm (halfway between systolic and diastolic); pressure maintained for 5 min
0–8 petechiae in 6-cm circle (50 mm Hg for 15 min)
10–20 petechiae in 5-cm circle (80 mm Hg)

SI:
<5–10 petechiae in 2.5-cm circle on forearm (halfway between systolic and diastolic); pressure maintained for 5 min
0–8 petechiae in 6-cm circle (50 mm Hg for 15 min)
10–20 petechiae in 5-cm circle (80 mm Hg)

Triglycerides — S after ≥12-hr fast — × 0.01

	M (mg/dl)	F (mg/dl)		M (g/L)	F (g/L)
Cord blood	10–98	10–98		0.10–0.98	0.10–0.98
0–5 yr	30–86	32–99		0.30–0.86	0.32–0.99
6–11 yr	31–108	35–114		0.31–1.08	0.35–1.14
12–15 yr	36–138	41–138		0.36–1.38	0.41–1.38
16–19 yr	40–163	40–128		0.40–1.63	0.40–1.28
20–29 yr	44–185	40–128		0.44–1.85	0.40–1.28

Adults: Recommended (desirable) levels

	M	F		M	F
	40–160 mg/dl			0.40–1.60 g/L	
	35–135 mg/dl			0.35–1.35 g/L	

Urea nitrogen — S, P — × 0.357

	Conventional	SI
Cord blood	21–40 mg/dl	7.5–14.3 mmol urea/L
Premature (1 wk)	3–25 mg/dl	1.1–9 mmol urea/L
Neonate	3–12 mg/dl	1.1–4.3 mmol urea/L
Infant/child	5–18 mg/dl	1.8–6.4 mmol urea/L
Thereafter	7–18 mg/dl	2.5–6.4 mmol urea/L

Urine, volume — U (24-hr) — × 0.001

	Conventional	SI
Neonate	50–300 ml/24 hr	0.050–0.300 L/24 hr
Infant	350–550 ml/24 hr	0.350–0.550 L/24 hr
Child	500–1,000 ml/24 hr	0.500–1.000 L/24 hr
Adolescent	700–1,400 ml/24 hr	0.700–1.400 L/24 hr
Thereafter		
M	800–1,800 ml/24 hr	0.800–1.800 L/24 hr
F	600–1,600 ml/24 hr	0.600–1.600 L/24 hr
	(varies with intake and other factors)	

WBC. See Leukocytes.

Therapeutic and Toxic Ranges (Peak and Trough) of Antibiotics

Antibiotic	Specimen	Reference Range				Factor	Reference Range (SI)				Comments
		Peak		Trough			SI Peak		SI Trough		
		Therapeutic (µg/ml)	Toxic (µg/ml)	Therapeutic (µg/ml)	Toxic (µg/ml)		Therapeutic (µmol/ml)	Toxic (µmol/ml)	Therapeutic (µmol/ml)	Toxic (µmol/ml)	
Amikacin	S	20–25	>30	1–4	>8	×1.708	34–43	>51	1.7–6.8	>14	i c
Chloramphenicol	S	10–20	>25			×3.095	31–62	>77			c
Gentamicin	S	6–10	>12	0.5–2.0	>2.0	×2.064	12–21	>25	1.0–4.1	>4.1	c i
Netilmicin	S	6–10	>12	0.5–2.0	>2	×2.103	13–21	>25	1.1–4.2	>4.2	c i
Tobramycin	S	6–10	>12	0.5–2.0	>2	×2.139	13–21	>26	1.1–4.3	>4.3	c i
Vancomycin	S	30–40	>60	5–10	>20	×0.303	9.1–12.1	>18.2	1.5–3.0	>6.1	c i

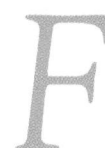

Childhood Immunizations

Recommended Childhood Immunization Schedule, United States, January–December 1999

Vaccines[1] are listed under routinely recommended ages. Bars *indicate range of recommended ages for immunization. Any dose not given at the recommended age should be given as a "catch-up" immunization at any subsequent visit when indicated and feasible.* Ovals *indicate vaccines to be given if previously recommended doses were missed or given earlier than the recommended minimum age.*

Age ▶ Vaccine ▼	Birth	1 mo	2 mo	4 mo	6 mo	12 mo	15 mo	18 mo	4–6 yr	11–12 yr	14–16 yr
Hepatitis B[2]		Hep B									
			Hep B			Hep B				Hep B	
Diphtheria, tetanus, pertussis[3]			DTaP	DTaP	DTaP		DTaP[3]		DTaP	Td	
H. influenzae type b[4]			Hib	Hib	Hib	Hib					
Polio[5]			IPV	IPV		Polio[5]			Polio		
Rotavirus[6]			Rv[6]	Rv[6]	Rv[6]						
Measles, mumps, rubella[7]						MMR			MMR[7]	MMR[7]	
Varicella[8]						Var				Var[8]	

[1] This schedule indicates the recommended ages for routine administration of currently licensed childhood vaccines. Combination vaccines may be used whenever any components of the combination are indicated and its other components are not contraindicated. Providers should consult the manufacturers' package inserts for detailed recommendations.

[2] **Infants born to HBsAg-negative mothers** should receive the 2nd dose of hepatitis B vaccine at least 1 month after the 1st dose. The 3rd dose should be administered at least 4 months after the 1st dose and at least 2 months after the 2nd dose, but not before 6 months of age for infants.
Infants born to HBsAg-positive mothers should receive hepatitis B vaccine and 0.5 ml hepatitis B immune globulin (HBIG) within 12 hours of birth at separate sites. The 2nd dose is recommended at 1–2 months of age and the 3rd dose at 6 months of age.
Infants born to mothers whose HBsAg status is unknown should receive hepatitis B vaccine within 12 hours of birth. Maternal blood should be drawn at the time of delivery to determine the mother's HBsAg status; if the HBsAg test is positive, the infant should receive HBIG as soon as possible (no later than 1 week of age).
All children and adolescents (through 18 years of age) who have not been immunized against hepatitis B may begin the series during any visit. Special efforts should be made to immunize children who were born in or whose parents were born in areas of the world with moderate or high endemicity of HBV infection.

[3] DTaP (diphtheria and tetanus toxoids and acellular pertussis vaccine) is the preferred vaccine for all doses in the immunization series, including completion of the series in children who have received one or more doses of whole-cell DTP vaccine. Whole-cell DTP is an acceptable alternative to DTaP. The 4th dose (DTP or DTaP) may be administered as early as 12 months of age, provided 6 months have elapsed since the 3rd dose and if the child is unlikely to return at age 15–18 months. Td (tetanus and diphtheria toxoids) is recommended at 11–12 years of age if at least 5 years have elapsed since the last dose of DTP, DTaP, or DT. Subsequent routine Td boosters are recommended every 10 years.

[4] Three H. influenzae type b (Hib) conjugate vaccines are licensed for infant use. If PRP-OMP (PedvaxHIB and COMVAX [Merck]) is administered at 2 and 4 months of age, a dose at 6 months is not required. Because clinical studies in infants have demonstrated that using some combination products may induce a lower immune response to the Hib vaccine component, DTaP/Hib combination products should not be used for primary immunization in infants at 2, 4, or 6 months of age, unless FDA-approved for these ages.

[5] Two poliovirus vaccines currently are licensed in the United States: inactivated poliovirus vaccine (IPV) and oral poliovirus vaccine (OPV). The ACIP, AAP, and AAFP now recommend that the first two doses of poliovirus vaccine should be IPV. The ACIP continues to recommend a sequential schedule of two doses of IPV administered at ages 2 and 4 months, followed by two doses of OPV at 12–18 months and 4–6 years. Use of IPV for all doses also is acceptable and is recommended for immunocompromised persons and their household contacts. OPV is no longer recommended for the first two doses of the schedule and is acceptable only for special circumstances such as children of parents who do not accept the recommended number of injections, late initiation of immunization which would require an unacceptable number of injections, and imminent travel to polio-endemic areas. OPV remains the vaccine of choice for mass immunization campaigns to control outbreaks due to wild poliovirus.

[6] Rotavirus (Rv) vaccine is shaded and italicized to indicate: (1) health care providers may require time and resources to incorporate this new vaccine into practice; and (2) the AAFP feels that the decision to use rotavirus vaccine should be made by the parent or guardian in consultation with their physician or other health care provider. The first dose of Rv vaccine should not be administered before 6 weeks of age, and the minimum interval between doses is 3 weeks. The Rv vaccine series should not be initiated at 7 months of age or older, and all doses should be completed by the first birthday.

[7] The 2nd dose of measles, mumps, and rubella vaccine (MMR) is recommended routinely at 4–6 years of age but may be administered during any visit, provided at least 4 weeks have elapsed since receipt of the 1st dose and that both doses are administered beginning at or after 12 months of age. Those who have not previously received the 2nd dose should complete the schedule by the 11- to 12-year-old visit.

[8] Varicella vaccine is recommended at any visit on or after the first birthday for susceptible children, i.e. those who lack a reliable history of chicken pox (as judged by a health care provider) and who have not been immunized. Susceptible persons 13 years of age or older should receive two doses, given at least 4 weeks apart.

Approved by the Advisory Committee on Immunization Practices (ACIP), the American Academy of Pediatrics (AAP), and the American Academy of Family Physicians (AAFP). From American Academy of Pediatrics, Committee on Infectious Diseases (1996). Recommended childhood immunization schedule, United States, July–December 1996. *Pediatrics*, 97, 158–160.

Summary of Rules for Childhood Immunization*

Vaccine	Ages Usually Given; Other Guidelines	If Child Falls Behind—Minimum Intervals	Contraindications (Remember, Mild Illness Is Not a Contraindication)
DTaP (contains acellular pertussis) **DTP** (contains whole-cell pertussis) Give IM	• DTaP is preferred over DTP for all doses in the series. • Give at 2 mo, 4 mo, 6 mo, 15–18 mo, 4–6 yr of age. • May give dose 1 as early as 6 wk of age. • May give dose 4 as early as 12 mo of age if 6 mo has elapsed since dose 3 and the child is unlikely to return at age 15–18 mo. • If started with DTP, complete the series with DTaP. • Do not give DTaP or DTP to children ≥7 yr of age (give Td). • DTaP/DTP may be given with all other vaccines but at a separate site. • It is preferable but not mandatory to use the same DTaP product for all doses.	• Doses 2 and 3 may be given 4 wk after previous dose. • Dose 4 may be given 6 mo after dose 3. • If dose 4 is given before 4th birthday, wait at least 6 mo for dose 5. • If dose 4 is given after 4th birthday, dose 5 is not needed. • Don't restart series, no matter how long since previous dose.	(DTaP and DTP have the same contraindications and precautions.) • Anaphylactic reaction to a prior dose or to any vaccine component. • Moderate or severe acute illness. Don't postpone for minor illness. • Previous encephalopathy within 7 days after DTP/DTaP. • Unstable progressive neurologic problem. **Precautions:** The following are precautions, not contraindications. Generally when these conditions are present, the vaccine shouldn't be given. But there are situations when the benefit outweighs risk, so vaccination should be considered (e.g., pertussis outbreak). • Previous T ≥ 105°F (40.5°C) within 48 hr after dose. • Previous continuous crying lasting 3 or more hr within 48 hr after dose. • Previous convulsion within 3 days after immunization. • Previous pale or limp episode, or collapse within 48 hr after dose.
DT Give IM	• Give to children <7 yr of age if the child has had a serious reaction to the "P" in DTaP/DTP, or if the parents refuse the pertussis component. • DT can be given with all other vaccines but at a separate site.	For children who have fallen behind, use information in box directly above.	• Anaphylactic reaction to a prior dose or to any vaccine component. • Moderate or severe acute illness. Don't postpone for minor illness.
Td Give IM	• Use for persons ≥7 yr of age. • A booster dose is recommended for children 11–12 yr of age if 5 yr has elapsed since last dose. Then boost every 10 yr. • Td may be given with all other vaccines but at a separate site.	For those never vaccinated or behind schedule, or if the vaccination history is unknown: give dose 1 now; dose 2 is given 4 wk later; dose 3 is given 6 mo after dose 2; and then boost every 10 years.	• Anaphylactic reaction to a prior dose or to any vaccine component. • Moderate or severe acute illness. Don't postpone for minor illness.

Polio
IPV and **OPV**
Give IPV SQ
or IM
Give OPV PO

- Give at 2 mo, 4 mo, 6–18 mo, and 4–6 yr of age.
- Give IPV for doses 1 and 2 (except in special circumstances, e.g., parent's refusal, imminent travel to polio-endemic area).
- ACIP says for dose 3, give OPV at 12–18 mo, and for dose 4, give OPV at 4–6 yr. An all-IPV schedule is also acceptable. If an all-IPV or all-OPV schedule is used, dose 3 may be given as early as 6 mo of age.
- AAP/AAFP say give either IPV or OPV for doses 3 and 4. Dose 3 is given at 6–18 mo of age and dose 4 at 4–6 yr. ACIP/AAP/AAFP say IPV is acceptable for all 4 doses.
- Not routinely given to anyone ≥18 yr of age (except certain travelers).
- IPV may be given with all other vaccines but at a separate site.
- OPV may be given with all other vaccines.

- Doses 1, 2, and 3 (IPV or OPV) should be separated by at least 4 wk.
- All IPV: a 6-mo interval is preferred between doses 2 and 3 for best response.
- Dose 4 (IPV or OPV) is given between 4 and 6 yr of age.
- If dose 3 of an all-IPV or all-OPV series is given at ≥4 yr of age, dose 4 is not needed.
- Children who receive any combination of IPV and OPV doses must receive all 4 doses, regardless of the age when first initiated.
- Don't restart series, no matter how long since previous dose.

- Anaphylactic reaction to a prior dose or to any vaccine component.
- Moderate or severe acute illness. Don't postpone for minor illness.
- Use IPV when an adult in the household or other close contact has never been vaccinated against polio.
- In pregnancy, if immediate protection is needed, see the ACIP recommendations on the use of polio vaccine.

The following are contraindications for OPV (so use IPV in these situations):
- Cancer, leukemia, lymphoma, immunodeficiency, including HIV/AIDS.
- Taking a drug that lowers resistance to infection, e.g., anticancer drugs, high-dose steroids.
- Someone in the household has any of the above medical problems.

Varicella (Var)
Give SQ

- Routinely give at 12–18 mo.
- Vaccinate all children ≥12 mo of age, including all adolescents who have not had prior infection with chickenpox.
- If Var and MMR (and/or yellow fever vaccine) are not given on the same day, space them ≥28 days apart.
- Var may be given with all other vaccines but at a separate site.

- Do not give to children <12 mo of age.
- Susceptible children <13 yr of age receive 1 dose.
- Susceptible persons ≥13 yr of age receive 2 doses 4–8 wk apart.
- Don't restart series, no matter how long since previous dose.

- Anaphylactic reaction to a prior dose or to any vaccine component.
- Moderate or severe acute illness. Don't postpone for minor illness.
- Pregnancy, or possibility of pregnancy within 1 month.
- If blood, plasma, or immune globulin (IG or VZIG) were given in past 5 months, see ACIP recommendations or AAP's 1997 *Red Book* (p. 353) re: time to wait before vaccinating.
- Immunocompromised persons due to high doses of systemic steroids, cancer, leukemia, lymphoma, immunodeficiency. *Note:* For patients taking high doses of systemic steroids or for patients with leukemia, consult ACIP recommendations.

Note: Manufacturer recommends "no salicylates" for 6 wk following this vaccine.

---

* Hepatitis A, influenza, pneumococcal, and Lyme disease vaccines are indicated for many children and teens, so make sure you provide these vaccines to at-risk children. The newer combination vaccines are not listed on this table but may be used whenever administration of any component is indicated and none is contraindicated.

Table continued on following page

Vaccine	Ages Usually Given; Other Guidelines	If Child Falls Behind—Minimum Intervals	Contraindications (Remember, Mild Illness Is Not a Contraindication)
MMR Give SQ	• Give dose 1 at 12–15 mo. Give dose 2 at 4–6 yr. • Make sure that all children (and teens) over 4–6 yr have received both doses of MMR. • If a dose was given before 12 mo of age, give dose 1 at 12–15 mo of age with a minimum interval of 4 wk between these doses. • If MMR and Var (and/or yellow fever vaccine) are not given on the same day, space them ≥28 days apart. • May give with all other vaccines but at a separate site.	• Two doses of MMR are recommended for all children ≤18 yr of age. • Give whenever behind. *Exception:* If MMR and Var (and/or yellow fever vaccine) are not given on the same day, space them ≥28 days apart. • There should be a minimum interval of 28 days between MMR dose 1 and MMR dose 2. • Dose 2 can be given at any time if at least 28 days have elapsed since dose 1, and both doses are administered after 1 yr of age. • Don't restart series, no matter how long since previous dose.	• Anaphylactic reaction to a prior dose or to any vaccine component. • Pregnancy or possible pregnancy within next 3 mo (use contraception). • Moderate or severe acute illness. Don't postpone for minor illness. • If blood, plasma, or immune globulin was given in past 11 mo, see ACIP recommendations or *1997 Red Book* (p. 353) re: time to wait before vaccinating. • HIV is *not* a contraindication unless severely immunocompromised. • Immunocompromised persons, e.g., those with cancer, leukemia, lymphoma. *Note:* For patients on high-dose immunosuppressive therapy, consult ACIP recommendations regarding delay time. *Note:* MMR is *not* contraindicated if a PPD test was done recently, but PPD should be delayed if MMR was given 1–30 days before the PPD.
Hib Give IM	• HibTITER (HbOC) and ActHib (PRP-T): give at 2 mo, 4 mo, 6 mo, 12–15 mo. • PedvaxHiB (PRP-OMP): give at 2 mo, 4 mo, 12–15 mo. • Dose 1 of Hib vaccine may be given as early as 6 wk of age, but not earlier. • May give with all other vaccines, but at a separate site. • All Hib products licensed for the primary series are interchangeable. • Any Hib vaccine may be used for the booster dose. • Hib is not routinely given to children ≥5 yr of age.	**Rules for all Hib vaccines:** • The last dose (booster dose) is given no earlier than 12 mo of age and a minimum of 2 mo has elapsed since the previous dose. • For children ≥15 mo and <5 yr who have *never* received Hib vaccine, only 1 dose is needed. • Don't restart series, no matter how long since previous dose. **Rules for HbOC (HibTITER) and PRP-T (ActHib) only:** • Doses 2 and 3 may be given 4 wk after previous dose. • If dose 1 was given at 7–11 mo, only 3 doses are needed: dose 2 is given 4–8 wk after dose 1, then boost at 12–15 mo. • If dose 1 was given at 12–14 mo, give a booster dose in 2 mo. **Rules for PRP-OMP (PedvaxHib) only:** • Dose 2 may be given 4 wk after dose 1. • If dose 1 was given at 12–14 mo, boost 8 wk later.	• Anaphylactic reaction to a prior dose or to any vaccine component. • Moderate or severe acute illness. Don't postpone for minor illness.

Hep-B
Give IM

- Vaccinate all infants at 0–2 mo, 1–4 mo, 6–18 mo.
- Vaccinate all children 0–18 yr of age.
- For older children/teens, spacing options include: 0 mo, 1 mo, 6 mo; 0 mo, 2 mo, 4 mo; or 0 mo, 1 mo, 4 mo.
- Children who were born or whose parents were born in countries of high HBV endemicity or who have other risk factors should be vaccinated as soon as possible.
- If mother is HBsAg positive: give HBIG and hep-B dose 1 within 12 hr of birth, dose 2 at 1–2 mo, and dose 3 at 6 mo of age.
- If mother's HBsAg status is unknown: give hep-B dose 1 within 12 hr of birth, dose 2 at 1–2 mo, and dose 3 at 6 mo of age. If mother is later found to be HBsAg-positive, her infant should receive the additional protection of HBIG within the first 7 days of life.
- May give with all other vaccines, but at a separate site.
- Hepatitis B vaccine brands are interchangeable.

- Don't restart series, no matter how long since previous dose.
- Three-dose series can be started at any age.
- Minimum spacing for children and teens: 4 wk between doses 1 and 2, and 2 mo between doses 2 and 3. Overall there must be 4 mo between doses 1 and 3.
- Dose 3 should not be given earlier than 6 mo of age.

Dosing of hepatitis B vaccines:
- For Engerix-B, use 10 µg (0.5 ml) for 0 through 19 yr of age.
- For Recombivax HB, use 5 µg (0.5 ml) for 0 through 19 yr of age.

- Anaphylactic reaction to a prior dose or to any vaccine component.
- Moderate or severe acute illness. Don't postpone for minor illness.

Rotavirus
(Rv)
Give PO

- Give at 2 mo, 4 mo, and 6 mo.
- Dose 1 should not be given before 6 wk or at ≥7 mo.
- No dose should be given on or after the first birthday.
- Do not readminister a regurgitated dose.
- May give with all other vaccines.

- Minimum interval is 3 wk between doses.
- Use minimum intervals to achieve protection prior to rotavirus season or if behind schedule.
- Don't restart the series, no matter how long since previous dose.

- Moderate or severe acute illness, including persistent vomiting. Don't postpone for minor illness.
- Anaphylactic reaction to a prior dose or to any vaccine component.
- Known or suspected altered immunity, including infants born to HIV+ mothers unless it is known that the child is not HIV infected.
- For infants with preexisting chronic GI conditions, see ACIP statement.

Read the package inserts. For full immunization information, see recent ACIP statements published in *MMWR*; and for the latest recommendations of the AAP's Committee on Infectious Diseases, see the AAP's *1997 Red Book* and the journal, *Pediatrics*.

The Immunization Action Coalition developed this table to combine the recommendations for childhood immunization onto one page and to assist health care workers in determining the appropriate use and scheduling of vaccines. It can be posted in immunization clinics or clinicians' offices.

Thank you to the following individuals for their review: William Atkinson, MD, Harold Margolis, MD, Linda Moyer, RN, Jane Seward, MBBS, Robert Sharrar, MD, Thomas Vernon, MD, Richard Zimmerman, MD. Final responsibility for errors lies with the editors.

Comments? e-mail: medinfo@immunize.org, call: 651-647-9009, or mail to IAC at 1573 Selby Avenue, St. Paul, MN 55104.

This table is revised yearly. The most recent edition of this table is available on our website at www.immunize.org.

Adapted from ACIP, AAP, and AAFP by the Immunization Action Coalition, March 1999.

G

Recommendations
for Preventive
Pediatric Health
Care

Each child and family is unique; therefore, these **Recommendations for Preventive Pediatric Health Care** are designed for the care of children who are receiving competent parenting, have no manifestations of any important health problems, and are growing and developing in satisfactory fashion. **Additional visits may become necessary** if circumstances suggest variations from normal.

These guidelines represent a consensus by the Committee on Practice and Ambulatory Medicine in consultation with national committees and sections of the American Academy of Pediatrics. The Committee emphasizes the great importance of **continuity of care** in comprehensive health supervision and the need to avoid **fragmentation of care.**

A **prenatal visit** is recommended for parents who are at high risk, for first-time parents, and for those who request a conference. The prenatal visit should include anticipatory guidance and pertinent medical history. Every infant should have a newborn evaluation after birth.

AGE[4]	NEWBORN[1]	2-4d[2]	By 1mo	2mo	4mo	6mo	9mo	12mo	15mo	18mo	24mo	3y	4y	5y	6y	8y	10y	11y	12y	13y	14y	15y	16y	17y	18y	19y	20y	21y
		INFANCY[3]							EARLY CHILDHOOD[3]					MIDDLE CHILDHOOD[3]				ADOLESCENCE[3]										
HISTORY Initial/Interval	•	•	•	•	•	•	•	•	•	•	•	•	•	•	•	•	•	•	•	•	•	•	•	•	•	•	•	•
MEASUREMENTS Height and Weight	•	•	•	•	•	•	•	•	•	•	•	•	•	•	•	•	•	•	•	•	•	•	•	•	•	•	•	•
Head Circumference	•	•	•	•	•	•	•	•	•	•	•																	
Blood Pressure												•	•	•	•	•	•	•	•	•	•	•	•	•	•	•	•	•
SENSORY SCREENING Vision	S	S	S	S	S	S	S	S	S	S	S	O⁵	O	O	O	O	O	S	O	S	S	O	S	S	O	S	S	S
Hearing[6]	S/O	S	S	S	S	S	S	S	S	S	S	O	O	O	O	O	O	S	O	S	S	O	S	S	O	S	S	S
DEVELOPMENTAL/ BEHAVIORAL ASSESSMENT[7]	•	•	•	•	•	•	•	•	•	•	•	•	•	•	•	•	•	•	•	•	•	•	•	•	•	•	•	•
PHYSICAL EXAMINATION[8]	•	•	•	•	•	•	•	•	•	•	•	•	•	•	•	•	•	•	•	•	•	•	•	•	•	•	•	•
PROCEDURES – GENERAL[9] Hereditary/Metabolic Screening[10]		•←→																										
Immunization[11]				•	•	•		•	•	•			•					•			•		•					
Lead Screening[12]							←•																					
Hematocrit or Hemoglobin						←—•—→												←—•—→										
Urinalysis								←—→						•				←—•—→										
PROCEDURES – PATIENTS AT RISK Tuberculin Test[15]								*	*	*	*	*	*	*	*	*	*	*	*	*	*	*	*	*	*	*	*	*
Cholesterol Screening[16]													*	*	*	*	*	*	*	*	*	*	*	*	*	*	*	*
STD Screening[17]																		*	*	*	*	*	*	*	*	*	*	*
Pelvic Exam[18]																		*	*	*	*	*	*	*	•←→	*	*	*→
ANTICIPATORY GUIDANCE[19]	•	•	•	•	•	•	•	•	•	•	•	•	•	•	•	•	•	•	•	•	•	•	•	•	•	•	•	•
INJURY PREVENTION[20]	•	•	•	•	•	•	•	•	•	•	•	•	•	•	•	•	•	•	•	•	•	•	•	•	•	•	•	•
INITIAL DENTAL REFERRAL[21]												•																

1. Breastfeeding encouraged and instruction and support offered.
2. For newborns discharged in less than 48 hours after delivery.
3. Developmental, psychosocial, and chronic disease issues for children and adolescents may require frequent counseling and treatment visits separate from preventive care visits.
4. If a child comes under care for the first time at any point on the schedule, or if any items are not accomplished at the suggested age, the schedule should be brought up to date at the earliest possible time.
5. If the patient is uncooperative, rescreen within six months.
6. Some experts recommend objective appraisal of hearing in the newborn period. The Joint Committee on Infant Hearing has identified patients at significant risk for hearing loss. All children meeting these criteria should be objectively screened. See the Joint Committee on Infant Hearing 1994 Position Statement.
7. By history and appropriate physical examination; if suspicious, by specific objective developmental testing.
8. At each visit, a complete physical examination is essential, with infant totally unclothed, older child undressed and suitably draped.
9. These may be modified, depending upon entry point into schedule and individual need.
10. Metabolic screening (eg, thyroid, hemoglobinopathies, PKU, galactosemia) should be done according to state law.
11. Schedule(s) per the Committee on Infectious Diseases, published periodically in *Pediatrics*. Every visit should be an opportunity to update and complete a child's immunizations.
12. Blood lead screen per AAP statement "Lead Poisoning: From Screening to Primary Prevention" (1993).
13. All menstruating adolescents should be screened.
14. Conduct dipstick urinalysis for leukocytes for male and female adolescents.
15. TB testing per AAP statement "Screening for Tuberculosis in Infants and Children" (1994). Testing should be done upon recognition of high risk factors. If results are negative but high risk situation continues, testing should be repeated on an annual basis.
16. Cholesterol screening for high risk patients per AAP "Statement on Cholesterol" (1992). If family history cannot be ascertained and other risk factors are present, screening should be at the discretion of the physician.
17. All sexually active patients should be screened for sexually transmitted diseases (STDs).
18. All sexually active females should have a pelvic examination. A pelvic examination and routine pap smear should be offered as part of preventive health maintenance between the ages of 18 and 21 years.
19. Appropriate discussion and counseling should be an integral part of each visit for care.
20. From birth to age 12, refer to AAP's injury prevention program (TIPP[®]) as described in "A Guide to Safety Counseling in Office Practice" (1994).
21. Earlier initial dental evaluations may be appropriate for some children. Subsequent examinations as prescribed by dentist.

Key: • = to be performed   * = to be performed for patients at risk   S = subjective, by history   O = objective, by a standard testing method   = the range during which a service may be provided, with the dot indicating the preferred age.

NB: Special chemical, immunologic, and endocrine testing is usually carried out upon specific indications. Testing other than newborn (eg, inborn errors of metabolism, sickle disease, etc.) is discretionary with the physician. Variations, taking into account individual circumstances, may be appropriate.

The recommendations in this publication do not indicate an exclusive course of treatment or serve as a standard of medical care.

H

Growth Charts

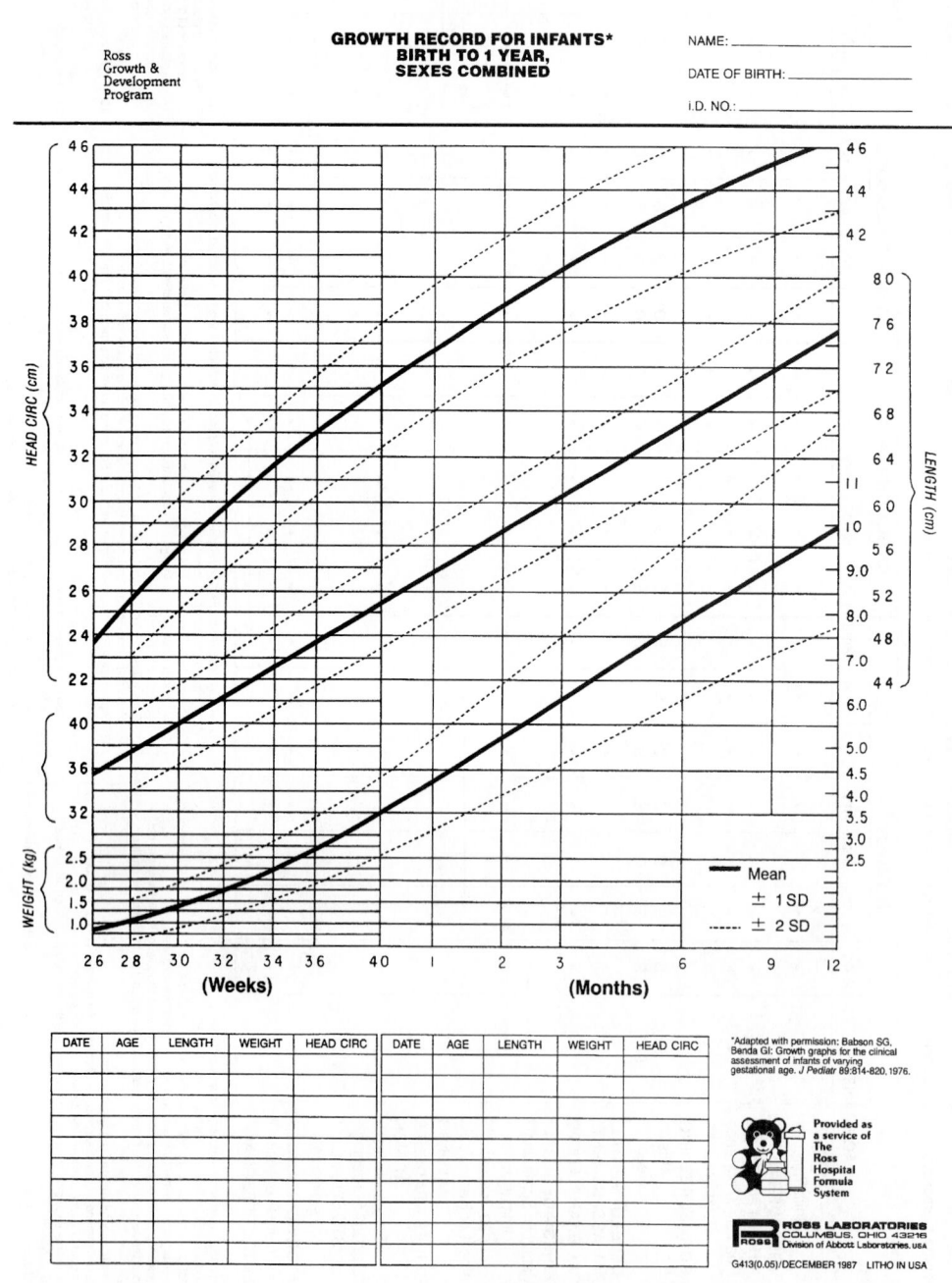

Ross
Growth &
Development
Program

GROWTH RECORD FOR INFANTS*
BIRTH TO 1 YEAR,
SEXES COMBINED

NAME: _____

DATE OF BIRTH: _____

I.D. NO.: _____

HEAD CIRC (cm)

LENGTH (cm)

WEIGHT (kg)

— Mean
± 1 SD
----- ± 2 SD

26 28 30 32 34 36 40
(Weeks)

1 2 3 6 9 12
(Months)

DATE	AGE	LENGTH	WEIGHT	HEAD CIRC	DATE	AGE	LENGTH	WEIGHT	HEAD CIRC

*Adapted with permission: Babson SG,
Benda GI: Growth graphs for the clinical
assessment of infants of varying
gestational age. *J Pediatr* 89:814-820, 1976.

Provided as
a service of
The
Ross
Hospital
Formula
System

ROSS LABORATORIES
COLUMBUS, OHIO 43216
Division of Abbott Laboratories, USA

G413(0.05)/DECEMBER 1987   LITHO IN USA

GIRLS: BIRTH TO 36 MONTHS; PHYSICAL GROWTH NCHS PERCENTILES*

NAME_____ RECORD #_____

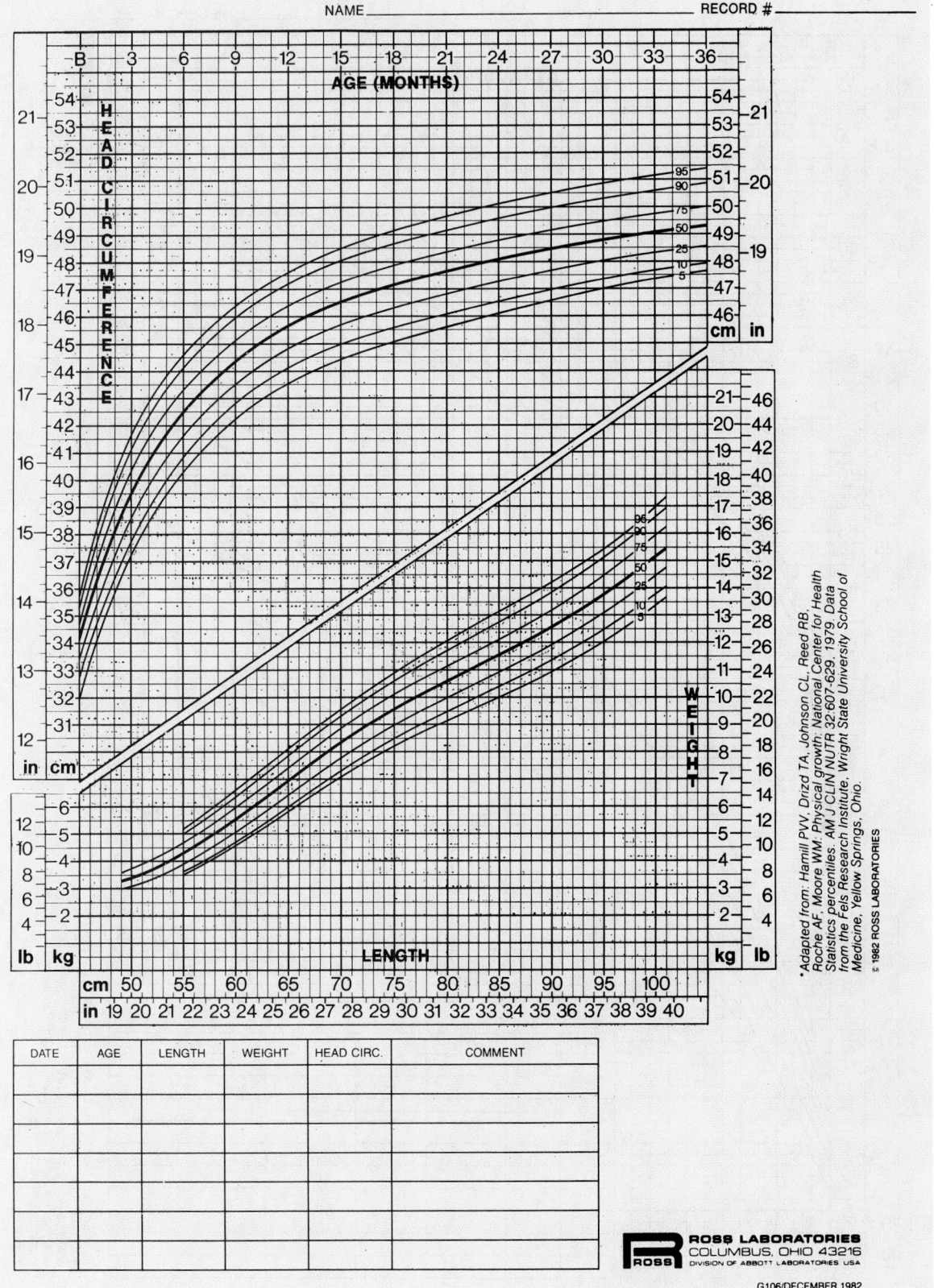

DATE	AGE	LENGTH	WEIGHT	HEAD CIRC.	COMMENT

*Adapted from: Hamill PVV, Drizd TA, Johnson CL, Reed RB, Roche AF, Moore WM: Physical growth: National Center for Health Statistics percentiles. AM J CLIN NUTR 32:607-629, 1979. Data from the Fels Research Institute, Wright State University School of Medicine, Yellow Springs, Ohio.
© 1982 ROSS LABORATORIES

ROSS LABORATORIES
COLUMBUS, OHIO 43216
DIVISION OF ABBOTT LABORATORIES USA

G106/DECEMBER 1982

Girls: Birth to 36 Months; Physical Growth NCHS Percentiles*

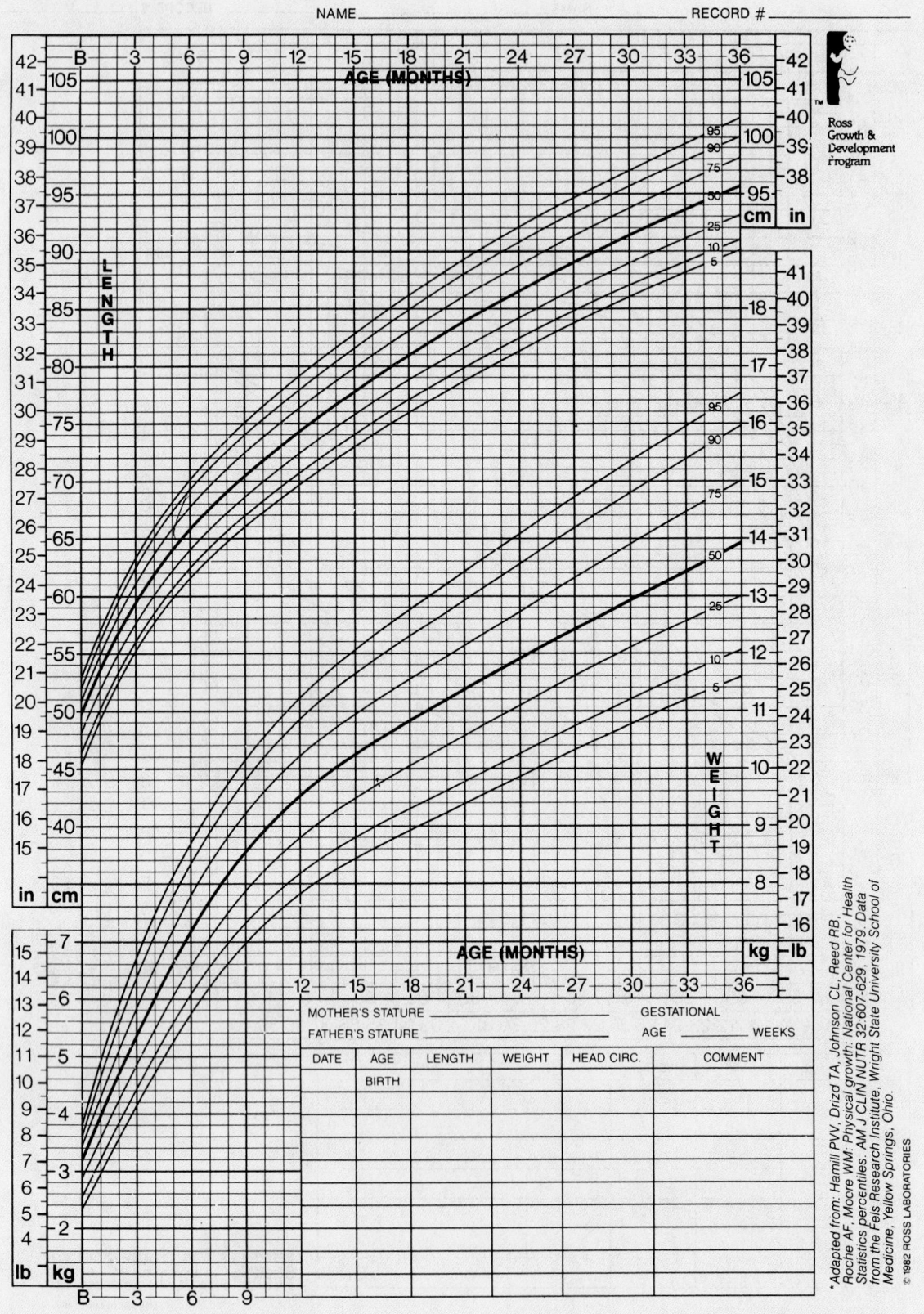

NAME _____ RECORD # _____

* Adapted from: Hamill PVV, Drizd TA, Johnson CL, Reed RB,
Roche AF, Moore WM: Physical growth: National Center for Health
Statistics percentiles. AM J CLIN NUTR 32:607-629, 1979. Data
from the Fels Research Institute, Wright State University School of
Medicine, Yellow Springs, Ohio.
© 1982 ROSS LABORATORIES

Ross
Growth &
Development
Program

MOTHER'S STATURE _____ GESTATIONAL
FATHER'S STATURE _____ AGE _____ WEEKS

DATE	AGE	LENGTH	WEIGHT	HEAD CIRC.	COMMENT
	BIRTH				

GIRLS: 2 TO 18 YEARS; PHYSICAL GROWTH NCHS PERCENTILES*

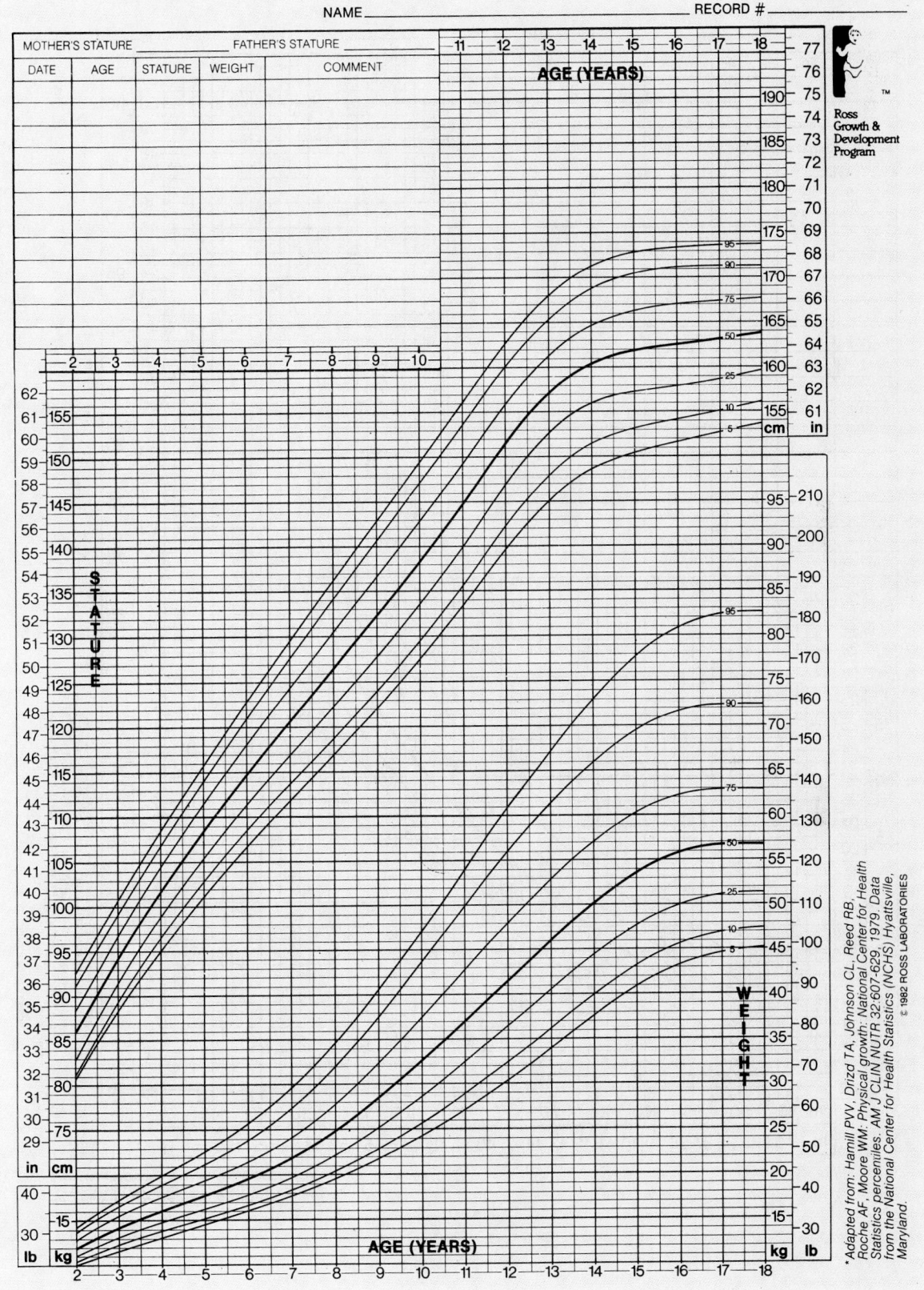

NAME_____ RECORD #_____

Ross
Growth &
Development
Program

*Adapted from: Hamill PVV, Drizd TA, Johnson CL, Reed RB, Roche AF, Moore WM. Physical growth: National Center for Health Statistics percentiles. AM J CLIN NUTR 32:607-629, 1979. Data from the National Center for Health Statistics (NCHS) Hyattsville, Maryland.

© 1982 ROSS LABORATORIES

Girls: Prepubescent; Physical Growth NCHS Percentiles*

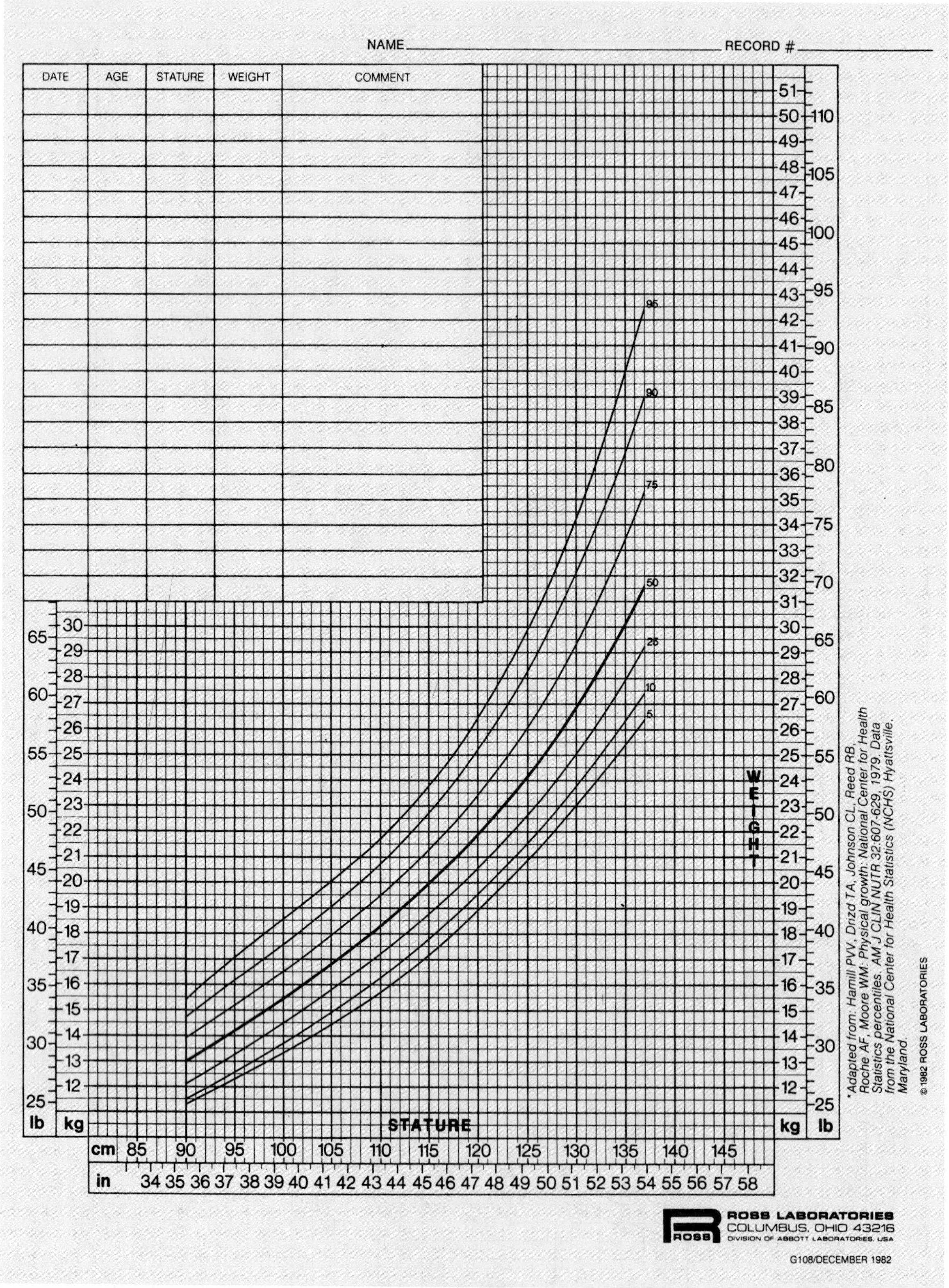
NAME
RECORD #
DATE
AGE
STATURE
WEIGHT
COMMENT
95
90
75
50
25
10
5
WEIGHT
STATURE
lb
kg
cm
in
*Adapted from: Hamill PVV, Drizd TA, Johnson CL, Reed RB, Roche AF, Moore WM: Physical growth: National Center for Health Statistics percentiles. AM J CLIN NUTR 32:607-629, 1979. Data from the National Center for Health Statistics (NCHS) Hyattsville, Maryland.
© 1982 ROSS LABORATORIES
ROSS LABORATORIES
COLUMBUS, OHIO 43216
DIVISION OF ABBOTT LABORATORIES, USA
G108/DECEMBER 1982

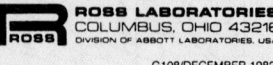

BOYS: BIRTH TO 36 MONTHS; PHYSICAL GROWTH NCHS PERCENTILES*

NAME _____ RECORD # _____

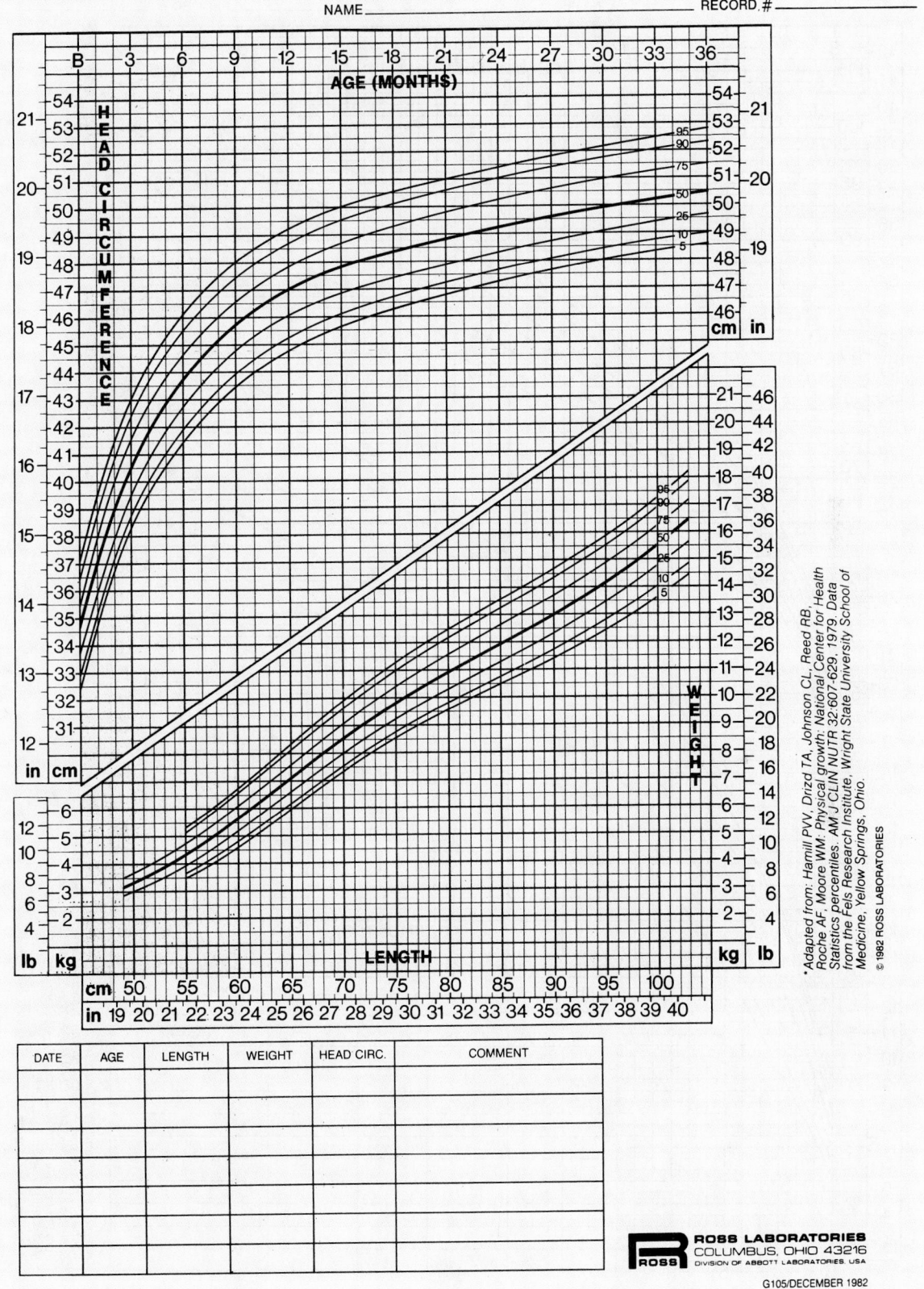

DATE	AGE	LENGTH	WEIGHT	HEAD CIRC.	COMMENT

*Adapted from: Hamill PVV, Drizd TA, Johnson CL, Reed RB, Roche AF, Moore WM: Physical growth: National Center for Health Statistics percentiles. AM J CLIN NUTR 32:607-629, 1979. Data from the Fels Research Institute, Wright State University School of Medicine, Yellow Springs, Ohio.

© 1982 ROSS LABORATORIES

ROSS LABORATORIES
COLUMBUS, OHIO 43216
DIVISION OF ABBOTT LABORATORIES, USA

G105/DECEMBER 1982

Boys: Birth to 36 Months; Physical Growth NCHS Percentiles*

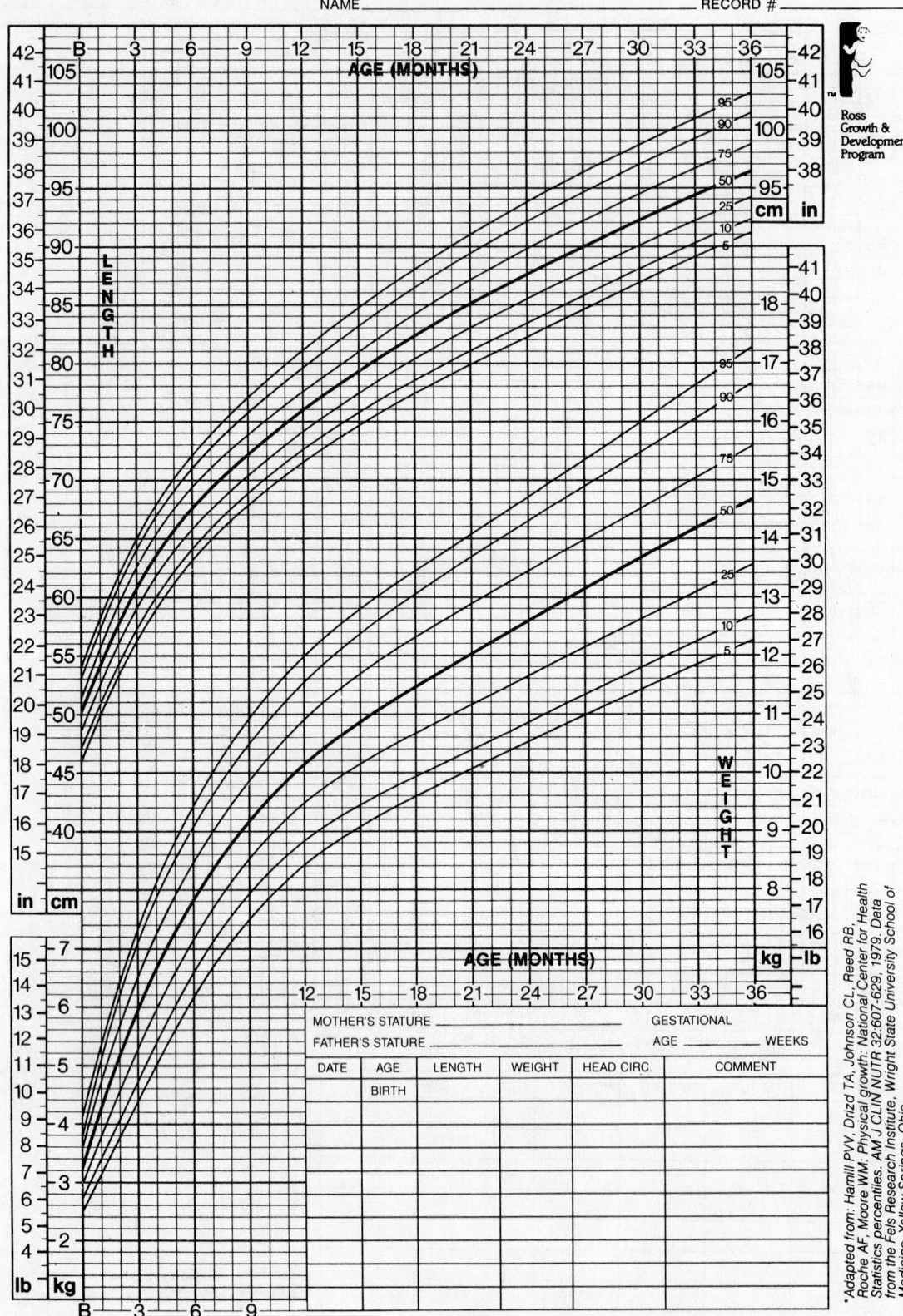

NAME _____ RECORD # _____

Ross
Growth &
Development
Program

*Adapted from: Hamill PVV, Drizd TA, Johnson CL, Reed RB,
Roche AF, Moore WM. Physical growth: National Center for Health
Statistics percentiles. AM J CLIN NUTR 32:607-629, 1979. Data
from the Fels Research Institute, Wright State University School of
Medicine, Yellow Springs, Ohio.

© 1982 ROSS LABORATORIES

MOTHER'S STATURE _____ GESTATIONAL

FATHER'S STATURE _____ AGE _____ WEEKS

DATE	AGE	LENGTH	WEIGHT	HEAD CIRC.	COMMENT
	BIRTH				

BOYS: 2 TO 18 YEARS; PHYSICAL GROWTH NCHS PERCENTILES*

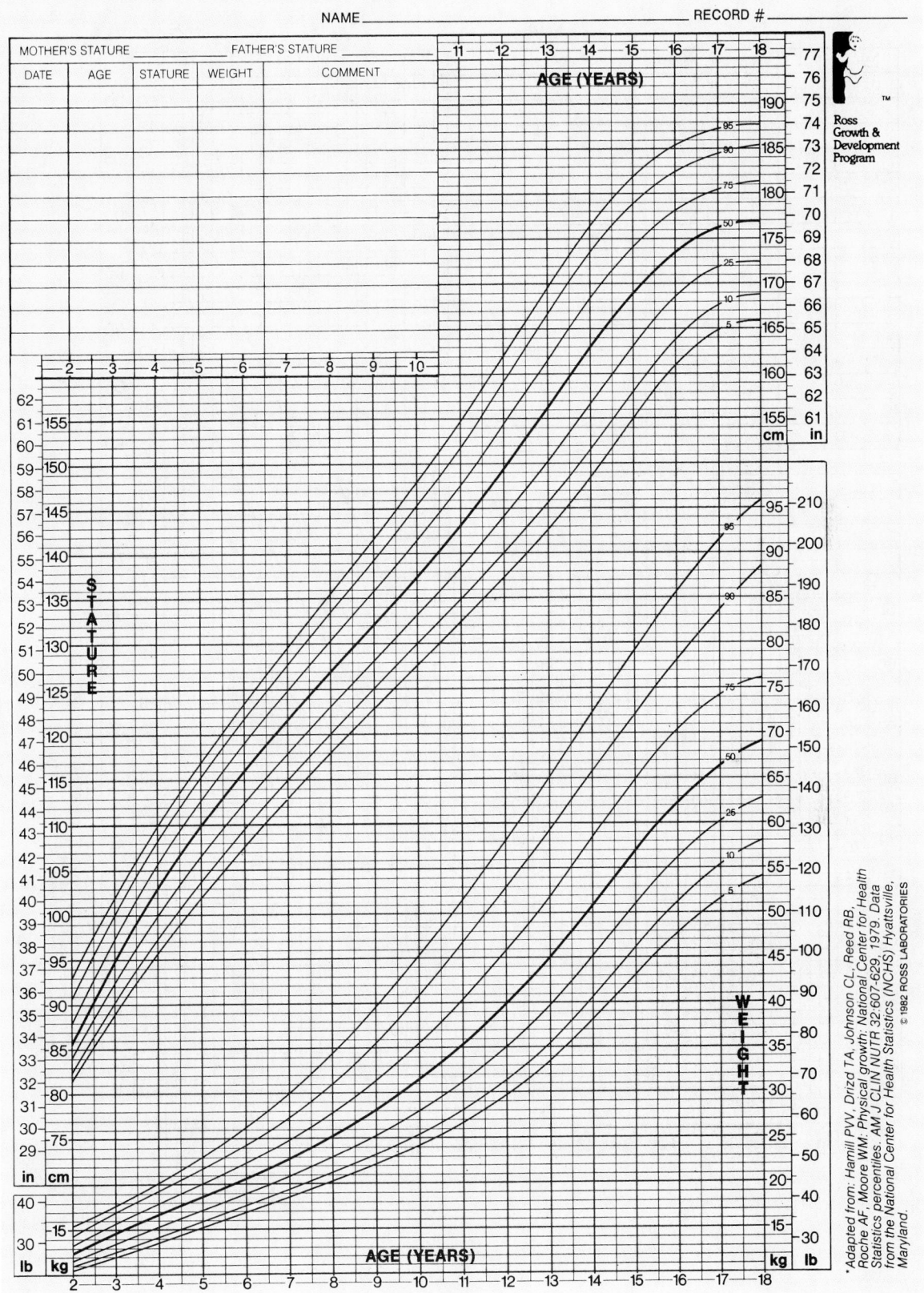

*Adapted from: Hamill PVV, Drizd TA, Johnson CL, Reed RB, Roche AF, Moore WM. Physical growth: National Center for Health Statistics percentiles. AM J CLIN NUTR 32:607-629, 1979. Data from the National Center for Health Statistics (NCHS), Hyattsville, Maryland.

© 1982 ROSS LABORATORIES

Ross
Growth &
Development
Program

BOYS: PREPUBESCENT; PHYSICAL GROWTH NCHS PERCENTILES*

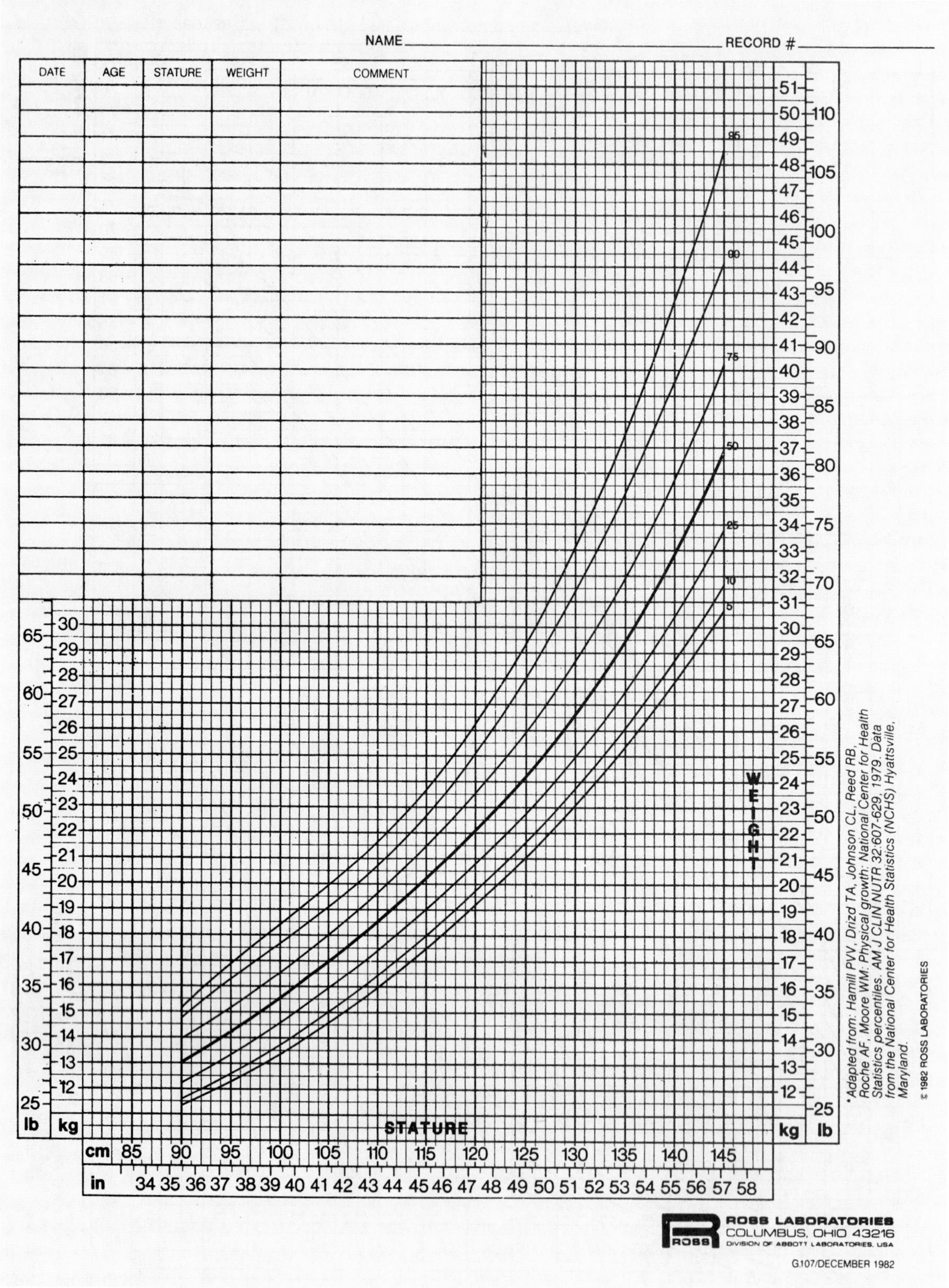

NAME_____ RECORD #_____

DATE	AGE	STATURE	WEIGHT	COMMENT

STATURE

cm 85 90 95 100 105 110 115 120 125 130 135 140 145

in 34 35 36 37 38 39 40 41 42 43 44 45 46 47 48 49 50 51 52 53 54 55 56 57 58

WEIGHT

Percentile curves: 95 90 75 50 25 10 5

*Adapted from: Hamill PVV, Drizd TA, Johnson CL, Reed RB, Roche AF, Moore WM. Physical growth: National Center for Health Statistics percentiles. AM J CLIN NUTR 32:607-629, 1979. Data from the National Center for Health Statistics (NCHS) Hyattsville, Maryland.

© 1982 ROSS LABORATORIES

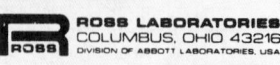
ROSS LABORATORIES
COLUMBUS, OHIO 43216
DIVISION OF ABBOTT LABORATORIES, USA

G.107/DECEMBER 1982

I

Denver
Developmental
Screening
Test II

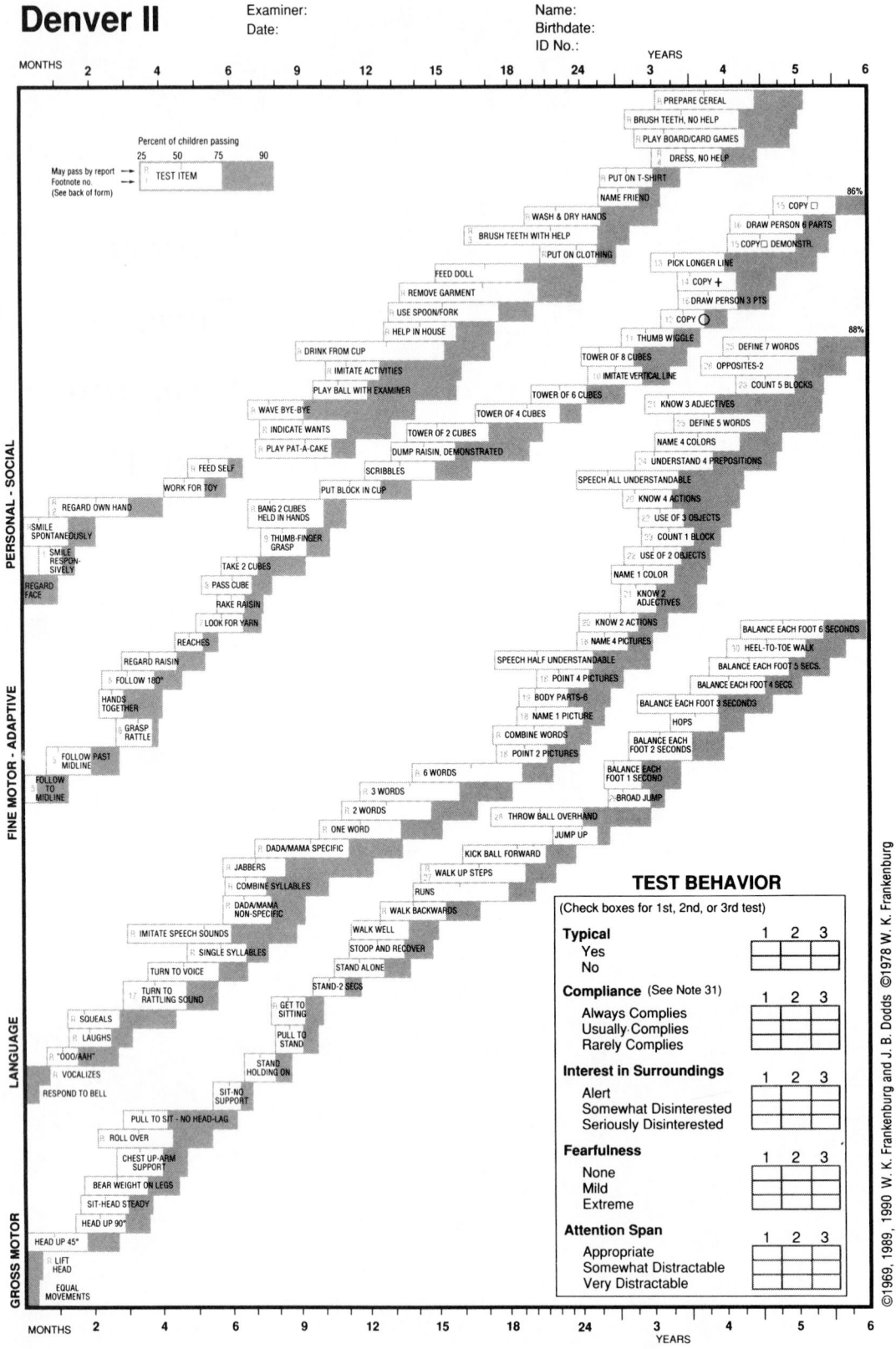

Note: The *Denver II Training Manual* is required to administer the test. The manual and other Denver II materials (kits, forms, training videotapes) can be obtained from Denver Developmental Materials, P.O. Box 6919, Denver, Colorado 80206-0910. Telephone: 303-355-4729 or 800-419-4729.

DIRECTIONS FOR ADMINISTRATION

1. Try to get child to smile by smiling, talking or waving. Do not touch him/her.
2. Child must stare at hand several seconds.
3. Parent may help guide toothbrush and put toothpaste on brush.
4. Child does not have to be able to tie shoes or button/zip in the back.
5. Move yarn slowly in an arc from one side to the other, about 8" above child's face.
6. Pass if child grasps rattle when it is touched to the backs or tips of fingers.
7. Pass if child tries to see where yarn went. Yarn should be dropped quickly from sight from tester's hand without arm movement.
8. Child must transfer cube from hand to hand without help of body, mouth, or table.
9. Pass if child picks up raisin with any part of thumb and finger.
10. Line can vary only 30 degrees or less from tester's line. |/
11. Make a fist with thumb pointing upward and wiggle only the thumb. Pass if child imitates and does not move any fingers other than the thumb.

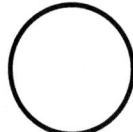

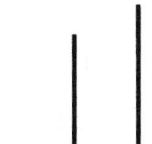

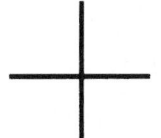

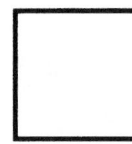

12. Pass any enclosed form. Fail continuous round motions.

13. Which line is longer? (Not bigger.) Turn paper upside down and repeat. (pass 3 of 3 or 5 of 6)

14. Pass any lines crossing near midpoint.

15. Have child copy first. If failed, demonstrate.

When giving items 12, 14, and 15, do not name the forms. Do not demonstrate 12 and 14.

16. When scoring, each pair (2 arms, 2 legs, etc.) counts as one part.
17. Place one cube in cup and shake gently near child's ear, but out of sight. Repeat for other ear.
18. Point to picture and have child name it. (No credit is given for sounds only.)
    If less than 4 pictures are named correctly, have child point to picture as each is named by tester.

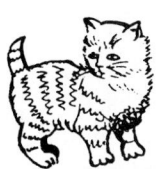 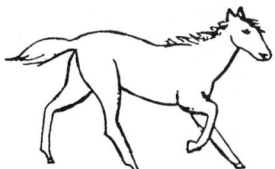 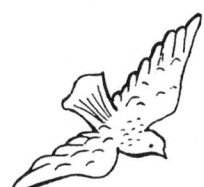 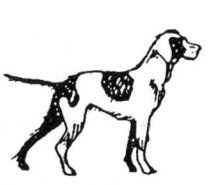 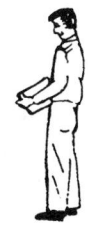

19. Using doll, tell child: Show me the nose, eyes, ears, mouth, hands, feet, tummy, hair. Pass 6 of 8.
20. Using pictures, ask child: Which one flies?... says meow?... talks?... barks?... gallops? Pass 2 of 5, 4 of 5.
21. Ask child: What do you do when you are cold?... tired?... hungry? Pass 2 of 3, 3 of 3.
22. Ask child: What do you do with a cup? What is a chair used for? What is a pencil used for?
    Action words must be included in answers.
23. Pass if child correctly places <u>and</u> says how many blocks are on paper. (1, 5).
24. Tell child: Put block **on** table; **under** table; **in front of** me, **behind** me. Pass 4 of 4.
    (Do not help child by pointing, moving head or eyes.)
25. Ask child: What is a ball?... lake?... desk?... house?... banana?... curtain?... fence?... ceiling? Pass if defined in terms of use, shape, what it is made of, or general category (such as banana is fruit, not just yellow). Pass 5 of 8, 7 of 8.
26. Ask child: If a horse is big, a mouse is __? If fire is hot, ice is __? If the sun shines during the day, the moon shines during the __? Pass 2 of 3.
27. Child may use wall or rail only, not person. May not crawl.
28. Child must throw ball overhand 3 feet to within arm's reach of tester.
29. Child must perform standing broad jump over width of test sheet (8 1/2 inches).
30. Tell child to walk forward, ⌒⌒⌒⌒⌒► heel within 1 inch of toe. Tester may demonstrate.
    Child must walk 4 consecutive steps.
31. In the second year, half of normal children are non-compliant.

OBSERVATIONS:

DENVER ARTICULATION SCREENING EXAM
for children 2 1/2 to 6 years of age

Instructions: Have child repeat each word after
you. Circle the underlined sounds that he pro-
nounces correctly. Total correct sounds is the
Raw Score. Use charts on reverse side to score
results.

NAME

HOSP. NO.

ADDRESS

Date: _____ Child's Age: _____ Examiner: _____ Raw Score: _____
Percentile: _____ Intelligibility: _____ Result: _____

1. table	6. zipper	11. sock	16. wagon	21. leaf
2. shirt	7. grapes	12. vacuum	17. gum	22. carrot
3. door	8. flag	13. yarn	18. house	
4. trunk	9. thumb	14. mother	19. pencil	
5. jumping	10. toothbrush	15. twinkle	20. fish	

Intelligibility: (circle one)   1. Easy to understand   3. Nct understandable
                                2. Understandable 1/2   4. Can't evaluate
                                       the time.

Comments:

Date: _____ Child's Age: _____ Examiner: _____ Raw Score _____
Percentile: _____ Intelligibility: _____ Result: _____

1. table	6. zipper	11. sock	16. wagon	21. leaf
2. shirt	7. grapes	12. vacuum	17. gum	22. carrot
3. door	8. flag	13. yarn	18. house	
4. trunk	9. thumb	14. mother	19. pencil	
5. jumping	10. toothbrush	15. twinkle	20. fish	

Intelligibility: (circle one)   1. Easy to understand   3. Not understandable
                                2. Understandable 1/2   4. Can't evaluate
                                       the time.

Comments:

Date: _____ Child's Age: _____ Examiner: _____ Raw Score_____
Percentile: _____ Intelligibility: _____ Result: _____

1. table	6. zipper	11. sock	16. wagon	21. leaf
2. shirt	7. grapes	12. vacuum	17. gum	22. carrot
3. door	8. flag	13. yarn	18. house	
4. trunk	9. thumb	14. mother	19. pencil	
5. jumping	10. toothbrush	15. twinkle	20. fish	

Intelligibility: (circle one)   1. Easy to understand   3. Not understandable
                                2. Understandable 1/2   4. Can't evaluate
                                       the time.

To score DASE words: Note raw score for child's performance. Match raw score line (extreme left of chart) with column representing child's age (to the closest *previous* age group). Where raw score line and age column meet denotes percentile rank of child's performance when compared with other children that age. Percentiles above heavy line are *abnormal,* below heavy line are *normal.*

PERCENTILE RANK

Raw Score	2.5 yr	3.0 yr	3.5 yr	4.0 yr	4.5 yr	5.0 yr	5.5 yr	6 yr
2	1							
3	2							
4	5							
5	9							
6	16							
7	23							
8	31	2						
9	37	4	1					
10	42	6	2					
11	48	7	4					
12	54	9	6	1	1			
13	58	12	9	2	3	1	1	
14	62	17	11	5	4	2	2	
15	68	23	15	9	5	3	2	
16	75	31	19	12	5	4	3	
17	79	38	25	15	6	6	4	
18	83	46	31	19	8	7	4	
19	86	51	38	24	10	9	5	1
20	89	58	45	30	12	11	7	3
21	92	65	52	36	15	15	9	4
22	94	72	58	43	18	19	12	5
23	96	77	63	50	22	24	15	7
24	97	82	70	58	29	29	20	15
25	99	87	78	66	36	34	26	17
26	99	91	84	75	46	43	34	24
27		94	89	82	57	54	44	34
28		96	94	88	70	68	59	47
29		98	98	94	84	84	77	68
30		100	100	100	100	100	100	100

To score intelligibility:

	NORMAL	ABNORMAL
2.5 years	Understandable half of the time or easy to understand	Not understandable
3 years and older	Easy to understand	Understandable half of the time or not understandable

Test result: 1. Normal on DASE and intelligibility = *normal*
2. Abnormal on DASE or intelligibility = *abnormal**

* If abnormal on initial screening, rescreen within 2 weeks. If abnormal again, child should be referred for complete speech evaluation.

J

Normal Blood Pressure Readings for Children

Normal Blood Pressure Readings for Girls

Age	Systolic Blood Pressure Percentile					Age	Diastolic Blood Pressure* Percentile				
	5th	10th	50th	90th	95th		5th	10th	50th	90th	95th
1 day	46	50	65	80	84	1 day	38	42	55	68	72
3 days	53	57	72	86	90	3 days	38	42	55	68	71
7 days	60	64	78	93	97	7 days	38	41	54	67	71
1 mo	65	69	84	98	102	1 mo	35	39	52	65	69
2 mo	68	72	87	101	106	2 mo	34	38	51	64	68
3 mo	70	74	89	104	108	3 mo	35	38	51	64	68
4 mo	71	75	90	105	109	4 mo	35	39	52	65	68
5 mo	72	76	91	106	110	5 mo	36	39	52	65	69
6 mo	72	76	91	106	110	6 mo	36	40	53	66	69
7 mo	72	76	91	106	110	7 mo	36	40	53	66	70
8 mo	72	76	91	106	110	8 mo	37	40	53	66	70
9 mo	72	76	91	106	110	9 mo	37	41	54	67	70
10 mo	72	76	91	106	110	10 mo	37	41	54	67	71
11 mo	72	76	91	105	110	11 mo	38	41	54	67	71
1 yr	72	76	91	105	110	1 yr	38	41	54	67	71
2 yr	71	76	90	105	109	2 yr	40	43	56	69	73
3 yr	72	76	91	106	110	3 yr	40	43	56	69	73
4 yr	73	78	92	107	111	4 yr	40	43	56	69	73
5 yr	75	79	94	109	113	5 yr	40	43	56	69	73
6 yr	77	81	96	111	115	6 yr	40	44	57	70	74
7 yr	78	83	97	112	116	7 yr	41	45	58	71	75
8 yr	80	84	99	114	118	8 yr	43	46	59	72	76
9 yr	81	86	100	115	119	9 yr	44	48	61	74	77
10 yr	83	87	102	117	121	10 yr	46	49	62	75	79
11 yr	86	90	105	119	123	11 yr	47	51	64	77	81
12 yr	88	92	107	122	126	12 yr	49	53	66	78	82
13 yr	90	94	109	124	128	13 yr	46	50	64	78	82
14 yr	92	96	110	125	129	14 yr	49	53	67	81	85
15 yr	93	97	111	126	130	15 yr	49	53	67	82	86
16 yr	93	97	112	127	131	16 yr	49	53	67	81	85
17 yr	93	98	112	127	131	17 yr	48	52	66	80	84
18 yr	94	98	112	127	131	18 yr	48	52	66	80	84

* K4 was used for ages less than 13; K5 was used for ages 13 and over.

Reprinted with permission from the Second Task Force on Blood Pressure Control in Children, National Heart, Lung and Blood Institute, Bethesda, MD. Tabular data prepared by Dr. B. Rosner, 1987.

Normal Blood Pressure Readings for Boys

	Systolic Blood Pressure Percentile						Diastolic Blood Pressure* Percentile				
Age	5th	10th	50th	90th	95th	Age	5th	10th	50th	90th	95th
1 day	54	58	73	87	92	1 day	38	42	55	68	72
3 days	55	59	74	89	93	3 days	38	42	55	68	71
7 days	57	62	76	91	95	7 days	37	41	54	67	71
1 mo	67	71	86	101	105	1 mo	35	39	52	64	68
2 mo	72	76	91	106	110	2 mo	33	37	50	63	66
3 mo	72	76	91	106	110	3 mo	33	37	50	63	66
4 mo	72	76	91	106	110	4 mo	34	37	50	63	67
5 mo	72	76	91	105	110	5 mo	35	39	52	65	68
6 mo	72	76	90	105	109	6 mo	36	40	53	66	70
7 mo	71	76	90	105	109	7 mo	37	41	54	67	71
8 mo	71	75	90	105	109	8 mo	38	42	55	68	72
9 mo	71	75	90	105	109	9 mo	39	43	55	68	72
10 mo	71	75	90	105	109	10 mo	39	43	56	69	73
11 mo	71	76	90	105	109	11 mo	39	43	56	69	73
1 yr	71	76	90	105	109	1 yr	39	43	56	69	73
2 yr	72	76	91	106	110	2 yr	39	43	56	68	72
3 yr	73	77	92	107	111	3 yr	39	42	55	68	72
4 yr	74	79	93	108	112	4 yr	39	43	56	69	72
5 yr	76	80	95	109	113	5 yr	40	43	56	69	73
6 yr	77	81	96	111	115	6 yr	41	44	57	70	74
7 yr	78	83	97	112	116	7 yr	42	45	58	71	75
8 yr	80	84	99	114	118	8 yr	43	47	60	73	76
9 yr	82	86	101	115	120	9 yr	44	48	61	74	78
10 yr	84	88	102	117	121	10 yr	45	49	62	75	79
11 yr	86	90	105	119	123	11 yr	47	50	63	76	80
12 yr	88	92	107	121	126	12 yr	48	51	64	77	81
13 yr	90	94	109	124	128	13 yr	45	49	63	77	81
14 yr	93	97	112	126	131	14 yr	46	50	64	78	82
15 yr	95	99	114	129	133	15 yr	47	51	65	79	83
16 yr	98	102	117	131	136	16 yr	49	53	67	81	85
17 yr	100	104	119	134	138	17 yr	51	55	69	83	87
18 yr	102	106	121	136	140	18 yr	52	56	70	84	88

* K4 was used for ages less than 13; K5 was used for ages 13 and over.

Reprinted with permission from the Second Task Force on Blood Pressure Control in Children, National Heart, Lung and Blood Institute, Bethesda, MD. Tabular data prepared by Dr. B. Rosner, 1987.

K

*Skin Fold
Thickness by
Age and Sex*

50th Percentiles

Skin fold thickness by age and sex, as measured by Harpenden skin fold calipers over triceps and under scapula. Scale is in millimeters on the left side and logarithmic transformation units on the right side. The lines shown are the 50th percentiles for British children.

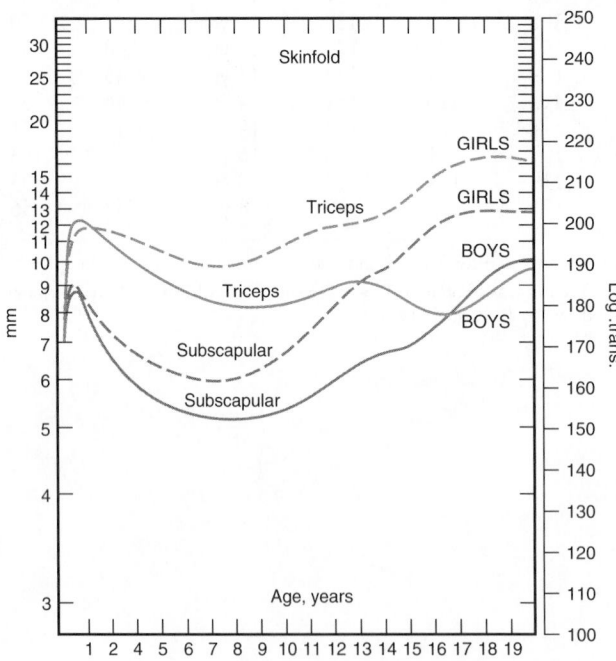

Reprinted by permission from Tanner, J. M. (1978). *Fetus into man: Physical growth from conception to maturity.* Cambridge, MA: Harvard University Press.

PROFESSIONAL ORGANIZATIONS

American Academy of Pediatrics
141 Northwest Point Boulevard
Elk Grove Village, IL 60007-1098
800-433-9016 or 847-228-5005
Fax: 847-228-5097
Website: www.aap.org

American College of Nurse-Midwives
818 Connecticut Avenue, NW
Suite 900
Washington, DC 20006
202-728-9860
Fax: 728-9897
e-mail: info@midwife.org
Website: www.midwife.org

American College of Obstetricians and Gynecologists
409 12th Street, SW
P.O. Box 96920
Washington, DC 20090-6920
Website: www.acog.org

Association of Women's Health, Obstetric, and Neonatal
    Nurses (AWHONN)
2000 L Street, NW
Suite 740
Washington, DC 20036
800-673-8499 (US)
800-245-0231 (Canada)
Fax: 202-728-0575
Website: www.awhonn.org

National Association of Neonatal Nurses
1304 Southpoint Boulevard
Suite 280
Petaluma, CA 94954-6861
800-451-3795
Fax: 707-762-0401
e-mail: nannmbrs@aol.com
Website: www.nann.org

National Association of Pediatric Nurse Associates and
    Practitioners (NAPNAP)
1101 Kings Highway North
Suite 206
Cherry Hill, NJ 08034-1912
609-667-1773
e-mail: info@napnap.org
Website: www.napnap.org

National Association of School Nurses
P.O. Box 1300
Scarborough, ME 04070-1300
207-338-2177
Fax: 207-338-2685
e-mail: nasnweb@aol.com
Website: www.vmedia.com/Nurses

Society of Pediatric Nurses
2170 South Parker Road
Suite 350
Denver, CO 80231-5711
800-723-2902
Fax: 303-750-3212
e-mail: bwoodward@aorn.org
Website: www.pedinurse.org

L

◆ ◆ ◆ ◆ ◆ ◆ ◆ ◆ ◆ ◆ ◆

Resources for Health Care Providers and Families

GENERAL MATERNAL-NEWBORN, WOMEN'S HEALTH, AND PEDIATRIC RESOURCES

National Center for Education in Maternal and Child
    Health
2000 15th Street, N
Suite 701
Arlington, VA 22201-2617
703-524-7802
Fax: 703-524-9335
e-mail: info@ncemch.org
Website: www.ncemch.org

National Center for Health Statistics
Centers for Disease Control and Prevention
Website: www.cdc.gov/nchswww/nchshome

National Health Information Center
Department of Health and Human Services
Website: nhic-nt.health.org
Has a health information database.

National Health Promotion and Disease Prevention Ob-
    jectives
Website: www.odphp.osophs.dhhs.gov/pubs/hp2000
Contains text of *Healthy People 2000* and 2010 objectives.

ABUSE, PHYSICAL OR SEXUAL

See also *Domestic Violence*

National Committee to Prevent Child Abuse (NCPCA)
200 South Michigan Avenue
17th Floor
Chicago, IL 60604-4357
312-663-3520
Fax: 312-939-8962
Website: www.childabuse.org

Parents Anonymous
675 West Foothill Boulevard
Suite 220
Claremont, CA 91711
909-621-6184
Fax: 909-625-6304
e-mail: www.parentsanon@msn.com

AIDS/HIV

The Names Project Foundation
310 Townsend Street
Suite 310
San Francisco, CA 94107
415-882-5500
Fax: 415-882-6200
Website: www.aidsquilt.org

ATTENTION DEFICIT-HYPERACTIVITY DISORDER

Children and Adults with Attention Deficit Disorders
    (CHADD)
8181 Professional Place
Suite 201
Landover, MD 20785
800-233-4050 or 301-306-7070
Fax: 301-306-7090
Website: www.chadd.org

National Attention Deficit Disorder Association
P.O. Box 1303
Northbrook, IL 60065-1303
440-350-9595
e-mail: DearADD@aol.com
Website: www.add.org

AUTISM

Autism Society of America
7910 Woodmont Avenue
Suite 300
Bethesda, MD 20814-3015
800-3AUTISM or 301-657-0881
Fax: 301-657-0869
Website: www.autism-society.org

Center for the Study of Autism
P.O. Box 4538
Salem, OR 97302
Website: www.autism.org

National Institute of Mental Health
6001 Executive Boulevard
Room 8184, MSC 9663
Bethesda, MD 20892-9663
301-443-4513
Fax: 301-443-4279
e-mail: nimhinfo@nih.gov
Website: www.nimh.nih.gov

BLINDNESS, VISUAL IMPAIRMENT

American Council of the Blind
1155 15th Street, NW
Suite 720
Washington, DC 20005
800-424-8666 or 202-467-5081
Fax: 202-467-5085
Website: www.acb.org

American Foundation for the Blind
1615 M Street, NW
Suite 250
Washington, DC 20036
202-347-8888 (voice), 202-347-0947 (TTY)
Fax: 202-347-0947
Website: www.dccare.org

The Blind Children's Center
4120 Marathon Street
Los Angeles, CA 90029-3584
800-222-3566 or 800-222-3567 (California) or 323-664-2153
Fax: 323-665-3828
Website: www.blindctr.org

Helen Keller National Center for Deaf-Blind Youth and
    Adults
111 Middleneck Road
Sands Point, NY 11050
516-944-8900 (voice, TTY) or 516-944-8637 (TTY)
Fax: 516-944-7302
Website: www.helenkeller.org

National Association for Parents of the Visually Handi-
    capped
P.O. Box 317
Watertown, MA 02472
800-562-6265 or 617-972-7441

BREAST-FEEDING

International Lactation Consultant Association (ILCA)
4101 Lake Boone Trail
Raleigh, NC 27607
919-787-5181
Fax: 919-787-4916
Website: www.ilca.org

LaLeche League International
1400 North Meacham Road
Schaumburg, IL 60173-4840
800-525-3243 or 847-519-7730
Fax: 847-519-0035
Website: www.lalecheleague.org

BURNS

American Burn Association
625 North Michigan Avenue
Suite 1530
Chicago, IL 60611
Website: www.ameriburn.org

Camp I-Thonka-Chi
Parkland Health and Hospital System
Medicine and Rehabilitation Department
5201 Harry Hines Boulevard
Dallas, TX 75235
214-590-8139

Website: www.swmed.edu/home_pages/parkland/burncamp
One of 32 camps in the United States that focus on children, ages 6–17 years, who have been hospitalized for burns.

International Shriners Headquarters
2900 Rocky Point Drive
Tampa, FL 33607-1435
800-237-5055 or 800-282-9161 (Florida) or 813-281-0300
Website: www.shriners.com
The Shriners maintain hospitals for children who have suffered burns.

CANCER

The Alpha Book on Cancer and Living
Alpha Institute
800-866-4111
Lists resources relating to children and cancer.

American Cancer Society
1599 Clifton, NE
Atlanta, GA 30329
800-ACS-2345 or 404-320-3333
Website: www.cancer.org

Association of Pediatric Oncology Nurses
4700 West Lake Avenue
Glenview, IL 60025
847-375-4724
Fax: 847-375-4777
e-mail: apon@amtec.com
Website: www.apon.org

Candlelighters Childhood Cancer Foundation
7910 Woodmont Avenue
Suite 460
Bethesda, MD 20814-3015
800-366-2223 or 301-657-8401
Fax: 301-718-2686
Website: www.candlelighters.org

The Center for Attitudinal Healing
33 Buchanan Drive
Sausalito, CA 94965
415-331-6161
Fax: 415-331-4545
Website: www.healingcenter.org
Provides support and bereavement services to children with cancer and other terminal illnesses.

Corporate Angel Network
Westchester County Airport
Building One
White Plains, NY 10604
914-328-1313
Website: www.corpangelnetwork.org
Nonprofit organization that coordinates free air transportation for ambulatory cancer patients traveling to and from treatment, checkups, and consultations.

Leukemia Society of America
600 3rd Avenue
New York, NY 10016
800-955-4572
Website: www.leukemia.org

Offers information and support to patients with leukemia, Hodgkin's disease, and lymphoma.

Make-A-Wish Foundation of America
100 West Clarendon
Suite 2200
Phoenix, AZ 85013
800-722-WISH (9474)
Fax: 602-279-0855
Website: www.wish.org
Grants wishes to children with life-threatening illnesses.

National Childhood Cancer Foundation
440 East Huntington Drive
Suite 300
Arcadia, CA 91066-6012
800-458-6223
Fax: 800-723-2822
Website: www.nccf.org

Ronald McDonald House Charities
1 Croc Drive
Oak Brook, IL 60523
630-623-7048
Website: www.rmhc.com
Provides housing near treatment centers for children with life-threatening diseases and their families.

Sunshine Kids Foundation
2814 Virginia
Houston, TX 77098
800-594-5756
Fax: 713-524-7165
e-mail: sunshine@hti.net
Website: www.hti.net/sunshine

CARDIOVASCULAR DISORDERS

American Heart Association
7272 Greenville Avenue
Dallas, TX 75231
214-373-6300
Website: www.americanheart.org

March of Dimes Birth Defects Foundation
1275 Mamaroneck Avenue
White Plains, NY 10605
914-428-7100
Website: www.modimes.org

CHILDBIRTH EDUCATION

American Academy of Husband-Coached Childbirth
P.O. Box 5224
Sherman Oaks, CA 91413-5224
800-4-A-BIRTH
Website: www.bradleybirth.org

International Childbirth Education Association (ICEA)
P.O. Box 20048
Minneapolis, MN 55420
612-854-8660
Fax: 612-854-8772
Website: www.icea.org

Lamaze International
1200 19th Street, NW
Suite 300
Washington, DC 20036-2422
800-368-4404 or 202-857-1128
Fax: 202-223-4579
e-mail: lamaze@dc.sba.com
Website: www.lamaze-childbirth.com

COMMUNICATION WITH CHILDREN

Association for the Care of Children's Health
19 Mantua Road
Mount Royal, NJ 08061
609-224-1742

Child Life Council, Inc.
11820 Parklawn Drive
Suite 202
Rockville, MD 20852-2529
301-881-7090
Fax: 301-881-7092
Website: www.childlife.org

Institute for Family-Centered Care
7900 Wisconsin Avenue
Suite 405
Bethesda, MD 20814
301-652-0281
Fax: 301-652-0186
Website: www.familycenteredcare.org

National Association for the Education of Young Children
1509 16th Street, NW
Washington, DC 20036-1426
800-424-2460
e-mail: naeyc@naeyc.org
Website: www.naeyc.org

Zero to Three
National Center for Infants, Toddlers, and Families
734 15th Street, NW
Suite 1000
Washington, DC 20005
202-638-1144
Fax: 202-638-0851
Website: www.zerotothree.org

CONTRACEPTION

Planned Parenthood Foundation of America
810 7th Avenue
New York, NY 10019
800-230-PLAN (directs callers to their nearest center)
Fax: 212-261-4560
Website: www.plannedparenthood.org

DEAFNESS, HEARING IMPAIRMENT

Alexander Graham Bell Association for the Deaf
3417 Volta Place, NW
Washington, DC 20007-2778
202-337-5220
Website: www.agbell.org

American Society for Deaf Children
1820 Tribute Road
Suite A
Sacramento, CA 95815
800-942-ASDC (parent hotline) or 916-641-6084 (voice, TTY)
Fax: 916-641-6085
Website: www.deafchildren.org

Helen Keller National Center for Deaf-Blind Youth and Adults
111 Middleneck Road
Sands Point, NY 11050
516-944-8900 (voice, TTY) or 516-944-8637 (TTY)
Fax: 516-944-7302
Website: www.helenkeller.org

National Information Center on Deafness
Gallaudet University
800 Florida Avenue, NE
Washington, DC 20002-3695
Website: www.gallaudet.edu/~nicd

DENTAL CARE

American Dental Association
Bureau of Health Education and Audiovisual Services
211 East Chicago Avenue
Chicago, IL 60611
312-440-2500
Fax: 312-440-2800
e-mail: online@ada.org
Website: www.ada.org

American Society of Dentistry for Children
211 East Chicago Avenue
Suite 920
Chicago, IL 69611
Website: www.cudental.creighton.edu/asdc

National Foundation of Dentistry for the Handicapped
1800 15th Street
Unit 100
Denver, CO 80202
303-534-5360
Fax: 303-534-5290

DEVELOPMENTAL MATERIALS

Denver Developmental Materials, Inc.
P.O. Box 6919
Denver, CO 80206-0919

DIABETES

American Association of Diabetes Educators
100 West Monroe Street
4th Floor
Chicago, IL 60603-1901
800-338-DMED or 312-424-2426
e-mail: aade@aadenet.org
Website: www.aadenet.org

American Diabetes Association
1660 Duke Street
Alexandria, VA 22314
800-DIABETES (800-342-2383) or 703-549-1500
Website: www.diabetes.org

Human Biological Database Interchange
1880 John F. Kennedy Boulevard
6th Floor
Philadelphia, PA 19103
800-222-6374 or 800-345-4234
Fax: 215-557-7154
Website: www.hbdi.org

International Diabetes Center
5000 West 39th Street
Minneapolis, MN 55416
612-927-3393
Website: www.idcdiabetes.com

Juvenile Diabetes Foundation International
120 Wall Street
New York, NY 10005
800-JDF-CURE or 212-785-9500
Fax: 212-785-9595
e-mail: info@jdfcure.com
Website: www.jdfcure.com

DOMESTIC VIOLENCE

See also *Abuse*

American Bar Association Commission on Domestic Violence
740 15th Street, NW
9th Floor
Washington, DC 20005-1002
Website: www.abanet.org/domviolence

Center for the Prevention of Sexual and Domestic Violence
936 North 34th
No. 200
Seattle, WA 98103
206-634-1903
Fax: 206-634-0115
Website: www.cpsdv.org
Provides educational materials for social service agencies, counselors, schools, lay and religious leaders, churches and synagogues, libraries, health care providers, law enforcement, and women's programs.

Domestic Violence Awareness Handbook
Website: www.usda.gov/da/shmd/aware
An online handbook distributed to government workers, but useful to all readers.

Domestic Violence Handbook
Website: www.domesticviolence.org
An online handbook for those who may be victims of domestic violence.

National Domestic Violence Hotline
P.O. Box 161810
Austin, TX 78716
800-799-SAFE (7233)
800-787-3224 (TTY)
e-mail: ndvh@ndvh.org (*E-mail is not confidential or secure!*)
Website: www.ndvh.org

GASTROINTESTINAL ALTERATIONS

American Celiac Society/Dietary Support Coalition
58 Musano Court
West Orange, NJ 07052
201-325-8837
Website: www.bentleac@umdnj.edu

American Cleft Palate–Craniofacial Association and
   Cleft Palate Foundation
104 South Estes Drive
Suite 204
Chapel Hill, NC 27514
919-933-9044
Fax: 919-933-9604
Website: www.cleft.com

American Pseudo-obstruction and Hirschsprung Disease Society
158 Pleasant Street
North Andover, MA 01845-2797
508-685-4477
Fax: 508-685-4488
e-mail: aphs@mail.tiac.net

Celiac-Sprue Association USA
P.O. Box 31700
Omaha, NE 68131-0700
402-558-0600
Fax: 402-558-1347
Website: www.csaceliacs.org

Crohn's and Colitis Foundation of America
386 Park Avenue South
17th Floor
New York, NY 10015
800-932-2423 or 212-685-3440
Fax: 212-779-4098
Website: www.ccfa.org

Directory of Digestive Diseases Organizations for Patients
National Digestive Diseases Information Clearinghouse
National Institute of Diabetes and Digestive and Kidney Diseases
National Institutes of Health
Website: www.niddk.nih.gov

Gluten Intolerance Group of North America
15110 10th Avenue, SW
Suite A
Seattle, WA 98166-1820
206-246-6652
Fax: 206-246-6531
e-mail: gig@accessone.com

March of Dimes Birth Defects Foundation
1275 Mamaroneck Avenue
White Plains, NY 10605
914-428-7100
Website: www.modimes.org

Pull-Thru Network
4 Woody Lane
Westport, CT 06880
203-221-7530
e-mail: pullthrunw@aol.com
Website: www.members.aol.com/pullthrunw/pullthru.htm
Information for parents of a child having a pull-through type of ostomy.

HEMATOLOGIC ALTERATIONS

Aplastic Anemia Foundation of America
P.O. Box 613
Annapolis, MD 21404
800-747-2820 or 410-867-0242
e-mail: aafacenter@aol.com
Website: www.aplastic.org

Cooley's Anemia Foundation and Thalassemia Action
  Group
129-90 26th Avenue
No. 203
Flushing, NY 11354
800-522-7222 or 718-321-CURE
Fax: 718-321-3340
e-mail: ncaf@aol.com
Website: www.thalassemia.org

The ITP Society*
333 East 38th Street
Room 830
New York, NY 10016
Website: www.ultranet.com/itpsoc
* Idiopathic Thrombocytopenic Purpura; formerly The
  Children's Blood Foundation.

National Hemophilia Foundation
116 West 32nd Street, 11th Floor
New York, NY 10001
HANDI phone: 800-42-HANDI or 212-328-3700
HANDI fax: 212-328-3799 or 212-328-3777
Website: www.hemophilia.org
HANDI is the National Hemophilia Foundation's information center to obtain facts on recommended treatment of bleeding disorders, practical issues of living
  with hemophilia or von Willebrand disease, hepatitis,
  HIV drugs and nutritional therapy, and financial issues. Services include Internet and MEDLINE searches,
  referrals to hemophilia treatment centers, and free
  publications for those with bleeding disorders. Hours
  are 9 A.M. to 5 P.M. Eastern time, Monday through
  Friday.

Sickle Cell Disease Association of America
200 Corporate Pointe
Suite 495
Culver City, CA 90230
800-421-8153 or 310-216-6363
Fax: 310-215-3722
Website: www.SickleCellDisease.org

INFERTILITY

RESOLVE, the National Infertility Association
1310 Broadway
Somerville, MA 02144
617-623-0744
e-mail: resolveinc@aol.com
Website: www.resolve.org

Society for Reproductive Medicine*
1209 Montgomery Highway
Birmingham, AL 35216-2809
205-978-5000
Fax: 205-978-5005
e-mail: asrm@asrm.org
Website: www.asrm.org
Has a nurse special interest group as well as patient infor-
  mation and links to other related websites.
* Formerly the American Fertility Society.

LATEX ALLERGY

Latex Allergy Information Service
176 Roosevelt Avenue
Torrington, CT 06790
860-482-6867
Fax: 860-482-7640
Website: www.familyvillage.wisc.edu
Publishes *Latex Allergy Newsletter* 11 times a year.

MENTAL RETARDATION

American Association of Mental Retardation
444 North Capitol Street, NW
Suite 846
Washington, DC 20001-1512
800-424-3688 or 202-387-1968
Fax: 202-387-2193
e-mail: mailbox@aamr.org
Website: www.aamr.org

The ARC*
800 East Border Street
Suite 300
Arlington, TX 76010
817-261-6003
Fax: 817-277-3491
e-mail: thearc@metronet.com
Website: www.thearc.org
* Formerly Association of Retarded Citizens.

National Down Syndrome Society
666 Broadway
8th Floor
New York, NY 10012-2317
800-221-4602 or 212-460-9330
Fax: 212-979-2873
Website: www.ndss.org

National Fragile-X Foundation
1441 York Street
Suite 303
Denver, CO 80206
800-688-8765 or 303-333-6155
Fax: 303-333-4369
e-mail: info@fragileX.org
Website: www.nfxf.org

MUSCULOSKELETAL ALTERATIONS

Arthritis Foundation
1300 West Peachtree Street
Atlanta, GA 30309
404-872-7100
Website: www.arthritis.org

Arthritis Society (Canada)
393 University Avenue
Suite 1700
Toronto, Ontario, Canada M5G 1E6
416-979-7228

Muscular Dystrophy Association of America, Inc.
3300 East Sunrise Drive
Tucson, AZ 85718
800-572-1717
e-mail: mda@mdausa.org
Website: www.mdausa.org

Muscular Dystrophy Association of Canada
2345 Yonge Street
Suite 900
Toronto, Ontario, Canada M4P 2E5
800-567-3873 or 416-488-0030
Fax: 416-488-7523
Website: www.mdac.ca

National Scoliosis Foundation, Inc.
5 Cabot Place
Stoughton, MA 02072
617-341-6333
Fax: 617-341-8333
e-mail: scoliosis@aol.com

Scoliosis Association, Inc.
P.O. Box 811705
Boca Raton, FL 33481-1705
800-800-0669

Osteogenesis Imperfecta Foundation, Inc.
804 West Diamond Avenue
Suite 210
Gaithersburg, MD 20878
301-947-0083
Fax: 301-947-0456
e-mail: bonelink@aol.com
Website: www.oif.org

NEUROLOGIC ALTERATIONS

Epilepsy Foundation
4351 Garden City Drive
Landover, MD 20785
800-EFA-1000 or 301-459-3700
Fax: 301-577-4941
e-mail: info@efa.org
Website: www.efa.org
Foundation has a special section on epilepsy and women.

Hydrocephalus Association
870 Market Street
Suite 955
San Francisco, CA 94102
415-732-7040
Fax: 415-732-7044
e-mail: hydroassoc@aol.com
Website: www.neurosurgery.mgh.harvard.edu

Hydrocephalus Foundation, Inc.
910 Rear Broadway
Saugus, MA 01906
Website: www.hydrocephalus.org

Spina Bifida Association
800-621-3141 or 202-944-3285
Fax: 202-944-3295
e-mail: ir@sbaa.org
Website: www.sbaa.org
Contains information and links to related sites. Also contains information on Agent Orange and latex allergy.

United Cerebral Palsy
1660 L Street, NW
Suite 700
Washington, DC 20036

800-872-5827
Fax: 202-776-0414
Website: www.ucpa.org/ucpnatl@upca.org
Related resource: Website that has links to other websites related to spina bifida: www.spinabifida.net

NUTRITION

American Dietetic Association
216 West Jackson Boulevard
Suite 800
Chicago, IL 60606-6995
800-877-1600 or 312-899-0040
Fax: 312-899-1979
Website: www.eatright.org

Clearinghouse on Infant Feeding and Maternal Nutrition
American Public Health Association
1015 15th Street, NW
Suite 300
Washington, DC 20005
202-789-5600
Fax: 202-789-5661
Website: www.apha.org

Food Research and Action Center
1875 Connecticut Avenue, NW
Suite 540
Washington, DC 20009
202-986-2200
Fax: 202-986-2525
Website: www.frac.org

International Lactation Consultant Association
4101 Lake Boone Trail
Raleigh, NC 27607
919-787-5181
Fax: 919-787-4916
Website: www.ilca.org

LaLeche League International
1400 North Meacham Road
Schaumburg, IL 60173-4840
800-525-3243 or 847-519-7730
Fax: 847-519-0035
Website: www.lalecheleague.org

National Dairy Council
O'Hare International Center
10255 West Higgins Road
Suite 900
Rosemont, IL 60018
800-426-8271
Website: www.nationaldairycouncil.org

PAIN IN CHILDREN

The Association for the Care of Children's Health
19 Mantua Road
Mt. Royal, NJ 08061
800-888-ACCH

Center for Research Dissemination and Liaison
AHCPR Publications Clearinghouse
P.O. Box 8547
Silver Spring, MD 20907
800-325-9295

City of Hope National Medical Center
Department of Nursing Research and Education
c/o Pain Resource Center
1500 East Duarte Road
Duarte, CA 91010
626-359-8111, ext. 2825 (Dir. Betty Ferrell)
Website: http://mayday.coh.org

International Association for the Study for Pain
IASP Secretary
909 NE 43rd Street
Room 306
Seattle, WA 98105-6021
206-547-6409
e-mail: IASP@locke.hs.washington.edu

Pediatric Pain Listserv
MAILSERV@ac.dal.ca.
First line of the message should read as follows: subscribe
  PEDIATRIC-PAIN

Books

A Child in Pain: How to Help, What To Do (1996)
L. Kuttner
Harltey & Marks, Publishers
Vancouver, British Columbia
Canada

Pain in Infants, Children, and Adolescents: An Overview
  (1993)
N. Schechter, C. Berde, and M. Yaster (Eds.)
Baltimore: Williams & Wilkins

Assessment Tools

Nancy Hester, PhD, RN, FAAN
Professor, School of Nursing
Campus Box 288-10
University of Colorado Health Sciences Center
4200 East 9th Avenue
Denver, CO 80262
e-mail: nancy.hester@uchsc.edu
Poker chip pain assessment tool.

Marilyn Savedra, DNS, RN
Professor Emeritus
University of California, San Francisco, School of Nursing
Box 0606, N411Y
San Francisco, CA 94143
General e-mail: data_at_nursing@ccmail.ucsf.edu
Website: www.nurseweb.ucsf.edu
Adolescent pain assessment tool.

PREGNANCY AND BIRTH

American Society for Psychoprophylaxis in Obstetrics
1200 19th Street, NW
Suite 300
Washington, DC 20036
800-368-4404 or 202-857-1128
Fax: 202-223-4579

Healthy Start National Resource Center
National Center for Education in Maternal and Child
  Health

Georgetown University
2000 15th Street, N
Suite 701
Arlington, VA 22201-2617
703-524-7802
Fax: 703-524-9335
e-mail: HealthyStart@ncemch.org
Website: www.healthystart.net

RESPIRATORY ALTERATIONS

General

American Academy of Allergy and Immunology
611 East Wells Street
Milwaukee, WI 53202
800-822-2762 or 414-272-6071
Website: www.aaaai.org

American Allergy Association
P.O. Box 7273
Menlo Park, CA 94026
415-272-6071
e-mail: allergyaid@aol.com

American Lung Association
1740 Broadway
New York, NY 10019
800-LUNG-USA (800-586-4872) or 212-315-8704
Website: www.lungusa.org

American SIDS Institute
6065 Roswell Road
Suite 876
Atlanta, GA 30328
404-843-1030
Fax: 404-843-0577
Website: www.sids.org

Asthma and Allergy Foundation of America
1125 15th Street, NW
Suite 502
Washington, DC 20005
800-7-ASTHMA or 202-466-7643
Fax: 202-466-8940
Website: www.aafa.org

National Jewish Medical Research Center
1400 Jackson Street
Denver, CO 80206
800-222-LUNG or 303-388-4461
Website: www.njc.org

National Allergy and Asthma Network
Mothers of Asthmatics
2715 Prosperity Avenue
Suite 150
Fairfax, VA 22031
800-878-4403 or 703-641-9595
Fax: 703-573-7794
Website: www.aanma.org

National Asthma Education and Prevention Program
National Heart, Lung and Blood Institute Information
  Center
National Institutes of Health

P.O. Box 30105
Bethesda, MD 20824-0105
301-251-1222
Fax: 301-251-1223
Website: www.nhlbisupport.com/asthma

National Sudden Infant Death Syndrome Resource Center
Health Resources and Services Administration
Tycon Courthouse
2070 Chain Bridge Road
Suite 450
Vienna, VA 22182
703-821-8955, extension 249
Fax: 703-821-2098
Website: www.circsol.com/SIDS

Resources for Self-Management of Respiratory Problems

Asthma Care Training for Kids
Asthma and Allergy Foundation of America
Ordering address:
220 Boylston Street
Chestnut Hill, MA 02176
617-965-7771
Fax: 617-965-8886

CALM: Childhood Asthma: Learning to Manage
Asthma and Allergy Foundation of America
(see contact information under *Asthma and Allergy Foundation of America*)

Children with Asthma: A Manual for Parents
Pedipress, Inc.
125 Redgate Lane
Amherst, MA 01002
800-611-6081 or 413-549-4095
Fax: 413-549-4095
Website: www.pedipress.com

Superstuff
American Lung Association
(see contact information under *American Lung Association*)

SAFETY

American Academy of Pediatrics
The Injury Prevention Program
141 Northwest Point Boulevard
Elk Grove Village, IL 60007-1098
800-433-9016 or 847-228-5005
Fax: 847-228-5097
Website: www.aap.org
The Injury Prevention Program (TIPP) is a multipart parent and child safety education program consisting of age-related parent surveys, brochures and handouts related to common causes of childhood accidents, child activity sheets, and first aid care.

American Spinal Injury Association
250 East Superior Street
Room 1436
Chicago, IL 60611
312-908-1242
Fax: 312-503-0869
Website: www.asia-spinalinjury.org

American Trauma Society
8903 Presidential Parkway
Suite 512
Upper Marlboro, MD 20772-2652
800-556-7890 or 301-420-4189
Website: www.amtrauma.org

Consumer Product Safety Commission
Washington, DC 20207
800-638-CPSC
Website: www.cpsc.gov

Harborview Injury Prevention and Research Center
University of Washington
325 9th Avenue
P.O. Box 359960
Seattle, WA 98104
206-521-1520
Fax: 206-521-1562
Website: www.weber.u.washington.edu/~hiprc

National Head Injury Foundation
1776 Massachusetts Avenue, NW
Suite 100
Washington, DC 20036
800-444-6443 or 202-296-6443

National Head and Spinal Cord Injury Prevention Program
American Association of Neurological Surgeons and Congress of Neurosurgical Surgeons
22 South Washington Street
Park Ridge, IL 60068
708-692-9500
Website: www.aans.org

National Highway Traffic Safety Administration
400 7th Street, SW
Washington, DC 20590
Website: www.nhtsa.dot.gov/nhtsa

National Rifle Association of America
Safety and Education Department
1600 Rhode Island Avenue, NW
Washington, DC 20036
Website: www.nra.org

National Safekids Campaign
1301 Pennsylvania Avenue, NW
Suite 1000
Washington, DC 20004-1707
202-662-0600
Fax: 202-393-2072

National Safety Council
1121 Spring Lake Drive
Itasca, IL 60143-3201
630-285-1121
Fax: 630-285-1315
Website: nsc.org

SCIPP/Statewide Comprehensive Injury Prevention Program
Massachusetts Department of Public Health
Division of Family Health Services
150 Tremont Street
Boston, MA 02111
617-727-1246
Website: www.magnet.state.ma.us/dph/unipp

SELF-CARE, CHILDREN (BOOKS)

Latchkey Kids: Unlocking Doors for Children and Their Families (1998)
Suzanne Lamorey and Bryan E. Robinson
Sage Publications
ISBN: 0761912606

Self-Care for Children
Mississippi Cooperative Extension Service
Website: www. exnet.iastate.edu/Pages/families/nncc/
  Choose.Quality.Care/selfcare.html

Teaching Your Child to Be Home Alone (1994)
Earl A. Grollman and Gerri L. Sweder
Jossey-Bass, Inc.
ISBN: 0029127513

TERMINAL ILLNESS SUPPORT, GRIEF, AND BEREAVEMENT

Association Resources
638 Prospect Avenue
Hartford, CT 06105-4250
860-586-7523
Fax: 860-586-7550
Website: www.associationresources.com
Professional organization for death education and
  counseling.

Bereavement/RTS*
Gunderson Lutheran Medical Center
1910 South Avenue
LaCrosse, WI 54601
800-362-9567, extension 4747
Organization for support of parents experiencing
  pregnancy loss or loss of a child during early
  infancy.
* Formerly Resolve Through Sharing.

The Center for Attitudinal Healing
33 Buchanan Drive
Sausalito, CA 94965
415-331-6161
Fax: 415-331-4545
Website: www.healingcenter.org
Provides support and bereavement services to children
  with cancer and other terminal illnesses.

Children's Hospice International
2202 Mt. Vernon Avenue
Suite 3C
Alexandria, VA 22301
703-684-0330
Fax: 703-684-0226

Compassionate Friends
P.O. Box 3696
Oak Brook, IL 60522-3696
630-990-0010
Fax: 630-990-0246
Website: www.compassionatefriends.org
Provides support for parents who have lost children
  through death.

Dougy Center for Grieving Children and Families
3909 SE 52nd Avenue
P.O. Box 86852
Portland, OR 97286
503-775-5683
Fax: 503-777-3097

Hospicelink
Hospice Education Institute
190 Westbrook Road
Essex, CT 06426-1511
800-331-1620 or 203-767-1620
Fax: 203-767-2746
Website: www.hospiceworld.org

Make-A-Wish Foundation of America
100 West Clarendon
Suite 2200
Phoenix, AZ 85013
800-722-WISH (9474)
Fax: 602-279-0855
Website: www.wish.org
Grants wishes to children with life-threatening illnesses.

Ronald McDonald House Charities
1 Croc Drive
Oak Brook, IL 60523
630-623-7048
Website: www.rmhc.com
Provides housing near treatment centers for children with
  life-threatening diseases and their families.

SHARE: Pregnancy and Infant Loss Support, Inc.
St. Joseph Health Center
300 First Capitol Drive
St. Charles, MO 63301-2893
800-821-6819 or 314-974-6164
Fax: 314-947-7486
e-mail: share@nationalshareoffice.com
Website: www.nationalshareoffice.com

Starlight Foundation
12424 Wilshire Boulevard
Suite 1050
Los Angeles, CA 90025
800-274-STAR
Fax: 310-207-2554
Website: www.starlight.org
Grants wishes and provides in-hospital entertainment for
  children with life-threatening illnesses.

The Warm Place
1510 Cooper Street
Fort Worth, TX 76104

Periodicals and On-Line Services

Bereavement: A Magazine of Hope and Healing
Bereavement Publishing, Inc.
5125 North Union Boulevard
Suite 4
Colorado Springs, CO 80918
719-266-0006
e-mail: grief@usa.net
Website: www.bereavementmag.com

Inside Fernside and *Fernside Online*
Fernside: A Center for Grieving Children
2303 Indian Mound Avenue
Cincinnati, OH 45212
513-841-1012
Fax: 513-841-1546
e-mail: info@fernside.org
Website: www.fernside.org
Newsletter and on-line service for children affected
by loss.

The Forum Newsletter
Association for Death Education and Counseling
533 Stagg Lane
Santa Cruz, CA 95062
408-475-6527
Website: www.adec.org

Professional Journals

Death Studies
Robert A. Neimeyer, Ed.
Taylor & Francis Books
47 Runway Road
Suite G
Levittown, PA 19057-4000
800-821-8312 (orders)
215-269-0368 (faxed orders)
Website: www.taylorandfrancis.com
Available as an on-line publication.

WOMEN'S HEALTH

JAMA Women's Health Information Center
Website: www.ama-assn.org/special/womh/womh.htm

National Women's Health Information Center
United States Public Health Service Office on Women's
Health
United States Department of Health and Human Ser-
vices
800-994-WOMAN
Website: www.forwoman.org

M

Nutrient Charts

Food and Nutrition Board, National Academy of Sciences—National Research Council Recommended Dietary Allowances,[a] Revised 1989 (Abridged)

Designed for the maintenance of good nutrition of practically all healthy people in the United States

Category	Age (years) or Condition	Weight[b] (kg)	(lb)	Height[b] (cm)	(in)	Protein (g)	Vitamin A (µg RE)[c]	Vitamin E (mg α-TE)[d]	Vitamin K (µg)	Vitamin C (mg)	Iron (mg)	Zinc (mg)	Iodine (µg)	Selenium (µg)
Infants	0.0–0.5	6	13	60	24	13	375	3	5	30	6	5	40	10
	0.5–1.0	9	20	71	28	14	375	4	10	35	10	5	50	15
Children	1–3	13	29	90	35	16	400	6	15	40	10	10	70	20
	4–6	20	44	112	44	24	500	7	20	45	10	10	90	20
	7–10	28	62	132	52	28	700	7	30	45	10	10	120	30
Males	11–14	45	99	157	62	45	1,000	10	45	50	12	15	150	40
	15–18	66	145	176	69	59	1,000	10	65	60	12	15	150	50
	19–24	72	160	177	70	58	1,000	10	70	60	10	15	150	70
	25–50	79	174	176	70	63	1,000	10	80	60	10	15	150	70
	51+	77	170	173	68	63	1,000	10	80	60	10	15	150	70
Females	11–14	46	101	157	62	46	800	8	45	50	15	12	150	45
	15–18	55	120	163	64	44	800	8	55	60	15	12	150	50
	19–24	58	128	164	65	46	800	8	60	60	15	12	150	55
	25–50	63	138	163	64	50	800	8	65	60	15	12	150	55
	51+	65	143	160	63	50	800	8	65	60	10	12	150	55
Pregnant						60	800	10	65	70	30	15	175	65
Lactating	1st 6 mo					65	1,300	12	65	95	15	19	200	75
	2nd 6 mo					62	1,200	11	65	90	15	16	200	75

Note: This table does not include nutrients for which dietary reference intakes have recently been established (see *Dietary Reference Intakes for Calcium, Phosphorus, Magnesium, Vitamin D, and Fluoride* [1997] and *Dietary Reference Intakes for Thiamin, Riboflavin, Niacin, Vitamin B₆, Folate, Vitamin B₁₂, Pantothenic Acid, Biotin, and Choline* [1998]).

[a] The allowances, expressed as average daily intakes over time, are intended to provide for individual variations among most normal persons as they live in the United States under usual environmental stresses. Diets should be based on a variety of common foods in order to provide other nutrients for which human requirements have been less well defined.

[b] Weights and heights of reference adults are actual medians for the U.S. population of the designated age, as reported by NHANES II. The median weights and heights of those under 19 years of age were taken from Hamill et al. (1979). The use of these figures does not imply that the height-to-weight ratios are ideal.

[c] Retinol equivalents. 1 retinol equivalent = 1 µg retinol or 6 µg β-carotene.

[d] α-Tocopherol equivalents. 1 mg d-α tocopherol = 1 α-TE.

Food and Nutrition Board, Institute of Medicine—National Academy of Sciences Dietary Reference Intakes: Recommended Intakes for Individuals

Life-Stage Group	Calcium (mg/d)	Phosphorus (mg/d)	Magnesium (mg/d)	Vitamin D (μg/d)[a,b]	Fluoride (mg/d)	Thiamin (mg/d)	Riboflavin (mg/d)	Niacin (mg/d)[c]	Vitamin B_6 (mg/d)	Folate (μg/d)[d]	Vitamin B_{12} (μg/d)	Pantothenic Acid (mg/d)	Biotin (μg/d)	Choline (mg/d)[e]
Infants														
0–6 mo	210*	100*	30*	5*	0.01*	0.2*	0.3*	2*	0.1*	65*	0.4*	1.7*	5*	125*
7–12 mo	270*	275*	75*	5*	0.5*	0.3*	0.4*	4*	0.3*	80*	0.5*	1.8*	6*	150*
Children														
1–3 yr	500*	460	80	5*	0.7*	0.5	0.5	6	0.5	150	0.9	2*	8*	200*
4–8 yr	800*	500	130	5*	1*	0.6	0.6	8	0.6	200	1.2	3*	12*	250*
Males														
9–13 yr	1,300*	1,250	240	5*	2*	0.9	0.9	12	1.0	300	1.8	4*	20*	375*
14–18 yr	1,300*	1,250	410	5*	3*	1.2	1.3	16	1.3	400	2.4	5*	25*	550*
19–30 yr	1,000*	700	400	5*	4*	1.2	1.3	16	1.3	400	2.4	5*	30*	550*
31–50 yr	1,000*	700	420	5*	4*	1.2	1.3	16	1.3	400	2.4	5*	30*	550*
51–70 yr	1,200*	700	420	10*	4*	1.2	1.3	16	1.7	400	2.4[f]	5*	30*	550*
>70 yr	1,200*	700	420	15*	4*	1.2	1.3	16	1.7	400	2.4[f]	5*	30*	550*
Females														
9–13 yr	1,300*	1,250	240	5*	2*	0.9	0.9	12	1.0	300	1.8	4*	20*	375*
14–18 yr	1,300*	1,250	360	5*	3*	1.0	1.0	14	1.2	400[g]	2.4	5*	25*	400*
19–30 yr	1,000*	700	310	5*	3*	1.1	1.1	14	1.3	400[g]	2.4	5*	30*	425*
31–50 yr	1,000*	700	320	5*	3*	1.1	1.1	14	1.3	400[g]	2.4	5*	30*	425*
51–70 yr	1,200*	700	320	10*	3*	1.1	1.1	14	1.5	400	2.4[f]	5*	30*	425*
>70 yr	1,200*	700	320	15*	3*	1.1	1.1	14	1.5	400	2.4[f]	5*	30*	425*
Pregnancy														
≤18 yr	1,300*	1,250	400	5*	3*	1.4	1.4	18	1.9	600[h]	2.6	6*	30*	450*
19–30 yr	1,000*	700	350	5*	3*	1.4	1.4	18	1.9	600[h]	2.6	6*	30*	450*
31–50 yr	1,000*	700	360	5*	3*	1.4	1.4	18	1.9	600[h]	2.6	6*	30*	450*
Lactation														
≤18 yr	1,300*	1,250	360	5*	3*	1.5	1.6	17	2.0	500	2.8	7*	35*	550*
19–30 yr	1,000*	700	310	5*	3*	1.5	1.6	17	2.0	500	2.8	7*	35*	550*
31–50 yr	1,000*	700	320	5*	3*	1.5	1.6	17	2.0	500	2.8	7*	35*	550*

Note: This table presents recommended dietary allowances (RDAs) in **bold type** and adequate intakes (AIs) in ordinary type followed by an asterisk (*). RDAs and AIs may both be used as goals for individual intake. RDAs are set to meet the needs of almost all (97% to 98%) individuals in a group. For healthy breast-fed infants, the AI is the mean intake. The AI for other life-stage and gender groups is believed to cover needs of all individuals in the group, but lack of data or uncertainty in the data prevent being able to specify with confidence the percentage of individuals covered by this intake.

a As cholecalciferol. 1 μg cholecalciferol = 40 IU vitamin D.

b In the absence of adequate exposure to sunlight.

c As niacin equivalents (NE). 1 mg of niacin = 60 mg of tryptophan; 0–6 months = preformed niacin (not NE).

d As dietary folate equivalents (DFE). 1 DFE = 1 μg food folate = 0.6 μg of folic acid (from fortified food or supplement) consumed with food = 0.5 μg of synthetic (supplemental) folic acid taken on an empty stomach.

e Although AIs have been set for choline, there are few data to assess whether a dietary supply of choline is needed at all stages of the life cycle, and it may be that the choline requirement can be met by endogenous synthesis at some of these stages.

f Because 10% to 30% of older people may malabsorb food-bound B_{12}, it is advisable for those older than 50 years to meet their RDA mainly by consuming foods fortified with B_{12} or a supplement containing B_{12}.

g In view of evidence linking folate intake with neural tube defects in the fetus, it is recommended that all women capable of becoming pregnant consume 400 μg of synthetic folic acid from fortified foods and/or supplements in addition to intake of food folate from a varied diet.

h It is assumed that women will continue consuming 400 μg of folic acid until their pregnancy is confirmed and they enter prenatal care, which ordinarily occurs after the end of the periconceptional period—the critical time for formation of the neural tube.

• • • • • • • • •

Estimated Safe and Adequate Daily Dietary Intakes of Selected Vitamins and Minerals*

Category	Age (years)	Vitamins	
		Biotin (μg)	Pantothenic Acid (mg)
Infants	0–0.5	10	2
	0.5–1	15	3
Children and adolescents	1–3	20	3
	4–6	25	4–1
	7–10	30	4–5
	11+	30–100	4–7
Adults		30–100	4–7

Category	Age (years)	Trace Elements†				
		Copper (mg)	Manganese (mg)	Fluoride (μg)	Chromium (μg)	Molybdenum (mg)
Infants	0–0.5	0.4–0.6	0.3–0.6	0.1–0.5	10–40	15–30
	0.5–1	0.6–0.7	0.6–1.0	0.2–1.0	20–60	20–40
Children and adolescents	1–3	0.7–1.0	1.0–1.5	0.5–1.5	20–80	25–50
	4–6	1.0–1.5	1.5–2.0	1.0–2.5	30–120	30–75
	7–10	1.0–2.0	2.0–3.0	1.5–2.5	50–200	50–150
	11+	1.5–2.5	2.0–5.0	1.5–2.5	50–200	75–250
Adults		1.5–3.0	2.0–5.0	1.5–4.0	50–200	75–250

* Because there is less information on which to base allowances, these figures are not given in the main table of RDA and are provided here in the form of ranges of recommended intakes.

† Since the toxic levels for many trace elements may be only several times usual intakes, the upper levels for the trace elements given in this table should not be habitually exceeded.

Data from National Research Council, Food and Nutrition Board, National Academy of Sciences, 1989. Williams, S. R. (1994). *Essentials of nutrition and diet therapy* (6th ed.). St. Louis: Mosby.

• • • • • • • • •

Estimated Sodium, Chloride, and Potassium Minimum Requirements of Healthy Persons*

Age	Weight (kg)*	Sodium (mg)*,†	Chloride (mg)*,†	Potassium (mg)‡
Months				
0–5	4.5	120	180	500
6–11	8.9	200	300	700
Years				
1	11.0	225	350	1,000
2–5	16.0	300	500	1,400
6–9	25.0	400	600	1,600
10–18	50.0	500	750	2,000
>18§	70.0	500	750	2,000

* No allowance has been included for large, prolonged losses from the skin through sweat.

† There is no evidence that higher intakes confer any health benefit.

‡ Desirable intakes of potassium may considerably exceed these values (>3,500 mg for adults).

§ No allowance included for growth. Values for those below 18 years assume a growth rate at 50th percentile reported by the National Center for Health Statistics and averaged for males and females.

Data from National Research Council, Food and Nutrition Board, National Academy of Sciences, 1989. Williams, S. R. (1994). *Essentials of nutrition and diet therapy* (6th ed.). St. Louis: Mosby.

Note: Page numbers in *italics* refer to figures; page numbers followed by d refer to displayed material; page numbers followed by p refer to procedures; page numbers followed by t refer to tables.

Index

Nursing process *(Continued)*
nursing diagnosis in, 37
planning in, 36d, 37
collaborative problems in, 38
Nursing research, 38
Nutrient density, definition of, 310
Nutrients, definition of, 54
Nutrition, 74d, 74–76. See also *Diet; Feeding; Food(s).*
assessment of, 75–76
culture and, family adjustment to newborn and, 507
dietary guidelines for, 74–75, 75d
during pregnancy, 311–326
abnormal prepregnancy weight and, 325
age and, 321
anemia and, 325
culture and, 319–321, 320t
eating disorders and, 325
energy requirements for, 312–313
folic acid for, 316
Food Guide Pyramid and, *318,* 318–319, 319t
in adolescents, 321–323
lactose intolerance and, 325
minerals for, 316d, 316–317
multiparity and, 326
nausea and vomiting and, 325
nursing care plan for, 328–331
nutritional supplementation for, 317–318
pica and, 325–326
protein requirements for, 313
recommended dietary allowances for, 312, 312t, 1638–1640
socioeconomic status and, 321
substance use and abuse and, 326
to prevent preterm birth, 698
vegetarianism and, 324t, 324–325
vitamins for, 313, 314t–315t, 316, 316d
water in, 318
weight gain and, 311t, 311–312, *312*
pediatric, growth and development and, 58
in biliary atresia, 1155
in bronchopulmonary dysplasia, 1236
in diabetes mellitus, 1451
in Hirschsprung disease, 1146
in postpartum period, teaching about, 495
of adolescents, 163, 164t, 166, 166d
of dying children, 941–942
of infants, 91t, 93–96, 94d
failure to thrive and. See *Failure to thrive.*
of newborns, 589, 589d
of preschoolers, 116t, 118d, 118–119
of preterm infants, 743–748
in cases of hyperbilirubinemia, 765
of school-age children, 139, 140t–141t, 142
of toddlers, 116t, 118d, 118–119
postpartum, 326–328
for lactating mothers, 327–328
for nonlactating mothers, 328
recommended dietary allowances for, 1638–1640
resources for, 1633
Nystagmus, definition of, 1555
end-stage, 841

Obesity, in school-age children, 141–142
Object permanence, 83, 110
Oblique fractures, in pediatric patients, 1410d
Oblique lie, 359
Observation, 24-hour, 902
Obstetric history, in antepartum care, 275
Obtundation, definition of, 824
Occult bleeding, definition of, 1106

Occult blood test, in pediatric patients, 1110d, 1598
Occult prolapse. See *Prolapsed cord.*
Occupational Safety and Health Administration, 19
Occupational therapy, for juvenile arthritis, 1419
Oculomotor nerve, assessment of, in pediatric patients, 860t
Oedipal stage, 59t
Ofloxacin, during pregnancy and lactation, 1583
Olfactory nerve, assessment of, in pediatric patients, 860t
Oligohydramnios, 183, 255, 337
definition of, 453, 686
Oligospermia, definition of, 190
Oliguria, definition of, 1085
Omphalocele, 1120t–1123t
Onlooker play, 69, *69*
Oogenesis, 239t, 239–240, *240*
definition of, 238
Oophoritis, 726
Open fractures, 1410d
Open head injury, 1488
Ophthalmia neonatorum, 542, 1564
definition of, 562, 1555
Ophthalmic medications, administration of, to pediatric patients, 1002, 1002p
Ophthalmoscopic examination, 843
Opiate(s), abuse of, during pregnancy, 616t, 618, 620
in pediatric patients, 1521t
definition of, 607
Opioid analgesics, during pregnancy and lactation, 1580–1581
for labor pain, 437t, 437–438, 449t
epidural, 438–440, *439,* 449t
intrathecal, 440–441, 449t
for pediatric pain, 1023–1024
Opioid antagonists, in labor, 437t, 438
Optic chiasm, 1466
Optic nerve, assessment of, in pediatric patients, 860t
Oral care, for dying children, 941–942
Oral contraceptives, 192t, 193t, 197–199, 198d, 198t, 199t
definition of, 190
during pregnancy and lactation, 1585
Oral feeding. See also *Breast-feeding; Formula-feeding.*
for preterm infants, 745, *745*
Oral glucose tolerance test, in gestational diabetes mellitus, 664
Oral hygiene, for infants and children, 954
Oral hypoglycemic agents, during pregnancy and lactation, 1582
Oral rehydration therapy, for pediatric patients, with diarrhea, 1097–1098
for vomiting, in pediatric patients, 1103
Oral route, medication absorption and, in pediatric patients, 992
medication administration by, in pediatric patients, 996–997, *997*
Oral stage, 59t
Oral temperature measurement, in pediatric patients, 956
Orientation, in newborns, assessment of, 559
Oropharyngeal airways, assessment of, 887d
Oropharynx, 1192
assessment of, in pediatric patients, 839
Orthopnea, definition of, 1191
Orthoses, definition of, 1384
Osgood-Schlatter disease, 1413–1414
nursing care for, 1413–1414
Osmolality, in pediatric patients, 1598

Osmotic diuresis, definition of, 631
Ossification, definition of, 1384
Osteoblastic, definition of, 1384
Osteochondritis deformans juvenilis, 1406d, 1406–1408
nursing care for, 1407–1408
Osteochondrosis, definition of, 1384
Osteoclastic, definition of, 1384
Osteogenesis imperfecta, 1414, 1414d
Osteomyelitis, 1391
in pediatric patients, 1414–1416, 1415d
nursing care for, 1415–1416
Osteoporosis, 795, 795–796
definition of, 778
Osteosarcoma, in pediatric patients, 1337–1339
nursing care for, 1338–1339
Osteotomy, definition of, 1384
Ostomy care, in pediatric patients, 975, 976p
Otic medications, administration of, to pediatric patients, 1002, 1003p
Otitis media, in pediatric patients, 1200–1204
diagnostic evaluation of, 1200
etiology and incidence of, 1200
management of, 1202–1203
manifestations of, 1200, *1202*
nursing care for, 1203–1204
pathophysiology of, 1201d
Otoacoustic emissions, evoked, as hearing test, in infants, 1570d
Otoscopic examination, 843, *844*
Oucher pain scale, 1019, 1019t, 1020t
Outcomes, expected, establishing, 37
Outcomes management, 8
Outer ear, 1556, 1557
Outpatient clinics, in postpartum period, 512
Outpatient facilities, as care setting, 903
for pediatric patients, 903
Ovarian artery, 231
Ovarian cycle, 233
Ovarian cysts, 798
Ovarian hyperstimulation syndrome, 213
Ovarian ligaments, 231
Ovarian veins, 231
Ovaries, *228,* 230, 1432
during pregnancy, 262
Overhydration, in preterm infants, signs of, 740–741, 741d
Overinvolvement, 814
signs of, 814d
Overstimulation, in preterm infants, 742–743
signs of, 742d
Oviduct(s), *228,* 229–230
disorders of, infertility and, 208–209
ligation of, 196
definition of, 190
pregnancy in. See *Pregnancy, ectopic.*
Ovovegetarians, definition of, 310
Ovulation, definition of, 238
detection of, for natural family planning, 201, 203, 203p–205p
disorders of, infertility and, 208
induction of, 213
inhibition of, by breast-feeding, 206
prediction of, in infertility, 212t
resumption of, following delivery, 480
Ovulation method, for natural family planning, 203
Ovulatory phase, of ovarian cycle, 233
Ovum(a), fusion with sperm, 242
release of, 241
sperm's entry into, 242
transport of, 241
Oxygen, partial pressure, in pediatric patients, 1598
Oxygen consumption, during pregnancy, 265
Oxygen hoods, for pediatric oxygen therapy, 977

Normal Vital Signs by Age

Age	Temperature*		Pulse Rate (BPM)	Respiratory Rate (breaths/min)	Blood Pressure (mm Hg)
	Fahrenheit	Celsius			
Newborn	96.8–99 (axillary)	36–37.2 (axillary)	120–160	30–60	Systolic: 46–92 Diastolic: 38–71
3 Years	97.5–98.6 (axillary)	36.4–37 (axillary)	80–125	20–30	Systolic: 72–110 Diastolic: 40–73
10 Years	97.5–98.6 (oral)	36.4–37 (oral)	70–110†	16–22	Systolic: 83–121 Diastolic: 45–79
16 Years	97.5–98.6 (oral)	36.4–37 (oral)	55–90	15–20	Systolic: 93–131‡ Diastolic: 49–85

* The normal range of the child's temperature will depend on the measuring method used. Temperatures exhibit circadian rhythms at all ages.

† After age 12 years, a boy's pulse is 5 BPM slower than a girl's.

‡ After age 14 years, blood pressure in boys is higher than in girls.

Temperature Equivalents: Celsius and Fahrenheit

Celsius	Fahrenheit	Celsius	Fahrenheit
34.0	93.2	38.4	101.1
34.2	93.6	38.6	101.4
34.4	93.9	38.8	101.8
34.6	94.3	39.0	102.2
34.8	94.6	39.2	102.5
35.0	95.0	39.4	102.9
35.2	95.4	39.6	103.2
35.4	95.7	39.8	103.6
35.6	96.1	40.0	104.0
35.8	96.4	40.2	104.3
36.0	96.8	40.4	104.7
36.2	97.1	40.6	105.1
36.4	97.5	40.8	105.4
36.6	97.8	41.0	105.8
36.8	98.2	41.2	106.1
		41.4	106.5
37.0	98.6	41.6	106.8
		41.8	107.2
		42.0	107.6
37.2	98.9	42.2	108.0
37.4	99.3	42.4	108.3
37.6	99.6	42.6	108.7
37.8	100.0	42.8	109.0
38.0	100.4		
38.2	100.7		

Conversion formulas:

Fahrenheit to Celsius $(°F - 32) \times (5/9) = °C$

Celsius to Fahrenheit $(°C) \times (9/5) + 32 = °F$